Unit 5
Foundations for Nursing Practice

UNIT 6
Psychosocial Basis for Nursing Practice

ice

FUNDAMENTALS OF NURSING

EIGHTH EDITION

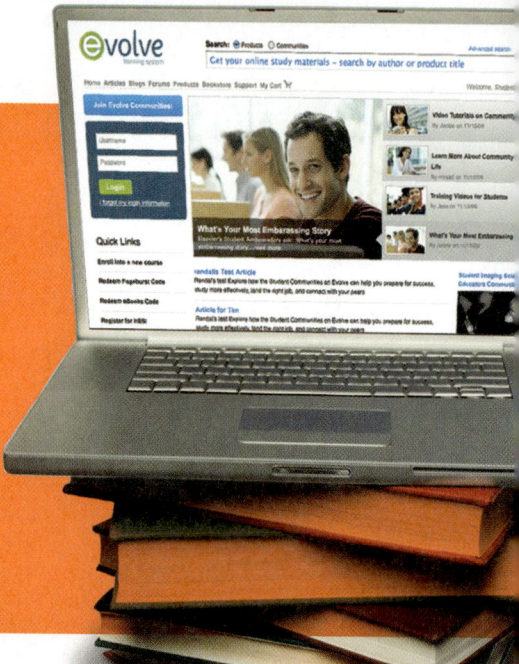

FUNDAMENTALS OF NURSING

EIGHTH EDITION

Patricia A. Potter, RN, MSN, PhD, FAAN
Director of Research
Patient Care Services
Barnes-Jewish Hospital
St. Louis, Missouri

Anne Griffin Perry, RN, EdD, FAAN
Professor and Associate Dean
School of Nursing
Southern Illinois University Edwardsville
Edwardsville, Illinois

Patricia A. Stockert, RN, BSN, MS, PhD
President of the College
Saint Francis Medical Center College of Nursing
Peoria, Illinois

Amy M. Hall, RN, BSN, MS, PhD, CNE
Chair and White Family Endowed Professor of Nursing
Dunigan Family Department of Nursing and Health Sciences
University of Evansville
Evansville, Indiana

ELSEVIER

ELSEVIER
MOSBY

3251 Riverport Lane
St. Louis, Missouri 63043

FUNDAMENTALS OF NURSING **ISBN 978-0-323-07933-4**

International Standard Book Number: 978-0-323-07933-4

Senior Content Strategist: Tamara Myers
Content Development Specialist: Tina Kaemmerer
Content Coordinator: Melissa Rawe
Publishing Services Manager: Deborah L. Vogel
Senior Project Manager: Jodi M. Willard
Design Direction: Brian Salisbury

Printed in Canada

Last digit is the print number: 9 8 7 6 5 4 3 2

CONTRIBUTORS

Paulette M. Archer, RN, EdD
Professor
Saint Francis Medical Center College of Nursing
Peoria, Illinois

Marjorie Baier, PhD, RN
Associate Professor
School of Nursing
Southern Illinois University Edwardsville
Edwardsville, Illinois

Karen Balakas, PhD, RN, CNE
Professor and Director
Clinical Research Partnerships
Goldfarb School of Nursing at Barnes-Jewish College
St. Louis, Missouri

Jeri Burger, PhD, RN
Assistant Professor
University of Southern Indiana
Evansville, Indiana

Linda Cason, MSN, RN-BC, NE-BC, CNRN
Manager Employee Education and Development Department
Deaconess Hospital
Evansville, Indiana

Janice Colwell, RN, MS, CWOCN, FAAN
Advance Practice Nurse
University of Chicago
Chicago, Illinois

Rhonda W. Comrie, PhD, RN, CNE, AE-C
Associate Professor
School of Nursing
Southern Illinois University-Edwardsville
Edwardsville, Illinois

Ruth M. Curchoe, RN, MSN, CIC
Director, Infection Prevention
Unity Health System
Rochester, New York

Marinetta DeMoss, RN, MSN
Manager of Staff Development
St. Mary's Medical Center
Evansville, Indiana

Christine R. Durbin, PhD, JD, RN
Assistant Professor
School of Nursing
Southern Illinois University Edwardsville
Edwardsville, Illinois

Margaret Ecker, RN, MS
Director, Nursing Quality
Kaiser Permanente Los Angeles Medical Center
Los Angeles, California

Linda Felver, PhD, RN
Associate Professor
School of Nursing
Oregon Health & Sciences University
Portland, Oregon

Susan Jane Fetzer, PhD, RN, MBA
Associate Professor
University of New Hampshire
Durham, New Hampshire

Victoria N. Folse, PhD, APN, PMHCNS-BC, LCPC
Director and Associate Professor
School of Nursing
Illinois Wesleyan University
Bloomington, Illinois

Kay E. Gaehle, PhD, RN
Associate Professor of Nursing
School of Nursing
Southern Illinois University Edwardsville
Edwardsville, Illinois

Lori Klingman, MSN, RN
Nursing Faculty and Advisor
Ohio Valley General Hospital School of Nursing
McKees Rocks, Pennsylvania

Mary S. Koithan, PhD, RN, CNS-BS
Associate Professor
College of Nursing
University of Arizona
Tucson, Arizona

Karen Korem, RN-BC, MA
Professional Practice Specialist
Geriatric Nurse Clinician
OSF Saint Francis Medical Center
Peoria, Illinois

Jerrilee LaMar, PhD, RN, CNE
Assistant Professor of Nursing
University of Evansville
Evansville, Indiana

Kathy Lever, MSN, WHNP-C
Associate Professor of Nursing
University of Evansville
Evansville, Indiana

Frank Lyerla, PhD, RN
Assistant Professor
School of Nursing
Southern Illinois University Edwardsville
Edwardsville, Illinois

Deborah Marshall, MSN
Assistant Professor of Nursing
Dunigan Family Department of Nursing
University of Evansville
Evansville, Indiana

Jill Parsons, RN, MSN, PCCN
Assistant Professor
MacMurray College
Jacksonville, Illinois

Patsy L. Ruchala, DNSc, RN
Director and Professor
University of Nevada-Reno
Reno, Nevada

Carrie Sona, RN, MSN, CCRN, ACNS, CCNS
Surgical Critical Care CNS
Barnes Jewish Hospital
St. Louis, Missouri

Ann B. Tritak, EdD, MA, BSN, RN
Dean and Professor of Nursing
School of Nursing
Saint Peter's College
Jersey City, New Jersey

Terry L. Wood, PhD, RN, CNE
Assistant Clinical Professor
School of Nursing
Southern Illinois University Edwardsville
Edwardsville, Illinois

Rita Wunderlich, PhD, RN
Associate Professor
Director Baccalaureate Program
Saint Louis University
St. Louis, Missouri

Valerie Yancey, PhD, RN
Associate Professor
School of Nursing
Southern Illinois University Edwardsville
Edwardsville, Illinois

REVIEWERS

Marianne Adam, MSN, CRNP
Assistant Professor
Moravian College
Bethlehem, Pennsylvania

Amy S. Adams, MSN, RN
Associate Professor
St. Elizabeth School of Nursing
Lafayette, Indiana

Rebecca Appleton, RN, PhD
Professor of Nursing
Marshall University
Huntington, West Virginia

Mary Dell Armwood, MSN, RN
Assistant Professor of Nursing
Southern Arkansas University
Magnolia, Arkansas

Suzanne Bailey, MSN, PMHCNS-BC
Associate Professor of Nursing
University of Evansville
Evansville, Indiana

Martha C. Baker, PhD, RN, APRN-BC
Director, BSN Program
Professor of Nursing
St. John's College of Nursing
Southwest Baptist University
Bolivar, Missouri

Margaret E. Barnes, RN, MSN
Assistant Professor
Indiana Wesleyan University
Marion, Indiana

Nicole Bartow, RN, MSN, BA
Director of Clinical Simulation Learning Center
University of Missouri-Columbia
Columbia, Missouri

Janet E. Bitzan, RN, PhD
Clinical Associate Professor
School of Nursing
University of Wisconsin-Milwaukee
Milwaukee, Wisconsin

Joanne Bonesteel, MS, RN
Nursing Faculty
Excelsior College
Albany, New York

Leigh Ann Bonney, MSN, RN
Instructor
OSF Saint Francis Medical Center
College of Nursing
Peoria, Illinois

Joy M. Boyd, RN, MSN
Assistant Professor of Nursing
Jackson State Community College
Jackson, Tennessee

Janet Witucki Brown, PhD, RN, CNE
Associate Professor
Knoxville College of Nursing
The University of Tennessee
Knoxville, Tennessee

Anna Bruch, RN, MSN
Professor of Nursing
Illinois Valley Community College
Oglesby, Illinois

Pat Callard, MSN, RN, CNE
Assistant Professor of Nursing
College of Graduate Nursing
Western University of Health Sciences
Pomona, California

Linda Cason, MSN, RN, CNRN, BC
Manager, Employee Education and Development and Health Science Library
Deaconess Hospital
Evansville, Indiana

Kim Clevenger, EdDc, MSN, RN, BC
Associate Professor of Nursing
Morehead State University
Morehead, Kentucky

Christine M. Corcoran, RN, MS, FNP-BC
Instructor
Coordinator NP Programs
College of Mount Saint Vincent
Bronx, New York

Suzanne M. Costello, RN, BSN, MSN
Professional Nurse Educator
Educational Specialist-Allied Health
Jameson Health System
New Castle, Pennsylvania

Graciela Lopez Cox, MSN, RN
Assistant Professor
School of Nursing
Sacramento Regional Learning Center
Samuel Merritt University
Sacramento, California

Vicki R. Crews, RN, MBA, MSN
Nursing Faculty
Hillsborough Community College
Tampa, Florida

Michele C. Curry, MS, RN
Senior Lecturer
Indiana University East School of Nursing
Indiana University
Richmond, Indiana

Judith L. Dedeker, RN, MSN, CNE
Associate Professor of Nursing
Southern Adventist University
Collegedale, Tennessee

Lauren Deichmann, MSN, FNP-BC
Family Nurse Practitioner
BJH Center for Preoperative Assessment and Planning
St. Louis, Missouri

Barbara Derwinski, MSN, RNC, WH, BC
Associate Professor
Bozeman College of Nursing
Montana State University-Billings Campus
Billings, Montana

Melinda Dicken, MSN, RN, CNS
Nursing Instructor
Azusa Pacific University
Azusa, California

Holly Johanna Diesel, RN, BSN, MSN, PhD
Associate Professor
Goldfarb School of Nursing
Barnes Jewish College
St. Louis, Missouri

Kimberly Dudas, PhD(c), MS, RN, ANP-BC, CNE
Assistant Professor
Accelerated Nursing Program Coordinator
New Jersey City University
Jersey City, New Jersey

Dawna Egelhoff, MSN, RN
Assistant Professor
School of Nursing
Lewis & Clark Community College
Godfrey, Illinois

Amber Essman, MSN, RN, CNE, CFRN
Assistant Professor
Chamberlain College of Nursing
Columbus, Ohio

Maryann Forbes, PhD, RN
Associate Professor
Adelphi University
Garden City, New York

Margie L. Francisco, EdD (c), RN, MSN
Nursing Professor
Illinois Valley Community College
Oglesby, Illinois

Narsis E. Garner, RN, BSN, MSN
Post Master Certification in Nursing Education
Assistant Professor of Nursing
Wilbur Wright College
Chicago, Illinois

Jacklyn Gentry, MSN, RN
Nursing Faculty
Brookline College
Phoenix, Arizona

Kathy L. Ham, RN, MSN, EdD
Assistant Professor
Southeast Missouri State University
Cape Girardeau, Missouri

Linda Hansen-Kyle, PhD, RN, CCM
Director, Nursing, San Diego Regional Center
Azusa Pacific University
San Diego, California

Martina Sherese Harris, BSN, MSN, EdD
Assistant Professor
School of Nursing
University of Tennessee at Chattanooga
Chattanooga, Tennessee

Mary Ann Helms, RN, MSN, MRE, EdD
Assistant Professor of Nursing
Coordinator at Volunteer State Community College
School of Nursing
Tennessee State University
Nashville, Tennessee

Patricia N. Hendrix, MS, BSN
Associate Professor
Motlow State Community College
Lynchburg, Tennessee

Deborah O. Himes, RN, MSN, ANP-BC
Instructor of Nursing
Brigham Young University
Provo, Utah

Mary Ann Jessee, RN, MSN
Instructor of Nursing
Vanderbilt University School of Nursing
Nashville, Tennessee

Sarah L. Keeling, RN, BSN, MN
Associate Professor
Georgia Perimeter College
Clarkston, Georgia

Lori Kelly, MSN, MBA
Instructor
Aquinas College
Nashville, Tennessee

Shari Kist, RN, PhD
Assistant Professor
Goldfarb School of Nursing
St. Louis, Missouri

Pamela D. Korte, RN, MS
Professor of Nursing
Monroe Community College
Rochester, New York

Stephen D. Krau, PhD, RN, CNE, CT
Associate Professor
School of Nursing
Vanderbilt University Medical Center
Nashville, Tennessee

Rebecca LaMont, MSN, APN, RN
Instructor of Nursing
Family Nurse Practitioner
Heartland Community College
Normal, Illinois

Scharmaine Lawson-Baker, DNP, FNP-BC
CEO and Founder
Advanced Clinical Consultants
New Orleans, Louisiana

Virginia Lester, RN, BSN, MSN
Assistant Professor in Nursing
Angelo State University
San Angelo, Texas

Norma J. Line, RN
Case Manager
Healing Touch International/St. Louis
Barnes Jewish Hospital
St. Louis, Missouri

Tami Kathleen Little, MS, RN
Nursing Faculty
Brookline College
Phoenix, Arizona

Laura Logan, MSN, RN
Clinical Instructor for School of Nursing
Stephen F. Austin State University
Nacogdoches, Texas

Mary M. Lopez, PhD, RN
Assistant Professor
Director MSNE Program
Director, Simulation Science Center
College of Graduate Nursing
Western University of Health Sciences
Pomona, California

Sharon L. Marquard, MSN, RN, CCRN
Assistant Professor of Nursing
St. Ambrose University
Davenport, Iowa

B. Gail Marshall, RN, BSN, MSM, MEd, CNE
Professor
Luzerne County Community College
Nanticoke, Pennsylvania

Laura Szopo Martin, MSN, RN
Professor of Nursing and Fundamentals Course Coordinator
College of Southern Nevada
Las Vegas, Nevada

Janis Longfield McMillan, RN, MSN
Nursing Faculty
Coconino Community College
Flagstaff, Arizona

Pamela S. Merida, MSN, RN
Assistant Professor
Nursing
St. Elizabeth School of Nursing
Lafayette, Indiana

Jeanie F. Minneci Mitchel, RNc, MSN, MA
Nursing Faculty
South Suburban College
South Holland, Illinois

Joseph Molinatti, EdD, RN
Assistant Professor of Nursing
College of Mount Saint Vincent
Bronx, New York

Pamela Molnar, RN, CEN
Clinical Instructor
Tennessee Technology Center
Pulaski, Tennessee

Cindy Mulder, RNC, MS, MSN, WHNP-BC, FNP-BC
Associate Professor
The University of South Dakota
Sioux Falls, South Dakota

Rebecca Otten, RN, EdD
Assistant Professor, Nursing
Assistant Director, Prelicensure Programs
California State University-Fullerton
Fullerton, California

Catherine J. Pagel, MSN, RN
Assistant Professor of Nursing
Mercy College of Health Sciences
Des Moines, Iowa

Whitney Payne, BA, MS, RN, FNP-BC
Family Nurse Practitioner
Barnes Jewish Hospital
St. Louis, Missouri

Elaine U. Polan, RNC, MS, PhD
Nursing Program Supervisor
Vocational Education & Extension Board Practical Nursing Program
Uniondale, New York

Susan Porterfield, PhD, FNP-C
NP Coordinator
Assistant Professor
Florida State University
Tallahassee, Florida

Cherie R. Rebar, MSN, MBA, RN, FNP, ND
Associate Director, Division of Nursing
Chair, Associate Degree Nursing Program
Associate Professor
Kettering College of Medical Arts
Kettering, Ohio

Anita K. Reed, MSN, RN
Clinical Instructor
St. Elizabeth School of Nursing/St. Joseph's College
Lafayette, Indiana

Rhonda J. Reed, RN, MSN, CRRN
Instructor
College of Nursing, Health, and Human Services
Indiana State University
Terre Haute, Indiana

Nila Reimer, PhD(c), MS, RN
Acting Director of Undergraduate Nursing Program
Indiana University
Purdue University
Fort Wayne, Indiana

Kristine A. Rose, RN, MSN
Instructor
St. Francis Medical Center College of Nursing
Peoria, Illinois

Carol A. Rueter, RN, MSN
USF Clinical Faculty
VA Nursing Academy Instructor
University of South Florida
James A. Haley VA
Tampa, Florida

Julie Ryhal, RN, MEd, LCEE
Education Coordinator
Grove City Medical Center
Grove City, Pennsylvania

Megan Sary, RN, BSN, MSN
Professor of Nursing
Merritt College
Oakland, California

Maura C. Schlairet, EdD, MSN, RN, CNL
Associate Professor
College of Nursing
Valdosta State University
Valdosta, Georgia

Susan Parnell Scholtz, PhD, RN
Associate Professor of Nursing
St. Luke's School of Nursing at Moravian College
Bethlehem, Pennsylvania

Gale Sewell, RN, MSN, CNE
Assistant Professor of Nursing
School of Nursing
Indiana Wesleyan University
Marion, Indiana

Cynthia M. Sheppard, RN, MSN, ACNS-BC
Associate Professor of Nursing
Schoolcraft College
Livonia, Michigan

Elaine R. Shingleton, RN, MSN, PHN
Faculty/Lecturer
California State University Eastbay-Concord Campus
Concord, California

Lorie Shobe-Hacker, MSN, RN
Associate Professor
Ivy Tech Community College
Indianapolis, Indiana

Elizabeth Sibson-Tuan, RN, MS
Bay Area Clinical Coordinator
Samuel Merritt University
Oakland, California

Mary Rado Simpson, PhD, RN
Professor of Nursing
Chair, Division of Nursing
Pikeville College
Pikeville, Kentucky

Emily G. Smith, MSN, RN, CRRN
Assistant Professor
School of Nursing
Endicott College
Beverly, Massachusetts

Janet Somlyay, MSN, CNS, CNE, CPNP-AC/PC, PMHNP-BC
Assistant Lecturer
Fay W. Whitney School of Nursing
University of Wyoming
Laramie, Wyoming

Ann D. Sprengel, EdD, MSN, RN
Professor
Department of Nursing
Southeast Missouri State University
Cape Girardeau, Missouri

Mary Strong, RN, BSN, MSN
Professor
Kirkwood Community College
Cedar Rapids, Iowa

Scott Carter Thigpen, RN, MSN, CCRN, CEN
Associate Professor of Nursing
South Georgia College
Douglas, Georgia

Sharon S. Thompson, MSN, RN, BC
Assistant Professor of Nursing
Tennessee Technological University
Cookeville, Tennessee

Kimberly Valich, MSN, RN
Department of Nursing Chairperson
Nursing Faculty
South Suburban College
South Holland, Illinois

Patricia Voelpel, RN, MS, ANP, CCRN
Clinical Assistant Professor
Director, 12 Month Accelerated Baccalaureate Nursing Program
Stony Brook University
Stony Brook, New York

Mary Walton, PhD, RN, ANP
Nursing Faculty
GateWay Community College, Maricopa Nursing
Phoenix, Arizona

Kathleen S. Whalen, PhD, RN, CNE
Assistant Professor of Nursing
Loretto Heights School of Nursing
Regis University
Denver, Colorado

Janet C. Whitworth, RN, DNP, FNP-BC
Assistant Professor
Goldfarb School of Nursing at Barnes Jewish College
St. Louis, Missouri

Angela Shirlean Williams, RN
Registered Nurse
Maury Regional Medical Center
Columbia, Tennessee

Janet E. Willis, MS, RN
Senior Professor
Harrisburg Area Community College
Harrisburg, Pennsylvania

Paige Wimberley, MSN, CNS, CNE
Assistant Professor of Nursing
Arkansas State University
Jonesboro, Arkansas

Janice P. Womack, RN
Nurse Executive Associate DSU
Northwest Georgia Regional Hospital
Rome, Georgia

Lea Wood, RN, BSN
Coordinator of the Clinical Simulation Learning Center
University of Missouri-Columbia
Columbia, Missouri

Toni C. Wortham, RN, BSN, MSN
Professor
Madisonville Community College
Madisonville, Kentucky

Jean Yockey, MSN, FNP-BC, CNE
Associate Professor
University of South Dakota
Vermillion, South Dakota

Damien Zsiros, MSN, RN, CNE, CRNP
Nursing Instructor
Fayette-Eberly Campus
The Pennsylvania State University
Uniontown, Pennsylvania

CONTRIBUTORS TO PREVIOUS EDITIONS

Jeanette Adams, PhD, MSN, APRN, CRNI
Coconut Grove, Florida

Myra. A. Aud, PhD, RN
Columbia, Missouri

Sylvia K. Baird, RN, BSN, MM
Grand Rapids, Michigan

Lois Bentler-Lampe, RN, MS
Peoria, Illinois

Janice Boundy, RN, PhD
Peoria, Illinois

Anna Brock, PhD, MSN, MEd, BSN
Hattiesburg, Mississippi

Sheryl Buckner, RN-BC, MS, CNE
Oklahoma City, Oklahoma

Pamela L. Cherry, RN, BSN, MSN, DNSc
Arcata, California

Eileen Costantinou, MSN, RN
St. Louis, Missouri

Martha Keene Elkin, RN, MS, IBCLC
Sumner, Maine

Leah W. Frederick, MS, RN, CIC
Scottsdale, Arizona

Mimi Hirshberg, RN, MSN
St. Louis, Missouri

Steve Kilkus, RN, MSN
Madison, Wisconsin

Judith Ann Kilpatrick, RN, DNSc
Chester, Pennsylvania

Anahid Kulwicki, RN, DNS, FAAN
Rochester, Michigan

Joyce Larson, PhD, MS, RN
Tampa, Florida

Kristine M. L'Ecuyer, RN, MSN, CCNS
St. Louis, Missouri

Ruth Ludwick, BSN, MSN, PhD, RNC
Kent, Ohio

Annette G. Lueckenotte, MS, RN, BC, GNP, GCNS
St. Louis, Missouri

Barbara Maxwell, RN, BSN, MS, MSN, CNS
Stone Ridge, New York

Elaine K. Neel, RN, BSN, MSN
Canton, Illinois

Wendy Ostendorf, BSN, MS, EdD
Aston, Pennsylvania

Dula Pacquiao, BSN, MA, EdD
Union, New Jersey

Nancy C. Panthofer, RN, MSN
Kent, Ohio

Elaine U. Polan, RNC, BSN, MS
Uniondale, New York

Debbie Sanazaro, RN, MSN, GNP
St. Louis, Missouri

Marilyn Schallom, RN, MSN, CCRN, CCNS
St. Louis, Missouri

Marshelle Thobaben, RN, MS, PHN, APNP, FNP
Arcata, California

Janis Waite, RN, MSN, EdD
Peoria, Illinois

Mary Ann Wehmer, RN, MSN, CNOR
Evansville, Indiana

Pamela Becker Weilitz, RN, MSN(R), BC, ANP, M-SCNS
St. Louis, Missouri

Joan Domigan Wentz, BSN, MSN
St. Louis, Missouri

Katherine West, BSN, MSEd, CIC
Manassas, Virginia

The ongoing writing and review of a text requires the support of many people. I dedicate this book to the many professional colleagues who have contributed, reviewed, and critiqued our texts over the years and have always elevated the quality of our work. And I dedicate this book to my very dear friends, who offer consistent support and understanding.

Patricia A. Potter

To the nursing faculty at Southern Illinois University Edwardsville and Saint Louis University. Your commitment to nursing and nursing education inspires us all to be the guardians of the discipline.
To my grandchildren, Cora Elizabeth Bryan, Amalie Mary Bryan, and Shepherd Charles Bryan.

Anne Griffin Perry

To my family and friends: Thank you for all your love and support as my passion for nursing has taken me on different pathways over the years. And to the faculty and staff of Saint Francis Medical Center College of Nursing: I am proud to be a part of such a great group of people who, through your caring and dedication to education and nursing, prepare excellent entry-level and advanced practice nurses for health care today and in the future.

Patricia A. Stockert

To Greg, the love of my life. Your never-ending love and support and ready supply of 4-cookbook casseroles have enabled me to achieve more than I could have ever imagined. Thank you for giving me the time to read, write, edit, travel, and think. And to the nursing faculty and staff at the University of Evansville. Your commitment to excellence in nursing education provides life-transforming experiences that are vital to shaping the nurses of the future. Thank you for your passion and most of all for your friendship. I am so blessed to have all of you in my life.

Amy M. Hall

STUDENT PREFACE

Fundamentals of Nursing provides you with all of the fundamental nursing concepts and skills you will need as a beginning nurse in a visually appealing, easy-to-use format. We know how busy you are and how precious your time is. As you begin your nursing education, it is very important that you have a resource that includes all the information you need to prepare for lectures, classroom activities, clinical assignments, and exams—and nothing more. We've written this text to meet all of those needs. This book was designed to help you succeed in this course and prepare you for more advanced study. In addition to the readable writing style and abundance of full-color photographs and drawings, we've incorporated numerous features to help you study and learn. We have made it easy for you to pull out important content. **Check out the following special learning aids:**

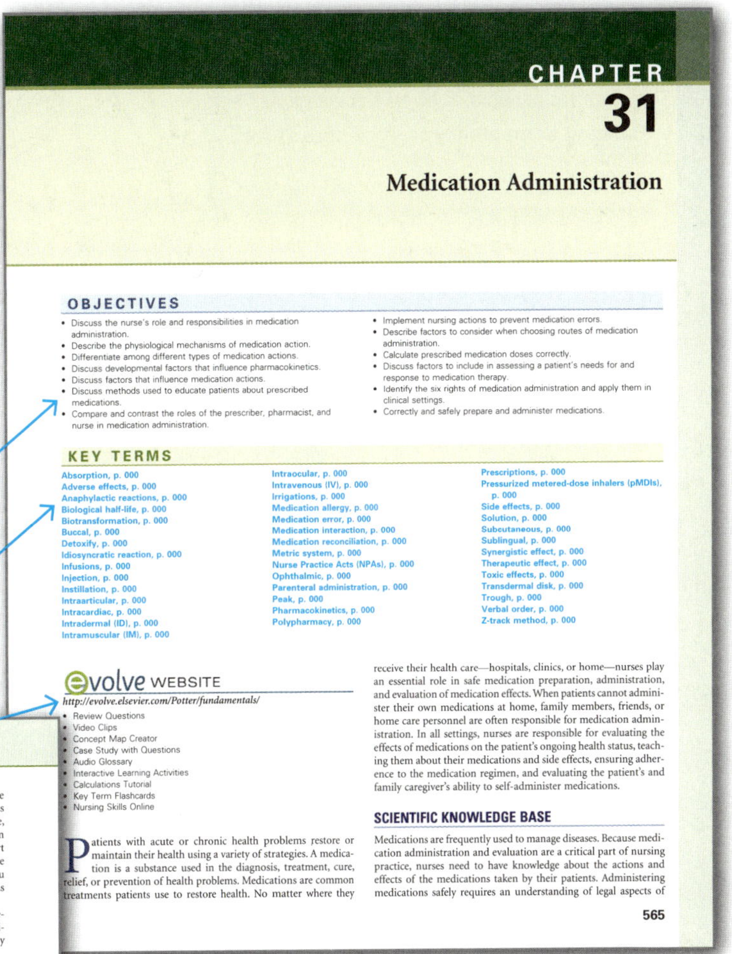

CHAPTER 31

Medication Administration

OBJECTIVES

- Discuss the nurse's role and responsibilities in medication administration.
- Describe the physiological mechanisms of medication action.
- Differentiate among different types of medication actions.
- Discuss developmental factors that influence pharmacokinetics.
- Discuss factors that influence medication actions.
- Discuss methods used to educate patients about prescribed medications.
- Compare and contrast the roles of the prescriber, pharmacist, and nurse in medication administration.
- Implement nursing actions to prevent medication errors.
- Describe factors to consider when choosing routes of medication administration.
- Calculate prescribed medication doses correctly.
- Discuss factors to include in assessing a patient's needs for and response to medication therapy.
- Identify the six rights of medication administration and apply them in clinical settings.
- Correctly and safely prepare and administer medications.

KEY TERMS

Absorption, p. 000
Adverse effects, p. 000
Anaphylactic reactions, p. 000
Biological half-life, p. 000
Biotransformation, p. 000
Buccal, p. 000
Detoxify, p. 000
Idiosyncratic reaction, p. 000
Infusions, p. 000
Injection, p. 000
Instillation, p. 000
Intraarticular, p. 000
Intracardiac, p. 000
Intradermal (ID), p. 000
Intramuscular (IM), p. 000
Intraocular, p. 000
Intravenous (IV), p. 000
Irrigations, p. 000
Medication allergy, p. 000
Medication error, p. 000
Medication interaction, p. 000
Medication reconciliation, p. 000
Metric system, p. 000
Nurse Practice Acts (NPAs), p. 000
Ophthalmic, p. 000
Parenteral administration, p. 000
Peak, p. 000
Pharmacokinetics, p. 000
Polypharmacy, p. 000
Prescriptions, p. 000
Pressurized metered-dose inhalers (pMDIs), p. 000
Side effects, p. 000
Solution, p. 000
Subcutaneous, p. 000
Sublingual, p. 000
Synergistic effect, p. 000
Therapeutic effect, p. 000
Toxic effects, p. 000
Transdermal disk, p. 000
Trough, p. 000
Verbal order, p. 000
Z-track method, p. 000

evolve WEBSITE

http://evolve.elsevier.com/Potter/fundamentals/

- Review Questions
- Video Clips
- Concept Map Creator
- Case Study with Questions
- Audio Glossary
- Interactive Learning Activities
- Calculations Tutorial
- Key Term Flashcards
- Nursing Skills Online

Patients with acute or chronic health problems restore or maintain their health using a variety of strategies. A medication is a substance used in the diagnosis, treatment, cure, relief, or prevention of health problems. Medications are common treatments patients use to restore health. No matter where they receive their health care—hospitals, clinics, or home—nurses play an essential role in safe medication preparation, administration, and evaluation of medication effects. When patients cannot administer their own medications at home, family members, friends, or home care personnel are often responsible for medication administration. In all settings, nurses are responsible for evaluating the effects of medications on the patient's ongoing health status, teaching them about their medications and side effects, ensuring adherence to the medication regimen, and evaluating the patient's and family caregiver's ability to self-administer medications.

SCIENTIFIC KNOWLEDGE BASE

Medications are frequently used to manage diseases. Because medication administration and evaluation are a critical part of nursing practice, nurses need to have knowledge about the actions and effects of the medications taken by their patients. Administering medications safely requires an understanding of legal aspects of

565

Learning Objectives begin each chapter to help you focus on the key information that follows.

Key Terms are listed at the beginning of each chapter and are boldfaced in the text. Page numbers help you quickly find where each term is defined.

Evolve Resources sections detail what electronic resources are available to you for every chapter.

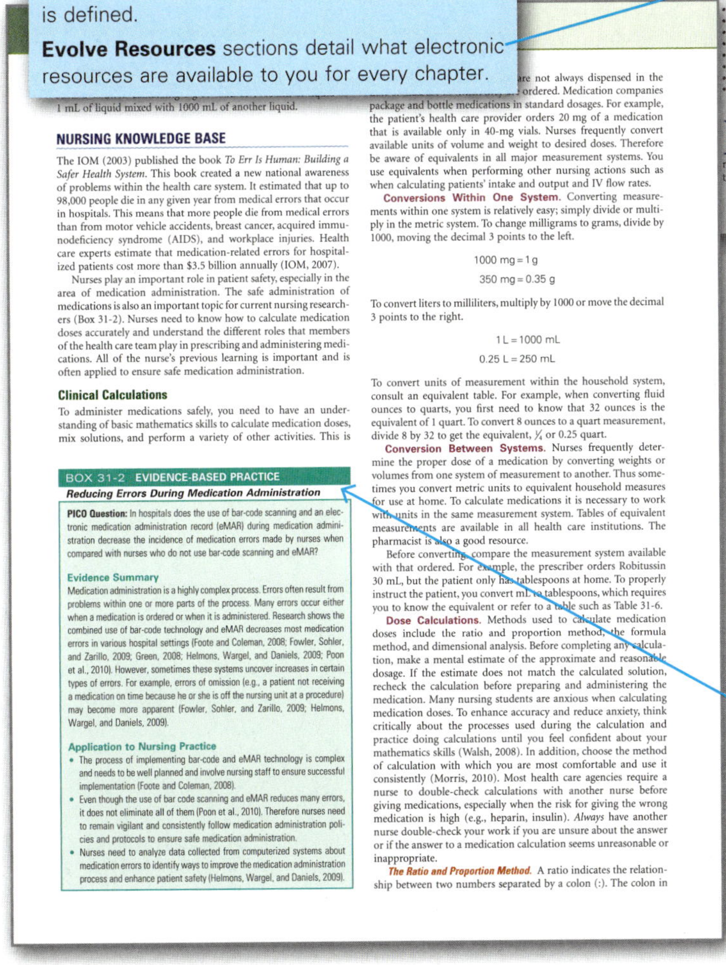

1 mL of liquid mixed with 1000 mL of another liquid.

NURSING KNOWLEDGE BASE

The IOM (2003) published the book *To Err Is Human: Building a Safer Health System*. This book created a new national awareness of problems within the health care system. It estimated that up to 98,000 people die in any given year from medical errors that occur in hospitals. This means that more people die from medical errors than from motor vehicle accidents, breast cancer, acquired immunodeficiency syndrome (AIDS), and workplace injuries. Health care experts estimate that medication-related errors for hospitalized patients cost more than $3.5 billion annually (IOM, 2007).

Nurses play an important role in patient safety, especially in the area of medication administration. The safe administration of medications is also an important topic for current nursing research-ers (Box 31-2). Nurses need to know how to calculate medication doses accurately and understand the different roles that members of the health care team play in prescribing and administering medications. All of the nurse's previous learning is important and is often applied to ensure safe medication administration.

Clinical Calculations

To administer medications safely, you need to have an understanding of basic mathematics skills to calculate medication doses, mix solutions, and perform a variety of other activities. This is

BOX 31-2 EVIDENCE-BASED PRACTICE

Reducing Errors During Medication Administration

PICO Question: In hospitals does the use of bar-code scanning and an electronic medication administration record (eMAR) during medication administration decrease the incidence of medication errors made by nurses when compared with nurses who do not use bar-code scanning and eMAR?

Evidence Summary

Medication administration is a highly complex process. Errors often result from problems within one or more parts of the process. Many errors occur either when a medication is ordered or when it is administered. Research shows the combined use of bar-code technology and eMAR decreases most medication errors in various hospital settings (Foote and Coleman, 2008; Fowler, Sohler, and Zarillo, 2009; Green, 2008; Helmons, Wargel, and Daniels, 2009; Poon et al., 2010). However, sometimes these systems uncover increases in certain types of errors. For example, errors of omission (e.g., a patient not receiving a medication on time because he or she is off the nursing unit at a procedure) may become more apparent (Fowler, Sohler, and Zarillo, 2009; Helmons, Wargel, and Daniels, 2009).

Application to Nursing Practice

- The process of implementing bar-code and eMAR technology is complex and needs to be well planned and involve nursing staff to ensure successful implementation (Foote and Coleman, 2008).
- Even though the use of bar code scanning and eMAR reduces many errors, it does not eliminate all of them (Poon et al., 2010). Therefore nurses need to remain vigilant and consistently follow medication administration policies and protocols to ensure safe medication administration.
- Nurses need to analyze data collected from computerized systems about medication errors to identify ways to improve the medication administration process and enhance patient safety (Helmons, Wargel, and Daniels, 2009).

...re not always dispensed in the ... ordered. Medication companies package and bottle medications in standard dosages. For example, the patient's health care provider orders 20 mg of a medication that is available only in 40-mg vials. Nurses frequently convert available units of volume and weight to desired doses. Therefore be aware of equivalents in all major measurement systems. You use equivalents when performing other nursing actions such as when calculating patients' intake and output and IV flow rates.

Conversions Within One System. Converting measurements within one system is relatively easy; simply divide or multiply in the metric system. To change milligrams to grams, divide by 1000, moving the decimal 3 points to the left.

1000 mg = 1 g

350 mg = 0.35 g

To convert liters to milliliters, multiply by 1000 or move the decimal 3 points to the right.

1 L = 1000 mL

0.25 L = 250 mL

To convert units of measurement within the household system, consult an equivalent table. For example, when converting fluid ounces to quarts, you first need to know that 32 ounces is the equivalent of 1 quart. To convert 8 ounces to a quart measurement, divide 8 by 32 to get the equivalent, ¼ or 0.25 quart.

Conversion Between Systems. Nurses frequently determine the proper dose of a medication by converting weights or volumes from one system of measurement to another. Thus sometimes you convert metric units to equivalent household measures for use at home. To calculate medications it is necessary to work with units in the same measurement system. Tables of equivalent measurements are available in all health care institutions. The pharmacist is also a good resource.

Before converting, compare the measurement system available with that ordered. For example, the prescriber orders Robitussin 30 mL, but the patient only has tablespoons at home. To properly instruct the patient, you convert mL to tablespoons, which requires you to know the equivalent or refer to a table such as Table 31-6.

Dose Calculations. Methods used to calculate medication doses include the ratio and proportion method, the formula method, and dimensional analysis. Before completing any calculation, make a rough estimate of the approximate and reasonable dosage. If the estimate does not match the calculated solution, recheck the calculation before preparing and administering the medication. Many nursing students are anxious when calculating medication doses. To enhance accuracy and reduce anxiety, think critically about the processes used during the calculation and practice doing calculations until you feel confident about your mathematics skills (Walsh, 2008). In addition, choose the method of calculation with which you are most comfortable and use it consistently (Morris, 2010). Most health care agencies require a nurse to double-check calculations with another nurse before giving medications, especially when the risk for giving the wrong medication is high (e.g., heparin, insulin). *Always* have another nurse double-check your work if you are unsure about the answer or if the answer to a medication calculation seems unreasonable or inappropriate.

The Ratio and Proportion Method. A ratio indicates the relationship between two numbers separated by a colon (:). The colon in

Evidence-Based Practice boxes summarize the results of a research study and indicate how that research can be applied to nursing practice.

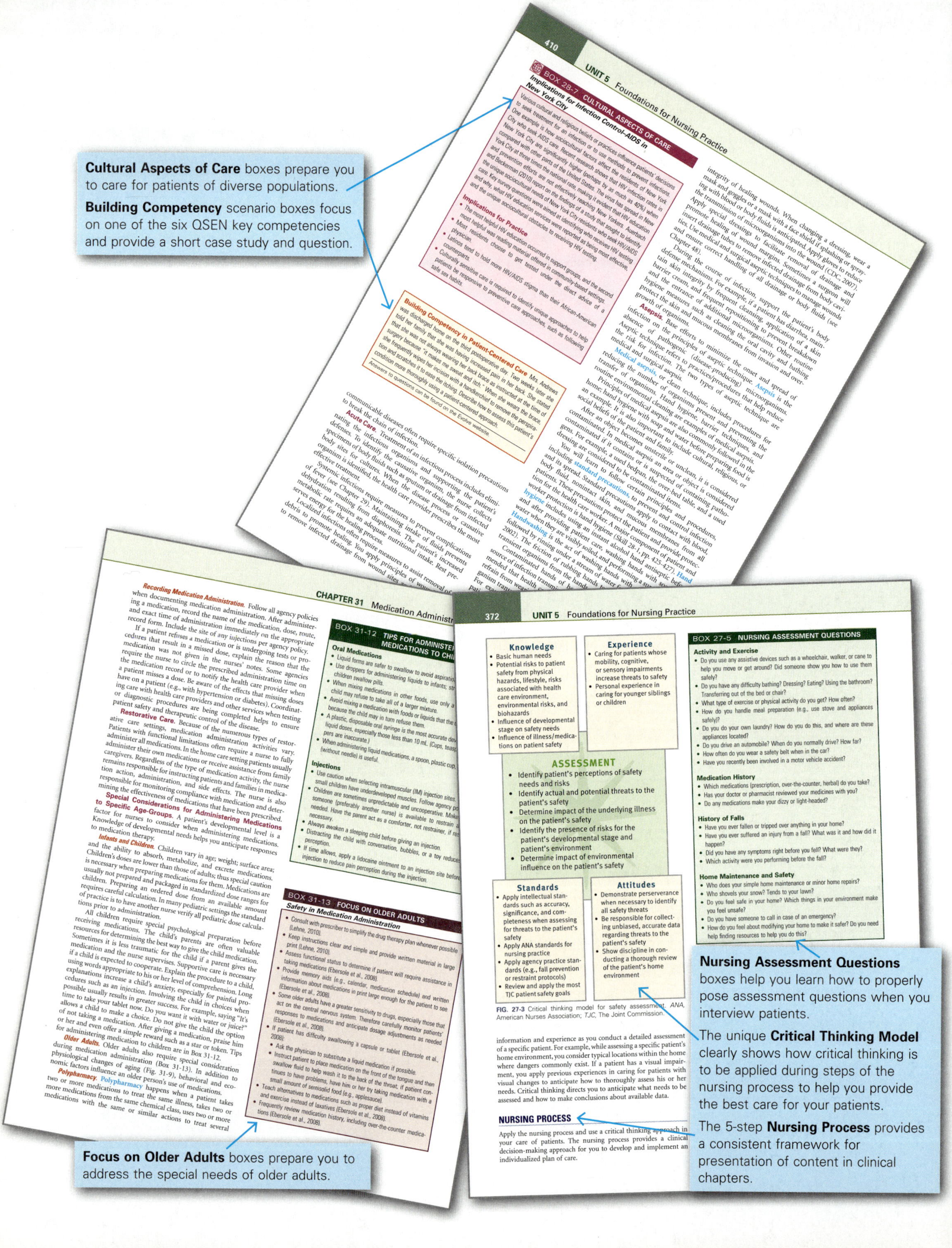

Cultural Aspects of Care boxes prepare you to care for patients of diverse populations.

Building Competency scenario boxes focus on one of the six QSEN key competencies and provide a short case study and question.

Nursing Assessment Questions boxes help you learn how to properly pose assessment questions when you interview patients.

The unique **Critical Thinking Model** clearly shows how critical thinking is to be applied during steps of the nursing process to help you provide the best care for your patients.

The 5-step **Nursing Process** provides a consistent framework for presentation of content in clinical chapters.

Focus on Older Adults boxes prepare you to address the special needs of older adults.

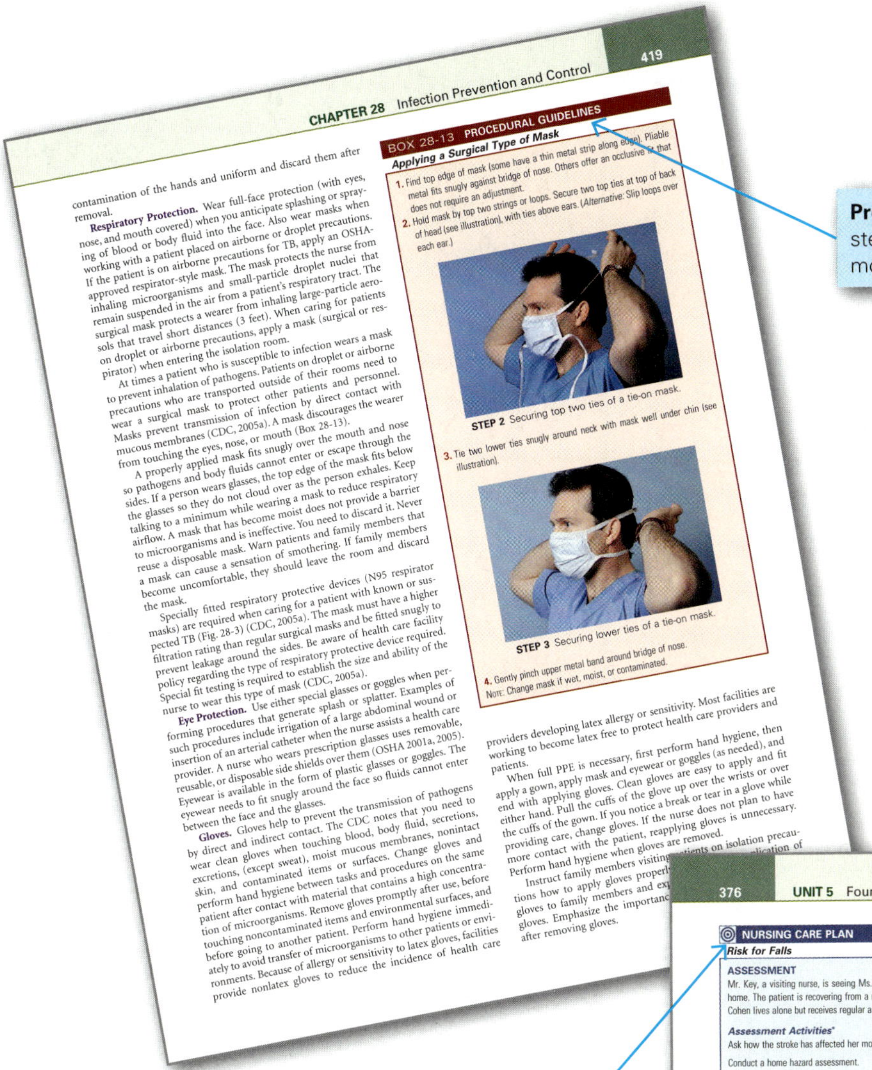

contamination of the hands and uniform and discard them after removal.

Respiratory Protection. Wear full-face protection (with eyes, nose, and mouth covered) when you anticipate splashing or spraying of blood or body fluid into the face. Also wear masks when working with a patient placed on airborne or droplet precautions. If the patient is on airborne precautions for TB, apply an OSHA-approved respirator-style mask. The mask protects the nurse from inhaling microorganisms and small-particle droplet nuclei that remain suspended in the air from a patient's respiratory tract. The surgical mask protects a wearer from inhaling large-particle aerosols that travel short distances (3 feet). When caring for patients on droplet or airborne precautions, apply a mask (surgical or respirator) when entering the isolation room.

At times a patient who is susceptible to infection wears a mask to prevent inhalation of pathogens. Patients on droplet or airborne precautions who are transported outside of their rooms need to wear a surgical mask to protect other patients and personnel. Masks prevent transmission of infection by direct contact with mucous membranes (CDC, 2005a). A mask discourages the wearer from touching the eyes, nose, or mouth (Box 28-13).

A properly applied mask fits snugly over the mouth and nose so pathogens and body fluids cannot enter or escape through the sides. If a person wears glasses, the top edge of the mask fits below the glasses so they do not cloud over as the person exhales. Keep talking to a minimum while wearing a mask to reduce respiratory airflow. A mask that has become moist does not provide a barrier to microorganisms and is ineffective. You need to discard it. Never reuse a disposable mask. Warn patients and family members that a mask can cause a sensation of smothering. If family members become uncomfortable, they should leave the room and discard the mask.

Specially fitted respiratory protective devices (N95 respirator masks) are required when caring for a patient with known or suspected TB (Fig. 28-3) (CDC, 2005a). The mask must have a higher filtration rating than regular surgical masks and be fitted snugly to prevent leakage around the sides. Be aware of health care facility policy regarding the type of respiratory protective device required. Special fit testing is required to establish the size and ability of the nurse to wear this type of mask (CDC, 2005a).

Eye Protection. Use either special glasses or goggles when performing procedures that generate splash or splatter. Examples of such procedures include irrigation of a large abdominal wound or insertion of an arterial catheter when the nurse assists a health care provider. A nurse who wears prescription glasses uses removable, reusable, or disposable side shields over them (OSHA 2001a, 2005). Eyewear is available in the form of plastic glasses or goggles. The eyewear needs to fit snugly around the face so fluids cannot enter between the face and the glasses.

Gloves. Gloves help to prevent the transmission of pathogens by direct and indirect contact. The CDC notes that you need to wear clean gloves when touching blood, body fluid, secretions, excretions, (except sweat), moist mucous membranes, nonintact skin, and contaminated items or surfaces. Change gloves and perform hand hygiene between tasks and procedures on the same patient after contact with material that contains a high concentration of microorganisms. Remove gloves promptly after use, before touching noncontaminated items and environmental surfaces, and before going to another patient. Perform hand hygiene immediately to avoid transfer of microorganisms to other patients or environments. Because of allergy or sensitivity to latex gloves, facilities provide nonlatex gloves to reduce the incidence of health care providers developing latex allergy or sensitivity. Most facilities are working to become latex free to protect health care providers and patients.

When full PPE is necessary, first perform hand hygiene, then apply a gown, apply mask and eyewear or goggles (as needed), and end with applying gloves. Clean gloves are easy to apply and fit either hand. Pull the cuffs of the glove up over the wrists or over the cuffs of the gown. If you notice a break or tear in a glove while providing care, change gloves. If the nurse does not plan to have more contact with the patient, reapplying gloves is unnecessary. Perform hand hygiene when gloves are removed.

Instruct family members visiting ...tients on isolation precautions how to apply gloves properl... ...lication of gloves to family members and ex... gloves. Emphasize the importanc... after removing gloves.

BOX 28-13 PROCEDURAL GUIDELINES

Applying a Surgical Type of Mask

1. Find top edge of mask (some have a thin metal strip along edge). Pliable metal fits snugly against bridge of nose. Others offer an occlusive fit that does not require an adjustment.
2. Hold mask by top two strings or loops. Secure two top ties at top of back of head (see illustration), with ties above ears. (*Alternative:* Slip loops over each ear.)

STEP 2 Securing top two ties of a tie-on mask.

3. Tie two lower ties snugly around neck with mask well under chin (see illustration).

STEP 3 Securing lower ties of a tie-on mask.

4. Gently pinch upper metal band around bridge of nose.

NOTE: Change mask if wet, moist, or contaminated.

Procedural Guidelines provide streamlined, step-by-step instructions for performing the most basic skills.

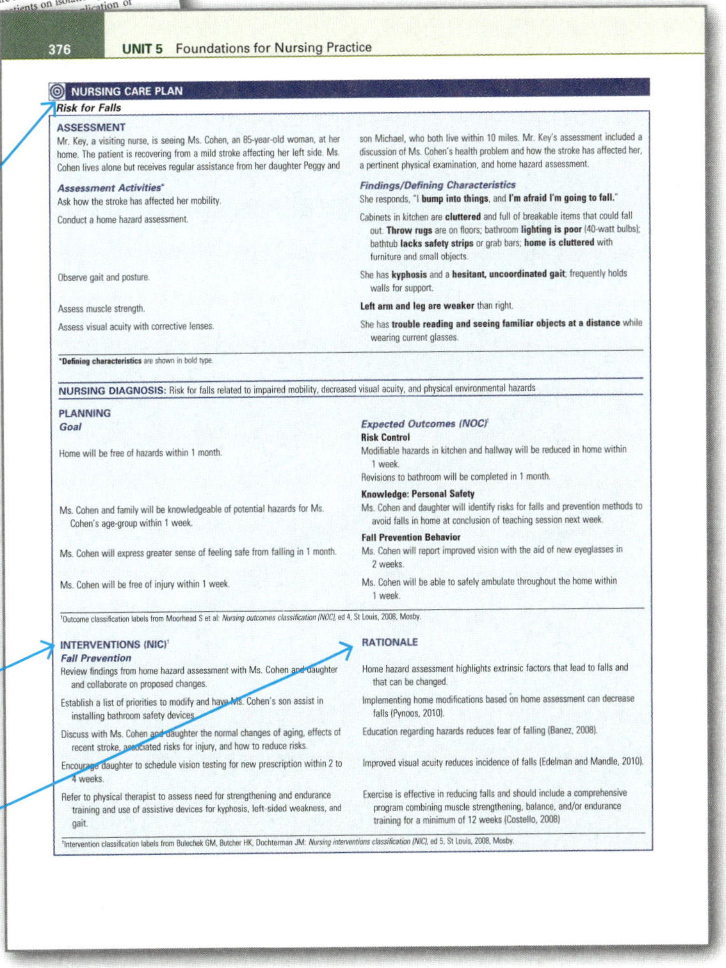

NURSING CARE PLAN

Risk for Falls

ASSESSMENT

Mr. Key, a visiting nurse, is seeing Ms. Cohen, an 85-year-old woman, at her home. The patient is recovering from a mild stroke affecting her left side. Ms. Cohen lives alone but receives regular assistance from her daughter Peggy and son Michael, who both live within 10 miles. Mr. Key's assessment included a discussion of Ms. Cohen's health problem and how the stroke has affected her, a pertinent physical examination, and home hazard assessment.

Assessment Activities[*]	*Findings/Defining Characteristics*
Ask how the stroke has affected her mobility.	She responds, "I **bump into things**, and **I'm afraid I'm going to fall.**"
Conduct a home hazard assessment.	Cabinets in kitchen are **cluttered** and full of breakable items that could fall out. **Throw rugs** are on floors; bathroom **lighting is poor** (40-watt bulbs); bathtub **lacks safety strips** or grab bars; **home is cluttered** with furniture and small objects.
Observe gait and posture.	She has **kyphosis** and a **hesitant, uncoordinated gait**; frequently holds walls for support.
Assess muscle strength.	**Left arm and leg are weaker** than right.
Assess visual acuity with corrective lenses.	She has **trouble reading and seeing familiar objects at a distance** while wearing current glasses.

*__Defining characteristics__ are shown in bold type.

NURSING DIAGNOSIS: Risk for falls related to impaired mobility, decreased visual acuity, and physical environmental hazards

PLANNING

Goal	*Expected Outcomes (NOC)*[†]
	Risk Control
Home will be free of hazards within 1 month.	Modifiable hazards in kitchen and hallway will be reduced in home within 1 week.
	Revisions to bathroom will be completed in 1 month.
	Knowledge: Personal Safety
Ms. Cohen and family will be knowledgeable of potential hazards for Ms. Cohen's age-group within 1 week.	Ms. Cohen and daughter will identify risks for falls and prevention methods to avoid falls in home at conclusion of teaching session next week.
	Fall Prevention Behavior
Ms. Cohen will express greater sense of feeling safe from falling in 1 month.	Ms. Cohen will report improved vision with the aid of new eyeglasses in 2 weeks.
Ms. Cohen will be free of injury within 1 week.	Ms. Cohen will be able to safely ambulate throughout the home within 1 week.

†Outcome classification labels from Moorhead S et al: *Nursing outcomes classification (NOC)*, ed 4, St Louis, 2008, Mosby.

INTERVENTIONS (NIC)[‡]	RATIONALE
Fall Prevention	
Review findings from home hazard assessment with Ms. Cohen and daughter and collaborate on proposed changes.	Home hazard assessment highlights extrinsic factors that lead to falls and that can be changed.
Establish a list of priorities to modify and have Ms. Cohen's son assist in installing bathroom safety devices.	Implementing home modifications based on home assessment can decrease falls (Pynoos, 2010).
Discuss with Ms. Cohen and daughter the normal changes of aging, effects of recent stroke, associated risks for injury, and how to reduce risks.	Education regarding hazards reduces fear of falling (Banez, 2008).
Encourage daughter to schedule vision testing for new prescription within 2 to 4 weeks.	Improved visual acuity reduces incidence of falls (Edelman and Mandle, 2010).
Refer to physical therapist to assess need for strengthening and endurance training and use of assistive devices for kyphosis, left-sided weakness, and gait.	Exercise is effective in reducing falls and should include a comprehensive program combining muscle strengthening, balance, and/or endurance training for a minimum of 12 weeks (Costello, 2008)

‡Intervention classification labels from Bulechek GM, Butcher HK, Dochterman JM: *Nursing interventions classification (NIC)*, ed 5, St Louis, 2008, Mosby.

Nursing Care Plans demonstrate how comprehensive a plan of care should be for a patient. Each plan helps you understand the process of assessment, the association of assessment findings with defining characteristics in the formation of nursing diagnoses, the identification of goals and outcomes, selection of nursing interventions, and the process for evaluating care.

Nursing Intervention Classification (NIC) and **Nursing Outcomes Classification (NOC)** terminologies are used in the care plans to build your knowledge of nursing concepts.

Rationales for each of the interventions in the care plans demonstrate the evidence to support nursing care approaches.

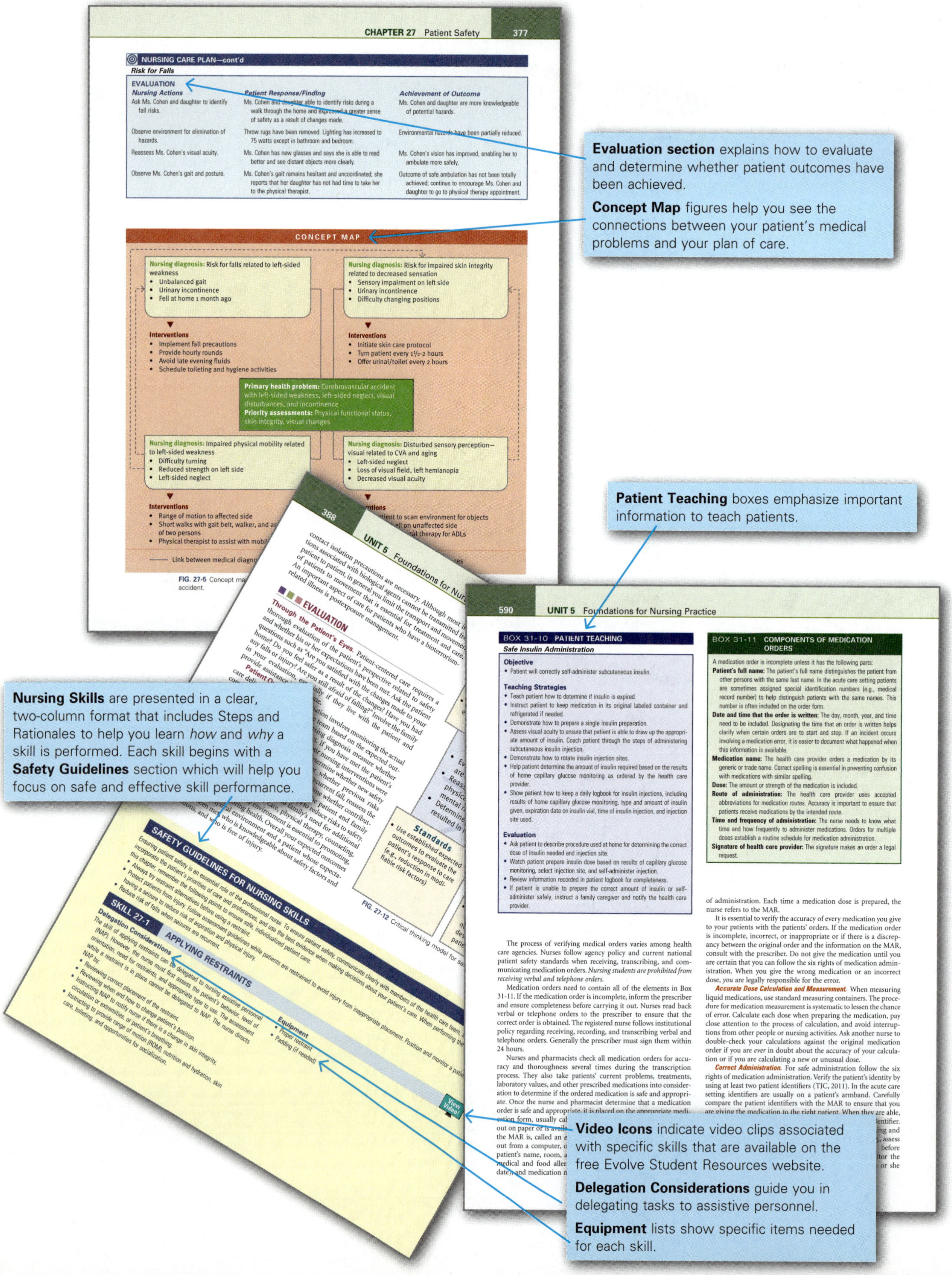

Evaluation section explains how to evaluate and determine whether patient outcomes have been achieved.

Concept Map figures help you see the connections between your patient's medical problems and your plan of care.

Patient Teaching boxes emphasize important information to teach patients.

Nursing Skills are presented in a clear, two-column format that includes Steps and Rationales to help you learn *how* and *why* a skill is performed. Each skill begins with a **Safety Guidelines** section which will help you focus on safe and effective skill performance.

Video Icons indicate video clips associated with specific skills that are available on the free Evolve Student Resources website.

Delegation Considerations guide you in delegating tasks to assistive personnel.

Equipment lists show specific items needed for each skill.

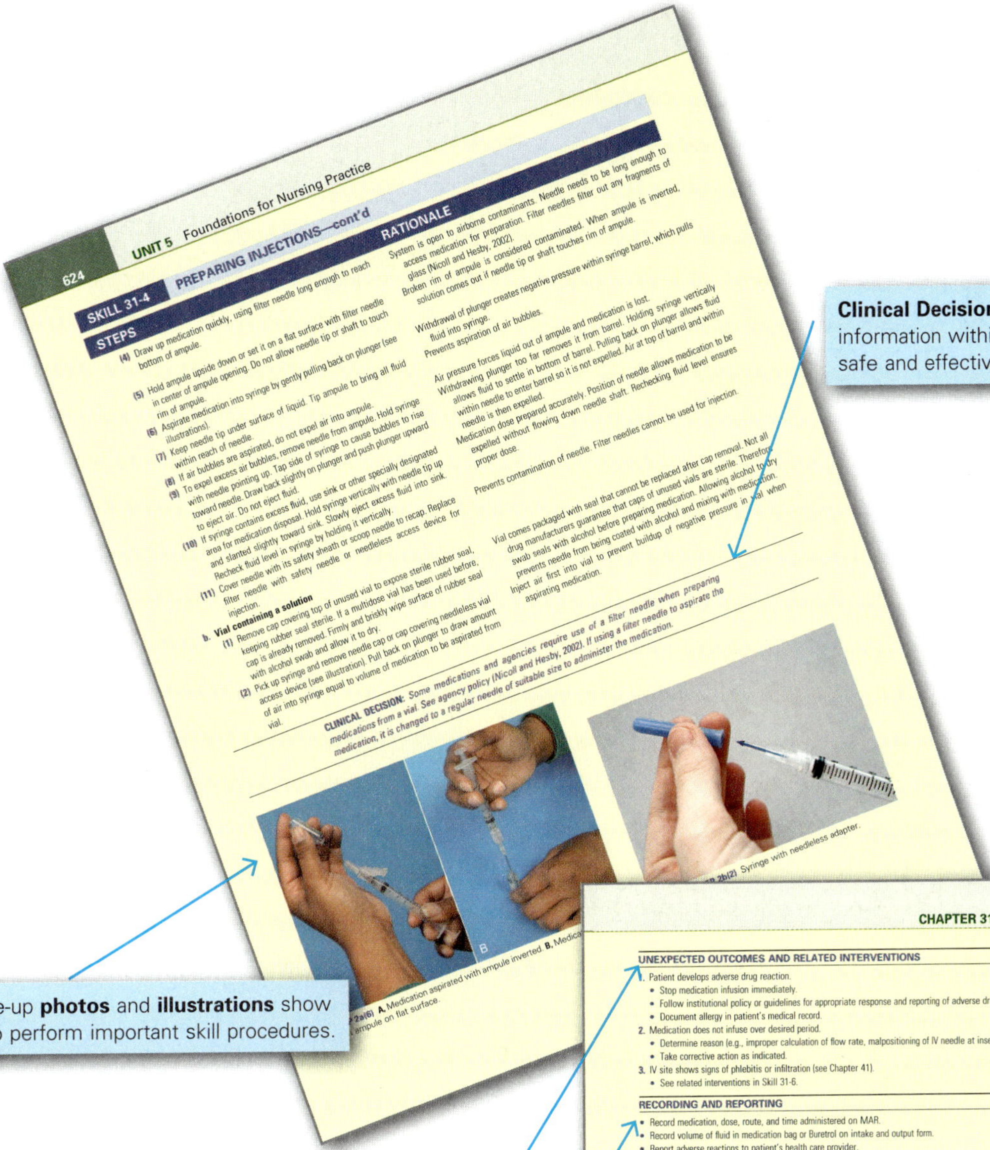

624 UNIT 5 Foundations for Nursing Practice

SKILL 31-4 PREPARING INJECTIONS—cont'd

STEPS	RATIONALE
(4) Draw up medication quickly, using filter needle long enough to reach bottom of ampule.	System is open to airborne contaminants. Needle needs to be long enough to access medication for preparation. Filter needles filter out any fragments of glass (Nicoll and Hesby, 2002).
(5) Hold ampule upside down or set it on a flat surface with filter needle in center of ampule opening. Do not allow needle tip or shaft to touch rim of ampule.	Broken rim of ampule is considered contaminated. When ampule is inverted, solution comes out if needle tip or shaft touches rim of ampule.
(6) Aspirate medication into syringe by gently pulling back on plunger (see illustrations).	Withdrawal of plunger creates negative pressure within syringe barrel, which pulls fluid into syringe.
(7) Keep needle tip under surface of liquid. Tip ampule to bring all fluid within reach of needle.	Prevents aspiration of air bubbles.
(8) If air bubbles are aspirated, do not expel air into ampule.	Air pressure forces liquid out of ampule and medication is lost.
(9) To expel excess air bubbles, remove needle from ampule. Hold syringe with needle pointing up. Tap side of syringe to cause bubbles to rise toward needle. Draw back slightly on plunger and push plunger upward to eject air. Do not eject fluid.	Withdrawing plunger too far removes it from barrel. Holding syringe vertically allows fluid to settle in bottom of barrel. Pulling back on plunger allows fluid within needle to enter barrel so it is not expelled. Air at top of barrel and within needle is then expelled.
(10) If syringe contains excess fluid, use sink or other specially designated area for medication disposal. Hold syringe vertically with needle tip up and slanted slightly toward sink. Slowly eject excess fluid into sink. Recheck fluid level in syringe by holding it vertically.	Medication dose prepared accurately. Position of needle allows medication to be expelled without flowing down needle shaft. Rechecking fluid level ensures proper dose.
(11) Cover needle with its safety sheath or scoop needle to recap. Replace filter needle with safety needle or needleless access device for injection.	Prevents contamination of needle. Filter needles cannot be used for injection.
b. Vial containing a solution	
(1) Remove cap covering top of unused vial to expose sterile rubber seal, keeping rubber seal sterile. If a multidose vial has been used before, cap is already removed. Firmly and briskly wipe surface of rubber seal with alcohol swab and allow it to dry.	Vial comes packaged with seal that cannot be replaced after cap removal. Not all drug manufacturers guarantee that caps of unused vials are sterile. Therefore swab seals with alcohol before preparing medication. Allowing alcohol to dry prevents needle from being coated with alcohol and mixing with medication.
(2) Pick up syringe and remove needle cap or cap covering needleless vial access device (see illustration). Pull back on plunger to draw amount of air into syringe equal to volume of medication to be aspirated from vial.	Inject air first into vial to prevent buildup of negative pressure in vial when aspirating medication.

CLINICAL DECISION: *Some medications and agencies require use of a filter needle when preparing medications from a vial. See agency policy (Nicoll and Hesby, 2002). If using a filter needle to aspirate the medication, it is changed to a regular needle of suitable size to administer the medication.*

STEP 2a(6) A, Medication aspirated with ampule inverted. B, Medication aspirated with ampule on flat surface.

STEP 2b(2) Syringe with needleless adapter.

Clear, close-up **photos** and **illustrations** show you how to perform important skill procedures.

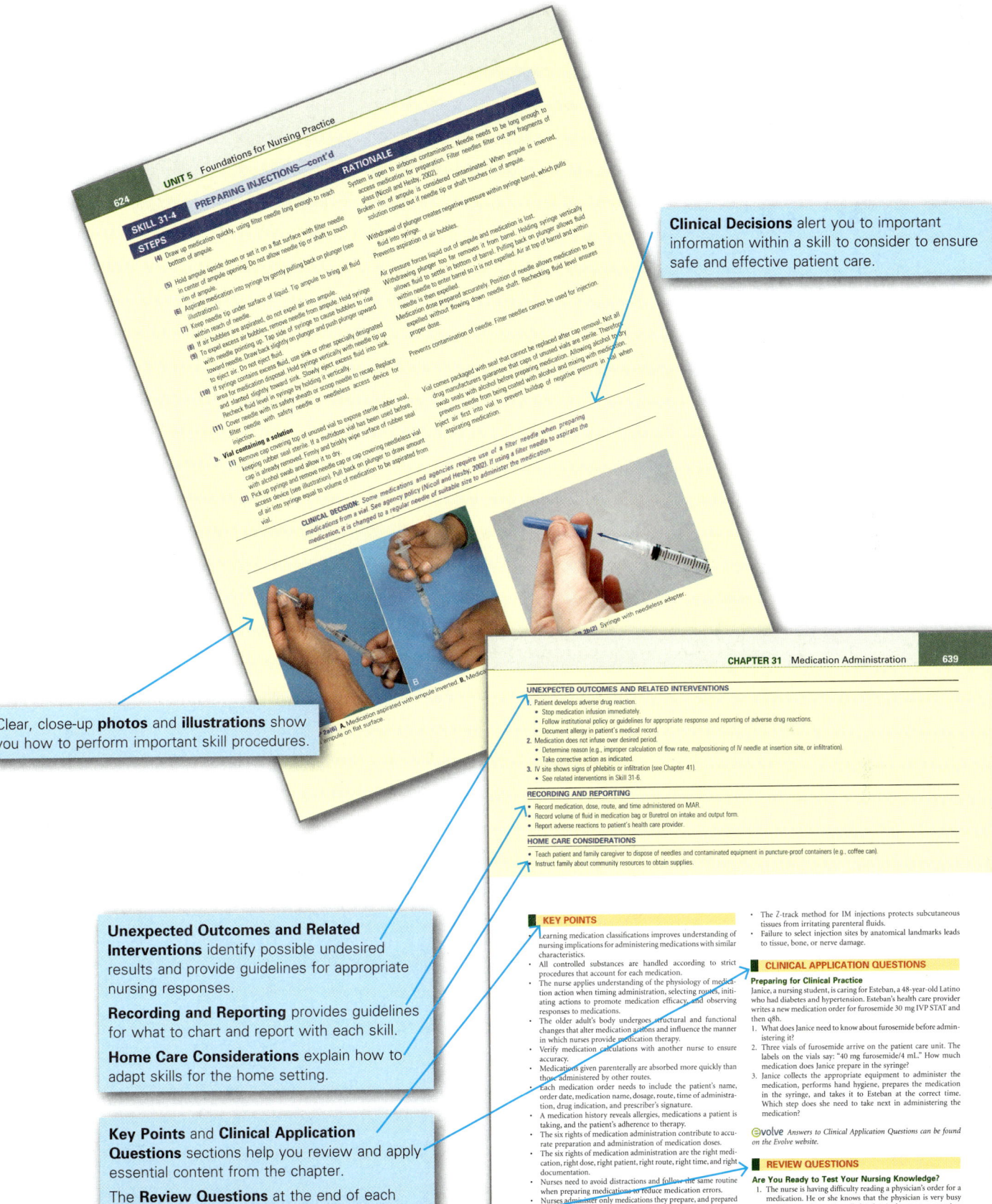

Clinical Decisions alert you to important information within a skill to consider to ensure safe and effective patient care.

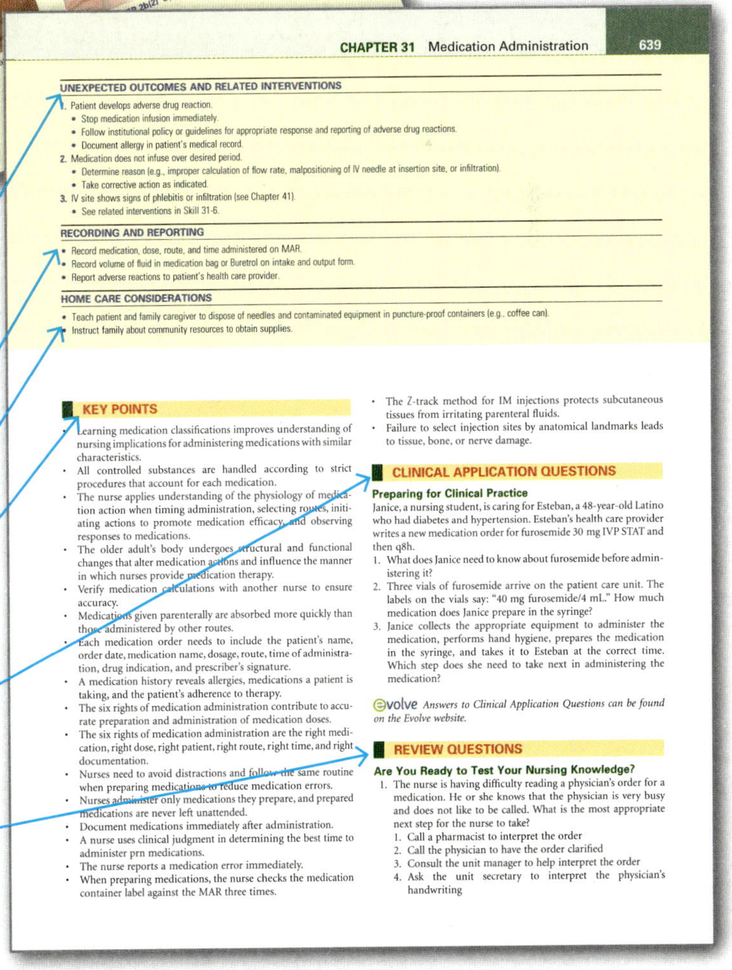

CHAPTER 31 Medication Administration 639

UNEXPECTED OUTCOMES AND RELATED INTERVENTIONS

1. Patient develops adverse drug reaction.
   - Stop medication infusion immediately.
   - Follow institutional policy or guidelines for appropriate response and reporting of adverse drug reactions.
   - Document allergy in patient's medical record.
2. Medication does not infuse over desired period.
   - Determine reason (e.g., improper calculation of flow rate, malpositioning of IV needle at insertion site, or infiltration).
   - Take corrective action as indicated.
3. IV site shows signs of phlebitis or infiltration (see Chapter 41).
   - See related interventions in Skill 31-6.

RECORDING AND REPORTING

- Record medication, dose, route, and time administered on MAR.
- Record volume of fluid in medication bag or Buretrol on intake and output form.
- Report adverse reactions to patient's health care provider.

HOME CARE CONSIDERATIONS

- Teach patient and family caregiver to dispose of needles and contaminated equipment in puncture-proof containers (e.g., coffee can).
- Instruct family about community resources to obtain supplies.

KEY POINTS

- Learning medication classifications improves understanding of nursing implications for administering medications with similar characteristics.
- All controlled substances are handled according to strict procedures that account for each medication.
- The nurse applies understanding of the physiology of medication action when timing administration, selecting routes, initiating actions to promote medication efficacy, and observing responses to medications.
- The older adult's body undergoes structural and functional changes that alter medication actions and influence the manner in which nurses provide medication therapy.
- Verify medication calculations with another nurse to ensure accuracy.
- Medications given parenterally are absorbed more quickly than those administered by other routes.
- Each medication order needs to include the patient's name, order date, medication name, dosage, route, time of administration, drug indication, and prescriber's signature.
- A medication history reveals allergies, medications a patient is taking, and the patient's adherence to therapy.
- The six rights of medication administration contribute to accurate preparation and administration of medication doses.
- The six rights of medication administration are the right medication, right dose, right patient, right route, right time, and right documentation.
- Nurses need to avoid distractions and follow the same routine when preparing medications to reduce medication errors.
- Nurses administer only medications they prepare, and prepared medications are never left unattended.
- Document medications immediately after administration.
- A nurse uses clinical judgment in determining the best time to administer prn medications.
- The nurse reports a medication error immediately.
- When preparing medications, the nurse checks the medication container label against the MAR three times.
- The Z-track method for IM injections protects subcutaneous tissues from irritating parenteral fluids.
- Failure to select injection sites by anatomical landmarks leads to tissue, bone, or nerve damage.

CLINICAL APPLICATION QUESTIONS

Preparing for Clinical Practice

Janice, a nursing student, is caring for Esteban, a 48-year-old Latino who had diabetes and hypertension. Esteban's health care provider writes a new medication order for furosemide 30 mg IVP STAT and then q8h.

1. What does Janice need to know about furosemide before administering it?
2. Three vials of furosemide arrive on the patient care unit. The labels on the vials say: "40 mg furosemide/4 mL." How much medication does Janice prepare in the syringe?
3. Janice collects the appropriate equipment to administer the medication, performs hand hygiene, prepares the medication in the syringe, and takes it to Esteban at the correct time. Which step does she need to take next in administering the medication?

evolve *Answers to Clinical Application Questions can be found on the Evolve website.*

REVIEW QUESTIONS

Are You Ready to Test Your Nursing Knowledge?

1. The nurse is having difficulty reading a physician's order for a medication. He or she knows that the physician is very busy and does not like to be called. What is the most appropriate next step for the nurse to take?
   1. Call a pharmacist to interpret the order
   2. Call the physician to have the order clarified
   3. Consult the unit manager to help interpret the order
   4. Ask the unit secretary to interpret the physician's handwriting

Unexpected Outcomes and Related Interventions identify possible undesired results and provide guidelines for appropriate nursing responses.

Recording and Reporting provides guidelines for what to chart and report with each skill.

Home Care Considerations explain how to adapt skills for the home setting.

Key Points and **Clinical Application Questions** sections help you review and apply essential content from the chapter.

The **Review Questions** at the end of each chapter, with the answer key included, help you evaluate learning and prepare for the examination.

PREFACE TO THE INSTRUCTOR

The nursing profession is always responding to dynamic change and continual challenges. Today nurses need a broad knowledge base from which to provide care. More important, nurses require the ability to know how to apply best evidence in practice to assure the best outcomes for their patients. The role of the nurse includes assuming the lead in preserving nursing practice and demonstrating its contribution to the health care of our nation. Nurses of tomorrow, therefore, need to become critical thinkers, patient advocates, clinical decision makers, and patient educators within a broad spectrum of care services.

The eighth edition of ***Fundamentals of Nursing*** was revised to prepare today's students for the challenges of tomorrow. This textbook is designed for beginning students in all types of professional nursing programs. The comprehensive coverage provides fundamental nursing concepts, skills, and techniques of nursing practice and a firm foundation for more advanced areas of study.

Fundamentals of Nursing provides a contemporary approach to nursing practice, discussing the entire scope of primary, acute, and restorative care. This new edition addresses a number of key current practice issues, including an emphasis on patient-centered care and evidence-based practice. Evidence-based practice is one of the most important initiatives in health care today. The increased focus on applying current evidence in skills and patient care plans helps students understand how the latest research findings should guide their clinical decision making.

KEY FEATURES

We have carefully developed this eighth edition with the student in mind. We have designed this text to welcome the new student to nursing, communicate our own love for the profession, and promote learning and understanding. Key features of the text include the following:

- Students will appreciate the **clear, engaging writing style.** The narrative actually addresses the reader, making this textbook more of an active instructional tool than a passive reference. Students will find that even complex technical and theoretical concepts are presented in a language that is easy to understand.
- **Comprehensive** coverage and readability of all fundamental nursing content.
- The **attractive, functional design** will appeal to today's visual learner. The clear, readable type and bold headings make the content easy to read and follow. Each special element is consistently color-keyed so students can readily identify important information.
- Hundreds of **large, clear, full-color photographs and drawings** reinforce and clarify key concepts and techniques.
- **Nursing process** format provides a consistent organizational framework for clinical chapters.
- **Learning aids** to help students identify, review, and apply important content in each chapter include Objectives, Key Terms, Key Points, Clinical Application Questions, and Review Questions.
- **Evolve Resources** lists detail the electronic resources available for the student at the beginning of every chapter.
- Covers **health promotion, acute and continuing care** to address today's practice in various settings.
- A **health promotion/wellness** thread is used consistently throughout the text.
- **Cultural diversity,** care of the **older adult,** and **patient teaching** are stressed throughout chapter narratives, as well as highlighted in special boxes.
- **Concept Maps** included in each clinical chapter show you the association between multiple nursing diagnoses for a patient with a selected medical diagnosis and the relationship between nursing interventions.
- **Nursing Care Plans** guide students on how to conduct an assessment and analyze the defining characteristics that indicate nursing diagnoses. The plans include NIC and NOC classifications to familiarize students with this important nomenclature. The evaluation sections of the plans show students how to evaluate and then determine the outcomes of care.
- A **critical thinking model provides a framework** for all clinical chapters, showing how elements of critical thinking, including knowledge, critical thinking attitudes, intellectual and professional standards, and experience, are integrated throughout the nursing process for making clinical decisions.
- **More than 55 nursing skills and 25 procedural guidelines** are presented. Nursing skills appear in a clear, two-column format with steps and supporting rationales that are often supported with current, evidenced-based research. Procedural guidelines boxes provide more streamlined, step-by-step instructions for performing very basic skills.
- **Delegation Considerations** guide when it is appropriate to delegate tasks to assistive personnel.
- **Unexpected Outcomes and Related Interventions** are highlighted within nursing skills to help students anticipate and appropriately respond to possible problems faced while performing skills.
- **Video Icons** indicate video clips associated with specific skills that are available on the Evolve Student Resources.
- **Printed endpapers** on the inside back cover provide information on locating specific assets in the book, including Skills, Procedure Guidelines, Nursing Care Plans, and Concept Maps.

NEW TO THIS EDITION

- **Safety Guidelines** section precedes each skill section. This helps students focus on safe and effective skill performance.
- **Skills sections** were moved to the end of the chapter for easier use, better text flow, and readability. In-text page callouts and colorful page bleeds help in locating these important sections.
- **Ongoing case studies** in each clinical chapter introduce "real-world" patients, families, and nurses. The chapter follows the same patient through the Nursing Care Plan, Concept Map, and meets them again in the Clinical Application Questions at the end of the chapter. These help students see how to apply the nursing process, along with critical thinking, to the care of patients. Cases take place in both acute and community settings, and include patients and nurses from a variety of cultural backgrounds.

- Information related to the **Quality and Safety Education for Nurses (QSEN)** initiative is highlighted by headings that coordinate with the key competencies. Building Competency scenarios for each chapter incorporate one of the six key competencies in QSEN.
- New **progressive case study** follows the same patient through each of the Nursing Process chapters (Chapters 16-20). This brings to life the framework of the process moving from Assessment, Diagnosis, Planning, Implementation, and Evaluation.
- Includes the latest **NANDA 2012-2014** diagnoses for up-to-date content.
- **New Skills** cover Blood Glucose Monitoring and Patient-Controlled Analgesia.
- **Expanded Review Questions** in each chapter resulting in an additional 250 questions. Answers are provided with questions and rationales are on Evolve.
- **Evidence-Based Practice** boxes now include a PICO question, provide a summary of nursing research evidence related to that specific topic, and then explain its implications for nursing practice. These have been updated to reflect current research topics and trends.
- Both ***Healthy People 2020*** and The Joint Commission's **2011 National Patient Safety Goals** are covered in this new edition promoting the importance of current research.
- **Chapter 41, *Fluid, Electrolyte, and Acid-Base Balance,*** has been completely rewritten and revised for better understanding of a complex topic.

LEARNING SUPPLEMENTS FOR STUDENTS

- The **Evolve Student Resources** are available online at http://evolve.elsevier.com/Potter/fundamentals/ and include the following valuable learning aids organized by chapter:
  - Chapter Review Questions from the book in an interactive format! Includes 750 questions to prepare for examinations
  - Answers and rationales to Chapter Review Questions
  - Answers and rationales to Clinical Application Questions
  - Answers and rationales to Building Competency scenario questions
  - Video clips highlight common skills
  - Animations
  - Concept Map Creator included in each clinical chapter
  - Case Study with questions
  - Audio glossary
  - Fluids & Electrolytes Tutorial
  - Interactive Learning Activities
  - Calculation Tutorial
  - Key Term Flashcards
  - Printable versions of Chapter Key Points
  - Nursing Skills Online reading assignments
  - Interactive Skills Performance Checklists are included for each skill in the text
  - Three practice quizzes cover all Fundamentals content for further study
- A thorough ***Study Guide*** by Geralyn Ochs provides an ideal supplement to help students understand and apply the content of the text. New to this edition is the inclusion of answers in the printed Study Guide. Each chapter includes multiple sections:
  - Preliminary Reading includes a chapter assignment from the text.
  - Comprehensive Understanding provides a variety of activities to reinforce the topics and main ideas from the text.
  - Review Questions are multiple-choice questions that require students to provide rationales for their answers. Answers and rationales are also provided on the Evolve site.
  - Clinical chapters include an Application of Critical Thinking Synthesis Model that expands the case study from the chapter's Care Plan and asks students to develop a step in the synthesis model based on the nurse and patient in the scenario. This helps students learn to apply both content learned and the critical thinking synthesis model.
- The handy ***Clinical Companion: Just the Facts*** complements, rather than abbreviates, the textbook. Content is presented in tabular, list, and outline format that equips your students with a concise, portable guide to all the facts and figures they'll need to know in their early clinical experiences.
- **Virtual Clinical Excursions** is an exciting workbook and CD-ROM experience that brings learning to life in a virtual hospital setting. The workbook guides students as they care for patients, providing ongoing challenges and learning opportunities. Each lesson in *Virtual Clinical Excursions* complements the textbook content and provides an environment for students to practice what they are learning. This CD/workbook is available separately or packaged at a special price with the textbook.

TEACHING SUPPLEMENTS FOR INSTRUCTORS

- The **Evolve Instructor Resources** (available online at http://evolve.elsevier.com/Potter/fundamentals) are a comprehensive collection of the most important tools instructors need, including the following:
  - **TEACH for Nurses** ties together every chapter resource you need for the most effective class presentations, with sections dedicated to objectives, teaching focus, nursing curriculum standards (including QSEN, BSN Essentials, and Concepts), instructor chapter resources, student chapter resources, answers to chapter questions, and an in-class case study discussion. Teaching strategies include content highlights, student activities, online activities, and large group activities.
  - The **Test Bank** contains a completely new set of more than 1350 questions with text page references and answers coded for NCLEX Client Needs category, nursing process, and cognitive level. Each question was involved in an instructor piloting process to ensure the best possible exam for students. The ExamView software allows instructors to create new tests; edit, add, and delete test questions; sort questions by NCLEX category, cognitive level, nursing process step, and question type; and administer/grade online tests.
  - Completely revised **PowerPoint Presentations** includes over 1500 slides for use in lectures. New to this edition are the inclusion of art within the slides and progressive case studies that include discussion questions and answers.
  - The **Image Collection** contains more than 1100 illustrations from the text for use in lectures.
  - **Simulation Learning System** is an online toolkit that helps instructors and facilitators effectively incorporate medium- to high-fidelity simulation into their nursing curriculum. Detailed patient scenarios promote and enhance the clinical decision-making skills of students at all levels. The system provides detailed instructions for preparation and implementation of the simulation experience, debriefing questions that encourage critical thinking, and learning resources to reinforce student comprehension. Each

scenario in *Simulation Learning System* complements the textbook content and helps bridge the gap between lectures and clinicals. This system provides the perfect environment for students to practice what they are learning in the text for a true-to-life, hands-on learning experience.

MULTIMEDIA SUPPLEMENTS FOR INSTRUCTORS AND STUDENTS

- **Nursing Skills Online 2.0** contains 18 modules rich with animations, videos, interactive activities, and exercises to help students prepare for their clinical lab experience. The instructionally designed lessons focus on topics that are difficult to master and pose a high risk to the patient if done incorrectly. Lesson quizzes allow students to check their learning curve and review as needed, and the module exams feed out to an instructor grade book. Modules cover Airway Management, Blood Therapy, Bowel Elimination/Ostomy Care, Chest Tubes, Enteral Nutrition, Infection Control, Injections, IV Fluid Administration, IV Fluid Therapy Management, IV Medication Administration, Nonparenteral Medication Administration, Safe Medication Administration, Safety, Specimen Collection, Urinary Catheterization, Vascular Access, Vital Signs, and Wound Care. Available alone or packaged with the text.
- **Mosby's Nursing Video Skills: Basic, Intermediate, Advanced version 3.0** provides 126 skills with overview information covering skill purpose, safety, and delegation guides; equipment lists; preparation procedures; procedure videos with printable step-by-step guidelines; appropriate follow-up care; documentation guidelines; and interactive review questions. Available online, as a student DVD set, or as a networkable DVD set for the institution.

ACKNOWLEDGMENTS

The eighth edition of *Fundamentals of Nursing* is the result of a continuing collaboration with Dr. Amy M. Hall and Dr. Patricia A. Stockert, which began with the seventh edition of *Basic Nursing*. Their insight, professionalism, attention to detail, and commitment to a quality textbook are unmatched. Their calm demeanor, sense of humor, and work ethic have made writing this textbook a pleasure.

- The editorial and production professionals at Mosby/Elsevier are supportive, creative, dedicated, and hard working. While there are many professionals involved in preparing this text, we wish to acknowledge the following persons:
    - Tamara Myers, Senior Content Strategist, for her vision, organization, professionalism, energy, and support in assisting us to develop a text that offers a state-of-the-art approach to the design, organization, and presentation of *Fundamentals of Nursing*. Her skill is in motivating and supporting a writing team so it can be creative and innovative while retaining the characteristics of a high-quality textbook.
    - Tina Kaemmerer made her maiden voyage as Content Development Specialist of *Fundamentals of Nursing*. She is an amazingly organized and talented individual who has done considerable behind-the-scenes work that has improved the accuracy and consistency in how we present content within the textbook. She, too, has limitless energy and is always willing to go the extra mile.
    - Jodi Willard, Senior Project Manager, is an accomplished production editor. Jodi approaches her work very professionally and is able to coordinate the multiple aspects of completing a well-designed finished product. She is talented and calm under pressure, and through her sense of humor and commitment to excellence guided this text to completion.
- Mike DeFilippo, St. Louis, Missouri, for his excellent photography.
- Goldfarb School of Nursing at Barnes-Jewish College, St. Louis, Missouri, for making their simulation lab available to us for photographs.
- To our contributors, clinicians, and educators who share their expertise and knowledge about nursing practice in helping to create informative, accurate, and current information. Knowledge of their clinical specialties ensures we have a state-of-the-art textbook. We are fortunate to be associated with excellent nurse authors who are able to convey standards of nursing excellence.
- To our many reviewers for their expertise, candor, knowledge of the literature, and astute comments that assist us in developing a text with high standards that reflect excellent professional nursing practice through the printed word.
- And special recognition to our professional colleagues at Barnes-Jewish Hospital, Southern Illinois University Edwardsville, Saint Francis Medical Center College of Nursing, and the University of Evansville.

After more than 28 years of collaboration we find ourselves very fortunate and humble. *Fundamentals of Nursing* and our other textbooks allow us to contribute to nursing knowledge and help shape the practice of nursing. Nursing excellence belongs to all of us, and we are happy to have the opportunity to continue the work we love.

Patricia A. Potter
Anne Griffin Perry

CONTENTS

Any updates to this textbook can be found in the Content Updates folder on Evolve at http://evolve.elsevier.com/Potter/fundamentals/.

UNIT 1 NURSING AND THE HEALTH CARE ENVIRONMENT

UNIT 2 CARING THROUGHOUT THE LIFE SPAN

UNIT 6 PSYCHOSOCIAL BASIS FOR NURSING PRACTICE

UNIT 7 PHYSIOLOGICAL BASIS FOR NURSING PRACTICE

CHAPTER

1

Nursing Today

OBJECTIVES

- Discuss the development of professional nursing roles.
- Describe educational programs available for professional registered nurse education.
- Describe the roles and career opportunities for nurses.
- Discuss the influence of social, political, and economic changes on nursing practices.

KEY TERMS

Advanced practice registered nurse (APRN), p. 7
American Nurses Association (ANA), p. 1
Caregiver, p. 7
Certified nurse-midwife (CNM), p. 8
Certified registered nurse anesthetist (CRNA), p. 8
Clinical nurse specialist (CNS), p. 8
Code of ethics, p. 4
Continuing education, p. 5
Genomics, p. 10
In-service education, p. 5
International Council of Nurses (ICN), p. 9
National League for Nursing (NLN), p. 9
Nurse administrator, p. 8
Nurse educator, p. 8
Nurse practitioner (NP), p. 8
Nurse researcher, p. 8
Nursing, p. 1
Patient advocate, p. 7
Professional organization, p. 9
Quality and Safety Education for Nurses (QSEN), p. 9
Registered nurse (RN), p. 5

evolve WEBSITE

http://evolve.elsevier.com/Potter/fundamentals/

- Review Questions
- Case Study with Questions
- Audio Glossary
- Interactive Learning Activities
- Key Term Flashcards
- Content Updates

Nursing is an art and a science. As a professional nurse you will learn to deliver care artfully with compassion, caring, and respect for each patient's dignity and personhood. As a science nursing practice is based on a body of knowledge that is continually changing with new discoveries and innovations. When you integrate the science and art of nursing into your practice, the quality of care you provide to your patients is at a level of excellence that benefits patients and their families.

Your opportunities for a nursing career are limitless. There are a variety of career paths, including clinical practice, education, research, management, administration, and even entrepreneurship. As a student it is important for you to understand the scope of nursing practice and how nursing influences the lives of your patients.

The patient is the center of your practice. The patient includes the individual, family, and/or community. Patients have a wide variety of health care needs, experiences, vulnerabilities, and expectations; but this is what makes nursing both challenging and rewarding. Making a difference in your patients' lives is fulfilling (e.g., helping a dying patient find relief from pain, helping a young mother learn parenting skills, and finding ways for older adults to remain independent in their homes). Nursing offers personal and professional rewards every day. This chapter presents a contemporary view of the evolution of nursing and nursing practice and the historical, practical, social, and political influences on the discipline of nursing.

When giving care, it is essential to provide a specified service according to standards of practice and to follow a code of ethics (American Nurses Association [ANA], 2008, 2010b). Professional practice includes knowledge from social and behavioral sciences, biological and physiological sciences, and nursing theories. In addition, nursing practice incorporates ethical and social values, professional autonomy, and a sense of commitment and community. The **American Nurses Association (ANA)** defines **nursing** as *the protection, promotion, and optimization of health and abilities; prevention of illness and injury; alleviation of suffering through the diagnosis and treatment of human response; and advocacy in the care of individuals, families, communities, and populations* (ANA, 2010b). The International Council of Nurses (ICN, 2010) has another definition: *Nursing encompasses autonomous and collaborative care of individuals of all ages, families, groups and communities, sick or well and in all settings. Nursing includes the promotion of health; prevention of illness; and the care of ill, disabled, and dying people. Advocacy, promotion of a safe environment, research, participation in shaping health policy and in patient and health systems management, and education are also key nursing roles.* Both of these definitions support the prominence and importance that nursing holds in providing safe, patient-centered health care to the global community.

Expert clinical nursing practice is a commitment to the application of knowledge, ethics, aesthetics, and clinical experience. Your ability to interpret clinical situations and make complex decisions is the foundation for your nursing care and the basis for the advancement of nursing practice and the development of nursing science (Benner, 1984; Benner, Tanner, and Chesla, 1997; Benner et al., 2010). Critical thinking skills are essential to nursing (see Chapter 15). When providing nursing care, you need to make clinical judgments and decisions about your patients' health care needs based on knowledge, experience, and standards of care. Use critical thinking skills and reflections to help you gain and interpret scientific knowledge, integrate knowledge from clinical experiences, and become a lifelong learner (Benner et al., 2010).

HISTORICAL HIGHLIGHTS

Nursing has responded and always will respond to the needs of its patients. In times of war the nursing response was to meet the needs of the wounded in combat zones and military hospitals in the United States and abroad. When communities face health care crises such as disease outbreaks or insufficient health care resources, nurses establish community-based immunization and screening programs, treatment clinics, and health promotion activities. Our patients are most vulnerable when they are injured, sick, or dying.

Since the beginning of the profession, nurses have studied and tested new and better ways to help their patients. A classic article described Florence Nightingale's work during the Crimean War. She studied and implemented methods to improve battlefield sanitation, which ultimately reduced illness, infection, and mortality (Cohen, 1984). Take time to reflect about Nightingale's actions centuries ago and think about the impact of her actions. She set the stage for using evidence to direct practice.

Today nurses are active in determining the best practices for skin care management, pain control, nutritional management, and care of older adults, to cite just a few examples. Nurse researchers are leaders in expanding knowledge in nursing and other health care disciplines. Their work provides evidence for practice to ensure that nurses have the best available evidence to support their practices (see Chapter 5).

Nursing is a combination of knowledge from the physical sciences, humanities, and social sciences, along with clinical competencies needed for safe, quality patient-centered care (Gugliemi, 2010). It continuously responds and adapts to new challenges. Nurses are in a unique position to refine and shape the future of health care.

Nurses are active in social policy and political arenas. Nurses and their professional organizations lobby for health care legislation to meet the needs of patients, particularly the medically underserved. For example, nurses in communities provide home visits to newborns of high-risk mothers (e.g., adolescent, poorly educated mothers or medically underserved). These visits result in fewer emergency department visits, fewer newborn infections, and reduced infant mortality (Mason et al., 2012).

Knowledge of the history of our profession increases your ability to understand the social and intellectual origins of the discipline. Although it is not practical to describe all of the historical aspects of professional nursing, some of the more significant milestones are described in the following paragraphs.

Florence Nightingale

In *Notes on Nursing: What It Is and What It Is Not*, Florence Nightingale established the first nursing philosophy based on health maintenance and restoration (Nightingale, 1860). She saw the role of nursing as having "charge of somebody's health" based on the knowledge of "how to put the body in such a state to be free of disease or to recover from disease" (Nightingale, 1860). During the same year she developed the first organized program for training nurses, the Nightingale Training School for Nurses at St. Thomas' Hospital in London.

Nightingale was the first practicing nurse epidemiologist (Cohen, 1984). Her statistical analyses connected poor sanitation with cholera and dysentery. She volunteered during the Crimean War in 1853 and traveled the battlefield hospitals at night carrying her lamp; thus she was known as the "lady with the lamp." The sanitary, nutrition, and basic facilities in the battlefield hospitals were poor at best. Eventually she was given the task to organize and improve the quality of the sanitation facilities. As a result, the mortality rate at the Barracks Hospital in Scutari, Turkey, was reduced from 42.7% to 2.2% in 6 months (Donahue, 2011).

The Civil War to the Beginning of the Twentieth Century

The Civil War (1860 to 1865) stimulated the growth of nursing in the United States. Clara Barton, founder of the American Red Cross, tended soldiers on the battlefields, cleansing their wounds, meeting their basic needs, and comforting them in death. The U.S. Congress ratified the American Red Cross in 1882 after 10 years of lobbying by Barton. Dorothea Lynde Dix, Mary Ann Ball (Mother Bickerdyke), and Harriet Tubman also influenced nursing during the Civil War (Donahue, 2011). As superintendent of the female nurses of the Union Army, Dix organized hospitals, appointed nurses, and oversaw and regulated supplies to the troops. Mother Bickerdyke organized ambulance services and walked abandoned battlefields at night, looking for wounded soldiers. Harriet Tubman was active in the Underground Railroad movement and assisted in leading over 300 slaves to freedom (Donahue, 2011).

The first professionally trained African American nurse was Mary Mahoney. She was concerned with relationships between cultures and races; and as a noted nursing leader she brought forth an awareness of cultural diversity and respect for the individual, regardless of background, race, color, or religion.

Isabel Hampton Robb helped found the Nurses' Associated Alumnae of the United States and Canada in 1896. This organization became the ANA in 1911. She authored many nursing textbooks, including *Nursing: Its Principles and Practice for Hospital and Private Use* (1894), *Nursing Ethics* (1900), and *Educational Standards for Nurses* (1907) and was one of the original founders of the *American Journal of Nursing* (AJN) (Donahue, 2011).

Nursing in hospitals expanded in the late nineteenth century. However, nursing in the community did not increase significantly until 1893, when Lillian Wald and Mary Brewster opened the Henry Street Settlement, which focused on the health needs of poor people who lived in tenements in New York City (Donahue, 2011). Nurses working in this settlement were some of the first to demonstrate autonomy in practice because they frequently encountered situations that required quick and innovative problem solving and critical thinking without the supervision or direction of a health care provider.

Twentieth Century

In the early twentieth century a movement toward developing a scientific, research-based defined body of nursing knowledge and practice was evolving. Nurses began to assume expanded and advanced practice roles. Mary Adelaide Nutting was instrumental in the affiliation of nursing education with universities. She became the first professor of nursing at Columbia University Teachers College in 1906 (Donahue, 2011). In addition, the Goldmark

Report concluded that nursing education needed increased financial support and suggested that university schools of nursing receive the money.

As nursing education developed, nursing practice also expanded, and the Army and Navy Nurse Corps were established. By the 1920s nursing specialization was developing. Graduate nurse-midwifery programs began; in the last half of the century specialty-nursing organizations were created. Examples of these specialty organizations include the American Association of Critical Care Nurses; Association of Operating Room Nurses (AORN); Emergency Nurses Association (ENA); Infusion Nurses Society (INS); Oncology Nursing Society (ONS); and Wound, Ostomy, Continence Nurses Society (WOCN).

Twenty-First Century

Nursing practice and education continue to evolve to meet the needs of society. In 1990 the ANA established the Center for Ethics and Human Rights (see Chapter 22). The Center provides a forum to address the complex ethical and human rights issues confronting nurses and designs activities and programs to increase ethical competence in nurses (ANA, 2010c).

Today the profession faces multiple challenges. Nurses and nurse educators are revising nursing practice and school curricula to meet the ever-changing needs of society, including bioterrorism, emerging infections, and disaster management. Advances in technology and informatics (see Chapter 26), the high acuity level of care of hospitalized patients, and early discharge from health care institutions require nurses in all settings to have a strong and current knowledge base from which to practice. In addition, nursing and the Robert Wood Johnson Foundation are taking a leadership role in developing standards and policies for end-of-life care through the *Last Acts Campaign* (see Chapter 36). The End-of-Life Nursing Education Consortium (ELNEC) offered collaboratively by the American Association of Colleges of Nursing (AACN) and the City of Hope Medical Center has brought end-of-life care and practices into nursing curricula and professional continuing-education programs for practicing nurses (Tilden and Thompson, 2009).

INFLUENCES ON NURSING

Multiple external forces affect nursing, including demographic changes of the population, human rights, increasing numbers of medically underserved, and the threat of bioterrorism.

Health Care Reform

Health care reform not only affects how health care is paid for but how it is delivered. There will be greater emphasis on health promotion, disease prevention, and illness management in the future. This model impacts the delivery of nursing care. More services will be in community-based care settings. As a result, more nurses will be needed to practice in community care centers, schools, and senior centers. This will require nurses to be more adept at assessing for resources, service gaps, and how the patient adapts to returning to the community. Nursing must respond to such changes by exploring new methods to provide care, changing nursing education, and revising practice standards (O'Neil, 2009).

Demographic Changes

The U.S. Census Bureau (2008a) predicts that between 2010 and 2050 there will be a steady rise in the population. This change alone requires expanded health care resources. Add to the population change a steady increase in the population of people 65 years and older (U.S. Census Bureau, 2008b). To effectively meet all the health care needs of the expanding and aging population, changes need to occur as to how care is provided, especially in the area of public health, to address health care reform and meet the needs of the changing population. The population is still shifting from rural areas to urban centers, and more people are living with chronic and long-term illness (Presley, 2010). Not only are there expansions of outpatient settings, but more and more people want to receive outpatient and community-based care and remain in their homes or community (see Chapters 2 and 3).

Medically Underserved

The rising rates of unemployment, underemployment and low-paying jobs, mental illness, and homelessness and rising health care costs all contribute to increases in the medically underserved population. Caring for the medically underserved population is a global issue; the social, political, and economic factors of a country affect both access to care and resources to provide and pay for these services (Huicho et al., 2010). In the United States some of the medically underserved population are poor and on Medicaid. Others are part of the working poor (i.e., they cannot afford their own insurance, but they make too much money to qualify for Medicaid and as a result do not receive any health care). In addition, the number of underserved patients who require home-based palliative care services is increasing. This is a group of patients whose physical status does not improve and heath care needs increase. As a result, the cost for home-based care continues to rise, to the point that some patients opt out of all palliative services because of costs (Fernandes et al., 2010). Today nurses and schools of nursing are developing partnerships to improve health outcomes in underserved communities. Nurses work in these community-based settings providing health promotion and disease prevention to the homeless, mentally ill, and others who have limited access to health care or who lack health care insurance (McCann, 2010).

Threat of Bioterrorism

The world is a changing place; the threats of bioterrorism are continuous. Many health care agencies, schools, and communities have educational programs to prepare for nuclear, chemical, or biological attack. Nurses are active in disaster preparedness. The ICN works alongside national nursing associations to determine how to best educate and prepare nurses for future disasters (Robinson, 2010). For example, public health emergency simulation exercises allow nurses and students to work with community disaster-preparedness groups and hospitals to determine what specific nursing activities are needed (Morrison and Catanzaro, 2010). These activities sometimes range from participation in vaccine research, decontamination in the event of biological attack, and triage for mass casualty to crisis response units. If a disaster were to occur, nurses would be essential in evaluating the strengths and weaknesses of any disaster plan.

Rising Health Care Costs

Skyrocketing health care costs present challenges to the profession, consumer, and the health care delivery system. As a nurse you are responsible for providing the patient with the best-quality care in an efficient and economically sound manner. The challenge is to use health care and patient resources wisely. Chapter 2 summarizes reasons for the rise in health care costs and its implications for nursing.

Nursing Shortage

There is an ongoing global nursing shortage, which results from insufficient qualified registered nurses (RNs) to fill vacant positions and the loss of qualified RNs to other professions (Flinkman et al., 2010). This shortage affects all aspects of nursing such as patient care, administration, and nursing education (Tanner and Bellack, 2010), but it also represents challenges and opportunities for the profession. Many health care dollars are invested in strategies aimed at recruiting a well-educated, critically thinking, motivated, and dedicated nursing workforce (Benner et al., 2010). There is a direct link between registered nurses' care and positive patient outcomes, reduced complication rates, and a more rapid return of the patient to an optimal functional status (Aiken, 2010; Lucero et al., 2009).

Professional nursing organizations predict that there will continue to be a diminishing pipeline of RNs in the future (AACN, 2008b; Aiken, 2010). Like it or not, the nursing shortage affects the needs of the consumer (Block and Sredl, 2006). With fewer nurses in the workplace, it is important for you to learn to use your patient contact time efficiently and professionally. Time management, therapeutic communication, patient education, and compassionate implementation of psychomotor skills are just a few of the essential skills you need. Most important, your patients leave the health care setting with a positive image of nursing and a feeling that they received quality care. In a rapid-discharge and high-tech health care environment nurses need to relate to their patients on a human, caring level (Manthey, 2008). Your patient should never feel rushed or that he or she was unimportant. If a certain aspect of patient care requires 15 minutes of contact, it will take the same time to deliver the care in an organized manner as it would in a rushed, harried manner.

NURSING AS A PROFESSION

Nursing is not simply a collection of specific skills, and you are not simply a person trained to perform specific tasks. Nursing is a profession. No one factor absolutely differentiates a job from a profession, but the difference is important in terms of how you practice. To act professionally you administer quality patient-centered care in a safe, conscientious, and knowledgeable manner. You are responsible and accountable to yourself and your patients and peers. A profession has the following primary characteristics:

- It requires a basic liberal foundation and an extended education of its members.
- It has a theoretical body of knowledge leading to defined skills, abilities, and norms.
- It provides a specific service.
- Members of a profession have autonomy in decision making and practice.
- The profession as a whole has a code of ethics for practice.

Scope and Standards of Practice

Since 1960 the ANA has engaged in documenting the scope of nursing and developing standards of practice (ANA, 2010b). Within this document are the Standards of Practice and Standards of Professional Performance. It is important that you know and apply these standards in your practice. The document is usually available in most schools of nursing and practice settings. The goal of this document is to improve the health and well-being of all individuals, communities, and populations through the significant and visible contributions of registered nursing using standard-based practice (ANA, 2010b).

BOX 1-1 ANA STANDARDS OF NURSING PRACTICE

1. **Assessment:** The registered nurse collects comprehensive data pertinent to the patient's health and/or the situation.
2. **Diagnosis:** The registered nurse analyzes the assessment data to determine the diagnoses or issues.
3. **Outcomes Identification:** The registered nurse identifies expected outcomes for a plan individualized to the patient or the situation.
4. **Planning:** The registered nurse develops a plan that prescribes strategies and alternatives to attain expected outcomes.
5. **Implementation:** The registered nurse implements the identified plan.

5a. **Coordination of Care:** The registered nurse coordinates care delivery.

5b. **Health Teaching and Health Promotion:** The registered nurse uses strategies to promote health and a safe environment.

5c. **Consultation:** The graduate level–prepared specialty nurse or advanced practice registered nurse provides consultation to influence the identified plan, enhance the abilities of others, and effect change.

5d. **Prescriptive authority and treatment:** The advanced practice registered

nurse uses prescriptive authority, procedures, referrals, treatment, and therapies in accordance with state and federal laws and regulations.

6. **Evaluation:** The registered nurse evaluates progress toward attainment of outcomes.

Standards of Practice. The Standards of Practice describe a competent level of nursing care (Box 1-1). The levels of care are demonstrated by the critical thinking model known as the nursing process: assessment, diagnosis, outcomes identification and planning, implementation, and evaluation (ANA, 2010b). The nursing process is the foundation of clinical decision making and includes all significant actions taken by nurses in providing care to patients (see Unit 3).

Standards of Professional Performance. The ANA Standards of Professional Performance (Box 1-2) describe a competent level of behavior in the professional role (ANA, 2010b). These standards provide objective guidelines for nurses to be accountable for their actions, their patients, and their peers. The standards provide a method to assure patients that they are receiving high-quality care, that the nurses know exactly what is necessary to provide nursing care, and that measures are in place to determine whether care meets the standards.

Code of Ethics. The **code of ethics** is the philosophical ideals of right and wrong that define the principles you will use to provide care to your patients. It is important for you to also incorporate your own values and ethics into your practice. As you incorporate these values, you explore what type of nurse you will be and how you will function within the discipline (ANA, 2008, 2010c). Ask yourself: how do your ethics, values, and practice compare with established standards? The ANA has a number of publications that address ethics and human rights in nursing. The *Code of Ethics for Nurses with Interpretive Statements* is a guide for carrying out nursing responsibilities that provide quality nursing care; it also outlines the ethical obligations of the profession (ANA, 2008). Chapter 22 provides a review of the nursing code of ethics and ethical principles for everyday practice.

BOX 1-2 ANA STANDARDS OF PROFESSIONAL PERFORMANCE

7. **Ethics:** The registered nurse practices ethically.
8. **Education:** The registered nurse attains knowledge and competency that reflects current nursing practice.
9. **Evidence-Based Practice and Research:** The registered nurse integrates evidence and research findings into practice.
10. **Quality of Practice:** The registered nurse contributes to quality nursing practice.
11. **Communication:** The registered nurse communicates effectively in all areas of practice.
12. **Leadership:** The registered nurse demonstrates leadership in the professional practice setting and the profession.
13. **Collaboration:** The registered nurse collaborates with health care consumer, family, and others in the conduct of nursing practice.
14. **Professional Practice Evaluation:** The registered nurse evaluates her or his own nursing practice in relation to professional practice standards and guidelines, relevant statutes, rules, and regulations.
15. **Resources:** The registered nurse uses appropriate resources to plan and provide nursing services that are safe, effective, and financially responsible.
16. **Environmental Health:** The registered nurse practices in an environmentally safe and healthy manner.

NURSING EDUCATION

Nursing requires a significant amount of formal education. The issues of standardization of nursing education and entry into practice remain a major controversy. In 1965 the ANA published a position paper on nursing education that emphasizes the role of education for the advancement of the science of the profession (ANA, 1965). Most nurses agree that nursing education is important to practice and that education needs to respond to changes in health care created by scientific and technological advances. There are various education preparations for an individual intending to be an RN. In addition, there is graduate nurse education and continuing and in-service education for practicing nurses.

Professional Registered Nurse Education

Currently in the United States the most frequent way to become a **registered nurse (RN)** is either through completion of an associate or baccalaureate degree program. Graduates of both programs are eligible to take the National Council Licensure Examination for Registered Nurses (NCLEX-RN®) to become RNs in the state in which they will practice.

The associate degree program in the United States is a 2-year program that is usually offered by a university or community college. This program focuses on the basic sciences and theoretical and clinical courses related to the practice of nursing.

The baccalaureate degree program usually includes 4 years of study in a college or university. The program focuses on the basic sciences; theoretical and clinical courses; and courses in the social sciences, arts, and humanities to support nursing theory. In Canada the degree of Bachelor of Science in Nursing (BScN) or Bachelor in Nursing (BN) is equivalent to the degree of Bachelor of Science in Nursing (BSN) in the United States. The *Essentials of Baccalaureate Education for Professional Nursing* (AACN, 2008a) delineates essential knowledge, practice and values, attitudes, personal qualities, and professional behavior for the baccalaureate-prepared nurse and guides faculty on the structure and evaluation of the curriculum. The National League for Nursing Accreditation Council (NLNAC) published the *NLNAC Standards and Criteria Baccalaureate Programs in Nursing—2008*. This document identifies core competencies for the professional nurse and supports the Pew Health Commission and the competencies of the Institute of Medicine (IOM) for health professionals (NLNAC, 2008). In addition, one of the IOM's recommendations is that 80% of nurses be prepared with a baccalaureate in nursing by 2020 (IOM, 2010) (see Chapter 2).

Graduate Education

After obtaining a baccalaureate degree in nursing, you can pursue graduate education leading to a master's or doctoral degree in any number of graduate fields, including nursing. A nurse completing a graduate program can receive a master's degree in nursing. The graduate degree provides the advanced clinician with strong skills in nursing science and theory, with emphasis on the basic sciences and research-based clinical practice. A master's degree in nursing is important for the roles of nurse educator and nurse administrator, and it is required for an advanced practice registered nurse (APRN).

Doctoral Preparation. Professional doctoral programs in nursing (DSN or DNSc) prepare graduates to apply research findings to clinical nursing. Other doctoral programs emphasize more basic research and theory and award the research-oriented Doctor of Philosophy (PhD) in nursing. Recently the AACN recommended the Doctor of Nursing Practice (DNP) as the terminal practice degree and required preparation for all APRNs by 2015 (Chase and Pruitt, 2006). The DNP is a practice-focused doctorate. It provides skills in obtaining expanded knowledge through the formulation and interpretations of evidence-based practice (Chism, 2010).

The need for nurses with doctoral degrees is increasing. Expanding clinical roles and continuing demand for well-educated nursing faculty, nurse administrators, and APRNs in the clinical settings and new areas of nursing specialties such as nursing informatics are just a few reasons for increasing the number of doctorally prepared nurses.

Continuing and In-Service Education

Nursing is a knowledge-based profession, and technological expertise and clinical decision making are qualities that our health care consumers demand and expect. Continuing education programs are one way to promote and maintain current nursing skills, gain new knowledge and theory, and obtain new skills reflecting the changes in the health care delivery system (Hale et al., 2010). **Continuing education** involves formal, organized educational programs offered by universities, hospitals, state nurses associations, professional nursing organizations, and educational and health care institutions. An example is a program on caring for older adults with dementia offered by a university or a program on safe medication practices offered by a hospital. Continuing education updates your knowledge about the latest research and practice developments, helps you to specialize in a particular area of practice, and teaches you new skills and techniques (Hale et al., 2010).

In-service education programs are instruction or training provided by a health care agency or institution. An in-service program is held in the institution and is designed to increase the knowledge, skills, and competencies of nurses and other health care professionals employed by the institution. Often in-service programs are focused on new technologies such as how to correctly use the newest safety syringes. Many in-service programs are designed to fulfill required competencies of an organization. For example, a hospital might offer an in-service program on safe principles for administering chemotherapy or a program on cultural sensitivity.

NURSING PRACTICE

You will have an opportunity to practice in a variety of settings, in many roles within those settings, and with caregivers in other related health professions. Administrators in health care agencies and institutions guide the practice of nursing only in part. State and provincial Nurse Practice Acts (NPAs) establish specific legal regulations for practice, and professional organizations establish standards of practice as criteria for nursing care. The ANA is concerned with legal aspects of nursing practice, public recognition of the significance of nursing practice to health care, and implications for nursing practice regarding trends in health care. The ANA definition of nursing illustrates the consistent orientation of nurses to providing care to promote the well-being of their patients individually or in groups and communities (ANA, 2010a).

Nurse Practice Acts

In the United States the State Boards of Nursing oversee NPAs. NPAs regulate the scope of nursing practice and protect public health, safety, and welfare. This protection includes shielding the public from unqualified and unsafe nurses. Although each state defines for itself the scope of nursing practice, most have similar NPAs. The definition of nursing practice published by the ANA is representative of the scope of nursing practice as defined in most states. However, in the last decade many states have revised their NPAs to reflect the growing autonomy of nursing and the expanded roles of nurses in practice. For example, NPAs expanded their scope to include minimum education requirements, required certifications, and practice guidelines for APRNs such as nurse practitioners and certified RN anesthetists. The expansion of scope of practice includes skills unique to the advanced practice role (e.g., advanced assessment, prescriptive authority for certain medications and diagnostic procedures, and some invasive procedures).

Licensure and Certification

Licensure. In the United States RN candidates must pass the NCLEX-RN® examination administered by the individual State Boards of Nursing. Regardless of educational preparation, the examination for RN licensure is exactly the same in every state in the United States. This provides a standardized minimum knowledge base for nurses.

Certification. Beyond the NCLEX-RN®, the nurse may choose to work toward certification in a specific area of nursing practice. Minimum practice requirements are set, based on the certification the nurse seeks. National nursing organizations such as the ANA have many types of certification to enhance your career such as certification in medical surgical or geriatric nursing. After passing the initial examination, you maintain your certification by ongoing continuing education and clinical or administrative practice.

Science and Art of Nursing Practice

Because nursing is both an art and a science, nursing practice requires a blend of the most current knowledge and practice standards with an insightful and compassionate approach to patient care. Your patients' health care needs are multidimensional. Thus your care will reflect the needs and values of society and professional standards of care and performance, meet the needs of each patient, and integrate evidence-based findings to provide the highest level of care. Nursing has a specific body of knowledge; however, it is essential that you socialize within the profession and practice to fully understand and apply the nursing knowledge base and develop professional expertise. Clinical expertise takes time and commitment. According to Benner et al. (2010), an expert nurse passes through five levels of proficiency when acquiring and developing generalist or specialized nursing skills (Box 1-3).

BOX 1-3 BENNER: FROM NOVICE TO EXPERT

Novice: Beginning nursing student or any nurse entering a situation in which there is no previous level of experience (e.g., an experienced operating room nurse chooses to now practice in home health). The learner learns via a specific set of rules or procedures, which are usually stepwise and linear.

Advanced Beginner: A nurse who has had some level of experience with the situation. This experience may only be observational in nature, but the nurse is able to identify meaningful aspects or principles of nursing care.

Competent: A nurse who has been in the same clinical position for 2 to 3 years. This nurse understands the organization and specific care required by the type of patients (e.g., surgical, oncology, or orthopedic patients). This nurse is a competent practitioner who is able to anticipate nursing care and establish long-range goals. In this phase the nurse has usually had experience with all types of psychomotor skills required by this specific group of patients.

Proficient: A nurse with more than 2 to 3 years of experience in the same clinical position. This nurse perceives a patient's clinical situation as a whole, is able to assess an entire situation, and can readily transfer knowledge gained from multiple previous experiences to a situation. This nurse focuses on managing care as opposed to managing and performing skills.

Expert: A nurse with diverse experience who has an intuitive grasp of an existing or potential clinical problem. This nurse is able to zero in on the problem and focus on multiple dimensions of the situation. He or she is skilled at identifying both patient-centered problems and problems related to the health care system or perhaps the needs of the novice nurse.

Data from Benner P: *From novice to expert: excellence and power in clinical nursing practice,* Menlo Park, Calif, 1984, Addison-Wesley.

Use the competencies of critical thinking in your practice. This includes integrating knowledge from basic science and nursing knowledge bases, applying knowledge from past and present experiences, applying critical thinking attitudes to a clinical situation, and implementing intellectual and professional standards (see Chapter 15). When you provide well–thought out care with compassion and caring, you provide each of your patients the best of the science and art of nursing care (see Chapter 7).

PROFESSIONAL RESPONSIBILITIES AND ROLES

As a nurse, you are responsible for obtaining and maintaining specific knowledge and skills for a variety of professional roles and responsibilities. Nurses provide care and comfort for patients in all health care settings. Nurses' concern for meeting the patient's needs remains the same whether care focuses on health promotion and illness prevention, disease and symptom management, family support, or end-of-life care.

Autonomy and Accountability

Autonomy is an essential element of professional nursing that involves the initiation of independent nursing interventions without medical orders. For example, you independently implement coughing and deep-breathing exercises for a patient who recently had surgery. You actively collaborate with other health professionals to pursue the best treatment plan for a patient. With increased autonomy comes greater responsibility and accountability. Accountability means that you are responsible, professionally and legally, for the type and quality of nursing care provided. You need to keep current and competent in nursing and scientific knowledge and technical skills. The nursing profession also regulates accountability through nursing audits and standards of practice.

Caregiver

As **caregiver,** you help patients maintain and regain health, manage disease and symptoms, and attain a maximal level function and independence through the healing process. You provide healing through both physical and interpersonal skills. Healing involves more than achieving improved physical well-being. You need to meet all health care needs of the patient by providing measures that restore a patient's emotional, spiritual, and social well-being. As a caregiver, you help the patient and family set goals and assist them with meeting these goals with minimal financial cost, time, and energy.

Advocate

As a **patient advocate,** you protect your patient's human and legal rights and provide assistance in asserting these rights if the need arises. As an advocate you act on behalf of your patient and secure your patient's health care rights and stand up for them (Hanks, 2010). For example, you provide additional information to help a patient decide whether or not to accept a treatment, or you find an interpreter to help family members communicate their concerns. You sometimes need to defend patients' rights in a general way by speaking out against policies or actions that put patients in danger or conflict with their rights.

Educator

As an educator you explain concepts and facts about health, describe the reason for routine care activities, demonstrate procedures such as self-care activities, reinforce learning or patient behavior, and evaluate the patient's progress in learning. Some of your patient teaching is unplanned and informal. For example, during a casual conversation you respond to questions about the reason for an intravenous infusion, a health issue such as smoking cessation, or necessary lifestyle changes. Other teaching activities are planned and more formal such as when you teach your patient to self-administer insulin injections. Always use teaching methods that match your patient's capabilities and needs and incorporate other resources such as the family in teaching plans (see Chapter 25).

Communicator

Your effectiveness as a communicator is central to the nurse-patient relationship. It allows you to know your patients, including their strengths and weaknesses, and their needs. Communication is essential for all nursing roles and activities. You will routinely communicate with patients and families, other nurses and health care professionals, resource persons, and the community. Without clear communication, it is impossible to give comfort and emotional support, give care effectively, make decisions with patients and families, protect patients from threats to well-being, coordinate and manage patient care, assist the patient in rehabilitation, or provide patient education. The quality of communication is a critical factor in meeting the needs of individuals, families, and communities (see Chapter 24).

Manager

Today's health care environment is fast paced and complex. Nurse managers need to establish an environment for collaborative patient-centered care to provide safe, quality care with positive patient outcomes. A manager coordinates the activities of members of the nursing staff in delivering nursing care and has personnel, policy, and budgetary responsibility for a specific nursing unit or agency. The manager uses appropriate leadership styles to create a nursing environment for the patients and staff that reflect the mission and values of the health care organization (see Chapter 21).

Career Development

Innovations in health care, expanding health care systems and practice settings, and the increasing needs of patients have been stimuli for new nursing roles. Today the majority of nurses practice in hospital settings, followed by community-based care, ambulatory care, and nursing homes/extended care settings.

Nursing provides an opportunity for you to commit to lifelong learning and career development to provide patients the state-of-the-art care they need. Career roles are specific employment positions or paths. Because of increasing educational opportunities for nurses, the growth of nursing as a profession, and a greater concern for job enrichment, the nursing profession offers expanded roles and different kinds of career opportunities. Your career path is limitless. You will probably switch career roles more than once. Take advantage of the different clinical practice and professional opportunities. These career opportunities include APRNs, nurse researchers, nurse risk managers, quality improvement nurses, consultants, and even business owners.

Provider of Care. Most nurses provide direct patient care in an acute care setting. As health care returns to the home care setting, there are increased opportunities for you to provide direct care in the patient's home or community. Use the nursing process and critical thinking skills to provide care that is both restorative and curative. Educate your patients and families to promote health maintenance and self-care. In collaboration with other health care team members, focus your care on returning the patient to his or her home at an optimal functional status.

In the hospital you may choose to practice in a medical-surgical setting or concentrate on a specific area of specialty practice such as pediatrics, critical care, or emergency care. Most specialty care areas require some experience as a medical-surgical nurse and additional continuing or in-service education. Many intensive care unit and emergency department nurses are required to have certification in advanced cardiac life support and critical care, emergency nursing, or trauma nursing.

Advanced Practice Registered Nurses. The **advanced practice registered nurse (APRN)** is the most independently functioning nurse. An APRN has a master's degree in nursing; advanced education in pathophysiology, pharmacology, and physical assessment; and certification and expertise in a specialized area of practice (APRN, 2008). There are four core roles for the APRN: clinical nurse specialist (CNS), certified nurse practitioner (CNP), certified nurse midwife (CNM), and certified RN anesthetist (CRNA). The educational preparation for the four roles is in at least one of the following six populations: adult-gerontology, pediatrics, neonatology, women's health/gender related, family/individual across life span, and psychiatric mental health (APRN, 2008). APRNs

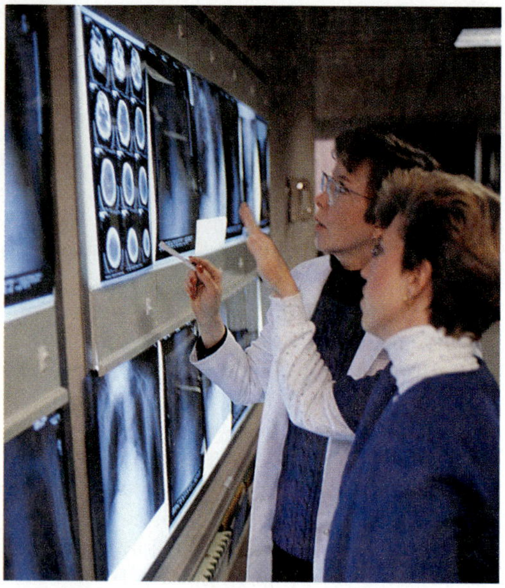

FIG. 1-1 Nurse specialist consults on a difficult patient case.

function as a clinician, educator, case manager, consultant, and researcher within his or her area of practice to plan or improve the quality of nursing care for the patient and family.

Clinical Nurse Specialist. The **clinical nurse specialist (CNS)** is an APRN who is an expert clinician in a specialized area of practice (Fig. 1-1). The specialty may be identified by a population (e.g., geriatrics), a setting (e.g., critical care), a disease specialty (e.g., diabetes), a type of care (e.g., rehabilitation), or a type of problem (e.g., pain) (National CNS Competency Task Force, 2010). The CNS practice is in all health care settings.

Nurse Practitioner. The **nurse practitioner (NP)** is an APRN who provides health care to a group of patients, usually in an outpatient, ambulatory care, or community-based setting. NPs provide care for patients with complex problems and a more holistic approach than physicians. The NP provides comprehensive care, directly managing the medical care of patients who are healthy or who have chronic conditions. A significant percentage of primary care visits by patients result from health-related problems that extend beyond the boundaries of medicine and demand the expertise of a nurse. The NP is able to establish a collaborative provider-patient relationship, working with a specific group of patients or with patients of all ages and health care needs. The major NP categories are acute care, adult, family, pediatric, women's, psychiatric mental health, and geriatric. An NP has the knowledge and skills necessary to detect and manage self-limiting acute and chronic stable medical conditions such as asthma, diabetes mellitus, and hypertension.

Certified Nurse-Midwife. A **certified nurse-midwife (CNM)** is an APRN who is also educated in midwifery and is certified by the American College of Nurse-Midwives. The practice of nurse-midwifery involves providing independent care for women during normal pregnancy, labor, and delivery and care for the newborn. It includes some gynecological services such as routine Papanicolaou (Pap) smears, family planning, and treatment for minor vaginal infections. A CNM practices with a health care agency that provides medical consultation, collaborative management, and referral.

Certified Registered Nurse Anesthetist. A **certified registered nurse anesthetist (CRNA)** is an APRN with advanced education in a nurse anesthesia accredited program. Nurse anesthetists provide surgical anesthesia under the guidance and supervision of an anesthesiologist, who is a physician with advanced knowledge of surgical anesthesia.

Nurse Educator. A **nurse educator** works primarily in schools of nursing, staff development departments of health care agencies, and patient education departments. Nurse educators need experience in clinical practice to provide them with practical skills and theoretical knowledge. A faculty member in a school of nursing educates students to become professional nurses. Nursing faculty members are responsible for teaching current nursing practice, trends, theory, and necessary skills in laboratories and clinical settings. Nurse educators in schools of nursing usually have graduate degrees in nursing and additional education. Many hold doctorate or advanced degrees in nursing, education, or administration such as a master's degree in business administration (MBA). Generally they have a specific clinical, administrative, or research specialty and advanced clinical experience.

Nurse educators in staff development departments of health care institutions provide educational programs for nurses within their institution. These programs include orientation of new personnel, critical care nursing courses, assisting with clinical skill competency, safety training, and instruction about new equipment or procedures. These nursing educators often participate in the development of nursing policies and procedures.

The primary focus of the nurse educator in the patient education department of an agency is to teach patients who are ill or disabled and their families how to self-manage their illness or disability. These nurse educators are usually specialized and certified such as a certified diabetes educator (CDE) or an ostomy care nurse and see only a specific population of patients.

Nurse Administrator. A **nurse administrator** manages patient care and the delivery of specific nursing services within a health care agency. Nursing administration begins with positions such as the assistant nurse manager. Experience and additional education sometimes lead to a middle-management position such as nurse manager of a specific patient care area or house supervisor or to an upper-management position such as assistant or associate director or director of nursing services.

Nurse manager positions usually require at least a baccalaureate degree in nursing, and director and nurse executive positions generally require a master's degree. Chief nurse executive and vice president positions in large health care organizations often require preparation at the doctoral level. Nurse administrators often have advanced degrees such as an MBA or a master's degree in hospital administration (MHA), public health (MPH), or health service administration.

In today's health care organizations directors may have responsibility for more than nursing units. Often directors manage a particular service or product line such as medicine or cardiology. Management of a service line often includes directing supportive functions and the health care personnel within areas such as medicine clinics, diagnostic departments, or outpatient.

Vice presidents of nursing or chief nurse executives often have responsibilities for all clinical functions within the hospital. This may include all ancillary personnel who provide and support patient care services. The nurse administrator needs to be skilled in business and management and understand all aspects of nursing and patient care. Functions of administrators include budgeting, staffing, strategic planning of programs and services, employee evaluation, and employee development.

Nurse Researcher. The **nurse researcher** investigates problems to improve nursing care and further define and expand the scope of nursing practice (see Chapter 5). The nurse researcher often works in an academic setting, hospital, or independent professional or community service agency. The preferred educational requirement is a doctoral degree, with at least a master's degree in nursing.

PROFESSIONAL NURSING ORGANIZATIONS

A **professional organization** deals with issues of concern to those practicing in the profession. In North America the major professional nursing organizations are the **National League for Nursing (NLN)** and the ANA. The NLN advances excellence in nursing education to prepare nurses to meet the needs of a diverse population in a changing health care environment. The NLN (2008) sets standards for excellence and innovation in nursing education.

The purpose of the ANA is to improve standards of health and the availability of health care, to foster high standards for nursing, and to promote the professional development and general and economic welfare of nurses. The ANA is part of the **International Council of Nurses (ICN)**. The objectives of the ICN parallel those of the ANA: promoting national associations of nurses, improving standards of nursing practice, seeking a higher status for nurses, and providing an international power base for nurses.

The ANA is active in political, professional, and financial issues affecting health care and the nursing profession. It is a strong lobbyist in professional practice issues such as limits of overtime hours. For example, ANA extensively lobbied state legislatures to restrict the length of overtime any one nurse's shift can be extended. When nurses' shifts last longer than 12 to 16 hours, both the patient's and nurse's safety is at risk. The risk for treatment errors and nurse injury is increased when the nurse's workday is extended.

Nursing students take part in organizations such as the National Student Nurses Association (NSNA) in the United States and the Canadian Student Nurses Association (CSNA) in Canada. These organizations consider issues of importance to nursing students such as career development and preparation for licensing. The NSNA often cooperates in activities and programs with the professional organizations.

Some professional organizations focus on specific areas such as critical care, nursing administration, nursing research, or nurse-midwifery. These organizations seek to improve the standards of practice, expand nursing roles, and foster the welfare of nurses within the specialty areas. In addition, professional organizations present educational programs and publish journals.

TRENDS IN NURSING

Nursing is a dynamic profession that grows and evolves as society and lifestyles change, as health care priorities and technologies change, and as nurses themselves change. The current philosophies and definitions of nursing have a holistic focus, which addresses the needs of the whole person in all dimensions, in health and illness, and in interaction with the family and community. In addition, there continues to be an increasing awareness for patient safety in all care settings.

Quality and Safety Education for Nurses

The Robert Wood Johnson Foundation sponsored the **Quality and Safety Education for Nurses (QSEN)** initiative to respond to reports about safety and quality patient care by the IOM (Barton et al., 2009). QSEN addresses the challenge to prepare nurses with the competencies needed to continuously improve the quality of care in their work environments (Table 1-1). The QSEN initiative encompasses the competencies of: patient-centered care, teamwork and collaboration, evidence-based practice, quality improvement, safety, and informatics (Cronenwett et al., 2007). For each competency there are targeted knowledge, skills, and attitudes

TABLE 1-1 Quality and Safety Education for Nurses

COMPETENCY	DEFINITION WITH EXAMPLES
Patient-Centered Care	Recognize the patient or designee as the source of control and full partner in providing compassionate and coordinated care based on respect for patient's preferences, values, and needs. ***Examples:*** *Involve family and friends in care. Elicit patient values and preferences. Provide care with respect for diversity of the human experience.*
Teamwork and Collaboration	Function effectively within nursing and interprofessional teams, fostering open communication, mutual respect, and shared decision making to achieve quality patient care. ***Examples:*** *Recognize the contributions of other health team members and patient's family members. Discuss effective strategies for communicating and resolving conflict. Participate in designing methods to support effective teamwork.*
Evidence-Based Practice	Integrate best current evidence with clinical expertise and patient/family preferences and values for delivery of optimal health care. ***Examples:*** *Demonstrate knowledge of basic scientific methods. Appreciate strengths and weaknesses of scientific bases for practice. Appreciate the importance of regularly reading relevant journals.*
Quality Improvement	Use data to monitor the outcomes of care processes and use improvement methods to design and test changes to continuously improve the quality and safety of health care systems. ***Examples:*** *Use tools such as flow charts and diagrams to make process of care explicit. Appreciate how unwanted variation in outcomes affects care. Identify gaps between local and best practices.*
Safety	Minimize risk of harm to patients and providers through both system effectiveness and individual performance. ***Examples:*** *Examine human factors and basic safety design principles and commonly used unsafe practices. Value own role in preventing errors.*
Informatics	Use information and technology to communicate, manage knowledge, mitigate error, and support decision-making. ***Examples:*** *Navigate an electronic health record. Protect confidentiality of protected health information in electronic health records.*

Adapted from Cronenwett L et al: Quality and safety education for nurses, *Nurs Outlook* 57:122, 2007.

BOX 1-4 EVIDENCE-BASED PRACTICE

Safety Competencies and Patient-Centered Care

PICO Question: What is the impact of communication strategies in developing competency in teamwork and collaboration in new graduates?

Evidence Summary

Patient care needs are increasingly complex, and this trend is expected to continue well into the future. The American Association of Colleges of Nursing (AACN, 2008a) endorsed a new set of guidelines, which parallel the QSEN competencies, to direct the preparation of baccalaureate nurses to provide safe, high-quality patient care (Barton et al., 2009). Collaboration and teamwork are essential competencies in delivering safe, effective patient-centered care.

Students need more than classroom and clinical experiences to understand the intricacies of effective teamwork and collaboration (Sullivan et al., 2009). They need to be able to practice teamwork in safe, clinical simulations. For teamwork and collaboration to be successful, there must be strong and clear communication between and among all health care professions. Adverse events, omission of care, and confusion are serious events in today's health care environments. Inaccurate communication among health care providers leads to serious events (Manojlovich and DeCicco, 2007). Teaching effective communication strategies across the disciplines is an effective method to help bridge this gap (Robinson et al., 2010).

Application to Nursing Practice

- Communicate with clarity and precision when designing multidisciplinary plans of care (Robinson et al., 2010).
- Seek out the skills and expertise of other disciplines.
- Develop a culture of mutual respect for all disciplines and professionals within the discipline (Manojilovich and DeCicco, 2007).
- Recognize that electronic communication may be quick, but in some situations it may not be effective (Robinson et al., 2010). When patient care issues are at stake, a focused, well-organized interdisciplinary meeting is more effective than a series of "round-robin" e-mails.
- It usually takes the same amount of time to communicate and collaborate ineffectively as it does to do it effectively.

(KSAs). The KSAs are elements that are integrated in a nursing prelicensure program (Jarzemsky et al., 2010). As you gain experience in clinical practice, you will encounter situations in which your education helps you to make a difference in improving patient care (Box 1-4).

Whether that difference in care is to provide evidence for implementing care at the bedside, identify a safety issue, or study patient data to identify trends in outcomes, each of these situations requires competence in patient-centered care, safety, or informatics. Although it is not within the scope of this textbook to present the QSEN initiative in its entirety, subsequent clinical chapters will provide you an opportunity to address how to build competencies in one or more of these areas.

Genomics

Genetics is the study of inheritance, or the way traits are passed down from one generation to another. Genes carry the instructions for making proteins, which in turn direct the activities of cells and functions of the body that influence traits such as hair and eye color. **Genomics** is a newer term that describes the study of all the genes in a person and interactions of these genes with one another and with that person's environment (CDC, 2010). Using genomic information allows health care providers to determine how genomic changes contribute to patient conditions and influence treatment decisions (Badzek et al., 2008). For example, when a family member has colon cancer before the age of 50, it is likely that other family members are at risk for developing this cancer. Knowing this information is important for family members who will need a colonoscopy before the age of 50 and repeat colonoscopies more often than the patient who is not at risk. In this case nurses are key in identifying the patients' risk factors through assessment and counseling patients about what this genomic finding means to them personally and to their family.

Public Perception of Nursing

Nursing is a pivotal health care profession. As frontline health care providers, nurses practice in all health care settings and constitute the largest number of health care professionals. They are essential to providing skilled, specialized, knowledgeable care; improving the health status of the public; and ensuring safe, effective quality care (ANA, 2010b).

Consumers of health care are more informed than ever, and with the Internet consumers have access to more health care and treatment information. This information affects the perception the public has of nursing. For example, the media frequently highlights incidents of preventable medical errors such as medication and surgical errors. Publications such as *To Err Is Human* (IOM, 2000) describe strategies for government, health care providers, industry, and consumers to reduce preventable medical errors. When you care for patients, realize how your approach to care influences public opinion. Always act in a competent professional manner.

Impact of Nursing on Politics and Health Policy

Political power or influence is known as the ability to influence or persuade an individual holding a government office to exert the power of that office to affect a desired outcome. Nurses' involvement in politics is receiving greater emphasis in nursing curricula, professional organizations, and health care settings. Professional nursing organizations have employed lobbyists to urge state legislatures and the U.S. Congress to improve the quality of health care (Mason et al., 2012).

The ANA works for the improvement of health standards and the availability of health care services for all people, fosters high standards of nursing, stimulates and promotes the professional development of nurses, and advances their economic and general welfare. The purposes are unrestricted by considerations of nationality, race, creed, lifestyle, color, gender, or age. The ANA employs RNs as lobbyists at the federal level. State nursing organizations also hire lobbyists and legislative specialists to work on state nursing issues and assist with federal efforts. Finally, lobbyists working on behalf of nursing are employed in Washington, DC, by professional organizations such as the American Federation of Teachers, the NLN, the American College of Nurse-Midwives, the American Public Health Association, and the AACN. These groups aim to remove financial barriers to health care, increase the quality of nursing care available, increase economic rewards to nurses, and expand professional nursing roles.

You can influence policy decisions at all governmental levels. One way to get involved is by participating in local and national efforts (Mason et al., 2012). This effort is critical to exerting nurses' influence early in the political process. When nurses become serious students of social needs, activists in influencing policy to meet those needs, and generous contributors of time and money to nursing organizations and to candidates working for universal good health care, the future is bright indeed (Mason et al., 2012).

KEY POINTS

- Nursing responds to the health care needs of society, which are influenced by economic, social, and cultural variables of a specific era.
- Changes in society such as increased technology, new demographic patterns, consumerism, health promotion, and the women's and human rights movements lead to changes in nursing.
- Nursing definitions reflect changes in the practice of nursing and help bring about changes by identifying the domain of nursing practice and guiding research, practice, and education.
- Nursing standards provide the guidelines for implementing and evaluating nursing care.
- Professional nursing organizations deal with issues of concern to specialist groups within the nursing profession.
- Nurses are becoming more politically sophisticated and, as a result, are able to increase the influence of nursing on health care policy and practice.

CLINICAL APPLICATION QUESTIONS

Preparing for Clinical Practice

Mrs. Langman is in the hospital recovering from hip replacement surgery. Her surgery involved insertion of a new type of hip replacement prosthesis and newer postsurgical care. The advanced practice registered nurse is preparing her discharge medication and rehabilitation prescriptions. The staff nurse is preparing to transfer Mrs. Langman to a rehabilitation facility. The nurse educator is conducting bedside rounds to explain the new prosthesis and related postoperative care.

1. Identify similarities and differences in the roles of the staff nurse, advanced practice registered nurse, and nurse educator.
2. What is the educational preparation for each role?
3. Use information in this chapter to consider career objectives for yourself over the next 5 years. Obviously the first would be to complete your nursing program. But decide what you want to do as a professional nurse and then outline strategies to achieve these goals.

evolve *Answers to Clinical Application Questions can be found on the Evolve website.*

REVIEW QUESTIONS

Are You Ready to Test Your Nursing Knowledge?

1. You are participating in a clinical care coordination conference for a patient with terminal cancer. You talk with your colleagues about using the nursing code of ethics for professional registered nurses to guide care decisions. A nonnursing colleague asks about this code. Which of the following statements best describes this code?
   1. Improves self–health care
   2. Protects the patient's confidentiality
   3. Ensures identical care to all patients
   4. Defines the principles of right and wrong to provide patient care
2. An 18-year-old woman is in the emergency department with fever and cough. The nurse obtains her vital signs, auscultates her lung sounds, listens to her heart sounds, determines her level of comfort, and collects blood and sputum samples for analysis. Which standard of practice is performed?
   1. Diagnosis
   2. Evaluation
   3. Assessment
   4. Implementation
3. A patient in the emergency department has developed wheezing and shortness of breath. The nurse gives the ordered medicated nebulizer treatment now and in 4 hours. Which standard of practice is performed?
   1. Planning
   2. Evaluation
   3. Assessment
   4. Implementation
4. A nurse is caring for a patient with end-stage lung disease. The patient wants to go home on oxygen and be comfortable. The family wants the patient to have a new surgical procedure. The nurse explains the risk and benefits of the surgery to the family and discusses the patient's wishes with the family. The nurse is acting as the patient's:
   1. Educator
   2. Advocate
   3. Caregiver
   4. Case manager
5. Evidence-based practice is defined as:
   1. Nursing care based on tradition
   2. Scholarly inquiry of nursing and biomedical research literature
   3. A problem-solving approach that integrates best current evidence with clinical practice
   4. Quality nursing care provided in an efficient and economically sound manner
6. The examination for registered nurse licensure is exactly the same in every state in the United States. This examination:
   1. Guarantees safe nursing care for all patients
   2. Ensures standard nursing care for all patients
   3. Ensures that honest and ethical care is provided
   4. Provides a minimal standard of knowledge for a registered nurse in practice
7. Contemporary nursing requires that the nurse has knowledge and skills for a variety of professional roles and responsibilities. Which of the following are examples? (Select all that apply.)
   1. Caregiver
   2. Autonomy and accountability
   3. Patient advocate
   4. Health promotion
   5. Lobbyist
8. Advanced practice registered nurses generally:
   1. Function independently
   2. Function as unit directors
   3. Work in acute care settings
   4. Work in the university setting.
9. Health care reform will bring changes in the emphasis of care. Which of the following models is expected from health care reform?
   1. Moving from an acute illness to a health promotion, illness prevention model
   2. Moving from illness prevention to a health promotion model
   3. Moving from an acute illness to a disease management model
   4. Moving from a chronic care to an illness prevention model

10. Which of the following nursing roles may have prescriptive authority in their practice? (Select all that apply.)
    1. Critical care nurse
    2. Nurse practitioner
    3. Certified clinical nurse specialist
    4. Charge nurse
11. A critical care nurse is using a computerized decision support system to correctly position her ventilated patients to reduce pneumonia caused by accumulated respiratory secretions. This is an example of which Quality and Safety in the Education of Nurses (QSEN) competency?
    1. Patient-centered care
    2. Safety
    3. Teamwork and collaboration
    4. Informatics
12. A nurse is caring for an older-adult couple in a community-based assisted living facility. During the family assessment he notes that the couple has many expired medications and multiple medications for their respective chronic illnesses. They note that they go to two different health care providers. The nurse begins to work with the couple to determine what they know about their medications and helps them decide on one care provider rather than two. This is an example of which Quality and Safety in the Education of Nurses (QSEN) competency?
    1. Patient-centered care
    2. Safety
    3. Teamwork and collaboration
    4. Informatics
13. A nurse is working with a young childbearing family who has one child with a congenital heart disease. The parents are trying to determine the risks of a second child being born with congenital heart disease. Describe why genomics information is important in assisting the parents in this decision.
14. The nurses on an acute care medical floor notice an increase in pressure ulcer formation in their patients. A nurse consultant decides to compare two types of treatment. The first is the procedure currently used to assess for pressure ulcer risk. The second uses a new assessment instrument to identify at-risk patients. Given this information, the nurse consultant exemplifies which career?
    1. Clinical nurse specialist
    2. Nurse administrator
    3. Nurse educator
    4. Nurse researcher
15. Nurses at a community hospital are in an education program to learn how to use a new pressure-relieving device for patients at risk for pressure ulcers. This is which type of education?
    1. Continuing education
    2. Graduate education
    3. In-service education
    4. Professional Registered Nurse Education

Answers: **1.** 4; **2.** 3; **3.** 4; **4.** 2; **5.** 3; **6.** 4; **7.** 1, 2, 3, 4; **8.** 1; **9.** 1; **10.** 2, 3; **11.** 4; **12.** 2; **13.** See Evolve; **14.** 4; **15.** 3.

REFERENCES

Aiken LH: Economics of nursing, *Policy Politics Nurs* 9(93):73, 2010.

American Association of Colleges of Nursing: *Essentials of baccalaureate education for professional nursing*, Washington, DC, 2008a, The Association.

American Association of Colleges of Nursing: *Joint statement from the Tri-Council for Nursing on Recent Registered Nurse Supply and Demand Projections, News Release*, Washington, DC, 2008b, The Association, http://www.aacn.nche.edu/Media/NewsReleases/2010/tricouncil.html. Accessed July 2010.

American Nurses Association: *A position paper: educational preparation for nurse practitioners and assistants to nurses*, Kansas City, Mo, 1965, The Association.

American Nurses Association: *Code for of ethics for nurses with interpretive statements*, Silver Spring, Md, 2008, The Association.

American Nurses Association: *Nursing's social policy statement: the Essence of the Profession*, Silver Spring, Md, 2010a, American Nurses Publishing.

American Nurses Association: *Nursing: scope and standards of practice*, ed 2, Silver Spring, Md, 2010b, The Association.

American Nurses Association: *Guide to the code of ethics for nurses: interpretation and application*, Silver Spring, Md, 2010c, The Association.

APRN Consensus Work Group and National Council of State Boards of Nursing, APRN Joint Dialogue Report, July 7, 2008, http://nursingworld.org/consensusmodeltoolkit. Accessed July 16, 2010.

Badzek LB, et al: Genomics and nursing practice: advancing the nursing profession, *Online J Issues Nurs* 13(1):1, 2008.

Benner P: *From novice to expert: excellence and power in clinical nursing practice*, Menlo Park, Calif, 1984, Addison-Wesley.

Benner P, Tanner CA, Chesla CA: The social fabric or nursing knowledge, *Am J Nurs* 97(7):16, 1997.

Benner P, et al: *Educating nurses: a call for radical transformation*, Stanford, Calif, 2010, Carnegie Foundation for the Advancement of Teaching.

Block V, Sredl D: Nursing education and professional practice, *J Staff Dev* 22(1):23, 2006.

Centers for Disease Control and Prevention: *Genomics and health frequently asked questions*, 2010, http://www.cdc.gov/genomics/public/faq.htm. Accessed Sept 17, 2010.

Chase SK, Pruitt RH: The practice doctorate: innovation or disruption? *J Nurs Educ* 45(5):158, 2006.

Chism LA: *The doctor of nursing practice: a guidebook for role development and professionals' issues*, Sudbury Mass, 2010, Jones & Bartlett Publishers.

Cohen IB: Florence Nightingale, *Sci Am* 250(128):137, 1984.

Cronenwett L, et al: Quality and safety education for nurses, *Nurs Outlook* 57:122, 2007.

Donahue MP: *Nursing: the finest art—an illustrated history*, ed 3, St Louis, 2011, Mosby.

Fernandes R, et al: Home-based palliative care services for underserved populations, *J Palliative Med* 13(4):413, 2010.

Gugliemi M: Celebrating the freedom to leverage the power of nursing, *AORN* 91(5):533, 2010.

Hale MA, et al: Continuing education needs of nurses in a voluntary continuing nursing education state, *J Cont Educ Nurs* 41(3):107, 2010.

Huicho L, et al: Increasing access to health workers in underserved areas: a conceptual framework for measuring results, *Bull World Health Org* 88:357, 2010.

Institute of Medicine: *To err is human*, Washington, DC, 2000, The Institute.

Institute of Medicine: *The future of nursing: Leading change, advancing health*, Washington DC, 2010, National Academy Press.

International Council of Nurses: *ICN definition of nursing*, 2010, http://icn.ch/definition.htm. Accessed September 15, 2010.

Jarzemsky P, et al: Incorporating quality and safety education for nurses' competencies in simulation scenario design, *Nurse Educator* 35(2):90, 2010.

Manthey M: *The invisible power of nursing*, *Creative Nurs* 14(1):3, 2008.

Mason DJ, et al: *Policy & politics in nursing and health care*, ed 6, Philadelphia, 2012, Saunders.

McCann E: Building a community-academic partnership to improve health outcomes in an underserved community, *Public Health Nurs* 27(1):32, 2010.

Morrison AM, Catanzaro AM: High-fidelity simulation and emergency preparedness, *Pub Health Nurs* 27(2):164, 2010.

O'Neil E: Four factors that guarantee health care change, *J Prof Nurs* 25(6):317, 2009.

National CNS Competency Task Force, Core Competencies, National Association of Clinical Nurse Specialists: *Core Competencies*, Philadelphia, 2010, The Association.

National League for Nursing Accrediting Commission: *Standards and Criteria Baccalaureate Degree Programs in Nursing*, New York, 2008, The League. http://nlnac.org/manuals/SC2008_BACCALAUREATE.htm. Accessed July 7, 2010.

Nightingale F: *Notes on nursing: what it is and what it is not*, London, 1860, Harrison and Sons.

Presley S: Rural NPs embrace private practice, *Am J Nurs* 115(5):21, 2010.

Robinson JJA: Nursing and disaster preparedness, *Int Nurs Rev* 57(2):148, 2010.

Tanner CA, Bellack JP: Our faculty for the future, *J Nurs Educ* 49(3):123, 2010.

Tilden VP, Thompson S: Policy issues in end-of-life care, *J Prof Nurs* 25(6):363, 2009.

US Census Bureau, Population Division: *Projections of the Population and Components of change for the United States: 2010 to 2050 (NP2008-T1)*, release date Aug 14, 2008a, http://www.census.gov/population/www/projections/summarytables.html. Accessed July 5, 2010.

US Census Bureau, Population Division: *Projections of the Population by selected age-groups and sex for the United States: 2010 to 2050 (NP2008-T2)*, Release date Aug 14, 2008b, http://www.census.gov/population/www/projections/summarytables.html. Accessed July 5, 2010.

RESEARCH REFERENCES

Barton AJ, et al: A national Delphi to determine developmental progression of quality and safety competencies in nursing education, *Nurs Outlook* 57(6):313, 2009.

Flinkman M, et al: Nurses' intention to leave the profession: integrative review, *J Adv Nurs* 66(7):1422, 2010.

Hanks RG: Development and testing of an instrument to measure protective nursing advocacy, *Nurs Ethics* 17(2):255, 2010.

Lucero RJ, et al: Variations in nursing care quality across hospitals, *J Adv Nurs* 65(11):2299, 2009.

Manojlovich M, DeCicco B: Healthy work environments, nurse-physician communication, and patients' outcomes, *AJCC* 16(6):536, 2007.

Robinson FP, et al: Perceptions of effective and ineffective nurse-physician communication in hospitals, *Nurs Forum* 45(3):206, 2010.

Sullivan DT, et al: Assessing quality and safety competencies of graduating prelicensure nursing students, *Nurs Outlook* 57(6):323, 2009.

CHAPTER 2

The Health Care Delivery System

OBJECTIVES

- Compare the various methods for financing health care.
- Explain the advantages and disadvantages of managed health care.
- Discuss the types of settings that provide various health care services.
- Discuss the role of nurses in different health care delivery settings.
- Differentiate primary care from primary health care.
- Explain the impact of quality and safety initiatives on delivery of health care.
- Discuss the implications that changes in the health care system have on nursing.
- Discuss opportunities for nursing within the changing health care delivery system.

KEY TERMS

Acute care, p. 18
Adult day care centers, p. 22
Assisted living, p. 21
Capitation, p. 15
Diagnosis-related groups (DRGs), p. 15
Discharge planning, p. 19
Extended care facility, p. 20
Globalization, p. 27
Home care, p. 20
Hospice, p. 22
Independent practice association (IPA), p. 16
Integrated delivery networks (IDNs), p. 17
Managed care, p. 15
Medicaid, p. 20
Medicare, p. 20
Minimum Data Set (MDS), p. 21
Nursing informatics, p. 26
Nursing-sensitive outcomes, p. 26
Patient-centered care, p. 24
Pay for performance, p. 24
Primary health care, p. 17
Professional standards review organizations (PSROs), p. 15
Prospective payment system (PPS), p. 15
Rehabilitation, p. 20
Resource utilization groups (RUGs), p. 15
Respite care, p. 22
Restorative care, p. 20
Skilled nursing facility, p. 21
Utilization review (UR) committees, p. 15
Vulnerable populations, p. 27
Work redesign, p. 18

evolve WEBSITE

http://evolve.elsevier.com/Potter/fundamentals/

- Review Questions
- Case Study with Questions
- Audio Glossary
- Interactive Learning Activities
- Key Term Flashcards
- Content Updates

The U.S. health care system is complex and constantly changing. A broad variety of services are available from different disciplines of health professionals, but gaining access to services is often very difficult for those with limited health care insurance. Uninsured patients present a challenge to health care and nursing because they are more likely to skip or delay treatment for acute and chronic illnesses and die prematurely (Thompson and Lee, 2007). The continuing development of new technologies and medications, which shortens length of stay (LOS), also causes health care costs to increase. Thus health care institutions are managing health care more as businesses than as service organizations. Challenges to health care leaders today include reducing health care costs while maintaining high-quality care for patients, improving access and coverage for more people, and encouraging healthy behaviors (Knickman and Kovner, 2009). Health care providers are discharging patients sooner from hospitals, resulting in more patients needing nursing homes or home care. Often families provide care for their loved ones in the home setting. Nurses face major challenges to prevent gaps in health care across health care settings so individuals remain healthy and well within their own homes and communities.

Nursing is a caring discipline. Values of the nursing profession are rooted in helping people to regain, maintain, or improve health; prevent illness; and find comfort and dignity. The health care system of the new millennium is less service oriented and more business oriented because of cost-saving initiatives, which often causes tension between the caring and business aspects of health care (Knickman and Kovner, 2009). The Institute of Medicine (IOM) (2001) calls for a health care delivery system that is safe, effective, patient centered, timely, efficient, and equitable. The National Priorities Partnership is a group of 28 organizations from a variety of health care disciplines that have joined together to work toward transforming health care (National Priorities Partnership, 2008). The group has set the following national priorities:

- Patient and Family Engagement—Providing patient-centered, effective care
- Population Health—Bringing increased focus on wellness and prevention

- Safety—Eliminating errors whenever and wherever possible
- Care Coordination—Providing patient-centered, high-value care
- Palliative Care—Providing appropriate and compassionate care for patients experiencing advanced illnesses
- Overuse—Reducing waste to achieve effective, affordable care

The Institute of Medicine and Robert Woods Johnson Foundation (2011) put forth a vision for a transformed health care delivery system. The health care system of the future makes quality care accessible to all populations, focuses on wellness and disease prevention, improves health outcomes, and provides compassionate care across the life span. Transformations in health care are changing the practice of nursing. Nursing continues to lead the way in change and retain values for patient care while meeting the challenges of new roles and responsibilities. These changes challenge the nurse to provide evidence-based, compassionate care and continue in the role as patient advocate (Singleton, 2010). According to the IOM (2011) report, nurses need to be transformed by:

- Practicing to the full extent of their education and training.
- Achieving higher levels of education and training through an improved education system that provides seamless progression.
- Becoming full partners, with physicians and other health care providers, in redesigning the health care system.
- Improving data collection and information infrastructure for effective workforce planning and policy making.

HEALTH CARE REGULATION AND COMPETITION

Through most of the twentieth century, few incentives existed for controlling health care costs. Insurers or third-party payers paid for whatever the health care providers ordered for a patient's care and treatment. As health care costs continued to rise out of control, regulatory and competitive approaches had to control health care spending. The federal government, the biggest consumer of health care, which paid for Medicare and Medicaid, created **professional standards review organizations (PSROs)** to review the quality, quantity, and cost of hospital care (Sultz and Young, 2006). Medicare-qualified hospitals had physician-supervised **utilization review (UR) committees** to review the admissions and to identify and eliminate overuse of diagnostic and treatment services ordered by physicians caring for patients on Medicare.

One of the most significant factors that influenced payment for health care was the **prospective payment system (PPS).** Established by Congress in 1983, the PPS eliminated cost-based reimbursement. Hospitals serving patients who received Medicare benefits were no longer able to charge whatever a patient's care cost. Instead, the PPS grouped inpatient hospital services for Medicare patients into **diagnosis-related groups (DRGs).** Each group has a fixed reimbursement amount with adjustments based on case severity, rural/urban/regional costs, and teaching costs. Hospitals receive a set dollar amount for each patient based on the assigned DRG, regardless of the patient's length of stay or use of services. Most health care providers (e.g., health care networks or managed care organizations) now receive capitated payments. **Capitation** means that the providers receive a fixed amount per patient or enrollee of a health care plan (Jonas et al., 2007). Capitation aims to build a payment plan for select diagnoses or surgical procedures that consists of the best standards of care at the lowest cost.

Capitation and prospective payment influences the way health care providers deliver care in all types of settings. Many now use DRGs in the rehabilitation setting, and **resource utilization groups (RUGs)** in long-term care. In all settings health care providers try to manage costs so the organizations remain profitable. For example, when patients are hospitalized for lengthy periods, hospitals have to absorb the portion of costs that are not reimbursed. This simply adds more pressure to ensure that patients are managed effectively and discharged as soon as is reasonably possible. Thus hospitals started to increase discharge planning activities, and hospital lengths of stay began to shorten. Because patients are discharged home as soon as possible, home care agencies now provide complex technological care, including mechanical ventilation and long-term parenteral nutrition.

Managed care describes health care systems in which the provider or health care system receives a predetermined capitated payment for each patient enrolled in the program. In this case the managed care organization assumes financial risk in addition to providing patient care. The focus of care of the organization shifts from individual illness care to prevention, early intervention, and outpatient care. If people stay healthy, the cost of medical care declines. Systems of managed care focus on containing or reducing costs, increasing patient satisfaction, and improving the health or functional status of individuals (Sultz and Young, 2006). Table 2-1 summarizes the most common types of health care insurance plans.

In 2006 the National Quality Forum defined a list of 28 "Never Events" that are devastating and preventable. Examples of Never Events include patient death or serious injury related to a medication error or the administration of incompatible blood products. In 2007 Medicare ruled it would no longer pay for medical costs associated with these errors. Many states now require mandatory reporting of these events when they occur (Agency for Healthcare Research and Quality Patient Safety Network, n.d.).

Major health care reform came in 2010 with the signing into law of the Patient Protection and Affordable Care Act (Public Law No. 111-148). Health care reform of this magnitude has not occurred in the United States since the 1960s when Medicare and Medicaid were signed into law. The Patient Protection and Affordable Care Act focuses on the major goals of increasing access to health care services for all, reducing health care costs, and improving health care quality. Provisions in the law include insurance industry reforms that increase insurance coverage and decrease costs, increased funding for community health centers, increased primary care services and providers, and improved coverage for children (Adashi et al., 2010; HealthReform.gov, 2010).

EMPHASIS ON POPULATION WELLNESS

The United States health care delivery system faces many issues such as rising costs, increased access to services, a growing population, and improved quality of outcomes. As a result, the emphasis of the health care industry today is shifting from managing illness to managing health of a community and the environment.

The Health Services Pyramid developed by the Core Functions Project serves as a model for improving the health care of U.S. citizens (Fig. 2-1). The pyramid shows that population-based health care services provide the basis for preventive services. These services include primary, secondary, and tertiary health care. Achievements in the lower tiers of the pyramid contribute to the improvement of health care delivered by the higher tiers. Health care in the United States is moving toward health care practices that emphasize managing health rather than managing illness. The premise is that in the long term, health promotion reduces health

TABLE 2-1 Examples of Health Care Plans

TYPE	DEFINITION	CHARACTERISTICS
Managed care organization (MCO)	Provides comprehensive preventive and treatment services to a specific group of voluntarily enrolled people. Structures include a variety of models: *Staff model:* Physicians are salaried employees of the MCO. *Group model:* MCO contracts with single group practice *Network model:* MCO contracts with multiple group practices and/or integrated organizations. **Independent practice association (IPA):** The MCO contracts with physicians who usually are not members of groups and whose practices include fee-for-service and capitated patients.	Focus is on health maintenance, primary care. All care is provided by a primary care physician. Referral is needed for access to specialist and hospitalization. It may use capitated payments.
Preferred provider organization (PPO)	Type of managed care plan that limits an enrollee's choice to a list of "preferred" hospitals, physicians, and providers. An enrollee pays more out-of-pocket expenses for using a provider not on the list.	Contractual agreement exists between a set of providers and one or more purchasers (self-insured employers or insurance plans). Comprehensive health services are at a discount to companies under contract. Focus is on health maintenance.
Medicare	A federally administrated program by the Commonwealth Fund or the Centers for Medicare and Medicaid Services (CMS); a funded national health insurance program in the United States for people 65 years and older. Part A provides basic protection for medical, surgical, and psychiatric care costs based on diagnosis-related groups (DRGs); also provides limited skilled nursing facility care, hospice, and home health care. Part B is a voluntary medical insurance; covers physician, certain other specified health professional services, and certain outpatient services. Part C is a managed care provision that provides a choice of three insurance plans. Part D is a voluntary Prescription Drug Improvement (Jonas et al, 2007).	Payment for plan is deducted from monthly individual Social Security check. It covers services of nurse practitioners. It does not pay full cost of certain services. Supplemental insurance is encouraged.
Medicaid	Federally funded, state-operated program that provides: (1) health insurance to low-income families; (2) health assistance to low-income people with long-term care (LTC) disabilities; and (3) supplemental coverage and LTC assistance to older adults and Medicare beneficiaries in nursing homes. Individual states determine eligibility and benefits.	It finances a large portion of care for poor children, their parents, pregnant women, and disabled very poor adults. It reimburses for nurse-midwifery and other advanced practice nurses (varies by state). It reimburses nursing home funding.
Private insurance	Traditional fee-for-service plan. Payment is computed after patient receives services on basis of number of services used.	Policies are typically expensive. Most policies have deductibles that patients have to meet before insurance pays.
LTC insurance	Supplemental insurance for coverage of LTC services. Policies provide a set amount of dollars for an unlimited time or for as little as 2 years.	It is very expensive. A good policy has a minimum waiting period for eligibility; payment for skilled nursing, intermediate, or custodial care and home care.
State Children's Health Insurance Programs (SCHIP)	Federally funded, state-operated program to provide health coverage for uninsured children. Individual states determine participation eligibility and benefits.	It covers children not poor enough for Medicaid.

care costs. A wellness perspective focuses on the health of populations and the communities in which they live rather than just on finding a cure for an individual's disease. Life expectancy for Americans is 77.9 years, which has shown a steady increase in the past century. Along with increased life expectancy, adult deaths related to coronary heart disease and stroke continue a long-term decreasing trend, and there is a decreasing trend in deaths of children since 1900 (Centers for Disease Control and Prevention, [CDC], 2007). The reduction in mortality rates has been credited to advancements in sanitation and prevention of infectious diseases (e.g., water, sewage, immunization, and crowded living conditions); patient teaching (e.g., dietary habits, decrease in tobacco use, and blood pressure control); and injury prevention programs (e.g., seat belt restraints, child seats, and helmet laws).

HEALTH CARE SETTINGS AND SERVICES

Currently the U.S. health care system has five levels of care for which health care providers offer services: disease prevention; health promotion; and primary, secondary, and tertiary health care. The health care settings within which the levels of care are provided include preventive, primary, secondary, tertiary, restorative, and

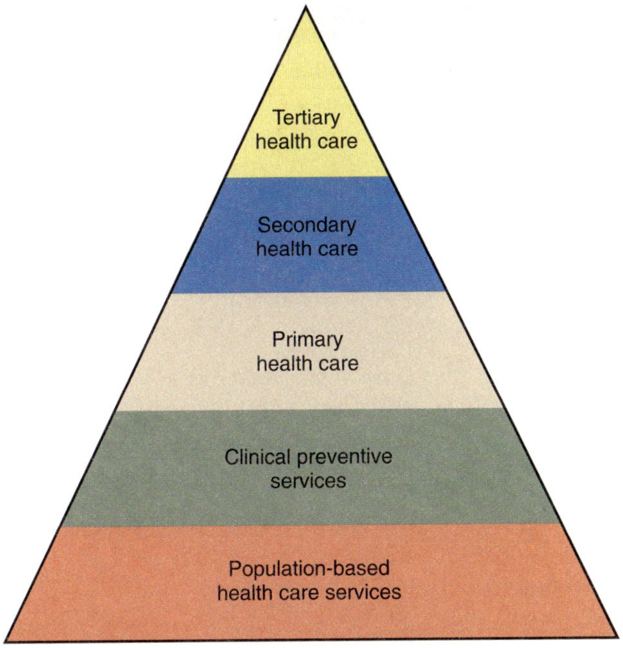

FIG. 2-1 Health services pyramid. (US Public Health Service: *The core functions project*, Washington, DC, 1994/update 2000, Office of Disease Prevention and Health Promotion. From Stanhope M, Lancaster J: *Public health nursing: population-centered health care in the community*, ed 7, St. Louis, 2008, Mosby.)

continuing care settings (Box 2-1). Larger health care systems have **integrated delivery networks (IDNs)** that include a set of providers and services organized to deliver a continuum of care to a population of patients at a capitated cost in a particular setting (Jonas et al., 2007). An integrated system reduces duplication of services across levels or settings of care to ensure that patients receive care in the most appropriate settings.

Changes unique to each setting of care have developed because of health care reform. For example, many health care providers now place greater emphasis on wellness, directing more resources toward primary and preventive care services. Nurses are especially important as patient advocates in maintaining continuity of care throughout the levels of care. They have the opportunity to provide leadership to communities and health care systems. The ability to find strategies that better address patient needs at all levels of care is critical to improving the health care delivery system.

Health care agencies seek accreditation and certification as a way to demonstrate quality and safety in the delivery of care and to evaluate the performance of the organization based on established standards. Accreditation is earned by the entire organization; specific programs or services within an organization earn certifications (The Joint Commission [TJC], 2011). The Joint Commission (formerly The Joint Commission on Accreditation of Healthcare Organizations) accredits health care organizations across the continuum of care, including hospitals and ambulatory care, long-term care, home care, and behavioral health agencies. Other accrediting agencies have a specific focus such as the Commission on Accreditation of Rehabilitation Facilities (CARF) and the Community Health Accrediting Program (CHAP). Disease-specific certifications are available in most all chronic diseases (TJC, 2011). Accreditation and certification survey processes help organizations identify problems and develop solutions to improve the safety and quality of delivered care and services.

BOX 2-1 EXAMPLES OF HEALTH CARE SERVICES

Primary Care (Health Promotion)
- Prenatal and well-baby care
- Nutrition counseling
- Family planning
- Exercise classes

Preventive Care
- Blood pressure and cancer screening
- Immunizations
- Mental health counseling and crisis prevention
- Community legislation (e.g., seat belts, air bags, bike helmets)

Secondary Acute Care
- Emergency care
- Acute medical-surgical care
- Radiological procedures for acute problems (e.g., x-rays, CT scans)

Tertiary Care
- Intensive care
- Subacute care

Restorative Care
- Cardiovascular and pulmonary rehabilitation
- Sports medicine
- Spinal cord injury programs
- Home care

Continuing Care
- Assisted living
- Psychiatric and older adult day care

Preventive and Primary Health Care

Primary health care focuses on improved health outcomes for an entire population. It includes primary care and health education, proper nutrition, maternal/child health care, family planning, immunizations, and control of diseases. Primary health care requires collaboration among health professionals, health care leaders, and community members. This collaboration needs to focus on improving health care equity, making health care systems person centered, developing reliable and accountable health care leaders, and promoting and protecting the health of communities (WHO, 2008). Successful community-based health programs take societal and environmental factors into consideration when addressing the health needs of communities (WHO, 2008). In settings in which patients receive preventive and primary care such as schools, physician's offices, occupational health clinics, community health centers, and nursing centers, health promotion is a major theme (Table 2-2). Health promotion programs lower the overall costs of health care by reducing the incidence of disease, minimizing complications, and thus reducing the need to use more expensive health care resources. In contrast, preventive care is more disease oriented and focused on reducing and controlling risk factors for disease through activities such as immunization and occupational health programs. Chapter 3 provides a more comprehensive discussion of primary health care in the community.

Secondary and Tertiary Care

In secondary and tertiary care the diagnosis and treatment of illnesses are traditionally the most common services. With the arrival of managed care, many now deliver these services in primary care

TABLE 2-2 **Preventive and Primary Care Services**

TYPE OF SERVICE	PURPOSE	AVAILABLE PROGRAMS/SERVICES
School health	These are comprehensive programs that include health promotion principles throughout a school curriculum. They emphasize program management, interdisciplinary collaboration, and community health principles.	Positive life skills Nutritional planning Health screening Counseling Communicable disease prevention Crisis intervention
Occupational health	This is a comprehensive program designed for health promotion and accident or illness prevention in the workplace setting. It aims to increase worker productivity, decrease absenteeism, and reduce use of expensive medical care	Environmental surveillance Physical assessment Health screening Health education Communicable disease control Counseling
Physicians' offices	They provide primary health care (diagnosis and treatment). Many focus on health promotion practices. Nurse practitioners often partner with a physician in managing patient population.	Routine physical examination Health screening Diagnostics Treatment of acute and chronic ailments
Nurse-managed clinics	These clinics provide nursing services with a focus on health promotion and education, chronic disease assessment management, and support for self-care and caregivers.	Day care Health risk appraisal Wellness counseling Employment readiness Acute and chronic care management
Block and parish nursing	Nurses living within a neighborhood provide services to older patients or those unable to leave their homes. It fills in gaps not available in traditional health care system.	Running errands Transportation Respite care Homemaker aides Spiritual health
Community health centers	These are outpatient clinics that provide primary care to a specific patient population (e.g., well-baby, mental health, diabetes) that lives in a specific community. They are often associated with a hospital, medical school, church, or other community organization.	Physical assessment Health screening Disease management Health education Counseling

settings. Disease management is the most common and expensive service of the health care delivery system. The acutely and chronically ill represent about 20% of the people in the United States, who consume about 80% of health care spending (CDC, 2007). Over 80% of adults 65 years of age have at least one chronic health condition that causes multiple health problems (Missouri Families, 2008).

Uninsured individuals are an increasing problem in health care. The fastest growing age-group of uninsured citizens is young adults between the ages of 19 and 34 (Billings and Cantor, 2009). Young adults turning 19 years of age from low-income families are in danger of being uninsured because of the inability to attend college and find employment with health care benefits. Coverage for young adults is important for various reasons. This age-group has a high incidence of obesity, pregnancy, and human immunodeficiency virus (HIV). People in this age-group are also less likely to see a doctor on a regular basis and follow up on a problem if they do not have health insurance. Lack of insurance rates varies by race. Statistics show that 34% of Hispanics, 19% of African Americans, and 10% of the white or Caucasian population do not have health insurance (CDC, 2010).

People who do not have health care insurance often wait longer before presenting for treatment; thus they are usually sicker and need more health care. As a result, secondary and tertiary care (also called **acute care**) is more costly. With the arrival of more advanced technology and managed care, physicians now perform simple surgeries in office surgical suites instead of in the hospital. Cost to the patient is lower in the office because the general overhead cost of the facility is lower.

Hospitals. Hospital emergency departments, urgent care centers, critical care units, and inpatient medical-surgical units provide secondary and tertiary levels of care. Quality, safe care is the focus of most acute care organizations; satisfaction with health care services is important to them. Patient satisfaction becomes a priority in a busy, stressful location such as the inpatient nursing unit. Patients expect to receive courteous and respectful treatment, and they want to be involved in daily care decisions. As a nurse, you play a key role in bringing respect and dignity to the patient (Vlasses and Smeltzer, 2007). Acute care nurses need to be responsive to learning patient needs and expectations early to form effective partnerships that ultimately enhance the level of nursing care given.

Because of managed care, the number of days patients can expect to be hospitalized is limited based on their DRGs on admission. Therefore nurses need to use resources efficiently to help patients successfully recover and return home. To contain costs, many hospitals have redesigned nursing units. Because of **work redesign,** more services are available on nursing units, thus minimizing the need to transfer and transport patients across multiple diagnostic and treatment areas.

Hospitalized patients are acutely ill and need comprehensive and specialized tertiary health care. The services provided by hospitals vary considerably. Some small rural hospitals offer only limited emergency and diagnostic services and general inpatient services. In comparison, large urban medical centers offer comprehensive, up-to-date diagnostic services, trauma and emergency care, surgical intervention, intensive care units (ICUs), inpatient services, and rehabilitation facilities. Larger hospitals also offer professional staff from a variety of specialties such as social service, respiratory therapy, physical and occupational therapy, and speech therapy. The focus in hospitals is to provide the highest quality of care possible so patients are discharged early but safely to home or another health care facility that will adequately manage remaining health care needs.

Discharge planning begins the moment a patient is admitted to a health care facility. Nurses play an important role in **discharge planning** in the hospital, where continuity of care is important. To achieve continuity of care, nurses use critical thinking skills and apply the nursing process (see Unit 3). To anticipate and identify the patient's needs, nurses work with all members of the interdisciplinary health care team. They take the lead to develop a plan of care that moves the patient from the hospital to another level of health care such as the patient's home or a nursing home. Discharge planning is a centralized, coordinated, interdisciplinary process that ensures that the patient has a plan for continuing care after leaving a health care agency.

Because patients leave hospitals as soon as their physical conditions allow, they often have continuing health care needs when they go home or to another facility. For example, a surgical patient requires wound care at home after surgery. A patient who has had a stroke requires ambulation training. Patients and families worry about how they will care for unmet needs and manage over the long term. Nurses help by anticipating and identifying patients' continuing needs before the actual time of discharge and by coordinating health care team members in achieving an appropriate discharge plan.

Some patients are more in need of discharge planning because of the risks they present (e.g., patients with limited financial resources, limited family support, and long-term disabilities or chronic illness). However, any patient who is being discharged from a health care facility with remaining functional limitations or who has to follow certain restrictions or therapies for recovery needs discharge planning. All caregivers who care for a patient with a specific health problem participate in discharge planning. The process is truly interdisciplinary. For example, patients with diabetes visiting a diabetes management center requires the group effort of a diabetes nurse educator, dietitian, and physician to ensure that they return home with the right information to manage their condition. A patient who has experienced a stroke will not be discharged from a hospital until the team has established plans with physical and occupational therapists to begin a program of rehabilitation.

Effective discharge planning often requires referrals to various health care disciplines. In many agencies a health care provider's order is necessary for a referral, especially when planning specific therapies (e.g., physical therapy). It is best to have patients and families participate in referral processes so they are involved early in any necessary decision making. Some tips on making the referral process successful include the following:

- Make a referral as soon as possible.
- Give the care provider receiving the referral as much information about the patient as possible. This avoids duplication of effort and exclusion of important information.
- Involve the patient and family in the referral process, including selecting the necessary referral. Explain the service that the referral will provide, the reason for the referral, and what to expect from the services of the referral.
- Determine what the referral discipline recommends for the patient's care and include this in the treatment plan as soon as possible.

The nurse provides resources to improve the long-term outcomes of patients with limitations. Discharge planning depends on comprehensive patient and family education (see Chapter 25). Patients need to know what to do when they get home, how to do it, and for what to observe when problems develop. Patients require the following instruction before they leave health care facilities:

- Safe and effective use of medications and medical equipment
- Instruction in potential food-drug interactions and counseling on nutrition and modified diets
- Rehabilitation techniques to support adaptation to and/or functional independence in the environment
- Access to available and appropriate community resources
- When and how to obtain further treatment
- The patient's and family's responsibilities in the patient's ongoing health care needs and the knowledge and skills needed to carry out those responsibilities
- When to notify their health care provider for changes in functioning or new symptoms

Intensive Care. An ICU or critical care unit is a hospital unit in which patients receive close monitoring and intensive medical care. ICUs have advanced technologies such as computerized cardiac monitors and mechanical ventilators. Although many of these devices are on regular nursing units, the patients hospitalized within ICUs are monitored and maintained on multiple devices. Nursing and medical staff have special knowledge about critical care principles and techniques. An ICU is the most expensive health care delivery site because each nurse usually cares for only one or two patients at a time and because of all the treatments and procedures the patients in the ICU require.

Psychiatric Facilities. Patients who suffer emotional and behavioral problems such as depression, violent behavior, and eating disorders often require special counseling and treatment in psychiatric facilities. Located in hospitals, independent outpatient clinics, or private mental health hospitals, psychiatric facilities offer inpatient and outpatient services, depending on the seriousness of the problem. Patients enter these facilities voluntarily or involuntarily. Hospitalization involves relatively short stays with the purpose of stabilizing patients before transfer to outpatient treatment centers. Patients with psychiatric problems receive a comprehensive multidisciplinary treatment plan that involves them and their families. Medicine, nursing, social work, and activity therapy work together to develop a plan of care that enables patients to return to functional states within the community. At discharge from inpatient facilities, patients usually receive a referral for follow-up care at clinics or with counselors.

Rural Hospitals. Access to health care in rural areas has been a serious problem. Most rural hospitals have experienced a severe shortage of primary care providers. Many have closed because of economic failure. In 1989 the Omnibus Budget Reconciliation Act (OBRA) directed the U.S. Department of Health and Human Services (USDHHS) to create a new health care organization, the rural primary care hospital (RPCH). The Balanced Budget Act of 1997 changed the designation for rural hospitals to Critical Access

Hospital (CAH) if certain criteria were met (American Medical Association, 2009). A CAH is located in a rural area and provides 24-hour emergency care, with no more than 25 inpatient beds for providing temporary care for 96 hours or less to patients needing stabilization before transfer to a larger hospital. Physicians, nurse practitioners, or physician assistants staff a CAH. The CAH provides inpatient care to acutely ill or injured people before transferring them to better-equipped facilities. Basic radiological and laboratory services are also available.

With health care reform, more big-city health care systems are branching out and establishing connections or mergers with rural hospitals. The rural hospitals provide a referral base to the larger tertiary care medical centers. With the development of advanced technologies such as telemedicine, rural hospitals have increased access to specialist consultations. Nurses who work in rural hospitals or clinics require competence in physical assessment, clinical decision making, and emergency care. Having a culture of evidence-based practice is important in rural hospitals so nurses practice using the best evidence to achieve optimal patient outcomes (Burns et al., 2009). Advanced practice nurses (e.g., nurse practitioners and clinical nurse specialists) use medical protocols and establish collaborative agreements with staff physicians.

Restorative Care

Patients recovering from an acute or chronic illness or disability often require additional services to return to their previous level of function or reach a new level of function limited by their illness or disability. The goals of **restorative care** are to help individuals regain maximal functional status and enhance quality of life through promotion of independence and self-care. With the emphasis on early discharge from hospitals, patients usually require some level of restorative care. For example, some patients require ongoing wound care and activity and exercise management until they have recovered enough following surgery to independently resume normal activities of daily living.

The intensity of care has increased in restorative care settings because patients leave hospitals earlier. The restorative health care team is an interdisciplinary group of health professionals and includes the patient and family or significant others. In restorative settings nurses recognize that success depends on effective and early collaboration with patients and their families. Patients and families require a clear understanding of goals for physical recovery, the rationale for any physical limitations, and the purpose and potential risks associated with therapies. Patients and families are more likely to follow treatment plans and achieve optimal functioning when they are involved in restorative care.

Home Health Care (Home Care). **Home care** is the provision of medically related professional and paraprofessional services and equipment to patients and families in their homes for health maintenance, education, illness prevention, diagnosis and treatment of disease, palliation, and rehabilitation. Nursing is one service most patients use in home care. However, home care also includes medical and social services; physical, occupational, speech, and respiratory therapy; and nutritional therapy. These services usually occur once or twice a day for as long as 7 days a week. A home care service also coordinates the access to and delivery of home health equipment, or durable medical equipment, which is any medical product adapted for home use.

Health promotion and education are traditionally the primary objectives of home care, yet at present most patients receive home care because they need nursing or medical care. Examples of home nursing care include monitoring vital signs; assessment; administering parenteral or enteral nutrition, medications, and IV or blood therapy; and wound or respiratory care. The focus is on patient and family independence. Nurses address recovery and stabilization of illness in the home and identify problems related to lifestyle, safety, environment, family dynamics, and health care practices.

Approved home care agencies usually receive reimbursement for services from the government (such as **Medicare** and **Medicaid** in the United States), private insurance, and private pay. The government has strict regulations that govern reimbursement for home care services. An agency cannot simply charge whatever it wants for a service and expect to receive full reimbursement. Government programs set the cost of reimbursement for most professional services.

Nurses in home care provide individualized care. They have a caseload and assist patients in adapting to permanent or temporary physical limitations so they are able to assume a more normal daily home routine. Home care requires a strong knowledge base in many areas such as family dynamics (see Chapter 10), cultural practices (see Chapter 9), spiritual values (see Chapter 35), and communication principles (see Chapter 24).

Rehabilitation. **Rehabilitation** restores a person to the fullest physical, mental, social, vocational, and economic potential possible. Patients require rehabilitation after a physical or mental illness, injury, or chemical addiction. Specialized rehabilitation services such as cardiovascular, neurological, musculoskeletal, pulmonary, and mental health rehabilitation programs help patients and families adjust to necessary changes in lifestyle and learn to function with the limitations of their disease. Drug rehabilitation centers help patients become free from drug dependence and return to the community.

Rehabilitation services include physical, occupational, and speech therapy and social services. Ideally rehabilitation begins the moment a patient enters a health care setting for treatment. For example, some orthopedic programs now have patients perform physical therapy exercises before major joint repair to enhance their recovery after surgery. Initially rehabilitation usually focuses on the prevention of complications related to the illness or injury. As the condition stabilizes, rehabilitation helps to maximize the patient's functioning and level of independence.

Rehabilitation occurs in many health care settings, including special rehabilitation agencies, outpatient settings, and the home. Frequently patients needing long-term rehabilitation (e.g., patients who have had strokes and spinal cord injuries) have severe disabilities affecting their ability to carry out the activities of daily living. When rehabilitation services occur in outpatient settings, patients receive treatment at specified times during the week but live at home the rest of the time. Health care providers apply specific rehabilitation strategies to the home environment. Nurses and other members of the health care team visit homes and help patients and families learn to adapt to illness or injury.

Extended Care Facilities. An **extended care facility** provides intermediate medical, nursing, or custodial care for patients recovering from acute illness or those with chronic illnesses or disabilities. Extended care facilities include intermediate care and skilled nursing facilities. Some include long-term care and assisted living facilities. At one point extended care facilities primarily cared for older adults. However, because hospitals discharge their patients sooner, there is a greater need for intermediate care settings for patients of all ages. For example, health care providers transfer a young patient who has experienced a traumatic brain injury resulting from a car accident to an extended care facility for rehabilitative or supportive care until discharge to the home becomes a safe option.

An intermediate care or **skilled nursing facility** offers skilled care from a licensed nursing staff. This often includes administration of IV fluids, wound care, long-term ventilator management, and physical rehabilitation. Patients receive extensive supportive care until they are able to move back into the community or into residential care. Extended care facilities provide around-the-clock nursing coverage. Nurses who work in a skilled nursing facility need nursing expertise similar to that of nurses working in acute care inpatient settings, along with a background in gerontological nursing principles (see Chapter 14).

Continuing Care

Continuing care describes a variety of health, personal, and social services provided over a prolonged period. These services are for people who are disabled, who were never functionally independent, or who suffer a terminal disease. The need for continuing health care services is growing in the United States. People are living longer, and many of those with continuing health care needs have no immediate family members to care for them. A decline in the number of children families choose to have, the aging of care providers, and the increasing rates of divorce and remarriage complicate this problem. Continuing care is available within institutional settings (e.g., nursing centers or nursing homes, group homes, and retirement communities), communities (e.g., adult day care and senior centers), or the home (e.g., home care, home-delivered meals, and hospice) (Meiner, 2011).

Nursing Centers or Facilities. The language of long-term care is confusing and constantly changing. The nursing home has been the dominant setting for long-term care (Meiner, 2011). With the 1987 OBRA, the term *nursing facility* became the term for nursing homes and other facilities that provided long-term care. Now *nursing center* is the most appropriate term. A nursing center typically provides 24-hour intermediate and custodial care such as nursing, rehabilitation, dietary, recreational, social, and religious services for residents of any age with chronic or debilitating illnesses. In some cases patients stay in nursing centers for room, food, and laundry services only. Most persons living in nursing centers are older adults. A nursing center is a resident's temporary or permanent home, with surroundings made as homelike as possible (Sorrentino, 2007). The philosophy of care is to provide a planned, systematic, and interdisciplinary approach to nursing care to help residents reach and maintain their highest level of function (Resnick and Fleishell, 2002).

According to the U.S. Bureau of the Census, just over 5% of people 65 years of age and older live in nursing centers and other facilities (Missouri Families, 2008). The nursing center industry is one of the most highly regulated industries in the United States. These regulations have raised the standard of services provided (Box 2-2). One regulatory area that deserves special mention is that of resident rights. Nursing facilities have to recognize residents as active participants and decision makers in their care and life in institutional settings (Meiner, 2011). This also means that family members are active partners in the planning of residents' care.

Interdisciplinary functional assessment of residents is the cornerstone of clinical practice within nursing centers (Meiner, 2011). Government regulations require that staff comprehensively assess each resident and make care planning decisions within a prescribed period. A resident's functional ability (e.g., ability to perform activities of daily living) and long-term physical and psychosocial well-being are the focus. Staff must complete the Resident Assessment Instrument (RAI) on all residents. The RAI consists of the **Minimum Data Set (MDS)** (Box 2-3), Resident Assessment Protocols, and utilization guidelines of each state. The RAI provides a national database for nursing facilities so policy makers will better understand the health care needs of the long-term care population. The MDS is a rich resource for nurses in determining the best interventions to support the health care needs of this growing population.

Assisted Living. Assisted living is one of the fastest growing industries within the United States. There are approximately 38,000 assisted living facilities that house more than 975,000 people in the United States (National Center for Assisted Living [NCLA], 2010). **Assisted living** offers an attractive long-term care setting with an environment more like home and greater resident autonomy. Residents require some assistance with activities of daily living but remain relatively independent within a partially protective setting. A group of residents live together, but each resident has his or her own room and shares dining and social activity

BOX 2-2 MAJOR REGULATORY REQUIREMENTS DEFINED BY THE 1987 OMNIBUS BUDGET RECONCILIATION ACT

- Resident rights
- Admission, transfer, and discharge rights
- Resident behavior and facility practices
- Quality of life
- Resident assessment
- Quality of care
- Nursing services
- Dietary services
- Physician services
- Specialized rehabilitative services
- Dental services
- Pharmacy services
- Infection control
- Physical environment
- Administration

From Health Care Financing Administration, Department of Health and Human Services: *Requirements for states and long-term care facilities,* 42 CFR 483 Subpart B (483.1-75), October 1, 2004. http://ecfr.gpoaccess.gov/cgi/t/text/text-idx?c=ecfr&tpl=/ecfrbrowse/Title42/42cfr483_main_02.tpl. Accessed June 18, 2011.

BOX 2-3 MINIMUM DATA SET AND EXAMPLES OF RESIDENT ASSESSMENT PROTOCOLS

Minimum Data Set

- Resident's background
- Cognitive, communication/hearing, and vision patterns
- Physical functioning and structural problems
- Mood, behavior, and activity patterns
- Psychosocial well-being
- Bowel and bladder continence
- Health conditions
- Disease diagnoses
- Oral/nutritional and dental status
- Skin condition
- Medication use
- Special treatments and procedures

Resident Assessment Protocols (Examples)

- Delirium
- Falls
- Pressure ulcers
- Psychotropic drug use

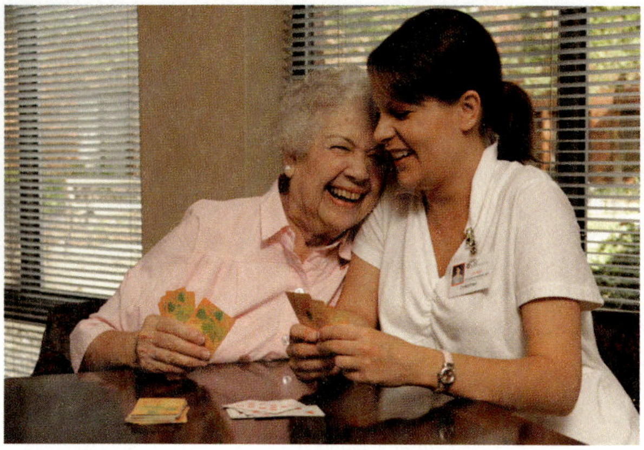

FIG. 2-2 Providing nursing services in assisted living facilities promotes physical and psychosocial health.

areas. Usually people keep all of their personal possessions in their residences. Facilities range from hotel-like buildings with hundreds of units to modest group homes that house a handful of seniors. Assisted living provides independence, security, and privacy all at the same time (Ebersole et al., 2008). These facilities promote physical and psychosocial health (Fig. 2-2). Services in an assisted living facility include laundry, assistance with meals and personal care, 24-hour oversight, and housekeeping (NCAL, 2010). Some facilities provide assistance with medication administration. Nursing care services are not always directly available, although home care nurses can visit patients in assisted living facilities. Unfortunately most residents of assisted living facilities pay privately. The average monthly fee is $3022 for a private unit (NCAL, 2010). With no government fee caps and little regulation, assisted living is not always an option for individuals with limited financial resources.

Respite Care. The need to care for family members within the home creates great physical and emotional problems for family caregivers, especially if the people for whom they care have either physical or cognitive limitations. The family caregiver usually not only has the responsibility for providing care to a loved one but often has to maintain a full-time job, raise a family, and manage the routines of daily living as well. **Respite care** is a service that provides short-term relief or "time off" for people providing home care to an ill, disabled, or frail older adult (Meiner, 2011). Respite care is offered in the home, a day care setting, or a health care institution that provides overnight care. The family caregiver is able to leave the home for errands or some social time while a responsible person stays in the home to care for the loved one. There are few formal respite care programs in the United States because of cost. Currently Medicare does not cover respite care, and Medicaid has strict requirements for services and eligibility (Sultz and Young, 2006).

Adult Day Care Centers. **Adult day care centers** provide a variety of health and social services to specific patient populations who live alone or with family in the community. Services offered during the day allow family members to maintain their lifestyles and employment and still provide home care for their relatives (Meiner, 2011). Day care centers are associated with a hospital or nursing home or exist as independent centers. Frequently the patients need continuous health care services (e.g., physical therapy or counseling) while their families or support persons work. The centers usually operate 5 days per week during typical business hours and usually charge on a daily basis. Adult day care centers allow patients to retain more independence by living at home, thus potentially reducing the costs of health care by avoiding or delaying an older adult's admission to a nursing center. Nurses working in day care centers provide continuity between care delivered in the home and the center. For example, nurses ensure that patients continue to take prescribed medication and administer specific treatments. Knowledge of community needs and resources is essential in providing adequate patient support (Ebersole et al., 2008).

Hospice. A **hospice** is a system of family-centered care that allows patients to live and remain at home with comfort, independence, and dignity while easing the pains of terminal illness. The focus of hospice care is palliative care, not curative treatment (see Chapter 43). The interdisciplinary team in the hospice works continuously with the patient's health care provider to develop and maintain a patient-directed individualized plan of care. Many hospice programs provide respite care, which is important in maintaining the health of the primary caregiver and family.

ISSUES IN HEALTH CARE DELIVERY

The climate in health care today influences both health care professionals and consumers. Because those who provide patient care are the most qualified to make changes in the health care delivery system, nurses need to participate fully and effectively within all aspects of health care. As nursing faces issues of how to maintain health care quality while reducing costs, nurses need to acquire the knowledge, skills, and values necessary to practice competently and effectively. It will also become more important than ever before to collaborate with other health care professionals to design new approaches for patient care delivery.

Nursing Shortage

There are more than 3.1 million nurses in the United States, making nursing the largest health care profession in the country (American Association of Colleges of Nursing [AACN], 2011). Although nearly 57% of the nurses work in medical-surgical hospitals, they are involved in delivering health care at all levels, including primary and preventive care (AACN, 2011). In spite of the large number of practicing nurses, a critical shortage of nurses is projected in the United States. It is expected that this shortage will worsen with increased need for health care services by the aging baby-boomer generation (AACN, 2010). It is estimated that over 500,000 new nursing positions will be created by 2018, resulting in a 22% increase in the size of the nursing workforce (U.S. Department of Labor, 2009). The economic climate and recession had brought about an easing of the nursing shortage (Buerhaus et al., 2009). This easing is not expected to last, mainly because of the aging nursing workforce and potential retirements. The average age of nurses is projected to be 44.5 years by 2012 (AACN, 2010). One other factor contributing to the shortage is the slow growth in nursing school enrollments, often because of nursing faculty shortages, space limitations, and clinical site availability (AACN, 2010; Buerhaus et al., 2009). Buerhaus et al. (2009) estimate that by 2025 the shortage will grow to 260,000 nurses.

Competency

The Pew Health Professions Commission, a national and interdisciplinary group of health care leaders, recommended 21

BOX 2-4 INSTITUTE OF MEDICINE COMPETENCIES FOR THE TWENTY-FIRST CENTURY

Provide Patient-Centered Care
- Recognize and respect differences in patients' values, preferences, and needs.
- Relieve pain and suffering.
- Coordinate continuous care.
- Effectively communicate with and educate patients.
- Share decision making and management.
- Advocate for disease prevention and health promotion.

Work in Interdisciplinary Teams
- Cooperate, collaborate, and communicate.
- Integrate care to ensure that care is continuous and reliable.

Use Evidence-Based Practice
- Integrate best research with clinical practice and patient values.
- Participate in research activities as possible.

Apply Quality Improvement
- Identify errors and hazards in care.
- Practice using basic safety design principles.
- Measure quality in relation to structure, process, and outcomes.
- Design and test interventions to change processes.

Use Informatics
- Use information technology to communicate, manage knowledge, reduce error, and support decision-making.

Adapted from Institute of Medicine (IOM): *Crossing the quality chasm: a new health system for the 21st century,* Washington DC, 2001, National Academies Press; and Institute of Medicine: *Health professions education: a bridge to quality,* Washington, DC, 2003, National Academies Press.

BOX 2-5 TEN RULES OF PERFORMANCE IN A REDESIGNED HEALTH CARE SYSTEM

1. Care is based on continuous healing relationships.
2. Care is individualized based on patient needs and values.
3. The patient is the source of control participating in shared decision making.
4. Knowledge is shared, and information flows freely.
5. Decision making is evidence based, with care based on the best available scientific knowledge.
6. Safety is a system property and focused on reducing errors.
7. Transparency is necessary through sharing information with patients and families.
8. Patient needs are anticipated through planning.
9. Waste is continuously decreased.
10. Cooperation and communication among clinicians are priorities.

Adapted from Institute of Medicine (IOM): *Crossing the quality chasm: a new health system for the 21st century,* Washington DC, 2001, National Academies Press; and Institute of Medicine: *Health professions education: a bridge to quality,* Washington, DC, 2003, National Academies Press.

competencies for health care professionals in the twenty-first century (Pew Health Professions Commission, 1998). The competencies emphasize the importance of public service, caring for the health of communities, and developing ethically responsible behaviors. In addressing the continued challenge facing the health care system, the IOM (2001) identified five interrelated competencies that are essential for all health care workers in the twenty-first century (Box 2-4). Shifts to an emphasis on prevention and management place increased importance on the competencies of care management and coordination, patient education, public health, and transitional care (IOM, 2011). The IOM also identified 10 important rules of performance for a health care system to follow to better meet patient needs (Box 2-5) (IOM, 2003).

The health care practitioner competencies are an excellent tool for measuring how well a nurse practices nursing and serve as a guide for the development of a professional nursing career. A consumer of health care expects that the standards of nursing care and practice in any health care setting are appropriate, safe, and efficacious. Health care organizations ensure quality care by establishing policies, procedures, and protocols that are evidence based and follow national accrediting standards. A nurse's responsibility is to follow policies and procedures and know the most current practice standards. Ongoing competency is a nurse's responsibility. It is also the nurse's responsibility to obtain necessary continuing education, follow an established code of ethics, and earn certifications in specialty areas (Jordan et al., 2008). Development of a professional practice portfolio that shows learning activities and professional accomplishments is one way to show competency in nursing (Scott-Tilley, 2008).

Evidence-Based Practice

As professionals, nurses are challenged to stay familiar with new information to provide the highest quality of patient care. Nursing practice is dynamic and always changing because of new information coming from research studies, practice trends, technological development, and social issues affecting patients. Nurses need to analyze new knowledge to make sound and informed decisions about patient care (Kotzer and Arellana, 2008). Evidence-based practice is a problem-solving approach to clinical practice that involves the conscientious use of current best evidence, along with clinical expertise and patient preferences and values in making decisions about patient care (Melnyk and Fineout-Overholt, 2010). Evidence-based practice, research-based practice, and best practice are terms that are often used interchangeably. However, research-based practice refers to the use of knowledge based on the results of research studies; whereas evidence-based practice adds a nurse's clinical experience, practice trends, and patient preferences (Melnyk and Fineout-Overholt, 2010). Chapter 5 offers a thorough review of evidence-based practice.

Quality and Safety in Health Care

Nursing plays an important role in quality and safety in health care (Box 2-6). Quality health care is the "degree to which health services for individuals and populations increase the likelihood of desired health outcomes and are consistent with current professional knowledge" (IOM, 2001). Safety is a critical part of quality health care (Tzeng and Yin, 2007). The National Quality Forum (NQF) (2010) identified 34 health care practices, organized in seven functional areas that improve patient safety by decreasing the occurrence of adverse events. Examples of NQF practices include hand hygiene, teamwork, training, influenza prevention, catheter-associated urinary tract infection prevention, fall prevention, and medication reconciliation (NQF, 2010). Health care providers define the quality of their services by measuring health care outcomes that show how a patient's health status has changed. Examples of outcomes that are monitored are readmission rates for patients who have had surgery, functional health status of patients

BOX 2-6 EVIDENCE-BASED PRACTICE

Nursing Work Environment and Patient Safety

PICO Question: What nursing factors in the nursing work environment contribute to patient safety in hospitals?

Evidence Summary

Studies examined a variety of factors within the nursing work environment that contribute to patient safety. Nurses working in Magnet hospitals were more likely to participate in problem solving to reduce errors (Hughes et al., 2009). Environments that empowered nurses gave them control over their own practice and participation in decision making on the unit. These nurses had greater involvement in identifying patient safety issues, communicated more about safety issues, and found solutions for problems that jeopardized patient safety (Hughes et al., 2009; Spence Laschinger, 2008). Key to the development of empowering work environments were the nurse leaders and managers. Spence Laschinger (2008) found that nursing work groups that were committed to patient safety were a positive characteristic of the safety climate on the nursing unit. Research also showed that the percentage of certified registered nurses on a unit was directly related to patient safety (Kendall-Gallagher and Blegen, 2009). Greater safety compliance was also found on smaller nursing units that had less patient and work complexity (Hughes et al., 2009). Continued research is needed to validate the effect that nursing has on patient safety.

Application to Nursing Practice

- Seek out health care institutions that have empowering environments, such as shared governance, on nursing units (Spence Laschinger, 2008).
- Work toward obtaining certification in your specialty nursing area (Kendall-Gallagher and Blegen, 2009).
- Become involved in committees and decision-making processes on the unit (Spence Laschinger, 2008).
- Develop nursing work groups that are committed to patient safety (Hughes et al., 2009).
- Open channels of communication that involve the staff nurse in identifying patient safety issues (Hughes et al., 2009).

after discharge (e.g., ability and time frame for returning to work), and the rate of infection after surgery. Nurses play an important role in gathering and analyzing quality outcome data. Within a rural hospital setting, knowledge of the rural culture and connectedness to the community are unique features related to quality care (Baernholdt et al., 2010).

Pay for performance programs and public reporting of hospital quality data are designed to promote quality, effective, and safe patient care by physicians and health care organizations. These programs are quality improvement strategies that reward excellence through financial incentives to motivate change to achieve measurable improvements (Lindenauer et al., 2007). Nurses play an important role in helping hospitals meet the measure for quality, efficiency, and patient satisfaction (Lutz and Root, 2007). They are often the health care provider who ensures that performance measures occur. For example, one performance measure is the standard that any patient admitted with a possible myocardial infarction receives an aspirin. In an acute care setting a nurse is the one who obtains an order for the aspirin and ensures that the patient receives it in a timely manner (Bodrock and Mion, 2008). Research shows that financial incentives modestly increase quality improvement efforts in hospitals that do public reporting (Lindenauer et al., 2007). Some health care organizations use balanced scorecards to report data on their key performance indicators. These scorecards are reported publicly so health care consumers can use the information when choosing health care services.

More and more health care institutions are focused on improving processes as a way to improve quality and safety. Many use strategies such as Six Sigma, Lean Six Sigma, or Value Stream Analysis. Six Sigma is a data-driven approach to process improvement that reduces variation in process. It is a measure of quality (isixsigma, 2010). For example, a nursing unit sets up a project to collect data on the process of administering the first dose of an ordered chemotherapy. The audit reveals delays in getting the drug from the pharmacy to the nursing unit. Using Six Sigma, the collected data are analyzed, and unnecessary steps in the process are identified. On the basis of this analysis the process is streamlined to decrease time from ordering to administration. Lean Six Sigma and value stream analysis are two other methods that focus on improvement of processes through studying each step of a process to determine if the step adds value and reduces the health care organization's time, costs, and resources (Burger, 2008; Carey, 2010). The aim of both is to eliminate unnecessary, nonvalue-added costly steps to reduce waste.

Health plans throughout the United States rely on the Healthcare Effectiveness Data and Information Set (HEDIS) as a quality measure. The National Committee for Quality Assurance (NCQA) created HEDIS to collect various data to measure the quality of care and services provided by different health plans. It is the database of choice for the Centers for Medicare and Medicaid Services (CMS). HEDIS compares how well health plans perform on 71 measures across eight domains of care in the key areas of quality and effectiveness of care, access to care, and patient satisfaction with the health plan and doctors (NCQA, 2010). For accreditation purposes The Joint Commission requires health care organizations to determine how well an organization meets patient needs and expectations. Organizations are using outcomes such as patient satisfaction to redesign how they manage and deliver care in hopes of improving quality in the long term.

Patient Satisfaction. Every major health care organization measures certain aspects of patient satisfaction. The Hospital Consumer of Assessment of Healthcare Providers and Systems (HCAHPS) is a standardized survey developed to measure patient perceptions of their hospital experience (HCAHPS, 2010). HCAHPS was developed by the CMS and the Agency for Healthcare Research and Quality as a way for hospitals to collect and report data publicly for comparison purposes. The survey is administered to a randomly selected sample of adults who were discharged from a hospital between 48 hours and 6 weeks ago. The survey has 27 questions that ask patients to respond about communication with nurses and physicians, responsiveness of hospital staff, pain management, communication about medications, discharge planning, cleanliness and quietness of the environment, overall satisfaction, and willingness to recommend the hospital (HCAHPS, 2010). Nursing environments affect HCAHPS scores. Research found that hospitals that improved the nursing work environment and lowered nurse-patient ratios by one patient had higher patient satisfaction levels and patients who were more likely to recommend the hospital to others (Kutney-Lee et al., 2009).

The Picker Institute identified eight dimensions of **patient-centered care** (Box 2-7) that most affect patients' experiences with health care. The eight dimensions cover most of the scope of nursing practice. This is not a surprise because nurses are involved in almost every aspect of a patient's care in a hospital. A close look shows that many of the aspects reflected in patient satisfaction apply to almost any health care setting.

BOX 2-7 THE DIMENSIONS OF PATIENT-CENTERED CARE

Respect Values, Preferences, and Expressed Needs
- Patients expect to be treated with dignity, respect, and sensitivity to cultural beliefs, values, and quality-of-life issues.
- Patients want to be informed and share in decisions about their care.
- Patients' perceptions of needs should not be completely different from those identified by a care provider.

Coordination and Integration of Care
- A competent and caring staff reduces feelings of powerlessness.
- Patients look for someone to be in charge of care and communicate clearly with other health care team members.
- Patients expect to have services and care well coordinated. This includes areas of clinical care, front-line patient care, and ancillary and support services.
- Patients need to know at all times whom to call for help.

Information, Communication, and Education
- Patients expect to receive accurate and timely information about their clinical status, progress, or prognosis.
- Patients and families need to be informed of major changes in therapies or status.
- Patients need tests and procedures explained clearly in language they understand.
- Patients and family members want to know how to manage care on their own.

Physical Comfort
- Physical care needs to provide comfort for pain management.
- Nurses need to respond in a timely and effective way to any request for pain medication, explain the extent of pain patients can expect, and offer alternatives for pain management.
- Patients expect privacy and to have their cultural values respected.
- Patients often need help to complete activities of daily living.
- The health care setting environment needs to be clean and comfortable, with accessibility for visits by family.

Emotional Support and Relief of Fear and Anxiety
- Patients look to care providers to share their fears and concerns.
- Patients need to understand the impact that illness will have on their ability to care for themselves and their family.
- Patients worry about their ability to pay for their medical care. Identify staff that will help alleviate this worry.

Involvement of Family and Friends
- Care providers need to recognize, respect, and meet the needs of patients, family, and friends.
- Patients have the right to determine if family members are to be involved in decisions about their care.
- Patients expect family or friends who will provide physical support and care after discharge to be properly informed.

Transition and Continuity
- Patients want information about medications to take, physical limitations, dietary or treatment plans to follow, and danger signals for which to look after hospitalization or treatment.
- Patients expect to have their continuing health care needs met after discharge with well-coordinated services.
- Patients and family members expect access to necessary health care resources on a continuing basis.

Access to Care
- Patients want to get to hospitals, clinics, and physicians' offices easily and without hassle.
- Patients need to be able to find transportation when going to different health care settings.
- Patients want to schedule appointments at convenient times without difficulty.
- Patients want to be able to see a specialist when a referral is made.
- Patients expect to receive clear instructions on how to obtain referrals to other health care providers.

Adapted from Picker Institute: *Principles of patient-centered care,* 2011, http:pickerinstitute.org/about/picker-principles. Accessed December 28, 2011.

The survey tool from The Picker Institute measures patient satisfaction along the eight dimensions. The survey looks globally at patient perceptions of care in an attempt to understand how all hospital departments influence patient satisfaction. The program mails surveys to patients after they leave a health care setting. Many other companies have developed similar patient satisfaction surveys that are distributed in the mail to patients. Staff involved in patient care receive the satisfaction scores as feedback regarding their success in meeting patient expectations. The nursing staff is responsible for identifying unique issues that influence patient satisfaction on their unit. For example, nurses working on an oncology unit have different patient satisfaction issues around physical comfort than nurses caring for new mothers. Patient satisfaction findings become the basis for many quality improvement studies.

It is important for nurses to recognize the need to provide patient- and family-centered care. Identifying patient and family expectations, knowledge, preferences, cultural beliefs, and values is an important part of patient-centered care (Cronenwett et al., 2007; Institute for Patient- and Family-Centered Care [IPFCC], 2010). Concepts of patient-centered care include respect and dignity, sharing of information, participation in care and care decisions, and collaboration (IPFCC, 2010). By learning early what a patient expects with regard to information, comfort, and availability of family and friends, nurses are able to better plan patient care. They should ask about the patient's expectations when the patient first enters a health care setting, while care continues, and when a patient is discharged. Patient expectations are an important measure of the evaluation of nursing care. A Patient and Family Advisory Council is one strategy that is effective in obtaining patient and family feedback to develop patient- and family-centered care (Zarubi et al., 2008).

Magnet Recognition Program

The American Nurses Credentialing Center (ANCC) established the Magnet Recognition Program to recognize health care organizations that achieve excellence in nursing practice (ANCC, 2010c). In the United States approximately 6.4% of health care organizations have achieved Magnet status (ANCC, 2010b). Health care organizations that apply for Magnet status must demonstrate quality patient care, nursing excellence, and innovations in professional practice. The professional work environment must allow

BOX 2-8 MAGNET MODEL AND FORCES OF MAGNETISM

MAGNET MODEL COMPONENTS	FORCES OF MAGNETISM
Transformational Leadership—A vision for the future and the systems and resources to achieve the vision are created by nursing leaders.	• Quality of Nursing Leadership • Management Style
Structural Empowerment—Structures and processes provide an innovative environment in which staff are developed and empowered and professional practice flourishes.	• Organizational Structure • Personnel Policies and Programs • Community and the Health Organization • Image of Nursing • Professional Development
Exemplary Professional Practice—Strong professional practice is established, and accomplishments of the practice are demonstrated.	• Professional Models of Care • Consultation and Resources • Autonomy • Nurses as Teachers • Interdisciplinary Relationships
New Knowledge, Innovations, and Improvements—Contributions are made to the profession in the form of new models of care, use of existing knowledge, generation of new knowledge, and contributions to the science of nursing.	• Quality Improvement
Empirical Quality Outcomes—Focus is on structure and processes and demonstration of positive clinical, work force, and patient and organizational outcomes.	• Quality of Care

Adapted from American Nurses Credentialing Center: *A new model for ANCC's Magnet Recognition Program*, 2010a, http://www.nursecredentialing.org/Magnet/ProgramOverview/NewMagnetModel.aspx.

BOX 2-9 NURSING QUALITY INDICATORS

- Patient falls
- Patient falls with injury
- Pressure ulcers—community acquired, hospital acquired, unit acquired
- Staff mix
- Nursing hours per patient day
- Registered nurse (RN) surveys on job satisfaction and practice environment scale
- RN education and certification
- Pediatric pain assessment cycle
- Pediatric intravenous infiltration rate
- Psychiatric patient assault rate
- Restraint prevalence
- Nurse turnover
- Hospital-acquired infections of ventilator-associated pneumonia, central line–associated bloodstream infection, catheter-associated urinary tract infection

Data from National Database of Nursing Quality Indicators (NDNQI): NDNQI: transforming data into quality care, 2010, http://www.nursingquality.org. Accessed June 18, 2011.

nurses to practice with a sense of empowerment and autonomy to deliver quality nursing care. The revised Magnet model has five components that are affected by global issues that are challenging nursing today (ANCC, 2010a) (Box 2-8). The five components are Transformational Leadership; Structural Empowerment; Exemplary Professional Practice; New Knowledge, Innovation, and Improvements; and Empirical Quality Results. Institutions achieve Magnet status through an appraisal process that requires them to present evidence showing achievement of the 14 forces of magnetism (see Box 2-8). Magnet status requires nurses to collect data on specific nursing-sensitive quality indicators or outcomes and compare their outcomes against a national, state, or regional database to demonstrate quality of care.

Nursing-Sensitive Outcomes. **Nursing-sensitive outcomes** are patient outcomes and select nursing workforce characteristics that are directly related to nursing care such as changes in patients' symptom experiences, functional status, safety, psychological distress, registered nurse (RN) job satisfaction, total nursing hours per patient day, and costs. Nurses assume accountability and responsibility for achieving and accepting the consequences of these outcomes. The National Database of Nursing Quality Indicators (NDNQI) was developed by the American Nurses Association to measure and evaluate nursing-sensitive outcomes with the purpose of improving patient safety and quality care (NDNQI, 2010) (Box 2-9). The NDNQI reports quarterly results on nursing outcomes at the nursing unit level. This provides a database for individual hospitals to compare their performance against nursing performance nationally (Kurtzman and Jennings, 2008). The evaluation of patient outcomes and nursing workforce characteristics remains important to nursing and the health care delivery system. Chapter 5 describes approaches for measuring outcomes.

Because of the importance of nursing-sensitive outcomes, the Agency for Healthcare Research Quality funded several nursing research studies that looked at the relationship of nurse staffing levels to adverse patient outcomes. These studies found a connection between higher levels of staffing by registered nurses (RNs) in hospitals and fewer negative patient outcomes. For example, the incidence of hospital-acquired pneumonia was highly sensitive to RN staffing levels. Adding just 30 minutes of RN staffing per patient day greatly reduced the incidence of pneumonia in patients following surgery. These studies also found that increased levels of nurse staffing positively impacted nurse satisfaction. Future studies will examine how nurses' workloads affect patient safety and how their working conditions affect medication safety. Measuring and monitoring nursing-sensitive outcomes reveal the interventions that improve patients' outcomes. Nurses and health care facilities use nursing-sensitive outcomes to improve nurses' workloads, enhance patient safety, and develop sound policies related to nursing practice and health care.

Nursing Informatics and Technological Advancements

Quality and Safety Education for Nurses (QSEN) identified informatics as a competency for nurses (Cronenwett et al., 2007). **Nursing informatics** "uses information and technology to communicate, manage knowledge, mitigate error, and support decision-making" (Cronenwett et al., 2007). Data are individually distinct pieces of reality. Examples of data nurses collect and use to deliver safe patient care include a patient's blood pressure or the measurement of a patient's wound. Nurses gain or use *information* when they organize, structure, or interpret data. A nurse uses information when looking at trends in a patient's blood pressure readings over the past 24 hours or when evaluating the changes in the size of a wound over the past 3 weeks. *Knowledge* develops when nurses combine and identify relationships between different pieces of information. For example, nurses know that diet plays an important role in blood pressure control and wound healing. They use this knowledge to teach patients at risk for developing high blood pressure to limit their salt intake and to teach patients who have wounds the importance of eating a well-rounded diet that includes adequate protein, vitamins, and minerals. Knowledge and skills in informatics also provides the nurse ability to access quality electronic sources of health care information to plan and coordinate patient care (Cronenwett et al., 2007). The focus of nursing informatics is not on the technology or the computer; rather, its focus is on the organization, analysis, and dissemination of information (American Nurses Association, 2008). Chapter 26 provides a thorough review of how nursing informatics improves the way nurses provide health care through use of the electronic health record.

Advances in technology are constantly evolving. People work, play, and view the world much differently because of these advances. Technological advancements also influence where and how nurses provide care to patients. Technological advances help nurses improve direct care processes, patient outcomes, and work environments (Zuzelo et al., 2008). Sophisticated equipment such as electronic IV infusion devices, cardiac telemetry (a device that monitors a patient's heart rate wherever the patient is on a nursing unit), and computerized medication dispensation systems (see Chapter 31) are just a few examples that have changed health care. In many ways, technology makes the nurse's work easier, but it does not replace nursing judgment. For example, it is the nurse's responsibility when managing a patient's IV therapy to monitor the infusion to be sure that it infuses on time and without complications. An electronic infusion device provides a constant rate of infusion, but nurses need to be sure that they calculate the rate correctly. The device sets off an alarm if the infusion slows, making it important for the nurse to respond to the alarm and troubleshoot the problem. Technology does not replace a nurse's critical eye and clinical judgment. Challenges arise for nurses when technologies create inefficient delivery systems or uses or need repairs. These problems increase the nurses' workload (Zuzelo et al., 2008).

Technology also affects the way we communicate with others. Personal computers, cell phones, and personal digital assistants (PDAs) allow us to communicate and share information or data with others in a variety of formats around the world. People expect accurate information to be delivered to them as it develops. Managing communication, information, and data is challenging in health care. Health care agencies use data to measure their outcomes and improve patient care. Accrediting bodies, insurance companies, and Medicare/Medicaid all require collection and reporting of accurate data. Furthermore, nurses need accurate, up-to-date information to make the best decisions about patient care. Therefore it is crucial that nurses help health care agencies develop an effective way to manage the collection, interpretation, and distribution of information.

Nurses need to play a role in evaluating and implementing new technological advances. They use technology and informatics to improve the effectiveness of nursing care, enhance safety, and improve patient outcomes. Most important, it is essential for nurses to remember that the focus of nursing care is not the machine or the technology; it is the patient. Therefore nurses need to constantly attend to and connect with their patients and ensure that their dignity and rights are preserved at all levels of care.

Globalization of Health Care

Globalization, the increasing connectedness of the world's economy, culture, and technology, is one of the forces reshaping the health care delivery system (Oulton, 2012). Advances in communication, primarily through the Internet, allow nurses, patients, and other health care providers to talk with others worldwide about health care issues. Improved communication, easier air travel, and easing of trade restrictions are making it easier for people to engage in "health tourism." Health tourism is the travel to other nations to seek out health care.

Many problems affect the health status of people around the world. For example, poverty is still deadlier than any disease and is the most frequent reason for death in the world today. Poverty increases the disparities in health care services among vulnerable populations (Crigger, 2008). Nations and communities that experience poverty have limited access to vaccines, clean water, and standard medical care. The growth of urbanization also currently is affecting global health. As cities become more densely populated, problems with pollution, noise, crowding, inadequate water, improper waste disposal, and other environmental hazards become more apparent. Children, women, and older adults are **vulnerable populations** most threatened by urbanization. Nurses work toward improving the health of all populations (Crigger, 2008). Although globalization of trade, travel, and culture improves the availability of health care services, the spread of communicable diseases such as tuberculosis and severe acute respiratory syndrome has become more common. Finally, the results of global environmental changes and disasters affect health. Changes in climate and natural disasters threaten food supplies and often allow infectious diseases to spread more rapidly.

Nurses need to understand how worldwide communication and globalization of health care influence nursing practice. Health care consumers demand quality and service and have become more knowledgeable. They often have searched the Internet about their health concerns and medical conditions. They also use the Internet to select their health care providers. As a result of **globalization,** health care providers have to make their services more accessible. Because of advances in communication, nurses and other health care providers practice across state and national boundaries. In response to the nursing shortage in the early 2000s, health care institutions recruited nurses from around the world to work in the United States. This was an effort to continue to provide quality, safe patient care. This trend is expected to continue to fill vacant nursing positions (Buerhaus et al., 2009). The hiring of nurses from other nations has required American hospitals to better understand and work with nurses from different cultures and with different needs.

As a leader in health care, remain aware of what is happening in the community, nation, and around the world. The International Council of Nurses (ICN), based in Switzerland, represents nursing worldwide. The purpose of the ICN is to advance the nursing profession worldwide and influence health policy (ICN, 2010). The goals of ICN are to bring nursing together, advance the nursing profession, and influence health policy worldwide (ICN, 2010). The unique focus of nursing on caring helps nurses address the issues presented by globalization. Nurses and the nursing profession are able to help overcome these issues by working together to improve nursing education throughout the world, retaining nurses and recruiting people to be nurses, and being advocates for changes that will improve the delivery of health care. Be prepared for future health care issues. Globalization has influenced many other industries. As a leader, nursing has to take control and be proactive in developing solutions before someone outside of nursing takes control.

THE FUTURE OF HEALTH CARE

This discussion of the health care delivery system began with the issue of change. Change is often threatening, but it also opens up opportunities for improvement. The ultimate issue in designing and delivering health care is ensuring the health and welfare of the population. Health care in the United States and around the world is not perfect. Patients do not receive continuity of care when they see multiple health care providers. Often patients are uninsured or underinsured and do not have access to necessary services. However, health care organizations are trying to become better prepared to deal with the challenges in health care. Increasingly, health care organizations are changing how they provide their services, reducing unnecessary costs, improving access to care, and trying to provide high-quality patient care. Professional nursing is an important player in the future of health care delivery. The solutions necessary to improve the quality of health care depend largely on the active participation of nurses.

KEY POINTS

- Increasing costs and decreasing reimbursement are forcing health care institutions to deliver care more efficiently without sacrificing quality.
- In a managed care system the provider of care receives a predetermined capitated payment regardless of the services a patient uses.
- The Medicare prospective reimbursement system is based on payment calculated on the basis of DRG assignment.
- Levels of health care describe the range of services and settings in which health care is available to patients in all stages of health and illness.
- Health promotion occurs in home, work, and community settings.
- Nurses are facing the challenge of keeping populations healthy and well within their own homes and communities.
- Successful community-based health programs involve building relationships with the community and incorporating cultural and environmental factors.
- Hospitalized patients are acutely ill, requiring better coordination of services before discharge.
- Rehabilitation allows an individual to return to a level of normal or near-normal function after a physical or mental illness, injury, or chemical dependency.
- Home care agencies provide a wide variety of health care services with an emphasis on patient and family independence.
- Discharge planning begins at admission to a health care facility and helps in the transition of a patient's care from one environment to another.
- Health care organizations are being evaluated on the basis of outcomes such as prevention of complications, patients' functional outcomes, and patient satisfaction.
- Nurses need to remain knowledgeable and proactive about issues in the health care delivery system to provide quality patient care and positively affect health.

CLINICAL APPLICATION QUESTIONS

Preparing for Clinical Practice

Community Hospital is a 400-bed urban hospital, one of six hospitals in a health care system. The system also operates a local community clinic that primarily serves a poor multicultural population. The nursing department of the hospital is considering making application to the American Nurses Credentialing Center for Magnet status. Nursing units are working on a number of projects to prepare for the Magnet application process.

1. You are a staff nurse on a medical-surgical floor at the hospital. The unit is trying to improve its culture in patient safety. How would you go about helping to improve the culture of safety on the unit?
2. Discuss three strategies that the community clinic can use to deliver patient- and family-centered care.
3. You are asked by a nurse at another hospital what it means to be a "Magnet hospital." Describe the Magnet model of nursing to answer the nurse's question.

evolve *Answers to Clinical Application Questions can be found on the Evolve website.*

REVIEW QUESTIONS

Are You Ready to Test Your Nursing Knowledge?

1. Which of the following is an example of the principle of patient-centered care focused on continuity and transition?
   1. The nurse asks the patient who in the family should have access to patient information
   2. The nurse is teaching the patient how to change the wound dressing at home
   3. The nurse responds promptly to the patient's request for pain medication
   4. The nurse schedules the patient's diagnostic scan following the physical therapy session
2. Which activity performed by the nurse is related to maintaining competency in nursing practice?
   1. Asking another nurse about how to change the settings on a medication pump
   2. Regularly attending unit staff meetings
   3. Participating as a member of the professional nursing council
   4. Attending a review course in preparation for the certification examination
3. The patient tells the nurse that she is enrolled in a preferred provider organization (PPO) but does not understand what this is. What is the nurse's best explanation of a PPO?
   1. This health plan is for people who cannot afford their own health insurance
   2. This health plan is operated by the government to provide health care to older adults
   3. This health plan provides you with a preferred list of physicians, hospitals, and providers from which you can choose
   4. This is a fee-for-service plan in which you can choose any physician or hospital
4. Which of the following is an example of the nurse participating in primary care activities?
   1. Providing prenatal teaching on nutrition to a pregnant woman during the first trimester
   2. Working with patients in a cardiac rehabilitation program

3. Assessing a patient at an emergent care facility
4. Providing home wound care to a patient

5. Nurses on a nursing unit are discussing the processes that led up to a near-miss error on the clinical unit. They are outlining strategies that will prevent this in the future. This is an example of nurses working on what issue in the health care system?
   1. Patient safety
   2. Evidence-based practice
   3. Patient satisfaction
   4. Maintenance of competency
6. Which of the following statements is true regarding Magnet status recognition for a hospital?
   1. Nursing is run by a Magnet manager who makes decisions for the nursing units
   2. Nurses in Magnet hospitals make all of the decisions on the clinical units
   3. Magnet is a term that is used to describe hospitals that are able to hire the nurses they need
   4. Magnet is a special designation for hospitals that achieve excellence in nursing practice
7. Which statement made by the nurse is an example of applying the principle of patient-centered care while focusing on alleviation of a patient's fear and anxiety?
   1. "Let's talk about the concerns that you have about going home."
   2. "I'll get the medication prescriptions for you before discharge"
   3. "I'll be back in 30 minutes to help you get cleaned up"
   4. "I'll make a referral to the home health nurse for you"
8. Which of the following is/are characteristics of managed care systems? (Select all that apply.)
   1. Provider receives a predetermined payment for each patient in the program.
   2. Payment is based on a set fee for each service provided.
   3. System includes a voluntary prescription drug program for an additional cost.
   4. System tries to reduce costs while keeping patients healthy.
   5. Focus of care is on prevention and early intervention.
9. Which of the following nursing activities is found in a tertiary health care environment?
   1. Administering influenza immunizations at the senior independent living facility
   2. Providing well-baby care in the clinic run by the local community health department
   3. Admitting a patient following open heart surgery to the cardiovascular intensive care unit
   4. Working the triage desk in the emergency department
10. Which of the following activities performed by the nurse is/are focused on the patient-centered care principle of physical comfort? (Select all that apply.)
    1. Asking the patient what a tolerable level of pain is for him or her following surgery
    2. Providing a back rub at bedtime
    3. Offering the patient a warm washcloth for his or her hands before eating
    4. Teaching the patient about the new antihypertensive medication ordered
    5. Scheduling the patient's follow-up appointments on discharge
    6. Changing the bed linens for a patient who is experiencing diaphoresis
11. The nursing staff is developing a quality program for the floor. Which of the following are nursing-sensitive indicators from the National Database of Nursing Quality Indicators that the nurses can use to measure patient safety and quality for the unit? (Select all that apply.)
    1. Number of medication errors committed by registered nurses (RNs)
    2. Turnover rate of nurses on the unit
    3. Incidence of patient falls
    4. Number of certified RNs
    5. Number of emergency department admissions per year
12. The nurse is providing restorative care to a patient following an extended hospitalization for an acute illness. Which of the following is an appropriate goal for restorative care?
    1. Patient will be able to walk 200 feet without shortness of breath
    2. Wound will heal without signs of infection
    3. Patient will express concerns related to return to home
    4. Patient will identify strategies to improve sleep habits
13. A nurse is presenting information to a management class of nursing students on the topic of groups of inpatient hospital services that have a fixed reimbursement amount, with adjustments made on the basis of case severity and regional costs. The nurse is presenting information to the class on which topic?
    1. Utilization review committee
    2. Resource utilization group
    3. Capitation payment system
    4. Diagnosis-related groups
14. When a nurse uses information and technology to communicate, locate and use knowledge, reduce and eliminate errors, and help make decisions, the nurse is working in which area?
    1. Integrated delivery system
    2. Health care patient system
    3. Nursing informatics
    4. Computerized nursing network
15. Which of the following are examples of the principle of patient-centered care that is focused on respect, values, preferences, and expressed needs? (Select all that apply.)
    1. Administer antihypertensive medications to patient daily.
    2. Pulling the curtain around the patient bed before changing the wound dressing on the patient's leg
    3. Allowing the patient to ask questions and express his or her concern about surgery
    4. Explaining a colonoscopy procedure to the patient
    5. Working with the family to bring in ethnic foods that the patient prefers

Answers: **1.** 2; **2.** 4; **3.** 3; **4.** 1; **5.** 1; **6.** 4; **7.** 1; **8.** 1, 4, 5; **9.** 3; **10.** 1, 2, 3, 6; **11.** 2, 3, 4; **12.** 1; **13.** 4; **14.** 3; **15.** 2, 3, 5.

REFERENCES

Adashi EY, et al: Health care reform and primary care—the growing importance of the community health center, *N Engl J Med* 362(22):2047, 2010.

Agency for Healthcare Research and Quality Patient Safety Network (AHRQ PSNet): *Patient safety primer: Never events*, n.d., http://psnet.ahrq.gov/printviewPrimer.aspx?primerID=3. Accessed September 5, 2011.

American Association of Colleges of Nursing: *Nursing fact sheet*, 2011, http://www.aacn.nche/edu/Media/FactSheets/nursfact.htm. Accessed June 20, 2011.

American Association of Colleges of Nursing: *Nursing shortage*, 2010, http://www.aacn.nche.edu/Media/FactSheets/NursingShortage.htm. Accessed June 18, 2011.

American Medical Association: *Critical access hospital fact sheet*, 2009, http://www.aacvpr.org/Portals/0/policy/resources/CAH_factsheet_june2009.pdf. Accessed June 20, 2011.

American Nurses Association: *Nursing informatics scope and standards of practice*, Silver Springs, Md, 2008, The Association.

American Nurses Credentialing Center: *A new model for ANCC's Magnet Recognition Program*, 2010a, http://www.nursecredentialing.org/Magnet/ProgramOverview/NewMagnetModel.aspx. Accessed May 5, 2010.

American Nurses Credentialing Center: *Growth of the program*, 2010b, http://www.nursecredentialing.org/Magnet/ProgramOverview/GrowthoftheProgram.aspx, Accessed June 18, 2011.

American Nurses Credentialing Center: *Magnet program overview*, 2010c, http://www.nursecredentialing.org/Magnet/ProgramOverview.aspx. Accessed June 18, 2011.

Billings J, Cantor JC: *Access to care*. In Kovner AR, Knickman JR, editors: *Health care delivery in the United States*, ed 9, New York, 2009, Springer.

Bodrock JA, Mion LC: Pay for performance in hospitals: implications for nurses and nursing care, *Qual Manage Health Care* 17(2):102, 2008.

Burger G: *The 5 Whys: A Simple Tool in Value Stream Analysis*, 2008, http://www.isixigma.com/library/content/c070910a.asp. Accessed June 18, 2011.

Carey G: *Comparing and blending ISO9000 and lean six sigma*, 2010, http://www.isixsigma.com/index.php?option=comk2&view=item&id=67&Itemid=1&Itemid=1. Accessed January 10, 2012.

Centers for Disease Control and Prevention: *Fast facts: life expectancy. Deaths: final data for 2007*, 2007, http://www.cdc.gov/nchs/fastats/lifexpec.htm. Accessed June 18, 2011.

Centers for Disease Control and Prevention: *Health risks in the United States: behavioral risk factor surveillance system at a glance*, 2010, http://www.cdc.gov/chronicdisease/resources/publications/AAG/brfss.htm. Accessed June 18, 2011.

Crigger NJ: Towards a viable and just global nursing ethics, *Nurs Ethics* 15(1):17, 2008.

Cronenwett L, et al: Quality and safety education for nurses, *Nurs Outlook* 55:122, 2007.

Ebersole P, et al: *Toward healthy aging: human needs and nursing response*, ed 7, St Louis, 2008, Mosby.

HCAHPS: *Fact sheet (CAHPS hospital survey, July 2010)*, 2010, http://www.hcahpsonline.org/facts.aspx. Accessed June 18, 2011.

HealthReform.gov: *Key provisions that take effect immediately*, 2010, http://www.healthreform.gov/reports/keyprovisions.html. Accessed June 18, 2011.

Institute for Patient and Family Centered Care [IPFCC]: *FAQ*, 2010, http://www.ipfcc.org/faq.html. Accessed June 18, 2011.

Institute of Medicine (IOM): *Crossing the quality chasm: a new health system for the 21st century*, Washington DC, 2001, National Academies Press.

Institute of Medicine: *Health professions education: a bridge to quality*, Washington, DC, 2003, National Academies Press.

Institute of Medicine (IOM): *The future of nursing: leading change, advancing health*, Washington DC, 2011, National Academies Press.

International Council of Nurses [ICN]: *Our mission*, 2010, http://www.icn.ch/about-icn/icns-mission/.

isixsigma: *Statistical Six Sigma definition*, 2010, http://www.isixsigma.com/index/php?option=com_k2&view=item&layout=item&id=1254&Itemid=110. Accessed June 18, 2011.

Jonas S, et al: *An introduction to the US health care system*, ed 6, New York, 2007, Springer.

Jordan C, et al: Public policy on competency: how will nursing address this complex issue? *J Cont Educ Nurs* 39(2):86, 2008.

Knickman JR, Kovner AR: Overview: the state of health care delivery in the United States. In Kovner AR, Knickman JR, editors: *Health care delivery in the United States*, ed 9, New York, 2009, Springer.

Kotzer AM, Arellana K: Defining an evidenced-based work environment for nursing in the USA, *J Clin Nurs* 17(12):1652, 2008.

Kurtzman ET, Jennings BM: Trends in transparency: nursing performance measurement and reporting, *J Nurs Admin* 38(7):349, 2008.

Lutz SL, Root D: Nurses, consumer satisfaction, and pay for performance, *Healthcare Finance Manage* 61(10):57, 2007.

Meiner SE: *Gerontologic nursing*, ed 4, St. Louis, 2011, Mosby.

Melnyk BM, Fineout-Overholt E: *Evidence-based practice in nursing and health care: a guide to best practice*, ed 2, Philadelphia, 2010, Lippincott, Williams & Wilkins.

Missouri Families: *Aging*, 2008, http://missourifamilies.org/quick/agingqa/agingqa30.htm. Accessed June 18, 2011.

National Center for Assisted Living [NCAL]: *Assisted living facility profile*, 2010, http://www.ahcancal.org/ncal/resources/Pages/ALFacilityProfile.aspx. Accessed June 18, 2011.

National Committee for Quality Assurance [NCQA]: *HEDIS and quality compass*, 2010, http://www.ncqa.org/tabid/187/Default.aspx. Accessed June 18, 2011.

National Database of Nursing Quality Indicators (NDNQI): *NDNQI: transforming data into quality care*, 2010, http://www.nursingquality.org. Accessed June 18, 2011.

National Priorities Partnership: *National priorities and goals: aligning our efforts to transform America's healthcare*, Washington, DC, 2008, National Quality Forum.

National Quality Forum [NQF]: *Safe practices for better healthcare—2010 update: a consensus report*, Washington, DC, 2010, National Quality Forum.

Oulton J: Nursing in the international community: a broader view of nursing issues. In Mason DJ et al: *Policy and politics in nursing and health care*, ed 6, St Louis, 2012, Saunders.

Pew Health Professions Commission, The Fourth Report of the Pew Health Professions Commission: *Recreating health professional practice for a new century*, 1998, The Commission.

Resnick B, Fleishell A: Developing a restorative care program: a five step approach that involves the resident, *Am J Nurs* 102(7):95, 2002.

Scott-Tilley DD: Competency in nursing: a concept analysis, *J Cont Educ Nurs* 39(2):58, 2008.

Singleton KA: Lead, follow, and get in the way: the medical-surgical nurse's role in health care reform, *Medsurg Nurs* 19(1):5, 2010.

Sorrentino S: *Mosby's textbook for nursing assistants*, ed 7, St Louis, 2007, Mosby.

Sultz HA, Young KM: *Health care USA: understanding its organization and delivery*, ed 5, Sudbury, 2006, Jones & Bartlett.

The Joint Commission: *Accreditation Process Overview*, 2011. http://www.jointcommission.org/accreditation_process_overview/. Accessed June 20, 2011.

Thompson JA, Lee V: The effect of health insurance disparities on the health care system, *AORN J* 86(5):745, 2007.

US Department of Labor. *Bureau of Labor Statistics: Employment projections: occupations with the largest job growth*,2009,http://www.bls.gov/emp/ep_table_104.htm. Accessed June 20, 2011.

Vlasses FR, Smeltzer CH: Toward a new future for health-care and nursing practice, *J Nurs Admin* 37(9):375, 2007.

World Health Organization [WHO]: *The WHO report 2008: primary health care now more than ever*, Geneva, Switzerland, 2008, WHO.

RESEARCH REFERENCES

Baernholdt M, et al: What does quality care mean to nurses in rural hospitals? *J Adv Nurs* 66(6):1346, 2010.

Buerhaus PI, et al: The recent surge in nurse employment: causes and implications, *Health Affairs* 28(4):w657, 2009, published online 12 June 2009, doi:10.1377/hlthaff.28.4.w657.

Burns HK, et al: Building an evidence-based practice infrastructure and culture: a model for rural and community hospitals, *J Nurs Admin* 39(7/8):321, 2009.

Hughes LC, et al: Quality and strength of patient safety climate on medical-surgical units, *Health Care Manage Rev* 34(1):28, 2009.

Kendall-Gallagher D, Blegen, MA: Competence and certification of registered nurses and safety of patients in intensive care units, *Am J Crit Care* 18(2):106, 2009.

Kutney-Lee A, et al: Nursing: a key to patient satisfaction, *Health Affairs* 28(4):w669, 2009, published online 12 June 2009, doi:10.1377/hlthaff.28.4.w669.

Lindenauer PK, et al: Public reporting and pay for performance in hospital quality improvement, *New Engl J Med* 356(5):486, 2007.

Spence Laschinger HK: Effect of empowerment on professional practice environments, work satisfaction, and patient care quality: further testing the nursing work life mode, *J Nurs Care Qual* 23(4):322, 2008.

Tzeng H, Yin C: No safety, no quality: synthesis of research on hospital and patient safety (1996-2007), *J Nurs Care Qual* 22(4):229, 2007.

Zarubi KL, et al: Putting patients and families at the center of care, *J Nurs Admin* 38(6):278, 2008.

Zuzelo PR, et al: Describing the influence of technologies on registered nurses' work, *Clin Nurse Spec* 22(3):132, 2008.

CHAPTER

3

Community-Based Nursing Practice

OBJECTIVES

- Explain the relationship between public health and community health nursing.
- Differentiate community health nursing from community-based nursing.
- Discuss the role of the community health nurse.
- Discuss the role of the nurse in community-based practice.
- Identify characteristics of patients from vulnerable populations that influence the community-based nurse's approach to care.
- Describe the competencies important for success in community-based nursing practice.
- Describe elements of a community assessment.

KEY TERMS

Community-based nursing, p. 33
Community health nursing, p. 32
Incident rates, p. 32
Population, p. 32
Public health nursing, p. 32
Vulnerable populations, p. 33

evolve WEBSITE

http://evolve.elsevier.com/Potter/fundamentals/

- Review Questions
- Case Study with Questions
- Audio Glossary
- Interactive Learning Activities
- Key Term Flashcards
- Content Updates

Community-based care focuses on health promotion, disease prevention, and restorative care. Because patients move quickly from acute care settings, there is a growing need to organize health care delivery services where people live, work, socialize, and learn (Swiadek, 2009). One way to achieve this goal is through a community-based health care model. Community-based health care is a collaborative, evidence-based model designed to meet the health care needs of a community (Downie, Ogilve, and Wichmann, 2005). A healthy community includes elements that maintain a high quality of life and productivity. For example, safety and access to health care services are elements that enable people to function productively in their community (U.S. Department of Health and Human Services [USDHHS], 2010). As community health care partnerships develop, nurses are in a strategic position to play an important role in health care delivery and improve the health of the community.

The focus of health promotion and disease prevention continues to be essential for the holistic practice of professional nursing. The history of nursing documents the roles of nurses in establishing and meeting the public health goals of their patients. Within community health settings, nurses are leaders in assessing, diagnosing, planning, implementing, and evaluating the types of public and community health services needed. Community health nursing and community-based nursing are components of a health care delivery system that improve the health of the general public.

COMMUNITY-BASED HEALTH CARE

It is important to understand the focus of community-based health care. Community-based health care is a model of care that reaches everyone in the community (including the poor and underinsured), focuses on primary rather than institutional or acute care, and provides knowledge about health and health promotion and models of care to the community. Community-based health care occurs outside traditional health care institutions such as hospitals. It provides services to individuals and families within the community for acute and chronic conditions (Stanhope and Lancaster, 2010).

Today the challenges in community-based health care are numerous. Social lifestyles, political policy, and economics all influence public health problems and subsequent health care services. Some of these problems include an increase in homeless and immigrant populations, an increase in sexually transmitted infections, underimmunization of infants and children, patients with chronic illnesses, and life-threatening diseases (e.g., patients living with human immunodeficiency virus [HIV] and other emerging infections). More than ever before, health care reform is necessary to bring attention to the health care needs of all communities.

Achieving Healthy Populations and Communities

The U.S. Department of Health and Human Services Public Health Service designed a program to improve the overall health status of people living in this country. The *Healthy People Initiative* was created to establish ongoing health care goals (see Chapter 6). The 2020 document strives to ensure that *Healthy People 2020* is relevant to diverse public health needs and seizes opportunities to achieve its goals. Since its inception, *Healthy People* has become a broad-based, public engagement initiative with thousands of citizens helping to shape it at every step along the way. The overall goals of *Healthy People 2020* are to increase life expectancy and quality of life and eliminate health disparities through an improved delivery of health care services (USDHHS, 2010).

Improved delivery of health care occurs through assessment of health care needs of individuals, families, and communities; development and implementation of public health policies; and improved access to care. For example, assessment includes systematic data collection on the population, monitoring the health status of the population, and accessing available information about the health of the community (Stanhope and Lancaster, 2010). A comprehensive community assessment can lead to community health programs such as adolescent smoking prevention, sex education, and proper nutrition. Some examples of assessment include gathering information on **incident rates** for identifying and reporting new infections or diseases, determining adolescent pregnancy rates, and reporting the number of motor vehicle accidents by teenage drivers.

Health professionals provide leadership in developing public policies to support the health of the population (Stanhope and Lancaster, 2010). Strong policies are driven by community assessment. For example, assessing the level of lead poisoning in young children often leads to a lead cleanup program to reduce the incidence of lead poisoning. Likewise more people are choosing to remain in their homes for end-of-life care. Assessing the numbers of people in the community who need end-of-life care can lead to evidence-based practices for addressing both the needs of the nurses and the home care needs of these patients (Smith and Porock, 2009) (Box 3-1).

BOX 3-1 EVIDENCE-BASED PRACTICE

Managing Chronic Leg Ulcers in a Community Setting

PICO Question: What is the effect on quality of life (QOL) in community-dwelling patients with chronic leg ulcers who participate in leg ulcer support group compared to patients who do not participate in a support group?

Evidence Summary

Healing chronic venous leg ulcers is expensive and time consuming and impacts a patient's level of function and QOL. In addition, pain and in some cases odor are associated with the leg wound. As a result, patients and their families are socially isolated. Patients also experience depression and anxiety related to the chronic impact and the long healing process (Jones et al., 2006). Each and all of these factors impact patients' perception of QOL. When nursing resources and support groups are available in a community setting, the costs of treatment are reduced, and QOL and function and activity increase (Edwards et al., 2009; Gordon et al., 2006).

Application to Nursing Practice

- The presence of chronic wound support groups provides patients and families an opportunity to interact with individuals who experience similar situations (Edwards et al., 2009).
- Nursing wound care specialists who make home visits to patients in their community settings are able to track the healing process as the patient's level of activity and function change and offer suggestions to improve the patient's level of independence (Gordon et al., 2006).
- It is necessary to understand that some patients and family members have depression and anxiety related to the chronic nature of the wound and the slow healing process (Jones et al., 2006).
- During the early phases of healing the patient and family may report that their QOL is very low; however, let them know that, as the wound heals, their ability and desire to socialize with others may increase, the cost of care may decline, and pain may decline or resolve. All of these factors can improve the patient's QOL reports (Hareendran et al., 2005).

Improved access to care ensures that essential community-wide health services are available and accessible to the total community (Stanhope and Lancaster, 2010). Examples include prenatal care programs for the uninsured and educational programs to ensure the competency of public health professionals. Population-based public health programs focus on disease prevention, health protection, and health promotion. This focus provides the foundation for health care services at all levels (see Chapter 2).

The five-level health services pyramid is an example of how to provide community-based services within existing health care services in a community (see Fig. 2-1 on p. 17). In this population-focused health care services model, the goals of disease prevention, health protection, and health promotion provide a foundation for primary, secondary, and tertiary health care services.

A rural community often has a hospital to meet the acute care needs of its citizens. However, a community assessment might reveal that there are minimal services to meet the needs of expectant mothers, reduce teenage smoking, or provide nutritional support for older adults. Community-based programs are able to provide these services and are effective in improving the health of the community. On the other hand, when a community has the resources for providing childhood immunizations, flu vaccines, primary preventive care services are able to focus on child developmental problems and child safety.

Public health services aim at achieving a healthy environment for all individuals. Health care providers apply these principles for individuals, families, and the communities in which they live. Nursing plays a role in all levels of the health services pyramid. By using public health principles you are better able to understand the types of environments in which patients live and the types of interventions necessary to help keep patients healthy.

COMMUNITY HEALTH NURSING

Frequently the terms *community health nursing* and *public health nursing* are used interchangeably, although they are different. A **public health nursing** focus requires understanding the needs of a **population** or a collection of individuals who have one or more personal or environmental characteristics in common (Stanhope and Lancaster, 2010). Examples of populations include high-risk infants, older adults, or a cultural group such as Native Americans. A public health nurse understands factors that influence health promotion and health maintenance, the trends and patterns influencing the incidence of disease within populations, environmental factors contributing to health and illness, and the political processes used to affect public policy. For example, the nurse uses data on increased incidence of playground injuries to lobby for a policy to use shock-absorbing material rather than concrete for new public playgrounds.

Public health nursing requires preparation at the basic entry level and sometimes requires a baccalaureate degree in nursing that includes educational preparation and clinical practice in public health nursing. A specialist in public health has a graduate level education with a focus in the public health sciences (American Nurses Association [ANA], 2007).

Community health nursing is nursing practice in the community, with the primary focus on the health care of individuals, families, and groups in a community. The goal is to preserve, protect, promote, or maintain health (Stanhope and Lancaster, 2010). The emphasis of such nursing care is to improve the quality of health and life within that community. In addition, the community health nurse provides direct care services to subpopulations within a community. These subpopulations often have a clinical focus in which the nurse has expertise. For example, a case manager follows older adults recovering from stroke and sees the need for community rehabilitation services, or a nurse practitioner gives immunizations to patients with the objective of managing communicable disease within the community. By focusing on subpopulations, the community health nurse cares for the community as a whole and considers the individual or family as only one member of a group at risk.

Competence as a community health nurse requires the ability to use interventions that include the broad social and political context of the community (Stanhope and Lancaster, 2010). The educational requirements for entry-level nurses practicing in community health nursing roles are not as clear as those for public health nurses. Not all hiring agencies require an advanced degree. However, nurses with a graduate degree in nursing who practice in community settings are considered community health nurse specialists, regardless of their public health experience (Stanhope and Lancaster, 2010).

Nursing Practice in Community Health

Community-focused nursing practice requires a unique set of skills and knowledge. In the health care delivery system nurses who become expert in community health practice usually have advanced nursing degrees, yet the baccalaureate-prepared generalist is also quite competent in formulating and applying population-focused assessments and interventions. The expert community health nurse understands the needs of a population or community through experience with individual families and working through their social and health care issues. Critical thinking is important in applying knowledge of public health principles, community health nursing, family theory, and communication in finding the best approaches in partnering with families.

Successful community health nursing practice involves building relationships with the community and being responsive to changes within the community. For example, when there is an increase in the incidence of grandparents assuming child care responsibilities, the community health nurse becomes an active part of a community by establishing an instructional program in cooperation with local schools and assists and supports grandparents in this caregiving role. The nurse knows the community members, needs, and resources and then works in collaboration with community leaders to establish effective health promotion and disease prevention programs. This requires working with highly resistant systems (e.g., welfare system) and trying to encourage them to be more responsive to the needs of a population. Skills of patient advocacy, communicating people's concerns, and designing new systems in cooperation with existing systems help to make community nursing practice effective.

COMMUNITY-BASED NURSING

Community-based nursing care takes place in community settings such as the home or a clinic, where the focus is on the needs of the individual or family. It involves the safety needs and acute and chronic care of individuals and families, enhances their capacity for self-care, and promotes autonomy in decision making (Stanhope and Lancaster, 2010). You use critical thinking and decision making for the individual patient and family—assessing health status, diagnosing health problems, planning care, implementing interventions, and evaluating outcomes of care. Because nurses provide direct care services where patients live, work, and play, it is important that nursing care remains focused on the individual and family and that the values of the individual, family, and the community are respected and incorporated (Reynolds, 2009).

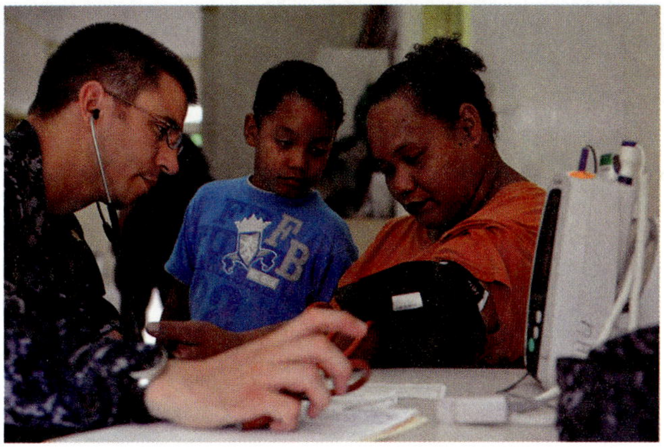

FIG. 3-1 Patient and family receiving care in a community-based care center. (Courtesy Mass Communication Specialist 2nd Class Daniel Viramontes.)

Community-based nursing centers function as the first level of contact between members of a community and the health care delivery system (Fig. 3-1). Ideally health care services are provided near where patients live. This approach helps to reduce the cost of health care for the patient and the stress associated with the financial burdens of care. In addition, these centers offer direct access to nurses and patient-centered health services and readily incorporate the patient and the patient's family or friends into a plan of care. Community-based nursing centers often care for the most vulnerable of the population (Kaiser et al., 2009).

With the individual and family as the patients, the context of community-based nursing is family-centered care within the community. This focus requires a strong knowledge base in family theory (see Chapter 10), principles of communication (see Chapter 24), group dynamics, and cultural diversity (see Chapter 9). You learn to partner with your patients and families so ultimately the patient and family assume responsibility for their health care decisions.

Vulnerable Populations

In a community setting nurses care for patients from diverse cultures and backgrounds and with various health conditions. However, changes in the health care delivery system have made high-risk groups the principal patients. For example, you are not likely to visit low-risk mothers and babies. Instead, adolescent mothers or mothers with drug addiction are more likely to receive home care services. **Vulnerable populations** are groups of patients who are more likely to develop health problems as a result of excess health risks, who are limited in access to health care services, or who depend on others for care. Individuals living in poverty, older adults, people who are homeless, immigrant populations, individuals in abusive relationships, substance abusers, and people with severe mental illnesses are examples of vulnerable populations. Public and community health nursing and primary care providers share health care responsibility for health promotion, screening, and early detection and disease prevention for vulnerable populations. These patients have intense health care needs that are unmet or ignored or require more care than can be provided in outpatient or hospital settings (Kaiser et al., 2009). Vulnerable individuals and their families often belong to more than one of these

BOX 3-2 GUIDELINES FOR ASSESSING MEMBERS OF VULNERABLE POPULATION GROUPS

Setting the Stage

- Learn as much as you can about the culture of the patients with whom you work so you will understand cultural practices and values that influence their health care practices.
- Provide culturally and linguistically competent assessment by understanding the meaning of language and nonverbal behavior in a patient's culture.
- Be sensitive to the fact that the individual or family you are assessing has other priorities that are more important to them. These may include financial or legal problems. Do not provide financial or legal advice, but make sure to connect the patient with someone who will help them.

Nursing History of an Individual or Family

- You often have only one opportunity to work with a vulnerable person or family. Conduct an organized, complete history that provides all the essential information you need to help the individual or family.
- Use a modified comprehensive assessment form to focus on the special needs of the vulnerable population group.
- Include questions about social support, economic status, resources for health care, developmental issues, current health problems, medication, and how the person or family manages their health status.
- Determine if the individual has any acute, chronic, or communicable conditions.

Physical Examination or Home Assessment

- Complete a thorough physical examination (on an individual) or home assessment. Collect only useful data.
- Be alert for indications of mental and physical abuse, changes from normal physical examination findings (see Chapter 30), or substance use (e.g., underweight, being inadequately clothed).
- Observe a family's living environment. Is the environment safe and clean? Is there adequate plumbing? Are there cooking or laundry facilities? Is ventilation adequate? Is the family exposed to raw sewage or animal waste? What does the neighborhood look like?

From Sebastian JG: Vulnerability and vulnerable populations: an overview. In Stanhope M, Lancaster J: *Foundations of nursing in the community: community-oriented practice,* ed 3, St Louis, 2010, Mosby.

groups. In addition, health care vulnerability affects all age-groups (Sebastian, 2010).

Vulnerable patients often come from varied cultures, have different beliefs and values, face language and literacy barriers, and have few sources of social support. Their special needs will be a challenge for you as you care for increasingly complex acute and chronic health conditions.

To provide competent care for vulnerable populations, you need to assess these patients accurately (Box 3-2). In addition, you need to evaluate and understand a patient's and family's cultural beliefs, values, and practices to determine their specific needs and the interventions that will most likely be successful in improving their state of health (see Chapter 9). It is important not to judge or evaluate your patient's beliefs and values about health in terms of your own culture, beliefs, and values. Communication and caring practices are critical in learning a patient's perceptions of his or her problems and then planning health care strategies that will be meaningful, culturally appropriate, and successful.

Barriers to access and use of services often lead to adverse health outcomes for vulnerable populations (Rew et al., 2009). Because of these poorer outcomes, vulnerable populations have shorter life spans and higher morbidity rates. Members of vulnerable groups frequently have multiple risks, which make them more sensitive to the cumulative effects of individual risk factors. It is essential for community-based nurses to assess members of vulnerable populations by taking into account the multiple stressors that affect their patients' lives. It is also important to learn the patients' strengths and resources for coping with stressors. Complete assessment of vulnerable populations enables a community health nurse to design interventions within the context of a community (Rew et al., 2009).

Immigrant Population. Researchers predict that the immigrant population will reach a 54% majority by 2050 (U.S. Census Bureau, 2009). Immigrant populations face multiple diverse health issues that cities, counties, and states need to address. These health care needs pose significant legal and policy issues. For some immigrants access to health care is limited because of language barriers and lack of benefits, resources, and transportation. Immigrant populations often have higher rates of hypertension, diabetes mellitus, and infectious diseases; decreased outcomes of care; and shorter life expectancies (Stanhope and Lancaster, 2010).

Frequently the immigrant population practices nontraditional healing practices (see Chapter 9). Although many of these healing practices are effective and complement traditional therapies, it is important that you know and understand all of your patient's health care practices.

Certain immigrant populations left their homes as a result of oppression, war, or natural disaster (e.g., Afghans, Bosnians, and Somalis). Be sensitive to these physical and psychological stressors and consequences and identify the appropriate resources to help understand your patients and their health care needs (Stanhope and Lancaster, 2010).

Effects of Poverty and Homelessness. People who live in poverty are more likely to live in hazardous environments, work at high-risk jobs, eat less nutritious diets, have multiple stressors in their lives, and be at risk for homelessness. Patients with low income levels not only lack financial resources but also live in poor environments and face practical problems such as poor or unavailable transportation. Homeless patients have even fewer resources than the poor. They are often jobless and do not have the advantage of shelter and must continually cope with finding a place to sleep at night and finding food. Chronic health problems tend to worsen because of poor nutrition and the inability to store nutritional foods. In addition, the homeless population is usually walking the streets and neighborhoods to seek shelter, and they lack a balance of rest and activity (Schanzer et al., 2007). There is a startling increase in adolescent homelessness. The homeless adolescent is usually without a nuclear family and has greater health care risks because of immaturity, which increases the prevalence of risky behaviors (Rew et al., 2008).

Patients Who Are Abused. Physical, emotional, and sexual abuse and neglect are major public health problems affecting older adults, women, and children. Risk factors for abusive relationships include mental health problems, substance abuse, socioeconomic stressors, and dysfunctional family relationships (Landenburger and Campbell, 2010). For some, risk factors may not be present. When dealing with patients at risk for or who have suffered abuse, it is important to provide protection. Interview patients you suspect are abused at a time when the patient has privacy and the individual suspected of being the abuser is not present. Patients who are abused may fear retribution if they discuss their problems with a health care provider. Most states have abuse hot lines that nurses

TABLE 3-1 Common Health Problems in Community-Dwelling Older Adults

PROBLEM	NURSING ROLES AND INTERVENTIONS
Hypertension	Monitor blood pressure and weight; educate about nutrition and antihypertensive drugs; teach stress management techniques; promote an optimal balance between rest and activity; establish blood pressure screening programs; assess patient's current lifestyle and promote lifestyle changes; promote dietary modifications by using techniques such as a diet diary.
Cancer	Obtain health history; promote monthly breast self-examinations and annual Papanicolaou (Pap) smears and mammograms for older women; promote regular physical examinations; encourage smokers to stop smoking; correct mistaken beliefs about processes of aging; provide emotional support and quality of care during diagnostic and treatment procedures.
Arthritis	Educate adult about management of activities, correct body mechanics, availability of mechanical appliances, and adequate rest; promote stress management; counsel and assist family in improving communication, role negotiation, and use of community resources; teach adult to be cautious of false advertisements that promise a cure for arthritis.
Confusional states	Provide for a protective environment; promote activities that reinforce reality; assist with adequate personal hygiene, nutrition, and hydration; provide emotional support to the family; recommend applicable community resources such as adult day care, home care aides, and homemaker services.
Dementia	Maintain the best possible functioning, protection, and safety; foster human dignity; demonstrate to the primary family caregiver techniques to dress, feed, and toilet adult; provide frequent encouragement and emotional support to caregiver; act as an advocate for patient when dealing with respite care and support groups; protect patient's rights; provide support to maintain family members' physical and mental health; maintain family stability; recommend financial services if needed.
Medication use and abuse	Obtain drug history; educate adult about safe medication storage, the danger of polypharmacy, the risks of drug-drug and drug-food interactions, and general information about drug (e.g., drug name, purpose, side effects, dosage); instruct adult about presorting techniques (using small containers with one dose of drug that are labeled with specific administration times).

Data from Stanhope M, Lancaster J: *Foundations of nursing in the community: community-oriented practice,* ed 3, St Louis, 2010, Mosby; and Meiner S, Lueckenotte AG: *Gerontologic nursing,* ed 3, St Louis, 2006, Mosby.

and other health care providers must notify when they identify an individual as being at risk.

Patients Who Abuse Substances. *Substance abuse* is a term that describes more than the use of illegal drugs. It also includes the abuse of alcohol and prescribed medications such as antianxiety agents and opioid analgesics. A patient with substance abuse often has health and socioeconomic problems. The socioeconomic problems result from the financial strain of the cost of drugs, criminal convictions from illegal activities used to obtain drugs, communicable disease from sharing drug paraphernalia, and family breakdown. For example, health problems for cocaine users often include nasal and sinus disorders and cardiac alterations that are sometimes fatal (Decker et al., 2006; Schanzer et al., 2007). Objectively assess your patient's substance use in terms of the amount, frequency, and type of use to gain useful information to assist the patient. Frequently these patients avoid health care for fear of judgmental attitudes and concerns over being arrested by the police.

Patients with Mental Illnesses. When a patient has a severe mental illness such as schizophrenia or bipolar disorder, multiple health and socioeconomic problems need to be explored. Many patients with severe mental illnesses are homeless or live in poverty. Others lack the ability to remain employed or even to care for themselves on a daily basis (Cunningham et al., 2006). Patients suffering from mental illness often require medication therapy, counseling, housing, and vocational assistance. In addition, they are at a greater risk for abuse and assault.

Patients with mental illnesses are no longer routinely hospitalized in long-term psychiatric institutions. Instead, resources are offered within the community. Although comprehensive service networks are in every community, many patients still go untreated. Many patients are left with fewer and more fragmented services, with little skill in surviving and functioning within the community. Collaboration with multiple community resources is essential when helping patients with severe mental illness to obtain adequate health care.

Older Adults. With the increasing older-adult population, simultaneous increases in the number of patients suffering from chronic diseases and a greater demand for health care services are seen. You need to view health promotion in the older adult from a broad context. Take time to understand what health means to older-adult patients and the steps they take to maintain their own health and improve their level of function (Meiner and Leuckenotte, 2006). Thorough assessment and appropriate community-based interventions provide an opportunity to improve the lifestyle and quality of life of older adults (Table 3-1).

Competency in Community-Based Nursing

Nurses in community-based practices need a variety of skills and talents to successfully assist patients to meet their health care needs. To be successful in this setting you will be a caregiver, case manager, change agent, patient advocate, collaborator, educator, counselor, and epidemiologist (Teeley et al., 2006). These skills work together to help the patient remain in the home near his or her family and support system.

Caregiver. First and foremost is the role of caregiver. In the community setting you manage and care for the health of the community. You apply the nursing process (see Unit 3) in a critical thinking approach to ensure appropriate, individualized nursing care for specific patients and their families. In addition, you individualize care within the context of the patient's community so long-term success is more likely. Together with the patient and family you develop a caring partnership to recognize actual and potential health care needs and identify needed community resources. As a caregiver, you also help to build a healthy community, which is one that is safe and includes elements to enable people to achieve and maintain a high quality of life and function.

Case Manager. In community-based practice, case management is an important competency (see Chapter 2). It is the ability to establish an appropriate plan of care based on assessment of patients and families and to coordinate needed resources and services for the patient's well-being across a continuum of care. Generally a community-based case manager assumes responsibility for the case management of multiple patients. The greatest challenge is coordinating the activities of multiple providers and payers in different settings throughout a patient's continuum of care. An effective case manager eventually learns the obstacles, limits, and even the opportunities that exist within the community that influence the ability to find solutions for patients' health care needs.

Change Agent. A community-based nurse is also a change agent. This involves identifying and implementing new and more effective approaches to problems. You act as a change agent within a family system or as a mediator for problems within a patient's community. You identify any number of problems (e.g., quality of community child care services, availability of older-adult day care services, or the status of neighborhood violence). As a change agent you empower individuals and their families to creatively solve problems or become instrumental in creating change within a health care agency. For example, if your patient has difficulty keeping regular health care visits, you determine why. Maybe the health clinic is too far and difficult to reach, or perhaps the hours of service are incompatible with the patient's transportation resourses. You work with the patient to solve the problem and help identify an alternative site such as a nursing clinic that is closer and has more convenient hours.

To effect change you gather and analyze facts before you implement the program. This requires you to be very familiar with the community itself. Many communities resist change, preferring to provide services in the established manner. Before analyzing facts, it is often necessary to manage conflict among the health care providers, clarify their roles, and clearly identify the needs of the patients. If the community has a history of poor problem solving, you will have to focus on developing problem-solving capabilities (Stanhope and Lancaster, 2010).

Patient Advocate. Patient advocacy is more important today in community-based practice because of the confusion surrounding access to health care services. Your patients often need someone to help them walk through the system and identify where to go for services, how to reach individuals with the appropriate authority, what services to request, and how to follow through with the information they receive. It is important to provide the information necessary for patients to make informed decisions in choosing and using services appropriately. In addition, it is important for you to support and at times defend your patients' decisions.

Collaborator. In a community-based nursing practice you need to be competent in working not only with individuals and their families but also with other related health care disciplines. Collaboration, or working in a combined effort with all those involved in care delivery, is necessary to develop a mutually acceptable plan that will achieve common goals (Stanhope and Lancaster, 2010). For example, when your patient is discharged home with terminal cancer, you collaborate with hospice staff, social workers, and pastoral care to initiate a plan to support end-of-life care for the patient and support the family. For collaboration to be effective, you will need mutual trust and respect for each professional's abilities and contributions.

Counselor. Knowing community resources is a critical factor in becoming an effective patient counselor. A counselor helps patients identify and clarify health problems and choose appropriate courses of action to solve those problems. For example, in employee assistance programs or women's shelters, a major amount of nurse-patient interaction is through counseling. As a counselor you are responsible for providing information, listening objectively, and being supportive, caring, and trustworthy. You do not make decisions but rather help your patients reach decisions that are best for them (Stanhope and Lancaster, 2010). Patients and families often require assistance in first identifying and clarifying health problems. For example, a patient who repeatedly reports a problem in following a prescribed diet is actually unable to afford nutritious foods or has family members who do not support good eating habits. You need to discuss with your patient factors that block or aid problem resolution, identify a range of solutions, and then discuss which solutions are most likely to be successful. You also encourage your patient to make decisions and express your confidence in the choice the patient makes.

Educator. In a community-based setting you have an opportunity to work with single individuals and groups of patients. Establishing relationships with community service organizations offers educational support to a wide range of patient groups. Prenatal classes, infant care, child safety, and cancer screening are just some of the health education programs provided in a community practice setting.

When the goal is to help your patients assume responsibility for their own health care, your role as an educator takes on greater importance (Stanhope and Lancaster, 2010). Patients and families must gain the skills and knowledge needed to learn how to care for themselves. Assess your patient's learning needs and readiness to learn within the context of the individual, the systems with which the individual interacts (e.g., family, business, and school), and the resources available for support. Adapt your teaching skills so you can instruct the patient within the home setting and make the learning process meaningful. In this practice setting you have the opportunity to follow patients over time. Planning for return demonstration of skills, using follow-up phone calls, and referring to community support and self-help groups give you an opportunity to provide continuity of instruction and reinforce important instructional topics (see Chapter 25).

Epidemiologist. As a community health nurse, you also apply principles of epidemiology. Your contacts with families, community groups such as schools and industries, and health care agencies place you in a unique position to initiate epidemiological activities. As an epidemiologist, you are involved in case finding, health teaching, and tracking incident rates of an illness. For example, a cafeteria worker in the local high school is diagnosed with active tuberculosis (TB). As a community health nurse, you help find new TB exposures or active disease within the worker's home, employment network, and community.

Nurse epidemiologists are responsible for community surveillance for risk factors (e.g., tracking incidence of elevated lead levels in children and identifying increased fetal and infant mortality rates, increases in adolescent pregnancy, presence of infectious and communicable diseases, and outbreaks of head lice). Nurse epidemiologists protect the level of health of the community, develop sensitivity to changes in the health status of the community, and help identify the cause of these changes.

COMMUNITY ASSESSMENT

When practicing in a community setting, you need to learn how to assess the community at large. Community assessment is the systematic data collection on the population, monitoring the health status of the population, and making information available about the health of the community (Stanhope and Lancaster, 2010). This is the environment in which patients live and work. Without an adequate understanding of that environment, any effort to promote a patient's health and institute necessary change is unlikely to be successful. The community has three components: structure or locale, the people, and the social systems. To develop a complete community assessment, take a careful look at each of the three components to identify needs for health policy, health programs, and needed health services (Box 3-3).

When assessing the structure or locale, you travel around the neighborhood or community and observe its design, the location of services, and the locations where residents meet. You obtain the demographics of the population by accessing statistics on the community from a local public health department or public library. Acquire information about existing social systems such as schools or health care facilities by visiting various sites and learning about their services.

BOX 3-3 COMMUNITY ASSESSMENT

Structure
- Name of community or neighborhood
- Geographical boundaries
- Emergency services
- Water and sanitation
- Housing
- Economic status (e.g., average household income, number of residents on public assistance)
- Transportation

Population
- Age distribution
- Sex distribution
- Growth trends
- Density
- Education level
- Predominant ethnic groups
- Predominant religious groups

Social System
- Education system
- Government
- Communication system
- Welfare system
- Volunteer programs
- Health system

Once you have a good understanding of the community, perform all individual patient assessments against that background. For example, when assessing a patient's home for safety, you consider the following: does the patient have secure locks on doors? Are windows secure and intact? Is lighting along walkways and entryways operational? As you conduct the patient assessment, it is important to know the level of community violence and the resources available when help is necessary. Always assess an individual in the context of the community.

CHANGING PATIENTS' HEALTH

In community-based practice, nurses care for patients from diverse backgrounds and in diverse settings. It is relatively easy over time to become familiar with the available resources within a particular community practice setting. Likewise, with practice you learn how to identify the unique needs of individual patients. However, the challenge is promoting and protecting a patient's health within the context of the community. For example, can a patient with lung disease have the quality of life necessary in a community that has a serious environmental pollution problem? Similarly, nurses bring together the resources necessary to improve the continuity of care that patients receive. You are a key figure in reducing the duplication of health care services and locating the best services for a patient's needs.

Perhaps the most important theme to consider is how well you understand your patients' lives. This begins by establishing strong, caring relationships with patients and their families (see Chapter 7). As you gain experience, after being accepted by a patient's family you are able to advise, counsel, and teach effectively and understand what truly makes the patient unique. The day-to-day activities of family life are the variables that influence how you will adapt nursing interventions. The time of day a patient goes to work, the availability of the spouse and patient's parents to provide child care, and the family values that shape views about health are just a few examples of the many factors you will consider in community-based practice. Once you acquire a picture of a patient's life, you then design interventions to promote health and prevent disease within the community-based practice setting.

KEY POINTS

- Principles of public health nursing practice focus on assisting individuals and communities with achieving a healthy living environment.
- Essential public health functions include community assessment, policy development, and access to resources.
- When population-based health care services are effective, there is a greater likelihood that the higher levels of services will contribute efficiently to health improvement of the population.
- The community health nurse cares for the community as a whole and assesses the individual or family within the context of the community.
- Successful community health nursing practice involves building relationships with the community and being responsive to changes within the community.
- The community-based nurse's competence is based on decision making at the level of the individual patient.
- The special needs of vulnerable populations are a challenge that nurses face in caring for these patients' increasingly complex acute and chronic health conditions.

- A community-based nurse is competent as a caregiver, collaborator, educator, counselor, change agent, patient advocate, case manager, and epidemiologist.
- Patients are more likely to accept a change if it is more advantageous, compatible, realistic, and easy to adopt.

CLINICAL APPLICATION QUESTIONS

Preparing for Clinical Practice

You are managing community care for Katie, age 17, who has cerebral palsy and is severely disabled. Because of the impact of this adolescent's disability, you are also providing care to Monica, age 50, who is a single parent. Katie is the youngest of three children. Her siblings are Josh, age 22, and Marilyn, age 19. Katie attends the special education program of the local school district, and Monica works as a teachers' aide in another school in the district. Katie will remain in the special education program until she is 21. Monica does not know what will happen when Katie is 21, and she has not investigated any other community resources for Katie in the last 10 years. Both siblings are in college and live in the home and are helpful in Katie's care. Josh will graduate from college, and his mother is encouraging him to move from the home.

1. What do you need to assess in the community to identify resources that provide family support in the care of a disabled child?
2. What resources do you need to identify for the family to assist Katie's siblings in moving from the home and beginning their careers?
3. What can you do to help the family begin to envision the new family structure as Josh and Marilyn move out of the home?

evolve *Answers to Clinical Application Questions can be found on the Evolve website.*

REVIEW QUESTIONS

Are You Ready to Test Your Nursing Knowledge?

1. A community nurse in a diverse community is working with health care professionals to provide prenatal care for underemployed and underinsured South African women. Which overall goal of *Healthy People 2020* does this represent?
   1. Assess the health care needs of individuals, families, or communities
   2. Develop and implement public health policies and improve access to care
   3. Gather information on incident rates of certain diseases and social problems
   4. Increase life expectancy and quality of life and eliminate health disparities
2. Using *Healthy People 2020* as a guide, which of the following would improve delivery of care to a community? (Select all that apply.)
   1. Community assessment
   2. Implementing public health policies
   3. Increasing access to care
   4. Determining rates of specific illnesses
   5. Reducing the number of fast food restaurants in the community
3. A nursing student in the last semester of the baccalaureate nursing program is beginning the community health practicum and will be working in a community-based clinic with a focus on asthma and allergies. What is the focus of the community health nurse in this clinic setting? (Select all that apply.)
   1. Decreasing the incidence of asthma attacks in the community
   2. Increasing healthy food choices for school lunches
   3. Assessing for factors that contribute to asthmatic attacks in the community
   4. Providing asthma education programs for the teachers in the local schools
4. A nurse caring for a Bosnian community identifies that the children are undervaccinated and the community is unaware of resources. The nurse assesses the community and determines that there is a health clinic within a 5-mile radius. The nurse meets with the community leaders and explains the need for immunizations, the location of the clinic, and the process of accessing health care resources. Which of the following practices is the nurse providing? (Select all that apply.)
   1. Educating about community resources
   2. Teaching the community about illness prevention
   3. Promoting autonomy in decision making
   4. Improving the health care of the children in the community
5. Vulnerable populations of patients are those who are more likely to develop health problems as a result of:
   1. Chronic diseases and homelessness
   2. Poverty and acute illness
   3. Lack of transportation, ability to perform self-care but are homeless
   4. Excess health risks, limits in access to health care services, and dependency on others for care
6. Which of the following are major public health problems commonly affecting older adults? (Select all that apply.)
   1. Substance abuse
   2. Dementia
   3. Financial limitations
   4. Communicable diseases
   5. Chronic physical illnesses
7. The local health department received information from the Centers for Disease Control and Prevention that the flu was expected to be very contagious this season. The nurses set up flu vaccine clinics in local churches and senior citizen centers. This activity is an example of which level of prevention?
8. A neighborhood with old homes is undergoing a lot of restoration. Lead paint was used in the buildings. The clinic is initiating a lead screening program. This activity is an example of which level of prevention?
9. In an occupational health setting, the nurse determines that a large number of employees smoke and designs an employee assistance program for smoking cessation. This is an example of which nursing role:
   1. Educator
   2. Counselor
   3. Collaborator
   4. Case manager
10. The nurse in a community health clinic notices an increase in the number of positive tuberculosis skin tests from students in a local high school during the most recent academic year. After comparing these numbers to the previous years, a 10% increase in positive tests was found. The nurse contacts the school nurse and the director of the health department. Together they begin to expand their assessment to all students and employees of

the school district. The community health nurse is acting in which nursing role(s)? (Select all that apply.)
1. Epidemiologist
2. Counselor
3. Collaborator
4. Case manager

11. In the community clinic the nurse provides care for a 40-year-old woman who takes insulin to manage her diabetes. The patient is having increased difficulty managing her disease, and the nurse wants her to consider a new insulin pump to help her control it. Which of the following increases the likelihood that the patient will accept this new insulin pump? (Select all that apply.)
    1. Supporting the patient as she tries the insulin pump on a limited basis
    2. Identifying why the patient is reluctant to use the insulin pump
    3. Telling the patient that many other patients you know use the insulin pump successfully
    4. The patient's perception that the insulin pump is more consistent with her health care goals than insulin administration
12. The nurse in a new community-based clinic is requested to complete a community assessment. Order the steps for completing this assessment.
    1. Structure or locale
    2. Social systems
    3. Population
13. On the basis of an assessment, the nurse identifies an increase in the immigrant population group in the community. How would he or she determine some of the health needs of this population? (Select all that apply.)
    1. Identify which two health needs the immigrant population views as most important
    2. Apply information from *Healthy People 2020*
    3. Determine how the population uses available health care resources
    4. Identify perceived barriers for health care
    5. Implement an exercise program to help with weight loss
14. A patient is worried about her 76-year-old grandmother who is in very good health and wants to live at home. The patient's concerns are related to her grandmother's safety. The neighborhood does not have a lot of crime. Using this scenario, which of the following are the most relevant to assess for safety?
    1. Crime rate, locks, lighting, neighborhood traffic
    2. Lighting, locks, clutter, medications
    3. Crime rate, medications, support system, clutter
    4. Locks, lighting, neighborhood traffic, crime rate
15. The nurse is working with the county health department on a task force to fully integrate the goals of *Healthy People 2020*. How does the nurse determine which goals need to be included or updated? (Select all that apply.)
    1. Assesses the health care resources within the community
    2. Assesses the existing health care programs offered by the county health department
    3. Compares existing resources and programs with *Healthy People 2020* goals
    4. Initiates new programs to meet *Healthy People 2020* goals.

Answers: **1.** 4; **2.** 1, 2, 3, 4; **3.** 1, 2, 4; **4.** 1, 2, 4; **5.** 4; **6.** 1, 2, 3, 5; **7.** Tertiary intervention; **8.** Secondary intervention; **9.** 2; **10.** 1, 3; **11.** 1, 2, 4; **12.** 1, 3, 2; **13.** 1, 2, 3, 4; **14.** 2; **15.** 1, 2, 3.

REFERENCES

American Nurses Association: *Standards of public health nursing practice*, Washington, DC, 2007, The Association.

Cunningham P, et al: The struggle to provide community-based care to low-income people with mental illnesses, *Health Affairs* 25(3):694, 2006.

Edwards H, et al: A randomized controlled trial of a community nursing intervention: improved quality of life and healing for clients with chronic leg ulcers, *J Clin Nurs* 18:1541, 2009.

Gordon LG, et al: A cost-effectiveness analysis of two community models of nursing care for managing chronic venous leg ulcers, *J Wound Care* 15:348, 2006.

Hareendran A, et al: Measuring the impact of venous leg ulcers on quality of life, *J Wound Care* 14:53, 2005.

Jones J, et al: Depression in patients with chronic venous ulceration, *Br J Nurs* 15:S17, 2006.

Landenburger KM, Campbell JC: Violence and human abuse. In Stanhope M, Lancaster J: *Foundations of nursing in the community: community-oriented practice*, ed 3, St. Louis, 2010, Mosby.

Meiner S, Lueckenotte AG: *Gerontologic nursing*, ed 3, St Louis, 2006, Mosby.

Reynolds J: Undertaking risk management in community nursing practice, *J Commun Nurs* 23(110):24, 2009.

Sebastian JG: Vulnerability and vulnerable populations: an overview. In Stanhope M, Lancaster J: *Foundations of nursing in the community: community-oriented practice*, ed 3, St Louis, 2010, Mosby.

Stanhope M, Lancaster J: *Foundations of nursing in the community: community-oriented practice*, ed 3, St Louis, 2010, Mosby.

Swiadek JW: The impact of healthcare issues on the future of the nursing profession: the resulting increased influence of community-based and public health nursing, *Nurs Forum* 44(1):19, 2009.

Teeley K et al: Incorporating quality improvement concepts and practice into a community health-nursing course, *J Nurs Educ* 45(2):86, 2006.

US Census Bureau, US Population Projections, 2009 National Population Projections, updated 2009, http://www.census.gov/population/www/projections/index.html. Accessed December 2010.

US Department of Health and Human Services, Public Health Service: *Healthy People 2020: a systematic approach to health improvement*, Washington, DC, 2010, US Government Printing Office, http://www.healthypeople.gov/2020/about/new2020.aspx. Accessed August 2010.

RESEARCH REFERENCES

Decker S, et al: From the streets to assisting living: perceptions of vulnerable population, *J Psychoc Nurs Mental Health Serv* 44(6):18, 2006.

Downie J, Ogilve S, Wichmann H: A collaborative model of community health nursing, *Contemp Nurse* 20:180, 2005.

Kaiser L, et al: Public and community health nursing interventions with vulnerable primary care clients: a pilot study, *J Comm Health Nurs* 26:87, 2009.

Rew L, et al: Interaction of duration of homelessness and gender in adolescent sexual health indicators, *J Nurs Scholarship* 40:109, 2008.

Rew L, et al: Development of a dynamic model to guide health disparities research, *Nursing Outlook* 57(3):132, 2009.

Schanzer B, et al: Homelessness, health status, and health care use, *Am J Public Health* 97:464, 2007.

Smith R, Porock D: Caring for people dying at home a research study into the need of community nurses, *Int J Palliative Nurs* 15(12):601, 2009.

CHAPTER

4

Theoretical Foundations of Nursing Practice

OBJECTIVES

- Explain the influence of nursing theory on a nurse's approach to practice.
- Describe types of nursing theories.
- Describe the relationship between nursing theory, the nursing process, and patient needs.
- Discuss selected theories from other disciplines.
- Discuss selected nursing theories.
- Describe theory-based nursing practice.

KEY TERMS

Assumptions, p. 42
Concepts, p. 41
Content, p. 43
Descriptive theory, p. 42
Domain, p. 40
Environment/situation, p. 41
Feedback, p. 43
Grand theories, p. 42
Health, p. 41
Input, p. 43
Interdisciplinary theory, p. 43
Middle-range theories, p. 42
Nursing, p. 41
Nursing paradigm, p. 40
Nursing theory, p. 41
Output, p. 43
Paradigm, p. 40
Person, p. 40
Phenomenon, p. 41
Prescriptive theories, p. 42
Theory, p. 41

evolve WEBSITE

http://evolve.elsevier.com/Potter/fundamentals/

- Review Questions
- Case Study with Questions
- Audio Glossary
- Interactive Learning Activities
- Key Term Flashcards
- Content Updates

Providing patient-centered nursing care is an expectation for all nurses. As you progress through your curriculum, you will learn to apply knowledge from nursing science, social sciences, physical sciences, biobehavioral sciences, ethics, and health policy. To address individual and family responses to health problems, theory-based nursing practice is important for designing and implementing nursing interventions. Initially you might find nursing theory difficult to understand or appreciate. However, as you increase your knowledge about theories, you will find that they help to describe, explain, predict, and/or prescribe nursing care measures. For example, a theory about caring gives you a way to communicate with your patients and their families and individualize care to meet their needs (Watson, 2010; Sumner, 2010). The scientific work used in developing theories expands the scientific knowledge of the profession. Theories offer well-grounded rationales for how and why nurses perform specific interventions and for predicting patient behaviors and outcomes.

Expertise in nursing is a result of knowledge and clinical experience. The expertise required to interpret clinical situations and make clinical judgments is the essence of nursing care and the basis for advancing nursing practice and nursing science (Benner et al., 2010). As you progress through your courses, reflect and learn from your experiences to grow professionally and use well-developed theories as a basis for your approach to patient care.

THE DOMAIN OF NURSING

The **domain** is the perspective of a profession. It provides the subject, central concepts, values and beliefs, phenomena of interest, and central problems of a discipline. The domain of nursing provides both a practical and theoretical aspect of the discipline. It is the knowledge of nursing practice as well as the knowledge of nursing history, nursing theory, education, and research. The domain of nursing gives nurses a comprehensive perspective that allows you to identify and treat patients' health care needs at all levels and in all health care settings.

A **paradigm** is a pattern of thought that is useful in describing the domain of a discipline. A paradigm links the knowledge of science, philosophy, and theories accepted and applied by the discipline. The paradigm of nursing includes four links: the person, health, environment/situation, and nursing. The elements of the **nursing paradigm** direct the activity of the nursing profession, including knowledge development, philosophy, theory, educational experience, research, and practice (Alligood and Tomey, 2010).

Person is the recipient of nursing care, including individual patients, groups, families, and communities. The person is central to the nursing care you provide. Because each person's needs are often complex, it is important to provide individualized patient-centered care.

Health has different meanings for each patient, the clinical setting, and the health care profession (see Chapter 6). It is dynamic and continuously changing. Your challenge as a nurse is to provide the best possible care based on the patient's level of health and health care needs at the time of care delivery.

Environment/situation includes all possible conditions affecting patients and the settings in which their health care needs occur. There is a continuous interaction between a patient and the environment. This interaction has positive and negative effects on the person's level of health and health care needs. Factors in the home, school, workplace, or community all influence a patient's level of health and health care needs. For example, an adolescent girl with type 1 diabetes needs to adapt her treatment plan to adjust for physical activities of school, the demands of a part-time job, and the timing of social events such as her prom.

Nursing is the "… diagnosis and treatment of human responses to actual or potential health problems …" (American Nurses Association, 2010). The scope of nursing is broad. For example, a nurse does not medically diagnose a patient's health condition as heart failure. However, a nurse will assess a patient's response to the decrease in activity tolerance as a result of the disease and develop nursing diagnoses of fatigue, activity intolerance, and ineffective coping. From these nursing diagnoses the nurse creates a patient-centered plan of care for each of the patient's health problems (see Unit 3). Use critical thinking skills to integrate knowledge, experience, attitudes, and standards into the individualized plan of care for each of your patients (see Chapter 15).

THEORY

Theories are designed to explain a phenomenon such as self-care or caring. For example, the nurse using Orem's self-care deficit theory helps to explain how patients meet their own therapeutic self-care demands. In this theory, nurses assist patients by acting for them or guiding necessary physical and/or psychological support (Alligood, 2010). Orem's theory contains a detailed framework of self-care concepts that are linked in such a way as to explain, describe, or predict the type of nursing care that helps patients achieve a better level of health (McEwen and Willis, 2011). A theory is a way of seeing through a "set of relatively concrete and specific concepts and the propositions that describe or link the concepts" (Fawcett, 2005).

A **nursing theory** is a conceptualization of some aspect of nursing that describes, explains, predicts, or prescribes nursing care (Meleis, 2011). For example, Orem's self-care deficit theory (2001) explains the factors within a patient's living situation that support or interfere with his or her self-care ability. As a result, a nurse who practices using this theory can anticipate such factors when designing an education plan for the patient. This theory has value in helping nursing design interventions to promote the patient's self-care in managing an illness such as asthma, heart failure, diabetes, or arthritis.

Theories constitute much of the knowledge of a discipline. Theory and scientific inquiry are vital links to one another, providing guidelines for decision making, problem solving, and nursing interventions (Selanders, 2010). Theories give us a perspective for assessing our patients' situations and organizing data and methods for analyzing and interpreting information. For example, if you use Orem's theory in practice, you assess and interpret data to determine patients' self-care needs, self-care deficits, and self-care

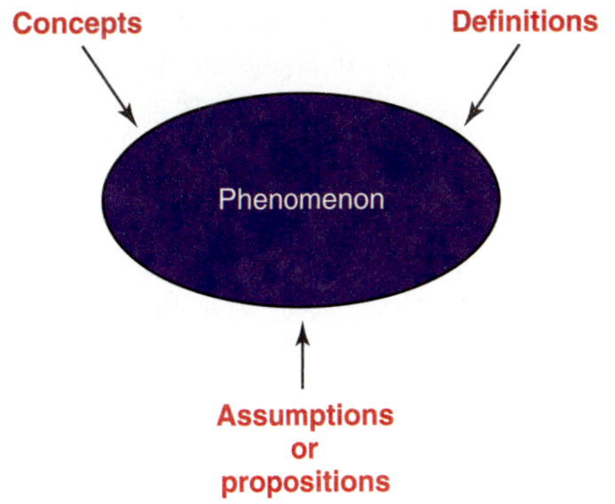

FIG. 4-1 Components of a nursing theory.

abilities in the management of their disease. The theory then guides the design of patient-centered nursing interventions. Application of nursing theory in practice depends on the knowledge of nursing and other theoretical models, how they relate to one another, and their use in designing nursing interventions.

Nursing is a science and an art. Nurses need a theoretical base to demonstrate knowledge about the science and art of the profession when they promote health and wellness for their patients, whether the patient is an individual, a family, or a community (Porter, 2010). A nursing theory helps to identify the focus, means, and goals of practice. Common theories enhance communication and increase autonomy and accountability for care to our patients (Meleis, 2011).

Components of a Theory

A **theory** contains a set of concepts, definitions, and assumptions or propositions that explain a phenomenon. The theory explains how these elements are uniquely related in the phenomenon (Fig. 4-1). For example, Kristin Swanson developed her theory about the phenomenon of caring by conducting extensive interviews with patients and their professional caregivers (Swanson, 1991). Swanson's theory of caring defines five components of caring: knowing, being with, doing for, enabling, and maintaining belief (see Chapter 7). These components provide a foundation of knowledge for nurses to direct and deliver caring nursing practices. Researchers test theories, and as a result they get a clearer perspective of all parts of a phenomenon. Swanson's theory of caring is one that provides a basis for identifying and testing nurse caring behaviors to determine if caring improves patient health outcomes (Watson, 2010).

Phenomenon. Nursing theories focus on the phenomena of nursing and nursing care. A **phenomenon** is the term, description, or label given to describe an idea or responses about an event, a situation, a process, a group of events, or a group of situations (Meleis, 2011). This phenomenon may be temporary or permanent. Examples of phenomena of nursing include caring, self-care, and patient responses to stress. For example, in Neuman's systems model (2011), phenomena focus on stressors perceived by the patient or caregiver. The theoretical model is an open systems model that views nursing as being primarily concerned with nursing actions in stress-related situations. These stressors may include, but are not limited to, patient responses, internal and external environmental factors, and nursing actions.

Concepts. A theory also consists of interrelated concepts. These **concepts** can be simple or complex and relate to an object or event that comes from individual perceptual experiences (Alligood and Tomey, 2010). Think of concepts as ideas and mental images. They help describe or label phenomena. Again, using Neuman's systems model (2011) as an example, there are concepts that affect the patient system. The patient system can be an individual, a group, a family, or a community. This system is an open structure that includes internal and external environmental factors. These concepts are physiological, psychological, sociocultural, developmental, and spiritual and may relate to health and wellness, illness prevention, stressors, and defense mechanisms (Meleis, 2011).

Definitions. The definitions within a theory communicate the general meaning of the concepts. These definitions describe the activity necessary to measure the concepts within a theory (Alligood and Tomey, 2010). For example, Neuman's model uses an open systems approach to describe how patient systems deal with stressors in their environments. A stressor is any stimuli that can produce tension and cause instability within the system. The environment includes internal and external factors that have the potential to affect the patient system. Internal factors exist within the patient system (e.g., the physiological and behavioral responses to illnesses). External factors are outside the patient system (e.g., changes in health care policy or an increase in the crime rate). It is important that nurses using Neuman's theory in practice focus their care on the system's responses to the stressors (Meleis, 2011). For example, when patients receive a new diagnosis and perceive the diagnosis to be stressful, they may react by withdrawing or eating an improper diet. In this situation the nurse focuses on both the illness process and the patient's response to the stressors and designs appropriate interventions.

Assumptions. Assumptions are the "taken-for-granted" statements that explain the nature of the concepts, definitions, purpose, relationships, and structure of a theory (Meleis, 2011). For example, in Neuman's systems model the assumptions include the following: patients are dynamic; the relationships between the concepts of a theory influence a patient's protective mechanisms and determine a patient's response; patients have a normal range of responses; stressors attack flexible lines of defense followed by the normal lines of defense; and the nurse's actions focus on primary, secondary, and tertiary prevention (Neuman, 2011).

Types of Theory

The general purpose of a theory is important because it specifies the context and situation in which the theory applies (Chinn and Kramer, 2011). For example, theories about pain focus on pain: its cause, effects, and alleviation measures. Theories have different purposes and are sometimes classified by levels of abstraction (grand theories versus middle-range theories) or the goals of the theory (descriptive or prescriptive). For example, a descriptive theory describes a phenomenon such as grief or caring. A predictive theory identifies conditions or factors that predict a phenomenon. A prescriptive theory details nursing interventions for a specific phenomenon and the expected outcome of the care. Box 4-1 summarizes goals of theoretical nursing models.

Grand theories are systematic and broad in scope, complex, and therefore require further specification through research. A grand theory does not provide guidance for specific nursing interventions; but it provides the structural framework for broad, abstract ideas about nursing. For example, Neuman's systems model is a grand theory that provides a comprehensive foundation for scientific nursing practice, education, and research (Walker and Avant, 2009).

Middle-range theories are more limited in scope and less abstract. They address a specific phenomenon and reflect practice (administration, clinical, or teaching). A middle-range theory tends to focus on a specific field of nursing, such as uncertainty, incontinence, social support, quality of life, and caring, rather than reflect on a wide variety of nursing care situations (Meleis, 2011). For example, Mishel's theory of uncertainty in illness (1990; 1997) focuses on patients' experiences with cancer while living with continual uncertainty. The theory provides a basis to help nurses understand how patients cope with uncertainty and the illness response.

Descriptive theories are the first level of theory development. They describe phenomena, speculate on why they occur, and describe their consequences. These theories explain, relate, and in some situations predict nursing phenomena (Meleis, 2011). For example, theories of growth and development describe the maturation processes of an individual at various ages (see Chapter 11). Descriptive theories do not direct specific nursing activities but help to explain patient assessments.

Prescriptive theories address nursing interventions for a phenomenon, describe the conditions under which the prescription (i.e., nursing interventions) occurs, and predict the consequences (Meleis, 2011). Prescriptive theories are action oriented and test the validity and predictability of a nursing intervention. These theories guide nursing research to develop and test specific nursing interventions (George, 2011). For example, Mishel's theory of uncertainty predicts that increasing the coping skills of patients with gynecological cancer assists their ability to deal with the uncertainty of the cancer diagnosis and treatment (Mishel, 1997). Thus the theory provides a framework to design interventions that support and strengthen patients' coping resources.

BOX 4-1 GOALS OF THEORETICAL NURSING MODELS

- Identify domain and goals of nursing.
- Provide knowledge to improve nursing administration, practice, education, and research.
- Guide research and expand the knowledge base of nursing.
- Identify research techniques and tools used to validate nursing interventions.
- Formulate legislation governing nursing practice, research, and education.
- Formulate regulations interpreting nurse practice acts.
- Develop curriculum plans for nursing education.
- Establish criteria for measuring quality of nursing care, education, and research.
- Guide development of a nursing care delivery system.
- Provide systematic structure and rationale for nursing activities.

Theory-Based Nursing Practice

Nursing is a practice-oriented discipline. Nursing knowledge is derived from basic and nursing sciences, experience, aesthetics, nurses' attitudes, and standards of practice. As nursing continues to grow as a profession, knowledge is needed to prescribe specific interventions to improve patient outcomes. Nursing theories and related concepts continue to evolve. Florence Nightingale spoke with firm conviction about the "nature of nursing as a profession that requires knowledge distinct from medical knowledge" (Nightingale, 1860; Selanders, 2010). The overall goal of nursing knowledge is to explain the practice of nursing as different and distinct from the practice of medicine, psychology, and other health care disciplines. Theory generates nursing knowledge for use

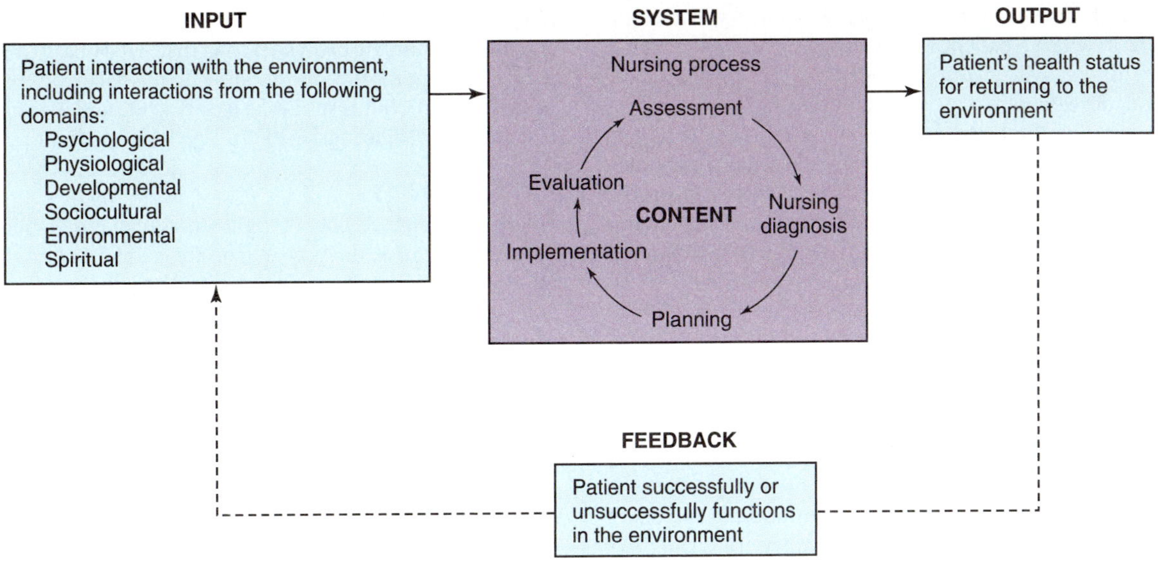

FIG. 4-2 Nursing process as a system.

in practice, thus supporting evidence-based practice. The integration of theory into practice is the basis for professional nursing (McEwen and Wills, 2011).

The nursing process is used in clinical settings to determine individual patient needs (see Unit 3). Although the nursing process is central to nursing, it is not a theory. It provides a systematic process for the delivery of nursing care, not the knowledge component of the discipline. However, a theory can direct how a nurse uses the nursing process. For example, the theory of caring influences what to assess, how to determine patient needs, how to plan care, how to select individualized nursing interventions, and how to evaluate patient outcomes.

INTERDISCIPLINARY THEORIES

To practice in today's health care systems, nurses need a strong scientific knowledge base from nursing and other disciplines such as the physical, social, and behavioral sciences. Knowledge from these other disciplines includes relevant theories that explain phenomena. An **interdisciplinary theory** explains a systematic view of a phenomenon specific to the discipline of inquiry. For example, Piaget's theory of cognitive development helps to explain how children think, reason, and perceive the world (see Chapter 11). Knowledge and use of this theory helps pediatric nurses design appropriate therapeutic play interventions for ill toddlers or school-age children.

Systems Theory

A system is composed of separate components. The components are interrelated and share a common purpose to form a whole. There are two types of systems, open and closed. An open system such as a human organism or a process such as the nursing process interacts with the environment, exchanging information between the system and the environment. Factors that change the environment also affect an open system. Neuman's systems theory (2011) defines a total-person model of wholism and an open-systems approach. A closed system such as a chemical reaction within a test tube does not interact with the environment.

Like all systems, the nursing process has a specific purpose or goal (see Unit 3). The goal of the nursing process is to organize and deliver patient-centered care. As a system the nursing process has the following components: input, output, feedback, and content (Fig. 4-2). **Input** for the nursing process is the data or information that comes from a patient's assessment (e.g., how the patient interacts with the environment and the patient's physiological function). **Output** is the end product of a system; and in the case of the nursing process it is whether the patient's health status improves, declines, or remains stable as a result of nursing care.

Feedback serves to inform a system about how it functions. For example, in the nursing process the outcomes reflect the patient's responses to nursing interventions. The outcomes are part of the feedback system to refine the plan of care. Other forms of feedback in the nursing process include responses from family members and consultation from other health care professionals.

The **content** is the product and information obtained from the system. Again, using the nursing process as an example, the content is the information about the nursing interventions for patients with specific health care problems. For example, patients with impaired bed mobility have common skin care needs and interventions (e.g., hygiene and scheduled positioning changes) that are very successful in reducing the risk for pressure ulcers.

Basic Human Needs

Maslow's hierarchy of needs is an interdisciplinary theory that is useful for designating priorities of nursing care (see Fig. 6-3, p. 69.) The hierarchy of basic human needs includes five levels of priority. The most basic, or first level, includes physiological needs such as air, water, and food. The second level includes safety and security needs, which involve physical and psychological security. The third level contains love and belonging needs, including friendship, social relationships, and sexual love. The fourth level encompasses esteem and self-esteem needs, which involve self-confidence, usefulness, achievement, and self-worth. The final level is the need for self-actualization, the state of fully achieving potential and having the ability to solve problems and cope realistically with situations of life. When using this hierarchy, basic physiological and safety needs are usually the first priority, especially when a patient is severely dependent physically. However, you will encounter situations in which a patient has no emergent physical or safety needs. Instead, you will give high priority to the psychological, sociocultural, developmental, or spiritual needs of the patient.

Patients entering the health care system generally have unmet needs. For example, a person brought to an emergency department experiencing acute pneumonia has an unmet need for oxygen, the most basic physiological need. An older woman in a high-crime area is concerned about physical safety. A widowed homemaker whose children have moved away feels that she does not belong or is not loved. The hierarchy of needs is a way to plan for individualized patient care.

Developmental Theories

Human growth and development are orderly predictive processes that begin with conception and continue through death. A variety of well-tested theoretical models describe and predict behavior and development at various phases of the life continuum. Chapter 11 details these developmental theories, and Chapters 12 through 14 demonstrate changes in growth and development in various age-groups.

Psychosocial Theories

Nursing is a diverse discipline that strives to meet the physiological, psychological, sociocultural, developmental, and spiritual needs of patients. Theoretical models to explain and/or predict patient responses exist in each of these domains. For example, Chapter 9 discusses models for understanding cultural diversity and implementing care to meet the diverse needs of the patient. Chapter 10 describes family theory and how to meet the needs of the family when the family is the patient or when the family is the caregiver. Chapter 36 discusses several models of grieving and demonstrates how to assist patients through loss, death, and grief.

SELECTED NURSING THEORIES

Definitions and theories of nursing can help you understand the practice of nursing. The following sections describe, in chronological order of theory development, selected theories and their concepts (Table 4-1).

Nightingale's Theory

Florence Nightingale's work was an initial model for nursing. Meleis (2011) notes that Nightingale's concept of the environment was the focus of nursing care and her suggestion that nurses need not know all about the disease process differentiated nursing from medicine. The focus of nursing is caring through the environment and helping the patient deal with the symptoms and changes in function related to an illness (Selanders, 2010).

Nightingale did not view nursing as limited to the administration of medications and treatments but oriented toward providing fresh air, light, warmth, cleanliness, quiet, and adequate nutrition (Nightingale, 1860). Through observation and data collection, she linked the patient's health status with environmental factors and initiated improved hygiene and sanitary conditions during the Crimean War.

Nightingale's "descriptive theory" provides nurses with a way to think about patients and their environment. Her letters and writings direct the nurse to act on behalf of the patient. Her visionary principles included the areas of practice, research, and education. Most important, her concepts and principles shaped and defined nursing practice (Alligood and Tomey, 2010). Nightingale taught and used the nursing process, noting that "vital observation [assessment] ... is not for the sake of piling up miscellaneous information or curious facts, but for the sake of saving life and increasing health and comfort (Nightingale, 1860)."

Peplau's Theory

Hildegard Peplau's theory (1952) focuses on interpersonal relations between the nurse, the patient, and the patient's family and developing the nurse-patient relationship. The patient is an individual with a need, and nursing is an interpersonal and therapeutic process. This nurse-patient relationship is influenced by both the nurse's and the patient's perceptions and preconceived ideas (George, 2011).

In developing a nurse-patient relationship, the nurse can serve as a resource person, counselor, and surrogate. For example, when the patient seeks help, the nurse and patient first discuss the nature of any problems, and the nurse explains the services available. As the nurse-patient relationship develops, the nurse and patient mutually define the problems and potential solutions. The patient gains from this relationship by using available services to meet needs, and the nurse helps the patient reduce anxiety related to the health care problems.

Peplau's theory is unique: the collaborative nurse-patient relationship creates a "maturing force" through which interpersonal effectiveness meets the patient's needs. This theory is useful in establishing effective nurse-patient communication when obtaining a nursing history, providing patient education, or counseling patients and their families (see Chapter 24). When the patient's original needs are resolved, new needs sometimes emerge. According to Peplau, the following phases characterize the nurse-patient interpersonal relationship: orientation, working phase, and termination (George, 2011).

Henderson's Theory

Virginia Henderson defines nursing as "assisting the individual, sick or well, in the performance of those activities that will contribute to health, recovery, or a peaceful death and that the individual would perform unaided if he or she had the necessary strength, will, or knowledge" (Harmer and Henderson, 1955; Henderson, 1966). Henderson organized the theory into 14 basic needs of the whole person and includes phenomena from the following domains of the patient: physiological, psychological, sociocultural, spiritual, and developmental. The interpersonal relationship between the nurse and the patient creates a caring environment to identify the patient's needs, plan the goals of care, and provide patient-centered nursing care (George, 2011). Framing nursing care around the needs of the individual allows you to use Henderson's theory for a variety of patients across the life span and in multiple settings along the health care continuum.

Orem's Theory

Dorothea Orem's self-care deficit theory (2001) focuses on the patient's self-care needs. Orem defines self-care as a learned, goal-oriented activity directed toward the self in the interest of maintaining life, health, development, and well-being. The goal of Orem's theory is to help the patient perform self-care and manage his or her health problems. Nursing care is necessary when the patient is unable to fulfill biological, psychological, developmental, or social needs. This theory works well in all steps of the nursing process (George, 2011). The nurse assesses and determines why a patient is unable to meet these needs, identifies goals to assist the

TABLE 4-1 Summary of Nursing Theories

THEORIST	GOAL OF NURSING	FRAMEWORK FOR PRACTICE
Nightingale—1860	Facilitate the reparative processes of the body by manipulating patient's environment	Nurse manipulates patient's environment to include appropriate noise, nutrition, hygiene, light, comfort, socialization, and hope.
Peplau—1952	Develop interaction between nurse and patient	Nursing is a significant, therapeutic, interpersonal process. Nurses participate in structuring health care systems to facilitate interpersonal relationships.
Henderson—1955	Work interdependently with other health care workers, assisting patient in gaining independence as quickly as possible; help patient gain lacking strength	Nurses help patient perform Henderson's 14 basic needs.
Orem—1971	Care for and help patient attain total self-care	Nursing care is necessary when the patient is unable to fulfill biological, psychological, developmental, or social needs.
King—1971	Use communication to help patient reestablish positive adaptation to environment	Nursing is a dynamic interpersonal process among nurse, patient, and health care system.
Neuman—1974	Help individuals, families, and groups attain and maintain maximal level of total wellness by purposeful interventions	Stress reduction is goal of systems model of nursing practice. Nursing actions are in primary, secondary, or tertiary level of prevention.
Leininger—1978	Provide care consistent with nursing's emerging science and knowledge with caring as central focus	With this transcultural care theory, caring is the central and unifying domain for nursing knowledge and practice.
Roy—1970	Identify types of demands placed on patient, assess adaptation to demands, and help patient adapt	This adaptation model is based on the physiological, psychological, sociological, and dependence-independence adaptive modes.
Watson—1979	Promote health, restore patient to health, and prevent illness	Involves the philosophy and science of caring. Caring is an interpersonal process comprising interventions to meet human needs.
Benner and Wrubel—1989	Focus on patient's need for caring as a means of coping with stressors of illness	Caring is central to the essence of nursing. It creates the possibilities for coping and enables possibilities for connecting with and concern for others.

Modified from Chinn PL, Kramer ML: *Integrated knowledge development in nursing,* ed 8, St. Louis, 2011, Mosby.

patient, intervenes to help the patient perform self-care, and evaluates how much self-care the patient is able to perform. According to Orem's theory, the goal of nursing is to increase the patient's ability to independently meet these needs (George, 2011; Orem, 2001).

Leininger's Theory

Leininger used her background in anthropology to form her theory of cultural care diversity and universality (Alligood, 2010). Human caring varies among cultures in its expressions, processes, and patterns. Social structure factors such as the patient's religion, politics, culture, and traditions are significant forces affecting care and influencing the patient's health and illness patterns. While reading the chapter on culture, think about the diversity of the patients and their nursing care needs (see Chapter 9). The major concept of Leininger's theory is cultural diversity, and the goal of nursing care is to provide the patient with culturally specific nursing care (Alligood, 2010; Leininger, 1991). To provide care to patients of unique cultures, the nurse safely integrates the patient's cultural traditions, values, and beliefs into the plan of care. Leininger's theory recognizes the importance of culture and its influence on everything that involves the patient and the providers of nursing care (George, 2011). For example, some cultures believe that the leader in the community needs to be present during health care decisions. As a result, the health care team may need to reschedule when rounds occur to include the community leader. In addition, symptom expression also differs among cultures. A person with an Irish background might be stoic and not complain about pain, whereas a person from a Middle Eastern culture might be very vocal about pain. In both cases the nurse needs to skillfully incorporate the patient's cultural practices in assessing the patient's level of pain (e.g., is the pain getting worse or remaining the same?).

Betty Neuman's Theory

The Neuman systems model is based on stress and the client's reaction to the stressor (George, 2011). In this model the client is the individual, group, family, or community. The system is composed of five concepts that interact with one another: physiological, psychological, sociocultural, developmental, and spiritual (Neuman, 2011). These concepts interact with both internal and external environmental factors and all levels of prevention (primary, secondary, and tertiary) to achieve optimal wellness (Neuman and Reed, 2007). Neuman considers any internal and external factors as stressors (Alligood, 2010) that affect the patient's stability and any or all of the five system concepts. The role of nursing is to stabilize the patient or situation. When you apply the Neuman systems model, you assess the stressor and the patient's response to the stressor, identify nursing diagnoses, plan patient-centered care, implement interventions, evaluate the patient's response, and determine if the stressor is resolved.

BOX 4-2 EVIDENCE-BASED PRACTICE

Theory-Based Practice in the Management of Heart Failure

PICO Question: What impact does applying the Roy adaptation model have on improved functional status in patients with heart failure?

Evidence Summary

The Roy adaptation model is a nursing discipline-specific theoretical model used to guide practice (Roy et al., 2009). The model is applicable in multiple settings with patients across the life span. According to this theory people adapt to changing environmental stimuli, and this adaptation is useful in assisting patients toward recovery (DeSanto-Madeya and Fawcett, 2009). An experimental study was designed to determine the effects of the Roy adaptation model on patient education, exercise, and social support systems in patients with heart failure (Bakan and Akyol, 2008). Patients were taught how medications, diet, and exercise improved their activity tolerance. They learned how to adapt their exercise prescription so they gradually increased their tolerance. In addition, the patients' support system also participated in the education and exercise program and became part of the patients' adaptation resources. The study documented that the patients in the experimental group benefited from application of the Roy adaptation model in their cardiac rehabilitation.

Application to Nursing Practice

- When using a nursing theory such as Roy's adaptation model, patients can learn techniques to improve their ability to adapt to an illness or condition.
- Involving a patient's support system increases the patient's ability to use adaptive techniques.
- Nursing theories readily support theory-based nursing practices and define the specific interventions for patients.
- Use of literature resources supports theory-based interventions.

Roy's Theory

The Roy adaptation model (Roy, 1989; Roy et al., 2009) views the patient as an adaptive system. According to Roy's model, the goal of nursing is to help the person adapt to changes in physiological needs, self-concept, role function, and interdependent relations during health and illness (Alligood and Tomey, 2010). The need for nursing care occurs when the patient cannot adapt to internal and external environmental demands. All individuals must adapt to the following demands: meeting basic physiological needs, developing a positive self-concept, performing social roles, and achieving a balance between dependence and independence.

The nurse determines which demands are causing problems for a patient and assesses how well the patient is adapting to them. Nurses direct care at helping the patient adapt to the changes (George, 2011; Alligood, 2010). For example, a patient recovering from a worsening of heart failure needs nursing interventions to assist in adapting to the resultant activity in tolerance (Box 4-2).

Watson's Theory

Jean Watson's theory of transpersonal caring (2005, 2008) defines the outcome of nursing activity in regard to the humanistic aspects of life (Alligood and Tomey, 2010). The purpose of nursing action is to understand the interrelationship among health, illness, and human behavior. Thus nursing is concerned with promoting and restoring health and preventing illness.

Watson designed the model around the caring process, assisting patients in attaining or maintaining health or dying peacefully (Watson, 2005). This caring process requires the nurse to be knowledgeable about human behavior and human responses to actual or potential health problems (see Chapter 7). The nurse also needs to know individual patient needs, how to respond to others, and strengths and limitations of the patient and family and those of the nurse. In addition, the nurse comforts and offers compassion and empathy to patients and their families. Caring represents all factors the nurse uses to deliver care to the patient (Watson, 1996).

Benner and Wrubel's Theory

The primacy of caring is a model proposed by Patricia Benner and Judith Wrubel (1989). Caring is central to nursing and creates possibilities for coping, enables possibilities for connecting with and concern for others, and allows for giving and receiving help (Chinn and Kramer, 2011). Caring means that persons, events, projects, and things matter to people. It presents a connection and represents a wide range of involvement (e.g., caring about one's family, one's friendships, and one's patients). Benner and Wrubel see the personal concern as an inherent feature of nursing practice. In caring for one's patients, nurses help patients recover by noticing interventions that are successful and that guide future caregiving.

• • •

Application of nursing theory in practice depends on nurses having knowledge of the theories and an understanding of how they relate to one another. Theories are the organizing frameworks for the science of nursing and the substantive approaches for nursing care. They provide critical thinking structures to guide clinical reasoning and problem solving.

LINK BETWEEN THEORY AND KNOWLEDGE DEVELOPMENT IN NURSING

Nursing has its own body of knowledge that is both theoretical and experiential. Theoretical knowledge includes and "reflects on the basic values, guiding principles, elements, and phases of a conception of nursing" (Meleis, 2011). The goals of theoretical knowledge stimulate thinking and create a broad understanding of the "science" and practices of the nursing discipline.

Experiential knowledge is not organized in the same manner as theoretical knowledge. This type of knowledge or the "art" of nursing is based on nurses' experience in providing care to patients. You achieve this through personal knowledge gained through reflection on care experiences, synthesis, and integration of the art and science of nursing.

Nursing theories help direct nursing practice. When using theory-based nursing practice, you apply the principles of the theory in delivering nursing interventions in your practice. Theory-based nursing practice improves nurse satisfaction and patient outcomes because the basic values, guiding principles, and elements from the foundation of a particular nursing theory give meaning to the practice and influence how patient care is provided (Veo, 2010).

Relationship Between Nursing Theory and Nursing Research

The relationship between nursing theory and nursing research builds the scientific knowledge base of nursing, which is then applied to practice. As more research is conducted, the discipline learns to what extent a given theory is useful in providing information to improve patient care. The relationships of components in a theory often help drive the research questions. For example, the components within Orem's self-care deficit theory have led nurse researchers to test interventions for improving self-care. In one study, older hospitalized adults were able to learn their medication schedules and improve their activities of daily living before discharge, were discharged earlier, and had fewer complications (Glasson et al., 2006).

Sometimes research is used to identify new theories. Theory-generating research tries to discover and describe relationships of phenomena without imposing preconceived notions (e.g., hypotheses) of what the phenomena under study mean (George, 2011). In theory-generating research the investigator makes observations to view a phenomenon in a new way. For example, a researcher wants to understand end-of-life decision making. In this example, the researcher interviews surrogate decision makers. From these interviews he or she makes objective observations about the surrogate's decision-making process, resulting in an initial theory of surrogate decision making (Loomis, 2009).

Theory-testing research determines how accurately a theory describes a nursing phenomenon. Testing helps to develop the evidence for describing or predicting patient outcomes. The researcher has some preconceived idea as to how patients describe or respond to a phenomenon and generates research questions or hypotheses to test the assumptions of the theory. No one study tests all components of a theory; researchers test the theory through a variety of research activities. Referring to the previous example of surrogate decision making, the researcher tests elements of the theory. For example, interviews of decision makers indicated that there was a need for more knowledge about end-of-life care expectations (Loomis, 2009). The researcher then designs and tests an educational program that incorporates end-of-life expectation with one that does not to determine which is most effective for groups of surrogate caregivers. Theory-generating or theory-testing research refines the knowledge base of nursing. As a result, nurses incorporate research-based interventions into theory-based practice. As research activities continue, not only does the knowledge and science of nursing increase, but patients are the recipients of the best evidence-based nursing practice (see Chapter 5).

As an art, nursing relies on knowledge gained from practice and reflection on past experiences. As a science, nursing draws on scientifically tested knowledge applied in the practice setting (Kikuchi, Simmons, and Romyn, 1996). But it is the "expert nurse" who transports the art and science of nursing into the scientific realm of creative caring.

KEY POINTS

- A nursing theory is a conceptualization of some aspect of nursing communicated for the purpose of describing, explaining, predicting, and/or prescribing nursing care.
- Grand theories are the complex structural framework for broad, abstract ideas.
- Middle-range theories are more limited in scope and less abstract. These theories address specific phenomena or concepts and reflect practice.
- The paradigm of nursing identifies four links of interest to the profession: the person, health, environment/situation, and nursing. Nurse theorists agree that these four components are essential to the development of theory.
- Theory is the generation of nursing knowledge used for practice. Nursing process is the method for applying the theory or knowledge. The integration of theory and nursing process is the basis for professional nursing.
- Theories from nursing and other disciplines help explain how the roles and actions of nurses fit together in nursing.
- Theory-generating research tries to discover and describe relationships without imposing preconceived notions (e.g., hypotheses) of what the phenomenon under study means.
- Theory-testing research determines how accurately a theory describes nursing phenomena.

CLINICAL APPLICATION QUESTIONS

Preparing for Clinical Practice

1. Kathy Jones and Sheri Walker are sophomores in a college program. Next week they will have their first clinical practice. Kathy will be in a community health setting, and Sheri will be in an acute health care agency. They need to prepare general assessment questions applicable to both settings using Orem's self-care deficit theory. Explain how the theory might apply for patient assessment in different health care settings.
   a. Acute care
   b. Community-based care
2. In a classroom setting you are given the following examples of questions that lead either to theory-generating or theory-testing research. Identify whether they are theory testing or theory generating and explain.
   a. Do patients who receive a prescribed exercise program wean more quickly from the mechanical ventilator?
   b. What are the perspectives of patients who are weaned from mechanical ventilation?

evolve *Answers to Clinical Application Questions can be found on the Evolve website.*

REVIEW QUESTIONS

Are You Ready to Test Your Nursing Knowledge?

1. Which of the following are components of the paradigm of nursing?
   1. The person, health, environment, and theory
   2. Health, theory, concepts, and environment
   3. Nurses, physicians, health, and patient needs
   4. The person, health, environment/situation, and nursing
2. A theory is a set of concepts, definitions, relationships, and assumptions that:
   1. Formulate legislation.
   2. Explain a phenomenon.
   3. Measure nursing functions.
   4. Reflect the domain of nursing practice.
3. A patient with diabetes is controlling the disease with insulin and diet. The nursing health care provider is focusing efforts to teach the patient self-management. Which of the following nursing theories is useful in promoting self management?
   1. Neuman
   2. Orem
   3. Roy
   4. Peplau
4. While working in a community health clinic, it is important to obtain nursing histories and get to know the patients. Part of history taking is to develop the nurse-patient relationship. Which of the following apply to Peplau's theory when establishing the nurse-patient relationship? (Select all that apply.)
   1. An interaction between the nurse and patient must develop.
   2. The patient's needs must be clarified and described.

3. The nurse-patient relationship is influenced by patient and nurse preconceptions.
4. The nurse-patient relationship is influenced only by the nurse's preconceptions.

5. Theory-based nursing practice uses a theoretical approach for nursing care. This approach moves nursing forward as a science. This suggests that:
   1. One theory will guide nursing practice.
   2. Scientists will decide nursing decisions.
   3. Nursing will only base patient care on the practice of other sciences.
   4. Theories will be tested to describe or predict patient outcomes.
6. To practice in today's health care environment, nurses need a strong scientific knowledge base from nursing and other disciplines such as the physical, social, and behavioral sciences. This statement identifies the need for which of the following?
   1. Systems theories
   2. Developmental theories
   3. Interdisciplinary theories
   4. Health and wellness models
7. Which of the following theories describe the life processes of an older adult facing chronic illness?
   1. Systems theories
   2. Developmental theories
   3. Interdisciplinary theories
   4. Health and wellness models
8. Match the following components of systems theory with the definition of that component.

1. Feedback	A. Data entering the system
2. Input	B. End product
3. Content	C. Data related to system functioning
4. Output	D. Product and information obtained from the system

9. A patient is admitted to an acute care area. The patient is an active business man who is worried about getting back to work. He has had severe diarrhea and vomiting for the last week. He is weak, and his breathing is labored. Using Maslow's hierarchy of needs, identify this patient's immediate priority.
   1. Self-actualization
   2. Air, water, and nutrition
   3. Safety
   4. Esteem and self-esteem needs
10. Which of the following is closely aligned with Leininger's theory?
    1. Caring for patients from unique cultures
    2. Understanding the humanistic aspects of life
    3. Variables affecting a patient's response to a stressor
    4. Caring for patients who cannot adapt to internal and external environmental demands
11. Match the following theories with their definitions.

1. Grand theory	A. Addresses specific phenomena and reflect practice
2. Middle-range theory	B. First level in theory development and describes a phenomenon
3. Descriptive theory	C. Provides a structural framework for broad concepts about nursing
4. Prescriptive theory	D. Linked to outcomes (consequences of specific nursing interventions)

12. A nurse is applying Henderson's theory as a basis for theory based-nursing practice. Which other elements are important for theory-based nursing practice? (Select all that apply.)
    1. Knowledge of nursing science
    2. Knowledge of related sciences
    3. Knowledge about current health care issues
    4. Knowledge of standards of practice
13. Which of the following statements apply to theory generation? (Select all that apply.)
    1. Builds scientific knowledge base of nursing
    2. Discovers relationships of phenomena to practice
    3. Tests specific phenomena
    4. Identifies observations about a phenomenon
14. Which of the following statements about theory-based nursing practice is incorrect?
    1. Contributes to evidence-based practice
    2. Provides a systematic process for designing nursing interventions
    3. Is not linked to nursing outcomes
    4. Guides the nurse's assessment
15. As an art nursing relies on knowledge gained from practice and reflection on past experiences. As a science nursing relies on (select all that apply):
    1. Experimental research.
    2. Nonexperimental research.
    3. Research from other disciplines.
    4. Professional opinions.

Answers: **1.** 4; **2.** 2; **3.** 2; **4.** 1, 2, 3; **5.** 4; **6.** 3; **7.** 2; **8.** 1 C, 2 A, 3 D, 4 B; **9.** 2; **10.** 1; **11.** 1 C, 2 A, 3 B, 4 D; **12.** 1, 2, 4; **13.** 1, 2, 4; **14.** 3; **15.** 1, 2, 3.

REFERENCES

Alligood MR: *Nursing theory utilization & application*, ed 4, St Louis, 2010, Mosby.

Alligood MR, Tomey AM: *Nursing theorists and their work*, ed 7, St Louis, 2010, Mosby.

American Nurses Association: *Nursing's social policy statement: the essence of the profession*, Silver Spring, Md, 2010, American Nurses Publishing.

Benner P, Wrubel J: *The primacy of caring: stress and coping in health and illness*, Menlo Park, Calif, 1989, Addison-Wesley.

Benner P, et al: *Educating nurses: a call for radical transformation*, Stanford, Calif, 2010, Carnegie Foundation for the Advancement of Teaching.

Chinn PL, Kramer MK: *Integrated knowledge development in nursing*, ed 8, St Louis, 2011, Mosby.

DeSanto-Madeya S, Fawcett J: Toward understanding and measuring adaptation level in the context of the Roy adaptation model, *Nurs Sci Q* 22(4):355, 2009.

Fawcett J: *Contemporary nursing knowledge: analysis and evaluation of conceptual models of nursing*, ed 2, Philadelphia, 2005, FA Davis.

George J: *Nursing theories: a base for professional nursing practice*, ed 6, Saddle River, NJ, 2011, Pearson.

Harmer D, Henderson V: *Textbook of the principles and practice of nursing*, ed 5, Riverside, NJ, 1955, Macmillan.

Henderson V: *The nature of nursing*, New York, 1966, Macmillan.

Kikuchi JF, Simmons H, Romyn D: *Truth in nursing inquiry*, Thousand Oaks, Calif, 1996, Sage Publications.

King IM: *Toward a theory for nursing*, New York, 1971, John Wiley & Sons.

Leininger M: *Transcultural nursing: concepts, theories, and practice*, 1978, John Wiley & Sons.

Leininger MM: *Culture care diversity and universality: a theory of nursing, Pub No 15-2402*, New York, 1991, National League for Nursing Press.

McEwen M, Wills EM: *Theoretical basis for nursing*, ed 3, Philadelphia, 2011, Lippincott Williams & Wilkins.

Meleis AI: *Theoretical nursing: development and progress*, ed 5, Philadelphia, 2011, Lippincott Williams & Wilkins.

Neuman B: (1974). The Betty Neuman health-care systems model: A total person aproach to patient problems. In JP Riehl and C Roy, editors: *Conceptual models for nursing practice*, ed 2, Norwalk, CT, 1974, Appleton-Century-Crofts.

Neuman BM: *The Neuman systems model*, ed 5, Norwalk, Conn, 2011, Pearson, Prentice Hall.

Neuman BM, Reed KS: A Neuman systems model perspective on nursing in 2050, *Nurs Sci Q* 20:111, 2007.

Nightingale F: *Notes on nursing: what it is and what it is not*, London, 1860, Harrison & Sons.

Orem DE: *Nursing: concepts of practice*, New York, 1971, McGraw-Hill.

Orem DE: *Nursing: concepts of practice*, ed 6, New York, 2001, McGraw-Hill.

Peplau HE: *Interpersonal relations in nursing*, New York, 1952, GP Putnam's Sons.

Porter S: Fundamentals patterns of knowing in nursing: the challenge of evidenced-based practice, *Adv Nurs Sci* 33(1):3, 2010.

Roy C: Adaptation: A conceptual framework for nursing. *Nurs Outlook* 18:42, 1970.

Roy C: Relating nursing theory to nursing education: A new era, *Nurse Educator* 4:16, 1979.

Roy C: The Roy adaptation model. In Riehl JP, Roy C, editors: *Conceptual models for nursing practice*, ed 3, New York, 1989, Appleton-Century-Crofts.

Roy R, et al: The Roy adaptation model and research, *Nurs Sci Q* 21:209, 2009.

Selanders LC: The power of environmental adaptation: Florence Nightingale's original theory for nursing practice, *J Holistic Nurs* 28(1):81, 2010.

Walker LO, Avant KC: *Strategies for theory construction in nursing*, ed 5, Upper Saddle River, NJ, 2009, Prentice Hall.

Watson J: *Nursing: the philosophy and science of caring*, Boston, 1979, Little, Brown.

Watson J: *Watson's theory of transpersonal care, In Walker PH, Neuman B: Blueprint for use of nursing models: education, research, practice, and administration, Pub NO 14-2696*, New York, 1996, National League of Nursing Press.

Watson J: *Caring science as sacred science*, Philadelphia, 2005, FA Davis.

Watson J: *The philosophy and science of caring*, Boulder, 2008, University Press of Colorado.

Watson J: Caring science and the next decade of holistic healing: transforming self and system from the inside out, *Am Holistic Nurses Assoc* 30(2):14, 2010.

RESEARCH REFERENCES

Bakan G, Akyol AD: Theory-guided interventions for adaptation to heart failure, *J Adv Nurs* 61(6):596, 2008.

Glasson J, et al: Evaluation of a model of nursing care for older patients using participatory action research in an acute medical ward, *J Clin Nurs* 15(5):588, 2006.

Loomis B: End-of-life issues: difficult decisions and dealing with grief, *Nurs Clin North Am* 44:223, 2009.

Mishel MH: Reconceptualization of the uncertainty in illness theory, *Image J Nurs Sch* 22(4):256, 1990.

Mishel MH: Uncertainty in acute care, *Annu Rev Nurs Res* 15:57, 1997.

Sumner J: A critical lens on the instrumentation of caring in nursing research, *Adv Nurs Sci* 33(1): E17, 2010.

Swanson KM: Empirical development of a middle-range theory of caring, *Nurs Res* 40(3):161, 1991.

Veo P: Concept mapping for applying theory to nursing practice, *J Nurses Staff Dev* 26(1):22, 2010.

CHAPTER 5

Evidence-Based Practice

OBJECTIVES

- Discuss the benefits of evidence-based practice.
- Describe the five steps of evidence-based practice.
- Develop a PICOT question.
- Explain the levels of evidence available in the literature.
- Discuss ways to apply evidence in practice.
- Explain how nursing research improves nursing practice.
- Discuss the steps of the research process.
- Discuss priorities for nursing research.
- Explain the relationship between evidence-based practice and performance improvement.
- Describe the components of a quality improvement program.

KEY TERMS

evolve WEBSITE

http://evolve.elsevier.com/Potter/fundamentals/

- Review Questions
- Case Study with Questions
- Audio Glossary
- Interactive Learning Activities
- Key Term Flashcards
- Content Updates

Rick has been a registered nurse (RN) on a surgical unit for over 5 years. During that time standard nursing care for patients following abdominal surgery has included getting the patient out of bed, sitting in a chair, and walking within the first postoperative day. Patients are encouraged to walk farther and more frequently each day until they begin to pass gas or have a bowel movement. Rick has noticed lately that several of his patients who have had abdominal surgery have experienced a postoperative ileus. This happens when the patient's gastrointestinal tract fails to begin moving after surgery (see Chapter 50). When patients have a postoperative ileus, they have increased pain and are in the hospital longer. Rick raises the question with the other RNs in the department, "What if we had our patients sit and rock in a rocking chair instead of sitting in a regular high-back chair after abdominal surgery? Is it possible that rocking after surgery will decrease the incidence of postoperative ileus?"

Most nurses like Rick practice nursing according to what they learn in nursing school, their experiences in practice, and the policies and procedures of their institution. Such an approach to practice does not guarantee that nursing practice is always based on up-to-date scientific information. Sometimes nursing practice is based on tradition and not on current evidence. If Rick went to the scientific literature for articles about how to prevent postoperative ileus, he would find some studies that indicate that simple changes in activity such as encouraging patients to rock in a rocking chair following surgery may help them recover more quickly. The evidence from research and the opinions of nursing experts provide a basis for Rick and his colleagues to make evidence-based changes to their care of patients following abdominal surgery. The use of evidence in practice enables clinicians like Rick to provide the highest quality of care to their patients and families.

A CASE FOR EVIDENCE

Nurses practice in an "age of accountability" in which quality and cost issues drive the direction of health care (Makadon et al., 2010; Moore et al., 2010). The general public is more informed about their own health and the incidence of medical errors within health care institutions across the country. Greater scrutiny is being given as to why certain health care approaches are used, which ones work, and which ones do not. As a result, evidence-based practice (EBP) is a guide to help nurses make effective, timely, and appropriate clinical decisions in response to the broad political, professional, and societal forces that nurses and other health professionals are confronted with daily (Scott and McSherry, 2009).

Nurses face important clinical decisions when caring for patients (e.g., what to assess in a patient and what interventions are best to use). It is important to translate best evidence into best practices at a patient's bedside. For example, changing how patients are cared for after abdominal surgery is one way that Rick (see previous case study) can use evidence at the bedside. **Evidence-based practice (EBP)** is a problem-solving approach to clinical practice that integrates the conscientious use of best evidence in combination with a clinician's expertise and patient preferences and values in making decisions about patient care (Fig. 5-1) (Melnyk and Fineout-Overholt, 2011; Sackett et al., 2000). Today EBP is becoming a goal of all health care institutions and an expectation of professional nurses who are expected to use current evidence when caring for patients (Ingersoll et al., 2010).

Nurses find evidence in different places. A good textbook incorporates evidence into the practice guidelines and procedures it describes. However, a textbook relies on scientific literature, which is sometimes outdated by the time the book is published. Articles from nursing and the health care literature are available on almost any topic involving nursing practice in either journals or on the Internet. Although the scientific basis of nursing practice has grown, some practices are not yet "research based" (Titler et al., 2001). The challenge is to obtain the very best, most current accurate information at the right time, when you need it for patient care.

The best information is the evidence that comes from well-designed, systematically conducted research studies, mostly found in scientific journals. Unfortunately much of that evidence never reaches the bedside. Nurses in practice settings, unlike in educational settings, do not always have easy access to databases for scientific literature. Instead, they often care for patients on the basis of tradition or convenience. Another source of information comes from nonresearch evidence, including quality improvement and risk management data; international, national, and local standards; infection control data; benchmarking, retrospective, or concurrent chart reviews; and clinicians' expertise. It is important to rely more on research evidence rather than solely on nonresearch evidence. When you face a clinical problem, always ask yourself where you can find the best evidence to help you find the best solution in caring for patients.

Even when you use the best evidence available, application and outcomes will differ based on your patient's values, preferences, concerns, and/or expectations (Oncology Nursing Society [ONS], n.d.). As a nurse, you develop critical thinking skills to determine whether evidence is relevant and appropriate to your patients and to a clinical situation. For example, a single research article suggests that the use of therapeutic touch is effective in reducing abdominal incision pain. However, if your patient's cultural beliefs prevent the use of touch, you will likely need to search for a better evidence-based therapy that patients will accept. Using your clinical expertise and considering patient values and preferences ensures that you apply the evidence available in practice both safely and appropriately.

Steps of Evidence-Based Practice

EBP is a systematic approach to rational decision making that facilitates achievement of best practices. A step-by-step approach ensures that you obtain the strongest available evidence to apply in patient care (Oh et al., 2010). There are six steps of EBP (Melnyk and Fineout-Overholt, 2011):

1. Ask a clinical question.
2. Collect the most relevant and best evidence.
3. Critically appraise the evidence you gather.
4. Integrate all evidence with one's clinical expertise and patient preferences and values in making a practice decision or change.
5. Evaluate the practice decision or change.
6. Share the outcomes of EBP changes with others.

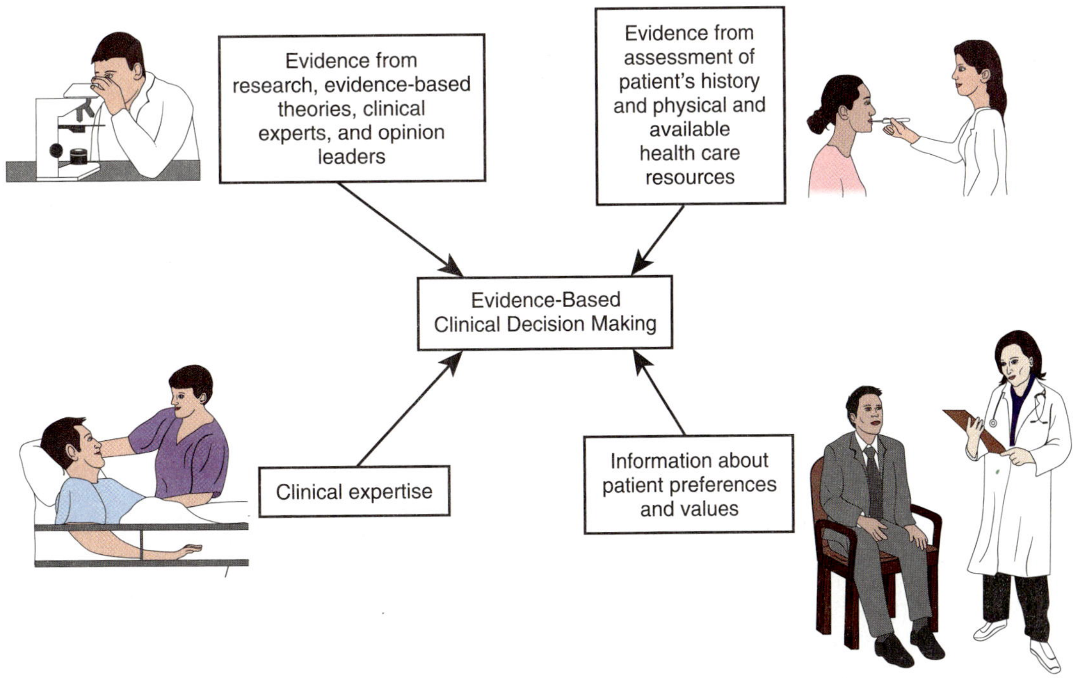

FIG. 5-1 Model for evidence-based clinical decision making.

Ask a Clinical Question. Always think about your practice when caring for patients. Question what does not make sense to you and what needs to be clarified. Think about a problem or area of interest that is time consuming, costly, or not logical (Stilwell et al., 2010). Use problem- and knowledge-focused triggers to think critically about clinical and operational nursing unit issues (Titler et al., 2001). A problem-focused trigger is one you face while caring for a patient or a trend you see on a nursing unit. For example, while Rick is caring for patients following abdominal surgery, he wonders, "If we changed our patients' activity levels after surgery, would they experience fewer episodes of postoperative ileus?" Other examples of problem-focused trends include the increasing number of patient falls or incidence of urinary tract infections on a nursing unit. Such trends lead you to ask, "How can I reduce falls on my unit?" or "What is the best way to prevent urinary tract infections in postoperative patients?"

A knowledge-focused trigger is a question regarding new information available on a topic. For example, "What is the current evidence to improve pain management in patients with migraine headaches?" Important sources of this type of information are standards and practice guidelines available from national agencies such as the Agency for Healthcare Research and Quality (AHRQ), the American Pain Society (APS), or the American Association of Critical Care Nurses (AACN). Other sources of knowledge-focused triggers include recent research publications and nurse experts within an organization.

Sometimes you use data gathered from a health care setting to examine clinical trends to develop clinical questions. For example, most hospitals keep monthly records on key quality of care or performance indicators such as medication errors or infection rates. All magnet-designated hospitals maintain the National Database of Nursing Quality Improvement (NDNQI) (see Chapter 2). The database includes information on falls, pressure ulcer incidence, and nurse satisfaction. Typically quality and risk management data do not give you evidence in finding a solution to a problem, but the data inform you about the nature or severity of problems that then allow you to form practice questions.

The questions you ask eventually lead you to the evidence for an answer. When you ask a question and then go to the scientific literature, you do not want to read 100 articles to find the handful that are most helpful. You want to be able to read the best four-to-six articles that specifically address your practice question. Melnyk and Fineout-Overholt (2011) suggest using a PICOT format to state your question. The five elements of a **PICOT question** are summarized in Box 5-1. The more focused a question you ask, the easier it becomes to search for evidence in the scientific literature. For example, Rick develops the following PICOT question: *Do patients who have had abdominal surgery (P) and who rock in a rocking chair (I) have a reduced incidence of postoperative ileus (O) during hospitalization (T) when compared with patients who receive standard nursing care following surgery (C)?* Another example is: *Is an adult patient's (P) blood pressure more accurate (O) when measuring with the patient's legs crossed (I) versus the patient's feet flat on the floor (C)?*

Proper question formatting allows you to identify key words to use when conducting your literature search. Note that a well-designed PICOT question does not have to follow the sequence of P, I, C, O, and T. In addition, intervention (I), comparison (C), and time (T) are not appropriate to be used in every question. The aim is to ask a question that contains as many of the PICOT elements as possible. For example, here is a meaningful question that contains only a P and O: *How do patients with cystic fibrosis (P) rate their quality of life (O)?*

Inappropriately formed questions (e.g., What is the best way to reduce wandering? What is the best way to improve family's satisfaction with patient care?) are background questions that will likely lead to many irrelevant sources of information, making it difficult to find the best evidence. Sometimes a background question is needed to identify a more specific PICOT question. The PICOT format allows you to ask questions that are intervention focused. For questions that are not intervention focused, the meaning of the letter *I* can be an area of interest (Melnyk and Fineout-Overholt, 2011). For example, *What is the difference in retention (O) of new nursing graduates (P) who have previous experience as nurse assistants (I) versus those who do not (C)?*

The questions you ask using a PICOT format help to identify knowledge gaps within a clinical situation. When you raise well–thought-out questions, you should understand the evidence that is missing to guide clinical practice. Remember: do not be satisfied with clinical routines. Always question and use critical thinking to consider better ways to provide patient care.

BOX 5-1 DEVELOPING A PICOT QUESTION

P = Patient population of interest
Identify patients by age, gender, ethnicity, and disease or health problem.
I = Intervention of interest
Which intervention is worthwhile to use in practice (e.g., a treatment, diagnostic test, prognostic factor)?
C = Comparison of interest
What is the usual standard of care or current intervention used now in practice?
O = Outcome
What result do you wish to achieve or observe as a result of an intervention (e.g., change in patient behavior, physical finding, patient perception)?
T = Time
What amount of time is needed for an intervention to achieve an outcome (e.g., the amount of time needed to change quality of life or patient behavior)?

Building Competency in Evidence-Based Practice While attending a professional nursing conference about the care of surgical patients, Rick hears a report about a research study in which nurses at one hospital had their patients chew gum following abdominal surgery. The results of the research study indicated that patients who chewed peppermint gum three times a day had reduced nausea and a return of bowel sounds sooner after surgery compared with patients who did not chew gum. Using this information, develop a PICOT question that Rick could use to further investigate this intervention. Identify each part of the PICOT question.

Answers to questions can be found on the Evolve website.

Collect the Best Evidence. Once you have a clear and concise PICOT question, you are ready to search for evidence. You can find the evidence you need in a variety of sources: agency policy and procedure manuals, quality improvement data, existing clinical practice guidelines, or computerized bibliographical databases. Do not hesitate to ask for help to find appropriate evidence. Your faculty is always a key resource. When you are assigned to a health

TABLE 5-1 Searchable Scientific Literature Databases and Sources

DATABASES	SOURCES
AHRQ	Agency for Healthcare Research and Quality; includes clinical guidelines and evidence summaries http://www.ahrq.gov
CINAHL	Cumulative Index of Nursing and Allied Health Literature; includes studies in nursing, allied health, and biomedicine http://www.cinahl.com
MEDLINE	Includes studies in medicine, nursing, dentistry, psychiatry, veterinary medicine, and allied health http://www.ncbi.nim.nih.gov
EMBASE	Biomedical and pharmaceutical studies http://www.embase.com
PsycINFO	Psychology and related health care disciplines http://www.apa.org/psycinfo/
Cochrane Database of Systematic Reviews	Full text of regularly updated systematic reviews prepared by the Cochrane Collaboration; includes completed reviews and protocols http://www.cochrane.org/reviews
National Guidelines Clearinghouse	Repository for structured abstracts (summaries) about clinical guidelines and their development; also includes condensed version of guideline for viewing http://www.guideline.gov
PubMed	Health science library at the National Library of Medicine; offers free access to journal articles http://www.nlm.nih.gov
World Views on Evidence-Based Nursing	Electronic journal containing articles that provide a synthesis of research and an annotated bibliography for selected references

care setting, use agency experts such as advanced practice nurses, staff educators, risk managers, and infection control nurses.

When using the scientific literature for evidence, seek the assistance of a medical librarian. He or she knows the various databases that are available to you (Table 5-1). The databases contain large collections of published scientific studies, including peer-reviewed research. A **peer-reviewed** article is one reviewed by a panel of experts familiar with the topic or subject matter of the article before it was published. The librarian is available to help translate your PICOT question into the language or key words that will yield the best evidence search. When conducting a search, it is necessary to enter and manipulate different key words until you get the combination that gives you the key articles that you want to read about your question. When you enter a word to search into a database, be prepared for some confusion with the evidence you obtain. The vocabulary within published articles is often vague. The word you select sometimes has one meaning to one author and a very different meaning to another.

When Rick searches for evidence to answer his PICOT question, he asks for help from a medical librarian. The medical librarian helps him learn how to choose alternative words or terms that identify his PICOT question. During their search Rick identifies three research articles published since 1990 that address the effects of rocking in a rocking chair on return of bowel function following abdominal surgery (Massey, 2010; Moore et al., 1995; Thomas et al., 1990).

MEDLINE and the Cumulative Index of Nursing and Allied Health Literature (CINAHL) are among the best-known comprehensive databases to search for scientific knowledge in health care (Melnyk and Fineout-Overholt, 2011). Among the many databases, some are available through vendors at a cost, some are free of charge, and some offer both options. As a student you have access to an institutional subscription through a vendor purchased by your school. One of the more common vendors is OVID, which offers several different databases. Databases are also available free on the Internet. The Cochrane Database of Systematic Reviews is a valuable source of high-quality evidence. It includes the full text of regularly updated systematic reviews and protocols for reviews currently under way. Collaborative review groups prepare and maintain the reviews. The protocols provide the background, objectives, and methods for reviews in progress (Melnyk and Fineout-Overholt, 2011). The National Guidelines Clearinghouse (NGC) is a database supported by the AHRQ. It contains **clinical guidelines,** systematically developed statements about a plan of care for a specific set of clinical circumstances involving a specific patient population. Examples of clinical guidelines on NCG include care of children and adolescents with type 1 diabetes and practice guidelines for the treatment of adults with low back pain. The NGC is invaluable when developing a plan of care for a patient (see Chapter 18).

Fig. 5-2 represents the hierarchy of available evidence. The level of rigor or amount of confidence you can have in a study's findings decreases as you move down the pyramid. At this point in your nursing career, you cannot be an expert on all aspects of the types of studies conducted. But you can learn enough about the types of studies to help you know which ones have the best scientific evidence. At the top of the pyramid are systematic reviews or meta-analyses, which are state-of-the-art summaries from an individual researcher or panel of experts. Meta-analyses and systematic reviews are the perfect answers to PICOT questions because they rigorously summarize current evidence.

During either a meta-analysis or a systematic review, a researcher asks a PICOT question, reviews the highest level of evidence available (e.g., randomized controlled trials [RCTs]), summarizes what is currently known about the topic, and reports if current evidence

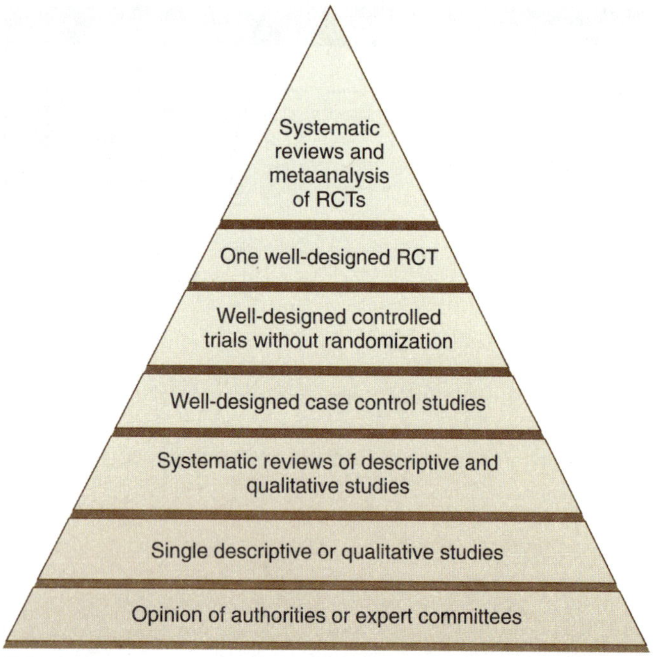

FIG. 5-2 Hierarchy of evidence. *RCTs,* Randomized controlled trials. (Modified from Guyatt G, Rennie D: *User's guide to the medical literature,* Chicago, 2002, American Medical Association; Harris RP et al: Current methods of the US Prevention Services Task Force: a review of the process, *Am J Prev Med* 20:21, 2001; Melnyk BM, Fineout-Overholt E: *Evidence-based practice in nursing and healthcare: a guide to best practice,* ed 2, Philadelphia, 2011, Lippincott Williams & Wilkins.)

supports a change in practice or if further study is needed. The main difference is that in a meta-analysis the researcher uses statistics to show the effect of an intervention on an outcome, whereas in a systematic review no statistics are used to draw conclusions about the evidence. In the Cochrane Library all entries include information on meta-analyses and systematic reviews. If you use MEDLINE or CINAHL, enter a textword such as "meta-analysis" or "systematic review" or the MeSH heading of *evidence-based medicine* to obtain scientific reviews on your PICOT question.

The RCT is the most precise form of experimental study and therefore is the gold standard for research. A single RCT is not as conclusive as a review of several RCTs on the same question. However, a single RCT that tests the intervention included in your question yields very useful evidence. If RCTs are not available, you can use results from other research studies such as descriptive or qualitative studies to help answer your PICOT question. The use of clinical experts may be at the bottom of the evidence pyramid, but do not consider clinical experts to be a poor source of evidence. Expert clinicians use evidence frequently as they build their own practice, and they are rich sources of information for clinical problems.

Critically Appraise the Evidence. Perhaps the most difficult step in the EBP process is critiquing or analyzing the available evidence. Critiquing evidence involves evaluating it, which includes determining the value, feasibility, and usefulness of evidence for making a practice change (ONS, n.d.). When critiquing evidence, first evaluate the scientific merit and clinical applicability of the findings of each study. Then with a group of studies and expert opinion determine what findings have a strong enough basis for use in practice. After critiquing the evidence you will be able to answer the following questions. Do the articles together offer evidence to explain or answer my PICOT question? Do the articles show support for the reliability and validity of the evidence? Can I use the evidence in practice?

As a student new to nursing, it takes time to acquire the skills to critique evidence like an expert. When you read an article, do not put it down and walk away because of the statistics and technical language. Know the elements of an article and use a careful approach when reviewing each one. Evidence-based articles include the following elements:

- *Abstract.* An abstract is a brief summary of the article that quickly tells you if it is research or clinically based. An abstract summarizes the purpose of the article. It also includes the major themes or findings and the implications for nursing practice.
- *Introduction.* The introduction contains more information about the purpose of the article. There is usually brief supporting evidence as to why the topic is important.

  Together the abstract and introduction help you decide if you want to continue to read the entire article. You will know if the topic of the article is similar to your PICOT question or related closely enough to provide useful information. If you decide that this article may help answer your question, continue to read the next elements of the article.
- *Literature review or background.* A good author offers a detailed background of the level of science or clinical information that exists about the topic. The literature review offers an argument about what led the author to conduct a study or report on a clinical topic. This section of an article is very valuable. Even if the article itself does not address your PICOT question the way you desire, the literature review will possibly lead you to other more useful articles. After reading a literature review, you should have a good idea of how past research led to the researcher's question. For example, a study designed to test an educational intervention for older adult family caregivers reviews literature that describes characteristics of caregivers, the type of factors influencing caregivers' ability to cope with stressors of caregiving, and any previous educational interventions used with families.
- *Manuscript narrative.* The "middle section" or narrative of an article differs according to the type of evidence-based article it is (Melnyk and Fineout-Overholt, 2011). A clinical article describes a clinical topic, which often includes a description of a patient population, the nature of a certain disease or health alteration, how patients are affected, and the appropriate nursing therapies. An author sometimes writes a clinical article to explain how to use a therapy or new technology. A research article contains several subsections within the narrative, including the following:
  - *Purpose statement:* Explains the focus or intent of a study. It includes research questions or **hypotheses**—predictions made about the relationship or difference between study **variables** (concepts, characteristics, or traits that vary within or among subjects). An example of a research question is: What environmental characteristics are common among young adults who experience frequent exacerbations of asthma?
- *Methods or design:* Explains how a research study was organized and conducted to answer the research question or test the hypothesis. This is when you learn the type of study that

was conducted (e.g., RCT, case control study, or qualitative study). You also learn how many subjects or persons were in a study. In health care studies subjects may include patients, family members, or health care staff. The language in the methods section is sometimes confusing because it explains details about how the researcher designed the study to obtain the most accurate results possible. Use your faculty member as a resource to help interpret this section.

- *Results or conclusions.* Clinical and research articles have a summary section. In a clinical article the author explains the clinical implications for the topic presented. In a research article the author details the results of the study and explains whether a hypothesis is supported or how a research question is answered. This section includes a statistical analysis if it is a quantitative research study. A qualitative study summarizes the descriptive themes and ideas that arise from the researcher's analysis of data. Do not let the statistical analysis in an article overwhelm you. Read carefully and ask these questions: Does the researcher describe the results? Were the results significant? A good author also discusses any limitations to a study in this section. The information on limitations is valuable in helping you decide if you want to use the evidence with your patients. Have a faculty member or an expert nurse help you interpret statistical results.
- *Clinical implications.* A research article includes a section that explains if the findings from the study have clinical implications. The researcher explains how to apply findings in a practice setting for the type of subjects studied.

After Rick critiques each article for his PICOT question, he combines the findings from the three articles he found about the use of rocking chairs to determine the state of the evidence. He uses critical thinking to consider the scientific rigor of the evidence and how well it answers his PICOT question. He also considers the evidence in light of his patients' concerns and preferences. As a clinician Rick judges whether to use the evidence for the group of patients for whom he normally cares on the surgical unit. Patients frequently have complex medical histories and patterns of responses (Melnyk and Fineout-Overholt, 2011). Ethically it is important for Rick to consider evidence that will benefit patients and do no harm. He needs to decide if the evidence is relevant, is easily applicable in his setting of practice, and has the potential for improving patient outcomes.

Integrate the Evidence. Once you decide that the evidence is strong and applicable to your patients and clinical situation, incorporate it into practice. Your first step is simply to apply the research in your plan of care for a patient (see Chapter 18). Use the evidence you find as a rationale for an intervention you plan to try. For instance, you learned about an approach to bathe older adults who are confused and decide to use the technique during your next clinical assignment. You use the bathing technique with your own assigned patients, or you work with a group of other students or nurses to revise a policy and procedure or develop a new clinical protocol.

The literature Rick found reveals that rocking in a rocking chair after bowel surgery usually results in a quicker return of bowel function following surgery when compared with standard nursing care (Massey, 2010; Moore et al., 1995; Thomas et al., 1990). Rick then meets with his colleagues on the unit practice committee to recommend a protocol for patients who have abdominal surgery. The protocol outlines guidelines to have patients routinely sit in rocking chairs when they get out of bed after surgery.

Evidence is integrated in a variety of ways through teaching tools, clinical practice guidelines, policies and procedures, and new assessment or documentation tools. Depending on the amount of change needed to apply evidence in practice, it becomes necessary to involve a number of staff from a given nursing unit. It is important to consider the setting where you want to apply the evidence. Is there support from all staff? Does the practice change fit with the scope of practice in the clinical setting? Are resources (time, secretarial support, and staff) available to make a change? When evidence is not strong enough to apply in practice, your next option is to conduct a pilot study to investigate your PICOT question. A pilot study is a small-scale research study or one that includes a quality or performance improvement project.

Evaluate the Practice Decision or Change. After applying evidence in your practice, your next step is to evaluate the outcome. How does the intervention work? How effective was the clinical decision for your patient or practice setting? Sometimes your evaluation is as simple as determining if the expected outcomes you set for an intervention are met (see Chapters 18 and 20). For example, after the use of a transparent intravenous (IV) dressing, does the IV dislodge, or does the patient develop the complication of phlebitis? When using a new approach to preoperative teaching, does the patient learn what to expect after surgery?

When an EBP change occurs on a larger scale, an evaluation is more formal. For example, evidence showing factors that contribute to pressure ulcers might lead a nursing unit to adopt a new skin care protocol. To evaluate the protocol, nurses track the incidence of pressure ulcers over a course of time (e.g., 6 months to a year). In addition, they collect data to describe both patients who develop ulcers and those who do not. This comparative information is valuable in determining the effects of the protocol and whether modifications are necessary.

When evaluating an EBP change, determine if the change was effective, if modifications in the change are needed, or if the change needs to be discontinued. Events or results that you do not expect may occur. For example, a hospital that implements a new method of cleaning IV line puncture sites discovers an increased rate of IV line infections and reevaluates the new cleaning method to determine why infections have increased. If the hospital does not evaluate this change in practice, more patients will develop IV site infections. *Never* implement a practice change without evaluating its effect.

In Rick's case the unit practice committee collects evaluation data after 3 months of implementing the rocking chair protocol to determine if patients experienced a lower incidence of postoperative ileus following abdominal surgery. After completing chart reviews, the committee discovers that patients who used the rocking chairs following abdominal surgery experienced fewer incidences of postoperative ileus compared with patients who did not use rockers before the protocol was implemented. The protocol patients went home 1 to 2 days sooner than the patients who did not use the rocking chairs. Patient interviews revealed that the patients were satisfied with the rocking movement and that, not only did the rocking chairs help them pass gas faster, but the patients also felt less anxious because of the rocking motion. After talking with the committee, Rick discovered that not all patients were able to use rocking chairs during this time because the unit did not have enough rocking chairs. He presented these data to his manager who approved the purchase of more rocking chairs.

Share the Outcomes with Others. After implementing an EBP change, it is important to communicate the results. If you implement an evidence-based intervention with one patient, you and the patient determine the effectiveness of that intervention. When a practice change occurs on a nursing unit level, the first group to discuss the outcomes of the change is often the clinical staff on that unit. To enhance professional development and promote positive patient outcomes beyond the unit level, share the results with various groups of nurses or other care providers such as the nursing practice council or the research council. Clinicians enjoy and appreciate seeing the results of a practice change. In addition, the practice change will more likely be sustainable and remain in place when staff are able to see the benefits of an EBP change.

As a professional nurse it is critical to contribute to the growing knowledge of nursing practice, especially if he or she is involved in an EBP change. Nurses often communicate the outcomes of EBP changes at professional conferences and meetings. Being involved in professional organizations allows them to present EBP changes in scientific abstracts, poster presentations, or even podium presentations.

After evaluating the results of the EBP change, Rick decides to present the outcomes to the nursing research committee at his hospital. The chief nursing officer hears Rick's presentation and encourages him to submit an abstract about his EBP change to a national professional nursing conference. Rick submits his abstract for consideration as a poster presentation at the annual Midwest Nursing Research Society conference, and it is accepted. During the conference Rick tells other nurses about his EBP change and is contacted by several nurses after the conference who are thinking about implementing the use of rocking chairs on their patient care units.

NURSING RESEARCH

After completing a thorough review and critique of the scientific literature, you might not have enough strong evidence to make a practice change. Instead you may find a gap in knowledge that makes your PICOT question go unanswered. When this happens, the best way to answer your PICOT question is to conduct a research study. At this time in your career you will not be conducting research. However, it is important for you to understand the process of nursing research and how it generates new knowledge.

The International Council of Nurses (ICN) (2007) supports the need for nursing research as a means for improving the health and welfare of people. **Nursing research** is a way to identify new knowledge, improve professional education and practice, and use resources effectively. Research means to search again or to examine carefully. It is a systematic process that asks and answers questions to generate knowledge. The knowledge provides a scientific basis for nursing practice and validates the effectiveness of nursing interventions. Nursing research improves professional education and practice and helps nurses use resources effectively. The scientific knowledge base of nursing continues to grow today, thus furnishing evidence nurses can use to provide safe and effective patient care. Many professional and specialty nursing organizations support the conduct of research for advancing nursing science.

An example of how research can expand our practice can be seen in the work of Dr. Norma Metheny who has spent many years asking questions about how to prevent the aspiration of tube feeding in patients who receive feeding through nasogastric tubes (Metheny et al., 1988, 1989, 1990, 1994, 2000). Through her research she identified factors that increase the risk for aspiration and approaches to use in determining tube feeding placement. Dr. Metheny's findings are incorporated into this textbook and have changed the way nurses administer tube feedings to patients. Through research Dr. Metheny has contributed to the scientific body of knowledge that has saved patients' lives and helped to prevent the serious complication of aspiration.

Outcomes Management Research

The management of care delivery outcomes is a growing concern for nurse clinicians and researchers (Melnyk and Fineout-Overholt, 2011). Outcomes research assesses and documents the effectiveness of health care services and interventions. It responds to the increased demands from policy makers, insurers, and the public to justify care practices and systems in terms of improved patient outcomes and costs (Polit and Beck, 2007). For example, studying the effects of an outpatient education program on the ability of older adult patients to follow a nutrition and exercise program is an outcome study.

Care delivery outcomes are the observable or measurable effects of some intervention or action (Melnyk and Fineout-Overholt, 2011). As is the case with the expected outcomes you develop in a plan of care (see Chapter 18), a care delivery outcome focuses on the recipient of service (e.g., patient, family, or community) and not the provider (e.g., nurse or physician). For example, an outcome of a diabetes education program is that patients are able to self-administer insulin, not the nurses' success in instructing all patients newly diagnosed with diabetes.

A problem in outcomes research is the clear definition or selection of measurable outcomes. Components of an outcome include the outcome itself, how it is observed (the indicator), its critical characteristics (how it is measured), and its range of parameters (Melnyk and Fineout-Overholt, 2011). For example, health care settings commonly measure the outcome of patient satisfaction when they introduce new services (e.g., new care delivery model or outpatient clinic). The outcome is patient satisfaction, observed through patients' responses to a patient satisfaction instrument, including characteristics such as nursing care, physician care, support services, and the environment. Patients complete the instrument, responding to a scale (parameter) designed to measure their degree of satisfaction (e.g., scale of 1 to 5). The combined score on the instrument yields a measure of patient satisfaction, an outcome that the facility can track over time.

Although the nursing literature now addresses the identification of "nursing-sensitive outcomes" (Box 5-2), or outcomes that are sensitive to nursing practice (Ingersoll et al., 2010; Montalvo, 2007), researchers frequently choose outcomes that do not measure a true impact of care delivery, particularly nursing care delivery. For example, common outcome measures include morbidity, mortality, readmission rate, or length of stay. Although important outcomes to understand, they do not always measure the true effect of a specific nursing intervention on care delivery. For example, if a nurse researcher intends to measure the success of a nurse-initiated protocol to manage blood glucose levels in critically ill patients, the researcher will not likely measure mortality because it is too broad and susceptible to many factors (e.g., the selection of medical therapies, the patients' acuity of illness) other than the nurse-initiated protocol. Instead, he or she will have a better idea of the effects of the protocol by measuring the outcome of patients' blood glucose ranges. The nurse researcher obtains the blood glucose level of patients placed on the protocol and compares them to a desired range that represents good blood glucose control.

BOX 5-2 EXAMPLES OF NURSING-SENSITIVE OUTCOME MEASURES

- Nursing hours per patient day and skill mix
- Patient falls, with and without injury
- Pediatric pain assessment, intervention, and reassessment cycle
- Pediatric peripheral intravenous infiltration rate
- Pressure ulcer prevalence
- Psychiatric physical/sexual assault rate
- Restraint prevalence
- Registered nurse (RN) education, certification, and satisfaction
- Voluntary nurse turnover and vacancy rate
- Nosocomial infections:
  - Catheter-associated urinary tract infection (UTI)
  - Central-line catheter-associated blood stream infection (CABSI)
  - Ventilator-associated pneumonia (VAP)

Data from Montalvo I: The National Database of Nursing Quality Indicators (NDNQI), *Online J Issues Nurs* 12(3), 2007, http://www.nursingworld.org/MainMenuCategories/ANAMarketplace/ANAPeriodicals/OJIN/TableofContents/Volume122007/No3Sept07/NursingQualityIndicators.aspx. Accessed October 14, 2010.

Scientific Method

The **scientific method** is the foundation of research and the most reliable and objective of all methods of gaining knowledge. This method is an advanced, objective means of acquiring and testing knowledge. Aspects of the method guide you in applying research evidence in practice and in conducting research. When using research findings to change practice, you need to understand the process that a researcher uses to guide a study. For example, when Rick considered whether to have the patients on his unit use a rocking chair following abdominal surgery, he needed to know if this had been tested on similar patients and the outcomes or results. The scientific method is a systematic, step-by-step process that provides support that the findings from a study are **valid, reliable,** and **generalizable** to subjects similar to those researched.

Researchers use the scientific method to understand, explain, predict, or control a nursing phenomenon (Polit and Beck, 2007). Systematic, orderly procedures characterize this method to limit the possibility for error, although it is not without fault. The scientific method minimizes the chance that **bias** or opinion by a researcher will influence the results of research and thus the knowledge gained. The characteristics of scientific research are as follows (Polit and Beck, 2007):

- The research identifies the problem area or area of interest to study.
- The steps of planning and conducting a research study occur in a systematic and orderly way.
- Researchers try to control external factors that are not being studied but can influence a relationship between the phenomena they are studying. For example, if a nurse is studying the relationship between diet and heart disease, he or she controls other characteristics among subjects such as stress or smoking history because they are contributing factors to this disease. Patients on a study diet and those on a regular diet would both have to have similar levels of stress and smoking histories to test the true effect of the diet.
- Researchers gather **empirical data** through the use of observations and assessments and use the data to discover new knowledge.
- The goal is to understand phenomena to apply the knowledge generally to a broad group of patients.

Nursing and the Scientific Approach

In the past much of the information used in nursing practice was borrowed from other disciplines such as biology, physiology, and psychology. Often nurses applied this information to their practice without testing it. For example, nurses use several methods to help patients sleep. Interventions such as giving a patient a back rub, making sure that the bed is clean and comfortable, and preparing the environment by dimming the lights are nursing measures that are used frequently and in general are logical, commonsense approaches. However, when these measures are considered in greater depth, questions arise about their applications. For example, are they the best methods to promote sleep? Do different patients in different situations require other interventions to promote sleep?

Research provides a way to study nursing questions and problems in greater depth within the context of nursing. If nurses do not use an evidence-based approach to practice, they often rely on personal experience or the statements of nursing experts alone. If an intervention works for most patients, you may become satisfied with this success without questioning whether there might be a better way for other patients. If the intervention is not successful, you might use an approach practiced by a colleague or try a different sequence of accepted measures. Even if an intervention discovered with this approach is effective for one or more patients, it is not always appropriate for other patients in other settings. Nursing interventions must be tested through research to determine the measures that work best with specific patients.

Nursing research addresses issues important to the discipline of nursing. Some of these issues relate to the profession itself, education of nurses, patient and family needs, and issues within the health care delivery system. Once research is completed, it is important to disseminate or communicate the findings. One method of dissemination is through publication of the findings in professional journals. Nursing research uses many methods to study clinical problems (Box 5-3). There are two broad approaches to research: quantitative and qualitative methods.

Quantitative Research. **Quantitative nursing research** is the study of nursing phenomena that offers precise measurement and quantification. For example, a study dealing with pain therapies quantitatively measures pain severity. A study testing different forms of surgical dressings measures the extent of wound healing. Quantitative research is the precise, systematic, objective examination of specific concepts. It focuses on numerical data, statistical analysis, and controls to eliminate bias in findings (Polit and Beck, 2007). Although there are many quantitative methods, the following sections briefly describe experimental, nonexperimental, survey, and evaluation research.

Experimental Research. An RCT is a true **experimental study** that tightly controls conditions to eliminate bias and ensure that findings can be generalizable to similar groups of subjects. Researchers test an intervention (e.g., new drug, therapy, or education method) against the usual standard of care (Box 5-4). They randomly assign subjects to either a control or treatment group. In other words, all subjects in a study have an equal chance to be in either group. The treatment group receives the experimental intervention, and the control group receives the usual standard of care. The researchers measure both groups for the same outcomes to see if there is a difference. When an RCT is completed, the researcher will know if the intervention leads to better outcomes than the standard of care.

BOX 5-3 TYPES OF RESEARCH

Historical research: Studies designed to establish facts and relationships concerning past events. *Example:* Study examining the societal factors that led to the acceptance of advanced practice nurses by patients.

Exploratory research: Initial study designed to develop or refine the dimensions of phenomena or to develop or refine a hypothesis about the relationships among phenomena. *Example:* Pilot study testing the benefits of a new exercise program for older adults with dementia.

Evaluation research: Study that tests how well a program, practice, or policy is working. *Example:* Study measuring the outcomes of an informational campaign designed to improve parents' ability to follow immunization schedules for their children.

Descriptive research: Study that measures characteristics of persons, situations, or groups and the frequency with which certain events or characteristics occur. *Example:* Study to examine RNs' biases toward caring for obese patients.

Experimental research: Study in which the investigator controls the study variable and randomly assigns subjects to different conditions to test the variable. *Example:* RCT comparing chlorhexidine with Betadine in reducing the incidence of IV-site phlebitis.

Correlational research: Study that explores the interrelationships among variables of interest without any active intervention by the researcher. *Example:* Study examining the relationship between RNs' educational levels and their satisfaction in the nursing role.

RNs, Registered nurses; *RCT,* randomized controlled trial; *IV,* intravenous.

BOX 5-4 EXAMPLE OF A RANDOMIZED CONTROLLED TRIAL

Research question: Will the use of a formal education program for patients at risk for diabetes compared with a traditional educational pamphlet improve patient's blood glucose level and weight control?

Subjects: 130 adult patients with risk factors for diabetes who visit a local medicine clinic

Randomization: Patients are randomly assigned to one of two groups using a random numbers table.

Treatment group: 65 patients attend an 8-hour class on diabetes prevention, with group discussion, lecture, and interactive computer program use.

Control group: 65 patients receive a printed pamphlet outlining risks for diabetes and health promotion strategies.

Outcome measure: Both groups have blood glucose levels and weight measured before receiving education and every month for 3 months after receiving education.

Analysis: Statistical tests comparing the blood glucose levels and weight for the two groups will show if the treatment has the predicted effect.

Controlled trials without randomization are studies that test interventions, but researchers have not randomized the subjects into control or treatment groups. Thus there is bias in how the study is conducted. Some findings are distorted because of how the study was designed. A researcher wants to be as certain as possible when testing an intervention that the intervention is the reason for the desired outcomes. In a nonrandomized controlled trial the way in which subjects fall into the control or treatment group sometimes influences the results. This suggests that the intervention tested was not the only factor affecting the results of the study. Careful critique allows you to determine if bias were present in a study and what effect, if any, the bias had on the results of the study.

Although RCTs investigate cause and effect and are excellent for testing drug therapies or medical treatments, this approach is not always the best for testing nursing interventions. The nature of nursing care causes nurse researchers to ask questions that are not always answered best by an RCT. For example, nurses help patients with problems such as knowledge deficits and symptom management. Learning to understand how patients experience health problems cannot always be addressed through an RCT. Therefore nonexperimental descriptive studies are often used in nursing research.

Nonexperimental Research. Nonexperimental descriptive studies describe, explain, or predict phenomena such as factors that lead to an adolescent's decision to smoke cigarettes and those that lead patients with dementia to fall in a hospital setting.

A case control study is one in which researchers study one group of subjects with a certain condition (e.g., asthma) at the same time as another group of subjects who do not have the condition. A case control study determines if there is an association between one or more predictor variables and the condition (Melnyk and Fineout-Overholt, 2011). For example, is there an association between predictor variables such as family history or environmental exposure to dust and the incidence of asthma? Often a case control study is conducted retrospectively, or after the fact. Researchers look back in time and review available data about their two groups of subjects to understand what variables explain the condition. These studies involve a small number of subjects, creating a risk of bias. Sometimes the subjects in the two groups differ on certain other variables (e.g., amount of stress or history of contact allergies) that also influence the incidence of the condition, more so than the variables being studied. Correlational studies describe the relationship between two variables (e.g., the age of the adolescent and if the adolescent smokes). The researcher determines if the two variables are correlated or associated with one another and to what extent.

Many times researchers use findings from descriptive studies to develop studies that test interventions. For example, if the researcher determines that adolescents 15 years old and older tend to smoke, he or she might test if participation in a program about smoking for older adolescents is effective in helping adolescents stop smoking.

Surveys. Surveys are common in quantitative research. They obtain information from populations regarding the frequency, distribution, and interrelation of variables among subjects in the study (Polit and Beck, 2007). An example is a survey designed to measure nurses' perceptions of physicians' willingness to collaborate in practice. Surveys obtain information about practices, education, experience, opinions, and other characteristics of people. The most basic function of a survey is description. Surveys gather a large amount of data to describe the population and the topic of study. It is important in survey research that the population sampled be large enough to keep sampling error at a minimum.

Evaluation Research. **Evaluation research** is a form of quantitative research that determines how well a program, practice, procedure, or policy is working (Polit and Beck, 2007). An example is outcomes management research. Evaluation research determines why a program or some components of the program are successful or unsuccessful. When programs are unsuccessful, evaluation

TABLE 5-2 **Comparison of Steps of the Nursing Process with the Research Process**

NURSING PROCESS	RESEARCH PROCESS
Problem identification	Identify area of interest or clinical problem: • Review literature. • Formulate theoretical framework. • Identify study variables. • Devise research question(s)/hypotheses.
Study design	Design study protocol: • Select research design/methodology. • Identify sample population: number, recruitment, assignment to groups. • Select data collection methods. • Select instrumentation: questionnaires, physiological measures, interviews, treatments. • Formulate proposed analysis: statistical methods to answer research questions/hypotheses.
Conducting the study	Obtain necessary approvals. Recruit subjects. Implement the study protocol/collect data: • Pilot study may be done initially. • Continually assess study methodology. Is study consistently carried out? Are all investigators following study protocol?
Data analysis	Analyze results of the study: • Interpret demographics of study population. • Analyze each research question/hypothesis. • Interpret results, including conclusions, limitations.
Use of the findings	Formulate recommendations for further research. Determine implications for nursing. Disseminate the findings: presentations, publications, research use in practice.

research identifies problems with the program and opportunities for change or barriers to program implementation.

Qualitative Research. **Qualitative nursing research** is the study of phenomena that are difficult to quantify or categorize such as patients' perceptions of illness. This method describes information obtained in a nonnumerical form (e.g., data in the form of written transcripts from a series of interviews). Qualitative research offers answers when trying to understand patients' experiences with health problems and the contexts in which the experiences occur. Patients have the opportunity to tell their stories and share their experiences in these studies. The findings are in depth because patients are usually very descriptive in what they choose to share. Examples of qualitative studies include "patient's perceptions of nurses' caring in a palliative care unit," and "the perceptions of stress by family members of critically ill patients."

Qualitative research involves **inductive reasoning** to develop generalizations or theories from specific observations or interviews (Polit and Beck, 2007). For example, a nurse extensively interviews cancer survivors and then summarizes the common themes from all of the interviews to inductively determine the characteristics of cancer survivors' quality of life. Qualitative research involves the discovery and understanding of important behavioral characteristics or phenomena. An example is a qualitative research study conducted by Nixon and Narayanasamy (2010) that described the spiritual needs of patients with brain tumors and how well nurses support these needs.

There are a number of different qualitative research methods, including ethnography, phenomenology, and grounded theory. Each is based on a different philosophical or methodological view of how to collect, summarize, and analyze qualitative data.

RESEARCH PROCESS

The **research process** is an orderly series of steps that allow a researcher to move from asking the research question to finding the answer. Usually the answer to the initial research question leads to new questions and other areas of study. The research process builds knowledge for use in other similar situations. For example, a nurse researcher might seek knowledge about why a particular event happens or the best way to provide care for patients with a certain health problem. The research process provides knowledge that a nurse can apply repeatedly to a whole group or class of patients. Table 5-2 summarizes steps of the research process. Initially the researcher identifies an area of inquiry (identifying a problem), which often results from clinical practice. For example, after speaking with a researcher at a professional nursing conference, Rick decides he wants to conduct a pilot study on the nursing unit to determine if chewing peppermint gum following colon surgery prevents patients from having nausea and reduces the incidence of postoperative ileus. He reviews the relevant literature to determine what is known about chewing peppermint gum and its effect on bowel mobility and nausea following abdominal surgery. Rick notes that, although many patients report problems with nausea and return of bowel function, there is limited research on the effects of chewing gum on these two outcomes.

Following identification of the problem and review of the literature, Rick designs a study with the help of a nurse researcher. The sample includes all patients who are having elective colon resections. Subjects are excluded if they need to have surgery because of an emergency situation. Rick places each subject into one of the two groups (experimental or control) based on random assignment. The control group receives standard postoperative care. The experimental or treatment group receives standard postoperative care, and they chew gum for 5 minutes three times a day. Subjects have a 50-50 chance of being in each group. Rick selects appropriate instruments to measure postoperative nausea and decides to use patient assessment data to determine when nurses first hear bowel sounds and when patients first pass flatus and have a bowel movement after surgery.

Before conducting any study with human subjects, the researcher obtains approvals from the agency's human subjects committee or institutional review board (IRB). An IRB includes scientists and laypersons who review all studies conducted in the institution to ensure that ethical principles, including the rights of human subjects, are followed. **Informed consent** means that research subjects (1) are given full and complete information about the purpose of a study, procedures, data collection, potential harm and benefits, and alternative methods of treatment; (2) are capable of fully understanding the research and the implications of participation; (3) have the power of free choice to voluntarily consent or decline participation in the research; and (4) understand how the researcher maintains confidentiality or anonymity. **Confidentiality** guarantees that any information a subject provides will not be reported in any manner that identifies the subject and will not be accessible to people outside the research team.

Once Rick's study begins, the nurses on his unit collect data as indicated in the study protocol. The team analyzes the data from the nausea instrument and the chart review about bowel function from the two groups studied. With the help of a statistician from the hospital, a comparison of the results determines whether patients who chewed peppermint gum experienced less nausea and a quicker return of bowel function than the patients who had standard nursing care. The results from this study will advance postoperative nursing care.

In any study a researcher must consider study limitations. Limitations are factors that affect study findings such as a small sample of subjects, a unique setting where the study was conducted, or the failure of the study to include representative cultural groups or age-groups. Rick's team conducted a pilot study because little data were available about the benefits of chewing gum following abdominal surgery. The sample size only included 20 patients in each group, and it was challenging to collect all the data from the patient charts because of inconsistencies in documentation. Therefore the results of Rick's study have limited generalizability to other patients who are experiencing abdominal surgery. The limitations in this study help Rick decide how to refine or adapt it for further investigation in the future.

A researcher also addresses the implications for nursing practice. This ultimately helps fellow researchers, clinicians, educators, and administrators know how to apply findings from a study in practice. At the conclusion of Rick's study, the research team recommends that patients who have elective colon resections be offered the opportunity to chew peppermint gum following surgery. The surgeons on the unit agreed to the change in practice. The team decides to consider conducting future studies to investigate this intervention with patients who have other types of abdominal surgeries. In addition, the team suggests ways to effectively introduce the use of chewing gum into other surgical units following surgery.

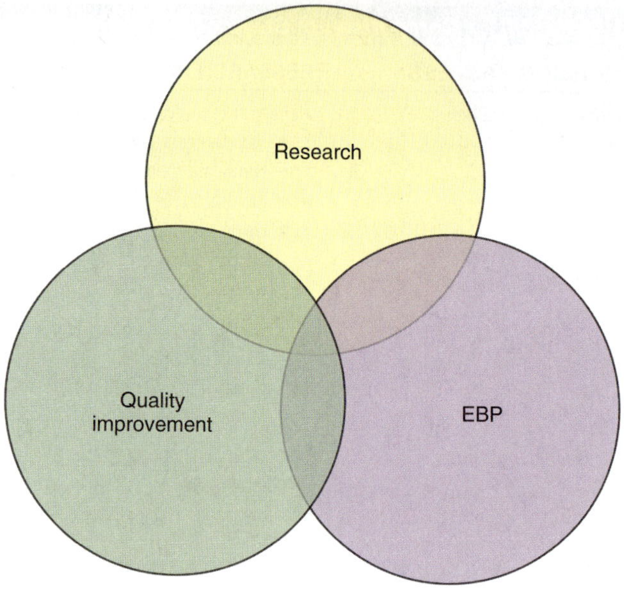

FIG. 5-3 The overlapping relationship among research, evidence-based practice, and quality improvement. *EBP,* Evidence-based practice.

QUALITY AND PERFORMANCE IMPROVEMENT

Every health care organization gathers data on a number of health outcome measures as a way to gauge its quality of care. This is the focus of outcomes management. Examples of quality data include fall rates, number of medication errors, incidence of pressure ulcers, and infection rates. Health care organizations actively promote efforts for improving patient care and outcomes, particularly with respect to reducing medical errors and enhancing patient safety. Quality data are the outcome of both quality improvement (QI) and performance improvement (PI) initiatives. The Joint Commission (TJC, 2010a) defines **quality improvement (QI)** as an approach to the continuous study and improvement of the processes of providing health care services to meet the needs of patients and others and inform health care policy. The QI program of an institution focuses on improvement of health care–related processes (e.g., medication delivery or fall prevention). Performance measurement analyzes what an institution does and how well it does it. In **performance improvement (PI)** an organization analyzes and evaluates current performance and uses the results to develop focused improvement actions. PI activities are typically clinical projects conceived in response to identified clinical problems and designed to use research findings to improve clinical practice (Melnyk and Fineout-Overholt, 2011).

EBP, research, and quality improvement are closely interrelated (Fig. 5-3). Although you use all of these in nursing practice, it is important to know the similarities and differences between them (Table 5-3). When implementing an EBP project, it is important to first review evidence from appropriate research and QI data. The information helps you better understand the extent of a problem in practice and within your organization. QI data inform you about how processes work within an organization and thus offer information about how to make EBP changes. When implementing a research project, EBP and QI can inform opportunities for research.

TABLE 5-3 Similarities and Differences Among Evidence-Based Practice, Research, and Quality Improvement

	EVIDENCE-BASED PRACTICE	RESEARCH	QUALITY IMPROVEMENT
Purpose	Use of information from research, professional experts, personal experience, and patient preferences to determine safe and effective nursing care with the goal of improving patient care and outcomes	Systematic inquiry answers questions, solves problems, and contributes to the generalizable knowledge base of nursing; it may or may not improve patient care.	Improves work processes to improve patient outcomes and efficiency of health systems
Focus	Implementation of evidence already known into practice	Evidence is generated to find answers for questions that are not known about nursing practice.	Measures effects of practice and/or practice change on specific patient population
Data sources	Multiple research studies, expert opinion, personal experience, patients	Subjects or participants have predefined characteristics that include or exclude them from the study; researcher collects and analyzes data from subjects.	Data from patient records or patients who are in a specific area such as on a patient care unit or admitted to a particular hospital
Who conducts the activity?	Practicing nurses and possibly other members of the health care team	Researchers may or may not be employed by the health care agency and usually are not a part of the clinical health care team.	Employees of a health care agency, such as nurses, physicians, pharmacists
Is activity part of regular clinical practice?	Yes	No	Yes
Is IRB approval needed?	No	Yes	Sometimes
Funding sources	Internal, from health care agency	Usually external, such as a grant	Internal, from health care agency

IRB, Institutional review board.

Rapid-cycle improvements measured through QI often identify gaps in evidence. Similarly EBP literature reviews often identify gaps in scientific evidence. Thus the two processes help to identify topics for research. When implementing a QI project, you consider information from research and EBP that aims to improve or better understand practice, thus helping to identify worthy processes to evaluate. Here is an example of how the three processes can merge to improve nursing practice. A nursing unit has an increase in the number of patient falls over the last several months. QI data identifies the type of patients who fall, time of day of falls, and possible precipitating factors (e.g., efforts to reach the bathroom, multiple medications, or patient confusion). A thorough analysis of QI data then leads clinicians to conduct a literature review and implement the best evidence available to prevent patient falls for the type of patients on the unit. Once the staff apply the evidence in a fall-prevention protocol, they implement the protocol (in this case, focusing efforts on care approaches during evening hours) and evaluate its results. Recurrent problems with falls may lead staff to conduct a research study.

Quality Improvement Programs

A well-organized QI program focuses on processes or systems that contribute to patient, staff, or system outcomes. A systematic approach ensures that all employees support a continuous QI philosophy. An organizational culture in which all staff members understand their responsibility toward maintaining and improving quality is essential. Typically in health care many individuals are involved in single processes of care. For example, medication delivery involves the nurse who prepares and administers the drugs, the health care provider who prescribes medications, the pharmacist who prepares the dosage, the secretary who communicates about new orders being written, and the transporter who delivers medications. All members of the health care team collaborate together in QI activities. As a member of the nursing team, you participate in recognizing trends in practice, identifying when recurrent problems develop, and initiating opportunities to improve the quality of care.

The QI process begins at the staff level, where problems are defined. This requires staff members to know the practice standards or guidelines that define quality. Unit QI committees review activities or services considered to be most important in providing quality care to patients. To identify the greatest opportunity for improving quality, the committees consider activities that are high-volume (greater than 50% of the activity of a unit), high-risk (potential for trauma or death), and problem areas (potential for patient, staff, or institution). TJC's annual National Patient Safety Goals provide another focus for QI committees to explore and identify problem areas (TJC, 2010b) (see Chapter 38). Sometimes the problem is presented to a committee in the form of a sentinel event (i.e., an unexpected occurrence involving death or serious physical or psychological injury). Once a committee defines the problem, it applies a formal model for exploring and resolving quality concerns. There are many models for QI and PI. One model is the PDSA cycle: plan, do, study, and act:

Plan—Review available data to understand existing practice conditions or problems to identify the need for change.

Do—Select an intervention on the basis of the data reviewed and implement the change.

Study—Study (evaluate) the results of the change.

Act—If the process change is successful with positive outcomes, act on the practices by incorporating them into daily unit performance.

Six Sigma or Lean is another quality improvement model. In this model organizations carefully evaluate processes to reduce costs, enhance quality and revenue, and improve teamwork while using the talents of existing employees and the fewest resources. In a lean organization all employees are responsible and accountable for integrating quality improvement methodologies and tools into daily work (Kimsey, 2010).

Some organizations use a quality improvement model called rapid-cycle improvement or rapid-improvement event (RIE). RIEs are very intense, usually week-long events, in which a group gets together to evaluate a problem with the intent of making radical changes to current processes (Kimsey, 2010). Changes are made within a very short time. The effects of the changes are measured quickly, results are evaluated, and further changes are made when necessary. RIE is appropriate to use when a serious problem exists that greatly affects patient safety and needs to be solved quickly.

Once a QI committee makes a practice change, it is important to communicate results to staff in all appropriate organizational departments. Practice changes will likely not last when QI committees fail to report findings and results of interventions. Regular discussions of QI activities through staff meetings, newsletters, and memos are good communication strategies. Often a QI study reveals information that prompts organization-wide change. An organization must be responsible for responding to the problem with the appropriate resources. Revision of policies and procedures, modification of standards of care, and implementation of new support services are examples of ways an organization responds.

KEY POINTS

- A challenge in EBP is to obtain the very best, most current information at the right time, when you need it for patient care.
- Using your clinical expertise and considering patients' values and preferences ensures that you will apply the evidence in practice both safely and appropriately.
- The five steps of EBP provide a systematic approach to rational clinical decision making.
- The more focused a PICOT question is, the easier it will become to search for evidence in the scientific literature.
- The hierarchy of available evidence offers a guide to the types of literature or information that offer the best scientific evidence.
- A randomized controlled trial is the highest level of experimental research.
- Expert clinicians are a rich source of evidence because they use it frequently to build their own practice and solve clinical problems.
- The critique or evaluation of evidence includes determining the value, feasibility, and usefulness of evidence for making a practice change.
- After critiquing all articles for a PICOT question, synthesize or combine the findings to consider the scientific rigor of the evidence and whether it has application in practice.
- When you decide to apply evidence, consider the setting and whether there is support from staff and available resources.
- Research is a systematic process that asks and answers questions that generate knowledge, which provides a scientific basis for nursing practice.
- Outcomes research is designed to assess and document the effectiveness of health care services and interventions.
- Nursing research involves two broad approaches for conducting studies: quantitative and qualitative methods.
- The research process usually consists of the following steps: identifying the problem, designing the study, conducting the study, analyzing the data, and using the findings.
- A thorough analysis of QI data leads clinicians to understand work processes and the need to change practice.

CLINICAL APPLICATION QUESTIONS

Preparing for Clinical Practice

The nursing staff on Rick's postsurgical unit have been reviewing their patients' medical records and have seen a steady increase in the incidence of pressure ulcers over the last 3 months, especially in patients who are incontinent. Rick speaks with the wound care specialist in the hospital about this issue. The specialist recommends that the nurses try using special wipes that include an emollient to clean patients who are incontinent.

1. Rick and the nursing staff decide to approach this practice change using evidence-based practice. What would be a PICOT question for this group to ask? Identify each part of the PICOT question.
2. Rick conducts a literature search and gathers research articles about the PICOT question. He evaluates the scientific merit of each of the articles and determines that he has sufficient evidence to answer the PICOT question. Which step of the evidence-based practice process has Rick completed?
3. Rick and the staff on the postsurgical unit implemented a new skin care protocol for patients who are incontinent after surgery. The protocol has been implemented for 4 months. Rick needs to determine if this practice change has been effective. What outcome does Rick need to measure? Describe one method he could use to measure this outcome.

evolve *Answers to Clinical Application Questions can be found on the Evolve website.*

REVIEW QUESTIONS

Are You Ready to Test Your Nursing Knowledge?

1. A nurse researcher interviews parents of children who have diabetes and asks them to describe how they deal with their child's illness. The analysis of the interviews yields common themes and stories describing the parents' coping strategies. This is an example of which type of study?
   1. Historical
   2. Qualitative
   3. Correlational
   4. Experimental
2. A nurse who works in a newborn nursery asks, "I wonder if the moms who breastfeed their babies would be able to breastfeed more successfully if we played peaceful music while they were breastfeeding." In this example of a PICOT question, the *I* is:
   1. Breastfeeding moms.
   2. Infants.
   3. Peaceful music.
   4. The nursery.
3. A nurse researcher conducts a study that randomly assigns 100 patients who smoke and attend a wellness clinic into two groups. One group receives the standard smoking cessation handouts; the other group takes part in a new educational program that includes a smoking cessation support group. The nurse plans to compare the effectiveness of the standard

treatment with the educational program. What type of a research study is this?
1. Qualitative
2. Descriptive
3. Correlational
4. Randomized controlled trial

4. A group of nurses have implemented an evidence-based practice (EBP) change and have evaluated the effectiveness of the change. Their next step is to:
1. Conduct a literature review.
2. Share the findings with others.
3. Conduct a statistical analysis.
4. Create a well-defined PICOT question.

5. Arrange the following steps of evidence-based practice (EBP) in the appropriate order:
1. Integrate the evidence.
2. Ask the burning clinical question.
3. Evaluate the practice decision or change.
4. Share the results with others.
5. Critically appraise the evidence you gather.
6. Collect the most relevant and best evidence.

6. When recruiting subjects to participate in a study about the effects of an exercise program on balance, the researcher provides full and complete information about the purpose of the study and gives the subjects the choice to participate or not participate in the study. This is an example of:
1. Bias.
2. Anonymity.
3. Confidentiality.
4. Informed consent.

7. Nurses on a pediatric nursing unit are discussing ways to improve patient care. One nurse asks a colleague, "I wonder how best to measure pain in a child who has sickle cell disease?" This question is an example of a/an:
1. Hypothesis.
2. PICOT question.
3. Problem-focused trigger.
4. Knowledge-focused trigger.

8. The nurses on a medical unit have seen an increase in the number of pressure ulcers that develop in their patients. They decide to initiate a quality improvement project using the PDSA model. Which of the following is an example of "Do" from that model?
1. Implement the new skin care protocol on all medicine units.
2. Review the data collected on patients cared for using the protocol.
3. Review the QI reports on the six patients who developed ulcers over the last 3 months.
4. Based on findings from patients who developed ulcers, implement an evidence-based skin care protocol.

9. A nurse researcher decides to complete a study to evaluate how Florence Nightingale improved patient outcomes in the Crimean War. This is an example of what type of research?
1. Historical
2. Evaluation
3. Exploratory
4. Experimental

10. A group of nurses on the research council of a local hospital are measuring nursing-sensitive outcomes. Which of the following is a nursing-sensitive outcome that the nurses need to consider measuring?
1. Incidence of asthma among children of parents who smoke
2. Frequency of low blood sugar episodes in children at a local school
3. Number of patients who fall and experience subsequent injury on the evening shift
4. Number of sexually active adolescent girls who attend the community-based clinic for birth control

11. A group of staff nurses notice an increased incidence of medication errors on their unit. After further investigation it is determined that the nurses are not consistently identifying the patient correctly. A change is needed quickly. What type of quality improvement method would be most appropriate?
1. PDSA
2. Six Sigma
3. Rapid-improvement event
4. A randomized controlled trial

12. A nurse is providing care to a patient who is experiencing major abdominal trauma following a car accident. The patient is losing blood quickly and needs a blood transfusion. The nurse finds out that the patient is a Jehovah's Witness and cannot have blood transfusions because of religious beliefs. He or she notifies the patient's health care provider and receives an order to give the patient an alternative to blood products. This is an example of:
1. A quality improvement study.
2. An evidence-based practice change.
3. A time when calling the hospital's ethics committee is essential.
4. Considering the patient's preferences and values while providing care.

13. A group of staff educators are reading a research study together at a journal club meeting. While reviewing the study, one of the nurses states that it evaluates if newly graduated nurses progress through orientation more effectively when they participate in patient simulation exercises. Which part of the research process is reflected in this nurse's statement?
1. Introduction
2. Purpose statement
3. Methods
4. Results

14. A research study is investigating the following research question: What is the effect of the diagnosis of breast cancer on the roles of the family? In this study "the diagnosis of breast cancer" and "family roles" are examples of:
1. Surveys
2. The sample
3. Variables
4. Data collection points

15. A nurse researcher is developing a research proposal and is in the process of selecting an instrument to measure anxiety. In which part of the research process is this nurse?
1. Analyzing the data
2. Designing the study
3. Conducting the study
4. Identifying the problem

Answers: **1.** 2; **2.** 3; **3.** 4; **4.** 2; **5.** 2, 6, 5, 1, 3, 4; **6.** 4; **7.** 4; **8.** 1; **9.** 1; **10.** 3; **11.** 3; **12.** 4; **13.** 2; **14.** 3; **15.** 2.

REFERENCES

Ingersoll GL, et al: Meeting Magnet® research and evidence-based practice expectations through hospital-based research centers, *Nurs Econ* 28(4):226, 2010.

International Council of Nurses: *Nursing research: ICN position statement, 2007*, http://www.icn.ch/images/stories/documents/publications/position_statements/B05_Nsg_Research.pdf. Accessed June 23, 2011.

Kimsey DB: Lean methodology in health care, *AORN J* 92(1):53, 2010.

Makadon HJ, et al: Value management: optimizing quality, service, and cost, *J Healthc Qual* 32(1):29, 2010.

Melnyk BM, Fineout-Overholt E: *Evidence-based practice in nursing and healthcare: a guide to best practice*, ed 2, Philadelphia, 2011, Lippincott Williams & Wilkins.

Montalvo I: The National Database of Nursing Quality Indicators (NDNQI), *Online J Issues Nurs* 12(3), 2007, http://www.nursingworld.org/MainMenuCategories/ANAMarketplace/ANAPeriodicals/OJIN/TableofContents/Volume122007/No3Sept07/NursingQualityIndicators.aspx. Accessed October 14, 2010.

Oncology Nursing Society: *Evidence-based practice resource area*, n.d., http://onsopcontent.ons.org/toolkits/evidence/. Accessed October 2010.

Polit DF, Beck CT: *Nursing research: generating and assessing evidence for nursing practice*, ed 8, Philadelphia, 2007, Lippincott Williams & Wilkins.

Sackett DL, et al: *Evidence-based medicine: how to practice and teach EBM*, London, 2000, Churchill Livingstone.

Stilwell SB, et al: Asking the clinical question: a key step in evidence-based practice, *Am J Nurs* 110(3):58, 2010.

The Joint Commission (TJC): *Performance measurement*, 2010a, http://www.jointcommission.org/PerformanceMeasurement/. Accessed October 16, 2010.

The Joint Commission (TJC): *2010 National Patient Safety Goals (NPSGs)*, 2010b, http://www.jointcommission.org/PatientSafety/NationalPatientSafetyGoals/. Accessed October 16, 2010.

RESEARCH REFERENCES

Massey RL: A randomized trial of rocking-chair motion on the effect of postoperative ileus duration in patients with cancer recovering from abdominal surgery, *Appl Nurs Res* 23(2):59, 2010.

Metheny N, et al: Measures to test placement of nasogastric and nasointestinal feeding tubers: a review, *Nurs Res* 37:324, 1988.

Metheny N, et al: Effectiveness of pH measurement in predicting feeding tube placement, *Nurs Res* 38(5):262, 1989.

Metheny N, et al: Effectiveness of the auscultatory method in predicting feeding tube location, *Nurs Res* 39(5):262, 1990.

Metheny N, et al: Visual characteristics of aspirates from feeding tubes as a method for predicting tube location, *Nurs Res* 43:282, 1994.

Metheny N, et al: Development of a reliable and valid bedside test for bilirubin and its utilization for improving prediction of feeding tube location, *Nurs Res* 49(6):202, 2000.

Moore CL, et al: Clinical process variation: effect on quality and cost of care, *Am J Managed Care* 16(5):385, 2010.

Moore L, et al: Investigation of rocking as a postoperative intervention to promote gastrointestinal motility, *Gastroenterol Nurs* 18(3):87, 1995.

Nixon A, Narayanasamy A: The spiritual needs of neuro-oncology patients from patients' perspective, *J Clin Nurs* 19(15–16):2259, 2010.

Oh EG, et al: Integrating evidence-based practice into RN-to-BSN clinical nursing education, *J Nurs Ed* 49(7):387, 2010.

Scott K, McSherry R: Evidence-based nursing: clarifying the concepts for nurses in practice, *J Clin Nurs* 18(8):1085, 2009.

Thomas L, et al: The effects of rocking, diet modifications, and antiflatulant medication of postcesarean section gas pain, *J Perinatal Neonatal Nurs* 4(3):12, 1990.

Titler MG, et al: The Iowa model of evidence-based practice to promote quality care, *Crit Care Clin North Am* 13(4):497, 2001.

CHAPTER

6

Health and Wellness

OBJECTIVES

- List the two general *Healthy People 2020* public health goals for Americans.
- Discuss the definition of health.
- Discuss the health belief, health promotion, basic human needs, and holistic health models to understand the relationship between the patient's attitudes toward health and health practices.
- Describe variables influencing health beliefs and practices.
- Describe health promotion, wellness, and illness prevention activities.
- Discuss the three levels of preventive care.
- Describe four types of risk factors.
- Discuss risk factor modification and changing health behaviors.
- Describe variables influencing illness behavior.
- Describe the impact of illness on the patient and family.
- Discuss the nurse's role in health and illness.

KEY TERMS

Active strategies of health promotion, p. 71
Acute illness, p. 74
Chronic illness, p. 74
Health, p. 66
Health behavior change, p. 73
Health behaviors, p. 66
Health belief model, p. 66
Health promotion, p. 70
Holistic health model, p. 67
Illness, p. 73
Illness behavior, p. 74
Illness prevention, p. 71
Passive strategies of health promotion, p. 71
Primary prevention, p. 71
Risk factor, p. 71
Secondary prevention, p. 71
Tertiary prevention, p. 71
Wellness, p. 71

evolve WEBSITE

http://evolve.elsevier.com/Potter/fundamentals/

- Review Questions
- Case Study with Questions
- Audio Glossary
- Interactive Learning Activities
- Key Term Flashcards
- Content Updates

In the past most individuals and societies viewed good health, or wellness, as the opposite or absence of disease. This simple attitude ignores states of health between disease and good health. Health is a multidimensional concept and is viewed from a broader perspective. An assessment of the patient's state of health is an important aspect of nursing.

Models of health offer a perspective to understand the relationships between the concepts of health, wellness, and illness. Nurses are in a unique position to help patients achieve and maintain optimal levels of health. They need to understand the challenges of today's health care system and embrace the opportunities to promote health and wellness and prevent illness. In an era of cost containment and advanced technology, nurses are a vital link to the improved health of individuals and society. They identify actual and potential risk factors that predispose a person or a group to illness. In addition, the nurse uses risk factor modification strategies to promote health and wellness and prevent illness.

Different attitudes cause people to react in different ways to illness or the illness of a family member. Medical sociologists call this reaction *illness behavior*. Nurses who understand how patients react to illness can minimize its effects and help patients and their families maintain or return to the highest level of functioning.

HEALTHY PEOPLE DOCUMENTS

Healthy People provides science-based, 10-year national objectives for promoting health and preventing disease. In 1979 an influential document, *Healthy People: the Surgeon General's Report on Health Promotion and Disease Prevention,* was published; it introduced a goal for improving the health of Americans by 1990. The report outlined priority objectives for preventive services, health protection, and health promotion that addressed improvements in health status, risk reduction, public and professional awareness of prevention, health services and protective measures, and surveillance and evaluation. The report served as a framework for the 1990s as the United States increased the focus on health promotion and disease prevention instead of illness care. The strategy announced by the Secretary of Health and Human Services required a cooperative effort by government, voluntary and professional organizations, businesses, and individuals. Widely cited by popular media, in professional journals, and at health conferences, it has inspired health promotion programs throughout the country.

Healthy People 2000: National Health Promotion and Disease Prevention Objectives, published in 1990, identified health improvement goals and objectives to be reached by the year 2000 (U.S. Department of Health and Human Services [USDHHS, Public Health Service], 1990). *Healthy People 2010,* published in 2000, served as a road map for improving the health of all people in the United States for the first decade of the twenty-first century (USDHHS, 2000). This edition emphasized the link between individual health and community health and the premise that the health of communities determines the overall health status of the nation. *Healthy People 2020* was approved in December 2010. *Healthy People 2020* promotes a society in which all people live long, healthy lives. There are four overarching goals: (1) attain high-quality, longer lives free of preventable disease, disability, injury, and premature death; (2) achieve health equity, eliminate disparities, and improve the health of all groups; (3) create social and physical environments that promote good health for all; and (4) promote quality of life, healthy development, and healthy behaviors across all life stages (USDHHS, 2011).

DEFINITION OF HEALTH

Defining health is difficult. The World Health Organization (WHO) defines **health** as a "state of complete physical, mental, and social well-being, not merely the absence of disease or infirmity" (WHO, 1947). Many other aspects of health need to be considered. Health is a state of being that people define in relation to their own values, personality, and lifestyle. Each person has a personal concept of health. Pender, Murdaugh, and Parsons (2011) define health as the actualization of inherent and acquired human potential through goal-directed behavior, competent self-care, and satisfying relationships with others while adjustments are made as needed to maintain structural integrity and harmony with the environment.

Individuals' views of health vary among different age-groups, genders, races, and cultures (Pender, Murdaugh, and Parsons, 2011). Pender (1996) explains that "all people free of disease are not equally healthy." Views of health have broadened to include mental, social, and spiritual well-being and a focus on health at the family and community levels (Pender, Murdaugh, and Parsons, 2006).

To help patients identify and reach health goals, nurses discover and use information about their concepts of health. Pender, Murdaugh, and Parsons (2011) suggest that for many people conditions of life rather than pathological states define health. Life conditions can have positive or negative effects on health long before an illness is evident (Pender, Murdaugh, and Parsons, 2011). Life conditions include socioeconomic variables such as environment, diet, and lifestyle practices or choices and many other physiological and psychological variables.

Health and illness are defined according to individual perception. Health often includes conditions previously considered to be illness. For example, a person with epilepsy who has learned to control seizures with medication and who functions at home and work may no longer consider himself or herself ill. Nurses need to consider the total person and the environment in which the person lives to individualize nursing care and enhance meaningfulness of the patient's future health status.

MODELS OF HEALTH AND ILLNESS

A model is a theoretical way of understanding a concept or idea. Models represent different ways of approaching complex issues. Because health and illness are complex concepts, models are used to understand the relationships between these concepts and the patient's attitudes toward health and **health behaviors.**

Health beliefs are a person's ideas, convictions, and attitudes about health and illness. They may be based on factual information or misinformation, common sense or myths, or reality or false expectations. Because health beliefs usually influence health behavior, they can positively or negatively affect a patient's level of health. Positive health behaviors are activities related to maintaining, attaining, or regaining good health and preventing illness. Common positive health behaviors include immunizations, proper sleep patterns, adequate exercise, stress management, and nutrition. Negative health behaviors include practices actually or potentially harmful to health such as smoking, drug or alcohol abuse, poor diet, and refusal to take necessary medications.

Nurses developed the following health models to understand patients' attitudes and values about health and illness and to provide effective health care. These nursing models allow you to understand and predict patients' health behavior, including how they use health services and adhere to recommended therapy.

Health Belief Model

Rosenstoch's (1974) and Becker and Maiman's (1975) **health belief model** (Fig. 6-1) addresses the relationship between a person's beliefs and behaviors. The health belief model helps you understand factors influencing patients' perceptions, beliefs, and behavior to plan care that will most effectively assist patients in maintaining or restoring health and preventing illness (Box 6-1).

The first component of this model involves an individual's perception of susceptibility to an illness. For example, a patient needs to recognize the familial link for coronary artery disease. After this link is recognized, particularly when one parent and two siblings have died in their fourth decade from myocardial infarction, the patient may perceive the personal risk of heart disease.

The second component is an individual's perception of the seriousness of the illness. This perception is influenced and modified by demographic and sociopsychological variables, perceived threats of the illness, and cues to action (e.g., mass media campaigns and advice from family, friends, and medical professionals). For example, a patient may not perceive his heart disease to be serious, which may affect the way he takes care of himself.

The third component—the likelihood that a person will take preventive action—results from a person's perception of the benefits of and barriers to taking action. Preventive actions include lifestyle changes, increased adherence to medical therapies, or a search for medical advice or treatment. A patient's perception of susceptibility to disease and his or her perception of the seriousness of an illness help to determine the likelihood that the patient will or will not partake in healthy behaviors.

Health Promotion Model

The health promotion model (HPM) proposed by Pender (1982; revised, 1996) was designed to be a "complementary counterpart to models of health protection" (Fig. 6-2). It defines health as a positive, dynamic state, not merely the absence of disease (Pender, Murdaugh, and Parsons, 2011). Health promotion is directed at increasing a patient's level of well-being. The HPM describes the multidimensional nature of persons as they interact within their environment to pursue health (Pender, 1996; Pender, Murdaugh, and Parsons, 2011). The model focuses on the following three areas: (1) individual characteristics and experiences, (2) behavior-specific knowledge and affect, and (3) behavioral outcomes. The

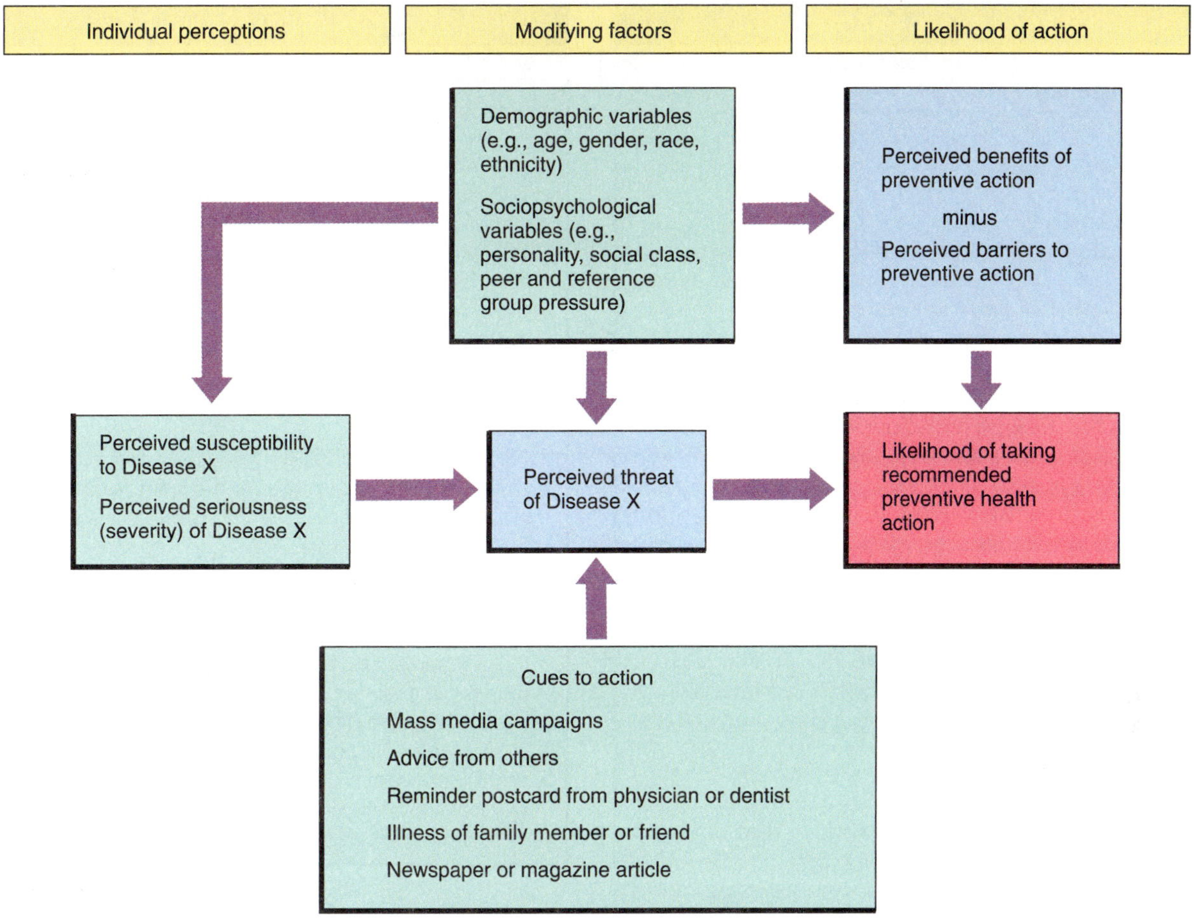

FIG. 6-1 Health belief model. (Data from Becker M, Maiman L: Sociobehavioral determinants of compliance with health and medical care recommendations, *Med Care* 13[1]:10, 1975.)

HPM notes that each person has unique personal characteristics and experiences that affect subsequent actions. The set of variables for behavioral-specific knowledge and affect have important motivational significance. These variables can be modified through nursing actions. Health-promoting behavior is the desired behavioral outcome and is the end point in the HPM. Health-promoting behaviors result in improved health, enhanced functional ability, and better quality of life at all stages of development (Pender, Murdaugh, and Parsons, 2011) (Box 6-2).

Maslow's Hierarchy of Needs

Basic human needs are elements that are necessary for human survival and health (e.g., food, water, safety, and love). Although each person has other unique needs, all people share the basic human needs, and the extent to which basic needs are met is a major factor in determining a person's level of health.

Maslow's hierarchy of needs is a model that nurses use to understand the interrelationships of basic human needs (Fig. 6-3). According to this model, certain human needs are more basic than others (i.e., some needs must be met before other needs [e.g., fulfilling the physiological needs before the needs of love and belonging]). Self-actualization is the highest expression of one's individual potential and allows for continual discovery of self. Maslow's model takes into account individual experiences, always unique to the individual (Ebersole et al., 2008).

The hierarchy of needs model provides a basis for nurses to care for patients of all ages in all health settings. However, when applying the model, the focus of care is on the patient's needs rather than on strict adherence to the hierarchy. It is unrealistic to always expect a patient's basic needs to occur in the fixed hierarchical order. In all cases an emergent physiological need takes precedence over a higher-level need. In other situations a psychological or physical safety need takes priority. For example, in a house fire fear of injury and death takes priority over self-esteem issues. Although it would seem that a patient who has just had surgery might have the strongest need for pain control in the psychosocial area, if the patient just had a mastectomy, her main need may be in the areas of love, belonging, and self-esteem. It is important not to assume the patient's needs just because other patients reacted in a certain way. Maslow's hierarchy can be very useful when applied to each patient individually. To provide the most effective care, you need to understand the relationships of different needs and the factors that determine the priorities for each patient.

Holistic Health Models

Health care has begun to take a more holistic view of health by considering emotional and spiritual well-being and other dimensions of an individual as important aspects of physical wellness. The **holistic health model** of nursing attempts to create conditions that promote optimal health. In this model, nurses using the

BOX 6-1 EVIDENCE-BASED PRACTICE

Mammography Practices in Asian-American Immigrant Women

PICO Question: What sociocultural factors affect mammography screening practices in women who are Asian-American?

Evidence Summary

Breast cancer is a leading cause of cancer deaths in women. Routine screening with mammograms is the recommended practice for early breast cancer detection. Asian women are more likely to not use mammograms for screening, to have breast cancer diagnosed at a later stage, and to have larger tumors at diagnosis (Lee et al., 2009; Lee-Lin et al., 2007; Wu and Ronis, 2009). The health belief model was used to examine the women's knowledge and perceptions about developing breast cancer and preventive actions taken such as mammography. Results showed that only approximately 50% of the women studied had a mammogram in the last year (Lee et al., 2009; Lee-Lin et al., 2007; Wu and Ronis, 2009). Findings showed that the length of time the woman lived in the United States, having a recommendation from a health care provider, and insurance coverage were significantly related to having a mammogram (Lee-Lin et al., 2007). Other factors that contributed to having a mammogram included age, education, a higher perceived benefit to having the test, and higher levels of perceived risk of cancer (Wu and Ronis, 2009). The top three identified barriers to having a mammogram were remembering to have one, a belief that a mammogram is painful, and worry about radiation exposure (Lee-Lin et al., 2007).

Application to Nursing Practice

- Assess misconceptions that women hold related to breast cancer and mammogram screening (Wu and Ronis, 2009).
- Develop culturally tailored interventions for immigrants who speak limited English (Lee et al., 2009).
- Primary health care workers need to educate women about the American Cancer Society guidelines for mammogram screening (Lee-Lin et al., 2007).
- Assess the barriers that the women identified to increase likelihood of obtaining mammograms (Lee-Lin et al., 2007).
- Develop strategies to increase screening rates for at-risk subgroups such as recent immigrants (Wu and Ronis, 2009).
- Consider the woman's perceived susceptibility to breast cancers and perceived benefit of screening when planning education (Lee et al., 2009).

BOX 6-2 FOCUS ON OLDER ADULTS

Health Promotion

- Promote healthy lifestyles by encouraging regular physical activity, accepting responsibility for one's own health, using stress management strategies, focusing on self-care abilities, and practicing relaxation (Lee and Park, 2006; Pender, Murdaugh, and Parsons, 2011).
- Consider the older adult's social environment and strengthening social support to promote health and provide access to resources (Callaghan, 2005; Ebersole et al., 2008).
- Use a holistic approach to promoting health. The focus is not on absence of disease but on achieving the highest level of health in the presence of disease (Ebersole et al., 2008).
- Injury prevention is a key strategy to promote and improve health (Ebersole et al., 2008).
- Fear of falling is a significant risk related to older adults' avoidance of physical activity. Assess for the fear and provide support, make environmental changes to help decrease falls, and provide assistive devices as needed (Bertera and Bertera, 2008).
- Factors that have been reported to affect older adults' willingness to engage in health promotion activities may include socioeconomic factors, beliefs and attitudes for patients and providers, encouragement by a health care professional, specific motivation based on efficacy beliefs, access to resources, age, number of chronic illnesses, mental and physical health, marital status, ability for self-care, gender, education, and support system presence (Byam-Williams and Salyer, 2010; Callaghan, 2005).
- Scientific evidence increasingly indicates that physical activity can extend years of active independent life, reduce disability, and improve the quality of life for older persons (Chodzko-Zajko et al., 2009).

nursing process consider patients to be the ultimate experts concerning their own health and respect patients' subjective experience as relevant in maintaining health or assisting in healing. In the holistic health model patients are involved in their healing process, thereby assuming some responsibility for health maintenance (Edelman and Mandle, 2010).

Nurses using the holistic nursing model recognize the natural healing abilities of the body and incorporate complementary and alternative interventions such as music therapy, reminiscence, relaxation therapy, therapeutic touch, and guided imagery because they are effective, economical, noninvasive, nonpharmacological complements to traditional medical care (see Chapter 32). These holistic strategies, which can be used in all stages of health and illness, are integral in the expanding role of nursing.

Nurses use holistic therapies either alone or in conjunction with conventional medicine. For example, they use reminiscence in the geriatric population to help relieve anxiety for a patient dealing with memory loss or for a cancer patient dealing with the difficult side effects of chemotherapy. Music therapy in the operating room creates a soothing environment. Relaxation therapy is frequently useful to distract a patient during a painful procedure such as a dressing change. Breathing exercises are commonly taught to help patients deal with the pain associated with labor and delivery.

VARIABLES INFLUENCING HEALTH AND HEALTH BELIEFS AND PRACTICES

Many variables influence a patient's health beliefs and practices. Internal and external variables influence how a person thinks and acts. As previously stated, health beliefs usually influence health behavior or health practices and likewise positively or negatively affect a patient's level of health. Therefore understanding the effects of these variables allows you to plan and deliver individualized care.

Internal Variables

Internal variables include a person's developmental stage, intellectual background, perception of functioning, and emotional and spiritual factors.

Developmental Stage. A person's thought and behavior patterns change throughout life. The nurse considers the patient's level of growth and development when using his or her health beliefs and practices as a basis for planning care. The study of development involves finding patterns or general principles that apply to most people most of the time (Murray et al., 2008). The concept of illness for a child, adolescent, or adult depends on the

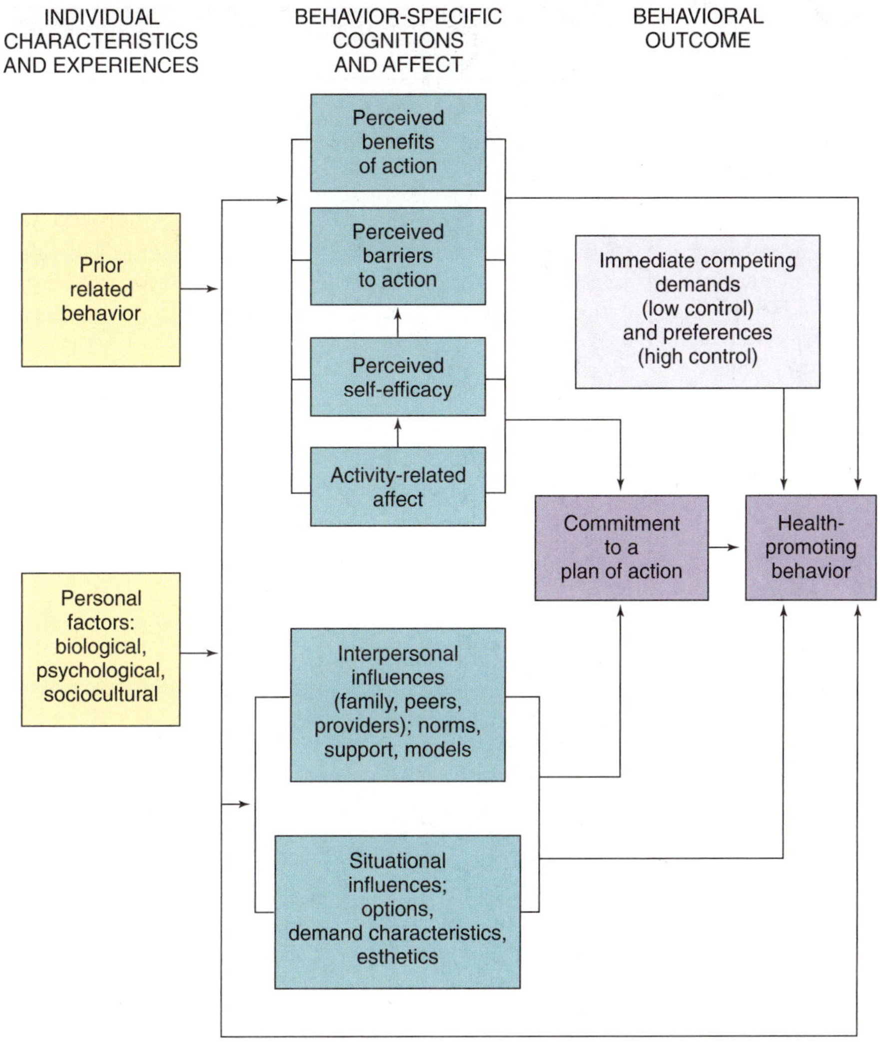

FIG. 6-2 Health promotion model (revised). (Redrawn from Pender NJ, Murdaugh CL, Parsons MA: *Health promotion in nursing practice,* ed 5, Upper Saddle River, NJ, 2006, Prentice Hall.)

individual's developmental stage. Fear and anxiety are common among ill children, especially if thoughts about illness, hospitalization, or procedures are based on lack of information or lack of clarity of information. Emotional development may also influence personal beliefs about health-related matters. For example, you use different techniques for teaching about contraception to an adolescent than you use for an adult. Knowledge of the stages of growth and development helps predict the patient's response to the present illness or the threat of future illness. Adapt the planning of nursing care to these expectations and to the patient's abilities to participate in self-care.

Intellectual Background. A person's beliefs about health are shaped in part by the person's knowledge, lack of knowledge, or incorrect information about body functions and illnesses, educational background, and past experiences. These variables influence how a patient thinks about health. In addition, cognitive abilities shape the *way* a person thinks, including the ability to understand factors involved in illness and apply knowledge of health and illness to personal health practices. Cognitive abilities also relate to a person's developmental stage. A nurse considers intellectual background so these variables can be incorporated into nursing care (Edelman and Mandle, 2010).

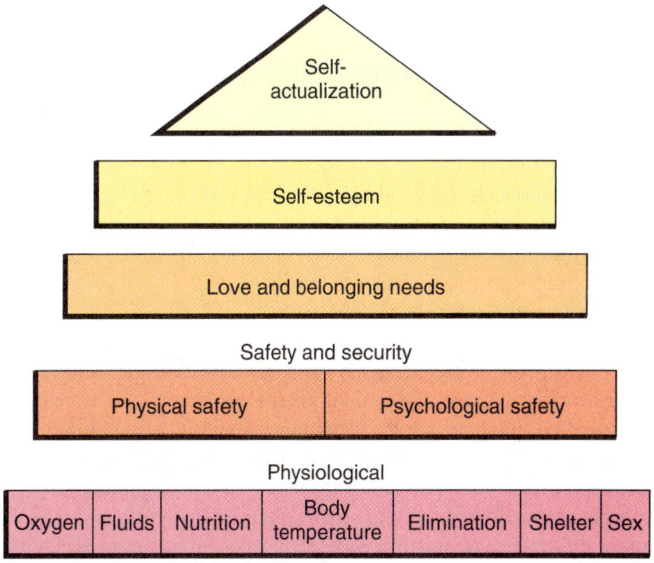

FIG. 6-3 Maslow's hierarchy of needs. (Redrawn from Maslow AH: *Motivation and personality,* ed 3, Upper Saddle River, NJ, 1970, Prentice Hall.)

Perception of Functioning. The way people perceive their physical functioning affects health beliefs and practices. When you assess a patient's level of health, gather subjective data about the way the patient perceives physical functioning such as level of fatigue, shortness of breath, or pain. Then obtain objective data about actual functioning such as blood pressure, height measurements, and lung sound assessment. This information allows you to more successfully plan and implement individualized care.

Emotional Factors. The patient's degree of stress, depression, or fear can influence health beliefs and practices. The manner in which a person handles stress throughout each phase of life influences the way he or she reacts to illness. A person who generally is very calm may have little emotional response during illness, whereas an individual unable to cope emotionally with the threat of illness may either overreact to it and assume that it is life threatening or deny the presence of symptoms and not take therapeutic action (see Chapter 37).

Spiritual Factors. Spirituality is reflected in how a person lives his or her life, including the values and beliefs exercised, the relationships established with family and friends, and the ability to find hope and meaning in life. Spirituality serves as an integrating theme in people's lives (see Chapter 35). Religious practices are one way that people exercise spirituality. Some religions restrict the use of certain forms of medical treatment. You need to understand patients' spiritual dimensions to involve patients effectively in nursing care.

External Variables

External variables influencing a person's health beliefs and practices include family practices, socioeconomic factors, and cultural background.

Family Practices. The way that patients' families use health care services generally affects their health practices. Their perceptions of the seriousness of diseases and their history of preventive care behaviors (or lack of them) influence how patients think about health. For example, if a young woman's mother never had annual gynecological examinations or Papanicolaou (Pap) smears, it is unlikely that the daughter will have annual Pap smears.

Socioeconomic Factors. Social and psychosocial factors increase the risk for illness and influence the way that a person defines and reacts to illness. Psychosocial variables include the stability of the person's marital or intimate relationship, lifestyle habits, and occupational environment. A person generally seeks approval and support from social networks (neighbors, peers, and co-workers), and this desire for approval and support affects health beliefs and practices.

Social variables partly determine how the health care system provides medical care. The organization of the health care system determines how patients can obtain care, the treatment method, the economic cost to the patient, and potential reimbursement to the health care agency or patient.

Like social variables, economic variables often affect a patient's level of health by increasing the risk for disease and influencing how or at what point the patient enters the health care system. A person's compliance with a treatment designed to maintain or improve health is also affected by economic status. A person who has high utility bills, a large family, and a low income tends to give a higher priority to food and shelter than to costly drugs or treatment or expensive foods for special diets. Some patients decide to take medications every other day rather than every day as prescribed to save money, which greatly affects the effectiveness of the medications.

BOX 6-3 CULTURAL ASPECTS OF CARE

Cultural Health Beliefs

The cultural and ethnic backgrounds of patients shape their views of health, how to treat and prevent illness, and what constitutes good care (Narayan, 2010). Health and illness beliefs often fall into magicoreligious, biomedical, and deterministic beliefs (Singleton and Krause, 2009). The magicoreligious belief is often seen in Latin American, African American, and Middle Eastern cultures. These beliefs focus on hexes (i.e., supernatural forces that cause illness) (Yeo, 2009). Illness may also be viewed as a punishment for sins, or it can focus on evil spirits or disease-bearing foreign objects. The biomedical belief system, seen in the United States, believes that health and illness are related to physical and biochemical processes, with disease being a breakdown of the processes. The belief of determinism focuses on outcomes that are externally preordained and cannot be changed (Singleton and Krause, 2009). Other examples of cultural beliefs that affect health care practices include yin/yang balance, free flow of chi, influence of humors, the importance of hexes, and spirits and soul loss (Yeo, 2009). Recognizing the patient's health beliefs helps the nurse provide holistic nursing care that considers the physical, psychological, social, emotional, and spiritual needs of each patient (Maier-Lorentz, 2008).

Implications for Practice

- Be aware of the impact of culture on a patient's view and understanding of illness.
- Focus on understanding the patient's traditions, values, and beliefs and how these dimensions may affect health, wellness, and illness.
- Do not stereotype a patient based on his or her culture and assume that they will adopt all cultural beliefs and practices (Narayan, 2010).
- When teaching patients about their illness and treatment regimens, it is important for nurses to understand that unique cultural perceptions exist regarding the cause of an illness and its treatment.
- Use a trained interpreter if possible when the patient and family do not speak English to avoid misinterpretation of information (Yeo, 2009).
- Be aware of your own cultural background and recognize prejudices that may lead to stereotyping and discrimination (Maier-Lorentz, 2008).

Cultural Background. Cultural background influences beliefs, values, and customs. It influences the approach to the health care system, personal health practices, and the nurse-patient relationship. Cultural background also influences an individual's beliefs about causes of illness and remedies or practices to restore health (Box 6-3). If you are not aware of your own cultural patterns of behavior and language, you will have difficulty recognizing and understanding your patient's behaviors and beliefs. You will also probably have difficulty interacting with patients. As with family and socioeconomic variables, you need to incorporate cultural variables into a patient's care plan (see Chapter 9).

HEALTH PROMOTION, WELLNESS, AND ILLNESS PREVENTION

Health care has become increasingly focused on health promotion, wellness, and illness prevention. The rapid rise of health care costs has motivated people to seek ways of decreasing the incidence and minimizing the results of illness or disability.

The concepts of health promotion, wellness, and illness prevention are closely related and in practice overlap to some extent. All are focused on the future; the difference among them involves motivations and goals. **Health promotion** activities such as routine exercise and good nutrition help patients maintain or enhance their present levels of health. They motivate people to act positively to reach more stable levels of health. **Wellness** education teaches people how to care for themselves in a healthy way and includes topics such as physical awareness, stress management, and self-responsibility. Wellness strategies help people achieve new understanding and control of their lives. **Illness prevention** activities such as immunization programs protect patients from actual or potential threats to health. They motivate people to avoid declines in health or functional levels.

Nurses emphasize health promotion activities, wellness-enhancing strategies, and illness prevention activities as important forms of health care because they assist patients in maintaining and improving health. The goal of a total health program is to improve a patient's level of well-being in all dimensions, not just physical health. Total health programs are based on the belief that many factors can affect a person's level of health.

Examples of the health topics and objectives as defined by *Healthy People 2020* include physical activity, adolescent health, tobacco use, substance abuse, sexually transmitted diseases, mental health and mental disorders, injury and violence prevention, environmental health, immunization and infectious disease, and access to health care (USDHHS, 2011). A complete list of topics and objectives is available on the *Healthy People* website (www.healthypeople.gov). These objectives and topics show the importance of health promotion and illness prevention and encourage all to participate in the improvement of health.

Individual practices such as poor eating habits and little or no exercise influence health. Physical stressors such as a poor living environment, exposure to air pollutants, and an unsafe environment also affect health. Hereditary and psychological stressors such as emotional, intellectual, social, developmental, and spiritual factors influence one's level of health. Total health programs are directed at individuals' changing their lifestyles by developing habits that improve their level of health.

Other programs are aimed at specific health care problems. For example, support groups help people with human immunodeficiency virus (HIV) infection. Exercise programs encourage participants to exercise regularly to reduce their risk of cardiac disease. Stress-reduction programs teach participants to cope with stressors and reduce their risks for multiple illnesses such as infections, gastrointestinal disease, and cardiac disease.

Some health promotion, wellness education, and illness prevention programs are operated by health care agencies; others are operated independently. Many businesses have on-site health promotion activities for employees. Likewise, colleges and community centers offer health promotion and illness prevention programs. Some nurses actively participate in these programs, providing direct care, and others act as consultants or refer patients to these programs. The goal of these activities is to improve a patient's level of health through preventive health services, environmental protection, and health education.

Health care professionals who work in the field of health promotion use proactive attempts to prevent illness or disease. Health promotion activities are passive or active. With **passive strategies of health promotion,** individuals gain from the activities of others without acting themselves. The fluoridation of municipal drinking water and the fortification of homogenized milk with vitamin D are examples of passive health promotion strategies. With **active strategies of health promotion,** individuals are motivated to adopt specific health programs. Weight-reduction and smoking-cessation programs require patients to be actively involved in measures to improve their present and future levels of wellness while decreasing the risk of disease.

Health promotion is a process of helping people improve their health to reach an optimal state of physical, mental, and social well-being (WHO, 2009). An individual takes responsibility for health and wellness by making appropriate lifestyle choices. Lifestyle choices are important because they affect a person's quality of life and well-being. Making positive lifestyle choices and avoiding negative lifestyle choices also plays a role in preventing illness. In addition to improving quality of life, preventing illness has an economic impact because it decreases health care costs.

Levels of Preventive Care

Nursing care oriented to health promotion, wellness, and illness prevention is described in terms of health activities on primary, secondary, and tertiary levels (Table 6-1).

Primary Prevention. **Primary prevention** is true prevention; it precedes disease or dysfunction and is applied to patients considered physically and emotionally healthy. Primary prevention aimed at health promotion includes health education programs, immunizations, and physical and nutritional fitness activities. Primary prevention includes all health promotion efforts and wellness education activities that focus on maintaining or improving the general health of individuals, families, and communities (Edelman and Mandle, 2010). Primary prevention includes specific protection such as immunization for influenza and hearing protection in occupational settings.

Secondary Prevention. **Secondary prevention** focuses on individuals who are experiencing health problems or illnesses and are at risk for developing complications or worsening conditions. Activities are directed at diagnosis and prompt intervention, thereby reducing severity and enabling the patient to return to a normal level of health as early as possible (Edelman and Mandle, 2010). A large portion of nursing care related to secondary prevention is delivered in homes, hospitals, or skilled nursing facilities. It includes screening techniques and treating early stages of disease to limit disability by averting or delaying the consequences of advanced disease. Screening activities also become a key opportunity for health teaching as a primary prevention intervention (Edelman and Mandle, 2010).

Tertiary Prevention. **Tertiary prevention** occurs when a defect or disability is permanent and irreversible. It involves minimizing the effects of long-term disease or disability by interventions directed at preventing complications and deterioration (Edelman and Mandle, 2010). Activities are directed at rehabilitation rather than diagnosis and treatment. Care at this level helps patients achieve as high a level of functioning as possible, despite the limitations caused by illness or impairment. This level of care is called preventive care because it involves preventing further disability or reduced functioning.

RISK FACTORS

A **risk factor** is any situation, habit, social or environmental condition, physiological or psychological condition, developmental or intellectual condition, spiritual condition, or other variable that increases the vulnerability of an individual or group to an illness or accident. Risk factors, behavior, risk factor modification, and behavior modification are integral components of health promotion, wellness, and illness prevention activities. Nurses in all areas of practice often have opportunities to help patients adopt activities to promote health and decrease risks of illness.

TABLE 6-1 Three Levels of Prevention

PRIMARY PREVENTION		SECONDARY PREVENTION		TERTIARY PREVENTION
HEALTH PROMOTION	SPECIFIC PROTECTION	EARLY DIAGNOSIS AND PROMPT TREATMENT	DISABILITY LIMITATIONS	RESTORATION AND REHABILITATION
Health education Good standard of nutrition adjusted to developmental phases of life Attention to personality development Provision of adequate housing and recreation and agreeable working conditions Marriage counseling and sex education Genetic screening Periodic selective examinations	Use of specific immunizations Attention to personal hygiene Use of environmental sanitation Protection against occupational hazards Protection from accidents Use of specific nutrients Protection from carcinogens Avoidance of allergens	Case-finding measures: individual and mass screening activities Selective examinations to cure and prevent disease process, prevent spread of communicable disease, prevent complications and sequelae, and shorten period of disability	Adequate treatment to arrest disease process and prevent further complications and sequelae Provision of facilities to limit disability and prevent death	Provision of hospital and community facilities for retraining and education to maximize use of remaining capacities Education of public and industry to use rehabilitated persons to fullest possible extent Selective placement Work therapy in hospitals Use of sheltered colony

Data from Leavell H, Clark AE: *Preventive medicine for the doctors in his community,* ed 3, New York, 1965, McGraw-Hill; and modified from Edelman CL, Mandle CL: *Health promotion throughout the life span,* ed 7, St Louis, 2010, Mosby.

The presence of risk factors does not mean that a disease will develop, but risk factors increase the chances that the individual will experience a particular disease or dysfunction. Nurses and other health care professionals are concerned with risk factors, sometimes called *health hazards,* for several reasons. Risk factors play a major role in how a nurse identifies a patient's health status. They can also influence health beliefs and practices if a person is aware of their presence. Risk factors are often placed in the following interrelated categories: genetic and physiological factors, age, physical environment, and lifestyle.

Genetic and Physiological Factors

Physiological risk factors involve the physical functioning of the body. Certain physical conditions such as being pregnant or overweight place increased stress on physiological systems (e.g., the circulatory system), increasing susceptibility to illness. Heredity, or genetic predisposition to specific illness, is a major physical risk factor. For example, a person with a family history of diabetes mellitus is at risk for developing the disease later in life. Other documented genetic risk factors include family histories of cancer, heart disease, kidney disease, or mental illness.

Age

Age affects a person's susceptibility to certain illnesses. For example, premature infants and neonates are more susceptible to infections. As a person ages, the risk of heart disease and many types of cancers increases. Age risk factors are often closely associated with other risk factors such as family history and personal habits. Nurses need to educate their patients about the importance of regularly scheduled checkups for their age-group. Various professional organizations and federal agencies develop and update recommendations for health screenings, immunizations, and counseling. Access to scientific evidence, recommendations for clinical prevention services, and information on how to incorporate recommended preventive services into practice can be found at www.ahrq.gov/clinic/prevenix.htm.

Environment

Where we live and the condition of that area (its air, water, and soil) determine how we live, what we eat, the disease agents to which we are exposed, our state of health, and our ability to adapt (Murray et al., 2008). The physical environment in which a person works or lives can increase the likelihood that certain illnesses will occur. For example, some kinds of cancer and other diseases are more likely to develop when industrial workers are exposed to certain chemicals or when people live near toxic waste disposal sites. Nursing assessments extend from the individual to the family and the community in which they live (Murray et al., 2008).

Lifestyle

Many activities, habits, and practices involve risk factors. Lifestyle practices and behaviors often have positive or negative effects on health. Lifestyle choices contribute to seven of the ten leading causes of death (Table 6-2). Practices with potential negative effects are risk factors. Some habits are risk factors for specific diseases. For example, excessive sunbathing increases the risk of skin cancer; smoking increases the risk of lung diseases, including cancer; and a poor diet and being overweight increase the risk of cardiovascular disease. Because of lifestyle choices, there is an increased emphasis on preventive care. Lifestyle choices lead to health problems that cause a huge impact on the economics of the health care system. Therefore it is important to understand the effect of lifestyle behaviors on health status. Nurses educate their patients and the public on wellness-promoting lifestyle behaviors.

Stress is a lifestyle risk factor if it is severe or prolonged or if the person is unable to cope with life events adequately. Stress threatens both mental health (emotional stress) and physical well-being (physiological stress). Both play a part in the development of an illness and affect the ability to adapt to potential changes associated with the illness and survive a life-threatening illness. Stress also interferes with health promotion activities and the ability to implement needed lifestyle modifications. Some emotional stressors result from life events such as divorce, pregnancy, death of a spouse

TABLE 6-2 Causes of Death in the United States in 2007 and Contributing Lifestyle Choices

LEADING CAUSES OF DEATH	NUMBER (%)*	LIFESTYLE CHOICES
Heart disease	616,067 (25.4)	Physical inactivity, poor nutrition, use of tobacco
Cancer	562,875 (23.2)	Use of tobacco, poor nutrition, excess sun exposure, no use of preventive screenings
Stroke (cerebrovascular diseases)	135,952 (5.6)	Use of tobacco, poor nutrition, physical inactivity
Chronic lower respiratory diseases	127,924 (5.3)	Use of tobacco
Accidents (unintentional injuries)	123,706 (5.1)	Use of alcohol and drugs, no use of seat belt or motorcycle helmet
Alzheimer's disease	74,632 (3.1)	
Diabetes	71,382 (2.9)	Obesity, poor nutrition
Influenza and pneumonia	52,717 (2.2)	Use of tobacco, lack of immunizations
Nephritis, nephrotic syndrome, nephrosis	46,448 (1.9)	
Septicemia	34,828 (1.4)	

*Data from Centers for Disease Control and Prevention: *Deaths and mortality*, http://www.cdc.gov/nchs/fastats/deaths.htm. Accessed June 30, 2009.

or family member, and financial instabilities. For example, job-related stressors overtax a person's cognitive skills and decision-making ability, leading to "mental overload" or "burnout" (see Chapter 37). Stress also threatens physical well-being and is associated with illnesses such as heart disease, cancer, and gastrointestinal disorders (Pender, Murdaugh, and Parsons, 2011). Always review life stressors as part of a comprehensive risk factor analysis.

The goal of risk factor identification is to help patients visualize the areas in their life that can be modified, controlled, or even eliminated to promote wellness and prevent illness. A variety of available health risk appraisal forms can be used to estimate a person's specific health threats based on the presence of various risk factors (Edelman and Mandle, 2010). Implementation of a health risk appraisal tool needs to be linked with educational programs and other community resources if it is to result in necessary lifestyle changes and risk reduction (Pender, Murdaugh, and Parsons, 2011).

RISK-FACTOR MODIFICATION AND CHANGING HEALTH BEHAVIORS

Identifying risk factors is the first step in health promotion, wellness education, and illness prevention. Discuss health hazards with the patient following a comprehensive nursing assessment, then help the patient decide if he or she wants to maintain or improve his or her health status by taking risk-reduction actions (Edelman and Mandle, 2010). Risk-factor modification, health promotion or illness prevention activities, or any program that attempts to change unhealthy lifestyle behaviors is a wellness strategy. Emphasize wellness strategies that teach patients to care for themselves in a healthier way because they have the ability to increase the quality of life and decrease the potential high costs of unmanaged health problems.

Some attempts to change are aimed at the cessation of a health-damaging behavior (e.g., tobacco use or alcohol misuse) or the adoption of a healthy behavior (e.g., healthy diet or exercise) (Pender, Murdaugh, and Parsons, 2011). It is difficult to change health behavior, especially when the behavior is ingrained in a person's lifestyle patterns. The importance of nurses using an HPM to identify risky behaviors and implement the change process cannot be overemphasized because it is the nurse who spends the greatest amount of time in direct contact with patients. In addition, leading causes of death continue to relate to health behaviors that require a change, and nurses are able to motivate and facilitate important health behavior change when working with individuals, families, and communities (Edelman and Mandle, 2010).

Understanding the process of changing behaviors will help you support difficult **health behavior changes** in patients. It is believed that change involves movement through a series of stages. DiClemente and Prochaska (1998) describe the stages of change in the transtheoretical model of change (Table 6-3). These stages range from no intention to change (precontemplation), considering a change within the next 6 months (contemplation), making small changes (preparation), and actively engaging in strategies to change behavior (action) to maintaining a changed behavior (maintenance stage). As individuals attempt a change in behavior, relapse followed by recycling through the stages frequently occurs. When relapse occurs, the person will return to the contemplation or precontemplation stage before attempting the change again. Relapse is a learning process, and the lessons learned from relapse can be applied to the next attempt to change. It is important to understand what happens at the various stages of the change process to time the implementation of interventions (wellness strategies) adequately and provide appropriate care at each stage.

Once an individual identifies a stage of change, the change process facilitates movement through the stages. To be most effective, you choose nursing interventions that match the stage of change (DiClemente and Prochaska, 1998). Most behavior-change programs are designed for (and have a chance of success when) people are ready to take action regarding their health behavior problems. Only a minority of people are actually in this action stage (Prochaska, 1991). Changes are maintained over time only if they are integrated into an individual's overall lifestyle (Box 6-4). Maintaining healthy lifestyles can prevent hospitalizations and potentially lower the cost of health care.

ILLNESS

Illness is a state in which a person's physical, emotional, intellectual, social, developmental, or spiritual functioning is diminished or impaired. Cancer is a disease process, but one patient with leukemia who is responding to treatment may continue to function as usual, whereas another patient with breast cancer who is preparing for surgery may be affected in dimensions other than the physical. Therefore illness is not synonymous with disease. Although nurses need to be familiar with different types of diseases and their treatments, they often are concerned more with illness, which may include disease but also includes the effects on functioning and well-being in all dimensions.

TABLE 6-3 **Stages of Health Behavior Change**

STAGE	DEFINITION	NURSING IMPLICATIONS
Precontemplation	Not intending to make changes within the next 6 months	Patient is not interested in information about the behavior and may be defensive when confronted with it.
Contemplation	Considering a change within the next 6 months	Ambivalence may be present, but patients will more likely accept information since they are developing more belief in the value of change.
Preparation	Making small changes in preparation for a change in the next month	Patient believes that advantages outweigh disadvantages of behavior change; needs assistance in planning for the change.
Action	Actively engaged in strategies to change behavior; lasts up to 6 months	Previous habits may prevent taking action relating to new behaviors; identify barriers and facilitators of change.
Maintenance stage	Sustained change over time; begins 6 months after action has started and continues indefinitely	Changes need to be integrated into the patient's lifestyle.

Data from Prochaska JO, DiClemente CC: Stages of change in the modification of problem behaviors, *Prog Behav Modif* 28:184, 1992; and Conn VS: A staged-based approach to helping people change health behaviors, *Clin Nurs Spec* 8(4):187, 1994.

BOX 6-4 **PATIENT TEACHING**

Lifestyle Changes

Objective

- Patient will reduce health risks related to poor lifestyle habits (e.g., high-fat diet, sedentary lifestyle) through behavior change.

Teaching Strategies

- Practice active listening, and ask the patient how he or she prefers to learn (Cornett, 2009).
- Begin with determining what information the patient knows regarding health risks related to poor lifestyle.
- Ask which barriers the patient perceives with the planned lifestyle change.
- Assist the patient in establishing goals for change.
- In collaboration with the patient, establish time lines for modification of eating and exercise lifestyle habits.
- Reinforce the process of change.
- Use written resources at an appropriate reading level (Villaire and Mayer, 2009).
- Ensure that the education materials are culturally appropriate (Villaire and Mayer, 2009).
- Include family members to support the lifestyle change.

Evaluation

- Have the patient maintain an exercise and eating calendar to track adherence and provide positive reinforcement.
- Ask the patient to discuss success with lifestyle changes such as minutes spent in activity or actual number of fruits and vegetables eaten.

Acute and Chronic Illness

Acute and chronic illness are two general classifications of illness used in this chapter. Both acute and chronic illnesses have the potential to be life threatening. An **acute illness** is usually reversible, has a short duration, and is often severe. The symptoms appear abruptly, are intense, and often subside after a relatively short period. An acute illness may affect functioning in any dimension. A **chronic illness** persists, usually longer than 6 months, is irreversible, and affects functioning in one or more systems. Patients often fluctuate between maximal functioning and serious health relapses that may be life threatening. A person with a chronic illness is similar to a person with a disability in that both have varying degrees of functional limitations that result from either a pathological process or an injury (Larsen, 2009a). In addition, the social surroundings and physical environment in which the individual lives frequently affect the abilities, motivation, and psychological maintenance of the person with a chronic illness or disability.

Chronic illnesses and disabilities remain a leading health problem in North America for older adults and children. Issues of coping and living with a chronic illness can be complex and overwhelming. Chronic illnesses are related to four modifiable health behaviors: physical inactivity, poor nutrition, use of tobacco, and excessive alcohol consumption (CDC, 2009). A major role for nursing is to provide patient education aimed at helping patients manage their illness or disability. The goal of managing a chronic illness is to reduce the occurrence or improve the tolerance of symptoms. By enhancing wellness, nurses improve the quality of life for patients living with chronic illnesses or disabilities.

Patients with chronic diseases and their families continually adjust and adapt to their illnesses. How an individual perceives an illness influences the type of coping responses. In response to a chronic illness, an individual develops an illness career. The illness career is flexible and changes in response to changes in health, interactions with health professionals, psychological changes related to grief, and stress related to the illness (Larsen, 2009b).

Illness Behavior

People who are ill generally act in a way that medical sociologists call **illness behavior.** It involves how people monitor their bodies, define and interpret their symptoms, take remedial actions, and use the resources in the health care system (Mechanic, 1995). Personal history, social situations, social norms, and past experiences affect illness behavior (Larsen, 2009b). How people react to illness varies widely; illness behavior displayed in sickness is often used to manage life adversities (Mechanic, 1995). In other words, if people perceive themselves to be ill, illness behaviors become coping mechanisms. For example, illness behavior results in a patient being released from roles, social expectations, or responsibilities. A homemaker views the "flu" as either an added stressor or a temporary release from child care and household responsibilities.

Variables Influencing Illness and Illness Behavior

Internal and external variables influence both health and health behavior and illness and illness behavior. The influences of these variables and the patient's illness behavior often affect the likelihood of seeking health care, compliance with therapy, and health outcomes. Nurses plan individualized care based on an understanding of these variables and behaviors to help patients cope with their illness at various stages. The goal is to promote optimal functioning in all dimensions throughout an illness.

Internal Variables. Internal variables, such as patient perceptions of symptoms and the nature of the illness, influence patient behavior. If patients believe that the symptoms of their illnesses disrupt their normal routine, they are more likely to seek health care assistance than if they do not perceive the symptoms to be disruptive. Patients are also more likely to seek assistance if they believe the symptoms are serious or life threatening. Persons awakened by crushing chest pains in the middle of the night generally view this symptom as potentially serious and life threatening, and they will probably be motivated to seek assistance. However, such a perception can also have the opposite effect. Individuals may fear serious illness, react by denying it, and not seek medical assistance.

The nature of the illness, either acute or chronic, also affects a patient's illness behavior. Patients with acute illnesses are likely to seek health care and comply readily with therapy. On the other hand, a patient with a chronic illness in which symptoms are not cured but only partially relieved may not be motivated to comply with the therapy plan. Some patients who are chronically ill become less actively involved in their care, experience greater frustration, and comply less readily with care. Because nurses generally spend more time than other health care professionals with chronically ill patients, they are in the unique position of being able to help these patients overcome problems related to illness behavior. A patient's coping skills and his or her locus of control are other internal variables that affect the way the patient behaves when ill (see Chapter 37).

External Variables. External variables influencing a patient's illness behavior include the visibility of symptoms, social group, cultural background, economic variables, accessibility of the health care system, and social support. The visibility of the symptoms of an illness affects body image and illness behavior. A patient with a visible symptom is often more likely to seek assistance than a patient with no visible symptoms.

Patients' social groups either assist in recognizing the threat of illness or support the denial of potential illness. Families, friends, and co-workers all potentially influence patients' illness behavior. Patients often react positively to social support while practicing positive health behaviors. A person's cultural and ethnic background teaches the person how to be healthy, how to recognize illness, and how to be ill. The effects of disease and its interpretation vary according to cultural circumstances. Ethnic differences influence decisions about health care and the use of diagnostic and health care services. Dietary practices among ethnic groups, occupations held by certain cultural groups, and cultural beliefs are other factors that contribute to illness and the distribution of disease (Giger and Davidhizar, 2008).

Economic variables influence the way a patient reacts to illness. Because of economic constraints, some patients delay treatment and in many cases continue to carry out daily activities. Patients' access to the health care system is closely related to economic factors. The health care system is a socioeconomic system that patients enter, interact within, and exit. For many patients entry into the system is complex or confusing, and some patients seek nonemergency medical care in an emergency department because they do not know how otherwise to obtain health services or do not have access to care. The physical proximity of patients to a health care agency often influences how soon they enter the system after deciding to seek care.

Impact of Illness on the Patient and Family

Illness is never an isolated life event. The patient and family deal with changes resulting from illness and treatment. Each patient responds uniquely to illness, requiring you to individualize nursing interventions. The patient and family commonly experience behavioral and emotional changes and changes in roles, body image and self-concept, and family dynamics.

Behavioral and Emotional Changes. People react differently to illness or the threat of illness. Individual behavioral and emotional reactions depend on the nature of the illness, the patient's attitude toward it, the reaction of others to it, and the variables of illness behavior.

Short-term, nonlife-threatening illnesses evoke few behavioral changes in the functioning of the patient or family. For example, a father who has a cold lacks the energy and patience to spend time in family activities. He becomes irritable and prefers not to interact with his family. This is a behavioral change, but the change is subtle and does not last long. Some may even consider such a change a normal response to illness.

Severe illness, particularly one that is life threatening, leads to more extensive emotional and behavioral changes such as anxiety, shock, denial, anger, and withdrawal. These are common responses to the stress of illness. You can develop interventions to help the patient and family cope with and adapt to this stress when the stressor itself usually cannot be changed.

Impact on Body Image. Body image is the subjective concept of physical appearance (see Chapter 33). Some illnesses result in changes in physical appearance. Patients' and families' reactions differ and usually depend on the type of changes (e.g., loss of a limb or an organ), their adaptive capacity, the rate at which changes takes place, and the support services available.

When a change in body image such as results from a leg amputation occurs, the patient generally adjusts in the following phases: shock, withdrawal, acknowledgment, acceptance, and rehabilitation. Initially the patient is in shock because of the change or impending change. He or she depersonalizes the change and talks about it as though it were happening to someone else. As the patient and family recognize the reality of the change, they become anxious and often withdraw, refusing to discuss it. Withdrawal is an adaptive coping mechanism that helps the patient adjust. As the patient and family acknowledge the change, they move through a period of grieving. At the end of the acknowledgment phase, they accept the loss. During rehabilitation the patient is ready to learn how to adapt to the change in body image through use of prosthesis or changing lifestyles and goals.

Impact on Self-Concept. Self-concept is a mental self-image of strengths and weaknesses in all aspects of personality. Self-concept depends in part on body image and roles but also includes other aspects of psychology and spirituality (see Chapters 33 and 35). The effect of illness on the self-concepts of patients and family members is usually more complex and less readily observed than role changes.

Self-concept is important in relationships with other family members. For example, a patient whose self-concept changes because of illness may no longer meet family expectations, leading to tension or conflict. As a result, family members change their interactions with the patient. In the course of providing care, you observe changes in the patient's self-concept (or in the self-concepts of family members) and develop a care plan to help him or her adjust to the changes resulting from the illness.

Impact on Family Roles. People have many roles in life such as wage earner, decision maker, professional, child, sibling, or parent. When an illness occurs, parents and children try to adapt to the major changes that result. Role reversal is common (see Chapter 10). If a parent of an adult becomes ill and cannot carry out usual activities, the adult child often assumes many of the parent's responsibilities and in essence becomes a parent to the parent. Such a reversal of the usual situation can lead to stress, conflicting responsibilities for the adult child, or direct conflict over decision making.

Such a change may be subtle and short term or drastic and long term. An individual and family generally adjust more easily to subtle, short-term changes. In most cases they know that the role change is temporary and will not require a prolonged adjustment. However, long-term changes require an adjustment process similar to the grief process (see Chapter 36). The patient and family often require specific counseling and guidance to help them cope with role changes.

Impact on Family Dynamics. As a result of the effects of illness on the patient and family, family dynamics often change. Family dynamics are the processes by which the family functions, makes decisions, gives support to individual members, and copes with everyday changes and challenges. When a parent in a family becomes ill, family activities and decision making often come to a halt as the other family members wait for the illness to pass, or the family members delay action because they are reluctant to assume the ill person's roles or responsibilities. Women living with spouses who have chronic illness experience a feeling of detachment from the spouse, a sense of loneliness, and a change in their relationship (Eriksson and Svedlund, 2006). The nurse views the whole family as a patient under stress, planning care to help the family regain the maximal level of functioning and well-being (see Chapter 10).

KEY POINTS

- Health and wellness are not merely the absence of disease and illness.
- A person's state of health, wellness, or illness depends on individual values, personality, and lifestyle.
- The health belief model considers the relationship between a person's health beliefs and health behaviors.
- The health promotion model highlights factors that increase individual well-being and self-actualization.
- Maslow's hierarchy of needs model emphasizes identifying a patient's individual needs, prioritizing the needs, and encouraging the patient's individual discovery of self (self-actualization).
- Holistic health models of nursing promote optimal health by incorporating active participation of patients in improving their health state.
- Health beliefs and practices are influenced by internal and external variables and should be considered when planning care.
- Health promotion activities help maintain or enhance health.
- Wellness education teaches patients how to care for themselves.
- Illness prevention activities protect against health threats and thus maintain an optimal level of health.
- Nursing incorporates health promotion activities, wellness education, and illness prevention activities rather than simply treating illness.
- The three levels of preventive care are primary, secondary, and tertiary.
- Risk factors threaten health, influence health practices, and are important considerations in illness prevention activities.
- Improvement in health may involve a change in health behaviors.
- The transtheoretical model of change describes a series of changes through which patients progress for successful behavior change rather than simply assuming that all patients are in an action stage.
- Illness behavior, like health practices, is influenced by many variables and must be considered by the nurse when planning care.
- Illness can have many effects on the patient and family, including changes in behavior and emotions, family roles and dynamics, body image, and self-concept.

CLINICAL APPLICATION QUESTIONS

Preparing for Clinical Practice

Mrs. Hillman is a 28-year-old divorced woman who is a single parent. She has two children, a 2-year-old boy and a 4-year-old girl. She currently does not have a job. She smokes one pack of cigarettes per day. The father of the children has limited involvement in the care of the children and gives her money when he can. Her mother lives 500 miles away, but her sister lives close by. She occasionally stops by to help with the children. Mrs. Hillman regularly takes the children to the local health clinic for care but she has not seen a health care provider since the delivery of her last child. She is experiencing a persistent cough and fatigue.

1. Identify internal and external variables that are impacting Mrs. Hillman's ability to care for herself.
2. What primary intervention activities are important for Mrs. Hillman and her family?
3. Using the transtheoretical model of change, which question could you ask Mrs. Hillman to determine how to target smoking cessation?

evolve *Answers to Clinical Application Questions can be found on the Evolve website.*

REVIEW QUESTIONS

Are You Ready to Test Your Nursing Knowledge?

1. The nurse is participating at a health fair at the local mall giving influenza vaccines to senior citizens. What level of prevention is the nurse practicing?
   1. Primary prevention
   2. Secondary prevention
   3. Tertiary prevention
   4. Quaternary prevention
2. A patient experienced a myocardial infarction 4 weeks ago and is currently participating in the daily cardiac rehabilitation sessions at the local fitness center. In what level of prevention is the patient participating?

1. Primary prevention
2. Secondary prevention
3. Tertiary prevention
4. Quaternary prevention

3. Based on the transtheoretical model of change, what is the most appropriate response to a patient who states: "Me, exercise? I haven't done that since junior high gym class, and I hated it then!"
   1. "That's fine. Exercise is bad for you anyway."
   2. "OK. I want you to walk 3 miles 4 times a week, and I'll see you in 1 month."
   3. "I understand. Can you think of one reason why being more active would be helpful for you?"
   4. "I'd like you to ride your bike 3 times this week and eat at least four fruits and vegetables every day."
4. A patient comes to the local health clinic and states: "I've noticed how many people are out walking in my neighborhood. Is walking good for you?" What is the best response to help the patient through the stages of change for exercise?
   1. "Walking is OK. I really think running is better."
   2. "Yes, walking is great exercise. Do you think you could go for a 5-minute walk next week?"
   3. "Yes, I want you to begin walking. Walk for 30 minutes every day and start to eat more fruits and vegetables."
   4. "They probably aren't walking fast enough or far enough. You need to spend at least 45 minutes if you are going to do any good."
5. A male patient has been laid off from his construction job and has many unpaid bills. He is going through a divorce from his marriage of 15 years and has been seeing his pastor to help him through this difficult time. He does not have a primary health care provider because he has never really been sick and his parents never took him to the physician when he was a child. Which external variables influence the patient's health practices? (Select all that apply.)
   1. Difficulty paying his bills
   2. Seeing his pastor as a means of support
   3. Family practice of not routinely seeing a health care provider
   4. Stress from the divorce and the loss of a job
6. The nurse is conducting a home visit with an older adult couple. She assesses that the lighting in the home is poor and there are throw rugs throughout the home and a low footstool in the living room. She discusses removing the rugs and footstool and improving the lighting with the couple. The nurse is addressing which level of need according to Maslow?
   1. Physiological
   2. Safety and security
   3. Love and belonging
   4. Self-actualization
7. When taking care of patients, the nurse routinely asks them if they take any vitamins or herbal medications, encourages family members to bring in music that the patient likes to help the patient relax, and frequently prays with her patients if that is important to them. The nurse is practicing which model?
   1. Holistic
   2. Health belief
   3. Transtheoretical
   4. Health promotion
8. When illness occurs, different attitudes about it cause people to react in different ways. What do medical sociologists call this reaction to illness?
   1. Health belief
   2. Illness behavior
   3. Health promotion
   4. Illness prevention
9. A patient at the community clinic asks the nurse about health promotion activities that she can do because she is concerned about getting diabetes mellitus since her grandfather and father both have the disease. This statement reflects that the patient is in what stage of the health belief model?
   1. Perceived threat of the disease
   2. Likelihood of taking preventive health action
   3. Analysis of perceived benefits of preventive action
   4. Perceived susceptibility to the disease.
10. A nurse works in a special care unit for children with severe immunology problems and is caring for a 3-year-old boy from Greece. The boy's father is with him while his mother and sister are back in Greece. The nurse is having difficulty communicating with the father. What action does the nurse take?
    1. Care for the boy as she would any other patient
    2. Ask the manager to talk with the father and keep him out of the unit
    3. Have another nurse care for the boy because maybe that nurse will do better with the father
    4. Search for help with interpretation and understanding of the cultural differences by contacting someone from the local Greek community
11. A patient with a 20-year history of diabetes mellitus had a lower leg amputation. Which statement made by the patient indicates that he is experiencing a problem with body image?
    1. "I just don't have any energy to get out of bed in the morning."
    2. "I've been attending church regularly with my wife since I got out of the hospital."
    3. "My wife has taken over paying the bills since I've been in the hospital."
    4. "I don't go out very much because everyone stares at me."
12. The patient states she joined a fitness club and attends the aerobics class three nights a week. The patient is in what stage of behavioral change?
    1. Precontemplation
    2. Contemplation
    3. Preparation
    4. Action
13. The nurse is developing a health promotion program on healthy eating and exercise for high school students using the health belief model as a framework. Which statement made by a nursing student is related to the individual's perception of susceptibility to an illness?
    1. "I don't have time to exercise because I have to work after school every night."
    2. "I'm worried about becoming overweight and getting diabetes because my father has diabetes."
    3. "The statistics of how many teenagers are overweight is scary."
    4. "I've decided to start a walking club at school for interested students."
14. The nurse assesses the following risk factors for coronary artery disease (CAD) in a male patient. Which factors are classified as genetic and physiological? (Select all that apply.)

1. Sedentary lifestyle
2. Father died from CAD at age 50
3. History of hypertension
4. Eats diet high in sodium
5. Elevated cholesterol level
6. Age is 44 years

15. Which activity represents secondary prevention?
    1. A home health care nurse visits a patient's home to change a wound dressing.
    2. A 50-year-old woman with no history of disease attends the local health fair and has her blood pressure checked.
    3. The school health nurse provides a program to the first-year students on healthy eating.
    4. The patient attends cardiac rehabilitation sessions weekly.

Answers: **1.** 1; **2.** 3; **3.** 3; **4.** 2; **5.** 1, 3, 4; **6.** 2; **7.** 1; **8.** 2; **9.** 4; **10.** 4; **11.** 4; **12.** 4; **13.** 2; **14.** 2, 3, 5, 6; **15.** 1.

REFERENCES

Becker M, Maiman L: Sociobehavioral determinants of compliance with health and medical care recommendations, *Med Care* 13(1):10, 1975.

Centers for Disease Control and Prevention [CDC]: *Chronic diseases and health promotion*, National Center for Chronic Disease Prevention and Health Promotion, 2009, http://www.cdc.gov/chronicdisease/overview/index.htm. Accessed June 17, 2011.

Chodzko-Zajko W, et al: American College of Sports Medicine position stand. Exercise and physical activity for older adults, *Medicine & Science in Sports & Exercise* 41(7):1510, 2009.

Cornett S: Assessing and addressing health literacy, *Online J Issues Nurs* 14(3):10913734, 2009.

DiClemente C, Prochaska J: Toward a comprehensive trans-theoretical model of change. In Miller WR, Healther N, editors: *Treating addictive behaviors*, New York, 1998, Plenum Press.

Ebersole P, et al: *Toward healthy aging: human needs and nursing response*, ed 7, St Louis, 2008, Mosby.

Edelman CL, Mandle CL: *Health promotion throughout the life span*, ed 7, St Louis, 2010, Mosby.

Giger JN, Davidhizar RE: *Transcultural nursing: assessment and intervention*, St Louis, 2008, Mosby.

Larsen PD: Chronicity. In Lubkin IM, Larsen PD, editors: *Chronic illness: impact and intervention*, ed 7, Boston, 2009a, Jones & Bartlett.

Larsen PD: Illness behavior. In Lubkin IM, Larsen PD, editors: *Chronic illness: impact and intervention*, ed 7, Boston, 2009b, Jones & Bartlett.

Maier-Lorentz MM: Transcultural nursing; its importance in nursing practice, *J Cult Diversity* 15(1):37, 2008.

Mechanic D: Sociological dimensions of illness behavior, *Soc Sci Med* 41(9):1207, 1995.

Murray RB, et al: *Health promotion strategies through the lifespan*, ed 8, Upper Saddle River, NJ, 2008, Prentice Hall.

Narayan MC: Culture's effects on pain assessment and management, *Am J Nurs* 110(4):38, 2010.

Pender NJ: *Health promotion and nursing practice*, Norwalk, Conn, 1982, Appleton-Century-Crofts.

Pender NJ: *Health promotion and nursing practice*, ed 3, Stamford, Conn, 1996, Appleton & Lange.

Pender NJ, Murdaugh CL, Parsons MA: *Health promotion in nursing practice*, ed 5, Upper Saddle River, NJ, 2006, Prentice Hall.

Pender NJ, Murdaugh CL, Parsons MA: *Health promotion in nursing practice*, ed 6, Upper Saddle River, NJ, 2011, Prentice Hall.

Prochaska JO: Assessing how people change, *Cancer* 67(3:suppl):805, 1991.

Rosenstoch I: Historical origin of the health belief model, *Health Educ Monogr* 2:334, 1974.

Singleton K, Krause EMS: Understanding cultural and linguistic barriers to health literacy, *Online J Issues Nurs* 3(2):2, 2009.

US Department of Health and Human Services: *Healthy People 2010: understanding and improving health*, ed 2, Washington, DC, 2000, U.S. Government Printing Office.

US Department of Health and Human Services: *HealthyPeople.gov, 2011*. Accessed June 17, 2011.

US Department of Health and Human Services, Public Health Service: *Healthy People 2000: national health promotion and disease prevention objectives*, Washington, DC, 1990, US Government Printing Office.

Villaire M, Mayer G: Health literacy: the low hanging fruit in health care reform, *J Healthcare Finance* 36(2):55, 2009.

World Health Organization Interim Commission: *Chronicle of WHO*, Geneva, 1947, The Organization.

World Health Organization: *Milestones in health promotion: statement from global conferences*, Geneva, Switzerland, 2009, WHO Press.

Yeo G: How will the US healthcare system meet the challenge of the ethnogeriatric imperative? *J Am Geriatr Soc* 57(7):1278, 2009.

RESEARCH REFERENCE

Bertera EM, Bertera RL: Fear of falling and activity avoidance in a national sample of older adults in the United States, *Health Social Work* 33(1):54, 2008.

Byam-Williams J, Salyer J: Factors influencing the health-related lifestyle of community-dwelling older adults, *Home Healthcare Nurse* 28(2):115, 2010.

Callaghan D: Health behaviors, self-efficacy, self-care, and basic conditioning factors in older adults, *Journal of Community Health Nursing* 22(3):169, 2005.

Eriksson M, Svedlund M: "The intruder": spouses' narratives about life with a chronically ill partner, *J Clin Nurs* 15:324, 2006.

Lee H, et al: Do cultural factors predict mammography behavior among Korean immigrants in the USA? *J Adv Nurs* 65(12):2574, 2009.

Lee Y, Park K: Health practices that predict recovery from functional limitations in older adults, *Am J Prev Med* 31(1):25, 2006.

Lee-Lin F, et al: Screening practices among Chinese American immigrants, *J Obstet Gynecol Neonatal Nurs* 36:212, 2007.

Wu TY, Ronis D: Correlates of recent and regular mammography screening among Asian-American women, *J Adv Nurs* 65(11):2434, 2009.

CHAPTER 7

Caring in Nursing Practice

OBJECTIVES

- Discuss the role that caring plays in building the nurse-patient relationship.
- Compare and contrast theories on caring.
- Discuss the evidence that exists about patients' perceptions of caring.
- Explain how an ethic of care influences nurses' decision making.
- Describe ways to express caring through presence and touch.
- Describe the therapeutic benefit of listening to patients.
- Explain the relationship between knowing a patient and clinical decision making.

KEY TERMS

Caring, p. 80
Comforting, p. 84
Ethic of care, p. 83
Presence, p. 83
Transcultural, p. 80
Transformative, p. 81

evolve WEBSITE

http://evolve.elsevier.com/Potter/fundamentals/

- Review Questions
- Case Study with Questions
- Audio Glossary
- Interactive Learning Activities
- Key Term Flashcards
- Content Updates

Caring is central to nursing practice, but it is even more important in today's hectic health care environment. The demands, pressure, and time constraints in the health care environment leave little room for caring practice, which results in nurses and other health professionals becoming dissatisfied with their jobs and cold and indifferent to patient needs (Watson, 2006, 2009). Increasing use of technological advances for rapid diagnosis and treatment often causes nurses and other health care providers to perceive the patient relationship as less important. Technological advances become dangerous without a context of skillful and compassionate care. Despite these challenges, more professional organizations are stressing the importance of caring in health care. *Nursing's Agenda for the Future* (ANA, 2002) states that "Nursing is the pivotal health care profession highly valued for its specialized knowledge, skill, and caring in improving the health status of the individual, family, and the community." The American Organization of Nurse Executives (AONE, 2005) describes caring and knowledge as the core of nursing, with caring being a key component of what a nurse brings to a patient experience (Fig. 7-1).

It is time to value and embrace caring practices and expert knowledge that are the heart of competent nursing practice (Benner and Wrubel, 1989; Benner et al., 2010). When you engage patients in a caring and compassionate manner, you learn that the therapeutic gain in caring makes enormous contributions to the health and well-being of your patients.

Have you ever been ill or experienced a problem requiring health care intervention? Think about that experience. Then consider the following two scenarios and select the situation that you believe most successfully demonstrates a sense of caring.

A nurse enters a patient's room, greets the patient warmly while touching him or her lightly on the shoulder, makes eye contact, sits down for a few minutes and asks about the patient's thoughts and concerns, listens to the patient's story, looks at the intravenous (IV) solution hanging in the room, briefly examines the patient, and then checks the vital sign summary on the bedside computer screen before departing the room.

A second nurse enters the patient's room, looks at the IV solution hanging in the room, checks the vital sign summary sheet on the bedside computer screen, and acknowledges the patient but never sits down or touches him or her. The nurse makes eye contact from above while the patient is lying in bed. He or she asks a few brief questions about the patient's symptoms and leaves.

There is little doubt that the first scenario presents the nurse in specific acts of caring. The nurse's calm presence, parallel eye contact, attention to the patient's concerns, and physical closeness all express a person-centered, comforting approach. In contrast, the second scenario is task-oriented and expresses a sense of indifference to patient concerns. Both of these scenarios take approximately the same amount of time but leave very different patient perceptions. It is important to remember that, during times of illness or when a person seeks the professional guidance of a nurse,

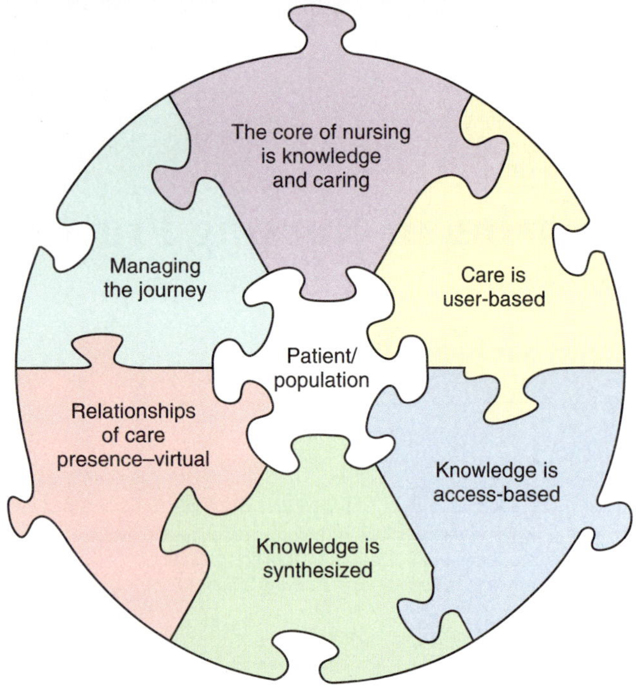

FIG. 7-1 AONE guiding principles for future care delivery. (Copyright © 2005 by the American Organization of Nurse Executives [AONE]. All rights reserved.)

caring is essential in helping the individual reach positive outcomes.

THEORETICAL VIEWS ON CARING

Caring is a universal phenomenon influencing the ways in which people think, feel, and behave in relation to one another. Since Florence Nightingale, nurses have studied caring from a variety of philosophical and ethical perspectives. A number of nursing scholars have developed theories on caring because of its importance to nursing practice. This chapter does not detail all of the theories of caring, but it is designed to help you understand how caring is at the heart of a nurse's ability to work with all patients in a respectful and therapeutic way.

Caring Is Primary

Benner offers nurses a rich, holistic understanding of nursing practice and caring through the interpretation of expert nurses' stories. After listening to nurses' stories and analyzing their meaning, she described the essence of excellent nursing practice, which is caring. The stories revealed the nurses' behaviors and decisions that expressed caring. Caring means that persons, events, projects, and things matter to people (Benner and Wrubel, 1989; Benner et al., 2010). It is a word for being connected.

Caring determines what matters to a person. It underlies a wide range of interactions, from parental love to friendship, from caring for one's work to caring for one's pet, to caring for and about one's patients. Benner and Wrubel (1989) note: "Caring creates possibility." Personal concern for another person, an event, or thing provides motivation and direction for people to care. Caring as a professional framework has practical implications for transforming nursing practice (Drenkard, 2008). Through caring, nurses help patients recover in the face of illness, give meaning to their illness, and maintain or reestablish connection. Understanding how to provide humanistic caring and compassion begins early in nursing education and continues to mature through experiential practice (Gallagher-Lepak and Kubsch, 2009).

Patients are not all the same. Each person brings a unique background of experiences, values, and cultural perspectives to a health care encounter. Caring is always specific and relational for each nurse-patient encounter. As nurses acquire more experience, they typically learn that caring helps them to focus on the patients for whom they care. Caring facilitates a nurse's ability to know a patient, allowing the nurse to recognize a patient's problems and find and implement individualized solutions.

BOX 7-1 CULTURAL ASPECTS OF CARE

Nurse Caring Behaviors

Caring includes knowing a patient's cultural values and beliefs (Suliman et al., 2009). Although the need for human caring is universal, its application is based on cultural norms. As a result, expectations may change across cultures. For example, providing time for family presence is often more valuable to traditional Asian families than a nursing presence. Using touch to convey caring sometimes crosses cultural norms. Sometimes gender-congruent caregivers or the patient's family need to provide caring touch. When listening to the patient, some cultures view eye contact as disrespectful.

Implications for Practice

- Know the patient's cultural norms for caring practices.
- Know the patient's cultural practices regarding end-of-life care. In some cultures it is considered insensitive to tell the patient that he or she is dying (Suliman et al., 2009).
- Determine if a member of the patient's family or cultural group is the best resource to use for caring practices such as providing presence or touching (Galanti, 2008).
- Know the patient's cultural practices regarding the removal of life support (Galanti, 2008).

Leininger's Transcultural Caring

From a transcultural perspective, Madeleine Leininger (1991) describes the concept of care as the essence and central, unifying, and dominant domain that distinguishes nursing from other health disciplines (see Chapter 4). Care is an essential human need, necessary for the health and survival of all individuals. Care, unlike cure, helps an individual or group improve a human condition. Acts of caring refer to nurturing and skillful activities, processes, and decisions to assist people in ways that are empathetic, compassionate, and supportive. An act of caring depends on the needs, problems, and values of the patient. Leininger's studies of numerous cultures around the world found that care helps protect, develop, nurture, and provide survival to people. It is needed for people of all cultures to recover from illness and to maintain healthy life practices.

Leininger (1991) stresses the importance of nurses' understanding cultural caring behaviors. Even though human caring is a universal phenomenon, the expressions, processes, and patterns of caring vary among cultures (Box 7-1). Caring is very personal; thus its expression differs for each patient. For caring to be effective, nurses need to learn culturally specific behaviors and words that reflect human caring in different cultures to identify and meet the needs of all patients (see Chapter 9).

Watson's Transpersonal Caring

Patients and their families expect a high quality of human interaction from nurses. Unfortunately many conversations between patients and their nurses are very brief and disconnected. Watson's theory of caring is a holistic model for nursing that suggests that a conscious intention to care promotes healing and wholeness (Watson, 2005, 2010). The theory integrates the human caring processes with healing environments, incorporating the life-generating and life-receiving processes of human caring and healing for nurses and their patients (Watson, 2006). The theory describes a consciousness that allows nurses to raise new questions about what it means to be a nurse, to be ill, and to be caring and healing. The transpersonal caring theory rejects the disease orientation to health care and places care before cure (Watson, 1996, 2008). The practitioner looks beyond the patient's disease and its treatment by conventional means. Instead, transpersonal caring looks for deeper sources of inner healing to protect, enhance, and preserve a person's dignity, humanity, wholeness, and inner harmony (see also Chapter 4).

In Watson's view caring becomes almost spiritual. It preserves human dignity in the technological, cure-dominated health care system (Watson, 2006). The emphasis is on the nurse-patient relationship. The focus is on the people behind the patient and nurse and the caring relationship (Table 7-1). A nurse communicates caring-healing to the patient through the consciousness of the nurse. This takes place during a single caring moment between nurse and patient. A connection forms between the one cared for and the one caring. The model is **transformative** because the relationship influences both the nurse and the patient for better or for worse (Watson, 2006, 2010). Caring-healing consciousness promotes healing. Application of Watson's caring model in practice enhances nurses' caring practices (Box 7-2).

TABLE 7-1 Watson's 10 Carative Factors (Watson, 2005, 2008)

CARATIVE FACTOR	EXAMPLE IN PRACTICE
Forming a human-altruistic value system	Use loving kindness to extend yourself. Use self-disclosure appropriately to promote a therapeutic alliance with your patient.
Instilling faith-hope	Provide a connection with the patient that offers purpose and direction when trying to find the meaning of an illness.
Cultivating a sensitivity to one's self and to others	Learn to accept yourself and others for their full potential. A caring nurse matures into becoming a self-actualized nurse.
Developing a helping, trusting, human caring relationship	Learn to develop and sustain helping, trusting, authentic, caring relationships through effective communication with your patients.
Promoting and expressing positive and negative feelings	Support and accept your patients' feelings. In connecting with your patients you show a willingness to take risks in sharing in the relationship.
Using creative problem-solving, caring processes	Apply the nursing process in systematic, scientific problem-solving decision making in providing patient-centered care.
Promoting transpersonal teaching-learning	Learn together while educating the patient to acquire self-care skills. The patient assumes responsibility for learning.
Providing for a supportive, protective, and/or corrective mental, physical, societal, and spiritual environment	Create a healing environment at all levels, physical and nonphysical. This promotes wholeness, beauty, comfort, dignity, and peace.
Meeting human needs	Assist patients with basic needs with an intentional care and caring consciousness.
Allowing for existential-phenomenological-spiritual forces	Allow spiritual forces to provide a better understanding of yourself and your patient.

Swanson's Theory of Caring

Kristen Swanson (1991) studied patients and professional caregivers in an effort to develop a theory of caring for nursing practice. This middle-range theory of caring was developed from three perinatal studies that interviewed women who miscarried, parents and health care professionals in a newborn intensive care unit, and socially at-risk mothers who received long-term public health intervention. All groups were in a perinatal (before, during, or after the birth of a child) setting or context and experienced the phenomenon of caring. Researchers asked each group questions regarding how they experienced or expressed caring in their situations (Swanson, 1999a, 1999b). After analyzing the stories and descriptions of the three groups, Swanson developed a theory of caring. The theory describes caring as consisting of five categories or processes (Table 7-2). Swanson (1991) defines caring as a nurturing way of relating to a valued other toward whom one feels a personal sense of commitment and responsibility. This theory supports the claim that caring is a central nursing phenomenon but not necessarily unique to nursing practice.

Swanson's work (1991) provides direction for how to develop useful and effective caring strategies. Each of the caring processes has definitions and subdimensions that serve as the basis for nursing interventions. Nursing care and caring are crucial in making positive differences in patients' health and well-being outcomes (Swanson, 1999a). Thus research findings develop and refine the theory and continue to guide clinical nursing practice (Andershed and Olsson, 2009). For example, Swanson (1999b) tested the effects of caring-based counseling on women's emotional well-being in the first year after miscarrying. Caring-based counseling was significant in reducing women's depression and anger, particularly for women in the first 4 months following miscarriage.

Summary of Theoretical Views

Nursing caring theories have common themes. Duffy, Hoskins, and Seifert (2007) identify these commonalities as human interaction or communication, mutuality, appreciating the uniqueness of individuals, and improving the welfare of patients and their families. Caring is highly relational. The nurse and the patient enter into a relationship that is much more than one person simply "doing tasks for" another. There is a mutual give-and-take that develops as nurse and patient begin to know and care for one another (Hudacek, 2008; Sumner, 2010). Caring theories are valuable when assessing patient perceptions of being cared for in a multicultural environment (Suliman et al., 2009). Frank (1998) described a

BOX 7-2 EVIDENCE-BASED PRACTICE

Enhancing Caring

PICO Question: Do patient satisfaction rates among hospitalized adult patients improve when carative nursing practices are used?

Evidence Summary

Patient satisfaction is an important indicator for the quality of health care. Caring facilitates healing and improves patient satisfaction with nursing care (Rush et al., 2008; Osterman et al., 2010). Researchers integrated human science caring into a professional practice model in a large health care system. This model was designed to increase nurses' presence and help them know their patients better. In turn the nurses implemented practice changes. Patient satisfaction increased, and patients indicated a willingness to return to the health care system in the event hospitalization was needed in the future (Drenkard, 2008). When using carative nursing practices, the interaction between the nurse and patient is essential and contributes to patient-centered care (Hobbs, 2009).

Application to Nursing Practice

- Setting a specific dedicated time to meet one-on-one with a patient during each nursing shift encourages the patient to be an active partner in care and helps the nurse understand the patient's perception of the need for caring (Drenkard, 2008).
- The use of caring in nursing practice encourages a more holistic approach to nursing care.
- As nurses use caring, they get to know their patients and therefore better meet their needs (Drenkard, 2008).
- The caring model involves a closeness, commitment, and involvement in the nurse-patient relationship, which contributes to patient-centered care (Hobbs, 2009).

TABLE 7-2 Swanson's Theory of Caring (Swanson, 1991)

CARING PROCESS	DEFINITIONS	SUBDIMENSIONS
Knowing	Striving to understand an event as it has meaning in the life of the other	Avoiding assumptions Centering on the one cared for Assessing thoroughly Seeking cues Engaging the self or both
Being with	Being emotionally present to the other	Being there Conveying ability Sharing feelings Not burdening
Doing for	Doing for the other as he or she would do for self if it were at all possible	Comforting Anticipating Performing skillfully Protecting Preserving dignity
Enabling	Facilitating the other's passage through life transitions (e.g., birth, death) and unfamiliar events	Informing/explaining Supporting/allowing Focusing Generating alternatives Validating/giving feedback
Maintaining belief	Sustaining faith in the other's capacity to get through an event or transition and face a future with meaning	Believing in/holding in esteem Maintaining a hope-filled attitude Offering realistic optimism "Going the distance"

personal situation when he was suffering from cancer: "What I wanted when I was ill was a mutual relationship of *persons* who were also clinician and patient." It was important for Frank to be seen as one of two fellow human beings, not the dependent patient being cared for by the expert technical clinician.

Caring seems highly invisible at times when a nurse and patient enter a relationship of respect, concern, and support. The nurse's empathy and compassion become a natural part of every patient encounter. However, when caring is absent, it becomes very obvious. For example, if the nurse shows disinterest or chooses to avoid a patient's request for help, his or her inaction quickly conveys an uncaring attitude. Benner and Wrubel (1989) relate the story of a clinical nurse specialist who learned from a patient what caring is all about: "I felt that I was teaching him a lot, but actually he taught me. One day he said to me (probably after I had delivered some well-meaning technical information about his disease), 'You're doing an OK job, but I can tell that every time you walk in that door you're walking out.'" In this nurse's story the patient perceived that the nurse was simply going through the motions of teaching and showed little caring toward the patient. Patients quickly know when nurses fail to relate to them.

As you practice caring, your patient will sense your commitment and willingness to enter into a relationship that allows you to understand the patient's experience of illness. In a study of oncology patients, one patient described a nurse's caring as "putting the heart in it" and "having an investment" that makes "patients feel that you are with them" (Radwin, 2000). Thus the nurse becomes a coach and partner rather than a detached provider of care.

One aspect of caring is enabling, when a nurse and patient work together to identify alternatives in approaches to care and resources. Consider a nurse working with a patient recently diagnosed with diabetes mellitus who must learn how to administer daily insulin injections. The nurse enables the patient by providing instruction in a manner that allows the patient to successfully adapt diabetes management strategies such as self-medication, exercise, and diet to his own lifestyle.

Another common theme of caring is to understand the context of a person's life and illness. It is difficult to show caring for another individual without gaining an understanding of who the person is and his or her perception of the illness. Exploring the following questions with your patients helps you understand their perceptions of illness: How was your illness first recognized? How do you feel about the illness? How does your illness affect your daily life practices? Knowing the context of a patient's illness helps you choose and individualize interventions that will actually help the patient. This approach is more successful than simply selecting interventions on the basis of your patient's symptoms or disease process.

PATIENTS' PERCEPTIONS OF CARING

Leininger's, Watson's, and Swanson's theories provide an excellent beginning to understanding the behaviors and processes that characterize caring. Researchers explored nursing care behaviors as perceived by patients (Table 7-3). Their findings emphasize what

TABLE 7-3 Comparison of Research Studies Exploring Nurse Caring Behaviors (as Perceived by Patients)

PATIENT FALLS: ACUTE CARE NURSES' EXPERIENCES (RUSH ET AL [2008])	EXPLORATORY STUDY OF NURSES' PRESENCE IN DAILY CARE ON AN ONCOLOGY UNIT (OSTERMAN ET AL [2010])	IMPORTANCE OF KNOWING THE PATIENT IN WEANING FROM MECHANICAL VENTILATION (CROCKER AND SCHOLES [2009])
Using compassion when identifying risk factors associated with falling Using nursing presence to know the patient and identify patient-centered factors that promote or impede patient risk of falls Communicating effectively between nurses and patient/family Incorporating patients and families into the solution	Being compassionate and patient is important. Developing patient-nurse trust and responsiveness to patient is critical to the emergence of full presence. Maintaining presence is a way to provide emotional support to patients who are experiencing overwhelming stressors and decisions. Morning care provides an opportunity for nurses to be present with their patients.	Nursing presence contributes to knowing the patient. Patients indicated that "knowing" the patient was essential to patient-centered care. Maintaining a balance of continuity of care and nursing expertise. The inexperienced nurse was more likely to be away from the patient or provide care in a hurried manner. Creating a trusting relationship between patient and nurse is important.

patients expect from their caregivers and thus provide useful guidelines for your practice. Patients continue to value nurses' effectiveness in performing tasks; but clearly patients value the affective dimension of nursing care.

The study of patients' perceptions is important because health care is placing greater emphasis on patient satisfaction (see Chapter 2). Duffy, Hoskins, and Seifert (2007) developed the Caring Assessment Tool (CAT) to measure caring from a patient's perspective. This tool and other caring assessments help you, as a beginning professional, to appreciate the type of behaviors that hospitalized patients identify as caring. When patients sense that health care providers are sensitive, sympathetic, compassionate, and interested in them as people, they usually become active partners in the plan of care (Gallagher-Lepak and Kubsch, 2009). Suliman et al. (2009) studied the impact of Watson's caring theory as an assessment framework in a multicultural environment. Patients in the study indicated that they did not perceive any cultural bias when they perceived nurses to be caring. Radwin (2000) found that oncology patients associated excellent nursing care with attentiveness, partnership, individualization, rapport, and caring. As institutions look to improve patient satisfaction, creating an environment of caring is a necessary and worthwhile goal. Patient satisfaction with nursing care is an important factor in their decision to return to a hospital.

As you begin clinical practice, consider how patients perceive caring and the best approaches to provide care. Behaviors associated with caring offer an excellent starting point. It is also important to determine an individual patient's perceptions and unique expectations. Frequently patients and nurses differ in their perceptions of caring (Hudacek, 2008). For that reason focus on building a relationship that allows you to learn what is important to your patients (Gallagher-Lepak and Kubsch, 2009). For example, your patient is fearful of having an intravenous catheter inserted, and you are still a novice at catheter insertion. Instead of giving a lengthy description of the procedure to relieve anxiety, you decide that the patient will benefit more if you obtain assistance from a skilled staff member. Knowing who patients are helps you select caring approaches that are most appropriate to their needs.

ETHIC OF CARE

Caring is a moral imperative, not a commodity to be bought and sold. Caring for other human beings protects, enhances, and preserves human dignity. It is a professional, ethical covenant that nursing has with its public (Watson, 2010). Caring science provides a disciplinary foundation from which you deliver patient-centered care (Watson, 2005, 2008). Chapter 22 explores the importance of ethics in professional nursing. The term *ethics* refers to the ideals of right and wrong behavior. In any patient encounter a nurse needs to know what behavior is ethically appropriate. An ethic of care is unique so professional nurses do not make professional decisions based solely on intellectual or analytical principles. Instead, an ethic of care places caring at the center of decision making. For example, what resources should be used to care for an indigent patient? Is it caring to place a disabled relative in a long-term care facility?

An **ethic of care** is concerned with relationships between people and with a nurse's character and attitude toward others. Nurses who function from an ethic of care are sensitive to unequal relationships that lead to an abuse of one person's power over another—intentional or otherwise. In health care settings patients and families are often on unequal footing with professionals because of the patient's illness, lack of information, regression caused by pain and suffering, and unfamiliar circumstances. An ethic of care places the nurse as the patient's advocate, solving ethical dilemmas by attending to relationships and by giving priority to each patient's unique personhood.

CARING IN NURSING PRACTICE

It is impossible to prescribe ways that guarantee whether or when a nurse becomes a caring professional. Experts disagree as to whether caring is teachable or more fundamentally a way of being in the world. For those who find caring a normal part of their lives, it is a product of their culture, values, experiences, and relationships with others. Persons who do not experience care in their lives often find it difficult to act in caring ways. As you deal with health and illness in your practice, you grow in your ability to care. Caring behaviors include providing presence, offering a caring touch, and listening.

Providing Presence

Providing **presence** is a person-to-person encounter conveying a closeness and sense of caring. Fredriksson (1999) explains that presence involves "being there" and "being with." "Being there" is not only a physical presence; it also includes communication and understanding. Presence is an interpersonal process that is characterized by sensitivity, holism, intimacy, vulnerability, and adaptation to unique circumstances. It results in improved mental well-being for nurses and patients and improved physical well-being in patients (Finfgeld-Connett, 2006). The interpersonal relationship of "being there" depends on the fact that a nurse is attentive to the patient. Presence can be translated into an actual caring art that affects the healing and well-being of both the nurse and patient. It is often used in conjunction with other nursing interventions such as establishing the nurse-patient relationship, providing comfort measures, providing patient education, and listening. The outcomes of nursing presence include alleviating suffering, decreasing a sense of isolation and vulnerability, and personal growth (Zyblock, 2010). This type of presence is something the nurse offers to the patient in achieving patient care goals.

Nursing requires being present with patients at a moment of crisis or need (Zyblock, 2010). "Being with" is also interpersonal. The nurse gives himself or herself, which means being available and at a patient's disposal. If patients accept the nurse, they will invite him or her to see, share, and touch their vulnerability and suffering. One's human presence never leaves one unaffected (Watson, 2008). The nurse then enters the patient's world. In this presence the patient is able to put words to feelings and understand himself or herself in a way that leads to identifying solutions, seeing new directions, and making choices.

When a nurse establishes presence, eye contact, body language, voice tone, listening, and a positive and encouraging attitude act together to create openness and understanding. The message conveyed is that the other's experience matters to the one caring (Swanson, 1991). Establishing presence enhances the nurse's ability to learn from the patient. This strengthens the nurse's ability to provide adequate and appropriate nursing care.

It is especially important to establish presence and caring when patients are experiencing stressful events or situations. Awaiting a physician's report of test results, preparing for an unfamiliar procedure, and planning for a return home after serious illness are just a few examples of events in the course of a person's illness that can create unpredictability and dependency on care providers. The nurse's presence and caring help to calm anxiety and fear related to stressful situations (Finfgeld-Connett, 2008a, 2008b). Giving reassurance and thorough explanations about a procedure, remaining at the patient's side, and coaching the patient through the experience all convey a presence that is invaluable to the patient's well-being.

Touch

Patients face situations that are embarrassing, frightening, and painful. Whatever the feeling or symptom, patients look to nurses to provide comfort. The use of touch is one **comforting** approach that reaches out to patients to communicate concern and support. Touch is relational and leads to a connection between nurse and patient. It involves contact and noncontact touch. Contact touch involves obvious skin-to-skin contact, whereas noncontact touch refers to eye contact. It is difficult to separate the two. Both in turn are described within three categories: task-oriented touch, caring touch, and protective touch (Fredriksson, 1999).

Nurses use task-oriented touch when performing a task or procedure. The skillful and gentle performance of a nursing procedure conveys security and a sense of competence. An expert nurse learns that any procedure is more effective when administered carefully and in consideration of any patient concern. For example, if a patient is anxious about having a procedure such as the insertion of a nasogastric tube, the nurse offers comfort through a full explanation of the procedure and what the patient will feel. Then the nurse performs the procedure safely, skillfully, and successfully. This is done as the nurse prepares the supplies, positions the patient, and gently manipulates and inserts the nasogastric tube. Throughout a procedure the nurse talks quietly with the patient to provide reassurance and support.

Caring touch is a form of nonverbal communication, which successfully influences a patient's comfort and security, enhances self-esteem, increases confidence of the caregivers, and improves mental well-being (Osterman et al, 2010). You express this in the way you hold a patient's hand, give a back massage, gently position a patient, or participate in a conversation. When using a caring touch, you connect with the patient physically and emotionally (Zyblock, 2010).

Protective touch is a form of touch that protects the nurse and/or patient (Fredriksson, 1999). The patient views it either positively or negatively. The most obvious form of protective touch is preventing an accident (e.g., holding and bracing the patient to avoid a fall). Protective touch is also a kind of touch that protects the nurse emotionally. A nurse withdraws or distances herself or himself from a patient when he or she is unable to tolerate suffering or needs to escape from a situation that is causing tension. When used in this way, protective touch elicits negative feelings in a patient (Fredriksson, 1999).

Because touch conveys many messages, use it with discretion. Touch itself is a concern when crossing cultural boundaries of either the patient or the nurse (Benner et al., 2010; Benner, 2004). The patient generally permits task-orientated touch because most individuals give nurses and physicians a license to enter their personal space to provide care (see Box 7-1, p. 80). Know and understand if patients accept touch and how they interpret your intentions.

Listening

Caring involves an interpersonal interaction that is much more than two persons simply talking back and forth (Bunkers, 2010). Listening is a critical component of nursing care and is necessary for meaningful interactions with patients (Shipley, 2010). It is a planned and deliberate act in which the listener is present and engages the patient in a nonjudgmental and accepting manner. It includes "taking in" what a patient says and interpreting and understanding what the patient is saying and then giving back that understanding to the patient (Shipley, 2010). Listening to the meaning of what a patient says helps create a mutual relationship. True listening leads to truly knowing and responding to what really matters to the patient and family.

When an individual becomes ill, he or she usually has a story to tell about the meaning of the illness. Any critical or chronic illness affects all of a patient's life choices and decisions, sometimes the individual's identity. Being able to tell that story helps the patient break the distress of illness. Thus a story needs a listener. Frank (1998) described his own feelings during his experience with cancer: "I needed a [health care professional's] gift of listening in order to make my suffering a relationship between *us,* instead of an iron cage around *me.*" He needed to be able to express what he needed when he was ill. The personal concerns that are part of a patient's illness story determine what is at stake for the patient. Caring through listening enables the nurse to be a participant in the patient's life.

To listen effectively you need to silence yourself and listen with openness (Fredriksson, 1999). Fredriksson describes silencing one's mouth and also the mind. It is important to remain intentionally silent and concentrate on what the patient has to say. Give patients your full, focused attention as they tell their stories.

When an ill person chooses to tell his or her story, it involves reaching out to another human being. Telling the story implies a relationship that develops only if the clinician exchanges his or her stories as well. Frank (1998) argues that professionals do not routinely take seriously their own need to be known as part of a clinical relationship. Yet, unless the professional acknowledges this need, there is no reciprocal relationship, only an interaction. There is pressure on the clinician to know as much as possible about the patient, but it isolates the clinician from the patient. By contrast, in knowing and being known, each supports the other (Frank, 1998).

Through active listening you begin to truly know your patients and what is important to them (Bernick, 2004). Learning to listen to a patient is sometimes difficult. It is easy to become distracted by tasks at hand, colleagues shouting instructions, or other patients waiting to have their needs met. However, the time you take to listen effectively is worthwhile, in both the information gained and the strengthening of the nurse-patient relationship. Listening involves paying attention to the individual's words and tone of voice and entering his or her frame of reference (see Chapter 24). By observing the expressions and body language of the patient, you find cues to help the patient explore ways to achieve greater peace.

Knowing the Patient

One of the five caring processes described by Swanson (1991) is knowing the patient. Knowing the patient comprises both the nurse's understanding of a specific patient and his or her subsequent selection of interventions (Radwin, 2000). It is essential when providing patient-centered care. Two elements that facilitate knowing are continuity of care and clinical expertise. When patient care is fragmented, knowing the patient declines, and patient-centered care is compromised (Crocker and Scholes, 2009).

Knowing develops over time as a nurse learns the clinical conditions within a specialty and the behaviors and physiological responses of patients. Intimate knowing helps the nurse respond to what really matters to the patient. To know a patient means that the nurse avoids assumptions, focuses on the patient, and engages in a caring relationship with the patient that reveals information and cues that facilitate critical thinking and clinical judgments (see Chapter 15). Knowing the patient is at the core of the clinical decision-making process.

Factors that contribute to knowing the patient include time, continuity of care, team work of the nursing staff, trust, and experience. Barriers to knowing the patient are often related to the organizational structure of the organization and economic constraints. Organizational changes often result in decreasing the amount of time that registered nurses are able to spend with their patients, which in turn affects the nurse-patient relationships. Decreased length of stay also reduces the interactions' between nurses and their patients (Crocker and Scholes 2009; MacDonald, 2008).

Consequences of not knowing the patient are many. In the acute care setting, not knowing the patient contributes to risk for falls and actual falls (Rush et al., 2008). Patients and their families don't understand the complexities of treatment and their participation in care (MacDonald, 2008). Finally, patients do not adequately understand their discharge guidelines and may administer their home medications or treatments incorrectly. By establishing a caring relationship, the understanding that develops helps the nurse to better know the patient as a unique individual and choose the most appropriate and efficacious nursing therapies (Hobbs, 2009).

The caring relationships that a nurse develops over time, coupled with the nurse's growing knowledge and experience, provide a rich source of meaning when changes in a patient's clinical status occur. Expert nurses develop the ability to detect changes in patients' conditions almost effortlessly (Benner et al., 2010). Clinical decision making, perhaps the most important responsibility of the professional nurse, involves various aspects of knowing the patient: responses to therapies, routines and habits, coping resources, physical capacities and endurance, and body typology and characteristics. Experienced nurses know additional facts about their patients such as their experiences, behaviors, feelings, and perceptions (Benner et al., 2010; MacDonald, 2008). When you make clinical decisions accurately in the context of knowing a patient well, improved patient outcomes result. When a nurse bases care on knowing a patient, the patient perceives care as personalized, comforting, supportive, and healing.

The most important thing for a beginning nurse to recognize is that knowing a patient is more than simply gathering data about the patient's clinical signs and condition. Success in knowing the patient lies in the relationship you establish. To know a patient is to enter into a caring, social process, which results in a nurse-patient relationship whereby the patient comes to feel known by the nurse (Bunkers, 2010; MacDonald, 2008).

Spiritual Caring

Spiritual health occurs when a person finds a balance between his or her own life values, goals, and belief systems and those of others (see Chapter 35). Research shows a link between spirit, mind, and body. An individual's beliefs and expectations have effects on the person's physical well-being.

Establishing a caring relationship with a patient involves interconnectedness between the nurse and the patient. This interconnectedness is why Watson (2008, 2009, 2010) describes the caring relationship in a spiritual sense. Spirituality offers a sense of connectedness: intrapersonally (connected with oneself), interpersonally (connected with others and the environment), and transpersonally (connected with the unseen, God, or a higher power). In a caring relationship the patient and the nurse come to know one another so both move toward a healing relationship by (Watson, 2008):

- Mobilizing hope for the patient and the nurse.
- Finding an interpretation or understanding of illness, symptoms, or emotions that is acceptable to the patient.
- Assisting the patient in using social, emotional, or spiritual resources.
- Recognizing that caring relationships connect us human to human, spirit to spirit.

Relieving Pain and Suffering

Relieving pain and suffering is more than giving pain medications, repositioning the patient, or cleaning a wound. The relief of pain and suffering encompasses caring nursing actions that give a patient comfort, dignity, respect, and peace. Ensuring that the patient care environment is clean and pleasant and includes personal items makes the physical environment a place that soothes and heals the mind, body, and spirit (Gallagher-Lepak and Kubsch, 2009).

Through skillful and accurate assessment of a patient's level and type of pain you are able to design patient-centered care to improve the patient's level of comfort. There are multiple interventions for

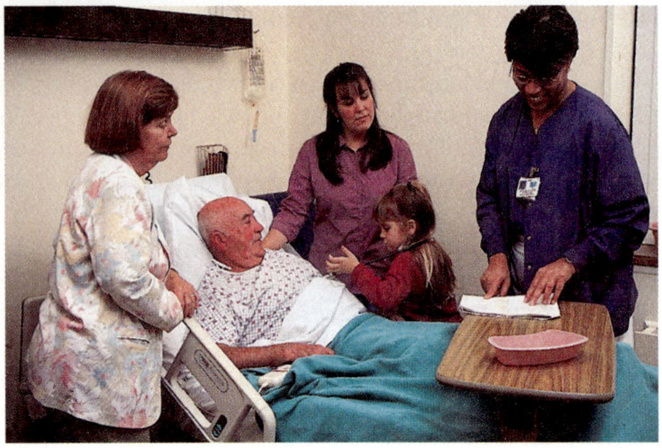

FIG. 7-2 Nurse discusses patient's health care needs with the family.

BOX 7-3 NURSE CARING BEHAVIORS AS PERCEIVED BY FAMILIES

- Being honest
- Advocating for patient's care preferences
- Giving clear explanations
- Keeping family members informed
- Asking permission before doing something to a patient
- Providing comfort (e.g., offering warm blanket, rubbing a patient's back)
- Reading patient passages from religious texts, favorite book, cards, or mail
- Providing for and maintaining patient privacy
- Assuring the patient that nursing services will be available
- Helping patients do as much for themselves as possible
- Teaching the family how to keep the relative physically comfortable

Data from Brown CL et al: Caring in action: the patient care facilitator role, *Int J Hum Caring* 9(3):51, 2005; Radwin L: Oncology patients' perceptions of quality nursing care, *Res Nurs Health* 23(3):179, 2000; and Carr T: Mapping the processes and qualities of spiritual nursing care, *Qual Health Res* 18(5):686, 2008.

pain relief, but knowing about the patient and the meaning of his or her pain guides your care (see Chapter 43). Often conveying a quiet caring presence, touching a patient, or listening helps you to assess and understand the meaning of your patient's pain or discomfort. The caring presence helps you and your patient design goals for pain relief.

Human suffering is multifaceted, affecting a patient physically, emotionally, socially, and spiritually. It also affects the patient's family and friends. You may find yourself working with a young family whose newborn baby has multiple developmental challenges. Their emotional suffering encompasses anger, guilt, fear, or grief. You cannot fix it, but you can provide comfort through a listening, nonjudgmental caring presence. Patients and their families are comforted by a caring listener (Hudacek, 2008).

Family Care

People live in their worlds in an involved way. Each person experiences life through relationships with others. Thus caring for an individual cannot occur in isolation from that person's family. As a nurse it is important to know the family almost as thoroughly as you know a patient (Fig. 7-2). The family is an important resource. Success with nursing interventions often depends on their willingness to share information about the patient, their acceptance and understanding of therapies, whether the interventions fit with their daily practices, and whether they support and deliver the therapies recommended.

Families of patients with cancer perceived many nurse caring behaviors to be most helpful (Box 7-3). It is critical that the nurse ensures the patient's well-being and helps the family members to be active participants. Although specific to families of patients with cancer, these behaviors offer useful guidelines for developing a caring relationship with all families. Begin a relationship by learning who makes up the patient's family and what their roles are in the patient's life. Showing the family that you care for and are concerned about the patient creates an openness that then enables a relationship to form with the family. Caring for the family takes into consideration the context of the patient's illness and the stress it imposes on all members (see Chapter 10).

THE CHALLENGE OF CARING

Assisting individuals during a time of need is the reason many enter nursing. When nurses are able to affirm themselves as caring individuals, their lives achieve a meaning and purpose (Benner, 2004; Benner et al., 2010). Caring is a motivating force for people to become nurses, and it becomes a source of satisfaction when nurses know that they have made a difference in their patients' lives.

It is becoming more of a challenge to care in today's health care system. Being a part of the helping professions is difficult and demanding. Nurses are torn between the human caring model and the task-oriented biomedical model and institutional demands that consume their practice (Watson and Foster, 2003). Nurses have increasingly less time to spend with patients, making it much harder to know who they are. A reliance on technology and cost-effective health care strategies and efforts to standardize and refine work processes all undermine the nature of caring. Too often patients become just a number, with their real needs either overlooked or ignored.

The American Nurses Association (ANA), National League for Nursing (NLN), American Organization of Nurse Executives (AONE), and American Association of Colleges of Nursing (AACN) recommend strategies to reverse the current nursing shortage. A number of these strategies have potential for creating work environments that enable nurses to demonstrate more caring behaviors. Environmental factors promote a more artful nursing and caring presence that further enhances patient-centered care (Finfgeld-Connett, 2008a; Hobbs, 2009). Strategies include introducing greater flexibility into the work environment structure, rewarding experienced nurse mentors, improving nurse staffing, and providing nurses with autonomy over their practice (Brown et al., 2005; Watson, 2009).

If health care is to make a positive difference in their lives, patients cannot be treated like machines or robots. Instead, health care must become more holistic and humanistic. Nurses play an important role in making caring an integral part of health care delivery. This begins by making caring a part of the philosophy and environment in the workplace. Incorporating caring concepts into standards of nursing practice establishes the guidelines for professional conduct. Finally, during day-to-day practice with patients and families, nurses need to be committed to caring and willing to establish the relationships necessary for personal, competent, compassionate, and meaningful nursing care. "Consistent with the wisdom and vision of Nightingale, nursing is a lifetime journey of caring and healing, seeking to understand and preserve the wholeness of human existence and to offer compassionate, informed knowledgeable human caring …" (Watson, 2009).

KEY POINTS

- Caring is the heart of a nurse's ability to work with people in a respectful and therapeutic way.
- Caring is specific and relational for each nurse-patient encounter.
- For caring to achieve cure, nurses need to learn the culturally specific behaviors and words that reflect human caring in different cultures.
- Because illness is the human experience of loss or dysfunction, any treatment or intervention given without consideration of its meaning to the individual is likely to be worthless.
- Caring involves a mutual give and take that develops as nurse and patient begin to know and care for one another.
- It is difficult to show caring to individuals without gaining an understanding of who they are and their perception of their illness.
- Presence involves a person-to-person encounter that conveys closeness and a sense of caring that involves "being there" and "being with" patients.
- Research shows that touch, both contact and noncontact, includes task-orientated touch, caring touch, and protective touch.
- The skillful and gentle performance of a nursing procedure conveys security and a sense of competence in the nurse.
- Listening is not only "taking in" what a patient says; it also includes interpreting and understanding what the patient is saying and giving back that understanding.
- Knowing the patient is at the core of the process that nurses use to make clinical decisions.

CLINICAL APPLICATION QUESTIONS

Preparing for Clinical Practice

1. Mrs. Lowe is a 52-year-old patient being treated for lymphoma (cancer of the lymph nodes) that occurred 6 years after a lung transplant. Mrs. Lowe is discouraged about her current health status and has a lot of what she describes as muscle pain. The unit where Mrs. Lowe is receiving care has a number of very sick patients and is short staffed.
   a. You enter her room to do a morning assessment and find Mrs. Lowe crying. How are you going to use caring practices to help her, knowing that your day has just begun and you have many nursing interventions to complete?
   b. When you listen to Mrs. Lowe, she explains that her muscle pain is very bothersome and it was worse when she was alone. Both you and Mrs. Lowe determine that an injection for her pain would be beneficial. In what way can you show caring in the way you administer the injection to Mrs. Lowe?
   c. Mrs. Lowe's day is getting better. She seems more comfortable and is crying less. You find that your day is more controlled. What else can you do for Mrs. Lowe?
2. During your next clinical practicum, select a patient to talk with for at least 15 to 20 minutes. Ask the patient to tell you about his or her illness. Review the skills of listening in this chapter and in Chapter 24. Immediately after your discussion, reflect on the discussion with the patient and determine if you have enough information about him or her to answer the following questions:
   a. What do you believe the patient was trying to tell you about his or her illness?
   b. Why was it important for the patient to share his or her story?
   c. What did you do that made it easy or difficult for the patient to talk with you? What did you do well? What could you have done better?
   d. Would you rate yourself a good listener? How can you listen better?

evolve *Answers to Clinical Application Questions can be found on the Evolve website.*

REVIEW QUESTIONS

Are You Ready to Test Your Nursing Knowledge?

1. A nurse hears a colleague tell a nursing student that she never touches a patient unless she is performing a procedure or doing an assessment. The nurse tells the student that from a caring perspective:
   1. She does not touch the patients either.
   2. Touch is a type of verbal communication.
   3. There is never a problem with using touch.
   4. Touch forms a connection between nurse and patient.
2. Of the five caring processes described by Swanson, which describes "knowing the patient"?
   1. Anticipating the patient's cultural preferences
   2. Determining the patient's physician preference
   3. Establishing an understanding of a specific patient
   4. Gathering task-oriented information during assessment
3. A Muslim woman enters the clinic to have a woman's health examination for the first time. Which nursing behavior applies Swanson's caring process of "knowing the patient?"
   1. Sharing feelings about the importance of having regular woman's health examinations
   2. Gaining an understanding of what a woman's health examination means to the patient
   3. Recognizing that the patient is modest; obtaining gender-congruent caregiver
   4. Explaining the risk factors for cervical cancer
4. Helping a new mother through the birthing experience demonstrates which of Swanson's five caring processes?
   1. Knowing
   2. Enabling
   3. Doing for
   4. Being with
5. A patient is fearful of upcoming surgery and a possible cancer diagnosis. He discusses his love for the Bible with his nurse, who recommends a favorite Bible verse. Another nurse tells the patient's nurse that there is no place in nursing for spiritual caring. The patient's nurse replies:
   1. "Spiritual care should be left to a professional."
   2. "You are correct, religion is a personal decision."
   3. "Nurses should not force their religious beliefs on patients."
   4. "Spiritual, mind, and body connections can affect health."
6. Which of the following is a strategy for creating work environments that enable nurses to demonstrate more caring behaviors?
   1. Increasing the working hours of the staff
   2. Increasing salary benefits of the staff
   3. Creating a setting that allows flexibility and autonomy for staff
   4. Encouraging increased input concerning nursing functions from physicians

7. When a nurse helps a patient find the meaning of cancer by supporting beliefs about life, this is an example of:
   1. Instilling hope and faith.
   2. Forming a human-altruistic value system.
   3. Cultural caring.
   4. Being with.
8. An example of a nurse caring behavior that families of acutely ill patients perceive as important to patients' well-being is:
   1. Making health care decisions for patients.
   2. Having family members provide a patient's total personal hygiene.
   3. Injecting the nurse's perceptions about the level of care provided.
   4. Asking permission before performing a procedure on a patient.
9. A nurse demonstrates caring by helping family members:
   1. Become active participants in care.
   2. Provide activities of daily living (ADLs).
   3. Remove themselves from personal care.
   4. Make health care decisions for the patient.
10. Listening is not only "taking in" what a patient says; it also includes:
    1. Incorporating the views of the physician.
    2. Correcting any errors in the patient's understanding.
    3. Injecting the nurse's personal views and statements.
    4. Interpreting and understanding what the patient means.
11. A nurse is caring for an older adult who needs to enter an assisted-living facility following discharge from the hospital. Which of the following is an example of listening that displays caring?
    1. The nurse encourages the patient to talk about his concerns while reviewing the computer screen in the room.
    2. The nurse sits at the patient's bedside, listens as he relays his fear of never seeing his home again, and then asks if he wants anything to eat.
    3. The nurse listens to the patient's story while sitting on the side of the bed and then summarizes the story.
    4. The nurse listens to the patient talk about his fears of not returning home and then tells him to think positively.
12. Presence involves a person-to-person encounter that:
    1. Enables patients to care for self.
    2. Provides personal care to a patient.
    3. Conveys a closeness and a sense of caring.
    4. Describes being in close contact with a patient.
13. A nurse enters a patient's room, arranges the supplies for a Foley catheter insertion, and explains the procedure to the patient. She tells the patient what to expect; just before inserting the catheter, she tells the patient to relax and that, once the catheter is in place, she will not feel the bladder pressure. The nurse then proceeds to skillfully insert the Foley catheter. This is an example of what type of touch?
    1. Caring touch
    2. Protective touch
    3. Task-oriented touch
    4. Interpersonal touch
14. A hospice nurse sits at the bedside of a male patient in the final stages of cancer. He and his parents made the decision that he would move home and they would help him in the final stages of his disease. The family participates in his care, but lately the nurse has increased the amount of time she spends with the family. Whenever she enters the room or approaches the patient to give care, she touches his shoulder and tells him that she is present. This is an example of what type of touch?
    1. Caring touch
    2. Protective touch
    3. Task-oriented touch
    4. Interpersonal touch
15. Match the following caring behaviors with their definitions.

1. Knowing	a. Sustaining faith in one's capacity to get through a situation
2. Being with	b. Striving to understand an event's meaning for another person
3. Doing for	c. Being emotionally there for another person
4. Maintaining belief	d. Providing for another as he or she would do for themselves.

Answers: 1. 4; 2. 3; 3. 2; 4. 2; 5. 4; 6. 3; 7. 1; 8. 4; 9. 1; 10. 4; 11. 3; 12. 3; 13. 3; 14. 1; 15. 1 b, 2 c, 3 d, 4 a.

REFERENCES

American Nurses Association: *Nursing's agenda for the future: a call to the nation,* 2002, http://www.nursingworld.org/naf. Accessed May 9, 2008.

American Organization of Nurse Executives: *Guiding principles for patient care delivery toolkit,* 2005, http://www.aone.org. Accessed July 3, 2011.

Bernick L: Caring for older adults: practice guided by Watson's care-healing model, *Nurs Sci Q* 17(2):128, 2004.

Benner P: Relational ethics of comfort, touch, solace-endangered arts, *Am J Critical Care* 13(4):346, 2004.

Benner P, Wrubel J: *The primacy of caring: stress and coping in health and illness,* Menlo Park, Calif, 1989, Addison Wesley.

Benner P, et al: *Educating nurses: a call for radical transformation,* Stanford, Calif, 2010, Carnegie Foundation for the Advancement of Teaching.

Bunkers SS: The power and possibility in listening, *Nurs Sci Quarterly* 23(1):22, 2010.

Crocker C, Scholes J: The importance of knowing the patient in weaning from mechanical ventilation, *Nurs Crit Care* 14(6):289, 2009.

Drenkard KN: Integrating human caring science into a professional nursing practice model, *Crit Care Nurs Clin North Am* 20:403, 2008.

Frank AW: Just listening: narrative and deep illness, *Fam Syst Health* 16(3):197, 1998.

Galanti GA: *Caring for patients from different cultures,* ed 4, Philadelphia, 2008, University of Pennsylvania Press.

Gallagher-Lepak S, Kubsch S: Transpersonal caring: a nursing practice guideline, *Holisitic Nurs Pract* 23(3):171, 2009.

Leininger MM: *Culture care diversity and universality: a theory of nursing,* Pub No 15-2402, New York, 1991, National League for Nursing Press.

MacDonald M: Technology and its effect on knowing the patient: a clinical issue analysis, *Clin Nurse Spec* 22(3):149, 2008.

Shipley SD: Listening a: a concept analysis, *Nurs Forum* 45(2):125, 2010.

Swanson K: What is known about caring in nursing science. In Hinshaw AS, et al, editor: *Handbook of clinical nursing research,* Sherman Oaks, Calif, 1999a, Sage Publications.

Watson J: *Caring science as sacred science,* Philadelphia, 2005, FA Davis.

Watson J: Caring theory as an ethical guide to administrative and clinical practices, *Nurs Adm Q* 30(1):8, 2006.

Watson J: *The philosophy and science of caring,* Boulder, 2008, University Press of Colorado.

Watson J: Caring science and human caring theory: transforming personal and professional practices of nursing and health care, *J Health Human Services Admin* 31(4):466, 2009.

Watson J: Caring science and the next decade of holistic healing: transforming self and system from the inside out, *Am Holistic Nurses Assoc* 30(2):14, 2010.

Zyblock DM: Nursing presence in contemporary nursing practice, *Nurs Forum* 45(2):120, 2010.

RESEARCH REFERENCES

Andershed B, Olsson K: Review of research related to Kristen Swanson's middle-range theory of caring, *Scand J Caring Sci* 23:598, 2009.

Brown CL, et al: Caring in action: the patient care facilitator role, *Int J Human Caring* 9(3):51, 2005.

Duffy JR, Hoskins L, Seifert RF: Dimensions of caring: psychometric evaluation of the caring assessment tool, *Adv Nurs Sci* 30(3):235, 2007.

Finfgeld-Connett D: Meta-synthesis of caring in nursing, *J Clin Nurs* 17:196, 2006.

Finfgeld-Connett D: Qualitative convergence of three nursing concepts: art of nursing, presence, and caring, *J Adv Nurs* 63(5):527, 2008a.

Finfgeld-Connett D: Qualitative comparison and synthesis of nursing presence and caring, *Intl J Nurs Terminol Classifications* 19(3):111, 2008b.

Fredriksson L: Modes of relating in a caring conversation: a research synthesis on presence, touch, and listening, *J Adv Nurs* 30(5):1167, 1999.

Hobbs JL: A dimensional analysis of patient-centered care, *Nurs Res* 58(1):52, 2009.

Hudacek SS: Dimensions of caring: a qualitative analysis of nurses' stories, *J Nurs Educ* 47(3):124, 2008.

Osterman PLC, et al: An exploratory study of nurses' presence in daily care on an oncology unit, *Nurs Forum* 45(3):197, 2010.

Radwin L: Oncology patients' perceptions of quality nursing care, *Res Nurs Health* 23(3):179, 2000.

Rush KL, et al: Patient falls: acute care nurses' experiences, *J Clin Nurs* 18:357, 2008.

Suliman WA, et al: Applying Watson's nursing theory to assess patient perceptions of being cared for in a multicultural environment, *J Nurs Res* 17(4):293, 2009.

Sumner J: A critical lens on the instrumentation of caring in nursing theory, *Adv Nurs Sci* 33(1):E17, 2010.

Swanson KM: Empirical development of a middle-range theory of caring, *Nurs Res* 40(3):161, 1991.

Swanson, KM: Effects of caring, measurement, and time on miscarriage impact and women's well being, *Nurs Res* 48(6):288, 1999b.

Watson J, Foster R: The Attending Nurse Caring Model: integrating theory, evidence and advanced caring-healing therapeutics for transforming professional practice, *J Clin Nurs* 12:360, 2003.

CHAPTER

8

Caring for the Cancer Survivor

OBJECTIVES

- Discuss the concept of cancer survivorship.
- Describe the influence of cancer survivorship on patients' quality of life.
- Discuss the effects cancer has on the family.
- Explain the nursing implications related to cancer survivorship.
- Discuss the essential components of survivorship care.

KEY TERMS

Biological response modifiers (biotherapy), p. 90
Cancer-related fatigue (CRF), p. 92
Cancer survivor, p. 90
Chemotherapy, p. 90
Chemotherapy-related cognitive impairment (CRCI), p. 92
Hormone therapy, p. 90
Neuropathy, p. 92
Oncology, p. 97
Paresthesias, p. 92
Posttraumatic stress disorder (PTSD), p. 93
Radiation therapy, p. 90

evolve WEBSITE

http://evolve.elsevier.com/Potter/fundamentals/

- Review Questions
- Case Study with Questions
- Audio Glossary
- Interactive Learning Activities
- Key Term Flashcards
- Content Updates

Currently there are 16 million cancer survivors in the United States; the number of survivors will continue to grow since more than 1.5 million new cases of cancer are diagnosed each year (National Cancer Institute [NCI], 2010; American Cancer Society [ACS], 2011). Among children diagnosed with cancer, 81.46% survive for at least 5 years. Of adults diagnosed with cancer, 68% survive at least 5 years. The number of people surviving cancer will continue to increase as new cases are diagnosed and those already treated live longer. Cancer survivors' health care problems have largely been ignored or misunderstood because of the belief that health problems are over for those who receive treatment, survive, and are given a "clean bill of health." There are many different trajectories or courses for cancer survival (Box 8-1). With the advances made in early diagnosis and improved treatment, more patients are becoming long-term survivors of cancer. The major forms of cancer therapy—surgery, **chemotherapy, hormone therapy, biological response modifiers (biotherapy),** and **radiation therapy**—often create unwanted long-term effects on tissues and organ systems that impair a person's health and quality of life in many ways (Institute of Medicine [IOM], 2006). Thus cancer survivorship has enormous implications for the way these individuals monitor and manage their health throughout their lives. As a nurse, you will care for these patients when they seek care for their cancer and for other medical conditions.

The National Coalition for Cancer Survivorship (2004) offers a definition of a **cancer survivor:** "An individual is considered a cancer survivor from the time of diagnosis, through the balance of his or her life." Family members and friends are also survivors because they experience the effects that cancer has on their loved ones. Cancer truly is a life-changing event. Although progress is being made, evidence shows that there is a neglected phase of cancer care (i.e., the period following first diagnosis and initial treatment and before the development of a recurrence of the initial cancer or death) (IOM, 2006). In this phase many survivors do not have consistent health care follow-up. Once treatment is completed, contact with a cancer care provider often stops, and survivors' needs go unnoticed or untreated. Despite the incredible advances made in cancer care, many long-term survivors suffer unnecessarily and die from delayed second cancer diagnoses or treatment-related chronic disease (Curtis et al., 2006).

Nurses have the responsibility to better understand the needs of cancer survivors and provide the most current evidence-based approaches for managing late and long-term effects of cancer and cancer treatment. Evidence suggests that survivors among racial and ethnic minorities and other underserved populations have more posttreatment symptoms and poorer treatment outcomes than Caucasians (Centers for Disease Control and Prevention [CDC], 2004). The disparities in health among ethnic groups are related to a complex interplay of economic, social, and cultural factors, with poverty being a key factor (IOM, 2006). Being able to provide comprehensive care to a cancer survivor begins with recognizing the effects of cancer and its treatment and learning about the survivor's own meaning of health.

BOX 8-1 THE SEASONS OF CANCER SURVIVAL

Acute survival: Starts with the diagnosis of cancer. Diagnostic and therapeutic efforts dominate. Fear and anxiety are constant elements of this phase.

Extended survival: Period during which a patient goes into remission or has ended the basic, rigorous course of treatment and enters a phase of watchful waiting. Patient undergoes periodic examinations and/or intermittent therapy. Fear of recurrence is common. This is usually a period of physical limitations. Diminished strength, fatigue, pain, nausea, reduced tolerance for exercise, or hair loss often occurs in the acute phase; but patients now have to deal with cancer in the home, community, and workplace.

Permanent survival: This phase is roughly equated with "cure," but the experience permanently affects the survivor. Problems with employment and insurance are common. The long-term secondary effects of cancer treatment on health represent an area in which permanent survivors are at risk.

Modified from Mullan F: Seasons of survival: reflections of a physician with cancer, *N Engl J Med* 313(4):270, 1985; and Institute of Medicine and National Research Council, Hewitt M, Greenfield S, Stovall E, editors: *From cancer patient to cancer survivor: lost in transition,* Washington, DC, 2006, National Academies Press.

THE EFFECTS OF CANCER ON QUALITY OF LIFE

As people live longer after diagnosis and treatment for cancer, it becomes important to understand the types of distress that many survivors experience and how it affects their quality of life (Fig. 8-1). Quality of life in cancer survivorship means having a balance between the experience of increased dependence while seeking both independence and interdependence. Of course there are always exceptions in regard to the level of distress that survivors face. For some, cancer becomes an experience of self-reflection and an enhanced sense of what life is about (Box 8-2). Regardless of each survivor's journey with cancer, having cancer affects each person's physical, social, psychological, and spiritual well-being.

Physical Well-Being and Symptoms

Cancer survivors are at increased risk for cancer (either a recurrence of the cancer for which they were treated or a second cancer) and for a wide range of treatment-related problems (IOM, 2006). The increased risk for developing a second cancer is the result of cancer treatment, genetic factors or other susceptibility, or an interaction between treatment and susceptibility (Curtis et al., 2006). The risk for treatment-related problems is associated with the complexity of the cancer itself (e.g., type of tumor and stage of disease); the type, variety, and intensity of treatments used (e.g., chemotherapy and radiation combined); and the age and underlying health status of the patient. The following description shows how a cancer survivor's physical health problems can be complex and burdensome.

Susan was an Army nurse who learned 7 months after discharge from the Army that she had Hodgkin's disease. Hodgkin's is a malignancy of lymphoid tissue. Susan received an aggressive course of treatment that included surgery, 6 months of chemotherapy, and 3 months of total lymph node irradiation. It took many months for her bone marrow to heal and blood values to return to normal. After a few years she had bilateral mastectomies for treatment-related breast cancer. She also received 3 years of immunotherapy for cancer in situ

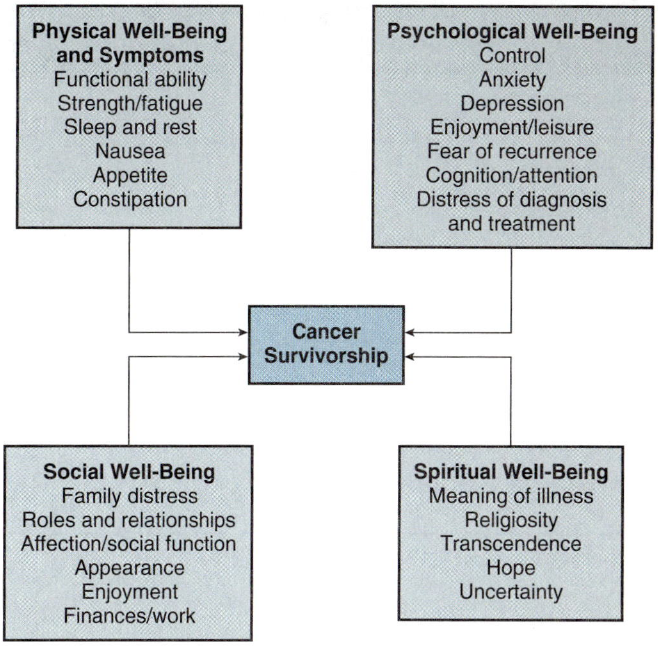

FIG. 8-1 Dimensions of quality of life affected by cancer. (From Ferrell B: *Introduction to cancer survivorship strategies for success, survivorship education for quality cancer care,* Pasadena, Calif, 2006, City of Hope National Medical Center.)

BOX 8-2 EVIDENCE-BASED PRACTICE

Cultural Aspects of Being a Cancer Survivor

PICO Question: Does the life experience of being a cancer survivor differ based on culture?

Evidence Summary

A number of different researchers have explored the cultural differences in patients who are cancer survivors. Low acculturated Hispanic cancer survivors have higher life satisfaction as compared to high acculturated Hispanic survivors because of high spirituality and positive social support (Stephens et al., 2010). Latina breast cancer survivors experience lower levels of social support and quality of life than comparable Caucasian women (Sammarco and Konecny, 2010). Mexican American female caregivers fear the cancer diagnosis, see cancer as a punishment, value maintenance of hope, believe in God and the doctor, and selectively disclose medical information (Cagle and Wolff, 2009). Older African American survivors report that social support is influenced by fears and stigma expressed by family and friends, the desire to decrease the burden and disruption on the lives of family and friends, and treatment and side effects (Hamilton et al., 2010). Some of these survivors withdrew from traditional support systems because of fear of being ostracized.

Application to Nursing Practice

- Although cancer survivors go through similar steps of cancer diagnosis and treatment, they experience cancer and the long-term impact differently based on their cultural beliefs.
- Nurses need to be aware and respect patients' cultural differences regarding the cancer experience.
- Assess patients' social support and their beliefs about cancer and incorporate these beliefs into nursing care approaches.
- Spiritual beliefs often significantly impact the patient's cancer experience.

TABLE 8-1 Examples of Late Effects of Surgery Among Adult Cancer Survivors

PROCEDURE	LATE EFFECT
Any surgical procedure	Pain, psychosocial distress, impaired wound healing
Surgery involving brain or spinal cord	Impaired cognitive function, motor sensory alterations, altered vision, swallowing, language, bowel and bladder control
Head and neck surgery	Difficulties with communication, swallowing, and breathing
Abdominal surgery	Risk of intestinal obstruction, hernia, altered bowel function
Lung resection	Difficulty breathing, fatigue, generalized weakness
Prostatectomy	Urinary incontinence, sexual dysfunction, poor body image

Modified from Institute of Medicine and National Research Council, Hewitt M, Greenfield S, Stovall E, editors: *From cancer patient to cancer survivor: lost in transition,* Washington, DC, 2006, National Academies Press.

(tumor not metastasized) of the bladder. She continues to experience many noncancer conditions: premature menopause, early osteoporosis, hypothyroidism, lung fibrosis, and atrophy of neck and upper chest muscles (Leigh, 2006).

This story is not unusual among survivors and highlights the long disease course that many cancer survivors face. A number of tissues and body systems are impaired as a result of cancer and its treatment (Table 8-1). Late effects of chemotherapy and/or radiation include osteoporosis, heart failure, diabetes, amenorrhea in women, sterility in men and women, impaired gastrointestinal motility, abnormal liver function, impaired immune function, **paresthesias,** hearing loss, and problems with thinking and memory (IOM, 2006). Some cancer treatments cause painful peripheral **neuropathy** (Pignataro and Swisher, 2010). Certain conditions resolve over time, but tissue damage causes some symptoms to persist indefinitely, especially when patients receive high-dose chemotherapy. Health care professionals do not always recognize these conditions as delayed problems. Often conditions such as osteoporosis, hearing loss, or change in memory are instead considered to be age related. It is common for patients with cancer to have multiple symptoms, and more attention is being given to the existence of symptom clusters. A symptom cluster is a group of several related and coexisting symptoms such as pain-insomnia-fatigue or pain-depression-fatigue (Kirkova et al., 2010; Xiao, 2010). Researchers are trying to better understand symptom clusters, their effects on patients, and whether clusters require a different treatment approach than current symptom management.

Cancer-related fatigue (CRF) and associated sleep disturbances are among the most frequent and disturbing complaints of people with cancer. The symptoms often last many months after chemotherapy and radiation. The National Comprehensive Cancer Network Clinical Practice Guidelines for CRF treatment includes interventions for controlling fatigue through routine physical exercise, development of good sleep habits, eating a balanced diet, and counseling for depression that often accompanies CRF. Acupuncture may also help control CRF in cancer survivors (Johnston, Xiao, and Hui, 2007; Escalante and Manzullo, 2009).

Chemotherapy-related cognitive impairment (CRCI) is estimated to occur in 17% to 75% of persons who receive standard-dose chemotherapy for cancer treatment (Myers, 2009). These cognitive changes occur during all phases of the cancer treatment, ranging from subtle symptoms such as a decreased attention span and being easily distracted to more obvious symptoms such as difficulty walking and significant behavior changes (Evans and Eschiti, 2009). There is no way to predict if a person will have CRCI. Some people who experience this symptom have difficulty working and processing information in their day-to-day lives, which affects daily functioning and the quality of their work and social life (Boykoff, Moieni, and Subramanian, 2009).

Often health care providers wrongly attribute the symptoms of cancer or the symptoms from the side effects of treatment to aging. This often leads to late diagnosis or a failure to provide aggressive and effective treatment of symptoms. Cancer is a chronic disease because of the serious consequences and the persistent nature of some of its late effects (IOM, 2006). The range of effects that patients suffer varies greatly. For example, a 46-year-old woman with early-stage melanoma on the right arm underwent successful surgery and only had an inconspicuous scar. In contrast, Susan, the Army nurse diagnosed with Hodgkin's disease, underwent intensive chemotherapy followed by an extended course of radiation. She faced serious and substantial long-term health problems from her treatment. Patients living with cancer present significant variations in the type of conditions they develop and the length of time the conditions persist.

Numerous factors contribute to survivors not receiving timely and appropriate treatment for the physical effects they suffer. Survivors often delay reporting symptoms because they fear being perceived as ungrateful for being disease free or they fear cancer recurrence (Polomano and Farrar, 2006). Survivors are not always aware that painful conditions or syndromes are common and frequently believe that pain relief is not possible (see Chapter 43). Health care providers have limited awareness of the prevalence and incidence of pain and other symptoms among survivors and frequently have limited education in symptom management. In the case of pain management, health care providers do not always acknowledge the potential for chronic pain following curative cancer therapies, or they sometimes fail to inform patients about potential long-term consequences of cancer treatment (Polomano and Farrar, 2006). Few health care settings track the health-related quality of life and symptomatology of patients over time. Researchers are beginning to recognize the need to identify the long-term patterns of symptoms most commonly associated with types of cancer and its treatment.

Psychological Well-Being

The physical effects of cancer and its treatment sometimes extend to cause serious psychological distress (see Chapter 37). Research suggests that some long-term (10-year) cancer survivors have impaired mood but also demonstrate aspects of psychological well-being compared to a cancer-free comparison group (Costanzo, Ryff, and Singer, 2009). In addition, older survivors show resilient social well-being, spirituality, and personal growth compared to younger survivors. What creates the individual response to having cancer is unclear. Research in culturally diverse long-term adult colorectal cancer survivors associates the belief in curability of the cancer with survival of over 15 years (Soler-Vilá et al., 2009). This does not mean that, just because someone believes that his or her cancer is cured, it is; however, perhaps these people had more positive coping strategies when dealing with their cancer.

Fear of cancer recurrence is common among cancer survivors (Simard, Savard, and Ivers, 2010). Use of positive coping strategies seems to help make this fear less troublesome. The levels of this fear are higher in survivors with more negative intrusive thoughts about their illness. When cancer recurs, patients and families face new challenges and distress (Vivar et al., 2009).

Another common psychological problem for survivors is **post-traumatic stress disorder (PTSD).** PTSD is a psychiatric disorder characterized by an acute emotional response to a traumatic event or situation. Approximately 3% to 4% of patients recently diagnosed with early-stage cancer experience symptoms of PTSD (e.g., grief, intrusive thoughts about the disease, nightmares, relational difficulties, or fear). This percentage increases to 35% in patients evaluated after treatment (NCI, 2009). Being unmarried or less educated or having a lower income and less social and emotional support increases the risk for PTSD (Stuber et al., 2010). The following description is an example of a cancer survivor's response to the stressors of cancer treatment:

The first question I asked my radiation oncologist after completing treatment for nonmetastatic breast and ovarian cancer was: "When can I go back to my job?" I remember him looking at me skeptically and replying, "Considering the work you do, I would think that 8 weeks of rest and recovery is the minimum." I left the clinic excited that my treatments were over and I could get on with my life. Eight weeks later I woke up tired after sleepless nights. I was bald and had peripheral neuropathy in my hands and feet that was crippling, and the drug I was taking made me feel like I had arthritis all over my body. Where was my energy and soft blond hair? Why couldn't I think straight? There is no way I could do my job like this. I felt like I was drowning (Bush, 2009).

The disabling effects of chronic cancer symptoms disrupt family and personal relationships, impair individuals' work performance, and often isolate survivors from normal social activities. Such changes in lifestyle create serious implications for a survivor's psychological well-being. When cancer changes a patient's body image or alters sexual function, the survivor frequently experiences significant anxiety and depression in interpersonal relationships. In the case of breast-cancer survivors, studies show that poorer self-ratings of quality of life are associated with poor body image, coping strategies, and a lack of social support (IOM, 2006).

Some factors ease the psychological stress associated with having cancer. A survivor who sees cancer as a challenging experience and a controllable threat has less stress (Jacobsen, 2006). Patients who use problem-oriented, active, and emotionally expressive coping processes also manage stress well (see Chapter 37). Survivors who have social and emotional support systems and maintain open communication with their treatment providers will also likely have less psychological distress (Jacobsen, 2006).

Social Well-Being

Cancer affects any age-group (Fig. 8-2). The developmental effects of cancer are perhaps best seen in the social impact that occurs across the life span. For adolescents and young adults, cancer seriously alters a young person's social skills, sexual development, body image, and the ability to think about and plan for the future (see Chapter 11). Cancer interrupts their lives, causing young survivors either to feel out of touch with the interests of their peers or to perceive interests as superficial (Blum, 2006). In addition, because cancer makes them feel different, young survivors, out of fear of

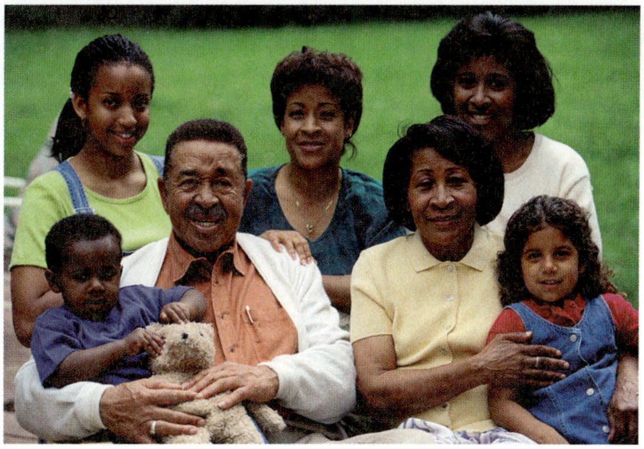

FIG. 8-2 A family representing young and old. Each member could be a cancer survivor.

rejection, have problems with dating and developing new relationships. Often the course of cancer or its treatment causes young adults to delay leaving their parents. The natural separation that occurs when young adults finish school and plan to start their careers is postponed or stopped. Often a young adult then feels ill equipped to take on the real world.

Adults (ages 30 to 59) who have cancer experience significant changes in their families. Once a member of the family is diagnosed with cancer, every family member's role, plans, and abilities changes (Blum, 2006). The healthy spouse often takes on added job responsibilities to provide additional income for the family. A spouse, sibling, grandparent, or child often assumes caregiving responsibilities for the patient. Patients who experience changes in sexuality, intimacy, and fertility see their marriages affected, often resulting in divorce.

A history of cancer significantly affects employment opportunities and the ability of a survivor to obtain and retain health and life insurance (IOM, 2006). Often a survivor experiences health-related work limitations that require a reduced work schedule or a complete change in employment. Between 64% and 84% of cancer survivors who worked before their diagnosis return to work (Steiner, Nowels, and Main, 2010). The most common problems reported by survivors who return to work are physical effort, heavy lifting, stooping, concentration, and keeping up with the work pace. Factors that affect a return to work include cancer site, prognosis, type of treatment, socioeconomic status, and characteristics of the work to be done. Middle-age cancer survivors have disability rates similar to those of people with chronic illnesses other than cancer (Short, Vasey, and Belue, 2008). The economic burden of cancer is enormous. If a survivor's illness affects his or her ability to work, less income goes to the individual and family. In addition, high out-of-pocket expenses for prescription drugs, medical devices and supplies and expenses for coinsurance and copayments usually increase (IOM, 2006). The problems are even greater for low-income survivors if they are uninsured or underinsured. Some Americans have health insurance that provides insurance coverage for most cancer-related care. However, approximately 42 million Americans have no health insurance at all. The uninsured do not receive the care they need, they suffer from a poorer state of health, and they are more likely to die earlier than those who have insurance (IOM, 2006).

Older adults face many social concerns as a result of cancer. The disease causes some survivors to retire prematurely or decrease work hours, thus decreasing income. The older adult faces a fixed income and the limitations of Medicare reimbursement. Many older survivors see their retirement pensions erode away quickly. They often have to use their income for basic expenses and cancer care costs, thus limiting opportunities for social activities. Many older adults have moved to retirement residences in other states and find themselves isolated from the social support of their families. Older adults also face a high level of disability as a result of cancer and cancer treatment and report a higher incidence of limitations in activities of daily living than older adults without cancer (IOM, 2006). As a result, many older cancer survivors require ongoing caregiving support either from family members or professional caregivers.

Spiritual Well-Being

Cancer challenges a person's spiritual well-being (see Chapter 35). Key features of spiritual well-being include a harmonious interconnectedness, creative energy, and a faith in a higher power or life force (Brown-Saltzman, 2006). Cancer and its treatment create physical and psychological changes that cause survivors to question, "Why me?" and wonder if perhaps their disease is some form of punishment. They often experience a level of spiritual distress, a disruption in a person's spirit or life principle. Survivors most at risk for spiritual distress are those with energy-consuming anxiety, an inability to forgive, low self-esteem, maturational losses, and mental illness (Brown-Saltzman, 2006). Additional risk factors include poor relationships and situational losses.

Relationships with a God, a higher power, nature, family, or community are critical for survivors. Cancer threatens relationships because it makes it difficult for survivors to maintain a connection and a sense of belonging. Cancer isolates survivors from meaningful interaction and support, which then threatens their ability to maintain hope. Long-term treatment, the recurrence of cancer, and the lingering side effects of treatment all create a level of uncertainty for survivors.

CANCER AND FAMILIES

A survivor's family takes different forms: the traditional nuclear family, extended family, single-parent family, close friends, and blended families (see Chapter 10). Once cancer affects a member of the family, it affects all other members as well. Usually a member of the family becomes the patient's caregiver. Family caregiving is a stressful experience, depending on the relationship between patient and caregiver and the nature and extent of the patient's disease. Members of the "sandwich generation" (i.e., caregivers who are 30 to 50 years old) are often caught in the middle of caring for their own immediate family and a parent with cancer. The demands are many, from providing ongoing encouragement and support and assisting with household chores to providing hands-on physical care (e.g., bathing, assisting with toileting, or changing a dressing) when cancer is advanced. Caregiving also involves the psychological demands of communicating, problem solving, and decision making; social demands of remaining active in the community and work; and economic demands of meeting financial obligations.

Family Distress

Living through cancer and treatment is a stressful time for families. Many caregivers and cancer survivors attempt to hide cancer-related thoughts and concerns from one another, which increases adverse psychological outcomes (Langer, Brown, and Syrjala, 2009). Motivation for this behavior is often to protect one another from the distress that is experienced by each member of the family. Holding back emotions is sometimes a part of this effort to shield one another from true thoughts and feelings (Porter et al., 2009). Porter et al. found that, if cancer survivors and their partners participated in an educational program to teach the importance of disclosing feelings and then actually disclosed them, relationships and intimacy were improved. Encouraging honest communication within families is an important intervention for you to implement to enhance family relationships.

Families struggle to maintain core functions when one of their members is a cancer survivor. Core family functions include maintaining an emotionally and physically safe environment, interpreting and reducing the threat of stressful events (including the cancer) for family members, and nurturing and supporting the development of individual family members (Lewis, 2006). In child-rearing families, this means providing an attentive parenting environment for children and information and support to children when their sense of well-being becomes threatened. When a member of the family has cancer, these core functions become threatened. Spouses often do not know what to do to support the survivor, and they struggle with how to help. In the end family functions become fragmented, and family members develop an uncertainty about their roles.

IMPLICATIONS FOR NURSING

Cancer survivorship creates many implications for nurses who help survivors plan for optimal lifelong health. Much needs to be done to research appropriate interventions for the effects of cancer and its treatment. Nurses are in a strong position to take the lead in improving public health efforts to manage the long-term consequences of cancer. Improvement is also necessary in the education of nurses and survivors about the phenomenon of survivorship. As a nursing student, you too can make a difference. This section addresses approaches to incorporate cancer survivorship into your nursing practice.

Survivor Assessment

Knowing that there are many cancer survivors in the health care system, consider how to assess patients who report a history of cancer. It is important to assess a cancer survivor's needs as a standard part of your practice. When you are collecting a nursing history (see Chapter 30), explore with your patients their history of cancer, including the diagnosis and type of treatment they either are undergoing or have received in the past. Be aware that some patients do not always report that they have had cancer. Thus, when a patient tells you that he or she has had surgery, ask if it was cancer related. When a patient reveals a history of chemotherapy, radiation, biotherapy, or hormone therapy, you need to refer to resources to help you understand how these therapies typically affect patients in both the short and long term. Then extend your assessment to determine if these treatment effects exist for your patient. Consider not only the effects of the cancer and its treatment (such as potential symptoms) but how it will affect any other medical condition. For example, if a patient also has heart disease, how will cancer-related fatigue affect this individual?

Understanding the cancer experience comes from a patient's own story. Asking general, open-ended questions about the patient's survivor experience will help the patient reveal his or her story. For example, you might ask, "Having cancer is a journey for many. Tell me how the disease most affects you right now," or "What are the biggest problems that you are having from cancer?" or "What can

I do to help you at this point?" These types of questions focus on the area that is most important to the patient and communicate to patients your interest in their situation. Show a caring approach so patients know that their story will be accepted (see Chapter 7).

Symptom management is an ongoing problem for many cancer survivors. If cancer is their primary diagnosis, it will be natural for you to explore any presenting symptoms. Be sure to learn specifically how symptoms are affecting the patient. For example, is pain also causing fatigue, or is a neuropathy causing the patient to walk with an abnormal gait? If cancer is secondary, you do not want important symptoms to go unrecognized. Ask the patient, "Since your diagnosis of and treatment for cancer, what physical changes or symptoms have you had?" "How do these changes affect you now?" Depending on the symptoms a patient identifies, you explore each one to gain a complete picture of his or her health status (Table 8-2). Some patients are reluctant to report or discuss their symptoms. Be patient; and, once you identify a symptom, explore the extent to which the symptom is currently affecting the patient.

Because you know that cancer affects a patient's quality of life in many ways, be sure to explore the patient's psychological, social, and spiritual needs and resources. Sometimes you will not be able to conduct a thorough assessment when you perform an initial nursing history. If this is the case, incorporate your assessment into your ongoing patient care. Observe your patient's interactions with family members and friends. When you are administering care to patients, talk about their daily lives and determine the extent to which cancer has changed their lifestyle.

TABLE 8-2 Examples of Assessment Questions for Cancer Survivors

CATEGORY	EXAMPLES OF QUESTIONS
Symptoms	• Tell me about the symptoms you are having from your cancer treatment. • Describe any pain or discomfort in the area where you had surgery or radiation; discomfort, pain, or unusual sensations in your hands or feet; weakness in your legs or arms; or problems moving around. • Are you experiencing fatigue, sleeplessness, shortness of breath? If so, please describe. • Sometimes people believe that they are starting to have problems after chemotherapy such as paying attention, remembering things, or finding words. Have you noticed any changes like these?
Psychosocial problems	• How distressed are you feeling at this point on a scale of 0 to 10 with 10 being the worst distress that you could imagine? • Tell me how you think your family is doing with your cancer? • What do you see in your family members' responses to your cancer that concerns you?
Sexuality problems	• If you have had sexual changes, what strategies have you tried to make things better? Have these strategies worked? • Would you be open to a health care provider who knows how to help you? • Since your cancer, do you see yourself differently as a person?

One area that is often difficult for nurses to assess well is a patient's sexuality. Sexuality is more than simply the physical ability to perform a sex act or conceive a child. It also includes a person's body image, sexual response (e.g., interest and satisfaction), and sexual roles and relationships (see Chapter 34). Surgery for many cancers is disfiguring, and chemotherapy and radiation often alter a patient's sexual response (e.g., prostate, breast, and gynecological cancers). Cancer therapies have the potential to cause fatigue, apathy, nausea, vomiting, malaise, and sleep disturbances, all of which interfere with a patient's libido (Pelusi, 2006). It is important to simply realize that cancer often does influence the patient's sexuality. It helps to develop a comfort level in acknowledging with patients that sexual changes are common at any age level. Ask a patient, "Since your diagnosis of and treatment for cancer, has your ability or interest in sexual activity changed? If so, how?" Patients will appreciate your sensitivity and interest in their well-being. When patients begin to discuss their sexual problems, be familiar with the expert resources in your institution (e.g., psychologist or social worker) available for patient referral.

Patient Education

When you care for a cancer patient, it is important to understand whether the patient administers most of his or her own self-care or if support is required from a family caregiver. This is essential to provide the most appropriate patient education, both in the form of content and in your teaching approach. Schumacher et al. (2006) developed a conceptual model, the transactional model of cancer family caregiving skill, which describes the relationship among cancer patients and family caregivers in the performance of family caregiving skills (Fig. 8-3). The model offers a perspective on caregivers and cancer survivors both as individuals and as a team. Family caregiving skill is the ability to respond effectively and smoothly to the demands of an illness and pattern of care using multiple caregiving processes (Schumacher et al., 2006). Illness demands of cancer include dealing with symptoms, responding to illness behaviors (e.g., role changes, avoiding interaction), modifying activities for an illness situation, nutritional support, interpersonal care, use of community resources, managing acute illness episodes, and implementing treatments. The patient and caregiver follow a continuum of three patterns of care: the self-caregiving pattern (patients are mostly independent with caregivers in a standby role), the collaborative care pattern (patients and caregivers share care activities and respond together to illness demands), and the family caregiving pattern (patients are unable to perform independently and require extensive caregiver involvement) (Schumacher et al., 2006). A patient's and caregiver's response to a demand involves performing caregiving processes (e.g., monitoring [observing for problems], interpreting [identifying the problem], making decisions and adjustments, accessing resources, and providing hands-on care). In terms of providing hands-on care, family caregivers often provide complex nursing procedures in the home such as managing intravenous infusions or irrigating wounds. Knowledge about caregiving or self-care, previous experience, and emotions influence the way caregivers and survivors respond and acquire caregiving processes. Schumacher's model is a helpful resource for you to apply when initially assessing the patient and caregiver condition, identifying their learning needs, and recognizing the type of information to teach. Learn where the patient and caregiver are along the caregiving continuum and determine the information needed to support them in meeting caregiving demands and performing caregiving processes. Frequently this means that any education will involve

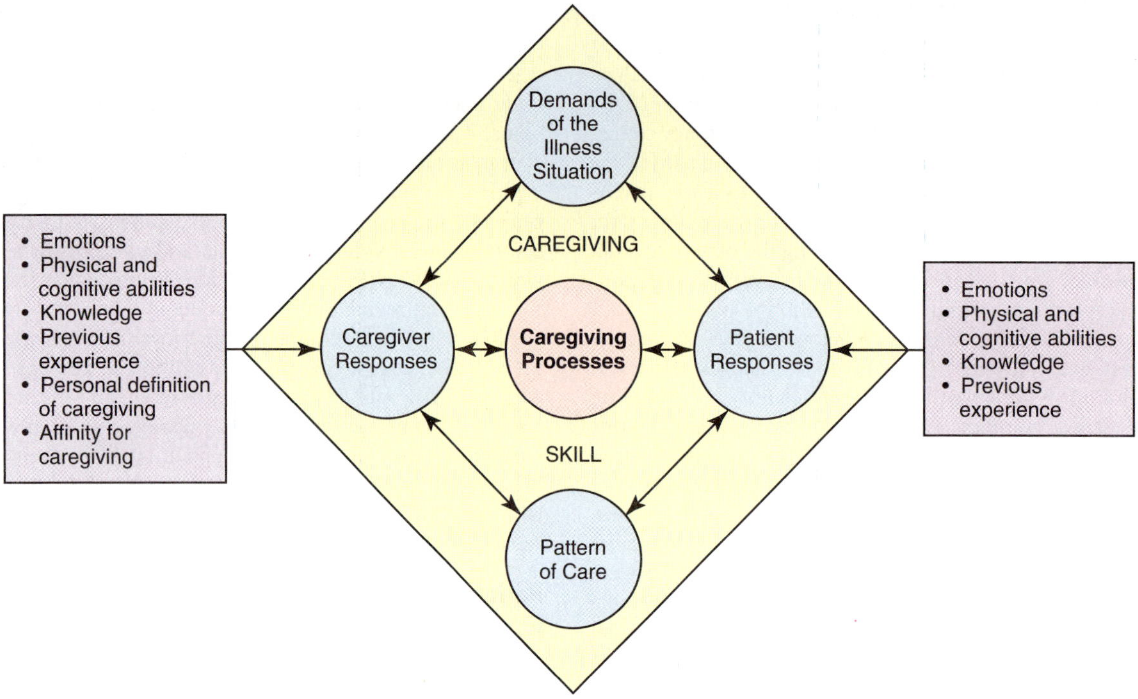

FIG. 8-3 Transactional model of cancer family caregiving skill. (From Schumacher KL et al: A transactional model of family caregiving skill, *Adv Nurs Sci* 29(3):271, 2006.)

both the patient and family caregiver together, unless the relationship is strained and the patient chooses not to have the caregiver involved.

It is a nurse's responsibility to educate cancer survivors and their families about the effects of cancer and cancer treatment. This means that, when you care for a cancer survivor, you need to understand the nature of the patient's particular disease and know the short- and long-term effects of each therapy. Cancer survivors who have an increased need for health-related information are younger and non-Caucasian, have less-than-excellent postcancer care, and have a history of other diseases (Beckford et al., 2008). When designing education that promotes self-management in caregiving, plan activities on the basis of the family caregiver's and cancer survivor's perceived disease-related problems and assist them with problem solving and gaining the self-efficacy or confidence to deal with these problems. Patient education helps survivors assume healthier lifestyle behaviors that will then give them control of aspects of their health and improve outcomes from cancer and chronic illness.

When caring for patients with an initial diagnosis of cancer, reinforce their health care provider's explanations of the risks related to their cancer and treatment, what they need to self-monitor (e.g., appetite, weight, and effects of fatigue), and what to discuss with health care providers in the future. If you teach patients and their family caregivers about the potential for treatment effects such as pain, neuropathy, or cognitive change, they are more likely to report their symptoms. It allows them to know what signs or changes to anticipate and monitor. Survivors need to learn how to manage problems related to persistent symptoms. For example, survivors with neuropathy need to learn how to protect the hands and feet, prevent falls, and avoid accidental burns.

Because survivors have an increased risk for developing a second cancer and/or chronic illness, it is important to educate them about lifestyle behaviors and the importance of participating in ongoing cancer screening and early detection practices. Lifelong cancer screening provides the opportunity to identify new cancers in early stages (Wilkins and Woodgate, 2008). When health care providers recommend follow-up screening in cancer survivors, there is a higher likelihood that the person will actually have the screening test (Mayer et al., 2007). Many survivors become interested in learning more about dietary supplements and nutritional complementary therapies to manage disease symptoms (IOM, 2006). Scientific evidence shows that several health promotion areas are of interest to cancer survivors: smoking cessation, physical activity, diet and nutrition (see Chapter 44), and the use of complementary and alternative medicine (see Chapter 32). Teach patients useful strategies to promote their health. Some health care providers wrongly attribute the symptoms of cancer or the side effects of treatment to aging. This often leads to late diagnosis or a failure to provide aggressive and effective treatment of symptoms.

Providing Resources

Numerous organizations and agencies provide resources to cancer survivors. However, many survivors do not receive timely and appropriate referrals to these resources. As a nurse, you will find that many people (e.g., friends, neighbors, and family members) come to you for advice about health care before they actually become a patient. It is important to know that cancer-related hospital and ambulatory care are not standardized. For example, when a patient with cancer is hospitalized, the availability of ancillary services for long-term care varies by care setting. Hospital-based oncologists are usually in larger hospitals and not in smaller ones. An NCI–designated cancer center offers the most comprehensive and up-to-date clinical care. NCI-designated centers also conduct important clinical trials to investigate the most current cancer therapies. Your role is to tell patients about the different resources available so they are able to make informed choices about their care. You can refer patients to the NCI website (http://www.cancer.gov/), which contains a current list of NCI-designated comprehensive cancer centers.

A wealth of cancer-related community support services is available to survivors through voluntary organizations such as the ACS (www.cancer.org), the Lance Armstrong Foundation (http://www.livestrong.org), and The National Coalition for Cancer Survivorship (NCCS) (http://www.canceradvocacy.org). Most offer their services at no cost. Many supportive services offer call centers and Internet-based information and discussion boards in addition to direct service delivery (IOM, 2006). Health care professionals are not consistent in referring patients to these valuable services. In addition, although community-based services help most survivors, there are gaps in service provision for assistance with transportation, home care, child care, and financial assistance. Become knowledgeable about the services within your community. There are several national agencies across the country, including the Cancer Support Community (http://www.thewellnesscommunity.org) and agencies targeted to racial groups such as the Sisters Network (http://www.sistersnetworkinc.org) and the Witness Program (http://www.acrc.uams.edu/patients/witness_project).

COMPONENTS OF SURVIVORSHIP CARE

Once primary cancer treatment ends, health care professionals need to develop an organized plan for survivorship care. This does not always occur because of inadequacies in the health care system, including a health care provider not assuming responsibility for coordinating care, fragmentation of care between specialists and general practitioners, and a lack of guidance on how survivors can improve their health outcomes (IOM, 2006). Patients with cancer often do not receive noncancer care (e.g., care for diabetes or heart conditions) when their cancer diagnosis shifts attention away from care that is routine but necessary. The IOM (2006) recommends four essential components of survivorship care: (1) prevention and detection of new cancers and recurrent cancer; (2) surveillance for cancer spread, recurrence, or second cancers; (3) intervention for consequences of cancer and its treatment (e.g., medical problems, symptoms, and psychological distress); and (4) coordination between specialists and primary care providers.

Survivorship Care Plan

To meet the health care needs of cancer survivors, it is essential for a "survivorship care plan" to be written by the principal provider who coordinates the patient's **oncology** treatment (Jacobsen, 2006; IOM, 2006). When the survivor is released from the oncologist, the internist and other health care providers provide and coordinate care based on knowledge of prior cancer history and treatment. The IOM (2006) also recommends that health insurance plans cover care outlined in a survivor care plan. Survivor plans are not always developed, and health insurance companies do not routinely cover this type of care. Ideally you review a survivorship care plan with a patient when he or she is formally discharged from a treatment program. The plan then becomes a guide for any future cancer or cancer-related care. Health care providers use the plan as a guide for patient education and screening for secondary cancers. Survivors use it to raise questions with health care providers to prompt appropriate care during follow-up visits. Box 8-3 highlights the components of a survivorship care plan.

Cancer organizations such as the Lance Armstrong Foundation (LiveStrong) and the Association of Cancer Online Resources (ACOR) (http://www.acor.org) provide Internet guides for the development of survivorship care plans. Several NCI-designated cancer centers and pediatric cancer centers provide survivorship care planning. Even though Internet guidelines for care plans exist, many survivors do not receive care at NCI-designated cancer centers and are discharged with no survivor plan. Thus nurses and other health care providers need to become more vigilant in recognizing cancer survivors and attempting to link them with the support and resources they require. Nurses make a difference when they consider the long-term issues that cancer survivors face after their time of diagnosis and in contributing to solutions to manage or relieve cancer-associated health problems. A strong interprofessional approach that includes nurses, oncology specialists, dietitians, social workers, pastoral care, and rehabilitation professionals is necessary. Together an interprofessional team provides a plan of care that addresses treatment-related problems and future health risks and offers a wellness focus to give patients a sense of hope as he or she enters the survivor experience.

BOX 8-3 A SURVIVORSHIP CARE PLAN

On discharge from cancer treatment, every patient and his or her primary health care provider should receive a record of all care received from the oncologist. In addition, the patient and health care provider should receive a follow-up plan incorporating available evidence-based standards of care.

Care Summary
- Diagnostic tests performed and results
- Tumor characteristics (e.g., site, stage, and grade)
- Dates when treatment started and stopped
- Surgery, chemotherapy, radiotherapy, transplant, hormone therapy, or gene therapy provided, including the specific agents used
- Psychosocial, nutritional, and other supportive services provided
- Full contact information for treating institutions and key providers
- Identification of a key point of contact and coordinator of care

Follow-up Plan
- Likely course of recovery
- Description of recommended cancer screening and other periodic testing/examinations
- Information about possible late and long-term effects of treatment and symptoms of such effects
- Information about possible signs of recurrence and second tumors
- Information about the possible effects of cancer on marital/partner relationship, sexual functioning, work, and parenting
- Information on the potential insurance, employment, and financial consequences of cancer and, as necessary, referral to counseling, legal aid, and financial assistance
- Specific recommendations for healthy behaviors
- Information about genetic counseling and testing as appropriate
- Information about known effective chemoprevention strategies for secondary prevention
- Referrals to specific follow-up care providers
- A listing of cancer-related resources and information

Modified from the President's Cancer Panel: Living beyond cancer: Finding a new balance, Bethesda, MD, 2004, National Cancer Institute; and Institute of Medicine and National Research Council, Hewitt M, Greenfield S, Stovall E, editors: *From cancer patient to cancer survivor: lost in transition,* Washington, DC, 2006, National Academies Press.

KEY POINTS

- Nurses care for cancer survivors when they seek care for their cancer and other medical conditions.
- Many cancer survivors have serious health problems that are related to their treatments.

- Cancer survivors among racial and ethnic minorities and other underserved populations have more posttreatment symptoms and poorer treatment outcomes than Caucasians.
- Survivors are often reluctant to report symptoms because of a fear of being perceived as ungrateful for being disease free or a fear of cancer recurrence.
- How well a survivor adapts to the cancer experience psychologically depends on predisposing factors, the person's current psychological status, the extent of his or her disease, and the presence of disruptive signs and symptoms.
- The disabling effects of chronic cancer symptoms disrupt family and personal relationships, impair individuals' work performance, and often isolate survivors from normal social activities.
- Adults who have cancer experience significant changes within their families, including a change in each member's role.
- Relationships among cancer survivors and family members become difficult to maintain because family members often do not know, understand, or have the skills or confidence to support the survivor's reactions to cancer.
- Because survivors are at an increased risk for developing a second cancer and/or chronic illness, it is important to educate them about lifestyle behaviors that will improve the quality of their lives.
- Once a patient's primary cancer treatment ends, health care professionals should develop an organized plan for survivorship care.
- Ideally you review a survivorship care plan with a patient when he or she is formally discharged from a treatment program, and it becomes a guide for any future cancer or cancer-related care.

CLINICAL APPLICATION QUESTIONS

Preparing for Clinical Practice

1. Do you have a friend or family member who has cancer and is willing to talk about it? If so, ask the individual to tell you what the experience has been like and what he or she would recommend to help you provide better care for survivors.
2. Ms. Ritter is a 32-year-old woman who visits the medical outpatient clinic for her final course of chemotherapy to treat breast cancer. She is married and has one child, a daughter, who is 6 years old. She and her husband hoped to have another child in the near future but now wonder if that will be possible. She shared with the nursing staff her concerns about the future and how cancer will affect her and her family. Her case manager talks with her about a survivorship care plan before discharge from the clinic. Identify two follow-up care plan components that would be important when considering Ms. Ritter's role as a wife and parent.
3. Ms. Ritter tells her nurse, "This chemotherapy has made me feel so tired, and there are many nights I can't sleep very well. I am looking forward to this ending." What is an appropriate response the nurse might give Ms. Ritter?

evolve *Answers to Clinical Application Questions can be found on the Evolve website.*

REVIEW QUESTIONS

Are You Ready to Test Your Nursing Knowledge?

1. Cancer survivors are at risk for treatment-related problems. Which of the patients listed below has the greatest risk for developing such a problem?
   1. An 80-year-old woman undergoing surgery for removal of a basal cell carcinoma on the face
   2. A 71-year-old man receiving high-dose chemotherapy and radiation for an advanced-stage lymphoma
   3. A 26-year-old man receiving chemotherapy for testicular cancer that is localized to the testicle
   4. A 48-year-old woman receiving radiation for Hodgkin's disease that involves lymph nodes extending above and below the diaphragm
2. Mr. Wallace is a 34-year-old who is a 5-year survivor of Hodgkin's disease. He continues to have symptoms related to his chemotherapy treatment. Mr. Wallace is a computer expert and enjoys Internet discussion groups. What is the best resource a nurse can recommend to help him access a survivorship care plan?
   1. Association of Cancer Online Resources
   2. National Coalition for Cancer Survivorship
   3. American Cancer Society
   4. National Cancer Institute
3. A nurse reviews the medical record of a 40-year-old patient newly admitted to the medical nursing unit for evaluation of diabetes. As the nurse reviews the patient's medical history, she notices that the patient had bladder surgery 3 years ago. Which of the following assessment questions is most appropriate for the nurse to ask to determine if the patient is a cancer survivor?
   1. Determining if the patient had additional surgeries recently
   2. Assessing the patient's medication history
   3. Determining if the surgery was cancer related
   4. Assessing if the patient's parents had cancer
4. A nurse working in a medicine clinic knows that it is important to recognize cancer survivors who are most at risk for posttreatment symptoms. Which of the following patients will likely be at greatest risk for posttreatment symptoms?
   1. A 50-year-old mother of three who was diagnosed with late-stage breast cancer and has hypertension
   2. A 20-year-old male college student diagnosed with leukemia whose father had lung cancer
   3. A 32-year-old Hispanic woman who has been diagnosed with local cervical cancer and receives Medicaid
   4. A 72-year-old African American male who had colorectal cancer with surgery, radiation, and a second round of chemotherapy because of failure of initial treatment and has diabetes
5. A 41-year-old man who underwent a craniotomy for the removal of a brain tumor 6 months ago comes to the clinic for his monthly follow-up visit. In planning your assessment, you anticipate that the patient may possibly experience which of the following late effects of surgery? (Select all that apply.)
   1. Pain
   2. Fatigue
   3. Blurred vision
   4. Difficulty breathing
   5. Poor attention span
6. To successfully assess if a patient is experiencing cognitive changes as a result of cancer treatment or complications of treatment, which of the following questions by a nurse is likely most relevant?
   1. Describe for me your medication schedule.
   2. How distressed are you feeling right now on a scale of 0 to 10?

3. Tell me about when you first noticed symptoms from your chemotherapy.
4. Tell me what you notice differently in your ability to get work done at your office.

7. A support group of cancer survivors is discussing cancer-related fatigue (CRF). The survivor most likely to gain relief from CRF is the survivor who does which of the following? (Select all that apply.)
   1. Takes naps during the day and evening
   2. Drinks energy drinks daily
   3. Exercises every other day
   4. Eats a balanced diet
8. Mr. Timmons has been receiving treatment for colon cancer on and off for a year. He received multiple chemotherapy regimens and a course of radiation. The 58-year-old patient is able to perform his own hygiene but needs assistance from his wife to move about safely in the home because of ongoing fatigue and weakness. His wife assists him with dressing when he becomes excessively tired. This caregiving skill pattern is best described as which of the following?
   1. The self-caregiving pattern
   2. The collaborative care pattern
   3. The family caregiving pattern
   4. The team caregiving pattern
9. Fill in the Blank. The period during which a cancer patient goes into remission following the basic, rigorous course of chemotherapy and enters a phase of watchful waiting, is called _______________.
10. A nurse in an oncology outpatient clinic has been seeing a woman and her husband since the woman was diagnosed with breast cancer. Sometimes the husband appears supportive, asking questions about his wife's care. At other times the husband seems easily distracted and uninterested. The nurse decides to reassess the psychosocial condition of the patient and her husband. Which of the following questions best elicits needed psychosocial information?
    1. "In what way does the pain you have affect you on a daily basis?"
    2. "Describe to me what you eat in a typical day."
    3. "Tell me how you think you and your husband are dealing with your cancer."
    4. "Are the two of you having any relational difficulties because of your cancer?"
11. Katie, a child in remission for leukemia, and her mother come to the pediatrician's office for a routine physical examination. The nurse asks Katie about whether she is having continued symptoms. Her mom says," I don't know why you want all of this information about Katie's cancer treatment. The leukemia is gone." The best response from the nurse in support of the child and mother would be:
    1. "The doctor likes to keep the records complete on all of her patients."
    2. "Just because Katie is in remission does not mean that it will stay that way."
    3. "It is common for children to have delayed effects from treatment, so we need to know this to plan Katie's care properly."
    4. "I understand your concern. If you don't want to provide the information, sign this release form."
12. Mr. Stewart is a 62-year-old patient diagnosed with prostate cancer who underwent surgical removal of the prostate 3 days ago. He lives with his wife at home. The nurse is planning to provide discharge instructions for the patient. What would be the most effective initial question to ask of the patient and family in determining the approach to discharge instructions?
    1. "Mr. Stewart, have you had surgery in the past?"
    2. "The doctor has ordered you to go home with a urinary catheter. Tell me how you think you can manage this."
    3. "Mrs. Stewart, do you find it difficult to look at your husband's incision? If so, tell me how you feel."
    4. "Mr. Stewart, describe for me how much your wife normally helps you at home and what you can do on your own."
13. A 62-year-old patient is being admitted to a surgical unit for a total hip replacement. The nurse reviews his medical record and learns that the patient has a history of impaired liver function and paresthesias in his feet. After assessing the patient's medical history further, the nurse is not sure what caused the liver impairment or paresthesia. To clarify, an appropriate question to ask the patient is which of the following?
    1. "Have you been treated for cancer in the past?"
    2. "What is the nature of your liver problem?"
    3. "Has the doctor discussed with you whether your liver problems will affect your recovery from surgery?"
    4. "How long have you had the numbness and tingling in your feet?"
14. Ben, a 31-year-old nursing student, is caring for Maria, a 45-year-old Latina woman who is receiving chemotherapy following surgery for breast cancer. Based on the evidence about cultural influences on cancer patients, Ben knows that which factor will likely influence this patient's ability to cope with her cancer?
    1. Transportation resources to the oncology clinic
    2. Whether the patient's physician is male or female
    3. The stigma family members place on cancer
    4. The level of social support available to the patient
15. Caring for a patient with cancer is unique because of the effects of the disease and associated treatment. An understanding of a patient's symptom experience is critical and best revealed by a nurse asking which of the following questions? (Select all that apply.)
    1. "What symptoms do you think you are having as a result of your cancer?"
    2. "Describe for me how the symptoms affect you in your daily life."
    3. "Let's focus on your pain. Tell me how it affects you."
    4. "Can you describe for me how your family provides care for your symptoms?"

Answers: **1.** 2; **2.** 1; **3.** 3; **4.** 4; **5.** 3, 5; **6.** 4; **7.** 3, 4; **8.** 2; **9.** Extended survival; **10.** 3; **11.** 3; **12.** 4; **13.** 1; **14.** 4; **15.** 1, 2, 3.

REFERENCES

American Cancer Society: *Facts and figures 2011*, 2011, http://www.cancer.org/Research/CancerFactsFigures/CancerFactsFigures/cancer-facts-figures-2011, Accessed June 19, 2011.

Blum D: *State of the science: social well being and survivorship*, Presentation at Survivorship Education for Quality Cancer Care, Pasadena, Calif, July 2006.

Brown-Saltzman K: *Spiritual well-being and survivorship*, Presentation at Survivorship Education for Quality Cancer Care, Pasadena, Calif, July 2006.

Bush N: Post-traumatic stress disorder related to the cancer experience, *Oncol Nurs Forum* 36(4):395, 2009.

Centers for Disease Control and Prevention: *The national action plan for cancer survivorship: advancing public health strategies*, 2004, http://www.cdc.gov/cancer/survivorship/pdf/plan.pdf. Accessed June 19, 2011.

Curtis RE, et al, editors: *New malignancies among cancer survivors: SEER Cancer Registries*, 1973-2000, NIH Pub 05-5302, Bethesda, Md, 2006, National Cancer Institute. http://www.seer.cancer.gov/publications/mpmono/FrontPages.pdf

Escalante CP, Manzullo EF: Cancer-related fatigue: the approach and treatment, *J Gen Intern Med* 24(suppl 2):412, 2009.

Evans K, Eschiti VS: Cognitive effects of cancer treatment: "chemo brain" explained, *Clin J Oncol Nurs* 13(6):661, 2009.

Institute of Medicine and National Research Council, Hewitt M, Greenfield S, Stovall E, editors: *From cancer patient to cancer survivor: lost in transition*, Washington, DC, 2006, National Academies Press.

Jacobsen P: *State of science: psychological well-being and survivorship*, Presentation at Survivorship Education for Quality Cancer Care, Pasadena, Calif, July 2006.

Leigh S: Cancer survivorship: a first-person perspective, *Am J Nurs* 106(3 suppl):12, 2006.

Lewis FM: The effects of cancer survivorship on families and caregivers, *Am J Nurs* 106(3 suppl):20, 2006.

National Cancer Institute (NCI): *Cancer trends progress report—2009/2010 Update*, NIH, DHHS, Bethesda, Md, April 2010, http://progressreport.cancer.gov/. Accessed June 19, 2011.

National Cancer Institute (NCI): *Post-traumatic stress disorder*, 2009, http://cancer.gov/cancertopics/pdq/supportivecare/post-traumatic-stress/health professional. Accessed August 30, 2010.

National Coalition for Cancer Survivorship: *Cancer survivorship*, 2004, NCCS, glossary at www.canceradvocacy.org.

Pelusi J: Sexuality and body image, *Am J Nurs* 106(3 suppl):32, 2006.

Polomano RC, Farrar JT: Pain and neuropathy in cancer survivors, *Am J Nurs* 106(3 suppl):39, 2006.

RESEARCH REFERENCES

Beckford EB, et al: Health-related information needs in a large and diverse sample of adult cancer survivors: implications for cancer care, *J Cancer Survivorship* 2:179, 2008.

Boykoff N, Moieni M, Subramanian SK: Confronting chemobrain: an in-depth look at survivors' reports of impact on work, social networks, and health care response, *J Cancer Survivorship* 3:223, 2009.

Cagle CS, Wolff E: Blending voices of Mexican American cancer caregivers and healthcare providers to improve care, *Oncol Nurs Forum* 36(5):555, 2009.

Costanzo E, Ryff C, Singer B: Psychosocial adjustment among cancer survivors: findings from a national survey of health and well-being, *Health Psychol* 28(2), 2009.

Hamilton JB, et al: Perceptions of support among older African American cancer survivors, *Oncol Nurs Forum* 37(4):484, 2010.

Johnston MF, Xiao B, Hui K: Acupuncture and fatigue: current basis for shared communication between breast cancer survivors and providers, *J Cancer Survivorship* 1:306, 2007.

Kirkova J, et al: Cancer symptom clusters: old concept but new data, *Am J Hosp Palliative Care* 27(4):282, 2010.

Langer SL, Brown JD, Syrjala KL: Intrapersonal and interpersonal consequences of protective buffering among cancer patients and caregivers, *Cancer* 115:4311, 2009.

Mayer D, et al: Screening practices in cancer survivors, *J Cancer Survivorship* 1:17, 2007.

Myers JS: Chemotherapy-related cognitive impairment: neuroimaging, neuropsychological testing, and the neuropsychologist, *Clin J Oncol Nurs* 13(4):413, 2009.

Pignataro RM, Swisher AK: Chemotherapy-induced peripheral neuropathy: risk factors, pathophysiology, assessment, and potential physical therapy interventions, *Rehabil Oncol* 28(2):10, 2010.

Porter LS, et al: Partner-assisted emotional disclosure for patients with gastrointestinal cancer, *Cancer* 115(S18):4326, 2009.

Sammarco A, Konecny LM: Quality of life, social support, and uncertainty among Latina and Caucasian breast cancer survivors: a comparative study, *Oncol Nurs Forum* 37(1):93, 2010.

Schumacher KL, et al: A transactional model of cancer family caregiving skill, *Adv Nurs Sci* 29(3):271, 2006.

Short PF, Vasey JJ, Belue R: Work disability associated with cancer survivorship and other chronic illnesses, *Psycho-Oncol* 17(1):91, 2008.

Simard S, Savard J, Ivers H: Fear of cancer recurrence: specific profiles and nature of intrusive thoughts, *J Cancer Survivorship* 4(4):361, 2010, DOI 10.1007/s11764-010-0136-8.

Soler-Vilá H, et al: Cancer-specific beliefs and survival in nonmetastatic colorectal cancer patients, *Cancer* 115:4270, 2009.

Steiner JF, Nowels CT, Main DS: Returning to work after cancer: quantitative studies and prototypical narratives, *Psycho-Oncol* 9(2):115, 2010.

Stephens C, Stein K, Landrine H: The role of acculturation in life satisfaction among Hispanic cancer survivors: results of the American Cancer Society's study of cancer survivors, *Psycho-Oncol* 19:376, 2010.

Stuber ML, et al: Prevalence and predictors of posttraumatic stress disorder in adult survivors of childhood cancer, *Pediatrics* 125(5):e1124, 2010.

Vivar CG, et al: The psychosocial impact of recurrence on cancer survivors and family members: a narrative review, *J Adv Nurs* 65(4):724, 2009.

Wilkins KL, Woodgate RLR: Preventing second cancers in cancer survivors, *Oncol Nurs Forum* 35(2):E12, 2008.

Xiao C: The state of science in the study of cancer symptom clusters, *Eur J Oncol Nurs* 14(5):417, 2010.

CHAPTER

9

Culture and Ethnicity

OBJECTIVES

- Describe social and cultural influences in health, illness, and caring patterns.
- Differentiate culturally congruent from culturally competent care.
- Describe steps toward developing cultural competence.
- Identify major components of cultural assessment.
- Use cultural assessment to identify significant values, beliefs, and practices critical to nursing care of individuals experiencing life transitions.
- Demonstrate nursing interventions that achieve culturally congruent care.
- Analyze outcomes of culturally congruent care.
- Apply research findings in culturally congruent care.

KEY TERMS

Acculturation, p. 103
Assimilation, p. 103
Biculturalism, p. 103
Bilineal, p. 111
Culture, p. 102
Cultural care accommodation or negotiation, p. 113
Cultural care preservation or maintenance, p. 113
Cultural care repatterning or restructuring, p. 113
Cultural competence, p. 103
Cultural imposition, p. 103
Cultural pain, p. 107
Culturally congruent care, p. 103
Culture-bound syndrome, p. 104
Emic worldview, p. 102
Enculturation, p. 103
Ethnicity, p. 102
Ethnohistory, p. 107
Ethnocentrism, p. 103
Etic worldview, p. 102
Fictive, p. 111
Matrilineal, p. 111
Naturalistic practitioners, p. 104
Patrilineal, p. 111
Personalistic practitioners, p. 104
Rites of passage, p. 105
Subcultures, p. 102
Transcultural nursing, p. 103

evolve WEBSITE

http://evolve.elsevier.com/Potter/fundamentals/

- Review Questions
- Case Study with Questions
- Audio Glossary
- Interactive Learning Activities
- Key Term Flashcards
- Content Updates

The demographic profile of the United States is changing dramatically as a result of immigration patterns and significant increases in culturally diverse populations already residing in the country. According to the U.S. Census Bureau, approximately 33% of the population currently belongs to a racial or ethnic minority group (Fig. 9-1). The U.S. Census also projects that this percentage will increase to 50% by the year 2050 (U.S. Census Bureau, 2010). Because it is important to care for people holistically, nurses need to integrate culturally congruent care within their nursing practice.

HEALTH DISPARITIES

Despite significant improvements in the overall health status of the U.S. population in the last few decades, disparities in health status among ethnic and racial minorities continues to be a serious local and national challenge. The Office of Minority Health and Health Disparities (2007a) reports that minority populations are more likely to have poor health and die at an earlier age because of a complex interaction among genetic differences, environmental and socioeconomic factors, and specific health behaviors such as the use of herbs to prevent or treat illnesses. Racial and ethnic minorities are more likely than white non-Hispanics to be poor or near poor. In addition, Hispanics, African Americans, and some Asian subgroups are less likely than white non-Hispanics to have a high school education. In general, racial and ethnic minorities often experience poorer access to health care and lower quality of preventive, primary, and specialty care. Eliminating such disparities in health status of people from diverse racial, ethnic, and cultural backgrounds has become one of the two most important priorities of *Healthy People 2020* (U.S. Department of Health and Human Services [USDHHS], 2010). Populations with health disparities

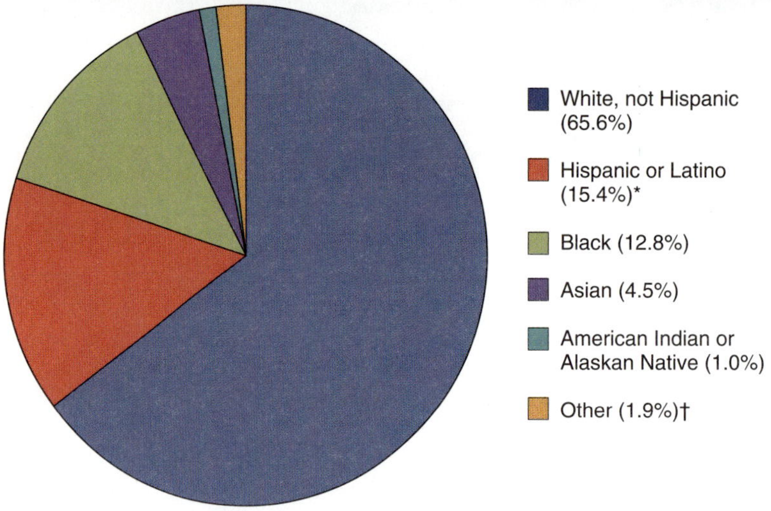

FIG. 9-1 Summary of U.S. Census Data. (Data from U.S. Census Bureau: *State and county quick facts*, 2010, http://quickfacts.census.gov/qfd/states/00000.html.) *Hispanics may be of any race, so they are also included in applicable race categories; therefore total percentages are greater than 100%. †Includes Native Hawaiian, Pacific Islander, and people reporting two or more races.

have a significantly increased incidence of diseases or increased morbidity and mortality when compared to the health status of the general population.

UNDERSTANDING CULTURAL CONCEPTS

The Office of Minority Health (OMH) (2005) describes **culture** as the thoughts, communications, actions, customs, beliefs, values, and institutions of racial, ethnic, religious, or social groups. Culture is a concept that applies to a group of people whose members share values and ways of thinking and acting that are different from those of people who are outside the group (Srivastava, 2007).

Culture has both visible (easily seen) and invisible (less observable) components. The invisible value-belief system of a particular culture is often the major driving force behind visible practices. For example, although an Apostolic Pentecostal woman can be identified by her long hair, no makeup, and the wearing of a skirt or dress, nurses cannot appreciate the meanings and beliefs associated with her appearance without further assessment. Apostolic Pentecostals believe that a woman's hair is her glory and should never be cut. Likewise, they believe that men and women need to dress differently and women need to be modest (wearing no makeup). These outward signs symbolize their belief in the scriptural definition of womanhood (United Pentecostal Church International, 2011). Cutting a woman's hair without consent of the individual or her family is sacrilegious and violates the ethnoreligious identity of the person. On the other hand, a woman of another faith who wears her hair long does not attach meaning to the length of her hair but wears it long because of a fashion preference.

In any society there is a dominant culture that exists along with other subcultures. Although subcultures have similarities with the dominant culture, they maintain their unique life patterns, values, and norms. In the United States the dominant culture is Anglo-American with origins from Western Europe. **Subcultures** such as the Appalachian and Amish cultures are examples of ethnic and religious groups with characteristics distinct from the dominant culture. Primary and secondary characteristics of culture are defined by the degree to which an individual identifies with his or her cultural group. Primary characteristics include nationality, race, gender, age, and religious beliefs. Secondary characteristics include socioeconomic and immigration status, residential patterns, personal beliefs, and political orientation.

Significant influences such as historical and social realities shape an individual's or group's worldview. Worldview is woven into the fabric of one's culture. It determines how people perceive others, how they interact and relate with reality, and how they process information (Walker et al., 2010). It is important that the nurse advocates for the patient based on the patient's worldview. Plan and provide nursing care in partnership with the patient to ensure that it is safe, effective, and culturally sensitive (McFarland and Eipperle, 2008).

Ethnicity refers to a shared identity related to social and cultural heritage such as values, language, geographical space, and racial characteristics. Members of an ethnic group feel a common sense of identity. Some declare their ethnic identity to be Irish, Vietnamese, or Brazilian. Ethnicity is different from race, which is limited to the common biological attributes shared by a group such as skin color (Dein, 2006). Examples of racial classifications include Asian and Caucasian.

Worldview refers to "the way people tend to look out upon the world or their universe to form a picture or value stance about life or the world around them" (Leininger, 2006). In any intercultural encounter there is an insider or native perspective **(emic worldview)** and an outsider perspective **(etic worldview).** For example, after giving birth, a Korean woman requests seaweed soup for her first meal. This request puzzles the nurse. Although the nurse has an emic view of professional postpartum care, as an outsider to the Korean culture he or she is not aware of the significance of the soup to the patient. Conversely, the Korean patient who has an etic view of American professional care assumes that seaweed soup is available in the hospital because it cleanses the blood and promotes healing and lactation (Edelstein, 2011). Unless the nurse seeks the patient's emic view, he or she is likely to suggest other varieties of soups available from the dietary department, disregarding the cultural meaning of the practice to the patient.

The processes of **enculturation** and **acculturation** facilitate cultural learning. Socialization into one's primary culture as a child is known as enculturation. In contrast, acculturation is a second-culture learning that occurs when the culture of a minority is gradually displaced by the culture of the dominant group in the process of **assimilation** (Cowan and Norman, 2006). When the process of assimilation occurs, members of an ethnocultural community are absorbed into another community and lose their unique characteristics such as language, customs, and ethnicity. Assimilation may be spontaneous, which is usually the case with immigrants, or forced, as is often the case of the assimilation of ethnic minority communities. **Biculturalism** (sometimes known as *multiculturalism)* occurs when an individual identifies equally with two or more cultures (Purnell and Paulanka, 2008).

It is easy for nurses to stereotype cultural groups after reading generalized information about various ethnic minority practices and beliefs (Dein, 2006). Avoid stereotypes or unwarranted generalizations about any particular group that prevents further assessment of the individual's unique characteristics. It is also important to determine how many of an individual's life patterns are consistent with his or her heritage (Armer and Radina, 2006).

Culturally Congruent Care

Leininger (2002) defines **transcultural nursing** as a comparative study of cultures to understand similarities (culture universal) and differences (culture-specific) across human groups. The goal of transcultural nursing is **culturally congruent care,** or care that fits the person's life patterns, values, and a set of meanings. Patterns and meanings are generated from people themselves rather than predetermined criteria. Culturally congruent care is sometimes different from the values and meanings of the professional health care system. Discovering patients' culture care values, meanings, beliefs, and practices as they relate to nursing and health care requires nurses to assume the role of learners and partner with patients and families in defining the characteristics of meaningful and beneficial care (Leininger and McFarland, 2002). Effective nursing care needs to integrate the cultural values and beliefs of individuals, families, and communities (Webber, 2008).

Cultural competence is the process of acquiring specific knowledge, skills, and attitudes to ensure delivery of culturally congruent care (Campinha-Bacote, 2002). This process has five interlocking components:

1. *Cultural awareness:* An in-depth self-examination of one's own background, recognizing biases, prejudices, and assumptions about other people
2. *Cultural knowledge:* Obtaining sufficient comparative knowledge of diverse groups, including their indigenous values, health beliefs, care practices, worldview, and bicultural ecology
3. *Cultural skills:* Being able to assess social, cultural, and biophysical factors influencing treatment and care of patients
4. *Cultural encounters:* Engaging in cross-cultural interactions that provide learning of other cultures and opportunities for effective intercultural communication development
5. *Cultural desire:* The motivation and commitment to caring that moves an individual to learn from others, accept the role as learner, be open and accepting of cultural differences, and build on cultural similarities

Specific knowledge, skills, and attitudes are required in the delivery of culturally congruent care to individuals and communities. Nurses who provide culturally competent care bridge cultural gaps to provide meaningful and supportive care for patients. For example, a nurse assigned to a female Egyptian patient decides to seek information about the Egyptian culture. On learning that Egyptians value female modesty and gender-congruent care, the nurse encourages female relatives to help the patient meet her needs for personal hygiene. The nurse's cultural encounter enhances understanding of the nonverbal cues of the patient's discomfort with lack of privacy.

Implementing culturally competent care requires support from health care agencies. For example, a nurse who is aware of Gypsy culture and skilled in dealing with Gypsy families is not able, as an individual, to provide for a Gypsy family's need to be present in groups near the bedside of a hospitalized family member. The nurse needs organizational support in adapting space resources to accommodate the volume of visitors who will remain with the patient for long periods.

Because patients who seek care could be from countless different world cultures, it is unlikely that a nurse could be competent in all cultures of the world. However, nurses can have general knowledge and skills to prepare them to provide culturally sensitive care, regardless of the patient's and family's culture (Purnell and Paulanka, 2008).

Cultural Conflicts

Culture provides the context for valuing, evaluating, and categorizing life experiences. Cultural groups transmit their values, morals, and norms from one generation to another, which predisposes members to **ethnocentrism,** a tendency to hold one's own way of life as superior to others. Ethnocentrism is the cause of biases and prejudices that associate negative permanent characteristics with people who are different from the valued group. When a person acts on these prejudices, discrimination occurs. For example, a nurse refuses to give prescribed pain medication to a young African male with sickle cell anemia because of the nurse's belief (stereotyped bias) that young male Africans are likely to be drug abusers. Nurses and other health care providers who have cultural ignorance or cultural blindness about differences generally resort to **cultural imposition** and use their own values and lifestyles as the absolute guide in dealing with patients and interpreting their behaviors. Thus a nurse who believes that people should bear pain quietly as a demonstration of strong moral character is annoyed when a patient insists on having pain medication and denies the patient's discomfort.

CULTURAL CONTEXT OF HEALTH AND CARING

Culture is the way in which groups of people make sense of their experiences relevant to life transitions such as birth, illness, and dying. For example, in most African groups a thin body is a sign of poor health. In some Hispanic cultures a plump baby is perceived as healthy. Traditionally in Arab culture pregnancy is not a medical condition but rather a normal life transition; thus a pregnant woman does not always go to a health care provider unless she has a problem (Purnell and Paulanka, 2008).

Table 9-1 provides a comparison of cultural contexts of health and illness in western and nonwestern cultures. Cultural beliefs highly influence what people believe to be the cause of illness. For example, many Hmong refugees (group of people who originated from the mountainous regions of Laos) believe that epilepsy is caused by the wandering of the soul. Treatment includes intervention by a shaman who performs a ritual to retrieve the patient's soul (Fadiman, 1997; Helsel et al., 2005). Their belief is distinct from the scientifically determined neurological abnormality

TABLE 9-1 Comparative Cultural Contexts of Health and Illness

	WESTERN CULTURES	NONWESTERN CULTURES
Cause of illness	Biomedical causes	Imbalance between humans and nature Supernatural Magico-religious
Method of diagnosis	Scientific, high-tech Specialty focused Organ-specific manifestations	Naturalistic, magico-religious Holistic Mixed Global, nonspecific symptomatology
Treatment	Specialty specific Pharmacological Surgery	Holistic Mixed (e.g., magico-religious, supernatural herbal, biomedical)
Practitioners/healers	Uniform standards and qualifications for practice	May be learned through apprenticeship Criteria for practice not uniform Reputation established in community
Caring pattern	Self-care Self-determination	Caring provided by others Group reliance and interdependence

Data from Foster G: Disease etiologies in non-Western medical systems, *Am Anthropol* 78:773, 1976; Kleinman A: *Patients and healers in the context of culture*, Berkeley, 1979, University of California Press; and Leininger MM, McFarland MR: *Transcultural nursing: concepts, theories, research and practice*, ed 3, New York, 2002, McGraw-Hill.

causing seizures. The biomedical orientation of western cultures emphasizing scientific investigation and reducing the human body to distinct parts is in conflict with the holistic conceptualization of health and illness in nonwestern cultures. Holism is evident in the belief in continuity between humans and nature and between human events and metaphysical and magico-religious phenomena. Therefore for the Hmong people epilepsy is connected to the magical and supernatural forces in nature. Establishing a diagnosis of epilepsy in western cultures requires scientifically proven techniques and confirmed criteria for the abnormality. Such medical criteria are meaningless to the Hmong, who believe in the global causation of the illness that goes beyond the mind and body of the person to forces in nature. A Hmong seeks a shaman, whereas a westerner seeks a neurologist. A shaman has an established reputation in the Hmong community, whose qualifications for healing are neither determined by published standardized criteria nor confined to specific bodily systems. A shaman uses rituals symbolizing the supernatural, spiritual, and naturalistic modalities of prayers, herbs, and incense burning.

The dominant value orientation in North American society is individualism and self-reliance in achieving and maintaining health. Caring approaches generally promote the patient's independence and ability for self-care. In collectivistic cultures that value group reliance and interdependence such as traditional Asians, Hispanics, and Africans, caring behaviors require actively providing physical and psychosocial support for family or community members. An adult patient is not expected to be solely responsible for his or her care and well-being; rather, family and kin are relied on to make decisions and provide care (Purnell and Paulanka, 2008). For example, a traditional older Chinese woman refuses to independently perform rehabilitation exercises after hip surgery until her daughter is present. The western health care provider interprets this as a lack of self-responsibility and motivation for her care. In contrast, the patient interprets the nurse's insistence on self-care as uncaring behavior.

Cultural Healing Modalities and Healers

Foster (1976) identified two distinct categories of healers cross-culturally. **Naturalistic practitioners** attribute illness to natural, impersonal, and biological forces that cause alteration in the equilibrium of the human body. Healing emphasizes use of naturalistic modalities, including herbs, chemicals, heat, cold, massage, and surgery. In contrast, **personalistic practitioners** believe that an external agent, which can be human (i.e., sorcerer) or nonhuman (e.g., ghosts, evil, or deity), causes health and illness. Personalistic beliefs emphasize the importance of humans' relationships with others, both living and deceased, and with their deities. For example, a voodoo priest uses modalities that combine supernatural, magical, and religious beliefs through the active facilitation of an external agent or personalistic practitioner. A Haitian woman who believes in voodoo attributes her illness to a curse placed by someone and seeks the services of a voodoo priest to remove the cause. Personalistic approaches also include naturalistic modalities such as massage, aromatherapy, and herbs (see Chapter 32). Some patients seek both types of practitioners and use a combination of modalities to achieve health and treat illness. Different cultural groups in the United States use a variety of cultural healers (Table 9-2).

Avoid making rash judgments about patients' practices when they use both healing systems at the same time. In addition, gain knowledge and understanding of remedies used by patients to prevent cultural imposition. For example, many Southeast Asian cultures practice folk remedies such as coining (rubbing a coin roughly on the skin), cupping (placing heated cups on the skin), pinching, and burning to relieve aches and pains and remove bad wind or noxious elements that cause illness. Other groups, including eastern Europeans, use cupping as treatment for respiratory ailments. These remedies leave peculiar visible markings on the skin in the form of ecchymosis, superficial burns, strap marks, or local tenderness. Cultural ignorance of these practices causes a practitioner to call authorities for suspicion of abuse.

Culture-Bound Syndrome

Human groups create their own interpretation and descriptions of biological and psychological malfunctions within their unique social and cultural context (Dein, 2006). **Culture-bound syndromes** are illnesses that are specific to one culture. They are used to explain personal and social reactions of the members of the culture. Culture-bound syndromes occur in any society. In the United States "going postal," which refers to extreme and uncontrollable anger in the workplace that may result in shooting people, is now considered a culture-bound syndrome (Flaskerud, 2009). *Hwa-byung* is a Korean culture-bound syndrome observed among middle-age, low-income women who are overwhelmed and frustrated by the burden of caregiving for their in-laws, husbands, and children. Symptoms are generally somatic manifestations consisting of insomnia, fatigue, anorexia, indigestion, feelings of an epigastric mass, palpitations, heat, panic, feelings of impending doom, and dyspnea. Women unconsciously avoid expressions of symptoms that counter the cultural ideal of females as the caretaker of older adults, husbands, and children. Symptoms reflect the cultural definition of illness as imbalance between heat (yang) and cold (yin) (Purnell and Paulanka, 2008).

TABLE 9-2 **Cultural Healers**

CULTURAL GROUP	HEALER	NATURE OF PRACTICE
Chinese and Southeast Asians	Herbalist	Combination of plant, animal, and mineral products in restoring balance based on yin/yang concepts
	Acupuncturist	Yin treatment using needles to restore balance and flow of *qi;* yang treatment using moxibustion or heat with acupuncture possibly indicated to restore yin/yang balance
	Fortune teller	Consultation to foretell outcomes of plans and seek spiritual advice to enhance good fortune and deal with misfortune
	Shaman	Combination of prayers, chanting, and herbs to treat illnesses caused by supernatural, psychological, and physical factors
Asian Indians	Ayurvedic practitioner	Combination of dietary, herbal, and other naturalistic therapies to prevent and treat illness
Native American	Shaman	Combination of prayers, chanting, and herbs to treat illnesses caused by supernatural, psychological, and physical factors
African American	Granny midwife	Consultation in diagnosing and treating common illnesses and care of women in childbirth and children
	Spiritualist	Spiritual advising, counseling, and praying to treat illness or cope with personal and psychosocial problems
	Voodoo practitioners *Hougan* (male) *Mambo* (female)	Combination of herbs, drumming, and symbolic offerings to cure illness, remove curses, and protect a person
Hispanic	*Curandero/a*	Combination of prayers, herbs, and other rituals to treat traditional illnesses, especially in children
	Parteras Lay midwives	Assistance for women in childbirth and newborn care
	Yerbero Herbalist	Consultation for herbal treatment of traditional illnesses
	Sabador Bonesetters	Massage and manipulation of bones and joints used to treat a variety of ailments, including musculoskeletal conditions
	Espiritista Spiritualist	Foretelling of future and interpretation of dreams; combination of prayers, herbs, potions, amulets, and prayers for curing illnesses, including witchcraft
	Santero/a	Combination of prayers, symbolic offerings, herbs, potions, and amulets against witchcraft and curses

Data from Hautman MA: Folk health and illness beliefs, *Nurse Pract* 4(4):23, 1976; Loustaunau MO, Sobo EJ: *The cultural context of health, illness and medicine,* Westport, Conn, 1997; Spector RE: *Cultural diversity in health and illness,* ed 6, Englewood Cliffs, NJ, 2004, Prentice Hall.

CULTURE AND LIFE TRANSITIONS

Cultures generally mark transitions to different phases of life by rituals that symbolize cultural values and meanings attached to these life passages. Van Gennep (1960) originated the concept of **rites of passage** as significant social markers of changes in a person's life. Examining the practices surrounding these life events provides a view of the cultural meanings and expressions relevant to these transitions. For example, sending flowers and get-well greetings to a sick person is a ritual showing love and care for the patient in the dominant American culture in which privacy is valued. In collectivistic groups such as the Hispanic culture, physical presence of loved ones with the patient during illness demonstrates caring.

Pregnancy

All cultures value reproduction because it promotes continuity of the family and community. Pregnancy is generally associated with caring practices that symbolize the significance of this life transition in women. Infertility in a woman is considered grounds for divorce and rejection among Arabs. Pregnancy that occurs outside of accepted societal norms is generally taboo. Among traditional Muslims pregnancy out of wedlock sometimes results in the family's imposing severe sanctions against the female member (Purnell and Paulanka, 2008).

Some cultures that subscribe to the hot and cold theory of illness such as many Asian and Hispanic cultures view pregnancy as a hot state; thus they encourage cold foods such as milk and milk products, yogurt, sour foods, and vegetables (Edelstein, 2011). They believe that hot foods such as chilies, ginger, and animal products cause miscarriage and fetal abnormality. Modesty is a strong value among Afghan (Omeri et al., 2006) and Arab women (Kulwicki et al., 2005). These women sometimes avoid or refuse to be examined by male health care providers because of embarrassment. Religious beliefs sometimes interfere with prenatal testing, as in the case of a Filipino couple refusing amniocentesis because they believe that the outcome of pregnancy is God's will and not subject to testing.

Childbirth

How individuals express pain and the expectation about how to treat suffering varies cross-culturally and in different religions. For example, Vietnamese women are often stoic regarding the pain of childbirth because their culture views childbirth pain as a normal part of life (McLachlan and Waldenstrom, 2005). Traditional Puerto Rican and Mexican women often vocalize their pain during labor and avoid breathing through their mouths because this causes the uterus to rise. Traditional Arab Americans are sometimes physically or verbally more expressive when experiencing pain. Fear of drug addiction and the belief that pain is a form of spiritual atonement for one's past deeds motivate most Filipino mothers to tolerate pain without much complaining or asking for medication. Religious beliefs sometimes prohibit the presence of males, including husbands, from the delivery room. This often occurs among devout Muslims, Hindus, and Orthodox Jews (Purnell and Paulanka, 2008).

Health care providers other than physicians attend childbirth in some groups such as *parteras* among Mexicans, herb doctors among Appalachian and southern African Americans, and *hilots* among Filipinos (Nelms and Gorski, 2006). Known in their communities, these practitioners are affordable and accessible in remote areas. They use a combination of naturalistic, religious, and supernatural modalities combining herbs, massage, and prayers.

Newborn

The definition of newborn and how age is counted in children varies in some cultures. Among traditional Vietnamese and Koreans a newborn is 1 year old at birth. Once acculturated to the U.S. culture, they assume a bicultural view, deducting 1 year from the age of the child when speaking to an outsider. Naming ceremonies vary by culture. In the Yoruba tribes in Nigeria, the baby is named at the official naming ceremony that occurs 8 days after birth and coincides with circumcision. Many cultures around the world greatly celebrate the birth of a son, including Chinese, Asian Indians, Islamic groups, and Igbos in West Africa.

The name of the child often reflects cultural values of the group. It is typical for a Hispanic baby to have several first names followed by the surnames of the father and mother (e.g., Maria Kristina Lourdes Lopez Vega). The bilineal tracing of descent from both the mother's and father's side in Hispanic groups differs from the patrilineal system, in which the last name of the father precedes the child's first name. In the Chinese culture individuals trace descent only from the paternal side. Thus the name Chen Lu means that Lu is the daughter of Mr. Chen.

Newborns and young children are often considered vulnerable, and societies use a variety of ways to prevent harm to the child. Among the mostly Catholic Filipinos, parents keep the newborn inside the home until after the baptism to ensure the baby's health and protection. Traditional Arabs and Iranians believe that babies are vulnerable to cold and wind; thus they wrap them in blankets.

Postpartum Period

In many nonwestern cultures the postpartum period is associated with vulnerability of the mother to cold. To restore balance mothers do not shower and take sponge baths. Some groups have special dietary practices to restore balance. Cultural groups have preferences in terms of what types of foods are appropriate to restore balance in women after birth. Some Chinese mothers prefer soups, rice, rice wine, and eggs; whereas Guatemalan women avoid beans, eggs, and milk during the postpartum period (Edelstein, 2011). The length of the postpartum period is generally much longer (30 to 40 days) in nonwestern cultures to provide support for the mother and her baby (Chin et al., 2010).

Filipino, Mexicans, and Pacific Islanders use an abdominal binder to prevent air from entering the woman's uterus and to promote healing (Purnell and Paulanka, 2008). Among Orthodox Jewish, Islamic, and Hindu cultures, bleeding is associated with pollution. A woman goes into a ritual bath after bleeding stops before she is able to resume relations with her husband (Lewis, 2003). In some African cultures such as in Ghana and Sierra Leone some women do not resume sexual relations with their husbands until the baby is weaned.

Grief and Loss

Dying and death bring traditions that are meaningful to groups of people for most of their lives (see Chapter 36). When traditional medical measures fail, cultural beliefs and practices that are religious and spiritual become the focus. Societies assign different meanings to death of a child, a young person, and an older adult (Box 9-1). In western cultures with strong future time orientation and in which a child is expected to survive his or her parents, death of a young person is devastating. However, in other cultures, in which infant mortality is very high, the emotional distress over a child's death is tempered by the reality of the commonly observed risks of growing up. Thus the untimely death of an adult is sometimes mourned more deeply.

People such as devout Hindus and Buddhists who believe in the concept of reincarnation view death as a step toward rebirth. Care of the dying focuses on supporting the patient's preparation for a good death. The family prays and reads religious scriptures to the patient to improve his or her chances in the next cycle. Buddhists generally believe that life is suffering and suffering ends when a person moves beyond the earthly desires and atones for past misdeeds. When a Hindu dies, the body is bathed, massaged in oil, dressed in clean clothes, and cremated before the next sunrise to ensure that the soul passes quickly from this life to the next (Lobar et al., 2006).

BOX 9-1 EVIDENCE-BASED PRACTICE

Cultural Beliefs and Rituals Surrounding Death

PICO Question: What intervention is best when planning culturally competent care for a dying patient?

Evidence Summary

Although culture and religion are important to people who are dying and their families, practices surrounding the death of a loved one vary among cultures and religions. Many cultures and religions use their beliefs to allow them to pray, talk, and remember their loved one. Rituals often accompany ceremonies and are used to delay death, ward off evil, ensure that the dying person is remembered, and help the family cope with the death. Respect for dying family members and protection of their souls are important. Many practices that surround death are influenced by religion and culture. Those who are Hispanic and Latino often have rituals that are heavily influenced by Catholicism. African Americans and Caribbeans identify the importance of faith, hope, and prayer. Similarities exist between Hindu and Buddhist beliefs about funeral arrangements, afterlife, family customs and Karma (Lobar et al., 2006). Although preparing for death is important for many Chinese individuals, many believe that talking about death brings evil spirits, bad luck, and a premature death (Chan and Yau, 2009-2010).

Application to Nursing Practice

- Be aware of religious and cultural preferences when helping patients and families prepare for death.
- Ask families about the rituals and ceremonies they use to help them cope with the death of a loved one.
- Allow patients and families the ability to participate in planning which rituals will be performed at the patient's bedside.
- Be sensitive to cultural perceptions regarding organ donation, viewing the body, and preparing for burial.

Culture strongly influences pain expression and need for pain medication. A typical American believes that individual freedom and autonomy are synonymous with freedom from pain and suffering, but other groups accept suffering. Do not assume that all people value pain relief equally. Patients suffer **cultural pain** when health care providers disregard values or cultural beliefs (Maputle and Jali, 2006). Inability of Orthodox Jews to pray in groups at the bedside with the dying patient because of limitations in the number of visitors allowed causes cultural pain in the patient and family. Working with the family and their religious/spiritual leader facilitates culturally congruent care (Purnell and Paulanka, 2008).

Organizational policies need to be sensitive to patients' cultural life patterns, especially during times of grief and loss. The dominant values in American society of individual autonomy and self-determination are often in direct conflict with diverse groups. Advance directives, informed consent, and consent for hospice are examples of mandates that sometimes violate patients' values. Informed consent and advance directives protect the right of the individual to know and make decisions ensuring continuity of these rights, even when the individual is incapacitated. However, in some cultures the designated family members assume decision making during illness and are trusted to make the right decision for the individual. Some groups such as African Americans, Asian Americans, and Hispanics expect their families to make decisions for them; and family members prefer to protect the individual from unnecessary suffering by knowing the reality of imminent death. These cultures value group interdependence and view individual autonomy as an unnecessary burden for a loved one who is ill (Purnell and Paulanka, 2008).

The meaning and expressions of grief vary from culture to culture. The color black is not always a symbol of grief. Hindu mourners wear white. Among the usually reserved East Asians, the extent to which mourners publicly express grief reflects the social position and status of the deceased. Muslims do not encourage wailing, but crying is permitted. Muslim women are discouraged from visiting cemeteries (Lobar et al., 2006). Korean families sometimes hire people to lead the open grieving. Loud crying and screaming are common.

Religious beliefs also affect attitudes toward cremation, organ donation, and the treatment of body parts. Devout Muslims refuse an autopsy or organ donation for fear of desecrating the dead and because of their belief that one has to be whole to appear in front of the creator. Many prefer burial over cremation (Lobar et al., 2006).

CULTURAL ASSESSMENT

Cultural assessment is a systematic and comprehensive examination of the cultural care values, beliefs, and practices of individuals, families, and communities. The goal of cultural assessment is to gather significant information from the patient that enables the nurse to implement culturally congruent and safe patient care (Box 9-2). For example, it allows the nurse to gather information about which foods are culturally acceptable and whether the person practices alternative medicine and to assess pain (Maier-Lorentz, 2008). There are several models for cultural assessment, each involving different levels of skill and knowledge. Leininger's Sunrise Model (2002) in Fig. 9-2 demonstrates the inclusiveness of culture in everyday life and helps to explain why cultural assessment needs to be comprehensive. The model assumes that cultural care values, beliefs, and practices are fixed in the cultural and social structural dimensions of society, which include environmental context, language, and ethnohistory. **Ethnohistory** refers to significant historical experiences of a particular group. For example, many older Americans tend to be frugal and save everything because of their experience with the Great Depression. These patient's stories reveal the broad picture of who they are and the cultural lifestyle they embrace. Leininger's model differentiates folk care, which is caring as defined by the people, from health care, which is provided by health care professionals and based on the scientific, biomedical caring system.

Census Data

A nurse begins cultural assessment by knowing population demographic changes in the community setting of practice. Having background knowledge of a culture assists the nurse in conducting a focused assessment. Gather demographics from the local and regional census data and from the demographic breakdown of patients who come to the health care setting. Population demographics include the distribution of ethnic groups, education, occupations, and incidence of the most common illnesses. Comprehensive cultural assessment requires skill and time; preparation and anticipation of need are important.

Asking Questions

One problem in cultural assessment is failing to assess the insider or emic perspective of patients and interpret information during the assessment. Use open-ended, focused, and contrast questions. The aim is to encourage patients to describe values, beliefs, and practices that are significant to their care that health care providers will take for granted unless otherwise uncovered. Culturally oriented questions are by nature broad and require many descriptions (Box 9-3).

Establishing Relationships

In contrast to other types of interviews, cultural assessment is intrusive and time consuming and requires a trusting relationship between participants. Miscommunication commonly occurs in intercultural interactions. This is because of language and

BOX 9-2 CULTURAL ASPECTS OF CARE

Understanding Cultural Safety

It is important for nurses and other health care providers to provide culturally safe care for patients and their families. Health care disparity in minority populations is an international problem, even in multicultural societies. A large body of research has identified that the health of an ethnic group is jeopardized when their cultural identity is demeaned or disempowered. Research has identified associations between perceived racial discrimination and hypertension, low birth weight, and mental disorders (Baker, 2007).

Culturally safe care can be defined as providing an environment in which people are treated with respect for their identity and dignity for who they are and in which a shared experience of listening and learning is created (Johnstone and Kanitsaki, 2007).

Implications for Practice

- Set culture care as a priority.
- Approach patients and families in a culturally sensitive manner.
- Engage in negotiated partnerships with patients and families.
- Enable the families and social networks of patients to serve as backup support.

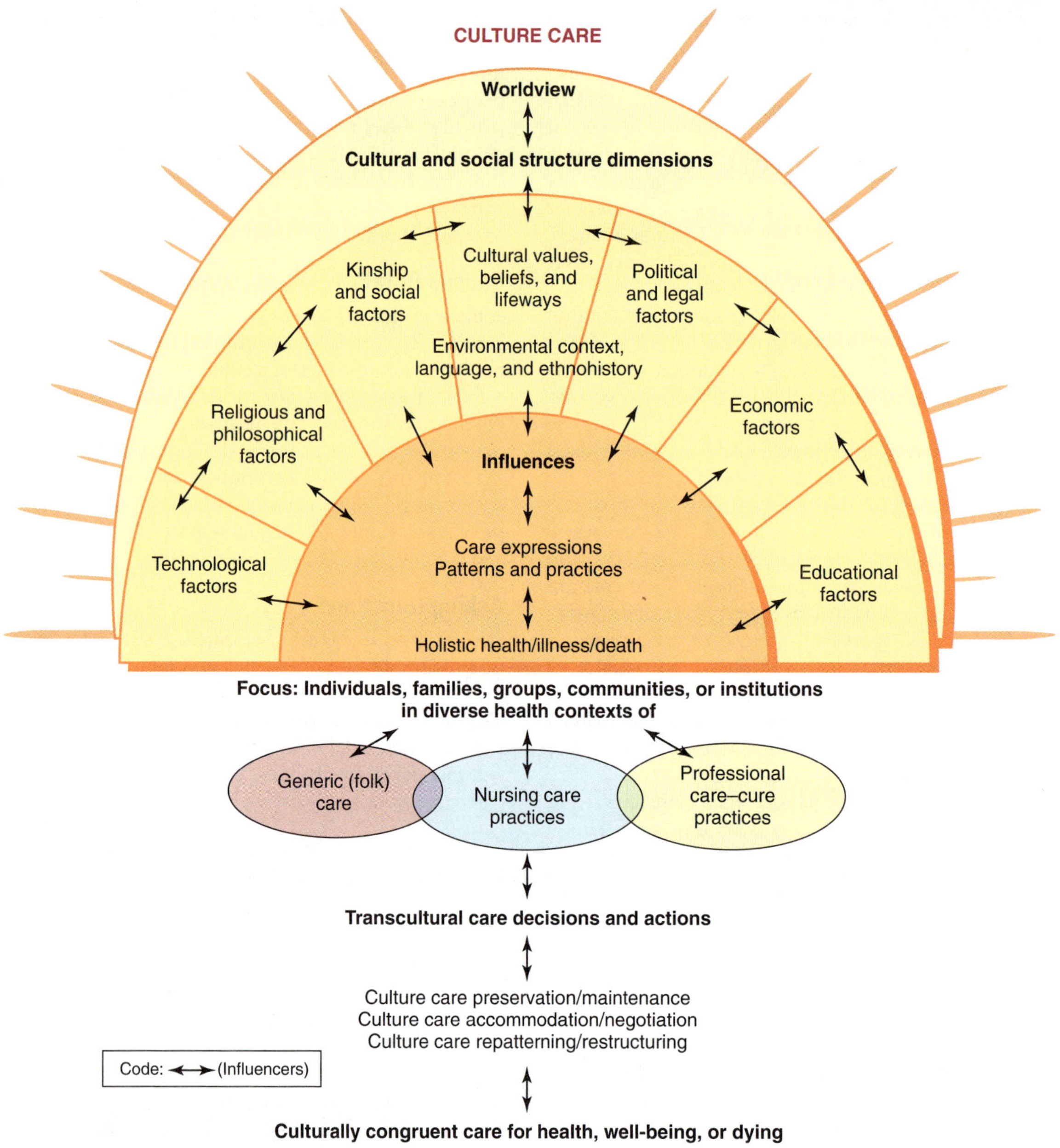

FIG. 9-2 Leininger's culture care theory and sunrise model. (Reprinted with permission from Leininger MM, McFarland MR: *Transcultural nursing: concepts, theories, research and practice,* ed 3, New York, 2002, McGraw-Hill.)

communication differences between and among participants and differences in interpreting each other's behaviors. Nurses use transcultural communication skills to interpret the patient's behavior within his or her own context of meanings and to behave in a culturally congruent way. Transcultural communication manages the impression the nurse makes on the patient to achieve desired outcomes of communication (Purnell and Paulanka, 2008). Transcultural communication requires linguistic skills, culturally congruent interpretation of behaviors of others, listening, and observation skills. In a cultural assessment the goal is to generate knowledge about the patient's values, beliefs, and practices about nursing and health care. If the nurse's behavior is offensive to the patient, he or she will not likely participate in the interaction.

To provide safe and effective patient care, you need to develop and use transcultural communication skills and be able to work with interpreters (Box 9-4). Interpreters are more effective when they have knowledge of the culture of the patient. They provide accurate accounts of what is said and, just as important, offer information regarding the cultural beliefs of the patient and family. Interpreters tactfully formulate culturally sensitive questions that provide the health care provider with needed information (Dysart-Gale, 2007). On admission nurses assess and document language(s)

BOX 9-3 NURSING ASSESSMENT QUESTIONS

Open-Ended
- What do you think caused your illness?
- How do you want us to help you with your problem?

Focused
- Did you have this problem before?
- Is there someone you want us to talk to about your care?

Contrast
- How different is this problem from the one you had previously?
- What is the difference between what we are doing and what you think we should be doing for you?

Ethnohistory
- How long have you/your parents resided in this country?
- What is your ethnic background or ancestry?
- How strongly does your culture influence you?
- Tell me why you left your homeland.

Social Organization
- Who lives with you?
- Whom do you consider members of your family?
- Where do other members of your family live?
- Who makes the decisions for you or your family?
- To whom do you go outside of your family for support?
- What expectations do you have of your family members who are males, females, old, or young?

Socioeconomic Status
- What do you do for a living?
- How different is your life here from back home?

Bicultural Ecology and Health Risks
- What caused your problem?
- How does this problem affect or how has it affected your life and your family?
- How do you treat this problem at home?
- What other problems do you have?

Language and Communication
- What language(s) do you speak at home?
- What language(s) do you use to read and write?
- How should we address you or what should we call you?
- What kinds of communication upset or offend you?

Caring Beliefs and Practices
- What do you do to keep yourself well?
- What do you do to show someone you care?
- How do you take care of sick family members?
- Which caregivers do you seek when you are sick?
- How different is what we do from what your family does for you when you are sick?

patients speak and write and determine if patients need an interpreter.

Federal mandates for culturally sensitive health care delivery require accommodation for language differences. According to the Office of Minority Health and Health Disparities (2007b), national standards regarding language services include:

BOX 9-4 RULES OF IMPRESSION MANAGEMENT

1. Greet patients and their visitors in their own language if possible.
2. Introduce yourself. Tell patients what to call you.
3. Welcome visitors and request them to introduce themselves and explain how they are related to the patient.
4. Thank the visitors for coming.
5. Ask to talk with the patient in private and offer to accompany visitors to the waiting room.
6. Inform visitors that you will call them when you finish with the patient.
7. Tell the patient your purpose.
8. Clarify if the patient wants someone else such as a family member to be present.
9. Avoid asking the patient questions in front of the family or spouse that will put him or her at risk with this group.
10. If the patient needs an interpreter:
    a. Introduce yourself to the interpreter.
    b. Determine the qualifications of the interpreter.
        (1) Make sure that the interpreter can speak the dialect of the patient.
        (2) Ensure gender, age, and ethnic compatibility of the interpreter with the patient's preference and topic of discussion.
        (3) Watch for differences in educational and socioeconomic status between the patient and interpreter.
        (4) Orient the interpreter to your purpose and expectation (e.g., assessment of the patient's level of pain, intent to explain procedure to the patient).
    c. Clarify your questions about the interpreter's training, compatibility with the patient, and the interpreter's understanding of your expectations beforehand.
    d. Introduce the interpreter to the patient.
    e. Pace your speech slowly and allow time for back translation.
    f. Direct your questions to the patient.
    g. Request the interpreter to ask the patient for feedback and clarification at regular intervals.
    h. Observe the patient's nonverbal and verbal behaviors.
    i. Thank both the patient and interpreter.
11. Ask the patient with whom you will need to consult for major decisions and how to contact this person.
12. Observe nonverbal behavior and match the degree of distance exhibited by the patient.

- Providing language assistance services free of charge to all patients with limited English at all points of contact.
- Notifying patients, both verbally and in writing, of their rights to receive language-assistance services.
- Using interpreters for patients with limited English proficiency (unless the patient requests that family or friends interpret for them).

The Joint Commission (2010) requires that informed consent materials be in the patient's language whenever possible and that an interpreter be available whenever discussing informed consent with a patient. If informed consent documents are not available in the patient's language, The Joint Commission also recommends that the health care provider obtain verbal consent from the patient via the interpreter and that this is thoroughly documented in the patient's medical record.

Nurses need to know their agencies' policies and procedures regarding these mandates. Working with interpreters and patients with little or no fluency in English requires skill development. In hospital settings use an interpreter to communicate information

BOX 9-5 LANGUAGE ACCESS SERVICES

- All health care organizations are required to offer free language assistance, including bilingual staff or interpreter services to each patient with limited English proficiency. These services must be offered in a timely manner at all hours of operation at all points of contact.
- Patients must be informed, in their preferred language, of their right to receive language assistance services both verbally and in written form.
- The competence of bilingual staff and interpreters providing language assistance must be ensured by the health care organization.
- Unless requested by the patient, family and friends should not be used to provide interpretation services.
- Interpreters are more effective when they have knowledge of the culture of the patient.
- Patient-related information and signage must be posted in the service area of the health care organization in the languages of the groups who are commonly served.

Data from Office of Minority Health US Department of Health and Human Services: A patient-centered guide to implementing language across services in healthcare organizations, 2005, http://minorityhealth.hhs.gov/Assets/pdf/Checked/HC-LSIG.pdf

about the patient's medical condition. It is not suitable for family members to translate health care information, but they can assist with ongoing interaction during the patient's care (Box 9-5).

Consider what needs to be discussed with a patient when selecting an interpreter. In some Hispanic and Asian groups a woman's breasts and genitals generally are not discussed with members of the opposite sex, including male members of one's family. In some societies, adults occupy a higher status than the young. Children in immigrant groups learn the English language faster than their parents because of their schooling experience in the new culture when they immigrate at a young age. However, assuming that children are ideal interpreters for their parents is an insult to the authority of the parent who has to take directions from a child.

Compatibility between the ethnic backgrounds of the interpreter and patient is another consideration to facilitate trust. An Israeli interpreter may cause much anxiety and distrust in a Palestinian immigrant who experienced violence from these groups in the home country. Socioeconomic and educational differences between interpreters and patients sometimes become barriers to effective interpretation. Interpreters need training not only in interpretation but also in knowing their role, which is to repeat back what the patient said without judging the content.

Selected Components of Cultural Assessment

Nurses learn various skills needed to gather an accurate and comprehensive cultural assessment. The following components of cultural assessment provide insight into the type of information that is useful in planning and delivering nursing care.

Family Structure. Integrate patients' and families' concepts of meaningful and supportive care into nursing care (see Chapter 7). Caring expressions integrate the central values of a culture. In collectivistic cultures caring means active involvement of the group, emphasizing mutual and reciprocal obligations of members to care for one another. When caring for patients from collective cultures, work with patients' families as a group, looking for ways the family can participate in basic care activities. Understand the family's social hierarchy and assume a collaborative role with patients and their families.

Culture differentiates caring roles of males and females. In many cultures caretaking tasks are the primary responsibility of women; men provide financial support and make major decisions. Age and position in the social hierarchy also influence caring roles and responsibilities. In some cultures older women are the first group consulted during illness of family members and in the care of women and children.

Ethnic Heritage and Ethnohistory. Knowledge of a patient's country of origin and its history and ecological contexts are significant to health care. For example, Haitian immigrants have linguistic and communication patterns distinct from those of Jamaicans, even though they both come from the Caribbean and have a common history of slavery. Differences come from their colonial history and intermingling with the local indigenous people. As a result of cultural differences between India and Jamaica, Hindu immigrants from Jamaica have different cultural characteristics from those originating from India. Hindu immigrants from Jamaica often have nutritional, communication, and health patterns more similar to African Jamaicans than South Asian Hindus. In caring for an Indian Hindu who grew up in Jamaica, expect the patient to interact more like a Jamaican, even though the person looks like he or she is from south India.

Immigration from one country to another occurs for various reasons. Refugees are relocated without any choice in their initial residence, in contrast to immigrants, who have options as to where they go. Refugees experience greater dislocation and deprivation than immigrants who enter a new country with specialized skills and education and have the option to return to their homeland. Age of immigration often determines the level of acculturation, with younger immigrants acculturating faster than older immigrants. Although acculturation and length of residence in the new culture are related, other factors such as education, racial characteristics, and familiarity with the language affect the extent of a person's acculturation. Ask patients about the condition or situation that brought them to the United States and how they think they are adjusting. Socioeconomic status in the new society is often not comparable to one's previous status in the country of origin. New immigrants often begin with small resources but keep the values and desires of their previous economic status. Assess for problems (such as financial hardships, becoming comfortable with the language, or understanding the routines used to set medical appointments) to make reasonable and appropriate adjustments to care. Refer patients to community resources when possible.

Bicultural Effects on Health. Identify patients' health risks related to sociocultural and biological history on admission. Some distinct health risks are the result of the ecological context of the culture. For example, immigrants originating from the region near the Nile River are generally at risk for parasitic infestations that are prevalent in that area. Immigrants from the Third World with poor sanitary conditions and water supply are at risk for infections such as hepatitis. Certain genetic disorders are also linked with specific ethnic groups such as Tay-Sachs among Ashkenazi Jews and malignant hypertension among African Americans. Lactose intolerance is frequently observed among Asians, Africans, and Hispanics (Office of Minority Health, 2005).

Social Organization. Cultural groups consist of units of organization defined by kinship, status, and appropriate roles for their members. In the dominant American society the most common unit of social organization is the nuclear family, in which married children and adults establish separate residences from their parents. Although different configurations of a family exist, the most common is the nuclear household made up of parents and their young children (see Chapter 10). In collectivistic cultures families are made up of distant blood relatives across three generations and **fictive** or nonblood kin. Kinship extends to both the father's and mother's side of the family **(bilineal)** or is limited to the side of either father **(patrilineal)** or mother **(matrilineal)**. Patrilineally extended families exist among Chinese and Hindus, in which a woman moves into her husband's clan after marriage and minimizes ties with her own parents and siblings. Consider all options when determining a patient's next of kin. This is especially relevant to new immigrants and refugees, who often have not relocated with all members of their family. Collectivistic groups often regard members of their ethnic group as closest kin and want to consult them for health care decisions and permit them to speak on their behalf.

A patient's status within the social hierarchy is generally linked with qualities such as age, gender, and achieved status such as education and position. The dominant culture in the United States emphasizes achievement as the determinant of status, whereas most collectivistic cultures give higher priority to age and gender. The eldest male is next to his father in terms of authority in many Asian and African cultures. A Korean mother is subject to the authority of her oldest son in the absence of her husband. Sometimes an adult Hispanic woman will not sign informed consent for surgery or other medical procedures without consulting her husband, oldest son, or brothers. Older adults occupy higher status in some societies, resulting in grandparents forcing their decisions over their married children regarding the care of the grandchildren. Determine who has authority for making decisions within the family and how to communicate with the proper individuals.

Culture defines the expected roles of its members. Certain behaviors are acceptable in children but not in adults. Gender also differentiates role expectations. For example, among devout Muslims females perform the task of caregiving, whereas males are the financial providers and major decision makers. Thus nurses need to anticipate that some Muslim women insist on staying at the bedside of their children, in-laws, or husbands. However, do not assume that, just because the woman is the primary caregiver, she will make decisions independently. Determine the family social hierarchy as soon as possible to prevent offending patients and their families. Working with established family hierarchy prevents delays and achieves better patient outcomes.

Religious and Spiritual Beliefs. Religious and spiritual beliefs frequently influence the patient's worldview about health and illness, pain and suffering, and life and death. Determine the patient's religious and spiritual beliefs and their effect on health care during admission. Also understand the emic perspective of your patients. For example, to a Hmong animist spirits are dead ancestors or forces external to the person. To some Americans spirituality means an inner, personal relationship with God. Although it is sometimes difficult to find the appropriate time to discuss religion and spirituality in a hospital setting, nurses need to assess what is important to the spiritual well-being of patients and learn as much as possible about their spiritual and religious practices (see Chapter 35).

Devout Muslims pray five times daily and undergo an obligatory ritual cleansing of some parts of their body before praying. Anticipate the ritual cleansing needs of the patient and provide privacy for praying. For example, reschedule diagnostic procedures to allow Buddhist patients to participate in the festivities of their New Year. Anticipating the needs of Orthodox Jewish patients during the Sabbath, when they refrain from using electrical appliances, requires creative accommodations by the staff such as placing articles of care near the patient so he or she does not need to use the call light or telephone to get assistance. Determine how to contact the patient's next of kin who are unreachable by telephone during the Sabbath in case emergencies arise.

BOX 9-6 PATIENT TEACHING

Cultural Considerations in Healthy Food Choices

Objective
- Patient will verbalize healthy foods that are culturally appropriate.

Teaching Strategies
- Refer patient to speak with a dietitian who is familiar with cultural food choices.
- Develop a diet plan that includes patient's cultural diet preferences.
- Provide culturally sensitive teaching brochures that describe healthy food choices.
- Include people in family who help shop for and prepare food in the home.

Evaluation
- Ask patient to keep a food diary for 1 week and evaluate food choices.
- Ask patient to describe how cultural food choices will fit within his or her prescribed diet.

Religious beliefs are evident in patients' dietary practices (Box 9-6). Devout Hindus avoid beef, and many are vegetarians. Many Buddhists are vegetarians as well. *Halal* foods, which include meat, fish, fresh fruit, vegetables, eggs, milk, and cheese, are permissible for Muslims. Halal meat comes from animals slaughtered during a prayer ritual. Prohibited, or *Haram,* foods include non-Halal meat, animals with fangs, pork products, gelatin products, and alcohol (Edelstein, 2011). Muslims fast during the daylight hours for the 28 days of *Ramadan,* which occurs during the ninth lunar month. Although children and sick and frail individuals are exempt from fasting, do not assume that these individuals eat regular meals during Ramadan. Rescheduling treatments and medications is often necessary to prevent complications such as hypoglycemia.

Jewish patients who follow a kosher diet avoid meat from carnivores, pork products, and fish without scales or fins. Kosher meat comes from permissible animals that are slaughtered with the least amount of suffering. Kosher foods must not be contaminated by nonkosher foods. Thus meat is served separately from dairy, and dishes used for serving and eating these products are also separated (Edelstein, 2011).

The nursing staff needs to have background information available about major holy days and practices for commonly encountered religions. Such information prevents scheduling nonemergency treatments and procedures on major holy days such as the Jewish holidays Yom Kippur, Rosh Hashanah, or Passover. Religious mandates followed by Jehovah's Witnesses require followers to have bloodless surgery and avoid blood transfusions. Identify and contact patients' religious and spiritual leaders before problems occur and work with these leaders to mediate in times of crisis.

Life transitions are often manifested in religious and spiritual beliefs. Male circumcision occurs among Jewish and Islamic groups. Female circumcision is common among some African and Muslim groups. Anointing of the sick is a Roman Catholic sacrament. Hospitalized Catholic patients often receive daily communion. The family of a critically ill Jewish patient turns his or her head eastward or to the right side. The family of a dying Hindu remains at the bedside to place a drop of the holy water from the River Ganges on the patient's lips immediately after death to help his or her soul to the next life. A dying Hispanic patient is not left alone so a close kin is able to hear the patient's wishes, allowing the soul to leave in peace.

Foods with Cultural Significance. Many foods have cultural significance and are adopted for traditional celebrations, medicinal purposes, and general nutritional health. For instance, in Italy it is a tradition to eat eel on Christmas Eve. It symbolizes a new beginning because eels replace their skin as they shed it. In Sweden the smorgasbord is an important part of special events such as holidays and weddings (Edelstein, 2011). Cake is a part of birthday and wedding celebrations in the United States. Russians consider honey to have healing qualities and use it to treat colds and coughs. Many Japanese follow traditional beliefs that food should be consumed as close to its natural state as possible, for instance raw fish *(sashimi)* used in making sushi.

Communication Patterns. Cultural groups have distinct linguistic and communication patterns. These patterns reflect core cultural values of a society. In the dominant American culture that supports individualism, people value assertive communication because it manifests the ideal of individual autonomy and self-determination. In collectivistic cultures the context of relationships among participants shapes communication. Promoting group harmony is a priority; thus participants interact based on their expected positions and relationships within the social hierarchy. Individuals are more likely to remain respectful and show deference to older adults or family leaders, even though they disagree on an issue. Differences in status and position, age, gender, and outsider versus insider determine the content and process of communication (Box 9-7). Among Asian cultures face-saving communication promotes harmony by indirect, ambiguous communication and conflict avoidance. In this culture spoken messages often have little to do with their meanings. Saying "no" to a superior or older person is not permissible. An affirmative response only means that "I heard you"; it is not full agreement. This type of response is likely to happen in a health care setting because a health care provider is perceived as a person of authority to some Asian, African, or Hispanic patients. Observing a patient's behavior and clarifying messages heard from a trusted insider prevents misinterpretation.

In cultural groups with distinct linear hierarchy, negotiation of conflict occurs among people within the same level of position or authority. Identifying and working with established family hierarchy prevents miscommunication. In cultures with highly differentiated gender roles some patients place more value on the advice of a man than a woman. By recognizing and working within this cultural context, nurses become more effective in achieving outcomes.

Culture also shapes nonverbal communication. It influences the distance between participants in an interaction, the degree of eye contact, the extent of touching, and how much private information the patient shares. Patients use less distance when speaking to trusted insiders and persons of the same age, gender, and position in the social hierarchy. Many ethnic groups tend to speak their own dialect with insiders for ease and privacy and as a marker of insider status. To minimize this distance when communicating with patients, nurses establish rapport and behave in a culturally congruent manner through impression management.

BOX 9-7 FOCUS ON OLDER ADULTS

Culturally Sensitive Communication

- Ask older adults how they like to be addressed. If in doubt, address them formally (e.g., Mr. Lin) (Meiner, 2011).
- Determine patient's preferences for touch (Meiner, 2011). For example, in the United States Americans often greet each other with a firm handshake. However, many Native Americans see this as a sign of aggression, and touch outside of marriage is sometimes forbidden in older adults from the Middle East.
- Investigate the patient's preferences for silence (Meiner, 2011). Generally Eastern cultures value silence, whereas Western cultures are uncomfortable with it.
- Be aware of the patient's beliefs about eye contact during conversation (Meiner, 2011). In European American cultures direct eye contact is a sign of honesty and truthfulness. However, eye contact with other groups such as older Native Americans is not allowed. Older Asian adults sometimes avoid eye contact with authority figures because it is considered disrespectful, and direct eye contact between genders in Middle Eastern cultures is sometimes forbidden except between spouses.

Time Orientation

All cultures have past, present, and future time dimensions. This information is useful in planning a day of care, setting up appointments for procedures, and helping a patient plan self-care activities in the home. The dominant American culture is future-time oriented, and people from this culture tend to schedule their time. When working with patients who are future-time oriented, it is important to plan and adhere to a schedule (Srivastava, 2007). Future-time orientation minimizes present time; thus communication tends to be direct and focused on task achievement. The rushed, hurried, and businesslike communication of a future-time oriented person may appear uncaring or disrespectful to those who are present or past-time oriented.

In some cultures time is oriented to the present, and events take place when the person arrives. Present-time orientation is in conflict with the dominant future-time orientation in health care that emphasizes punctuality and adherence to appointments. Within present-time oriented cultures it is acceptable to be late to appointments. When making appointments and referrals, explore and manage anticipated barriers to time adherence with the patient. Anticipate conflicts and make adjustments when caring for ethnic groups that value present-time orientation. African Americans, Puerto Ricans, Mexicans, Chinese, and Native Americans are some of the groups that value present-time orientation (Giger and Davidhizar, 2008). Past-time orientation is associated with adaptive cultures and populations who are exposed to situations that require immediate action such as immigrant populations (Crockett et al., 2009). Improving a patient's access to health services mandates culturally congruent time schedules that accommodate cultural patterns.

CARING BELIEFS AND PRACTICES

Obtain information about folk remedies and cultural healers that the patient uses. Assessment data yield information about the patient's beliefs about the illness and the meaning of the signs and symptoms. Focus assessment on the emic perspective of the patient. Allowing the patient to describe the meanings of care and identify caring behaviors is fundamental to culturally congruent care.

Experience with Professional Health Care

Understanding the emic perspective of the patient about professional health care is valuable in correcting misconceptions and preventing culturally offensive actions. Previous encounters with professional caregivers affect patients' adherence to therapies and continuing access of services. For example, if a patient previously had problems with male caregivers, assign female caregivers to the patient whenever possible. If a patient perceives an essential health care resource to be inaccessible, help to find a way to connect the patient with the resource. Partnership between health care professionals and the community provides proactive and open feedback from culturally diverse patient groups. Use of comparative assessment questions gives nurses insight into patients' perceptions and reactions to different aspects of the health care system and facilitates evaluation of patient outcomes.

Culturally Congruent Care

To provide culturally congruent care it is important to identify potential conflicts between patients' health care needs and their health care practices and cultural values. Leininger (2006) identified three nursing decision and action modes to achieve culturally congruent care. All three modes of professional decisions and actions assist, support, facilitate, or enable people of particular cultures.

1. **Cultural care preservation or maintenance**—Retain and/or preserve relevant care values so patients maintain their well-being, recover from illness, or face handicaps and/or death.
2. **Cultural care accommodation or negotiation**—Adapt or negotiate with others for a beneficial or satisfying health outcome.
3. **Cultural care repatterning or restructuring**—Reorder, change, or greatly modify patients' lifestyles for a new, different, and beneficial health care pattern.

Nurses are able to use any or all of these action modes simultaneously. These actions require that nurses have knowledge of patients' culture and the willingness, commitment, and skills to work with patients and families in decision making. The intended outcome of these actions and decisions is meaningful, supportive, and facilitative care as judged by the patient.

KEY POINTS

- Culture is the context for interpreting human experiences such as health and illness and provides direction to decisions and actions.
- Culturally congruent care is meaningful, supportive, and facilitative because it fits valued life patterns of patients.
- Nurses achieve culturally congruent care through cultural assessment and the application of cultural preservation, accommodation, and repatterning.
- Culturally competent care requires knowledge, attitudes, and skills supportive of implementation of culturally congruent care.
- Cultural assessment requires a comprehensive and thorough investigation of a patient's cultural values, beliefs, and practices.
- Transcultural nursing is a comparative study and understanding of cultures to identify specific and universal caring constructs across cultures.
- Impression management facilitates culturally congruent communication and intercultural relationships.

CLINICAL APPLICATION QUESTIONS

Preparing for Clinical Practice

A 43-year-old male patient, who is an Orthodox Jew, is hospitalized following a motor vehicle accident. The nurse caring for the patient notes that he has not touched most of the food on his plate and has only eaten his bread and fruit. In reviewing the patient's intake over the past 2 days, the nurse notes that this patient has eaten very little. The nurse reviews the patient's diet order and finds that his diet orders indicate that he is to receive no pork products. The patient was served meatloaf, macaroni and cheese, green beans, a dinner roll, and a fresh peach for lunch. For dinner he was served lasagna, breadsticks, a salad, and a pear for dessert.

1. Explain possible causes for the patient's poor appetite.
2. Identify nursing interventions to help increase the patient's food intake.
3. Of the three nursing decisions and action modes described by Leininger (2006), explain which one is the most appropriate for this patient.

evolve *Answers to Clinical Application Questions can be found on the Evolve website.*

REVIEW QUESTIONS

Are You Ready to Test Your Nursing Knowledge?

1. A 6-month-old child from Guatemala was adopted by an American family in Indiana. The child's socialization into the American midwestern culture is best described as:
   1. Assimilation.
   2. Acculturation.
   3. Biculturalism.
   4. Enculturation.
2. A 46-year-old woman from Bosnia came to the United States 6 years ago. Although she did not celebrate Christmas when she lived in Bosnia, she celebrates Christmas with her family now. This woman has experienced assimilation into the culture of the United States because she:
   1. Chose to be bicultural.
   2. Adapted to and adopted the American culture.
   3. Had an extremely negative experience with the American culture.
   4. Gave up part of her ethnic identity in favor of the American culture.
3. To enhance their cultural awareness, nursing students need to make an in-depth self-examination of their own:
   1. Motivation and commitment to caring.
   2. Social, cultural, and biophysical factors.
   3. Engagement in cross-cultural interactions.
   4. Background, recognizing personal biases and prejudices.
4. Which of the following is required in the delivery of culturally congruent care?
   1. Learning about vast cultures
   2. Motivation and commitment to caring
   3. Influencing treatment and care of patients
   4. Acquiring specific knowledge, skills, and attitudes
5. A registered nurse is admitting a patient of French heritage to the hospital. Which question asked by the nurse indicates that the nurse is stereotyping the patient?
   1. "What are your dietary preferences?"
   2. "What time do you typically go to bed?"
   3. "Do you bathe and use deodorant more than one time a week?"
   4. "Do you have any health issues that we should know about?"
6. When action is taken on one's prejudices:
   1. Discrimination occurs.
   2. Delivery of culturally congruent care is ensured.
   3. Effective intercultural communication develops.
   4. Sufficient comparative knowledge of diverse groups is obtained.

7. A nursing student is doing a community health rotation in an inner-city public health department. The student investigates sociodemographic and health data of the people served by the health department, and detects disparities in health outcomes between the rich and poor. This is an example of a(n):
   1. Illness attributed to natural and biological forces.
   2. Creation of the student's interpretation and descriptions of the data.
   3. Influence of socioeconomic factors in morbidity and mortality.
   4. Combination of naturalistic, religious, and supernatural modalities.
8. Culture strongly influences pain expression and need for pain medication. However, cultural pain is:
   1. Not expressed verbally or physically.
   2. Expressed only to others from a similar culture.
   3. Usually more intense than physical pain.
   4. Suffered by a patient whose valued way of life is disregarded by practitioners.
9. Which of the following best represents the dominant values in American society on individual autonomy and self-determination?
   1. Physician orders
   2. Advance directive
   3. Durable power of attorney
   4. Court-appointed guardian
10. The nurse at an outpatient clinic asks a patient who is Chinese American with newly diagnosed hypertension if he is limiting his sodium intake as directed. The patient does not make eye contact with the nurse but nods his head. What should the nurse do next?
    1. Ask the patient how much salt he is consuming each day
    2. Discuss the health implications of sodium and hypertension
    3. Remind the patient that many foods such as soy sauce contain "hidden" sodium
    4. Suggest some low-sodium dietary alternatives
11. A female Jamaican immigrant has been late to her last two clinic visits, which in turn had to be rescheduled. The best action that the nurse could take to prevent the patient from being late to her next appointment is:
    1. Give her a copy of the city bus schedule.
    2. Call her the day before her appointment as a reminder to be on time.
    3. Explore what has prevented her from being at the clinic in time for her appointment.
    4. Refer her to a clinic that is closer to her home.
12. A nursing student is taking postoperative vital signs in the postanesthesia care unit. She knows that some ethnic groups are more prone to genetic disorders. Which of the following patients is most at risk for developing malignant hypertension?
    1. Ashkenazi Jew
    2. Chinese American
    3. African American
    4. Filipino
13. A community health nurse is making a healthy baby visit to a new mother who recently emigrated to the United States from Ghana. When discussing contraceptives with the new mom, the mother states that she won't have to worry about getting pregnant for the time being. The nurse understands that the mom most likely made this statement because:
    1. She won't resume sexual relations until her baby is weaned.
    2. She is taking the medroxyprogesterone (Depo-Provera) shot.
    3. Her husband was recently deployed to Afghanistan.
    4. She has access to free condoms from the clinic.
14. During their clinical postconference meeting, several nursing students were discussing their patients with their instructor. One student from a middle-class family shared that her patient was homeless. This is an example of caring for a patient from a different:
    1. Ethnicity.
    2. Culture.
    3. Heritage.
    4. Religion.
15. When interviewing a Native American patient on admission to the hospital emergency department, which questions are appropriate for the nurse to ask? (Select all that apply.)
    1. Do you use any folk remedies?
    2. Do you have a family physician?
    3. Do you use a Shaman?
    4. Does your family have a history of alcohol abuse?

Answers: 1. 4; 2. 2; 3. 4; 4. 4; 5. 3; 6. 1; 7. 3; 8. 4; 9. 2; 10. 1; 11. 3; 12. 3; 13. 1; 14. 2; 15. 1, 2, 3.

REFERENCES

Baker C: Globalization and the cultural safety of an immigrant Muslim community, *J Adv Nurs* 57(3):296, 2007, DOI: 10.1111/j.1365-2648.2006.04104.x

Campinha-Bacote J: The process of cultural competence in the delivery of healthcare services: a model of care, *J Transcult Nurs* 13(3):181, 2002.

Dein S: Race, culture and ethnicity in minority research: a critical discussion, *J Cult Diversity* 13(2):68, 2006.

Dysart-Gale D: Clinicians and medical interpreters: negotiating culturally appropriate care for patients with limited English ability, *Family Commun Health* 30(3): 237, 2007.

Edelstein S: *Food, cuisine and cultural competency for culinary, hospitality and healthcare professionals*, Sudbury, Mass, 2011, Jones & Bartlett.

Fadiman A: *The spirit catches you and you fall down*, New York, 1997, Farrar, Straus & Giroux.

Flaskerud J: What do we need to know about the culture-bound syndromes? *Iss Ment Health Nurs* 30:406, 2009.

Foster G: Disease etiologies in non-Western medical systems, *Am Anthropol* 78:773, 1976.

Giger J, Davidhizar R: *Transcultural nursing: assessment and intervention*, ed 5, St Louis, 2008, Mosby.

Leininger MM: Culture care theory: a major contribution to advance transcultural nursing knowledge and practices, *J Transcult Nurs* 13(3):189, 2002.

Leininger MM, McFarland MR: *Transcultural nursing: concepts, theories, research and practice*, ed 3, New York, 2002, McGraw-Hill.

Leininger MM: Culture care diversity and universality theory and evolution of the ethnonursing method. In Leininger MM, McFarland MR, editors: *Culture care diversity and universality: a worldwide theory of nursing*, ed 2, Sudbury, Mass, 2006, Jones & Bartlett.

Lewis JA: Jewish perspectives on pregnancy and childbearing, *MCN Am J Matern Child Nurs* 28(5):306, 2003.

Lobar SL, et al: Cross-cultural beliefs, ceremonies, and rituals surrounding death of a loved one, *Pediatr Nurs* 32(1):44, 2006.

Maier-Lorentz MM: Transcultural nursing: its importance in nursing practice, *J Cult Diversity* 15(1):37, 2008.

McFarland MM, Eipperle MK: Culture care theory: A proposed practice theory guide for nurse practitioners in primary care settings, *Contemp Nurse* (28)1:48, 2008.

Meiner SE: *Gerontologic nursing*, ed 4, St Louis, 2011, Mosby.

Office of Minority Health, US Department of Health and Human Services: *A patient-centered guide to implementing language across services in healthcare organizations*, 2005, http://www.minorityhealth.hhs.gov/Assets/pdf/Checked/HC-LSIG.pdf. Accessed July 10, 2011.

Office of Minority Health and Health Disparities: *About minority health,* 2007a, http://www.cdc.gov/omhd/AMH/AMH.htm. Accessed July 10, 2011.

Office of Minority Health and Health Disparities: *National standards on culturally and linguistically appropriate services (CLAS),* 2007b, http://minorityhealth.hhs.gov/assets/pdf/checked/executive.pdf. Accessed July 10, 2011.

Purnell LD, Paulanka BJ: *Transcultural healthcare: a culturally competent approach,* ed 3, Philadelphia, 2008, FA Davis.

Srivastava RH: *The healthcare professional's guide to clinical competence,* Toronto, 2007, Elsevier.

The Joint Commission: *Advancing effective communication, cultural competence, and patient-and family-centered care: a roadmap for hospitals (monograph),* 2010, http://www.jointcommission.org//PatientSafety/HLC, accessed October 2, 2010.

US Census Bureau: *State and county quick facts,* 2010, http://quickfacts.census.gov/qfd/states/00000.html. Accessed July 10, 2011.

US Department of Health and Human Services: *Healthy People 2020,* Washington, DC, 2010, USDHHS.

United Pentecostal Church International: *Our doctrinal foundation,* 2011, http://www.upci.org/about-us/beliefs/21-about-us/beliefs/91. Accessed July 10, 2011.

Van Gennep A: *The rites of passage,* Chicago, 1960, University of Chicago Press (translated by Vizedom MB, Caffee GL).

Webber P: Yes, Virginia, nursing does have laws, *Nurs Sc Q* 21(1):68, 2008.

RESEARCH REFERENCES

Armer J, Radina M: Definition of health and health promotion behaviors, *J Multicult Nurs Health* 13(3):443, 2006.

Chan CKL, Yau MK: Death preparation among the ethnic Chinese well-elderly in Singapore: an exploratory study, *OMEGA* 60(3):225, 2009-2010.

Chin YM, et al: Zuo yuezi practice among Malaysian Chinese women: traditional versus modernity, *Br J Midwifery* 18(3):170, 2010.

Cowan DT, Norman I: Cultural competence in nursing: new meanings, *J Transcult Nurs* 17(1):82, 2006.

Crockett R, et al: Time orientation and health-related behaviour: measurement in general population samples, *Psychol Health* 24(3):333, 2009.

Helsel D, et al: Chronic illness and Hmong Shamans, *J Transcult Nurs* 16(4):150, 2005.

Johnstone MJ, Kanitsaki O: Health care provider and consumer understanding of cultural safety and cultural competency in health care: an Australian study, *J Cult Diversity* 14(2):96, 2007.

Kulwicki A, et al: Collaborative partnership for culture care: enhancing health services for the Arab community, *J Transcult Nurs* 11(1):31, 2005.

Lobar SL, et al: Cross-cultural beliefs, ceremonies, and rituals surrounding death of a loved one, *Pediatr Nurs* 32(1):44, 2006.

Maputle MS, Jali MN: Dealing with diversity: incorporating cultural sensitivity into midwifery practice in the tertiary hospital of Capricorn district, Limpopo province, *Curationis* 29(4):61, 2006.

McLachlan H, Waldenstrom U: Childbirth experiences in Australia of women born in Turkey, Vietnam and Australia, *Birth: Issues Perinatal Care* 34(4):272, 2005.

Nelms LW, Gorski J: The role of the African traditional healer in women's health, *J Transcult Nurs* 17(4):184, 2006.

Omeri A, et al: Beyond asylum: implications for nursing and health care delivery for Afghan refugees in Australia, *J Transcult Nurs* 17(1):30, 2006.

Walker RL, et al: Ethnic group differences in reasons for living and moderating role of cultural worldview, *Cult Diversity Ethnic Minority Psychol* 16(3):372, DOI:10.1037/a0019720, 2010.

CHAPTER

10

Caring for Families

OBJECTIVES

- Discuss how the term family reflects family diversity.
- Explain how the relationship between family structure and patterns of functioning affects the health of individuals within the family and the family as a whole.
- Discuss the way family members influence one another's health.
- Discuss the role of families and family members as caregivers.
- Discuss factors that promote or impede family health.
- Compare family as context to family as patient and explain the way these perspectives influence nursing practice.
- Use the nursing process to provide for the health care needs of the family.

KEY TERMS

Family, p. 116
Family as context, p. 121
Family as patient, p. 121
Family as system, p. 122
Family caregiving, p. 126
Family forms, p. 117
Hardiness, p. 121
Reciprocity, p. 127
Resiliency, p. 121

evolve WEBSITE

http://evolve.elsevier.com/Potter/fundamentals/

- Review Questions
- Case Study with Questions
- Audio Glossary
- Interactive Learning Activities
- Key Term Flashcards
- Content Updates

THE FAMILY

The family is a central institution in American society; however, the concept, structure, and functioning of the family unit continue to change over time. Families face many challenges, including the effects of health and illness, childbearing and childrearing, changes in family structure and dynamics, and caring for older parents. Family characteristics or attributes such as durability, resiliency, and diversity help families adapt to challenges.

Family durability is the term for the intrafamilial system of support and structure that extends beyond the walls of the household. For example, the parents may remarry or the children may leave home as adults, but in the end the "family" transcends long periods and inevitable lifestyle changes.

Family resiliency is the ability of the family to cope with expected and unexpected stressors. The family's ability to adapt to role and structural changes, developmental milestones, and crises shows resilience. For example, a family is resilient when the wage earner loses a job and another member of the family takes on that role. The family survives and thrives as a result of the challenges they encounter from stressors.

Family diversity is the uniqueness of each family unit. For example, some families experience marriage for the first time and then have children in later life. Another family may include parents with young children as well as grandparents living in the home. Every person within a family unit has specific needs, strengths, and important developmental considerations.

As you care for patients and their families, you are responsible for understanding family dynamics, which include the family makeup (configuration), structure, function, problem-solving, and coping capacity. Use this knowledge to build on the family's relative strengths and resources (Duhamel, 2010). The goal of family-centered nursing care is to promote, support, and provide for the well-being and health of the family and individual family members (Astedt-Kurki et al., 2002; Joronen and Astedt-Kurki, 2005).

Concept of Family

The term *family* brings to mind a visual image of adults and children living together in a satisfying, harmonious manner (Fig. 10-1). For some this term has the opposite image. Families represent more than a set of individuals, and a family is more than a sum of its individual members (Kaakinen et al., 2010). Families are as diverse as the individuals who compose them. Patients have deeply ingrained values about their families that deserve respect. You need to understand how your patients define their family. Think of the **family** as a set of relationships that the patient identifies as family or as a network of individuals who influence one another's lives, whether or not there are actual biological or legal ties.

Definition: What Is a Family?

Defining family initially appears to be a simple undertaking. However, different definitions result in heated debates among social scientists and legislators. The definition of family is significant and affects who is included on health insurance policies, who has access to children's school records, who files joint tax returns, and who is eligible for sick-leave benefits or public assistance

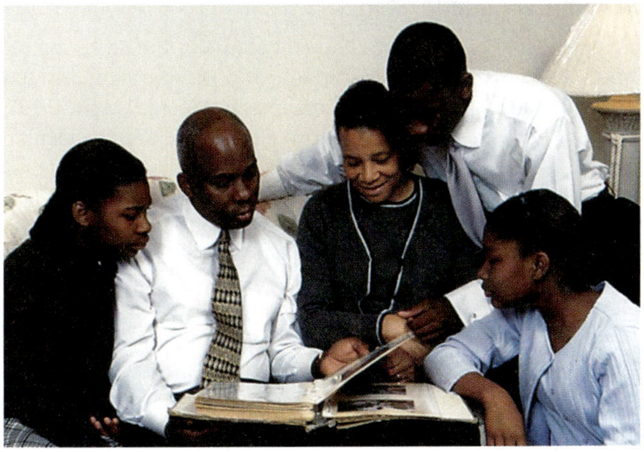

FIG. 10-1 Family celebrations and traditions strengthen the role of the family.

programs. The family is defined biologically, legally, or as a social network with personally constructed ties and ideologies. For some patients family includes only persons related by marriage, birth, or adoption. To others, aunts, uncles, close friends, cohabitating persons, and even pets are family. Your personal beliefs do not have to be the same as those of your patient. Understand that families take many forms and have diverse cultural and ethnic orientations. In addition, no two families are alike. Each has its own strengths, weaknesses, resources, and challenges.

CURRENT TRENDS AND NEW FAMILY FORMS

Family forms are patterns of people considered by family members to be included in the family (Box 10-1). Although all families have some things in common, each family form has unique problems and strengths. Maintain an open mind about what makes up a family so you do not overlook potential resources and concerns.

Although the institution of the family remains strong, the family itself is changing. The "typical" family (two biological parents and children) is no longer the norm. People are marrying later, women are delaying childbirth, and couples are choosing to have fewer children or none at all. The number of people living alone is expanding rapidly and represents approximately 26% of all households. Divorce rates continue to be high; it is estimated that 54% of marriages will end in divorce (U.S. Bureau of the Census, 2008). A number of divorced adults remarry; the median interval between divorce and remarriage is about 3 years. Remarriage often results in a blended family with a complex set of relationships among stepparents, stepchildren, half brothers and sisters, and extended family members.

Marital roles are also more complex as families increasingly comprise two wage earners. The majority of women work outside the home, and about 60% of mothers are in the workforce (U.S. Bureau of the Census, 2008). Balancing employment and family life creates a variety of challenges in terms of child care and household work for both parents. The balance for working parents between child care and household duties is positive when the working parents' job and life satisfactions remain high (Hill, 2005). There is no proof that maternal employment is damaging for children (Hill, 2005; Shpancer et al., 2006). However, finding quality child care is a major issue. Managing household tasks is another challenge. Although equal division of labor receives verbal approval, most household tasks remain "women's work." There is some evidence that the father's role is changing. Fathers now participate more fully in day-to-day parenting responsibilities. Twenty-four percent of children (ages 0 to 4) have their fathers as caretakers whether or not the fathers are employed (U.S. Bureau of the Census, 2008).

The number of single-parent families, which doubled from the 1970s to the 1990s, seems to be stabilizing. Forty-one percent of children are living with mothers who have never married; many of these children are a result of an adolescent pregnancy. Although mothers head most single-parent families, father-only families are on the rise.

Adolescent pregnancy is an ever-increasing concern. The majority of adolescent mothers continue to live with their families. A teenage pregnancy has long-term consequences for the mother. For example, adolescent mothers frequently quit high school and have inadequate job skills and limited health care resources. The overwhelming task of being a parent while still being a teenager often severely stresses family relationships and resources. In addition, there is an increased risk for subsequent adolescent pregnancy, inability to obtain quality job skills, and poor lifestyles (Harper et al., 2010). Stressors are also placed on teenage fathers when their partner becomes pregnant. These young men have poorer support systems and fewer resources to teach them how to parent. In addition, adolescent fathers report early adverse family relationships such as exposure to domestic violence and parental separation or divorce and lack positive fathering role models (Biello, Sipsma, and Kershaw, 2010). As a result, both adolescent parents often struggle with the normal tasks of development and identity but must accept a parenting role that they are not ready for physically, emotionally, socially, and/or financially.

Many homosexual couples define their relationship in family terms. Approximately half of all gay male couples live together compared with three fourths of lesbian couples. These couples are more open about their sexual preferences and more vocal about their legal rights. Some homosexual families include children,

BOX 10-1 FAMILY FORMS

Nuclear Family
The nuclear family consists of husband and wife (and perhaps one or more children).

Extended Family
The extended family includes relatives (aunts, uncles, grandparents, and cousins) in addition to the nuclear family.

Single-Parent Family
The single-parent family is formed when one parent leaves the nuclear family because of death, divorce, or desertion or when a single person decides to have or adopt a child.

Blended Family
The blended family is formed when parents bring unrelated children from prior adoptive or foster parenting relationships into a new, joint living situation.

Alternative Family
Relationships include multiadult households, "skip-generation" families (grandparents caring for grandchildren), communal groups with children, "nonfamilies" (adults living alone), cohabitating partners, and homosexual couples.

either through adoption or artificial insemination or from prior relationships.

The fastest-growing age-group in America is 65 years of age and over. For the first time in history the average American has more living parents than children, and children are more likely to have living grandparents and even great-grandparents. This "graying" of America continues to affect the family life cycle, particularly the "sandwich generation"—made up of the children of older adults (see section on restorative care). These individuals, who are usually in the middle years, have to meet their own needs along with those of their children and their aging parents. This balance of needs often occurs at the expense of their own well-being and resources. In addition, many of the family caregivers report that support from professional health professionals is lacking (Touhy and Jett, 2010). Most family caregivers are women; the average age is 46, with 13% being 65 years of age or older, and they frequently provide more than 20 hours of care per week (Schumacher, Beck, and Marren, 2006a). Caring for a frail or chronically ill relative is a primary concern for a growing number of families. It is not uncommon for people in their 60s and 70s to be the major caregivers for one another. Box 10-2 provides a list of family nursing gerontological concerns.

More grandparents are raising their grandchildren (U.S. Bureau of the Census, 2008). This new parenting responsibility is the result of a number of societal factors: the increase in the divorce rate, dual-income families, and single parenthood. Most often it is a consequence of legal intervention when parents are unfit or renounce their parental obligations.

Families face many challenges, including changing structures and roles in the changing economic status of society. In addition, social scientists identify four further trends as threats or concerns facing the family: (1) changing economic status (e.g., declining family income and lack of access to health care), (2) homelessness, (3) family violence, and (4) the presence of acute or chronic illnesses.

BOX 10-2 FOCUS ON OLDER ADULTS

Caregiver Concerns

- Assess the family for the existence of caregivers who provide daily or respite care for older adult family members. For example, determine the caregiving roles for members of the family (e.g., providing additional financial support, designating someone to obtain groceries and medications, providing hands-on physical care).
- Assess for caregiver burden such as tension in relationships between family caregivers and care recipients, changes in level of health, changes in mood, and anxiety and depression (Tamayo et al., 2010).
- Caregivers are most often spouses, who are sometimes older adults with declining physical stamina, or middle-age children, who often have other family responsibilities.
- Later-life families have a different social network than younger families because friends and same-generation family members often have died or been ill themselves. Look for social support within the community and church affiliation (Tamayo et al., 2010).
- Take time to individualize and reinforce instruction. The patient's status may change over time, and care specifics also change (Davidson, 2009).
- Abuse of older adults in families occurs across all social classes. Spouses are the most frequent abusers. Nurses need to report unexplained bruises and skin trauma to state protective agencies.

Changing Economic Status

Making ends meet is a daily concern because of the declining economic status of families. Although two-income families have become the norm, real family income has not increased since 1973. Families at the lower end of the income scale have been particularly affected, and single-parent families are especially vulnerable. Because of recent economic trends adult children are often faced with moving back home after college because they cannot find employment or in some cases lose their jobs.

The number of American children living below the poverty level continues to rise. The number of children living below poverty increased by 2 million since 2000, and 8.1 million children are uninsured (Children's Defense Fund [CDF], 2010). A majority of uninsured children have at least one parent who works but is unable to afford insurance. When caring for these families, the nurse needs to be sensitive to their desire for independence but also help them with obtaining appropriate financial and health care resources. For example, you inform the family where to go within the community to obtain assistance with energy bills, dental and health care, and assistance with school supplies.

Homelessness

Homelessness is a major public health issue. According to public health organizations, *absolute homelessness* describes people without physical shelter who sleep outdoors, in vehicles, in abandoned buildings, or in other places not intended for human habitation. *Relative homelessness* describes those who have a physical shelter, but one that does not meet the standards of health and safety (National Coalition for the Homeless, 2010).

The fastest growing section of the homeless population is families with children. This includes complete nuclear families and single-parent families. It is expected that 3.5 million people are homeless and 1.35 million are families with children. Poverty, mental and physical illness, and lack of affordable housing are primary causes of homelessness (National Coalition for the Homeless, 2010). Homelessness severely affects the functioning, health, and well-being of the family and its members. Children of homeless families are often in fair or poor health and have higher rates of asthma, ear infections, stomach problems, and mental illness (see Chapter 3). As a result, usually the only access to health care for these children is through an emergency department.

Children who are homeless face difficulties such as meeting residency requirements for public schools, inability to obtain previous enrollment records, and enrolling in and attending school. As a result, they are more likely to drop out of school and become unemployable (National Coalition for the Homeless, 2010). Homeless families and their children are at serious risk for developing long-term health, psychological, and socioeconomic problems. For example, the children are frequently underimmunized and at risk for childhood illnesses; they may fall behind in school and are at risk of dropping out; or they can develop risky behaviors.

Family Violence

The statistics regarding family violence are even more disturbing. Approximately 3.3 to 10 million children reported being abused or neglected in the period from 1991 to 2004 (Family Violence Prevention Fund, 2008a). Emotional, physical, and sexual abuse occurs toward spouses, children, and older adults and across all social classes. Factors associated with family violence are complex and include stress, poverty, social isolation, psychopathology, and learned family behavior. Other factors such as alcohol and drug abuse, pregnancy, sexual orientation, and mental illness increase the incidence of abuse within a family (Family Violence Prevention Fund, 2008b). Although abuse sometimes ends when one leaves a specific family environment, negative long-term physical and emotional consequences are often evident. One of the consequences includes moving from one abusive situation to another. For example, an adolescent girl sees marriage as a way to leave her parents' abusive home and in turn marries a person who continues the abuse in her marriage.

Acute or Chronic Illness

Any acute or chronic illness influences the entire family economically, emotionally, socially, and functionally and affects the family's decision-making and coping resources. Hospitalization of a family member is stressful for the whole family. Hospital environments are foreign, physicians and nurses are strangers, the medical language is difficult to understand or interpret, and family members are separated from one another.

During an acute illness such as a trauma, myocardial infarction, or surgery, family members are often left in waiting rooms to anticipate information about their loved one. Communication among family members may be misdirected from fear and worry. Sometimes previous family conflicts rise to the surface, whereas others are suppressed. When implementing a patient-centered care model, patients' family members and surrogate decision makers must become active partners in decision making and care (Davidson, 2009). Understand the family's cultural beliefs and values and need for communication and support.

Chronic illnesses are a global health problem. Adaptations to chronic illnesses pose unique challenges for the family (Weinert et al., 2008). Frequently family patterns and interactions, social activities, work and household schedules, economic resources, and other family needs and functions must be reorganized around the chronic illness or disability. Despite the stressors, families also learn how to manage many aspects of their loved one's illness or disability. Astute nursing care helps the family prevent and/or manage medical crises, control symptoms, learn how to provide specific therapies, adjust to changes over the course of the illness, avoid isolation, obtain community resources, and assist in helping the family resolve conflict.

Chronic illnesses are common in a majority of family units. Chronic illness impacts a family's quality of life. Families must work at developing working partnerships with the health care delivery system to identify available health care and community resources for disease management (Weinert et al., 2008). The chronic illness continuum ranges from newly diagnosed illness to end stages of the disease. The patient's level of independence changes over time, and family members need to adapt to changing caregiving needs (Tamayo et al., 2010). Common chronic illnesses include but are not limited to asthma, diabetes, cardiovascular illnesses, renal disease, human immunodeficiency virus (HIV), and cancer.

Trauma. Trauma is a sudden unplanned event. Family members often struggle to cope with the challenges of a severe, life-threatening event, which can include the stressors associated with a family member hospitalized in an intensive care environment, loss of a family member, or an acute psychiatric illness. The powerlessness that family members experience makes them very vulnerable and less able to make important decisions about the health of the family. In caring for family members, answer their questions honestly. When you do not know the answer, find someone who does. Provide realistic assurance; giving false hope breaks the nurse-patient trust and also affects how the family can adjust to "bad news." When the victim of trauma is hospitalized, take time to make sure that the family is comfortable. You can bring them something to eat or drink, give them a blanket, or encourage them to get a meal. Sometimes telling the family that you will stay with their loved one while they are gone is all they need to feel comfortable in leaving. Most family members have a cell phone and can be reached easily if their loved one's condition changes.

End-of-Life Care. You will encounter many families with a terminally ill member. Although people equate terminal illness with cancer, many diseases have terminal aspects (e.g., heart failure, pulmonary and renal diseases, and neuromuscular diseases). Although some family members may be prepared for their loved one's death, their need for information, support, assurance, and presence is great (see Chapter 36). The more you know about your patient's family, how they interact with one another, their strengths, and their weaknesses, the better. Each family approaches and copes with end-of-life decisions differently. Give the family information about the dying process. Help the family set up home care if they desire and obtain hospice and other appropriate resources, including grief support. Make sure that the family knows what to do at the time of death. If you are present at the time of death, be sensitive to the family's needs (e.g., provide for privacy and allow sufficient time for saying good-byes).

THEORETICAL APPROACHES: AN OVERVIEW

A number of different perspectives can be applied when caring for families. It is important that you understand some of the broader perspectives for family nursing. The family health system (FHS) and developmental theories are two perspectives used in this chapter to help you provide nursing care to the family as a whole and the individuals within the family structure. These theoretical perspectives and their concepts provide the foundation for family assessment and interventions.

Family Health System

When assessing the family, it is important to use a guide such as the FHS to identify all of their needs. The FHS is a holistic model that guides the assessment and care for families (Anderson, 2000; Anderson and Friedemann, 2010). The FHS includes five realms/processes of family life: interactive, developmental, coping, integrity, and health. The FHS approach is one method for family assessment to determine areas of concern and strengths, which helps you develop a plan of care with family nursing interventions and outcomes. As with all systems, the FHS has both unspoken and spoken goals, which vary according to the stage in the family life cycle, family values, and individual concerns of the family members. When working with families, the goal of care is to improve family health or well-being, assist in family management of illness conditions or transitions, and achieve health outcomes related to the family areas of concern.

Developmental Stages

Families, like individuals, change and grow over time. Although they are far from identical to one another, they tend to go through common stages. Each developmental stage has its own challenges, needs, and resources and includes tasks that need to be completed before the family is able to successfully move on to the next stage. Societal changes and an aging population have caused changes in the stages and transitions in the family life cycle. For example, adult children are not leaving the nest as predictably or as early as in the

TABLE 10-1 Stages of the Family Life Cycle

FAMILY LIFE-CYCLE STAGE	EMOTIONAL PROCESS OF TRANSITION: KEY PRINCIPLES	CHANGES IN FAMILY STATUS REQUIRED TO PROCEED DEVELOPMENTALLY
Unattached young adult	Accepting parent-offspring separation	Differentiation of self in relation to family of origin Development of intimate peer relationships Establishment of self in work
Joining of families through marriage: newly married couple	Committing to new system	Formation of marital system Realignment of relationships with extended families and friends to include spouse
Family with young children	Accepting new generation of members into system	Adjusting marital system to make space for children Taking on parental roles Realignment of relationships with extended family to include parenting and grandparenting roles
Family with adolescents	Increasing flexibility of family boundaries to include children's independence	Shifting of parent-child relationships to permit adolescents to move into and out of system Refocusing on midlife material and career issues Beginning shift toward concerns for older generation
Launching children and moving on	Accepting multitude of exits from and entries into family system	Adjusting to reduction in family size Developing adult-to-adult relationships between grown children and their parents Realigning relationships to include in-laws and grandchildren Dealing with disabilities and death of parents (grandparents)
Family in later life	Accepting shifting of generational roles	Maintaining own or couple functioning and interests in the face of physiological decline; exploring new familial and social role options Making room in system for wisdom and experience of older adults; supporting older generations without overfunctioning for them Dealing with retirement Dealing with loss of spouse, siblings, and other peers and preparation for own death; a life review, in which one reviews life experiences and decisions

From Duvall EM, Miller BC: *Marriage and family development,* ed 6, Boston, 2005, Allyn & Bacon. Printed and electronically reproduced by permission of Pearson Education, Inc, Upper Saddle River, NJ.

past, and many are returning home. In addition, more people are living into their 80s and 90s. Sixty-five is now considered the "backside of middle age," and the length of the midlife stage in the family life cycle has increased, as has the later stage in family life.

McGoldrick and Carter based their 1985 classic model of family life stages on expansion, contraction, and realignment of family relationships that support the entry, exit, and development of the members (Hanson et al., 2005). This model describes the emotional aspects of lifestyle transition and the changes and tasks necessary for the family to proceed developmentally (Table 10-1). Use this model to promote family behaviors to achieve essential tasks and help families prepare for later transitions such as when helping families prepare for a new baby (see Chapter 13).

ATTRIBUTES OF FAMILIES

Structure

Families have a structure and a way of functioning. Structure and function are closely related and continually interact with one another. Structure is based on the ongoing membership of the family and the pattern of relationships, which are often numerous and complex. For example, a woman's relationships frequently include wife-husband, mother-son, mother-daughter, employee-boss, and colleague-colleague, each with different demands, roles, and expectations. Patterns of relationships form power and role structures within the family. Determine a family's structures by observing family members' behaviors and interactions.

Structure promotes or impedes the family's ability to respond to stressors. Very rigid or very flexible structures impair functioning. A rigid structure specifically dictates who is able to accomplish a task and may limit the number of persons outside the immediate family who can assume these tasks. For example, in one family the mother is the only acceptable person to provide emotional support for the children, or the husband is the only one to provide financial support. A change in the health status of the person responsible for a task places a burden on the family because no other person is available or considered acceptable to assume that task. A family must adapt its structure. For example, when a homemaker is ill, the tasks of managing the household (e.g., preparing the meals, maintaining the house, and driving school-age children to appointments and events) need to be shared. The older children may help prepare the meals, and the other parent or a family member drives the children to the events, or perhaps the events are rescheduled.

An extremely open structure also presents problems for the family. When the family structure is extremely open, consistent patterns of behavior that lead to automatic action do not exist. An example is an inconsistent parenting role. The parent sometimes is a strict authoritarian figure and at other times treats the child as a "best friend and confidant." This type of conduct causes family members to become confused about what behavior is appropriate and who is reliable for support. During a crisis or rapid change, family members do not have a defined structure to "fall back on," and family disintegration is sometimes a result.

Function

Family functioning is what the family does. Specific functional aspects include the way a family reproduces, interacts to socialize its young, cooperates to meet economic needs, and relates to the larger society. Family functioning also focuses on the processes used by the family to achieve its goals. Some processes include communication among family members, goal setting, conflict resolution, caregiving, nurturing, and use of internal and external resources. Traditional reproductive, sexual, economic, and educational goals that were once universal family goals no longer apply to all families. For example, a married couple who decides not to have children still consider themselves a family. Another example includes a blended family whose spouses bring school-age children into the new marriage. However, the spouses decide not to co-mingle their finances and have separate educational goals for their minor children. As a result, this family does not have the traditional economic patterns of a nuclear family.

Families achieve goals more successfully when communication is clear and direct. Clear communication enhances problem solving and conflict resolution, and it facilitates coping with life-changing or life-threatening stressors. Another process to facilitate goal achievement includes the ability to nurture and promote growth. For example, families might have a specific celebration for a good report card, a job well done, or specific milestones. They also nurture by helping children know right and wrong. In this situation a family might have a specific form of discipline such as "time out" or taking away privilege, and the children know why the discipline is given. Thus when a situation occurs, the child is disciplined and learns not to behave like that again.

Families need to have multiple resources available. For example, a social network is an excellent resource. Social relationships such as friends or churches within the community are important for family celebrations but also act as buffers, particularly during times of stress, and reduce a family's vulnerability.

The Family and Health

Many factors influence the health of the family (e.g., its relative position in society, economic resources, and geographical boundaries). Although American families exist within the same culture, they live in very different ways as a result of race, values, social class, and ethnicity. In some minority groups multiple generations of single-parent families live together in one home. Class and ethnicity produce differences in the access of families to the resources and rewards of society. This access creates differences in family life, most significantly in different life chances for its members.

Distribution of wealth greatly affects the capacity to maintain health. Low educational preparation, poverty, and decreased social support compound one another, magnifying their effect *on* sickness in the family, and magnifying the amount of sickness *in* the family. Economic stability increases a family's access to adequate health care, creates more opportunity for education, increases good nutrition, and decreases stress (National Coalition of the Homeless, 2010; Children's Defense Fund, 2010).

The family is the primary social context in which health promotion and disease prevention take place. The family's beliefs, values, and practices strongly influence health-promoting behaviors of its members (Epley et al., 2010). In turn the health status of each individual influences how the family unit functions and its ability to achieve goals. When the family satisfactorily functions to meet its goals, its members tend to feel positive about themselves and their family. Conversely, when they do not meet goals, families view themselves as ineffective.

Some families do not place a high value on good health. In fact, some families accept harmful practices. In some cases a family member gives mixed messages about health. For example, a parent continues to smoke while telling children that smoking is bad for them. Family environment is crucial because health behavior reinforced in early life has a strong influence on later health practices. In addition, the family environment is a crucial factor in an individual's adjustment to a crisis. Although relationships are strained when confronted with illness, research indicates that family members can have the potential to be a primary force for coping (Bluvol and Ford-Gilboe, 2004).

Attributes of Healthy Families. The family is a dynamic unit; it is exposed to threats, strengths, changes, and challenges. Some families are crisis proof, whereas others are crisis prone. The crisis-proof, or effective, family is able to combine the need for stability with the need for growth and change. This type of family has a flexible structure that allows adaptable performance of tasks and acceptance of help from outside the family system. The structure is flexible enough to allow adaptability but not so flexible that the family lacks cohesiveness and a sense of stability. The effective family has control over the environment and influences the immediate environment of home, neighborhood, and school. The ineffective, or crisis-prone, family lacks or believes it lacks control over the environments.

Health promotion research often focuses on the stress-moderating effect of **hardiness** and **resiliency** as factors that contribute to long-term health. Family hardiness is the internal strengths and durability of the family unit. A sense of control over the outcome of life, a view of change as beneficial and growth producing, and an active rather than passive orientation in adapting to stressful events characterize family hardiness (McCubbin, McCubbin, and Thompson, 1996). Family resiliency is the ability to cope with expected and unexpected stressors. It helps to evaluate healthy responses when individuals and families are experiencing stressful events. Resources and techniques that a family or individuals within the family use to maintain a balance or level of health assist in understanding a family's level of resiliency.

FAMILY NURSING

To provide compassion and caring for your patients and their families, you need a scientific knowledge base in family theory and knowledge in family nursing. A focus on the family is necessary to safely discharge patients back to the family or community settings. The members of the family may need to assume the role of primary caregiver. Family caregivers have unique nursing and caregiving needs and too often feel abandoned by the health care system (Reinhard, 2006). When a life-changing illness occurs, the family has to make major adjustments to care for a family member. Often the psychological, social, and health care needs of the caregiver go unmet (Tamayo et al., 2010).

Family nursing is based on the assumption that all people, regardless of age, are members of some type of family form, such as the traditional nuclear family or an alternate family. The goal of family nursing is to help the family and its individual members reach and maintain maximum health throughout and beyond the illness experience (Box 10-3). Family nursing is the focus of the future across all practice settings and is important in all health care environments.

There are different approaches for family nursing practice. For the purposes of this chapter, family nursing practice has three levels of approaches: (1) **family as context;** (2) **family as patient;**

BOX 10-3 EVIDENCE-BASED PRACTICE

Social Support for the Family Caregiver

PICO Question: Does strengthening social support systems improve the emotional and physical health of family caregivers?

Evidence Summary

When a family member has an illness or trauma that changes his or her physical or cognitive function, it is often a major life-changing event for the spouse, parent, family, and loved ones. Illnesses include but are not limited to strokes, cancer, Parkinson's disease, or motor vehicle and sports-related injuries. As the patient moves through acute care and rehabilitation phases, families face major changes in family dynamics, social interactions, financial commitments, and emotional support systems (Davidson, 2009; Tamayo et al., 2010). When the patient returns home, existing disabilities affect the primary caregiver and other members of the family. Families face additional changes when adjusting to the physical, emotional, and psychological consequences of the illness or trauma. The family's and caregiver's social roles and activities, health-related activities and practices, and family dynamics all change (Rosenthal et al., 2008). As a result, family members note changes in their physical and emotional health and a decline in their quality of life. Identifying social support systems and structures help the caregiver maintain a sense of hope, maintain their own health status, engage in more social activities, and have some respite from the day-to-day caregiving tasks (Duggleby et al., 2010; Weinert et al., 2008).

Application to Nursing Practice

- Focus interventions on the family's strengths (e.g., if some family members are good at helping their loved one exercise, involve them in physical rehabilitation activities [Rosenthal et al., 2008]).
- Consider the primary caregiver's experience when designing intervention (e.g., has the caregiver observed any technical nursing care? Does the caregiver have a health care background? Has he or she provided care to another person?).
- Build on the strengths of the patient and the caregivers, including their sense of hope, rather than focusing solely on any weaknesses and challenges (Duggleby et al., 2010).
- Encourage the caregiver to set a routine time for respite. The caregiver then knows when he or she can have some relaxation time or spouses can have a "date night."
- Teach older children to be part of the support system. Show them how to participate in the care of a family member. Older children, especially grandchildren, enjoy listening to the stories of the family (Bluvol and Ford-Gilboe, 2004; Tamayo et al., 2010).
- Encourage the patient, caregivers, and family members to "tell their story" (Bluvol and Ford-Gilboe, 2004; Duggleby et al., 2010).

and (3) the newest model, called **family as system,** which includes both relational and transactional concepts. If only one family member receives nursing care, it is realistic and practical to view the family as context. When all family members are involved in the daily care of one another, nursing intervention with one individual necessitates some change in the activities of the others, suggesting that family as patient is the best approach. All three approaches are useful in providing effective nursing care.

Family As Context

When you view the family as context, the primary focus is on the health and development of an individual member existing within a specific environment (i.e., the patient's family). Although the focus is on the individual's health status, assess how much the family provides the individual's basic needs. Needs vary, depending on the individual's developmental level and situation. Because families provide more than just material essentials, you will also need to consider their ability to help the patient meet psychological needs. Some family members need direct interventions themselves.

Family As Patient

When the family as patient is the approach, family processes and relationships (e.g., parenting or family caregiving) are the primary focuses of nursing care. Focus your nursing assessment on family patterns versus individual member characteristics. Concentrate on patterns and processes that are consistent with reaching and maintaining family and individual health. Plan care to meet not only the patient's needs, but also the changing needs of the family. Dealing with very complex family problems often requires an interdisciplinary approach. Always be aware of the limits of nursing practice and make referrals when appropriate.

Family As System

It is important to understand that, although you are able to make theoretical and practical distinctions between the family as context and the family as patient, they are not necessarily mutually exclusive. When you care for the family as a system, you are caring for each family member (family as context) and the family unit (family as patient), using all available environmental, social, psychological, and community resources.

The following clinical scenario illustrates three levels of approaches to family care.

You are assisting with end-of-life care for David Daniels, who is 35 years old. David and his wife, Lisa, have three school-age children. David expressed a wish to die at home and not in a hospital or extended care facility. Lisa is on family leave from her job to help David through this period. Both Lisa and David are only children. David's parents are no longer living, but Lisa's mother is committed to stay with the family to help Lisa and David.

When you view this family as *context,* you focus on the patient (David) as an individual. You assess and meet David's comfort, hygiene, and nutritional needs. You also meet David's social and emotional needs. When viewing the family as *patient,* you assess and meet David's family's comfort and nutritional needs. You determine the family's need for rest and their stage of coping. It is important to determine the demands placed on David and the family. In addition, you need to continually evaluate the family's available resources such as time, finances, coping skills, and energy level to support David through the end of life.

When viewing the family as *system,* you use elements from both of the previous perspectives, but you also assess the resources available to the family. Using the knowledge of the family as context, patient, and a system, individualize care decisions based on the family assessment and your clinical judgment. For example, based on your assessment, you determine that the family is not eating adequately. You also determine that Lisa is experiencing more stress, not sleeping well, and trying to "do it all" regarding her children's school and after-school activities. In addition, Lisa does not want to leave David's bedside when members of their church come to help. You recognize that this family is under enormous stress and that their basic needs such as meals, rest, and school activities are not adequately met. As a result, you determine that (1) the family needs assistance with meals, (2) Lisa needs time to

BOX 10-4 FIVE REALMS OF FAMILY LIFE: FAMILY HEALTH SYSTEM—FAMILY ASSESSMENT PLAN

Interactive Processes
- Family relationships—Is the family a nuclear or blended family? Is it a single-parent family?
- Family communication—How do family members share ideas, concerns?
- Family nurturing—How are family values set and communicated? How are house rules established?
- Intimacy expression—Does the family hug, touch, laugh, or cry together?
- Social support—Who in the community, school, or workplace is close to the family?
- Conflict resolution—How does conflict resolution occur? Who initiates it?
- Roles (instrumental and expressive)—What are the formal roles such as wage earner, disciplinarian, problem solver? What are the informal roles (e.g., peacekeeper)?
- Family leisure life—Vacations: what does the family do to relax? Do the parents have "date night?"

Developmental Processes
- Current family transitions—Recent death, divorces, children leaving/returning home, new births
- Family stage task completion or progression—Childbearing years, empty nesters, grandparenting
- Individual developmental issues that affect family development—Individuals in the family with social issues such as difficulty in school or legal issues who cannot participate in family development
- Development of health issue and family impact—Acute or chronic illnesses, high-risk pregnancies, delayed physical development

Coping Processes
- Problem solving—How did the family solve previous problems? Is there a single problem solver or a family resolution?
- Use of resources—Does the family use family or individual therapists, Alcoholics Anonymous, conflict resolution resources, anger management resources?
- Family life stressors and daily hassles—These include financial concerns, overscheduled children, caregiver for older adults.
- Family coping strategies and effectiveness—How do the family and individuals cope (e.g., exercise, overeating, arguing)?
- Past experiences with handling crises—This includes information about past crisis such as financial stress, illness, legal problems.
- Family resistance resources—Does the family take measures to avoid stress such as adhering to a budget, obtaining tutoring resources for their children?

Integrity Processes
- Family values—What do the family consider as their important values (e.g., health, togetherness)?
- Family beliefs—For example, ask about beliefs about health/illness, end-of-life care, advance directives.
- Family meaning—For example, ask what the family means to each member.
- Family rituals—For example, ask about celebration of holidays, birthdays, weddings; coping with death (e.g., wakes, funerals).
- Family spirituality—Ask what spirituality means. How does the family define their spirituality?
- Family culture and practices—Identify cultural customs and practice that impact health care.

Health Processes
- Family health beliefs and beliefs about health concern or problem—Does the family practice health and illness prevention or wait until a problem occurs?
- Health behaviors of the family—How does the ill family member react? How does the family react to illness? Do the family members react the same way to an ill family member, or do they react differently when a homemaker is ill versus the wage earner?
- Health patterns and health management activities—How do the family members manage their health? How do they manage care?
- Family caretaking responsibilities—When someone is ill, who is the caregiver? Is it always the same person?
- Disease conditions, treatments, and consequences for the family—Obtain current disease and treatment history for the family.
- Family illness stressors—What are these stressors (e.g., worsening of a chronic illness or when "Mom" is sick and cannot run the household)?
- Relationship with health care providers and health system access—What type of health care provider does the family have (e.g., primary care, pediatrician)? How often does the family see the providers? Any hospitalizations?

Modified from Anderson KH, Friedemann ML: Strategies to teach family assessment and intervention through an online international curriculum, *J Fam Nurs* 16(2):213, 2010; and Anderson KH: The family health system approach to family systems nursing, *J Fam Nurs* 6(2):103, 2000.

rest, and (3) the family's church is eager to help with David's day-to-day care. On the basis of these decisions, you work with Lisa, David, and the family to set up a schedule among Lisa, her mother, and two close church members to provide Lisa with some time away from David's bedside. However, David and Lisa determine when this time will be. Because of the church involvement, members of the church begin to take responsibility for groceries and all meal preparation for the family. In addition, other members of the church help with the children's school and after-school activities.

NURSING PROCESS FOR THE FAMILY

Nurses interact with families in a variety of community-based and clinical settings. The nurse uses the nursing process to care for an individual within a family (e.g., the family as context) or the entire family (e.g., the family as patient). When initiating the care of families, three factors organize the family approach to the nursing process:

1. The nurse views all individuals within their family context.
2. Families have an impact on individuals.
3. Individuals have an impact on families.

Assessing the Needs of the Family

Family assessment is a priority in order to provide adequate family care and support. You have an essential role in helping families adjust to acute and chronic illness, but first you need to understand the family unit and what a patient's illness means to the family members and family functioning. You also need to understand how the illness has affected the family structure and the support the family requires (Kaakinen et al., 2010). Although the family as a whole differs from individual members, the measure of family health is more than a summary of the health of all members. The form, structure, function, and health of the family are areas unique to family assessment. Box 10-4 includes the five areas of family life to include in an assessment.

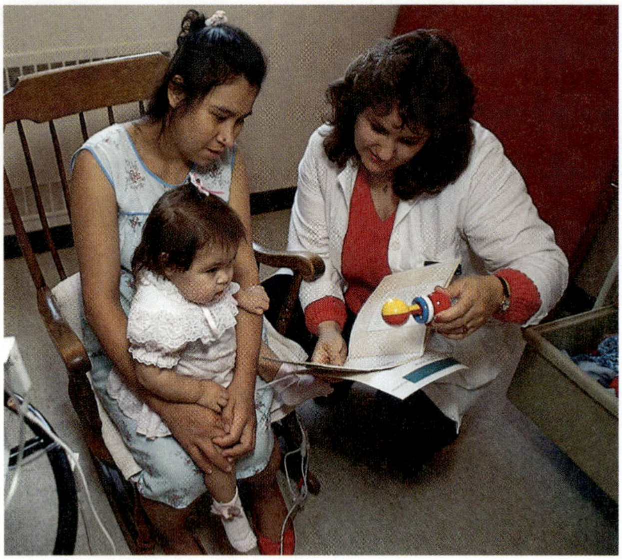

FIG. 10-2 Nurse providing family education. (From Hockenberry MJ, Wilson D: *Wong's nursing care of infants and children,* ed 9, St Louis, 2011, Mosby.)

During an assessment, incorporate knowledge of the patient's illness and assess the primary patient and the family. When focusing on the family, begin the family assessment by determining the patient's definition of and attitude toward the family. The concept of family is highly individualized. The patient's definition will influence how much you are able to incorporate the family into nursing care. To determine family form and membership, ask who the patient considers family or with whom the patient shares strong emotional feelings. If the patient is unable to express a concept of family, ask with whom the patient lives, spends time, and shares confidences and then ask whether the patient considers them to be family or like family. To further assess the family structure, ask questions that determine the power structure and patterning of roles and tasks (e.g., "Who decides where to go on vacation?" "How are tasks divided in your family?" "Who mows the lawn?" "Who usually prepares the meals?").

You need to assess family functions such as the ability to provide emotional support for members, the ability to cope with current health problems or situations, and the appropriateness of its goal setting and progress toward achievement of developmental tasks (Fig. 10-2). Also determine whether the family is able to provide and distribute sufficient economic resources and whether its social network is extensive enough to provide support.

Always recognize and respect the family's cultural background (see Chapter 9). Culture is an important variable when assessing the family because race and ethnicity affect structure, function, health beliefs, values, and the way the family perceives events (Box 10-5). The United States is increasingly more diverse. A large number of immigrants enter the country daily, adding to both the number and variety of the many ethnic groups that make up the population. American health care institutions tend to operate from a white, middle-class perspective; and immigrant populations have particular difficulty understanding and "fitting into" the system. Cultural assessment educators encourage the use of a "culturagram," which allows you to assess and empower culturally diverse families and encourages ethnic-sensitive practice. This tool assesses a variety of factors such as language spoken in the home; impact of crisis events; and values regarding family, education, and work.

BOX 10-5 CULTURAL ASPECTS OF CARE

Family Nursing

Families have unique perspectives and characteristics, and they have differences in values, beliefs, and philosophies. The cultural heritage of the family or member of the family affects religious practices, childrearing practices, recreational activities, and nutritional preferences. You need to be culturally sensitive and respectful when caring for multicultural patients. Incorporate individualized cultural preferences into your plan of care so it is culturally congruent. Design your care to integrate the personal values, life patterns, and beliefs of the patient and family into prescribed therapies.

Implications for Practice

- The dominant culture in the United States encourages self-care; however, collectivistic cultures such as traditional Asians, Hispanics, and Africans rely on family members to care for the ill (Giger and Davidhizar, 2008).
- In some cultures, including Gypsy, Asian, Middle Eastern, and Hispanic, males are traditionally the authority figures.
- The family structure sometimes includes multiple generations living together. For example, traditional Hispanic and Filipino families include distant blood relatives from the maternal and paternal sides of the family.
- In some cultures such as traditional Chinese or Japanese cultures, it is the custom for family members to take care of the patient's needs (Galanti, 2008).
- Intergenerational support and patterns of living arrangements are related to cultural background. For example, traditional Chinese, African American, Japanese, and Hispanic persons are more likely to live in extended family households than are their white counterparts (Giger and Davidhizar, 2008).
- In some cultures it is a sign of elder disrespect to place older adults in nursing homes, even when an older adult family member has severe dementia.
- Modesty is a strong value among Arab cultures. Many Arab women bring female family members to health care visits, and a female health care provider must examine the woman.
- In the presence of a critical or terminal illness, some cultures such as Orthodox Jews come in groups to pray together with the family at the patient's bedside (Galanti, 2008).
- Health beliefs differ among various cultures, which affect the decision of a family and its members about when and where to seek help. For example, traditional Asians rarely consider symptoms as psychological and are not likely to go to mental health clinics.

Drawing conclusions based on cultural backgrounds requires critical thinking and careful consideration. It is imperative to remember that categorical generalizations are misleading (e.g., all Asian Americans are good at mathematics). As many caution, overgeneralizations in terms of racial and ethnic group characteristics do not lead to greater understanding of the culturally diverse family. Culturally different families vary in meaningful and significant ways; however, neglecting to examine similarities leads to inaccurate assumptions and stereotyping. For example, more similarities than differences exist in parenting behaviors among white, African American, Hispanic, and Asian American parents. In addition, Asian American families use alternative therapies for illnesses and ailments. Other cultures such as Latino prefer to stay with their family members during illness (see Chapter 9). A comprehensive, culturally sensitive family assessment is critical in order for you to understand family life, the current changes within it, and the family's overall goals and expectations. These data provide the foundation for family-centered nursing care (Anderson and Friedemann, 2010).

Family-Focused Care

Use a family-focused approach to enhance your nursing care. When you establish a relationship with a patient and his or her family, it is important to identify potential and external resources. A complete patient and family assessment provides this information. Together with patients and their families, develop plans of care that all members clearly understand and mutually agree to follow. Goals that you establish need to be concrete and realistic, compatible with a family's developmental stage, and acceptable to family members.

Collaboration with family members is essential, whether the family is the patient or the context of care. Collaborate closely with all appropriate family members when determining what they hope to achieve with regard to the family's health. You base a positive collaborative relationship on mutual respect and trust. The family needs to feel "in control" as much as possible. By offering alternative actions and asking family members for their own ideas and suggestions, you help to reduce the family's feelings of powerlessness. For example, offering options for how to prepare a low-fat diet or how to rearrange the furnishings of a room to accommodate a family member's disability gives the family an opportunity to express their preferences, make choices, and ultimately feel as though they have contributed. Collaborating with other disciplines increases the likelihood of a comprehensive approach to the family's health care needs, and it ensures better continuity of care. Using other disciplines is particularly important when discharge planning from a health care facility to home or an extended care facility is necessary (Bluvol and Ford-Gilboe, 2004).

When you view the family as the patient, you need to support communication among all family members. This ensures that the family remains informed about the goals and interventions for health care. Often you participate in conflict resolution between family members so each member is able to confront and resolve problems in a healthy way. Help the family identify and use external and internal resources as necessary. For example, who in the family can run errands to get groceries while the patient is unable to drive? Are there members from the church who can come and provide respite care? Ultimately your aim is to help the family reach a point of optimal function, given the family's resources, capacities, and desire to become healthier.

Challenges for Family Nursing

If a patient has been hospitalized or is in a rehabilitation setting, discharge planning begins with the initiation of care and includes the family. You are responsible for an accurate assessment of what will be needed for care in the home at the time of discharge, along with any shortcomings in the home setting. For example, if a postoperative patient is discharged to home and the older adult husband does not feel comfortable with the dressing changes required, you need to find out if anyone else in the family or neighborhood is willing and able to do this. If not, you will need to arrange for a home care service referral. If the patient also needs exercise and strength training, you consult with the primary health care provider to recommend referral for physical therapy.

Cultural sensitivity (see Chapter 9) in family nursing requires recognizing not only the diverse ethnic, cultural, and religious backgrounds of patients but also the differences and similarities within the same family. When providing family-centered care, recognize and integrate cultural practices, religious ceremonies, and rituals. Using effective and respectful communication techniques enables you to collaborate with the family to determine how best to integrate their beliefs and practices within the prescribed health care plan. For example, traditional Asian and Mexican American cultures frequently want to remain at the bedside around the clock and provide personal care for their loved ones. Integrating the family's values and needs into the care plan involves teaching family members how to provide simple direct care measures, thus providing culturally sensitive and competent care. Together the nurse and the family blend the cultural and health care needs of the patient.

Implementing Family-Centered Care

Whether caring for a patient with the family as context, directing care to the family as patient, or providing care to the family as a system, nursing interventions aim to increase family members' abilities in certain areas, remove barriers to health care, and do things that the family is not able to do for itself. Assist the family in problem solving, provide practical services, and express a sense of acceptance and caring by listening carefully to family members' concerns and suggestions.

One of the roles you need to adopt is that of educator. Health education is a process by which the nurse and patient share information in a two-way fashion (see Chapter 25). Sometimes you recognize family/patient needs for information through direct questioning, but the methods for recognizing these needs are generally far more subtle. For example, you recognize that a new father is fearful of cleaning his newborn's umbilical cord or that an older adult woman is not using her cane or walker safely. Respectful communication is necessary. Often you find the subtle needs for information by saying, "I notice you are trying to not touch the umbilical cord; I see that a lot." Or "You use the cane the way I did before I was shown a way to keep from falling or tripping over it; do you mind if I show you?" When you are confident and skillful instead of coming across as an authority on the subject, your patient's defenses are down, making the patient more willing to listen without feeling embarrassed. You will also recognize patient and family learning needs on the basis of the patient's health condition and physical and mental limitations. Your focus as an educator may become the family caregiver, so that he or she can become prepared to manage the skills and processes needed to manage the patient's needs within the home. When educating patients and families, identify the best time to provide accurate health information about diagnosis, necessary self-care activities, and the projected course of the patient's condition. Such information helps the family caregiver to interpret behavior correctly and not to "blame" the patient (Schumacher, Beck, and Marren, 2006a).

Health Promotion. Although the family is the basic social context in which members learn health behaviors, the primary focus on health promotion has traditionally been on individuals. When implementing family nursing, health promotion interventions improve or maintain the physical, social, emotional, and spiritual well-being of the family unit and its members (Duhamel, 2010; Rosenthal et al., 2008). Health promotion behaviors need to be tied to the developmental stage of the family (e.g., adequate prenatal care for the childbearing family or adherence to immunization schedules for the childrearing family). Your interventions should be designed to enable individual members and the total family to reach their optimal levels of wellness.

One approach for meeting goals and promoting health is the use of family strengths. Families do not often look at their own system as one that has inherent, positive components. Family strengths include clear communication, adaptability, healthy childrearing practices, support and nurturing among family members, the use of crisis for growth, a commitment to one another and the family unit, and a sense of cohesiveness and spirituality (Schumacher, Beck, and Marren, 2006a). Help the family focus on their strengths instead of on problems and weaknesses. For example, point out that a couple's 10-year marriage has endured many crises and transitions. Therefore they are likely to be able to adapt to this latest challenge. Refer families to health promotion programs aimed at enhancing these attributes as needed. For example, some communities have low-cost fitness activities for school-age children designed to reduce the risk for obesity.

Acute Care. Because the family is becoming more of a focus in nursing care, you need to emphasize family needs within the context of today's health care delivery system. Be aware of the implication of early discharge for patients and their families. Remember that increasing numbers of people within the household are now being employed outside the home. These factors are challenges in preparing family members to assist with health care or locate appropriate community resources. Often when family members assume the role of caregiver, they lose support from significant others and are at risk for caregiver role strain (Schumacher, Beck, and Marren, 2006a). You need to be sure that families are willing to assume care responsibilities.

Family nursing requires a holistic view not only of the patient but also of the family. Nursing care in the acute environment is very complex, making it a challenge for the patient to feel cared for and to keep family members involved. A helpful tool is an independent journal in which patients and family members communicate their thoughts, ideas, and reactions. The patient or family members use the journal as an open communication tool, updating entries based on their needs and observations of the acute care experience. It is also helpful for a family member to use the journal as a record of care activities. It also provides data about when the patient was turned, who visited, when the last pain medication was administered, and any special patient requests. This information helps patients and families who are trying to "keep up" with what is happening in the acute care environment.

Restorative and Continuing Care. In restorative and continuing care settings the challenge in family nursing is in trying to maintain patients' functional abilities within the context of the family. This includes having home care nurses help patients remain in their homes following acute injuries or illnesses, surgery, or exacerbation of a chronic illness. It also requires finding ways to better the lives of chronically ill and disabled individuals and their families.

Family Caregiving. One way you provide family care is through support of family caregivers. In 2007, the economic value of family caregiving was estimated at $375 billion, which exceeded the total amount of 2007 Medicaid expenditures ($311 billion) and approached the total expenditures in Medicare ($432 billion) (AARP Public Policy Institute, 2008). Research shows that millions of Americans are taking on the burden of caregiving without acknowledging the effect that it has on their lives and without realizing that relief is available. Multiple national outreach programs such as the National Family Caregivers Association (www.thefamilycaregiver.org) and the National Alliance for Caregiving (www.caregiving.org) connect family caregivers to information and services that can help improve their lives and the level of care they can offer their loved ones.

Family caregiving is a family process that occurs in response to an illness and encompasses multiple cognitive, behavioral, and interpersonal processes (Schumacher et al., 2006b). It typically involves the routine provision of services and personal care activities for a family member by spouses, siblings, friends, or parents. Caregiving activities include finding resources, providing personal care (bathing, feeding, or grooming), monitoring for complications or side effects of an illness or treatments, providing instrumental activities of daily living (shopping or housekeeping), and the ongoing emotional support and decision making that is necessary (Schumacher, Beck, and Marren, 2006a). Family caregiving can create caregiver burden and strain. The physical and emotional demands are high, and the disease itself creates changes in the family structure and roles. Family caregivers often feel ill prepared to take on the demands of care for their loved ones (Tamayo et al., 2010). Providing education to the family caregiver helps relieve some of the stress of caregiving (Box 10-6).

BOX 10-6 PATIENT TEACHING

Family Caregiving: Caregiver Role Strain

Objective

- Patient/family will design two interventions to reduce caregiver role strain.

Teaching Strategies

- Explain to all members of the family involved in caregiving that role strain may be present when the following occur:
  - There is a change in caregiver's appetite/weight, sleeping, or leisure activities. In addition, social withdrawal, irritability, anger, or changes in the caregiver's overall level of health can occur.
  - The caregiver is fearful when learning new therapies or administering new medications to the disabled/ill family member.
  - The caregiver loses interest in his or her personal appearance.
  - Signs of caregiver role strain may intensify if the loved one's health status changes or when institutional care is considered.
- Interventions for caregiver role strain
  - Help family members set up alternating schedules to give the primary caregiver some rest.
  - Design a schedule or other methods to provide groceries, meals, and housekeeping for the caregiver and patient.
  - Identify community resources for transportation, respite care, and support groups.
- Offer an opportunity to ask questions, and when possible provide a phone number for questions and assistance.
- Provide family members with the contact information of the patient's health care provider, and instruct them to call if the caregiver has health problems, the caregiver seems overly exhausted, or they observe changes in the caregiver's interactions and attention to normal activities.

Evaluation

- Ask the family to identify two to three indicators for caregiver role strain.
- Review with the family their plan to provide groceries, meals, and occasional respite care for the caregiver and patient.
- Ask the family where they keep the contact information of the patient's health care provider and when they would call the health care provider.

Whenever an individual becomes dependent on another family member for care and assistance, significant stress affects both the caregiver and the care recipient. In addition, the caregiver needs to continue to meet the demands of his or her usual lifestyle (e.g., raising children, working full time, or dealing with personal problems or illness). In many instances adult children, the sandwich generation, are trying to take care of their parents while meeting the needs of their own family (Box 10-7). Without adequate preparation and support from health care providers, caregiving puts the family at risk for serious problems, including a decline in the health

BOX 10-7 SANDWICH GENERATION

- Usually a daughter or daughter-in-law
- Conflicting responsibilities for aging parents, children, spouse, and job
- Frequently tries to "do it all"
- May not recognize need for help or request help
- May not pursue own health care
- Potential interventions:
  - Help families establish realistic priorities
  - Suggest that family members use family leave plans or obtain some "flex time" from their employer
  - Explore resources (e.g., deliveries for meals, respite care)

of the caregiver and that of the care receiver and dysfunctional and even abusive relationships (Schumacher, Beck, and Marren, 2006a; Tamayo et al., 2010).

Despite its demands, family caregiving can be a positive and rewarding experience. It is more than simply a series of tasks and usually occurs within the context of a family. Whether it is a wife caring for a husband or a daughter caring for a mother, caregiving is an interactional process. The interpersonal dynamics among family members influence the ultimate quality of caregiving. Thus the nurse plays a key role in helping family members develop better communication and problem-solving skills to build the relationships needed for caregiving to be successful (Stajduhar et al., 2008; Tamayo et al., 2010).

Variables such as caregiver and care-recipient expectations of one another influence caregiving quality. Carruth (1996) studied the concept of **reciprocity,** acknowledging the importance of the capability of care recipients to share exchanges that contribute to a caregiver's perception of self-worth. When the caregiver knows that the care recipient appreciates his or her efforts and values the assistance provided, a healthier and more satisfying caregiving relationship exists. When a caregiver and patient solve problems together, this helps them avoid overprotection or oversolicitous behavior. Patients feel in control of their care and responsible for care decisions. The caregiver also feels very positive and enjoys the caregiving experience (Isaksen, Thuen, and Hanestad, 2003).

Providing care and support for family caregivers enhances patient safety and involves using available family and community resources. Establishing a caregiving schedule that enables all family members to participate, helping patients to identify extended family members who can share any financial burdens posed by caregiving, and having distant relatives send cards and letters communicating their support is very helpful. However, it is imperative for you to understand the relationship between potential caregivers and care recipients. If the relationship is not a supportive one, community services are often a better resource for the patient and family.

Use of community resources includes locating a service required by the family or providing respite care so the family caregiver has time away from the care recipient. Examples of services that are beneficial to families include caregiver support groups, housing and transportation services, food and nutrition services, housecleaning, legal and financial services, home care, hospice, and mental health resources. Before referring a family to a community resource, it is critical that the nurse understand the family's dynamics and know whether the family wants support. Often a family caregiver resists help, feeling obligated to be the sole source of support to the care recipient. Be sensitive to family relationships and help caregivers understand the normalcy of caregiving demands. Given the appropriate resources, caregivers are able to acquire the skills and knowledge necessary to effectively care for their loved ones within the context of the home while maintaining rich and rewarding personal relationships.

KEY POINTS

- Family structure and functions influence the lives of its individual members.
- Family members influence one another's health beliefs, practices, and status.
- The concept of family is highly individual; care focuses on the patient's attitude toward the family rather than on an inflexible definition of family.
- The family's structure, functioning, and relative position in society significantly influence its health and ability to respond to health problems.
- A nurse can view the family in three ways: as context, as the patient, or as a system.
- Measures of family health involve more than a summary of individual members' health.
- Family members as caregivers are often spouses who are either older adults themselves or adult children trying to work full-time, care for aging parents, and launch teenagers successfully.
- Cultural sensitivity is vital to family nursing. Some members have differing beliefs, traditions, and restrictions, even within the same generation.
- Family caregiving is an interactive process that occurs within the context of the relationships among its members.

CLINICAL APPLICATION QUESTIONS

Preparing for Clinical Practice

Kathy is a home health nurse working with the Kline family. This is a family of four: Carol, a 45-year-old single mother; her two adolescent sons, Matt and Kent; and Sara, her 76-year-old mother, who is in the last stages of Alzheimer's disease. The mother has lived with Carol and her children for 10 years. Sara was a great support to Carol when her husband died 11 years ago. She helped Carol raise Matt and Kent. The family has decided to care for Sara in the home until she dies. Kathy is helping the family care for Sara in the home.

1. What type of assessments are important to determine family functioning and structure?
2. What should Kathy assess to determine how the family can achieve their goal of caring for Sara?
3. How does Kathy help the family determine their strengths, weaknesses, and resources?

evolve *Answers to Clinical Application Questions can be found on the Evolve website.*

REVIEW QUESTIONS

Are You Ready to Test Your Nursing Knowledge?

1. The Collins family includes a mother, Jean; stepfather, Adam; two teenage biological daughters of the mother, Lisa and Laura; and a biological daughter of the father, 25-year-old Stacey. Stacey just moved home following the loss of her job in another city. The family is converting a study into Stacey's bedroom and is in the process of distributing household

chores. When you talk to members of the family, they all think that their family can adjust to lifestyle changes. This is an example of family:
1. Diversity.
2. Durability.
3. Resiliency.
4. Configuration.

2. The most common reason grandparents are called on to raise their grandchildren is because of:
1. Single parenthood.
2. Legal interventions.
3. Dual-income families.
4. Increased divorce rate.

3. A family's access to adequate health care, opportunity for education, sound nutrition, and decreased stress is affected by:
1. Development.
2. Family function.
3. Family structure.
4. Economic stability.

4. David Singer is a single parent of a 3-year-old boy, Kevin. Kevin has well-managed asthma and misses day care infrequently. David is in school studying to be an information technology professional. His income and time are limited, and he admits to going to fast-food restaurants frequently for dinner. However, he and his son spend a lot of time together. David receives state-supported health care for his son, but he does not have health insurance or a personal physician. He has his son enrolled in a government-assisted day care program. Which of the following are risks to this family's level of health? (Select all that apply.)
1. Economic status
2. Chronic illness
3. Underinsured
4. Government-assisted day care

5. The Cleric family, which includes a mother, stepfather, two teenage biological daughters of the mother, and a biological daughter of the father is an example of a(n):
1. Nuclear family.
2. Blended family.
3. Extended family.
4. Alternative family.

6. Which of the following are possible outcomes with clear family communication? (Select all that apply.)
1. Family goals
2. Decision making
3. Methods of discipline
4. Impaired coping

7. Communication among family members is an example of family:
1. Attributes.
2. Function.
3. Structure.
4. Development.

8. Which of the following contribute to family hardiness? (Select all that apply.)
1. Family meetings
2. Established family roles
3. Willingness to change in time of stress
4. Passive orientation to life

9. Which of the following demonstrate family resiliency? (Select all that apply.)
1. Resuming full-time work when spouse loses job
2. Arguing ways to deal with problems among siblings
3. Developing hobbies when children leave home
4. Placing blame on family members

10. When nurses view the family as context, their primary focus is on the:
1. Family members within a system.
2. Family process and relationships.
3. Family relational and transactional concepts.
4. Health needs of an individual member.

11. Diane is a hospice nurse who is caring for the Robinson family. This family is providing end-of-life care for their grandmother, who has terminal breast cancer. When Diane visits the home 3 times a week, she focuses on symptom management for the grandmother and assists the family with coping skills. Diane's approach is an example of which of the following?
1. Family as context
2. Family as patient
3. Family as system
4. Family as structure

12. Which of the following are included in a family function assessment? (Select all that apply.)
1. Cultural practices
2. Decision making
3. Rituals and celebrations
4. Neighborhood crime data

13. Karen Johnson is a single mother of a school-age daughter. Linda Brown is also a single mother of two teenage daughters. Karen and Linda are active professionals, have busy social lives, and date occasionally. Three years ago they decided to share a house and housing costs, living expenses, and child care responsibilities. The children consider one another as their family. This family form is considered a(n):
1. Diverse family relationship.
2. Blended family relationship.s
3. Extended family relationship.
4. Alternative family relationship.

14. During a visit to a family clinic the nurse teaches the mother about immunizations, car seat use, and home safety for an infant and toddler. Which type of nursing interventions are these?
1. Health promotion activities
2. Acute care activities
3. Restorative care activities
4. Growth and development–care activities

15. Which best defines family caregiving? (Select all that apply.)
1. Designing a nurturing family to raise children
2. Providing physical and emotional care for a family member
3. Establishing a safe physical environment for a family
4. Monitoring for side effects of illness and treatments

Answers: **1.** 3; **2.** 2; **3.** 4; **4.** 1, 3; **5.** 2; **6.** 1, 2, 3; **7.** 2; **8.** 1, 2, 3; **9.** 1, 3; **10.** 4; **11.** 2; **12.** 1, 2, 3; **13.** 4; **14.** 1; **15.** 2, 3, 4.

REFERENCES

AARP Public Policy Institute (2008): *Issue Brief: Valuing the invaluable: A new look at the economic value of family caregiving,* 2008 Update, http://assets.aarp.org/rgcenter/il/i13_caregiving.pdf. Accessed November 1, 2010.

Anderson KH, Friedemann ML: Strategies to teach family assessment and intervention through an online international curriculum, *J Fam Nurs* 16(2):213, 2010.

Children's Defense Fund: *State of America's Children—2010 Report,* Washington, DC, 2010, Children's Defense Fund, http://www.childrensdefense.org/child-research-data-publications/data/state-of-americas-children-2010-report.html. Accessed August 19, 2010.

Davidson JE: Family-centered care: meeting the needs of patients' families and helping families adapt to critical illness, *Crit Care Nurse* 29(3):28, 2009.

Duhamel F: Implementing family nursing: how do we translate knowledge into clinical practice? Part 2, *J Fam Nurs* 16(1):8, 2010.

Epley P, et al: Characteristics and trends in family-centered conceptualizations, *J Fam Social Work* 13:269, 2010.

Family Violence Prevention Fund: *Domestic violence is a serious widespread social problem in America: the facts,* 2008a, http://www.endabuse. Accessed August 19, 2010.

Family Violence Prevention Fund: The facts on children and domestic violence, 2008b, http://www.endabuse.org. Accessed August 19, 2010.

Galanti GA: *Caring for patients from different cultures,* ed 4, Philadelphia, 2008, University of Pennsylvania Press.

Giger JN; Davidhizar RE: *Transcultural nursing: assessment and intervention,* ed 5, St Louis, 2008, Mosby.

Hanson SM, et al: *Family health care nursing, theory, practice and research,* ed 3, Philadelphia, 2005, FA Davis.

Kaakinen JR, et al: *Family health care nursing: theory, practice, and research,* ed 4, Philadelphia, 2010, FA Davis.

National Coalition for the Homeless: *Homeless families with children: NCH fact sheet,* Washington, DC, 2010, The Coalition, http://www.nationalhomeless.org/publications/facts. Accessed August 19, 2010.

Reinhard SC: Wanted nurses who support caregivers, *Am J Nurs* 106(8):13, 2006.

Schumacher K, Beck C, Marren JM: Family caregivers, *Am J Nurs* 106(8):40, 2006a.

Stajduhar KI, et al: Factors influencing family caregivers' ability to cope with providing end-of-life cancer care at home, *Cancer Nurs* 31(1):77, 2008.

Touhy TA, Jett KF: *Ebersole and Hess: Gerontological nursing healthy aging,* ed 3, St Louis, 2010, Mosby.

US Bureau of the Census: *Population profile of the United States: 2008* (Internet release, 2008 update), Washington, DC, 2008, The Bureau, http://www.census.gov. Accessed August 15, 2010.

RESEARCH REFERENCES

Anderson KH: The family health system approach to family systems nursing, *J Fam Nurs* 6(2):103, 2000.

Astedt-Kurki P, et al: Development and testing of a family nursing scale, *West J Nurs Res* 24(5):567, 2002.

Biello KB, Sipsma HL, Kershaw T: Effect of teenage parenthood on mental health trajectories: does sex matter? *Am J Epidemiol* 162(3):279, 2010.

Bluvol A, Ford-Gilboe M: Hope, health work and quality of life in families of stroke survivors, *J Adv Nurs* 48(4):322, 2004.

Carruth AK: Development and testing of the caregiver reciprocity scale, *Nurs Res* 45:92, 1996.

Duggleby W, et al: Metasynthesis of the hope experience of family caregivers of persons with chronic illness, *Qual Health Res* 20(2):148, 2010.

Harper CC, et al: Abstinence and teenagers: prevention counseling practices of health care providers serving high-risk patients in the United States, *Perspect Sexual Reprod Health* 42(2):125, 2010.

Hill EJ: Work-family facilitation and conflict, working fathers and mothers, work-family stressors and support, *J Fam Issues* 26(6):793, 2005.

Isaksen AS, Thuen F, Hanestad B: Patients with cancer and their close relatives: experiences with treatment, care, and support, *Cancer Nurs* 26(1):68, 2003.

Joronen K, Astedt-Kurki P: Familial contribution to adolescent subjective well-being, *Int J Nurs Pract* 11:125, 2005.

McCubbin MA, McCubbin HI, Thompson AI: Family Hardiness Index (FHI). In McCubbin HI, Thompson AI, McCubbin MS, editors: *Family assessment: resiliency, coping, and adaptation, inventories for research and practice,* Madison, 1996, University of Wisconsin Press.

Rosenthal MS, et al: Family child care provider's experience in health promotion, *Fam Commun Health* 31(4):326, 2008.

Schumacher KL, et al: A transactional model of cancer family caregiving skill. *ANS* 29(3):271, 2006b.

Shpancer N, et al: Quality of care attributions to employed versus stay-at-home mothers, *Early Child Dev Care* 176(2):183, 2006.

Tamayo GJ, et al: Caring for the caregiver, *Oncol Nurs Forum* 37(1):E50, 2010.

Weinert C, et al: Evolution of a conceptual model for adaptation to chronic illness, *J Nurs Scholarship* 40(4):364, 2008.

CHAPTER

11

Developmental Theories

OBJECTIVES

- Discuss factors influencing growth and development.
- Describe biophysical developmental theories.
- Describe and compare the psychoanalytical/psychosocial theories proposed by Freud and Erikson.
- Describe Piaget's theory of cognitive development.
- Apply developmental theories when planning interventions in the care of patients throughout the life span.
- Discuss nursing implications for the application of developmental principles to patient care.

KEY TERMS

Biophysical development, p. 131
Conventional reasoning, p. 135
Erikson's theory of psychosocial development, p. 132
Freud's psychoanalytical model of personality development, p. 131
Kohlberg's theory of moral development, p. 135
Piaget's theory of cognitive development, p. 134
Postconventional reasoning, p. 136
Temperament, p. 133

evolve WEBSITE

http://evolve.elsevier.com/Potter/fundamentals/

- Review Questions
- Case Study with Questions
- Audio Glossary
- Interactive Learning Activities
- Key Term Flashcards
- Content Updates

Understanding normal growth and development helps nurses predict, prevent, and detect deviations from patients' own expected patterns. Growth encompasses the physical changes that occur from the prenatal period through older adulthood and also demonstrates both advancement and deterioration. Young children grow more quickly than older children, and by adulthood growth in height ceases. In late adulthood there is a loss of both muscle and bone, which may cause a decrease in height in some people (Santrock, 2009). Development refers to the biological, cognitive, and socioemotional changes that begin at conception and continue throughout a lifetime. Development is dynamic and includes progression. However, in some disease processes development is delayed or regresses. For example, older adults demonstrate cognitive development resulting in wisdom as they incorporate life experiences into decision making, but they do not perform as well as young adults when speed is required for information processing (Santrock, 2008).

Individuals have unique patterns of growth and development. The ability to progress through each developmental phase influences the overall health of the individual. The success or failure experienced within a phase affects the ability to complete subsequent phases. If individuals experience repeated developmental failures, inadequacies sometimes result. However, when the individual experiences repeated successes, health is promoted. For example, a child who does not walk by 20 months may demonstrate delayed gross motor ability that slows exploration and manipulation of the environment. In contrast, a child who walks by 10 months is able to explore and find stimulation in the environment.

Today nurses need to adopt a life span perspective of human development that takes into account all developmental stages of life. Traditionally development focused on childhood, but a comprehensive view of development also includes the changes that occur during the adult years. An understanding of growth and development throughout the life span assists in planning questions for health screening and health history and in health teaching for patients of all ages.

DEVELOPMENTAL THEORIES

Developmental theories provide a framework for examining, describing, and appreciating human development. For example, knowledge of Erikson's psychosocial theory of development helps caregivers understand the importance of supporting the development of basic trust in the infancy stage. Trust establishes the foundation for all future relationships. Developmental theories are also important in helping nurses assess and treat a person's response to an illness. Understanding the specific task or need of each developmental stage guides caregivers in planning appropriate individualized care for patients. Specific developmental theories that define the aging process for adults are discussed in Chapters 13 and 14.

Human development is a dynamic and complex process that cannot be explained by only one theory. This chapter presents biophysical, psychoanalytical/psychosocial, cognitive, and moral developmental theories. Chapters 25 and 35 cover the areas of learning theory for patient teaching and spiritual development.

Biophysical Developmental Theories

Biophysical development is how our physical bodies grow and change. Health care providers are able to quantify and compare the changes that occur as a newborn infant grows into adulthood against established norms. How does the physical body age? What are the triggers that move the body from the physical characteristics of childhood, through adolescence, to the physical changes of adulthood?

Gesell's Theory of Development. Fundamental to Gesell's theory of development is that each child's pattern of growth is unique and this pattern is directed by gene activity (Gesell, 1948). Gesell found the pattern of maturation follows a fixed developmental sequence in humans. Sequential development is evident in fetuses, in which there is a specified order of organ system development. Today we know that growth in humans is both cephalocaudal and proximodistal. The cephalocaudal pattern describes the sequence in which growth is fastest at the top (head and then down); proximodistal growth starts at the center of the body and moves toward the extremities.

Genes direct the sequence of development; but environmental factors also influence development, resulting in developmental changes. For example, genes may direct the growth rate for an individual, but that growth is only maximized if environmental conditions are adequate. Poor nutrition or chronic disease often affects the growth rate and results in smaller stature, regardless of the genetic blueprint. However, adequate nutrition and the absence of disease cannot result in stature beyond that determined by heredity.

Psychoanalytical/Psychosocial Theory

Theories of psychoanalytical/psychosocial development describe human development from the perspectives of personality, thinking, and behavior (Table 11-1). Psychoanalytical theory explains development as primarily unconscious and influenced by emotion. Psychoanalytical theorists maintain that these unconscious drives influence development through universal stages experienced by all individuals (Berger, 2007).

Sigmund Freud. **Freud's psychoanalytical model of personality development** states that individuals go through five stages of psychosexual development and that each stage is characterized by sexual pleasure in parts of the body: the mouth, the anus, and the genitals. Freud believed that adult personality is the result of how an individual resolved conflicts between these sources of pleasure and the mandates of reality (Berger, 2007; Santrock, 2009).

Stage 1: Oral (Birth to 12 to 18 Months). Initially sucking and oral satisfaction are not only vital to life but also extremely pleasurable in their own rights. Late in this stage the infant begins to realize that the mother/parent is something separate from self. Disruption in the physical or emotional availability of the parent (e.g., inadequate bonding or chronic illness) could affect an infant's development.

Stage 2: Anal (12 to 18 Months to 3 Years). The focus of pleasure changes to the anal zone. Children become increasingly aware of the pleasurable sensations of this body region with interest in the products of their effort. Through the toilet-training process the child delays gratification to meet parental and societal expectations.

Stage 3: Phallic or Oedipal (3 to 6 Years). The genital organs are the focus of pleasure during this stage. The boy becomes interested in the penis; the girl becomes aware of the absence of the penis, known as *penis envy*. This is a time of exploration and imagination as the child fantasizes about the parent of the opposite sex as his or her first love interest, known as the *Oedipus* or *Electra complex*. By the end of this stage the child attempts to reduce this conflict by identifying with the parent of the same sex as a way to win recognition and acceptance.

Stage 4: Latency (6 to 12 Years). In this stage Freud believed that sexual urges from the earlier oedipal stage are repressed and channeled into productive activities that are socially acceptable. Within the educational and social worlds of the child, there is much to learn and accomplish.

Stage 5: Genital (Puberty Through Adulthood). In this final stage sexual urges reawaken and are directed to an individual outside the family circle. Unresolved prior conflicts surface during adolescence. Once the individual resolves conflicts, he or she is then capable of having a mature adult sexual relationship.

Freud believed that the components of the human personality develop in stages and regulate behavior. These components are the

TABLE 11-1 Comparison of Major Developmental Theories

DEVELOPMENTAL STAGE/AGE	FREUD (PSYCHOSEXUAL DEVELOPMENT)	ERIKSON (PSYCHOSOCIAL DEVELOPMENT)	PIAGET (COGNITIVE/ MORAL DEVELOPMENT)	KOHLBERG (DEVELOPMENT OF MORAL REASONING)
Infancy (birth to 18 months)	Oral stage	Trust vs. mistrust Ability to trust others	Sensorimotor period Progress from reflex activity to simple repetitive actions	
Early childhood/toddler (18 months to 3 years)	Anal stage	Autonomy vs. shame and doubt Self-control and independence	Preoperational period—thinking using symbols Egocentric	Preconventional level Punishment-obedience orientation
Preschool (3-5 years)	Phallic stage	Initiative vs. guilt Highly imaginative	Use of symbols Egocentric	Preconventional level Premoral Instrumental orientation
Middle childhood (6-12 years)	Latent stage	Industry vs. inferiority Engaged in tasks and activities	Concrete operations period Logical thinking	Conventional level Good boy–nice girl orientation
Adolescence (12-19 years)	Genital stage	Identity vs. role confusion Sexual maturity, "Who am I?"	Formal operations period Abstract thinking	Postconventional level Social contract orientation

id, the ego, and the superego. The id (i.e., basic instinctual impulses driven to achieve pleasure) is the most primitive part of the personality and originates in the infant. The ego represents the reality component, mediating conflicts between the environment and the forces of the id. The ego helps people judge reality accurately, regulate impulses, and make good decisions. The third component, the superego, performs regulating, restraining, and prohibiting actions. Often referred to as the conscience, the superego is influenced by the standards of outside social forces (e.g., parent or teacher).

Some of Freud's critics contend that he based his analysis of personality development on biological determinants and ignored the influence of culture and experience. Other critics think that Freud's basic assumptions such as the Oedipus complex are not applicable across different cultures. Psychoanalysts today believe that the role of conscious thought is much greater than Freud imagined (Santrock, 2008).

Erik Erikson. Freud had a strong influence on his psychoanalytical followers, including Erik Erikson (1902-1994), who constructed a theory of development that differed from Freud's in two major views. Erikson maintained that development occurred throughout the life span and that it focused on psychosocial stages rather than psychosexual stages.

According to **Erikson's theory of psychosocial development,** individuals need to accomplish a particular task before successfully mastering the stage and progressing to the next one. Each task is framed with opposing conflicts, and tasks once mastered are challenged and tested again during new situations or at times of conflict (Hockenberry and Wilson, 2011). Erikson's eight stages of life are described here.

Trust versus Mistrust (Birth to 1 Year). Establishing a basic sense of trust is essential for the development of a healthy personality. The infant's successful resolution of this stage requires a consistent caregiver who is available to meet his needs. From this basic trust in parents, the infant is able to trust in himself, in others, and in the world (Hockenberry and Wilson, 2011). The formation of trust results in faith and optimism. A nurse's use of anticipatory guidance helps parents cope with the hospitalization of an infant and the infant's behaviors when discharged to home.

Autonomy versus Sense of Shame and Doubt (1 to 3 Years). By this stage a growing child is more accomplished in some basic self-care activities, including walking, feeding, and toileting. This newfound independence is the result of maturation and imitation. The toddler develops his or her autonomy by making choices. Choices typical for the toddler age-group include activities related to relationships, desires, and playthings. There is also opportunity to learn that parents and society have expectations about these choices. Limiting choices and/or enacting harsh punishment leads to feelings of shame and doubt. The toddler who successfully masters this stage achieves self-control and willpower. The nurse models empathetic guidance that offers support for and understanding of the challenges of this stage.

Initiative versus Guilt (3 to 6 Years). Children like to pretend and try out new roles. Fantasy and imagination allow them to further explore their environment. Also at this time they are developing their superego, or conscience. Conflicts often occur between the child's desire to explore and the limits placed on his or her behavior. These conflicts sometimes lead to feelings of frustration and guilt. Guilt also occurs if the caregiver's responses are too harsh. Preschoolers are learning to maintain a sense of initiative without imposing on the freedoms of others. Successful resolution of this stage results in direction and purpose. Teaching the child impulse control and cooperative behaviors helps the family avoid the risks of altered growth and development.

Industry versus Inferiority (6 to 11 Years). School-age children are eager to apply themselves to learning socially productive skills and tools. They learn to work and play with their peers. They thrive on their accomplishments and praise. Without proper support for learning new skills or if skills are too difficult, they develop a sense of inadequacy and inferiority. Children at this age need to be able to experience real achievement to develop a sense of competency. Erikson believed that the adult's attitudes toward work are traced to successful achievement of this task (Erikson, 1963). During hospitalization it is important for the school-age child to understand the routines and participate as actively as possible in his or her treatment. For example, some children enjoy keeping a record of their intake and output.

Identity versus Role Confusion (Puberty). Dramatic physiological changes associated with sexual maturation mark this stage. There is a marked preoccupation with appearance and body image. This stage, in which identity development begins with the goal of achieving some perspective or direction, answers the question, "Who am I?" Acquiring a sense of identity is essential for making adult decisions such as choice of a vocation or marriage partner. Each adolescent moves in his or her unique way into society as an interdependent member. There are also new social demands, opportunities, and conflicts that relate to the emergent identity and separation from family. Erikson held that successful mastery of this stage resulted in devotion and fidelity to others and to their own ideals (Hockenberry and Wilson, 2011). The nurse provides education and anticipatory guidance for the parent about the changes and challenges to the adolescent. Nurses also help hospitalized adolescents deal with their illness by giving them enough information to allow them to make decisions about their treatment plan.

Intimacy versus Isolation (Young Adult). Young adults, having developed a sense of identity, deepen their capacity to love others and care for them. They search for meaningful friendships and an intimate relationship with another person. Erikson portrayed intimacy as finding the self and then losing the self in another (Santrock, 2008). If the young adult is not able to establish companionship and intimacy, isolation results because he or she fears rejection and disappointment (Berger, 2007). Nurses must understand that hospitalization increases a young adults' need for intimacy; thus young adults benefit from the support of their partner or significant other during this time.

Generativity versus Self-Absorption and Stagnation (Middle Age). Following the development of an intimate relationship, the adult focuses on supporting future generations. The ability to expand one's personal and social involvement is critical to this stage of development. Middle-age adults achieve success in this stage by contributing to future generations through parenthood, teaching, and community involvement. Achieving generativity results in caring for others as a basic strength. Inability to play a role in the development of the next generation results in stagnation (Santrock, 2008). Nurses assist physically ill adults in choosing creative ways to foster social development. Middle-age persons often find a sense of fulfillment by volunteering in a local school, hospital, or church.

Integrity versus Despair (Old Age). Many older adults review their lives with a sense of satisfaction, even with their inevitable mistakes. Others see themselves as failures, with their lives marked by despair and regret. Older adults often engage in a retrospective appraisal of their lives. They interpret their lives as a meaningful whole or experience regret because of goals not achieved (Berger, 2007). Because the aging process creates physical and social losses,

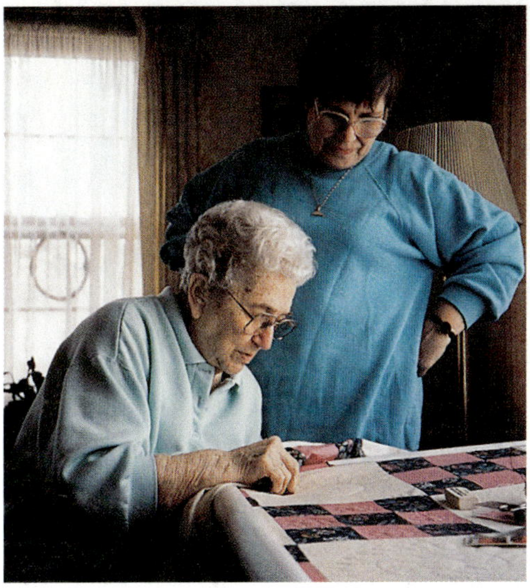

FIG. 11-1 Quilting keeps this older adult active.

some adults also suffer loss of status and function (e.g., through retirement or illness). These external struggles are also met with internal struggles such as the search for meaning in life. Meeting these challenges creates the potential for growth and the basic strength of wisdom (Fig. 11-1).

Nurses are in positions of influence within their communities to help people feel valued, appreciated, and needed. Erikson stated, "Healthy children will not fear life, if their parents have integrity enough not to fear death" (Erikson, 1963). Although Erikson believed that problems in adult life resulted from unsuccessful resolution of earlier stages, his emphasis on family relationships and culture offered a broad, life-span view of development. As a nurse, you will use this knowledge of development as you deliver care in any health care setting.

Theories Related to Temperament. **Temperament** is a behavioral style that affects an individual's emotional interactions with others (Santrock, 2008). Personality and temperament are often closely linked, and research shows that individuals possess some enduring characteristics into adulthood. The individual differences that children display in responding to their environment significantly influence the way others respond to them and their needs. Knowledge of temperament helps parents better understand their child (Hockenberry and Wilson, 2011).

Psychiatrists Stella Chess (1914-2007) and Alexander Thomas (1914-2003) conducted a 20-year longitudinal study that identified three basic classes of temperament:

- *The easy child*—Easygoing and even-tempered. This child is regular and predictable in his or her habits. An easy child is open and adaptable to change and displays a mild-to–moderately intense mood that is typically positive.
- *The difficult child*—Highly active, irritable, and irregular in habits. Negative withdrawal toward others is typical, and the child requires a more structured environment. A difficult child adapts slowly to new routines, people, or situations. Mood expressions are usually intense and primarily negative.
- *The slow-to-warm up child*—Typically reacts negatively and with mild intensity to new stimuli. The child adapts slowly with repeated contact unless pressured and responds with mild but passive resistance to novelty or changes in routine.

Research on temperament and its stability has continued, with an emphasis on the individual's ability to make thoughtful decisions about behavior in demanding situations. Knowledge of temperament and how it impacts the parent-child relationship is critical when providing anticipatory guidance for parents. With the birth of a second child, most parents find that the strategies that worked well with the first child no longer work at all. The nurse individualizes counseling to greatly improve the quality of interactions between parents and children (Hockenberry and Wilson, 2011).

Perspectives on Adult Development

Early study of development focused only on childhood because scholars throughout history regarded the aging process as one of inevitable and irreversible decline. However, we now know that, although the changes come more slowly, people continue to develop new abilities and adapt to shifting environments. The life span perspective suggests that understanding adult development requires multiple viewpoints. Two of the ways that researchers have studied adult development are through the stage-crisis view and the life span approach. The most well-known stage theory is the one developed by Erik Erikson that was discussed earlier. Another stage theory that contributed to understanding development throughout the life span was provided through the work of Robert Havinghurst.

Stage-Crisis Theory. Physicist, educator, and aging expert Robert Havinghurst (1900-1991) conducted extensive research and developed a theory of human development based on developmental tasks. Havinghurst's theory incorporates three primary sources for developmental tasks: tasks that surface because of physical maturation, tasks that evolve from personal values, and tasks that are a result of pressures from society. As with Erikson, Havinghurst believed that successful resolution of the developmental task was essential to successful progression throughout life. He identified six stages and six-to-ten developmental tasks for each stage: infancy and early childhood (birth to age 6), middle childhood (6 to 12 years), adolescence (13 to 18 years), early adulthood (19 to 30 years), middle adulthood (30 to 60 years), and late adulthood (60 and over). Havinghurst believed that the number of tasks differs in each age level for individuals because of the interrelationship among biology, society, and personal values. In later years Havinghurst turned his focus to the study of aging. In response to the view that older adults should gradually withdraw from society, Havinghurst proposed an *activity theory,* which states that continuing an active, involved lifestyle results in greater satisfaction and well-being in aging (see Chapter 14).

Life Span Approach. The contemporary life-events approach takes into consideration the variations that occur for each individual. This view considers the individual's personal circumstances (health and family support), how the person views and adjusts to changes, and the current social and historical context in which the individual is living (Santrock, 2009). Contemporary theorists such as Paul Baltes (1939-2006) and Laura Carstensen (1954-) have continued to study development in adulthood and proposed theories that support the need for a balance between the pursuit of active engagement and selection of activities that support personal enjoyment for successful aging. The selective optimization with compensation theory (Baltes, Freund, and Li, 2005) is based on the concept that, as individuals age, they are able to compensate for some decreases in physical or cognitive performance by developing new approaches. They are also able to optimize performance in some areas through continued practice or the use of new technology. Carstensen, Isaacowitz, and Charles (1999) developed the socioemotional selectivity theory suggesting that, as people age, they become more selective and invest their energies in meaningful relationships, goals, and activities. Current research on successful aging is much more consistent with a life span approach that emphasizes age-related goals that are relationship and socially oriented to support continued well-being (Reichstadt et al., 2010).

Cognitive Developmental Theory

Psychoanalytical/psychosocial theories focus on an individual's unconscious thought and emotions; cognitive theories stress how people learn to think and make sense of their world. As with personality development, cognitive theorists have explored both childhood and adulthood. Some of the theories highlight qualitative changes in thinking; others expand to include social, cultural, and behavioral dimensions.

Jean Piaget. Jean Piaget (1896-1980) was most interested in the development of children's intellectual organization: how they think, reason, and perceive the world. **Piaget's theory of cognitive development** includes four periods that are related to age and demonstrate specific categories of knowing and understanding. He built his theory on years of observing children as they explored, manipulated, and tried to make sense out of the world in which they lived. Piaget believed that individuals move from one stage to the other seeking cognitive equilibrium or a state of mental balance (Santrock, 2009). Within each of these primary periods of cognitive development are specific stages (see Table 11-1).

Period I: Sensorimotor (Birth to 2 Years). Infants develop a schema or action pattern for dealing with the environment. These schemas include hitting, looking, grasping, or kicking. Schemas become self-initiated activities (e.g., the infant learning that sucking achieves a pleasing result generalizes the action to suck fingers, blanket, or clothing). Successful achievement leads to greater exploration. During this stage the child learns about himself and his environment through motor and reflex actions. He or she learns that he or she is separate from the environment and that aspects of the environment (e.g., parents or favorite toy) continue to exist even though they cannot always be seen. Piaget termed this understanding that objects continue to exist even when they cannot be seen, heard, or touched *object permanence* and considered it one of the child's most important accomplishments.

Period II: Preoperational (2 to 7 Years). During this time children learn to think with the use of symbols and mental images. They exhibit "egocentrism" in that they see objects and persons from only one point of view, their own. They believe that everyone experiences the world exactly as they do. Early in this stage children demonstrate "animism" in which they personify objects. They believe that inanimate objects have lifelike thought, wishes, and feelings. Their thinking is influenced greatly by fantasy and magical thinking. Children at this stage have difficulty conceptualizing time. Play becomes a primary means by which they foster their cognitive development and learn about the world (Fig. 11-2). Nursing interventions during this period recognize the use of play as the way the child understands the events taking place.

Period III: Concrete Operations (7 to 11 Years). Children now are able to perform mental operations. For example, the child thinks about an action that before was performed physically. Children are now able to describe a process without actually doing it. At this time they are able to coordinate two concrete perspectives in social and scientific thinking so they are able to appreciate the difference between their perspective and that of a friend. Reversibility is one of the primary characteristics of concrete operational thought. Children can now mentally picture a series of steps and reverse the steps to get back to the starting point. The ability to mentally classify objects according to their quantitative dimensions, known as *seriation,* is achieved. They are able to correctly order or sort objects by length, weight, or other characteristics. Another major accomplishment of this stage is conservation, or the ability to see objects or quantities as remaining the same despite a change in their physical appearance (Santrock, 2009).

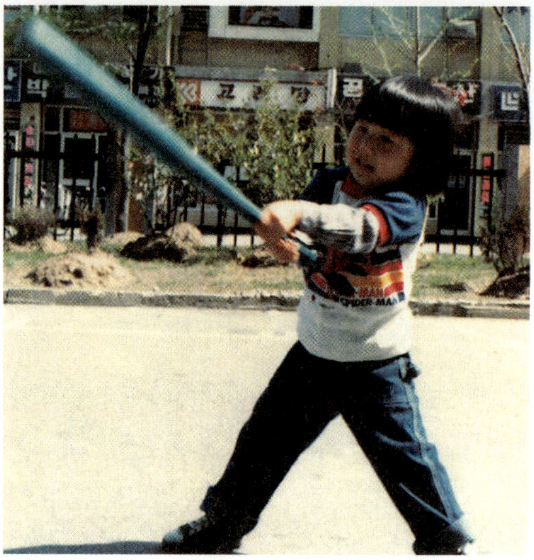

FIG. 11-2 Play is important to a child's development.

Period IV: Formal Operations (11 Years to Adulthood). The transition from concrete to formal operational thinking occurs in stages during which there is a prevalence of egocentric thought. This egocentricity leads adolescents to demonstrate feelings and behaviors characterized by self-consciousness, a belief that their actions and appearance are constantly being scrutinized (an "imaginary audience"), that their thoughts and feelings are unique (the "personal fable"), and that they are invulnerable (Santrock, 2008). These feelings of invulnerability frequently lead to risk-taking behaviors, especially in early adolescence. As adolescents share experiences with peers, they learn that many of their thoughts and feelings are shared by almost everyone, helping them to know that they are not so different. As adolescents mature, their thinking moves to abstract and theoretical subjects. They have the capacity to reason with respect to possibilities. For Piaget this stage marked the end of cognitive development.

Piaget's work has been challenged over the years as researchers have continued to study cognitive development. For example, some aspects of objective performance emerge earlier than Piaget believed, and other cognitive abilities can surface later than he predicted. We now know that many adults may not become formal operational thinkers and others have cognitive development that goes beyond the stages that Piaget proposed (Santrock, 2009). Assessment of cognitive ability becomes critical as the nurse engages in health care teaching for patients and families.

Research in Adult Cognitive Development. Research into cognitive development in adulthood began in the 1970s and continues today. Research supports that adults do not always arrive at one answer to a problem but frequently accept several possible solutions. Adults also incorporate emotions, logic, practicality, and flexibility when making decisions. On the basis of these observations, developmentalists proposed a fifth stage of cognitive development termed *postformal thought.* Within this stage adults

BOX 11-1 EVIDENCE-BASED PRACTICE

Applying Developmental Theory to Care of Chronically Ill Older Adults

PICO Question: Among older adult patients diagnosed with heart failure (HF), does screening for depression result in improved quality of life and improved physical symptoms?

Evidence Summary

Neglect of physical health, increased symptoms from chronic illness, and forgetfulness are frequently attributed to the aging process. However, older adults do not withdraw from society or lose their cognitive abilities as part of their normal development. Depression among older adults is common, especially in those with a chronic illness such as HF. Research has found the prevalence of depression in these individuals to be as high as 58% among hospitalized patients and up to 48% in those receiving outpatient treatments (Hägglund et al., 2008). Depression often contributes to poor physical and emotional health outcomes and is a major risk factor for poor prognosis and high mortality rates in patients with HF (Cully et al., 2010). It is difficult at times to differentiate between symptoms of depression and worsening signs of HF, especially fatigue. In a study conducted with older adults who were diagnosed with HF and those without HF but who reported general fatigue and reduced activity, the researchers found no difference in the prevalence of depression (Hägglund et al., 2008). Others have noted that, since physical disorders increase with age independent of depression, the decreased diagnosis of depression in older adults is sometimes a result of confusing depression with physical symptoms and lack of screening for depression (Kessler et al., 2010).

Screening for depression as part of the overall health assessment leads to treatment that would greatly improve older adults' physical, social, and emotional functioning. It is important that nurses apply developmental theory and recognize the need to identify depression so appropriate treatment can be provided.

Application to Nursing Practice

- Be aware of the symptoms of depression such as general fatigue or insomnia since older adults and family members may attribute these signs to "old age" and not recognize the potential for treatment.
- Understanding adult development and its implications for practice is essential in providing nursing care for older adult patients.
- Understanding the older adult's concept of depression and views on treatment for mental illness helps you explain complementary and alternative treatment measures.

demonstrate the ability to recognize that answers vary from situation to situation and that solutions need to be sensible.

One of the earliest to develop a theory of adult cognition was William Perry (1913-1998), who studied college students and found that continued cognitive development involved increasing cognitive flexibility. As adolescents were able to move from a position of accepting only one answer to realizing that alternative explanations could be right, depending on one's perspective, there was a significant cognitive change. Adults change how they use knowledge, and the emphasis shifts from attaining knowledge or skills to using knowledge for goal achievement (Box 11-1).

Moral Developmental Theory

Moral development refers to the changes in a person's thoughts, emotions, and behaviors that influence beliefs about what is right or wrong. It encompasses both *interpersonal* and *intrapersonal* dimensions as it governs how we interact with others (Santrock, 2009). Although various psychosocial and cognitive theorists address moral development within their respective theories, the theories of Piaget and Kohlberg are more widely known (see Table 11-1).

Lawrence Kohlberg's Theory of Moral Development. Kohlberg's theory of moral development expands on Piaget's cognitive theory. Kohlberg interviewed children, adolescents, and eventually adults and found that moral reasoning develops in stages. From an examination of responses to a series of moral dilemmas, he identified six stages of moral development under three levels (Kohlberg, 1981).

Level I: Preconventional Reasoning. This is the premoral level, in which there is limited cognitive thinking and the individual's thinking is primarily egocentric. At this stage thinking is mostly based on likes and pleasures. This stage progresses toward having punishment guide behavior. The person's moral reason for acting, the "why," eventually relates to the consequences that the person believes will occur. These consequences come in the form of punishment or reward. It is at this level that children view illness as a punishment for fighting with their siblings or disobeying their parents. Nurses need to be aware of this egocentric thinking and reinforce that the child does not become ill because of wrongdoing.

Stage 1: Punishment and Obedience Orientation. In this first stage a child's response to a moral dilemma is in terms of absolute obedience to authority and rules. A child in this stage reasons, "I must follow the rules; otherwise I will be punished." Avoiding punishment or the unquestioning deference to authority is characteristic motivation to behave. Physical consequences guide right and wrong choices. If the child is caught, it must be wrong; if he or she escapes, it must be right.

Stage 2: Instrumental Relativist Orientation. In this stage the child recognizes that there is more than one right view; a teacher has one view that is different from that of the child's parent. The decision to do something morally right is based on satisfying one's own needs and occasionally the needs of others. The child perceives punishment not as proof of being wrong (as in stage 1) but as something that one wants to avoid. Children at this stage follow their parent's rule about being home in time for supper because they do not want to be confined to their room for the rest of the evening if they are late.

Level II: Conventional Reasoning. At level II, conventional reasoning, the person sees moral reasoning based on his or her own personal internalization of societal and others' expectations. A person wants to fulfill the expectations of the family, group, or nation and also develop a loyalty to and actively maintain, support, and justify the order. Moral decision making at this level moves from, "What's in it for me?" to "How will it affect my relationships with others?" Emphasis now is on social rules and a community-centered approach (Berger, 2007). Nurses observe this when family members make end-of-life decisions for their loved ones. Individual members often struggle with this type of moral dilemma. Grief support involves an understanding of the level of moral decision making of each family member (see Chapter 36).

Stage 3: Good Boy–Nice Girl Orientation. The individual wants to win approval and maintain the expectations of one's immediate group. "Being good" is important and defined as having good motives, showing concern for others, and keeping mutual relationships through trust, loyalty, respect, and gratitude. One earns approval by "being nice." For example, a person in this stage stays after school and does odd jobs to win the teacher's approval.

Stage 4: Society-Maintaining Orientation. Individuals expand their focus from a relationship with others to societal concerns during stage 4. Moral decisions take into account societal perspectives. Right behavior is doing one's duty, showing respect for authority, and maintaining the social order. Adolescents choose not to attend a party where they know beer will be served, not because they are afraid of getting caught, but because they know that it is not right.

Level III: Postconventional Reasoning. The person finds a balance between basic human rights and obligations and societal rules and regulations in the level of **postconventional reasoning.** Individuals move away from moral decisions based on authority or conformity to groups to define their own moral values and principles. Individuals at this stage start to look at what an ideal society would be like. Moral principles and ideals come into prominence at this level (Berger, 2007).

Stage 5: Social Contract Orientation. Having reached stage 5, an individual follows the societal law but recognizes the possibility of changing the law to improve society. The individual also recognizes that different social groups have different values but believes that all rational people would agree on basic rights such as liberty and life. Individuals at this stage make more of an independent effort to determine what society *should* value rather than what the society as a group *would* value, as would occur in stage 4. The United States Constitution is based on this morality.

Stage 6: Universal Ethical Principle Orientation. Stage 6 defines "right" by the decision of conscience in accord with self-chosen ethical principles. These principles are abstract, like the Golden Rule, and appeal to logical comprehensiveness, universality, and consistency (Kohlberg, 1981). For example, the principle of justice requires the individual to treat everyone in an impartial manner, respecting the basic dignity of all people, and guides the individual to base decisions on an equal respect for all. Civil disobedience is one way to distinguish Stage 5 from Stage 6. Stage 5 emphasizes the basic rights, the democratic process, and following laws without question, whereas stage 6 defines the principles by which agreements will be most just. For example, a person in stage 5 follows a law, even if it is not fair to a certain racial group. An individual in stage 6 may not follow a law if it does not seem just to the racial group. For example, Martin Luther King believed that although we need laws and democratic processes, people who are committed to justice have an obligation to disobey unjust laws and accept the penalties for disobeying these laws (Crain, 1985).

Kohlberg's Critics. Kohlberg constructed a systemized way of looking at moral development and is recognized as a leader in moral developmental theory. However, critics of his work raise questions about his choice of research subjects. For example, most of Kohlberg's subjects were males raised in Western philosophical traditions. Research attempting to support Kohlberg's theory with individuals raised in the Eastern philosophies found that individuals raised in Eastern philosophies never rose above stages 3 or 4 of Kohlberg's model. To some, these findings suggest that people from Eastern philosophies have not reached higher levels of moral development, which is untrue. Others believe Kohlberg's research design did not allow a way to measure those raised within a different culture.

Kohlberg has also been criticized for age and gender bias. Carol Gilligan, an associate, criticizes Kohlberg for his gender biases. She believes that he developed his theory based on a justice perspective that focused on the rights of individuals. In contrast, Gilligan's research looked at moral development from a care perspective that viewed people in their interpersonal communications, relationships, and concern for others (Santrock, 2009). She believes that females are socialized to be nurturing and caring and thus are reluctant to make judgments based solely on justice (Berger, 2007). Other researchers have examined Gilligan's theory in studies with children and have not found evidence to support gender differences (Berger, 2007; Santrock, 2009).

Moral Reasoning and Nursing Practice. Nurses need to know their own moral reasoning level. Recognizing your own moral developmental level is essential in separating your beliefs from others when helping patients with their moral decision-making process. It is also important to recognize the level of moral reasoning used by other members of the health care team and its influence on a patient's care plan. Ideally all members of the health care team are on the same level, creating a unified outcome. This is exemplified in the following scenario: The nurse is caring for a homeless person and believes that all patients deserve the same level of care. The case manager, who is responsible for resource allocation, complains about the patient's length of stay and the amount of resources being expended on this one patient. The nurse and the case manager are in conflict because of their different levels of moral decision making within their practices. They decide to hold a health care team conference to discuss their differences and the ethical dilemma of ensuring that the patient receives an appropriate level of care.

Developmental theories help nurses to use critical thinking skills when asking how and why people respond as they do. From the diverse set of theories included in this chapter, the complexity of human development is evident. No one theory successfully describes all the intricacies of human growth and development. Today's nurse needs be knowledgeable about several theoretical perspectives when working with patients.

Your assessment of a patient requires a thorough analysis and interpretation of data to form accurate conclusions about his or her developmental needs. Accurate identification of nursing diagnoses relies on your ability to consider developmental theory in data analysis. You compare normal developmental behaviors with those projected by developmental theory. Examples of nursing diagnoses applicable to patients with developmental problems include *risk for delayed development, delayed growth and development,* and *risk for disproportionate growth.*

Growth and development, as supported by a life-span perspective, is multidimensional. The theories included are the basis for a meaningful observation of an individual's pattern of growth and development. They are important guidelines for understanding important human processes that allow nurses to begin to predict human responses and recognize deviations from the norm.

KEY POINTS

- Nurses administer care for individuals at various developmental stages. Developmental theory provides a basis for nurses to assess and understand the responses seen in their patients.
- Humans continue to develop throughout their lives. Development is not limited to childhood and adolescence; persons grow and develop throughout their life span.
- Theory is a way to account for how and why people grow up as they do. Theories provide a framework to clarify and organize existing observations to explain and try to predict human behavior.
- Growth refers to the quantitative changes that nurses measure and compare to norms.
- Development implies a progressive and continuous process of change, leading to a state of organized and specialized

functional capacity. These changes are quantitatively measurable but are more distinctly measured in qualitative changes.

- Biophysical development theory explores theories of why individuals age from a biological standpoint, why development follows a predictable sequence, and how environmental factors can influence development.
- Cognitive development focuses on the rational thinking processes that include the changes in how children, adolescents, and adults perform intellectual operations.
- Developmental tasks are age-related achievements, the success of which leads to happiness; whereas failure often leads to unhappiness, disapproval, and difficulty in achieving later tasks.
- Developmental crisis occurs when a person is having great difficulty meeting tasks of the current developmental period.
- Psychosocial theories describe human development from the perspectives of personality, thinking, and behavior with varying degrees of influence from internal biological forces and external societal/cultural forces.
- Temperament is a behavioral pattern that affects the individual's interactions with others.
- Moral development theory attempts to define how moral reasoning matures for an individual.

CLINICAL APPLICATION QUESTIONS

Preparing for Clinical Practice

1. Mrs. Banks is an 84-year-old woman who has recently been diagnosed with breast cancer. She also has severe cardiovascular disease that limits her choices of treatment. She has completed a series of radiation treatments that have left her exhausted and unable to participate in her usual activities. Her oncologist now recommends a cycle of chemotherapy treatments that her cardiologist believes would be fatal. Her family is urging her to do all that is recommended. The patient, who is in good spirits despite her diagnosis, decides against further medical treatment.
   a. How does Mrs. Banks' cognitive developmental stage impact her decision making related to her health care?
   b. Which of the psychosocial developmental theories helps explain her decision?
   c. Using your knowledge of her developmental stage, how can you help the family adjust to her choice?
2. Amanda Peters, 9 years old, was admitted to the unit yesterday with a new diagnosis of type I diabetes. Her mother has spent the night with her and is arranging the food on Amanda's breakfast tray when you enter the room to check her blood sugar and administer her insulin. Although the diabetes educator will be meeting with Amanda and her family, as part of her care today you want to begin her discharge teaching.
   a. According to Piaget's theory, how will Amanda's cognitive development direct your teaching?
   b. Using Erikson's theory as a basis, what psychosocial factors will you consider when discussing home care with Amanda and her family?
   c. Based on her developmental stage, how can Amanda's family support her active participation in care?
3. You have been assigned to care for Daniel Jackson, a 17-year-old male who was in an automobile accident several days ago and sustained a fractured pelvis. He has had a surgical repair and remains on bed rest. School is starting next month and he was scheduled to begin football practice next week. During bedside report he refuses to make eye contact with the nursing staff or respond to any questions to help direct his care.
   a. How will you incorporate your knowledge of adolescent development as you establish priorities for his care?
   b. Thinking about Erikson's theory, what psychosocial concerns do you anticipate that Daniel might experience during his hospitalization and recovery period?
   c. How will Daniel's cognitive development contribute to his future planning?

evolve *Answers to Clinical Application Questions can be found on the Evolve website.*

REVIEW QUESTIONS

Are You Ready to Test Your Nursing Knowledge?

1. The nurse is aware that preschoolers often display a developmental characteristic that makes them treat dolls or stuffed animals as if they have thoughts and feelings. This is an example of:
   1. Logical reasoning.
   2. Egocentrism.
   3. Concrete thinking.
   4. Animism.
2. An 18-month-old child is noted by the parents to be "angry" about any change in routine. This child's temperament is most likely to be described as:
   1. Slow to warm up.
   2. Difficult.
   3. Hyperactive.
   4. Easy.
3. Nine-year-old Brian has a difficult time making friends at school and being chosen to play on the team. He also has trouble completing his homework and, as a result, receives little positive feedback from his parents or teacher. According to Erikson's theory, failure at this stage of development results in:
   1. A sense of guilt.
   2. A poor sense of self.
   3. Feelings of inferiority.
   4. Mistrust.
4. The nurse teaches parents how to have their children learn impulse control and cooperative behaviors. This would be during which of Erickson's stages of development?
   1. Trust versus mistrust
   2. Initiative versus guilt
   3. Industry versus inferiority
   4. Autonomy versus sense of shame and doubt
5. When Ryan was 3 months old, he had a toy train; when his view of the train was blocked, he did not search for it. Now that he is 9 months old, he looks for it, reflecting the presence of:
   1. Object permanence.
   2. Sensorimotor play.
   3. Schemata.
   4. Magical thinking.
6. When preparing a 4-year-old child for a procedure, which method is developmentally most appropriate for the nurse to use?
   1. Allowing the child to watch another child undergoing the same procedure
   2. Showing the child pictures of what he or she will experience

3. Talking to the child in simple terms about what will happen
4. Preparing the child through play with a doll and toy medical equipment

7. A 35-year-old woman is speaking with you about her recent diagnosis of a chronic illness. She is concerned about her treatment options in relation to her ability to continue to care for her family. As she considers the options and alternatives, she incorporates information, her values, and emotions to decide which plan will be the best fit for her. She is using which form of cognitive development?
   1. Conventional reasoning
   2. Formal operations
   3. Integrity versus despair
   4. Postformal thought
8. You are caring for a recently retired man who appears withdrawn and says he is "bored with life." Applying the work of Havinghurst, you would help this individual find meaning in life by:
   1. Encouraging him to explore new roles.
   2. Encouraging relocation to a new city.
   3. Explaining the need to simplify life.
   4. Encouraging him to adopt a new pet.
9. Place the following stages of Freud's psychosexual development in the proper order by age progression.
   1. Oedipal
   2. Latency
   3. Oral
   4. Genital
   5. Anal
10. According to Piaget's cognitive theory, a 12-year-old child is most likely to engage in which of the following activities?
    1. Using building blocks to determine how houses are constructed
    2. Writing a story about a clown who wants to leave the circus
    3. Drawing pictures of a family using stick figures
    4. Writing an essay about patriotism
11. Allison, age 15 years, calls her best friend Laura and is crying. She has a date with John, someone she has been hoping to date for months, but now she has a pimple on her forehead. Laura firmly believes that John and everyone else will notice the blemish right away. This is an example of the:
    1. Imaginary audience.
    2. False-belief syndrome.
    3. Personal fable.
    4. Personal absorption syndrome.
12. Elizabeth, who is having unprotected sex with her boyfriend, comments to her friends, "Did you hear about Kathy? You know, she fools around so much; I heard she was pregnant. That would never happen to me!" This is an example of adolescent:
    1. Imaginary audience.
    2. False-belief syndrome.
    3. Personal fable.
    4. Sense of invulnerability.
13. Teaching an older adult how to use e-mail to communicate with a grandchild who lives in another state is an example of ____________, which aids cognitive performance by using new approaches.
    1. Cognitive development
    2. Activity theory
    3. Selective optimization with compensation
    4. Formal operations
14. Dave reports being happy and satisfied with his life. What do we know about Dave?
    1. He is in one of the later developmental periods, concerned with reviewing his life.
    2. He is atypical, since most people in any of the developmental stages report significant dissatisfaction with their lives.
    3. He is in one of the earlier developmental periods, concerned with establishing a career and satisfying long-term relationships.
    4. It is difficult to determine Dave's developmental stage since most people report overall satisfaction with their lives in all stages.
15. You are working in a clinic that provides services for homeless people. The current local regulations prohibit providing a service that you believe is needed by your patients. You adhere to the regulations but at the same time are involved in influencing authorities to change the regulation. This action represents which stage of moral development?
    1. Instrumental relativist orientation
    2. Social contract orientation
    3. Society-maintaining orientation
    4. Universal ethical principle orientation

Answers: **1.** 4; **2.** 2; **3.** 3; **4.** 2; **5.** 1; **6.** 4; **7.** 4; **8.** 1; **9.** 3, 5, 2, 1, 4; **10.** 2; **11.** 1; **12.** 4; **13.** 3; **14.** 4; **15.** 2.

REFERENCES

Baltes PB, Freund AM, Li S: The psychological science of human aging. In Johnson ML, editor: *The Cambridge handbook of age and aging*, New York, 2005, Cambridge University Press, p 47.

Berger KS: *The developing person: Through the life span*, ed 7, New York, 2007, Worth.

Carstensen LL, Isaacowitz DM, Charles ST: Taking time seriously: A theory of socioemotional selectivity, *Am Psychol* 54:165, 1999.

Crain WC: *Theories of development*, Upper Saddle River, NJ, 1985, Prentice Hall, http://faculty.plts.edu/gpence/html/kohlberg.htm. Accessed June 19, 2011.

Erikson E: *Childhood and society*, New York, 1963, Norton.

Gesell A: *Studies in child development*, New York, 1948, Harper.

Hockenberry MJ, Wilson D: *Wong's nursing care of infants and children*, ed 9, St Louis, 2011, Mosby.

Kohlberg L: *The philosophy of moral development: Moral stages and the idea of justice*, San Francisco, 1981, Harper & Row.

Reichstadt J, et al: Older adults' perspectives on successful aging: Qualitative interviews, *Am J Geriatr Psychiatry* 18(7):567, 2010.

Santrock JW: *Life span development*, ed 12, New York, 2008, McGraw-Hill.

Santrock JW: *A topical approach to life span development*, ed 5, New York, 2009, McGraw-Hill.

RESEARCH REFERENCES

Cully JA, et al: Predicting quality of life in veterans with heart failure: The role of disease severity, depression, and comorbid anxiety, *Behav Med* 36:70–76, 2010.

Hägglund L, et al: Depression among elderly people with and without heart failure, managed in a primary healthcare setting, *Scandinav J Caring Sci* 22:376–382, 2008.

Kessler RC, et al: Age differences in major depression: Results from the National Comorbidity Survey Replication (NCS-R), *Psychol Med* 40(2):225–237, 2010.

CHAPTER

12

Conception Through Adolescence

OBJECTIVES

- Discuss common physiological and psychosocial health concerns during the transition of the child from intrauterine to extrauterine life.
- Describe characteristics of physical growth of the unborn child and from birth to adolescence.
- Describe cognitive and psychosocial development from birth to adolescence.
- Explain the role of play in the development of a child.
- Discuss ways in which the nurse is able to help parents meet their children's developmental needs.

KEY TERMS

Adolescence, p. 151
Apgar score, p. 140
Attachment, p. 140
Embryo, p. 139
Embryonic stage, p. 139
Estrogen, p. 151
Fetal stage, p. 139
Fetus, p. 140
Fontanels, p. 141
Inborn errors of metabolism (IEMs), p. 142
Infancy, p. 143
Menarche, p. 152
Molding, p. 141
Neonatal period, p. 141
Placenta, p. 140
Preembryonic stage, p. 139
Preschool period, p. 147
Puberty, p. 151
School-age, p. 149
Sexually transmitted infection (STI), p. 151
Testosterone, p. 151
Toddlerhood, p. 146

evolve WEBSITE

http://evolve.elsevier.com/Potter/fundamentals/

- Review Questions
- Case Study with Questions
- Audio Glossary
- Interactive Learning Activities
- Key Term Flashcards
- Content Updates

STAGES OF GROWTH AND DEVELOPMENT

Human growth and development are continuous and complex processes that are typically divided into stages organized by age-groups such as from conception to adolescence. Although this chronological division is arbitrary, it is based on the timing and sequence of developmental tasks that the child must accomplish to progress to another stage. This chapter focuses on the various physical, psychosocial, and cognitive changes and health risks and health promotion concerns during the different stages of growth and development.

SELECTING A DEVELOPMENTAL FRAMEWORK FOR NURSING

Providing developmentally appropriate nursing care is easier when you base planning on a theoretical framework (see Chapter 11). An organized, systematic approach ensures that the plan of care assesses and meets the child's and family's needs. If you deliver nursing care only as a series of isolated actions, you will possibly overlook some of the child's developmental needs. A developmental approach encourages organized care directed at the child's current level of functioning to motivate self-direction and health promotion. For example, nurses encourage toddlers to feed themselves to advance their developing independence and thus promote their sense of autonomy. Another example involves a nurse understanding an adolescent's need to be independent and thus establishing a contract about the care plan and its implementation.

INTRAUTERINE LIFE

From the moment of conception until birth, human development proceeds at a predictive and rapid rate. During gestation or the prenatal period, the embryo grows from a single cell to a complex, physiological being. All major organ systems develop in utero, with some functioning before birth. Development proceeds in a cephalocaudal (head-to-toe) and proximal-distal (central-to-peripheral) pattern (Santrock, 2009).

Pregnancy that reaches full term is calculated to last an average of 38 to 40 weeks and is divided into three stages or trimesters. Beginning on the day of fertilization, the first 14 days are referred to as the preembryonic stage, followed by the embryonic stage that lasts from day 15 until the eighth week. These two stages are then followed by the fetal stage that lasts from the end of the eighth week until birth (Davidson et al., 2008). Gestation is commonly divided into equal phases of 3 months called trimesters.

The **placenta** begins development at the third week of the embryonic stage and produces essential hormones that help maintain the pregnancy. It functions as the fetal lungs, kidneys, gastrointestinal tract, and an endocrine organ. Because the placenta is extremely porous, noxious materials such as viruses, chemicals, and drugs also pass from mother to child. These agents are called teratogens and can cause abnormal development of structures in the embryo. The effect of teratogens on the **fetus** or unborn child depends on the developmental stage in which exposure takes place, individual genetic susceptibility, and the quantity of the exposure. The embryonic stage is the most vulnerable since all body organs are formed by the eighth week. Some maternal infections can cross the placental barrier and negatively influence the health of the mother, fetus, or both. It is important to educate women about avoidable sources of teratogens and help them make healthy lifestyle choices before and during pregnancy.

Health Promotion During Pregnancy

The diet of a woman both before and during pregnancy has a significant effect on fetal development. Women who do not consume adequate nutrients and calories during pregnancy may not be able to meet the fetus' nutritional requirements. An increase in weight does not always indicate an increase in nutrients. In addition, the pattern of weight gain is important for tissue growth in a mother and fetus. For women who are at normal weight for height, the recommended weight gain is 25 to 35 pounds over three trimesters (Davidson et al., 2008). As a nurse, you are in a key position to provide women with the education they need about nutrition before conception and throughout an expectant mother's pregnancy.

Pregnancy presents a developmental challenge that includes physiological, cognitive, and emotional states that are accompanied by stress and anxiety. The expectant woman will soon adopt a parenting role; and relationships within the family will change, whether or not there is a partner involved. Pregnancy can be a period of conflict or support; family dynamics impact fetal development. Parental reactions to pregnancy change throughout the gestational period, with most couples looking forward to the birth and addition of a new family member (Davidson et al., 2008). Listen carefully to concerns expressed by a mother and her partner and offer support through each trimester.

The age of the pregnant woman sometimes plays a role in the health of the fetus and the overall pregnancy. Fetuses of older mothers are at risk for chromosomal defects, and older women may have more difficulty in becoming pregnant (Santrock, 2009). Studies indicate that pregnant adolescents often seek out less prenatal care than women in their 20s and 30s and are at higher risk for complications of pregnancy and labor. Infants of teen mothers are at increased risk for prematurity; low birth weight; and exposure to alcohol, drugs, and tobacco in utero and early childhood (Davidson et al., 2008). Adolescents who have been able to participate in prenatal classes may have improved nutrition and healthier babies.

Fetal growth and hormonal changes during pregnancy often result in discomfort for the expectant mother. Common concerns expressed include problems such as nausea and vomiting, breast tenderness, urinary frequency, heartburn, constipation, ankle edema, and backache. Always anticipate these discomforts and provide self-care education throughout the pregnancy. Discussing the physiological causes of these discomforts and offering suggestions for safe treatment can be very helpful for expectant mothers and contribute to overall health during pregnancy (Davidson et al., 2008).

Some complementary and alternative therapies such as herbal supplements can be harmful during pregnancy. Your assessment should include questions about use of these substances when providing education during pregnancy (Davidson et al., 2008). You can promote maternal and fetal health by providing accurate and complete information about health behaviors that support positive outcomes for pregnancy and childbirth.

TRANSITION FROM INTRAUTERINE TO EXTRAUTERINE LIFE

The transition from intrauterine to extrauterine life requires profound physiological changes in the newborn and occurs during the first 24 hours of life. Assessment of the newborn during this period is essential to ensure that the transition is proceeding as expected. Gestational age and development, exposure to depressant drugs before or during labor, and the newborn's own behavioral style also influence the adjustment to the external environment.

Physical Changes

An immediate assessment of the newborn's condition to determine the physiological functioning of the major organ systems occurs at birth. The most widely used assessment tool is the **Apgar score.** Heart rate, respiratory effort, muscle tone, reflex irritability, and color are rated to determine overall status of the newborn. The Apgar assessment is generally conducted at 1 and 5 minutes after birth and is sometimes repeated until the newborn's condition stabilizes. The most extreme physiological change occurs when the newborn leaves the utero circulation and develops independent circulatory and respiratory functioning.

Nursing interventions at birth include maintaining an open airway, stabilizing and maintaining body temperature, and protecting the newborn from infection. The removal of nasopharyngeal and oropharyngeal secretions with suction or a bulb syringe ensures airway patency. Newborns are susceptible to heat loss and cold stress. Because hypothermia increases oxygen needs, it is essential to stabilize and maintain the newborn's body temperature. Healthy newborns may be placed directly on the mother's abdomen and covered in warm blankets or provided warmth via a radiant warmer. Preventing infection is a major concern in the care of the newborn, whose immune system is immature. Good handwashing technique is the most important factor in protecting the newborn from infection. You can help prevent infection by instructing parents and visitors to wash their hands before touching the infant.

Psychosocial Changes

After immediate physical evaluation and application of identification bracelets, the nurse promotes the parents' and newborn's need for close physical contact. Early parent-child interaction encourages parent-child **attachment.** Merely placing the family together does not promote closeness. Most healthy newborns are awake and alert for the first half-hour after birth. This is a good time for parent-child interaction to begin. Close body contact, often including breastfeeding, is a satisfying way for most families to start bonding. If immediate contact is not possible, incorporate it into the care plan as early as possible, which means bringing the newborn to an ill parent or bringing the parents to an ill or premature child. Attachment is a process that evolves over the infant's first 24 months of life, and many psychologists believe that a secure attachment is an important foundation for psychological development in later life (Santrock, 2009).

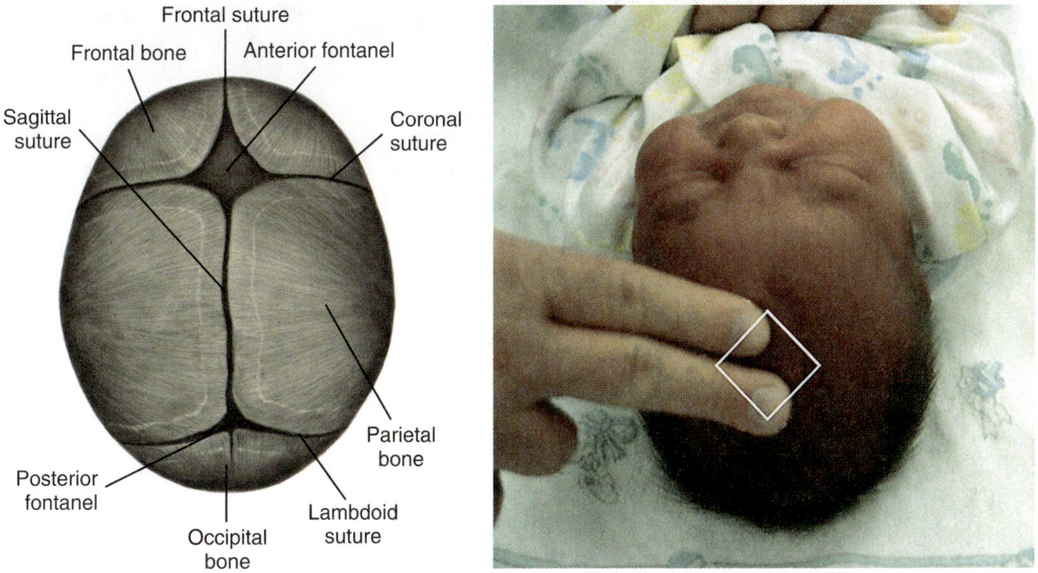

FIG. 12-1 Fontanels and suture lines. (From Hockenberry MJ, Wilson D: *Wong's nursing care of infants and children,* ed 9, St Louis, 2011, Mosby.)

NEWBORN

The **neonatal period** is the first 28 days of life. During this stage the newborn's physical functioning is mostly reflexive, and stabilization of major organ systems is the primary task of the body. Behavior greatly influences interaction among the newborn, the environment, and caregivers. For example, the average 2-week-old smiles spontaneously and is able to look at the mother's face. The impact of these reflexive behaviors is generally a surge of maternal feelings of love that prompt the mother to cuddle the baby. You apply knowledge of this stage of growth and development to promote newborn and parental health. For example, the newborn's cry is generally a reflexive response to an unmet need (such as hunger, fatigue, or discomfort). Thus you help parents identify ways to meet these needs by counseling them to feed their baby on demand rather than on a rigid schedule.

Physical Changes

You perform a comprehensive nursing assessment as soon as the newborn's physiological functioning is stable, generally within a few hours after birth. At this time the nurse measures height, weight, head and chest circumference, temperature, pulse, and respirations and observes general appearance, body functions, sensory capabilities, reflexes, and responsiveness. Following a comprehensive physical assessment, assess gestational age and interactions between infant and parent that indicate successful attachment (Hockenberry and Wilson, 2011).

The average newborn is 2700 to 4000 g (6 to 9 pounds), 48 to 53 cm (19 to 21 inches) in length, and has a head circumference of 33 to 35 cm (13 to 14 inches). Neonates lose up to 10% of birth weight in the first few days of life, primarily through fluid losses by respiration, urination, defecation, and low fluid intake. They usually regain birth weight by the second week of life; and a gradual pattern of increase in weight, height, and head circumference is evident. Accurate measurement as soon as possible after birth provides a baseline for future comparison (Hockenberry and Wilson, 2011).

Normal physical characteristics include the continued presence of lanugo on the skin of the back; cyanosis of the hands and feet for the first 24 hours; and a soft, protuberant abdomen. Skin color varies according to racial and genetic heritage and gradually changes during infancy. **Molding,** or overlapping of the soft skull bones, allows the fetal head to adjust to various diameters of the maternal pelvis and is a common occurrence with vaginal births. The bones readjust within a few days, producing a rounded appearance to the head. The sutures and **fontanels** are usually palpable at birth. Fig. 12-1 shows the diamond shape of the anterior fontanel and the triangular shape of the posterior fontanel between the unfused bones of the skull. The anterior fontanel usually closes at 12 to 18 months, whereas the posterior fontanel closes by the end of the second or third month.

Assess neurological function by observing the newborn's level of activity, alertness, irritability, and responsiveness to stimuli and the presence and strength of reflexes. Normal reflexes include blinking in response to bright lights, startling in response to sudden loud noises or movement, sucking, rooting, grasping, yawning, coughing, sneezing, palmar grasp, swallowing, plantar grasp, Babinski, and hiccoughing. Assessment of these reflexes is vital because the newborn depends largely on reflexes for survival and in response to its environment. Fig. 12-2 shows the tonic neck reflex in the newborn.

Normal behavioral characteristics of the newborn include periods of sucking, crying, sleeping, and activity. Movements are generally sporadic, but they are symmetrical and involve all four extremities. The relatively flexed fetal position of intrauterine life continues as the newborn attempts to maintain an enclosed, secure feeling. Newborns normally watch the caregiver's face; have a nonpurposeful reflexive smile; and respond to sensory stimuli, particularly the primary caregiver's face, voice, and touch.

In accordance with the recommendations of the American Academy of Pediatrics (AAP), position infants for sleep on their backs to decrease the risk of sudden infant death syndrome (SIDS) (Hockenberry and Wilson, 2011; Santrock, 2008). Newborns establish their individual sleep-activity cycle, and parents develop sensitivity to their baby's cues. Studies have found that parents position their infants at home in the same positions they observed in the hospital setting; thus nurses must demonstrate correct positioning on the back to reduce the incidence of SIDS (Davidson et al., 2008). Co-sleeping or bed sharing has also been reported to possibly be

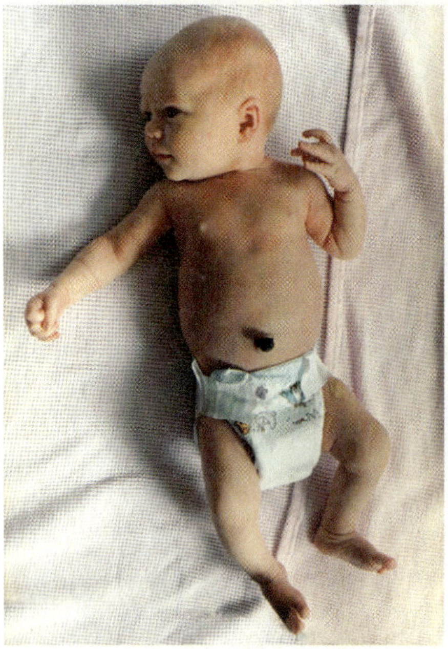

FIG. 12-2 Tonic neck reflex. Newborns assume this position while supine. (From Hockenberry MJ, Wilson D: *Wong's nursing care of infants and children,* ed 9, St Louis, 2011, Mosby.)

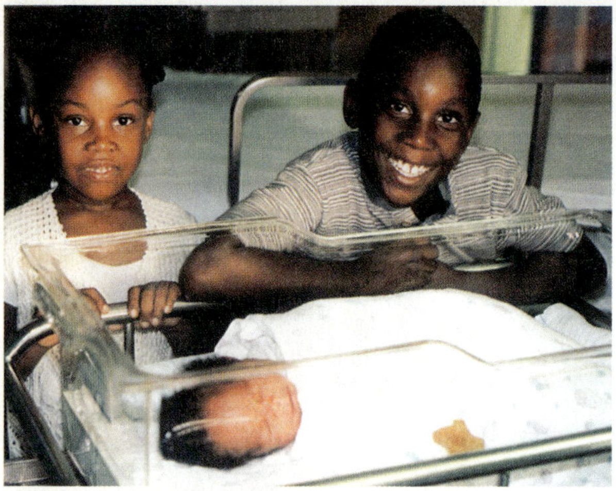

FIG. 12-3 Siblings should be involved in newborn care. (Courtesy Elaine Polan, RNC, BSN, MS.)

associated with an increased risk for SIDS (Hockenberry and Wilson, 2011; Santrock, 2008). Safeguards include proper positioning; removing stuffed animals, soft bedding, and pillows; and avoiding overheating the infant. Individuals should avoid smoking during pregnancy and around the infant because it places the infant at greater risk for SIDS (Hockenberry and Wilson, 2011).

Cognitive Changes

Early cognitive development begins with innate behavior, reflexes, and sensory functions. Newborns initiate reflex activities, learn behaviors, and learn their desires. At birth infants are able to focus on objects about 20 to 25 cm (8 to 10 inches) from their faces and perceive forms. A preference for the human face is apparent. Teach parents about the importance of providing sensory stimulation such as talking to their babies and holding them to see their faces. This allows infants to seek or take in stimuli, thereby enhancing learning and promoting cognitive development.

For newborns crying is a means of communication to provide cues to parents. Some babies cry because their diapers are wet or they are hungry or want to be held. Others cry just to make noise or because they need a change in position or activity. The crying frustrates the parents if they cannot see an apparent cause. With the nurse's help parents learn to recognize infants' cry patterns and take appropriate action when necessary.

Psychosocial Changes

During the first month of life most parents and newborns normally develop a strong bond that grows into a deep attachment. Interactions during routine care enhance or detract from the attachment process. Feeding, hygiene, and comfort measures consume much of infants' waking time. These interactive experiences provide a foundation for the formation of deep attachments. Early on older siblings need to have opportunity to be involved in the newborn's care. Family involvement helps support growth and development and promotes nurturing (Fig. 12-3).

If parents or children experience health complications after birth, this *may* compromise the attachment process. Infants' behavioral cues are sometimes weak or absent, and caregiving is possibly less mutually satisfying. Some tired or ill parents have difficulty interpreting and responding to their infants. Preterm infants and those born with congenital anomalies are often too weak to be responsive to parental cues and require special supportive nursing care. For example, infants born with heart defects tire easily during feedings. Nurses can support parental attachment by pointing out positive qualities and responses of the newborn and acknowledging how difficult the separation can be for parents and infant.

Health Promotion

Screening. Newborn screening tests are administered before babies leave the hospital to identify serious or life-threatening conditions before symptoms begin. Results of the screening tests are sent directly to the infant's pediatrician. If a screening test suggests a problem, the baby's physician usually follows up with further testing and may refer the infant to a specialist for treatment if needed. Blood tests help determine **inborn errors of metabolism (IEMs).** These are genetic disorders caused by the absence or deficiency of a substance, usually an enzyme, essential to cellular metabolism that results in abnormal protein, carbohydrate, or fat metabolism. Although IEMs are rare, they account for a significant proportion of health problems in children. Neonatal screening is done to detect phenylketonuria (PKU), hypothyroidism, galactosemia, and other diseases to allow appropriate treatment that prevents permanent mental retardation and other health problems.

The AAP recommends universal screening of newborn hearing before discharge since studies have indicated that the incidence of hearing loss is as high as 1 to 3 per 1000 normal newborns (Davidson et al., 2008). If health care providers detect the loss before 3 months of age and intervention is initiated by 6 months, children are able to achieve normal language development that matches their cognitive development through the age of 5 (Hockenberry and Wilson, 2011).

Car Seats. An essential component of discharge teaching is the use of a federally approved car seat for transporting the infant from the hospital or birthing center to home. Automobile injuries are a leading cause of death in children in the United States. Many of these deaths occur when the child is not properly restrained

TABLE 12-1 Gross- and Fine-Motor Development in Infancy

AGE	GROSS-MOTOR SKILL	FINE-MOTOR SKILL
Birth to 1 month	Complete head lag persists No ability to sit upright Inborn reflexes are predominant	Reflexive grasp
2 to 4 months	When prone, lifts head and chest and bears weight on forearms With support able to sit erect with good head control Can turn from side to back	Holds rattle for short periods Looks at and plays with fingers Able to bring objects from hand to mouth
4 to 6 months	Turns from abdomen to back at 5 months and then back to abdomen at 6 months Can support much of own weight when pulled to stand No head lag when pulled to sit	Grasps objects at will and can drop them to pick up another object Pulls feet to mouth to explore Can hold a baby bottle
6 to 8 months	Sits alone without support Bears full weight on feet and can hold on to furniture Can move from a sitting to kneeling position	Bangs objects together Pulls a string to obtain an object Transfers objects from hand to hand
8 to 10 months	Crawls or pulls entire body along floor using arms Pulls self to standing or sitting Creeps on hands and knees	Picks up small objects Uses pincer grasp well Shows hand preference
10 to 12 months	Stands alone Walks holding onto furniture Sits down from a standing position	Can place objects into containers Able to hold a crayon or pencil and make a mark on paper

Adapted from Hockenberry M, Wilson D: *Wong's nursing care of infants and children,* ed 8, St Louis, 2007, Mosby; Santrock JW: *Life-span development,* ed 12, New York, 2008, McGraw-Hill.

(Hockenberry and Wilson, 2011). Parents need to learn how to properly fit the restraint to the infant and how to properly install the car seat. All infants and toddlers should ride in a rear-facing car safety seat until they are 2 years of age or until they reach the highest weight or height allowed by the manufacturer or their car safety seat (American Academy of Pediatrics, 2011a). Placing an infant in a rear-facing restraint in the front seat of a vehicle is extremely dangerous in any vehicle with a passenger-side air bag. Nurses are responsible for providing education on the use of a car seat before discharge from the hospital.

Cribs and Sleep. Beginning June 28, 2011, new federal safety standards prohibit the manufacture or sale of drop-side rail cribs (American Academy of Pediatrics, 2011b). New cribs sold in the United States must meet these governmental standards for safety, but some older cribs were manufactured before the newer requirements were instituted. Unsafe cribs should be disassembled and thrown away (American Academy of Pediatrics, 2011b). Parents also need to inspect an older crib to make sure the slats are no more than 6 cm (2.4 inches) apart. The crib mattress should fit snugly, and crib toys or mobiles should be attached firmly with no hanging strings or straps. Instruct parents to remove mobiles as soon as the infant is able to reach them (Hockenberry and Wilson, 2011). Also consider using a portable play yard, as long as it is not a model that has been recalled.

INFANT

During **infancy,** the period from 1 month to 1 year of age, rapid physical growth and change occur. This is the only period distinguished by such dramatic physical changes and marked development. Psychosocial developmental advances are aided by the progression from reflexive to more purposeful behavior. Interaction between infants and the environment is greater and more meaningful for the infant. During this first year of life the nurse easily observes the adaptive potential of infants because changes in growth and development occur so rapidly.

Physical Changes

Steady and proportional growth of the infant is more important than absolute growth values. Charts of normal age- and gender-related growth measurements enable the nurse to compare growth with norms for a child's age. Measurements recorded over time are the best way to monitor growth and identify problems. Size increases rapidly during the first year of life; birth weight doubles in approximately 5 months and triples by 12 months. Height increases an average of 2.5 cm (1 inch) during each of the first 6 months and about 1.2 cm (½ inch) each month until 12 months (Hockenberry and Wilson, 2011).

Throughout the first year the infant's vision and hearing continue to develop. Some infants as young as 3½ months are able to link visual and auditory stimuli (Santrock, 2009). Patterns of body function also stabilize, as evidenced by predictable sleep, elimination, and feeding routines. Some reflexes that are present in the newborn such as blinking, yawning, and coughing remain throughout life; whereas others such as grasping, rooting, sucking, and the Moro or startle reflex disappear after several months.

Gross-motor skills involve large muscle activities and are usually closely monitored by parents who easily report recently achieved milestones. Newborns can only momentarily hold their heads up, but by 4 months most infants have no head lag. The same rapid development is evident as infants learn to sit, stand, and then walk. Fine-motor skills involve small body movements and are more difficult to achieve than gross-motor skills. Maturation of eye-and-hand coordination occurs over the first 2 years of life as infants move from being able to grasp a rattle briefly at 2 months to drawing an arc with a pencil by 24 months. Development proceeds at a variable pace for each individual but usually follows the same pattern and within the same time frame (Table 12-1).

Cognitive Changes

The complex brain development during the first year is demonstrated by the infant's changing behaviors. As he or she receives stimulation through the developing senses of vision, hearing, and touch, the developing brain interprets the stimuli. Thus the infant learns by experiencing and manipulating the environment. Developing motor skills and increasing mobility expand an infant's environment and, with developing visual and auditory skills, enhance cognitive development. For these reasons Piaget (1952) named his first stage of cognitive development, which extends until around the third birthday, the sensorimotor period. Today's researchers have many more methods available to study the cognitive development of infants, and they believe that infants are far more competent than Piaget was able to discern by observation alone (Santrock, 2009) (see Chapter 11).

Infants need opportunities to develop and use their senses. Nurses need to evaluate the appropriateness and adequacy of these opportunities. For example, ill or hospitalized infants sometimes lack the energy to interact with their environment, thereby slowing their cognitive development. Infants need to be stimulated according to their temperament, energy, and age. The nurse uses stimulation strategies that maximize the development of infants while conserving their energy and orientation. An example of this is a nurse talking to and encouraging an infant to suck on a pacifier while administering the infant's tube feeding.

Language. Speech is an important aspect of cognition that develops during the first year. Infants proceed from crying, cooing, and laughing to imitating sounds, comprehending the meaning of simple commands, and repeating words with knowledge of their meaning. By 1 year infants not only recognize their own names but are able to say three to five words and understand almost 100 words (Hockenberry and Wilson, 2011). The nurse promotes language development by encouraging parents to name objects on which their infant's attention is focused. The nurse also assesses the infant's language development to identify developmental delays or potential abnormalities.

Psychosocial Changes

Separation and Individuation. During their first year infants begin to differentiate themselves from others as separate beings capable of acting on their own. Initially, infants are unaware of the boundaries of self, but through repeated experiences with the environment they learn where the self ends and the external world begins. As they determine their physical boundaries, they begin to respond to others (Fig. 12-4).

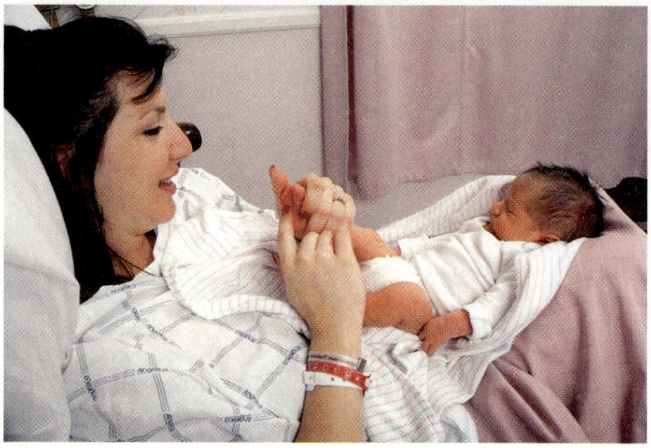

FIG. 12-4 Smiling at and talking to an infant encourage bonding. (From Murray SS, McKinney ES: *Foundations of maternal-newborn and women's health nursing,* ed 5, St Louis, 2010, Saunders.)

Two- and 3-month-old infants begin to smile responsively rather than reflexively. Similarly they recognize differences in people when their sensory and cognitive capabilities improve. By 8 months most infants are able to differentiate a stranger from a familiar person and respond differently to the two. Close attachment to their primary caregivers, most often parents, usually occurs by this age. Infants seek out these persons for support and comfort during times of stress. The ability to distinguish self from others allows infants to interact and socialize more within their environments. For example, by 9 months infants play simple social games such as patty-cake and peek-a-boo. More complex interactive games such as hide-and-seek involving objects are possible by age 1.

Erikson (1963) describes the psychosocial developmental crisis for the infant as trust versus mistrust. He explains that the quality of parent-infant interactions determines development of trust or mistrust. The infant learns to trust self, others, and the world through the relationship between the parent and child and the care the child receives (Hockenberry and Wilson, 2011). During infancy the child's temperament or behavioral style becomes apparent and influences the interactions between parent and child. You can help parents understand their child's temperament and determine appropriate childrearing practices (see Chapter 11).

Assess the availability and appropriateness of experiences contributing to psychosocial development. Hospitalized infants often have difficulty establishing physical boundaries because of repeated bodily intrusions and painful sensations. Limiting these negative experiences and providing pleasurable sensations are interventions that support early psychosocial development. Extended separations from parents complicate the attachment process and increase the number of caregivers with whom the infant must interact. Ideally the parents provide the majority of care during hospitalization. When parents are not present, either at home or in the hospital, make an attempt to limit the number of different caregivers who have contact with the infant and to follow the parents' directions for care. These interventions foster the infant's continuing development of trust.

Play. Play provides opportunities for development of cognitive, social, and motor skills. Much of infant play is exploratory as infants use their senses to observe and examine their own bodies and objects of interest in their surroundings. Adults facilitate infant learning by planning activities that promote the development of milestones and providing toys that are safe for the infant to explore with the mouth and manipulate with the hands such as rattles, wooden blocks, plastic stacking rings, squeezable stuffed animals, and busy boxes.

Health Risks

Injury Prevention. Injury from motor vehicle accidents, aspiration, suffocation, falls, or poisoning is a major cause of death in children 6 to 12 months old. An understanding of the major developmental accomplishments during this time period allows for injury-prevention planning. As the child achieves gains in motor development and becomes increasingly curious about the environment, constant watchfulness and supervision are critical for injury prevention.

Child Maltreatment. Child maltreatment includes intentional physical abuse or neglect, emotional abuse or neglect, and

BOX 12-1 WARNING SIGNS OF ABUSE

- Physical evidence of abuse or neglect, including previous injuries
- Conflicting stories about the accident/trauma
- Injury blamed on sibling or another party
- Injury inconsistent with the history such as a concussion and a broken arm from falling off the bed
- History inconsistent with the child's developmental age such as a 6-month-old burned by turning on the hot water
- An initial complaint not associated with the signs and symptoms present (e.g., bringing the child to the clinic for a cold when there is evidence of physical trauma)
- Inappropriate response of the child, especially an older child, such as not wanting to be touched, looking at caregiver before answering any questions
- Previous reports of abuse in the family
- Frequent emergency department or clinic visits

Adapted from Hockenberry MJ, Wilson D: *Wong's nursing care of infants and children*, ed 8, St Louis, 2007, Mosby.

sexual abuse (Hockenberry and Wilson, 2011). More children suffer from neglect than any other type of maltreatment. Children of any age can suffer from maltreatment, but the youngest are the most vulnerable. In addition, many children suffer from more than one type of maltreatment. No one profile fits a victim of maltreatment, and the signs and symptoms vary (Box 12-1).

A combination of signs and symptoms or a pattern of injury should arouse suspicion. It is important for the health care provider to be aware of certain disease processes and cultural practices. Lack of awareness of normal variants such as Mongolian spots causes the health care provider to assume that there is abuse. Children who are hospitalized for maltreatment have the same developmental needs as other children their age, and the nurse needs to support the child's relationship with the parents (Hockenberry and Wilson, 2011).

Health Promotion

Nutrition. The quality and quantity of nutrition profoundly influences the infant's growth and development. Many women have already selected a feeding method well before the infant's birth, yet others will have questions for the nurse later in the pregnancy. Nurses are in a unique position to help parents select and provide a nutritionally adequate diet for their infant. Understand that factors such as support, culture, role demands, and previous experiences influence feeding methods (Davidson et al., 2008).

Breastfeeding is recommended for infant nutrition because breast milk contains the essential nutrients of protein, fats, carbohydrates, and immunoglobulins that bolster the ability to resist infection. Both the AAP and the U.S. Department of Health and Human Services recommend human milk for the first year of life (Hockenberry and Wilson, 2011). However, if breastfeeding is not possible or if the parent does not desire it, an acceptable alternative is iron-fortified commercially prepared formula. Recent advances in the preparation of infant formula include the addition of nucleotides and long-chain fatty acids, which augment immune function and increase brain development. The use of whole cow's milk, 2% cow's milk, or alternate milk products before the age of 12 months is not recommended. The composition of whole cow's milk can cause intestinal bleeding, anemia, and increased incidence of allergies (Hockenberry and Wilson, 2011).

The average 1-month-old infant takes approximately 18 to 21 ounces of breast milk or formula per day. This amount increases slightly during the first 6 months and decreases after introducing solid foods. The amount of formula per feeding and the number of feedings vary among infants. The addition of solid foods is not recommended before the age of 6 months because the gastrointestinal tract is not sufficiently mature to handle these complex nutrients and infants are exposed to food antigens that produce food protein allergies. Developmentally, infants are not ready for solid food before 6 months. The extrusion (protrusion) reflex causes food to be pushed out of the mouth. The introduction of cereals, fruits, vegetables, and meats during the second 6 months of life provides iron and additional sources of vitamins. This becomes especially important when children change from breast milk or formula to whole cow's milk after the first birthday. Solid foods should be offered one new food at a time. This allows for identification if a food causes an allergic reaction. The use of fruit juices and nonnutritive drinks such as fruit-flavored drinks or soda should be avoided since these do not provide sufficient and appropriate calories during this period (Hockenberry and Wilson, 2011). Infants also tolerate well-cooked table foods by 1 year. The amount and frequency of feedings vary among infants; thus be sure to discuss differing feeding patterns with parents.

Supplementation. The need for dietary vitamin and mineral supplements depends on the infant's diet. Full-term infants are born with some iron stores. The breastfed infant absorbs adequate iron from breast milk during the first 4 to 6 months of life. After 6 months iron-fortified cereal is generally an adequate supplemental source. Because iron in formula is less readily absorbed than that in breast milk, formula-fed infants need to receive iron-fortified formula throughout the first year.

Adequate concentrations of fluoride to protect against dental caries are not available in human milk; therefore fluoridated water or supplemental fluoride is generally recommended. A recent concern is the use of complementary and alternative medical therapies in children that may or may not be safe. Inquire about the use of such products to help the parent determine whether or not the product is truly safe for the child (Hockenberry and Wilson, 2011).

Immunizations. The widespread use of immunizations has resulted in the dramatic decline of infectious diseases over the past 50 years and therefore is a most important factor in health promotion during childhood. Although most immunizations can be given to persons of any age, it is recommended that the administration of the primary series begin soon after birth and be completed during early childhood. Vaccines are among the safest and most reliable drugs used. Minor side effects sometimes occur; however, serious reactions are rare. Parents need instructions regarding the importance of immunizations and common side effects such as low-grade fever and local tenderness. The recommended schedule for immunizations changes as new vaccines are developed and advances are made in the field of immunology. Stay informed of the current policies and direct parents to the primary caregiver for their child's schedule. The AAP maintains the most current schedule on their Internet website, http://www.aap.org. Research over the past three decades has clearly indicated that infants experience pain with invasive procedures (e.g., injections) and that nurses need to be aware of measures to reduce or eliminate pain with any health care procedure (see Chapter 31).

Sleep. Sleep patterns vary among infants, with many having their days and nights reversed until 3 to 4 months of age. Thus it is common for infants to sleep during the day. By 6 months most infants are nocturnal and sleep between 9 and 11 hours at night.

Total daily sleep averages 15 hours. Most infants take one or two naps a day by the end of the first year. Many parents have concerns regarding their infant's sleep patterns, especially if there is difficulty such as sleep refusal or frequent waking during the night. Carefully assesses the individual problem before suggesting interventions to address their concern.

TODDLER

Toddlerhood ranges from the time children begin to walk independently until they walk and run with ease, which is from 12 to 36 months. The toddler has increasing independence bolstered by greater physical mobility and cognitive abilities. Toddlers are increasingly aware of their abilities to control and are pleased with successful efforts with this new skill. This success leads them to repeated attempts to control their environments. Unsuccessful attempts at control result in negative behavior and temper tantrums. These behaviors are most common when parents stop the initial independent action. Parents cite these as the most problematic behaviors during the toddler years and at times express frustration with trying to set consistent and firm limits while simultaneously encouraging independence. Nurses and parents can deal with the negativism by limiting the opportunities for a "no" answer. For example, the nurse does not ask the toddler, "Do you want to take your medicine now?" Instead, he or she tells the child that it is time to take medicine and offers a choice of water or juice to drink with it.

Physical Changes

The average toddler grows 6.2 cm (2.5 inches) in height and gains approximately 5 to 7 pounds each year (Santrock, 2009). The rapid development of motor skills allows the child to participate in self-care activities such as feeding, dressing, and toileting. In the beginning the toddler walks in an upright position with a broad stance and gait, protuberant abdomen, and arms out to the sides for balance. Soon the child begins to navigate stairs, using a rail or the wall to maintain balance while progressing upward, placing both feet on the same step before continuing. Success provides courage to attempt the upright mode for descending the stairs in the same manner. Locomotion skills soon include running, jumping, standing on one foot for several seconds, and kicking a ball. Most toddlers ride tricycles, climb ladders, and run well by their third birthday.

Fine-motor capabilities move from scribbling spontaneously to drawing circles and crosses accurately. By 3 years the child draws simple stick people and is usually able to stack a tower of small blocks. Children now hold crayons with their fingers rather than with their fists and can imitate vertical and horizontal strokes. They are able to manage feeding themselves with a spoon without rotating it and can drink well from a cup without spilling. Toddlers can turn pages of a book one at a time and can easily turn doorknobs (Hockenberry and Wilson, 2011).

Cognitive Changes

Toddlers increase their ability to remember events and begin to put thoughts into words at about 2 years of age. They recognize that they are separate beings from their mothers, but they are unable to assume the view of another. Toddlers reason based on their own experience of an event. They use symbols to represent objects, places, and persons. Children demonstrate this function as they imitate the behavior of another that they viewed earlier (e.g., pretend to shave like daddy), pretend that one object is another (e.g., use a finger as a gun), and use language to stand for absent objects (e.g., request bottle).

Language. The 18-month-old child uses approximately 10 words. The 24-month-old child has a vocabulary of up to 300 words and is generally able to speak in two-word sentences, although the ability to understand speech is much greater than the number of words acquired (Hockenberry and Wilson, 2011). "Who's that?" and "What's that?" are typical questions children ask during this period. Verbal expressions such as "me do it" and "that's mine" demonstrate the 2-year-old child's use of pronouns and desire for independence and control. By 36 months the child can use simple sentences, follow some grammatical rules, and learn to use five or six new words each day. Language development may seem to occur in early childhood, but it actually develops further into the later school years and adolescence (Santrock, 2009). Parents can facilitate language development best by talking to their children. Reading to children helps expand their vocabulary, knowledge, and imagination. Television is never used instead of parent-child interaction.

Psychosocial Changes

According to Erikson (1963) a sense of autonomy emerges during toddlerhood. Children strive for independence by using their developing muscles to do everything for themselves and become the master of their bodily functions. Their strong wills are frequently exhibited in negative behavior when caregivers attempt to direct their actions. Temper tantrums result when parental restrictions frustrate toddlers. Parents need to provide toddlers with graded independence, allowing them to do things that do not result in harm to themselves or others. For example, young toddlers who want to learn to hold their own cups often benefit from two-handled cups with spouts and plastic bibs with pockets to collect the milk that spills during the learning process.

Play. Socially toddlers remain strongly attached to their parents and fear separation from them. In their presence they feel safe, and their curiosity is evident in their exploration of the environment. The child continues to engage in solitary play during toddlerhood but also begins to participate in parallel play, which is playing *beside* rather than *with* another child. Play expands the child's cognitive and psychosocial development. It is always important to consider if toys support development of the child, along with the safety of the toy.

Health Risks

The newly developed locomotion abilities and insatiable curiosity of toddlers make them at risk for injury. Toddlers need close supervision at all times and particularly when in environments that are not childproofed (Fig. 12-5).

Poisonings occur frequently because children near 2 years of age are interested in placing any object or substance in their mouths to learn about it. The prudent parent removes or locks up all possible poisons, including plants, cleaning materials, and medications. These parental actions create a safer environment for exploratory behavior. Lead poisoning continues to be a serious health hazard in the United States, and children under the age of 6 years are most vulnerable (Hockenberry and Wilson, 2011).

Toddlers' lack of awareness regarding the danger of water and their newly developed walking skills make drowning a major cause of accidental death in this age-group. Limit setting is extremely important for toddlers' safety. Motor vehicle accidents account for half of all accidental deaths in children between the ages of 1 and 4 years. Some of these deaths are the result of unrestrained

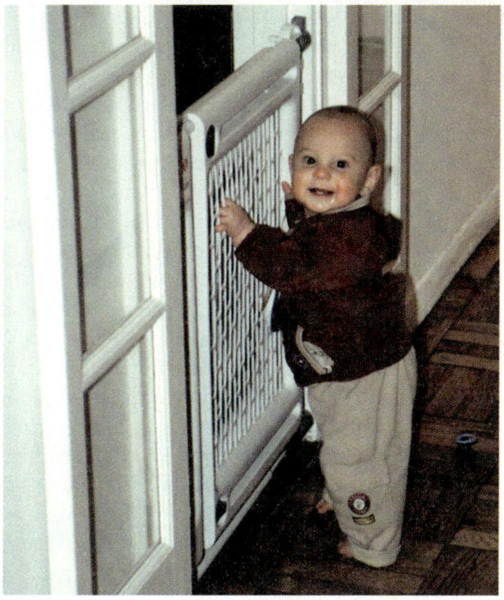

FIG. 12-5 Safety precautions should be provided for toddlers. (Courtesy Elaine Polan, RNC, BSN, MS.)

children, and some are attributed to injuries within the car resulting from not using car seat safety guidelines (Hockenberry and Wilson, 2011). Injury prevention is best accomplished by associating various injuries with the attainment of developmental milestones.

Toddlers who become ill and require hospitalization are most stressed by the separation from their parents. Nurses encourage parents to stay with their child as much as possible and actively participate in providing care. Creating an environment that supports parents helps greatly in gaining the cooperation of the toddler. Establishing a trusting relationship with the parents often results in toddler acceptance of treatment.

Health Promotion

Nutrition. Childhood obesity and the associated chronic diseases that result are sources of concern for all health care providers. Children establish lifetime eating habits in early childhood, and there is increased emphasis on food choices. They increasingly meet nutritional needs by eating solid foods. The healthy toddler requires a balanced daily intake of bread and grains, vegetables, fruit, dairy products, and proteins. Because the consumption of more than a quart of milk per day usually decreases the child's appetite for these essential solid foods and results in inadequate iron intake, advise parents to limit milk intake to 2 to 3 cups per day (Hockenberry and Wilson, 2011). Children are usually not offered low-fat or skim milk until age 2 because they need the fat for satisfactory physical and intellectual growth.

Mealtime has psychosocial and physical significance. If the parents struggle to control toddlers' dietary intake, problem behavior and conflicts can result. Toddlers often develop "food jags," or the desire to eat one food repeatedly. Rather than becoming disturbed by this behavior, encourage parents to offer a variety of nutritious foods at meals and to provide only nutritious snacks between meals. Serving finger foods to toddlers allows them to eat by themselves and to satisfy their need for independence and control. Small, reasonable servings allow toddlers to eat all of their meals.

Toilet Training. Increased locomotion skills, the ability to undress, and development of sphincter control allow toilet training if the toddler has developed the necessary language and cognitive abilities. Parents often consult nurses for an assessment of readiness for toilet training. Recognizing the urge to urinate and or defecate is crucial in determining the child's mental readiness. The toddler must also be motivated to hold on to please the parent rather than letting go to please the self to successfully accomplish toilet training (Hockenberry and Wilson, 2011). The nurse needs to remind parents that patience, consistency, and a nonjudgmental attitude, in addition to the child's readiness, are essential to successful toilet training.

PRESCHOOLERS

The **preschool period** refers to the years between ages 3 and 5. Children refine the mastery of their bodies and eagerly await the beginning of formal education. Many people consider these the most intriguing years of parenting because children are less negative, more accurately share their thoughts, and more effectively interact and communicate. Physical development occurs at a slower pace than cognitive and psychosocial development.

Physical Changes

Several aspects of physical development continue to stabilize in the preschool years. Children gain about 5 pounds per year; the average weight at 3 years is 32 pounds; at 4 years, 37 pounds; and at 5 years about 41 pounds. Preschoolers grow 6.2 to 7.5 cm (2½ to 3 inches) per year, double their birth length around 4 years, and stand an average of 107 cm (43 inches) tall by their fifth birthday. The elongation of the legs results in more slender-appearing children. Little difference exists between the sexes, although boys are slightly larger with more muscle and less fatty tissue. Most children are completely toilet trained by the preschool years (Hockenberry and Wilson, 2011).

Large and fine muscle coordination improves. Preschoolers run well, walk up and down steps with ease, and learn to hop. By 5 years they usually skip on alternate feet, jump rope, and begin to skate and swim. Improving fine-motor skills allows intricate manipulations. They learn to copy crosses and squares. Triangles and diamonds are usually mastered between ages 5 and 6. Scribbling and drawing help to develop fine muscle skills and the eye-hand coordination needed for the printing of letters and numbers.

Children need opportunities to learn and practice new physical skills. Nursing care of healthy and ill children includes an assessment of the availability of these opportunities. Although children with acute illnesses benefit from rest and exclusion from usual daily activities, children who have chronic conditions or who have been hospitalized for long periods need ongoing exposure to developmental opportunities. The parents and nurse weave these opportunities into the children's daily experiences, depending on their abilities, needs, and energy level.

Cognitive Changes

Maturation of the brain continues, with the most rapid growth occurring in the frontal lobe areas, where planning and organizing new activities and maintaining attention to tasks are paramount. Scientific advances in the use of brain-scanning techniques have demonstrated that patterns within the brain change significantly between the ages of 3 to 15 years (Santrock, 2009).

Preschoolers demonstrate their ability to think more complexly by classifying objects according to size or color and by questioning.

Children have increased social interaction, as is illustrated by the 5-year-old child who offers a bandage to a child with a cut finger. Children become aware of cause-and-effect relationships, as illustrated by the statement, "The sun sets because people want to go to bed." Early causal thinking is also evident in preschoolers. For example, if two events are related in time or space, children link them in a causal fashion. For example, the hospitalized child reasons, "I cried last night, and that's why the nurse gave me the shot." As children near age 5, they begin to use or learn to use rules to understand causation. They then begin to reason from the general to the particular. This forms the basis for more formal logical thought. The child now reasons, "I get a shot twice a day, and that's why I got one last night." Children in this stage also believe that inanimate objects have lifelike qualities and are capable of action, as seen through comments such as, "Trees cry when their branches get broken."

Preschoolers' knowledge of the world remains closely linked to concrete (perceived by the senses) experiences. Even their rich fantasy life is grounded in their perception of reality. The mixing of the two aspects often leads to many childhood fears, and adults sometimes misinterpret it as lying when children are actually presenting reality from their perspective. Preschoolers believe that, if a rule is broken, punishment results immediately. During these years they believe that a punishment is automatically connected to an act and do not yet realize that it is socially mediated (Santrock, 2008).

The greatest fear of this age-group appears to be that of bodily harm; this is evident in children's fear of the dark, animals, thunderstorms, and medical personnel. This fear often interferes with their willingness to allow nursing interventions such as measurement of vital signs. Preschoolers cooperate if they are allowed to help the nurse measure the blood pressure of a parent or to manipulate the nurse's equipment.

Language. Preschoolers' vocabularies continue to increase rapidly; and by the age of 6 children have 8000 to 14,000 words that they use to define familiar objects, identify colors, and express their desires and frustrations (Santrock, 2008). Language is more social, and questions expand to "Why?" and "How come?" in the quest for information. Phonetically similar words such as *die* and *dye* or *wood* and *would* cause confusion in preschool children. Avoid such words when preparing them for procedures and assess comprehension of explanations.

Psychosocial Changes

The world of preschoolers expands beyond the family into the neighborhood where children meet other children and adults. Their curiosity and developing initiative lead to actively exploring the environment, developing new skills, and making new friends. Preschoolers have a surplus of energy that permits them to plan and attempt many activities that are beyond their capabilities such as pouring milk from a gallon container into their cereal bowls. Guilt arises within children when they overstep the limits of their abilities and think that they have not behaved correctly. Children who in anger wished that their sibling were dead experience guilt if that sibling becomes ill. Children need to learn that "wishing" for something to happen does not make it occur. Erikson (1963) recommends that parents help their children strike a healthy balance between initiative and guilt by allowing them to do things on their own while setting firm limits and providing guidance.

Sources of stress for preschoolers can include changes in caregiving arrangements, starting school, the birth of a sibling, parental marital distress, relocation to a new home, or an illness. During these times of stress preschoolers sometimes revert to bed wetting or thumb sucking and want the parents to feed, dress, and hold them. These dependent behaviors are often confusing and embarrassing to parents. They benefit from the nurse's reassurance that they are the child's normal coping behaviors. Provide experiences that these children are able to master. Such successes help them return to their prior level of independent functioning. As language skills develop, encourage children to talk about their feelings. Play is also an excellent way for preschoolers to vent frustration or anger and is a socially acceptable way to deal with stress.

Play. The play of preschool children becomes more social after the third birthday as it shifts from parallel to associative play. Children playing together engage in similar if not identical activity; however, there is no division of labor or rigid organization or rules. Most 3-year-old children are able to play with one other child in a cooperative manner in which they make something or play designated roles such as mother and baby. By age 4 children play in groups of two or three, and by 5 years the group has a temporary leader for each activity.

Pretend play allows children to learn to understand others' points of view, develop skills in solving social problems, and become more creative. Some children have imaginary playmates. These playmates serve many purposes. They are friends when the child is lonely, they accomplish what the child is still attempting, and they experience what the child wants to forget or remember. Imaginary playmates are a sign of health and allow the child to distinguish between reality and fantasy.

Television, videos, electronic games, and computer programs also help support development and the learning of basic skills. However, these should be only one part of the child's total play activities. The AAP (2011c) advises no more than 1 to 2 hours per day of educational, nonviolent TV programs, which should be supervised by parents or other responsible adults in the home. Limiting TV viewing will provide more time for children to read, engage in physical activity, and socialize with others (Hockenberry and Wilson, 2011).

Health Risks

As fine- and gross-motor skills develop and the child becomes more coordinated with better balance, falls become much less of a problem. Guidelines for injury prevention in the toddler also apply to the preschooler. Children need to learn about safety in the home, and parents need to continue close supervision of activities. Children at this age are great imitators; thus parental example is important. For instance, parental use of a helmet while bicycling sets an appropriate example for the preschooler.

Health Promotion

Little research has explored preschoolers' perceptions of their own health. Parental beliefs about health, children's bodily sensations, and their ability to perform usual daily activities help children develop attitudes about their health. Preschoolers are usually quite independent in washing, dressing, and feeding. Alterations in this independence influence their feelings about their own health.

Nutrition. Nutrition requirements for the preschooler vary little from those of the toddler. The average daily intake is 1800 calories. Parents often worry about the amount of food their child is consuming, and this is a relevant concern because of the problem of childhood obesity. However, the quality of the food is more important than quantity in most situations. Preschoolers consume about half of average adult portion sizes. Finicky eating habits are characteristic of the 4-year-old; however, the 5-year-old is more interested in trying new foods.

Sleep. Preschoolers average 12 hours of sleep a night and take infrequent naps. Sleep disturbances are common during these years. Disturbances range from trouble getting to sleep to nightmares to prolonging bedtime with extensive rituals. Frequently children have had an overabundance of activity and stimulation. Helping them to slow down before bedtime usually results in better sleeping habits.

Vision. Vision screening usually begins in the preschool years and needs to occur at regular intervals. One of the most important tests is to determine the presence of nonbinocular vision or strabismus. Early detection and treatment of strabismus are essential by ages 4 to 6 to prevent amblyopia, the resulting blindness from disuse (Hockenberry and Wilson, 2011).

SCHOOL-AGE CHILDREN AND ADOLESCENTS

The developmental changes between ages 6 and 18 are diverse and span all areas of growth and development. Children develop, expand, refine, and synchronize physical, psychosocial, cognitive, and moral skills so the individual is able to become an accepted and productive member of society. The environment in which the individual develops skills also expands and diversifies. Instead of the boundaries of family and close friends, the environment now includes the school, community, and church. With age-specific assessment, you need to review the appropriate developmental expectations for each age-group. You can promote health by helping children and adolescents achieve a necessary developmental balance.

SCHOOL-AGE CHILDREN

During these "middle years" of childhood, the foundation for adult roles in work, recreation, and social interaction is laid. In industrialized countries this school-age period begins when the child starts elementary school around the age of 6 years. Puberty, around 12 years of age, signals the end of middle childhood. Children make great developmental strides during these years as they develop competencies in physical, cognitive, and psychosocial skills.

The school or educational experience expands the child's world and is a transition from a life of relatively free play to one of structured play, learning, and work. The school and home influence growth and development, requiring adjustment by the parents and child. The child learns to cope with rules and expectations presented by the school and peers. Parents have to learn to allow their child to make decisions, accept responsibility, and learn from the experiences of life.

Physical Changes

The rate of growth during these early school years is slow and consistent, a relative calm before the growth spurt of adolescence. The school-age child appears slimmer than the preschooler as a result of changes in fat distribution and thickness (Hockenberry and Wilson, 2011). The average increase in height is 5 cm (2 inches) per year, and weight increases by 4 to 7 pounds per year. Many children double their weight during these middle childhood years, and most girls exceed boys in both height and weight by the end of the school years (Hockenberry and Wilson, 2011).

School-age children become more graceful during the school years because their large muscle coordination improves and their strength doubles. Most children practice the basic gross-motor skills of running, jumping, balancing, throwing, and catching during play, resulting in refinement of neuromuscular function and skills. Individual differences in the rate of mastering skills and ultimate skill achievement become apparent during their participation in many activities and games. Fine-motor skills improve; and, as children gain control over fingers and wrists, they become proficient in a wide range of activities.

Most 6-year-old children are able to hold a pencil adeptly and print letters and words; by age 12 the child is able to make detailed drawings and write sentences in script. Painting, drawing, playing computer games, and modeling allow children to practice and improve newly refined skills. The improved fine-motor capabilities of youngsters in middle childhood allow them to become very independent in bathing, dressing, and taking care of other personal needs. They develop strong personal preferences in the way these needs are met. Illness and hospitalization threaten children's control in these areas. Therefore it is important to allow them to participate in care and maintain as much independence as possible. Children whose care demands restriction of fluids cannot be allowed to decide the amount of fluids they will drink in 24 hours, but they can help decide the type of fluids and help keep a record of their intake.

Assessment of neurological development is often based on fine-motor coordination. Fine-motor coordination is critical to success in the typical American school, where children have to hold pencils and crayons and use scissors and rulers. The opportunity to practice these skills through schoolwork and play is essential to learning coordinated, complex behaviors.

As skeletal growth progresses, body appearance and posture change. Earlier the child's posture was stoop shouldered, with slight lordosis and a prominent abdomen. The posture of a school-age child is more erect. It is essential to evaluate children, especially girls after the age of 12 years, for scoliosis, the lateral curvature of the spine.

Eye shape alters because of skeletal growth. This improves visual acuity, and normal adult 20/20 vision is achievable. Screening for vision and hearing problems is easier, and results are more reliable because school-age children more fully understand and cooperate with the test directions. The school nurse typically assesses the growth, visual, and auditory status of school-age children and refers those with possible deviations to a health care provider such as their family practitioner or pediatrician.

Cognitive Changes

Cognitive changes provide the school-age child with the ability to think in a logical manner about the here and now and to understand the relationship between things and ideas. They are now able to use their developed thinking abilities to experience events without having to act them out (Hockenberry and Wilson, 2011). Their thoughts are no longer dominated by their perceptions; thus their ability to understand the world greatly expands.

School-age children have the ability to concentrate on more than one aspect of a situation. They begin to understand that others do not always see things as they do and even begin to understand another viewpoint. They now have the ability to recognize that the amount or quantity of a substance remains the same even when its shape or appearance changes. For instance, two balls of clay of equal size remain the same amount of clay even when one is flattened and the other remains in the shape of a ball.

The young child is able to separate objects into groups according to shape or color, whereas the school-age child understands that the same element can exist in two classes at the same time. By 7 or 8 years these children develop the ability to place objects in order according to their increasing or decreasing size (Hockenberry and

Wilson, 2011; Santrock, 2009). School-age children frequently have collections such as baseball cards or stuffed animals that demonstrate this new cognitive skill.

Language Development. Language growth is so rapid during middle childhood that it is no longer possible to match age with language achievements. Children improve their use of language and expand their structural knowledge. They become more aware of the rules of syntax, the rules for linking words into phrases and sentences. They also identify generalizations and exceptions to rules. They accept language as a means for representing the world in a subjective manner and realize that words have arbitrary rather than absolute meanings. Children begin to think about language, which enables them to appreciate jokes and riddles. They are not as likely to use a literal interpretation of a word; rather they reason about its meaning within a context (Hockenberry and Wilson, 2011).

Psychosocial Changes

Erikson (1963) identifies the developmental task for school-age children as industry versus inferiority. During this time children strive to acquire competence and skills necessary for them to function as adults. School-age children who are positively recognized for success feel a sense of worth. Those faced with failure often feel a sense of mediocrity or unworthiness, which sometimes results in withdrawal from school and peers.

School-age children begin to define themselves on the basis of their internal characteristics more than external characteristics. They begin to define their self-concept and develop self-esteem, an overall self-evaluation. Interaction with peers allows them to define their own accomplishments in relation to others as they work to develop a positive self-image (Santrock, 2008).

Peer Relationships. Group and personal achievements become important to the school-age child. Success is important in physical and cognitive activities. Play involves peers and the pursuit of group goals. Although solitary activities are not eliminated, group play overshadows them. Learning to contribute, collaborate, and work cooperatively toward a common goal becomes a measure of success (Fig. 12-6).

The school-age child prefers same-sex peers to opposite-sex peers. In general, girls and boys view the opposite sex negatively.

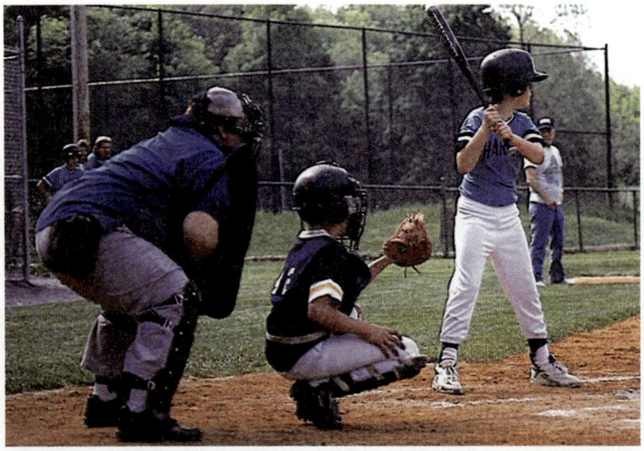

FIG. 12-6 School-age children gain a sense of achievement working and playing with peers. (From Hockenberry MJ, Wilson D: *Wong's nursing care of infants and children,* ed 9, St Louis, 2011, Mosby.)

Peer influence becomes quite diverse during this stage of development. Clubs and peer groups become prominent. School-age children often develop "best friends" with whom they share secrets and with whom they look forward to interacting on a daily basis. Group identity increases as the school-age child approaches adolescence.

Sexual Identity. Freud described middle childhood as the latency period because he believed that children of this period had little interest in their sexuality. Today many researchers believe that school-age children have a great deal of curiosity about their sexuality. Some experiment, but this play is usually transitory. Children's curiosity about adult magazines or meanings of sexually explicit words is also an example of their sexual interest. This is the time for children to have exposure to sex education, including sexual maturation, reproduction, and relationships (Hockenberry and Wilson, 2011).

Stress. Today's children experience more stress than children in earlier generations. Stress comes from parental expectations; peer expectations; the school environment; or violence in the family, school, or community. Some school-age children care for themselves before or after school without adult supervision. Latchkey children sometimes feel increased stress and are at greater risk for injury and unsafe behaviors (Hockenberry and Wilson, 2011). The nurse helps the child cope with stress by helping the parents and child to identify potential stressors and designing interventions to minimize stress and the child's stress response. Deep-breathing techniques, positive imagery, and progressive relaxation of muscle groups are interventions that most children can learn (see Chapter 32). Include the parent, child, and teacher in the intervention for maximal success.

Health Risks

Accidents and injuries are a major health problem affecting school-age children. They now have more exposure to various environments and less supervision, but their developed cognitive and motor skills make them less likely to suffer from unintentional injury. Some school-age children are risk takers and attempt activities that are beyond their abilities (Hockenberry and Wilson, 2007). Motor vehicle injuries as a passenger or pedestrian and bicycle injuries are among the most common in this age-group.

Infections account for the majority of all childhood illnesses; respiratory infections are the most prevalent. The common cold remains the chief illness of childhood. Certain groups of children are more prone to disease and disability, often as a result of barriers to health care. Poverty and the prevalence of illness are highly correlated. Access to care is often very limited, and health promotion and preventive health measures are minimal.

Health Promotion

Perceptions. During the school-age years identity and self-concept become stronger and more individualized. Perception of wellness is based on readily observable facts such as presence or absence of illness and adequacy of eating or sleeping. Functional ability is the standard by which personal health and the health of others are judged. Six-year-olds are aware of their body and modest and sensitive about being exposed. Nurses need to provide for privacy and offer explanations of common procedures.

Health Education. The school-age period is crucial for the acquisition of behaviors and health practices for a healthy adult life. Because cognition is advancing during the period, effective health education must be developmentally appropriate. Promotion of good health practices is a nursing responsibility. Programs directed at health education are frequently organized and conducted in the school. Effective health education teaches children about their bodies and how the choices they make impact their health (Hockenberry and Wilson, 2011). During these programs focus on the development of behaviors that positively affect children's health status.

Health Maintenance. Parents need to recognize the importance of annual health maintenance visits for immunizations, screenings, and dental care. When their school-age child reaches 10 years of age, parents need to begin discussions in preparation for upcoming pubertal changes. Topics include introductory information regarding menstruation, sexual intercourse, reproduction, and **sexually transmitted infections (STIs).** Human papilloma virus (HPV) is a widespread virus that will infect over 50% of males and females in their lifetime (AAP, 2010). For many individuals HPV clears spontaneously, but for others it can cause significant consequences. Females can develop cervical, vaginal, and vulvar cancers and genital warts; and males can develop genital warts. Since it is not possible to determine who or who will not develop disease from the virus, the Centers for Disease Control and Prevention (CDC) (2010a), along with the AAP, recommends routine HPV vaccination for girls ages 11 to 12 and for young women ages 13 through 26 who have not already been vaccinated. It is further recommended that HPV vaccine be given to boys and young men ages 9 to 26 years.

Safety. Because accidents such as fires and car and bicycle crashes are the leading cause of death and injury in the school-age period, safety is a priority health teaching consideration. Nurses contribute to the general health of children by educating them about safety measures to prevent accidents. At this age encourage children to take responsibility for their own safety.

Nutrition. Growth often slows during the school-age period as compared to infancy and adolescence. School-age children are developing eating patterns that are independent of parental supervision. The availability of snacks and fast-food restaurants makes it increasingly difficult for children to make healthy choices. The prevalence of obesity among children 6 to 11 years of age increased from 6.5% in 1980 to 19.6% in 2008 (CDC, 2010b). Childhood obesity has become a prominent health problem, resulting in increased risk for hypertension, diabetes, coronary heart disease, fatty liver disease, pulmonary complications such as sleep apnea, musculoskeletal problems, dyslipidemia, and potential for psychological problems. Studies have found that overweight children are teased more often, less likely to be chosen as a friend, and more likely to be thought of as lazy and sloppy by their peers (Hockenberry and Wilson, 2011). Nurses contribute to meeting national policy goals by promoting healthy lifestyle habits, including nutrition. School-age children need to participate in educational programs that enable them to plan, select, and prepare healthy meals and snacks. Children need adequate caloric intake for growth throughout childhood accompanied by activity for continued gross-motor development.

ADOLESCENTS

Adolescence is the period during which the individual makes the transition from childhood to adulthood, usually between ages 13 and 20 years. The term *adolescent* usually refers to psychological maturation of the individual, whereas **puberty** refers to the point at which reproduction becomes possible. The hormonal changes of puberty result in changes in the appearance of the young person, and cognitive development results in the ability to hypothesize and deal with abstractions. Adjustments and adaptations are necessary to cope with these simultaneous changes and the attempt to establish a mature sense of identity. In the past many referred to adolescence as a stormy and stressful period filled with inner turmoil, but today it is recognized that most teenagers successfully meet the challenges of this period.

The nurse's understanding of development provides a unique perspective for helping teenagers and parents anticipate and cope with the stresses of adolescence. Nursing activities, particularly education, promote healthy development. These activities occur in a variety of settings, and you can direct them at the adolescent, parents, or both. For example, the nurse conducts seminars in a high school to provide practical suggestions for solving problems of concern to a large group of students such as treating acne or making responsible decisions about drugs or alcohol use. Similarly a group education program for parents about how to cope with teenagers would promote parental understanding of adolescent development.

Physical Changes

Physical changes occur rapidly in adolescence. Sexual maturation occurs with the development of primary and secondary sexual characteristics. The four main focuses of the physical changes are:

1. Increased growth rate of skeleton, muscle, and viscera.
2. Sex-specific changes such as changes in shoulder and hip width.
3. Alteration in distribution of muscle and fat.
4. Development of the reproductive system and secondary sex characteristics.

Wide variation exists in the timing of physical changes associated with puberty between sexes and within the same sex. Girls tend to begin their physical changes approximately 2 years earlier than boys, usually between the ages of 11 to 14 years (Santrock, 2009). The rates of height and weight gain are usually proportional, and the sequence of pubertal growth changes is the same in most individuals.

Hormonal changes within the body create change when the hypothalamus begins to produce gonadotropin-releasing hormones that stimulate ovarian cells to produce **estrogen** and testicular cells to produce **testosterone.** These hormones contribute to the development of secondary sex characteristics such as hair growth and voice changes and play an essential role in reproduction. The changing concentrations of these hormones are also linked to acne and body odor. Understanding these hormonal changes enables you to reassure adolescents and educate them about body care needs.

Boys who mature early are more poised, relaxed, good-natured, skilled in athletic activities, and likely to be school leaders than boys who mature late. In contrast, girls who mature early are less satisfied with their figures by late adolescence. The reason for this is that early-maturing girls tend to be shorter and somewhat heavier than late-maturing girls, who tend to be taller and thinner (Santrock, 2008). Being like peers is extremely important for adolescents (Fig. 12-7). Any deviation in the timing of the physical changes is extremely difficult for adolescents to accept. Therefore provide emotional support for those undergoing early or delayed puberty. Even adolescents whose physical changes are occurring at the normal times seek confirmation of and reassurance about their normalcy.

Height and weight increases usually occur during the prepubertal growth spurt, which peaks in girls at about 12 years and in boys at about 14 years. Girls' height increases 5 to 20 cm (2 to 8 inches), and weight increases by 15 to 55 pounds. Boys' height increases

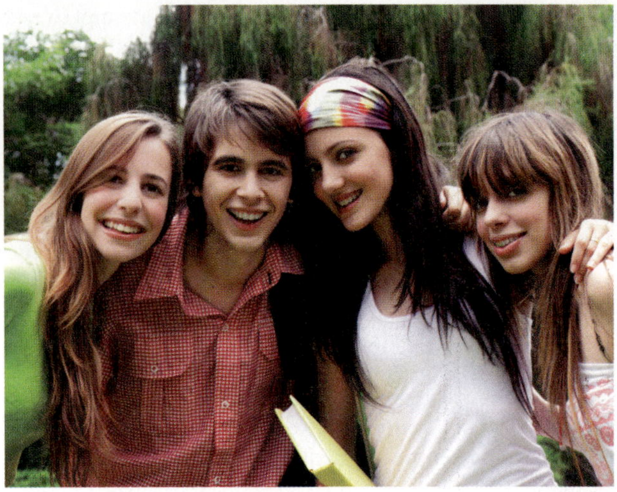

FIG. 12-7 Peer interactions help increase self-esteem during puberty. (© Petrenko Andriy.)

approximately 10 to 30 cm (4 to 12 inches), and weight increases by 15 to 65 pounds. Individuals gain the final 20% to 25% of their height and 50% of their weight during this time period (Hockenberry and Wilson, 2011).

Girls attain 90% to 95% of their adult height by **menarche** (the onset of menstruation) and reach their full height by 16 to 17 years of age, whereas boys continue to grow taller until 18 to 20 years of age. Fat is redistributed into adult proportions as height and weight increase, and gradually the adolescent torso takes on an adult appearance. Although individual and sex differences exist, growth follows a similar pattern for both sexes. Personal growth curves help the nurse assess physical development. However, the individual's sustained progression along the curve is more important than a comparison to the norm.

Cognitive Changes

The adolescent develops the ability to determine and rank possibilities, solve problems, and make decisions through logical operations. The teenager thinks abstractly and deals effectively with hypothetical problems. When confronted with a problem, the adolescent considers an infinite variety of causes and solutions. For the first time the young person moves beyond the physical or concrete properties of a situation and uses reasoning powers to understand the abstract. School-age individuals think about what is, whereas adolescents are able to imagine what might be.

Adolescents are now able to think in terms of the future rather than just current events. These newly developed abilities allow the individual to have more insight and skill in playing video, computer, and board games that require abstract thinking and deductive reasoning about many possible strategies. A teenager even solves problems requiring simultaneous manipulation of several abstract concepts. Development of this ability is important in the pursuit of an identity. For example, newly acquired cognitive skills allow the teenager to define appropriate, effective, and comfortable sex-role behaviors and to consider their impact on peers, family, and society. A higher level of cognitive functioning makes the adolescent receptive to more detailed and diverse information about sexuality and sexual behaviors. For example, sex education includes an explanation of physiological sexual changes and birth control measures.

Adolescents also develop the ability to understand how an individual's ideas or actions influence others. This complex development of thought leads them to question society and its values. Although adolescents have the capability to think as well as an adult, they do not have experiences on which to build. It is common for teenagers to consider their parents too narrow minded or too materialistic. At this time adolescents believe that they are unique and the exception, giving rise to their risk-taking behaviors. In other words, adolescents think that they are invincible. For example, an adolescent might state that he or she "is able to drive fast and not have an accident."

Language Skills. Language development is fairly complete by adolescence, although vocabulary continues to expand. The primary focus becomes communication skills that the adolescent uses effectively in various situations. Adolescents need to communicate thoughts, feelings, and facts to peers, parents, teachers, and other persons of authority. The skills used in these diverse communication situations vary. Adolescents need to select the person with whom to communicate, decide on the exact message, and choose the way to transmit the message. For example, how teenagers tell parents about failing grades is not the same as how they tell friends. Good communication skills are critical for adolescents in overcoming peer pressure and unhealthy behaviors. The following are some hints for communicating with adolescents:

- Do not avoid discussing sensitive issues. Asking questions about sex, drugs, and school opens the channels for further discussion.
- Ask open-ended questions.
- Look for the meaning behind their words or actions.
- Be alert to clues to their emotional state.
- Involve other individuals and resources when necessary.

Psychosocial Changes

The search for personal identity is the major task of adolescent psychosocial development. Teenagers establish close peer relationships or remain socially isolated. Erikson (1963) sees identity (or role) confusion as the prime danger of this stage and suggests that the cliquish behavior and intolerance of differences seen in adolescent behavior are defenses against identity confusion (Erikson, 1968). Adolescents work at becoming emotionally independent from their parents while retaining family ties. They are often described as being ambivalent. They love and hate their parents. In addition, they need to develop their own ethical systems based on personal values. They need to make choices about vocation, future education, and lifestyle. The various components of total identity evolve from these tasks and compose adult personal identity that is unique to the individual.

Sexual Identity. Physical changes of puberty enhance achievement of sexual identity. The physical evidence of maturity encourages the development of masculine and feminine behaviors. If these physical changes involve deviations, the person has more difficulty developing a comfortable sexual identity. Adolescents depend on these physical clues because they want assurance of maleness or femaleness and they do not wish to be different from peers. Without these physical characteristics, achieving sexual identity is difficult.

Group Identity. Adolescents seek a group identity because they need esteem and acceptance. Similarity in dress or speech is common in teenage groups. Peer groups provide the adolescent with a sense of belonging, approval, and the opportunity to learn acceptable behavior. Popularity with opposite-sex and same-sex peers is important. The strong need for group identity seems to conflict at times with the search for personal identity. It is as though adolescents require close bonds with peers so they later achieve a sense of individuality.

Family Identity. The movement toward stronger peer relationships is contrasted with adolescents' movements away from parents. Although financial independence for adolescents is not the norm in American society, many work part-time, using their income to bolster independence. When they cannot have a part-time job because of studies, school-related activities, and other factors, parents can provide allowances for clothing and incidentals, which encourage them to develop decision-making and budgeting skills.

Some adolescents and families have more difficulty during these years than others. Adolescents need to make choices, act independently, and experience the consequences of their actions. Nurses help families consider appropriate ways for them to foster the independence of their adolescent while maintaining family structure.

Health Identity. Another component of personal identity is perception of health. This component is of specific interest to health care providers. Healthy adolescents evaluate their own health according to feelings of well-being, ability to function normally, and absence of symptoms (Hockenberry and Wilson, 2011). They also often include health maintenance and health promotion behaviors as important concerns.

Therefore interventions to improve health perception concentrate on the adolescent period. The rapid changes during this period make health promotion programs especially crucial. Adolescents try new roles, begin to stabilize their identity, and acquire values and behaviors from which their adult lifestyle will evolve. They are able to identify behaviors such as smoking and substance abuse as threatening to health in general terms but frequently tend to underestimate the effect of the potentially negative consequences of their own actions (Hockenberry and Wilson, 2011).

Health Risks

Accidents. Accidents remain the leading cause of death in adolescence. Motor vehicle accidents, which are the most common cause of death, resulted in 74% of all unintentional deaths among teens 10 to 19 years (Hockenberry and Wilson, 2011). Such accidents are often associated with alcohol intoxication or drug abuse. Bicycling fatalities were 4 to 7 times more likely to occur in males than females. Other frequent causes of accidental death in teenagers are drowning and the use of firearms. Feelings of being indestructible lead to risk-taking behavior. The use of alcohol precedes many injuries, and adolescents continue to be both the victims and perpetrators of violence. A proposed objective for Healthy People 2020 is to reduce the percentage of middle and public high schools with a violent incident (U.S. Department of Health and Human Services [USDHHS], 2009a).

Violence and Homicide. Homicide is the second leading cause of death in the 15- to 24-year-old age-group, and for African American teenagers it is the most likely cause of death (National Institutes of Health, 2010). Results from the Youth Risk Behavior Surveillance System show that, in 2007, 18% of high school students had carried a weapon (e.g., gun, club, or knife) at some point during the preceding 30 days (USDHHS, 2009b). Individuals 12 years of age and older are most likely to be killed by an acquaintance or gang member, most often with a firearm. Because having a gun in the home raises the risk of homicide and suicide for adolescents, include assessment of gun presence in the home when counseling families (Hockenberry and Wilson, 2011).

BOX 12-2 EVIDENCE-BASED PRACTICE

Prevention Programs for School-Based Violence

PICO Question: For middle- and high-school students, are classroom-based curricular programs that promote prosocial behaviors and attitudes compared with efforts to improve the social and interpersonal climate of a school more effective in reducing school violence?

Evidence Summary

School violence is a serious problem that encompasses everyday events such as physical assaults and fighting, threats and intimidation, sexual harassment, bullying or cyberbullying, dating violence, and stalking (Theriot, 2008). Research shows that dating violence behaviors are the most common in schools and that adolescents involved in dating violence are more likely to be involved in violent relationships as adults (Theriot, 2008). In this current era of local school accountability, health care workers and educators are charged with the responsibility of assessing the prevalence of school violence, using evidence-based programs to address the behaviors, and monitoring the effectiveness of the programs (Benbenishty et al., 2008).

Currently two different approaches are used to reduce school violence. The first approach involves the delivery of classroom-based educational programs that focus on interpersonal skills, attitudes, and emotional literacy. These programs teach students to resolve conflicts and maintain peer relationships without resorting to aggressive or violent behavior (Park-Higgerson et al., 2008). The second approach is to establish efforts to improve the social and interpersonal climate of the school. These schools focus on the relationships among students, faculty, and administrators and the policies within the school that address violent behaviors (Greene, 2008; Johnson, 2009).

The research literature indicates that school-based curricular programs can be effective but need to be implemented in schools that have a positive school climate. Programs designed to prevent school violence have largely focused on reducing student-to-student aggressive behaviors and have not fully considered interpersonal relationships between students and adults in schools, student bonding to schools, and organizational factors that comprise school climate. Reducing school violence depends on implementation of both approaches.

Application to Nursing Practice

- Ongoing school violence assessment is critical to providing a healthy school environment.
- Including dating violence and stalking at school is essential and should be a part of nursing assessment.
- School nurses can work with educators to provide an environment that promotes adolescent health.
- Successful programs are those that are tailored to a specific school.
- Although the individual is the person responsible for violent behavior, violence occurs in context so health providers and educators can work together to ensure a healthy environment.

Violence among adolescents has become a national concern (Box 12-2). Statistics now show that 63 out of every 1000 high-school students are the victims of violence at school (Johnson, 2009; Kongsuwan et al., 2009). This violence is not just limited to physical assaults and fighting, threats and intimidation, sexual harassment, or bullying. It can also include adolescent dating violence and stalking at school (Theriot, 2008). Nurses working with adolescents need to be aware of the potential for school violence and include screening questions when providing health care, regardless of the setting.

Suicide. Suicide is the third leading cause of death in adolescents 13 to 19 years of age, and in a recent study by the National Center for Health Statistics, one fifth of high-school students indicated that they had contemplated suicide in the previous 12 months (Santrock, 2008). Depression and social isolation commonly precede a suicide attempt, but suicide probably results from a combination of several factors. Nurses must be able to identify the factors associated with adolescent suicide risk and precipitating events. The following warning signs often occur for at least a month before suicide is attempted:

- Decrease in school performance
- Withdrawal
- Loss of initiative
- Loneliness, sadness, and crying
- Appetite and sleep disturbances
- Verbalization of suicidal thought

Make immediate referrals to mental health professionals when assessment suggests that adolescents are considering suicide. Guidance helps them focus on the positive aspects of life and strengthen coping abilities.

Substance Abuse. Substance abuse is a concern for all who work with adolescents. Adolescents often believe that mood-altering substances create a sense of well-being or improve level of performance. All adolescents are at risk for experimental or recreational substance use, but those who have dysfunctional families are more at risk for chronic use and physical dependency. Some adolescents believe that substance use makes them more mature. They further believe that they will look and feel better with drug usage. Current statistics show that, by the end of their high-school years, 85% of adolescents have used alcohol, 65% have tried smoking, and 49% have experimented with marijuana (Hockenberry and Wilson, 2011). Tobacco use continues to be a problem among adolescents; and, although its use is declining, 3 out of 10 adolescents are active smokers at the time of high-school graduation.

Eating Disorders. Adolescent overweight and obesity are current concerns in the United States, and most teens try dieting at some time to control weight. Unfortunately the number of eating disorders is on the rise in adolescent girls; thus the benefits of a healthy diet should be discussed with all adolescents. Routine nutritional screening should be a part of the health care provided to all adolescents. Areas to include in the assessment are past and present diet history, food records, eating habits, attitudes, health beliefs, and socioeconomic and psychosocial factors (Hockenberry and Wilson, 2011).

Anorexia nervosa and bulimia are two eating disorders that appear in adolescence. Anorexia nervosa is a clinical syndrome with both physical and psychosocial components that involves the pursuit of thinness through starvation. Persons with anorexia nervosa have an intense fear of gaining weight and refuse to maintain body weight at the minimal normal weight for their age and height. Bulimia nervosa is most identified with binge eating and behaviors to prevent weight gain. Behaviors include self-induced vomiting, misuse of laxatives and other medications, and excessive exercise. Unlike anorexia, bulimia occurs within a normal weight range; thus it is much more difficult to detect. Because adolescents rarely volunteer information about behaviors to prevent weight gain, it is important to take a thorough dietary history. If left undetected and untreated, these disorders lead to significant morbidity and mortality (Hockenberry and Wilson, 2011; Santrock, 2008).

Sexually Transmitted Infections. STIs annually affect 3 million sexually active adolescents. This high degree of incidence makes it imperative that sexually active adolescents be screened for STIs, even when they have no symptoms. The annual physical examination of a sexually active adolescent includes a thorough sexual history and a careful examination of the genitalia so STIs are not missed. Be proactive by using the interview process to identify risk factors in the adolescent and provide education to prevent STIs, including human immunodeficiency virus (HIV), HPV, and unwanted pregnancies (Hockenberry and Wilson, 2011). As discussed earlier for school-age children, immunization for HPV infection should be considered at this time if not already administered.

Pregnancy. Adolescent pregnancy continues to be a major social challenge for our nation. The United States has the highest rate of teenage pregnancy and childbearing annually compared to other industrialized nations (Hockenberry and Wilson, 2011; Santrock, 2008). Adolescent pregnancy occurs across socioeconomic classes, in public and private schools, among all ethnic and religious backgrounds, and in all parts of the country. Teenage pregnancy with early prenatal supervision is less harmful to both mother and child than earlier believed. Pregnant teens need special attention to nutrition, health supervision, and psychological support. Adolescent mothers also need help in planning for the future and obtaining competent day care for their infants.

Health Promotion

Health Education. Community and school-based health programs for adolescents focus on health promotion and illness prevention. Nurses need to be sensitive to the emotional cues from adolescents before initiating health teaching to know when the teen is ready to discuss concerns. In addition, discussions with adolescents need to be private and confidential. Adolescents define health in much the same way as adults and look for opportunities to reach their physical, mental, and emotional potential. Large numbers of school-based clinics have been developed and implemented to respond to adolescents' needs. Adolescents are much more likely to use these health care services if they encounter providers who are caring and respectful (Hockenberry and Wilson, 2011).

Nurses play an important role in preventing injuries and accidental deaths. For example, urging adolescents to discuss alternatives to driving when under the influence of drugs or alcohol prepares them to consider alternatives when such an occasion arises. As a nurse, identify adolescents at risk for abuse, provide education to prevent accidents related to substance abuse, and provide counseling to those in rehabilitation.

Minority Adolescents. By the next century estimates predict that minorities as a group will become the majority. African American, Hispanic, Latino, Asian, Native American, and Alaska Native American adolescents are the fastest-growing segment in the U.S. population. Minority adolescents experience a greater percentage of health problems and barriers to health care (Hockenberry and Wilson, 2011). Issues of concern for these adolescents living in a high-risk environment include learning or emotional difficulties, death related to violence, unintentional injuries, increased rate for adolescent pregnancy, STIs, HIV infection, and acquired immunodeficiency syndrome (AIDS). Poverty is a major factor negatively affecting the lives of minority adolescents. Limited access to health services is common. Nurses are able to make a significant contribution to improving access to appropriate health care for adolescents. With knowledge about various cultures and the means to care for minority adolescents, the nurse acts as an advocate to ensure accessibility of appropriate services.

Gay, Lesbian, and Bisexual Adolescents. Researchers have studied development of a gay or lesbian identity in adults, but there are limited studies related to adolescents. It is widely known that, although some adolescents participate in same-gender sexual activity, they do not necessarily become homosexual as adults (Hockenberry and Wilson, 2011; Santrock, 2008). Adolescents who believe that they have a homosexual or bisexual orientation often try to keep it hidden to avoid any associated stigma. This increases their vulnerability to depression and suicide. The teens who choose to disclose a homosexual or bisexual orientation become at risk for violence, harassment, and family abuse. If a teen chooses to disclose sexual orientation to you, help the adolescent construct a safety plan before telling his or her family or friends in case the response is not supportive (Hockenberry and Wilson, 2011). One of the new additions to *Healthy People 2020* objectives is to increase the percentage of middle and high schools that prohibit harassment based on a student's sexual orientation or gender identity (USDHHS, 2009a).

KEY POINTS

- A developmental perspective helps the nurse understand commonalities and variations in each stage and the impact they have on the patient's health.
- During critical periods of development, a multitude of factors foster or hinder optimal physical, cognitive, and psychosocial development.
- Physiological, cognitive, and psychosocial development continue from conception through adolescence; thus be familiar with normal parameters to determine potential problems and identify ways to promote normal development.
- The most rapid period of growth and development occurs during infancy.
- The toddler's development of fine- and gross-motor skills support the move toward independence,
- Preschoolers interpret language literally and are unable to see another's point of view.
- Physical growth during the school years is slow and steady until the skeletal growth spurt just before puberty.
- The major psychosocial developmental task of the school-age child is the development of a sense of industry or competency.
- Adolescence begins with puberty, when primary sexual characteristics begin to develop and secondary sexual characteristics complete development.
- Adolescents are able to solve complex mental problems, which includes use of deductive reasoning.
- Accidents are the major cause of death in all age-groups.
- Sexually transmitted diseases are the most common communicable diseases among adolescents.

CLINICAL APPLICATION QUESTIONS

Preparing for Clinical Practice

You are caring for 12-year-old Elizabeth who has been hospitalized for an appendectomy. Her mother tells you that she is concerned about her lack of physical development compared to her peers. As a nurse you know that adolescents are preoccupied with their bodies and develop individual images of what they think they should look like. You are also aware that adolescents define health in terms of not just absence of illness but also being able to live up to one's physical, mental, and social potential.

1. What would you want to discuss concerning the onset of puberty with Elizabeth?
2. What psychosocial concerns may Elizabeth have in relation to her concerns about physical development?
3. How will Elizabeth's cognitive and psychosocial development direct your teaching?

evolve *Answers to Clinical Application Questions can be found on the Evolve website.*

REVIEW QUESTIONS

Are You Ready to Test Your Nursing Knowledge?

1. In an interview with a pregnant patient, the nurse discussed the three risk factors that have been cited as having a possible effect on prenatal development. They are:
   1. Nutrition, stress, and mother's age.
   2. Prematurity, stress, and mother's age.
   3. Nutrition, mother's age, and fetal infections.
   4. Fetal infections, prematurity, and placenta previa.
2. A parent has brought her 6-month-old infant in for a well-child check. Which of her statements indicates a need for further teaching?
   1. "I can start giving her whole milk at about 12 months."
   2. "I can continue to breastfeed for another 6 months."
   3. "I've started giving her plenty of fruit juice as a way to increase her vitamin intake."
   4. "I can start giving her solid food now."
3. The type of injury a child is most vulnerable to at a specific age is most closely related to which of the following?
   1. Provision of adult supervision.
   2. Educational level of the parent
   3. Physical health of the child
   4. Developmental level of the child
4. Which approach would be best for the nurse to use with a hospitalized toddler?
   1. Always give several choices.
   2. Set few limits to allow for open expression.
   3. Use noninvasive methods when possible.
   4. Gain cooperation before attempting treatment.
5. The nurse is providing information on prevention of sudden infant death syndrome (SIDS) to the mother of a young infant. Which of the following statements indicates that the mother has a good understanding? (Select all that apply.)
   1. "I won't use a pacifier to help my baby sleep."
   2. "I'll be sure my baby does not spend any time on her abdomen."
   3. "I'll place my baby on her back for sleep."
   4. "I'll be sure to keep my baby's room cold."
6. In evaluating the gross-motor development of a 5-month-old infant, which of the following would the nurse expect the infant to do?
   1. Roll from abdomen to back
   2. Move from prone to sitting unassisted
   3. Sit upright without support
   4. Turn completely over
7. Parents are concerned about their toddler's negativism and ask the nurse for guidance. Which is the most appropriate recommendation?
   1. Provide more attention.
   2. Reduce opportunities for a "no" answer.
   3. Be consistent with punishment.
   4. Provide opportunities for the toddler to make decisions.
8. When nurses are communicating with adolescents, they should:
   1. Be alert to clues to their emotional state.
   2. Ask closed-ended questions to get straight answers.

3. Avoid looking for meaning behind adolescents' words or actions.
4. Avoid discussing sensitive issues such sex and drugs.

9. Which of the following statements is most descriptive of the psychosocial development of school-age children?
   1. Boys and girls play equally with each other.
   2. Peer influence is not yet an important factor to the child.
   3. They like to play games with rigid rules.
   4. Children frequently have "best friends."
10. You are caring for a 4-year-old child who is hospitalized for an infection. He tells you that he is sick because he was "bad." Which is the most correct interpretation of his comment?
    1. Indicative of extreme stress
    2. Representative of his cognitive development
    3. Suggestive of excessive discipline at home
    4. Indicative of his developing sense of inferiority
11. At a well-child examination, the mother comments that her toddler eats little at mealtime, will only sit briefly at the table, and wants snacks all the time. Which of the following should the nurse recommend?
    1. Provide nutritious snacks.
    2. Offer rewards for eating at mealtimes.
    3. Avoid snacks so she is hungry at mealtime.
    4. Explain to her firmly why eating at mealtime is important.
12. An 8-year-old child is being admitted to the hospital from the emergency department with an injury from falling off her bicycle. Which of the following will most help her adjust to the hospital?
    1. Explain hospital routines such as meal times to her.
    2. Use terms such as "honey" and "dear" to show a caring attitude.
    3. Explain when her parents can visit and why siblings cannot come to see her.
    4. Since she is young, orient her parents to her room and hospital facility.
13. The school nurse is counseling an obese 10-year-old child. What factor would be important to consider when planning an intervention to support the child's health?
    1. Concentrate on the child only rather than the family since it is the child's responsibility.
    2. Consider the use of medications to suppress the appetite.
    3. First plan for weight loss through dieting and then add activity as tolerated.
    4. Plan food intake to allow for growth
14. You are working in an adolescent health center when a 15-year-old patient shares with you that she thinks she is pregnant and is worried that she may now have a sexually transmitted infection (STI). Her pregnancy test is negative. What is your next priority of care?
    1. Contact her parents to alert them of her need for birth control.
    2. Refer her to a primary health care provider to obtain a prescription for birth control.
    3. Counsel her on safe sex practices.
    4. Ask her to have her partner come to the clinic for STI testing.
15. While working in the high-school clinic, one of the students tells you that she is worried about her friend who has started to refuse to participate in group activities, no longer cares about how she looks at school, and is not going to all of her classes. Your assessment of these symptoms may indicate that:
    1. She has just broken up with her boyfriend and time will heal all.
    2. You will need to observe her over time to see if symptoms persist.
    3. School may be too difficult for her right now.
    4. She may be at increased risk for suicide.

Answers: **1.** 1; **2.** 3; **3.** 4; **4.** 4; **5.** 3, 4; **6.** 1; **7.** 2; **8.** 1; **9.** 4; **10.** 2; **11.** 1; **12.** 1; **13.** 4; **14.** 3; **15.** 4.

REFERENCES

American Academy of Pediatrics: Healthy Children: *Safety and prevention: HPV (Gardasil): What you need to know*, 2010, http://www.healthychildren.org/English/safety-prevention/immunizations/pages/Human-Papillomavirus-HPV-vaccine-what-you-need-to-know.aspx. Accessed December, 2010.

American Academy of Pediatrics: Healthy Children*: Safety and prevention: Car safety seats: Information for families in 2011*, 2011a, http://www.healthychildren.org/English/safety-prevention/on-the-go/Pages/Car-Safety-Seats-Information-for-Families.aspx?nfstatus=401&nftoken=00000000-0000-0000-0000-000000000000&nfstatusdescription=ERROR%3a+No+local+token. Accessed July 2011.

American Academy of Pediatrics: Healthy Children: *Safety and prevention: New crib standards: What parents need to know*, 2011b, http://www.healthychildren.org/english/safety-prevention/at-home/pages/new-crib-standards-what-parents-need-to-know.aspx?nfstatus. Accessed July 2011.

American Academy of Pediatrics: Healthy Children: *Family Life: Where we stand: TV viewing time.* 2011c, http://www.healthychildren.org/English/family-life/Media/pages/Where-We-Stand-TV-Viewing-Time.aspx?nfstatus. Accessed July 2011.

Centers for Disease Control and Prevention: *Vaccine information statement 3/30/2010,* 2010a, http://www.cdc.gov/vaccines/pubs/vis/downloads/vis-hpv-gardasil.pdf. Accessed November, 2010.

Centers for Disease Control and Prevention: *Healthy youth: Childhood obesity,* 2010b, http://www.cdc.gov/healthyyouth/obesity/. Accessed July 2011.

Davidson MR, et al: *Olds' maternal-newborn nursing & women's health across the lifespan*, ed 8, Upper Saddle River, NJ, 2008, Pearson Prentice Hall.

Erikson EH: *Childhood and society*, ed 2, New York, 1963, Norton.

Erikson EH: *Identity: youth and crises*, New York, 1968, Norton.

Hockenberry M, Wilson D: *Wong's nursing care of infants and children*, ed 9, St Louis, 2011, Mosby.

National Institutes of Health: US National Library of Medicine: *Death among children and adolescents,* 2010, http://www.nlm.nih.gov/medlineplus/ency/article/001915.htm. Accessed July 2011.

Piaget J: *The origins of intelligence in children*, New York, 1952, International Universities Press.

Santrock JW: *Life-span development*, ed 12, New York, 2008, McGraw-Hill.

Santrock JW: *A topical approach to lifespan development*, ed 5, New York, 2009, McGraw-Hill.

US Department of Health and Human Services: *Healthy People 2020 the road ahead,* 2009a, http://www.healthypeople.gov/hp2020/. Accessed January 6, 2011.

US Department of Health and Human Services, Health Resources and Services Administration: *Child Health USA 2008-2009,* 2009b, http://mchb.hrsa.gov/chusa08/pdfs/c08.pdf. Accessed July 2011.

RESEARCH REFERENCES

Benbenishty R, et al: School violence assessment: a conceptual framework, instruments, and methods, *Children Schools* 30(1):71, 2008.

Greene MB: Reducing school violence: school-based curricular programs and school climate, *Prevention Res* 15(1):12, 2008.

Johnson SL: Improving the school environment to reduce school violence: a review of the literature, *J School Health* 79(10):451, 2009.

Kongsuwan V, et al: Perspectives of adolescents, parents, and teachers on youth violence, *Self-Care Dependence-Care Nurs* 17(1):23, 2009.

Park-Higgerson HK, et al: The evaluation of school-based violence prevention programs: a meta-analysis, *J School Health* 78(9):465, 2008.

Theriot MT: Conceptual and methodological considerations for assessment and prevention of adolescent dating violence and stalking at school, *Children Schools* 30(4):223, 2008.

CHAPTER 13

Young and Middle Adults

OBJECTIVES

- Discuss developmental theories of young and middle adults.
- List and discuss major life events of young and middle adults and the childbearing family.
- Describe developmental tasks of the young adult, the childbearing family, and the middle adult.
- Discuss the significance of family in the life of the adult.
- Describe normal physical changes in young and middle adulthood and pregnancy.
- Discuss cognitive and psychosocial changes occurring during the adult years.
- Describe health concerns of the young adult, the childbearing family, and the middle adult.

KEY TERMS

Braxton Hicks contractions, p. 163
Climacteric, p. 164
Doula, p. 159
Infertility, p. 162
Lactation, p. 163
Menopause, p. 164
Millennial generation, p. 157
Prenatal care, p. 163
Puerperium, p. 163
Sandwich generation, p. 164

evolve WEBSITE

http://evolve.elsevier.com/Potter/fundamentals/

- Review Questions
- Case Study with Questions
- Audio Glossary
- Interactive Learning Activities
- Key Term Flashcards
- Content Updates

Young and middle adulthood is a period of challenges, rewards, and crises. Challenges may include the demands of working and raising families, although there are many rewards with these as well. Adults also face crises such as caring for their aging parents, the possibility of job loss in a changing economic environment, and dealing with their own developmental needs and those of their family members.

Classic works by developmental theorists such as Levinson et al (1978), Diekelmann (1976), Erikson (1963, 1982), and Havighurst (1972) attempted to describe the phases of young and middle adulthood and related developmental tasks (see Chapter 11 for an in-depth discussion of developmental theories).

Traditional masculine roles include providing and protecting. However, these roles are now shared with women. Faced with a societal structure that differs greatly from the norms of 20 or 30 years ago, both men and women are assuming different roles in today's society. Men were traditionally the primary supporter of the family. Today many women pursue careers and contribute significantly to their families' incomes. In 2006 60% of women participated in the U.S. labor force and constituted 46% of all U.S. workers in the U.S. labor force. Thirty-eight percent of employed women worked in management or professional and related occupations, 34% worked in sales and office occupations; and another 20% worked in service occupations (Business and Professional Women's Foundation, 2007). However, according to the American Federation of Labor and Congress of Industrial Organizations (AFL-CIO) (2008) workers' union, women in the United States are paid 77.6 cents for every dollar men receive for comparable work.

Developmental theories provide nurses with a basis for understanding the life events and developmental tasks of the young and middle adult. Patients present challenges to nurses who themselves are often young or middle adults coping with the demands of their respective developmental period. Nurses need to recognize the needs of their patients even if they are not experiencing the same challenges and events.

YOUNG ADULTS

Young adulthood is the period between the late teens and the mid to late 30s (Edelman and Mandle, 2010). In recent years young adults between the ages of 18 and 29 have been referred to as part of the **millennial generation.** In 2009 young adults made up approximately 33% of the population (U.S. Census Bureau, 2009). According to the Pew Research Center (2010), today's young adults are history's first "always connected" generation, with digital technology and social media major aspects of their lives. They adapt well to new experiences, are more ethnically and racially diverse than previous generations, and are the least overtly religious American generation in modern times. Young adults increasingly move away from their families of origin, establish career goals, and decide whether to marry or remain single and whether to begin families; however, often these goals may be delayed (e.g., because of the economic recession of recent years).

Physical Changes

The young adult usually completes physical growth by the age of 20. An exception to this is the pregnant or lactating woman. The physical, cognitive, and psychosocial changes and the health concerns of the pregnant woman and the childbearing family are extensive.

Young adults are usually quite active, experience severe illnesses less commonly than older age-groups, tend to ignore physical symptoms, and often postpone seeking health care. Physical characteristics of young adults begin to change as middle age approaches. Unless patients have illnesses, assessment findings are generally within normal limits.

Cognitive Changes

Critical thinking habits increase steadily through the young- and middle-adult years. Formal and informal educational experiences, general life experiences, and occupational opportunities dramatically increase the individual's conceptual, problem-solving, and motor skills.

Identifying an occupational direction is a major task of young adults. When people know their skills, talents, and personality characteristics, educational preparation and occupational choices are easier and more satisfying. A bachelor's or associate's degree is the most significant source of postsecondary education for 12 of the 20 fastest-growing occupations.

An understanding of how adults learn helps you to develop patient education plans (see Chapter 25). Adults enter the teaching-learning situation with a background of unique life experiences, including illness. Therefore always view adults as individuals. Their adherence to regimens such as medications, treatments, or lifestyle changes such as smoking cessation involves decision-making processes. When determining the amount of information that an individual needs to make decisions about the prescribed course of therapy, consider factors that possibly affect the individual's adherence to the regimen, including educational level, socioeconomic factors, and motivation and desire to learn.

Because young adults are continually evolving and adjusting to changes in the home, workplace, and personal lives, their decision-making processes need to be flexible. The more secure young adults are in their roles, the more flexible and open they are to change. Insecure persons tend to be more rigid in making decisions.

Psychosocial Changes

The emotional health of the young adult is related to the individual's ability to address and resolve personal and social tasks. The young adult is often caught between wanting to prolong the irresponsibility of adolescence and assume adult commitments. However, certain patterns or trends are relatively predictable. Between the ages of 23 and 28, the person refines self-perception and ability for intimacy. From 29 to 34 the person directs enormous energy toward achievement and mastery of the surrounding world. The years from 35 to 43 are a time of vigorous examination of life goals and relationships. People make changes in personal, social, and occupational areas. Often the stresses of this reexamination results in a "midlife crisis" in which marital partner, lifestyle, and occupation change.

Ethnic and gender factors have a sociological and psychological influence in an adult's life, and these factors pose a distinct challenge for nursing care. Each person holds culture-bound definitions of health and illness. Nurses and other health professionals bring with them distinct practices for the prevention and treatment of illness. Knowing too little about a patient's self-perception or beliefs regarding health and illness creates conflict between the nurse and the patient. Changes in the traditional role expectations of both men and women in young and middle adulthood also lead to greater challenges for nursing care. For example, women often continue to work during the childrearing years, and many women struggle with the enormity of balancing three careers: wife, mother, and employee. This is a potential source of stress for the adult working woman. Men are more aware of parental and household responsibilities and find themselves having more responsibilities at home while achieving their own career goals (Fortinash and Holoday Worret, 2008). An understanding of ethnicity, race, and gender differences enables a nurse to provide individualized care (see Chapter 9).

Support from a nurse, access to information, and appropriate referrals provide opportunities for achievement of a patient's potential. Health is not merely the absence of disease but involves wellness in all human dimensions. The nurse acknowledges the importance of the young adult's psychosocial needs and needs in all other dimensions. The young adult needs to make decisions concerning career, marriage, and parenthood. Although each person makes these decisions based on individual factors, a nurse needs to understand the general principles involved in these aspects of psychosocial development while assessing the young adult's psychosocial status.

Lifestyle. Family history of cardiovascular, renal, endocrine, or neoplastic disease increases a young adult's risk of illness. Your role in health promotion is to identify modifiable factors that increase the young adult's risk for health problems and provide patient education and support to reduce unhealthy lifestyle behaviors (Sanchez et al., 2009).

A personal lifestyle assessment (see Chapter 6) helps nurses and patients identify habits that increase the risk for cardiac, malignant, pulmonary, renal, or other chronic diseases. The assessment includes general life satisfaction, hobbies, and interests; habits such as diet, sleeping, exercise, sexual habits, and use of caffeine, tobacco, alcohol, and illicit drugs; home conditions and pets; economics, including type of health insurance; occupational environment, including type of work and exposure to hazardous substances; and physical or mental stress. Military records, including dates and geographical area of assignments, may also be useful in assessing the young adult for risk factors. Prolonged stress from lifestyle choices increases wear and tear on the adaptive capacities of the body. Stress-related diseases such as ulcers, emotional disorders, and infections sometimes occur (see Chapter 37).

Career. A successful vocational adjustment is important in the lives of most men and women. Successful employment not only ensures economic security, but it also leads to friendships, social activities, support, and respect from co-workers.

Two-career families are increasing. The two-career family has benefits and liabilities. In addition to increasing the family's financial base, the person who works outside the home is able to expand friendships, activities, and interests. However, stress exists in a two-career family as well. These stressors result from a transfer to a new city; increased expenditures of physical, mental, or emotional energy; child care demands; or household needs. To avoid stress in a two-career family, partners should share all responsibilities. For example, some families may decide to limit recreational expenses and instead hire someone to do routine housework. Others set up an equal division of household, shopping, and cooking duties.

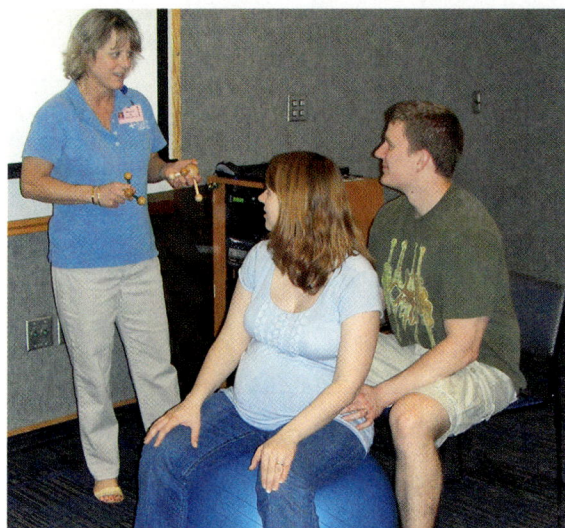

FIG. 13-1 Nurse providing Lamaze class for expectant young adults.

Sexuality. The development of secondary sex characteristics occurs during the adolescent years (see Chapter 12). Physical development is accompanied by the ability to perform sex acts. The young adult usually has emotional maturity to complement the physical ability and therefore is able to develop mature sexual relationships and establish intimacy. Young adults who have failed to achieve the developmental task of personal integration sometimes develop relationships that are superficial and stereotyped (Fortinash and Holoday Worret, 2008).

Masters and Johnson (1970) contributed important information about the physiological characteristics of the adult sexual response (see Chapter 34). The psychodynamic aspect of sexual activity is as important as the type or frequency of sexual intercourse to young adults. To maintain total wellness, encourage adults to explore various aspects of their sexuality and be aware that their sexual needs and concerns change. As the rate of early initiation of sexual intercourse continues to increase, young adults are at risk for sexually transmitted infections (STIs). Consequently there is an increased need for education regarding the mode of transmission, prevention, and symptom recognition and management for STIs.

Childbearing Cycle. Conception, pregnancy, birth, and the puerperium are major phases of the childbearing cycle. The changes during these phases are complex. Education such as Lamaze classes can prepare pregnant women, their partners, and other support persons to participate in the birthing process (Fig. 13-1). A current trend in some health care agencies is to provide either professional labor support (Sauls, 2006) or a lay **doula,** a support person to be present during labor to assist women who have no other source of support (Campbell et al., 2006). The stress that many women experience after childbirth has a significant impact on postpartum women's health (Box 13-1).

BOX 13-1 EVIDENCE-BASED PRACTICE

Assessing for Postpartum Depression

PICO Question: What psychosocial interventions affect a young adult woman's risk for postpartum depression (PPD)?

Evidence Summary

A woman often experiences dramatic physical and psychosocial changes during the postpartum period that impact health, with up to 85% of women experiencing some type of mood disturbance. For most women these transient symptoms are referred to as "postpartum blues" (Beck, 2006; USPSTF, 2009). Common symptoms of postpartum blues, including rapidly fluctuating mood, tearfulness, irritability, and anxiety, are generally mild (Beck, 2006; Doucet et al., 2009). A 10% to 15% group of women experience a more persistent form of PPD after the birth of a baby, and 0.1% to 0.2% of postpartum women experience postpartum psychosis (Robertson, 2010; USPSTF, 2009). The onset of postpartum psychosis carries a high risk of suicide and infanticide (murder of an infant). The onset of postpartum psychosis is abrupt and severe, with clinical manifestations of delusions, hallucinations, thoughts of harming or killing the baby, unwillingness to eat or sleep, frantic energy, risk of suicide, and severe depressive symptoms (Beacham et al., 2008).

Research findings indicate several risk factors for the development of postpartum mood disorder, including stress, fatigue, quality of relationship with the father of the baby, social support, birth of a preterm or low-birth-weight infant, and young maternal age (Akincigil et al., 2010; Bei et al., 2010). Studies also show that postpartum depression may have a negative impact on the maternal-infant relationship, infant development, and long-term child behavior (Knitzer et al., 2008; Poobalan et al., 2007). Postpartum psychosis is an extremely serious and rare postpartum mood disorder, and it is considered a psychiatric emergency.

Successful treatment of PPD depends on early identification and intervention. Clinical assessment of pregnant and postpartum women that is guided by the major predictors of PPD can help nurses identify women most at risk. Subsequently intervention can be initiated before the occurrence of depressive symptoms (Records et al., 2007).

Application to Nursing Practice

- Assess for potential postpartum stressors such as fatigue, first-time mother, previous postpartum stress, or feeling of social isolation.
- Identify sources of social support for new mothers after they are discharged from the hospital with their babies such as new-mother visits, young-mother groups, and mom's day out activities.
- Create culturally appropriate, primary prevention strategies for stressors that new mothers encounter.
- Educate new mothers and their families on the risks for and signs and symptoms of postpartum stress and depression.
- Provide new mothers with information on health care and community resources for use during the postpartum period.

Types of Families. During young adulthood most individuals experience singlehood and the opportunity to be on their own. Those who eventually marry encounter several changes as they take on new responsibilities. For example, many married couples choose to become parents (Fig. 13-2). Some young adults choose alternative lifestyles. Chapter 10 reviews forms of families.

Singlehood. Social pressure to get married is not as great as it once was, and many young adults do not marry until their late 20s or early 30s or not at all. For young adults who remain single, parents and siblings become the nucleus for a family. Some view close friends and associates as "family." One cause for the increased single population is the expanding career opportunities for women. Women enter the job market with greater career potential and have greater opportunities for financial independence. More single individuals are choosing to live together outside of marriage and become parents either biologically or through adoption. Similarly many married couples choose to separate or divorce if they find their marital situation unsatisfactory.

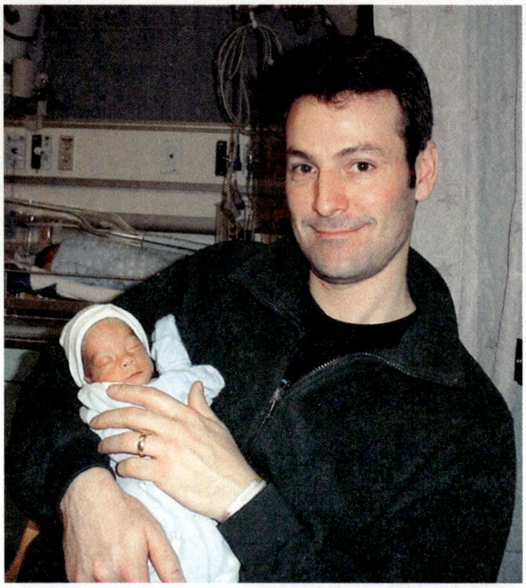

FIG. 13-2 Parent-child nurturing is important in adapting to a newborn. (From Hockenberry MJ, Wilson D: *Wong's nursing care of infants and children,* ed 9, St Louis, 2011, Mosby.)

Parenthood. The availability of contraception makes it easier for today's couples to decide when and if to start a family. Social pressures may encourage a couple to have a child or influence them to limit the number of children they have. Economic considerations frequently enter into the decision-making process because of the expense of childrearing. General health status and age are also considerations in decisions about parenthood because couples are getting married later and postponing pregnancies, which often results in smaller families.

Alternative Family Structures and Parenting. Changing norms and values about family life in the United States reveal basic shifts in attitudes about family structure. The trend toward greater acceptance of cohabitation without marriage is a factor in the greater numbers of infants being born to single women. In addition, approximately 1.5 million parents are gay or lesbian. More than one third of lesbians have given birth, and one in six gay men have fathered or adopted a child. Gay and lesbian parents are raising 3% of foster children in the United States (Gates et al., 2007). The American Academy of Pediatrics (AAP), in recognizing the needs of gay and lesbian parents and their children, published a policy statement supporting adoption of children and the parenting role by same-sex parents (AAP, 2002). However, many times parents from alternative family structures still feel a lack of support and even bias from the health care system (Makadon, 2006; McManus et al., 2006).

Hallmarks of Emotional Health. Most young adults have the physical and emotional resources and support systems to meet the many challenges, tasks, and responsibilities they face. During psychosocial assessment of young adults, assess for 10 hallmarks of emotional health (Box 13-2) that indicate successful maturation in this developmental stage.

BOX 13-2 TEN HALLMARKS OF EMOTIONAL HEALTH

1. A sense of meaning and direction in life
2. Successful negotiation through transitions
3. Absence of feelings of being cheated or disappointed by life
4. Attainment of several long-term goals
5. Satisfaction with personal growth and development
6. When married, feelings of mutual love for partner; when single, satisfaction with social interactions
7. Satisfaction with friendships
8. Generally cheerful attitude
9. No sensitivity to criticism
10. No unrealistic fears

Health Risks

Health risk factors for a young adult originate in the community, lifestyle patterns, and family history. The lifestyle habits that activate the stress response (see Chapter 37) increase the risk of illness. Smoking is a well-documented risk factor for pulmonary, cardiac, and vascular diseases in smokers and the individuals who receive secondhand smoke. Inhaled cigarette pollutants increase the risk of lung cancer, emphysema, and chronic bronchitis. The nicotine in tobacco is a vasoconstrictor that acts on the coronary arteries, increasing the risk of angina, myocardial infarction, and coronary artery disease. Nicotine also causes peripheral vasoconstriction and leads to vascular problems.

Family History. A family history of a disease puts a young adult at risk for developing it in the middle or older adult years. For example, a young man whose father and paternal grandfather had myocardial infarctions (heart attacks) in their 50s has a risk for a future myocardial infarction. The presence of certain chronic illnesses such as diabetes mellitus in the family increases the family member's risk of developing a disease. Regular physical examinations and screening are necessary at this stage of development.

Personal Hygiene Habits. As in all age-groups, personal hygiene habits in the young adult are risk factors. Sharing eating utensils with a person who has a contagious illness increases the risk of illness. Poor dental hygiene increases the risk of periodontal disease. Individuals avoid gingivitis (inflammation of the gums) and periodontitis (loss of tooth support) through oral hygiene (see Chapter 39).

Violent Death and Injury. Violence is a common cause of mortality and morbidity in the young-adult population. Factors that predispose individuals to violence, injury, or death include poverty, family breakdown, child abuse and neglect, drug involvement (dealing or illegal use), repeated exposure to violence, and ready access to guns. It is important for the nurse to perform a thorough psychosocial assessment, including such factors as behavior patterns, history of physical and substance abuse, education, work history, and social support systems to detect personal and environmental risk factors for violence. Death and injury occur from physical assaults, motor vehicle or other accidents, and suicide attempts. In 2007, homicides occurred at a higher rate among men and people ages 20 to 24 years than other violent deaths (USDHHS, CDC, 2010a).

Intimate partner violence (IPV), formerly referred to as domestic violence, is a global public health problem. It exists along a continuum from a single episode of violence to ongoing battering (USDHHS, CDC, 2009a). IPV often begins with emotional or mental abuse and may progress to physical or sexual assault. Each year women in the United States experience approximately 4.8 million intimate partner–related physical assaults and rapes, and men are the victims of approximately 2.9 intimate partner–related physical assaults. Physical injuries from IPV range from minor cuts and bruises to broken bones, internal bleeding, and head trauma.

IPV is linked to such harmful health behaviors as smoking, alcohol abuse, drug use, and risky sexual activity. Risk factors for the perpetration of IPV include using drugs or alcohol, especially drinking heavily; unemployment; low self-esteem; antisocial or borderline personality traits; desire for power and control in relationships; and being a victim of physical or psychological abuse (El-Bassel et al., 2007; Gil-Gonzalez et al., 2008). The greatest risk of violence occurs during the reproductive years. A pregnant woman has a 35.6% greater risk of being a victim of IPV than a nonpregnant woman. Women experiencing IPV may be more likely to delay prenatal care and are at increased risk for multiple poor maternal and infant health outcomes such as low maternal weight gain, infections, high blood pressure, vaginal bleeding, and delivery of a preterm or low-birth-weight infant (NACCHO, 2008).

Substance Abuse. Substance abuse directly or indirectly contributes to mortality and morbidity in young adults. Intoxicated young adults are often severely injured in motor vehicle accidents, resulting in death or permanent disability to other young adults as well.

Dependence on stimulant or depressant drugs sometimes results in death. Overdose of a stimulant drug ("upper") stresses the cardiovascular and nervous systems to the extent that death occurs. The use of depressants ("downers") leads to an accidental or intentional overdose and death.

Caffeine is a naturally occurring legal stimulant that is readily available in carbonated beverages; chocolate-containing foods; coffee and tea; and over-the-counter medications such as cold tablets, allergy and analgesic preparations, and appetite suppressants. It is the most widely ingested stimulant in North America. Caffeine stimulates catecholamine release, which in turn stimulates the central nervous system; it also increases gastric acid secretion, heart rate, and basal metabolic rate. This alters blood pressure, increases diuresis, and relaxes smooth muscle. Consumption of large amounts of caffeine results in restlessness, anxiety, irritability, agitation, muscle tremor, sensory disturbances, heart palpitations, nausea or vomiting, and diarrhea in some individuals.

Substance abuse is not always diagnosable, particularly in its early stages. Nonjudgmental questions about use of legal drugs (prescribed drugs, tobacco, and alcohol), soft drugs (marijuana), and more problematic drugs (cocaine or heroin) are a routine part of any health assessment. Obtain important information by making specific inquiries about past medical problems, changes in food intake or sleep patterns, or problems of emotional lability. Reports of arrests because of driving while intoxicated, wife or child abuse, or disorderly conduct are reasons to investigate the possibility of drug abuse more carefully.

Unplanned Pregnancies. Unplanned pregnancies are a continued source of stress that may result in adverse health outcomes for the mother, infant, and family. Often young adults have educational and career goals that take precedence over family development. Interference with these goals affects future relationships and parent-child relationships.

Determination of situational factors that affect the progress and outcome of an unplanned pregnancy is important. Exploration of problems such as financial, career, and living accommodations; family support systems; potential parenting disorders; depression; and coping mechanisms is important in assessing the woman with an unplanned pregnancy.

Sexually Transmitted Infections. STIs are a major health problem in young adults. Examples of STIs include syphilis, chlamydia, gonorrhea, genital herpes, and acquired immunodeficiency syndrome (AIDS). STIs have immediate physical effects such as genital discharge, discomfort, and infection. They also lead to chronic disorders, infertility, or even death. They remain a major public health problem for sexually active people, with almost half of all new infections occurring in men and women younger than 24 years of age (USDHHS, CDC, 2009b). In 2008 20- to 24-year-old men had the highest rate of chlamydia among men (1056.1 per 100,000 population); chlamydia rates in men of this age-group increased by 12.6% from the previous year.

TABLE 13-1 Occupational Hazards/Exposures Associated with Diseases and Cancers

JOB CATEGORY	OCCUPATIONAL HAZARD/ EXPOSURE	WORK-RELATED CONDITION/ CANCER
Agricultural workers	Pesticides, infectious agents, gases, sunlight	Pesticide poisoning, "farmer's lung," skin cancer
Anesthetists	Anesthetic gases	Reproductive effects, cancer
Automobile workers	Asbestos, plastics, lead, solvents	Asbestosis, dermatitis
Carpenters	Wood dust, wood preservatives, adhesives	Nasopharyngeal cancer, dermatitis
Cement workers	Cement dust, metals	Dermatitis, bronchitis
Dry cleaners	Solvents	Liver disease, dermatitis
Dye workers	Dyestuffs, metals, solvents	Bladder cancer, dermatitis
Glass workers	Heat, solvents, metal powders	Cataracts
Hospital workers	Infectious agents, cleansers, latex gloves, radiation	Infections, latex allergies, unintentional injuries
Insulators	Asbestos, fibrous glass	Asbestosis, lung cancer, mesothelioma
Jackhammer operators	Vibration	Raynaud's phenomenon
Lathe operators	Metal dusts, cutting oils	Lung disease, cancer
Office computer workers	Repetitive wrist motion on computers; eyestrain	Tendonitis, carpal tunnel syndrome, tenosynovitis

From Stanhope M, Lancaster J: *Foundations of nursing in the community,* ed 3, St Louis, 2010, Mosby.

Environmental or Occupational Factors. A common environmental or occupational risk factor is exposure to work-related hazards or agents that cause diseases and cancer (Table 13-1). Examples include lung diseases such as silicosis from inhalation of talcum and silicon dust and emphysema from inhalation of smoke. Cancers resulting from occupational exposures may involve the lung, liver, brain, blood, or skin. Questions regarding occupational exposure to hazardous materials should be a routine part of your assessment.

Health Concerns

Health Promotion. Lifestyles (e.g., use of tobacco or alcohol) of young adults may put them at risk for illnesses or disabilities during their middle- or older-adult years. Young adults are also genetically susceptible to certain chronic diseases such as diabetes mellitus and familial hypercholesterolemia (Huether and McCance,

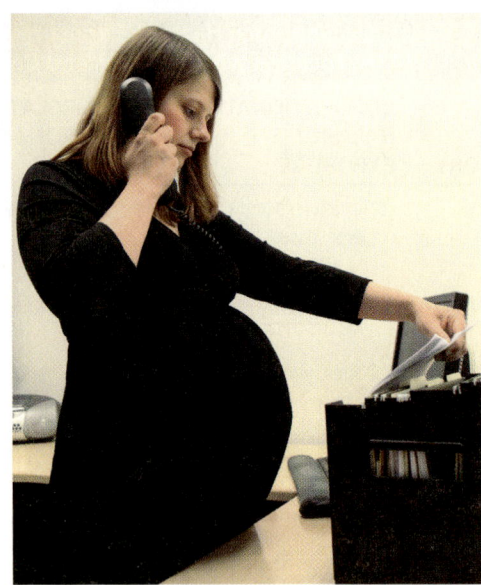

FIG. 13-3 The ability to handle day-to-day challenges at work minimizes stress.

2008). Some diseases that may appear in later years are avoidable if identified early. Encourage adults to perform monthly skin, breast, or male genital self-examination (see Chapter 30). Breast cancer is the most common major cancer among women in the United States, with a steadily increasing incidence. A nurse's role is extremely important in educating female patients about breast self-examinations (BSEs) and the current breast screening recommendations. Encourage routine assessment of the skin for recent changes in color or presence of lesions and changes in their appearance. Prolonged exposure to ultraviolet rays of the sun by adolescents and young adults increase the risk for development of skin cancer later in life. Crohn's disease, a chronic inflammatory disease of the small intestine, most commonly occurs between 15 and 35 years of age. Many young adults have misconceptions regarding transmission and treatment of STIs. Encourage partners to know one another's sexual history and practices. Be alert for STIs when patients come to clinics with complaints of urological or gynecological problems (see Chapter 34). Assess young adults for knowledge and use of safe-sex practices and genital self-examinations. Provide information on safe sex practice (e.g., use of condoms and having only one sex partner).

Psychosocial Health. The psychosocial health concerns of the young adult are often related to job and family stressors. As noted in Chapter 37, stress is valuable because it motivates a patient to change. However, if the stress is prolonged and the patient is unable to adapt to the stressor, health problems develop.

Job Stress. Job stress can occur every day or from time to time. Most young adults are able to handle day-to-day crises (Fig. 13-3). Situational job stress occurs when a new boss enters the workplace, a deadline is approaching, or the worker has new or greater numbers of responsibilities. A recent trend in today's business world and a risk factor for job stress is corporate downsizing, leading to increased responsibilities for employees with fewer positions within the corporate structure. Job stress also occurs when a person becomes dissatisfied with a job or the associated responsibilities. Because individuals perceive jobs differently, the types of job stressors vary from patient to patient. A nurse's assessment of a young adult includes a description of the usual work performed. Job assessment also includes conditions and hours, duration of employment, changes in sleep or eating habits, and evidence of increased irritability or nervousness.

Family Stress. Because of the multiplicity of changing relationships and structures in the emerging young adult family, stress is frequently high (see Chapter 10). Situational stressors occur during events such as births, deaths, illnesses, marriages, and job losses. Stress is often related to a number of variables, including the career paths of both husband and wife, and leads to dysfunction in the young adult family. This is reflected in the fact that the highest divorce rate occurs during the first 3 to 5 years of marriage for young adults under the age of 30. When a patient seeks health care and presents stress-related symptoms, the nurse needs to assess for the occurrence of a life-change event.

Each family member has certain predictable roles or jobs. These roles enable the family to function and be an effective part of society. When they change as a result of illness, a situational crisis often occurs. Assess environmental and familial factors, including support systems and coping mechanisms commonly used by family members.

Infertility. The term **infertility** refers to a prolonged time to conceive. An estimated 10% to 15% of reproductive couples are infertile, and many are young adults. However, approximately half of the couples evaluated and treated in infertility clinics become pregnant. In about 15% of infertile couples the cause is unknown. Female factors such as ovulatory dysfunction or a pelvic factor is responsible for infertility in 50% of couples, and infertility in 35% of couples is caused by a male factor such as sperm and semen abnormalities. For some infertile couples a nurse is the first resource they identify. Nursing assessment of the infertile couple includes both comprehensive histories of the male and female partners to determine factors that have affected fertility and pertinent physical findings (Lowdermilk and Perry, 2007).

Obesity. Obesity is a major health problem in young adults and is recognized as a risk factor for other health problems later in life. Obesity, influenced by poor diet and inactivity, has been linked to the development of conditions such as type 2 diabetes, hypertension, high cholesterol, asthma, joint problems, psoriatic arthritis, and poor health status (Ogdie and Gelfand, 2010; Soltani-Arabshashi et al., 2010; USDHHS, CDC, 2010b). Studies are linking time spent by young adults in sedentary behaviors such as watching television or being on the computer with increased abdominal obesity (Cleland et al, 2008). Nursing assessment of diet and physical activity of young adults is an important part of data collection. All young adults should be counseled about the benefits of a healthful diet and physical activity.

Exercise. People of all ages, both male and female, benefit from regular physical activity (USDHHS, 2002); however, young adults are spending increasingly more time with technology and less time engaged in physical activity. Exercise in young adults is important to prevent or decrease the development of chronic health conditions such as high blood pressure, obesity, and diabetes that develop later in life. Exercise improves cardiopulmonary function by decreasing blood pressure and heart rate; increases the strength and size of muscles; and decreases fatigability, insomnia, tension, and irritability. Conduct a thorough musculoskeletal assessment and exercise history to develop a realistic exercise plan. Encourage regular exercise within the patient's daily schedule.

Pregnant Woman and Childbearing Family. A developmental task for most young adult couples is the decision to begin a family. Although the physiological changes of pregnancy and childbirth occur only in the woman, cognitive and psychosocial changes and health concerns affect the entire childbearing family, including the baby's father, siblings, and grandparents. Single-parent families and young single mothers tend to be particularly vulnerable both economically and socially.

Health Practices. Women who are anticipating pregnancy benefit from good health practices before conception; these include a balanced diet, exercise, dental checkups, avoidance of alcohol, and cessation of smoking.

Prenatal Care. **Prenatal care** is the routine examination of the pregnant woman by an obstetrician or advanced practice nurse such as a nurse practitioner or certified nurse midwife. Prenatal care includes a thorough physical assessment of the pregnant woman during regularly scheduled intervals; provision of information regarding STIs, other vaginal infections, and urinary infections that adversely affect the fetus; and counseling about exercise patterns, diet, and child care. Regular prenatal care addresses health concerns that may arise during the pregnancy.

Physiological Changes. The physiological changes and needs of the pregnant woman vary with each trimester. Be familiar with them, their causes, and implications for nursing. All women experience some physiological changes in the first trimester. For example, they commonly have morning sickness, breast enlargement and tenderness, and fatigue. During the second trimester growth of the uterus and fetus results in some of the physical signs of pregnancy. During the third trimester increases in **Braxton Hicks contractions** (irregular, short contractions), fatigue, and urinary frequency occur.

Puerperium. The **puerperium** is a period of approximately 6 weeks after delivery. During this time the woman's body reverts to its prepregnant physical status. Determine the woman's knowledge of and ability to care for both herself and for her newborn baby. Assessment of parenting skills and maternal-infant interactions is particularly important. The process of **lactation** or breastfeeding offers many advantages to both the new mother and baby. For the inexperienced mother breastfeeding can be a source of anxiety and frustration. Be alert for signs that the mother needs information and assistance (Dunn et al., 2006).

Needs for Education. The entire childbearing family needs education about pregnancy, labor, delivery, breastfeeding, and integration of the newborn into the family structure.

Psychosocial Changes. Like the physiological changes of pregnancy, psychosocial changes occur at various times during the 9 months of pregnancy and in the puerperium. Table 13-2 summarizes the major categories of psychosocial changes and implications for nursing intervention.

Health Concerns. The pregnant woman and her partner have many health questions. For example, they wonder whether the pregnancy and baby will be normal. The majority of the health needs related to pregnancy are met with proper prenatal care.

Acute Care. Young adults typically require acute care for accidents, substance abuse, exposure to environmental and occupational hazards, stress-related illnesses, respiratory infections, gastroenteritis, influenza, urinary tract infections, and minor surgery. An acute minor illness causes a disruption in life activities of young adults and increases stress in an already hectic lifestyle. Dependency and limitations posed by treatment regimens also increase frustration. To give them a sense of maintaining control of their health care choices, it is important to keep them informed about their health status and involve them in health care decisions.

Restorative and Continuing Care. Chronic conditions are not common in young adulthood, but they sometimes occur. Chronic illnesses such as hypertension, coronary artery disease, and diabetes have their onset in young adulthood but may not be recognized until later in life. Causes of chronic illness and disability in the young adult include accidents, multiple sclerosis, rheumatoid arthritis, AIDS, and cancer. Chronic illness or disability threatens a young adult's independence and results in the need to change personal, family, and career goals. Nursing interventions for the young adult faced with chronic illness or disability need to focus on problems related to sense of identity, establishing independence, reorganizing intimate relationships and family structure, and launching a chosen career (Santacroce and Lee, 2006).

TABLE 13-2 Major Psychosocial Changes During Pregnancy

CATEGORY	IMPLICATIONS FOR NURSING
Body image	Morning sickness and fatigue contribute to poor body image. Woman feels big, awkward, and unattractive during third trimester when fetus is growing more rapidly. Increase in breast size sometimes makes the woman feel more feminine and sexually appealing. Woman takes extra time with hygiene and grooming, trying new hairstyles and makeup. Woman begins to "show" during the second trimester and starts to plan maternity wardrobe. Woman has general feeling of well-being when she feels the baby move and hears the heartbeat.
Role changes	Both partners think about and have feelings of uncertainty about impending role changes. Both partners have feelings of ambivalence about becoming parents and concern about ability to be parents.
Sexuality	Woman needs reassurance that sexual activity will not harm fetus. Woman's desire for sexual activity is influenced by body image. Woman desires cuddling and holding rather than sexual intercourse.
Coping mechanisms	Woman needs reassurance that childbirth and childrearing are natural and positive experiences but are also stressful. Woman is often unable to cope with particular stressors such as finding new housing, preparing the nursery, or participating in childbirth classes.
Stresses during puerperium	Woman returns home from hospital fatigued and unfamiliar with infant care. Woman experiences physical discomfort or feelings of anxiety or depression. Woman must return to work soon after delivery with subsequent feelings of guilt, anxiety, or, possibly a sense of freedom or relief.

MIDDLE ADULTS

In 2009 39.8% of the population was middle-age adults between the ages of 35 and 64, a slight increase over the 2005 data (U.S. Census Bureau, 2010). In middle adulthood the individual makes

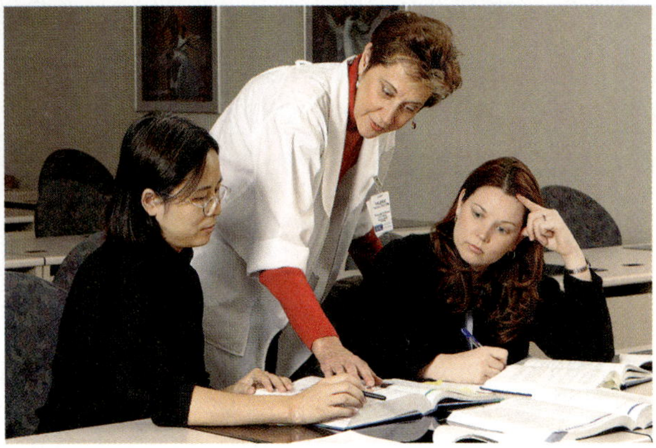

FIG. 13-4 Middle adults enjoy helping young people become productive and responsible adults.

lasting contributions through involvement with others. Generally the middle-adult years begin around the early to mid 30s and last through the late 60s, corresponding to Levinson's developmental phases of "settling down" and the "payoff years." During this period personal and career achievements have often already been experienced. Many middle adults find particular joy in helping their children and other young people become productive and responsible adults (Fig. 13-4). They also begin to help aging parents while being responsible for their own children, placing them in the **sandwich generation.** Using leisure time in satisfying and creative ways is a challenge that, if met satisfactorily, enables middle adults to prepare for retirement.

Although most middle adults have achieved socioeconomic stability, recent trends in corporate downsizing have left many either jobless or forced to accept lower-paying jobs. According to the U.S. Census Bureau (2009), the real median household income in the United States fell 3.6% between 2007 and 2008, and the number of people without health insurance coverage rose from 45.7 million in 2007 to 46.3 million in 2008. As a result, a greater proportion of the population became unable to afford adequate health care.

Men and women need to adjust to inevitable biological changes. As in adolescence, middle adults use considerable energy to adapt self-concept and body image to physiological realities and changes in physical appearance. High self-esteem, a favorable body image, and a positive attitude toward physiological changes occur when adults engage in physical exercise, balanced diets, adequate sleep, and good hygiene practices that promote vigorous, healthy bodies.

Physical Changes

Major physiological changes occur between 40 and 65 years of age. Because of this it is important to assess the middle adult's general health status. A comprehensive assessment offers direction for health promotion recommendations and planning and implementing any acutely needed interventions. The most visible changes during middle adulthood are graying of the hair, wrinkling of the skin, and thickening of the waist. Decreases in hearing and visual acuity are often evident during this period. Often these physiological changes during middle adulthood have an impact on self-concept and body image. Table 13-3 summarizes abnormal findings to consider when conducting a physical examination (see Chapter 30). The most significant physiological changes during middle age are menopause in women and the climacteric in men.

Perimenopause and Menopause. Menstruation and ovulation occur in a cyclical rhythm in women from adolescence into middle adulthood. Perimenopause is the period during which ovarian function declines, resulting in a diminishing number of ova and irregular menstrual cycles, and generally lasts 1 to 3 years. **Menopause** is the disruption of this cycle, primarily because of the inability of the neurohormonal system to maintain its periodic stimulation of the endocrine system. The ovaries no longer produce estrogen and progesterone, and the blood levels of these hormones drop markedly. Menopause typically occurs between 45 and 60 years of age (see Chapter 34). Approximately 10% of women have no symptoms of menopause other than cessation of menstruation, 70% to 80% are aware of other changes but have no problems, and approximately 10% experience changes severe enough to interfere with activities of daily living.

Climacteric. The **climacteric** occurs in men in their late 40s or early 50s (see Chapter 34). Decreased levels of androgens cause climacteric. Throughout this period and thereafter a man is still capable of producing fertile sperm and fathering a child. However, penile erection is less firm, ejaculation is less frequent, and the refractory period is longer.

Cognitive Changes

Changes in the cognitive function of middle adults are rare except with illness or trauma. Some middle adults enter educational or vocational programs to prepare themselves with new skills and information for entering the job market or changing jobs.

Psychosocial Changes

The psychosocial changes in the middle adult involve expected events such as children moving away from home and unexpected events such as a marital separation or the death of a close friend.

The nurse assesses major life changes occurring in any middle adult for whom he or she cares and the impact that the changes have on that person's state of health. Individual psychosocial factors such as coping mechanisms and sources of social support should also be included in the assessment.

In the middle-adult years, as children depart from the household, the family enters the postparental family stage. Time and financial demands on the parents decrease, and the couple faces the task of redefining their own relationship. It is during this period that many middle adults take on healthier lifestyles. Assessment of health promotion needs for the middle adult includes adequate rest, leisure activities, regular exercise, good nutrition, reduction or cessation in the use of tobacco or alcohol, and regular screening examinations. Assessment of the middle adult's social environment is also important, including relationship concerns; communication and relationships with children, grandchildren, and aging parents; and caregiver concerns with their own aging or disabled parents.

Career Transition. Career changes occur by choice or as a result of changes in the workplace or society. In recent decades middle adults change occupations more often for a variety of reasons, including limited upward mobility, decreasing availability of jobs, and seeking an occupation that is more challenging. In some cases downsizing, technological advances, or other changes force middle adults to seek new jobs. Such changes, particularly when unanticipated, result in stress that affects health, family relationships, self-concept, and other dimensions.

Sexuality. After the departure of their last child from the home, many couples recultivate their relationships and find increased marital and sexual satisfaction during middle age. The onset of menopause and the climacteric affect the sexual health of the middle adult. Some women may desire increased sexual activity because pregnancy is no longer possible. Menopausal women also

TABLE 13-3 **Abnormal Physical Assessment Findings in the Middle Adult**

BODY SYSTEM	ASSESSMENT FINDINGS
Integument	Very thin skin Rough, flaky, dry skin Lesions
Scalp and hair	Excessive generalized hair loss or patchy hair loss Excessive scaliness
Head and neck	Large, thick skull and facial bones Asymmetry in movement of head and/or neck Drooping of one side of the face
Eyes	Reduced peripheral vision Asymmetrical position of the light reflex Drooping of the upper lid (ptosis) Redness or crusting around the eyelids
Ears	Discharge of any kind Reddened, swollen ear canals
Nose, sinuses, and throat	Nasal tenderness Occlusion of nostril Swollen and pale pink or bluish-gray nasal mucosa Sinuses tender to palpation or on percussion Asymmetrical movement or loss of movement of uvula Tonsils red or enlarged
Thorax and lungs	Unequal chest expansion Unequal fremitus, hyperresonance, diminished or absent breath sounds Adventitious lung sounds such as crackles and wheezes
Heart and vascular system	Pulse inequality, weak pulses, bounding pulses, or variations in strength of pulse from beat to beat Bradycardia or tachycardia Hypertension Hypotension
Breasts—female	Recent increase in size of one breast Pigskinlike or orange-peel appearance Redness or painful breasts
Breasts—male	Soft, fatty enlargement of breast tissue
Abdomen	Bruises, areas of local discoloration; purple discoloration; pale, taut skin Generalized abdominal distention Hypoactive, hyperactive, decreased, or absent bowel sounds
Female genitalia	Asymmetrical labia Swelling, pain, or discharge from Bartholin's glands Decreased tone of vaginal musculature Cervical enlargement or projection into the vagina Reddened areas or lesions in the vagina
Male genitalia	Rashes, lesions, or lumps on skin of shaft of penis Discharge from penis Enlarged scrotal sac Bulges that appear at the external inguinal ring or femoral canal when the patient bears down
Musculoskeletal system	Uneven weight bearing Decreased range of joint motion; swollen, red, or enlarged joint; painful joints Decreased strength against resistance
Neurological system	Lethargy Inadequate motor responses Abnormal sensory system responses: inability to smell certain aromas, loss of visual fields, inability to feel and correctly identify facial stimuli, absent gag reflex

experience vaginal dryness and dyspareunia or pain during sexual intercourse (see Chapter 34).

During middle age a man may notice changes in the strength of his erection and a decrease in his ability to experience repeated orgasm. Other factors influencing sexuality during this period include work stress, diminished health of one or both partners, and the use of prescription medications. For example, antihypertensive agents have side effects that influence sexual desire or functioning. Sometimes both partners experience stresses related to sexual changes or a conflict between their sexual needs and self-perceptions and social attitudes or expectations (see Chapter 34).

Family Psychosocial Factors. Psychosocial factors involving the family include the stresses of singlehood, marital changes, transition of the family as children leave home, and the care of aging parents.

Singlehood. Many adults over 35 years of age in the United States have never been married. Many of these are college-educated people who have embraced the philosophy of choice and freedom, delayed marriage, and delayed parenthood. Some middle adults choose to remain single but also opt to become parents either biologically or through adoption. Many single middle adults have no relatives but share a family type of relationship with close friends or work associates. Consequently some single middle adults feel isolated during traditional "family" holidays such as Thanksgiving or Christmas. In times of illness middle adults who have chosen to remain single and childless have to rely on other relatives or friends, increasing caregiving demands of family members who also have other responsibilities. Nursing assessment of single middle adults needs to include a thorough assessment of psychosocial factors, including the individual's definition of family and available support systems.

Marital Changes. Marital changes occurring during middle age include death of a spouse, separation, divorce, and the choice of remarrying or remaining single. A widowed, separated, or divorced patient goes through a period of grief and loss in which it is necessary to adapt to the change in marital status. Normal grieving progresses through a series of phases, and resolution of grief often takes a year or more. You need to assess the level of coping of the middle adult to the grief and loss associated with certain life changes (see Chapter 36).

Family Transitions. The departure of the last child from the home is also a stressor. Many parents welcome freedom from childrearing responsibilities, whereas others feel lonely or without direction. *Empty nest syndrome* is the term used to describe the sadness and loneliness that accompany children leaving home. Eventually parents need to reassess their marriage and try to resolve conflicts and plan for the future. Occasionally this readjustment phase leads to marital conflicts, separation, and divorce (see Chapter 10).

Care of Aging Parents. Increasing life spans in the United States and Canada have led to increased numbers of older adults in the population. Therefore greater numbers of middle adults need to address the personal and social issues confronting their aging parents. Many middle adults find themselves caught between the responsibilities of caring for dependent children and those of caring for aging and ailing parents. These middle adults thus find themselves in the sandwich generation, in which the challenges of caregiving can be stressful. The needs of family caregivers are being given more emphasis in the health care system.

Housing, employment, health, and economic realities have changed the traditional social expectations between generations in families. The middle adult and older-adult parent often have conflicting relationship priorities while the older adult strives to remain independent. Negotiations and compromises help to define and resolve problems. Nurses deal with middle and older adults in the community, long-term care facilities, and hospitals. Help identify the health needs of both groups and assist the multigenerational family in determining the health and community resources available to them as they make decisions and plans. Evaluate family relationships to determine family members' perceptions of responsibility and loyalty in relation to caring for older-adult members. Assessment of environmental resources (e.g., number of rooms in the house or stairwells) in relation to the complexity of health care demands for the older adult is also important.

Health Concerns

Health Promotion and Stress Reduction. Because middle adults experience physiological changes and face certain health realities, their perceptions of health and health behaviors are often important factors in maintaining health. Today's complex world makes individuals more prone to stress-related illnesses such as heart attacks, hypertension, migraine headaches, ulcers, colitis, autoimmune disease, backache, arthritis, and cancer. When adults seek health care, nurses focus on the goal of wellness and guide patients to evaluate health behaviors, lifestyle, and environment.

Throughout life people have many stressors (see Chapter 37). After identifying these stressors, work with the patient to intervene and modify the stress response. Specific interventions for stress reduction fall into three categories. First minimize the frequency of stress-producing situations. Together with the patient identify approaches to preventing stressful situations such as habituation, change avoidance, time blocking, time management, and environmental modification. Second, increase stress resistance such as increasing self-esteem, improving assertiveness, redirecting goal alternatives, and reorienting cognitive appraisal. Finally, avoid the physiological response to stress. Use relaxation techniques, imagery, and biofeedback to recondition the patient's response to stress. Chapters 36 and 37 explain these general interventions in greater detail.

Obesity. Obesity is a growing, expensive health concern for middle adults. It can reduce quality of life and increases risk for many serious chronic diseases and premature death. In 2007 no state in the United States had met the Healthy People 2010 objective to reduce obesity prevalence among adults to 15% (USDHHS, CDC, 2010b). Health consequences of obesity include such ailments as high blood pressure, high blood cholesterol, type 2 (non-insulin dependent) diabetes, coronary heart disease, osteoarthritis, and obstructive sleep apnea. Continued focus on the goal of wellness helps patients evaluate health behaviors and lifestyle that contribute to obesity during the middle adult years. Counseling related to physical activity and nutrition is an important component of the plan of care for overweight and obese patients.

Forming Positive Health Habits. A habit is a person's usual practice or manner of behavior. Frequent repetition reinforces this behavior pattern until it becomes the individual's customary way of behaving. Some habits support health such as exercise and brushing and flossing the teeth each day. Other habits involve risk factors to health such as smoking or eating foods with little or no nutritional value.

During assessment a nurse frequently obtains data indicating positive and negative health behaviors by a patient. Examples of positive health behaviors include regular exercise, adherence to good dietary habits, avoidance of excess consumption of alcohol, participation in routine screening and diagnostic tests (e.g., laboratory screening for serum cholesterol or mammography) for disease prevention and health promotion, and lifestyle changes to reduce stress. The nurse helps the patient maintain habits that protect health and offers healthier alternatives to poor habits.

Health teaching and counseling often focus on improving health habits. The more you understand the dynamics of behavior and habits, the more likely it is that your interventions will help patients achieve or reinforce health-promoting behaviors.

To help patients form positive health habits, you act as a teacher and facilitator. By providing information about how the body functions and how patients form and change habits, patients' levels of knowledge regarding the potential impact of behavior on health are raised. You cannot change your patients' habits. They have control of and are responsible for their own behaviors. Explain psychological principles of changing habits and offer information about health risks. Offer positive reinforcement (such as praise and rewards) for health-directed behaviors and decisions. Such reinforcement increases the likelihood that the behavior will be repeated. However, ultimately the patient decides which behaviors will become habits of daily living.

Help middle adults consider factors such as prevention of STIs, substance abuse, and accident prevention in relation to decreasing health risks. For example, provide patients with factual information on STI causes, symptoms, and transmission. Discuss methods of protection during sexual activity with a patient in an open and nonjudgmental manner and reinforce the importance of practicing safe sex (see Chapter 34). Provide counseling and support for patients seeking treatment for substance abuse. Help them recognize and alter unsafe and potential health hazards. In addition, encourage them to express their feelings so they become proficient in solving problems and recognizing risk factors themselves. Barriers to change exist (Box 13-3). Unless you minimize or eliminate these barriers, it is futile to encourage the patient to take action.

Psychosocial Health

Anxiety. Anxiety is a critical maturational phenomenon related to change, conflict, and perceived control of the environment. Adults often experience anxiety in response to the physiological and psychosocial changes of middle age. Such anxiety motivates the adult to rethink life goals and stimulates productivity. However, for some adults this anxiety precipitates psychosomatic illness and preoccupation with death. In this case the middle adult views life as being half or more over and thinks in terms of the time left to live.

Clearly a life-threatening illness, marital transition, or job stressor increases the anxiety of a patient and family. Use crisis intervention or stress-management techniques to help a patient adapt to the changes of the middle-adult years (see Chapter 37).

Depression. Depression is a mood disorder that manifests itself in many ways. Although the most frequent age of onset is between ages 25 and 44, it is common among adults in the middle years and has many causes. The risk factors for depression include being female; disappointments or losses at work, at school, or in family relationships; departure of the last child from the home; and family history. In fact, the incidence of depression in women is twice that of men. Persons experiencing mild depression describe themselves as feeling sad, blue, downcast, down in the dumps, and tearful. Other symptoms include alterations in sleep patterns such as difficulty in sleeping (insomnia) or sleeping too much (hypersomnia), irritability, feelings of social disinterest, and decreased alertness. Physical changes such as weight gain or loss, headaches, or feelings of fatigue regardless of the amount of rest are also depressive symptoms. Individuals with depression that occurs during the middle years commonly experience moderate-to-high anxiety and have physical complaints. Mood changes and depression are common occurrences during menopause. The abuse of alcohol or other substances makes depression worse. Nursing assessment of the depressed middle adult includes focused data collection regarding individual and family history of depression, mood changes, cognitive changes, behavioral and social changes, and physical changes. Collect assessment data from both the patient and the patient's family because family data are often particularly important, depending on the level of depression the middle adult is experiencing.

Community Health Programs. Community health programs offer services to prevent illness, promote health, and detect disease in the early stages. Nurses make valuable contributions to the health of the community by taking an active part in planning screening and teaching programs and support groups for middle adults.

Family planning, birthing, and parenting skills are program topics in which adults are usually interested. Health screening for diabetes, hypertension, eye disease, and cancer is a good opportunity for the nurse to perform assessment and provide health teaching and health counseling.

Health education programs promote changes in behavior and lifestyle. As a health teacher, offer information that enables patients to make decisions about health practices within the context of health promotion for young-to-middle adults. Make sure that educational programs are culturally appropriate. Changes to more positive health practices during young and middle adulthood lead to fewer or less complicated health problems as an older adult. During health counseling, collaborate with the patient to design a plan of action that addresses the patient's health and well-being. Through objective problem solving, you can help the patient grow and change.

Acute Care. Acute illnesses and conditions experienced in middle adulthood are similar to those of young adulthood. However, injuries and acute illnesses in middle adulthood require a longer recovery period because of the slowing of healing processes. In addition, acute illnesses and injuries experienced in middle adulthood are more likely to become chronic conditions. For middle adults in the sandwich generation, stress levels also increase as he or she tries to balance responsibilities related to employment, family life, care of children, and care of aging parents while recovering from an injury or acute illness.

Restorative and Continuing Care. Chronic illnesses such as diabetes mellitus, hypertension, rheumatoid arthritis, or multiple sclerosis affect the roles and responsibilities of the middle adult. Some results of chronic illness are strained family relationships, modifications in family activities, increased health care tasks, increased financial stress, the need for housing adaptation, social isolation, medical concerns, and grieving. The degree of disability and the patient's perception of both the illness and the disability determine the extent to which lifestyle changes occur. A few examples of the problems experienced by patients who develop debilitating chronic illness during adulthood include role reversal,

BOX 13-3 BARRIERS TO CHANGE

External Barriers	Internal Barriers
• Lack of facilities	• Lack of knowledge
• Lack of materials	• Insufficient skills to effect change in health habits
• Lack of social supports	• Undefined short- and long-term goals
• Lack of motivation	

changes in sexual behavior, and alterations in self-image. Along with the current health status of the chronically ill middle adult, you need to assess the knowledge base of both the patient and family. This assessment includes the medical course of the illness and the prognosis for the patient. In addition, you must determine the coping mechanisms of the patient and family; adherence to treatment and rehabilitation regimens; and the need for community and social services, along with appropriate referrals.

KEY POINTS

- Adult development involves orderly and sequential changes in characteristics and attitudes that adults experience over time.
- Many changes experienced by the young adult are related to the natural process of maturation and socialization.
- Young adults are in a stable period of physical development, except for changes related to pregnancy.
- Cognitive development continues throughout the young- and middle-adult years.
- Emotional health of young adults is correlated with the ability to address and resolve personal and social problems.
- Young adults choose a career and decide whether to remain single or marry and begin a family.
- Pregnant women need to understand physiological changes occurring in each trimester.
- Psychosocial changes and health concerns during pregnancy and the puerperium affect the parents, the siblings, and often the extended family.
- Prenatal care reduces maternal and fetal mortality and morbidity.
- Midlife transition begins when a person becomes aware that physiological and psychosocial changes signify passage to another stage in life.
- Two significant physiological changes of the middle years are menopause in women and the climacteric in men.
- Cognitive changes are rare in middle age except in cases of illness or physical trauma.
- Psychosocial changes for middle adults are often related to career transition, sexuality, marital changes, family transition, and care of aging parents.
- Health concerns of middle adults commonly involve stress-related illnesses, health assessment, and adoption of positive health habits.

CLINICAL APPLICATION QUESTIONS

Preparing for Clinical Practice

A 24-year-old female patient who smokes two packs of cigarettes per day has come to the clinic to talk with the nurse about quitting smoking. She began smoking when she was 14 years old. She complains to the nurse at the clinic, "I just can't seem to kick the habit no matter how hard I try. I am smoking more now because of increased stress from my job."

1. What information does the nurse need to know to help this patient quit smoking?
2. Which factors will have the greatest impact on health promotion related to smoking cessation in this patient?
3. What steps should the nurse take to help this patient decrease her stress?

evolve *Answers to Clinical Application Questions can be found on the Evolve website.*

REVIEW QUESTIONS

Are You Ready to Test Your Nursing Knowledge?

1. With the exception of pregnant or lactating women, the young adult has usually completed physical growth by the age of:
   1. 18.
   2. 20.
   3. 25.
   4. 30.
2. The nurse is completing an assessment on a male patient, age 24. Following the assessment, the nurse notes that his physical and laboratory findings are within normal limits. Because of these findings, nursing interventions are directed toward activities related to:
   1. Instructing him to return in 2 years.
   2. Instructing him in secondary prevention.
   3. Instructing him in health promotion activities.
   4. Implementing primary prevention with vaccines.
3. When determining the amount of information that a patient needs to make decisions about the prescribed course of therapy, many factors affect the patient's compliance with the regimen, including educational level and socioeconomic factors. Which additional factor affects compliance?
   1. Gender
   2. Lifestyle
   3. Motivation
   4. Family history
4. A patient is laboring with her first baby, which is coming 2 weeks early. Her husband is in the military and might not get back in time, and both families are unable to be with her during labor. The doctor decides to call in which of the following people employed by the birthing area to be a support person to be present during labor?
   1. Nurse
   2. Midwife
   3. Assistant
   4. Lay doula
5. A single young adult female interacts with a group of close friends from college and work. They celebrate birthdays and holidays together. In addition, they help one another through many stressors. She views these individuals as:
   1. Family.
   2. Siblings.
   3. Substitute parents.
   4. Alternative family structure.
6. Sharing eating utensils with a person who has a contagious illness increases the risk of illness. This type of health risk arises from:
   1. Lifestyle.
   2. Community.
   3. Family history.
   4. Personal hygiene habits.
7. A 50-year-old woman has elevated cholesterol profile values that increase her cardiovascular risk factor. One method to control this risk factor is to identify current diet trends and describe dietary changes to reduce the risk. This nursing activity is a form of:
   1. Referral.
   2. Counseling.
   3. Health education
   4. Stress management techniques.

8. A 34-year-old female executive has a job with frequent deadlines. She notes that, when the deadlines appear, she has a tendency to eat high-fat, high-carbohydrate foods. She also explains that she gets frequent headaches and stomach pain during these deadlines. The nurse provides a number of options for the executive, and she chooses yoga. In this scenario yoga is used as a(n):
   1. Outpatient referral.
   2. Counseling technique.
   3. Health promotion activity.
   4. Stress-management technique.
9. A 50-year-old male patient is seen in the clinic. He tells the nurse that he has recently lost his job and his wife of 26 years has asked for a divorce. He has a flat affect. Family history reveals that his father committed suicide at the age of 53. The nurse should assess for the following:
   1. Cardiovascular disease
   2. Depression
   3. Sexually transmitted infection
   4. Iron deficiency anemia
10. Middle-age adults frequently find themselves trying to balance responsibilities related to employment, family life, care of children, and care of aging parents. People finding themselves in this situation are frequently referred to as being a part of:
   1. The sandwich generation.
   2. The millennial generation.
   3. Generation X.
   4. Generation Y.
11. Intimate partner violence (IPV) is linked to which of the following factors? (Select all that apply.)
   1. Alcohol abuse
   2. Pregnancy
   3. Unemployment
   4. Drug use
12. Sexually transmitted infections (STIs) continue to be a major health problem in young adults. Men ages 20 to 24 years have the highest rate of which STI?
   1. Chlamydia
   2. Syphilis
   3. Gonorrhea
   4. Herpes zoster
13. Formation of positive health habits may prevent the development of chronic illness later in life. Which of the following are examples of positive health habits? (Select all that apply.)
   1. Routine screening and diagnostic tests
   2. Unprotected sexual activity
   3. Regular exercise
   4. Excess alcohol consumption
14. Chronic illness (e.g., diabetes mellitus, hypertension, rheumatoid arthritis) may affect a person's roles and responsibilities during middle adulthood. When assessing the knowledge base of both the middle-age patient with a chronic illness and his family, the assessment should include which of the following? (Select all that apply.)
   1. The medical course of the illness
   2. The prognosis for the patient
   3. Coping mechanisms of the patient and family
   4. The need for community and social services
15. A 45-year-old obese woman tells the nurse that she wants to lose weight. After conducting a thorough assessment, the nurse concludes that which of the following may be contributing factors to the woman's obesity? (Select all that apply.)
   1. The woman works in an executive position that is very demanding.
   2. The woman works out at the corporate gym at 5 AM two mornings per week
   3. The woman says that she has little time to prepare meals at home and eats out at least four nights a week.
   4. The woman says that she tries to eat "low cholesterol" foods to help lose weight.

Answers: **1.** 2; **2.** 3; **3.** 3; **4.** 4; **5.** 1; **6.** 4; **7.** 3; **8.** 4; **9.** 2; **10.** 1; **11.** 1, 2, 3, 4; **12.** 1; **13.** 1, 3; **14.** 1, 2, 3, 4; **15.** 1, 3.

REFERENCES

AFL-CIO: *AFL-CIO celebrates international women's day,* March 7, 2008, http://www.aflcio.org/mediacenter/prsptm/pr03072008a.cfm. Accessed July 15, 2011.

American Academy of Pediatrics: Technical report: coparent or second-parent adoption by same-sex parents, *Pediatrics* 109(2):341, 2002, http://www.aappolicy.aappublications.org/cgi/content/full/pediatrics;102/2/339. Accessed October 12, 2011.

Beacham T, et al: Assessing postpartum depression in women, *Home Healthcare Nurse* 26(9):553, October 2008.

Beck C: Postpartum depression: it isn't just the blues, *Am J Nurs* 106(5):40, 2006.

Business and Professional Women's Foundation: *101 facts on the status of working women,* October 2007, http://www.bpusa.org/files/public/101factsPct07.pdf. Accessed July 15, 2011.

Diekelmann J: The young adult: the choice is health or illness, *Am J Nurs* 76:1276, 1976.

Dunn S, et al: The relationship between vulnerability factors and breastfeeding outcome, *J Obstet Gynecol Neonatal Nurs* 35(1):87, 2006.

Edelman C, Mandle C: *Health promotion throughout the life span,* ed 7, St Louis, 2010, Mosby.

Erikson E: *Childhood society,* ed 2, New York, 1963, WW Norton.

Erikson E: *The lifecycle completed: a review,* New York, 1982, WW Norton.

Fortinash K, Holoday Worret P: *Psychiatric mental health nursing,* ed 4, St Louis, 2008, Mosby.

Gates G, et al: Adoption and foster care by gay and lesbian parents in the United States, *The Williams Institute, UCLA School of Law,* March 2007, http://www.law.ucla.edu/williamsinstitute/publications/FinalAdoptionReport.pdf. Accessed July 15, 2011.

Gil-Gonzalez D, et al: Childhood experiences of violence in perpetrators as a risk factor of intimate partner violence: a systematic review, *J Public Health* 30(1):14, 2008.

Havighurst R: Successful aging. In Williams RH, Tibbits C, Donahue W, editors: *Process of aging,* vol 1, New York, 1972, Atherton.

Huether S, McCance K: *Understanding pathophysiology,* ed 4, St Louis, 2008, Mosby.

Knitzer J, Theberge S, Johnson K: Reducing maternal depression and its impact on young children, *National Center for Children in Poverty, Project THRIVE, Issue Brief No. 2,* January 2008, http://www.nccp.org/publications/pdf/text_791.pdf. Accessed July 15, 2011.

Levinson D, et al: *The seasons of a man's life,* New York, 1978, Knopf.

Lowdermilk D, Perry S: *Maternity and women's health care,* ed 9, St Louis, 2007, Mosby.

Makadon H: Improving health care for the lesbian and gay communities, *N Eng J Med* 354:895, 2006.

Masters W, Johnson V: *Human sexual response,* Boston, 1970, Little, Brown.

National Association of County & City Health Officials (NACCHO): *Intimate partner violence among pregnant and parenting women: local health department strategies for assessment, intervention, and prevention,* 2008, Washington, D.C., http://naccho.org/. Accessed July 15, 2011.

Pew Research Center: *Millennials: a portrait of generation,* February 2010, http://pewsocialtrends.org/assets/pdf/millennials-confident-connected-open-to-change.pdf. Accessed July 15, 2011.

Sanchez A, et al: Modeling innovative interventions for optimizing healthy lifestyle promotion in primary care, *BMC Health Services Research* 9(103), 2009, http://www.biomedcentral.com/content/pdf/1472-6963-9-103.pdf. Accessed July 15, 2011.

US Census Bureau: *Income, poverty and health insurance coverage in the United States,* 2008, September 2009, http://www.census.gov/prod/2009pubs/p60-236.pdf. Accessed July 15, 2011.

US Census Bureau: *Annual estimates of the white alone or in combination resident population by sex and age for the United States,* April 1, 2000 to July 1, 2009 (NC-EST2009-

04-WAC), August 2010, http://www.census.gov/popest/national/asrh/NC-EST2009-asrh.html. Accessed July 15, 2011.

US Department of Health and Human Services (USDHHS): *Healthy People 2010*, ed 2, McLean, Va, 2002, International Medical Publishing.

US Department of Health and Human Services (USDHHS), Centers for Disease Control and Prevention (CDC): *Understanding intimate partner violence fact sheet*, 2009a, http://www.cdc.gov/violenceprevention/pdf/IPV_factsheet-a.pdf. Accessed July 15, 2011.

US Department of Health and Human Services (USDHHS), Centers for Disease Control and Prevention (CDC): *Sexually transmitted disease surveillance, 2008*, November 2009b, http://www.cdc.gov/std/stats08/surv2008-Complete.pdf. Accessed July 15, 2011.

US Department of Health and Human Services (USDHHS), Centers for Disease Control and Prevention (CDC): Surveillance for violent deaths—national violent death reporting system, 16 states, 2007, *MMWR* 59(No SS-4) May 14, 2010a, www.cdc.gov/mmwr/PDF/ss/ss5904.pdf. Accessed July 15, 2011.

US Department of Health and Human Services (USDHHS), Centers for Disease Control and Prevention (CDC): Vital signs: State-specific prevalence of obesity among adults—United States, 2009, *MMWR* 59: 1, early release August 3, 2010b.

US Preventive Service Task Force (USPSTF): Screening for depression in adults: US preventive services task force recommendation statement, *Ann Intern Med* 151(11): 784, 2009.

RESEARCH REFERENCES

Akincigil A, et al: Predictors of maternal depression in the first year postpartum: marital status and mediating role of relationship quality, *Soc Work Health Care* 49(3):227, 2010.

Bei B, et al: Subjective perception of sleep, but not its objective quality, is association with immediate postpartum mood disturbances in health women, *Sleep* 33(4):531, 2010.

Campbell DA, et al: A randomized control trial of continuous support in labor by a lay doula, *J Obstet Gynecol Neonatal Nurs* 35(4):456, 2006.

Cleland V, et al: Television viewing and abdominal obesity in young adults: is the association mediated by food and beverage consumption during viewing time or reduced leisure-time physical activity? *Am J Clin Nutr* 87(5):1148, 2008.

Doucet S, et al: Differentiation and clinical implications of postpartum depression and postpartum psychosis, *J Obstet Gynecol Neonatal Nurs* 38(3):269, 2009.

El-Bassel N, et al: Perpetration of intimate partner violence among men in methadone treatment programs in New York City, *Am J Public Health* 97(7):1230, 2007.

McManus A, et al: Lesbian experiences and needs during childbirth: guidance for health care providers, *J Obstet Gynecol Neonatal Nurs* 35(1):13, 2006.

Ogdie A, Gelfand J: Identification of risk factors for psoriatic arthritis: scientific opportunity meets clinical need, *Arch Dermatol* 146:785, 2010.

Poobalan A, et al: Effects of treating postnatal depression on mother-infant interaction and child development, *Br J Psych* 191:378, 2007.

Records K, et al: Psychometric assessment of the Postpartum Depression Predictors Inventory-Revised, *J Nurs Measurement* 15(3):189, 2007.

Robertson K: Understanding the needs of women with postnatal depression, *Nurs Stand* 24(46):47, 2010.

Santacroce SJ, Lee YL: Uncertainty, posttraumatic stress, and health behavior in young adult childhood cancer survivors, *Nurs Res* 55(4):259, 2006.

Sauls DJ: Dimensions of professional labor support for intrapartum practice, *J Nurs Scholarsh* 38(1):36, 2006.

Soltani-Arabshashi R, et al: Obesity in early adulthood as a risk for psoriatic arthritis, *Arch Derm* 146(7):721, 2010.

CHAPTER

14

Older Adults

OBJECTIVES

- Identify common myths and stereotypes about older adults.
- Identify selected biological and psychosocial theories of aging.
- Discuss common developmental tasks of older adults.
- Describe common physiological changes of aging.
- Differentiate among delirium, dementia, and depression.
- Discuss issues related to psychosocial changes of aging.
- Describe selected health concerns of older adults.
- Identify nursing interventions related to the physiological, cognitive, and psychosocial changes of aging.

KEY TERMS

Activity theory, p. 173
Ageism, p. 172
Continuity theory, p. 173
Delirium, p. 178
Dementia, p. 178
Depression, p. 178
Developmental theories, p. 173
Disengagement theory, p. 173
Gerotranscendence, p. 173
Gerontological nursing, p. 174
Gerontology, p. 172
Nonstochastic theories, p. 173
Reality orientation, p. 186
Reminiscence, p. 187
Stochastic theories, p. 173
Validation therapy, p. 186

evolve WEBSITE

http://evolve.elsevier.com/Potter/fundamentals/

- Review Questions
- Case Study with Questions
- Audio Glossary
- Interactive Learning Activities
- Key Term Flashcards
- Content Updates

Age 65 is considered to be the lower boundary for "old age" in demographics and social policy within the United States. However many older adults consider themselves to be "middle-age" well into their seventh decade. Chronological age often has little relation to the reality of aging for an older adult. Each person ages in his or her own way. Every older adult is unique, and as a nurse you need to approach each one as an individual, even though this chapter makes generalizations about the aging process and its effect on individuals.

The number of older adults in the United States is growing, both absolutely and as a proportion of the total population. In 2009 there were 39.6 million adults over age 65 in the United States, representing 12.9% of the population or one in eight Americans (Administration on Aging [AOA], 2010). This represents an increase of 4.8 million since 1998. Part of that increase is the result of extension of the average life span. Women who were age 65 in 2007 could expect to live another 19.8 years, and men another 17.1 years. According to estimates, the number of older adults will increase to 72.1 million by 2030. Factors that contribute to the projected increase in the number of older adults are the aging of the baby-boom generation and the growth of the population segment over age 85. The baby boomers are the large group of adults born between 1946 and 1964. The first baby boomers reached age 65 in 2011. As the large number of baby boomers age, the social and health care programs necessary to meet their needs must dramatically reform their services. The diversity of the population over age 65 is also increasing. In 2008 minorities (African Americans, Hispanics, Asians, American Indians/Eskimos/Aleuts, and other Pacific Islanders) made up 19.6% of the population over age 65 (AOA, 2010). Nurses need to take the cultural, ethnic, and racial diversity represented by these numbers into account as they care for older adults from these groups. The challenge is to gain new knowledge and skills to provide culturally sensitive and linguistically appropriate care. Chapter 9 provides further information on culturally competent care.

VARIABILITY AMONG OLDER ADULTS

The nursing care of older adults poses special challenges because of great variation in their physiological, cognitive, and psychosocial health. Older adults also vary widely in their levels of functional ability. Most older adults are active and involved members of their communities. A smaller number have lost the ability to care for themselves, are confused or withdrawn, and/or are unable to make decisions concerning their needs. Most older adults live in noninstitutional settings. In 2008 54.6% of older adults in noninstitutional settings lived with a spouse (41.7% of older women, 72% of older men) (AOA, 2009); 30.5% lived alone (39.5% of older women, 18.5% of older men); and only 4.1% of all older adults resided in institutions such as nursing homes or centers.

Aging does not inevitably lead to disability and dependence. Most older people remain functionally independent despite the increasing prevalence of chronic disease. Nursing assessment provides valuable clues to the effects of a disease or illness on a patient's functional status. Chronic conditions add to the complexity of assessment and care of the older adult. Most older persons have at least one chronic condition, and many have multiple conditions. The most frequently diagnosed chronic conditions occurring in 2005 to 2007 were arthritis (49%), hypertension (41%), all types of heart disease (31%), any cancer (22%), and diabetes (18%) (AOA, 2009). The physical and psychosocial aspects of aging are closely related. A reduced ability to respond to stress, the experience of multiple losses, and the physical changes associated with normal aging combine to place people at high risk for illness and functional deterioration. Although the interaction of these physical and psychosocial factors is often serious, do not assume that all older adults have signs, symptoms, or behaviors representing disease and decline or that these are the only factors you need to assess. You also need to identify the older adult's strengths and abilities during the assessment and encourage independence as an integral part of your plan of care (Kresevic, 2008).

MYTHS AND STEREOTYPES

Despite ongoing research in the field of **gerontology,** myths and stereotypes about older adults persist. These include false ideas about their physical and psychosocial characteristics and lifestyles. When health care providers hold negative stereotypes about aging, they can negatively affect the quality of patient care. Although nurses are susceptible to these myths and stereotypes, they have the responsibility to replace them with accurate information.

Some people stereotype older adults as ill, disabled, and physically unattractive. Although many older adults have chronic conditions or have at least one disability that limits their performance of activities of daily living (ADLs), most noninstitutionalized older adults (39.1%) assess their health as excellent or very good (AOA, 2009). Some people believe that older adults are forgetful, confused, rigid, bored, and unfriendly and that they are unable to understand and learn new information. Yet specialists in the field of gerontology view centenarians, the oldest of the old, as having an optimistic outlook on life, good memories, broad social contacts and interests, and tolerance for others. Although changes in vision or hearing and reduced energy and endurance sometimes affect the process of learning, older adults are lifelong learners. Use teaching techniques to compensate for sensory changes, provide additional time for remembering and responding, and present concrete rather than abstract material to facilitate learning by older adults. Other effective teaching techniques draw on the older adult's past experiences and correspond to his or her identified interests rather than to the content areas that the health care professional believes are important. Box 14-1 presents additional teaching strategies to address the special learning needs of older adults.

BOX 14-1 PRINCIPLES FOR PROMOTING OLDER-ADULT LEARNING

- Make sure that the patient is ready to learn before trying to teach. Watch for clues that indicate that the patient is preoccupied or too anxious to comprehend the material.
- Is the patient physically well enough to be taught? Is he or she in pain?
- Sit facing the patient so he or she is able to watch your lip movements and facial expressions.
- Speak slowly and in a normal tone of voice.
- Present one idea or concept at a time.
- Emphasize concrete rather than abstract material.
- Give the patient enough time in which to respond because older adults process information slower than younger persons.
- Keep environmental distractions to a minimum. Provide appropriate lighting and a comfortable setting.
- Defer teaching if the patient becomes distracted or tired or cannot concentrate for other reasons.
- Invite another member of the household to join the discussion.
- Use audio, visual, and tactile cues to enhance learning and help the patient remember information.
- Ask for feedback to ensure that the patient understands the information.
- Use past experience; connect new learning to previous knowledge.

Modified from Parker P: Theories of aging. In Gilman P et al: *Nursing review and resource manual gerontological nursing*, ed 2, Silver Springs, MD, 2009, American Nurses Credentialing Center Institute for Credentialing Innovation; Ebersole et al: *Toward healthy aging: human needs and nursing response*, St Louis, 2008, Mosby.

Stereotypes about lifestyles include mistaken ideas about living arrangements and finances. Misconceptions about their financial status range from beliefs that many are affluent to beliefs that many are poor. According to the AOA (2009), 9.7% of persons over age 65 had incomes below the poverty level, with another 6.3% classified as near poor. The median income reported was $18,337, with 87% coming from Social Security.

In a society that values attractiveness, energy, and youth, these myths and stereotypes lead to the undervaluing of older adults. Some people equate worth with productivity; therefore they think that older adults become worthless after they leave the workforce. Others consider their knowledge and experience too outdated to have any current value. These ideas demonstrate **ageism,** which is discrimination against people because of increasing age, just as people who are racists and sexists discriminate because of skin color and gender. According to experts in the field of gerontology, unopposed ageism has the potential to undermine the self-confidence of older adults, limit their access to care, and distort caregivers' understanding of the uniqueness of each older adult. Older adults who have a positive image about aging actually live 7.5 years longer than those with a negative image (Levy et al., 2002). Nursing can help promote a positive perception regarding the aging process when working with these patients.

Today laws exist that ban discrimination on the basis of age. The economic and political power of older adults challenges ageist views. Older adults are a significant proportion of the consumer economy. As voters and activists in various issues, they have major influence in the formation of public policy. Their participation adds a unique perspective on social, economic, and technological issues because they have experienced almost a century of developments. In the past 100 years our nation has progressed from riding in horse-drawn carriages to tracking the adventures of the international space station. Gaslights and steam power have been replaced by electricity and nuclear power. Computers and copier machines replace typewriters and carbon paper. Many older adults lived through or were born during the Great Depression of 1929. They also experienced two world wars and wars in Korea, Vietnam, and the Persian Gulf and are now experiencing the war on terrorism. Older adults have seen changes in health care as the era of the family physician gave way to the age of specialization. After witnessing the government initiatives establishing the Social Security system, Medicare, and Medicaid, older adults are currently living with the changes imposed by health care reform and the uncertainty of the future of Social Security and Medicare. Living through all of these events and changes, they have stories and examples of coping with change to share.

NURSES' ATTITUDES TOWARD OLDER ADULTS

It is important for you to assess your own attitudes toward older adults; your own aging; and the aging of your family, friends, and patients. Nurses' attitudes come from personal experiences with older adults, education, employment experiences, and attitudes of co-workers and employing institutions. Given the increasing number of older adults in health care settings, forming positive attitudes toward them and gaining specialized knowledge about aging and their health care needs are priorities for all nurses. Positive attitudes are based in part on a realistic portrayal of the characteristics and health care needs of older adults. It is critical for you to learn to respect older adults and actively involve them in care decisions and activities. In the past institutional settings such as hospitals and nursing centers often treated older adults as objects rather than independent, dignified people. The time has come for nurses to recognize and address ageism by questioning prevailing negative attitudes and stereotypes and reinforcing the realities of aging as they care for older adults in all care settings.

THEORIES OF AGING

Various theories exist that describe the complex biopsychosocial processes of aging. However, there is no single, universally accepted theory that predicts and explains the complexities of the aging process. You need to be aware of the scientific attempts to explain the aging process and the concepts included in the theories. Although the theories are in various stages of development and have limitations, use them to increase your understanding of the phenomena affecting the health and well-being of older adults and to guide nursing care.

The biological theories of aging are either stochastic or nonstochastic. **Stochastic theories** view aging as the result of random cellular damage that occurs over time. The accumulated damage leads to the physical changes that are recognized as characteristic of the aging process. **Nonstochastic theories** view aging as the result of genetically programmed physiological mechanisms within the body that control the process of aging.

The psychosocial theories of aging, developed during the 1960s, explain changes in behavior, roles, and relationships that come with aging. These theories reflect the values that the theorist and society held at the time the theory was developed. A sample of theories follows. **Disengagement theory,** the oldest psychosocial theory, states that aging individuals withdraw from customary roles and engage in more introspective, self-focused activities (Cummings and Henry, 1961). The **activity theory,** unlike the disengagement theory, considers the continuation of activities performed during middle age as necessary for successful aging (Havighurst et al., 1963). **Continuity theory,** or **developmental theories,** suggests that personality remains stable and behavior becomes more predictable as people age (Neugarten, 1964). The personality and behavior patterns developed during a lifetime determine the degree of engagement and activity in older adulthood. The more recent theory of **gerotranscendence** proposes that the older adult experiences a shift in perspective with age (Wadensten, 2007). The person moves from a materialistic and national view of the world to a more cosmic and transcendent one, causing an increase in overall life satisfaction (Jett, 2008). Critics suggest that theories either fail in some measure to consider the many factors that affect an individual's response to aging or address those factors in a too-simplistic fashion. Rather, each individual ages uniquely.

BOX 14-2 DEVELOPMENTAL TASKS FOR OLDER ADULTS

- Adjusting to decreasing health and physical strength
- Adjusting to retirement and reduced or fixed income
- Adjusting to death of a spouse, children, siblings, friends
- Accepting self as aging person
- Maintaining satisfactory living arrangements
- Redefining relationships with adult children and siblings
- Finding ways to maintain quality of life

DEVELOPMENTAL TASKS FOR OLDER ADULTS

Theories of aging are closely linked to the concept of developmental tasks appropriate for distinct stages of life. Although no two individuals age in the same way, either biologically or psychosocially, researchers have developed frameworks outlining developmental tasks for older adults (Box 14-2). These developmental tasks are common to many older adults and are associated with varying degrees of change and loss. The more common losses are of health, significant others, a sense of being useful, socialization, income, and independent living. How older adults adjust to the changes of aging is highly individualized. For some adaptation and adjustment are relatively easy. For others coping with aging changes requires the assistance of family, friends, and health care professionals. Be sensitive to the effect of losses on older adults and their families and be prepared to offer support.

Older adults must adjust to the physical changes that accompany aging. The extent and timing of these changes vary from individual to individual; but, as body systems age, changes in appearance and functioning occur. These changes are not associated with a disease; they're normal. The presence of disease sometimes alters the timing of the changes or their impact on daily life. The section on physiological changes describes structural and functional changes of aging.

Some older adults, both men and women, find it difficult to accept aging. This is apparent when they understate their ages when asked, adopt younger styles of clothing, or attempt to hide physical evidence of aging with cosmetics. Others deny their aging in ways that are potentially problematic. For example, some older adults deny functional declines and refuse to ask for help with tasks that place their safety at great risk. Others avoid activities designed for their benefit such as senior citizens' centers and senior health promotion activities and thus do not receive the benefits these programs offer. Acceptance of personal aging does not mean retreat into inactivity, but it does require a realistic review of strengths and limitations.

Older adults retired from employment outside the home have to cope with the loss of a work role. Older adults who worked at home and the spouses of those who worked outside the home also face role changes. Some may welcome retirement as a time to pursue new interests and hobbies, volunteer in their community, continue their education, or start a new career. Retirement plans for others may include changing residence by moving to a different city or state or to a different type of housing within the same area.

Reasons other than retirement also lead to changes of residence. For example, physical impairments may require relocation to a smaller, single-level home or nursing center. A change in living arrangements for the older adult usually requires an extended period of adjustment, during which assistance and support from health care professionals, friends, and family members are necessary.

The majority of older adults cope with the death of a spouse. In 2008 almost half (42%) of all older women were widows, and 14% of older men were widowers (AOA, 2010). Some older adults must cope with the death of adult children and grandchildren. All experience the deaths of friends. These deaths represent both losses and reminders of personal mortality. Coming to terms with them is often difficult. By assisting older adults through the grieving process, you help them resolve the issues posed by these deaths.

The redefining of relationships with children that occurred as the children grew up and left home continues as older adults experience the challenges of aging. A variety of issues sometimes occur, including but not limited to control of decision making, dependence, conflict, guilt, and loss. How these issues surface in situations and how they are resolved depend in part on the past relationship between the older adult and their adult children. All the involved parties have past experiences and powerful emotions. When adult children become their parents' caregivers, they have to find ways to balance the demands of their own children and careers with the many challenges of family caregiving. As adult children and aging parents negotiate the aspects of changing roles, nurses are in the position to act as counselors to both the parents and the children. An aim is to help older adults find ways to maintain their quality of life. What defines quality of life is unique for each person.

COMMUNITY-BASED AND INSTITUTIONAL HEALTH CARE SERVICES

Nurses encounter older-adult patients in a wide variety of community and institutional health care settings. Outside of an acute care hospital, nurses care for older adults in private homes and apartments, retirement communities, adult day care centers, assisted-living facilities, and nursing centers (extended care, intermediate care, and skilled nursing facilities). Chapter 2 describes these settings and the services provided in detail.

Nurses help older adults and their families by providing information and answering questions as they make choices among care options. The assistance of the nurse is especially valuable when decisions about moving to a nursing center must be made. Some family caregivers consider nursing center placement when in-home care becomes increasingly difficult or when convalescence (recovery) from hospitalization requires more assistance than the family is able to provide. Although the decision to enter a nursing center is never final and a nursing center resident is sometimes discharged to home or another less-acute facility, many older adults may view the nursing center as their final residence. Results of state and federal inspections of nursing centers are available to the public at the nursing center, on-line, and at the inspectors' offices. The best way to evaluate the quality of a nursing center in a community is for the patient and family to visit that facility and inspect it personally. The Medicare website (http://www.Medicare.gov/NHcompare) is an excellent resource for you to learn about the quality rating of a nursing center based on the health inspections, staffing, and quality measures of the facility. It also offers a nursing center checklist. Box 14-3 summarizes some features to look for in a nursing center.

BOX 14-3 FOCUS ON OLDER ADULTS

Selection of a Nursing Center or Home

An important step in the process of selecting a nursing center is to visit it. A nursing home should meet these criteria (CMS, 2008; Rantz et al., 2001):

- Does not feel like a hospital. It is a home, a place where people live. Residents should be encouraged to personalize their rooms. Privacy is respected.
- Is Medicare and Medicaid certified.
- Has adequate, qualified staff members who have passed criminal background checks.
- Provides quality care, in addition to assistance with basic activities of daily living such as bathing, dressing, eating, oral hygiene, and toileting. Staff should assist residents with social and recreational activities.
- Offers quality food and mealtime choices.
- Families should be welcome when they visit the facility. Whether they wish to provide information, ask questions, participate in care planning, or assist with social activities or physical care, staff should encourage family involvement.
- Is clean. There should be no pervasive odors in the facility. The environment should be "homelike."
- Provides active communication from staff to patient and family.
- Members of the nursing home staff are attentive to resident requests and actively involved with assisting the residents. They focus on the person, not on the task.

ASSESSING THE NEEDS OF OLDER ADULTS

Gerontological nursing requires creative approaches for maximizing the potential of older adults. With comprehensive assessment information regarding strengths, limitations, and resources, the nurse and the older adult identify needs and problems. Together they select interventions to maintain the older adult's physical abilities and create an environment for psychosocial and spiritual well-being. A thorough assessment requires the nurse to actively engage older adults and provide them enough time to share important information about their health.

Nursing assessment takes into account five key points to ensure an age-specific approach: (1) the interrelation between physical and psychosocial aspects of aging, (2) the effects of disease and disability on functional status, (3) the decreased efficiency of homeostatic mechanisms, (4) the lack of standards for health and illness norms, and (5) altered presentation and response to a specific disease (Meiner, 2011). A comprehensive assessment of an older adult takes more time than the assessment of a younger adult because of the longer life and medical history and the potential complexity of the history. During the physical examination allow rest periods as needed or conduct the assessment in several sessions because of the reduced energy and limited endurance of some frail older adults. Remember to review both prescribed and over-the-counter medications carefully with the patient.

Sensory changes also affect data gathering. Your choice of communication techniques depends on visual or hearing impairments of the older adult. If older adults are unable to understand your visual or auditory cues, assessment data may be inaccurate or misleading. For example, if an older adult has difficulty hearing a nurse's questions, inappropriate responses might lead the nurse to believe that the person is confused. Chapter 49 explains in detail techniques to use when communicating with older adults who have a hearing impairment. When a person has a visual impairment, use these communication techniques:

BOX 14-4 CULTURAL ASPECTS OF CARE

Communication During Assessment

The older adult's cultural values and beliefs about health, illness, and treatment influence the quality of assessment data the nurse collects in an interview. For example, Sims (2010) found that health care providers' unfamiliarity with black women's ethnic notions can lead to misinterpretations and misunderstandings that influence their interactions. Be knowledgeable about the characteristics of an older adult's cultural group because it affects nurse-patient communication during the assessment process (Touhy and Jett, 2010).

Implications for Practice

- Use cultural interpreters when necessary,
- Use appropriate conventions of the handshake and silence during interactions (Meiner, 2011).
- Identify how the older adult wishes to be addressed; use culturally appropriate titles.
- Assess the health-related beliefs and practices of the older patient's culture group and adapt questions to obtain information on how the patient incorporates them into daily practice.
- Know beliefs and practices of the older patient's culture group regarding spatial requirements, eye contact, and touch and use them to establish rapport.
- Use a pain-rating scale for identifying and rating pain.
- Determine patient's use of folk remedies.

- Sit or stand at eye level, in front of the patient in full view.
- Face the older adult while speaking; do not cover your mouth.
- Provide diffuse, bright, nonglare lighting.
- Encourage the older adult to use his or her familiar assistive devices such as glasses or magnifiers.

Memory deficits, if present, affect the accuracy and completeness of an assessment. Information contributed by a family member or other caregiver is sometimes necessary to supplement the older adult's recollection of past medical events and information such as allergies and immunizations. Use tact when involving another person in the assessment interview. The additional person supplements the answers of the older adult with the consent of the older adult, but the older adult remains the focus of the interview.

During all aspects of the assessment you are responsible for providing culturally competent care. See Chapter 9 for a detailed description of the components of a cultural assessment. There are ways to provide culturally competent care while communicating with older adults during the assessment process (Box 14-4).

During assessment use caution when interpreting the signs and symptoms of diseases and laboratory values. Historically researchers have used younger populations to establish these signs and norms. However, the classic signs and symptoms of diseases are sometimes absent, blunted, or atypical in older adults (Gray-Miceli et al., 2010). This is especially true in the case of bacterial infection, pain, acute myocardial infarction, and heart failure. The masquerading of disease is possibly caused by age-related changes in organ systems and homeostatic mechanisms, progressive loss of physiological and functional reserves, or coexisting acute or chronic conditions. As a result the older adult with a urinary tract infection may present with confusion, incontinence, and an elevation of body temperature (within normal limits) instead of having fever, dysuria, frequency, or urgency. Some older adults with pneumonia have tachycardia, tachypnea, and confusion with decreased appetite and functioning, without the more common symptoms of fever and productive cough. Instead of crushing, substernal chest pain and diaphoresis, the older adult with a myocardial infarction experiences a sudden onset of dyspnea often accompanied by anxiety and confusion. Variations from the usual norms for laboratory values are sometimes caused by age-related changes in cardiac, pulmonary, renal, and metabolic function (Amella, 2006).

It is important to recognize early indicators of an acute illness in older adults. Note changes in mental status, occurrence and reason for falls, dehydration, decrease in appetite, loss of function, dizziness, and incontinence because these may be indicators not presented in younger adults. A key principle of providing age-appropriate nursing care is timely detection of these cardinal signs of illness so early treatment can begin (Box 14-5). Mental status

BOX 14-5 EXAMPLES OF ALTERED PRESENTATION OF ILLNESSES IN OLDER ADULTS OCCURRING IN VARIOUS HEALTH CARE SETTINGS

Hospital

- Confusion is not inevitable. Look for an acute illness, neurological events, new medication, or the presence of risk factors for delirium.
- Many hospitalized older adults suffer from chronic dehydration exacerbated by acute illness.
- Not all older adults have fevers with infection. Symptoms instead include increased respiratory rate, falls, incontinence, or confusion.

Nursing Home

- Health care providers often undertreat pain in older adults, especially those with dementia. Look for nonverbal cues or pain presence such as grimacing or resistance to care.
- Decline in functional ability (even a minor one such as the inability to sit upright in a chair) is a signal of new illness.
- Residents with less muscle mass—both the frail and the obese—are at a much higher risk for toxicity from protein-binding drugs such as phenytoin (Dilantin and others) and warfarin (Coumadin and others).
- New urinary and/or fecal incontinence is often a sign of the onset of a new illness.

Ambulatory Care

- Complaints of fatigue or decreased ability to do usual activities are signs of anemia, thyroid problems, depression, or neurological or cardiac problems.
- Severe gastrointestinal problems in older adults do not always present with the same acute symptoms seen in younger patients. Ask about constipation, cramping sensations, and changes in bowel habits.
- Older adults reporting increased dyspnea and confusion, especially those with a cardiac history, need to go to the emergency department because these are the most common manifestations of myocardial infarction in this population.
- Depression is common among older adults with chronic illnesses. Watch for lack of interest in former activities, significant personal losses, or changes in role or home life.

Home Care

- Investigate all falls, focusing on balance, gait, and neurological issues.
- Monitor older adults with late-stage heart disease for loss of appetite as an early symptom of impending failure.
- Drug-drug and drug-food interactions in older patients who are seeing more than one provider and taking multiple medications are common. Watch for signs.

Modified from Amella E: Presentation of illness in older adults, *AORN J* 83(2): 372, 377, 385, 2006.

changes commonly occur as a result of disease and psychological issues. Some mental changes are often drug related, caused by drug toxicity or adverse drug events. A fall can be a common event for an older adult and can be injury producing and costly (Ferrari et al., 2010). A fall is a complex event that needs careful investigation to find out if it was the result of environmental causes or the symptom of a new-onset illness. Problems with the cardiac, respiratory, musculoskeletal, neurological, urological, and sensory body systems can present with a fall as a chief symptom of a new-onset condition. Dehydration is common in older adults because of decreased oral intake related to a reduced thirst response and less free water as a consequence of a decrease in muscle mass. When vomiting and diarrhea accompany the onset of an acute illness, the older adult is at risk for further dehydration. Decrease in appetite is a common symptom with the onset of pneumonia, heart failure, and urinary tract infection. Loss of functional ability occurs in a subtle fashion over a period of time; or it occurs suddenly, depending on the underlying cause. Thyroid disease, infection, cardiac or pulmonary conditions, metabolic disturbances, and anemia are common causes of functional decline; thus nurses play an essential role in early identification, referral, and treatment of health problems.

Physiological Changes

Perception of well-being defines quality of life. Understanding the older adult's perceptions about health status is essential for accurate assessment and development of clinically relevant interventions. Their concepts of health generally depend on personal perceptions of functional ability. Therefore older adults engaged in ADLs usually consider themselves healthy; whereas those who have physical, emotional, or social impairments that limit their activities perceive themselves as ill.

Some frequently observed physiological changes in older adults are normal (Table 14-1). The changes are not always pathological processes in themselves, but they make older adults more vulnerable to some common clinical conditions and diseases. Some older

TABLE 14-1 Common Physiological Changes with Aging at a Glance

SYSTEM	COMMON CHANGES
Integumentary	Loss of skin elasticity with fat loss in extremities, pigmentation changes, glandular atrophy (oil, moisture, sweat glands), thinning hair, with hair turning gray-white (facial hair: decreased in men, increased in women), slower nail growth, atrophy of epidermal arterioles
Respiratory	Decreased cough reflex; decreased cilia; increased anterior-posterior chest diameter; increased chest wall rigidity; fewer alveoli, increased airway resistance; increased risk of respiratory infections
Cardiovascular	Thickening of blood vessel walls; narrowing of vessel lumen; loss of vessel elasticity; lower cardiac output; decreased number of heart muscle fibers; decreased elasticity and calcification of heart valves; decreased baroreceptor sensitivity; decreased efficiency of venous valves; increased pulmonary vascular tension; increased systolic blood pressure; decreased peripheral circulation
Gastrointestinal	Periodontal disease; decrease in saliva, gastric secretions, and pancreatic enzymes; smooth muscle changes with decreased esophageal peristalsis and small intestinal motility; gastric atrophy, decreased production of intrinsic factor, increased stomach pH, loss of smooth muscle in the stomach, hemorrhoids, anal fissures; rectal prolapse and impaired rectal sensation.
Musculoskeletal	Decreased muscle mass and strength, decalcification of bones, degenerative joint changes, dehydration of intervertebral disks
Neurological	Degeneration of nerve cells, decrease in neurotransmitters, decrease in rate of conduction of impulses
Sensory	
Eyes	Decreased accommodation to near/far vision (presbyopia), difficulty adjusting to changes from light to dark, yellowing of the lens, altered color perception, increased sensitivity to glare, smaller pupils
Ears	Loss of acuity for high-frequency tones (presbycusis), thickening of tympanic membrane, sclerosis of inner ear, buildup of earwax (cerumen)
Taste	Often diminished; often fewer taste buds
Smell	Often diminished
Touch	Decreased skin receptors
Proprioception	Decreased awareness of body positioning in space
Genitourinary	Fewer nephrons, 50% decrease in renal blood flow by age 80, decreased bladder capacity Male—enlargement of prostate Female—reduced sphincter tone
Reproductive	Male—sperm count diminishes, smaller testes, erections less firm and slow to develop Female—decreased estrogen production, degeneration of ovaries, atrophy of vagina, uterus, breasts
Endocrine	General—alterations in hormone production with decreased ability to respond to stress Thyroid—decreased secretions Cortisol, glucocorticoids—increased antiinflammatory hormone Pancreas—increased fibrosis, decreased secretion of enzymes and hormones
Immune System	Thymus involution T-cell function decreases

Modified from Touhy T, Jett K: *Ebersole and Hess' gerontological nursing and healthy aging,* ed 3, St Louis, 2010, Mosby.

adults experience all of these changes, and others experience only a few. The body changes continuously with age; and specific effects on particular older adults depend on health, lifestyle, stressors, and environmental conditions. The nurse needs to know about these normal, more common changes to provide appropriate care for older adults and assist with adaptation to the changes.

General Survey. The general survey begins during the initial nurse-patient encounter and includes a quick but careful head-to-toe scan of the older adult that the nurse writes in a brief description (see Chapter 30). An initial inspection reveals if eye contact and facial expression are appropriate to the situation and universal aging changes such as facial wrinkles, gray hair, loss of body mass in the extremities, and an increase of body mass in the trunk.

Integumentary System. With aging the skin loses resilience and moisture. The epithelial layer thins, and elastic collagen fibers shrink and become rigid. Wrinkles of the face and neck reflect lifelong patterns of muscle activity and facial expressions, the pull of gravity on tissue, and diminished elasticity. Spots and lesions are often present on the skin. Smooth, brown, irregularly shaped spots (age spots or senile lentigo) initially appear on the backs of the hands and on forearms. Small, round, red or brown cherry angiomas occur on the trunk. Seborrheic lesions or keratoses appear as irregular, round or oval, brown, watery lesions. Years of sun exposure contribute to the aging of the skin and lead to premalignant and malignant lesions. You need to rule out these three malignancies related to sun exposure when examining skin lesions: melanoma, basal cell carcinoma, and squamous cell carcinoma (see Chapter 30).

Head and Neck. The facial features of the older adult may become more pronounced from loss of subcutaneous fat and skin elasticity. Facial features appear asymmetrical because of missing teeth or improperly fitting dentures. In addition, common vocal changes include a rise in pitch and a loss of power and range.

Visual acuity declines with age. This is often the result of retinal damage, reduced pupil size, development of opacities in the lens, or loss of lens elasticity. Presbyopia, a progressive decline in the ability of the eyes to accommodate from near to far vision, is common. Ability to see in darkness and adapt to abrupt changes from dark to light areas (and the reverse) is reduced. More ambient light is necessary for tasks such as reading and other ADLs. Older adults have increased sensitivity to the effects of glare. Pupils are smaller and react slower. Objects do not appear bright, but the older adult has difficulty when coming from bright to dark environments. Changes in color vision and discoloration of the lens make it difficult to distinguish between blues and greens and among pastel shades. Dark colors such as blue and black appear the same. Diseases of the older eye include cataract, macular degeneration, diabetic retinopathy, and retinal detachment. Cataracts, a loss of the transparency of the lens, are a prevalent disorder among older adults. They normally result in blurred vision, sensitivity to glare, and gradual loss of vision. Chapter 49 outlines nursing interventions for adapting to a patient's visual changes.

Noise is the most prevalent risk factor for impaired hearing. Exposure earlier in life exacerbates hearing loss in old age. However, auditory changes are often subtle. Most of the time older adults ignore the early signs of hearing loss until friends and family members comment on compensatory attempts such as turning up the volume on televisions or avoiding social conversations. A common age-related change in auditory acuity is presbycusis. Presbycusis affects the ability to hear high-pitched sounds and sibilant consonants such as *s*, *sh*, and *ch*. Before the nurse assumes presbycusis, it is necessary to inspect the external auditory canal for the presence of cerumen. Impacted cerumen, a common cause of diminished hearing acuity, is easy to treat.

Salivary secretion is reduced, and taste buds atrophy and lose sensitivity. The older adult is less able to differentiate among salty, sweet, sour, and bitter tastes. The sense of smell also decreases, further reducing taste. Health conditions, treatments, and/or medications can alter taste. It is often a challenge to promote optimal nutrition in an older patient because of the loss of smell and changes in taste.

Thorax and Lungs. Because of changes in the musculoskeletal system, the configuration of the thorax sometimes changes. Respiratory muscle strength begins to decrease, and the anteroposterior diameter of the thorax increases. Vertebral changes caused by osteoporosis lead to dorsal kyphosis, the curvature of the thoracic spine. Calcification of the costal cartilage causes decreased mobility of the ribs. The chest wall gradually becomes stiffer. Lung expansion decreases, and the person is less able to cough deeply. If kyphosis or chronic obstructive lung disease is present, breath sounds become distant. With these changes the older adult is more susceptible to pneumonia and other bacterial or viral infections.

Heart and Vascular System. Decreased contractile strength of the myocardium results in decreased cardiac output. The decrease is significant when the older adult experiences anxiety, excitement, illness, or strenuous activity. The body tries to compensate for decreased cardiac output by increasing the heart rate during exercise. However, after exercise it takes longer for the older adult's rate to return to baseline. Systolic and/or diastolic blood pressures are sometimes abnormally high. Although a common chronic condition, hypertension is not a normal aging change and predisposes older adults to heart failure, stroke, renal failure, coronary heart disease, and peripheral vascular disease.

Peripheral pulses frequently are weaker, although still palpable, in the lower extremities. Older adults sometimes complain that their lower extremities are cold, particularly at night. Changes in the peripheral pulses in the upper extremities are less common.

Breasts. As estrogen production diminishes, the milk ducts of the breasts are replaced by fat, making breast tissue less firm. Decreased muscle mass, tone, and elasticity result in smaller breasts in older women. In addition, the breasts sag. Atrophy of glandular tissue, coupled with more fat deposits, results in a slightly smaller, less dense, and less nodular breast. Gynecomastia, enlarged breasts in men, is often the result of medication side effects, hormonal changes, or obesity. Both older men and women are at risk of breast cancer.

Gastrointestinal System and Abdomen. Aging leads to an increase in the amount of fatty tissue in the trunk. As a result, the abdomen increases in size. Because muscle tone and elasticity decrease, it also becomes more protuberant. Gastrointestinal function changes include a slowing of peristalsis and alterations in secretions. The older adult experiences these changes by becoming less tolerant of certain foods and having discomfort from delayed gastric emptying. Alterations in the lower gastrointestinal tract lead to constipation, flatulence, or diarrhea.

Reproductive System. Changes in the structure and function of the reproductive system occur in both sexes as the result of hormonal alterations. Female menopause is related to a reduced responsiveness of the ovaries to pituitary hormones and a resultant decrease in estrogen and progesterone levels. In men there is no definite cessation of fertility associated with aging. Spermatogenesis begins to decline during the fourth decade and continues into the ninth. However, the changes in reproductive structure and function do not affect libido; sexual desires, thoughts, and actions continue throughout all decades of life (Wallace, 2008). Less frequent sexual activity often results from illness, death of a sexual partner, or decreased socialization.

Urinary System. Hypertrophy of the prostate gland is frequently seen in older men. This hypertrophy enlarges the gland and places pressure on the neck of the bladder. As a result, urinary retention, frequency, incontinence, and urinary tract infections occur. In addition, prostatic hypertrophy results in difficulty initiating voiding and maintaining a urinary stream. Benign prostatic hypertrophy is different from cancer of the prostate. Cancer of the prostate is the second most common cause of cancer death in men over age 50. In 2010 the American Cancer Society estimated that one in six men will be diagnosed with prostate cancer and 1 in 36 will die (American Cancer Society, 2010).

Urinary incontinence is an abnormal condition that can occur in both older men and women. Men may be afraid to discuss incontinence with their physician because of embarrassment and because they think that urinary incontinence is a "woman's disease." Older women, particularly those who have had children, experience stress incontinence, an involuntary release of urine that occurs when they cough, laugh, sneeze, or lift an object. This is a result of a weakening of the perineal and bladder muscles. Other types of urinary incontinence are urge, overflow, functional, and mixed incontinence. The risk factors for urinary incontinence include age, menopause, diabetes, hysterectomy, stroke, and obesity.

Musculoskeletal System. With aging muscle fibers become smaller. Muscle strength diminishes in proportion to the decline in muscle mass. Beginning in the 30s, bone density and bone mass decline in men and women. Older adults who exercise regularly do not lose as much bone and muscle mass or muscle tone as those who are inactive. Osteoporosis is a major public health threat. An estimated 10 million Americans already have the disease, and an additional 34 million are at risk with low bone mass (National Osteoporosis Foundation, 2010). Postmenopausal women experience a greater rate of bone demineralization than older men. Women who maintain calcium intake throughout life and into menopause have less bone demineralization than women with low calcium intake. Older men with poor nutrition and decreased mobility are also at risk for bone demineralization.

Neurological System. A decrease in the number and size of neurons in the nervous system begins in the middle of the second decade. Neurotransmitters, chemical substances that enhance or inhibit nerve impulse transmission, change with aging as a result of the decrease in neurons. All voluntary reflexes are slower, and individuals often have less of an ability to respond to multiple stimuli. In addition, older adults frequently report alterations in the quality and the quantity of sleep (see Chapter 42), including difficulty falling asleep, difficulty staying asleep, difficulty falling asleep again after waking during the night, waking too early in the morning, and excessive daytime napping. These problems are believed to be caused by age-related changes in the sleep-wake cycle.

Functional Changes

Physical function is a dynamic process. It changes as individuals interact with their environments. Functional status in older adults includes the day-to-day ADLs involving activities within physical, psychological, cognitive, and social domains. A decline in function can often be linked to illness or disease and its degree of chronicity. However, ultimately it is the complex relationship among all of these areas that influences an older adult's functional abilities and overall well-being.

Keep in mind that it may be difficult for older adults to accept the changes that occur in all areas of their lives, which in turn have a profound effect on functional status. Some deny the changes and continue to expect the same performance from themselves, regardless of age. Conversely some overemphasize them and prematurely limit their activities and involvement in life. The fear of becoming dependent is an overwhelming one for the older adult who is experiencing functional decline as a result of aging. Educate older adults to promote understanding of age-related changes, appropriate lifestyle adjustments, and effective coping. Factors that promote the highest level of function in all the areas include a healthy, well-balanced diet; paced and appropriate activity; regularly scheduled visits with a health care provider; regular participation in meaningful activities; use of stress management techniques; and avoidance of alcohol, tobacco, or illicit drugs.

Functional status in older adults refers to the capacity and safe performance of ADLs and instrumental activities of daily living (IADLs). It is a sensitive indicator of health or illness in the older adult. ADLs (such as bathing, dressing, and toileting) and IADLs (such as the ability to write a check, shop, prepare meals, or make phone calls) are essential to independent living; therefore carefully assess whether or not the older adult has changed the way he or she completes these tasks. Occupational and physical therapists are your best resources for a comprehensive assessment. A sudden change in function, as evidenced by a decline or change in the older adult's ability to perform any one or combination of ADLs, is often a sign of the onset of an acute illness (e.g., pneumonia, urinary tract infection, or electrolyte imbalance) or worsening of a chronic problem (e.g., diabetes or cardiovascular disease) (Kresevic, 2008).

Health care providers who work in a range of different settings are able to perform functional assessment. Several standardized functional assessment tools are widely available. There is an online collection of the tools used most commonly with older adults at the geriatric nursing website of the American Nurses Association (ANA), www.geronurseonline.org. When you identify a decline in a patient's function, focus your nursing interventions on maintaining, restoring, and maximizing the older adult's functional status to maintain independence while preserving dignity.

Cognitive Changes

A common misconception about aging is that cognitive impairments are widespread among older adults. Because of this misconception, older adults often fear that they are, or soon will be, cognitively impaired. Younger adults often assume that older adults will become confused and no longer able to handle their affairs. Forgetfulness as an expected consequence of aging is a myth. Some structural and physiological changes within the brain are associated with cognitive impairment. Reduction in the number of brain cells, deposition of lipofuscin and amyloid in cells, and changes in neurotransmitter levels occur in older adults both with and without cognitive impairment. Symptoms of cognitive impairment such as disorientation, loss of language skills, loss of the ability to calculate, and poor judgment *are not* normal aging changes and require you to further assess patients for underlying causes. There are standard assessment forms for determining a patient's mental status, including the Mini-Mental State Exam (MMSE), the Confusion Assessment Method (CAM) and the NEECHAM Confusion Scale (Ebersole et al., 2008).

The three common conditions affecting cognition are **delirium, dementia,** and **depression** (Table 14-2). Distinguishing among these three conditions is challenging. Complete a careful and thorough assessment of older adults with cognitive changes to

TABLE 14-2 Comparison of Clinical Features of Delirium, Dementia, and Depression

CLINICAL FEATURE	DELIRIUM	DEMENTIA	DEPRESSION
Onset	Sudden/abrupt; depends on cause	Insidious/slow and often unrecognized	Happens with major life changes; often abrupt but can be gradual
Course	Short, daily fluctuations in symptoms; worse at night, in darkness, and on awakening	Long, no diurnal effects; symptoms progressive yet relatively stable over time; some deficits with increased stress	Diurnal effects, typically worse in the morning; situational fluctuations but less than with delirium
Progression	Abrupt	Slow but uneven	Variable; rapid or slow but even
Duration	Hours to less than 1 month; longer if unrecognized and untreated	Months to years	At least 6 weeks; sometimes several months to years
Consciousness	Reduced/disturbed	Clear	Clear
Alertness	Fluctuates; lethargic or hypervigilant	Generally normal	Normal
Attention	Impaired; fluctuates; inattention; distractible	Generally normal	Minimal impairment but is easily distracted
Orientation	Generally impaired; severity varies	Generally normal to person but not to place or time	Selective disorientation
Memory	Recent and immediate impaired; forgetful; many need instructions for simple tasks one step at a time	Recent and remote impaired	Selective or "patchy" impairment; "islands" of intact memory; evaluation often difficult because of low motivation
Thinking	Disorganized, distorted, fragmented, illogical; incoherent speech, either slow or accelerated	Difficulty with abstraction; thoughts diminished; judgment impaired; words difficult to find	Intact but with themes of hopelessness, helplessness, or self-deprecation
Perception	Distorted, illusions, delusions, and hallucinations; difficulty distinguishing between reality and misperceptions	Misperceptions usually absent	Intact; delusions and hallucinations absent except in severe cases
Psychomotor behavior	Variable; hypokinetic, hyperkinetic, and mixed	Normal; some have apraxia	Variable; psychomotor retardation or agitation
Sleep/wake cycle	Disturbed; cycle reversed	Fragmented	Disturbed; usually early morning awakening
Associated features	Variable affective changes; symptoms of autonomic hyperarousal; exaggeration of personality type; associated with acute physical illness	Affect tends to be superficial, inappropriate, and labile (changing); attempts to hide deficits in intellect; personality changes, aphasia, agnosia sometimes present; lacks insight	Affect depressed; dysphoric mood; exaggerated and detailed complaints; preoccupied with personal thoughts; insight present; verbal elaboration; somatic complaints, poor hygiene, neglect of self
Assessment	Distracted from task; makes numerous errors	Failings highlighted by family, frequent "near miss" answers; struggles with test; great effort to find an appropriate reply; frequent requests for feedback on performance	Failings highlighted by individual, frequent "don't knows"; little effort; frequently gives up; indifferent toward test; does not care or attempt to find answer

Modified from Braes T et al: Assessing cognitive function. In Capezuti E et al: *Evidence-based geriatric nursing protocols for best practice,* ed 3, New York, 2008, Springer.

distinguish among them. Select appropriate nursing interventions that are specific to the cause of the cognitive impairment.

Delirium. Delirium, or acute confusional state, is potentially a reversible cognitive impairment that often has a physiological cause. Physiological causes include electrolyte imbalances; cerebral anoxia; hypoglycemia; medication effects; tumors; subdural hematomas; and cerebrovascular infection, infarction, or hemorrhage. Delirium in older adults sometimes accompanies systemic infections and is often the presenting symptom for pneumonia or urinary tract infection. Sometimes it is also caused by environmental factors such as sensory deprivation or unfamiliar surroundings or psychosocial factors such as emotional distress or pain. Sleep deprivation is another possible reason for delirium. Although it occurs in any setting, an older adult in the acute care setting is especially at risk because of predisposing factors (physiological, psychosocial, and environmental) in combination with the underlying medical condition. Dementia is an additional risk factor that greatly increases the risk for delirium, and it is possible for delirium and dementia to occur in a patient at the same time. The presence of delirium is a medical emergency and requires prompt assessment and intervention. Nurses are at the bedside 24/7 and in a position to recognize delirium development and report it. The cognitive impairment usually reverses once health care providers identify and treat the cause of delirium.

Dementia. Dementia is a generalized impairment of intellectual functioning that interferes with social and occupational functioning. It is an umbrella term that includes Alzheimer's disease, Lewy body disease, frontal-temporal dementia, and vascular dementia. Cognitive function deterioration leads to a decline in the ability to perform basic ADLs and IADLs. Unlike delirium, a gradual, progressive, irreversible cerebral dysfunction characterizes dementia. Because of the similarity between delirium and dementia, you need to assess carefully to rule out the presence of delirium whenever you suspect dementia.

Nursing management of older adults with any form of dementia always considers the safety and physical and psychosocial needs of the older adult and the family. These needs change as the progressive nature of dementia leads to increased cognitive deterioration. To meet the needs of the older adult, individualize nursing care to enhance quality of life and maximize functional performance by improving cognition, mood, and behavior. Box 14-6 lists general nursing principles for care of older adults with cognitive changes. Support and education about Alzheimer's disease for patients, families, and professionals can be found at the Alzheimer's Association website (www.alz.org).

Depression. Approximately one third of older adults experience depressive symptoms (Mental Health America, 2011). Older adults sometimes experience late-life depression, but it is not a normal part of aging. Depression is the most common, yet most undetected and untreated, impairment in older adulthood. Co-occurring diseases may include stroke, dementia, Parkinson's disease, heart disease, cancer, and pain-provoking diseases such as arthritis. Loss of a significant loved one or a nursing center admission may precipitate depression. Clinical depression is treatable and includes medication, psychotherapy, or a combination of both. Of special note, suicide attempts in older adults are often successful. In fact, suicide in older adults comprises 20% of all suicides (Mental Health America, 2011).

BOX 14-6 NURSING CARE PRINCIPLES FOR CARE OF COGNITIVELY IMPAIRED OLDER ADULTS

- Institute medical measures to correct underlying physiological alterations.
- Maximize safe function. Keep a routine, limit choices (e.g., clothes for dressing, what to eat), allow for rest.
- Provide unconditional positive regard. Be respectful. Nonverbal communication also should be positive.
- Use behaviors to gauge activity and stimulation. Watch for facial signs of anxiety.
- Teach caregivers to listen to the behaviors that show stress (e.g., verbalizations such as repetition).
- Modify the environment.
- Promote social interaction based on abilities. Make sure that the environment is safe for mobility and promote way-finding with pictures or cues. Try to identify patients who wander and remove the cause (e.g., pain, thirst, unfamiliar surroundings, new noises).
- Compensate for any sensory deficits (e.g., hearing aids, glasses, dentures).
- Encourage fluid intake (make sure that fluids are accessible) and avoid long periods of giving nothing orally.
- Be vigilant for drug reactions or interactions; consider onset of new symptoms as an adverse reaction.
- Activate bed and chair alarms.
- Provide ongoing assistance to family caregivers; educate them in nursing care techniques and inform them about community resources.

Modified from Fletcher K: Dementia. In Capezuti et al: *Evidence-based geriatric nursing protocols for best practice,* ed 3, New York, 2008, Springer; Ebersole P et al: *Toward healthy aging: human needs and nursing response,* St Louis, 2008, Mosby.

Psychosocial Changes

The psychosocial changes occurring during aging involve life transitions and loss. The longer people live, the more transitions with which they must cope, and the more losses they experience. Life transitions, of which loss is a major component, include retirement and the associated financial changes, changes in roles and relationships, alterations in health and functional ability, changes in one's social network, and relocation. But the universal loss for older adults usually revolves around the loss of relationships through death.

It is important to assess both the nature of the psychosocial changes that occur in older adults as a result of life transitions and the loss and the adaptations to the changes. During the assessment ask how the older adult feels about self, self in relation to others, and self as one who is aging and what coping methods and skills have been beneficial. Areas to address during the assessment include family, intimate relationships, past and present role changes, finances, housing, social networks, activities, health and wellness, and spirituality. Specific topics related to these areas include retirement, social isolation, sexuality, housing and environment, and death.

Retirement. Many often mistakenly associate retirement with passivity and seclusion. In actuality it is a stage of life characterized by transitions and role changes. This transition requires letting go of certain habits and structure and developing new ones (Touhy and Jett, 2010). The psychosocial stresses of retirement are usually related to role changes with a spouse or within the family and to loss of the work role. Sometimes problems related to social isolation and finances are present. The age of retirement varies. But, whether it occurs at age 55, 65, or 75, it is one of the major turning points in life.

Preretirement planning is an important advisable task. People who plan in advance for retirement generally have a smoother transition. Preretirement planning is more than financial planning. Planning begins with consideration of the "style" of retirement desired and includes an inventory of interests, current skills, and general health. Meaningful retirement planning is critical as the population continues to age.

Retirement affects more than just the retired. It affects the spouse, adult children, and even grandchildren. When the spouse is still working, the retired person faces time alone. There may be new expectations of the retired person. For example, a working spouse might have new ideas about the amount of housework expected of the retired person. Problems develop when the plans of the retired person conflict with the work responsibilities of the working spouse. The roles of the retiree and the working spouse need clarification. Adult children may expect the retired person to always babysit for the grandchildren, forgetting that this is a time for the retired person to pursue other personal interests.

Loss of the work role has a major impact on some retired persons. When so much of life has revolved around work and the personal relationships at work, the loss of the work role can be devastating. Personal identity is often rooted in the work role, and with retirement individuals need to construct a new identity. Individuals also lose the structure imposed on daily life when they no longer have a work schedule. The social exchanges and interpersonal support that occur in the workplace are lost. In the adjustment to retirement the older adult has to develop a personally meaningful schedule and a supportive social network.

Factors that influence the retired person's satisfaction with life are health status and sufficient income. Positive preretirement expectations also contribute to satisfaction in retirement. The nurse can help the older adult and family prepare for retirement by discussing with them several key areas, including relations with spouse and children; meaningful activities and interests; building social networks; issues related to income; health promotion and maintenance; and long-range planning, including wills and advance directives.

Social Isolation. Many older adults experience social isolation. Isolation is sometimes a choice, the result of a desire not to interact with others. It is also a response to conditions that inhibit the ability or the opportunity to interact such as the lack of access to transportation. Although some older adults choose isolation or a lifelong pattern of reduced interaction with others, older adults who experience social isolation become vulnerable to its consequences. An older adult's vulnerability increases in the absence of the support of other adults, as occurs with loss of the work role or relocation to unfamiliar surroundings. Impaired sensory function, reduced mobility, and cognitive changes all contribute to reduced interaction with others and can place the older adult at risk for isolation.

You assess patients' potential for social isolation by identifying their social network, access to transportation, and willingness and desire to interact with others. Your findings assist you in helping a lonely older adult rebuild social networks and reverse patterns of isolation. Many communities have outreach programs designed to make contact with isolated older adults such as Meals on Wheels, which provides nutritional meals. Outreach programs such as daily telephone calls by volunteers or needs for activities such as social outings also meet socialization needs. Social service agencies in most communities welcome older adults as volunteers and provide the opportunity for them to serve while meeting their socialization or other needs. Churches, colleges, community centers, and libraries offer a variety of programs for older adults that increase the opportunity to meet people with similar activities, interests, and needs.

Sexuality. All older adults, whether healthy or frail, need to express their sexual feelings. Sexuality involves love, warmth, sharing, and touching, not just the act of intercourse. Sexuality plays an important role in helping the older adult maintain self-esteem. To help an older adult achieve or maintain sexual health, you need to understand the physical changes in a person's sexual response (Chapter 34). You need to provide privacy for any discussion of sexuality and maintain a nonjudgmental attitude. Open-ended questions inviting the older adult to explain sexual activities or concerns elicit more information than a list of closed-ended questions about specific activities or symptoms. Include information about the prevention of sexually transmitted infections when appropriate. Sexuality and the need to express sexual feelings remain throughout the human life span.

When considering the older adult's need for sexual expression, do not ignore the important need to touch and be touched. Touch is an overt expression with many meanings and is an important part of intimacy (Atkinson, 2006). Touch complements traditional sexual methods or serves as an alternative sexual expression when physical intercourse is not desired or possible. Knowing an older adult's sexual needs allows you to incorporate this information into the nursing care plan.

The sexual preferences of older adults are as diverse as those of the younger population. Clearly not all older adults are heterosexual, yet little research has been done on older adult homosexuals and their health care needs. A number of emerging issues have the potential to substantially affect caregiving in the future, including the demographic changes and the overall aging of the U.S. population, shifts in the nature of families, growing economic pressures, and the societal context of caregiving (Fredriksen-Goldsen et al., 2009). Nurses often find that they are called on to help other health care professionals understand the sexual needs of older adults and advise them. Not all nurses feel comfortable counseling older adults about sexual health and intimacy-related needs. Be prepared to refer older adults to an appropriate professional counselor.

Housing and Environment. The extent of an older adult's ability to live independently influences housing choices. Changes in social roles, family responsibilities, and health status influence their living arrangements. Some choose to live with family members. Others prefer their own homes or other housing options near their families. Leisure or retirement communities provide older people with living and social opportunities in a one-generation setting. Federally subsidized housing, where available, offers apartments with communal, social, and in some cases food-service arrangements.

The goal of your assessment of a patient's environment is to consider resources that promote independence and functional ability. When assisting older adults with housing needs, assess their activity level, financial status, access to public transportation and community activities, environmental hazards, and support systems (Touhy and Jett, 2010). When helping patients consider housing choice, anticipate their future needs as much as possible. For example, a housing unit with only one floor and without exterior steps is a prudent choice for the older adult with severe arthritis who has already had lower-extremity joint replacement surgery and anticipates the need for future operations. Assessment of safety, a major component of the older adult's environment, includes risks within the environment and the older adult's ability to recognize and respond to the risks (Chapter 27). Safety risks in the home include factors leading to injury such as water heaters set at excessively hot temperatures or environmental barriers such as throw rugs or slippery floor surfaces that could cause a fall. Assess if the person has a pet that could easily move around the person's feet to cause a fall. Lighting in the home must be assessed. Is the light bright enough to see walkways and stairs, and is there a lit path to the bathroom at night? Conduct a home and environmental check with the person's family caregiver present if possible.

Housing and environment affect the health of older adults. The environment can support or hinder physical and social functioning, enhance or drain energy, and complement or tax existing physical changes such as vision and hearing. For example, furnishings with red, orange, and yellow colors are easiest for older adults to see. Shiny waxed floors may appear to be wet or have a hole in them. Older adults have difficulty distinguishing between green and blue and among pastel shades. Door frames and baseboards should be a color that contrasts with the color of the wall to improve perception of the boundaries of halls and rooms. Stairs should have a color contrast at the edge of the step so the older person knows where the stair ends. Glare from highly polished floors, metallic fixtures, and windows is difficult for the older adult to tolerate.

Furniture must be comfortable and designed for the musculoskeletal changes of older adults. Older adults need to examine it carefully for size, comfort, and function before purchasing it. It must be easy to get into and out of and provide back support. Test dining room chairs for comfort during meals and for height in relation to the table. Armrests make it easier for patients to get in and out of a chair because they can use their arms to assist in lifting. Older adults often prefer transferring out of a wheelchair to another chair for meals because some styles of wheelchairs do not let older adults sit close enough to the table to eat comfortably. Raising the table to clear the wheelchair arms brings the table closer to the older adult but makes it too high for comfortable use. To make getting out of bed easier and safer, the height of the bed needs to allow the older adult's feet to be flat on the floor when he or she is sitting on the side of the bed.

Death. Part of one's life history is the experience of loss through the death of relatives and friends (see Chapter 36). This includes the loss of the older generations of families and sometimes, sadly, the loss of a child. However, death of a spouse is the loss that affects the lives of most older people. The death of a spouse affects older women more than men, a trend that will probably continue in the future. In spite of these experiences, it is wrong to assume that the older adult is comfortable with the idea of death. A key role of the nurse is to help older adults understand the meaning of the loss and cope with it.

Older people have a wide variety of attitudes and beliefs about death, but fear of their own death is uncommon (Friedman, 2006). Rather they are concerned with fear of being a burden, experiencing suffering, being alone, and the use of life-prolonging measures. The stereotype that the death of an older adult is a blessing does not apply to every older adult. Even as death approaches, many older adults still have unfinished business and are not prepared for it. Families and friends are not always ready to let go of him or her. The nurse is often the person to whom the older adult and family members or friends turn to for assistance. Knowledge of the grieving process (see Chapter 36), excellent communication skills; understanding of legal issues; familiarity with community resources; and awareness of one's own feelings, limitations, and strengths as they relate to care of those confronting death are critical.

ADDRESSING THE HEALTH CONCERNS OF OLDER ADULTS

As the population ages and life expectancy increases, emphasis on health promotion and disease prevention increases (see Chapter 6). The number of older adults becoming enthusiastic and motivated about these aspects of health is increasing. A number of national programs and projects address preventive practices in the older-adult population. The national initiative *Healthy People 2020* (HealthyPeople.gov), has a number of major goals affecting the older adult population, including increasing the number of older adults with one or more chronic conditions who report confidence in maintaining their conditions, reducing the proportion of older adults who have moderate-to-severe functional limitations, reducing the number of emergency department visits resulting from falls among older adults, increasing the number of older adults who live at home but have unmet long-term services and support; and increasing the proportion of older adults with reduced physical or cognitive function who engage in light, moderate, or vigorous leisure-term physical activities. Agencies that serve older adults will continue to collaborate in such efforts to promote health and prevent disease.

The challenges of health promotion and disease prevention for older adults are complex and affect health care providers as well. For the older adult, previous health care experiences, personal motivation, health beliefs, culture, and nonhealth-related factors such as transportation and finances can create barriers to participation. Barriers for health care providers include beliefs and attitudes about which services and programs to provide, their effectiveness and the lack of consistent guidelines, and absence of a coordinated approach. The nurse's role is to focus interventions on maintaining and promoting patients' function and quality of life. You can help older adults become empowered to make their own health care decisions and realize their optimum level of health, function, and quality of life (Resnick, 2006) Always be open to recognizing an older adult's concerns so you can adjust a plan of care accordingly. Although various interventions cross all three levels of care (i.e., health promotion, acute care, and restorative care), some approaches are unique to each level.

Health Promotion and Maintenance: Physiological Concerns

Older adults vary in their desire to participate in health promotion activities; therefore use an individualized approach, taking into account the person's beliefs about the importance of staying healthy and fit and remaining independent. Researchers have not fully identified the factors that lead to good health in advanced age, but three important factors seem to be genetics, good health habits, and preventive measures. Use creative approaches to incorporate health promotion activities in all health care settings.

The AOA (2009) reports that in 2008 38% of older persons had some type of disability (i.e., difficulty in hearing, vision, cognition, ambulation, self-care, or independent living). Some of these disabilities are relatively minor, but others cause people to require assistance to meet important personal needs. The incidence of disability increases with age. Limitations in ADLs limit the ability to live independently. The ADL limitations most often reported include walking, showering and bathing, getting in and out of bed and chair, dressing, toileting, and eating. There is a strong relationship between disability status and reported health status. The effect of chronic conditions on the lives of older adults varies widely, but in general chronic conditions further diminish well-being and a sense of independence. Direct nursing interventions at managing these conditions and educating family caregivers in ways to give appropriate support. It is also important to focus interventions on prevention. General preventive measures for you to recommend to older adults include:

- Participation in screening activities (e.g., blood pressure, mammography, Pap smears, depression, vision and hearing testing, colonoscopy)
- Regular exercise
- Weight reduction if overweight
- Eating a low-fat, well-balanced diet
- Moderate alcohol use
- Regular dental visits
- Smoking cessation
- Immunization for seasonal influenza, tetanus, diphtheria and pertussis, shingles, and pneumococcal disease

Those who die from influenza are predominately older adults. A debate currently centers about influenza deaths and the older adult. Do older adults die because of influenza or is the death related to worsening of a chronic illness and influenza? However, providers continue to strongly recommend annual immunization of all older adults for influenza, with special emphasis on residents of nursing homes or residential or long-term care facilities. Not all older adults are current with their booster injections, and some never

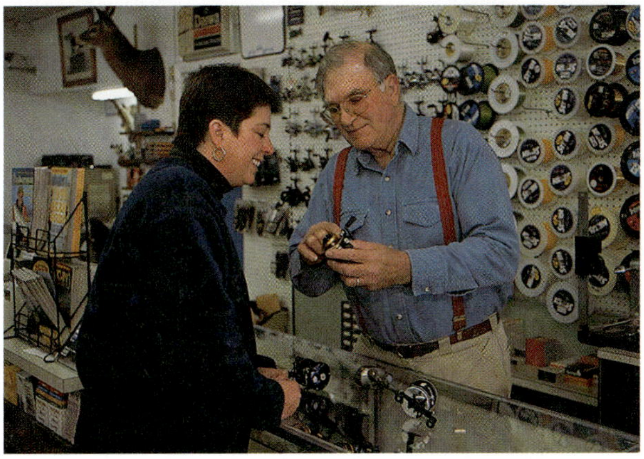

FIG. 14-1 This older adult works part time at a sporting goods store.

received the primary series of injections. Ask older adults about the current status of all immunizations, provide information about the immunizations, and make arrangements for the older adult to receive the immunizations as needed.

Most older adults are interested in their health and are capable of taking charge of their lives. They want to remain independent and prevent disability (Fig. 14-1). Initial screenings establish baseline data that you use to determine wellness, identify health needs, and design health maintenance programs. Following initial screening sessions, share with older adults information on nutrition, exercise, medications, and safety precautions. You can also provide information on specific conditions such as hypertension, arthritis, or self-care procedures such as foot and skin care. By providing information about health promotion and self-care, you significantly improve the health and well-being of older adults.

Heart Disease. Heart disease is the leading cause of death in older adults (CDC, 2010a). Common cardiovascular disorders are hypertension and coronary artery disease. Hypertension is a silent killer because often the person is unaware that his or her blood pressure is elevated (see Chapter 29). Although over half of Americans have elevated diastolic and/or systolic pressures, the fact that hypertension is common does not make it normal or harmless. Treatment of systolic pressures 160 mm Hg or higher is linked to reduced incidence of myocardial infarction, stroke, and heart failure. In coronary artery disease partial or complete blockage of one or more coronary arteries leads to myocardial ischemia and myocardial infarction. The risk factors for both hypertension and coronary artery disease include smoking, obesity, lack of exercise, and stress. Additional risk factors for coronary artery disease include hypertension, hyperlipidemia, and diabetes mellitus. Nursing interventions for hypertension and coronary artery disease address weight reduction, exercise, dietary changes, limiting salt and fat intake, stress management, and smoking cessation. Patient teaching also includes information about medication management, blood-pressure monitoring, and the symptoms indicating the need for emergency care.

Cancer. Malignant neoplasms are the second most common cause of death among older adults (CDC, 2010a). Nurses educate older adults about early detection, treatment, and cancer risk factors. Examples include smoking cessation, teaching breast self-examination (see Chapter 30), and encouraging all older adults to have annual screening for fecal occult blood with a rectal examination. It is also important to educate older adults about the signs of cancer and encourage prompt reporting of nonhealing skin lesions, unexpected bleeding, change in bowel habits, nagging cough, lump in breast or another part of body, change in a mole, difficulty swallowing, and unexplained weight loss. Cancer is difficult to detect because providers often mistake symptoms as part of the normal aging process or signs of a person's chronic disease. You need to carefully distinguish between signs of normal aging and signs of pathological conditions.

Stroke (Cerebrovascular Accident). Cerebrovascular accidents (CVAs) continue to be the third leading cause of death in the United States and occur as brain ischemia (inadequate blood supply to areas of brain caused by arterial blockage) or brain hemorrhage (subarachnoid or intercerebral bleeds) (CDC, 2010a). Risk factors for CVAs include hypertension, hyperlipidemia, diabetes mellitus, history of transient ischemic attacks, and family history of cardiovascular disease. CVAs often impair the functional abilities of older adults and lead to the inability to live independently. The scope of nursing interventions ranges from teaching older adults about risk-reduction strategies to teaching family caregivers the early warning signs of a stroke and ways to support a patient during recovery and rehabilitation.

Smoking. Cigarette smoking is a risk factor among the four most common causes of death: heart disease, cancer, stroke, and lung disease. Smoking is the most preventable cause of disease and death in the United States. As of 2009 an estimated 9.5% of people ages 65 and older smoked cigarettes (CDC, 2010b). Approximately 440,000 people die annually from smoking-related diseases, and 300,000 of those deaths occur in people ages 65 and older (CMS, 2010).

Smoking cessation is a health promotion strategy for older adults just as it is for younger adults. Older smokers still benefit from smoking cessation. In addition to reducing risk, it sometimes stabilizes existing conditions such as chronic obstructive pulmonary disease (COPD) and coronary artery disease. Smoking cessation after age 65 can add 2 to 3 years to life expectancy. Within a year of quitting, former smokers reduce their risk of coronary heart disease by 50% (National Cancer Institute, 2010). Smoking-cessation programs recommended by the CDC (2008) include individual, group, and telephone counseling and the use of nicotine (gum and patch) or nonnicotine medications. If the patient rejects smoking cessation, suggest at least a reduction in smoking. Finally, arrange with the older adult a quit or reduction date and a follow-up visit or contact to discuss the quit attempt. At follow-up visits, offer encouragement and assistance in modifying the plan as necessary.

Alcohol Abuse. Alcoholism can be found in older adults. Alcohol is inexpensive, legal, and accessible. Studies of alcohol abuse in older adults report two patterns: a lifelong pattern of heavy drinking that continues and a pattern when heavy drinking begins late in life. Frequently cited causes of excessive alcohol use are depression, loneliness, and lack of social support.

Alcohol abuse may be underidentified in older adults. The clues to creating suspicion of alcohol abuse are subtle, and coexisting dementia or depression sometimes complicates the assessment. Suspicion of alcohol abuse increases when there is a history of repeated falls and accidents, social isolation, recurring episodes of memory loss and confusion, failure to meet home and work obligations, a history of skipping meals or medications, and difficulty managing household tasks and finances. When you suspect that an older adult is abusing alcohol, realize that a variety of treatment needs are present. Treatment includes age-specific approaches that acknowledge the stresses experienced by the older adult and encourage involvement in activities that match the older adult's interests and increase feelings of self-worth. The identification and treatment of co-existing depression are also important. The continuum of interventions can range from simple education to formalized treatment programs that include pharmacotherapy, psychotherapy, and rehabilitation.

Nutrition. Lifelong eating habits and situational factors influence how older adults meet their needs for good nutrition. Lifelong eating habits based in tradition, ethnicity, and religion influence the choice of what foods are eaten and how they are prepared. Situational factors affecting nutrition include access to grocery stores, finances, physical and cognitive capability for food preparation, and a place to store food and prepare meals. Older adults' levels of activity and clinical conditions affect their nutritional needs. Level of activity has implications for the total amount of required calories. Older adults who are sedentary usually need fewer calories than those who are more active. However, activity alone does not determine caloric requirements. Additional calories are often necessary in clinical situations such as recovery from surgery, whereas fewer calories are necessary when the older adult has diabetes or is overweight.

Good nutrition for older adults includes appropriate caloric intake and limited intake of fat, salt, refined sugars, and alcohol. The nutritional guidelines displayed in the USDA's MyPlate (see Chapter 44) are the basic recommendations for older-adult nutrition. Protein intake is sometimes lower than recommended if older adults have reduced financial resources or limited access to grocery stores. Difficulty chewing meat because of poor dentition or poor-fitting dentures also limits protein intake. Fat intake is higher than usual because of the substitution of fast-food restaurant meals for meals prepared at home or because of methods of cooking featuring fried foods and sauces using butter and cream. Some use extra salt and sugar while cooking or at the table to compensate for a diminished sense of taste.

Older adults with dementia have special nutritional needs. As their memory and functional skills decline with the progression of dementia, they lose the ability to remember when to eat, how to prepare food, and how to feed themselves. Caloric needs may increase because of the energy expended in pacing and wandering activities. When caring for older adults with dementia, routinely monitor weight and food intake, serve food that is easy to eat such as finger foods (e.g., chicken strips, sandwiches, cut-up vegetables, and fruit), provide assistance with eating, and offer food supplements that are tasty and easy to swallow.

Dental Problems. Dental problems with natural teeth and dentures are common in older adults. Dental caries, gingivitis, broken or missing teeth, and ill-fitting or missing dentures affect nutritional adequacy, cause pain, and lead to infection. Dentures are a frequent problem because the cost is not covered by Medicare and dentures tend to be quite expensive. Help prevent dental and gum disease through education about routine dental care (see Chapter 39).

Exercise. Encourage older adults to maintain physical exercise and activity. The primary benefits of exercise include maintaining and strengthening functional ability and promoting a sense of enhanced well-being. Regular daily exercise such as walking builds endurance, increases muscle tone, improves joint flexibility, strengthens bones, reduces stress, and contributes to weight loss. Other benefits include improvement of cardiovascular function, improved plasma lipoprotein profiles, increased metabolic rate, increased gastrointestinal transit time, prevention of depressive illness, and improved sleep quality. Older adults who participate in group exercise programs or physical therapy may experience improved mobility, gait, and balance, resulting in fewer falls (Michael et al., 2010).

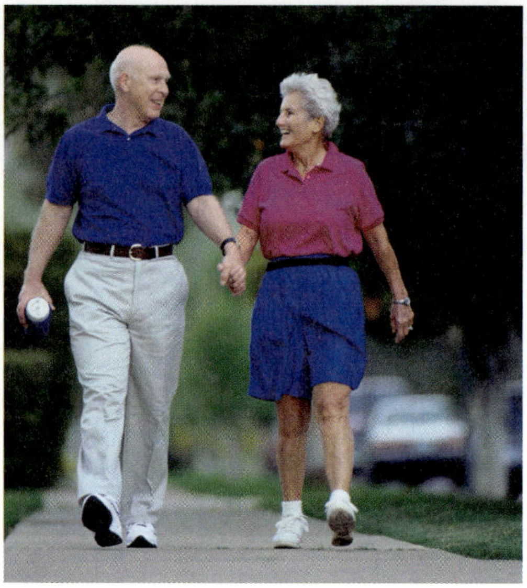

FIG.14-2 This couple enjoys walking together.

Consult with physical therapists and the patient's physician to plan an exercise program that meets physical needs and is one the patient enjoys. Consider the patient's physical limitations and encourage the older adult to stick with the exercise program. Many factors influence an individual's willingness to participate in an exercise program. These include general beliefs about benefits of exercise, past experiences with exercise, personal goals, personality, and any unpleasant sensations associated with exercise.

Walking is the preferred exercise of many older adults (Fig. 14-2). Walking and other low-impact exercises such as riding a stationary exercise bicycle or water exercises in a swimming pool protect the musculoskeletal system and joints. Other exercises can be included in the older adult's ADLs. For example, adults can perform arm and leg circles while watching television. Before beginning an exercise program, the older adult needs to have a physical examination. Exercise programs for sedentary older adults who have not been exercising regularly need to begin conservatively and progress slowly. Safety considerations include wearing good support shoes and clothing appropriate to the exercise, drinking water before and after exercising, avoiding outdoor exercise when the weather is very warm or very cold, and exercising with a partner. Instruct older adults to stop exercising and seek help if they experience chest pain or tightness, shortness of breath, dizziness or light-headedness, joint pain, or palpitations during exercise.

Falls. Falls are a safety concern of many older adults. One in three adults age 65 and older falls each year (CDC, 2010c). Fall-related injuries are often associated with a patient's preexisting medical conditions such as osteoporosis and bleeding tendencies. Hospitalization and placement in a nursing center for rehabilitation or long-term placement is sometimes necessary after a fall. In 2009 emergency departments treated 2.2 million nonfatal fall injuries among older adults; more than 582,000 of these patients had to be hospitalized (CDC, 2010c). The most common injuries in older adults include fractures of the spine, hip, forearm, leg, ankle, pelvis, upper arm, and hand. Older adults who fall may develop a fear of falling, which may in turn cause them to limit their

BOX 14-7 RISK FACTORS FOR FALLS IN OLDER ADULTS

Intrinsic Factors
- History of a previous fall
- Impaired vision
- Postural hypotension or syncope
- Conditions affecting mobility such as arthritis, muscle weakness, peripheral neuropathy, foot problems
- Conditions affecting balance and gait
- Alterations in bladder function such as frequency or urge incontinence and nocturia
- Cognitive impairment, agitation, and confusion
- Adverse medication reactions (sedatives, hypnotics, anticonvulsants, opioids)
- Slowed reaction times
- Deconditioning

Extrinsic Factors
- Environmental hazards outside and within the home such as poor lighting, slippery or wet flooring, items on floor that are easy to trip over, furniture placement and other obstacles to ambulation, and sidewalks and stairs in poor repair
- Inappropriate footwear
- Unfamiliar environment of a hospital room that contains barriers to movement (e.g., clutter, equipment, poor lighting at night)
- Improper use of assistive devices (e.g., canes, walkers, crutches)

activities, leading to reduced mobility and loss of physical fitness (CDC, 2010c). See Chapter 38 for a complete description of fall-prevention interventions. Box 14-7 summarizes both intrinsic and extrinsic risk factors leading to falls.

Sensory Impairments. Because of common sensory impairments experienced by an older adult, it is important to promote existing sensory function and to be sure that the patient lives in a safe environment. Whenever you provide care activities, make sure that the patient is wearing any assist devices such as a hearing aid or glasses so he or she can fully participate in care. Chapter 49 describes in detail the nursing interventions used to maintain and improve sensory function.

Pain. Pain is not a normal part of healthy aging. It is a symptom and a sensation of distress, alerting the person that something is wrong. It is prevalent in the older-adult population; it may be acute or chronic. The consequences of persistent pain include depression, loss of appetite, sleep difficulties, changes in gait and mobility, and decreased socialization. Many factors influence the management of pain, including cultural influences on the meaning and expression of pain for older adults, fears related to the use of analgesic medications, and the problem of pain assessment with cognitively impaired older adults. Nurses caring for older adults have to advocate for appropriate and effective pain management (see Chapter 43). Again, the goal of nursing management of pain in older adults is to maximize function and improve quality of life.

Medication Use. One of the greatest challenges for older adults is safe medication use. Although the elderly make up approximately 12% of the U.S. population, they consume 31% of the nation's prescribed drugs (Lehne, 2010). Some medication categories such as analgesics, antidepressants, antihistamines, antihypertensives, sedative-hypnotics, and muscle relaxants create a high likelihood of adverse effects in older adults. They are at risk for adverse medication effects because of age-related changes in the absorption, distribution, metabolism, and excretion of drugs, collectively referred to as the process of pharmacokinetics (see Chapter 31). Medications sometimes interact with one another, adding or negating the effect of another drug. Examples of adverse effects include confusion, impaired balance, dizziness, nausea, and vomiting. Because of these effects, some older adults are unwilling to take medications; others do not adhere to the prescribed dosing schedule, or they may try to medicate themselves with herbal and over-the-counter medications.

BOX 14-8 EVIDENCE-BASED PRACTICE

Polypharmacy in Older Adults

PICO Question: What adverse outcomes does polypharmacy versus limited medication use cause in older adults who live in the community?

Evidence Summary

Polypharmacy is an important factor in causing numerous health problems for older adults, including the risk for adverse drug events (ADEs), the inappropriate use of medications, and falls (Baranzini et al., 2009; Lau et al., 2010). A study of a sample of over 4500 older adults ages 65 and over living in the community found that 44% took more than five medications (Lau et al., 2010). When patients are near death, one study found an increase in medication use, with patients averaging 7.9 prescriptions (Chen et al., 2010). Patients with dementia are also vulnerable, experiencing a higher total prescription use and greater likelihood of having inappropriate prescriptions (Lau et al., 2010). Polypharmacy regimens that include at least one established fall-increasing drug group (e.g., antiarrhythmic and antiparkinson) may be a greater problem than polypharmacy alone (Baranzini et al., 2009). Although many prescriptions may be needed for some individuals, more prudent care is needed to lessen the risks. However, decreasing the number of medications alone may not effectively improve the quality of medication use (Lau et al., 2010). Certain medications will always be critical for managing patients' health conditions.

Application to Nursing Practice
- Have patients and family caregivers be sure that one physician (or nurse practitioner) knows all medications that a patient is prescribed. This is especially important if a patient sees several physicians.
- When a patient develops a new behavior or clinical change, consider a possible ADE; consult the physician and a clinical pharmacist.
- Older adults in long-term settings should have medications reviewed routinely (e.g., monthly).
- In long-term settings prescription of certain medications (e.g., laxatives for constipation) may occur without identifying underlying causes of the condition for which they are prescribed. Nurses should be aggressive in use of nonpharmacological treatments known to be effective.

Polypharmacy, the concurrent use of many medications, increases the risk for adverse drug effects (Box 14-8). Although polypharmacy may reflect inappropriate prescribing, the concurrent use of multiple medications is often necessary when an older adult has multiple acute and chronic conditions. For example, it is common for a patient to take more than one medication to control hypertension. The nurse's role is to ensure the greatest therapeutic benefit with the least amount of harm by educating patients about safe medication use. Nurses must question the efficacy and safety of combinations of prescribed medications and advocate for the older adult to prevent adverse reactions. Older adults may also use over-the-counter or herbal medications. The mix of over-the-counter and herbal medications with prescription medications can also create adverse reactions.

For some older adults safely managing medications is complex and often becomes overwhelming. Some older adults take their medications incorrectly because they do not understand the administration instructions, thereby complicating a nurse's assessment of effects and side effects. Medications that need to be taken more than once or twice a day are a concern because the patient may not remember to take them as scheduled. As a nurse you are in a position to assist older adult patients as they carry out this important self-care activity (see Chapter 31).

The cost of prescriptions can be prohibitive. You can advocate for patients who may need certain medications by working with pharmacies or drug companies to provide the needed medication at less cost. Often a generic medication that will provide the desired effect is available at a reduced cost.

Work collaboratively with older adults to ensure safe and appropriate use of all medications, both prescribed and over-the-counter. Teach an older adult the names of all medications that he or she is taking, when and how to take them, and desirable and undesirable effects. Explain how to avoid adverse effects and/or interactions of medications and how to establish and follow an appropriate self-administration pattern. Strategies for reducing the risk for an adverse medication effect in the older adult include reviewing the medications with the older adult at each visit; examining for potential interactions with food or other medications; simplifying and individualizing the medication regimen; taking every opportunity to inform the older adult and family about all aspects of medication use; and encouraging the older adult to question the physician, advanced practice nurse, and/or pharmacist about all prescribed medications and all over-the-counter medications.

When providers use medications to manage confusion, special care is necessary. The sedatives and tranquilizers sometimes prescribed for acutely confused older adults may cause or exacerbate confusion and increase risks for falls or other injuries. Carefully administer medications used to manage confused behaviors, taking into account age-related changes in body systems that affect pharmacokinetic activity. When confusion has a physiological cause (such as an infection), health care providers must treat the cause rather than the confused behavior. When confusion varies by time of day or is related to environmental factors, use creative, nonpharmacological measures such as making the environment more meaningful, providing adequate light, encouraging use of assistive devices, or even calling friends or family members to let older adults hear reassuring voices.

Health Promotion and Maintenance: Psychosocial Health Concerns

Interventions supporting the psychosocial health of older adults resemble those for other age-groups. However, some interventions are more crucial for older adults experiencing social isolation; cognitive impairment; or stresses related to retirement, relocation, or approaching death.

Therapeutic Communication. Therapeutic communication skills enable you to perceive and respect the older adult's uniqueness and health care expectations. Attentive nurses provide care in a timely fashion, meeting a patient's expressed or unexpressed needs. A caring nurse expresses attitudes of concern, kindness, and compassion. Knowledgeable nurses not only demonstrate procedural competence but recognize needs and relay information skillfully. Patients accept and respect nurses who meet these expectations and communicate effectively about concern for the older adult's welfare. However, you cannot simply enter an older adult's environment and immediately establish a therapeutic relationship. First you have to be knowledgeable and skilled in communication techniques (see Chapter 24).

Touch. Touch is a therapeutic tool that you use to help comfort older adults. A pilot study by Wang and Hermann (2006) showed that agitation levels were significantly lower in demented older adults who received a healing touch intervention. Touch provides sensory stimulation, induces relaxation, provides physical and emotional comfort, orients the person to reality, shows warmth, and communicates interest. It is a powerful physical expression of a relationship.

Older adults are often deprived of touching when separated from family or friends. An older adult who is isolated, dependent, or ill; who fears death; or who lacks self-esteem has a greater need for touch. You recognize touch deprivation by behaviors as simple as an older adult reaching for the nurse's hand or standing close to the nurse. Unfortunately older men are sometimes wrongly accused of sexual advances when they reach out to touch others. When you use touch, be aware of cultural variations and individual preferences (see Chapters 7 and 9). Touch should convey respect and sensitivity. Do not use it in a condescending way such as patting an older adult on the head. When you reach out to an older adult, do not be surprised if the older adult reciprocates.

Reality Orientation. **Reality orientation** is a communication technique that makes an older adult more aware of time, place, and person. The purposes of reality orientation include restoring a sense of reality; improving the level of awareness, promoting socialization; elevating independent functioning; and minimizing confusion, disorientation, and physical regression. Although you use reality orientation techniques in any health care setting, they are especially useful in the acute care setting. The older adult experiencing a change in environment, surgery, illness, or emotional stress is at risk for becoming disoriented. Environmental changes such as the bright lights, unfamiliar noises, and lack of windows in specialized units of a hospital often lead to disorientation and confusion. Absence of familiar caregivers is also disorienting. Using anesthesia, sedatives, tranquilizers, analgesics, and physical restraints with older patients increases disorientation. Anticipate and monitor for disorientation and confusion as possible consequences of hospitalization, relocation, surgery, loss, or illness and incorporate interventions based on reality orientation into the care plan.

The principles of reality orientation offer useful guidelines for communicating with acutely confused individuals. The key elements of reality orientation include frequent reminders of person, time, and place; the use of environmental aids such as clocks, calendars, and personal belongings; and stability of environment, routine, and staff. However, do not continue to reorient older adults with chronic cognitive impairment. Communication is always respectful, patient, and calm. Answer questions from the older adult simply and honestly with sensitivity and a caring attitude.

Validation Therapy. **Validation therapy** is an alternative approach to communication with a confused older adult. Whereas reality orientation insists that the confused older adult agree with our statements of time, place, and person, validation therapy accepts the description of time and place as stated by the confused older adult. Older adults with dementia are less likely to benefit and more likely to become agitated by a caregiver's insistence on the "correct" time, place, and person. In validation therapy you do not challenge or argue with statements and behaviors of the confused older adult. They represent an inner need or feeling. For example, the person might insist that the day is actually a different day because of high anxiety. The appropriate nursing intervention is to recognize and address that inner need or feeling. Validation does not involve reinforcing the confused older adult's misperceptions; it reflects sensitivity to hidden meanings in statements and behaviors. By listening with sensitivity and validating what the patient is expressing, you convey respect, reassurance, and understanding. Validating or respecting confused older adults' feelings in the time and place that is real to them is more important than insisting on the literally correct time and place.

Reminiscence. Reminiscence is recalling the past. Many older adults enjoy sharing past experiences. As a therapy, reminiscence uses the recollection of the past to bring meaning and understanding to the present and resolve current conflicts. Looking back to positive resolutions of problems reminds the older adult of coping strategies used successfully in the past. Reminiscing is also a way to express personal identity. Reflection on past achievements supports self-esteem. For some older adults the process of looking back on past events uncovers new meanings for those events.

During the assessment process use reminiscence to assess self-esteem, cognitive function, emotional stability, unresolved conflicts, coping ability, and expectations for the future. For example, have a patient talk about a previous loss to assess coping. You can also reminisce during direct care activities. Taking time to ask questions about past experiences and listening attentively conveys to an older adult your attitudes of respect and concern.

Although many use reminiscence in a one-on-one situation, it is also used as a group therapy for cognitively impaired or depressed older adults. The nurse organizes the group and selects strategies to start a conversation. For example, the nurse asks the group to discuss family activities or childhood memories. He or she adapts the group's size, structure, process, goals, and activities to meet its members' needs.

Body-Image Interventions. The way that older adults present themselves influences body image and feelings of isolation (Chapter 33). Some physical characteristics of older adulthood such as distinguished-looking gray hair are socially desirable. Other features such as a lined face that displays character or wrinkled hands that show a lifetime of hard work are also impressive. However, too often society sees older people as incapacitated, deaf, obese, or shrunken in stature. Consequences of illness and aging that threaten the older adult's body image include invasive diagnostic procedures, pain, surgery, loss of sensation in a body part, skin changes, and incontinence. The use of devices such as dentures, hearing aids, artificial limbs, indwelling catheters, ostomy devices, and enteral feeding tubes also affects body image.

The nurse needs to consider the importance to the older adult of presenting a socially acceptable image. When older adults have acute or chronic illnesses, the related physical dependence makes it difficult for them to maintain body image. You influence the older adult's appearance by helping with grooming and hygiene. It takes little effort to help the older adult comb hair, clean dentures, shave, or change clothing. He or she does not choose to have an objectionable appearance. Be sensitive to odors in the environment. Odors created by urine and some illnesses are often present. By controlling odors you may prevent visitors from shortening their stay or not coming at all.

OLDER ADULTS AND THE ACUTE CARE SETTING

Older adults in the acute care setting need special attention to help them adjust to the acute care environment and meet their basic needs. The acute care setting poses increased risk for adverse events such as delirium, dehydration, malnutrition, health care–associated infections (HAIs), urinary incontinence, and falls. The risk for delirium increases when hospitalized older adults experience immobilization, sleep deprivation, infection, dehydration, pain, sensory impairment, drug interactions, anesthesia, and hypoxia. Nonmedical causes of delirium include placement in unfamiliar surroundings and staff, bed rest, separation from supportive family members, and stress. Impaired vision or hearing contributes to confusion and interferes with attempts to reorient the older adult. When the prevention of delirium fails, nursing management begins with identifying and treating the cause. Supportive interventions include encouraging family visits, providing memory cues (clocks, calendars, and name tags), and compensating for sensory deficits. Reality orientation techniques are also useful.

Older adults are at greater risk for dehydration and malnutrition during hospitalization because of standard procedures such as limiting food and fluids in preparation for diagnostic tests and medications that decrease appetite. The risk for dehydration and malnutrition increases when older adults are unable to reach beverages or feed themselves while in bed or connected to medical equipment. Interventions include getting the patient out of bed, providing beverages and snacks frequently, and including favorite foods and beverages in the diet plan.

The increased risk for HAIs in older adults is associated with age-related reductions in immune system responses. In a study including 47 hospitals in 14 countries across four continents, adults over 64 years of age (prevalence 12%) suffered more HAIs than others (Manyon-White, 2009). Urinary catheter–related bacteriuria in older adults is the most common type. Other HAIs in this population include infection at the surgical site, pneumonia, and bloodstream infections. Prevention begins with hand hygiene and measures to minimize the risk of infection from procedures (see Chapter 28).

Older hospitalized adults in acute care are at risk for becoming incontinent of urine (transient incontinence). Causes of incontinence include delirium, untreated urinary tract infection, medications, restricted mobility or need for assistance to get to the bathroom, and constipation or stool impaction. Interventions to decrease incontinence include individualized care planning to provide voiding opportunities and modification of the environment to improve access to the toilet. Avoid indwelling urinary catheterization and promote measures to prevent skin breakdown (see Chapter 45).

The increased risk for skin breakdown and the development of pressure ulcers is related to changes in aging skin and to situations that occur in the acute care setting such as immobility, incontinence, and malnutrition. The key points in the prevention of skin breakdown are avoiding pressure with proper positioning and use of a support surface based on risk status, reducing shear forces and friction, providing meticulous skin care and moisture management, and providing nutritional support (see Chapter 48).

Older adults in the acute care setting are at risk for falling and sustaining injuries. The cause of a fall is typically multifactorial and composed of intrinsic or extrinsic factors (see Box 14-7). Sedative and hypnotic medications increase unsteadiness. Medications causing orthostatic hypotension also increase the risk for falls because of the blood pressure drop when the older adult gets out of a bed or chair. The increase in urine output from diuretics increases the risk for falling by increasing the number of attempts to get out of bed to void. Attempts to get out of bed when physically restrained sometimes lead to injury when the older adult becomes entangled in the restraint. Equipment such as wires from monitors, intravenous tubing, urinary catheters, and other medical devices become obstacles to safe ambulation. Impaired vision prevents the older adult from seeing tripping hazards such as trash cans. Interventions to reduce the risk for falling in a health care setting are discussed in Chapter 38.

OLDER ADULTS AND RESTORATIVE CARE

Restorative care refers to two types of ongoing care: the continuation of the recovery from acute illness or surgery that began in the acute care setting and support of chronic conditions that affect day-to-day functioning. Both types of restorative care take place in private homes and long-term care settings.

Direct interventions during convalescence from acute illness or surgery aim at regaining or improving patients' prior level of independence in ADLs. Continue interventions that began in the acute care setting and later modify them as convalescence progresses. To achieve this continuation, the discharge information provided by the acute care setting must include information on the ongoing interventions (e.g., exercise routines, wound care routines, medication schedules, and blood glucose monitoring). Interventions also need to address the restoration of interpersonal relationships and activities at either their previous level or at the level desired by the older adult. When restorative care addresses chronic conditions, the goals of care include stabilizing the chronic condition, promoting health, and promoting independence in ADLs.

Interventions to promote independence in ADLs address a person's physical ability, cognitive ability, and safety. The physical ability to perform ADLs requires strength, flexibility, and balance. You need to make accommodation for impairments of vision, hearing, and touch. The cognitive ability to perform ADLs requires the ability to recognize, judge, and remember. Cognitive impairments such as dementia interfere with safe performance of ADLs, although the older adult is still physically capable of the activities. Interventions to promote independence in ADLs should adapt these requirements to the needs and lifestyle of the older adult. You always consider safety because it is not enough just to be able to perform any of the ADLs. The older adult needs to be able to perform the ADLs with a level of risk that is acceptable to him or her.

Beyond the basic ADLs, you need to support an older adult's ability to perform IADLs such as using a telephone, doing laundry, cleaning the home or apartment, and driving an automobile. To remain living independently at home or in an apartment, older adults need to be able to perform IADLs, purchase services by outside workers, or have a supportive network of family and friends who assist with these tasks. Occupational therapists are an important resource for helping persons adapt when IADLs are difficult to perform.

Restorative care measures focus on activities to prevent, improve, reduce, or eliminate problems. You establish priorities of care and patient goals, determine expected outcomes, and select appropriate interventions. You do this with the older adult's participation so the patient understands interventions and to avoid conflicts in approaches or priorities. Consideration of the older adult's lifetime experiences and the values and sociocultural patterns developed serves as the basis for planning individual care. When the older adult's cognitive status prevents participation in health care decisions, you need to include the family. Family and friends are rich sources of data because they knew the older adult before the impairment. Frequently they provide explanations for the older adult's behaviors and suggest methods of management. Thoughtful assessment and planning lead to goals of care that consider the influence of normal aging changes, facilitate an optimal level of comfort and coping, and promote independence in self-care activities.

KEY POINTS

- Nursing care of older adults poses special challenges because of great variation in their physiological, cognitive, and psychosocial health.
- When health care providers hold negative stereotypes about aging, these stereotypes can negatively affect the quality of patient care.
- A developmental task of aging includes dealing with common losses, including loss of health, significant others, a sense of being useful, socialization, income, and independent living.
- The best way to evaluate the quality of a nursing center in a community is for the patient and family to visit that facility and inspect it personally.
- A comprehensive assessment of an older adult takes more time than the assessment of a younger adult because of the longer life and medical history and the potential complexity of the history.
- Classic signs and symptoms of diseases are sometimes absent, blunted, or atypical in older adults.
- Normal physiological changes of aging are not pathological processes, but they make older adults more vulnerable to some common clinical conditions and diseases.
- A sudden change in function, as evidenced by a decline or change in the older adult's ability to perform any one or combination of ADLs or IADLs, is often a sign of the onset of an acute illness.
- Symptoms of cognitive impairment such as disorientation, loss of language skills, and poor judgment are not normal aging changes and require you to further assess patients for underlying causes.
- Assess a patient's potential for social isolation by identifying his or her social network, access to transportation, and willingness and desire to interact with others.
- General preventive health measures for older adults include routine health screening; regular exercise; weight reduction if overweight; eating a low-fat, well-balanced diet; moderate alcohol use; regular dental visits; smoking cessation; and immunization.
- Polypharmacy, the concurrent use of many medications, increases the risk for adverse drug effects, inappropriate use of medications, and falls in older adults.
- Reminiscence uses the recollection of the past to bring meaning and understanding to the present and resolve current conflicts.
- Acute care settings place older adults at risk for delirium, dehydration, malnutrition, HAIs, and falls.
- Restorative nursing interventions stabilize chronic conditions, promote health, and promote independence in basic and instrumental activities of daily living.

CLINICAL APPLICATION QUESTIONS

Preparing for Clinical Practice

Mrs. Kaven is an 81-year-old woman who is admitted to the hospital following emergency surgery for a hip pinning of a hip fracture secondary to a fall at her home. Her other medical problems are hypertension, hypothyroidism, and anxiety disorder for which she takes a diuretic and thyroid replacement medication. She has had bilateral knee replacements in the past. Her home is "handicap" friendly. She is a retired bookkeeper, a widow living independently at her home, and usually very active. She drives, plays cards weekly with her friends, and participates in church activities twice a week. She hires help for household cleaning and yard work. She wears glasses, has uncorrected cataracts, and uses a cane.

You are assigned to care for her on her first postoperative day after the hip pinning. You learn in report that Mrs. Kaven has been receiving opioids for postoperative pain, with her last pain rating a 5 on a scale of 0 to 10. She has intravenous fluids for hydration for the first 24 hours. She has an indwelling urinary catheter. The night nurse reports that Mrs. Kaven was restless all night and slept very little and that she had even tried to get out of bed. You enter Mrs. Kaven's room and find her picking at the air and talking to herself as she tries to eat her breakfast. She is not wearing her glasses. She is oriented to self only. As you do your shift assessment, you recognize that she is delirious.

1. During your assessment what conditions prompt you to suspect that the patient has delirium? (Select all that apply.)
   1. Presence of indwelling urinary catheter
   2. Orientation status
   3. Presence of hypertension
   4. Distraction from being able to eat
2. Mrs. Kaven's good friend comes to visit. She is concerned that the patient seems confused. She asks the nurse if there is anything she can do to help the patient be less confused. The nurse's best suggestions would be to do which of the following: (Select all that apply.)
   1. Help her put on her glasses.
   2. Let her rest without the presence of a visitor.
   3. Have a conversation with her about activities of the day.
   4. Avoid giving her too many oral fluids.
3. Explain the approach that the patient's physician and other health care providers must use to reverse the patient's delirium. Give some examples of these approaches.

evolve *Answers to Clinical Application Questions can be found on the Evolve website.*

REVIEW QUESTIONS

Are You Ready to Test Your Nursing Knowledge?

1. A student nurse is caring for a 78-year-old patient with multiple sclerosis. The patient has had an indwelling Foley catheter in for 3 days. Eight hours ago the patient's temperature was 37.1° C (98.8° F). The student reports her recent assessment to the registered nurse (RN): the patient's temperature is 37.2° C (99° F); the Foley catheter is still in place, draining dark urine; and the patient is uncertain what time of day it is. From what the RN knows about presentation of symptoms in older adults, what should he recommend first?
   1. Tell the student that temporary confusion is normal and simply requires reorientation
   2. Tell the student to increase the patient's fluid intake since the urine is concentrated
   3. Tell the student that her assessment findings are normal for an older adult
   4. Tell the student that he will notify the physician of the findings
2. A patient's family member is considering having her mother placed in a nursing center. You have talked with the family before and know that this is a difficult decision. Which of the following criteria would you recommend in choosing a nursing center? (Select all that apply.)
   1. The center should be clean, and rooms should look like a hospital room.
   2. There should be adequate staffing on all shifts.
   3. Social activities should be available for all residents.
   4. Three meals should be served daily with a set menu and serving schedule.
   5. Family involvement in care planning and assisting with physical care is necessary.
3. A nurse has conducted an assessment of a new patient who has come to the medical clinic. The patient is 82 years old and has had osteoarthritis for 10 years and diabetes mellitus for 20 years. He is alert but becomes easily distracted during the nursing history. He recently moved to a new apartment, and his pet beagle died just 2 months ago. He is most likely experiencing:
   1. Dementia.
   2. Depression.
   3. Delirium.
   4. Disengagement.
4. A major life event such as the death of a loved one, a move to a nursing home, or a cancer diagnosis could precipitate:
   1. Dementia.
   2. Delirium.
   3. Depression.
   4. Stroke.
5. Sexuality is maintained throughout our lives. Which answer below best explains sexuality in an older adult?
   1. When the sexual partner passes away, the survivor no longer feels sexual.
   2. A decrease in an older adult's libido occurs.
   3. Any outward expression of sexuality suggests that the older adult is having a developmental problem.
   4. All older adults, whether healthy or frail, need to express sexual feelings.
6. Older adults experience a change in sexual activity. Which best explains this change?
   1. The need to touch and be touched is decreased.
   2. The sexual preferences of older adults are not as diverse.
   3. Physical changes usually do not affect sexual functioning.
   4. Frequency and opportunities for sexual activity may decline.
7. You see a 76-year-old woman in the outpatient clinic. Her chief complaint is vision. She states she has really noticed glare in the lights at home. Her vision is blurred; and she is unable to play cards with her friends, read, or do her needlework. You suspect that she may have:
   1. Presbyopia.
   2. Disengagement.
   3. Cataract(s).
   4. Depression.
8. A nurse is caring for a patient preparing for discharge from the hospital the next day. The patient does not read and has a hearing loss. His family caregiver will be visiting before discharge. What can you do to facilitate the patient's understanding of his discharge instructions? (Select all that apply.)
   1. Speak loudly so the patient can hear you.
   2. Sit facing the patient so he is able to watch your lip movements and facial expressions.
   3. Present one idea or concept at a time.

4. Send a written copy of the instructions home with him and tell him to have the family review them.
5. Include the family caregiver in the teaching session.

9. Taste buds atrophy and lose sensitivity, and appetite may decrease. As a result, the older adult is less able to discern:
   1. Spicy and bland foods.
   2. Salty, sour, and bitter tastes.
   3. Hot and cold food temperatures.
   4. Moist and dry food preparations.
10. Kyphosis, a change in the musculoskeletal system, leads to:
    1. Decreased bone density in the vertebrae and hips.
    2. Increased risk for pathological stress fractures in the hips.
    3. Changes in the configuration of the spine that affect the lungs and thorax.
    4. Calcification of the bony tissues of the long bones such as in the legs and arm.
11. A 63-year-old patient is retiring from his job at an accounting firm where he was in a management role for the past 20 years. He has been with the same company for 42 years and was a dedicated employee. His wife is a homemaker. She raised their five children, babysits for her grandchildren as needed, and belongs to numerous church committees. What are your major concerns for this patient? (Select all that apply.)
    1. The loss of his work role
    2. The risk of social isolation
    3. A determination if the wife will need to start working
    4. How the wife expects household tasks to be divided in the home in retirement
    5. The age the patient chose to retire
12. During a home health visit a nurse talks with a patient and his family caregiver about the patient's medications. The patient has hypertension and renal disease. Which of the following findings places him at risk for an adverse drug event? (Select all that apply.)
    1. Taking two medications for hypertension
    2. Taking a total of eight different medications during the day.
    3. Having one physician who reviews all medications
    4. Patient's health history
    5. Involvement of the caregiver in assisting with medication administration
13. You are caring for an 80-year-old man who recently lost his wife. He shares with you that he has been drinking more than he ever did in the past and feels hopeless without his wife. He reports that he rarely sees his children and feels isolated and alone. This patient is at risk for:
    1. Dementia.
    2. Liver failure.
    3. Dehydration.
    4. Suicide.
14. You are working with an older adult after an acute hospitalization. Your goal is to help this person be more in touch with time, place, and person. What might you try?
    1. Reminiscence
    2. Validation therapy
    3. Reality orientation
    4. Body image interventions
15. A 71-year-old patient enters the emergency department after falling down stairs in the home. The nurse is conducting a fall history with the patient and his wife. They live in a one-level ranch home. He has had diabetes for over 15 years and experiences some numbness in his feet. He wears bifocal glasses. His blood pressure is stable around 130/70. The patient does not exercise regularly and complains of weakness in his legs when climbing stairs. He is alert, oriented, and able to answer questions clearly. What are the fall risk factors for this patient? (Select all that apply.)
    1. Presence of a chronic disease
    2. Impaired vision
    3. Residence design
    4. Blood pressure
    5. Leg weakness
    6. Exercise history

Answers: **1.** 4; **2.** 2, 3, 5; **3.** 2; **4.** 3; **5.** 4; **6.** 4; **7.** 3; **8.** 2, 3, 5; **9.** 2; **10.** 3; **11.** 1, 4; **12.** 2, 4; **13.** 4; **14.** 3; **15.** 2, 5, 6.

REFERENCES

Administration on Aging (AOA): *A profile of older Americans,* 2009, http://www.aoa.gov/AoARoot/Aging_Statistics/Profile/2009/6.aspx. Accessed December 31, 2010.

Administration on Aging (AOA): *A profile of older Americans,* 2010, http://www.aoa.gov/AoARoot/Aging_Statistics/Profile/index.aspx. Accessed December 31, 2010.

Amella E: Presentation of illness in older adults, *AORN J* 83(2):372, 377, 385, 2006.

American Cancer Society, Prostate Cancer, 2010, http://www.cancer.org/Cancer/ProstateCancer/DetailedGuide/prostate-cancer-key-statistics. Accessed December 31, 2010.

Atkinson P: Intimacy and sexuality. In Meiner S, Lueckenotte A, editors: *Gerontologic nursing,* ed 3, St Louis, 2006, Mosby.

Centers for Disease Control and Prevention (CDC): *Clinical practice guideline: treating tobacco use and dependence,* update 2008, http://www.surgeongeneral.gov/tobacco/treating_tobacco_use08.pdf 2008. Accessed February 1, 2011.

Centers for Disease Control and Prevention (CDC): *Injury prevention and control, data and statistics,* Atlanta Ga, 2010a, CDC, http://www.cdc.gov/injury/wisqars/LeadingCauses.html. Accessed February 1, 2011.

Centers for Disease Control and Prevention (CDC): *Smoking and tobacco use,* Atlanta, Ga, 2010b, CDC, http://www.cdc.gov/tobacco/data_statistics/tables/adults/index.htm. Accessed February 1, 2011.

Centers for Disease Control and Prevention (CDC): *Injury prevention and control: home and recreational safety: cost of falls among older adults,* Atlanta, Ga, 2010c, CDC, http://www.cdc.gov/HomeandRecreationalSafety/Falls/fallcost.html. Accessed February 1, 2011.

Centers for Medicare & Medicaid Services (CMS): *Guide to choosing a nursing home,* Baltimore, Md, 2008, CMS, http://www.medicare.gov/nursing/checklist.as. Accessed January 9, 2011.

Centers for Medicare & Medicaid Services (CMS): *Smoking cessation overview,* Baltimore Md, 2010, CMS, http://www.cms.gov/SmokingCessation/. Accessed February 1, 2011.

Cummings E, Henry W: *Growing old: the process of disengagement,* New York, 1961, Basic Books.

Ebersole P, et al: *Toward healthy aging: human needs and nursing response,* St Louis, 2008, Mosby Elsevier.

Ferrari M, et al: Contributing factors associated with impulsivity-related falls in hospitalized, older adults, *J Nurs Care Quality* 25:320, 2010.

Fredriksen-Goldsen K, et al: Chronically ill midlife and older lesbians, gay men, and bisexuals and their informal caregivers: the impact of the social context, *Sex Res Social Policy* 6(4):52, 2009.

Friedman S: Loss and end-of-life issues. In Meiner S, Lueckenotte A, editors: *Gerontologic nursing,* ed 3, St Louis, 2006, Mosby.

Gray-Miceli D, et al: Teaching strategies for atypical presentation of illness in older adults, *J Gerontol Nurs* 36(7):38, 2010.

Havighurst RJ, et al: Disengagement, personality and life satisfaction in the later years. In Hansen P, editor: *Age with a future,* Copenhagen, 1963, Munksgoarsd.

Jett K: Theories of aging. In Ebersole P, et al: *Toward healthy aging; human needs & nursing response,* ed 7, St Louis, 2008, Mosby.

Kresevic D: Assessment of function. In Capezuti E and others: *Evidence-based geriatric nursing protocols for best practice,* ed 3, New York, 2008, Springer.

Lehne RA: *Pharmacology for nursing care,* ed 7, St Louis, 2010, Saunders.

Levy B, et al: Attitudes about aging affect longevity, *J Pers Social Psychol* 33(9):10, 2002.

Meiner S: *Gerontologic nursing,* ed 4, St Louis, 2011, Mosby.

Mental Health America—2011, http://www.mentalhealthamerica.net/index.cfm?objectid=C7DF94FF-1372-4D20-C8E34FC. Accessed January 2, 2011.
National Cancer Institute, US National Cancer Institute Fact Sheet: *Harms of smoking and benefits of quitting*, 2010, http://www.cancer.gov/cancertopics/factsheet/Tobacco/cessation. Accessed February 1, 2011.
National Osteoporosis Foundation: *Bone health basics*, 2010, http://www.nof.org/aboutosteoporosis/bonebasics/whybonehealth. Accessed December 29, 2010.
Neugarten B: *Personality in middle and late life*, New York, 1964, Atherton.
Rantz M, et al: *The new nursing homes: a 20-minute way to find great long-term care*, Minneapolis, 2001, Fairview Press.
Resnick B: Health promotion and illness/disability prevention. In Meiner S, Lueckenotte A, editors: *Gerontologic nursing*, ed 3, St Louis, 2006, Mosby.
Touhy TA, Jett KF: *Ebersole and Hess' gerontological nursing and healthy aging*, ed 3, St Louis, 2010, Mosby.
Wallace A: Assessment of sexual health in older adults, *Am J Nurs* 108(7):52, 2008.

RESEARCH REFERENCES

Baranzini F, et al: Fall-related injuries in a nursing home setting: is polypharmacy a risk factor? *BMC Health Services Res* 9:228, 2009.
Chen I, et al: Use of medication by nursing home residents nearing end of life: a preliminary report, *J Nurs Res* 18(3):199, 2010.
Lau DT, et al: Polypharmacy and potentially inappropriate medication use among community-dwelling elders with dementia, *Alzheimer Dis Assoc Disord* 24(1):56, 2010.
Manyon-White R, et al: An international survey of the prevalence of hospital-acquired infection, *J Hosp Infect* 11:43, 2009.
Michael YL, et al: Primary care-relevant interventions to prevent falling in older adults: a systematic evidence review for the US Preventive Services Task Force, *Ann Intern Med* 153(12):843, 2010.
Sims CM: Ethnic notions and healthy paranoias: understanding of the context of experience and interpretations of healthcare encounters among older black women, *Ethn Health* 15(5):495, 2010.
Wadensten B: The theory of gerotranscendence as applied to gerontological nursing, Part I, *Int J Older People Nurs* 2:296, 2007.
Wang KL, Hermann C: Pilot study to test the effectiveness of healing touch on agitation in people with dementia, *Geriatr Nurs* 27(1):34, 2006.

CHAPTER 15

Critical Thinking in Nursing Practice

OBJECTIVES

- Describe characteristics of a critical thinker.
- Discuss the nurse's responsibility in making clinical decisions.
- Discuss how reflection improves clinical decision making.
- Describe the components of a critical thinking model for clinical decision making.
- Discuss critical thinking skills used in nursing practice.
- Explain the relationship between clinical experience and critical thinking.
- Discuss the critical thinking attitudes used in clinical decision making.
- Explain how professional standards influence a nurse's clinical decisions.
- Discuss the relationship of the nursing process to critical thinking.

KEY TERMS

Clinical decision making, p. 196
Concept map, p. 202
Critical thinking, p. 193
Decision making, p. 195
Diagnostic reasoning, p. 196
Evidence-based knowledge, p. 193
Inference, p. 196
Nursing process, p. 197
Problem solving, p. 195
Reflection, p. 202
Scientific method, p. 195

evolve WEBSITE

http://evolve.elsevier.com/Potter/fundamentals/

- Review Questions
- Case Study with Questions
- Audio Glossary
- Interactive Learning Activities
- Key Term Flashcards
- Content Updates

Every day you think critically without realizing it. If it's hot outside, you take off a sweater. If your DVD doesn't start, you reposition the disc. If you decide to walk the dogs, you change to a pair of walking shoes. These examples involve critical thinking as you face each day and prepare for all possibilities. As a nurse, you will face many clinical situations involving patients, family members, health care staff, and peers. In each situation it is important to try to see the big picture and think smart. To think smart you have to develop critical thinking skills to face each new experience and problem involving a patient's care with open-mindedness, creativity, confidence, and continual inquiry. When a patient develops a new set of symptoms, asks you to offer comfort, or requires a procedure, it is important to think critically and make sensible judgments so the patient receives the best nursing care possible. Critical thinking is not a simple step-by-step, linear process that you learn overnight. It is a process acquired only through experience, commitment, and an active curiosity toward learning.

CLINICAL DECISIONS IN NURSING PRACTICE

Nurses are responsible for making accurate and appropriate clinical decisions. Clinical decision making separates professional nurses from technical personnel. For example, a professional nurse observes for changes in patients, recognizes potential problems, identifies new problems as they arise, and takes immediate action when a patient's clinical condition worsens. Technical personnel simply follow direction in completing aspects of care that the professional nurse has identified as necessary. A professional nurse relies on knowledge and experience when deciding if a patient is having complications that call for notification of a health care provider or decides if a teaching plan for a patient is ineffective and needs revision. Benner (1984) describes clinical decision making as judgment that includes critical and reflective thinking and action and application of scientific and practical logic. Most patients have health care problems for which there are no clear textbook solutions. Each patient's problems are unique, a product of the patient's physical health, lifestyle, culture, relationship with family and friends, living environment, and experiences. Thus as a nurse you do not always have a clear picture of a patient's needs and the appropriate actions to take when first meeting a patient. Instead you must learn to question, wonder, and explore different perspectives and interpretations to find a solution that benefits the patient.

Because no two patients' health problems are the same, you always apply critical thinking differently. Observe patients closely, gather information about them, examine ideas and inferences about patient problems, recognize the problems, consider scientific principles relating to the problems, and develop an approach to nursing care. With experience you learn to creatively seek new knowledge, act quickly when events change, and make quality decisions for patients' well-being. You will find nursing to be rewarding and fulfilling through the clinical decisions you make.

CRITICAL THINKING DEFINED

Mr. Jacobs is a 58-year-old patient who had a radical prostatectomy for prostate cancer yesterday. His nurse, Tonya, finds the patient lying supine in bed with arms extended along his sides but tensed. When Tonya checks the patient's surgical wound and drainage device, she notes that the patient winces when she gently places her hands to palpate around the surgical incision. She asks Mr. Jacobs when he last turned onto his side, and he responds, "Not since last night some time." Tonya asks Mr. Jacobs if he is having incisional pain, and he nods yes, saying, "It hurts too much to move." Tonya considers the information she has observed and learned from the patient to determine that he is in pain and has reduced mobility because of it. She decides that she needs to take action to relieve Mr. Jacobs' pain so she can turn him more frequently and begin to get him out of bed for his recovery.

In the case example the nurse observes the clinical situation, asks questions, considers what she knows about postoperative pain and risk for immobility, and takes action. The nurse applies **critical thinking,** a continuous process characterized by open-mindedness, continual inquiry, and perseverance, combined with a willingness to look at each unique patient situation and determine which identified assumptions are true and relevant (Heffner and Rudy, 2008). Critical thinking involves recognizing that an issue (e.g., patient problem) exists, analyzing information about the issue (e.g., clinical data about a patient), evaluating information (reviewing assumptions and evidence) and making conclusions (Settersten and Lauver, 2004). A critical thinker considers what is important in each clinical situation, imagines and explores alternatives, considers ethical principles, and makes informed decisions about the care of patients.

Critical thinking is a way of thinking about a situation that always asks "Why?", "What am I missing?", "What do I really know about this patient's situation?", and "What are my options?" (Heffner and Rudy, 2008; Paul and Heaslip, 1995). Tonya knew that pain was likely going to be a problem because the patient had extensive surgery. Her review of her observations and the patient's report of pain confirmed her knowledge that pain was a problem. Her options include giving Mr. Jacobs an analgesic and waiting until it takes effect so she is able to reposition and make him more comfortable. Once he has less acute pain, Tonya offers to teach Mr. Jacobs some relaxation exercises.

You begin to learn critical thinking early in your practice. For example, as you learn about administering baths and other hygiene measures, take time to read your textbook and the nursing literature about the concept of comfort. What are the criteria for comfort? How do patients from other cultures perceive comfort? What are the many factors that promote comfort? The use of **evidence-based knowledge,** or knowledge based on research or clinical expertise, makes you an informed critical thinker. Thinking critically and learning about the concept of comfort prepares you to better anticipate your patients' needs, identify comfort problems more quickly, and offer appropriate care. Critical thinking requires

TABLE 15-1 Critical Thinking Skills

SKILL	NURSING PRACTICE APPLICATIONS
Interpretation	Be orderly in data collection. Look for patterns to categorize data (e.g., nursing diagnoses [see Chapter 17]). Clarify any data you are uncertain about.
Analysis	Be open-minded as you look at information about a patient. Do not make careless assumptions. Do the data reveal what you believe is true, or are there other options?
Inference	Look at the meaning and significance of findings. Are there relationships between findings? Do the data about the patient help you see that a problem exists?
Evaluation	Look at all situations objectively. Use criteria (e.g., expected outcomes, pain characteristics, learning objectives) to determine results of nursing actions. Reflect on your own behavior.
Explanation	Support your findings and conclusions. Use knowledge and experience to choose strategies to use in the care of patients.
Self-regulation	Reflect on your experiences. Identify the ways you can improve your own performance. What will make you believe that you have been successful?

Modified from Facione P: *Critical thinking: a statement of expert consensus for purposes of educational assessment and instruction. The Delphi report: research findings and recommendations prepared for the American Philosophical Association,* ERIC Doc No. ED 315, Washington, DC, 1990, ERIC.

cognitive skills and the habit of asking questions, remaining well informed, being honest in facing personal biases, and always being willing to reconsider and think clearly about issues (Facione, 1990). When core critical thinking skills are applied to nursing, they show the complex nature of clinical decision making (Table 15-1). Being able to apply all of these skills takes practice. You also need to have a sound knowledge base and thoughtfully consider what you learn when caring for patients.

Nurses who apply critical thinking in their work are able to see the big picture from all possible perspectives. They focus clearly on options for solving problems and making decisions rather than quickly and carelessly forming quick solutions (Kataoka-Yahiro and Saylor, 1994). Nurses who work in crisis situations such as the emergency department often act quickly when patient problems develop. However, even these nurses exercise discipline in decision making to avoid premature and inappropriate decisions. Learning to think critically helps you care for patients as their advocate, or supporter, and make better-informed choices about their care. Facione and Facione (1996) identified concepts for thinking critically (Table 15-2). Critical thinking is more than just problem solving. It is a continuous attempt to improve how to apply yourself when faced with problems in patient care.

Thinking and Learning

Learning is a lifelong process. Your intellectual and emotional growth involves learning new knowledge and refining your ability to think, problem solve, and make judgments. To learn, you have to be flexible and always open to new information. The science of nursing is growing rapidly, and there will always be new information for you to apply in practice. As you have more clinical experiences and apply the knowledge you learn, you will become better

TABLE 15-2 Concepts for a Critical Thinker

CONCEPT	CRITICAL THINKING BEHAVIOR
Truth seeking	Seek the true meaning of a situation. Be courageous, honest, and objective about asking questions.
Open-mindedness	Be tolerant of different views; be sensitive to the possibility of your own prejudices; respect the right of others to have different opinions.
Analyticity	Analyze potentially problematic situations; anticipate possible results or consequences; value reason; use evidence-based knowledge.
Systematicity	Be organized, focused; work hard in any inquiry.
Self-confidence	Trust in your own reasoning processes.
Inquisitiveness	Be eager to acquire knowledge and learn explanations even when applications of the knowledge are not immediately clear. Value learning for learning's sake.
Maturity	Multiple solutions are acceptable. Reflect on your own judgments; have cognitive maturity.

Modified from Facione N, Facione P: Externalizing the critical thinking in knowledge development and clinical judgment, *Nurs Outlook* 44(3):129, 1996.

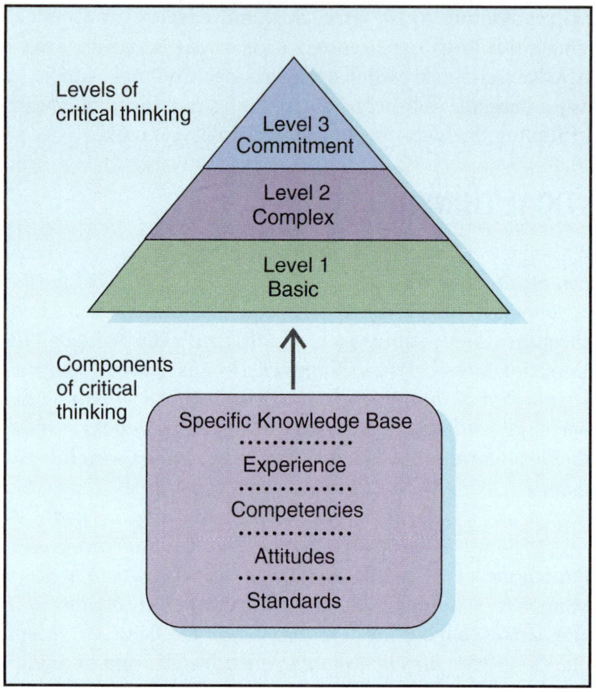

FIG. 15-1 Critical thinking model for nursing judgment. (Redrawn from Kataoka-Yahiro M, Saylor C: A critical thinking model for nursing judgment, *J Nurs Educ* 33(8):351, 1994. Modified from Glaser E: *An experiment in the development of critical thinking,* New York, 1941, Bureau of Publications, Teachers College, Columbia University; Miller M, Malcolm N: Critical thinking in the nursing curriculum, *Nurs Health Care* 11:67, 1990; Paul RW: The art of redesigning instruction. In Willsen J, Blinker AJA, editors: *Critical thinking: how to prepare students for a rapidly changing world,* Santa Rosa, Calif, 1993, Foundation for Critical Thinking; and Perry W: *Forms of intellectual and ethical development in the college years: a scheme,* New York, 1979, Holt, Rinehart, & Winston.)

at forming assumptions, presenting ideas, and making valid conclusions.

When you care for a patient, always think ahead and ask these questions: What is the patient's status now? How might it change and why? Which physiological and emotional responses do I anticipate? What do I know to improve the patient's condition? In which way will specific therapies affect the patient? What should be my first action? Do not let your thinking become routine or standardized. Instead, learn to look beyond the obvious in any clinical situation, explore the patient's unique responses to health alterations, and recognize which actions are needed to benefit the patient. With experience you are able to recognize patterns of behavior, see commonalities in signs and symptoms, and anticipate reactions to therapies. Thinking about these experiences allows you to better anticipate each new patient's needs and recognize problems when they develop.

LEVELS OF CRITICAL THINKING IN NURSING

Your ability to think critically grows as you gain new knowledge in nursing practice. Kataoka-Yahiro and Saylor (1994) developed a critical thinking model (Fig. 15-1) that includes three levels: basic, complex, and commitment. An expert nurse thinks critically almost automatically. As a beginning student you make a more conscious effort to apply critical thinking because initially you are more task oriented and trying to learn how to organize nursing care activities. At first you apply the critical thinking model at the basic level. As you advance in practice, you adopt complex critical thinking and commitment.

Basic Critical Thinking

At the basic level of critical thinking a learner trusts that experts have the right answers for every problem. Thinking is concrete and based on a set of rules or principles. For example, as a nursing student you use a hospital procedure manual to confirm how to insert a Foley catheter. You likely follow the procedure step by step without adjusting it to meet a patient's unique needs (e.g., positioning to minimize the patient's pain or mobility restrictions). You do not have enough experience to anticipate how to individualize the procedure. At this level answers to complex problems are either right or wrong (e.g., when no urine drains from the catheter, the catheter tip must not be in the bladder), and one right answer usually exists for each problem. Basic critical thinking is an early step in developing reasoning (Kataoka-Yahiro and Saylor, 1994). A basic critical thinker learns to accept the diverse opinions and values of experts (e.g., instructors and staff nurse role models). However, inexperience, weak competencies, and inflexible attitudes can restrict a person's ability to move to the next level of critical thinking.

Complex Critical Thinking

Complex critical thinkers begin to separate themselves from experts. They analyze and examine choices more independently. The person's thinking abilities and initiative to look beyond expert opinion begin to change. A nurse learns that alternative and perhaps conflicting solutions exist.

Consider the case of Mr. Rosen, a 36-year-old man who had hip surgery. The patient is having pain but is refusing his ordered analgesic. His health care provider is concerned that the patient will not progress as planned, delaying rehabilitation. While discussing the importance of rehabilitation with Mr. Rosen, the nurse, Edwin, realizes the patient's reason for not taking pain medication. Edwin learns that the patient practices meditation at home. As a complex critical thinker, Edwin recognizes that Mr. Rosen has options for pain relief. Edwin decides to discuss meditation and other nonpharmacological interventions with the patient as pain control options and how, when combined with analgesics, these interventions can potentially enhance pain relief.

In complex critical thinking each solution has benefits and risks that you weigh before making a final decision. There are options. Thinking becomes more creative and innovative. The complex critical thinker is willing to consider different options from routine procedures when complex situations develop. You learn a variety of different approaches for the same therapy.

Commitment

The third level of critical thinking is commitment (Kataoka-Yahiro and Saylor, 1994). At this level a person anticipates when to make choices without assistance from others and accepts accountability for decisions made. As a nurse you do more than just consider the complex alternatives that a problem poses. At the commitment level you choose an action or belief based on the available alternatives and support it. Sometimes an action is to not act or to delay an action until a later time. You choose to delay as a result of your experience and knowledge. Because you take accountability for the decision, you consider the results of the decision and determine whether it was appropriate.

CRITICAL THINKING COMPETENCIES

Kataoka-Yahiro and Saylor (1994) describe critical thinking competencies as the cognitive processes a nurse uses to make judgments about the clinical care of patients. These include general critical thinking, specific critical thinking in clinical situations, and specific critical thinking in nursing. General critical thinking processes are not unique to nursing. They include the scientific method, problem solving, and decision making. Specific critical thinking competencies in clinical health care situations include diagnostic reasoning, clinical inference, and clinical decision making. The specific critical thinking competency in nursing involves use of the nursing process. Each of the competencies is discussed in the following paragraphs.

General Critical Thinking

Scientific Method. The scientific method is a way to solve problems using reasoning. It is a systematic, ordered approach to gathering data and solving problems used by nurses, physicians, and a variety of other health care professionals. This approach looks for the truth or verifies that a set of facts agrees with reality. Nurse researchers use the **scientific method** when testing research questions in nursing practice situations (see Chapter 5). The scientific method has five steps:

1. Identifying the problem
2. Collecting data
3. Formulating a question or hypothesis
4. Testing the question or hypothesis
5. Evaluating results of the test or study

Consider the following example of the scientific method in nursing practice.

A nurse caring for patients who receive large doses of chemotherapy for ovarian cancer sees a pattern of patients developing severe inflammation in the mouth (mucositis) (identifies problem). The nurse reads research articles (collects data) about mucositis and learns that there is evidence to show that having patients keep ice in their mouths (cryotherapy) during the chemotherapy infusion reduces severity of mucositis after treatment. He or she asks (forms question), "Do patients with ovarian cancer who receive chemotherapy have less severe mucositis when given cryotherapy versus standard mouth rinse in the oral cavity?" The nurse then collaborates with colleagues to develop a nursing protocol for using ice with certain chemotherapy infusions. The nurses on the oncology unit collect information that allows them to compare the incidence and severity of mucositis for a group of patients who use cryotherapy versus those who use standard-practice mouth rinse (tests the question). They analyze the results of their project and find that the use of cryotherapy reduced the frequency and severity of mucositis in their patients (evaluating the results). They decide to continue the protocol for all patients with ovarian cancer.

Problem Solving. You face problems every day such as a computer program that doesn't function properly or a close friend who has lost a favorite pet. When a problem arises, you obtain information and use it, plus what you already know, to find a solution. Patients routinely present problems in practice. For example, a home care nurse learns that a patient has difficulty taking her medications regularly. The patient is unable to describe what medications she has taken for the last 3 days. The medication bottles are labeled and filled. The nurse has to solve the problem of why the patient is not adhering to or following her medication schedule. The nurse knows that the patient was discharged from the hospital and had five medications ordered. The patient tells the nurse that she also takes two over-the-counter medications regularly. When the nurse asks her to show the medications that she takes in the morning, the nurse notices that she has difficulty reading the medication labels. The patient is able to describe the medications that she is to take but is uncertain about the times of administration. The nurse recommends having the patient's pharmacy relabel the medications in larger lettering. In addition, the nurse shows the patient examples of pill organizers that will help her sort her medications by time of day for a period of 7 days.

Effective **problem solving** also involves evaluating the solution over time to make sure that it is effective. It becomes necessary to try different options if a problem recurs. From the previous example, during a follow-up visit the nurse finds that the patient has organized her medications correctly and is able to read the labels without difficulty. The nurse obtained information that correctly clarified the cause of the patient's problem and tested a solution that proved successful. Having solved a problem in one situation adds to a nurse's experience in practice, and this allows the nurse to apply that knowledge in future patient situations.

Decision Making. When you face a problem or situation and need to choose a course of action from several options, you are making a decision. **Decision making** is a product of critical thinking that focuses on problem resolution. Following a set of criteria helps to make a thorough and thoughtful decision. The criteria may be personal; based on an organizational policy; or, frequently in the case of nursing, a professional standard. For example, decision making occurs when a person decides on the choice of a health care provider. To make a decision, an individual has to recognize and define the problem or situation (need for a certain type of health care provider to provide medical care) and assess all options (consider recommended health care providers or choose one whose office is close to home). The person has to weigh each option against a set of personal criteria (experience, friendliness, and reputation), test possible options (talk directly with the different health care providers), consider the consequences of the decision (examine pros and cons of selecting one health care provider over another), and make a final decision. Although the set of criteria follows a sequence of steps, decision making involves moving back and forth when considering all criteria. It leads to informed conclusions that are supported by evidence and reason. Examples of decision making in the clinical area include determining which patient care priority requires the first response, choosing a type of dressing for a patient with a surgical wound, or selecting the best teaching approach for a family caregiver who will assist a patient who is returning home after a stroke.

Specific Critical Thinking

Diagnostic Reasoning and Inference. Once you receive information about a patient in a clinical situation, **diagnostic reasoning** begins. It is the analytical process for determining a patient's health problems (Harjai and Tiwari, 2009). Accurate recognition of a patient's problems is necessary before you decide on solutions and implement action. It requires you to assign meaning to the behaviors and physical signs and symptoms presented by a patient. Diagnostic reasoning begins when you interact with a patient or make physical or behavioral observations. An expert nurse sees the context of a patient situation (e.g., a patient who is feeling light-headed with blurred vision and who has a history of diabetes is possibly experiencing a problem with blood glucose levels), observes patterns and themes (e.g., symptoms that include weakness, hunger, and visual disturbances suggest hypoglycemia), and makes decisions quickly (e.g., offers a food source containing glucose). The information a nurse collects and analyzes leads to a diagnosis of a patient's condition. Nurses do not make medical diagnoses, but they do assess and monitor patients closely and compare the patients' signs and symptoms with those that are common to a medical diagnosis. This type of diagnostic reasoning helps health care providers pinpoint the nature of a problem more quickly and select proper therapies.

Part of diagnostic reasoning is clinical **inference,** the process of drawing conclusions from related pieces of evidence and previous experience with the evidence. An inference involves forming patterns of information from data before making a diagnosis. Seeing that a patient has lost appetite and experienced weight loss over the last month, the nurse infers that there is a nutritional problem. An example of diagnostic reasoning is forming a nursing diagnosis such as *imbalanced nutrition: less than body requirements* (see Chapter 17).

In diagnostic reasoning use patient data that you gather or collect to logically recognize the problem. For example, after turning a patient you see an area of redness on the right hip. You palpate the area and note that it is warm to the touch and the patient complains of tenderness. You press over the area with your finger; after you release pressure, the area does not blanch or turn white. After thinking about what you know about normal skin integrity and the effects of pressure, you form the diagnostic conclusion that the patient has a pressure ulcer. As a student, confirm your judgments with experienced nurses. At times you possibly will be wrong, but consulting with nurse experts gives you feedback to build on future clinical situations.

Often you cannot make a precise diagnosis during your first meeting with a patient. Sometimes you sense that a problem exists but do not have enough data to make a specific diagnosis. Some patients' physical conditions limit their ability to tell you about symptoms. Some choose to not share sensitive and important information during your initial assessment. Some patients' behaviors and physical responses become observable only under conditions not present during your initial assessment. When uncertain of a diagnosis, continue data collection. You have to critically analyze changing clinical situations until you are able to determine the patient's unique situation. Diagnostic reasoning is a continuous behavior in nursing practice. Any diagnostic conclusions that you make will help the health care provider identify the nature of a problem more quickly and select appropriate medical therapies.

Clinical Decision Making. As in the case of general decision making, clinical decision making is a problem-solving activity that focuses on defining a problem and selecting an appropriate action. In clinical decision making a nurse identifies a patient's problem and selects a nursing intervention. When you approach a clinical problem such as a patient who is less mobile and develops an area of redness over the hip, you make a decision that identifies the problem (impaired skin integrity in the form of a pressure ulcer) and choose the best nursing interventions (skin care and a turning schedule). Nurses make clinical decisions all the time to improve a patient's health or maintain wellness. This means reducing the severity of the problem or resolving the problem completely. **Clinical decision making** requires careful reasoning (i.e., choosing the options for the best patient outcomes on the basis of the patient's condition and the priority of the problem).

Improve your clinical decision making by knowing your patients. Nurse researchers found that expert nurses develop a level of knowing that leads to pattern recognition of patient symptoms and responses (White, 2003). For example, an expert nurse who has worked on a general surgery unit for many years is more likely able to detect signs of internal hemorrhage (e.g., fall in blood pressure, rapid pulse, change in consciousness) than a new nurse. Over time a combination of experience, time spent in a specific clinical area, and the quality of relationships formed with patients allow expert nurses to know clinical situations and quickly anticipate and select the right course of action. Spending more time during initial patient assessments to observe patient behavior and measure physical findings is a way to improve knowledge of your patients. In addition, consistently assessing and monitoring patients as problems occur help you to see how clinical changes develop over time. The selection of nursing therapies is built on both clinical knowledge and specific patient data, including:

- The identified status and situation you assessed about the patient, including data collected by actively listening to the patient regarding his or her health care needs.
- Knowledge about the clinical variables (e.g., age, seriousness of the problem, pathology of the problem, patient's preexisting disease conditions) involved in the situation, and how the variables are linked together.
- A judgment about the likely course of events and outcome of the diagnosed problem, considering any health risks the patient has; includes knowledge about usual patterns of any diagnosed problem or prognosis.
- Any additional relevant data about requirements in the patient's daily living, functional capacity, and social resources.

- Knowledge about the nursing therapy options available and the way in which specific interventions will predictably affect the patient's situation.

Always keep the patient your center of focus as you try to solve his or her clinical problems. Making an accurate clinical decision allows you to set priorities for the interventions to implement first (see Chapter 18). Because different patients bring different variables to a situation, a certain activity is sometimes a higher priority in one situation and less of a priority in another. For example, if a patient is physically dependent, unable to eat, and incontinent of urine, you recognize skin integrity as a greater priority than if the patient was immobile but continent of urine and able to eat a normal diet. Do not assume that certain health situations produce automatic priorities. For example, a patient who has surgery is anticipated to experience a certain level of postoperative pain, which often becomes a priority for care. However, if the patient is experiencing severe anxiety that increases pain perception, it becomes necessary for you to focus on ways to relieve the anxiety before pain-relief measures will be effective.

Critical thinking and clinical decision making are complicated because nurses care for multiple patients in fast-paced and unpredictable environments. When you work in a busy setting, use criteria such as the clinical condition of the patient, Maslow's hierarchy of needs (see Chapter 6), the risks involved in treatment delays, and patients' expectations of care to determine which patients have the greatest priorities for care. For example, a patient who is having a sudden drop in blood pressure along with a change in consciousness requires your attention immediately as opposed to a patient who needs you to collect a urine specimen or a patient who needs your help to walk down the hallway. Critical thinking allows a nurse to attend to the patient whose condition is changing quickly and delegate the specimen collection and ambulation to nursing assistive personnel (Box 15-1). For you to manage the wide variety of problems associated with groups of patients, skillful, prioritized clinical decision making is critical (Box 15-2).

Nursing Process as a Competency

Nurses apply the **nursing process** as a competency when delivering patient care (Kataoka-Yahiro and Saylor, 1994). The nursing process is a five-step clinical decision-making approach: assessment, diagnosis, planning, implementation, and evaluation. The purpose of the nursing process is to diagnose and treat human responses to actual or potential health problems (American Nurses Association, 2010). Human responses include patient symptoms and physiological reactions to treatment, the need for knowledge when health care providers make a new diagnosis or treatment plan, and a patient's ability to cope with loss. Use of the process allows nurses to help patients meet agreed-on outcomes for better health (Fig. 15-2). The nursing process requires a nurse to use the general and specific critical thinking competencies described earlier to focus on a particular patient's unique needs. The format for the nursing process is unique to the discipline of nursing and provides a common language and process for nurses to "think through" patients' clinical problems (Kataoka-Yahiro and Saylor, 1994). Unit 3 describes the nursing process.

The nursing process allows for flexibility for use in all clinical settings. When using it, identify a patient's health care needs by collecting thorough information and clearly defining all nursing diagnoses or collaborative problems. You plan care by determining priorities, setting goals and expected outcomes of care, and collaborating with family and health care team members. Then you deliver nursing interventions competently and evaluate the effects of your care. When you become more competent in using the nursing process, you will be able to focus not only on a single patient problem or diagnosis but on multiple problems and diagnoses. As a nurse, always be thinking and recognizing what step of

BOX 15-1 EVIDENCE-BASED PRACTICE

Critical Thinking and Delegation

PICO Question: Do nurses in acute care apply critical thinking to delegate nursing care?

Evidence Summary

Nurses synthesize large amounts of information and think through complex and often emergent clinical situations to make decisions about patient care, including delegation. In two separate studies nurses were asked to describe the process of delegation in their clinical practice (Bittner and Gravlin, 2009; Potter et al., 2010). An important delegation issue is the right circumstances. Registered nurses (RNs) are responsible for making clinical decisions when patients' conditions change, including determining what and when to delegate. RNs in one study were able to identify when to adjust their requests of nursing assistive personnel (NAP) according to patients' needs (Potter et al., 2010). When an RN makes the clinical decision to delegate care, there is the expectation that NAP will report significant findings and that the RN will follow up on tasks that have been delegated. Delegation is ineffective if RNs fail to carry out proper supervision and evaluation of care. When delegation is ineffective, often activities such as ambulation, feedings, and turning are missed by NAP. Successful delegation depends on good communication, developing a trusting and respectful relationship, and showing initiative.

Application to Nursing Practice

- Effective communication is needed between RNs and NAP for giving feedback and clarifying tasks and patient status.
- When patients' clinical conditions change, warranting attention by RNs, clear directions are necessary to avoid missed care.
- Applying critical thinking helps RNs make the decision about when to appropriately delegate care.

BOX 15-2 CLINICAL DECISION MAKING FOR GROUPS OF PATIENTS

- Identify the nursing diagnoses and collaborative problems of each patient (see Chapter 17).
- Analyze patients' diagnoses/problems and decide which are most urgent on the basis of basic needs, the patients' changing or unstable status, and problem complexity (see Chapter 18).
- Consider the time it will take to care for patients whose problems are of high priority (e.g., do you have the time to restart a critical intravenous (IV) line when medication is due for a different patient?).
- Consider the resources you have to manage each problem, nursing assistive personnel assigned with you, other health care providers, and patients' family members.
- Consider how to involve the patients as decision makers and participants in care.
- Decide how to combine activities to resolve more than one patient problem at a time.
- Decide which, if any, nursing care procedures to delegate to assistive personnel so you are able to spend your time on activities requiring professional nursing knowledge.
- Discuss complex cases with other members of the health care team to ensure a smooth transition in care requirements.

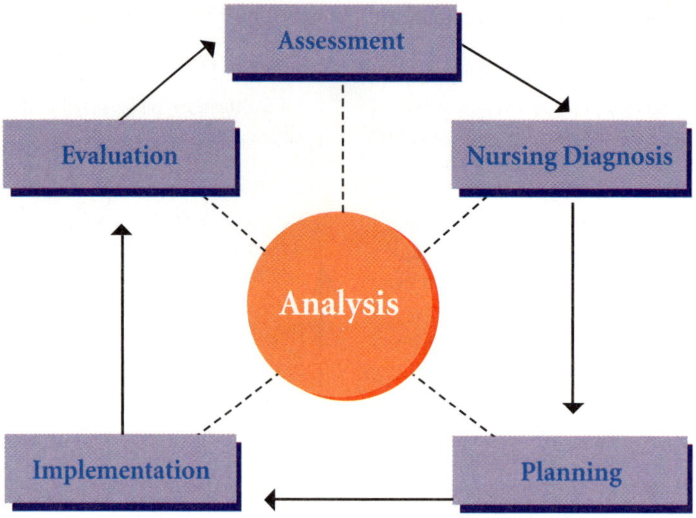

FIG. 15-2 Five-step nursing process model.

the process you are using. Within each step you apply critical thinking to provide the very best professional care to your patients.

A CRITICAL THINKING MODEL FOR CLINICAL DECISION MAKING

Thinking critically is at the core of professional nursing competence. The ability to think critically, improve clinical practice, and decrease errors in clinical judgments is the vision of nursing practice (Di Vito-Thomas, 2005). This text offers a model to help you develop critical thinking. Models help to explain concepts. Because critical thinking in nursing is complex, a model explains what is involved as you make clinical decisions and judgments about your patients. Kataoka-Yahiro and Saylor (1994) developed a model of critical thinking for nursing judgment based in part on previous work by a number of nurse scholars and researchers (Paul, 1993; Miller and Malcolm, 1990) (see Fig. 15-1). The model defines the outcome of critical thinking: nursing judgment that is relevant to nursing problems in a variety of settings. According to this model, there are five components of critical thinking: knowledge base, experience, critical thinking competencies (with emphasis on the nursing process), attitudes, and standards. The elements of the model combine to explain how nurses make clinical judgments that are necessary for safe, effective nursing care (see Box 15-2). Throughout this text the model shows you how to apply critical thinking as part of the nursing process. Graphic illustration of the critical thinking model in our clinical chapters shows you how to apply elements of critical thinking in assessing patients, planning the interventions you provide, and evaluating the results. If you learn to apply each element of this model in the way you think about patients, you will become a confident and effective professional.

Specific Knowledge Base

The first component of the critical thinking model is a nurse's specific knowledge base. Knowledge prepares you to better anticipate and identify patients' problems by understanding their origin and nature. Nurses' knowledge varies according to educational experience and includes basic nursing education, continuing education courses, and additional college degrees. In addition, it includes the initiative you show in reading the nursing literature to remain current in nursing science. A nurse's knowledge base is continually changing as science progresses (Swinny, 2010). As a nurse your knowledge base includes information and theory from the basic sciences, humanities, behavioral sciences, and nursing. Nurses use their knowledge base in a different way than other health care disciplines because they think holistically about patient problems. For example, a nurse's broad knowledge base offers a physical, psychological, social, moral, ethical, and cultural view of patients and their health care needs. The depth and extent of knowledge influence your ability to think critically about nursing problems.

Consider this scenario: Robert Perez previously earned a bachelor's degree in education and taught high school for 1 year. He is starting his third year of study in his nursing program. He has successfully completed the required courses in the sciences, health ethics, introduction to nursing concepts, and communication principles. His first clinical course is on health promotion with a clinical assignment at a general medical clinic. Although he is still new to nursing, his experiences as a teacher and his preparation and knowledge base in nursing help him know how to interview patients and begin to make clinical decisions about patients' health promotion practices.

Experience

Nursing is a practice discipline. Clinical learning experiences are necessary to acquire clinical decision-making skills. Swinny (2010) explains that knowledge itself is not necessarily related to the development of critical thinking. Instead knowledge combined with clinical expertise from experience defines critical thinking. In clinical situations you learn from observing, sensing, talking with patients and families, and reflecting actively on all experiences. Clinical experience is the laboratory for testing your nursing knowledge. You learn that "textbook" approaches form the basis for practice, but you make safe adaptations or revisions in approaches to fit the setting, the patient's unique qualities, and the experiences you have from caring for previous patients. With experience you begin to understand clinical situations, recognize cues of patients' health patterns, and interpret cues as relevant or irrelevant. Perhaps the best lesson a new nursing student can learn is to value all patient experiences, which become stepping-stones for building new knowledge and inspiring innovative thinking.

During the previous summer Robert worked as a nurse assistant in a nursing home. This experience provided valuable time for interacting with older-adult patients and giving basic nursing care. As Robert thinks about his clinical experience at the clinic, he recognizes that he still has a lot to learn. However, each patient has provided him valuable learning experiences. Specifically he has developed good interviewing skills, understands the importance of the family in an individual's health, and has learned how nurses are patient advocates. He has also learned that older adults need more time to perform activities such as eating, bathing, and grooming; therefore he has adapted these skill techniques. His time in the physical assessment laboratory and the time he worked in the nursing home have helped him begin to be a watchful observer. Finally Robert's previous experience as a teacher helps him apply educational principles in his nursing role.

Your practice improves from what you learn personally. The opportunities you have to experience different emotions, crises, and successes in your lives and relationships with others build your experience as a nurse.

The Nursing Process Competency

Competency, specifically the nursing process, is the third component of the critical thinking model. In your practice you apply critical thinking components during each step of the nursing process. Throughout the clinical chapters of this text, the relationship of critical thinking to the nursing process is emphasized.

Attitudes for Critical Thinking

The fourth component of the critical thinking model is attitudes. Eleven attitudes define the central features of a critical thinker and how a successful critical thinker approaches a problem (Paul, 1993) (Box 15-3). For example, when a patient complains of anxiety before a diagnostic procedure, the curious nurse explores possible reasons for the patient's concerns. The nurse shows discipline in collecting a thorough assessment to find the source of the patient's anxiety. Attitudes of inquiry involve an ability to recognize that problems exist and that there is a need for evidence to support the truth in what you think is true. Critical thinking attitudes are guidelines for how to approach a problem or decision-making situation. An important part of critical thinking is interpreting, evaluating, and making judgments about the adequacy of various arguments and available data. Knowing when you need more information, knowing when information is misleading, and recognizing your own knowledge limits are examples of how critical thinking attitudes guide decision making. Table 15-3 summarizes the use of critical thinking attitudes in nursing practice.

Confidence. When you are confident, you feel certain about accomplishing a task or goal such as performing a procedure or making a diagnostic decision. Confidence grows with experience in recognizing your strengths and limitations. You shift your focus from your own needs (e.g., remembering how to perform a procedure) to the patient's needs. When you are not confident in performing a nursing skill, you become anxious about not knowing what to do. This prevents you from giving attention to the patient. Always be aware of what you know and what you do not know. If you have a question about a procedure, discuss it with your nursing instructor first before attempting it on your patient. Never attempt anything on your patient unless you have the knowledge base and feel confident. Patient safety is of the upmost importance. When you show confidence, your patients recognize it by how you communicate and the way you perform nursing care. Confidence builds trust between you and your patients.

BOX 15-3 COMPONENTS OF CRITICAL THINKING IN NURSING

I. Specific knowledge base in nursing
II. Experience
III. Critical thinking competencies
  A. General critical thinking
  B. Specific critical thinking
  C. Specific critical thinking in nursing: nursing process
IV. Attitudes for critical thinking
  Confidence, Independence, Fairness, Responsibility, Risk taking, Discipline, Perseverance, Creativity, Curiosity, Integrity, Humility
V. Standards for critical thinking
  A. Intellectual standards
    Clear, Precise, Specific, Accurate, Relevant, Plausible, Consistent, Logical, Deep, Broad, Complete, Significant, Adequate (for purpose), Fair
  B. Professional standards
    1. Ethical criteria for nursing judgment
    2. Criteria for evaluation
    3. Professional responsibility

Modified from Kataoka-Yahiro M, Saylor C: A critical thinking model for nursing judgment, *J Nurs Educ* 33(8):351, 1994. Data from Paul RW: The art of redesigning instruction. In Willsen J, Blinker AJA, editors: *Critical thinking: how to prepare students for a rapidly changing world,* Santa Rosa, Calif, 1993, Foundation for Critical Thinking.

Thinking Independently. As you gain new knowledge, you learn to consider a wide range of ideas and concepts before forming an opinion or making a judgment. This does not mean that you ignore other people's ideas. Instead you learn to consider all sides of a situation. However, a critical thinker does not accept another person's ideas without question. When thinking independently, you challenge the ways others think and look for rational and logical answers to problems. Begin to raise important questions about your practice. For example, why is one type of surgical dressing ordered over another, why do your patients not get pain relief, and what can you do to help patients with literacy problems learn about their medications? When nurses ask questions and look for the evidence behind clinical problems, they are thinking independently; this is an important step in evidence-based practice (Chapter 5). Independent thinking and reasoning are essential to the improvement and expansion of nursing practice.

Fairness. A critical thinker deals with situations justly. This means that bias or prejudice does not enter into a decision. For example, regardless of how you feel about obesity, you do not allow personal attitudes to influence the way you care for a patient who is overweight. Look at a situation objectively and consider all viewpoints to understand the situation completely before making a decision. Having a sense of imagination helps you develop an attitude of fairness. Imagining what it is like to be in your patient's situation helps you see it with new eyes and appreciate its complexity.

TABLE 15-3 Critical Thinking Attitudes and Applications in Nursing Practice

CRITICAL THINKING ATTITUDE	APPLICATION IN PRACTICE
Confidence	Learn how to introduce yourself to a patient; speak with conviction when you begin a treatment or procedure. Do not lead a patient to think that you are unable to perform care safely. Always be well prepared before performing a nursing activity. Encourage a patient to ask questions.
Thinking independently	Read the nursing literature, especially when there are different views on the same subject. Talk with other nurses and share ideas about nursing interventions.
Fairness	Listen to both sides in any discussion. If a patient or family member complains about a co-worker, listen to the story and then speak with the co-worker as well. If a staff member labels a patient uncooperative, assume the care of that patient with openness and a desire to meet that patient's needs.
Responsibility and authority	Ask for help if you are uncertain about how to perform a nursing skill. Refer to a policy and procedure manual to review steps of a skill. Report any problems immediately. Follow standards of practice in your care.
Risk taking	If your knowledge causes you to question a health care provider's order, do so. Be willing to recommend alternative approaches to nursing care when colleagues are having little success with patients.
Discipline	Be thorough in whatever you do. Use known scientific and practice-based criteria for activities such as assessment and evaluation. Take time to be thorough and manage your time effectively.
Perseverance	Be cautious of an easy answer. If co-workers give you information about a patient and some fact seems to be missing, clarify the information or talk to the patient directly. If problems of the same type continue to occur on a nursing division, bring co-workers together, look for a pattern, and find a solution.
Creativity	Look for different approaches if interventions are not working for a patient. For example, a patient in pain may need a different positioning or distraction technique. When appropriate, involve the patient's family in adapting your approaches to care methods used at home.
Curiosity	Always ask why. A clinical sign or symptom often indicates a variety of problems. Explore and learn more about the patient so as to make appropriate clinical judgments.
Integrity	Recognize when your opinions conflict with those of a patient; review your position, and decide how best to proceed to reach outcomes that will satisfy everyone. Do not compromise nursing standards or honesty in delivering nursing care.
Humility	Recognize when you need more information to make a decision. When you are new to a clinical division, ask for an orientation to the area. Ask registered nurses (RNs) regularly assigned to the area for assistance with approaches to care.

Responsibility and Accountability. When caring for patients you are responsible for correctly performing nursing care activities based on standards of practice. Standards of practice are the minimum level of performance accepted to ensure high-quality care. For example, you do not take shortcuts (e.g., failing to identify a patient, prepare medication doses for multiple patients at the same time) when administering medications. A professional nurse is competent in performing nursing therapies and making clinical decisions about patients. As a nurse you are answerable or accountable for your decisions and the outcomes of your actions. This means that you are accountable for recognizing when nursing care is ineffective and you know the limits and scope of your practice

Risk Taking. Persons often associate taking risks with danger. Driving 30 miles an hour over the speed limit is a risk that sometimes results in injury to the driver and an unlucky pedestrian. But risk taking does not always have negative outcomes. Risk taking is desirable, particularly when the result is a positive outcome. A critical thinker is willing to take risks in trying different ways to solve problems. The willingness to take risks comes from experience with similar problems. Risk taking often leads to advances in patient care. Nurses in the past have taken risks in trying different approaches to skin and wound care and pain management, to name a few. When taking a risk, consider all options; follow safety guidelines; analyze any potential dangers to a patient; and act in a well-reasoned, logical, and thoughtful manner.

Discipline. A disciplined thinker misses few details and follows an orderly or systematic approach when collecting information, making decisions, or taking action. For example, you have a patient who is in pain. Instead of only asking the patient, "How severe is your pain on a scale of 0 to 10?" you also ask more specific questions about the character of pain. For example, "What makes the pain worse? Where does it hurt? How long have you noticed it?" Being disciplined helps you identify problems more accurately and select the most appropriate interventions.

Perseverance. A critical thinker is determined to find effective solutions to patient care problems. This is especially important when problems remain unresolved or recur. Learn as much as possible about a problem and try various approaches to care. Persevering means to keep looking for more resources until you find a successful approach. For example, a patient who is unable to speak following throat surgery poses challenges for the nurse to be able to communicate effectively. Perseverance leads the nurse to try different communication approaches (e.g., message boards or alarm bells) until he or she finds a method that the patient is able to use. A critical thinker who perseveres is not satisfied with minimal effort but works to achieve the highest level of quality care.

Creativity. Creativity involves original thinking. This means that you find solutions outside of the standard routines of care while still keeping standards of practice. Creativity motivates you to think of options and unique approaches. A patient's clinical problems, social support systems, and living environment are just a few examples of factors that make the simplest nursing procedure more complicated. For example, a home care nurse has to find a way to help an older patient with arthritis have greater mobility in the home. The patient has difficulty lowering and raising herself in a chair because of pain and limited range of motion in her knees. The nurse uses wooden blocks to elevate the chair legs so the patient is able to sit and stand with little discomfort while making sure the chair is safe to use.

Curiosity. A critical thinker's favorite question is "Why?" In any clinical situation you learn a great deal of information about a patient. As you analyze patient information, data patterns appear that are not always clear. Having a sense of curiosity motivates you to inquire further (e.g., question family, consult with a physician, or review the scientific literature) and investigate a clinical situation so you get all the information you need to make a decision.

Integrity. Critical thinkers question and test their own knowledge and beliefs. Your personal integrity as a nurse builds trust from your co-workers. Nurses face many dilemmas or problems in everyday clinical practice, and everyone makes mistakes at times. A person of integrity is honest and willing to admit to mistakes or inconsistencies in his or her own behavior, ideas, and beliefs. In addition, the professional nurse always tries to follow the highest standards of practice.

Humility. It is important for you to admit to any limitations in your knowledge and skill. Critical thinkers admit what they do not know and try to find the knowledge needed to make proper decisions. It is common for a nurse to be an expert in one area of clinical practice but a novice in another. That is because the knowledge in all areas of nursing is unlimited. A patient's safety and welfare are at risk if you do not admit your inability to deal with a practice problem. You have to rethink a situation; learn more; and use the new information to form opinions, draw conclusions, and take action.

The first patient Robert meets in the clinic is a young man who has signs and symptoms of chlamydia, a sexually transmitted disease. The patient has had the symptoms for over 3 weeks and voices concern about what it means to have the disease. Robert examines the young man and finds that the patient has redness and itching on the penis with a yellowish discharge. He uses discipline to check further and asks if the patient has pain on urination. He also checks him for fever. Robert has limited knowledge about chlamydia, so he consults with the clinic nurse practitioner, who explains the nature of the infection, the risks it poses to the patient, and the usual course of treatment. Robert returns and speaks more confidently with the patient about chlamydia, the reason for his symptoms, the need to tell sex partners about the infection, and the importance of wearing a condom.

Standards for Critical Thinking

The fifth component of the critical thinking model includes intellectual and professional standards (Kataoka-Yahiro and Saylor, 1994).

Intellectual Standards. Paul (1993) identified 14 intellectual standards (see Box 15-3) universal for critical thinking. An intellectual standard is a guideline or principle for rational thought. You apply these standards when you use the nursing process. When you consider a patient problem, apply the intellectual standards such as preciseness, accuracy, and consistency to make sure that all clinical decisions are sound. A thorough use of the intellectual standards in clinical practice makes certain that you do not perform critical thinking haphazardly.

Mrs. Lamar is an 82-year-old patient who comes to the medical clinic for a follow-up following the diagnosis of a diabetic foot ulcer. Robert finds the ulcer on the patient's left foot. A quick check of the patient's medical record reveals a description of the ulcer by one of the clinic nurses from 2 weeks earlier. The patient is receiving a topical medication for the ulcer. Robert uses the same assessment criteria applied during the last clinic visit to examine the patient's ulcer (consistent). He methodically inspects the affected area of the skin, measures the size of the ulcer, and notes the appearance of any drainage (complete). He asks the patient to describe how she has been caring for the ulcer to determine if she needs health teaching (relevant). When the patient explains that she washes the ulcer, Robert asks her to describe exactly what she has used to clean the ulcer and how often (precise). He documents the wound location and appearance in the clinic record using specific anatomical terms (accurate). By applying appropriate intellectual standards, Robert is able to determine that the ulcer is healing and has improved since the last assessment.

Professional Standards. Professional standards for critical thinking refer to ethical criteria for nursing judgments, evidence-based criteria used for evaluation, and criteria for professional responsibility (Paul, 1993). Application of professional standards requires you to use critical thinking for the good of individuals or groups (Kataoka-Yahiro and Saylor, 1994). Professional standards promote the highest level of quality nursing care.

Excellent nursing practice is a reflection of ethical standards (Chapter 22). Patient care requires more than just the application of scientific knowledge. Being able to focus on a patient's values and beliefs helps you make clinical decisions that are just, faithful to the patient's choices, and beneficial to the patient's well-being. Critical thinkers maintain a sense of self-awareness through conscious awareness of their beliefs; values; feelings; and the multiple perspectives that patients, family members, and peers present in clinical situations. Critical thinking also requires the use of evidence-based criteria for making clinical judgments. These criteria are sometimes scientifically based on research findings (see Chapter 5) or practice based on standards developed by clinical experts and performance improvement initiatives of the institution. Examples are the clinical practice guidelines developed by individual clinical agencies and national organizations such as the Agency for Healthcare Research Quality (AHRQ). A clinical practice guideline includes standards for the treatment of select clinical conditions such as stroke, deep vein thrombosis, and pressure ulcers. Another example is clinical criteria used to categorize clinical conditions such as the criteria for staging pressure ulcers (see Chapter 48) and rating phlebitis (see Chapter 41). Evidence-based evaluation criteria set the minimum requirements necessary to ensure appropriate and high-quality care.

Nurses routinely use evidence-based criteria to assess patients' conditions and determine the efficacy of nursing interventions. For example, accurate assessment of symptoms such as pain includes use of assessment criteria such as the duration, severity, location, aggravating or relieving factors, and effects on daily lifestyle (see Chapter 43). In this case assessment criteria allow you to accurately determine the nature of a patient's symptoms, select appropriate therapies, and evaluate if the therapies are effective. The standards of professional responsibility that a nurse tries to achieve are the standards cited in Nurse Practice Acts, institutional practice guidelines, and professional organizations' standards of practice (e.g., The American Nurses Association Standards of Professional Performance (see Chapter 1). These standards "raise the bar" for the responsibilities and accountabilities that a nurse assumes in guaranteeing quality health care to the public.

DEVELOPING CRITICAL THINKING SKILLS

To develop critical thinking skills, it is important to learn how to connect knowledge and theory with practice. Your ability to make sense of what you learn in the classroom, from reading, or from having dialogue with other students and then to apply it during patient care is always challenging.

Reflective Journaling

How often do you think back on a situation to consider the following: Why did that occur? How did I act? What could I have done differently? What knowledge could I have applied? **Reflection** is the process of purposefully thinking back or recalling a situation to discover its purpose or meaning. It is like rewinding a videotape. Reflection involves playing back a situation in your head and taking time to honestly review everything you remember about it. Reflective practice is a conscious process of thinking, analyzing, and learning from your work situations by way of journaling or regularly meeting with colleagues to explore work situations and self-evaluate (Cirocco, 2007). Critical thinking becomes more deliberate through reflection because it allows you to think about your previous thinking to make your future thinking better (Jackson, 2006).

Reflective journal writing is a tool for developing critical thought and reflection by clarifying concepts. Reflective writing gives you the opportunity to define and express the clinical experience in your own words (Di Vito-Thomas, 2005). By keeping a journal of each of your clinical experiences, you are able to explore personal perceptions or understanding of each experience and develop the ability to apply theory in practice. The use of a journal improves your observation and descriptive skills. Writing skills also improve through the development of conceptual clarity. The Circle of Meaning model adapted to nursing encourages concept clarification and a search for meaning in nursing practice (Bilinski, 2002). The model uses the following questions to help you journey through a clinical experience and find meaning:

1. Which experience, situation, or information in your clinical experience seems confusing, difficult, or interesting?
2. What is the meaning of the experience? What feelings did you have? What feelings did your patient have? What influenced the experience? Which guesses or questions developed with the first connection in question 1? Give examples.
3. Do the feelings, guesses, or questions remind you of any experience from the past or present or something that you think is a desirable future experience? How does it relate? What are the implications/significance?
4. What are the connections between what is being described and what you have learned about nursing science, research, and theory? What are some possible solutions? Which approach or solution would you choose and why? How is this approach effective?

Keeping a journal of your patient care experiences helps you become aware of how you make clinical decisions. Begin by recording notes after a clinical experience. Telling a story and drawing a picture are two additional ways to identify the experience on which you wish to reflect. Describe in detail what you felt, thought, and did. Analyze the experience by considering feelings, thoughts, and possible meaning. Challenge any preconceived ideas you have when you look at actual clinical situations. Describe the significance of the experience. Do not include patient identification in your journal, and refer to your journal when you care for patients in similar situations.

Meeting with Colleagues

Another way to develop critical thinking skills is regularly meeting with colleagues to discuss and examine work experiences. Having the chance to discuss anticipated and unanticipated outcomes in any clinical situation allows you to continually learn and develop your expertise and knowledge (Cirocco, 2007). When nurses have a formal means to discuss their experiences such as a staff meeting or unit practice council, the dialogue allows for questions, differing viewpoints, and sharing experiences. When they are able to discuss their practices, the process validates good practice and also offers challenges and constructive criticism. Much can be learned by drawing from others' experiences and perspectives to promote reflective critical thinking.

Concept Mapping

As a nurse you care for patients who have multiple nursing diagnoses or collaborative problems. A **concept map** is a visual representation of patient problems and interventions that shows their relationships to one another. It offers a nonlinear picture of a patient that can then be used for comprehensive care planning (Taylor and Wros, 2007). The primary purpose of concept mapping is to better synthesize relevant data about a patient, including assessment data, nursing diagnoses, health needs, nursing interventions, and evaluation measures (Hill, 2006). Through drawing a concept map, you learn to organize or connect information in a unique way so the diverse information that you have about a patient begins to form meaningful patterns and concepts. You begin to see a more holistic view of a patient. When you see the relationship between the various patient diagnoses and the data that support them, you better understand a patient's clinical situation. Concept maps become more detailed, integrated, and comprehensive as you learn more about the care of a patient and the care you provide similar patients (Ferrario, 2004). The similarities and differences that you see among patients build your decision-making skills. Unit 3 includes chapters that provide diagrams of actual concept maps and more detail on their development. Concept maps can also be found in Units 5 and 6.

CRITICAL THINKING SYNTHESIS

Critical thinking is a reasoning process by which you reflect on and analyze your own thoughts, actions, and knowledge. To be a good critical thinker requires dedication and a desire to grow intellectually. As a beginning nurse it is important to learn the steps of the nursing process and incorporate the elements of critical thinking (Fig. 15-3). The two processes go hand in hand in making quality decisions about patient care. This text provides a model to show you how important critical thinking is in nursing practice. Throughout the clinical chapters of this text, the components of

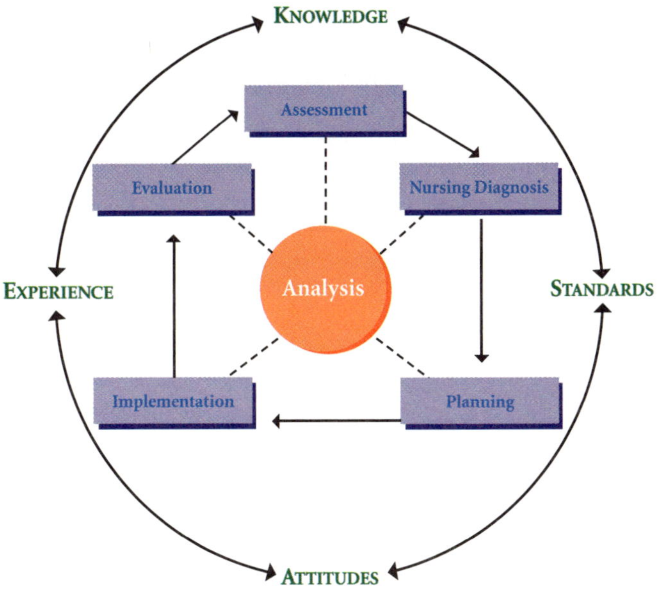

FIG. 15-3 Synthesis of critical thinking with the nursing process competency.

critical thinking are emphasized to help you better understand their relationship to the nursing process.

KEY POINTS

- Clinical decision making involves judgment that includes critical and reflective thinking and action and application of scientific and practical logic.
- Nurses who apply critical thinking in their work focus on options for solving problems and making decisions rather than rapidly and carelessly forming quick, single solutions.
- Following a procedure step by step without adjusting to a patient's unique needs is an example of basic critical thinking.
- In complex critical thinking a nurse learns that alternative and perhaps conflicting solutions exist.
- In diagnostic reasoning you collect patient data and analyze them to determine the patient's problems.
- The nursing process is a blueprint for patient care that involves both general and specific critical thinking competencies in a way that focuses on a particular patient's unique needs.
- The critical thinking model combines a nurse's knowledge base, experience, competence in the nursing process, attitudes, and standards to explain how nurses make clinical judgments that are necessary for safe, effective nursing care.
- Clinical learning experiences are necessary for you to acquire clinical decision-making skills.
- Critical thinking attitudes help you to know when more information is necessary and when it is misleading and to recognize your own knowledge limits.
- The use of intellectual standards during assessment ensures that you obtain a complete database of information.
- Professional standards for critical thinking refer to ethical criteria for nursing judgments, evidence-based criteria for evaluation, and criteria for professional responsibility.
- Meeting regularly with colleagues allows you to discuss anticipated and unanticipated outcomes in any clinical situation to continually learn and develop your expertise and knowledge.

CLINICAL APPLICATION QUESTIONS

Preparing for Clinical Practice

Josh is a second-year nursing student working in a surgical clinic. He is checking Mr. Isaac's surgical wound. After removing the gauze dressing, he notes in the nurses' notes from the last visit that the wound was 3 cm long and the skin around the wound was tender when palpated. When Josh examines the wound, he measures the length and width in centimeters with a tape measure, observes the character of the tissues, looks for drainage, and palpates around the wound for tenderness and an increase in drainage. He asks Mr. Isaac if he is having discomfort from the wound and if the pain is limiting his activity.

1. Explain which intellectual standards Josh used in the wound assessment and support your answers.
2. Mr. Isaac asks Josh if the wound is going to heal soon, stating, "I thought it would have healed by now." Josh responds by saying, "What did your doctor tell you about the time it would take to heal the wound? I plan to talk with him to let him know how the wound looks so we're sure we're using the right type of dressing." In this example Josh is displaying which of the following attitudes for critical thinking during his communication:
   1. Confidence
   2. Integrity
   3. Creativity
   4. Risk taking
3. Two weeks later Mr. Isaac again comes to the clinic. The wound has not progressed, but there are no signs of infection. Josh talks with Mr. Isaac about his activities. He also has Mr. Isaac describe the type of diet he has been eating and the amount of food intake. Josh's line of questioning is an example of which critical thinking competency? Explain.

evolve Answers to Clinical Application Questions can be found on the Evolve website.

REVIEW QUESTIONS

Are You Ready to Test Your Nursing Knowledge?

1. While assessing a patient, the nurse observes that the patient's intravenous (IV) line is not infusing at the ordered rate. The nurse assesses the patient for pain at the IV site, checks the flow regulator on the tubing, looks to see if the patient is lying on the tubing, checks the point of connection between the tubing and the IV catheter, and then checks the condition of the site where the intravenous catheter enters the patient's skin. After the nurse readjusts the flow rate, the infusion begins at the correct rate. This is an example of:
   1. Inference.
   2. Diagnostic reasoning.
   3. Competency.
   4. Problem solving.
2. The nurse sits down to talk with a patient who lost her sister 2 weeks ago. The patient reports she is unable to sleep, feels very fatigued during the day, and is having trouble at work. The nurse asks her to clarify the type of trouble. The patient explains she can't concentrate or even solve simple problems. The nurse records the results of the assessment, describing the patient as having ineffective coping. This is an example of:
   1. Diagnostic reasoning.
   2. Competency.

3. Inference.
4. Problem solving.

3. A patient on a surgical unit develops sudden shortness of breath and a drop in blood pressure. The staff respond, but the patient dies 30 minutes later. The manager on the nursing unit calls the staff involved in the emergency response together. The staff discusses what occurred over the 30-minute time frame, the actions taken, and whether other steps should have been implemented. The nurses in this situation are:
   1. Problem solving.
   2. Showing humility.
   3. Conducting reflective practice.
   4. Exercising responsibility.
4. A nurse has worked on an oncology unit for 3 years. One patient has become visibly weaker and states, "I feel funny." The nurse knows how patients often have behavior changes before developing sepsis when they have cancer. The nurse asks the patient questions to assess thinking skills and notices the patient shivering. The nurse goes to the phone, calls the physician, and begins the conversation by saying, "I believe that your patient is developing sepsis. I want to report symptoms I'm seeing." What examples of critical thinking concepts does the nurse show? (Select all that apply.)
   1. Experience
   2. Ethical
   3. Analyticity
   4. Self-confidence
   5. Risk taking
5. A nurse who is working on a surgical unit is caring for four different patients. Patient A will be discharged home and is in need of instruction about wound care. Patients B and C have returned from the operating room within an hour of each other, and both require vital signs and monitoring of their intravenous (IV) lines. Patient D is resting following a visit by physical therapy. Which of the following activities by the nurse represent(s) use of clinical decision making for groups of patients? (Select all that apply.)
   1. Consider how to involve patient A in deciding whether to involve the family caregiver in wound care instruction.
   2. Think about past experience with patients who develop postoperative complications.
   3. Decide which activities can be combined for patients B and C.
   4. Carefully gather any assessment information and identify patient problems.
6. The surgical unit has initiated the use of a pain-rating scale to assess patients' pain severity during their postoperative recovery. The registered nurse (RN) looks at the pain flow sheet to see the pain scores recorded for a patient over the last 24 hours. Use of the pain scale is an example of which intellectual standard?
   1. Deep
   2. Relevant
   3. Consistent
   4. Significant
7. During a home health visit the nurse prepares to instruct a patient in how to perform range-of-motion (ROM) exercises for an injured shoulder. The nurse verifies that the patient took an analgesic 30 minutes before arrival at the patient's home. After discussing the purpose for the exercises and demonstrating each one, the nurse has the patient perform them. After two attempts with only the second of three exercises, the patient stops and says, "This hurts too much. I don't see why I have to do this so many times." The nurse applies the critical thinking attitude of integrity in which of the following actions?"
   1. "I understand your reluctance, but the exercises are necessary for you to regain function in your shoulder. Let's go a bit more slowly and try to relax."
   2. "I see that you're uncomfortable. I'll call your doctor to decide the next step."
   3. "Show me exactly where your pain is and rate it for me on a scale of 0 to 10."
   4. "Is anything else bothering you? Other than the pain, is there any other reason you might not want to do the exercises?"
8. The nurse cared for a 14-year-old with renal failure who died near the end of the work shift. The health care team tried for 45 minutes to resuscitate the child with no success. The family was devastated by the loss, and, when the nurse tried to talk with them, the mother said, "You can't make me feel better; you don't know what it's like to lose a child." Which of the following examples of journal entries might best help the nurse reflect and think about this clinical experience? (Select all that apply.)
   1. Data entry of time of day, who was present, and condition of the child
   2. Description of the efforts to restore the child's blood pressure, what was used, and questions about the child's response
   3. The meaning the experience had for the nurse with respect to her understanding of dealing with a patient's death
   4. A description of what the nurse said to the mother, the mother's response, and how the nurse might approach the situation differently in the future
9. A nurse has been working on a surgical unit for 3 weeks. A patient requires a Foley catheter to be inserted, so the nurse reads the procedure manual for the institution to review how to insert it. The level of critical thinking the nurse is using is:
   1. Commitment.
   2. Scientific method.
   3. Basic critical thinking.
   4. Complex critical thinking.
10. A patient had hip surgery 16 hours ago. During the previous shift the patient had 40 mL of drainage in the surgical drainage collection device for an 8-hour period. The nurse refers to the written plan of care, noting that the health care provider is to be notified when drainage in the device exceeds 100 mL for the day. On entering the room, the nurse looks at the device and carefully notes the amount of drainage currently in it. This is an example of:
    1. Planning.
    2. Evaluation.
    3. Intervention.
    4. Diagnosis.
11. A 67-year-old patient will be discharged from the hospital in the morning. The health care provider has ordered three new medications for her. Place the following steps of the nursing process in the correct order.
    ____ 1. The nurse returns to the patient's room and asks her to describe the medicines she will be taking at home.
    ____ 2. The nurse talks with the patient and family about who will be available if the patient has difficulty taking

medicines and considers consulting with the health care provider about a home health visit.

____ 3. The nurse asks the patient if she is in pain, feels tired, and is willing to spend the next few minutes learning about her new medicines.

____ 4. The nurse brings the containers of medicines and information leaflets to the bedside and discusses each medication with her.

____ 5. The nurse considers what she learns from the patient and identifies the patient's nursing diagnosis.

12. The nurse asks a patient how she feels about her impending surgery for breast cancer. Before the discussion the nurse reviewed the description of loss and grief and therapeutic communication principles in his textbook. The critical thinking component involved in the nurse's review of the literature is:
    1. Experience.
    2. Problem solving.
    3. Knowledge application.
    4. Clinical decision making.
13. A nurse is working with a nursing assistive personnel (NAP) on a busy oncology unit. The nurse has instructed the NAP on the tasks that need to be performed, including getting patient A out of bed, collecting a urine specimen from patient B, and checking vital signs on patient C, who is scheduled to go home. Which of the following represent(s) successful delegation? (Select all that apply.)
    1. A nurse explains to the NAP the approach to use in getting the patient up and why the patient has activity limitations.
    2. A nurse is asked by a patient to help her to the bathroom; the nurse leaves the room and directs the NAP to assist the patient instead.
    3. The nurse sees the NAP preparing to help a patient out of bed, goes to assist, and thanks the NAP for her efforts to get the patient up early.
    4. The nurse is in patient B's room to check an intravenous (IV) line and collects the urine specimen while in the room.
    5. The nurse offers support to the NAP when needed but allows her to complete patient care tasks without constant oversight.
14. Which of the following is unique to the commitment level of critical thinking?
    1. Weighs benefits and risks when making a decision.
    2. Analyzes and examine choices more independently.
    3. Concrete thinking.
    4. Anticipates when to make choices without others' assistance.
15. In which of the following examples is the nurse not applying critical thinking skills in practice?
    1. The nurse considers personnel experience in performing intravenous (IV) line insertion and ways to improve performance.
    2. The nurse uses a fall risk inventory scale to determine a patient's fall risk.
    3. The nurse observes a change in a patient's behavior and considers which problem is likely developing.
    4. The nurse explains the procedure for giving a tube feeding to a second nurse who has floated to the unit to assist with care.

Answers: **1.** 4; **2.** 1; **3.** 3; **4.** 3, 4; **5.** 1, 3; **6.** 3; **7.** 1; **8.** 2, 3, 4; **9.** 3; **10.** 2; **11.** The correct order is 3 (assessment), 5 (nursing diagnosis), 2 (planning), 4 (intervention), 1 (evaluation); **12.** 3; **13.** 1, 3, 4; **14.** 4; **15.** 4.

REFERENCES

American Nurses Association: *Nursing's social policy statement: the essence of the profession*, Washington, DC, 2010, The Association.

Benner P: *From novice to expert: excellence and power in clinical nursing practice*, Menlo Park, Calif, 1984, Addison-Wesley.

Bilinski H: The mentored journal, *Nurs Educ* 27(1):37, 2002.

Facione N, Facione P: Externalizing the critical thinking in knowledge development and clinical judgment, *Nurs Outlook* 44:129, 1996.

Ferrario CG: Developing nurses' critical thinking skills with concept mapping, *J Nurses Staff Dev* 20(6):261, 2004.

Harjai PK, Tiwari R: Model of critical diagnostic reasoning: achieving expert clinician performance, *Nurs Educ Perspect* 30(5):305, 2009.

Heffner S, Rudy S: Critical thinking: what does it mean in the care of elderly hospitalized patients? *Crit Care Nurs Q* 31(1):73, 2008.

Hill C: Integrating clinical experiences into the concept mapping process, *Nurse Educ* 31(1):36, 2006.

Jackson M: Defining the concept of critical thinking. In Jackson M, Ignatavicius DD, Case B, editors: *Conversations in critical thinking and clinical judgment,* American Association of Critical Care Nurses, Sudbury, Mass, 2006, Jones & Bartlett.

Kataoka-Yahiro M, Saylor C: A critical thinking model for nursing judgment, *J Nurs Educ* 33(8):351, 1994.

Miller M, Malcolm N: Critical thinking in the nursing curriculum, *Nurs Health Care* 11:67, 1990.

Paul RW: The art of redesigning instruction. In Willsen J, Blinker AJA, editors: *Critical thinking: how to prepare students for a rapidly changing world*, Santa Rosa, Calif, 1993, Foundation for Critical Thinking.

Paul RW, Heaslip P: Critical thinking and intuitive nursing practice, *J Adv Nurs* 22:40, 1995.

Swinny B: Assessing and developing critical thinking skills in the intensive care unit, *Crit Care Nurs Q* 33(1):2, 2010.

Taylor J, Wros P: Concept mapping: a nursing model for care planning, *J Nurs Ed* 46(5):211, 2007.

RESEARCH REFERENCES

Bittner NP, Gravlin G: Critical thinking, delegation, and missed nursing care, *J Nurs Admin* 39(3):142, 2009.

Cirocco M: How reflective practice improves nurses' critical thinking ability, *Gastroenterol Nurs* 30(6):405, 2007.

Di Vito-Thomas P: Nursing student stories on learning how to think like a nurse, *Nurse Educ* 30(3):133, 2005.

Facione P: *Critical thinking: a statement of expert consensus for purposes of educational assessment and instruction. The Delphi report: research findings and recommendations prepared for the American Philosophical Association*, ERIC Doc No. ED 315-423, Washington, DC, 1990, ERIC.

Potter P, et al: Delegation practices between registered nurses and nursing assistive personnel, *J Nurs Manage* 18(2):157, 2010.

Settersten L, Lauver DR: Critical thinking, perceived health status, and participation in health behaviors, *Nurs Res* 53(1):11, 2004.

White AH: Clinical decision making among fourth year nursing students: an interpretive study, *J Nurs Educ* 42(3):113, 2003.

CHAPTER

16

Nursing Assessment

OBJECTIVES

- Discuss the relationship between critical thinking and nursing assessment.
- Explain the process of data collection.
- Differentiate between subjective and objective data.
- Describe the methods of data collection.
- Discuss the process of conducting a patient-centered interview.
- Describe the components of a nursing history.
- Explain the differences among comprehensive, problem-oriented, and focused assessments.
- Explain the relationship between data interpretation and validation.
- Conduct a nursing assessment.

KEY TERMS

Assessment, p. 207
Back channeling, p. 213
Closed-ended questions, p. 214
Concomitant symptoms, p. 215
Cue, p. 208
Database, p. 207
Functional health patterns, p. 208
Inference, p. 208
Nursing health history, p. 214
Nursing process, p. 206
Objective data, p. 210
Open-ended questions, p. 213
Review of systems (ROS), p. 216
Subjective data, p. 210
Validation, p. 217

evolve WEBSITE

http://evolve.elsevier.com/Potter/fundamentals/

- Review Questions
- Concept Map Creator
- Case Study with Questions
- Audio Glossary
- Interactive Learning Activities
- Key Term Flashcards
- Content Updates

The **nursing process** is a critical thinking process that professional nurses use to apply the best available evidence to caregiving and promoting human functions and responses to health and illness (American Nurses Association, 2010). It is the fundamental blueprint for how to care for patients. The nursing process is also a standard of practice, which, when followed correctly, protects nurses against legal problems related to nursing care (Austin, 2008). As a nursing student, you learn the five steps of the nursing process—assessment, diagnosis, planning, implementation, and evaluation—as if they were a linear process (Fig. 16-1). However, in fact the nursing process is dynamic and continuous; and, after more experience in practice, you learn to move back and forth among the various steps (Potter et al., 2005). Consider the following scenario that was also described in Chapter 15:

Mr. Jacobs is a 58-year-old patient who had a radical prostatectomy (removal of prostate gland) for prostate cancer yesterday. He is married to Martha, who has been at his bedside most of the morning. His nurse, Tonya Moore, just started the day shift on the surgical unit and finds the patient lying flat in bed with arms tensed and extended along his sides. When Tonya checks the surgical wound and drainage device, she notes that Mr. Jacobs winces when she gently places her hands to palpate around the incisional area. She asks Mr. Jacobs when he last turned onto his side, and he responds, "Not since last night some time." Tonya asks Mr. Jacobs if he is having incisional pain, and he nods yes, saying, "It hurts too much to move." Tonya clarifies, "On a scale of 0 to 10 with 0 being no pain and 10 being the worst pain you have ever had, rate how you feel now." Mr. Jacobs states, "Oh, this is at least a 7." Tonya considers the information she has observed and learned from Mr. Jacobs to determine that he is in pain and has reduced mobility because of it. She decides that she needs to take action to relieve Mr. Jacobs' pain so she can turn him more frequently and begin to get him out of bed for his recovery.

Each time you meet a patient, you apply the nursing process, as Tonya did while caring for Mr. Jacobs, to provide appropriate and effective nursing care. The process begins with the first step, assessment, the gathering and analysis of information about the patient's health status. You then make clinical judgments from the assessment to identify the patient's response to health problems in the form of nursing diagnoses. Once you define appropriate nursing diagnoses, you create a plan of care. Planning includes setting goals and expected outcomes for your care and selecting interventions (nursing and collaborative) individualized to each of the patient's nursing diagnoses. The next step, implementation, involves performing the planned interventions. After performing

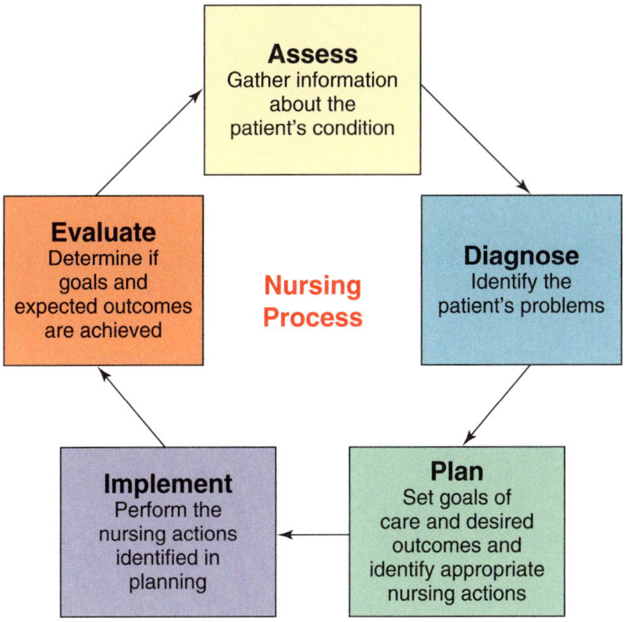

FIG. 16-1 Five-step nursing process.

interventions, you evaluate the patient's response and whether the interventions were effective. The nursing process is central to your ability to provide timely and appropriate care to your patients.

The nursing process is a variation of scientific reasoning. Practicing the five steps of the nursing process allows you to be organized and conduct your practice in a systematic way. You learn to make inferences about the meaning of a patient's response to a health problem or generalize about the patient's functional state of health. Through assessment a pattern begins to form. For example, if Mr. Jacobs is having incisional pain, the data allow Tonya to infer that his mobility is limited. Tonya gathers more information (e.g., palpating gently over the incision, having Mr. Jacobs rate the severity of discomfort, and noting that he limits movement) until an accurate classification of the patient's problem is determined such as the following nursing diagnosis: *acute pain related to trauma of incision* and the diagnosis of *impaired physical mobility related to incisional pain.* Clearly defining your patients' problems provides the basis for planning and implementing nursing interventions and evaluating the outcomes of care.

CRITICAL THINKING APPROACH TO ASSESSMENT

Assessment is the deliberate and systematic collection of information about a patient to determine his or her current and past health and functional status and his or her present and past coping patterns (Carpenito-Moyet, 2009). Nursing **assessment** includes two steps:

1. Collection of information from a primary source (the patient) and secondary sources (e.g., family members, health professionals, and medical record)
2. The interpretation and validation of data to ensure a complete database

The purpose of assessment is to establish a **database** about the patient's perceived needs, health problems, and responses to these problems. In addition, the data reveal related experiences, health practices, goals, values, and expectations about the health care system.

When a plumber comes to your home to repair a problem you describe as a "leaking faucet," the plumber checks the faucet, its attachments to the water line, and the water pressure in the system to determine the real problem. A patient presents an initial health problem to you. For example, Mr. Jacobs presents with signs of pain following surgery. You then proceed to observe his behaviors, ask questions about the nature of the problem, listen to the cues he provides, and conduct a physical examination (see Chapter 30). You also usually interview family members who are familiar with the patient's health problems and any existing medical record data. The data you collect fall into different sets or patterns of information that point to a diagnostic conclusion. Once a plumber knows the source of the leaking faucet, he is able to repair it. Once you know the nature and source of a patient's specific health problems (such as Mr. Jacob's incisional pain), you are able to provide interventions that will restore, maintain, or improve the patient's health.

Critical thinking is a vital part of assessment (see Chapter 15). It allows you to see the big picture when you form conclusions or make decisions about a patient's health condition. While gathering data about a patient, you synthesize relevant knowledge, recall prior clinical experiences, apply critical thinking standards and attitudes, and use standards of practice to direct your assessment in a meaningful and purposeful way (Fig. 16-2). Your knowledge from the physical, biological, and social sciences allows you to ask relevant questions and collect relevant history and physical assessment data related to the patient's presenting health care needs. For example, Tonya knows that Mr. Jacobs had his prostate gland removed. She reviewed her medical-surgical textbook and learned that a radical prostatectomy involves removal of a lot of tissue, including the prostate gland, seminal vesicles, part of the bladder neck, and lymph nodes. This knowledge helps her to recognize that considerable swelling can potentially create acute pain; thus she decides to inspect and palpate around Mr. Jacob's incisional area. She also questions Mr. Jacobs about how the discomfort affects his ability to turn or move in bed. Using good communication skills through interviewing and applying critical thinking intellectual standards (such as being precise and accurate in using a pain scale) enables Tonya to collect complete, accurate, and relevant data.

Prior clinical experience contributes to the skills of assessment. For example, Tonya cared for a patient with surgical incision pain in the past and knows that pain is often disabling and limits a patient's normal motion. This experience allows Tonya to thoroughly assess the extent to which pain affects the patient's ability to move and eventually get out of bed, an important step in Mr. Jacob's recovery. Validation of any abnormal assessment findings and personal observation of assessments performed by skilled professionals help you become competent in assessment. You also learn to apply standards of practice and accepted standards of "normal" for physical assessment data when assessing patients. Use of critical thinking attitudes such as curiosity, perseverance, and confidence ensure you complete a comprehensive database.

Data Collection

You perform assessment to gather information needed to make an accurate judgment about a patient's current condition (Magnan and Maklebust, 2009). Your information comes from:

- The patient, through interview, observations, and physical examination.
- Family members or significant others' reports and response to interviews.
- Other members of the health care team.

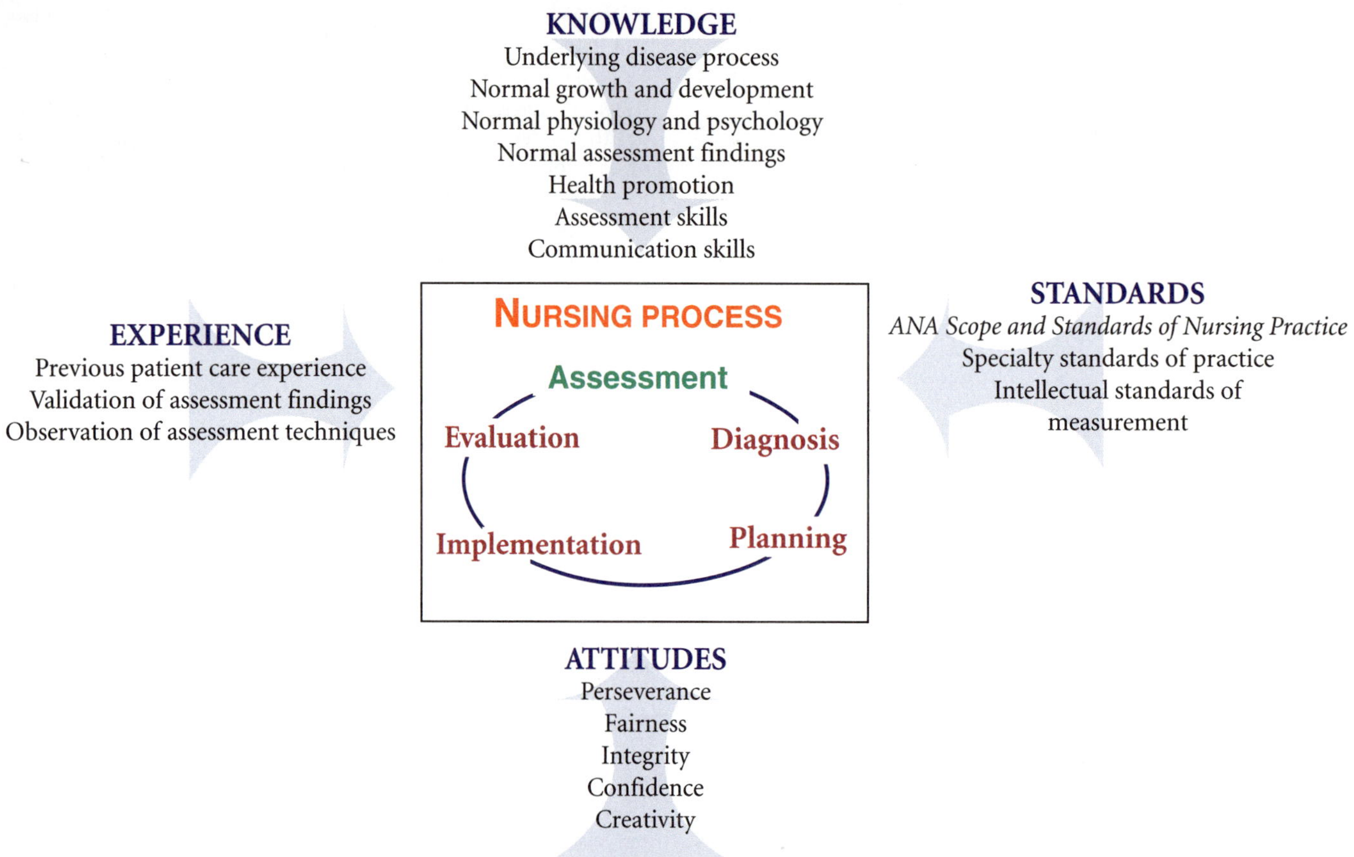

FIG. 16-2 Critical thinking and the assessment process.

- Medical record information (e.g., patient history, laboratory work, x-ray film results, multidisciplinary consultations).
- Scientific literature (evidence about assessment techniques and standards).

As you begin a patient assessment, think critically about what to assess for that specific patient. Determine which questions or measurements are appropriate based on your clinical knowledge and experience and your patient's health history and responses. When you first meet a patient, perform a quick screening. Usually your screening is based on a treatment situation. For example, a community health nurse assesses the patient's neighborhood and community; an emergency department nurse uses the ABC (airway-breathing-circulation) approach; and a surgical nurse focuses on the patient's symptoms following surgery, the expected healing response, and potential complications. For Mr. Jacobs, Tonya first focuses on the nature and severity of his pain, the risk of limited postoperative mobility, and the possibility that the wound is infected. She later expands her assessment to determine how Mr. Jacobs is adjusting emotionally to his surgery.

You learn to differentiate important data from the total data collected. A **cue** is information that you obtain through use of the senses. An **inference** is your judgment or interpretation of these cues (Fig. 16-3). For example, a patient crying is a cue that possibly implies fear or sadness. You ask the patient about any concerns and make known any nonverbal expressions you notice in an effort to direct the patient to share his or her feelings. It is possible to miss important cues when you conduct an initial overview. However, always try to interpret cues from the patient to know how in depth to make your assessment. Remember, thinking is human and imperfect. You acquire appropriate thinking processes when conducting assessments but expect to make mistakes in missing important cues (Lunney, 2006). Assessment is dynamic and allows you to freely explore relevant patient problems as you discover them.

After your observational screening, focus on the assessment cues and patterns of information that suggest problem areas. There are two approaches to a comprehensive assessment. One involves use of a structured database format, based on an accepted theoretical framework or practice standard. Gordon's model of 11 **functional health patterns** (1994) (Box 16-1) is an example. The theory or practice standard provides categories of information for you to assess. Gordon's functional health patterns model offers a holistic framework for assessment of any health problem. Tonya plans to direct her assessment of Mr. Jacobs to the cognitive-perceptual pattern to learn more about what the patient knows about the surgery and his prognosis and how he prefers to learn and make decisions about his care. Tonya is anticipating his need for education about postoperative recovery. She also plans to assess his sexuality-reproductive pattern to determine how he is accepting the potential change in sexual function resulting from surgery. A theoretical or standard-based assessment provides for a comprehensive review of a patient's health care problems.

An assessment moves from the general to the specific. For example, you assess all of Gordon's 11 functional health patterns and then determine if patterns or problems appear in your data. You then ask more focused questions about the health patterns that

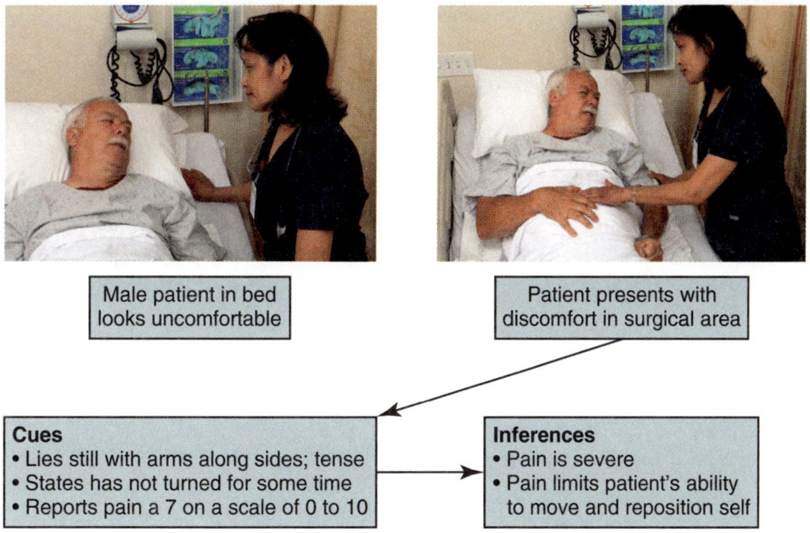

FIG. 16-3 Observational overview using cues and forming inferences.

BOX 16-1 TYPOLOGY OF 11 FUNCTIONAL HEALTH PATTERNS

Health perception–health management pattern: Describes patient's self-report of health and well-being; how patient manages health (e.g., frequency of health care provider visits, adherence to therapies at home); knowledge of preventive health practices

Nutritional-metabolic pattern: Describes patient's daily/weekly pattern of food and fluid intake (e.g., food preferences or restrictions, special diet, appetite); actual weight; weight loss or gain

Elimination pattern: Describes patterns of excretory function (bowel, bladder, and skin)

Activity-exercise pattern: Describes patterns of exercise, activity, leisure, and recreation; ability to perform activities of daily living

Sleep-rest pattern: Describes patterns of sleep, rest, and relaxation

Cognitive-perceptual pattern: Describes sensory-perceptual patterns; language adequacy, memory, decision-making ability

Self-perception–self-concept pattern: Describes patient's self-concept pattern and perceptions of self (e.g., self-concept/worth, emotional patterns, body image)

Role-relationship pattern: Describes patient's patterns of role engagements and relationships

Sexuality-reproductive pattern: Describes patient's patterns of satisfaction and dissatisfaction with sexuality pattern; patient's reproductive patterns; premenopausal and postmenopausal problems

Coping–stress tolerance pattern: Describes patient's ability to manage stress; sources of support; effectiveness of the patterns in terms of stress tolerance

Value-belief pattern: Describes patterns of values, beliefs (including spiritual practices), and goals that guide patient's choices or decisions

Data from Gordon M: *Nursing diagnosis: process and application*, ed 3, St Louis, 1994, Mosby; and Carpenito-Moyet LJ: *Nursing diagnosis: application to clinical practice*, ed 13, Philadelphia, 2009, Lippincott Williams & Wilkins.

suggest a problem exists. You organize patterns of behavior and physiological responses that relate to a functional health category. The complete assessment of the 11 functional health patterns represents the interaction of the patient and the environment, which Gordon calls biopsychosocial integration. According to Gordon (1994), you cannot understand one health pattern without

TABLE 16-1 Example of Problem-Focused Patient Assessment: Pain

PROBLEM AND ASSOCIATED FACTORS	QUESTIONS	PHYSICAL ASSESSMENT
Nature of pain	Describe your pain for me. Place your hand over the area that hurts or is uncomfortable.	Observe nonverbal cues. Observe where patient points to pain; note if it radiates or is localized.
Precipitating factors	Do you notice if pain worsens during any activities or specific time of day? Is pain associated with movement?	Observe if patient demonstrates nonverbal signs of pain during movement, positioning, swallowing.
Severity	Rate your pain on a scale of 0 to 10.	Inspect area of discomfort; palpate for tenderness.

knowledge of the other patterns. Ultimately your assessment identifies functional patterns (patient strengths) and dysfunctional patterns (nursing diagnoses) that help you develop the nursing care plan.

The second approach for conducting a comprehensive assessment is the problem-oriented approach. You focus on the patient's presenting situation and begin with problematic areas such as incisional pain or limited understanding of postoperative recovery. You ask the patient follow-up questions to clarify and expand your assessment so you can understand the full nature of the problem. Later your physical examination further confirms your observations. Tonya's assessment of Mr. Jacobs ensures that she knows the type of pain he is having and the extent to which it limits his activities. Table 16-1 offers an example of a problem-focused assessment. Once you complete the assessment, thoroughly analyze the extent and nature of a patient's problem so you are able to later develop a care plan.

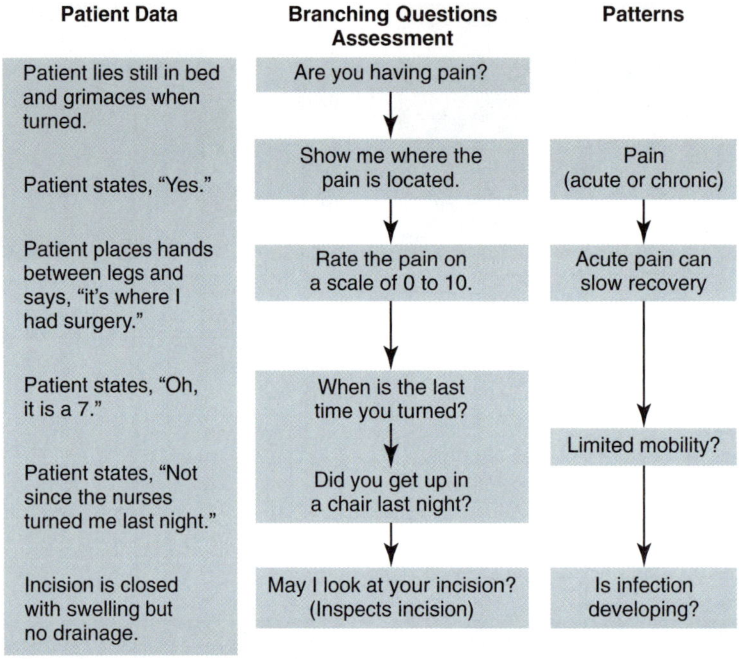

FIG. 16-4 Example of branching logic for selecting assessment questions.

Whatever approach you use to collect data, you begin to cluster cues, make inferences, and identify emerging patterns and potential problem areas. To do this well you critically anticipate, which means that you try to stay a step ahead of the assessment. Think about what the data tell you. Remember to always have supporting cues before you make an inference. Your inferences direct you to further questions. Once you ask a patient a question or make an observation, patterns form, and the information branches to an additional series of questions or observations (Fig. 16-4). Knowing how to probe and frame questions is a skill that grows with experience. You learn to decide which questions are relevant to a situation and to attend to accurate interpretations of data.

Types of Data. There are two primary sources of data: subjective and objective. **Subjective data** are your patients' verbal descriptions of their health problems. Only patients provide subjective data. For example, Mr. Jacobs's report of incision pain and his expression of concern about whether the pain means that he will not be able to go home as soon as he hoped are subjective findings. Subjective data usually include feelings, perceptions, and self-report of symptoms. Only patients provide subjective data relevant to their health condition. The data sometimes reflect physiological changes, which you further explore through objective data collection.

Objective data are observations or measurements of a patient's health status. Inspecting the condition of a surgical incision or wound, describing an observed behavior, and measuring blood pressure are examples of objective data. The measurement of objective data is based on an accepted standard such as the Fahrenheit or Celsius measure on a thermometer, inches or centimeters on a measuring tape, or known characteristics of behaviors (e.g., anxiety or fear). When you collect objective data, apply critical thinking intellectual standards (e.g., clear, precise, and consistent) so you can correctly interpret your findings.

Sources of Data. As a nurse you obtain data from a variety of sources that provide information about the patient's current level of wellness and functional status, anticipated prognosis, risk factors, health practices and goals, responses to previous treatment, and patterns of health and illness.

Patient. A patient is usually your best source of information. Patients who are conscious, alert, and able to answer questions correctly provide the most accurate information about their health care needs, lifestyle patterns, present and past illnesses, perception of symptoms, responses to treatment, and changes in activities of daily living. Always consider the setting for your assessment and your patient's condition. A patient experiencing acute symptoms in an emergency department will not offer as much information as one who comes to an outpatient clinic for a routine checkup. An older adult requires more time than someone younger, and often multiple visits are required to gather a complete database (Seidel et al., 2011) (Box 16-2). Always be attentive and show a caring presence with patients (see Chapter 7). Let a patient know you are interested in what he or she has to say. Patients are less likely to fully reveal the nature of their health care problems when nurses show little interest or are easily distracted by activities around them.

Family and Significant Others. Family members and significant others are primary sources of information for infants or children; critically ill adults; and patients who are mentally handicapped, disoriented, or unconscious. In cases of severe illness or emergency situations, families are often the only sources of information for nurses and other health care providers. The family and significant others are also important secondary sources of information. They confirm findings that a patient provides (e.g., whether he takes medications regularly at home or how well he sleeps or eats). Include the family when appropriate. Remember, a patient does not always want you to question or involve the family. You must obtain a patient's agreement to include family members or friends. Often spouses or close friends sit in during an assessment and provide their view of the patient's health problems or needs. Not only do they supply information about the patient's current health status, but they are also able to tell when changes in the patient's status occurred. Family members are often very well informed because of

BOX 16-2 FOCUS ON OLDER ADULTS

Approaches for Gathering an Older-Adult Assessment

- Listen patiently.
- Allow for pauses and time for patient to tell the story.
- Recognize normal changes associated with aging. These changes might be considered abnormal in a younger adult.
- If patient has a proxy (person who legally represents patient), gather history information from that individual.
- If patient has limited hearing or visual deficits, use nonverbal communication when conducting a patient-centered interview.
  - **Patient-directed eye gaze:** This allows the nurse or patient who is speaking to check whether information is understood. It is a signal for readiness to initiate interaction with a patient. Eye contact shows that you are interested in what the other person is saying.
  - **Affirmative head nodding:** This has an important social function. It helps to regulate an interaction (especially when alternate people speak), supports spoken language, and allows for comment on the interaction concerning the rapport and content of the communication.
  - **Smiling:** Smiling is positive and considered as a sign of good humor, warmth, and immediacy. It is most important when first establishing the nurse-patient relationship.
  - **Forward leaning:** This shows awareness, attention, and immediacy. During an interaction it also clearly suggests interest in that person.

their experiences living with the patient and observing how health problems affect daily living activities. Family and friends make important observations about the patient's needs that can affect the way care is delivered (e.g., how a patient eats a meal or how he or she makes choices).

Health Care Team. You frequently communicate with other health care team members in gathering information about patients. In the acute care setting the change-of-shift report is how nurses from one shift communicate information to nurses on the next shift (see Chapter 26). During the report you have the chance to collect the first set of information about patients assigned to your care. Researchers found that bedside rounds, also called *bedside handover,* promote patient-centered care (Chaboyer, McMurray, and Wallis, 2010). During bedside rounds, the nurse who is completing care for a shift, the patient, and the nurse assuming care for a shift share information about the patient's condition, status of problems, and treatment plan for the next shift. In some settings other health care team members participate in the rounds. When nurses, physicians, physical therapists, social workers, or other staff consult on a patient's condition, they share information about how the patient is interacting within the health care environment, the patient's reactions to treatment, and the result of diagnostic procedures or therapies. Every member of the team is a source of information for identifying and verifying information about the patient.

Medical Records. The medical record is a source for the patient's medical history, laboratory and diagnostic test results, current physical findings, and the primary health care provider's treatment plan. The record is a valuable tool for checking the consistency and similarities of your personal observations. Data in the records offer a baseline and ongoing information about the patient's response to illness and progress to date. The Health Insurance Portability and Accountability Act (HIPAA) of 1996 has a privacy rule that came into effect on April 14, 2003 to set standards for the protection of health information (USDHHS, 2003). Information in a patient's record is confidential. Each health care agency has policies governing how the patient's health information can be shared among health care providers (see Chapter 26). It is important to know organization policies for reviewing a patient's medical record for the purpose of assessment.

Other Records and the Scientific Literature. Educational, military, and employment records sometimes contain significant health care information (e.g., immunizations). If a patient received services at a community health center or different hospital, you need written permission from the patient or guardian to access the records. The HIPAA regulations protect access to patients' health information. The privacy rule allows health care providers to share protected information as long as they use reasonable safeguards. Check the policy of your agency for HIPAA guidelines.

Reviewing nursing, medical, and pharmacological literature about a patient's illness completes your assessment database. This review increases your knowledge about the patient's diagnosed problems, expected symptoms, treatment, prognosis, and established standards of therapeutic practice. The scientific literature offers evidence to direct you on how and why to conduct assessments for particular patient conditions. A knowledgeable nurse obtains relevant, accurate, and complete information for the assessment database.

Nurse's Experience. Through clinical experience a nurse observes other patients; recognizes clinical changes; and learns the types of questions to ask, choosing only the questions that will give the most useful information. A nurse's expertise develops after testing and refining inferences, questions, and principle- or standard-based expectations. For example, while caring for Mr. Jacobs, Tonya has learned what a prostatectomy incision looks like and how a patient responds to the associated discomfort. In the future Tonya will more quickly recognize the behavior of a patient in acute pain and how it affects normal mobility. Practical experience and the opportunity to make clinical decisions strengthen your critical thinking.

Methods of Data Collection

As a nurse you use patient-centered interviews, the nursing health history, physical examination, and results of laboratory and diagnostic tests to collect data for a patient's assessment database.

Patient-Centered Interview. A patient-centered *interview* is an approach for obtaining from patients the data that are needed to foster a caring nurse-patient relationship, adherence to interventions, and treatment effectiveness (Smith et al., 2006). The interview technique is the basis of a conceptual model used by nurse practitioners to form long-term therapeutic relationships with patients (Lein and Wills, 2007). However, the model has aspects that are useful to all nurses when conducting interviews for patient assessment. The partnership that forms in a patient-centered interview empowers a patient, promotes mutual decision making with the nurse, and ensures continuity of care (Dontje et al., 2004).

The expectation in a busy acute care setting such as a hospital nursing unit or clinic is for nurses to complete in a limited amount of time a patient history and nursing assessment. In the home health setting there is usually more time and fewer distractions; this allows a nurse to conduct a thorough interview. Agencies set standards for the type of information to be collected in health histories. However, there is a risk that standard assessments do not capture the patient's full story. In a patient-centered interview an organized conversation with the patient allows the patient to set the initial focus and initiate discussion about his or her chief problems or reasons for seeking health care (Lein and Wills, 2007).

A successful interview requires preparation. Collect available information about the patient before starting the interview. For example, review the information you learn during a change-of-shift report and then plan to interview the hospitalized patient as you make patient rounds and before you begin to provide ordered interventions. Create a favorable environment for the interview. A good interview environment is free of distractions, unnecessary noise, and interruptions. The patient is more likely to be open and honest if the interview is private (i.e., out of earshot of other patients, visitors, or staff). Timing is important in avoiding interruptions. If possible, set aside a 10- to 15-minute period when no other activities are planned. More time is even better but is difficult to plan when you have multiple patients. During the interview always observe your patient for signs of discomfort or fatigue and plan accordingly. Remember to let a patient decide whether to involve the family in the interview. After an initial interview, follow-up discussions allow you to learn more about a patient's situation and focus on specific problem areas. An initial patient-centered interview involves: (1) setting the stage, (2) gathering information about the patient's chief concerns or problems and setting an agenda, (3) collecting the assessment or a nursing health history, and (4) terminating the interview.

Setting the Stage. Greet the patient using his or her full name, introduce yourself and explain your role (if it is the first time you have met), and remove any barriers to privacy by closing a room curtain or shutting a door. This is the orientation phase of an interview. When you explain the reason for collecting a health history, also assure the patient that any information obtained remains confidential and is used only by health care professionals who provide his or her care. HIPAA regulations require patients to sign an authorization before you collect personal health data (USDHHS, 2003). Refer to your agency policy for the authorization process.

After giving Mr. Jacobs pain medication for his incisional pain, Tonya waits 30 minutes and decides to take the time to assess Mr. Jacobs more fully. She reviews the surgical summary in the chart and the last set of nurses' notes and enters the patient's room.

Tonya: Mr. Jacobs, I am Tonya Moore. I did not fully introduce myself earlier when you looked so uncomfortable. You look a bit more comfortable now. Can you rate your pain again for me on a scale of 0 to 10?"

Mr. Jacobs: "Yes, I think the medicine has helped. I would rate the pain a 4."

Tonya: "Good. If you're comfortable, I'd like to spend about 10 minutes to better understand what you know about your surgery and discuss it with you. Everything you share will be confidential between you and the persons providing your care. I will let nurses on the next shift know about your care."

Mr. Jacobs: "Ok, I would appreciate that."

Set an Agenda. You begin an interview by gathering information about the patient's current chief concerns or problems and setting an agenda. Remember, the best clinical interview focuses on the patient, not your agenda. Let the patient know your purpose (such as collecting an assessment or a nursing history) and ask the patient for his or her list of concerns or problems. This is the time that allows the patient to feel comfortable speaking with you and become an active partner in decisions about care. The professionalism and the competence that you show when interviewing patients strengthens the nurse-patient relationship.

Tonya: "I'm going to ask you questions about what you know about your surgery and what you need to do once you go home. But first tell me your main concerns."

Mr. Jacobs: "Concerns, you mean about the surgery?"

Tonya: "Yes, or any other health problems you would like to discuss."

Mr. Jacobs: "Well, I hope they got all of the cancer. I want to do what I need to do to get out of here as soon as I can."

Tonya: "Ok, Is there anything else?"

Mr. Jacobs: "I'm worried about my wife and me. My doctor told me that the surgery could change our ability to have sex."

Tonya: "Ok, your doctor will talk to you about your tumor. Don't be afraid to ask him questions. Which changes concern you?

Mr. Jacobs: "Well I worry that, you know, I may not be able to have intercourse."

Tonya: "It's true; that is a risk of surgery. It's important to learn from the doctor whether there was any nerve injury during surgery. It's something you need to ask him. And we can discuss it further when you know the results. Now let me ask you about your expectations after surgery so we can have a teaching plan for you. Does that sound reasonable?"

Mr. Jacobs: "Yes, I'm not sure what to expect before I get out of here."

Collect the Assessment or Nursing Health History. Start an assessment or a health history with open-ended questions that allow patients to describe more clearly their concerns and problems. For example, you can begin by having the patient explain symptoms or physical concerns, describe what he or she knows about the health problem, or ask him or her to describe health care expectations. Use attentive listening and other therapeutic communication techniques (see Chapter 24) that encourage a patient to tell his or her story. Observe verbal cues the patient expresses. Stay focused and orderly and do not rush. An initial interview (e.g., the one you conduct to collect a complete nursing history) is more extensive. You gather information about the patient's concerns and then complete all relevant sections of the nursing history (see the following dialogue). Ongoing interviews, which occur each time you interact with your patient, do not need to be as extensive. An ongoing interview allows you to update the patient's status and concerns, focus on changes previously identified, and review new problems. In the case study Tonya is gathering information to plan her postoperative teaching for Mr. Jacobs.

Tonya: "Mr. Jacobs, tell me what you expect over the next few days before you go home."

Mr. Jacobs: "Well, the doctor did tell me that I would have this catheter in my bladder after I go home. But I don't know if I have to do anything with this dressing over my stitches."

Tonya: "Un huh, go on."

Mr. Jacobs: "Will I have something to take for this pain as long as I am here, and what will I have to take at home?"

Tonya: "Yes, your doctor has ordered your pain medicine every 4 hours around the clock. You need to tell us when you begin to feel uncomfortable. You'll have a pain medicine prescribed when you go home. Do you have any other concerns or questions about your surgery?"

Mr. Jacobs: "No, I don't think so."

Tonya: "Ok. First you're right; the catheter will stay in your bladder, probably about 2 weeks. Your surgeon will have you come to the office to have it removed. We'll talk about how you and your wife can manage the catheter, and we'll probably recommend a visit by a home health nurse. I want to look at the dressing over your incision more closely. You have a small drain in the incision to make sure fluid drains and the tissues heal well. I want to talk with you and your wife about how to observe for signs of infection."

Mr. Jacobs: "Is infection common?"

Tonya: "No, but you need to know the signs of an infection; so, if something happens once you return home, you can call your doctor quickly."

Terminating the Interview. As in the other phases of the interview, termination requires skill. You summarize your discussion with the patient and check for accuracy of the information collected. Give your patient a clue that the interview is coming to an end. For example, say, "I have just two more questions. We'll be finished in a few more minutes." This helps the patient maintain direct attention without being distracted by wondering when the interview will end. This approach also gives the patient an opportunity to ask additional questions. End the interview in a friendly manner, telling the patient when you will return to provide care.

Tonya: "Thank you, Mr. Jacobs. I am just about finished with my questions. Can I get you anything?"

Mr. Jacobs: "No, I want to rest a bit."

Tonya: You have given me a good idea of which topics we need to cover to prepare you for going home. And we'll include your wife in these discussions. Pain control is our priority right now, and we can talk further about the medicines you'll be taking when you go home. I want to go over catheter and dressing care after you rest so you feel prepared to go home. I also plan to come back and talk to you more about the surgery and its effects on your sexual function. Is there anything I can do for you now?"

Mr. Jacobs: "No, you've been helpful already."

A skillful interviewer adapts interview strategies based on the patient's responses. You successfully gather relevant health data when you are prepared for the interview and able to carry out each interview phase with minimal interruption.

Interview Techniques. How you conduct the interview is just as important as the questions you ask. Always use good communication techniques (see Chapter 24). During the interview you are responsible for directing the flow of the discussion so your patient has the opportunity to freely contribute stories about his or her health problems to enable you to get as much detailed information as possible. Some interviews are focused; others are comprehensive. Listen and consider the information shared because this helps you direct the patient to provide more detail or discuss a topic that might reveal a possible problem. Because a patient's report includes subjective information, validate data from the interview later with objective data. For example, if the patient reports difficulty breathing, this will lead you to further assess respiratory rate and lung sounds during the physical examination.

During an interview obtain information (when appropriate) about a patient's physical, developmental, emotional, intellectual, social, and spiritual dimensions. Physical and developmental information reflects normal functioning and reveals pathological changes caused by illness, trauma, or developmental crisis. Emotional information includes the patient's behavioral responses to changes in health and patterns of living. Relevant emotional information includes mood, perceptions, body image, self-concept, and attitudes about sexuality. Intellectual information includes intellectual performance, problem-solving ability, educational level, communication patterns, and attention span. Social information involves environmental, cultural, ethnic, or social patterns that affect the present or future level of wellness. You also collect information about life goals and values and religious practices, part of a patient's spirituality.

Observe the patient's nonverbal communication such as use of eye contact, body language, or tone of voice. While observing a patient's nonverbal behavior, appearance, and interaction with the environment, determine whether the data you obtain are consistent with what the patient states verbally. Your observations lead you to pursue further objective information to form accurate conclusions. Patients also obtain information during interviews. If you establish a trusting nurse-patient relationship, the patient feels comfortable asking you questions about the health care environment, planned treatments, diagnostic testing, and available resources. The patient needs this information to make decisions about goals and the plan of care.

Open-ended Questions. In a patient-centered interview you try to find out, in the patient's own words, what the health problem is and its probable cause. Remember, patients are usually the best resources in talking about their symptoms or relating their health history. Begin by asking the patient an *open-ended question* to elicit his or her story (Box 16-3). An open-ended question does not presuppose a specific answer. For example, say, "So, why did you come to the hospital today?" or "Tell me about the problems you're having." The use of **open-ended questions** prompts patients to describe a situation in more than one or two words. This technique leads to a discussion in which patients actively describe their health status. The use of open-ended questions strengthens your relationship with a patient because it shows that you want to hear the patient's thoughts and feelings. Remember to encourage and let the patient tell the entire story.

Back Channeling. Reinforce your interest in what the patient has to say through the use of good eye contact and listening skills. In addition, you may use **back channeling,** which includes active listening prompts such as "all right," "go on," or "uh-huh." These indicate that you have heard what the patient says and are interested in hearing the full story. Back channeling encourages a patient to give more details.

Probing. As a patient tells his or her story, encourage a full description without trying to control the direction the story takes. This requires you to probe with further open-ended statements

BOX 16-3 EXAMPLES OF OPEN- AND CLOSED-ENDED QUESTIONS

Open-Ended Questions

- Tell me how you are feeling.
- Tell me how your health has been.
- Describe how your wife has been helping you.
- Give me an example of how you get relief from your pain at home.

Closed-Ended Questions

- Do you think the medication is helping you?
- Who helps you at home?
- Do you understand why you are having the x-ray examination?
- Are you having pain now?
- On a scale of 0 to 10, how would you rate your pain?

such as, "Is there anything else you can tell me?" or "What else is bothering you?" Ask as many questions as it takes until the patient has nothing else to say. Remember to be observant. If the patient becomes fatigued or uncomfortable, know when to postpone an interview.

Closed-ended Questions. Once a patient finishes his or her story, use a problem-seeking interview technique. This approach takes the information provided in the patient's story and more fully describes and identifies specific problem areas. For example, a patient reports experiencing indigestion over the course of several days and acknowledges having some diarrhea and loss of appetite. The patient's explanation for the cause relates to a recent series of trips that changed his eating habits. Focus on the symptoms the patient identifies and the general indigestion problem by asking **closed-ended questions** that limit answers to one or two words such as "yes" or "no" or a number or frequency of a symptom (see Box 16-3). For example, ask, "How often does the diarrhea occur?" or "Do you have pain or cramping?" Closed-ended questions require short answers and clarify previous information or provide additional information. The questions do not encourage the patient to volunteer more information than you request. This type of questioning helps you acquire specific information about health problems such as symptoms, precipitating factors, or relief measures.

A good interviewer leaves with a complete story that contains enough details for understanding a patient's perceptions of his or her health status and the information needed to help identify nursing diagnoses and/or collaborative health problems. Always clarify or validate any information about which you are unclear.

Cultural Considerations in Assessment

As a professional nurse it is important to conduct all assessments with cultural competence. This involves a conscientious understanding of your patient's culture so you can offer better care within differing value systems and act with respect and understanding without imposing your own attitudes and beliefs (Seidel et al., 2011). To conduct an accurate and complete assessment, you need to consider a patient's cultural background. When cultural differences exist between you and a patient, respect the unfamiliar and be sensitive to a patient's uniqueness. For clarity, explain the intent of any questions you have. Avoid making stereotypes; the assumptions tied to stereotypes can lead you to collect inaccurate information. Instead draw on knowledge from your assessment and ask questions in a constructive and probing way to allow you to truly know who the patient is. You must be sure that you grasp exactly what a patient means and know exactly what a patient thinks you mean in words and actions. If you are unsure about what a patient is saying, ask for clarification to prevent making the wrong diagnostic conclusion. Do not make assumptions about a patient's cultural beliefs and behaviors without validation from the patient (Seidel et al., 2011).

Communication and culture are interrelated in the way feelings are expressed verbally and nonverbally. If you learn the variations in how people of different cultures communicate, you will gather more accurate information from patients. For example, people from Spain and France make firm eye contact when speaking. However, this is considered rude or immodest by certain Asian or Middle Eastern cultures. Americans often tend to let the eyes wander (Seidel et al., 2011). Using the right approach with eye contact shows respect for your patient and likely results in the patient sharing more information. It is easier to explore cultural differences if you allow time for thoughtful answers and ask your questions in a comfortable order. Here are examples (Seidel et al., 2011; Swartz, 2010):

- When talking about a patient's illness:
  - What do you think is wrong with you?
  - What do you call your problem?
  - What worries you the most about your sickness?
- When talking about treatments:
  - What should be done to get rid of your problem?
  - People have told me that there are ways of treating sickness that doctors and nurses don't use. Do you know any of them? Have you ever tried them?
  - Has anyone else helped you with this problem?
  - What benefit will you get from the treatment?

Nursing Health History

You gather a **nursing health history** during either your initial or an early contact with a patient. The history is a major component of assessment. Most health history forms are structured. However, based on information you gained from your patient's story (during the patient-centered interview), you learn which components of the history to explore fully and which require less detail. A good assessor learns to refine and broaden questions as needed to correctly assess the patient's unique needs. Time and patient priorities determine how complete a history will be. A comprehensive history covers all health dimensions (Fig. 16-5), allowing you to develop a complete plan of care. A nursing history usually contains the same basic components.

Biographical Information. Biographical information is factual demographic data about the patient. The patient's age, address, occupation and working status, marital status, source of health care, and types of insurance are included. Admitting office staff usually collect this information.

Reason for Seeking Health Care. This is the information you gather when you initially set an agenda during the patient-centered interview. You learn the patient's chief concerns or problems. Compare what you learn from the patient with the "chief complaint," which is often typed on the patient's admission sheet. Often you learn much more. Ask a patient why he or she is seeking health care; for example, "Tell me, Mr. Lynn, what brought you to the clinic today?" You record the patient's response in quotations to indicate the subjective response. The patient's statement is not diagnostic; instead it is his or her perception of reasons for seeking health care. Clarification of the patient's perception identifies potential needs for symptom management, education, counseling, or referral to community resources.

Patient Expectations. The assessment of patient expectations is not the same as the reason for seeking medical care, although they are often related. It is important to assess the patient's understanding of why he or she is seeking health care. Failure to identify a patient's expectations of health care providers results in poor patient satisfaction. Patient satisfaction is a standard measure of quality for all hospitals throughout the country (see Chapter 2). Patients typically have expectations of receiving information about their treatments and prognosis and a plan of care for returning home. In addition, patients expect relief of pain and other symptoms and caring expressed by health care providers. During the initial interview a patient expresses expectations when entering the health care setting. Later, as the patient interacts with health care providers, it is valuable to assess whether these expectations have changed or been met.

Present Illness or Health Concerns. If a patient presents with an illness, collect essential and relevant data about

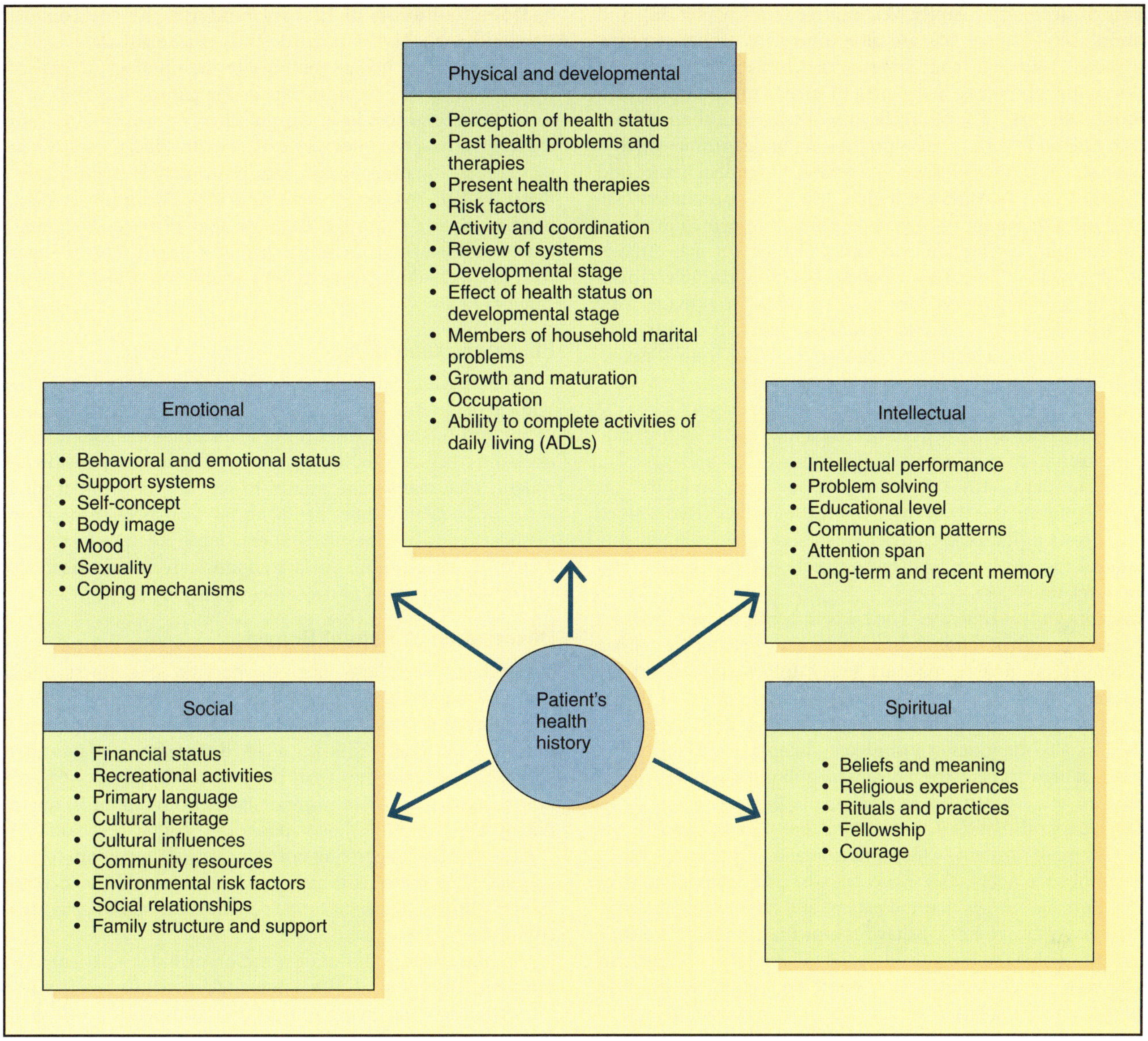

FIG. 16-5 Dimensions for gathering data for a health history.

the symptoms and their effects on the patient's health. Apply the critical thinking intellectual standards of complete and deep (see Box 15-3 on p. 199) by assessing these factors:

- Location—Where is the symptom located?
- Onset and duration—When did it start? How long has it lasted?
- Precipitating factors—What makes symptoms worse? Are there activities (e.g., exercise) that affect the symptoms?
- Relieving factors—What does the patient do to become more comfortable or relieve the symptoms?
- Quality—Have the patient describe what the symptom feels like.
- Severity—Have the patient rate the severity on a scale of 0 to 10. This gives you a baseline with which to compare in follow-up assessments.
- **Concomitant symptoms**—Does the patient experience other symptoms along with the primary symptom? For example, does nausea accompany pain?

Health History. The information in a patient's health history provides data on the patient's health care experiences and current health habits (see Fig. 16-5). Assess whether the patient has ever been hospitalized, injured, or had surgery. Include a complete medication history (including herbal and over-the-counter drugs). Also essential are descriptions of allergies, including allergic reactions to food, latex, drugs, or contact agents (e.g., soap). Asking patients if they have had problems with medications or food helps to clarify the type and amount of agent, the specific reaction, and whether the patient has required treatment. If the patient has an allergy, note the specific reaction and treatment on the assessment form.

The history also includes a description of the patient's habits and lifestyle patterns. Assessing for the use of alcohol, tobacco, caffeine, or recreational drugs (e.g., methamphetamine or cocaine) determines the patient's risk for diseases involving the liver, lungs, heart, or nervous system. Noting the type of habit and the frequency and duration of use provides essential data. Assessing patterns of sleep (see Chapter 42), exercise (see Chapter 38), and nutrition (see Chapter 44) are also important when planning nursing care. Ultimately your aim is to match the patient's lifestyle patterns with approaches in the plan of care as much as possible.

Family History. The family history obtains data about immediate and blood relatives. The objectives are to determine whether the patient is at risk for illnesses of a genetic or familial nature and to identify areas of health promotion and illness prevention (see Chapter 6). The family history also provides information about family structure, interaction, support, and function that often is useful in planning care (see Chapter 10). For example, Tonya assesses the level of support Mrs. Jacobs is willing to provide. Mrs. Jacobs tells Tonya that the two have been married 32 years and states, "I feel I can do whatever is needed for him." Tonya's assessment shows a pattern that Mrs. Jacob is supportive and able to help her husband adjust to any initial limitations in activity when he returns home. Her assessment ultimately allows her to incorporate Mrs. Jacobs into the patient teaching portion of the patient's plan of care (see Chapter 18). If a patient's family is not supportive, it is better to not involve them in care. Stressful family relationships are sometimes a significant barrier when you try to help patients with problems involving loss, self-concept, spiritual health, and personal relationships.

Environmental History. The environmental history provides data about a patient's home and working environments with a focus on determining the patient's safety. Information about the home environment includes function of utilities, layout of rooms in the house, and the presence of any barriers or risks for injury. The history also identifies exposure to pollutants in the workplace, existence of high crime in the patient's neighborhood, and available resources that assist patients in returning to the community.

Psychosocial History. A psychosocial history reveals the patient's support system, which often includes spouse, children, other family members, and close friends. The history includes information about ways that the patient and family typically cope with stress (see Chapter 37). Behaviors patients use at home to cope with stress, such as walking, reading, or talking with a friend, can also be used as nursing interventions if the patient experiences stress while receiving health care. In addition, you need to learn if the patient has experienced any recent losses that create a sense of grief (see Chapter 36).

Spiritual Health. Life experiences and events shape a person's spirituality. The spiritual dimension represents the totality of one's being and is difficult to assess quickly (see Chapter 35). Review with patients their beliefs about life, their source for guidance in acting on beliefs, and the relationship they have with family in exercising their faith. Also assess rituals and religious practices that patients use to express their spirituality.

Review of Systems. The review of systems (ROS) is a systematic approach for collecting the patient's self-reported data on all body systems (see Chapter 30). You probably will not cover all of the questions in each system every time you collect a history. Nevertheless, always include some questions about each system in the nursing history, but pay close attention when a patient mentions an unexpected sign or symptom. In this case explore the system more in depth. The systems you assess depend on the patient's condition and the urgency in starting care. During the ROS ask the patient about the normal functioning of each body system and any noted changes. Such changes are subjective data because they are described as perceived by the patient. Findings from the ROS are later confirmed during the physical examination.

Documentation of History Findings. As you conduct the nursing health history, record your assessment data in a clear, concise manner using appropriate terminology. Standardized forms make it easy to enter data as the patient responds to questions. In settings that have computerized documentation, entry of assessment data becomes very easy. A clear, concise record is necessary for use by other health care professionals (see Chapter 26). Regardless of the model used in a documentation system, you need to have a thorough database that provides historical and current information about the patient's health. This information then becomes the baseline against which you evaluate any future changes.

Physical Examination

A physical examination (see Chapter 30) is an investigation of the body to determine its state of health. The examination involves use of the techniques of inspection, palpation, percussion, auscultation, and smell. A complete examination includes a patient's height, weight, vital signs, and a head-to-toe examination of all body systems. The data from a hands-on physical assessment allow you to collect valuable objective information needed to form accurate diagnostic conclusions. Always conduct an examination competently with a caring and culturally sensitive approach.

Observation of Patient Behavior

Throughout a patient-centered interview and physical examination it is important for you to closely observe a patient's verbal and nonverbal behaviors. The information adds depth to your objective database. You learn to determine if data obtained by observation matches what the patient communicates verbally. For example, if a patient expresses no concern about an upcoming diagnostic test but shows poor eye contact, shakiness, and restlessness, all suggesting anxiety, verbal and nonverbal data conflict. Observations direct you to gather additional objective information to form accurate conclusions about the patient's condition.

An important aspect of observation includes a patient's level of function: the physical, developmental, psychological, and social aspects of everyday living. Observation of level of function differs from observation you make during an interview. Observation of level of function involves watching what a patient does such as eating or making a decision about preparing a medication rather than what the patient tells you he or she can do. Observation of function often occurs in the home or in a health care setting during a return demonstration.

Diagnostic and Laboratory Data

The results of diagnostic and laboratory tests provide further explanation of alterations or problems identified during the nursing health history and physical examination. For example, during the history the patient reports having a bad cold for 6 days and at present has a productive cough with brown sputum and mild shortness of breath. On physical examination you notice an elevated temperature, increased respirations, and decreased breath sounds in the right lower lobe. You review the results of a complete blood count and note that the white blood cell count is elevated (indicating an infection). You report your results to the patient's health care provider, who orders a chest x-ray film. When the results of the x-ray film show the presence of a right lower lobe infiltrate, the health care provider makes the medical diagnosis of pneumonia. Your assessment leads to the associated nursing diagnosis of *impaired gas exchange.*

Some patients collect and monitor laboratory data in the home. For example, patients with diabetes mellitus often measure blood glucose daily. Ask patients about their routine results to determine their response to illness and information about the effects of treatment measures. Compare laboratory data with the established norms for a particular test, age-group, and gender.

Interpreting and Validating Assessment Data

Whichever clinical situation you face, assessment involves the continuous interpretation of information. This is one critical thinking aspect of assessment. The successful interpretation and validation of assessment data ensure that you have collected a complete database for your patient. Ultimately this leads you to the second step of the nursing process, in which you make clinical decisions in your patient's care. These decisions are either in the form of nursing diagnoses or collaborative problems that require treatment from several disciplines (Carpenito-Moyet, 2009) (see Chapter 17).

Interpretation. When interpreting assessment information critically, you determine the presence of abnormal findings, recognize that further observations are needed to clarify information, and begin to identify the patient's health problems. As you form a database, you begin to see patterns of data that direct you to collect more information and clarify what you have. The patterns of data reveal meaningful and usable clusters. A data cluster is a set of signs or symptoms that you group together in a logical way (Box 16-4). The clusters begin to clearly identify the patient's health problems.

Data Validation. Before you complete data interpretation, validate the collected information you have to avoid making incorrect inferences. **Validation** of assessment data is the comparison of data with another source to determine data accuracy. For example, you observe a patient crying and logically infer that it is related to hospitalization or a medical diagnosis. Making such an initial inference is not wrong, but problems result if you do not validate the inference with the patient. Instead ask, "I notice that you have been crying. Can you tell me about it?" By validating you discover the real reason for the patient's crying behavior. Ask patients to validate unclear information obtained during an interview and history. Validate findings from the physical examination and observation of patient behavior by comparing data in the medical record and consulting with other nurses or health care team members. Often family or friends can validate your assessment information.

Validation opens the door for gathering more assessment data because it involves clarifying vague or unclear data. Occasionally you need to reassess previously covered areas of the nursing history or gather further physical examination data. Continually analyze and think about a patient's database to make concise, accurate, and meaningful interpretations. Critical thinking applied to assessment enables you to fully understand the patient's problems, judge the extent of the problems carefully, and discover possible relationships between the problems.

Tonya gathered initial data about the character of Mr. Jacob's incisional pain. She applied critical thinking in her assessment as she considered what she knew about a prostatectomy and the anticipated postoperative problems that can develop. As she assessed Mr. Jacobs, she applied intellectual standards, being precise (location of pain), consistent and accurate (use of pain-rating scale), and complete (probing for factors that worsen pain). However, Mr. Jacobs was also having trouble resting, showed irritability at times when questioned, and had poor eye contact when speaking. Tonya saw the need for more information. She directed her assessment to learn more about Mr. Jacob's concerns about the success of his surgery and what to expect during recovery. Tonya asks, "Mr. Jacobs, you earlier said that you hoped they got all of the cancer. You seem uneasy. Can you tell me how you feel about your surgery?" Mr. Jacobs tells Tonya, "My friend had prostate cancer. He had surgery, but it came back. He had a long fight." Tonya could make several inferences from this information, but she applies the critical thinking attitude of discipline and stays focused to ensure that her assessment is accurate and comprehensive. She validates her inferences with Mr. Jacobs, "You sound anxious about the outcome of your surgery. Your friend had a recurrence of his cancer. Are you uncertain about what to expect?" Mr. Jacobs validates Tonya's assessment, "Yes, I'm worried. My friend and family members have died from cancer. My wife depends on me; well, we depend on one another. I'm a person who likes to have information so I can make the right decisions and know what to do." Tonya now has more complete information to help her identify Mr. Jacob's health problems and make correct diagnostic conclusions.

BOX 16-4 RECOGNIZING DATA CLUSTERS

Interpret how data form patterns or trends.

- Patient uncomfortable: remains still in bed
  - Limits turning
  - Grimaces when moving
- Mobility limited: limits turning
  - Only out of bed once after surgery
- Knowledge about surgery: asks questions about pain control
  - Unsure about dressing care
  - Asks about risk of infection
- Appears anxious or uneasy: poor eye contact at times
  - Restless
  - Asks numerous questions

Data Documentation

Data documentation is the last part of a complete assessment. The timely, thorough, and accurate documentation of facts is required in recording patient data. If you do not record an assessment finding or problem interpretation, it is lost and unavailable to anyone else caring for the patient. If information is not specific, the reader is left with only general impressions. Observing and recording patient status are legal and professional responsibilities. The Nurse Practice Acts in all states and the American Nurses Association *Nursing's Social Policy Statement* (2010) require accurate data collection and recording as independent functions essential to the role of the professional nurse.

Being factual is easy after it becomes a habit. The basic rule is to record all observations succinctly. When recording data, pay attention to facts and be as descriptive as possible. Anything heard, seen, felt, or smelled should be reported exactly. Record objective information in accurate terminology (e.g., weighs 170 kg, abdomen is soft and nontender to palpation). Record subjective information from a patient in quotation marks. When entering data, do not generalize or form judgments through written communication. Conclusions about such data become nursing diagnoses and thus must be factual and accurate. As you gain experience and become familiar with clusters and patterns of signs and symptoms, you correctly conclude the existence of a problem. Review Chapter 26 for details on documentation.

Concept Mapping

Most of the patients for whom you care present with more than one health problem. A concept map is a visual representation that allows you to graphically show the connections between a patient's many health problems. Hinck et al. (2006) showed that concept mapping is an effective learning strategy to understand the relationships that exist among patient problems (Box 16-5). Concept maps help students evaluate their thinking patterns and see the reasons for nursing care (Taylor and Wros, 2007). Your first step in concept mapping is to organize the assessment data you collect for your patient. Placing all of the cues together into the clusters that form patterns leads you to the next step of the nursing process, nursing diagnosis (see Chapter 17). Through concept mapping you obtain a holistic perspective of your patient's health care needs, which ultimately leads you to making better clinical decisions. Fig. 16-6 shows the first step in a concept map that Tonya will develop for Mr. Jacobs as a result of her nursing assessment. Tonya begins to identify patterns reflecting the problems Mr. Jacobs faces. As a result of the assessment she has noted: a mobility restriction, discomfort over incision, need for instruction about surgical postoperative care, and the patient's concern over effects that surgery will have on relationship with wife. The next step (see Chapter 17) is to identify specific nursing diagnoses so appropriate nursing interventions can be provided.

BOX 16-5 EVIDENCE-BASED PRACTICE

Using Concept Maps as a Learning Strategy

PICO Question: Is a concept map an effective strategy for nurses and nursing students to use to identify nursing concepts (nursing diagnoses)?

Evidence Summary

Concept mapping is a learning strategy used to help nursing students and staff nurses understand key nursing concepts (such as nursing diagnoses and clinical problems) and the relationship among those concepts. For example, a learner is able to view various aspects of a patient's health problems and the cause-and-effect associations to enhance critical thinking. Studies have tested the effectiveness of concept mapping on the learning of nursing students and staff nurses. Research also has investigated satisfaction with the strategy. Results show that concept mapping significantly improves students' and nurses' abilities to see patterns and relationships in concepts to plan and evaluate nursing care. Maps are effective in helping nurses learn components of new clinical protocols. Evaluation also reveals positive student and staff satisfaction (Hinck et al., 2006; Phelps et al., 2009).

Application to Nursing Practice

- A concept map organizes and links information about a patient in unique and meaningful ways.
- The relationships seen among multiple nursing diagnoses or clinical concepts allow nursing students and nurses to plan interventions that are therapeutic for more than one problem area.
- Use of concept maps helps nursing students and nurses reflect and critically think about relationships among clinical information in a way that promotes clinical decision making.

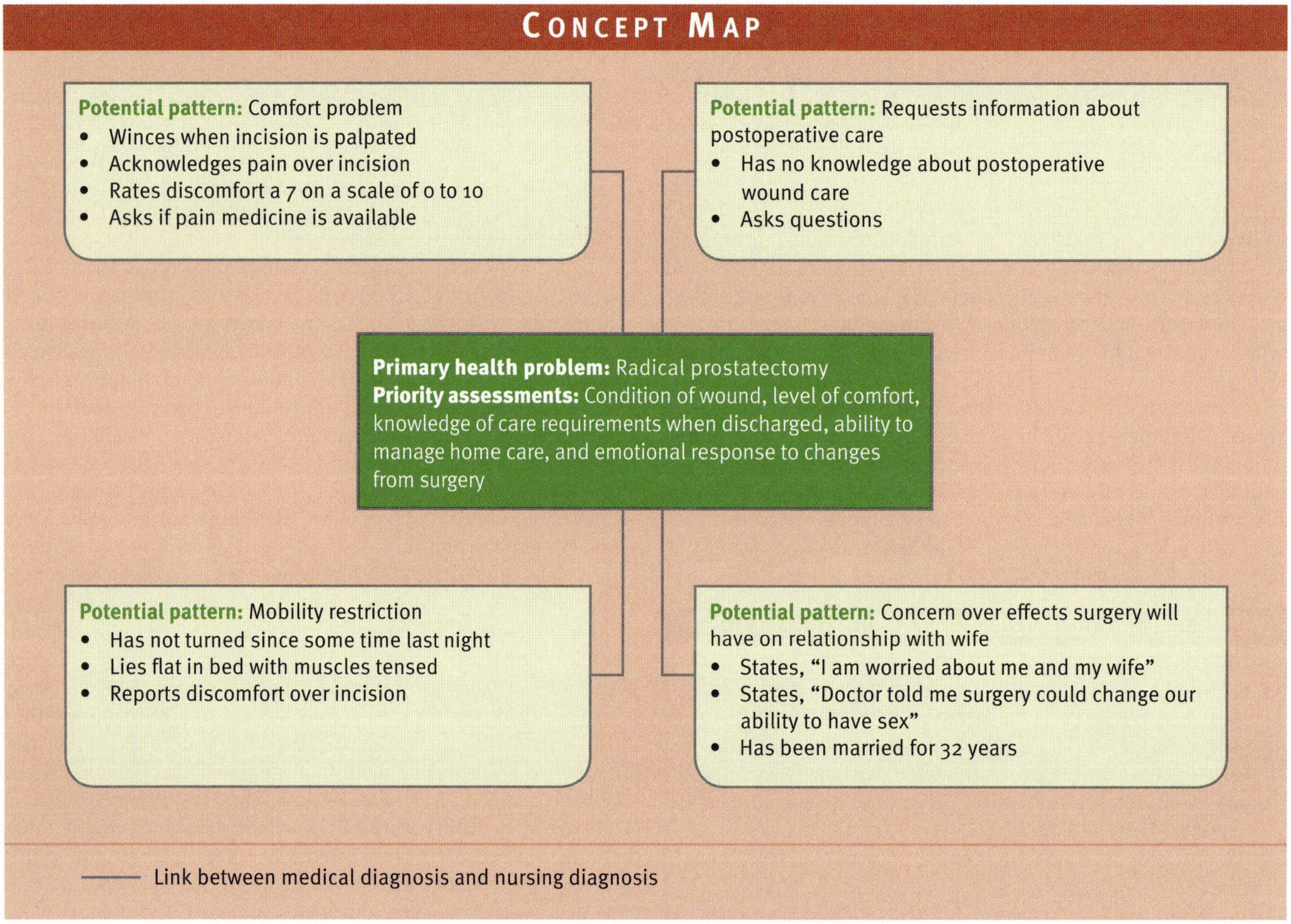
CONCEPT MAP
Potential pattern: Comfort problem
• Winces when incision is palpated
• Acknowledges pain over incision
• Rates discomfort a 7 on a scale of 0 to 10
• Asks if pain medicine is available
Potential pattern: Requests information about postoperative care
• Has no knowledge about postoperative wound care
• Asks questions
Primary health problem: Radical prostatectomy
Priority assessments: Condition of wound, level of comfort, knowledge of care requirements when discharged, ability to manage home care, and emotional response to changes from surgery
Potential pattern: Mobility restriction
• Has not turned since some time last night
• Lies flat in bed with muscles tensed
• Reports discomfort over incision
Potential pattern: Concern over effects surgery will have on relationship with wife
• States, "I am worried about me and my wife"
• States, "Doctor told me surgery could change our ability to have sex"
• Has been married for 32 years
Link between medical diagnosis and nursing diagnosis

FIG. 16-6 Concept map for Mr. Jacobs: Assessment.

KEY POINTS

- The nursing process is a variation of scientific reasoning that involves five steps: assessment, nursing diagnosis, planning, implementation, and evaluation.
- Assessment involves collecting information from the patient and secondary sources (e.g., family members) along with interpreting and validating the information to form a complete database.
- There are two approaches to gathering a comprehensive assessment: use of a structured database format and use of a problem-focused approach.
- Once a patient provides subjective data, explore the findings further by collecting objective data.
- During assessment critically anticipate and use an appropriate branching set of questions or observations to collect data and cluster cues of assessment information to identify emerging patterns and problems.
- In a patient-centered interview an organized conversation with the patient allows the patient to set the initial focus and initiate discussion about his or her health problems.
- A successful interview requires preparation, including reviewing all available information about the patient, preparing the interview environment, and timing to avoid interruptions.
- An initial patient-centered interview involves: (1) setting the stage, (2) gathering information about the patient's problems and setting an agenda, (3) collecting the assessment or a nursing health history, and (4) terminating the interview.
- The best clinical interview focuses on the patient, not your own agenda.
- During an assessment interview encourage patients to tell their stories about their illnesses or health care problems.
- It is easier to explore cultural differences if you allow time for thoughtful answers and ask your questions in a comfortable order.
- When collecting a complete nursing history, let the patient's story guide you in fully exploring the components related to his or her problems.
- Successful interpretation and validation of assessment data ensure that you have collected a complete database.

CRITICAL THINKING EXERCISES

Preparing for Clinical Practice

Tonya is planning to return to Mr. Jacob's room and spend more time discussing his concerns about going home and what to expect. She knows that Mrs. Jacobs usually comes in to visit around 11 AM, just before lunchtime. Tonya believes that Mrs. Jacobs will be an important source of support in providing Mr. Jacobs any ongoing home care. The surgeon has ordered home health for Mr. Jacobs since he is going home with an indwelling catheter. Tonya's assessment will be shared with the home health agency.

1. Tonya goes to Mr. Jacob's room and asks if it is okay to include Mrs. Jacobs in the discussion about his postoperative care. Explain why Tonya has asked for Mr. Jacob's consent.
2. Tonya and Mr. Jacobs have the following interaction:
   Tonya: Mr. Jacobs, I want to know what you understand about your urinary catheter.
   Mr. Jacobs: I think it helps me to pass urine until I heal.
   Tonya: Uh huh … go on.
   Mr. Jacobs: I think the doctor said it would still be in when I go home.
   Tonya's phrase "uh huh … go on" is an example of what interviewing technique? Explain why it is useful.
3. While in Mr. Jacob's room, Tonya discusses his knowledge about surgery and performs a routine assessment of his current condition. Tonya has collected information from her assessment of Mr. Jacobs. Identify each of the items in the assessment list as either subjective or objective data.
   1. Urine output for last 4 hours is 240 mL.
   2. Mr. Jacobs rates pain severity at a level 3.
   3. Incision is 15 cm long and without drainage.
   4. Mr. Jacobs states, "I don't know when I can start to drive when I go home".

evolve *Answers to Clinical Application Questions can be found on the Evolve website.*

REVIEW QUESTIONS

Are You Ready to Test Your Nursing Knowledge?

1. A nurse assesses a patient who comes to the pulmonary clinic. "I see that it's been over 6 months since you've been in, but your appointment was for every 2 months. Tell me about that. Also I see from your last visit that the doctor recommended routine exercise. Can you tell me how successful you have been following his plan?" The nurse's assessment covers which of Gordon's functional health patterns?
   1. Value-belief pattern
   2. Cognitive-perceptual pattern
   3. Coping–stress-tolerance pattern
   4. Health perception–health management pattern
2. The nurse asks a patient, "Describe for me your typical diet over a 24-hour day. What foods do you prefer? Have you noticed a change in your weight recently?" This series of questions would likely occur during which phase of a patient-centered interview?
   1. Setting the stage
   2. Gathering information about the patient's chief concerns
   3. Collecting the assessment
   4. Termination
3. What type of interview techniques does the nurse use when asking these questions, "Do you have pain or cramping?" "Does the pain get worse when you walk?" (Select all that apply.)
   1. Active listening
   2. Open-ended questioning
   3. Closed-ended questioning
   4. Problem-oriented questioning
4. What technique(s) best encourage(s) a patient to tell his or her full story? (Select all that apply.)
   1. Active listening
   2. Back channeling
   3. Validating
   4. Use of open-ended questions
   5. Use of closed-ended questions
5. A nurse gathers the following assessment data. Which of the following cues form(s) a pattern suggesting a problem? (Select all that apply.)
   1. The skin around the wound is tender to touch.
   2. Fluid intake for 8 hours is 800 mL.
   3. Patient has a heart rate of 78 and regular.
   4. Patient has drainage from surgical wound.
   5. Body temperature is 101° F (38.3° C).
   6. Patient asks, "I'm worried that I won't return to work when I planned."

6. The nurse makes the following statement during a change of shift report to another nurse. "I assessed Mr. Diaz, my 61-year-old patient from Chile. He fell at home and hurt his back 3 days ago. He has some difficulty turning in bed, and he says that he has pain that radiates down his leg. He rates his pain at a 6, but I don't think it's that severe. You know that back patients often have chronic pain. He seems fine when talking with his family. Have you cared for him before?" What does the nurse's conclusion suggest?
   1. The nurse is making an accurate clinical inference.
   2. The nurse has gathered cues to identify a potential problem area.
   3. The nurse has allowed stereotyping to influence her assessment.
   4. The nurse wants to validate her information with the other nurse.
7. A nurse checks a patient's intravenous (IV) line in his right arm and sees inflammation where the catheter enters the skin. She uses her finger to apply light pressure (i.e., palpation) just above the IV site. The patient tells her the area is tender. The nurse checks to see if the IV line is running at the correct rate. This is an example of what type of assessment?
   1. Agenda setting
   2. Problem-focused
   3. Objective
   4. Use of a structured database format
8. A patient who visits the allergy clinic tells the nurse practitioner that he is not getting relief from shortness of breath when he uses his inhaler. The nurse decides to ask the patient to explain how he uses the inhaler, when he should take a dose of medication, and what he does when he gets no relief. On the basis of Gordon's functional health patterns, which pattern does the nurse assess?
   1. Health perception–health management pattern
   2. Value-belief pattern
   3. Cognitive-perceptual pattern
   4. Coping–stress tolerance pattern
9. A nurse is conducting a patient-centered interview. Place the statements from the interview in the correct order.
   1. "You say you've lost weight. Tell me how much weight you have lost in the last month."
   2. "My name is Todd. I'll be the nurse taking care of you today. I'm going to ask you a series of questions to gather your health history."
   3. "I have no further questions. Thank you for your patience."
   4. "Tell me what brought you to the hospital."
   5. "So, to summarize, you've lost about 6 pounds in the last month, and your appetite has been poor—correct?"
10. Which of the following are examples of data validation? (Select all that apply.)
   1. The nurse assesses the patient's heart rate and compares the value with the last value entered in the medical record.
   2. The nurse asks the patient if he is having pain and then asks the patient to rate the severity.
   3. The nurse observes a patient reading a teaching booklet and asks the patient if he has questions about its content.
   4. The nurse obtains a blood pressure value that is abnormal and asks the charge nurse to repeat the measurement.
   5. The nurse asks the patient to describe a symptom by saying, "Go on."
11. A patient tells the nurse during a visit to the clinic that he has been sick to his stomach for 3 days and he vomited twice yesterday. Which of the following responses by the nurse is an example of probing?
   1. So you've had an upset stomach and began vomiting—correct?
   2. Have you taken anything for your stomach?
   3. Is anything else bothering you?
   4. Have you taken any medication for your vomiting?
12. The nurse is assessing the character of a patient's migraine headache and asks, "Do you feel nauseated when you have a headache?" The patient's response is "yes." In this case the finding of nausea is which of the following?
   1. An objective finding
   2. A clinical inference
   3. A validation
   4. A concomitant symptom
13. During the review of systems in a nursing history, a nurse learns that the patient has been coughing mucus. Which of the following nursing assessments would be best for the nurse to use to confirm a lung problem? (Select all that apply.)
   1. Family report
   2. Chest x-ray film
   3. Physical examination with auscultation of the lungs
   4. Medical record summary of x-ray film findings
14. A nurse working on a medicine nursing unit is assigned to a 78-year-old patient who just entered the hospital with symptoms of H1N1 flu. The nurse finds the patient to be short of breath with an increased respiratory rate of 30 breaths/min. He lost his wife just a month ago. The nurse's knowledge about this patient results in which of the following assessment approaches at this time? (Select all that apply.)
   1. A problem-focused approach
   2. A structured comprehensive approach
   3. Using multiple visits to gather a complete database
   4. Focusing on the functional health pattern of role-relationship
15. A 58-year-old patient with nerve deafness has come to his doctor's office for a routine examination. The patient wears two hearing aids. The advanced practice nurse who is conducting the assessment uses which of the following approaches while conducting the interview with this patient? (Select all that apply.)
   1. Maintain a neutral facial expression
   2. Lean forward when interacting with the patient
   3. Acknowledge the patient's answers through head nodding
   4. Limit direct eye contact

Answers: **1.** 4; **2.** 3; **3.** 3, 4; **4.** 1, 2, 4; **5.** 1, 4, 5; **6.** 3; **7.** 2; **8.** 1; **9.** 2, 4, 1, 5, 3; **10.** 1, 4; **11.** 3; **12.** 4; **13.** 3, 4; **14.** 1, 3; **15.** 2, 3.

REFERENCES

American Nurses Association: *Nursing's social policy statement: the essence of the profession*, ed 3, Washington, DC, 2010, The Association.

Austin S: Seven legal tips for safe nursing practice, *Nursing* 38(3):34, 2008.

Carpenito-Moyet LJ: *Nursing diagnosis: application to clinical practice*, ed 13, Philadelphia, 2009, Lippincott, Williams & Wilkins.

Dontje J, et al: A unique set of interactions: The MSU sustained partnership model of nurse practitioner primary care, *J Am Academy Nurs Pract* 16(2):63, 2004.

Gordon M: *Nursing diagnosis: process and application*, ed 3, St Louis, 1994, Mosby.

Lein C, Wills CE: Using patient-centered interviewing skills to manage complex patient encounters in primary care, *J Am Academy Nurs Pract* 19(5):215, 2007.

Lunney M: Helping nurses use NANDA, NOC, and NIC: novice to expert, *J Nurs Admin* 36(3):118, 2006.

Magnan MA, Maklebust J: The nursing process and pressure ulcer prevention: making the connection, *Adv Skin Wound Care* 22:83, 2009.

Seidel HM, et al: *Mosby's guide to physical examination*, ed 7, St Louis, 2011, Mosby.

Swartz MH: *Textbook of physical diagnosis*, ed 6, Philadelphia, 2010, Saunders.

Taylor J, Wros P: Concept mapping: a nursing model for care planning, *J Nurs Ed* 46(5):211, 2007.

U.S. Department of Health and Human Services: Summary of the HIPAA privacy rule, 2003, http://www.hhs.gov/ocr/privacy/hipaa/understanding/summary/privacysummary.pdf. Accessed January 17, 2012.

RESEARCH REFERENCES

Chaboyer W, McMurray A, Wallis M: Bedside nursing handover: a case study, *Int J Nurs Pract* 16(1):27, 2010.

Hinck SM, et al: Student learning with concept mapping of care plans in community-based education, *J Prof Nurs* 22(1):23, 2006.

Phelps SE, et al: Staff development story: concept mapping: a staff development strategy for enhancing oncology critical thinking, *J Nurses Staff Dev* 25(1):42, 2009.

Potter P, et al: Understanding the cognitive work of nursing in the acute care environment, *J Nurs Admin* 35(7/8):327, 2005.

Smith RC, et al: Primary care clinicians treat patients with medically unexplained symptoms: a randomized controlled trial, *J Gen Intern Med* 21:671, 2006.

CHAPTER

17

Nursing Diagnosis

OBJECTIVES

- Discuss the purposes of using nursing diagnosis in practice.
- Differentiate among a nursing diagnosis, medical diagnosis, and collaborative problem.
- Discuss the relationship of critical thinking to the nursing diagnostic process.
- Describe the steps of the nursing diagnostic process.
- Explain how defining characteristics and the etiological process individualize a nursing diagnosis.
- Describe sources of diagnostic errors.
- Identify nursing diagnoses from a nursing assessment.

KEY TERMS

evolve WEBSITE

http://evolve.elsevier.com/Potter/fundamentals/

- Review Questions
- Concept Map Creator
- Case Study with Questions
- Audio Glossary
- Interactive Learning Activities
- Key Term Flashcards
- Content Updates

During the nursing assessment process (see Chapter 16) a nurse gathers the information needed to make diagnostic conclusions about patient care. A diagnosis is a clinical judgment based on information. You review information collected about a patient, see cues and patterns in the data, and identify the patient's specific health care problems. Some of the conclusions lead to identifying nursing diagnoses, whereas others do not. Diagnostic conclusions include problems treated primarily by nurses (nursing diagnoses) and those requiring treatment by several disciplines (collaborative problems). Together nursing diagnoses and collaborative problems represent the range of patient conditions that require nursing care (Carpenito-Moyet, 2009).

When physicians refer to commonly accepted medical diagnoses such as diabetes mellitus or osteoarthritis, they all know the meaning of the diagnoses and the standard approaches for treatment. A **medical diagnosis** is the identification of a disease condition based on a specific evaluation of physical signs, symptoms, the patient's medical history and the results of diagnostic tests and procedures. Physicians are licensed to treat diseases and conditions described in medical diagnostic statements.

Nursing has a similar diagnostic language. Nursing diagnosis, the second step of the nursing process (Fig. 17-1), classifies health problems within the domain of nursing. A **nursing diagnosis** such as *acute pain* or *nausea* is a clinical judgment about individual, family, or community responses to actual and potential health problems or life processes that the nurse is licensed and competent to treat (NANDA International, 2012). What makes the nursing diagnostic process unique is having patients involved, when possible, in the process.

A **collaborative problem** is an actual or potential physiological complication that nurses monitor to detect the onset of changes in a patient's status (Carpenito-Moyet, 2009). When collaborative problems develop, nurses intervene in collaboration with personnel from other health care disciplines. Nurses manage collaborative problems such as hemorrhage, infection, and paralysis using medical, nursing, and allied health (e.g., physical therapy) interventions. For example, a patient with a surgical wound is at risk for developing an infection; thus a physician prescribes antibiotics. The nurse monitors the patient for fever and other signs of infection and implements appropriate wound care measures. A dietitian recommends a therapeutic diet high in protein and nutrients to promote wound healing.

Selecting the correct nursing diagnosis on the basis of an assessment involves diagnostic expertise (i.e., being able to make quick and accurate conclusions from patient data) (Cho, Staggers, and Park, 2010). This is essential because accurate diagnosis of patient problems ensures that you select more effective and efficient nursing interventions. Diagnostic expertise improves with time. Consider the case study involving Mr. Jacobs and his nurse, Tonya Moore.

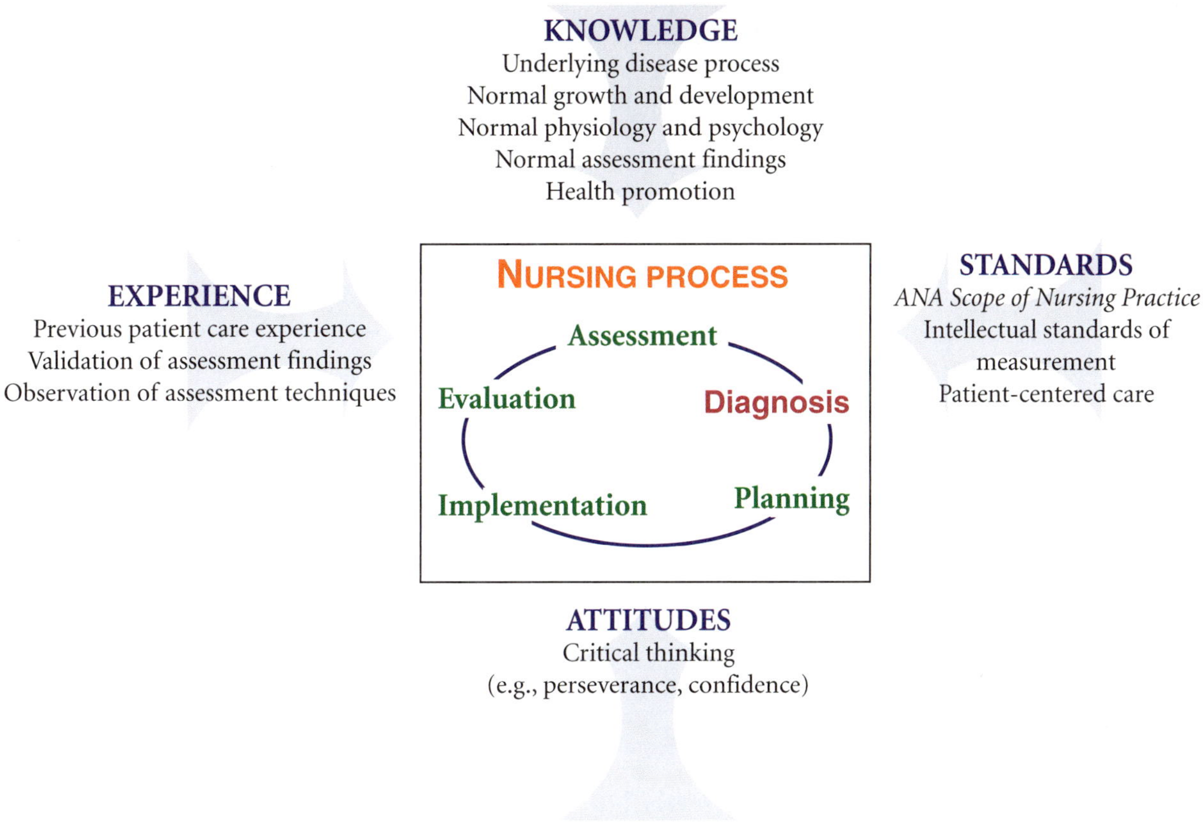

FIG. 17-1 Critical thinking and the nursing diagnostic process.

During her assessment Tonya gathers information suggesting that Mr. Jacobs possibly has a number of health problems. The data about Mr. Jacobs show patterns in four areas: comfort, requesting information about postoperative care, mobility restriction, and worries about his future and his relationship with Mrs. Jacobs. Selecting specific diagnostic labels for these problem areas allows Tonya to develop a relevant and appropriate plan of care. For example, with respect to Mr. Jacobs' request for information, there are two accepted nursing diagnostic labels for problems related to knowledge: ***deficient knowledge*** *and* ***readiness for enhanced knowledge.*** *Knowing the difference between these two diagnoses and identifying which one applies to Mr. Jacobs is key to selecting the right type of interventions for his problem. A physician needs to rule out rheumatoid arthritis versus osteoarthritis to be sure that a patient receives the right form of medical treatment. Tonya analyzes her information about Mr. Jacobs and identifies the factors that show the pattern that fits a specific diagnosis. This means that Tonya considers that the patient has no knowledge about or experience with postoperative wound care and freely asks questions. Tonya knows that these factors are defining characteristics that allow her to make an accurate nursing diagnosis.*

HISTORY OF NURSING DIAGNOSIS

Nursing diagnosis was first introduced in the nursing literature in 1950 (McFarland and McFarlane, 1989). Fry (1953) proposed the formulation of nursing diagnoses and an individualized nursing care plan to make nursing more creative. This emphasized the nurse's independent practice (e.g., patient education and symptom relief) compared with the dependent practice driven by physicians' orders (e.g., medication administration and intravenous fluids). Initially professional nursing did not support nursing diagnoses. The *Model Nurse Practice Act* of the American Nurses Association (ANA) (1955) excluded diagnosis or prescriptive therapies. As a result, few nurses used nursing diagnoses in their practice.

When Yura and Walsh (1967) developed the theory of the nursing process, it included four parts: assessment, planning, implementation, and evaluation. However, nurse leaders soon recognized that assessment data needed to be clustered into patterns and interpreted before nurses could complete the remaining steps of the process (NANDA International, 2012). You cannot plan and then intervene correctly if you do not know the problems with which you are dealing. In 1973 the first national conference to identify the interpretations of data that represent the health conditions that are of a concern to nursing was held. The first conference on nursing diagnosis identified and defined 80 nursing diagnoses (Gebbie, 1998). The list continues to grow on the basis of nursing research and the work of members of the North American Nursing Diagnosis Association International (NANDA-I) (NANDA International, 2012).

With use of the term *nursing diagnosis,* nurses make diagnostic conclusions and therefore the clinical decisions necessary for safe and effective nursing practice. The ANA's paper *Scope of Nursing Practice* (1987), which defined nursing as the diagnosis and treatment of human responses to health and illness, helped strengthen

BOX 17-1 EVIDENCE-BASED PRACTICE

Nursing Diagnosis Impact on Nursing Practice

PICO Question: Has the use of nursing diagnosis by nurses improved outcomes in nursing practice?

Evidence Summary

A total of 36 articles from the nursing literature were reviewed to identify the outcomes of nursing diagnosis (Muller-Staub et al., 2006). The articles included reports on the effects of nursing diagnosis on documentation of assessment, frequency, and accuracy of nursing diagnosis in practice and coherence between nursing diagnoses and selected interventions and outcomes. This systematic review found that the use of nursing diagnosis improved the quality of documented patient assessments in 14 of the studies. Coherence among nursing diagnosis and interventions improved in 8 of the studies. A total of 10 studies reported that nursing diagnosis improved identification of commonly occurring diagnoses in similar practice settings. Results varied since a total of 8 studies found no evidence that standardized electronic documentation of nursing diagnosis led to better nursing outcomes. Overall the trend shows that use of nursing diagnosis has favorable effects in nursing practice.

Application to Nursing Practice

- Develop a familiarity with agency documentation systems and the use of nursing diagnosis.
- Use of nursing diagnosis offers an approach to ensure more comprehensive nursing assessment.
- Use of nursing diagnosis can improve selection of nursing interventions by all nurses in a practice setting.

the definition of nursing diagnosis. In 1980 and 1995 the ANA included diagnosis as a separate activity in its publication *Nursing: a Social Policy Statement* (ANA, 2003). It continues today in the ANA's most recent policy statement (ANA, 2010). As a result, most state Nurse Practice Acts include nursing diagnosis as part of the domain of nursing practice.

Research in the field of nursing diagnosis continues to grow (Box 17-1). As a result, NANDA-I continually develops and adds new diagnostic labels to the NANDA International listing (Box 17-2). The use of standard formal nursing diagnostic statements serves several purposes in nursing practice:

- Provides a precise definition of a patient's problem that gives nurses and other members of the health care team a common language for understanding the patient's needs
- Allows nurses to communicate (e.g., written and electronic) what they do among themselves with other health care professionals and the public
- Distinguishes the nurse's role from that of the physician or other health care provider
- Helps nurses focus on the scope of nursing practice
- Fosters the development of nursing knowledge
- Promotes creation of practice guidelines that reflect the essence of nursing

CRITICAL THINKING AND THE NURSING DIAGNOSTIC PROCESS

The diagnostic process requires you to use critical thinking (see Chapter 15). In the practice of nursing it is important for you to know nursing diagnoses, their definitions and the defining characteristics for making diagnoses, related factors pertinent to the diagnoses, and the interventions suited for treating the diagnoses (NANDA International, 2012). This means that you need to know how to access this information easily within the agency in which you work because the information is much too extensive for you to memorize. Sources of information about nursing diagnoses include faculty, advanced practice nurses, documentation systems, and in some settings practice guidelines or protocols. Experience also plays a role in becoming adept at nursing diagnosis. Learn from the patients for whom you care because this helps you think more carefully about your assessment information and what it means. The application of critical thinking attitudes and standards helps you to be thorough, comprehensive, and accurate when identifying nursing diagnoses that apply to your patients.

The diagnostic reasoning process involves using the assessment data you gather about a patient to logically explain a clinical judgment, in this case a nursing diagnosis. The diagnostic process flows from the assessment process and includes decision-making steps (Fig. 17-2). These steps include data clustering, identifying patient health problems, and formulating the diagnosis.

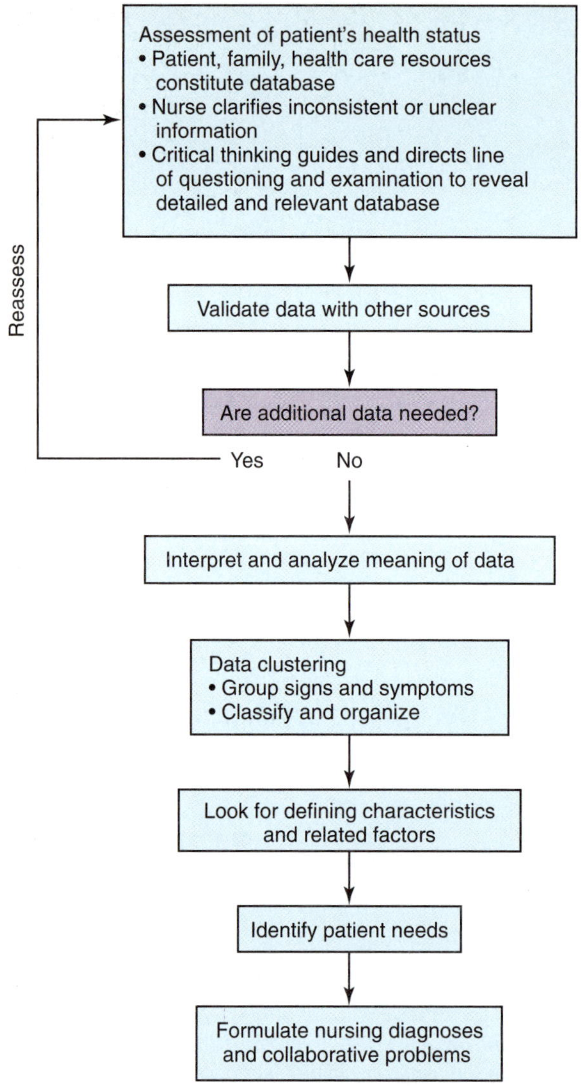

FIG. 17-2 Nursing diagnostic process.

BOX 17-2 NANDA INTERNATIONAL NURSING DIAGNOSES

Activity Intolerance
Risk for **Activity** Intolerance
Ineffective **Activity** Planning
Risk for Ineffective **Activity** Planning
Risk for **Adverse Reaction** to Iodinated Contrast Media
Ineffective **Airway** Clearance
Risk for **Allergy** Response
Anxiety
Risk for **Aspiration**
Risk for Impaired **Attachment**
Autonomic Dysreflexia
Risk for **Autonomic** Dysreflexia
Disorganized Infant **Behavior**
Readiness for Enhanced Organized Infant **Behavior**
Risk for Disorganized Infant **Behavior**
Risk for **Bleeding**
Risk for Unstable **Blood** Glucose Level
Disturbed **Body** Image
Risk for Imbalanced **Body** Temperature
Insufficient **Breast** Milk
Ineffective **Breastfeeding**
Interrupted **Breastfeeding**
Readiness for Enhanced **Breastfeeding**
Ineffective **Breathing** Pattern
Decreased **Cardiac** Output
Caregiver Role Strain
Risk for **Caregiver** Role Strain
Ineffective **Childbearing** Process
Readiness for Enhanced **Childbearing** Process
Risk for Ineffective **Childbearing** Process
Impaired **Comfort**
Readiness for Enhanced **Comfort**
Readiness for Enhanced **Communication**
Impaired **Verbal** Communication
Acute **Confusion**
Chronic **Confusion**
Risk for Acute **Confusion**
Constipation
Perceived **Constipation**
Risk for **Constipation**
Contamination
Risk for **Contamination**
Readiness for Enhanced Community **Coping**
Defensive **Coping**
Ineffective **Coping**
Readiness for Enhanced **Coping**
Ineffective Community **Coping**
Compromised Family **Coping**
Disabled Family **Coping**
Readiness for Enhanced Family **Coping**
Death Anxiety
Risk for Sudden Infant **Death** Syndrome
Decisional Conflict
Readiness for Enhanced **Decision-Making**
Ineffective **Denial**
Impaired **Dentition**
Risk for Delayed **Development**
Diarrhea
Risk for **Disuse** Syndrome
Deficient **Diversional** Activity
Risk for **Dry Eye**
Risk for **Electrolyte** Imbalance
Disturbed **Energy** Field
Impaired **Environmental** Interpretation Syndrome
Adult **Failure** to Thrive
Risk for **Falls**
Dysfunctional **Family** Processes
Interrupted **Family** Processes
Readiness for Enhanced **Family** Processes
Fatigue
Fear
Ineffective Infant **Feeding** Pattern
Readiness for Enhanced **Fluid** Balance
Risk for Imbalanced **Fluid** Volume
Deficient **Fluid** Volume
Excess **Fluid** Volume
Risk for Deficient **Fluid** Volume
Impaired **Gas** Exchange
Risk For Dysfunctional **Gastrointestinal** Motility
Dysfunctional **Gastrointestinal** Motility
Risk for Ineffective **Gastrointestinal** Perfusion
Grieving
Complicated **Grieving**
Risk for Complicated **Grieving**
Risk for Disproportionate **Growth**
Delayed **Growth** and Development
Deficient Community **Health**
Risk-Prone **Health** Behavior
Ineffective **Health** Maintenance
Impaired **Home** Maintenance
Readiness for Enhanced **Hope**
Hopelessness
Risk for Compromised **Human** Dignity
Hyperthermia
Hypothermia
Readiness for Enhanced **Immunization** Status
Ineffective **Impulse** Control
Functional Urinary **Incontinence**
Overflow Urinary **Incontinence**
Reflex Urinary **Incontinence**
Stress Urinary **Incontinence**
Urge Urinary **Incontinence**
Risk for Urge Urinary **Incontinence**
Bowel **Incontinence**
Risk for **Infection**
Risk for **Injury**
Insomnia
Decreased **Intracranial** Adaptive Capacity
Neonatal **Jaundice**
Risk for Neonatal **Jaundice**
Deficient **Knowledge**
Readiness for Enhanced **Knowledge**
Latex Allergy Response
Risk for **Latex** Allergy Response
Sedentary **Lifestyle**
Risk for Impaired **Liver** Function
Risk for **Loneliness**
Risk for Disturbed **Maternal–Fetal** Dyad

Continued

BOX 17-2 NANDA INTERNATIONAL NURSING DIAGNOSES—cont'd

Impaired **Memory**
Impaired Bed **Mobility**
Impaired Physical **Mobility**
Impaired Wheelchair **Mobility**
Moral Distress
Nausea
Unilateral **Neglect**
Noncompliance
Readiness for Enhanced **Nutrition**
Imbalanced **Nutrition**: Less Than Body Requirements
Risk for Imbalanced **Nutrition**: More Than Body Requirements
Imbalanced **Nutrition**: More Than Body Requirements
Impaired **Oral** Mucous Membrane
Acute **Pain**
Chronic **Pain**
Impaired **Parenting**
Readiness for Enhanced **Parenting**
Risk for Impaired **Parenting**
Risk for Perioperative **Positioning** Injury
Risk for **Peripheral** Neurovascular Dysfunction
Disturbed **Personal** Identity
Risk for Disturbed **Personal** Identity
Risk for **Poisoning**
Post-Trauma Syndrome
Risk for **Post-Trauma** Syndrome
Readiness for Enhanced **Power**
Powerlessness
Risk for **Powerlessness**
Ineffective **Protection**
Rape-Trauma Syndrome
Ineffective **Relationship**
Readiness for Enhanced **Relationship**
Risk for Ineffective **Relationship**
Impaired **Religiosity**
Readiness for Enhanced **Religiosity**
Risk for Impaired **Religiosity**
Relocation Stress Syndrome
Risk for **Relocation** Stress Syndrome
Risk for Ineffective **Renal** Perfusion
Impaired Individual **Resilience**
Readiness for Enhanced **Resilience**
Risk for Compromised **Resilience**
Parental **Role** Conflict
Ineffective **Role** Performance
Bathing **Self-Care** Deficit
Dressing **Self-Care** Deficit
Feeding **Self-Care** Deficit
Toileting **Self-Care** Deficit
Readiness for Enhanced **Self-Care**
Readiness for Enhanced **Self-Concept**
Chronic Low **Self-Esteem**
Situational Low **Self-Esteem**
Risk for Chronic Low **Self-Esteem**
Risk for Situational Low **Self-Esteem**
Ineffective **Self-Health** Management
Readiness for Enhanced **Self-Health** Management
Risk for **Self-Mutilation**
Self-Mutilation
Self-Neglect
Sexual Dysfunction
Ineffective **Sexuality** Pattern
Risk for **Shock**
Impaired **Skin** Integrity
Risk for Impaired **Skin** Integrity
Sleep Deprivation
Readiness for Enhanced **Sleep**
Disturbed **Sleep** Pattern
Impaired **Social** Interaction
Social Isolation
Chronic **Sorrow**
Spiritual Distress
Risk for **Spiritual** Distress
Readiness for Enhanced **Spiritual** Well-Being
Stress Overload
Risk for **Suffocation**
Risk for **Suicide**
Delayed **Surgical** Recovery
Impaired **Swallowing**
Ineffective Family **Therapeutic** Regimen Management
Risk for **Thermal** Injury
Ineffective **Thermoregulation**
Impaired **Tissue** Integrity
Ineffective Peripheral **Tissue** Perfusion
Risk for Decreased Cardiac **Tissue** Perfusion
Risk for Ineffective Cerebral **Tissue** Perfusion
Risk for Ineffective Peripheral Tissue Perfusion
Impaired **Transfer** Ability
Risk for **Trauma**
Impaired **Urinary** Elimination
Readiness for Enhanced **Urinary** Elimination
Urinary Retention
Risk for **Vascular** Trauma
Impaired Spontaneous **Ventilation**
Dysfunctional **Ventilatory** Weaning Response
Risk for Other-Directed **Violence**
Risk for Self-Directed **Violence**
Impaired **Walking**
Wandering

 In order to make safe and effective judgments using NANDA-I nursing diagnoses it is essential that nurses refer to the definitions and defining characteristics of the diagnoses listed in the work.

Data Clustering

A **data cluster** is a set of signs or symptoms gathered during assessment that you group together in a logical way. In the case of Mr. Jacobs, Tonya clustered together the signs and symptoms of "patient wincing when incision palpated," "patient acknowledges discomfort over incision," "patient rates discomfort a 7 on a scale of 0 to 10," and "pain increases with movement." Tonya analyzed these data to recognize the pattern of a comfort problem. Data clusters are patterns of data that contain **defining characteristics,** the clinical criteria that are observable and verifiable. Each **clinical criterion** is an objective or subjective sign, symptom, or risk factor that, when analyzed with other criteria, leads to a diagnostic conclusion.

BOX 17-3 EXAMPLES OF NANDA INTERNATIONAL–APPROVED NURSING DIAGNOSES WITH DEFINING CHARACTERISTICS

DIAGNOSIS: ACUTE PAIN	DIAGNOSIS: CHRONIC PAIN
Defining Characteristics	**Defining Characteristics**
Coded (scale of 0 to 10) report	Coded (scale of 0 to 10) report
Self-focus	Self-focusing
Sleep disturbance	Changes in sleep pattern
Verbal report of pain	Verbal report of pain
Protective gestures	Observed protective behavior
Guarding behavior	Guarding behavior
Change in blood pressure	Altered ability to continue previous activities
Diaphoresis	
Expressive behavior	Atrophy of involved muscle group
Positioning to avoid pain	Depression
Pupil dilation	Fatigue
	Fear of reinjury

Each NANDA-I–approved nursing diagnosis has an identified set of defining characteristics that support identification of a nursing diagnosis (NANDA International, 2012). You learn to recognize patterns of defining characteristics from your patient assessments and then readily select the corresponding diagnosis. Working with similar patients over a period of time helps you recognize clusters of defining characteristics, but remember that each patient is unique and requires an individualized diagnostic approach. Box 17-3 shows two examples of approved nursing diagnoses and their associated defining characteristics.

Interpretation—Identifying Health Problems

While analyzing clusters of data, you begin to consider the patient's health problems. Your interpretation of the information allows you to select among various diagnoses the ones that apply to your patient. It is critical to select the correct diagnostic label for a patient's need. Usually from assessment to diagnosis you move from general information to specific. It helps to think of the problem identification phase in assessment as the general health care problem and the formulation of the nursing diagnosis as the specific health problem. For example, after analyzing Mr. Jacob's problem with comfort, Tonya begins to identify data needed for a specific pain diagnosis.

Often a patient has defining characteristics that apply to more than one diagnosis. For example, Mr. Jacobs provided a verbal report of pain and showed protective behavior in minimizing movement while lying in bed. Both of these defining characteristics possibly indicates that the patient has either *acute pain* or *chronic pain* as nursing diagnoses. Knowing that there are similar diagnoses directs you to gather more information to clarify your interpretation. For example, Tonya checks Mr. Jacobs' blood pressure after he rates his discomfort a 7 on a 10-point rating scale. She notes that his blood pressure is elevated, a defining characteristic unique to the diagnosis of *acute pain*. When interpreting data to form a diagnosis, remember that the absence of certain defining characteristics suggests that you reject a diagnosis under consideration. Thus in the same example, if Tonya's assessment eliminates the signs of fatigue, fear of reinjury, and depression, it is less likely Mr. Jacobs' is having *chronic pain*. In addition, Tonya recognizes that the pain source is the patient's incision and not some underlying chronic problem. The correct diagnosis for Mr. Jacobs is *acute pain*. Always examine the defining characteristics in your database carefully to support or eliminate a nursing diagnosis. To be more accurate, review all characteristics, eliminate irrelevant ones, and confirm the relevant ones.

Formulating a Nursing Diagnosis

To individualize a nursing diagnosis further, you identify the associated related factor. A **related factor** is a condition, historical factor, or etiology that gives a context for the defining characteristics and shows a type of relationship with the nursing diagnosis (NANDA International, 2012). A related factor allows you to individualize a nursing diagnosis for a specific patient. For example, Mr. Jacobs has just undergone surgery and has an incision in the perineal area. This information is important in the context of the nature of his discomfort, and it is used in making a final diagnosis. Placing a diagnosis into the context of the patient's situation clarifies the nature of the patient's health problem. Tonya considers the nature of Mr. Jacobs' pain and identifies his diagnosis as *acute pain related to trauma of an incision*. When Tonya is ready to form her plan of care and select nursing interventions, this concise nursing diagnosis allows her to select therapies suited to postoperative pain management. For example, *acute pain related to trauma of an incision* is more prescriptive for Mr. Jacobs' situation than a nursing diagnosis of *acute pain related to muscular injury*.

While focusing on patterns of defining characteristics, you also compare a patient's pattern of data with data that are consistent with normal, healthful patterns. Use accepted norms as the basis for comparison and judgment. This includes using laboratory and diagnostic test values, professional standards, and normal anatomical or physiological limits. When comparing patterns, judge whether the grouped signs and symptoms are expected for the patient and whether they are within the range of healthful responses. Isolate any defining characteristics not within healthy norms to allow you to identify a specific problem.

Nursing diagnoses provide the basis for selection of nursing interventions to achieve outcomes for which you, as a nurse, are accountable (NANDA International, 2012). A nursing diagnosis focuses on a patient's actual or potential response to a health problem rather than on the physiological event, complication, or disease. A nurse cannot independently treat a medical diagnosis such as a tumor of the prostate. However, Tonya manages Mr. Jacobs' postoperative care, monitoring his postoperative progress and wound care, fluid administration, and medication therapy to prevent collaborative problems from developing. Collaborative problems occur or probably will occur in association with a specific disease, trauma, or treatment (Carpenito-Moyet, 2009). You need nursing knowledge to assess a patient's specific risk for these problems, identify the problems early, and take preventive action (Fig. 17-3). Critical thinking is necessary in identifying nursing diagnoses and collaborative problems so you appropriately individualize care for your patients.

Types of Nursing Diagnoses

NANDA-I (2012) identifies three types of nursing diagnoses: actual diagnoses, risk diagnoses, and health promotion diagnoses. An **actual nursing diagnosis** describes human responses to health conditions or life processes that exist in an individual, family, or

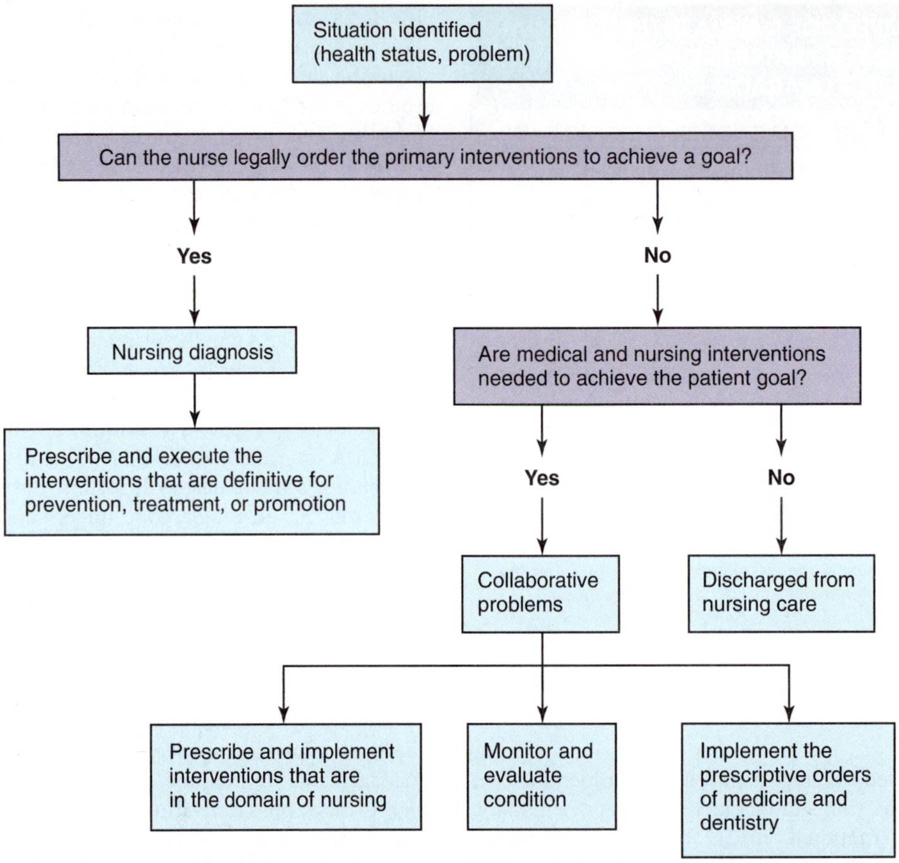

FIG. 17-3 Differentiating nursing diagnoses from collaborative problems. (©1990, 1988, 1985 Lynda Juall Carpenito. Redrawn from Carpenito LJ: *Nursing diagnosis: application to clinical practice* ed 6, Philadelphia, 1995, Lippincott.)

community. Defining characteristics support the diagnostic judgment (NANDA International, 2012). The selection of an actual diagnosis indicates that there are sufficient assessment data to establish the nursing diagnosis. Tonya assessed Mr. Jacobs as having discomfort from the prostatectomy incision with a severity rated at 7 on a 10-point rating scale. The pain increased with movement. As a result of the pain, Mr. Jacobs has limited movement in bed. *Acute pain* is an actual nursing diagnosis. Examples of other actual diagnoses include:

- Wandering
- Impaired social interaction
- Stress urinary incontinence

A **risk nursing diagnosis** describes human responses to health conditions or life processes that may develop in a vulnerable individual, family, or community (NANDA International, 2012). These diagnoses do not have related factors or defining characteristics because they have not occurred yet. Instead a risk diagnosis has risk factors. Risk factors are the environmental, physiological, psychological, genetic, or chemical elements that place a person at risk for a health problem. For example, after Mr. Jacobs' surgery, the presence of his incision, an open wound, poses a risk for a hospital-acquired infection. The key assessment for a risk diagnosis is the presence of risk factors (e.g., an incision and the hospital environment) that support a patient's vulnerability. The risk factors are the diagnostic-related factors that help in planning preventive health care measures. In Mr. Jacobs' case *risk for infection* is appropriate for his condition. Other examples of risk nursing diagnoses include:

- Risk for loneliness
- Risk for acute confusion

A **health promotion nursing diagnosis** is a clinical judgment of a person's, family's, or community's motivation, desire, and readiness to increase well-being and actualize human health potential as expressed in their readiness to enhance specific health behaviors such as nutrition and exercise. Health promotion diagnoses can be used in any health state and do not require current levels of wellness (NANDA International, 2012). A person's readiness is supported by defining characteristics. Examples of health promotion nursing diagnoses include:

- Readiness for enhanced family coping
- Readiness for enhanced nutrition

Components of a Nursing Diagnosis

When communicating a nursing diagnosis, through either discussions with health care colleagues or documentation of your care, it is important to use the language adopted within an agency. Most settings use a two-part format in labeling a nursing diagnosis: the NANDA-I diagnostic label followed by a statement of a related factor (Table 17-1). The two-part format provides a diagnosis meaning and relevance for a particular patient.

Diagnostic Label. The **diagnostic label** is the name of the nursing diagnosis as approved by NANDA International (see Box 17-2). It describes the essence of a patient's response to health conditions in as few words as possible. All NANDA-I approved diagnoses also have a definition. The definition describes the characteristics of the human response identified. You refer to

TABLE 17-1 NANDA International Two-Part Nursing Diagnosis Format

DIAGNOSTIC STATEMENT	EXAMPLES OF RELATED FACTORS
Acute pain	Biological, chemical, physical, or psychological injury agents (e.g., inflammation, edema, burn)
Anxiety	Change (economic status, environment, health status, role), familial association, maturational crisis, situational crisis, stress, threat of death, unmet needs
Impaired urinary elimination	Anatomical obstruction, urinary tract infection, sensory motor impairment)
Impaired skin integrity	Fluid retention, age extremes, hyperthermia, mechanical factors (e.g., shearing, pressure), medications, moisture, physical immobilization, impaired sensation

definitions of nursing diagnoses to assist in identifying a patient's correct diagnosis, which helps especially when selecting between two diagnoses with similar defining characteristics. The diagnostic labels include descriptors used to give additional meaning to the diagnosis. For example, the diagnosis *impaired physical mobility* includes the descriptor *impaired* to describe the nature or change in mobility that best describes the patient's response. Examples of other descriptors include *compromised, decreased, deficient, delayed, effective, imbalanced, impaired,* and *increased.*

Related Factors. The related factor is identified from the patient's assessment data and is the reason the patient is displaying the nursing diagnosis. The related factor is associated with a patient's actual or potential response to the health problem and can change by using specific nursing interventions. Related factors for NANDA-I diagnoses include four categories: pathophysiological (biological or psychological), treatment-related, situational (environmental or personal), and maturational (Carpenito-Moyet, 2009). The "related to" phrase is not a cause-and-effect statement. It indicates that the etiology contributes to or is associated with the patient's diagnosis (Fig. 17-4). The inclusion of the "related to" phrase requires you to use critical thinking to individualize the nursing diagnosis and then select nursing interventions (Table 17-2).

The **etiology** or related factor of a nursing diagnosis is always within the domain of nursing practice and a condition that responds to nursing interventions. Sometimes health care providers record medical diagnoses as the etiology of the nursing diagnosis. This is incorrect. Nursing interventions do not change a medical diagnosis. However, you direct nursing interventions at behaviors or conditions that you are able to treat or manage. For example, the nursing diagnosis *acute pain related to prostatectomy* is incorrect. Nursing actions do not affect the medical diagnosis of the surgical removal of the prostate gland. Rewording the diagnosis to read *acute pain related to trauma* of incision results in nursing interventions directed at appropriate wound care, using turning techniques to reduce stress on the suture line and offering nonpharmacological comfort measures (see Chapter 43). In the case of a risk nursing diagnosis, a risk factor is the related factor. Table 17-3 demonstrates the association between a nurse's assessment of a patient, the clustering of defining characteristics, and the formulation of nursing diagnoses. The diagnostic process results in the formation of a total diagnostic label that allows you to develop an appropriate, patient-centered plan of care. The

TABLE 17-2 Comparison of Interventions for Nursing Diagnoses with Different Related Factors

NURSING DIAGNOSES	RELATED FACTOR	INTERVENTIONS
Patient A		
Anxiety	Uncertainty over surgery	Provide detailed instructions about the surgical procedure, recovery process, and postoperative care activities. Plan formal time for patient to ask questions.
Impaired physical mobility	Acute pain	Administer analgesics 30 minutes before planned exercise. Instruct patient in technique to splint painful site during activity.
Patient B		
Anxiety	Loss of job	Consult with social worker to arrange for job counseling. Encourage patient to continue health promotion activities (e.g., exercise, routine social activities).
Impaired physical mobility	Musculoskeletal injury	Have patient perform active range-of-motion exercises to affected extremity every 2 hours. Instruct patient on use of three-point crutch gait.

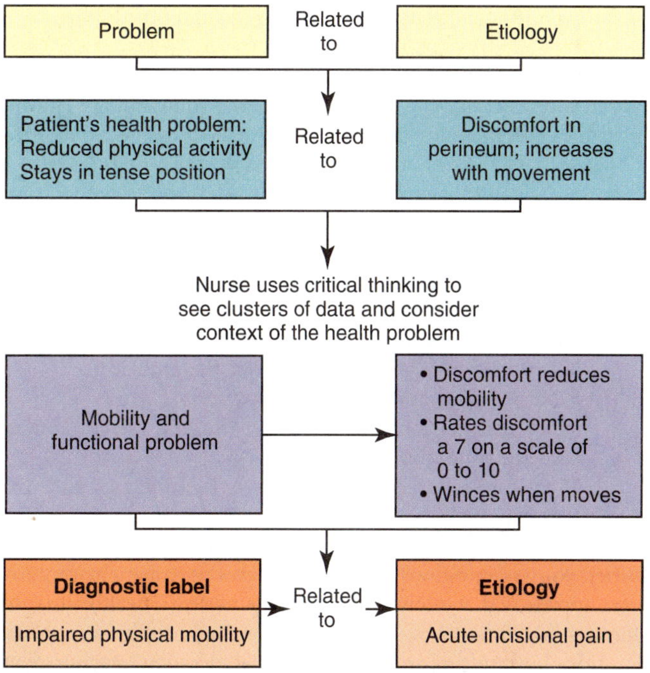

FIG. 17-4 Relationship between a diagnostic label and related factor (etiology).

defining characteristics and relevant etiologies are from NANDA International (2012).

The PES Format. Some agencies prefer a three-part nursing diagnostic label. In this case the diagnostic label consists of the NANDA-I label, the related factor, and the defining characteristics

TABLE 17-3 Developing a Two-Part Nursing Diagnosis Label

ASSESSMENT ACTIVITIES	DEFINING CHARACTERISTICS (CLUSTERING CUES)	ETIOLOGIES ("RELATED TO")	NURSING DIAGNOSIS
Ask patient to rate severity of pain on a scale from 0 to 10.	Verbal report of pain at a level of 7	Physical; swelling from incisional trauma	Acute pain related to trauma of incision
Observe patient's positioning in bed.	Lies flat, avoids turning		
Observe for any nonverbal signs of discomfort.	Winces when surgical wound is palpated		
Ask patient to describe what he knows about surgery.	Has no knowledge about postoperative wound care	Inexperience; first time to have surgery	Deficient knowledge related to inexperience with surgery
Observe his interactions.	Asks questions about pain control and what to expect.		
Question wife's role in postoperative care and her level of knowledge.	Wife to provide support within the home; no knowledge of how to manage wound		

(Ackley and Ladwig, 2011). This approach makes a diagnosis even more patient specific. The acronym PES stands for problem, etiology, and symptoms.

- **P** (problem)—NANDA-I label—Example: *impaired physical mobility*
- **E** (etiology or related factor)—Example: incisional pain
- **S** (symptoms or defining characteristics)—briefly lists defining characteristic(s) that show evidence of the health problem. Example: evidenced by restricted turning and positioning

PES diagnostic statement: *Impaired physical mobility related to incisional pain,* evidenced by restricted turning and positioning.

Cultural Relevance of Nursing Diagnoses

When you select nursing diagnoses, consider your patients' cultural diversity. This includes knowing the cultural differences that affect how a patient defines health and illness and wants to be treated (Smith, 2007). It is important to consider your own cultural competence so you are more sensitive to a patient's health care problems and the implications.

Here are examples of questions that contribute to making culturally competent nursing diagnoses (Smith, 2007):

- How has this health problem affected you and your family?
- What do you believe will help or fix the problem?
- What worries you the most about this problem?
- What do you expect from us, your nurses, to help maintain some of your cultural practices?
- What cultural practices do you do to keep yourself and your family well?
- Which practices within your culture are important to you?

When you ask questions such as these, you use a patient-centered care approach that allows you to see the patient's health situation through his or her eyes. When making a diagnosis, be sure to also consider how culture influences the related factor for your diagnostic statement. For example, *impaired verbal communication related to cultural differences* or *noncompliance related to patient value system* reflects diagnostic conclusions that consider a patient's unique cultural needs.

Your own culture potentially influences the cues and defining characteristics that you select from your assessment. In an older but still relevant study, Wieck (1996) examined how cultural differences among nurses influenced the choice of defining characteristics in making nursing diagnoses. The researchers studied the diagnosis of pain within six different cultural groups of nurses. Generally the nurses were consistent in selecting defining characteristics. However, when diagnosing pain, some of the nurses did not select restlessness or grimace as defining characteristics. The nurses were not familiar with such characteristics because they were not common to how their own culture expressed pain. Cultural awareness and sensitivity improve your accuracy in making nursing diagnoses.

CONCEPT MAPPING NURSING DIAGNOSES

When caring for a patient or groups of patients, think critically about their needs and how to prevent problems from developing. Your holistic view of a patient heightens the challenge of thinking about all patient needs and problems. Few patients have single problems. Often you care for a patient with multiple nursing diagnoses. Therefore a picture of each patient usually consists of several interconnections between sets of data, all associated with identified patient problems. A concept map diagrams the critical thinking associated with making accurate diagnoses. It is one way to graphically represent the connections between concepts (nursing diagnoses) and ideas that are related to a central subject (e.g., the patient's health problems). For each diagnosis you list defining characteristics and begin to see the connections or association among different diagnostic statements.

As you proceed in applying each step of the nursing process, your concept map expands with more detail about planned interventions (see Chapter 18). A concept map promotes critical thinking because you identify, graphically display, and link key concepts by organizing and analyzing information (Hsu and Hsieh, 2005).

Fig. 17-5 shows the next step in the development of Tonya's concept map for Mr. Jacobs. Tonya began during the assessment step of the nursing process (see Chapter 16) to gather a database for Mr. Jacobs. Her assessment included Mr. Jacobs' perspective of his health problems and the objective and subjective data she collected through observation and examination. She validated findings and added to the database as she learned new information. Data sources include physical, psychological, and sociocultural domains. Tonya applies clinical reasoning and intuition that reflect her own basic nursing knowledge, her past experiences with

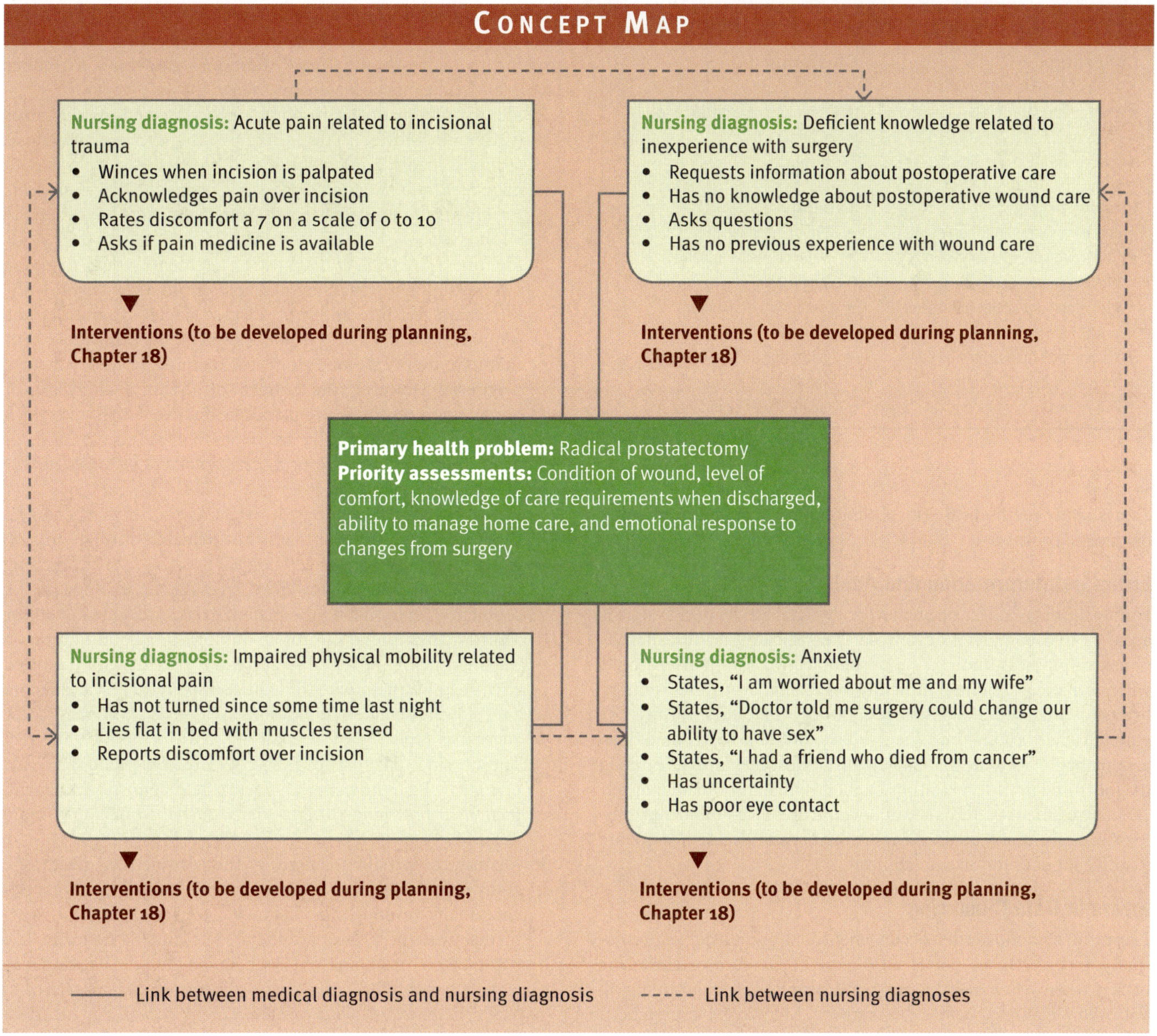
CONCEPT MAP
Nursing diagnosis: Acute pain related to incisional trauma
• Winces when incision is palpated
• Acknowledges pain over incision
• Rates discomfort a 7 on a scale of 0 to 10
• Asks if pain medicine is available
Interventions (to be developed during planning, Chapter 18)
Nursing diagnosis: Deficient knowledge related to inexperience with surgery
• Requests information about postoperative care
• Has no knowledge about postoperative wound care
• Asks questions
• Has no previous experience with wound care
Interventions (to be developed during planning, Chapter 18)
Primary health problem: Radical prostatectomy
Priority assessments: Condition of wound, level of comfort, knowledge of care requirements when discharged, ability to manage home care, and emotional response to changes from surgery
Nursing diagnosis: Impaired physical mobility related to incisional pain
• Has not turned since some time last night
• Lies flat in bed with muscles tensed
• Reports discomfort over incision
Interventions (to be developed during planning, Chapter 18)
Nursing diagnosis: Anxiety
• States, "I am worried about me and my wife"
• States, "Doctor told me surgery could change our ability to have sex"
• States, "I had a friend who died from cancer"
• Has uncertainty
• Has poor eye contact
Interventions (to be developed during planning, Chapter 18)
Link between medical diagnosis and nursing diagnosis
Link between nursing diagnoses

FIG. 17-5 Concept map for Mr. Jacobs: Nursing diagnoses.

patients, patterns seen in similar situations, and reference to institutional standards and procedures (e.g., pain-management policies or postoperative teaching protocols). As Tonya begins to see patterns of defining characteristics, she places labels to identify the four nursing diagnoses that apply to Mr. Jacobs. She is also able to see the relationship among the diagnoses and connects them on the concept map. If Mr. Jacobs does not receive pain relief, Tonya knows from her experience in caring for patients with pain that he will have continued problems in achieving necessary mobility for recovery. The diagnoses of *acute pain* and *impaired physical mobility* are closely related. In addition, if pain is unrelieved, it will be difficult for Mr. Jacobs' to be receptive to any patient teaching Tonya wants to provide about postoperative care, an intervention that will be later planned for *deficient knowledge*. If Mr. Jacobs' remains anxious about the outcome of his surgery and whether he can fulfill his role sexually with his wife, this *anxiety* can heighten pain perception and influence his ability to learn. Concept mapping organizes and links information to allow you to see new wholes and appreciate the complexity of patient care (Ferrario, 2004). Tonya's next step on the care map is to identify the appropriate nursing interventions for Mr. Jacobs' care (see Chapter 18).

The advantage of a concept map is its central focus on the patient rather than the patient's disease or health alteration. This encourages nursing students to concentrate on patients' specific health problems and nursing diagnoses. The focus also promotes patient participation with the eventual plan of care.

SOURCES OF DIAGNOSTIC ERRORS

Errors may occur in the nursing diagnostic process during data collection, interpretation, clustering, and labeling of the diagnosis (Box 17-4). Chapter 16 reviews how to conduct a systematic assessment so you have all of the data necessary for making accurate and timely nursing diagnoses and collaborative problems. As a nurse

BOX 17-4 SOURCES OF DIAGNOSTIC ERROR

Collecting
- Lack of knowledge or skill
- Inaccurate data
- Missing data
- Disorganization

Clustering
- Insufficient cluster of cues
- Premature or early closure
- Incorrect clustering

Interpreting
- Inaccurate interpretation of cues
- Failure to consider conflicting cues
- Using an insufficient number of cues
- Using unreliable or invalid cues
- Failure to consider cultural influences or developmental stage

Labeling
- Wrong diagnostic label selected
- Evidence that another diagnosis is more likely
- Condition a collaborative problem
- Failure to validate nursing diagnosis with patient
- Failure to seek guidance

always apply methodical critical thinking for an accurate nursing diagnostic process.

Errors in Interpretation and Analysis of Data

Following data collection, review your database to decide if it is accurate and complete. Review data to validate that measurable, objective physical findings support subjective data. For example, when a patient reports "difficulty breathing," you also want to listen to lung sounds, assess respiratory rate, and measure the patient's chest excursion. When you are not able to validate data, it signals an inaccurate match between clinical cues and the nursing diagnosis. Begin interpretation by identifying and organizing relevant assessment patterns to support the presence of patient problems. Be careful to consider conflicting cues or decide if there are insufficient cues to form a diagnosis.

Errors in Data Clustering

Errors in data clustering occur when data are clustered prematurely, incorrectly, or not at all. Premature closure of clustering occurs when you make the nursing diagnosis before grouping all data. For example, before his surgery, Mr. Jacobs experienced urinary incontinence and complained of urgency and nocturia. The nurse in the clinic clustered the available data and considered that *impaired urinary elimination* was a probable diagnosis. However, incorrect clustering occurs when you try to make a nursing diagnosis fit the signs and symptoms obtained. In this example further assessment revealed that the patient had bladder distention and dribbling and the type of incontinence was likely overflow incontinence. As a result of these findings the nurse was able to make a more accurate diagnosis, *urinary retention.* Always identify the nursing diagnosis from the data, not the reverse. An incorrect nursing diagnosis affects quality of patient care.

Errors in the Diagnostic Statement

Clinical reasoning leads to a higher quality of nursing diagnosis, which eventually leads to etiology-specific interventions and enhanced patient outcomes (Muller-Staub et al., 2008). The more competent you become in diagnostic reasoning, the more likely it is that you will correctly select diagnostic statements. This results in the appropriate selection of nursing interventions and patient outcomes during planning and implementation (see Chapters 18 and 19). Reduce errors by selecting appropriate, concise, and precise language using NANDA-I terminology. Be sure that the etiology portion of the diagnostic statement is within the scope of nursing to diagnose and treat. Additional guidelines to reduce errors in the diagnostic statement follow.

1. Identify the patient's response, not the medical diagnosis (Carpenito-Moyet, 2009). Because the medical diagnosis requires medical interventions, it is legally inadvisable to include it in the nursing diagnosis. Change the diagnosis *acute pain related to prostatectomy* to *acute pain related to trauma of an incision.*
2. Identify a NANDA-I diagnostic statement rather than the symptom. Identify nursing diagnoses from a cluster of defining characteristics and not just a single symptom. One symptom is insufficient for problem identification. For example, dyspnea alone does not definitively lead you to a diagnosis. However, the pattern of dyspnea, shortness of breath, pain on inspiration, and productive cough with thick secretions are defining characteristics that lead you to the diagnosis of *ineffective breathing pattern related to increased airway secretions.*
3. Identify a treatable etiology or risk factor rather than a clinical sign or chronic problem that is not treatable through nursing intervention. An accurate etiology allows you to select nursing interventions directed toward correcting the etiology of the problem or minimizing the patient's risk. A diagnostic test or a chronic dysfunction is not an etiology or a condition that a nursing intervention is able to treat. A patient with fractured ribs likely has pain when inhaling; impaired chest excursion; and slower, shallow respirations. An x-ray film may show atelectasis (collapse of alveolar air sacs) in the area affected. The nursing diagnosis of *ineffective breathing pattern related to shallow respirations* is an incorrect diagnostic statement. *Ineffective breathing pattern related to pain in chest* is more accurate.
4. Identify the problem caused by the treatment or diagnostic study rather than the treatment or study itself. Patients experience many responses to diagnostic tests and medical treatments. These responses are the area of nursing concern. The patient who has angina and is scheduled for a cardiac catheterization possibly has a nursing diagnosis of *anxiety related to lack of knowledge about cardiac catheterization.* An incorrect diagnosis is *anxiety related to cardiac catheterization.*
5. Identify the patient response to the equipment rather than the equipment itself. Patients are often unfamiliar with medical technology. The diagnosis of *deficient knowledge regarding the need for cardiac monitoring* is accurate compared with the statement *anxiety related to cardiac monitor.*
6. Identify the patient's problems rather than your problems with nursing care. Nursing diagnoses are always patient centered and form the basis for goal-directed care. *Potential intravenous complications related to poor vascular access* indicates a nursing problem in initiating and maintaining intravenous therapy. The diagnosis *risk for infection* properly centers attention on patient needs.
7. Identify the patient problem rather than the nursing intervention. You plan nursing interventions after identifying a nursing diagnosis. The statement, "offer bedpan frequently because of altered elimination patterns," changes to the correct diagnostic statement, *diarrhea related to food intolerance.* This corrects the misstatement and allows proper implementation of the nursing process. More appropriate interventions are selected rather than a single intervention that will not solve the problem.

8. Identify the patient problem rather than the goal of care. You establish goals during the planning step of the nursing process (see Chapter 18). Goals based on accurate identification of a patient's problems serve as a basis to determine problem resolution. Change the diagnostic statement, "Patient needs high-protein diet related to potential alteration in nutrition," to *imbalanced nutrition: less than body requirements related to inadequate protein intake.*
9. Make professional rather than prejudicial judgments. Base nursing diagnoses on subjective and objective patient data and do not include your personal beliefs and values. Remove your judgment from *impaired skin integrity related to poor hygiene habits* by changing the nursing diagnosis to read *impaired skin integrity related to inadequate knowledge about perineal care.*
10. Avoid legally inadvisable statements (Carpenito-Moyet, 2009). Statements that imply blame, negligence, or malpractice have the potential to result in a lawsuit. The statement, "recurrent angina related to insufficient medication," implies an inadequate prescription by the health care provider. Correct problem identification is *chronic pain related to improper use of medications.*
11. Identify the problem and etiology to avoid a circular statement. Circular statements are vague and give no direction to nursing care. Change the statement, "impaired breathing pattern related to shallow breathing," to identify the patient problem and cause, *ineffective breathing pattern related to incisional pain.*
12. Identify only one patient problem in the diagnostic statement. Every problem has different specific expected outcomes. Confusion during the planning step occurs when you include multiple problems in a nursing diagnosis. Restate *pain and anxiety related to difficulty in ambulating* as two nursing diagnoses such as *impaired physical mobility related to pain in right knee* and *anxiety related to difficulty in ambulating.* It is permissible to include multiple etiologies contributing to one patient problem, as in *complicated grieving related to diagnosed terminal illness and change in family role.*

Documentation and Informatics

Once you identify a patient's nursing diagnoses, enter them either on the written plan of care or in the electronic health information record of the agency. In the clinical facility list nursing diagnoses chronologically as you identify them. When initiating an original care plan, place the highest-priority nursing diagnoses first. This depends on the patient's condition and the nature of the nursing diagnosis (e.g., acute physical health problem versus a long-term chronic health management issue). Thereafter add nursing diagnoses to the list. Date a nursing diagnosis at the time of entry. When caring for a patient, review the list and identify nursing diagnoses with the greatest priority, regardless of chronological order.

In some settings data-driven computerized decision support systems are in place that allow you to be more accurate in making nursing diagnoses. A computer-based clinical decision support function involves use of the computer to bring relevant knowledge to bear for the health care of a patient (Cho, Staggers, and Park, 2010). The database within one of these systems includes diagnostic labels (e.g., NANDA-I diagnostic labels), defining characteristics, activities, and indicators for nursing. A nurse enters assessment data, and the computer helps by organizing the data into clusters that enhance the ability to select accurate diagnoses. Once diagnoses are selected, the computer system also directs the nurse to intervention options to select for a patient.

NURSING DIAGNOSES: APPLICATION TO CARE PLANNING

Nursing diagnosis is a mechanism for identifying the domain of nursing. Diagnoses direct the planning process and the selection of nursing interventions to achieve desired outcomes for patients. Just as the medical diagnosis of diabetes leads a physician to prescribe a low-carbohydrate diet and medication for blood glucose control, the nursing diagnosis of *impaired skin integrity* directs a nurse to apply certain support surfaces to a patient's bed and initiate a turning schedule. In Chapter 18 you will learn how unifying the languages of NANDA-I with the Nursing Interventions Classification (NIC) and Nursing Outcomes Classification (NOC) facilitates the process of matching nursing diagnoses with accurate and appropriate interventions and outcomes (Dochterman and Jones, 2003). The care plan (see Chapter 18) is a map for nursing care and demonstrates your accountability for patient care. By making accurate nursing diagnoses, your subsequent care plan communicates to other professionals the patient's health care problems and ensures that you select relevant and appropriate nursing interventions.

KEY POINTS

- The diagnostic process is a clinical judgment that involves reviewing assessment information, recognizing cues and patterns in the data, and identifying the patient's specific health care problems.
- The nursing diagnostic process is unique from that of medical diagnosis in that patients become involved in the diagnostic process when possible.
- Accurate diagnosis of patient problems ensures the selection of more effective and efficient nursing interventions.
- One purpose of nursing diagnosis is that it provides a precise definition of a patient's problem that gives nurses and other members of the health care team a common language for understanding the patient's needs.
- The nursing diagnostic process includes data clustering, identifying patient needs or problems, and formulating the nursing diagnosis or collaborative problem.
- Defining characteristics are subjective and objective clinical criteria that form clusters, leading to a diagnostic conclusion.
- When an assessment reveals defining characteristics that apply to more than one nursing diagnosis, gather more information to clarify your interpretation.
- Absence of defining characteristics suggests that you reject a proposed diagnosis.
- A nursing diagnosis is usually written in a two-part format, including a diagnostic label and an etiological or related factor.
- A three-part nursing diagnosis, using a PES format, includes a diagnostic label, etiological statement, and symptoms or defining characteristics.
- The "related to" factor of the diagnostic statement helps you to individualize a patient's nursing diagnoses and provides direction for your selection of appropriate interventions.
- Risk factors serve as cues to indicate that a risk nursing diagnosis applies to a patient's condition.
- A concept map is a visual representation of a patient's nursing diagnoses and their relationship with one another.
- Nursing diagnostic errors occur by errors in data collection, interpretation and analysis of data, clustering of data, or the diagnostic statement.

CLINICAL APPLICATION QUESTIONS

Preparing for Clinical Practice

Tonya discusses the concerns Mr. Jacobs has about his sexual relationship with his wife. She knows that a radical prostatectomy can cause nerve damage that impairs a man's ability to have a normal erection. Tonya says, "You've told me that you're worried about you and your wife. Can you tell me more?" Mr. Jacobs says, "I feel uncertain about my ability to have sex. The doctor said before the surgery that there is a risk of damaging a nerve that can affect my ability to perform sexually." Tonya observes that Mr. Jacobs has poor eye contact as they talk and his voice quivers. Tonya asks, "How would you describe your relationship with Mrs. Jacobs?" The patient responds, "Oh, it's been really good. We've had our ups and downs like anyone else, but she has been so good to me. I worry that I won't be able to be the husband she wants any more." Tonya clarifies, "Has the doctor visited since surgery to discuss your concerns?" Mr. Jacobs replies, "No, he hasn't been in yet."

1. Which of the following are defining characteristics from the assessment?
   1. Quiver in Mr. Jacobs' voice
   2. Nurse's statement, "You've told me that you're worried."
   3. Uncertainty about ability to have sex
   4. Poor eye contact
   5. Nurse's question, "Can you tell me more?"
2. Tonya clusters the defining characteristics to select the diagnostic label of *anxiety*. What would you identify as the related factor for this diagnosis?
3. If Tonya identified the diagnosis as *anxiety related to risk of nerve damage during surgery*, would this be an accurate nursing diagnosis? Explain.

evolve *Answers to Clinical Application Questions can be found on the Evolve website.*

REVIEW QUESTIONS

Are You Ready to Test Your Nursing Knowledge?

1. The nurse identified that the patient has pain on a scale of 7, he winces during movement, and he expresses discomfort over the incisional area. He guards the area by resisting movement. The incision appears to be healing, but there is natural swelling. Write a three-part nursing diagnostic statement using the PES format.
2. Review the following nursing diagnoses and identify the diagnoses that are stated correctly. (Select all that apply.)
   1. Anxiety related to fear of dying
   2. Fatigue related to chronic emphysema
   3. Need for mouth care related to inflamed mucosa
   4. Risk for infection
3. A nurse reviews data gathered regarding a patient's pain symptoms. The nurse compares the defining characteristics for *acute pain* with those for *chronic pain* and in the end selects *acute pain* as the correct diagnosis. This is an example of the nurse avoiding an error in:
   1. Data collection.
   2. Data clustering.
   3. Data interpretation.
   4. Making a diagnostic statement.
4. The nursing diagnosis *readiness for enhanced communication* is an example of a(n):
   1. Risk nursing diagnosis.
   2. Actual nursing diagnosis.
   3. Health promotion nursing diagnosis
   4. Wellness nursing diagnosis.
5. In the following examples, which nurses are making nursing diagnostic errors? (Select all that apply.)
   1. The nurse who listens to lung sounds after a patient reports "difficulty breathing"
   2. The nurse who considers conflicting cues in deciding which diagnostic label to choose
   3. The nurse assessing the edema in a patient's lower leg who is unsure how to assess the severity of edema
   4. The nurse who identifies a diagnosis on the basis of a single defining characteristic
6. A nurse is reviewing a patient's list of nursing diagnoses in the medical record. The most recent nursing diagnosis is *diarrhea related to intestinal colitis*. This is an incorrectly stated diagnostic statement, best described as:
   1. Identifying the clinical sign instead of an etiology.
   2. Identifying a diagnosis based on prejudicial judgment.
   3. Identifying the diagnostic study rather than a problem caused by the diagnostic study.
   4. Identifying the medical diagnosis instead of the patient's response to the diagnosis.
7. A nurse is assigned to a new patient admitted to the nursing unit following admission through the emergency department. The nurse collects a nursing history and interviews the patient. Place the following steps for making a nursing diagnosis in the correct order.
   _____ 1. Considers context of patient's health problem and selects a related factor
   _____ 2. Reviews assessment data, noting objective and subjective clinical criteria
   _____ 3. Clusters clinical criteria that form a pattern
   _____ 4. Chooses diagnostic label
8. Match the activity on the left with the source of diagnostic error on the right:

Activity	Source of Diagnostic Error
a. Nurse listens to lungs for first time and is not sure if abnormal lung sounds are present.	__ 1. Collecting data
b. After reviewing objective data, nurse selects diagnosis of *fear* before asking patient to discuss feelings.	__ 2. Interpreting
c. Nurse identifies incorrect diagnostic label.	__ 3. Clustering
d. Nurse does not consider patient's cultural background when reviewing cues.	__ 4. Labeling
e. Nurse prepares to complete decision on diagnosis and realizes that clinical criteria are grouped incorrectly to form a pattern.	

9. Review the following list of nursing diagnoses and identify those stated incorrectly. (Select all that apply.)
   1. Acute pain related to lumbar disk repair
   2. Sleep deprivation related to difficulty falling asleep
   3. Constipation related to inadequate intake of liquids
   4. Potential nausea related to nasogastric tube insertion
10. The nurse completed the following assessment: 63-year-old female patient has had abdominal pain for 6 days. She reports

not having a bowel movement for 4 days, whereas she normally has a bowel movement every 2 to 3 days. She has not been hospitalized in the past. Her abdomen is distended. She reports being anxious about upcoming tests. Her temperature was 37° C, pulse 82 and regular, blood pressure 128/72. Which of the following data form a cluster, showing a relevant pattern? (Select all that apply.)
   1. Vital sign results
   2. Abdominal distention
   3. Age of patient
   4. Change in bowel elimination pattern
   5. Abdominal pain
   6. No past history of hospitalization
11. In question 10, which additional data do you collect to add to the cluster of information? (Short answer)
12. The nurse in a geriatric clinic collects the following information from an 82-year-old patient and her daughter, the family caregiver. The daughter explains that the patient is "always getting lost." The patient sits in the chair but gets up frequently and paces back and forth in the examination room. The daughter says, "I just don't know what to do because I worry she will fall or hurt herself." The daughter states that, when she took her mother to the store, they became separated, and the mother couldn't find the front entrance. The daughter works part time and has no one to help watch her mother. Which of the data form a cluster, showing a relevant pattern?(Select all that apply.)
   1. Daughter's concern of mother's risk for injury
   2. Pacing
   3. Patient getting lost easily
   4. Daughter working part time
   5. Getting up frequently
13. Which of the following are examples of collaborative problems? (Select all that apply.)
   1. Nausea
   2. Hemorrhage
   3. Wound infection
   4. Fear
14. Two nurses are having a discussion at the nurses' station. One nurse is a new graduate who added, "Patient needs improved bowel function related to constipation" to a patient's care plan. The nurse's colleague, the charge nurse says, "I think your diagnosis is possibly worded incorrectly. Let's go over it together." A correctly worded diagnostic statement is:
   1. Need for improved bowel function related to change in diet.
   2. Patient needs improved bowel function related to alteration in elimination.
   3. Constipation related to inadequate fluid intake.
   4. Constipation related to hard infrequent stools.
15. The following nursing diagnoses all apply to one patient. As the nurse adds these diagnoses to the care plan, which diagnoses will not include defining characteristics?
   1. Risk for aspiration
   2. Acute confusion
   3. Readiness for enhanced coping
   4. Sedentary lifestyle

Answers: **1.** P, acute pain; E, related to incisional trauma; S, evidenced by pain reported at 7, with guarding, and restricted turning and positioning; **2.** 1, 4; **3.** 3; **4.** 3; **5.** 3, 4; **6.** 4; **7.** 2, 3, 4, 1; **8.** 1 a, 2 b and d, 3 e, 4 c; **9.** 1, 2, 4; **10.** 2, 4, 5; **11.** See Evolve; **12.** 2, 3, 5; **13.** 2, 3; **14.** 3; **15.** 1.

REFERENCES

Ackley BJ, Ladwig GB: *Nursing diagnosis handbook*, ed 9, St Louis, Mosby, 2011.

American Nurses Association: *Model nurse practice act*, Washington, DC, 1955, The Association.

American Nurses Association: *Scope of nursing practice*, Washington, DC, 1987, The Association.

American Nurses Association: *Nursing's social policy statement*, ed 2, Washington, DC, 2003, The Association.

American Nurses Association: *Nursing's social policy statement*, ed 3, Washington, DC, 2010, The Association.

Carpenito-Moyet LJ: *Nursing diagnoses: application to clinical practice*, ed 13, Philadelphia, 2009, Lippincott, Williams & Wilkins.

Dochterman JM, Jones DA: *Unifying nursing languages: the harmonization of NANDA, NIC, NOC*, Washington, DC, 2003, American Nurses Association.

Ferrario CG: Developing nurses' critical thinking skills with concept mapping, *J Nurses Staff Dev* 20(6):261, 2004.

Fry VS: The creative approach to nursing, *Am J Nurs* 53:301, 1953.

Gebbie K: Utilization of a classification of nursing diagnosis, *Nurs Diagn* 9(2 suppl):17, 1998.

McFarland GK, McFarlane EA: *Nursing diagnosis and intervention: planning for patient care*, St Louis, 1989, Mosby.

NANDA International *Nursing diagnoses: definitions and classification, 2012-2014*, Oxford, 2012, Wiley-Blackwell.

Smith LS: Documenting culturally competent psychosocial nursing diagnoses, *Nursing* 37(1):70, 2007.

Yura H, Walsh M: *The nursing process*, Norwalk, Conn, 1967, Appleton-Century-Crofts.

RESEARCH REFERENCES

Cho I, Staggers N, Park I: Nurses' responses to differing amounts and information content in a diagnostic computer-based decision support application, *Comput Inform Nurs* 28(2):95, 2010.

Hsu L, Hsieh S: Concept maps as an assessment tool in a nursing course, *J Prof Nurs* 21(3):141, 2005.

Muller-Staub M, et al: Nursing diagnoses, interventions and outcomes—application and impact on nursing practice: systematic review, *J Adv Nurs* 56(5):514, 2006.

Muller-Staub M, et al: Implementing nursing diagnostics effectively: cluster randomized trial. *J Adv Nurs* 63(3): 291, 2008.

Wieck KL: Diagnostic language consistency among multicultural English-speaking nurses, *Nurs Diagn* 7(2):70, 1996.

CHAPTER

18

Planning Nursing Care

OBJECTIVES

- Explain the relationship of planning to assessment and nursing diagnosis.
- Discuss criteria used in priority setting.
- Describe goal setting.
- Discuss the difference between a goal and an expected outcome.
- List the seven guidelines for writing an outcome statement.
- Develop a plan of care from a nursing assessment.
- Discuss the differences between nurse-initiated, physician-initiated, and collaborative interventions.
- Discuss the process of selecting nursing interventions during planning.
- Describe the role that communication plays in planning patient-centered care.
- Describe the consultation process.

KEY TERMS

Collaborative interventions, p. 242
Consultation, p. 249
Critical pathways, p. 247
Dependent nursing interventions, p. 242
Expected outcome, p. 238
Goal, p. 238
Independent nursing interventions, p. 242
Interdisciplinary care plans, p. 244
Long-term goal, p. 239
Nursing care plan, p. 244
Nursing-sensitive patient outcome, p. 240
Patient-centered goal, p. 239
Planning, p. 236
Priority setting, p. 237
Scientific rationale, p. 245
Short-term goal, p. 239

evolve WEBSITE

http://evolve.elsevier.com/Potter/fundamentals/

- Review Questions
- Concept Map Creator
- Case Study with Questions
- Audio Glossary
- Interactive Learning Activities
- Key Term Flashcards
- Content Updates

Tonya conducted a thorough assessment of Mr. Jacobs' health status and identified four nursing diagnoses: acute pain related to incisional trauma, deficient knowledge regarding postoperative recovery related to inexperience with surgery, impaired physical mobility related to incisional pain, and anxiety related to uncertainty over course of recovery. Tonya is responsible for planning Mr. Jacobs' nursing care from the time of her initial assessment in the morning until the end of her shift. The care that she plans will continue throughout the course of Mr. Jacobs' hospital stay by the other nurses involved in Mr. Jacobs' care. If Tonya plans well, the individualized interventions that she selects will prepare the patient for a smooth transition home. Collaboration with the patient is critical for a plan of care to be successful. Using input from Mr. Jacobs, Tonya identifies the goals and expected outcomes for each of his nursing diagnoses. The goals and outcomes direct Tonya in selecting appropriate therapeutic interventions. Tonya knows that Mrs. Jacobs' must be involved in the patient's care because of the ongoing support that she provides and because she will be a key care provider once Mr. Jacobs' returns home. In addition, Mr. Jacobs has told Tonya that his wife is the one who keeps their family together. Consultation with other health care providers such as social work or home health ensures that the right resources are used in planning care. Careful planning involves seeing the relationships among a patient's problems, recognizing that certain problems take precedence over others, and proceeding with a safe and efficient approach to care.

After you identify a patient's nursing diagnoses and collaborative problems, you begin planning, the third step of the nursing process. **Planning** involves setting priorities, identifying patient-centered goals and expected outcomes, and prescribing individualized nursing interventions. Ultimately during implementation your interventions resolve the patient's problems and achieve the expected goals and outcomes (see Chapter 19). Planning requires critical thinking applied through deliberate decision making and problem solving. It also involves working closely with patients, their families, and the health care team through communication and ongoing consultation. Patients benefit most when their care represents a collaborative effort from the expertise of all health care team members. A plan of care is dynamic and changes as the patient's needs change.

ESTABLISHING PRIORITIES

Remember that a single patient often has multiple nursing diagnoses and collaborative problems. In addition, once you enter into nursing practice, you do not care for just a single patient. Eventually you care for groups of patients. Being able to carefully and wisely set priorities for a single patient or group of patients ensures the timeliest, relevant, and appropriate care.

Priority setting is the ordering of nursing diagnoses or patient problems using determinations of urgency and/or importance to establish a preferential order for nursing actions (Hendry and Walker, 2004). In other words, as you care for a patient or a group of patients, you must deal with certain aspects of care before others. By ranking a patient's nursing diagnoses in order of importance, you attend to each patient's most important needs and better organize ongoing care activities. Priorities help you to anticipate and sequence nursing interventions when a patient has multiple nursing diagnoses and collaborative problems. Together with your patients, you select mutually agreed-on priorities based on the urgency of the problems, the patient's safety and desires, the nature of the treatment indicated, and the relationship among the diagnoses. Establishing priorities is not a matter of numbering the nursing diagnoses on the basis of severity or physiological importance. Nurses establish priorities in relation to clinical importance, but they also prioritize on the basis of time. On a given day the demands that exist within a health care setting require you to ration your time wisely.

Classify a patient's priorities as high, intermediate, or low importance. Nursing diagnoses that, if untreated, result in harm to a patient or others (e.g., those related to airway status, circulation, safety, and pain) have the highest priorities. One way to consider diagnoses of high priority is to consider Maslow's hierarchy of needs (see Chapter 6). For example, *risk for other-directed violence, impaired gas exchange,* and *decreased cardiac output* are examples of high-priority nursing diagnoses that drive the priorities of safety, adequate oxygenation, and adequate circulation. However, it is always important to consider each patient's unique situation. High priorities are sometimes both physiological and psychological and may address other basic human needs. Avoid classifying only physiological nursing diagnoses as high priority. Consider Mr. Jacobs' case. Among his nursing diagnoses, *acute pain* and *anxiety* are of the highest priority. Tonya knows that she needs to relieve Mr. Jacobs' acute pain and lessen his anxiety so he will be responsive to discharge education and be able to participate in postoperative care activities.

Intermediate priority nursing diagnoses involve nonemergent, nonlife-threatening needs of patients. In Mr. Jacobs' case, *deficient knowledge* and *impaired physical mobility* are both intermediate diagnoses. It is important for Mr. and Mrs. Jacobs' to understand potential problems that develop following surgery, know how to recognize the problems, and be able to continue appropriate care at home. Focused and individualized instruction from all members of the health care team is necessary throughout a patient's hospitalization. The diagnosis of impaired physical mobility is not life threatening and will likely resolve once Tonya and the other nurses collaborate with the surgeon to ensure effective pain control. Relief of pain will make Mr. Jacobs' more mobile and more active in his road to recovery.

Low-priority nursing diagnoses are not always directly related to a specific illness or prognosis but affect the patient's future wellbeing. Many low-priority diagnoses focus on the patient's long-term health care needs. Tonya has not yet identified a nursing diagnosis related to Mr. Jacobs' concern about his sexual function. At this point the patient's anxiety over the uncertainty of the success of surgery, the risk of cancer recurrence, and his concern about his sexual function are the predominant problems. If the patient learns from the surgeon that the procedure resulted in damage to the nerves affecting his sexual performance, a diagnosis more pertinent to this health problem is appropriate.

The order of priorities changes as a patient's condition changes, sometimes within a matter of minutes. Each time you begin a sequence of care such as at the beginning of a hospital shift or a patient's clinic visit, it is important to reorder priorities. For example, when Tonya first met Mr. Jacobs, his *acute pain* was rated at a 7, and it was apparent that the administration of an analgesic was more a priority than trying to reposition or use other nonpharmacological approaches (e.g., relaxation or distraction). Later, after receiving the analgesic, Mr. Jacobs' pain lessened to a level of 4; and Tonya was able to gather more assessment information and begin to focus on his problem of *deficient knowledge.* Ongoing patient assessment is critical to determine the status of your patient's nursing diagnoses. The appropriate ordering of priorities ensures that you meet a patient's needs in a timely and effective way.

Priority setting begins at a holistic level when you identify and prioritize a patient's main diagnoses or problems (Hendry and Walker, 2004). However, you also need to prioritize the specific interventions or strategies that you will use to help a patient achieve desired goals and outcomes. For example, as Tonya considers the high-priority diagnosis of *acute pain* for Mr. Jacobs, she decides during each encounter which intervention to do first among these options: administering an analgesic, repositioning, and teaching relaxation exercises. Critical thinking helps her to prioritize. Tonya knows that a certain degree of pain relief is necessary before a patient can participate in relaxation exercises. When she is in the patient's room, she might decide to turn and reposition Mr. Jacobs first and then prepare the analgesic. However, if Mr. Jacobs expresses that pain is a high level and is too uncomfortable to turn, Tonya chooses obtaining and administering the analgesic as her first priority. Later, with Mr. Jacobs' pain more under control, she considers whether relaxation is appropriate.

Involve patients in priority setting whenever possible. Patient-centered care requires you to know a patient's preferences, values, and expressed needs. Tonya must learn what Mr. Jacobs expects with regard to pain control to have a relevant plan of care in place. In some situations a patient assigns priorities different from those you select. Resolve any conflicting values concerning health care needs and treatments with open communication, informing the patient of all options and consequences. Consulting with and knowing the patient's concerns do not relieve you of the responsibility to act in a patient's best interests. Always assign priorities on the basis of good nursing judgment.

Ethical care is a part of priority setting. When ethical issues make priorities less clear, it is important to have open dialogue with the patient, the family, and other health care providers (Holmstrom and Hoglund, 2007). For example, when you care for a patient nearing death or one newly diagnosed with a chronic long-term disabling disease, you need to be able to discuss the situation fully with the patient, know his or her expectations, know your own professional responsibility in protecting the patient from harm, know the physician's therapeutic or palliative goals, and then form a plan of care. Chapter 22 outlines strategies for choosing a course of action when facing an ethical dilemma.

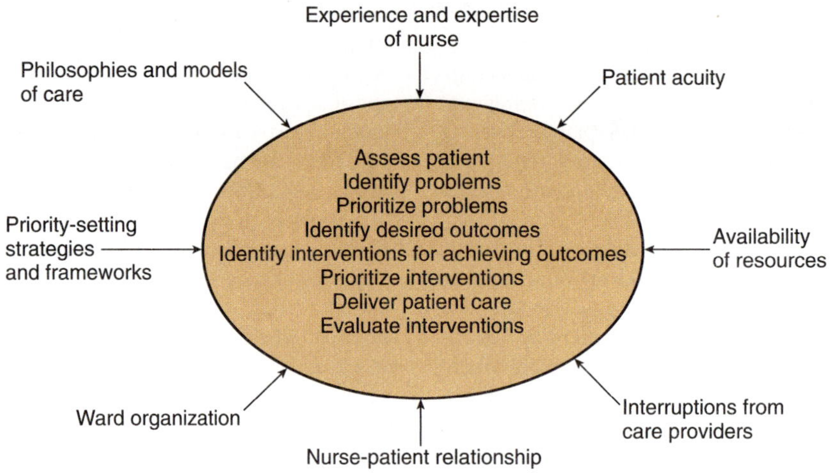

FIG. 18-1 A model for priority setting. (Modified from Hendry C, Walker A: Priority setting in clinical nursing practice, *J Adv Nurs* 47[4]:427, 2004.)

Priorities in Practice

Hendry and Walker (2004) address an important issue regarding priority setting (Fig. 18-1). Many factors within the health care environment affect your ability to set priorities. For example, in the hospital setting the model for delivering care (see Chapter 21), the organization of a nursing unit, staffing levels, and interruptions from other care providers affect the minute-by-minute determination of patient care priorities. Available resources (e.g., nurse specialists, laboratory technicians, and dietitians), policies and procedures, and supply access affect priorities as well. Finally, patients' conditions are always changing; thus priority setting is always changing.

The same factors that influence your minute-by-minute ability to prioritize nursing actions affect the ability to prioritize nursing diagnoses for groups of patients. The nature of nursing work challenges your ability to cognitively attend to a given patient's priorities when you care for more than one patient. The nursing care process is nonlinear (Potter et al., 2005). Often you complete an assessment and identify nursing diagnoses for one patient, leave the room to perform an intervention for a second patient, and move on to consult on a third patient. Nurses exercise "cognitive shifts" (i.e., shifts in attention from one patient to another during the conduct of the nursing process). This shifting of attention occurs in response to changing patient needs, new procedures being ordered, or environmental processes interacting (Potter et al., 2005). Because of these cognitive shifts, it becomes important to stay organized and know your patients' priorities. Always work from your plan of care and use your patients' priorities to organize the order for delivering interventions and organizing documentation of care.

CRITICAL THINKING IN SETTING GOALS AND EXPECTED OUTCOMES

Once you identify nursing diagnoses for a patient, ask yourself, "What is the best approach to address and resolve each problem? What do I plan to achieve?" Goals and expected outcomes are specific statements of patient behavior or physiological responses that you set to resolve a nursing diagnosis or collaborative problem. For example, Tonya chooses to administer ordered analgesics for Mr. Jacobs' *acute pain* and provide nursing measures that promote relaxation and minimize any other sources of discomfort. She hopes to achieve pain relief (goal). The specific patient behaviors or physiological responses (expected outcomes) include Mr. Jacobs' reporting pain at a level below 4, showing more freedom in movement and less grimacing, and being able to participate in education sessions.

During planning you select goals and outcomes for each nursing diagnosis to provide a clear focus for the type of interventions needed to care for your patient and to then evaluate the effectiveness of these interventions. A **goal** is a broad statement that describes a desired change in a patient's condition or behavior. Mr. Jacobs has the diagnosis of *deficient knowledge* regarding his postoperative recovery. A goal of care for this diagnosis includes, "Patient expresses understanding of postoperative risks." The goal requires making Mr. Jacobs aware of the risks associated with his type of surgery. It gives Tonya a clear focus on the topics to include in her instruction. An **expected outcome** is a measurable criterion to evaluate goal achievement. Once an outcome is met, you then know that a goal has been at least partially achieved. Sometimes several expected outcomes must be met for a single goal. Measurable outcomes for the goal of "understanding postoperative risks" include: "Patient identifies signs and symptoms of wound infection," and "Patient explains signs of urinary obstruction," both risks from a prostatectomy. After Tonya instructs Mr. Jacobs, she determines if he can identify signs and symptoms of wound infection; if so, the goal is partially met. If the patient can also explain signs of urinary obstruction, the goal is fully met.

Planning nursing care requires critical thinking (Fig. 18-2). Critically evaluate the identified nursing diagnoses, the urgency or priority of the problems, and the resources of the patient and the health care delivery system. You apply knowledge from the medical, sociobehavioral, and nursing sciences to plan patient care. The selection of goals, expected outcomes, and interventions requires consideration of your previous experience with similar patient problems and any established standards for clinical problem management. The goals and outcomes need to meet established intellectual standards by being relevant to patient needs, specific, singular, observable, measurable, and time limited. You also use critical thinking attitudes in selecting interventions with the greatest likelihood of success.

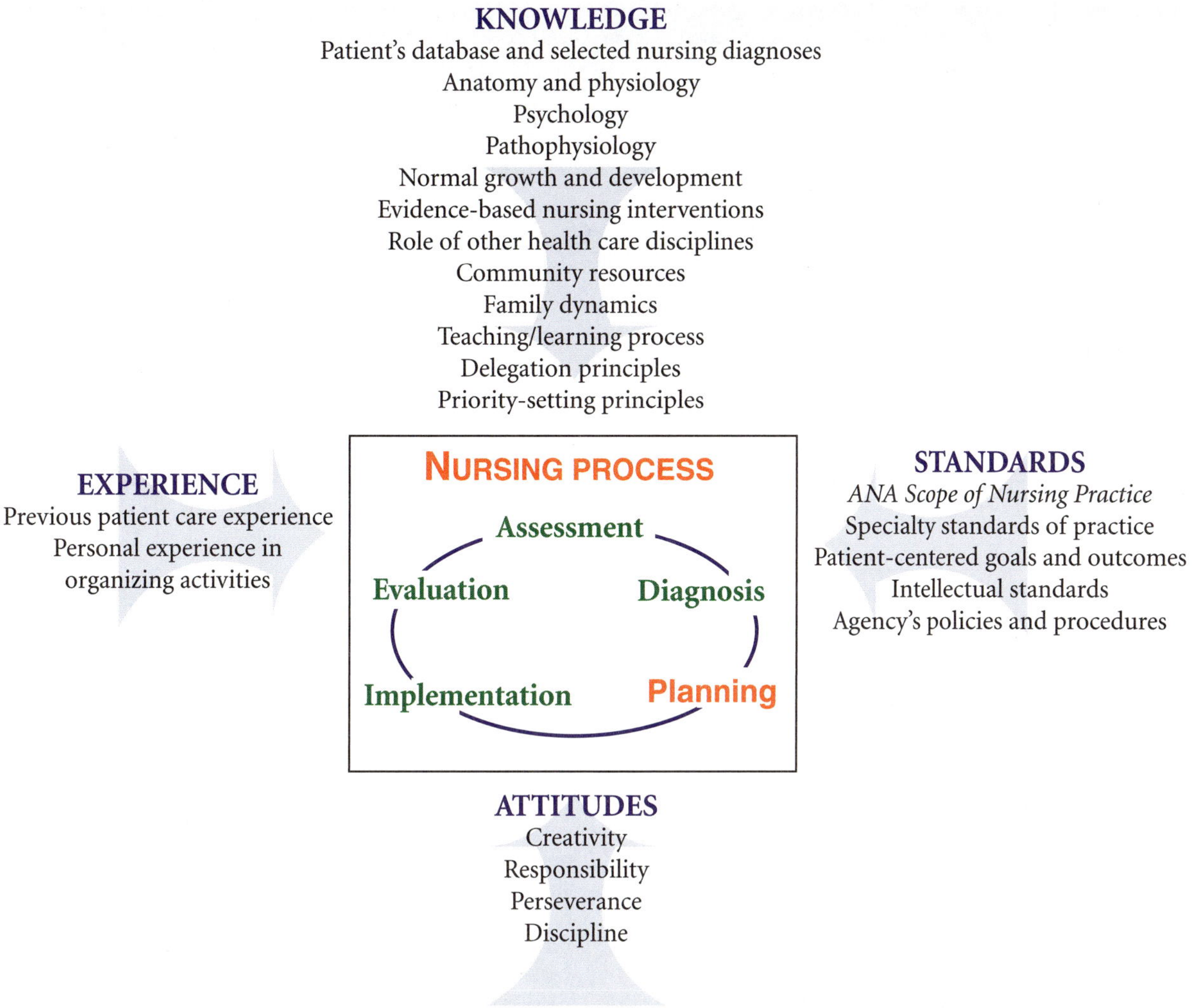

FIG. 18-2 Critical thinking and the process of planning care.

Goals of Care

A **patient-centered goal** reflects a patient's highest possible level of wellness and independence in function. It is realistic and based on patient needs and resources. For example, consider the diagnoses of *acute pain* versus *chronic pain.* A patient such as Mr. Jacobs with *acute pain* can realistically expect pain relief. In contrast, a patient with terminal bone cancer in *chronic pain* can only expect an acceptable level of pain control. A patient goal represents a predicted resolution of a diagnosis or problem, evidence of progress toward resolution, progress toward improved health status, or continued maintenance of good health or function (Carpenito-Moyet, 2009).

Each goal is time limited so the health care team has a common time frame for problem resolution. For example, the goal of "patient will achieve pain relief" for Mr. Jacobs is complete by adding the time frame "by day of discharge." With this goal in place, all efforts by the health care team are aimed at managing the patient's pain. At the time of discharge evaluation of expected outcomes (e.g., pain-rating score, signs of grimacing, level of movement) show if the goal was met. The time frame depends on the nature of the problem, etiology, overall condition of the patient, and treatment setting. A **short-term goal** is an objective behavior or response that you expect a patient to achieve in a short time, usually less than a week. In an acute care setting you often set goals for over a course of just a few hours. A **long-term goal** is an objective behavior or response that you expect a patient to achieve over a longer period, usually over several days, weeks, or months (e.g., "Patient will be tobacco free within 60 days"). Table 18-1 shows the progression from nursing diagnoses to goals and expected outcomes and the relationship to nursing interventions.

Role of the Patient in Goal Setting. Always partner with patients when setting their individualized goals. Mutual goal setting includes the patient and family (when appropriate) in prioritizing the goals of care and developing a plan of action. For patients to participate in goal setting, they need to be alert and have some degree of independence in completing activities of daily living, problem solving, and decision making. Unless goals are mutually set and there is a clear plan of action, patients fail to fully participate in the plan of care. Patients need to understand and see the value of nursing therapies, even though they are often totally dependent on you as the nurse. When setting goals, act as an advocate or support for the patient to select nursing interventions that promote his or her return to health or prevent further deterioration when possible.

TABLE 18-1 Examples of Goal Setting with Expected Outcomes for Mr. Jacobs

NURSING DIAGNOSES	GOALS	EXPECTED OUTCOMES
Acute pain related to incisional trauma	Mr. Jacobs achieves pain relief by day of discharge.	Mr. Jacobs reports pain at a level or 3 or below by discharge. Mr. Jacobs moves and turns freely in bed within 24 hours. Mr. Jacobs shows less grimacing during movement in 24 hours.
Anxiety related to uncertainty over course of recovery	Mr. Jacobs expresses acceptance of health status by day of discharge.	Mr. Jacobs discusses surgical outcomes with surgeon in 24 hours. Mr. Jacobs shares concerns with wife before discharge. Mr. Jacobs describes effects surgery will have on recovery.
Deficient knowledge regarding surgical recovery related to inexperience with surgery	Mr. Jacobs expresses understanding of postoperative risks in 24 hours.	Mr. Jacobs is able to identify signs and symptoms of wound infection in 48 hours. Mr. Jacobs or wife is able to demonstrate catheter care by discharge. Mr. Jacobs is able to identify problems to report to surgeon by discharge.
Impaired physical mobility related to incisional pain	Mr. Jacobs ambulates independently in 3 days.	Mr. Jacobs initiates turning in bed independently in 24 hours. Mr. Jacobs gets up to chair 3 times daily for next 2 days. Mr. Jacobs walks with assistance to hallway in 48 hours.

Tonya has a discussion with Mr. Jacobs and his wife together about setting the plan for the diagnosis of deficient knowledge. Tonya explains the topics that they need to discuss so the couple understands Mr. Jacobs' postoperative risks. They plan the instruction the next day just before lunch when Mrs. Jacobs' visits. Mr. Jacobs asks to have the instruction also include information on how the surgery can affect his sexual function. Tonya agrees and plans to clarify with the surgeon so the information is accurate and realistic. The surgeon has told Mr. Jacobs that there is a risk, but it is too early to know the extent of any possible nerve damage.

Expected Outcomes

An expected outcome is a specific measurable change in a patient's status that you expect to occur in response to nursing care. Outcomes as a result of Mr. Jacobs' postoperative instruction include his ability to describe signs of a surgical wound infection and identify when to call his surgeon with problems. Expected outcomes direct nursing care because they are the desired physiological, psychological, social, developmental, or spiritual responses that indicate resolution of a patient's health problems. A patient's willingness and capability to reach an expected outcome improves his or her likelihood of achieving it. Taken from both short- and long-term goals, outcomes determine when a specific patient-centered goal has been met.

Usually you develop several expected outcomes for each nursing diagnosis and goal because sometimes one nursing action is not enough to resolve a patient problem. In addition, a list of the step-by-step expected outcomes gives you practical guidance in planning interventions. Always write expected outcomes sequentially, with time frames (see Table 18-1). Time frames give you progressive steps in which to move a patient toward recovery and offer an order for nursing interventions. They also set limits for problem resolution.

Nursing Outcomes Classification. Much attention in the current health care environment is focused on measuring outcomes to gauge the quality of health care. If a chosen intervention repeatedly results in desired outcomes that benefit patients, it needs to become part of a standardized approach to a patient problem. For example, if the use of a chlorhexidine mouthwash (intervention) repeatedly results in a lower incidence of aspiration pneumonia (outcome) in critically ill patients, use of the mouthwash needs to become part of standard mouth care in critical care units.

Nursing plays an important role in monitoring and managing patient conditions and diagnosing problems that are amenable to nursing intervention. The clinical reasoning and decision making of nurses is a key part of quality health care (Moorhead et al., 2008). Thus it becomes important to identify and measure patient outcomes that are influenced by nursing care. A **nursing-sensitive patient outcome** is a measurable patient, family or community state, behavior, or perception largely influenced by and sensitive to nursing interventions (Moorhead et al., 2008). For the nursing profession to become a full participant in clinical evaluation research, policy development, and interdisciplinary work, nurses need to identify and measure patient outcomes influenced by nursing interventions. The Iowa Intervention Project has done just that. It published the Nursing Outcomes Classification (NOC) and linked the outcomes to NANDA International nursing diagnoses (Moorhead et al., 2008). For each NANDA International nursing diagnosis there are multiple NOC suggested outcomes. These outcomes have labels for describing the focus of nursing care and include indicators to use in evaluating the success with nursing interventions (Table 18-2). NOC contains outcomes for individuals, family caregivers, the family, and the community in all health care settings. Efforts to measure outcomes and capture the changes in the status of patients over time allow nurses to improve patient care quality and add to nursing knowledge (Moorhead et al., 2008). The use of a common set of outcomes allows nurses to study the effects of nursing interventions over time and across settings. The fourth edition of NOC standardizes the way to measure patient outcomes. It is an excellent resource for you to develop care plans and concept maps. NOC outcomes provide a common nursing language for continuity of care and measurement of the success of nursing interventions.

Guidelines for Writing Goals and Expected Outcomes

There are seven guidelines for writing goals and expected outcomes.

Patient-Centered. Outcomes and goals reflect patient behaviors and responses expected as a result of nursing interventions. Write a goal or outcome to reflect a patient's specific behavior, not to reflect your goals or interventions.

TABLE 18-2 Examples of NANDA International Nursing Diagnoses and Suggested NOC Linkages

NURSING DIAGNOSIS	SUGGESTED NOC OUTCOMES (EXAMPLES)	OUTCOME INDICATORS (EXAMPLES)
Deficient knowledge	Knowledge: Treatment Procedures	Description of treatment procedure Description of steps in procedure
	Knowledge: Disease Process	Effects of disease Specific disease process
Activity intolerance	Activity Tolerance	Oxygen saturation with activity Pulse rate with activity Respiratory rate with activity
	Self-Care Status	Bathes self Dresses self Prepares food and fluid for eating

NOC, Nursing Outcomes Classification.

- A correct goal statement: "Patient will ambulate independently in 3 days."
- A correct outcome statement: "Patient will ambulate in the hall 3 times a day by 4/22."
- A common error is to write an intervention: "Ambulate patient in the hall 3 times a day."

Singular Goal or Outcome. You want to be precise when you evaluate a patient's response to a nursing action. Each goal and outcome should address only one behavior or response. If an outcome reads, "Patient's lungs will be clear to auscultation, and respiratory rate will be 20 breaths per minute by 8/22," your measurement of outcomes will be complicated. When you evaluate that the lungs are clear but the respiratory rate is 28 breaths per minute, you do not know if the patient achieved the expected outcome. By splitting the statement into two parts, "Lungs will be clear to auscultation by 8/22," and "Respiratory rate will be 20 breaths per minute by 8/22," you are able to determine if and when the patient achieves each outcome. Singularity allows you to decide if there is a need to modify the plan of care.

A goal also contains only one behavior or response. The example, "Patient will administer a self-injection and demonstrate infection control measures," is incorrect because the statement includes two different behaviors, administer and demonstrate. Instead word the goal as follows, "Patient will administer a self-injection by discharge." The specific criteria you use to measure success of the goal are the singular expected outcomes. For example, "Patient will prepare medication dose correctly," and "Patient uses medical asepsis when preparing injection site."

Observable. You need to be able to observe if change takes place in a patient's status. Observable changes occur in physiological findings and in the patient's knowledge, perceptions, and behavior. You observe outcomes by directly asking patients about their condition or using assessment skills. For example, you observe the goal, "Patient will be able to self-administer insulin," through the outcome of watching, "Patient prepares insulin dosage correctly by 8/30." For the outcome, "Lungs will be clear on auscultation by 8/31," you auscultate the lungs following any therapy. The outcome statement, "Patient will appear less anxious," is not correct because there is no specific behavior observable for "will appear." A more correct outcome is, "Patient will show better eye contact during conversations."

Measurable. You learn to write goals and expected outcomes that set standards against which to measure the patient's response to nursing care. Examples such as, "Body temperature will remain 98.6° F," and, "Apical pulse will remain between 60 and 100 beats per minute," allow you to objectively measure changes in the patient's status. Do not use vague qualifiers such as "normal," "acceptable," or "stable" in an expected outcome statement. Vague terms result in guesswork in determining a patient's response to care. Terms describing quality, quantity, frequency, length, or weight allow you to evaluate outcomes precisely.

Time-Limited. The time frame for each goal and expected outcome indicates when you expect the response to occur. It is very important to collaborate with patients to set realistic and reasonable time frames. Time frames help you and the patient to determine if the patient is making progress at a reasonable rate. If not, you must revise the plan of care. Time frames also promote accountability in delivering and managing nursing care.

Mutual Factors. Mutually set goals and expected outcomes ensure that the patient and nurse agree on the direction and time limits of care. Mutual goal setting increases the patient's motivation and cooperation. As a patient advocate, apply standards of practice, evidence-based knowledge, safety principles, and basic human needs when assisting patients with setting goals. Your knowledge background helps you select goals and outcomes that should be met on the basis of typical responses to clinical interventions. Yet you must consider patients' desires to recover and their physical and psychological condition to set goals and outcomes to which they can agree.

Realistic. Set goals and expected outcomes that a patient is able to reach based on your assessment. This is a challenge when the time allotted for care is limited. But it also means that you must communicate these goals and outcomes to caregivers in other settings who will assume responsibility for patient care (e.g., home health, rehabilitation). Realistic goals provide patients a sense of hope that increases motivation and cooperation. To establish realistic goals, assess the resources of the patient, health care facility, and family. Be aware of the patient's physiological, emotional, cognitive, and sociocultural potential and the economic cost and resources available to reach expected outcomes in a timely manner.

CRITICAL THINKING IN PLANNING NURSING CARE

Part of the planning process is to select nursing interventions for meeting the patient's goals and outcomes. Once nursing diagnoses have been identified and goals and outcomes are selected, you choose interventions individualized for the patient's situation. Nursing interventions are treatments or actions based on clinical judgment and knowledge that nurses perform to meet patient outcomes (Bulechek et al., 2008). During planning you select interventions designed to help a patient move from the present level of health to the level described in the goal and measured by the expected outcomes. The actual implementation of these interventions occurs during the implementation phase of the nursing process (see Chapter 19).

Choosing suitable nursing interventions involves critical thinking and your ability to be competent in three areas: (1) knowing the scientific rationale for the intervention, (2) possessing the necessary psychomotor and interpersonal skills, and (3) being able to function within a particular setting to use the available health care resources effectively (Bulechek et al., 2008).

Types of Interventions

There are three categories of nursing interventions: nurse-initiated, physician-initiated, and collaborative interventions. Some patients require all three categories, whereas other patients need only nurse- and physician-initiated interventions.

Nurse-initiated interventions are the **independent nursing interventions,** or actions that a nurse initiates. These do not require an order from another health care professional. As a nurse you act independently on a patient's behalf. Nurse-initiated interventions are autonomous actions based on scientific rationale. Examples include elevating an edematous extremity, instructing patients in side effects of medications, or repositioning a patient to achieve pain relief. Such interventions benefit a patient in a predicted way related to nursing diagnoses and patient goals (Bulechek et al., 2008). Nurse-initiated interventions require no supervision or direction from others. Each state within the United States has Nurse Practice Acts that define the legal scope of nursing practice (see Chapter 23). According to the Nurse Practice Acts in a majority of states, independent nursing interventions pertain to activities of daily living, health education and promotion, and counseling. For Mr. Jacobs Tonya selects anxiety-reduction interventions such as using a calm and reassuring approach, listening attentively, and providing factual information.

Physician-initiated interventions are **dependent nursing interventions,** or actions that require an order from a physician or another health care professional. The interventions are based on the physician's or health care provider's response to treat or manage a medical diagnosis. Advanced practice nurses who work under collaborative agreements with physicians or who are licensed independently by state practice acts are also able to write dependent interventions. As a nurse you intervene by carrying out the provider's written and/or verbal orders. Administering a medication, implementing an invasive procedure (e.g., inserting a Foley catheter, starting an intravenous [IV] infusion), changing a dressing, and preparing a patient for diagnostic tests are examples of physician-initiated interventions.

Each physician-initiated intervention requires specific nursing responsibilities and technical nursing knowledge. You are often the one performing the intervention, and you must know the types of observations and precautions to take for the intervention to be delivered safely and correctly. For example, when administering a medication you are responsible for not only giving the medicine correctly, but also knowing the classification of the drug, its physiological action, normal dosage, side effects, and nursing interventions related to its action or side effects (see Chapter 31). You are responsible for knowing when an invasive procedure is necessary, the clinical skills necessary to complete it, and its expected outcome and possible side effects. You are also responsible for adequate preparation of the patient and proper communication of the results. You perform dependent nursing interventions, like all nursing actions, with appropriate knowledge, clinical reasoning, and good clinical judgment.

Collaborative interventions, or interdependent interventions, are therapies that require the combined knowledge, skill, and expertise of multiple health care professionals. Typically when you plan care for a patient, you review the necessary interventions and determine if the collaboration of other health care disciplines is necessary. A patient care conference with an interdisciplinary health care team results in selection of interdependent interventions.

In the case study involving Mr. Jacobs, Tonya plans independent interventions to help calm Mr. Jacobs' anxiety and begin teaching him about postoperative care activities. Among the dependent interventions Tonya plans to implement are the administration of an analgesic and ordered wound care. Tonya's collaborative intervention involves consulting with the unit discharge coordinator, who will help Mr. and Mrs. Jacobs plan for their return home and consult with the home health department to ensure that the Jacobs have home health visits.

When preparing for physician-initiated or collaborative interventions, do not automatically implement the therapy but determine whether it is appropriate for the patient. Every nurse faces an inappropriate or incorrect order at some time. The nurse with a strong knowledge base recognizes the error and seeks to correct it. The ability to recognize incorrect therapies is particularly important when administering medications or implementing procedures. Errors occur in writing orders or transcribing them to a documentation form or computer screen. Clarifying an order is competent nursing practice, and it protects the patient and members of the health care team. When you carry out an incorrect or inappropriate intervention, it is as much your error as the person who wrote or transcribed the original order. You are legally responsible for any complications resulting from the error (see Chapter 23).

Selection of Interventions

During planning do not select interventions randomly. For example, patients with the diagnosis of *anxiety* do not always need care in the same way with the same interventions. You treat *anxiety related to the uncertainty of surgical recovery* very differently than *anxiety related to a threat to loss of family role function.* When choosing interventions, consider six important factors: (1) characteristics of the nursing diagnosis, (2) goals and expected outcomes, (3) evidence base (e.g., research or proven practice guidelines) for the interventions, (4) feasibility of the intervention, (5) acceptability to the patient, and (6) your own competency (Bulechek et al., 2008) (Box 18-1). When considering a plan of care, review resources such as the nursing literature, standard protocols or guidelines, the Nursing Interventions Classification (NIC), critical pathways, policy or procedure manuals, or textbooks. Collaboration with other health professionals is also useful. As you select interventions, review your patient's needs, priorities, and previous experiences to select the interventions that have the best potential for achieving the expected outcomes.

Nursing Interventions Classification. Just as with the standardized NOC, the Iowa Intervention Project has also developed a set of nursing interventions that provides a level of standardization to enhance communication of nursing care across all health care settings and to compare outcomes (Bulechek et al., 2008). The NIC model includes three levels: domains, classes, and interventions for ease of use. The domains are the highest level (level 1) of the model, using broad terms (e.g., safety and basic physiological) to organize the more specific classes and interventions (Table 18-3). The second level of the model includes 30 classes, which offer useful clinical categories to reference when selecting interventions. The third level of the model includes the 542 interventions, defined as any treatment based on clinical judgment and knowledge that a nurse performs to enhance patient outcomes (Bulechek et al., 2008) (Box 18-2). Each intervention then includes a variety of

BOX 18-1 CHOOSING NURSING INTERVENTIONS

Characteristics of the Nursing Diagnosis

- Interventions should alter the etiological (related to) factor or signs and symptoms associated with the diagnostic label. ***Example: Acute pain related to incisional trauma—choose interventions that relieve swelling and strain on incision site (positioning and turning measures) and lower pain reception (analgesic).***
- When an etiological factor cannot change, direct the interventions toward treating the signs and symptoms (e.g., defining characteristics for a diagnosis). ***Example: Deficient knowledge regarding surgical recovery related to inexperience—choose interventions directed toward providing information that answer patient's questions about recovery procedures and relieve anxiety.***
- For potential or high-risk diagnoses, direct interventions at altering or eliminating risk factors for the diagnosis.

Expected Outcomes

- State outcomes in terms used to evaluate the effect of an intervention. This language assists in selecting the intervention. ***Example: For the outcome "patient will perform urinary catheter care by discharge," the nurse will evaluate skills instruction by observing the patient perform catheter care.***
- Nursing Interventions Classification (NIC) is designed to show the link to Nursing Outcomes Classification (NOC) (Moorhead et al., 2008). Use these resources in developing care plans.

Research Base

- Research evidence in support of a nursing intervention will indicate the effectiveness of using the intervention with certain types of patients.
- Refer to the evidence (e.g., research articles or evidence-based practice protocols that describe the use of evidence in similar clinical situations and settings) in selecting interventions.
- When research is not available, use scientific principles (e.g., infection control) or consult a clinical expert about your patient.

Feasibility

- A specific intervention has the potential to interact with other interventions.
- Be knowledgeable about the total plan of care.
- Consider cost: Is the intervention clinically effective and cost efficient?
- Consider time: Are time and personnel resources available? ***Example: If you plan to get a patient up into a chair 3 times a day, will there be staff to assist with the transfer?***

Acceptability to the Patient

- A treatment plan needs to be acceptable to the patient and family and match the patient's goals, health care values, and culture.
- Promote informed choice; help a patient know how to participate in and anticipate the effect of interventions.

Capability of the Nurse

- Be prepared to carry out the intervention.
- Have the necessary psychosocial and psychomotor skills to complete the intervention.
- Be able to function within the specific setting and effectively and efficiently use health care resources.

Modified from Bulechek GM et al: *Nursing interventions classification (NIC),* ed 5, St Louis, 2008, Mosby.

BOX 18-2 EXAMPLE OF INTERVENTIONS FOR PHYSICAL COMFORT PROMOTION

Class: Physical Comfort Promotion

Interventions to promote comfort using physical techniques

Interventions (Examples)

Aromatherapy
Cutaneous Stimulation
Environmental Management
Heat/Cold Application
Nausea Management
Pain Management
Progressive Muscle Relaxation
Simple Massage

Examples of Linked Nursing Diagnoses

Acute Pain
Chronic Pain

From Bulechek GM et al: *Nursing interventions classification (NIC),* ed 5, St Louis, 2008, Mosby.

BOX 18-3 EXAMPLE OF AN INTERVENTION AND ASSOCIATED NURSING ACTIVITIES

Intervention—Environmental Management: Comfort

Examples of Activities

- Create a calm and supportive environment.
- Provide a safe and clean environment.
- Adjust room temperature to that most comfortable for the individual.
- Avoid unnecessary exposure, drafts, overheating, or chilling.
- Prevent unnecessary interruptions and allow for rest period.
- Monitor skin, especially over bony prominences, for signs of pressure or irritation.
- Provide prompt attention to call bells, which should always be within reach.

From Bulechek GM et al: *Nursing interventions classification (NIC),* ed 5, St Louis, 2008, Mosby.

nursing activities from which to choose (Box 18-3) and which a nurse commonly uses in a plan of care. NIC interventions are also linked with NANDA International nursing diagnoses for ease of use (NANDA International, 2012). For example, if a patient has a nursing diagnosis of *acute pain,* there are 21 recommended interventions, including pain management, cutaneous stimulation, and anxiety reduction. Each of the recommended interventions has a variety of activities for nursing care. NIC is a valuable resource for selecting appropriate interventions and activities for your patient. It is evolving and practice oriented. The classification is comprehensive, including independent and collaborative interventions. It remains your decision to determine which interventions and activities best suit your patient's individualized needs and situation.

SYSTEMS FOR PLANNING NURSING CARE

In any health care setting a nurse is responsible for providing a nursing plan of care for all patients. The plan of care sometimes takes several forms (e.g., nursing Kardex, standardized care plans, and computerized plans). More hospitals today are adopting

TABLE 18-3 Nursing Interventions Classification (NIC) Taxonomy

DOMAIN 1	DOMAIN 2	DOMAIN 3
Level 1 Domains		
1. Physiological: Basic Care that supports physical functioning	**2. Physiological: Complex** Care that supports homeostatic regulation	**3. Behavioral** Care that supports psychosocial functioning and facilitates lifestyle changes
Level 2 Classes		
A *Activity and Exercise Management:* Interventions to organize or assist with physical activity and energy conservation and expenditure	G *Electrolyte and Acid-Base Management:* Interventions to regulate electrolyte/acid-base balance and prevent complications	O *Behavior Therapy:* Interventions to reinforce or promote desirable behaviors or alter undesirable behaviors
B *Elimination Management:* Interventions to establish and maintain regular bowel and urinary elimination patterns and manage complications caused by altered patterns	H *Drug Management:* Interventions to facilitate desired effects of pharmacological agents	P *Cognitive Therapy:* Interventions to reinforce or promote desirable cognitive functioning or alter undesirable cognitive functioning
C *Immobility Management:* Interventions to manage restricted body movement and the sequelae	I *Neurological Management:* Interventions to optimize neurological functions	Q *Communication Enhancement:* Interventions to facilitate delivering and receiving verbal and nonverbal messages
D *Nutrition Support:* Interventions to modify or maintain nutritional status	J *Perioperative Care:* Interventions to provide care before, during, and immediately after surgery	R *Coping Assistance:* Interventions to assist another to build on own strengths, adapt to a change in function, or achieve a higher level of function
E *Physical Comfort Promotion:* Interventions to promote comfort using physical techniques	K *Respiratory Management:* Interventions to promote airway patency and gas exchange	S *Patient Education:* Interventions to facilitate learning
F *Self-Care Facilitation:* Interventions to provide or assist with routine activities of daily living	L *Skin/Wound Management:* Interventions to maintain or restore tissue integrity	T *Psychological Comfort Promotion:* Interventions to promote comfort using psychological techniques
	M *Thermoregulation:* Interventions to maintain body temperature within a normal range	
	N *Tissue Perfusion Management:* Interventions to optimize circulation of blood and fluids to the tissue	

From Bulechek GM et al: *Nursing interventions classification (NIC),* ed 5, St Louis, 2008, Mosby.

electronic health records (EHRs) and a documentation system that includes software programs for nursing care plans (Hebda et al., 2009). Generally a **nursing care plan** includes nursing diagnoses, goals and/or expected outcomes, specific nursing interventions, and a section for evaluation findings so any nurse is able to quickly identify a patient's clinical needs and situation. Nurses revise a plan when a patient's status changes. Electronic care plans often follow a standardized format, but you can individualize each plan to a unique patient's needs (see Chapter 26). The standardized format is usually based on nursing diagnoses or select problem areas, which nurses are able to individualize for a specific patient. In hospitals and community-based settings, patients receive care from more than one nurse, physician, or allied health professional. Thus more institutions are developing **interdisciplinary care plans,** which include contributions from all disciplines involved in patient care. The interdisciplinary plan is designed to improve the coordination of all patient therapies and communication among all disciplines.

A nursing care plan reduces the risk for incomplete, incorrect, or inaccurate care. As the patient's problems and status change, so does the plan. A nursing care plan is a guideline for coordinating nursing care, promoting continuity of care, and listing outcome criteria to be used later in evaluation (see Chapter 20). The plan of care communicates nursing care priorities to nurses and other health care professionals. It also identifies and coordinates resources for delivering nursing care. For example, in a care plan you list specific supplies necessary to use in a dressing change or names of clinical nurse specialists who are providing consultation for a patient.

The nursing care plan enhances the continuity of nursing care by listing specific nursing interventions needed to achieve the goals of care. All nurses who care for a given patient carry out these nursing interventions (e.g., throughout each day during a patient's length of stay [in a hospital] or during weekly visits to the home [home health nursing]). A correctly formulated nursing care plan makes it easy to continue care from one nurse to another. The Nursing Care Plan provides an example of a care plan for Mr. Jacobs, using the format found throughout this text.

A care plan includes a patient's long-term needs. Incorporating the goals of the care plan into discharge planning is important. Thus it is beneficial to involve the family in planning care if the patient is agreeable. The family is often a resource to help the patient meet health care goals. In addition, meeting some of the family's needs will possibly improve the patient's level of wellness. Discharge planning is especially important for a patient undergoing long-term rehabilitation in the community and who will require ongoing home care. Same-day surgeries and earlier discharges from hospitals require you to begin planning discharge from the moment the patient enters the health care agency. The complete care plan is the blueprint for nursing action. It provides direction for implementation of the plan and a framework for evaluation of the patient's response to nursing actions.

Change of Shift

The change-of-shift report is the standard practice used for off-going nurses leaving a shift to communicate information about the patient's plan of care to oncoming patient care personnel. At the

DOMAIN 4	DOMAIN 5	DOMAIN 6	DOMAIN 7
4. **Safety** Care that supports protection against harm	5. **Family** Care that supports the family	6. **Health System** Care that supports effective use of the health care delivery system	7. **Community** Care that supports the health of the community
U *Crisis Management:* Interventions to provide immediate short-term help in both psychological and physiological crises	W *Childbearing Care:* Interventions to assist in understanding and coping with the psychological and physiological changes during the childbearing period	Y *Health System Mediation:* Interventions to facilitate the interface between patient/family and the health care system	c *Community Health Promotion:* Interventions that promote the health of the whole community
V *Risk Management:* Interventions to initiate risk-reduction activities and continue monitoring risks over time	Z *Childrearing Care:* Interventions to assist in rearing children	a *Health System Management:* Interventions to provide and enhance support services for the delivery of care	d *Community Risk Management:* Interventions that assist in detecting or preventing health risks to the whole community
	X *Life Span Care:* Interventions to facilitate family unit functioning and promote the health and welfare of family members throughout the life span	b *Information Management:* Interventions to facilitate communication among health care providers	

end of a shift you discuss your patients' plans of care and their overall progress with the next caregivers. Thus all nurses are able to discuss current and relevant information about each patient's plan of care. The newest term used to describe this process is *nursing handoff*. It is a critical time when nurses collaborate and share important information that ensures the continuity of care for a patient and prevents errors or delays in providing nursing interventions. In the past the change-of-shift report typically involved nurses leaving their report on an audiotape recorder, which would be heard by the oncoming nursing staff. This approach did not consistently allow staff from both shifts to share information one on one, ask questions, clarify misunderstandings, and validate the patients' priority problems. Audiotapes are often difficult to hear, and frequently nurses omit information. In some agencies, the nursing handoff process occurs during walking rounds when nurses exchange information about patients at the bedside, giving patients the opportunity to also ask questions and confirm information. Recent research identifies approaches to use for effective handoffs and barriers to their effectiveness. However, there is no evidence for one best nursing hand-off practice (Riesenberg et al., 2010) (Box 18-4). Written care plans organize information exchanged by nurses in change-of-shift reports (see Chapter 26). You learn to focus your reports on the nursing care, treatments, and expected outcomes documented in the care plans. Avoid adding personal opinions about the patient since these are not relevant and could unnecessarily influence the oncoming nurse's perception of him or her as an individual.

Student Care Plans

Student care plans are useful for learning the problem-solving technique, the nursing process, skills of written communication, and organizational skills needed for nursing care. Most important, a student care plan helps you apply knowledge gained from the nursing and medical literature and the classroom to a practice situation. Students typically write a care plan for each nursing diagnosis. The student care plan is more elaborate than a care plan used in a hospital or community agency because its purpose is to teach the process of planning care. Each school uses a different format for student care plans. Often, the format used is similar to the one used by the health care agency that provides students from that school their clinical experiences.

One example of a form of care plan developed by students is the six-column format. Starting from left to right, the six columns include: (1) assessment data relevant to corresponding diagnosis, (2) goals, (3) outcomes identified for the patient, (4) implementation for the plan of care, (5) a **scientific rationale** (the reason that you chose a specific nursing action, based on supporting evidence), and (6) a section to evaluate your care. In the implementation section you select the interventions appropriate for the patient. The following questions help you design a plan:

- *What* is the intervention?
- *When* should each intervention be implemented?
- *How* should the intervention be performed for this specific patient?
- *Who* should be involved in each aspect of intervention?

NURSING CARE PLAN

Anxiety

ASSESSMENT

Mr. Jacobs is a 58-year-old patient who had a radical prostatectomy for prostate cancer yesterday. The patient has a surgical incision in the retropubic area, which is a low midline abdominal incision. The surgery involves removal of the prostate gland, seminal vesicles, and part of the bladder neck. After the surgery there are risks of the patient having erectile dysfunction and incontinence. Before surgery Mr. Jacobs' doctor told him that the surgery could change his ability to have sex and there was also a chance of some urinary incontinence. The surgeon has not discussed this topic with Mr. Jacobs since the patient came to the surgical nursing unit. Mr. Jacobs' wife has been with the patient and is the person who will provide care and support in the home.

*Assessment Activities**	*Findings/Defining Characteristics*
Ask patient what concerns he has about surgery.	Patient **states being worried** about his wife and himself and the risk of sexual dysfunction. Patient also worries because he has a friend who had cancer.
Observe patient's facial expression.	Patient shows **poor eye contact** when discussing condition.
Observe body movements.	Patient shows **tenseness** in way he **clenches hands** and in **facial expression.**

*__Defining characteristics__ are shown in bold type.

NURSING DIAGNOSIS: Anxiety related to uncertainty over course of recovery

PLANNING

Goals	*Expected Outcomes (NOC)*†
	Acceptance: Health Status
Mr. Jacobs expresses acceptance of health status by day of discharge.	Patient discusses surgical outcomes with surgeon in 24 hours. Patient shares concerns with wife before day of discharge. Patient describes effects surgery will have on recovery by day of discharge.
	Anxiety Level
Mr. Jacobs expresses relief of concerns by day of discharge.	Patient maintains eye contact during instructional discussions in 24 hours. Patient shows less facial tension during discussions in 24 hours. Patient is able to concentrate and attend to instructions in 48 hours.

†Outcomes classification labels from Moorhead S et al: *Nursing outcomes classification (NOC),* ed 4, St Louis, 2008, Mosby.

INTERVENTIONS (NIC)‡	RATIONALE
Anxiety Reduction	
Use a calm, reassuring approach in discussions	For patient to be able to express concerns, he must see nurse as being nonthreatening, reliable, and understanding (Vacarolis and Halter, 2009).
When pain is under control, have patient verbalize his perceptions, feelings, and fears.	Pain relief allows patient to attend to issues causing anxiety and discuss them more.
Encourage Mrs. Jacobs to stay with her husband as much as possible; include her in discussions.	A support system benefits a patient experiencing stress. Strong families tend to have good problem-solving skills and a commitment to one another (Schumacher et al., 2006).
Instruct Mr. Jacobs in use of progressive relaxation techniques.	Techniques teach patient how to effectively rest and reduce muscle tension, reduce symptom distress, and improve well-being (Hui et al., 2006).
Collaborate with physician to provide factual information concerning diagnosis, treatment, and prognosis.	The nurse often clarifies information provided by health care providers and is often the primary source of information needed for a patient to adjust to health problems (Bastable, 2006).

‡Intervention classification labels from Bulechek GM, Butcher HK, and Dochterman JM: *Nursing interventions classification (NIC),* ed 5, St Louis, 2008, Mosby.

EVALUATION

Nursing Actions	*Patient Response/Finding*	*Achievement of Outcome*
Ask Mr. Jacobs to describe what he understands about the result of his surgery and how it will affect his recovery.	Mr. Jacobs reports that his surgeon has told him the nerve affecting his ability to have sex was saved. He knows he has to have the catheter in for about a week but is not sure if incontinence is likely.	Outcomes partially met. Will discuss likelihood of incontinence more fully with surgeon. Adjust instructional plan as needed.
Observe Mr. Jacob's facial expressions.	Mr. Jacobs assumes more comfortable position in bed with less clenching of hands and a more relaxed facial expression. He maintains eye contact during discussions.	Patient's level of tension is declining.

BOX 18-4 EVIDENCE-BASED PRACTICE

Nursing Hand-Offs

PICO Question: Does the use of handoff communication compared with traditional report between nurses in acute care settings reduce errors?

Evidence Summary

A nursing handoff or change-of-shift report involves a nurse-to-nurse verbal exchange of information about patients (Athwal et al., 2009). The process involves communicating essential information to oncoming nurses, which occurs in the form of patient bedside rounds and taped or verbal reports in a conference room. Athwal et al. (2009) found that a combination of a written update along with a bedside shift report reduced the total time expended for shift report, reduced nurse overtime hours, and led to fewer times patients used call lights. In a systematic review of scientific articles discussing nursing handoffs, Riesenberg, Leisch, and Cunningham (2010) identified a number of strategies for effective handoffs and barriers to effective handoffs. However, the researchers stress that no evidence points to best nursing handoff practices and whether errors are reduced. There are risks in implementing interventions when strong evidence is lacking. Thus nurses need to carefully consider the strategies that this study found useful and decide if they fit their own institutional setting and resources.

Application to Nursing Practice

Strategies for Effective Nursing Handoffs

- Manage your time so you are prepared to give report and be concise.
- Keep report patient-centered; ask questions and clarify.
- Standardize the process using tools, forms, and checklists and be sure that essential information is consistently included.
- During walking rounds include patient and family in discussion of goals.
- Limit interruptions and distraction.

Barriers to Effective Nursing Handoffs

- Communication barriers, including omissions (missing or incomplete information), errors (incorrect, extraneous, duplicate), disorganized report or one that is routine and not individualized
- Social problems, including a culture of blame on unit that inhibits questioning
- Complexity of cases and high patient care load—increased volume of patient information and inadequate time to report

Each scientific rationale that you use to support a nursing intervention needs to include a reference, whenever possible, to document the source from the scientific literature. This reinforces the importance of evidence-based nursing practice. It is also important that each intervention be specific and unique to a patient's situation. Nonspecific nursing interventions result in incomplete or inaccurate nursing care, lack of continuity among caregivers, and poor use of resources. Common omissions that nurses make in writing nursing interventions include action, frequency, quantity, method, or person to perform them. These errors occur when nurses are unfamiliar with the planning process. Table 18-4 illustrates these types of errors by showing incorrect and correct statements of nursing interventions. The sixth column of the care plan includes a section for you to evaluate the plan of care: was each outcome fully or only partially met? Use the evaluation column to document whether the plan requires revision or when outcomes are met, thus indicating when a particular nursing diagnosis is no longer relevant to the patient's plan of care (see Chapter 20).

Care Plans for Community-Based Settings. Planning care for patients in community-based settings (e.g., clinics, community centers, or patients' homes) involves using the same principles of nursing practice. However, in these settings you need to complete a more comprehensive community, home, and family assessment. Ultimately the patient/family unit must be able to independently provide the majority of health care. You design a plan to (1) educate the patient/family about the necessary care techniques and precautions, (2) teach the patient/family how to integrate care within family activities, and (3) guide the patient/family on how to assume a greater percentage of care over time. Finally the plan includes nurses' and the patient's/family's evaluation of expected outcomes.

Critical Pathways. Critical pathways are patient care management plans that provide the multidisciplinary health care team with the activities and tasks to be put into practice sequentially (over time); their main purpose is to deliver timely care at each phase of the care process for a specific type of patient (Espinosa-Aguilar et al., 2008). A critical pathway clearly defines transition points in patient progress and draws a coordinated map of activities by which the health care team can help to make these transitions as efficient as possible. A pathway allows staff from all

TABLE 18-4 Frequent Errors in Writing Nursing Interventions

TYPE OF ERROR	INCORRECTLY STATED NURSING INTERVENTION	CORRECTLY STATED NURSING INTERVENTION
Failure to precisely or completely indicate nursing actions	Turn patient every 2 hours.	Turn patient every 2 hours, using the following schedule: 8 AM—supine 10 AM—left side; Noon—prone 2 PM—right side } Repeat at 4 PM and 2 AM
Failure to indicate frequency	Perform blood glucose measurements.	Measure blood glucose before each meal: 7 AM—11 AM—5 PM.
Failure to indicate quantity	Irrigate wound once a shift: 6 AM—2 PM—8 PM.	Irrigate wound with 100 mL normal saline until clear: 6 AM—2 PM—8 PM.
Failure to indicate method	Change patient's dressing once a shift: 6 AM—2 PM—10 PM.	Replace patient's dressing with Neosporin ointment to wound and two dry 4 × 4 dressings secured with hypoallergenic tape once a shift: 2 PM—10 PM—6 AM.

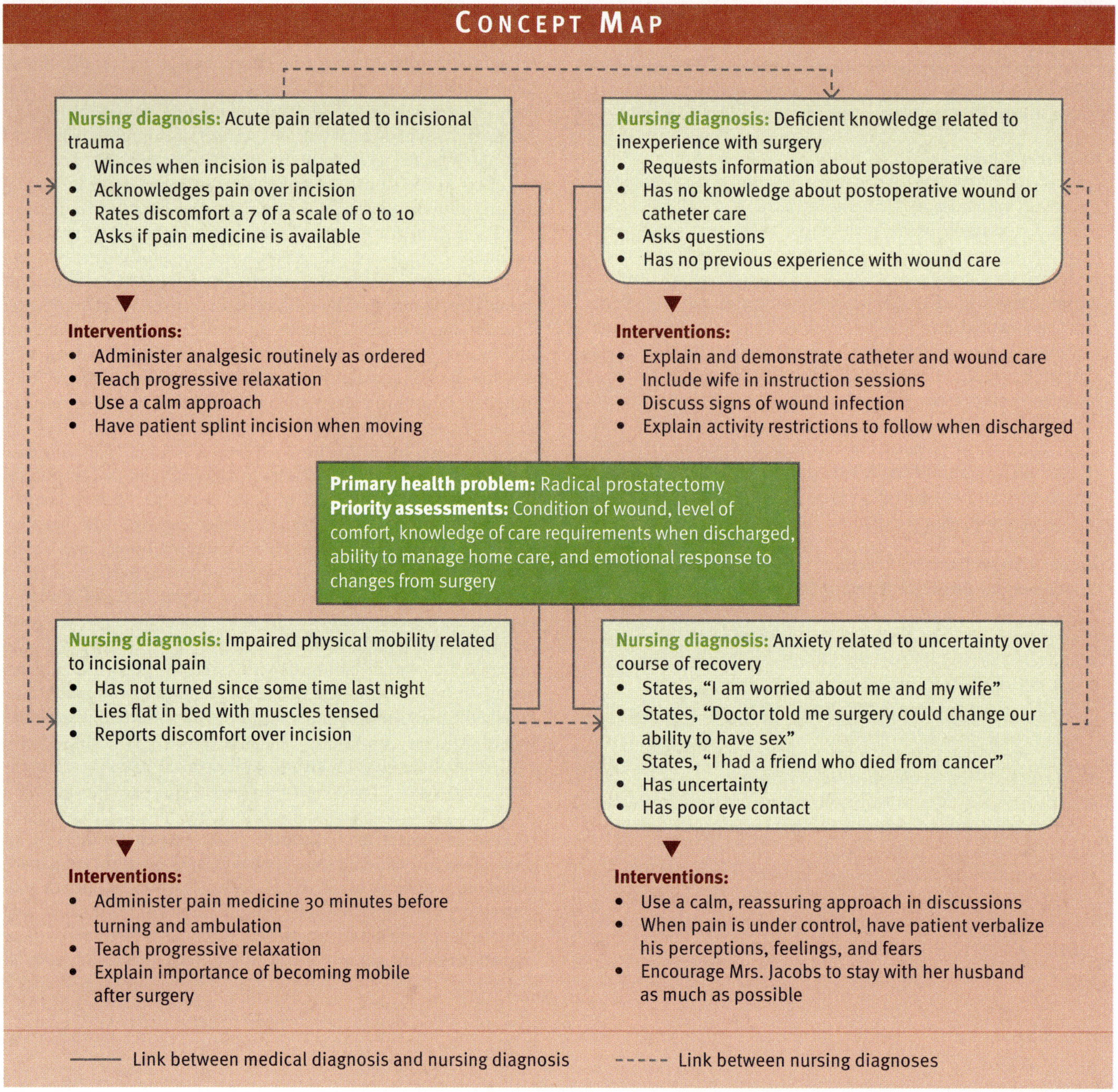
CONCEPT MAP
Nursing diagnosis: Acute pain related to incisional trauma
• Winces when incision is palpated
• Acknowledges pain over incision
• Rates discomfort a 7 of a scale of 0 to 10
• Asks if pain medicine is available
Interventions:
• Administer analgesic routinely as ordered
• Teach progressive relaxation
• Use a calm approach
• Have patient splint incision when moving
Nursing diagnosis: Deficient knowledge related to inexperience with surgery
• Requests information about postoperative care
• Has no knowledge about postoperative wound or catheter care
• Asks questions
• Has no previous experience with wound care
Interventions:
• Explain and demonstrate catheter and wound care
• Include wife in instruction sessions
• Discuss signs of wound infection
• Explain activity restrictions to follow when discharged
Primary health problem: Radical prostatectomy
Priority assessments: Condition of wound, level of comfort, knowledge of care requirements when discharged, ability to manage home care, and emotional response to changes from surgery
Nursing diagnosis: Impaired physical mobility related to incisional pain
• Has not turned since some time last night
• Lies flat in bed with muscles tensed
• Reports discomfort over incision
Interventions:
• Administer pain medicine 30 minutes before turning and ambulation
• Teach progressive relaxation
• Explain importance of becoming mobile after surgery
Nursing diagnosis: Anxiety related to uncertainty over course of recovery
• States, "I am worried about me and my wife"
• States, "Doctor told me surgery could change our ability to have sex"
• States, "I had a friend who died from cancer"
• Has uncertainty
• Has poor eye contact
Interventions:
• Use a calm, reassuring approach in discussions
• When pain is under control, have patient verbalize his perceptions, feelings, and fears
• Encourage Mrs. Jacobs to stay with her husband as much as possible
Link between medical diagnosis and nursing diagnosis
Link between nursing diagnoses

FIG. 18-3 Concept map for Mr. Jacobs: Planning.

disciplines to develop integrated care plans for a projected length of stay or number of visits. Critical pathways improve continuity of care because they clearly define the responsibility of each health care discipline. Well-developed pathways include evidence-based interventions and therapies.

Concept Maps

Chapter 16 first described concept maps and their use in care planning. Because you care for patients who present with multiple health problems and related nursing diagnoses, it is often not realistic to have a written columnar plan developed for each nursing diagnosis. In addition, the columnar plans do not contain a means to show the association between different nursing diagnoses and different nursing interventions. A concept map offers you a visual representation of all patient nursing diagnoses and allows you to diagram interventions for each. You quickly see the relationship between the diagnoses and often how a single intervention often applies to more than one health problem. Concept maps group and categorize nursing concepts to give you a holistic view of your patient's health care needs and help you make better clinical decisions in planning care.

In Chapter 17 you learned how to add nursing diagnostic labels to a concept map. When planning care for each nursing diagnosis, analyze the relationships among the diagnoses. Draw dotted lines between nursing diagnoses to indicate their relationship to one another (Fig. 18-3). It is important for you to make meaningful associations between one concept and another. The links need to be accurate, meaningful, and complete so you can explain why nursing diagnoses are related. For example, Mr. Jacobs' *anxiety* and *acute pain* are interrelated; in addition, pain has an influence on his reduced mobility. Pain and anxiety both influence his ability to respond to instruction for his deficient knowledge.

Finally, on a separate sheet of paper or on the map itself, list nursing interventions to attain the outcomes for each nursing diagnosis. This step corresponds to the planning phase of the nursing process. While caring for the patient, use the map to write the patient's responses to each nursing activity. Also write your clinical impressions and inferences regarding the patient's progress toward expected outcomes and the effectiveness of interventions. Keep the concept map with you throughout the clinical day. As you revise the plan, take notes and add or delete nursing interventions. Use the information recorded on the map for your documentation of patient care. Critical thinkers learn by organizing and relating cognitive concepts. Concept maps help you learn the interrelationships among nursing diagnoses to create a unique meaning and organization of information.

CONSULTING OTHER HEALTH CARE PROFESSIONALS

Planning involves consultation with members of the health care team. Consultation occurs at any step in the nursing process, but you consult most often during planning and implementation. During these times you are more likely to identify a problem requiring additional knowledge, skills, or resources. This requires you to be aware of your strengths and limitations as a team member. **Consultation** is a process by which you seek the expertise of a specialist such as your nursing instructor, a physician, or a clinical nurse educator to identify ways to handle problems in patient management or the planning and implementation of therapies. The consultation process is important so all health care providers are focused on common patient goals. Always be prepared before you make a consult. Consultation is based on the problem-solving approach, and the consultant is the stimulus for change.

Often an experienced nurse is a valuable consultant when you face an unfamiliar patient care situation such as a new procedure or a patient presenting a set of symptoms that you cannot identify. In clinical nursing, consultation helps to solve problems in the delivery of nursing care. For example, a nursing student consults a clinical specialist for wound care techniques or an educator for useful teaching resources. Nurses are consulted for their clinical expertise, patient education skills, or staff education skills. Nurses also consult with other members of the health care team such as physical therapists, nutritionists, and social workers. Again, the consultation focuses on problems in providing nursing care.

When to Consult

Consultation occurs when you identify a problem that you are unable to solve using personal knowledge, skills, and resources. The process requires good intrapersonal and interprofessional collaboration. Consultation with other care providers increases your knowledge about the patient's problems and helps you learn skills and obtain resources. A good time to consult with another health care professional is when the exact problem remains unclear. An objective consultant enters a clinical situation and more clearly assesses and identifies the nature of a problem, whether it is patient, personnel, or equipment oriented. Most often you consult with health care providers who are working in your clinical area. However, sometimes you consult over the telephone (Box 18-5).

BOX 18-5 TIPS FOR MAKING PHONE CONSULTATIONS

- Have the information you need available BEFORE you make a call. At a minimum have the medical record, any medication sheets (if the consultation is about a medicine), and any notes on recent care activities.
- Assess the patient yourself before making the call. For example, when you consult with physicians, they rely heavily on your assessment so they can give appropriate advice.
- Understand why you are calling for consultation and think through some possible solutions. Your experience in caring for the patient probably allows you to make useful suggestions. This also gives you ownership of the care of patients.
- Be prepared to summarize what you think the problem is.

Data from Maison D: Effective communications are more important than ever: a physician's perspective, *J Home Care Hospice Professional* 24(3):178, 2006.

How to Consult

Begin with your own understanding of a patient's clinical problems. The first step in making a consultation is to identify the general problem area. Second, direct the consultation to the right professional such as another nurse or social worker. Third, provide the consultant with relevant information about the problem area. Include a brief summary of the problem, methods used to resolve the problem so far, and outcomes of these methods. Also share information from the patient's medical record, conversations with other nurses, and the patient's family.

Fourth, do not prejudice or influence consultants. Consultants are in the clinical setting to help identify and resolve a nursing problem, and biasing or prejudicing them blocks problem resolution. Avoid bias by not overloading consultants with subjective and emotional conclusions about the patient and the problem.

Fifth, be available to discuss the consultant's findings and recommendations. When you request a consultation, provide a private, comfortable atmosphere for the consultant and patient to meet. However, this does not mean that you leave the environment. A common mistake is turning the whole problem over to the consultant. The consultant is not there to take over the problem but to help you resolve it. When possible, request the consultation for a time when both you and the consultant are able to discuss the patient's situation with minimal interruptions or distractions. Finally, incorporate the consultant's recommendations into the care plan. The success of the advice depends on the implementation of the problem-solving techniques. Always give the consultant feedback regarding the outcome of the recommendations.

KEY POINTS

- During planning determine patient goals, set priorities, develop expected outcomes of nursing care, and select interventions for the nursing care plan.
- Priorities help you anticipate and sequence nursing interventions when a patient has multiple nursing diagnoses and collaborative problems.
- Goals and expected outcomes provide clear direction for the selection and use of nursing interventions and the evaluation of the effectiveness of the interventions.

- In setting goals the time frame depends on the nature of the problem, etiology, overall condition of the patient, and treatment setting.
- A patient-centered goal is singular, observable, measurable, time limited, mutual, and realistic.
- An expected outcome is an objective criterion for goal achievement.
- Nurse-initiated interventions require no order and no supervision or direction from others.
- Physician-initiated interventions require specific nursing responsibilities and technical nursing knowledge.
- During a nursing handoff nurses collaborate and share important information that ensures the continuity of care for a patient and prevents errors or delays in providing nursing interventions.
- Care plans and critical pathways increase communication among nurses and facilitate the continuity of care from one nurse to another and from one health care setting to another.
- A concept map provides a visually graphic way to show the relationship between patients' nursing diagnoses and interventions.
- The NIC taxonomy provides a standardization to help nurses select suitable interventions for patients' problems.
- Correctly written nursing interventions include actions, frequency, quantity, method, and the person to perform them.
- Consultation increases your knowledge about a patient's problem and helps in learning skills and obtaining the resources needed to solve the problem.
- When making a consultation, first identify the general problem, direct the consultation to the right professional, and provide the consultant with relevant information about the problem.

CLINICAL APPLICATION QUESTIONS

Preparing for Clinical Practice

Tonya sets out to formally plan Mr. Jacobs' care. For the nursing diagnosis of *impaired physical mobility related to incisional pain*, Tonya identifies the goal of "Patient will walk 100 yards three times a day"; and the outcome she lists is, "Patient will report pain below level of 4 and will not splint incision when moving within 48 hours." The interventions she selects for her plan include administering the ordered analgesic, progressive relaxation, and splinting the incision when the patient gets out of bed. The following three questions apply to the case study.

1. Critique the goal and outcomes that Tonya set and explain if they were written correctly.
2. Among the interventions that Tonya selected, which ones are independent, dependent, and collaborative?
3. What interventions will possibly increase the likelihood that the patient's goals of care and outcomes will be met?

evolve *Answers to Clinical Application Questions can be found on the Evolve website.*

REVIEW QUESTIONS

Are You Ready to Test Your Nursing Knowledge?

1. A nurse is assigned to a patient who has returned from the recovery room following surgery for a colorectal tumor. After an initial assessment the nurse anticipates the need to monitor the patient's abdominal dressing, intravenous (IV) infusion, and function of drainage tubes. The patient is in pain, reporting 6 on a scale of 0 to 10, and will not be able to eat or drink until intestinal function returns. The family has been in the waiting room for an hour, wanting to see the patient. The nurse establishes priorities first for which of the following situations? (Select all that apply.)
   1. The family comes to visit the patient.
   2. The patient expresses concern about pain control.
   3. The patient's vital signs change, showing a drop in blood pressure.
   4. The charge nurse approaches the nurse and requests a report at end of shift.
2. A patient signals the nurse by turning on the call light. The nurse enters the room and finds the patient's drainage tube disconnected, 100 mL of fluid in the intravenous (IV) line, and the patient asking to be turned. Which of the following does the nurse perform first?
   1. Reconnect the drainage tubing
   2. Inspect the condition of the IV dressing
   3. Improve the patient's comfort and turn onto her side.
   4. Obtain the next IV fluid bag from the medication room
3. A nurse assesses a 78-year-old patient who weighs 240 pounds (108.9 kg) and is partially immobilized because of a stroke. The nurse turns the patient and finds that the skin over the sacrum is very red and the patient does not feel sensation in the area. The patient has had fecal incontinence on and off for the last 2 days. The nurse identifies the nursing diagnosis of *risk for impaired skin integrity*. Which of the following goals are appropriate for the patient? (Select all that apply.)
   1. Patient will be turned every 2 hours within 24 hours.
   2. Patient will have normal bowel function within 72 hours.
   3. Patient's skin will remain intact through discharge.
   4. Patient's skin condition will improve by discharge.
4. Setting a time frame for outcomes of care serves which of the following purposes?
   1. Indicates which outcome has priority
   2. Indicates the time it takes to complete an intervention
   3. Indicates how long a nurse is scheduled to care for a patient
   4. Indicates when the patient is expected to respond in the desired manner
5. A patient has been in the hospital for 2 days because of newly diagnosed diabetes. His medical condition is unstable, and the medical staff is having difficulty controlling his blood sugar. The physician expects that the patient will remain hospitalized at least 3 more days. The nurse identifies one nursing diagnosis as *deficient knowledge regarding insulin administration related to inexperience with disease management*. Which of the following patient care goals are long term?
   1. Patient will explain relationship of insulin to blood glucose control.
   2. Patient will self-administer insulin.
   3. Patient will achieve glucose control.
   4. Patient will describe steps for preparing insulin in a syringe.
6. A patient has been in the hospital for 2 days because of newly diagnosed diabetes. His medical condition is unstable, and the medical staff is having difficulty controlling his blood sugar. The physician expects that the patient will remain hospitalized at least 3 more days. The nurse identifies one nursing diagnosis as *deficient knowledge regarding insulin administration related to inexperience with disease management*. What does the nurse

need to determine before setting the goal of "patient will self-administer insulin?" (Select all that apply.)
1. Goal within reach of the patient
2. The nurse's own competency in teaching about insulin
3. The patient's cognitive function
4. Availability of family members to assist

7. The nurse writes an expected-outcome statement in measurable terms. An example is:
   1. Patient will be pain free.
   2. Patient will have less pain.
   3. Patient will take pain medication every 4 hours.
   4. Patient will report pain acuity less than 4 on a scale of 0 to 10.
8. A patient has the nursing diagnosis of *nausea*. The nurse develops a care plan with the following interventions. Which are examples of collaborative interventions?
   1. Provide frequent mouth care.
   2. Maintain intravenous (IV) infusion at 100 mL/hr.
   3. Administer prochlorperazine (Compazine) via rectal suppository.
   4. Consult with dietitian on initial foods to offer patient.
   5. Control aversive odors or unpleasant visual stimulation that triggers nausea.
9. A 72-year-old patient has come to the health clinic with symptoms of a productive cough, fever, increased respiratory rate, and shortness of breath. His respiratory distress increases when he walks. He lives alone and did not come to the clinic until his neighbor insisted. He reports not getting his pneumonia vaccine this year. Blood tests show the patient's oxygen saturation to be lower than normal. The physician diagnoses the patient as having pneumonia. Match the priority level with the nursing diagnoses identified for this patient:

Nursing Diagnoses	**Priority Level**
1. Impaired gas exchange _____	a. Long term
2. Risk for activity intolerance _____	b. Short term
3. Ineffective self-health management _____	c. Intermediate

10. An 82-year-old patient who resides in a nursing home has the following three nursing diagnoses: *risk for fall, impaired physical mobility related to pain,* and *wandering related to cognitive impairment.* The nursing staff identified several goals of care. Match the goals on the left with the appropriate outcome statements on the right.

Goals	**Outcomes**
1. Patient will ambulate independently in 3 days. _____	a. Patient will express fewer nonverbal signs of discomfort.
2. Patient will be injury free for 1 month. _____	b. Patient will follow a set care routine.
3. Patient will be less agitated. _____	c. Patient will walk correctly using a walker.
4. Patient will achieve pain relief. _____	d. Patient will exit a low bed without falling.

11. A nurse is preparing for change-of-shift rounds with the nurse who is assuming care for his patients. Which of the following statements or actions by the nurse are characteristics of ineffective handoff communication?
    1. This patient is anxious about his pain after surgery; you need to review the information I gave him about how to use a patient-controlled analgesia (PCA) pump this evening.
    2. The nurse refers to the electronic care plan in the electronic health record (EHR) to review interventions for the patient's care.
    3. During walking rounds the nurse talks about the problem the patient care technicians created by not ambulating the patient.
    4. The nurse gives her patient a pain medication before report so there is likely to be no interruption during rounding.
12. Which of the following outcome statements for the goal, "Patient will achieve a gain of 10 lbs (4.5 kg) in body weight in a month" are worded incorrectly? (Select all that apply.)
    1. Patient will eat at least three fourths of each meal by 1 week.
    2. Patient will verbalize relief of nausea and have no episodes of vomiting in 1 week.
    3. Patient will eat foods with high-calorie content by 1 week.
    4. Give patient liquid supplements 3 times a day.
13. A nurse from home health is talking with a nurse who works on an acute medical division within a hospital. The home health nurse is making a consultation. Which of the following statements describes the unique difference between a nursing care plan from a hospital versus one for home care?
    1. The goals of care will always be more long term.
    2. The patient and family need to be able to independently provide most of the health care.
    3. The patient's goals need to be mutually set with family members who will care for him or her.
    4. The expected outcomes need to address what can be influenced by interventions.
14. Which outcome allows you to measure a patient's response to care more precisely?
    1. The patient's wound will appear normal within 3 days.
    2. The patient's wound will have less drainage within 72 hours.
    3. The patient's wound will reduce in size to less than 4 cm (1½ inches) by day 4.
    4. The patient's wound will heal without redness or drainage by day 4.
15. A nurse identifies several interventions to resolve the patient's nursing diagnosis of *impaired skin integrity*. Which of the following are written in error? (Select all that apply.)
    1. Turn the patient regularly from side to back to side.
    2. Provide perineal care, using Dove soap and water, every shift and after each episode of urinary incontinence.
    3. Apply a pressure-relief device to bed.
    4. Apply transparent dressing to sacral pressure ulcer.

Answers: **1.** 2, 3; **2.** 1; **3.** 2, 3; **4.** 4; **5.** 3; **6.** 1, 3, 4; **7.** 4; **8.** 4; **9.** 1b, 2c, 3a; **10.** 1c, 2d, 3b, 4a; **11.** 3; **12.** 2, 4; **13.** 2; **14.** 3; **15.** 1, 3.

REFERENCES

Bastable SB: *Essentials of patient education*, Sudbury, Mass, 2006, Jones & Bartlett.

Bulechek GM, et al: *Nursing interventions classification (NIC)*, ed 5, St Louis, 2008, Mosby.

Carpenito-Moyet LJ: *Nursing diagnoses: application to clinical practice*, ed 13, Philadelphia, 2009, Lippincott Williams & Wilkins.

Espinosa-Aguilar A, et al: Design and validation of a critical pathway for hospital management of patients with severe traumatic brain injury, *J Trauma* 64(5):1327, 2008.

Hebda T, et al: *Handbook of informatics for nurses and health care professionals*, ed 4, Upper Saddle River, NJ, 2009, Pearson Prentice Hall.

Moorhead S, et al: *Nursing outcomes classification*, ed 4, St Louis, 2008, Mosby.

NANDA International: *Nursing diagnoses: definitions and classification 2012-2014*, United Kingdom, 2012, Wiley-Blackwell.

Schumacher K, et al: Family caregivers, *Am J Nurs* 106(8):40, 2006.

Vacarolis EM, Halter MJ: *Essentials of psychiatric mental health nursing: a communication approach to evidence-based care*, St Louis, 2009, Saunders.

RESEARCH REFERENCES

Athwal P, et al: Standardization of change-of-shift report, *J Nurs Care Qual* 24(2):143, 2009.

Hendry C, Walker A: Priority setting in clinical nursing practice: literature review, *J Adv Nurs* 47(4):427, 2004.

Holmstrom I, Hoglund AT: The faceless encounter: ethical dilemmas in telephone nursing, *J Clin Nurs* 17(16):2237, 2007.

Hui PN, et al: An evaluation of two behavioral rehabilitation programs, qigong versus progressive relaxation, in improving the quality of life in cardiac patients, *J Altern Complement Med* 12(4):351, 2006.

Potter P, et al: Understanding the cognitive work of nursing in the acute care environment, *J Nurs Admin* 35(7/8):327, 2005.

Riesenberg LA, Leisch J, Cunningham JM: Nursing hand-offs: a systematic review of the literature, *Am J Nurs* 110(4):24, 2010.

CHAPTER

19

Implementing Nursing Care

OBJECTIVES

- Explain the relationship of implementation to the nursing diagnostic process.
- Describe the association between critical thinking and selecting nursing interventions.
- Discuss the differences between protocols and standing orders.
- Identify preparatory activities to use before implementation.
- Discuss the value of the Nursing Interventions Classification system in documenting nursing care.
- Discuss the steps for revising a plan of care before performing implementation.
- Define the three implementation skills.
- Describe and compare direct and indirect nursing interventions.
- Select appropriate interventions for an assigned patient.

KEY TERMS

Activities of daily living (ADLs), p. 259
Adverse reaction, p. 261
Clinical practice guideline, p. 255
Counseling, p. 260
Direct care, p. 253
Implementation, p. 253
Indirect care, p. 253
Instrumental activities of daily living (IADLs), p. 260
Interdisciplinary care plans, p. 262
Lifesaving measure, p. 260
Nursing intervention, p. 253
Patient adherence, p. 262
Preventive nursing actions, p. 261
Standing order, p. 256

evolve WEBSITE

http://evolve.elsevier.com/Potter/fundamentals/

- Review Questions
- Concept Map Creator
- Case Study with Questions
- Audio Glossary
- Interactive Learning Activities
- Key Term Flashcards
- Content Updates

You first met Tonya and Mr. Jacobs in Chapter 16. The two have collaborated during the nursing process to develop a relevant and appropriate plan of care. During implementation Tonya works with fellow health care colleagues and Mr. and Mrs. Jacobs to provide the safest and most effective nursing interventions for the patient's health care problems. Implementation is circular, like all steps of the nursing process. This means that, during the course of Mr. Jacobs' hospitalization, as his clinical condition changes Tonya reassesses the status of existing nursing diagnoses, confirms that these diagnoses are still appropriate, evaluates the patient's responses to planned interventions (see Chapter 20), and continues to deliver interventions in a timely and competent manner. Critical thinking, which includes good clinical decision making, is important for the successful implementation of nursing interventions.

Implementation, the fourth step of the nursing process, formally begins after the nurse develops a plan of care. With a care plan based on clear and relevant nursing diagnoses, the nurse initiates interventions that are designed to achieve the goals and expected outcomes needed to support or improve the patient's health status. A **nursing intervention** is any treatment based on clinical judgment and knowledge that a nurse performs to enhance patient outcomes (Bulechek et al., 2008). Ideally the interventions a nurse uses are evidenced based (see Chapter 5), providing the most current, up-to-date, and effective approaches for managing patient problems. Interventions include direct and indirect care measures aimed at individuals, families, and/or the community.

Direct care interventions are treatments performed through interactions with patients (Bulechek et al., 2008). For example, a patient receives direct intervention in the form of medication administration, insertion of an intravenous (IV) infusion, or counseling during a time of grief. **Indirect care** interventions are treatments performed away from the patient but on behalf of the patient or group of patients (Bulechek et al., 2008). For example, indirect care measures include actions for managing the patient's environment (e.g., safety and infection control), documentation, and interdisciplinary collaboration. Both direct and indirect care measures fall under the intervention categories described in Chapter 18: nurse-initiated, physician-initiated, and collaborative. For example, the direct intervention of patient education is a nurse-initiated intervention. The indirect intervention of consultation is a collaborative intervention.

Benner (1984) defined the domains of nursing practice, which help to explain the nature and intent of the many ways nurses intervene for patients (Box 19-1). These domains are current today. The extent of organizational and work role competencies has

BOX 19-1 DOMAINS OF NURSING PRACTICE

- The Helping Role
- The Teaching-Coaching Function
- The Diagnostic and Patient-Monitoring Function
- Effective Management of Rapidly Changing Situations
- Administering and Monitoring Therapeutic Interventions and Regimens
- Monitoring and Ensuring the Quality of Health Care Practices
- Organizational and Work-Role Competencies

From Benner P: *From novice to expert,* Menlo Park, Calif, 1984, Addison Wesley.

become more complex; thus it is important that the focus of implementation always be the patient. Nursing is an art and a science. It is not simply a task-based profession. Thus you learn to intervene for a patient within the context of his or her unique situation. Examples of factors to consider during intervention follow. Who is the patient? What does this illness mean to the patient and his or her family? What clinical situation requires you to intervene? How does the patient perceive the interventions that you will deliver? Will any cultural considerations influence your approach? In what way do you best support or show caring as you intervene? The answers to these questions enable you to deliver care compassionately and effectively with the best outcomes for your patients.

CRITICAL THINKING IN IMPLEMENTATION

The delivery of nursing interventions is a complex decision-making process that involves critical thinking. The context in which you deliver care to each patient and the many interventions required result in decision-making approaches for each clinical situation. Critical thinking is necessary to consider the complexity of interventions, including the number of alternative approaches and the amount of time available to act.

Tonya indentified four relevant nursing diagnoses for Mr. Jacobs: ***acute pain*** *related to incisional trauma,* ***deficient knowledge*** *regarding postoperative recovery related to inexperience with surgery,* ***impaired physical mobility*** *related to incisional pain, and* ***anxiety*** *related to uncertainty over the course of recovery. The diagnoses are interrelated, and sometimes a planned intervention (e.g., administering pain medication) treats or modifies more than one of the patient's health problems (pain and impaired physical mobility). Tonya applies critical thinking and uses her time with Mr. Jacobs wisely by anticipating his priorities, applying the knowledge she has about his problems and the interventions planned, and implementing care strategies skillfully.*

Before implementing a planned intervention, use critical thinking to confirm whether the intervention is correct and still appropriate for the patient's clinical situation. Even though you have planned a set of interventions for a patient, you have to exercise good judgment and decision making before actually delivering each intervention. Always think before you act. Patients' conditions often change minute to minute. You need to consider the scheduling of activities on a nursing unit, which often dictates when and how to complete an intervention. Thus many factors influence your decision on how and when to intervene. You are responsible for having the necessary knowledge and clinical competency to perform interventions for your patients safely and effectively. Some tips for making decisions during implementation follow.

- Review the set of all possible nursing interventions for the patient's problem (e.g., for Mr. Jacobs' pain Tonya considers analgesic administration, positioning and splinting, progressive relaxation, and other nonpharmacological approaches).
- Review all possible consequences associated with each possible nursing action (e.g., Tonya considers that the analgesic will either relieve pain; have little or insufficient effect; or cause an adverse reaction, including sedating the patient and increasing the risk of falling).
- Determine the probability of all possible consequences (e.g., if Mr. Jacobs' pain has decreased with analgesia and positioning in the morning and there have been no side effects, it is unlikely that adverse reactions will occur, and the intervention will be successful; however, if the patient continues to remain highly anxious, his pain may not be relieved, and Tonya needs to consider an alternative).
- Make a judgment of the value of the consequence to the patient (e.g., if the administration of an analgesic is effective, Mr. Jacobs will likely become less anxious and more responsive to postoperative instruction and counseling about his anxiety).

The selection and performance of nursing interventions for a patient are part of clinical decision making. The critical thinking model described in Chapter 15 provides a framework for how to make decisions when implementing nursing care (Fig. 19-1). You learn how to implement nursing care using appropriate knowledge. For example, as you proceed with an intervention, you consider what you know about the purpose of the intervention, the steps in performing the intervention correctly, the medical condition of the patient, and his or her expected response. It is important to prepare well before first caring for any patient. With experience you become more proficient in anticipating what to expect in a given clinical situation and how to modify your approach. As you gain clinical experience, you are able to consider which interventions worked previously, which have not, and why. It also helps to know the clinical standards of practice for your agency. For example, one hospital has a different set of standards for patient education than another. The standards of practice offer guidelines for selection of interventions and their frequency and whether you are able to delegate the procedures.

As you perform a nursing intervention, apply intellectual standards, which are the guidelines for rational thought and responsible action. For example, before Tonya begins to teach Mr. Jacobs, she considers how to make her instructions relevant, clear, logical, and complete to promote patient learning. She knows that it will be helpful to involve Mrs. Jacobs so any instruction is relevant to their home situation. Using simple, clear explanations and repeated instructions promote learning for Mr. Jacobs, who is inexperienced with postoperative recovery. Making an instructional DVD on wound care available to the family is a valuable resource for repeated viewing in the home.

As a critical thinker, apply critical thinking attitudes when you intervene. For example, show confidence in performing an intervention. When you are unsure of how to perform a procedure, be responsible in seeking assistance from others. Confidence in performing interventions builds trust with patients. Creativity and self-discipline are attitudes that guide you in reviewing, modifying, and implementing interventions. As a beginning nursing student, seek out supervision from instructors or experienced nurses to guide you in the decision-making process for implementation.

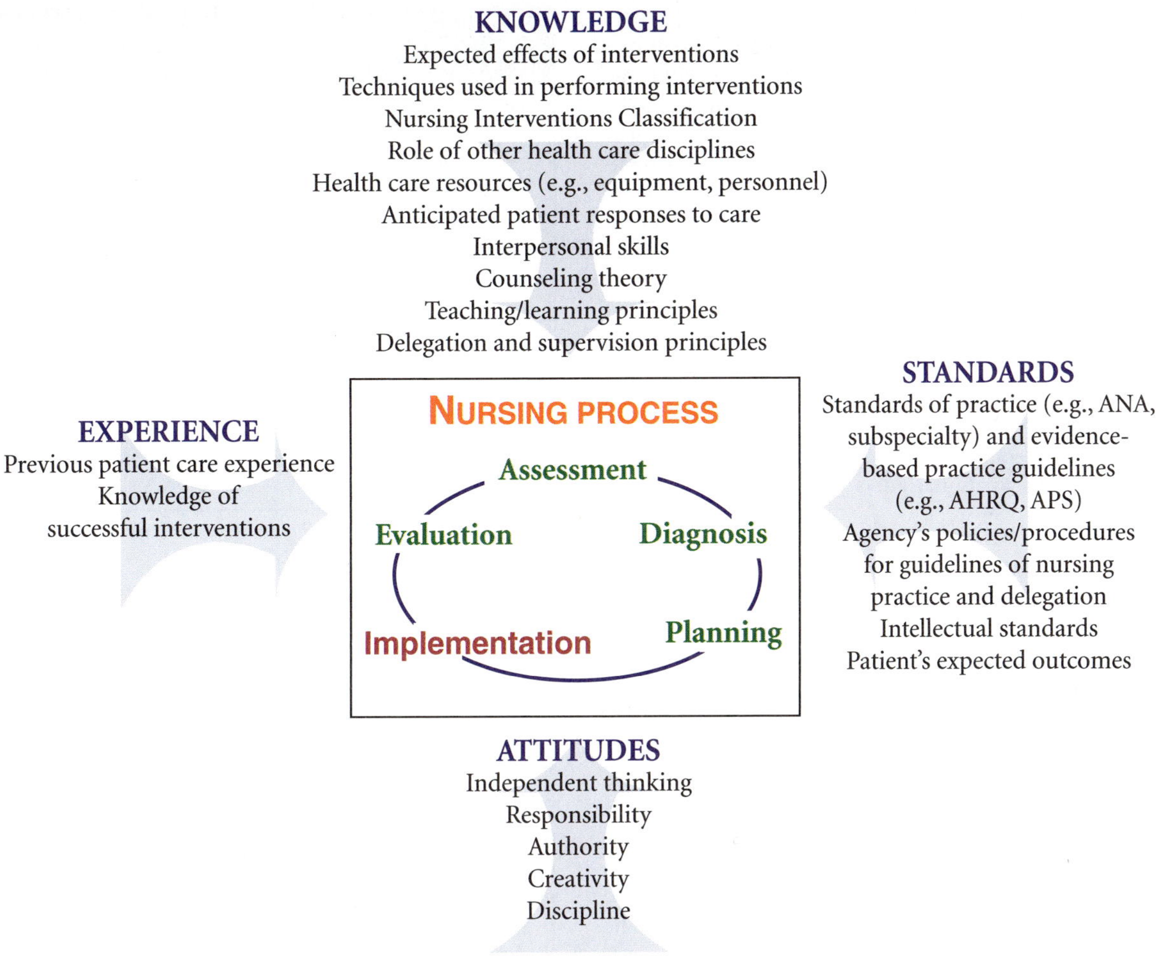

FIG. 19-1 Critical thinking and the process of implementing care. *AHRQ,* Agency for Healthcare Research Quality; *ANA,* American Nurses Association; *APS,* American Pain Society.

STANDARD NURSING INTERVENTIONS

Health care settings present various ways for nurses to create and individualize a patient's plan of care. Each plan of care is totally unique to that patient, with interventions individualized on the basis of his or her specific health problems. In certain situations a nurse develops the plan on the basis of personal knowledge and clinical experience. However, systems are available that provide standardized interventions for nurses to use in their plan of care. Many patients have common health care problems; thus standardized interventions for these health problems make it quicker and easier for nurses to intervene. More important, if the standards are evidence based, the nurse is more likely to deliver the most clinically effective interventions to improve patient outcomes (see Chapter 5). Standardized interventions most often set a level of clinical excellence for practice. Nurse- and physician-initiated standardized interventions are available in the form of clinical guidelines or protocols, preprinted (standing) orders, and Nursing Interventions Classification (NIC) interventions. At a professional level the American Nurses Association (ANA) defines standards of professional nursing practice, which include standards for the implementation step of the nursing process. These standards are authoritative statements of the duties that all registered nurses are expected to perform competently, regardless of role, patient population they serve, or specialty (ANA, 2010) (see Chapter 1).

Clinical Practice Guidelines and Protocols

A **clinical practice guideline** or protocol is a systematically developed set of statements that helps nurses, physicians, and other health care providers make decisions about appropriate health care for specific clinical situations (Manchikanti et al., 2010). A guideline guides interventions for specific health care problems or conditions such as low back pain, dizziness, or deep vein thrombosis. The guideline is developed on the basis of an authoritative examination of current scientific evidence (National Guideline Clearinghouse [NGC], 2010). Guidelines are now seen as key tools for improving the quality of health care and bridging the gap between the growth of research findings and actual clinical practice (Rosenbrand et al., 2008).

Clinicians within a health care agency sometimes choose to review the scientific literature and their own standard of practice to develop guidelines and protocols in an effort to improve their standard of care. For example, a hospital develops a rapid-assessment protocol to improve the identification and early treatment of patients suspected of having a stroke. However, clinical practice guidelines have already been developed by national health groups such as the National Institutes of Health and the National Guideline Clearinghouse. These guidelines are readily available to any clinician or health care institution that wishes to adopt evidence-based guidelines in the care of patients with specific health problems. One valuable source for nursing practice guidelines is the Gerontological Nursing Interventions Research Center (GNIRC) at the University of Iowa. The center has numerous clinical guidelines, including ones for acute confusion and delirium, acute pain management, and fall prevention for older adults (GNIRC, 2010).

Advanced practice nurses who provide primary care for patients in outpatient settings frequently follow diagnostic and treatment protocols. In such a setting nurses assess the patient and identify abnormalities. The protocol outlines the conditions that nurses are permitted to treat such as controlled hypertension and the types of treatment that they are permitted to administer such as antihypertensive medications. In acute care settings it is common to find clinical protocols that outline independent nursing interventions for specific conditions. Examples include protocols for admission and discharge, pressure ulcer care, and incontinence management. Protocols are also used in interdisciplinary settings for diagnostic testing and physical, occupational, and speech therapies.

Standing Orders

A **standing order** is a preprinted document containing orders for the conduct of routine therapies, monitoring guidelines, and/or diagnostic procedures for specific patients with identified clinical problems. A standing order directs the conduct of patient care in a specific clinical setting. Licensed prescribing health care providers in charge of care at the time of implementation approve and sign standing orders. These orders are common in critical care settings and other specialized practice settings where patients' needs change rapidly and require immediate attention. An example of such a standing order is one specifying certain medications such as lidocaine or propranolol for an irregular heart rhythm. After assessing the patient and identifying the irregular rhythm, the critical care nurse gives the specified medication without first notifying the physician. The physician's initial standing order covers the nurse's action. After completing a standing order, the nurse notifies the physician. Standing orders are common in the community health setting, where the nurse faces situations that do not permit immediate contact with a health care provider. Standing orders give the nurse legal protection to intervene appropriately in the patient's best interest.

NIC Interventions

The NIC system developed by the University of Iowa helps to differentiate nursing practice from that of other health care professionals (Box 19-2). The NIC interventions offer a level of standardization to enhance communication of nursing care across settings and to compare outcomes. By using NIC nurses learn the common interventions recommended for various NANDA International nursing diagnoses. Nurses also learn the numerous care activities for each NIC intervention. Recently the NIC interventions have been used for work complexity assessment, a process that helps nurses identify interventions performed on a routine basis for their patient populations (Scherb and Weydt, 2009). Chapter 18 describes the NIC system in more detail.

Standards of Practice

The ANA Standards of Professional Nursing Practice (ANA, 2010) are to be used as evidence of the standard of care that registered nurses provide their patients (see Chapter 1). The standards are formally reviewed on a regular basis. The newest standards include competencies for establishing professional and caring relationships, using evidence-based interventions and technologies, providing holistic care across the life span to diverse groups, and using community resources and systems. In addition, the standards emphasize implementing a timely plan following patient safety goals (ANA, 2010).

BOX 19-2 PURPOSES OF THE NURSING INTERVENTIONS CLASSIFICATION

1. Standardization of the nomenclature (e.g., labeling, describing) of nursing interventions; standardizes the language nurses use to describe sets of actions in delivering patient care
2. Expanding nursing knowledge about connections among nursing diagnoses, treatments, and outcomes; connections determined through the study of actual patient care using a database that the classification generates
3. Developing nursing and health care information systems
4. Teaching decision making to nursing students; defining and classifying nursing interventions to teach beginning nurses how to determine a patient's need for care and to respond appropriately
5. Determining the cost of services provided by nurses
6. Planning for resources needed in all types of nursing practice settings
7. Language to communicate the unique functions of nursing
8. Link with the classification systems of other health care providers

From Bulechek GM et al: *Nursing interventions classification (NIC)*, ed 5, St Louis, 2008, Mosby.

IMPLEMENTATION PROCESS

Preparation for implementation ensures efficient, safe, and effective nursing care. Five preparatory activities include reassessing the patient, reviewing and revising the existing nursing care plan, organizing resources and care delivery, anticipating and preventing complications, and implementing nursing interventions.

Tonya returns to Mr. Jacobs' room 30 minutes after administering a dose of IV morphine for his incisional pain. She notices that he is more relaxed and turning a bit on his own. She asks him to rate his pain on a scale of 0 to 10, and he responds that it is now a 3. With the pain currently under control, Tonya decides to get the patient up in a chair to begin increasing his activity level. While Mr. Jacobs is in the chair, Tonya gets the teaching booklets she wants to use to prepare the patient for wound and catheter care in the home. She knows that Mrs. Jacobs is due to arrive at any time; thus she plans to include her in the discussion. Tonya also knows that this is Mr. Jacobs' first time up in the chair; thus she anticipates monitoring him closely and judging if he is alert and comfortable enough to begin the planned instruction.

Reassessing the Patient

Assessment is a continuous process that occurs each time you interact with a patient. When you collect new data about a patient, you sometimes identify a new nursing diagnosis or determine the need to modify the care plan. During the initial phase of implementation reassess the patient. The reassessment often focuses on one primary nursing diagnosis, or one dimension of the patient such as level of comfort, or one system such as the cardiovascular system. The reassessment helps you decide if the proposed nursing actions are still appropriate for the patient's level of wellness. Reassessment is not the evaluation of care (see Chapter 20), but it is the gathering of additional information to ensure that the plan of care is appropriate. *For example, Tonya plans to talk with Mr. Jacobs*

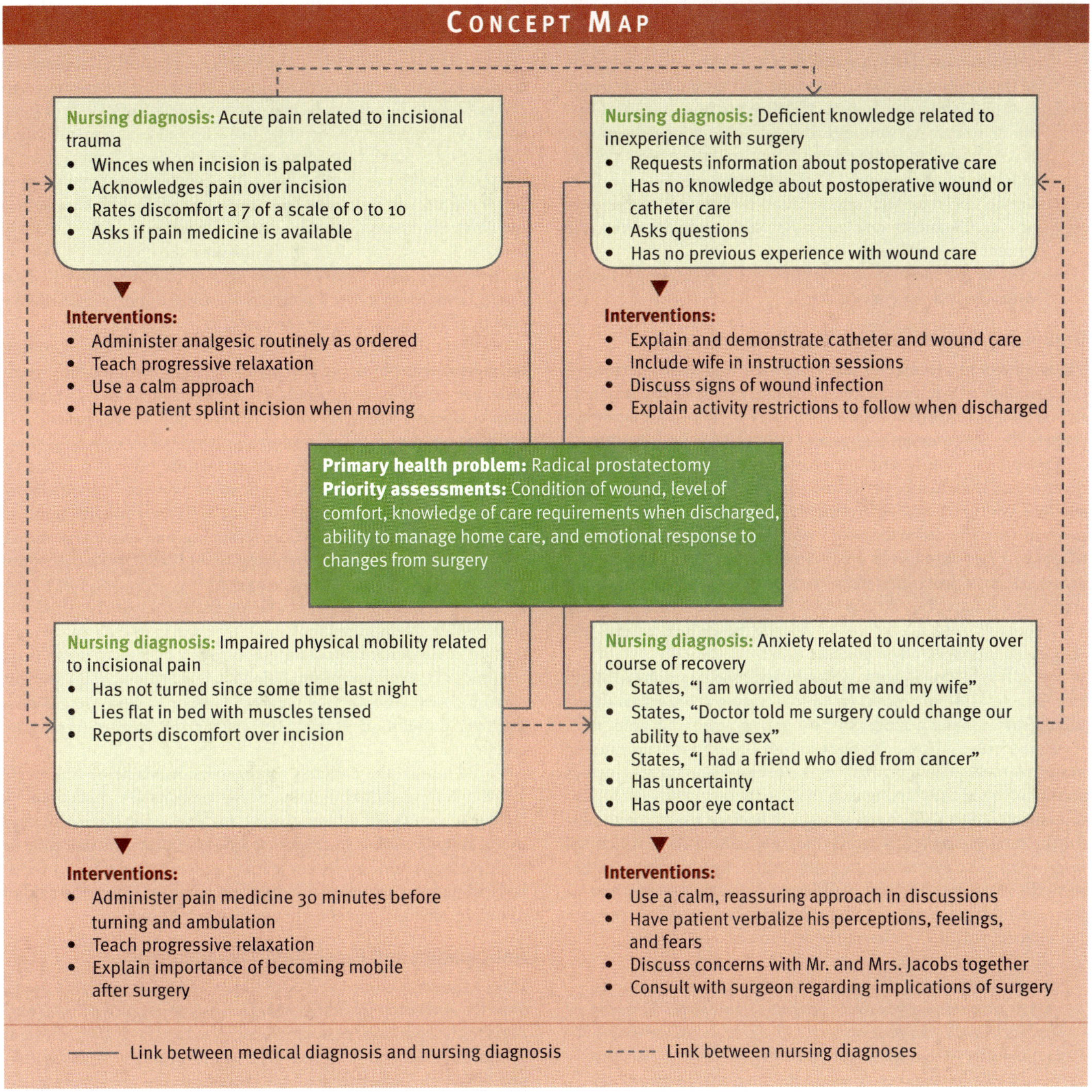
CONCEPT MAP
Nursing diagnosis: Acute pain related to incisional trauma
• Winces when incision is palpated
• Acknowledges pain over incision
• Rates discomfort a 7 of a scale of 0 to 10
• Asks if pain medicine is available
Interventions:
• Administer analgesic routinely as ordered
• Teach progressive relaxation
• Use a calm approach
• Have patient splint incision when moving
Nursing diagnosis: Deficient knowledge related to inexperience with surgery
• Requests information about postoperative care
• Has no knowledge about postoperative wound or catheter care
• Asks questions
• Has no previous experience with wound care
Interventions:
• Explain and demonstrate catheter and wound care
• Include wife in instruction sessions
• Discuss signs of wound infection
• Explain activity restrictions to follow when discharged
Primary health problem: Radical prostatectomy
Priority assessments: Condition of wound, level of comfort, knowledge of care requirements when discharged, ability to manage home care, and emotional response to changes from surgery
Nursing diagnosis: Impaired physical mobility related to incisional pain
• Has not turned since some time last night
• Lies flat in bed with muscles tensed
• Reports discomfort over incision
Interventions:
• Administer pain medicine 30 minutes before turning and ambulation
• Teach progressive relaxation
• Explain importance of becoming mobile after surgery
Nursing diagnosis: Anxiety related to uncertainty over course of recovery
• States, "I am worried about me and my wife"
• States, "Doctor told me surgery could change our ability to have sex"
• States, "I had a friend who died from cancer"
• Has uncertainty
• Has poor eye contact
Interventions:
• Use a calm, reassuring approach in discussions
• Have patient verbalize his perceptions, feelings, and fears
• Discuss concerns with Mr. and Mrs. Jacobs together
• Consult with surgeon regarding implications of surgery
—— Link between medical diagnosis and nursing diagnosis
----- Link between nursing diagnoses

FIG. 19-2 Concept map for Mr. Jacobs: Implementation.

about surgery and what to expect during recovery. However, she learns from Mr. Jacobs that Mrs. Jacobs' visit has been delayed until lunchtime. She knows that Mrs. Jacobs is an important resource for Mr. Jacobs' recovery, but she decides to get Mr. Jacobs up in a chair and focus on how he tolerates the activity anyway. Pain control is still a priority. Tonya will help Mr. Jacobs back to bed after about 30 minutes, allow him to rest until lunchtime, and then begin her instruction.

Reviewing and Revising the Existing Nursing Care Plan

After reassessing a patient, review the care plan and compare assessment data to validate the nursing diagnoses and determine whether the nursing interventions remain the most appropriate for the clinical situation. If the patient's status has changed and the nursing diagnosis and related nursing interventions are no longer appropriate, modify the nursing care plan. An out-of-date or incorrect care plan compromises the quality of nursing care. Review and modification enable you to provide timely nursing interventions to best meet the patient's needs.

After reviewing the care plan, Tonya made a few revisions to Mr. Jacobs' concept map (Fig. 19-2). Tonya notices that eye contact with Mr. Jacobs has improved; trust is building. Mr. Jacobs' pain has also lessened. She modifies her plan for reducing anxiety by planning a discussion with Mr. and Mrs. Jacobs together and consulting with the surgeon.

Modification of an existing written care plan includes four steps:

1. Revise data in the assessment column to reflect the patient's current status. Date any new data to inform other members of the health care team of the time that the change occurred.
2. Revise the nursing diagnoses. Delete nursing diagnoses that are no longer relevant and add and date any new diagnoses. It is necessary to revise related factors and the patient's goals, outcomes, and priorities. Date any revisions.
3. Revise specific interventions that correspond to the new nursing diagnoses and goals. Revisions need to reflect the patient's present status.
4. Choose the method of evaluation for determining whether you achieved patient outcomes.

Organizing Resources and Care Delivery

The resources of a facility include equipment and skilled personnel. Organization of equipment and personnel makes timely, efficient, skilled patient care possible (see Chapter 21). It is also important to prepare the environment and patient for a nursing intervention.

Equipment. Most nursing procedures require some equipment or supplies. Before performing an intervention, decide which supplies you need and determine their availability. Is the equipment in working order to ensure safe use, and do you know how to use it? Place supplies in a convenient location to provide easy access during a procedure. Keep extra supplies available in case of errors or mishaps, but do not open them unless you need them. This controls health care costs. After a procedure return any unopened supplies to storage areas.

Personnel. Nursing care delivery models vary among facilities (see Chapter 21). The model by which nursing is organized determines how nursing personnel deliver patient care. For example, a registered nurse's (RN's) accountabilities differ in a team nursing model from those in a primary nursing model. A primary nurse is accountable for the nursing care that a patient receives during his or her length of stay or course of visits. A team nurse is accountable for the care that a patient receives for a specific shift in which the nurse works. As a nurse you are responsible for deciding whether to perform an intervention or delegate it to another member of the nursing team. Your ongoing assessment of a patient, and not the intervention alone, directs the decision about delegation.

For example, Tonya knows that nursing assistive personnel (NAP) can competently assist patients to ambulate. However, she has learned that patients who transfer to a chair or ambulate the first time after surgery are often less stable; the NAP should not be the one to assess the patient's response. She decides to personally help Mr. Jacobs get up and into a chair to evaluate his response. Tonya thus redirects the NAP to perform more suitable care activities such as helping Tonya make Mr. Jacobs' bed or assisting a different patient with oral hygiene.

Nursing staff work together as patients' needs demand it. If a patient makes a request such as use of a bedpan or assistance in feeding, help the patient if you have time rather than trying to find the NAP who is in a different room. Nursing staff respect colleagues who show initiative; collaborate together; and communicate with one another on an ongoing, reciprocal basis as patients' needs change (Potter et al., 2010). When interventions are complex or physically difficult, you probably need assistance from colleagues. For example, you and the NAP more effectively change a dressing in a large gaping wound when you apply the dressing and the NAP assists with patient positioning and handing off of supplies.

Environment. A patient's care environment needs to be safe and conducive to implementing therapies. Patient safety is your first concern. If the patient has sensory deficits, physical disabilities, or an alteration in level of consciousness, arrange the environment to prevent injury. For example, provide a patient's assist devices (e.g., walker or eyeglasses), rearrange furniture and equipment when ambulating a patient, or make sure that the water temperature is not too warm before a bath. The patient benefits most from nursing interventions when surroundings are compatible with care activities. When you need to expose a patient's body parts, do so privately by closing room doors or curtains because the patient will then be more relaxed. Ask visitors to leave as you complete care. Reduce distractions to enhance a patient's learning opportunities. Make sure that lighting is adequate to perform procedures correctly.

Patient. Before you implement interventions, make sure that the patient is as physically and psychologically comfortable as possible. For example, symptoms such as nausea, dizziness, fatigue, or pain frequently interfere with a patient's full concentration and ability to cooperate. Offer comfort measures before initiating interventions to help the patient participate more fully. If you need a patient to be alert, administer a dose of pain medication strong enough to relieve discomfort but not to impair mental faculties (e.g., ability to follow instruction, reasoning, and communication). If a patient is fatigued, delay ambulation or transfer to a chair until after he or she has had a chance to rest.

Even if symptoms are not a factor, make the patient physically comfortable during interventions. Start any intervention by controlling environmental factors, taking care of physical needs (e.g., elimination), avoiding interruptions, and positioning the patient correctly. Also consider the patient's level of endurance and plan only the amount of activity that he or she is able to tolerate comfortably.

Awareness of the patient's psychosocial needs helps you create a favorable emotional climate. Some patients feel reassured by having a significant other present to lend encouragement and moral support. Other strategies include planning sufficient time or multiple opportunities for the patient to work through and ventilate feelings and anxieties. Adequate preparation allows the patient to obtain maximal benefit from each intervention.

Anticipating and Preventing Complications

Risks to patients come from both illness and treatment. As a nurse, look for and recognize these risks, adapt your choice of interventions to the situation, evaluate the relative benefit of the treatment versus the risk, and take risk-prevention measures. Many conditions place the patient at risk for complications. For example, the patient with preexisting left-sided paralysis following a stroke 2 years earlier is at risk for developing a pressure ulcer following orthopedic surgery because it requires traction and bed rest. A patient with obesity and diabetes who has major abdominal surgery is at risk for poor wound healing and developing the complications of a fistula or dehiscence. Nurses are often the first ones to detect and document changes in a patient's condition. In her classic research Benner (1984) notes that expert nurses learn to anticipate breakdown and deterioration of patients even before confirming diagnostic signs develop.

Your knowledge of pathophysiology and experience with previous patients help in identifying the risk of complications that can occur. A thorough assessment reveals the level of a patient's current risk. The evidence or scientific rationales for how certain interventions (e.g., pressure-relief devices, repositioning, or wound care) prevent or minimize complications help you select the preventive measures that likely are most useful. For example, if a patient who is obese has uncontrolled postoperative pain, the risk for pressure ulcer development increases because the patient is unwilling or unable to change position frequently. The nurse anticipates when the patient's pain will be aggravated, administers ordered analgesics, and then positions the patient to remove pressure on the skin and underlying tissues. If the patient continues to have difficulty turning or repositioning, the nurse selects a pressure-relief device to place on the patient's bed.

Some nursing procedures pose risks. Be aware of potential complications and take precautionary measures. For example, the patient who has a feeding tube is at risk for aspiration. Position the patient in high-Fowler's position and check the tube position before administering a feeding.

Identifying Areas of Assistance. Certain nursing situations require you to obtain assistance by seeking additional personnel, knowledge, and/or nursing skills. Before beginning care, review the plan to determine the need for assistance and the type required. Sometimes you need assistance in performing a procedure, providing comfort measures, or preparing the patient for a diagnostic test. Do not take shortcuts if assistance is not immediately available since this increases risk of injury to you and the patient. For example, when you care for a patient who is overweight and immobilized, you require additional personnel and transfer equipment to turn and position the patient safely. Be sure to determine the number of additional personnel and if you need them in advance. Discuss your need for assistance with other nurses or NAP.

You require additional knowledge and skills in situations in which you are less experienced. Because of the continual growth in health care technology, you may lack the skills to perform a procedure. When you are asked to administer a new medication, operate a new piece of equipment, or administer a procedure with which you are unfamiliar, follow these steps.

- Seek information you need to be informed about the procedure. Check the scientific literature for evidence-based information, review resource manuals and the procedure book of the agency, or consult with experts (e.g., pharmacists, clinical nurse specialists) who are familiar with the procedure.
- Collect all equipment necessary for the procedure.
- Have another nurse who has completed the procedure correctly and safely provide assistance and guidance. The assistance can come from another staff nurse, a supervisor, an educator, or a nurse specialist. Requesting assistance occurs frequently in all types of nursing practice and is a learning process that continues throughout educational experiences and into professional development. One tip is to verbalize with an instructor or staff nurse the steps you will take before actually performing the procedure to improve your confidence.

Implementation Skills

Nursing practice includes cognitive, interpersonal, and psychomotor (technical) skills. You need each type of skill to implement direct and indirect nursing interventions. You are responsible for knowing when one type of implementation skill is preferred over another and for having the necessary knowledge and skill to perform each.

Cognitive Skills. Cognitive skills involve the application of critical thinking in the nursing process. Always use good judgment and sound clinical decision making when performing any intervention. This ensures that no nursing action is automatic. Always think and anticipate so you individualize patient care appropriately. Know the rationale for therapeutic interventions and understand normal and abnormal physiological and psychological responses. In addition, know the evidence in nursing science to ensure that you deliver the most current and relevant nursing interventions. You learn to integrate different concepts and relate them to each other while recollecting facts, situations, and patients for whom you have cared previously (Di Vito-Thomas, 2005).

Tonya knows the pathophysiology of prostate cancer, the anatomy of the prostate gland and surrounding structures, and the normal mechanisms for pain. She considers each of these as she observes Mr. Jacobs, noting how the patient's movement and position either aggravate or lessen his incisional pain. Tonya focuses on relieving Mr. Jacobs' acute pain with an analgesic but then considers the noninvasive interventions needed to provide even greater pain relief so the patient can gain needed rest and relaxation.

Interpersonal Skills. Interpersonal skills are essential for effective nursing action. Develop a trusting relationship, express a level of caring, and communicate clearly with a patient and his or her family (see Chapter 24). Good interpersonal communication is critical for keeping patients informed, providing individualized patient teaching, and effectively supporting patients with challenging emotional needs. Proper use of interpersonal skills enables you to be perceptive of the patient's verbal and nonverbal communication. As a member of the health care team, communicate patient problems and needs clearly, intelligently, and in a timely manner.

Psychomotor Skills. Psychomotor skills require the integration of cognitive and motor activities. For example, when giving an injection you need to understand anatomy and pharmacology (cognitive) and use good coordination and precision to administer the injection correctly (motor). With time and practice you learn to perform skills correctly, smoothly, and confidently. This is critical in establishing patient trust. You are responsible for acquiring necessary psychomotor skills through your experience in the nursing laboratory, the use of interactive instructional technology, or actual hands-on care of patients. When attempting a new skill, always assess your level of competency and obtain the necessary resources to ensure that the patient receives safe treatment.

DIRECT CARE

Nurses provide a wide variety of direct care measures (i.e., activities that nurses perform through patient interactions). How a nurse interacts affects the success of any direct care activity. Remain sensitive to a patient's clinical condition, values and beliefs, expectations, and cultural views. All direct care measures require competent and therefore safe practice. Show a caring approach each time you provide direct care.

Activities of Daily Living

Activities of daily living (ADLs) are activities usually performed in the course of a normal day, including ambulation, eating, dressing, bathing, and grooming (see Chapter 39). A patient's need for assistance with ADLs is temporary, permanent, or rehabilitative. For example, a patient with impaired physical mobility because of bilateral arm casts has a temporary need for assistance. After the casts are removed, the patient gradually regains the strength and range of motion needed to perform ADLs. In contrast, a patient with an irreversible injury to the cervical spinal cord is paralyzed and has a permanent need for assistance. It is unrealistic to plan rehabilitation with a goal of becoming independent with ADLs for this patient. Instead the patient learns new ways to perform ADLs independently through rehabilitation. Occupational and physical therapists play a key role in rehabilitation to restore ADL function.

When your assessment reveals that a patient is experiencing fatigue, a limitation in mobility, confusion, and pain, assistance with ADLs is likely. For example, a patient who experiences shortness of breath avoids eating because of the associated fatigue. Help the patient by setting up meals and offering to cut up food and plan for more frequent, small meals to maintain the patient's nutrition. Assistance with ADLs ranges from partial assistance to complete care. Remember to always respect the patient's wishes and determine his or her preferences. Patients from some cultures prefer receiving assistance with ADLs from family members. As long as a patient is stable and alert, it is appropriate to allow family to assist with care. Most patients want to remain independent in meeting their basic needs. Allow the patient to participate to the level that he or she is able. Involving the patient in planning the timing and types of interventions boosts the patient's self-esteem and willingness to become more independent.

Instrumental Activities of Daily Living

Illness or disability sometimes alters a patient's ability to be independent in society. **Instrumental activities of daily living (IADLs)** include such skills as shopping, preparing meals, house cleaning, writing checks, and taking medications. Nurses within the home care and community health setting frequently help patients adapt ways to perform IADLs. Occupational therapists are specially trained to know how to adapt approaches for patients to use when performing IADLs. Often family and friends are excellent resources for assisting patients. In acute care it is important for you to anticipate how a patient's illness affects the ability to perform IADLs so you can make appropriate referrals.

Physical Care Techniques

You routinely perform a variety of physical care techniques when caring for a patient. Physical care techniques involve the safe and competent administration of nursing procedures (e.g., turning and positioning, performing invasive procedures, administering medications, and providing comfort measures). The specific knowledge and skills needed to perform these procedures are in subsequent clinical chapters of this text. Common methods for administering physical care techniques appropriately include protecting you and the patient from injury, using safe patient handling techniques, using proper infection control practices, staying organized, and following applicable practice guidelines.

To carry out a procedure you need to be knowledgeable about the procedure itself, the standard frequency, the steps, and the expected outcomes. In a hospital you perform many procedures each day, often for the first time. Before conducting a new procedure, always assess the situation and your personal competencies to determine if you need assistance, new knowledge, or new skills. Benner (1984) made an important observation about physical care techniques. Nurses always need to make varied and thoughtful adaptations when administering and monitoring patient therapies. For example, when you change a complicated dressing, you can choose from many dressing materials and cleansing solutions, and the patient's size affects how to secure a dressing. Performing any procedure correctly requires critical thinking and thoughtful decision making.

Lifesaving Measures

A **lifesaving measure** is a physical care technique that you use when a patient's physiological or psychological state is threatened (see Chapter 40). The purpose of lifesaving measures is to restore physiological or psychological homeostasis. Such measures include administering emergency medications, instituting cardiopulmonary resuscitation, intervening to protect a confused or violent patient, and obtaining immediate counseling from a crisis center for a severely anxious patient. If an inexperienced nurse faces a situation requiring emergency measures, the proper nursing actions are to stay with the patient, maintain support, and have another staff member obtain an experienced professional.

Counseling

Counseling is a direct care method that helps a patient use a problem-solving process to recognize and manage stress and facilitate interpersonal relationships. As a nurse, you counsel patients to accept actual or impending changes resulting from stress (see Chapter 37). Examples include patients who are facing terminal illness or chronic disease. Counseling involves emotional, intellectual, spiritual, and psychological support. A patient and family who need nursing counseling have normal adjustment difficulties and are upset or frustrated, but they are not necessarily psychologically disabled. A good example is the stress that a young woman faces when caring for her aging mother. Family caregivers need assistance in adjusting to the physical and emotional demands of caregiving. Sometimes they need respite (i.e., a break from providing care). The recipient of care also needs assistance in adjusting to his or her disability. Patients with psychiatric diagnoses require therapy from nurses specializing in psychiatric nursing or social workers, psychiatrists, or psychologists.

Many counseling techniques foster cognitive, behavioral, developmental, experiential, and emotional growth in patients. Most of the techniques listed in Box 19-3 require additional knowledge beyond the scope of this text. Counseling encourages individuals to examine available alternatives and decide which choices are

BOX 19-3 COUNSELING STRATEGIES AND SELECTED EXAMPLES USED BY NURSES

Behavior Modification
- Encourage alternative behavior (e.g., meditation instead of smoking to relieve stress).
- Develop a chart to record and track eating habit changes.
- Use social skills training (e.g., role playing) to change behaviors (e.g., anger or aggression).

Bereavement Counseling
- Assist patient in productive reminiscing of loved one.
- Support patient in removing loved one's belongings from home.

Relaxation Exercises
- Progressive muscle relaxation exercises and guided imagery

Crisis Intervention
- Therapy designed to assist in coping with crisis
- Anticipatory guidance to recognize and avoid modifiable crises

Play Therapy
- Help children through play to cope with loss and grief.
- Help children cope with chronic illness.
- Help children become competent in self-care activities.

useful and appropriate. When patients are able to examine alternatives, they develop a sense of control and are able to better manage stress.

Teaching

Teaching is an important nursing responsibility because education is key to patient-centered care (see Chapter 25). A teaching plan is essential, especially when patients are inexperienced and being asked to manage health problems they are facing for the first time. Counseling and teaching closely align. Both involve using good interpersonal skills to create a change in the patient. However, with counseling the change results in the development of new attitudes and feelings, whereas in teaching the focus of change is intellectual growth or the acquisition of new knowledge or psychomotor skills (Redman, 2005).

When you educate patients, respect the diversity of their human experiences, know their values and preferences as to how they learn, and respect their expertise with their own health management. As an educator you present health care principles, procedures, and techniques to inform patients about their health status and help them achieve self-care within their capabilities. The types of teaching topics that you address with patients are unlimited. However, be aware that teaching is also an ongoing process of keeping patients informed. Patients want to know why you do what you do. For example, incorporate into your interventions explanations of procedures, why they are being done, what the expected outcomes are, and what the patient can expect. A simple application is informing a patient about his or her IV infusion: explain what the IV fluid bag contains, how long the bag should last, the sensations the patient will feel if the IV site becomes inflamed, the fact that a small flexible catheter is in the arm, and any potential side effects of medications in the bag.

Teaching takes place in all health care settings (Fig. 19-3). As a nurse you are accountable for the quality of education you deliver. Know your patient; be aware of the cultural and social factors that influence a patient's willingness and ability to learn. It is also important to know your patient's health literacy level. Can he or she read directions or make calculations that sometimes are necessary with self-care skills? The teaching-learning process is an interaction between you and the learner, and it offers an organizational structure and framework for successful patient education. Don't assume that patients understand their illness or disease. If they seem uneasy or refuse a treatment, simply ask what concerns them. This gives you the opportunity to provide further teaching and correct knowledge deficiencies.

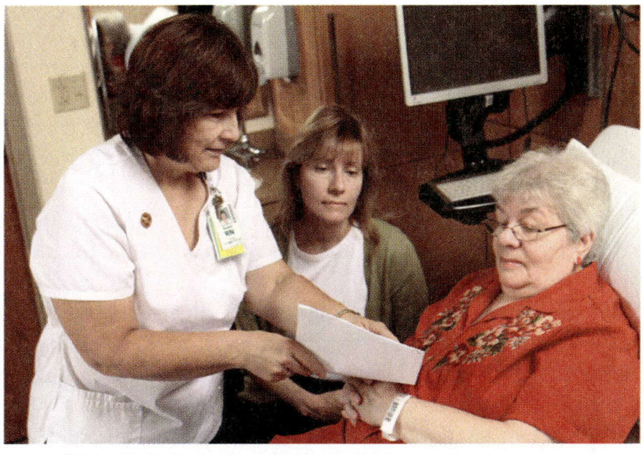

FIG. 19-3 Teaching patient discharge instructions.

Controlling for Adverse Reactions

An **adverse reaction** is a harmful or unintended effect of a medication, diagnostic test, or therapeutic intervention. Adverse reactions can possibly follow any nursing intervention; thus learn to anticipate and know which adverse reactions to expect. Nursing actions that control for adverse reactions reduce or counteract the reaction. For example, when applying a moist heat compress, you want to prevent burning the patient's skin. First assess the condition of the area where you plan to place the compress. Following application of the compress, inspect the area every 5 minutes for any adverse reaction such as excessive reddening of the skin from the heat or skin maceration from the moisture. When completing a health care provider–directed intervention such as medication administration, you need to understand the potential side effects of the drug. After you administer the medication, evaluate the patient for any adverse effects. Also be aware of drugs that counteract the side effects. For example, a patient has an unknown hypersensitivity to penicillin and develops hives after three doses. You record the reaction, stop further administration of the drug, and consult with the physician. You then administer an ordered dose of diphenhydramine (Benadryl), an antihistamine and antipruritic medication, to reduce the allergic response and relieve the itching.

When caring for a patient who is undergoing a particular diagnostic test, you need to understand the test and any potential adverse effects. For example, a patient has not had a bowel movement in 24 hours after a barium enema. Because bowel impaction is a potential side effect of a barium enema, you increase fluid intake and instruct the patient to let nursing personnel know when a bowel movement occurs. Although adverse effects are not common, they do occur. It is important that you recognize the signs and symptoms of an adverse reaction and intervene in a timely manner.

Preventive Measures

Preventive nursing actions promote health and prevent illness to avoid the need for acute or rehabilitative health care (see Chapter 1). Changes in the health care system are leading to greater emphasis on health promotion and illness prevention. Primary prevention aimed at health promotion includes health education programs, immunizations, and physical and nutritional fitness activities. Secondary prevention focuses on people who are experiencing health problems or illnesses and who are at risk for developing complications or worsening conditions. It includes screening techniques and treating early stages of disease. Tertiary prevention involves minimizing the effects of long-term illness or disability, including rehabilitation measures.

INDIRECT CARE

Indirect care measures include nurse actions aimed at management of the patient care environment and interdisciplinary collaborative actions that support the effectiveness of direct care interventions (Bulechek et al., 2008). Many of the measures are managerial in nature such as emergency cart maintenance and environmental and supply management (Box 19-4). Nurses spend much time in indirect and unit management activities. Communication of information about patients (e.g., change-of-shift report and consultation) is critical, ensuring that direct care activities are planned, coordinated, and performed with the proper resources. Delegation of care to NAP is another indirect care activity (see Chapter 21). When performed correctly, delegation ensures that the right care provider performs the right tasks so the nurse and NAP work most efficiently together for the patient's benefit.

BOX 19-4 EXAMPLES OF INDIRECT CARE ACTIVITIES

- Documentation (electronic or written)
- Delegation of care activities to nursing assistive personnel
- Medical order transcription
- Infection control (e.g., proper handling and storage of supplies, use of protective isolation)
- Environmental safety management (e.g., make patient rooms safe, strategically assigning patients in a geographical proximity to a single nurse)
- Telephone consultations with physicians and other health care providers
- Change-of-shift report
- Collecting, labeling, and transporting specimens
- Transporting patients to procedural areas and other nursing units

From Bulechek GM et al: *Nursing interventions classification (NIC)*, ed 5, St Louis, 2008, Mosby.

Communicating Nursing Interventions

Any intervention that you provide for a patient is communicated in a written (or electronic) and oral format. Written interventions are part of the nursing care plan (see Chapter 18) and a patient's permanent medical record. Staff in many institutions develop **interdisciplinary care plans** (i.e., plans representing the contributions of all disciplines caring for a patient). After completing any nursing interventions, you document the treatment and patient's response in the appropriate part of the record (see Chapter 26). The record entry usually includes a brief description of pertinent assessment findings, the specific intervention(s), and the patient's response. A written record validates that you performed the procedure and provides valuable information to subsequent caregivers about the approaches needed to provide successful care.

You also communicate nursing interventions verbally to other health care professionals. Unless communication is timely and accurate, caregivers can be uninformed, interventions may be duplicated needlessly, procedures may be delayed, or tasks may be left undone. Patients can quickly tell when members of the health care team communicate inconsistent messages, indicating that no one is in charge. Nurses commonly communicate orally when conferring with colleagues, during a change of shift, transferring a patient to another unit, or discharging a patient to another health care agency. Always be clear, concise, and to the point when you communicate nursing interventions.

Delegating, Supervising, and Evaluating the Work of Other Staff Members

Depending on the system of health care delivery, the nurse who develops the care plan frequently does not perform all of the nursing interventions. Some activities you coordinate and delegate to other members of the health care team (see Chapter 21). For example, an RN delegates components of care but not the nursing process itself (American Nurses Association [ANA], 2006). Noninvasive and frequently repetitive interventions such as skin care, ambulation, grooming, vital signs on stable patients, and hygiene measures are examples of care activities that you delegate to NAP such as a nurse assistant. When a nurse delegates aspects of a patient's care to another staff member, the nurse who assigns the tasks is responsible for ensuring that each task is appropriately assigned and completed according to the standard of care. You are responsible for delegating direct care interventions to personnel who are competent. Recently the ANA and the National Council of State Boards of Nursing (NCSBN) released a joint statement outlining 10 principles for delegation (Trossman, 2006). The principles are a blueprint to help RNs better understand delegation, keep patients safe, and protect their professional practice.

ACHIEVING PATIENT GOALS

Regardless of the type of interventions, you implement nursing care to achieve patient goals and outcomes. In most clinical situations multiple interventions are necessary to achieve select outcomes. In addition, patients' conditions often change minute by minute. Therefore it is important for you to apply principles of care coordination such as good time management, organizational skills, and appropriate use of resources to ensure that you deliver interventions effectively and meet desired outcomes (see Chapter 21). Priority setting is critical in successful implementation. Priorities help you to anticipate and sequence nursing interventions when a patient has multiple nursing diagnoses and collaborative problems (see Chapter 18).

Another way to achieve patient goals is to help them adhere to their treatment plan. **Patient adherence** means that patients and families invest time in carrying out required treatments. To ensure patients a smooth transition across different health care settings (e.g., hospital to home and clinic to home to assisted living), it becomes important to introduce interventions that patients are willing and able to follow. Adequate and timely discharge planning and education of the patient and family are the first steps in promoting a smooth transition from one health care setting to another or to the home. To be effective with discharge planning and education, you individualize your care and take into consideration the various factors that influence a patient's health beliefs. For example, for Tonya to effectively help Mr. Jacobs follow the activity limitations required after surgery, she needs to know if Mr. Jacobs understands the risks to wound healing if limitations are not followed. Chapter 6 reviews the principles of the health belief model, which influence how patients adhere to health care recommendations. You are responsible for delivering interventions in a way that reflects your understanding of a patient's health beliefs, culture, lifestyle pattern, and patterns of wellness. In addition, reinforcing successes with the treatment plan encourages the patient to follow the care plan.

KEY POINTS

- Implementation is the fourth step of the nursing process in which nurses initiate interventions that are designed to achieve the goals and expected outcomes of the patient's plan of care.
- A direct-care intervention is a treatment performed through interactions with a patient that can include nurse-initiated, physician-initiated, and collaborative approaches.
- Always think first and determine if an intervention is correct and appropriate and if you have the resources needed to implement it.
- Clinical guidelines or protocols are evidence-based documents that guide decisions and interventions for specific health care problems.
- When preparing to perform an intervention, reassess the patient, review and revise the existing nursing care plan, organize resources and care delivery approaches, anticipate and prevent complications, and implement the intervention.
- The implementation of nursing care often requires additional knowledge, nursing skills, and personnel resources.

- Before beginning to perform interventions, make sure that the patient is as physically and psychologically comfortable as possible.
- Use good judgment and sound clinical decision making when performing any intervention to ensure that no nursing action is automatic.
- To anticipate and prevent complications, identify risks to the patient, adapt interventions to the situation, evaluate the relative benefit of a treatment versus the risk, and initiate risk-prevention measures.
- Methods used to ensure that you administer physical care techniques appropriately include protecting you and the patient from injury, using proper infection control practices, staying organized, and following applicable practice guidelines.
- When you delegate aspects of a patient's care, you are responsible for ensuring that each task is assigned appropriately and completed according to the standard of care.
- To complete any nursing procedure, you need to know the procedure, its frequency, the steps, and the expected outcomes.

CLINICAL APPLICATION QUESTIONS

Preparing for Clinical Practice

Tonya is preparing to change the dressing over Mr. Jacobs' wound, and Mrs. Jacobs is present to observe. Tonya determines Mr. Jacob's level of pain to be sure that he is comfortable. She decides to include discussion of wound and urinary catheter care during her time with the family. Before beginning instruction with the Jacobs, Tonya asks Mr. Jacobs if he is ready to learn about wound and catheter care. She observes Mr. and Mrs. Jacobs' behaviors to note their receptivity to instruction. She prepares all of her supplies before the dressing change. She also assesses the condition of the dressing before she starts.

1. When Tonya asks Mr. Jacobs about his readiness for instruction, which aspect of the implementation process is she performing?
2. When changing Mr. Jacobs' dressing, Tonya cleans the wound following clinical practice guidelines for her nursing unit and checks the incision for signs of infection. Explain the benefit of cleansing the wound on the basis of practice guidelines.
3. When Tonya begins instructing the Jacobs about wound care, what implementation skill most likely ensures good outcomes, specifically that the patient is able to learn how to change his dressing correctly at home?

evolve *Answers to Clinical Application Questions can be found on the Evolve website.*

REVIEW QUESTIONS

Are You Ready to Test Your Nursing Knowledge?

1. The nurse enters a patient's room and finds that the patient was incontinent of liquid stool. The patient has recurrent redness in the perineal area, and there is concern that he is developing a pressure ulcer. The nurse cleanses the patient, inspects the skin, and applies a skin barrier ointment to the perineal area. She calls the ostomy and wound care specialist and asks that he visit the patient to recommend skin care measures. Which of the following describe the nurse's actions? (Select all that apply.)
   1. The application of the skin barrier is a dependent care measure.
   2. The call to the ostomy and wound care specialist is an indirect care measure.
   3. The cleansing of the skin is a direct care measure.
   4. The application of the skin barrier is a direct care measure.
2. During the implementation step of the nursing process, a nurse reviews and revises the nursing plan of care. Place the following steps of review and revision in the correct order:
   1. Review the care plan.
   2. Decide if the nursing interventions remain appropriate.
   3. Reassess the patient.
   4. Compare assessment findings to validate existing nursing diagnoses.
3. A nurse checks a physician's order and notes that a new medication was ordered. The nurse is unfamiliar with the medication. A nurse colleague explains that the medication is an anticoagulant used for postoperative patients with risk for blood clots. The nurse's best action before giving the medication is to:
   1. Have the nurse colleague check the dose with her before giving the medication.
   2. Consult with a pharmacist to obtain knowledge about the purpose of the drug, the action, and the potential side effects.
   3. Ask the nurse colleague to administer the medication to her patient.
   4. Administer the medication as prescribed and on time.
4. When does implementation begin as the fourth step of the nursing process?
   1. During the assessment phase
   2. Immediately in some critical situations
   3. After the care plan has been developed
   4. After there is mutual goal setting between nurse and patient
5. Before consulting with a physician about a patient's need for urinary catheterization, the nurse considers the fact that the patient has urinary retention and has been unable to void on her own. The nurse knows that evidence for alternative measures to promote voiding exists, but none has been effective, and that before surgery the patient was voiding normally. This scenario is an example of which implementation skill?
   1. Cognitive
   2. Interpersonal
   3. Psychomotor
   4. Consultative
6. The nurse enters a patient's room, and the patient asks if he can get out of bed and transfer to a chair. The nurse takes precautions to use safe patient handling techniques and transfers the patient. This is an example of which physical care technique?
   1. Meeting the patient's expressed wishes
   2. Indirect care measure
   3. Protecting a patient from injury
   4. Staying organized when implementing a procedure
7. In which of the following examples is a nurse applying critical thinking attitudes when preparing to insert an intravenous (IV) catheter? (Select all that apply.)
   1. Following the procedural guideline for IV insertion
   2. Seeking necessary knowledge about the steps of the procedure from a more experienced nurse
   3. Showing confidence in performing the correct IV insertion technique
   4. Being sure that the IV dressing covers the IV site completely
8. Which steps does the nurse follow when he or she is asked to perform an unfamiliar procedure? (Select all that apply.)

1. Seeks necessary knowledge
2. Reassesses the patient's condition
3. Collects all necessary equipment
4. Delegates the procedure to a more experienced staff member
5. Considers all possible consequences of the procedure

9. For each of the following interventions, note which are direct and which are indirect nursing interventions. Place a D for direct or I for indirect in the space provided
   1. A nurse checks the monthly performance improvement report on fall occurrences on a unit. ______________
   2. A nurse discusses with the patient exercise restrictions to follow on return home. ______________
   3. A nurse consults with a dietitian about a patient's therapeutic diet food choices. ______________
   4. A nurse administers a tube feeding. ______________
   5. A nurse assists a colleague in applying a complex dressing to a patient's wound. ______________
10. A nurse is talking with a patient who is visiting a neighborhood health clinic. The patient came to the clinic for repeated symptoms of a sinus infection. During their discussion the nurse checks the patient's medical record and realizes that he is due for a tetanus shot. Administering the shot is an example of what type of preventive intervention?
    1. Tertiary
    2. Direct care
    3. Primary
    4. Secondary
11. A nurse is orienting a new graduate nurse to the unit. The graduate nurse asks, "Why do we have standing orders for cases when patients develop life-threatening arrhythmias? Is not each patient's situation unique?" What is the nurse's best answer?
    1. Standing orders are used to meet our physician's preferences.
    2. Standing orders ensure that we are familiar with evidence-based guidelines for care of arrhythmias.
    3. Standing orders allow us to respond quickly and safely to a rapidly changing clinical situation.
    4. Standing orders minimize the documentation we have to provide.
12. A nurse on a cancer unit is reviewing and revising the written plan of care for a patient who has the nursing diagnosis of nausea. Place the following steps in their proper order:
    1. The nurse revises approaches in the plan for controlling environmental factors that worsen nausea.
    2. The nurse enters data in the assessment column showing new information about the patient's nausea.
    3. The nurse adds the current date to show that the diagnosis of nausea is still relevant.
    4. The nurse decides to use the patient's self-report of appetite and fluid intake as evaluation measures.
13. When a nurse properly positions a patient and administers an enema solution at the correct rate for the patient's tolerance, this is an example of what type of implementation skill?
    1. Interpersonal
    2. Cognitive
    3. Collaborative
    4. Psychomotor
14. The nurse reviews a patient's medical record and sees that tube feedings are to begin after a feeding tube is inserted. In recent past experiences the nurse has seen patients on the unit develop diarrhea from tube feedings. The nurse consults with the dietitian and physician to determine the initial rate that will be ordered for the feeding to lessen the chance of diarrhea. This is an example of what type of direct care measure?
    1. Preventive
    2. Controlling for an adverse reaction
    3. Consulting
    4. Counseling
15. A nurse is starting on the evening shift and is assigned to care for a patient with a diagnosis of *impaired skin integrity related to pressure and moisture on the skin.* The patient is 72 years old and had a stroke. The patient weighs 250 pounds and is difficult to turn. As the nurse makes decisions about how to implement skin care for the patient, which of the following actions does the nurse implement? (Select all that apply.)
    1. Review the set of all possible nursing interventions for the patient's problem
    2. Review all possible consequences associated with each possible nursing action
    3. Consider own level of competency
    4. Determine the probability of all possible consequences

Answers: **1.** 2, 3, 4; **2.** 3, 1, 4, 2; **3.** 2; **4.** 3; **5.** 1; **6.** 3; **7.** 2, 3; **8.** 1, 3, 5; **9.** 1 (I), 2 (D), 3 (I) 4 (D), 5 (D); **10.** 3; **11.** 3; **12.** 2, 3, 1, 4; **13.** 4; **14.** 2; **15.** 1, 2, 4.

REFERENCES

American Nurses Association: *Principles for delegation,* 2006, http://nursingworld.org/staffing/lawsuit/PrinciplesDelegation.pdf. Accessed October 15, 2006.

American Nurses Association: *Scope and standards of practice: nursing,* ed 2, Silver Spring, Md, 2010, American Nurses Association.

Bulechek GM, et al: *Nursing interventions classification (NIC),* ed 5, St Louis, 2008, Mosby.

Gerontological Nursing Interventions Research Center: *Evidence-based practice guidelines,* 2010, University of Iowa, http://www.nursing.uiowa.edu/Hartford/nurse.ebp.htm based.htm. Accessed December 28, 2010.

Manchikanti L, et al: A critical review of the American Pain Society clinical practice guidelines for interventional techniques. Part 1, Diagnostic interventions, *Pain Physician* 13(3):E141, 2010.

National Guideline Clearinghouse: *Guidelines,* 2010, Agency for Healthcare Research and Quality, 2010, http://www.guideline.gov. Accessed December 29, 2010.

Redman BK: *The practice of patient education,* ed 10, St Louis, 2005, Mosby.

Rosenbrand K, et al: Guideline development, *Studies Health Technol Informatics* 139:3, 2008.

Scherb CA, Weydt AP: Work complexity assessment, nursing interventions classification, and nursing outcomes classification: making connections, *Creative Nurs* 15(1):16, 2009.

Trossman S: Getting a clearer picture on delegation, *Am Nurs Today* 1(1):54, 2006.

RESEARCH REFERENCES

Benner P: *From novice to expert,* Menlo Park, Calif, 1984, Addison-Wesley.

Di Vito-Thomas P: Nursing student stories on learning how to think like a nurse, *Nurse Educ* 30(3):133, 2005.

Potter P, et al: Delegation practices between registered nurses and nursing assistive personnel, *J Nurs Manag* 18(2):157, 2010.

CHAPTER

20

Evaluation

OBJECTIVES

- Discuss the relationship between critical thinking and evaluation.
- Describe the standards of professional nursing practice for evaluation.
- Explain the relationship among goals of care, expected outcomes, and evaluative measures when evaluating nursing care.
- Give examples of evaluation measures for determining a patient's progress toward outcomes.
- Evaluate the outcomes of care for a patient.
- Describe how evaluation leads to discontinuation, revision, or modification of a plan of care.

KEY TERMS

Evaluation, p. 265
Evaluative measures, p. 268
Nursing-sensitive outcome, p. 267
Standard of care, p. 271

evolve WEBSITE

http://evolve.elsevier.com/Potter/fundamentals/

- Review Questions
- Case Study with Questions
- Audio Glossary
- Interactive Learning Activities
- Key Term Flashcards
- Content Updates

When a repairman comes to a home to fix a leaking faucet, he turns the faucet on to determine the problem, changes or adjusts parts, and rechecks the faucet to determine if the leak is fixed. After a patient diagnosed with pneumonia completes a course of antibiotics, the health care provider often has him or her return to the office to have a chest x-ray examination to determine if the pneumonia has cleared. When a nurse provides wound care, including application of a warm compress, several steps are involved. He or she assesses the appearance of the wound, determines its severity, applies the appropriate form of compress, and returns later to determine if the condition of the wound has improved. These three scenarios depict what ultimately occurs during the process of evaluation. The repairman rechecks the faucet, the physician orders a chest x-ray film, and the nurse reinspects the patient's wound. Evaluation involves two components: an examination of a condition or situation and a judgment as to whether change has occurred. Ideally after an intervention takes place, evaluation reveals an improvement, a desired outcome.

The previous chapters on the nursing process describe how you apply critical thinking to gather patient data, form nursing diagnoses, develop a plan of care, and implement interventions in the care plan. **Evaluation,** the final step of the nursing process, is crucial to determine whether, after application of the nursing process, the patient's condition or well-being improves. You apply all that you know about a patient and his or her condition and your experiences with previous patients to evaluate whether nursing care was effective. *You conduct evaluative measures to determine if your patients met expected outcomes, not if nursing interventions were completed.* The expected outcomes established during planning are the standards against which the nurse judges whether goals have been met and if care is successful.

In the continuing case study, Tonya has instructed Mr. Jacobs about necessary wound care. Mrs. Jacobs also participates in the education session. Tonya discusses with the family the importance of wound care in preventing infection and has Mr. and Mrs. Jacobs observe the dressing change. During the dressing change Tonya uses safe and appropriate intervention techniques to protect the integrity of the wound and minimize transmission of infection. She also discusses how physical stress such as bending and lifting strains a suture line; thus Mr. Jacobs needs to limit activity for the first few weeks after surgery. Tonya encourages the Jacobs to ask any questions they have about wound care. Tonya returns to Mr. Jacobs' room an hour later to evaluate the results of her instruction. For the nursing diagnosis of deficient knowledge, Tonya set the expected outcomes of: "Patient and wife will describe the signs and symptoms of a wound infection, explain how activity affects wound healing, and demonstrate a dressing change correctly." Mr. Jacobs is resting in bed, and Mrs. Jacobs is reading one of the instruction brochures as Tonya enters the room. Tonya says, "Mrs. Jacobs, I see that you're reviewing the booklet I gave you. Do you have any questions"? Mrs. Jacobs responds, "I guess I understand what to look for with an infection. I hope I can recognize changes." Tonya asks, "Tell me the signs of infection."

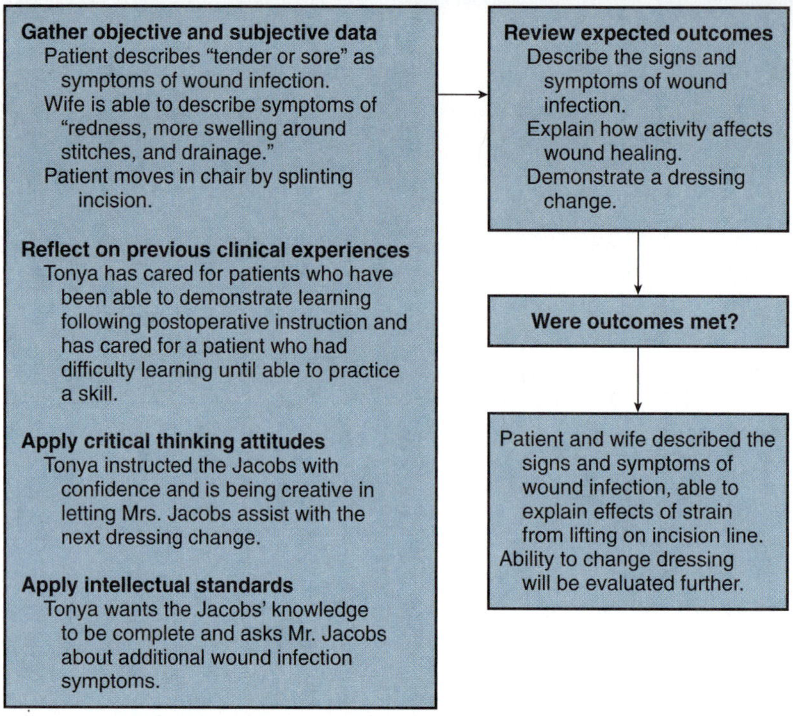

Gather objective and subjective data
Patient describes "tender or sore" as symptoms of wound infection.
Wife is able to describe symptoms of "redness, more swelling around stitches, and drainage."
Patient moves in chair by splinting incision.
Reflect on previous clinical experiences
Tonya has cared for patients who have been able to demonstrate learning following postoperative instruction and has cared for a patient who had difficulty learning until able to practice a skill.
Apply critical thinking attitudes
Tonya instructed the Jacobs with confidence and is being creative in letting Mrs. Jacobs assist with the next dressing change.
Apply intellectual standards
Tonya wants the Jacobs' knowledge to be complete and asks Mr. Jacobs about additional wound infection symptoms.
Review expected outcomes
Describe the signs and symptoms of wound infection.
Explain how activity affects wound healing.
Demonstrate a dressing change.
Were outcomes met?
Patient and wife described the signs and symptoms of wound infection, able to explain effects of strain from lifting on incision line.
Ability to change dressing will be evaluated further.

FIG. 20-1 Critical thinking and the evaluation process.

Mrs. Jacobs replies, "Redness, more swelling around the stitches, and drainage." Tonya asks Mr. Jacobs, "Are there any other signs of infection?" Mr. Jacobs responds, "You said that my incision would feel more tender or sore and that I might have a fever." "That's right," Tonya remarks. "Tell me why your doctor has limited your lifting for a month." Mr. Jacobs answers, "So I don't strain my incision and pull out the stitches." "Right again," Tonya affirms," I think that before you go home tomorrow we should let you watch one more dressing change and even let your wife help me."

Evaluation is an ongoing process that occurs whenever you have contact with a patient. Once you deliver an intervention, you gather subjective and objective data from the patient, family, and health care team members. You also review knowledge regarding the patient's current condition, treatment, resources available for recovery, and expected outcomes. By referring to previous experiences caring for similar patients, you are in a better position to know how to evaluate your patient. You can anticipate what to evaluate. Apply critical thinking attitudes and standards to determine whether outcomes of care are achieved (Fig. 20-1). If outcomes are met, the overall goals for the patient also are met. Compare patient behavior and responses that you assessed before delivering nursing interventions with behavior and responses that occur after administering nursing care. Critical thinking directs you to analyze the findings from evaluation (Fig. 20-2). Has the patient's condition improved? Is the patient able to improve, or are there physical factors preventing recovery? To what degree does this patient's motivation or willingness to pursue healthier behaviors influence responses to therapies?

During evaluation you make clinical decisions and continually redirect nursing care. For example, when Tonya evaluates the Jacobs' learning, she applies knowledge of patient education principles and postoperative wound healing to interpret whether learning has occurred and whether further instruction is needed. Tonya knows that repetition is important in learning and thus plans another instruction session with the family during a dressing change the next day. Evaluative findings determine Tonya's next course of action. In the Jacobs' case Tonya knows that this is the first time Mr. Jacobs has had major surgery. Mrs. Jacobs voiced concern about recognizing the signs of infection. To meet the outcomes of care, Tonya plans to discuss the appearance of the wound during normal healing and specifically how signs of infection present. She reinforces this explanation during the dressing change so Mr. and Mrs. Jacobs can look at the wound closely again under Tonya's instruction.

Positive evaluations occur when the patient meets desired outcomes, which leads you to conclude that the nursing intervention(s) were effective. For example, in the case study Tonya notes that Mrs. Jacobs identified three signs and symptoms of infection and Mr. Jacobs identified two. Therefore Tonya determines the expected outcome of "describing signs and symptoms of wound infection" was partially met by the patient. However, further instruction is necessary. Unmet or undesirable outcomes such as incorrect or incomplete knowledge indicate that interventions are not effective in minimizing or resolving the actual problem or avoiding an at-risk problem. An unmet outcome reveals that the patient has not responded to interventions as planned. As a result, the nurse changes the plan of care by trying different therapies or changing the frequency or approach of existing therapies.

This sequence of critically evaluating and revising therapies continues until you and the patient successfully and appropriately resolve the problems defined by nursing diagnoses. Remember that evaluation is dynamic and ever changing, depending on the patient's nursing diagnoses and conditions. As problems change, so do expected outcomes. A patient whose health status continuously changes requires more frequent evaluation. In addition, you evaluate priority diagnoses first. For example, Tonya continues to evaluate Mr. Jacobs' *acute pain* before evaluating the status of his *deficient knowledge*.

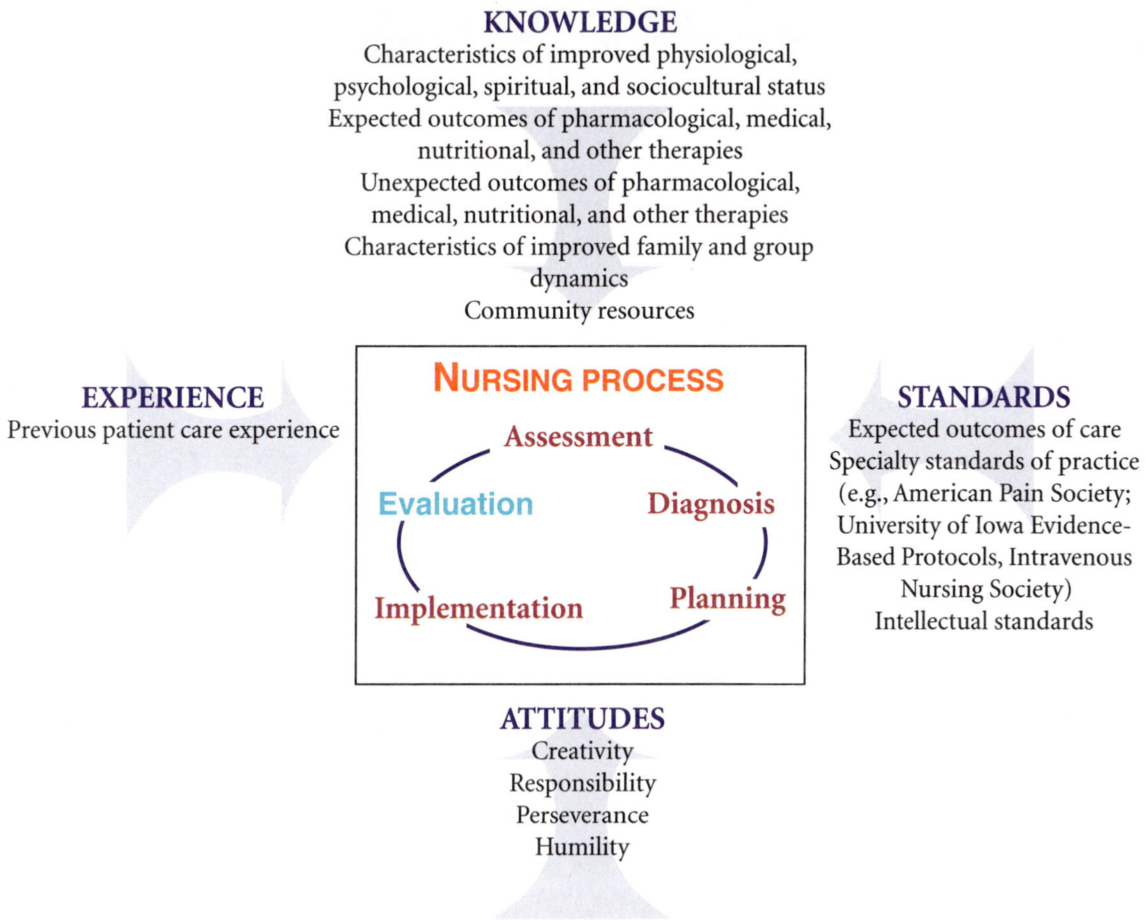

FIG. 20-2 Critical thinking and evaluation.

STANDARDS FOR EVALUATION

Nursing care helps patients resolve actual health problems, prevent the occurrence of potential problems, and maintain a healthy state. The evaluation process is an integral step to that end. The American Nurses Association (ANA) defines standards of professional nursing practice, which include standards for the evaluation step of the nursing process (see Chapter 1). The standards are authoritative statements of the duties that all registered nurses, regardless of role, patient population they serve, or specialty, are expected to perform competently (ANA, 2010). The competencies for evaluation include being systematic and using criterion-based evaluation, collaborating with patients and other professionals, using ongoing assessment data to revise the plan, and communicating results to patients and families. It is also important to ensure the responsible and appropriate use of interventions to minimize unwarranted or unwanted treatment (ANA, 2010).

Criterion-Based Evaluation

You evaluate nursing care by knowing what to look for as described in the criterion-based standards included in a patient's goals and expected outcomes. The goals and outcomes are objective criteria needed to judge a patient's response to care.

Goals. A goal is the expected behavior or response that indicates resolution of a nursing diagnosis or maintenance of a healthy state. It is a summary statement of what will be accomplished when the patient has met all expected outcomes. For Mr. Jacobs Tonya selected the goal of, "Patient expresses acceptance of health status by day of discharge" for the nursing diagnosis of *anxiety* (see Chapter 18). Successful achievement of this goal depends on Tonya delivering interventions selected from the Nursing Interventions Classification (NIC), including acceptance of health status and anxiety level (see Nursing Care Plan, Chapter 18).

Goals often are also based on standards of care or guidelines established for minimal safe practice. For example, the Infusion Nurses Society (INS) has standards of care for prevention of the intravenous (IV) complication phlebitis (INS, 2006). When a nurse cares for a patient with a peripheral IV line, the goal, "The IV site will remain free of phlebitis," is established on the basis of sound practice standards. The INS phlebitis scale contains physical criteria for determining phlebitis (see Chapter 41).

Expected Outcomes. An expected outcome is an end result that is measurable, desirable, and observable and translates into observable patient behaviors (ANA, 2010). It is a measure that tells you if the interventions applied in patient care led to successful goal achievement. When nurses apply the nursing process, a **nursing-sensitive outcome** is a measurable patient or family state, behavior, or perception largely influenced by and sensitive to nursing interventions (Moorhead et al., 2008). The interventions must be within the scope of nursing practice and integral to the processes of nursing care. Examples of nursing-sensitive outcomes include reduction in pain frequency, incidence of pressure ulcers, and incidence of falls (Box 20-1). In comparison, medical outcomes are largely influenced by medical interventions. Examples

BOX 20-1 EVIDENCE-BASED PRACTICE

Nursing-Sensitive Outcomes

PICO Question: In hospitals does the use of nursing-sensitive outcomes improve the quality of nursing care?

Evidence Summary

The current climate in health care is to increase the accountability of health care organizations for the quality of the care they provide (Loan et al., 2011). Nursing-sensitive outcomes are providing benchmarks for hospitals to gauge the quality of their care. The use of nursing-sensitive outcomes such as pressure ulcer prevalence, symptom frequency (pain, nausea, fatigue), medication administration errors, and fall and fall injury incidence offer hospitals an opportunity to compare their performance with specificity (Brown et al., 2010). In addition, these outcome measures offer a way to measure staffing effectiveness (Loan et al., 2011). Doran et al. (2006) showed that nursing-sensitive outcomes are sensitive to changes in patients' conditions and thus are a potential measure of quality of care.

Application to Nursing Practice

- Nursing care is a key factor in the outcomes of hospitalized patients.
- The collection of nursing-sensitive outcomes offers important feedback to nurses about whether nursing interventions lead to patient care improvement.
- The selection of nursing-sensitive outcomes in a plan of care makes nurses accountable for the care delivered to patients and whether there is an improvement in their health status.

include patient mortality, surgical wound infection, and hospital readmissions. Outcomes are statements of progressive, step-by-step physical, emotional, or behavioral responses that the patient needs to accomplish to achieve the goals of care. When you achieve outcomes, the related factors for a nursing diagnosis usually no longer exist. Two of the expected outcomes for Mr. Jacobs' goal of, "Patient expresses acceptance of health status by day of discharge," are "Patient describes surgical outcomes in discussion with surgeon in 24 hours," and "Patient shares concerns with wife before day of discharge." Tonya evaluates Mr. Jacobs by observing for behaviors that reflect anxiety and discussing what the patient has learned from the surgeon and discussed with his wife. The related factor of "uncertainty over recovery" no longer exists if Mr. Jacobs is able to relate surgical outcomes discussed with the surgeon and reports having had a discussion about those outcomes with his wife.

Evaluation is not a description of the achievement of an intervention. Evaluation of Mr. Jacobs *does not* involve observing his ability to perform relaxation exercises for his anxiety. Evaluation *does* involve observation of the patient's behavior (facial expression) during discussions about his recovery.

A valuable resource for selecting outcomes is the Nursing Outcomes Classification (NOC) (see Chapter 18). It offers a language for the evaluation step of the nursing process. The purposes of NOC are (1) to identify, label, validate, and classify nurse-sensitive patient outcomes; (2) to field test and validate the classification; and (3) to define and test measurement procedures for the outcomes and indicators using clinical data (Moorhead et al., 2008). Within the NOC taxonomy you can select outcomes specific for nursing interventions that relate to nursing diagnoses. The NOC project complements the work of NANDA International (NANDA-I) and the NIC project. The NOC classification offers nursing-sensitive outcomes for NANDA-I nursing diagnoses (Table 20-1).

TABLE 20-1 **Linkages Between Nursing Outcomes Classification and Nursing Diagnoses**

NURSING DIAGNOSIS	SUGGESTED OUTCOMES	INDICATORS (EXAMPLES)
Acute pain	Comfort level	Reports physical well-being Reports satisfaction with symptom control Expresses satisfaction with pain control
	Pain control	Recognizes pain onset Uses analgesics appropriately Reports pain controlled
	Pain level	Reports pain severity Frequency of pain Muscle tension
Deficient knowledge	Knowledge: treatment procedures	Description of treatment procedures
	Knowledge: illness care	Description of disease process Description of prescribed activity

For each outcome there are specific recommended evaluation indicators (i.e., the patient behaviors or responses that are measures of outcome achievement).

Collaborate and Evaluate Effectiveness of Interventions

An important aspect of patient-centered care and evaluation is collaboration. A nurse must respect the patient and family as a core member of the health care team, meaning that the patient and family must be actively involved in the evaluation process. When you develop patient care goals and expected outcomes with a patient, he or she becomes an important resource for being able to tell you if outcomes are being met. For example, a patient knows best if pain has lessened or if breathing is easier. The same holds true for the family, who often can recognize changes in patient behavior sooner than you can because of their familiarity with the patient. Members of the health care team who contribute to the patient's care also gather evaluative findings.

Proper evaluation determines the effectiveness of nursing interventions, allowing you to answer the following questions: What is the patient's response to nursing care? Was the therapy effective in improving the patient's physical or emotional health? It is important to evaluate whether each patient reaches a level of wellness or recovery that the health care team and patient established in the goals of care. In addition, have you met the patient's expectations of care? Ask patients about their perceptions of care such as, "Did you receive the type of pain relief you expected?" "Did you receive enough information to change your dressing when you return?" This level of evaluation determines the patient's satisfaction with care and strengthens partnering between you and the patient.

Evaluative Measures. Evaluating a patient's response to nursing care requires the use of **evaluative measures,** which are assessment skills and techniques (e.g., observations, physiological measurements, patient interview) (Fig. 20-3). In fact, evaluative measures are the same as assessment measures, but you perform them at the point of care when you make decisions about the patient's status and progress. The intent of assessment is to identify

TABLE 20-2 **Evaluative Measures to Determine the Success of Goals and Expected Outcomes**

GOALS	EVALUATIVE MEASURES	EXPECTED OUTCOMES
Patient's pressure ulcer will heal within 7 days.	Inspect color, condition, and location of pressure ulcer. Measure diameter of ulcer daily. Note odor and color of drainage from ulcer.	Erythema will be reduced in 2 days. Diameter of ulcer will decrease in 5 days. Ulcer will have no drainage in 2 days. Skin overlying ulcer will be closed in 7 days.
Patient will tolerate ambulation to end of hall by 11/20.	Palpate patient's radial pulse before exercise. Palpate patient's radial pulse 10 minutes after exercise. Assess respiratory rate during exercise. Observe patient for dyspnea or breathlessness during exercise.	Pulse will remain below 110 beats per minute during exercise. Pulse rate will return to resting baseline within 10 minutes after exercise. Respiratory rate will remain within two breaths of patient's baseline rate. Patient will deny feeling of breathlessness.

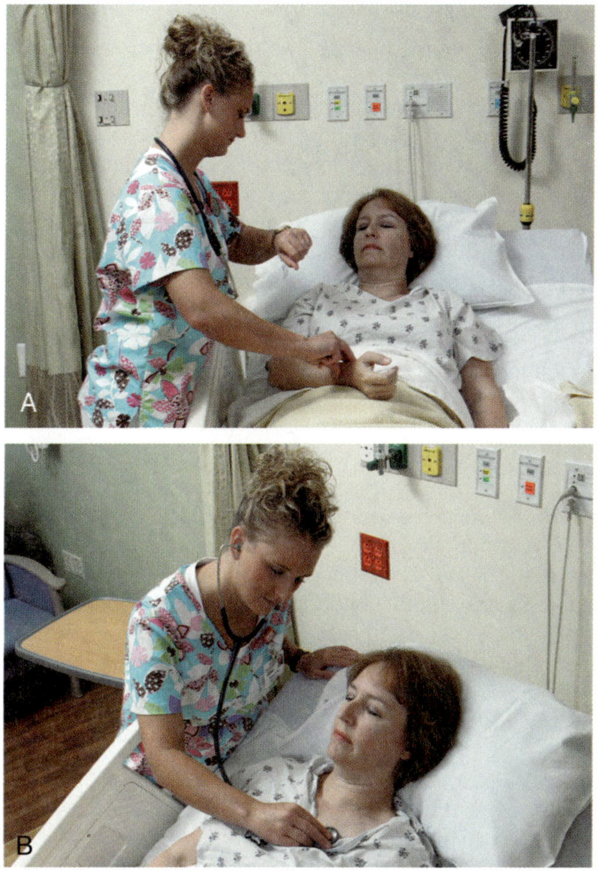

FIG. 20-3 Evaluative measures. **A,** Nurse evaluates patient's vital signs. **B,** Nurse evaluates patient's lung sounds.

which, if any, problems exist. The intent of evaluation is to determine if the known problems have remained the same, improved, worsened, or otherwise changed.

In many clinical situations it is important to collect evaluative measures over a period of time to determine if a pattern of improvement or change exists. A one-time observation of a pressure ulcer is insufficient to determine that the ulcer is healing. It is important to note a consistency in change. For example, over a period of 2 days is the pressure ulcer gradually decreasing in size, is the amount of drainage declining, and is the redness of inflammation resolving? Recognizing a pattern of improvement or deterioration allows you to reason and decide whether the patient's problems (expressed in nursing diagnoses) are resolved. This is very important in the home care or nursing home setting. It may take weeks or even months to determine if interventions led to a pattern of improvement. For example, when evaluating a patient's risk for falls over time, has the patient, family, or health care team successfully reduced fall risks in the home such as eliminating barriers in the home, removing factors impairing the person's vision, or providing direction for proper use of assistive devices?

Interpreting and Summarizing Findings. A patient's clinical condition often changes during an acute illness. In contrast, chronic illness results in slow, subtle changes. When you evaluate the effect of interventions, you interpret or learn to recognize relevant evidence about a patient's condition, even evidence that sometimes does not match clinical expectations. By applying your clinical knowledge and experience, you recognize complications or adverse responses to illness and treatment in addition to expected outcomes.

Careful monitoring and early detection of problems are a patient's first line of defense. Always make clinical judgments on your observations of what is occurring with a specific patient and not merely on what happens to patients in general. Frequently changes are not obvious. Evaluations are patient specific, based on a close familiarity with each patient's behavior, physical status, and reaction to caregivers. Critical thinking skills promote accurate evaluation, which leads to the appropriate revision of ineffective care plans and discontinuation of therapy that has successfully resolved a problem.

Using evidence, you make judgments about a patient's condition. To develop clinical judgment you match the results of evaluative measures with expected outcomes to determine whether or not a patient's status is improving. When interpreting findings, you compare the patient's behavioral responses and the physiological signs and symptoms you expect to see with those actually seen from your evaluation. Comparing expected and actual findings allows you to interpret and judge the patient's condition and whether predicted changes have occurred (Table 20-2). To objectively evaluate the degree of success in achieving outcomes of care, perform the following steps:

1. Examine the outcome criteria to identify the exact desired patient behavior or response.
2. Evaluate the patient's actual behavior or response.
3. Compare the established outcome criteria with the actual behavior or response.
4. Judge the degree of agreement between outcome criteria and the actual behavior or response.
5. If there is no agreement (or only partial agreement) between the outcome criteria and the actual behavior or response, what is/are the barrier(s)? Why did they not agree?

TABLE 20-3 Examples of Objective Evaluation of Goal Achievement

GOALS	OUTCOME CRITERIA	PATIENT RESPONSE	EVALUATION FINDINGS
Patient will change surgical dressing correctly by 12/18.	Patient demonstrates correct hand hygiene by 12/16. Patient describes material to use in dressing change by 12/17. Patient demonstrates dressing change by 12/18.	Patient used antiseptic hand rub correctly to wash hands. Patient applied clean gauze correctly and taped securely in place over incision.	Patient shows progression toward outcomes and achieved desired behavior.
Patient's lungs will be free of secretions by 11/30.	Coughing will be nonproductive by 11/29. Lungs will be clear to auscultation by 11/30. Respirations will be 20 per minute by 11/30.	Patient coughed frequently and productively on 11/29 following nebulization. Lungs were clear to auscultation on 11/30. Respirations were 18 per minute on 11/29.	Patient will require continued nebulizer therapy. Condition is improving.

Evaluation is easier to perform after you care for a patient over a long period. You are then able to make subtle comparisons of patient responses and behaviors. When you have not cared for a patient over an extended time, evaluation improves by referring to previous experiences or asking colleagues who are familiar with the patient to confirm evaluation findings. The accuracy of any evaluation improves when you are familiar with the patient's behavior and physiological status or have cared for more than one patient with a similar problem.

Remember to evaluate each expected outcome and its place in the sequence of care. If not, it is difficult to determine which outcome in the sequence was not met. Thus you cannot revise and redirect the plan of care at the most appropriate time. If the patient achieves the expected outcomes, you either continue the care plan to maintain a therapeutic status or discontinue interventions because the goal of care is met. If evaluation determines that the expected outcomes were not met or only partially met, you begin reassessment and revision of the care plan. If the patient's behavior begins to show changes but does not yet meet criteria set, the goal is partially met. If there is no progress, the goal is not met (Table 20-3).

Document Results

Documentation and reporting are important parts of evaluation. Accurate information needs to be present in a patient's medical record and shared during handoff communication so nurses and other health care team members know if a patient is progressing and to make ongoing clinical decisions. In settings in which the same nurse will not be providing care throughout a patient's stay, it becomes very important to have consistent, thorough documentation of the patient's progress towards expected outcomes. The use of nursing diagnostic language and the NIC and NOC is becoming more common in electronic medical records (Hendrix, 2009). The use of standardized nursing languages can improve the quality, consistency, and accuracy of what is documented by providing a broad base of nursing knowledge at the point of care (Lunney, 2006). In addition, electronic systems provide linkages to make it easier to interpret cues regarding whether interventions led to expected patient outcomes. When documenting a patient's response to your interventions, describe the interventions, the evaluative measures used, the outcomes achieved, and the continued plan of care. For example:

1430: Instructed patient on importance of handwashing and need to change surgical dressing if it becomes soiled, moist, or loosened. Asked patient to describe when it is necessary to change a surgical dressing. Patient was able to identify a soiled or moist dressing. Discussed further the need for a dressing to be secure. Provided pamphlet with outline of dressing change principles. Will discuss wound care with patient and wife one more time before discharge.

Your aim in documenting is to present a clear argument from the evaluative data as to whether a patient is progressing or not.

Disseminate results to patients and families. One of the ANA standards for evaluation is to share results of care with patients and their families according to federal and state regulations (ANA, 2010). Keep patients and families informed about the patients' progress. Be aware of guidelines of your agency for the type of clinical information (e.g., diagnostic findings, results of treatment) that you can communicate.

Care Plan Revision

Each time you evaluate a patient you determine if the plan of care continues or whether revisions are necessary. If your patient meets a goal successfully, discontinue that portion of the care plan. Unmet and partially met goals require you to continue intervention. It may be appropriate to modify or add nursing diagnoses for a new plan of care with appropriate goals, expected outcomes, and interventions. You must also redefine priorities. An important step in critical thinking is knowing how the patient is progressing and how problems either resolve or worsen.

Tonya's evaluation of Mr. Jacobs' interventions for deficient knowledge revealed the following: The patient and wife are able to identify signs and symptoms of wound infection, and the patient knows that strain on the suture line can affect healing. Tonya sees that the outcomes of care are partially met. She still hopes to evaluate Mr. and Mrs. Jacobs' ability to continue wound care at home through a demonstration planned for tomorrow. However, she also recognizes that, although Mr. Jacobs knows that strain on his incision can pull out the stitches, he may not realize which activities that he normally does at home would strain it. Thus she decides to modify her instructional approach by reassessing the types of activities Mr. Jacobs does at home (e.g., type of lifting, exercise, manual work) and incorporate that information into her teaching strategies.

Discontinuing a Care Plan. After you determine that expected outcomes and goals have been met, confirm this evaluation with the patient when possible. If you and the patient agree, you discontinue that portion of the care plan. Documentation of a discontinued plan ensures that other nurses will not unnecessarily continue interventions for that portion of the plan of care.

Continuity of care assumes that care provided to patients is relevant and timely. You waste much time when you do not communicate achieved goals.

Modifying a Care Plan. When goals are not met, you identify the factors that interfere with their achievement. Usually a change in the patient's condition, needs, or abilities makes alteration of the care plan necessary. For example, when teaching self-administration of insulin, a nurse discovers that the patient has developed a new problem, a tremor associated with a side effect of a medication. The patient is unable to draw medication from a syringe or inject the needle safely. As a result, the original outcomes, "Patient will correctly prepare insulin in a syringe," and "Patient will administer insulin injection independently," cannot be met. The nurse introduces new interventions (instructing a family member in insulin preparation and administration) and revises outcomes, "Family caregiver will correctly prepare insulin in syringe," and "Family caregiver will administer insulin injection correctly," to meet the goal of care.

At times a lack of goal achievement results from an error in nursing judgment or failure to follow each step of the nursing process. Patients often have multiple and complex problems. Always remember the possibility of overlooking or misjudging something. When a goal is not met, no matter what the reason, repeat the entire nursing process sequence for that nursing diagnosis to identify necessary changes to the plan. Reassess the patient, determine accuracy of the nursing diagnosis, establish new goals and expected outcomes, and select new interventions.

Reassessment. A complete reassessment of all patient factors relating to the nursing diagnosis and etiology is necessary when modifying a plan. Reassessment requires critical thinking as you compare new data about the patient's condition with previously assessed information. Knowledge from previous experiences helps you direct the reassessment process. Caring for patients and families who have had similar health problems gives you a strong background of knowledge to use for anticipating patient needs and knowing what to assess. Reassessment ensures that the database is accurate and current. It also reveals a missing link (i.e., a critical piece of new information that was overlooked and thus interfered with goal achievement). You sort, validate, and cluster all new data to analyze and interpret differences from the original database. You also document reassessment data to alert other nursing staff to the patient's status.

Redefining Diagnoses. After reassessment, determine which nursing diagnoses are accurate for the situation. Ask whether you selected the correct diagnosis and whether the diagnosis and the etiological factor are current. Then revise the problem list to reflect the patient's changed status. Sometimes you make a new diagnosis. You base your nursing care on an accurate list of nursing diagnoses. Accuracy is more important than the number of diagnoses selected. As the patient's condition changes, the diagnoses also change.

Goals and Expected Outcomes. When revising a care plan, review the goals and expected outcomes for necessary changes. In addition, examine the goals for unchanged nursing diagnoses for their appropriateness because a change in one problem sometimes affects the goals in others. Determining that each goal and expected outcome is realistic for the problem, etiology, and time frame is particularly important. Unrealistic expected outcomes and time frames make goal achievement difficult.

Clearly document goals and expected outcomes for new or revised nursing diagnoses so all team members are aware of the revised care plan. When the goal is still appropriate but has not yet been met, try changing the evaluation data to allow more time. You may also decide at this time to change interventions. For example, when a patient's pressure ulcer does not show signs of healing, you choose to use a different support surface or a different type of wound cleanser.

Interventions. The evaluation of interventions examines two factors: the appropriateness of the intervention selected and the correct application of the intervention. Appropriateness is based on the standard of care for a patient's health problem. A **standard of care** is the minimum level of care accepted to ensure high quality of care to patients. Standards of care define the types of therapies typically administered to patients with defined problems or needs. For example, if a patient who is receiving chemotherapy for leukemia has the nursing diagnosis *nausea related to pharyngeal irritation,* the standard of care established by the nursing department for this problem might include pain-control measures, mouth care guidelines, and diet therapy. The nurse reviews the standard of care to determine whether the right interventions have been chosen or whether additional ones are required.

Increasing or decreasing the frequency of interventions is another approach to ensure appropriate application of an intervention. You adjust interventions on the basis of the patient's actual response to therapy and your previous experience with similar patients. For example, if a patient continues to have congested lung sounds, you increase the frequency of coughing and deep-breathing exercises to remove secretions.

During evaluation you find that some planned interventions are designed for an inappropriate level of nursing care. If you need to change the level of care, substitute a different action verb, such as *assist* in place of *provide* or *demonstrate* in place of *instruct.* For example, assisting a patient to walk requires a nurse to be at the patient's side during ambulation, whereas providing an assistive device (e.g., a cane or walker) suggests that the patient is more independent. In addition, demonstration requires you to show a patient how a skill is performed rather than simply telling the patient how to perform it. Sometimes the level of care is appropriate, but the interventions are unsuitable because of a change in the expected outcome. In this case discontinue the interventions and plan new ones.

Make any changes in the plan of care based on the nature of the patient's unfavorable response. Consulting with other nurses often yields suggestions for improving the care delivery approach. Experienced nurses are often excellent resources. Simply changing the care plan is not enough. Implement the new plan and reevaluate the patient's response to the nursing actions. *Evaluation is continuous.*

Occasionally during evaluation you discover unmet patient needs. This is normal. The nursing process is a systematic, problem-solving approach to individualized patient care, but there are many factors affecting each patient with health care problems. Patients with the same health care problem are not treated the same way. As a result, you sometimes make errors in judgment. The systematic use of evaluation provides a way for you to catch these errors. By consistently incorporating evaluation into practice you minimize errors and ensure that the patient's plan of care is appropriate and relevant. The evaluation of nursing care is a professional responsibility, and it is a crucial component of nursing care.

KEY POINTS

- Evaluation is a step of the nursing process that includes two components: an examination of a condition or situation and a judgment as to whether change has occurred.

- During evaluation apply critical thinking to make clinical decisions and redirect nursing care to best meet patient needs.
- Positive evaluations occur when you meet desired outcomes and they lead you to conclude that your interventions were effective.
- Criterion-based standards for evaluation are the physiological, emotional, and behavioral responses that are a patient's goals and expected outcomes.
- Evaluative measures are assessment skills or techniques that you use to collect data for determining if outcomes were met.
- It sometimes becomes necessary to collect evaluative measures over time to determine if a pattern of change exists.
- When interpreting findings, you compare the patient's behavioral responses and physiological signs and symptoms that you expect to see with those actually seen from your evaluation and judge the degree of agreement.
- Documentation of evaluative findings allows all members of the health care team to know whether or not a patient is progressing.
- A patient's nursing diagnoses, priorities, and interventions sometimes change as a result of evaluation.
- Evaluation examines two factors: the appropriateness of the interventions selected and the correct application of the intervention.

CLINICAL APPLICATION QUESTIONS

Preparing for Clinical Practice

Tonya examines Mr. Jacobs' surgical incision and notices a 1.25-cm (0.5-inch) circle of yellowish drainage on the gauze dressing. On close inspection of the suture line, she also observes an area of swelling around two stitches. Mr. Jacobs notices Tonya's expression as she looks at the dressing and asks, "Is anything wrong?" Tonya responds, "A small amount of drainage is coming from your incision. Don't be alarmed." As Tonya applies mild pressure over the incision, she asks Mr. Jacobs if the area is tender. He grimaces a bit and says, "Yes, a little." Tonya says, "I'm going to let your surgeon know about this." After she consults with the physician, an intravenous (IV) antibiotic is ordered. While in Mr. Jacobs' room, Tonya notices that the patient is breathing faster and looks up to the ceiling and sighs.

1. When Tonya evaluated the surgical incision, two components of evaluation occurred. Describe each.
2. Based on this clinical scenario, how might Tonya need to modify the patient's care plan? Refer to the concept map (Fig. 19-2) on p. 257 in Chapter 19.
3. Identify two evaluative measures that Tonya used to evaluate the condition of Mr. Jacobs' wound.

evolve *Answers to Clinical Application Questions can be found on the Evolve website.*

REVIEW QUESTIONS

Are You Ready to Test Your Nursing Knowledge?

1. A nurse caring for a patient with pneumonia sits the patient up in bed and suctions his airway. After suctioning, the patient describes some discomfort in his abdomen. The nurse auscultates the patient's lung sounds and gives him a glass of water. Which of the following is an evaluative measure used by the nurse?
   1. Suctioning the airway
   2. Sitting patient up in bed
   3. Auscultating lung sounds
   4. Patient describing type of discomfort
2. A nurse caring for a patient with pneumonia sits the patient up in bed and suctions the patient's airway. After suctioning, the patient describes some discomfort in his abdomen. The nurse auscultates the patient's lung sounds and gives him a glass of water. Which of the following would be appropriate evaluative criteria used by the nurse? (Select all that apply.)
   1. Patient drinks contents of water glass.
   2. Patient's lungs are clear to auscultation in bases.
   3. Patient reports abdominal pain on scale of 0 to 10.
   4. Patient's rate and depth of breathing are normal with head of bed elevated.
3. The evaluation process includes interpretation of findings as one of its five elements. Which of the following is an example of interpretation?
   1. Evaluating the patient's response to selected nursing interventions
   2. Selecting an observable or measurable state or behavior that reflects goal achievement
   3. Reviewing the patient's nursing diagnoses and establishing goals and outcome statements
   4. Matching the results of evaluative measures with expected outcomes to determine patient's status
4. A goal specifies the expected behavior or response that indicates:
   1. The specific nursing action was completed.
   2. The validation of the nurse's physical assessment.
   3. The nurse has made the correct nursing diagnoses.
   4. Resolution of a nursing diagnosis or maintenance of a healthy state.
5. A patient is recovering from surgery for removal of an ovarian tumor. It is 1 day after her surgery. Because she has an abdominal incision and dressing and a history of diabetes, the nurse has selected a nursing diagnosis of *risk for infection.* Which of the following is an appropriate goal statement for the diagnosis?
   1. Patient will remain afebrile to discharge.
   2. Patient's wound will remain free of infection by discharge.
   3. Patient will receive ordered antibiotic on time over next 3 days.
   4. Patient's abdominal incision will be covered with a sterile dressing for 2 days.
6. Unmet and partially met goals require the nurse to do which of the following? (Select all that apply.)
   1. Redefine priorities
   2. Continue intervention
   3. Discontinue care plan
   4. Gather assessment data on a different nursing diagnosis
   5. Compare the patient's response with that of another patient
7. A patient comes to a medical clinic with the diagnosis of asthma. The nurse practitioner decides that the patient's obesity adds to the difficulty of breathing; the patient is 5 feet 7 inches tall and weighs 200 pounds (90.7 kg). Based on the nursing diagnosis of *imbalanced nutrition: more than body requirements,* the practitioner plans to place the patient on a therapeutic diet. Which of the following are evaluative measures for determining if the patient achieves the goal of a desired weight loss? (Select all that apply.)
   1. The patient eats 2000 calories a day.
   2. The patient is weighed during each clinic visit.

3. The patient discusses factors that increase the risk of an asthma attack.
4. The patient's food diary that tracks intake of daily meals is reviewed.

8. The nurse follows a series of steps to objectively evaluate the degree of success in achieving outcomes of care. Place the steps in the correct order.
   1. The nurse judges the extent to which the condition of the skin matches the outcome criteria.
   2. The nurse tries to determine why the outcome criteria and actual condition of skin do not agree.
   3. The nurse inspects the condition of the skin.
   4. The nurse reviews the outcome criteria to identify the desired skin condition.
   5. The nurse compares the degree of agreement between desired and actual condition of the skin.
9. The nurse checks the intravenous (IV) solution that is infusing into the patient's left arm. The IV solution of 9% NS is infusing at 100 mL/hr as ordered. The nurse reviews the nurses' notes from the previous shift to determine if the dressing over the site was changed as scheduled per standard of care. While in the room, the nurse inspects the condition of the dressing and notes the date on the dressing label. In what ways did the nurse evaluate the IV intervention? (Select all that apply.)
   1. Checked the IV infusion location in left arm
   2. Checked the type of IV solution
   3. Confirmed from nurses' notes the time of dressing change and checked label
   4. Inspected the condition of the IV dressing
10. Which of the following statements correctly describe the evaluation process? (Select all that apply.)
    1. Evaluation is an ongoing process.
    2. Evaluation usually reveals obvious changes in patients.
    3. Evaluation involves making clinical decisions.
    4. Evaluation requires the use of assessment skills.
11. A clinic nurse assesses a patient who reports a loss of appetite and a 15-pound weight loss since 2 months ago. The patient is 5 feet 10 inches tall and weighs 135 pounds (61.2 kg). She shows signs of depression and does not have a good understanding of foods to eat for proper nutrition. The nurse makes the nursing diagnosis of *imbalanced nutrition: less than body requirements related to reduced intake of food*. For the goal of, "Patient will return to baseline weight in 3 months," which of the following outcomes would be appropriate? (Select all that apply.)
    1. Patient will discuss source of depression by next clinic visit.
    2. Patient will achieve a calorie intake of 2400 daily in 2 weeks.
    3. Patient will report improvement in appetite in 1 week.
    4. Patient will identify food protein sources.
12. A patient is being discharged after abdominal surgery. The abdominal incision is healing well with no signs of redness or irritation. Following instruction, the patient has demonstrated effective care of the incision, including cleansing the wound and applying dressings correctly to the nurse. These behaviors are an example of:
    1. Evaluative measure.
    2. Expected outcome.
    3. Reassessment.
    4. Standard of care.
13. A patient has limited mobility as a result of a recent knee replacement. The nurse identifies that he has altered balance and assists him in ambulation. The patient uses a walker presently as part of his therapy. The nurse notes how far the patient is able to walk and then assists him back to his room. Which of the following is an evaluative measure?
    1. Uses walker during ambulation
    2. Presence of altered balance
    3. Limited mobility in lower extremities
    4. Observation of distance patient is able to walk
14. A patient is being discharged today. In preparation the nurse removes the intravenous (IV) line from the right arm and documents that the site was "clean and dry with no signs of redness or tenderness." On discharge the nurse reviews the care plan for goals met. Which of the following goals can be evaluated with what you know about this patient?
    1. Patient expresses acceptance of health status by day of discharge.
    2. Patient's surgical wound will remain free of infection.
    3. Patient's IV site will remain free of phlebitis.
    4. Patient understands when to call physician to report possible complications.
15. A nursing student is talking with one of the staff nurses who works on a surgical unit. The student's care plan is to include nursing-sensitive outcomes for the nursing diagnosis of *acute pain*. A nursing-sensitive outcome suitable for this diagnosis would be:
    1. Patient will achieve pain relief by discharge.
    2. Patient will be free of a surgical wound infection by discharge.
    3. Patient will report reduced pain severity in 2 days.
    4. Patient will describe purpose of pain medicine by discharge.

Answers: **1.** 3; **2.** 2, 4; **3.** 4; **4.** 4; **5.** 2; **6.** 1, 2; **7.** 2, 4; **8.** 4, 3, 5, 1, 2; **9.** 3, 4; **10.** 1, 3, 4; **11.** 2, 3; **12.** 2; **13.** 4; **14.** 3; **15.** 3.

REFERENCES

American Nurses Association: *Scope and standards of practice: nursing*, ed 2, Silver Spring Md, 2010, American Nurses Association.

Brown DS, et al: Nursing-sensitive benchmarks for hospitals to gauge high-reliability performance, *J Healthc Qual* 32(6):9, 2010.

Hendrix SE: An experience with implementation of NIC and NOC in a clinical information system, *CIN: Comput Inform Nurs* 27(1):7, 2009.

Infusion Nurses Society (INS): 2006 Infusion nursing standards of practice, *J Infus Nurs* 29(suppl 1):S1, 2006.

Lunney M. Helping nurses use NANDA, NOC, and NIC: novice to expert, *Nurse Educator* 31(1):40, 2006.

Moorhead S, et al: *Nursing outcomes classification (NOC)*, ed 4, St Louis, 2008, Mosby.

RESEARCH REFERENCES

Doran DM, et al: Nursing-sensitive outcomes data collection in acute care and long-term care settings, *Nursing Research* 55(2S):S75, 2006.

Loan LA, et al: Participation in a national outcomes database: monitoring outcomes over time, *Nurs Admin Q* 35(1):72, 2011.

CHAPTER

21

Managing Patient Care

OBJECTIVES

- Differentiate among the types of nursing care delivery models.
- Describe the elements of decentralized decision making.
- Discuss the ways in which a nurse manager supports staff involvement in a decentralized decision-making model.
- Discuss ways to apply clinical care coordination skills in nursing practice.
- Discuss principles to follow in the appropriate delegation of patient care activities.

KEY TERMS

Accountability, p. 277
Authority, p. 277
Autonomy, p. 277
Case management, p. 276
Decentralized management, p. 277
Delegation, p. 281
Empowered, p. 274
Primary nursing, p. 276
Responsibility, p. 277
Shared governance, p. 278
Team nursing, p. 276
Total patient care, p. 276

evolve WEBSITE

http://evolve.elsevier.com/Potter/fundamentals/

- Review Questions
- Case Study with Questions
- Audio Glossary
- Interactive Learning Activities
- Key Term Flashcards
- Content Updates

As a nursing student it is important for you to acquire the necessary knowledge and competencies that ultimately allow you to practice as an entry-level staff nurse. The National Council of State Boards of Nursing (NCSBN) identified competencies that registered nurses (RNs) and licensed practical/vocational nurses need on entry to practice (Kearney, 2009) (Box 21-1). Regardless of the type of setting in which you eventually choose to work as a staff nurse, you will be responsible for using organizational resources, participating in organizational routines while providing direct patient care, using time productively, collaborating with all members of the health care team, and using certain leadership characteristics to manage others on the nursing team. The delivery of nursing care within the health care system is a challenge because of the changes that influence health professionals, patients, and health care organizations (see Chapter 2). However, change offers opportunities. As you develop the knowledge and skills to become a staff nurse, you learn what it takes to effectively manage the patients for whom you care and to take the initiative in becoming a leader among your professional colleagues.

BUILDING A NURSING TEAM

Nurses are self-directed and, with proper leadership and motivation, are able to solve most complex problems. A nurse's education and commitment to practicing within established standards and guidelines ensures a rewarding professional career. As a nurse it is also important to work in an empowering environment as a member of a solid and strong nursing team. A strong nursing team works together to achieve the best outcomes for patients (Batcheller et al., 2004).

Building an **empowered** nursing team begins with the nurse executive, who is often vice president or director of nursing. The executive's position within an organization is critical in uniting the strategic direction of an organization with the philosophical values and goals of nursing. The nurse executive is both a clinical and business leader who is concerned with maximizing quality of care and cost-effectiveness while maintaining relationships and professional satisfaction of the staff. The relationship between the nurse and nurse manager contributes to job satisfaction and retention (Ulrich et al., 2005). Perhaps the most important responsibility of the nurse executive is to establish a philosophy for nursing that enables managers and staff to provide quality nursing care. In this environment staff members have high levels of productivity and make contributions to the success of the organization (Feltner et al., 2008). Box 21-2 identifies the characteristics of an effective nurse leader.

It takes an excellent nurse manager and an excellent nursing staff to make an empowering work environment. Together a manager and the nursing staff have to share a philosophy of care for their work unit. A philosophy of care includes the professional

BOX 21-1 ENTRY-LEVEL NURSE COMPETENCIES

- Possess a systems focus to see the big picture.
- Understand the environment of care.
- Manage the care of patients.
- Be able to critically think as demonstrated by assessment of problem, identification of solution, implementation of solution, evaluation of care, and follow-up of care.
- Communicate effectively with physicians and health care team members.
- Demonstrate nursing knowledge and display confidence in knowledge base.
- Work as a team member collaborating with health care team members.
- Have a patient orientation and focus with actions focused on patient and patient needs.
- Respect the rights, beliefs, wishes, and values of patients.
- Be a patient advocate.
- Recognize own limitations and see support of validation of decisions as needed.
- Demonstrate knowledge of roles, responsibilities, and functions of a nurse.

Modified from Kearney MH: *Report of the findings from the post-entry competence study,* Chicago, 2009, National Council of State Boards of Nursing; National Council of State Boards of Nursing: *2009 tuning analysis: a comparison of US and international nursing educational competences*, Chicago, 2010, National Councils State Boards of Nursing.

BOX 21-2 CHARACTERISTICS OF AN EFFECTIVE LEADER

- Is an effective communicator
- Is consistent in managing conflict
- Is knowledgeable and competent in all aspects of delivery of care
- Is a role model for staff
- Uses participatory approach in decision making
- Delegates work appropriately
- Sets objectives and guides staff
- Displays caring, understanding, and empathy for others
- Motivates others
- Is proactive and flexible

Modified from Dunham-Taylor J: Quantum leadership: love one another. In Dunham-Taylor J, Pinczak JZ: *Financial management for nurse managers*, ed 2, Boston, 2010, Jones & Bartlett Publishers; Feltner A et al: Nurses' views on the characteristics of an effective leader, *AORN J* 87(2):363, 2008.

nursing staff's values and concerns for the way they view and care for patients. For example, a philosophy addresses the purpose of the nursing unit, how staff works with patients and families, and the standards of care for the work unit. Selection of a nursing care delivery model and a management structure that supports professional nursing practice are essential to the philosophy of care.

Magnet Recognition

One way of creating an empowering work environment is through the Magnet Recognition Program (see Chapter 2). A Magnet hospital has a transformed culture with a practice environment that is dynamic, autonomous, collaborative, and positive for nurses. The culture focuses on concern for patients. Typically a Magnet hospital has clinical promotion systems and research and evidence-based practice programs. The nurses have professional autonomy over their practice and control over the practice environment (Upenieks and Sitterding, 2008). A Magnet hospital empowers the nursing team to make changes and be innovative. Professional nurse councils at the organizational and unit level are one way to create an empowerment model. An effective empowerment model leads to a staff that feels valued and has increased autonomy and a work environment that promotes job satisfaction (Gokenbach, 2007). This culture and empowerment combine to produce a strong collaborative relationship among team members and improve patient quality outcomes (Box 21-3).

BOX 21-3 EVIDENCE-BASED PRACTICE

Magnet Hospital Work Environment Characteristics and Outcomes

PICO Question: Do hospital work environment characteristics and outcomes differ between Magnet and non-Magnet hospitals?

Evidence Summary

The Magnet Recognition Program recognizes nursing services that build programs of excellence for the delivery of nursing care, promote quality in environments that support professional nursing practice, and promote achievement of positive patient outcomes (American Nurses Credentialing Center, 2010). Several studies examined specific work environment characteristics and outcomes to determine if they are different in Magnet versus non-Magnet hospitals. Nurses in Magnet hospitals place a high value on quality patient care, are focused on patient safety, and are more likely to communicate about errors and participate in problem solving related to errors (Hughes et al., 2009; Ulrich et al., 2009). Characteristics of Magnet hospitals were found to be positively related to climates of patient safety (Armstrong et al., 2009). Nurses in Magnet hospitals or Magnet-aspiring hospitals had higher levels of current job satisfaction, were more likely to stay with their organization, and felt empowered (Armstrong et al., 2009; Lacey et al., 2007; Lacey et al., 2009; Ulrich et al., 2009). A positive perception of support for nursing was found in Magnet hospitals or Magnet-aspiring hospitals (Lacey et al., 2007). Other identified characteristics of Magnet hospitals included increased efforts to encourage teamwork, increased recognition and reward of nurses, provision of mentoring programs for new graduates, and increased support for nursing continuing education efforts (Ulrich et al., 2009).

Application to Nursing Practice

- Seek employment in institutions that provide mentoring for new graduate nurses.
- Work on developing effective communication with peers and members of the health care team.
- Openly communicate with peers on the nursing unit related to patient safety issues.
- Develop problem-solving skills to be able to find solutions to patient safety issues.
- Participate as a member of the professional governance council of your unit or organization.
- Attend workshops and conferences to develop nursing competencies such as collaboration skills and communication.
- Seek work environments in which nursing is valued and supported.

Nursing Care Delivery Models

Since the time of Florence Nightingale nurses have used a variety of nursing care delivery models to provide care for patients. Ideally the philosophy that nurses establish for the quality care of patients guides the selection of a care delivery model. However, too often a lack of nursing resources and business plans from the health care organization influences the final decision. A care delivery model needs to help nurses achieve desirable outcomes for their patients, either in the way work is organized or in the way a nurse's responsibilities are defined. Important factors contributing to success of a care delivery model are decision-making authority for nurses who provide direct care, autonomy, collaborative practice, and effective methods of communicating with colleagues, physicians, and other health care providers (Tiedeman and Lookinland, 2004). In effective nursing models, the experienced RN provides faster diagnosis and intervention, which promotes a safe patient environment (Berkow et al., 2007).

Three common models are team nursing, total patient care, and primary nursing. **Team nursing** developed in response to the severe nursing shortage following World War II. By 2000 the interdisciplinary team was a more common model (Marriner Tomey, 2009). **Total patient care** delivery was the original care delivery model developed during Florence Nightingale's time. The model disappeared in the 1930s and became popular again during the 1970s and 1980s, when the number of RNs increased (Tiedeman and Lookinland, 2004). The **primary nursing** model of care delivery was developed to place RNs at the bedside and improve the accountability of nursing for patient outcomes and the professional relationships among staff members (Marriner Tomey, 2009). The model became more popular in the 1970s and early 1980s as hospitals began to employ more RNs. Primary nursing supports a philosophy regarding nurse and patient relationships. Table 21-1 summarizes the three nursing models.

Case management is a care management approach that coordinates and links health care services to patients and their families while streamlining costs and maintaining quality (Marriner Tomey, 2009) (see Chapter 2). The Case Management Society of America (2010) defines case management as "a collaborative process of assessment, planning, facilitation, and advocacy for options and services to meet an individual's health needs through communication and available resources to promote quality cost-effective outcomes." Case management is unique because clinicians, either as individuals or as part of a collaborative group, oversee the management of patients with specific, complex health problems or are held accountable for some standard of cost management and quality.

For example, a case manager coordinates a patient's acute care in the hospital and follows up with the patient after discharge home. Case managers do not always provide direct care but instead work with and supervise the care delivered by other staff and health care team members and actively coordinate patient discharge planning. Ongoing communication with team members facilitates the patient's transition to home (Carr, 2007). In this situation the case manager helps the patient identify health needs, determine the services and resources that are available, and make cost-efficient choices (Marriner Tomey, 2009). The case manager frequently oversees a caseload of patients with complex nursing and medical problems. Often he or she is an advanced practice nurse who, through specific interventions, helps to improve patient outcomes, optimize patient safety by facilitating care transitions, decrease length of stay, and lower health care costs (Carr, 2007; Thomas, 2008).

TABLE 21-1 Nursing Care Delivery Models

NURSING MODEL	CHARACTERISTICS	ADVANTAGES	DISADVANTAGES
Team nursing	• Registered nurse (RN) leads team of other RNs, practical nurses, and unlicensed assistive personnel (UAP). • Team members provide direct patient care under supervision of RN. • Team leader develops patient care plans, coordinates care among team members, and provides care requiring complex nursing skills. • There is hierarchical communication from charge nurse to charge nurse, charge nurse to team leader, and team leader to team members.	• Care is provided through a collaborative style that encourages each member of team to work with and help the other members. • Model has a high level of autonomy for the team leader. • Decision making occurs at clinical level. • Nursing care conferences help to solve patient problems • Patient care coordinator has time to manage unit issues.	• RN team leader does not spend time with patients; thus patients may not see RN often. • Team leader needs to take time to delegate work.
Total patient care	• RN is responsible for all aspects of care for one or more patients during a shift of care. • Care can be delegated. • RN works directly with patient, family, and health care team members.	• Patient satisfaction with model is high. • RNs plan care. • There is a high degree of collaboration with other health care team members.	• Continuity of care is often a problem if RNs do not communicate patient needs to one another. • Model may not be cost effective because of high number of RNs needed to provide care.
Primary nursing	• One primary RN assumes responsibility for a caseload of patients. • When an RN is working, he or she provides care for the same patients during their stay in a facility. • RN assesses patient, develops plan of care, and delivers appropriate nursing interventions. • Communication is lateral from nurse to nurse and caregiver to caregiver.	• Model is flexible and uses a variety of staffing levels and mixes. • Model has a high level of autonomy and authority. • Model promotes collaboration with physician. • Model provides continuity of care if facilitated. • Model reduces number of errors that occur when relaying orders.	• Associate nurse cannot change care plan without discussing with primary nurse. • Model does not necessarily decrease cost of care, even with staff mix.

Modified from Marriner Tomey A: *Guide to nursing management and leadership,* ed 8, St Louis, 2009, Mosby; Tiedeman ME, Lookinland S: Traditional models of care delivery: what have we learned? *J Nurs Adm* 34(6):291, 2004.

Many organizations use critical pathways or CareMaps in a case management delivery system (see Chapter 18). These are multidisciplinary treatment plans for specific cases. The case manager, along with members of the health care team, uses the critical pathways or CareMaps to implement timely interventions in a coordinated plan of care. The plans eliminate the guesswork in patient care because all members of the health care team work from the same plan.

Decision Making

With a philosophy for nursing established, it is the manager who directs and supports staff in the realization of that philosophy. The nurse executive supports managers by establishing a structure that helps to achieve organizational goals and provide appropriate support to care delivery staff. It takes a committed nurse executive, an excellent manager, and an empowered nursing staff to create an enriching work environment in which nursing practice thrives.

Decentralized management, in which decision making is moved down to the level of staff, is very common within health care organizations. This type of management structure has the advantage of creating an environment in which managers and staff become more actively involved in shaping the identity and determining the success of a health care organization. Working in a decentralized structure has the potential for greater collaborative effort, increased competency of staff, increased staff motivation, and ultimately a greater sense of professional accomplishment and satisfaction.

Progressive organizations achieve more when employees at all levels are actively involved. As a result, the role of a nurse manager is critical in the management of effective nursing units or groups. Box 21-4 highlights the diverse responsibilities of nursing managers. To make decentralized decision making work, managers need to know how to move it down to the lowest level possible. On a nursing unit it is important for all nursing staff members (RNs, licensed practical nurses [LPNs], and licensed vocational nurses [LVNs]), nurse assistants, and unit secretaries to become involved. They need to be kept well informed. They also need to be given the opportunity by managers to participate in problem-solving activities, including opportunities in direct patient care and unit activities such as committee participation. Important elements of the decision-making process are responsibility, autonomy, authority, and accountability (Anders and Hawkins, 2006).

Responsibility refers to the duties and activities that an individual is employed to perform. A position description outlines a professional nurse's responsibilities. Nurses meet these responsibilities through participation as members of the nursing unit.

Responsibility reflects ownership. The individual who manages the employee has to distribute responsibility, and the employee has to accept it. Managers have to be sure that staff clearly understand their responsibilities, particularly in the face of change. For example, when hospitals participate in work redesign, patient care delivery models change significantly. A manager is responsible for clearly defining the RN's role within the new care delivery model. If decentralized decision making is in place, professional staff have a voice in identifying the new RN role. Each RN on the work team is responsible for knowing his or her role and how to perform that role on the busy nursing unit. For example, primary nurses are responsible for completing a nursing assessment of all assigned patients and developing a plan of care that addresses each of the patient's nursing diagnoses (see Chapters 15 to 20). As the staff delivers the plan of care, the primary nurse evaluates whether the plan is successful. This responsibility becomes a work ethic for the nurse in delivering excellent patient care.

Autonomy is freedom of choice and responsibility for the choices (Marriner Tomey, 2009). Autonomy consistent with the scope of professional nursing practice maximizes your effectiveness as a nurse (Weston, 2008). With clinical autonomy a professional nurse makes independent decisions about patient care, planning nursing care for the patient within the scope of professional nursing practice. The nurse implements independent nursing interventions (Weston, 2008) (see Chapter 18). Another type of autonomy for nurses is work autonomy. In work autonomy the nurse makes independent decisions about the work of the unit such as scheduling or unit governance (Weston, 2008). Autonomy is not an absolute; it occurs in degrees. For example, a nurse has the autonomy to develop and implement a discharge teaching plan based on specific patient needs for any hospitalized patient. He or she also provides nursing care that complements the prescribed medical therapy.

Authority refers to legitimate power to give commands and make final decisions specific to a given position (Anders and Hawkins, 2006; Marriner Tomey, 2009). For example, a primary nurse managing a caseload of patients discovers that members of the nursing team did not follow through on a discharge teaching plan for an assigned patient. The primary nurse has the authority to consult other nurses to learn why the team did not follow recommendations on the plan of care and to choose appropriate teaching strategies for the patient that all members of the team will follow. The primary nurse has the final authority in selecting the best course of action for the patient's care.

Accountability refers to individuals being answerable for their actions. It means that as a nurse you accept the commitment to provide excellent patient care and the responsibility for the outcomes of the actions in providing that care (Anders and Hawkins, 2006). A primary nurse is accountable for his or her patients' outcomes and for ensuring that each patient learns the information necessary to improve self-care. The nurse demonstrates accountability by checking on the patient and family after discharge and reviewing with the nursing team whether continuity in teaching occurred.

BOX 21-4 RESPONSIBILITIES OF THE NURSE MANAGER

- Assist staff in establishing annual goals for the unit and systems needed to accomplish goals.
- Monitor professional nursing standards of practice on the unit.
- Develop an ongoing staff development plan, including one for new employees.
- Recruit new employees (interview and hire).
- Conduct routine staff evaluations.
- Establish self as a role model for positive customer service (customers include patients, families, and other health care team members).
- Submit staffing schedules for the unit.
- Conduct regular patient rounds and problem solve patient or family complaints.
- Establish and implement a unit quality improvement plan.
- Review and recommend new equipment for the unit.
- Conduct regular staff meetings.
- Make rounds with health care providers.
- Establish and support staff and interdisciplinary committees.

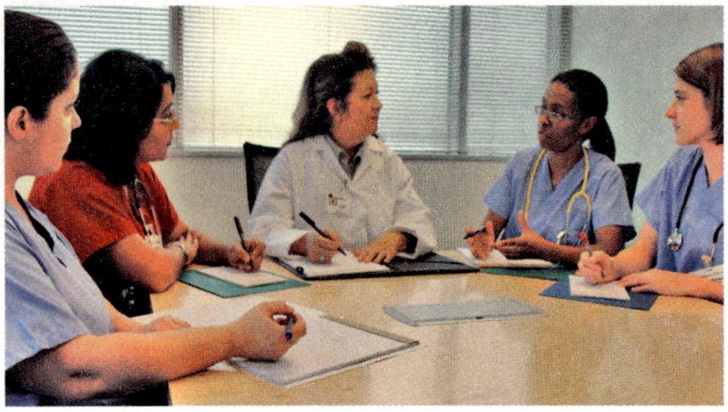

FIG. 21-1 Staff collaborating on practice issues. (From Yoder-Wise P: *Leading and managing in nursing*, ed 5, St Louis, 2010, Mosby.)

A successful decentralized nursing unit supports the four elements of decision making: responsibility, autonomy, authority, and accountability. An effective manager sets the same expectations for the staff in how decisions are made. Staff routinely meet to discuss and negotiate how to maintain an equality and balance in the elements. Staff members need to feel comfortable in expressing differences of opinion and challenging ways in which the team functions while recognizing their own responsibility, autonomy, authority, and accountability. Ultimately decentralized decision making helps create the philosophy of professional nursing care for the unit.

Staff Involvement. When decentralized decision making exists on a nursing unit, all staff members actively participate in unit activities (Fig. 21-1). The influence and control that nurses have over their practice contribute to job satisfaction (Schmalenberg and Kramer, 2008). Because the work environment promotes participation, all staff members benefit from the knowledge and skills of the entire work group. If the staff learns to value knowledge and the contributions of co-workers, better patient care is an outcome. Experienced RNs provide leadership and mentoring on a nursing unit while promoting collaborative practice (Berkow et al., 2007). The nursing manager supports staff involvement through a variety of approaches:

1. *Establishing nursing practice or problem-solving committees or professional* shared governance *councils.* Chaired by senior clinical staff, these groups establish and maintain care standards for nursing practice on their work unit. Shared governance councils promote empowerment in staff nurses and enable them to control their nursing practice (Kramer et al., 2008, 2010). The committees review and establish standards of care, develop policy and procedures, resolve patient satisfaction issues, or develop new documentation tools. It is important for the committees to focus on patient outcomes rather than only work issues to ensure quality care on the unit. Quality of care is further improved when nurses control their own practice (Anders and Hawkins, 2006). The committee establishes methods to ensure that all staff have input or participation on practice issues. Managers do not always sit on a committee, but they receive regular reports of committee progress. The nature of work on the nursing unit determines committee membership. At times members of other disciplines (e.g., pharmacy, respiratory therapy, or clinical nutrition) participate in practice committees or shared governance councils.
2. *Nurse/physician collaborative practice.* Collaboration is a process between individuals. There is a sharing of different perspectives that are then synthesized to better understand complex problems. An outcome of collaboration is a shared solution that could not have been accomplished by a single person or organization. Nurse-physician collaboration improves patient safety and outcomes and reduces errors (Manojlovich et al., 2008; Seago, 2008). The care delivery model of the nursing unit, an environment that supports teamwork, and organizational values influence how nurses and physicians collaborate. An open communication system that fosters respect, trust, shared decision making, and teamwork among all team members is critical to achieving quality patient care (Cronenwett et al., 2007). Physicians sometimes attend practice committees when clinical problems arise and present timely in-service programs.
3. *Interdisciplinary collaboration.* The emphasis on efficiency in health care delivery brings all members of the health care team together. Teamwork decreases mistakes because team members commit to shared knowledge, skills, and attitudes (Baker et al., 2006). Interdisciplinary collaboration leads to decreased patient mortality, decreased health care costs, and increased nurse job satisfaction (Manojlovich et al., 2008). Mutual respect is a critical part of any collaborative relationship (Ulrich et al., 2005). Essential characteristics for effective teams include having a common purpose, communicating frequently, anticipating one another, trust, managing conflict well, and providing feedback to one another (Baker et al., 2006). Use your judgment to decide which problems are complex and require a collaborative process. At the patient care level, staff recognize the importance of prompt referrals and timely communication with other health professionals. Participating in interdisciplinary patient care rounds, use of protocols and critical pathways, and holding interdisciplinary training for collaboration development are strategies that promote interdisciplinary collaboration (Kramer et al., 2010). Other strategies include having representatives of the various disciplines together in practice projects, in-service programs, conferences, and staff meetings.
4. *Staff communication.* A manager's greatest challenge, especially if a work group is large, is communication with staff. It is difficult to make sure that all staff members receive the same message: the correct message. In the present health care environment, staff quickly become uneasy and distrusting if they fail to hear about planned changes on their work unit. However, a manager cannot assume total responsibility for all communication. An effective manager uses a variety of approaches to communicate quickly and accurately to all staff. For example, many managers distribute biweekly or monthly newsletters of ongoing unit or agency activities. Minutes of committee meetings are usually in an accessible location for all staff to read. When the team needs to discuss important issues regarding the operations of the unit, the manager conducts staff meetings. When the unit has practice or quality improvement committees, each committee member has the responsibility to communicate directly to a select number of staff members. Thus all staff members are contacted and given the opportunity for input.
5. *Staff education.* A professional nursing staff needs to always grow in knowledge. It is impossible to remain knowledgeable about current medical and nursing practice trends without ongoing education. The nurse manager is responsible for making learning opportunities available so staff members remain competent in their practice. This involves planning in-service programs, sending staff to continuing education classes and professional conferences, and having staff present

case studies or practice issues during staff meetings. Staff members are responsible for pursuing educational opportunities when they know that their competencies are lacking.

LEADERSHIP SKILLS FOR NURSING STUDENTS

It is important that as a nursing student you prepare yourself for leadership roles. This does not mean that you have to quickly learn how to lead a team of nursing staff. Instead first learn to become a dependable and competent provider of patient care. As a nursing student you are responsible and accountable for the care you give to your patients. Learn to become a leader by consulting with instructors and nursing staff to obtain feedback in making good clinical decisions, learning from mistakes and seeking guidance, working closely with professional nurses, and trying to improve your performance during each patient interaction. These skills require you to think critically and solve problems in the clinical setting. Thinking critically allows nurses to provide higher quality care, meet the needs of patients while considering their preferences, consider alternatives to problems, understand the rationale for performing nursing interventions, and evaluate the effectiveness of interventions (Benner et al., 2008). Clinical experiences develop these critical thinking skills (Toofany, 2008). Important leadership skills to learn include clinical care coordination, team communication, delegation, and knowledge building.

Clinical Care Coordination

You acquire necessary skills so you can deliver patient care in a timely and effective manner. In the beginning this often involves only one patient, but eventually it will involve groups of patients. Clinical care coordination includes clinical decision making, priority setting, use of organizational skills and resources, time management, and evaluation. The activities of clinical care coordination require use of critical reflection, critical reasoning, and clinical judgment (Benner et al., 2008). They are important first steps in developing a caring relationship with a patient. Use a critical thinking approach, applying previous knowledge and experience to the decision-making process (see Chapter 15).

Clinical Decisions. Your ability to make clinical decisions depends on application of the nursing process (see Chapters 16 to 20). When you begin a patient assignment, the first activity involves a focused but complete assessment of the patient's condition so you are able to make an accurate judgment about his or her nursing diagnoses and collaborative health problems (see Chapter 16). This initial contact is an important first step in developing a caring relationship with a patient. Following the identification of a patient's diagnoses and problems, you develop a plan of care, implement nursing interventions, and evaluate patient outcomes. The process requires clinical decision making, using a critical thinking approach (see Chapter 15).

If you do not make accurate clinical decisions about a patient, undesirable outcomes will probably occur. The patient's condition worsens or remains the same when you lose the potential for improvement. An important lesson in organizational skills is to be thorough. Learn to attend and listen to the patient, look for any cues (obvious or subtle) that point to a pattern of findings, and direct the assessment to explore the pattern further. Accurate clinical decision making keeps you focused on the proper course of action. Never hesitate to ask for assistance when a patient's condition changes.

Priority Setting. After forming a picture of the patient's total needs, you set priorities by deciding which patient needs or problems need attention first (see Chapter 18). It is important to prioritize in all caregiving situations because it allows you to see relationships among patient problems and avoid delays in taking action that possibly leads to serious complications for a patient (Hendry and Walker, 2004). If a patient is experiencing serious physiological or psychological problems, the priority becomes clear. You need to act immediately to stabilize his or her condition. Hendry and Walker (2004) classify patient problems in three priority levels:

- *High priority*—An immediate threat to a patient's survival or safety such as a physiological episode of obstructed airway, loss of consciousness, or a psychological episode of an anxiety attack.
- *Intermediate priority*—Nonemergency, non–life-threatening actual or potential needs that the patient and family members are experiencing. Anticipating teaching needs of patients related to a new drug and taking measures to decrease postoperative complications are examples of intermediate priorities.
- *Low priority*—Actual or potential problems that are not directly related to the patient's illness or disease. These problems are often related to developmental needs or long-term health care needs. An example of a low priority problem is a patient at admission who will eventually be discharged and needs teaching for self-care in the home.

Many patients have all three types of priorities, requiring you to make careful judgments in choosing a course of action. Obviously high-priority needs demand immediate attention. When a patient has diverse priority needs, it helps to focus on his or her basic needs. For example, a patient who is in traction reports being uncomfortable from being in the same position. The dietary assistant arrives in the room to deliver a meal tray. Instead of immediately assisting the patient with the meal, you reposition him and offer basic hygiene measures. The patient likely becomes more interested in eating after he is more comfortable. He also is more receptive to any instruction you want to provide.

Eventually you will be required to meet the priority needs of a group of patients. This means that you need to know the priority needs of each patient within the group, assessing each patient's needs as soon as possible while addressing high priorities first. To identify which patients require assessment first, rely on information from the change-of-shift report, the classification system of the agency that identifies patient acuity, and information from the medical record. Over time you learn to spontaneously rank patients' needs by priority or urgency. Priorities do not remain stable but change as a patient's condition changes. It is important to think about the resources available, be flexible in recognizing that priority needs often change, and consider how to use time wisely.

You also make priorities on the basis of patient expectations. Sometimes you have established an excellent plan of care; however, if the patient is resistant to certain therapies or disagrees with the approach, you have very little success. Working closely with the patient and showing a caring attitude are important. Share the priorities you have defined with the patient to establish a level of agreement and cooperation.

Organizational Skills. Implementing a plan of care requires you to be effective and efficient. Effective use of time means doing the right things, whereas efficient use of time means doing things right. Learn to become efficient by combining various nursing activities—in other words, doing more than one thing at a time. For example, during medication administration or while obtaining a specimen, combine therapeutic communication, teaching interventions, and assessment and evaluation. Always try to establish and strengthen relationships with patients and use any patient contact as an opportunity to convey important information. Patient interaction gives you the chance to show caring and interest. Always attend to the patient's behaviors and responses to therapies to assess if new problems are developing and evaluate responses to interventions.

A well-organized nurse approaches any planned procedure by having all of the necessary equipment available and making sure that the patient is prepared. If the patient is comfortable and well informed, the likelihood that the procedure will go smoothly increases. Sometimes you require the assistance of colleagues to perform or complete a procedure. It is always wise to have the work area organized and preliminary steps completed before asking co-workers for assistance.

As you begin to deliver care based on established priorities, events sometimes occur within the health care setting that interfere with plans. For example, just as you begin to provide morning hygiene for a hospitalized patient, an x-ray technician enters to take a chest x-ray film. Once the technician completes the x-ray examination, a phlebotomist arrives to draw a blood sample. In this case your priorities seem to conflict with the priorities of other health care personnel. It is important to always keep the patient's needs at the center of attention. If the patient experienced symptoms earlier that required a chest x-ray film and laboratory work, it is important to be sure that the diagnostic tests are completed. In another example a patient is waiting to visit family, and a chest x-ray film is a routine order from 2 days earlier. The patient's condition has stabilized, and the x-ray technician is willing to return later to shoot the film. In this case attending to the patient's hygiene and comfort so family members can visit is more of a priority.

Use of Resources. Appropriate use of resources is an important aspect of clinical care coordination. Resources in this case include members of the health care team. In any setting the administration of patient care occurs more smoothly when staff members work together. Never hesitate to have staff assist you, especially when there is an opportunity to make a procedure or activity more comfortable and safer for the patient. For example, assistance in turning, positioning, and ambulating patients is frequently necessary when patients are unable to move. Having a staff member, such as nursing assistive personnel (NAP), assist with handling equipment and supplies during more complicated procedures such as catheter insertion or dressing change helps make procedures more efficient. In addition, you often have to recognize personal limitations and use professional resources for assistance. For example, you assess a patient and find relevant clinical signs and symptoms but are unfamiliar with the physical condition. Consulting with an RN confirms findings and ensures that you take the proper course of action for the patient. A leader knows his or her limitations and seeks professional colleagues for guidance and support.

Time Management. Changes in health care and increasing complexity of patients create stress for nurses as they work to meet patient needs (Marriner Tomey, 2009). One way to manage this stress is through the use of time management skills. These skills involve learning how, where, and when to use your time. Because you have a limited amount of time with patients, it is essential to remain goal oriented and use it wisely. You quickly learn the importance of using patient goals as a way to identify priorities. However, also learn how to establish personal goals and time frames. For example, you are caring for two patients on a busy surgical nursing unit. One had surgery the day before, and the other will be discharged the next day. Clearly the first patient's goals center on restoring physiological function impaired as a result of the stress of surgery. The second patient's goals center on adequate preparation to assume self-care at home. In reviewing the therapies required for both patients, you learn how to organize your time so the activities of care and patient goals are achieved. You need to anticipate when care will be interrupted for medication administration and diagnostic testing and when is the best time for planned therapies such as dressing changes, patient education, and patient ambulation. Delegation of tasks is another way to help improve time management.

One useful time-management skill involves making a priority to-do list (Hackworth, 2008). When you first begin working with a patient or patients, it helps to make a list that sequences the nursing activities you need to perform. The change-of-shift report helps to sequence activities based on what you learn about the patient's condition and the care provided before you arrive on the unit. It is helpful to consider activities that have specific time limits in terms of addressing patient needs such as administering a pain medication before a scheduled procedure or instructing patients before their discharge home. You also analyze the items on the list that are scheduled by agency policies or routines (e.g., medications or intravenous [IV] tubing changes). Note which activities need to be done on time and which activities you can do at your discretion. You have to administer medication within a specific schedule, but you are also able to perform other activities while in the patient's room. Finally, estimate the amount of time needed to complete the various activities. Activities requiring the assistance of other staff members usually take longer because you have to plan around their schedules.

Good time management also involves setting goals to help you complete one task before starting another (Hackworth, 2008). If possible complete the activities started with one patient before moving on to the next. Care is then less fragmented, and you are better able to focus on what you are doing for each patient. As a result, it is less likely that you will make errors. Time management requires an ability to anticipate the activities of the day and combine activities when possible. Other strategies to help you manage your time are keeping your work area clean and clutter free and trying to decrease interruptions as you are completing tasks (Pearce, 2007). Box 21-5 summarizes principles of time management.

Evaluation. Evaluation is one of the most important aspects of clinical care coordination (see Chapter 20). It is a mistake to think that evaluation occurs at the end of an activity. It is an ongoing process. Once you assess a patient's needs and begin therapies directed at a specific problem area, immediately evaluate whether therapies are effective and the patient's response. The process of evaluation compares actual patient outcomes with expected outcomes. For example, a clinic nurse assesses a foot ulcer of a patient who has diabetes to determine if healing has progressed since the last clinic visit. When expected outcomes are not met, evaluation reveals the need to continue current therapies for a longer period, revise approaches to care, or introduce new therapies. As you care for a patient throughout the day, anticipate when to return to the bedside to evaluate care (e.g., 30 minutes after a medication was administered, 15 minutes after an IV line has begun infusing, or 60 minutes after discussing discharge instructions with the patient and family).

Keeping a focus on evaluation of the patient's progress lessens the chance of becoming distracted by the tasks of care. It is common

BOX 21-5 PRINCIPLES OF TIME MANAGEMENT

Goal setting: Review the patient's goals of care for the day and any goals you have for activities such as completing documentation, attending a patient care conference, giving a staff report, or preparing medications for administration.

Time analysis: Reflect on how you use your time. While working on a clinical area, keep track of how you use your time in different activities. This provides valuable information to reveal how well organized you really are.

Priority setting: Set the priorities that you have established for patients within set time frames. For example, determine when is the best time to have teaching sessions, plan ambulation, and provide rest periods based on what you know about the patient's condition. For example, if a patient is nauseated or in pain, it is not a good time for a teaching session.

Interruption control: Everyone needs time to socialize or discuss issues with colleagues. However, do not let this interrupt important patient care activities such as medication administration. Use time during report, mealtime, or team meetings to the best of your advantage. In addition, plan time to assist fellow colleagues so it complements your patient care schedule.

Evaluation: At the end of each day take time to think and reflect about how effectively you used your time. If you are having difficulties, discuss them with an instructor or a more experienced staff member.

to assume that staying focused on planned activities ensures that you will perform care appropriately. However, task orientation does not ensure good patient outcomes. Learn that at the heart of good organizational skills is the constant inquiry into the patient's condition and progress toward an improved level of health.

Team Communication

As a part of a nursing team, you are responsible for open, professional communication. Regardless of the setting, an enriching professional environment is one in which staff members respect one another's ideas, share information, and keep one another informed. On a busy nursing unit this means keeping colleagues informed about patients with emerging problems, physicians who have been called for consultation, and unique approaches that solved a complex nursing problem. Strategies to improve your communication with physicians include addressing the physician by name, having the patient and chart available when discussing patient issues, focusing on the patient problem, and being professional and not aggressive (Nadzam, 2009). In a clinic setting it may mean sharing unusual diagnostic findings or conveying important information regarding a patient's source of family support. One way of fostering good team communication is by setting expectations of one another. A nurse treats colleagues with respect, listens to the ideas of other staff members without interruption, explores the way other staff members think, and is honest and direct while communicating. Part of good communication is clarifying what others are saying and building on the merits of co-workers' ideas (Marriner Tomey, 2009). An efficient team knows that it is able to count on all members when needs arise. Sharing expectations of what, when, and how to communicate is a step toward establishing a strong work team. Structured communication techniques that improve communication include briefings or short discussions among team members, group rounds on patients, and the use of Situation-Background-Assessment-Recommendation (SBAR) when sharing information (see Chapter 26) (Nadzam, 2009).

Delegation

The art of effective delegation is a skill you need to observe and practice to improve your own management skills. The American Nurses Association (1995) defined **delegation** as transferring responsibility for the performance of an activity or task while retaining accountability for the outcome. Delegation results in achievement of quality patient care, improved efficiency, increased productivity, empowered staff, and development of others (Huston, 2009; Marriner Tomey, 2009). Asking a staff member to obtain an ordered specimen while you attend to a patient's pain medication request effectively prevents a delay in the patient gaining pain relief and accomplishes two tasks related to the patient. Delegation also provides job enrichment. You show trust in colleagues by delegating tasks to them and showing staff members that they are important players in the delivery of care. Successful delegation is important to the quality of the RN-NAP relationship and their willingness to work together (Bittner and Gravlin, 2009; Potter et al., 2010). Never delegate a task that you dislike doing or would not do independently because this creates negative feelings and poor working relationships (Huston, 2009). For example, if you are in the room when a patient asks to be placed on a bedpan, you assist the patient rather than leave the room to find the nurse assistant. Remember that, even though the delegation of a task transfers the responsibility and authority to another person, you are accountable for the delegated task.

As a nurse you are responsible and accountable for providing care to patients and delegating care activities to NAP. However, the nurse does not delegate the steps of the nursing process of assessment, diagnosis, planning, and evaluation because these steps require nursing judgment (American Nurses Association [ANA] and National Council of State Boards of Nursing [NCSBN], 2005). Recognize that when you delegate to NAP, you delegate tasks, not patients. Do not give NAP sole responsibility for the care of patients. Instead, it is you as the professional nurse in charge of patient care who decides which activities NAP perform independently and which the RN and NAP perform in partnership. One way to accomplish this is to have the RN and technician or NAP conduct rounds together. You assess each patient as the technician helps to attend to basic patient needs. Care is delegated based on assessment findings and priority setting. As an RN, you are always responsible for the assessment of a patient's ongoing status; but if a patient is stable you delegate vital sign monitoring to NAP.

The RN is the one in most settings who decides when delegation is appropriate. The LPN directs care in many long-term care facilities. The National Council of State Boards of Nursing (1995) has provided some guidelines for delegation of tasks in accordance with an RN's legal scope of practice (Box 21-6). As the leader of the health care team, the RN gives clear instructions, effectively prioritizes patient needs and therapies, and gives staff timely and meaningful feedback. NAP respond positively when you include them as part of the nursing team.

Appropriate delegation begins with knowing which skills you are able to delegate. This requires you to be familiar with the Nurse Practice Act of the state, institutional policies and procedures, and job description for NAP provided by the institution. These standards help to define the necessary level of competency of NAP.

An institution's policies, procedures, and job description for NAP contain specific guidelines regarding which tasks or activities a nurse is able to delegate. The job description identifies any required education and the types of tasks NAP can perform, either independently or with RN direct supervision. Institutional policy defines the amount of training required of NAP while employed.

BOX 21-6 THE FIVE RIGHTS OF DELEGATION

Right Task
The right task is one that you delegate for a specific patient such as tasks that are repetitive, require little supervision, are relatively noninvasive, have results that are predictable, and have potential minimal risk.

Right Circumstances
Consider the appropriate patient setting, available resources, and other relevant factors. In an acute care setting patients' conditions often change quickly. Use good clinical decision making to determine what to delegate.

Right Person
The right person is delegating the right tasks to the right person to be performed on the right person.

Right Direction/Communication
You give a clear, concise description of the task, including its objective, limits, and expectations. Communication needs to be ongoing between the registered nurse and NAP during a shift of care.

Right Supervision/Evaluation
Provide appropriate monitoring, evaluation, intervention as needed, and feedback. NAP need to feel comfortable asking questions and seeking assistance.

Modified from National Council of State Boards of Nursing: *Delegation: concepts and decision-making process,* Chicago, 1995, The Council; National Council of State Boards of Nursing, *The five rights of delegation*, Chicago, 1997, The Council; and American Nurses Association (ANA) and National Council of State Boards of Nursing (NCSBN): *Joint statement on delegation,* http://www.ncsbn.org/pdfs/Joint_statement.pdf, 2006.

Procedures detail who is qualified to perform a given nursing procedure, whether supervision is necessary, and the type of reporting required. You need to have a means to easily access policies or have supervisory staff who inform you about NAP's job duties.

As a professional nurse you cannot simply assign NAP to tasks without considering the implications. Assess a patient and determine a plan of care before identifying which tasks someone else is able to perform. When directing NAP, determine how much supervision is necessary. Is it the first time a staff member performed the task? Does the patient present a complicating factor that makes the RN's assistance necessary? Does the staff member have prior experience with a particular type of patient in addition to having received training on skill performance? The final responsibility is to evaluate whether NAP performed a task properly and whether desired outcomes were met.

Efficient delegation requires constant communication (i.e., sending clear messages and listening so all participants understand expectations regarding patient care) (Gravlin and Bittner, 2010). Provide clear instructions when delegating tasks. These instructions initially focus on the procedure itself, what will be accomplished, and the unique needs of a patient. The RN also communicates when and what information to report such as expected observations and specific patient concerns (NCSBN, 2005). Communication is a two-way process in delegation; thus NAP need to have the chance to ask questions and have your expectations made clear (ANA and NCSBN, 2005; NCSBN, 2005). Conflict often occurs between RNs and NAP when there is little or poor communication (Potter et al., 2010). Handoff disconnects, lack of knowledge about the workload of team members, and difficulty dealing with conflict are examples of communication failures that often result in delegation ineffectiveness and omissions of nursing care (Gravlin and Bittner, 2010). As you become more familiar with a staff member's competency, trust builds, and staff need fewer instructions; but clarification of patients' specific needs is always necessary.

Another important step in delegation is evaluation of the staff member's performance, achievement of the patient's outcomes, the communication process used, and any problems or concerns that occurred (NCSBN, 2005). When an NAP performs a task correctly and does a good job, it is important to provide praise and recognition. If the staff member's performance is not satisfactory, give constructive and appropriate feedback. As a nurse, always give specific feedback regarding any mistakes that staff members make, explaining how to avoid the mistake or a better way to handle the situation. Giving feedback in private is the professional way and preserves the staff member's dignity. When giving feedback, make sure to focus on things that can be changed, choose only one issue at a time, and give specific details. Frequently when the NAP's performance does not meet expectations, it is the result of inadequate training or assignment of too many tasks. You discover the need to review a procedure with staff and offer demonstration or even recommend that additional training be scheduled with the education department. If too many tasks are being delegated, this might be a nursing practice issue. All staff need to discuss the appropriateness of delegation on their unit. Sometimes NAP need help in learning how to prioritize. In some cases you discover that you are overdelegating.

Once you delegate the task appropriately, it is important to monitor and supervise NAP in task performance. Clear directions and statement of desired outcomes increase the likelihood of successful completion of the task. If you observe a change in patient status, if the task is not being performed as directed or by agency policy and procedures, or if the NAP is having difficulty completing the task, you need to intervene and follow up as needed (ANA and NCSBN, 2005; NCSBN, 2005). It is your responsibility to complete documentation of the delegated task. Here are a few tips on appropriate delegation (Huston, 2009):

- *Assess the knowledge and skills of the delegatee:* Assess the knowledge and skills of the NAP by asking open-ended questions that elicit conversation and details about what he or she knows; for example, "How do you usually apply the cuff when you measure a blood pressure?" or "Tell me how you prepare the tubing before you give an enema."
- *Match tasks to the delegatee's skills:* Know which tasks and skills are in the scope of practice and job description for the team members to whom you delegate in your facility. Determine if personnel have learned critical thinking skills such as knowing when a patient is in harm or the difference between normal clinical findings and changes to report.
- *Communicate clearly:* Always provide clear directions by describing a task, the desired outcome, and the time period within which NAP need to complete the task. Never give instructions through another staff member. Make the person feel as though he or she is part of the team. Begin requests for help with *please* and end with *thank you.* For example, "I'd like you to please help me by getting Mr. Floyd up to ambulate before lunch. Be sure to check his blood pressure before he stands and write your finding on the graphic sheet. OK? Thanks."
- *Listen attentively:* Listen to NAP's response after you provide directions. Do they feel comfortable in asking questions or

requesting clarification? If you encourage a response, listen to what the person has to say. Be especially attentive if the staff member has a deadline to meet for another nurse. Help sort out priorities.
- *Provide feedback:* Always give NAP feedback regarding performance, regardless of outcome. Let them know of a job well done. A thank you increases the likelihood of the NAP helping in the future. If an outcome is undesirable, find a private place to discuss what occurred, any miscommunication, and how to achieve a better outcome in the future.

Knowledge Building

As a professional nurse, recognize the importance of pursuing knowledge to remain competent. You need to maintain and improve your knowledge and skills. Lifelong learning is needed to be able to continuously provide safe, effective, quality care to patients (Josiah Macy Jr. Foundation, 2008). A leader recognizes that there is always something new to learn. Opportunities for learning occur with each patient interaction, each encounter with a professional colleague, and each meeting or class session in which health care professionals meet to discuss clinical care issues. People always have different experiences and knowledge to share. Ongoing development of skills in delegation, communication, and teamwork helps maintain and build competency (Gravlin and Bittner, 2010). In-service programs, workshops, professional conferences, and collegiate courses offer innovative and current information on the rapidly changing world of health care. To become a leader, actively pursue learning opportunities, both formal and informal, and learn to share knowledge with the professional colleagues you encounter.

KEY POINTS

- A manager sets a philosophy for a work unit, ensures appropriate staffing, mobilizes staff and institutional resources to achieve objectives, motivates staff members to carry out their work, sets standards of performance, and makes decisions to achieve objectives.
- Consideration communicates mutual trust, respect, and rapport between a manager and staff members.
- Empowering staff members brings out the best in a manager and allows him or her to concentrate on effective patient care systems, support risk taking and innovation, and focus on results and rewards.
- An empowered nursing staff has decision-making authority to change how they practice.
- Nursing care delivery models vary according to the responsibility and autonomy of the RN in coordinating care delivery and the roles other staff members play in assisting with care.
- Critical to the success of decision making is making staff members aware that they have the responsibility, authority, autonomy, and accountability for the care they give and the decisions they make.
- A nurse manager encourages decentralized decision making by establishing nursing practice committees, supporting nurse-physician and interdisciplinary collaboration, setting and implementing quality improvement plans, and maintaining timely staff communication.
- Clinical care coordination involves accurate clinical decision making, establishing priorities, efficient organizational skills, appropriate use of resources and time management skills, and an ongoing evaluation of care activities.
- In an enriched professional environment, each member of a nursing work team is responsible for open, professional communication.
- Effective delegation requires the use of good communication skills.
- When done correctly, delegation improves job efficiency, productivity, and job enrichment.
- An important responsibility for the nurse who delegates nursing care is evaluation of the staff member's performance and patient outcomes.

CLINICAL APPLICATION QUESTIONS

Preparing for Clinical Practice

You are a staff nurse on a 32-bed cardiac step-down unit. The hospital obtained Magnet recognition last year. You are assigned as the preceptor for Tony, RN, who is a new graduate nurse, who just started his nursing career on your floor.

1. You and Tony just received morning shift report on your patients. You are assigned the following patients. Which patient do you and Tony need to see first? Explain your answer.
    1. Mr. Dodson, a 52-year-old patient who was admitted yesterday with a diagnosis of angina pectoris. He is scheduled for a cardiac stress test at 0900.
    2. Mrs. Wallace, a 60-year-old patient who was transferred out of intensive care at 0630 today. She had uncomplicated coronary artery bypass surgery yesterday.
    3. Mr. Workman, a 45-year-old patient who experienced a myocardial infarction 2 days ago. He is complaining of chest pain rated as 6 on a scale of 0 to 10.
    4. Mrs. Harris, a 76-year-old patient who had a permanent pacemaker inserted yesterday. She is complaining of incision pain rated as a 5 on a scale of 0 to 10.
2. As you work with Tony, you notice that he has trouble with organizational skills when providing patient care. What strategies will you suggest to Tony to help him improve in organizing his delivery of patient care?
3. Marianne, a NAP, is paired to work with you and Tony. You overhear Tony giving Marianne directions for what she needs to do. Tony says, "Marianne, in the next hour please assist Mrs. Harris in room 418 with her afternoon walk. She needs to walk 200 feet, which is from her room down the hall to the nurses' station and back to her room. Take her pulse before and after she walks and record it in her chart. I'll check with you when you're finished to see how she did. Do you have any questions before you walk her? Thank you for your help." Based on what you know about delegation, did Tony give appropriate or inappropriate directions to Marianne? Provide rationale for your answer.

evolve *Answers to Clinical Application Questions can be found on the Evolve website.*

REVIEW QUESTIONS

Are You Ready to Test Your Nursing Knowledge?

1. After the 0700 shift report the registered nurse (RN) delegates three tasks to the nursing assistant. At 1300 the RN tells the nursing assistant that he would like to talk to her about the first task that was delegated, which was walking the patient, Mrs. Taylor, earlier that morning. The RN says, "You did a good job walking Mrs. Taylor by 0930. I saw that you recorded her pulse before and after the walk. I saw that Mrs. Taylor walked

in the hallway barefoot. For safety, the next time you walk a patient, you need to make sure that the patient wears slippers or shoes. Please walk Mrs. Taylor again by 1500." Which characteristics of good feedback did the RN use when talking to the nursing assistant? (Select all that apply.)
   1. Feedback is given immediately.
   2. Feedback focuses on one issue.
   3. Feedback offers concrete details.
   4. Feedback identifies ways to improve.
   5. Feedback focuses on changeable things.
   6. Feedback is specific about what is done incorrectly only.
2. As the nurse, you need to complete all of the following. Which task do you complete first?
   1. Administer the oral pain medication to the patient who had surgery 3 days ago
   2. Make a referral to the home care nurse for a patient who is being discharged in 2 days
   3. Complete wound care for a patient with a wound drain that has an increased amount of drainage since last shift
   4. Notify the health care provider of the decreased level of consciousness in the patient who had surgery 2 days ago
3. You are the charge nurse on a surgical unit. You are doing staff assignments for the 3-to-11 shift. Which patient do you assign to the licensed practical nurse (LPN)?
   1. The patient who transferred out of intensive care an hour ago
   2. The patient who requires teaching on new medications before discharge
   3. The patient who had a vaginal hysterectomy 2 days ago and is being discharged tomorrow
   4. The patient who is experiencing some bleeding problems following surgery earlier today
4. The type of care management approach that coordinates and links health care services to patients and their families while streamlining costs and maintaining quality is:
   1. Primary nursing.
   2. Total patient care.
   3. Functional nursing.
   4. Case management.
5. While administering medications, the nurse realizes that she has given the wrong dose of medication to a patient. She acts by completing an incident report and notifying the patient's health care provider. The nurse is exercising:
   1. Authority.
   2. Responsibility.
   3. Accountability.
   4. Decision making.
6. Your nursing manager distributes biweekly newsletters of ongoing unit or health care agency activities and posts minutes of committee meetings on a bulletin board in the staff break room. This is an example of:
   1. Staff communication.
   2. Problem-solving committees.
   3. Interdisciplinary collaboration.
   4. Nurse-physician collaborative practice.
7. The nurse asks the nursing assistant to hold the legs of a female patient during a Foley catheter insertion. This is an example of a nurse displaying:
   1. Organizational skills.
   2. Use of resources.
   3. Time management.
   4. Evaluation.
8. The nurse is assisting the patient with coughing and deep-breathing exercises following abdominal surgery. This is which priority nursing need for this patient?
   1. Low priority
   2. High priority
   3. Intermediate priority
   4. Nonemergency priority
9. The registered nurse (RN) checks on a patient who was admitted to the hospital with pneumonia. The patient is coughing profusely and requires nasotracheal suctioning. Orders include an intravenous (IV) infusion of antibiotics. The patient is febrile and asks the RN if he can have a bath because he has been perspiring profusely. Which task is appropriate to delegate to the nursing assistant?
   1. Assessing vital signs
   2. Changing IV dressing
   3. Nasotracheal suctioning
   4. Administering a bed bath
10. Which task is appropriate for a registered nurse (RN) to delegate to the nursing assistant?
   1. Explaining to the patient the preoperative preparation before the surgery in the morning
   2. Administering the ordered antibiotic to the patient before surgery
   3. Obtaining the patient's signature on the surgical informed consent
   4. Assisting the patient to the bathroom before leaving for the operating room
11. Which of the following strategies focus on improving nurse-physician collaborative practice? (Select all that apply.)
   1. Inviting the physician to attend the practice council meeting
   2. Participating in physician morning rounds
   3. Placing physician photos and names in unit newsletter
   4. Contacting physician promptly to discuss patient problems
   5. Providing a list of physician contact numbers to all staff nurses
12. The nurses on the unit developed a system for self-scheduling of work shifts. This is an example of:
   1. Responsibility.
   2. Autonomy.
   3. Accountability.
   4. Authority.
13. Which example demonstrates the nurse performing the skill of evaluation?
   1. The nurse explains the side effects of the new blood pressure medication ordered for the patient.
   2. The nurse asks the patient to rate pain on a scale of 0 to 10 before administering the pain medication.
   3. After completing the teaching, the nurse observes the patient draw up and administer an insulin injection.
   4. The nurse changes the patient's leg ulcer dressing using aseptic technique.
14. The nurse is explaining the case management model to a group of nursing students. Which characteristics best describe the model? (Select all that apply.)
   1. Case managers provide all patient care.
   2. Multidisciplinary care plans are used.
   3. Case managers coordinate discharge planning.
   4. Staffing is expensive and may not decrease care costs.
   5. Communication with health care team members is important.
   6. Model helps to improve patient safety and quality.

15. The nurse collects the supplies for the dressing change for the patient in bed 1 and signs out the capillary blood glucose monitoring equipment to test the glucose of the patient in bed 2 before walking down the hall to the room. The nurse is displaying:
    1. Organizational skills.
    2. Use of resources.
    3. Priority setting.
    4. Clinical decision making.

Answers: 1. 2, 3, 4, 5; 2. 4; 3. 3; 4. 4; 5. 3; 6. 1; 7. 2; 8. 3; 9. 4; 10. 4; 11. 1, 2, 4; 12. 2; 13. 3; 14. 2, 3, 5, 6; 15. 1.

REFERENCES

American Nurses Association: Position statement on registered nurse utilization of assistive personnel, *Am Nurse* 25(2):7, 1995.

American Nurses Association (ANA), National Council of State Boards of Nursing (NCSBN): *Joint statement on delegation,* 2005, http://www.ncsbn.org/pdfs/Joint_statement.pdf. Accessed August 4, 2011.

American Nurses Credentialing Center (ANCC). Magnet Recognition Program, 2010, http://www.nursecredentialing.org/Magnet.aspx. Accessed August 4, 2011.

Anders RL, Hawkins JA: *Mosby's nursing leadership and management online*, St Louis, 2006, Mosby.

Baker DP, et al: Teamwork as an essential component of high-reliability organizations, *Health Service Res* 41(4): 1576, 2006.

Batcheller J, et al: A practice model for patient safety: the value of the experienced registered nurse, *J Nurs Admin* 34(4):200, 2004.

Benner P, et al: Clinical reasoning, decision making, and action: thinking critically and clinically. In Agency for Healthcare Research and Quality: *Patient safety and quality: an evidence-based handbook for nurses*, AHRQ Pub No. 08-0043, Rockville, Md, 2008, The Agency.

Carr DD: Case managers optimize patient safety by facilitating effective care transitions, *Prof Case Manage* 12(2):70, 2007.

Case Management Society of America: *What is a case manager?* 2010, http://www.cmsa.org/Home/CMSA/whatisacasemanager/tabid/224/Default.aspx. Accessed August 4, 2011.

Cronenwett L, et al: Quality and safety education for nurses, *Nurs Outlook* 55(3):122, 2007.

Gokenbach V: Professional nurse councils: a new model to create excitement and improve value and productivity, *J Nurs Admin* 37(10):440, 2007.

Hackworth T: Time management for the nurse leader, *Nurs 2008 Crit Care* 3(2):10, 2008.

Huston CJ: 10 tips for successful delegation, *Nursing* 39(3):54, 2009.

Josiah Macy Jr. Foundation: Continuing education in the health professions: improving healthcare through lifelong learning, *J Cont Educ Nurs* 34(3):112, 2008.

Manojlovich M, et al: Nursing practice and work environment issues in the 21st century, *Nurs Res* 57(1S):S11, 2008.

Marriner Tomey A: *Guide to nursing management and leadership*, ed 8, St Louis, 2009, Mosby.

Nadzam DM: Nurses' role in communication and patient safety, *J Nurs Care Qual* 24(3):184, 2009.

National Council of State Boards of Nursing (NCSBN): *Delegation: concepts and decision-making process*, Chicago, 1995, The Council.

National Council of State Boards of Nursing: *Working with others: a position paper*, Chicago, 2005, The Council.

Pearce C: Ten steps to managing time, *Nurs Manage* 14(1):23, 2007.

Seago JA: Professional communication. In Agency for Health Research and Quality: *Patient safety and quality: an evidence-based handbook for nurses*, AHRQ Pub No. 08-0043, Rockville, Md, 2008, The Agency.

Tiedeman ME, Lookinland S: Traditional models of care delivery: what have we learned? *J Nurs Admin* 34(6):291, 2004.

Toofany S: Critical thinking among nurses, *Nurs Manage* 14(9):28, 2008.

Upenieks VV, Sitterding M: Achieving Magnet redesignation: a framework for cultural change, *J Nurs Admin* 38(10):419, 2008.

Weston MJ: Defining control over nursing practice and autonomy, *J Nurs Admin* 38(9):404, 2008.

RESEARCH REFERENCES

Armstrong K, et al: Workplace empowerment and Magnet hospital characteristics as predictors of patient safety climate, *J Nurs Care Qual* 24(1):55, 2009.

Berkow S, et al: Fourteen unit attributes to guide staffing, *J Nurs Admin* 37(3):150, 2007.

Bittner NP, Gravlin G: Critical thinking, delegation, and missed care in nursing practice, *J Nurs Admin* 39(3):142, 2009.

Feltner A, et al: Nurses' views on the characteristics of an effective leader, *AORN J* 87(2):363, 2008.

Gravlin G, Bittner NP: Nurses' and nursing assistants' reports of missed care and delegation, *J Nurs Admin* 40(7/8):329, 2010.

Hendry C, Walker A: Priority setting in clinical nursing practice: literature review, *J Adv Nurs* 47(4):427, 2004.

Hughes LC, et al: Quality and strength of patient safety climate on medical-surgical units, *Health Care Manage Rev* 34(1):19, 2009.

Kearney MH: *Report of the findings from the post-entry competence study*, Chicago, 2009, National Council of State Boards of Nursing.

Kramer M, et al: Structures and practices enabling staff nurses to control their practice, *West J Nurs Res* 30(5):539, 2008.

Kramer M, et al: Nine structures and leadership practices essential for a magnetic (healthy) work environment, *Nurs Admin Q* 34(1):4, 2010.

Lacey SR, et al: Nursing support, workload, and intent to stay in Magnet, Magnet-aspiring, and non-Magnet hospitals, *J Nurs Admin* 37(4):199, 2007.

Lacey SR, et al: Differences between pediatric registered nurses' perception of organizational support, intent to stay, workload, and overall satisfaction, and years employed as a nurse in Magnet and non-Magnet pediatric hospitals: implications for administrators, *Nurs Admin Q* 33(1):6, 2009.

Potter PA, et al: Delegation practices between registered nurses and nursing assistive personnel, *J Nurs Manage* 18:157, 2010.

Schmalenberg C, Kramer M: Clinical units with the healthiest work environments, *Critical Care Nurse*, 28(3):65, 2008

Thomas PL: Case manager role definition: do they make an organizational impact? *Prof Case Manage* 13(2):61, 2008.

Ulrich BT, et al: How RNs view the work environment: results of a national survey of registered nurses, *J Nurs Admin* 33(9):389, 2005.

Ulrich BT, et al: Magnet status and registered nurse views of the work environment and nursing as a career, *J Nurs Admin* 39(7/8):S54, 2009.

CHAPTER

22

Ethics and Values

OBJECTIVES

- Discuss the role of ethics in professional nursing.
- Discuss the role of values in the study of ethics.
- Examine and clarify personal values.
- Understand basic philosophies of health care ethics.
- Explain a nursing perspective in ethics.
- Apply critical thinking to ethical dilemmas.
- Discuss contemporary ethical issues.

KEY TERMS

Accountability, p. 287
Advocacy, p. 287
Autonomy, p. 286
Beneficence, p. 286
Code of ethics, p. 287
Confidentiality, p. 287
Consequentialism, p. 289
Deontology, p. 288
Ethics, p. 286
Ethics of care, p. 290
Fidelity, p. 287
Justice, p. 287
Nonmaleficence, p. 287
Responsibility, p. 287
Teleology, p. 289
Utilitarianism, p. 289
Value, p. 288

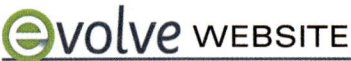

evolve WEBSITE

http://evolve.elsevier.com/Potter/fundamentals/

- Review Questions
- Case Study with Questions
- Audio Glossary
- Interactive Learning Activities
- Key Term Flashcards
- Content Updates

On your unit you are taking care of a 35-year-old female patient admitted in the final stages of her struggle with brain cancer. She is a single mother and has two young children at home. She received conventional and even experimental treatment, but the tumor has continued to grow. The medical team decides that further treatment would be futile. In an especially open discussion with you, she expresses her wish to explore a "do not resuscitate" (DNR) order. The attending physician reviews the clinical data and agrees that the patient is entering the terminal stages of her disease. However, in his opinion she is not ready to discuss end-of-life issues. He says that he has asked her about a DNR order, but she declines to discuss it. You suggest that he convene a family conference to discuss DNR options, but he dismisses the proposal at this time since his opinion is that the patient is not ready to participate.

Ethics is the study of conduct and character. It is concerned with determining what is good or valuable for individuals, for groups of individuals, and for society at large. Acts that are ethical reflect a commitment to standards beyond personal preferences (i.e., standards that individuals, professions, and societies strive to meet). However, when decisions must be made about health care, differing values and opinions among individuals can result in disagreement about the right thing to do, as the previous scenario illustrates. Understandable conflict occurs among health care providers, families, patients, friends, and people in the community about the right thing to do when ethics, values, and perceptions about health care collide. This chapter describes tools for you to use to embrace the role of ethics in your professional life and to participate and promote resolution when ethical dilemmas develop.

BASIC TERMS IN HEALTH ETHICS

For a discussion of ethics, it is helpful to establish a basic vocabulary. Your understanding of the terms common in ethical discourse helps you to shape your own thoughts about ethical issues and situations and participate thoughtfully in discussions.

Autonomy

When applied to politics or government, **autonomy** refers to freedom from external control. Similarly in health care, respect for autonomy refers to the commitment to include patients in decisions about all aspects of care as a way of acknowledging and protecting a patient's independence. For example, when a patient faces surgery, the surgeon has an obligation to review the surgical procedure, including risks and benefits, out of respect for the patient's autonomy. The consent that patients read and sign before surgery documents this respect for autonomy.

Beneficence

Beneficence refers to taking positive actions to help others. The principle of beneficence is fundamental to the practice of nursing and medicine. The agreement to act with beneficence implies that the best interests of the patient remain more important than self-interest. It implies that nurses practice primarily as a service to others, even in the details of daily work.

Nonmaleficence

Maleficence refers to harm or hurt; thus **nonmaleficence** is the avoidance of harm or hurt. In health care, ethical practice involves not only the will to do good, but the equal commitment to do no harm. The health care professional tries to balance the risks and benefits of care while striving at the same time to do the least harm possible. A bone marrow transplant procedure may offer a chance at cure; but the process involves periods of suffering, and it may not be possible to guarantee a positive outcome. Decisions about the best course of action can be difficult and full of uncertainty, precisely because nurses agree to avoid harm at the same time as they commit to promoting benefit.

Justice

Justice refers to fairness. The term is most often used in discussions about access to health care resources, including the just distribution of resources. Discussions about health insurance, hospital locations and services, even organ transplants generally refer to issues of justice. The term *just culture* refers to the promotion of open discussion whenever mistakes occur, or nearly occur, without fear of recrimination. By fostering open discussion about errors, members of the health care team become informed participants, able to design new systems that prevent harm.

Fidelity

Fidelity refers to the agreement to keep promises. As a nurse you keep promises by following through on your actions and interventions. If you assess a patient for pain and offer a plan to manage the pain, the standard of fidelity encourages you to monitor the patient's response to the plan. Professional behavior includes revision of the plan as necessary to try to keep the promise to reduce pain. Fidelity also refers to the unwillingness to abandon patients even when care becomes controversial or complex.

PROFESSIONAL NURSING CODE OF ETHICS

A **code of ethics** is a set of guiding principles that all members of a profession accept. It is a collective statement about the group's expectations and standards of behavior. Codes serve as guidelines to assist professional groups when questions arise about correct practice or behavior. The American Nurses Association (ANA) established the first code of nursing ethics decades ago. The ANA reviews and revises the code regularly to reflect changes in practice. However, basic principles of responsibility, accountability, advocacy, and confidentiality remain constant (Box 22-1).

Advocacy

Advocacy refers to the support of a particular cause. As a nurse you advocate for the health, safety, and rights of patients, including their right to privacy. Your special relationship with patients provides you with knowledge that is specific to your role as a registered nurse and as such provides you the opportunity to make a unique contribution to understanding a patient's point of view.

Responsibility

The word **responsibility** refers to a willingness to respect one's professional obligations and follow through on promises. As a nurse you are responsible for your actions and for the actions of those to whom you delegate tasks. You strive to remain competent to practice so you are able to follow through on your responsibilities reliably.

BOX 22-1 ANA CODE OF ETHICS

A nurse, in all professional relationships, practices with compassion and respect for the inherent dignity, worth, and uniqueness of every individual, unrestricted by considerations of social or economic status, personal attributes, or the nature of health problems.

- The nurse's primary commitment is to the patient, whether an individual, family, group, or community.
- The nurse promotes, advocates for, and strives to protect the health, safety, and rights of the patient.
- The nurse is responsible and accountable for individual nursing practice and determines the appropriate delegation of tasks consistent with the nurse's obligation to provide optimum patient care.
- The nurse owes the same duties to self as to others, including the responsibility to preserve integrity and safety, to maintain competence, and to continue personal and professional growth.
- The nurse participates in establishing, maintaining, and improving health care environments and conditions of employment conducive to the provision of quality health care and consistent with the values of the profession through individual and collective action.
- The nurse participates in the advancement of the profession through contributions to practice, education, administration, and knowledge development.
- The nurse collaborates with other health professionals and the public in promoting community, national, and international efforts to meet health needs.

The profession of nursing, as represented by associations and their members, is responsible for articulating nursing values, for maintaining the integrity of the profession and its practice, and for shaping social policy.

Accountability

Accountability refers to the ability to answer for one's actions. You learn to ensure that your professional actions are explainable to your patients and your employer. Health care institutions also exercise accountability by monitoring individual and institutional compliance with national standards established by agencies such as The Joint Commission (TJC) and the ANA. Compliance officers in most health care facilities provide compliance oversight. TJC establishes national guidelines to ensure patient and workplace safety through consistent, effective nursing practices (TJC, 2011). ANA sets national standards for continuing education and curriculum development for nursing schools (ANA, 2011). TJC and ANA promote ethical decision making by requiring health care institutions to create a multidisciplinary forum, or ethics committee, for discussion of ethical issues.

Confidentiality

The concept of **confidentiality** in health care is widely respected. Federal legislation known as the Health Insurance Portability and Accountability Act of 1996 (HIPAA) mandates the protection of patients' personal health information. The legislation defines the rights and privileges of patients for protection of privacy. It establishes fines for violations (US Department of Health and Human

Services, 2011). See Chapter 26 for details on HIPAA regulations governing communication of patient information contained in medical records, both hardcopy and electronic.

VALUES

Nursing is a work of intimacy. Nursing practice requires you to be in contact with patients physically, emotionally, psychologically, and spiritually. In most other intimate relationships you choose to enter the relationship precisely because you anticipate that your values will be shared with the other person. But as a nurse you agree to provide care to your patients solely on the basis of their need for your services. As discussed previously, the ethical principles of beneficence and fidelity shape the practice of health care and distinguish it from other common human relationships.

A **value** is a personal belief about the worth of a given idea, attitude, custom, or object that sets standards that influence behavior. Inevitably you will work with patients and colleagues whose values differ from yours. To negotiate differences of opinion and value, it is important to be clear about your own values: what you value, why, and how you respect your own values even as you try to respect those of others whose values differ from yours. The values that an individual holds reflect cultural and social influences, and these values vary among people and develop and change over time. For example, in some cultures decisions about health care flow from group or family-based discussion rather than independent decisions by one person. Such a practice challenges your commitment to respect patient autonomy. Your effort to resolve differing opinions and maintain your cultural competence becomes the hallmark of your commitment to ethical practice (Box 22-2).

BOX 22-2 CULTURAL ASPECTS OF CARE

Culturally Competent Care: End-of-Life Decisions

Research about end-of-life care shows that the standard of autonomous decision making is not necessarily universal. Some older-adult patients may defer to their children to make decisions for them as a sign of respect. Still others defer to a group elder to make decisions, even when the patient is competent to make them (Crawley, 2002). Although respect for autonomy has a strong presence in Western philosophy, especially in health care ethics, other cultures may express a preference for group process in making important decisions. For example, Pottinger et al. (2007) explain that "in some Asian cultures, the family is the smallest unit of identity and value is placed on interdependence as opposed to individualism . . . their strong desire to carry out this responsibility evokes equally strong feelings in Western health care providers who value autonomy in decision making."

Volker (2005) summarizes findings from several surveys of patients from different ethnic backgrounds about preferences at the end of life. The goal of the surveys was to identify cultural differences so health care providers could provide more culturally sensitive care. One survey showed that European Americans, Mexican Americans, and African Americans agreed with the concept of an advance directive. However, Mexican Americans and African Americans were "less receptive" than European Americans to the need for a written advance directive. In another survey European Americans were less likely than Mexican Americans to want life-sustaining treatments at the end of life. Korean Americans were knowledgeable about end-of-life technologies but would not choose them personally.

Implications for Practice

Volker points out that research that tries to predict behaviors based on ethnicity can be hindered by the lack of uniform definitions for various ethnic groups and by the infinite variety of human beings, even if they do seem to come from a particular ethnicity or culture. Therefore culturally competent care requires respect and patience. According to Volker, the American College of Physicians proposes the following ground rules:

- Acknowledgment of and respect for cultural differences
- A willingness to negotiate and compromise when world views differ
- Being aware of one's own values and biases
- Using communication skills that enhance empathy
- Knowing cultural practices of patient groups regularly seen
- Understanding that all patients are individuals and they may not share the same views as others within their own ethnic group

Value Formation

Development of values begins in childhood, shaped by experiences within the family unit. Variations in childrearing result in variations in values and behaviors as children grow. The fundamental urge to love and nurture children takes on different expressions within each of the wide variety of cultures in our world.

Schools, governments, religious traditions, and other social institutions play a role in the formation of values, reinforcing or sometimes challenging family values. Over time an individual acquires values by choosing some that the community holds strongly and perhaps discarding or transforming others.

Finally, individual experiences (i.e., the unpredictable twists and turns that occur in life) influence value formation. A person who suffers great loss early in life can grow to value things differently from someone whose life has been free from suffering.

Values Clarification

Ethical dilemmas almost always occur in the presence of conflicting values. To resolve ethical dilemmas one needs to distinguish among value, fact, and opinion. Sometimes people have such strong values that they consider them to be facts, not just opinion. Sometimes people are so passionate about their values that they provoke judgmental attitudes during conflict. Clarifying values—your own, your patients', your co-workers'—is an important and effective part of ethical discourse. In the process of values clarification, you learn to tolerate differences in a way that often (although not always) becomes the key to the resolution of ethical dilemmas.

Examine the cultural values exercise in Box 22-3. The values in the exercise conflict are in neutral terms so you can appreciate how differing values need not indicate "right" or "wrong." For example, for some people it is important to remain silent and stoic in the presence of great pain, and for others it is important to talk about it to understand and control it. Identifying values as something separate from facts can help you find tolerance for others, even when differences among you seem worlds apart.

ETHICS AND PHILOSOPHY

Historically health care ethics constituted a search for fixed standards that would determine right action. Over time ethics has grown into a complex field of study, more flexible than fixed, filled with differences of opinion and deeply meaningful efforts to understand human interaction. The following review introduces to you a variety of philosophies that you may encounter during ethical discussions in health care settings.

Deontology

A traditional ethical theory, deontology proposes a system of ethics that is perhaps most familiar to health care practitioners. Its foundations come from the work of an eighteenth-century philosopher, Immanuel Kant (1724-1804). **Deontology** defines actions as right or wrong based on their "right-making characteristics" such as

BOX 22-3 CULTURAL VALUES EXERCISE

The column on the right contains statements describing an opinion; the column on the left contains statements describing the opposite opinion. Neither statement is right, nor is it wrong. These statements reflect opinion, not necessarily fact. If persons from a variety of cultures were given this questionnaire, some would strongly agree with the beliefs on the right, and others with the opinions on the left. Read each statement and reflect on your own values and opinions. Circle 1 if you strongly agree with the statement on the left, 2 if you moderately agree. Circle 4 if you strongly agreement with the statement on the right and 3 if you moderately agree.

STATEMENT	RANK	STATEMENT
Preparing for the future is an important activity and reflects maturity.	1 2 3 4	Life has a predestined course. The individual should follow that course.
Vague answers are dishonest and confusing.	1 2 3 4	Vague answers are sometimes preferred because they avoid embarrassment and confrontation.
Punctuality and efficiency are characteristics of a person who is both intelligent and concerned.	1 2 3 4	Punctuality is not as important as maintaining a relaxed atmosphere, enjoying the moment, and being with family and friends.
When in severe pain, it is important to remain strong and not to complain too much.	1 2 3 4	When in severe pain, it is better to talk about the discomfort and express frustration.
It is self-centered and unwise to accept a gift from someone you do not know well.	1 2 3 4	It is an insult to refuse a gift when it is offered.
Addressing someone by his or her first name shows friendliness.	1 2 3 4	Addressing someone by his or her first name is disrespectful.
Direct questions are usually the best way to gain information.	1 2 3 4	Direct questioning is rude and could cause embarrassment.
Direct eye contact shows interest.	1 2 3 4	Direct eye contact is intrusive.
Ultimately the independence of the individual must come before the needs of the family.	1 2 3 4	The needs of the individual are always less important than the needs of the family.

Modified from Renwick GW, Rhinesmith SH: *An exercise in cultural analysis for managers,* Chicago, 1995, Intercultural Press.

fidelity to promises, truthfulness, and justice (Beauchamp and Childress, 2008). It specifically does not look to consequences of actions to determine right or wrong. Instead it examines a situation for the existence of essential right or wrong. For example, if you try to make a decision about the ethics of a controversial medical procedure, deontology guides you to focus on how the procedure ensures fidelity to the patient, truthfulness, justice, and beneficence. You focus less on the consequences (ethically speaking). If an act is just, respects autonomy, and provides good, it will be right, and it will be ethical according to this philosophy. Deontology depends on a mutual understanding and acceptance of these principles.

Often people in ethical dilemmas have to choose between conflicting principles. For example, application of the principle of respect for autonomy is sometimes confusing when dealing with children. The health care team may recommend a certain course of treatment, but the parent disagrees or even refuses the recommendation. Whose autonomy should receive the respect—the parent's? Who should speak for the child's best interest? Communities struggle to decide who ultimately is responsible for the well-being of children. A commitment to respect the "rightness" of autonomy is a guiding principle in deontology, but adherence to the principle alone may not provide clear answers to ethical dilemmas.

Utilitarianism

A utilitarian system of ethics proposes that the value of something is determined by its usefulness. This philosophy is also known as **consequentialism** because its main emphasis is on the outcome or consequence of action. A third term associated with this philosophy is **teleology,** from the Greek word telos, meaning "end," or the study of ends or final causes. John Stuart Mill (1806-1873), a British philosopher, first proposed its philosophical foundations. The greatest good for the greatest number of people is the guiding principle for determining right action in this system. As with deontology, **utilitarianism** relies on the application of a certain principle, (i.e., measures of "good" and "greatest") (Beauchamp and Childress, 2008). The difference between utilitarianism and deontology is the focus on outcomes. Utilitarianism measures the effect that an act will have; deontology looks to the presence of principle regardless of outcome.

People have conflicting definitions of "greatest good." For example, research suggests that education about safe sex practices reduces the spread of human immunodeficiency virus (HIV). Reducing incidence of HIV is good for a great number of people. For some, education about sex is best provided within a family setting rather than in school because it promotes family values. However, for others the greater good is educating the greatest number of people in the most effective way possible; therefore sex education in the public schools would ensure the greatest good. As with deontology, utilitarianism provides guidance, but it does not guarantee agreement.

Feminist Ethics

Feminist ethics critiques conventional ethics such as deontology and utilitarianism. It looks to the nature of relationships to guide participants in making difficult decisions, especially relationships in which power is unequal or in which a point of view has become ignored or invisible (Brody, 2009). Writers with a feminist perspective tend to concentrate more on practical solutions than on theory.

Feminist ethicists propose that the natural human urge to be influenced by relationships is a positive value. Critics of feminist ethics are concerned about the lack of focus on universal principals. Without guidance from universal principals, they argue, solutions depend completely on the situation itself.

Ethics of Care

The ethics of care and feminist ethics are closely related. Both promote a philosophy that focuses on understanding relationships, especially personal narratives.

An early proponent of the ethics of care, Nel Noddings (1984), used the term *the one-caring* to identify the individual who provides care, and *the cared-for* to refer to the patient. In adopting this language Noddings hoped to emphasize the role of feelings. Contemporary writers such as Virginia Held (2005) continue to build on Noddings' foundations by making a case for a focus on the fundamental nature of relationships in understanding ethical issues. **Ethics of care** may even address issues beyond individual relationships such as ethical concerns about the structures within which individual caring occurs such as health care facilities.

Consensus in Bioethics

Bringing different points of view to agreement and harmony, or consensus, requires skill and patience. Building consensus is essentially an act of discovery, in which "collective wisdom" guides a group to the best possible decision. It encourages respect for unusual points of view while striving for agreement among all participants (Dressler, 2006). As a strategy for solving dilemmas, consensus building promotes respect and agreement rather than a particular philosophy or moral system itself. In the example of the processing of the ethical dilemma described in this chapter, the process is basically one of consensus building.

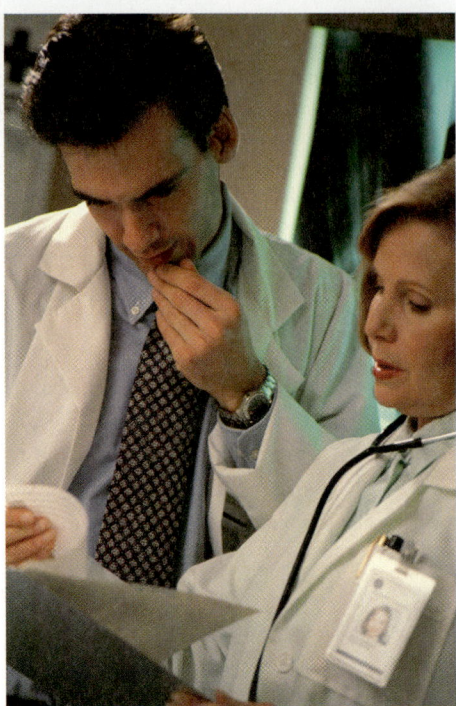

FIG. 22-1 Nurses collaborate with other professionals in making ethical decisions. (Copyright 2007 Jupiter Images Corporation.)

NURSING POINT OF VIEW

All patients in the health care system interact with a nurse at some point, and they interact in ways that are unique to nursing. Nurses generally engage with patients over longer periods of time than other disciplines. Because nurses are involved in intimate physical acts such as bathing, feeding, and special procedures, patients and families may feel safer or more comfortable in revealing information not always shared with physicians, health care providers, or others. Details about family life, information about coping styles, personal preferences, and details about fears and insecurities are likely to come out during the course of nursing interventions. Your ability to recognize these aspects of a patient's situation and express your professional concerns accordingly provides critical value to the discussion.

On the other hand, it is important to remember that care of any patient involves many disciplines. Managers and administrators from many different professional backgrounds contribute to ethical discourse with their knowledge of systems, distribution of resources, financial possibilities, or limits (Fig. 22-1).

Processing an Ethical Dilemma

Ethical dilemmas cause distress and controversy for both patients and caregivers. To minimize distress, you learn to process ethical issues carefully and deliberately. The process should promote the free expression of feelings and opinions. However, you do not resolve an ethical dilemma by considering only what people want and feel (Zoloth, 2010).

Resolving an ethical dilemma is similar to the nursing process in its methodical approach to a clinical issue. But it differs from the nursing process in that it requires negotiation of differences of opinion. As Zoloth (2010) suggests, the resolution of conflicting opinions works best when the following elements are part of the process: the presumption of good will on the part of all participants, strict adherence to confidentiality, patient-centered decision making, and the welcome participation of families and primary caregivers.

The process begins with gathering all pertinent information for an assessment and continues with planning, implementation, and evaluation. To distinguish an ethical problem from other kinds of problems, Curtin (2004) proposes that, if the issue is an ethical one, it entails at least one of the following:

- You are unable to resolve it solely through a review of scientific data.
- It is perplexing. You cannot easily think logically or make a decision about the problem.
- The answer to the problem will have a profound relevance for areas of human concern.

Participants begin the process with a clear statement of the ethical problem. Agreement about the nature of the problem facilitates constructive discussion. Next, listing possible courses of action helps the group explore options and identify dissent. As a group you consider and evaluate alternatives with respect for all differences of opinion. Most of the time people in an ethical conflict come to a resolution and implement a plan. Evaluation of the plan follows (Box 22-4).

If the process involves a family conference or changes in the management plan, you document the process in the medical record. Some institutions use a special ethics consultation form to structure documentation. However, if the ethical concern does not directly affect patient care, you may document the discussion in meeting minutes or in a memorandum to those involved in the discussion.

Now that we have established basic vocabulary terms and reviewed a variety of ethics philosophies, let us return to the patient care scenario at the beginning of this chapter to illustrate how methodical processing can help to resolve an ethical dilemma.

You are caring for a patient with a terminal illness. The patient has discussed with you her desire to explore DNR orders. However, she expresses conflicting sentiments to the admitting physician, and you are challenged with how to proceed.

BOX 22-4 KEY STEPS IN THE RESOLUTION OF AN ETHICAL DILEMMA

Step 1: Ask the question, is this an ethical dilemma? If a review of scientific data does not resolve the question, if the question is perplexing, and if the answer will have relevance for areas of human concern, an ethical dilemma probably exists.
Step 2: Gather information relevant to the case. Patient, family, institutional, and social perspectives are important sources of relevant information.
Step 3: Clarify values. Distinguish among fact, opinion, and values.
Step 4: Verbalize the problem. A clear, simple statement of the dilemma is not always easy, but it helps to ensure effectiveness in the final plan and facilitates discussion.
Step 5: Identify possible courses of action.
Step 6: Negotiate a plan. Negotiation requires a confidence in one's own point of view and a deep respect for the opinions of others.
Step 7: Evaluate the plan over time.

Step 1. Is this situation an ethical dilemma? If the question remains perplexing and the answer will have profound relevance for several areas of human concern, an ethical dilemma exists.

Your situation meets the criteria for an ethical dilemma. The disagreement does not revolve around whether the patient is in a terminally ill state; thus further clinical information will not change the basic question: Should the patient have an opportunity to discuss DNR orders at this time? The question is perplexing. Two professional team members, you and the attending physician, disagree on an assessment of a patient's readiness to confront difficult issues related to dying. The answer to the question, "Is this patient ready to discuss end of life?" has important human implications. If she is not ready, raising the issues could cause anguish and fear in the patient and her family. If she is ready and the team avoids discussion, she could suffer unnecessarily in silence. If she is very close to death, the lack of a DNR order necessitates the application of cardiopulmonary resuscitation (CPR) in a futile situation. As a nurse you know that CPR can cause pain. If applied when an extension of life is unlikely, it could prolong suffering and reduce dignity. On the other hand, if the patient or her loved ones prefer to ensure that all actions to preserve life are taken, regardless of the outcome, a DNR order would violate the patient's wishes.

Step 2. Gather as much information as possible that is relevant to the case. Because resolution of dilemmas often comes from unlikely sources, it is helpful to incorporate as much knowledge as possible. Helpful information includes laboratory and test results, the clinical state of the patient in question, and current literature about the diagnosis or condition of the patient. A patient's religious, cultural, and family situations are part of the assessment.

Since the dilemma exists because two professionals disagree about a patient's state of mind, it is helpful to reassess the patient. An independent assessment could help resolve differences of opinion. Family members or significant others in the patient's life often hold important clues to a patient's state of mind.

Step 3. Examine and determine your values about the issues. Part of the goal is to accurately identify your own opinion. An equally critical goal is to form respect for others' opinions.

Reflect on your values. You think that this patient wants a DNR order in place. But does this opinion accurately represent the patient's wishes? Let's say that your religious beliefs would allow you to obtain DNR status if you were in the patient's condition. After talking with the patient, you learn that her religion discourages acts that diminish life in any way. You realize that she may have come to view a DNR order as "giving up" or "acting like God." In addition, you understand that the attending physician has not had time to know this patient well. You continue to believe that the patient is capable of a discussion, in spite of her statements to the physician. In fact, you believe that she will benefit from a discussion, regardless of the final decision. Perhaps the combination of an unfamiliar caretaker and declining physical health has silenced her, even though her fears and concerns persist.

Step 4. Verbalize the problem. By agreeing to a statement of the problem, the group is able to conduct a focused discussion.

Is a DNR order right or wrong thing for this patient? Is she ready to discuss the options?

Step 5. Consider possible courses of action. What options are possible in this situation?

Do you initiate a discussion with the patient independent of the physician? Is this outside of your professional domain, and is it in the patient's best interest for you to facilitate a DNR order from another physician? What if your assessment of the patient is incorrect? Do you contribute to the dignity or the distress of the patient? The answers to these questions can be elusive because they depend on an understanding of patient feelings and values that are not necessarily obvious. Even if you cannot write a DNR order legally, it does not relieve you of troubling questions because the ability to influence a physician's or patient's decision regarding DNR remains.

Step 6. Negotiate the outcome. Negotiations happen informally at the bedside or in a conference room. Sometimes a formal ethics meeting is necessary. Wherever negotiations occur, the nurse has an obligation to articulate a personal point of view.

If an ethics committee meeting occurs, the discussion usually involves participants from several disciplines. A facilitator or chairperson ensures that the group examines all points of view and identifies all relevant issues. In the best circumstances participants discover a course of action that meets criteria for consensus, or acceptance by all. However, occasionally they leave the discussion disappointed or even opposed to the decision. But in a successful discussion all members will have agreed on an action.

The principles involved during the discussion include beneficence and nonmaleficence: Which plan would provide the most good for this patient, a DNR order or no order? A separate question addresses the patient's point of view and a respect for autonomy: Would a discussion with the patient promote well-being or anguish? The commitment to respect a patient's autonomy reveals that a troublesome question remains: Does the patient want something different from what she is expressing?

With several members of the health care team present, the discussion proceeds. You present your point of view. You continue to sense that the patient is ready to discuss DNR orders. But you also respect the attending physician and his perception that the patient is reluctant to talk freely about it. In the end the team proposes the following: a formal meeting with the patient in which you, the attending physician, and a respected family member are present. You support this proposal because you believe that it maximizes comfort from the patient's network of friends and family. In addition, you recognize that in a trusting environment the patient is most likely to express herself freely. You suggest that, rather than asking if the patient wants a DNR order, perhaps the team could wait for her to initiate the discussion. In this way the team would be sure of her consent and willingness to address the difficult questions about dying.

Step 7. Evaluate the action.

At the meeting the patient brings up the DNR order. She expresses relief at the chance to explore her options and feelings. The physician clarifies pain management issues that she broaches. She wants to discuss a DNR order but requests a visit from her priest before making a final decision.

Institutional Resources

Health care institutions establish ethics committees to process ethical dilemmas. Ethics committees are usually multidisciplinary and serve several purposes: education, policy recommendation, and case consultation. Any person involved in an ethical dilemma, including nurses, physicians, health care providers, patients, and family members, can request access to an ethics committee.

You also process ethical issues in settings other than a committee. Nurses provide insight about ethical problems at family conferences, staff meetings, or even in one-on-one meetings.

Many ethical problems begin when people feel misled or are not aware of their options and do not know when to speak up about their concerns. You address such concerns in a variety of constructive settings. Ethics committees serve to complement relationships within the workplace and the community and offer a valuable resource for strengthening these relationships (Box 22-5).

> **BOX 22-5 EVIDENCE-BASED PRACTICE**
>
> ***Moral Distress***
>
> **PICO Question:** Which ethical actions diminish distress and promote compassionate care for nurses experiencing moral distress when caring for dying patients?
>
> **Evidence Summary**
>
> Fully 45% of nurses interviewed for this study considered leaving their positions to alleviate the burden of moral distress (Hamric, 2007). Moral distress describes the anguish experienced when a person feels unable to act according to closely held core values. Evidence from interviews with nurses and physicians in 14 intensive care units (ICUs) shed light on moral distress. The interviews revealed that physicians are as capable of experiencing moral distress as are nurses. For both nurses and physicians the highest levels of distress were experienced when caregivers felt pressured to continue unwarranted aggressive treatments for patients in the ICU.
>
> **Application to Nursing Practice**
>
> - Since moral distress is a shared experience, efforts to alleviate distress are most successful when the efforts are also shared. The authors recommend:
>   - Interdisciplinary ethics education, in which nurses and physicians learn together about ethical discourse.
>   - Sharing stories about professional perspectives regarding difficult clinical decisions.
>   - Increasing opportunities for collegial practice such as routine multidisciplinary rounds.
>   - Recurrent situations of moral distress indicate underlying systemic problems of poor communication, inadequate collaboration, and perceived powerlessness must be addressed if nurses and physicians are to minimize this phenomenon in clinical settings (Ulrich, Hamric, and Grady, 2010). Willingness to speak up if they experience moral distress takes courage, but engaging in constructive conversation is key to the management of moral distress in the workplace.

ISSUES IN HEALTH CARE ETHICS

You will face professional ethical issues in all kinds of settings throughout your career. Issues change as society and technologies change, but common denominators remain: the basic process used to address the issues and your responsibility to maintain skill and patience in dealing with them. The following section describes examples of current issues in which ethical concerns can occur.

Quality of Life

Quality of life represents something deeply personal. Health care researchers work to develop quality-of-life measures to define scientifically the value and benefits of certain medical interventions. Statistical analyses help scientists apply the measures in research and other settings (Walters, 2009). These measures take into account the age of the patient, the patient's ability to live independently, his or her ability to contribute to society in a gainful way, and other nuanced measures of quality. The question of quality of life is central to discussions about futile care, cancer therapy, health care provider–assisted suicide, and DNR discussions.

The population of disabled persons in the United States and elsewhere has reshaped the discussion about quality of life. The national movement to respect the abilities of the "disabled" has raised the visibility of quality-of-life issues and forced a reconsideration of the definition of quality. For example, many school districts no longer separate physically or mentally challenged children but rather integrate them into mainstream classrooms. Public places such as restaurants and buses are accessible to people who use wheelchairs. Antidiscrimination laws enhance the economic security of people with physical, mental, or emotional challenges. These changes have increased the integration of disabled persons into general society. The changes remind society, including health care workers, that definitions of quality are deeply based in individual experience.

Genetic Screening

Genetic testing can alert a patient to a condition that may not yet be evident but that is certain to develop in the future. What are the risks and benefits to individuals and to society of learning about the presence of a disease that has not yet caused symptoms or for which a cure is not yet available? The presence of Huntington's disease, an incurable disease for now, is detectable by genetic testing. Huntington's disease is a degenerative neurological disease that affects cognitive, emotional, and physical function. Symptoms usually do not appear until the third or fourth decade of life. If a parent or grandparent has the disease, offspring are at risk for developing it (National Institute of Neurological Disorders and Stroke, 2010). Patients may be eager to learn if they will develop the disease so they are able to make decisions about childbearing, career, and retirement planning. Others are reluctant to face the knowledge that they have the disease before symptoms begin, unwilling to compromise healthy years with anxieties about pending emotional and intellectual losses (Wexler, 2010).

Care at the End of Life

Predictions about health outcomes are not always accurate. Even when they are, opinions about the value or worth of the outcome differ. For example, patients at risk for breast cancer occasionally request a mastectomy before any symptoms of breast disease have appeared, fearful of a family history and thinking that it will prevent future suffering. Physicians may be understandably reluctant to provide this intervention, based on knowledge of risk factors and their commitment to "do no harm." On the other hand, a physician might recommend that a patient undergo a liver transplantation for end-stage liver disease even though the likelihood of a cure is uncertain. The patient may hold the opinion that the transplant is pointless: unlikely to produce benefit that justifies the suffering he or she anticipates. Agreement on what is best is often elusive.

The term *futile* refers to something that is hopeless or serves no useful purpose. In health care discussions the term refers to interventions unlikely to produce benefit for a patient. The concept is slippery when applied to clinical situations.

If a patient is dying, in a condition with little or no hope of recovery, almost any intervention beyond symptom management and comfort measures is seen as futile. In this situation an agreement to label an intervention as futile can help providers, families, and patients turn to palliative care measures as a more constructive approach to the situation (see Chapter 36).

When an aging patient is at the end of life, issues may be complicated by his or her ability to make competent decisions because of conditions such as dementia or stroke. How and when to respect the wishes of older patients whose cognitive capacities are in doubt or dispute can complicate clinical decisions and necessitate ethical discourse (Box 22-6).

BOX 22-6 FOCUS ON OLDER ADULTS

Ethical Issues and Aging

- Older people usually are not as familiar with the concept of autonomy as people from younger generations. As a result, older adults are sometimes uncomfortable disagreeing with physicians, health care providers, or nurses. They view assertiveness as a violation of trust.
- As people age, they develop clinical conditions that affect the communication process: hearing and vision deficits, memory impairments, and chronic illness. Some patients become incapacitated by stroke or disease. Most older adults take multiple medications, some of which affect cognitive skills in subtle ways. It is important to evaluate the competence of a patient to make decisions and provide assistance when necessary, especially when treatment choices conflict or ethical issues arise (Burke and Laramie, 2003).
- Consensus about medical goals for the older adult is hard to achieve. When is a person so diminished by old age that a treatment plan not only prolongs life but also prolongs suffering? Working to ensure dignity and comfort is as important as achieving medical success (Burke and Laramie, 2003).

Access to Care

The number of uninsured in the United States grew from 39 million people in 2000 to more than 46.3 million people by 2008, over 15% of the total population (US Census Bureau, 2009). Many of the uninsured are women or children. The Kaiser Family Foundation reports that young adults ages 19 to 29 have the highest uninsured rate of any age-group in the United States and represent 30% of the overall uninsured population (Schwartz and Schwartz, 2010). Although two thirds of the uninsured are poor, nearly 80% come from working families (Holahan, Cook, and Dubay, 2007). Access to care and health care reform may seem distantly related to your daily job or a specific patient care assignment. But as a nurse you will certainly deal with ethical issues related to access to care. You may care for a patient about to be discharged from the hospital when you find that he or she cannot afford to fill a prescription. Do you advocate for a delay in discharge? Do you have time to find financial resources to subsidize the prescription costs? Your involvement with issues such as these and others requires a dedication to your professional ethics, a personal commitment to continuing education, and continuing engagement.

• • •

The courage and intelligence to act as both an advocate for patients and a professional member of the health care community come from a committed effort to learn and understand ethical principles. As a professional nurse you provide a unique point of view regarding patients, the systems that support patients, and the institutions that make up the health care system. You have a duty and a privilege to articulate that point of view. Learning the language of ethical discourse is a part of the skill necessary to exercise this privilege. Review and consideration of various ethical principles helps you form personal points of view, a necessary factor in the negotiation of difficult ethical situations.

KEY POINTS

- Ethics is the study of conduct and character. It is concerned with determining what is good or valuable for individuals and society at large.
- The ANA code of ethics provides a foundation for professional nursing.
- Professional nursing promotes accountability, responsibility, advocacy, and confidentiality.
- Standards of ethics in health care include autonomy, beneficence, nonmaleficence, justice, and fidelity.
- The process of values clarification helps you to explore values and feelings and decide how to act on personal beliefs and respect values of others, even if they differ from yours.
- Ethical problems arise in the presence of differences in values, changing professional roles, technological advances, and social issues that influence quality of life.
- A process for resolving ethical dilemmas that respects differences of opinions and all participants equally helps health care providers resolve conflict about right actions.
- A nurse's point of view offers a unique voice in the resolution of ethical dilemmas.

CLINICAL APPLICATION QUESTIONS

Preparing for Clinical Practice

You are caring for a 17-year-old female African American patient with sickle cell disease who has been admitted for treatment of sickle cell crisis. Sickle cell disease is a genetic abnormality that affects hemoglobin in the red blood cells. The defect is found primarily in African Americans. In a sickle cell crisis weakened red blood cells clump together and impede blood flow, causing extreme pain. To prevent stroke and manage the pain of the crisis, your patient needs aggressive fluid and comfort management. Even though she is receiving pain medication around the clock, she continues to report acute pain, a level of 10 on a scale of 0 to 10. In her distress she complains about almost everything: her roommate, the food, even the intravenous line that delivers the fluids and pain medications. Her home is far from the hospital, and neither her parents nor her friends are able to visit. She has an older brother who has been convicted of possession of illegal drugs.

1. Examine and describe your values and opinions about pain, pain management, and addiction.
2. Describe any ethical concerns you might have about this patient's autonomy.
3. How can you apply the principals of beneficence and fidelity in this situation? What about nonmaleficence?

evolve *Answers to Clinical Application Questions can be found on the Evolve website.*

REVIEW QUESTIONS

Are You Ready to Test Your Nursing Knowledge?

1. The patient for whom you are caring needs a liver transplant to survive. This patient has been out of work for several months and doesn't have health insurance or enough cash. What principles would be a priority in a discussion about ethics?
   1. Accountability because you as the nurse are accountable for the well-being of this patient
   2. Respect for autonomy because this patient's autonomy will be violated if he does not receive the liver transplant
   3. Ethics of care because the caring thing that a nurse could provide this patient is resources for a liver transplant
   4. Justice because the first and greatest question in this situation is how to determine the just distribution of resources
2. The point of the ethical principal to "do no harm" is an agreement to reassure the public that in all ways the health care team not only works to heal patients but agree to do this in the least painful and harmful way possible. Which principle describes this agreement?
   1. Beneficence
   2. Accountability
   3. Nonmaleficence
   4. Respect for autonomy
3. A child's immunization may cause discomfort during administration, but the benefits of protection from disease, both for the individual and society, outweigh the temporary discomforts. Which principle is involved in this situation?
   1. Fidelity
   2. Beneficence
   3. Nonmaleficence
   4. Respect for autonomy
4. When a nurse assesses a patient for pain and offers a plan to manage the pain, which principal is used to encourage the nurse to monitor the patient's response to the pain?
   1. Fidelity
   2. Beneficence
   3. Nonmaleficence
   4. Respect for autonomy
5. What is the best example of the nurse practicing patient advocacy?
   1. Seek out the nursing supervisor in conflicting procedural situations
   2. Document all clinical changes in the medical record in a timely manner
   3. Work to understand the law as it applies to an error in following standards of care
   4. Assess the patient's point of view and prepare to articulate it
6. Successful ethical discussion depends on people who have a clear sense of personal values. When a group of people share many of the same values, it may be possible to refer for guidance to philosophical principals of utilitarianism. This philosophy proposes which of the following?
   1. The value of something is determined by its usefulness to society.
   2. People's values are determined by religious leaders.
   3. The decision to perform a liver transplant depends on a measure of the moral life that the patient has led so far.
   4. The best way to determine the solution to an ethical dilemma is to refer the case to the attending physician or health care provider.
7. The philosophy sometimes called the *ethics of care* suggests that ethical dilemmas can best be solved by attention to which of the following?
   1. Patients
   2. Relationships
   3. Ethical principles
   4. Code of ethics for nurses
8. In most ethical dilemmas in health care, the solution to the dilemma requires negotiation among members of the health care team. Why is the nurse's point of view valuable?
   1. Nurses understand the principle of autonomy to guide respect for patient's self-worth.
   2. Nurses have a scope of practice that encourages their presence during ethical discussions.
   3. Nurses develop a relationship to the patient that is unique among all professional health care providers.
   4. The nurse's code of ethics recommends that a nurse be present at any ethical discussion about patient care.
9. Ethical dilemmas often arise over a conflict of opinion. What is the critical first step in negotiating the difference of opinion?
   1. Consult a professional ethicist to ensure that the steps of the process occur in full.
   2. Gather all relevant information regarding the clinical, social, and spiritual aspects of the dilemma.
   3. Ensure that the attending physician or health care provider has written an order for an ethics consultation to support the ethics process.
   4. List the ethical principles that inform the dilemma so negotiations agree on the language of the discussion.
10. The ANA code of nursing ethics articulates that the nurse "promotes, advocates for, and strives to protect the health, safety, and rights of the patient." This includes the protection of patient privacy. On the basis of this principal, if you participate in a public online social network such as Facebook, could you post images of a patient's x-ray film if you deleted all patient identifiers?
    1. Yes because patient privacy would not be violated as long as the patient identifiers were removed
    2. Yes because respect for autonomy implies that you have the autonomy to decide what constitutes privacy

3. No because, even though patient identifiers are removed, someone could identify the patient based on other comments that you make online about his or her condition and your place of work
4. No because the principal of justice requires you to allocate resources fairly

11. When an ethical dilemma occurs on your unit, can you resolve the dilemma by taking a vote?
    1. Yes because ethics is essentially a democratic process, with all participants sharing an equal voice
    2. No because an ethical dilemma involves the resolution of conflicting values and principals rather than simply the identification of what people want to do
    3. Yes because ethical dilemmas otherwise take up time and energy that is better spent at the bedside performing direct patient care
    4. No because most ethical dilemmas are resolved by deferring to the medical director of the ethics department
12. Resolution of an ethical dilemma involves discussion with the patient, the patient's family, and participants from all health care disciplines. Which of the following describes the role of the nurse in the resolution of ethical dilemmas?
    1. To articulate his or her unique point of view, including knowledge based on clinical and psychosocial observations
    2. To await new clinical orders from the physician
    3. To limit discussions about ethical principals
    4. To allow the patient and the physician to resolve the dilemma without regard to personally held values or opinions regarding the ethical issues
13. A precise definition for the word *quality* is difficult to articulate when it comes to quality of life. Why? (Select all that apply.)
    1. Quality of life is measured by potential income, and average income varies in different regions of the country.
    2. Community values are subject to change, and communities influence definitions of "quality."
    3. Individual experiences influence perceptions of quality in potentially different ways, making consensus difficult.
    4. Placing measurable value on elusive elements such as cognitive skills, ability to perform meaningful work, and relationship to family is challenging.
14. Which of the following explain how health care reform is an ethical issue? (Select all that apply.)
    1. Access to care is an issue of beneficence, a fundamental principal in health care ethics.
    2. Reforms promote the principle of beneficence, a hallmark of health care ethics.
    3. Purchasing health care insurance may become an obligation rather than a choice, a potential conflict between autonomy and beneficence.
    4. Lack of access to affordable health care causes harm, and nonmaleficence is a basic principal of health care ethics.
15. Which is the best method of negotiating or processing difficult ethical situations?
    1. Ethical issues arise between dissenting providers and can be best resolved by deference to an independent arbitrator such a chaplain.
    2. Since ethical issues usually affect policy and procedure, a legal expert is the best consultant to help resolve disputes.
    3. Institutional ethics committees help to ensure that all participants involved in the ethical dilemma get a fair hearing and an opportunity to express values, feelings, and opinions as a way to find consensus.
    4. Medical experts are best able to resolve conflicts about outcome predictions.

Answers: **1.** 4; **2.** 3; **3.** 2; **4.** 1; **5.** 4; **6.** 1; **7.** 2; **8.** 3; **9.** 2; **10.** 3; **11.** 2; **12.** 1; **13.** 2, 3, 4; **14.** 2, 3, 4; **15.** 3.

REFERENCES

American Nurses Association (ANA): *Education and competence*, 2011, http://www.nursingworld.org/. Accessed January 20, 2011.

Beauchamp T, Childress J: *Principles of biomedical ethics*, ed 4, New York, 2008, Oxford University Press.

Brody H: *Future of bioethics*, New York, 2009, Oxford University Press.

Burke MM, Laramie JA: *Primary care of the older adult: a multidisciplinary approach*, St Louis, 2003, Mosby.

Curtin L: Ethics in management: the ethical handling of ethical issues, *J Clin Syst Manage* 2004 6(4):14, 2004.

Dressler L: *Consensus through conversation: how to achieve high-commitment decisions*, San Francisco, 2006, Barrett-Koehler.

Held V: *The ethics of care*, Oxford, 2005, Oxford University Press.

Holahan J, Cook A, Dubay L: *Characteristics of the uninsured: who is eligible for public coverage and who needs help affording coverage*, Menlo Park, CA, 2007, Henry J. Kaiser Family Foundation. http://www.kff.org/uninsured/upload/7613.pdf.

National Institute of Neurological Disorders and Stroke: *Huntington's disease information page*, 2010, http://www.ninds.nih.gov/disorders/huntington/huntington.htm. Accessed January 20, 2011.

Noddings N: *Caring: a feminist approach to ethics and moral education*, Berkeley, 1984, University of California Press.

Pottinger A, et al: The end of life. In Srivaastava RH, editor: *Guide to clinical cultural competence*, Toronto, 2007, Elsevier.

Schwartz K, Schwartz T: *How will health reform impact young adults?* Menlo Park, CA, May 2010, Henry J. Kaiser Family Foundation. http://www.kff.org/healthreform/upload/7785-03.pdf.

The Joint Commission (TJC): *Joint Commission requirements and 2011 summary of national patient safety goals*, 2011, http://www.jointcommission.org/standards_information/npsgs.aspx. Accessed January 20, 2011.

US Census Bureau: *Income, poverty, and health insurance coverage in the United States*, 2009, http://www.census.gov/prod/2010pubs/p60-238.pdf. Accessed January 20, 2011.

US Department of Health and Human Services, Office for Civil Rights: *HIPAA medical privacy, national standards to protect the privacy of personal health information*, 2011, http://www.hhs.gov/ocr/hipaa/. Accessed January 20, 2011.

Walters SJ: *Quality of life outcomes in clinical trials and health care evaluation*, New Jersey, 2009, John Wiley and Sons.

Wexler A: *The woman who walked into the sea: Huntington's and the making of a genetic disease*, New Haven, 2010, Yale University Press.

Zoloth L: Learning a practice of uncertainty: clinical ethics and the nurse. In Cowen PS, Moorhead S, editors: *Current issues in nursing*, ed 7, St Louis, 2010, Mosby.

RESEARCH REFERENCES

Crawley LM, et al: Strategies for culturally effective end-of-life care, *Ann Intern Med* 136:673, 2002.

Hamric AB, Blackhall LB: Nurse-physician perspectives on the care of dying patients in intensive care units: Collaboration, moral distress, and ethical climate, *Crit Care Med* 35(2):422, 2007.

Ulrich CM, Hamric AB, Grady C: Moral distress: a growing problem in the health professions? *Hastings Cent Rep* 40(1):20, 2010.

Volker DL: Control and end-of-life care: does ethnicity matter? *Am J Hosp Palliat Care* 22(6):442, 2005.

CHAPTER

23

Legal Implications in Nursing Practice

OBJECTIVES

- Explain the legal concept of standard of care.
- Discuss the nurse's role in witnessing the informed consent process.
- Describe the legal responsibilities and obligations of nurses regarding the following federal statutes: Americans with Disabilities Act (ADA), Emergency Medical Treatment and Active Labor Act (EMTALA), Health Insurance Portability and Accountability Act of 1996 (HIPAA), and the Patient Self-Determination Act (PSDA).
- List sources for standards of care for nurses.
- Describe the nurse's role regarding a "do not resuscitate" (DNR) order.
- Define legal aspects of nurse-patient, nurse–health care provider, nurse-nurse, and nurse-employer relationships.
- List the elements needed to prove negligence.
- Describe the nursing implications associated with legal issues that occur in nursing practice.

KEY TERMS

Administrative law, p. 296
Assault, p. 301
Battery, p. 301
Civil laws, p. 297
Common law, p. 297
Confidentiality, p. 299
Criminal laws, p. 297
Defamation of character, p. 302
Durable power of attorney for health care (DPAHC), p. 299
Felony, p. 297
Informed consent, p. 302
Intentional torts, p. 301
Libel, p. 302
Living wills, p. 298
Malpractice, p. 302
Misdemeanor, p. 297
Negligence, p. 302
Nurse Practice Acts, p. 296
Occurrence report, p. 305
Privacy, p. 299
Regulatory law, p. 296
Risk management, p. 305
Slander, p. 302
Standards of care, p. 297
Statutory law, p. 296
Tort, p. 301

evolve WEBSITE

http://evolve.elsevier.com/Potter/fundamentals/

- Review Questions
- Case Study with Questions
- Audio Glossary
- Interactive Learning Activities
- Key Term Flashcards
- Content Updates

Safe nursing practice requires understanding the legal framework of health care. Understanding the legal implications of nursing practice demands critical reasoning skills to protect the patient's rights and the nurse from liability. Society expects safe health care delivery, especially from nurses who are typically perceived as the most trusted profession. As patient care practice innovations and new health care technologies emerge, the principles of negligence and malpractice liability are being applied to challenging new situations. Nurses should not fear the law but instead practice nursing armed with the judgment skills that are the outcomes of informed critical thinking.

LEGAL LIMITS OF NURSING

As a professional nurse you need to understand the legal limits influencing your practice. This, along with good judgment and sound decision making, ensures that your patients receive safe and appropriate nursing care.

Sources of Law

The legal guidelines that nurses follow come from statutory law, regulatory law, and common law. Elected legislative bodies such as state legislatures and the U.S. Congress create **statutory law.** An example of state statutes are the Nurse Practice Acts found in all 50 states (see Chapter 1). **Nurse Practice Acts** describe and define the legal boundaries of nursing practice within each state. An example of a federal statute enacted by the U.S. Congress is the Americans with Disabilities Act (ADA) (1990). The ADA protects the rights of individuals who are disabled in the workplace, in educational institutions, and throughout our society. **Regulatory law,** or **administrative law,** reflects decisions made by administrative bodies such as State Boards of Nursing when they pass rules and regulations. An example of a regulatory law is the requirement to report incompetent or unethical nursing conduct to the State

Board of Nursing. **Common law** results from judicial decisions made in courts when individual legal cases are decided. Examples of common law include informed consent, the patient's right to refuse treatment, negligence, and malpractice.

Statutory law is either civil or criminal. **Civil laws** protect the rights of individuals within our society and provide for fair and equitable treatment when civil wrongs or violations occur (Garner, 2006). The consequences of civil law violations are damages in the form of fines or specific performance of good works such as public service. An example of a civil law violation for a nurse is negligence or malpractice. **Criminal laws** protect society as a whole and provide punishment for crimes, which are defined by municipal, state, and federal legislation (Garner, 2006). There are two classifications of crimes. A **felony** is a crime of a serious nature that has a penalty of imprisonment for longer than 1 year or even death. A **misdemeanor** is a less serious crime that has a penalty of a fine or imprisonment for less than 1 year. An example of criminal conduct for nurses is misuse of a controlled substance.

Standards of Care

Standards of care are the legal requirements for nursing practice that describe minimum acceptable nursing care. Standards reflect the knowledge and skill ordinarily possessed and used by nurses actively practicing in the profession (Guido, 2010) (see Chapter 1). The American Nurses Association (ANA) (2010) develops standards for nursing practice, policy statements, and similar resolutions. These standards outline the scope, function, and role of the nurse in practice. Nursing standards of care are described in the Nurse Practice Act of every state, in the federal and state laws regulating hospitals and other health care institutions, by professional and specialty nursing organizations, and by the policies and procedures established by the health care facility where nurses work (Guido, 2010). In a malpractice lawsuit a nurse's actual conduct is compared to nursing standards of care to determine whether the nurse acted as any reasonably prudent nurse would act under the same or similar circumstances. For example, if a patient receives a burn from a warm compress application, negligence is determined by reviewing if the nurse followed the correct procedure for applying the compress. A breach of the nursing standard of care is one element that must be proven in the tort of nursing negligence or malpractice (Daller, 2010).

Nurse Practice Acts define the scope of nursing practice, distinguishing between nursing and medical practice and establishing education and licensure requirements for nurses. The rules and regulations enacted by a State Board of Nursing define the practice of nursing more specifically. For example, State Boards develop rules regarding intravenous therapy. Another example involves the use of nursing assistive personnel (NAP) (e.g., nurse assistants). Some State Boards of Nursing define the registered nurse's responsibilities specifically and develop position statements and guidelines to help licensed nurses delegate safely to NAP (National Council of State Boards of Nursing [NCSBN], 2005). All nurses are responsible for knowing the provisions of the Nurse Practice Act of the state in which they work and the rules and regulations enacted by the State Board of Nursing and other regulatory administrative bodies.

The Joint Commission (TJC) (2011a) requires accredited hospitals to have written nursing policies and procedures. These internal standards of care are specific and need to be accessible on all nursing units. For example, a policy/procedure outlining the steps to follow when changing a dressing or administering medication provides specific information about how nurses are to perform these tasks. Some hospitals are also now using commercially published procedural textbooks to reference the general policies and procedures of the institution. You need to know the policies, procedures, and protocols of your employing institution so you use the same standard of care as the other nurses in your institution. Institutional policies and procedures need to conform to state and federal laws and community standards and cannot conflict with legal guidelines that define acceptable standards of care (Guido, 2010).

In a lawsuit for malpractice or nursing negligence, a nursing expert testifies to the jury about the standards of nursing care as applied to the facts of the case (Box 23-1). A nurse may be requested

BOX 23-1 ANATOMY OF A LAWSUIT

Pleadings Phase

Petition—elements of the claim: The plaintiff outlines what the defendant nurse did wrong and how, as a result of that alleged negligence, the plaintiff was injured.

Answer: The nurse admits or denies each allegation in the petition. The prosecutor must prove anything that the nurse does not admit.

Discovery

Interrogatories: Written questions requiring answers under oath. Usual questions concern witnesses, insurance experts, and which health care providers the plaintiff has seen before and after the incident.

Medical records: The defendant obtains all of the plaintiff's relevant medical records for treatment before and after the incident.

Witnesses' depositions: Questions are posed to the witness under oath to obtain all relevant, nonprivileged information about the case.

Parties' depositions: The plaintiff and defendants (physician, nurse, hospital personnel) are almost always deposed.

Other witnesses: Factual witnesses, both neutral and biased, including family members on the plaintiff's side and other medical personnel (e.g., nurses) on the defendant's side, are deposed to obtain information and their version of the case.

Treating physicians' or health care providers' depositions: Before subsequent treating, physicians' or health care providers' depositions are taken to establish issues such as those concerning preexisting conditions, causation, the nature and extent of injuries, and permanency.

Experts: The plaintiff selects experts to establish the essential legal elements of the case against the defendant. The defendant selects experts to establish the appropriateness of the nursing care.

Trial

Following discovery phase of 1 to 3 years or longer, trial may last days to months.

Proof of Negligence

The nurse owed a duty to the patient.

The nurse did not carry out the duty or breached it (failure to use the degree of skill and learning ordinarily used under the same or similar circumstances by members of his or her profession).

The patient was injured:
- Medical bills, lost wages
- Pain and suffering
- Perinatal damages
- Wrongful death damages

The patient's injury was caused by the nurse's failure to carry out that duty ("but for" the breach of duty, the patient would not have been injured).

to give evidence in a deposition; this appearance needs to be taken seriously (Scott, 2009). The jury uses the standards of care to determine whether the nurse acted appropriately. Nurse experts base their opinions on existing standards of practice established by Nurse Practice Acts, professional organizations, institutional policies and procedures, federal and state hospital licensing laws, TJC standards, job descriptions, and current nursing research literature (Guido, 2010). Usually nurses are responsible for meeting the same standards as other nurses practicing in similar settings. Specialized nurses such as nurse anesthetists, operating room (OR) nurses, intensive care nurses, or certified nurse-midwives have specially defined standards of care and skills. Ignorance of the law or of standards of care is not a defense against malpractice. The best way for nurses to keep up with the current legal issues affecting nursing practice is to maintain familiarity with standards of care and the policies and procedures of their employing agency and to read current nursing literature in their practice area (ANA, 2010).

One of the first and most important cases to discuss a nurse's liability was *Darling v Charleston Community Memorial Hospital.* It involved an 18-year-old man with a fractured leg. The emergency department physician applied a cast with insufficient padding. The man's toes became swollen and discolored, and he developed decreased sensation. He complained to the nursing staff many times. Although the nurses recognized the symptoms as signs of impaired circulation, they failed to tell their supervisor that the physician did not respond to their calls or the patient's needs. Gangrene developed, and the man's leg was amputated. Although the physician was held liable for incorrectly applying the cast, the nursing staff was also held liable for failing to adhere to the standards of care for monitoring and reporting the patient's symptoms. Even though the nurses attempted to contact the physician, this case holds that, when the physician fails to respond, the nurse must go over the health care provider's head to make sure that he or she is appropriately treated. Almost every state uses this 1965 Illinois Supreme Court case as legal precedence.

FEDERAL STATUTORY ISSUES IN NURSING PRACTICE

Americans with Disabilities Act

The Americans with Disabilities Act (ADA) (1990) is a broad civil rights statute that protects the rights of people with physical or mental disabilities (Grohar-Murray and Langan, 2011). The ADA prohibits discrimination and ensures for persons with disabilities equal opportunities in employment, state and local government services, public accommodations, commercial facilities, and transportation. It is also the most extensive law on how employers must treat health care workers and patients infected with the human immunodeficiency virus (HIV). The Supreme Court ruled in 1998 in *Bragdon v Abbott* that even asymptomatic HIV constitutes a disability within the meaning of the ADA. This means that the ADA protects a person who is HIV positive but does not have acquired immunodeficiency syndrome (AIDS). The ADA regulations protect the privacy of infected people by giving individuals the opportunity to decide whether to disclose their disability. However, several cases have held that the health care provider has to disclose the fact that he or she has HIV. Despite these rulings, ADA protects health care workers in the workplace with disabilities such as HIV infection. Likewise, health care workers cannot discriminate against HIV-positive patients (Guido, 2010).

Emergency Medical Treatment and Active Labor Act

As a result of patients being transferred from private to public hospitals without appropriate screening and stabilization (referred to as *patient dumping*), Congress enacted the Emergency Medical Treatment and Active Labor Act (EMTALA) (1986). This act provides that, when a patient comes to the emergency department or the hospital, an appropriate medical screening occurs within the capacity of the hospital. If an emergency condition exists, the hospital is not to discharge or transfer the patient until the condition stabilizes. Exceptions to this provision include if the patient requests transfer or discharge in writing after receiving information about the benefits and risks or if a health care provider certifies that the benefits of transfer outweigh the risks.

Mental Health Parity Act

Health insurance plans are free to eliminate coverage for certain specialties and impose limits on the amount of coverage that they will pay for certain illnesses. However, if health insurance plans provide mental health benefits, the Mental Health Parity Act of 1996 forbids health plans from placing lifetime or annual limits on mental health coverage that are less generous than those placed on medical or surgical benefits.

Admission of a patient to a mental health unit occurs involuntarily or on a voluntary basis. Involuntary detention occurs when an individual files with the court within 96 hours of the patient's initial detention. A judge may determine that the patient is a danger to self or others; then the judge will grant the involuntary detention, and the patient can be detained for 21 more days for psychiatric treatment.

Potentially suicidal patients are admitted to mental health units. If the patient's history and medical records indicate suicidal tendencies, the patient must be kept under supervision. Lawsuits result from patients' attempts at suicide within the hospital. The allegations in the lawsuits are that the health care provider failed to provide adequate supervision and safeguard the facilities. Documentation of precautions against suicide is essential.

Advance Directives

Advance directives include living wills, health care proxies, and durable powers of attorney for health care (Blais et al., 2006). They are based on values of informed consent, patient autonomy over end-of-life decisions, truth telling, and control over the dying process. The Patient Self-Determination Act (PSDA) (1991) requires health care institutions to provide written information to patients concerning their rights under state law to make decisions, including the right to refuse treatment and formulate advance directives. Under the act the patient's record needs to document whether or not the patient has signed an advance directive. For living wills or durable powers of attorney for health care to be enforceable, the patient must be legally incompetent or lack the capacity to make decisions regarding health care treatment. A judge makes the determination of legal competency, and the health care provider and family usually make the determination of decisional capacity. Decisional capacity is the ability to make right choices for oneself as they relate to medical care. Be familiar with the policies of your institution complying with the act. Likewise, check the state laws to see if a state honors an advance directive that originates in another state.

Living Wills. **Living wills** represent written documents that direct treatment in accordance with a patient's wishes in the event of a terminal illness or condition. With this legal document the patient is able to declare which medical procedures he or she wants or does not want when terminally ill or in a persistent vegetative state. Living wills are often difficult to interpret and not clinically specific in unforeseen circumstances. Each state providing for living wills has its own requirements for executing them. If health care workers follow the directions of the living will, they should be immune from liability (Bross, 2006).

Health Care Proxies or Durable Power of Attorney for Health Care. A health care proxy or **durable power of attorney for health care (DPAHC)** is a legal document that designates a person or persons of one's choosing to make health care decisions when the patient is no longer able to make decisions on his or her own behalf. This agent makes health care treatment decisions based on the patient's wishes (Blais et al., 2006).

In addition to federal statutes, the ethical doctrine of autonomy ensures the patient the right to refuse medical treatment. Courts upheld the right to refuse medical treatment in the 1986 *Bouvia v Superior Court* case. They have also upheld the right of a legally competent patient to refuse medical treatment for religious reasons. Christian Scientists may refuse medical treatment based on religious beliefs, and Jehovah's Witnesses may accept medical treatment but may refuse blood transfusions based on personal religious beliefs. The U.S. Supreme Court stated in the *Cruzan v Director of Missouri Department of Health* case in 1990 that "we assume that the U.S. Constitution would grant a constitutionally protected competent person the right to refuse lifesaving hydration and nutrition." In cases involving the patient's right to refuse or withdraw medical treatment, the courts balance the patient's interest with the interest of the state in protecting life, preserving medical ethics, preventing suicide, and protecting innocent third parties. Children are generally the innocent third parties. Although the courts will not force adults to undergo treatment refused for religious reasons, they will grant an order allowing hospitals and health care providers to treat children of Christian Scientists or Jehovah's Witnesses who have denied consent for treatment of their minor children.

In addition to patient refusals of treatment, the nurse frequently encounters a DNR order. DNR means "do not resuscitate" or "no code." Documentation that the health care provider has consulted with the patient and/or family is required before attaching a DNR order to the patient's medical record (Guido, 2010).The health care provider needs to review DNR orders routinely in case the patient's condition demands a change. If a patient does not have a DNR order, health care providers need to make every effort to revive the patient. Some states such as Ohio offer DNR Comfort Care and DNR Comfort Care Arrest protocols. Protocols in these instances list specific actions that health care providers will take when providing cardiopulmonary resuscitation (CPR).

CPR is an emergency treatment provided without patient consent. Health care providers perform CPR on an appropriate patient unless there is a DNR order in the patient's chart. The New York law, the first adopted legislation regarding DNR, is one of the most comprehensive in the United States (New York DNR Statute, 1988). The statutes assume that all patients will be resuscitated unless there is a written DNR order in the chart. Legally competent adult patients consent to a DNR order verbally or in writing after receiving the appropriate information by the health care provider. Be familiar with the DNR protocols of your state.

Uniform Anatomical Gift Act

An individual who is at least 18 years of age has the right to make an organ donation (defined as a "donation of all or part of a human body to take effect upon or after death"). Donors need to make the gift in writing with their signature. In many states adults sign the back of their driver's license, indicating consent to organ donation.

In most states Required Request laws mandate that, at the time of admission to a hospital, a qualified health care provider has to ask each patient over age 18 whether he or she is an organ or tissue donor. If the answer is affirmative, the health care provider obtains a copy of the document. If the answer is negative, the health care provider discusses the option to make or refuse an organ donation and places such documentation in the patient's medical record. The health care provider who certifies death is not involved in the removal or transplantation of organs (see Chapter 36).

The National Organ Transplant Act of 1984 prohibits the purchase or sale of organs. The act provides civil and criminal immunity to the hospital and health care provider who performs in accordance with the act. The act also protects the donor's estate from liability for injury or damage that results from the use of the gift. Organ transplantation is extremely expensive. Patients in end-stage renal disease are eligible for Medicare coverage for a kidney transplant, but private insurance pays for other transplants. The United Network for Organ Sharing (UNOS) has a contract with the federal government and sets policies and guidelines for the procurement of organs. Patients who require organ transplantation are on a waiting list for an organ in their geographical area that gives priority to patients who demonstrate the greatest need. Be familiar with the policies and procedures of your employing institution regarding organ donation.

Health Insurance Portability and Accountability Act

The Health Insurance Portability and Accountability Act of 1996 (HIPAA) represents one of the more recent federal statutory acts affecting nursing care. This law provides rights to patients and protects employees. It protects individuals from losing their health insurance when changing jobs by providing portability. It allows employees to change jobs without losing coverage as a result of preexisting coverage exclusion as long as they have had 12 months of continuous group health insurance coverage (Carter, 2010).

In the privacy section of the HIPAA, there are standards regarding accountability in the health care setting (Carter, 2010). These rules create patient rights to consent to the use and disclosure of their protected health information, to inspect and copy one's medical record, and to amend mistaken or incomplete information. It limits who is able to access a patient's record. It establishes the basis for privacy and confidentiality concerns, viewed as two basic rights within the U.S. health care setting. **Privacy** is the right of patients to keep personal information from being disclosed. **Confidentiality** protects private patient information once it has been disclosed in health care settings. Patient confidentiality is a sacred trust. Nurses help organizations protect patients' rights to confidentiality. Although the HIPAA does not require such measures as soundproof rooms in hospitals, it does mean that nurses and all health care providers need to avoid discussing patients in public hallways and provide reasonable levels of privacy in communicating with and about patients in any manner. Message boards used in patients' hospital rooms to post daily nursing care information can no longer contain information revealing the patient's medical condition. With the increased use of technology in the health care setting such as with the use of electronic health records, nurses have a challenging task to maintain patient privacy and confidentiality. HIPAA violations have civil and criminal sanctions.

Health care information privacy is also protected by standards set by the Health Care Financing Administration (HCFA) for hospitals and health care providers who participate in Medicare and Medicaid (Guido, 2010). These standards require that hospitals and health care providers give notice to patients of their rights to decisions about their care, grievances regarding their care management, personal freedom and safety, confidentiality, access to their own medical records, and freedom from restraints that are not clinically necessary. In addition, many state laws allow patients to access their medical records. Exceptions to the ability to access medical records apply to psychotherapy notes or when the health care provider has determined that access would result in harm to the patient or another party (Privacy Rights Clearinghouse, 2011).

Restraints

The Federal Nursing Home Reform Act (1987) gave residents in certified nursing homes the right to be free of unnecessary and inappropriate restraints. The use of physical restraints is a safety strategy that has been used in hospitals and long-term care settings to protect patients from injury. However, the Centers for Medicare and Medicaid Services (2007) and The Joint Commission (2011a) have set standards for reducing the use of restraints in health care settings and for using them only with extreme caution. The risks associated with the use of restraints are serious. A restraint-free environment is the first goal of care for all patients. *There are many alternatives to the use of restraints, and you should try all of them before using restraints.* Restraints can be used (1) only to ensure the physical safety of the resident or other residents, (2) when less restrictive interventions are not successful, and (3) only on the written order of a health care provider (TJC, 2011a). Written orders include a specific episode with start and end times. Litigation from improper restraint use is a common nursing legal issue (Evans and Cotter, 2008). Nurses are negligent for failure to initiate safety procedures when the patient condition necessitates it. Knowing when and how to use restraints correctly is key (Chapter 27). Liability for improper or unlawful restraint and for patient injury from unprotected falls lies with the nurse and the health care institution. Nurses who apply restraints in violation of state and federal regulations may be charged with abuse, battery, or false imprisonment.

STATE STATUTORY ISSUES IN NURSING PRACTICE

Licensure

A State Board of Nursing licenses all registered nurses in the state in which they practice. The requirements for licensure vary among states, but most states have minimum education requirements and require a licensure examination. All states use the National Council Licensure Examinations (NCLEX®) for registered nurse and licensed practical nurse examinations. Licensure permits people to offer special skills to the public, and it also provides legal guidelines for protection of the public.

The State Board of Nursing suspends or revokes a license if a nurse's conduct violates provisions in the licensing statute based on administrative law rules that implement and enforce the statute. For example, nurses who perform illegal acts such as selling or taking controlled substances jeopardize their license status. Because a license is a property right, the State Board has to follow due process before revoking or suspending a license. Due process means that nurses must be notified of the charges brought against them and have an opportunity to defend against them in a hearing. Hearings for suspension or revocation of a license do not occur in court. Usually a panel of professionals conducts the hearing. Some states provide administrative and judicial review of such cases after nurses have exhausted all other forms of appeal.

Good Samaritan Laws

Nurses act as Good Samaritans by providing emergency assistance at an accident scene (Good Samaritan Act, 1997). All states have Good Samaritan laws enacted to encourage health care professionals to assist in emergencies (Dachs and Elias, 2008). These laws limit liability and offer legal immunity if a nurse helps at the scene of an accident. For example, if you stop at the scene of an automobile accident and give appropriate emergency care such as applying pressure to stop hemorrhage, you are acting within accepted standards, even though proper equipment is not available. If the patient subsequently develops complications as a result of your actions, you are immune from liability as long as you acted without gross negligence (Good Samaritan Act, 1997). Although Good Samaritan laws provide immunity to the nurse who does what is reasonable to save a person's life, if you perform a procedure for which you have no training, you are liable for any injury resulting from that act. You should only provide care that is consistent with your level of expertise. In addition, once you have committed to providing emergency care to a patient, you must stay with that patient until you can safely transfer his or her care to someone who can provide needed care such as emergency medical technicians (EMTs) or emergency department staff. If you leave the patient without properly transferring or handing him or her off to a capable person, you may be liable for patient abandonment and responsible for any injury suffered after you leave him or her (Dachs, 2008). Three states (Louisiana, Minnesota, and Vermont) have enacted "failure-to-act" laws that make it a crime not to provide Good Samaritan care (Dachs and Elias, 2008).

Public Health Laws

Nurses, especially those employed in community health settings, need to understand public health laws. State legislatures enact statutes under health codes, which describe the reporting laws for communicable diseases and school immunizations and those intended to promote health and reduce health risks in communities. The Centers for Disease Control and Prevention (CDC) (http://www.CDC.gov) and the Occupational Health and Safety Act (OHSA) (http://www.osha.gov) provide guidelines on a national level for safe and healthy communities and work environments. The purposes of public health laws are protection of public health, advocating for the rights of people, regulating health care and health care financing, and ensuring professional accountability for care provided. Community and public health nurses have the legal responsibility to enforce laws enacted to protect public health (see Chapter 3). These laws include reporting suspected abuse and neglect such as child abuse, elder abuse, or domestic violence; reporting communicable diseases; ensuring that patients in the community have received required immunizations; and reporting other health-related issues enacted to protect public health. To encourage reports of suspected cases, states provide legal immunity for the reporter if the report is made in good faith. Any health care professional who does not report suspected child abuse or neglect may be liable for civil or criminal legal action.

The Uniform Determination of Death Act

Many legal issues surround the event of death, including a basic definition of the actual point at which a person is legally dead. There are essentially two standards for the determination of death. The cardiopulmonary standard requires irreversible cessation of circulatory and respiratory functions. The whole-brain standard requires irreversible cessation of all functions of the entire brain, including the brainstem. The reason for the development of different definitions is to facilitate recovery of organs for transplantation. Even though the patient is legally "brain dead," the patient's organs are sometimes healthy for donation to other patients. Most states have adopted the Uniform Determination of Death Act (1980). It states that health care providers can use either the cardiopulmonary or the whole-brain definition to determine death. Be aware of legal definitions of death because you need to document all events that occur when the patient is in your care. Nurses have a specific legal obligation to treat the deceased person's remains with dignity (see Chapter 36). Wrongful handling of a deceased person's remains causes emotional harm to the surviving family.

Autopsy

An autopsy or postmortem examination may be requested by the patient or patient's family, as a part of an institutional policy; or it may be required by law. When a patient's death has occurred under suspicious circumstances or if the patient died within 24 hours of admission to a health care facility, the decision to conduct a postmortem examination is made by the medical examiner (Autopsy Consent, 1998). When the patient's death is not subject to a medical examiner review, consent must be obtained. The priority for giving consent is (1) the patient in writing before death; (2) durable power of attorney; (3) surviving spouse; (4) surviving child, parent, or sibling in the order named.

Physician-Assisted Suicide

Providing end-of-life care in today's world is challenging for health care professionals because people are living longer. The Oregon Death with Dignity Act (1994) was the first statute that permitted physician or health care provider–assisted suicide. The statute stated that a competent individual with a terminal disease could make an oral and written request for medication to end his or her life in a humane and dignified manner. A terminal disease is an "incurable and irreversible disease that has been medically confirmed and will, within reasonable medical judgment, produce death within 6 months."

The American Nurses Association (ANA) (2008) has held that nurses' participation in assisted suicide violates the code of ethics for nurses. The American Association of Colleges of Nursing (AACN) supports the International Council of Nurses' mandate to ensure an individual's peaceful end of life (Guido, 2010). The positions of these two national organizations are not contradictory and require nurses to approach a patient's end of life with openness to listening to the patient's expressions of fear and to attempt to control the patient's pain.

CIVIL AND COMMON LAW ISSUES IN NURSING PRACTICE

Torts

A **tort** is a civil wrong made against a person or property. Torts are classified as intentional, quasi-intentional, or unintentional. **Intentional torts** are willful acts that violate another's rights such as assault, battery, and false imprisonment. Quasi-intentional torts are acts in which intent is lacking but volitional action and direct causation occur such as in invasion of privacy and defamation of character. The third classification of tort is the unintentional tort, which includes negligence or malpractice.

Intentional Torts

Assault. **Assault** is any action that places a person in apprehension of a harmful or offensive contact without consent. No actual contact is necessary. It is an assault for a nurse to threaten to give a patient an injection or to threaten to restrain a patient for an x-ray procedure when the patient has refused consent. Likewise, it is an assault for a patient to threaten a nurse (Guido, 2010).

Battery. **Battery** is any intentional touching without consent. The contact can be harmful to the patient and cause an injury, or it can be merely offensive to the patient's personal dignity. In the example of a nurse threatening to give a patient an injection without the patient's consent, if the nurse actually gives the injection, it is battery. Battery also results if the health care provider performs a procedure that goes beyond the scope of the patient's consent. For example, if the patient gives consent for an appendectomy and the surgeon performs a tonsillectomy, battery has occurred. The key component is the patient's consent.

In some situations consent is implied. For example, if a patient gets into a wheelchair or transfers to a stretcher after receiving advice that it is time to be taken for an x-ray procedure, the patient has given implied consent to the procedure. If the patient learns that he or she will have an x-ray film of the head instead of the foot and the patient refuses to have the x-ray film taken, the consent has been revoked or withdrawn.

False Imprisonment. The tort of false imprisonment occurs with unjustified restraint of a person without legal warrant. This occurs when nurses restrain a patient in a confined area to keep the person from freedom. False imprisonment requires that the patient be aware of the confinement. An unconscious patient has not been falsely imprisoned (Guido, 2010).

Quasi-Intentional Torts

Invasion of Privacy. The tort of invasion of privacy protects the patient's right to be free from unwanted intrusion into his or her private affairs. HIPAA privacy standards have raised awareness of the need for health care professionals to provide confidentiality and privacy. Typically invasion of privacy is the release of a patient's medical information to an unauthorized person such as a member of the press, the patient's employer, or the patient's family. The information that is in a patient's medical record is a confidential communication that may be shared with health care providers for the purpose of medical treatment only.

Do not disclose the patient's confidential medical information without his or her consent. A patient must authorize the release of information and designate to whom the health care information may be released. For example, respect the wish not to inform the patient's family of a terminal illness. Similarly, do not assume that a patient's spouse or family members know all of the patient's history, particularly with respect to private issues such as mental illness, medications, pregnancy, abortion, birth control, or sexually transmitted infections. When a family asks to see a patient's medical record, you must instead establish a relationship that allows for open communication so you can discuss the family's concerns.

An individual's right to privacy sometimes conflicts with the public's right to know. In one case a television crew filmed a married couple who were participating in a hospital program. The couple had previously told no one but their immediate family that they were involved in the in vitro fertilization program and had received assurance that there would be no publicity or public exposure. After the newscast they received phone calls and embarrassing questions. The couple filed a lawsuit. The court held that the husband and wife stated a claim for invasion of privacy and that, even though the in vitro fertilization program was of public interest, the identity of the plaintiffs was a private matter (*YG v Jewish Hospital,* 1990).

Many states, through their respective public health departments, require that hospitals report certain infectious or communicable diseases. Sometimes the patient is a public figure whose physical condition is newsworthy (Guido, 2010). There are also cases in which information about a scientific discovery or a major medical breakthrough is newsworthy, as with the first heart transplant case or the first artificial heart recipient. If an event falls into any of these categories, guide information through the public relations department of the institution to ensure that invasion of privacy does not occur. It is not the nurse's responsibility to decide independently the legality of disclosing information.

Defamation of Character. **Defamation of character** is the publication of false statements that result in damage to a person's reputation. **Slander** occurs when one speaks falsely about another. For example, if a nurse tells people erroneously that a patient has gonorrhea and the disclosure affects the patient's business, the nurse is liable for slander. **Libel** is the written defamation of character (e.g., charting false entries in a medical record).

Unintentional Torts

Negligence. **Negligence** is conduct that falls below a standard of care. The law establishes the standard of care for the protection of others against an unreasonably great risk of harm (Garner, 2006). For example, if a driver of a car acts unreasonably in failing to stop at a stop sign, it is negligence. In general, courts define negligence in car accident cases and other negligence cases as that degree of care that an ordinarily careful and prudent person would use under the same or similar circumstances. Negligent acts such as hanging the wrong intravenous solution for a patient or allowing a NAP to administer a medication often lead to disciplinary action by the state board of nursing.

Malpractice. **Malpractice** is one type of negligence and often referred to as professional negligence. When nursing care falls below a standard of care, nursing malpractice results. Certain criteria are necessary to establish nursing malpractice: (1) the nurse (defendant) owed a duty to the patient (plaintiff), (2) the nurse did not carry out that duty, (3) the patient was injured, and (4) the nurse's failure to carry out the duty caused the injury. Even though nurses do not intend to injure patients, some patients file claims of malpractice if nurses give care that does not meet the appropriate standards. Malpractice sometimes involves failing to check a patient's identification correctly before administering blood and then giving the blood to the wrong patient. It also involves administering a medication to a patient even though the medical record contains documentation that the patient has an allergy to that medication. In general, courts define nursing malpractice as the failure to use that degree of skill or learning ordinarily used under the same or similar circumstances by members of the nursing profession (Box 23-2) (Austin, 2006).

The best way for nurses to avoid malpractice is to follow standards of care, give competent health care, and communicate with other health care providers. You also avoid malpractice by developing a caring rapport with the patient and documenting assessments, interventions, and evaluations fully. Nurses need to know the current nursing literature in their areas of practice. Know and follow the policies and procedures of the institution where you work. Be sensitive to common sources of patient injury such as falls and medication errors. Finally, communicate with the patient, explain tests and treatments, document that you provided specific explanations to him or her, and listen to his or her concerns about treatments. You are accountable for reporting any significant changes in the patient's condition to the health care provider and documenting these changes in the chart (see Chapter 26). Timely and truthful documentation is important to provide the communication necessary among health care team members. Be certain that documentation is legible and signed (Austin, 2006).

BOX 23-2 COMMON NEGLIGENT ACTS

- Failure to assess and/or monitor, including making a nursing diagnosis
  - Failure to monitor in timely fashion
  - Failure to use proper equipment to monitor the patient
  - Failure to document the monitoring
- Failure to notify the health care provider of problems
- Failure to follow orders
- Failure to follow the six rights of medication administration
- Failure to convey discharge instructions
- Failure to ensure patient safety, especially patients who have a history of falling, are heavily sedated, have disequilibrium problems, are frail, are mentally impaired, get up in the night, and are uncooperative
- Failure to follow policies and procedures
- Failure to properly delegate and supervise

A number of courts have stated that, when a health care provider negligently alters or loses medical records relevant to a malpractice claim, the health care provider needs to demonstrate why these events occurred. An institution has a duty to maintain nursing records. Statutes and accreditation regulations establish these duties. Nursing notes contain substantial evidence needed to understand the care received by a patient. If records are lost or incomplete, there is a presumption that the care was negligent and therefore the cause of the patient's injuries. In addition, incomplete or illegible records make the health care provider less credible or believable.

Consent

A signed consent form is required for all routine treatment, hazardous procedures such as surgery, some treatment programs such as chemotherapy, and research involving patients (TJC, 2011a). A patient signs general consent forms when admitted to the hospital or other health care facility. The patient or his or her representative needs to sign separate special consent or treatment forms before the performance of a specialized procedure. State statutes provide the designation of individuals who are legally able to give consent to medical treatment (Medical Patient Rights Act, 1994). Nurses need to know the law in their states and be familiar with the policies and procedures of their employing institution regarding consent (Box 23-3). If a patient is deaf or illiterate or speaks a foreign language, an official interpreter must be present to explain the terms of consent. A family member or acquaintance who speaks a patient's language should not interpret health information. Make every effort to assist the patient in making an informed choice.

Informed Consent. **Informed consent** is a person's agreement to allow something to happen such as surgery or an invasive diagnostic procedure, based on a full disclosure of risks, benefits, alternatives, and consequences of refusal (Garner, 2006). Informed consent creates a legal duty for the health care provider to disclose material facts in terms the patient is able to understand to make an informed choice (Guido, 2010). Failure to obtain consent in situations other than emergencies will possibly result in a claim of battery. Without informed consent a patient may bring a lawsuit against the health care provider for negligence.

BOX 23-3 STATUTORY GUIDELINES FOR LEGAL CONSENT FOR MEDICAL TREATMENT

Those who consent to medical treatment are governed by state law but generally include the following:

I. Adults
   A. Any competent individual 18 years of age or older for himself or herself
   B. Any parent for his or her unemancipated minor
   C. Any guardian for his or her ward
   D. Any adult for the treatment of his or her minor brother or sister (if an emergency and parents are not present)
   E. Any grandparent for a minor grandchild (if an emergency and parents are not present)

II. Minors
   A. For his or her child and any child in his or her legal custody
   B. For himself or herself in the following situations:
      1. Lawfully married or a parent (emancipated)
      2. Pregnancy (excluding abortions)
      3. Venereal disease
      4. Drug or substance abuse
   C. Unemancipated minors may not consent to abortions without one of the following:
      1. Consent of one parent
      2. Self-consent granted by court order
      3. Consent specifically given by a court

Informed consent is part of the health care provider–patient relationship. It must be obtained and witnessed when the patient is not under the influence of medication such as opioids. Because nurses do not perform surgery or direct medical procedures, in most situations obtaining patients' informed consent does not fall within the nursing duty. The person responsible for performing the procedure has the responsibility to obtain the informed consent.

Key elements of responsibility for the health care provider include the following: (1) the patient receives a brief, complete explanation of the procedure or treatment; (2) the patient receives the names and qualifications of persons performing and assisting in the procedure; (3) the patient receives a description of the serious harm, including death, that may occur as a result of the procedure and anticipated pain and/or discomfort; (4) the patient receives an explanation of alternative therapies to the proposed procedure/treatment and the risks of doing nothing; (5) the patient knows that he or she has the right to refuse the procedure/treatment without discontinuing other supportive care; (6) the patient knows that he or she may refuse the procedure/treatment even after the procedure has begun.

The nurse's signature witnessing the consent means that the patient voluntarily gave consent, the patient's signature is authentic, and the patient appears to be competent to give consent (Guido, 2010). When nurses provide consent forms for patients to sign, they must ask the patients if they understand the procedure for which they are giving consent. If patients deny understanding or you suspect that they do not understand, notify the health care provider or nursing supervisor. Health care providers must inform a patient refusing surgery or other medical treatment about any harmful consequences of refusal. If the patient persists in refusing the treatment, this rejection needs to be written, signed, and witnessed. It is important to note that nursing students cannot and should not be responsible for or asked to witness consent forms because of the legal nature of the document.

Parents are usually the legal guardians of pediatric patients; therefore they typically are the persons who sign consent forms for treatment. If the parents are divorced, the parent with legal custody gives consent. Occasionally a parent or guardian refuses treatment for a child. In these cases the court sometimes intervenes on the child's behalf.

In some instances obtaining informed consent is difficult. For example, if the patient is unconscious, you must obtain consent from a person legally authorized to give it on the patient's behalf. Sometimes the patient has legally designated other surrogate decision makers through special power of attorney documents or court guardianship procedures. In emergencies, if it is impossible to obtain consent from the patient or an authorized person, a health care provider may perform a procedure required to benefit the patient or save a life without liability for failure to obtain consent. In such cases the law assumes that the patient would wish to be treated.

Patients with mental illnesses must also give consent. They retain the right to refuse treatment until a court has legally determined that they are incompetent to decide for themselves.

Abortion Issues

In 1973 in the case of *Roe v Wade,* the U.S. Supreme Court ruled that there is a fundamental right to privacy, which includes a woman's decision to have an abortion. The court ruled that during the first trimester a woman could end her pregnancy without state regulation because the risk of natural mortality from abortion is less than with normal childbirth. During the second trimester the state has an interest in protecting maternal health, and it enforces regulations regarding the person performing the abortion and the abortion facility. By the third trimester, when the fetus becomes viable, the state's interest is to protect the fetus; therefore it prohibits abortion except when necessary to save the mother.

In 1989 in the case of *Webster v Reproductive Health Services* the court substantially narrowed the *Roe v Wade* case. Some states require viability tests before conducting abortions if the fetus is over 28 weeks' gestational age. Some states also require a minor's parental consent or a judicial decision that the minor is mature and can self-consent.

Nursing Students

Nursing students are liable if their actions cause harm to patients. If a student harms a patient as a direct result of his or her actions or lack of action, the student, instructor, hospital, or health care facility and the university or educational institution generally share the liability for the incorrect action. Nursing students should never be assigned to perform tasks for which they are unprepared, and instructors should supervise them carefully as they learn new skills. Although nursing students are not employees of the hospital, the institution has a responsibility to monitor their acts. They are expected to perform as professional nurses would in providing safe patient care. Faculty members are usually responsible for instructing and observing students, but in some situations staff nurses serving as preceptors share these responsibilities. Every nursing school should provide clear definitions of preceptor and faculty responsibility.

When students work as nursing assistants or nurse's aides when not attending classes, they should not perform tasks that do not appear in a job description for a nurse's aide or assistant. For example, even if a student has learned to administer intramuscular medications in class, the student now working as a nurse's aide may not perform this task. If a staff nurse overseeing the nursing assistant or aide knowingly assigns work without regard for the person's ability to safely conduct the task defined in the job description, the staff nurse is also liable. If someone requests students employed as nurse's aides to perform tasks that they are not prepared to complete safely, they need to bring this information to the supervisor's attention so they are able to obtain the needed help.

Malpractice Insurance

Malpractice or professional liability insurance is a contract between the nurse and the insurance company. Malpractice insurance provides for a defense when a nurse is in a lawsuit involving professional negligence or medical malpractice. As part of the insurance contract, the insurance company pays for any judgment or settlement of the case and for the attorney's fees generated in the representation of the nurse. Nurses employed by health care institutions generally are covered by insurance provided by the institution and do not need to purchase any supplemental insurance unless the nurse plans to practice nursing outside of the employing institution. However, the insurance provided by the employing institution only covers nurses while they are working within the scope of their employment. Because nurses are professionals and it is often difficult to separate their private lives from their professional skills, they need to consider purchasing individual professional liability insurance, even if the employing institution has coverage. For example, a hospital policy does not cover a nurse when neighbors and friends ask him or her to provide nursing care on a volunteer basis if the neighbor or friend files suit (Guido, 2010). Nursing students need to check with their educational institutions regarding the need for liability insurance.

Nurses need to consult their lawyers on which types of policies to purchase and which rights or duties, if any, exist under the policy. If both the employing institution and the nurse are sued in a professional liability case, even though the nurse has insurance with the hospital, he or she needs to notify his or her private insurance carrier of the lawsuit. If both the hospital policy and the private policy are considered primary and the hospital loses as a result of the nurse's acts, theoretically the hospital could sue the nurse's private insurer to recover its losses. However, most private insurance policies for nurses are excess policies and only begin covering the nurse after all of the primary (hospital) insurance coverage has been exhausted. Because hospital insurance coverage is generally much broader and has higher monetary limits than private insurance coverage, hospitals very rarely sue nurses' private insurers.

Abandonment and Assignment Issues

Short Staffing. During nursing shortages or staff downsizing periods, the issue of inadequate staffing occurs. The Community Health Accreditation Program (CHAP) and other state and federal standards require institutions to have guidelines for determining the number (staffing ratios) of nurses required to give care to a specific number of patients. Legal problems occur if there are not enough nurses to provide competent care or if nurses work excessive overtime (Box 23-4). One such example is in a class-action suit, *Spires v Hospital Corporation of America,* filed on April 10, 2006. The wife claims that there was poor patient care related to insufficient registered nurse staffing and that the poor nurse-staffing levels led to the resultant death of her husband. This suit emphasizes the potential seriousness of short staffing and the importance of nurses' asserting employee rights. In an attempt to address the short-staffing problem, 15 states and the District of Columbia have legislation to mandate fixed nurse-patient ratios for all areas of acute care nursing. The safe staffing ratio debate is occurring throughout the country and demands close attention by all nurses (ANA, 2011).

BOX 23-4 EVIDENCE-BASED PRACTICE

Consequences of Working Overtime

PICO Question: Does excess shift work by nurses have a negative effect on patient safety?

Evidence Summary

As hospitals struggle with the nurse shortage, nurses find themselves working more and longer hours and taking care of more patients. In a survey of more than 2000 nurses, 28% stated that they worked longer than 12 hours per day, including overtime; one third said that they worked more than 40 hours per week; and 23% rotated shifts (Trinkoff et al., 2006). Nurses' level of alertness changes when their work extends to off-shift work. Cognitive and psychomotor skills are impaired as indicated by delayed reaction time and decreased coordination (Berger and Hobbs, 2006). Poor patient outcomes as evidenced by increased rates of catheter-associated urinary tract infections and pressure ulcers are related to increased nursing overtime (Stone et al., 2007). As nurse staffing levels decrease, the incidence of patient falls, medication errors, and restraint application duration rate increases (Garrett, 2008).

Application to Nursing Practice

- The longer a nurse stays at work, especially if over 12.5 hours a shift, the greater is the likelihood that he or she will make an error or near error related to patient care.
- When a nurse agrees to work longer than 40 or 50 hours per week, it increases the chance of making an error affecting patient care.
- Nurses who volunteer to work overtime are subjecting themselves to potentially making medical errors.

If nurses are assigned to care for more patients than is reasonable, they need to bring this information to the attention of the nursing supervisor (Guido, 2010). If nurses have to accept unreasonable assignments, they need to make written protests to nursing administrators. Although these protests do not relieve nurses of responsibility if a patient suffers an injury because of inattention, it shows that the nurses were attempting to act reasonably. Whenever you make a written protest, keep a copy of this document in your personal file. Most administrators recognize that knowledge of a potential problem shifts some of the responsibility to the institution. Do not walk out when staffing is inadequate because you may be charged with patient abandonment. A nurse who refuses to accept an assignment may be considered insubordinate. It is important to know the policies and procedures of the institution on how to handle such reports before the situation occurs.

Floating. Nurses are sometimes required to "float" from the area in which they normally practice to other nursing units based on census load and patient acuities. In one case a nurse in obstetrics was assigned to an emergency department. A patient entered the emergency department and complained of chest pain. The patient received an incorrect dose of lidocaine by the obstetrical nurse and died after suffering irreversible brain damage and cardiac arrest. The nurse lost the malpractice lawsuit. Nurses who float need to inform the supervisor of any lack of experience in caring for the type of patients on the nursing unit. They also need to request and receive an orientation to the unit. Supervisors are liable if they give a staff nurse an assignment that he or she cannot safely handle. Before accepting employment, learn the policies of the institution regarding floating and have an understanding as to what is expected (Kane-Urrabazo, 2006).

Health Care Providers' Orders. The health care provider (physician or advanced practice nurse) is responsible for directing medical treatment. Nurses follow health care providers' orders unless they believe the orders are in error or harm patients. Therefore you need to assess all orders; if you find one to be erroneous or harmful, further clarification from the health care provider is necessary. If the health care provider confirms an order and you still believe that it is inappropriate, inform the supervising nurse or follow the established chain of command. The supervising nurse should help resolve the questionable order. A medical consultant sometimes helps clarify its appropriateness or inappropriateness. A nurse carrying out an inaccurate or inappropriate order is legally responsible for any harm the patient suffers.

In a malpractice lawsuit against a health care provider and a hospital, one of the most frequently litigated issues is whether the nurse kept the health care provider informed of the patient's condition. To inform a health care provider properly, you perform a competent nursing assessment of the patient to determine the signs and symptoms that are significant in relation to the attending health care provider's tasks of diagnosis and treatment. Be certain to document that you notified the health care provider and his or her response, your follow-up, and the patient's response.

The health care provider should write all orders. The nurse is responsible for transcribing written orders correctly. If a verbal order is necessary (e.g., during an emergency), it is signed by the health care provider as soon as possible, usually within 24 hours. Nurses verify the complete order or test results by reading verbal orders back to the health care provider. Nursing students *never* take verbal orders. Be familiar with the policy and procedures of the institution regarding verbal orders.

RISK MANAGEMENT

Risk management is an organization's system of ensuring appropriate nursing care by identifying potential hazards and eliminating them before harm occurs (Guido, 2010). The steps involved in risk management include identifying possible risks, analyzing them, acting to reduce the risks, and evaluating the steps taken. One tool used in risk management is the **occurrence report.** Occurrence reports are sometimes called *incident reports.*

Occurrence reporting provides a database for further investigation in an attempt to determine deviations from standards of care and corrective measures needed to prevent recurrence and to alert risk management to a potential claim situation. Examples of an occurrence include patient or visitor falls or injury; failure to follow health care provider orders; significant complaint by patient, family, health care provider, or other hospital department; error in technique or procedure; and malfunctioning device or product. Institutions generally have specific guidelines to direct health care providers in how to complete the occurrence report. The report is confidential and separate from the medical record. As a nurse, you are responsible for providing information in the medical record about the occurrence. *Never document in the patient's medical record that you completed an occurrence report.*

Risk management also requires complete documentation. A nurse's documentation is often the evidence of care received by a patient and serves as proof that the nurse acted reasonably and safely. When a lawsuit is filed, very often the nurses' notes are the first thing an attorney reviews (Austin, 2006). The nurse's assessments and the reporting of significant changes in the assessments are very important factors in defending a lawsuit. Therefore, it is critical for you to document the health care provider contacted, the information communicated to the health care provider, and the health care provider's response.

For nurses in practice the underlying rationale for quality improvement and risk management programs is the highest possible quality of care. Some insurance companies, medical and nursing organizations, and TJC require the use of quality improvement and risk management procedures (TJC, 2011a).

One area of potential risk is associated with the use of electronic monitoring devices. No monitor is reliable at all times; therefore do not depend on them completely. Continual assessment of a patient is necessary to help document the accuracy of electronic monitoring. There are also electrical hazards to the nurse and the patient. Biomedical engineers check equipment to ensure that it is in proper working order and that a patient will not receive an electrical shock.

All nurses need to be risk managers. For example, surgeons rely on operating room nurses to compare the consent form with the indicated and prepped surgical site for accuracy. Because of errors with patients undergoing the wrong surgery or having surgery performed on the wrong site, The Joint Commission's Universal Protocol includes guidelines for preventing such mishaps (TJC, 2011b). Implement this protocol whenever an invasive surgical procedure is to be performed, regardless of the location (hospital, ASC, or health care provider office). The three principles of the protocol include a preoperative verification that ensures all relevant documents and studies are available before the start of the procedure and are consistent with the patient's expectations; marking of the operative site with indelible ink to mark left and right distinction, multiple structures (e.g., fingers), and levels of the spine; and a "time out" just before starting the procedure for final verification of the correct patient, procedure, site, and any implants.

In the OR sponge, needle, and instrument counts are routine surgical standards to prevent patient injury and lawsuits. Health care providers rely on nurses to provide an accurate count of sponges and instruments inserted at the end of a procedure, even though it is the health care provider who inserts sponges and instruments into the surgical wound. Generally, when the chart records a correct sponge count and the patient suffers an injury because of a retained sponge, the hospital is liable because the nurse charted a correct count when it, in fact, was incorrect.

Professional Involvement

As a nurse you should stay involved in professional organizations and on committees that define the standards of care for nursing practice. If current laws, rules and regulations, or policies under which nurses practice do not reflect reality, you need to become involved as an advocate to see that the scope of nursing practice is defined accurately. Be willing to represent nursing and the patient's perspective in the community as well. The voice of nursing is powerful and effective when the organizing focus is the protection and welfare of the public entrusted to nurses' care (Blais et al., 2006).

KEY POINTS

- Registered nurses and licensed practical nurses are licensed by the state in which they practice; licensing is based on educational requirements, the passing of an examination, and other criteria.
- The civil law system is concerned with the protection of a person's private rights, and the criminal law system deals with the rights of individuals and society as defined by legislative statutes.

- A nurse is liable for malpractice if the nurse (defendant) owed a duty to the patient (plaintiff), the nurse did not carry out that duty, the patient was injured, and the nurse's failure to carry out the duty caused the patient's injury.
- All patients are entitled to confidential health care and freedom from unauthorized release of information.
- Under the law practicing nurses must follow standards of care, the guidelines of professional organizations, and the written policies and procedures of employing institutions.
- Nurses who witness consents are responsible for confirming that patients have voluntarily given informed consent for any surgery or other medical procedure before the procedure is performed.
- Nurses are responsible for performing all procedures correctly and exercising professional judgment as they carry out health care providers' orders.
- Nurses follow health care providers' orders unless they believe the orders to be in error or harmful to patients.
- Staffing standards determine the ratio of nurses to patients; if the nurse has to care for more patients than is reasonable, he or she needs to make a formal protest to the nursing administration.
- Legal issues involving death include documenting all events surrounding the death and treating a deceased person with dignity.
- All nurses need to know the laws that apply to their area of practice.
- Depending on state laws, nurses are required to report possible criminal activities such as child abuse and certain communicable diseases.
- Nurses are patient advocates and ensure quality of care through risk management and lobbying for safe nursing practice standards.
- Nurses file incident/occurrence reports for all errors even when someone is not injured.

CLINICAL APPLICATION QUESTIONS

Preparing for Clinical Practice

You are working the first shift on the hematology-oncology unit and receive report on your assigned team of four patients. You have a nursing assistive personnel assigned to help you with routine care. You make quick rounds on your patients to ensure that there are no immediate needs before you begin checking medications. Patient No. 1 is scheduled for surgery later in the morning for a biopsy and needs the surgical consent signed. Patient No. 2 is receiving blood products for an HIV complication and needs frequent vital sign monitoring. You find patient No. 3, an 83-year-old confused man, lying on the floor. He states that he needed to go to the restroom and no one was there to help. You call for help to get the patient back in bed and assess for further injuries.

1. The nurse prepares the surgical consent form for patient No. 1. What key points does he or she need to ensure that the patient received before witnessing informed consent?
2. The son of patient No. 2 calls to talk to the nurse caring for his father. The son asks questions about the reason for the blood administration. What guidelines does the nurse follow in responding to the son's questions about the father's condition? What federal statutes are involved in this scenario?
3. One week after discharge from the hospital, the hospital received a written complaint from the family of patient No. 3 about the incident related to the fall and the intent to take legal action.
    a. What must patient No. 3 establish to prove negligence against the nurse?
    b. Describe situations in which restraints may be legally applied to prevent falls.

evolve *Answers to Clinical Application Questions can be found on the Evolve website.*

REVIEW QUESTIONS

Are You Ready to Test Your Nursing Knowledge?

1. A nurse is caring for a patient who recently had coronary bypass surgery. Which are legal sources of standards of care the nurse uses to deliver safe health care? (Select all that apply.)
    1. Information provided by the head nurse
    2. Policies and procedures of the employing hospital
    3. State Nurse Practice Act
    4. Regulations identified in The Joint Commission's manual
    5. The American Nurses Association standards of nursing practice
2. A nurse is sued for failure to monitor a patient appropriately after a procedure. Which of the following statements are correct about this lawsuit? (Select all that apply.)
    1. The nurse represents the plaintiff.
    2. The defendant must prove injury, damage, or loss.
    3. The person filing the lawsuit has the burden of proof.
    4. The plaintiff must prove that a breach in the prevailing standard of care caused an injury.
3. A nurse stops to help in an emergency at the scene of an accident. The injured party files a suit, and the nurse's employing institution insurance does not cover the nurse. What would probably cover the nurse in this situation?
    1. The nurse's automobile insurance
    2. The nurse's homeowner's insurance
    3. The Good Samaritan laws, which grant immunity from suit if there is no gross negligence
    4. The Patient Care Partnership, which may grant immunity from suit if the injured party consents
4. A nurse is planning care for a patient going to surgery. Who is responsible for informing the patient about the surgery along with possible risks, complications, and benefits?
    1. Family member
    2. Surgeon
    3. Nurse
    4. Nurse Manager
5. A woman who is a Jehovah's Witness has severe life-threatening injuries and is hemorrhaging following a car accident. The health care provider ordered 2 units of packed red blood cells to treat the woman's anemia. The woman's husband refuses to allow the nurse to give his wife the blood. What is the nurse's responsibility?
    1. Obtain a court order to give the blood
    2. Coerce the husband into giving the blood
    3. Call security and have the husband removed from the hospital
    4. Abide by the husband's wishes and inform the health care provider
6. The nurse notes that an advance directive is on a patient's medical record. Which statement represents the best description of an advance directive guideline the nurse will follow?
    1. A living will allows an appointed person to make health care decisions when the patient is in an incapacitated state.

2. A living will is invoked only when the patient has a terminal condition or is in a persistent vegetative state.
3. The patient cannot make changes in the advance directive once admitted to the hospital.
4. A durable power of attorney for health care is invoked only when the patient has a terminal condition or is in a persistent vegetative state.

7. A nurse notes that the health care unit keeps a listing of the patient names at the front desk in easy view for health care providers to more efficiently locate the patient. The nurse talks with the nursing manager because this action is a violation of which act?
   1. Mental Health Parity Act
   2. Patient Self-Determination Act (PSDA)
   3. Health Insurance Portability and Accountability Act (HIPAA)
   4. Emergency Medical Treatment and Active Labor Act
8. Which of the following actions, if performed by a registered nurse, would result in both criminal and administrative law sanctions against the nurse? (Select all that apply.)
   1. Taking or selling controlled substances
   2. Refusing to provide health care information to a patient's child
   3. Reporting suspected abuse and neglect of children
   4. Applying physical restraints without a written physician's order
9. The nurse received a hand-off report at the change of shift in the conference room from the night shift nurse. The nursing student assigned to the nurse asks to review the medical records of the patients assigned to them. The nurse begins assessing the assigned patients and lists the nursing care information for each patient on each individual patient's message board in the patient rooms. The nurse also lists the patients' medical diagnoses on the message board. Later in the day the nurse discusses the plan of care for a patient who is dying with the patient's family. Which of these actions describes a violation of the Health Insurance Portability and Accountability Act (HIPAA)?
   1. Discussing patient conditions in the nursing report room at the change of shift
   2. Allowing nursing students to review patient charts before caring for patients to whom they are assigned
   3. Posting medical information about the patient on a message board in the patient's room
   4. Releasing patient information regarding terminal illness to family when the patient has given permission for information to be shared
10. The patient has a fractured femur that is placed in skeletal traction with a fresh plaster cast applied. The patient experiences decreased sensation and a cold feeling in the toes of the affected leg. The nurse observes that the patient's toes have become pale and cold but forgets to document this because one of the nurse's other patients experienced cardiac arrest at the same time. Two days later the patient in skeletal traction has an elevated temperature, and he is prepared for surgery to amputate the leg below the knee. Which of the following statements regarding a breach of duty apply to this situation? (Select all that apply.)
    1. Failure to document a change in assessment data
    2. Failure to provide discharge instructions
    3. Failure to follow the six rights of medication administration
    4. Failure to use proper medical equipment ordered for patient monitoring
    5. Failure to notify a health care provider about a change in the patient's condition
11. A homeless man enters the emergency department seeking health care. The health care provider indicates that the patient needs to be transferred to the City Hospital for care. This action is most likely a violation of which of the following laws?
    1. Health Insurance Portability and Accountability Act (HIPAA)
    2. Americans with Disabilities Act (ADA)
    3. Patient Self-Determination Act (PSDA)
    4. Emergency Medical Treatment and Active Labor Act (EMTALA)
12. You are the night shift nurse and are caring for a newly admitted patient who appears to be confused. The family asks to see the patient's medical record. What is the first nursing action to take?
    1. Give the family the record
    2. Give the patient the record
    3. Discuss the issues that concern the family with them
    4. Call the nursing supervisor
13. A home health nurse notices significant bruising on a 2-year-old patient's head, arms, abdomen, and legs. The patient's mother describes the patient's frequent falls. What is the best nursing action for the home health nurse to take?
    1. Document her findings and treat the patient
    2. Instruct the mother on safe handling of a 2-year-old child
    3. Contact a child abuse hotline
    4. Discuss this story with a colleague
14. A new graduate nurse is being mentored by a more experienced nurse. They are discussing the ways nurses need to remain active professionally. Which of the statements below indicates the new graduate understands ways to remain involved professionally? (Select all that apply.)
    1. "I am thinking about joining the health committee at my church."
    2. "I need to read newspapers, watch news broadcasts, and search the Internet for information related to health."
    3. "I will join nursing committees at the hospital after I have several years of experience and better understand the issues affecting nursing."
    4. "Nurses do not have very much voice in legislation in Washington, DC, because of the shortage of nurses.
15. You are floated to work on a nursing unit where you are given an assignment that is beyond your capability. What is the best nursing action to take first?
    1. Call the nursing supervisor to discuss the situation
    2. Discuss the problem with a colleague
    3. Leave the nursing unit and go home
    4. Say nothing and begin your work

Answers: **1.** 2, 3, 4, 5; **2.** 3, 4; **3.** 3; **4.** 2; **5.** 4; **6.** 2; **7.** 3; **8.** 1, 4; **9.** 3; **10.** 1, 5; **11.** 4; **12.** 3; **13.** 3; **14.** 1, 2; **15.** 1.

REFERENCES

American Nurses Association: *Guide to the code of ethics for nurses: interpretation and application*, Silver Spring, Md, 2008, The Association.

American Nurses Association: *Nursing: scope and standards of practice*, ed 2, Silver Spring, Md, 2010, The Association.

American Nurses Association: Nurse staffing laws enacted in the states, http://www.safestaffingsaveslives.org/WhatisANADoing/StateLegislation/StaffingPlansandRatios.aspx, 2011. Accessed August 21, 2011.

Austin S: Ladies of the jury, I present the nursing documentation, *Nursing* 36(1):56, 2006.

Blais K, et al: *Professional nursing practice: concepts and perspectives*, ed 5, Upper Saddle River, NJ, 2006, Pearson Prentice Hall.

Bross W: Healthcare issues: patient self determination acts and informed consent, *Ala Nurse* 32(4):9, 2006.

Carter P: *HIPAA compliance handbook*, Austin, 2010, Wolters Kluwer.

Centers for Medicare and Medicaid Services: *Revisions to Medicare conditions of participation, 482.13*, Bethesda, Md, 2007, US Department of Health and Human Services.

Dachs R, Elias J: What you need to know when called upon to be a good Samaritan, *Fam Pract Manag* 15(4):37, 2008.

Daller M: *Tort law desk reference*, 2010, Wolters Kluwer.

Evans K, Cotter V: Avoiding restraints in patients with dementia, *Am J Nurs* 108(3):40, 2008.

Garner B: *Black's law dictionary*, pocket ed 3, St Paul, 2006, West Publishing.

Grohar-Murray M, Langan J: *Leadership and management in nursing*, ed 4, Boston, Mass, 2011, Pearson.

Guido G: *Legal and ethical issues in nursing*, ed 5, Upper Saddle River, NJ, 2010, Prentice Hall.

Kane-Urrabazo C: Said another way: our obligation to float, *Nurs Forum* 41(2):95, 2006.

National Council of State Boards of Nursing: *Working with others: a position paper*, 2005, http://www.ncsbn.org/pdfs/Working_with_Others.pdf. Accessed August 21, 2011.

Privacy Rights Clearinghouse: Medical privacy FAQ, https://www.privacyrights.org/fs/fs8b-MedFAQ.htm, 2011. Accessed August 21, 2011.

Scott R: *Promoting legal and ethical awareness: a primer for health professionals and patients*, St Louis, 2009, Mosby.

The Joint Commission (TJC): *Comprehensive accreditation manual for hospitals: the official handbook (E-dition)*, Oak Brook Terrace, IL, 2011a, The Joint Commission.

The Joint Commission (TJC): Critical Access Hospital National Patient Safety Goals, 2011b, http://www.jointcommission.org. Retrieved August 7, 2011.

RESEARCH REFERENCES

Berger, A, Hobbs B: Impact of shift work on the health and safety of nurses and patients, *Clin J Oncol Nurs* 10(4):465, 2006.

Garrett C: The effect of nurse staffing patterns on medical errors and nurse burnout, *AORN J* 87(6):1191, 2008.

Stone PA, et al: Nurse working conditions and patient safety outcome, *Med Care* 45(6):571, 2007.

Trinkoff A, et al: How long and how much are nurses now working? *Am J Nurs* 106(4):60, 2006.

STATUTES

Americans with Disabilities Act (ADA), 42 USC §§121.010-12213 (1990)

Autopsy Consent, Mo Rev Stat, {194.115 (1998)

Emergency Medical Treatment and Active Labor Act (EMTALA), 42 USC §1395 (dd) (1986)

Federal Nursing Home Reform Act from the Omnibus Budget Reconciliation Act of 1987

Good Samaritan Act, IL Compiled Statutes, 745 ILCS 49/ (1997)

Health Insurance Portability and Accountability Act of 1996 (HIPAA), Public Law No. 104 (1996)

Medical Patient Rights Act, IL Compiled Statutes, 410 ILCS 50 (1994)

Mental Health Parity Act of 1996, 29 USC §1885 (1996)

National Organ Transplant Act, Public Law 98–507 (1984)

New York DNR Statute, NY Public Health Laws §2962 (1988)

Oregon Death with Dignity Act, Ore Rev Stat §§127.800-127.897 (1994)

Patient Self-Determination Act, 42 CFR 417 (1991)

Uniform Anatomical Gift Act (1987)

Uniform Determination of Death Act (1980)

CASES

Bouvia v Superior Court, 225 Cal Rptr 297 (1986)

Bragdon v Abbott, 524 U.S. 624 (1998)

Cruzan v Director Missouri Department of Health, 497 U.S. 261 (1990)

Darling v Charleston Community Memorial Hospital, 33 Ill 2d 326 (Ill 1965)

Roe v Wade, 410 U.S. 113 (1973)

Spires v Hospital Corporation of America, 28 U.S.C. §1391(b) Kansas (2006), http://www.kansas.com/multimedia/kansas/archive/pdfs/041106spireshca.pdf

Webster v Reproductive Health Services, 492 U.S. 490 (1989)

YG v Jewish Hospital, 795 SW2d 488 (Mo App 1990)

CHAPTER

24

Communication

OBJECTIVES

- Describe aspects of critical thinking that are important to the communication process.
- Describe the five levels of communication and their uses in nursing.
- Describe the basic elements of the communication process.
- Identify significant features and therapeutic outcomes of nurse-patient helping relationships.
- Identify a nurse's communication approaches within the four phases of a nurse-patient helping relationship.
- Identify significant features and desired outcomes of nurse–health care team member relationships.
- Describe qualities, behaviors, and communication techniques that affect professional communication.
- Discuss effective communication techniques for older patients.
- Identify patient health states that contribute to impaired communication.
- Discuss nursing care measures for patients with special communication needs.

KEY TERMS

evolve WEBSITE

http://evolve.elsevier.com/Potter/fundamentals/

- Review Questions
- Case Study with Questions
- Audio Glossary
- Interactive Learning Activities
- Key Term Flashcards
- Content Updates

COMMUNICATION AND NURSING PRACTICE

Communication is a lifelong learning process. Nurses make the intimate journey with patients and their families from the miracle of birth to the mystery of death. As a nurse you communicate with patients and families to collect meaningful assessment data, provide education, and interact using therapeutic communication to promote personal growth and attainment of health-related goals. Despite the complexity of technology and the multiple demands on nurses' time, it is the intimate moment of connection that makes all the difference in the quality of care and meaning for a patient and a nurse.

Communication is an essential part of patient-centered nursing care. Patient safety also requires effective communication among members of the health care team as patients move from one caregiver to another or from one care setting to another. Breakdown in communication among the health care team is a major cause of errors in the workplace and threatens professional credibility (World Health Organization, 2007). Effective team communication and collaboration skills are essential to ensure patient safety and high-quality patient care (Cronenwett et al., 2007). Competency in communication helps maintain effective relationships within the entire sphere of professional practice and meets legal, ethical, and clinical standards of care.

The qualities, behaviors, and therapeutic communication techniques described in this chapter characterize professionalism in helping relationships. Although the term *patient* is often used, the same principles apply when communicating with any person in any nursing situation.

Communication and Interpersonal Relationships

Caring relationships formed among a nurse and those affected by a nurse's practice are at the core of nursing (see Chapter 7). Communication is the means of establishing these helping-healing relationships. All behavior communicates, and all communication influences behavior. For these reasons communication is essential to the nurse-patient relationship.

Nurses with expertise in communication express caring by the following (Watson, 1985):

- Becoming sensitive to self and others
- Promoting and accepting the expression of positive and negative feelings
- Developing helping-trust relationships
- Instilling faith and hope
- Promoting interpersonal teaching and learning
- Providing a supportive environment
- Assisting with gratification of human needs
- Allowing for spiritual expression

A nurse's ability to relate to others is important for interpersonal communication. This includes the ability to take initiative in establishing and maintaining communication, to be authentic (one's self), and to respond appropriately to the other person. Effective interpersonal communication also requires a sense of mutuality, a belief that the nurse-patient relationship is a partnership and that both are equal participants. Nurses honor the fact that people are very complex and ambiguous. Often more is communicated than first meets the eye, and patient responses are not always what you expect. By giving all of your attention to a patient, you attend to the patient's needs and aid the healing process (Tavernier, 2006). Most nurses embrace the profession's view of the holistic nature of people and experience synergy in human interaction. When patients and nurses work together, much can be accomplished.

Therapeutic communication occurs within a healing relationship between a nurse and patient (Arnold and Boggs, 2011). Like any powerful therapeutic agent, the nurse's communication can result in both harm and good. Every nuance of posture, every small expression and gesture, every word chosen, every attitude held—all have the potential to hurt or heal, affecting others through the transmission of human energy. Knowing that intention and behavior directly influence health gives nurses tremendous ethical responsibility to do no harm to those entrusted to their care. Respect the potential power of communication and do not carelessly misuse communication to hurt, manipulate, or coerce others. Skilled communication empowers others and enables people to know themselves and make their own choices, an essential aspect of the healing process. Nurses have wonderful opportunities to bring about good things for themselves, their patients, and their colleagues through this kind of therapeutic communication.

Developing Communication Skills

Gaining expertise in communication requires both an understanding of the communication process and reflection about one's communication experiences as a nurse. Nurses who develop critical thinking skills make the best communicators. They draw on theoretical knowledge about communication and integrate this knowledge with knowledge previously learned through personal experience. They interpret messages received from others, analyze their content, make inferences about their meaning, evaluate their effect, explain rationale for communication techniques used, and self-examine personal communication skills (Balzer-Riley, 2007).

Critical thinking in nursing, based on established standards of nursing care and ethical standards, promotes effective communication. When you consider a patient's problems, it is important to apply critical thinking standards to ensure sound effective communication (Chitty, 2010). For example, curiosity motivates a nurse to communicate and know more about a person. Patients are more likely to communicate with nurses who express an interest in them. Perseverance and creativity are also attitudes conducive to communication because they motivate a nurse to communicate and identify innovative solutions. A self-confident attitude is important because a nurse who conveys confidence and comfort while communicating more readily establishes an interpersonal helping-trusting relationship. In addition, an independent attitude encourages a nurse to communicate with colleagues and share ideas about nursing interventions. Such an attitude often involves risk taking because colleagues sometimes question suggested nursing interventions. At the same time, an attitude of fairness goes a long way in the ability to listen to both sides in any discussion. Integrity allows nurses to recognize when their opinions conflict with those of their patients, review positions, and decide how to communicate to reach mutually beneficial decisions. It is also very important for a nurse to communicate responsibly and ask for help if uncertain or uncomfortable about an aspect of patient care. An attitude of humility is necessary to recognize and communicate the need for more information before making a decision (Paul, 1993).

It is challenging to understand human communication within interpersonal relationships. Each individual bases his or her perceptions about information received through the five senses of sight, hearing, taste, touch, and smell (Arnold and Boggs, 2011). An individual's culture and education also influence perception. Critical thinking helps nurses overcome **perceptual biases,** or human tendencies that interfere with accurately perceiving and interpreting messages from others. People often assume that others think, feel, act, react, and behave as they would in similar circumstances. They tend to distort or ignore information that goes against their expectations, preconceptions, or stereotypes (Beebe et al., 2010). By thinking critically about personal communication habits, you learn to control these tendencies and become more effective in interpersonal relationships.

As communication skills develop, competence in the nursing process also grows. You need to integrate communication skills throughout the nursing process as you collaborate with patients and health care team members to achieve goals (Box 24-1). Use communication skills to gather, analyze, and transmit information and accomplish the work of each step of the process. Assessment, diagnosis, planning, implementation, and evaluation all depend on effective communication among nurse, patient, family, and others on the health care team. Although the nursing process is a reliable framework for patient care, it does not work well unless you master the art of effective interpersonal communication.

The nature of the communication process requires you to constantly make decisions about what, when, where, why, and how to convey a message. A nurse's decision making is always contextual (i.e., the unique features of any situation influence the nature of the decisions made). For example, the explanation of the importance of following a prescribed diet to a patient with a newly diagnosed medical condition differs from the explanation to a patient who has repeatedly chosen not to follow diet restrictions. Effective communication techniques are easy to learn, but their application is more difficult. Deciding which techniques best fit each unique nursing situation is challenging. Communication about specific diagnoses such as cancer or end of life and dealing with patient and family emotions can be challenging, and some nurses struggle to cope with their own reactions and emotions (Sheldon et al., 2006).

Throughout this chapter brief clinical examples guide you in the use of effective communication techniques. Situations that challenge a nurse's decision-making skills and call for careful use of therapeutic techniques often involve the types of persons described in Box 24-2. Because the best way to acquire skill is through practice, it is useful for you to discuss and role-play these scenarios before experiencing them in the clinical setting. Consider

BOX 24-1 COMMUNICATION THROUGHOUT THE NURSING PROCESS

Assessment
- Verbal interviewing and history taking
- Visual and intuitive observation of nonverbal behavior
- Visual, tactile, and auditory data gathering during physical examination
- Written medical records, diagnostic tests, and literature review

Nursing Diagnosis
- Intrapersonal analysis of assessment findings
- Validation of health care needs and priorities via verbal discussion with patient
- Documentation of nursing diagnosis

Planning
- Interpersonal or small-group health care team planning sessions
- Interpersonal collaboration with patient and family to determine implementation methods
- Written documentation of expected outcomes
- Written or verbal referral to health care team members

Implementation
- Delegation and verbal discussion with health care team
- Verbal, visual, auditory, and tactile health teaching activities
- Provision of support via therapeutic communication techniques
- Contact with other health resources
- Written documentation of patient's progress in medical record

Evaluation
- Acquisition of verbal and nonverbal feedback
- Comparison of actual and expected outcomes
- Identification of factors affecting outcomes
- Modification and update of care plan
- Verbal and/or written explanation of revisions of care plan to patient

BOX 24-2 CHALLENGING COMMUNICATION SITUATIONS

- People who are silent, withdrawn, and have difficulty expressing feelings or needs
- People who are sad and depressed
- People with special needs
- People who are angry or confrontational and cannot listen to explanations
- People who are uncooperative and resent being asked to help others
- People who are talkative or lonely and want someone else to be with them all the time
- People who are demanding and expect others to meet their requests
- People who are frightened, anxious, and having difficulty coping
- People who have difficulty seeing or hearing
- People who are confused and disoriented
- People who speak and/or understand little English
- People who are flirtatious or sexually inappropriate

who is involved in the situation to decide which communication will be most effective.

Levels of Communication

Nurses use different levels of communication in their professional role. A competent nurse uses a variety of techniques in each level.

Intrapersonal communication is a powerful form of communication that occurs within an individual. This level of communication is also called *self-talk, self-verbalization,* or *inner thought.* People's thoughts strongly influence perceptions, feelings, behavior, and self-concept. You need to be aware of the nature and content of your own thinking. Self-talk provides a mental rehearsal for difficult tasks or situations so individuals deal with them more effectively and with increased confidence (Gibson and Foster, 2007; White, 2008). Nurses and patients use intrapersonal communication to develop self-awareness and a positive self-concept that enhances appropriate self-expression. For example, you improve your health and self-esteem through positive self-talk by replacing negative thoughts with positive assertions.

Interpersonal communication is one-on-one interaction between a nurse and another person that often occurs face to face. It is the level most frequently used in nursing situations and lies at the heart of nursing practice. It takes place within a social context and includes all the symbols and cues used to give and receive meaning. Because meaning resides in persons and not in words, messages received are sometimes different from intended messages. Nurses work with people who have different opinions, experiences, values, and belief systems; thus it is important to validate meaning or mutually negotiate it between participants. For example, use interaction to assess understanding and clarify misinterpretations when teaching a patient about a health concern. Meaningful interpersonal communication results in exchange of ideas, problem solving, expression of feelings, decision making, goal accomplishment, team building, and personal growth.

Transpersonal communication is interaction that occurs within a person's spiritual domain. Study of the influence of religion and spirituality has increased dramatically in recent years, and ongoing research helps us understand the role of nurses in addressing a patient's spiritual needs (Pesut et al., 2008). Many people use prayer, meditation, guided reflection, religious rituals, or other means to communicate with their "higher power." Nurses have a responsibility to assess a patient's spiritual needs and intervene to meet those needs (see Chapter 35).

Small-group communication is interaction that occurs when a small number of persons meet. This type of communication is usually goal directed and requires an understanding of group dynamics. When nurses work on committees, lead patient support groups, form research teams, or participate in patient care conferences, they use a small-group communication process. Small groups are most effective when they are cohesive and committed and have an appropriate meeting place with suitable seating arrangements (Arnold and Boggs, 2011). A nurse's role varies with the function of a group. He or she frequently coordinates the group, provides recognition and acceptance of the contributions of each group member, and provides encouragement and motivation to help the group meet its goals (Townsend, 2009).

Public communication is interaction with an audience. Nurses have opportunities to speak with groups of consumers about health-related topics, present scholarly work to colleagues at conferences, or lead classroom discussions with peers or students. Public communication requires special adaptations in eye contact, gestures, voice inflection, and use of media materials to communicate messages effectively. Effective public communication increases audience knowledge about health-related topics, health issues, and other issues important to the nursing profession.

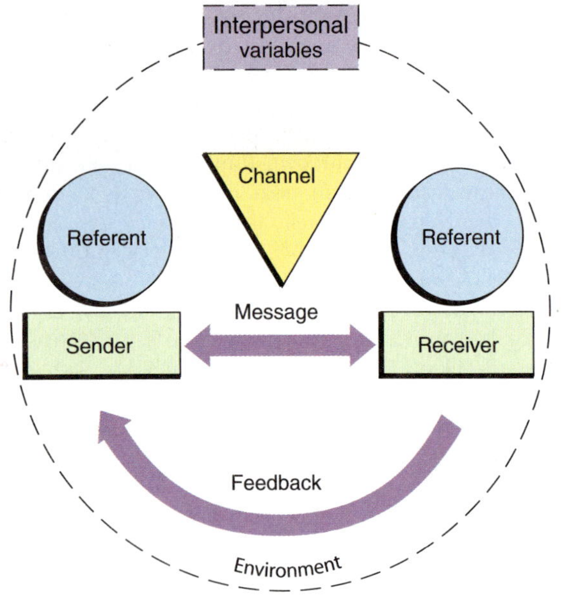

FIG. 24-1 Communication as active process between sender and receiver.

BASIC ELEMENTS OF THE COMMUNICATION PROCESS

Communication is an ongoing, dynamic, and multidimensional process. Fig. 24-1 shows the basic elements of the communication process. This simple linear model represents a very complex process with its essential components. Nursing situations have many unique aspects that influence the nature of communication and interpersonal relationships. As a professional, you will use critical thinking to focus on each aspect of communication so your interactions are purposeful and effective.

Referent

The **referent** motivates one person to communicate with another. In a health care setting sights, sounds, odors, time schedules, messages, objects, emotions, sensations, perceptions, ideas, and other cues initiate communication. Knowing which stimulus initiates communication enables you to develop and organize messages more efficiently and better perceive meaning in another's message. A patient request for help prompted by difficulty breathing brings a different nursing response than a request prompted by hunger.

Sender and Receiver

The **sender** is the person who encodes and delivers the message, and the **receiver** is the person who receives and decodes the message. The sender puts ideas or feelings into a form that is transmitted and is responsible for the accuracy of its content and emotional tone. The sender's message acts as a referent for the receiver, who is responsible for attending to, translating, and responding to the sender's message. Sender and receiver roles are fluid and change back and forth as two persons interact; sometimes sending and receiving occurs simultaneously. The more the sender and receiver have in common and the closer the relationship, the more likely they will accurately perceive one another's meaning and respond accordingly.

Messages

The **message** is the content of the communication. It contains verbal, nonverbal, and symbolic language. Personal perceptions sometimes distort the receiver's interpretation of the message. Two nurses can provide the same information yet convey very different messages because of their personal communication styles. Two persons understand the same message differently. You send effective messages by expressing clearly, directly, and in a manner familiar to the receiver. You determine the need for clarification by watching the listener for nonverbal cues that suggest confusion or misunderstanding. Communication is difficult when participants have different levels of education and experience. "Your incision is well approximated without purulent drainage" means the same as "Your wound edges are close together, and there are no signs of infection," but the latter is easier to understand. You can also send messages in writing, but make sure that patients are able to read.

Channels

Channels are means of conveying and receiving messages through visual, auditory, and tactile senses. Facial expressions send visual messages, spoken words travel through auditory channels, and touch uses tactile channels. Individuals usually understand a message more clearly when the sender uses more channels to convey it. For example, when teaching about insulin self-injection, the nurse talks about and demonstrates the technique, gives the patient printed information, and encourages hands-on practice with the vial and syringe. Nurses use verbal, nonverbal, and mediated (technological) communication channels. They send and receive information in person, by informal or formal writing, over the telephone or pager, by audiotape and videotape, through fax and electronic mail, and through interactive and informational websites.

Feedback

Feedback is the message the receiver returns. It indicates whether the receiver understood the meaning of the sender's message. Senders seek verbal and nonverbal feedback to evaluate the effectiveness of communication. The sender and receiver need to be sensitive and open to one another's messages, clarify the messages, and modify behavior accordingly. In a social relationship both persons assume equal responsibility for seeking openness and clarification, but the nurse assumes primary responsibility in the nurse-patient relationship.

Interpersonal Variables

Interpersonal variables are factors within both the sender and receiver that influence communication. Perception is one such variable that provides a uniquely personal view of reality formed by an individual's expectations and experiences. Each person senses, interprets, and understands events differently. A nurse says, "You have been very quiet since your family left. Is there something on your mind?" One patient may perceive the nurse's question as caring and concerned; another perceives the nurse as invading privacy and is less willing to talk. Other interpersonal variables include educational and developmental levels, sociocultural backgrounds, values and beliefs, emotions, gender, physical health status, and roles and relationships. Variables associated with illness such as pain, anxiety, and medication effects also affect nurse-patient communication.

Environment

The **environment** is the setting for sender-receiver interaction. For effective communication the environment needs to meet participant needs for physical and emotional comfort and safety.

Noise, temperature extremes, distractions, and lack of privacy or space create confusion, tension, and discomfort. Environmental distractions are common in health care settings and interfere with messages sent between people. You control the environment as much as possible to create favorable conditions for effective communication.

FORMS OF COMMUNICATION

Messages are conveyed verbally and nonverbally, concretely and symbolically. As people communicate, they express themselves through words, movements, voice inflection, facial expressions, and use of space. These elements work in harmony to enhance a message or conflict with one another to contradict and confuse it.

Verbal Communication

Verbal communication uses spoken or written words. Verbal language is a code that conveys specific meaning through a combination of words. The most important aspects of verbal communication are presented in the following paragraphs.

Vocabulary. Communication is unsuccessful if senders and receivers cannot translate one another's words and phrases. When a nurse cares for a patient who speaks another language, an interpreter is often necessary. Even those who speak the same language use subcultural variations of certain words (e.g., *dinner* means a noon meal to one person and the last meal of the day to another). Medical jargon (technical terminology used by health care providers) sounds like a foreign language to patients unfamiliar with the health care setting. Limiting use of medical jargon to conversations with other health care team members improves communication. Children have a more limited vocabulary than adults. They may use special words to describe bodily functions or a favorite blanket or toy. Teenagers often use words in unique ways that are unfamiliar to adults.

Denotative and Connotative Meaning. Some words have several meanings. Individuals who use a common language share the denotative meaning: *baseball* has the same meaning for everyone who speaks English, but *code* denotes cardiac arrest primarily to health care providers. The connotative meaning is the shade or interpretation of the meaning of a word influenced by the thoughts, feelings, or ideas people have about the word. For example, health care providers tell a family that a loved one is in serious condition, and they believe that death is near; but to nurses *serious* simply describes the nature of the illness. You need to carefully select words, avoiding easily misinterpreted words, especially when explaining a patient's medical condition or therapy. Even a much-used phrase such as "I'm going to take your vital signs" may be unfamiliar to an adult or frightening to a child.

Pacing. Conversation is more successful at an appropriate speed or pace. Speak slowly and enunciate clearly. Talking rapidly, using awkward pauses, or speaking slowly and deliberately conveys an unintended message. Long pauses and rapid shifts to another subject give the impression that you are hiding the truth. Think before speaking and develop an awareness of the rhythm of your speech to improve pacing.

Intonation. Tone of voice dramatically affects the meaning of a message. Depending on intonation, even a simple question or statement expresses enthusiasm, anger, concern, or indifference. Be aware of voice tone to avoid sending unintended messages. For example, a patient interprets a nurse's patronizing tone of voice as condescending, and this inhibits further communication. A patient's tone of voice often provides information about his or her emotional state or energy level.

Clarity and Brevity. Effective communication is simple, brief, and direct. Fewer words result in less confusion. Speaking slowly, enunciating clearly, and using examples to make explanations easier to understand improve clarity. Repeating important parts of a message also clarifies communication. Phrases such as "you know" or "OK?" at the end of every sentence detract from clarity. Use short sentences and words that express an idea simply and directly. "Where is your pain?" is much better than "I would like you to describe for me the location of your discomfort."

Timing and Relevance. Timing is critical in communication. Even though a message is clear, poor timing prevents it from being effective. For example, you do not begin routine teaching when a patient is in severe pain or emotional distress. Often the best time for interaction is when a patient expresses an interest in communicating. If messages are relevant or important to the situation at hand, they are more effective. When a patient is facing emergency surgery, discussing the risks of smoking is less relevant than explaining presurgical procedures.

Nonverbal Communication

Nonverbal communication includes the five senses and everything that does not involve the spoken or written word. Researchers have estimated that approximately 7% of meaning is transmitted by words, 38% is transmitted by vocal cues, and 55% is transmitted by body cues. Thus nonverbal communication is unconsciously motivated and more accurately indicates a person's intended meaning than the spoken words (Jones, 2009). When there is incongruity between verbal and nonverbal communication, the receiver usually "hears" the nonverbal message as the true message.

All kinds of nonverbal communication are important, but interpreting them is often problematic. Sociocultural background is a major influence on the meaning of nonverbal behavior. In the United States, with its diverse cultural communities, nonverbal messages between people of different cultures are easily misinterpreted. Because the meaning attached to nonverbal behavior is so subjective, it is imperative that you verify it (Stuart, 2009). Assessing nonverbal messages is an important nursing skill.

Personal Appearance. Personal appearance includes physical characteristics, facial expression, and manner of dress and grooming. These factors help communicate physical well-being, personality, social status, occupation, religion, culture, and self-concept. First impressions are largely based on appearance. Nurses learn to develop a general impression of patient health and emotional status through appearance, and patients develop a general impression of the nurse's professionalism and caring in the same way.

Posture and Gait. Posture and gait (way of walking) are forms of self-expression. The way people sit, stand, and move reflects attitudes, emotions, self-concept, and health status. For example, an erect posture and a quick, purposeful gait communicate a sense of well-being and confidence. Leaning forward conveys attention. A slumped posture and slow shuffling gait indicates depression, illness, or fatigue.

Facial Expression. The face is the most expressive part of the body. Facial expressions convey emotions such as surprise, fear, anger, happiness, and sadness. Some people have an expressionless face, or flat affect, which reveals little about what they are thinking or feeling. An inappropriate affect is a facial expression that does not match the content of a verbal message (e.g., smiling when describing a sad situation). People are sometimes unaware of the messages their expressions convey. For example, a nurse frowns in concentration while doing a procedure, and the patient interprets this as anger or disapproval. Patients closely observe nurses. Consider the impact a nurse's facial expression has on a person who asks, "Am I going to die?" The slightest change in the eyes, lips, or facial muscles reveals the nurse's feelings. Although it is hard to control all facial expressions, try to avoid showing shock, disgust, dismay, or other distressing reactions in a patient's presence.

Eye Contact. People signal readiness to communicate through eye contact. Maintaining eye contact during conversation shows respect and willingness to listen. Eye contact also allows people to closely observe one another. Lack of eye contact may indicate anxiety, defensiveness, discomfort, or lack of confidence in communicating. However, persons from some cultures consider eye contact intrusive, threatening, or harmful and minimize or avoid its use (see Chapter 9). Always consider a person's culture when interpreting the meaning of eye contact. Eye movements communicate feelings and emotions. Looking down on a person establishes authority, whereas interacting at the same eye level indicates equality in the relationship. Rising to the same eye level as an angry person helps establish autonomy.

Gestures. Gestures emphasize, punctuate, and clarify the spoken word. Gestures alone carry specific meanings, or they create messages with other communication cues. A finger pointed toward a person communicates several meanings; but, when accompanied by a frown and stern voice, the gesture becomes an accusation or threat. Pointing to an area of pain is sometimes more accurate than describing its location.

Sounds. Sounds such as sighs, moans, groans, or sobs also communicate feelings and thoughts. Combined with other nonverbal communication, sounds help to send clear messages. They have several interpretations: moaning conveys pleasure or suffering, and crying communicates happiness, sadness, or anger. Validate nonverbal messages with the patient to interpret them accurately.

Territoriality and Personal Space. Territoriality is the need to gain, maintain, and defend one's right to space. Territory is important because it provides people with a sense of identity, security, and control. It is sometimes separated and made visible to others such as a fence around a yard or a bed in a hospital room. Personal space is invisible, individual, and travels with the person. During interpersonal interaction, people maintain varying distances between each other, depending on their culture, the nature of their relationship, and the situation. When personal space becomes threatened, people respond defensively and communicate less effectively. Situations dictate whether the interpersonal distance between nurse and patient is appropriate. Box 24-3 provides examples of nursing actions within zones of personal space and touch (Kneisl and Trigoboff, 2009; Stuart, 2009). Nurses frequently move into patients' territory and personal space because of the nature of caregiving. You need to convey confidence, gentleness, and respect for privacy, especially when your actions require intimate contact or involve a patient's vulnerable zone.

Symbolic Communication

Good communication requires awareness of **symbolic communication,** the verbal and nonverbal symbolism used by others to convey meaning. Art and music are forms of symbolic communication used by nurses to enhance understanding and promote healing. Lane (2006) found that creative expressions such as art, music, and dance have a healing effect on patients. Patients reported decreased pain and a greater sense of joy and hope.

BOX 24-3 ZONES OF PERSONAL SPACE AND TOUCH

Zones of Personal Space

Intimate Zone (0 to 18 Inches)
- Holding a crying infant
- Performing physical assessment
- Bathing, grooming, dressing, feeding, and toileting a patient
- Changing a patient's dressing

Personal Zone (18 Inches to 4 Feet)
- Sitting at a patient's bedside
- Taking a patient's nursing history
- Teaching an individual patient
- Exchanging information at change of shift

Social Zone (4 to 12 Feet)
- Making rounds with a physician
- Sitting at the head of a conference table
- Teaching a class for patients with diabetes
- Conducting a family support group

Public Zone (12 Feet and Greater)
- Speaking at a community forum
- Testifying at a legislative hearing
- Lecturing to a class of students

Zones of Touch

Social Zone (Permission not Needed)
- Hands, arms, shoulders, back

Consent Zone (Permission Needed)
- Mouth, wrists, feet

Vulnerable Zone (Special Care Needed)
- Face, neck, front of body

Intimate Zone (Great Sensitivity Needed)
- Genitalia, rectum

Metacommunication

Metacommunication is a broad term that refers to all factors that influence communication. Awareness of influencing factors helps people better understand what is communicated (Arnold and Boggs, 2011). For example, a nurse observes a young patient holding his body rigidly, and his voice is sharp as he says, "Going to surgery is no big deal." The nurse replies, "You say having surgery doesn't bother you, but you look and sound tense. I'd like to help." Awareness of the tone of the verbal response and the nonverbal behavior results in further exploration of the patient's feelings and concerns.

PROFESSIONAL NURSING RELATIONSHIPS

A nurse's application of knowledge, understanding of human behavior and communication, and commitment to ethical behavior help create professional relationships. Having a philosophy based on caring and respect for others helps you be more successful in establishing relationships of this nature.

Nurse-Patient Helping Relationships

Helping relationships are the foundation of clinical nursing practice. In such relationships you assume the role of professional helper and come to know a patient as an individual who has unique health needs, human responses, and patterns of living. Therapeutic relationships promote a psychological climate that facilitates positive change and growth. Therapeutic communication between you and your patients allows the attainment of health-related goals (Arnold and Boggs, 2011). The goals of a therapeutic relationship focus on a patient achieving optimal personal growth related to personal identity, ability to form relationships, and ability to satisfy needs and achieve personal goals (Stuart, 2009). There is an explicit time frame, a goal-directed approach, and a high expectation of confidentiality. A nurse establishes, directs,

BOX 24-4 PHASES OF THE HELPING RELATIONSHIP

Preinteraction Phase

Before meeting a patient:

- Review available data, including the medical and nursing history.
- Talk to other caregivers who have information about the patient.
- Anticipate health concerns or issues that arise.
- Identify a location and setting that fosters comfortable, private interaction.
- Plan enough time for the initial interaction.

Orientation Phase

When the nurse and patient meet and get to know one another:

- Set the tone for the relationship by adopting a warm, empathetic, caring manner.
- Recognize that the initial relationship is often superficial, uncertain, and tentative.
- Expect the patient to test your competence and commitment.
- Closely observe the patient and expect to be closely observed by the patient.
- Begin to make inferences and form judgments about patient messages and behaviors.
- Assess the patient's health status.
- Prioritize the patient's problems and identify his or her goals.
- Clarify the patient's and your roles.
- Form contracts with the patient that specify who will do what.
- Let the patient know when to expect the relationship to be terminated.

Working Phase

When the nurse and patient work together to solve problems and accomplish goals:

- Encourage and help the patient express feelings about his or her health.
- Encourage and help the patient with self-exploration.
- Provide information needed to understand and change behavior.
- Encourage and help the patient set goals.
- Take action to meet the goals set with the patient.
- Use therapeutic communication skills to facilitate successful interactions.
- Use appropriate self-disclosure and confrontation.

Termination Phase

During the ending of the relationship:

- Remind the patient that termination is near.
- Evaluate goal achievement with the patient.
- Reminisce about the relationship with the patient.
- Separate from the patient by relinquishing responsibility for his or her care.
- Achieve a smooth transition for the patient to other caregivers as needed.

and takes responsibility for the interaction; and a patient's needs take priority over a nurse's needs. Your nonjudgmental acceptance of a patient is an important characteristic of the relationship. Acceptance conveys a willingness to hear a message or acknowledge feelings. It does not mean that you always agree with the other person or approve of the patient's decisions or actions. A helping relationship between you and a patient does not just happen—you create it with care, skill, and trust.

A natural progression of four goal-directed phases characterizes the nurse-patient relationship. The relationship often begins before you meet a patient and continues until the caregiving relationship ends (Box 24-4). Even a brief interaction uses an abbreviated version of the same preinteraction, orientation, working, and termination phases (Stuart, 2009). For example, the nursing student gathers patient information to prepare in advance for caregiving, meets the patient and establishes trust, accomplishes health-related goals through use of the nursing process, and says goodbye at the end of the day.

Socializing is an important initial component of interpersonal communication. It helps people get to know one another and relax. It is easy, superficial, and not deeply personal; whereas therapeutic interactions are often more intense, difficult, and uncomfortable. A nurse often uses social conversation to lay a foundation for a closer relationship: "Hi, Mr. Simpson, I hear it's your birthday today. How old are you?" A friendly, informal, and warm communication style helps establish trust, but you have to get beyond social conversation to talk about issues or concerns affecting the patient's health. During social conversation some patients ask personal questions such as those about your family or place of residence. Students often wonder whether it is appropriate to reveal such information. The skillful nurse uses judgment about what to share and provides minimal information or deflects such questions with gentle humor and refocuses conversation back to the patient.

Creating a therapeutic environment depends on your ability to communicate, comfort, and help patients meet their needs. Comfort is a critical value inherent in the practice of nursing. Therapeutic interactions increase feelings of personal control by helping a person feel secure, informed, and valued. Optimizing personal control facilitates emotional comfort, which minimizes physical discomfort and enhances recovery activities (Williams and Irurita, 2006).

In a therapeutic relationship it is important to encourage patients to share personal stories. Sharing stories is called *narrative interaction*. Through narrative interactions you begin to understand the context of others' lives and learn what is meaningful for them from their perspective. For example, a nurse uses narratives to understand a patient's perception of risk and the meaning of risk when taking medication that increases the risk of bleeding (Andreas et al., 2010) and to explore patient experiences of dignity in care (Dawood and Gallini, 2010). It is important to listen to patient stories to better understand their concerns, experiences, and challenges. This information is not usually revealed using a standard history form that elicits short answers.

Nurse-Family Relationships

Many nursing situations, especially those in community and home care settings, require you to form helping relationships with entire families. The same principles that guide one-on-one helping relationships also apply when the patient is a family unit, although communication within families requires additional understanding of the complexities of family dynamics, needs, and relationships (see Chapter 10).

Nurse–Health Care Team Relationships

Communication with other members of the health care team affects patient safety and the work environment. Breakdown in communication is a frequent cause of serious injuries in health care settings (World Health Organization, 2007). When patients move from one nursing unit to another or from one provider to another, also known as *hand-offs*, there is a risk for miscommunication. Accurate communication is essential to prevent errors (Cronenwett et al., 2007).

Use of common language when communicating critical information helps prevent misunderstandings. SBAR is a popular

BOX 24-5 EVIDENCE-BASED PRACTICE

Safe and Effective Interprofessional Communication

PICO Question: Do hand-off communication techniques in health care team communication improve patient outcomes?

Evidence Summary

Mutual respect and trust enable clarification and unambiguous communication. Establishing a relationship and face-to-face communication are important for teamwork. Practitioners need an understanding and appreciation of unique professional roles to work together as a team, collaborating to provide patient-centered care (Robinson et al., 2010; Sutter et al., 2009). Scorning others, making others feel incompetent, linguistic and cultural barriers, and overdependence on electronic communication systems contribute to ineffective communication (Sutter et al., 2009).

Use of communication techniques such as SBAR (Situation, Background, Assessment, Recommendation) provides a framework for a conversation among health care providers that fosters patient safety. Consistent communication practices minimize risk with hand-off communication (Amato-Vealey, Barba, and Vealey, 2008; Cronenwett et al., 2007).

Application to Nursing Practice

- Work in interdisciplinary teams to develop understanding and respect for other disciplines.
- Develop common language for critical information.
- Use a standardized SBAR format for report when patients are transferred to other units or facilities.
- Provide the opportunity for questions and confirmation of understanding of communication.

communication tool that helps standardize communication among health care providers. SBAR stands for Situation, Background, Assessment, and Recommendation (Pope et al., 2008). Research indicates that effective communication between health care providers and other members of the health care team ensures patient safety and promotes optimal patient outcomes (Amato-Vealey, Barba, and Vealey, 2008). Evidence identifies nursing actions that increase effectiveness of nurse-to-nurse interaction and interprofessional communication (Box 24-5).

Building Competency in Teamwork and Collaboration You are caring for Jane, a 78-year-old who was admitted this morning from home with pneumonia. On assessment you find that Jane has a temperature of 38.7° C (101.6° F) and an oxygen saturation of 88% on 3 L of oxygen and is confused and restless. Jane's daughter reports that Jane is usually alert and oriented, functions well, and lives alone. The health care provider has not seen Jane. Using SBAR (Situation-Background-Assessment-Recommendation), describe how you will communicate with the on-call physician to effectively address your concerns about Jane's condition.

Answers to questions can be found on the Evolve website.

Professional nursing care requires nurses to interact with members of the nursing team and interdisciplinary health care providers. Effective communication leads to a healthy work environment (Triola, 2006). Communication focuses on team building, facilitating group processes, collaborating, consulting, delegating, supervising, leading, and managing (see Chapter 21). Social, informational, and therapeutic interactions help team members build morale, accomplish goals, and strengthen working relationships. Lateral violence between colleagues sometimes occurs and includes behaviors such as withholding information, backbiting, making snide remarks, and nonverbal expressions of disapproval such as raising eyebrows or making faces. Lateral violence has an adverse effect on the work environment, leading to job dissatisfaction, poor retention of qualified nurses, nurses leaving the profession, and poor teamwork (Sheridan-Leos, 2008). It interferes with effective health care team communication and jeopardizes patient safety (Harter and Moody, 2010). Intimidation decreases the likelihood that a nurse will report a near-miss, question an order, or take action to improve the quality of patient care. There must be zero tolerance of lateral violence. Develop skill in conflict management and assertive communication to stop the spread of lateral violence in the workplace (Patterson, 2007).

Nurse-Community Relationships

Many nurses form relationships with community groups by participating in local organizations, volunteering for community service, or becoming politically active. You need to establish relationships with your community to be an effective change agent (see Chapter 3). Effective health communication requires awareness of language, nonverbal communication, and respect for contextual and cultural influences (Greef et al., 2009). Communication within the community occurs through channels such as neighborhood newsletters, health fairs, public bulletin boards, newspapers, radio, television, and electronic information sites. Use these forms of communication to share information and discuss issues important to community health.

ELEMENTS OF PROFESSIONAL COMMUNICATION

Professional appearance, demeanor, and behavior are important in establishing trustworthiness and competence. They communicate that you have assumed the professional helping role, are clinically skilled, and are focused on your patients. Nothing harms the professional image of nursing like an individual nurse's inappropriate appearance or behavior.

A professional is expected to be clean, neat, well groomed, conservatively dressed, and odor free. Visible tattoos and piercings are not acceptable in the professional setting. Professional behavior reflects warmth, friendliness, confidence, and competence. Professionals speak in a clear, well-modulated voice; use good grammar; listen to others; help and support colleagues; and communicate effectively. Being on time, organized, well prepared, and equipped for the responsibilities of the nursing role also communicate professionalism.

Courtesy

Common courtesy is part of professional communication. To practice courtesy, say hello and goodbye to patients and knock on doors before entering. State your purpose, address people by name, and say "'please" and "thank you" to team members. When a nurse is discourteous, others perceive him or her as rude or insensitive. It sets up barriers between nurse and patient and causes friction among team members.

Use of Names

Always introduce yourself. Failure to give your name and status (e.g., nursing student, registered nurse, or licensed practical nurse) or acknowledge a patient creates uncertainty about the interaction and conveys an impersonal lack of commitment or caring. Making eye contact and smiling recognizes others. Addressing people by name conveys respect for human dignity and uniqueness. Because using last names is respectful in most cultures, nurses usually use a patient's last name in an initial interaction and then use the first name if the patient requests it. Ask how your patients and co-workers prefer to be addressed and honor their personal preferences. Using first names is appropriate for infants, young children, patients who are confused or unconscious, and close team members. Avoid terms of endearment such as "honey," "dear," "grandma," or "sweetheart." Avoid referring to patients by diagnosis, room number, or other attribute, which is demeaning and sends the message that you do not care enough to know the person as an individual.

Trustworthiness

Trust is relying on someone without doubt or question. Being trustworthy means helping others without hesitation. To foster trust, communicate warmth and demonstrate consistency, reliability, honesty, competence, and respect. Sometimes it isn't easy for a patient to ask for help. Trusting another person involves risk and vulnerability; but it also fosters open, therapeutic communication and enhances the expression of feelings, thoughts, and needs. Without trust a nurse-patient relationship rarely progresses beyond social interaction and superficial care. Avoid dishonesty at all costs. Withholding key information, lying, or distorting the truth violates both legal and ethical standards of practice. Sharing personal information or gossiping about others sends the message that you cannot be trusted and damages interpersonal relationships.

Autonomy and Responsibility

Autonomy is being self-directed and independent in accomplishing goals and advocating for others. Professional nurses make choices and accept responsibility for the outcomes of their actions (Townsend, 2009). They take initiative in problem solving and communicate in a way that reflects the importance and purpose of the therapeutic conversation (Arnold and Boggs, 2011). Professional nurses also recognize a patient's autonomy.

Assertiveness

Assertiveness allows you to express feelings and ideas without judging or hurting others. Assertive behavior includes intermittent eye contact; nonverbal communication that reflects interest, honesty, and active listening; spontaneous verbal responses with a confident voice; and culturally sensitive use of touch and space. An assertive nurse communicates self-assurance; communicates feelings; takes responsibility for choices; and is respectful of others' feelings, ideas, and choices (Stuart, 2009; Townsend, 2009). Assertive behavior increases self-esteem and self-confidence, increases the ability to develop satisfying interpersonal relationships, and increases goal attainment. Assertive individuals make decisions and control their lives more effectively than nonassertive individuals. They deal with criticism and manipulation by others, learn to say no, set limits, and resist intentionally imposed guilt. Assertive responses contain "I" messages such as "I want," "I need," "I think," or "I feel" (Townsend, 2009).

NURSING PROCESS

Apply the nursing process and use a critical thinking approach in your care of patients. The nursing process provides a clinical decision-making approach for you to develop and implement an individualized plan of care. It guides care for patients who need special assistance with communication. Use therapeutic communication techniques as an intervention in an interpersonal nursing situation.

BOX 24-6 ASSESSMENT: FACTORS INFLUENCING COMMUNICATION

Psychophysiological Context

Internal factors influencing communication:
- Physiological status (e.g., pain, hunger, weakness, dyspnea)
- Emotional status (e.g., anxiety, anger, hopelessness, euphoria)
- Growth and development status (e.g., age, developmental tasks)
- Unmet needs (e.g., safety/security, love/belonging)
- Attitudes, values, and beliefs (e.g., meaning of illness experience)
- Perceptions and personality (e.g., optimist/pessimist, introvert/extrovert)
- Self-concept and self-esteem (e.g., positive or negative)

Relational Context

Nature of the relationship among participants:
- Social, helping, or working relationship
- Level of trust among participants
- Level of caring expressed
- Level of self-disclosure among participants
- Shared history of participants
- Balance of power and control

Situational Context

Reason for communication:
- Information exchange
- Goal achievement
- Problem resolution
- Expression of feelings

Environmental Context

Physical surroundings in which communication takes place:
- Privacy level
- Noise level
- Comfort and safety level
- Distraction level

Cultural Context

Sociocultural elements that affect an interaction:
- Educational level of participants
- Language and self-expression patterns
- Customs and expectations

ASSESSMENT

During the assessment process thoroughly assess each patient and critically analyze findings to ensure that you make patient-centered clinical decisions required for safe nursing care.

Through the Patient's Eyes. Patient-centered care requires careful assessment of a patient's values, preferences, and cultural, ethnic, and social backgrounds (Cronenwett et al., 2007). Internal and external factors affect a patient's ability to communicate (Box 24-6). Assessing these factors keeps the focus on the patient and helps you make patient-centered decisions during the communication process.

Physical and Emotional Factors. It is especially important to assess the psychophysiological factors that influence communication. Many altered health states and human responses limit communication. Persons with hearing or visual impairments often have difficulty receiving messages (see Chapter 49). Facial trauma, laryngeal cancer, or endotracheal intubation often prevents movement of air past vocal cords or mobility of the tongue, resulting in inability to articulate words. An extremely breathless person needs to use oxygen to breathe rather than speak. Persons with aphasia after a stroke or in late-stage Alzheimer's disease often cannot understand or form words. Some mental illnesses such as psychoses or depression cause patients to jump from one topic to another, constantly verbalize the same words or phrases, or exhibit a slowed speech pattern. Persons with high anxiety are sometimes unable to perceive environmental stimuli or hear explanations. Finally, patients who are unresponsive or heavily sedated cannot send or respond to verbal messages.

Review of a patient's medical record provides relevant information about his or her ability to communicate. The medical history and physical examination document physical barriers to speech, neurological deficits, and pathophysiology affecting hearing or vision. Reviewing a patient's medication record is also important. For example, opiates, antidepressants, neuroleptics, hypnotics, or sedatives may cause a patient to slur words or use incomplete sentences. The nursing progress notes sometimes reveal other factors that contribute to communication difficulties such as the absence of family members to provide more information about a confused patient.

Assessment includes communicating directly with patients to determine their ability to attend to, interpret, and respond to stimuli. If patients have difficulty communicating, it is important to assess the effect of the problem. Patients who cannot communicate effectively often have difficulty expressing needs and responding appropriately to the environment. Patients who are unable to speak are at risk for injury unless nurses identify an alternate communication method. If barriers exist that make it difficult to communicate directly with patients, family or friends become important sources concerning the patients' communication patterns and abilities.

Developmental Factors. Aspects of a patient's growth and development also influence nurse-patient interaction. For example, an infant's self-expression is limited to crying, body movement, and facial expression; whereas older children express their needs more directly. Adapt communication techniques to the special needs of infants and children. Communicating with children and their parents requires special consideration. Depending on the child's age, include the parents, child, or both as sources of information about the child's health. Giving a young child toys or other distractions allows parents to give you their full attention. Children are especially responsive to nonverbal messages; sudden movements, loud noises, or threatening gestures are frightening. They often prefer to make the first move in interpersonal contacts and do not like adults to stare or look down at them. A child who has received little environmental stimulation possibly is behind in language development, thus making communication more challenging.

Age alone does not determine an adult's capacity for communication. Hearing loss and visual impairments are common changes that occur during aging that contribute to communication barriers (Lubinski, 2010). Communicate with older adults on an adult level and avoid patronizing or speaking in a condescending manner. Simple measures facilitate communication with older individuals who have hearing loss (Box 24-7).

Sociocultural Factors. Culture influences thinking, feeling, behaving, and communicating. Be aware of the typical patterns of interaction that characterize various cultures. For example, European Americans are more open and willing to discuss private family matters; whereas Hispanics, African Americans, and Asian Americans are sometimes reluctant to reveal personal or family information to strangers. Hispanics and Asian Americans value a quiet demeanor and self-restraint; to be open or argumentative reflects negatively on family honor. Native Americans also value silence and are comfortable with it.

Foreign-born persons do not always speak or understand English. Those who speak English as a second language often experience difficulty with self-expression or language comprehension. To practice cultural sensitivity in communication, understand that persons of different cultures use different degrees of eye contact, personal space, gestures, loudness of voice, pace of speech, touch, silence, and meaning of language. Make a conscious effort not to interpret messages through your cultural perspective, but consider the communication within the context of the other individual's background. Avoid stereotyping, patronizing, or making fun of other cultures. Language and cultural barriers are not only frustrating but also dangerous, causing delay in care (Box 24-8).

BOX 24-7 FOCUS ON OLDER ADULTS

Tips for Improved Communication with Older Adults Who Have Hearing Loss

- Make sure the patient knows that you are talking.
- Face the patient, be sure that your face/mouth is visible to him or her, and do not chew gum or talk while chewing.
- Speak clearly but do not exaggerate lip movement or shout.
- Speak a little more slowly but not excessively slow.
- Check for hearing aids and glasses or use of adaptive equipment.
- Choose a quiet, well-lit environment with minimal distractions.
- Allow time for the patient to respond. Do not assume that patient is being uncooperative if he or she does not reply or takes a long time to reply.
- Give the patient a chance to ask questions.
- Keep communication short and to the point. Do not ramble and change subjects (Swann, 2007).

BOX 24-8 CULTURAL ASPECTS OF CARE

Communication with Non–English-Speaking Patients

Patients who speak little or no English present challenges for nurse-patient communication. Federal and state laws require that consumers of health care have access to interpreter services, but these services are costly; thus use is often limited to crucial interactions. Sometimes there is a delay in interpreter services, yet some patients require urgent care. Use of family members, children, or auxiliary personnel poses legal liabilities. Language is not the only barrier. Cultural differences also lead to misunderstanding. Developing cultural competence increases understanding (Regenstein et al., 2009; Cobb, 2010).

Implications for Practice

- Understand your own cultural values and biases.
- Assess the patient's primary language and level of fluency in English.
- Provide an interpreter for the patient and health care providers to communicate with each other.
- Speak directly to the patient even if an interpreter is present.
- Nodding or statements such as "OK" do not necessarily mean that the patient understands.
- Provide written information in English and primary language.
- Learn about other cultures, especially those commonly encountered in your work area.

Gender. Gender is another factor influencing how we think, act, feel, and communicate. Men tend to use less verbal communication but are more likely to initiate communication and address issues more directly. They are also more likely to talk about issues. Women tend to disclose more personal information and use more active listening, answering with responses that encourage the other person to continue the conversation. It is important for you to recognize a patient's gender communication pattern. Being insensitive blocks therapeutic nurse-patient relationships. Newer research questions the differences between male and female communication patterns (Arnold and Boggs, 2011). Assess communication patterns of each individual and do not make assumptions simply based on gender.

NURSING DIAGNOSIS

Most individuals experience difficulty with some aspect of communication. Patients sometimes lack skills in attending, listening, responding, and self-expression as a result of illness or the effects of treatment. You will use creative communication techniques with individuals who experience more serious impairments in communication.

The primary nursing diagnostic label used to describe a patient with limited or no ability to communicate verbally is *impaired verbal communication.* This is the state in which an individual experiences a decreased, delayed, or absent ability to receive, process, transmit, and use symbols (Doenges et al., 2010). A patient has defining characteristics such as the inability to articulate words, inappropriate verbalization, difficulty forming words, and difficulty comprehending, which you cluster together to form the diagnosis. This diagnosis is useful for a wide variety of patients with special problems and needs related to communication such as impaired perception, reception, and articulation. Although a patient's primary problem is impaired verbal communication, the associated difficulty in self-expression or altered communication patterns may also contribute to other nursing diagnoses:

- Anxiety
- Social isolation
- Ineffective coping
- Compromised family coping
- Powerlessness
- Impaired social interaction

The related factors for a nursing diagnosis focus on the causes of the communication disorder. In the case of impaired verbal communication, these are physiological, mechanical, anatomical, psychological, cultural, or developmental in nature. Accuracy in identifying related factors is necessary so you select interventions that effectively resolve the diagnostic problem. For example, you manage the diagnosis of *impaired verbal communication related to cultural difference (Hispanic heritage)* very differently than the diagnosis of *impaired verbal communication related to hearing loss.*

PLANNING

Once you have identified the nature of a patient's communication dysfunction, consider several factors when designing the care plan. Motivation is a factor in improving communication, and patients often require encouragement to try different approaches that involve significant change. It is especially important to involve the patient and family in decisions about the plan of care to determine whether suggested methods are acceptable. Meet basic comfort and safety needs before introducing new communication methods and techniques. Allow adequate time for practice. Participants need to be patient with themselves and one another to achieve effective communication. When the focus is on practicing communication, arrange for a quiet, private place that is free of distractions such as television or visitors. Communication aids such as a writing or picture board for a patient with a tracheostomy or a special call system for a paralyzed patient enhance communication.

Goals and Outcomes. In general, the goal of effective nursing care is that the patient experiences a sense of trust in the nurse and health care team. Expected outcomes for the patient with impaired communication are also important to identify. Outcomes are very specific and measurable and a way to determine if the broader goal is met. For example, outcomes for the patient possibly include the following:

- Patient initiates conversation about diagnosis or health care problem.
- Patient is able to attend to appropriate stimuli.
- Patient conveys clear and understandable messages with health care team.
- Patient expresses increased satisfaction with the communication process.

At times you care for patients whose difficulty in sending, receiving, and interpreting messages interferes with healthy interpersonal relationships. In this case impaired communication is a contributing factor to other nursing diagnoses such as *impaired social interaction* or *ineffective coping.* Plan interventions to help these patients improve their communication skills. Expected outcomes for a patient in this situation possibly include demonstrating the ability to appropriately express needs, feelings, and concerns; communicating thoughts and feelings more clearly; engaging in appropriate social conversation with peers and staff; and increasing feelings of autonomy and assertiveness.

Setting Priorities. It is essential to always maintain an open line of communication so a patient is able to express emergent needs or problems. This sometimes involves an intervention as simple as keeping a call light in reach for a patient restricted to bed or providing communication augmentative devices (e.g., message board or Braille computer). When you plan to have lengthy interactions with a patient, it is important to address physical care priorities so the discussion is not interrupted. Make the patient comfortable by ensuring that any symptoms are under control and elimination needs have been met.

Teamwork and Collaboration. To ensure an effective plan of care, you sometimes need to collaborate with other health care team members who have expertise in communication strategies. Speech therapists help patients with aphasia, interpreters are often necessary for patients who speak a foreign language, and mental health nurse specialists help angry or highly anxious patients to communicate more effectively.

IMPLEMENTATION

In carrying out any plan of care, use communication techniques that are appropriate for a patient's individual needs. Before learning how to adapt communication methods to help patients with serious communication impairments, it is necessary to learn the communication techniques that serve as the foundation for professional communication. It is also important to understand communication techniques that create barriers to effective interaction.

Therapeutic Communication Techniques. Therapeutic communication techniques are specific responses that encourage the expression of feelings and ideas and convey acceptance and respect. Learning these techniques helps you develop awareness of the variety of nursing responses available for use in different situations. Although some of the techniques seem artificial at first, skill and comfort increase with practice. Tremendous satisfaction results from developing therapeutic relationships and achieving desired patient outcomes.

Active Listening. Active listening means being attentive to what a patient is saying both verbally and nonverbally. Active listening facilitates patient communication. Inexperienced nurses sometimes feel the need to talk to prove they know what they are doing or to decrease anxiety (Stuart, 2009). It is often difficult at first to be quiet and really listen. Active listening enhances trust because you communicate acceptance and respect for a patient. Several nonverbal skills facilitate attentive listening. You identify them by the acronym SOLER (Townsend, 2009):

S—Sit facing the patient. This posture conveys the message that you are there to listen and are interested in what the patient is saying.

O—Observe an open posture (i.e., keep arms and legs uncrossed). This posture suggests that you are "open" to what the patient says. A "closed" position conveys a defensive attitude, possibly provoking a similar response in the patient.

L—Lean toward the patient. This posture conveys that you are involved and interested in the interaction.

E—Establish and maintain intermittent eye contact. This behavior conveys your involvement in and willingness to listen to what the patient is saying. Absence of eye contact or shifting the eyes gives the message that you are not interested in what the patient is saying.

R—Relax. It is important to communicate a sense of being relaxed and comfortable with the patient. Restlessness communicates a lack of interest and a feeling of discomfort to the patient.

Sharing Observations. Nurses make observations by commenting on how the other person looks, sounds, or acts. Stating observations often helps a patient communicate without the need for extensive questioning, focusing, or clarification. This technique helps start a conversation with quiet or withdrawn persons. Do not state observations that will embarrass or anger a patient, such as telling someone, "You look a mess!" Even if you make such an observation with humor, the patient can become resentful.

Sharing observations differs from making assumptions, which means drawing unnecessary conclusions about the other person without validating them. Making assumptions puts a patient in the position of having to contradict the nurse. Examples include the nurse interpreting fatigue as depression or assuming that untouched food indicates lack of interest in meeting nutritional goals. Making observations is a gentler and safer technique: "You look tired …," "You seem different today …," or "I see you haven't eaten anything."

Sharing Empathy. Empathy is the ability to understand and accept another person's reality, accurately perceive feelings, and communicate this understanding to the other. To convey empathy, accurately perceive the patient's situation, communicate that understanding to the patient, and act on your understanding to help the patient (Varcarolis and Halter, 2009). To express empathy, you reflect that you understand and feel the importance of the other person's communication. Such empathetic understanding requires you to be both sensitive and imaginative, especially if you have not had similar experiences. Strive to be empathetic in every situation because it is a key to unlocking concern and communicating support for others. Statements reflecting empathy are highly effective because they tell a person that you heard both the emotional and the factual content of the communication. Empathetic statements are neutral and nonjudgmental and help establish trust in difficult situations. For example, the nurse says to an angry patient who has low mobility after a stroke, "It must be very frustrating to know what you want and not be able to do it."

Sharing Hope. Nurses recognize that hope is essential for healing and learn to communicate a "sense of possibility" to others. Appropriate encouragement and positive feedback are important in fostering hope and self-confidence and for helping people achieve their potential and reach their goals. You give hope by commenting on the positive aspects of the other person's behavior, performance, or response. Sharing a vision of the future and reminding others of their resources and strengths also strengthen hope. Reassure patients that there are many kinds of hope and that meaning and personal growth can come from illness experiences. For example, the nurse says to a patient discouraged about a poor prognosis, "I believe that you'll find a way to face your situation because I've seen your courage and creativity."

Sharing Humor. Humor is an important but often underused resource in nursing interactions. It is a coping strategy that adds perspective and helps a nurse and patient adjust to stress. The Association for Applied and Therapeutic Humor (2008) defines therapeutic humor as "any intervention that promotes health and wellness by stimulating a playful discovery, expression or appreciation of the absurdity or incongruity of life's situations." Humor provides emotional support to patients and humanizes the illness experience. Patients use humor to establish relationships with care providers; relieve anxiety about illness, diagnostic procedures, or treatments; and release anger in a socially acceptable manner (Buxman, 2008). The goals of using humor as a health care provider are to bring hope and joy to the situation and enhance a patient's well-being and the therapeutic relationship. You use humor during the orientation phase of a relationship to establish a therapeutic relationship and during the working phase as you help a patient cope with a situation.

Today it is common that nurses care for patients from different cultures. When you interact with patients who do not have a full grasp of the language, it is important to realize that they may misunderstand or misinterpret jokes and statements meant to be humorous. It is also important to recognize that, when either a nurse or patient tries to speak in another language, mistakes sometimes occur.

Dean and Major (2008) found that humor enhances teamwork, relieves tension, and helps nurses reframe difficult situations, allowing them to gain perspective. It also increases emotional flexibility, allowing nurses to shift rapidly from one situation to another. Huntley (2009) noted that humor helps nurses cope with serious situations and improves the work environment. Laughter provides a diversion from stress-related tension.

Health care professionals sometimes use a kind of dark, negative humor after difficult or traumatic situations as a way to deal with unbearable tension and stress. This coping humor has a high potential for misinterpretation as uncaring by persons not involved in the situation. For example, nursing students are sometimes offended and wonder how staff are able to laugh and joke after unsuccessful resuscitation efforts. When nurses use coping humor within earshot of patients or their loved ones, great emotional distress results.

Sharing Feelings. Emotions are subjective feelings that result from one's thoughts and perceptions. Feelings are not right, wrong, good, or bad, although they are pleasant or unpleasant. If individuals do not express feelings, stress and illness may worsen. You help patients express emotions by making observations, acknowledging feelings, encouraging communication, giving permission to express "negative" feelings, and modeling healthy emotional self-expression. At times patients will direct their anger or frustration prompted by their illness toward you. Do not take such expressions personally. Acknowledging patients' feelings communicates that you listened to and understood the emotional aspects of their illness situation.

When you care for patients, be aware of your own emotions because feelings are difficult to hide. Students sometimes wonder whether it is helpful to share feelings with patients. Sharing emotion makes nurses seem more human and brings people closer. It is appropriate to share feelings of caring or even cry with others, as long as you are in control of the expression of these feelings and expresses them in a way that does not burden the patient or break confidentiality. Patients are perceptive and sense your emotions. It is usually inappropriate to discuss negative personal emotions such as anger or sadness with patients. A social support system of colleagues is helpful; and employee assistance programs, peer group meetings, and the use of interdisciplinary teams such as social work and pastoral care provide other means for nurses to safely express feelings away from patients.

Using Touch. Because of modern fast-paced technical environments, nurses are required more than ever to bring the sense of caring and human connection to their patients (see Chapter 7). Touch is one of the most potent forms of communication. Historically physical touch played a central role in healing (Leder and Krucoff, 2008). Nurses are privileged to experience more of this intimate form of personal contact than almost any other professional. Touch is used during procedures and assessment or to convey emotion (Playfair, 2010). It conveys many messages such as affection, emotional support, encouragement, tenderness, and personal attention. Comfort touch such as holding a hand is especially important for vulnerable patients who are experiencing severe illness with its accompanying physical and emotional losses (Fig. 24-2). When people are ill, they may feel detached from their body and become isolated from others. Touch helps them increase awareness of their body and gain connection with another person (Leder and Krucoff, 2008).

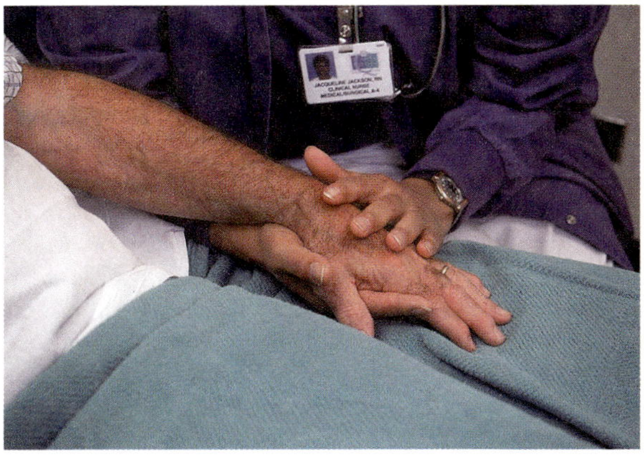

FIG. 24-2 The nurse uses touch to communicate.

Students often initially find giving intimate care to be stressful, especially when caring for patients of the opposite gender. They learn to cope with intimate contact by changing their perception of the situation. Since much of what nurses do involves touching, you need to learn to be sensitive to others' reactions to touch and use it wisely. It should be as gentle or as firm as needed and delivered in a comforting, nonthreatening manner. Sometimes you withhold touch (e.g., highly suspicious or angry persons respond negatively or even violently to a nurse's touch).

Using Silence. It takes time and experience to become comfortable with silence. Most people have a natural tendency to fill empty spaces with words, but sometimes these spaces really allow time for a nurse and patient to observe one another, sort out feelings, think about how to say things, and consider what has been communicated. Silence prompts some people to talk. It allows a patient to think and gain insight (Stuart, 2009). In general, allow a patient to break the silence, particularly when he or she has initiated it.

Silence is particularly useful when people are confronted with decisions that require much thought. For example, it helps a patient gain the necessary confidence to share the decision to refuse medical treatment. It also allows the nurse to pay particular attention to nonverbal messages such as worried expressions or loss of eye contact. Remaining silent demonstrates patience and a willingness to wait for a response when the other person is unable to reply quickly. Silence is especially therapeutic during times of profound sadness or grief.

Providing Information. Providing relevant information tells other people what they need or want to know so they are able to make decisions, experience less anxiety, and feel safe and secure. It is also an integral aspect of health teaching. It usually is not helpful to hide information from patients, particularly when they seek it. If a health care provider withholds information, the nurse clarifies the reason with him or her. Patients have a right to know about their health status and what is happening in their environment. Information of a distressing nature needs to be communicated with sensitivity, at a pace appropriate to a patient's ability to absorb it, and in general terms at first: "John, your heart sounds have changed from earlier today, and so has your blood pressure. I'll let your doctor know." A nurse provides information that enables others to understand what is happening and what to expect: "Mrs. Evans, John is getting an echocardiogram right now. This test uses painless sound waves to create a moving picture of his heart structures and valves and should tell us what is causing his murmur."

Clarifying. To check whether understanding is accurate, restate an unclear or ambiguous message to clarify the sender's meaning. In addition, ask the other person to rephrase it, explain further, or give an example of what the person means. Without clarification you may make invalid assumptions and miss valuable information. Despite efforts at paraphrasing, sometimes you do not understand the patient's message. You need to let the patient know if this is the case: "I'm not sure I understand what you mean by 'sicker than usual.' What is different now?"

Focusing. Focusing centers on key elements or concepts of a message. If conversation is vague or rambling or patients begin to repeat themselves, focusing is a useful technique. Do not use focusing if it interrupts patients while they are discussing an important issue. Rather use it to guide the direction of conversation to important areas: "We've talked a lot about your medications; now let's look more closely at the trouble you're having in taking them on time."

Paraphrasing. Paraphrasing is restating another's message more briefly using one's own words. Through paraphrasing you send feedback that lets a patient know that he or she is actively involved in the search for understanding. Practice is required to paraphrase accurately. If the meaning of a message is changed or distorted through paraphrasing, communication becomes ineffective. For example, a patient says, "I've been overweight all my life and never had any problems. I can't understand why I need to be on a diet." Paraphrasing this statement by saying, "You don't care if you're overweight," is incorrect. It is more accurate to say, "You're not convinced that you need a diet because you've stayed healthy."

Asking Relevant Questions. Nurses ask relevant questions to seek information needed for decision making. Ask only one question at a time and fully explore one topic before moving to another area. During patient assessment questions follow a logical sequence and usually proceed from general to more specific. Open-ended questions allow patients to take the conversational lead and introduce pertinent information about a topic. For example, "What's your biggest problem at the moment?" Use focused questions when more specific information is needed in an area: "How has your pain affected your life at home?" Allow patients to respond fully to open-ended questions before asking more-focused questions. Closed-ended questions elicit a yes, no, or one-word response: "How many times a day are you taking pain medication?" Although they are helpful during assessment, they are generally less useful during therapeutic exchanges.

Asking too many questions is sometimes dehumanizing. Seeking factual information does not allow a nurse or patient to establish a meaningful relationship or deal with important emotional issues. It is a way for a nurse to ignore uncomfortable areas in favor of more comfortable, neutral topics. A useful exercise is to try conversing without asking the other person a single question. By using techniques such as giving general leads ("tell me about it . . ."), making observations, paraphrasing, focusing, and providing information, you discover important information that would have remained hidden if you limited the communication process to questions alone.

Summarizing. Summarizing is a concise review of key aspects of an interaction. It brings a sense of satisfaction and closure to an individual conversation and is especially helpful during the termination phase of a nurse-patient relationship. By reviewing a conversation, participants focus on key issues and add relevant information as needed. Beginning a new interaction by summarizing a previous one helps a patient recall topics discussed and shows him or her that you analyzed their communication. Summarizing also clarifies expectations, as in this example of a nurse manager who has been working with an unsatisfied employee: "You've told me a lot of things about why you don't like this job and how unhappy you've been. We've also come up with some possible ways to make things better, and you've agreed to try some of them and let me know if any help."

Self-Disclosure. Self-disclosures are subjectively true personal experiences about the self that are intentionally revealed to another person. This is not therapy for a nurse; rather it shows patients that the nurse understands their experiences and their experiences are not unique. You choose to share experiences or feelings that are similar to those of the patient and emphasize both the similarities and differences. This kind of self-disclosure is indicative of the closeness of the nurse-patient relationship and involves a particular kind of respect for the patient. You offer it as an expression of sincerity and honesty, and it is an aspect of empathy (Stuart, 2009). Self-disclosures need to be relevant and appropriate and made to benefit the patient rather than yourself. Use them sparingly so the patient is the focus of the interaction: "That happened to me once, too. It was devastating, and I had to face some things about myself that I didn't like. I went for counseling, and it really helped. . . . What are your thoughts about seeing a counselor?"

Confrontation. When you confront someone in a therapeutic way, you help the other person become more aware of inconsistencies in his or her feelings, attitudes, beliefs, and behaviors (Stuart, 2009). This technique improves patient self-awareness and helps him or her recognize growth and deal with important issues. Use confrontation only after you have established trust, and do it gently with sensitivity: "You say you've already decided what to do, yet you're still talking a lot about your options."

Nontherapeutic Communication Techniques. Certain communication techniques hinder or damage professional relationships. These specific techniques are referred to as *nontherapeutic* or *blocking* and often cause recipients to activate defenses to avoid being hurt or negatively affected. Nontherapeutic techniques discourage further expression of feelings and ideas and engender negative responses or behaviors in others.

Asking Personal Questions. "Why don't you and John get married?" Asking personal questions that are not relevant to the situation simply to satisfy your curiosity is not appropriate professional communication. Such questions are nosy, invasive, and unnecessary. If patients wish to share private information, they will. To learn more about a patient's interpersonal roles and relationships, ask a question such as: "How would you describe your relationship with John?"

Giving Personal Opinions. "If I were you, I'd put your mother in a nursing home." When a nurse gives a personal opinion, it takes decision making away from the other person. It inhibits spontaneity, stalls problem solving, and creates doubt. Personal opinions differ from professional advice. At times people need suggestions and help to make choices. Suggestions that you present are options; the other person makes the final decision. Remember that the problem and its solution belong to the other person and not to you. A much better response is, "Let's talk about which options are available for your mother's care."

Changing the Subject. "Let's not talk about your problems with the insurance company. It's time for your walk." Changing the subject when another person is trying to communicate their story is rude and shows a lack of empathy. It tends to block further communication, and the sender then withholds important messages or fails to openly express feelings. Thoughts and spontaneity are interrupted, ideas become tangled, and information provided is sometimes inadequate. In some instances changing the subject serves as a face-saving maneuver. If this happens, reassure the patient that you will return to his or her concerns: "After your walk let's talk some more about what's going on with your insurance company."

Automatic Responses. "Older adults are always confused." "Administration doesn't care about the staff." Stereotypes are generalized beliefs held about people. Making stereotyped remarks about others reflects poor nursing judgment and threatens nurse-patient or team relationships. A cliché is a stereotyped comment such as, "You can't win them all," that tends to belittle the other person's feelings and minimize the importance of his or her message. These automatic phrases communicate that you are not taking concerns seriously or responding thoughtfully. Another kind of automatic response is parroting (i.e., repeating what the other person has said word for word). Parroting is easily overused and is not as effective as paraphrasing. A simple "oh?" gives you time to think if the other person says something that takes one by surprise.

A nurse who is task oriented automatically makes the task or procedure the entire focus of interaction with patients, missing opportunities to communicate with them as individuals and meet their needs. Task-oriented nurses are often perceived as cold, uncaring, and unapproachable. When students first perform technical skills, it is difficult to integrate therapeutic communication because of the need to focus on the procedure. In time you learn to integrate communication with high-visibility tasks and accomplish several goals simultaneously.

False Reassurance. "Don't worry, everything will be all right." When a patient is seriously ill or distressed, you may be tempted to offer hope to the patient with statements such as "You'll be fine" or "There's nothing to worry about." When a patient is reaching for understanding, false reassurance discourages open communication. Offering reassurance not supported by facts or based in reality does more harm than good. Although you are trying to be kind, it has the secondary effect of helping you avoid the other person's distress, and it tends to block conversation and discourage further expression of feelings. A more facilitative response is, "It must be difficult not to know what the surgeon will find. What can I do to help?"

Sympathy. "I'm so sorry about your mastectomy; it must be terrible to lose a breast." Sympathy is concern, sorrow, or pity felt for a patient. The nurse takes on a patient's problems as if they were his or her own. Sympathy is a subjective look at another person's world that prevents a clear perspective of the issues confronting that person. If a nurse overidentifies with a patient, objectivity is lost, and the nurse is not able to help the patient work through the situation (Townsend, 2009). Although sympathy is a compassionate response to another's situation, it is not as therapeutic as empathy. A nurse's own emotional issues sometimes prevent effective problem solving and impair good judgment. A more empathetic approach is: "The loss of a breast is a major change. How do you think it will affect your life?"

Asking for Explanations. "Why are you so anxious?" Some nurses are tempted to ask the other person to explain why the person believes, feels, or has acted in a certain way. Patients frequently interpret "why" questions as accusations or think the nurse knows the reason and is simply testing them. Regardless of patient perception of your motivation, "why" questions cause resentment, insecurity, and mistrust. If you need additional information, it is best to phrase a question to avoid using the word "why." "You seem upset. What's on your mind?" is more likely to help the anxious patient communicate.

Approval or Disapproval. "You shouldn't even think about assisted suicide; it's not right." Do not impose your own attitudes, values, beliefs, and moral standards on others while in the professional helping role. Other people have the right to be themselves and make their own decisions. Judgmental responses often contain terms such as *should, ought, good, bad, right,* or *wrong.* Agreeing or disagreeing sends the subtle message that you have the right to make value judgments about patient decisions. Approving implies that the behavior being praised is the only acceptable one. Often a patient shares a decision with you, not in an effort to seek approval but to provide a means to discuss feelings. Disapproval implies that the patient needs to meet your expectations or standards. Instead help patients explore their own beliefs and decisions. The response, "I'm surprised you're considering assisted suicide. Tell me more about it," gives the patient a chance to express ideas or feelings without fear of being judged.

Defensive Responses. "No one here would intentionally lie to you." Becoming defensive in the face of criticism implies that the other person has no right to an opinion. The sender's concerns are ignored when the nurse focuses on the need for self-defense, defense of the health care team, or defense of others. When patients express criticism, listen to what they have to say. Listening does not imply agreement. You need to listen uncritically to discover reasons for a patient's anger or dissatisfaction. By avoiding a defensive attitude you are able to defuse anger and uncover deeper concerns: "You believe that people have been dishonest with you. It must be hard to trust anyone."

Passive or Aggressive Responses. "Things are bad, and there's nothing I can do about it." "Things are bad, and it's all your fault." Passive responses serve to avoid conflict or sidestep issues. They reflect feelings of sadness, depression, anxiety, powerlessness, and hopelessness. Aggressive responses provoke confrontation at the other person's expense. They reflect feelings of anger, frustration, resentment, and stress. Nurses who lack assertive skills also use triangulation, complaining to a third party rather than confronting the problem or expressing concerns directly to the source. This lowers team morale and draws others into the conflict situation. Assertive communication is a far more professional approach for the nurse to take.

Arguing. "How can you say you didn't sleep a wink when I heard you snoring all night long?" Challenging or arguing against perceptions denies that they are real and valid to the other person. It implies that the other person is lying, misinformed, or uneducated. The skillful nurse gives information or presents reality in a way that avoids argument: "You feel like you didn't get any rest at all last night, even though I thought you slept well since I heard you snoring."

Adapting Communication Techniques for the Patient with Special Needs. With our aging population more patients have difficulty communicating. Hearing loss increases with age; 47% of Americans age 75 or older have a hearing impairment (NIDCD, 2010). Vision loss affects communication and presents a challenge for the 6.5 million Americans age 65 and older who report significant vision loss (AFB, 2010). Interacting with people who have conditions that impair communication requires special thought and sensitivity. Such patients benefit greatly when you adapt communication techniques to their unique circumstances or developmental level. For example, a nurse caring for a patient with *impaired verbal communication related to cultural differences* provides a table of simple words in the patient's language. The nurse and patient use the table to help communicate about basic needs such as food, water, toileting, pain relief, and sleep. Environmental considerations and adaptive equipment improve communication with hearing-impaired individuals (Swann, 2007). Research findings suggest that many of the difficulties in communicating with patients with severe communication impairment come from the lack of an understandable nurse-patient communication system (Hemsley et al., 2001). Further research in care of adults with cerebral palsy found that successful communication between nurses and patients with complex communication needs requires the nurse's knowledge of communication assistive devices and collaboration with the patient and family (Balandin et al., 2007).

A nurse directs actions toward meeting the goals and expected outcomes identified in the plan of care, addressing both the communication impairment and its contributing factors. Box 24-9 lists many methods available to encourage, enhance, restore, or substitute for verbal communication. Be sure that a patient is physically able to use the chosen method and that it does not cause frustration by being too complicated or difficult.

BOX 24-9 COMMUNICATING WITH PATIENTS WHO HAVE SPECIAL NEEDS

Patients Who Cannot Speak Clearly (Aphasia, Dysarthria, Muteness)
- Listen attentively, be patient, and do not interrupt.
- Ask simple questions that require "yes" or "no" answers.
- Allow time for understanding and response.
- Use visual cues (e.g., words, pictures, and objects) when possible.
- Allow only one person to speak at a time.
- Encourage patient to converse.
- Let patient know if you have not understood him or her.
- Collaborate with speech therapist as needed.
- Use communication aids:

Patients Who Are Cognitively Impaired
- Use simple sentences and avoid long explanations.
- Ask one question at a time.
- Allow time for patient to respond.
- Be an attentive listener.
- Include family and friends in conversations, especially in subjects known to patient.

Patients Who Are Hearing Impaired
- Check for hearing aids and glasses.
- Reduce environmental noise.
- Get patient's attention before speaking.
- Face patient with mouth visible.
- Do not chew gum.
- Speak at normal volume—do not shout.
- Rephrase rather than repeat if misunderstood.
- Provide a sign language interpreter if indicated.

Patients Who Are Visually Impaired
- Check for use of glasses or contact lenses.
- Identify yourself when you enter room and notify patient when you leave room.
- Speak in a normal tone of voice.
- Do not rely on gestures or nonverbal communication.
- Use indirect lighting, avoiding glare.
- Use at least 14-point print.

Patients Who Are Unresponsive
- Call patient by name during interactions.
- Communicate both verbally and by touch.
- Speak to patient as though he or she can hear.
- Explain all procedures and sensations.
- Provide orientation to person, place, and time.
- Avoid talking about patient to others in his or her presence.

Patients Who Do Not Speak English
- Speak to patient in normal tone of voice.
- Establish method for patient to ask for assistance (call light or bell).
- Provide an interpreter as needed.
- Avoid using family members, especially children, as interpreters.
- Use communication board, pictures, or cards.
- Translate words from native language into English list for patient to make basic requests.
- Have dictionary (e.g., English/Spanish) available if patient can read.

Because nursing care of the older adult is ideally delivered through an interdisciplinary model, the primary goal is to establish a reliable communication system that all health care team members can understand easily. Effective communication involves adapting to special needs resulting from sensory, motor, or cognitive impairments. Encouraging older adults to share life stories and reminisce about the past has a therapeutic effect and increases their sense of well-being. Avoid sudden shifts from subject to subject. It is helpful to include a patient's family and friends and become familiar with a patient's favorite topics for conversation.

EVALUATION

Evaluate the effectiveness of your own communication by videotaping practice sessions with peers or by making process recordings—written records of your verbal and nonverbal interactions with patients. Process recording analysis reveals how to improve personal communication techniques to make them more effective. Box 24-10 contains a sample communication analysis of such a record. Analysis of a process recording enables you to evaluate the following:

- Determine whether you encouraged openness and allowed the patient to "tell his story," expressing both thoughts and feelings
- Identify any missed verbal or nonverbal cues or conversational themes
- Examine whether nursing responses blocked or facilitated the patient's efforts to communicate
- Determine whether nursing responses were positive and supportive or superficial and judgmental
- Examine the type and number of questions asked
- Determine the type and number of therapeutic communication techniques used
- Discover any missed opportunities to use humor, silence, or touch

Through the Patient's Eyes. You and your patient determine the success of the plan of care by evaluating patient communication outcomes together. You also evaluate nursing interventions to determine what strategies or interventions were effective and what patient changes resulted because of the interventions. Ask the patient if you and other members of the interdisciplinary health care team met his or her expectations. Successful nursing care related to patients' communication needs results in clear and effective communication between patients and all members of the health care team. Other outcomes include patient satisfaction and the delivery of safe care.

Patient Outcomes. If expected outcomes are not met or if progress is not satisfactory, you determine what factors influenced the outcomes, then modify the plan of care. If your evaluation data indicate a patient perceives difficulty in communicating, you explore contributing factors so they can be addressed. For example, if using a pen and paper is frustrating for a nonverbal patient whose handwriting is shaky, you revise the care plan to include use of a picture board instead. Possible questions you ask when a patient does not meet expected outcomes include:

- You seem to be having difficulty communicating right now. What do you think is contributing to this?
- You are telling me that you do not feel anxious right now, but your face appears tense. Help me better understand how you are feeling right now.

BOX 24-10 SAMPLE COMMUNICATION ANALYSIS

Nurse: "Good morning, Mr. Simpson."
(Smiles, approaches bed holding clipboard)
Acknowledged by name, social greeting to begin conversation

Patient: "What's good about it?"
(Arms crossed over chest, frowning, direct stare)
Nonverbal signs of anger

Nurse: "You sound unhappy."
(Pulls up chair and sits at bedside)
Sharing observation, nonverbal communication of availability

Patient: "You'd be unhappy, too, if nobody would answer your questions. That girl wouldn't tell me my blood sugar."
(Angry voice tone, challenging expression)
Further expression of feelings facilitated by nurse making accurate observation

Nurse: "This hospital has a fine staff, Mr. Simpson. I'm sure no one would intentionally keep information from you."
Feeling threatened and being defensive, a nontherapeutic technique

Nurse: "I'm going to test your glucose in a minute, and I'll tell you the results."
(Does test) "Your blood sugar was 350."
Providing information, demonstrating trustworthiness

Patient: "I'm so afraid complications will set in since my blood sugar is high."
(Stares out window)
Feels free to express deeper concerns, but they are hard to face

Nurse: "What kinds of things are you worried about?"
Open-ended question to seek information

Patient: "I could lose a leg, like my mother did, or go blind or have to live hooked up to a kidney machine for the rest of my life.

Nurse: "You've been thinking about all kinds of things that could go wrong, and it adds to your worry not to be told what your blood sugar is."
Summarizing to let patient "hear" what he has communicated

Patient: "I always think the worst."
(Shakes head in exasperation)
Expressing insight into his "inner dialogue"

Nurse: "I'll pass along to the tech that it's OK to tell you your glucose levels. And later this afternoon I'd like us to talk more about some things you can do to help avoid these complications and set some goals for controlling your glucose."
Providing information, encouraging collaboration and goal setting

- You seem frustrated with the use of pencil and paper to communicate. Would you like to try a letter board or a picture board and see if either of these is easier for you to use?

Evaluation of the communication process helps nurses gain confidence and competence in interpersonal skills. Becoming an effective communicator greatly increases the nurse's professional satisfaction and success. There is no skill more basic, no tool more powerful.

KEY POINTS

- Communication is a powerful therapeutic tool and an essential nursing skill that influences others and achieves positive health outcomes.
- Effective interdisciplinary communication is essential to provide safe transitions and care.
- Effective communication is critical in promoting collaboration and teamwork providing patient-centered care.
- Critical thinking facilitates communication through creative inquiry, focused self-awareness and awareness of others, purposeful analysis, and control of perceptual biases.
- Communication is most effective when the receiver and sender accurately perceive the meaning of one another's messages.
- The sender's and receiver's physical and developmental status, perceptions, values, emotions, knowledge, sociocultural background, roles, and environment all influence message transmission.
- Effective verbal communication requires appropriate intonation, clear and concise phrasing, proper pacing of statements, and proper timing and relevance of a message.
- Effective nonverbal communication complements and strengthens the message conveyed by verbal communication.
- Nurses use intrapersonal, interpersonal, transpersonal, small-group, and public interaction to achieve positive change and health goals.
- Nurses strengthen helping relationships by establishing trust, empathy, autonomy, confidentiality, and professional competence.
- Effective communication techniques are facilitative and tend to encourage the other person from openly expressing ideas, feelings, or concerns.
- Ineffective communication techniques are inhibiting and tend to block the other person's willingness to openly express ideas, feelings, or concerns.
- Blend social and informational interactions with therapeutic communication techniques to help your patients explore feelings and manage health issues.
- Older adults with sensory, motor, or cognitive impairments require the adaptation of communication techniques to compensate for their loss of function and special needs.
- Patients with impaired verbal communication require special consideration and alterations in communication techniques to facilitate sending, receiving, and interpreting messages.
- Desired outcomes for patients with impaired verbal communication include increased satisfaction with interpersonal interactions, the ability to send and receive clear messages, and attention to and accurate interpretation of verbal and nonverbal cues.

CLINICAL APPLICATION QUESTIONS

Preparing for Clinical Practice

Mr. Simpson is a 78-year-old patient whose wife died last year. He has been living alone. He has limited cooking skills; thus he eats out a lot. Since his wife died, his blood sugar has been poorly controlled. To help Mr. Simpson gain better blood sugar control, the dietitian came to see him. After she left, Mr. Simpson was angry and stated his desire to leave the hospital right now. He stated, "That diet person came to see me, and she doesn't know anything."

1. How would you approach Mr. Simpson? What communication techniques would you use and what would you avoid?
2. You talk with the dietitian and learn that she gave the patient information about his diet and recipes he could try. As you talk with him, you learn that the physician told him he might not be able to live alone anymore. You realize that he doesn't know how to cook. Knowing this, how would you respond to him?

3. After talking with Mr. Simpson, you determine that he is able to care for himself at home but will need some assistance. He is willing to consider various options for meal preparation. You call the physician to discuss this. Your hospital has established SBAR (Situation-Background-Assessment-Recommendation) as a standard communication tool. How do you effectively communicate your concerns and the patient's need to the physician using SBAR?

evolve *Answers to Clinical Application Questions can be found on the Evolve website.*

REVIEW QUESTIONS

Are You Ready to Test Your Nursing Knowledge?

1. The nurse summarizes the conversation with the patient to determine if the patient has understood him or her. This is what element of the communication process?
   1. Referent
   2. Channel
   3. Environment
   4. Feedback
2. Mrs. Jones states that she gets anxious when she thinks about giving herself insulin. How do you use your understanding of intrapersonal communication to help with this?
   1. Provide her the opportunity to practice drawing up insulin
   2. Coach her to give herself positive messages about her ability to do this
   3. Bring her written material that clearly describes the steps of insulin administration
   4. Use therapeutic communication to help her express her feeling about giving herself an injection
3. The nurse has a patient who is short of breath and calls the health care provider using SBAR (Situation-Background-Assessment-Recommendation) to help with the communication. What does the nurse first address?
   1. The respiratory rate is 28.
   2. The patient has a history of lung cancer.
   3. The patient is short of breath.
   4. He or she requests an order for a breathing treatment.
4. You are caring for Mr. Smith, who is facing amputation of his leg. During the orientation phase of the relationship, what would you do?
   1. Summarize what you have talked about in the previous sessions
   2. Review his medical record and talk to other nurses about how he is reacting
   3. Explore his feelings about losing his leg
   4. Talk with him about his favorite hobbies
5. The nurse states, "When you tell me that you're having a hard time living up to expectations, are you talking about your family's expectations?" The nurse is using which therapeutic communication technique?
   1. Providing information
   2. Clarifying
   3. Focusing
   4. Paraphrasing
6. Which of the following statements would be most likely to block communication?
   1. "You look kind of tired today."
   2. "Why do you always put so much salt on your food?"
   3. "It sounds like this has been a hard time for you."
   4. "If you use your oxygen when you walk, you may be able to walk farther."
7. You are caring for an 80-year-old woman, and you ask her a question while you are across the room washing your hands. She does not answer. What is your next action?
   1. Leave the room quietly since she evidently does not want to be bothered right now
   2. Repeat the question in a loud voice, speaking very slowly
   3. Move to her bedside, get her attention, and repeat the question while facing her
   4. Bring her a communication board so she can express her needs
8. You ask another nurse how to collect a laboratory specimen. The nurse raises her eyebrows and asks, "Why don't you figure it out?" What would be the best response?
   1. Say nothing and walk away. Find a different nurse to help you.
   2. "When you brush me off like that, it takes me even longer to do my job."
   3. "Why do you always put me down like that?"
   4. "I guess I just enjoy having you make fun of me."
9. When the nurse takes the patient's nursing history, he or she sits:
   1. Next to the patient.
   2. 4 to 12 feet from the patient.
   3. 18 inches to 4 feet from the patient.
   4. 12 inches to 3 feet from the patient.
10. When working with an older adult, the nurse remembers to avoid:
    1. Touching the patient.
    2. Allowing the patient to reminisce.
    3. Shifting quickly from subject to subject.
    4. Asking the patient how he or she feels.
11. The statement that best explains the role of collaboration with others for the patient's plan of care is which of the following?
    1. The professional nurse consults the health care provider for direction in establishing goals for patients.
    2. The professional nurse depends on the latest literature to complete an excellent plan of care for patients.
    3. The professional nurse works independently to plan and deliver care and does not depend on other staff for assistance.
    4. The professional nurse works with colleagues and the patient's family to provide combined expertise in planning care.
12. Identify behaviors that foster the development of trust. (Select all that apply.)
    1. Answer the call light promptly.
    2. Call the patient by first name unless requested otherwise.
    3. Do all the care as quickly as possible and leave the room so the patient can rest.
    4. Answer questions honestly.
    5. Demonstrate competence when doing treatments.
13. A patient with limited English proficiency is going to be discharged on new medication. How does the nurse complete the discharge teaching?
    1. Uses a dictionary to give directions for medication administration
    2. Explains the directions to the patient's 14-year-old daughter

3. Obtains an interpreter to facilitate communication of medication information
4. Uses a picture board and visual aids to communicate medication administration information

14. Your patient has just been told that she has cancer, and she is crying. Which actions facilitate therapeutic communication? (Select all that apply.)
    1. Turning on the television to her favorite show
    2. Pulling the curtain to provide privacy
    3. Offering to discuss information about her condition
    4. Asking her why she is crying
    5. Sitting quietly by her bed and hold her hand

15. Mr. Sakda emigrated from Thailand. When taking care of him, you note that he looks relaxed and smiles but seldom looks at you directly. How do you respond?
    1. Use therapeutic communication to assess for increased anxiety
    2. Sit down and position yourself closer so you are at eye level
    3. Deflect your eyes downward to show respect
    4. Continue to maintain eye contact

Answers: **1.** 4; **2.** 2; **3.** 3; **4.** 4; **5.** 2; **6.** 2; **7.** 3; **8.** 2; **9.** 3; **10.** 3; **11.** 4; **12.** 1, 4, 5; **13.** 3; **14.** 2, 3, 5; **15.** 3.

REFERENCES

American Foundation for the Blind (AFB: Facts and figures on adults with vision loss, http://www.afb.org/Section.asp?SectionID=15&TopicID=413&DocumentID=4900, 2010. Accessed August 16, 2011.

Amato-Vealey EJ, Barba MP, Vealey RJ: Hand-off communication: a requisite for perioperative patient safety, *AORN J* 88(5):763, 2008.

Arnold E, Boggs KU: *Interpersonal relationships: professional communication skills for nurses*, ed 6, St Louis, 2011, Saunders.

Association for Applied and Therapeutic Humor: Home page, 2008, http://www.aath.org/. Accessed August 16, 2011.

Balzer-Riley J: *Communication in nursing*, ed 6, St Louis, 2007, Mosby.

Beebe SA, et al: *Interpersonal communication: relating to others*, ed 6, Boston, 2010, Allyn & Bacon.

Buxman K: Humor in the OR: a stitch in time? *AORN J* 88(1):67, 2008.

Chitty KK: *Professional nursing concepts and challenges*, ed 6, St Louis, 2010, Saunders.

Cobb TG: Strategies for providing cultural competent health care for Hmong Americans, *J Cultural Diversity* 17(3):79, 2010.

Cronenwett L, et al: Quality and safety education for nurses, *Nurs Outlook* 55(3):122, 2007.

Doenges ME, et al: *Nursing diagnosis manual: planning, individualizing, and documenting client care*, ed 3, Philadelphia, 2010, FA Davis.

Gibson AS, Foster C: The role of self-talk in the awareness of physiological state and physical performance, *Sports Med* 37(12):1029, 2007.

Harter M, Moody C: The cost of lateral violence: all pain and no gain, *SC Nurse* 17(1):4, 2010.

Huntley MJ: Take time for laughter, *Creat Nurs* 15(1):39, 52, 2009.

Jones L: The healing relationship, *Nurs Standard* 24(3):64, 2009.

Kneisl CR, Trigoboff E: *Contemporary psychiatric–mental health nursing*, ed 2, Upper Saddle River, NJ, 2009, Pearson Education.

Lane MR: Arts in health care: a new paradigm for holistic nursing practice, *J Holistic Nurs* 24(1):70, 2006.

Leder D, Krucoff MW: The touch that heals: the uses and meanings of touch in the clinical encounter, *J Altern Complement Med* 14(3):321, 2008.

Lubinski R: Communicating effectively with elders and their families, *The ASHA Leader*, March 16, 2010.

National Institute on Deafness and other Communication Disorders (NIDCD): *Quick statistics*, http://www.nidcd.nih.gov/health/statistics/quick.htm, 2010. Accessed August 16, 2011.

Patterson P: Lateral violence: why it's serious and what OR managers can do, *OR Manager* 23(12):1, 2007.

Paul R: The art of redesigning instruction. In Willsen J, Blinker AJA, editors: *Critical thinking: how to prepare students for a rapidly changing world*, Santa Rosa, Calif, 1993, Foundation for Critical Thinking.

Playfair C: Human relationships: an exploration of loneliness and touch, *Br J Nurs* 19(2):122, 2010.

Pope B, et al: Raising the SBAR: how better communication improves patient outcomes, *Nursing* 38(3):41, 2008.

Sheridan-Leos N: Understanding lateral violence in nursing, *Clin J Oncol Nurs* 12(3):399, 2008.

Stuart GW: *Principles and practice of psychiatric nursing*, ed 9, St Louis, 2009, Mosby.

Swann J: Helpful vibrations: assistive devices in hearing loss, *Nurs Residential Care* 9(11):531, 2007.

Tavernier SS: An evidence-based conceptual analysis of presence, *Holistic Nurs Pract* 20(3):152, 2006.

Townsend MC: *Psychiatric mental health nursing: concepts of care*, Philadelphia, 2009, FA Davis.

Varcarolis EM, Halter MJ: *Essentials of psychiatric mental health nursing: a communication approach to evidence based care*, St Louis, 2009, Elsevier.

Watson J: *Nursing: human science and health care*, Norwalk, Conn, 1985, Appleton-Century-Crofts.

White SJ: Using self-talk to embrace career satisfaction and performance, *Am J Health Syst Pharm* 65(6):514, 516, 519, 2008.

World Health Organization: Communication during patient hand-overs, *Patient Safety Solutions* 1(solution 3):1, www.who.int/entity/patientsafety/solutions/patientsafety/PS-Solution3.pdf, May 2007. Accessed August 17, 2011.

RESEARCH REFERENCES

Andreas DC, et al: Understanding risk communication through patient narratives about complex antithrombotic therapies, *Qual Health Res* 20(8):1155, 2010.

Balandin S, et al: Communicating with nurses: the experiences of 10 adults with cerebral palsy and complex communication needs, *Appl Nurs Res* 20(2):56, 2007.

Dawood M, Gallini A: Using discovery interviews to understand the patient experience, *Nurs Manage* 17(1):26, 2010.

Dean RAK, Major JE: From critical care to comfort care: the sustaining value of humour, *J Clin Nurs* 17:1088, 2008.

Greef M, et al: Students' community health service delivery: experiences of involved parties, *Curationis* 32(1):33, 2009.

Hemsley B, et al: Nursing the patient with severe communication impairment, *J Adv Nurs* 35(6):827, 2001.

Pesut B, et al: Conceptualizing spirituality and religion for healthcare, *J Clin Nurs* 17(21):2803, 2008.

Regenstein M, et al: Challenges in language services: identifying and responding to patients' needs, *J Immigrant Minority Health* 11:476, 2009.

Robinson FP, et al: Perceptions of effective and ineffective nurse-physician communication in hospitals, *Nurs Forum* 45(3):206, 2010.

Sheldon LK, et al: Difficult communication in nursing, *J Nurs Scholarsh* 38(2):141, 2006.

Sutter E, et al: Role understanding and effective communication as core competencies for collaborative practice, *J Interprofessional Care* 23(1):41, 2009.

Triola N: Dialogue and discourse: are we having the right conversations? *Crit Care Nurse* 26(1):60, 2006.

Williams AM, Irurita VF: Emotional comfort: the patient's perspective of a therapeutic context, *Int J Nurs Stud* 43(4):405, 2006.

CHAPTER

25

Patient Education

OBJECTIVES

- Identify the appropriate topics that address a patient's health education needs.
- Describe the similarities and differences between teaching and learning.
- Identify the role of the nurse in patient education.
- Identify the purposes of patient education.
- Use communication principles when providing patient education.
- Describe the domains of learning.
- Identify basic learning principles.
- Discuss how to integrate education into patient-centered care.
- Differentiate factors that determine readiness to learn from those that determine ability to learn.
- Compare and contrast the nursing and teaching processes.
- Write learning objectives for a teaching plan.
- Establish an environment that promotes learning.
- Include patient teaching while performing routine nursing care.
- Use appropriate methods to evaluate learning.

KEY TERMS

Affective learning, p. 331
Analogies, p. 341
Cognitive learning, p. 330
Functional illiteracy, p. 337
Health literacy, p. 337
Learning, p. 329
Learning objective, p. 330
Motivation, p. 332
Psychomotor learning, p. 331
Reinforcement, p. 340
Return demonstration, p. 341
Self-efficacy, p. 332
Teaching, p. 329

evolve WEBSITE

http://evolve.elsevier.com/Potter/fundamentals/

- Review Questions
- Case Study with Questions
- Audio Glossary
- Interactive Learning Activities
- Key Term Flashcards
- Content Updates

Patient education is one of the most important roles for a nurse in any health care setting. Shorter hospital stays, increased demands on nurses' time, an increase in the number of chronically ill patients, and the need to give acutely ill patients meaningful information quickly emphasize the importance of quality patient education. As nurses try to find the best way to educate patients, the general public has become more assertive in seeking knowledge, understanding health, and finding resources available within the health care system. Nurses provide patients with information needed for self-care to ensure continuity of care from the hospital to the home (Falvo, 2010).

Patients have the right to know and be informed about their diagnoses, prognoses, and available treatments to help them make intelligent, informed decisions about their health and lifestyle. Part of patient-centered care is to integrate educational approaches that acknowledge patients' expertise with their own health. Creating a well-designed, comprehensive teaching plan that fits a patient's unique learning needs reduces health care costs, improves the quality of care, and ultimately changes behaviors to improve patient outcomes. Ultimately this helps patients make informed decisions about their care and become healthier and more independent (Edelman and Mandle, 2010; Villablanca et al., 2010).

STANDARDS FOR PATIENT EDUCATION

Patient education has long been a standard for professional nursing practice. All state Nurse Practice Acts recognize that patient teaching falls within the scope of nursing practice (Bastable, 2006). In addition, various accrediting agencies set guidelines for providing patient education in health care institutions. For example, The Joint Commission (TJC, 2011) sets standards for patient and family education. These standards require nurses and the health care team to assess patients' learning needs and provide education about many topics, including medications, nutrition, the use of medical equipment, pain, and the patient's plan of care. Successful accomplishment of the standards requires collaboration among health care professionals and enhances patient safety. Educational efforts should be patient-centered by taking into consideration patients' own education and experience, their desire to actively participate in the educational process, and their psychosocial, spiritual, and cultural values. It is important to document evidence of successful patient education in patients' medical records. Standards such as these help to direct your patient education.

PURPOSES OF PATIENT EDUCATION

The goal of educating others about their health is to help individuals, families, or communities achieve optimal levels of health (Edelman and Mandle, 2010). Patient education is an essential component of providing safe, patient-centered care (QSEN, 2010). In addition, providing education about preventive health care helps reduce health care costs and hardships on individuals, families, and communities. Patients now know more about health and want to be involved in health maintenance. Provide education about health and health care in places that are convenient and familiar to patients. Comprehensive patient education includes three important purposes, each involving a separate phase of health care.

Maintenance and Promotion of Health and Illness Prevention

As a nurse you are a visible, competent resource for patients who want to improve their physical and psychological well-being. In the school, home, clinic, or workplace you provide information and skills that enable patients to assume healthier behaviors. For example, in childbearing classes you teach expectant parents about physical and psychological changes in the woman and fetal development. After learning about normal childbearing, the mother who applies new knowledge is more likely to eat healthy foods, engage in physical exercise, and avoid substances that can harm the fetus. Promoting healthy behavior through education allows patients to assume more responsibility for their health (Longo et al., 2010). Greater knowledge results in better health maintenance habits. When patients become more health conscious, they are more likely to seek early diagnosis of health problems (Hawkins et al., 2011; Redman, 2007).

Restoration of Health

Injured or ill patients need information and skills to help them regain or maintain their levels of health. Patients recovering from and adapting to changes resulting from illness or injury often seek information about their condition. For example, a woman who recently had a hysterectomy asks about her pathology reports and expected length of recovery. However, some patients find it difficult to adapt to illness and become passive and uninterested in learning. As the nurse you learn to identify patients' willingness to learn and motivate interest in learning (Redman, 2007). The family often is a vital part of a patient's return to health. Family caregivers often require as much education as the patient, including information on how to perform skills within the home. If you exclude the family from a teaching plan, conflicts can occur. However, do not assume that the family should be involved; assess the patient-family relationship before providing education for family caregivers.

Coping with Impaired Functions

Not all patients fully recover from illness or injury. Many have to learn to cope with permanent health alterations. New knowledge and skills are often necessary for patients to continue activities of daily living. For example, a patient loses the ability to speak after larynx surgery and has to learn new ways of communicating. Changes in function are physical or psychosocial. In the case of serious disability such as following a stroke or a spinal cord injury, the patient's family needs to understand and accept many changes in his or her physical capabilities. The family's ability to provide support results in part from education, which begins as soon as you identify the patient's needs and the family displays a willingness to help. Teach family members to help the patient with health care management (e.g., giving medications through gastric tubes and doing passive range-of-motion exercises). Families of patients with alterations such as alcoholism, mental retardation, or drug dependence learn to adapt to the emotional effects of these chronic conditions and provide psychosocial support to facilitate the patient's health. Comparing the desired level of health with the actual state of health enables you to plan effective teaching programs.

TEACHING AND LEARNING

It is impossible to separate teaching from learning. **Teaching** is an interactive process that promotes learning. It consists of a conscious, deliberate set of actions that help individuals gain new knowledge, change attitudes, adopt new behaviors, or perform new skills (Billings and Halstead, 2009). A teacher provides information that prompts the learner to engage in activities that lead to a desired change.

Learning is the purposeful acquisition of new knowledge, attitudes, behaviors, and skills (Bastable, 2008). Complex patterns are required if the patient is to learn new skills, change existing attitudes, transfer learning to new situations, or solve problems (Redman, 2007). A new mother exhibits learning when she demonstrates how to bathe her newborn. The mother shows transfer of learning when she uses the principles she learned about bathing a newborn when she bathes her older child. Generally teaching and learning begin when a person identifies a need for knowing or acquiring an ability to do something. Teaching is most effective when it responds to the learner's needs (Redman, 2007). The teacher assesses these needs by asking questions and determining the learner's interests. Interpersonal communication is essential for successful teaching to occur (see Chapter 24).

Role of the Nurse in Teaching and Learning

Nurses have an ethical responsibility to teach their patients (Heiskell, 2010). In *The Patient Care Partnership,* the American Hospital Association (2003) indicates that patients have the right to make informed decisions about their care. The information required to make informed decisions must be accurate, complete, and relevant to patients' needs.

TJC's *Speak Up Initiatives* helps patients understand their rights when receiving medical care (TJC, 2010). The assumption is that patients who ask questions and are aware of their rights have a greater chance of getting the care they need when they need it. The program offers the following ***Speak Up*** tips to help patients become more involved in their treatment:

- **S**peak up if you have questions or concerns. If you still do not understand, ask again. It is your body, and you have a right to know.
- **P**ay attention to the care you get. Always make sure that you are getting the right treatments and medicines by the right health care professionals. Do not assume anything.
- **E**ducate yourself about your illness. Learn about the medical tests that are prescribed and your treatment plan.
- **A**sk a trusted family member or friend to be your advocate (advisor or supporter).
- **K**now which medicines you take and why you take them. Medication errors are the most common health care mistakes.
- **U**se a hospital, clinic, surgery center, or other type of health care organization that has been carefully evaluated.
- **P**articipate in all decisions about your treatment. You are the center of the health care team.

In addition, patients are advised that they have a right to be informed about the care they will receive, obtain information about care in their preferred language, know the names of their caregivers, receive treatment for pain, receive an up-to-date list of current medications, and expect that they will be heard and treated with respect.

Teach information that patients and their families need. You frequently clarify information provided by health care providers and are the primary source of information that patients need to adjust to health problems (Bastable, 2006). However, it is also important to understand patients' preferences for what they wish to learn. For example, a patient requests information about a new medication, or family members question the reason for their mother's pain. Identifying the need for teaching is easy when patients request information. However, a patient's need for teaching is often less obvious. To be an effective educator, the nurse has to do more than just pass on facts. Carefully determine what patients need to know and find the time when they are ready to learn. When nurses value and provide education, patients are better prepared to assume health care responsibilities. Nursing research about patient education supports the positive impact of patient education on patient outcomes (Box 25-1).

BOX 25-1 EVIDENCE-BASED PRACTICE

The Effectiveness of Patient Education in Self-Management of Heart Failure

PICO Question: Do patients who participate in nurse-led educational programs manage their heart failure (HF) at home better when compared with patients who do not receive formalized health education about HF management?

Evidence Summary

Patients who live with HF need education about their diagnosis and its effects on daily living to prevent multiple hospitalizations and promote optimal functioning. However, many patients do not clearly understand why they have HF or how to control it effectively. HF, especially when it is poorly controlled, negatively influences quality of life (While and Kiek, 2009). Research shows that patient education provided by nurses positively influences patient outcomes and reduces hospitalizations. Individualized patient education helps patients better manage their HF, which improves their function and quality of life. Quality nurse-directed patient education includes the following components: basic facts about HF; managing stress, depression, and social interactions; making healthy food choices; improving activity level; and managing fluid balance (Boren et al., 2009). However, successful HF management requires more than patient education. Nurses also need to implement interventions that empower patients to make informed decisions about their care. Enhancing self-efficacy positively influences quality of life and improves the ability to manage HF (Evangelista and Shinnick, 2008; While and Kiek, 2009; Yehle and Plake, 2010).

Application to Nursing Practice

- Nurse-directed patient education about lifestyle choices and management of the physical and psychosocial aspects of health and exercise, coupled with interventions that improve self-efficacy, enhance quality of life in patients with HF.
- Nurses must ensure that educational interventions and instructions match patients' health literacy abilities.
- Improving quality of life enhances functional ability in patients with HF.
- Patients who receive nurse-directed patient education improve their ability to manage their health and experience better outcomes, both physically and emotionally.

Teaching as Communication

The teaching process closely parallels the communication process (see Chapter 24). Effective teaching depends in part on effective interpersonal communication. A teacher applies each element of the communication process while providing information to learners. Thus the teacher and learner become involved together in a teaching process that increases the learner's knowledge and skills.

The steps of the teaching process are similar to those of the communication process. You use patient requests for information or perceive a need for information because of a patient's health restrictions or the recent diagnosis of an illness. Then you identify specific **learning objectives** to describe what the learner will be able to do after successful instruction.

The nurse is the sender who conveys a message to the patient. Many intrapersonal variables influence your style and approach. Attitudes, values, emotions, cultural perspective, and knowledge influence the way information is delivered. Past experiences with teaching are also helpful for choosing the best way to present necessary content.

The receiver in the teaching-learning process is the learner. A number of intrapersonal variables affect motivation and ability to learn. Patients are ready to learn when they express a desire to do so and are more likely to receive the message when they understand the content. Attitudes, anxiety, and values influence the ability to understand a message. The ability to learn depends on factors such as emotional and physical health, education, cultural perspective, patients' values about their health, the stage of development, and previous knowledge.

Effective communication involves feedback. An effective teacher provides a mechanism for evaluating the success of a teaching plan and then provides positive reinforcement (Bastable, 2008; Redman, 2007). Examples of ways to evaluate teaching sessions through feedback include having a patient demonstrate a newly learned skill or asking a patient to describe how the correct dosage schedule for a new medication will be incorporated into a daily routine. Feedback needs to show the success of the learner in achieving objectives (i.e., the learner verbalizes information or provides a return demonstration of skills learned).

DOMAINS OF LEARNING

Learning occurs in three domains: cognitive (understanding), affective (attitudes), and psychomotor (motor skills) (Bloom, 1956; Bastable, 2008). Any health topic involves one or all domains or any combination of the three. You often work with patients who need to learn in each domain. For example, patients diagnosed with diabetes need to learn how diabetes affects the body and how to control blood glucose levels for healthier lifestyles (cognitive domain). In addition, patients begin to accept the chronic nature of diabetes by learning positive coping mechanisms (affective domain). Finally, many patients living with diabetes learn to test their blood glucose levels at home. This requires learning how to use a glucose meter (psychomotor domain). The characteristics of learning within each domain influence the teaching and evaluation methods used. Understanding each learning domain prepares the nurse to select proper teaching techniques and apply the basic principles of learning (Box 25-2).

Cognitive Learning

Cognitive learning includes all intellectual behaviors and requires thinking (Bastable, 2008). In the hierarchy of cognitive behaviors the simplest behavior is acquiring knowledge, whereas the

most complex is evaluation. Cognitive learning includes the following:
- Knowledge: Learning new facts or information and being able to recall them
- Comprehension: The ability to understand the meaning of learned material
- Application: Using abstract, newly learned ideas in a concrete situation
- Analysis: Breaking down information into organized parts
- Synthesis: The ability to apply knowledge and skills to produce a new whole
- Evaluation: A judgment of the worth of a body of information for a given purpose

BOX 25-2 APPROPRIATE TEACHING METHODS BASED ON DOMAINS OF LEARNING

Cognitive
- Discussion (one-on-one or group)
  - Involves nurse and one patient or a nurse with several patients
  - Promotes active participation and focuses on topics of interest to patient
  - Allows peer support
  - Enhances application and analysis of new information
- Lecture
  - Is more formal method of instruction because it is teacher controlled
  - Helps learner acquire new knowledge and gain comprehension
- Question-and-answer session
  - Addresses patient's specific concerns
  - Assists patient in applying knowledge
- Role play, discovery
  - Allows patient to actively apply knowledge in controlled situation
  - Promotes synthesis of information and problem solving
- Independent project (computer-assisted instruction), field experience
  - Allows patient to assume responsibility for completing learning activities at own pace
  - Promotes analysis, synthesis, and evaluation of new information and skills

Affective
- Role play
  - Allows expression of values, feelings, and attitudes
- Discussion (group)
  - Allows patient to receive support from others in group
  - Helps patient learn from others' experiences
  - Promotes responding, valuing, and organization
- Discussion (one-on-one)
  - Allows discussion of personal, sensitive topics of interest or concern

Psychomotor
- Demonstration
  - Provides presentation of procedures or skills by nurse
  - Permits patient to incorporate modeling of nurse's behavior
  - Allows nurse to control questioning during demonstration
- Practice
  - Gives patient opportunity to perform skills using equipment in a controlled setting
  - Provides repetition
- Return demonstration
  - Permits patient to perform skill as nurse observes
  - Provides excellent source of feedback and reinforcement
- Independent projects, games
  - Requires teaching method that promotes adaptation and origination of psychomotor learning
  - Permits learner to use new skills

Affective Learning

Affective learning deals with expression of feelings and acceptance of attitudes, opinions, or values. Values clarification (see Chapter 22) is an example of affective learning. The simplest behavior in the hierarchy is receiving, and the most complex is characterizing (Krathwohl et al., 1964). Affective learning includes the following:
- Receiving: Being willing to attend to another person's words
- Responding: Active participation through listening and reacting verbally and nonverbally
- Valuing: Attaching worth to an object or behavior demonstrated by the learner's behavior
- Organizing: Developing a value system by identifying and organizing values and resolving conflicts
- Characterizing: Acting and responding with a consistent value system

Psychomotor Learning

Psychomotor learning involves acquiring skills that require the integration of mental and muscular activity such as the ability to walk or use an eating utensil (Redman, 2007). The simplest behavior in the hierarchy is perception, whereas the most complex is origination. Psychomotor learning includes the following:
- Perception: Being aware of objects or qualities through the use of sense organs
- Set: A readiness to take a particular action; there are three sets: mental, physical, and emotional
- Guided response: The performance of an act under the guidance of an instructor involving imitation of a demonstrated act
- Mechanism: A higher level of behavior by which a person gains confidence and skill in performing a behavior that is more complex or involves several more steps than a guided response
- Complex overt response: Smoothly and accurately performing a motor skill that requires a complex movement pattern
- Adaptation: The ability to change a motor response when unexpected problems occur
- Origination: Using existing psychomotor skills and abilities to perform a highly complex motor act that involves creating new movement patterns

BASIC LEARNING PRINCIPLES

To teach effectively and efficiently, you first need to understand how people learn (Eshleman, 2008). Motivation addresses a person's desire or willingness to learn (Redman, 2007). The patient's willingness to become involved in learning influences your teaching approach. Previous knowledge, experience, attitudes, and sociocultural factors influence a person's motivation. The ability to learn depends on physical and cognitive attributes, developmental level, physical wellness, and intellectual thought processes. An ideal learning environment allows a person to attend to instruction.

A person's learning style affects preferences for learning. People process information in the following ways: by seeing and hearing, reflecting and acting, reasoning logically and intuitively, and analyzing and visualizing. Some people learn information gradually, whereas others learn more sporadically. Effective teaching plans include a combination of approaches that meet multiple learning styles (Billings and Halstead, 2009).

Motivation to Learn

Attentional Set. An attentional set is the mental state that allows the learner to focus on and comprehend a learning activity. Before learning anything, patients must give attention to, or concentrate on, the information to be learned. Physical discomfort, anxiety, and environmental distractions influence the ability to attend. Therefore determine the patient's level of comfort before beginning a teaching plan and ensure that the patient is able to focus on the information.

As anxiety increases, the patient's ability to pay attention often decreases. Anxiety is uneasiness or worry resulting from anticipating a threat or danger. When faced with change or the need to act differently, a person feels anxious. Learning requires a change in behavior and thus produces anxiety. A mild level of anxiety motivates learning. However, a high level of anxiety prevents learning from occurring. It incapacitates a person, creating an inability to focus on anything other than relieving the anxiety. Manage the patient's anxiety (see Chapter 37) before educating to improve the patient's comprehension and understanding of the information given (Fredericks et al., 2008).

Motivation. **Motivation** is a force that acts on or within a person (e.g., an idea, emotion, or a physical need) to cause the person to behave in a particular way (Redman, 2007). If a person does not want to learn, it is unlikely that learning will occur. Motivation sometimes results from a social, task mastery, or physical motive.

A social motive is a need for connection, social approval, or self-esteem. People normally seek out others with whom they can compare opinions, abilities, and emotions. For example, new parents often seek validation of ideas and parenting techniques from others whom they have identified as role models in their social environment or health care workers with whom they have established a relationship.

Task mastery motives are based on needs such as achievement and competence. For example, a high school senior who has diabetes begins to test blood glucose levels and make decisions about insulin dosages in preparation for leaving home and establishing independence. The ability to successfully manage diabetes provides the motivation to master the task or skill. After a person succeeds at a task, he or she is usually motivated to achieve more.

Often patient motives are physical. Some patients are motivated to return to a level of physical normalcy. For example, a patient with a below-the-knee amputation is motivated to learn how to walk with assistive devices. Knowledge that is necessary for survival, problem recognition, and critical decision making creates a stronger stimulus for learning than knowledge that merely promotes health (Bastable, 2006).

You assess a patient's motivation to learn and what the patient needs to know to promote compliance with their prescribed therapy. Unfortunately not all people are interested in maintaining health. Many do not adopt new health behaviors or change unhealthy behaviors unless they perceive a disease as a threat, overcome barriers to changing health practices, and see the benefits of adopting a healthy behavior. For example, some patients with lung disease continue to smoke. No therapy has an effect unless a person believes that health is important.

Use of Theory to Enhance Motivation and Learning. Health education often involves changing attitudes and values that are not easy to change by simply teaching facts. Therefore it is important for you to use various interventions based on theory when developing patient education plans. Because of the complexity of the patient education process, different theories and models are available to guide patient education. Using a theory that matches the patient's needs in practice will provide more effective patient education. Social learning theory provides one of the most useful approaches to patient education because it explains the characteristics of the learner and guides the educator in developing effective teaching interventions that result in enhanced learning and improved motivation (Bandura, 2001; Stonecypher, 2009).

According to social learning theory, people continuously attempt to control events that affect their lives. This allows them to attain desired outcomes and avoid undesired outcomes, resulting in improved motivation. **Self-efficacy,** a concept included in social learning theory, refers to a person's perceived ability to successfully complete a task. When people believe that they are able to execute a particular behavior, they are more likely to perform the behavior consistently and correctly (Bandura, 1997).

Self-efficacy beliefs come from four sources: enactive mastery experiences, vicarious experiences, verbal persuasion, and physiological and affective states (Bandura, 1997). Understanding the four sources of self-efficacy allows you to develop interventions to help patients adopt healthy behaviors. For example, a nurse who is wishing to teach a child recently diagnosed with asthma how to correctly use an inhaler expresses personal belief in the child's ability to use the inhaler (verbal persuasion). Then the nurse demonstrates how to use the inhaler (vicarious experience). Once the demonstration is complete, the child uses the inhaler (enactive mastery experience). As the child's wheezing and anxiety decrease after the correct use of the inhaler, he or she experiences positive feedback, further enhancing his or her confidence to use it (physiological and affective states). Interventions such as these enhance perceived self-efficacy, which in turn improves the achievement of desired outcomes.

Self-efficacy is a concept included in many health promotion theories because it often is a strong predictor of healthy behaviors and because many interventions improve self-efficacy, resulting in improved lifestyle choices (Bandura, 1997). Because of its use in theories and research studies, many evidence-based teaching interventions include a focus on self-efficacy. When nurses implement interventions to enhance self-efficacy, their patients frequently experience positive outcomes. For example, researchers associated interventions that include self-efficacy with effective management of heart failure (While and Kiek, 2009; Yehle and Plake, 2010), participation in physical activity (Ashford et al., 2010), self-management of arthritis (Nunez et al., 2009), and improved management of asthma in children (Coffman et al., 2009).

Psychosocial Adaptation to Illness. A temporary or permanent loss of health is often difficult for patients to accept. They need to grieve, and the process of grieving gives them time to adapt psychologically to the emotional and physical implications of illness. The stages of grieving (see Chapter 36) include a series of responses that patients experience during a loss such as illness. They experience these stages at different rates and sequences, depending on their self-concept before illness, the severity of the illness, and the changes in lifestyle that the illness creates. Effective, supportive care guides the patient through the grieving process.

Readiness to learn is related to the stage of grieving (Table 25-1). Patients cannot learn when they are unwilling or unable to accept the reality of illness. However, properly timed teaching facilitates adjustment to illness or disability. Identify the patient's stage of

TABLE 25-1 **Relationship Between Psychosocial Adaptation to Illness, Grief, and Learning**

STAGE	PATIENT'S BEHAVIOR	LEARNING IMPLICATIONS FOR NURSE AND FAMILY CAREGIVER	RATIONALE
Denial or disbelief	Patient avoids discussion of illness ("I'm fine; there's nothing wrong with me"), withdraws from others, and disregards physical restrictions. Patient suppresses and distorts information that has not been presented clearly.	Provide support, empathy, and careful explanations of all procedures while they are being done. Let patient know that you are available for discussion. Explain situation to family or significant other if appropriate. Teach in present tense (e.g., explain current therapy).	Patient is not prepared to deal with problem. Any attempt to convince or tell patient about illness results in further anger or withdrawal. Provide only information patient pursues or absolutely requires.
Anger	Patient blames and complains and often directs anger toward nurse or others.	Do not argue with patient but listen to concerns. Teach in present tense. Reassure family and significant others of patient's normalcy.	Patient needs opportunity to express feelings and anger; he or she is still not prepared to face future.
Bargaining	Patient offers to live better life in exchange for promise of better health. ("If God lets me live, I promise to quit smoking.")	Continue to introduce only reality. Teach only in present tense.	Patient is still unwilling to accept limitations.
Resolution	Patient begins to express emotions openly, realizes that illness has created changes, and begins to ask questions.	Encourage expression of feelings. Begin to share information needed for future and set aside formal times for discussion.	Patient begins to perceive need for assistance and is ready to accept responsibility for learning.
Acceptance	Patient recognizes reality of condition, actively pursues information, and strives for independence.	Focus teaching on future skills and knowledge required. Continue to teach about present occurrences. Involve family/significant other in teaching information for discharge.	Patient is more easily motivated to learn. Acceptance of illness reflects willingness to deal with its implications.

grieving on the basis of his or her behaviors. When the patient enters the stage of acceptance, the stage compatible with learning, introduce a teaching plan. Continuous assessment of the patient's behaviors determines the stages of grieving. Teaching continues as long as the patient remains in a stage conducive to learning.

Active Participation. Learning occurs when the patient is actively involved in the educational session (Edelman and Mandle, 2010). A patient's involvement in learning implies an eagerness to acquire knowledge or skills. It also improves the opportunity for the patient to make decisions during teaching sessions. For example, when teaching car seat safety during a parenting class, hold a teaching session in the parking lot where the participants park their cars. Encourage active participation by providing the learners with several different car seats for them to place in their cars. At the completion of this session, the parents are able to determine which type of car seat fits in their cars and which is the easiest to use. This provides participants with the information needed to purchase the appropriate car seat.

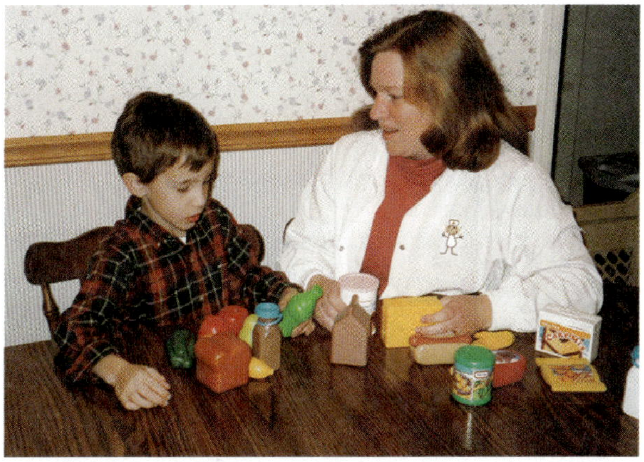

FIG. 25-1 The nurse uses developmentally appropriate food models to teach healthy eating behaviors to the school-age child.

Ability to Learn

Developmental Capability. Cognitive development influences the patient's ability to learn. You can be a competent teacher, but if you do not consider the patient's intellectual abilities, teaching is unsuccessful. Learning, like developmental growth, is an evolving process. You need to know the patient's level of knowledge and intellectual skills before beginning a teaching plan. Learning occurs more readily when new information complements existing knowledge. For example, measuring liquid or solid food portions requires the ability to perform mathematical calculations. Reading a medication label or discharge instructions requires reading and comprehension skills. Learning to regulate insulin dosages requires problem-solving skills.

Learning in Children. The capability for learning and the type of behaviors that children are able to learn depend on the child's maturation. Without proper physiological, motor, language, and social development, many types of learning cannot take place. However, learning occurs in children of all ages. Intellectual growth moves from the concrete to the abstract as the child matures. Therefore information presented to children needs to be understandable, and the expected outcomes must be realistic, based on the child's developmental stage (Box 25-3). Use teaching aids that are developmentally appropriate (Fig. 25-1). Learning occurs when behavior changes as a result of experience or growth (Hockenberry and Wilson, 2011).

BOX 25-3 TEACHING METHODS BASED ON PATIENT'S DEVELOPMENTAL CAPACITY

Infant
- Keep routines (e.g., feeding, bathing) consistent.
- Hold infant firmly while smiling and speaking softly to convey sense of trust.
- Have infant touch different textures (e.g., soft fabric, hard plastic).

Toddler
- Use play to teach procedure or activity (e.g., handling examination equipment, applying bandage to doll).
- Offer picture books that describe story of children in hospital or clinic.
- Use simple words such as *cut* instead of *laceration* to promote understanding.

Preschooler
- Use role play, imitation, and play to make learning fun.
- Encourage questions and offer explanations. Use simple explanations and demonstrations.
- Encourage children to learn together through pictures and short stories about how to perform hygiene.

School-Age Child
- Teach psychomotor skills needed to maintain health. (Complicated skills such as learning to use a syringe take considerable practice.)
- Offer opportunities to discuss health problems and answer questions.

Adolescent
- Help adolescent learn about feelings and need for self-expression.
- Use teaching as collaborative activity.
- Allow adolescents to make decisions about health and health promotion (safety, sex education, substance abuse).
- Use problem solving to help adolescents make choices.

Young or Middle Adult
- Encourage participation in teaching plan by setting mutual goals.
- Encourage independent learning.
- Offer information so adult understands effects of health problem.

Older Adult
- Teach when patient is alert and rested.
- Involve adult in discussion or activity.
- Focus on wellness and person's strength.
- Use approaches that enhance sensorially impaired patient's reception of stimuli (see Chapter 49).
- Keep teaching sessions short.

Adult Learning. Teaching adults differs from teaching children. Adults are able to critically reflect on their current situation and sometimes need help to see their problems and change their perspectives (Redman, 2007). Because adults become independent and self-directed as they mature, they are often able to identify their own learning needs (Billings and Halstead, 2009). Learning needs come from problems or tasks that result from real-life situations. Although adults tend to be self-directed learners, they often become dependent in new learning situations. The amount of information provided and the amount of time that is spent with the adult patient vary, depending on the patient's personal situation and readiness to learn. An adult's readiness to learn is often associated with his or her developmental stage and other events that are occurring in his or her life. Resolve any needs or issues that the patient perceives as extremely important so learning can occur.

Adults have a wide variety of personal and life experiences on which to draw. Therefore enhance adult learning by encouraging them to use these experiences to solve problems (Eshleman, 2008). Furthermore, make education patient-centered by developing educational topics and goals in collaboration with the adult patient. Adult patients are ultimately responsible for changing their own behavior. Assessing what the adult patient currently knows, teaching what the patient wants to know, and setting mutual goals improve the outcomes of patient education (Bastable, 2008).

Physical Capability. The ability to learn often depends on the patient's level of physical development and overall physical health. To learn psychomotor skills, a patient needs to possess a certain level of strength, coordination, and sensory acuity. For example, it is useless to teach a patient to transfer from a bed to a wheelchair if he or she has insufficient upper body strength. An older patient with poor eyesight or the inability to grasp objects tightly cannot learn to apply an elastic bandage. Therefore do not overestimate the patient's physical development or status. The following physical characteristics are necessary to learn psychomotor skills:
- Size (height and weight match the task to perform or the equipment to use [e.g., crutch walking])
- Strength (ability of the patient to follow a strenuous exercise program)
- Coordination (dexterity needed for complicated motor skills such as using utensils or changing a bandage)
- Sensory acuity (visual, auditory, tactile, gustatory, and olfactory; sensory resources needed to receive and respond to messages taught)

Any condition (e.g., pain or fatigue) that depletes a person's energy also impairs the ability to learn. For example, a patient who spends a morning having rigorous diagnostic studies is unlikely to be able to learn because of fatigue. Postpone teaching when an illness becomes aggravated by complications such as a high fever or respiratory difficulty. After working with a patient, assess the patient's energy level by noting the patient's willingness to communicate, the amount of activity initiated, and his or her responsiveness toward questions. Temporarily stop teaching if the patient needs rest. You achieve greater teaching success when patients are physically able to actively participate in learning.

Learning Environment

Factors in the physical environment where teaching takes place make learning either a pleasant or a difficult experience (Bastable, 2008). The ideal setting helps the patient focus on the learning task. The number of persons that the nurse teaches, the need for privacy, the room temperature, the room lighting, noise, the room ventilation, and the room furniture are important factors when choosing the setting. The ideal environment for learning is a room that is well lit and has good ventilation, appropriate furniture, and a comfortable temperature. A darkened room interferes with the patient's ability to watch your actions, especially when demonstrating a skill or using visual aids such as posters or pamphlets. A room that is cold, hot, or stuffy makes the patient too uncomfortable to focus on the information being presented.

It is also important to choose a quiet setting. A quiet setting offers privacy; infrequent interruptions are best. Provide privacy even in a busy hospital by closing cubicle curtains or taking the patient to a quiet spot. Family caregivers often need to share in discussions in the home. However, patients who are reluctant to discuss the nature of the illness when others are in the room benefit from receiving education in a room separate from household activities such as a bedroom.

Teaching a group of patients requires a room that allows everyone to be seated comfortably and within hearing distance of the teacher. Make sure that the size of the room does not overwhelm the group. Arranging the group to allow participants to observe one another further enhances learning. More effective communication occurs as learners observe others' verbal and nonverbal interactions.

NURSING PROCESS

Apply the nursing process and use a critical thinking approach in your care of patients. The nursing process provides a clinical decision-making approach for you to develop and implement an individualized plan of care. A relationship exists between the nursing and teaching processes (Redman, 2007). During the assessment phase of the nursing process, determine the patient's health care needs (see Unit 3). At times assessment reveals a patient's need for health care information. Individualize nursing diagnoses to a patient's situation and establish a plan of care to meet desired goals and outcomes and prescribe evidence-based nursing interventions for improving or maintaining a patient's health. Evaluation determines the level of success in meeting goals of care.

While diagnosing a patient's health care problems, you often identify the need for education. When education becomes a part of the care plan, the teaching process begins. Like the nursing process, the teaching process requires assessment—in this case, analyzing the patient's learning needs, motivation, and ability to learn. A diagnostic statement specifies the information or skills that the patient requires. Develop specific learning objectives, implement appropriate patient-centered teaching strategies, and use learning principles to ensure that the patient acquires the necessary knowledge and skills. Finally, the teaching process requires an evaluation of learning based on learning objectives.

The nursing and teaching processes are not the same. The nursing process requires assessment of all sources of data to determine a patient's total health care needs. The teaching process focuses on the patient's learning needs and willingness and capability to learn. Table 25-2 compares the teaching and nursing processes.

ASSESSMENT

Through the Patient's Eyes. When providing patient education, it is important to partner with the patient to ensure safe, compassionate, and coordinated care (QSEN, 2010). During the assessment process, thoroughly assess a patient and critically analyze your findings to ensure that you make patient-centered clinical decisions required for safe nursing care. To be successful in teaching a patient, you need to assess all factors influencing the choice of relevant content, the patient's ability to learn, and the resources available for instruction. By seeing health care situations "through patients' eyes," you gain a better appreciation of their knowledge, expectations, and preferences for learning. Learning needs, identified by both you and a patient, determine the choice of teaching content. An effective assessment provides the basis for individualized patient teaching (Olsen, 2010). Box 25-4 summarizes examples of specific assessment questions to use in determining a patient's unique learning needs.

Sometimes nurses use formal educational assessment tools to determine their patients' perceived learning needs. Other times they simply identify their patients' expectations during routine assessments. Patients identify their own learning needs based on the implications of living with their illness. To meet these learning needs, assess what patients view as important information to know. When a patient feels a need to know something, he or she is likely to be receptive to information presented. For example, many parents need to know how to care for their new baby. Therefore they are often very receptive to information about baby care (e.g., how to feed the baby and make sure that he or she gets enough sleep).

Learning Needs. Determine information that is critical for patients to learn. Learning needs change, depending on a patient's current health status. Because the health status is dynamic, assessment is an ongoing activity. Assess the following:

- Information or skills needed by the patient to perform self-care and to understand the implications of a health problem—Health care team members anticipate learning needs related to specific health problems. For example, you teach a young man who has just entered high school how to perform testicular self-examination.
- Patient experiences (e.g., new or recurring problem, past hospitalization) that influence the need to learn

TABLE 25-2 Comparison of the Nursing and Teaching Processes

BASIC STEPS	NURSING PROCESS	TEACHING PROCESS
Assessment	Collect data about patient's physical, psychological, social, cultural, developmental, and spiritual needs from patient, family, diagnostic tests, medical record, nursing history, and literature.	Gather data about patient's learning needs, motivation, ability to learn, and teaching resources from patient, family, learning environment, medical record, nursing history, and literature.
Nursing diagnosis	Identify appropriate nursing diagnoses based on assessment findings.	Identify patient's learning needs on basis of three domains of learning.
Planning	Develop an individualized care plan. Set diagnosis priorities based on patient's immediate needs, expected outcomes, and patient-centered goals. Collaborate with patient on care plan.	Establish learning objectives stated in behavioral terms. Identify priorities regarding learning needs. Collaborate with patient about teaching plan. Identify type of teaching method to use.
Implementation	Perform nursing care therapies. Include patient as active participant in care. Involve family/significant other in care as appropriate.	Implement teaching methods. Actively involve patient in learning activities. Include family caregiver as appropriate.
Evaluation	Identify success in meeting desired outcomes and goals of nursing care. Alter interventions as indicated when goals are not met.	Determine outcomes of teaching-learning process. Measure patient's achievement of learning objectives. Reinforce information as needed.

BOX 25-4 NURSING ASSESSMENT QUESTIONS

Previous Learning and Identification of Learning Needs and Preferences
- What do you want to know about _____________?
- What do you know about your illness and your treatment plan?
- Which experiences have you had in the past that are similar to those you are experiencing now?
- Together we can choose the best way for you to learn about your disease. How can I best help you?
- When you learn new information, do you prefer to have it given to you in pictures or written down in words?
- When you give someone directions to your house, do you tell the person how to get there, write out the instructions, or draw a map?

Self-Management
- How does (or will) your illness affect your current lifestyle?
- Which barriers currently exist that prevent you from managing your illness the way you would like to manage it?
- What role do you believe your health care providers should take in helping you manage your illness or maintain health?
- How involved do you want a family member to be in the management of your illness? Who is that family member?

Culture and Spiritual Influences
- Which cultural or spiritual beliefs do you have regarding your illness and the prescribed treatment?

For Family Caregivers
- When are you available to help, and how do you plan to help your loved one?
- Your spouse needs some help. How do you feel about learning how to assist him or her?
- Tell me how you feel about performing the care activities that your family member requires.

- Information that family caregivers require to support the patient's needs—The amount of information needed depends on the extent of the family member's role in helping the patient.

Motivation to Learn. Ask questions that identify and define the patient's motivation. These questions help to determine if the patient is prepared and willing to learn. Assess the following motivational factors:
- Behavior (e.g., attention span, tendency to ask questions, memory, and ability to concentrate during the teaching session)
- Health beliefs and sociocultural background—Sociocultural norms, values, and traditions all influence a patient's beliefs and values about health and various therapies, communication patterns, and perceptions of time (see Chapter 9).
- Perception of the severity and susceptibility of a health problem and the benefits and barriers to treatment
- Perceived ability to perform health behaviors
- Desire to learn
- Attitudes about health care providers (e.g., role of patient and nurse in making decisions)
- Learning style preference—Patients who are visual learners learn best when you use pictures and diagrams to explain information. Patients who prefer auditory learning are distracted by pictures and prefer listening to information (e.g., podcasts). Kinesthetic learners learn best while they are moving and participating in hands-on activities. Demonstrations and role playing work well with these learners (Eshleman, 2008). Patients who learn best by reasoning logically and intuitively learn better if presented with a case study that requires careful analysis and discussion with others to arrive at conclusions.

Ability to Learn. Determine the patient's physical and cognitive ability to learn. Health care providers often underestimate patients' cognitive deficits. Many factors impair the ability to learn, including fatigue, body temperature, electrolyte levels, oxygenation status, and blood glucose level. In any health care setting several of these factors often influence a patient at the same time. Assess the following factors related to the ability to learn:
- Physical strength, endurance, movement, dexterity, and coordination—Determine the extent to which the patient can perform skills. For example, have the patient manipulate equipment that will be used in self-care at home.
- Sensory deficits (see Chapter 49) that affect the patient's ability to understand or follow instruction
- Patient's reading level—This is often difficult to assess because patients who are functionally illiterate are often able to conceal it by using excuses such as not having the time or not being able to see. One way to assess a patient's reading level and level of understanding is to ask the patient to read instructions from an educational handout and then explain their meaning (see the discussion of health literacy, p. 337).
- Patient's developmental level—This influences the selection of teaching approaches (see Box 25-3).
- Patient's cognitive function, including memory, knowledge, association, and judgment
- Pain, fatigue, anxiety, or other physical symptoms that interfere with the ability to maintain attention and participate—In acute care settings a patient's physical condition can easily prevent a patient from learning.

Teaching Environment. The environment for a teaching session needs to be conducive to learning. Assess the following environmental factors:
- Distractions or persistent noise—A quiet area is essential for effective learning.
- Comfort of the room, including ventilation, temperature, lighting, furniture, and size
- Room facilities and available equipment

Resources for Learning. A patient frequently requires the support of family members or significant others. If this support is necessary, assess the readiness and ability of a family caregiver to learn the information necessary for the care of the patient. Also review resources within the home environment. Assess the following:
- Patient's willingness to have family caregivers involved in the teaching plan and provide health care—Information about the patient's health care is confidential unless the patient chooses to share it. Sometimes it is difficult for the patient to accept the help of family caregivers, especially when bodily functions are involved.
- Family caregiver's perceptions and understanding of the patient's illness and its implications—Family caregivers' perceptions should match those of the patient; otherwise conflicts occur in the teaching plan.
- Family caregiver's willingness and ability to participate in care—If the patient chooses to share information about his or her health status with family members, they need to be responsible, willing, and physically and cognitively

able to assist in care activities such as bathing or administering medications. Not all family members meet these requirements.

- Resources—These include financial or material resources such as having the ability to obtain health care equipment.
- Teaching tools, including brochures, audiovisual materials, or posters—Printed material needs to present current information that is written clearly and logically and matches the patient's reading level.

Health Literacy and Learning Disabilities. Current research shows that health literacy is a strong predictor of a person's health status (Kim and Yu, 2010; Wolf et al., 2010). The World Health Organization (2011) defines **health literacy** as the cognitive and social skills that determine the motivation and ability of individuals to gain access to, understand, and use information in ways that promote and maintain good health. Health literacy includes patients' reading and mathematics skills, comprehension, ability to make health-related decisions, and successful functioning as a consumer of health care (Speros, 2005). Persons most likely to be at risk for low health literacy include the elderly (age 65 years and older), minority populations, immigrant populations, persons of low income (approximately half of Medicare/Medicaid recipients read below the fifth-grade level), and people with chronic mental and/or physical health conditions (National Network of Libraries of Medicine, 2011).

Functional illiteracy, the inability to read above a fifth-grade level, is a major problem in America today. The National Assessment of Adult Literacy Survey (NAALS), conducted in 2003 by the National Center for Education Statistics, assessed the extent of literacy skills in Americans over the age of 16 (Kutner et al., 2006). Results from the NAALS reflected that over 75 million American adults had basic or below-basic levels of health literacy. Approximately 14% of adults could not understand a basic patient education pamphlet, and 36% could not perform moderately difficult tasks (e.g., reading a childhood vaccination chart or determining possible medication interactions from a prescription label). Older adults, men, people who did not speak English before entering school, people living below poverty level, and people without a high school education tended to have lower health literacy scores. White and Asian/Pacific Islander adults had higher literacy levels than African American, Native American/Alaska Native, and multiracial adults. Hispanic adults had the lowest levels of health literacy.

To compound the problem, the readability of printed health education material ranges from elementary school to college level. Currently printed educational materials are often above the patient's reading level (Clauson et al., 2010; MacDonald et al., 2010). Removing medical terms from health information lowers the reading level, but this often does not bring it to an acceptable level. Unfortunately health care professionals do not always address the gap between the patient's reading level and the readability of educational materials (Attwood, 2008; Rothman et al., 2009). This results in unsafe care. To ensure patient safety, all health care providers need to ensure that information is presented clearly and in a culturally sensitive manner (TJC, 2010).

Because health literacy influences how you deliver teaching strategies, it is critical for you to assess a patient's health literacy before providing instruction. Assessing health literacy is challenging, especially in busy clinical settings where there is often little time to conduct a thorough health literacy assessment. However, all health care providers need to identify problems and provide appropriate education to people who have special health literacy needs (TJC, 2010). Research shows that many Americans read and understand information that is 3 to 5 years below their last year of formal education.

Try asking patients to perform simple literacy skills. For example, can a patient read back to you a medication label correctly? After you give a simple 1-minute explanation of a diet or exercise program, can the patient explain it back to you? Can a patient correctly describe in his or her own words the information in a written handout? Most people with low health literacy say they are good readers even if they cannot read (Lee et al., 2010). You can use a variety of screening tools to test literacy. The Wide Range Achievement Test (WRAT 3) evaluates reading, spelling, and arithmetic skills for patients from 5 to 74 years of age. The Rapid Estimate of Adult Literacy in Medicine (REALM) uses pronunciation of health care terms to determine approximate reading level. The Cloze test, a test of reading comprehension, asks patients to fill in the blanks that are in a written paragraph. You also need to assess the patient's ability to understand mathematical calculations in addition to reading skills.

In addition to illiteracy, assess patients for learning disabilities that impair the ability to learn. For example, many self-care behaviors require an understanding of mathematics, including computation and fractions. If a patient's learning disability impairs the ability to effectively use mathematics skills, teaching is challenging, especially when trying to teach him or her about complex medication dosages and frequencies. Another learning disability that affects a patient's ability to learn includes attention-deficit/hyperactivity disorder (ADHD). Patients with ADHD frequently have a low threshold of frustration and difficulty recalling information and staying focused during educational sessions.

Patients who have low health literacy or learning disabilities may be ashamed of not being able to understand you and often try to mask their inability to comprehend information. Therefore make sure that you are sensitive and maintain a therapeutic relationship with your patients while assessing their ability to learn. Appreciating the unique qualities of your patients helps to ensure safe and effective patient care (QSEN, 2010).

NURSING DIAGNOSIS

After assessing information related to the patient's ability and need to learn, interpret data and cluster-defining characteristics to form diagnoses that reflect his or her specific learning needs (Box 25-5). This ensures that teaching will be goal directed and individualized. If a patient has several learning needs, the nursing diagnoses guide priority setting. When the nursing diagnosis is *deficient knowledge,* the diagnostic statement describes the specific type of learning

BOX 25-5 NURSING DIAGNOSTIC PROCESS

Deficient Knowledge (Psychomotor) Regarding Use of Crutches Related to Lack of Experience

ASSESSMENT ACTIVITIES	DEFINING CHARACTERISTICS
Have patient describe how to walk with crutches.	Patient states that he or she has not received information about use of crutches. Patient asks questions about how to use crutches.
Have patient demonstrate three-point crutch walking on level surfaces and up stairs.	Patient uses crutches inappropriately. Patient cannot go up or down stairs on crutches.

need and its cause (e.g., *deficient knowledge regarding psychomotor learning related to inexperience with medication self-administration).* Classifying diagnoses by the three learning domains helps you to focus specifically on subject matter and teaching methods. Patients often require education to support resolution of their various health problems. Examples of nursing diagnoses that indicate a need for education include the following:

- Deficient knowledge (affective, cognitive, psychomotor)
- Ineffective health maintenance
- Impaired home maintenance
- Ineffective family therapeutic regimen management
- Ineffective self-health management
- Noncompliance (with medications)

When you can manage or eliminate health care problems through education, the related factor of a diagnostic statement is *deficient knowledge.* For example, an older adult is having difficulty managing a medication regimen that involves a number of newly prescribed medications she has to take at different times of the day. The nursing diagnosis is *Ineffective self-health management* related to deficient knowledge. In this case educating the patient about her medications and the correct dosage schedules improves her ability to schedule and take them as directed. When you identify conditions that cause barriers to effective learning (e.g., nursing diagnosis of *acute pain* or *activity intolerance*), teaching is inappropriate. In these cases delay teaching until the nursing diagnosis is resolved or the health problem controlled.

PLANNING

After determining the nursing diagnoses that identify a patient's learning needs, develop a teaching plan, determine goals and expected outcomes, and involve the patient in selecting learning experiences (see the Nursing Care Plan). Expected outcomes (or learning objectives) guide the choice of teaching strategies and approaches with a patient. Patient participation ensures a more relevant, meaningful plan.

Goals and Outcomes. Goals of patient education indicate that a patient achieves a better understanding of the information provided and is able to attain health or better manage illness. If possible, include the patient when establishing learning goals and outcomes and serve as a resource in setting the minimum criteria for success. Outcomes often describe a behavior that identifies the patient's ability to do something on completion of teaching such as *will empty* colostomy bag, or *will administer* an injection. When developing outcomes, conditions or time frames need to be realistic and meet the patient's needs (e.g., "will identify the side effects of aspirin by discharge"). Consider conditions under which the patient or family will typically perform the behavior (e.g., "will walk from bedroom to bathroom using crutches").

In some health care settings nurses develop written teaching plans. The teaching plan includes topics for instruction, resources (e.g., equipment, teaching booklets, and referrals to special educational programs), recommendations for involving family, and objectives of the teaching plan. Some plans are very detailed, whereas others are in outline form. Use the plan to provide continuity of instruction. The more specific the plan, the easier it is to follow.

The setting influences the complexity of any teaching plan. In an acute care setting plans are concise and focused on the primary learning needs of the patient because there is limited time for teaching. Home care and outpatient clinic teaching plans are usually more comprehensive in scope because you often have more time to instruct patients and patients are often less anxious in outpatient settings.

Setting Priorities. Include the patient when determining priorities for patient education. Base priorities on the patient's immediate needs, nursing diagnoses, and the goals and outcomes established for him or her. Priorities also depend on what the patient perceives to be most important, his or her anxiety level, and the amount of time available to teach. A patient's learning needs are set in order of priority. For example, a patient recently diagnosed with coronary artery disease has deficient knowledge related to the illness and its implications. The patient benefits most by first learning about the correct way to take nitroglycerin and how long to wait before calling for help when chest pain occurs. Once you assist in meeting patient needs related to basic survival, you can discuss other topics such as exercise and nutritional changes.

Timing. When is the right time to teach? Before a patient enters a hospital? When a patient first enters a clinic? At discharge? At home? Each is appropriate because patients continue to have learning needs and opportunities as long as they stay in the health care system. Plan teaching activities for a time when the patient is most attentive, receptive, and alert and organize the patient's activities to provide time for rest and teaching-learning interactions.

Timing is sometimes difficult because the emphasis is often on a patient's early discharge from a hospital. For example, it takes several days after surgery for a patient to be alert and comfortable enough to learn. By the time a patient feels ready to learn, sometimes discharge is already scheduled. Therefore, to improve patient outcomes, anticipate patients' educational needs before they occur.

Although prolonged sessions cause concentration and attentiveness to decrease, make sure that teaching sessions are not too brief. The patient needs time to comprehend the information and give feedback. It is easier for him or her to tolerate and retain interest in the material during frequent sessions lasting 10 to 15 minutes. However, factors such as shorter hospital stays and lack of insurance reimbursement for outpatient education sessions often necessitate longer teaching sessions.

The frequency of sessions depends on the learner's abilities and the complexity of the material. For example, a child newly diagnosed with diabetes requires more visits to an outpatient center than the older adult who has had diabetes for 15 years and lives in a nursing home. Make sure that intervals between teaching sessions are not so long that the patient forgets information. Home care nurses frequently reinforce learning during home visits when patients are discharged from the hospital.

Organizing Teaching Material. An effective teacher carefully considers the order of information to present. When a nurse has an ongoing relationship with a patient, as in the case of home health or case management, an outline of content helps organize information into a logical sequence. Material needs to progress from simple to complex ideas because a person must learn the simple facts and concepts before learning how to make associations or complex interpretations of ideas. Staff nurses in an acute care setting will often focus on the simpler, more essential concepts, whereas home health nurses can better address complex issues. For example, to teach a woman how to feed her husband who has a gastric tube, the nurse first teaches the wife how to measure the tube feeding and manipulate the equipment. Once the wife has accomplished this, the process of administering the feeding occurs.

Begin instruction with essential content because patients are more likely to remember information that you teach early in the teaching session. For example, immediately after surgical removal of a malignant breast tumor, the patient has many learning needs. Start

NURSING CARE PLAN

Deficient Knowledge: Surgical Procedure

ASSESSMENT

Connie, a nurse in a surgeon's office, is preparing Mr. Holland for a colon resection, which is scheduled in 1 week. Mr. Holland is 75 years old and has recently been diagnosed with colorectal cancer. Connie's assessment focuses on Mr. Holland's readiness to learn and factors that affect his ability to understand the procedure and related postoperative care.

*Assessment Activities**	*Findings/Defining Characteristics*
Assess Mr. Holland's readiness to learn and ask what the surgeon has already told him about the surgery.	Mr. Holland responds, "**I can't remember what the doctor told me** at my last appointment, but **I need to know how to take care of myself.** My surgery is scheduled for next week."
Ask Mr. Holland to explain what he knows about postoperative care, including performing a return demonstration of deep breathing and coughing.	Mr. Holland is **unable to describe postoperative care or provide a return demonstration of deep breathing and coughing.**
Observe Mr. Holland's behavior during the office visit.	Mr. Holland states he is anxious but asks appropriate questions. He maintains good contact with the nurse.

*__Defining characteristics__ are shown in bold type.

NURSING DIAGNOSIS: Deficient Knowledge: surgical procedure related to lack of recall and exposure to information

PLANNING

Goals	*Expected Outcomes (NOC)*†
	Knowledge: Treatment Procedure
Mr. Holland will describe preoperative and postoperative care activities before surgery.	Mr. Holland will verbalize understanding of the surgical procedure, postoperative monitoring, and activity planned on the day of surgery.
Mr. Holland will participate in postoperative care during hospitalization.	Mr. Holland will demonstrate deep breathing and coughing and advance his level of physical activity after his surgery.

†Outcome classification labels from Moorhead S et al: *Nursing outcomes classification (NOC),* ed 4, St Louis, 2008, Mosby.

INTERVENTIONS (NIC)‡	RATIONALE
Learning Readiness Enhancement	
Provide a nonthreatening environment in the consultation area. Sit with the patient and encourage any questions during instruction.	The adult patient's learning is enhanced when the patient is ready to learn and when he or she perceives the information to be important. (Bastable, 2008).
Learning Facilitation	
Offer Mr. Holland multiple teaching modalities (e.g., brochure and audiotape describing preoperative and postoperative care) while explaining preoperative and postoperative care.	Providing patients with educational methods that use multiple senses is effective in educating older adults. Older adults prefer written handouts in large fonts (Meiner, 2011).
Explain postoperative care activities, including frequent monitoring and demonstrate deep breathing and coughing, and have Mr. Holland perform return demonstration.	Improving self-efficacy by using role modeling and having the patient perform behaviors enhances the successful adoption of healthy behaviors (Bandura, 1997).

‡Intervention classification labels from Bulechek GM, Butcher HK, and Dochterman JM: *Nursing interventions classification (NIC),* ed 5, St Louis, 2008, Mosby.

EVALUATION

Nursing Actions	*Patient Response/Finding*	*Achievement of Outcome*
Ask Mr. Holland to describe what will happen before and after surgery.	Mr. Holland is able to state understanding of preoperative and postoperative care activities.	Mr. Holland's anxiety level has decreased, and he reports that he is ready for surgery.
Observe patient as he demonstrates deep breathing and coughing and advances his activity after surgery.	Mr. Holland is able to deep breathe and cough after surgery, but he is hesitant to advance his activity level.	Patient has not totally achieved outcome of advancing activity after surgery. Manage barriers inhibiting attainment of this outcome (e.g., pain), and continue to encourage and educate patient.

with essential information such as how to monitor the incision site for signs of infection; deal with the emotional aspects of a cancer diagnosis and complete the teaching session with informative but less critical content, including the warning signs of cancer. Repetition reinforces learning. A concise summary of key topics helps the learner remember the most important information (Bastable, 2008).

Teamwork and Collaboration. During planning choose appropriate teaching methods, encourage the patient to offer suggestions, and make referrals to other health care professionals (e.g., dietitians and physical, speech, or occupational therapists) when appropriate. The nurse is the member of the health care team primarily responsible for ensuring that all patient educational needs are met. However, sometimes patient needs are highly complex. In these cases identify appropriate health education resources within the health care system or the community during planning. Examples of resources for patient education include diabetes education clinics, cardiac rehabilitation programs, prenatal classes, and support groups. When patients receive education and support from these types of resources, the nurse obtains a referral order when necessary, encourages patients to attend educational sessions, and reinforces information taught. Resources that specialize in a particular health need (e.g., wound care or ostomy specialists) are integral to successful patient education.

IMPLEMENTATION

The implementation of patient education depends on your ability to critically analyze assessment data when identifying learning needs and developing the teaching plan (see Care Plan). Carefully evaluate the learning objectives and determine which teaching and learning principles most effectively and efficiently assist the patient in meeting expected goals and outcomes. Implementation involves believing that each interaction with a patient is an opportunity to teach. Use evidence-based interventions to create an effective learning environment.

Maintaining Learning Attention and Participation. Active participation is key to learning. Persons learn better when more than one of the senses is stimulated. Audiovisual aids and role play are good teaching strategies. By actively experiencing a learning event, the person is more likely to retain knowledge. A teacher's actions also increase learner attention and interest. When conducting a discussion with a learner, the teacher stays active by changing the tone and intensity of his or her voice, making eye contact, and using gestures that accentuate key points of discussion. An effective teacher engages learners and talks and moves among a group rather than remaining stationary behind a lectern or table. A learner remains interested in a teacher who is actively enthusiastic about the subject under discussion.

Building on Existing Knowledge. A patient learns best on the basis of preexisting cognitive abilities and knowledge. Thus a teacher is more effective when he or she presents information that builds on a learner's existing knowledge. A patient quickly loses interest if a nurse begins with familiar information. For example, a patient who has lived with multiple sclerosis for several years is beginning a new medication that is given subcutaneously. Before teaching the patient how to prepare the medication and give the injection, the nurse asks him or her about previous experience with injections. On assessment the nurse learns that the patient's father had diabetes and the patient administered the insulin injections. The nurse individualizes the teaching plan by building on the patient's previous knowledge and experience with insulin injections.

Teaching Approaches. A nurse's approach in teaching is different from teaching methods. Some situations require a teacher to be directive. Others require a nondirective approach. An effective teacher concentrates on the task and uses teaching approaches according to the learner's needs. A learner's needs and motives frequently change over time. Thus the effective teacher is always aware of the need to modify teaching approaches.

Telling. Use the telling approach when teaching limited information (e.g., preparing a patient for an emergent diagnostic procedure). If a patient is highly anxious but it is vital for information to be given, telling is effective. When using telling, the nurse outlines the task the patient will perform and gives explicit instructions. There is no opportunity for feedback with this method.

Participating. In the participating approach the nurse and patient set objectives and become involved in the learning process together. The patient helps decide content, and the nurse guides and counsels the patient with pertinent information. In this method there is opportunity for discussion, feedback, mutual goal setting, and revision of the teaching plan. For example, a parent caring for a child with leukemia learns how to care for the child at home and recognize problems that need to be reported immediately. The parent and nurse collaborate on developing an appropriate teaching plan. After each teaching session is completed, the parent and nurse review the objectives together, determine if the objectives were met, and plan what will be covered in the next session.

Entrusting. The entrusting approach provides the patient the opportunity to manage self-care. The patient accepts responsibilities and performs tasks correctly and consistently. The nurse observes the patient's progress and remains available to assist without introducing more new information. For example, a patient has been managing diabetes well for 10 years. Because of the development of a complication, the patient now has to walk instead of jog during exercise. The patient understands how to adjust insulin when exercising to prevent hypoglycemia. The nurse instructs the patient about the newly prescribed exercise therapy and allows him or her to adjust insulin dosages independently.

Reinforcing. **Reinforcement** requires using a stimulus that increases the probability for a response. A learner who receives reinforcement before or after a desired learning behavior is likely to repeat the behavior. Feedback is a common form of reinforcement. Reinforcers are positive or negative. Positive reinforcement such as a smile or spoken approval produces desired responses. Although negative reinforcement such as frowning or criticizing decreases an undesired response, people usually respond better to positive reinforcement (Bastable, 2008). The effects of negative reinforcement are less predictable and often undesirable.

Three types of reinforcers are social, material, and activity. When a nurse works with a patient, most reinforcers are social, used to acknowledge a learned behavior (e.g., smiles, compliments, or words of encouragement). Examples of material reinforcers are food, toys, and music. These work best with young children. Activity reinforcers rely on the principle that a person is motivated to engage in an activity if he or she has the opportunity to engage in a more desirable activity after completion of the task. For example, a patient is more likely to go to a mental health counseling session if he or she is given the chance to go outside for a walk afterward.

Choosing an appropriate reinforcer involves giving careful thought and attention to individual preferences. Observing behavior often helps reveal the best reinforcer to use. Do not use reinforcers as threats. They are not effective with every patient. A young child responds more to social reinforcers than do older children or adults. In adults reinforcement is more effective when the nurse establishes a therapeutic relationship with the patient.

Incorporating Teaching with Nursing Care. Many nurses find that they are able to teach more effectively while delivering nursing care. This becomes easier as you gain confidence in your clinical skills. For example, while hanging blood you explain to the patient why the blood is necessary and the symptoms of a transfusion reaction that need to be reported immediately. Another example is explaining the side effects of a medication while administering it. An informal, unstructured style relies on the positive therapeutic relationship between nurse and patient, which fosters spontaneity in the teaching-learning process. Teaching during routine care is efficient and cost-effective (Fig. 25-2).

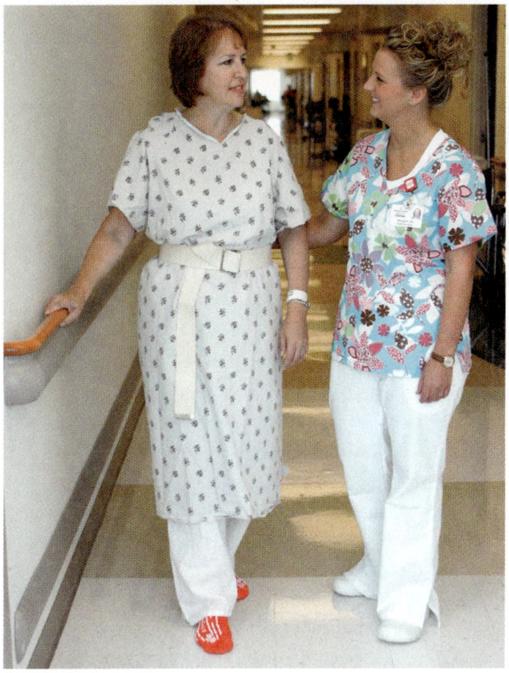

FIG. 25-2 Teaching postoperative care while walking with the patient uses time efficiently.

Instructional Methods. Choose instructional methods that match a patient's learning needs, the time available for teaching, the setting, the resources available, and your comfort level with teaching. Skilled teachers are flexible in altering teaching methods according to the learner's responses. An experienced teacher uses a variety of techniques and teaching aids. Do not expect to be an expert educator when first entering nursing practice. Learning to become effective in teaching takes time and practice.

When first starting to teach patients, it helps to remember that patients perceive you as an expert. However, this does not mean that they expect you to have all of the answers. It simply means that they expect that you will keep them appropriately informed. Effective nurses keep the teaching plan simple and focused on patients' needs.

One-on-One Discussion. Perhaps the most common method of instruction is one-on-one discussion. When teaching a patient at the bedside, in a physician's office, or in the home, the nurse shares information directly. You usually give information in an informal manner, allowing the patient to ask questions or share concerns. Use various teaching aids such as models or diagrams during the discussion, depending on the patient's learning needs. Use unstructured and informal discussions when helping patients understand the implications of illness and ways to cope with health stressors.

Group Instruction. Some nurses choose to teach patients in groups because of the advantages associated with group teaching. Groups are an economical way to teach a number of patients at one time, and patients are able to interact with one another and learn from the experiences of others. Learning in a group of six or less is more effective and avoids outburst behaviors. Groups also foster the development of positive attitudes that help patients meet learning objectives (Bezalel et al., 2010). Group instruction often involves both lecture and discussion. Lectures are highly structured and efficient in helping groups of patients learn standard content about a subject. A lecture does not ensure that learners are actively thinking about the material presented; thus discussion and practice sessions are essential. After a lecture, learners need the opportunity to share ideas and seek clarification. Group discussions allow patients and families to learn from one another as they review common experiences. A productive group discussion helps participants solve problems and arrive at solutions toward improving each member's health. To be an effective group leader, the nurse guides participation. Acknowledging a look of interest, asking questions, and summarizing key points foster group involvement. However, not all patients benefit from group discussions, and sometimes the physical or emotional level of wellness makes participation difficult or impossible.

Preparatory Instruction. Patients frequently face unfamiliar tests or procedures that create significant anxiety. Providing information about procedures often decreases anxiety because patients have a better idea of what to expect during the procedure, which helps to give them a sense of control. The known is less threatening than the unknown. Use the following guidelines for giving preparatory explanations:

- Describe physical sensations during a procedure. For example, when drawing a blood specimen, explain that the patient will feel a sticking sensation as the needle punctures the skin.
- Describe the cause of the sensation, preventing misinterpretation of the experience. For example, explain that a needlestick burns because the alcohol used to clean the skin enters the puncture site.
- Prepare patients only for aspects of the experience that others have commonly noticed. For example, explain that it is normal for a tight tourniquet to cause a person's hand to tingle and feel numb.

Demonstrations. Use demonstrations when teaching psychomotor skills such as preparation of a syringe, bathing an infant, crutch walking, or taking a pulse. Demonstrations are most effective when learners first observe the teacher and then, during a **return demonstration,** have the chance to practice the skill. Combine a demonstration with discussion to clarify concepts and feelings. An effective demonstration requires advanced planning:

1. Be sure that the learner can easily see each step of the demonstration. Position the learner to provide a clear view of the skill being performed.
2. Assemble and organize the equipment. Make sure that all equipment works.
3. Perform each step slowly and accurately in sequence while analyzing the knowledge and skills involved and allow the patient to handle the equipment
4. Review the rationale and steps of the procedure.
5. Encourage the patient to ask questions so he or she understands each step.
6. Judge proper speed and timing of the demonstration based on the patient's cognitive abilities and anxiety level.
7. To demonstrate mastery of the skill, have the patient perform a return demonstration under the same conditions that will be experienced at home or in the place where the skill is to be performed. For example, when a patient needs to learn to walk with crutches, the nurse simulates the home environment. If the patient's home has stairs, the patient practices going up and down a staircase in the hospital.

Analogies. Learning occurs when a teacher translates complex language or ideas into words or concepts that the patient understands. **Analogies** supplement verbal instruction with familiar images that make complex information more real and understandable. For example, when explaining arterial blood pressure, use an analogy of the flow of water through a hose. Follow these general principles when using analogies:

- Be familiar with the concept.
- Know the patient's background, experience, and culture.
- Keep the analogy simple and clear.

Role Play. During role play people are asked to play themselves or someone else. Patients learn required skills and feel more confident in being able to perform them independently. The technique involves rehearsing a desired behavior. For example, a nurse who is teaching a parent how to respond to a child's behavior pretends to be a child who is having a temper tantrum. The parent responds to the nurse who is pretending to be the child. Afterward the nurse evaluates the parent's response and determines whether an alternative approach would have been more appropriate.

Simulation. Simulation is a useful technique for teaching problem solving, application, and independent thinking. During individual or group discussion you pose a pertinent problem or situation for patients to solve. For example, patients with heart disease plan a meal that is low in cholesterol and fat. The patients in the group decide which foods are appropriate. You ask the group members to present their diet, providing an opportunity to identify mistakes and reinforce correct information.

Illiteracy and Other Disabilities. It is important to use words that a patient is able to understand. Medical jargon is confusing. Implications of low health literacy, illiteracy, and learning disabilities include an impaired ability to analyze instructions or synthesize information. In addition, many of these patients have not acquired the problem-solving skills of drawing conclusions and inferences from experience, and they do not ask questions to obtain or clarify information that has been presented. Box 25-6 summarizes nursing interventions that nurses use when caring for patients who have literacy or learning disability problems.

Sometimes patients have sensory deficits that affect how the nurse presents information (see Chapter 49). For example, patients who are deaf require a sign language interpreter. Not all people who are deaf read lips. Therefore it is very important to provide clear written materials that match the patients' reading level. Visual impairments also impact the teaching strategy used by the nurse. Many people who are blind have acute listening skills. Avoid shouting and announce your presence to patients with visual impairments before approaching them. If the patient has partial vision, use colors and a print font size (14-point font or greater) that the patient is able to see. Be sure to use proper lighting. Other helpful interventions include audiotaping teaching sessions and providing structured, well-organized instructions (Bastable, 2008).

Building Competency in Patient-Centered Care You are caring for Bob, a 47-year-old patient with type 1 diabetes who is having difficulty following a complicated medication schedule at home. He needs to take different medications, including insulin injections, several times a day. During your assessment, you find he has difficulty understanding printed teaching sheets. He admits, "I had to drop out of school when I was in eighth grade, and my vision is not as good as it used to be." What additional assessment questions and teaching strategies, approaches, and tools do you use to enhance Bob's learning and ability to take his medications as they are ordered?

Answers to questions can be found on the Evolve website.

Cultural Diversity. You must have knowledge of a patient's cultural background and beliefs and his or her ability to understand instructions in a language different from his or her native language (see Chapter 9 and Box 25-7). Cultural diversity poses a

BOX 25-6 PATIENT TEACHING

Teaching an Illiterate Patient or Patient with a Learning Disability

Objective
- Patient will perform desired behaviors accurately.

Teaching Strategies
- Establish trust with patient before beginning the teaching-learning session.
- Use simple terminology to enhance patient's understanding.
- Avoid medical jargon. If necessary, explain medical terms using basic one- or two-syllable words.
- Keep teaching sessions short and to the point and minimize distractions.
- Include the most important information at the beginning of the session.
- Relate practical information to personal experiences or real-life situations.
- Use visual cues and simple analogies when appropriate.
- Frequently ask patient for feedback to determine if he or she comprehends information.
- Ask for return demonstrations and clarify instructions when needed.
- Provide teaching materials that reflect reading level of patient, with attention given to short words and sentences, large type, and simple format (generally information written on a fifth-grade reading level is recommended for adult learners).
- Reinforce most important information at the end of the session.
- Schedule teaching sessions at frequent intervals.
- Model appropriate behavior and use role-play to help patient learn how to ask questions and ask for help effectively.

Evaluation
- Ask patient to verbalize understanding of information taught.
- Observe and evaluate patient's ability to perform desired behaviors.

Data from Bastable S: *Nurse as educator: principles of teaching and learning for nursing practice,* ed 3, Sudbury, Mass, 2008, Jones & Bartlett.

BOX 25-7 CULTURAL ASPECTS OF CARE

Patient Education

Patient education needs to be patient-centered and culturally sensitive for learning to occur. Assessing patients' preferred learning approaches and adapting education to meet patients' needs facilitates the attainment of educational outcomes. Sociocultural norms, values, and traditions often determine the importance of different health education topics and the preference of one learning approach over another. Educational efforts are especially challenging when patients and educators do not speak the same language or when written materials are not culturally sensitive and are written above patients' reading abilities.

Implications for Practice
- Establish rapport with culturally diverse patients before starting teaching sessions (Campinha-Bacote, 2009).
- Sociocultural background influences a patient's desire to learn and which information the patient perceives as important to learn (Campinha-Bacote, 2009).
- Carefully assess a patient's preference for educational delivery method to ensure successful learning.
- Nurses must have a wide variety of culturally sensitive educational resources available to them to meet the needs of diverse populations.
- When you and the patient do not speak the same language, accurate translators are necessary.

great challenge when you are trying to provide culturally sensitive care. When educating patients of different ethnic groups, be aware of the distinctive aspects of each culture, being careful not to stereotype patients (Campinha-Bacote, 2009). Collaborate with other nurses and educators to present appropriate teaching approaches, and ask the people in the cultural group to help by sharing their values and beliefs. Ethnic nurses are excellent resources who are able to provide input through their experiences to improve the care provided to members of their own community (Bastable, 2008). When patients cannot understand English, use trained and certified health care interpreters to provide health care information.

In addition, be aware of intergenerational conflict of values. This occurs when immigrant parents uphold their traditional values and their children, who are exposed to American values in social encounters, develop beliefs similar to those of their American peers. Consider this conflict in values when providing information to families or groups who have members from different generations. To enhance patient education in culturally diverse populations, know when and how to provide education while respecting cultural values. Modify teaching regarding interventions or desired behaviors to accommodate for cultural differences. Effective educational strategies often require the nurse to use different patterns of communication (Campinha-Bacote, 2009).

Using Teaching Tools. Many teaching tools are available for patient education. Selection of the right tool depends on the instructional method, the patient's learning needs, and his or her ability to learn (Table 25-3). For example, a printed pamphlet is not the best tool to use for a patient with poor reading comprehension, but an audiotape is a good choice for a patient with visual impairment.

Special Needs of Children and Older Adults. Children, adults, and older adults learn differently. You adapt teaching strategies to each learner. Children pass through several developmental stages (see Unit 2). In each developmental stage children acquire new cognitive and psychomotor abilities that respond to different types of teaching methods (Fig. 25-3). Incorporate parental input in planning health education for children.

Older adults experience numerous physical and psychological changes as they age (see Chapter 14). These changes not only increase their educational needs but also create barriers to learning unless adjustments are made in nursing interventions. Sensory changes such as visual and hearing changes require adaptation of

TABLE 25-3 Teaching Tools for Instruction

DESCRIPTION	LEARNING IMPLICATIONS
Written Materials	
Printed Material and Online Materials	
Written teaching tools available in print or online as pamphlets, booklets, brochures	Material must be easy to read. Information must be accurate and current. Method is ideal for understanding complex concepts and relationships.
Programmed Instruction	
Written sequential presentation of learning steps requiring that learners answer questions and teachers tell them whether they are right or wrong	Instruction is primarily verbal, but teacher sometimes uses pictures or diagrams. Method requires active learning, giving immediate feedback, correcting wrong answers, and reinforcing right answers. Learner works at own pace.
Computer Instruction	
Use of programmed instruction format in which computers store response patterns for learners and select further lessons on basis of these patterns (programs can be individualized)	Method requires reading comprehension, psychomotor skills, and familiarity with computer.
Nonprint Materials	
Diagrams	
Illustrations that show interrelationships by means of lines and symbols	Method demonstrates key ideas, summarizes, and clarifies key concept.
Graphs (Bar, Circle, or Line)	
Visual presentations of numerical data	Graphs help learner grasp information quickly about single concept.
Charts	
Highly condensed visual summary of ideas and facts that highlights series of ideas, steps, or events	Charts demonstrate relationship of several ideas or concepts. Method helps learners know what to do.
Pictures	
Photographs or drawings used to teach concepts in which the third dimension of shape and space is not important	Photographs are more desirable than diagrams because they more accurately portray the details of the real item.
Physical Objects	
Use of actual equipment, objects, or models to teach concepts or skills	Models are useful when real objects are too small, large, or complicated or are unavailable. Allows learners to manipulate objects that they will use later in skill.
Other Audiovisual Materials	
Slides, audiotapes, television, and videotapes used with printed material or discussion	Materials are useful for patients with reading comprehension problems and visual deficits.

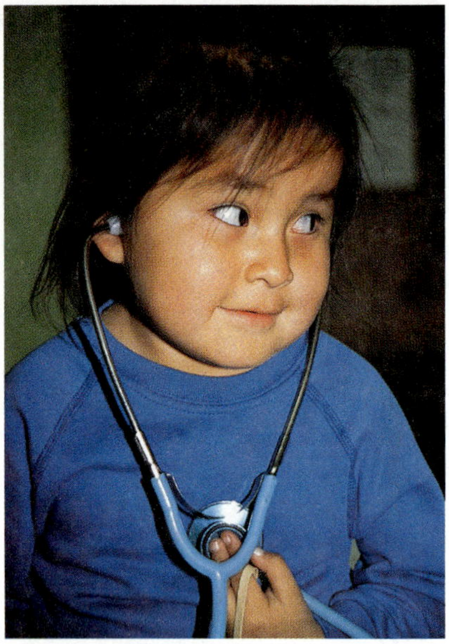

FIG. 25-3 The preschool child learns not to be afraid of medical equipment by being allowed to handle the stethoscope and imitating its use.

teaching methods to enhance functioning. Older adults learn and remember effectively if the nurse paces the learning properly and if the material is relevant to the learner's needs and abilities. Although many older adults have slower cognitive function and reduced short-term memory, you facilitate learning in several ways to support behaviors that maximize the individual's capacity for self-care (Box 25-8).

Establish short-term goals when teaching older patients. Include family members who assume care for the patient. However, be sensitive to the patient's desire for assistance because offering unwanted support often results in negative outcomes and perceptions of nagging and interference. Furthermore, not all relationships between older adults and other family members are therapeutic. Because of the high incidence of abuse and neglect of older adults, assess family dynamics before including family members in educational sessions.

BOX 25-8 FOCUS ON OLDER ADULTS

Providing Patient Education

You facilitate learning by using the following interventions when providing patient education to older adults:

- Begin and end each teaching session with the most important information.
- Present information slowly.
- Speak in a low tone of voice (lower tones are easier to hear than higher tones).
- Allow enough time for understanding the material.
- Emphasize concrete material that applies to current situations.
- Present only crucial information to avoid overwhelming the learner.
- Provide specific information in frequent, small amounts.
- Repeat important information.
- Relate new material to previous life experiences.
- Build on existing knowledge.
- Allow patients to progress at their own pace (older adults are more cautious; thus it may take longer to adopt a behavior change).
- Use group experiences if appropriate to enhance problem solving.
- If using written material, assess patient's ability to read and use information that is printed in large type and in a color that contrasts highly with the background (e.g., black 14-point print on buff-colored paper). Avoid blues and greens because they are more difficult to see.

Data from Ebersole P et al: *Toward healthy aging,* ed 7, St Louis, 2008, Mosby; Edelman CL, Mandle CL: *Health promotion throughout the lifespan,* ed 7, St Louis, 2010, Mosby.

EVALUATION

Through the Patient's Eyes. Patient education is not complete until you evaluate outcomes of the teaching-learning process (see Care Plan). Engage patients in the evaluation process to determine if they have learned essential material. It is also important to determine if patients believe they have the information necessary to continue self-care activities within the home. This is why it is important to evaluate through the patient's eyes, respecting the type of situations patients return to after receiving care. Evaluation reinforces correct behavior, helps learners realize how to change incorrect behavior, and helps the teacher determine adequacy of teaching (Redman, 2007).

Patient Outcomes. The nurse is legally responsible for providing accurate, timely patient information that promotes continuity of care; therefore it is essential to document the outcomes of teaching. Documentation of patient teaching also supports quality improvement efforts, meets TJC's standards, and promotes third-party reimbursement. Teaching flow sheets and written plans of care (e.g., CareMaps) are excellent records that document the plan, implementation, and evaluation of learning.

You evaluate success by observing a patient's performance of each expected behavior. Success depends on a patient's ability to meet the established outcome and goals. Carefully phrase questions to ensure that the learner understands them and that objectives are truly measured. Questions to ask when evaluating patient education include the following:

- Were the patient's goals or outcomes realistic and observable?
- Did the patient value the information provided?
- Was the patient willing to change an existing or adopt a new behavior?
- What barriers prevented learning or change in behaviors?
- Is the patient able to perform the behavior or skill in the natural setting (e.g., home)?
- How well is the patient able to answer questions about the topic?
- If the patient is completing a log, how well does the log match what was taught?
- Does the patient continue to have problems understanding the information or performing a skill? If so, how can the nurse change the interventions to enhance knowledge or skill performance?

KEY POINTS

- The nurse ensures that patients, families, and communities receive information needed to promote, restore, and maintain optimal health.
- Teaching is most effective when it is responsive to a learner's needs.
- Teaching is a form of interpersonal communication, with the teacher and learner actively involved in a process that increases the learner's knowledge and skills.

- The ability to learn depends on a person's physical and cognitive attributes.
- The ability to attend to the learning process depends on physical comfort and anxiety levels and the presence of environmental distraction.
- A person's health beliefs influence the willingness to gain knowledge and skills necessary to maintain health.
- Use of a theory (e.g., social learning theory) or theoretical concepts (e.g., self-efficacy) enhances learning.
- Time teaching so it occurs when a patient is ready to learn.
- Patients of different age-groups require different teaching strategies because of developmental capabilities.
- Involve patients actively in all aspects of teaching plans.
- Nurses use learning objectives to set learning priorities.
- A combination of teaching methods improves the learner's attentiveness and involvement.
- A teacher is more effective when presenting information that builds on a learner's existing knowledge.
- Effective teachers use positive reinforcement.
- Older adults learn most effectively when information is paced slowly and presented in small amounts.
- Evaluate a patient's learning by observing performance of expected learning behaviors under desired conditions.
- Effective documentation describes the entire process of patient education, promotes continuity of care, and demonstrates that educational standards have been met.

CLINICAL APPLICATION QUESTIONS

Preparing for Clinical Practice

While Connie is providing preoperative teaching, she provides Mr. Holland with several teaching brochures that explain what colorectal cancer is and what to expect before, during, and after the surgery. Mr. Holland reads through the brochures and nods his head as if he understands the material.

1. To evaluate Mr. Holland's learning, Connie asks him to verbalize what he read in his own words. He has trouble describing it. Connie asks him questions about information in the brochures and discovers that he misunderstood much of the information. What do these assessment data suggest about Mr. Holland's health literacy? What special considerations does Connie need to implement at this time?
2. The surgeon comes to see Mr. Holland after surgery. A new nurse, John, is in the hospital room at this time. The surgeon tells Mr. Holland that his cancer is aggressive and that he will probably need to have chemotherapy once the incision is healed. The surgeon leaves the room. John turns to Mr. Holland. He states, "I'm sure the doctor is wrong. After all, he's a surgeon, not an oncologist." Which stage of grieving is Mr. Holland experiencing? What approach should John take in planning education for him?
3. Mr. Holland has been discharged. In planning discharge teaching, John reviews the medications Mr. Holland will be taking at home. He notices that his physician has prescribed three new medications. When John asks Mr. Holland what he understands about them, he states, "I've never heard of these medications." When John asks him to explain when he should take the medications, Mr. Holland is unable to do so correctly. What is the nursing diagnosis for this situation?

evolve Answers to Clinical Application Questions can be found on the Evolve website.

REVIEW QUESTIONS

Are You Ready to Test Your Nursing Knowledge?

1. A patient needs to learn to use a walker. Which domain is required for learning this skill?
   1. Affective domain
   2. Cognitive domain
   3. Attentional domain
   4. Psychomotor domain
2. The nurse is planning to teach a patient about the importance of exercise. When is the best time for teaching to occur? (Select all that apply.)
   1. When there are visitors in the room
   2. When the patient's pain medications are working
   3. Just before lunch, when the patient is most awake and alert
   4. When the patient is talking about current stressors in his or her life
3. A patient newly diagnosed with cervical cancer is going home. The patient is avoiding discussion of her illness and postoperative orders. What is the nurse's best plan in teaching this patient?
   1. Teach the patient's spouse
   2. Focus on knowledge the patient will need in a few weeks
   3. Provide only the information that the patient needs to go home
   4. Convince the patient that learning about her health is necessary
4. The school nurse is about to teach a freshman-level high school health class about nutrition. What is the best instructional approach to ensure that the students meet the learning outcomes?
   1. Provide information using a lecture
   2. Use simple words to promote understanding
   3. Develop topics for discussion that require problem solving
   4. Complete an extensive literature search focusing on eating disorders
5. A nurse is going to teach a patient how to perform breast self-examination. Which behavioral objective does the nurse set to best measure the patient's ability to perform the examination?
   1. The patient will verbalize the steps involved in breast self-examination within 1 week.
   2. The nurse will explain the importance of performing breast self-examination once a month.
   3. The patient will perform breast self-examination correctly on herself before the end of the teaching session.
   4. The nurse will demonstrate breast self-examination on a breast model provided by the American Cancer Society.
6. A patient with chest pain is having an emergency cardiac catheterization. Which teaching approach does the nurse use in this situation?
   1. Telling approach
   2. Selling approach
   3. Entrusting approach
   4. Participating approach
7. The nurse is teaching a parenting class to a group of pregnant adolescents. The nurse pretends to be the baby's father, and the adolescent mother is asked to show how she would respond to the father if he gave her a can of beer. Which teaching approach did the nurse use?
   1. Role play
   2. Discovery

3. An analogy
4. A demonstration

8. An older adult is being started on a new antihypertensive medication. In teaching the patient about the medication, the nurse:
   1. Speaks loudly.
   2. Presents the information once.
   3. Expects the patient to understand the information quickly.
   4. Allows the patient time to express himself or herself and ask questions.
9. A patient needs to learn how to administer a subcutaneous injection. Which of the following reflects that the patient is ready to learn?
   1. Describing difficulties a family member has had in taking insulin
   2. Expressing the importance of learning the skill correctly
   3. Being able to see and understand the markings on the syringe
   4. Having the dexterity needed to prepare and inject the medication
10. A patient who is hospitalized has just been diagnosed with diabetes. He is going to need to learn how to give himself injections. Which teaching method does the nurse use?
    1. Simulation
    2. Demonstration
    3. Group instruction
    4. One-on-one discussion
11. When a nurse is teaching a patient about how to administer an epinephrine injection in case of a severe allergic reaction, he or she tells the patient to hold the injection like a dart. Which of the following instructional methods did the nurse use?
    1. Telling
    2. Analogy
    3. Demonstration
    4. Simulation
12. A nurse needs to teach a young woman newly diagnosed with asthma how to manage her disease. Which of the following topics does the nurse teach first?
    1. How to use an inhaler during an asthma attack
    2. The need to avoid people who smoke to prevent asthma attacks
    3. Where to purchase a medical alert bracelet that says she has asthma
    4. The importance of maintaining a healthy diet and exercising regularly
13. A nurse is teaching a group of young college-age women the importance of using sunscreen when going out in the sun. What type of content is the nurse providing?
    1. Simulation
    2. Restoring health
    3. Coping with impaired function
    4. Health promotion and illness prevention
14. A nurse is planning a teaching session about healthy nutrition with a group of children who are in first grade. The nurse determines that after the teaching session the children will be able to name three examples of foods that are fruits. This is an example of:
    1. A teaching plan.
    2. A learning objective.
    3. Reinforcement of content.
    4. Enhancing the children's self-efficacy.
15. A nurse is teaching a 27-year-old gentleman how to adjust his insulin dosages based on his blood sugar results. What type of learning is this?
    1. Cognitive
    2. Affective
    3. Adaptation
    4. Psychomotor

Answers: **1.** 4; **2.** 2; **3.** 3; **4.** 3; **5.** 3; **6.** 1; **7.** 1; **8.** 4; **9.** 2; **10.** 2; **11.** 2; **12.** 1; **13.** 4; **14.** 2; **15.** 1.

REFERENCES

American Hospital Association: *The patient care partnership: understanding expectations, rights, and responsibilities,* 2003, http://www.aha.org/aha/issues/Communicating-With-Patients/pt-care-partnership.html. Accessed October 23, 2010.

Attwood CA: Health literacy: do your patients really understand? *AACN Viewpoint* 30(2):3, 2008.

Bandura A: *Self-efficacy: the exercise of control,* New York, 1997, WH Freeman.

Bandura A: Social cognitive theory: an agentic perspective, *Annu Rev Psychol* 52:1, 2001.

Bastable SB: *Essentials of patient education,* Sudbury, Mass, 2006, Jones & Bartlett.

Bastable SB: *Nurse as educator: principles of teaching and learning for nursing practice,* ed 3, Sudbury, Mass, 2008, Jones & Bartlett.

Billings DM, Halstead JA: *Teaching in nursing,* ed 3, St Louis, 2009, Saunders.

Bloom BS, editor: Taxonomy of educational objectives, *Cognitive domain,* vol 1, New York, 1956, Longman.

Campinha-Bacote J: A culturally competent model of care for African Americans, *Urol Nurs* 29(1):49, 2009.

Edelman CL, Mandle CL: *Health promotion throughout the life span,* ed 7, St Louis, 2010, Mosby.

Eshleman KY: Adapting teaching styles to accommodate learning preferences for effective hospital development, *Prog Transplant* 18(4):2008.

Falvo DR: *Effective patient education: a guide to increased compliance,* ed 4, Sudbury, Mass, 2010, Jones & Bartlett.

Heiskell H: Ethical decision-making for the utilization of technology-based patient/family education, *Online J Nurs Informatics* 14(1), 2010.

Hockenberry M, Wilson D: *Wong's nursing care of infants and children,* ed 9, St Louis, 2011, Mosby.

Krathwohl DR, et al: *Taxonomy of educational objectives: the classification of educational goals. Handbook II, affective domain,* New York, 1964, David McKay.

Meiner SA: *Gerontologic nursing,* ed 4, St Louis, 2011, Mosby.

National Network of Libraries of Medicine: *Health Literacy,* 2011, http://nnlm.gov/outreach/consumer/hlthlit.html. Accessed August 12, 2011.

Olsen L: Patient assessment: building a foundation for optimal patient discharge outcomes, *Care Manage* 16(3): 11, 2010.

QSEN: *Competency KSAs (pre-licensure),* 2010, http://www.qsen.org/ksas_prelicensure.php#patient-centered_care. Accessed October 23, 2010.

Redman BK: *The practice of patient education,* ed 10, St Louis, 2007, Mosby.

Rothman RL, et al: Health literacy and quality: focus on chronic illness care and patient safety, *Pediatrics* 124(Suppl 3):S315, 2009.

Stonecypher K: Creating a patient education tool, *J Contin Educ Nurs* 40(10):462, 2009.

The Joint Commission: *Speak up initiatives,* 2010, http://www.jointcommission.org/PatientSafety/SpeakUp/. Accessed October 23, 2010.

The Joint Commission (TJC): *Comprehensive accreditation manual for hospitals: the official handbook* (E-dition), The Joint Commission, 2011.

World Health Organization: *Health Promotion: Track 2: Health literacy and health behaviour* 2011, http://www.who.int/healthpromotion/conferences/7gchp/track2/en/. Accessed August 12, 2011.

RESEARCH REFERENCES

Ashford S, et al: What is the best way to change self-efficacy to promote lifestyle and recreational physical activity? A systematic review with meta-analysis, *Br J Health Psychol* 15:265, 2010.

Bezalel T, et al: The effect of a group education programme on pain and function through knowledge acquisition and home-based exercise among patients with knee osteoarthritis: a parallel randomized single-blind clinical trial, *Physiotherapy* 96(2):137, 2010.

Boren SA, et al: Heart failure self-management education: a systematic review of the evidence, *Int J Evid Based Healthc* 7(3):159, 2009.

Clauson KA, et al: Readability of patient- and health care professional–targeted dietary supplement leaflets used for diabetes and chronic fatigue syndrome, *J Altern Complement Med* 16(1):119, 2010.

Coffman JM, et al: Do school-based asthma education programs improve self-management and health outcomes? *Pediatrics* 124(2):729, 2009.

Evangelista LS, Shinnick MA: What do we know about adherence and self-care? *J Cardiovasc Nurs* 23(3):250, 2008.

Fredericks S, et al: The effect of anxiety on learning outcomes post-CABG, *Can J Nurs Res* 40(1):127, 2008.

Hawkins N, et al: Why the PAP test? Awareness and use of the PAP test among women in the United States, *J Womens Health* 20(4):511, 2011, doi: 10.1089/jwh2011.2730.

Kim SH, Yu X: The mediating effect of self-efficacy on the relationship between health literacy and health status in Korean older adults: a short report, *Aging Ment Health* 14(7):870, 2010.

Kutner M, et al: *The health literacy of America's adults: results from the 2003 National Assessment of Adult Literacy* (NCES 2006-2483), Washington, DC, 2006, US Department of Education, National Center for Education Statistics, http://nces.ed.gov/pubs2006/2006483.pdf.

Lee SY, et al: Short assessment of health literacy—Spanish and English: a comparable test of health literacy for Spanish and English speakers, *Health Serv Res* 45(4):1105, 2010.

Longo DR, et al: Health information seeking, receipt, and use in diabetes self-management, *Ann Fam Med* 8:334, 2010, doi: 10.1370/afm.1115.

MacDonald S, et al: Readability of information leaflets given to attenders at hospital with a head injury, *Emerg Med J* 27(4):279, 2010.

Nunez DE, et al: A review of the efficacy of the self-management model on health outcomes in community-residing older adults with arthritis, *Worldviews on Evid Based Nurs* 6(3):130, 2009.

Speros C: Health literacy: concept analysis, *J Adv Nurs* 50(6):633, 2005.

Villablanca AC, et al: Outcomes of comprehensive heart care programs in high-risk women, *J Women's Health* 19(7): 1313, 2010.

While A, Kiek F: Chronic heart failure: promoting quality of life, *Br J Commun Nurs* 14(2):54, 2009.

Wolf MS, et al: In search of 'low health literacy': threshold vs. gradient effect of literacy on health status and mortality, *Soc Sci Med* 70(9):1335, 2010.

Yehle KS, Plake KS: Self-efficacy and educational interventions in heart failure: a review of the literature, *J Cardiovasc Nurs* 25(3):175, 2010.

CHAPTER

26

Documentation and Informatics

OBJECTIVES

- Describe methods for interdisciplinary communication within the health care team.
- Identify purposes of a health care record.
- Discuss legal guidelines for documentation.
- Identify ways to maintain confidentiality of electronic and written records.
- Describe five quality guidelines for documentation and reporting.
- Discuss the relationship between documentation and financial reimbursement for health care.
- Describe the different methods used in record keeping.
- Discuss the advantages of standardized documentation forms.
- Identify elements to include when documenting a patient's discharge plan.
- Identify the important aspects of home care and long-term care documentation.
- Describe the purpose and content of a hand-off report.
- Explain when to take and how to verify telephone orders.
- Discuss the relationship between informatics and quality health care.
- Describe the advantages of a nursing information system.
- Identify ways to reduce data entry errors.

KEY TERMS

Accreditation, p. 349
Acuity records, p. 356
Case management, p. 355
Charting by exception (CBE), p. 354
Clinical decision support system (CDSS), p. 360
Computerized provider order entry (CPOE), p. 361
Consultations, p. 349
Critical pathways, p. 355
DAR, p. 354
Diagnosis-related group (DRG), p. 350
Documentation, p. 348
Electronic health record (EHR), p. 353
Electronic medical record (EMR), p. 353
Firewall, p. 361
Flow sheets, p. 356
Focus charting, p. 354
Hand-off reports, p. 357
Health informatics, p. 359
Incident (occurrence) report, p. 358
Information technology (IT), p. 359
Kardex, p. 356
Nursing informatics, p. 359
PIE, p. 354
Problem-oriented medical record (POMR), p. 353
Referrals, p. 349
SOAP, p. 354
SOAPIE, p. 354
Source record, p. 354
Standardized care plans, p. 356
Variances, p. 355

evolve WEBSITE

http://evolve.elsevier.com/Potter/fundamentals/

- Review Questions
- Case Study with Questions
- Audio Glossary
- Interactive Learning Activities
- Key Term Flashcards
- Content Updates

Documentation is anything written or printed on which you rely as record or proof of patient actions and activities. Documentation in a patient's medical record is a vital aspect of nursing practice. Nursing documentation must be accurate, comprehensive, and flexible enough to retrieve clinical data, maintain continuity of care, track patient outcomes, and reflect current standards of nursing practice. Information in the patient record provides a detailed account of the level of quality of care delivered to patients. Effective documentation ensures continuity of care, saves time, and minimizes the risk of errors.

There are several documentation systems for recording patient data. Regardless whether documentation is entered electronically or on paper, as a member of the health care team you communicate information about patients in an accurate, timely, and effective manner. The quality of patient care depends on your ability to communicate with other members of the health care team. All health care providers require the same information about patients to develop an organized, comprehensive plan of care. When a plan is not communicated to all members of the health care team, care becomes fragmented, tasks are repeated, and often delays or omissions in therapy occur.

The health care environment creates many challenges for accurately documenting and reporting the care delivered to patients. The quality of care, the standards of regulatory agencies and nursing practice, the reimbursement structure in the health care system, and legal guidelines make documentation and reporting an extremely important responsibility of a nurse. Whether the transfer of patient information occurs through verbal reports, written documents, or electronically, you need to follow basic principles to maintain confidentiality of information.

CONFIDENTIALITY

Nurses are legally and ethically obligated to keep information about patients confidential. They may not discuss a patient's examination, observation, conversation, diagnosis, or treatment with other patients or staff not involved in the patient's care. Only staff directly involved in a patient's care have legitimate access to the records. Patients frequently request copies of their medical records, and they have the right to read them. Each institution has policies to control the manner for sharing records. In most situations patients are required to give written permission for release of medical information.

Legislation to protect patient privacy for health information, the Health Insurance Portability and Accountability Act (HIPAA), governs all areas of patient information and management of that information. To eliminate barriers that could delay access to care, providers are required to notify patients of their privacy policy and make a reasonable effort to obtain written acknowledgment of this notification. HIPAA requires that disclosure or requests regarding health information are limited to the minimum necessary. This includes only the specific information required for a particular purpose. For example, if you need a patient's home telephone number to reschedule an appointment, access to the medical records is limited solely to telephone information.

Sometimes nurses use health care records for data gathering, research, or continuing education. As long as a nurse uses a record as specified and permission is granted, this is permitted. When you are a student in a clinical setting, confidentiality and compliance with HIPAA are part of professional practice. You can review your patients' medical records only for information needed to provide safe and effective patient care. For example, when you are assigned to care for a patient, you need to review the patient's medical record and plan of care. You *do not* share this information with classmates (except for clinical conferences) and *do not* access the medical records of other patients on the unit. Access to electronic health records is traceable through user log-in information. Not only is it unethical to view medical records of other patients, but breaches of confidentiality can lead to disciplinary action by employers and dismissal from work or nursing school. To protect patient confidentiality, ensure that written or electronic materials used in your student clinical practice *do not* include patient identifiers (e.g., room number, date of birth, demographic information) and *never* print material from an electronic health record for personal use.

STANDARDS

Within a health care organization there are standards that govern the type of information you document and for which you are accountable. Institutional standards or policies often dictate the frequency of documentation such as how often you record a nursing assessment or a patient's level of pain. Know the standards of your health care organization to ensure complete and accurate documentation. Nurses are expected to meet the standard of care for every nursing task they perform. Patient records can be used as evidence in a court of law if standards are not met (ANA, 2005).

In addition, your documentation needs to conform to the standards of the National Committee for Quality Assurance (NCQA) and accrediting bodies such as The Joint Commission (TJC) to maintain institutional **accreditation** and minimize liability. Usually an organization incorporates accreditation standards into its policies and revises documentation forms to suit these standards. Current documentation standards require that all patients admitted to a health care facility have an assessment of physical, psychosocial, environmental, self-care, knowledge level, and discharge planning needs. TJC standards require that your documentation be within the context of the nursing process, including evidence of patient and family teaching and discharge planning (TJC, 2011). Other standards such as HIPAA include those directed by state and federal regulatory agencies and are enforced through the Department of Justice and the Centers for Medicare and Medicaid Services (ANA, 2005).

INTERDISCIPLINARY COMMUNICATION WITHIN THE HEALTH CARE TEAM

Patient care requires effective communication among members of the health care team. Effective communication takes place along two approaches. A patient's record or chart is a confidential, permanent legal documentation of information relevant to his or her health care. The record is a continuing account of the patient's health care status and is available to all members of the health care team. All records contain the following information:

- Patient identification and demographic data
- Informed consent for treatment and procedures
- Admission data
- Nursing diagnoses or problems and nursing or interdisciplinary care plan
- Record of nursing care treatment and evaluation
- Medical history
- Medical diagnoses
- Therapeutic orders
- Medical and health discipline progress notes
- Physical assessment findings
- Diagnostic study results
- Patient education
- Summary of operative procedures
- Discharge plan and summary

Reports are oral, written, or audiotaped exchanges of information among caregivers. Common reports given by nurses include change-of-shift reports, telephone reports, hand-off reports, and incident reports. A health care provider calls a nursing unit to receive a verbal report on a patient's condition. The laboratory submits a written report providing the results of diagnostic tests and often notifies the nurse by telephone if results are critical.

Team members communicate information through discussions or conferences. For example, a discharge planning conference involves members of all disciplines (e.g., nursing, social work, dietary, medicine, and physical therapy) who meet to discuss the patient's progress toward established discharge goals. **Consultations** are another form of discussion in which one professional caregiver gives formal advice about the care of a patient to another caregiver. For example, a nurse caring for a patient with a chronic wound consults with a wound care specialist. Nurses document **referrals** (an arrangement for services by another care provider), consultations, and conferences in a patient's permanent record to allow all caregivers to plan care accordingly.

PURPOSES OF RECORDS

The patient record is a valuable source of data for all members of the health care team. Its purposes include communication, legal documentation, financial billing, education, research, and auditing/monitoring.

Communication

The patient's record is one way that health care team members communicate patient needs and progress, individual therapies, content of consultations, patient education, and discharge planning. The plan of care needs to be clear to anyone reading the chart (see Unit 3). The record is the most current and accurate continuous source of information about a patient's health care status. Information communicated in the patient's record allows health care providers to know a patient thoroughly, facilitating safe, effective, and timely patient-centered decisions. To enhance communication and promote safe patient care, you base communication on assessment findings and document patient information as you provide care (e.g., immediately after providing a nursing intervention or completing a patient assessment).

Legal Documentation

Accurate documentation is one of the best defenses for legal claims associated with nursing care (see Chapter 23). To limit nursing liability nursing documentation must indicate clearly that a patient received individualized, goal-directed nursing care based on the nursing assessment. The record must describe exactly what happened to a patient and follow agency standards. This is best achieved when you chart immediately after providing care. Even though nursing care may have been excellent, in a court of law "care not documented is care not provided."

Common charting mistakes that result in malpractice include: (1) failing to record pertinent health or drug information, (2) failing to record nursing actions, (3) failing to record that medications have been given, (4) failing to record drug reactions or changes in patients' conditions, (5) writing illegible or incomplete records, and (6) failing to document discontinued medications. Table 26-1 provides guidelines for legally sound documentation.

Reimbursement

Diagnosis-related groups (DRGs) are the basis for establishing reimbursement for patient care. A DRG is a classification based on patients' medical diagnoses. Hospitals are reimbursed a predetermined dollar amount by Medicare for each DRG. Detailed recording establishes diagnoses for determining a DRG. Your documentation clarifies the type of treatment a patient receives and supports reimbursement to the health care agency.

A medical record audit reviews financial charges used in the patient's care. Private insurance carriers and auditors from federal agencies review records to determine the reimbursement that a patient or a health care agency receives. Accurate documentation of supplies and equipment used assists in accurate and timely reimbursement.

Education

A patient's record contains a variety of information, including diagnoses, signs and symptoms of disease, successful and unsuccessful therapies, diagnostic findings, and patient behaviors. One way to learn the nature of an illness and the individual patient's response to it is to read the patient care record. No two patients have identical records, but you can identify patterns of information in records of patients who have similar health problems. With this information you learn to anticipate the type of care required for a patient.

Research

After obtaining appropriate agency approvals, nurse researchers often use patients' records for research studies to gather statistical data on the frequency of clinical disorders, complications, use of specific medical and nursing therapies, recovery from illness, and deaths. Researchers also use this information to investigate nursing interventions or health problems. For example, a nurse wants to compare a new method of pain control with a standard pain protocol using two groups of patients. The records provide data on the two types of interventions: the new method and the standard pain control. The nurse researcher collects data from the records that describe the type and dose of analgesic medications used, objective assessment data, and patients' subjective reports of pain relief. The researcher then compares the findings to determine if the new method was more effective than the standard pain control protocol. Analysis of the data contributes to evidence-based nursing practice and quality health care (see Chapter 5).

Auditing and Monitoring

Hospitals establish quality improvement programs for conducting objective, ongoing reviews of patient care. Quality improvement programs keep nurses informed of standards of nursing practice to maintain excellence in nursing care. Accrediting agencies such as TJC (2011) require quality improvement programs and set standards for the information located in a patient's record, including indications that a plan of care is developed with the patient as a participant and that discharge planning and patient education have occurred. Institutions and accrediting groups establish standards for quality care. Nurses audit records throughout the year to determine the degree to which standards of care are met and identify areas needing improvement and staff development (see Chapter 5). Nurses share deficiencies identified during monitoring with all members of the nursing staff to make changes in policy or practice.

GUIDELINES FOR QUALITY DOCUMENTATION AND REPORTING

High-quality documentation and reporting are necessary to enhance efficient, individualized patient care. Quality documentation and reporting have five important characteristics: they are factual, accurate, complete, current, and organized.

Factual

A factual record contains descriptive, objective information about what a nurse sees, hears, feels, and smells. An objective description is the result of direct observation and measurement. For example, "B/P 80/50, patient diaphoretic, heart rate 102 and regular." Avoid vague terms such as *appears, seems,* or *apparently* because these words suggest that you are stating an opinion, do not accurately communicate facts, and do not inform another caregiver of the details regarding the behaviors exhibited by a patient. Objective documentation includes observations of a patient's behaviors. For example, instead of documenting "the patient seems anxious," provide objective signs of anxiety and document "the patient's pulse rate is elevated at 110 beats/min, respiratory rate is slightly labored at 22 breaths/min, and the patient reports increased restlessness."

The only subjective data included in the record are what the patient says. When recording subjective data, document the patient's exact words within quotation marks whenever possible. For example, when he or she exhibits anxiety, you record, "Patient states, 'I feel very nervous.'" Include objective data to support subjective data so your charting is as descriptive as possible.

TABLE 26-1 Legal Guidelines for Recording

GUIDELINES	RATIONALE	CORRECT ACTION
Do not erase, apply correction fluid, or scratch out errors made while recording.	Charting becomes illegible: it appears as if you were attempting to hide information or deface a written record.	Draw single line through error, write word *error* above it, and sign your name or initials and date it. Then record note correctly.
Do not document retaliatory or critical comments about patient or care by other health care professionals. Do not enter personal opinions.	Statements can be used as evidence for nonprofessional behavior or poor quality of care.	Enter only objective and factual observations of patient's behavior; quote all patient comments.
Correct all errors promptly.	Errors in recording can lead to errors in treatment or may imply an attempt to mislead or hide evidence.	Avoid rushing to complete charting; be sure that information is accurate and complete.
Record all facts.	Record must be accurate, factual, and objective.	Be certain entry is factual and thorough. A person reading the documentation should be able to determine that patient had adequate care.
Do not leave blank spaces in nurses' notes.	Another person can add incorrect information in space.	Chart consecutively, line by line; if space is left, draw line horizontally through it and sign your name at end.
Record all written entries legibly and in black ink. Do not use felt-tip pens or erasable ink.	Illegible entries can be misinterpreted, causing errors and lawsuits; ink from felt-tip pen smudges or runs when wet and may destroy documentation; erasures are not permitted in patient charting; black ink is more legible when records are photocopied or scanned.	Never erase entries or use correction fluid and never use pencil.
If an order is questioned, record that clarification was sought.	If you perform order known to be incorrect, you are just as liable for prosecution as the health care provider.	Do not record "physician made error." Instead, chart that "Dr. Smith was called to clarify order for analgesic." Include the date and time of phone call, with whom you spoke, and the outcome.
Chart only for yourself.	You are accountable for information that you enter into a patient's record.	Never chart for someone else (exception: if caregiver has left unit for day and calls with information that needs to be documented; include date and time of entry and reference specific date and time to which you are referring and name of source of information in entry; include that information was provided via telephone).
Avoid using generalized, empty phrases such as "status unchanged" or "had good day."	This type of documentation is subjective and does not reflect patient assessment.	Use complete, concise descriptions of care so documentation is objective and factual.
Begin each entry with date and time and end with your signature and title.	This guideline ensures that correct sequence of events is recorded; signature documents who is accountable for care delivered.	Do not wait until end of shift to record important changes that occurred several hours earlier; be sure to sign each entry (e.g., Mary Marcus, RN).
For computer documentation keep your password to yourself.	This maintains security and confidentiality.	Once logged into computer, do not leave computer screen unattended. Log out when you leave the computer. Make sure that computer screen is not accessible for public viewing.

Accurate

The use of exact measurements establishes accuracy. For example, a description such as "Intake, 360 mL of water" is more accurate than "Patient drank an adequate amount of fluid." Charting that an abdominal wound is "5 cm in length without redness, drainage, or edema" is more descriptive than "large wound healing well." Accurate measurements help you determine if a patient's condition has changed.

Documentation of concise data is clear and easy to understand. It is essential to avoid the use of unnecessary words and irrelevant detail. For example, the fact that the patient is watching television is only necessary when this activity is significant to the patient's status and plan of care.

To ensure patient safety use abbreviations carefully to avoid misinterpretation. TJC's "do not use" list of abbreviations (see Chapter 31) is used by all health care providers to promote patient safety. In addition, TJC (2011) requires that health care institutions develop a list of standard abbreviations, symbols, and acronyms to be used by all members of the health care team when documenting or communicating patient care and treatment. To minimize errors spell out abbreviations in their entirety when they become confusing.

Correct spelling demonstrates a level of competency and attention to detail. Many terms can easily be misinterpreted (e.g., *dysphagia* or *dysphasia* and *dram* or *gram*). Some spelling errors result in serious treatment errors (e.g., the names of certain medications such as Lamictal and Lamisil or morphine and Numorphan are similar). Transcribe such terms carefully to ensure that the patient receives the correct medication.

All entries in medical records must be dated, and there must be a method to identify the authors of all entries (TJC, 2011). Each entry in a patient's record ends with the caregiver's full name or initials and status such as "Jane Woods, RN." When initials are used, the full name and status of the individual are found in the medical record to allow others to readily identify the individual. As a nursing student, enter your full name and nursing student (NS) abbreviation, such as "David Jones, NS. The abbreviation for *nursing student* varies between *NS* for *nursing student* or *SN* for *student nurse.* Include your educational institution when required by agency policy.

Complete

The information within a recorded entry or a report must be complete, containing appropriate and essential information. Criteria for thorough communication exist for certain health problems or nursing activities (Table 26-2). Your written entries in a patient's medical record describe the nursing care you administer and the patient's response. An example of a thorough nurse's note follows:

1915 Verbalizes sharp, throbbing pain localized along lateral side of right ankle, beginning approximately 15 minutes ago after twisting his foot on the stairs. Rates pain as 8 on a scale of 0-10. Pain increased with movement, slightly relieved with elevation. Pedal pulses equal bilaterally. Right ankle circumference 1 cm larger than left. Bilateral lower extremities warm, pale pink, skin intact, responds to tactile stimulation and capillary refill less than 3 seconds. Ice applied to right ankle. Percocet 2 tabs (PO) given for pain. States pain somewhat relieved with ice, rates pain as 6 on a scale of 0-10. Dr. M. Smith notified. Lee Turno, RN

1945 Rates pain as a 3 on a scale of 0-10. States, "The pain medication really helped." Lee Turno, RN

You frequently use flow sheets or graphic records when documenting routine activities such as daily hygiene care, vital signs, and pain assessments. Describe these data in greater detail when they are relevant such as when a change in functional ability or status occurs. For example, if your patient's blood pressure, pulse, and respirations are elevated above expected values following a walk down the hall, document additional description about the patient's status and response to the walk in the appropriate place in the medical record (e.g., nurse's notes).

Current

Timely entries are essential in a patient's ongoing care. Delays in documentation lead to unsafe patient care. To increase accuracy and decrease unnecessary duplication, many health care agencies keep records or computers near a patient's bedside to facilitate immediate documentation of information as it is collected from a patient. Document the following activities or findings at the time of occurrence:

- Vital signs
- Pain assessment
- Administration of medications and treatments
- Preparation for diagnostic tests or surgery, including preoperative checklist

TABLE 26-2 Examples of Criteria for Reporting and Recording

TOPIC	CRITERIA TO REPORT OR RECORD
Assessment	
Subjective data	Patient's description of episode in quotation marks (e.g., "I feel like an elephant is sitting on my chest, and I can't catch my breath.") Describe in patient's own words the onset, location, description of condition (severity, duration, frequency, precipitating, aggravating and relieving factors) (e.g., "The pain in my left knee started last week after I knelt on the ground. Every time I bend my knee I have a shooting pain on the inside of the knee.")
Patient behavior (e.g., anxiety, confusion, hostility)	Onset, behaviors exhibited, precipitating factors, patient's verbal behavior (e.g., pacing in room, avoiding eye contact with nurse, and repeatedly stating, "I have to go home now.")
Objective data (e.g., rash, tenderness, breath sounds)	Onset, location, description of condition (see previous criteria) (e.g., 1100: 2-cm raised pale red area noted on back of left hand)
Nursing Interventions and Evaluation	
Treatments (e.g., enema, bath, dressing change)	Time administered, equipment used (if appropriate), patient's response (objective and subjective changes) compared to previous treatment (e.g., denied incisional pain during abdominal dressing change, ambulated 300 feet in hallway without assistance)
Medication administration	Immediately after administration document: time medication given, preliminary assessment (e.g., pain level, vital signs), patient response or effect of medication; for example: 1500: Reports a "throbbing headache all over my head." Rates pain at 6 (scale 0-10). Tylenol 650 mg given PO. 1530: Patient reports pain level 2 (scale 0-10) and states "the throbbing has stopped."
Patient teaching	Information presented, method of instruction (e.g., discussion, demonstration, videotape, booklet), and patient response, including questions and evidence of understanding such as return demonstration or change in behavior
Discharge planning	Measurable patient goals or expected outcomes, progress toward goals, need for referrals

- Change in patient's status and who was notified (e.g., physician, manager, patient's family)
- Admission, transfer, discharge, or death of a patient
- Treatment for sudden change in patient's status
- Patient's response to treatment or intervention

Most health care agencies use military time, a 24-hour system that avoids misinterpretation of AM and PM times (Fig. 26-1). Instead of two 12-hour cycles in standard time, the military clock is one 24-hour time cycle. The military clock ends with midnight at 2400 and begins at 1 minute after midnight as 0001. For example, 10:22 AM is 1022 military time; 1:00 PM is 1300 military time.

Organized

Communicate information in a logical order. It is also more effective when notes are concise, clear, and to the point. To document notes about complex situations in an organized fashion think about the situation and make a list of what you need to include before beginning to enter data in the medical record. Applying critical thinking skills and the nursing process gives logic and order to nursing documentation. For example, an organized entry describes the patient's pain, your assessment and interventions, and the patient's response. Use the nursing process to give logic and organization to your documentation.

METHODS OF DOCUMENTATION

There are several documentation systems for recording patient data. Regardless whether documentation is entered electronically or on paper, each health care agency selects a documentation system that reflects its philosophy of nursing. The same system is used throughout a specific agency and may be used throughout a health care system as well.

Paper and Electronic Health Records

Traditionally health care professionals documented on paper medical records. Paper records are episode oriented, with a separate record for each patient visit to a health care agency (Hebda et al., 2009). Key information such as patient allergies, current medications, and complications from treatment may be lost from one episode of care (e.g., hospitalization or clinic visit) to the next, jeopardizing a patient's safety.

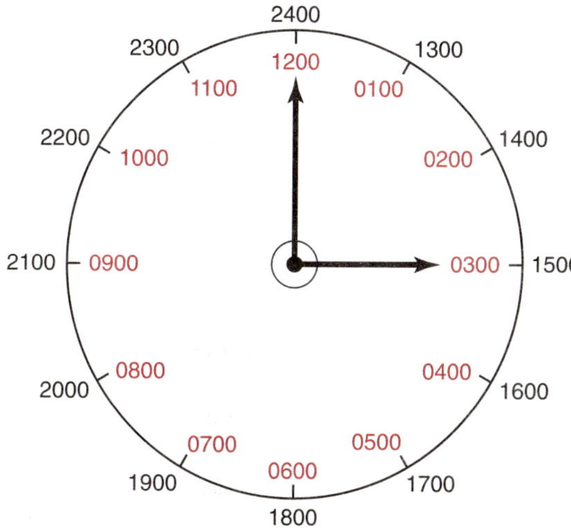

FIG. 26-1 Comparison of 24 hours of military time with the hourly positions for civilian time on the clock face.

To enhance communication among health care providers and thus patient safety, the American Recovery and Reinvestment Act of 2009 set a goal that all medical records will be kept electronically as of 2014. Many professional organizations and accrediting body initiatives also support initiation of the **electronic health record (EHR).** The EHR is an electronic record of patient health information generated whenever a patient accesses medical care in any health care delivery setting (HIMSS, 2003). Although the **electronic medical record (EMR)** contains patient data gathered in a health care setting at a specific time and place and is a part of the EHR, the two terms are frequently used interchangeably (Garets and Davis, 2005; Hebda et al., 2009).

The EHR provides access to a patient's health record information at the time and place that clinicians need it. A unique feature of an EHR is its ability to integrate all pertinent patient information into one record, regardless of the number of times a patient enters a health care system. An EHR also includes results of diagnostic studies that may include images and sound and decision support software programs. Because an unlimited number of patient records potentially can be stored within an EHR system, health care providers can access clinical data to identify quality issues, link interventions with positive outcomes, and make evidence-based decisions.

The EHR improves continuity of health care from one episode of illness to another. A clinician accesses relevant and timely information about a patient and focuses on the priority problems of care to make timely, well-informed clinical decisions. An EHR is a powerful tool because of the decision support resources it contains. For example, in a hospital setting an EHR gathers data and performs checks to support regulatory and accreditation requirements. An EHR includes tools to guide and critique medication administration (see Chapter 31) and basic decision support tools such as physician order sets and interdisciplinary treatment plans.

The ultimate development of an EHR for all patients will affect the entire health care community. Currently the American Medical Association, American Nurses Association, the HIMSS, and the American Medical Informatics Association are just some of the organizations gathering information from health care professionals to support the adoption of EHR standards (Hebda et al., 2009). All disciplines and health care organizations will benefit from the implementation of an EHR. The key advantages of an EHR for nursing include providing a means to compare ongoing clinical data about a patient with original baseline information and maintaining an ongoing record of a patient's health education. In addition, the EHR offers easier access to quality data for research and automates evidence-based guidelines.

Narrative Documentation

Narrative documentation is the traditional method for recording nursing care. It is simply the use of a story-like format to document information specific to patient conditions and nursing care. However, narrative charting has many disadvantages, including the tendency to be repetitious and time consuming and to require the reader to sort through much information to locate desired data (Box 26-1).

Problem-Oriented Medical Record

The **problem-oriented medical record (POMR)** is a method of documentation that emphasizes patients' problems. Data are organized by problem or diagnosis. Ideally each member of the health care team contributes to a single list of identified patient problems. This approach coordinates a common plan of care. The POMR has

BOX 26-1 EXAMPLES OF PROGRESS NOTES WRITTEN IN DIFFERENT FORMATS

Narrative Note

Stated "I'm dreading surgery. Last time I had a lot of pain when I got out of bed." Discussed alternatives for pain control and importance of postoperative activity. Encouraged to ask for pain medication before pain becomes severe. Stated, "I feel better prepared now." Verbalized positive effect of activity on healing and circulation.

SOAP (Subjective—Objective—Assessment—Plan)

S—"I'm worried about what it will be like after surgery."

O—Asking frequent questions about surgery. Has had no previous experience with surgery. Wife present and supportive.

A—Deficient knowledge regarding surgery related to inexperience. Patient also expressing anxiety.

P—Explain routine preoperative preparation. Demonstrate and explain rationale for turning, coughing, and deep breathing (TCDB) exercises. Provide explanation and teaching booklet on postoperative nursing care.

PIE (Problem—Intervention—Evaluation)

P—Deficient knowledge regarding surgery related to inexperience.

I—Explained normal preoperative preparations for surgery. Demonstrated TCDB exercises. Provided booklet on postoperative nursing care.

E—Demonstrated TCDB exercises correctly. Needs review of postoperative nursing care.

Focus Charting (Data—Action—Response)

D—Stated, "I'm worried about what it will be like after surgery." Asking frequent questions about surgery. Has had no previous experience with surgery. Wife present and is supportive.

A—Explained normal preoperative preparations for surgery. Demonstrated TCDB exercises. Provided booklet on postoperative nursing care.

R—Demonstrates TCDB exercises correctly. Needs review of postoperative nursing care. States, "I feel better knowing a little bit of what to expect."

the following major sections: database, problem list, care plan, and progress notes.

Database. The database section contains all available assessment information pertaining to a patient (e.g., history and physical examination, the nurse's admission history and ongoing assessment, the dietitian's assessment, laboratory reports, and radiological test results). It is the foundation for identifying patient problems and planning care. As new data become available, you revise the database. It accompanies patients through successive hospitalizations or clinic visits.

Problem List. After analyzing data, health care team members identify problems and make a single problem list. The problem list includes the patient's physiological, psychological, social, cultural, spiritual, developmental, and environmental needs. Team members list the problems in chronological order and file the list in the front of the patient's record to serve as an organizing guide for his or her care. Add new problems as you identify them. When a problem is resolved, record the date and highlight it or draw a line through the problem and its number.

Care Plan. Disciplines involved in the patient's care develop a care plan or plan of care for each problem (see Chapter 18). Nurses document the plan of care in a variety of formats. Generally these plans of care include nursing diagnoses, expected outcomes, and interventions.

Progress Notes. Health care team members monitor and record the progress of a patient's problems. Progress notes come in various formats or structured notes. One method is SOAP charting (see Box 26-1). The acronym SOAP stands for:

S—Subjective data (verbalizations of the patient)
O—Objective data (that which is measured and observed)
A—Assessment (diagnosis based on the data)
P—Plan (what the caregiver plans to do).

An I and E are sometimes added (i.e., SOAPIE) in some institutions. The I stands for intervention, and the E represents evaluation. The logic for SOAPIE notes is similar to that of the nursing process. You collect data about a patient's problems, draw conclusions, and develop a plan of care. The nurse numbers each SOAP note and titles it according to the problem on the list.

A second progress note method is the PIE format. It is similar to SOAP charting in its problem-oriented nature. However, PIE charting differs from the SOAP method in that it has a nursing origin, whereas SOAP originated from medical records. The format simplifies documentation by unifying the care plan and progress notes. PIE differs from SOAP notes because the narrative does not include assessment information. A nurse's daily assessment data appear on flow sheets, preventing duplication of data. The narrative note includes P—Problem, I—Intervention, and E—Evaluation. The PIE notes are numbered or labeled according to the patient's problems. Resolved problems are dropped from daily documentation after the nurse's review. Continuing problems are documented daily.

A third narrative format is focus charting. It involves use of DAR notes, which include D—Data (both subjective and objective), A—Action or nursing intervention, and R—Response of the patient (i.e., evaluation of effectiveness). A DAR note addresses patient concerns: a sign or symptom, condition, nursing diagnosis, behavior, significant event, or change in a patient's condition (see Box 26-1). Documentation follows the nursing process. Nurses broaden their thinking to include any patient concerns, not just problem areas. Focus charting incorporates all aspects of the nursing process, highlights a patient's concerns, and can be integrated into any clinical setting (Mosby, 2006).

Source Records

In a source record a patient's chart has a separate section for each discipline (e.g., nursing, medicine, social work, or respiratory therapy) to record data. Caregivers can easily locate the proper section of the record in which to make entries. Table 26-3 lists the components of a source record. Details about a specific problem are distributed throughout the record. For example, the nurse describes the character of abdominal pain and the use of relaxation therapy and analgesic medication in the nurses' notes. The health care provider describes the progress of the patient's bowel obstruction and the plan for surgery in a separate section of the record. The results of x-ray film examinations that show the location of the bowel obstruction are in the test results section of the record. The method by which source records are organized does not show how information from the disciplines is related or how care is coordinated to meet all of the patient's needs.

Charting by Exception

Charting by exception (CBE) focuses on documenting deviations from established norms. This approach reduces documentation time and highlights trends or changes in a patient's condition (Mosby, 2006). It is a shorthand method for documenting normal findings and routine care based on clearly defined standards of

TABLE 26-3 Organization of Traditional Source Record

SECTIONS	CONTENTS
Admission sheet	Specific demographic data about patient: legal name, identification number, gender, age, birth date, marital status, occupation and employer, health insurance, nearest relative to notify in an emergency, religious preference, name of attending physician, date and time of admission
Physician's order sheet	Record of physician's or other health care provider's orders for treatment and medications with date, time, and signature
Nurse's admission assessment	Summary of nursing history and physical examination
Graphic sheet and flow sheet	Record of repeated observations and measurements such as vital signs, daily weights, and intake and output
Medical history and examination	Results of initial examination performed by physician, including findings, family history, confirmed diagnoses, and medical plan of care
Nurses' notes	Narrative record of nursing process: assessment, nursing diagnosis, planning, implementation, and evaluation of care
Medication records	Accurate documentation of all medications administered to patient: date, time, dose, route, and nurse's signature
Progress notes	Ongoing record of patient's progress and response to medical therapy and review of disease process; often is interdisciplinary and includes documentation from health-related disciplines (e.g., health care providers, physical therapy, social work)
Other health care records	Includes results from diagnostic tests (e.g., laboratory and x-ray film results), consent forms, and sometimes documentation from health-related disciplines (e.g., radiology, social work); organization of information varies per policies of health care agency
Discharge summary	Summary of patient's condition, progress, prognosis, rehabilitation, and teaching needs at time of dismissal from hospital or health care agency

practice and predetermined criteria for nursing assessments and interventions. With standards integrated into documentation forms such as predefined normal assessment findings or predetermined interventions, a nurse then only documents significant findings or exceptions to the predefined norms. The nurse writes a progress note only when the standardized statement on the form is not met. Assessments are standardized on forms so all caregivers evaluate and document findings consistently.

The assumption with charting by exception is that all standards are met unless otherwise documented. When you see entries in the chart, you know that something out of the ordinary has occurred. Thus, when changes in a patient's condition have developed, it is easy to track them. When patients' conditions change, enter thorough and precise descriptions of the effects of these changes on patients and the actions taken.

BOX 26-2 EXAMPLE OF VARIANCE DOCUMENTATION

A 56-year-old patient is on a surgical unit 1 day after surgery. He has an elevated temperature, his breath sounds are decreased bilaterally in the bases of both lobes of the lungs, and he is slightly confused. Ordinarily 1 day after surgery the patient should be afebrile with lungs clear. The following is an example of the variance documentation for this patient.

Breath sounds diminished bilaterally at the bases. T, 100.4; P, 92; R, 28/min; oxygen sat, 84%. Daughter states he is "confused" and did not recognize her when she arrived a few minutes ago. Oxygen started at 2 L per standing orders. Will monitor pulse oximetry and vital signs every 15 minutes. Physician notified of change in status. Daughter at bedside.

Case Management Plan and Critical Pathways

The case management model of delivering care (see Chapter 2) incorporates an interdisciplinary approach to documenting patient care. Many organizations summarize the standardized plan of care into critical pathways for a specific disease or condition. Critical pathways are interdisciplinary care plans that include patient problems, key interventions, and expected outcomes within an established time frame. All health care team members use the same critical pathway to monitor a patient's progress during each shift or, in the case of home care, every visit.

Critical pathways eliminate nurses' notes, flow sheets, and nursing care plans because the document integrates all relevant information. Unexpected outcomes, unmet goals, and interventions not specified within the critical pathway are called variances. A variance occurs when the activities on the critical pathway are not completed as predicted or the patient does not meet the expected outcomes. An example of a variance is when a patient develops pulmonary complications after surgery, requiring oxygen therapy and monitoring with pulse oximetry. A positive variance occurs when a patient progresses more rapidly than expected (e.g., use of a Foley catheter is discontinued a day early). A variance analysis is necessary to review the data for trends and for developing and implementing an action plan to respond to the identified patient problems (Box 26-2). In addition, variances often result from changes in the patient's health or because of other health complications not associated with the primary reason for which the patient requires care. Once you identify a variance, you modify the patient's care to meet the needs associated with the variance. Over time health care teams sometimes revise critical pathways if similar variances reoccur.

COMMON RECORD-KEEPING FORMS

A variety of paper or electronic forms are available for the type of information nurses routinely document. The categories within a form are usually derived from institutional standards of practice or guidelines established by accrediting agencies.

Admission Nursing History Forms

A nurse completes a nursing history form when a patient is admitted to a nursing unit. The form guides the nurse through a complete assessment to identify relevant nursing diagnoses or problems (see Chapter 16). Data provide baseline data to compare with changes in the patient's condition.

Flow Sheets and Graphic Records

Flow sheets allow you to quickly and easily enter assessment data about a patient, including vital signs and routine repetitive care such as hygiene measures, ambulation, meals, weights, and safety and restraint checks. They provide current patient information that is accessible to all members of the health care team. Because there is a coding system for data entry, flow sheets help team members quickly see patient trends over time and decrease time spent on writing narrative notes. If an occurrence on a flow sheet is unusual or changes significantly, enter a focus note. For example, if a patient's blood pressure becomes dangerously high, first complete a focus assessment. You record your assessment and the action taken in the progress notes. Critical and acute care units commonly use flow sheets for all types of physiological data.

Patient Care Summary or Kardex

Many hospitals now have computerized systems that provide information in the form of a patient care summary that is often printed for each patient during each shift. The summary automatically updates as nurses make decisions and data (e.g., orders) are entered into the computer. In some settings a **Kardex,** a portable "flip-over" file or notebook, is kept at the nurses' station. Most Kardex forms have an activity and treatment section and a nursing care plan section that organize information for quick reference. An updated Kardex eliminates the need for repeated referral to the chart for routine information throughout the day. The patient care summary or Kardex includes the following information:

- Basic demographic data (e.g., age, religion)
- Health care provider's name
- Primary medical diagnosis
- Medical and surgical history
- Current orders from health care provider (e.g., dressing changes, ambulation, glucose monitoring)
- Nursing care plan
- Nursing orders (e.g., education sessions, symptom relief measures, counseling)
- Scheduled tests and procedures
- Safety precautions used in the patient's care
- Factors related to activities of daily living
- Nearest relative/guardian or person to contact in an emergency
- Emergency code status (e.g., indication of "do not resuscitate" order)
- Allergies

Standardized Care Plans

Some institutions use **standardized care plans** to make documentation more efficient. The plans, based on the institution's standards of nursing practice, are preprinted, established guidelines used to care for patients who have similar health problems. After completing a nursing assessment, the nurse identifies the standard care plans that are appropriate for the patient and places the plans in his or her medical record. The nurse modifies the plans to individualize the therapies. Most standardized care plans also allow a nurse to add specific goals or desired outcomes of care and the dates by which these outcomes should be achieved.

Standardized care plans are useful when conducting quality improvement audits. They also improve continuity of care among professional nurses. When they are used in a health care facility, the nurse remains responsible for providing individualized care to each patient. Standardized care plans cannot replace a nurse's professional judgment and decision making. Update care plans on a regular basis to ensure that they are current and appropriate.

Discharge Summary Forms

To save costs and ensure appropriate reimbursement, it is important to prepare patients for an effective, timely discharge from a health care institution. A patient's discharge also needs to result in desirable outcomes. Interdisciplinary discharge planning ensures that a patient leaves the hospital in a timely manner with the necessary resources (Box 26-3).

Ideally discharge planning begins at admission. By identifying discharge needs early, nursing and other health care professionals can begin planning for home care, support services, and any equipment needs at home. Nurses revise a plan of care as a patient's condition changes. Involve the patient and family in the discharge planning process so they have the necessary information and resources to return home. Discharge documentation includes medications, diet, community resources, follow-up care, and who to contact in case of an emergency or for questions.

Acuity Records

Although **acuity records** are not part of a patient's medical record, they are useful for determining the hours of care and staff required for a given group of patients. A patient's acuity level, usually determined by a computer program, is based on the type and number of nursing interventions (e.g., intravenous [IV] therapy, wound care, or ambulation assistance) required over a 24-hour period. The acuity level rates patients compared with one another. For example, an acuity system rates bathing patients from 1 (totally dependent) to 5 (independent). A patient returning from surgery requiring frequent monitoring and extensive care has an acuity level of 1 compared with another patient awaiting discharge after a successful recovery from surgery who has an acuity level of 5. Accurate acuity ratings justify overtime and the number and qualifications of staff needed to safely care for patients. The patient-to-staff ratios established for a unit depend on a composite gathering of 24-hour acuity data for each patient receiving care.

BOX 26-3 DISCHARGE SUMMARY INFORMATION

- Use clear, concise descriptions in the patient's own language.
- Provide step-by-step description of how to perform a procedure (e.g., home medication administration). Reinforce explanation with printed instructions.
- Identify precautions to follow when performing self-care or administering medications.
- Review signs and symptoms of complications that should be reported to the health care provider.
- List names and phone numbers of health care providers and community resources that the patient can contact.
- Identify any unresolved problem, including plans for follow-up and continuous treatment.
- List actual time of discharge, mode of transportation, and who accompanied the patient.

HOME CARE DOCUMENTATION

When providing home care, nurses use astute assessment skills to develop a plan of care and gather the needed information about changes in a patient's health care status. This information frequently comes from patient family members. Documentation in the home care system is different from other areas of nursing. Medicare has specific guidelines to establish eligibility for home care reimbursement. Information used for reimbursement comes from a patient's medical record. In addition, home care documentation systems provide the entire health care team with the information needed to enhance teamwork. Documentation is both the quality control and the justification for reimbursement from Medicare, Medicaid, or private insurance companies. Nurses must document all their services for payment (e.g., direct skilled care, patient instructions, skilled observation, and evaluation visits) (TJC, 2011). Information in the home care medical record includes patient assessment, referral and intake forms, interprofessional plan of care, a list of medications, and reports to third-party payers.

Some parts of the record remain in the home with the patient; other information is needed in an office setting. Thus duplication of documentation is often necessary. Agency policies indicate which forms nurses need to leave at their office versus which forms must be taken into the home. Computerized patient records are evolving to address these different needs. With the use of laptop computers, it is becoming possible for the records to be available in multiple locations, which allows greater access to information about a patient's interdisciplinary needs.

LONG-TERM HEALTH CARE DOCUMENTATION

Increasing numbers of older adults and people with disabilities in the United States require care in long-term health care facilities. Nursing personnel often face documentation challenges much different from those in the acute care setting. The Centers for Medicare and Medicaid Services (CMS) establishes guidelines related to accidents and supervision of residents of long-term care facilities. The guidelines require careful documentation for appropriate reimbursement in long-term care agencies (Senft, 2008). You assess each resident in a long-term care agency receiving funding from Medicare and Medicaid programs using the Resident Assessment Instrument/Minimum Data Set (RAI/MDS). This documentation provides standardized protocols for assessment and care planning and a minimum data set to promote quality improvement within and across facilities (Dellefield, 2007). When residents' records are reviewed for reimbursement, there is an expectation that these protocols such as skin assessments, wound care, and assisted ambulation are met. Documentation supports an interdisciplinary approach to the assessment and planning process for patients. Communication among nurses, social workers, recreational therapists, and dietitians is essential in the regulated documentation process. The fiscal support for long-term care residents hinges on the justification of nursing care as demonstrated in sound documentation of the services rendered (Dellefield, 2007).

REPORTING

Nurses communicate information about patients to help team members make appropriate decisions about patient care. It is important that any form of verbal report be timely, accurate, and relevant. Reports commonly used by nurses include hand-off, telephone, and incident reports.

Hand-Off Report

Hand-off reports happen any time one health care provider transfers care of a patient to another health care provider. The purpose of hand-off reports is to provide better continuity and individualized care for patients. For example, if you find that a patient breathes better in a certain position, you relay that information to the next nurse caring for the patient (Table 26-4). Examples of hand-off reports include change-of-shift reports and transfer reports.

Standardizing communication during hand-off reports helps ensure patient safety. Hand-off communications include up-to-date information about a patient's condition, required care, treatments, medications, services, and any recent or anticipated changes. Information during patient hand-off can be given face-to-face, in

TABLE 26-4 Comparison of Do's and Don'ts of Hand-Off Reports

DO'S	DON'TS
Provide only essential background information about patient (i.e., name, gender, medical diagnosis, and history).	Don't review all routine care procedures or tasks (e.g., bathing, scheduled changes).
Identify patient's nursing diagnoses or health care problems and their related causes.	Don't review all biographical information already available in written form.
Describe objective measurements or observations about patient's condition and response to health problem; emphasize recent changes.	Don't use critical comments about patient's behavior such as "Mrs. Wills is so demanding."
Share significant information about family members as it relates to patient's problems.	Don't make assumptions about relationships among family members.
Continuously review ongoing discharge plan (e.g., need for resources, patient's level of preparation to go home).	Don't engage in idle gossip.
Relay significant changes to staff in the way therapies are to be given (e.g., different position for pain relief, new medication).	Don't describe basic steps of a procedure.
Describe instructions given in teaching plan and patient's response.	Don't explain detailed content unless staff members ask for clarification.
Evaluate results of nursing or medical care measures (e.g., effect of back rub or analgesic administration).	Don't simply describe results as "good" or "poor." Be specific.
Be clear about priorities to which oncoming staff must attend.	Don't force oncoming staff to guess what to do first.

writing, or verbally such as over the telephone or via audiorecording. Regardless of the way hand-off reports are given, it is essential for staff to have an opportunity for last-minute updates, to clarify information, or to receive information on care events or changes in a patient's condition. Properly performed, a hand-off report provides an opportunity to share essential information to ensure patient safety and continuity of care (Schroeder, 2006).

An effective hand-off report is quick and efficient. A good report provides a baseline for comparisons and indicates the kind of care anticipated for the next nurse who will be caring for the patient. An organized and concise approach helps you set goals and anticipate patient needs and lessens the chance of overlooking important information. A sample format follows: background information (name, age, and medical diagnosis); primary health problem; unusual occurrences; discharge planning issues; identification of significant changes in measurable terms (e.g., pain scale); observations; findings; time when new, STAT, or prn medications were given; care required such as medications that need to be started, when to assess the effectiveness of STAT/prn medications, or when a dressing needs to be changed next; progress with teaching; interventions; and family involvement. It is especially important to report any recent changes or priority situations concerning a patient's condition. Report elements do not include normal findings or routine information retrievable from other sources or derogatory or inappropriate comments about a patient or family, which could possibly lead to legal charges if overheard by the patient or family (Benson et al., 2007). This type of language contributes to prejudicial opinions about a patient.

Telephone Reports and Orders

Telephone Reports. A registered nurse makes a telephone report when significant events or changes in a patient's condition have occurred. A telephone report needs to include clear, accurate, and concise information. About 60% of the worst type of medical errors, called *sentinel events,* relate to communication problems that often arise during telephone reports (Hemmila, 2006). Thus some institutions use SBAR, an acronym that stands for Situation-Background-Assessment-Recommendation. SBAR standardizes telephone communication of significant events or changes in a patient's condition and is a communication strategy designed to improve patient safety. For example, when describing the *situation,* you include both the admitting and secondary diagnoses and the problem your patient is having as the current issue. *Background* information includes pertinent medical history, previous laboratory tests and treatments, psychosocial issues, allergies, and current code status. For *assessment* data include significant findings in your head-to-toe physical assessment, recent vital signs, current treatment measures, restrictions, recent laboratory results and diagnostics, and pain status. Then provide your *recommendation,* in which you suggest a plan of care and what needs to be addressed (Hemmila, 2006).

Document every phone call you make to a health care provider. Documentation includes when the call was made, who made it (if you did not make the call), who was called, to whom information was given, what information was given, what information was received, and verification of the information with the provider. Health care institutions have a process for a verification "read back" when receiving information or critical test results. An example follows: "Laboratory technician J. Ignacio reported a potassium level of 5.9. Dr. Wade notified at 2030. Information transcribed and read back for verification. Ordered change in IV fluids. D_5NS 1000 mL to run at 125 mL per hour. D. Markle, RN, read back."

BOX 26-4 GUIDELINES FOR TELEPHONE AND VERBAL ORDERS

- Clearly determine the patient's name, room number, and diagnosis.
- Repeat any prescribed orders back to the physician or health care provider.
- Use clarification questions to avoid misunderstandings.
- Write TO (telephone order) or VO (verbal order), including date and time, name of patient, the complete order; sign the name of the physician or health care provider and nurse.
- Follow agency policies; some institutions require telephone (and verbal) orders to be reviewed and signed by two nurses.
- The health care provider must co-sign the order within the time frame required by the institution (usually 24 hours).

Telephone and Verbal Orders. A telephone order (TO) occurs when a health care provider gives an order over the phone to a registered nurse. A verbal order (VO) involves the health care provider giving orders to a nurse while they are standing near each other. TOs and VOs usually occur at night or during emergencies and frequently cause medical errors (Bombard, 2008). The nurse receiving a TO or VO writes down the complete order or enters it into the computer as it is being given. Then he or she reads the order back to the health care provider, called *read back,* and receives confirmation from the person who gave the order that it is correct (Bombard, 2008). An example follows: "10/16/2011: 0815, Tylenol 3, 2 tablets, every 6 hours for incisional pain. TO Dr. Knight/J. Woods, RN, read back." The health care provider later verifies the TO or VO legally by signing it within a set time (e.g., 24 hours) as set by hospital policy. TOs and VOs are used only when absolutely necessary and not for the sake of convenience. In some situations it is prudent to have a second person listen to TOs. Check agency policy. Box 26-4 provides guidelines that promote accuracy when receiving TOs.

Incident or Occurrence Reports

An incident or occurrence is any event that is not consistent with the routine operation of a health care unit or routine care of a patient. Examples of incidents include patient falls, needlestick injuries, a visitor having symptoms of illness, medication administration errors, accidental omission of ordered therapies, and circumstances that lead to injury or a risk for patient injury. Analysis of incident reports helps with the identification of trends in systems and unit operations that provide justification for changes in policies and procedures or for in-service seminars. **Incident (or occurrence) reports** are an important part of the quality improvement program of a unit (see Chapter 5).

Always contact the patient's health care provider whenever an incident happens. Note that you do not mention the incident report in the patient's medical record. Instead you document an objective description of what happened, what you observed, and the follow-up actions taken in the patient's medical record. It is important to evaluate and document the patient's response to the error or incident.

Follow agency policy when making an incident report. These reports are an important part of quality improvement. The overall goal is to identify changes needed to prevent future recurrence. File the report with the appropriate risk-management department of the agency. Analysis of incident or occurrence reports helps identify trends in an organization that provide justification for changes in policies and procedures or for in-service programs.

HEALTH INFORMATICS

Health informatics is defined by the American Medical Informatics Association (AMIA) as, "The application of computer and information science in all basic and applied biomedical sciences to facilitate the acquisition, processing, interpretation, optimal use, and communication of health-related data. The focus is the patient and the process of care, and the goal is to enhance the quality and efficiency of care provided" (Hebda et al., 2009). Nursing competence in health care informatics is becoming a priority as health care facilities adopt EMRs/EHRs and other technologies. A recent survey found that only 28% of primary care physicians in the United States used EMRs in practice (Davis et al., 2009). Another survey of 2952 hospitals in the United States reported that only 1.5% of U.S. hospitals have a comprehensive EHR system in place and 10.9% were using a basic EHR (Jha et al., 2009). Use of EMRs/EHRs is increasing as a result of the creation of the federal Health Information Technology for Economic and Clinical Health Act (HITECH) in 2009. The government will make incentive payments totaling over $27 billion over a 10-year period to health care agencies and provider's offices that adopt EHRs and use data meaningfully from the EHR to promote safe, high-quality patient care resulting in positive patient outcomes (Blumenthal, 2010). In addition, penalties will be assessed to health care facilities that do not adopt EHRs or show meaningful use of data generated from EHRs.

NURSING INFORMATICS

All nurses deal with data, information, and knowledge (Hebda et al., 2009). It is important that you know how to record, interpret, and report data and critically think and apply knowledge to use information for patient care. Data include numbers, characters, or facts that you collect according to a perceived need for analysis and possible action. You gain knowledge from gathering and using information from several sources (Hebda et al., 2009). An example is a nurse's observation of a wound's edges, color of drainage, and measurement of the length of a wound. When a nurse examines data describing the condition of the wound over time, a pattern develops showing that the wound is not healing (information). On the basis of evidence available in the scientific literature, the nurse applies knowledge of wound care principles and intervenes to manage the patient's wound.

In health care settings it is a challenge to easily access data and information about patients. This is especially true when information is recorded manually on printed forms. For example, a nurse working in risk management who is interested in investigating patient falls has to review page by page the records of patients who have fallen to identify the common factors contributing to falls. Remember that three important purposes of medical records are communication, education, and research. When a health care organization relies on handwritten patient records, the process of locating, summarizing, and comparing information is slow and difficult. Thus it becomes even more difficult to access information in a timely manner to provide or improve patient care. It also becomes difficult to locate data sources for research purposes. Furthermore, when data about patients are compared manually, it is more difficult to see the trends that help educate staff about patient care. The most efficient way to use data and information to improve quality of care, complete research, and provide education is through information technology (Institute of Medicine, 2001).

Information technology (IT) refers to the management and processing of information, generally with the assistance of computers (Hebda et al., 2009). Advances in technology allow health care agencies to move from paper-based medical records to computer-based records. A health care information system (HIS) is a group of systems used within a health care organization to support and enhance health care (Hebda et al., 2009). A HIS consists of two major types of information systems: clinical information systems (CISs) and administrative information systems. Together the two systems operate to make the entry and communication of data and information more efficient. You will find that any single health care agency uses one or several CISs and administrative information systems. For example, a small community hospital uses a nursing information system (NIS); an order entry system; and laboratory, radiology, and pharmacy systems to coordinate their core patient care services. A nurse working in such a hospital documents nursing care on a computer, locates and reviews laboratory test results, orders sterile supplies, and enters health care provider orders for x-ray films and patients' medications.

Many hospitals now use NISs to support the documentation of nursing process activities and offer resources for managing nursing care delivery. A reliable NIS is the product of nursing informatics. **Nursing informatics** is a specialty that integrates nursing science, computer science, and information science to manage and communicate data, information, and knowledge in nursing practice (American Nurses Association, 2008). It facilitates the integration of data, information, and knowledge to support patients, nurses, and other providers in decision making in all roles and settings. The application of nursing informatics results in an efficient and effective NIS. An expertly designed CIS based on nursing informatics integrates and supports clinical judgments with up-to-date evidence-based practice. An effective NIS meets two goals. First, it supports the way that nurses function and work by providing them the flexibility to use the system to view data and collect information, provide patient care, and document a patient's condition and care provided. Second, it supports and enhances nursing practice through improved access to information and clinical decision-making tools (Hebda et al., 2009).

In the fast-paced world of nursing, nursing informatics plays an important role in helping nurses make decisions more rapidly and accurately. It has revolutionized how health care providers locate or mine patient data to look for trends and patterns between patient outcomes and care provided by nurses. New technologies also allow nurses to study the effect of systems on error reduction and patient safety. Through the application of nursing informatics, practical applications of technology enhance bedside care and education.

Numerous groups, including the ANA (2008), recommend that all nurses acquire a minimal level of awareness and competence in informatics and use of IT. Competence in informatics is not the same as computer competency. To become competent in informatics you need to be able to use evolving methods of discovering, retrieving, and using information in practice (Hebda et al., 2009). This means that you learn to recognize when information is needed and have the skills to find, evaluate, and use that information effectively. For example, you need to know how to acquire, critique, and apply scientific evidence from literature databases (see Chapter 5). As a nurse you also need to know how to use clinical databases within your institution and apply the information so you can deliver high-quality, appropriate patient care.

Nursing Information Systems

A good information system that incorporates principles of nursing informatics supports the work you do. As a nurse you need to access a computer program easily, review the patient's medical history and health care provider orders, and then go to the patient's bedside to conduct a comprehensive assessment. Once you have completed the assessment, you enter data into the computer terminal at the patient's bedside and develop a plan of care from the information gathered. This allows you to quickly share the plan of care with the patient. Periodically you return to the computer to check on laboratory test results and document the therapies you administer. The computer screens and optional pop-up windows make it easy to locate information, enter and compare data, and make changes.

NISs have two designs. The nursing process design is the most traditional. It organizes documentation within well-established formats such as admission and postoperative assessment problem lists, care plans, discharge planning instructions, and intervention lists or notes. More advanced systems incorporate standardized nursing languages such as the North American Nursing Diagnosis Association (NANDA) International nursing diagnoses, the Nursing Interventions Classification (NIC), and the Nursing Outcomes Classification (NOC) into the software. For example, the documentation of nursing admission assessment findings relies on a menu-driven approach. A menu lists related commands that you select from the computer screen to complete the patient assessment. The commands direct you through various assessment categories such as a patient's medication history, nutritional status, psychosocial history, and review of systems. After you enter assessment data into a computer, a program offers menu lists for the selection of nursing diagnoses and interventions, allowing you to individualize a patient's care plan. Another example is a program for discharge instructions. After you enter the necessary information for a patient's discharge instructions, follow-up appointments, and medication information, the system generates printed copies of the instructions for you to review and give to patients on discharge. You place a copy in the patient's record. This information is also available for home care staff and the patient's health care provider.

The nursing process design includes formats for the following:

- Generation of a nursing work list that indicates routine scheduled activities related to the care of each patient
- Documentation of routine aspects of patient care such as hygiene, positioning, fluid intake and output, wound care measures, and blood glucose measurements
- Progress note entries using narrative notes, charting by exception, and flow-sheet charting
- Documentation of medication administration (see Chapter 31)

The second design model for a NIS is the protocol or critical pathway design (Hebda et al., 2009). This design offers an interdisciplinary format to manage information. All health care providers use a protocol system to document the care they provide. Evidence-based clinical protocols or critical pathways provide the formatting or design for the type of information that clinicians enter into the system. The information system allows a user to select one or more appropriate protocols for a patient. An advanced system merges multiple protocols, using a master protocol or path to direct patient care activities. Standard health care provider order sets are included in the protocols and automatically processed. The system integrates appropriate information into the medication delivery process to enhance patient safety. In addition, the system identifies variances of the anticipated outcomes on the protocols as they are charted.

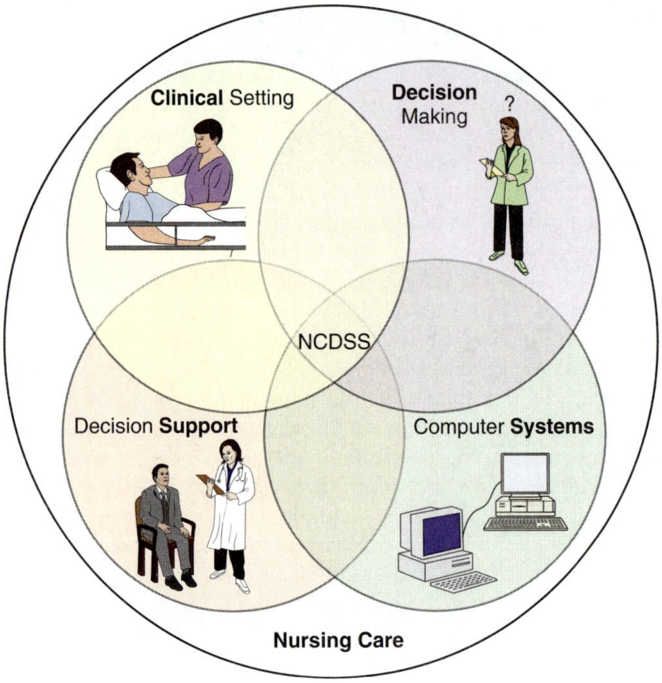

FIG. 26-2 Model of a nursing clinical decision support system (NCDSS). (Courtesy Frank Lyerla.)

This provides all caregivers the ability to analyze variances and offer an accurate clinical picture of a patient's progress.

Clinical decision support systems (CDSSs) are computerized programs used within the health care setting to support decision making (Lyerla, 2008). When used to support nursing decisions it is called a *nursing CDSS* (Fig. 26-2). A CDSS is based on "rules" and "if-then" statements, linking information and/or producing alerts, warnings, or other information to the user. The information within a CDSS is current, is evidence based, and has the ability to be updated. Information provided by a CDSS is given to the right person at the right time. For example, an effective CDSS notifies health care providers of patient allergies before ordering a medication. This enhances patient safety during the medication ordering process. CDSSs also improve nursing care. When patient assessment data are combined with patient care guidelines, nurses are better able to implement evidence-based nursing care, resulting in improved patient outcomes (Box 26-5).

Advantages of a Nursing Information System. Anecdotal reports and descriptive studies suggest that NISs offer important advantages to nurses in practice. Hebda et al. (2009) outline some specific advantages:

- Increased time to spend with patients
- Better access to information
- Enhanced quality of documentation
- Reduced errors of omission
- Reduced hospital costs
- Increased nurse job satisfaction
- Compliance with requirements of accrediting agencies (e.g., TJC)
- Development of a common clinical database

The transition to computerized documentation presents both opportunities and challenges to nurses and nurse managers. A barrier to the successful implementation of a CIS is the reluctance of some nurses and other clinical staff to accept technological advances. Often clinicians fail to understand how technology can improve the way they deliver care and enhance clinical decision

BOX 26-5 EFFECT OF CLINICAL DECISION SUPPORT SYSTEMS (CDSS) ON PATIENT OUTCOMES

PICO Question: Do nurses who work at health care agencies that use CDSS provide safer and more effective patient care when compared with nurses who work at agencies that do not use CDSS?

Evidence Summary

Nurses who provide evidence-based care at the bedside provide safe and effective care. However, one barrier to evidence-based nursing care is getting information to nurses at the bedside when they need it. Several studies investigated the effect of CDSS on patient outcomes. For example, Lyerla et al. (2010) found that nurses are more likely to follow evidence-based guidelines when caring for patients who are on ventilators when the CDSS combined interventions for ventilator-associated pneumonia with nursing assessment data. The use of CDSS is also linked with adherence to implementation of evidence-based sepsis care in intensive care units (Giuliano, Lecardo, and Staul, 2011) and completion of screening for osteoporosis in primary care settings (DeJesus et al., 2011). These studies show that CDSS that provide automatic decision support at the time and place nurses need it enhances the quality and safety of patient care. CDSS also help nurses initiate evidence-based care faster and with more accuracy, improving patient outcomes.

Application to Nursing Practice

- CDSS enhance the implementation of evidence-based practice into nursing care because they remind nurses which interventions need to be implemented for specific patients at the time the care is needed.
- Nurses need to be involved in the design and selection of CDSS to ensure that clinical decision support is provided effectively and efficiently.
- Nurses need to evaluate patient outcomes when CDSS are used. They also need to be involved in developing solutions to improve the effectiveness of CDSS when opportunities for improvement are identified.

processes. The successful implementation of a NIS requires preparation, involvement, and commitment of the entire nursing staff. The process is complex and includes more than just implementing a new technology. It is important to address educating staff, changing attitudes and cultures, and standardizing documentation and health care practices (Oroviogoicoechea et al., 2007). Successful integration requires nurses to understand the potential of informatics and IT. Although promoters of NISs suggest that adoption of computerized charting provides time saving for nursing workload, currently there is inconsistent evidence of time saved with use of electronic patient records (Choi et al., 2006).

Privacy, Confidentiality, and Security Mechanisms. Computerized documentation has legal risks. It is possible for anyone to access a computer station within a health care agency and gain information about almost any patient. Therefore protection of information and computer systems is a top priority. Confidentiality of access to computerized records is a major issue, particularly with the implementation of HIPAA. HIPAA was the first federal legislation to protect automated patient records and uniform personal health information (PHI) nationwide (Hebda et al., 2009). PHI includes individually identifiable health information such as demographic data; facts that relate to an individual's past, present, or future physical or mental health condition; provision of care; and payment for the provision of care that identifies the individual (Hebda et al., 2009).

Most security mechanisms for information systems use a combination of logical and physical restrictions to protect information and computer systems. They include measures such as firewalls and the installation of antivirus and spyware-detection software. A **firewall** is a combination of hardware and software that protects private network resources (e.g., the information system of the hospital) from outside hackers, network damage, and theft or misuse of information. For example, an automatic sign-off is a safety mechanism that logs a user off the computer system after a specified period of inactivity (Hebda et al., 2009). An automatic sign-off is used in most patient care areas and other departments that handle sensitive data.

Physical security measures include placing computers or file servers in restricted areas or using privacy filters for computer screens visible to visitors or others without access. This form of security has limited benefit, especially if an organization uses mobile wireless devices such as notebooks, tablet personal computers (PCs), and personal digital assistants (PDAs). These devices are easily misplaced or lost, falling into the wrong hands. Some organizations use motion detectors or alarms with these devices to help prevent theft.

Access or log-in codes along with passwords are frequently used for authenticating access to electronic records. A password is a collection of alphanumeric characters that a user types into a computer before accessing a program. A user usually needs to enter a password after the entry and acceptance of an access code or user name. A password does not appear on the computer screen when it is typed, nor should it be known to anyone but the user and information system administrators (Hebda et al., 2009). Strong passwords use combinations of letters, numbers, and symbols that are difficult to guess. When using a health care agency computer system, it is essential that you do not share your computer password with anyone under any circumstances. A good system requires frequent and random changes in personal passwords to prevent unauthorized persons from tampering with records. In addition, most staff have access only to patients in their work area. Some staff (e.g., administrators or risk managers) have authority to access all patient records. To protect patient privacy, health care agencies track who accesses patient records and when they access them. Disciplinary action, including loss of employment, occurs when nurses or other health care personnel inappropriately access patient information.

Handling and Disposal of Information. It is extremely important to keep medical records confidential. However, it is equally important to safeguard the information that is printed from the record or extracted for report purposes. For example, you print a copy of a nursing activities work list to use as a day planner while administering care to patients. You refer to information on the list and write notes to enter later into the computer. Information on the list is PHI, must be kept confidential, and cannot be left out for view by unauthorized persons. You destroy (e.g., shred) anything that is printed when the information is no longer needed.

Printing and faxing information from a patient's record is a primary source for the unauthorized release of information. All papers containing PHI (e.g., Social Security number, date of birth or age, patient's name or address) must be destroyed. Most agencies have shredders or locked receptacles for shredding and later incineration. Nurses also work in settings where they are responsible for erasing computer files from the hard drive that contain calendars, surgery or diagnostic procedure schedules, or other daily records that contain PHI (Hebda et al., 2009). Know and follow the disposal policies for records in the institution where you work.

Institutions need to have sound policies for the use of fax machines, specifically which type of information can be sent and to which departments. Information that you send by fax should not exceed that requested or required for immediate clinical needs. The following are some steps to take to enhance fax security (Hebda et al., 2009):

- Confirm that fax numbers are correct before sending to be sure that you direct information properly.
- Use a cover sheet, especially if a fax machine serves a number of different users.
- Authenticate at both ends before data transmission to verify that source and destination are correct.
- Use programmed speed-dial keys to eliminate the chance of a dialing error and misdirected information.
- Place fax machines in a secure area.
- Limit machine access to designated individuals.
- Log fax transmissions. This feature is often available electronically on the machine.

Clinical Information Systems

Any clinician, including nurses, physicians, pharmacists, social workers, and therapists, uses programs available on a Clinical Information System (CIS). These programs include monitoring systems; order entry systems; and laboratory, radiology, and pharmacy systems. A monitoring system includes devices that automatically monitor and record biometric measurements (e.g., vital signs, oxygen saturation, cardiac index, and stroke volume) in critical care and specialty areas. The devices electronically send measurements directly to the nursing documentation system.

Order-entry systems allow nurses to order supplies and services from another department. An example is the ability to order sterile supplies from the central supply department. This eliminates written order forms and expedites the delivery of needed supplies to a nursing unit. **Computerized provider order entry (CPOE)** is a process by which a health care provider directly enters orders for patient care into the hospital information system. In advanced systems CPOE has built-in reminders and alerts that help a health care provider select the most appropriate medication or diagnostic test. The Institute of Medicine has instituted major initiatives to improve the quality of care and reduce medication errors. Many believe that CPOE is one answer. The direct entry of orders eliminates issues related to illegible handwriting and transcription errors. In addition, a CPOE system potentially speeds the implementation of ordered diagnostic tests and treatments, which improves staff productivity and saves money (Hebda et al., 2009) because the unit secretary no longer transcribes a written order onto a nursing order form. Orders made through CPOE are integrated within the record and sent to the appropriate departments (e.g., pharmacy or radiology).

KEY POINTS

- The medical record is a legal document and requires information describing the care that is delivered to a patient.
- The computerized health record (or electronic health record) is a digital version of a patient's medical record.
- All information pertaining to a patient's health care management that is gathered by examination, observation, conversation, or treatment is confidential.
- Access to patient records is limited to individuals involved in the care of the patient.
- Interdisciplinary communication is essential within the health care team.
- Accurate record keeping requires an objective interpretation of data with precise measurements, correct spelling, and proper use of abbreviations.
- A nurse's signature on an entry in a record designates accountability for the contents of that entry.
- Any change in a patient's condition warrants immediate documentation about the event and the action that was taken to keep a record accurate.
- The medical record is a financial record that serves as the basis for reimbursement.
- Problem-oriented medical records are organized by the patient's health care problems.
- The intent of SOAP, SOAPIE, PIE, or DAR charting formats is to organize entries in the progress notes according to the nursing process.
- Medicare guidelines for establishing a patient's home care cost reimbursement is the basis for documentation by home care nurses.
- Long-term care documentation is interdisciplinary and closely linked with fiscal requirements of outside agencies.
- Computerized Information Systems (CIS) provide information about patients in an organized and easily accessible fashion.
- The major purpose of the hand-off report is to maintain continuity of care.
- Rounds allow nurses to perform needed assessments, evaluate patients' progress, and determine the best interventions for a patient's needs.
- Always verify patient care information communicated by telephone using the "read back" process.
- A hospital information system consists of two major types of information systems: CIS and administrative information systems.
- Nursing informatics facilitates the integration of data, information, and knowledge to support patients, nurses, and other providers in decision making in all roles and settings.
- Protection of the confidentiality of patients' health information and the security of computer systems are top priorities that include log-in processes, audit trails, firewalls, data recovery processes, and policies about handling and disposing of data to protect patient information.

CLINICAL APPLICATION QUESTIONS

Preparing for Clinical Practice

David Page, an 80-year-old man, is admitted to the hospital with a diagnosis of possible pneumonia. He states that he is not feeling well and has a frequent productive cough, which is worse at night. Vital signs are: blood pressure, 150/90 mm Hg; pulse rate, 92 beats/min; respirations, 22 breaths/min. During your initial assessment he coughs violently for 40 to 45 seconds. His lungs have wheezes and rhonchi in both bases and are otherwise clear. He states, "My chest hurts when I cough, and the pain radiates into my arm."

1. Which data do you document as objective?
2. Which data are subjective?
3. The nurse documents assessment findings in an electronic documentation system in narrative format. Discuss the problems associated with this style of documentation.

evolve *Answers to Clinical Application Questions can be found on the Evolve website.*

REVIEW QUESTIONS

Are You Ready to Test Your Nursing Knowledge?

1. A manager who is reviewing the nurses' notes in a patient's medical record finds the following entry, "Patient is difficult to care for, refuses suggestion for improving appetite." Which of the following directions does the manager give to the staff nurse who entered the note?
   1. Avoid rushing when charting an entry.
   2. Use correction fluid to remove the entry.
   3. Draw a single line through the statement and initial it.
   4. Enter only objective and factual information about the patient.
2. A new graduate nurse is providing a telephone report to a patient's health care provider and accepting telephone orders from the provider. Which of the following actions requires the new nurse's preceptor to intervene? The new nurse:
   1. Uses SBAR (Situation-Background-Assessment-Recommendation) as a format when providing the report.
   2. Gives a newly ordered medication before entering the order in the patient's medical record.
   3. Reads the orders back to the health care provider after receiving them and verifies their accuracy.
   4. Asks the preceptor to listen in on the phone conversation.
3. As you enter the patient's room, you notice that he is anxious to say something. He quickly states, "I don't know what's going on; I can't get an explanation from my doctor about my test results. I want something done about this." Which of the following is the most appropriate documentation of the patient's emotional status?
   1. The patient has a defiant attitude and is demanding his test results.
   2. The patient appears to be upset with his nurse because he wants his test results immediately.
   3. The patient is demanding and complains frequently about his doctor.
   4. The patient stated that he felt frustrated by the lack of information he received regarding his tests.
4. You are reviewing Health Insurance Portability and Accountability Act (HIPAA) regulations with your patient during the admission process. The patient states, "I've heard a lot about these HIPAA regulations in the news lately. How will they affect my care?" Which of the following is the best response?
   1. HIPAA allows all hospital staff access to your medical record.
   2. HIPAA limits the information that is documented in your medical record.
   3. HIPAA provides you with greater control over your personal health care information.
   4. HIPAA enables health care institutions to release all of your personal information to improve continuity of care.
5. A patient asks for a copy of her medical record. The best response by the nurse is to:
   1. State that only her family may read the record.
   2. Indicate that she has the right to read her record.
   3. Tell her that she is not allowed to read her record.
   4. Explain that only health care workers have access to her record.
6. Which of the following charting entries is most accurate?
   1. Patient walked up and down hallway with assistance, tolerated well.
   2. Patient up, out of bed, walked down hallway and back to room, tolerated well.
   3. Patient up, walked 50 feet and back down hallway with assistance from nurse. Spouse also accompanied patient during the walk.
   4. Patient walked 50 feet and back down hallway with assistance from nurse; HR 88 and regular before exercise, 94 and regular following exercise.
7. Match the correct entry with the appropriate SOAP (Subjective—Objective—Assessment—Plan) category.
   1. S   a. Repositioned patient on right side. Encouraged patient to use patient-controlled analgesia (PCA) device.
   2. O   b. "The pain increases every time I try to turn on my left side."
   3. A   c. Acute pain related to tissue injury from surgical incision.
   4. P   d. Left lower abdominal surgical incision, 3 inches in length, closed, sutures intact, no drainage. Pain noted on mild palpation.
8. On the nursing unit you are able to access a patient's medical record and review the education that other nurses provided to the patient during an initial hospitalization and three subsequent clinic visits. This type of feature is most common in what type of record system?
   1. Information technology.
   2. Electronic health record.
   3. Personal health information.
   4. Administrative information system.
9. You are giving a hand-off report to another nurse who will be caring for your patient at the end of your shift. Which of the following pieces of information do you include in the report? (Select all that apply.)
   1. The patient's name, age, and admitting diagnosis
   2. Allergies to food and medications
   3. Your evaluation that the patient is "needy"
   4. How much the patient ate for breakfast
   5. That the patient's pain rating went from 8 to 2 on a scale of 1 to 10 after receiving 650 mg of Tylenol
10. You are supervising a beginning nursing student who is documenting patient care. Which of the following actions requires you to intervene? The nursing student:
    1. Documented medication given by another nursing student.
    2. Included the date and time of all entries in the chart.
    3. Stood with his back against the wall while documenting on the computer.
    4. Signed all documentation electronically.
11. A group of nurses is discussing the advantages of using computerized provider order entry (CPOE). Which of the following statements indicates that the nurses understand the major advantage of using CPOE?
    1. "CPOE reduces transcription errors."
    2. "CPOE reduces the time necessary for health care providers to write orders."
    3. "Health care providers can write orders from any computer that has Internet access."
    4. "CPOE reduces the time nurses use to communicate with health care providers."

12. You are helping to design a new patient discharge teaching sheet that will go home with patients who are discharged to home from your unit. Which of the following do you need to remember when designing the teaching sheet?
    1. The new federal laws require that teaching sheets be e-mailed to patients after they are discharged.
    2. You need to use words the patients can understand when writing the directions.
    3. The form needs to be given to patients in a sealed envelope to protect their health information.
    4. The names of everyone who cared for the patient in the hospital need to be included on the form in case the patient has questions at home.
13. A nurse caring for a patient on a ventilator electronically documents the head of bed elevated at 20 degrees. Suddenly an alert warning appears on the screen warning the nurse that this patient is at a high risk for aspiration because the head of the bed is not elevated high enough. This warning is known as what type of system?
    1. Electronic health record
    2. Clinical documentation
    3. Clinical decision support system
    4. Computerized physician order entry
14. While reviewing the pulmonary section of a patient's electronic chart, the physician notices blank spaces since the initial assessment the previous day when the nurse documented that the lung assessment was within normal limits. There also are no progress notes about the patient's respiratory status in the nurse's notes. The most likely reason for this is because:
    1. The nurses forgot to document on the pulmonary system.
    2. The nurses were charting by exception.
    3. The computer is not working correctly.
    4. The physician does not have authorization to view the nursing assessment.
15. What is an appropriate way for a nurse to dispose of printed patient information?
    1. Rip several times and place in a standard trash can
    2. Place in the patient's paper-based chart
    3. Place in a secure canister marked for shredding
    4. Burn the documents

Answers: **1.** 4; **2.** 2; **3.** 4; **4.** 3; **5.** 2; **6.** 4; **7.** 1b, 2d, 3c, 4a; **8.** 2; **9.** 1, 2, 5; **10.** 1; **11.** 1; **12.** 2; **13.** 3; **14.** 2; **15.** 3.

REFERENCES

American Nurses Association: *Principles for documentation, principles for practice: a resource package for registered nurses*, Silver Spring, Md, 2005, The Association.

American Nurses Association: *Scope and standards of nursing informatics practice*, Washington, DC, 2008, American Nurses Publishing.

Benson E, et al: Improving nursing shift-to-shift report, *J Nurs Care Qual* 22(1):80, 2007.

Blumenthal D: The "meaningful use" regulation for electronic health records, *N Engl J Med* 363(6):501, 2010.

Bombard C: Lines of communication, *Nurs Spectr (Gt Chic Ne Ill NW Indiana Ed)* 21(4):24, 2008.

Choi WH, et al: Comparison of direct and indirect nursing-care times between physician order entry system and electronic medical records, *Stud Health Technol Inform* 122:288, 2006.

Davis K, et al: Health information technology and physician perceptions of quality of care and satisfaction, *Health Policy* 90:239, 2009.

Dellefield M: Implementation of the resident assessment instrument/minimum data set in the nursing home as organization: implications for quality improvement in RN clinical assessment, *Geriatr Nurs* 28(6):377, 2007.

Garets D, Davis M: *Electronic medical records vs. electronic health records: yes, there is a difference;* White Paper, August 26, HIMSS Analytics LLC, 2005, www.himssanalytics.com/docs/WP_EMR_EHR.pdf. Accessed August 24, 2011.

Healthcare Information and Management Systems Society (HIMSS): *EHR definition, attributes, and essential requirements*, version 1.1, September 24, 2003, http://www.himss.org/content/files/ehrattributes070703.pdf. Accessed July 28, 2010.

Hebda T, et al: *Handbook of informatics for nurses and health care professionals*, ed 4, Upper Saddle River, NJ, 2009, Pearson Prentice Hall.

Hemmila D: Talking the talk: hospitals use SBAR to standardize communication, *NurseWeek* 7(17):26, 2006.

Institute of Medicine: *Crossing the quality chasm: a new health system for the twenty-first century*, Washington, DC, 2001, National Academies Press.

Lyerla F: Design and implementation of a nursing clinical decision support system to promote guideline adherence, *Computers Inform Nurs* 26(4):227, 2008.

Mosby's surefire documentation: how, what, and when nurses need to document, ed 2, St Louis, 2006, Mosby.

Oroviogoicoechea C, et al: Review: evaluating information systems in nursing, *J Clin Nurs* 17(5):567, 2007.

Schroeder S: Picking up the PACE: a new template for shift report, *Nursing* 36(10):22, 2006.

Senft D: Accidents and supervision: new CMS F-tag guidance, *Geriatr Nurs* 29(1):12, 2008.

The Joint Commission (TJC): *Comprehensive accreditation manual for hospitals: the official handbook* (E-dition), The Joint Commission, 2011.

RESEARCH REFERENCES

DeJesus RS, et al: Predictors of osteoporosis screening completion rates in a primary care practice, *Popul Health Manage* 14(5):243, 2011.

Giuliano KK, Lecardo M, Staul L: Impact of protocol watch on compliance with the Surviving Sepsis campaign, *Am J Crit Care* 20(4):313, 2011.

Jha A, et al: Use of electronic health records in US hospitals, *N Engl J Med* 360(16):1628, 2009.

Lyerla F, et al: A nursing clinical decision support system and potential predictors of head-of-bed position for patients receiving mechanical ventilation, *Am J Crit Care* 19(1):39, 2010.

CHAPTER 27

Patient Safety

OBJECTIVES

- Discuss the importance of consensus standards for public reporting of patient safety events.
- Describe environmental hazards that pose risks to a person's safety.
- Discuss methods to reduce physical hazards and the transmission of pathogens.
- Discuss the specific risks to safety related to developmental age.
- Identify the factors to assess when a patient is in restraints.
- Describe the four categories of safety risks in a health care agency.
- Describe assessment activities designed to identify patients' physical, psychosocial, and cognitive status as it pertains to their safety.
- Identify relevant nursing diagnoses associated with risks to safety.
- Develop a nursing care plan for patients whose safety is threatened.
- Describe nursing interventions specific to a patients' age for reducing risk of falls, fires, poisonings, and electrical hazards.
- Define the knowledge, skills, and attitudes necessary to promote safety in a health care setting.

KEY TERMS

Aura, p. 387
Food and Drug Administration (FDA), p. 366
Immunization, p. 367
Pathogen, p. 367
Poison, p. 367
Pollutant, p. 368
Restraint, p. 384
Seizure, p. 387
Seizure precautions, p. 387
Status epilepticus, p. 387

evolve WEBSITE

http://evolve.elsevier.com/Potter/fundamentals/

- Review Questions
- Video Clips
- Concept Map Creator
- Case Study with Questions
- Skills Performance Checklists
- Audio Glossary
- Interactive Learning Activities
- Key Term Flashcards
- Content Updates

Safety, often defined as freedom from psychological and physical injury, is a basic human need. Health care provided in a safe manner and a safe community environment is essential for a patient's survival and well-being. A safe environment reduces the risk for illness and injury and helps to contain the cost of health care by preventing extended lengths of treatment and/or hospitalization, improving or maintaining a patient's functional status, and increasing the patient's sense of well-being. The Institute of Medicine's report *To Err Is Human: Building a Safer Health System* (2000) was a pivotal publication that brought patient safety to the forefront of health care in the United States. This report indicated that 44,000 to 98,000 people die each year as a result of preventable medical errors. In an effort to improve patient safety, many organizations have become devoted to developing and monitoring key health care safety initiatives and providing information to health care organizations and the public. Health care organizations foster a patient-centered safety culture by continually focusing on performance improvement endeavors, risk management findings, and safety reports; providing current reliable technology; integrating evidence-based practice into procedures; designing a safe work environment and atmosphere; and providing continuing education and access to appropriate resources for staff (Box 27-1). As part of the health care team, the nurse has the professional responsibility to be engaged in activities that support a patient-centered safety culture. Considerable emphasis has also been placed on improving the education of student nurses so they become more competent in promoting safe health care practices. The Quality and Safety Education for Nurses (QSEN) project was developed to meet the challenge of preparing future nurses who will have the knowledge, skills, and attitudes necessary to continuously improve the quality and safety of the health care systems within which they work (QSEN, 2011). The QSEN safety competency for a nurse is defined as "Minimizes risk of harm to patients and providers through both system effectiveness and individual performance." As a nurse you are responsible for incorporating critical thinking skills when using the nursing process, assessing each patient and his or her environment for hazards that threaten safety, and planning and intervening appropriately to maintain a safe environment. By doing this, you become a provider of safe acute, restorative, and continuing care and an active participant in health promotion.

SCIENTIFIC KNOWLEDGE BASE

Environmental Safety

A patient's environment includes all of the many physical and psychosocial factors that influence or affect the life and survival of that patient. This broad definition of environment crosses the

BOX 27-1 RESOURCES RELATED TO SAFETY AND SAFETY INITIATIVES

- The Joint Commission http://www.jointcommission.org/PatientSafety
- The Agency for Healthcare Research and Quality http://www.psnet.ahrq.gov/
- The Institute for Healthcare Improvement http://www.ihi.org/ihi
- The U.S. Department of Veterans Affairs http://www.patientsafety.gov
- Centers for Medicare and Medicaid Services http://www.cms.gov
- Quality Improvement Organization Support Center http://www.qualitynet.org
- ECRI Institute http://www.ecri.org
- U.S. Department of Health and Human Services http://www.hospitalcompare.hhs.gov

continuum of care for settings in which the nurse and patient interact such as the hospital, long-term care facility, clinic, community center, school, and home. A safe environment protects the staff as well, allowing them to function optimally. Vulnerable groups who often require help in achieving a safe environment include infants, children, older adults, the ill, the physically and mentally disabled, the illiterate, and the poor. A safe environment includes meeting basic needs, reducing physical hazards and the transmission of pathogens, and controlling pollution.

Basic Needs. Physiological needs, including the need for sufficient oxygen, nutrition, and optimum temperature, influence a person's safety. According to Maslow's hierarchy of needs, these basic needs must be met before physical and psychological safety and security can be addressed (see Chapter 6).

Oxygen. Supplemental oxygen is sometimes required to meet a person's oxygenation needs. Oxygen is not flammable, but fire needs oxygen to start and to keep burning. When more oxygen is in the air, a fire burns hotter and faster. Strict codes regulate the use and storage of medical oxygen in health care facilities. This is not necessarily true in the home environment. Hospital emergency departments see approximately 1190 thermal burns per year caused by ignitions associated with home medical oxygen (National Fire Protection Association, 2008). Smoking is by far the leading cause of burns, reported fires, deaths, and injuries involving home medical oxygen.

Be aware of factors in a patient's environment that decrease the amount of available oxygen. A common environmental hazard in the home is an improperly functioning heating system. A furnace, stove, or fireplace that is not properly vented introduces carbon monoxide into the environment. Carbon monoxide affects a person's oxygenation by binding with hemoglobin, preventing the formation of oxyhemoglobin and thus reducing the supply of oxygen delivered to tissues (see Chapter 40). Low concentrations cause nausea, dizziness, headache, and fatigue. Very high concentrations cause death after 1 to 3 minutes of exposure (National Fire Protection Association, 2010a).

Nutrition. Meeting nutritional needs adequately and safely requires environmental controls and knowledge (see Chapter 44). Health care facilities and restaurants are required to meet State Board of Health regulations. To protect consumers, commercially processed and packaged foods are subject to **Food and Drug Administration (FDA)** regulations. The FDA is a federal agency responsible for the enforcement of federal regulations regarding the manufacture, processing, and distribution of foods, drugs, and cosmetics to protect consumers against the sale of impure or dangerous substances. Although food supply in the United States is one of the safest in the world, each year about 76 million illnesses occur, more than 300,000 persons are hospitalized, and 5,000 die from foodborne illness (Centers for Disease Control and Prevention, 2009). Groups at the highest risk are children, pregnant women, older adults, and people with compromised immune systems. Foods that are inadequately prepared or stored or subject to unsanitary conditions increase the patient's risk for infections and food poisoning.

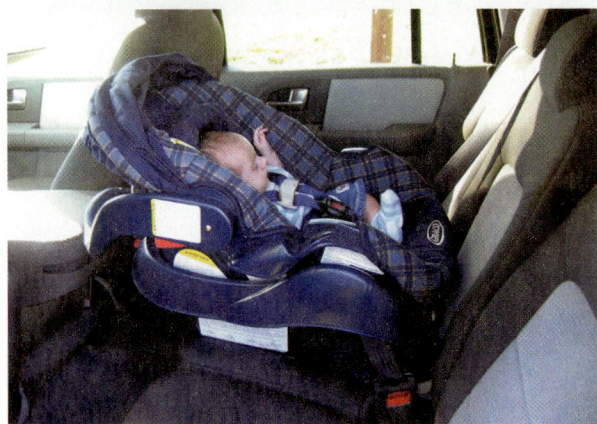

FIG. 27-1 Infant car seat. (Courtesy Brian and Mayannyn Sallee, Las Vegas, Nevada.)

Temperature. A person's comfort zone is usually between 18.3° and 23.9° C (65° and 75° F). Temperature extremes that frequently occur during the winter and summer affect comfort, productivity, and safety. Exposure to severe cold for prolonged periods causes frostbite and accidental hypothermia. Frostbite occurs when a surface area of the skin freezes as a result of exposure to extremely cold temperatures. Hypothermia occurs when the core body temperature is 35° C (95° F) or below. Older adults, the young, patients with cardiovascular conditions, patients who have ingested drugs or alcohol in excess, and people who are homeless are at high risk for hypothermia. Exposure to extreme heat changes the electrolyte balance of the body and raises the core body temperature, resulting in heatstroke or heat exhaustion. Chronically ill patients, older adults, and infants are at greatest risk for injury from extreme heat. These patients need to avoid extremely hot, humid environments (see Chapter 29).

Physical Hazards. On average 33.5 million injuries take place each year, with the majority occurring inside or outside of the home (Centers for Disease Control and Prevention, 2010a). Physical hazards in the environment threaten a person's safety and often result in physical or psychological injury or death. Unintentional injuries are the fifth leading cause of death for Americans of all ages (National Center for Injury Prevention, 2010a). Motor vehicle accidents are the leading cause, followed by poisonings and falls. Additional hazards consist of fire and disasters. A nurse plays a role in educating patients about common safety hazards and how to prevent injury while placing emphasis on hazards to which patients are more vulnerable.

Motor Vehicle Accidents. Vehicle design and equipment such as seat belts, air bags, and laminated windshields (remain in one piece when impacted) have improved safety for vehicle occupants. State specific laws relating to young driver licensing, safety belt use, child restraint use, and motorcycle helmets exist for protection. Child safety seats and booster seats appropriate for the child's age and weight and the type of car need to be used (Fig. 27-1). The American Academy of Pediatrics (2011) recommends that all infants and toddlers ride in the back seat with a rear-facing car safety seat until they are 2 years of age or they reach the highest weight or height allowed by the manufacturer of the car safety seat. The website of the Academy, Healthy Children, http://www.aap.org/healthtopics/carseatsafety.cfm, has information for children of all ages and the type of safety seat to use. The back seat of a car is the safest part of the vehicle in the event of a crash and prevents injury from deployment of passenger and side air bags. According to the Centers for Disease Control and Prevention (2010b), the risk of motor vehicle accidents is higher among 16- to 19-year-old drivers than any other age-group. Teens are more likely to underestimate dangerous situations or not be able to recognize hazardous situations, speed and allow shorter headways, ride with intoxicated drivers, and drive after using alcohol and drugs. Teens also have the lowest rate of seat belt use. Older drivers are keeping their licenses longer and driving more miles than in the past. Per mile traveled, fatal crash rates increase starting at age 75 and increase markedly after age 80 (Insurance Institute for Highway Safety, 2008). An older adult is not always able to quickly observe situations in which an accident is likely to occur. Decreased hearing acuity alters the ability to hear emergency vehicle sirens or vehicle horns. Because of decreased nervous system response, older adults are unable to react as quickly as they once could to avoid an accident. A decline in these skills accounts for the most common types of accidents, including right-of-way and turning accidents.

Poison. A **poison** is any substance that impairs health or destroys life when ingested, inhaled, or absorbed by the body. Almost any substance is poisonous if too much is taken. Sources in a person's home include drugs, medicines, other solid and liquid substances, and gases and vapors. Poisons often impair the function of every major organ system. Health care providers are at risk from chemicals such as toxic cleaning agents. In the home accidental poisoning is a greater risk for toddlers, preschoolers, and young school-age children, who often ingest household cleaning solutions, medications, or personal hygiene products. Emergency treatment is necessary when a person ingests a poisonous substance or comes in contact with a chemical that is absorbed through the skin. In 2008 more than 2000 people a day were seen in emergency departments after a poison incident (Centers for Disease Control and Prevention, 2010c). Specific antidotes or treatments are available only for some types of poisons. A poison control center is the best resource for patients and parents needing information about the treatment of an accidental poisoning.

Although lead has not been used in house paint or plumbing materials since the U.S. Consumer Product Safety Commission banned it in 1978, older homes in poorer communities continue to contain high lead levels. Soil and water systems are sometimes contaminated. Poisoning occurs from swallowing or inhaling lead. Fetuses, infants, and children are more vulnerable to lead poisoning than adults because their bodies absorb lead more easily and small children are more sensitive to the damaging effects of lead. Exposure to excessive levels of lead affects a child's growth or causes learning and behavioral problems and brain and kidney damage (Agency for Toxic Substances and Disease Registry, 2010).

Falls. Falls are a major public health problem. Among adults 64 years and older, falls are the leading cause of unintentional death (Centers for Disease Control and Prevention, 2010a). Numerous factors increase the risk of falls, including a history of falling, being age 65 or over, reduced vision, orthostatic hypotension, gait and balance problems, urinary incontinence, use of walking aids, and the effects of various medications (e.g., anticonvulsants, hypnotics, sedatives, certain analgesics) (Deandrea et al., 2010). Common physical hazards that lead to falls include inadequate lighting, barriers along normal walking paths and stairways, and a lack of safety devices in the home. Often a fall leads to serious injury such as fractures or internal bleeding. Patients most at risk for injury are those with bleeding tendencies resulting from disease or medical treatments and osteoporosis. Injuries frequently result from accidental contact with objects on stairs, floors, bedside tables, closet shelves, refrigerator tops, and bookshelves. Children fall from anywhere (i.e., trees, wall/fences, playground equipment, furniture, and moving objects such as skateboards and bicycles). Forces from falls lead to injury with variable severity, depending on the height of the fall, body position on impact, and impact surface.

Fire. A total of 386,500 home fires were reported in the United States in 2008, resulting in 2,755 deaths and 13,160 injuries (National Fire Protection Association, 2010b). The leading cause of fire-related death is careless smoking, especially when people smoke in bed at home. The improper use of cooking equipment and appliances, particularly stoves, is the main source for in-home fires and fire injuries. Smoke detectors and carbon monoxide detectors need to be placed strategically throughout a home. Multipurpose fire extinguishers need to be near the kitchen and any workshop areas.

Disasters. When they strike, natural disasters such as floods, tsunamis, hurricanes, tornadoes, and wildfires are a major cause of death and injury. These types of disasters result in death and leave many people homeless. Every year millions of Americans face disaster and its terrifying consequences (FEMA, 2010). Bioterrorism is another cause of disaster. Threats of this type come in the form of biological, chemical, and radiological attacks. Bioterrorism, or the use of biological agents to create fear and threat, is the most likely form of a terrorist attack to occur. Although terrorists could use any agent, health officials are most concerned with biological agents such as anthrax, smallpox, pneumonic plague, botulism, tularemia, and viral hemorrhagic fevers (American Medical Association, 2010).

Transmission of Pathogens. Pathogens and parasites pose a threat to patient safety (see Chapter 28). A **pathogen** is any microorganism capable of producing an illness. The most common means of transmission of pathogens is by the hands. For example, if an individual infected with hepatitis A does not wash his or her hands thoroughly after having a bowel movement, the risk for transmitting the disease during food preparation is great. One of the most effective methods for limiting the transmission of pathogens is the medically aseptic practice of hand hygiene (see Chapter 28). The human immunodeficiency virus (HIV), the pathogen that causes acquired immunodeficiency syndrome (AIDS), and the hepatitis B virus are transmitted through blood and other select body fluids. High-risk behaviors that include sexual contact and drug use are common risk factors for HIV. People who abuse drugs often share syringes and needles, which increase the risk of acquiring these viruses. Some states and many nonprofit organizations fund syringe exchange programs as a means to slow down the spread of infectious diseases obtained through needle sharing (Coalition for Safe Community Needle Disposal, 2010).

Immunization also reduces, and in some cases prevents, the transmission of disease from person to person. Individuals acquire active immunity by an injection of a small amount of attenuated (weakened) or dead organisms or modified toxins from the organism (toxoids) into the body. Passive immunity occurs when antibodies produced by other persons or animals are introduced into a person's bloodstream for protection against a pathogen.

Insects and rodents often carry pathogens. For example, some mosquitoes are carriers of malaria and West Nile virus. Rats and mice carry rat-bite fever. Uncontrolled mosquito and rodent populations increase the risk for these diseases. People living at the poverty level sometimes live in unmaintained homes or housing. Rat and roach infestations are common problems. Mosquito repellant and rodent traps help eliminate this risk.

Proper disposal of human waste controls the transmission of disease and parasites. Without a satisfactory sewer and waste system in a community, the population is at risk for illnesses such as typhoid fever and hepatitis.

Pollution. A healthy environment is free of pollution. A **pollutant** is a harmful chemical or waste material discharged into the water, soil, or air. People commonly think of pollution only in terms of air, land, or water pollution; but excessive noise is also a form of pollution that presents health risks. Air pollution is the contamination of the atmosphere with a harmful chemical. Prolonged exposure to it increases the risk of pulmonary disease. In urban areas industrial waste and vehicle exhaust are common contributors to air pollution. In the home, school, or workplace, cigarette smoke is the primary cause of air pollution. Improper disposal of radioactive and bioactive waste products (e.g., dioxin) can cause land pollution. Water pollution is the contamination of lakes, rivers, and streams, usually by industrial pollutants. Water treatment facilities filter harmful contaminants from the water, but these systems sometimes contain flaws. If water becomes contaminated, the public needs to use bottled or boiled water for drinking and cooking. Flooding frequently causes damage to water treatment stations and also requires the use of bottled or boiled water.

NURSING KNOWLEDGE BASE

Factors Influencing Patient Safety

In addition to being knowledgeable about the home and health care environment and the inherent safety risks, nurses need to be familiar with a patient's developmental level; mobility, sensory, and cognitive status; lifestyle choices; and knowledge of common safety precautions. They also need to be aware of the special risks to safety that are found in health care settings.

Risks at Developmental Stages. A patient's developmental stage creates threats to safety as a result of lifestyle, cognitive and mobility status, sensory impairments, and safety awareness. With this information, you tailor safety prevention programs to the needs, preferences, and life circumstances of particular age-groups. Unfortunately all age-groups are subject to abuse. Child abuse, domestic violence, and elder abuse are serious threats to safety. Chapters 12 through 14 discuss these topics.

Infant, Toddler, and Preschooler. Injuries are the leading cause of death in children over age 1 and cause more death and disabilities than do all diseases combined (Hockenberry and Wilson, 2009). The nature of the injury sustained is closely related to normal growth and development. For example, the incidence of lead poisoning is highest in late infancy and toddlerhood. Children at this stage explore the environment and, because of their increased level of oral activity, put objects in their mouth. This increases risk for poisoning and choking. Fire often results from their curiosity in playing with matches. In addition, limited physical coordination contributes to falls from bicycles and playground equipment. Additional injuries at this age are related to riding unrestrained in a motor vehicle, drowning, and head trauma from objects. Accidents involving children are largely preventable, but parents need to be aware of specific dangers at each stage of growth and development. Accident prevention thus requires health education for parents and the removal of dangers whenever possible.

School-Age Child. When a child enters school, the environment expands to include the school, transportation to and from school, school friends, and after-school activities. School-age children are learning how to perform more complicated motor activities and often are uncoordinated. Parents, teachers, and nurses need to instruct children in safe practices to follow at school or play, including what to do if approached by strangers. Teach school-age children involved in team and contact sports the rules for playing safely and how to use protective safety equipment such as helmets and other protective gear. Head injuries are a major cause of death, with bicycle accidents being one of the major causes of such injuries (Hockenberry and Wilson, 2009). Bikes need to be the proper size for the child, and helmets must be worn (Fig. 27-2). Additional injuries in this age-group are decreased by properly using seat belts and booster seats in motor vehicles and providing pedestrian safety education.

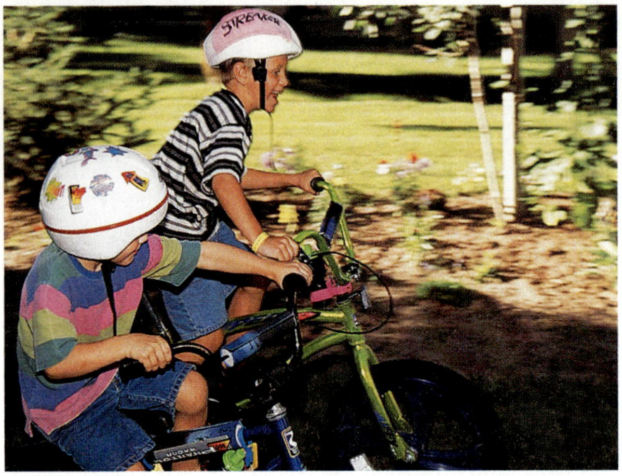

FIG. 27-2 Proper bicycle safety equipment for school-age child.

Adolescent. As children enter adolescence, they develop greater independence and begin to develop a sense of identity and their own values. The adolescent begins to separate emotionally from his or her family, and peers generally have a stronger influence. Wide variations that swing from childlike to mature behavior are characteristic of adolescent behavior (Hockenberry and Wilson, 2009). In an attempt to relieve the tensions associated with physical and psychosocial changes and peer pressures, some adolescents engage in risk-taking behaviors such as smoking, drinking alcohol, and using drugs. This increases the incidence of accidents such as drowning and motor vehicle accidents. When adolescents learn to drive, their environment expands, and so does their potential for injury. Fortunately teen motor vehicle crashes are preventable by avoiding distractions such as using cell phones, texting, eating, and drinking while driving.

To assess for possible substance abuse, have parents look for environmental and psychosocial clues from their children. Environmental clues include the presence of drug-oriented magazines, beer and liquor bottles, drug paraphernalia and blood spots on clothing and the continual wearing of long-sleeved shirts in hot weather and dark glasses indoors. Psychosocial clues include failing grades, change in dress, increased absenteeism from school, isolation, increased aggressiveness, and changes in interpersonal relationships. Because adolescence is a time when mature sexual physical characteristics develop, some adolescents begin to have physical relationships with others that present the risk of sexually transmitted diseases.

Adult. The threats to an adult's safety are frequently related to lifestyle habits. For example, a person who uses alcohol excessively is at greater risk for motor vehicle accidents. People who smoke long-term have a greater risk of cardiovascular or pulmonary disease as a result of the inhalation of smoke and the effect of nicotine on the circulatory system. Likewise, the adult experiencing a high level of stress is more likely to have an accident or illness such as headaches, gastrointestinal (GI) disorders, and infections.

Older Adult. The physiological changes associated with aging, effects of multiple medications, psychological factors, and acute or chronic disease increase the older adult's risk for falls and other types of accidents. Falls often result in bruises, hip fractures, or head trauma. The risk of being seriously injured in a fall increases with age. Older patients are more likely to fall in the bedroom, bathroom, and kitchen. Environmental factors such as broken stairs, icy sidewalks, inadequate lighting, throw rugs, and exposed electrical cords cause many of the accidents. Inside falls most often occur while transferring from beds, chairs, and toilets; getting into or out of bathtubs; tripping over items such as cords covered by rugs or carpets, carpet edges, or doorway thresholds; slipping on wet surfaces; and descending stairs. Fear of falling is a concern of community-dwelling older adults, and many avoid activities because of their fear (Zijlstra et al., 2007). Falls can be decreased by multiple-component group exercise, Tai Chi, having a physician or pharmacist review all medications, having an eye examination annually, and decreasing hazards in the home that increase falls (Gillespie et al., 2009).

Individual Risk Factors. Other risk factors posing threats to safety include lifestyle, impaired mobility, sensory or communication impairment, and the lack of safety awareness.

Lifestyle. Some lifestyle choices increase safety risks. People who drive or operate machinery while under the influence of chemical substances (drugs or alcohol), work at inherently dangerous jobs, or are risk takers are at greater risk of injury. In addition, people experiencing stress, anxiety, fatigue, or alcohol or drug withdrawal or those taking prescribed medications are sometimes more accident prone. Because of these factors, some people are too preoccupied to notice the source of potential accidents such as cluttered stairs or a stop sign.

Impaired Mobility. A patient with impaired mobility has many kinds of safety risks. Muscle weakness, paralysis, and poor coordination or balance are major factors in falls. Immobilization predisposes patients to additional physiological and emotional hazards, which in turn further restrict mobility and independence. Persons who are physically challenged are at greater risk for injury when entering motor vehicles and buildings that are not handicapped accessible.

Sensory or Communication Impairment. Cognitive impairments associated with delirium, dementia, and depression place patients at greater risk for injury. These conditions contribute to altered concentration and attention span, impaired memory, and orientation changes. Patients with these alterations become easily confused about their surroundings and are more likely to have falls and burns. Patients with visual, hearing, tactile, or communication impairment such as aphasia or a language barrier are not always able to perceive a potential danger or express their need for assistance (see Chapter 49).

Lack of Safety Awareness. Some patients are unaware of safety precautions such as keeping medicine or poisons away from children or reading the expiration date on food products. A complete nursing assessment, including a home inspection, helps you identify the patient's level of knowledge regarding home safety so you can correct deficiencies with an individualized nursing care plan.

Risks in the Health Care Agency. Patient safety continues to be one of the most pressing health care challenges in the nation.

BOX 27-2 THE JOINT COMMISSION 2011 NATIONAL PATIENT SAFETY GOALS FOR HOSPITALS

- Identify patients correctly.
  - Use at least two patient identifiers.
  - Eliminate transfusion errors.
- Improve staff communication.
  - Report important test results in a timely manner.
- Use medicines safely.
  - Label medications.
  - Reduce harm to patients who take anticoagulation therapy.
- Reduce the risk of health care–associated infections.
  - Meet hand hygiene guidelines.
  - Prevent multidrug-resistant organism infections.
  - Prevent central line–associated bloodstream infections.
  - Use safe practices to treat the part of the body where surgery was performed.
- Check patient medicines.
  - Identify current medicines and make sure that it is okay for patients to take any new medicines with current medicines.
  - Give a list of patient's medicines to the next provider before discharge.
  - Give a list of patient's medicines to patient and family before discharge; explain the list.
- Identify patient safety risks.
  - Identify individuals at risk for suicide.

Medical errors are the eighth leading cause of death (Agency for Healthcare Research and Quality, 2010). Medical errors happen when something that was planned as part of medical care doesn't work out or when the wrong plan was used. They occur in all health care settings. You must be aware of regulatory and organizational safety initiatives and individual patient risk factors. The Joint Commission (TJC) and the Centers for Medicare and Medicaid Services (CMS) have placed an increased emphasis on error prevention and patient safety. Their "Speak Up" campaign encourages patients to take a role in preventing health care errors by becoming active, involved, and informed participants on the health care team. For example, patients are encouraged to ask health care workers if they have washed their hands before providing care. National Patient Safety Goals of TJC (2011b) are specifically directed to reduce the risk of medical errors (Box 27-2). The goals are designed to promote specific improvements in patient safety and highlight ongoing problematic areas in health care. These evidence-based recommendations require health care facilities to focus their attention on a series of specific actions.

The National Quality Forum (NQF) (2011a) has the mission of improving the quality of health care in America by:

- Building consensus on national priorities and goals for performance improvement and working in partnership to achieve them;
- Endorsing national consensus standards for measuring and publicly reporting on performance; and
- Promoting the attainment of national goals through education and outreach programs.

Recently the NQF released its National Voluntary Consensus Standards for Public Reporting of Patient Safety Events (NQF, 2011b). The report provides a framework for publicly reporting patient safety information—including events, indicators, and

BOX 27-3 THE NATIONAL QUALITY FORUM LIST OF SERIOUS REPORTABLE EVENTS

Surgical Events

A. Surgery performed on the wrong body part
B. Surgery performed on the wrong patient
C. Wrong surgical procedure performed on a patient
D. Unintended retention of foreign object in a patient after surgery or procedure
E. Intraoperative or immediately postoperative death

Product or Device Events

A. Patient death or serious disability associated with use of contaminated drugs, devices, or biologicals provided by the health care facility
B. Patient death or serious disability associated with use or function of a device in patient care when the device is used or functions other than as intended
C. Patient death or serious disability associated with intravascular air embolism that occurs during care in a health care facility

Patient-Protection Events

A. Infant discharged to wrong person
B. Patient death or serious disability associated with patient elopement
C. Patient suicide or attempted suicide resulting in serious disability during care in a health care facility

Care-Management Events

A. Patient death or serious disability associated with medication error
B. Patient death or serious disability associated with hemolytic reaction as a result of administration of ABO/HLA-incompatible blood or blood products
C. Maternal death or serious disability associated with labor or delivery in a low-risk pregnancy during care in a health care facility
D. Patient death or serious disability associated with hypoglycemia, the onset of which occurs during care in a health care facility
E. Death or serious disability associated with failure to identify and treat hyperbilirubinemia in neonates
F. Stage III or IV pressure ulcers acquired after admission to a health care facility
G. Patient death or serious disability caused by spinal manipulative therapy
H. Artificial insemination with wrong donor sperm or wrong egg

Environmental Events

A. Patient death or serious disability associated with an electric shock during care in a health care facility
B. Any incident in which a line designated for oxygen or other gas to be delivered to a patient contains the wrong gas or is contaminated by toxic substances
C. Patient death or serious disability associated with burn incurred from any source during care in a health care facility
D. Patient death or serious disability associated with fall during care in a health care facility
E. Patient death or serious disability associated with use of restraints or bed rails during care in a health care facility

Criminal Events

A. Care provided by someone impersonating a health care provider
B. Abduction of patient of any age
C. Sexual assault on patient within or on the grounds of a health care facility
D. Death or significant injury resulting from a physical assault that occurs within or on the grounds of the facility

From National Quality Forum (NQF): *Serious reportable events in healthcare 2006 update: a consensus report,* Washington, DC, 2007, NQF p 6, accessed May 25, 2011, from http://www.qualityforum.org/Publications/2007/03/Serious_Reportable_Events_in_Healthcare-2006_Update.aspx.

measures—about health care organizations to consumers. It is important for nurses to understand the NQF standards and their intent since ultimately they influence the types of priorities that patient care organizations (e.g., hospitals, community health centers) set to improve the quality of care delivered to patients. Many of the NQF measures of patient safety (e.g., patient falls with injury, incidence of pressure ulcers, and central line bloodstream infection) are standards for judging the quality of care of health care organizations. The measures are also used by other organizations such as TJC and the CMS. Among the safety measures, the NQF endorsed a select list of serious reportable events (SREs), which was updated in 2006. The 28 events (Box 27-3) are a major focus of health care providers for patient safety initiatives. The CMS names select SREs as *Never Events* (i.e., adverse events that should never occur in a health care setting) (Department of Health and Human Services, 2008). The CMS now denies hospitals higher payment for any hospital-acquired condition resulting from or complicated by the occurrence of certain Never Events (Box 27-4). Many of the hospital-acquired conditions (e.g., fall or stage III pressure ulcer) are nurse-sensitive indicators, meaning that a nurse directly affects their development. The NQF (2010) also released 34 safe practices for better health care. Evidence supports the effectiveness of these practices in reducing the occurrence of adverse health care events.

Being aware of and engaged in activities focused on the prevention of these conditions not only enhances patient safety but also contributes to the overall success of the health care facility. The

BOX 27-4 THE 2009 CENTERS FOR MEDICARE AND MEDICAID SERVICES HOSPITAL-ACQUIRED CONDITIONS (PRESENT-ON-ADMISSION INDICATORS)

- Foreign object retained after surgery
- Air embolism
- Blood incompatibility
- Pressure ulcer stages III and IV
- Falls and trauma (fracture, dislocation, intracranial injury, crushing injury, burn, electric shock)
- Catheter-associated urinary tract infections
- Vascular catheter-associated infections
- Manifestations of poor glycemic control (diabetic ketoacidosis, nonketotic hyperosmolar coma, hypoglycemic coma, secondary diabetes with ketoacidosis, secondary diabetes with hyperosmolarity)
- Surgical site infections following:
  - Mediastinitis following coronary artery bypass graft
  - Certain orthopedic procedures (spine, neck, shoulder, elbow)
  - Bariatric surgery for obesity (laparoscopic gastric bypass, gastroenterostomy, laparoscopic gastric restrictive surgery)
- Deep vein thrombosis and pulmonary embolism following certain orthopedic procedures (total knee replacement, hip replacement)

From Centers for Medicare and Medicaid Services: *Hospital-acquired conditions,* 2010, accessed May 25, 2011, from http://www.cms.gov/HospitalAcqCond/06_Hospital-Acquired_Conditions.asp.

CMS believes that the Never Events will strengthen incentives by hospitals to develop safety practices and reduce health care costs in the long term. Health care facilities often conduct a failure mode and effect analysis (FMEA) to identify problems with processes and products before they occur.

When an actual or potential adverse event occurs, the nurse or health care provider involved completes an incident or occurrence report. An incident report is a confidential document that completely describes any patient accident occurring on the premises of a health care agency (see Chapter 23). Reporting allows the organization to identify trends/patterns throughout the facility and areas to improve. Focusing on the root cause of an event instead of the individual involved promotes a "culture of safety" that helps in specifically identifying what contributed to an error. The probability of an accident occurring declines with adherence to evidence-based principles of safety (Taylor-Adams et al., 2009).

Nurses face specific environmental risks in health care facilities. An example is the various forms of chemicals used. Chemicals found in some medications (e.g., chemotherapy), anesthetic gases, cleaning solutions, and disinfectants are potentially toxic if ingested, absorbed into the skin, or inhaled. Material safety data sheets (MSDSs) are required resources available in any health care agency (Occupational Safety and Health Administration, 1996). The MSDS provides detailed information about the chemical, health hazards imposed, first aid guidelines, and precautions for safe handling and use. MSDSs give information on the steps to take in case the material is released or spilled. Be aware of the location of the MSDSs and be knowledgeable about hazardous chemicals in your environment. Spread of pathogens also presents a risk to both nurses and other patients. Therefore always follow standard and transmission-based isolation precautions, along with proper hand hygiene (see Chapter 28).

Specific risks to a patient's safety within the health care environment include falls, patient-inherent accidents, procedure-related accidents, and equipment-related accidents. The nurse assesses for these four potential problem areas and, considering the developmental level of the patient, takes steps to prevent or minimize accidents.

Falls. Falls result in minor to severe injuries such as hip fractures or head trauma that result in reduced mobility and independence and increase the risk for premature death. Patients who have underlying disease states are more susceptible to fall-related injuries (Hughes, 2008). For example, a patient with a bleeding disorder is more likely to have an intracranial bleed; a patient with osteoporosis has a greater chance for fracture. The unfamiliar environment, acute illness, surgery, mobility status, medications, treatments, and placement of various tubes and catheters are common challenges that place patients of any age at risk of falling. Factors the nurse can influence include assessment and communication about patient risks, information access, signage, the environment, teamwork, and involving the patient and family (Dykes et al., 2009). Falls that result in injuries often extend a patient's length of stay in the health care environment, placing them at an even greater risk for other complications.

Patient-Inherent Accidents. Patient-inherent accidents are accidents (other than falls) in which the patient is the primary reason for the accident. Examples include self-inflicted cuts, injuries, and burns; ingestion or injection of foreign substances; self-mutilation or fire setting; and pinching fingers in drawers or doors. One of the more common precipitating factors for a patient-inherent accident is a seizure.

Procedure-Related Accidents. Procedure-related accidents are caused by health care providers and include medication and fluid administration errors, improper application of external devices, and accidents related to improper performance of procedures such as dressing changes or urinary catheter insertion. Nurses are able to prevent many procedure-related accidents by adhering to organizational policy and procedures and standards of nursing practice. For example, proper preparation and administration of medications, use of patient and medication bar coding, and "Smart" intravenous (IV) pumps reduce medication errors (see Chapters 31 and 41). All staff need to be aware that distractions and interruptions contribute to procedure-related accidents and need to be limited, especially during high-risk procedures such as medication administration. The potential for infection is reduced when surgical asepsis is used for sterile dressing changes or any invasive procedure such as insertion of a urinary catheter. Finally, correct use of safe patient handling techniques and equipment reduces the risk of injuries when moving and lifting patients (see Chapter 47).

Equipment-Related Accidents. Accidents that are equipment related result from the malfunction, disrepair, or misuse of equipment or from an electrical hazard. To avoid rapid infusion of IV fluids, all general-use and patient-controlled analgesic pumps need to have free-flow protection devices. To avoid accidents, do not operate monitoring or therapy equipment without adequate instruction. If faulty equipment is discovered, place a tag on it to prevent it from being used on another patient and promptly report any malfunctions. Assess potential electrical hazards to reduce the risk of electrical fires, electrocution, or injury from faulty equipment. In health care settings the clinical engineering staff make regular safety checks of equipment. Facilities must report all suspected medical device—related deaths to both the FDA and the manufacturer of the product if known (FDA, 2009). This is usually done in conjunction with the risk management department after tagging and removing the piece of equipment.

Building Competency in Safety The nurse manager on an oncology unit learns that the hospital purchased new intravenous (IV) infusion pumps or "smart pumps" that provide a mechanism to deliver chemotherapy drugs more safely. To promote a culture of safety, what does the manager do next to ensure quality safe patient care?

Answers to questions can be found on the Evolve website.

CRITICAL THINKING

Successful critical thinking requires a synthesis of knowledge, experience, information gathered from patients, critical thinking attitudes, and intellectual and professional standards. Clinical judgments require the nurse to anticipate necessary information, analyze the data, and make decisions regarding patient care. Critical thinking is an ongoing process. During assessment (Fig. 27-3) you consider all critical thinking elements and information about the specific patient to make appropriate nursing diagnoses.

In the case of safety, the nurse integrates knowledge from nursing and other scientific disciplines, previous experiences in caring for patients who had an injury or were at risk, critical thinking attitudes such as responsibility and discipline, and any standards of practice that are applicable. For example, the American Nurses Association (ANA) standards for nursing practice address the nurse's responsibility in maintaining patient safety. TJC (2011b) also provides standards for safety. You refer to all of this

Knowledge
- Basic human needs
- Potential risks to patient safety from physical hazards, lifestyle, risks associated with health care environment, environmental risks, and biohazards
- Influence of developmental stage on safety needs
- Influence of illness/medications on patient safety

Experience
- Caring for patients whose mobility, cognitive, or sensory impairments increase threats to safety
- Personal experience in caring for younger siblings or children

ASSESSMENT
- Identify patient's perceptions of safety needs and risks
- Identify actual and potential threats to the patient's safety
- Determine impact of the underlying illness on the patient's safety
- Identify the presence of risks for the patient's developmental stage and patient's environment
- Determine effect of environmental influence on the patient's safety

Standards
- Apply intellectual standards such as accuracy, significance, and completeness when assessing for threats to the patient's safety
- Apply ANA standards for nursing practice
- Apply agency practice standards (e.g., fall prevention or restraint protocols)
- Review and apply the most current TJC patient safety goals

Attitudes
- Demonstrate perserverance when necessary to identify all safety threats
- Be responsible for collecting unbiased, accurate data regarding threats to the patient's safety
- Show discipline in conducting a thorough review of the patient's home environment

FIG. 27-3 Critical thinking model for safety assessment. *ANA*, American Nurses Association; *TJC*, The Joint Commission.

information and experience as you conduct a detailed assessment of a specific patient. For example, while assessing a specific patient's home environment, you consider typical locations within the home where dangers commonly exist. If a patient has a visual impairment, you apply previous experiences in caring for patients with visual changes to anticipate how to thoroughly assess his or her needs. Critical thinking directs you to anticipate what needs to be assessed and how to make conclusions about available data.

NURSING PROCESS

Apply the nursing process and use a critical thinking approach in your care of patients. The nursing process provides a clinical decision-making approach for you to develop and implement an individualized plan of care.

BOX 27-5 NURSING ASSESSMENT QUESTIONS

Activity and Exercise
- Do you use any assistive devices such as a wheelchair, walker, or cane to help you move or get around? Did someone show you how to use them safely?
- Do you have any difficulty bathing? Dressing? Eating? Using the bathroom? Transferring out of the bed or chair?
- What type of exercise or physical activity do you get? How often?
- How do you handle meal preparation (e.g., use stove and appliances safely)?
- Do you do your own laundry? How do you do this, and where are these appliances located?
- Do you drive an automobile? When do you normally drive? How far?
- How often do you wear a safety belt when in the car?
- Have you recently been involved in a motor vehicle accident?

Medication History
- Which medications (prescription, over-the-counter, herbal) do you take?
- Has your doctor or pharmacist reviewed your medicines with you?
- Do any medications make your dizzy or light-headed?

History of Falls
- Have you ever fallen or tripped over anything in your home?
- Have you ever suffered an injury from a fall? What was it and how did it happen?
- Did you have any symptoms right before you fell? What were they?
- Which activity were you performing before the fall?

Home Maintenance and Safety
- Who does your simple home maintenance or minor home repairs?
- Who shovels your snow? Tends to your lawn?
- Do you feel safe in your home? Which things in your environment make you feel unsafe?
- Do you have someone to call in case of an emergency?
- How do you feel about modifying your home to make it safer? Do you need help finding resources to help you do this?

ASSESSMENT

During the assessment process thoroughly assess each patient and critically analyze findings to ensure that you make patient-centered clinical decisions required for safe nursing care.

Through the Patient's Eyes. Patients generally expect to be safe in health care settings and in their homes. However, there are times when a patient's view of what is safe does not agree with that of the nurse and the standards he or she hopes to enforce. For this reason your assessment needs to be patient centered and include the patient's own perceptions of his or her risk factors, knowledge of how to adapt to such risks, and previous experience with any accidents. This is important if you need to make changes in the patient's environment. Patients usually do not purposefully put themselves in jeopardy. When they are uninformed or inexperienced, threats to their safety occur. You always need to consult patients or family members about ways to reduce hazards in their environment. To conduct a thorough patient assessment, consider possible threats to a patient's safety, including the immediate environment and any individual risk factors. Ask the patient specific questions related to safety (Box 27-5).

Nursing History. A nursing history includes data about a patient's level of wellness to determine if any underlying conditions

TABLE 27-1 Fall Assessment Tool

Fall Risk Factor Category Scoring not completed for the following reason(s) (check any that apply). ☐ Complete paralysis or completely immobilized. Implement basic safety (low fall risk) interventions. ☐ Patient has a history of more than one fall within 6 months before admission. Implement high–fall risk interventions throughout hospitalization. ☐ Patient has experienced a fall during this hospitalization. Implement high–fall risk interventions throughout hospitalization. ☐ Patient is deemed high fall risk per protocol (e.g., seizure precautions). Implement high fall-risk interventions per protocol.	
COMPLETE THE FOLLOWING AND CALCULATE FALL RISK SCORE.	
IF NO BOX IS CHECKED, SCORE FOR CATEGORY IS 0	**POINTS**
Age (single-select) ☐ 60-69 years (1 point) ☐ 70-79 years (2 points) ☐ ≥80 years (3 points)	
Fall History (single-select) ☐ One fall within 6 months before admission (5 points)	
Elimination (Bowel and Urine) (single-select) ☐ Incontinence (2 points) ☐ Urgency or frequency (2 points) ☐ Urgency/frequency and incontinence (4 points)	
Medications: Includes PCA/Opiates, Anticonvulsants, Antihypertensives, Diuretics, Hypnotics, Laxatives, Sedatives, and Psychotropics (single-select) ☐ On one high fall–risk drug (3 points) ☐ On two or more high fall–risk drugs (5 points) ☐ Sedated procedure within past 24 hours (7 points)	
Patient Care Equipment: Any Equipment That Tethers Patient (e.g., IV Infusion, Chest Tube, Indwelling Catheters, SCDs) (single-select) ☐ One present (1 point) ☐ Two present (2 points) ☐ 3 or more present (3 points)	
Mobility (Multi-select, Choose All That Apply and Add Points Together) ☐ Requires assistance or supervision for mobility, transfer, or ambulation (2 points) ☐ Unsteady gait (2 points) ☐ Visual or auditory impairment affecting mobility (2 points)	
Cognition (Multi-select, Choose All That Apply and Add Points Together) ☐ Altered awareness of immediate physical environment (1 point) ☐ Impulsive (2 points) ☐ Lack of understanding of one's physical and cognitive limitations (4 points)	
TOTAL Moderate risk = 6-13 total points High risk = >13 total points	

IV, Intravenous.

exist that pose threats to safety. For example, give special attention to assessing a patient's gait, lower-body muscle strength and coordination, balance, and vision. Consider a review of the patient's developmental status as you analyze assessment information. Also review if the patient is taking any medications or undergoing any procedures that pose risks. For example, use of diuretics increases the frequency of voiding and results in the patient having to use toilet facilities more often. Falls often occur with patients who have to get out of bed quickly because of urinary urgency.

Health Care Environment. When the patient is cared for within a health care facility, you need to determine if any hazards exist in the immediate care environment. Does the placement of equipment (e.g., drainage bags, IV pumps) or furniture pose barriers when the patient attempts to ambulate? Does positioning of the patient's bed allow him or her to easily reach items on a bedside table or stand? Does the patient need assistance with ambulation? Are there multiple tubes or IV lines? Is the call bell within reach? The nurse collaborates with clinical engineering staff to make sure that equipment functions properly and is in good condition.

Risk for Falls. Assessment of a patient's risk factors for falling is essential in determining specific needs and developing targeted interventions to prevent falls. Many different fall assessment instruments are available; use the tool chosen by your health care agency. A fall assessment tool (Table 27-1) helps you assess important risk factors. At a minimum the assessment needs to be completed on admission, following a change in the patient's condition, after a fall, and when transferred. If it is determined that the patient is at risk for falling, regular assessment always continues. In many cases family members are important resources in assessing a patient's fall risk. Families often are able to report on the patient's level of confusion and ability to ambulate. Based on the results of a fall risk assessment, you implement multiple evidence-based interventions. It is very important to inform a patient and family members about the patient's risks. Often younger patients are not aware of how medications and treatments cause dizziness, orthostatic hypotension, or changes in balance. When patients are unaware of their risks, they are less likely to ask for assistance. If family members are informed, they will often call for help (when they are visiting patients) to be sure that patients are appropriately assisted.

Risk for Medical Errors. Be alert to factors within your own work environment that create conditions in which medical errors are more likely to occur. Studies show that overwork and fatigue cause a significant decrease in alertness and concentration, leading to errors (Trinkoff et al., 2006). It is important for you to be aware of these factors and include checks and balances when working under stress. For example, to reduce the potential for a medical error, it is essential for you to check the patient's identification by using two identifiers (e.g., name and birthday or name and account number) according to facility policy before beginning any procedure or administering a medication (see Chapter 31).

Disasters. Hospitals must be prepared to respond and care for a sudden influx of patients at the time of a community disaster. Guidelines for a disaster response are included in a facility emergency management plan. All hospitals conduct disaster drills on a routine basis. Communication is a key to any emergency management plan. Nurses must know what happened, how many patients to expect, and when patients will begin to arrive so they can prepare both themselves and their facility. Although the occurrence of a bioterrorist attack has been limited to the anthrax deaths following September 11, 2001, the threat is very real. Be prepared to make accurate and timely assessments in any type of setting. A bioterrorist attack will likely resemble a natural outbreak initially. Acutely ill patients representing the earliest cases after a covert attack seek care in emergency departments. Patients less ill at the onset of an illness possibly seek care in primary care settings. Basic epidemiological principles exist to assess whether a patient's presentation of symptoms is typical of an endemic disease or an unusual event that raises concern. Features that alert nurses to the possibility of a bioterrorism-related outbreak include the following (Dire, 2008):

- Disease (or strain) not endemic
- Unusual antibiotic resistance patterns
- Atypical clinical presentation
- Case distribution geographically (from same location) and/or temporally inconsistent
- Other inconsistent elements (e.g., number of cases, mortality and morbidity rates, deviations from disease occurrence baseline)

Patient's Home Environment. When caring for a patient in the home, a home hazard assessment is necessary. See http://homesafetycouncil.org/safetyguide for a sample home assessment guide. A thorough hazard assessment covers topics such as adequacy of lighting (inside and outdoors), presence of safety devices, placement of furniture or other items that can create barriers, condition of flooring, and safety in the kitchen and bathrooms. Know where medications and cleaning supplies are located. Walk through the home with the patient and discuss how he or she normally conducts daily activities and whether the environment poses problems. Assess for the presence of locks on doors and windows that make the home less susceptible to intruders. When assessing the adequacy of lighting, inspect the areas where the patient moves and works such as outside walkways, steps, interior halls, and doorways. Getting a sense of the patient's routines helps you recognize less obvious hazards.

Assessment for risk of food infection or poisoning includes assessing a patient's knowledge of food preparation and storage practices. For example, does a patient know to check expiration dates of prepared food and milk products? Does he or she keep foods in the refrigerator that are fresh and not spoiled? Does the patient clean fresh fruits and vegetables correctly before eating them? Assess for clinical signs of infection by conducting an examination of GI and central nervous system function, observing for a fever, and analyzing the results of cultures of feces and emesis. In the home inspect suspected food and water sources and assess the patient's handwashing practices. It is useful to ask patients when they routinely wash their hands. This then prompts a helpful discussion about the purpose and importance of handwashing.

Assessment of the environmental comfort of a patient's home includes a review of when the patient normally has heating and cooling systems serviced. Does the patient have a functional furnace or space heater? Does the home have air conditioning or fans? You need to inform patients who use space heaters of the risk for fires. Are smoke detectors, carbon monoxide detectors, and fire extinguishers present and placed strategically throughout the home and checked routinely?

When patients live in older homes, encourage them to have inspections for the presence of lead in paint, dust, or soil. Because lead also comes from the solder or plumbing fixtures in a home, patients need to have water from each faucet tested. Local health offices will help homeowners locate a trained lead inspector who takes samples from various locations and has them analyzed at a laboratory for lead content.

It is important that your assessment help individuals focus on avoiding losses and reducing their risk for injury associated with disasters. The FEMA (http://www.fema.gov/) and the American Red Cross (http://www.redcross.org/) provide nationwide education to help community members prepare for disasters of all types.

NURSING DIAGNOSIS

Gather data from your nursing assessment and analyze clusters of defining characteristics to identify relevant nursing diagnoses. Include specific related or contributing factors to individualize your nursing care (Box 27-6). For example, the nursing diagnosis *risk for injury* is sometimes related to altered mobility or sensory alteration (e.g., visual). Altered mobility leads you to select such nursing interventions as range-of-motion (ROM) exercises or teaching the proper use of safety devices such as side rails, canes, or crutches. Visual impairment as the related factor leads you to select different interventions such as keeping the area well lit; orienting the patient to the surrounding; or keeping eye glasses clean, handy, and well protected. When you do not identify the correct related factor, the use of inappropriate interventions increases a patient's risk for injury. For example, not evaluating the home environment for hazards possibly results in sending a hospitalized patient home only to return with an additional

BOX 27-6 NURSING DIAGNOSTIC PROCESS

Risk for Injury

ASSESSMENT ACTIVITIES	DEFINING CHARACTERISTICS
Observe patient's posture, range of motion, strength, balance, and body alignment.	Uncoordinated, shuffling gait Stooped posture
Ask about patient's visual acuity.	Reports difficulty seeing at night Reports "tripping" over rugs and furniture
Complete a home hazard appraisal.	Poorly lighted home Rooms filled with small items Excessive amount of furniture for size of room Rugs not secure

injury. Nursing diagnoses for patients with safety risk include the following:

- Risk for falls
- Impaired home maintenance
- Risk for injury
- Deficient knowledge
- Risk for poisoning
- Risk for suffocation
- Risk for trauma

PLANNING

Patients with actual or potential risks to safety require a nursing care plan with interventions that prevent and minimize threats to their safety. Design your interventions to help a patient feel safe to move about and interact freely within the environment. The total plan of care addresses all aspects of patient needs and uses resources of the health care team and the community when appropriate. Critically synthesize information from multiple sources (Fig. 27-4). Critical thinking ensures that the patient's plan of care integrates all that you learned about the patient and the key critical thinking elements. For example, you reflect on knowledge regarding the services that other disciplines (e.g., occupational therapy, case management) provide in helping patients return to their home environments safely. Also reflect on any previous experience when a patient benefited from safety interventions. Such experience helps you adapt approaches with each new patient. Applying critical thinking attitudes such as creativity helps you to collaborate with the patient in planning interventions that are relevant and most useful, particularly when making changes in the home environment.

Goals and Outcomes. You collaborate with the patient, family, and other members of the health care team when setting goals and expected outcomes during the planning process (see the Nursing Care Plan). The patient who is an active participant in reducing threats to safety becomes more alert to potential hazards and is more likely to adhere to the plan. Make sure that goals and outcomes for each nursing diagnosis are measurable and realistic, with consideration of the resources available to the patient. For example, in the case of the nursing diagnosis of *impaired physical mobility related to left-sided paralysis*, the goal is the patient "remains free of injury by discharge." Examples of expected outcomes include:

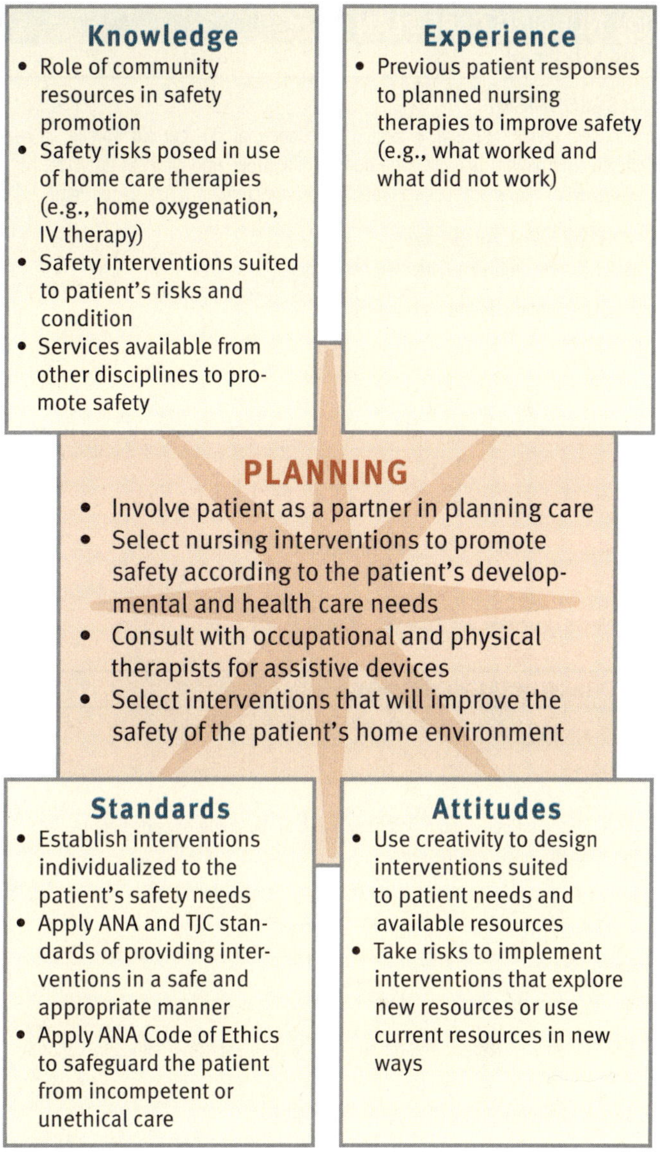
Knowledge
• Role of community resources in safety promotion
• Safety risks posed in use of home care therapies (e.g., home oxygenation, IV therapy)
• Safety interventions suited to patient's risks and condition
• Services available from other disciplines to promote safety
Experience
• Previous patient responses to planned nursing therapies to improve safety (e.g., what worked and what did not work)
PLANNING
• Involve patient as a partner in planning care
• Select nursing interventions to promote safety according to the patient's developmental and health care needs
• Consult with occupational and physical therapists for assistive devices
• Select interventions that will improve the safety of the patient's home environment
Standards
• Establish interventions individualized to the patient's safety needs
• Apply ANA and TJC standards of providing interventions in a safe and appropriate manner
• Apply ANA Code of Ethics to safeguard the patient from incompetent or unethical care
Attitudes
• Use creativity to design interventions suited to patient needs and available resources
• Take risks to implement interventions that explore new resources or use current resources in new ways

FIG. 27-4 Critical thinking model for safety planning. *ANA,* American Nurses Association; *TJC,* The Joint Commission.

- Patient uses tripod cane correctly within 24 hours.
- Patient describes approach to rise up from bed correctly with assistance by end of the teaching session today.

Setting Priorities. Prioritize a patient's nursing diagnoses and interventions to provide safe and efficient care. For example, the patient described in the concept map (Fig. 27-5) has several nursing diagnoses. The patient's mobility problem is an obvious priority because of its influence on risk for falls and skin integrity. Plan individualized interventions based on the severity of risk factors and the patient's developmental stage, level of health, lifestyle, and cultural needs (Box 27-7). Planning involves an understanding of the patient's need to maintain independence within physical and cognitive capabilities. Collaborate to establish ways of maintaining the patient's active involvement within the home and health care environment. Education of the patient and family is also an important intervention to plan for reducing safety risks over the long term.

NURSING CARE PLAN

Risk for Falls

ASSESSMENT

Mr. Key, a visiting nurse, is seeing Ms. Cohen, an 85-year-old woman, at her home. The patient is recovering from a mild stroke affecting her left side. Ms. Cohen lives alone but receives regular assistance from her daughter Peggy and son Michael, who both live within 10 miles. Mr. Key's assessment included a discussion of Ms. Cohen's health problem and how the stroke has affected her, a pertinent physical examination, and home hazard assessment.

*Assessment Activities**	*Findings/Defining Characteristics*
Ask how the stroke has affected her mobility.	She responds, "I **bump into things,** and **I'm afraid I'm going to fall.**"
Conduct a home hazard assessment.	Cabinets in kitchen are **cluttered** and full of breakable items that could fall out. **Throw rugs are on floors;** bathroom **lighting is poor** (40-watt bulbs); bathtub **lacks safety strips** or grab bars; **home is cluttered** with furniture and small objects.
Observe gait and posture.	She has **kyphosis** and a **hesitant, uncoordinated gait;** frequently holds walls for support.
Assess muscle strength.	**Left arm and leg are weaker** than right.
Assess visual acuity with corrective lenses.	She has **trouble reading and seeing familiar objects at a distance** while wearing current glasses.

*__Defining characteristics__ are shown in bold type.

NURSING DIAGNOSIS: Risk for falls

PLANNING

Goals	*Expected Outcomes (NOC)*†
	Risk Control
Mrs. Cohen's family will modify the home to eliminate hazards within 1 month.	Family members will reduce modifiable hazards in kitchen and hallway within 1 week. Family members will make revisions to bathroom in 1 month.
	Knowledge: Personal Safety
Ms. Cohen and family will be knowledgeable of potential hazards for Ms. Cohen's age-group within 1 week.	Ms. Cohen and daughter will identify risks for falls and prevention methods to avoid falls in home at conclusion of teaching session next week.
	Fall Prevention Behavior
Ms. Cohen will express greater sense of feeling safe from falling in 1 month.	Ms. Cohen will report improved vision with the aid of new eyeglasses in 2 weeks.
Ms. Cohen will be free of injury within 1 week.	Ms. Cohen will safely ambulate throughout the home within 1 week.

†Outcome classification labels from Moorhead S et al: *Nursing outcomes classification (NOC),* ed 4, St Louis, 2008, Mosby.

INTERVENTIONS (NIC)‡	RATIONALE
Fall Prevention	
Review findings from home hazard assessment with Ms. Cohen and her children and collaborate on proposed changes.	Home hazard assessment highlights extrinsic factors that lead to falls and that can be changed.
Establish a list of priorities to modify and have Ms. Cohen's son assist in installing bathroom safety devices.	Implementing home modifications based on home assessment decreases falls (Pynoos, 2010).
Discuss with Ms. Cohen and daughter the normal changes of aging, effects of recent stroke, associated risks for injury, and how to reduce risks.	Education regarding hazards reduces fear of falling (Banez, 2008).
Encourage daughter to schedule vision testing for new prescription within 2 to 4 weeks.	Improved visual acuity reduces incidence of falls (Edelman and Mandle, 2010).
Refer to physical therapist to assess need for strengthening and endurance training and use of assistive devices for kyphosis, left-sided weakness, and gait.	Exercise is effective in reducing falls and needs to include a comprehensive program combining muscle strengthening, balance, and/or endurance training for a minimum of 12 weeks (Costello, 2008)

‡Intervention classification labels from Bulechek GM, Butcher HK, Dochterman JM: *Nursing interventions classification (NIC),* ed 5, St Louis, 2008, Mosby.

NURSING CARE PLAN

***Risk for Falls*—cont'd**

EVALUATION

Nursing Actions	*Patient Response/Finding*	*Achievement of Outcome*
Ask Ms. Cohen and family to identify fall risks.	Ms. Cohen and family are able to identify risks during a walk through the home and expressed a greater sense of safety as a result of changes made.	Ms. Cohen and family are more knowledgeable of potential hazards.
Observe environment for elimination of hazards.	Throw rugs were removed. Lighting increased to 75 watts except in bathroom and bedroom.	Environmental hazards are partially reduced.
Reassess Ms. Cohen's visual acuity.	Ms. Cohen has new glasses and says she is able to read better and see distant objects more clearly.	Ms. Cohen's vision has improved, enabling her to ambulate more safely.
Observe Ms. Cohen's gait and posture.	Ms. Cohen's gait remains hesitant and uncoordinated; she reports that her daughter has limited time to take her to the physical therapist.	Outcome of safe ambulation is not totally achieved; help daughter develop a schedule that allows her time to take her mother to physical therapy appointments.

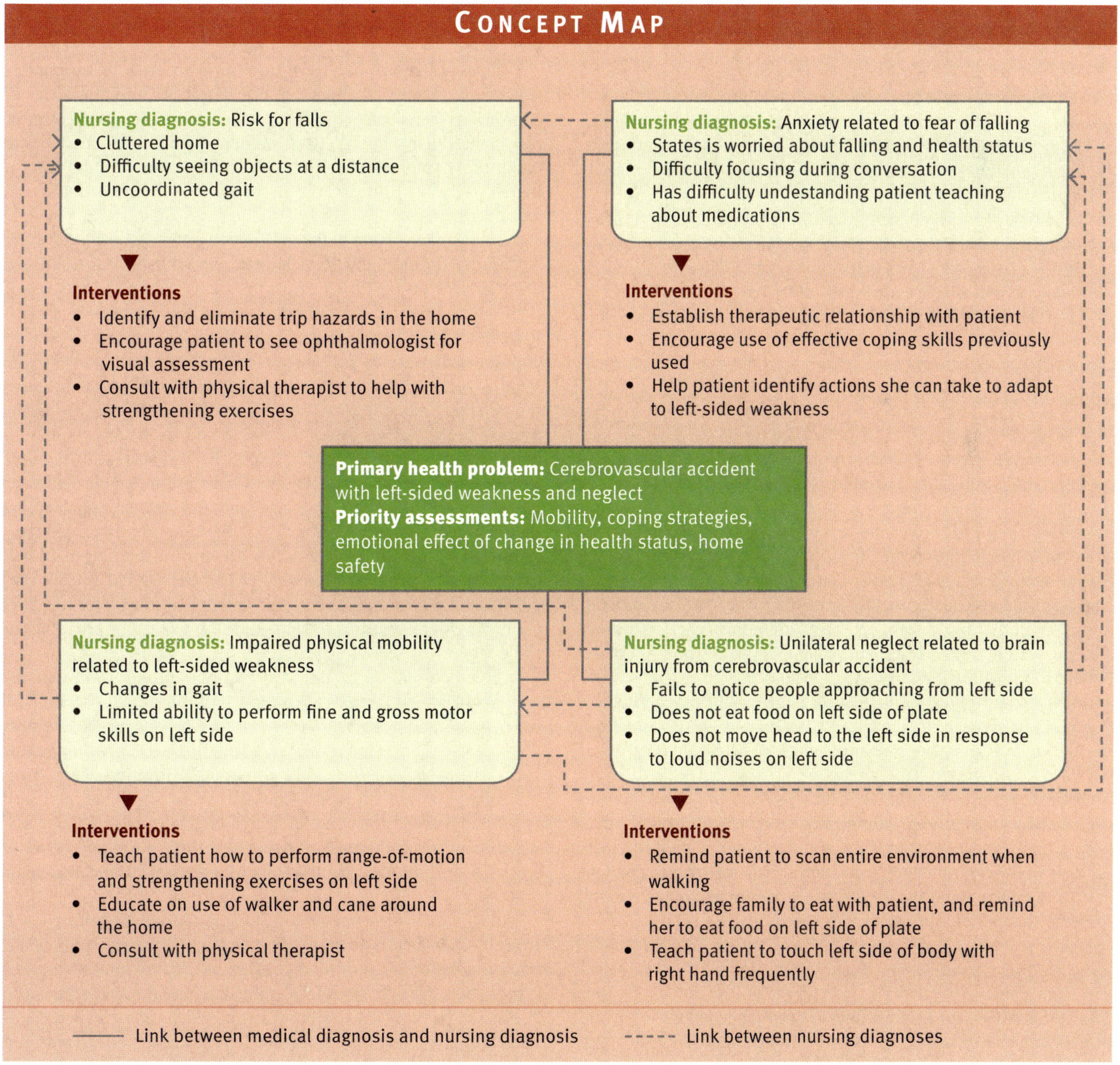
CONCEPT MAP
Nursing diagnosis: Risk for falls
• Cluttered home
• Difficulty seeing objects at a distance
• Uncoordinated gait
Interventions
• Identify and eliminate trip hazards in the home
• Encourage patient to see ophthalmologist for visual assessment
• Consult with physical therapist to help with strengthening exercises
Nursing diagnosis: Anxiety related to fear of falling
• States is worried about falling and health status
• Difficulty focusing during conversation
• Has difficulty undestanding patient teaching about medications
Interventions
• Establish therapeutic relationship with patient
• Encourage use of effective coping skills previously used
• Help patient identify actions she can take to adapt to left-sided weakness
Primary health problem: Cerebrovascular accident with left-sided weakness and neglect
Priority assessments: Mobility, coping strategies, emotional effect of change in health status, home safety
Nursing diagnosis: Impaired physical mobility related to left-sided weakness
• Changes in gait
• Limited ability to perform fine and gross motor skills on left side
Interventions
• Teach patient how to perform range-of-motion and strengthening exercises on left side
• Educate on use of walker and cane around the home
• Consult with physical therapist
Nursing diagnosis: Unilateral neglect related to brain injury from cerebrovascular accident
• Fails to notice people approaching from left side
• Does not eat food on left side of plate
• Does not move head to the left side in response to loud noises on left side
Interventions
• Remind patient to scan entire environment when walking
• Encourage family to eat with patient, and remind her to eat food on left side of plate
• Teach patient to touch left side of body with right hand frequently
Link between medical diagnosis and nursing diagnosis
Link between nursing diagnoses

FIG. 27-5 Concept map for Ms. Cohen. *ADLs,* Activities of daily living; *CVA,* cerebrovascular accident.

BOX 27-7 CULTURAL ASPECTS OF CARE

A Patient-Centered Care Approach

Hospitalization places patients at risk for injury in an unfamiliar and confusing environment. The experience is usually at least minimally frightening. Normal life cues such as a bed without side rails and the direction one usually takes to the bathroom are absent. Thought processes and coping mechanisms are affected by illness and its accompanying emotions. Thus patients are more vulnerable to injury. This vulnerability is often intensified for patients of diverse backgrounds. It is a nurse's responsibility to diligently protect all patients, regardless of their socioeconomic status and cultural background. Most untoward events are related to failures of communication. This is especially important during assessment. Ensure you use an approach that recognizes a patient's cultural background so you ask appropriate questions to reveal health behaviors and risks. You also need to be aware of cultural beliefs about restraints when caring for patients who need restraints. Safety is enhanced when you consider patients in light of the whole person and value seeing each care situation through "the patient's eyes" and not just through your own perspective. Some specific patient-centered safety guidelines about the use of restraints follow.

Implications for Practice

- When restraints are needed, assess their meaning to the patient and the family. For example, some Asian families view the restraining of older adults as disrespectful. Similarly some survivors of war or persecution view restraints as imprisonment or punishment.
- Collaborate with family members in accommodating a patient's cultural perspectives about restraints. Removing the restraints when family members are present shows respect and caring for the patient.
- Define the protocol of the nursing unit on the use of restraints. Identify potential areas for negotiation with the patient's/family's preferences such as using a jacket versus arm restraints.

Teamwork and Collaboration. Collaboration with the patient, family, and other disciplines such as social work and occupational and physical therapy become an important part of the patient's plan of care. For example, a hospitalized patient may need to go to a rehabilitation facility to gain strength and endurance before being discharged home. Communication is essential. You communicate risk factors and the plan of care with the patient, family, and other health care providers, including other disciplines and nurses on other shifts. Permanent dry-erase boards in the patient room with patient information such as activity and level of assistance communicate information to all health care providers. A standard approach to communication such as SBAR (Situation, *B*ackground, *A*ssessment, *R*ecommendation) helps you obtain and organize information (see Chapter 26).

Patients need to be able to identify, select, and know how to use resources within their community (e.g., neighborhood block homes, local police departments, and neighbors willing to check on their well-being) that enhance safety. Make sure that the patient and family understand the need for these resources and are willing to make changes that promote their safety.

IMPLEMENTATION

The QSEN (2011) project outlines recommended skills to ensure nurse competency in patient safety. Among these skills are those involving safe nursing practice during direct care:

- Demonstrate effective use of technology and standardized practices that support safety and quality.
- Demonstrate effective use of strategies to reduce risk of harm to self or others.
- Use appropriate strategies to reduce reliance on memory (such as forcing functions, checklists).

Direct your nursing interventions toward maintaining the patient's safety in all types of settings. You implement health promotion and illness prevention measures in the community setting, whereas prevention is a priority in the acute care setting.

Health Promotion. To promote an individual's health, it is necessary for the individual to be in a safe environment and practice a lifestyle that minimizes risk of injury. Edelman and Mandle (2010) describe passive and active strategies aimed at health promotion. Passive strategies include public health and government legislative interventions (e.g., sanitation and clean water laws) (see Chapter 3). Active strategies are those in which the individual is actively involved through changes in lifestyle (e.g., wearing seat belts or installing outdoor lighting) and participation in wellness programs.

Nurses participate in health promotion activities by supporting legislation, acting as positive role models, and working in community-based settings. Because environmental and community values have the greatest influence on health promotion, community and home health nurses are able to assess and recommend safety measures in the home, school, neighborhood, and workplace.

Developmental Interventions

Infant, Toddler, and Preschooler. Growing, curious children need adults to protect them from injury. Children are trusting of their environment and do not perceive themselves to be in danger. Educate parents or guardians about reducing risks of injuries to children and ways to promote safety in the home (Table 27-2). Nurses working in prenatal and postpartum settings easily incorporate safety into the care plan of the childbearing family. Community health nurses assess the home and show parents how to promote safety. Educate parents about the importance of immunizations and how they protect a child from life-threatening disease.

School-Age Child. School-age children increasingly explore their environment (see Chapter 12). They have friends outside their immediate neighborhood; and they become more active in school, church, and community activities. The school-age child needs specific teaching regarding safety in school and at play. See Table 27-2 for nursing interventions to help guide the parent in providing for the safety of the school-age child.

Adolescent. Risks to the safety of adolescents involve many factors outside the home because much of their time is spent away from home and with their peer group (see Chapter 12). Adults serve as role models for adolescents and, through providing examples, setting expectations, and providing education, help them minimize risks to their safety. This age-group has a high incidence of suicide because of feelings of decreased self-worth and hopelessness. Be aware of the risks posed at this time and be prepared to teach adolescents and their parents measures to prevent accidents and injury.

Adult. Risks to young and middle-age adults frequently result from lifestyle factors such as childrearing, high stress levels, inadequate nutrition, use of firearms, excessive alcohol intake, and substance abuse (see Chapter 13). In this fast-paced society there also appears to be more expression of anger, which can quickly precipitate accidents related to "road rage." Help adults understand their safety risks and guide them in making lifestyle modifications by

TABLE 27-2 Interventions to Promote Safety for Children and Adolescents

INTERVENTION	RATIONALE
Infants and Toddlers	
Have infants sleep on their back or side. Teach parents the mnemonic "back to sleep."	Placing infants on their back confers the lowest risk of sudden infant death syndrome (SIDS) and is the preferred position (American Academy of Pediatrics, 2005).
Do not fill cribs with pillows, large stuffed toys, or comforters. Use snug-fitting sheets.	Possibility exists for infants to become entwined in sheets and other bedding and suffocate.
Do not attach pacifiers to string or ribbon and place around a child's neck.	String or ribbon around the neck increases risk for choking.
Follow all instructions for preparing and storing formula.	Proper formula preparation and storage prevent contamination. Following product directions ensures proper concentration of formula. Undiluted formula causes fluid and electrolyte disturbances; very diluted formula does not provide sufficient nutrients.
Use large, soft toys without small parts such as buttons.	Small parts become dislodged, and choking and aspiration can occur.
Do not leave the mesh sides of playpens lowered; spaces between crib slats need to be less than 2⅜ inches (6 cm) apart.	Possibility exists for a child's head becoming wedged in the lowered mesh side or between crib slats, and asphyxiation may occur.
Never leave crib sides down or babies unattended on changing tables or in infant seats, swings, strollers, or high chairs.	Infants and toddlers roll or move and fall from changing tables or out of accessories such as infant seats or swings.
Discontinue using accessories such as infant seats and swings when the child becomes too active or physically too big and/or according to the manufacturer's directions.	When physically active or too big, the child can fall out of or tip over these accessories and suffer an injury.
Never leave a child alone in the bathroom, tub, or near any water source (e.g., pool).	Supervision reduces risk for accidental drowning.
Baby-proof the home; remove small or sharp objects and toxic or poisonous substances, including plants; install safety locks on floor-level cabinets.	Babies explore their world with their hands and mouth. Choking and poisoning can occur.
Remove plastic bags from the cleaners or grocery store from the home.	Removal reduces risk for suffocation from plastic bags.
Cover electrical outlets.	Covers reduce opportunity for crawling babies to insert objects into outlets and experience an electrical shock.
Place window guards on all windows.	Guards prevent children from falling out of windows.
Install keyless locks (e.g., deadbolts) on doors above a child's reach, even when they are standing on a chair.	Deadbolts prevent a toddler from leaving the house and wandering off. Death from exposure, car accidents, and drowning can occur. Keyless locks allow for rapid exit in case of fire.
Put children weighing less than 80 pounds or under 8 years of age in an age/weight-appropriate car seat that has been installed according to manufacturer's instructions (see Fig. 27-1). This includes car seats and booster seats. In cars with a passenger air bag, children under 12 need to be in the back seat. All passengers need to wear seat belts.	In case of a sudden stop or crash, an unrestrained child suffers severe head injuries and death.
Caregivers need to learn cardiopulmonary resuscitation (CPR) and the Heimlich maneuver.	Caregivers need to be prepared to intervene in acute emergencies such as choking.
Preschoolers	
Teach children to swim at an early age but always provide supervision near water.	Learning to swim is a useful skill that can someday save a child's life. However, all children need constant supervision near water.
Teach children how to cross streets and walk in parking lots. Instruct them to never run out after a ball or toy.	Pedestrian accidents involving young children are common.
Teach children not to talk to, go with, or accept any item from a stranger.	Avoiding strangers reduces the risk of injury and stranger abduction.
Teach children basic physical safety rules such as proper use of safety scissors, never running with an object in their mouth or hand, and never attempting to use the stove or oven unassisted.	Risk of injury is lower if children know basic safety procedures.
Teach children not to eat items found in the street or grass.	Avoiding these items reduces risk for possible poisoning.
Remove doors from unused refrigerators and freezers. Instruct children not to play or hide in a car trunk or unused appliances.	If a child cannot freely exit from appliances and car trunks, asphyxiation can occur.

Continued

TABLE 27-2 Interventions to Promote Safety for Children and Adolescents—cont'd

INTERVENTION	RATIONALE
School-Age Children	
Teach children the safe use of equipment for play and work.	The child needs to learn the safe, appropriate use of implements to avoid injury.
Teach children proper bicycle safety, including use of helmet and rules of the road.	Reduces injuries from falling off a bike or being hit by a car.
Teach children proper techniques for specific sports and the need to wear proper safety gear (e.g., helmets, eyewear, mouth guards).	Using proper sports techniques, correct equipment, and protective gear prevents injuries.
Teach children not to operate electrical equipment while unsupervised.	If an electrical mishap were to occur, no one would be available to help.
Do not allow children access to firearms or other weapons. Keep all firearms in locked cabinets.	Children are often fascinated by firearms and weapons and sometimes attempt to play with them.
Adolescents	
Encourage enrollment in driver's education classes.	Many injuries in this age-group are related to motor-vehicle accidents.
Provide information about the effects of using alcohol and drugs.	Adolescents are prone to risk-taking behaviors and are subject to peer pressures.
Refer adolescents to community and school-sponsored activities.	The adolescent needs to socialize with peers yet needs some supervision.
Encourage mentoring relationships between adults and adolescents.	Adolescents are in need of role models after whom they can pattern their behavior.
Teach them safe use of the Internet.	Avoids overuse and possible exposure to inappropriate websites.

Modified from Hockenberry M, Wilson D: *Wong's nursing care of infants and children,* ed 9, St Louis, 2011, Mosby.

BOX 27-8 FOCUS ON OLDER ADULTS

Physiological Changes of Aging and Their Effect on Patient Safety

- Older adults experience visual and hearing alterations. Encourage annual vision and hearing examinations and frequent cleaning of glasses and hearing aids as a means of preventing falls and burns.
- Some older adults have slowed reaction time. Teach patients safety tips for avoiding automobile accidents. Sometimes driving needs to be restricted to daylight hours or temporarily or permanently suspended.
- Range of motion, flexibility, and strength decrease. Encourage supervised exercise classes for older adults and teach them to seek assistance with household tasks as needed. Safety features such as grab bars in the bathroom are often necessary.
- Reflexes are slowed, and the ability to respond to multiple stimuli is reduced. Provide adequate, meaningful stimuli but prevent sensory overload.
- Nocturia and incontinence are more frequent in older adults. Institute a regular toileting schedule for the patient. A recommended frequency is every 3 hours. Give diuretics in the morning. Provide assistance, along with adequate lighting, to patients who need to go to the bathroom at night.
- Memory is sometimes impaired. Patients need to use medication organizers, which can be purchased at any drugstore at a very reasonable cost. Fill these dispensers once a week with the proper medications to be taken at a specific time during the day.
- The family plays a significant role in the care of older adults. There are 65.7 million unpaid caregivers for adults, who are mostly family members (National Alliance for Caregiving, 2011). These family caregivers spend an average of 19 hours per week providing care (National Alliance for Caregiving, 2009). Encourage the family to allow the older adult to remain as independent as possible and provide help only for those things that are especially stressful or depleted.
- The high prevalence of chronic conditions in older adults results in the use of a high number of prescription and over-the-counter medications. Coupled with age-related changes in pharmacokinetics, there is a greater risk of serious adverse effects. Medications typically prescribed for older adults include anticholinergics, diuretics, anxiolytic and hypnotic agents, antidepressants, antihypertensives, vasodilators, analgesics, and laxatives, all of which pose risks or interact to increase the risk for falls. Review the patient's drug profile to ensure that these drugs are used cautiously and assess the patient regularly for any adverse effects that increase fall risk.

referring them to resources such as classes to help quit smoking and for stress management, including employee-assistance programs. Also encourage adults to exercise regularly, maintain a healthy diet, practice relaxation techniques, and get adequate sleep.

Older Adult. Nursing interventions for older adults reduce the risk of falls and other accidents and compensate for the physiological changes of aging (Box 27-8). Most injuries to older adults involve falls, automobile accidents, and those related to burns or fires (National Center for Injury Prevention and Control, 2010b). Advancing age and the concurrent physiological changes in vision, hearing, mobility, reflexes, circulation, and the ability to make quick judgments all predispose older adults to falls (see Chapter 14). Certain disease states common to older adults such as arthritis or strokes and the effects of many medications such as sedatives, diuretics, and anticoagulants also increase the chance of injury. The American Geriatric Society (2009) developed an algorithm on prevention of falls (Fig. 27-6). Hospitalization or any unfamiliar environment, confusion, multiple medical problems, various medications, immobility concerns, urinary urgency, age-related sensory changes, and postural instability are major contributors to falling (Meiner, 2011). Provide information about neighborhood resources to help the older adult maintain an independent lifestyle. Older

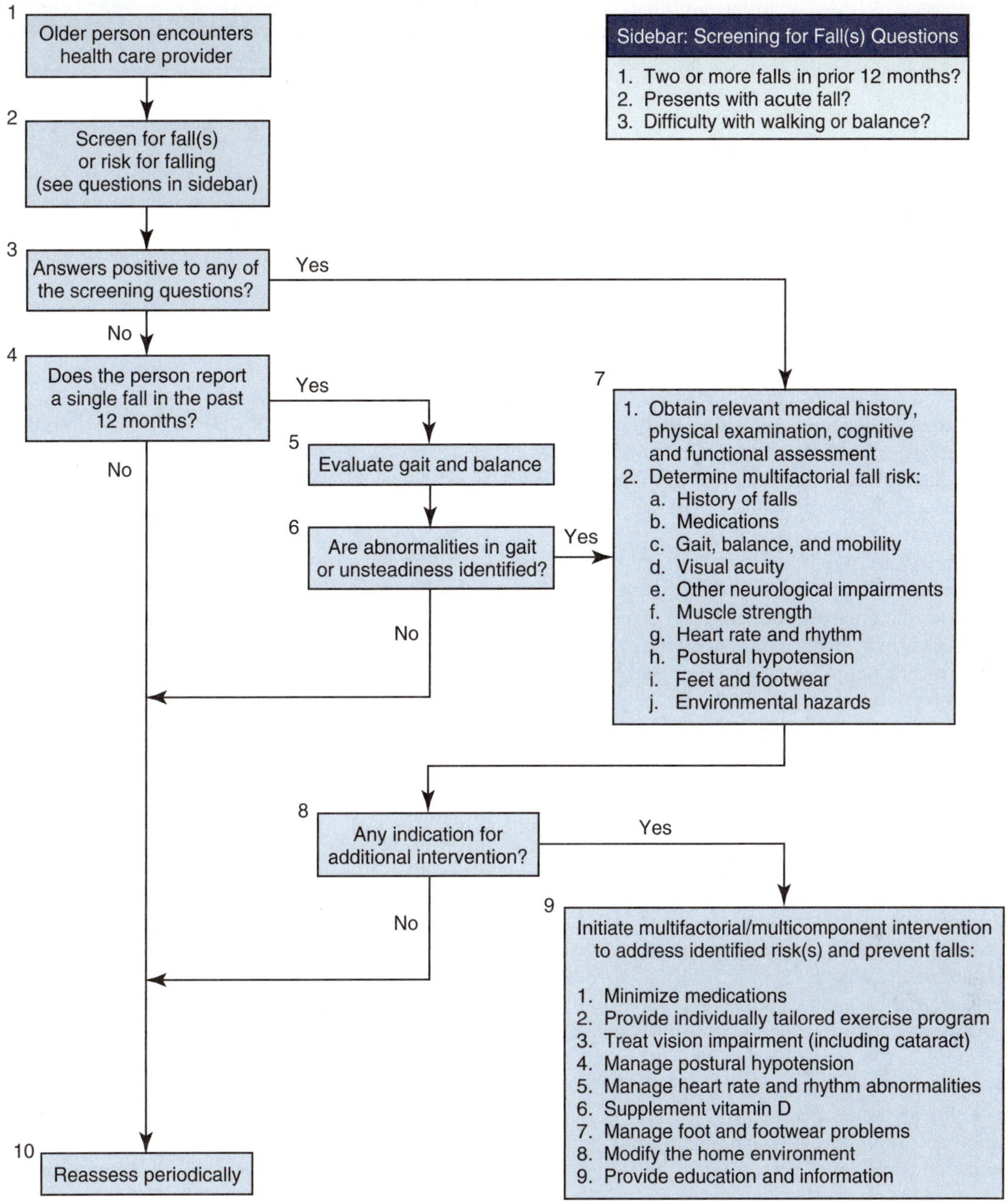

FIG. 27-6 American Geriatrics Society Clinical Practice Guideline Fall Prevention Algorithm 2010. (From American Geriatrics Society/British Geriatrics Society: *Clinical practice guideline for prevention of falls in older persons,* 2010, accessed May 25, 2011, from http://www.medcats.com/FALLS/frameset.htm.)

adults frequently relocate to new neighborhoods and need to become acquainted with new resources such as modes of transportation, church schedules, and food resources (e.g., Meals on Wheels).

Building Competency in Patient-Centered Care A 68-year-old male patient experienced a stroke 2 weeks ago. He has weakness and reduced sensation in his right leg and arm. He is returning home from the hospital and will have ongoing rehabilitation. What are this patient's risks for injury on returning home, and how does the nurse involve the family in the patient's care?

Answers to questions can be found on the Evolve website.

Educate patients regarding safe driving tips (e.g., driving shorter distances or only in daylight, using side and rearview mirrors carefully, and looking behind them toward their "blind spot" before changing lanes). If hearing is a problem, encourage the patient to keep a window rolled down while driving or reduce the volume of the radio or CD player. Counseling is often necessary to help older patients make the decision of when to stop driving. At that time help locate resources in the community that provide transportation.

Burns and scalds are also more apt to occur with older people because they sometimes forget and leave hot water running or become confused when turning the dials on a stove or other heating appliance. Nursing measures for preventing burns minimize the risk from impaired vision. Hot water faucets and dials are color coded to make it easier for the adult to know which is hot and which is cold. Reducing the temperature of the hot water heater is also very beneficial.

Many older adults love to walk. Reduce pedestrian accidents for older adults and all other age-groups by persuading people to wear reflectors on garments when walking at night; stand on the sidewalk and not in the street when waiting to cross a street; always cross at corners and not in the middle of the block (particularly if the street is a major one); cross with the traffic light and not against it; and look left, right, and left again before entering the street or crosswalk.

Environmental Interventions. Nursing interventions directed at eliminating environmental threats include those associated with a person's basic needs and general preventive measures.

Basic Needs. Nurses contribute to a safer environment by helping patients meet basic needs related to oxygen, nutrition, and temperature. When oxygen is in use, precautions must be taken to prevent fire. Contact with heat or a spark is required to trigger combustion; therefore certain precautions are necessary, regardless of the setting where oxygen is in use. Post "No Smoking" and "Oxygen in Use" signs in patient rooms. Do not use oxygen around electrical equipment or flammable products. Store oxygen tanks upright in carts or stands to prevent tipping or falling or place the tanks flat on the floor when not in use. Check tubing for kinks that would affect the oxygen flow. Maintain oxygen at the prescribed liter flow and do not change without a health care provider's order. Additional precautions are indicated for liquid or pressurized oxygen and when traveling with home oxygen. Refer to the oxygen supplier. In the home recommend that the patient be sure to have annual inspections of heating systems, chimneys, and fuel-burning appliances. Carbon monoxide detectors are available at a reasonable cost but are not a replacement for proper use and maintenance of fuel-burning appliances.

Teach basic techniques for food handling and preparation so nutritional needs are met safely:

- Proper refrigeration, storage, and preparation of food decrease the risk of foodborne illness. Store perishable foods in refrigerators to maintain freshness.
- Wash hands before preparing foods.
- Rinse fruits and vegetables thoroughly.
- Pay attention to prevent cross-contamination of one food with another during food preparation, especially with poultry.
- Use a separate cutting board for vegetables, meats, and poultry.
- Adequately cook foods to kill any residual organisms. Refrigerate leftovers promptly. Bacteria grow quickly at room temperature.
- Have family caregivers label the date when leftovers are saved.

General Preventive Measures. Adequate lighting and security measures in and around the home, including the use of nightlights, exterior lighting, and locks on windows and doors, enable patients to reduce the risk of injury from crime. The local police department and community organizations often have safety classes available for residents to learn how to take precautions to minimize the chance of becoming involved in a crime. For example, some useful tips include always parking the car near a bright light or busy public area, carrying a whistle attached to the car keys, keeping car doors locked while driving, and always paying attention while driving to notice if anyone starts to follow the car.

BOX 27-9 PATIENT TEACHING

Prevention of Electrical Hazards

Objective

- Patient will recognize and eliminate electrical hazards in the home.

Teaching Strategies

- Discuss importance of checking for grounding of electrical appliances and other equipment.
- Provide examples of common hazards: frayed cords, damaged equipment, and overloaded outlets.
- Discuss guidelines to prevent electrical shocks:
  - Use extension cords only when necessary and use electrical tape to secure the cord to the floor, preferably against baseboards.
  - Do not run wires under carpeting.
  - Grasp the plug, not the cord, when unplugging items.
  - Keep electrical items away from water.
  - Do not operate unfamiliar equipment.
  - Disconnect items before cleaning.

Evaluation

- Have patient list electrical hazards existing in the home.
- Review steps the patient will take to eliminate these hazards.
- Check the home after the patient has had an opportunity to eliminate hazards.

Modifications in the environment easily reduce the risk of falls. To reduce the risk of injury in the home, remove all obstacles from halls and other heavily traveled areas. Necessary objects such as clocks, glasses, or tissues remain on bedside tables within reach of the patient but out of the reach of children. Take care to ensure that end tables are secure and have stable, straight legs. Place nonessential items in drawers to eliminate clutter. If small area rugs are used, secure them with a nonslip pad or skid-resistant adhesive strips. Make sure that carpeting on the stairs is secured with carpet tacks. If patients have a history of falling and live alone, recommend that they wear an electronic safety alert device. When activated by the wearer, this device alerts a monitoring site to call emergency services for assistance.

Accidental home fires typically result from smoking in bed, placing cigarettes in trash cans, grease fires, improper use of candles or space heaters, or electrical fires resulting from faulty wiring or appliances. Teach patients and families how to reduce the risk of electrical injury in the home (Box 27-9) and how to use a home fire extinguisher (Box 27-10). To reduce the risk of fires in the home, instruct patients to quit smoking or smoke outside the home. Have them inspect the condition of cooking equipment and appliances, particularly irons and stoves. For patients with visual deficits, it helps to have dials installed with large numbers or symbols on temperature controls. Make sure that smoke detectors are in strategic positions throughout the home so the alarm will alert the occupants in a home in case of fire. Make sure that all patients, even young children, are familiar with the phrase "stop, drop, and roll," which describes what to do when a person's clothing or skin is burning.

Help parents reduce the risk of accidental poisoning by teaching them to keep hazardous substances such as medications, cleaning fluids, and batteries out of the reach of children. Drug and other substance poisonings in adolescents and adults are commonly related to suicide attempts or drug experimentation. Teach parents that calling a poison control center for information before

BOX 27-10 PATIENT TEACHING

Correct Use of a Fire Extinguisher in the Home

Objective

- Patient will use a fire extinguisher in the home correctly.

Teaching Strategies

- Discuss how to choose a correct location for an extinguisher. It is recommended that one be placed on each level of the home, near an exit, in clear view, away from stoves and heating appliances, and above the reach of small children. Keep a fire extinguisher in the kitchen, near the furnace, and in the garage. Make sure that patients read instructions after purchasing the extinguisher and keep them for periodic review.
- Describe the steps to take before using the extinguisher. Attempt to fight the fire only when all occupants have left the home, the fire department has been called, the fire is confined to a small area, there is an exit route readily available, the extinguisher is the right type for the fire (see discussion in text for a description of the types of extinguishers), and the patient knows how to use it.
- Instruct the patient to memorize the mnemonic PASS: *P*ull the pin to unlock handle, *A*im low at the base of the fire, *S*queeze the handles, and *S*weep the unit from side to side (see Fig. 27-11).

Evaluation

- Patient is able to describe when it is appropriate to use a home fire extinguisher.
- Patient correctly lists the steps to take before attempting to use an extinguisher.
- Patient demonstrates correct use of the extinguisher while reciting the instructions with the mnemonic PASS.

BOX 27-11 INTERVENING IN ACCIDENTAL POISONING

1. Assess for signs or symptoms of ingestion of harmful substance such as nausea, vomiting, foaming at the mouth, drooling, difficulty breathing, sweating, and lethargy.
2. Terminate exposure to the poison by having the person empty his or her mouth of pills, plant parts, or other material.
3. If poisoning is caused by skin or eye contact, irrigate the skin or eye with copious amounts of cool tap water for 15 to 20 minutes. In the case of an inhalation exposure, safely remove the victim from the potentially dangerous environment.
4. Identify the type and amount of substance ingested to help determine the correct type and amount of antidote needed.
5. If the victim is conscious and alert, call the local poison control center or the national toll-free poison control center number (1-800-222-1222) before attempting any intervention. Poison control centers have information needed to treat poisoned patients or offer referral to treat.

   The administration of ipecac syrup is no longer recommended for routine home treatment of poisoning.
6. If the victim has collapsed or stopped breathing, call 911 for emergency transportation to the hospital. Initiate CPR if indicated until emergency personnel arrive. Ambulance personnel can provide emergency measures if needed. In addition, a parent or guardian is sometimes too upset to drive safely.
7. Position the victim with head turned to side to reduce risk for aspiration.
8. Never induce vomiting if the victim has ingested the following poisonous substances: lye, household cleaners, hair care products, grease or petroleum products, furniture polish, paint thinner, or kerosene.
9. Never induce vomiting in an unconscious or convulsing victim because vomiting increases risk for aspiration.

Modified from Hockenberry MJ, Wilson D: *Wong's essentials of pediatric nursing*, ed 8, St Louis, 2009, Mosby; American Academy of Pediatrics, Committee on Injury, Violence and Poison Prevention: Poison treatment in the home, *Pediatrics* 112 (5):1182, 2003.

CPR, Cardiopulmonary resuscitation.

attempting home remedies will save their child's life. Guidelines for accepted interventions for accidental poisonings are available to teach a parent or guardian (Box 27-11). Older adults are also at risk for poisoning because diminished eyesight may cause an accidental ingestion of a toxic substance. In addition, the impaired memory of some older adults results in an accidental overdose of prescription medications.

Be sure that medications are kept in their original containers and labeled in large print. Recommend the use of medication organizers that are filled once a week by the patient and/or family. Have patients keep poisonous substances out of the bathroom and discard old or unused medications. In the health care setting it is important for you to know how to respond when exposure to a poisonous substance occurs. In addition, adhere to guidelines for intervening in accidental poisoning. Ensure the poison control center phone number is visible near the telephone in homes with young children. In all cases of suspected poisoning, patients need to call this number immediately.

To prevent the transmission of pathogens, nurses teach aseptic practices. Medical asepsis, which includes hand hygiene and environmental cleanliness, reduces the transfer of organisms (see Chapter 28). Patients and family members need to learn thorough hand hygiene (handwashing or use of hand rub) and when to use it (e.g., before and after caring for a family member, before food preparation, before preparing a medication for a family member, after using the bathroom, and after contacting any body fluids). Patients also need to know how to dispose of infected material such as wound dressings and used needles in the home setting. Heavy plastic containers such as hard, colored plastic liquid detergent bottles are excellent for needle disposal. The Environmental Protection Agency (EPA) encourages disposal of used needles by way of community drop-off programs, household hazardous waste facilities, sharps mail-back programs, or home needle destruction devices (Coalition for Safe Community Needle Disposal, 2010). Teach patients "safe sex" practices, including abstinence, correct use of condoms, and engaging in monogamous relationships to reduce the risk for sexually transmitted infections.

Acute Care. Nurses use standard precautions for all patients to protect themselves from contact with blood and other potentially infectious body fluids (see Chapter 28). Additional specific safety measures are applicable to patients in the acute care environment. Nurses are responsible for making a patient's bedside safe. Explain and demonstrate to patients how to use the call light or intercom system and always place the call device close to the patient at the conclusion of every nurse-patient interaction. Respond quickly to call lights and bed/chair alarms. Keep the environment free from clutter around the bedside. Many health care organizations are implementing hourly rounding to reduce falls (Box 27-12). In addition, nurses sometimes apply color-coded wristbands to patients' wrists to communicate a patient's fall risk. In 2008 the American Hospital Association issued an advisory recommending that hospitals standardize wristband colors; red for patient allergies, yellow for fall risk, and purple for do-not-resuscitate preferences. This recommendation came after a

BOX 27-12 EVIDENCE-BASED PRACTICE

Effects of Nursing Rounds on Patient Safety

PICO Question: In the hospitalized adult patient, will hourly rounding compared with standard practice decrease patient falls and pressure ulcer development?

Evidence Summary

Patient falls and development of pressure ulcers are nurse-sensitive indicators. Nurses have the opportunity to reduce these adverse outcomes based on evidence-based nursing actions. Hospitalized patients often require assistance with basic activities of daily living such as eating, toileting, and mobility. Not meeting patient needs in a timely fashion decreases patient satisfaction and places patients at greater risk for injury (Meade et al., 2006). Current evidence supports a patient-centered approach to nursing care by implementing purposeful hourly rounding (Weisgram and Raymond, 2008; Ford, 2010). Hourly nursing rounds are conducted hourly during the day and evening shift and are completed at least every 2 hours during the night. Every-2-hour rounds entail rounding every 2 hours throughout the entire 24-hour period. Evidence-based nursing rounds influence safety outcomes such as checking patients for the 5 Ps: *p*ain, *p*otty, *p*osition, *p*ossessions, and *p*lan of care.

Application to Nursing Practice

- Implementation of purposeful, hourly nursing rounds improves outcomes in reducing patient falls (Weisgram and Raymond, 2008; Ford, 2010). However, in one study every-2-hour rounds did not significantly reduce falls (Meade et al., 2006).
- Implementation of hourly nursing rounds also reduces patient development of pressure ulcers (Studer Group, 2007).
- Purposeful rounding includes specific nursing actions such as addressing toileting, turning, and ensuring that possessions are within reach.
- Nurses and NAPs often share rounding responsibilities.

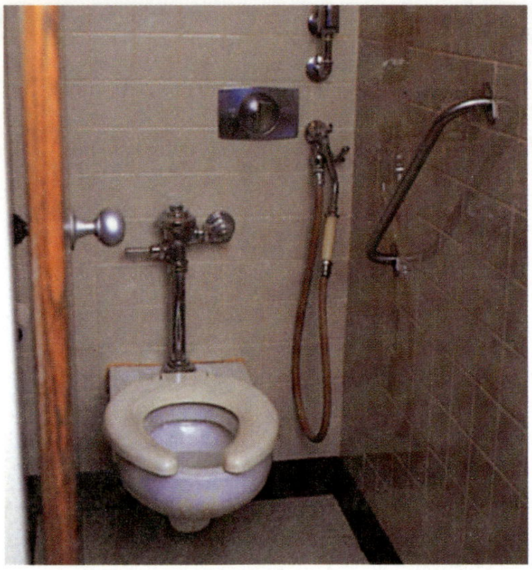

FIG. 27-7 Safety bars around toilets and showers.

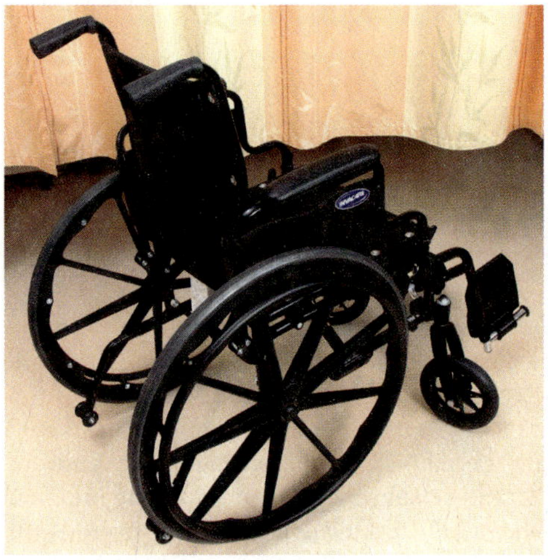

FIG. 27-8 Wheelchair with safety locks and anti-tip bars.

near-miss incident in which a nurse working in two different hospitals placed a wrong-colored band on a patient. Many state hospital associations and communities are now standardizing colors to reduce confusion both within and across the health care organizations (American Hospital Association, 2008). The nurse takes measures to help patients avoid falls, injuries from use of restraints and side rails, fires, poisoning, and electrical hazards. Special precautions are necessary to prevent injury in patients susceptible to having seizures. Radiation injuries are also a specific safety concern. Finally be prepared to respond to a disaster emergency, including a bioterrorist attack.

Falls. Most hospitals have fall prevention protocols instituted for patients at risk for falling. For example, a patient receives a fall risk identification bracelet (yellow in color), is given information about fall risks, and receives additional nursing interventions (e.g., hourly rounding, placement on a low safety bed, yellow gown). Include family members in safety discussions. A gait belt provides a secure way to steady or guide patients who need assistance with ambulation when transferring or walking. Use additional safety equipment as needed when moving patients (see Chapter 47). When patients use assistive aids such as canes, crutches, or walkers, it is important to routinely check the condition of rubber tips and the integrity of the aid. Remove excess furniture and equipment and make sure that patients wear rubber-soled shoes or slippers for walking or transferring. Safety bars near toilets (Fig. 27-7), locks on beds and wheelchairs (Fig. 27-8), and call lights are additional safety features found in health care settings. In the health care environment frequent observations of the patient at risk for falls are important to reduce the potential for injury (Meade et al., 2006).

Restraints. Patients who are confused, disoriented, or repeatedly fall or try to remove medical devices (e.g., oxygen equipment, IV lines, or dressings) often require the temporary use of restraints to keep them safe. Restraints are not a solution to a patient problem but rather a temporary means to maintain patient safety. They are either chemical or physical. Chemical restraints are medications such as anxiolytics and sedatives used to manage a patient's behavior and are not a standard treatment or dosage for the patient's condition. A physical **restraint** is any manual method, physical or mechanical device, material, or equipment that immobilizes or reduces the ability of a patient to move his or her arms, legs, body, or head freely (TJC, 2011a). A restraint does not include devices such as orthopedically prescribed devices, surgical dressings or bandages, protective helmets, or other methods that involve physically holding a patient to conduct routine physical examinations or tests, protecting the patient from falling out of bed, or permitting the patient to participate in activities without the risk of physical harm (TJC, 2011a).

BOX 27-13 ALTERNATIVES TO RESTRAINTS

- Orient patients and families to environment; explain all procedures and treatments.
- Provide companionship and supervision; use trained sitters; adjust staffing and involve family.
- Offer diversionary activities such as music or something to hold; enlist support and input from family.
- Assign confused or disoriented patients to rooms near nurses' station and observe them frequently.
- Use calm, simple statements and physical cues as needed.
- Use de-escalation, time-out, and other verbal intervention techniques when managing aggressive behaviors.
- Provide appropriate visual and auditory stimuli (e.g., family pictures, clock, radio).
- Remove cues that promote leaving (e.g., elevators, stairs, or street clothes).
- Promote relaxation techniques and normal sleep patterns.
- Institute exercise and ambulation schedules as allowed by patient's condition; consult physical therapist for mobility and exercise programs.
- Attend frequently to needs for toileting, food, and liquid.
- Camouflage intravenous lines with clothing, stockinette, or Kling dressing.
- Evaluate all medications patient is receiving and ensure effective pain management.
- Reassess physical status and review laboratory findings.

Modified from The Joint Commission Resources: *Strategies for avoiding restraint related errors*, 2006, http://www.jcrinc.com; and Geriatric nursing resources for care of older adults: *Physical restraints*, 2006, http://www.geronurseonline.org/index.

The use of restraints is associated with serious complications resulting from immobilization such as pressure ulcers, pneumonia, constipation, and incontinence. In some cases death has resulted because of restricted breathing and circulation. Patients have been strangled while trying to get out of bed while restrained in a jacket or vest restraint. As a result, many health care facilities have eliminated the use of the jacket (vest) restraint (Capezuti et al., 2008). Loss of self-esteem, humiliation, and agitation are also serious concerns. Because of these risks, legislation emphasizes reducing the use of restraints. Regulatory agencies such as TJC and the CMS enforce standards for the safe use of restraint devices. The optimal goal for all patients is a restraint-free environment. Always consider and implement alternatives to restraints first. Individualize your approaches for each patient. Restraint alternatives include more frequent observations, involvement of family during visitation, frequent reorientation, and the introduction of familiar and meaningful stimuli (e.g., knitting or crocheting or looking at family photos) within the environment to reduce behaviors such as wandering that often leads to restraint use (Box 27-13).

In nursing homes, evidence shows that outcomes related to behavior issues, cognitive performance, falls, walking dependence, activities of daily living, pressure ulcers, and contractures are significantly worse when a restraint is used compared to no restraint (Castle, 2009). An interdisciplinary approach that includes individualized assessments and development of structured treatment plans reduces restraint use.

The use of restraints involves a psychological adjustment for the patient and family. If restraints are necessary, the nurse assists family members and patients by explaining their purpose, expected care while the patient is restrained, precautions taken to avoid injury, and that the restraint is temporary and protective. Informed consent from family members is sometimes required before using restraints (e.g., in long-term care settings).

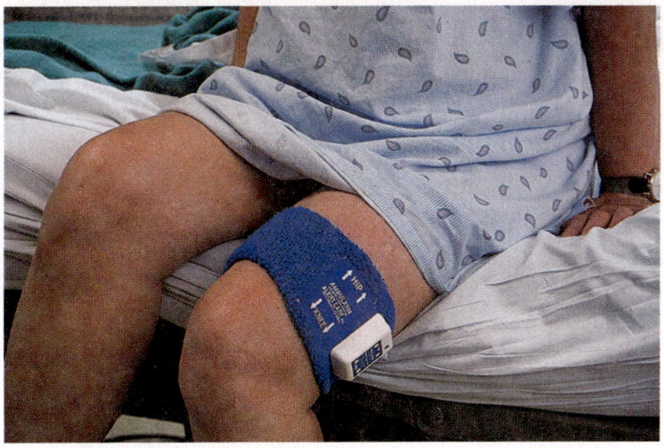

FIG. 27-9 Patient wearing an Ambularm device.

For legal purposes know agency-specific policy and procedures for appropriate use and monitoring of restraints. The use of a restraint must be clinically justified and a part of the patient's prescribed medical treatment and plan of care. A physician's order is required, based on a face-to-face assessment of the patient. The order must be current, state the type and location of restraint, and specify the duration and circumstances under which it will be used. These orders need to be renewed within a specific time frame according to the policy of the agency. In the hospital each original restraint order and renewal is limited to 4 hours for adults, 2 hours for ages 9 through 17, and 1 hour for children under age 9 (CMS, 2009; TJC, 2011a). Orders may be renewed to the time limits for a maximum of 24 consecutive hours. Restraints are not to be ordered prn (as needed). You must conduct ongoing assessment of patients who are restrained. Proper documentation, including the behaviors that necessitated the application of restraints, the procedure used in restraining, the condition of the body part restrained (e.g., circulation to hand), and the evaluation of the patient response, is essential. Restraints must be removed periodically, and the nurse assesses the patient to determine if they continue to be necessary. Skill 27-1 on pp. 388-392 includes guidelines for the proper use and application of restraints. Use of restraints must meet one of the following objectives:

- Reduce the risk of patient injury from falls
- Prevent interruption of therapy such as traction, IV infusions, nasogastric (NG) tube feeding, or Foley catheterization
- Prevent patients who are confused or combative from removing life-support equipment
- Reduce the risk of injury to others by the patient

In keeping with current safety trends, electronic devices are also sometimes used as alternatives to restraints. For example, the Ambularm, worn on the leg, signals when the leg is in a dependent position such as over the side rail or on the floor (Fig. 27-9). You also sometimes place weight-sensitive sensor mats on patients' mattresses or in the chair. An audible alarm sounds at the bedside when pressure is released off the sensor mat. The alarm often signals at the central nurses' station so staff is alerted quickly when a patient is up and out of bed. Alarms on doors also alert staff or family members when a patient who is confused, disoriented, or prone to wandering opens a door.

A less-restrictive restraint is the Posey bed (Fig. 27-10). It is a soft-sided, self-contained enclosed bed that is much less restrictive than chemical or physical restraints. It allows for freedom of

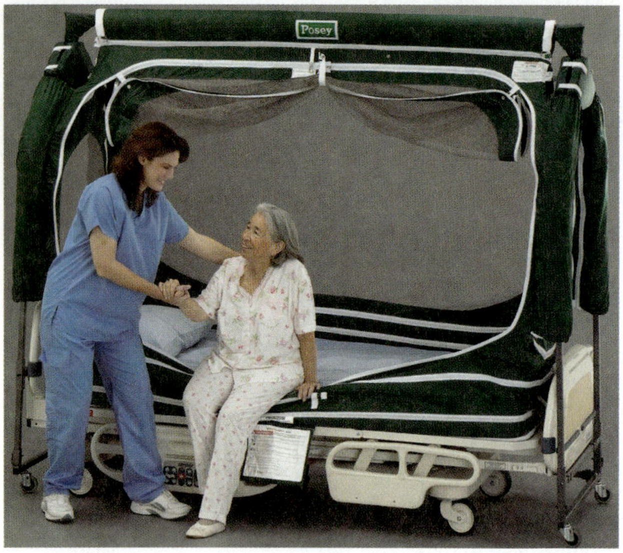

FIG. 27-10 The Posey Bed All Care Model. (Courtesy JT Posey Co, Arcadia, Calif.)

movement and thus reduces the side effects such as pressure ulcers and loss of dignity caused by physical restraints. A vinyl top covers the padded upper frame of the bed, and the nylon-net canopy surrounds the mattress and completely encloses the patient in the bed. Zippers on the four sides of the enclosure provide access to the patient. The Posey bed enclosure works well for patients who are restless and unpredictable, cognitively impaired, and at risk for injury if they were to fall or get out of bed such as patients on anticoagulant therapy at risk for intracranial bleed. The bed is also a safer alternative to side rails.

Side Rails. Side rails help to increase a patient's mobility and/or stability when in bed or moving from bed to chair. They are the most commonly used physical restraint. There are a variety of beds with different side rail designs. Basically the patient needs to have a route to exit a bed safely and maneuver freely within the bed; in this case side rails are not considered a restraint. For example, raising only the top two side rails so the lower part of the bed is open gives the patient room to exit a bed safely. Side rails used to prevent a patient such as one who is sedated from falling out of bed are not considered a restraint. Always check agency policy about the use of side rails. Be sure that a bed is in the lowest position possible when side rails are raised. Always assess the risk of using side rails compared to not using them. Check their condition; bars between the bed rails need to be closely spaced to prevent entrapment, the space between bed rails and mattress and between headboard and mattress is filled to prevent patients from falling in between, and latches securing bed rails are stable.

The use of side rails alone for a patient who is disoriented usually causes more confusion and further injury. A patient who is determined to get out of bed attempts to climb over the side rail or climbs out at the foot of the bed. Either attempt usually results in a fall or injury. Nursing interventions to reduce a patient's confusion first focus on determining and eliminating the cause of the confusion such as a response to a new medication, dehydration, or pain. Frequently nurses mistake a patient's attempt to explore his or her environment or to self-toilet as confusion. Additional safety measures include the use of a low bed with a nonskid mat placed alongside the bed on the floor. A low bed reduces the distance between the bed and floor, facilitating a roll rather than a fall from the bed.

BOX 27-14 FIRE INTERVENTION GUIDELINES FOR NURSES WORKING IN HEALTH CARE AGENCIES

- Keep the phone number for reporting fires visible on the telephone at all times.
- Know the fire drill and evacuation plan of the agency.
- Know the location of all fire alarms, exits, extinguishers, and oxygen shut-off.
- Use the mnemonic RACE to set priorities in case of fire:
  R—Rescue and remove all patients in immediate danger.
  A—Activate the alarm. Always do this before attempting to extinguish even a minor fire.
  C—Confine the fire by closing doors and windows and turning off oxygen and electrical equipment.
  E—Extinguish the fire using an appropriate extinguisher (see Fig. 27-11).

Fires. Although smoking is usually not allowed in hospital settings, smoking-related fires continue to pose a significant risk because of unauthorized smoking in the bed or bathroom. Institutional fires typically result from an electrical or anesthetic-related fire. The best intervention is to prevent fires. Nursing measures include complying with the smoking policies of the agency and keeping combustible materials away from heat sources. Box 27-14 discusses additional fire intervention guidelines for nurses in health care agencies. Regardless of where a fire occurs, it is important to have an evacuation plan in place. Know where fire extinguishers and gas shut-off valves are located and how to activate a fire alarm.

If a fire occurs in a health care agency, protect patients from immediate injury, report the exact location of the fire, contain it, and extinguish it if possible. Some agencies have fire doors that are held open by magnets and close automatically when a fire alarm sounds. It is important to keep equipment away from blocking these doors. All personnel evacuate patients when appropriate. Patients who are close to the fire, regardless of its size, are at risk of injury and need to be moved to another area. If the patient is on life support, you need to maintain his or her respiratory status manually with a bag-valve-mask device (e.g., Ambu-bag) (see Chapter 40) until he or she is moved away from the fire. Direct all ambulatory patients to walk by themselves to a safe area. In some cases they are able to help move patients in wheelchairs. You generally move bedridden patients from the scene of a fire by a stretcher, their bed, or a wheelchair. If none of these methods is appropriate, they need to be carried from the area. If you have to carry a patient, do so correctly (e.g., two-man carry). If you overextend your physical limits for lifting, injuring yourself results in further injury to the patient. If fire department personnel are on the scene, they help evacuate the patients.

After a fire is reported and patients are out of danger, nurses and other personnel take measures to contain or extinguish it such as closing doors and windows, placing wet towels along the base of doors, turning off sources of oxygen and electrical equipment, and using a fire extinguisher. Fire extinguishers are categorized as type A, used for ordinary combustibles (e.g., wood, cloth, paper, and many plastic items); type B, used for flammable liquids (e.g., gasoline, grease, paint, and anesthetic gas); and type C, used for electrical equipment. Fig. 27-11 demonstrates the process of using an extinguisher.

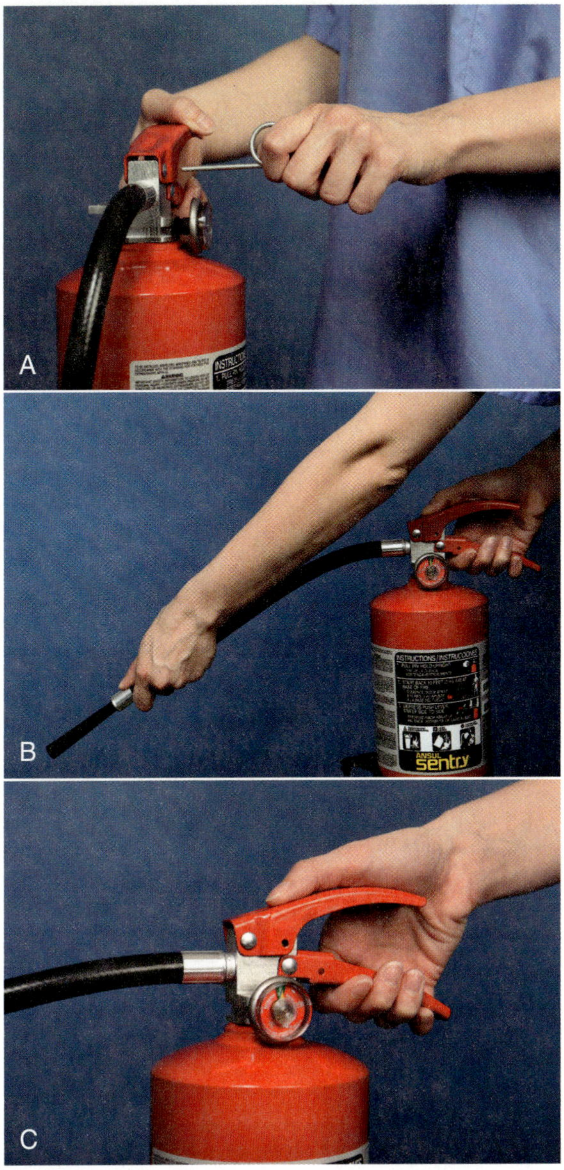

FIG. 27-11 Correct use of a fire extinguisher. A, ***P***ull pin. B, ***A***im at base of fire. C, ***S***queeze handles and ***S***weep from side to side to coat area evenly.

Electrical Hazards. Much of the equipment used in health care settings is electrical and must be well maintained. The clinical engineering departments of hospitals inspect biomedical equipment such as hospital beds, infusion pumps, or ventilators regularly. You know that a piece of equipment is safe to use when you see a safety inspection sticker with an expiration date. Decrease the risk for electrical injury and fire by using properly grounded and functional electrical equipment. The ground prong of an electrical outlet carries any stray electrical current back to the ground. Remove equipment that is not in proper working order or that sparks when plugged in for service and notify the appropriate hospital staff.

Seizures. Patients who have experienced some form of neurological injury or metabolic disturbance are at risk for a seizure. A **seizure** is hyperexcitation and disorderly discharge of neurons in the brain leading to a sudden, violent, involuntary series of muscle contractions that is paroxysmal and episodic, causing loss of consciousness, falling, tonicity (rigidity of muscles), and clonicity (jerking of muscles). A generalized tonic-clonic, or grand mal, seizure lasts approximately 2 minutes (no longer than 5) and is characterized by a cry and loss of consciousness with falling, tonicity, clonicity, and incontinence. During a fall or as a result of muscle jerking, musculoskeletal injuries can occur. Before a convulsive episode a few patients report an aura, which serves as a warning or sense that a seizure is about to occur. An **aura** is often a bright light, smell, or taste. During the seizure activity the patient often experiences shallow breathing, cyanosis, and loss of bladder and bowel control. A postictal phase follows the seizure, during which the patient has amnesia or confusion and falls into a deep sleep. A person in the community needs to be taken to a medical facility immediately if he or she has repeated seizures; if a single seizure lasts longer than 5 minutes without any sign of slowing down or is unusual in some way; if the person has trouble breathing afterwards or appears to be injured or in pain; or if recovery is different from usual (Epilepsy Foundation, 2010). Prolonged or repeated seizures indicate **status epilepticus.** This condition is a medical emergency and requires intensive monitoring and treatment. It is important that you observe the patient carefully before, during, and after the seizure so you are able to document the episode accurately. **Seizure precautions** encompass all nursing interventions to protect the patient from traumatic injury, position for adequate ventilation and drainage of oral secretions, and provide privacy and support following the seizure (see Skill 27-2 on pp. 392-294).

Radiation. Radiation is a health hazard in health care settings where radiation and radioactive materials are used in the diagnosis and treatment of patients. Hospitals have strict guidelines concerning the care of patients who are receiving radiation and radioactive materials. Be familiar with established agency protocols. To reduce your exposure to radiation, limit the time spent near the source, make the distance from the source as great as possible, and use shielding devices such as lead aprons. Staff regularly working near radiation wear devices that track the accumulative exposure to radiation.

Disasters. As a nurse, you need to be prepared to respond and care for a sudden influx of patients during a disaster. TJC (2011b) requires hospitals to have an emergency management plan that addresses identifying possible emergency situations and their probable impact, maintaining adequate amount of supplies, and a formal response plan that includes actions to be taken by staff and steps to restore essential services and resume normal operations following the emergency.

Infection control practices are critical in the event of a biological attack. Therefore you manage all patients with suspected or confirmed bioterrorism-related illnesses using standard precautions (see Chapter 28). For certain diseases such as smallpox or pneumonic plague, additional precautions such as airborne or contact isolation precautions are necessary. Most infections associated with biological agents are not transmissible from patient to patient. However, limit the transport and movement of patients to movement that is essential for treatment and care. An important aspect of care for patients who have a bioterrorism-related illness is postexposure management.

EVALUATION

Through the Patient's Eyes. Patient-centered care requires a thorough evaluation of the patient's perspective related to safety and whether his or her expectations have been met. Ask the patient questions such as "Are you satisfied with the changes made to your home? Do you feel safer as a result of the changes? Have you had any falls or injury? Are you still afraid of falling?" Involve the family in your evaluation, especially if they live with the patient and provide assistance in the home.

Patient Outcomes. Evaluation involves monitoring the actual care delivered by the health care team based on the expected outcomes (Fig. 27-12). For each nursing diagnosis measure whether the outcomes of care have been met. If you have met the patient's goals the diagnosis is resolved, and your nursing interventions were effective and appropriate. If not, you determine whether new safety risks to the patient have developed or whether previous risks remain. For example, if the patient has a recurrent fall, reassess the conditions surrounding that fall and determine whether contributing factors can be removed or managed. The patient and family need to participate to find permanent ways to reduce risks to safety.

When patient outcomes are not met, ask the following questions:

- What factors led to your fall?
- Help me understand what makes you feel unsafe in your environment.
- What questions do you have about your safety?
- Has your health care provider recently changed your medications?
- Do you need help locating community resources to help make your home safer?
- What changes have you recently experienced that you believe contributes to your risk for falling or lack of safety?

Continually assesses the patient's and family's need for additional support services such as home care, physical therapy, counseling, and further teaching. A safe environment is essential to promoting, maintaining, and restoring health. Overall your expected outcomes include a safe physical environment and a patient whose expectations have been met, who is knowledgeable about safety factors and precautions, and who is free of injury.

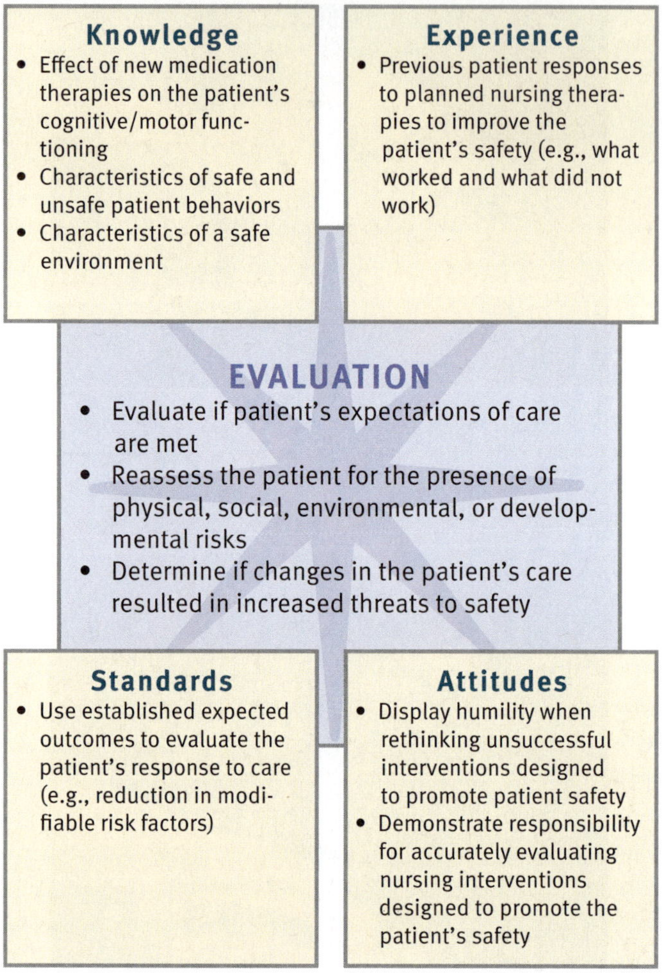

Knowledge
• Effect of new medication therapies on the patient's cognitive/motor functioning
• Characteristics of safe and unsafe patient behaviors
• Characteristics of a safe environment
Experience
• Previous patient responses to planned nursing therapies to improve the patient's safety (e.g., what worked and what did not work)
EVALUATION
• Evaluate if patient's expectations of care are met
• Reassess the patient for the presence of physical, social, environmental, or developmental risks
• Determine if changes in the patient's care resulted in increased threats to safety
Standards
• Use established expected outcomes to evaluate the patient's response to care (e.g., reduction in modifiable risk factors)
Attitudes
• Display humility when rethinking unsuccessful interventions designed to promote patient safety
• Demonstrate responsibility for accurately evaluating nursing interventions designed to promote the patient's safety

FIG. 27-12 Critical thinking model for safety evaluation.

SAFETY GUIDELINES FOR NURSING SKILLS

Ensuring patient safety is an essential role of the professional nurse. To ensure patient safety, communicate clearly with members of the health care team, assess and incorporate the patient's priorities of care and preferences, and use the best evidence when making decisions about your patient's care. When performing the skills in this chapter, remember the following points to ensure safe, individualized patient care:

- Always try restraint alternatives before using a restraint. Involve familly in your approach.
- Protect patients from injury. Follow assessment guidelines while patients are restrained to avoid injury from inappropriate placement. Position and monitor a patient having a seizure to reduce risk of aspiration and physical injury.
- Protect patients from falling by implementing fall prevention protocols and providing patient and family education about fall prevention.

SKILL 27-1 APPLYING RESTRAINTS

View Video!

Delegation Considerations

The skill of applying restraints can be delegated to nursing assistive personnel (NAP). However, the nurse must first assess the patient's behavior, level of orientation, need for restraints, and appropriate type to use. The assessment while a restraint is in place cannot be delegated to NAP. The nurse directs NAP by:

- Reviewing correct placement of the restraint.
- Reviewing when and how to change patient's position.
- Instructing NAP to notify nurse if there is a change in skin integrity, circulation in extremities, or patient's breathing.
- Instructing to provide range of motion (ROM), nutrition and hydration, skin care, toileting, and opportunities for socialization.

Equipment

- Proper restraint
- Padding (if needed)

STEP	RATIONALE
ASSESSMENT	
1 Assess patient's behavior such as confusion; disorientation; agitation; restlessness; combativeness; repeated removal of tubing, dressing, or other therapeutic devices; creating a risk to other patients; and inability to follow directions.	If patient's behavior continues despite treatment or restraint alternatives, use of restraint is indicated. You use the least restrictive type of restraint.
2 Determine failure of restraint alternatives. Review agency policies regarding restraints. Check health care provider's order for purpose, type, location, and duration of restraint. Determine if signed consent for use of restraint is necessary.	A physician or licensed independent practitioner who is responsible for the care of the patient orders restraints. The physician must be authorized to order restraints by the policy of the hospital. Consult the attending physician as soon as possible if he or she did not write the original order. Unless state law is more restrictive, orders for the use of restraint for the management of violent or self-destructive behavior that jeopardizes the immediate physical safety of the patient, staff, or others is renewed within the following time frame: 4 hours for adults, 2 hours for children ages 9 through 17, and 1 hour for children under age 9. Orders are renewed to the time limits for a maximum of 24 consecutive hours (CMS, 2009; TJC, 2011a).

CLINICAL DECISION: *A physician, clinical psychologist, or other licensed independent practitioner responsible for the care of the patient evaluates the patient in person within 1 hour of the initiation of restraint used for the management of violent or self-destructive behavior that jeopardizes the physical safety of the patient, staff, or others. A registered nurse or a physician assistant may conduct the in-person evaluation if trained in accordance with the requirements and consults with the above health care provider after the evaluation as determined by hospital policy (TJC, 2011a).*

STEP	RATIONALE
3 Review manufacturer's instructions for restraint application before entering patient's room. Determine most appropriate size restraint.	You need to be familiar with all devices used for patient care and protection. Incorrect application of restraint device results in patient injury or death.
4 Inspect area where restraint is to be placed. Note if there is any nearby tubing or device. Assess condition of skin, sensation, adequacy of circulation, and range of joint motion.	Restraints sometimes compress and interfere with functioning of devices or tubes. Assessment provides baseline to monitor patient's response to restraint.
PLANNING	
1 Gather equipment and perform hand hygiene.	Promotes organization and reduces transmission of microorganisms.
2 Approach patient in a calm, confident manner. Identify patient using two identifiers (e.g., name and birthday or name and account number) according to facility policy.	Ensures correct patient; complies with a recommended National Patient Safety Goal (TJC, 2011a).
3 Explain what you plan to do. Provide privacy. Be sure that patient is comfortable and in correct anatomical position.	Reduces patient anxiety and promotes cooperation; positioning prevents contractures and neurovascular impairment.
IMPLEMENTATION	
1 Adjust bed to proper height and lower side rail on side of patient contact.	Allows nurse to use proper body mechanics and prevents injury during restraint application.
2 Pad skin and bony prominences (as necessary) that will be under restraint.	Reduces friction and pressure from restraint to skin and underlying tissue.
3 Apply proper-size restraint:	
Note: Refer to manufacturer's directions.	
a. *Belt restraint:* Have patient in sitting position. Apply belt over clothes, gown, or pajamas. Make sure that you place restraint at waist, not chest or abdomen. Remove wrinkles or creases in clothing. Bring ties through slots in belt. Help patient lie down if in bed. Avoid applying belt too tightly (see illustrations).	Restrains center of gravity and prevents patient from rolling off stretcher or sitting up while on stretcher or from falling out of bed. Tight application interferes with ventilation if belt moves up over abdomen or chest.
b. *Extremity (ankle or wrist) restraint:* Restraint designed to immobilize one or all extremities. Commercially available limb restraints are made of sheepskin with foam padding. Wrap limb restraint around wrist or ankle with soft part toward skin and secure snugly (not tightly) in place by Velcro straps or buckle. Insert two fingers under secured restraint (see illustration).	Maintain immobilization of extremity to protect patient from fall or accidental removal of therapeutic device (e.g., IV tube, Foley catheter). Tight application interferes with circulation and potentially causes neurovascular injury.

SKILL 27-1 APPLYING RESTRAINTS—cont'd

STEP	RATIONALE
CLINICAL DECISION: *Patient with wrist and ankle restraints is at risk for aspiration if placed in bed in supine position. Place patient in lateral position rather than supine.*	
c. *Mitten restraint:* Thumbless mitten device restrains patient's hands. Place hand in mitten, being sure Velcro strap(s) are around wrist and not forearm (see illustration).	Prevents patient from dislodging invasive equipment, removing dressings, or scratching but allows greater movement than a wrist restraint.
d. *Elbow restraint (freedom splint):* Restraint consists of piece of fabric with slots in which you place tongue blades. Insert patient's arm so elbow joint rests against padded area with tongue blades, keeping joint rigid (see illustration).	Commonly used with infants and children to prevent elbow flexion (e.g., when IV line placed in antecubital fossa).
CLINICAL DECISION: *This text does not address application of vest restraints. Many health care agencies ban the use of jacket (vest) restraints because of their association with fatal injuries.*	

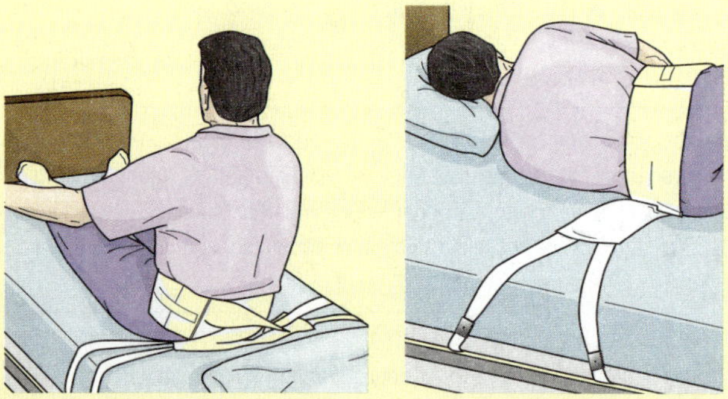

STEP 3a *Left,* Apply belt restraint with patient sitting. *Right,* Properly applied belt restraint allows patient to turn in bed. (From Sorrentino SA: *Mosby's textbook for long-term care nursing assistants,* ed 6, St Louis, 2011, Mosby).

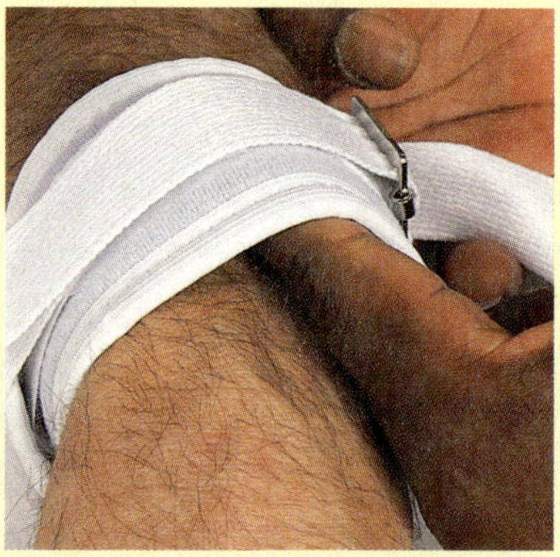

STEP 3b Securing an extremity restraint. Check restraint for constriction by inserting two fingers under restraint.

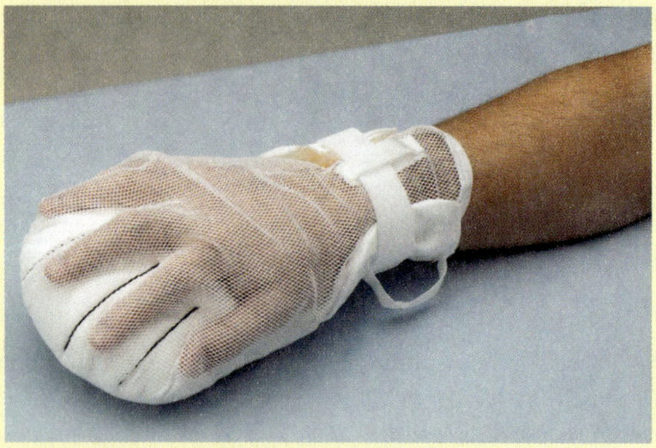

STEP 3c Mitten restraint. (Courtesy Posey Company, Arcadia, Calif.)

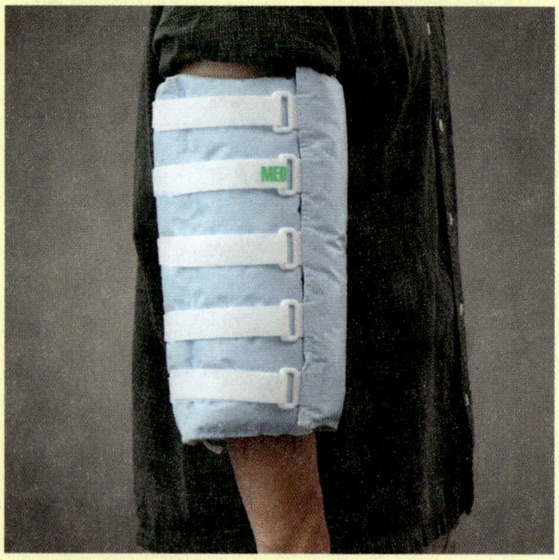

STEP 3d Freedom elbow restraint. (Courtesy Posey Company, Arcadia, Calif.)

STEP	RATIONALE
4 Attach restraint straps to portion of bed frame that moves when raising or lowering head of bed. **Do not** attach to side rails. Attach restraint to chair frame for patient in chair or wheelchair, being sure tie is out of patient's reach.	Patient will be injured if restraint is secured to side rail and it is lowered.
5 Secure restraints with quick-release tie (see illustrations). Do not tie in a knot. Be sure that tie is out of patient reach.	Allows for quick release in an emergency.

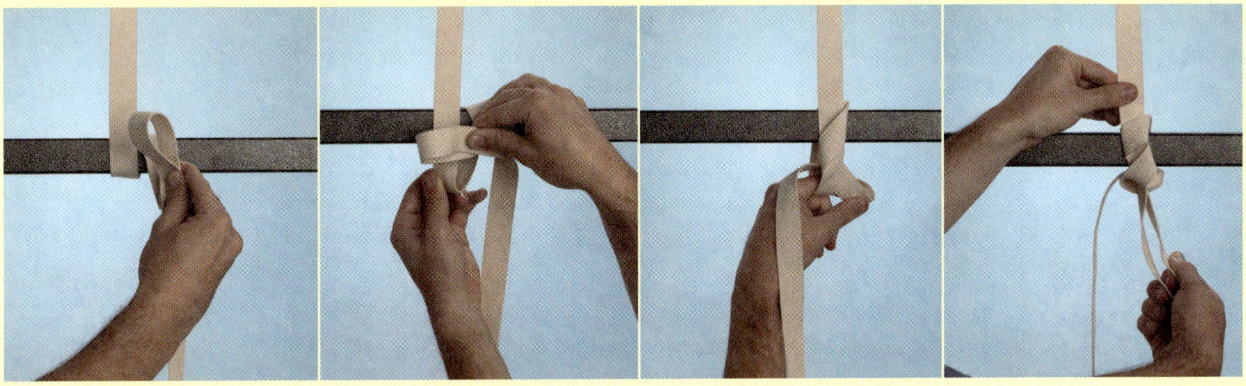

STEP 5 Posey quick-release tie. (Courtesy Posey Company, Arcadia, Calif.)

STEP	RATIONALE
6 Assess proper placement of restraint, skin integrity, pulses, skin temperature and color, and sensation of restrained body part.	Provides baseline to later evaluate if injury develops from restraint.
7 Remove restraint at least every 2 hours (TJC, 2011a) or more frequently as determined by agency policy. If patient is violent or noncompliant, remove one restraint at a time and/or have staff assistance while removing restraints.	Removal provides opportunity to change patient's position, offer nutrients, perform full ROM, toilet, exercise patient, and assess condition of site and need for continuation.

CLINICAL DECISION: *Do not leave a patient who is violent or aggressive unattended while restraints are off.*

STEP	RATIONALE
8 Secure call light or intercom system within reach.	Allows patient, family, or caregiver to obtain assistance quickly.
9 Leave bed or chair with wheels locked. Keep bed in lowest position.	Locked wheels prevent bed or chair from moving if patient tries to get out. If patient falls with bed in lowest position, this reduces chance of injury.
10 Perform hand hygiene.	Reduces transmission of microorganisms.

EVALUATION

STEP	RATIONALE
1 Following application, monitor patient's condition according to facility policy. Use judgment and consider patient's condition and type of restraint when selecting physical assessment measures (e.g., circulation, nutrition and hydration, ROM in extremities, vital signs, hygiene and elimination, physical and psychological status, and readiness for discontinuation). Perform visual checks if patient is too agitated (TJC, 2011a).	Frequent assessments prevent injury to patient and ensure removal of restraint at earliest possible time. Frequency of monitoring guides staff in determining appropriate intervals for evaluation based on patient's needs and condition, type of restraint used, risk associated with use of chosen intervention, and other relevant factors.
2 The physician, licensed independent practitioner (LIP), or registered nurse trained according to CMS requirements needs to evaluate patient within either 1 or 4 hours after initiation of restraints, depending on Medicare status of hospital (see agency policy).	Determines patient's immediate situation, reaction to restraints, medical and behavioral condition, and need to continue or terminate restraints (CMS, 2007)
3 After 24 hours, before writing a new order, a physician or LIP who is responsible for patient's care must see and assess patient.	Ensures that restraint application continues to be medically appropriate.
4 Observe IV catheters, urinary catheters, and drainage tubes to determine that they are positioned correctly and that therapy remains uninterrupted.	Reinsertion is uncomfortable and increases risk for infection or interrupts therapy.

SKILL 27-1 APPLYING RESTRAINTS—cont'd

UNEXPECTED OUTCOMES AND RELATED INTERVENTIONS

1 Patient experiences impaired skin integrity.
- Reassess need for continued use of restraint and if you can use alternative measures. If restraint is necessary to protect patient or others from injury, ensure that you applied restraint correctly and provided adequate padding.
- Check skin under restraint for abrasions and remove restraints more frequently.
- Institute appropriate skin/wound care (see Chapter 48).
- Change wet or soiled restraints to prevent skin maceration.

2 Patient has altered neurovascular status of an extremity such as cyanosis, pallor, and coldness of skin or complains of tingling, pain, or numbness.
- Remove restraint immediately and notify health care provider.

3 Patient releases restraint and suffers a fall or other traumatic injury.
- Attend to patient's immediate physical needs, inform health care provider of fall or injury, and reassess type of restraint and its correct application.

RECORDING AND REPORTING

- Record patient's behavior before restraints were applied.
- Record restraint alternatives attempted and patient's response.
- Record patient's level of orientation and patient's or family member's understanding of purpose of restraint and consent (when required).
- Record reason for restraint, type of restraint used, time of starting and ending restraints, times restraint was released, and routine observations (e.g., skin color, pulses, sensation, vital signs, behavior) in nurses' notes and flow sheets.

HOME CARE CONSIDERATIONS

- A physical restraint is a device that requires a physician's order. Do not send a patient home with intent of restraining unless device is necessary to protect patient from injury. If patient's family wishes to use restraint at home, a physician's order is required, and you need to give clear instructions regarding proper application, care needed while in restraints, and complications for which to look. Carefully assess the family for competency and understanding of intent for using restraint.

SKILL 27-2 SEIZURE PRECAUTIONS

Delegation Considerations

The skill of seizure precautions cannot be delegated to nursing assistive personnel (NAP). However, the skills for making the environment safe can be delegated. The nurse directs NAP by:
- Explaining patient's prior seizure history and factors that typically trigger a seizure.
- Emphasizing not to try to restrain patient or place anything in patient's mouth.

Equipment
- Suction machine
- Oral airway
- Oral Yankauer suction catheter
- Oxygen via nasal cannula or face mask
- Stethoscope, sphygmomanometer, pulse oximeter
- Equipment for intravenous (IV) access
- Emergency medications (e.g., IV diazepam, lorazepam, valproate, phenytoin)
- Clean gloves

STEP	RATIONALE
ASSESSMENT	
1 Assess patient's seizure history and knowledge of precipitating factors. Note frequency of past seizures, presence and type of typical aura (e.g., metallic taste, perception of breeze blowing on face, or noxious odor), and body parts affected if known. Use family as resource if necessary.	Knowledge about seizure history enables you to anticipate onset of seizure activity and take appropriate safety measures.
2 Assess for medical and surgical conditions, including electrolyte disturbances such as hypoglycemia, hyperkalemia; heart disease; excess fatigue; alcohol or caffeine consumption.	These are common conditions that lead to seizures or exacerbate existing seizure condition.
3 Assess medication history and patient's adherence. Assess therapeutic drug levels of anticonvulsants if test results available.	Not taking seizure medications as prescribed and stopping them suddenly often precipitate seizure activity.
4 Inspect patient's environment for potential safety hazards (e.g., extra furniture) if seizure occurs. Keep bed in low position, side rails up at head of bed, patient in side-lying position when possible.	Protect patient from injury sustained by striking head or body on furniture or equipment.
5 Assess patient's cultural perspective about the meaning of seizures and their treatment.	Some cultures follow different caring practices for a person with seizures.
PLANNING	
1 For patients with a history of generalized seizures, have oxygen setup, suction apparatus, and clean gloves available for immediate use.	This ensures prompt intervention directed toward maintaining a patent airway.

STEP	RATIONALE
IMPLEMENTATION	
1 When seizure begins, note time, stay with patient, and call for help. Track duration of seizure. Notify health care provider immediately. Have staff member bring emergency cart to bedside.	Documents the episode accurately. Provides for patient safety. Provides access to emergency medications and IV equipment as needed.
2 Position patient safely. If standing or sitting, guide patient to floor and protect head by cradling in nurse's lap or placing a pad under head. Do not lift patient from floor to bed while seizure is in progress. Clear surrounding area of furniture. If patient is in bed, remove pillows and raise side rails.	Prevents traumatic injury. Suffocation often occurs with use of pillow.
3 If possible, turn patient onto one side, head tilted slightly forward.	Allow tongue to fall away from the airway and allow drainage of saliva.
4 If possible, provide privacy. Have staff control flow of visitors in area.	Embarrassment is common after a seizure, especially if others witnessed the seizure.
5 Do not restrain patient; hold limbs loosely if they are flailing. Place something soft under head. Loosen clothing such as collar or belt.	Prevent musculoskeletal injury. Promote free ventilatory movement of chest and abdomen.

CLINICAL DECISION: *Because injury results from forcible insertion of objects into mouth, never force apart a patient's clenched teeth. Do not place any objects into patient's mouth such as fingers, medicine, tongue depressor, or airway when teeth are clenched. Insert a bite-block or oral airway in advance if you recognize the possibility of a tonic-clonic seizure.*

STEP	RATIONALE
6 Maintain patient's airway and suction as needed. Check level of consciousness and oxygen saturation. Check vital signs. Provide oxygen by nasal cannula or mask if ordered. Use oral airway only if you can easily access oral cavity.	Prevent hypoxia during seizure activity.
7 Stay with patient, observing sequence and timing of seizure activity. Note the following: type of seizure; parts of body affected; if there was a loss of consciousness; presence of autonomic signs of lip smacking, mastication, or grimacing; rolling of eyes; presence of incontinence or diaphoresis; presence of apnea.	Continued observation assists in documentation, diagnosis, and treatment of seizure disorder.
8 As patient regains consciousness, reorient and reassure. Explain what happened and answer patient's questions. Stay with patient until full recovery.	Informing patients of type of seizure activity experienced assists them in participating knowledgeably in their care. Some patients remain confused for a period of time or become violent.
9 Following seizure, assist patient to position of comfort in bed with side rails up (one rail down for easy exit) and bed in lowest position (see illustration). Place call light or intercom system within reach and provide a quiet, nonstimulating environment.	Provide for continued safety. Patients are often confused and sleepy following a seizure.

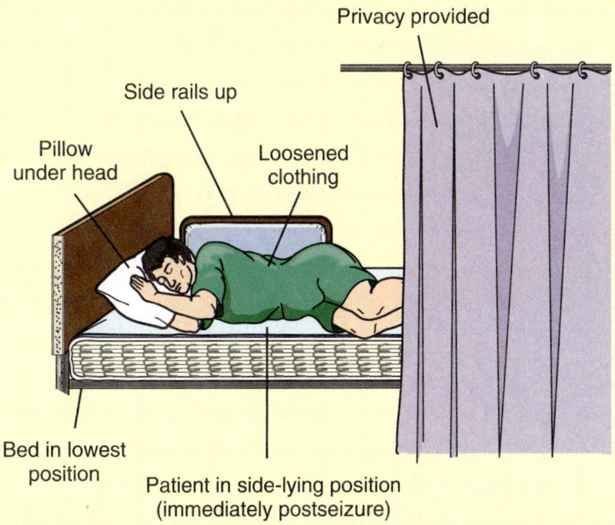

STEP 9 Position of patient following seizure and when on seizure precautions.

STEP	RATIONALE
10 Offer psychosocial support; provide time for patient to express feelings and concerns.	Patients who accept the reality of their disease integrate it into their own self-concept and have higher levels of self-esteem.
11 Perform hand hygiene.	Reduce transmission of microorganisms.

SKILL 27-2 SEIZURE PRECAUTIONS—cont'd

STEP	RATIONALE
EVALUATION	
1 Conduct a head-to-toe evaluation, including an inspection of oral cavity for breaks in mucous membranes from bites or broken teeth; look for bruising of skin or injury to bones and joints.	Determine presence of any traumatic injuries resulting from seizure activity.

CLINICAL DECISION: *If onset of seizure was not witnessed and you suspect patient fell and struck head, treat as a closed head injury or spinal injury. Place a cervical collar on patient before attempting to turn.*

STEP	RATIONALE
2 Evaluate patient's mental status after seizure (level of consciousness, confusion, hallucinations).	Temporary mental status changes are common following a seizure.
3 Check patient's oxygen saturation and vital signs.	Determine stability of oxygenation and circulation.
4 If possible, ask patient to verbalize feelings after seizure.	Therapeutic interaction enables patient to recognize feelings associated with having a seizure disorder.

UNEXPECTED OUTCOMES AND RELATED INTERVENTIONS

1 Patient suffers traumatic injury.
- Continue to protect patient from further injury.
- Notify the health care provider immediately.
- Ensure environment is free of safety hazards.

2 Seizure lasts more than 5 minutes or patient has repeated seizures over 30 minutes, indicating status epilepticus.
- Establish or maintain patient's airway and administer oxygen.
- Notify health care provider immediately.
- Be prepared to call rapid response team or code blue.

3 Patient verbalizes feelings of embarrassment and humiliation.
- Offer support and allow patient to verbalize feelings.
- Encourage patient and family to participate in decision making and planning of care.

RECORDING AND REPORTING

- Record thoroughly in nurses' notes your observations before, during, and after seizure. Provide detailed description of type of seizure activity and sequence of events (e.g., presence of aura [if any], level of consciousness, posture, color, movement of extremities, incontinence, and patient's status immediately following seizure).
- Report to primary health care provider immediately as seizure begins. Status epilepticus is an emergency situation requiring immediate medical therapy.

HOME CARE CONSIDERATIONS

- Instruct family members in steps to take when patient experiences a seizure.
- Assess patient's home for environmental hazards in light of seizure condition.
- Until seizure condition is well controlled (usually for at least 1 year), make sure patient does not take a tub bath or engage in activities such as swimming unless knowledgeable family member is present. Driving is restricted until permitted by state regulations.
- Refer patient to the Epilepsy Foundation or a similar community resource for support groups.

KEY POINTS

- In the community a safe environment means that basic needs are achievable, physical hazards are reduced, transmission of pathogens and parasites is reduced, pollution is controlled, and sanitation is maintained.
- A safe health care environment is one that reduces the risk of injury, including minimizing falls, patient-inherent accidents, procedure-inherent accidents, and equipment-related accidents.
- Reduction of physical hazards in the environment includes providing adequate lighting, decreasing clutter, and securing the home.
- Reduce the transmission of pathogens through medical and surgical asepsis, immunization, adequate food sanitation, insect and rodent control, and appropriate disposal of human waste.
- Every developmental age involves specific safety risks.
- Children younger than 5 years of age are at greatest risk for home accidents that result in severe injury and death.
- The school-age child is at risk for injury at home, at school, and while traveling to and from school.
- Adolescents are at risk for injury from automobile accidents, suicide, and substance abuse.
- Threats to an adult's safety are frequently associated with lifestyle habits.
- Risks for injury for older patients are directly related to the physiological changes of the aging process.
- Nursing interventions for promoting safety are individualized for patients' developmental stage, lifestyle, and environment.
- Continually evaluate the patient's safety risk and update the nursing care plan appropriately.
- Use physical restraints only as a last resort, when patients' behavior places them or others at risk for injury.

CLINICAL APPLICATION QUESTIONS

Preparing for Clinical Practice

Ms. Cohen is hospitalized for repair of a fractured hip after a fall at home. Ms. Cohen requires intravenous (IV) antibiotics after surgery. Shortly after the first dose, she became restless and started picking at her IV line and frequently attempting to get out of bed. Several restraint alternatives were attempted but, because of Ms. Cohen's restlessness, she was successful at pulling out her IV line and getting out of bed. It becomes necessary to restrain Ms. Cohen.

1. You know that a health care provider's order is required for the restraint. What are essential components of the restraint order?
2. What assessments do you need to perform on Ms. Cohen while she is restrained?
3. The physician orders a belt restraint. Your assessment of Ms. Cohen the next day reveals that during the day she is alert and pleasantly confused but not attempting to get out of bed. Do you continue use of the restraint? Explain.

evolve *Answers to Clinical Application Questions can be found on the Evolve website.*

REVIEW QUESTIONS

Are You Ready to Test Your Nursing Knowledge?

1. The nurse's first action after discovering an electrical fire in a patient's room is to:
   1. Activate the fire alarm.
   2. Confine the fire by closing all doors and windows.
   3. Remove all patients in immediate danger.
   4. Extinguish the fire by using the nearest fire extinguisher.
2. A parent calls the pediatrician's office frantic about the bottle of cleaner that her 2-year-old son drank. Which of the following is the most important instruction the nurse gives to this parent?
   1. Give the child milk.
   2. Give the child syrup of ipecac.
   3. Call the poison control center.
   4. Take the child to the emergency department.
3. The nursing assessment on a 78-year-old woman reveals shuffling gait, decreased balance, and instability. On the basis of the patient's data, which one of the following nursing diagnoses indicates an understanding of the assessment findings?
   1. Activity intolerance
   2. Impaired bed mobility
   3. Acute pain
   4. Risk for falls
4. A couple is with their adolescent daughter for a school physical and state they are worried about all the safety risks affecting this age. What is the greatest risk for injury for an adolescent?
   1. Home accidents
   2. Physiological changes of aging
   3. Poisoning and child abduction
   4. Automobile accidents, suicide, and substance abuse
5. The nurse found a 68-year-old female patient wandering in the hall. The patient says she is looking for the bathroom. Which interventions are appropriate to ensure the safety of the patient? (Select all that apply.)
   1. Insert a urinary catheter.
   2. Leave a night light on in the bathroom.
   3. Ask the physician to order a restraint.
   4. Keep the bed in low position with upper and lower side rails up.
   5. Assign a staff member to stay with the patient.
   6. Provide scheduled toileting during the night shift.
   7. Keep the pathway from the bed to the bathroom clear.
6. The family of a patient who is confused and ambulatory insists that all four side rails be up when the patient is alone. What is the best action to take in this situation? (Select all that apply.)
   1. Contact the nursing supervisor.
   2. Restrict the family's visiting privileges.
   3. Ask the family to stay with the patient if possible.
   4. Inform the family of the risks associated with side-rail use.
   5. Thank the family for being conscientious and put the four rails up.
   6. Discuss alternatives with the family that are appropriate for this patient.
7. A physician writes an order to apply a wrist restraint to a patient who has been pulling out a surgical wound drain. Place the following steps for applying the restraint in the correct order.
   ___ 1. Explain what you plan to do.
   ___ 2. Wrap a limb restraint around wrist or ankle with soft part toward skin and secure.
   ___ 3. Determine that restraint alternatives fail to ensure patient's safety.
   ___ 4. Identify the patient using proper identifier.
   ___ 5. Pad the patient's wrist.
8. A child in the hospital starts to have a grand mal seizure while playing in the playroom. What is your most important nursing intervention during this situation?
   1. Begin cardiopulmonary respiration.
   2. Restrain the child to prevent injury.
   3. Place a tongue blade over the tongue to prevent aspiration.
   4. Clear the area around the child to protect the child from injury.
9. A 62-year-old woman is being discharged home with her husband after surgery for a hip fracture from a fall at home. When providing discharge teaching about home safety to this patient and her husband, the nurse knows that:
   1. A safe environment promotes patient activity.
   2. Assessment focuses on environmental factors only.
   3. Teaching home safety is difficult to do in the hospital setting.
   4. Most accidents in the older adult are caused by lifestyle factors.
10. A fragile, 87-year-old nursing home resident is admitted to the hospital with dehydration and increased confusion. The patient has upper limb restraints to prevent her from pulling out her nasogastric tube. What instructions does the nurse give to nursing assistive personnel (NAP)?
11. The nursing assessment of an 80-year-old patient who demonstrates some confusion but no anxiety reveals that the patient is a fall risk because she continues to get out of bed without help despite frequent reminders. The initial nursing intervention to prevent falls for this patient is to:
    1. Place a bed alarm device on the bed.
    2. Place the patient in a belt restraint.
    3. Provide one-on-one observation of the patient.
    4. Apply wrist restraints.
12. To ensure the safe use of oxygen in the home by a patient, which of the following teaching points does the nurse include? (Select all that apply.)

1. Smoking is prohibited around oxygen.
2. Demonstrate how to adjust the oxygen flow rate based on patient symptoms.
3. Do not use electrical equipment around oxygen.
4. Special precautions may be required when traveling with oxygen

13. How does the nurse support a culture of safety? (Select all that apply.)
    1. Completing incident reports when appropriate
    2. Completing incident reports for a near miss
    3. Communicating product concerns to an immediate supervisor
    4. Identifying the person responsible for an incident
14. You are admitting Mr. Jones, a 64-year-old patient who had a right hemisphere stroke and a recent fall. The wife stated that he has a history of high blood pressure, which is controlled by an antihypertensive and a diuretic. Currently he exhibits left-sided neglect and problems with spatial and perceptual abilities and is impulsive. He has moderate left-sided weakness that requires the assistance of two and the use of a gait belt to transfer to a chair. He currently has an intravenous (IV) line and a urinary catheter in place. What factors increase his fall risk at this time? (Select all that apply.)
    1. Smokes a pack a day
    2. Used a cane to walk at home
    3. Takes antihypertensive and diuretics
    4. History of recent fall
    5. Neglect, spatial and perceptual abilities, impulsive
    6. Requires assistance with activity, unsteady gait
    7. IV line, urinary catheter
15. At 3 AM the emergency department nurse hears that a tornado hit the east side of town. What action does the nurse take first?
    1. Prepare for an influx of patients
    2. Contract the American Red Cross
    3. Determine how to restore essential services
    4. Evacuate patients per the disaster plan

Answers: **1.** 3; **2.** 3; **3.** 4; **4.** 4; **5.** 2, 6, 7; **6.** 3, 4, 6; **7.** 3, 4, 1, 5, 2; **8.** 4; **9.** 1; **10.** See Evolve; **11.** 1; **12.** 1, 3, 4; **13.** 1, 2, 3; **14.** 3, 4, 5, 6, 7; **15.** 1.

REFERENCES

Agency for Healthcare Research and Quality: *Navigating the health care system: Where medical errors occur and how to avoid them*, Rockville, Md, May 2010, http://www.ahrq.gov/video/healthcolumns/errors/errors.htm. Accessed August 20, 2011.

Agency for Toxic Substances and Disease Registry: *Lead: toxFAQs*, 2010, accessed from http://www.atsdr.cdc.gov/toxfaqs/tf.asp?id=93&tid=22. Accessed August 20, 2011.

American Academy of Pediatrics: Task force on sudden infant death syndrome, *Pediatrics* 116(5):1245, 2005.

American Academy of Pediatrics: *Car safety seats: information for families for 2011. Healthy Children*, 2011, http://www.aap.org/healthtopics/carseatsafety.cfm. Accessed April 25, 2011.

American Geriatric Society: *Clinical practice guideline falls prevention in older persons*, 2009, accessed from http://www.medcats.com/FALLS/frameset.htm. Accessed August 20, 2011.

American Hospital Association: *Quality advisory: implementing standardized colors for patient alert wristbands*, 2008, http://www.aha.org/advocacy-issues/tools-resources/advisory/2008/080904-quality-adv.pdf. Accessed October 4, 2011.

American Medical Association: *Bioterrorism—frequently asked questions*, 2010, http://www.ama-assn.org/ama1/pub/upload/mm/415/bioterrorism_faqs.pdf. Accessed August 20, 2011.

Capezuti E, et al: Least restrictive or least understood? Waist restraints, provider practices, and risk of harm, *J Aging Soc Policy* 20(3):305, 2008.

Centers for Disease Control and Prevention (CDC): *Food safety*, 2009, accessed from http://www.cdc.gov/foodsafety/. Accessed August 20, 2011.

Centers for Disease Control and Prevention (CDC): *Percentage distribution of injuries by place of occurrence, among males and females—National health interview survey, United States, 2004-2007*, (Morbidity and Mortality Weekly Report) Atlanta, Ga, 2010a, Office of Surveillance, Epidemiology and Laboratory Services, Centers for Disease Control and Prevention, United States, Department of Health and Human Services.

Centers for Disease Control and Prevention (CDC): *Injury prevention and control: motor vehicle safety*, 2010b, http://www.cdc.gov/Motorvehiclesafety/teen_drivers/teendrivers_factsheet.html. Accessed April 23, 2011.

Centers for Disease Control and Prevention (CDC): *Poison prevention*, 2010c, accessed from http://www.cdc.gov/Features/PoisonPrevention. Accessed August 20, 2011.

Centers for Medicare and Medicaid Services (CMS): *Revisions to Medicare conditions of participation*, 482.13, Bethesda, Md, 2007, US Department of Health and Human Services.

Centers for Medicare and Medicaid Services (CMS): *State Operations Manual, Appendix A—Survey protocol, regulations, and interpretive guidelines for hospitals*, 2009, accessed from http://www.cms.gov/manuals/downloads/som107ap_a_hospitals.pdf. Accessed August 20, 2011.

Coalition for Safe Community Needle Disposal: *Types of sharps disposal programs*, 2010, accessed from http://www.safeneedledisposal.org/index.cfm?load=page&page=43. Accessed October 4, 2011.

Department of Health and Human Services, Office of Inspector General: *Adverse events in hospitals: overview of key issues, OEI-06-07-00470*, Washington DC, 2008, DHHS.

Dire DJ: *CBRNE—Biological warfare agents*, 2008, accessed from http://emedicine.medscape.com/article/829613-overview. Accessed October 4, 2011.

Edelman CL, Mandle CL: *Health promotion throughout the life span*, ed 7, St Louis, 2010, Mosby.

Epilepsy Foundation: First aid for seizures, 2010, accessed from http://www.epilepsyfoundation.org/aboutepilepsy/firstaid/index.cfm. Accessed August 20, 2011.

Federal Emergency Management Agency (FEMA): *About FEMA*, 2010, accessed from http://www.fema.gov/about/index.shtm. Accessed August 20, 2011.

Food and Drug Administration (FDA): *Reporting serious problems to the FDA: how to report*. 2009, accessed from http://www.fda.gov/MedicalDevices/Safety/ReportaProblem/default.htm. Accessed August 20, 2011.

Hockenberry MJ, Wilson D: *Wong's essentials of pediatric nursing*, ed 8, St Louis, 2009, Mosby.

Hughes RG, editor: *Patient safety and quality: an evidenced-based handbook for nurses*, AHRQ Publication No. 08-0043, Rockville, Md, 2008, Agency for Healthcare Research and Quality.

Institute of Medicine Committee on Quality of Health Care in America: *To err is human: building a safer health system*, Washington, DC, 2000, National Academies Press.

Insurance Institute for Highway Safety (2008). *Fatality facts 2008 older people*, 2008, accessed from http://www.iihs.org/research/fatality_facts_2008/olderpeople.html. Accessed August 20, 2011.

Meiner S: *Gerontologic nursing*, ed 4, St Louis, 2011, Mosby.

National Alliance for Caregiving: *Caring in the US: a focused look at those caring for someone age 50 or older*, 2009, accessed from http.//www.caregiving.org/data/FINALRegularExSum50plus.pdf. Accessed October 4, 2011.

National Alliance for Caregiving: *Research*, 2011, accessed April 22, 2011 from http://www.caregiving.org/research.

National Center for Injury Prevention and Control: *10 leading causes of death, United States 1999-2007*, 2010a, accessed from http://webappa.cdc.gov/sasweb/ncipc/leadcaus10.html. Accessed August 20, 2011.

National Center for Injury Prevention and Control: *1999-2007, United States unintentional injuries ages 65-85+, all races, both sexes*, 2010b, accessed from http://webappa.cdc.gov/sasweb/ncipc/leadcaus10.html. Accessed October 4, 2011.

National Fire Protection Association: *Fires and burns involving home medical oxygen*, Quincy, Mass, 2008, NFPA, http://www.nfpa.org/assets/files/PDF/OS.Oxygen.pdf.

National Fire Protection Association: *Symptoms of carbon monoxide poisoning*, 2010a, accessed from http://www.nfpa.org/itemDetail.asp?categoryID=1733&URL=Safety%20information?For%20consumers/Fire%20&%20safety%20equipment/Carbon%20monoxide/Symptoms%20of%20CO%20poisoning. Accessed August 20, 2011.

National Fire Protection Association: *The U.S. Fire Problem*, 2010b, http://www.nfpa.org/categoryList.asp?categoryID=953&URL=Research%20&%20Reports/Fire%20statistics/The%20U.S.%20fire%20problem&cookie%5Ftest=1. Accessed October 4, 2011.

National Quality Forum (NQF): *National Quality Forum safe practices for better healthcare-2010 update*, Washington DC, 2010, http://www.qualityforum.org/Publications/2010/04/Safe_Practices_for_Better_Healthcare_-_2010_Update.aspx. Accessed May 30, 2011.

National Quality Forum (NQF): *Mission and vision*, Washington DC, 2011a, http://www.qualityforum.org/About_NQF/Mission_and_Vision.aspx. Accessed April 12, 2011.

National Quality Forum (NQF): *National voluntary consensus standards for public reporting of patient safety events,* Washington DC, 2011b, http://www.qualityforum.org/Publications/2011/02/National_Voluntary_Consensus_Standards_for_Public_Reporting_of_Patient_Safety_Event_Information.aspx. Accessed May 30, 2011.

Occupational Safety and Health Administration (OSHA): *Hazardous communication,* 1996, www.osha.gov/pls/oshaweb/owadisp.show_document?p_table=STANDARDS&p_id=10099. Accessed August 20, 2011.

Pynoos J, et al: Environmental assessment and modification as fall prevention strategies for older adults, *Clin Geriatr Med* 26(4):633, 2010.

Quality and Safety Education for Nurses (QSEN): *University of North Carolina at Chapel Hill, Chapel Hill, NC,* 2011, http://www.qsen.org/. Accessed April 23, 2011.

Studer Group: *Hourly rounding: Supplement,* The Studer Group, Gulf Breeze, FL, 2007, http://www.mc.vanderbilt.edu/root/pdfs/nursing/hourly_rounding_supplement-studer_group.pdf. Accessed January 28, 2012.

Taylor-Adams S, et al: Safety skills for clinicians: an essential component of patient safety, *J Patient Safety* 4(3):141, 2009.

The Joint Commission (TJC): *Comprehensive accreditation manual for hospitals,* Chicago, 2011a, TJC.

The Joint Commission: *2011 National Patient Safety Goals (NPSGs),* 2011b, TJC. Available at http://www.jointcommission.org/standards_information/npsgs.aspx.

RESEARCH REFERENCES

Banez C, et al: Development, implementation and evaluation of an interprofessional falls prevention program for older adults, *J Am Geriatr Soc* 56(8):1549, 2008.

Castle NG: The health consequences of using physical restraints in nursing homes, *Med Care* 47(11):1164, 2009.

Costello E, Edelstein JE: Update on falls prevention for community-dwelling older adults: review of single and multifactorial intervention programs, *J Rehabil Res Dev* 45(8):1135, 2008.

Deandrea S, et al: Risk factors for falls in community dwelling older people: a systematic review and meta-analysis, *Epidemiology* 21(5):658, 2010.

Dykes PC, et al: Why do patients in acute care hospitals fall? Can falls be prevented? *J Nurs Admin* 39(6):299, 2009.

Ford BM: Hourly rounding: a strategy to improve patient satisfaction scores, *Medsurg Nurs* 19(3):188, 2010.

Gillespie LD, et al: *Interventions for preventing falls in older people living in the community,* Cochrane Database Systematic Reviews, CD007146, vol 15, no 2, 2009.

Meade CM, et al: Effects of nursing rounds on patients' call light use, satisfaction and safety, *Am J Nurs* 106(9):58, 2006.

Trinkoff A, et al: How long and how much are nurses working? *Am J Nurs* 106(4):60, 2006.

Weisgram B, Raymond S: Using evidence-based nursing rounds to improve patient outcomes, *Medsurg Nurs* 17(6):429, 2008.

Zijlstra GA, et al: Prevalence and correlates of fear of falling, and associated avoidance of a population of community-living older people, *Age Ageing* 36(3):304, 2007.

CHAPTER

28

Infection Prevention and Control

OBJECTIVES

- Explain the relationship between the chain and transmission of infection.
- Give an example of preventing infection for each element of the infection chain.
- Identify the normal defenses of the body against infection.
- Discuss the events in the inflammatory response.
- Identify patients most at risk for infection.
- Describe the signs/symptoms of a localized infection and those of a systemic infection.
- Explain conditions that promote the transmission of health care–associated infection.
- Explain the difference between medical and surgical asepsis.
- Explain the rationale for standard precautions.
- Perform proper procedures for hand hygiene.
- Explain how infection control measures differ in the home versus the hospital.
- Properly don a surgical mask, sterile gown, and sterile gloves.
- Explain procedures for each isolation category.
- Understand the definition of occupational exposure.
- Explain the postexposure process.

KEY TERMS

Aerobic, p. 399
Anaerobic, p. 399
Asepsis, p. 410
Asymptomatic, p. 399
Bactericidal, p. 400
Bacteriostasis, p. 400
Broad-spectrum antibiotics, p. 402
Colonization, p. 399
Communicable disease, p. 399
Cough etiquette, p. 413
Disinfection, p. 412
Edema, p. 403
Endogenous infection, p. 403
Epidemiology, p. 421
Exogenous infection, p. 403
Exudates, p. 403
Granulation tissue, p. 403
Hand hygiene, p. 410
Handwashing, p. 410
Health care–associated infections (HAIs), p. 403
Iatrogenic infections, p. 403
Immunocompromised, p. 399
Infection, p. 399
Infectious, p. 399
Invasive, p. 398
Leukocytosis, p. 403
Localized, p. 401
Medical asepsis, p. 410
Microorganisms, p. 399
Necrotic, p. 402
Normal floras, p. 402
Pathogens, p. 399
Phagocytosis, p. 403
Purulent, p. 403
Reservoir, p. 399
Sanguineous, p. 403
Serous, p. 403
Standard precautions, p. 410
Sterile field, p. 423
Sterilization, p. 412
Suprainfection, p. 402
Surgical asepsis, p. 421
Susceptibility, p. 401
Suppurative, p. 407
Symptomatic, p. 399
Systemic, p. 401
Vector, p. 401
Virulence, p. 399

evolve WEBSITE

http://evolve.elsevier.com/Potter/fundamentals/

- Review Questions
- Video Clips
- Animations
- Concept Map Creator
- Case Study with Questions
- Skills Performance Checklists
- Audio Glossary
- Interactive Learning Activities
- Key Term Flashcards
- Content Updates

The incidence of patients developing infections as the direct result of contact during health care is increasing. Current trends, public awareness, and rising costs of health care have increased the importance of infection prevention and control. The Joint Commission (TJC) (2011) views this as a patient safety issue. Infection prevention and control are essential for creating a safe health care environment for patients, families, and staff. Nurses play a primary role in infection prevention and control. Patients in all health care settings are at risk for acquiring infections because of lower resistance to pathogens; increased exposure to pathogens, some of which may be resistant to most antibiotics; and **invasive** procedures. Health care workers are at risk for exposure to infections as a result of contact with patient blood, body fluids, and contaminated equipment and surfaces. By practicing basic infection prevention and control techniques, you avoid spreading pathogens to patients and sustaining an exposure when providing direct care.

Patients and their families need to be able to recognize sources of infection and understand measures used to protect themselves. Patient teaching must include basic information about infection, the various modes of transmission, and appropriate methods of prevention.

Health care workers protect themselves from contact with infectious material, sharps injury, and/or exposure to a communicable disease by applying knowledge of the infectious process and using appropriate personal protective equipment (PPE). Diseases such as hepatitis B and C, human immunodeficiency virus (HIV) infection, acquired immunodeficiency syndrome (AIDS), tuberculosis (TB), and multidrug-resistant organisms require a greater emphasis on infection prevention and control techniques (Centers for Disease Control and Prevention [CDC], 2004, 2006).

SCIENTIFIC KNOWLEDGE BASE

Nature of Infection

An **infection** is the invasion of a susceptible host by **pathogens** or **microorganisms,** resulting in disease. It is important to know the difference between an infection and colonization. **Colonization** is the presence and growth of microorganisms within a host but without tissue invasion or damage (Tweeten, 2009). Disease or infection results only if the pathogens multiply and alter normal tissue function. Some **infectious** diseases such as viral meningitis and pneumonia have a low or no risk for transmission. Although these illnesses can be serious for the patient, they do not pose a risk to others, including caregivers.

If an infectious disease can be transmitted directly from one person to another, it is termed a **communicable disease** (Tweeten, 2009). If the pathogens multiply and cause clinical signs and symptoms, the infection is **symptomatic.** If clinical signs and symptoms are not present, the illness is termed **asymptomatic.** Hepatitis C is an example of a communicable disease that can be asymptomatic. It is most efficiently transmitted through the direct passage of blood into the skin from a percutaneous exposure, even if the source patient is asymptomatic (CDC, 2010c).

Chain of Infection

The presence of a pathogen does not mean that an infection will occur. Infection occurs in a cycle that depends on the presence of all of the following elements:

- An infectious agent or pathogen
- A reservoir or source for pathogen growth
- A port of exit from the reservoir
- A mode of transmission
- A port of entry to a host
- A susceptible host

Infection can develop if this chain remains uninterrupted (Fig. 28-1). Preventing infections involves breaking the chain of infection.

Infectious Agent. Microorganisms include bacteria, viruses, fungi, and protozoa (Table 28-1). Microorganisms on the skin are either resident or transient flora. Resident organisms (normal flora) are permanent residents of the skin, where they survive and multiply without causing illness (CDC, 2002; WHO, 2009). The potential for microorganisms or parasites to cause disease depends on the number of microorganisms present; their **virulence,** or ability to produce disease; their ability to enter and survive in the host; and the susceptibility of the host. Resident skin microorganisms are not virulent. However, they sometimes cause serious infection when surgery or other invasive procedures allow them to enter deep tissues or when a patient is severely **immunocompromised** (has an impaired immune system).

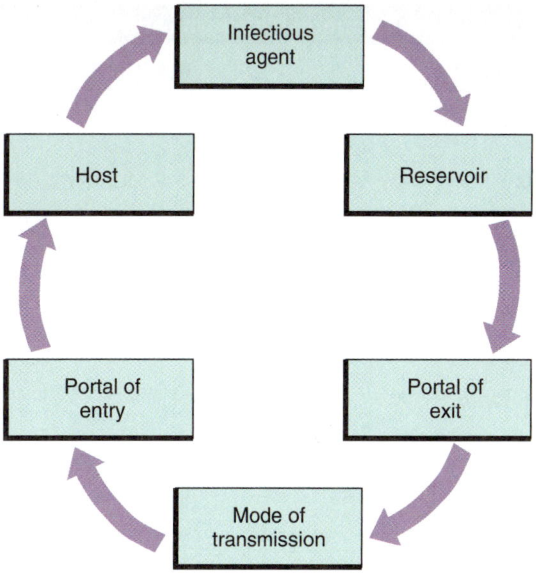

FIG. 28-1 Chain of infection.

Transient microorganisms attach to the skin when a person has contact with another person or object during normal activities. For example, when you touch a contaminated gauze dressing, transient bacteria adhere to your skin. These organisms may be readily transmitted unless removed using hand hygiene (Larson, 2005). If hands are visibly soiled with proteinaceous material, washing with soap and water is the preferred practice. If hands are not visibly soiled, use of an alcohol-based hand product or handwashing with soap and water is acceptable for disinfecting hands of health care workers (CDC, 2002; WHO, 2009).

Reservoir. A **reservoir** is a place where microorganisms survive, multiply, and await transfer to a susceptible host. Common reservoirs are humans and animals (hosts), insects, food, water, and organic matter on inanimate surfaces (fomites). Frequent reservoirs for health care–associated infections (HAIs) include health care workers, especially their hands; patients; equipment; and the environment. Human reservoirs are divided into two types: those with acute or symptomatic disease and those who show no signs of disease but are carriers of it. Humans can transmit microorganisms in either case. Animals, food, water, insects, and inanimate objects can also be reservoirs for infectious organisms. To thrive, organisms require a proper environment, including appropriate food, oxygen, water, temperature, pH, and light.

Food. Microorganisms require nourishment. Some such as *Clostridium perfringens,* the microbe that causes gas gangrene, thrive on organic matter. Others such as *Escherichia coli* consume undigested foodstuff in the bowel. Carbon dioxide and inorganic material such as soil provide nourishment for other organisms.

Oxygen. **Aerobic** bacteria require oxygen for survival and for multiplication sufficient to cause disease. Aerobic organisms cause more infections in humans than anaerobic organisms. An example of an aerobic organism is *Staphylococcus aureus.* **Anaerobic** bacteria thrive where little or no free oxygen is available. Infections deep within the pleural cavity, in a joint, or in a deep sinus tract are typically caused by anaerobes. An example of an anaerobic organism is *Clostridium difficile,* an organism that causes antibiotic-induced diarrhea.

Water. Most organisms require water or moisture for survival. For example, a frequent place for microorganisms is the moist

TABLE 28-1 Common Pathogens and Some Infections or Diseases They Produce

ORGANISM	MAJOR RESERVOIR(S)	MAJOR INFECTIONS/DISEASES
Bacteria		
Escherichia coli	Colon	Gastroenteritis, urinary tract infection
Staphylococcus aureus	Skin, hair, anterior nares, mouth	Wound infection, pneumonia, food poisoning, cellulitis
Streptococcus (beta-hemolytic group A) organisms	Oropharynx, skin, perianal area	"Strep throat," rheumatic fever, scarlet fever, impetigo, wound infection
Streptococcus (beta-hemolytic group B) organisms	Adult genitalia	Urinary tract infection, wound infection, postpartum sepsis, neonatal sepsis
Mycobacterium tuberculosis	Droplet nuclei from lungs, larynx	Tuberculosis
Neisseria gonorrhoeae	Genitourinary tract, rectum, mouth	Gonorrhea, pelvic inflammatory disease, infectious arthritis, conjunctivitis
Rickettsia rickettsii	Wood tick	Rocky Mountain spotted fever
Staphylococcus epidermidis	Skin	Wound infection, bacteremia
Viruses		
Hepatitis A virus	Feces	Hepatitis A
Hepatitis B virus	Blood and certain body fluids, sexual contact	Hepatitis B
Hepatitis C virus	Blood, certain body fluids, sexual contact	Hepatitis C
Herpes simplex virus (type 1)	Lesions of mouth or skin, saliva, genitalia	Cold sores, aseptic meningitis, sexually transmitted disease, herpetic whitlow
Human immunodeficiency virus (HIV)	Blood, semen, vaginal secretions via sexual contact	Acquired immunodeficiency syndrome (AIDS)
Fungi		
Aspergillus organisms	Soil, dust, mouth, skin, colon, genital tract	Aspergillosis, pneumonia, sepsis
Candida albicans	Mouth, skin, colon, genital tract	Candidiasis, pneumonia, sepsis
Protozoa		
Plasmodium falciparum	Blood	Malaria

Modified from Moore V: Microbiology basics. In Carrico R, editor: *APIC text of infection control and epidemiology,* Washington, DC, 2009, Association for Professionals in Infection Control and Epidemiology.

drainage from a surgical wound. Some bacteria assume a form, called a *spore,* which is resistant to drying. A common spore-forming bacterium is *C. difficile,* an organism that causes antibiotic-induced diarrhea.

Temperature. Microorganisms can live only in certain temperature ranges. Each species of bacteria has a specific temperature at which it grows best. The ideal temperature for most human pathogens is 20° to 43° C (68° to 109° F). For example, *Legionella pneumophila* grows best in water at 25° to 42° C (77° to 108° F) (Moore, 2009; Ritter, 2005). Cold temperatures tend to prevent growth and reproduction of bacteria **(bacteriostasis).** A temperature or chemical that destroys bacteria is **bactericidal.**

pH. The acidity of an environment determines the viability of microorganisms. Most microorganisms prefer an environment within a pH range of 5.0 to 7.0. Bacteria in particular thrive in urine with an alkaline pH.

Light. Microorganisms thrive in dark environments such as those under dressings and within body cavities.

Port of Exit. After microorganisms find a site to grow and multiply, they need to find a port of exit if they are to enter another host and cause disease. Ports of exit include sites such as blood, skin and mucous membranes, respiratory tract, genitourinary tract, gastrointestinal tract, and transplacental (mother to fetus).

Skin and Mucous Membranes. The skin is considered a port of exit because any break in the integrity of the skin and mucous membranes allows pathogens to exit the body. This may be exhibited by the creation of purulent drainage. The presence of purulent drainage is a potential port of exit.

Respiratory Tract. Pathogens that infect the respiratory tract such as the influenza virus are released from the body when an infected person sneezes or coughs.

Urinary Tract. Normally urine is sterile. However, when a patient has a urinary tract infection (UTI), microorganisms exit during urination.

Gastrointestinal Tract. The mouth is one of the most bacterially contaminated sites of the human body, but most of the organisms are normal floras. Organisms that are normal floras in one person can be pathogens in another. For example, organisms exit when a person expectorates saliva. In addition, gastrointestinal ports of exit include bowel elimination, drainage of bile via surgical wounds, or drainage tubes.

Reproductive Tract. Organisms such as *Neisseria gonorrhoeae* and HIV exit through a man's urethral meatus or a woman's vaginal canal during sexual contact.

Blood. The blood is normally a sterile body fluid; however, in the case of communicable diseases such as hepatitis B or C or HIV, it becomes a reservoir for pathogens.

Modes of Transmission. Each disease has a specific mode of transmission. Many times you are able to do little about the infectious agent or the susceptible host, but by practicing infection

BOX 28-1 MODES OF TRANSMISSION

Contact

Direct

- Person-to-person (fecal, oral) physical contact between source and susceptible host (e.g., touching patient feces and then touching your inner mouth or consuming contaminated food)

Indirect

- Personal contact of susceptible host with contaminated inanimate object (e.g., needles or sharp objects, dressings, environment)

Droplet

- Large particles that travel up to 3 feet during coughing, sneezing, or talking and come in contact with susceptible host

Airborne

- Droplet nuclei or residue or evaporated droplets suspended in air during coughing or sneezing or carried on dust particles

Vehicles

- Contaminated items
- Water
- Drugs, solutions
- Blood
- Food (improperly handled, stored, or cooked; fresh or thawed meats)

Vector

- External mechanical transfer (flies)
- Internal transmission such as parasitic conditions between vector and host such as:
  - Mosquito
  - Louse
  - Flea
  - Tick

Modified from Tweeten S: General principles of epidemiology. In Carrico R, editor: *APIC text of infection control and epidemiology,* Washington, DC, 2005, Association for Professionals in Infection Control and Epidemiology.

prevention and control techniques such as hand hygiene, you interrupt the mode of transmission (Box 28-1). The same microorganism is sometimes transmitted by more than one route. For example, varicella zoster (chickenpox) is spread by the airborne route in droplet nuclei or by direct contact.

The major route of transmission for pathogens identified in the health care setting is the unwashed hands of the health care worker (CDC, 2002; Cipriano, 2007; WHO, 2009). Equipment used within the environment (e.g., a stethoscope, blood pressure cuff, or bedside commode) often becomes a source for the transmission of pathogens.

Port of Entry. Organisms enter the body through the same routes they use for exiting. For example, when a needle pierces a patient's skin, organisms enter the body if proper skin preparation is not performed first. Factors such as a depressed immune system that reduce body defenses enhance the chances of pathogens entering the body.

Susceptible Host. Susceptibility to an infectious agent depends on the individual's degree of resistance to pathogens. Although everyone is constantly in contact with large numbers of microorganisms, an infection does not develop until an individual becomes susceptible to the strength and numbers of the microorganisms. A person's natural defenses against infection and certain risk factors (e.g., age, nutritional status, presence of chronic disease, trauma, and smoking) affect susceptibility (resistance) (Fardo, 2009). Organisms such as *S. aureus* with resistance to key antibiotics are becoming more common in all health care settings, but especially acute care. The increased resistance is associated with the frequent and sometimes inappropriate use of antibiotics over the years in all settings (i.e., acute care, ambulatory care, clinics, and long-term care) (Arnold, 2009).

BOX 28-2 COURSE OF INFECTION BY STAGE

Incubation Period

Interval between entrance of pathogen into body and appearance of first symptoms (e.g., chickenpox, 10 to 21 days after exposure; common cold, 1 to 2 days; influenza, 1 to 5 days; mumps, 12 to 26 days).

Prodromal Stage

Interval from onset of nonspecific signs and symptoms (malaise, low-grade fever, fatigue) to more specific symptoms. (During this time microorganisms grow and multiply, and patient may be capable of spreading disease to others.) For example, herpes simplex begins with itching and tingling at the site before the lesion appears.

Illness Stage

Interval when patient manifests signs and symptoms specific to type of infection. For example, strep throat is manifested by sore throat, pain, and swelling; mumps is manifested by high fever, parotid and salivary gland swelling.

Convalescence

Interval when acute symptoms of infection disappear. (Length of recovery depends on severity of infection and patient's host resistance; recovery may take several days to months.)

THE INFECTIOUS PROCESS

By understanding the chain of infection, you have knowledge that is vital in preventing infections. When the patient acquires an infection, observe for signs and symptoms of infection and take appropriate actions to prevent its spread. Infections follow a progressive course (Box 28-2).

If an infection is localized (e.g., a wound infection), the patient usually experiences localized symptoms such as pain, tenderness, and redness at the wound site. Use standard precautions, appropriate PPE, and hand hygiene when assessing the wound. The use of these precautions and hand hygiene blocks the spread of infection to other sites or other patients. An infection that affects the entire body instead of just a single organ or part is systemic and can become fatal if undetected and untreated.

The course of an infection influences the level of nursing care provided. The nurse is responsible for properly administering antibiotics, monitoring the response to drug therapy (see Chapter 31), using proper hand hygiene, and standard precautions. Supportive therapy includes providing adequate nutrition and rest to bolster defenses against the infectious process. The course of care for the patient often has additional effects on body systems affected by the infection.

Defenses Against Infection

The body has natural defenses that protect against infection. Normal floras, body system defenses, and inflammation are all nonspecific defenses that protect against microorganisms

TABLE 28-2 Normal Defense Mechanisms Against Infection

DEFENSE MECHANISMS	ACTION	FACTORS THAT MAY ALTER DEFENSE MECHANISMS
Skin		
Intact multilayered surface (first line of defense body against infection)	Provides barrier to microorganisms and antibacterial activity	Cuts, abrasions, puncture wounds, areas of maceration
Shedding of outer layer of skin cells	Removes organisms that adhere to outer layers of skin	Failure to bathe regularly, improper handwashing technique
Sebum	Contains fatty acid that kills some bacteria	Excessive bathing
Mouth		
Intact multilayered mucosa	Provides mechanical barrier to microorganisms	Lacerations, trauma, extracted teeth
Saliva	Washes away particles containing microorganisms Contains microbial inhibitors (e.g., lysozyme)	Poor oral hygiene, dehydration
Eye		
Tearing and blinking	Provides mechanisms to reduce entry (blinking) or assist in washing away (tearing) particles containing pathogens, thus reducing dose of organisms	Injury, exposure—splash/splatter of blood or other potentially infectious material into eye
Respiratory Tract		
Cilia lining upper airway, coated by mucus	Traps inhaled microbes and sweeps them outward in mucus to be expectorated or swallowed	Smoking, high concentration of oxygen and carbon dioxide, decreased humidity, cold air
Macrophages	Engulf and destroy microorganisms that reach alveoli of lung	Smoking
Urinary Tract		
Flushing action of urine flow	Washes away microorganisms on lining of bladder and urethra	Obstruction to normal flow by urinary catheter placement, obstruction from growth or tumor, delayed micturition
Intact multilayered epithelium	Provides barrier to microorganisms	Introduction of urinary catheter, continual movement of catheter in urethra
Gastrointestinal Tract		
Acidity of gastric secretions	Prevents retention of bacterial contents	Administration of antacids
Rapid peristalsis in small intestine		Delayed motility resulting from impaction of fecal contents in large bowel or mechanical obstruction by masses
Vagina		
At puberty, normal flora causing vaginal secretions to achieve low pH	Inhibit growth of many microorganisms	Antibiotics and oral contraceptives disrupting normal flora

regardless of prior exposure. If any body defenses fail, an infection usually occurs and leads to a serious health problem.

Normal Floras. The body normally contains microorganisms that reside on the surface and deep layers of skin, in the saliva and oral mucosa, and in the gastrointestinal and genitourinary tracts. A person normally excretes trillions of microbes daily through the intestines. **Normal floras** do not usually cause disease when residing in their usual area of the body but instead participate in maintaining health.

Normal floras of the large intestine exist in large numbers without causing illness. They also secrete antibacterial substances within the walls of the intestine. The normal floras of the skin exert a protective, bactericidal action that kills organisms landing on the skin. The mouth and pharynx are also protected by floras that impair growth of invading microbes. Normal floras maintain a sensitive balance with other microorganisms to prevent infection. Any factor that disrupts this balance places a person at increased risk for acquiring a disease. For example, the use of **broad-spectrum antibiotics** for the treatment of infection can lead to **suprainfection.** A suprainfection develops when broad-spectrum antibiotics eliminate a wide range of normal flora organisms, not just those causing infection. When normal bacterial floras are eliminated, body defenses are reduced, which allows for disease-producing microorganisms to multiply, causing illness (Arnold, 2009).

Body System Defenses. A number of body organ systems have unique defenses against infection (Table 28-2). The skin, respiratory tract, and gastrointestinal tract are easily accessible to microorganisms. Pathogenic organisms can adhere to the surface skin, be inhaled into the lungs, or be ingested with food. Each organ system has defense mechanisms physiologically suited to its specific structure and function. For example, the lungs cannot completely control the entrance of microorganisms. However, the airways are lined with moist mucous membranes and hairlike projections, or cilia, that rhythmically beat to move mucus or cellular debris up to the pharynx to be expelled through swallowing.

Inflammation. The cellular response of the body to injury, infection, or irritation is termed *inflammation.* Inflammation is a protective vascular reaction that delivers fluid, blood products, and nutrients to an area of injury. The process neutralizes and eliminates pathogens or dead **(necrotic)** tissues and establishes a means of repairing body cells and tissues. Signs of localized inflammation include swelling, redness, heat, pain or tenderness, and loss of function in the affected body part. When inflammation becomes systemic, other signs and symptoms develop, including fever, leukocytosis, malaise, anorexia, nausea, vomiting, lymph node enlargement, or organ failure.

Physical agents, chemical agents, or microorganisms trigger the inflammatory response. Mechanical trauma, temperature extremes, and radiation are examples of physical agents. Chemical agents include external and internal irritants such as harsh poisons or gastric acid. Sometimes microorganisms also trigger this response.

After tissues are injured, a series of well-coordinated events occurs. The inflammatory response includes the following:

1. Vascular and cellular responses
2. Formation of inflammatory **exudates** (fluid and cells that are discharged from cells or blood vessels [e.g., pus or serum])
3. Tissue repair

Vascular and Cellular Responses. Acute inflammation is an immediate response to cellular injury. Rapid vasodilation occurs, allowing more blood near the location of the injury. The increase in local blood flow causes the redness and localized warmth at the site of inflammation.

Injury causes tissue damage and possibly necrosis. As a result the body releases chemical mediators that increase the permeability of small blood vessels; and fluid, protein, and cells enter interstitial spaces. The accumulation of fluid appears as localized swelling **(edema).** Another sign of inflammation is pain. The swelling of inflamed tissues increases pressure on nerve endings, causing pain. As a result of physiological changes occurring with inflammation, the involved body part may have a temporary loss of function. For example, a localized infection of the hand causes the fingers to become swollen, painful, and discolored. Joints become stiff as a result of swelling, but function of the fingers returns when inflammation subsides.

The cellular response of inflammation involves white blood cells (WBCs) arriving at the site. WBCs pass through blood vessels and into the tissues. **Phagocytosis** is a process that involves the destruction and absorption of bacteria. Through the process of phagocytosis, specialized WBCs, called *neutrophils* and *monocytes,* ingest and destroy microorganisms or other small particles. If inflammation becomes systemic, other signs and symptoms develop. **Leukocytosis,** or an increase in the number of circulating WBCs, is the response of the body to WBCs leaving blood vessels. A serum WBC count is normally 5,000 to 10,000/mm^3 but typically rise to 15,000 to 20,000/mm^3 and higher during inflammation. Fever is caused by phagocytic release of pyrogens from bacterial cells, which causes a rise in the hypothalamic set point (see Chapter 29).

Inflammatory Exudate. Accumulation of fluid and dead tissue cells and WBCs forms an exudate at the site of inflammation. Exudate may be **serous** (clear, like plasma), **sanguineous** (containing red blood cells), or **purulent** (containing WBCs and bacteria). Usually the exudate is cleared away through lymphatic drainage. Platelets and plasma proteins such as fibrinogen form a meshlike matrix at the site of inflammation to prevent its spread.

Tissue Repair. When there is injury to tissue cells, healing involves the defensive, reconstructive, and maturative stages (see Chapter 48). Damaged cells are eventually replaced with healthy new cells. The new cells undergo a gradual maturation until they take on the same structural characteristics and appearance as the previous cells. If inflammation is chronic, tissue defects sometimes fill with fragile **granulation tissue.** Granulation tissue is not as strong as tissue collagen and assumes the form of scar tissue.

Health Care–Associated Infections

Patients in health care settings, especially hospitals and long-term care facilities, have an increased risk of acquiring infections. **Health care–associated infections (HAIs),** formerly called *nosocomial* or *health care–acquired infections,* result from the delivery of health services in a health care facility. They occur as the result of invasive procedures, antibiotic administration, the presence of multidrug-resistant organisms, and breaks in infection prevention and control activities.

Patients who develop HAIs often have multiple illnesses, are older adults, and are poorly nourished; thus they are more susceptible to infections. In addition, many patients have a lowered resistance to infection because of underlying medical conditions (e.g., diabetes mellitus or malignancies) that impair or damage the immune response of the body. Invasive treatment devices such as intravenous (IV) catheters or indwelling urinary catheters impair or bypass the natural defenses of the body against microorganisms. Critical illness increases patients' susceptibility to infections, especially multidrug-resistant bacteria. Meticulous hand hygiene practices, the use of chlorhexidine washes, and other advances in intensive care unit (ICU) infection prevention help to prevent these infections (Doyle et al., 2011).

Iatrogenic infections are a type of HAI from a diagnostic or therapeutic procedure. For example, procedures such as a bronchoscopy and treatment with broad-spectrum antibiotics increase the risk for certain infections (Arnold, 2009; Stricof, 2009). Use critical thinking when practicing aseptic techniques and follow basic infection prevention and control policies and procedures to reduce the risk of HAIs. Always consider the patient's risks for infection and anticipate how the approach to care increases or decreases the risk.

Health care–associated infections are exogenous or endogenous. An **exogenous infection** comes from microorganisms found outside the individual such as *Salmonella, Clostridium tetani,* and *Aspergillus.* They do not exist as normal floras. **Endogenous infection** occurs when part of the patient's flora becomes altered and an overgrowth results (e.g., staphylococci, enterococci, yeasts, and streptococci). This often happens when a patient receives broad-spectrum antibiotics that alter the normal floras. When sufficient numbers of microorganisms normally found in one body site move to another site, an endogenous infection develops. The number of microorganisms needed to cause a health care–associated infection depends on the virulence of the organism, the susceptibility of the host, and the body site affected.

The number of health care employees having direct contact with a patient, the type and number of invasive procedures, the therapy received, and the length of hospitalization influence the risk of infection. Major sites for HAIs include surgical or traumatic wounds, urinary and respiratory tracts, and the bloodstream (Box 28-3).

Health care–associated infections significantly increase costs of health care. Older adults have increased susceptibility to these infections because of their affinity to chronic disease and the aging process itself (Box 28-4). Extended stays in health care institutions, increased disability, increased costs of antibiotics, and prolonged recovery times add to the expenses both of the patient and the health care institution and funding bodies (e.g., Medicare). Often costs for HAIs are not reimbursed; as a result, prevention has a beneficial financial impact and is an important part of managed care. TJC (2011) lists several national safety goals focusing on the care of older adults (e.g., ensuring that older adults receive influenza and pneumonia vaccine or preventing infection after surgery).

BOX 28-3 SITES FOR AND CAUSES OF HEALTH CARE–ASSOCIATED INFECTIONS

Improperly performing hand hygiene increases patient risk for all types of health care–associated infections.

Urinary Tract
- Unsterile insertion of urinary catheter
- Improper positioning of the drainage tubing
- Open drainage system
- Catheter and tube becoming disconnected
- Drainage bag port touching contaminated surface
- Improper specimen collection technique
- Obstructing or interfering with urinary drainage
- Urine in catheter or drainage tube being allowed to reenter bladder (reflux)
- Repeated catheter irrigations

Surgical or Traumatic Wounds
- Improper skin preparation before surgery (e.g., shaving vs. clipping hair; not performing a preoperative bath or shower)
- Failure to clean skin surface properly
- Failure to use aseptic technique during dressing changes
- Use of contaminated antiseptic solutions

Respiratory Tract
- Contaminated respiratory therapy equipment
- Failure to use aseptic technique while suctioning airway
- Improper disposal of secretions

Bloodstream
- Contamination of intravenous (IV) fluids by tubing
- Insertion of drug additives to IV fluid
- Addition of connecting tube or stopcocks to IV system
- Improper care of needle insertion site
- Contaminated needles or catheters
- Failure to change IV access site when inflammation first appears
- Improper technique during administration of multiple blood products
- Improper care of peritoneal or hemodialysis shunts
- Improperly accessing an IV port

BOX 28-4 FOCUS ON OLDER ADULTS

Risks for Infection

- An age-related decline in immune system function, termed *immune senescence,* increases the susceptibility of the body to infection and slows overall immune response (Lesser, Paiusi, and Leips, 2006).
- Older adults are less capable of producing lymphocytes to combat challenges to the immune system. When antibodies are produced, the duration of their response is shorter, and fewer cells are produced (Fardo, 2009).
- Risks associated with the development of health care–associated infections in older patients include poor nutrition, unintentional weight loss, and low serum albumin levels (Meiner and Lueckenotte, 2006).
- After age 70 older adults appear likely to produce autoantibodies that attack parts of the body itself instead of infections (Fardo, 2009).
- Older adults experience loss and stress along with suppressed immunity related to bereavement, depression, and poor social support (Fardo, 2009).

NURSING KNOWLEDGE BASE

Body substances such as feces, urine, and wound drainage contain potentially infectious microorganisms. Health care workers are at risk for exposure to microorganisms in the hospital and/or home setting (Fauerbach, 2009). They follow specific infection prevention practices to reduce the risk of cross-contamination and transmission to other patients when caring for a patient with a known or suspected infection (CDC, 2007).

The experience of having a serious infection creates feelings of anxiety, frustration, loneliness, and anger in patients and/or their families (Calfree et al., 2008). These feelings worsen when patients are isolated to prevent transmission of a microorganism to other patients or health care staff. Isolation disrupts normal social relationships with visitors and caregivers. Patient safety is usually an additional risk for the patient on isolation precautions (Murphy, 2009). For example, an older patient with dementia is at increased risk for falling when confined in a room with the door closed. When family members fear the possibility of developing the infection, they avoid contact with the patient. Some patients perceive the simple procedures of proper hand hygiene and gown and glove use as evidence of rejection. Help patients and families reduce some of these feelings by discussing the disease process, explaining isolation procedures, and maintaining a friendly, understanding manner.

When establishing a plan of care, it is important for you to know how a patient reacts to an infection or infectious disease. The challenge is to identify and support behaviors that maintain human health or prevent infection.

Factors Influencing Infection Prevention and Control

Multiple factors influence a patient's susceptibility to infection. It is important to understand how each of these factors alone or in combination increases this risk. When more than one factor is present, the patient's susceptibility often increases, which affects length of stay, recovery time, and/or overall level of health following an illness. Understanding these factors assists in assessing and caring for a patient who has an infection or is at risk for one.

Age. Throughout life, susceptibility to infection changes. For example, an infant has immature defenses against infection. Born with only the antibodies provided by the mother, the infant's immune system is incapable of producing the necessary immunoglobulins and WBCs to adequately fight some infections. However, breastfed infants often have greater immunity than bottle-fed infants because they receive their mother's antibodies through the breast milk. As the child grows, the immune system matures; but the child is still susceptible to organisms that cause the common cold, intestinal infections, and infectious diseases such as mumps, measles, and chickenpox (if not vaccinated).

The young or middle-age adult has refined defenses against infection. Viruses are the most common cause of communicable illness in young or middle-age adults. Since 2000 there has been a major effort to vaccinate all children against all infectious diseases for which vaccines are available. Vaccine-preventable disease levels are at or near record lows (CDC, 2011). For example; hepatitis B infection in children and adolescents decreased by 89% in 2005 (CDC, 2005b).

Defenses against infection change with aging (Lesser, Paiusi, and Leips, 2006). The immune response, particularly cell-mediated immunity, declines. Older adults also undergo alterations in the structure and function of the skin, urinary tract, and

TABLE 28-3 **Assessing the Risk of Infection in Adults**

RISK FACTOR	CAUSES	OUTCOME
Chronic disease	COPD, heart failure, diabetes	Pneumonia, skin breakdown, venous stasis ulcers
Lifestyle—high-risk behaviors	Exposure to communicable/infectious diseases, use of IV drugs and other drugs/substances	STIs, HIV, HBV, HCV, opportunistic infections, viral infections, yeast infections, liver failure
Occupation	Miner, unemployed, homeless	Black lung disease, pneumonia, TB, poor nutritional intake, lack of access to medical care, stress
Diagnostic procedures	Invasive radiology, transplant	Multiple IV lines, immunosuppressive drugs
Heredity	Sickle cell disease, diabetes	Anemia, delayed healing
Travel history	West Nile virus, SARS, avian flu, *Hantavirus*	Meningitis, acute respiratory distress
Trauma	Fractures, internal bleeding	Sepsis, secondary infection
Nutrition	Obesity, anorexia	Impaired immune response

Modified from Tweeten SM: General principles of epidemiology. In Carrico R, editor: *APIC text of infection control and epidemiology,* Washington, DC, 2009, Association for Professionals in Infection Control and Epidemiology.
COPD, Chronic obstructive pulmonary disease; *HBV,* hepatitis B virus; *HCV,* hepatitis C virus; *HIV,* human immunodeficiency virus; *IV,* intravenous; *SARS,* severe acute respiratory syndrome; *STIs,* sexually transmitted infections; *TB,* tuberculosis.

lungs. For example, the skin loses its turgor, and the epithelium thins. As a result it is easier to tear or abrade the skin, which increases the potential for invasion by pathogens. In addition, older adults who are hospitalized or reside in an assisted-living or residential care facility are at risk for airborne infections. Ensuring that health care workers are vaccinated against influenza reduces the transmission of this illness in older adults (Thomas et al., 2010).

Nutritional Status. A patient's nutritional health directly influences susceptibility to infection. A reduction in the intake of protein and other nutrients such as carbohydrates and fats reduces body defenses against infection and impairs wound healing (see Chapter 48). Patients with illnesses or problems that increase protein requirements, such as extensive burns and conditions causing fever, are at further risk. Patients who have undergone surgery, for example, require increased protein. A thorough diet history is necessary. Determine a patient's normal daily nutrient intake and whether preexisting problems such as nausea, impaired swallowing, or oral pain alter food intake. Confer with a dietitian to assist in calculating the calorie count of foods ingested.

Stress. The body responds to emotional or physical stress by the general adaptation syndrome (see Chapter 37). During the alarm stage the basal metabolic rate increases as the body uses energy stores. Adrenocorticotropic hormone increases serum glucose levels and decreases unnecessary antiinflammatory responses through the release of cortisone. If stress continues or becomes intense, elevated cortisone levels result in decreased resistance to infection. Continued stress leads to exhaustion, which causes depletion in energy stores, and the body has no resistance to invading organisms. The same conditions that increase nutritional requirements such as surgery or trauma also increase physiological stress.

Disease Process. Patients with diseases of the immune system are at particular risk for infection. Leukemia, AIDS, lymphoma, and aplastic anemia are conditions that compromise a host by weakening defenses against infectious organisms. For example, patients with leukemia are unable to produce enough WBCs to ward off infection. Patients with HIV are often unable to ward off simple infections and are prone to opportunistic infections.

Patients with chronic diseases such as diabetes mellitus and multiple sclerosis are also more susceptible to infection because of general debilitation and nutritional impairment. Diseases that impair body system defenses such as emphysema and bronchitis (which impair ciliary action and thicken mucus), cancer (which alters the immune response), and peripheral vascular disease (which reduces blood flow to injured tissues) increase susceptibility to infection. Patients with burns have a high susceptibility to infection because of the damage to skin surfaces. The greater the depth and extent of the burns, the higher the risk for infection.

NURSING PROCESS

Apply the nursing process and use a critical thinking approach in your care of patients. The nursing process provides a clinical decision-making approach for you to develop and implement an individualized plan of care.

ASSESSMENT

During the assessment process, thoroughly assess each patient and critically analyze findings to ensure that you make patient-centered clinical decisions required for safe nursing care. Determine how the patient feels about the illness or risk for infection. Assess his or her defense mechanisms, susceptibility, and knowledge of how infections are transmitted (Table 28-3). Conduct a review of systems and travel history with the patient and family to reveal any risks for exposure to a communicable disease. Immunization and vaccination history are also very useful. It is important to be thorough in assessing a patient's clinical condition. A medication history is necessary to identify medications that increase a patient's susceptibility to infection. An analysis of laboratory findings provides information about a patient's defense against infection. The early recognition of infection or risk factors helps you make the correct nursing diagnosis and establish a treatment plan.

Through the Patient's Eyes. Some patients with infection have a variety of problems. It is important to ask specific questions to determine the patient's and family's needs related to the risk for infection or disease status (Box 28-5). These needs vary from

BOX 28-5 NURSING ASSESSMENT QUESTIONS

Risk Factors
- Do you have any recent cuts or lacerations? Show me the location.
- Describe for me any illnesses or diseases that you have and those for which you receive treatment.
- Have you had any recent diagnostic testing such as cystoscopy performed?

Possible Existing Infections
- Do you have or feel like you have a fever?
- Do you have any cuts or wounds with drainage?
- Do you have any pain/burning during urination?

Medication History
- List for me the medications you are currently taking.
- Describe any over-the-counter medications or herbals that you are currently taking.

Stressors
- Tell me about any major lifestyle change occurring such as the loss of employment or place of residence, divorce, or disability.

patient to patient and include physical, psychological, social, or economic needs. Patients with chronic or serious infection, especially communicable infections such as TB or AIDS, experience psychological and social problems from self-imposed isolation or rejection by friends and family. Ask the patient how the infection affects the ability to maintain relationships and perform activities of daily living. Determine whether chronic infection has drained the patient's financial resources. Ask about his or her expectations of care and determine how much he or she wants to be involved in planning care. Some patients and their families wish to know more about the disease process, whereas others only want to know the interventions necessary to treat the infection. Encourage patients to verbalize their expectations so you are able to establish interventions to meet patients' priorities.

Status of Defense Mechanisms. Review physical assessment findings and the patient's medical condition to determine the status of normal defense mechanisms against infection. For example, any break in the skin such as an ulcer on the foot of a patient who has diabetes is a potential site for infection. Any reduction in the primary or secondary defenses of the body against infection, such as a weakened ability to cough, places a patient at increased risk.

Patient Susceptibility. As noted in a previous section, age, nutritional status, stress, and disease process are factors that influence susceptibility to infection. Gather information about each factor through your interview and the patient's and family's medical history.

Medical Therapy. Some drugs and medical therapies compromise immunity to infection. Assess your patient's medication history to determine whether he or she takes any medications that increase infection susceptibility. These include any over-the-counter medications and herbal supplements. A review of therapies received within the health care setting further reveals risks. For example, adrenal corticosteroids, prescribed for several conditions, are antiinflammatory drugs that cause protein breakdown and impair the inflammatory response against bacteria and other pathogens. Cytotoxic and antineoplastic drugs attack cancer cells but also cause the side effects of bone marrow depression and normal cell toxicity, which affects the body's response against pathogens.

Clinical Appearance. The signs and symptoms of infection may be local or systemic. Localized infections are most common in areas of skin or mucous membrane breakdown such as surgical and traumatic wounds, pressure ulcers, oral lesions, and abscesses.

To assess an area for localized infection, first inspect it for redness and swelling caused by inflammation. Because there may be drainage from open lesions or wounds, wear clean gloves. Infected drainage may be yellow, green, or brown, depending on the pathogen. For example, green nasal secretions often indicate a sinus infection. Ask the patient about pain or tenderness around the site. Some patients complain of tightness and pain caused by edema. If the infected area is large enough, movement is restricted. Gentle palpation of an infected area usually results in some degree of tenderness. Wear protective eyewear and a surgical mask when there is a risk for splash or spray with blood or body fluids.

Systemic infections cause more generalized symptoms than local infection. These symptoms often include fever, fatigue, nausea/vomiting, and malaise. Lymph nodes that drain the area of infection often become enlarged, swollen, and tender during palpation. For example, an abscess in the peritoneal cavity causes enlargement of lymph nodes in the groin. An infection of the upper respiratory tract causes cervical lymph node enlargement. If an infection is serious and widespread, all major lymph nodes may enlarge.

Systemic infections sometimes develop after treatment for localized infection has failed. Be alert for changes in the patient's level of activity and responsiveness. As systemic infections develop, an elevation in body temperature can lead to episodes of increased heart and respiratory rates and low blood pressure. Involvement of major body systems produces specific symptoms. For example, a pulmonary infection results in a productive cough with purulent sputum. A UTI results in cloudy, foul-smelling urine.

An infection does not always present with typical signs and symptoms in all patients. For example, some older adults have an advanced infection before it is identified. Because of the aging process, there is a reduced inflammatory and immune response. Older adults have increased fatigue and diminished pain sensitivity. A reduced or absent fever response often occurs from chronic use of aspirin or nonsteroidal antiinflammatory drugs. Atypical symptoms such as confusion, incontinence, or agitation may be the only symptoms of an infectious illness (Fardo, 2009). For example, as many as 20% of older adults with pneumonia do not have the typical signs and symptoms of fever, shaking, chills, and rusty productive sputum. Often the only symptoms are an unexplained increase in heart rate, confusion, or generalized fatigue. A pneumonia vaccine is available and recommended for all persons with chronic respiratory problems and those over 65 years of age.

Laboratory Data. Review laboratory data as soon as they are available. Laboratory values such as increased WBCs and/or a positive blood culture often indicate infection (Table 28-4). However, laboratory values are not enough to detect infection. You need to assess other clinical signs. A culture result may show growth of an organism in the absence of infection. For example, in the older adult bacterial growth in urine without clinical symptoms does not always indicate the presence of a UTI (Gantz, 2009). It is also important to note that laboratory values often vary from laboratory to laboratory. Be sure to know the standard range of laboratory values for the laboratory in your facility.

TABLE 28-4 **Laboratory Tests to Screen for Infection**

LABORATORY VALUE	NORMAL (ADULT) VALUES	INDICATION OF INFECTION
White blood cell (WBC) count	5000-10,000/mm^3	Increased in acute infection, decreased in certain viral or overwhelming infections
Erythrocyte sedimentation rate	Up to 15 mm/hr for men and 20 mm/hr for women	Elevated in presence of inflammatory process
Iron level	60-90 g/100 mL	Decreased in chronic infection
Cultures of urine and blood	Normally sterile, without microorganism growth	Presence of infectious microorganism growth
Cultures and Gram stain of wound, sputum, and throat	No WBCs on Gram stain, possible normal flora	Presence of infectious microorganism growth and WBCs on Gram stain
Differential Count (Percentage of Each Type of White Blood Cell)		
Neutrophils	55%-70%	Increased in acute **suppurative** (pus-forming) infection, decreased in overwhelming bacterial infection (older adult)
Lymphocytes	20%-40%	Increased in chronic bacterial and viral infection, decreased in sepsis
Monocytes	5%-10%	Increased in protozoan, rickettsial, and tuberculosis infections
Eosinophils	1%-4%	Increased in parasitic infection
Basophils	0.5%-1.5%	Normal during infection

BOX 28-6 **NURSING DIAGNOSTIC PROCESS**

Risk for Infection

ASSESSMENT ACTIVITIES	DEFINING CHARACTERISTICS
Check results of laboratory tests.	WBC count 5000/mm^3
Review current medications.	Patient receiving antibiotics and oral antidiabetic medications
Identify potential sites of infection.	IV catheter in right forearm, in place for 3 days Foley catheter draining cloudy amber-colored urine

IV, Intravenous; *WBC,* white blood cell.

NURSING DIAGNOSIS

During assessment gather objective data such as inspection of an open incision or a reduced caloric intake record and subjective data such as a patient's complaint of tenderness over a surgical wound site. Review the data carefully, looking for clusters of defining characteristics or risk factors that create a pattern. This pattern suggests a specific nursing diagnosis (Box 28-6). The following are examples of nursing diagnoses that often apply:

- Risk for infection
- Imbalanced nutrition: less than body requirements
- Impaired oral mucous membrane
- Risk for impaired skin integrity
- Social isolation
- Impaired tissue integrity
- Readiness for enhanced immunization status

It is necessary to validate data such as inspecting the integrity of a wound more carefully and to review laboratory findings to confirm a diagnosis. Success in planning appropriate nursing interventions depends on the accuracy of the diagnosis and the ability to meet the patient's needs. This requires an accurate related to factor in the diagnostic statement. For example, minimizing the risk for infection in a patient with a diagnosis of *impaired oral mucous membrane related to mouth breathing* requires proper hygiene measures, including frequent oral care. Minimizing the risk for infection in a patient with a nursing diagnosis of *imbalanced nutrition: less than body requirements related to inability to absorb nutrients* requires good nutritional support and fluid balance. The correct "related to" factor will ensure relevant and appropriate interventions for a patient.

PLANNING

Goals and Outcomes. The patient's care plan is based on each nursing diagnosis and related factor (see the Nursing Care Plan). Develop a plan that sets realistic outcomes so interventions are purposeful, direct, and measurable. When you care for a patient with broken skin who has a nursing diagnosis of *risk for infection,* implement skin and wound care measures to promote healing. The expected outcome of "absence of drainage" sets a target for measuring the patient's improvement. Common goals of care applicable to patients with infection often include the following:

- Preventing exposure to infectious organisms
- Controlling or reducing the extent of infection
- Maintaining resistance to infection
- Verbalizing understanding of infection prevention and control techniques (e.g., hand hygiene)

Patients often have multiple nursing diagnoses that are interrelated, and one diagnosis impacts on another diagnosis. A concept map for Mrs. Andrews helps to show the relationships between multiple nursing diagnoses (Fig. 28-2).

Setting Priorities. Establish priorities for each diagnosis and related goals of care. For example, you are caring for a patient with cancer who develops an open wound and is unable to tolerate solid foods. The priority of administering therapies to promote wound healing such as improved nutritional intake overrides the goal of educating the patient to assume self-care therapies at home. When the patient's condition improves, the priorities change, and patient education becomes an essential intervention.

Teamwork and Collaboration. The development of a care plan includes prevention and infection control practices from multiple disciplines. Select interventions in collaboration with the patient, the family, and others on the health care team such as the dietitian or respiratory therapist. Know the patient's sociocultural

NURSING CARE PLAN

Risk for Infection

ASSESSMENT

Mrs. Andrews has diabetes mellitus and degenerative disk disease. She had surgery on her spine late last night. She is currently experiencing pain along her incision and is having difficulty walking. Cody is the nursing student assigned to care for Mrs. Andrews. During hand-off report, Cody finds out that Mrs. Andrews needs to wear a brace when she is out of bed and is having difficulty turning herself when she is in bed. The physical therapist plans to help Mrs. Andrews transfer into a chair after breakfast.

Assessment Activities	*Findings/Defining Characteristics**
Review Mrs. Andrew's chart for laboratory data that reflects infection (e.g., white blood cell [WBC] count).	The **WBC count is 9500.**
Inspect incision area.	**Incision** edges are slightly pink; edges approximated; no drainage noted.
Review risk factors for infection.	Has had **diabetes mellitus** for past 16 years; states blood sugars have been "poorly controlled" for the past year. Dietary assessment reflects malnutrition preoperatively. Is **taking a glucocorticosteroid,** which reduces inflammation and suppresses the immune system.

***Defining characteristics** are shown in bold type.

NURSING DIAGNOSIS: Risk for infection

PLANNING

Goals	*Expected Outcomes (NOC)†*
	Immune Status
Mrs. Andrews will remain free from symptoms of infection.	Mrs. Andrews will remain afebrile. Mrs. Andrews will have no signs or symptoms of infection (e.g., incision intact; edges approximated; no redness, swelling, or drainage)
	Knowledge: Infection Management
Mrs. Andrews describes ways to prevent infection before discharge.	Mrs. Andrews will identify signs and symptoms of infection by the end of today. Mrs. Andrews will demonstrate appropriate hand hygiene before discharge. Mrs. Andrews will identify who will help assess incisional site when she goes home.

†Outcome classification labels from Moorhead S et al: *Nursing outcomes classification (NOC),* ed 4, St Louis, 2008, Mosby.

INTERVENTIONS (NIC)‡	RATIONALE
Infection Protection	
Teach Mrs. Andrews and family how to perform hand hygiene correctly.	Meticulous hand hygiene reduces bacterial counts on the hands (Larson, 2005). Patient can easily come in contact with organisms in the environment that can cause infection.
Instruct Mrs. Andrews to report the following to the caregiver: temperature greater than 38° C (100° F), persistent pain or redness, swelling and drainage from incision.	Signs and symptoms indicate infection.
Help Mrs. Andrews identify a family member to check the incision until it is healed, and teach the family member signs and symptoms of infection.	Mrs. Andrews will be unable to visualize incision since it is on her back; she will need a family member to help monitor healing of the surgical site.

‡Intervention classification labels from Bulecheck GM, Butcher HK, and Dochterman JM: *Nursing interventions classification (NIC),* ed 5, St Louis, 2008, Mosby,

EVALUATION

Nursing Actions	*Patient Response/Finding*	*Achievement of Outcome*
Compare Mrs. Andrews's body temperature with baseline.	Mrs. Andrews remains afebrile and has no drainage from incision.	Mrs. Andrews has no active infection at this time.
Ask Mrs. Andrews to describe signs and symptoms to report to health care provider.	Mrs. Andrews able to identify temperature range to report. Unable to identify signs of wound infection.	Mrs. Andrews has partial understanding of signs and symptoms to report. Will require additional instruction. Offer information sheet.
Observe for signs of infection at incisional site (e.g., redness, warmth, and wound discharge).	Incision shows no signs of infection.	Incision is showing signs of healing.

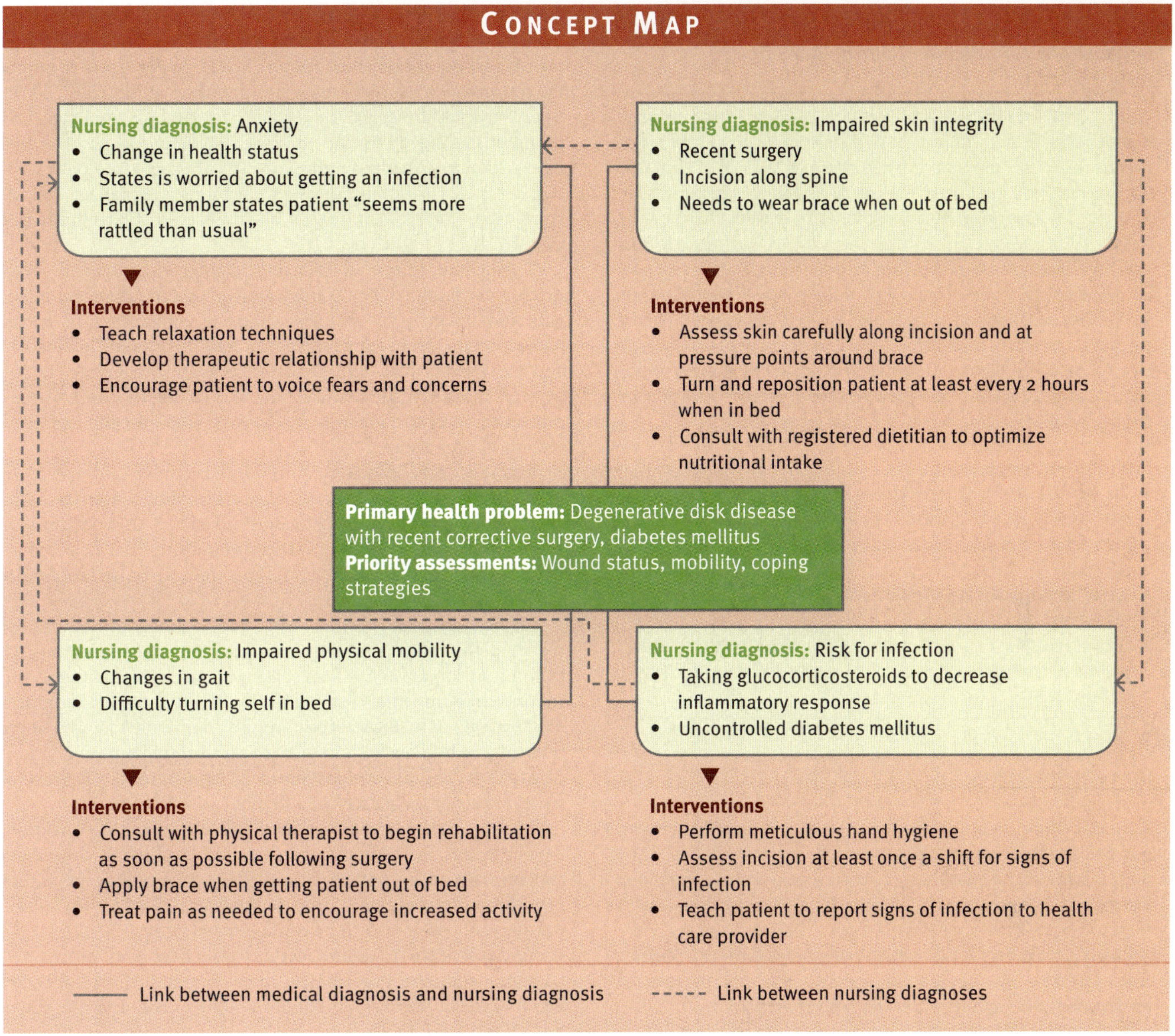
CONCEPT MAP
Nursing diagnosis: Anxiety
• Change in health status
• States is worried about getting an infection
• Family member states patient "seems more rattled than usual"
Interventions
• Teach relaxation techniques
• Develop therapeutic relationship with patient
• Encourage patient to voice fears and concerns
Nursing diagnosis: Impaired skin integrity
• Recent surgery
• Incision along spine
• Needs to wear brace when out of bed
Interventions
• Assess skin carefully along incision and at pressure points around brace
• Turn and reposition patient at least every 2 hours when in bed
• Consult with registered dietitian to optimize nutritional intake
Primary health problem: Degenerative disk disease with recent corrective surgery, diabetes mellitus
Priority assessments: Wound status, mobility, coping strategies
Nursing diagnosis: Impaired physical mobility
• Changes in gait
• Difficulty turning self in bed
Interventions
• Consult with physical therapist to begin rehabilitation as soon as possible following surgery
• Apply brace when getting patient out of bed
• Treat pain as needed to encourage increased activity
Nursing diagnosis: Risk for infection
• Taking glucocorticosteroids to decrease inflammatory response
• Uncontrolled diabetes mellitus
Interventions
• Perform meticulous hand hygiene
• Assess incision at least once a shift for signs of infection
• Teach patient to report signs of infection to health care provider
Link between medical diagnosis and nursing diagnosis
Link between nursing diagnoses

FIG. 28-2 Concept map for Mrs. Andrews.

preferences to help you in identifying the most appropriate types of interventions (Box 28-7). In addition, consult with an expert in infection control in planning the patient's care. Before discharge consult with case management to complete a home assessment and identify home health needs. Case managers work with the patient, family, and home care services to ensure that a safe discharge plan is in place.

When care continues into the patient's home, the home care nurse plans to ensure that the home environment supports good infection prevention and control practices. For example, if a patient does not have running water yet requires wound care, even simple hand hygiene with soap and water is difficult to achieve. Home health nurses instruct patients to perform hand hygiene with either bottled water and soap or alcohol-based hand products.

IMPLEMENTATION

By identifying and assessing a patient's risk factors and implementing appropriate measures, you can effectively reduce the risk of infection.

Health Promotion. Use your critical thinking skills to prevent an infection from developing or spreading. In the home and community settings, strengthen the defenses of a potential host against infection. Nutrition support, rest, maintenance of physiological protective mechanisms, and recommended immunizations protect patients. For example, an annual vaccination to protect against influenza is an important element of risk reduction.

In health care settings, implement procedures to minimize the numbers and kinds of organisms that are transmitted. Eliminating reservoirs of infection, controlling ports of exit and entry, and avoiding actions that transmit microorganisms prevent bacteria from finding a new site in which to grow. Proper use of sterile supplies, barrier precautions, standard precautions, transmission-based precautions, and hand hygiene are examples of methods to control the spread of microorganisms.

Having an infection prevention and control conscience helps you apply principles of medical and surgical asepsis. When a patient develops an infection, implement techniques and procedures to reduce the opportunity for health care personnel and other patients to be exposed to the infection. Patients with

BOX 28-7 CULTURAL ASPECTS OF CARE

Implications for Infection Control–AIDS in New York City

Various cultural and religious beliefs or practices influence patients' decisions to seek treatment for an infection or to use methods to prevent infections. One example is how sociocultural factors affect the residents of New York City who seek AIDS care. Recent research shows that HIV infection rates in New York City are significantly higher (perhaps by as much as 40%) when compared with other parts of the United States. The virus has spread in New York City at three times the national rate, making it evident that HIV education and prevention efforts are not effectively reaching New Yorkers. Auerbach and Beckerman (2010) report on the findings of a study that sought to identify the unique sociocultural needs of New York City residents who seek HIV/AIDS care. Key survey questions were aimed at identifying who receives HIV testing and why, what HIV education services were reported as being most effective, and the unique sociocultural obstacles to receiving HIV testing.

Implications for Practice

- The most helpful HIV education occurred in support groups, and the second most helpful was reading material offered in community-based settings.
- Most residents choose to get tested under the direct advice of a physician.
- Latinos tend to hold more HIV/AIDS stigma than their African-American counterparts.
- Culturally sensitive care is required to identify unique approaches to help patients be responsive to preventive care approaches, such as following safe sex habits.

Building Competency in Patient-Centered Care Mrs. Andrews was discharged home on the third postoperative day. Two weeks later she told her family that she was having increased pain in her back. She stated that she was not always wearing her back brace as instructed at the time of surgery because "it makes me sweat and itch." When she wears the brace, she frequently wipes her incision with a handkerchief to remove the perspiration and scratches it to ease the itching. Describe how to assess this patient's condition more thoroughly using a patient-centered approach.

Answers to questions can be found on the Evolve website.

communicable diseases often require specific isolation precautions to break the chain of infection.

Acute Care. Treatment of an infectious process includes eliminating the infectious organisms and supporting the patient's defenses. To identify the causative organism, the nurse collects specimens of body fluids such as sputum or drainage from infected body sites for cultures. When the disease process or causative organism is identified, the health care provider prescribes the most effective treatment.

Systemic infections require measures to prevent complications of fever (see Chapter 29). Maintaining intake of fluids prevents dehydration resulting from diaphoresis. The patient's increased metabolic rate requires an adequate nutritional intake. Rest preserves energy for the healing process.

Localized infections often require measures to assist removal of debris to promote healing. You apply principles of wound care to remove infected drainage from wound sites and support the integrity of healing wounds. When changing a dressing, wear a mask and goggles or a mask with a face shield if splashing or spraying with blood or body fluids is anticipated. Apply gloves to reduce the transmission of microorganisms into the wound (CDC, 2007). Apply special dressings to facilitate removal of drainage and promote healing of wound margins. Sometimes a surgeon will insert drainage tubes to remove infected drainage from body cavities. Use medical and surgical aseptic techniques to manage wounds and ensure correct handling of all drainage or body fluids (see Chapter 48).

During the course of infection, support the patient's body defense mechanisms. For example, if a patient has diarrhea, maintain skin integrity by frequent cleansing, application of a skin barrier cream, and frequent repositioning to prevent breakdown and the entrance of additional microorganisms. Other routine hygiene measures such as cleaning the oral cavity and bathing protect the skin and mucous membranes from invasion and overgrowth of organisms.

Asepsis. Base efforts to minimize the onset and spread of infection on the principles of aseptic technique. **Asepsis** is the absence of pathogenic (disease-producing) microorganisms. Aseptic technique refers to practices/procedures that help reduce the risk for infection. The two types of aseptic technique are medical and surgical asepsis.

Medical asepsis, or clean technique, includes procedures for reducing the number of organisms present and preventing the transfer of organisms. Hand hygiene, barrier techniques, and routine environmental cleaning are examples of medical asepsis.

Principles of medical asepsis are also commonly followed in the home; hand hygiene with soap and water before preparing food is an example. It is also important to include cultural, religious, or social beliefs of the patient and family.

After an object becomes unsterile or unclean, it is considered contaminated. In medical asepsis an area or object is considered contaminated if it contains or is suspected of containing pathogens. For example, a used bedpan, the over-bed table, and a used dressing are considered to be contaminated items.

You will learn to follow certain principles and procedures, including **standard precautions,** to prevent and control infection and its spread. Standard precautions apply to contact with blood, body fluid, nonintact skin, and mucous membranes from all patients. These precautions protect the patient and provide protection for the health care worker. A major component of patient and worker protection is hand hygiene (Skill 28-1, pp. 425-427). **Hand hygiene** includes using an instant alcohol hand antiseptic before and after providing patient care, washing hands with soap and water when they are visibly soiled, and performing a surgical scrub. **Handwashing** is the act of washing hands with soap and water, followed by rinsing under a stream of water for 15 seconds (CDC, 2002). The friction of rubbing hands together removes soil and transient organisms from the hands.

Contaminated hands of health care workers are a primary source of infection transmission in health care settings. It is recommended that health care workers have well-manicured nails and refrain from wearing artificial nails (Box 28-8) to reduce microorganism transmission. Transmission of infection occurs very easily. For example, you are performing a dressing change, and the patient's roommate asks for assistance with a blocked IV line. If you do not perform hand hygiene before handling the IV line, you transfer organisms from the patient's wound to the roommate's IV site. TJC has identified compliance with proper hand hygiene as a National Patient Safety Goal (TJC, 2011).

BOX 28-8 EVIDENCE-BASED PRACTICE

Pathogens and Artificial Fingernails

PICO Question: What are the bacterial counts on the hands of health care workers who wear artificial nails versus natural nails?

Evidence Summary

The effectiveness of hand hygiene is reduced by type and length of fingernails. Evidence shows health care workers wearing artificial nails carry more pathogenic organisms, especially gram-negative organisms and yeast, on their fingertips and at the junction of natural nail and the artificial nail. Studies also show that health care workers with chipped nail polish or artificial nails have higher numbers of bacteria on their fingertips than those without artificial nails (Rothrock, 2006). For this reason the Centers for Disease Control (CDC) hand hygiene guideline recommends that artificial nails and extenders not be worn when working with high-risk patients (CDC, 2002). In response to this recommendation, health care providers prohibit health care workers who provide direct patient care from wearing artificial nails (Rothrock, 2006; CDC 2002).

The American Association of Operating Room Nurses (AORN) also recommends prohibiting the wearing of artificial nails and extenders because their presence negatively affects the effectiveness of the surgical scrub (AORN, 2007).

The Joint Commission (TJC) listed the reduction of health care–associated infections as a National Patient Safety Goal 7 in 2007. Referring to the CDC's hand hygiene guideline of 2002, the TJC cites that avoiding the wearing of artificial nails is a category 1A recommendation. Category 1A recommendations are those backed by strong evidentiary support.

Application to Nursing Practice

- Do not wear artificial nails or extenders when performing patient care (CDC, 2002).
- Keep natural nails clean, well manicured at ¼ inch long, and free of nail gels and acrylic products.

The use of alcohol-based hand rubs is recommended by the CDC (2002) to improve hand hygiene practices, protect health care worker's hands, and reduce transmission of pathogens to patients and personnel in health care settings. Alcohols have excellent germicidal activity and are as effective as soap and water.

The CDC (2002; WHO, 2009) recommends the following:

1. When hands are visibly dirty, when soiled with blood or other body fluids, before eating, and after using the toilet, wash hands with water and either a nonantimicrobial or antimicrobial soap.
2. Wash hands if exposed to spore-forming organisms such as *Clostridium difficile* or *Bacillus anthracis.*
3. If hands are not visibly soiled (WHO, 2009), use an alcohol-based waterless antiseptic agent for routinely decontaminating hands in the following clinical situations:
   a. Before, after, and between direct patient contact (e.g., taking a pulse, lifting a patient, performing a procedure)
   b. After contact with body fluids or excretions, mucous membranes, nonintact skin, or wound dressings
   c. When moving from a contaminated to a clean body site during patient care
   d. After contact with inanimate surfaces or objects in the patient's room (e.g., over-bed table, bed linen, IV pump)
   e. Before caring for patients with severe neutropenia or other forms of severe immune suppression
   f. Before putting on sterile gloves and before inserting indwelling urinary catheters, peripheral vascular catheters, or other invasive devices
   g. After removing gloves

Instruct patients and visitors about the proper technique and times for hand hygiene. Teaching hand hygiene is particularly important if health care is to continue at home. Patients need to wash their hands before eating or handling food; after handling contaminated equipment, linen, or organic material; and after elimination. Encourage visitors to wash their hands before eating or handling food; after coming in contact with infected patients; and after handling contaminated equipment, patient furniture, or organic material (Gould et al., 2011).

You are responsible for providing the patient with a safe environment. Many hospitals are encouraging patients to follow the recommendations of The Joint Commission's "Speak Up" campaign. The Joint Commission, together with the Centers for Medicare and Medicaid Services, launched a national campaign in 2002 to urge patients to take a role in preventing health care errors by becoming active, involved, and informed participants on the health care team. The program features brochures, posters, and buttons on a variety of patient safety topics. One recommendation is to have patients speak up to be sure the health care provider has cleaned his or her hands or wears gloves.

The effectiveness of infection prevention practices depends on the conscientiousness and consistency in using effective aseptic technique by all health care providers. It is human nature to forget key procedural steps or, when hurried, to take shortcuts that break aseptic procedures. However, failure to comply with basic procedures places the patient at risk for an infection that can seriously impair recovery or lead to death.

Cleaning, Disinfection, and Sterilization. Proper cleaning, disinfection, and sterilization of contaminated objects significantly reduce and often eliminate microorganisms. In health care facilities a sterile processing department is responsible for the disinfection and sterilization of reusable supplies and equipment. However, in the home care setting sometimes the nurse has to perform these functions. Many principles of cleaning and disinfection also apply to the home.

Cleaning. Cleaning is the removal of all soil (e.g., organic and inorganic material) from objects and surfaces (Rutala and Weber, 2008, 2009). Generally cleaning involves use of water and mechanical action with detergents or enzymatic products. When an object comes in contact with an infectious or potentially infectious material, it is contaminated. If the object is disposable, it is discarded. Reusable objects need to be cleaned thoroughly before reuse and then either disinfected or sterilized according to manufacturer recommendations. Failure to follow manufacturer recommendations transfers liability from the manufacturer to the health care facility or agency if an infection results from improper processing.

Apply protective eyewear (or a face shield) and utility (dishwashing style) gloves when cleaning equipment that is soiled by organic material such as blood, fecal matter, mucus, or pus. Protective barriers provide protection from potentially infectious organisms. A brush and detergent or soap are necessary for cleaning. The following steps ensure that an object is clean:

1. Rinse contaminated object or article with cold running water to remove organic material. Hot water causes the protein in organic material to coagulate and stick to objects, making removal difficult.
2. After rinsing, wash the object with soap and warm water. Soap or detergent reduces the surface tension of water and

emulsifies dirt or remaining material. Rinse the object thoroughly.
3. Use a brush to remove dirt or material in grooves or seams. Friction dislodges contaminated material for easy removal. Open hinged items for cleaning.
4. Rinse the object in warm water.
5. Dry the object and prepare it for disinfection or sterilization if indicated by classification of the item—critical, semicritical, or noncritical.
6. The brush, gloves, and sink used to clean the equipment are considered contaminated and are cleaned and dried according to policy.

Disinfection and Sterilization. **Disinfection** describes a process that eliminates many or all microorganisms, with the exception of bacterial spores, from inanimate objects (Rutala and Weber, 2008, 2009). There are two types of disinfection: the disinfection of surfaces and high-level disinfection, which is required for some patient care items such as endoscopes and bronchoscopes. You accomplish disinfection using a chemical disinfectant or wet pasteurization (used for respiratory therapy equipment). Examples of disinfectants are alcohols, chlorines, glutaraldehydes, hydrogen peroxide, and phenols. Glutaraldehydes are caustic and toxic to tissues and pose a potential health risk. **Sterilization** is the complete elimination or destruction of all microorganisms, including spores. Steam under pressure, ethylene oxide (ETO) gas, hydrogen peroxide plasma, and chemicals are the most common sterilizing agents. ETO poses a potential health risk to staff processing with this agent, and exposure must be monitored.

The decision to clean, clean and disinfect, or sterilize depends on the intended use of the item. There are three categories of device classification (Box 28-9). Be familiar with the health care facility or agency policy and procedures for cleaning, handling, and delivering care items for eventual disinfection and sterilization. Workers in the central processing area who are specially trained in disinfection and sterilization perform most of the procedures. The following factors influence the efficacy of the disinfecting or sterilizing method:

- *Concentration of solution and duration of contact*—A weakened concentration or shortened exposure time lessens its effectiveness.
- *Type and number of pathogens*—The greater the number of pathogens on an object, the longer the required disinfecting time.
- *Surface areas to treat*—All dirty surfaces and areas need to be fully exposed to disinfecting and sterilizing agents. The type of surface is an important factor. Is the surface porous or nonporous?
- *Temperature of the environment*—Disinfectants tend to work best at room temperature.
- *Presence of soap*—Soap causes certain disinfectants to be ineffective. Thorough rinsing of an object is necessary before disinfecting.
- *Presence of organic materials*—Disinfectants become inactivated unless blood, saliva, pus, or body excretions are washed off.

Table 28-5 lists processes for disinfection and sterilization and their characteristics. Some delicate instruments requiring sterilization cannot tolerate steam and must be processed using gas or plasma.

Infection Prevention and Control—Patient Safety. Effective prevention and control of infection requires you to remain aware of the modes of transmission and ways to control them (Box 28-10). In the hospital, home, or extended care facility a patient needs a personal set of care items. Sharing bedpans, urinals, bath basins, and eating utensils easily leads to cross-infection. In facilities where health care–associated diarrhea occurs, electronic thermometers are not recommended for rectal temperatures. You usually use oral or tympanic thermometers to assess temperature (Ackley and Ladwig, 2011). Do not use electronic thermometers for patients on contact isolation.

Always be careful when handling exudate such as urine, feces, emesis, and blood. Contaminated fluids easily splash while being discarded in toilets or hoppers. These containers need to be emptied at water level to reduce the risk of splash or splatter, and gloves and protective eyewear are worn. Appropriately dispose of disposable soiled items in trash bags. Dispose of items contaminated with large amounts of blood in biohazard bags. Check the location of the biohazard bags because it varies depending on the health care facility. Handle laboratory specimens from all patients as if they were infectious and place them in designated biohazard containers or bags for transport or disposal.

Even though there is no science to show that medical waste poses a health risk, you need to be aware of the state regulations for the handling and disposal of medical (infectious) waste. Occupational Safety and Health Administration (OSHA) regulations address the handling and disposal of blood and body fluids

BOX 28-9 CATEGORIES FOR STERILIZATION, DISINFECTION, AND CLEANING

Critical Items

Items that enter sterile tissue or the vascular system present a high risk of infection if they are contaminated with microorganisms, especially bacterial spores. *Critical items* must be *sterile*. These items include:

- Surgical instruments
- Cardiac or intravascular catheters
- Urinary catheters
- Implants

Semicritical Items

Items that come in contact with mucous membranes or nonintact skin also present a risk. These objects must be free of all microorganisms (except bacterial spores). *Semicritical items* must be *high-level disinfected (HLD)* or *sterilized*. These items include:

- Respiratory and anesthesia equipment
- Endoscopes
- Endotracheal tubes
- Gastrointestinal endoscopes
- Diaphragm fitting rings

After rinsing, dry items and store in a manner to protect from damage and contamination.

Noncritical Items

Items that come in contact with intact skin but not mucous membranes must be clean. *Noncritical items* must be *disinfected*. These items include:

- Bedpans
- Blood pressure cuffs
- Bed rails
- Linens
- Stethoscopes
- Bedside trays and patient furniture
- Food utensils

TABLE 28-5 Examples of Disinfection and Sterilization Processes

CHARACTERISTICS	EXAMPLES OF USE
Moist Heat	
Steam is moist heat under pressure. When exposed to high pressure, water vapor reaches temperature above boiling point to kill pathogens and spores.	Autoclave sterilizes heat-tolerant surgical instruments and semicritical patient care items.
Chemical Sterilants—High-Level Disinfection (HLD)	
A number of chemical disinfectants are used in health care. These include alcohols, chlorines, formaldehyde, glutaraldehyde, hydrogen peroxide, iodophors, phenolics, and quaternary ammonium compounds. Each product performs in a unique manner and is used for a specific purpose.	Chemicals disinfect heat-sensitive instruments and equipment such as endoscopes, respiratory therapy equipment.
Ethylene Oxide (ETO) Gas	
This gas destroys spores and microorganisms by altering metabolic processes of cells. Fumes are released within an autoclave-like chamber. Ethylene oxide gas is toxic to humans, and aeration time varies with products.	This gas sterilizes most medical materials.
Boiling Water	
Boiling is least expensive for use in home. Bacterial spores and some viruses resist boiling. It is not used in health care facilities.	Commonly used in the home for items such as urinary catheters, suction tubes, and drainage collection devices.

that potentially pose a risk for the transmission of bloodborne pathogens. These regulations defer to state laws and regulations (OSHA, 2001a).

To control organisms exiting via the respiratory tract, cover your mouth or nose when coughing or sneezing. Teach patients, health care staff, patient's families, and visitors respiratory hygiene or **cough etiquette** (Table 28-6). The use of posters and written material explaining cough etiquette to learners is beneficial. Cough etiquette has become more important because of concerns for transmission of respiratory infections such as *Mycobacterium tuberculosis,* severe acute respiratory syndrome (SARS), and H1N1 influenza (CDC, 2005a, 2007, 2010b). The elements of a respiratory hygiene or cough etiquette include (1) covering your nose/mouth with a tissue when you cough and promptly disposing of the contaminated tissue; (2) placing a surgical mask on a patient if it does not compromise respiratory function or is applicable, which may not be feasible in pediatric populations; (3) hand hygiene after contact with contaminated respiratory secretions; and (4) spatial separation greater than 3 feet from persons with respiratory infections (CDC, 2007).

Health care personnel with upper respiratory tract infections are often placed on work restriction. Working when ill poses an additional risk to patients and co-workers. Work restriction for non–work-related illness requires the use of sick time. Work-related illness or exposures are covered by workers' compensation. Employee health and infection prevention and control services are often responsible for ensuring compliance with these guidelines.

To prevent transmission of microorganisms through indirect contact, you keep soiled items and equipment from touching your clothing. A common error is to carry dirty linen in the arms against the uniform. Use fluid-resistant linen bags or carry soiled linen with hands held out from the body. Cover laundry hampers and empty them before they become overloaded.

Many measures that control the exit of microorganisms likewise control the entrance of pathogens. Maintaining the integrity of skin and mucous membranes reduces the chances of microorganisms reaching a host. Keep the patient's skin well lubricated by using lotion as appropriate. Patients who are immobilized and debilitated are particularly susceptible to skin breakdown. Do not

BOX 28-10 INFECTION PREVENTION AND CONTROL TO REDUCE RESERVOIRS OF INFECTION

Bathing
- Use soap and water to remove drainage, dried secretions, or excess perspiration.

Dressing Changes
- Change dressings that become wet and/or soiled (see Chapter 48).

Contaminated Articles
- Place tissues, soiled dressings, or soiled linen in fluid-resistant bags for proper disposal.

Contaminated Sharps
- Place all needles, safety needles, and needleless systems into puncture-proof containers, which should be located at the site of use. Federal law requires the use of needle-safe technology. Blood tube holders are single use only (OSHA: Needlestick Safety Prevention Act of 2000, 2001b).

Bedside Unit
- Keep table surfaces clean and dry.

Bottled Solutions
- Do not leave bottled solutions open.
- Keep solutions tightly capped.
- Date bottles when opened and discard in 24 hours.

Surgical Wounds
- Keep drainage tubes and collection bags patent to prevent accumulation of serous fluid under the skin surface.

Drainage Bottles and Bags
- Wear gloves and protective eyewear if splashing or spraying with contaminated blood or body fluids is anticipated.
- Empty and dispose of drainage suction bottles according to facility policy.
- Empty all drainage systems on each shift unless otherwise ordered by a physician.
- Never raise a drainage system (e.g., urinary drainage bag) above the level of the site being drained unless it is clamped off.

TABLE 28-6 Centers for Disease Control and Prevention Isolation Guidelines

The CDC (2002; WHO, 2009) recommends the following:

1. When hands are visibly dirty, when soiled with blood or other body fluids, before eating, and after using the toilet, wash hands with either a nonantimicrobial soap or antimicrobial soap and water.
2. Wash hands if exposed to spore-forming organisms such as *Clostridium difficile* or *Bacillus anthracis.*

Standard Precautions (Tier One) for Use with All Patients

- Standard precautions apply to blood, blood products, all body fluids, secretions, excretions (except sweat), nonintact skin, and mucous membranes.
- Perform hand hygiene before, after, and between direct contact with patients. (Examples of between-contact activities are cleaning hands after a patient care activity, moving to a nonpatient care activity, and cleaning hands again before returning to perform patient contact.)
- Perform hand hygiene after contact with blood, body fluids, mucous membranes, nonintact skin, secretions, excretions or wound dressings; after contact with inanimate surfaces or articles in a patient room; and immediately after gloves are removed.
- When hands are visibly soiled or contaminated with blood or body fluids, wash them with either a nonantimicrobial soap or an antimicrobial soap and water.
- When hands are not visibly soiled or contaminated with blood or body fluids, use an alcohol-based, waterless antiseptic agent to perform hand hygiene (WHO, 2009).
- Wash hands with nonantimicrobial soap and water if contact with spores (e.g., *Clostridium difficile*) is likely to have occurred.
- Do not wear artificial fingernails or extenders if duties include direct contact with patients at high risk for infection and associated adverse outcomes.
- Wear gloves when touching blood, body fluids, secretions, excretions, nonintact skin, mucous membranes, or contaminated items or surfaces is likely. Remove gloves and perform hand hygiene between patient care encounters and when going from a contaminated to a clean body site.
- Wear personal protective equipment when the anticipated patient interaction indicates that contact with blood or body fluids may occur.
- A private room is unnecessary unless the patient's hygiene is unacceptable (e.g., uncontained secretions, excretions, or wound drainage).
- Discard all contaminated sharp instruments and needles in a puncture-resistant container. Health care facilities must make available needleless devices. Any needles should be disposed of uncapped, or a mechanical safety device is activated for recapping.
- Respiratory hygiene/cough etiquette: Have patients cover the nose/mouth when coughing or sneezing; use tissues to contain respiratory secretions and dispose in nearest waste container; perform hand hygiene after contacting respiratory secretions and contaminated objects/materials; contain respiratory secretions with procedure or surgical mask; sit at least 3 feet away from others if coughing.

Transmission-Based Precautions (Tier Two) for Use with Specific Types of Patients

CATEGORY	INFECTION/CONDITION	BARRIER PROTECTION
Airborne precautions (droplet nuclei smaller than 5 microns)	Measles, chickenpox (varicella), disseminated varicella zoster, pulmonary or laryngeal tuberculosis	Private room, negative-pressure airflow of at least 6 to 12 exchanges per hour via high-efficiency particulate air (HEPA) filtration; mask or respiratory protection device, N95 respirator (depending on condition)
Droplet precautions (droplets larger than 5 microns; being within 3 feet of the patient)	Diphtheria (pharyngeal), rubella, streptococcal pharyngitis, pneumonia or scarlet fever in infants and young children, pertussis, mumps, *Mycoplasma* pneumonia, meningococcal pneumonia or sepsis, pneumonic plague	Private room or cohort patients; mask or respirator required (depending on condition) (refer to agency policy)
Contact precautions (direct patient or environmental contact)	Colonization or infection with multidrug-resistant organisms such as VRE and MRSA, *C. difficile*, shigella, and other enteric pathogens; major wound infections; herpes simplex; scabies; varicella zoster (disseminated); respiratory syncytial virus in infants, young children or immunocompromised adults	Private room or cohort patients (see agency policy), gloves, gowns
Protective environment	Allogeneic hematopoietic stem cell transplants	Private room; positive airflow with 12 or more air exchanges per hour; HEPA filtration for incoming air; mask to be worn by patient when out of room during times of construction in area

Modified from Centers for Disease Control and Prevention, Hospital Infection Control Practice Advisory Committee: Guidelines for isolation precautions in hospitals, *MMWR Morb Mortal Wkly Rep* 57/RR-16:39, 2007.
MRSA, Methicillin-resistant *Staphylococcus aureus; VRE,* vancomycin-resistant enterococcus.

position patients on tubes or objects that cause breaks in the skin. Dry, wrinkle-free linen reduces the chances of skin breakdown. It is important to turn and position patients before their skin becomes reddened. Frequent oral hygiene prevents drying of mucous membranes. A water-soluble ointment keeps the patient's lips well lubricated.

After elimination instruct women to clean the rectum and perineum by wiping from the urinary meatus toward the rectum. Cleaning in a direction from the least to the most contaminated area helps reduce genitourinary infections. Meticulous and frequent perineal care is especially important in older adult women who wear disposable incontinence pads.

Another cause for entrance of microorganisms into a host is improper handling and management of urinary catheters and drainage sets (see Chapter 45). Keep the point of connection between a catheter and drainage tube closed and intact. As long as such systems are closed, their contents are considered sterile. Outflow spigots on drainage bags should also remain closed to

BOX 28-11 INFECTION PREVENTION AND CONTROL: PROTECTING THE SUSCEPTIBLE HOST

Protecting Normal Defense Mechanisms

- Regular bathing removes transient microorganisms from the surface of the skin. Lubrication helps keep the skin hydrated and intact.
- Perform regular oral hygiene. Saliva contains enzymes that promote digestion and has a bactericidal action to maintain control of bacteria. Flossing removes tartar and plaque that cause germ infection.
- Maintenance of adequate fluid intake promotes normal urine formation and a resultant outflow of urine to flush the bladder and urethral lining of microorganisms.
- For patients who are physically dependent or immobilized, encourage routine coughing and deep breathing to keep lower airways clear of mucus.
- Encourage proper immunization of children or adult patients who are exposed to certain infectious microorganisms. Children are vaccinated for measles, mumps, rubella, chickenpox, diphtheria, and other vaccine-preventable diseases. Adults receive one booster of tetanus-diphtheria-acellular pertussis (Tdap), annual flu vaccine, and others as recommended by the Centers for Disease Control and Prevention (CDC) (2010a). Older adults should receive pneumococcal vaccine and annual influenza vaccine.

Maintaining Healing Processes

- Promote intake of adequate fluids and a well-balanced diet containing essential proteins, vitamins, carbohydrates, and fats. The nurse also uses measures to increase the patient's appetite.
- Promote a patient's comfort and sleep so energy stores are replaced daily.
- Help the patient learn techniques to reduce stress.

prevent entrance of bacteria. Minimize movement of the catheter at the urethra by stabilizing it with tape or a securing device to reduce chances of microorganisms ascending the urethra into the bladder. Do not share urine-measuring containers among patients. Perform hand hygiene when caring for urinary drainage systems. Sometimes you care for patients with closed drainage systems that collect wound drainage, bile, or other body fluids. Make sure that the site from which a drainage tube exits remains clear of excess moisture or accumulated drainage. Keep all tubing connected throughout use and only open drainage receptacles when it is necessary to discard or measure the volume of drainage (see Chapter 48).

As a nurse you sometimes obtain specimens from drainage tubes or IV tubing ports. Disinfect tubes and ports by scrubbing the surface with alcohol or a chlorhexidine solution for 15 seconds before entering the system.

A final method for reducing the entry of microorganisms is the technique for wound cleaning. The surgical wound is considered to be sterile. To prevent entry of microorganisms into the wound, always clean outward from a wound site. When applying an antiseptic or cleaning with soap and water, wipe around the wound edge first and then clean outward away from the wound (see Chapter 48). Use clean gauze for each revolution around the circumference of the wound. A patient's resistance to infection improves as you protect normal body defenses against infection. Intervene to maintain the normal reparative processes of the body (Box 28-11). Nurses also protect themselves and others through the use of isolation precautions.

The risk of transmitting HAIs or infectious disease among patients is high, especially with an organism such as methicillin-resistant *S. aureus* (MRSA). When a patient has a suspected or known infection, health care workers are alerted and follow infection prevention and control practices. However, they are not always aware that patients have an infection. Body substances such as feces, saliva, mucus, and wound drainage always contain potentially infectious organisms.

Isolation and Isolation Precautions. Isolation is the separation and restriction of movement of ill persons with contagious diseases. Health care facilities are required to have the capability of isolating patients. For example, patients with suspected or confirmed active TB are usually placed in an airborne infection isolation room (CDC, 2007). However, not all communicable diseases require placing a patient in a special private room. You can conduct many isolation practices in standard rooms using barrier precautions.

Barrier precautions include the appropriate use of personal protective equipment (PPE) such as gowns, gloves, masks, eyewear, and other protective devices or clothing. The choice of barriers depends on the task being performed. Barrier protection applies to all patients because every patient has the potential to transmit infection via blood and body fluids and the risk for infection transmission is unknown. The CDC issued new isolation guidelines in 2007 that build on the two-tiered approach established in the 1996 guidelines.

The first and most important tier is standard precautions. The second tier addresses isolation precautions, which are based on the mode of transmission of a disease (see Table 28-6). Isolation precautions are termed *airborne, droplet, contact,* and *protective environment.* The precautions are for patients with highly transmissible pathogens. The protective environment category is designed for patients who have undergone transplants and gene therapy (CDC, 2007).

- *Contact precautions:* Used for direct and indirect contact with patients and their environment. Direct contact refers to the care and handling of contaminated body fluids. An example includes blood or other body fluids from an infected patient that enter the health care worker's body through direct contact with compromised skin or mucous membranes. Indirect contact involves the transfer of an infectious agent through a contaminated intermediate object such as contaminated instruments or hands of health care workers. The health care worker may transmit microorganisms from one patient site to another if hand hygiene is not performed between patients (CDC, 2007).
- *Droplet precautions:* Focus on diseases that are transmitted by large droplets expelled into the air and travel 3 to 6 feet from the patient. Droplet precautions require the wearing of a surgical mask when within 3 feet of the patient, proper hand hygiene, and some dedicated-care equipment. An example is a patient with influenza.
- *Airborne precautions:* Focus on diseases that are transmitted by smaller droplets, which remain in the air for longer periods of time. This requires a specially equipped room with a negative air flow referred to as an *airborne infection isolation room.* Air is not returned to the inside ventilation system but is filtered through a high-efficiency particulate air (HEPA) filter and exhausted directly to the outside. All health care personnel wear an N95 respirator every time they enter the room.
- *Protective environment:* Focuses on a very limited patient population. This form of isolation requires a specialized room with positive airflow. The airflow rate is set at greater

than 12 air exchanges per hour, and all air is filtered through a HEPA filter. Patients are not allowed to have dried or fresh flowers or potted plants in these rooms (CDC, 2007).
- When using the isolation guidelines of the CDC, refer to additional CDC documents to prevent health care–associated aspergillosis and Legionnaires' disease in immunocompromised patients and the spread of multidrug-resistant organisms (CDC, 2007).

Regardless of the type of isolation system, follow these basic principles:
- Use thorough hand hygiene before entering and leaving the room of a patient in isolation.
- Dispose of contaminated supplies and equipment in a manner that prevents spread of microorganisms to other persons as indicated by the mode of transmission of the organism.
- Apply knowledge of a disease process and the mode of infection transmission when using protective barriers.
- Protect all persons who might be exposed during transport of a patient outside the isolation room.

Psychological Implications of Isolation. When a patient requires isolation in a private room, a sense of loneliness sometimes develops because normal social relationships become disrupted. This situation can be psychologically harmful, especially for children. A recent study noted that patients in isolation suffered more depression and anxiety and were less satisfied with their care (Abad et al., 2010). Patients' body images become altered as a result of the infectious process. Some feel unclean, rejected, lonely, or guilty. Infection prevention and control practices further intensify these beliefs of difference or undesirability. Isolation disrupts normal social relationships with visitors and caregivers. Take the opportunity to listen to a patient's concerns or interests. If you rush care or show a lack of interest in a patient's needs, he or she feels rejected and even more isolated.

Before you institute isolation measures, the patient and family need to understand the nature of the disease or condition, the purposes of isolation, and steps for carrying out specific precautions. If they are able to participate in maintaining infection prevention and control practices, the chances of reducing the spread of infection increase. Teach the patient and family to perform hand hygiene and use barrier protection if appropriate. Demonstrate each procedure; be sure to give the patient and family an opportunity for practice. It is also important to explain how infectious organisms are transmitted so the patient and family understand the difference between contaminated and clean objects. Explaining and demonstrating these procedures, especially hand hygiene, helps the family to consistently practice correct hand hygiene and prescribed isolation measures (Gould et al., 2011).

Take measures to improve the patient's sensory stimulation during isolation. Make sure that the room environment is clean and pleasant. Open drapes or shades and remove excess supplies and equipment. Listen to the patient's concerns or interests. Mealtime is a particularly good opportunity for conversation. Providing comfort measures such as repositioning, a back massage, or a warm sponge bath increase physical stimulation. Depending on the patient's condition, encourage him or her to walk around the room or sit up in a chair. Recreational activities such as board games or cards are an option to keep the patient mentally stimulated.

Explain to the family the patient's risk for depression or loneliness (Abad et al., 2010). Encourage visiting family members to avoid expressions or actions that convey revulsion or disgust related to infection prevention and control practices. Discuss ways to provide meaningful stimulation.

The Isolation Environment. Private rooms used for isolation sometimes provide negative-pressure airflow to prevent infectious particles from flowing out of a room to other rooms and the air handling system. Special rooms with positive-pressure airflow are also used for highly susceptible immunocompromised patients such as recipients of transplanted organs. On the door or wall outside the room the nurse posts a card listing precautions for the isolation category in use according to health care facility policy. The card is a handy reference for health care personnel and visitors and alerts anyone who might enter the room accidentally that special precautions must be followed.

The isolation room or an adjoining anteroom needs to contain hand hygiene and PPE supplies. Soap and antiseptic (antimicrobial) solutions need to be available. Personnel and visitors perform hand hygiene before approaching the patient's bedside and again before leaving the room. If toilet facilities are unavailable, there are special procedures for handling portable commodes, bedpans, or urinals.

All patient care rooms, including those used for isolation; contain an impervious bag for soiled or contaminated linen and a trash container with plastic liners. Impervious receptacles prevent transmission of microorganisms by preventing leaking and soiling of the outside surface. A disposable rigid container needs to be available in the room to discard used sharps such as safety needles and syringes.

Remain aware of infection prevention and control techniques while working with patients in protected environments. You need to feel comfortable performing all procedures and yet remain conscious of infection prevention and control principles. Depending on the microorganism and mode of transmission, evaluate which articles or equipment to take into an isolation room. For example, the CDC (2007) recommends the dedicated use of articles such as stethoscopes, sphygmomanometers, or rectal thermometers in the isolation room of a patient infected or colonized with vancomycin-resistant enterococci. Do not use these devices on other patients unless they are first adequately cleaned and disinfected. Box 28-12 describes the procedures to perform when using shared equipment.

Personal Protective Equipment. PPE, specialized clothing or equipment worn by a health care worker for protection against infectious materials (gowns, masks or respirators, protective eyewear, and gloves), should be readily available for personnel performing patient care (CDC, 2004). The equipment to be used is task based.

Gowns. The primary reason for gowning is to prevent soiling clothes during contact with a patient. Gowns or cover-ups protect health care personnel and visitors from coming in contact with infected material and blood or body fluids. Gowns are often required depending on the expected amount of exposure to infectious material. Gowns used for barrier protection are made of a fluid-resistant material. Change gowns immediately if damaged or heavily contaminated. Isolation gowns are disposable or reusable.

Isolation gowns usually open at the back and have ties or snaps at the neck and waist to keep the gown closed and secure. Gowns need to be long enough to cover all outer garments. Long sleeves with tight-fitting cuffs provide added protection. No special technique is required for applying clean gowns as long as they are fastened securely. However, carefully remove gowns to minimize

BOX 28-12 PROCEDURAL GUIDELINES

View Video!

Caring for a Patient on Isolation Precautions

Delegation Considerations

The skill of caring for a patient on isolation precautions can be delegated to nursing assistive personnel (NAP). However, it is the nurse who assesses the patient's status and isolation indications. Instruct NAP about:

- Special precautions regarding individual patient needs such as transportation to diagnostic tests.
- Precautions about bringing equipment into the patient's room

Equipment

Barrier protection determined by type of isolation—gloves, gowns, masks, protective eyewear, or face shield—that may be needed; supplies depend on procedures performed in room; sharps container; disposable blood pressure (BP) cuff

1. Assess isolation indications (e.g., patient's medical history for exposure, laboratory tests, wound drainage).
2. Review agency policies and precautions necessary for the specific isolation system and consider care measures you will perform while in patient's room.
3. Review nurses' notes or speak with colleagues regarding patient's emotional state and adjustment to isolation.
4. Perform hand hygiene and prepare all equipment that you need to take into patient's room. In some cases equipment remains in the room (stethoscope or BP cuff). Decide which isolation equipment is necessary before entering the patient's room. For example, decide if you need a gown and gloves for a patient in contact precautions or a special respirator mask for a patient on airborne precautions.
5. Prepare for entrance into isolation room:
   a. Apply cover gown, being sure that it covers all outer garments. Pull sleeves down to wrist. Tie securely at neck and waist (see illustration).

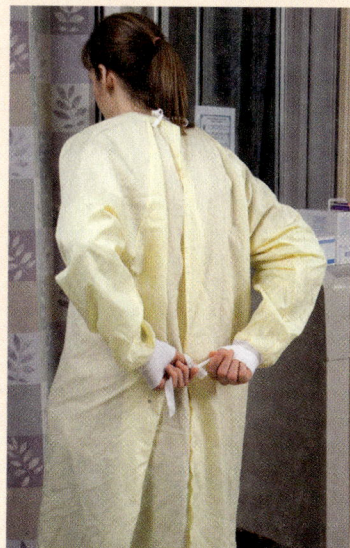

STEP 5a Tie gown at waist.

   b. Apply either surgical mask or respirator around mouth and nose. (Type depends on type of precautions and facility policy.) The nurse must have a medical evaluation and be fit tested before using a respirator (OSHA, 1995).
   c. If needed, apply eyewear or goggles snugly around face and eyes. If prescription glasses are worn, side shield may be used.
   d. Apply clean gloves. (NOTE: Wear unpowdered latex-free gloves if patient has a history of latex allergy.) Wear gloves within gown; bring glove cuffs over edge of gown sleeves (see illustration).

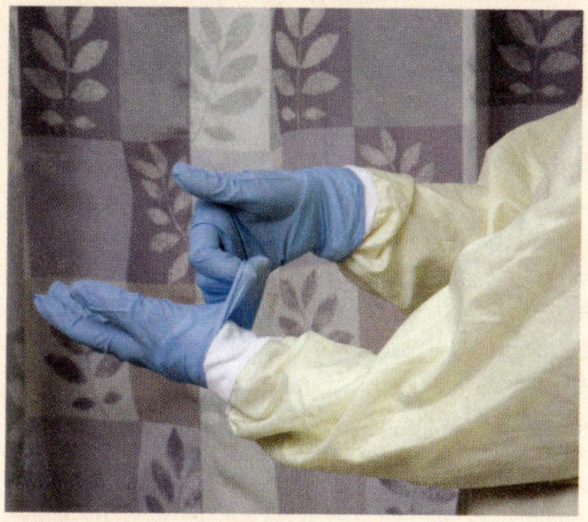

STEP 5d Apply gloves over gown sleeves.

6. Enter patient's room. Arrange supplies and equipment. (If equipment will be removed from room for reuse, place on clean paper towel.)
7. Explain purpose of isolation and necessary precautions to patient and family. Offer opportunity to ask questions. Assess for evidence of emotional problems that can occur from isolation.
8. Assess vital signs.
   a. If patient is infected or colonized with a resistant organism (e.g., vancomycin-resistant enterococcus [VRE], methicillin-resistant *Staphylococcus aureus* [MRSA]), equipment remains in room whenever possible. This includes stethoscope and BP cuff.
   b. If stethoscope is to be reused, clean diaphragm or bell with alcohol. Set aside on clean surface.
   c. Use individual electronic or disposable thermometer.

CLINICAL DECISION: If disposable thermometer indicates a fever, assess for other signs/symptoms. Confirm fever using an electronic thermometer (Ackley and Ladwig, 2011).

9. Administer medications (see Chapter 31).
   a. Give oral medication in wrapper or cup.
   b. Dispose of wrapper or cup in plastic-lined receptacle.
   c. Administer injection.
   d. Discard safety needle and syringe or needle into sharps container.
   e. If you are not wearing gloves and hands come into contact with contaminated article or body fluids, perform hand hygiene as soon as possible.
10. Administer hygiene, encouraging patient to discuss questions or concerns about isolation. Provide informal teaching at this time.
   a. Avoid allowing gown to become wet. Carry wash basin out away from gown; avoid leaning against any wet surface.
   b. Remove linen from bed; avoid contact with gown. Place in linen bag according to agency policy.
   c. Remove gloves and perform hand hygiene. Reglove if further care is necessary.
11. Collect specimens.
   a. Place specimen containers on clean paper towel in patient's bathroom. Follow procedure for collecting specimen of body fluids.
   b. Transfer specimen to container without soiling outside of container. Place container in plastic bag and place label on outside of bag or per

Continued

BOX 28-12 PROCEDURAL GUIDELINES

Caring for a Patient on Isolation Precautions—cont'd

facility policy. Label specimen in front of patient (TJC, 2011). Perform hand hygiene and reglove if additional procedures are needed.

12. Dispose of linen and trash bags as they become full.
    a. Use sturdy, moisture-resistant single bags to contain soiled articles. Use double bag if outside of bag is contaminated.
    b. Tie bags securely at top in knot (see illustration).

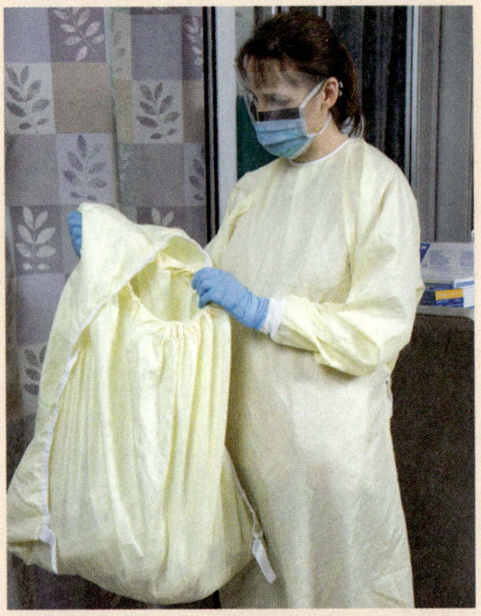

STEP 12b Tie trash bag securely.

13. Remove all reusable equipment. Clean any contaminated surfaces (see health care facility or agency policy).
14. Resupply room as needed. Have a staff member outside isolation room hand you new supplies.
15. Explain to patient when you plan to return to room. Ask whether patient requires any personal care items, books, or magazines.
16. Leave isolation room. The order for removing personal protective equipment (PPE) depends on what was needed for the type of isolation. The sequence listed is based on full PPE being required.
    a. Remove gloves. Remove one glove by grasping cuff and pulling glove inside out over hand. Discard glove. With ungloved hand tuck finger inside cuff of remaining glove and pull it off, inside out (see illustration).

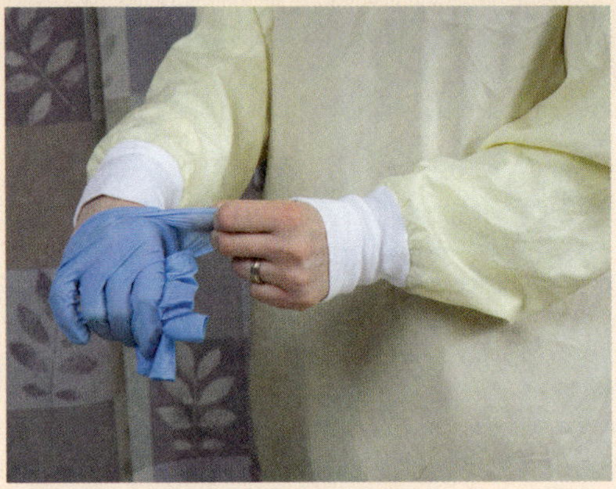

STEP 16a Remove glove.

    b. Remove eyewear/face shield or goggles.
    c. Untie waist and neck strings of gown. Allow gown to fall from shoulders. Remove hands from sleeves without touching outside of gown. Hold gown inside at shoulder seams and fold inside out. Discard in laundry bag if fabric or in trash can if gown is disposable.
    d. Remove mask: If mask loops over your ears, remove from ears and pull away from face. For a tie-on mask, untie *top* mask strings; hold strings; and then untie bottom strings, pull mask away from face, and drop it into trash receptacle. Do not touch outer surface of mask (see illustrations).

CLINICAL DECISION: If a patient is in isolation for airborne precautions, wait to remove mask until after you leave the patient's room and close the door.

    e. Perform hand hygiene.
    f. Leave room and close door if necessary. (Make sure that door is closed if patient is on airborne precautions.)
    g. Dispose of all contaminated supplies and equipment in a manner that prevents spread of microorganisms to other persons (see health care facility or agency policy).

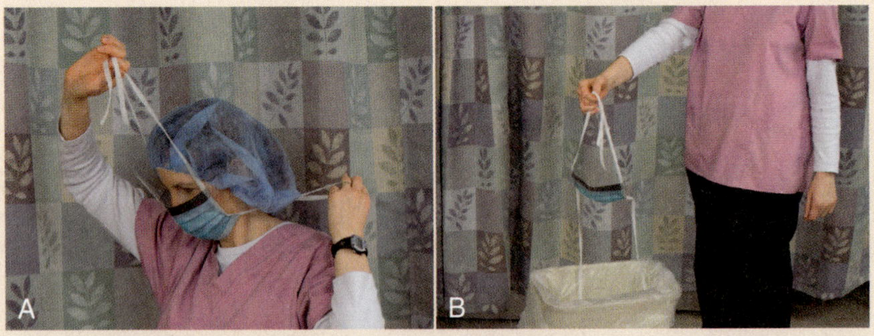

STEP 16d A, Untie top strings of mask. **B,** Drop mask into trash.

contamination of the hands and uniform and discard them after removal.

Respiratory Protection. Wear full-face protection (with eyes, nose, and mouth covered) when you anticipate splashing or spraying of blood or body fluid into the face. Also wear masks when working with a patient placed on airborne or droplet precautions. If the patient is on airborne precautions for TB, apply an OSHA-approved respirator-style mask. The mask protects the nurse from inhaling microorganisms and small-particle droplet nuclei that remain suspended in the air from a patient's respiratory tract. The surgical mask protects a wearer from inhaling large-particle aerosols that travel short distances (3 feet). When caring for patients on droplet or airborne precautions, apply a mask (surgical or respirator) when entering the isolation room.

At times a patient who is susceptible to infection wears a mask to prevent inhalation of pathogens. Patients on droplet or airborne precautions who are transported outside of their rooms need to wear a surgical mask to protect other patients and personnel. Masks prevent transmission of infection by direct contact with mucous membranes (CDC, 2005a). A mask discourages the wearer from touching the eyes, nose, or mouth (Box 28-13).

A properly applied mask fits snugly over the mouth and nose so pathogens and body fluids cannot enter or escape through the sides. If a person wears glasses, the top edge of the mask fits below the glasses so they do not cloud over as the person exhales. Keep talking to a minimum while wearing a mask to reduce respiratory airflow. A mask that has become moist does not provide a barrier to microorganisms and is ineffective. You need to discard it. Never reuse a disposable mask. Warn patients and family members that a mask can cause a sensation of smothering. If family members become uncomfortable, they should leave the room and discard the mask.

Specially fitted respiratory protective devices (N95 respirator masks) are required when caring for patients on airborne precautions, such as patients with known or suspected TB (Fig. 28-3) (CDC, 2005a). The mask must have a higher filtration rating than regular surgical masks and be fitted snugly to prevent leakage around the sides. Be aware of health care facility policy regarding the type of respiratory protective device required. Special fit testing is required to establish the size and ability of the nurse to wear this type of mask (CDC, 2005a).

Eye Protection. Use either special glasses or goggles when performing procedures that generate splash or splatter. Examples of such procedures include irrigation of a large abdominal wound or insertion of an arterial catheter when the nurse assists a health care provider. A nurse who wears prescription glasses uses removable, reusable, or disposable side shields over them (OSHA, 2001a). Eyewear is available in the form of plastic glasses or goggles. The eyewear needs to fit snugly around the face so fluids cannot enter between the face and the glasses.

Gloves. Gloves help to prevent the transmission of pathogens by direct and indirect contact. The CDC notes that you need to wear clean gloves when touching blood, body fluid, secretions, excretions, (except sweat), moist mucous membranes, nonintact skin, and contaminated items or surfaces. Change gloves and perform hand hygiene between tasks and procedures on the same patient after contact with material that contains a high concentration of microorganisms. Remove gloves promptly after use, before touching noncontaminated items and environmental surfaces, and before going to another patient. Perform hand hygiene immediately to avoid transfer of microorganisms to other patients or environments. Because of allergy or sensitivity to latex gloves, facilities provide nonlatex gloves to reduce the incidence of health care providers developing latex allergy or sensitivity. Most facilities are working to become latex free to protect health care providers and patients.

When full PPE is necessary, first perform hand hygiene, then apply a gown, apply mask and eyewear or goggles (as needed), and end with applying gloves. Clean gloves are easy to apply and fit either hand. Pull the cuffs of the glove up over the wrists or over the cuffs of the gown. If you notice a break or tear in a glove while providing care, change gloves. If the nurse does not plan to have more contact with the patient, reapplying gloves is unnecessary. Perform hand hygiene when gloves are removed.

Instruct family members visiting patients on isolation precautions how to apply gloves properly. Demonstrate application of gloves to family members and explain the reason for the use of gloves. Emphasize the importance of performing hand hygiene after removing gloves.

BOX 28-13 PROCEDURAL GUIDELINES

Applying a Surgical Type of Mask

1. Find top edge of mask (some have a thin metal strip along edge). Pliable metal fits snugly against bridge of nose. Others offer an occlusive fit that does not require an adjustment.
2. Hold mask by top two strings or loops. Secure two top ties at top of back of head (see illustration), with ties above ears. (*Alternative:* Slip loops over each ear.)

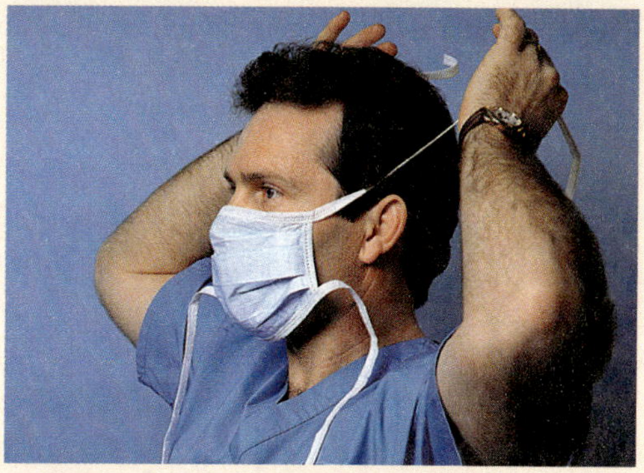

STEP 2 Securing top two ties of a tie-on mask.

3. Tie two lower ties snugly around neck with mask well under chin (see illustration).

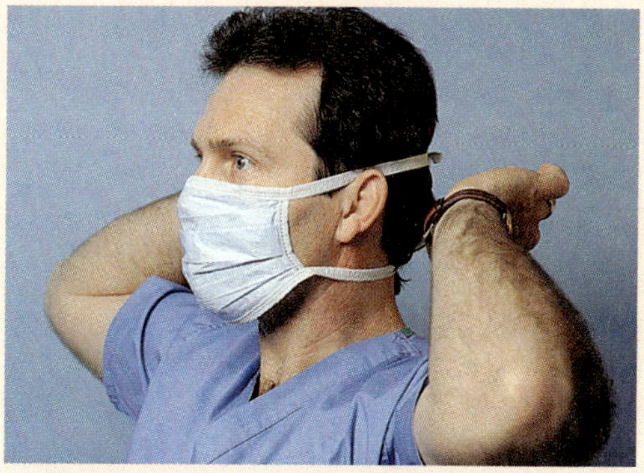

STEP 3 Securing lower ties of a tie-on mask.

4. Gently pinch upper metal band around bridge of nose.

NOTE: Change mask if wet, moist, or contaminated.

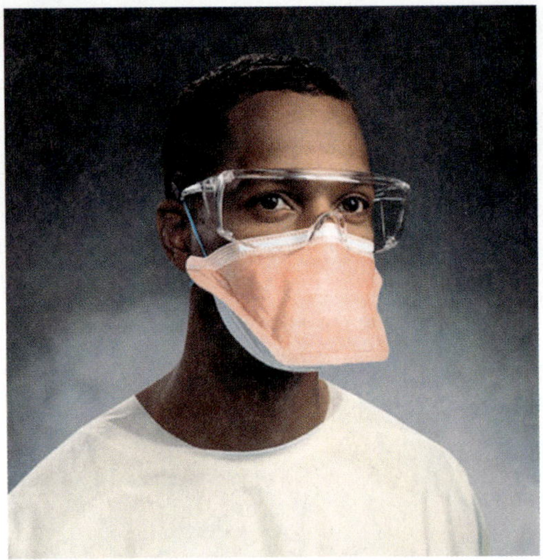

FIG. 28-3 N95 respirator mask with protective eyewear. (Courtesy Kimberly-Clark Health Care, Roswell, Ga.)

Specimen Collection. Many laboratory studies are often necessary when a patient is suspected of having an infectious or communicable disease (Box 28-14). You collect body fluids and secretions suspected of containing infectious organisms for culture and sensitivity tests. After a specimen is sent to a laboratory, the laboratory technologist identifies the microorganisms growing in the culture. Additional test results indicate antibiotics to which the organisms are resistant or sensitive. Sensitivity reports determine which antibiotics used in treatment are effective and need to be ordered for treatment.

You obtain all culture specimens using clean gloves and sterile equipment. Collecting fresh material such as wound drainage from the site of infection ensures that neighboring microbes do not contaminate a specimen. Seal all specimen containers tightly to prevent spillage and contamination of the outside of the container.

Bagging Trash or Linen. Bagging contaminated items prevents accidental exposure of personnel and contamination of the surrounding environment. Double bagging is not recommended. Studies demonstrate that this procedure is not necessary to prevent and control infection (CDC, 2007). The use of a single, intact, standard-size linen bag that is not overfilled and tied securely is adequate to prevent infection transmission. Check the color code of bag that your facility uses for bagging these items.

Transporting Patients. Before transferring patients to wheelchairs or stretchers, give them clean gowns to serve as robes. Patients infected with organisms transmitted by the airborne route normally leave their rooms only for essential purposes such as diagnostic procedures or surgery. When a patient has an airborne infection, he or she must wear a mask when leaving the room. Notify personnel in diagnostic or procedural areas or the operating room of the type of isolation precautions the patient requires. Some patients being transported drain body fluids onto a stretcher or wheelchair. Use an extra layer of sheets to cover the stretcher or seat of the wheelchair. Be sure to clean the equipment with an approved germicide after patient use and before another patient uses the shared equipment.

Role of the Infection Control Professional. An infection control professional is a valuable resource for assisting nurses in controlling HAIs. These professionals are specially trained in infection prevention and control. They are responsible for advising health care personnel regarding infection prevention and control practices and monitoring infections within the hospital. An infection control professional's responsibilities often include:

- Providing staff and patient education on infection prevention and control
- Developing and reviewing infection prevention and control policies and procedures
- Recommending appropriate isolation procedures
- Screening patient records for community-acquired infections that are reportable to the public health department
- Consulting with employee health departments concerning recommendations to prevent and control the spread of infection among personnel, such as TB testing

BOX 28-14 SPECIMEN COLLECTION TECHNIQUES*

View Video!

Ensure that all specimen containers used have the biohazard symbol on the outside (Pagana and Pagana, 2010).

Wound Specimen

Clean site with sterile water or saline before wound specimen collection (see Chapter 48). Apply gloves and use cotton-tipped swab or syringe to collect as much drainage as possible. Have clean test tube or culture tube on clean paper towel. After swabbing center of wound site, grasp collection tube with a paper towel. Carefully insert swab without touching outside of tube. After securing top of tube, transfer tube into biohazard bag for transport and perform hand hygiene.

Blood Specimen *(This procedure is often performed by a laboratory technician.)*

Wearing gloves, use a needle-safe syringe and culture media bottles to collect up to 10 mL of blood per culture bottle (check health care facility or agency policy). After prepping, perform venipuncture at two different sites at two different times (a minimum of 15 to 30 minutes between sets) to decrease likelihood of both specimens being contaminated with skin flora. Place blood culture bottles on a clean paper towel on bedside table or other surface; swab off bottle tops with alcohol. Inject an appropriate and equal amount of blood into the aerobic bottle (first) and anaerobic bottle (second). Transfer specimen into clean, labeled biohazard bag for transport. Remove gloves and perform hand hygiene.

Stool Specimen

Wearing gloves, use clean cup with seal top (need not be sterile) and tongue blade to collect a small amount, approximately 1 inch (2 to 3 cm), of stool. Place cup on clean paper towel in patient's bathroom. Using tongue blade, collect needed amount of feces from patient's bedpan. Transfer feces to cup without touching outside surface of cup. Dispose of tongue blade and place seal on cup. Transfer specimen into clean biohazard bag for transport. Remove gloves and perform hand hygiene.

Urine Specimen

Apply gloves and use sterile cup to collect 1 to 5 mL of urine. Place cup or tube on clean towel in patient's bathroom. If patient has a urinary catheter, use a needleless safety syringe to collect specimen from the sampling port on the catheter (see manufacturer instructions). Instruct patient to follow procedure to obtain a clean voided specimen (see Chapter 45) if not catheterized. Secure top of transfer container, label container in front of patient, and place in a biohazard bag with label attached. Remove gloves and perform hand hygiene.

*Health care facility or agency policies may differ on type of containers and amount of specimen material required.

BOX 28-15 PATIENT TEACHING

Infection Prevention and Control

Objective

- Patient will assume self-care using proper infection prevention and control techniques.

Teaching Strategies

- Instruct patient about cleaning equipment using soap and water and disinfecting with an appropriate disinfectant such as diluted bleach.
- Demonstrate proper hand hygiene, explaining that patient needs to perform before and after all treatments and when infected body fluids are contacted.
- Instruct patient in the signs and symptoms of wound infection and when to notify the health care provider.
- For patients who receive tube feedings at home, explain the importance of preparing enough formula for only 8 hours (commercially prepared) or 4 hours (home prepared). Tell patient that contaminated enteral feeding sometimes causes infections. Rinse feeding bag and tubing with mild soap and water daily and dry.
- Instruct patient to place contaminated dressings and other disposable items containing infectious body fluids in impervious plastic or brown paper bags. Place needles in metal or hard plastic containers such as coffee cans or laundry detergent bottles and tape the openings shut. *Some states have specific requirements for sharps disposal. Check local regulations.*
- Clean noticeably soiled linen separate from other laundry. Wash in warm water with detergent. There are no special recommendations for setting a dryer temperature (CDC, 2007).

Evaluation

- Ask patient or family member to describe techniques used to reduce transmission of infection.
- Have patient demonstrate select techniques.
- Ask patient to explain the risks of infection based on his or her condition.

- Gathering statistics regarding the epidemiology (cause and effect) of health care–associated infections
- Notifying the public health department of incidences of communicable diseases within the facility
- Consulting with all hospital departments to investigate unusual events or clusters of infection
- Monitoring antibiotic-resistant organisms in the institution

Infection Prevention and Control for Hospital Personnel. Health care workers are continually at risk for exposure to infectious microorganisms. OSHA and CDC publish rules, regulations, and guidelines to protect employees from bloodborne pathogens in the workplace. The OSHA regulations and CDC guidelines are incorporated into the policies and procedures of health care institutions and are part of regularly scheduled staff education programs.

Patient Education. Often patients need to learn to use infection prevention and control practices at home (Box 28-15). Preventive technique becomes almost second nature to the nurse who practices it daily. However, the patient is less aware of factors that promote the spread of infection or ways to prevent its transmission. The home environment may not always lend itself to infection prevention and control. Often you help a patient adapt according to the resources available to maintain hygienic techniques. Generally patients in a home care setting have a decreased risk of infection because of decreased exposure to resistant organisms such as those found in a health care facility and fewer invasive procedures. However, it is important to educate patients about infection prevention and control techniques.

Surgical Asepsis. Surgical asepsis or sterile technique prevents contamination of an open wound, serves to isolate the operative area from the unsterile environment, and maintains a sterile field for surgery. Surgical asepsis includes procedures used to eliminate all microorganisms, including pathogens and spores, from an object or area (Rutala and Weber, 2008, 2009). In surgical asepsis an area or object is considered contaminated if touched by any object that is not sterile. It demands the highest level of aseptic technique and requires that all areas be kept free of infectious microorganisms.

Use surgical asepsis in the following situations:

- During procedures that require intentional perforation of the patient's skin such as insertion of IV catheters or central lines
- When the integrity of the skin is broken as a result of trauma, surgical incision, or burns
- During procedures that involve insertion of catheters or surgical instruments into sterile body cavities such as insertion of a urinary catheter

Although surgical asepsis is common in the operating room, labor and delivery area, and major diagnostic areas, you also use surgical aseptic techniques at the patient's bedside (e.g., when inserting IV or urinary catheters, suctioning the tracheobronchial airway, and reapplying sterile dressings). A nurse in an operating room follows a series of steps to maintain sterile technique, including applying a mask, protective eyewear, and a cap; performing a surgical hand scrub; and applying a sterile gown and gloves. In contrast, a nurse performing a dressing change at a patient's bedside only performs hand hygiene and applies sterile gloves. For certain procedures (e.g., changing a central line dressing) the nurse also uses a mask. Regardless of the procedures followed or the setting, the nurse always recognizes the importance of strict adherence to aseptic principles (Iwamoto, 2009).

Patient Preparation. Because surgical asepsis requires exact techniques, you need to have the patient's cooperation. Certain patients fear moving or touching objects during a sterile procedure, whereas others try to assist. Explain how you will perform a procedure and what the patient can do to avoid contaminating sterile items, including the following:

- Avoid sudden movements of body parts covered by sterile drapes.
- Refrain from touching sterile supplies, drapes, or the nurse's gloves and gown.
- Avoid coughing, sneezing, or talking over a sterile area.

Certain sterile procedures last an extended time. The nurse assesses a patient's needs and anticipates factors that may disrupt a procedure. If a patient is in pain, administer ordered analgesics about a half an hour before a sterile procedure begins. Ask a patient if he or she needs to use the bathroom or a bedpan. Often patients have to assume relatively uncomfortable positions during sterile procedures. Help a patient assume the most comfortable position possible. Finally, a patient's condition sometimes results in actions or events that contaminate a sterile field. For example, a patient with a respiratory infection transmits organisms by coughing or talking. Anticipate such a problem and place a surgical mask on him or her before the procedure begins.

Principles of Surgical Asepsis. Performing sterile aseptic procedures requires a work area in which objects can be handled with minimal risk of contamination. A sterile field provides a sterile surface for placement of sterile equipment. It is an area considered free of microorganisms and consists of a sterile kit or tray, a work surface draped with a sterile towel or wrapper, or a table covered with a large sterile drape (Church and Bjerke, 2009). When beginning a surgically aseptic procedure, nurses follow certain principles to ensure maintenance of asepsis. Failure to follow these principles places patients at risk for infection. The following principles are important:

1. *A sterile object remains sterile only when touched by another sterile object.* This principle guides a nurse in placement of sterile objects and how to handle them.
   a. Sterile touching sterile remains sterile (e.g., use sterile gloves or sterile forceps to handle objects on a sterile field).
   b. Sterile touching clean becomes contaminated (e.g., if the tip of a syringe or other sterile object touches the surface of a clean disposable glove, the object is contaminated).
   c. Sterile touching contaminated becomes contaminated (e.g., when a nurse touches a sterile object with an ungloved hand, the object is contaminated).
   d. Sterile state is questionable (e.g., when you find a tear or break in the covering of a sterile object). Discard it regardless of whether the object itself appears untouched.
2. *Only sterile objects may be placed on a sterile field.* All items are properly sterilized before use. Sterile objects are kept in clean, dry storage areas. The package or container holding a sterile object must be intact and dry. A package that is torn, punctured, wet, or open is considered unsterile.
3. *A sterile object or field out of the range of vision or an object held below a person's waist is contaminated.* Nurses never turn their back on a sterile field or a sterile tray or leave it unattended. Contamination can occur accidentally by a dangling piece of clothing, falling hair, or an unknowing patient touching a sterile object. Any object held below waist level is considered contaminated because it cannot be viewed at all times. Keep sterile objects in front with the hands as close together as possible.
4. *A sterile object or field becomes contaminated by prolonged exposure to air.* Avoid activities that create air currents such as excessive movements or rearranging linen after a sterile object or field becomes exposed. When you open sterile packages, it is important to minimize the number of people walking into an area. Microorganisms also travel by droplet through the air. Do not talk, laugh, sneeze, or cough over a sterile field or when gathering and using sterile equipment. When opening sterile packages, hold the item or piece of equipment as close as possible to the sterile field without touching the sterile surface.
5. *When a sterile surface comes in contact with a wet, contaminated surface, the sterile object or field becomes contaminated by capillary action.* If moisture leaks through the protective covering of a sterile package, microorganisms travel to the sterile object. When stored sterile packages become wet, discard the objects immediately or send the equipment for resterilization. When working with a sterile field or tray, you may have to pour sterile solutions. Any spill is a source of contamination unless on a sterile surface that moisture cannot penetrate. Urinary catheterization trays contain sterile supplies that rest in a sterile, plastic container. In contrast, if you place a piece of sterile gauze in its wrapper on a patient's bedside table and the table surface is wet, the gauze is considered contaminated.

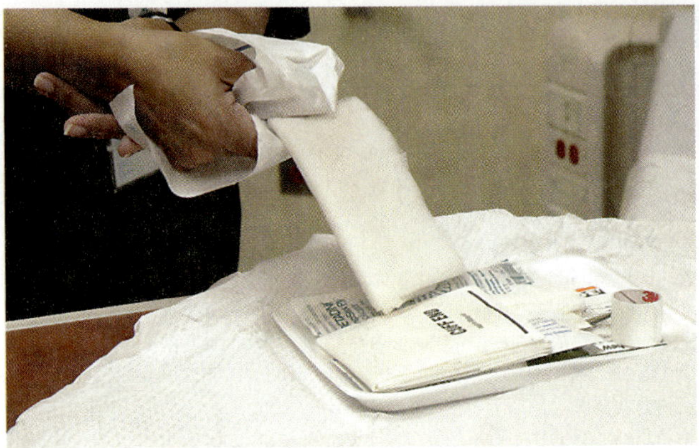

FIG. 28-4 Placing sterile item on sterile field.

6. *Fluid flows in the direction of gravity.* A sterile object becomes contaminated if gravity causes a contaminated liquid to flow over the surface of the object. To avoid contamination during a surgical hand scrub, hold your hands above your elbows. This allows water to flow downward without contaminating your hands and fingers. The principle of water flow by gravity is also the reason for drying from fingers to elbows, with hands held up, after the scrub.
7. *The edges of a sterile field or container are considered to be contaminated.* Frequently you place sterile objects on a sterile towel, drape, or tray (Fig. 28-4). Because the edge of the drape touches an unsterile surface such as a table or bed linen, a 2.5-cm (1-inch) border around the drape is considered contaminated. Objects placed on the sterile field need to be inside this border. The edges of sterile containers become exposed to air after they open and thus are contaminated. After you remove a sterile needle from its protective cap or after you remove forceps from a container, the objects must not touch the edge of the container.

Performing Sterile Procedures. Assemble all of the equipment that will be needed before a procedure. Have a few extra supplies available in case objects accidentally become contaminated. Do not leave a sterile area. Before a sterile procedure, explain each step so the patient can cooperate fully. If an object becomes contaminated during the procedure, do not hesitate to discard it immediately.

Donning and Removing Caps, Masks, and Eyewear. Wear a surgical mask and eyewear without a cap for any sterile procedures on a general nursing unit. Eyewear is worn as a part of standard precautions if there is a risk of fluid or blood splashing into your eyes. For sterile surgical procedures, you first apply a clean cap that covers all of your hair and then the surgical mask and eyewear. A mask must fit snugly around the face and nose. After wearing a mask for several hours, the area over the mouth and nose often becomes moist. Because moisture promotes the growth of microorganisms, change the mask if it becomes moist.

Protective glasses or goggles fit snugly around the forehead and face to fully protect the eyes. Wear eyewear only for procedures that create the risk of body fluids splashing into the eyes. Remove PPE in the following order: gloves, face shield or goggles, gown, and then mask or respirator (CDC, 2005b). After removing all PPE, perform hand hygiene.

Opening Sterile Packages. Sterile items such as syringes, gauze dressings, or catheters are packaged in paper or plastic containers and are impervious to microorganisms as long as they are dry and intact. Some institutions wrap reusable supplies (e.g., operating

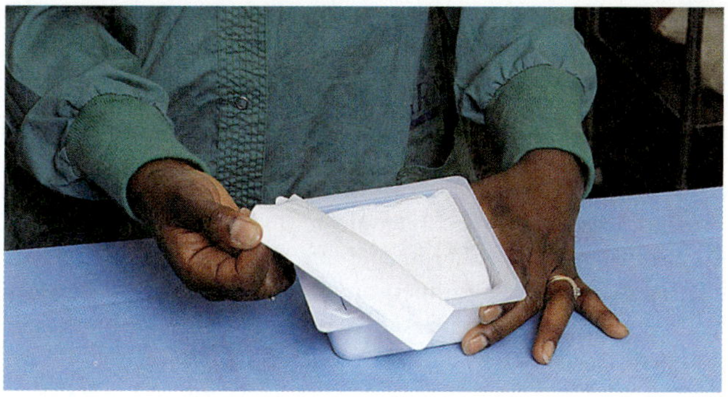

FIG. 28-5 Nurse opens sterile package on work area above waist level.

room instruments) in a double thickness of paper, linen, or muslin. These packages are permeable to steam and thus allow for steam autoclaving. Sterile items are kept in clean, enclosed storage cabinets and separated from dirty equipment.

Sterile supplies have chemical tapes indicating that a sterilization process has taken place. The tapes change color during the process. Failure of the tapes to change color means that the item is not sterile. Health care facilities follow the principles of event-related sterility, a concept that items are considered sterile if the packaging is uncompromised (Jefferson, 2009). Never use a sterile item if the packaging is open or soiled or shows evidence that the package had been wet. Before opening a sterile item, perform hand hygiene. Inspect the supplies for package integrity and sterility and assemble the supplies in the work area such as the bedside table or treatment room before opening packages. A bedside table or countertop provides a large, clean working area for opening items. Keep the work area above waist level. Do not open sterile supplies in a confined space where contamination might occur.

Opening a Sterile Item on a Flat Surface. You must open sterile packages without contaminating the contents. Commercially packaged items are usually designed so you only have to tear away or separate the paper or plastic cover. Hold the item in one hand while pulling the wrapper away with the other (Fig. 28-5). Take care to keep the inner contents sterile before use. You may use a sterile wrapper from a commercial kit or a sterile paper or linen wrapper from an institutional pack to create a sterile field on which to work. Use the inner surface of the package (except for the 1-inch (2.5-cm) border around the edges) as a sterile field to add sterile items. You can grasp the 1-inch border to maneuver the field on a table surface. See Skill 28-2 on pp. 427-431 for the steps to follow in preparing a sterile field.

Opening a Sterile Item While Holding It. To open a small sterile item, hold the package in your nondominant hand while opening the top flap and pulling it away from you. Using the dominant hand, carefully open the sides and innermost flap away from the enclosed sterile item in the same order previously mentioned. You open the item in a hand so you can pass the item to a person wearing sterile gloves or transfer the item to a sterile field.

Preparing a Sterile Field. When performing sterile procedures, you need a sterile work area that provides room for handling and placing of sterile items. A **sterile field** is an area free of microorganisms and prepared to receive sterile items. You prepare the field by using the inner surface of a sterile wrapper as the work surface or by using a sterile drape or dressing tray. After creating the surface for the sterile field, add sterile items by placing them directly on the field or transferring them with a sterile forceps (see Skill 28-2). Discard an object that comes in contact with the 1-inch (2.5-cm) border.

Sometimes you will wear sterile gloves while preparing items on a sterile field. If you do this, you can touch the entire drape, but sterile items must be handed over by an assistant. The gloves cannot touch the wrappers of sterile items.

Pouring Sterile Solutions. Often you have to pour sterile solutions into sterile containers. A bottle containing a sterile solution is sterile on the inside and contaminated on the outside; the neck of the bottle is also contaminated, but the inside of the bottle cap is considered sterile. After you remove the cap or lid, you hold it in your hand or place its sterile side (inside) up on a clean surface. This means that you are able to see the inside of the lid as it rests on the table surface. Never rest a bottle cap or lid on a sterile surface, even though the inside of the cap is sterile. The outer edge of the cap is unsterile and contaminates the surface. Placing a sterile cap down on an unsterile surface increases the chances of the inside of the cap becoming contaminated.

Hold the bottle with its label in the palm of the hand to prevent the possibility of the solution wetting and fading the label. Before pouring the solution into the container, pour a small amount (1 to 2 mL) into a disposable cap or plastic-lined waste receptacle. The discarded solution cleans the lip of the bottle. Keep the edge of the bottle away from the edge or inside of the receiving container. Pour the solution slowly to avoid splashing the underlying drape or field. Never hold the bottle so high above the container that even slow pouring causes splashing. Hold the bottle outside the edge of the sterile field.

Surgical Scrub. Patients undergoing operative procedures are at an increased risk for infection. Nurses working in operating rooms perform surgical hand antisepsis (Skill 28-3, pp. 431-433) to decrease and suppress the growth of skin microorganisms in case of glove tears. For maximum elimination of bacteria, remove all jewelry and keep the nails clean and short. Do not wear artificial nails or extenders because they often hold a greater number of bacteria (AORN, 2007; WHO, 2009). Nurses who have active skin infections, open lesions or cuts, or respiratory infections should be excluded from the surgical team.

During surgical hand antisepsis the nurse scrubs from fingertips to elbows with an antiseptic soap before each operation. The optimum duration of the surgical hand scrub is unclear, although research indicates that it probably depends on the type of antimicrobial product (CDC, 2002). The traditional scrub time in the United States for both the initial and the subsequent scrub is 5 minutes. Follow manufacturer recommendation for scrub solutions. For many years preoperative handwashing protocols required nurses to scrub with a brush. However, this practice can damage the skin. Scrubbing with a disposable sponge or combination sponge-brush reduces bacterial counts on the hands as effectively as scrubbing with a brush. However, several studies suggest that neither a brush nor a sponge is necessary to reduce bacterial counts on the hands, especially when using an alcohol-based product (CDC, 2002).

Applying Sterile Gloves. Sterile gloves are an additional barrier to bacterial transfer. There are two gloving methods: open and closed. Nurses who work on general nursing units use open gloving before procedures such as dressing changes or urinary catheter insertions. The closed-gloving method, which you perform after applying a sterile gown, is practiced in operating rooms and special treatment areas. Skills 28-4 and 28-5 (pp. 434-437) review the steps of each sterile gloving technique. Make sure to select the proper glove size; the glove should not stretch so tightly that it can easily tear, yet it must be tight enough that you can pick up objects easily.

Donning a Sterile Gown. Nurses wear sterile gowns when assisting at the sterile field in the operating room, delivery room, and special treatment areas. It allows the nurse to handle sterile objects and also be comfortable with less risk of contamination. The sterile gown acts as a barrier to decrease shedding of microorganisms from skin surfaces into the air and thus prevents wound contamination. Nurses caring for patients with large open wounds or assisting physicians during major invasive procedures (e.g., inserting an arterial catheter) also wear sterile gowns. The circulating nurse generally does not wear one.

The nurse does not apply a sterile gown until after applying a mask and surgical cap and performing surgical handwashing. He or she picks up the gown from a sterile pack, or an assistant hands the gown to the nurse. Only a certain portion of the gown (i.e., the area from the anterior waist to, but not including, the collar and the anterior surface of the sleeves) is considered sterile. The back of the gown, the area under the arms, the collar, the area below the waist, and the underside of the sleeves are not sterile because the nurse cannot keep these areas in constant view and ensure their sterility. Skill 28-4 reviews the steps for applying a sterile gown.

EVALUATION

Measure the success of infection prevention and control techniques by determining whether you achieved the goals for reducing or preventing infection. Document the patient's response to therapies for infection prevention and control. A clear description of any signs and symptoms of systemic or local infection is necessary to give all nurses a baseline for comparative evaluation.

Through the Patient's Eyes. The patient at risk for infection needs to understand the measures needed to reduce or prevent microorganism growth and spread. Providing patients and/or family members the opportunity to discuss infection prevention and control measures or to demonstrate procedures such as hand hygiene reveals their ability to comply with therapy. Be sure that you understand the patient's perceptions of how infection spreads and how it can affect him or her as you evaluate the results of your instruction. Sometimes patients require new information, or previously instructed information needs reinforcement.

Patient Outcomes. A comparison of the patient's response such as absence of fever or wound infection are examples of expected outcomes for measuring the success of nursing interventions. Observe wounds during dressing changes to determine the degree of wound healing. Monitor patients, especially those at risk, for signs and symptoms of infection. For example, a patient who has undergone a surgical procedure is at risk for infection at the surgical site and other invasive sites such as the venipuncture site or central line sites. In addition, the patient is at risk for a respiratory tract infection as a result of decreased mobility and for a UTI if an indwelling catheter is present. Observe all invasive and surgical sites for swelling, erythema, or purulent drainage. Monitor breath sounds for changes and observe sputum character for change in color or consistency. Review laboratory test results for leukocytes. For example, leukocytosis in the urine often indicates a UTI. The absence of signs or symptoms of infection is the expected outcome of infection prevention and control.

Exposure Issues. Patients and health care personnel, including housekeepers and maintenance personnel, are at risk for acquiring infections from accidental needlesticks. After administering an injection or inserting an IV catheter, place the used needle safety device in a puncture-resistant box (see Chapter 31). Sharps boxes must be at the site of use; this is an OSHA requirement. With the passage of the Needlestick Safety and Prevention Act in 2000 (OSHA, 2001b) and the implementation of safety needle devices, incidence rate of sharps injuries decreased. All sharps must now be either needle safe or needleless. In the past a stray needle lying in bed linen or carelessly thrown into a wastebasket served as a prime source for exposure to bloodborne pathogens. Hepatitis B and C are the infections most commonly transmitted by contaminated needles (Box 28-16). Report any

BOX 28-16 HEPATITIS B VACCINATION AND FOLLOW-UP AFTER HEPATITIS C AND HUMAN IMMUNODEFICIENCY VIRUS EXPOSURE

1. Health care employers shall make available the hepatitis B vaccine and vaccination series to all employees who may have occupational exposures. If an employee declines the vaccine, he or she must sign a declination form. Evaluation and follow-up care is available to all employees who have been exposed.
2. Hepatitis B vaccinations are made available to employees within 10 working days of assignment—this means before starting to provide patient care and after receiving education and training on the vaccine.
3. A blood test (titer) is offered in some facilities 1 to 2 months after completing the three-dose vaccine series (check the health care facility or agency policy).
4. Vaccine is offered at no cost to employees. At present the vaccine does not require any boosters.
5. After exposure, no treatment is needed if there is a positive blood titer on file. If no positive titer is on file, follow the CDC guidelines.

Exposure to Hepatitis C Virus

1. If the source patient is positive for hepatitis C virus (HCV), the employee receives a baseline test.
2. At 4 weeks after exposure the employee should be offered an HCV-RNA test to determine if he or she contracted HCV.
3. If positive, the employee starts treatment.
4. There is no prophylactic treatment for HCV after exposure.
5. Early treatment for infection can prevent chronic infection.

Exposure to Human Immunodeficiency Virus

1. If the patient is positive for human immunodeficiency virus (HIV) infection, a viral load study should be performed to determine the amount of virus present in the blood.
2. If the exposure meets the CDC criteria for HIV prophylactic treatment (PEP), it should be started as soon as possible, preferably within 24 hours after the exposure (CDC, 2005b).

All medical evaluations and procedures, including the vaccine and vaccination series and evaluation after exposure (prophylaxis), are made available at no cost to at-risk employees.

A confidential written medical evaluation will be available to employees with exposure incidents.

From Occupational Safety and Health Administration: Occupational Safety and Health Act of 2001, 2001, 2005, *http://www.cdc.gov.*
CDC, Centers for Disease Control and Prevention; *RNA,* ribonucleic acid; *PEP,* postexposure prophylaxis.

contaminated needlestick immediately. Additional criteria for exposure reporting include blood or other potentially infectious materials (OPIMs) in direct contact with an open area of the skin, blood or OPIM that is splashed into a health care worker's eye or mouth or up the nose, and cuts with a sharp object that is covered with blood or OPIM.

Follow-up for risk of acquiring infection begins with source patient testing. Access to testing the source patient is stated in the testing law for each state. Some states have deemed consent, which means that the state has granted the patients consent to be tested. Other states require that the patient consent to testing for the presence of bloodborne pathogens. Know the testing policies in the facility and state where you practice. Health care facilities, agencies, and workers' compensation require the exposed employee to complete an injury report and seek appropriate treatment if needed. The need for treatment is linked to the results of a risk assessment and the testing of the patient. Test the patient for HIV, hepatitis B virus (HBV), and hepatitis C virus (HCV). If positive for HIV or HCV, testing for syphilis may be indicated because of the incidence of co-infection (CDC, 2005b, 2010c). It is required that an exposed employee be given the patient's testing results. This is *not* a violation of the Health Insurance Portability and Accountability Act (HIPAA) of 1996. Both the CDC and OSHA state that this information must be given to the exposed health care worker contingent on the health care worker's willingness to be tested.

Testing the exposed employee at the time of the exposure is not needed immediately unless required by the state testing law. If the patient tests positive for a bloodborne pathogen or if the source patient is unknown, prophylactic treatment is recommended for the employee.

Exposures also occur involving non-bloodborne pathogens. Airborne and droplet diseases also pose a risk to the non-immune nurse. The CDC (2010a) published a list of recommended immunizations and vaccinations for health care workers. The recommended vaccinations and immunizations include hepatitis B vaccine; TB testing; annual influenza vaccine; measles, mumps, rubella (MMR); chickenpox vaccine; and tetanus, diphtheria, and pertussis. Employee health should review your health history and offer appropriate prevention. Declination forms are needed if these are declined (OSHA, 2001a).

SAFETY GUIDELINES FOR NURSING SKILLS

Ensuring patient safety is an essential role of the professional nurse. To ensure patient safety, communicate clearly with members of the health care team, assess and incorporate the patient's priorities of care and preferences, and use the best evidence when making decisions about your patient's care. When performing the skills in this chapter, remember the following points to ensure safe, individualized patient care.

- Use clean gloves when you anticipate contact with body fluids and nonintact skin or mucous membranes when there is a risk of drainage.
- Use gown, mask, and eye protection when there is a risk for splash.
- Keep bedside table surfaces clutter free, clean, and dry when performing aseptic procedures.
- Clean all equipment that is shared between patients.
- Ensure that patients cover mouth and nose when coughing or sneezing, use tissues to contain respiratory secretions, and dispose of tissues in waste receptacle.

SKILL 28-1 HAND HYGIENE

View Video!

Delegation Considerations

The skill of hand hygiene is performed by all caregivers. Instruct all caregivers to use proper hand hygiene.

Equipment

- Antiseptic hand rub
  - Alcohol-based, waterless, antiseptic-containing emollient
- Handwashing
  - Easy-to-reach sink with warm running water
  - Antimicrobial or non-antimicrobial soap
  - Paper towels or air dryer
  - Disposable nail cleaner (optional)

STEP	RATIONALE
1 Inspect surface of your hands for breaks or cuts in skin or cuticles. Cover any skin lesions with a dressing before providing care. If lesions are too large to cover, you may be restricted from direct patient care (CDC, 2002).	Open cuts or wounds can harbor high concentrations of microorganisms. Health care facility or agency policy often prevents nurses from caring for high-risk patients if open lesions are present on hands.
2 Inspect hands for visible soiling.	If hands are visibly soiled, use soap and water until soil is removed.
3 Inspect condition of nails. Natural tips should be ¼ inch from fingertip and smooth. DO NOT WEAR artificial nails or extensions.	Subungual areas of hands harbor high concentrations of bacteria. Long nails and chipped or old polish increase the number of bacteria residing on hands. Artificial applications increase microbial load on hands (Boyce and Pittet, 2008; CDC, 2002) (see Box 28-8).
4 Push wristwatch and long uniform sleeves above wrists. Avoid wearing rings.	Provides complete access to fingers, hands, and wrists. Some studies show that skin underneath rings carry a higher bacterial load. Gram-negative bacilli, enterobacteria, and *Staphylococcus aureus* are more common under rings (Boyce and Pittet, 2008; Fagernes and Lingaas, 2009).

SKILL 28-1 HAND HYGIENE—cont'd

STEP	RATIONALE
5 Antiseptic hand rub	
a. Apply an ample amount of product to palm of one hand (see illustration).	Enough product is needed to thoroughly cover the hands.
b. Rub hands together, covering all surfaces of hands and fingers with antiseptic (see illustration).	Covering all aspects of the hands kills transient bacteria; ensures complete antimicrobial action.
c. Rub hands together for several seconds until alcohol is dry. Allow hands to dry before applying gloves.	Provides enough time for antimicrobial solution to work.
6 Handwashing using antiseptic soap	
a. Stand in front of sink, keeping hands and uniform away from sink surface. (If hands touch sink during handwashing, repeat process.)	Inside of sink is a contaminated area. Reaching over sink increases risk of touching edge, which is contaminated.
b. Turn on water. Turn faucet on or push knee pedals laterally or press pedals with foot to regulate flow and temperature (see illustration).	Knee pads within the operating room and treatment areas are preferred to prevent hand contact with faucet. Faucet handles are likely to be contaminated with organic debris and microorganisms (AORN, 2007).
c. Avoid splashing water against uniform.	Microorganisms travel and grow in moisture.
d. Regulate flow of water so temperature is warm.	Warm water removes less of the protective oils than hot water.
e. Wet hands and wrists thoroughly under running water. Keep hands and forearms lower than elbows during washing.	Hands are the most contaminated parts to be washed. Water flows from least to most contaminated area, rinsing microorganisms into the sink.
f. Apply 3 to 5 mL of antiseptic soap and rub hands together vigorously, lathering thoroughly (see illustration).	Ensures that all surface areas of the hands and fingers are cleaned.

CLINICAL DECISION: *The decision whether to use a non-antimicrobial soap, antimicrobial soap, or alcohol-based hand antiseptic depends on the procedure, the patient's immune status, and the type of infection the patient has (CDC, 2002).*

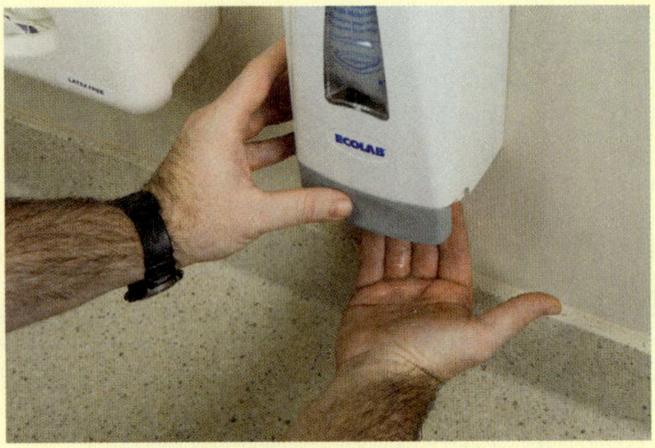

STEP 5a Apply waterless antiseptic to hands.

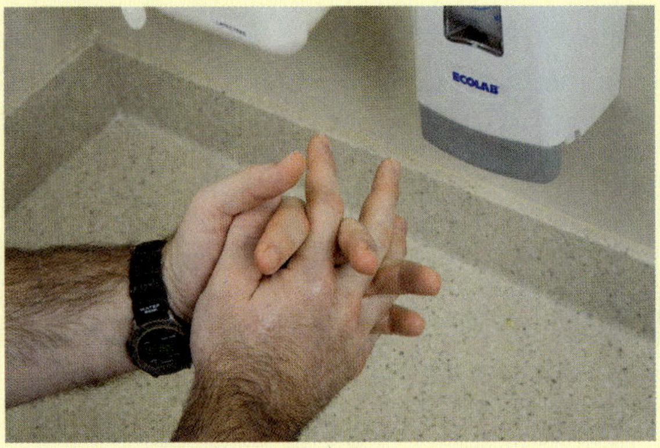

STEP 5b Rub hands thoroughly.

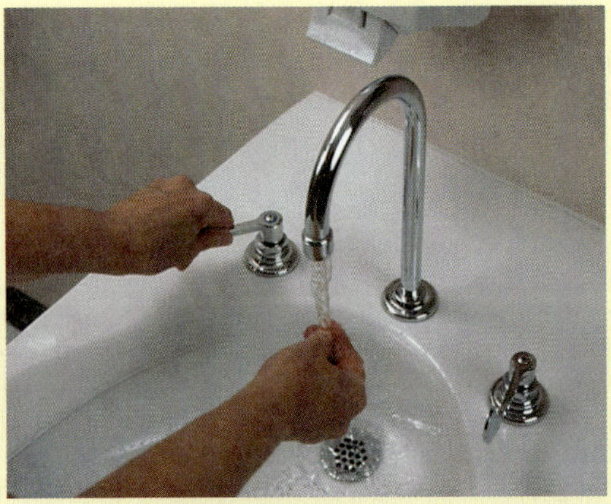

STEP 6b Turn on water.

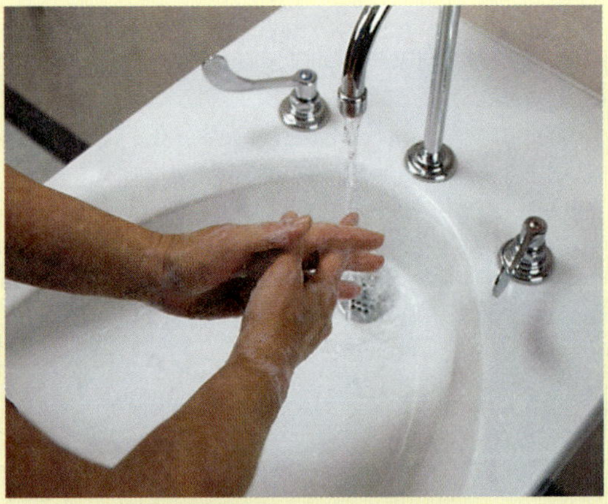

STEP 6f Lather hands thoroughly.

STEP	RATIONALE
g. Wash hands using plenty of lather and friction for at least 15 seconds. Interlace fingers and rub palms and back of hands with circular motion at least 5 times each. Keep fingertips down to facilitate removal of microorganisms.	Soap cleans by emulsifying fat and oil and lowering surface tension. Friction and rubbing mechanically loosen and remove dirt and transient bacteria. Interlacing fingers and thumbs ensures that all surfaces are cleansed. Adequate time is needed to expose skin surfaces to antimicrobial agent.
h. Areas under fingernails are often soiled. Clean them with fingernails of other hand and additional soap with an orangewood stick (optional).	Areas under nails are often highly contaminated, which increases the risk of infection for the nurse or patient.
i. Rinse hands and wrists thoroughly, keeping hands down and elbows up (see illustration).	Rinsing mechanically washes away dirt and microorganisms.
j. Dry hands thoroughly from fingers to wrists and forearms with paper towel, single-use cloth, or warm air dryer.	Drying from cleanest (fingertips) to least clean (forearms) area avoids contamination. Drying hands prevents chapping and roughened skin.
k. If used, discard paper towel in proper receptacle.	Prevents transfer of microorganisms.
l. Turn off water with foot or knee pedals. To turn off hand faucet, using clean, dry paper towel; avoid touching handles with hands (see illustration).	Wet towel and hands allow transfer of pathogens from faucet to hands. Faucet handles are contaminated.

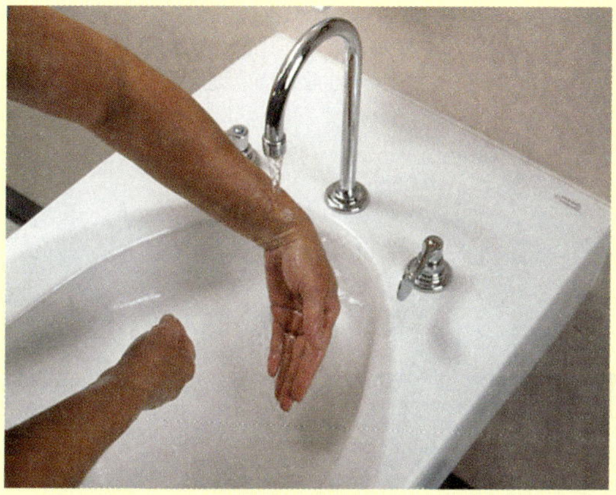

STEP 6i Rinse hands.

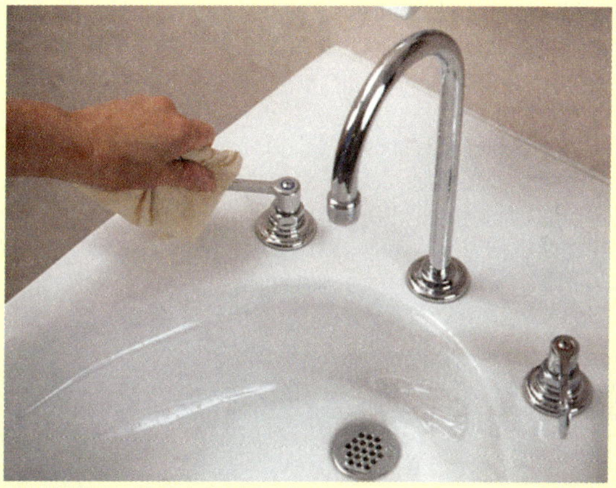

STEP 6l Turn off faucet.

HOME CARE CONSIDERATIONS

- Evaluate the handwashing facilities in the home to determine the potential for contamination, how close the facilities are to the patient, and available supplies in the area.
- Evaluate the availability of warm running water and soap when conducting home visits and anticipate the need for alternative handwashing products such as alcohol-based hand rubs and/or detergent-containing towels.
- Instruct the patient and primary caregiver in proper techniques and situations for handwashing.

SKILL 28-2 PREPARATION OF STERILE FIELD

View Video!

Delegation Considerations

The skill of preparing a sterile field cannot be delegated to nursing assistive personnel (NAP). A surgical technician may prepare a sterile field as indicated by health care facility policy.

Equipment

- Sterile pack (commercial or institution wrapped)
- Sterile drape to be used as a sterile field
- Sterile gloves (optional, check agency policy)
- Sterile solution and equipment specific to the procedure
- Waist-high table or countertop surface
- Appropriate PPE (see agency policy)

STEP	RATIONALE
1 Apply personal protective equipment as needed (consult agency policy).	Controls the spread of microorganisms.
2 Complete all priority care tasks before beginning procedure.	Sterile field should be prepared as close as possible to time of use (AORN, 2007).
3 Ask visitors to step out of room briefly during procedure.	Traffic and movement increase potential for spread of microorganisms through air currents.

SKILL 28-2 PREPARATION OF STERILE FIELD—cont'd

STEP	RATIONALE
4 Select a clean, dry work surface above waist level.	A sterile object held below the waist is contaminated.
5 Assemble necessary equipment and check expiration dates or labels and condition of supply packaging for sterility of equipment.	Preparation of equipment in advance prevents break in technique. Equipment that has evidence of previously being open, soiled, or wet is considered unsterile.
6 Perform hand hygiene.	Reduces transmission of microorganisms.
7 Prepare sterile field.	
a. Sterile commercial kit or tray containing sterile items	
(1) Place sterile kit or pack containing sterile items on work surface.	Ensures sterility of packaged drape.
(2) Open outside cover and remove kit from dust cover. Place on work surface.	Inner kit remains sterile.
(3) Grasp outer edge of tip of outermost flap.	Outer surface of package is considered unsterile. There is a 2.5-cm (1-inch) border around any sterile drape or wrap that is considered unsterile.
(4) Open outermost flap away from body, keeping arm outstretched and away from the sterile field (see illustration).	Reaching over sterile field contaminates it.
(5) Grasp outer edge of first side of flap.	Outer border is considered unsterile.
(6) Open side flap, pulling to side and allowing it to lie flat on table surface (see illustration). Keep arm to the side and do not extend it over the sterile surface.	Drape or flap should lie flat so it will not accidentally rise up and contaminate inner surface or the sterile items placed on its surface.
(7) Grasp outer edge of second side flap. Repeat for opening second side of package, pulling out to side (see illustration).	
(8) Grasp outer edge of last and innermost flap.	
(9) Stand away from sterile package and pull flap back, allowing it to fall flat on work surface (see illustration).	Reaching over sterile field contaminates it.

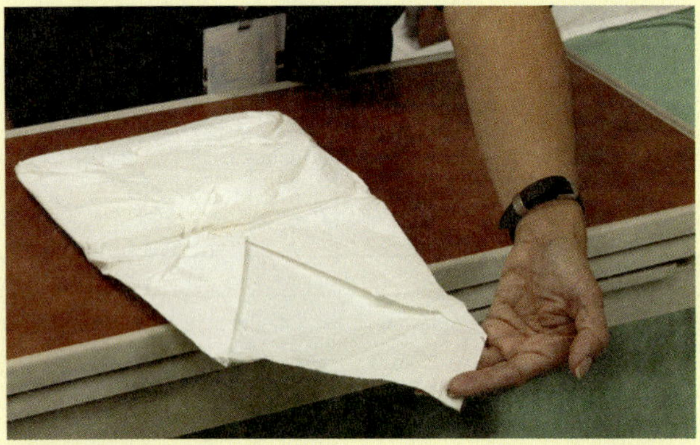

STEP 7a(4) Open outermost flap of sterile kit away from body.

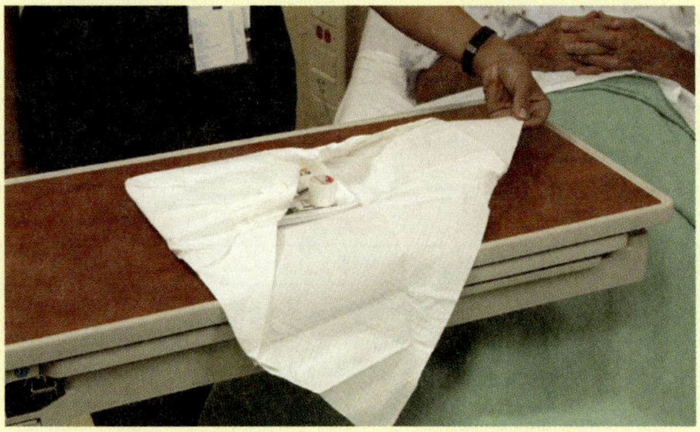

STEP 7a(6) Open first side flap, pulling to side.

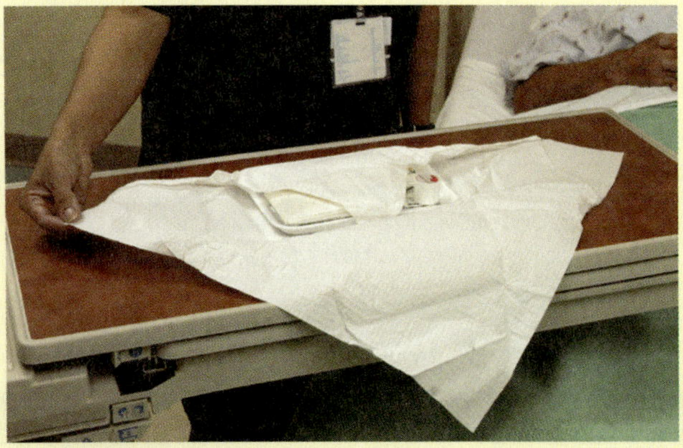

STEP 7a(7) Open second side flap, pulling to side.

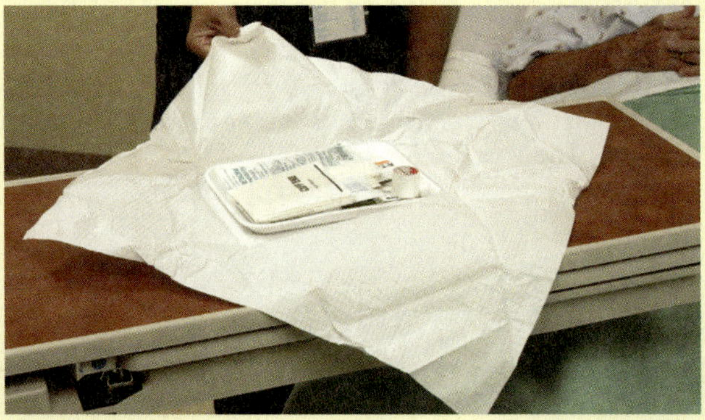

STEP 7a(9) Open last and innermost flap, standing away from sterile field.

STEP	RATIONALE
b. Sterile linen-wrapped package	
(1) Place package on work surface.	
(2) Remove sterilization tape and seal and unwrap both layers, following Steps 7a (1) to (9) as with sterile kit (see illustrations).	
(3) Use opened package wrapper as a sterile field.	Inner surface of wrapper is considered sterile.

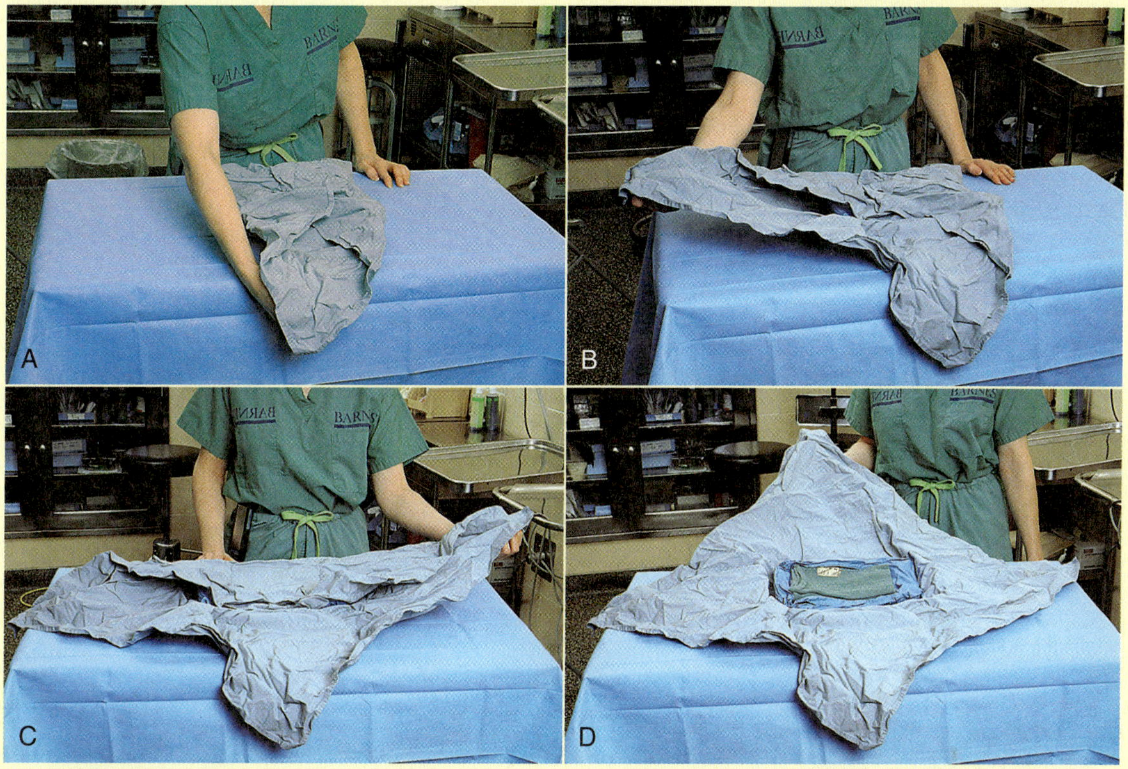

STEP 7b(2) A, Nurse opens the top flap away from the body. **B,** Nurse's arm is kept out away from the sterile field while opening a side flap. **C,** Nurse opens second side flap, keeping arm away from sterile field. **D,** Nurse opens back flap.

STEP	RATIONALE
c. Sterile drape	
(1) Place pack containing sterile drape on work surface. Follow Steps 7a (1) to (9) to open.	Ensures sterility of packaged drape.
(2) Apply sterile glove.	
Note: This is an option, depending on health care facility policy. You may touch outer 1-inch border of drape without wearing gloves.	
(3) Grasp folded top edge of drape with fingertips of one hand. Gently lift drape up from its wrapper without touching any object.	If sterile object touches any nonsterile object, it becomes contaminated.
(4) Allow drape to unfold, keeping it above waist, and work surface and away from body. (Carefully discard outer wrapper with other hand.)	Object held below person's waist or above chest is contaminated.

SKILL 28-2 PREPARATION OF STERILE FIELD—cont'd

STEP	RATIONALE
(5) With other hand grasp adjacent corner of drape. Hold drape straight over work surface (see illustration).	Drape can now be properly placed with two hands.
(6) Holding drape, first position bottom half over top half of intended work surface (see illustration).	Prevents nurse from reaching over sterile field.
(7) Allow top half of drape to be placed over bottom half of work surface (see illustration).	A flat sterile surface is now available for placement of sterile items.
8 Adding sterile items	
a. Open sterile item (following package directions) while holding outside wrapper in nondominant hand.	Frees dominant hand for unwrapping outer wrapper.
b. Carefully peel wrapper onto nondominant hand.	Item remains sterile. Inner surface of wrapper covers hand, making it sterile.
c. Being sure wrapper does not fall down on sterile field, place item onto field at angle. *Do not hold arm over sterile field* (see illustration).	Prevents reaching over field and contaminating its surface.
d. Dispose of outer wrapper.	Prevents accidental contamination of sterile field.

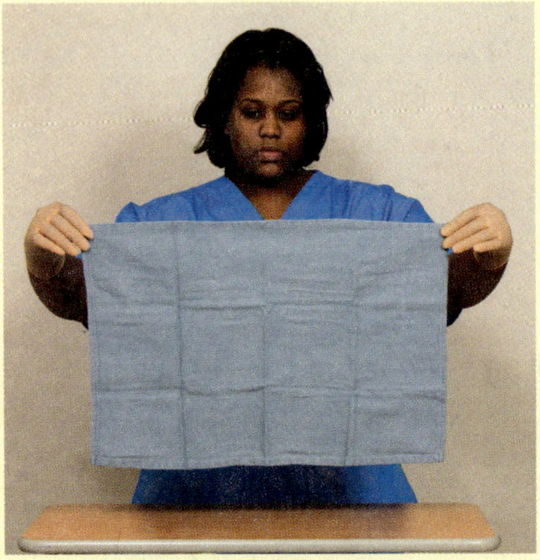
STEP 7c(5) Hold drape straight up and away from body.

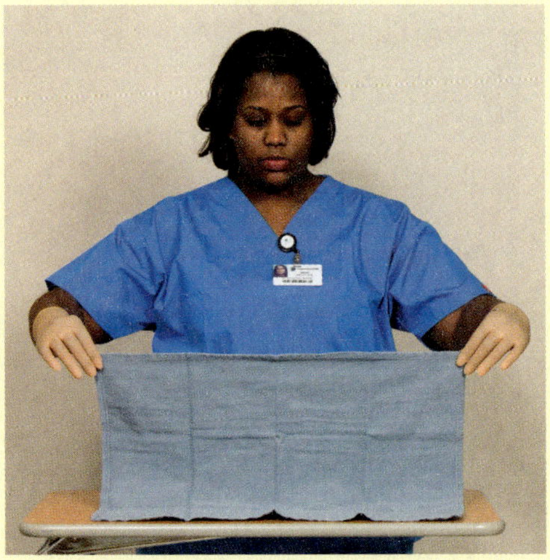
STEP 7c(6) Lay bottom half over work surface.

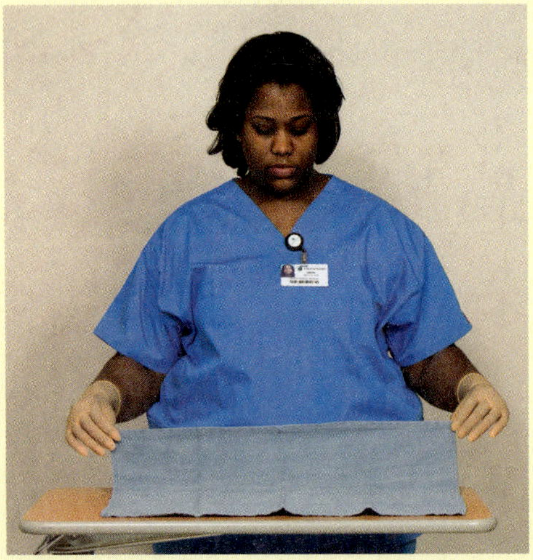
STEP 7c(7) Place top half of drape over work surface.

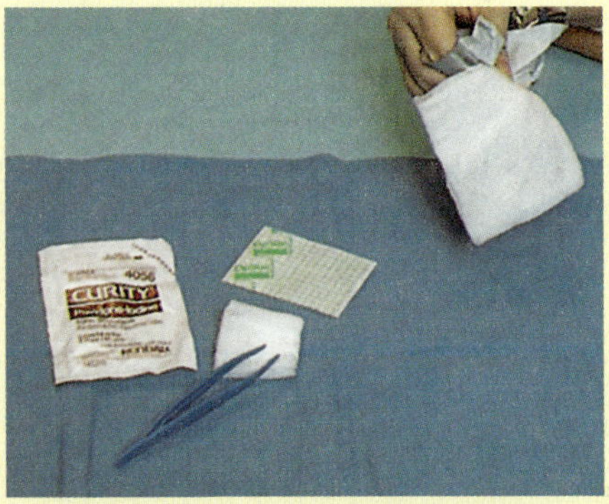

STEP 8c Add item to sterile field.

STEP	RATIONALE
9 Pour sterile solution	
a. Verify contents and expiration date of solution.	Ensures proper solution and sterility of contents.
b. Be sure receptacle for solution is located near or on sterile work surface edge. Sterile kits have cups or plastic molded sections into which you can pour fluids.	Prevents reaching over sterile field.
c. Remove sterile seal and cap from bottle in an upward motion. With solution bottle held away from sterile field, with the label facing up and the bottle lip 1 to 2 inches above inside of receiving container, slowly pour contents into container (see illustration).	Prevents contamination of bottle lip and keeps inside of cap sterile. Edge and outside of bottle are considered contaminated. Slow pouring prevents splashing liquids, which causes fluid permeation of sterile barrier (called *strike through*) and results in contamination

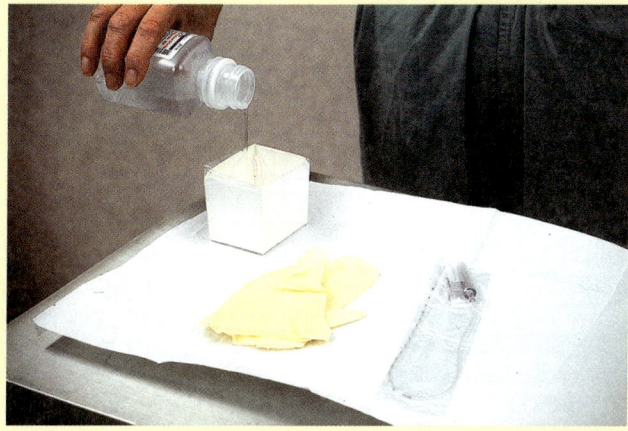

STEP 9c Pour solution into receiving container on sterile field.

STEP	RATIONALE
10 Perform procedure using sterile technique.	Prevents transmission of infection to patient.

RECORDING AND REPORTING

- It is not necessary to record or report this procedure.

SKILL 28-3 SURGICAL HAND ASEPSIS

Delegation Considerations

The skill of surgical hand asepsis can be delegated to properly trained surgical technicians (know the state Nurse Practice Act).

Equipment

- Deep sink with foot or knee controls for dispensing water and soap (faucets should be high enough for hands and forearms to fit comfortably)
- Antimicrobial agent approved by the health care facility
- Surgical scrub sponge with plastic nail pick (optional)
- Paper face mask, cap or hood, surgical shoe covers
- Sterile towel
- Sterile pack containing sterile gown
- Protective eyewear (glasses or goggles)

STEP	RATIONALE
1 Consult manufacturer policy regarding required length of time and antiseptic to use for hand antisepsis.	Guidelines vary regarding ideal time needed and antiseptic to use for surgical scrub.
2 Remove bracelets, rings, and watches.	Jewelry may harbor or protect microorganisms from removal. Allergic skin reactions may occur as a result of scrub agent or glove powder accumulating under jewelry.
3 Be sure that fingernails are short, clean, and healthy. Artificial nails should be removed. Natural nails should be less than ¼ inch long.	Long nails and chipped or old polish increase number of bacteria residing on nails. Long fingernails can puncture gloves, causing contamination. Artificial nails are known to harbor gram-negative microorganisms and fungus (AORN, 2007; CDC, 2002).

CLINICAL DECISION: *Remove nail polish if chipped or worn longer than 4 days because it likely will harbor microorganisms (AORN, 2007).*

SKILL 28-3 SURGICAL HAND ASEPSIS—cont'd

STEP	RATIONALE
4 Inspect condition of cuticles, hands, and forearms for abrasions, cuts, or open lesions.	These conditions increase likelihood of more microorganisms residing on skin surfaces. Broken skin permits microorganisms to enter layers of the skin, providing deeper microbial breeding grounds (AORN, 2007).
5 Apply surgical shoe covers, cap or hood, face mask, and protective eyewear.	Mask prevents escape into air of microorganisms that can contaminate hands. Other protective wear prevents exposure to blood and body fluid splashes during the procedure.
6 Turn on water using knee or foot controls and adjust to comfortable temperature.	Knee or foot controls prevent contamination of hands after scrub.
7 Prescrub wash/rinse: Wet hands and arms under running lukewarm water and lather with detergent to 5 cm (2 inches) above elbows. (Hands need to be above elbows at all times.)	Water runs by gravity from fingertips to elbows. Hands become cleanest part of upper extremity. Keeping hands elevated allows water to flow from least to most contaminated areas. Washing a wide area reduces risk of contaminating overlying gown that the nurse later applies.
8 Rinse hands and arms thoroughly under running water. **Remember to keep hands above elbows.**	Rinsing removes transient bacteria from fingers, hands, and forearms.
9 Under running water clean under nails of both hands with nail pick. Discard after use (see illustration).	Removes dirt and organic material that harbor large numbers of microorganisms.
10 Surgical hand scrub (with brush)	
a. Wet clean sponge and apply antimicrobial agent. Visualize each finger, hand, and arm as having four sides. Wash all four sides effectively. Scrub the nails of one hand with 15 strokes. Scrub the palm, each side of thumb and fingers, and posterior side of hand with 10 strokes each (see illustration).	Friction loosens resident bacteria that adhere to skin surfaces. Ensures coverage of all surfaces. Scrubbing is performed from cleanest area (hands) to marginal area (upper arms).
b. Divide the arm mentally into thirds: scrub each third 10 times (AORN, 2007) (see illustration). Some health care facility policies require scrub by time rather than 10 strokes. Rinse brush and repeat sequence for the other arm. A two-brush method may be substituted (check health care facility policy).	Eliminates transient microorganisms and reduces resident hand flora.
c. Discard brush. Flex arms and rinse from fingertips to elbows in one continuous motion, allowing water to run off at elbow (see illustration).	Hands remain the cleanest part of upper extremities.

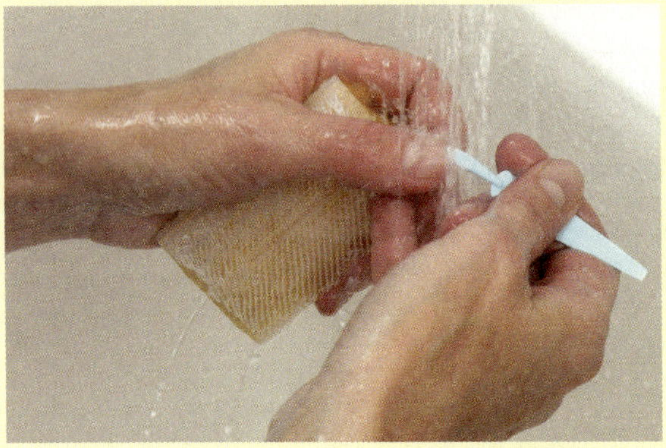

STEP 9 Clean under fingernails.

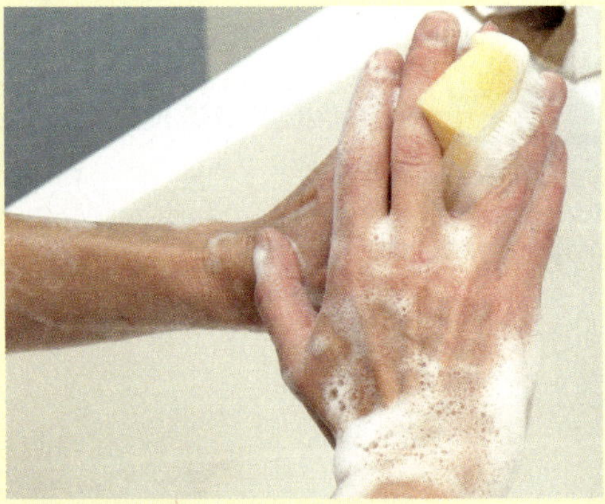

STEP 10a Scrub side of fingers.

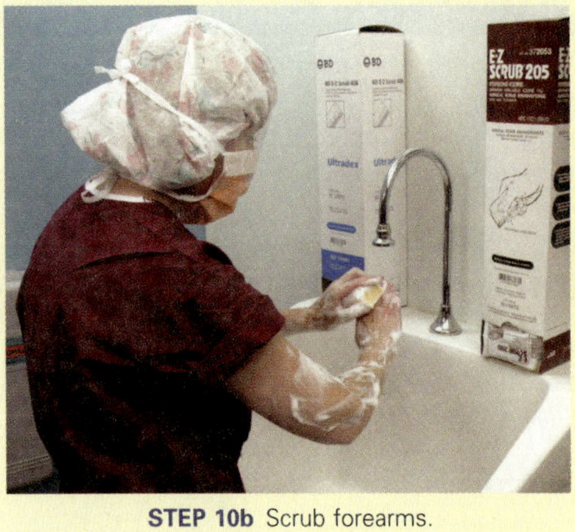

STEP 10b Scrub forearms.

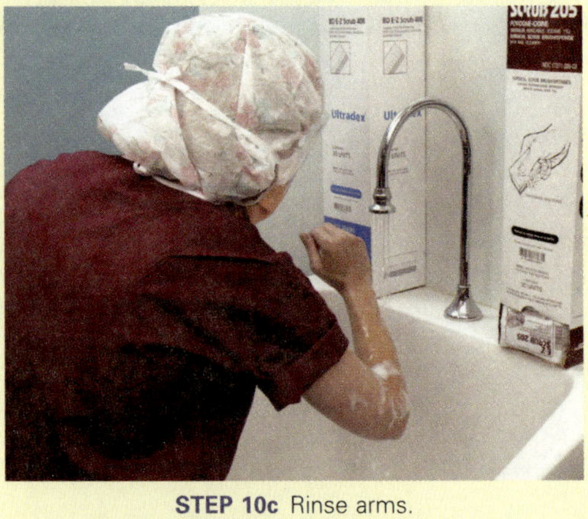

STEP 10c Rinse arms.

STEP	RATIONALE
d. Turn off water with foot or knee control, with hands elevated in front of and away from body. Enter operating room suite by backing into room.	Keeps hands free of microorganisms.
e. Approach sterile setup; grasp sterile towel, taking care not to drip water onto sterile setup.	Water contaminates sterile setup.
f. Bending slightly at waist, keeping hands and arms above waist and outstretched, grasp one end of sterile towel and dry one hand, moving from fingers to elbow in a rotating motion (see illustration).	Avoids sterile towel from contacting unsterile scrub attire and transferring contamination to hands. Dry skin from cleanest (hands) to least clean (elbows).
g. Repeat drying method for other hand by carefully reversing towel or using a new sterile towel.	Prevents accidental contamination.
h. Drop towel into linen hamper or circulating nurse's hand.	Prevents accidental contamination.
11 *Optional:* Brushless antiseptic hand rub	
a. After prescrub wash, dry hands and forearms thoroughly with paper towel.	Promotes reduction in microorganisms on all surfaces of hands and arms.
b. Dispense 2 mL of antimicrobial agent hand preparation into palm of one hand. Dip fingertips of opposite hand into hand preparation and work it under nails. Spread remaining hand preparation over hand and up to just above elbow, covering all surfaces (see illustration).	
c. Using another 2 mL of hand preparation, repeat with other hand.	
d. Dispense another 2 mL of hand preparation into either hand and reapply to all aspects of both hands up to wrist. Allow to dry before donning gloves.	Ensures complete antiseptic coverage of all hand surfaces.
12 Proceed with sterile gowning (see Skill 28-4).	

RECORDING AND REPORTING

- It is not necessary to record or report this procedure.
- Report any skin dermatitis to employee health or infection control per agency policy.

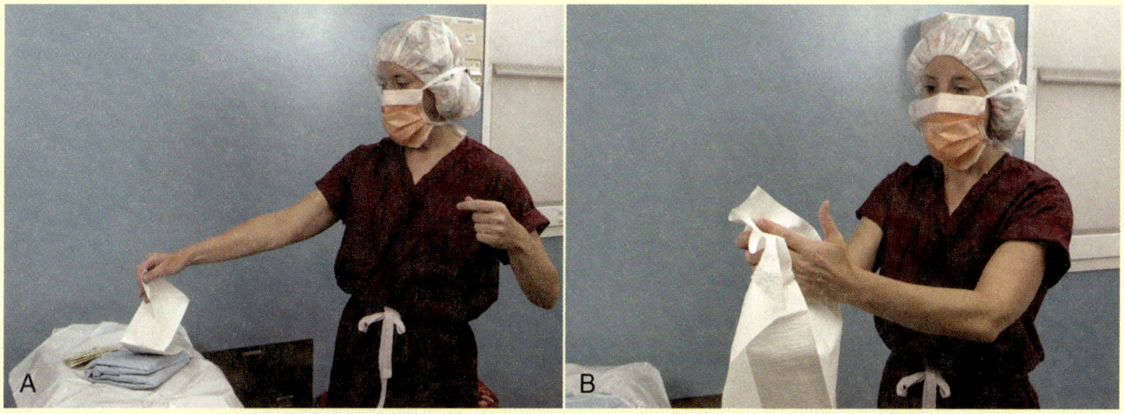

STEP 10f A, Grasp sterile towel. **B,** Drying sequence.

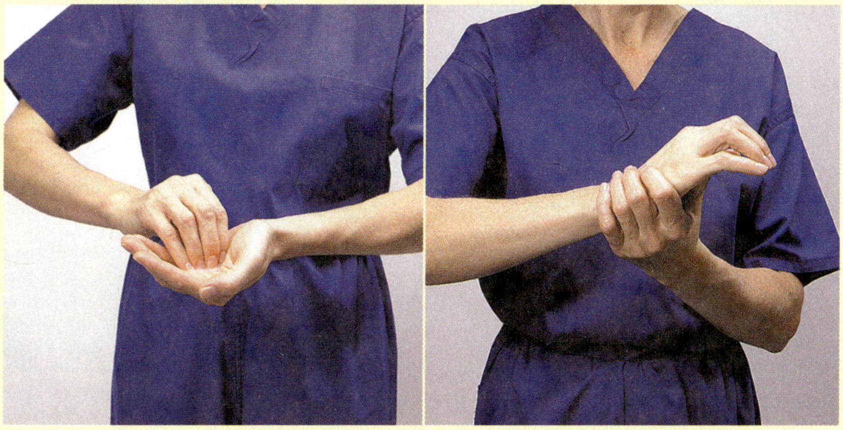

STEP 11b Application of antimicrobial agent for brushless hand scrub. Nurse using 3M Avagard. (Photos courtesy of 3M Health Care.)

SKILL 28-4 APPLYING A STERILE GOWN AND PERFORMING CLOSED GLOVING

Delegation Considerations

Applying a sterile gown and closed gloving can be delegated to a properly trained surgical technician (know the state Nurse Practice Act).

Equipment

- Package of proper-size sterile gloves (latex free if nurse or patient has sensitivity or allergy)
- Sterile pack containing sterile gown
- Clean, flat, dry surface
- Paper face masks, cap or hood, surgical shoe covers
- Protective eyewear/face shield

STEP	RATIONALE
APPLYING STERILE GOWN	
1 Before entering operating room or treatment area, apply cap, face mask, eyewear, and foot covers (paper or cloth covers fit over work shoes).	Prevents hair and air droplet nuclei from contaminating sterile work areas. Eyewear protects mucous membranes of eye. Foot covers reduce contamination from shoes.
2 Perform thorough surgical hand wash (see Skill 28-3).	Removes transient and resident bacteria from fingers, hands, and forearms.
3 Circulating nurse assists by opening sterile pack containing sterile gown (folded inside out).	Outer surface of gown remains sterile.
4 Circulating nurse prepares glove package by peeling outer wrapper open while keeping inner contents sterile. Places inner glove package on sterile field created by sterile outer wrapper.	Keeps gloves sterile and allows nurse who has scrubbed to handle sterile items.
5 Reach down to sterile gown package; lift folded gown directly upward and step back away from table.	Provides wide margin of safety, avoiding contamination of gown.
6 Holding folded gown, locate neckband. With both hands grasp inside front of gown just below neckband.	Clean hands can touch inside of gown without contaminating outer surface.
7 Allow gown to unfold, keeping inside of gown toward body. Do not touch outside of gown with bare hands.	Outside of gown is sterile surface.
8 With hands at shoulder level, slip both arms into armholes simultaneously (see illustration). Ask circulating nurse to bring gown over your shoulders by reaching inside to arm seams and pulling gown on, leaving sleeves covering hands.	Careful application prevents contamination. Gown covers hands to prepare for closed gloving.
9 Have circulating nurse securely tie back of gown at neck and waist (see illustration). (If gown is wraparound style, do not touch sterile flap to cover it until you are gloved.)	Gown must completely enclose underlying garments.

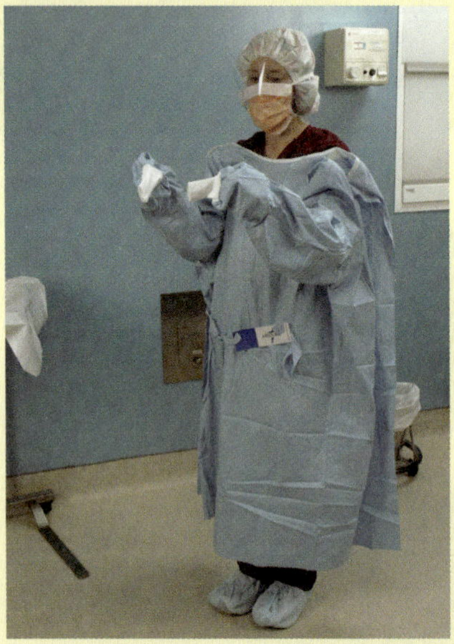

STEP 8 Place arms in sleeves.

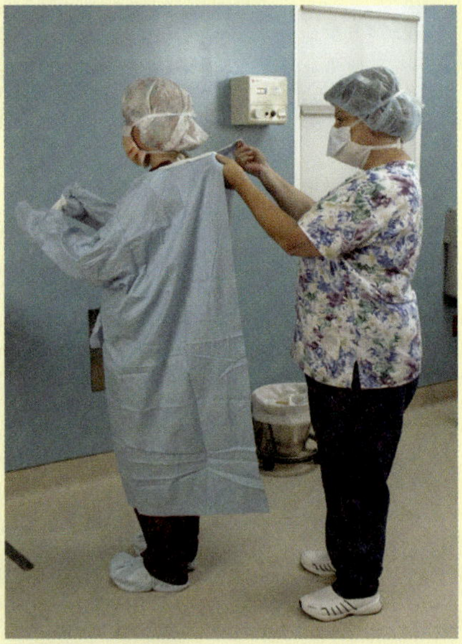

STEP 9 Circulating nurse ties scrub gown.

STEP	RATIONALE
PERFORMING CLOSED GLOVING	
10 Closed gloving	
a. With hands covered by gown sleeves, open inner sterile glove package (see illustration).	Hands remain clean. Sterile gown cuff touches sterile glove surface.
b. With dominant hand inside gown cuff, pick up glove for nondominant hand by grasping folded cuff.	Sterile gown touches sterile glove.
c. Extend nondominant forearm with palm up and place palm of glove against palm of nondominant hand. Glove fingers point toward elbow.	Positions glove for application over cuffed hand, keeping glove sterile.
d. Grasp back of glove cuff with covered dominant hand and turn glove cuff over end of nondominant hand and gown cuff (see illustration).	Seal created by glove cuff over gown prevents exit of microorganisms over operative sterile field.
e. Grasp top of glove and underlying gown sleeve with covered dominant hand. Carefully extend fingers into glove, being sure that glove cuff covers gown cuff.	
f. Glove dominant hand in same manner, reversing hands (see illustration). Use gloved nondominant hand to pull on glove. Keep hand inside sleeve (see illustrations).	Sterile touches sterile.
g. Be sure that fingers are fully extended into both gloves.	Ensures that nurse has full dexterity while using gloved hand.

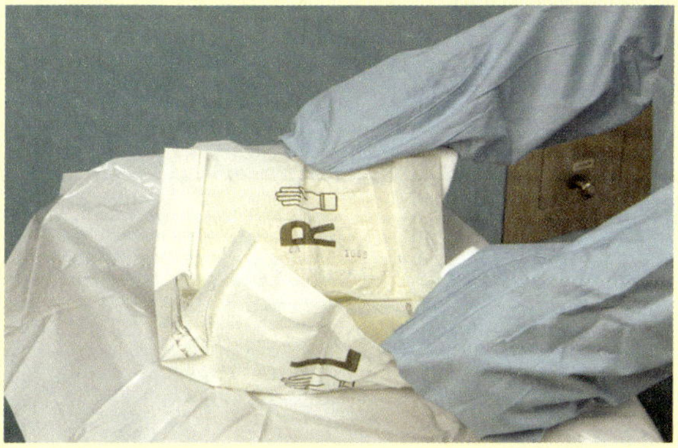

STEP 10a Scrub nurse opens glove package.

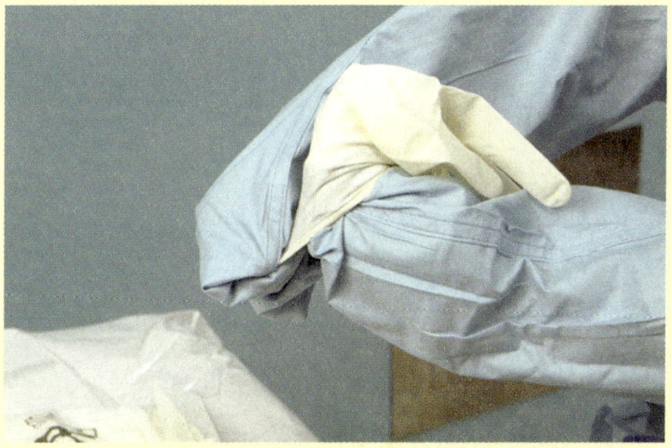
STEP 10d Glove is applied to left hand as right hand remains inside cuff.

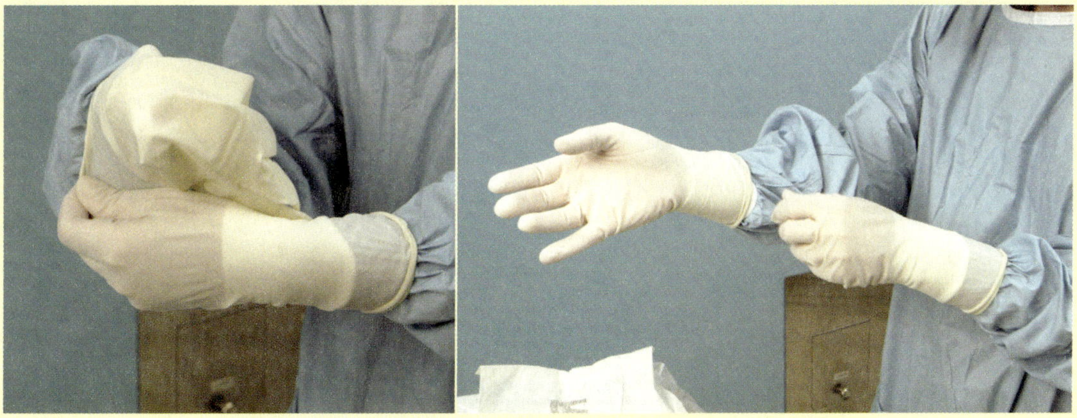
STEP 10f Second glove is applied.

SKILL 28-4 APPLYING A STERILE GOWN AND PERFORMING CLOSED GLOVING—cont'd

STEP	RATIONALE
11 For wraparound sterile gowns: take gloved hand and release fastener or ties in front of gown.	Front of gown is sterile.
12 Hand paper tab connected to sterile tie to circulating nurse, who is nonsterile (see illustration). Circulating nurse stands still as you turn completely around to left, allowing for margin of safety as gown wraps around and covers your back. Take back sterile tie from circulating nurse and secure tie to gown.	Contact with team member could contaminate gown and gloves. Gown must enclose undergarments.

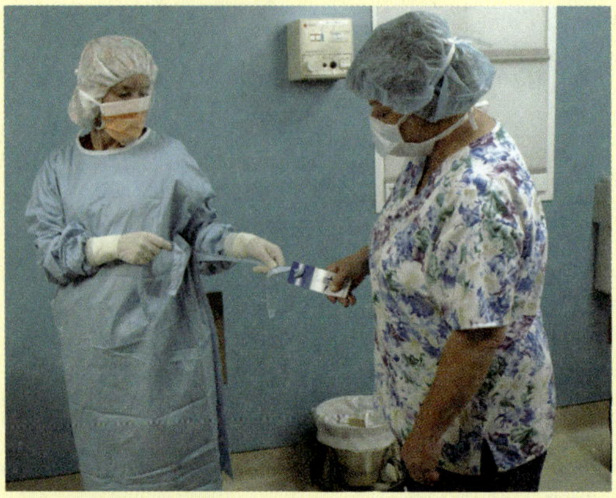

STEP 12 Hand tie to sterile team member.

RECORDING AND REPORTING

- It is not necessary to record or report this procedure.

SKILL 28-5 OPEN GLOVING

View Video!

Delegation Considerations

The skill of open gloving can be delegated when personnel are trained to perform a sterile procedure.

Equipment

- Sterile gloves (proper size)

STEP	RATIONALE
1 Perform thorough hand hygiene.	Removes bacteria from skin surfaces and reduces transmission of infection.
2 Remove outer glove package wrapper by carefully separating and peeling apart sides.	Prevents inner glove package from accidentally opening and touching contaminated objects.
3 Grasp inner package and lay it on clean, flat surface just above waist level. Open package, keeping gloves on wrappers inside surface (see illustration).	Sterile object held below waist is contaminated. Inner surface of glove package is sterile.

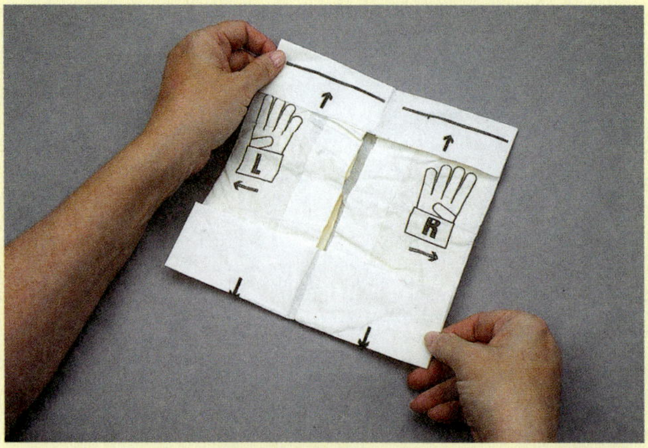

STEP 3 Open package.

STEP	RATIONALE
4 Identify right and left glove. Each glove has cuff approximately 5 cm (2 inches) wide. Glove dominant hand first.	Proper identification of gloves prevents contamination by improper fit. Gloving of dominant hand first improves dexterity.
5 With thumb and first two fingers of nondominant hand, grasp edge of cuff of glove for dominant hand. Touch only inside surface of glove.	Inner edge of cuff lies against skin and thus is not sterile.
6 Carefully pull glove over dominant hand, leaving cuff and being sure that it does not roll up wrist. Be sure that thumb and fingers are in proper spaces (see illustration).	If outer surface of glove touches hand or wrist, it is contaminated.
7 With gloved dominant hand, slip fingers underneath cuff of second glove (see illustration).	Cuff protects gloved fingers. Sterile touching sterile prevents glove contamination.
8 Carefully pull second glove over nondominant hand. Do not allow fingers and thumb of gloved dominant hand to touch any part of exposed nondominant hand. Keep thumb of dominant hand abducted back (see illustration).	Contact of gloved hand with exposed hand results in contamination.
9 After second glove is on, interlock fingers of gloved hands and hold away from body above waist level until beginning procedure (see illustration).	Prevents accidental contamination from hand movement.

GLOVE DISPOSAL

10 Grasp outside of one cuff with other gloved hand; avoid touching wrist. Pull halfway down palm of hand. Take thumb of half-ungloved hand and place under cuff of other glove.	Minimizes contamination of underlying skin.
11 Pull glove off, turning it inside out. Discard in receptacle.	Outside of glove does not touch skin surface.
12 Take fingers of bare hand and tuck inside remaining glove cuff. Peel glove off, inside out. Discard in receptacle.	

RECORDING AND REPORTING

- It is not necessary to record or report this procedure.

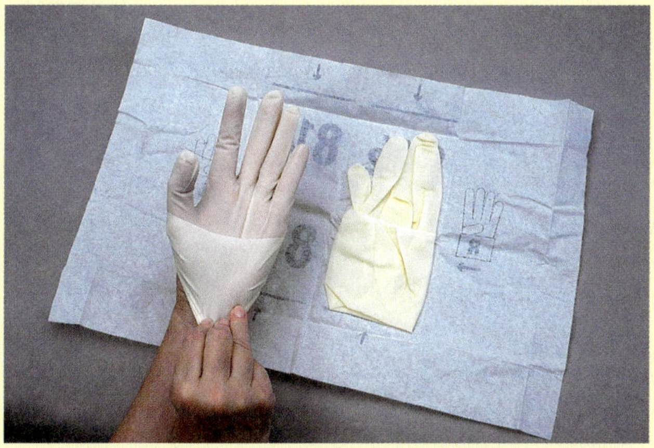

STEP 6 Pull glove over dominant hand.

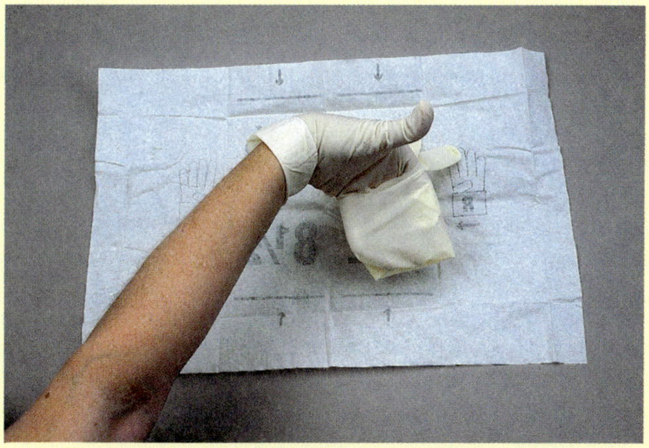

STEP 7 Slip fingers underneath cuff of second glove.

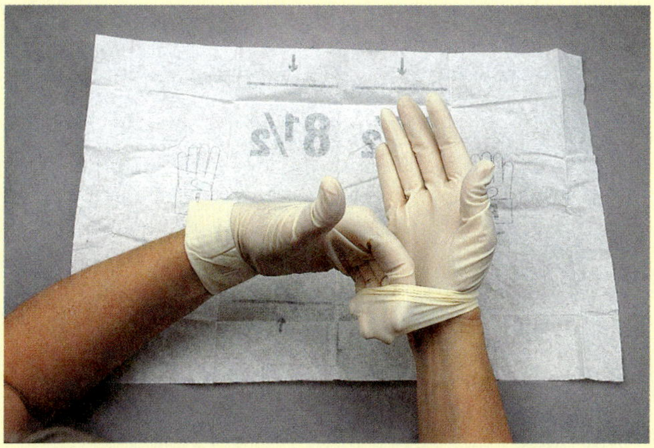

STEP 8 Pull second glove over nondominant hand.

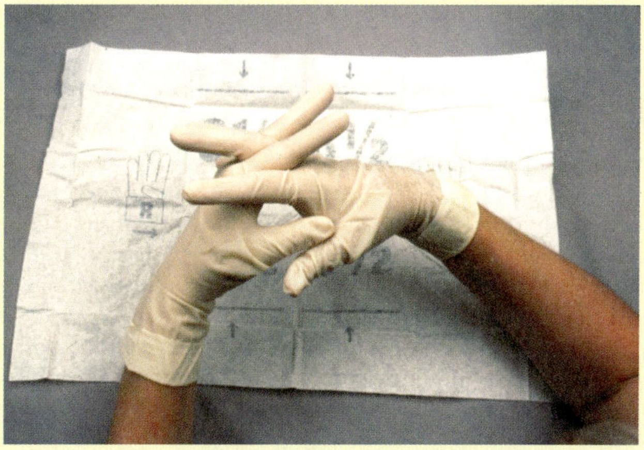

STEP 9 Hands are interlocked.

KEY POINTS

- Hand hygiene is the most important technique to use in preventing and controlling transmission of infection.
- The potential for microorganisms to cause disease depends on the number of organisms, virulence, ability to enter and survive in a host, and susceptibility of the host.
- Normal body floras help to resist infection by releasing antibacterial substances and inhibiting multiplication of pathogenic microorganisms.
- The signs of local inflammation and infection are identical.
- An infection can develop as long as the six elements composing the infection chain are uninterrupted.
- Microorganisms are transmitted by direct and indirect contact, airborne spread, and vectors and contaminated articles.
- Increasing age, poor nutrition, stress, inherited conditions, chronic disease, and treatments or conditions that compromise the immune response increase susceptibility to infection.
- The major sites for health care–associated infections include the urinary and respiratory tracts, bloodstream, and surgical or traumatic wounds.
- The CDC now recommends use of alcohol-based waterless antiseptics as an alternative to handwashing unless hands are visibly soiled.
- Invasive procedures, medical therapies, long hospitalization, and contact with health care personnel increase a hospitalized patient's risk for acquiring a health care–associated infection.
- Isolation practices may prevent personnel and patients from acquiring infections and transmission of microorganisms to other persons.
- Standard precautions use generic barrier techniques when caring for all patients.
- Proper cleaning requires mechanical removal of all soil from an object or area.
- A patient in isolation is subject to sensory deprivation because of the restricted environment.
- An infection prevention and control professional monitors the incidence of infection within an institution and provides educational and consulting services.
- Surgical asepsis requires more stringent techniques than medical asepsis and is directed at eliminating microorganisms.
- If the skin is broken or if an invasive procedure into a body cavity normally free of microorganisms is performed, follow surgical aseptic practices.

CLINICAL APPLICATION QUESTIONS

Preparing for Clinical Practice

Mrs. Andrews did well after her spinal surgery and was discharged home on the third postoperative day. Two weeks later she told her family that she was having increased pain in her back. She stated that she was not always wearing her back brace as instructed at the time of surgery because "it makes me sweat and itch." When she wears the brace, she frequently wipes over her incision with a handkerchief to remove the perspiration and scratches it to ease the itching. Her daughter noted that the incision was reddened with a small amount of drainage coming from the site. Mrs. Andrews was readmitted, and an incision and drainage of the back wound were performed.

1. What do you need to include when assessing the wound for infection?
2. If Mrs. Andrews were to develop a systemic infection as a result of the localized wound infection, which assessments would you expect to find? Explain your answers.
3. Which methods of infection control do you need to use when caring for Mrs. Andrews?

evolve *Answers to Clinical Application Questions can be found on the Evolve website.*

REVIEW QUESTIONS

Are You Ready to Test Your Nursing Knowledge?

1. If an infectious disease can be transmitted directly from one person to another, it is a:
   1. Susceptible host.
   2. Communicable disease.
   3. Port of entry to a host.
   4. Port of exit from the reservoir.
2. Which is the most likely means of transmitting infection between patients?
   1. Exposure to another patient's cough
   2. Sharing equipment among patients
   3. Disposing of soiled linen in a shared linen bag
   4. Contact with a health care worker's hands
3. Identify the interval when a patient progresses from nonspecific signs to manifesting signs and symptoms specific to a type of infection.
   1. Illness stage
   2. Convalescence
   3. Prodromal stage
   4. Incubation period
4. Which of the following is the most *effective* way to break the chain of infection?
   1. Hand hygiene
   2. Wearing gloves
   3. Placing patients in isolation
   4. Providing private rooms for patients
5. A family member is providing care to a loved one who has an infected leg wound. What would you instruct the family member to do after providing care and handling contaminated equipment or organic material?
   1. Wear gloves before eating or handling food.
   2. Place any soiled materials into a bag and double bag it.
   3. Have the family member check with the doctor about need for immunization.
   4. Perform hand hygiene after care and/or handling contaminated equipment or material.
6. A patient is isolated for pulmonary tuberculosis. The nurse notes that the patient seems to be angry, but he knows that this is a normal response to isolation. Which is the best intervention?
   1. Provide a dark, quiet room to calm the patient.
   2. Reduce the level of precautions to keep the patient from becoming angry.
   3. Explain the reasons for isolation procedures and provide meaningful stimulation.
   4. Limit family and other caregiver visits to reduce the risk of spreading the infection.
7. The nurse wears a gown when:
   1. The patient's hygiene is poor.
   2. The nurse is assisting with medication administration.

3. The patient has acquired immunodeficiency syndrome (AIDS) or hepatitis.
4. Blood or body fluids may get on the nurse's clothing from a task that he or she plans to perform.

8. The nurse has redressed a patient's wound and now plans to administer a medication to the patient. Which is the correct infection control procedure?
   1. Leave the gloves on to administer the medication.
   2. Remove gloves and administer the medication.
   3. Remove gloves and perform hand hygiene before administering the medication.
   4. Leave the medication on the bedside table to avoid having to remove gloves before leaving the patient's room.
9. When a nurse is performing surgical hand asepsis, the nurse must keep hands:
   1. Below elbows.
   2. Above elbows.
   3. At a 45-degree angle.
   4. In a comfortable position.
10. What is the best method to sterilize a straight urinary catheter and suction tube in the home setting?
    1. Use an autoclave.
    2. Use boiling water.
    3. Use ethylene oxide gas.
    4. Use chemicals for disinfection.
11. A patient has an indwelling urinary catheter. Why does an indwelling urinary catheter present a risk for urinary tract infection?
    1. It keeps an incontinent patient's skin dry.
    2. It can get caught in the linens or equipment.
    3. It obstructs the normal flushing action of urine flow.
    4. It allows the patient to remain hydrated without having to urinate.
12. Put the following steps for removal of protective barriers after leaving an isolation room in order:
    1. Untie top, then bottom mask strings and remove from face.
    2. Untie waist and neck strings of gown. Allow gown to fall from shoulders and discard. Remove gown, rolling it onto itself without touching the contaminated side.
    3. Remove gloves.
    4. Remove eyewear or goggles.
    5. Perform hand hygiene.
13. Your ungloved hands come in contact with the drainage from your patient's wound. What is the correct method to clean your hands?
    1. Wash them with soap and water.
    2. Use an alcohol-based hand cleaner.
    3. Rinse them and use the alcohol-based hand cleaner.
    4. Wipe them with a paper towel.
14. A patient's surgical wound has become swollen, red, and tender. You note that the patient has a new fever and leukocytosis. What is the best immediate intervention?
    1. Notify the health care provider and use surgical technique to change the dressing.
    2. Reassure the patient and recheck the wound later.
    3. Notify the health care provider and support the patient's fluid and nutritional needs.
    4. Alert the patient and caregivers to the presence of an infection to ensure care after discharge.
15. While preparing to do a sterile dressing change, a nurse accidentally sneezes over the sterile field that is on the over-the-bed table. Which of the following principles of surgical asepsis, if any, has the nurse violated?
    1. When a sterile field comes in contact with a wet surface, the sterile field is contaminated by capillary action.
    2. Fluid flows in the direction of gravity.
    3. A sterile field becomes contaminated by prolonged exposure to air.
    4. None of the principles were violated.

Answers: 1. 2; 2. 4; 3. 3; 4. 1; 5. 4; 6. 3; 7. 4; 8. 3; 9. 2; 10. 2; 11. 3; 12. 3, 4, 2, 1, 5; 13. 1; 14. 3; 15. 3.

REFERENCES

Ackley B, Ladwig G: *Nursing diagnosis handbook, evidence-based guide to planning care*, ed 10, St Louis, 2011, Mosby.

Arnold F: Antimicrobials and resistance. In Carrico R, editor: *APIC text of infection control and epidemiology*, Washington, DC, 2009, Association for Professionals in Infection Control and Epidemiology.

Boyce JM, Pittet D: *HICPAC/SHEA/APIC/IDSA Hand Hygiene Task Force and the CDC Healthcare Control Practices Advisory Committee guidelines for hand hygiene in healthcare settings*, Atlanta, 2008.

Calfree D, et al: Strategies to prevent transmission of methicillin-resistant *Staphylococcus aureus* in acute care hospitals, *Infect Control Hosp Epidemiol* 29(suppl 1): S62–S80, 2008.

Centers for Disease Control and Prevention, US Department of Health & Human Services: *Guidance for the selection and use of personal protective equipment (PPE) in the health care setting, CDC*, 2004, http://www.cdc.gov/ncidod/dhqp/pdf/ppe/PPEslides6-29-04.ppt. Accessed December 2, 2005.

Centers for Disease Control and Prevention (CDC): *Guideline for preventing the transmission of Mycobacterium tuberculosis in health-care facilities*, Washington, DC, 2005a, CDC.

Centers for Disease Control and Prevention (CDC): *Updated US Public Health Service guidelines for the management of occupational exposures to HIV and recommendations for post exposure prophylaxis*, Washington, DC, 2005b, CDC.

Centers for Disease Control and Prevention (CDC): *Management of multidrug-resistant organisms in healthcare settings*, 2006, CDC.

Centers for Disease Control and Prevention (CDC): *Guideline for isolation precautions: preventing transmission of infectious agents in healthcare settings—recommendations to the Healthcare Infection Control Practices Advisory Committee (HICPAC)*, Washington, DC, 2007, CDC, www.cdc.gov/ncidod/dhap/pdf/guidelines/Isolation2007. Accessed September 1, 2010.

Centers for Disease Control and Prevention: Immunization Schedules, CDC, 2010a, http://www.cdc.gov/vaccines/recs/schedules/default.htm. Accessed August 20, 2011.

Centers for Disease Control and Prevention (CDC): *Interim guidance for infection control for care of patients with confirmed or suspected swine influenza A (H1N1) virus infection in a healthcare setting*, 2010b, http://www.cdc.gov/h1n1flu/guideline_infectioncontrol.htm. Accessed January 31, 2012.

Centers for Disease Control and Prevention (CDC): Sexually transmitted diseases treatment guidelines (includes chapter on hepatitis C), *MMWR Morb Mortal Wkly Rep* 59(RR-12):1, 2010c.

Centers for Disease Control and Prevention: Vaccines and preventable diseases, CDC, 2011, http://www.cdc.gov/vaccines/vpd-vac/default.htm. Accessed August 20, 2011.

Church N, Bjerke N: Surgical services. In Carrico R, editor: *APIC text of infection control and epidemiology*, Washington, DC, 2009, Association for Professionals in Infection Control and Epidemiology.

Cipriano P: Save a life—wash your hands, *Am Nurse Today* 2(1):10, 2007, http://www.AmericanNurseToday.com.

Fardo R: Geriatrics. In Carrico R, editor: *APIC text of infection control and epidemiology*, Washington, DC, 2009, Association for Professionals in Infection Control and Epidemiology.

Fauerbach L: Risk factors for infection transmission. In Carrico R, editor: *APIC text of infection control and epidemiology*, Washington, DC, 2009, Association for Professionals in Infection Control and Epidemiology.

Gantz NM: Geriatric infections. In Carrico R, editor: *APIC text of infection control and epidemiology*, Washington,

DC, 2009, Association for Professionals in Infection Control and Epidemiology.

Iwamoto P: Aseptic technique. In Carrico R, editor: *APIC text of infection control and epidemiology*, Washington, DC, 2009, Association for Professionals in Infection Control and Epidemiology.

Jefferson J: Central services. In Carrico R, editor: *APIC text of infection control and epidemiology*, Washington, DC, 2009, Association for Professionals in Infection Control and Epidemiology.

Larson E: APIC guideline for hand washing and hand antisepsis in health-care settings. In *APIC infection control and applied epidemiology: principles and practice*, St Louis, 2005, Mosby.

Lesser KJ, Paiusi IC, Leips J: Naturally occurring genetic variation in the age-specific immune response of *Drosophila melanogaster*, *Aging Cell* 5(4):293, 2006.

Meiner S, Lueckenotte AG: *Gerontologic nursing*, ed 3, St Louis, 2006, Mosby.

Moore V: Microbiology basics. In Carrico R, editor: *APIC text of infection control and epidemiology*, Washington, DC, 2009, Association for Professionals in Infection Control and Epidemiology.

Murphy D: Patient safety. In Carrico R, editor: *APIC text of infection control and epidemiology*, Washington, DC, 2009, Association for Professionals in Infection Control and Epidemiology.

Occupational Safety and Health Administration (OSHA): Respiratory protective devices: Final rules and notice. *Fed Regis* 60:30336, 1995.

Occupational Safety and Health Administration (OSHA): Enforcement procedures for the occupational exposure to bloodborne injury final rule, *Fed Reg* 66:5318, 2001a.

Occupational Safety and Health Administration (OSHA): *Needlestick Safety and Prevention Act, Public Law* 106-430, 2001b.

Pagana KD, Pagana TJ: *Manual of diagnostic testing and laboratory results*, ed 4, St Louis, 2010, Mosby.

Ritter H: Microbiology/laboratory diagnostics. In Carrico R, editor: *APIC text of infection control and epidemiology*, Washington, DC, 2005, Association for Professionals in Infection Control and Epidemiology.

Rutala W, Weber DJ: Centers for Disease Control and Prevention, Hospital Infection Control Practices Advisory Committee: *Guideline for disinfection and sterilization in healthcare facilities*, 2008, http://www.cdc.gov/hicpac/Disinfection_Sterilization/toc.html. Accessed August 25, 2011.

Rutala W, Weber DJ: Cleaning, disinfection and sterilization. In Carrico R, editor: *APIC text of infection control and epidemiology*, Washington, DC, 2009, Association for Professionals in Infection Control and Epidemiology.

Stricof R: Endoscopy. In Carrico R, editor: *APIC text of infection control and epidemiology*, Washington, DC, 2009, Association for Professionals in Infection Control and Epidemiology.

The Joint Commission: *2011 National Patient Safety Goals (NPSGs)*, 2011, The Commission. Available at http://www.jointcommission.org/standards_information/npsgs.aspx.

Tweeten SM: General principles of epidemiology. In Carrico R, editor: *APIC text of infection control and epidemiology*, Washington, DC, 2009, Association for Professionals in Infection Control and Epidemiology.

World Health Organization (WHO): *Guidelines on hand hygiene*, Geneva, Switzerland, 2009, WHO Press.

RESEARCH REFERENCES

Abad C, et al: Adverse effects of isolation in hospitalised patients: a systematic review, *J Hosp Infect* 76(2):97, 2010.

Association of Operating Room Nurses (AORN): *Standards, recommended practices, and guidelines*, Denver, 2007, The Association.

Auerbach C, Beckerman NL: HIV/AIDS prevention in New York City: Identifying sociocultural needs of the community, *Soc Work Health Care* 49(2):109, 2010.

Centers for Disease Control and Prevention, Hospital Infection Control Practices Advisory Committee: *Guideline for hand hygiene in health-care settings*, Volume 51/RR16 October 25, 2002, http://www.cdc.gov/handhygiene/Guidelines.html. Accessed August 25, 2011.

Doyle JS, et al: Epidemology of infections acquired in intensive care units, *Sem Resp Crit Care Med* 32(2):115, 2011.

Fagernes M, Lingaas E: Impact of finger rings on transmission of bacteria during hand contact, *Infect Control Hosp Epidemiol* 30(5):427, 2009.

Gould D, et al: *Interventions to improve hand hygiene compliance in patient care, Cochrane Database of Systematic Reviews*, volume 8, The Cochrane Library, 2011, The Cochrane Collaboration.

Rothrock J: *What are the current guidelines about wearing artificial nails and nail polish in the healthcare setting?* 2006, http://www.medscape.com/viewarticle/547793. Accessed August 25, 2011.

Thomas RE, et al: Influenza vaccination for healthcare workers who work with the elderly: Systematic review, *Vaccine* 29(2):344, 2010.

CHAPTER 29

Vital Signs

OBJECTIVES

- Explain the principles and mechanisms of thermoregulation.
- Describe nursing measures that promote heat loss and heat conservation.
- Discuss physiological changes associated with fever.
- Accurately assess body temperature, pulse, respirations, oxygen saturation, and blood pressure.
- Explain the physiology of normal regulation of blood pressure, pulse, oxygen saturation, and respirations.
- Describe factors that cause variations in body temperature, pulse, oxygen saturation, respirations, and blood pressure.
- Describe cultural and ethnic variations with blood pressure assessment.
- Identify ranges of acceptable vital sign values for an infant, a child, and an adult.
- Explain variations in technique used to assess an infant's, a child's, and an adult's vital signs.
- Describe the benefits and precautions involving self-measurement of blood pressure.
- Identify when to take vital signs.
- Accurately record and report vital sign measurements.
- Appropriately delegate measurement of vital signs to nursing assistive personnel.

KEY TERMS

Afebrile, p. 445
Antipyretics, p. 452
Auscultatory gap, p. 463
Basal metabolic rate (BMR), p. 443
Blood pressure, p. 458
Bradycardia, p. 455
Cardiac output, p. 452
Celsius, p. 447
Conduction, p. 443
Convection, p. 444
Core temperature, p. 442
Diaphoresis, p. 444
Diastolic pressure, p. 458
Diffusion, p. 456
Dysrhythmia, p. 455
Eupnea, p. 456
Evaporation, p. 444
Fahrenheit, p. 447
Febrile, p. 445
Fever, p. 445
Fever of unknown origin (FUO), p. 445
Frostbite, p. 446
Heat exhaustion, p. 446
Heatstroke, p. 446
Hematocrit, p. 459
Hypertension, p. 460
Hyperthermia, p. 446
Hypotension, p. 461
Hypothermia, p. 446
Hypoxemia, p. 456
Malignant hyperthermia, p. 446
Nonshivering thermogenesis, p. 443
Orthostatic hypotension, p. 461
Oxygen saturation, p. 457
Perfusion, p. 456
Postural hypotension, p. 461
Pulse deficit, p. 455
Pulse pressure, p. 459
Pyrexia, p. 445
Pyrogens, p. 445
Radiation, p. 443
Shivering, p. 443
Sphygmomanometer, p. 461
Systolic pressure, p. 458
Tachycardia, p. 454
Thermoregulation, p. 446
Ventilation, p. 456
Vital signs, p. 441

evolve WEBSITE

http://evolve.elsevier.com/Potter/fundamentals/

- Review Questions
- Video Clips
- Animations
- Case Study with Questions
- Skills Performance Checklists
- Audio Glossary
- Interactive Learning Activities
- Key Term Flashcards
- Content Updates

The most frequent measurements obtained by health care providers are those of temperature, pulse, blood pressure (BP), respiratory rate, and oxygen saturation. As indicators of health status, these measures indicate the effectiveness of circulatory, respiratory, neural, and endocrine body functions. Because of their importance they are referred to as **vital signs.** Pain, a subjective symptom, is often called the fifth vital sign and is frequently measured with the others (see Chapter 43). Measurement of vital signs provides data to determine a patient's usual state of health (baseline data). Many factors such as the temperature of the environment, the patient's physical exertion, and the effects of illness cause vital signs to change, sometimes outside an acceptable range. Assessment of vital signs provides data to identify nursing diagnoses, implement planned interventions, and evaluate outcomes of care. An alteration in vital signs signals a change in physiological function and the need for medical or nursing intervention.

Vital signs are a quick and efficient way of monitoring a patient's condition or identifying problems and evaluating his or her response to intervention. When you learn the physiological variables influencing vital signs and recognize the relationship of their changes to other physical assessment findings, you can make precise

BOX 29-1 VITAL SIGNS

Acceptable Ranges for Adults

Temperature Range: 36° to 38° C (96.8° to 100.4° F)
Average oral/tympanic: 37° C (98.6° F)
Average rectal: 37.5° C (99.5° F)
Average axillary: 36.5° C (97.7° F)

Pulse
60 to 100 beats/min

Respirations
12 to 20 breaths/min

Blood Pressure
Average: <120/<80 mm Hg
Pulse pressure: 30 to 50 mm Hg

BOX 29-2 WHEN TO MEASURE VITAL SIGNS

- On admission to a health care facility
- When assessing a patient during home care visits
- In a hospital on a routine schedule according to the health care provider's order or hospital standards of practice
- Before and after a surgical procedure or invasive diagnostic procedure
- Before, during, and after a transfusion of blood products
- Before, during, and after the administration of medication or therapies that affect cardiovascular, respiratory, or temperature-control functions
- When a patient's general physical condition changes (e.g., loss of consciousness or increased intensity of pain)
- Before and after nursing interventions influencing a vital sign (e.g., before a patient previously on bed rest ambulates or before a patient performs range-of-motion exercises)
- When a patient reports nonspecific symptoms of physical distress (e.g., feeling "funny" or "different")

determinations about a patient's health problems. Vital signs and other physiological measurements are the basis for clinical decision making and problem solving.

GUIDELINES FOR MEASURING VITAL SIGNS

Vital signs are a part of the assessment database. You include them in a complete physical assessment (see Chapter 30) or obtain them individually to assess a patient's condition. Establishing a database of vital signs during a routine physical examination serves as a baseline for future assessments. The patient's needs and condition determine when, where, how, and by whom vital signs are measured. You need to measure them correctly, and at times you appropriately delegate their measurement. You also need to know expected values (Box 29-1), interpret your patient's values, communicate findings appropriately, and begin interventions as needed. Use the following guidelines to incorporate measurements of vital signs into nursing practice:

- The nurse caring for the patient is responsible for measurement of vital signs. Although you sometimes delegate measurement of selected vital signs (i.e., in stable patients), as a nurse you need to analyze them to interpret their significance and make decisions about interventions.
- Ensure that equipment is functional and appropriate for the size and age of the patient. Equipment used to measure vital signs (e.g., a thermometer) needs to work properly to obtain accurate findings.
- Select equipment based on the patient's condition and characteristics (e.g., do not use an adult-size BP cuff for a child).
- Know the patient's usual range of vital signs. These values can differ from the acceptable range for that age or physical state. The patient's usual values serve as a baseline for comparison with later findings. Thus you are able to detect a change in condition over time.
- Determine the patient's medical history, therapies, and prescribed medications. Some illnesses or treatments cause predictable changes in vital signs. Some medications affect one or more vital signs.
- Control or minimize environmental factors that affect vital signs. For example, assessing the patient's temperature in a warm, humid room may yield a value that is not a true indicator of his or her condition.
- Use an organized, systematic approach when taking vital signs. Each procedure requires a step-by-step approach to ensure accuracy.
- Based on the patient's condition, collaborate with health care providers to decide the frequency of vital sign assessment. In the hospital, health care providers order a minimum frequency of vital sign measurements for each patient. Following surgery or treatment intervention you measure vital signs more frequently to detect complications. In a clinic or outpatient setting you take vital signs before the health care provider examines the patient and after any invasive procedures. As a patient's physical condition worsens, it is often necessary to monitor vital signs as often as every 5 to 10 minutes. The nurse is responsible for judging whether more frequent assessments are necessary (Box 29-2).
- Use vital sign measurements to determine indications for medication administration. For example, give certain cardiac drugs only within a range of pulse or BP values. Administer antipyretics when temperature is elevated outside of the acceptable range for the patient. Know the acceptable ranges for your patients before administering medications.
- Analyze the results of vital sign measurement. Vital signs are not interpreted in isolation. You need to also know related physical signs or symptoms and be aware of the patient's ongoing health status.
- Communicate significant changes in vital signs to the patient's health care provider or the charge nurse. Document findings and compare with baseline measurements to identify significant changes. When vital signs appear abnormal, have another nurse or health care provider repeat the measurement to verify readings.
- Instruct the patient or family caregiver in vital sign assessment and the significance of findings.

BODY TEMPERATURE

Physiology

Body temperature is the difference between the amount of heat produced by body processes and the amount of heat lost to the external environment.

$$\text{Heat produced} - \text{Heat lost} = \text{Body temperature}$$

Despite extremes in environmental conditions and physical activity, temperature-control mechanisms of humans keep body **core temperature** (temperature of the deep tissues) relatively constant (Fig. 29-1). However, surface temperature varies, depending on blood flow to the skin and the amount of heat lost to the external environment. Because of these surface temperature changes, the

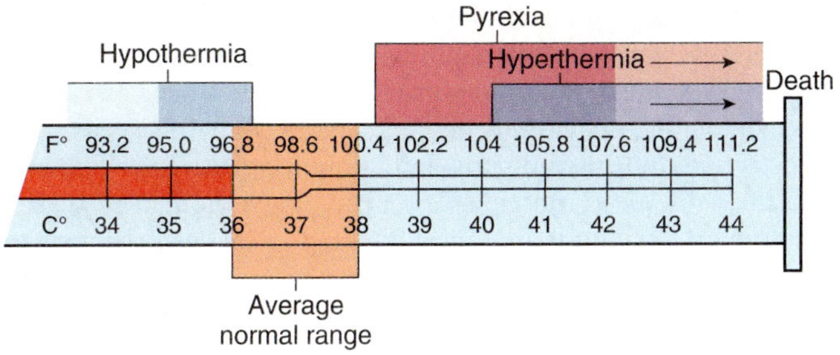

FIG. 29-1 Ranges of normal temperature values and abnormal body temperature alterations.

acceptable temperature of humans ranges from 36° to 38° C (96.8° to 100.4° F). Bodily tissues and cells function best within the relatively narrow temperature range.

The site of temperature measurement (oral, rectal, axillary, tympanic membrane, temporal artery, esophageal, pulmonary artery, or even urinary bladder) is one factor that determines a patient's temperature. For healthy young adults the average oral temperature is 37° C (98.6° F). In clinical practice you learn the temperature range of individual patients. No single temperature is normal for all people.

The measurement of body temperature aims to obtain a representative average temperature of core body tissues. Sites reflecting core temperatures are more reliable indicators of body temperature than those reflecting surface temperatures. In addition, the temperature value obtained often differs, depending on the measurement site.

Regulation. Physiological and behavioral mechanisms regulate the balance between heat lost and heat produced, or **thermoregulation.** For the body temperature to stay constant and within an acceptable range, various mechanisms maintain the relationship between heat production and heat loss. Apply knowledge of temperature-control mechanisms to promote temperature regulation.

Neural and Vascular Control. The hypothalamus, located between the cerebral hemispheres, controls body temperature the same way a thermostat works in the home. A comfortable temperature is the "set point" at which a heating system operates. In the home a drop in environmental temperature activates the furnace, whereas a rise in temperature shuts the system down.

The hypothalamus senses minor changes in body temperature. The anterior hypothalamus controls heat loss, and the posterior hypothalamus controls heat production. When nerve cells in the anterior hypothalamus become heated beyond the set point, impulses are sent out to reduce body temperature. Mechanisms of heat loss include sweating, vasodilation (widening) of blood vessels, and inhibition of heat production. The body redistributes blood to surface vessels to promote heat loss.

If the posterior hypothalamus senses that body temperature is lower than the set point, the body initiates heat-conservation mechanisms. Vasoconstriction (narrowing) of blood vessels reduces blood flow to the skin and extremities. Compensatory heat production is stimulated through voluntary muscle contraction and muscle shivering. When vasoconstriction is ineffective in preventing additional heat loss, shivering begins. Disease or trauma to the hypothalamus or the spinal cord, which carries hypothalamic messages, causes serious alterations in temperature control.

Heat Production. Thermoregulation depends on the normal function of heat production processes. Heat produced by the body is a by-product of metabolism, which is the chemical reaction in all body cells. Food is the primary fuel source for metabolism. Activities requiring additional chemical reactions increase the metabolic rate. As metabolism increases, additional heat is produced. When metabolism decreases, less heat is produced. Heat production occurs during rest, voluntary movements, involuntary shivering, and nonshivering thermogenesis.

- Basal metabolism accounts for the heat produced by the body at absolute rest. The average **basal metabolic rate (BMR)** depends on the body surface area. Thyroid hormones also affect the BMR. By promoting the breakdown of body glucose and fat, thyroid hormones increase the rate of chemical reactions in almost all cells of the body. When large amounts of thyroid hormones are secreted, the BMR can increase 100% above normal. The absence of thyroid hormones reduces the BMR by half, causing a decrease in heat production. The male sex hormone testosterone increases BMR. Men have a higher BMR than women.
- Voluntary movements such as muscular activity during exercise require additional energy. The metabolic rate increases during activity, sometimes causing heat production to increase up to 50 times normal.
- **Shivering** is an involuntary body response to temperature differences in the body. The skeletal muscle movement during shivering requires significant energy. Shivering sometimes increases heat production 4 to 5 times greater than normal. The heat that is produced helps equalize the body temperature, and the shivering ceases. In vulnerable patients shivering seriously drains energy sources, resulting in further physiological deterioration.
- **Nonshivering thermogenesis** occurs primarily in neonates. Because neonates cannot shiver, a limited amount of vascular brown tissue, present at birth, is metabolized for heat production.

Heat Loss. Heat loss and heat production occur simultaneously. Skin structure and exposure to the environment result in constant, normal heat loss through radiation, conduction, convection, and evaporation.

Radiation is the transfer of heat from the surface of one object to the surface of another without direct contact between the two. As much as 85% of the surface area of the human body radiates heat to the environment. Peripheral vasodilation increases blood flow from the internal organs to the skin to increase radiant heat loss. Peripheral vasoconstriction minimizes radiant heat loss. Radiation increases as the temperature difference between the objects increases. Radiation heat loss can be considerable during surgery when the patient's skin is exposed to a cool environment. However, if the environment is warmer than the skin, the body absorbs heat through radiation.

The patient's position enhances radiation heat loss (e.g., standing exposes a greater radiating surface area, and lying in a fetal position minimizes heat radiation). Help promote heat loss through radiation by removing clothing or blankets. Covering the body with dark, closely woven clothing decreases the amount of heat lost from radiation.

Conduction is the transfer of heat from one object to another with direct contact. Solids, liquids, and gases conduct heat through contact. When the warm skin touches a cooler object, heat is lost. Conduction normally accounts for a small amount of heat loss. Applying an ice pack or bathing a patient with a cool cloth increases conductive heat loss. Applying several layers of clothing reduces conductive loss. The body gains heat by conduction when it makes contact with materials warmer than skin temperature (e.g., application of an aquathermia pad).

Convection is the transfer of heat away by air movement. A fan promotes heat loss through convection. Convective heat loss increases when moistened skin comes into contact with slightly moving air.

Evaporation is the transfer of heat energy when a liquid is changed to a gas. The body continuously loses heat by evaporation. Approximately 600 to 900 mL a day evaporates from the skin and lungs, resulting in water and heat loss. By regulating perspiration or sweating, the body promotes additional evaporative heat loss. When body temperature rises, the anterior hypothalamus signals the sweat glands to release sweat through tiny ducts on the surface of the skin. Sweat evaporates, resulting in heat loss. During physical exercise over 80% of the heat produced is lost by evaporation (Lim, Byrne, and Lee, 2008).

Diaphoresis is visible perspiration primarily occurring on the forehead and upper thorax, although you can see it in other places on the body. For each hour of exercise in hot conditions approximately 1 L of body fluid is lost in sweat (Lim, Byrne, and Lee, 2008). Excessive evaporation causes skin scaling and itching and drying of the nares and pharynx. A lowered body temperature inhibits sweat gland secretion. People who have a congenital absence of sweat glands or a serious skin disease that impairs sweating are unable to tolerate warm temperatures because they cannot cool themselves adequately.

Skin in Temperature Regulation. The skin regulates temperature through insulation of the body, vasoconstriction (which affects the amount of blood flow and heat loss to the skin), and temperature sensation. The skin, subcutaneous tissue, and fat keep heat inside the body. Persons with more body fat have more natural insulation than do slim and muscular people.

The way the skin controls body temperature is similar to the way an automobile radiator controls engine temperature. An automobile engine generates a great deal of heat. Water is pumped through the engine to collect the heat and carry it to the radiator, where a fan transfers the heat from the water to the outside air. In the human body the internal organs produce heat; during exercise or increased sympathetic stimulation the amount of heat produced is greater than the usual core temperature. Blood flows from the internal organs, carrying heat to the body surface. The skin has many blood vessels, especially the areas of the hands, feet, and ears. Blood flow through these vascular areas of the skin varies from minimal flow to as much as 30% of the blood ejected from the heart. Heat transfers from the blood, through vessel walls, to the surface of the skin and is lost to the environment through the heat-loss mechanisms. The core temperature of the body remains within safe limits.

The degree of vasoconstriction determines the amount of blood flow and heat loss to the skin. If the core temperature is too high, the hypothalamus inhibits vasoconstriction. As a result, blood vessels dilate, and more blood reaches the surface of the skin. On a hot, humid day the blood vessels in the hands are dilated and easily visible. In contrast, if the core temperature becomes too low, the hypothalamus initiates vasoconstriction, and blood flow to the skin lessens to conserve heat.

Behavioral Control. Healthy individuals are able to maintain comfortable body temperature when exposed to temperature extremes. The ability of a person to control body temperature depends on (1) the degree of temperature extreme, (2) the person's ability to sense feeling comfortable or uncomfortable, (3) thought processes or emotions, and (4) the person's mobility or ability to remove or add clothes. Individuals are unable to control body temperature if any of these abilities is lost. For example, infants are able to sense uncomfortable warm conditions but need assistance in changing their environment. Older adults sometimes need help in detecting cold environments and minimizing heat loss. Illnesses, a decreased level of consciousness, or impaired thought processes result in an inability to recognize the need to change behavior for temperature control. When temperatures become extremely hot or cold, health-promoting behaviors such as removing or adding clothing have a limited effect on controlling temperature.

Factors Affecting Body Temperature

Many factors affect body temperature. Changes in body temperature within an acceptable range occur when physiological or behavioral mechanisms alter the relationship between heat production and heat loss. Be aware of these factors when assessing temperature variations and evaluating deviations from normal.

Age. At birth the newborn leaves a warm, relatively constant environment and enters one in which temperatures fluctuate widely. Temperature-control mechanisms are immature. An infant's temperature responds drastically to changes in the environment. Take extra care to protect newborns from environmental temperatures. Provide adequate clothing, and avoid exposing infants to temperature extremes. A newborn loses up to 30% of body heat through the head and therefore needs to wear a cap to prevent heat loss. When protected from environmental extremes, the newborn's body temperature is usually within 35.5° to 37.5° C (95.9° to 99.5° F).

Temperature regulation is unstable until children reach puberty. The usual temperature range gradually drops as individuals approach older adulthood. The older adult has a narrower range of body temperatures than the younger adult. Oral temperatures of 35° C (95° F) are sometimes found in older adults in cold weather. However, the average body temperature of older adults is approximately 36° C (96.8° F). Older adults are particularly sensitive to temperature extremes because of deterioration in control mechanisms, particularly poor vasomotor control (control of vasoconstriction and vasodilation), reduced amounts of subcutaneous tissue, reduced sweat gland activity, and reduced metabolism.

Exercise. Muscle activity requires an increased blood supply and carbohydrate and fat breakdown. Any form of exercise increases metabolism and heat production and thus body temperature. Prolonged strenuous exercise such as long-distance running temporarily raises body temperature.

Hormone Level. Women generally experience greater fluctuations in body temperature than men. Hormonal variations during the menstrual cycle cause body temperature fluctuations. Progesterone levels rise and fall cyclically during the menstrual cycle. When progesterone levels are low, the body temperature is a few tenths of a degree below the baseline level. The lower temperature persists until ovulation occurs. During ovulation greater amounts of progesterone enter the circulatory system and raise the body temperature to previous baseline levels or higher. These temperature variations help to predict a woman's most fertile time to achieve pregnancy.

Body temperature changes also occur in women during menopause (cessation of menstruation). Women who have stopped menstruating often experience periods of intense body heat and sweating lasting from 30 seconds to 5 minutes. During these periods often intermittent skin temperature increases up to 4° C (7.2° F), referred to as hot flashes. This is caused by the instability of the vasomotor controls for vasodilation and vasoconstriction.

Circadian Rhythm. Body temperature normally changes 0.5° to 1° C (0.9° to 1.8° F) during a 24-hour period. However, temperature is one of the most stable rhythms in humans. The temperature is usually lowest between 1:00 and 4:00 AM (Fig. 29-2). During the day body temperature rises steadily until a maximum temperature value at about 4:00 PM and then declines to early-morning levels (Henker and Carlson, 2007). Temperature patterns are not automatically reversed in people who work at night and sleep during the day. It takes 1 to 3 weeks for the cycle to reverse. In general, the circadian temperature rhythm does not change with age.

Stress. Physical and emotional stress increase body temperature through hormonal and neural stimulation. These physiological changes increase metabolism, which increases heat production. A patient who is anxious about entering a hospital or a health care provider's office often has a higher normal temperature.

Environment. Environment influences body temperature. When placed in a warm room a patient may be unable to regulate body temperature by heat-loss mechanisms, and the body temperature may elevate. If the patient were outside in the cold without warm clothing, body temperature may be low as a result of extensive radiant and conductive heat loss. Environmental temperatures affect infants and older adults more often because their temperature-regulating mechanisms are less efficient.

Temperature Alterations. Changes in body temperature outside the usual range are related to excessive heat production, excessive heat loss, minimal heat production, minimal heat loss, or any combination of these alterations.

Fever. **Fever,** or **pyrexia,** occurs because heat-loss mechanisms are unable to keep pace with excessive heat production, resulting in an abnormal rise in body temperature. A fever is usually not harmful if it stays below 39° C (102.2° F). A single temperature reading does not always indicate a fever. In addition to physical signs and symptoms of infection, fever determination is based on several temperature readings at different times of the day compared with the usual value for that person at that time.

A true fever results from an alteration in the hypothalamic set point. **Pyrogens** such as bacteria and viruses elevate body temperature. Pyrogens act as antigens, triggering immune system responses. The hypothalamus reacts to raise the set point, and the body responds by producing and conserving heat. Several hours pass before the body temperature reaches the new set point. During this period a person experiences chills, shivers, and feels cold, even though the body temperature is rising (Fig. 29-3). The chill phase resolves when the new set point, a higher temperature, is achieved. During the next phase, the plateau, the chills subside, and the person feels warm and dry. If the new set point is "overshot" or the pyrogens are removed (e.g., destruction of bacteria by antibiotics), the third phase of a **febrile** episode occurs. The hypothalamus set point drops, initiating heat loss responses. The skin becomes warm and flushed because of vasodilation. Diaphoresis assists in evaporative heat loss. When the fever "breaks," the patient becomes **afebrile.**

Fever is an important defense mechanism. Mild temperature elevations as high as 39° C (102.2° F) enhance the immune system of the body. During a febrile episode white blood cell production is stimulated. Increased temperature reduces the concentration of iron in the blood plasma, suppressing the growth of bacteria. Fever also fights viral infections by stimulating interferon, the natural virus-fighting substance of the body.

Fevers and fever patterns serve a diagnostic purpose. Fever patterns differ, depending on the causative pyrogen (Box 29-3). The increase or decrease in pyrogen activity results in fever spikes and declines at different times of the day. The duration and degree of fever depend on the strength of the pyrogen and the ability of the individual to respond. The term **fever of unknown origin (FUO)** refers to a fever with an undetermined cause.

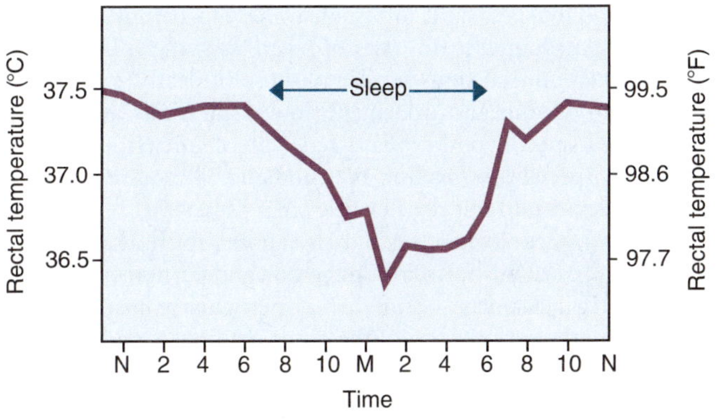

FIG. 29-2 Temperature cycle for 24 hours.

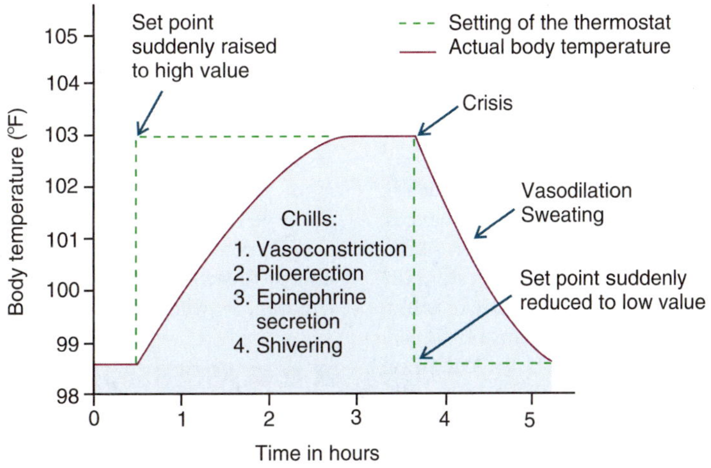

FIG. 29-3 Effect of changing set point of hypothalamic temperature control during a fever. (Modified from Guyton AC, Hall JE: *Textbook of medical physiology,* ed 12, Philadelphia, 2011, Saunders.)

BOX 29-3 PATTERNS OF FEVER

Sustained: A constant body temperature continuously above 38° C (100.4° F) that has little fluctuation

Intermittent: Fever spikes interspersed with usual temperature levels (Temperature returns to acceptable value at least once in 24 hours.)

Remittent: Fever spikes and falls without a return to normal temperature levels.

Relapsing: Periods of febrile episodes and periods with acceptable temperature values (Febrile episodes and periods of normothermia are often longer than 24 hours.)

During a fever cellular metabolism increases, and oxygen consumption rises. Body metabolism increases 10% for every degree Celsius of temperature elevation (Henker and Carlson, 2007). Heart and respiratory rates increase to meet the metabolic needs of the body for nutrients. The increased metabolism uses energy that produces additional heat. If a patient has a cardiac or respiratory problem, the stress of a fever is great. A prolonged fever weakens a patient by exhausting energy stores. Increased metabolism requires additional oxygen. If the body cannot meet the demand for additional oxygen, cellular hypoxia (inadequate oxygen) occurs. Myocardial hypoxia produces angina (chest pain). Cerebral hypoxia produces confusion. Interventions during a fever include oxygen therapy. When water loss through increased respiration and diaphoresis is excessive, the patient is at risk for fluid volume deficit. Dehydration is a serious problem for older adults and children with low body weight. Maintaining optimum fluid volume status is an important nursing action (see Chapter 41).

Hyperthermia. An elevated body temperature related to the inability of the body to promote heat loss or reduce heat production is **hyperthermia.** Whereas fever is an upward shift in the set point, hyperthermia results from an overload of the thermoregulatory mechanisms of the body. Any disease or trauma to the hypothalamus impairs heat-loss mechanisms. **Malignant hyperthermia** is a hereditary condition of uncontrolled heat production that occurs when susceptible people receive certain anesthetic drugs.

Heatstroke. Heat depresses hypothalamic function. Prolonged exposure to the sun or a high environmental temperature overwhelms the heat-loss mechanisms of the body. These conditions cause **heatstroke,** defined as a body temperature of 40° C (104° F) or more (Lewis, 2007). Heatstroke is a dangerous heat emergency with a high mortality rate. Patients at risk include the very young or very old and those who have cardiovascular disease, hypothyroidism, diabetes, or alcoholism. Also at risk are those who take medications that decrease the ability of the body to lose heat (e.g., phenothiazines, anticholinergics, diuretics, amphetamines, and beta-adrenergic receptor antagonists) and those who exercise or work strenuously (e.g., athletes, construction workers, and farmers).

Signs and symptoms of heatstroke include giddiness, confusion, delirium, excess thirst, nausea, muscle cramps, visual disturbances, and even incontinence. Vital signs reveal a body temperature sometimes as high as 45° C (113° F), with an increase in heart rate (HR) and lowering of BP. The most important sign of heatstroke is hot, dry skin. Victims of heatstroke do not sweat because of severe electrolyte loss and hypothalamic malfunction. If the condition progresses, the patient with heatstroke becomes unconscious, with fixed, nonreactive pupils. Permanent neurological damage occurs unless cooling measures are rapidly started.

Heat Exhaustion. **Heat exhaustion** occurs when profuse diaphoresis results in excess water and electrolyte loss. Caused by environmental heat exposure, the patient exhibits signs and symptoms of fluid volume deficit (see Chapter 41). First aid includes transporting him or her to a cooler environment and restoring fluid and electrolyte balance.

TABLE 29-1 Classification of Hypothermia

	CELSIUS	FAHRENHEIT
Mild	34°-36°	93.2°-96.8°
Moderate	30°-34°	86.0°-93.2°
Severe	<30°	<86°

Hypothermia. Heat loss during prolonged exposure to cold overwhelms the ability of the body to produce heat, causing hypothermia. **Hypothermia** is classified by core temperature measurements (Table 29-1). It is sometimes unintentional such as falling through the ice of a frozen lake. Occasionally hypothermia is intentionally induced during surgical or emergency procedures to reduce metabolic demand and the need of the body for oxygen.

Accidental hypothermia usually develops gradually and goes unnoticed for several hours. When skin temperature drops below 35° C (95° F), the patient suffers uncontrolled shivering, loss of memory, depression, and poor judgment. As the body temperature falls below 34.4° C (94° F), HR, respiratory rate, and BP fall. The skin becomes cyanotic. Patients experience cardiac dysrhythmias, loss of consciousness, and unresponsiveness to painful stimuli if hypothermia progresses. In cases of severe hypothermia a person demonstrates clinical signs similar to those of death (e.g., lack of response to stimuli and extremely slow respirations and pulse). When you suspect hypothermia, assessment of core temperature is critical. A special low-reading thermometer is required because standard devices do not register below 35° C (95° F).

Frostbite occurs when the body is exposed to subnormal temperatures. Ice crystals form inside the cell, and permanent circulatory and tissue damage occurs. Areas particularly susceptible to frostbite are the earlobes, tip of the nose, and fingers and toes. The injured area becomes white, waxy, and firm to the touch. The patient loses sensation in the affected area. Interventions include gradual warming measures, analgesia, and protection of the injured tissue.

NURSING PROCESS

Apply the nursing process and use a critical thinking approach in your care of patients. The nursing process provides a clinical decision-making approach for you to develop and implement an individualized plan of care. Knowledge of the physiology of body temperature regulation is essential to assess and evaluate a patient's response to temperature alterations and intervene safely. Implement independent measures to increase or minimize heat loss, promote heat conservation, and increase comfort. These measures complement the effects of medically ordered therapies during illness. You also provide education to family members, parents of children, or other caregivers.

ASSESSMENT

Through the Patient's Eyes. During the assessment process thoroughly assess each patient, explore his or her beliefs and experiences, and critically analyze findings to ensure that you make patient-centered clinical decisions required for safe nursing care.

Sites. Core and surface body temperature can be measured at several sites. Intensive care units use the core temperatures of the pulmonary artery, esophagus, and urinary bladder. These measurements require the use of continuous invasive devices placed in body cavities or organs and continually display readings on an electronic monitor.

Use a thermometer to obtain intermittent temperature measurements from the mouth, rectum, tympanic membrane, temporal artery, and axilla. You can also apply noninvasive chemically prepared thermometer patches to the skin. Oral, rectal, axillary, and skin temperature sites rely on effective blood circulation at the measurement site. The heat of the blood is conducted to the thermometer probe. Tympanic temperature relies on the radiation of body heat to an infrared sensor. Because the tympanic membrane shares the same arterial blood supply as the hypothalamus, it is a core temperature. Temporal artery measurements detect the temperature of cutaneous blood flow.

To ensure accurate temperature readings, measure each site correctly (see Skill 29-1 on pp. 467-471). The temperature obtained varies, depending on the site used, but it is usually between 36° C (96.8° F) and 38° C (100.4° F). Rectal temperatures are usually 0.5° C (0.9° F) higher than oral temperatures, and axillary temperatures are usually 0.5° C (0.9° F) lower than oral temperatures. Each of the common temperature measurement sites has advantages and disadvantages (Box 29-4). Choose the safest and most accurate site for the patient. When possible, use the same site when repeated measurements are necessary.

Thermometers. Two types of thermometers are available for measuring body temperature: electronic and disposable. The mercury-in-glass thermometer, once the standard device, has been eliminated from health care facilities because of the environmental hazards of mercury. However, some patients still use mercury-in-glass thermometers at home. When you find a mercury-in-glass thermometer in the home, teach the patient about safer temperature devices and encourage the disposal of mercury products at appropriate neighborhood hazardous disposal locations.

Each device measures temperature using the **Celsius** or **Fahrenheit** scale. Electronic thermometers convert the temperature scales by activating a switch. When it is necessary to convert temperature readings, use the following formulas:

1. To convert Fahrenheit to Celsius, subtract 32 from the Fahrenheit reading and multiply the result by 5/9.

$$C = (F - 32) \times 5/9$$

$$\text{Example: } 40° \text{ C} = (104° \text{ F} - 32) \times 5/9$$

2. To convert Celsius to Fahrenheit, multiply the Celsius reading by 9/5 and add 32 to the product.

$$F = (9/5 \times °C) + 32$$

$$\text{Example: } 104° \text{ F} = (9/5 \times 40° \text{ C}) + 32°$$

Electronic Thermometer. The electronic thermometer consists of a rechargeable battery-powered display unit, a thin wire cord, and a temperature-processing probe covered by a disposable probe cover (Fig. 29-4). Separate unbreakable probes are available for oral and rectal use. You can also use the oral probe for axillary temperature measurement. Electronic thermometers provide two modes of operation: a 4-second predictive temperature and a 3-minute standard temperature. In day-to-day clinical situations most nurses use the 4-second predictive mode. A sound signals, and a reading appears on the display unit when the peak temperature reading has been measured.

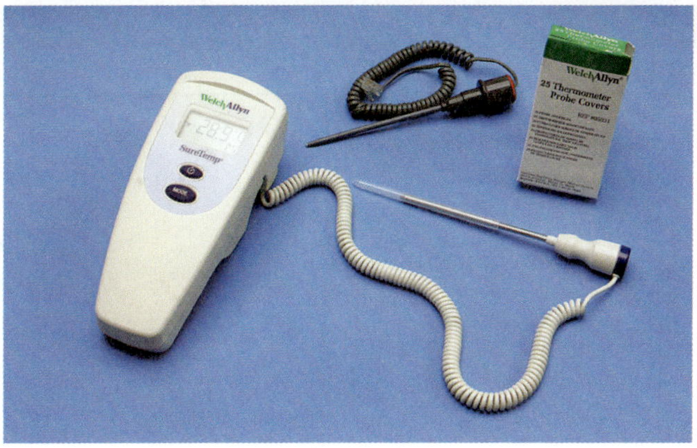

FIG. 29-4 Electronic thermometer. Blue probe is for oral or axillary use. Red probe is for rectal use.

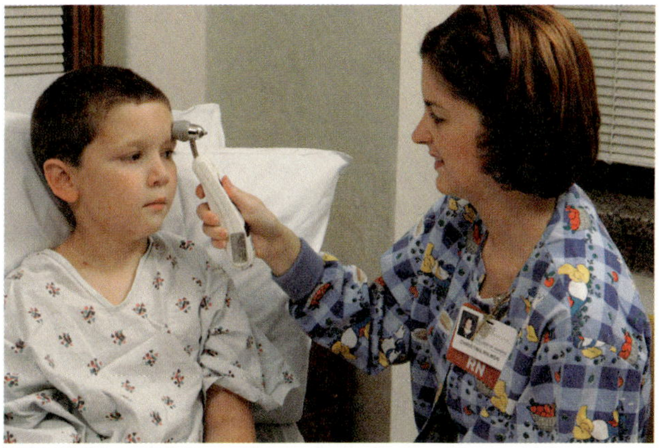

FIG. 29-5 Temporal artery thermometer scanning child's forehead.

Another form of electronic thermometer is used exclusively for tympanic temperature. An otoscope-like speculum with an infrared sensor tip detects heat radiated from the tympanic membrane. Within seconds of placement in the auditory canal, a sound signals, and a reading appears on the display unit when the peak temperature reading has been measured (Box 29-5).

Another form of electronic thermometer measures the temperature of the superficial temporal artery. A handheld scanner with an infrared sensor tip detects the temperature of cutaneous blood flow by sweeping the sensor across the forehead and just behind the ear (Fig. 29-5). After scanning is complete, a reading appears on the display unit. Temporal artery temperature is a reliable noninvasive measure of core temperature (Box 29-6).

The greatest advantages of electronic thermometers are that their readings appear within seconds and they are easy to read. The plastic sheath is unbreakable and ideal for children. Their expense is a major disadvantage. Maintaining cleanliness of the probes is an important consideration. For example, if not properly cleaned between patients, gastrointestinal contamination of the rectal probe causes disease transmission. Wipe the thermometer daily with alcohol and the thermometer probe with an alcohol swab after each patient, paying particular attention to the ridges where the probe cover is secured to the probe.

Chemical Dot Thermometers. Single-use or reusable chemical dot thermometers (Fig. 29-6) are thin strips of plastic with a

BOX 29-4 ADVANTAGES AND DISADVANTAGES OF SELECT TEMPERATURE MEASUREMENT SITES

SITE ADVANTAGES	SITE LIMITATIONS
Oral	
Easily accessible—requires no position change Comfortable for patient Provides accurate surface temperature reading Reflects rapid change in core temperature Reliable route to measure temperature in patients who are intubated	Causes delay in measurement if patient recently ingested hot/cold fluids or foods, smoked, or is receiving oxygen by mask/cannula Not for patients who had oral surgery, trauma, history of epilepsy, or shaking chills Not for infants, small children, or patients who are confused, unconscious, or uncooperative Risk of body fluid exposure
Tympanic Membrane	
Easily accessible site Minimal patient repositioning required Obtained without disturbing, waking, or repositioning patients Used for patients with tachypnea without affecting breathing Provides accurate core reading because eardrum close to hypothalamus; sensitive to core temperature changes Very rapid measurement (2 to 5 seconds) Unaffected by oral intake of food or fluids or smoking Used in newborns to reduce infant handling and heat loss	More variability of measurement than with other core temperature devices (Lawson, Bridges, and Ballou, 2007) Requires removal of hearing aids before measurement Requires disposable sensor cover with only one size available Otitis media and cerumen impaction distorts readings (Lawson et al., 2007) Not used in patients who have had surgery of the ear or tympanic membrane Does not accurately measure core temperature changes during and after exercise Does not obtain continuous measurement Affected by ambient temperature devices such as incubators, radiant warmers, and facial fans When used in neonates, infants, and children under 3 years old, use care to position device correctly because anatomy of ear canal makes it difficult to position Inaccuracies reported caused by incorrect positioning of handheld unit
Rectal	
Sometimes considered to be more reliable when oral temperature cannot be obtained	Lags behind core temperature during rapid temperature changes (Henker and Carlson, 2007) Not for patients with diarrhea, rectal disorders, or bleeding tendencies or those who had rectal surgery Requires positioning and is often source of patient embarrassment and anxiety Risk of body fluid exposure Requires lubrication Not for routine vital signs in newborns Readings influenced by impacted stool
Axilla	
Safe and inexpensive Used with newborns and unconscious patients	Long measurement time Underestimates core temperature (Lawson et al., 2007) Requires continuous positioning by nurse Measurement lags behind core temperature during rapid temperature changes Not recommended to detect fever in infants and young children (Lim, Byrne, and Lee, 2008) Requires exposure of thorax, which results in temperature loss, especially in newborns Affected by exposure to environment, including time to place thermometer
Skin	
Inexpensive Provides continuous reading Safe and noninvasive Used for neonates	Measurement lags behind other sites during temperature changes, especially during hyperthermia Adhesion impaired by diaphoresis or sweat Reading affected by environmental temperature Cannot be used for patients with allergy to adhesive
Temporal Artery	
Easy to access without position change Very rapid measurement No risk of injury to patient or nurse Eliminates need to disrobe or be unbundled Comfortable for patient Used in premature infants, newborns, and children Reflects rapid change in core temperature Sensor cover not required	Inaccurate with head covering or hair on forehead Affected by skin moisture such as diaphoresis or sweating

BOX 29-5 EVIDENCE-BASED PRACTICE

Comparing Temperatures at Different Measurement Sites

PICO Question: Are tympanic thermometers compared with oral or temporal thermometers accurate in measuring body temperature in hospitalized patients?

Evidence Summary

Numerous devices and sites for measuring temperature allow you to select the best approach for the clinical condition of the patient. As the patient's condition changes, obtaining a temperature using a different temperature device for a different site is sometimes needed. Oral, tympanic, and temporal thermometers are the most frequently used devices for medical and surgical adult and pediatric patients. To safely substitute a temperature measurement from one site to another, the temperature agreement needs to be within 1° C (1.8° F). The reliability of the tympanic membrane thermometer has been questioned (Lawson et al., 2007). A study of postoperative patients reported that nearly 20% of the patients had at least a 2° C (3.6° F) difference between tympanic and oral temperature measurements (Frommelt, Ott, and Hays, 2008). In a study of the tympanic and temporal temperatures of 178 acute care patients, over 40% of the patients' two temperatures differed more than 1° C (1.8° F) (Woodrow et al., 2006). In another study five trained data collectors obtained tympanic and temporal temperatures of over 200 preoperative and postoperative patients. Although 63% of the temperatures were within a 0.5° C (0.9° F) difference, the temperatures varied by over 1° C (1.8° F) in 13% of patients (Fetzer and Lawrence, 2008).

The unreliability of the tympanic thermometer is attributed to errors in technique and patient characteristics such as the presence of cerumen. Research shows a lack of agreement among commonly used temperature devices. Selection of the site to obtain a patient's temperature is a nursing responsibility. When evaluating temperature over time, measurements obtained from different sites are not interchangeable. Use values from a consistent site when trending temperatures.

Application to Nursing Practice

- Always record the site of a temperature measurement with the temperature.
- Do not compare an oral temperature taken at one time with a tympanic or temporal artery temperature taken earlier or later.
- There is no agreement as to the most accurate noninvasive temperature measurement site.

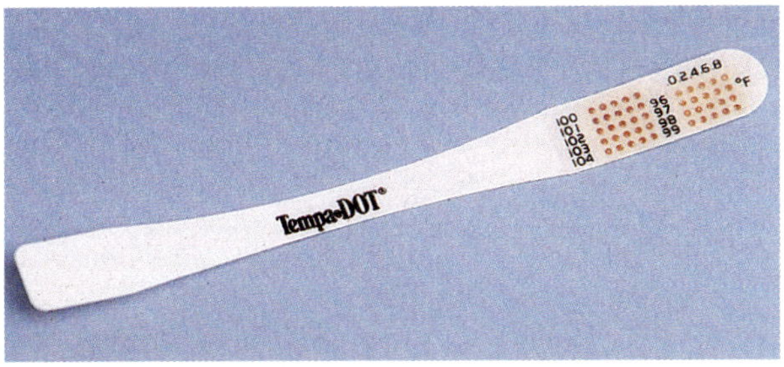

FIG. 29-6 Disposable, single-use thermometer strip.

temperature sensor at one end. The sensor consists of a matrix of chemically impregnated dots that change color at different temperatures. In the Celsius version there are 50 dots, each representing a temperature increment of 0.1° C, over a range of 35.5° C to 40.4° C. The Fahrenheit version has 45 dots with increments of 0.2° F and a range of 96° F to 104.8° F. Chemical dots on the

BOX 29-6 PROCEDURAL GUIDELINES

Measurement of Temporal Artery Temperature

Delegation Considerations

The skill of measuring temporal artery temperature can be delegated to nursing assistive personnel (NAP). Instruct the NAP to:

- Obtain temperature for select patient with ordered frequency.
- Report abnormalities to the nurse for further assessment.

Equipment

Temporal artery thermometer, alcohol wipes (optional), probe cover (optional).

1. Identify the patient using two identifiers (e.g., name and birth date or name and account number) according to facility policy.
2. Perform hand hygiene.
3. Ensure that forehead is dry; wipe with towel if needed.
4. Place probe flush on patient's forehead to avoid measuring ambient temperature.
5. Press red scan button with your thumb. Continuous scanning for highest temperature occurs until you release button.
6. Slowly slide thermometer straight across forehead while keeping probe flush on skin.
7. Keeping scan button pressed, lift probe from forehead and touch it to neck just behind earlobe (area where perfume is typically applied).
8. While scanning, a clicking sound occurs and stops when peak temperature is reached.
9. Release scan button; read and record temperature. Reading remains on for 15 seconds after you release the button.
10. Clean probe with alcohol wipe or remove and dispose of probe cover if used.
11. Perform hand hygiene.
12. Discuss findings with patient as needed.
13. Compare measurement with patient baseline and acceptable values.
14. Record temperature on nurses' notes, vital sign flow sheet, or electronic medical record.

thermometer change color to reflect temperature reading, usually within 60 seconds. Most are for single use. In one reusable brand for a single patient the chemical dots return to the original color within a few seconds. Chemical dot thermometers are usually for oral temperatures. You also use them at axillary or rectal sites, covered by a plastic sheath at the latter site, with a placement time of 3 minutes. Chemical dot thermometers are useful for screening temperatures, especially in infants and young children and patients who are intubated. Because chemical dot thermometers often underestimate oral temperature by 0.4° C (0.7° F) or more, use electronic thermometers to confirm measurements made with a chemical dot thermometer when treatment decisions are involved. Chemical dot thermometers are useful when caring for patients on protective isolation to avoid the need to take electronic instruments into patient rooms (see Chapter 28).

Another disposable thermometer useful for screening temperature is a temperature-sensitive patch or tape. Applied to the forehead or abdomen, chemical sensitive areas of the patch change color at different temperatures.

NURSING DIAGNOSIS

After concluding your assessment, cluster defining characteristics to form a nursing diagnosis (Box 29-7). For example, an increase in body temperature, flushed skin, skin warm to touch, and tachycardia indicate the diagnosis of *hyperthermia.* State the nursing diagnosis as either an at-risk or actual temperature alteration.

BOX 29-7 NURSING DIAGNOSTIC PROCESS

Ineffective Thermoregulation Related to Aging and Inability to Adapt to Environmental Temperature

ASSESSMENT ACTIVITIES	DEFINING CHARACTERISTICS
Obtain vital signs, including temperature, pulse (see Skill 29-2), respirations (see Skill 29-3), SpO_2 (see Skill 29-4).	Increased body temperature above usual range Tachycardia Tachypnea Hypoxemia
Palpate skin.	Warm, dry skin
Observe patient's appearance and behavior while talking and resting.	Restlessness Confusion Flushed appearance
Review medical history.	Found in unventilated apartment during heat wave; 85 years old with history of dementia

Implement actions to minimize or eliminate the risk factors if the patient has risk factors for temperature alterations. Examples of nursing diagnoses for patients with body temperature alterations include the following:

- Risk for imbalanced body temperature
- Hyperthermia
- Hypothermia
- Ineffective thermoregulation

Once you determine a diagnosis, accurately select the related factor or etiology. The related factor allows you to select appropriate nursing interventions. In the example of hyperthermia, a related factor of vigorous activity results in much different interventions than a related factor of decreased ability to perspire.

PLANNING

During planning integrate the knowledge gathered from assessment and the patient history to develop an individualized plan of care (see the Nursing Care Plan). Match the patient's needs with interventions that are supported and recommended in the clinical research literature.

Goals and Outcomes. The plan of care for a patient with alteration in temperature includes realistic and individualized goals along with relevant outcomes. This requires collaboration with the patient and family in setting goals and outcomes and selecting nursing interventions. Establish expected outcomes to gauge progress toward returning the body temperature to an acceptable range. In cases in which the temperature alteration requires helping patients modify their environment, goals may be long term (e.g., obtaining appropriate clothing to wear in cold weather). Short-term goals such as regaining normal range of body temperature improve patient health. In the example of a patient who has an elevated fever and excessive diaphoresis, the goal of care is attaining fluid and electrolyte balance. The outcome is that patient intake and output will be equal for the next 24 hours.

Setting Priorities. Set priorities of care with regard to the extent that the temperature alteration affects a patient. The severity of a temperature alteration and its effects, together with the patient's general health status, influence your priorities in his or her care. Safety is a top priority. Often other medical problems complicate the care plan. For instance, body temperature imbalance affects body requirements for fluids. Patients with heart problems often have difficulty tolerating required fluid replacement therapy.

Teamwork and Collaboration. Patients at risk for imbalanced body temperature require an individualized care plan directed at maintaining normothermia and reducing risk factors. For example, it is important to establish the outcome that the patient can explain appropriate actions to take and available community resources to use (e.g., cooling stations) during a heat wave. Teach the patient and caregiver the importance of thermoregulation and actions to take during excessive environmental heat. Education is particularly important for parents, who need to know how to take action at home and whom to call (e.g., health care provider's office, home care nurse) when an infant or child develops a temperature imbalance.

IMPLEMENTATION

Health Promotion. By maintaining balance between heat production and heat loss you promote the health of patients at risk for imbalanced body temperature. Consider patient activity, temperature of the environment, and clothing. Teach patients to avoid strenuous exercise in hot, humid weather; drink fluids such as water or clear fruity juices before, during, and after exercise; and wear light, loose-fitting, light-colored clothes. Also teach patients to avoid exercising in areas with poor ventilation, wear a protective covering over the head when outdoors, and expose themselves to hot climates gradually.

Prevention is the key for patients at risk for hypothermia. It involves educating patients, family members, and friends. Patients at risk include the very young; the very old; and people debilitated by trauma, stroke, diabetes, drug or alcohol intoxication, and sepsis. Patients who are mentally ill or handicapped sometimes fall victim to hypothermia because they are unaware of the dangers of cold conditions. People without adequate home heating, shelter, diet, or clothing are also at risk. Fatigue, dark skin color, malnutrition, and hypoxemia also contribute to the risk of frostbite.

Acute Care

Fever. When an elevated body temperature develops, initiate interventions to treat fever. The objective of therapy is to increase heat loss, reduce heat production, and prevent complications. The choice of interventions depends on the cause; adverse effects; and the strength, intensity, and duration of the temperature elevation. Nurses are essential in assessing and implementing temperature-reducing strategies (Box 29-8). The health care provider attempts to determine the cause of the elevated temperature by isolating the causative pyrogen. Sometimes it is necessary to obtain culture specimens for laboratory analysis such as urine, blood, sputum, and wound sites (see Chapter 28). Some antibiotic medications are ordered to be given after the cultures have been obtained. Administering antibiotics destroys pyrogenic bacteria and eliminates body stimulus for the elevated temperature.

Most fevers in children are of a viral origin, last only briefly, and have limited effects. However, children still have immature temperature-control mechanisms, and temperatures can rise rapidly. Dehydration and febrile seizures occur during rising temperatures of children between 6 months and 3 years of age. Febrile seizures are unusual in children more than 5 years of age. The extent of the temperature, often exceeding 38.8° C (101.8° F), seems to be a more important factor than the rapidity of the temperature increase. Children are at particular risk for fluid volume deficit because they can quickly lose large amounts of fluids in proportion

NURSING CARE PLAN

Hyperthermia

ASSESSMENT

Mr. Coburn is a 56-year-old school teacher who arrives at the outpatient clinic with malaise. His medical history includes a past urinary tract infection. Several of his students have been out of school lately with colds. He has been feeling poorly for the past 3 days.

Assessment Activities	*Findings/Defining Characteristics**
Palpate skin.	Mr. Coburn's skin is **warm and dry** to touch.
Observe patient's behavior while talking and resting.	Mr. Coburn appears to have labored breathing. His face is **flushed.**
Obtain vital signs.	Blood pressure right arm 116/62 mm Hg, left arm 114/64 mm Hg; right radial pulse **128 beats/min,** regular and bounding; respiratory rate **26 breaths/min;** SpO_2 98% on room air; oral temperature **39.2° C** (102.6° F).
Review medical history.	He admits to smoking one pack of cigarettes per day and recently began expectorating **yellow-green sputum.** He has been **tired** for the past 3 days and on rising in the morning has been dizzy.

***Defining characteristics** are shown in bold type.

NURSING DIAGNOSIS: Hyperthermia related to infectious process

PLANNING

Goals	*Expected Outcomes (NOC)*† **Thermoregulation**
Mr. Coburn will regain normal range of body temperature within next 24 hours.	Body temperature will decline at least 1° C (1.8° F) within next 8 hours.
Mr. Coburn will state a sense of comfort and rest within next 48 hours.	Patient will verbalize increased satisfaction with rest and sleep pattern. Patient will report increase in energy level within next 3 days.
Mr. Coburn's fluid and electrolyte balance will be maintained during next 3 days.	Intake will equal output within next 24 hours. No evidence of postural hypotension during ambulation.

†Outcome classification labels from Moorhead S et al: *Nursing outcomes classification (NOC),* ed 4, St Louis, 2008, Mosby.

INTERVENTIONS (NIC)‡ *Fever Treatment*	**RATIONALE**
Instruct Mr. Coburn to reduce external coverings and keep clothing and bed linen dry.	Promotes heat loss through conduction and convection.
Instruct Mr. Coburn to use ordered antipyretic medications safely when needed for comfort.	Antipyretics reduce set point (Lehne, 2010).
Instruct Mr. Coburn to limit physical activity and increase frequency of rest periods over next 2 days.	Activity and stress increase metabolic rate, contributing to heat production.
Instruct Mr. Coburn to increase oral fluids of choice to 8 to 10 8-oz glasses of fluid daily.	Increased metabolic rate and diaphoresis associated with fever causes loss of body fluids (Hockenberg, 2008).

‡Intervention classification labels from Bulechek GM, Butcher HK, and Dochterman JM: *Nursing interventions classification (NIC),* ed 5, St Louis, 2008, Mosby.

EVALUATION

Nursing Actions	*Patient Response/Finding*	*Achievement of Outcome*
Obtain body temperature measurement.	Body temperature 37.8° C (100.0° F).	Body temperature within normal limits.
Obtain orthostatic blood pressure measurements.	Blood pressure measurements lying, sitting, and standing are within 5 mm Hg of each other.	No evidence of postural hypotension.
Ask Mr. Coburn if his energy level has changed since the last visit.	He responds, "I am sleeping much better and have returned to work with a lot more energy."	Improved rest and sleep pattern and increased energy level.

BOX 29-8 NURSING INTERVENTIONS FOR PATIENTS WITH A FEVER

Interventions (Unless Contraindicated)

- Obtain blood cultures (before beginning antibiotics) if ordered. Obtain blood specimens to coincide with temperature spikes when the antigen-producing organism is most prevalent.
- Minimize heat production: reduce the frequency of activities that increase oxygen demand such as excessive turning and ambulation; allow rest periods; limit physical activity.
- Maximize heat loss: reduce external covering on patient's body without causing shivering; keep clothing and bed linen dry.
- Satisfy requirements for increased metabolic rate: provide supplemental oxygen therapy as ordered to improve oxygen delivery to body cells; provide measures to stimulate appetite and offer well-balanced meals; provide fluids (at least 8 to 10 8-oz glasses for patients with normal cardiac and renal function) to replace fluids lost through insensible water loss and sweating.
- Promote patient comfort: encourage oral hygiene because oral mucous membranes dry easily from dehydration; control temperature of the environment without inducing shivering; apply damp cloth to patient's forehead.
- Identify onset and duration of febrile episode phases: examine previous temperature measurements for trends.
- Initiate health teaching as indicated.
- Control environmental temperature to 21° to 27° C (70° to 80° F).

to their body weight. It is important to maintain accurate intake and output records, weigh the patient daily, and encourage fluids.

Sometimes a fever is a hypersensitivity response to a drug. Drug fevers are often accompanied by other allergy symptoms such as rash or pruritus (itching). Treatment involves withdrawing the medication.

Antipyretics are medications that reduce fever. Nonsteroidal antiinflammatory drugs such as acetaminophen, salicylates, indomethacin, and ketorolac reduce fever by increasing heat loss. Corticosteroids reduce heat production by interfering with the immune system and mask signs of infection. They are not used to treat a fever. However, they can suppress fever in response to a pyrogen.

Nonpharmacological therapy for fever uses methods that increase heat loss by evaporation, conduction, convection, or radiation. Make sure that nursing measures to enhance body cooling do not stimulate shivering. Shivering is counterproductive and increases energy expenditure up to 400%. Tepid sponge baths, bathing with alcohol-water solutions, applying ice packs to axillae and groin areas, and cooling fans were previously used to reduce fever; however, avoid these therapies because they lead to shivering. There is no advantage of these methods over antipyretic medications.

Blankets cooled by circulating water delivered by motorized units increase conductive heat loss. Follow manufacturer instructions for applying these hypothermia blankets because of the risk for skin breakdown and "freeze burns." Placing a bath blanket between the patient and the hypothermia blanket and wrapping distal extremities (fingers, toes, and genitalia) reduces the risk of injury to the skin and tissue from hypothermia therapy. Wrapping the patient's extremities reduces the incidence and intensity of shivering. Medications such as meperidine or butorphanol reduce shivering.

Heatstroke. Heatstroke is an emergency situation. First aid treatment includes moving the patient to a cooler environment, removing excess body clothing, placing cool wet towels over the skin, and using oscillating fans to increase convective heat loss. Emergency medical treatment includes intravenous (IV) fluids, irrigating the stomach and lower bowel with cool solutions, and hypothermia blankets.

Hypothermia. The priority treatment for hypothermia is to prevent a further decrease in body temperature. Removing wet clothes, replacing them with dry ones, and wrapping patients in blankets are key nursing interventions. In emergencies away from a health care setting, have the patient lie under blankets next to a warm person. A conscious patient benefits from drinking hot liquids such as soup and avoiding alcohol and caffeinated fluids. It is also helpful to keep the head covered, place the patient near a fire or in a warm room, or place heating pads next to areas of the body (head and neck) that lose heat the quickest.

Restorative and Continuing Care. Educate the patient with a fever about the importance of taking and continuing any antibiotics as directed until the course of treatment is completed. Children and older adults are at risk for fluid volume deficit because they can quickly lose large amounts of fluids in proportion to their body weight. Identifying preferred fluids and encouraging oral fluid intake is an important ongoing nursing intervention.

EVALUATION

Through the Patient's Eyes. Evaluate your patient's perspectives about the care provided. Is he or she satisfied with the outcomes of care or does the care plan need to be modified? Including the patient in the evaluation demonstrates that you value his or her perspective and contributes to patient safety.

Patient Outcomes. Evaluate all nursing interventions by comparing the patient's actual response to the expected outcomes of the care plan. Determine if goals of care were met and make revisions to the care plan when necessary. After any intervention measure the patient's temperature to evaluate for change. In addition, use other evaluative measures such as palpating the skin and assessing pulse and respirations. If therapies are effective, body temperature returns to an acceptable range, other vital signs stabilize, and the patient reports a sense of comfort.

PULSE

The pulse is the palpable bounding of blood flow noted at various points on the body. Blood flows through the body in a continuous circuit. The pulse is an indicator of circulatory status.

Physiology and Regulation

Electrical impulses originating from the sinoatrial (SA) node travel through heart muscle to stimulate cardiac contraction. Approximately 60 to 70 mL of blood enters the aorta with each ventricular contraction (stroke volume). With each stroke volume ejection, the walls of the aorta distend, creating a pulse wave that travels rapidly toward the distal ends of the arteries. The pulse wave moves 15 times faster through the aorta and 100 times faster through the small arteries than the ejected volume of blood. When a pulse wave reaches a peripheral artery, you can feel it by palpating the artery lightly against underlying bone or muscle. The pulse is the palpable bounding of the blood flow in the peripheral artery. The number of pulsing sensations occurring in 1 minute is the pulse rate.

The volume of blood pumped by the heart during 1 minute is the **cardiac output,** the product of HR and the stroke volume (SV) of the ventricle. In an adult the heart normally pumps 5000 mL of blood per minute. A change in HR or stroke volume does not

TABLE 29-2 Pulse Sites

SITE	LOCATION	ASSESSMENT CRITERIA
Temporal	Over temporal bone of head, above and lateral to eye	Easily accessible site used to assess pulse in children
Carotid	Along medial edge of sternocleidomastoid muscle in neck	Easily accessible site used during physiological shock or cardiac arrest when other sites are not palpable
Apical	Fourth to fifth intercostal space at left midclavicular line	Site used to auscultate for apical pulse
Brachial	Groove between biceps and triceps muscles at antecubital fossa	Site used to assess status of circulation to lower arm and auscultate blood pressure
Radial	Radial or thumb side of forearm at wrist	Common site used to assess character of pulse peripherally and assess status of circulation to hand
Ulnar	Ulnar side of forearm at wrist	Site used to assess status of circulation to hand; also used to perform an Allen's test
Femoral	Below inguinal ligament, midway between symphysis pubis and anterior superior iliac spine	Site used to assess character of pulse during physiological shock or cardiac arrest when other pulses are not palpable; used to assess status of circulation to leg
Popliteal	Behind knee in popliteal fossa	Site used to assess status of circulation to lower leg
Posterior tibial	Inner side of ankle, below medial malleolus	Site used to assess status of circulation to foot
Dorsalis pedis	Along top of foot, between extension tendons of great and first toe	Site used to assess status of circulation to foot

always change the output of the heart or the amount of blood in the arteries. For example, if a person's HR is 70 beats/min and the stroke volume is 70 mL, the cardiac output is 4900 mL per minute (70 beats/min times 70 mL per beat). If the HR drops to 60 beats/min and the stroke volume rises to 85 mL per beat, the cardiac output increases to 5100 mL or 5.1 L per minute (60 beats/min times 85 mL per beat).

Mechanical, neural, and chemical factors regulate the strength of ventricular contraction and its stroke volume. But when these factors are unable to alter stroke volume, a change in HR results in a change in cardiac output, which affects BP. As HR increases, there is less time for the heart to fill. As HR increases without a change in stroke volume, BP decreases. As HR slows, filling time is increased, and BP increases. The inability of BP to respond to increases or decreases in HR indicates a possible health problem. Report this to the health care provider.

An abnormally slow, rapid, or irregular pulse alters cardiac output. Assess the ability of the heart to meet the demands of body tissue for nutrients by palpating a peripheral pulse or using a stethoscope to listen to heart sounds (apical rate).

Assessment of Pulse

You can assess any artery for pulse rate, but you typically use the radial artery because it is easy to palpate. When a patient's condition suddenly worsens, the carotid site is recommended for quickly finding a pulse. The heart continues delivering blood through the carotid artery to the brain as long as possible. When cardiac output declines significantly, peripheral pulses weaken and are difficult to palpate.

The radial and apical locations are the most common sites for pulse rate assessment. Use the radial pulse to teach patients how to monitor their own HRs (e.g., athletes, persons taking heart medications, and patients starting a prescribed exercise regimen). If the radial pulse is abnormal or intermittent resulting from dysrhythmias or if it is inaccessible because of a dressing or cast, assess the apical pulse. When a patient takes medication that affects the HR, the apical pulse provides a more accurate assessment of heart function. The brachial or apical pulse is the best site for assessing an infant's or young child's pulse because other peripheral pulses are deep and difficult to palpate accurately.

Assessment of other peripheral pulse sites such as the brachial or femoral artery is unnecessary when routinely obtaining vital signs. You assess other peripheral pulses when conducting a complete physical, when surgery or treatment has impaired blood flow to a body part, or when there are clinical indications of impaired peripheral blood flow (see Chapter 30). Table 29-2 summarizes pulse sites and criteria for measurement. Skill 29-2 on pp. 472-475 outlines pulse rate assessment.

Use of a Stethoscope. Assessing the apical rate requires a stethoscope. The five major parts of the stethoscope are the earpieces, binaurals, tubing, bell chest piece, and diaphragm chest piece (Fig. 29-7).

The plastic or rubber earpieces should fit snugly and comfortably in your ears. The binaurals should be angled and strong enough so the earpieces stay firmly in the ears without causing discomfort. To ensure the best reception of sound, the earpieces follow the contour of the ear canal pointing toward the face when the stethoscope is in place.

The polyvinyl tubing is flexible and 30 to 40 cm (12 to 18 inches) in length. Longer tubing decreases the transmission of sound waves. Thick-walled and moderately rigid tubing eliminates transmission of environmental noise and prevents the tubing from kinking, which distorts sound wave transmission. Stethoscopes have single or dual tubes.

The chest piece consists of a bell and a diaphragm that you rotate into position. The diaphragm or bell needs to be in proper position during use to hear sounds through the stethoscope. To test the position of the chest piece, tap lightly on the diaphragm to determine which side is functioning. The diaphragm is the circular, flat portion of the chest piece covered with a thin plastic disk. It transmits high-pitched sounds created by the high-velocity movement of air and blood. Auscultate bowel, lung, and heart sounds

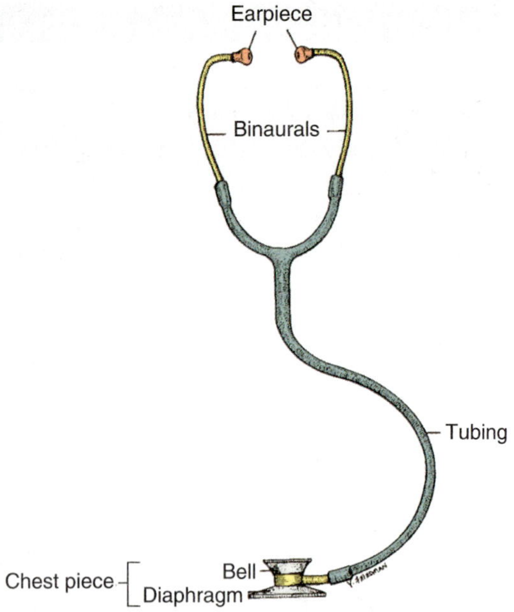

FIG. 29-7 Parts of stethoscope.

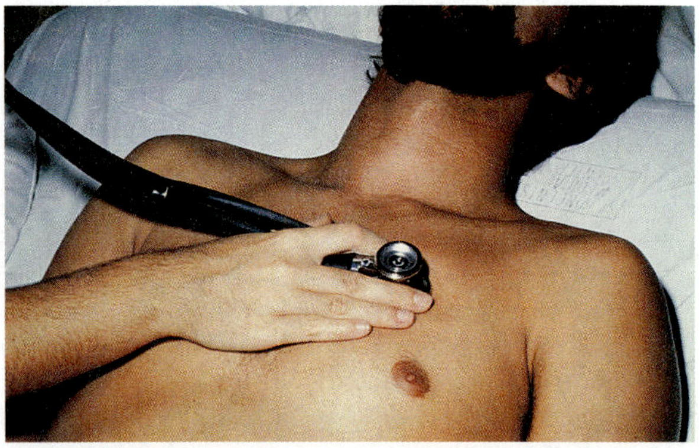

FIG. 29-8 Positioning diaphragm of stethoscope firmly and securely when auscultating high-pitched heart sounds.

using the diaphragm. Always place the stethoscope directly on the skin because clothing obscures the sound. Position the diaphragm to make a tight seal and press firmly against the patient's skin (Fig. 29-8).

The bell is the bowl-shaped chest piece usually surrounded by a rubber ring. The ring avoids chilling patients with cold metal when placed on the skin. The bell transmits low-pitched sounds created by the low-velocity movement of blood. Auscultate heart and vascular sounds using the bell. Apply the bell lightly, resting the chest piece on the skin (Fig. 29-9).

Compressing the bell against the skin reduces low-pitched sound amplification and creates a "diaphragm of skin." Some stethoscopes have one chest piece that combines features of the bell and diaphragm. When you use light pressure, the chest piece is a bell; exerting more pressure converts the bell into a diaphragm.

The stethoscope is a delicate instrument and requires proper care for optimal function. Remove the earpieces regularly and clean them of cerumen (earwax). Clean the bell and diaphragm of dust, lint, and body oils. Clean the tubing with mild soap and water between patients.

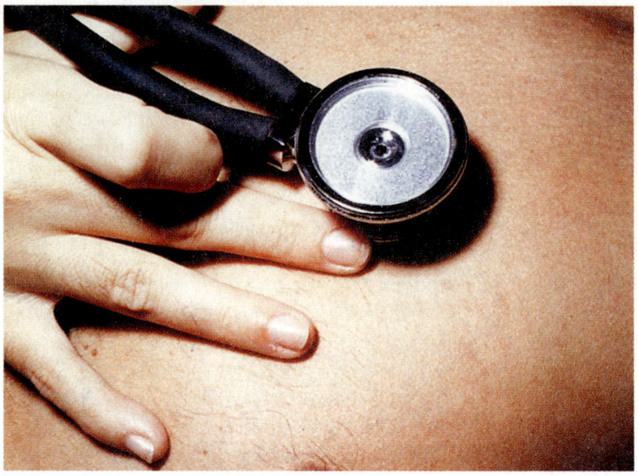

FIG. 29-9 Positioning bell of stethoscope lightly on skin to hear low-pitched heart sounds.

TABLE 29-3 Acceptable Ranges of Heart Rate

AGE	HEART RATE (BEATS/MIN)
Infant	120-160
Toddler	90-140
Preschooler	80-110
School-age child	75-100
Adolescent	60-90
Adult	60-100

Character of the Pulse

Assessment of the radial pulse includes measuring the rate, rhythm, strength, and equality. When auscultating an apical pulse, assess rate and rhythm only.

Rate. Before measuring a pulse, review the patient's baseline rate for comparison (Table 29-3). Some practitioners prefer to make baseline measurements of the pulse rate as a patient assumes a sitting, standing, and lying position. Postural changes affect the pulse rate because of alterations in blood volume and sympathetic activity. The HR temporarily increases when a person changes from a lying to a sitting or standing position.

When assessing the pulse, consider the variety of factors influencing the pulse rate (Table 29-4). A single factor or a combination of these factors often causes significant changes. If you detect an abnormal rate while palpating a peripheral pulse, the next step is to assess the apical rate. The apical rate requires auscultation of heart sounds, which provides a more accurate assessment of cardiac contraction.

Assess the apical rate by listening to heart sounds (see Chapter 30). Identify the first and second heart sounds (S_1 and S_2). At normal slow rates S_1 is low pitched and dull, sounding like a "lub." S_2 is higher pitched and shorter, creating the sound "dub." Count each set of "lub-dub" as one heartbeat. Using the diaphragm or bell of the stethoscope, count the number of lub-dubs occurring in 1 minute.

Peripheral and apical pulse rate assessment often reveals variations in HR. Two common abnormalities in pulse rate are tachycardia and bradycardia. Tachycardia is an abnormally elevated HR,

TABLE 29-4 **Factors Influencing Pulse Rate**

FACTOR	INCREASES PULSE RATE	DECREASES PULSE RATE
Exercise	Short-term exercise	Heart conditioned by long-term exercise, resulting in lower resting pulse and quicker return to resting level after exercise
Temperature	Fever and heat	Hypothermia
Emotions	Sympathetic stimulation increased by acute pain and anxiety, affecting heart rate; effect of chronic pain on heart rate varies	Parasympathetic stimulation increased by unrelieved severe pain affecting heart rate; relaxation
Drugs	Positive chronotropic drugs such as epinephrine	Negative chronotropic drugs such as digitalis; beta-adrenergic and calcium channel blockers
Hemorrhage	Sympathetic stimulation increased by loss of blood	
Postural changes	Standing or sitting	Lying down
Pulmonary conditions	Diseases causing poor oxygenation such as asthma, chronic obstructive pulmonary disease (COPD)	

above 100 beats/min in adults. **Bradycardia** is a slow rate, below 60 beats/min in adults.

An inefficient contraction of the heart that fails to transmit a pulse wave to the peripheral pulse site creates a **pulse deficit.** To assess a pulse deficit you and a colleague assess radial and apical rates simultaneously and then compare rates. The difference between the apical and radial pulse rates is the pulse deficit. For example, an apical rate of 92 with a radial rate of 78 leaves a pulse deficit of 14 beats. Pulse deficits are often associated with abnormal rhythms.

Rhythm. Normally a regular interval occurs between each pulse or heartbeat. An interval interrupted by an early or late beat or a missed beat indicates an abnormal rhythm or **dysrhythmia.** A dysrhythmia threatens the ability of the heart to provide adequate cardiac output, particularly if it occurs repetitively. You identify a dysrhythmia by palpating an interruption in successive pulse waves or auscultating an interruption between heart sounds. If a dysrhythmia is present, assess the regularity of its occurrence and auscultate the apical rate (see Chapter 30). Dysrhythmias are described as regularly irregular or irregularly irregular.

To document a dysrhythmia, the health care provider often orders an electrocardiogram, Holter monitor, or telemetry monitor. An electrocardiogram records the electrical activity of the heart for a 12-second interval. This test requires placement of electrodes across a patient's chest followed by recording of the heart rhythm. The patient wears the Holter monitor, which records and stores 24 hours of electrical activity. Access to the information recorded is not available until after the 24 hours have passed and the data are reviewed. Cardiac telemetry provides continuous monitoring of the electrical activity of the heart transmitted to a stationary monitor. Telemetry permits continuous observation of heart rhythm during all of a patient's daily activities and thus allows for immediate treatment if the rhythm becomes erratic or unstable.

Children often have a sinus dysrhythmia, which is an irregular heartbeat that speeds up with inspiration and slows with expiration. This is a normal finding that you can verify by having the child hold his or her breath; the HR usually becomes regular.

Strength. The strength or amplitude of a pulse reflects the volume of blood ejected against the arterial wall with each heart contraction and the condition of the arterial vascular system leading to the pulse site. Normally the pulse strength remains the same with each heartbeat. Document the pulse strength as bounding (4+); full or strong (3+); normal and expected (2+); diminished or barely palpable (1+); or absent (0). Include assessment of pulse strength in the assessment of the vascular system (see Chapter 30).

Equality. Assess radial pulses on both sides of the peripheral vascular system, comparing the characteristics of each. A pulse in one extremity is sometimes unequal in strength or absent in many disease states (e.g., thrombus [clot] formation, aberrant blood vessels, cervical rib syndrome, or aortic dissection). Assess all symmetrical pulses simultaneously except for the carotid pulse. Never measure the carotid pulses simultaneously because excessive pressure occludes blood supply to the brain.

Nursing Process and Pulse Determination

Pulse assessment determines the general state of cardiovascular health and the response of the body to other system imbalances. Tachycardia, bradycardia, and dysrhythmias are defining characteristics of many nursing diagnoses, including the following:

- Activity intolerance
- Anxiety
- Decreased cardiac output
- Fear
- Deficient/excess fluid volume
- Impaired gas exchange
- Hyperthermia
- Hypothermia
- Acute pain
- Ineffective peripheral tissue perfusion

The nursing care plan includes interventions based on the nursing diagnosis identified and the related factors. For example, the defining characteristics of an abnormal HR, exertional dyspnea, and a patient's verbal report of fatigue lead to a diagnosis of *activity intolerance.* When the related factor is *inactivity following a prolonged illness,* interventions focus on increasing the patient's daily exercise routine. Once the plan is implemented, evaluate patient outcomes by assessing his or her pulse.

RESPIRATION

Human survival depends on the ability of oxygen (O_2) to reach body cells and carbon dioxide (CO_2) to be removed from the cells. Respiration is the mechanism the body uses to exchange gases between the atmosphere and the blood and the blood and the cells. Respiration involves **ventilation** (the movement of gases in and out of the lungs), **diffusion** (the movement of oxygen and carbon dioxide between the alveoli and the red blood cells), and **perfusion** (the distribution of red blood cells to and from the pulmonary capillaries). Analyzing respiratory efficiency requires integrating assessment data from all three processes. Assess ventilation by determining respiratory rate, depth, and rhythm. Assess diffusion and perfusion by determining oxygen saturation.

Physiological Control

Breathing is generally a passive process. Normally a person thinks little about it. The respiratory center in the brainstem regulates the involuntary control of respirations. Adults normally breathe in a smooth, uninterrupted pattern 12 to 20 times a minute.

The body regulates ventilation using levels of CO_2, O_2, and hydrogen ion concentration (pH) in the arterial blood. The most important factor in the control of ventilation is the level of CO_2 in the arterial blood. An elevation in the CO_2 level causes the respiratory control system in the brain to increase the rate and depth of breathing. The increased ventilatory effort removes excess CO_2 (hypercarbia) by increasing exhalation. However, patients with chronic lung disease have ongoing hypercarbia. For these patients chemoreceptors in the carotid artery and aorta become sensitive to **hypoxemia,** or low levels of arterial O_2. If arterial oxygen levels fall, these receptors signal the brain to increase the rate and depth of ventilation. Hypoxemia helps to control ventilation in patients with chronic lung disease. Because low levels of arterial O_2 provide the stimulus that allows a patient to breathe, administration of high oxygen levels is fatal for patients with chronic lung disease.

Mechanics of Breathing

Although breathing is normally passive, muscular work is involved in moving the lungs and chest wall. Inspiration is an active process. During inspiration the respiratory center sends impulses along the phrenic nerve, causing the diaphragm to contract. Abdominal organs move downward and forward, increasing the length of the chest cavity to move air into the lungs. The diaphragm moves approximately 1 cm (4/10 inch), and the ribs retract upward from the midline of the body approximately 1.2 to 2.5 cm (½ to 1 inch). During a normal, relaxed breath, a person inhales 500 mL of air. This amount is referred to as the tidal volume. During expiration the diaphragm relaxes, and the abdominal organs return to their original positions. The lung and chest wall return to a relaxed position (Fig. 29-10). Expiration is a passive process. Sighing interrupts the normal rate and depth of ventilation, **eupnea.** The sigh, a prolonged deeper breath, is a protective physiological mechanism for expanding small airways and alveoli not ventilated during a normal breath.

The accurate assessment of respirations depends on the recognition of normal thoracic and abdominal movements. During quiet breathing the chest wall gently rises and falls. Contraction of the intercostal muscles between the ribs or contraction of the muscles in the neck and shoulders (the accessory muscles of breathing) is not visible. During normal quiet breathing diaphragmatic movement causes the abdominal cavity to rise and fall slowly.

Assessment of Ventilation

Respirations are the easiest of all vital signs to assess, but they are often the most haphazardly measured. Do not estimate respirations. Accurate measurement requires observation and palpation of chest wall movement.

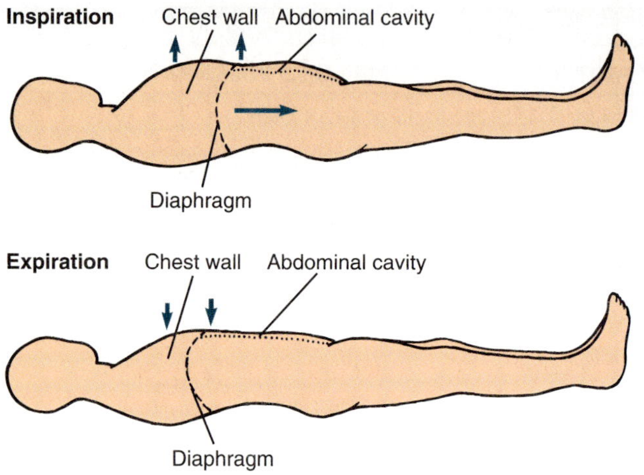

FIG. 29-10 Illustration of diaphragmatic and chest wall movement during inspiration and expiration.

A sudden change in the character of respirations is important. Because respiration is tied to the function of numerous body systems, consider all variables when changes occur (Box 29-9). For example, a drop in respirations occurring in a patient after head trauma often signifies injury to the brainstem. Abdominal trauma injures the phrenic nerve, which is responsible for diaphragmatic contraction.

Do not let a patient know that you are assessing respirations. A patient aware of the assessment can alter the rate and depth of breathing. Assess respirations immediately after measuring pulse rate, with your hand still on the patient's wrist as it rests over the chest or abdomen. When assessing a patient's respirations, keep in mind the patient's usual ventilatory rate and pattern, the influence any disease or illness has on respiratory function, the relationship between respiratory and cardiovascular function, and the influence of therapies on respirations. The objective measurements of respiratory status include the rate and depth of breathing and the rhythm of ventilatory movements (Skill 29-3 on pp. 476-478).

Respiratory Rate. Observe a full inspiration and expiration when counting ventilation or respiration rate. The usual respiratory rate varies with age (Table 29-5). The usual range of respiratory rate declines throughout life.

The apnea monitor is a device that aids respiratory rate assessment. This device uses leads attached to a patient's chest wall that sense movement. The absence of chest wall movement triggers the apnea alarm. Apnea monitoring is used frequently with infants in the hospital and at home to observe patients at risk for prolonged apneic events.

Ventilatory Depth. Assess the depth of respirations by observing the degree of excursion or movement in the chest wall. Describe ventilatory movements as deep, normal, or shallow. A deep respiration involves a full expansion of the lungs with full exhalation. Respirations are shallow when only a small quantity of air passes through the lungs and ventilatory movement is difficult to see. Use more objective techniques if you observe that chest excursion is unusually shallow (see Chapter 30). Table 29-6 summarizes types of breathing patterns.

Ventilatory Rhythm. Determine breathing pattern by observing the chest or the abdomen. Diaphragmatic breathing results from the contraction and relaxation of the diaphragm, and you observe it best by watching abdominal movements. Healthy

BOX 29-9 FACTORS INFLUENCING CHARACTER OF RESPIRATIONS

Exercise
- Exercise increases rate and depth to meet the body's need for additional oxygen and to rid the body of CO_2.

Acute Pain
- Pain alters rate and rhythm of respirations; breathing becomes shallow.
- Patient inhibits or splints chest wall movement when pain is in area of chest or abdomen.

Anxiety
- Anxiety increases respiration rate and depth as a result of sympathetic stimulation.

Smoking
- Chronic smoking changes pulmonary airways, resulting in increased rate of respirations at rest when not smoking.

Body Position
- A straight, erect posture promotes full chest expansion.
- A stooped or slumped position impairs ventilatory movement.
- Lying flat prevents full chest expansion.

Medications
- Opioid analgesics, general anesthetics, and sedative hypnotics depress rate and depth.
- Amphetamines and cocaine sometimes increase rate and depth.
- Bronchodilators slow rate by causing airway dilation.

Neurological Injury
- Injury to brainstem impairs respiratory center and inhibits respiratory rate and rhythm.

Hemoglobin Function
- Decreased hemoglobin levels (anemia) reduce oxygen-carrying capacity of the blood, which increases respiratory rate.
- Increased altitude lowers amount of saturated hemoglobin, which increases respiratory rate and depth.
- Abnormal blood cell function (e.g., sickle cell disease) reduces ability of hemoglobin to carry oxygen, which increases respiratory rate and depth.

TABLE 29-5 Acceptable Ranges of Respiratory Rate

AGE	RATE (BREATHS/MIN)
Newborn	35-40
Infant (6 months)	30-50
Toddler (2 years)	25-32
Child	20-30
Adolescent	16-20
Adult	12-20

men and children usually demonstrate diaphragmatic breathing. Women tend to use thoracic muscles to breathe, assessed by observing movements in the upper chest. Labored respirations usually involve the accessory muscles of respiration visible in the neck. When something such as a foreign body interferes with the movement of air in and out of the lungs, the intercostal spaces retract

TABLE 29-6 Alterations in Breathing Pattern

ALTERATION	DESCRIPTION
Bradypnea	Rate of breathing is regular but abnormally slow (less than 12 breaths/min).
Tachypnea	Rate of breathing is regular but abnormally rapid (greater than 20 breaths/min).
Hyperpnea	Respirations are labored, increased in depth, and increased in rate (greater than 20 breaths/min) (occurs normally during exercise).
Apnea	Respirations cease for several seconds. Persistent cessation results in respiratory arrest.
Hyperventilation	Rate and depth of respirations increase. Hypocarbia sometimes occurs.
Hypoventilation	Respiratory rate is abnormally low, and depth of ventilation is depressed. Hypercarbia sometimes occurs.
Cheyne-Stokes respiration	Respiratory rate and depth are irregular, characterized by alternating periods of apnea and hyperventilation. Respiratory cycle begins with slow, shallow breaths that gradually increase to abnormal rate and depth. The pattern reverses; breathing slows and becomes shallow, climaxing in apnea before respiration resumes.
Kussmaul's respiration	Respirations are abnormally deep, regular, and increased in rate.
Biot's respiration	Respirations are abnormally shallow for two to three breaths followed by irregular period of apnea.

during inspiration. A longer expiration phase is evident when the outward flow of air is obstructed (e.g., asthma).

With normal breathing a regular interval occurs after each respiratory cycle. Infants tend to breathe less regularly. The young child often breathes slowly for a few seconds and then suddenly breathes more rapidly. While assessing respirations, estimate the time interval after each respiratory cycle. Respiration is regular or irregular in rhythm.

Building Competency in Safety You are caring for Mrs. Larkam, a 28-year-old patient with type 1 diabetes who is admitted for pneumonia. Mrs. Larkam is also 7½ months' pregnant with her first child. She requires oxygen via humidified face mask at 28%. Which vital signs do you delegate to nursing assistive personnel (NAP), and in what order should the vital signs be obtained? Which device should be used to obtain her temperature? Positioning is important for Mrs. Larkam to improve her lung function. How do you reposition her when vital signs are obtained?

Answers to questions can be found on the Evolve website.

Assessment of Diffusion and Perfusion

Evaluate the respiratory processes of diffusion and perfusion by measuring the **oxygen saturation** of the blood. Blood flow through the pulmonary capillaries provides red blood cells for oxygen attachment. After oxygen diffuses from the alveoli into the pulmonary blood, most of the oxygen attaches to hemoglobin molecules

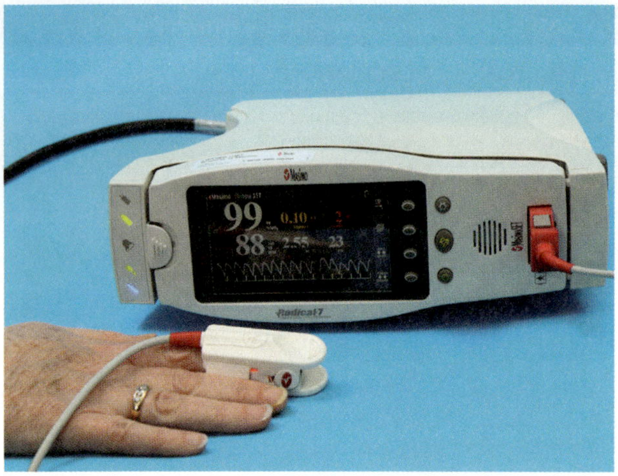
FIG. 29-11 Portable pulse oximeter with digit probe.

in red blood cells. Red blood cells carry the oxygenated hemoglobin molecules through the left side of the heart and out to the peripheral capillaries, where the oxygen detaches, depending on the needs of the tissues.

The percent of hemoglobin that is bound with oxygen in the arteries is the percent of saturation of hemoglobin (or SaO_2). It is usually between 95% and 100%. SaO_2 is affected by factors that interfere with ventilation, perfusion, or diffusion (see Chapter 40). The saturation of venous blood (SvO_2) is lower because the tissues have removed some of the oxygen from the hemoglobin molecules. Factors that interfere with or increase tissue oxygen demand affect the usual value for SvO_2, which is 70%.

Measurement of Arterial Oxygen Saturation. A pulse oximeter permits the indirect measurement of oxygen saturation (Skill 29-4 on pp. 478-480). The pulse oximeter is a probe with a light-emitting diode (LED) and photodetector connected by cable to an oximeter (Fig. 29-11). The LED emits light wavelengths that the oxygenated and deoxygenated hemoglobin molecules absorb differently. The photodetector detects the amount of oxygen bound to hemoglobin molecules, and the oximeter calculates the pulse saturation (SpO_2). SpO_2 is a reliable estimate of SaO_2 when the SaO_2 is over 70%. Values obtained with pulse oximetry are less accurate at saturations less than 70%.

The photodetector is in the oximeter probe. Selecting the appropriate probe is important to reduce measurement error. Digit probes are spring loaded and conform to various sizes. Earlobe probes have greater accuracy at lower saturations and are least affected by peripheral vasoconstriction. You can apply disposable sensor pads to a variety of sites, including the bridge of an adult's nose or the sole of an infant's foot. Factors that affect light transmission or peripheral arterial pulsations affect the ability of the photodetector to measure SpO_2 (Box 29-10). An awareness of these factors allows accurate interpretation of abnormal SpO_2 measurements.

Nursing Process and Respiratory Vital Signs

Measurement of respiratory rate, pattern, and depth, along with SpO_2, assesses ventilation, diffusion, and perfusion. You also conduct other assessments to measure respiratory status (see Chapter 30). Use assessment data to determine the nature of a patient's problem. Respiratory assessment data are defining characteristics of many nursing diagnoses, including the following:

- Activity intolerance
- Ineffective airway clearance
- Anxiety
- Ineffective breathing pattern
- Impaired gas exchange
- Acute pain
- Ineffective peripheral tissue perfusion
- Dysfunctional ventilatory weaning response

The nursing care plan includes interventions based on the nursing diagnosis identified and the related factors. For example, the defining characteristics of tachycardia, changes in depth of respirations, use of accessory muscles, dyspnea, and a decline in SpO_2 lead to a diagnosis of *impaired gas exchange.* Related factors could include an infectious process or a history of chronic obstructive lung disease with a 30–pack-year history of smoking. You select interventions based on the related factor. After intervening, evaluate patient outcomes by assessing the respiratory rate, ventilatory depth, rhythm, and SpO_2.

BOX 29-10 FACTORS AFFECTING DETERMINATION OF PULSE OXYGEN SATURATION (SpO_2)

Interference with Light Transmission

- Outside light sources interfere with ability of oximeter to process reflected light.
- Carbon monoxide (caused by smoke inhalation or poisoning) artificially elevates SpO_2 by absorbing light similar to oxygen.
- Patient motion interferes with ability of oximeter to process reflected light.
- Jaundice interferes with ability of oximeter to process reflected light.
- Intravascular dyes (methylene blue) absorb light similar to deoxyhemoglobin and artificially lower saturation.
- Nail polish, artificial nails, or metal studs in nails can interfere with light absorption and the ability of the oximeter to process reflected light (Cicek et al., 2010).
- Dark skin pigment sometimes results in signal loss or overestimation of saturation.

Interference with Arterial Pulsations

- Peripheral vascular disease (atherosclerosis) reduces pulse volume.
- Hypothermia at assessment site decreases peripheral blood flow.
- Pharmacological vasoconstrictors (e.g., epinephrine) decrease peripheral pulse volume.
- Low cardiac output and hypotension decrease blood flow to peripheral arteries.
- Peripheral edema obscures arterial pulsation.
- Tight probe records venous pulsations in finger that compete with arterial pulsations.

BLOOD PRESSURE

Blood pressure is the force exerted on the walls of an artery by the pulsing blood under pressure from the heart. Blood flows throughout the circulatory system because of pressure changes. It moves from an area of high pressure to one of low pressure. Systemic or arterial BP, the BP in the system of arteries in the body, is a good indicator of cardiovascular health. The contraction of the heart forces the blood under high pressure into the aorta. The peak of maximum pressure when ejection occurs is the **systolic pressure.** When the ventricles relax, the blood remaining in the arteries exerts a minimum or **diastolic pressure.** Diastolic pressure is the minimal pressure exerted against the arterial walls at all times.

The standard unit for measuring BP is millimeters of mercury (mm Hg). The measurement indicates the height to which the BP raises a column of mercury. Record BP with the systolic reading before the diastolic reading (e.g., 120/80). The difference between systolic and diastolic pressure is the **pulse pressure.** For a BP of 120/80, the pulse pressure is 40.

Physiology of Arterial Blood Pressure

Blood pressure reflects the interrelationships of cardiac output, peripheral vascular resistance, blood volume, blood viscosity, and artery elasticity. Your knowledge of these hemodynamic variables helps in the assessment of BP alterations.

Cardiac Output. The BP depends on the cardiac output. When volume increases in an enclosed space such as a blood vessel, the pressure in that space rises. Thus, as cardiac output increases, more blood is pumped against arterial walls, causing the BP to rise. Cardiac output increases as a result of an increase in HR, greater heart muscle contractility, or an increase in blood volume. Changes in HR occur faster than changes in heart muscle contractility or blood volume. A rapid or significant increase in HR decreases the filling time of the heart. As a result BP decreases.

Peripheral Resistance. The BP depends on peripheral vascular resistance. Blood circulates through a network of arteries, arterioles, capillaries, venules, and veins. Arteries and arterioles are surrounded by smooth muscle that contracts or relaxes to change the size of the lumen. The size of arteries and arterioles changes to adjust blood flow to the needs of local tissues. For example, when a major organ needs more blood, the peripheral arteries constrict, decreasing their supply of blood. More blood becomes available to the major organ because of the resistance change in the periphery. Normally arteries and arterioles remain partially constricted to maintain a constant flow of blood. Peripheral vascular resistance is the resistance to blood flow determined by the tone of vascular musculature and diameter of blood vessels. The smaller the lumen of a vessel, the greater is the peripheral vascular resistance to blood flow. As resistance rises, arterial BP rises. As vessels dilate and resistance falls, BP drops.

Blood Volume. The volume of blood circulating within the vascular system affects BP. Most adults have a circulating blood volume of 5000 mL. Normally the blood volume remains constant. However, an increase in volume exerts more pressure against arterial walls. For example, the rapid, uncontrolled infusion of IV fluids elevates BP. When circulating blood volume falls, as in the case of hemorrhage or dehydration, BP falls.

Viscosity. The thickness or viscosity of blood affects the ease with which blood flows through small vessels. The **hematocrit,** or percentage of red blood cells in the blood, determines blood viscosity. When the hematocrit rises and blood flow slows, arterial BP increases. The heart contracts more forcefully to move the viscous blood through the circulatory system.

Elasticity. Normally the walls of an artery are elastic and easily distensible. As pressure within the arteries increases, the diameter of vessel walls increases to accommodate the pressure change. Arterial distensibility prevents wide fluctuations in BP. However, in certain diseases such as arteriosclerosis, the vessel walls lose their elasticity and are replaced by fibrous tissue that cannot stretch well. Reduced elasticity results in greater resistance to blood flow. As a result, when the left ventricle ejects its stroke volume, the vessels no longer yield to pressure. Instead a given volume of blood is forced through the rigid arterial walls, and the systemic pressure rises. Systolic pressure is more significantly elevated than diastolic pressure as a result of reduced arterial elasticity.

TABLE 29-7 Average Optimal Blood Pressure for Age

AGE	BLOOD PRESSURE (mm Hg)
Newborn (3000 g [6.6 lb])	40 (mean)
1 month	85/54
1 year	95/65
6 years*	105/65
10-13 years*	110/65
14-17 years*	119/75
18 years and older	<120/<80

From National High Blood Pressure Education Program (NHBPEP); National Heart, Lung, and Blood Institute; National Institutes of Health: The seventh report of the Joint National Committee on Detection, Evaluation, and Treatment of High Blood Pressure, *JAMA* 289(19):2560, 2003.

*In children and adolescents hypertension is defined as blood pressure that on repeated measurement is at the 95th percentile or greater adjusted for age, height, and gender (NHBPEP, 2003).

Each hemodynamic factor significantly affects the others. For example, as arterial elasticity declines, peripheral vascular resistance increases. The complex control of the cardiovascular system normally prevents any single factor from permanently changing the BP. For example, if the blood volume falls, the body compensates with an increased vascular resistance.

Factors Influencing Blood Pressure

BP is not constant. Many factors continually influence it. One measurement cannot adequately reflect a patient's usual BP. Even under the best conditions, it changes from heartbeat to heartbeat. Blood pressure trends, not individual measurements, guide nursing interventions. Understanding these factors ensures a more accurate interpretation of BP readings.

Age. Normal BP levels vary throughout life (Table 29-7). BP increases during childhood. Evaluate the level of a child's or adolescent's BP with respect to body size and age. An infant's BP ranges from 65 to 115/42 to 80 mm Hg. The normal BP for a 7-year-old is 87 to 117/48 to 64 mm Hg. Larger children (heavier and/or taller) have higher BPs than smaller children of the same age. During adolescence BP continues to vary according to body size.

An adult's BP tends to rise with advancing age. The optimal BP for a healthy, middle-age adult is less than 120/80 mm Hg. Values of 120 to 139/80 to 89 mm Hg are considered prehypertension (NHBPEP, 2003) (Table 29-8). Older adults often have a rise in systolic pressure related to decreased vessel elasticity; however, BP greater than 140/90 is defined as hypertension and increases an older adult's risk for hypertension-related illness.

Stress. Anxiety, fear, pain, and emotional stress result in sympathetic stimulation, which increases HR, cardiac output, and vascular resistance. The effect of sympathetic stimulation increases BP. Anxiety raises BP as much as 30 mm Hg.

Ethnicity. The incidence of hypertension (high BP) is higher in African Americans than in European Americans. African Americans tend to develop more severe hypertension at an earlier age and have twice the risk for complications such as stroke and heart attack. Genetic and environmental factors are often contributing factors. Hypertension-related deaths are also higher among African Americans.

Gender. There is no clinically significant difference in BP levels between boys and girls. After puberty males tend to have higher BP readings. After menopause women tend to have higher BP levels than men of similar age.

Daily Variation. Blood pressure varies throughout the day, with lower BP during sleep between midnight and 3:00 AM. Between 3:00 AM and 6:00 AM there is a slow and steady rise in BP. When a patient awakens, there is an early-morning BP surge. It is highest during the day between 10:00 AM and 6 PM. No two persons have the same pattern or degree of variation.

Medications. Some medications directly or indirectly affect BP. Before BP assessment ask whether the patient is receiving antihypertensive or other cardiac medications, which lower BP (Table 29-9). Another class of medications affecting BP is opioid analgesics, which can lower it. Vasoconstrictors and an excess volume of IV fluids increase it.

Activity and Weight. A period of exercise can reduce BP for several hours afterwards. Older adults often experience a 5- to 10-mm fall in BP about 1 hour after eating. An increase in oxygen demand by the body during activity increases BP. Inadequate exercise frequently contributes to weight gain, and obesity is a factor in the development of hypertension.

Smoking. Smoking results in vasoconstriction, a narrowing of blood vessels. BP rises when a person smokes and returns to baseline about 15 minutes after stopping smoking.

Hypertension

The most common alteration in BP is **hypertension.** Hypertension is often asymptomatic. Prehypertension is diagnosed in adults when an average of two or more diastolic readings on at least two subsequent visits are between 80 and 89 mm Hg or when the average of multiple systolic BPs on two or more subsequent visits is between 120 and 139 mm Hg. Diastolic readings greater than 90 mm Hg and systolic readings greater than 140 mm Hg (NHBPEP, 2003) define hypertension. Categories of hypertension have been developed (see Table 29-8) and determine medical intervention. One elevated BP measurement does not qualify as a diagnosis of hypertension. However, if a high reading during the first BP measurement (e.g., 150/90 mm Hg) is obtained, the patient is encouraged to return for another checkup within 2 months (Table 29-10).

TABLE 29-8 Classification of Blood Pressure for Adults Ages 18 and Older

CATEGORY	SYSTOLIC (mm Hg)*		DIASTOLIC (mm Hg)*
Normal	<120		<80
Prehypertension†	120-139	or	80-89
Stage 1 hypertension	140-159	or	90-99
Stage 2 hypertension	≥160	or	≥100

Data from National High Blood Pressure Education Program (NHBPEP); National Heart, Lung, and Blood Institute; National Institutes of Health: The seventh report of the Joint National Committee on Detection, Evaluation and Treatment of High Blood Pressure, *JAMA* 289(19):2560, 2003.

*Treatment based on highest category.

†Based on the average of two or more readings taken at each of two or more visits after an initial screening. Patient should not be taking antihypertensive drugs or be acutely ill. When systolic and diastolic blood pressures fall into different categories, select the higher category to classify the individual's blood pressure status. For example, classify 160/92 mm Hg as stage 2 hypertension.

TABLE 29-10 Recommendations for Blood Pressure Follow-up

INITIAL BLOOD PRESSURE	FOLLOW-UP RECOMMENDED*
Normal	Recheck in 2 years.
Prehypertension	Recheck in 1 year.†
Stage 1 hypertension	Confirm within 2 months.†
Stage 2 hypertension	Evaluate or refer to source of care within 1 month. For those with higher pressure (e.g., >180/110 mm Hg), evaluate and treat immediately or within 1 week, depending on clinical situation and complications.

Data from National High Blood Pressure Education Program (NHBPEP); National Heart, Lung, and Blood Institute; National Institutes of Health: The seventh report of the Joint National Committee on Detection, Evaluation and Treatment of High Blood Pressure, *JAMA* 289(19):2560, 2003.

*Modify the scheduling of follow-up according to reliable information about past blood pressure measurements, other cardiovascular risk factors, or target organ damage.

†Provide advice about lifestyle modifications.

TABLE 29-9 Antihypertensive Medications

MEDICATION TYPE	NAMES	ACTION
Diuretics	Furosemide (Lasix), spironolactone (Aldactone), metolazone, polythiazide, benzthiazide	Lowers blood pressure by reducing resorption of sodium and water by the kidneys, thus lowering circulating fluid volume
Beta-adrenergic blockers	Atenolol (Tenormin), nadolol (Corgard), timolol maleate (Blocadren), propranolol (Inderal)	Combines with beta-adrenergic receptors in the heart, arteries, and arterioles to block response to sympathetic nerve impulses; reduces heart rate and thus cardiac output
Vasodilators	Hydralazine hydrochloride (Apresoline), minoxidil (Loniten)	Acts on arteriolar smooth muscle to cause relaxation and reduce peripheral vascular resistance
Calcium channel blockers	Diltiazem (Cardizem, Dilacor XR), verapamil hydrochloride (Calan SR), nifedipine (Procardia), nicardipine (Cardene)	Reduces peripheral vascular resistance by systemic vasodilation
Angiotensin-converting enzyme (ACE) inhibitors	Captopril (Capoten), enalapril (Vasotec), lisinopril (Prinivil, Zestril), benazepril (Lotensin)	Lowers blood pressure by blocking the conversion of angiotensin I to angiotensin II, preventing vasoconstriction; reduces aldosterone production and fluid retention, lowering circulating fluid volume
Angiotensin-II receptor blockers (ARBs)	Losartan (Cozaar), olmesartan (Benicar)	Lowers blood pressure by blocking the binding of angiotensin II, which prevents vasoconstriction

Hypertension is associated with thickening and loss of elasticity in the arterial walls. Peripheral vascular resistance increases within thick and inelastic vessels. The heart continually pumps against greater resistance. As a result blood flow to vital organs such as the heart, brain, and kidney decreases.

Persons with a family history of hypertension are at significant risk. Modifiable risk factors include obesity, cigarette smoking, heavy alcohol consumption, and high sodium (salt) intake. Sedentary lifestyle and continued exposure to stress are also linked to hypertension. The incidence of hypertension is greater in patients with diabetes, older adults, and African Americans. It is a major factor underlying deaths from strokes and is a contributing factor to myocardial infarctions (heart attacks). When patients are diagnosed with hypertension, educate them about BP values, long-term follow-up care and therapy, the usual lack of symptoms (the fact that it may not be "felt"), the ability of therapy to control but not cure it, and a consistently followed treatment plan that ensures a relatively normal lifestyle (NHBPEP, 2003).

Hypotension

Hypotension is present when the systolic BP falls to 90 mm Hg or below. Although some adults have a low BP normally, for most people low BP is an abnormal finding associated with illness.

Hypotension occurs because of the dilation of the arteries in the vascular bed, the loss of a substantial amount of blood volume (e.g., hemorrhage), or the failure of the heart muscle to pump adequately (e.g., myocardial infarction). Hypotension associated with pallor, skin mottling, clamminess, confusion, increased HR, or decreased urine output is life threatening and is reported to a health care provider immediately.

Orthostatic hypotension, also referred to as **postural hypotension,** occurs when a normotensive person develops symptoms and low BP when rising to an upright position. When a healthy individual changes from a lying–to sitting–to standing position, the peripheral blood vessels in the legs constrict. When standing the lower-extremity vessels constrict, preventing the pooling of blood in the legs caused by gravity. Thus an individual normally does not feel any symptoms when standing. In contrast, when patients have a decreased blood volume, their blood vessels are already constricted. When a patient with volume depletion stands, there is a significant drop in BP with an increase in HR to compensate for the drop in cardiac output. Patients who are dehydrated, anemic, or have experienced prolonged bed rest or recent blood loss are at risk for orthostatic hypotension. Some medications cause orthostatic hypotension if misused, especially in older adults or young patients. Always measure BP before administering such medications.

Assess for orthostatic hypotension during measurements of vital signs by obtaining BP and pulse with the patient supine, sitting, and standing. Obtain BP readings 1 to 3 minutes after the patient changes position. In most cases orthostatic hypotension is detected within a minute of standing. If it occurs, assist the patient to a lying position and notify the health care provider or nurse in charge. While obtaining orthostatic measurements, observe for other symptoms of hypotension such as fainting, weakness, or light-headedness. When recording orthostatic BP measurements, record the patient's position in addition to the BP measurement (e.g., 140/80 mm Hg supine, 132/72 mm Hg sitting, 108/60 mm Hg standing). The skill of orthostatic measurements requires critical thinking and ongoing nursing judgment when determining a patient's response to repositioning. Do not delegate this procedure.

Measurement of Blood Pressure

Arterial BP measurements are obtained either directly (invasively) or indirectly (noninvasively). The direct method requires the insertion of a thin catheter into an artery. Tubing connects the catheter with electronic hemodynamic monitoring equipment. The monitor displays a constant arterial pressure waveform and reading. Because of the risk of sudden blood loss from an artery, invasive BP monitoring is used only in intensive-care settings. The common indirect method requires a sphygmomanometer and stethoscope. Auscultation or palpation with auscultation is the most widely used technique (Skill 29-5 on pp. 480-484).

Blood Pressure Equipment. Before assessing BP, make sure that you are comfortable using a sphygmomanometer and stethoscope. A **sphygmomanometer** includes a pressure manometer, an occlusive cloth or vinyl cuff that encloses an inflatable rubber bladder, and a pressure bulb with a release valve that inflates the bladder (Fig. 29-12). The aneroid manometer has a glass-enclosed circular gauge containing a needle that registers millimeter calibrations. Before using the aneroid model, make sure that the needle points to zero and that the manometer is correctly calibrated. Aneroid sphygmomanometers require biomedical calibration every 6 months to verify their accuracy.

Cloth or disposable vinyl compression cuffs contain an inflatable bladder and come in different sizes. The size selected is proportional to the circumference of the limb being assessed (Fig. 29-13). Ideally the width of the cuff is 40% of the circumference (or 20% wider than the diameter) of the midpoint of the limb on which the cuff is used to measure BP. The bladder, enclosed by the cuff, encircles at least 80% of the upper arm of an adult and the entire arm of a child. Place the lower edge of the cuff above the antecubital fossa, allowing room for positioning the stethoscope bell or diaphragm. Many adults require a large adult cuff. Using the forearm when a larger cuff is not readily available is not recommended. An improperly fitting cuff causes inaccurate BP measurements (Table 29-11).

The release valve of the sphygmomanometer needs to be clean and freely movable in either direction. A closed valve holds the pressure constant. A sticky valve makes pressure cuff deflation hard to regulate.

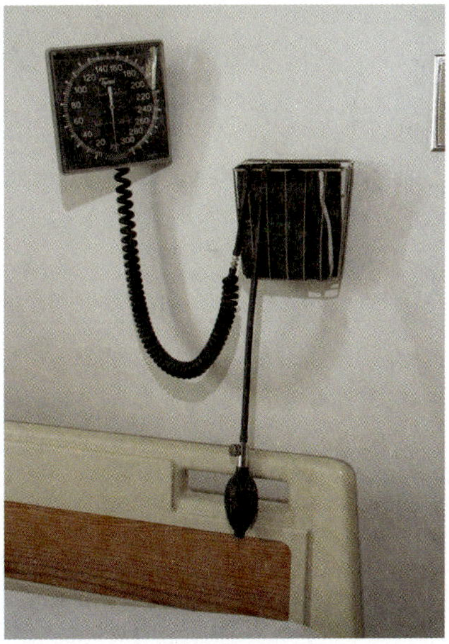

FIG. 29-12 Wall-mounted aneroid sphygmomanometer.

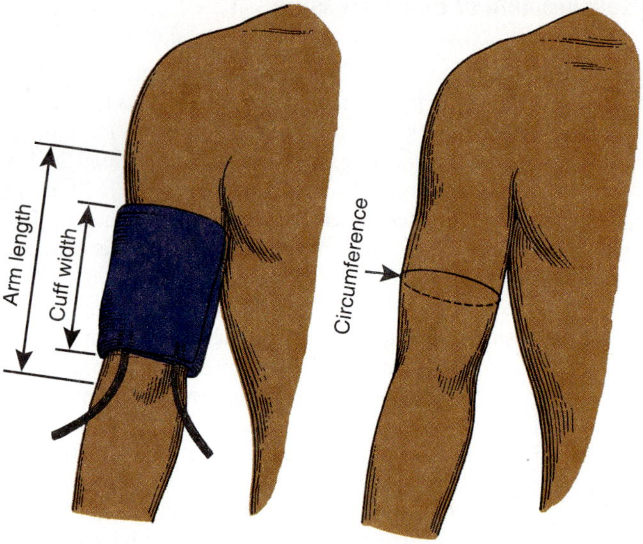

FIG. 29-13 Guidelines for proper blood pressure cuff size. Cuff width 20% more than upper-arm diameter or 40% of circumference and two thirds of arm length.

TABLE 29-11 Common Errors in Blood Pressure Assessment

ERROR	EFFECT
Bladder or cuff too wide	False-low reading
Bladder or cuff too narrow or too short	False-high reading
Cuff wrapped too loosely or unevenly	False-high reading
Deflating cuff too slowly	False-high diastolic reading
Deflating cuff too quickly	False-low systolic and false-high diastolic reading
Arm below heart level	False-high reading
Arm above heart level	False-low reading
Arm not supported	False-high reading
Stethoscope that fits poorly or impairment of examiner's hearing, causing sounds to be muffled	False-low systolic and false-high diastolic reading
Stethoscope applied too firmly against antecubital fossa	False-low diastolic reading
Inflating too slowly	False-high diastolic reading
Repeating assessments too quickly	False-high systolic reading
Inadequate inflation level	False-low systolic reading
Multiple examiners using different Korotkoff sounds for diastolic readings	False-high systolic and false-low diastolic reading

Auscultation. The best environment for BP measurement by auscultation is a quiet room at a comfortable temperature. Although the patient may lie or stand, sitting is the preferred position. In most cases BP readings obtained with the patient in the supine, sitting, and standing positions are similar.

The patient's position during routine BP determination needs to be the same during each measurement to permit a meaningful comparison of values. Before obtaining the patient's BP, attempt to control factors responsible for artificially high readings such as pain, anxiety, or exertion. The patient's perception that the physical or interpersonal environment is stressful affects the BP measurement. BP measurements taken at the patient's place of employment or in a health care provider's office are higher than those taken at the patient's home.

During the initial assessment obtain and record the BP in both arms. Normally there is a difference of 5 to 10 mm Hg between the arms. In subsequent assessments measure the BP in the arm with the higher pressure. Pressure differences greater than 10 mm Hg indicate vascular problems and are reported to the health care provider or nurse in charge.

Ask the patient to state his or her usual BP. If the patient does not know, inform him or her after measuring and recording it. This is a good opportunity to educate a patient about optimal values of BP, risk factors for developing hypertension, and dangers of hypertension.

Indirect measurement of arterial BP works on a basic principle of pressure. Blood flows freely through an artery until an inflated cuff applies pressure to tissues and causes the artery to collapse. After releasing the cuff pressure, the point at which blood flow returns and sound appears through auscultation is the systolic pressure.

In 1905 Korotkoff, a Russian surgeon, first described the sounds heard over an artery distal to the BP cuff. The first Korotkoff sound is a clear rhythmical tapping corresponding to the pulse rate that gradually increases in intensity. *Onset of the sound corresponds to the systolic pressure.* A blowing or swishing sound occurs as the cuff continues to deflate, resulting in the second Korotkoff sound. As the artery distends there is turbulence in blood flow. The third Korotkoff sound is a crisper and more intense tapping. The fourth Korotkoff sound becomes muffled and low pitched as the cuff is further deflated. At this point the cuff pressure has fallen below the pressure within the vessel walls; *this sound is the diastolic pressure in infants and children.* The fifth Korotkoff sound marks the disappearance of sound. *In adolescents and adults the fifth sound corresponds with the diastolic pressure* (Fig. 29-14). In some patients the sounds are clear and distinct. In others only the beginning and ending sounds are clear.

The American Heart Association recommends recording two numbers for a BP measurement: the point on the manometer when you hear the first sound for systolic and the point on the manometer when you hear the fifth sound for diastolic. Some institutions recommend recording the point when you hear the fourth sound as well, especially for patients with hypertension. Divide the numbers by slashed lines (e.g., 120/70 or 120/100/70). Note the arm used to measure the BP (e.g., right arm [RA] 130/70) and the patient's position (e.g., sitting).

BP assessment results in many medical decisions and nursing interventions. Obtaining an accurate measurement is essential. There are several sources for error (see Table 29-11). When you are unsure of a reading, have a colleague reassess the BP.

Assessment in Children. All children 3 years of age through adolescence need to have BP checked at least annually. BP in children changes with growth and development. Help parents understand the importance of this routine screening to detect children who are at risk for hypertension. The measurement of BP in infants and children is difficult for several reasons:

- Different arm size requires careful and appropriate cuff size selection. Do not choose a cuff based on the name of the cuff. An "infant" cuff is often too small for some infants.
- Readings are difficult to obtain in restless or anxious infants and children. Allow at least 15 minutes for children to

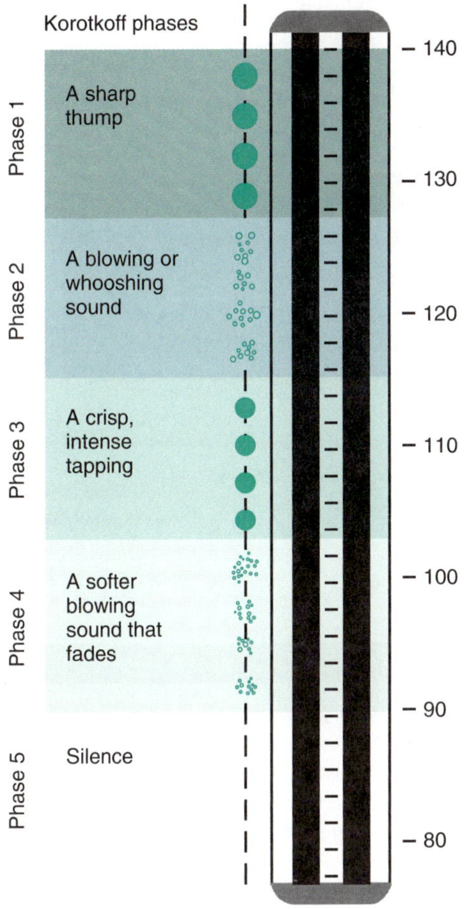

FIG. 29-14 The sounds auscultated during blood pressure measurement can be differentiated into five Korotkoff phases. In this example blood pressure is 140/90 mm Hg.

recover from recent activities and become less apprehensive. Preparing the child for the unusual sensation of the BP cuff increases cooperation. Most children understand the analogy of a "tight hug on your arm."

- Placing the stethoscope too firmly on the antecubital fossa causes errors in auscultation.
- Korotkoff sounds are difficult to hear in children because of low frequency and amplitude. A pediatric stethoscope bell is often helpful.

Ultrasonic Stethoscope. When you are unable to auscultate sounds because of a weakened arterial pulse, you can use an ultrasonic stethoscope (see Chapter 30). This stethoscope allows you to hear low-frequency systolic sounds. You frequently use this device when measuring the BP of infants and children and low BP in adults.

Palpation. Indirect measurement of BP by palpation is useful for patients whose arterial pulsations are too weak to create Korotkoff sounds. Severe blood loss and decreased heart contractility are examples of conditions that result in BPs too low to auscultate accurately. In these cases you can assess the systolic BP by palpation (Box 29-11). The diastolic BP is difficult to determine by palpation. When using the palpation technique, record the systolic value and how you measured it (e.g., RA 90/-, palpated, supine).

You can use the palpation technique along with auscultation. In some patients with hypertension the sounds usually heard over the brachial artery when the cuff pressure is high disappear as pressure is reduced and then reappear at a lower level. This temporary disappearance of sound is the **auscultatory gap.** It typically occurs between the first and second Korotkoff sounds. The gap in sound covers a range of 40 mm Hg and thus causes an underestimation of systolic pressure or overestimation of diastolic pressure. The examiner needs to be certain to inflate the cuff high enough to hear the true systolic pressure before the auscultatory gap. Palpation of the radial artery helps to determine how high to inflate the cuff. The examiner inflates the cuff 30 mm Hg above the pressure at which the radial pulse was palpated. Record the range of pressures in which the auscultatory gap occurs (e.g., BP RA 180/94 mm Hg with an auscultatory gap from 180 to 160 mm Hg, sitting).

BOX 29-11 PROCEDURAL GUIDELINES

Palpating Systolic Blood Pressure

Delegation Considerations

The skill of palpation of blood pressure (BP) cannot be delegated to nursing assistive personnel.

Equipment

Sphygmomanometer

1. Identify the patient using two identifiers (i.e., name and birth date or name and account number) according to facility policy.
2. Perform hand hygiene.
3. Apply BP cuff to extremity selected for measurement.
4. Continually palpate pulse of brachial, radial, or popliteal artery with fingertips of one hand.
5. Inflate BP cuff 30 mm Hg above point at which you no longer can palpate the pulse.
6. Slowly release valve and deflate cuff, allowing manometer needle mercury to fall 2 mm Hg per second.
7. Note point on manometer when pulse is again palpable; this is the systolic BP.
8. Deflate cuff rapidly and completely. Remove cuff from patient extremity unless you need to repeat the measurement.
9. Perform hand hygiene.
10. Record BP as systolic/-, palpated (e.g., BP 108/-, palpated) on vital sign flow sheet, in nurses' notes, or electronic medical record. Report abnormal findings to nurse in charge or health care provider.

Lower-Extremity Blood Pressure. Dressings, casts, IV catheters, or arteriovenous fistulas or shunts make the upper extremities inaccessible for BP measurement. You then need to obtain the BP in a lower extremity. Comparing upper-extremity BP with that in the legs is also necessary for patients with certain cardiac and BP abnormalities. The popliteal artery, palpable behind the knee in the popliteal space, is the site for auscultation. The cuff needs to be wide and long enough to allow for the larger girth of the thigh. Placing the patient in a prone position is best. If such a position is impossible, ask the patient to flex the knee slightly for easier access to the artery. Position the cuff 2.5 cm (1 inch) above the popliteal artery, with the bladder over the posterior aspect of the midthigh (Fig. 29-15). The procedure is identical to brachial artery auscultation. Systolic pressure in the legs is usually higher by 10 to 40 mm Hg than in the brachial artery, but the diastolic pressure is the same.

Electronic Blood Pressure Devices. Many different styles of electronic BP machines are available to determine BP automatically (Fig. 29-16). Electronic BP machines rely on an electronic sensor to detect the vibrations caused by the rush of blood through an artery (Box 29-12). Use electronic devices when frequent BP assessment is necessary such as in patients who are critically ill or unstable, during or after invasive procedures, or when therapies

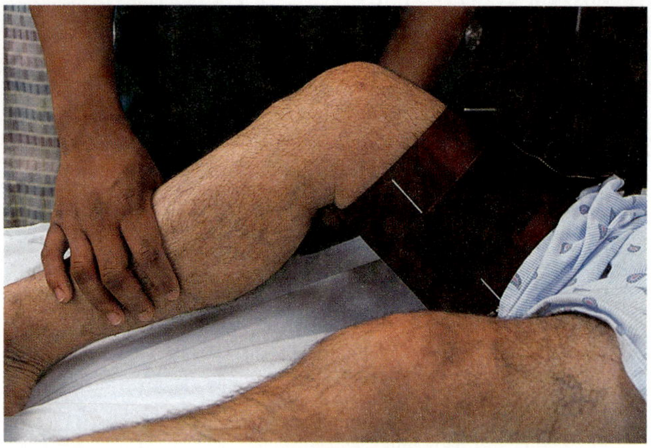

FIG. 29-15 Lower-extremity blood pressure cuff positioned above popliteal artery at midthigh with knee flexed.

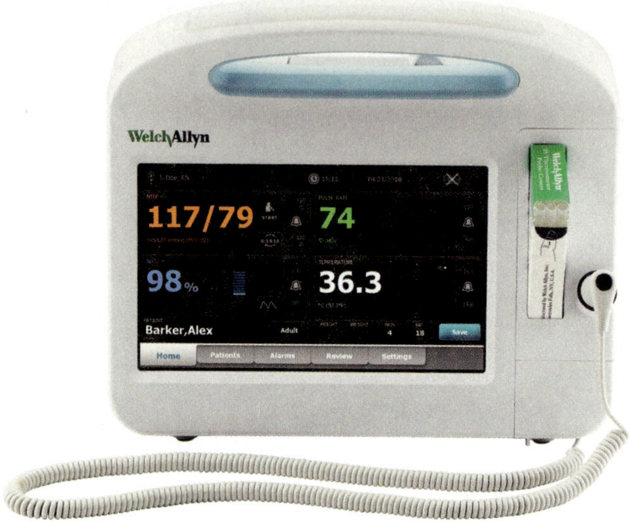

FIG. 29-16 Automatic blood pressure monitor. (Courtesy Welch Allyn.)

BOX 29-12 PROCEDURAL GUIDELINES

Electronic Blood Pressure Measurement

Delegation Considerations

The skill of obtaining an electronic blood pressure (BP) measurement can be delegated to nursing assistive personnel (NAP). However, an RN must first verify that the patient is stable and does not need to be closely monitored for evaluating response to medications. Instruct the NAP to:

- Select appropriate limb for BP measurement.
- Select appropriate-size BP cuff for designated limb.
- Obtain BP measurement for select patient with ordered frequency.
- Report abnormalities to nurse for further assessment.

Equipment

Electronic BP machine, BP cuff of appropriate size as recommended by manufacturer.

1. Identify the patient using two identifiers (i.e., name and birth date or name and account number) according to facility policy.
2. Determine appropriateness of using electronic BP measurement. Patients with irregular heart rate, peripheral vascular disease, seizures, tremors, and shivering are not candidates for this device (Bern et al., 2007).
3. Determine best site for cuff placement (see Skill 29-5, Step 3).
4. Perform hand hygiene. Assist patient to comfortable position, either lying or sitting. Plug in device and place it near patient, ensuring that connector hose between cuff and machine will reach.
5. Locate on/off switch and turn machine on to enable device to self-test computer systems.
6. Select appropriate cuff size for patient extremity (see Table 29-11) and appropriate cuff for machine. Electronic BP machines are vulnerable to error among older adults and obese patients (Heinemann et al., 2008). Electronic BP cuff and machine are matched by the manufacturer and are not interchangeable.
7. Expose extremity for measurement by removing restrictive clothing to ensure proper cuff application. Do not place BP cuff over clothing.
8. Prepare BP cuff by manually squeezing all the air out of cuff and connecting it to connector hose.
9. Wrap flattened cuff snugly around extremity, verifying that only one finger fits between cuff and patient's skin. Make sure that "artery" arrow marked on outside of cuff is placed correctly (see illustration for Skill 29-5, Step 4).
10. Verify that connector hose between cuff and machine is not kinked. Kinking prevents proper inflation and deflation of cuff.
11. Following manufacturer directions, set frequency control of automatic or manual and press start button. The first BP measurement pumps cuff to pressure of approximately 180 mm Hg. After this pressure is reached, the machine begins a deflation sequence that determines BP. The first reading determines peak pressure inflation for additional measurements.

    CLINICAL DECISION: If unable to obtain BP with electronic device, verify machine connections (e.g., plugged into working electrical outlet, hose-cuff connections tight, machine on, correct cuff). Repeat electronic BP; if unable to obtain, use auscultatory technique (see Skill 29-5).

12. When deflation is complete, digital display provides most recent values and flash time in minutes that has elapsed since measurement occurred.
13. Set frequency of BP measurements and upper and lower alarm limits for systolic, diastolic, and mean BP readings. Intervals between BP measurements are set from 1 to 90 minutes. Determine measurement frequency and alarm limits based on patient's acceptable range of BP, nursing judgment, and health care provider order.
14. Obtain additional readings at any time by pressing start button. (Sometimes you need these for unstable patients.) Pressing cancel button immediately deflates cuff.
15. If frequent BP determinations are necessary, leave cuff in place. Remove cuff at least every 2 hours to assess underlying skin integrity and, if possible, alternate BP sites. Patients with abnormal bleeding tendencies are at risk for microvascular rupture from repeated inflations. When patient no longer requires electronic BP machine, clean BP cuff according to facility policy to reduce transmission of microorganisms.
16. Compare electronic BP readings with auscultatory BP to verify accuracy of electronic BP device.
17. Record BP and site assessed on vital sign flow sheet, in nurses' notes, or electronic medical record (per agency policy). Record any signs of BP alterations in nurses' notes. Report abnormal findings to nurse in charge or health care provider.

BOX 29-13 PATIENT CONDITIONS NOT APPROPRIATE FOR ELECTRONIC BLOOD PRESSURE MEASUREMENT

- Irregular heart rate
- Peripheral vascular obstruction (e.g., clots, narrowed vessels)
- Shivering
- Seizures
- Excessive tremors
- Inability to cooperate
- Blood pressure less than 90 mm Hg systolic

require frequent monitoring (e.g., IV heart and BP medications). Box 29-13 lists conditions that are not appropriate for automatic BP devices.

The advantages of automatic devices are the ease of use and efficiency when repeated or frequent measurements are indicated. The ability to use a stethoscope is not necessary. However, automatic devices are more sensitive to outside interference and susceptible to error. Most electronic BP devices are unable to process sounds or vibrations of low BP. The range of device sophistication also makes BP measurement comparisons difficult. The use of automatic BP devices permits assessment of BP during interpersonal interactions. Talking to a patient while assessing the BP increases readings 10% to 40%.

Self-Measurement of Blood Pressure. Improved technology in electronic monitoring devices allows individuals to measure their own BPs in their home with the push of a button. The portable home devices include the aneroid sphygmomanometer and electronic digital readout devices that do not require use of a stethoscope. The electronic devices are easier to manipulate but require frequent recalibration, more than once a year. Because of their sensitivity, improper cuff placement or movement of the arm causes electronic devices to give incorrect readings.

Stationary automatic BP devices are often found in public places such as grocery stores, fitness clubs, airports, or work sites. Users simply rest their arms within the inflatable cuff of the machine, which contains a pressure sensor. The cuff fits over clothing. A visual display tells users their BP within 60 to 90 seconds. The reliability of the stationary machines is limited. BP values vary by 5 to 10 mm Hg or more (for both systolic and diastolic values) compared with pressures taken with a manual sphygmomanometer.

Self-measurement of BP has several benefits. Sometimes elevated BP is detected in persons previously unaware of a problem. Persons with prehypertension provide information about the pattern of BP values to their health care provider. Patients with hypertension benefit from participating actively in their treatment through self-monitoring, which helps adherence with treatment. The disadvantages of self-measurement include improper use of the device and risk of inaccurate readings. Some patients are needlessly alarmed with one elevated reading. Some patients with hypertension become overly conscious of their BP and inappropriately self-adjust medications.

Consumers can learn to use self-measurement devices if they have the information needed to perform the procedure correctly and if they know when to seek medical attention. Advise patients of possible inaccuracies in the BP devices, help them understand the meaning and implications of readings, and teach them proper measurement techniques. Encourage them to record the date of their BP readings to assess BP over time and share findings with their health care provider.

BOX 29-14 PATIENT TEACHING

Health Promotion

Objective

- Patient verbalizes measures to promote health.

Teaching Strategies

- Explain measures to prevent body temperature alterations.
- Instruct patients on risk factors for hypothermia, frostbite, and heat stroke. Demonstrate self-assessment of heart rate using the carotid pulse. Patients taking certain prescribed cardiac medications need to learn to assess their own pulse rate to detect side effects of medications. Patients undergoing cardiac rehabilitation need to learn to assess their own pulse rate to determine their response to exercise.
- Instruct patients on normal blood pressure values, risk factors for hypertension, usual lack of hypertension symptoms, ability of therapy to control but not cure, and benefits of a consistently followed hypertension treatment plan.
- Demonstrate how to obtain blood pressure to the patient's family caregiver using an appropriate-size blood pressure cuff for home use at the same time each day, after patient has had a brief rest, and the same position and arm each time pressure is taken.
- Instruct patient on signs and symptoms of hypoxemia.
- Instruct patient on the effect of cigarette smoking on oxygen saturation.

Evaluation

- Observe patient's ability to initiate preventive health measures to prevent body temperature alterations.
- Assess patient's accuracy in obtaining pulse rate.
- Assess family caregiver's accuracy in obtaining blood pressure.

Nursing Process and Blood Pressure Determination

The assessment of BP along with pulse assessment evaluates the general state of cardiovascular health and responses to other system imbalances. Hypotension, hypertension, orthostatic hypotension, and narrow or wide pulse pressures are defining characteristics of certain nursing diagnoses, including the following:

- Activity intolerance
- Anxiety
- Decreased cardiac output
- Deficient/excess fluid volume
- Risk for injury
- Acute pain
- Ineffective peripheral tissue perfusion

The nursing care plan includes interventions based on the nursing diagnosis identified and the related factors. For example, the defining characteristics of hypotension, dizziness, pulse deficit, and dysrhythmia lead to a diagnosis of *decreased cardiac output.* Related factors might include poor oral intake, excessive heat exposure, and a history of valvular heart disease. The related factor guides the choice of nursing interventions. Evaluate patient outcomes by assessing the BP following each intervention.

HEALTH PROMOTION AND VITAL SIGNS

The emphasis on health promotion and maintenance and discharge from hospital settings has resulted in an increase in the need for patients and their families to monitor vital signs in the home. Teaching considerations affect all vital sign measurements. Incorporate them within the patient's plan of care (Box 29-14).

BOX 29-15 FOCUS ON OLDER ADULTS

Factors Affecting Vital Signs of Older Adults

Temperature

- The temperature of older adults is at the lower end of the normal temperature range, 36° to 36.8° C (96.8° to 98.3° F) orally and 36.6° to 37.2° C (98° to 99° F) rectally. Therefore temperatures considered within normal range sometimes reflect a fever in an older adult. In an older adult fever is present when a single oral temperature is over 37.8° C (100° F); repeated oral temperatures are over 37.2° C (99° F); rectal temperatures are over 37.5° C (99.5° F); or temperature has increased more than 1° C (2° F) over baseline (High et al., 2009).
- Older adults are very sensitive to slight changes in environmental temperature because their thermoregulatory systems are not as efficient.
- A decrease in sweat gland reactivity in the older adult results in a higher threshold for sweating at high temperatures, which leads to hyperthermia and heatstroke.
- Be especially attentive to subtle temperature changes and other manifestations of fever in this population such as tachypnea, anorexia, falls, delirium, and overall functional decline.
- With aging loss of subcutaneous fat reduces the insulating capacity of the skin; older men are especially high risk for hypothermia.

Pulse Rate

- If it is difficult to palpate the pulse of an obese older adult, a Doppler device provides a more accurate reading.
- The older adult has a decreased heart rate at rest.
- It takes longer for the heart rate to rise in the older adult to meet sudden increased demands that result from stress, illness, or excitement. Once elevated, the pulse rate of an older adult takes longer to return to normal resting rate.
- When assessing the apical rate of an older woman, the breast tissue is gently lifted, and the stethoscope placed at the fifth intercostal space (ICS) or the lower edge of the breast.
- Heart sounds are sometimes muffled or difficult to hear in older adults because of an increase in air space in the lungs.

Blood Pressure

- Older adults often have decreased upper arm mass, which requires special attention to selection of blood pressure cuff size.
- Older adults sometimes have an increase in systolic pressure related to decreased vessel elasticity while the diastolic pressure remains the same, resulting in a wider pulse pressure.
- Instruct older adults to change position slowly and wait after each change to avoid postural hypotension and prevent injuries.

Respirations

- Aging causes ossification of costal cartilage and downward slant of ribs, resulting in a more rigid rib cage, which reduces chest wall expansion. Kyphosis and scoliosis that occur in older adults also restrict chest expansion and decrease tidal volume.
- Older adults depend more on accessory abdominal muscles during respiration than on weaker thoracic muscles.
- The respiratory system matures by the time a person reaches 20 years of age and begins to decline in healthy people after the age of 25. Despite this decline older adults are able to breathe effortlessly as long as they are healthy. However, sudden events that require an increased demand for oxygen (e.g., exercise, stress, illness) create shortness of breath in the older adult.
- Identifying an acceptable pulse oximeter probe site is difficult with older adults because of the likelihood of peripheral vascular disease, decreased cardiac output, cold-induced vasoconstriction, and anemia.

When considering how to teach patients and their families about vital sign measurements and their importance and significance, a patient's age is an important factor. With an increase in the older-adult population there is a greater need for family caregivers to be aware of changes that are unique to older adults. Box 29-15 identifies some of these variations.

RECORDING VITAL SIGNS

Special electronic and paper graphic flow sheets exist for recording vital signs (see Chapter 26). Identify institution procedure for documenting on a graphic. In addition to the actual vital sign values, record in the nurses' notes any accompanying or precipitating symptoms such as chest pain and dizziness with abnormal BP, shortness of breath with abnormal respirations, cyanosis with hypoxemia, or flushing and diaphoresis with elevated temperature. Document any interventions initiated as a result of vital sign measurement such as administration of oxygen therapy, hydration, or an antihypertensive medication.

Patients being managed on critical paths or CareMaps often have vital sign values listed as outcomes. If a vital sign value is above or below the anticipated outcomes, write a variance note to explain the nature of the variance and the nursing course of action. For example, a CareMap for a patient who has undergone lung surgery often has an outcome during the postoperative period of "afebrile." If the patient has a fever, the nurse's variance note addresses possible sources of fever (e.g., retained pulmonary secretions) and nursing interventions (e.g., increased suctioning, postural drainage, or hydration).

SAFETY GUIDELINES FOR NURSING SKILLS

Ensuring patient safety is an essential role of the professional nurse. To ensure patient safety, communicate clearly with the members of the health care team, assess and incorporate the patient's priorities of care and preferences, and use the best evidence when making decisions about your patient's care. When performing the skills in this chapter, remember the following points to ensure safe, individualized patient-centered care.

- Devices for measuring vital signs are often shared among patients. Cleaning each device carefully between patients decreases patients' risk of infection.
- BP cuffs and pulse oximetry sensors can apply excessive pressure on fragile skin. Rotating sites during repeated measurements decreases risk for skin breakdown.
- Analyze the trends for measuring vital signs and report abnormal findings to the health care provider.
- Determine frequency of measuring vital signs based on the patient's condition.

SKILL 29-1 MEASURING BODY TEMPERATURE

View Video!

Delegation Considerations

The skill of temperature measurement can be delegated to nursing assistive personnel (NAP). Instruct the NAP to:

- Select appropriate route and device to measure temperature.
- Take appropriate precautions when properly positioning the patient for rectal temperature measurement.
- Consider specific patient-related factors that falsely raise or lower temperature.
- Obtain temperature measurement at ordered frequency.
- Be aware of the usual values for patient.
- Report abnormalities to the nurse for further assessment.

Equipment

- Appropriate thermometer (see Box 29-4)
- Soft tissue or wipe
- Lubricant (for rectal measurements only)
- Pen, vital sign flow sheet, or record or patient's electronic medical record
- Clean gloves, plastic thermometer sleeve, disposable probe or sensor cover
- Towel

STEP	RATIONALE
ASSESSMENT	
1 Assess for signs and symptoms of temperature alterations and factors that influence body temperature.	Physical signs and symptoms indicate abnormal temperature. Enables you to accurately assess the nature of variations.
2 Determine previous activity that interferes with accuracy of temperature measurement. When taking oral temperature, wait 20 to 30 minutes before measuring temperature if patient has smoked or ingested hot or cold liquids or foods.	Smoking, mouth breathing, and oral intake cause false oral temperature readings (Henker and Carlson, 2007).
3 Determine appropriate temperature site and device for patient.	Site is chosen based on advantages and disadvantages of each site (see Box 29-4). Use disposable single-use thermometer for patient on isolation precautions.
PLANNING	
1 Identify the patient using two identifiers (i.e., name and birth date or name and account number) according to facility policy.	Ensures correct patient. Complies with recommended National Patient Safety Goal (TJC, 2011).
2 Explain route by which temperature will be taken and importance of maintaining proper position until reading is complete.	Patients are often curious about such measurements and need to be cautioned against prematurely removing thermometer to read results.
IMPLEMENTATION	
1 Perform hand hygiene.	Reduces transmission of microorganisms.
2 Assist patient in assuming comfortable position that provides easy access to temperature measurement site.	Ensures comfort and accuracy of temperature reading.
3 Obtain temperature reading.	
a. **Oral temperature measurement with electronic thermometer**	
(1) Apply clean gloves (optional).	Use of oral probe cover, which you can remove without physical contact, minimizes need to wear gloves.
(2) Remove thermometer pack from charging unit. Attach oral thermometer probe stem (blue tip) to thermometer unit. Grasp top of probe stem, being careful not to apply pressure on the ejection button.	Charging provides battery power. Ejection button releases plastic probe cover from probe stem.

SKILL 29-1 MEASURING BODY TEMPERATURE—cont'd

STEP	RATIONALE
(3) Slide disposable plastic probe cover over thermometer probe stem until cover locks in place (see illustrations).	Soft plastic cover will not break in patient's mouth and prevents transmission of microorganisms between patients.
(4) Ask patient to open mouth; gently place thermometer probe under tongue in posterior sublingual pocket lateral to center of lower jaw (see illustration).	Heat from superficial blood vessels in sublingual pocket produces temperature reading. With electronic thermometer, temperatures in right and left posterior sublingual pocket are significantly higher than in area under front of tongue.
(5) Ask patient to hold thermometer probe with lips closed.	Closed lips maintain proper position of thermometer during recording.
(6) Leave thermometer probe in place until audible signal indicates completion and temperate reading appears on digital display; remove thermometer probe from under patient's tongue.	Probe needs to stay in place until signal occurs to ensure accurate reading.
(7) Push ejection button on thermometer probe stem to discard plastic probe cover into appropriate receptacle.	Reduces transmission of microorganisms.
(8) Return thermometer probe stem to storage position of recording unit.	Storage position protects probe stem. Returning probe stem automatically causes digital reading to disappear.
(9) If gloves are worn, remove and dispose in appropriate receptacle. Perform hand hygiene.	Hand hygiene reduces transmission of microorganisms.
(10) Return thermometer to charger.	Charger maintains battery charge.

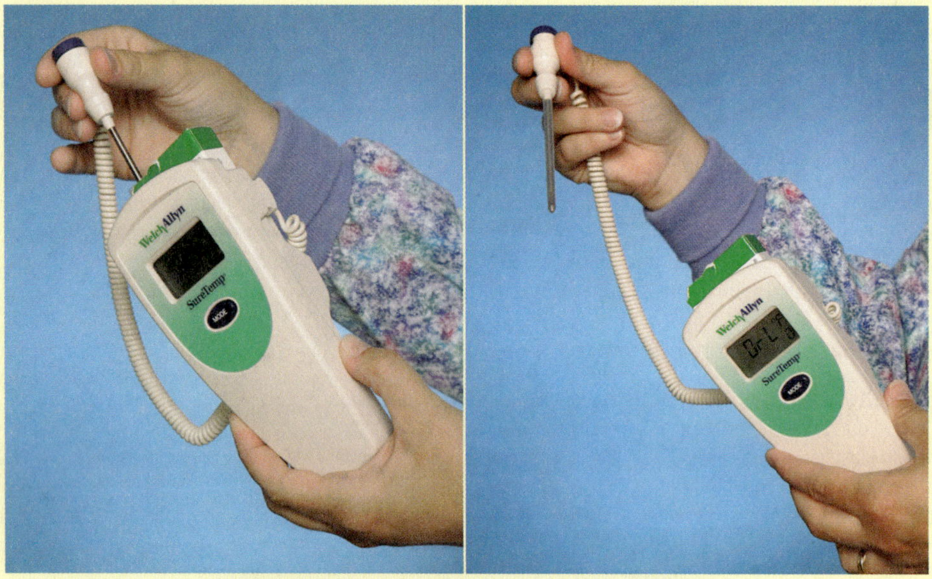

STEP 3a(3) Disposable plastic cover is placed over probe.

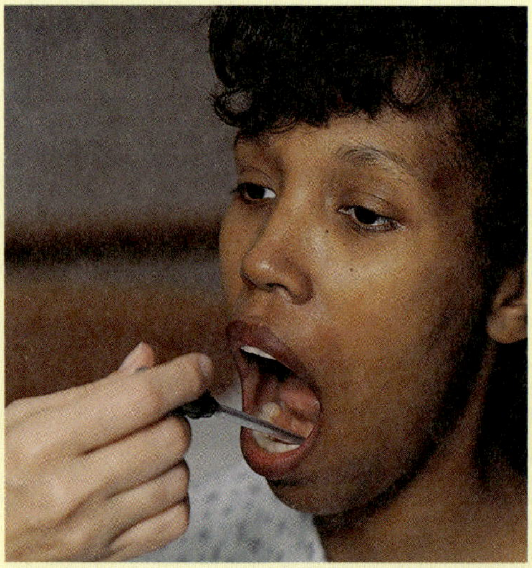

STEP 3a(4) Probe under tongue in posterior sublingual pocket.

STEP	RATIONALE
b. Rectal temperature measurement with electronic thermometer	
(1) Draw curtain around bed and/or close room door. Assist patient to Sims' position with upper leg flexed. Move aside bed linen to expose only anal area. Keep patient's upper body and lower extremities covered with sheet or blanket.	Maintains patient's privacy, minimizes embarrassment, and promotes comfort. Exposes anal area for correct thermometer placement.
(2) Apply clean gloves.	Maintains standard precautions when exposed to items soiled with body fluids (e.g., feces).
(3) Remove thermometer pack from charging unit. Attach rectal probe stem (red tip) to thermometer unit. Grasp top of probe stem, being careful not to apply pressure on the ejection button.	Charging provides battery power. Ejection button releases plastic cover from probe stem.
(4) Slide disposable plastic probe cover over thermometer probe stem until cover locks in place.	Soft plastic probe cover prevents transmission of microorganisms between patients.
(5) Squeeze liberal portion of lubricant on tissue. Dip end of probe cover into lubricant, covering 2.5 to 3.5 cm (1 to 1½ inches) for adult.	Lubrication minimizes trauma to rectal mucosa during insertion. Tissue avoids contamination of remaining lubricant in container.
(6) With nondominant hand, separate patient's buttocks to expose anus. Ask patient to breathe slowly and relax.	Fully exposes anus for thermometer insertion. Relaxes anal sphincter for easier thermometer insertion.
(7) Gently insert thermometer probe into anus in direction of umbilicus 2.5 to 3.5 cm (1 to 1½ inches) for adult. Do not force thermometer.	Ensures adequate exposure against blood vessels in rectal wall.

CLINICAL DECISION: *If you cannot adequately insert thermometer into rectum, remove it and consider alternative method for obtaining temperature.*

STEP	RATIONALE
(8) Once positioned, hold thermometer probe in place (see illustration) until audible signal indicates completion and patient's temperature appears on digital display; remove thermometer probe from anus.	Probe needs to stay in place until signal occurs to ensure accurate reading.

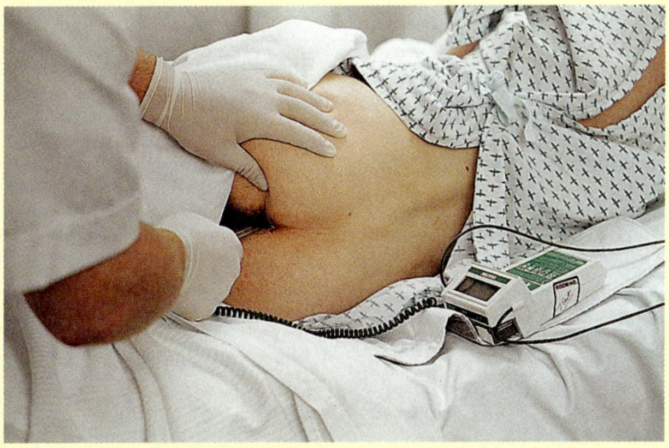

STEP 3b(8) Probe position in anus.

STEP	RATIONALE
(9) Push ejection button on thermometer stem to discard plastic probe cover into appropriate receptacle. Wipe probe stem with alcohol swab, paying particular attention to ridges where probe stem cover connects to probe.	Reduces transmission of microorganisms.
(10) Return thermometer probe stem to storage position of recording unit.	Protects probe stem from damage. Returning probe stem automatically causes digital reading to disappear.
(11) Wipe patient's anal area with soft tissue to remove lubricant or feces and discard tissue. Help patient assume a comfortable position.	Provides for comfort and hygiene.
(12) Remove and dispose of gloves in appropriate receptacle. Perform hand hygiene.	Reduces transmission of microorganisms.
(13) Return thermometer to charger. Verify that charger and probes are wiped with alcohol daily.	Maintains battery charge of thermometer unit. Reduces transmission of microorganisms.
c. Axillary temperature measurement with electronic thermometer	
(1) Draw curtain around bed and/or close door. Assist patient to a supine or sitting position. Move clothing or gown away from shoulder and arm.	Maintains patient's privacy, minimizes embarrassment. Position provides easy access to axilla. Exposes axilla for correct thermometer probe placement.
(2) Remove thermometer pack from charging unit. Be sure that oral probe stem (blue tip) is attached to thermometer unit. Grasp top of thermometer probe stem, being careful not to apply pressure on ejection button.	Charging provides battery power. Ejection button releases plastic cover from probe.
(3) Slide disposable plastic probe cover over thermometer stem until cover locks in place.	Soft plastic probe cover prevents transmission of microorganisms between patients.

SKILL 29-1 MEASURING BODY TEMPERATURE—cont'd

STEP	RATIONALE
(4) Raise patient's arm away from torso; inspect for skin lesion and excessive perspiration. Insert thermometer probe into center of axilla, lower arm over probe, and place arm across patient's chest (see illustration).	Maintains proper position of probe against blood vessels in axilla.

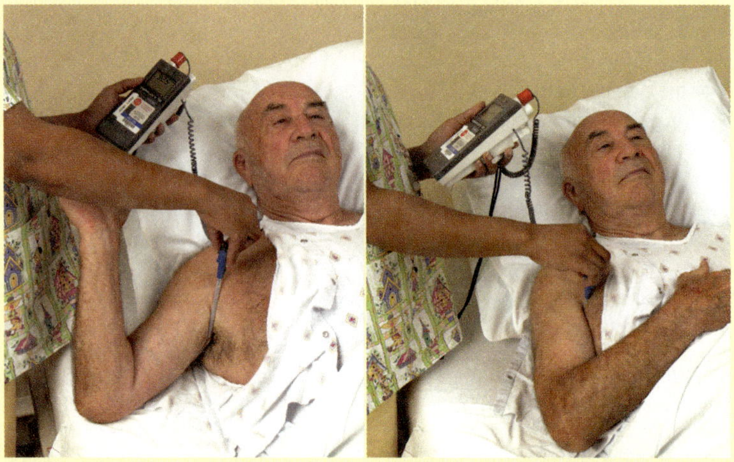

STEP 3c(4) Thermometer tip in axilla.

CLINICAL DECISION: *Do not use axilla if skin lesions are present because lesions alter local temperature and areas are painful to touch.*

STEP	RATIONALE
(5) Once positioned, hold thermometer probe in place until audible signal occurs and temperature appears on digital display. Remove thermometer probe from axilla.	Thermometer probe needs to stay in place until signal occurs to ensure accurate reading.
(6) Push ejection button on thermometer stem to discard plastic probe cover into appropriate receptacle.	Reduces transmission of microorganisms.
(7) Return thermometer stem to storage position of recording unit.	Storage position protects stem. Returning probe automatically causes digital reading to disappear.
(8) Help patient assume a comfortable position, replacing linen or gown.	Restores comfort and promotes privacy.
(9) Perform hand hygiene.	Reduces transmission of microorganisms.
(10) Return thermometer to charger.	Maintains battery charge.
d. Tympanic membrane temperature with electronic infrared thermometer	
(1) Help patient assume comfortable position with head turned toward side away from you. If patient has been lying on one side, use upper ear.	Ensures comfort and exposes auditory canal for accurate temperature measurement. Heat trapped in lower ear causes false-high temperature readings.
(2) Note if there is obvious earwax in patient's ear canal.	Earwax on lens cover blocks a clear optical pathway. It can lower tympanic temperature by 0.3° C (0.6° F). Switch to other ear or select alternative measurement site if needed.
(3) Remove thermometer handheld unit from charging base, being careful not to apply pressure to ejection button.	Base provides battery power. Removal of handheld unit from base prepares it to measure temperature. Ejection button releases plastic probe cover from thermometer tip.
(4) Slide clean disposable speculum cover over otoscope-like lens tip until it locks into place. Do not touch lens cover.	Soft plastic probe cover prevents transmission of microorganisms between patients. Lens cover needs to be free of dust, fingerprints, or earwax to ensure clear optical pathway.
(5) If right-handed, obtain temperature from patient's right ear; left-handed people obtain temperature from patient's left ear.	The less acute the angle of approach, the better the probe will seal inside the auditory canal.
(6) Insert infrared speculum into ear canal following manufacturer instructions for tympanic probe positioning:	Ear tug straightens external auditory canal, allowing maximum exposure of the tympanic membrane (Hockenberry and Wilson, 2007).
a. Pull ear pinna backward, up, and out for an adult. For children 3 years and younger, point covered probe toward midpoint between eyebrow and side burns. For children older than 3 years, pull pinna up and back (Hockenberry and Wilson, 2007).	Correctly positioning speculum tip with respect to ear canal ensures accurate readings.

STEP	RATIONALE
b. Move thermometer in a figure-eight pattern.	Some manufacturers recommend movement of the speculum tip in a figure-eight pattern, which allows the sensor to detect maximum tympanic membrane heat radiation.
c. Fit speculum tip snugly into canal and do not move (see illustration), pointing speculum tip toward nose.	Gentle pressure seals ear canal from ambient temperature, which alters readings as much as 2.8° C (5° F). Operator error leads to false-low temperatures.

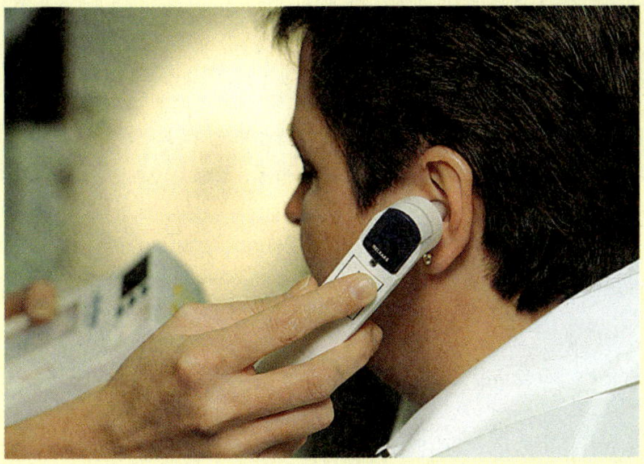

STEP 3d(6)c Tympanic thermometer with probe cover inserted into auditory canal.

STEP	RATIONALE
(7) Once positioned, press scan button on handheld unit. Leave speculum in place until audible signal indicates completion and patient's temperature appears on digital display.	Pressing scan button causes detection of infrared energy. Speculum needs to stay in place until signal occurs to ensure accurate reading.
(8) Carefully remove speculum from auditory meatus.	Prevents rubbing of sensitive outer ear lining.
(9) Push ejection button on handheld unit to discard speculum cover into appropriate receptacle.	Reduces transmission of microorganisms. Automatically causes digital reading to disappear.
(10) If temperature is abnormal or a second reading is necessary, replace speculum cover and wait 2 to 3 minutes before repeating measurement in same ear. Repeat measurement in other ear or try an alternative temperature site or instrument.	Time allows ear canal to regain usual temperature.
(11) Return handheld unit to charging base.	Protects sensor tip from damage.
(12) Help patient to get into a comfortable position.	Restores comfort and sense of well-being.
(13) Perform hand hygiene.	Reduces transmission of microorganisms.
4 Discuss findings with patient as needed.	Promotes participation in care and understanding of health status.

EVALUATION

STEP	RATIONALE
1 If temperature is assessed for first time, establish temperature as baseline if it is within normal range.	Used to compare future temperature measurements.
2 Compare temperature reading with patient's previous baseline and acceptable temperature range for his or her age-group.	Body temperature fluctuates within narrow range; comparison reveals presence of abnormality. Improper placement or movement of thermometer causes inaccuracies. Second measurement confirms initial findings of abnormal body temperature.

UNEXPECTED OUTCOMES AND RELATED INTERVENTIONS

1 Temperature 1° C (1.8° F) above usual range
- Assess possible sites (e.g., central line catheter, wounds) for localized infection and related data suggesting a systemic infection.
- Follow interventions listed in Box 29-8.

2 Fever persists or reaches unacceptable level as defined by health care provider.
- Notify health care provider and administer antipyretics and antibiotics as ordered.

3 Temperature 1° C (1.8° F) below usual range
- Remove any drafts, wet clothing, or linen.
- Apply extra blankets and, unless contraindicated, offer warm liquids.
- Monitor apical pulse rate and rhythm because hypothermia causes bradycardia and dysrhythmias.

RECORDING AND REPORTING

- Record temperature in nurses' notes or vital sign flow sheet. Document measurement of temperature after administration of specific therapies in narrative form in nurses' notes.
- Report abnormal findings to nurse in charge or health care provider.

HOME CARE CONSIDERATIONS

- Assess temperature and ventilation of patient's environment to determine existence of any environmental condition that influences patient's temperature.

SKILL 29-2 ASSESSING THE RADIAL AND APICAL PULSES

View Video!

Delegation Considerations

The skill of pulse measurement can be delegated to nursing assistive personnel (NAP) if the patient is stable and not at high risk for acute or serious cardiac problems. Instruct the NAP to:

- Consider specific factors related to patient history, usual values, or risk for irregular pulse.
- Obtain appropriate pulse measurements and position for select patient.
- Report specific abnormalities to the nurse for further assessment.

Equipment

- Stethoscope (apical pulse only)
- Wristwatch with second hand or digital display
- Pen, vital sign flow sheet, or patient's electronic health record
- Alcohol swab

STEP	RATIONALE
ASSESSMENT	
1 Determine need to assess radial or apical pulse:	Nurse uses clinical judgment to determine need for assessment.
a. Assess for any risk factors for pulse alterations. • History of heart disease • Cardiac dysrhythmias • Onset of sudden chest pain or acute pain from any site • Invasive cardiovascular diagnostic tests • Surgery • Sudden infusion of large volume of intravenous (IV) fluid • Internal or external hemorrhage, dehydration • Administration of medications that alter cardiac function	These conditions place patients at risk for pulse alterations. A history of peripheral vascular disease often alters pulse rate and quality.
b. Assess for signs and symptoms of altered stroke volume and cardiac output such as dyspnea, fatigue, chest pain, orthopnea, syncope, palpitations (person's unpleasant awareness of heartbeat), jugular venous distention, edema of dependent body parts, cyanosis, or pallor of skin (see Chapter 40).	Physical signs and symptoms indicate alteration in cardiac function.
c. Assess for signs and symptoms of peripheral vascular disease such as pale, cool extremities; thin, shiny skin with decreased hair growth; thickened nails.	Physical signs and symptoms indicate alteration in local arterial blood flow.
2 Assess for factors that influence pulse rate and rhythm: age, exercise, position changes, fluid balance, medications, temperature, and sympathetic stimulation.	Allows for accurate assessment of presence and significance of pulse alterations. Acceptable range of pulse rate changes with age (see Table 29-3).
3 Determine patient's previous baseline pulse rate if available in his or her medical record.	Allows for accurate assessment of change in condition and provides comparison with future apical pulse measurements.
4 Determine if patient has latex allergy.	If patient has latex allergy, verify that stethoscope is latex free.
PLANNING	
1 Explain that you will assess pulse or heart rate. Encourage patient to relax and not speak. If patient was active, wait 5 to 10 minutes before assessing pulse.	Activity and anxiety elevate heart rate. Patient's voice interferes with your ability to hear sound when assessing apical rate. Obtaining pulse rates at rest allows for objective comparison of values.
2 Identify the patient using two identifiers (i.e., name and birth date or name and account number) according to facility policy.	Ensures correct patient. Complies with recommended National Patient Safety Goals (TJC, 2011).
IMPLEMENTATION	
1 Perform hand hygiene.	Reduces transmission of microorganisms.
2 If necessary, draw curtain around bed and/or close door.	Maintains privacy.
3 Obtain pulse measurement.	

STEP	RATIONALE
a. Radial pulse	
(1) Help patient get into supine or sitting position.	Provides easy access to pulse sites.
(2) If supine, place patient's forearm straight alongside body or across lower chest or upper abdomen with wrist extended straight (see illustration). If sitting, bend patient's elbow 90 degrees and support lower arm on chair or on your arm.	Relaxed position of lower arm and slight flexion of wrist promote exposure of artery to palpation without restriction.
(3) Place tips of first two or middle three fingers of hand over groove along radial or thumb side of patient's inner wrist. Slightly extend wrist with palm down until you note strongest pulse (see illustration).	Fingertips are most sensitive parts of hand to palpate arterial pulsation. Your thumb has a pulsation that interferes with accuracy.
(4) Lightly compress against radius, obliterate pulse initially, and then relax pressure so pulse becomes easily palpable.	Pulse is more accurately assessed with moderate pressure. Too much pressure occludes pulse and impairs blood flow.
(5) Determine strength of pulse. Note whether thrust of vessel against fingertips is bounding (4+), full/strong (3+), normal/expected (2+), diminished or barely palpable (1+), or absent (0).	Strength reflects volume of blood ejected against arterial wall with each heart contraction. Accurate description of strength improves communication among nurses and other health care providers.
(6) After feeling a regular pulse, look at the second hand of a watch and begin to count rate: count the first beat after the second hand hits the number on the dial; count as one, then two, and so on.	Determine rate only after knowing that you can palpate pulse. Timing begins with zero. Count of one is first beat palpated after timing begins.
(7) If pulse is regular, count rate for 30 seconds and multiply total by 2.	A 30-second count is accurate for rapid, slow, or regular pulse rates.
(8) If pulse is irregular, count rate for 1 minute (60 seconds). Assess frequency and pattern of irregularity. Compare radial pulses bilaterally.	Inefficient contraction of heart fails to transmit pulse wave, interfering with cardiac output, resulting in irregular pulse. Longer time ensures accurate count.

CLINICAL DECISION: *If pulse is irregular, do an apical/radial pulse assessment to detect a pulse deficit. Count apical pulse (see Step 3b) while a colleague counts radial pulse. Begin apical pulse count out loud to simultaneously assess pulses. If pulse count differs by more than 2, a pulse deficit exists, which sometimes indicates alterations in cardiac output.*

STEP	RATIONALE
b. Apical pulse	
(1) Clean earpieces and diaphragm of stethoscope with alcohol swab.	Reduces transmission of microorganisms.
(2) Draw curtain around bed and/or close door.	Provides privacy and minimizes embarrassment.
(3) Help patient to supine or sitting position. Move aside bed linen and gown to expose sternum and left side of chest.	Exposes portion of chest wall for selection of auscultatory site.
(4) Locate anatomical landmarks to identify the point of maximal impulse (PMI), also called the apical impulse (see illustrations A-D). Heart is located behind and to left of sternum with base at top and apex at bottom. Find angle of Louis just below suprasternal notch between sternal body and manubrium; feels like a bony prominence (illustration A). Slip fingers down each side of angle to find second intercostal space (ICS) (illustration B). Carefully move fingers down left side of sternum to fifth ICS (illustration C) and laterally to the left midclavicular line (MCL) (illustration D). A light tap felt within an area 1 to 2 cm (½ to 1 inch) of the PMI is reflected from the apex of the heart.	Use of anatomical landmarks allows correct placement of stethoscope over apex of heart, enhancing ability to hear heart sounds clearly. If unable to palpate the PMI, reposition patient on left side. In the presence of serious heart disease, the PMI is located to the left of the MCL or at the sixth ICS.

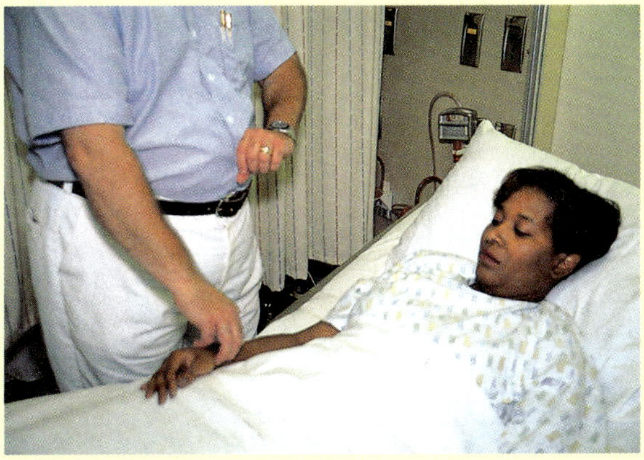

STEP 3a(2) Pulse check with patient's forearm at side with wrist extended.

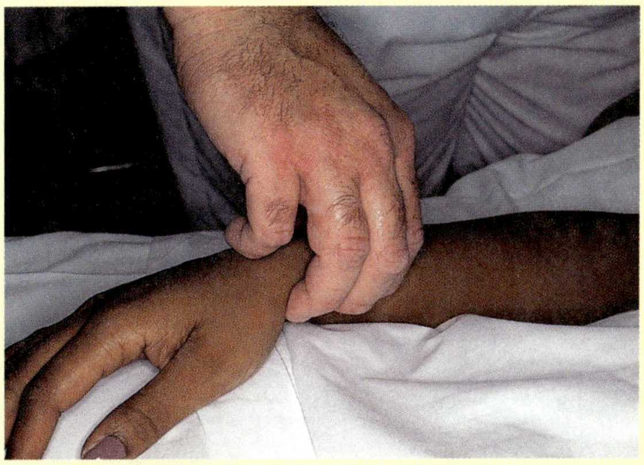

STEP 3a(3) Hand placement for pulse checks.

SKILL 29-2 ASSESSING THE RADIAL AND APICAL PULSES—cont'd

STEP	RATIONALE
(5) Place diaphragm of stethoscope in palm of hand for 5 to 10 seconds.	Warming of metal or plastic diaphragm prevents patient from being startled and promotes comfort.
(6) Place diaphragm of stethoscope over PMI at fifth ICS at left MCL and auscultate for normal S_1 and S_2 heart sounds (heard as "lub-dub") (see illustrations).	Allow stethoscope tubing to extend straight without kinks that would distort sound transmission. Normal sounds S_1 and S_2 are high pitched and best heard with the diaphragm.

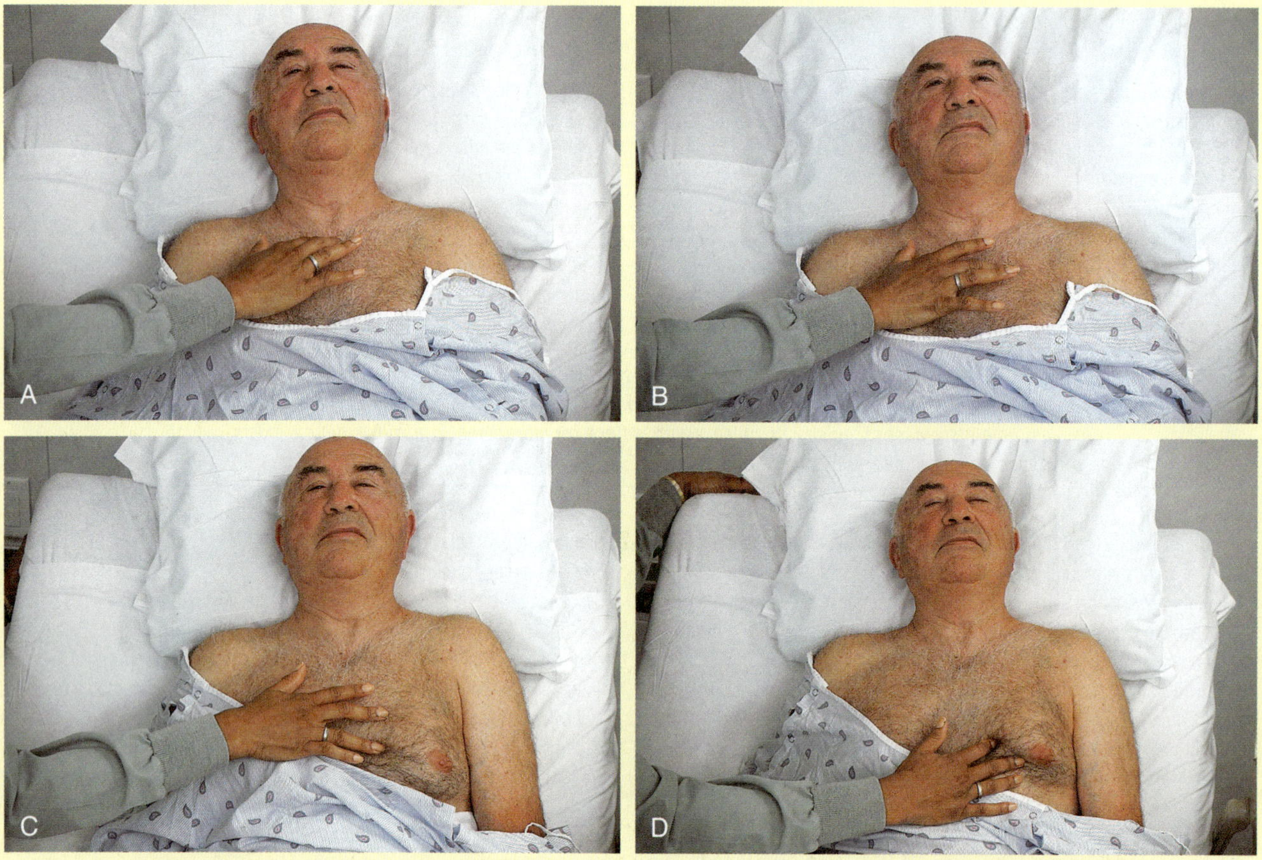

STEP 3b(4) A, Locating angle of Louis. **B,** Locating second intercostal space (ICS). **C,** Locating fifth ICS. **D,** Identifying midclavicular line (MCL).

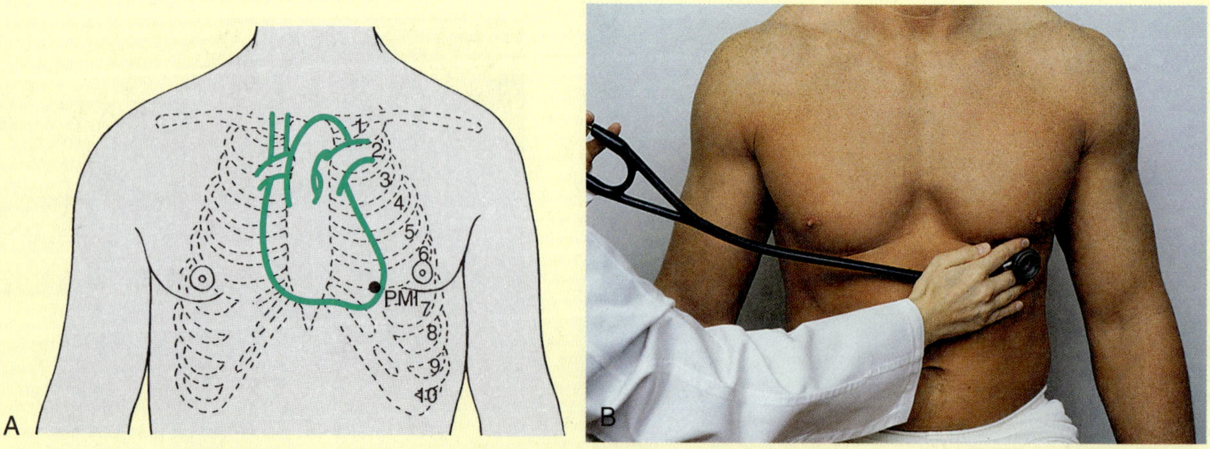

STEP 3b(6) A, Location of point of maximal impulse (PMI) in adult. **B,** Stethoscope over PMI.

STEP	RATIONALE
(7) When you hear S_1 and S_2 with regularity, use second hand of watch and begin to count rate: when sweep hand hits number 12 on dial, start counting with zero, then one, two, and so on.	Determine apical rate accurately only after you are able to auscultate sounds clearly. Timing begins with zero. Count of one is first sound auscultated after timing begins.
(8) If apical rate is regular, count for 30 seconds and multiply by 2.	Regular rate is accurate when measured for 30 seconds.

CLINICAL DECISION: *If heart rate is irregular or patient is receiving cardiovascular medication, count for 1 minute (60 seconds). Irregular rate is more accurately assessed when measured over a longer interval.*

STEP	RATIONALE
(9) Note if heart rate is irregular and describe pattern or irregularity (S_1 and S_2 occurring early or later after previous sequence of sounds [e.g., every third or every fourth beat is skipped]).	Regular occurrence of dysrhythmia within 1 minute indicates inefficient contraction of heart and alteration in cardiac output.
(10) Replace patient's gown and bed linen; help patient return to comfortable position.	Restores comfort and promotes sense of well-being.
(11) Perform hand hygiene.	Reduces transmission of microorganisms.
(12) Clean earpieces and diaphragm of stethoscope with alcohol swab routinely after each use.	Prevents transmission of microorganisms.
4 Perform hand hygiene.	Reduces transmission of microorganisms.
5 Discuss findings with patient as needed.	Promotes participation in care and understanding of health status.

EVALUATION

STEP	RATIONALE
1 Compare readings with previous baseline and/or acceptable range of heart rate for patient's age (see Table 29-3).	Evaluates for change in condition and alterations.
2 Compare peripheral pulse rate with apical rate and note discrepancy.	Differences between measurements indicate pulse deficit and warn of cardiovascular compromise. Abnormalities often require therapy.
3 Compare radial pulse equality and note discrepancy.	Differences between radial arteries indicate compromised peripheral vascular system.
4 Correlate pulse rate with data obtained from blood pressure and related signs and symptoms (palpitations, dizziness).	Pulse rate and blood pressure are interrelated.

UNEXPECTED OUTCOMES AND RELATED INTERVENTIONS

1 Radial pulse is weak, thready, or difficult to palpate.
- Assess both radial pulses and compare findings. Local obstruction to one extremity (e.g., clot, edema) decreases peripheral blood flow.
- Assess for swelling in surrounding tissues or other reason causing decreased peripheral blood flow (e.g., dressing, cast).
- Perform complete assessment of all peripheral pulses (see Chapter 30).
- Observe for symptoms associated with decreased tissue perfusion, including pallor and cool skin temperature of tissue distal to the weak pulse.
- Measure apical and radial pulse simultaneously to determine presence of pulse deficit.
- Assess for signs and symptoms associated with altered tissue perfusion, including pallor and cool skin temperature distal to the weak pulse.
- Have a second nurse assess pulses.

2 Apical pulse is greater than expected normal value (e.g., rate greater than 100 beats/min [tachycardia] in an adult; see Table 29-3).
- Identify related data, including fever, anxiety, pain, recent exercise, hypotension, decreased oxygenation, or dehydration.
- Observe for signs and symptoms of inadequate cardiac output, including fatigue, chest pain, orthopnea, cyanosis, and dizziness.

3 Apical pulse is less than expected normal value (e.g., rate less than 60 beats/min [bradycardia] in an adult; see Table 29-3).
- Observe for factors that alter heart rate such as digoxin and antidysrhythmics: it is sometimes necessary to withhold prescribed medications until the health care provider is able to evaluate the need to adjust dosage.
- Observe for signs and symptoms of inadequate cardiac output, including fatigue, chest pain, orthopnea, cyanosis, dizziness.

RECORDING AND REPORTING

- Record pulse rate with assessment site in nurses' notes or vital signs flow sheet. Document pulse rate after administration of specific therapies in narrative form in nurses' notes.
- Report abnormal findings to nurse in charge or health care provider immediately.

HOME CARE CONSIDERATIONS

- Assess home environment to determine room that affords quiet environment for auscultating apical rate.

SKILL 29-3 ASSESSING RESPIRATIONS

View Video!

Delegation Considerations

The skill of respiration measurement can be delegated to nursing assistive personnel (NAP) unless the patient is considered unstable. Instruct NAP to:

- Consider specific factors related to patient history that increase risk for increased, decreased, or irregular respirations.
- Obtain respiration measurements at appropriate times as determined by agency policy, health care provider's order, or patient condition such as onset of labored breathing or statement of breathing difficulty.
- Report respiratory abnormalities to the nurse immediately for further assessment.

Equipment

- Wristwatch with second hand or digital display
- Pen, vital sign flow sheet or record, or electronic health record

STEP	RATIONALE
ASSESSMENT	
1 Determine need to assess patient's respirations:	Nurse uses clinical judgment to determine need for assessment.
a. Identify risk factors for respiratory alterations, including: • Fever, pain, anxiety • Diseases of chest wall or muscles • Constrictive chest or abdominal dressings • Gastric distention • Pulmonary disease (emphysema, bronchitis, asthma, pneumonia, acute bronchitis) • Traumatic injury to chest wall with or without collapse of underlying lung tissue • Presence of a chest tube • Pulmonary edema and emboli • Head injury with damage to brainstem • Anemia	Conditions that place patient at risk for ventilatory and respiratory alterations are detected by changes in respiratory rate, depth, and rhythm.
b. Assess for signs and symptoms of respiratory alterations such as bluish or cyanotic appearance of nail beds, lips, mucous membranes, and skin; restlessness, irritability, confusion, reduced level of consciousness; pain during inspiration; labored or difficult breathing; adventitious breath sounds (see Chapter 30) or inability to breathe spontaneously; thick, frothy, blood-tinged, or copious sputum produced on coughing.	Physical signs and symptoms indicate alterations in respiratory status.
2 Assess pertinent laboratory values:	
a. Arterial blood gases (ABGs): Normal ABGs (values vary slightly among institutions): • pH: 7.35-7.45 • $PaCO_2$: 35-45 mm Hg • PaO_2: 80-100 mm Hg • SaO_2: 95%-100%	Arterial blood gases measure arterial blood pH; partial pressure of O_2 and CO_2; and arterial O_2 saturation, which reflects patient's oxygenation status.
b. Pulse oximetry (SpO_2): Acceptable SpO_2 ranges from 95% to 100%; however, a value of less than 90% is considered hypoxemia; values below 90% are acceptable for certain chronic disease conditions (see Skill 29-4).	SpO_2 less than 90% is often accompanied by changes in respiratory rate, depth, and rhythm.
c. Complete blood count (CBC): Normal CBC for adults (values vary among institutions): • *Hemoglobin:* 14 to 18 g/100 mL, males; 12 to 16 g/100 mL, females • *Hematocrit:* 42% to 52%, males; 37% to 47%, females • *Red blood cell count:* 4.7 to 6.1 million/mm^3, males; 4.2 to 5.4 million/mm^3, females (Pagana and Pagana, 2011)	Complete blood count measures red blood cell count; volume of red blood cells; and concentration of hemoglobin, which reflects patient's capacity to carry O_2.
3 Assess for factors that influence respirations (see Box 29-9).	Allows you to control for factors that can affect measurement.
4 Determine previous baseline respiratory rate (if available) from patient's record.	Allows you to assess for change in condition. Provides comparison with future respiratory measurements.
PLANNING	
1 Identify the patient using two identifiers (i.e., name and birth date or name and account number) according to facility policy.	Ensures correct patient. Complies with recommended National Patient Safety Goal (TJC, 2011).
2 Plan to assess respirations after measuring pulse in an adult.	Inconspicuous assessment of respirations immediately after pulse assessment prevents patient from consciously or unintentionally altering rate and depth of breathing.

STEP	RATIONALE
IMPLEMENTATION	
1 Perform hand hygiene. Draw curtain around bed and/or close door.	Prevents transmission of microorganisms. Maintains privacy.
2 Be sure that patient is in comfortable position, preferably sitting or lying with head of bed elevated 45 to 60 degrees. Be sure that patient's chest is visible. If necessary, move bed linen or gown.	Sitting erect promotes full ventilatory movement. Ensures clear view of chest wall and abdominal movements.
3 Place patient's arm in relaxed position across abdomen or lower chest or place your hand directly over patient's upper abdomen (see illustration).	A similar position used during pulse assessment allows respiratory rate assessment to be inconspicuous. Patient's hand or your hand rises and falls during respiratory cycle.

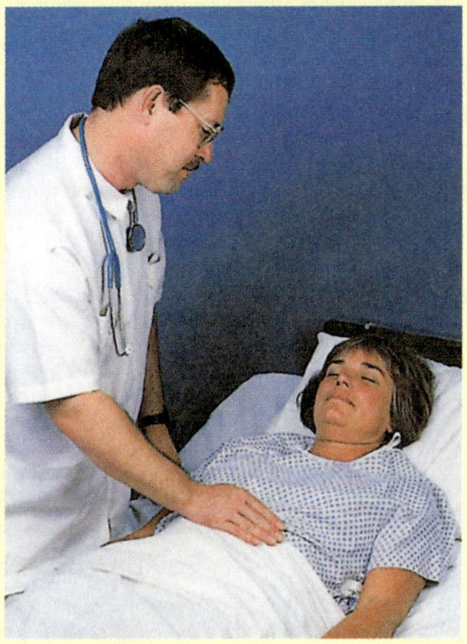

STEP 3 Nurse's hand over patient's abdomen to check respiration.

STEP	RATIONALE
4 Observe complete respiratory cycle (one inspiration and one expiration).	Rate is accurately determined only after you have observed a respiratory cycle.
5 After you observe a cycle, look at second hand of watch and begin to count rate: when sweep hand hits number on dial, begin time frame, counting one with first full respiratory cycle.	Timing begins with count of one. Respirations occur more slowly than pulse; thus timing does not begin with zero.
6 If rhythm is regular, count number of respirations in 30 seconds and multiply by 2. If rhythm is irregular, less than 12, or greater than 20, count for 1 full minute.	Respiratory rate is equivalent to number of respirations per minute. Suspected irregularities require assessment for at least 1 minute (see Table 29-6).
7 Note depth of respirations subjectively assessed by observing degree of chest wall movement while counting rate. You also objectively assess depth by palpating chest wall excursion or auscultating the posterior thorax after rate has been counted (see Chapter 30). Describe depth as shallow, normal, or deep.	Character of ventilatory movement reveals specific disease states that restrict volume of air from moving into and out of the lungs.
8 Note rhythm of ventilatory cycle. Normal breathing is regular and uninterrupted. Do not confuse sighing with abnormal rhythm.	Character of ventilations reveals specific types of alterations. Periodically people unconsciously take single deep breaths or sighs to expand small airways prone to collapse.

CLINICAL DECISION: *An irregular respiratory pattern or occurrence of periods of apnea (cessation of respiration for several seconds) is a symptom of underlying disease in the adult and must be reported to the nurse in charge or health care provider. The patient requires further assessment (see Chapter 30) and needs immediate intervention. An irregular respiratory rate and short apneic spells are normal for newborns.*

STEP	RATIONALE
9 Replace bed linen and patient's gown.	Restores comfort and promotes sense of well-being.
10 Perform hand hygiene.	Reduces transmission of microorganisms.
11 Discuss findings with patient as needed.	Promotes participation in care and understanding of health status.
EVALUATION	
1 If assessing respirations for first time, establish rate, rhythm, and depth as baseline if within normal range.	Used to compare future respiratory assessment.
2 Compare respirations with patient's previous baseline and normal rate, rhythm, and depth.	Allows nurse to assess for changes in patient's condition and presence of respiratory alterations.
3 Correlate respiratory rate, depth, and rhythm with data obtained from pulse oximetry and arterial blood gas measurements if available.	Ventilation, perfusion, and diffusion are interrelated.

SKILL 29-3 ASSESSING RESPIRATIONS—cont'd

UNEXPECTED OUTCOMES AND RELATED INTERVENTIONS

1 Patient has respiratory rate that is outside of expected normal values (e.g., less than 12 (bradypnea) or above 20 (tachypnea) breaths/min in an adult; see Table 29-5). Breathing pattern is irregular. Depth of respirations increase or decrease: patient feels short of breath.
- Observe for related factors, such as obstructed airway; assess for abnormal breath sounds, productive cough, restlessness, irritability, anxiety, confusion (see Chapter 30).
- Assist patient to supported sitting position (semi- or high-Fowler's) unless contraindicated, which improves ventilation.
- Provide oxygen as ordered (see Chapter 30).
- Assess for environmental factors that influence patient's respiratory rate such as secondhand smoke and poor room ventilation, and make corrections.

RECORDING AND REPORTING

- Record respiratory rate and character in nurses' notes or vital sign flow sheet.
- Record abnormal depth and rhythm in narrative form in nurses' notes.
- Document measurement of respiratory rate after administration of specific therapies in narrative form in nurses' notes.
- Indicate type and amount of oxygen therapy if used by patient during assessment. Document respiratory assessment after administration of specific therapies in narrative form in nurses' notes.
- Report abnormal findings to nurse in charge or health care provider immediately.

HOME CARE CONSIDERATIONS

- Assess for environmental factors in the home that influence patient's respiratory rate such as secondhand smoke, poor ventilation, or gas fumes.

SKILL 29-4 MEASURING OXYGEN SATURATION (PULSE OXIMETRY)

View Video!

Delegation Considerations

The skill of oxygen saturation measurement can be delegated to nursing assistive personnel (NAP) unless patient is unstable. Instruct the NAP to:
- Report to the nurse immediately any SpO_2 reading lower than 90%, which the nurse confirms.
- Obtain oxygen saturation at appropriate times as determined by agency policy, health care provider's order, or patient condition such as onset of labored breathing or cyanosis.
- Select appropriate sensor site, probe, and patient position for measurement of oxygen saturation.
- Refrain from using pulse oximetry as an assessment of heart rate because the oximeter does not detect an irregular pulse.

Equipment
- Oximeter
- Oximeter probe appropriate for patient and recommended by manufacturer
- Acetone or nail polish remover if needed
- Pen, vital sign flow sheet or record form, or patient's electronic medical record

STEP	RATIONALE
ASSESSMENT	
1 Determine need to measure patient's oxygen saturation:	Clinical judgment determines need for assessment.
a. Identify risk factors of decreased oxygen saturation, including: acute or chronic compromised respiratory function, recovery from general anesthesia or conscious sedation, traumatic injury to chest wall with or without collapse of underlying lung tissue, ventilator dependence, changes in supplemental oxygen therapy.	Certain conditions place patients at risk for decreased oxygen saturation.
b. Assess for signs and symptoms of alterations in oxygen saturation such as altered respiratory rate, depth, or rhythm; adventitious breath sounds (see Chapter 30); cyanotic appearance of nail beds, lips, mucous membranes, and skin; restlessness, irritability, confusion; reduced level of consciousness; labored or difficult breathing.	Physical signs and symptoms often indicate abnormal oxygen saturation.
2 Assess for factors that normally influence measurement of SpO_2 (see Box 29-10) in addition to oxygen therapy, hemoglobin level, body temperature, and medications such as bronchodilators.	Allows nurse to accurately assess oxygen saturation variations.
3 Determine previous baseline SpO_2 (if available) from patient's record.	Baseline information provides basis for comparison and assists in assessment of current status and evaluation of interventions.
4 Determine most appropriate patient-specific site (e.g., finger, earlobe) for sensor probe placement by measuring capillary refill (see Chapter 30). If capillary refill is greater than 3 seconds, select alternate site.	Sensor requires pulsating vascular bed to identify hemoglobin molecules that absorb emitted light. Changes in SpO_2 are reflected in circulation of finger capillary bed within 30 seconds and capillary bed of earlobe within 5-10 seconds.

STEP	RATIONALE
a. Site needs to have adequate local circulation and be free of moisture.	Moisture prevents the sensor from detecting SpO_2 levels.
b. Place probe on finger free of polish or artificial nail.	Artificial nails and certain nail polish colors alter readings (Cicek et al., 2010).
c. If tremors are present, use earlobe as site.	Motion artifact is most common cause of inaccurate readings (Mininni, 2009).
d. If patient is obese, clip-on probe may not fit properly; obtain a single-use (tape-on) probe.	
5 **Determine if patient has a latex allergy.**	Do not use adhesive sensors if patient has a latex allergy.
PLANNING	
1 Identify patient using two identifiers (i.e., name and birth date or name and account number) according to facility policy.	Ensures correct patient. Complies with recommended National Patient Safety Goal (TJC, 2011).
2 Explain purpose of procedure and how you measure oxygen saturation to patient. Instruct patient to breathe normally.	Promotes patient cooperation and increases compliance. Prevents large fluctuations in minute ventilation and possible error in SpO_2 readings.
IMPLEMENTATION	
1 Perform hand hygiene.	Reduces transmission of microorganisms.
2 Position patient comfortably. When using finger as monitoring site, support lower arm.	Ensures probe positioning and decreases motion artifact that interferes with SpO_2 determination.
3 Instruct patient to breathe normally.	Prevents large fluctuations in respiratory rate and depth and possible changes in SpO_2.
4 When using finger as monitoring site, remove any fingernail polish with acetone. Acrylic nails without polish do not interfere with SpO_2 determination.	Ensures accurate readings. Opaque coatings decrease light transmission; nail polish containing blue pigment absorbs light emissions and falsely alters saturation.
5 Attach sensor probe to monitoring site. Instruct patient that clip-on probe feels like a clothespin on finger but will not hurt.	Pressure spring tension of sensor probe on peripheral digit or earlobe is unexpected.

CLINICAL DECISION: *Do not attach probe to finger, ear, or bridge of nose if area is edematous or skin integrity is compromised. Do not attach probe to fingers that are hypothermic. Select ear or bridge of nose if adult patient has history of peripheral vascular disease. Do not use earlobe and bridge of nose sensors for infants and toddlers because of skin fragility. Do not use disposable adhesive probes if patient has latex allergy. Do not place sensor on same extremity as electronic blood pressure cuff because blood flow to finger is temporarily interrupted when cuff inflates and causes inaccurate readings that trigger alarms.*

STEP	RATIONALE
6 Once sensor is in place, turn on oximeter by activating power. Observe pulse waveform/intensity display and audible beep. Correlate oximeter pulse rate with patient's radial pulse. Differences require reevaluation of oximeter probe placement and may require reassessment of pulse rates.	Pulse waveform/intensity display enables detection of valid pulse or presence of interfering signal. Pitch of audible beep is proportional to SpO_2 value. Double-checking pulse rate ensures oximeter accuracy. Oximeter pulse rate, patient's radial pulse, and apical pulse rate should be the same. Any difference requires reevaluation of oximeter sensor probe placement and reassessment of pulse rates.
7 Leave probe in place until oximeter readout reaches constant value and pulse display reaches full strength during each cardiac cycle. Inform patient that oximeter will alarm if probe falls off or patient moves probe. Read SpO_2 on digital display.	Reading takes 10 to 30 seconds, depending on site selected.
8 If continuous SpO_2 monitoring is necessary, verify SpO_2 alarm limits and volume, which are preset by the manufacturer at a low of 85% and a high of 100%. Determine limits for SpO_2 and pulse rate alarms based on each patient's condition. Verify that alarms are on. Assess skin integrity every 2 hours under sensor probe. Relocate sensor probe at least every 24 hours or more frequently if skin integrity is altered or tissue perfusion compromised.	Alarms are set at appropriate limits and volumes to avoid frightening patients and visitors. Sensor probe tension and sensitivity to disposable sensor probe adhesive cause skin irritation and lead to disruption of skin integrity.
9 Help patient return to comfortable position.	Restores comfort and promotes sense of well-being.
10 Perform hand hygiene.	Reduces transmission of microorganisms.
11 Discuss findings with patient as needed.	Promotes participation in care and understanding of health status.
12 If planning intermittent or spot-checking SpO_2 measurements, remove probe and turn oximeter power off. Store probe in appropriate location.	Batteries will run out if oximeter is left on. Sensor probes are expensive and vulnerable to damage.
EVALUATION	
1 Compare SpO_2 readings with patient baseline and acceptable values.	Comparison reveals presence of abnormality.
2 Correlate SpO_2 with SaO_2 obtained from arterial blood gas measurements (see Chapter 41) if available.	Documents reliability of noninvasive assessment.
3 Correlate SpO_2 reading with data obtained from respiratory rate, depth, and rhythm assessment (see Skill 29-3).	Measurements assessing ventilation, perfusion, and diffusion are interrelated.
4 During continuous monitoring assess skin integrity underneath probe at least every 2 hours based on patient's peripheral circulation.	Prevents tissue ischemia.

SKILL 29-4 MEASURING OXYGEN SATURATION (PULSE OXIMETRY)—cont'd

UNEXPECTED OUTCOMES AND RELATED INTERVENTIONS

1 SpO_2 is less than 90%.
- Verify that oximeter probe is intact and outside light transmission does not influence measurement.
- Observe for signs and symptoms of decreased oxygenation: anxiety, restlessness, tachycardia, cyanosis.
- Verify that supplemental oxygen delivery system is delivered as ordered and functioning properly.
- Observe for and minimize factors that decrease SpO_2 such as lung secretions, increased activity, and hyperthermia.
- Assist patient to a position that maximizes ventilatory effort (e.g., place an obese patient in a high-Fowler's position).
- Notify nurse in charge or health care provider immediately.

2 Pulse rate indicated on the oximeter is less than patient's radial or apical pulse.
- Reposition sensor probe to an alternative site with increased blood flow.
- Assess patient for signs of altered cardiac output (e.g., decreased blood pressure, cool skin, confusion).

RECORDING AND REPORTING

- Record SpO_2 value on nurses' notes or vital sign flow sheet.
- Indicate type and amount of oxygen therapy used by patient during assessment.
- Record signs and symptoms of oxygen desaturation in nurses' notes.
- Report abnormal findings to nurse in charge or health care provider immediately.
- Document oxygen saturation after administration of specific therapies in narrative form in nurses' notes.
- Record in nurses' notes patient's use of continuous or intermittent pulse oximetry. Documents use of equipment for third-party payers.

HOME CARE CONSIDERATIONS

- Pulse oximetry is used in home care to noninvasively monitor oxygen therapy or changes in oxygen therapy.
- Instruct family caregivers to examine oximeter site before applying sensor.
- Instruct family caregivers on procedure to implement when oxygen saturation is not within acceptable values.

SKILL 29-5 MEASURING BLOOD PRESSURE

View Video!

Delegation Considerations

The skill of blood pressure (BP) measurement can be delegated to nursing assistive personnel (NAP) unless the patient is considered unstable. Instruct the NAP to:
- Obtain BP measurement at appropriate times as determined by agency policy, health care provider's order, or patient condition.
- Select appropriate limb for BP measurement.
- Select appropriate-size BP cuff for designated limb.
- Consider specific patient-related factors that influence BP and risk of orthostatic hypotension.
- Report abnormalities to the nurse for further assessment immediately.

Equipment

- Aneroid sphygmomanometer
- Cloth or disposable vinyl pressure cuff of appropriate size for patient's extremity
- Stethoscope
- Alcohol swab
- Pen, vital sign flow sheet or record form, or electronic medical record

STEP	RATIONALE
ASSESSMENT	
1 Determine need to assess patient's BP:	Nurse uses clinical judgment to determine need for assessment.
a. Identify risk factors, including: • History of cardiovascular or renal disease, diabetes • Circulatory shock (hypovolemic, septic, cardiogenic, or neurogenic) • Acute or chronic pain • Rapid intravenous infusion of fluids or blood products • Increased intracranial pressure • Toxemia of pregnancy	Conditions place patients at risk for BP alteration.
b. Observe for signs and symptoms of BP alterations:	Physical signs and symptoms often indicate alterations in BP.
(1) High BP (hypertension): headache (usually occipital), flushing of face, nosebleed, and fatigue in older adults	High BP is often asymptomatic until pressure is very high.
(2) Low BP (hypotension): dizziness, mental confusion; restlessness; pale, dusky, or cyanotic skin and mucous membranes; cool, mottled skin over extremities	

STEP	RATIONALE
2 Assess for factors that affect BP (see Table 29-11)	Allows you to ensure that BP measurement is accurate.
3 Determine best site for BP assessment. Avoid applying cuff to extremity when intravenous fluids are infusing, an arteriovenous shunt or fistula is present, breast or axillary surgery has been performed on that side, or extremity has been traumatized or diseased or requires a cast or bulky bandage. Use lower extremities when brachial arteries are inaccessible.	Inappropriate site selection results in poor amplification of sounds, causing inaccurate readings. Application of pressure from inflated bladder temporarily restricts blood flow and further compromises circulation in extremity that already has impaired blood flow.
4 Determine previous baseline BP (if available) from patient's record.	Allows nurse to assess for change in condition. Provides comparison with future BP measurements.
5 Determine if patient has latex allergy.	Verify that stethoscope and BP cuff are latex free if patient has latex allergy.
PLANNING	
1 Identify patient using two identifiers (i.e., name and birth date or name and account number) according to facility policy.	Ensures correct patient. Complies with recommended National Patient Safety Goal (TJC, 2011).
2 Explain to patient that you will assess BP. Have patient rest at least 5 minutes before measuring BP sitting or lying down; wait 1 minute if patient is standing. When possible, have patient sit in a chair (NHBPEP, 2003). Ask patient not to speak while measuring BP.	Allows patient to relax and helps to avoid falsely elevated readings. When assessed at rest, BP readings taken at different times are comparable. Talking to patient when assessing BP increases readings 10% to 40%.
3 Be sure that patient has not ingested caffeine or smoked for 30 minutes before BP measurement.	Caffeine or nicotine causes false BP elevations. Smoking immediately increases BP and lasts up to 15 minutes; caffeine increases BP up to 3 hours.
4 Assist patient to sitting position if appropriate. Be sure that room is warm, quiet, and relaxing.	Maintains patient comfort during measurement. Sitting is preferred to lying. Diastolic pressure measured with sitting is approximately 5 mm Hg higher than when measured supine. Patient perceptions of stressful environment affect BP measurement. Talking and background noise result in inaccurate measurements.
5 Select appropriate cuff size.	Improper cuff size results in inaccurate readings (see Table 29-11). If cuff is too small, it tends to come loose when being inflated or results in false-high readings. If the cuff is too large, you may obtain false-low readings.
IMPLEMENTATION	
1 Perform hand hygiene and clean stethoscope earpieces and diaphragm with alcohol swab.	Reduces transmission of microorganisms.
2 Position patient.	
a. Arm: Position patient sitting or lying, position his or her forearm at heart level. Turn palm up (see illustration). If sitting, instruct patient to keep feet flat on floor without crossing legs.	If arm is extended and not supported, patient performs isometric exercise that increases diastolic pressure. Placing arm above level of heart causes false-low reading 2 mm Hg for each inch above heart level. Leg crossing falsely increases systolic BP. Even in the supine position a diastolic pressure increases BP up to 3 to 4 mm Hg for each 5-cm (1.97-in) change in heart level.
b. Thigh: Position patient lying with thigh flat (provide support as needed). Have knee slightly flexed.	
3 Expose extremity (arm or leg) fully by removing constricting clothing.	Ensures proper cuff application. Do not place BP cuff over clothing. Tight clothing causes congestion of blood and can falsely elevate BP readings.

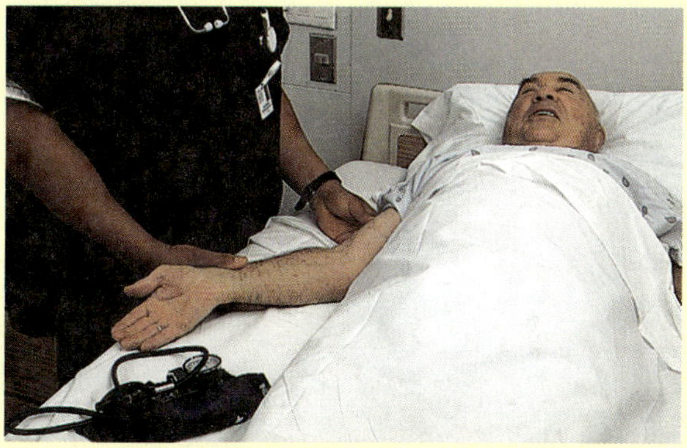

STEP 2a Patient's forearm supported in bed.

SKILL 29-5 MEASURING BLOOD PRESSURE—cont'd

STEP	RATIONALE
4 Palpate brachial artery (arm) (see illustration) or popliteal artery (leg). With cuff fully deflated, apply bladder of cuff above artery by centering arrows marked on cuff over artery. If there are no center arrows on cuff, estimate the center of the bladder and place it over artery. Position cuff 2.5 cm (1 inch) above site of pulsation (antecubital or popliteal space). Wrap cuff evenly and snugly around extremity (see illustrations).	Inflating bladder directly over artery ensures that proper pressure is applied during inflation. Loose-fitting cuff causes false-high readings.
5 Position manometer gauge no farther than 1 m (approximately 1 yard) away.	Looking up or down at scale results in inaccurate readings.
6 Measure BP.	
a. Two-step methods	
(1) Relocate brachial pulse. Palpate artery distal to cuff with fingertips of nondominant hand while inflating cuff rapidly to pressure 30 mm Hg above point at which pulse disappears. Slowly deflate cuff and note point when pulse reappears. Deflate cuff fully and wait 30 seconds.	Estimating systolic pressure prevents false low readings. Determine maximal inflation point for accurate reading by palpation. If unable to palpate artery because of weakened pulse, use an ultrasonic stethoscope (see Chapter 30). Completely deflating cuff prevents venous congestion and false-high readings.
(2) Place stethoscope earpieces in ears and be sure that sounds are clear, not muffled.	Each earpiece follows angle of ear canal to facilitate hearing.

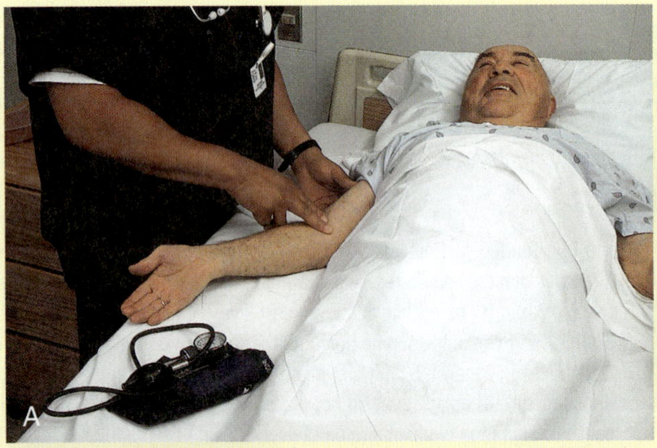

A

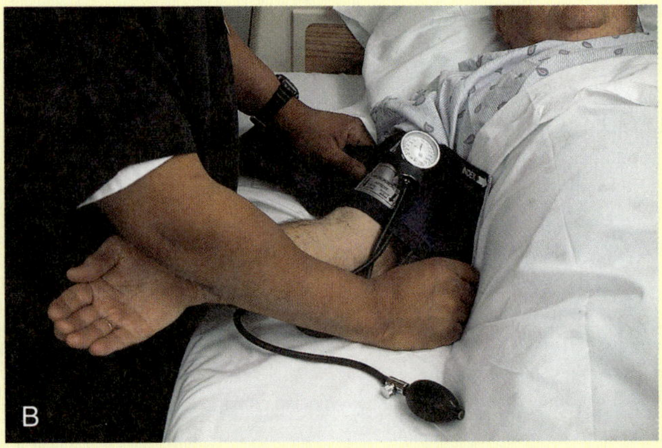

B

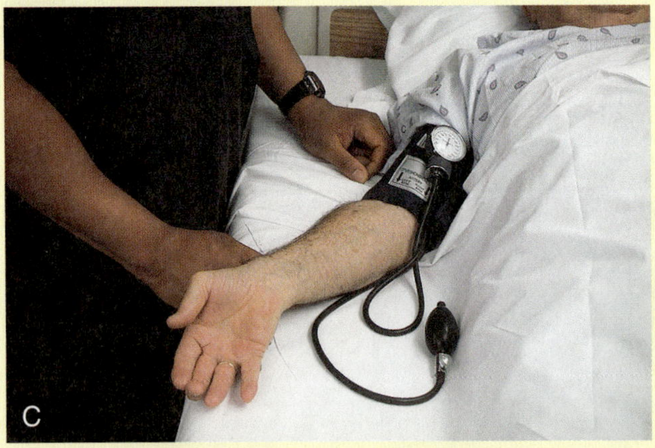

C

STEP 4 A, Nurse palpating patient's brachial artery. **B,** Center bladder cuff above artery. **C,** Blood pressure cuff wrapped around upper arm.

STEP	RATIONALE
(3) Relocate brachial or popliteal artery and place bell or diaphragm chest piece of stethoscope over it. Do not allow chest piece to touch cuff or clothing (see illustration).	Proper stethoscope placement ensures best sound reception. Stethoscope improperly positioned causes muffled sounds that often result in false-low systolic and false-high diastolic readings.
(4) Close valve of pressure bulb clockwise until tight.	Tightening valve prevents air leak during inflation.
(5) Quickly inflate cuff to 30 mm Hg above palpated systolic pressure (patient's estimated systolic pressure) (see illustration).	Rapid inflation ensures accurate measurement of systolic pressure.
(6) Slowly release pressure bulb valve and allow needle of manometer gauge to fall at rate of 2 to 3 mm Hg/sec. Make sure that there are no extraneous sounds.	Too-rapid or too-slow decline in pressure causes inaccurate readings. Noise interferes with precise determination of Korotkoff phases.
(7) Note point on manometer when you hear first clear sound. Sound slowly increases in intensity.	First Korotkoff sound reflects systolic BP.
(8) Continue to deflate cuff, noting point at which muffled or dampened sound appears.	Fourth Korotkoff sound involves distinct muffling of sounds and is an indicator of diastolic pressure in children (NHBPEP, 2003).
(9) Continue to deflate cuff gradually, noting point at which sound disappears in adults. Listen for 10 to 20 mm Hg after last sound and allow remaining air to escape quickly.	Beginning of fifth Korotkoff sound is indicator of diastolic pressure in adults (NHBPEP, 2003). Continuous cuff inflation causes arterial occlusion, resulting in numbness and tingling of patient's arm.
b. One-step method	
(1) Place stethoscope earpieces in ears and be sure sounds are clear, not muffled.	Each earpiece follows angle of ear canal to facilitate hearing.
(2) Relocate brachial or popliteal artery and place bell or diaphragm chest piece of stethoscope over it. Do not allow chest piece to touch cuff or clothing.	Proper stethoscope placement ensures optimal sound reception. Stethoscope improperly positioned causes muffled sounds that result in false-low systolic and false-high diastolic readings.
(3) Close valve of pressure bulb clockwise until tight. Quickly inflate cuff to 30 mm Hg above patient's usual systolic pressure.	Tightening of valve prevents air leak during inflation. Inflation above systolic level ensures accurate measurement of systolic BP.
(4) Slowly release pressure bulb valve and allow needle of manometer gauge to fall at rate of 2 to 3 mm Hg/sec.	Too-rapid or too-slow decline in pressure causes inaccurate readings.
(5) Note point on manometer when you hear first clear sound. Sound slowly increases in intensity.	First Korotkoff sound reflects systolic pressure.
(6) Continue to deflate cuff, noting point at which muffled or dampened sound appears.	Fourth Korotkoff sound involves distinct muffling of sounds and indicates diastolic pressure in children (NNBPEP, 2003).
(7) While gradually deflating cuff, note point at which sound disappears in adults. Listen for 10 to 20 mm Hg after last sound and allow remaining air to escape quickly.	Beginning of fifth Korotkoff sound indicates diastolic pressure in adults (NHBPEP, 2003). Continuous cuff inflation causes arterial occlusion, resulting in numbness and tingling of patient's arm.
7 American Heart Association recommends average of two sets of BP measurement, 2 minutes apart. Use second set of BP measurements as baseline. If readings are different by more than 5 mm Hg, additional readings are necessary.	Two sets of BP measurements help to prevent false positives based on patient's sympathetic response (alert reaction). Averaging minimizes effect of anxiety, which often causes first reading to be higher than subsequent measurements.
8 Remove cuff from extremity unless you need to repeat measurement. If this is first assessment of patient, repeat BP assessment on other extremity.	Comparison of BP in both extremities detects circulation problems. (Normal difference of 5 to 10 mm Hg exists between extremities.)
9 Help patient return to comfortable position and cover upper arm if previously clothed.	Restores comfort and promotes sense of well-being.
10 Discuss findings with patient as needed.	Promotes participation in care and understanding of health status.
11 Perform hand hygiene.	Reduces transmission of microorganisms.

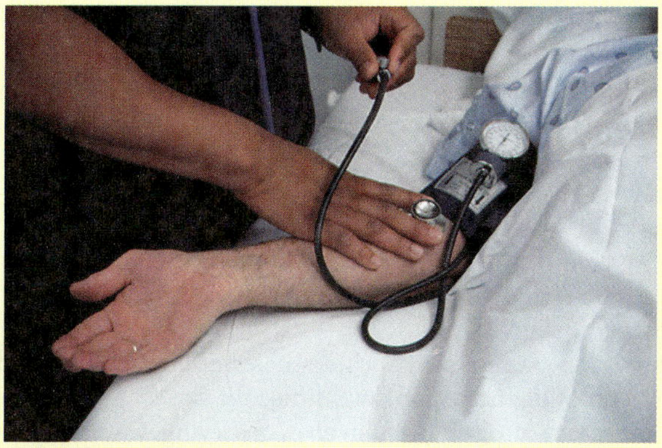

STEP 6a(3) Stethoscope over brachial artery to measure BP.

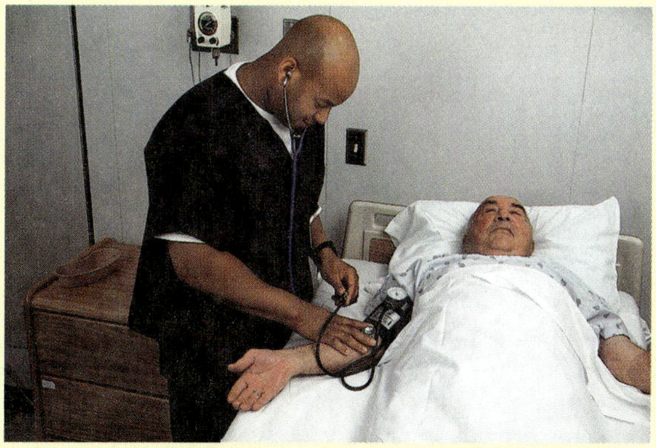

STEP 6a(5) Inflating BP cuff.

SKILL 29-5 MEASURING BLOOD PRESSURE—cont'd

STEP	RATIONALE
EVALUATION	
1 Compare reading with previous baseline and/or acceptable value of BP for patient's age.	Evaluates for change in condition and cardiovascular alterations.
2 Compare BP in both arms or both legs.	If using upper extremities, use arm with higher pressure for subsequent assessments unless contraindicated.
3 Correlate BP with data obtained from pulse assessment and related cardiovascular signs and symptoms.	BP and heart rate are interrelated.

UNEXPECTED OUTCOMES AND RELATED INTERVENTIONS

1 Unable to obtain BP reading
- Determine that no immediate crisis is present by obtaining pulse and respiratory rate.
- Assess for signs of decreased cardiac output; if present, notify nurse in charge or health care provider immediately.
- Use alternative sites or procedures to obtain BP: auscultate BP in lower extremity, use a Doppler ultrasonic instrument, implement palpation method to obtain systolic BP.
- Repeat BP measurement with sphygmomanometer. Electronic BP devices are less accurate in low–blood flow conditions.

2 BP is not sufficient for adequate perfusion and oxygenation of tissues.
- Compare BP value to baseline. A systolic reading of 90 mm Hg is an acceptable value for some patients.
- Position patient in supine position to enhance circulation and restrict activity if it is decreasing BP.
- Assess for signs and symptoms of hypotension such as tachycardia; weak, thready pulse; weakness, dizziness, confusion; cool, pale, dusky or cyanotic skin.
- Notify nurse in charge or health care provider immediately.
- Increase rate of intravenous infusion or administer vasoconstricting drugs if ordered.

3 BP is above acceptable range.
- Repeat BP measurement in other arm and compare findings. Verify correct selection and placement of cuff.
- Ask nurse colleague to repeat measurement in 1 to 2 minutes.
- Observe for related symptoms, although symptoms are sometimes not apparent until BP is extremely elevated.
- Report elevated BP to nurse in charge or health care provider to initiate appropriate evaluation and treatment.
- Administer antihypertensive medications as ordered.

4 Patent has a difference of more than 20 mm Hg systolic or diastolic when comparing BP measurements on upper extremities.
- Report abnormal findings to nurse in charge or health care provider.

RECORDING AND REPORTING

- Record BP in nurses' notes or vital sign flow sheet. BP measurement after administration of specific therapies needs to be documented in narrative form in nurses' notes.
- Record any signs or symptoms of BP alterations in narrative form in nurses' notes.
- Document measurement of BP after administration of specific therapies in narrative form in nurses' notes.
- Report abnormal findings to nurse in charge or health care provider immediately.

HOME CARE CONSIDERATIONS

- Assess home noise level to determine room that provides most quiet environment for assessing BP.
- Consider electronic BP cuff for home if patient has hearing difficulties, sufficient financial resources, and adequate dexterity.

KEY POINTS

- Measurement of vital signs includes the physiological measurement of temperature, pulse, BP, respirations, and oxygen saturation.
- Nurses measure vital signs as part of a complete physical examination or in a review of a patient's condition.
- Nurses assess changes in vital signs with other physical assessment findings, using clinical judgment to determine measurement frequency.
- Knowledge of the factors influencing vital signs assists in determining and evaluating abnormal values.
- Vital signs provide a basis for evaluating response to nursing interventions.
- Measure vital signs when the patient is inactive and the environment is controlled for comfort.
- Nurses help patients maintain body temperature by initiating interventions that promote heat loss, production, or conservation.
- A fever is one of the normal defense mechanisms of the body.
- Measurement of temperature using the temporal artery is the least invasive, most accurate method of obtaining core temperature.
- Respiratory assessment includes determining the effectiveness of ventilation, perfusion, and diffusion.
- Assessment of respiration involves observing ventilatory movements through the respiratory cycle.

- Variables affecting ventilation, perfusion, and diffusion influence oxygen saturation.
- To assess cardiac function, it is easy to measure pulse rate and rhythm using the radial or apical pulses.
- Hypertension is diagnosed only after an average of readings made during two or more subsequent visits reveals an elevated BP.
- Improper selection and application of the BP measurement cuff results in errors in BP measurement.
- Changes in one vital sign often influence characteristics of the other vital signs.

CLINICAL APPLICATION QUESTIONS

Preparing for Clinical Practice

Mr. Coburn, the 56-year-old school teacher who was seen earlier in the week for hyperthermia, arrives at the walk-in health center complaining of feeling dizzy and nauseated. You immediately note that he appears to be having some difficulty catching his breath during coughing spells. A new graduate nurse takes Mr. Coburn's admitting vital signs as: pulse 122, RR 14, BP 88/50 RA, tympanic temperature 38° C (100.4° F), SpO_2 92%. As you enter Mr. Coburn's room the electronic BP machine alarm is sounding. You note that it is flashing "72 systolic" with no diastolic reading. Mr. Coburn is turned on his right side, and his eyes are closed. His respirations appear labored.

1. List in order of priority your first five interventions.
2. Which vital signs should you reassess and which methods should you use?
3. Which hourly vital signs should you delegate to a NAP?

evolve *Answers to Clinical Application Questions can be found on the Evolve website.*

REVIEW QUESTIONS

Are You Ready to Test Your Nursing Knowledge?

1. A 52-year-old woman is admitted with dyspnea and discomfort in her left chest with deep breaths. She has smoked for 35 years and recently lost over 10 pounds. Her vital signs on admission are: HR 112, BP 138/82, RR 22, tympanic temperature 36.8° C (98.2° F), and oxygen saturation 94%. She is receiving oxygen at 2 L via a nasal cannula. Which vital sign reflects a positive outcome of the oxygen therapy?
   1. Temperature: 37° C (98.6° F)
   2. Radial pulse: 112
   3. Respiratory rate: 24
   4. Oxygen saturation: 96%
   5. Blood pressure: 134/78
2. The licensed practice nurse (LPN) provides you with the change-of-shift vital signs on four of your patients. Which patient do you need to assess first?
   1. 84-year-old man recently admitted with pneumonia, RR 28, SpO_2 89%
   2. 54-year-old woman admitted after surgery for fractured arm, BP 160/86 mm Hg, HR 72
   3. 63-year-old man with venous ulcers from diabetes, temperature 37.3° C (99.1° F), HR 84
   4. 77-year-old woman with left mastectomy 2 days ago, RR 22, BP 148/62
3. A 56-year-old patient with diabetes admitted for community-acquired pneumonia has a temperature of 38.2° C (100.8° F) via the temporal artery. Which additional assessment data are needed in planning interventions for the patient's infection? (Select all that apply.)
   1. Heart rate
   2. Presence of diaphoresis
   3. Smoking history
   4. Respiratory rate
   5. Recent bowel movement
   6. Blood pressure in right arm
   7. Patient's normal temperature
   8. Blood pressure in distal extremity
4. A 55-year-old widowed patient was in a motor vehicle accident and is admitted to a surgical unit after repair of a fractured left arm and left leg. She also has a laceration on her forehead. An intravenous (IV) line is infusing in the right antecubital fossa, and pneumatic compression stockings are on the right lower leg. She is receiving oxygen via a simple face mask. What sites do you instruct the nursing assistant to use for obtaining the patient's blood pressure and temperature?
   1. Right antecubital and tympanic membrane
   2. Right popliteal and right axillae
   3. Left antecubital and oral
   4. Left popliteal and temporal artery
5. A patient has been transferred to your unit from the respiratory intensive care unit, where he has been for the past 2 weeks recovering from pneumonia. He is receiving oxygen via 4 L nasal cannula. His respiratory rate is 26 breaths/min, and his oxygen saturation is 92%. In planning his care, which information is most helpful in determining your priority nursing interventions?
   1. Activity order
   2. Medication list
   3. Baseline vital signs
   4. Patient's perception of dyspnea
6. During a patient's routine annual physical, she tells you that she has noted that her heart feels like it's "racing," usually in the later morning, early afternoon, or just before she goes to bed. Her radial pulse rate is 68 beats/min and regular; her blood pressure is 134/82 mm Hg. What additional information is helpful in evaluating the patient's racing heart? (Select all that apply.)
   1. Dietary habits
   2. Medication list
   3. Exercise regimen
   4. Age, weight, and height
7. You observe a nursing student taking a blood pressure (BP) on a patient. The patient's BP range over the past 24 hours is 132/64 to 126/72 mm Hg. The student used a BP cuff that was too narrow for the patient. Which of the following BP readings made by the student is most likely caused by the incorrect choice of BP cuff?
   1. 96/40 mm Hg
   2. 110/66 mm Hg
   3. 130/70 mm Hg
   4. 156/82 mm Hg
8. As you are obtaining the oxygen saturation on a 19-year-old college student with severe asthma, you note that she has black nail polish on her nails. You remove the polish from one nail, and she asks you why her nail polish had to be removed. Your best reply is:
   1. Nail polish attracts microorganisms and contaminates the finger sensor.
   2. Nail polish increases oxygen saturation.
   3. Nail polish interferes with sensor function.
   4. Nail polish creates excessive heat in sensor probe.

9. A patient has been hospitalized for the past 48 hours with a fever of unknown origin. His medical record indicates tympanic temperatures of 38.7° C (101.6° F) (0400), 36.6° C (97.9° F) (0800), 36.9° C (98.4° F) (1200), 37.6° C (99.6° F) (1600), and 38.3° C (100.9° F) (2000). How would you describe this pattern of temperature measurements?
   1. Usual range of circadian rhythm measurements
   2. Sustained fever pattern
   3. Intermittent fever pattern
   4. Resolving fever pattern
10. A patient presents in the clinic with dizziness and fatigue. The nursing assistant reports a very slow radial pulse of 44. What is your priority intervention?
   1. Request that the nursing assistant repeat the pulse check
   2. Call for a stat electrocardiogram (ECG)
   3. Assess the patient's apical pulse and evidence of a pulse deficit
   4. Prepare to administer cardiac-stimulating medications
11. Which of the following patients is most at risk for tachycardia?
   1. A healthy professional tennis player
   2. A patient admitted with hypothermia
   3. A patient with a fever of 39.4° C (103° F)
   4. A 90-year-old male taking beta blockers
12. Which of the following patients is at most risk for tachypnea? (Select all that apply.)
   1. Patient just admitted with four rib fractures
   2. Woman who is 9 months' pregnant
   3. Adult who has consumed alcoholic beverages
   4. Adolescent awaking from sleep
13. The following blood pressures, taken 6 months apart, were recorded from patients screened by the nurse at the assisted-living facility. Which patient should be referred to the health care provider for hypertension evaluation?
   1. 120/80, 118/78, 124/82
   2. 128/84, 124/86, 128/88
   3. 148/82, 148/78, 134/86
   4. 154/78, 118/76, 126/84
14. A patient is admitted for dehydration caused by pneumonia and shortness of breath. He has a history of heart disease and cardiac dysrhythmias. The nursing assistant tells you his admitting vital signs. Which measurement should you reassess? (Select all that apply.)
   1. Right arm BP: 120/80
   2. Radial pulse rate: 72 and irregular
   3. Temporal temperature: 37.4° C (99.3° F)
   4. Respiratory rate: 28
   5. Oxygen saturation: 99%
15. A patient returns to your postoperative unit following surgery for right shoulder rotator cuff repair. The licensed practical nurse (LPN) reports that she had difficulty obtaining the patient's heart rate from his right radial pulse. What is your best response?
   1. Assess the patient's apical pulse to obtain the heart rate.
   2. Obtain the heart rate from right and left radial sites.
   3. Obtain the heart rate using the oximeter probe.
   4. Perform a complete assessment of all pulses.

Answers: 1. 4; 2. 1; 3. 1, 2, 4, 7; 4. 2; 5. 3; 6. 1, 2; 7. 4; 8. 3; 9. 3; 10. 3; 11. 3; 12. 1, 2; 13. 3; 14. 2, 4, 5; 15. 4.

REFERENCES

Henker R, Carlson KK: Fever: applying research to bedside practice, *AACN Adv Crit Care* 18(1):76, 2007.

High KP, et al: Clinical practice guideline for the evaluation of fever and infection in older adult residents of long-term care facilities: 2008 update by the Infectious Diseases Society of America, *Clin Infect Dis* 48(2):149, 2009.

Hockenberry MJ, Wilson D: *Wong's nursing care of infants and children*, ed 8, St Louis, 2007, Mosby.

Lehne R: *Pharmacology for nursing care*, ed 7, Philadelphia, 2010, Elsevier.

Lewis M: Heatstroke in older adults, *Am J Nurs* 107(6):52, 2007.

Mininni NC, et al: Pulse oximetry: an essential tool for the busy med-surg nurse, *Am Nurs Today* 4 (9):31, 2009.

National High Blood Pressure Education Program (NHBPEP); National Heart, Lung, and Blood Institute; National Institutes of Health (NIH): The seventh report of the Joint National Committee on Detection, Evaluation, and Treatment of High Blood Pressure, *JAMA* 289(19):2560, 2003.

Pagana KD, Pagana TJ: *Diagnostic and laboratory test reference*, ed 10, St Louis, 2011, Mosby.

The Joint Commission (TJC): *2011 National Patient Safety Goals (NPGs)*, 2011, TJC; available at http://www.jointcommission.org/standards_information/npsgs.aspx.

RESEARCH REFERENCES

Bern L, et al: Differences in BP values obtained with automated and manual methods in medical inpatients, *MedSurg Nurs* 16(6):356, 2007.

Cicek HS, et al: Effect of nail polish and henna on oxygen saturation determined by pulse oximetry in healthy young adult females, *Emerg Med J* 28(9):783, 2010.

Fetzer SJ, Lawrence A: Tympanic membrane versus temporal artery temperatures of adult perianesthesia patients, *J Peri Anesth Nurs* 3(4):230, 2008.

Frommelt T, Ott C, Hays V: Accuracy of different devices to measure temperature, *MedSurg Nurs* 17(3):171, 2008.

Heinemann M, et al: Automated versus manual BP measurement: a randomized crossover trial, *Int J Nurs Pract* 14:296, 2008.

Hockenberg G: Febrile response: management: evidence summaries—Joanna Briggs Institute, July 2008.

Lawson L, Bridges EJ, Ballou I: Accuracy and precision of noninvasive core temperature measurement in adult intensive care patients, *Am J Crit Care* (16):485, 2007.

Lim CH, Byrne C, Lee JK: Human thermoregulation and measurement of body temperature in exercise and clinical settings, *Ann Acad Med Singapore* 37:347, 2008.

Woodrow P, et al: Comparing no touch and tympanic thermometer temperature recordings, *Br J Nurs* 15:1010, 2006.

CHAPTER

30

Health Assessment and Physical Examination

OBJECTIVES

- Discuss the purposes of physical assessment.
- Discuss how cultural diversity influences a nurse's approach to and findings from a health assessment.
- List techniques for preparing a patient physically and psychologically before and during an examination.
- Describe interview techniques used to enhance communication during history taking.
- Make environmental preparations before an examination.
- Identify data to collect from the nursing history before an examination.
- Demonstrate the techniques used with each physical assessment skill.
- Discuss normal physical findings in a young, middle-age, and older adult.
- Discuss ways to incorporate health promotion and health teaching into the examination.
- Identify ways to use physical assessment skills during routine nursing care.
- Describe physical measurements made in assessing each body system.
- Identify self-screening examinations commonly performed by patients.
- Identify preventive screenings and the appropriate age(s) for each screening to occur.

KEY TERMS

Adventitious sounds, p. 525
Alopecia, p. 504
Aphasia, p. 557
Apical impulse or point of maximal impulse (PMI), p. 527
Arcus senilis, p. 511
Atrophied, p. 554
Auscultation, p. 494
Borborygmi, p. 544
Bruit, p. 532
Cerumen, p. 513
Clubbing, p. 536
Conjunctivitis, p. 511
Cyanosis, p. 500
Distention, p. 543
Dysrhythmia, p. 530
Ectropion, p. 510
Entropion, p. 510
Edema, p. 502
Erythema, p. 501
Excoriation, p. 516
Goniometer, p. 553
Hypertonicity, p. 554
Hypotonicity, p. 554
Indurated, p. 502
Inspection, p. 493
Integumentary system, p. 498
Jaundice, p. 501
Kyphosis, p. 551
Lordosis, p. 552
Malignancy, p. 519
Murmurs, p. 530
Nystagmus, p. 509
Olfaction, p. 493
Orthopnea, p. 524
Osteoporosis, p. 552
Ototoxicity, p. 514
Palpation, p. 493
Percussion, p. 494
Peristalsis, p. 544
PERRLA, p. 511
Petechiae, p. 502
Pigmentation, p. 500
Polyps, p. 516
Ptosis, p. 510
Scoliosis, p. 552
Stenosis, p. 531
Striae, p. 543
Syncope, p. 531
Thrill, p. 530
Turgor, p. 502
Ventricular gallop, p. 530
Vocal or tactile fremitus, p. 524

evolve WEBSITE

http://evolve.elsevier.com/Potter/fundamentals/

- Review Questions
- Video Clips
- Animations
- Case Study with Questions
- Audio Glossary
- Interactive Learning Activities
- Key Term Flashcards
- Content Updates

The health assessment and physical examination are the first steps toward providing safe and competent nursing care. The nurse is in a unique position to determine each patient's current health status, distinguish variations from the norm, and recognize improvements or deterioration in his or her condition. As a nurse, you must be able to recognize and interpret each patient's behavioral and physical presentation. By performing health assessments and physical examinations, you will identify health patterns and evaluate each patient's response to treatments and therapies.

Nurses gather assessment data about patients' past and current health conditions in a variety of ways, using a comprehensive or focused approach, depending on the patient situation. Assessments are performed at health fairs, at screening clinics, in a health provider's office, in acute care agencies, or in patients' homes. Depending on the outcome of an assessment, a nurse considers evidence-based recommendations for care based on a patient's values, the health provider's clinical expertise, or own personal experience.

A complete health assessment involves a nursing history (see Chapter 16) and behavioral and physical examination. Through the health history interview you gather subjective data about a patient's condition. You obtain objective data while observing a patient's behavior and overall presentation. You identify additional objective data through a head-to-toe body system review during the physical examination. Your clinical judgments are based on all of the gathered data to create a plan of care for each situation. With accurate data you create a patient-centered care plan, identifying the nursing diagnoses, desired patient outcomes, and nursing interventions. Continuity in health care improves when you evaluate a patient by making ongoing, objective, and comprehensive assessments.

PURPOSES OF THE PHYSICAL EXAMINATION

A physical examination is conducted as an initial evaluation in triage for emergency care; for routine screening to promote wellness behaviors and preventive health care measures; to determine eligibility for health insurance, military service, or a new job; or to admit a patient to a hospital or long-term care facility. After considering the patient's current condition, a nurse selects a focused physical examination on a specific system or area. For example, when a patient is having a severe asthma episode, the nurse first focuses on the pulmonary and cardiovascular systems so treatments can begin immediately. When the patient is no longer at risk for a bad outcome or injury, the nurse performs a more comprehensive examination of other body systems.

For patients who are hospitalized, a nurse integrates the collection of physical assessment data during routine patient care, validating findings with what is known about the patient's health history. For example, on entering a patient's room a nurse may notice behavioral patient cues that indicate comfort, anxiety, or sadness; assess the skin during the bed bath; or assess physical movements and swallowing abilities while administering medications. Use physical examination to do the following:

- Gather baseline data about the patient's health status.
- Support or refute subjective data obtained in the nursing history.
- Identify and confirm nursing diagnoses.
- Make clinical decisions about a patient's changing health status and management.
- Evaluate the outcomes of care.

Cultural Sensitivity

Respect the cultural differences among patients from a variety of backgrounds when completing an examination. It is important to remember that cultural differences influence patient behaviors. Consider the patient's health beliefs, use of alternative therapies, nutrition habits, relationships with family, and comfort with physical closeness during the examination and history. These factors will affect your approach as well as the type of findings you might expect.

Be culturally aware and avoid stereotyping on the basis of gender or race. There is a difference between cultural characteristics and physical characteristics. Learn to recognize common characteristics and disorders among members of ethnic populations within the community. It is equally important to recognize variations in physical characteristics such as in the skin and musculoskeletal system, which are related to racial variables. By recognizing cultural diversity, you show respect for each patient's uniqueness, leading to higher-quality care and improved clinical outcomes (see Chapter 9).

PREPARATION FOR EXAMINATION

Physical examination is a routine part of a nurse's patient assessment. In many care settings a head-to-toe physical assessment is required daily. You perform a reassessment when a patient's condition changes as it improves or worsens. In some health care settings such as during a home health visit a focused physical examination is preferred. Proper preparation of the environment, equipment, and patient ensures a smooth physical examination with few interruptions. A disorganized approach causes errors and incomplete findings. Safety for confused patients should be a priority; never leave a confused or combative patient alone during an examination.

Infection Control

Some patients present with open skin lesions, infected wounds, or other communicable diseases. Use standard precautions throughout an examination (see Chapter 28). When an open sore or microorganism is present, wear gloves to reduce contact with contaminants. If a patient has excessive drainage or there is a risk of splattering from a wound, additional personal protective equipment such as an isolation gown or eye shield should be used. Follow agency hand hygiene policies before initiating and after completing a physical assessment.

Although most health care agencies make nonlatex gloves available, it is your responsibility to identify latex allergies in patients and use equipment items that are latex free. By recognizing risk factors for latex allergies, the patient remains free of a natural rubber latex (NRL) allergy response. Two types of allergic responses appear with NRL. The most immediate is an immunological reaction type 1 response, for which the body develops antibodies known as *immunoglobulin E* that can lead to an anaphylactic response. Atopy occurs when there is an increased tendency for the body to form antibodies as a result of the immune response. The second is the allergic contact dermatitis type 4 response, which causes a delayed reaction that appears 12 to 48 hours after exposure (Bundesen, 2008). Both require prior exposure to the substance to which the body reacts. The severity of the response varies among individuals. Table 30-1 provides a short list of products that contain latex and suggests available alternatives.

Environment

A respectful, considerate physical examination requires privacy. In the acute setting, nurses perform assessments in a patient's room. Examination rooms are used in clinics or office settings. In the home the examination is performed in a space where privacy can be established such as the patient's bedroom.

Examination spaces need to be well equipped for any procedures. Adequate lighting is necessary to properly illuminate body parts. The hospital patient room can be secured for privacy so patients are comfortable discussing their condition. Eliminate extra noise and take precautions to prevent interruptions from others. The room must be warm enough to maintain comfort.

Depending on the body part being assessed, it may be difficult to perform a selected assessment skill when a patient is in bed or on a stretcher. Special examination tables make positioning easier and body areas more easily accessible. By assisting patients on and off the examination table, injury can be avoided, and falls prevented. Examination tables can be uncomfortable; elevate the head of the table about 30 degrees. A small pillow helps with head and neck comfort. If the examination is completed in the patient room, raise the patient's bed to be able to reach him or her more easily.

TABLE 30-1 Products Containing Latex and Nonlatex Substitutes*

PRODUCTS CONTAINING LATEX	NONLATEX SUBSTITUTES
Medical Equipment	
Disposable gloves	Vinyl, nitrile, or neoprene gloves
Blood pressure cuffs	Covered cuffs
Stethoscope tubing	Covered tubing
Intravenous injection ports	Needleless system, stopcocks, covered latex ports
Tourniquets	Latex-free or cloth-covered tourniquets
Syringes	Glass syringes
Adhesive tape	Nonlatex tapes
Oral and nasal airways	Nonlatex tubes
Endotracheal tubes	Hard plastic tubes
Catheters	Silicone catheters
Eye goggles	Silicone eye goggles
Anesthesia masks	Silicone masks
Respirators	Nonlatex respirators
Rubber aprons	Cloth-covered aprons
Wound drains	Silicone drains
Medication vial stoppers	Stoppers removed
Household Items	
Rubber bands	String; latex-free bands
Erasers	Silicone erasers
Motorcycle and bicycle handgrips	Handgrips removed or covered
Carpeting	Other types of flooring
Swimming goggles	Silicone construction
Shoe soles	Leather shoes
Expandable fabric (e.g., waistbands)	Fabric removed or covered
Dishwashing gloves	Vinyl gloves
Condoms	Nonlatex condoms
Diaphragms	Synthetic rubber diaphragms
Balloons	Mylar balloons
Pacifiers and baby bottle nipples	Silicone, plastic, or nonlatex pacifiers and nipples

Modified from American Latex Allergy Association: *Literature review on latex-food cross-reactivity, 1991-2006*, 2011, http://www.latexallergyresources.org/topics/CrossReactiveAllergens.cfm. Accessed September 8, 2011; and Seidel HM et al: *Mosby's guide to physical examination*, ed 7, St Louis, 2011, Mosby;
*This list is intended to provide examples of products and alternatives. It is not complete.

Equipment

Perform hand hygiene thoroughly before handling equipment and starting an examination. Arrange any necessary equipment so that it is readily available and easy to use. Prepare equipment as appropriate (e.g., warm the diaphragm of the stethoscope between the hands before applying it to the skin). Be sure that equipment functions properly before using it (e.g., ensure that the ophthalmoscope and otoscope have good batteries and light bulbs). Box 30-1 lists typical equipment used during a physical examination.

BOX 30-1 EQUIPMENT AND SUPPLIES FOR PHYSICAL ASSESSMENT

- Cervical brush or broom devices (if needed)
- Cotton applicators
- Disposable pad/paper towels
- Drapes/cover
- Eye chart (e.g., Snellen chart)
- Flashlight and spotlight
- Forms (e.g., physical, laboratory)
- Nonlatex gloves (clean)
- Gown for patient
- Ophthalmoscope
- Otoscope
- Papanicolaou (Pap) liquid preparation (if needed)
- Percussion (reflex) hammer
- Pulse oximeter
- Ruler
- Scale with height measurement rod
- Specimen containers, slides, wooden or plastic spatula, and cytological fixative (if needed)
- Sphygmomanometer and cuff
- Sterile swabs
- Stethoscope
- Tape measure
- Thermometer
- Tissues
- Tongue depressors
- Tuning fork
- Vaginal speculum (if needed)
- Water-soluble lubricant
- Watch with second hand or digital display

Physical Preparation of the Patient

To show respect for a patient, ensure that physical comfort needs are met. Before starting, ask if the patient needs to use the restroom. An empty bladder and bowel facilitate examination of the abdomen, genitalia, and rectum. Collection of urine or fecal specimens occurs at this time if needed.

Physical preparation involves making certain that patient privacy is maintained with proper dress and draping. The patient in the hospital likely is wearing only a simple gown. In the clinic or health care provider's office the patient needs to undress and usually is provided a disposable paper cover or paper gown. If the examination is limited to certain body systems, it is not always necessary for the patient to undress completely. Provide the patient privacy and plenty of time to undress to avoid embarrassment. After changing into the recommended gown or cover, the patient sits or lies down on the examination table with a light drape over the lap or lower trunk. Make sure that he or she stays warm by eliminating drafts, controlling room temperature, and providing warm blankets. Routinely ask if he or she is comfortable.

Positioning. During the examination ask the patient to assume proper positions so body parts are accessible and he or she stays comfortable. Table 30-2 lists the preferred positions for each part of the examination and contains figures illustrating the positions. Patients' abilities to assume positions depend on their physical strength, mobility, ease of breathing, age, and degree of wellness. After explaining the positions, help the patient to assume them. Take care to maintain respect and show consideration by adjusting the drapes so that only the area examined is accessible. During the examination a patient may need to assume more than one position. To decrease the number of position changes, organize the examination so all techniques requiring a sitting position are completed first, followed by those that require a supine position next, and so forth. Use extra care when positioning older adults with disabilities and limitations.

TABLE 30-2 Positions for Examination

POSITION	AREAS ASSESSED	RATIONALE	LIMITATIONS
Sitting 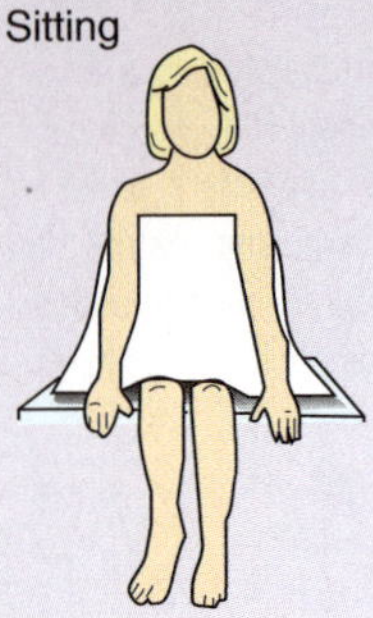	Head and neck, back, posterior thorax and lungs, anterior thorax and lungs, breasts, axillae, heart, vital signs, and upper extremities	Sitting upright provides full expansion of lungs and better visualization of symmetry of upper body parts.	Physically weakened patient is sometimes unable to sit. Use supine position with head of bed elevated instead.
Supine 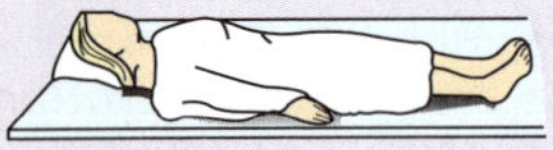	Head and neck, anterior thorax and lungs, breasts, axillae, heart, abdomen, extremities, pulses	This is most normally relaxed position. It provides easy access to pulse sites.	If patient becomes short of breath easily, raise the head of bed.
Dorsal recumbent 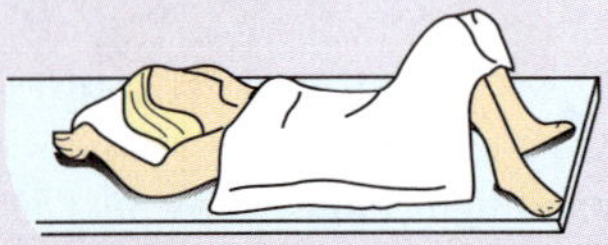	Head and neck, anterior thorax and lungs, breasts, axillae, heart, abdomen	Position is for abdominal assessment because it promotes relaxation of abdominal muscles.	Patients with painful disorders are more comfortable with knees flexed.
Lithotomy* 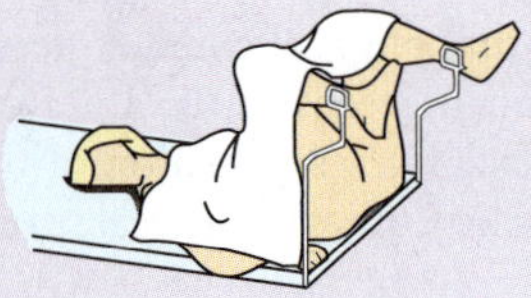	Female genitalia and genital tract	Position provides maximal exposure of female genitalia and facilitates insertion of vaginal speculum.	Lithotomy position is embarrassing and uncomfortable; thus examiner minimizes time that patient spends in it. Keep patient well draped.
Sims' 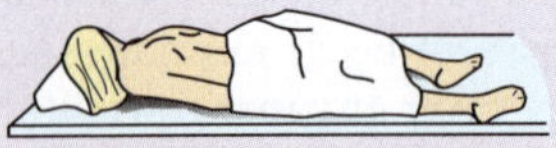	Rectum and vagina	Flexion of hip and knee improves exposure of rectal area.	Joint deformities hinder patient's ability to bend hip and knee.
Prone 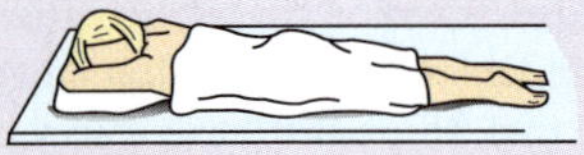	Musculoskeletal system	Position is only for assessing extension of hip joint, skin, buttocks.	Patients with respiratory difficulties do not tolerate this position well.
Lateral recumbent 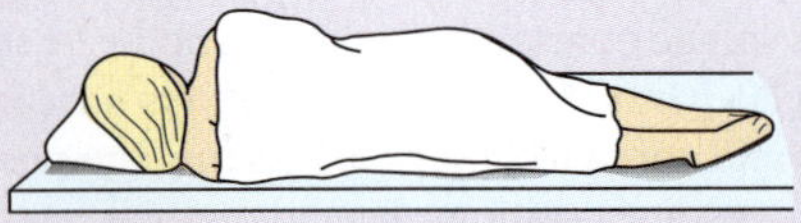	Heart	Position aids in detecting murmurs.	Patients with respiratory difficulties do not tolerate this position well.
Knee-chest* 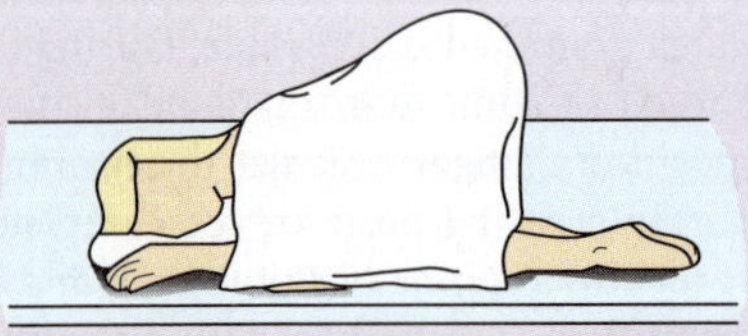	Rectum	Position provides maximal exposure of rectal area.	This position is embarrassing and uncomfortable.

*Some patients with arthritis or other joint deformities are unable to assume this position.

Psychological Preparation of a Patient

Many patients find an examination stressful or tiring, or they experience anxiety about possible findings. A thorough explanation of the purpose and steps of each assessment lets a patient know what to expect and how to cooperate. Adapt explanations to the patient's level of understanding and encourage him or her to ask questions and comment on any discomfort. Convey an open, professional approach while remaining relaxed. A quiet, formal demeanor inhibits the patient's ability to communicate, but a style that is too casual may cause him or her to doubt an examiner's competence (Seidel et al., 2011).

Consider cultural or social norms when performing an examination on a person of the opposite gender. When this situation occurs, another person of the patient's gender or a culturally approved family member needs to be in the room. By taking this step you demonstrate cultural awareness for a patient's individual needs. As a side benefit, the second person acts as a witness to the conduct of the examiner and the patient should any question arise.

During the examination, watch the patient's emotional responses by observing whether his or her facial expressions show fear or concern or if body movements indicate anxiety. When you remain calm, the patient is more likely to relax. Especially if the patient is weak or elderly, it is necessary to pace the examination, pausing at intervals to ask how he or she is tolerating the assessment. If the patient feels alright, the examination can proceed. However, do not force the patient to cooperate based on your schedule. Postponing the examination is advantageous because the findings may be more accurate when the patient can cooperate and relax.

Assessment of Age-Groups

It is necessary to use different interview styles and approaches to physical examination for patients of different age-groups. Your approach will vary with each group. When assessing children, show sensitivity and anticipate the child's perception of the examination as a strange and unfamiliar experience. Routine pediatric examinations focus on health promotion and illness prevention, particularly for the care of well children who receive competent parenting and have no serious health problems (Josephson and AACAP Work Group, 2007). This examination focuses on growth and development, sensory screening, dental examination, and behavioral assessment. Children who are chronically ill or disabled and foster, foreign-born, or adopted children sometimes require additional examination visits. When examining children, the following tips help in data collection:

- Gather all or part of the history on infants and children from parents or guardians.
- Perform the examination in a nonthreatening area; provide time for play to become acquainted.
- Because parents sometimes think the examiner is testing them, offer support during the examination and do not pass judgment.
- Call children by their first name and address the parents as "Mr., Mrs., or Ms." rather than by their first name unless instructed differently.
- Use open-ended questions to allow parents to share more information and describe more of the children's problems. This also allows observation of parent-child interactions. You can interview older children, who often provide details about their health history and severity of symptoms.
- Treat adolescents as adults and individuals because they tend to respond best when treated as such.
- Remember that adolescents have the right to confidentiality. After talking with parents about historical information, speak alone with adolescents.

A comprehensive health assessment and examination of older adults includes physical data, developmental stage, family relationships, religious and occupational pursuits, and a review of the patient's cognitive, affective, and social level (Kresevic, 2008). An important aspect is to assess the patient's ability to perform basic activities of daily living (e.g., bathing, grooming) and complex instrumental activities of daily living (e.g., making phone call).

Throughout the examination recognize that with advancing age the body does not demonstrate obvious injury or disease as vigorously as younger patients and older adults do not always exhibit the expected signs and symptoms (Meiner, 2011). Characteristically older adults present with subtle or atypical signs and symptoms. Principles to follow during examination of an older adult include the following:

- Do not stereotype about aging patients' level of cognition. Most older adults are able to adapt to change and learn about their health. Similarly most are reliable historians.
- Recognize that some older adults have sensory or physical limitations that affect how quickly they can be interviewed and examinations can be conducted. It might be necessary to plan for more than one examination session. Sometimes it helps to give patients an initial health questionnaire before they come to a clinic or office.
- Perform the examination with adequate space; this is especially important for patients with mobility aids such as a cane or walker.
- During the examination use patience, allow for pauses, and observe for details. Recognize normal physiological and behavioral changes that are characteristic of later life.
- Certain types of health information are stressful for older patients to give. Some view illness as a threat to independence and a step toward institutionalization.
- Be aware of the location of the closest bathroom facility in case the patient has an urgent need to eliminate.
- Be alert to signs of increasing fatigue such as sighing, grimacing, irritability, leaning against objects for support, and drooping head and shoulders.

ORGANIZATION OF THE EXAMINATION

You will conduct a physical examination by assessing each body system. Use judgment to ensure that an examination is relevant and includes the correct assessments. Patients with focused symptoms or needs require only parts of an examination; thus, when a patient comes to a clinic with symptoms of a severe chest cold, a neurological assessment should not be required. A patient entering the emergency department with acute abdominal symptoms requires assessment of the body systems most at risk for being abnormal. However, when a patient is admitted to the hospital, you will perform a complete examination at the time of admission and at least once each day. Agency guidelines may define the components of a complete examination (see agency policy). A patient in the community seeks screening for specific conditions, often dependent on the patient's age or health risks listed in Table 30-3.

Any physical examination should follow a systematic routine to avoid missing important findings. A head-to-toe approach includes all body systems, and the examiner recalls and performs each step in a predetermined order. For an adult the examination begins with an assessment of the head and neck and progresses methodically

TABLE 30-3 Recommended Preventive Screenings

DISEASE/CONDITION	AGE-GROUP	SCREENING MEASURES
Breast cancer*	Ages 20 to 39	Monthly breast self-examination (BSE). Clinical breast examination by health care professional every 3 years
	Ages 40 and up	Monthly BSE Annual clinical breast examination by health care professional Annual mammograms (Women at increased risk need to speak to health care provider regarding screening options.)
Colon/rectal cancer*	Ages 50 and up	Men and women need to have one of the following: fecal occult blood test (FOBT) or fecal immunochemical test (FIT) annually or flexible sigmoidoscopy (FSIG) every 5 years; the combination of FOBT or FIT annually and an FSIG every 5 years is preferred over either of the previous options; or double-contrast barium enema every 5 years; or colonoscopy every 10 years. They also need a digital rectal examination at the same time. Earlier screening is necessary if risk factors exist.
Ear disorders	All ages	Periodic hearing checks as needed
	Over age 65	Regular hearing checks
Eye disorders	Age 40 and under	Complete eye examination every 3 to 5 years (more if positive history for eye disease [e.g., diabetes])
	Ages 40 to 64	Complete eye examination every 2 years to screen for conditions that may go unnoticed (e.g., glaucoma)
	Age 65 and up	Complete eye examination every year
Heart/vascular disorders	Men age 45 to 65 Women age 45 to 65	Regular measurement of total blood cholesterol levels, lipids, and triglycerides; blood pressure screenings (If patient has risk factors for coronary artery disease [CAD], blood pressure screening needs to begin at age 20-35 for men, 20-45 for women.)
Obesity	All ages	Periodic height and weight measurements
Oral cavity/pharyngeal disorders/cancer	All ages (children, adults, older adults)	Regular dental examinations every 6 months
Ovarian cancer*	Age 18 and up or on becoming sexually active	Annual pelvic examinations by health care provider (This screening occasionally detects ovarian cancer in its advanced stage. Those at high risk need to have a thorough pelvic examination, a transvaginal ultrasound, and a blood test [tumor marker CA 125]).
Prostate cancer*	Ages 50 and up	Men who have at least a 10-year life expectancy need to have a digital rectal examination (DRE) and prostate-specific antigen (PSA) blood test annually. Men at high risk require earlier screening.
Skin cancer*	Ages 20 to 40	See specialist every 3 years
	Over 40	Annual skin checkups with biopsy of suspicious lesions
Testicular cancer*	Age 15 and up	Monthly testicular self-examination (TSE)
Uterine cancer*	Screening begins 3 years after having vaginal intercourse but not later than age 21	Annual pelvic examination by health care provider plus annual Papanicolaou (Pap) test
Cervical cancer	Screening begins 3 years after vaginal intercourse but not later than age 21	Annual pelvic examination by health care provider, plus an annual Pap test (At age 30 or after, those who have had three normal tests consecutively may be screened every 2 to 3 years. If patient has risk factors, screening needs to occur more frequently. Contact health care provider.)
Endometrial cancer	Same as for cervical cancer	Endometrial biopsy at age 35 for high-risk patients (those with or at risk for hereditary nonpolyposis colon cancer [HNPCC]) (At menopause women at average and high risk need to be informed about signs and symptoms to report.)

*Data from American Cancer Society: *Cancer facts and figures 2011,* Atlanta, 2011, The Society; website for further information on preventative screenings: *Guide to clinical preventive services,* AHRQ Publication No. 05-0570, Rockville, Md, 2011, Agency for Healthcare Research and Quality, http://www.ahrp.gov/.

down the body to incorporate all body systems. The following tips help keep an examination well organized:

- Compare both sides of the body for symmetry. A degree of asymmetry is normal (e.g., the biceps muscles in the dominant arm are sometimes more developed than the same muscles in the nondominant arm).
- If the patient is seriously ill, first assess the systems of the body most at risk for being abnormal. For example, a patient with chest pain first undergoes a cardiovascular assessment.
- If the patient becomes fatigued, offer rest periods between assessments.
- Perform painful procedures near the end of an examination.
- Record assessments in specific terms in the electronic or paper record. A standard form allows for recording information in the same sequence that it is gathered.
- Use common and accepted medical terms and abbreviations to keep notes accurate, brief, and concise.
- Record quick notes during the examination to avoid delays. Complete any larger documentation notes at the end of the examination.

TECHNIQUES OF PHYSICAL ASSESSMENT

The four techniques used in a physical examination are inspection, palpation, percussion, and auscultation.

Inspection

To inspect, carefully look, listen, and smell to distinguish normal from abnormal findings. To do so, you must be aware of any personal visual, hearing, or olfactory deficits. It is important to deliberately practice this skill and learn to recognize all of the possible pieces of data that can be gathered through inspection alone. **Inspection** occurs when interacting with a patient, watching for nonverbal expressions of emotional and mental status. Physical movements and structural components can also be identified in such an informal way. Most important, be deliberate and pay attention to detail. Follow these guidelines to achieve the best results during inspection:

- Make sure that adequate lighting is available, either direct or tangential.
- Use a direct lighting source (e.g., a penlight or lamp) to inspect body cavities.
- Inspect each area for size, shape, color, symmetry, position, and abnormality.
- Position and expose body parts as needed so all surfaces can be viewed but privacy can be maintained.
- When possible, check for side-to-side symmetry by comparing each area with its match on the opposite side of the body.
- Validate findings with the patient.

While assessing a patient, recognize the nature and source of body odors (Table 30-4). An unusual odor often indicates an underlying pathology. **Olfaction** helps to detect abnormalities that cannot be recognized by any other means. For example, when a patient's breath has a sweet, fruity odor, assess for signs of diabetes. Continue to inspect various parts of the body during the physical examination. Palpation may be used concurrently with inspection, or it may follow in a more deliberate fashion.

Palpation

Palpation involves using the sense of touch to gather information. Through touch you make judgments about expected and unexpected findings of the skin or underlying tissue, muscle, and bones.

TABLE 30-4 Assessment of Characteristic Odors

ODOR	SITE OR SOURCE	POTENTIAL CAUSES
Alcohol	Oral cavity	Ingestion of alcohol, diabetes
Ammonia	Urine	Urinary tract infection, renal failure
Body odor	Skin, particularly in areas where body parts rub together (e.g., underarms and under breasts)	Poor hygiene, excess perspiration (hyperhidrosis), foul-smelling perspiration (bromhidrosis)
	Wound site	Wound abscess
	Vomitus	Abdominal irritation, contaminated food
Feces	Vomitus/oral cavity (fecal odor)	Bowel obstruction
	Rectal area	Fecal incontinence
Foul-smelling stools in infant	Stool	Malabsorption syndrome
Halitosis	Oral cavity	Poor dental and oral hygiene, gum disease
Sweet, fruity ketones	Oral cavity	Diabetic acidosis
Stale urine	Skin	Uremic acidosis
Sweet, heavy, thick odor	Draining wound	*Pseudomonas* (bacterial) infection
Musty odor	Casted body part	Infection inside cast
Fetid, sweet odor	Tracheostomy or mucus secretions	Infection of bronchial tree (*Pseudomonas* bacteria)

For example, you palpate the skin for temperature, moisture, texture, turgor, tenderness, and thickness and the abdomen for tenderness, distention, or masses. Use different parts of the hand to detect different characteristics (Table 30-5). The palmar surface of the hand and finger pads is more sensitive than the fingertips and should be used to determine position, texture, size, consistency, masses, fluid, and crepitus (Fig. 30-1, *A*). Assess body temperature by using the dorsal surface or back of the hand (Fig. 30-1, *B*). The palmar surface of the hand and fingers (Fig. 30-1, *C*) is more sensitive to vibration. Measure position, consistency, and turgor by lightly grasping the body part with the fingertips (Fig. 30-1, *D*).

Touching the patient is a personal experience for both you and the patient. Display respect and concern throughout the examination. Before palpating consider the patient's condition and ability to tolerate the assessment techniques, paying close attention to areas that are painful or tender. In addition, always be conscious of the environment and any threats to the patient's safety.

Prepare for palpation by warming hands, keeping fingernails short and using a gentle approach. Palpation proceeds slowly, gently, and deliberately. The patient needs to be guided to relax and feel comfortable since tensed muscles make assessment more difficult. To promote relaxation, have him or her take slow, deep breaths and place both arms along the sides of the body. Ask the patient to point to more sensitive areas, watching for nonverbal signs of discomfort. *Palpate tender areas last.*

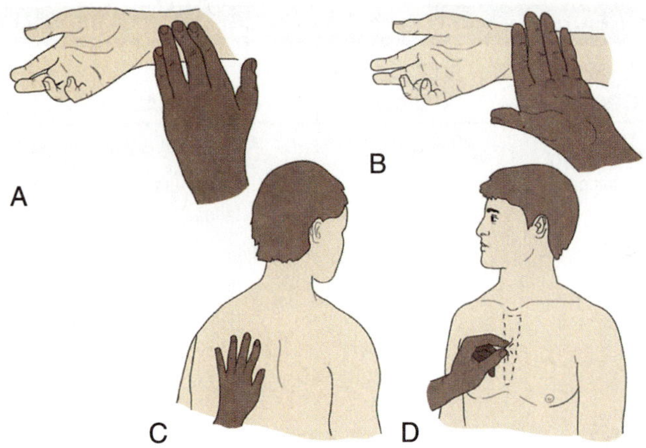

FIG. 30-1 **A,** Radial pulse is detected with the pads of fingertips, the most sensitive part of the hand. **B,** Dorsum of the hand detects temperature variations in skin. **C,** The bony part of the palm at the base of the fingers detects vibrations. **D,** Skin is grasped with the fingertips to assess turgor.

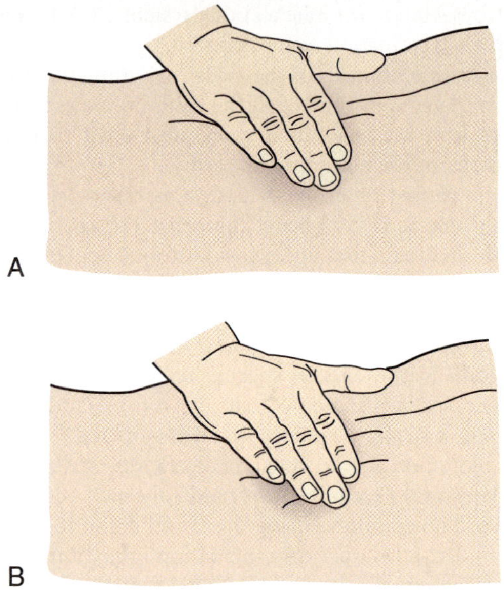

FIG. 30-2 **A,** During light palpation gentle pressure against underlying skin and tissues can detect areas of irregularity and tenderness. **B,** During deep palpation depress tissue to assess the condition of underlying organs.

TABLE 30-5 Examples of Characteristics Measured by Palpation

AREA EXAMINED	CRITERIA MEASURED	PORTION OF HAND TO USE
Skin	Temperature	Dorsum of hand/fingers
	Moisture	Palmar surface
	Texture	
	Turgor and elasticity	Grasping with fingertips
	Tenderness	
	Thickness	Palmar surface
Organs (e.g., liver and intestine)	Size Shape Tenderness Absence of masses	Entire palmar surface of hand or palmar surface of fingers
Glands (e.g., thyroid and lymph)	Swelling Symmetry and mobility	Pads of fingers
Blood vessels (e.g., carotid or femoral artery)	Pulse amplitude Elasticity Rate Rhythm	Palmar surface/pads of fingertips
Thorax	Excursion	Palmar surface
	Tenderness	Finger pads/palmar surface of fingers
	Fremitus	Palmar or ulnar surface of entire hand

Two types of palpation are used for physical examination, light and deep. Light palpation is performed by placing the hand on the body part being examined; it also involves pressing inward about 1 cm (½ inch). Light, superficial palpation of structures such as the abdomen gives the patient the chance to identify areas of tenderness (Fig. 30-2, *A*). Inquire about areas of tenderness and assess them further for potentially serious pathologies. Deep palpation is used to examine the condition of organs such as those in the abdomen (Fig. 30-2, *B*). Depress the area under examination approximately 4 cm (2 inches) (Seidel et al., 2011), using one or both hands (bimanually). When using bimanual palpation, relax one hand (sensing hand) and place it lightly over the patient's skin. The other hand (active hand) helps apply pressure to the sensing hand. The lower hand does not exert pressure directly and thus remains sensitive to detect organ characteristics. For safety deep palpation should be observed by your clinical instructor when you first attempt the procedure.

Percussion

Percussion involves tapping the skin with the fingertips to vibrate underlying tissues and organs. The vibration travels through body tissues, and the character of the resulting sound reflects the density of the underlying tissue. The denser the tissue, the quieter the sound. By knowing how various densities influence sound, it is possible to locate organs or masses, map their edges, and determine their size. An abnormal sound suggests a mass or substance such as air or fluid within an organ or body cavity. The skill of percussion is used more often by advanced practice nurses than by nurses in daily practice at the bedside.

Auscultation

Auscultation involves listening to sounds the body makes to detect variations from normal. Some sounds such as speech and coughing can be heard without additional equipment, but a stethoscope is necessary to hear internal body sounds.

Internal body sounds are created by blood, air, or gastric contents as they move against the body structures. For example, normal heart sounds are created when the heart valves close, moving blood to the next portion of the cardiovascular system. Normal sounds for each body system are discussed later in this chapter. Learn to recognize abnormal sounds after learning normal variations. Becoming more proficient in auscultation occurs by knowing the types of sounds each body structure makes and the location in which the sounds are heard best.

To auscultate internal sounds you need to hear well, have a good stethoscope, and know how to use it properly. Nurses with hearing disorders can obtain stethoscopes with extra sound amplification.

Chapter 29 describes the parts of the stethoscope and its general use. The bell is best for hearing low-pitched sounds such as vascular and certain heart sounds, and the diaphragm is best for listening to high-pitched sounds such as bowel and lung sounds.

By practicing with the stethoscope, you become proficient at using it and realize when sounds are clear and when there are extraneous sounds. Extraneous sounds created by rubbing against the tubing or chest piece interfere with auscultation of body organ sounds. By deliberately producing these sounds, you learn to recognize and disregard them during the actual examination. Box 30-2 contains ways to practice using and techniques for caring for the stethoscope. Describe any sound you hear using the following characteristics:

- Frequency indicates the number of sound wave cycles generated per second by a vibrating object. The higher the frequency, the higher the pitch of a sound and vice versa.
- Loudness refers to the amplitude of a sound wave. Auscultated sounds range from soft to loud.
- Quality refers to sounds of similar frequency and loudness from different sources. Terms such as *blowing* or *gurgling* describe the quality of sound.
- Duration means the length of time that sound vibrations last. The duration of sound is short, medium, or long. Layers of soft tissue dampen the duration of sounds from deep internal organs.

Auscultation requires concentration and practice. While listening, know which sounds are normally produced in certain parts of the body and what causes the sounds. Normal sounds will be discussed in each body system section of this chapter. After understanding the cause and character of normal auscultated sounds, it becomes easier to recognize abnormal sounds and their origins.

BOX 30-2 USE AND CARE OF THE STETHOSCOPE

- Ensure that the earpiece follows the contour of the ear canals. Learn which fit is best for you by comparing amplification of sounds with the earpieces in both directions.
- Place the earpieces in your ears with the tips turned toward the face. *Lightly* blow into the diaphragm. Again place the earpieces in your ears, this time with the ends turned toward the back of the head. *Lightly* blow into the diaphragm. You will find that you hear clearer sounds with the earpiece turned toward the face. After you have learned the right fit for the loudest amplification, wear the stethoscope the same way each time.
- Put on the stethoscope and *lightly* blow into the diaphragm. If the sound is barely audible, *lightly* blow into the bell. Sound is carried through only one part of the chest piece at a time. If the sound is greatly amplified through the diaphragm, the diaphragm is in position for use. If the sound is barely audible through the diaphragm, the bell is in position for use. Rotation of the diaphragm and bell places the chest piece in the desired position. Leave the diaphragm in position for the next exercise.
- Place the diaphragm over the anterior part of your chest. Ask a friend to speak in a normal conversational tone. Environmental noise seriously detracts from hearing the noise created by body organs. When using a stethoscope, the patient and the examiner need to remain quiet.
- Put on the stethoscope and gently tap the tubing. It is often difficult to avoid stretching or moving the stethoscope tubing. The examiner is in a position so the tubing hangs free. Moving or touching the tubing creates extraneous sounds.
- *Care of the stethoscope:* Remove earpieces regularly and clean; remove cerumen (earwax). Keep the bell and diaphragm free of dust, lint, and body oils. Keep the tubing away from any body oils. Avoid draping the stethoscope around the neck next to the skin. Clean by wiping the entire stethoscope (e.g., diaphragm, tubing) with alcohol or soapy water. Be sure to dry all parts thoroughly. Follow the manufacturer's recommendations.
- *Infection control:* Harmful bacteria such as gram-positive bacilli, methicillin-resistant *Staphylococcus aureus* (MRSA), nonaureus *Staphylococcus, Enterobacter cloacae,* and methicillin-sensitive *S. aureus* can be transferred from patient to patient when using portable equipment such as stethoscopes. Clean the stethoscope (diaphragm/bell) *before* reuse on another patient. Using a disinfectant such as isopropyl alcohol (with or without chlorhexidine), benzalkonium, or sodium hypochlorite is effective in reducing the number of bacterial colonies. Hand foam serves this purpose well. Earpieces of stethoscopes are sources of transferable bacteria. When you inadvertently touch your ears and care for the patient, potential pathogens could contaminate the earpieces. Using hand hygiene before and after patient contact decreases the risk of transmitting microorganisms from your ear to your patient. Follow institution infection control guidelines, especially contact precautions, to decrease this risk (Lecat et al., 2009).

GENERAL SURVEY

When a patient first enters the examination room, observe his or her walk and general appearance and be attentive to his or her behavior and dress. A general survey, or appraisal, of the patient's presentation and behavior provides information about characteristics of an illness, the patient's ability to function independently, body image, emotional state, recent changes in weight, and developmental status. If there are abnormalities or problems, assess the affected body system more closely during the full examination.

General Appearance and Behavior

Assess appearance and behavior while preparing the patient for the examination. For this review include:

- *Gender and race:* A person's gender affects the type of examination performed and the order of the assessments. Different physical features are related to gender and race. Certain illnesses are more likely to affect a specific gender or race (e.g., the incidence of skin cancer is more common in whites than in blacks, prostate cancer is higher in black men than in white men, and cancer of the bladder is four times higher in men than women) (American Cancer Society [ACS], 2011).
- *Age:* Age influences normal physical characteristics and a person's ability to participate in some parts of the examination.
- *Signs of distress:* Sometimes obvious signs or symptoms indicate pain (grimacing, splinting painful area), difficulty breathing (shortness of breath, sternal retractions), or anxiety. Set priorities and examine the related physical areas first.
- *Body type:* Observe if the patient appears trim and muscular, obese, or excessively thin. Body type reflects the level of health, age, and lifestyle.
- *Posture:* Normal standing posture shows an upright stance with parallel alignment of the hips and shoulders. Normal sitting posture involves some degree of rounding of the shoulders. Observe whether the patient has a slumped, erect, or bent posture, which reflects mood or pain. Changes in older adult physiology often result in a stooped, forward-bent posture, with the hips and knees somewhat flexed and the arms bent at the elbows.

- *Gait:* Observe as the patient walks into the room or stands at the bedside (if the patient is ambulatory). Note whether movements are coordinated or uncoordinated. A person normally walks smoothly, with the arms swinging freely at the sides and the head and face leading the body.
- *Body movements:* Observe whether movements are purposeful, noting any tremors involving the extremities. Determine if any body parts are immobile.
- *Hygiene and grooming:* Note the patient's level of cleanliness by observing the appearance of the hair, skin, and fingernails. Determine if his or her clothes are clean. Grooming depends on the patient's cognitive and emotional function, daily or social activities, and occupation. Observe for excessive use of cosmetics or colognes that could indicate a change in self-perception.
- *Dress:* Culture, lifestyle, socioeconomic level, and personal preference affect the selection and wearing of clothing. However, you should assess whether or not the clothing is appropriate for the temperature, weather conditions, or setting. Depressed or mentally ill people may not be able to select proper clothing, and an older adult might tend to wear extra clothing because of sensitivity to cold.
- *Body odor:* An unpleasant body odor can result from physical exercise, poor hygiene, or certain disease states. Validate any odors that might indicate a health problem.
- *Affect and mood:* Affect is a person's feelings as he or she appears to others. Patients express mood or emotional state verbally and nonverbally. Determine whether or not verbal expressions match nonverbal behavior and if the mood is appropriate for the situation. By maintaining eye contact you can observe facial expressions while asking questions.
- *Speech:* Normal speech is understandable and moderately paced and shows an association with the person's thoughts. However, emotions or neurological impairment sometimes causes rapid or slowed speech. Observe whether the patient speaks in a normal tone with clear inflection of words.
- *Signs of patient abuse:* During the examination observe if the patient fears his or her spouse or partner, a caregiver, a parent, or an adult child. Abuse of children, women, and older adults is a growing health problem. Consider any obvious physical injury or neglect as signs of possible abuse (e.g., evidence of malnutrition or presence of bruising on the extremities or trunk). Abuse occurs in many forms: physical, mental or emotional, sexual, social, and financial or economic. Observe the behavior of the individual for any signs of frustration, explanations that do not fit his or her physical presentation, or signs of injury. Most states mandate a report to a social service center when abuse or neglect is suspected (Box 30-3). It is difficult to detect abuse because victims often do not complain or report that they are in an abusive situation (Cohen et al., 2007). If abuse is suspected, find a way to interview the patient in private; patients are more likely to reveal any problems when the suspected abuser is absent from the room. It is imperative that you help the patient find safe housing or seek protection from the abuser since the risk for further abuse is high once the victim has reported it or tries to leave the abusive situation.
- *Substance abuse:* Unusual or inconsistent behavior may be an indicator of substance abuse, which can affect all socioeconomic groups. Although a single patient visit to a clinic does not always reveal the problem, unusual behaviors should be investigated further to reveal behaviors that should be confirmed with a well-focused history and physical examination. Always approach the patient in a caring and nonjudgmental way; substance abuse involves both emotional and lifestyle issues. Box 30-4 lists characteristics of patients who should be further assessed for potential substance abuse. The CAGE questionnaire provides a useful set of questions to guide assessment. CAGE is an acronym for the following:
  - Have you ever felt the need to **Cut down** on your drinking or drug use?
  - Have people **Annoyed** you by criticizing your drinking or drug use?
  - Have you ever felt bad or **Guilty** about your drinking or drug use?
  - Have you ever used or had a drink first thing in the morning as an **Eye-opener** to steady your nerves or feel normal?

If two or more of the CAGE questions are positive, be aware that substance abuse is likely and the patient needs guidance and encouragement to seek treatment. Among older adults risk factors for development of alcohol-related problems include chronic medical disorders, sleep disorders, social isolation, loneliness, bereavement, and acute or chronic pain. Older women appear to abuse alcohol more often than elderly men (Boyle and Davis, 2006).

Vital Signs

After completing the general survey, measure the patient's vital signs (see Chapter 29). Measurement of vital signs is more accurate if completed before beginning positional changes or movements. If there is a chance that the vital signs are skewed when first measured, recheck them later during the rest of the examination. Pain, considered the fifth vital sign, should also be assessed.

Height and Weight

Height and weight reflect a person's general health status. Standardized tables help reveal the normal expected adult weight for a given height (Table 30-6). Assess every patient to identify if he or she is at a healthy weight, overweight, or obese. Weight is routinely measured during health screenings, visits to physicians' offices or clinics, and on admission to the hospital. Infants and children are measured for both height and weight at each health care visit to assess for healthy growth and development. If older adults are underweight, difficulty with feeding and other functional activities is a possibility. Measuring height and weight of older adults, along with obtaining a dietary history, shows risk factors for chronic diseases (Box 30-5).

Assess trends in weight changes compared with height for signs of poor health. Assessments screen for abnormal weight changes. A patient's weight normally varies daily because of fluid loss or retention. However, a downward trend in a frail older adult indicates that there is a serious reduction in nutritional reserves. The nursing history helps to focus on possible causes for a change in weight (Table 30-7). Ask the patient to report current height and weight, along with a history of any substantial weight gain or loss. A weight gain of 5 pounds (2.3 kg) in 1 day indicates fluid-retention problems. A weight loss is considered significant if the patient has lost more than 5% of body weight in a month or 10% in 6 months.

When a patient is hospitalized, daily weight is measured at the same time of day, on the same scale, with approximately the same clothes. This allows an objective comparison of subsequent weights. Accuracy of weight measurement is important because health care

BOX 30-3 CLINICAL INDICATORS OF ABUSE

PHYSICAL FINDINGS	BEHAVIORAL FINDINGS
Child Abuse	
Blood on underclothing	Fear of certain people or places
Pain, itching, or unusual odor in genital area	Play activities recreate the abuse situation
Genital injuries	Regressed behavior
Difficulty sitting or walking	Sexual acting out
Pain while urinating; recurrent urinary tract infections	Knowledge of explicit sexual matters
Foreign bodies in rectum, urethra, or vagina	Preoccupation with others' or own genitals
Sexually transmitted infections	Profound and rapid personality changes
Pregnancy in young adolescent	Rapidly declining school performance
	Poor relationship with peers
Intimate Partner Violence	
Injuries and trauma inconsistent with reported cause	Overuse of health services
Multiple injuries involving head, face, neck, breasts, abdomen, and genitalia (black eyes, orbital fractures, broken nose, fractured skull, lip lacerations, broken teeth, vaginal tears)	Attempted suicide
	Eating or sleeping disorders
X-ray films showing old and new fractures in different stages of healing	Anxiety and panic attacks
Abrasions, lacerations, bruises/welts	Pattern of substance abuse (follows physical abuse)
Burns from cigarettes or other	Low self-esteem
Human bites	Depression
Unexplained injuries (e.g., bruises, fractures, and welts)	Sense of helplessness
Strangulation marks on neck from rope burns or bruises; throat pain, voice changes, trouble swallowing; damage to hyoid bone	Guilt
	Increased forgetfulness
	Stress-related complaints (headache, anxiety)
	Financial dependence on abuser
	Isolation from others
Older-Adult Abuse	
Injuries and trauma inconsistent with reported cause (scratch, bruise, or bite)	Dependent on caregiver
Hematomas, bruises at various stages of resolution	Physically and/or cognitively impaired
Unexplained bruises or welts, pattern bruises	Combative, verbally aggressive
Immersion burns	Wandering
Bruises, chafing, excoriation on wrist or legs (restraints)	Minimal social support
Burns from cigarettes or ropes	Prolonged interval between injury and medical treatment
Fractures inconsistent with cause described	Life circumstances do not match size of the patient's estate
Dried blood	Uncommunicative or isolated
Overmedication or undermedication	
Exposure to severe weather, cold or hot	
Torn, bloody underwear or vaginal and anal bruises	
Sunken eyes or loss of weight	
Extreme thirst	
Bed sores	

Data from Hockenberry MJ, Wilson P: *Wong's nursing care of infants and children*, ed 9, St Louis, 2011, Mosby; Krieger CL: Intimate partner violence, *Nurs Women's Health* 12(3):225, 2008; Muehlbauer M, Crane PA: Elder abuse and neglect, *J Psychosocial Nurs* 44(11):43; Westley C: Elder mistreatment: a self-learning module, *Medsurg Nurs* 14(2):133, 2005.

providers base medical and nursing decisions (e.g., drug dosage, medications) on changes.

Several different scales are available for use. Patients capable of bearing their own weight use a standing scale. The standard platform scale is calibrated by moving the large and small weights to zero. By adjusting the calibrating knob, the balance beam is leveled and steadied. The patient stands on the scale platform and remains still as the nurse adjusts the largest solid weight to the 50-pound or 22.5-kg increment under the patient's weight. Next the smaller weight is moved to balance the scale at the nearest ¼ pound or 0.1 kg (Seidel et al., 2011). Electronic scales automatically display the weight within seconds. They are calibrated automatically each time they are used.

Bed and chair scales are available for patients who are unable to bear weight. Newer electronic hospital beds have built-in electronic scales for weighing patients who are not able to get out of bed.

You can use a basket or platform scale to weigh infants. After removing the infant's clothing, weigh him or her in dry disposable diapers. Adjust the measurement later for the weight of the diaper, ensuring an accurate reading. Keep the room warm to prevent chills. Place a light cloth or paper on the surface of the infant scale to prevent cross-infection from urine or feces. When placing an infant in a basket or on a platform, hold a hand lightly above him or her to detect movements and prevent accidental falls. Measure an infant's weight in both ounces and grams.

BOX 30-4 BEHAVIORS THAT ARE SUSPICIOUS FOR SUBSTANCE ABUSE

Among Adolescents: Agitation, inappropriate behavior, poor coordination, seizure, respiratory depression, coma, asphyxiation, aspiration, pulmonary edema, cardiac arrhythmias, immune system impairment, self-inflicted trauma, and suicidal ideation

Red Flags:

- The risk of suicide, seizures, and violent behavior is high among substance abusers.
- Intoxicated patients—particularly those with phencyclidine (PCP) or methamphetamine intoxication—are at significant risk for becoming agitated and violent, placing themselves and others at risk for injury.

Observe for combinations or repetition of these behaviors:

- Frequently misses appointments
- Frequently requests written excuses for absence from work
- Chief complaints of insomnia, "bad nerves," or pain that does not fit a particular pattern
- Reports lost prescriptions (e.g., tranquilizers or pain medications) or asks for frequent refills
- Frequent emergency department visits
- History of changing health care providers or brings in medication bottles prescribed by several different providers
- History of gastrointestinal bleeds, peptic ulcers, pancreatitis, cellulitis, or frequent pulmonary infections
- Frequent sexually transmitted infections (STIs), complicated pregnancies, multiple abortions, or sexual dysfunction
- Complaints of chest pains or palpitations or has a history of admissions to rule out heart attacks
- History of activities that place the patient at risk for human immunodeficiency virus (HIV) infections (multiple partners, multiple rapes)
- Family history of addiction; history of childhood sexual, physical, or emotional abuse; or social and financial or marital problems
- Intimate partner violence

Data from American Psychiatric Association: *Diagnostic and statistical manual of mental disorders,* ed 4, text revision, Washington, DC, 2000, The Association; American Society of Addiction Medicine and Widlitz M, Marin D: Substance abuse in older adults: an overview, *Geriatrics* 57(12):29, 2002; and Walsh K et al: Examining the interface between substance misuse and intimate partner violence, *Substance Abuse Res Treatment* 3:25, 2009.

BOX 30-5 DIETARY HISTORY FOR OLDER ADULTS

- Does the older adult need or have help shopping for or preparing meals?
- Is income adequate for food purchasing? Food stamps or public assistance required?
- Does the patient ever skip meals?
- Are the five primary food groups from the food guide pyramid represented in the daily diet (see Chapter 44) (USDA and USDHHS, 2010)?
- Does the older adult take nutritional supplements such as multivitamins?
- Does the older adult take any medication affecting appetite or absorption of nutrients?
- Does the older adult have any religious or cultural beliefs and practices that influence diet?
- Does the older adult have a special diet, food intolerances, or allergies? Does the patient's diet contain an unusual amount of alcohol, sweets, or fried food?
- Does the older adult have problems with chewing, swallowing, or salivation?
- Does the older adult have gastrointestinal problems that interfere with food intake?

Data from Meiner SE: *Gerontologic nursing,* ed 4, St Louis, 2011, Mosby; Moore MC: *Pocket guide to nutritional assessment and care,* ed 5, St Louis, 2005, Mosby; and US Department of Agriculture and US Department of Health and Human Services: *Dietary guidelines for Americans, 2010,* ed 7, Washington, DC, 2010, US Government Printing Office.

Measure height in patients capable of standing by having them remove their shoes. The standing surface should be clean. Use a measuring rod attached vertically to a weight scale, or use a tape ruler on the wall. As the patient stands erect, place a flat surface on his or her head that is even with the vertical measure. Then read the number on the scale or ruler that indicates his or her height in centimeters or inches.

Remove the shoes of a nonweight-bearing patient and position the patient (such as an infant) supine on a firm surface. When measuring an infant, hold his or her head and make sure that his or her legs are straight at the knees. After positioning the infant, use a tape measure to measure length from the head to the bottom of the feet (Fig. 30-3). Record the infant's length to the nearest 0.5 cm or ¼ inch.

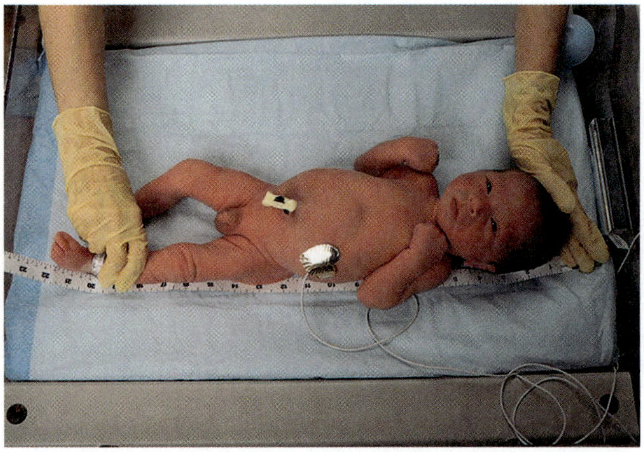

FIG. 30-3 Measurement of infant length. (From Murray SS, McKinney ES: *Foundations of maternal-newborn and women's health nursing,* ed 5, St Louis, 2010, Saunders.)

SKIN, HAIR, AND NAILS

The **integumentary system** refers to the skin, hair, scalp, and nails. To assess the integument, you first gather a health history to guide your examination and use the techniques of inspection and palpation.

Skin

Begin an assessment of the skin by focusing on the health history questions found in Table 30-8. The physical examination begins with an inspection of all visible skin surfaces; the less visible surfaces are assessed when you examine other body systems. Use the senses of sight, smell, and touch while performing inspection and palpation of the skin.

Assessment of the skin reveals the patient's health status related to oxygenation, circulation, nutrition, local tissue damage, and hydration. Check the condition of the patient's integument to determine the need for nursing care. For example, assessment findings can help determine the type of hygiene measures required to maintain integrity of the integument (see Chapter 39). Adequate

TABLE 30-6 Height and Weight Table: Weights for Persons 25 to 59 Years According to Build*

MEN					WOMEN				
HEIGHT					HEIGHT[†]				
FEET	INCHES	SMALL FRAME	MEDIUM FRAME	LARGE FRAME	FEET	INCHES	SMALL FRAME	MEDIUM FRAME	LARGE FRAME
5	2	128-134	131-141	138-150	4	10	102-111	109-121	118-131
5	3	130-136	133-143	140-153	4	11	102-111	111-123	120-134
5	4	132-138	135-145	142-156	5	0	103-113	113-126	122-137
5	5	134-140	137-148	144-160	5	1	104-115	115-129	125-140
5	6	136-142	139-151	146-164	5	2	106-118	118-132	128-143
5	7	138-145	142-154	149-168	5	3	108-121	121-135	131-147
5	8	140-148	145-157	152-172	5	4	111-124	124-138	134-151
5	9	142-151	148-160	155-176	5	5	114-127	127-141	137-155
5	10	144-154	151-163	158-180	5	6	117-130	130-144	140-159
5	11	146-157	154-166	161-184	5	7	120-133	133-147	143-163
6	0	149-160	157-170	164-188	5	8	123-136	136-150	146-167
6	1	152-164	160-174	168-192	5	9	126-139	139-153	149-170
6	2	155-168	164-178	172-197	5	10	129-142	142-156	152-173
6	3	158-172	167-182	176-207	5	11	132-145	145-159	155-176
6	4	162-176	171-187	181-207	6	0	138-151	148-162	158-179

Courtesy Metropolitan Life Insurance Company: *Statistical bulletin,* New York, 2010, Metropolitan.
*Indoor clothing weighing 5 pounds for men and 3 pounds for women.
†Shoes with 1-inch heels.

TABLE 30-7 Nursing History for Weight Assessment

ASSESSMENT	RATIONALE
Ask about total weight lost or gained; compare with usual weight; note time period for loss (e.g., gradual, sudden, desired, or undesired).	Assessment determines severity of problem and reveals if weight change is related to disease process, change in eating pattern, or pregnancy.
If weight loss desired, ask about eating habits, diet plan followed, food preparation, calorie intake, appetite, exercise pattern, support group participation, weight goal.	Assessment helps to determine appropriateness of diet plan followed.
If weight loss undesired, ask about anorexia; vomiting; diarrhea; thirst; frequent urination; and change in lifestyle, activity, and stress levels.	Assessment focuses on problems that cause weight loss (e.g., gastrointestinal problems).
Assess if patient has noted changes in social aspects of eating: more meals in restaurants, rushing to eat meals, stress at work, or skipping meals.	Lifestyle changes sometimes contribute to weight changes.
Assess if patient takes chemotherapy, diuretics, insulin, fluoxetine, prescription and nonprescription appetite suppressants, laxatives, oral hypoglycemics, or herbal supplements (weight loss); steroids, oral contraceptives, antidepressants, insulin (weight gain).	Weight gain or loss is a side effect of these medications.
Assess for preoccupation with body weight or body shape such as fasting, never feeling thin enough, unusually strict caloric intake or restrictions, laxative abuse, induced vomiting, amenorrhea, excessive exercise, alcohol intake.	Excesses indicate an eating disorder.

nutrition and hydration become goals of therapy if there is an alteration in the integumentary status (see Chapter 44).

Every patient has a risk for skin impairment during administration of care in a hospital setting. Risk increases if there is pressure against the skin when the patient is immobile, from reactions to various medications used in treatment, and from moisture if the patient is incontinent. At high risk are patients who are neurologically impaired or chronically ill or have had orthopedic or vascular injuries. Also at higher risk are patients with diminished mental status, poor tissue oxygenation, low cardiac output, or inadequate nutrition. Patients who are homebound, in nursing homes, or extended care facilities are often at risk for similar problems, depending on their level of mobility and the presence of chronic illness. Routinely assess the skin of all at-risk patients to look for primary or initial lesions that develop. Without proper care primary lesions can deteriorate to become secondary lesions that require

TABLE 30-8 Nursing History for Skin Assessment

ASSESSMENT	RATIONALE
Ask patient about history of changes in skin: dryness, pruritus, sores, rashes, lumps, color, texture, odor, and lesion that does not heal.	Patient is best source to recognize change. Usually skin cancer is first noticed as a localized change in skin color.
Consider if patient has the following history: fair, freckled, ruddy complexion; light-colored hair or eyes; tendency to burn easily.	Characteristics are risk factors for skin cancer.
Determine whether patient works or spends excessive time outside. If so, ask whether patient wears sunscreen and the level of protection.	Exposed areas such as face and arms are more pigmented than rest of body. The American Cancer Society (2011) recommends use of sunscreen.
Determine whether patient has noted lesions, rashes, or bruises.	Most skin changes do not develop suddenly. Change in character of lesion possibly indicates cancer. Bruising indicates trauma or bleeding disorder.
Question patient about frequency of bathing and type of soap used.	Excessive bathing and use of harsh soaps cause dry skin.
Ask if patient has had recent trauma to skin.	Some injuries cause bruising and changes in skin texture.
Determine whether patient has history of allergies.	Skin rashes commonly occur from allergies.
Ask if patient uses topical medications or home remedies on skin.	Incorrect use of topical agents causes inflammation or irritation.
Ask if patient goes to tanning parlors, uses sunlamps, or takes tanning pills.	Overexposure of skin to these irritants can cause skin cancer.
Ask if patient has family history of serious skin disorders such as skin cancer or psoriasis.	Family history can reveal information about patient's condition.
Determine if patient works with creosote, coal, tar, petroleum products, arsenic compounds, or radium.	Exposure to these agents creates risk for skin cancer.

more extensive nursing care. For example, the development of a pressure ulcer lengthens a hospital stay unless it is prevented or discovered and treated early (see Chapter 48).

Adequate lighting is required when assessing the skin. Daylight is the best choice to identify variations in skin color, especially for detecting skin changes in dark-skinned patients. When sunlight is not available, fluorescent lighting is the next best choice. Room temperature also affects skin assessment. A room that is too warm causes superficial vasodilation, resulting in increased redness of the skin. A cool environment causes the sensitive patient to develop cyanosis around the lips and nail beds (Seidel et al., 2011).

Although you inspect the skin over each part of the body during an examination, it is helpful to make a brief but careful overall visual sweep of the entire body. This approach provides a good idea of the distribution and extent of any lesions and the overall symmetry of skin color. Inspect all skin surfaces, making a point to do so when examining other body systems. Often overlooked, inspection of the feet is absolutely essential for patients with poor circulation or diabetes. If any abnormalities are found during an examination, palpate the involved areas. Use disposable gloves for palpation if open, moist, or draining lesions are present.

Throughout the examination remain alert for skin odors. White and black adolescents and adults ordinarily have body odor because they have a greater number of functioning apocrine glands. In contrast, Asians and Native Americans/American Indians often do not (Seidel et al., 2011). Fig. 30-4 illustrates a normal cross-section of the skin.

Color. Skin color varies from body part to body part and from person to person. Despite individual variations, it is usually uniform over the body. Table 30-9 lists common variations. Normal skin pigmentation ranges in tone from ivory or light pink to ruddy pink in light skin and from light to deep brown or olive in dark skin. In older adults **pigmentation** increases unevenly, causing discolored skin. While inspecting the skin be aware that cosmetics or tanning agents sometimes mask normal skin color.

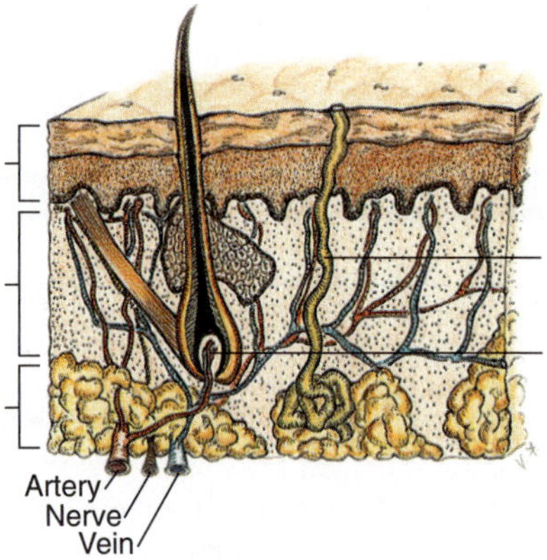

FIG. 30-4 A cross-section of the skin reveals three layers: epidermis, dermis, and subcutaneous fatty tissues.

The assessment of color first involves areas of the skin not exposed to the sun such as the palms of the hands. Note if the skin is unusually pale or dark. Areas exposed to the sun such as the face and arms are darker. It is more difficult to note changes such as pallor or cyanosis in patients with dark skin. Usually color hues are most evident in the palms, soles of the feet, lips, tongue, and nail beds. Areas of increased color (hyperpigmentation) and decreased color (hypopigmentation) are common. Skin creases and folds are darker than the rest of the body in the dark-skinned patient.

Inspect sites where abnormalities are more easily identified. For example, pallor is more evident in the face, buccal (mouth) mucosa, conjunctiva, and nail beds. Observe for **cyanosis** (bluish discoloration) in the lips, nail beds, palpebral conjunctivae, and palms. In recognizing pallor in the dark-skinned patient, observe that normal brown skin appears to be yellow-brown and normal black skin appears to be ashen gray. Also assess the lips, nail beds, and mucous membranes for generalized pallor; if pallor is present, the mucous

TABLE 30-9 **Skin Color Variations**

COLOR	CONDITION	CAUSES	ASSESSMENT LOCATIONS
Bluish (cyanosis)	Increased amount of deoxygenated hemoglobin (associated with hypoxia)	Heart or lung disease, cold environment	Nail beds, lips, mouth, skin (severe cases)
Pallor (decrease in color)	Reduced amount of oxyhemoglobin Reduced visibility of oxyhemoglobin resulting from decreased blood flow	Anemia Shock	Face, conjunctivae, nail beds, palms of hands Skin, nail beds, conjunctivae, lips
Loss of pigmentation	Vitiligo	Congenital or autoimmune condition causing lack of pigment	Patchy areas on skin over face, hands, arms
Yellow-orange (jaundice)	Increased deposit of bilirubin in tissues	Liver disease, destruction of red blood cells	Sclera, mucous membranes, skin
Red (erythema)	Increased visibility of oxyhemoglobin caused by dilation or increased blood flow	Fever, direct trauma, blushing, alcohol intake	Face, area of trauma, sacrum, shoulders, other common sites for pressure ulcers
Tan-brown	Increased amount of melanin	Suntan, pregnancy	Areas exposed to sun: face, arms, areolas, nipples

membranes are ashen gray. Assessment of cyanosis in the dark-skinned patient requires observing areas where pigmentation occurs the least (conjunctiva, sclera, buccal mucosa, tongue, lips, nail beds, and palms and soles). In addition, verify these findings with clinical manifestations (Seidel et al., 2011).

The best site to inspect for **jaundice** (yellow-orange discoloration) is on the patient's sclera. You can see normal reactive hyperemia, or redness, most often in regions exposed to pressure such as the sacrum, heels, and greater trochanter. Inspect for any patches or areas of skin color variation. Localized skin changes such as pallor or **erythema** (red discoloration) indicate circulatory changes. For example, an area of erythema is caused by localized vasodilation resulting from a sunburn, inflammation, or fever. It is difficult to observe erythema in the dark-skinned patient; thus palpate the area for heat and warmth to note the presence of skin inflammation. Compare the area with a different part of the skin to detect a difference in temperature. An area of an extremity that appears unusually pale results from arterial occlusion or edema. Be sure to ask if the patient has noticed any changes in skin coloring.

There is also a pattern of findings associated with patients who are chemically dependent or intravenous (IV) drug abusers (Table 30-10). It is sometimes difficult to recognize signs and symptoms through an isolated examination. A patient who takes repeated IV injections has edematous, reddened, and warm areas along the arms and legs. This pattern suggests recent injections. Evidence of old injection sites appears as hyperpigmented and shiny or scarred areas.

Moisture. The hydration of skin and mucous membranes helps to reveal body fluid imbalances, changes in the environment of the skin, and regulation of body temperature. Moisture refers to wetness and oiliness. The skin is normally smooth and dry. Skinfolds such as the axillae are normally moist. Minimal perspiration or oiliness is often present (Seidel et al., 2011). Increased perspiration can be associated with activity, exposure to warm environments, obesity, anxiety, or excitement. Use ungloved fingertips to palpate skin surfaces. Observe for dullness, dryness, crusting, and flaking that resembles dandruff when the skin surface is lightly rubbed. Excessively dry skin is common in older adults and persons who use excessive amounts of soap during bathing (Meiner, 2011). Other factors causing dry skin include lack of humidity, exposure to sun, smoking, stress, excessive perspiration, and dehydration. Excessive dryness worsens existing skin conditions such as eczema and dermatitis.

TABLE 30-10 **Physical Findings of the Skin Indicative of Substance Abuse**

SKIN FINDING	COMMONLY ASSOCIATED DRUG
Diaphoresis	Sedative hypnotic (including alcohol)
Spider angiomas	Alcohol, stimulants
Burns (especially fingers)	Alcohol
Needle marks	Opioids
Contusion, abrasions, cuts, scars	Alcohol, other sedative hypnotics, intravenous (IV) opioids
"Homemade" tattoos	Cocaine, IV opioids (prevents detection of injection sites)
Vasculitis	Cocaine
Red, dry skin	Phencyclidine (PCP)

Data from Brewer JD et al: Cocaine abuse: dermatologic manifestations and therapeutic approaches, *J Am Acad Dermatol* 59:483, 2008; McKenry L et al: *Mosby's pharmacology in nursing*, ed 22, St Louis, 2006, Mosby; and Smith DE, Seymour RB: *Clinician's guide to substance abuse*, New York, 2001, McGraw-Hill.

Temperature. The temperature of the skin depends on the amount of blood circulating through the dermis. Increased or decreased skin temperature indicates an increase or decrease in blood flow. An increase in skin temperature often accompanies localized erythema or redness of the skin. A reduction in skin temperature often accompanies pallor and reflects a decrease in blood flow. It is important to remember that a cold exam room can cause changes in the patient's skin temperature and color.

Accurately assess temperature by palpating the skin with the dorsum or back of the hand. Compare symmetrical body parts. Normally the skin temperature is warm. Sometimes it is the same throughout the body, and other times it varies in one area. Always assess skin temperature for patients at risk of having impaired circulation such as after a cast application or vascular surgery. You can identify a stage I pressure ulcer early by noting warmth over an area of erythema on the skin (see Chapter 48).

Texture. Texture refers to the character of the surface of the skin and how the deeper layers feel. By palpating lightly with the fingertips, you determine whether the patient's skin is smooth or rough, thin or thick, tight or supple, and **indurated** (hardened) or soft. The texture of the skin is normally smooth, soft, even, and flexible in children and adults. However, the texture is usually not uniform throughout, with thicker texture over the palms of the hand and soles of the feet. In older adults the skin becomes wrinkled and leathery because of a decrease in collagen, subcutaneous fat, and sweat glands.

Localized skin changes result from trauma, surgical wounds, or lesions. When there are irregularities in texture such as scars or indurations, ask the patient about recent injury to the skin. Deeper palpation sometimes reveals irregularities such as tenderness or localized areas of induration, which can be caused by repeated injections.

Turgor. **Turgor** refers to the elasticity of the skin. Normally the skin loses its elasticity with age, but fluid balance can also affect skin turgor. Edema or dehydration diminishes turgor. To assess skin turgor, grasp a fold of skin on the back of the forearm or sternal area with the fingertips and release (Fig. 30-5). Since the skin on the back of the hand is normally loose and thin, turgor is not reliably assessed at that site (Seidel et al., 2011). Normally the skin lifts easily and falls immediately back to its resting position. When turgor is poor, it stays pinched and shows tenting. Evaluate the ease with which the skin moves and the speed at which it returns to its resting state. Failure of the skin to reassume its normal contour or shape indicates dehydration. The patient with poor skin turgor does not have resilience to the normal wear and tear on the skin, and a decrease in turgor predisposes the patient to skin breakdown.

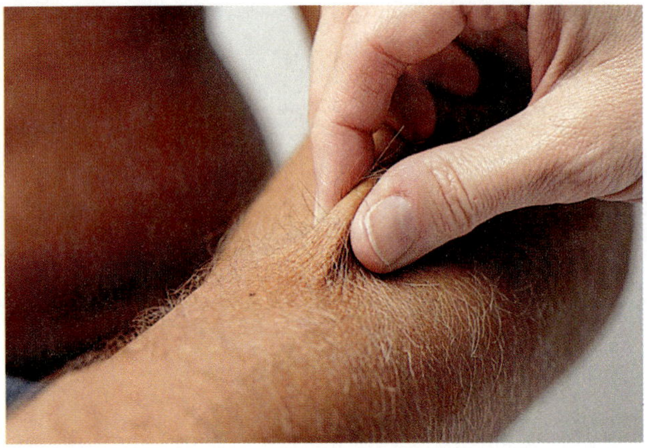

FIG. 30-5 Assessment for skin turgor. (From Seidel HM et al: *Mosby's guide to physical examination,* ed 7, St Louis, 2011, Mosby.)

Vascularity. The circulation of the skin affects color in localized areas and leads to the appearance of superficial blood vessels. Vascularity occurs in localized pressure areas when patients remain in one position. Vascularity appears reddened, pink or pale (see Chapter 48). With aging, capillaries become fragile and more easily injured. **Petechiae** are nonblanching, pinpoint-size, red or purple spots on the skin caused by small hemorrhages in the skin layers. Many petechiae have no known cause, but some may indicate serious blood-clotting disorders, drug reactions, or liver disease.

Edema. Areas of the skin become swollen or edematous from a buildup of fluid in the tissues. Direct trauma and impairment of venous return are two common causes of **edema.** Inspect edematous areas for location, color, and shape. The formation of edema separates the surface of the skin from the pigmented and vascular layers, masking skin color. Edematous skin also appears stretched and shiny. Palpate edematous areas to determine mobility, consistency, and tenderness. When pressure from the examiner's fingers leaves an indentation in the edematous area, it is called *pitting edema.* To assess the degree of pitting edema, press the edematous area firmly with the thumb for several seconds and release. The depth of pitting, recorded in millimeters, determines the degree of edema (Seidel et al., 2011). For example, 1+ edema equals a 2-mm depth, 2+ edema equals a 4-mm depth, 3+ equals 6 mm, and 4+ equals 8 mm (Fig. 30-6).

Lesions. The term *lesion* refers broadly to any unusual finding of the skin surface. Normally the skin is free of lesions, except for common freckles or age-related changes such as skin tags, senile keratosis (thickening of skin), cherry angiomas (ruby red papules), and atrophic warts. Lesions that are primary occur as an initial spontaneous sign of a pathological process such as with an insect bite. Secondary lesions result from later formation or trauma to a primary lesion such as occurs with a pressure ulcer. When you find a lesion, collect standard information about its color, location, texture, size, shape, type, grouping (clustered or linear), and distribution (localized or generalized). Next observe for any exudate, odor, amount, and consistency. Measure the size of the lesion in centimeters by using a small, clear, flexible ruler. Measure each lesion for height, width, and depth.

Palpation helps determine the mobility, contour (flat, raised, or depressed), and consistency (soft or indurated) of a lesion. Certain types of lesions present characteristic patterns. For example, a tumor is usually an elevated, solid lesion larger than 2 cm. Primary

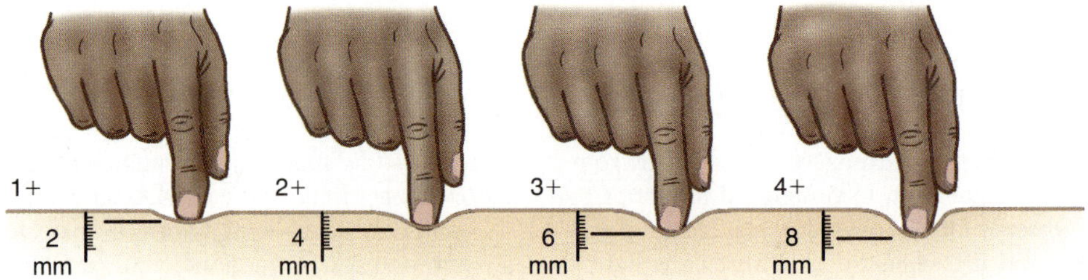

FIG. 30-6 Assessing for pitting edema. (From Seidel HM et al: *Mosby's guide to physical examination,* ed 7, St Louis, 2011, Mosby.)

lesions such as macules and nodules come from some stimulus to the skin (Box 30-6). Secondary lesions such as ulcers occur as alterations in primary lesions. After you identify a lesion, closely inspect it in good lighting. Palpate gently, covering the entire area of the lesion. If it is moist or draining fluid, wear gloves during palpation and pay attention to whether or not the patient identifies any areas of tenderness.

Skin (cutaneous) malignancies are the most common neoplasms in patients. For this reason the examiner should incorporate a thorough skin assessment on all patients. Cancerous lesions have distinct features and over time undergo changes in color and size (Box 30-7). Basal cell carcinoma is most common in sun-exposed areas and frequently occurs with a history of sun-damaged skin; it almost never spreads to other parts of the body. Squamous cell carcinoma is more serious than basal cell and develops on the outer layers of sun-exposed skin; these cells may travel to lymph nodes and throughout the body. Malignant melanoma, a skin cancer that develops from melanocytes, begins as a mole or other area that has changed in appearance and is usually located on normal skin; in African Americans (more than in other races), it can also appear under fingernails or on the palms of the hands and soles of the feet. Use the *ABCD* mnemonic to assess the skin for any type of carcinoma (ACS, 2011):

- *A*symmetry—look for an uneven shape
- *B*order irregularity—look for edges that are blurred, notched, or ragged
- *C*olor—look for pigmentation that is not uniform; variegated areas of blue, black, and brown and areas of pink, white, gray, blue, or red are abnormal
- *D*iameter—look for areas greater than the size of a typical pencil eraser

Report abnormal lesions to the health care provider for further examination. Since ultraviolet light of the sun or tanning beds increase the risk for development of skin cancers, teach patients about the risks that exist. They should be taught how to perform a skin self-examination, using the best-quality teaching materials (Box 30-8).

Hair and Scalp

Two types of hair cover the body: soft, fine, vellus hair, which covers the body; and coarse, long, thick terminal hair, which is easily visible on the scalp, axillae, and pubic areas and in the beard on men. First,

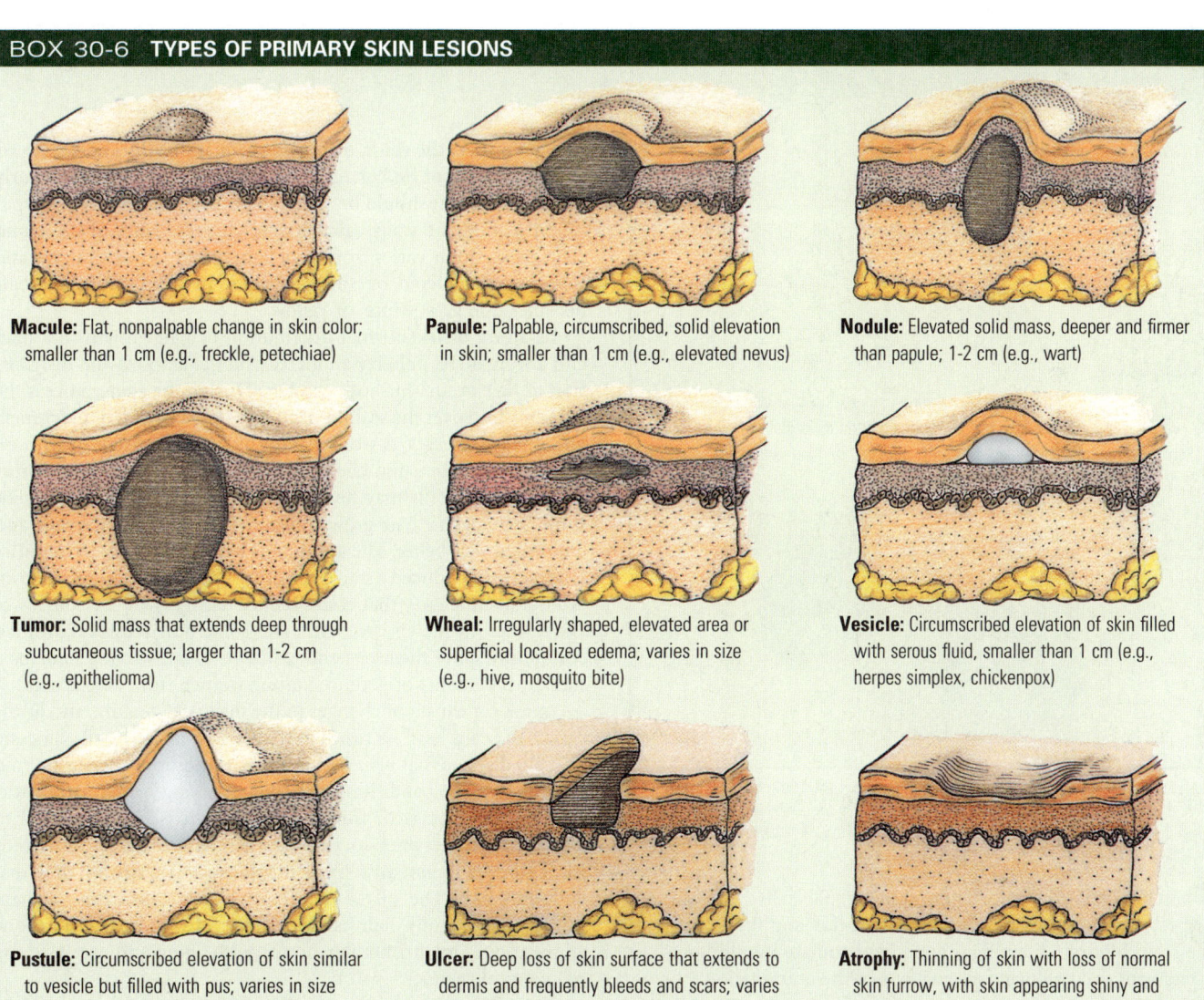

BOX 30-6 TYPES OF PRIMARY SKIN LESIONS

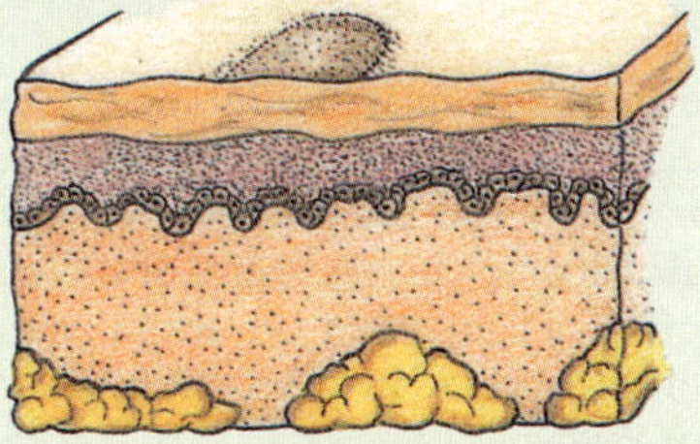

Macule: Flat, nonpalpable change in skin color; smaller than 1 cm (e.g., freckle, petechiae)

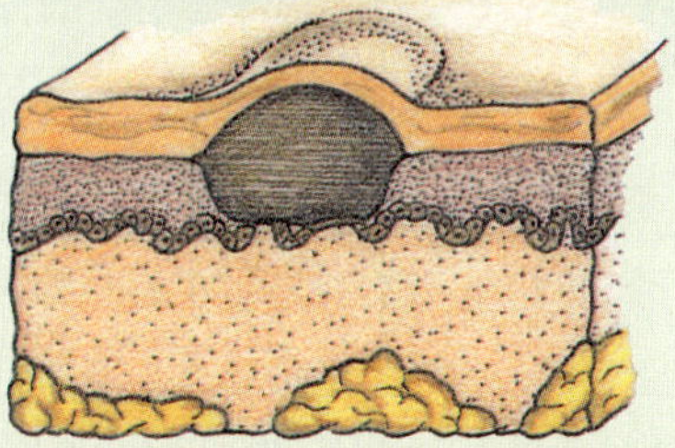

Papule: Palpable, circumscribed, solid elevation in skin; smaller than 1 cm (e.g., elevated nevus)

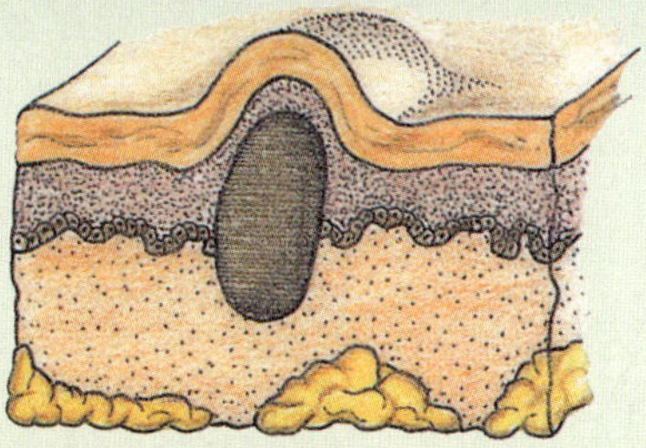

Nodule: Elevated solid mass, deeper and firmer than papule; 1-2 cm (e.g., wart)

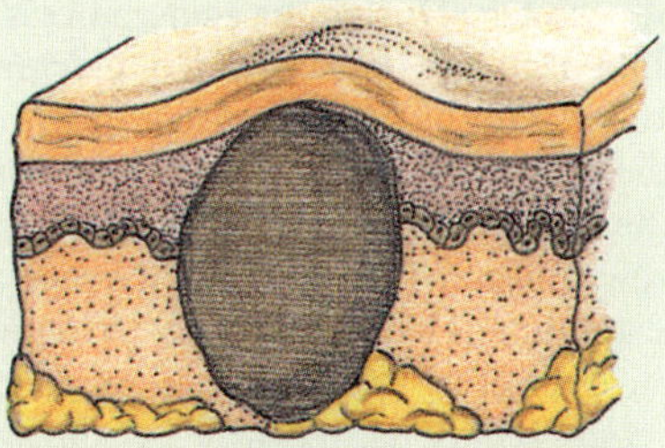

Tumor: Solid mass that extends deep through subcutaneous tissue; larger than 1-2 cm (e.g., epithelioma)

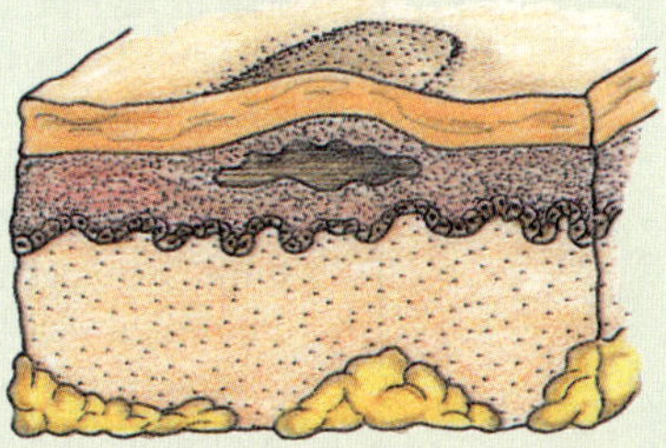

Wheal: Irregularly shaped, elevated area or superficial localized edema; varies in size (e.g., hive, mosquito bite)

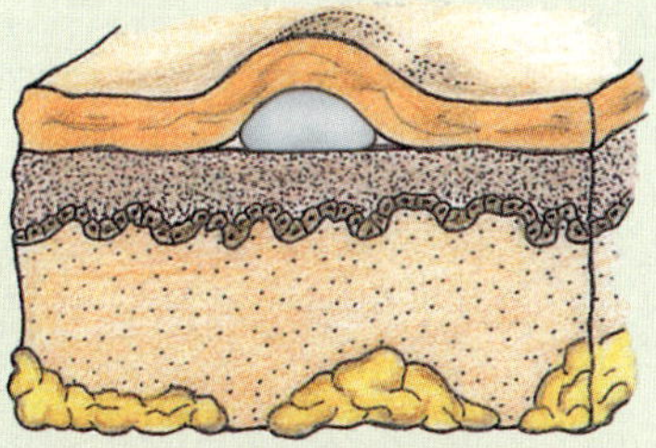

Vesicle: Circumscribed elevation of skin filled with serous fluid, smaller than 1 cm (e.g., herpes simplex, chickenpox)

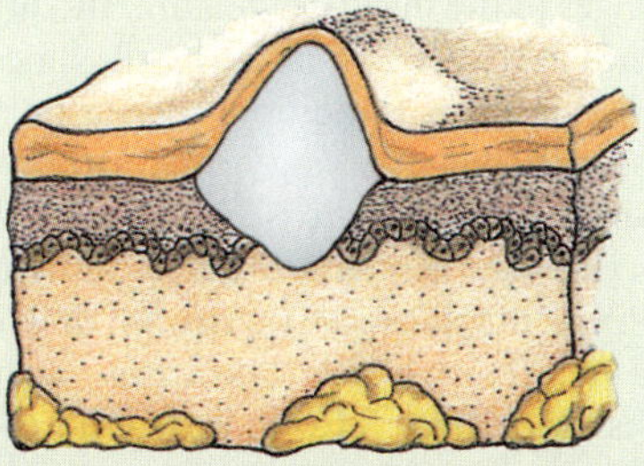

Pustule: Circumscribed elevation of skin similar to vesicle but filled with pus; varies in size (e.g., acne, staphylococcal infection)

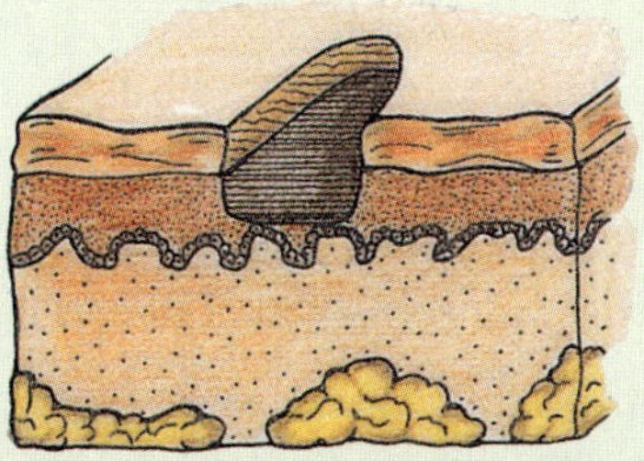

Ulcer: Deep loss of skin surface that extends to dermis and frequently bleeds and scars; varies in size (e.g., venous stasis ulcer)

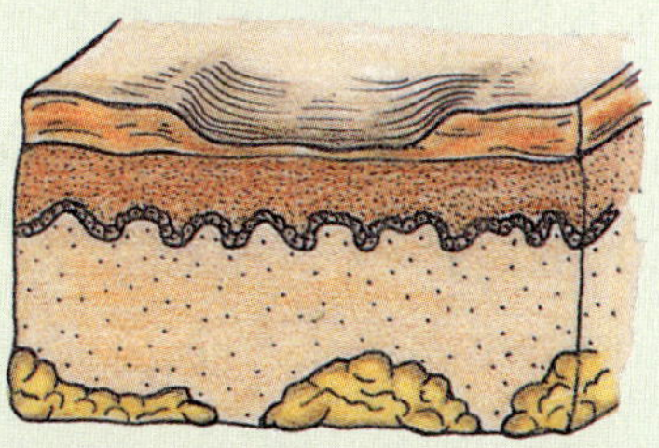

Atrophy: Thinning of skin with loss of normal skin furrow, with skin appearing shiny and translucent; varies in size (e.g., arterial insufficiency)

BOX 30-7 SKIN MALIGNANCIES

Basal Cell Carcinoma

0.5- to 1-cm crusted lesion that is flat or raised and has a rolled, somewhat scaly border

Frequently appearance of underlying, widely dilated blood vessels within the lesion

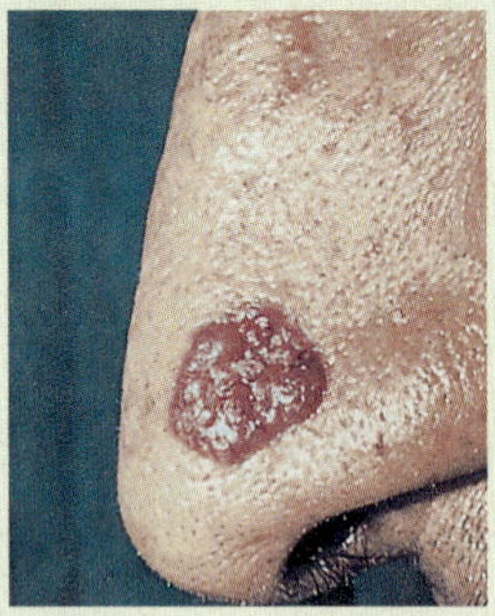

Squamous Cell Carcinoma

Occurs more often on mucosal surfaces and nonexposed areas of skin than basal cell

0.5- to 1.5-cm scaly lesion sometimes ulcerated or crusted; appears frequently and grows more rapidly than basal cell

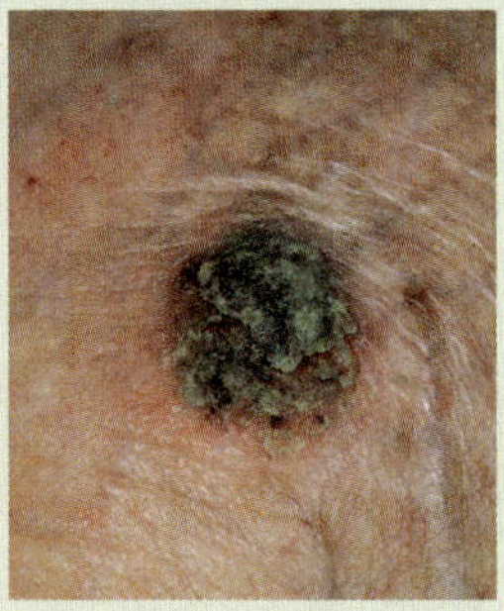

Melanoma

0.5- to 1-cm brown, flat lesion; appears on sun-exposed or nonexposed skin; variegated pigmentation, irregular borders, and indistinct margins

Ulceration, recent growth, or recent changes in long-standing mole are ominous signs

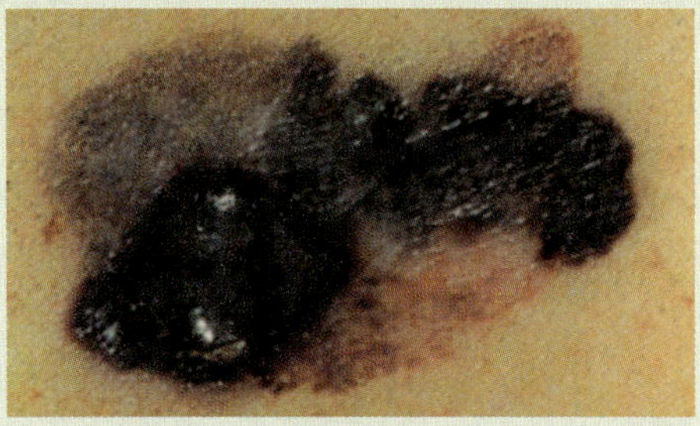

Illustrations from Belcher AE: *Cancer nursing*, St Louis, 1992, Mosby; Habif TP: *Clinical dermatology: a color guide to diagnosis and therapy*, ed 3, St Louis, 1996, Mosby; and Zitelli B, Davis H: *Atlas of pediatric physical diagnosis*, ed 2, St Louis, 1991, Mosby.

obtain health history information listed in Table 30-11. Prepare to inspect the condition and distribution of hair and the integrity of the scalp by first obtaining a good light source. In addition, hair assessment occurs during all portions of the examination.

Inspection. During inspection explain that it is necessary to separate parts of the hair to detect abnormalities. Wear a pair of clean gloves if open lesions or lice are noted.

TABLE 30-11 Nursing History for Hair and Scalp Assessment

ASSESSMENT	RATIONALE
Ask patient if he or she is wearing a wig or hairpiece and ask him or her to remove it.	Wigs or hairpieces interfere with inspection of hair and scalp. (Patient sometimes requests to omit this part of examination.)
Determine if patient has noted change in growth or loss of hair; change in texture or color.	Change often occurs slowly over time.
Identify type of hair care products used for grooming.	Excessive use of chemical agents and burning of hair causes drying and brittleness.
Determine if patient has recently had chemotherapy (drugs that cause hair loss) or taken a vasodilator (minoxidil) for hair growth.	Chemotherapeutic agents kill cells that rapidly multiply such as tumor and normal hair cells. Minoxidil causes excessive hair growth.
Has patient noted changes in diet or appetite?	Nutrition influences condition of hair.

First inspect the color, distribution, quantity, thickness, texture, and lubrication of body hair. Scalp hair is coarse or fine and curly or straight; and it should be shiny, smooth, and pliant. While separating sections of scalp hair, observe characteristics of color and coarseness. Color varies from very light blond to black to gray and is sometimes altered by rinses or dyes. In older adults the hair becomes dull gray, white, or yellow.

Be aware of the normal distribution of hair growth in a man and a woman. At puberty an increase in the amount and distribution of hair occurs for both genders. During the aging process the hair may thin over the scalp, axillae, and pubic areas. For older men, facial hair decreases. A woman with hirsutism has hair growth on the upper lip, chin, and cheeks, with vellus hair becoming coarser over the body. This may be related to an endocrine disorder. For some a change in hair growth negatively affects body image and emotional well-being. The amount of hair covering the extremities is sometimes reduced as a result of aging, or it could result from arterial insufficiency that could reduce hair growth over the lower extremities. In the United States and some other cultures, women commonly shave their legs and axilla, although shaving remains a matter of personal preference among women from all cultures.

Assess for causes of changes in the thickness, texture, and lubrication of scalp hair. At times these are a result of febrile illnesses or scalp diseases that result in hair loss. Conditions such as thyroid disease alter the condition of the hair, making it fine and brittle. Hair loss (alopecia) or thinning of the hair is usually related to genetic tendencies or endocrine disorders such as diabetes, thyroiditis, and even menopause. Poor nutrition causes stringy, dull, dry, and thin hair. The oil of sebaceous glands lubricates the hair, but excessively oily hair is associated with androgen hormone stimulation. Dry, brittle hair occurs with aging and excessive use of chemical agents.

Normally the scalp is smooth and inelastic, with even coloration. Carefully separate strands of hair and thoroughly inspect the scalp for lesions, which are not easy to notice in thick hair. Note

BOX 30-8 EVIDENCE-BASED PRACTICE

Skin Assessment

PICO Question: Is skin cancer detected early in patients at high risk for melanoma when they undergo annual full body skin examinations by health providers versus being taught self-examination with periodic check-ups?

Evidence Summary

The rates of melanoma and nonmelanoma skin cancers have been steadily increasing for the past 30 years, probably a result of increased cumulative ultraviolet exposure (ACS, 2011; Ridky, 2007). By identifying, treating, and removing nonmelanoma types early, the patient avoids repeated or extensive surgery (American Cancer Society [ACS], 2011).

In contrast, melanoma is the leading cause of death from skin cancer. Melanoma is most treatable when it is found in its thin, early stage, although patients who experience melanoma are at risk for future recurrence (Wolff et al., 2009). If the cancer spreads beyond the lymph nodes to body organs, the disease is fatal.

The ACS (2011) recommends that people engage in regular skin self-examination (SSE) for early identification and treatment. Comprehensive SSE may lead to earlier diagnosis of new or recurrent disease. Women who have positive body image and older women are more likely to perform skin SSE (Chait et al., 2009). Whole body screening by a health care provider is often recommended.

According to the U.S. Preventive Services Task Force, evidence showing that there is a benefit to whole body screening as a way to effectively reduce morbidity and mortality from melanoma is lacking (Wolff et al., 2009). The National Guideline Clearinghouse suggests that full-body screening may be beneficial for people who have a high risk because a first-degree relative had melanoma or because there is a personal history of skin cancer, organ transplantation, or long-term treatment with ultraviolet light for psoriasis (Marret et al., 2007). Further study needs to be done to fully know whether the cost, time, and accuracy of skin cancer screening warrant recommending it for the general public.

Application to Nursing Practice

- Instruct patient to conduct a complete monthly SSE, noting moles, blemishes, and birthmarks. Instruct to inspect all skin surfaces:
    - Perform the examination after a bath or shower, including a head-to-toe check.
    - Use a well-lit room and mirrors to examine all skin surfaces; enlisting a partner's help significantly increases the chance that the self-examination is thorough (Loescher et al., 2006).
- Instruct patient to report to their health care provider any change in size or color of moles or skin lesions or a sore that does not heal, starts to bleed, ooze or feel different (swollen, hard, lumpy, itchy, or tender to the touch). Especially instruct older adults, who tend to have delayed wound healing.
- Use supportive communication (Glanz et al., 2010, Mujumdar et al., 2009) to inform your patients of ways to prevent skin cancer by avoiding overexposure to the sun.
- Wear wide-brimmed hats and long sleeves.
- Apply broad-spectrum sunscreens with skin protection factor (SPF) of 15 or greater to protect against ultraviolet B (UVB) and ultraviolet A (UVA) rays approximately 15 minutes before going into the sun and after swimming or perspiring.
- Avoid tanning under the direct sun at midday (10 AM to 4 PM).
- Do not use indoor sunlamps, tanning parlors, or tanning pills.
- Inform patients who are on medications that make the skin more sensitive to the sun (e.g., oral contraceptives, antibiotics, antiinflammatories, antihypertensives, immunosuppressives) to take extra precautions when spending time in the sun.
- Inform patients to protect their children from the sun. Severe sunburns in childhood greatly increase melanoma risk later in life (ACS, 2011).
- Encourage all women to perform SSE, show respect for those who have a poorer body image as it relates to body mass index, and encourage and support feelings surrounding self-inspection (Chait et al., 2009).
- Teach patients to avoid very dry skin by avoiding hot water, harsh soaps, and drying agents such as rubbing alcohol; using a super-fatted (Dove) soap; and patting, not rubbing, the skin after bathing.
- Apply moisturizers to the skin regularly to reduce itching and drying and wear cotton clothing.

the characteristics of any scalp lesion. For lumps or bruises, ask if the patient has experienced recent head trauma. Moles on the scalp are common, but they can bleed as a result of vigorous combing or brushing. Dandruff or psoriasis frequently causes scaliness or dryness of the scalp.

Careful inspection of hair follicles on the scalp and pubic areas can reveal lice or other parasites. The three types of lice are *Pediculus humanus capitis* (head lice), *Pediculus humanus corporis* (body lice), and *Pediculus pubis* (crab lice). The presence of lice does not mean a person practices poor hygiene. Lice spread easily, especially among children who play closely together. Head and crab lice attach their eggs to hair. The tiny eggs look like oval particles of dandruff, although the lice themselves are difficult to see (Fig. 30-7). Head and body lice are very small with grayish-white bodies, whereas crab lice have red legs. To better identify infestations, observe for small, red, pustular eruptions in the hair follicles and areas where skin surfaces meet, such as behind the ears and in the groin. A person often has intense itching of the scalp, especially on the back of the head or neck. Combing with a fine-tooth comb reveals the small oval-shaped lice; discovery of lice requires immediate treatment. Teach the patient to perform best hair and scalp hygiene practices (Box 30-9).

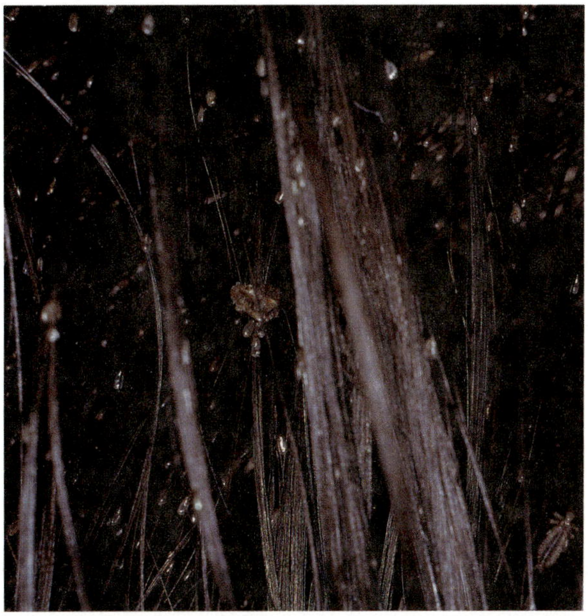

FIG. 30-7 Head lice. Numerous white nits attached to hairs. (From Weston WL et al: *Color textbook of pediatric dermatology,* ed 4, St Louis, 2007, Mosby.)

BOX 30-9 PATIENT TEACHING

Hair and Scalp Assessment

Objective

- Patient will perform proper hygiene practices for care of the hair and scalp.

Teaching Strategies

- Instruct patient about basic hygiene practices for hair and scalp care.
- Instruct patients who have head lice to shampoo thoroughly with pediculicide (shampoo available at drugstores) in cold water at a basin or sink. Do not use a tub or shower, where the medication can reach other body parts. Comb thoroughly with a fine-tooth comb (following product directions), and discard comb. *Caution: Do not use products containing Lindane, a toxic ingredient known to cause adverse reactions.* Repeat shampoo treatment 12 to 24 hours later.
- After shampooing, remove any detectable nits or nit cases with tweezers or a metal nit comb. A dilute solution of vinegar and water helps loosen nits.
- Instruct patients and parents about ways to reduce transmission of lice:
  - Do not share hair brushes, combs, hair pieces, hats, bedding, towels, or clothing with someone who has head lice.
  - Vacuum all rugs, car seats, pillows, furniture, and flooring thoroughly and discard vacuum bag.
  - Seal nonwashable items in plastic bags for 14 days if unable to dry-clean or vacuum.
  - Use thorough hand hygiene practices.
  - Launder all clothing, linen, and bedding in hot water and detergent, then dry in a hot dryer for at least 30 minutes. Dry-clean nonwashable items.
  - Do not use insecticide.
  - Instruct patient to notify his or her partner if lice were sexually transmitted.
  - Avoid physical contact with infested individuals and their belongings, especially clothing and bedding.
  - Soak any comb or brush used to remove lice for 15 minutes in very hot ammonia water (1 tsp ammonia to 2 cups hot water) or boiling water for 10 minutes.

Evaluation

- Have patient describe methods used to care for the hair and scalp.
- Have patient explain the steps to take to reduce lice transmission in the home.

Data from Heyman DL, editor: *Control of communicable diseases manual,* Washington, DC, 2009, American Public Health Association; and National Pediculosis Association: *Child care provider's guide to controlling head lice,* 2005, http://www.headlice.org. Accessed September 8, 2011.

TABLE 30-12 Nursing History for Nail Assessment

ASSESSMENT	RATIONALE
Ask if patient has experienced recent trauma or changes in nails (splitting, breaking, discoloration, thickening).	Trauma changes shape and growth of nail. Systemic conditions cause changes in color, growth, and shape.
Has the patient had other symptoms of pain, swelling, presence of systemic disease with fever, or psychological or physical stress?	Alterations sometimes occur slowly over time.
Question patient's nail care practices. Determine if patient has acrylic nails or silk wraps.	Change in nails can be caused by local or systemic problem. Acrylic nails and silk wraps are areas for fungal growth.
Determine if patient has risks for nail or foot problems (e.g., diabetes, peripheral vascular disease, older adulthood, obesity).	Chemical agents cause drying of nails. Improper care damages nails and cuticles. Vascular changes associated with diabetes and peripheral vascular disease reduce blood flow to peripheral tissues; foot lesions and thickened nails are common. Some older adults have trouble performing foot and nail care because of poor vision, lack of coordination, or inability to bend over. Obese patients have difficulty bending.

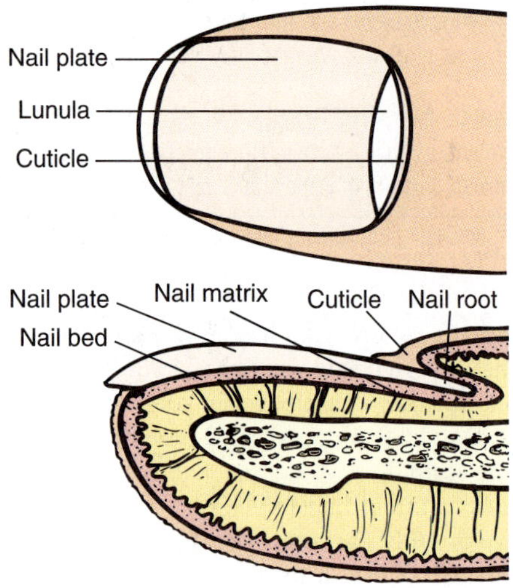

FIG. 30-8 Components of nail unit. (From Lewis SL et al: *Medical-surgical nursing,* ed 8, St Louis, 2011, Mosby.)

Nails

The condition of the nails reflects general health, state of nutrition, a person's occupation, and habits of self-care. Before assessing the nails, gather a brief history (Table 30-12). The most visible portion of the nail is the nail plate, the transparent layer of epithelial cells covering the nail bed (Fig. 30-8). The vascularity of the nail bed creates the underlying color of the nail. The semilunar whitish area at the base of the nail bed is called the *lunula,* from which the nail plate grows.

Inspection and Palpation. Inspect the nail bed for color, length, symmetry, cleanliness, and configuration. The shape and condition of the nails can give clues to pathophysiological problems. Assess the thickness and shape of the nail, the texture of the nail, the angle between the nail and the nail bed, and the condition of the lateral and proximal nail folds around the nail. When inspecting the nails, you gather a sense about the patient's hygiene practices. The nails are normally transparent, smooth, well rounded, and convex, with a nail bed angle of about 160 degrees (Box 30-10). A larger angle and softening of the nail bed indicate chronic oxygenation problems. The surrounding cuticles are smooth, intact, and without inflammation. When you assess for basic care of the nails, you recognize that nail biting, stains, and jagged edges either represent poor nail care or are caused by habits or occupational exposure to grease or dirt. Jagged, bitten, or broken nail edges or cuticles predispose a patient to localized infection.

BOX 30-10 ABNORMALITIES OF THE NAIL BED

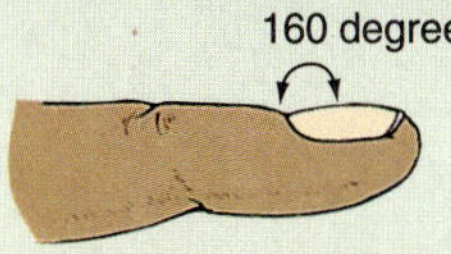

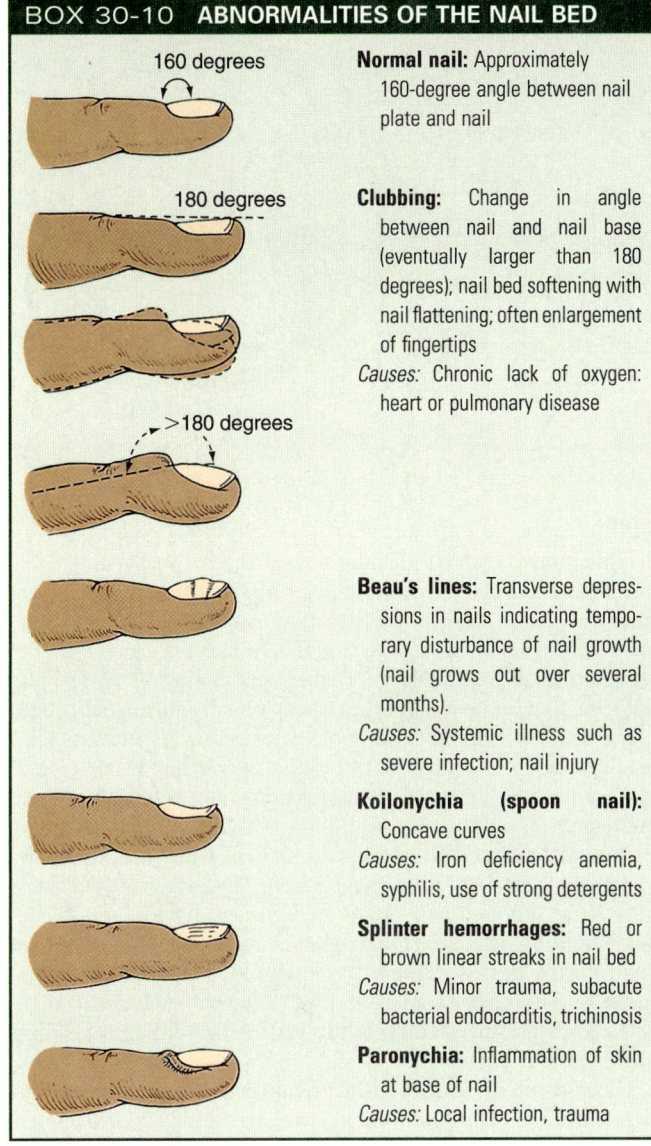

Normal nail: Approximately 160-degree angle between nail plate and nail

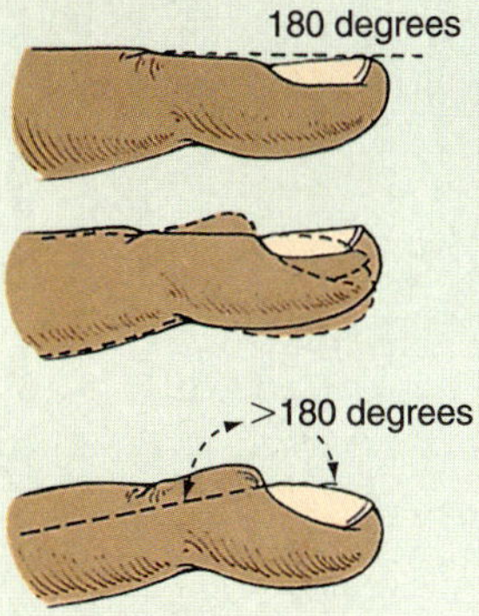

Clubbing: Change in angle between nail and nail base (eventually larger than 180 degrees); nail bed softening with nail flattening; often enlargement of fingertips
Causes: Chronic lack of oxygen: heart or pulmonary disease

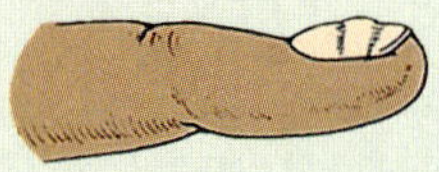

Beau's lines: Transverse depressions in nails indicating temporary disturbance of nail growth (nail grows out over several months).
Causes: Systemic illness such as severe infection; nail injury

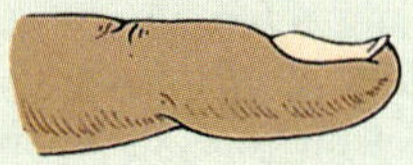

Koilonychia (spoon nail): Concave curves
Causes: Iron deficiency anemia, syphilis, use of strong detergents

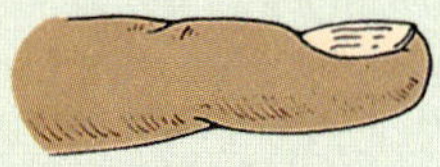

Splinter hemorrhages: Red or brown linear streaks in nail bed
Causes: Minor trauma, subacute bacterial endocarditis, trichinosis

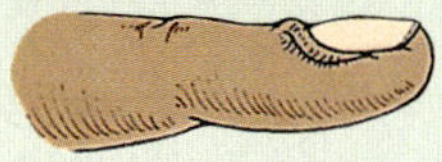

Paronychia: Inflammation of skin at base of nail
Causes: Local infection, trauma

When palpating, expect to find a firm nail base and check for any abnormalities such as erythema or swelling. For patients with impaired circulation, especially observe for early signs of infection or open lesions. To palpate, gently grasp the patient's finger and observe the color of the nail bed. The nail bed and nails appear pink with white nail tips in white patients. In darker-skinned patients the nail beds are darkly pigmented with a blue or reddish hue. A brown or black pigmentation is normal with longitudinal streaks (Fig. 30-9). Trauma, cirrhosis, diabetes mellitus, and hypertension cause splinter hemorrhages. Vitamin, protein, and electrolyte changes cause various lines or bands to form on the nail beds.

Nails normally grow at a constant rate, but direct injury or generalized disease changes growth patterns. With aging the nails of the fingers and toes become harder and thicker. Longitudinal striations develop, and the rate of nail growth slows. Nails become more brittle, dull, and opaque and turn yellow in older adults with insufficient calcium. In addition, the cuticle becomes less thick and wide.

Calluses and corns are commonly found on the toes or fingers. A callus is flat and painless, resulting from a thickening of the epidermis. Friction and pressure from shoes cause corns, usually over bony prominences. During the examination instruct the patient in proper nail care (Box 30-11).

BOX 30-11 PATIENT TEACHING

Nail Assessment

Objective

- Patient will properly care for fingernails, feet, and toenails.

Teaching Strategies

- Instruct patient to cut nails only after soaking them about 10 minutes in warm water. (**Exception:** Patients with diabetes or peripheral vascular disease are warned against soaking nails because this dries out the hands and feet; dry skin leads to infection.)
- Caution patient against over-the-counter preparations to treat corns, calluses, or ingrown toenails.
- Instruct patient to cut nails straight across and even with tops of fingers or toes. If patient has diabetes, tell him or her to file rather than cut nails (see Chapter 39).
- Instruct patient to shape nails with a file or emery board.
- If patient has diabetes:
  - Wash feet daily in warm water and carefully dry them, especially between the toes. Inspect feet each day in good lighting, looking for dry places and cracks in skin. Soften dry feet by applying a cream or lotion such as Nivea, Eucerin, or Alpha Keri.
  - Do not put lotion between toes; moisture between toes allows microorganisms to grow, leading to infections.
  - Caution patient against using sharp objects to poke or dig under toenail or around the cuticle.
  - Have patient see a podiatrist for treatment of ingrown toenails and nails that are thick or tend to split.

Evaluation

- Inspect nails during the next home visit.
- Have patient explain steps to take to avoid injury.

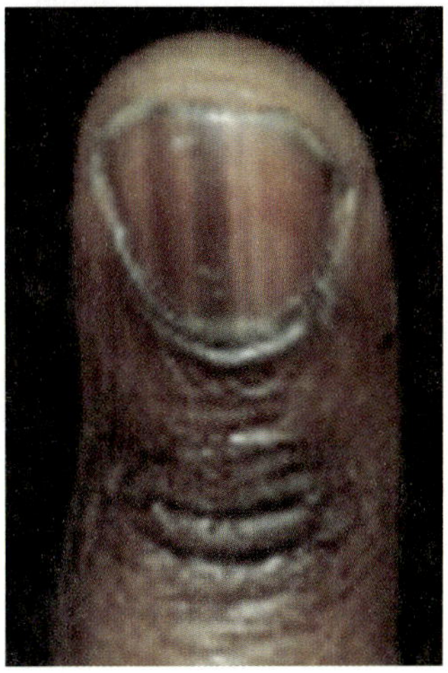

FIG. 30-9 Pigmented bands in nail of patient with dark skin. (From Habif TP: *Clinical dermatology: a color guide to diagnosis and therapy,* ed 5, St Louis, 2010, Mosby.)

HEAD AND NECK

An examination of the head and neck includes assessment of the head, eyes, ears, nose, mouth, pharynx, and neck (lymph nodes, carotid arteries, thyroid gland, and trachea). During assessment of

TABLE 30-13 Nursing History for Head Assessment

ASSESSMENT	RATIONALE
Determine if patient experienced recent head trauma. If so, assess state of consciousness after injury (immediately on return and 5 minutes later), duration of unconsciousness, and predisposing factors (e.g., seizure, poor vision, blackout).	Trauma is major cause for lumps, bumps, cuts, bruises, or deformities of scalp or skull. Loss of consciousness following head injury indicates possible brain injury.
Ask if patient has history of headache; note onset, duration, character, pattern, and associated symptoms.	Character of headache helps to reveal causative factors such as sinus infection, migraine, or neurological disorders.
Determine length of time patient has experienced neurological symptoms.	Duration of signs or symptoms reveals severity of problem.
Review patient's occupational history for use of safety helmets.	Nature of some occupations creates a risk for head injury.
Ask if patient participates in contact sports, cycling, rollerblading, or skateboarding.	These activities require use of safety helmets.

peripheral arteries also assess the carotid arteries. Assessment of the head and neck uses inspection, palpation, and auscultation, with inspection and palpation often used simultaneously.

Head

Inspection and Palpation. The nursing history screens for intracranial injury and local or congenital deformities (Table 30-13). Inspect the patient's head, noting the position, size, shape, and contour. The head is normally held upright and midline to the trunk. Holding it tilted to one side acts as a behavioral indicator of a potential unilateral hearing or visual loss or is a physical indicator of muscle weakness in the neck. A horizontal jerking or bobbing indicates a tremor.

Note the patient's facial features, looking at the eyelids, eyebrows, nasolabial folds, and mouth for shape and symmetry. It is normal for slight asymmetry to exist. If there is facial asymmetry, note if all features on one side of the face are affected or if only a portion of the face is involved. Various neurological disorders (e.g., facial nerve paralysis) affect different nerves that innervate muscles of the face.

Examine the size, shape, and contour of the skull. The skull is generally round with prominences in the frontal area anteriorly and the occipital area posteriorly. Trauma typically causes local skull deformities. In infants a large head results from congenital anomaly or the buildup of cerebrospinal fluid in the ventricles (hydrocephalus). Some adults have enlarged jaws and facial bones resulting from acromegaly, a disorder caused by excessive secretion of growth hormone. Palpate the skull for nodules or masses. Gently rotate the fingertips down the midline of the scalp and along the sides of the head to identify abnormalities. Palpate the temporomandibular joint (TMJ) space bilaterally. Place the fingertips just anterior to the tragus of each ear. The fingertips should slip into the joint space as the patient's mouth opens to gently palpate the joint spaces. Normally the movements should be smooth, although it is not unusual to hear or feel a clicking or snapping in the TMJ (Seidel et al., 2011).

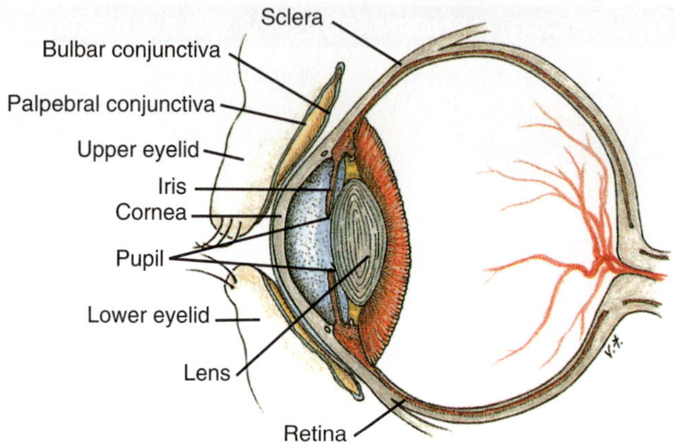

FIG. 30-10 Cross-section of eye.

Eyes

Examination of the eyes includes assessment of visual acuity, visual fields, extraocular movements, and external and internal eye structures. Fig. 30-10 shows a cross-section of the eye. The eye assessment detects visual alterations and determines the general level of assistance that patients require when ambulating or performing self-care activities. Some patients with visual problems also need special aids for reading educational materials or instructions (e.g., medication labels). Table 30-14 reviews the nursing history for an eye examination. Box 30-12 describes common types of visual problems.

Visual Acuity. The assessment of visual acuity (i.e., the ability to see small details) tests central vision. The easiest way to assess near vision is to ask patients to read printed material under adequate lighting. If patients wear glasses, make sure that they wear them during the assessment. Determine the language the patient speaks and his or her reading ability. Asking patients to read aloud helps to determine literacy. If the patient has difficulty reading, move to the next step.

Assessment of distant vision requires using a Snellen chart (paper chart or projection screen). The chart should be well lighted. Test vision without corrective lenses first. Have the patient sit or stand 6.1 m (20 feet) away from the chart and try to read all of the letters beginning at any line with both eyes open. Then have the patient read the line with each eye separately (patient covers the opposite eye with an index card or eye cover to avoid applying pressure to the eye). Note the smallest line for which the patient is able to read all of the letters correctly and record the visual acuity for that line. Repeat the test with the patient wearing corrective lenses. Complete the test rapidly enough so the patient does not memorize the chart (Seidel et al., 2011). If a patient is unable to read, use an *E* chart or one with pictures of familiar objects. Instead of reading letters, patients tell which direction each *E* is pointing or the name of the object.

The Snellen chart has standardized numbers at the end of each line of the chart. The numerator is the number 20, or the distance the patient stands from the chart. The denominator is the distance from which the normal eye is able to read the chart. Normal visual acuity is 20/20. The larger the denominator, the poorer the patient's visual acuity. For example, a value of 20/40 means that the patient, standing 20 feet away, can read a line that a person with normal vision can read from 40 feet away. Record visual acuity for each eye and both eyes, and record whether the test was performed with or without correction (including glasses or contact lenses).

TABLE 30-14 Nursing History for Eye Assessment

ASSESSMENT	RATIONALE
Determine if patient has history of eye disease, (e.g., glaucoma, retinopathy, cataracts), eye trauma, diabetes, hypertension, or eye surgery.	Some diseases or trauma cause risk for partial or complete visual loss. Patient may have had surgery for a visual disorder.
Determine problems that prompted patient to seek health care. Ask patient about eye pain, photophobia (sensitivity to light), burning or itching, excess tearing or crusting, diplopia (double vision) or blurred vision, awareness of a "film" or "curtain" over field of vision, floaters (small, black spots that seem to float across field of vision), flashing lights, or halos around lights.	Common symptoms of eye disease indicate need for health care provider.
Determine whether there is family history of eye disorders or diseases.	Certain eye problems such as glaucoma or retinitis pigmentosa are inherited.
Review patient's occupational history and recreational hobbies. Are safety glasses worn?	Performance of close, intricate work causes eye fatigue. Working with computers causes eye strain. Certain occupational tasks (e.g., working with chemicals) and recreational activities (e.g., fencing, motorcycle riding) place people at risk for eye injury unless they take precautions.
Ask patient if he or she wears glasses or contacts and, if so, how often.	Patients need to wear glasses or contacts during certain portions of examination for accurate assessment.
Determine when patient last visited ophthalmologist or optometrist.	Date of last eye examination reveals level of preventive care patient takes.
Assess medications patient is taking, including eye drops or ointment.	Determines need to assess patient's knowledge of medications. Certain medications cause visual symptoms.

If patients cannot read even the largest letters or figures of a Snellen chart, test their ability to count upraised fingers or distinguish light. Hold a hand 30 cm (1 foot) from the patient's face and have him or her count the upraised fingers. To check light perception shine a penlight into the eye and turn off the light. If the patient notes when the light is turned on or off, light perception is intact.

Assess near vision by asking the patient to read a handheld card containing a vision screening chart. The patient holds the card a comfortable distance (5 to 6 cm [about 12½ to 14 inches]) from the eyes and reads the smallest line possible. This portion of the examination is a good time to discuss the need for routine eye examinations (Box 30-13).

BOX 30-12 COMMON EYE AND VISION PROBLEMS

Hyperopia
Hyperopia is farsightedness, a refractive error in which rays of light enter the eye and focus behind the retina. Persons are able to clearly see distant objects but not close objects.

Myopia
Myopia is nearsightedness, a refractive error in which rays of light enter the eye and focus in front of the retina. Persons are able to clearly see close objects but not distant objects.

Presbyopia
Presbyopia is impaired near vision in middle-age and older adults, caused by loss of elasticity of the lens and associated with the aging process.

Retinopathy
Retinopathy is a noninflammatory eye disorder resulting from changes in retinal blood vessels. It is a leading cause of blindness.

Strabismus
Strabismus is a (congenital) condition in which both eyes do not focus on an object simultaneously; these eyes appear crossed. Impairment of the extraocular muscles or their nerve supply causes strabismus.

Cataracts
A cataract is an increased opacity of the lens, which blocks light rays from entering the eye. Cataracts sometimes develop slowly and progressively after age 35 or suddenly after trauma. Cataracts are one of the most common eye disorders. Most older adults (65 years old and older) have some evidence of visual impairment from cataracts.

Glaucoma
Glaucoma is intraocular structural damage resulting from elevated intraocular pressure. Obstruction of the outflow of aqueous humor causes this. Without treatment the disorder leads to blindness.

Macular Degeneration
Macular degeneration is blurred central vision often occurring suddenly, caused by a progressive degeneration of the center of the retina. It is the most common visual impairment of individuals over age 50 and the most common cause of blindness in older adults. There is no cure.

Extraocular Movements. Six small muscles guide the movement of each eye. Both eyes move parallel to one another in each of the six directions of gaze (Fig. 30-11). To assess extraocular movements the patient sits or stands, and the nurse faces the patient from 60 cm (2 feet) away. The nurse holds a finger at a comfortable distance (15 to 30 cm [6 to 12 inches]) from the patient's eyes. While the patient maintains his or her head in a fixed position facing forward, the nurse directs him or her to follow with the eyes only as the nurse's finger moves to the right, left, and diagonally up and down to the left and right. The nurse moves the finger smoothly and slowly within the normal field of vision.

As the patient gazes in each direction, observe for parallel eye movement, the position of the upper eyelid in relation to the iris, and the presence of abnormal movements. As the eyes move through each direction of gaze, the upper eyelid covers the iris only slightly. Nystagmus, an involuntary, rhythmical oscillation of the eyes, occurs as a result of local injury to eye muscles and supporting structures or a disorder of the cranial nerves innervating the

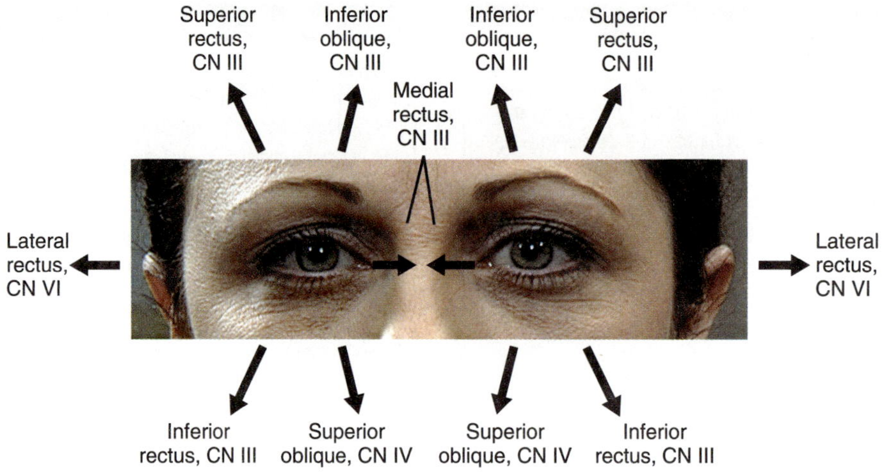

FIG. 30-11 Six directions of gaze. Direct patient to follow finger movement through each gaze. *CN,* Cranial nerve. (From Seidel HM et al: *Mosby's guide to physical examination,* ed 7, St Louis, 2011, Mosby.)

BOX 30-13 PATIENT TEACHING

Eye Assessment

Objective

- Patient will follow recommendations for regular eye examinations and prevention of injury.

Teaching Strategies

- Explain recommended frequency for eye testing with a Snellen chart and examination (see Table 30-3).
- Describe the typical symptoms of eye disease.
- Instruct older adult to take the following precautions because of normal vision changes: avoid or use caution while driving at night, increase lighting in the home to reduce risk of falls, and paint the first and last steps of a staircase and the edge of each of the other steps a bright color to aid depth perception.
- Remind patient that wearing protective eyewear prevents injury from debris and splashes.

Evaluation

- Ask patient or family member to report on patient's most recent visit to an ophthalmologist.
- Have patient describe when to have an eye examination.
- Ask patient to describe common symptoms of eye disease.
- Observe the home environment of a patient with visual deficits.

Modified from Agency for Healthcare Research and Quality: *Guide to clinical preventive services,* Rockville, Md, 2010, AHRQ, http://www.uspreventiveservicestaskforce.org/uspstf09/visualscr/viseldrs.pdf.

muscles. Initiate nystagmus in patients with normal eye movements by having them gaze to the far left or right.

Visual Fields. As a person looks straight ahead, he or she is normally able to see all objects in the periphery. To assess visual fields direct the patient to stand or sit 60 cm (2 feet) away at eye level. The patient gently closes or covers one eye (e.g., the left) and looks at your eye directly opposite. You close your opposite eye (in this case the right) so the field of vision is superimposed on that of the patient. Next move a finger equidistant between you and the patient outside the field of vision and slowly bring it back into the visual field. The patient reports when he or she is able to see the finger. If you see the finger before the patient does, a portion of the patient's visual field is reduced. To test temporal field vision, hold an object or your finger slightly behind the patient. Repeat the procedure for each field of vision for the other eye. Patients with visual field problems are at risk for injury because they cannot see all of the objects in front of them. Older adults commonly have loss of peripheral vision caused by changes in the lens.

External Eye Structures. To inspect external eye structures, stand directly in front of the patient at eye level and ask him or her to look at your face.

Position and Alignment. Assess the position of the eyes in relation to one another. Normally they are parallel to one another. Bulging eyes (exophthalmos) usually indicate hyperthyroidism. Crossed eyes (strabismus) result from neuromuscular injury or inherited abnormalities. Tumors or inflammation of the orbit often cause abnormal eye protrusion.

For the remainder of the eye examination have the patient remove contact lenses.

Eyebrows. Inspect the eyebrows for size, extension, texture of hair, alignment, and movement. Normally the eyebrows are symmetrical. Coarseness of hair and failure to extend beyond the temporal canthus possibly reveals hypothyroidism. Thin brows possibly are a result of waxing or plucking. Aging causes loss of the lateral third of the eyebrows. To assess movement, ask the patient to raise and lower the eyebrows. The brows normally raise and lower symmetrically. An inability to move the eyebrows indicates a facial nerve paralysis (cranial nerve VII).

Eyelids. Inspect the eyelids for position; color; condition of the surface; condition and direction of the eyelashes; and the patient's ability to open, close, and blink. When the eyes are open in a normal position, the lids cover the sclera above the iris but not the pupil. The lids are also close to the eyeball. An abnormal drooping of the lid over the pupil is called **ptosis** (pronounced "toe-sis"), caused by edema or impairment of the third cranial nerve. In the older adult ptosis results from a loss of elasticity that accompanies aging. The nurse observes for defects in the position of the lid margins. An older adult frequently has lid margins that turn out **(ectropion)** or in **(entropion).** Entropion sometimes leads to the lashes of the lid irritating the conjunctiva and cornea, increasing

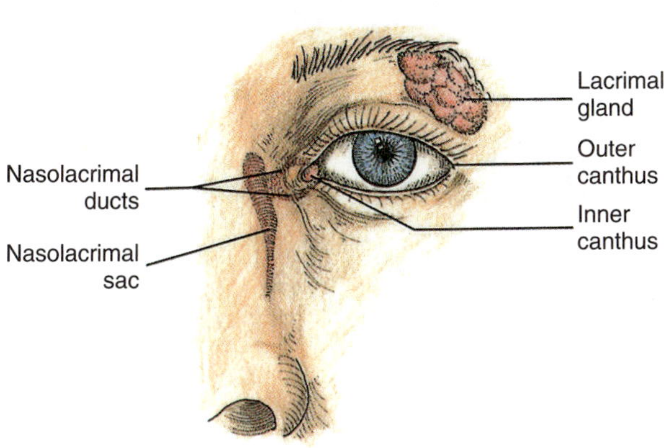

FIG. 30-12 The lacrimal apparatus secretes and drains tears, which moisten and lubricate eye structures.

the risk of infection. Normally the eyelashes are distributed evenly and curved outward away from the eye. An erythematous or yellow lump (hordeolum or sty) on the follicle of an eyelash indicates an acute suppurative inflammation.

To inspect the surface of the upper lids ask the patient to close his or her eyes while observing for tremors of the lids. The lids are normally smooth and the same color as the surrounding skin. Redness indicates inflammation or infection. Lid edema is sometimes caused by allergies or heart or kidney failure. Edema of the eyelids prevents them from closing. Inspect any lesions for typical characteristics and discomfort or drainage. Wear clean gloves if drainage is present.

The lids normally close symmetrically. Their failure to close exposes the cornea to drying. This condition is common in unconscious patients or those with facial nerve paralysis. To inspect the lower lids, ask the patient to open the eyes again while the nurse looks for the same characteristics noted for the upper lids. Normally a patient blinks involuntarily and bilaterally up to 20 times a minute. The blink reflex lubricates the cornea. Report absent, infrequent, rapid, or monocular (one-eyed) blinking.

Lacrimal Apparatus. The lacrimal gland (Fig. 30-12), located in the upper outer wall of the anterior part of the orbit, is responsible for tear production. Tears flow from the gland across the surface of the eye to the lacrimal duct, which is in the nasal corner or inner canthus of the eye. The lacrimal gland is sometimes the site of tumors or infections and should be inspected for edema and redness. Palpate the gland gently to detect tenderness; normally tenderness cannot be felt.

The nasolacrimal duct sometimes becomes obstructed, blocking the flow of tears. Observe for evidence of edema in the inner canthus. Gentle palpation of the duct at the lower eyelid just inside the lower orbital rim causes a regurgitation of tears.

Conjunctivae and Sclerae. The bulbar conjunctiva covers the exposed surface of the eyeball up to the outer edge of the cornea. Observe the sclera under the bulbar conjunctiva; it normally has the color of white porcelain in light-skinned patients and is light yellow in dark-skinned patients. Sclerae become pigmented and appear either yellow or green if liver disease is present.

Take care when inspecting the conjunctivae. For adequate exposure of the bulbar conjunctiva, retract the eyelids without placing pressure directly on the eyeball. Gently retract both lids, with the thumb and index finger pressed against the lower and upper bony orbits. Ask the patient to look up, down, and from side to side. Many patients begin to blink, making the examination difficult.

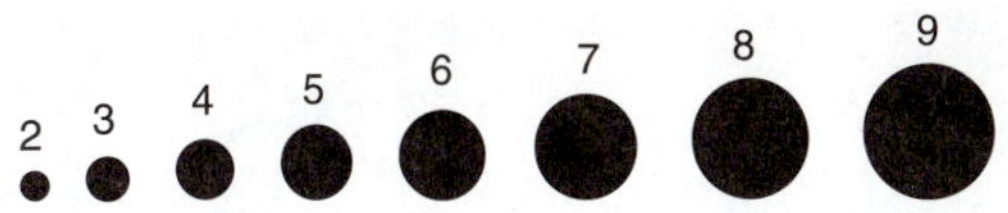

FIG. 30-13 Chart depicting pupillary size in millimeters.

Inspect for color, texture, and the presence of edema or lesions. Normally the conjunctivae are free of erythema. The presence of redness indicates an allergic or infectious **conjunctivitis.** Bright red blood in a localized area surrounded by normal-appearing conjunctiva usually indicates subconjunctival hemorrhage. Conjunctivitis is a highly contagious infection. It is easy to spread the crusty drainage that collects on eyelid margins from one eye to the other. Wear clean gloves during the examination. Performing proper hand hygiene is necessary before and after the examination.

Corneas. The cornea is the transparent, colorless portion of the eye covering the pupil and iris. From a side view, it looks like the crystal of a wristwatch. While the patient looks straight ahead, inspect the cornea for clarity and texture while shining a penlight obliquely across its entire surface. The cornea is normally shiny, transparent, and smooth. In older adults it loses its luster. Any irregularity in the surface indicates an abrasion or tear that requires further examination by a health care provider. Both conditions are very painful. Note the color and details of the underlying iris. In an older adult the iris becomes faded. A thin white ring along the margin of the iris, called an **arcus senilis,** is common with aging but is abnormal in anyone under age 40. To test for the corneal blink reflex, see the cranial nerve test section of this chapter.

Pupils and Irises. Observe the pupils for size, shape, equality, accommodation, and reaction to light. They are normally black, round, regular, and equal in size (3 to 7 mm in diameter) (Fig. 30-13). The iris should be clearly visible.

Cloudy pupils indicate cataracts. Dilated pupils result from glaucoma, trauma, neurological disorders, eye medications (e.g., atropine), or withdrawal from opioids. Inflammation of the iris or use of drugs (e.g., pilocarpine, morphine, or cocaine) causes constricted pupils. Pinpoint pupils are a common sign of opioid intoxication. Shining a beam of light through the pupil and onto the retina stimulates the third cranial nerve, causing the muscles of the iris to constrict. Any abnormality along the nerve pathways from the retina to the iris alters the ability of the pupils to react to light. Changes in intracranial pressure, lesions along the nerve pathways, locally applied ophthalmic medications, and direct trauma to the eye alter pupillary reaction.

Test pupillary reflexes (to light and accommodation) in a dimly lit room. Instruct the patient to avoid looking directly at the light. While the patient looks straight ahead, bring a penlight from the side of his or her face, directing the light onto the pupil (Fig. 30-14). A directly illuminated pupil constricts, and the opposite pupil constricts consensually. Observe the quickness and equality of the reflex. Repeat the examination for the opposite eye.

To test for accommodation, ask the patient to gaze at a distant object (the far wall) and then at a test object (finger or pencil) held approximately 10 cm (4 inches) from the bridge of his or her nose. The pupils normally converge and accommodate by constricting when looking at close objects. The pupillary responses are equal. Testing for accommodation is only important if the patient has a defect in the pupillary response to light (Seidel et al., 2011). If assessment of pupillary reaction is normal in all tests, record the abbreviation **PERRLA** (pupils equal, round, reactive to light, and accommodation).

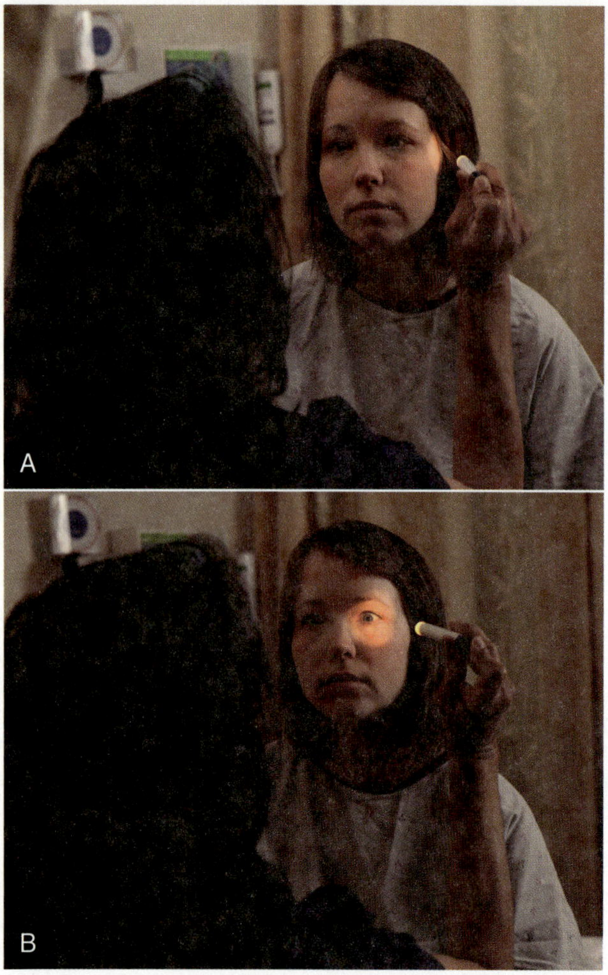

FIG. 30-14 **A,** To check pupillary reflexes the nurse first holds the penlight to the side of the patient's face. **B,** Illumination of the pupil causes pupillary constriction.

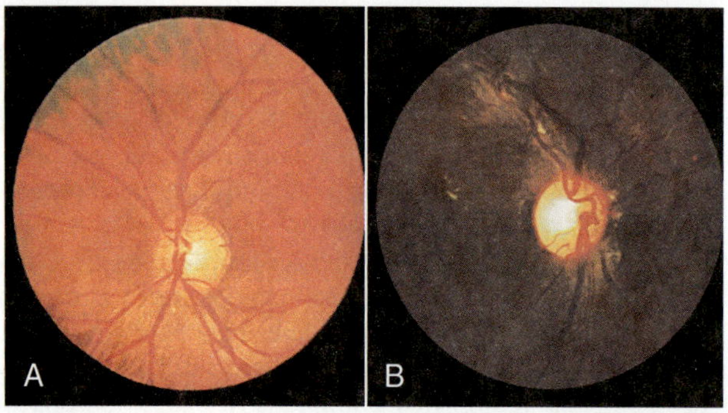

FIG. 30-15 Fundus of white patient **(A)** and black patient **(B)**. (Courtesy MEDCOM, Cypress, Calif.)

Internal Eye Structures. The examination of the internal eye structures through the use of an ophthalmoscope is beyond the scope of new graduate nurses' practice. Advanced nurse practitioners use the ophthalmoscope to inspect the fundus (Fig. 30-15), which includes the retina, choroid, optic nerve disc, macula, fovea centralis, and retinal vessels. Patients in greatest need of an examination are those with diabetes, hypertension, and intracranial disorders.

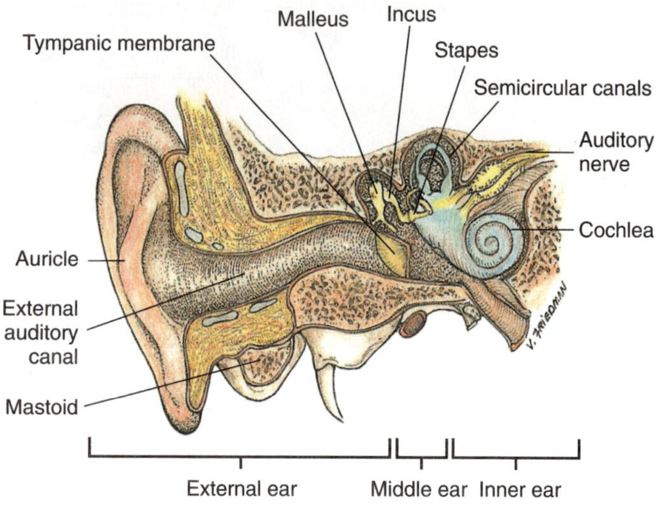

FIG. 30-16 Structures of external, middle, and inner ear.

Ears

The ear assessment determines the integrity of ear structures and hearing acuity. The three parts of the ear are the external, middle, and inner ear (Fig. 30-16). Inspect and palpate external ear structures, which consist of the auricle, outer ear canal, and tympanic membrane (eardrum). The ear canal is normally curved and approximately 2.5 cm (1 inch) long in an adult. It is lined with skin containing fine hairs, nerve endings, and glands secreting cerumen. The middle ear is inspected with an otoscope. It is an air-filled cavity containing the three bony ossicles (malleus, incus, and stapes). The eustachian tube connects the middle ear to the nasopharynx. Pressure between the outer atmosphere and the middle ear is stabilized through the eustachian tube. Finally the inner ear is tested by measuring the patient's hearing acuity. The inner ear contains the cochlea, vestibule, and semicircular canals. Assessing the ears determines the integrity of ear structures and the condition of hearing. Use nursing history data to identify patients' risks for hearing disorders (Table 30-15).

Understanding the mechanisms for sound transmission helps identify the nature of hearing disorders. Sound travels through the ear by air and bone conduction. Nerve impulses from the cochlea travel to the auditory (eighth cranial nerve) and the cerebral cortex. Disorders of the ear result from several types of problems, including mechanical dysfunction (blockage by cerumen or foreign body), trauma (foreign bodies or noise exposure), neurological disorders (auditory nerve damage), acute illnesses (viral infection), and toxic effects of medications.

Auricles. With the patient sitting comfortably, inspect the size, shape, symmetry, landmarks, position, and color of the auricle (Fig. 30-17). The auricles are normally of equal size and level with one another. The upper point of attachment is in a straight line with the lateral canthus, or corner of the eye. The position of the auricle is almost vertical. Ears that are low set or at an unusual angle are a sign of chromosome abnormality such as Down syndrome. Ear color is usually the same as that of the face, without moles, cysts, deformities, or nodules. Redness is a sign of inflammation or fever. Extreme pallor indicates frostbite.

Palpate the auricles for texture, tenderness, and skin lesions. Auricles are normally smooth and without lesions. If the patient complains of pain, gently pull the auricle, press on the tragus, and palpate behind the ear over the mastoid process. If palpating the

TABLE 30-15 Nursing History for Ear Assessment

ASSESSMENT	RATIONALE
Ask if patient has experienced ear pain, itching, discharge, vertigo, tinnitus (ringing in ears), or change in hearing.	These signs and symptoms indicate infection or hearing loss.
Assess risks for hearing problem. *Infants/children:* Hypoxia at birth, meningitis, birth weight less than 1500 g, family history of hearing loss, congenital anomalies of skull or face, nonbacterial intrauterine infections (rubella, herpes), maternal drug use, excessively high bilirubin, head trauma *Adults:* Exposure to industrial or recreational noise, genetic disease (Ménière's disease), neurodegenerative disorder	Risk factors predispose patient to permanent hearing loss. It is difficult to assess infant's hearing status with examination only.
Determine patient's exposure to loud noises at work and availability of protective devices.	Prolonged noise exposure causes temporary or permanent hearing loss.
Note behaviors indicative of hearing loss such as failure to respond when spoken to, requests to repeat comments, leaning forward to hear, and child's inattentiveness or use of monotonous voice tone.	Persons with hearing loss cope with sensory deficit through a variety of behavioral cues.
Assess if patient takes large doses of aspirin or other ototoxic drugs (e.g., aminoglycosides, furosemide, streptomycin, cisplatin, ethacrynic acid).	Medications have side effects of hearing loss.
Determine whether patient uses hearing aid.	Determination allows nurse to assess ability to care for device and adjust voice tone to communicate.
If patient had recent hearing problem, note onset, contributing factors, affected ear, and effect on activities of daily living.	Helps determine nature and severity of hearing problem.
Determine whether patient has repeated history of cerumen buildup in ear.	Cerumen impaction is common cause for conduction deafness.

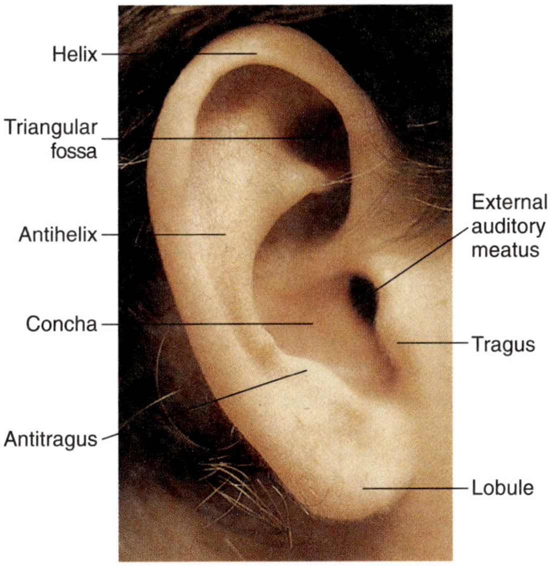

FIG. 30-17 Anatomical structures of auricle. (From Seidel HM et al: *Mosby's guide to physical examination,* ed 7, St Louis, 2011, Mosby.)

external ear increases the pain, an external ear infection is likely. If palpating the auricle and tragus does not influence the pain, the patient possibly has a middle ear infection. Tenderness in the mastoid area indicates mastoiditis.

Inspect the opening of the ear canal for size and presence of discharge. If discharge is present, wear clean gloves. A swollen or occluded meatus is not normal. A yellow, waxy substance called **cerumen** is common. Yellow or green, foul-smelling discharge indicates infection or a foreign body.

Ear Canals and Eardrums. Observe the deeper structures of the external and middle ear with the use of an otoscope. A special ear speculum attaches to the handle of the ophthalmoscope. For best visualization select the largest speculum that fits comfortably in the patient's ear. Before inserting the speculum, check for foreign bodies in the opening of the auditory canal.

Make sure that the patient avoids moving the head during the examination to avoid damage to the canal and tympanic membrane. Infants and young children might need to be held securely to prevent movement. Lay infants supine with head turned to one side and arms held securely at the sides. Have young children sit on their parents' laps with their legs held between the parents' knees.

Turn on the otoscope by rotating the dial at the top of the handle. To insert the speculum properly, ask the patient to tip the head slightly toward the opposite shoulder. Hold the handle of the otoscope in the space between the thumb and index finger, supported on the middle finger. This leaves the ulnar side of the hand to rest against the patient's head, stabilizing the otoscope as you insert it into the canal (Seidel et al., 2011). There are two ways to grip the otoscope: (1) hold the handle along the patient's face with the fingers against the face or neck; and (2) lightly brace the inverted otoscope against the side of the patient's head or cheek. This latter grip, used with children, prevents accidental movement of the otoscope deeper into the ear canal. Insert the scope while pulling the auricle upward and backward in the adult and older child (Fig. 30-18). This maneuver straightens the ear canal. For infants the auricle should be pulled down and back.

Insert the speculum slightly down and forward 1 to 1.5 cm (½ inch) into the ear canal. Take care not to scrape the sensitive lining, which is painful. The ear canal normally has little cerumen and is uniformly pink with tiny hairs in the outer third of the canal. Observe for color, discharge, scaling, lesions, foreign bodies, and

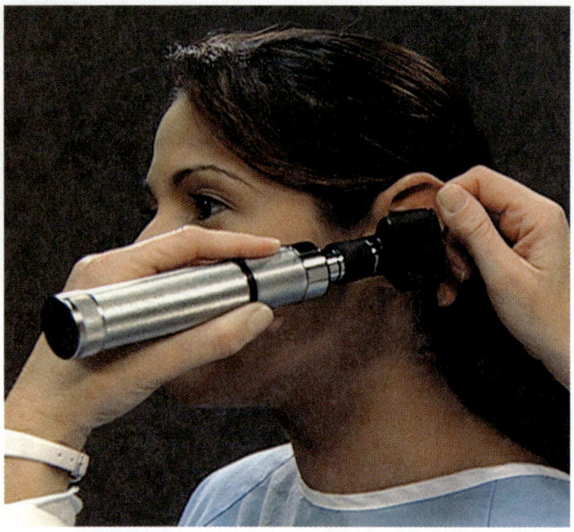

FIG. 30-18 Otoscopic examination. (From Seidel HM et al: *Mosby's guide to physical examination,* ed 7, St Louis, 2011, Mosby.)

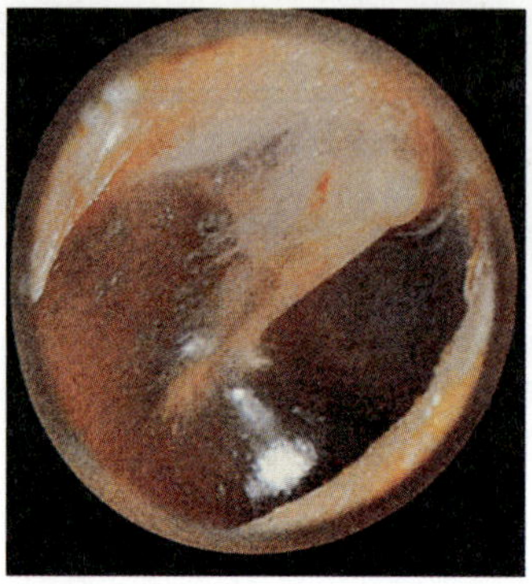

FIG. 30-19 Normal right tympanic membrane. (Courtesy Dr. Richard A. Buckingham, Abraham Lincoln School of Medicine, University of Illinois, Chicago.)

BOX 30-14 PATIENT TEACHING

Ear Assessment

Objective

- Patient will follow preventive guidelines for screening of hearing loss and proper cleaning technique for the ears.

Teaching Strategies

- Instruct patient in the proper way to clean the outer ear (see Chapter 39), avoiding use of cotton-tipped applicators and sharp objects such as hairpins, which cause impaction of cerumen deep in the ear canal or trauma.
- Tell patient to avoid inserting pointed objects into the ear canal.
- Encourage patients over age 65 to have regular hearing checks. Explain that a reduction in hearing is a normal part of aging (see Chapter 49).
- Instruct family members of patients with hearing loss to avoid shouting, speak in low tones, and be sure that patient is able to see the speaker's face.

Evaluation

- Ask patient to explain the proper technique for cleaning the ears.
- In a follow-up visit question patient about frequency of hearing checks.
- Observe patient with hearing loss interacting with family members.

cerumen. Normally cerumen is dry (light brown to gray and flaky) or moist (dark yellow or brown) and sticky. Dry cerumen is common in Asians and Native Americans (Seidel et al., 2011). A reddened canal with discharge is a sign of inflammation or infection. In other adults accumulated cerumen is a common problem; buildup creates a mild hearing loss. During the examination ask the patient about methods he or she uses to clean the ear canal (Box 30-14).

The light from the otoscope allows visualization of the tympanic membrane. Know the common anatomical landmarks and their appearances (Fig. 30-19). Gently move the otoscope so the entire tympanic membrane and its periphery are visible. Because the tympanic membrane is angled away from the ear canal, the light from the otoscope appears as a cone shape rather than a circle. A ring of fibrous cartilage surrounds the oval membrane. The umbo is near the center of the membrane, behind which is the attachment of the malleus. The underlying short process of the malleus creates a knoblike structure at the top of the drum. Check carefully to make sure that there are no tears or breaks in the membrane. The normal tympanic membrane is translucent, shiny, and pearly gray. It is free from tears or breaks. A pink or red bulging membrane indicates inflammation. A white color reveals pus behind it. The membrane is taut, except for the small triangular pars flaccida near the top. If cerumen is blocking the tympanic membrane, warm water irrigation safely removes the wax.

Hearing Acuity. A patient with a hearing loss often fails to respond to conversation. The three types of hearing loss are conduction, sensorineural, and mixed. A conduction loss interrupts sound waves as they travel from the outer ear to the cochlea of the inner ear because the sound waves are not transmitted through the outer and middle ear structures. For example, causes of a conduction loss include swelling of the auditory canal and tears in the tympanic membrane. A sensorineural loss involves the inner ear, auditory nerve, or hearing center of the brain. Sound is conducted through the outer and middle ear structures, but the continued transmission of sound becomes interrupted at some point beyond the bony ossicles. A mixed loss involves a combination of conduction and sensorineural loss. Patients working or living around loud noises are at risk for hearing loss. In addition, adolescents are at risk for premature hearing loss from continued exposure to loud music in their car or home or at concert events. Hearing loss among adolescents is increasing, especially among those with high levels of noise exposure such as from loud music (Shargorodsky et al., 2010).

Older adults experience an inability to hear high-frequency sounds and consonants (e.g., *S, Z, T,* and *G*). Deterioration of the cochlea and thickening of the tympanic membrane cause older adults to gradually lose hearing acuity. They are especially at risk for hearing loss caused by **ototoxicity** (injury to auditory nerve) resulting from high maintenance doses of antibiotics (e.g., aminoglycosides).

To conduct a hearing assessment, have the patient remove any hearing aid if worn. Note his or her response to questions. Normally he or she responds without excessive requests to have the questions repeated. If a hearing loss is suspected, check the patient's response to the whispered voice. Test one ear at a time while the patient occludes the other ear with a finger. Ask him or her to gently move the finger up and down during the test in response to the whispered sound. While standing 30 to 60 cm (1 to 2 feet) from the testing ear, speak while covering the mouth so the patient is

TABLE 30-16 Tuning Fork Tests

TESTS AND STEPS	RATIONALE
Weber's Test (Lateralization of Sound)	
Hold fork at its base and tap it lightly against heel of palm. Place base of vibrating fork on midline vertex of patient's head or middle of forehead (see illustration *A*). Ask patient if he or she hears the sound equally in both ears or better in one ear (lateralization).	Patient with normal hearing hears sound equally in both ears. In conduction deafness sound is heard best in impaired ear. In sensorineural hearing loss, sound is heard better in normal ear.
Rinne Test (Comparison of Air and Bone Conduction)	
Place stem of vibrating tuning fork against patient's mastoid process (see illustration *B*). Begin counting the interval with your watch. Ask patient to tell you when he or she no longer hears the sound; note number of seconds. Quickly place still-vibrating tines 1 to 2 cm (½ to 1 inch) from ear canal and ask patient to tell you when he or she no longer hears the sound (see illustration *C*). Continue counting time the sound is heard by air conduction. Compare number of seconds the sound is heard by bone conduction versus air conduction.	Patient should hear air-conducted sound twice as long as bone-conducted sound (2:1 ratio). For example, if patient hears bone-conducted sound for 10 seconds, he or she should hear air-conducted sound for an additional 10 seconds. In conduction deafness, patient hears bone conduction longer than air conduction in affected ear. In sensorineural loss, patient hears air conduction longer than bone conduction in affected ear, but at less than a 2:1 ratio (Seidel et al., 2011).

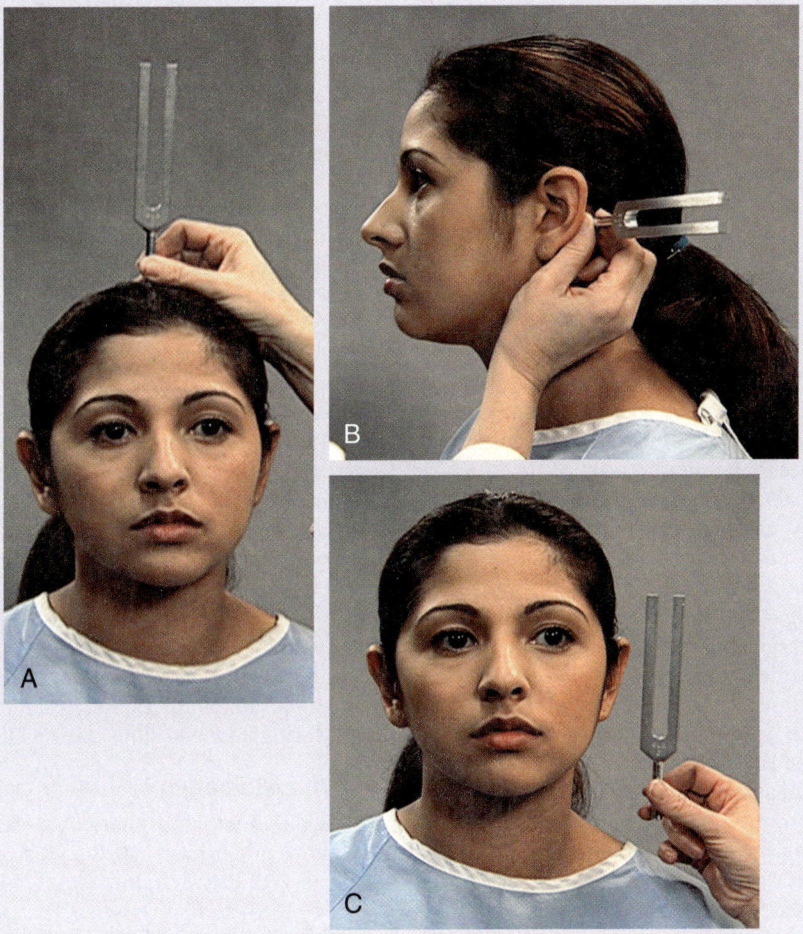

Illustrations from Seidel HM et al: *Mosby's guide to physical examination,* ed 7, St Louis, 2011, Mosby.

unable to read lips. After exhaling fully, whisper softly toward the unoccluded ear, reciting random numbers with equally accented syllables such as *nine-four-ten.* If necessary, gradually increase voice intensity until the patient correctly repeats the numbers. Then test the other ear for comparison. Seidel et al. (2011) report that patients normally hear numbers clearly when whispered, responding correctly at least 50% of the time.

If a hearing loss is present, test the hearing using a tuning fork. A tuning fork of 256 to 512 hertz (Hz) is most commonly used. The tuning fork allows for comparison of hearing by bone conduction with that of air conduction. Hold the base of the tuning fork with one hand without touching the tines. Tap the fork lightly against the palm of the other hand to set the fork in vibration (Table 30-16).

TABLE 30-17 Nursing History for Nose and Sinus Assessment

ASSESSMENT	RATIONALE
Ask if patient has had trauma to nose.	Trauma causes septal deviation and asymmetry of external nose.
Ask if patient has history of allergies, nasal discharge, epistaxis (nosebleeds), or postnasal drip.	History is useful in determining source or nature of nasal and sinus drainage.
If there is history of nasal discharge, assess color, amount, odor, duration, and associated symptoms (e.g., sneezing, nasal congestion, obstruction, or mouth breathing).	Aids in ruling out presence of infection, allergy, or drug use.
Assess for history of nosebleed, including site, frequency, amount of bleeding, treatment, and difficulty stopping bleeding.	Characteristics sometimes reveal trauma, medication use, or excessive dryness as causative factors.
Ask if patient uses nasal spray or drops, including amount, frequency, and duration of use.	Overuse of over-the-counter nasal preparations causes physical change in mucosa.
Ask if patient snores at night or has difficulty breathing.	Difficulty breathing or snoring indicates septal deviation or obstruction.

Nose and Sinuses

Assess the integrity of the nose and sinuses by using inspection and palpation. The patient sits during the examination. A penlight allows for gross examination of each naris. A more detailed examination requires use of a nasal speculum to inspect the deeper nasal turbinates. Do not use a speculum unless a qualified practitioner such as a nurse educator or an advanced practice nurse is present. Table 30-17 lists components of the nursing history.

Nose. When inspecting the external nose, observe for shape, size, skin, color, and the presence of deformity or inflammation. The nose is normally smooth and symmetrical with the same skin color as the face. Recent trauma sometimes causes edema and discoloration. If swelling or deformities exist, gently palpate the ridge and soft tissue of the nose by placing one finger on each side of the nasal arch and gently moving the fingers from the nasal bridge to the tip. Note any tenderness, masses, or underlying deviations. Nasal structures are usually firm and stable.

Air normally passes freely through the nose when a person breathes. To assess patency of the nares, place a finger on the side of the patient's nose and occlude one naris. Ask the patient to breathe with the mouth closed. Repeat the procedure for the other naris.

While illuminating the anterior nares, inspect the mucosa for color, lesions, discharge, swelling, and evidence of bleeding. If discharge is present, apply gloves. Normal mucosa is pink and moist without lesions. Pale mucosa with clear discharge indicates allergy. A mucoid discharge indicates rhinitis. A sinus infection results in yellowish or greenish discharge. Habitual use of intranasal cocaine and opioids causes puffiness and increased vascularity of the nasal mucosa. For the patient with a nasogastric tube, routinely check for local skin breakdown **(excoriation)** of the naris, characterized by redness and skin sloughing.

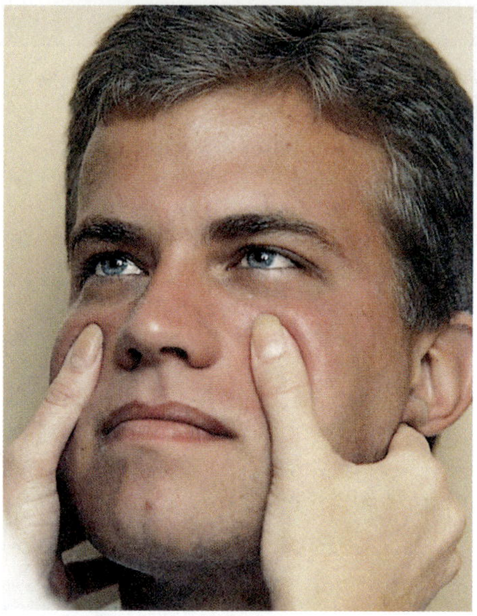

FIG. 30-20 Palpation of maxillary sinuses.

To view the septum and turbinates, have the patient tip the head back slightly to provide a clear view. Illuminate the septum and observe for alignment, perforation, or bleeding. Normally the septum is close to the midline and thicker anteriorly than posteriorly. The turbinates are covered with mucous membranes that warm and moisten inspired air. Normal mucosa is pink and moist, without lesions. A deviated septum obstructs breathing and interferes with passage of a nasogastric tube. Perforation of the septum often occurs after repeated use of intranasal cocaine. Note any **polyps** (tumorlike growths) or purulent drainage.

Sinuses. Examination of the sinuses involves palpation. In cases of allergies or infection, the interior of the sinuses becomes inflamed and swollen. The most effective way to assess for tenderness is by externally palpating the frontal and maxillary facial areas (Fig. 30-20). Palpate the frontal sinus by exerting pressure with the thumb up and under the patient's eyebrow. Gentle, upward pressure elicits tenderness easily if sinus irritation is present. Do not apply pressure to the eyes. If sinus tenderness is present, the sinuses may be transilluminated. However this procedure requires advanced experience. Box 30-15 describes teaching guidelines during nose and sinus assessment.

Mouth and Pharynx

Assess the mouth and pharynx to detect signs of overall health; determine oral hygiene needs; and determine therapies needed for patients with dehydration, restricted intake, oral trauma, or oral airway obstruction. To assess the oral cavity use a penlight and tongue depressor or gauze square. Wear clean gloves during the examination. Have the patient sit or lie down. Assess the oral cavity also while administering oral hygiene (see Chapter 39). Table 30-18 describes the nursing history for assessment of the mouth and pharynx.

Lips. Inspect the lips for color, texture, hydration, contour, and lesions. With the patient's mouth closed, view the lips from end to end. Normally they are pink, moist, symmetrical, and smooth (Fig. 30-21). Lip color in the dark-skinned patient varies from pink to plum. Have female patients remove their lipstick before the examination. Anemia causes pallor of the lips, with cyanosis caused by

TABLE 30-18 Nursing History for Mouth and Pharyngeal Assessment

ASSESSMENT	RATIONALE
Determine if patient wears dentures or retainers and if they are comfortable.	Patient needs to remove dentures to visualize and palpate gums. Ill-fitting dentures chronically irritate mucosa and gums.
Determine if patient has had recent change in appetite or weight.	Symptoms result from painful mouth conditions or poor hygiene.
Determine if patient uses tobacco products:	
• Smoking cigarette, cigar, or pipe	Smoking these products increases risk for lung, oral cavity, larynx, and esophageal cancers (American Cancer Society [ACS], 2011).
• Smokeless tobacco: use of chewing tobacco and snuff	Smokeless tobacco causes various cancers and noncancerous oral disorders. Long-term snuff users have increased risk for cancer of the gums and cheeks (ACS, 2011).
Review history for alcohol consumption.	Oral and pharyngeal cancers are more common in alcohol users than nonalcohol users. Combine tobacco with heavy use of alcohol, the risk is significantly increased, as the two act synergistically. Those who both smoke and drink, have a 15 times greater risk of developing oral cancer than others (Oral Cancer Foundation, 2011). Effects of alcohol are also independent of tobacco use.
Assess dental hygiene practices, including use of fluoride toothpaste, frequency of brushing and flossing, and frequency of dental visits.	Assessment reveals patient's need for education and/or financial support. Periodontal disease has a higher prevalence in older adults who have history of high plaque buildup, use tobacco, and visit the dentist infrequently.
Ask if patient has pain from chewing or eating. If so, ask if mouth lesions are present, including duration and associated symptoms.	Pain is often associated with broken tooth, teeth grinding, or temporomandibular joint problems. Extra care is needed during oral hygiene administration.
Review the patient's medical history for a previous diagnosis of the human papilloma virus.	The human papilloma virus, particularly HPV16, has been definitively implicated in oral cancers, particularly those that occur in the back of the mouth (oropharynx, base of tongue, tonsillar pillars and crypt, as well as the tonsils themselves) (Oral Cancer Foundation, 2011).

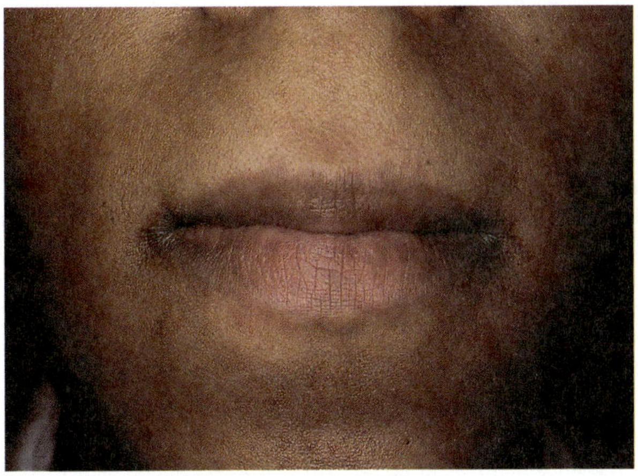

FIG. 30-21 Lips are normally pink, symmetrical, smooth, and moist.

respiratory or cardiovascular problems. Cherry-colored lips indicate carbon monoxide poisoning. Any lesions should be evaluated for the potential of being an infection, irritation, or skin cancer.

Buccal Mucosa, Gums, and Teeth. Ask the patient to clench the teeth and smile to observe teeth occlusion. The upper molars normally rest directly on the lower molars, and the upper incisors slightly override the lower incisors. A symmetrical smile reveals normal facial nerve function.

BOX 30-15 **PATIENT TEACHING**

Nose and Sinus Assessment

Objective

- Patient will explain self-care measures to address and minimize loss of olfaction.

Teaching Strategies

- Caution patient against overuse of over-the-counter nasal sprays, which leads to "rebound" effect, causing excess nasal congestion.
- Instruct parents in care of a child with nosebleeds: have child sit up and lean forward to avoid aspiration of blood, apply pressure to the anterior nose with the thumb and forefinger as the child breathes through the mouth, and apply ice or a cold cloth to the bridge of the nose if pressure fails to stop bleeding.
- Instruct older adults with loss of olfaction to follow safety precautions:
  - Install smoke detectors on each floor of their home.
  - Ask others to advise them when food smells pungent.
- Instruct older adults to always check dated labels on food to ensure against spoilage.

Evaluation

- Have patient explain proper use of over-the-counter nasal sprays.
- Have parents demonstrate and describe technique for stopping a nosebleed.
- Inspect patient's home during visit and look for smoke detectors. Ask to check some food items in the refrigerator.

BOX 30-16 **PATIENT TEACHING**

Mouth and Pharyngeal Assessment

Objective

- Patient will practice proper oral hygiene/dental care measures and identify symptoms of oral cancer.

Teaching Strategies

- Discuss proper techniques for oral hygiene, including brushing and flossing (see Chapter 39).
- Explain the early warning signs of oral cavity and pharynx cancer that should be checked by a health care professional, including a mouth sore that bleeds easily and does not heal, a lump or thickening in the cheek, a white or red patch on the mucosa that persists, a sore throat or a feeling that something is caught in the throat, numbness of the tongue or other area of the mouth, or a swelling of the jaw that causes dentures to not fit (Oral Cancer Foundation, 2011).
- Late symptoms of oral cancer are difficulty chewing, swallowing, or moving the tongue or jaw (ACS, 2011).
- Encourage regular dental examination every 6 months for children, adults, and older adults.

Evaluation

- Ask patient to demonstrate brushing.
- Have patient identify when to have regular dental checkups.
- Have patient identify the warning signs of oral cavity and pharynx cancer that require further evaluation by a health care provider.

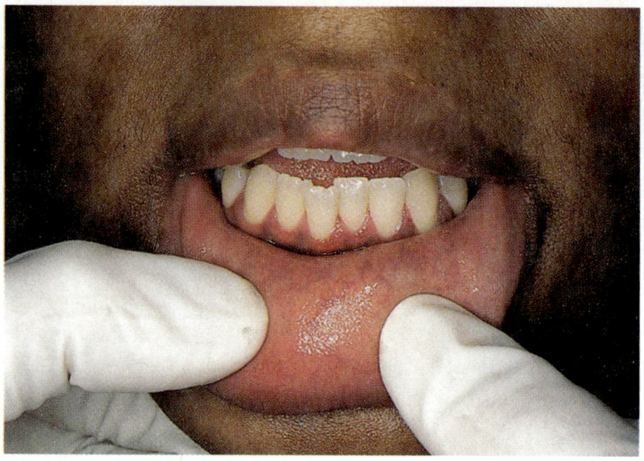

FIG. 30-22 Inspection of inner oral mucosa of lower lip.

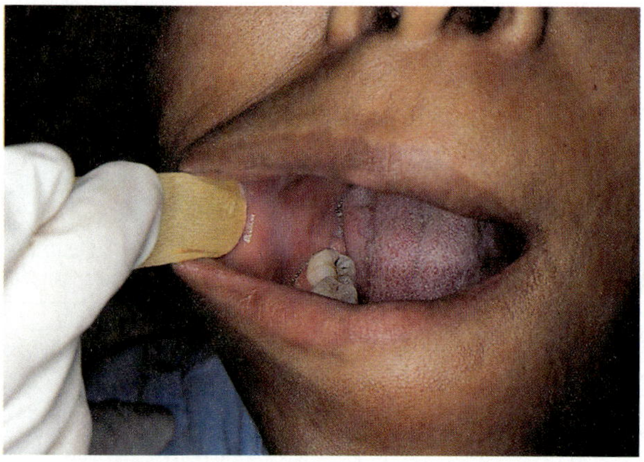

FIG. 30-23 Retraction of buccal mucosa allows for clear visualization.

Inspect the teeth to determine the quality of dental hygiene (Box 30-16). Note the position and alignment of the teeth. To examine the posterior surface of the teeth, have the patient open the mouth with the lips relaxed. Use a tongue depressor to retract the lips and cheeks, especially when viewing the molars. Note the color of teeth and presence of dental caries (cavities), tartar, and extraction sites. Normal, healthy teeth are smooth, white, and shiny. A chalky white discoloration of the enamel is an early indication of caries formation. Brown or black discolorations indicate the formation of caries. A stained yellow color is from tobacco use; coffee, tea, and colas cause a brown stain. In the older adult loose or missing teeth are common because bone resorption increases. An older adult's teeth often feel rough when tooth enamel calcifies. Yellow or darkened teeth are also common in the older adult because of the general wear and tear that exposes the darker underlying dentin.

To view the mucosa and gums, ask the patient to first remove any dental appliance. View the inner oral mucosa by having the patient open and relax the mouth slightly and then gently retract his or her lower lip away from the teeth (Fig. 30-22). Repeat this process for the upper lip. Inspect the mucosa for color; hydration; texture; and lesions such as ulcers, abrasions, or cysts. Normally the mucosa is glistening, pink, smooth, and moist. Some common small, yellow-white raised lesions on the buccal mucosa and lips are Fordyce spots, or ectopic sebaceous glands (Seidel et al., 2011). If lesions are present, palpate them gently with a gloved hand for tenderness, size, and consistency.

To inspect the buccal mucosa, ask the patient to open the mouth and then gently retract the cheeks with a tongue depressor (Fig. 30-23). View the surface of the mucosa from right to left and top to bottom. A penlight illuminates the most posterior portion of the mucosa. Normal mucosa is glistening, pink, soft, moist, and smooth. Varying shades of hyperpigmentation are normal in 10% of whites after age 50 and as many as 90% of blacks by the same age. For patients with normal pigmentation, the buccal mucosa is a good site to inspect for jaundice and pallor. In older adults the mucosa is normally dry because of reduced salivation. Thick white patches (leukoplakia) are often a precancerous lesion seen in heavy smokers and alcoholics. Palpate for any buccal lesions by placing the index finger within the buccal cavity and the thumb on the outer surface of the cheek. Patients who smoke cigarettes, cigars, or pipes and those who use smokeless tobacco have an increased risk of oral, pharyngeal, laryngeal, and esophageal cancer. These individuals may have leukoplakia or other lesions anywhere in their oral cavity (e.g., lips, gums, or tongue) at an early age.

Inspect the gums (gingivae) for color, edema, retraction, bleeding, and lesions while retracting the cheeks. Healthy gums are pink, smooth, and moist and fit tightly around each tooth. Dark-skinned patients often have patchy pigmentation. In older adults the gums are usually pale. Using clean gloves, palpate the gums to assess for lesions, thickening, or masses. Normally there is no tenderness. Spongy gums that bleed easily indicate periodontal disease and vitamin C deficiency. If the patient has loose or mobile teeth, swollen gums, or pockets containing debris at the tooth margins, a dental referral should be considered to check for periodontal disease or gingivitis.

Tongue and Floor of Mouth. Carefully inspect the tongue on all sides and the floor of the mouth. Have the patient relax the

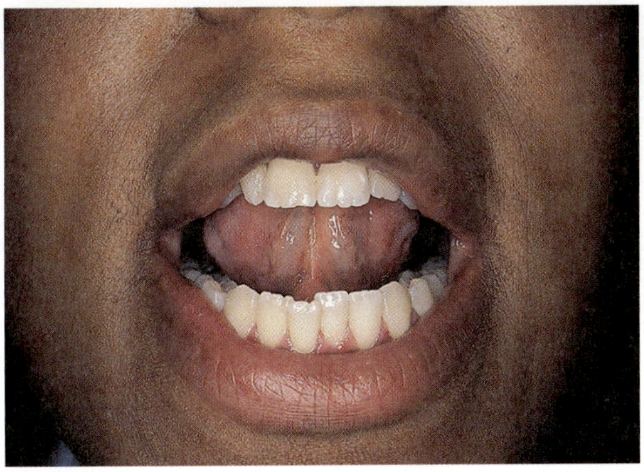

FIG. 30-24 The undersurface of the tongue is highly vascular.

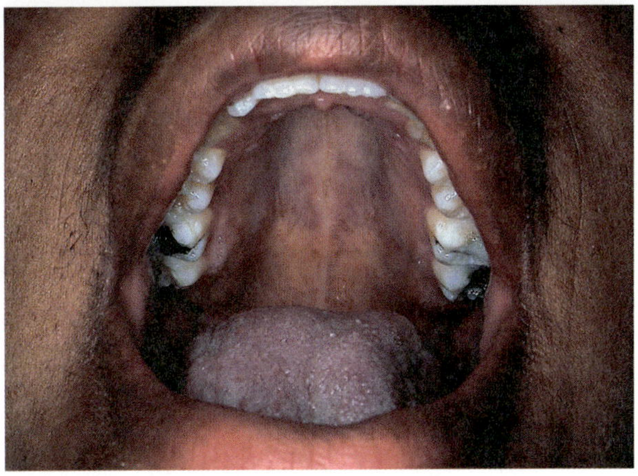

FIG. 30-25 The hard palate is located anteriorly in the roof of the mouth.

mouth and stick the tongue out halfway. Note any deviation, tremor, or limitation in movement. This tests hypoglossal nerve function. If the patient protrudes the tongue too far, it elicits the gag reflex. When the tongue protrudes, it lays midline. To test for tongue mobility, ask the patient to raise it up and move it from side to side. It should move freely.

Using a penlight for illumination, examine the tongue for color, size, position, texture, and coatings or lesions. A normal tongue is medium or dull red in color, moist, slightly rough on the top surface, and smooth along the lateral margins. The undersurface of the tongue and the floor of the mouth are highly vascular (Fig. 30-24). Take extra care to inspect this area, a common site for oral cancer lesions. The patient lifts the tongue by placing its tip on the palate behind the upper incisors. Inspect for color, swelling, and lesions such as nodules or cysts. The ventral surface of the tongue is pink and smooth, with large veins between the frenulum folds. To palpate the tongue, explain the procedure and ask the patient to protrude it. Grasp the tip with a gauze square and gently pull it to one side. With a gloved hand palpate the full length of the tongue and the base for any areas of hardening or ulceration. Varicosities (swollen, tortuous veins) are common in the older adult and rarely cause problems.

Palate. Have the patient extend the head backward, holding the mouth open to inspect the hard and soft palates. The hard palate, or roof of the mouth, is located anteriorly. The whitish hard palate is dome shaped. The soft palate extends posteriorly toward the pharynx. It is normally light pink and smooth. Observe the palates for color, shape, texture, and extra bony prominences or defects (Fig. 30-25). A bony growth, or exostosis, between the two palates is common.

Pharynx. Perform an examination of pharyngeal structures to rule out infection, inflammation, or lesions. Have the patient tip the head back slightly, open the mouth wide, and say "ah" while you place the tip of a tongue depressor on the middle third of the tongue. Take care not to press the lower lip against the teeth. By placing the tongue depressor too far anteriorly, the posterior part of the tongue mounds up, obstructing the view. Placing the tongue depressor on the posterior tongue elicits the gag reflex.

With a penlight, first inspect the uvula and soft palate (Fig. 30-26). Both structures, which are innervated by the tenth cranial (vagus) nerve, should rise centrally as the patient says "ah." Examine the anterior and posterior pillars, soft palate, and uvula. View the tonsils in the cavities between the anterior and posterior pillars and note the presence or absence of tissue. The posterior pharynx is

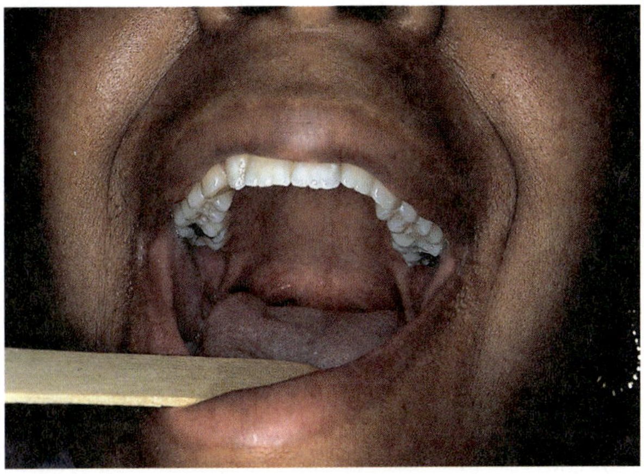

FIG. 30-26 A penlight and tongue depressor allow the visualization of the uvula and posterior soft palate.

behind the pillars. Normally pharyngeal tissues are pink and smooth and well hydrated. Small irregular spots of lymphatic tissue and small blood vessels are normal. Note edema, petechiae (small hemorrhages), lesions, or exudate. The back of the pharynx is a common site for oral cancer (Oral Cancer Foundation, 2011). Patients with chronic sinus problems frequently exhibit a clear exudate that drains along the wall of the posterior pharynx. Yellow or green exudate indicates infection. A patient with a typical sore throat has a red and edematous uvula and tonsillar pillars with possible presence of yellow exudate.

Neck

Assessment of the neck includes assessing the neck muscles, lymph nodes of the head and neck, carotid arteries, jugular veins, thyroid gland, and trachea (Fig. 30-27). You may postpone the examination of the jugular veins and carotid arteries until the vascular system assessment. Inspect and palpate the neck to determine the integrity of its structures and examine the lymphatic system. An abnormality of superficial lymph nodes sometimes reveals the presence of an infection or malignancy. Examine the lymphatic system region by region during the assessment of other body systems (head and neck, breast, genitalia, and extremities). Examination of the thyroid gland and trachea also aids in ruling out malignancies. Perform this examination with the patient sitting. The sternocleidomastoid

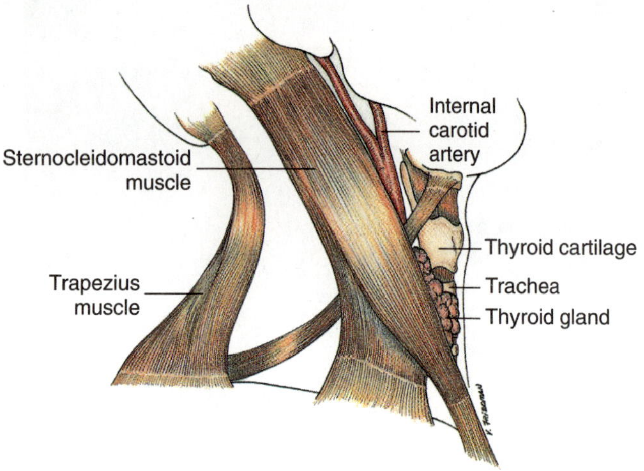

FIG. 30-27 Anatomical position of major neck structures. Note triangles formed by the sternocleidomastoid muscle, lower jaw, and anterior neck anteriorly and the sternocleidomastoid muscle, trapezius muscle, and lower neck posteriorly.

and trapezius muscles outline the areas of the neck, dividing each side of the neck into two triangles. The anterior triangle contains the trachea, thyroid gland, carotid artery, and anterior cervical lymph nodes. The posterior triangle contains the posterior lymph nodes. Table 30-19 reviews the nursing history for the head and neck examination.

Neck Muscles. First inspect the neck in the usual anatomical position, with slight hyperextension. Observe for symmetry of the neck muscles. Ask the patient to flex the neck with the chin to the chest, hyperextend the neck backward, and move the head laterally to each side and then sideways with the ear moving toward the shoulder. This tests the sternocleidomastoid and trapezius muscles. The neck normally moves without discomfort. Perform other tests for muscle strength and function during assessment of the musculoskeletal system.

Lymph Nodes. An extensive system of lymph nodes collects lymph from the head, ears, nose, cheeks, and lips (Fig. 30-28). The immune system protects the body from foreign antigens, removes damaged cells from the circulation, and provides a partial barrier to growth of malignant cells within the body. Assessing the lymph nodes requires competence when caring for patients with suspected immunoincompetence, which is often linked to allergies, human immunodeficiency virus (HIV) infection, autoimmune disease (e.g., lupus erythematosus), or serious infection.

With the patient's chin raised and head tilted slightly, first inspect the area where lymph nodes are distributed and compare both sides. This position stretches the skin slightly over any possible enlarged nodes. Inspect visible nodes for edema, erythema, or red streaks. Nodes are not normally visible.

Use a methodical approach to palpate the lymph nodes to avoid overlooking any single node or chain. The patient relaxes with the neck flexed slightly forward. Inspect and palpate both sides of the neck for comparison. During palpation either face or stand to the side of the patient for easy access to all nodes. Use the pads of the middle three fingers of each hand to gently palpate in a circular motion over the nodes (Fig. 30-29). Check each node methodically in the following sequence: occipital nodes at the base of the skull, postauricular nodes over the mastoid, preauricular nodes just in front of the ear, retropharyngeal nodes at the angle of the mandible, submandibular nodes, and submental nodes in the midline behind the mandibular tip. Try to detect enlargement and note the location, size, shape, surface characteristics, consistency, mobility, tenderness, and warmth of the nodes. If the skin is mobile, move it over the area of the nodes. It is important to press underlying tissue in each area and not simply move the fingers over the skin. However, if you apply excessive pressure, you miss small nodes and destroy palpable nodes.

TABLE 30-19 Nursing History for Neck Assessment

ASSESSMENT	RATIONALE
Assess for history of recent cold, infection, or enlarged lymph nodes or exposure to radiation or toxic chemicals.	Colds or infections cause temporary or permanent lymph node enlargement. Lymph nodes are also enlarged in various diseases such as cancer.
If there is an enlarged lymph node, consider reviewing history of intravenous drug use, hemophilia, sexual contact with persons infected with human immunodeficiency virus (HIV), history of blood transfusion, multiple and indiscriminate sexual contacts, or male with homosexual or bisexual activities.	These are risk factors for HIV infection.
Ask if patient has had history of neck pain with restriction in movement.	This indicates muscle strain, head injury, local nerve injury, or enlarged or swollen lymph node.
Ask if patient has had change in temperature preference (more or less clothing); swelling in neck; change in texture of hair, skin, or nails; or change in emotional stability.	Symptoms indicate thyroid disease.
Ask if patient has history of hypothyroidism or hyperthyroidism, takes thyroid medication, or has a family history of thyroid disease.	Disease or medications influence tissue growth of gland.
Review medical history of pneumothorax (collapsed lung) or bronchial tumor.	Conditions place patient at risk for tracheal displacement or lateral deviation.

To palpate supraclavicular nodes, ask the patient to bend the head forward and relax the shoulders. Palpate these nodes by hooking the index and third finger over the clavicle lateral to the sternocleidomastoid muscle. Palpate the deep cervical nodes only with the fingers hooked around the sternocleidomastoid muscle.

Normally lymph nodes are not easily palpable. However, small, mobile, nontender nodes are common. Lymph nodes that are large, fixed, inflamed, or tender indicate a problem such as local infection, systemic disease, or neoplasm (Seidel et al., 2011) (Box 30-17). When you find enlarged nodes, explore the adjacent areas and regions drained by the nodes. Tenderness almost always indicates inflammation. A problem involving a lymph node of the head and neck means an abnormality in the mouth, throat, abdomen, breasts, thorax, or arms. These are the areas drained by the head and neck nodes.

Thyroid Gland. The thyroid gland lies in the anterior lower neck, in front of and to both sides of the trachea. The gland is fixed

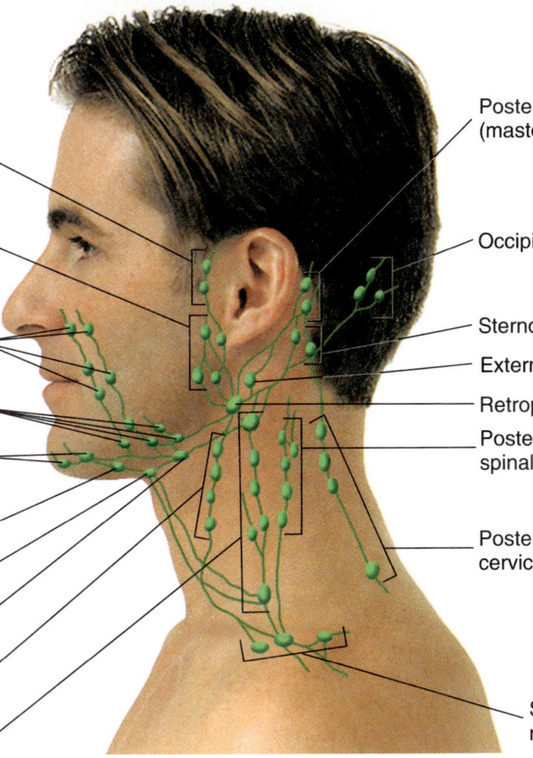

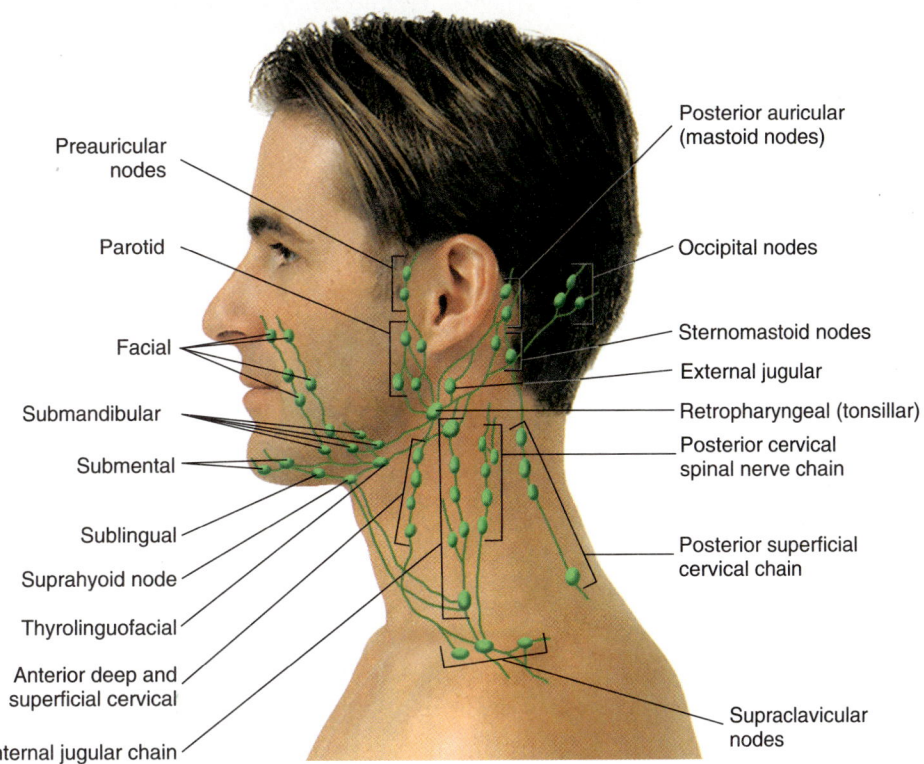

FIG. 30-28 Palpable lymph nodes in the head and neck. (From Seidel HM et al: *Mosby's guide to physical examination,* ed 7, St Louis, 2011, Mosby.)

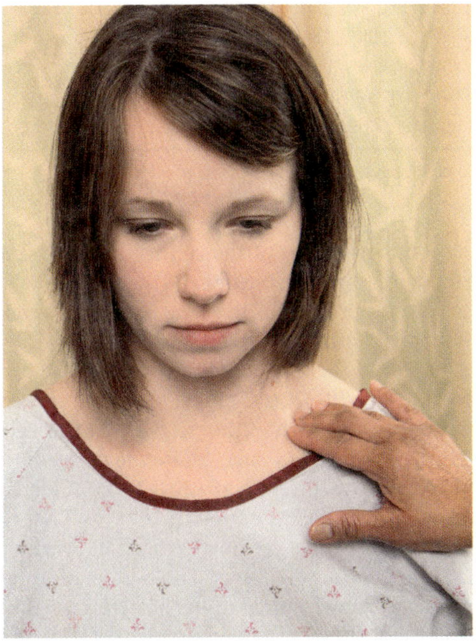

FIG. 30-29 Supraclavicular lymph node palpation.

to the trachea, with the isthmus overlying the trachea and connecting the two irregular, cone-shaped lobes (Fig. 30-30). Inspect the lower neck overlying the thyroid gland for obvious masses, symmetry, and any subtle fullness at the base of the neck. Ask the patient to hyperextend the neck, which helps tighten the skin for better visualization. Offer the patient a glass of water, and, while observing the neck, have him or her swallow. This maneuver helps to visualize an abnormally enlarged thyroid. Normally the thyroid cannot be visualized.

Advanced practice nurses examine the thyroid by palpating for more subtle masses; this technique is not discussed here.

Carotid Artery and Jugular Vein. This portion of the examination is described under examination of the vascular system (see later section).

BOX 30-17 PATIENT TEACHING

Neck Assessment

Objective

- Patient will take proper preventive action if he or she notices a mass in the neck.

Teaching Strategies

- Stress importance of regular compliance with medication schedule to patients with thyroid disease.
- Instruct patient about the lymph nodes and how infection commonly causes node tenderness and mild enlargement.
- Instruct patient to call a health care provider when he or she notices a fixed, enlarged lump or mass in the neck.
- Teach patient risk factors for HIV infection and other sexually transmitted diseases.

Evaluation

- Have patient explain when to notify a physician about a neck mass.

HIV, Human immunodeficiency virus.

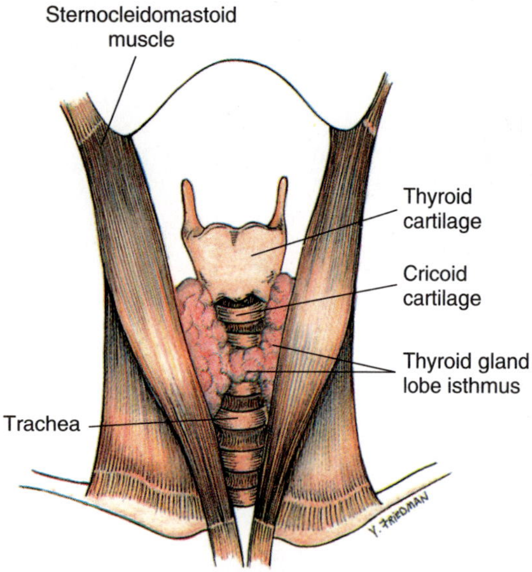

FIG. 30-30 Anatomical position of thyroid gland.

Trachea. The trachea is a part of the upper respiratory system that you directly palpate. It is normally located in the midline above the suprasternal notch. Masses in the neck or mediastinum and pulmonary abnormalities cause displacement laterally. Have the patient sit or lie down during palpation. Determine the position of the trachea by palpating at the suprasternal notch, slipping the thumb and index fingers to each side. Note if the finger and thumb shift laterally. Do not apply forceful pressure because this elicits coughing.

THORAX AND LUNGS

Accurate physical assessment of the thorax and lungs requires review of the ventilatory and respiratory functions of the lungs. If disease is affecting the lungs, it affects other body systems as well. For example, reduced oxygenation causes changes in mental alertness because of the sensitivity of the brain to lowered oxygen levels. Use data from all body systems to determine the nature of pulmonary alterations. You will use inspection, palpation, and auscultation to examine the thorax and lungs. Diagnostic equipment such as x-ray films, magnetic resonance imaging (MRI, and computed tomography (CT) scans create little need for the use of percussion as an assessment measure. Risk factors for lung disease are reviewed at the time of respiratory assessment (Box 30-18).

Before assessing the thorax and lungs, be familiar with the landmarks of the chest (Fig. 30-31, *A* to *C*). These landmarks help you identify findings and use assessment skills correctly. The patient's nipples, angle of Louis, suprasternal notch, costal angle, clavicles, and vertebrae are key landmarks that provide a series of imaginary lines for sign identification. Keep a mental image of the location of the lobes of the lung and the position of each rib (Fig. 30-32, *A* to *C*). The proper orientation to anatomical structures ensures a thorough assessment of the anterior, lateral, and posterior thorax.

Locating the position of each rib is critical to visualizing the lobe of the lung being assessed. To begin, locate the angle of Louis at the manubriosternal junction. The angle is a visible and palpable angulation of the sternum and is the point at which the second rib articulates with the sternum. Count the ribs and intercostal spaces (between the ribs) from this point. The number of each intercostal space corresponds with that of the rib just above it. The spinous process of the third thoracic vertebra and the fourth, fifth, and sixth ribs help to locate the lobes of the lung laterally. The lower lobes project laterally and anteriorly (Fig. 30-32, *B*). Posteriorly the tip or inferior margin of the scapula lies approximately at the level of the seventh rib (Fig. 30-32, *C*). After identifying the seventh rib, count upward to locate the third thoracic vertebra and align it with the inner borders of the scapula to locate the posterior lobes.

The examination requires the patient to be undressed to the waist, with good lighting. Assess patients at risk for pulmonary problems such as the patient confined to bed rest or with chest pain who cannot fully expand the lungs. The examination begins with the patient sitting for assessment of the posterior and lateral chest. Have him or her sit or lie down for assessment of the anterior chest. Table 30-20 reviews the nursing history for lung examination.

BOX 30-18 PATIENT TEACHING

Lung Assessment

Objective

- Patients of all age-groups will practice preventive care measures for lung health.

Teaching Strategies

- Explain risk factors for chronic lung disease and lung cancer, including cigarette smoking, history of smoking for over 20 years; exposure to environmental pollution; and radiation exposure from occupational, medical, and environmental sources. Exposure to radon and asbestos also increases risk. Other risk factors include exposure to certain metals (e.g., arsenic, cadmium, chromium), some organic chemicals, and tuberculosis. Exposure to secondhand cigarette smoke increases risk for nonsmokers (ACS, 2011).
- Share brochures on lung cancer, asthma, and COPD from American Cancer Society with patient and family.
- Instruct patient with asthma to identify and tell which triggers cause asthma episodes.
- Discuss warning signs of lung cancer such as a persistent cough, sputum streaked with blood, chest pains, and recurrent attacks of pneumonia or bronchitis.
- Counsel older adult on benefits of receiving influenza and pneumonia vaccinations because of a greater susceptibility to respiratory infection.
- Instruct patient with COPD in coughing and pursed-lip breathing exercises.
- Refer persons at risk for tuberculosis who visit clinics or health care centers for skin testing.

Evaluation

- Have patient describe risk factors for lung disease and cancer.
- Ask patient to identify any known risks for cancer.
- Ask patient to name warning signs of lung cancer.
- In a follow-up visit review patient's immunization record.
- Observe patient performing breathing exercises and coughing.

COPD, chronic obstructive pulmonary disease.

Posterior Thorax

Begin examination of the posterior thorax by observing for any signs or symptoms in other body systems that indicate pulmonary problems. Reduced mental alertness, nasal flaring, somnolence, and cyanosis are examples of assessed signs that indicate oxygenation problems. Inspect the posterior thorax by observing the shape and symmetry of the chest from the patient's back and front.

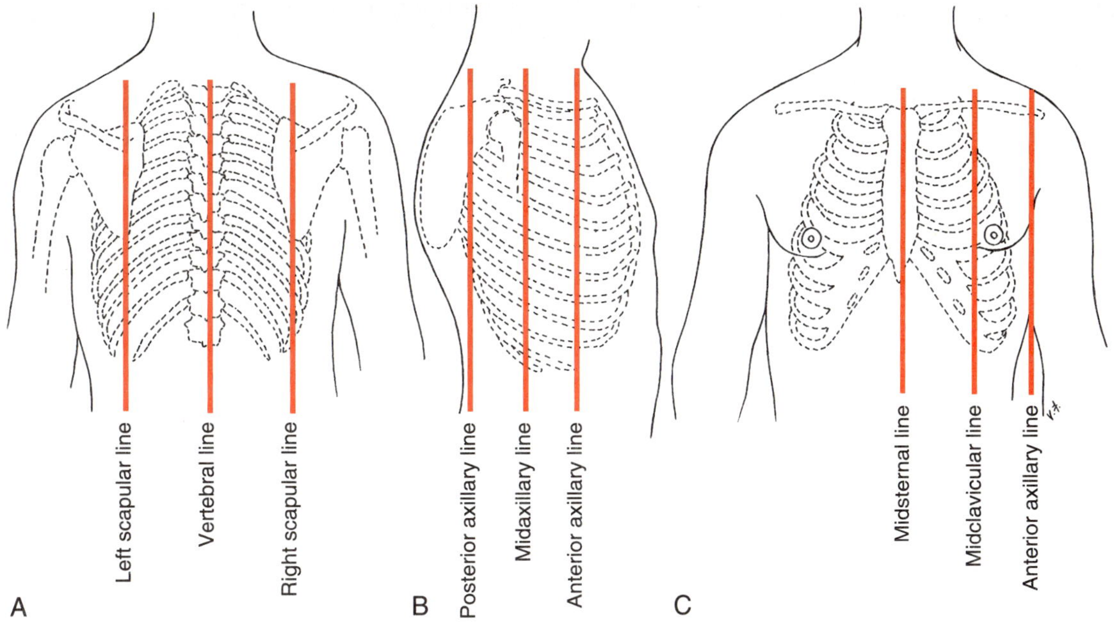

FIG. 30-31 Anatomical chest wall landmarks. **A,** Posterior chest landmarks. **B,** Lateral chest landmarks. **C,** Anterior chest landmarks.

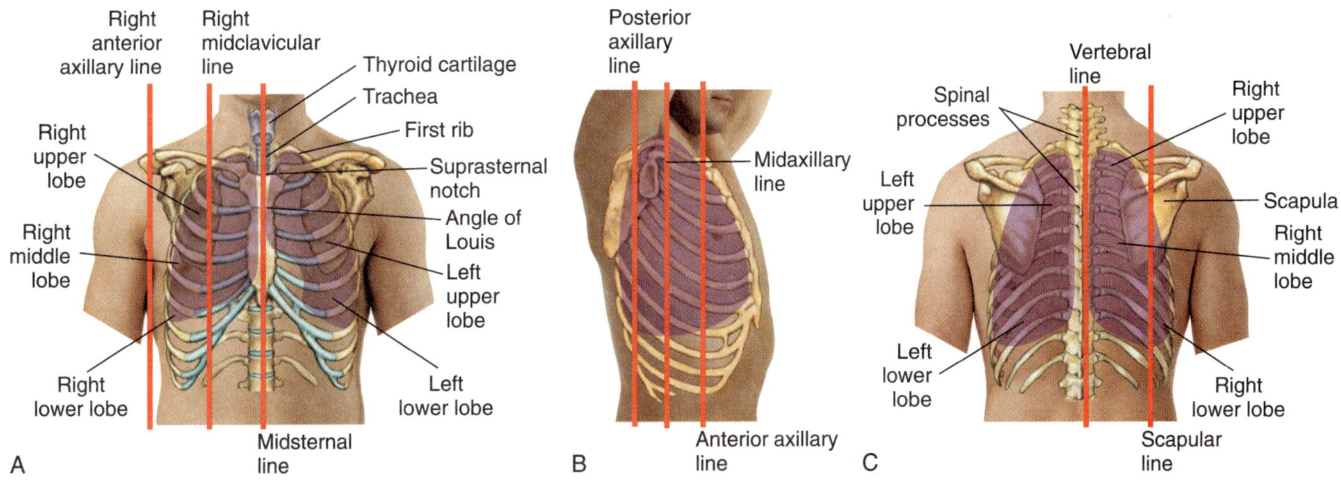

FIG. 30-32 Position of lung lobes in relation to anatomical landmarks. **A,** Anterior position. **B,** Lateral position. **C,** Posterior position. (From Seidel HM, et al: *Mosby's guide to physical examination, ed 7,* St Louis, 2011, Mosby.)

Note the anteroposterior diameter. Body shape or posture significantly impairs ventilatory movement. Normally the chest contour is symmetrical, with the anteroposterior diameter one third to one half of the transverse, or side-to-side, diameter. A barrel-shaped chest (anteroposterior diameter equals transverse diameter) characterizes aging and chronic lung disease. Infants have an almost round shape. Congenital and postural alterations cause abnormal contours. Some patients lean over a table or splint the side of the chest because of a breathing problem. Splinting or holding the chest wall because of pain causes a patient to bend toward the side affected. Such a posture impairs ventilatory movement.

Standing at a midline position behind the patient, look for deformities, position of the spine, slope of the ribs, retraction of the intercostal spaces during inspiration, and bulging of the intercostal spaces during expiration. The scapulae are normally symmetrical and closely attached to the thoracic wall. The normal spine is straight without lateral deviation. Posteriorly the ribs tend to slope across and down. The ribs and intercostal spaces are easier to see in a thin person. Normally no bulging or active movement occurs within the intercostal spaces during breathing. Bulging indicates that the patient is using great effort to breathe.

Also assess the rate and rhythm of breathing (see Chapter 29). Observe the thorax as a whole. It normally expands and relaxes regularly with equality of movement bilaterally. In healthy adults the normal respiratory rates vary from 12 to 20 respirations per minute.

Palpation of the posterior thorax provides further information about a patient's health status. Palpate the thoracic muscles and skeleton for lumps, masses, pulsations, and unusual movement. If the patient voices pain or tenderness, avoid deep palpation. Fractured rib fragments could be displaced against vital organs. Normally the chest wall is not tender. If there is a suspicious mass or

TABLE 30-20 Nursing History for Lung Assessment

ASSESSMENT	RATIONALE
Assess history of tobacco or marijuana use, including type of tobacco, duration and amount (Pack-years = Number of years smoking × Number of packs per day), age started, and efforts to quit and length of time since smoking stopped.	Smoking is a risk factor for lung cancer, heart disease, cerebrovascular disease, emphysema, or chronic bronchitis. It accounts for a significant percentage of all cancer deaths. It increases the risk for 15 types of cancer (American Cancer Society, 2010).
Ask if patient has had a *persistent cough* (productive or nonproductive), *sputum streaked with blood, voice change, chest pain,* shortness of breath, **orthopnea,** dyspnea during exertion or at rest, poor activity tolerance, or *recurrent attacks of pneumonia or bronchitis.*	Symptoms of cardiopulmonary alterations help localize objective physical findings. (Warning signals for lung cancer are in italic type.) The diaphragm of the lungs expands more easily when the individual is sitting upright, as for patients who must be in an upright position to breathe.
Determine if patient works in environment containing pollutants (e.g., asbestos, arsenic, coal dust) or requiring exposure to radiation. Does patient have exposure to secondhand smoke?	These risk factors increase chance for various lung diseases.
Review history for known or suspected human immunodeficiency virus (HIV) infection; substance abuse; low income; or being a resident or employee of nursing home or shelter, homeless, recent prison inmate, family member of tuberculosis (TB) patient, or immigrant to the United States from a country where TB is prevalent (Frakes and Evans, 2004).	These are risk factors for TB.
Ask if patient has history of persistent cough, hemoptysis, unexplained weight loss, fatigue, night sweats, or fever.	These are risk factors for both TB and HIV infection.
Does patient have history of chronic hoarseness?	Hoarseness indicates laryngeal disorder or abuse of cocaine or opioids (sniffing).
Assess history of allergies to pollens, dust, or other airborne irritants and to foods, drugs, or chemical substances.	Symptoms such as choking feeling, bronchospasm with respiratory stridor, wheezes on auscultation, and dyspnea are often caused by allergic response.
Review family history for cancer, TB, allergies, or chronic obstructive pulmonary disease.	Conditions place patient at risk for lung disease.
Ask if patient has had a pneumonia or influenza vaccine and a TB test; if not, educate him or her on need to do so.	The very young, the very old, and those with chronic respiratory problems or immunosuppressive diseases are at increased risk for respiratory disease.

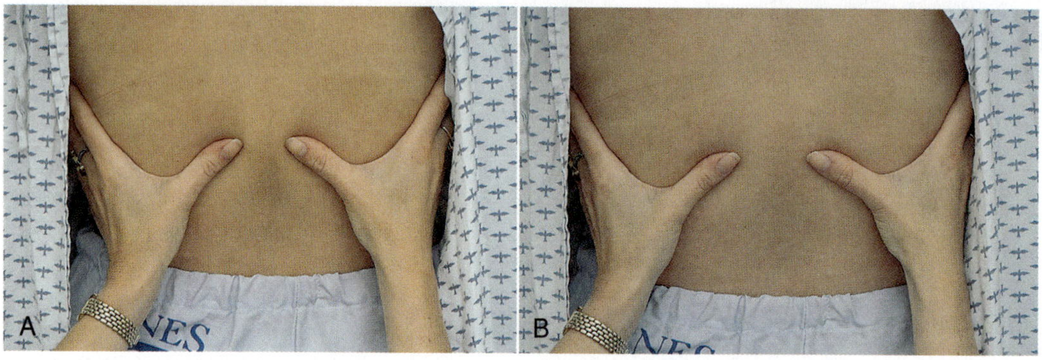

FIG. 30-33 A, Hand position for palpation of posterior thorax excursion. **B,** As patient inhales, movement of chest excursion separates thumbs.

swollen area, lightly palpate it for size, shape, and the typical qualities of a lesion.

To measure chest excursion or depth of breathing, stand behind the patient and place the thumbs along the spinal processes at the tenth rib, with the palms lightly contacting the posterolateral surfaces. Place thumbs 5 cm (2 inches) apart, pointing toward the spine with fingers pointing laterally (Fig. 30-33, *A*). Press the hands toward the spine so a small skinfold appears between the thumbs. Do not slide the hands over the skin. Instruct the patient to exhale and then take a deep breath. Note movement of the thumbs during inhalation (Fig. 30-33, *B*). Chest excursion is symmetrical, separating the thumbs 3 to 5 cm (1¼ to 2 inches). Reduced chest excursion may be caused by pain, postural deformity, or fatigue. In older adults chest movement normally declines because of costal cartilage calcification and respiratory muscle atrophy.

During speech the sound created by the vocal cords is transmitted through the lung to the chest wall. The sound waves create vibrations that you palpate externally. These vibrations are called **vocal or tactile fremitus.** The accumulation of mucus, the collapse of lung tissue, or the presence of one or more lung lesions blocks the vibrations from reaching the chest wall.

To palpate for tactile fremitus, place the palmar surfaces of the fingers or the ulnar part of the hand over symmetrical intercostal spaces, beginning at the lung apex (Fig. 30-34, *A*) and using a firm,

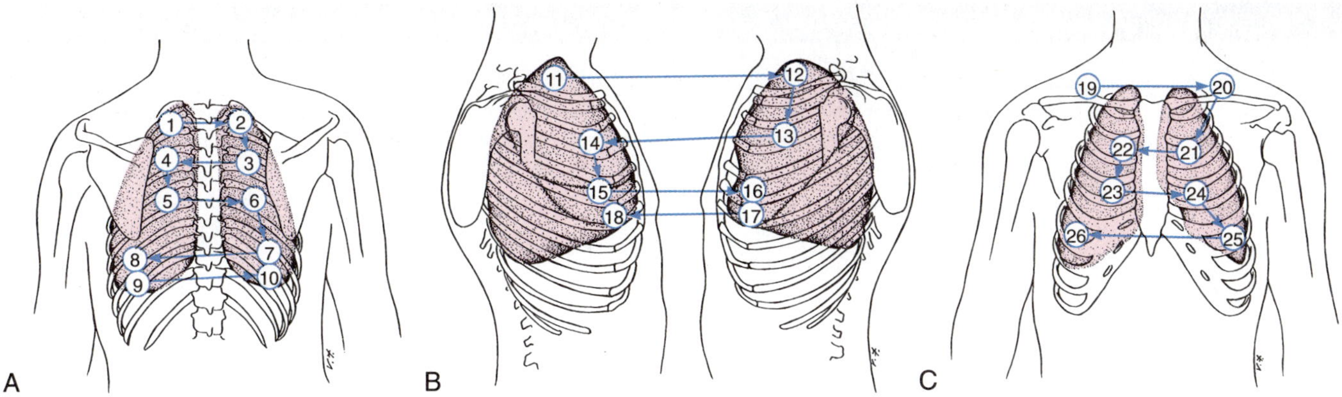

FIG. 30-34 **A** to **C,** A systematic pattern (posterior-lateral-anterior) is followed when palpating and auscultating the thorax.

light touch. Ask the patient to say "ninety-nine" or "one-one-one." Palpate both sides simultaneously and symmetrically (from top to bottom) for comparison or use one hand, quickly alternating between the two sides (Seidel et al., 2011). Normally a faint vibration is present as the patient speaks. If fremitus is faint, ask the patient to speak in a louder or lower tone of voice. Normally fremitus is symmetrical. Vibrations are strongest at the top, near the level of the tracheal bifurcation. Strong vibrations through the chest wall occur in crying infants.

Auscultation assesses the movement of air through the tracheobronchial tree and detects mucus or obstructed airways. Normally air flows through the airways in an unobstructed pattern. Recognizing the sounds created by normal airflow allows you to detect sounds caused by airway obstruction. Follow the same systematic approach when listening that was used for palpation (see Fig. 30-34, *A*).

Place the diaphragm of the stethoscope firmly on the skin, over the posterior chest wall between the ribs (Fig. 30-35). The patient folds the arms in front of the chest and keeps the head bent forward while taking slow, deep breaths with the mouth slightly open. Listen to an entire inspiration and expiration at each position of the stethoscope. If sounds are faint, as in the obese patient, ask the patient to breathe harder and faster temporarily. Breath sounds are much louder in children because of their thin chest walls. The bell works best in children because of a child's small chest. Auscultate for normal breath sounds and abnormal or **adventitious sounds.** Normal breath sounds differ in character, depending on the area you are auscultating. Bronchovesicular and vesicular sounds are normally heard over the posterior thorax (Table 30-21).

Abnormal sounds result from air passing through moisture, mucus, or narrowed airways. They also result from alveoli suddenly reinflating or an inflammation between the pleural linings of the lung. Adventitious sounds often occur superimposed over normal sounds. The four types of adventitious sounds are crackles, rhonchi, wheezes, and pleural friction rub. A specific entity causes each sound, and each has typical auditory features (Table 30-22). During auscultation note the location and characteristics of the sounds and listen for the absence of breath sounds (found in patients with collapsed or surgically removed lobes).

If there are abnormalities in tactile fremitus or auscultation, perform the vocal resonance tests (spoken and whispered voice sounds). Place the stethoscope over the same locations used to assess breath sounds and have the patient say "ninety-nine" in a normal voice tone. Normally the sound is muffled. If fluid is

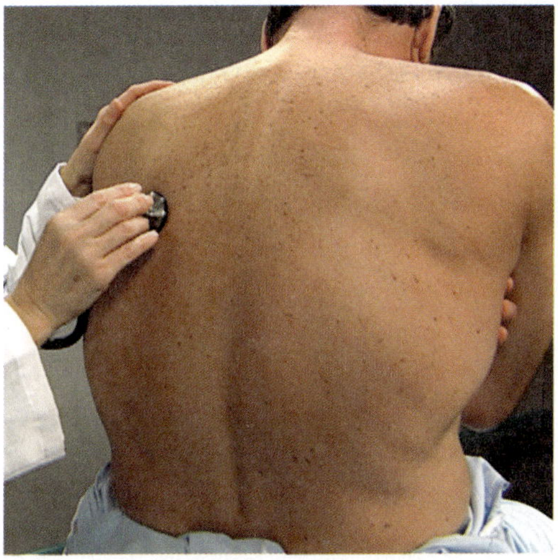

FIG. 30-35 Use the diaphragm of the stethoscope to auscultate breath sounds. (From Seidel HM et al: *Mosby's guide to physical examination,* ed 7, St Louis, 2011, Mosby.)

TABLE 30-21 Normal Breath Sounds

DESCRIPTION	LOCATION	ORIGIN
Vesicular		
Vesicular sounds are soft, breezy, and low pitched. Inspiratory phase is 3 times longer than expiratory phase.	Best heard over periphery of lung (except over scapula)	Created by air moving through smaller airways
Bronchovesicular		
Bronchovesicular sounds are blowing sounds that are medium pitched and of medium intensity. Inspiratory phase is equal to expiratory phase.	Best heard posteriorly between scapulae and anteriorly over bronchioles lateral to sternum at first and second intercostal spaces	Created by air moving through large airways
Bronchial		
Bronchial sounds are loud and high pitched with hollow quality. Expiration lasts longer than inspiration (3:2 ratio).	Heard only over trachea	Created by air moving through trachea close to chest wall

TABLE 30-22 Adventitious Breath Sounds

SOUND	SITE AUSCULTATED	CAUSE	CHARACTER
Crackles 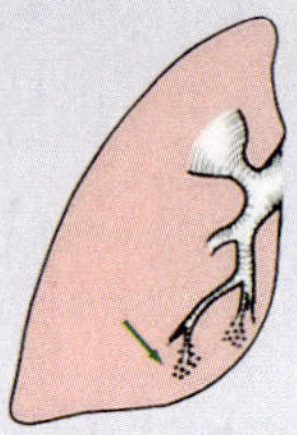	Are most common in dependent lobes: right and left lung bases	Random, sudden reinflation of groups of alveoli; disruptive passage of air through small airways	Fine crackles are high-pitched fine, short; interrupted crackling sounds heard during end of inspiration; usually not cleared with coughing. Medium crackles are lower; moister sounds heard during middle of inspiration; not cleared with coughing. Coarse crackles are loud, bubbly sounds heard during inspiration; not cleared with coughing.
Rhonchi (sonorous wheeze) 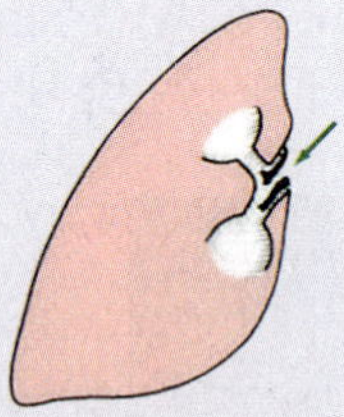	Are primarily heard over trachea and bronchi; if loud enough, able to be heard over most lung fields	Muscular spasm, fluid, or mucus in larger airways; new growth or external pressure causing turbulence	Loud, low-pitched, rumbling coarse sounds are heard either during inspiration or expiration; sometimes cleared by coughing.
Wheezes (sibilant wheeze) 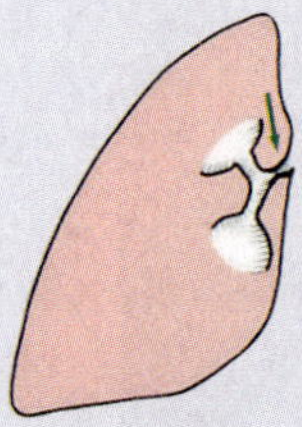	Heard over all lung fields	High-velocity airflow through severely narrowed or obstructed airway	High-pitched, continuous musical sounds are like a squeak heard continuously during inspiration or expiration; usually louder on expiration.
Pleural friction rub 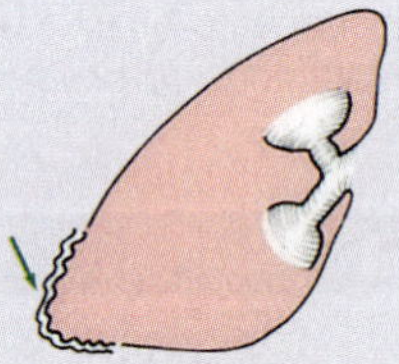	Heard over anterior lateral lung field (if patient is sitting upright)	Inflamed pleura; parietal pleura rubbing against visceral pleura	Dry, rubbing, or grating quality is heard during inspiration or expiration; does not clear with coughing; heard loudest over lower lateral anterior surface.

Data from Seidel HM et al: *Mosby's guide to physical examination,* ed 7, St Louis, 2011, Mosby.

compressing the lung, the vibrations from the patient's voice are transmitted to the chest wall, and the sound becomes clear (bronchophony). Then ask the patient to whisper "ninety-nine." The whispered voice is usually faint and indistinct. Certain lung abnormalities cause the whispered voice to become clear and distinct (whispered pectoriloquy).

Lateral Thorax

Extend the assessment of the posterior thorax to the lateral sides of the chest. The patient sits during examination of the lateral chest. Have the patient raise the arms to improve access to lateral thoracic structures. Use inspection, palpation, and auscultation skills to examine the lateral thorax (see Fig. 30-34, *B*). Do not assess excursion laterally. Normally the breath sounds you hear are vesicular.

Anterior Thorax

Inspect the anterior thorax for the same features as the posterior thorax. The patient sits or lies down with the head elevated. Observe the accessory muscles of breathing: sternocleidomastoid, trapezius, and abdominal muscles. The accessory muscles move little with normal passive breathing. However, patients who use a great deal of effort to breathe as a result of strenuous exercise or pulmonary disease (e.g., chronic obstructive pulmonary disease) rely on the accessory and abdominal muscles to contract, thereby leading to inspiration and expiration. Some patients who require great effort produce a grunting sound.

Observe the width of the costal angle. It is usually larger than 90 degrees between the two costal margins. Observe the breathing pattern. Normal breathing is quiet and barely audible near the open mouth. You most often assess respiratory rate and rhythm

TABLE 30-23 Nursing History for Heart Assessment

ASSESSMENT	RATIONALE
Determine history of smoking, alcohol intake, caffeine intake, use of prescriptive and recreational drugs, exercise habits, and dietary patterns and intake (including fat and sodium intake).	Smoking; alcohol ingestion; cocaine use; lack of regular exercise; intake of foods high in carbohydrates, fats, and cholesterol are risk factors for cardiovascular disease. Caffeine can cause heart dysrhythmias.
Determine if patient is taking medications for cardiovascular function (e.g., antidysrhythmics, antihypertensives) and if he or she knows their purpose, dosage, and side effects.	Knowledge allows nurse to assess compliance with drug therapies. Medications sometimes affect vital sign values.
Assess for chest pain or discomfort, palpitations, excess fatigue, cough, dyspnea, leg pain or cramps, edema of feet, cyanosis, fainting, and orthopnea. Ask if symptoms occur at rest or during exercise.	These are key symptoms of heart disease. Cardiovascular function is sometimes adequate during rest but not during exercise. Positions affect how well lungs can expand.
If patient reports chest pain, determine if it is cardiac in nature. Anginal pain is usually a deep pressure or ache that is substernal and diffuse, radiating to one or both arms, neck, or jaw.	Assessment determines nature of pain and need to initiate care immediately.
Determine whether patient has a stressful lifestyle. What physical demands and/or emotional stress exist?	Repeated exposure to stress increases risk for heart disease.
Assess family history for heart disease, diabetes, high cholesterol levels, hypertension, stroke, or rheumatic heart disease.	Factors increase risk for heart disease.
Ask patient about history of heart trouble (e.g., heart failure, congenital heart disease, coronary artery disease, dysrhythmias, murmurs).	Knowledge reveals patient's level of understanding of condition. Preexisting condition influences examination techniques used and findings to expect.
Determine whether patient has preexisting diabetes, lung disease, obesity, or hypertension.	These disorders alter heart function.

anteriorly (see Chapter 29). The male patient's respirations are usually diaphragmatic, whereas a female's are more costal. Accurate assessment occurs as the patient breathes passively.

Palpate the anterior thoracic muscles and skeleton for lumps, masses, tenderness, or unusual movement. The sternum and xiphoid are relatively inflexible. Place the thumbs parallel approximately along the costal margin 6 cm (2½ inches) apart with the palms touching the anterolateral chest. Push the thumbs toward the midline to create a skinfold. As the patient inhales deeply, the thumbs normally separate approximately 3 to 5 cm (1¼ to 2 inches), with each side expanding equally.

Assess tactile fremitus over the anterior chest wall. Anterior findings differ from posterior findings because of the heart and female breast tissue. Fremitus is felt next to the sternum at the second intercostal space, at the level of the bronchial bifurcation. It decreases over the heart, lower thorax, and breast tissue.

Auscultation of the anterior thorax follows a systematic pattern (see Fig. 30-34, *C*) comparing right and left sides. This is important so lung sounds in one region on one side of the body can be compared with sounds in the same region on the opposite side of the body.

If possible, have the patient sit to maximize chest expansion. Give special attention to the lower lobes, where mucus secretions commonly gather. Listen for bronchovesicular and vesicular sounds above and below the clavicles and along the lung periphery. In addition, auscultate for bronchial sounds, which are loud, high pitched, and hollow sounding, with expiration lasting longer than inspiration (3:2 ratio). This sound is normally heard over the trachea.

HEART

Compare the assessment of heart function with findings from the vascular assessment (see later section). Alterations in either system sometimes manifest as changes in the other. Some patients with signs or symptoms of heart (cardiac) problems have a life-threatening condition requiring immediate attention. In this case act quickly and conduct only the portions of the examination that are absolutely necessary. Conduct a more thorough assessment when the patient is more stable. The nursing history (Table 30-23) provides data to help interpret physical findings.

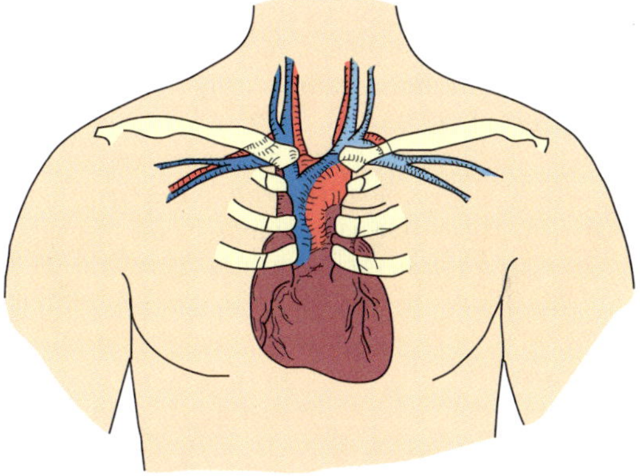

FIG. 30-36 Anatomical position of heart.

Assess cardiac function through the anterior thorax. Form a mental image of the exact location of the heart (Fig. 30-36). In the adult it is located in the center of the chest (precordium), behind and to the left of the sternum, with a small section of the right atrium extending to the right of the sternum. The base of the heart is the upper portion, and the apex is the bottom tip. The surface of the right ventricle composes most of the anterior surface of the heart. A section of the left ventricle shapes the left anterior side of the apex. The apex actually touches the anterior chest wall at approximately the fourth to fifth intercostal space just medial to the left midclavicular line. This is the **apical impulse or point of maximal impulse (PMI).**

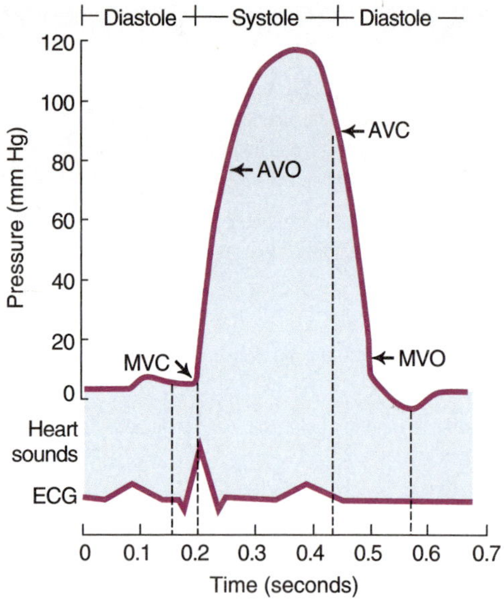

FIG. 30-37 Cardiac cycle. *AVC,* Aortic valve closes; *AVO,* aortic valve opens; *ECG,* electrocardiogram; *MVC,* mitral valve closes; *MVO,* mitral valve opens.

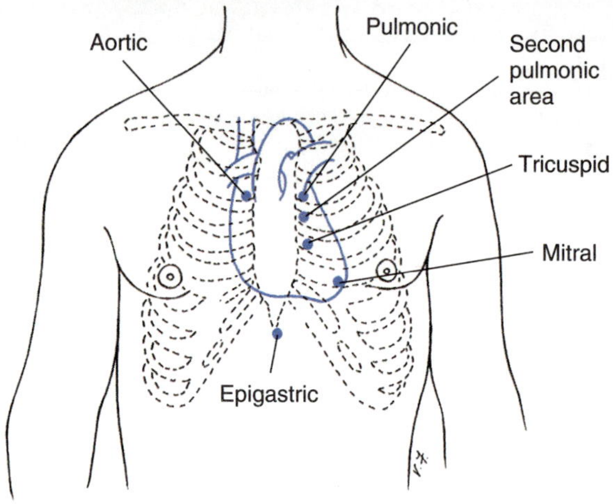

FIG. 30-38 Anatomical sites for assessment of cardiac function.

An infant's heart is positioned more horizontally. The apex of the heart is at the third or fourth intercostal space, just to the left of the midclavicular line. By the age of 7 a child's PMI is in the same location as the adult's. In tall, slender persons the heart hangs more vertically and is positioned more centrally. In shorter or stockier individuals the heart tends to lie more to the left and horizontally (Seidel et al., 2011).

To assess heart function, a clear understanding of the cardiac cycle and associated physiological events is of utmost importance (Fig. 30-37). The heart normally pumps blood through its four chambers in a methodical, even sequence. Events on the left side occur just before those on the right. As blood flows through each chamber, the valves open and close, the pressures within chambers rise and fall, and the chambers contract. Each event creates a physiological sign. Both sides of the heart function in a coordinated fashion.

There are two phases to the cardiac cycle: systole and diastole. During systole the ventricles contract and eject blood from the left ventricle into the aorta and from the right ventricle into the pulmonary artery. During diastole the ventricles relax, and the atria contract to move blood into the ventricles and fill the coronary arteries.

Heart sounds occur in relation to physiological events in the cardiac cycle. As systole begins, ventricular pressure rises and closes the mitral and tricuspid valves. Valve closure causes the first heart sound (S_1), often described as "lub." The ventricles then contract, and blood flows through the aorta and pulmonary circulation. After the ventricles empty, ventricular pressure falls below that in the aorta and pulmonary artery. This allows the aortic and pulmonic valves to close, causing the second heart sound (S_2), described as "dub." As ventricular pressure continues to fall, it drops below that of the atria. The mitral and tricuspid valves reopen to allow ventricular filling. When the heart attempts to fill an already distended ventricle, a third heart sound (S_3) can be heard, as with heart failure. An S_3 is considered abnormal in adults over 30 years of age but can often be heard normally in children and young adults. It can also be present among women in the late stages of pregnancy. A fourth heart sound (S_4) occurs when the atria contract to enhance ventricular filling. An S_4 is often heard in healthy older adults, children, and athletes; but it is not normal in adults. Because S_4 also indicates an abnormal condition, report it to a health care provider.

Inspection and Palpation

Make the patient relaxed and comfortable before the examination. Explain the procedure to relieve his or her anxiety. An anxious or uncomfortable patient has mild tachycardia, which leads to inaccurate findings.

Use the skills of inspection and palpation simultaneously. Begin the examination with the patient in the supine position or the upper body elevated 45 degrees because patients with heart disease frequently suffer shortness of breath while lying flat. Stand at the patient's right side. Do not let the patient talk, especially when auscultating heart sounds. Good lighting in the room is essential.

Direct your attention to the anatomical sites best suited for assessment of cardiac function. During inspection and palpation look for visible pulsations and exaggerated lifts and palpate for the apical impulse and any source of vibrations (thrills). Follow an orderly sequence, beginning with assessment of the base of the heart and moving toward the apex. First inspect the angle of Louis, which lies between the sternal body and manubrium, and feel the ridge in the sternum approximately 5 cm (2 inches) below the sternal notch. Slip the fingers along the angle on each side of the sternum to feel adjacent ribs. The intercostal spaces are just below each rib. The second intercostal space allows identification of each of the six anatomical landmarks (Fig. 30-38). The second intercostal space on the right is the aortic area, and the left second intercostal space is the *pulmonic area.* You need to use deeper palpation to feel the spaces in obese or heavily muscled patients. After locating the pulmonic area, move the fingers down the patient's left sternal border to the third intercostal space, called the *second pulmonic area.* The *tricuspid area* is located at the fourth or fifth intercostal space along the sternum. To find the *apical or mitral area,* locate the fifth intercostal space just to the left of the sternum and move the fingers laterally to the left midclavicular line. Locate the apical area with the palm of the hand or the fingertips. Normally you feel the apical impulse as a light tap in an area 1 to 2 cm (½ to ¾ inch) in diameter at the apex (Fig. 30-39). Another

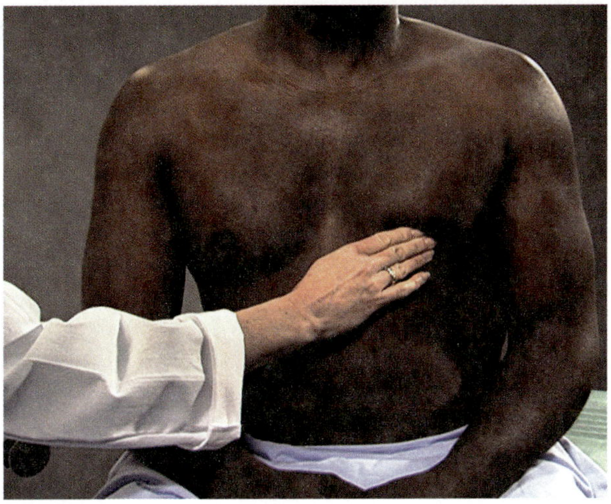

FIG. 30-39 Palpation of apical pulse. (From Seidel HM et al: *Mosby's guide to physical examination,* ed 7, St Louis, 2011, Mosby.)

landmark is the epigastric area at the tip of the sternum. Palpate there if you suspect aortic abnormalities.

Locate the six anatomical landmarks of the heart and inspect and palpate each area. Look for the appearance of pulsations, viewing each area over the chest at an angle to the side. Normally pulsations are not seen, except perhaps at the PMI in thin patients or at the epigastric area as a result of abdominal aorta pulsation. Use the proximal halves of the four fingers together and alternate this with the ball of the hand to palpate for pulsations. Touch the areas gently to allow movements to lift the hand. Normally no pulsations or vibrations are felt in the second, third, or fourth intercostal spaces. Loud murmurs cause a vibration. Time palpated pulsations or vibrations and their occurrence in relation to systole or diastole by auscultating heart sounds simultaneously.

The apical impulse or PMI is easily felt. If you cannot locate it with the patient in a supine position, have him or her roll onto the left side, moving the heart closer to the chest wall. Estimate the size of the heart by noting the diameter of the PMI and its position relative to the midclavicular line. In cases of serious heart disease, the cardiac muscle enlarges, with the PMI found to the left of the midclavicular line. The PMI is sometimes difficult to find in the older adult because the chest deepens in its anteroposterior diameters. It is also difficult to find in muscular or overweight patients. An infant's PMI is located near the third or fourth intercostal space. It is easy to palpate because of the child's thin chest wall.

Auscultation

Auscultation of the heart detects normal heart sounds, extra heart sounds, and murmurs. Concentrate on detecting low-intensity sounds created by valve closures. To begin auscultation eliminate all sources of room noise and explain the procedure to reduce the patient's anxiety. Follow a systematic pattern, beginning at the aortic area and inching the stethoscope across each of the anatomical sites. Listen for the complete cycle ("lub-dub") of heart sounds clearly at each location. Repeat the sequence using the bell of the stethoscope. Sometimes you will have a patient assume three different positions during the examination to hear sounds clearly (Fig. 30-40, *A* to *C*): sitting up and leaning forward (good for all areas and to hear high-pitched murmurs), supine (good for all areas), and left lateral recumbent (good for all areas; best position to hear low-pitched sounds in diastole).

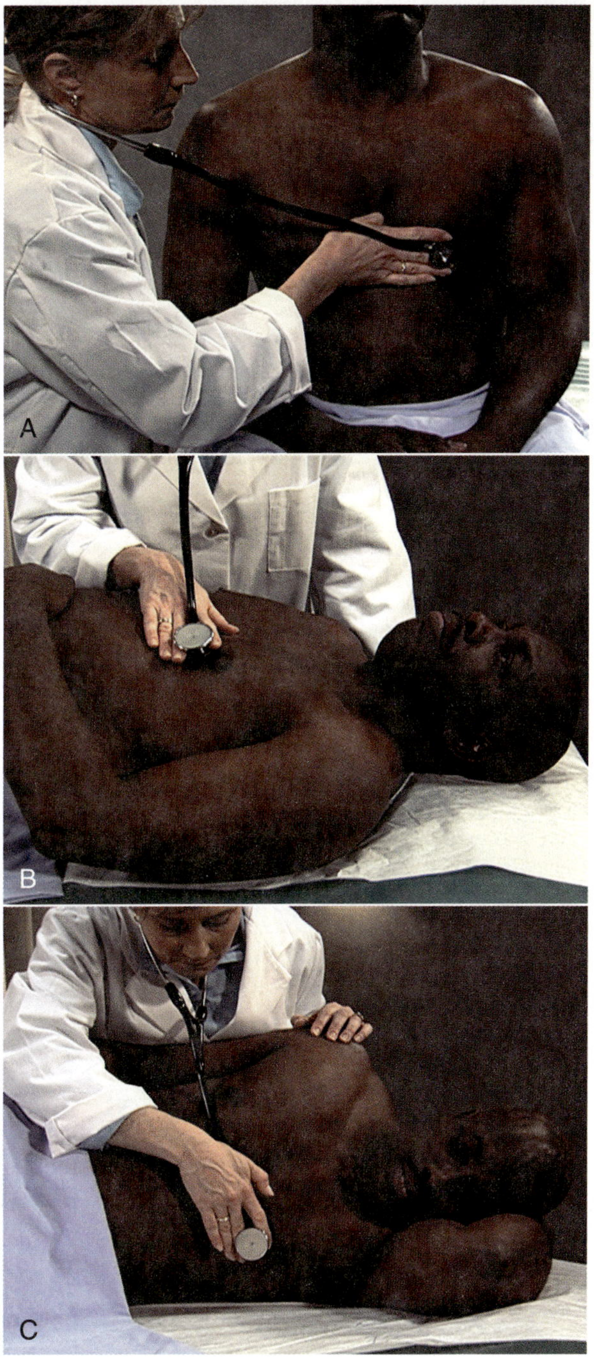

FIG. 30-40 Sequence of patient positions for heart auscultation. **A,** Sitting. **B,** Supine. **C,** Left lateral recumbent. (From Seidel HM et al: *Mosby's guide to physical examination,* ed 7, St Louis, 2011, Mosby.)

Learn to identify the first (S_1) and second (S_2) heart sounds. At normal rates S_1 occurs after the long diastolic pause and preceding the short systolic pause. S_1 is high pitched, dull in quality, and heard best at the apex. If it is difficult to hear S_1, time it in relation to the carotid pulsation. S_2 follows the short systolic pause and precedes the long diastolic pause; it is best heard at the aortic area.

Auscultate for rate and rhythm after hearing both sounds clearly. Each combination of S_1 and S_2 or "lub-dub" counts as one heartbeat. Count the rate for 1 minute and listen for the interval between S_1 and S_2 and then the time between S_2 and the next S_1. A regular rhythm involves regular intervals of time between each sequence of beats. There is a distinct silent pause between S_1 and S_2. Failure of the heart to beat at regular successive intervals is a **dysrhythmia.** Some dysrhythmias are life threatening.

When assessing an irregular heart rhythm, compare apical and radial pulse rates simultaneously to determine if a pulse deficit exists. Auscultate the apical pulse first and then immediately palpate the radial pulse (one-examiner technique). Assess the apical and radial rates at the same time when two examiners are present. When a patient has a pulse deficit, the radial pulse is slower than the apical pulse because ineffective contractions fail to send pulse waves to the periphery. Report a difference in pulse rates to the health care provider immediately.

Assess for extra heart sounds at each auscultatory site. Use the bell of the stethoscope and listen for low-pitched extra heart sounds such as S_3 and S_4 gallops, clicks, and rubs. Auscultate over all anatomical areas. S_3, or a **ventricular gallop,** occurs after S_2. It is caused by a premature rush of blood into a ventricle that is stiff or dilated as a result of heart failure and hypertension. The combination of S_1, S_2, and S_3 sounds like "Ken-tuck'-y."

S_4, or an atrial gallop, occurs just before S_1 or ventricular systole. The sound of an S_4 is similar to that of "Ten'-es-see." Physiologically it is caused by an atrial contraction pushing against a ventricle that is not accepting blood because of heart failure or other alterations. You can hear extra heart sounds more easily with the patient lying on the left side and the stethoscope at the apical site.

The final portion of the examination includes assessment for heart murmurs. **Murmurs** are sustained swishing or blowing sounds heard at the beginning, middle, or end of the systolic or diastolic phase. They are caused by increased blood flow through a normal valve, forward flow through a stenotic valve or into a dilated vessel or heart chamber, or backward flow through a valve that fails to close. A murmur is asymptomatic or a sign of heart disease (Box 30-19). They are common in children. Keep the following factors in mind when auscultating to detect murmurs:

- When a murmur is detected, auscultate the mitral, tricuspid, aortic, and pulmonic valve areas for placement in the cardiac cycle (timing); the place it is heard best (location); radiation; loudness; pitch; and quality.
- If a murmur occurs between S_1 and S_2, it is a systolic murmur.
- If it occurs between S_2 and the next S_1, it is a diastolic murmur.
- The location of a murmur is not necessarily directly over the valves. Experience with hearing murmurs helps with better understanding of where each type of murmur is best heard. For example, mitral murmurs are best heard at the apex of the heart.
- To assess for radiation, listen over areas in addition to where it is heard best. Murmurs can also be heard over the neck or back.
- Intensity or loudness is related to the rate of blood flow through the heart or the amount of blood regurgitated. Feel for a thrust or intermittent palpable sensation at the auscultation site in serious murmurs. A **thrill** is a continuous palpable sensation that resembles the purring of a cat. Intensity is recorded using the following grades (Seidel et al., 2011):

  Grade 1: Barely audible in a quiet room
  Grade 2: Clearly audible but quiet
  Grade 3: Moderately loud
  Grade 4: Loud, with associated thrill
  Grade 5: Very loud, thrill easily palpable
  Grade 6: Louder, may be heard without stethoscope; thrill palpable and visible
- A murmur is low, medium, or high in pitch, depending on the velocity of blood flow through the valves. A low-pitched murmur is best heard with the bell of the stethoscope. If the murmur is best heard with the diaphragm, the murmur is high pitched.

The quality of a murmur refers to its characteristic pattern and sound. A crescendo murmur starts softly and builds in loudness. A decrescendo murmur starts loudly and becomes less intense.

BOX 30-19 PATIENT TEACHING

Heart Assessment

Objective

- Patient will describe risk factors for heart disease and take appropriate steps to eliminate risks from lifestyle.

Teaching Strategies

- Explain risk factors for heart disease, including high dietary intake of saturated fat or cholesterol, lack of regular aerobic exercise, smoking, excess weight, stressful lifestyle, hypertension, and family history of heart disease.
- Refer patient (if appropriate) to resources available for controlling or reducing risks (e.g., nutritional counseling, exercise class, stress reduction programs).
- Teach patient to reduce dietary intake of cholesterol and saturated fats. Explain that approximately 70% to 75% of saturated fatty acids come from meats, poultry, fish, and dairy products. The American Heart Association (2011) recommends a diet that includes an intake that limits total fat to less than 25% to 35% of total calories, saturated fats to less than 7% of daily calories, trans fats to less than 1% of calories, and cholesterol to less than 300 mg/day.
- Encourage patient to have total blood cholesterol levels and triglycerides measured regularly. Desirable levels are less than 200 mg/100 mL. You need more than one cholesterol measurement to assess the blood cholesterol level accurately. Low-density lipoprotein (LDL) cholesterol is the major component of atherosclerotic plaques. Separate measurement of LDL cholesterol is wise in a patient with high total blood cholesterol levels. In an individual with no other risk factors, an LDL cholesterol level of 160 mg/100 mL or higher is high risk (Moore, 2005).
- Encourage patient to discuss with health care provider the need for periodic C-reactive protein (CRP) testing. CRP levels assess a patient's risk for cardiovascular disease.
- Advise patient to avoid cigarette smoke because nicotine causes vasoconstriction.
- Advise patient to quit smoking because this lowers the risk for coronary heart disease and coronary vascular disease (ACS, 2011).
- Patients who are at risk benefit from taking a daily low dose of aspirin. Consult health care provider before starting therapy.

Evaluation

- Ask patient to identify risk factors for heart disease.
- Have patient develop a meal plan low in saturated fat and cholesterol.
- Check patient's cholesterol level during follow-up appointments at the clinic or physician's office.
- Ask patient to describe ways he or she has chosen to reduce cardiac risk factors.

TABLE 30-24 Nursing History for Vascular Assessment

ASSESSMENT	RATIONALE
Determine if patient experiences leg cramps; numbness or tingling in extremities; sensation of cold hands or feet; pain in legs; or swelling or cyanosis of feet, ankles, or hand.	These signs and symptoms indicate vascular disease.
If patient experiences leg pain or cramping in lower extremities, ask if walking or standing for long periods or during sleep aggravate or relieve it.	Relationship of symptoms to exercise clarifies whether problem is vascular or musculoskeletal. Pain caused by vascular condition tends to increase with activity. Musculoskeletal pain usually is not relieved when exercise ends.
Ask patients if they wear tight-fitting garters, socks, or hosiery and sit or lie in bed with legs crossed.	Tight hosiery around lower extremities and crossing legs can impair venous return.
Reconsider previous heart risk factors (e.g., smoking, exercise, nutritional problems).	These predispose patient to vascular disease.
Assess medical history for heart disease, hypertension, phlebitis, diabetes, or varicose veins.	Circulatory and vascular disorders influence findings gathered during examination.

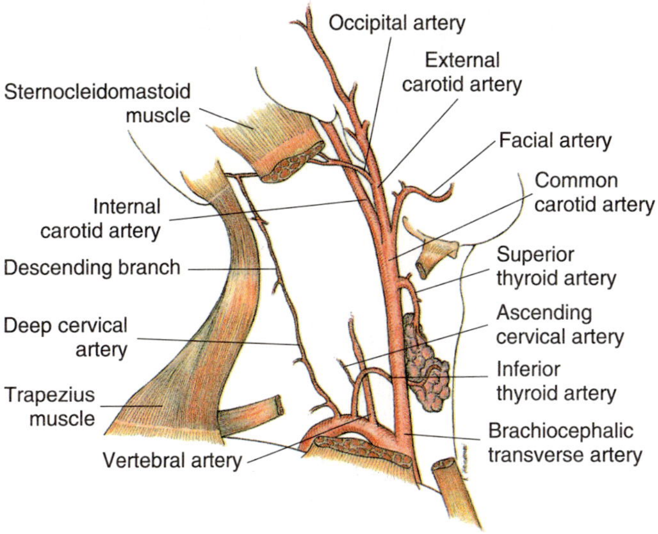

FIG. 30-41 Anatomical position of carotid artery.

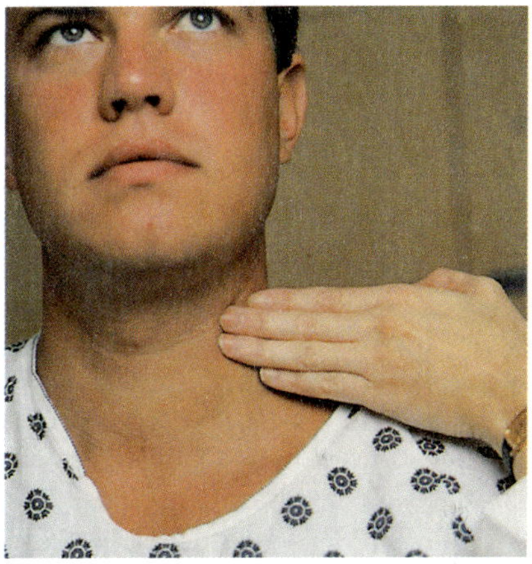

FIG. 30-42 Palpation of internal carotid artery along margin of sternocleidomastoid muscle.

VASCULAR SYSTEM

Examination of the vascular system includes measuring the blood pressure (see Chapter 29) and assessing the integrity of the peripheral vascular system. Table 30-24 reviews the nursing history data collected before the examination. Use the skills of inspection, palpation, and auscultation. Perform portions of the vascular examination during other body system assessments. For example, check the carotid pulse after palpating the cervical lymph nodes. Note signs and symptoms of arterial and venous insufficiency when assessing the skin.

Blood Pressure

When auscultating blood pressure, know that readings between the arms vary by as much as 10 mm Hg and tend to be higher in the right arm (Seidel et al., 2011). Always record the higher reading. Repeated systolic readings that differ by 15 mm Hg or more suggest atherosclerosis or disease of the aorta.

Carotid Arteries

When the left ventricle pumps blood into the aorta, the arterial system transmits pressure waves. The carotid arteries reflect heart function better than peripheral arteries because their pressure correlates with that of the aorta. The carotid artery supplies oxygenated blood to the head and neck (Fig. 30-41). The overlying sternocleidomastoid muscle protects it.

To examine the carotid arteries, have the patient sit or lie supine with the head of the bed elevated 30 degrees. Examine one carotid artery at a time. If both arteries are occluded simultaneously during palpation, the patient loses consciousness as a result of inadequate circulation to the brain. Do not palpate or massage the carotid arteries vigorously because the carotid sinus is located at the bifurcation of the common carotid arteries in the upper third of the neck. This sinus sends impulses along the vagus nerve. Its stimulation causes a reflex drop in heart rate and blood pressure, which causes **syncope** or circulatory arrest. This is a particular problem for older adults.

Begin inspection of the neck for obvious pulsation of the artery. Have the patient turn the head slightly away from the artery being examined. Sometimes the wave of the pulse is visible. The carotid is the only site for assessing the quality of a pulse wave. An absent pulse wave indicates arterial occlusion (blockage) or **stenosis** (narrowing).

To palpate the pulse ask the patient to look straight ahead or turn the head slightly toward the side you are examining. Turning relaxes the sternocleidomastoid muscle. Slide the tips of the index and middle fingers around the medial edge of the sternocleidomastoid muscle. Gently palpate to avoid occlusion of circulation (Fig. 30-42).

The normal carotid pulse is localized and strong rather than diffuse. It has a thrusting quality. As the patient breathes,

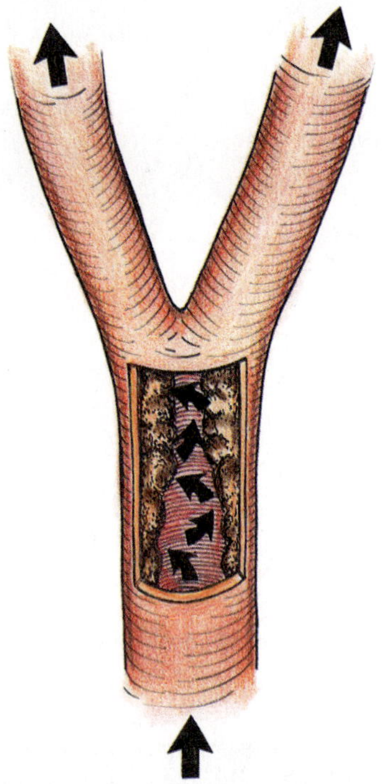

FIG. 30-43 Occlusion or narrowing of the carotid artery disrupts normal blood flow. The resultant turbulence creates a sound (bruit) that is auscultated.

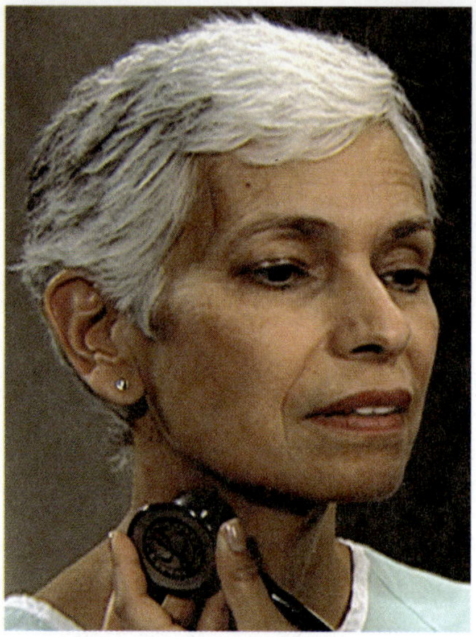

FIG. 30-44 Auscultation for carotid artery bruit. (From Seidel HM et al: *Mosby's guide to physical examination,* ed 7, St Louis, 2011, Mosby.)

no change occurs. Rotation of the neck or a shift from a sitting to a supine position does not change the quality of the carotid impulse. Both carotid arteries are normally equal in pulse rate, rhythm, and strength and are equally elastic. Diminished or unequal carotid pulsations indicate atherosclerosis or other forms of arterial disease.

The carotid is the most commonly auscultated pulse. Auscultation is especially important for middle-age or older adults or patients suspected of having cerebrovascular disease. When the lumen of a blood vessel is narrowed, it disturbs blood flow. As blood passes through the narrowed section, it creates turbulence, causing a blowing or swishing sound. The blowing sound is called a **bruit** (pronounced "brew-ee") (Fig. 30-43).

Place the bell of the stethoscope over the carotid artery at the lateral end of the clavicle and the posterior margin of the sternocleidomastoid muscle. Have the patient turn his or her head slightly away from the side being examined (Fig. 30-44). Ask him or her to hold the breath for a moment so breath sounds do not obscure a bruit. Normally you do not hear any sounds during carotid auscultation. Palpate the artery lightly for a thrill (palpable bruit) if you hear a bruit.

Jugular Veins

The most accessible veins for examination are the internal and external jugular veins in the neck. Both veins drain bilaterally from the head and neck into the superior vena cava. The external jugular vein lies superficially and is just above the clavicle. The internal jugular vein lies deeper, along the carotid artery.

It is best to examine the right internal jugular vein because it follows a more direct anatomical path to the right atrium of the heart. The column of blood inside the internal jugular vein serves as a manometer, reflecting pressure in the right atrium. The higher the column, the greater is the venous pressure. Raised venous pressure reflects right-sided heart failure.

Normally, when a patient lies in the supine position, the external jugular vein distends and becomes easily visible. In contrast, the jugular veins normally flatten when the patient changes to a sitting or standing position. However, for some patients with heart disease the jugular veins remain distended when sitting.

To measure venous pressure, first inspect the jugular veins. Venous pressure is influenced by blood volume, the capacity of the right atrium to receive blood and send it to the right ventricle and the ability of the right ventricle to contract and force blood into the pulmonary artery. Any factor resulting in greater blood volume within the venous system results in elevated venous pressure. Assess venous pressure by using the following steps:

1. Ask the patient to lie supine with the head elevated 30 to 45 degrees (semi-Fowler's position).
2. Expose the neck and upper thorax. Use a pillow to align the head. Avoid neck hyperextension or flexion to ensure that the vein is not stretched or kinked (Fig. 30-45).
3. Usually pulsations are not evident with the patient sitting up. As he or she slowly leans back into a supine position, the level of venous pulsations begins to rise above the level of the manubrium as much as 1 or 2 cm ($\frac{1}{2}$ to 1 inch) as the patient reaches a 45-degree angle. Measure venous pressure by measuring the vertical distance between the angle of Louis and the highest level of the visible point of the internal jugular vein pulsation.
4. Use two rulers. Line up the bottom edge of a regular ruler with the top of the area of pulsation in the jugular vein. Then take a centimeter ruler and align it perpendicular to the first ruler at the level of the sternal angle. Measure in centimeters the distance between the second ruler and the sternal angle (Fig. 30-46).
5. Repeat the same measurement on the other side. Bilateral pressures higher than 2.5 cm (1 inch) are considered elevated and are a sign of right-sided heart failure. One-sided pressure elevation is caused by obstruction.

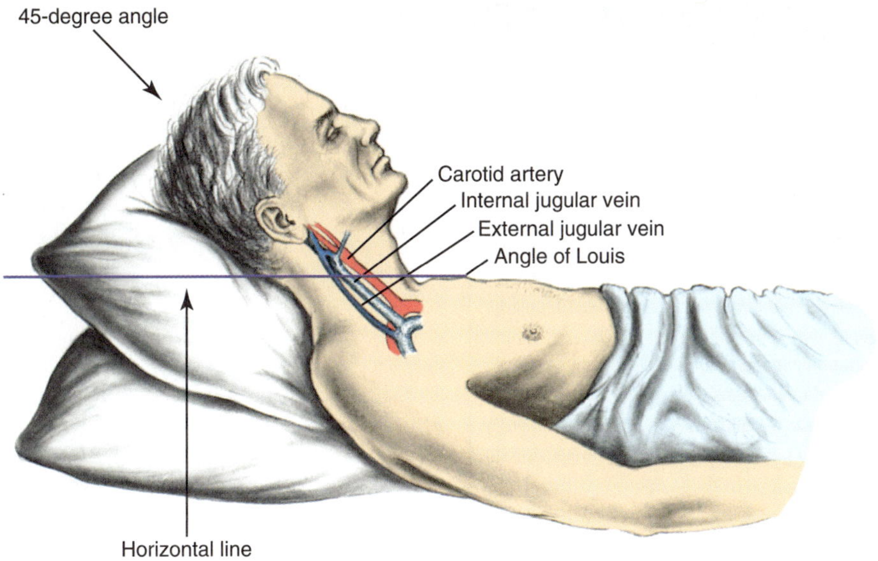

FIG. 30-45 Position of patient to assess jugular vein distention. (From Thompson JM et al: *Mosby's manual of clinical nursing,* ed 5, St Louis, 2001, Mosby.)

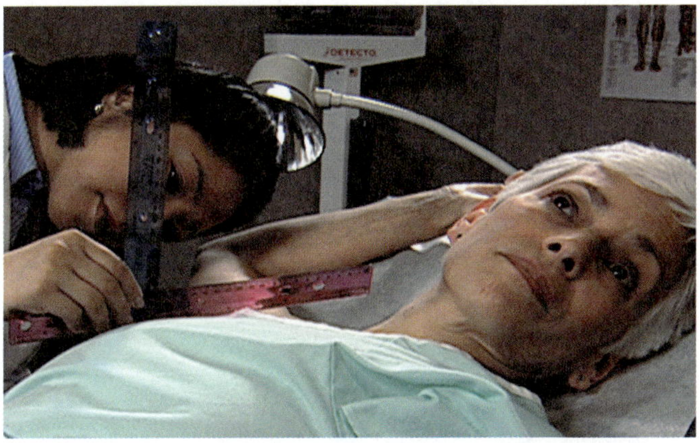

FIG. 30-46 Measuring jugular venous pressure. (From Seidel HM et al: *Mosby's guide to physical examination,* ed 7, St Louis, 2011, Mosby.)

TABLE 30-25 Indicators for Assessing Local Blood Flow

INDICATOR	RATIONALE
Systemic diseases (e.g., arteriosclerosis, atherosclerosis, diabetes).	Diseases result in changes in integrity of walls of arteries and smaller blood vessels.
Coagulation disorders (e.g., thrombosis, embolus).	Blood clot causes mechanical obstruction to blood flow.
Local trauma or surgery (e.g., contusion, fracture, vascular surgery).	Direct manipulation of vessels or localized edema impairs blood flow.
Application of constricting devices (e.g., casts, dressings, elastic bandages, restraints).	Constriction causes tourniquet effect, impairing blood flow to areas below site of constriction.

Peripheral Arteries and Veins

To examine the peripheral vascular system, first assess the adequacy of blood flow to the extremities by measuring arterial pulses and inspecting the condition of the skin and nails. Next, assess the integrity of the venous system. Assess the arterial pulses in the extremities to determine sufficiency of the entire arterial circulation.

Factors such as coagulation disorders, local trauma or surgery, constricting casts or bandages, and systemic diseases impair circulation to the extremities (Table 30-25). Discuss risk factors and ways to monitor for circulatory problems with the patient (Box 30-20).

Peripheral Arteries. Examine each peripheral artery using the distal pads of your second and third fingers. The thumb helps anchor the brachial and femoral artery. Apply firm pressure but avoid occluding a pulse. When a pulse is difficult to find, it helps to vary pressure and feel all around the pulse site. Be sure not to palpate your own pulse.

Routine vital signs usually include assessment of the rate and rhythm of the radial artery because it is easily accessible. Count the pulse for either 30 seconds or a full minute, depending on the character of the pulse (see Chapter 29). Always count an irregular pulse for 60 seconds. With palpation, normally feel the pulse wave at regular intervals. When an interval is interrupted by an early, a late, or a missed beat, the pulse rhythm is irregular. During cardiac emergencies health care providers usually assess the carotid artery because it is accessible and most useful in evaluating heart activity. To check local circulatory status of tissues (e.g., when a leg cast is in place or following vascular surgery), palpate the peripheral arteries long enough to note that a pulse is present.

Assess each peripheral artery for elasticity of the vessel wall, strength, and equality. The arterial wall is normally elastic, making it easily palpable. After depressing the artery, it springs back to shape when releasing the pressure. An abnormal artery is hard, inelastic, or calcified.

The strength of a pulse is a measurement of the force at which blood is ejected against the arterial wall. Some examiners use a scale rating from 0 to 4+ for the strength of a pulse (Seidel et al., 2011):

BOX 30-20 PATIENT TEACHING

Vascular Assessment

Objective

- Patient with vascular insufficiency will avoid activities that worsen circulatory status.

Teaching Strategies

- Instruct patient with risk or evidence of vascular insufficiency in the lower extremities to avoid tight clothing over the lower body or legs, avoid sitting or standing for long periods, avoid sitting with legs crossed, walk regularly, and elevate feet when sitting.
- Advise patient to avoid or stop cigarette smoking because nicotine causes vasoconstriction. Offer a referral to a reliable stop smoking program.
- Identify patient with hypertension about the benefits of regular monitoring of blood pressure (daily, weekly, or monthly). Teach patient how to use home monitoring kits.

Evaluation

- Ask patient to identify if blood pressure reading is within normal limits for age.
- Have patient with vascular insufficiency describe precautions to take to avoid further circulatory deficiency.
- Have patient demonstrate self-monitoring of blood pressure.

0: Absent, not palpable
1+: Pulse diminished, barely palpable
2+: Expected/normal
3+: Full pulse, increased
4+: Bounding pulse

Measure all peripheral pulses for equality and symmetry. Compare the left radial pulse with that of the right and so on. Lack of symmetry indicates impaired circulation such as a localized obstruction or an abnormally positioned artery.

In the upper extremities the brachial artery channels blood to the radial and ulnar arteries of the forearm and hand. If circulation in this artery becomes blocked, the hands do not receive adequate blood flow. If circulation in the radial or ulnar arteries becomes impaired, the hand still receives adequate perfusion. An interconnection between the radial and ulnar arteries guards against arterial occlusion (Fig. 30-47).

To locate pulses in the arm have the patient sit or lie down. Find the radial pulse along the radial side of the forearm at the wrist. Thin individuals have a groove lateral to the flexor tendon of the wrist. Feel the radial pulse with light palpation in the groove (Fig. 30-48). The ulnar pulse is on the opposite side of the wrist and feels less prominent (Fig. 30-49). Palpate the ulnar pulse only when evaluating arterial insufficiency to the hand.

To palpate the brachial pulse, find the groove between the biceps and triceps muscle above the elbow at the antecubital fossa (Fig. 30-50). The artery runs along the medial side of the extended arm. Palpate it with the fingertips of the first three fingers in the muscle groove.

The femoral artery is the primary artery in the leg, delivering blood to the popliteal, posterior tibial, and dorsalis pedis arteries (Fig. 30-51). An interconnection between the posterior tibial and dorsalis pedis arteries guards against local arterial occlusion.

Find the femoral pulse with the patient lying down with the inguinal area exposed (Fig. 30-52). The femoral artery runs below the inguinal ligament, midway between the symphysis pubis and the anterosuperior iliac spine. Sometimes deep palpation is necessary to feel the pulse. Bimanual palpation is effective in obese patients. Place the fingertips of both hands on opposite sides of the pulse site. Feel a pulsatile sensation when the arterial pulsation pushes the fingertips apart.

The popliteal pulse runs behind the knee. Have the patient slightly flex the knee with the foot resting on the examination table or assume a prone position with the knee slightly flexed (Fig. 30-53). Instruct him or her to keep leg muscles relaxed. Palpate with the fingers of both hands deeply into the popliteal fossa, just lateral to the midline. The popliteal pulse is difficult to locate.

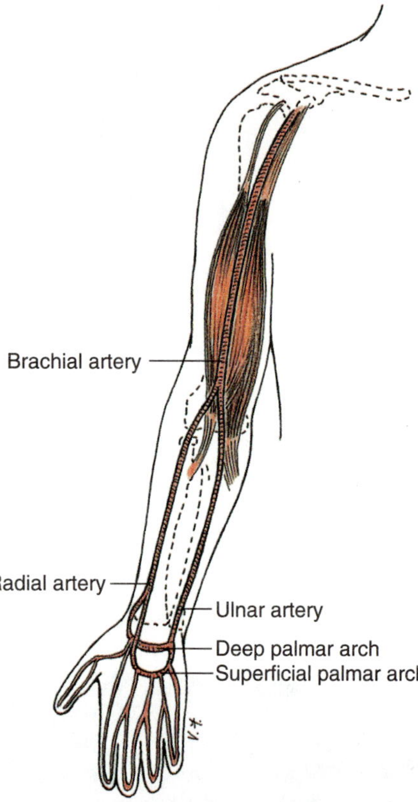

FIG. 30-47 Anatomical positions of brachial, radial, and ulnar arteries.

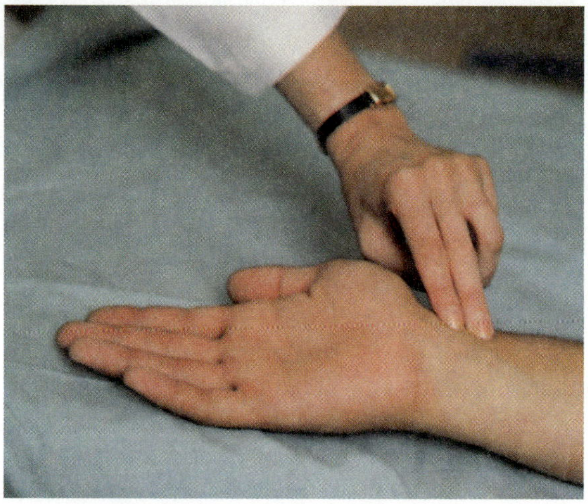

FIG. 30-48 Palpation of radial pulse.

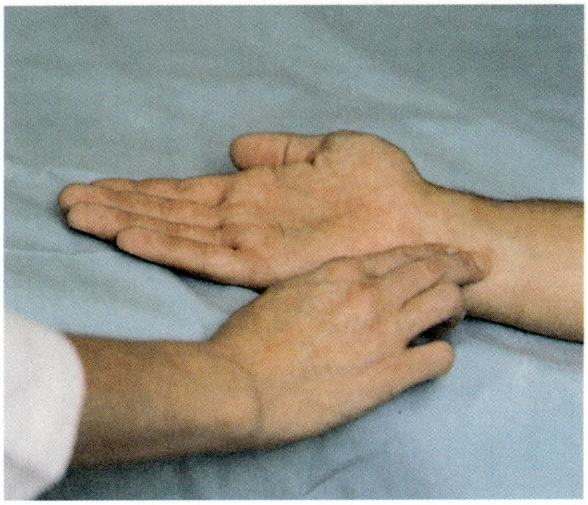

FIG. 30-49 Palpation of ulnar pulse.

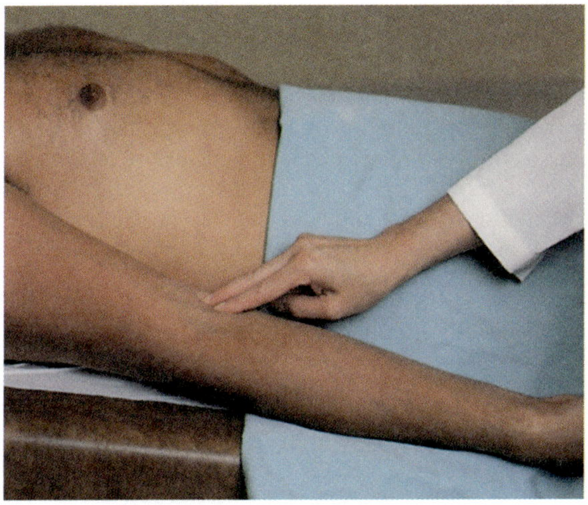

FIG. 30-50 Palpation of brachial pulse.

With the patient's foot relaxed, locate the dorsalis pedis pulse. The artery runs along the top of the foot in line with the groove between the extensor tendons of the great toe and first toe (Fig. 30-54). To find the pulse, place the fingertips between the first and second toes and slowly move up the dorsum of the foot. This pulse is sometimes congenitally absent.

Find the posterior tibial pulse on the inner side of each ankle (Fig. 30-55). Place the fingers behind and below the medial malleolus (ankle bone). With the foot relaxed and slightly extended, palpate the artery.

Ultrasound Stethoscopes. If a pulse is difficult to palpate, an ultrasound (Doppler) stethoscope is a useful tool that amplifies the sounds of a pulse wave. Factors that weaken a pulse or make palpation difficult include obesity, reduction in the stroke volume of the heart, diminished blood volume, or arterial obstruction. Apply a thin layer of transmission gel to the patient's skin at the pulse site or directly onto the transducer tip of the probe. Turn on the volume control and place the tip of the transducer at a 45- to 90-degree angle on the skin (Fig. 30-56). Move the transducer until you hear a pulsating "whooshing" sound that indicates that arterial blood flow is present.

Tissue Perfusion. The condition of the skin, mucosa, and nail beds offers useful data about the status of circulatory blood flow.

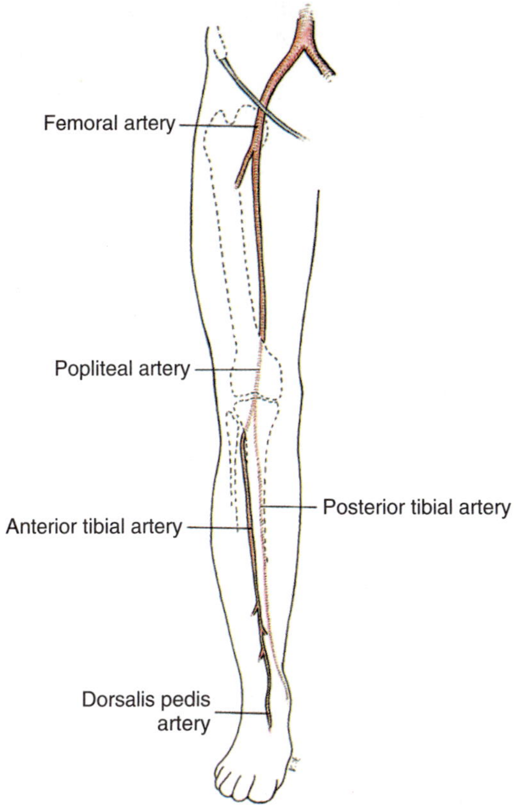

FIG. 30-51 Anatomical position of femoral, popliteal, dorsalis pedis, and posterior tibial arteries.

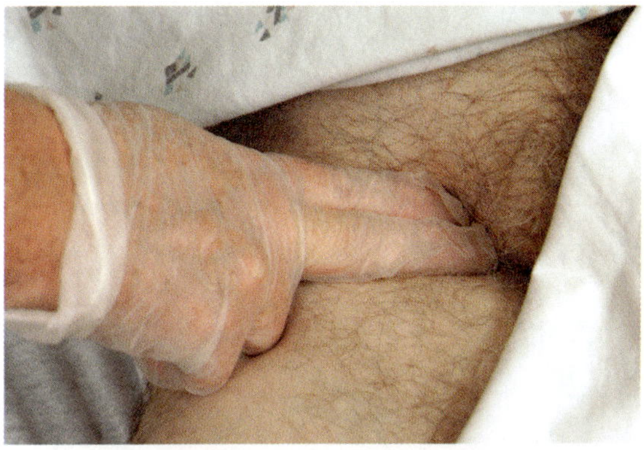

FIG. 30-52 Palpation of femoral pulse.

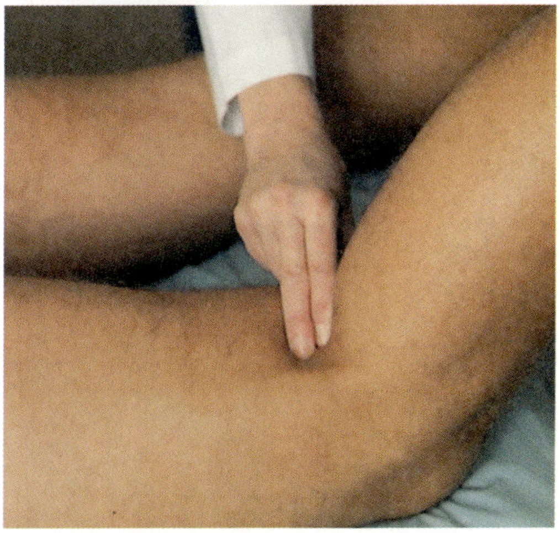

FIG. 30-53 Palpation of popliteal pulse.

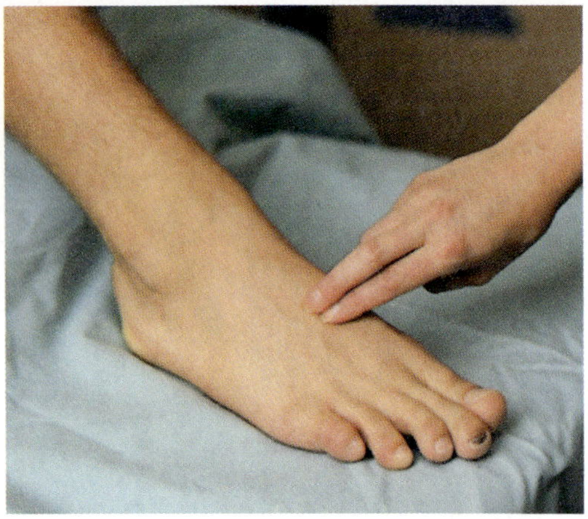

FIG. 30-54 Palpation of dorsalis pedis pulse.

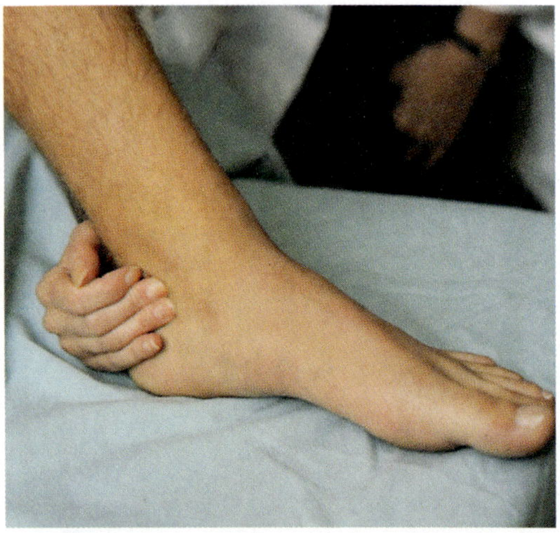

FIG. 30-55 Palpation of posterior tibial pulse.

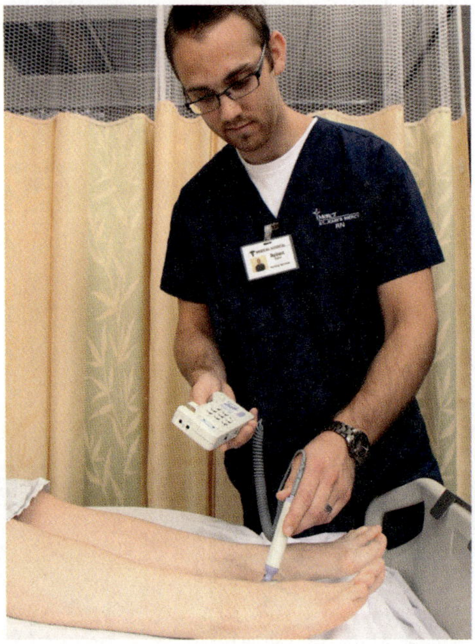

FIG. 30-56 Ultrasound stethoscope in position on the pedal pulse.

TABLE 30-26 Signs of Venous and Arterial Insufficiency

ASSESSMENT CRITERION	VENOUS	ARTERIAL
Color	Normal or cyanotic	Pale; worsened by elevation of extremity; dusky red when extremity is lowered
Temperature	Normal	Cool (blood flow blocked to extremity)
Pulse	Normal	Decreased or absent
Edema	Often marked	Absent or mild
Skin changes	Brown pigmentation around ankles	Thin, shiny skin; decreased hair growth; thickened nails

Examine the face and upper extremities, looking at the color of the skin, mucosa, and nail beds. The presence of cyanosis requires special attention. Heart disease sometimes causes central cyanosis, which indicates poor arterial oxygenation. Some characteristics of this are a bluish discoloration of the lips, mouth, and conjunctivae. Blue lips, earlobes, and nail beds are signs of peripheral cyanosis, which indicates peripheral vasoconstriction. When cyanosis is present, consult with a health care provider to request laboratory testing of oxygen saturation to determine the severity of the problem. Examination of the nails involves inspection for **clubbing,** a bulging of the tissues at the nail base. Clubbing is caused by insufficient oxygenation at the periphery resulting from conditions such as chronic emphysema and congenital heart disease.

Inspect the lower extremities for changes in color, temperature, and condition of the skin, indicating either arterial or venous alterations (Table 30-26). This is a good time to ask the patient about any history of pain in the legs. If an arterial occlusion is present, the patient has signs resulting from an absence of blood flow. Pain is distal to the occlusion. The five *Ps*—pain, pallor, pulselessness, paresthesias, and paralysis—characterize an occlusion. Venous congestion causes tissue changes that indicate an inadequate circulatory flow back to the heart.

During examination of the lower extremities, also inspect skin and nail texture; hair distribution on the lower legs, feet, and toes; the venous pattern; and scars, pigmentation, or ulcers. Palpate the legs and feet for color and temperature. Capillary refill, traditionally used to determine adequacy of peripheral blood flow to the digits, has limited value. More useful information is gained from grading pulses, assessing for color and warmth, and assessing pulses with a Doppler (Dufault et al., 2008).

The absence of hair growth over the legs indicates circulatory insufficiency. Remember not to confuse absence of hair on the legs with shaved legs. In addition, men who wear tight-fitting dress socks or jeans may have less hair on their calves. Chronic recurring ulcers of the feet or lower legs are a serious sign of circulatory insufficiency and require a health care provider's intervention.

Peripheral Veins. Assess the status of the peripheral veins by asking the patient to assume sitting and standing positions. Assessment includes inspection and palpation for varicosities, peripheral edema, and phlebitis. Varicosities are superficial veins that become dilated, especially when the legs are in a dependent position. They are common in older adults because the veins normally fibrose, dilate, and stretch. They are also common in people who stand for prolonged periods. Varicosities in the anterior or medial part of the thigh and the posterolateral part of the calf are abnormal.

Dependent edema around the area of the feet and ankles is a sign of venous insufficiency or right-sided heart failure. It is common in older adults and people who spend a lot of time standing (e.g., waitresses, security guards, and nurses). To assess for pitting edema, use the index finger to press firmly for several seconds and release over the medial malleolus or the shins. A depression left in the skin indicates edema. Grading 1+ through 4+ characterizes the severity of the edema (see Fig. 30-6).

Phlebitis is an inflammation of a vein that occurs commonly after trauma to the vessel wall, infection, immobilization, and prolonged insertion of IV catheters. To assess for phlebitis in the leg, inspect the calves for localized redness, tenderness, and swelling over vein sites. Gentle palpation of calf muscles reveals warmth, tenderness, and firmness of the muscle. Unilateral edema of the affected leg is one of the most reliable findings of phlebitis. Determine if dorsiflexion of the foot (Homans' sign) causes pain in the calf. However, Homans' sign is not always a reliable indicator of phlebitis or deep vein thrombosis (DVT) and is present in other conditions (Seidel et al., 2011). Performing the Homans' sign test is contraindicated in patients with DVT. If a clot is present in the leg, it may become dislodged from its original site during this test, resulting in a pulmonary embolism.

Lymphatic System

Assess the lymphatic drainage of the lower extremities during examination of the vascular system or during the female or male genital examination. Superficial and deep nodes drain the legs, but only two groups of superficial nodes are palpable. With the patient supine, palpate the area of the superficial inguinal nodes in the groin area (Fig. 30-57, *A*). Then move the fingertips toward the inner thigh, feeling for any inferior nodes. Use a firm but gentle pressure when palpating over each lymphatic chain. Multiple nodes are not normally palpable, although a few soft, nontender nodes are not unusual. Enlarged, hardened, tender nodes reveal potential sites of infection or metastatic disease.

In the upper extremities lymph is carried by the collecting ducts from the upper extremities to the subclavian lymphatic trunk. To assess this lymph system, gently palpate the epitrochlear nodes, located on the medial aspect of the arms near the antecubital fossa (Fig. 30-57, *B*). The proximal portion of the upper-extremity lymph system is located in the axilla and is usually assessed during examination of the breasts.

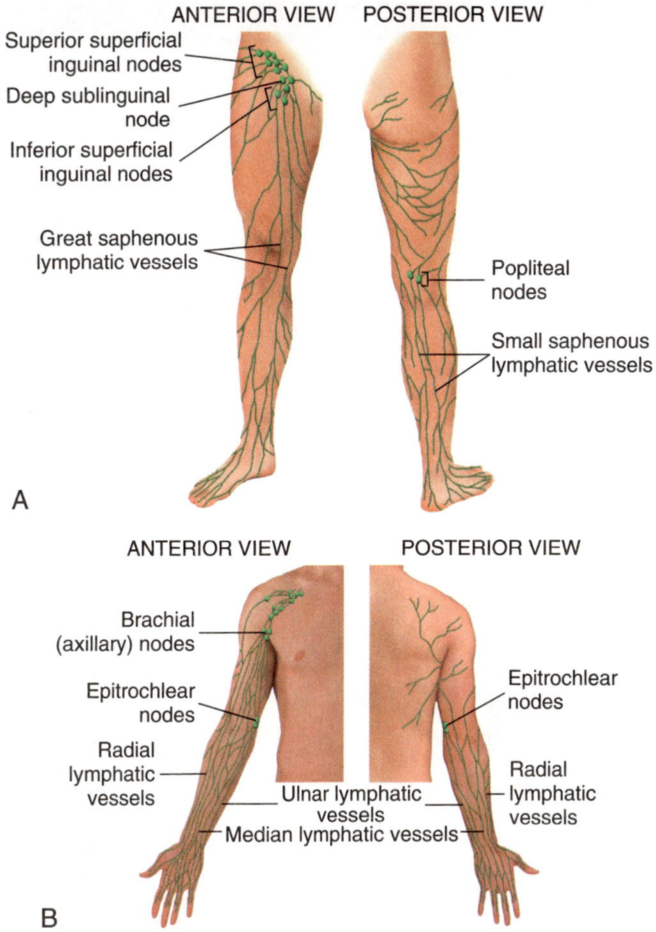

FIG. 30-57 A, Lymphatic drainage for the lower extremities. **B,** Lymphatic drainage for upper extremities. (From Seidel HM et al: *Mosby's guide to physical examination,* ed 7, St Louis, 2011, Mosby.)

BREASTS

It is important to examine the breasts of both female and male patients. Men have a small amount of glandular tissue, a potential site for the growth of cancer cells, in the breast. In contrast, the majority of the female breast is glandular tissue.

Female Breasts

New cases of invasive breast cancer were predicted to affect 230,480 women in the United States in 2011, with 2140 new cases expected in men (ACS, 2011). The disease is second to lung cancer as the leading cause of death in women with cancer. Early detection is the key to cure. A major responsibility for nurses is to teach patients health behaviors such as breast self-examination (BSE) (Box 30-21).

If the patient already performs BSE, assess the method she uses and times she does the examination in relation to her menstrual cycle. The best time for a BSE is the fourth through seventh day of the menstrual cycle or right after the menstrual cycle ends, when the breast is no longer swollen or tender from hormone elevations. If the woman is postmenopausal, advise her to check her breasts on the same day each month. The pregnant woman should also check her breasts on a monthly basis.

Older women require special attention when reviewing the need for regular BSE. Fixed incomes limit many older women; thus they fail to pursue regular clinical breast examination and mammography. Unfortunately many older women ignore changes in their breasts, assuming that they are a part of aging. In addition, physiological factors affect the ease with which older women perform a BSE. Musculoskeletal limitations, diminished peripheral sensation, reduced eyesight, and changes in joint range of motion (ROM) limit palpation and inspection abilities. Find resources for older women, including free screening programs. Teach family members to perform the patient's examination.

The American Cancer Society (ACS, 2011) recommends the following guidelines for the early detection of breast cancer:

- Monthly BSE is an option for women in their 20s.
- Women 20 years of age and older need to report any breast changes to a health care provider immediately.
- Women need a clinical breast examination by a health care provider every 3 years from ages 20 to 40 and annually for women over age 40.

BOX 30-21 BREAST SELF-EXAMINATION

Patients should perform breast self-examination (BSE) once a month to become familiar with the usual appearance and feel of both breasts. Familiarity makes it easier to notice any changes in the breast from one month to another. Early discovery of a change from baseline is the purpose of BSE.

If menstruating, the best time to do BSE is 2 or 3 days after the monthly period ends, when breasts are least likely to be tender or swollen. If no longer menstruating, pick a day such as the first day of the month as a reminder to do BSE. Instructions for BSE:

1. Stand before a mirror. Inspect both breasts for anything unusual such as discharge from the nipples, puckering, dimpling, or scaling of the skin.

The next two steps are designed to emphasize any change in the shape or contour of the breasts. During each step the patient will feel chest muscles tighten.

2. Watching closely in the mirror, clasp hands behind the head, and swing elbows forward.
3. Press hands firmly on hips and bow slightly toward the mirror while pulling shoulders and elbows forward.

Some women do the next part of the examination in the shower. Fingers glide over soapy skin, making it easy to appreciate the texture underneath.

4. Raise the left arm. Use three or four fingers of the right hand to explore the left breast firmly, carefully, and thoroughly. Beginning at the outer edge, press the flat part of the fingers in small circles, moving the circles slowly around the breast. Gradually work toward the nipple. Be sure to cover the entire breast. Pay special attention to the area between the breast and the armpit, including the armpit itself. Feel for any unusual lump or mass under the skin.
5. Gently squeeze the nipple and look for discharge. Repeat the examination on the right breast.
6. Repeat steps 4 and 5 lying down. Lie flat on back, right arm over the head and a pillow or folded towel under the right shoulder. This position flattens the breast and makes it easier to examine. Use the same circular motion described earlier.
7. Repeat on the right breast.

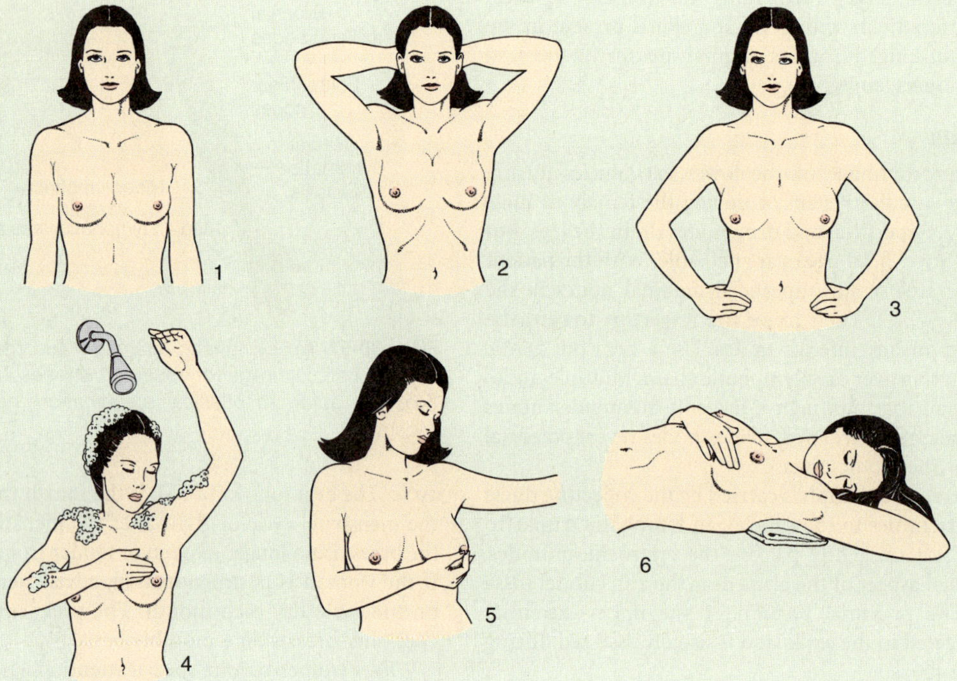

From Seidel HM et al: *Mosby's guide to physical examination,* ed 7, St Louis, 2011, Mosby.

- Women with a family history of breast cancer need an annual examination by a health care provider.
- Asymptomatic women need a screening mammogram by age 40; women age 40 and over need to have a mammogram annually.
- For women at increased risk, the ACS recommends talking with the health care provider for screening options and additional testing.

The patient's history (Table 30-27) reveals normal developmental changes and signs of breast disease. Because of its glandular structure, the breast undergoes changes during a woman's life. Knowing these changes (Box 30-22) allows complete and accurate assessment. Encourage both men and women to observe their breasts for changes.

Inspection. Have the patient remove the top gown or drape to allow simultaneous visualization of both breasts. Have her stand or sit with her arms hanging loosely at her sides. If possible, place a mirror in front of her during inspection so she sees what to look for when performing a BSE. To recognize abnormalities the patient needs to be familiar with the normal appearance of her breasts. Describe observations or findings in relation to imaginary lines that divide the breast into four quadrants and a tail. The lines cross at the center of the nipple. Each tail extends outward from the upper outer quadrant (Fig. 30-58).

Inspect the breasts for size and symmetry. Normally they extend from the third to the sixth ribs, with the nipple at the level of the fourth intercostal space. It is common for one breast to be smaller. However, inflammation or a mass causes a difference in size. As a

TABLE 30-27 Nursing History for Breast Assessment

ASSESSMENT	RATIONALE
Determine if woman is over age 40; has a personal or family history of breast cancer, early-onset menarche (before age 13), or late-age menopause (after age 50); has never had children or gave birth to first child after age 30; or has recently used oral contraceptives.	These are risk factors for breast cancer (American Cancer Society [ACS], 2011).
Ask if patient (both sexes) has noticed lump, thickening, pain, or tenderness of breast; discharge, distortion, retraction, or scaling of the nipple; or change in size of breast.	Potential signs and symptoms of breast cancer allow nurse to focus on specific areas of breast during assessment.
Determine patient's use of medications (oral contraceptives, digitalis, diuretics, steroids, or estrogen). Determine his or her caffeine intake.	Some medications cause nipple discharge. Hormones and caffeine cause fibrocystic changes in breast.
Determine patient's level of activity, alcoholic intake, and weight.	Breast cancer incidence rates correlate with being overweight or obese (postmenopausal), physical inactivity, and consumption of one or more alcoholic beverages per day (ACS, 2011).
Ask if patient performs monthly breast self-examination (BSE). If so, determine time of month she performs examination in relation to menstrual cycle. Have her describe or demonstrate method used.	Nurse's role is to educate patient about breast cancer and techniques for BSE.
If patient reports a breast mass, ask about length of time since she first noticed the lump. Does lump come and go, or is it always present? Have there been changes in the lump (e.g., size, relationship to menses), and are there associated symptoms?	Assessment helps to determine nature of mass (e.g., breast cancer vs. fibrocystic disease).

woman becomes older, the ligaments supporting the breast tissue weaken, causing the breasts to sag and the nipples to lower.

Observe the contour or shape of the breasts and note masses, flattening, retraction, or dimpling. Breasts vary in shape from convex to pendulous or conical. Retraction or dimpling can result from invasion of underlying ligaments by tumors. The ligaments fibrose and pull the overlying skin inward toward the tumor. Edema also changes the contour of the breasts. To bring out retraction or changes in the shape of breasts, ask the patient to assume three positions: raise arms above the head, press hands against the hips, and extend arms straight ahead while sitting and leaning forward. Each maneuver causes a contraction of the pectoral muscles, which accentuates the presence of any retraction.

Carefully inspect the skin for color; venous pattern; and the presence of lesions, edema, or inflammation. Lift each breast when necessary to observe lower and lateral aspects for color and texture

BOX 30-22 NORMAL CHANGES IN THE BREAST DURING A WOMAN'S LIFE SPAN

Puberty (8 to 20 Years)
Breasts mature in five stages. One breast may grow more rapidly than the other. The ages at which changes occur and rate of developmental progression vary.

Stage 1 (Preadolescent)
This stage involves elevation of the nipple only.

Stage 2
The breast and nipple elevate as a small mound, and the areolar diameters enlarge.

Stage 3
There is further enlargement and elevation of the breast and areola, with no separation of contour.

Stage 4
The areola and nipple project into the secondary mound above the level of the breast (does not occur in all girls).

Stage 5 (Mature Breast)
Only the nipple projects, and the areola recedes (varies in some women).

Young Adulthood (20 to 30 Years)
Breasts reach full (nonpregnant) size. Shape is generally symmetrical. Breasts are sometimes unequal in size.

Pregnancy
Breast size gradually enlarges to 2 to 3 times the previous size. Nipples enlarge and become erect. Areolas darken, and diameters increase. Superficial veins become prominent. The nipples expel a yellowish fluid (colostrum).

Menopause
Breasts shrink. Tissue becomes softer, sometimes flabby.

Older Adulthood
Breasts become elongated, pendulous, and flaccid as a result of glandular tissue atrophy. The skin of the breasts tends to wrinkle, appearing loose and flabby.

Nipples become smaller and flatter and lose erectile ability. They sometimes invert because of shrinkage and fibrotic changes.

Data from Ebersole P et al: *Toward healthy aging*, ed 7, St Louis, 2008, Mosby; Hockenberry MJ, Wilson D: *Wong's nursing care of infants and children*, ed 9, St Louis, 2011, Mosby; and Seidel HM et al: *Mosby's guide to physical examination*, ed 7, St Louis, 2011, Mosby.

changes. The breasts are the color of neighboring skin, and venous patterns are the same bilaterally. Venous patterns are easily visible in thin or pregnant women. Women with large breasts often have redness and excoriation of the undersurfaces caused by rubbing of skin surfaces.

Inspect the nipple and areola for size, color, shape, discharge, and the direction in which the nipples point. The normal areolas are round or oval and nearly equal bilaterally. Color ranges from pink to brown. In light-skinned women the areola turns brown during pregnancy and remains dark. In dark-skinned women the areola is brown before pregnancy (Seidel et al., 2011). Normally the nipples point in symmetrical directions, are everted, and have

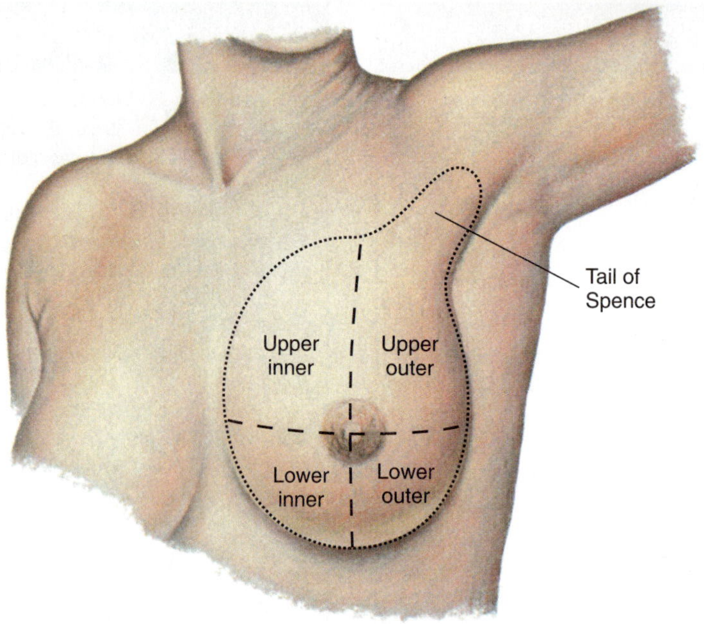

FIG. 30-58 Quadrants of left breast and axillary tail of Spence. (From Seidel HM et al: *Mosby's guide to physical examination*, ed 6, St Louis, 2006, Mosby.)

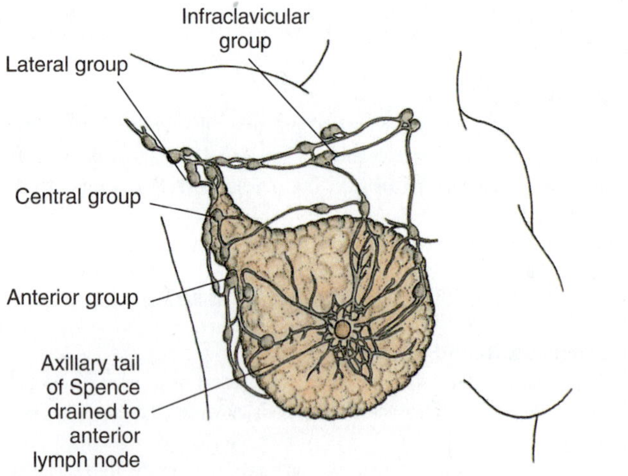

FIG. 30-59 Anatomical position of axillary and clavicular lymph nodes.

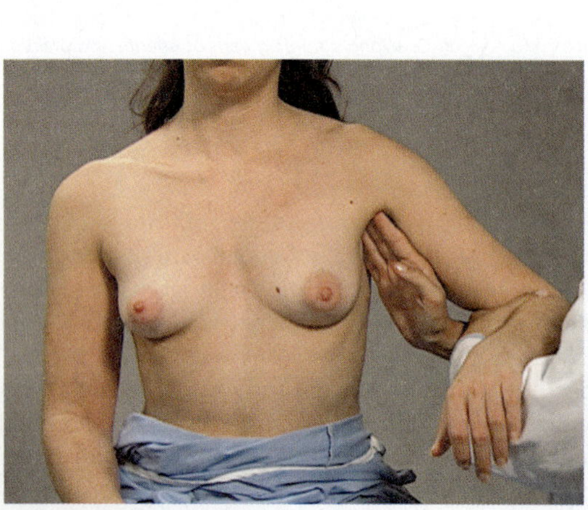

FIG. 30-60 Support patient's arm and palpate axillary lymph nodes. (From Seidel HM et al: *Mosby's guide to physical examination*, ed 7, St Louis, 2011, Mosby.)

no drainage. If the nipples are inverted, ask if this has been a lifetime history. A recent inversion or inward turning of the nipple indicates an underlying growth. Rashes or ulcerations are not normal on the breast or nipples. Note any bleeding or discharge from the nipple. Clear yellow discharge 2 days after childbirth is common. While inspecting the breasts, explain the characteristics you see. Teach the patient the significance of abnormal signs or symptoms.

Palpation. Palpation assesses the condition of underlying breast tissue and lymph nodes. Breast tissue consists of glandular tissue, fibrous supportive ligaments, and fat. Glandular tissue is organized into lobes that end in ducts that open onto the surface of the nipple. The largest portion of glandular tissue is in the upper outer quadrant and tail of each breast. Suspensory ligaments connect to skin and fascia underlying the breast to support the breast and maintain its upright position. Fatty tissue is located superficially and to the sides of the breast.

A large portion of lymph from the breasts drains into axillary lymph nodes. If cancerous lesions metastasize (spread), the nodes commonly become involved. Study the location of supraclavicular, infraclavicular, and axillary nodes (Fig. 30-59). The axillary nodes drain lymph from the chest wall, breasts, arms, and hands. A tumor of one breast sometimes involves nodes on the same and opposite sides.

To palpate the lymph nodes have the patient sit with her arms at her sides and muscles relaxed. While facing the patient and standing on the side you are examining, support her arm in a flexed position, and abduct it from the chest wall. Place the free hand against the patient's chest wall and high in the axillary hollow. With the fingertips press gently down over the surface of the ribs and muscles. Palpate the axillary nodes with the fingertips, gently rolling soft tissue (Fig. 30-60). Palpate four areas of the axilla: at the edge of the pectoralis major muscle along the anterior axillary line, the chest wall in the midaxillary area, the upper part of the humerus, and the anterior edge of the latissimus dorsi muscle along the posterior axillary line.

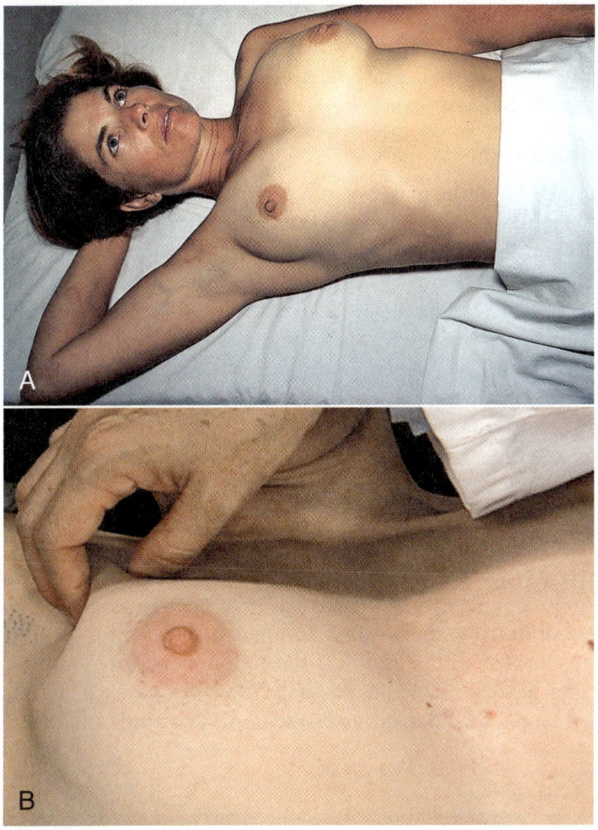

FIG. 30-61 **A,** The patient lies flat with arm abducted and hand under head to help flatten breast tissue evenly over the chest wall. **B,** Each breast is palpated in a systematic fashion. (**B** from Seidel HM et al: *Mosby's guide to physical examination,* ed 6, St Louis, 2006, Mosby.)

Normally lymph nodes are not palpable. Carefully assess each area and note their number, consistency, mobility, and size. One or two small, soft, nontender palpable nodes are normal. An abnormal palpable node feels like a small mass that is hard, tender, and immobile. Continue to palpate along the upper and lower clavicular ridges. Reverse the procedure for the patient's other side.

It is sometimes difficult for a patient to learn to palpate for lymph nodes. Lying down with the arm abducted makes the area more accessible. Instruct the patient to use her left hand for the right axillary and clavicular areas. Take the patient's fingertips and move them in the proper fashion. Then have the patient use her right hand to palpate for nodes on the left side.

With the patient lying supine and one arm under the head and neck (alternating with each breast), palpate her breast tissue. The supine position allows the breast tissue to flatten evenly against the chest wall. The position of the arm and hand further stretches and positions breast tissue evenly (Fig. 30-61, *A*). Place a small pillow or towel under the patient's shoulder blade to further position breast tissue. Palpate the tail of Spence (Fig. 30-61, *B*).

The consistency of normal breast tissue varies widely. The breasts of a young patient are firm and elastic. In an older patient the tissue sometimes feels stringy and nodular. A patient's familiarity with the texture of her own breasts is very important. Patients gain familiarity through monthly BSE (Box 30-23).

If the patient complains of a mass, examine the opposite breast to ensure an objective comparison of normal and abnormal tissue. Use the pads of the first three fingers to compress breast tissue gently against the chest wall, noting tissue consistency. Perform palpation systematically in one of three ways: (1) clockwise or counterclockwise, forming small circles with the fingers along each quadrant and the tail; (2) using a vertical technique with the fingers moving up and down each quadrant; or (3) palpating from the center of the breast in a radial fashion, returning to the areola to begin each spoke (Fig. 30-62, *A* to *C*). Whichever approach you use, be sure to cover the entire breast and tail, directing attention to any areas of tenderness. Use a bimanual technique when palpating large, pendulous breasts. Support the inferior portion of the breast in one hand while using the other hand to palpate breast tissue against the supporting hand.

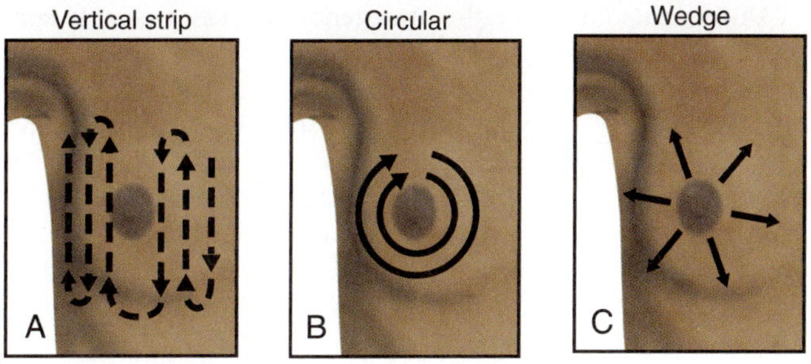

FIG. 30-62 Various methods for palpation of breast. **A,** Palpate from top to bottom in vertical strips. **B,** Palpate in concentric circles. **C,** Palpate out from center in wedge sections. (From Seidel HM et al: *Mosby's guide to physical examination,* ed 7, St Louis, 2011, Mosby.)

BOX 30-23 PATIENT TEACHING

Female Breast Assessment

Objective

- Patient will follow prevention and detection practices to ensure breast health.

Teaching Strategies

- Have patient perform return demonstration of breast self-examination (BSE) and offer the opportunity to ask questions.
- Explain recommended frequency of mammography and assessment by a health care provider.
- Discuss signs and symptoms of breast cancer.
- Discuss signs and symptoms of benign (fibrocystic) breast disease.
- Inform a woman who is obese or has a family history of breast cancer that she is at higher risk for the disease (ACS, 2011). Encourage dietary changes, including limiting meat consumption to well-trimmed, lean beef, pork, or lamb; removing skin from cooked chicken before eating it; selecting tuna and salmon packed in water and not oil; and using low-fat dairy products.
- Encourage patient to reduce intake of caffeine and theophyllines. Although this approach is controversial, it can reduce symptoms of benign (fibrocystic) breast disease.

Evaluation

- Have patient demonstrate BSE.
- During follow-up visit, determine whether patient has had mammography performed.
- Ask patient to explain frequency of mammography.
- Have patient describe signs and symptoms of breast cancer compared with benign (fibrocystic) breast disease.

During palpation note the consistency of breast tissue. It normally feels dense, firm, and elastic. With menopause breast tissue shrinks and becomes softer. The lobular feel of glandular tissue is normal. The lower edge of each breast sometimes feels firm and hard. This is the normal inframammary ridge and not a tumor. It helps to move the patient's hand so she can feel normal tissue variations. Palpate abnormal masses to determine location in relation to quadrants, diameter in centimeters, shape (e.g., round or discoid), consistency (soft, firm, or hard), tenderness, mobility, and discreteness (clear or unclear boundaries).

Cancerous lesions are hard, fixed, nontender, irregular in shape, and usually unilateral. A common benign condition of the breast is benign (fibrocystic) breast disease. Bilateral lumpy, painful breasts and sometimes nipple discharge characterize this condition. Symptoms are more apparent during the menstrual period. When palpated the cysts (lumps) are soft, well differentiated, and movable. Deep cysts feel hard.

Give special attention to palpating the nipple and areola. Palpate the entire surface gently. Use the thumb and index finger to compress the nipple and note any discharge. During the examination of the nipple and areola, the nipple sometimes becomes erect with wrinkling of the areola. These changes are normal. Continue by positioning the patient and examining the other breast.

After completing the examination, have the patient demonstrate self-palpation. Observe the patient's technique and emphasize the importance of a systematic approach. Urge the patient to see her health care provider if she discovers an abnormal mass during routine monthly BSE. She also needs to know all of the signs and symptoms of breast cancer.

Male Breasts

Examination of the male breast is relatively easy. Inspect the nipple and areola for nodules, edema, and ulceration. An enlarged male breast results from obesity or glandular enlargement. Breast enlargement in young males results from steroid use. Fatty tissue feels soft, whereas glandular tissue is firm. Use the same techniques to palpate for masses used in examination of the female breast. Because breast cancer in men is relatively rare, routine self-examinations are unnecessary. However, men who have a first-degree relative (e.g., mother or sister) with breast cancer, are at risk for breast cancer and need to palpate their breasts at regular intervals. Men at high risk may be scheduled by their health care provider for routine mammograms.

ABDOMEN

The abdominal examination is complex because of the number of organs located within and near the abdominal cavity. A thorough nursing history (Table 30-28) helps interpret physical signs. The examination includes an assessment of structures of the lower

TABLE 30-28 Nursing History for Abdominal Assessment

ASSESSMENT	RATIONALE
If patient has abdominal or low back pain, assess character of pain in detail (location, onset, frequency, precipitating factors, aggravating factors, type of pain, severity, course).	Pattern of characteristics of pain helps determine its source.
Carefully observe patient's movement and position, including lying still with knees drawn up, moving restlessly to find comfortable position, and lying on one side or sitting with knees drawn to chest.	Positions assumed by patient reveal nature and source of pain, including peritonitis, renal stone, and pancreatitis.
Assess normal bowel habits and stool character; ask if patient uses laxatives.	Data compared with physical findings help identify cause and nature of elimination problems.
Determine if patient has had abdominal surgery, trauma, or diagnostic tests of gastrointestinal (GI) tract.	Surgical or traumatic alterations of abdominal organs cause changes in expected findings (e.g., position of underlying organs). Diagnostic tests change character of stool.
Assess if patient has had recent weight changes or intolerance to diet (e.g., nausea, vomiting, cramping, especially in last 24 hours).	Data possibly indicate alterations in upper GI tract (stomach or gallbladder) or lower colon.
Assess for difficulty in swallowing, belching, flatulence (gas), bloody emesis (hematemesis), black or tarry stools (melena), heartburn, diarrhea, or constipation.	These characteristic signs and symptoms indicate GI alterations.
Ask if patient takes antiinflammatory medication (e.g., aspirin, ibuprofen, steroids) or antibiotics.	Pharmacological agents cause GI upset or bleeding.
Ask patient to locate tender areas before examination begins.	Assess painful areas last to minimize discomfort and anxiety.
Inquire about family history of cancer, kidney disease, alcoholism, hypertension, or heart disease.	Data possibly reveal risk for alterations identifiable during examination.
Determine if female patient is pregnant; note last menstrual period.	Pregnancy causes changes in abdominal shape and contour.
Assess patient's usual intake of alcohol.	Chronic alcohol ingestion causes gastrointestinal and liver problems.
Review patient's history for the following: health care occupation, hemodialysis, intravenous drug user, household or sexual contact with hepatitis B virus (HBV) carrier, heterosexual person with more than one sex partner in previous 6 months, sexually active homosexual or bisexual male, international traveler in area of high HBV infection rate.	Risk factors for HBV exposure.

gastrointestinal (GI) tract in addition to the liver, stomach, uterus, ovaries, kidneys, and bladder. Abdominal pain is one of the most common symptoms that patients report when seeking medical care. An accurate assessment requires matching patient history data with a careful assessment of the location of physical symptoms.

Assess the organs anteriorly and posteriorly. A system of landmarks help map out the abdominal region. The xiphoid process (tip of the sternum) is the upper boundary of the anterior abdominal region. The symphysis pubis marks the lower boundary. Divide the abdomen into four imaginary quadrants (Fig. 30-63, *A*); refer to assessment findings and record them in relation to each quadrant. Posteriorly the lower ribs and heavy back muscles protect the kidneys, which are located from the T12 to L3 vertebrae (Fig. 30-63, *B*). The costovertebral angle formed by the last rib and vertebral column is a landmark used during kidney palpation.

During the abdominal examination the patient needs to relax. A tightening of abdominal muscles hinders palpation. Ask the patient to void before beginning. Be sure that the room is warm and drape upper chest and legs. The patient lies supine or in a dorsal recumbent position with the arms at the sides and knees slightly bent. Place small pillows beneath the knees. If the patient places the arms under the head, the abdominal muscles tighten. Proceed calmly and slowly, being sure that there is adequate lighting. Expose the abdomen from just above the xiphoid process down to the symphysis pubis. Warm hands and stethoscope further promote relaxation. Ask the patient to report pain and point out tender areas. Assess tender areas last.

The order of an abdominal examination differs slightly from previous assessments. Begin with inspection and follow with auscultation. By using auscultation before palpation there is less chance of altering the frequency and character of bowel sounds. Be sure to have a tape measure and marking pen available during the examination.

Inspection

Make it a habit to observe the patient during routine care activities. Note his or her posture and look for evidence of abdominal splinting: lying with the knees drawn up or moving restlessly in bed. A patient free from abdominal pain does not guard or splint the abdomen. To inspect the abdomen for abnormal movement or shadows, stand on the patient's right side and inspect from above the abdomen. After sitting or stooping down to look across the abdomen, assess abdominal contour. Direct the examination light over the abdomen.

Skin. Inspect the skin over the abdomen for color, scars, venous patterns, lesions, and **striae** (stretch marks). The skin is subject to the same color variations as the rest of the body. Venous patterns are normally faint, except in thin patients. Striae result from stretching of tissue by obesity or pregnancy. Artificial openings indicate drainage sites resulting from surgery (see Chapter 50) or an ostomy (see Chapters 45 and 46). Scars reveal evidence of past trauma or surgery that has created permanent changes in underlying organ anatomy. Bruising indicates accidental injury, physical abuse, or a type of bleeding disorder. If needle marks or bruises are present, ask if the patient self-administers injections (e.g., low-molecular-weight heparin or insulin). Unexpected findings include generalized color changes such as jaundice or cyanosis. Shiny abdominal skin with a taut (tight) appearance can indicate ascites.

Umbilicus. Note the position; shape; color; and signs of inflammation, discharge, or protruding masses. A normal umbilicus is flat or concave with the color the same as that of the surrounding skin. Underlying masses cause displacement of the umbilicus. An everted (pouched-out) umbilicus usually indicates distention. Hernias (protrusion of abdominal organs through the muscle wall) cause upward protrusion of the umbilicus. Normally the umbilical area does not emit discharge.

Contour and Symmetry. Inspect for contour, symmetry, and surface motion of the abdomen, noting any masses, bulging, or distention. A flat abdomen forms a horizontal plane from the xiphoid process to the symphysis pubis. A round abdomen protrudes in a convex sphere from the horizontal plane. A concave abdomen appears to sink into the muscular wall. Each of these findings is normal if the shape of the abdomen is symmetrical. In older adults there is often an overall increased distribution of adipose tissue. The presence of masses on only one side, or asymmetry, possibly indicates an underlying pathological condition.

Intestinal gas, a tumor, or fluid in the abdominal cavity causes **distention** (swelling). When distention is generalized, the entire abdomen protrudes. The skin often appears taut, as if it were stretched over the abdomen. When gas causes distention, the flanks (side muscles) do not bulge. However, if fluid is the source of the problem, the flanks bulge. Ask the patient to roll onto one side. A protuberance forms on the dependent side if fluid is the cause of the distention. Ask the patient if the abdomen feels unusually tight.

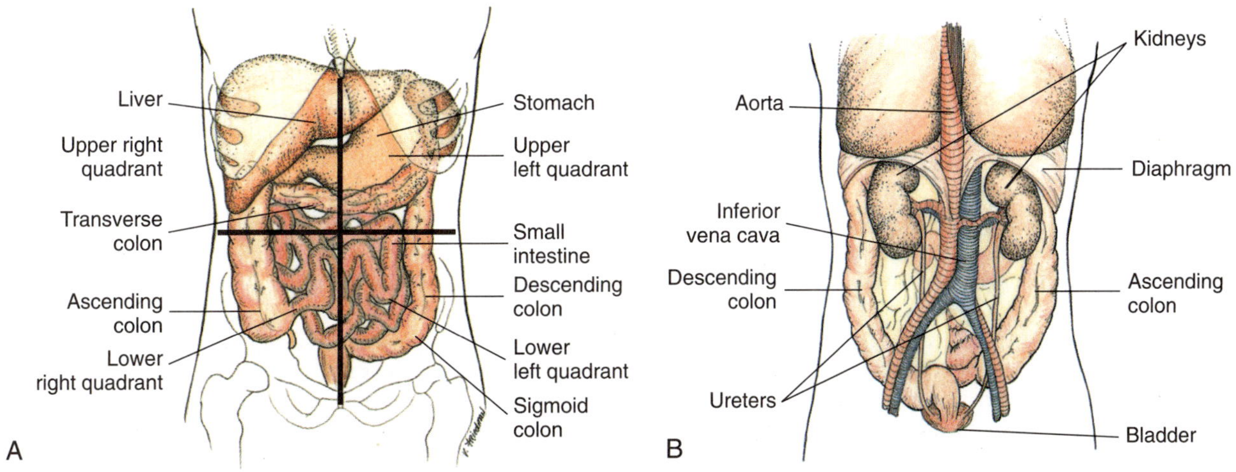

FIG. 30-63 **A,** Anterior view of abdomen divided by quadrants. **B,** Posterior view of abdominal section.

Be careful not to confuse distention with obesity. In obesity the abdomen is large, rolls of adipose tissue are often present along the flanks, and the patient does not complain of tightness in the abdomen. If distention is expected, measure the abdomen by placing a tape measure around it at the level of the umbilicus (this may require the patient to roll side-to-side as you position the tape measure). Consecutive measurements show any increase or decrease in distention. Use a marking pen to indicate the location of the tape measure.

Enlarged Organs or Masses. Observe the contour of the abdomen while asking the patient to take a deep breath and hold it. Normally the contour remains smooth and symmetrical. This maneuver forces the diaphragm downward and reduces the size of the abdominal cavity. Any enlarged organs in the upper abdominal cavity (e.g., liver or spleen) descend below the rib cage to cause a bulge. Perform a closer examination with palpation. To evaluate the abdominal musculature have the patient raise the head. This position causes superficial abdominal wall masses, hernias, and muscle separations to become more apparent.

Movement or Pulsations. Inspect for movement. Normally men breathe abdominally, and women breathe more costally. A patient with severe pain has diminished respiratory movement and tightens the abdominal muscles to guard against the pain. Closely inspect for peristaltic movement and aortic pulsation by looking across the abdomen from the side. These movements are visible in thin patients; otherwise no movement is present.

Auscultation

Auscultate before palpation during the abdominal assessment because manipulation of the abdomen alters the frequency and intensity of bowel sounds. Ask patients not to talk. Patients with GI tubes connected to suction need them temporarily turned off before beginning an examination.

Bowel Motility. **Peristalsis,** or the movement of contents through the intestines, is a normal function of the small and large intestine. Bowel sounds are the audible passage of air and fluid that peristalsis creates. Place the warmed diaphragm of the stethoscope lightly over each of the four quadrants. Normally air and fluid move through the intestines, creating soft gurgling or clicking sounds that occur irregularly 5 to 35 times per minute (Seidel et al., 2011). Sounds usually last ½ second to several seconds. It normally takes 5 to 20 seconds to hear a bowel sound. However, it takes 5 minutes of continuous listening before determining that bowel sounds are absent (Seidel et al., 2011). Auscultate all four quadrants to be sure that you do not miss any sounds. The best time to auscultate is between meals. Sounds are generally described as normal, audible, absent, hyperactive, or hypoactive. Absent sounds indicate a lack of peristalsis, possibly the result of late-stage bowel obstruction; paralytic ileus; or peritonitis. Normally absent or hypoactive bowel sounds occur after surgery following general anesthesia. Hyperactive sounds are loud, "growling" sounds called **borborygmi,** which indicate increased GI motility. Inflammation of the bowel, anxiety, diarrhea, bleeding, excessive ingestion of laxatives, and reaction of the intestines to certain foods cause increased motility. Teach patients practices to promote normal elimination patterns (Box 30-24).

Vascular Sounds. Bruits indicate narrowing of the major blood vessels and disruption of blood flow. The presence of bruits in the abdominal area can reveal aneurysms or stenotic vessels. Use the bell of the stethoscope to auscultate in the epigastric region and each of the four quadrants. Normally there are no vascular sounds over the aorta (midline through the abdomen) or femoral arteries (lower quadrants). You can hear renal artery bruits by placing the stethoscope over each upper quadrant anteriorly or over the costovertebral angle posteriorly. Report a bruit immediately to a health care provider.

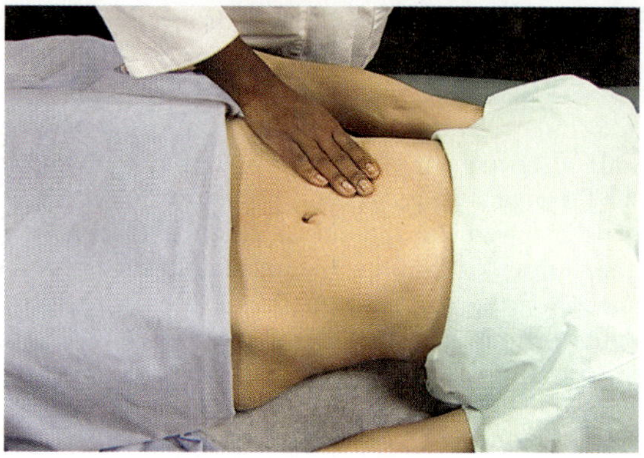

FIG. 30-64 Light palpation of abdomen. (From Seidel HM et al: *Mosby's guide to physical examination,* ed 7, St Louis, 2011, Mosby.)

BOX 30-24 PATIENT TEACHING

Abdominal Assessment

Objective

- Patient will maintain normal bowel elimination.

Teaching Strategies

- Explain factors that promote normal bowel elimination such as diet, regular exercise, limited use of over-the-counter drugs causing constipation, establishment of regular elimination schedule, and a good fluid intake (see Chapter 46). Stress importance for older adults.
- Caution patients about dangers of excessive use of laxatives or enemas.
- Instruct patient to have acute abdominal pain evaluated by a health care provider.

Evaluation

- Reassess patient's bowel elimination pattern and stool character after therapies begin.
- Observe patient using pain-relief measures and reassess character of pain.

Kidney Tenderness. With the patient sitting or standing erect, use direct or indirect percussion to assess for kidney inflammation. You might require an advanced practice nurse to help you with this skill. With the ulnar surface of the partially closed fist, percuss posteriorly the costovertebral angle at the scapular line. If the kidneys are inflamed, the patient feels tenderness during percussion.

Palpation

Palpation primarily detects areas of abdominal tenderness, distention, or masses. As your skill base increases, learn to palpate for specific organs by using light and deep palpation.

Use light palpation over each abdominal quadrant to detect areas of tenderness. Initially avoid areas previously identified as problem spots. Lay the palm of the hand with fingers extended and approximated lightly on the abdomen. Explain the maneuver to the patient and, with the palmar surface of the fingers, depress approximately 1.3 cm (½ inch) in a gentle dipping motion (Fig. 30-64). Avoid quick jabs and use smooth, coordinated movements. If the

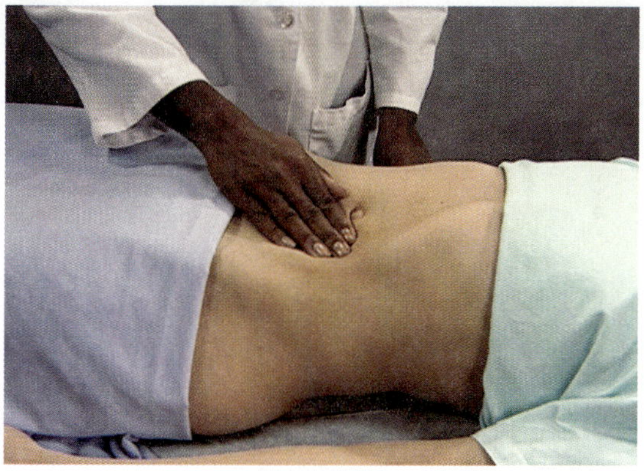

FIG. 30-65 Deep palpation of abdomen. (From Seidel HM et al: *Mosby's guide to physical examination,* ed 7, St Louis, 2011, Mosby.)

patient is ticklish, first place his or her hand on the abdomen with your hand on the patient's; continue this until the patient tolerates palpation.

Use a systematic palpation approach for each quadrant and assess for muscular resistance, distention, tenderness, and superficial organs or masses. Observe the patient's face for signs of discomfort. The abdomen is normally smooth with consistent softness and nontender without masses. In contrast to firm muscles found among young adults, an older adult often lacks abdominal tone. Guarding or muscle tenseness sometimes occurs while palpating a sensitive area. If tightening remains after the patient relaxes, peritonitis, acute cholecystitis, or appendicitis is sometimes the cause. It is easy to detect a distended bladder with light palpation. Normally the bladder lies below the umbilicus and above the symphysis pubis. Routinely check for a distended bladder if the patient has been unable to void (e.g., because of anesthesia or sedation) or has been incontinent or if an indwelling urinary catheter is not draining well.

With practice and experience perform deep palpation to delineate abdominal organs and detect less obvious masses. You need short fingernails. It is important for the patient to be relaxed while the hands depress approximately 2.5 to 7.5 cm (1 to 3 inches) into the abdomen (Fig. 30-65). Never use deep palpation over a surgical incision or over extremely tender organs. It is also unwise to use palpation on abnormal masses. Deep pressure causes tenderness in a healthy patient over the cecum, sigmoid colon, aorta, and the midline near the xiphoid process (Seidel et al., 2011).

Survey each quadrant systematically. Palpate masses for size, location, shape, consistency, tenderness, pulsation, and mobility. Test for rebound tenderness by pressing a hand slowly and deeply into the involved area and letting go quickly. The test is positive if the patient feels pain with the release of the hand. Rebound tenderness occurs in patients with peritoneal irritation such as occurs in appendicitis; pancreatitis; or any peritoneal injury causing bile, blood, or enzymes to enter the peritoneal cavity.

Aortic Pulsation. Palpate with the thumb and forefinger of one hand deeply into the upper abdomen just left of the midline to assess aortic pulsation. Normally a pulsation is transmitted forward. If the aorta is enlarged because of an aneurysm (localized dilation of a vessel wall), the pulsation expands laterally. Do not palpate a pulsating abdominal mass. When enlargement from an aneurysm is present, only lightly palpate this area, referring the finding to the health care provider. In obese patients it is often necessary to palpate with both hands, one on each side of the aorta.

FEMALE GENITALIA AND REPRODUCTIVE TRACT

Examination of the female genitalia is embarrassing to a patient unless you use a calm, relaxed approach. The gynecological examination is one of the most difficult experiences for adolescents. A person's cultural background further adds to apprehension. For example, female Mexican Americans have a strong social value that women do not expose their bodies to men or even to other women. Similarly, Chinese Americans believe that the examination of genitalia is offensive. Provide a thorough explanation of the reason for the procedures used in the examination. The lithotomy position assumed during the examination is an added source of embarrassment. A patient is more comfortable when you use correct positioning and draping. Be sure to explain each portion of the examination in advance so patients anticipate necessary actions. Adolescents sometimes choose to have parents present in the examination room.

Sometimes a patient requires a complete examination of the female reproductive organs, including assessing the external genitalia and performing a vaginal examination. You can examine external genitalia while performing routing hygiene measures or when preparing to insert a urinary catheter. An internal examination is part of each woman's preventive health care because ovarian cancer causes more deaths than any other cancer of the female reproductive system (ACS, 2011).

Adolescents and young adults are examined because of the growing incidence of sexually transmitted infections (STIs). The average age of menarche among young girls has declined, and the majority of male and female teenagers are sexually active by age 19 (Hockenberry and Wilson, 2011). It is important to assess a patient's level of anxiety when obtaining the nursing history (Table 30-29). Combine rectal and anal assessments with the pelvic examination since the patient is situated in a lithotomy or dorsal recumbent position.

Preparation of the Patient

The beginning nurse is often responsible for assisting a patient's health care provider with the examination. For a complete examination the following equipment is needed: examination table with stirrups, vaginal speculum of correct size, adjustable light source, sink, clean disposable gloves, sterile cotton swabs, glass slides, plastic or wooden spatula, cervical brush or broom device, cytological fixative, and culture plates or media (Seidel et al., 2011).

Make sure that the equipment is ready before the examination begins. Ask the patient to empty her bladder so the uterus and ovaries are readily palpable. Often it is necessary to collect a urine specimen. Assist the patient to the lithotomy position in bed or on an examination table for the external genitalia assessment. Assist her into stirrups for a speculum examination. Have a woman stabilize each foot in a stirrup and have her slide the buttocks down to the edge of the examining table. Place a hand at the edge of the table and instruct the patient to move until touching the hand. The patient's arms should be at her sides or folded across the chest to prevent tightening of abdominal muscles.

Some women suffering from pain or deformity of the joints are unable to assume a lithotomy position. In this situation it is necessary to have the patient abduct only one leg or have another assist in separating the patient's thighs. In addition, use the side-lying position with the patient on the left side with the right thigh and knee drawn up to her chest.

Give a square drape or sheet to the patient. She holds one corner over her sternum, the adjacent corners fall over each knee, and the

TABLE 30-29 Nursing History for Female Genitalia and Reproductive Tract Assessment

ASSESSMENT	RATIONALE
Determine if patient has had previous illness or surgery involving reproductive organs, including STIs.	Illness or surgery influences appearance and position of organs being examined.
Determine if patient has received HPV vaccine.	HPV increases patient's risk for development of cervical cancer.
Review menstrual history, including age at menarche, frequency and duration of menstrual cycle, character of flow (e.g., amount, presence of clots), presence of dysmenorrhea (painful menstruation), pelvic pain, dates of last two menstrual periods, and premenstrual symptoms.	This information helps to reveal level of reproductive health, including normalcy of menstrual cycle.
Ask patient to describe obstetrical history, including each pregnancy and history of abortions or miscarriages.	Observed physical findings vary, depending on woman's history of pregnancy.
Determine whether patient uses safe sex practices; have patient describe current and past contraceptive practices and problems encountered. Discuss risk of STIs and HIV infection.	Use of certain types of contraceptives influences reproductive health (e.g., sensitivity reaction to spermicidal jelly). Sexual history reveals risk for and understanding of STIs.
Assess if patient has signs and symptoms of vaginal discharge, painful or swollen perianal tissues, or genital lesions.	These signs and symptoms may indicate STI or other pathological condition.
Determine if patient has symptoms or history of genitourinary problems, including burning during urination, frequency, urgency, nocturia, hematuria, incontinence, or stress incontinence (see Chapter 45).	Urinary problems are associated with gynecological disorders, including STIs.
Ask if patient has had signs of bleeding outside of normal menstrual period or after menopause or has had unusual vaginal discharge.	These are warning signs for cervical and endometrial cancer or vaginal infection.
Determine if patient has history of HPV (condyloma acuminatum, herpes simplex, or cervical dysplasia); has multiple sex partners; smokes cigarettes; has had multiple pregnancies; or was young at first intercourse.	These are risk factors for cervical cancer (ACS, 2011).
Determine if patient is older than 40, obese, and has history of ovarian dysfunction, breast or endometrial cancer, irradiation of pelvic organs, or endometriosis; has family history of ovarian, breast, or colon cancer; has history of infertility or nulliparity; or use of estrogen (alone) hormone replacement therapy.	These are risk factors for ovarian cancer (ACS, 2011).
Determine if patient is postmenopausal, obese, or infertile; had early menarche; had late menopause; has history of hypertension, diabetes, gallbladder disease, or polycystic ovary disease; has family history of endometrial, breast, or colon cancer; or has a history of estrogen-related exposure (estrogen replacement therapy, tamoxifen use).	These are risk factors for endometrial cancer (ACS, 2011).

HIV, Human immunodeficiency virus; *HPV,* human papillomavirus (HPV) vaccine; *STI,* sexually transmitted infection.

fourth corner covers the perineum. After the examination begins, lift the drape over the perineum. A male examiner always needs to have a female attendant present during the examination, whereas a female examiner may choose to work alone. An additional female should be present if the patient requests it.

External Genitalia

Make sure that the perineal area is well illuminated. Follow standard precautions and wear clean gloves to prevent contact with infectious organisms. The perineum is sensitive and tender; do not touch the area suddenly without warning the patient. It is best to touch the inner thigh first before touching it.

While sitting at the end of the examination table or bed, inspect the quantity and distribution of hair growth. Preadolescents have no pubic hair. During adolescence hair grows along the labia, becoming darker, coarser, and curlier. In an adult hair grows in a triangle over the female perineum and along the medial surfaces of the thighs. The underlying skin is free of inflammation, irritation, or lesions.

Inspect surface characteristics of the labia majora. The skin of the perineum is smooth, clean, and slightly darker than other skin. The mucous membranes appear dark pink and moist. The labia majora can be gaping or closed, appear dry or moist, and are usually symmetrical. After childbirth the labia majora separate, causing the labia minora to become more prominent. When a woman reaches menopause, the labia majora become thinned; they become atrophied in older age. The labia majora are normally without inflammation, edema, lesions, or lacerations.

To inspect the remaining external structures, use your nondominant hand and gently place the thumb and index finger inside the labia minora and retract the tissues outwardly (Fig. 30-66). Be sure to have a firm hold to avoid repeated retraction against the sensitive tissues. Use the other hand to palpate the labia minora between the thumb and second finger. On inspection the labia minora are normally thinner than the labia majora, and one side is sometimes larger. The tissue feels soft on palpation and without tenderness. The size of the clitoris varies, but it normally does not exceed 2 cm in length and 0.5 cm in width. Look for atrophy, inflammation, or adhesions. If inflamed, the clitoris is a bright cherry red. In young women it is a common site for syphilitic lesions, or chancres, which appear as small open ulcers that drain serous material.

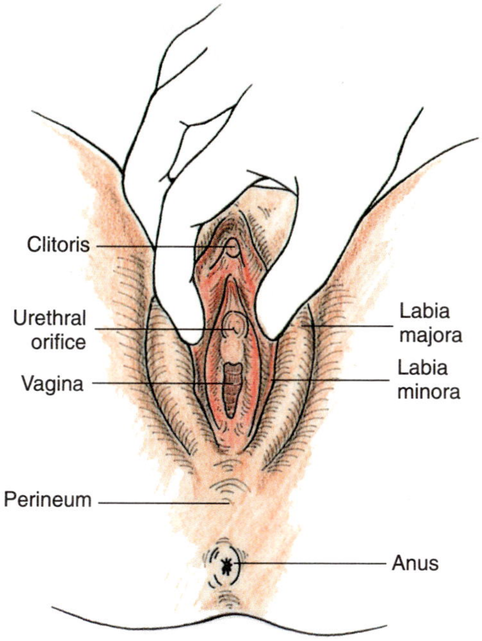

FIG. 30-66 Female external genitalia.

Inspect the urethral orifice carefully for color and position. It is normally intact without inflammation. The urethral meatus is anterior to the vaginal orifice and is pink. It appears as a small slit or pinhole opening just above the vaginal canal. Note any discharge, polyps, or fistulas.

Inspect the vaginal orifice for inflammation, edema, discoloration, discharge, and lesions. Normally the opening is a thin, vertical slit; and the tissue is moist. While inspecting the vaginal orifice, note the condition of the hymen, which is just inside the opening. In the virgin female the hymen restricts the opening of the vagina, but the tissue retracts or disappears after sexual intercourse.

Inspect the anus, looking for lesions and hemorrhoids (see rectal examination). After completion of the external examination, dispose of examination gloves and offer the patient soft disposable cloths for perineal hygiene.

Patients who are at risk for contracting an STI need to learn to perform a genital self-examination (Box 30-25). The purpose of the examination is to detect any signs or symptoms of an STI. Many persons do not know that they have an STI (e.g., chlamydia), and some STIs (e.g., syphilis) remain undetected for years.

Speculum Examination of Internal Genitalia

An examination of the internal genitalia requires much skill and practice. Advanced nurse practitioners and primary care providers perform this examination. As a nursing student you observe the procedure or assist the examiner by helping the patient with positioning, handing off specimen supplies, and providing emotional support for the patient.

The examination involves use of a plastic or metal speculum consisting of two blades and an adjustment device. The examiner inserts the speculum into the vagina to assess the internal genitalia for cancerous lesions and other abnormalities. During the examination the examiner collects a specimen for a Papanicolaou (Pap) test for cervical and vaginal cancer. The cervix is inspected for color, position, size, surface characteristics, and discharge (Seidel et al., 2011).

BOX 30-25 PATIENT TEACHING

Female Genitalia and Reproductive Tract Assessment

Objective

- Patient will use measures to maintain sexual health and prevent acquisition and transmission of sexually transmitted infections (STIs).

Teaching Strategies

- Instruct patient about purpose and recommended frequency of Papanicolaou (Pap) smears and gynecological examinations. Explain that the Pap smear is relatively painless and needed annually with a pelvic examination for women who are sexually active or over the age of 21. Patients are screened more often if certain risk factors exist such as a weak immune system, multiple sex partners, smoking, and a history of infections (e.g., human papillomavirus [HPV]).
- Counsel patient with an STI about the implications of diagnosis and treatment.
- Recommend the HPV vaccine for females ages 9 to 26 years to prevent cervical cancer (American Cancer Society [ACS], 2011; Centers for Disease Control and Prevention, 2011). The HPV vaccine prevents the most common types of HPV that cause cervical cancer and genital warts. It is given as a 3-dose vaccine.
- Instruct in genital self-examination (GSE). Using a mirror, position self to examine the area covered by the pubic hair. Spread the hair apart, looking for bumps, sores, or blisters. Also look for any warts, which appear as small, bumpy spots and enlarge to fleshy, cauliflower-like lesions. Next spread the outer vaginal lips apart and look at the clitoris for bumps, blisters, sores, or warts. Look at both sides of the inner vaginal lips. Inspect the area around the urinary and vaginal opening for bumps, blisters, sores, or warts.
- Explain warning signs of STIs: pain or burning on urination, pain during sex, pain in pelvic area, bleeding between menstruation, itchy rash around vagina, and abnormal vaginal discharge.
- Teach measures to prevent STIs: male partner's use of condoms, restricting number of sexual partners, avoiding sex with persons who have several other partners, and perineal hygiene measures.
- Tell patients with an STI to inform sexual partners of the need for an examination.
- Reinforce the importance of performing perineal hygiene (as appropriate).

Evaluation

- Ask patient to explain when she should routinely have a gynecological examination and Pap test.
- Have patient describe ways to prevent transmission of STIs.
- For patient with an STI, determine during follow-up visit if patient has followed safe sexual practices (use nonthreatening inquiry).

MALE GENITALIA

An examination of the male genitalia assesses the integrity of the external genitalia (Fig. 30-67), inguinal ring, and canal. Because the incidence of STIs in adolescents and young adults is high, an assessment of the genitalia needs to be a routine part of any health maintenance examination for this age-group (Box 30-26). The examination begins by having the patient void. Make sure the examination room is warm. Have the patient lie supine with the chest, abdomen, and lower legs draped or stand during the examination. Apply clean gloves.

Use a calm, gentle approach to lessen the patient's anxiety. The position and exposure of the body during the examination is embarrassing for some men. To minimize his anxiety, it often helps

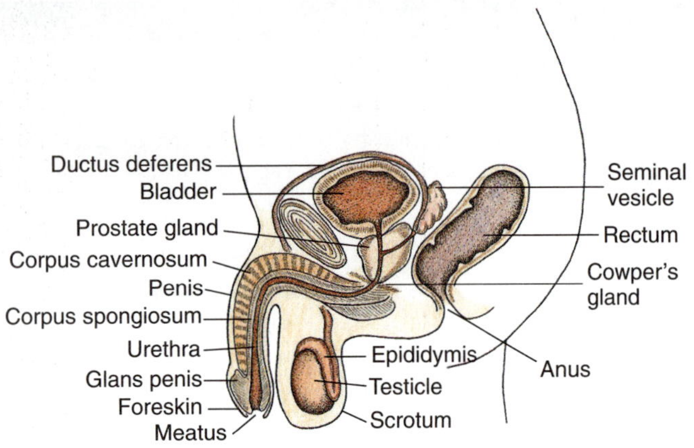

FIG. 30-67 External and internal male sex organs.

BOX 30-26 PATIENT TEACHING

Male Genitalia Assessment

Objective

- Patient will use measures to maintain sexual health and prevent acquisition and transmission of sexually transmitted infections (STIs).

Teaching Strategies

- Teach patient how to perform genital self-examination (see Box 30-27).
- Counsel patient who has an STI about diagnosis implications and treatment.
- Explain warning signs of STIs: pain on urination and during sex, abnormal penile discharge (different from usual), swollen lymph nodes, or rash or ulcer on skin or genitalia.
- Teach measures to prevent STIs: use of condoms, avoiding sex with infected partner, restricting number of sexual partners, avoiding sex with persons who have multiple partners, and using regular perineal hygiene.
- Recommend HPV vaccine for males ages 9 to 26 years. Boys and young men may choose to get this vaccine to prevent genital warts and anal cancer (CDC, 2011).
- Tell patients with an STI to inform their sexual partners of the need to have an examination.
- Instruct patient to seek treatment as soon as possible if partner becomes infected with an STI.

Evaluation

- Ask patient to describe methods for preventing and treating STIs.
- During a follow-up visit determine whether patient with an STI has used safe sex practices.

TABLE 30-30 Nursing History for Male Genitalia Assessment

ASSESSMENT	RATIONALE
Review normal urinary elimination pattern, including frequency of voiding; history of nocturia; character and volume of urine; daily fluid intake; symptoms of burning, urgency, and frequency; difficulty starting stream; and hematuria (see Chapter 45).	Urinary problems are directly associated with genitourinary problems because of anatomical structure of men's reproductive and urinary systems.
Assess patient's sexual history and use of safe sex habits (multiple partners, infection in partners, failure to use condom).	Sexual history reveals risk for and understanding of sexually transmitted diseases (STIs) and human immunodeficiency virus (HIV).
Determine if patient has received the HPV vaccine.	HPV is associated with genital warts in men and can lead to cervical cancer in females (CDC, 2011).
Determine if patient has had previous surgery or illness involving urinary or reproductive organs, including STI.	Alterations resulting from disease or surgery are sometimes responsible for symptoms or changes in organ structure or function.
Ask if patient has noted penile pain or swelling, genital lesions, or urethral discharge.	These signs and symptoms may indicate STI.
Determine if patient has noticed heaviness or painless enlargement of testis or irregular lumps.	These signs and symptoms are early warning signs for testicular cancer.
If patient reports an enlargement in inguinal area, assess if it is intermittent or constant, associated with straining or lifting, and painful and whether pain is affected by coughing, lifting, or straining at stool.	Signs and symptoms reflect potential inguinal hernia.
Ask if patient has difficulty achieving erection or ejaculation; also review whether patient is taking diuretics, sedatives, antihypertensives, or tranquilizers.	These medications influence sexual performance.

to offer explanations of the steps of examination so he anticipates all actions. Manipulate the genitalia gently to avoid causing erection or discomfort. Obtain a thorough history (Table 30-30) before the examination, ensuring that the assessment is complete.

Sexual Maturity

First note the sexual maturity of the patient by observing the size and shape of the penis and testes; the size, color, and texture of the scrotal skin; and the character and distribution of pubic hair. The testes first increase in size in preadolescence. During this time there is no pubic hair. By the end of puberty, the testes and penis enlarge to adult size and shape, and scrotal skin darkens and becomes wrinkled. With puberty hair is coarse and abundant in the pubic area. The penis has no hair, and the scrotum has very little hair (Fig. 30-68, *A* and *B*). Also inspect the skin covering the genitalia for lice, rashes, excoriations, or lesions. Normally it is clear, without lesions.

Penis

To inspect penile surfaces, manipulate the genitalia or have the patient assist. Inspect the shaft, corona, prepuce (foreskin), glans, and urethral meatus. The dorsal vein is apparent on inspection. In uncircumcised males retract the foreskin to reveal the glans and urethral meatus. The foreskin usually retracts easily. A small amount of white, thick smegma sometimes collects under this

BOX 30-27 MALE GENITAL SELF-EXAMINATION

All men 15 years and older need to perform this examination monthly using the following steps.

Genital Examination

- Perform the examination after a warm bath or shower when the scrotal skin is less thick.
- Stand naked in front of a mirror, hold the penis in your hand, and examine the head. Pull back the foreskin if uncircumcised to expose the glans.
- Inspect and palpate the entire head of the penis in a clockwise motion, looking carefully for any bumps, sores, or blisters (bumps and blisters may be light colored or red, resemble pimples).
- Look also for any genital warts (see illustration).
- Look at the opening (urethral meatus) at the end of the penis for discharge.
- Look along the entire shaft of the penis for the same signs.
- Be sure to separate pubic hair at the base of the penis and carefully examine the skin underneath.

Testicular Self-Examination

- Look for swelling or lumps in the skin of the scrotum while looking in the mirror.
- Use both hands, placing the index and middle fingers under the testicles and the thumb on top (see illustration).
- Gently roll the testicle, feeling for lumps, swelling, soreness, or a harder consistency.
- Find the epididymis (a cordlike structure on the top and back of the testicle; it is not a lump).
- Feel for small, pea-size lumps on the front and side of the testicle. Abnormal lumps are usually painless.
- Call your health care provider for abnormal findings.

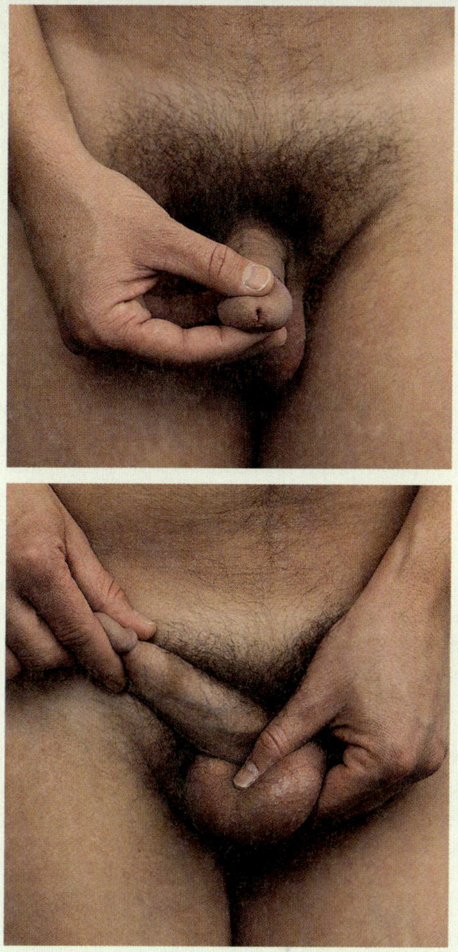

Illustrations from Seidel HM et al: *Mosby's guide to physical examination,* ed 7, St Louis, 2011, Mosby.

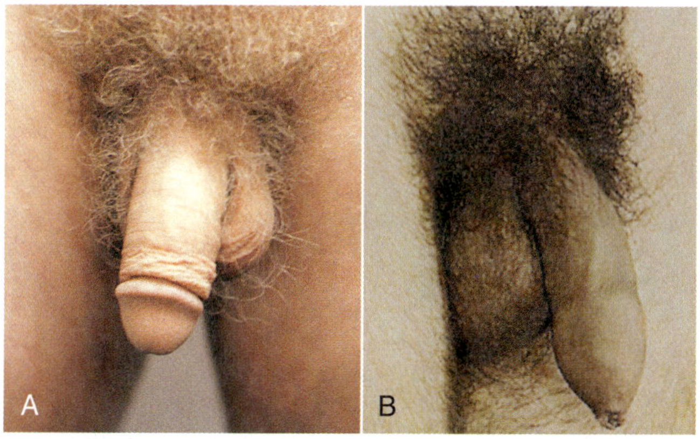

FIG. 30-68 Appearance of male genitalia. **A,** Circumcised. **B,** Uncircumcised. (From Seidel HM et al: *Mosby's guide to physical examination,* ed 7, St Louis, 2011, Mosby.)

foreskin. Obtain a culture if abnormal discharge is present. The urethral meatus is slitlike in appearance and positioned on the ventral surface just millimeters from the tip of the glans. In some congenital conditions the meatus is displaced along the penile shaft. The area between the foreskin and glans is a common site for venereal lesions. Gently compress the glans between the thumb and index finger; this opens the urethral meatus for inspection of lesions, edema, and inflammation. Normally the opening is glistening and pink without discharge. Palpate any lesion gently to note tenderness, size, consistency, and shape. When inspection and palpation of the glans is complete, pull the foreskin down to its original position.

Continue by inspecting the entire shaft of the penis, including the undersurface, looking for lesions, scars, or edema. Palpate the shaft between the thumb and first two fingers to detect localized areas of hardness or tenderness. A patient who has lain in bed for a prolonged time sometimes develops dependent edema in the penis shaft.

It is important for any male patient to learn to perform a genital self-examination to detect signs or symptoms of STIs, especially men who have had more than one sexual partner or whose partner has had other partners. Men may have an STI but not be aware of it; self-examination is a routine part of self-care (Box 30-27).

Scrotum

Be particularly cautious while inspecting and palpating the scrotum because the structures lying within the scrotal sac are very sensitive. The scrotum is divided internally into two halves. Each half contains a testicle, epididymis, and the vas deferens, which travels upward into the inguinal ring. Normally the left testicle is lower than the right. Inspect the size, shape, and symmetry of the scrotum while observing for lesions or edema. Gently lift the scrotum to view the posterior surface. The scrotal skin is usually loose, and the surface is coarse. The scrotal skin is more deeply pigmented than body skin. Tightening of the skin or loss of wrinkling reveals edema. The size of the scrotum normally changes with temperature variations because the dartos muscle contracts in cold and relaxes in warm temperatures. Lumps in the scrotal skin are commonly sebaceous cysts.

Testicular cancer is a solid tumor common in young men ages 18 to 34 years. Early detection is critical. Explain testicular self-examination (see Box 30-27) while examining the patient. The testes are normally sensitive but not tender. The underlying testicles are normally ovoid and approximately 2 to 4 cm (1 to 1½ inch) in size. Gently palpate the testicles and epididymis between the thumb and first two fingers. The testes feel smooth, rubbery, and free of nodules. The epididymis is resilient. Note the size, shape, and consistency of the organs. The most common symptoms of testicular cancer are a painless enlargement of one testis and the appearance of a palpable, small, hard lump, about the size of a pea, on the front or side of the testicle. In the older adult the testicles decrease in size and are less firm during palpation. Continue to palpate the vas deferens separately as it forms the spermatic cord toward the inguinal ring, noting nodules or swelling. It normally feels smooth and discrete.

Inguinal Ring and Canal

The external inguinal ring provides the opening for the spermatic cord to pass into the inguinal canal. The canal forms a passage through the abdominal wall, a potential site for hernia formation. A hernia is a protrusion of a portion of intestine through the inguinal wall or canal. Sometimes an intestinal loop enters the scrotum. Have the patient stand during this part of the examination.

During inspection ask the patient to strain or bear down. The maneuver helps to make a hernia more visible. Look for obvious bulging in the inguinal area.

Complete the examination by palpating for inguinal lymph nodes. Normally small, nontender, mobile horizontal nodes are palpable. Any abnormality indicates local or systemic infection or malignant disease.

RECTUM AND ANUS

A good time to perform the rectal examination is after the genital examination. Usually this examination is not performed for young children or adolescents. It detects colorectal cancer in its early stages. The rectal examination also detects prostatic tumors in men. Collect a health history (Table 30-31) to detect the patient's risk for bowel or rectal disease (men and women) or prostatic disease (men). Teach the patient about the purpose of the examination (Box 30-28).

The rectal examination is uncomfortable; thus explaining all steps helps a patient relax. Use a calm, slow-paced, gentle approach during the examination. Female patients remain in the dorsal recumbent position following genitalia examination or they assume a side-lying (Sims') position. The best way to examine men is to have the patient stand and bend over forward with hips flexed and upper body resting across an examination table. Examine a nonambulatory patient in the Sims' position. Use nonlatex clean gloves.

TABLE 30-31 Nursing History for Rectal and Anal Assessment

ASSESSMENT	RATIONALE
Determine whether patient has experienced bleeding from rectum, black or tarry stools (melena), rectal pain, or change in bowel habits (constipation or diarrhea).	These are warning signs of colorectal cancer* or other gastrointestinal alterations.
Determine whether patient has personal or strong family history of colorectal cancer, polyps, or chronic inflammatory bowel disease. Ask if patient is over age 40.	These are risk factors for colorectal cancer.*
Assess dietary habits, including high fat intake, diet high in processed or red meats, or deficient fiber content (inadequate fruits and vegetables).	Bowel cancer is often linked to dietary intake of fat or insufficient fiber intake.*
Determine if patient is obese, is physically inactive, smokes, or consumes alcohol.	These are risk factors for colorectal cancer.
Determine whether patient has undergone screening for colorectal cancer (digital examination, fecal occult blood test, flexible sigmoidoscopy, and colonoscopy).	Undergoing this screening reflects understanding and compliance with preventive health care measures.
Assess medication history for use of laxatives or cathartic medications.	Repeated use causes diarrhea and eventual loss of intestinal muscle tone.
Assess for use of codeine or iron preparations.	Codeine causes constipation. Iron turns the color of feces black and tarry.
Ask male patient if he has experienced weak or interrupted urine flow, inability to urinate, difficulty in starting or stopping urine flow, polyuria, nocturia, hematuria, or dysuria. Does patient have continuing pain in lower back, pelvis, or upper thighs?	These are warning signs of prostatic cancer.* Symptoms also suggest infection or prostate enlargement.

*Data from American Cancer Society: *Cancer facts and figures 2006,* Atlanta, 2010, The Society.

Inspection

Using the nondominant hand, gently retract the buttocks to view the perianal and sacrococcygeal areas. Perianal skin is smooth, more pigmented, and coarser than skin over the buttocks. Inspect anal tissue for skin characteristics, lesions, external hemorrhoids (dilated veins that appear as reddened protrusions), ulcers, fissures and fistulas, inflammation, rashes, or excoriation. Anal tissues are moist and hairless, and the voluntary external muscle sphincter holds the anus closed. Next ask a patient to bear down as though having a bowel movement. Any internal hemorrhoids or fissures appear at this time. Use clock reference (e.g., 3 o'clock or 8 o'clock) to describe location of findings. Normally there is no protrusion of tissue.

Digital Palpation

Examine the anal canal and sphincters with digital palpation, and in male patients palpate the prostate gland to rule out enlargement. Usually advanced practitioners perform this portion of the examination. This technique is not discussed here.

BOX 30-28 PATIENT TEACHING

Rectal and Anal Assessment

Objective

- Patient will be able to identify symptoms of colorectal and prostatic cancer.

Teaching Strategies

- Discuss the guidelines of the American Cancer Society (ACS) (2011) for early detection of colorectal cancer.
- Beginning at age 50, both men and women should follow one of these testing schedules:
  - Tests that find polyps and cancer
    - Flexible sigmoidoscopy every 5 years, or
    - Colonoscopy every 10 years, or
    - Double-contrast barium enema every 5 years, or
    - CT colonography (virtual colonoscopy) every 5 years
  - Tests that primarily find cancer
    - Yearly fecal occult blood test (gFOBT), or
    - Yearly fecal immunochemical test (FIT) every year, or
    - Stool DNA test (sDNA), interval uncertain
- Individuals at increased risk should discuss options with their health care provider.
- Discuss warning signs of colorectal cancer (see Table 30-31).
- Discuss with male patient the ACS guidelines (2011) for early detection of prostate cancer:
  - Digital rectal examination performed annually after age 50
  - Annual prostate-specific antigen (PSA) blood test for men age 50 and over
  - Prostate ultrasound testing if results of either digital rectal examination or PSA test is suspicious
  - Need for African American men or those with a first-degree relative diagnosed with prostate cancer to begin testing at age 45
- Discuss warning signs of prostate cancer.

Evaluation

- During follow-up visit determine whether patient has had a rectal examination performed.
- Have patient explain warning signs of colorectal and prostate cancer.

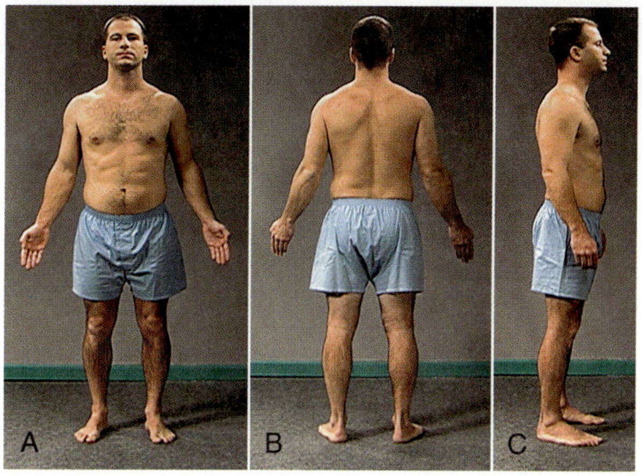

FIG. 30-69 Inspection of overall body posture. **A,** Anterior view. **B,** Posterior view. **C,** Lateral view. (From Seidel HM et al: *Mosby's guide to physical examination,* ed 7, St Louis, 2011, Mosby.)

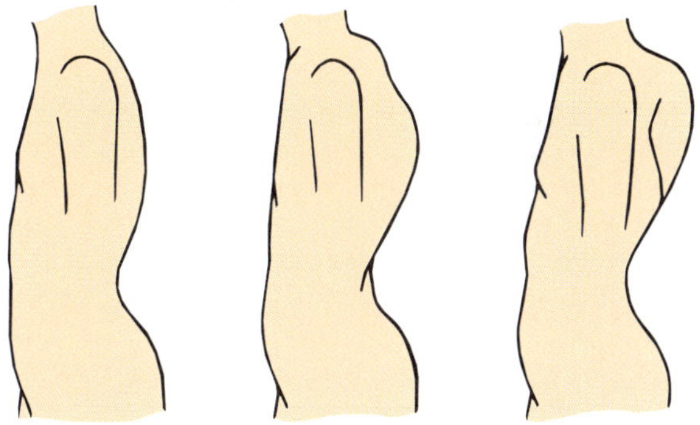

FIG. 30-70 Common postural abnormalities. **A,** Lordosis. **B,** Kyphosis. **C,** Scoliosis.

MUSCULOSKELETAL SYSTEM

The musculoskeletal assessment can be performed as a separate examination or integrated with other parts of the total physical examination. In addition, you can assess the patient's movements while performing other nursing care measures such as bathing or positioning. The assessment of musculoskeletal function focuses on determining range of joint motion, muscle strength and tone, and joint and muscle condition. Assessing musculoskeletal integrity is especially important when a patient reports pain or loss of function in a joint or muscle. Because muscular disorders are often the result of neurological disease, you may choose to perform a simultaneous neurological assessment.

While examining a patient's musculoskeletal function, visualize the anatomy of bone and muscle placement and joint structure (see Chapter 47). Joints vary in degree of mobility, depending on the type of joint.

For a complete examination expose the muscles and joints so they are free to move. Have the patient assume a sitting, supine, prone, or standing position while assessing specific muscle groups. Table 30-32 lists the information gathered in the nursing history.

General Inspection

Observe the patient's gait when entering the examination room. When the patient is unaware of the nature of your observation, gait is more natural. Later, a more formal test has the patient walk in a straight line away from and return to the point of origin. Note how the patient walks, sits, and rises from a sitting position. Normally patients walk with the arms swinging freely at the sides and the head leading the body. Older adults often walk with smaller steps and a wider base of support. Note foot dragging, limping, shuffling, and the position of the trunk in relation to the legs.

Observe the patient from the side and while facing the patient in a standing position. The normal standing posture is upright with parallel alignment of the hips and shoulders (Fig. 30-69, *A* to *C*). There is an even contour of the shoulders, level scapulae and iliac crests, alignment of the head over the gluteal folds, and symmetry of extremities. While observing from the side of the patient, note the normal cervical, thoracic, and lumbar curves. Holding the head erect is normal. As the patient sits, some degree of rounding of the shoulders is normal. Older adults tend to assume a stooped, forward-bent posture with the hips and knees somewhat flexed and arms bent at the elbows, raising the level of the arms.

Common postural abnormalities include lordosis, kyphosis, and scoliosis (Fig. 30-70, *A* to *C*). **Kyphosis,** or hunchback, is an

TABLE 30-32 Nursing History for Musculoskeletal Assessment

ASSESSMENT	RATIONALE
Determine if patient is involved in competitive sports (particularly involving collision and contact), fails to warm up adequately, is in poor physical condition, or has had a rapid growth spurt (adolescents).	These are risk factors for sports injury.
Review patient history for use of alcohol and/or caffeine; cigarette smoking; constant dieting; calcium intake less than 500 mg daily; thin and light body frame; nulliparous status; menopause before age 45; estrogen deficiency; postmenopause status; family history of osteoporosis; white, Asian, Native American, or northern European ancestry; advanced age; history of fractures/falls; inadequate calcium intake and vitamin D; sedentary lifestyle; chronic diseases (Cushing's hyperthyroidism and hypothyroidism, malabsorption/malnutrition disorders, neoplasm); long-term use of corticosteroids, methotrexate, phenytoin, aluminum-containing antacids; lack of weight-bearing exercise; lack of exposure to sunlight (Walker, 2010).	These are risk factors for osteoporosis.
Ask patient to describe history of problems in bone, muscle, or joint function (e.g., recent fall, trauma, lifting of heavy objects, history of bone or joint disease with sudden or gradual onset, location of alteration).	History helps to assess nature of musculoskeletal problem.
Assess nature and extent of pain, including location, duration, severity, predisposing and aggravating factors, relieving factors, and type.	Pain frequently accompanies alterations in bone, joints, or muscle. This has implications not only for comfort, but also for ability to perform activities of daily living.
Assess patient's normal activity pattern, including type of exercise routinely performed.	Provides baseline in assessment. Sedentary lifestyle and lack of appropriate exercise increase bone loss and risk of fractures.
Determine how alteration influences ability to perform activities of daily living (e.g., bathing, feeding, dressing, toileting, ambulating) and social functions (e.g., household chores, work, recreation, sexual activities).	The extent to which patient is able to perform self-care determines the level of nursing care. Type and degree of restriction in continuing social activities influence topics for patient education and ability of nurse to identify alternative ways to maintain function.
Assess height loss of woman over age 50 by subtracting current height from recall of maximum adult height.	Measurement is useful screening tool to predict osteoporosis.

BOX 30-29 PATIENT TEACHING

Health Promotion to Prevent Osteoporosis in Women

Objective

- Patient will follow measures to prevent or minimize osteoporosis.

Teaching Strategies

- Recommend women age 65 and older for routine screening for osteoporosis. Recommend men for screening as well; they are equally at risk for development of osteoporosis as they age.
- To reduce bone demineralization, instruct older adults in a proper exercise program (e.g., weight-bearing, muscle-strengthening, and balance-training exercises) to be followed 3 or more times a week.
- Encourage intake of calcium to meet the recommended daily allowance. Increased vitamin D aids calcium absorption.
- Recommendation for calcium supplements for adults over age 25 is 1000 to 1500 mg/day. Instruct patient to take no more than 600 mg of calcium at one time.
- Instruct older adults and those with osteoporosis in proper body mechanics and range-of-motion and moderate weight-bearing exercises (e.g., swimming and walking) to minimize trauma and subsequent fracture of bones.
- Instruct older patients to pace activities to compensate for loss in muscle strength.

Evaluation

- Observe patient's posture.
- Ask patient to describe therapies for preventing osteoporosis.
- Observe patient perform range-of-motion exercises.
- Have patient keep log of regular weight-training exercises.

exaggeration of the posterior curvature of the thoracic spine. This postural abnormality is common in older adults. **Lordosis,** or swayback, is an increased lumbar curvature. A lateral spinal curvature is called **scoliosis.** Loss of height is frequently the first clinical sign of osteoporosis, in which height loss occurs in the trunk as a result of vertebral fracture and collapse. **Osteoporosis** is a systemic skeletal condition that is noted to have both decreased bone mass and deterioration of bone tissue, making bones fragile and at risk for fracture (Nelson et al., 2010). Osteopenia, characterized by low bone mass of the hip, puts persons at risk for osteoporosis, fractures, and potential complications later in life. Approximately 80% of people with osteoporosis are women; approximately 20% of the time the disease affects men. It affects any age-group, including children. Patients should be taught ways to reduce the chance of developing this disease (Box 30-29).

During general inspection look at the extremities for overall size, gross deformity, bony enlargement, alignment, and symmetry. Normally there is bilateral symmetry in length, circumference, alignment, and position and in the number of skinfolds (Seidel et al., 2011). A general review pinpoints areas requiring specialized assessment.

Palpation

Apply gentle palpation to all bones, joints, and surrounding muscles during a complete examination. For a focused assessment only examine the involved area. Note any heat, tenderness, edema, or resistance to pressure. The patient should not feel any discomfort when you palpate. Muscles should be firm.

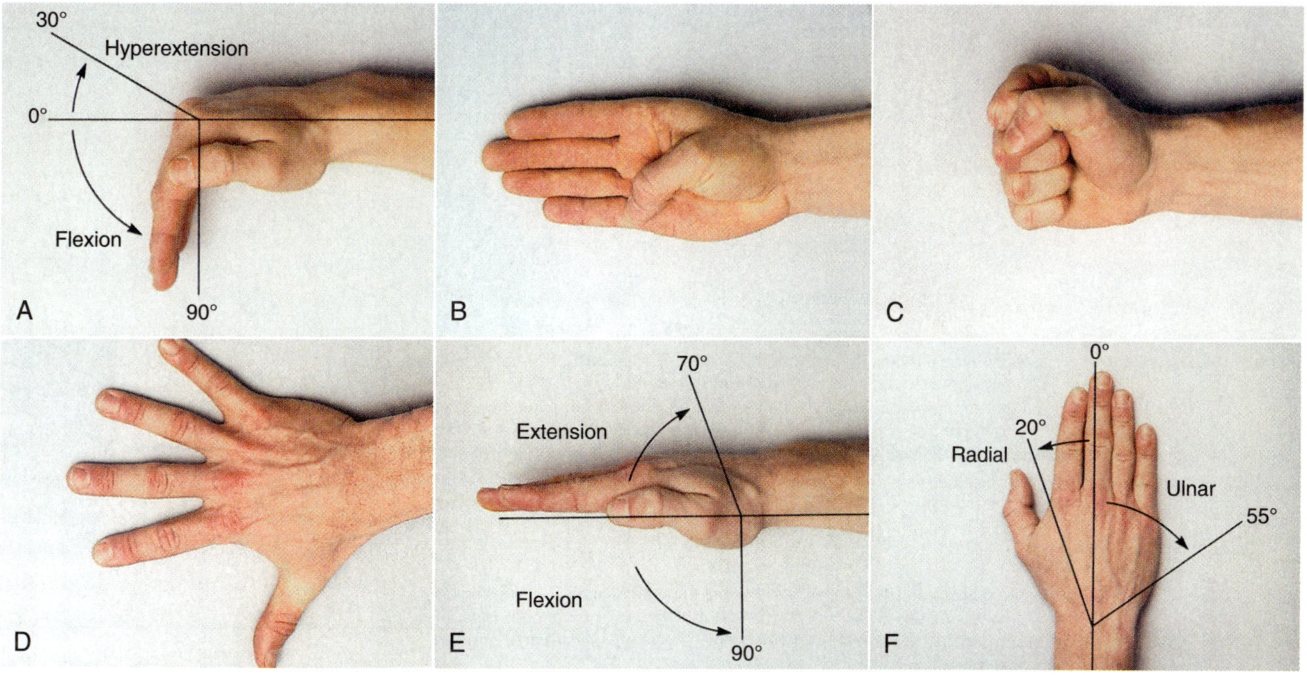

FIG. 30-71 Range of motion of hand and wrist. **A,** Metacarpophalangeal flexion and hyperextension. **B,** Finger flexion: thumb to each fingertip and to the base of the little finger. **C,** Finger flexion, fist formation. **D,** Finger abduction. **E,** Wrist flexion and hyperextension. **F,** Wrist radial and ulnar movement. (From Seidel HM et al: *Mosby's guide to physical examination,* ed 7, St Louis, 2011, Mosby.)

Range of Joint Motion

The examination includes comparison of both active and passive ROM. Ask the patient to put each major joint through active and passive full ROM (see Chapter 47). Learn the correct terminology for the movements that the joints are capable of making (Table 30-33) and teach the patient how to move through each ROM. Demonstrate ROM to the patient when possible. To assess ROM passively, ask the patient to relax and then passively move the extremities through their ROM. Compare the same body parts for equality in movement. Fig. 30-71, *A* to *F,* shows an example of ROM positions for the hand and wrist. Do not force a joint into a painful position. Know the normal range of each joint and the extent to which you can move the patient's joints. ROM is equal between contralateral joints. Ideally assess the patient's normal range to determine a baseline for assessing later change.

A **goniometer,** frequently used by physical and occupational therapists, measures the precise degree of motion in a particular joint and is mainly for patients who have a suspected reduction in joint movement. The instrument has two flexible arms with a 180-degree protractor in the center. Position the center of the protractor at the center of the joint you are measuring (Fig. 30-72). The arms extend along the body parts on each side of the protractor. Measure the joint angle before moving the joint. After taking the joint through a full ROM, measure the angle again to determine the degree of movement. Compare the reading with the normal degree of joint movement.

Joints are typically free from stiffness, instability, swelling, or inflammation. There should be no discomfort when applying pressure to bones and joints. In older adults joints often become swollen and stiff with reduced ROM resulting from cartilage erosion and fibrosis of synovial membranes (see Chapter 47). If a joint appears swollen and inflamed, palpate it for warmth.

TABLE 30-33 Terminology for Normal Range-of-Motion Positions

TERM	RANGE OF MOTION	EXAMPLES OF JOINTS
Flexion	Movement decreasing angle between two adjoining bones; bending of limb	Elbow, fingers, knee
Extension	Movement increasing angle between two adjoining bones	Elbow, knee, fingers
Hyperextension	Movement of body part beyond its normal resting extended position	Head
Pronation	Movement of body part so front or ventral surface faces downward	Hand, forearm
Supination	Movement of body part so front or ventral surface faces upward	Hand, forearm
Abduction	Movement of extremity away from midline of body	Leg, arm, fingers
Adduction	Movement of extremity toward midline of body	Leg, arm, fingers
Internal rotation	Rotation of joint inward	Knee, hip
External rotation	Rotation of joint outward	Knee, hip
Eversion	Turning of body part away from midline	Foot
Inversion	Turning of body part toward midline	Foot
Dorsiflexion	Flexion of toes and foot upward	Foot
Plantar flexion	Bending of toes and foot downward	Foot

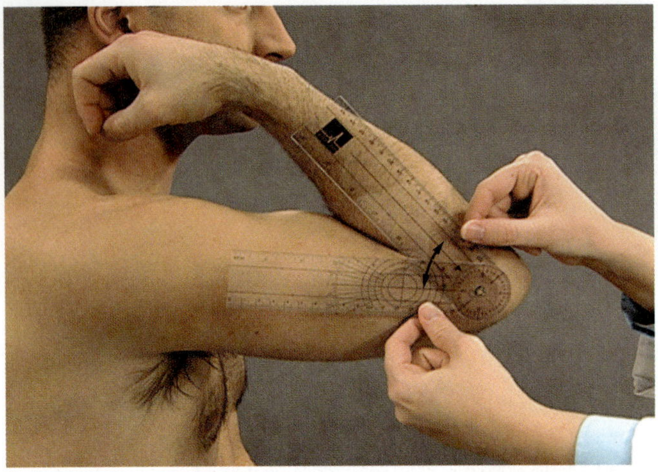

FIG. 30-72 The patient flexes the arm; the goniometer measures joint range of motion. (From Seidel HM et al: *Mosby's guide to physical examination,* ed 7, St Louis, 2011, Mosby.)

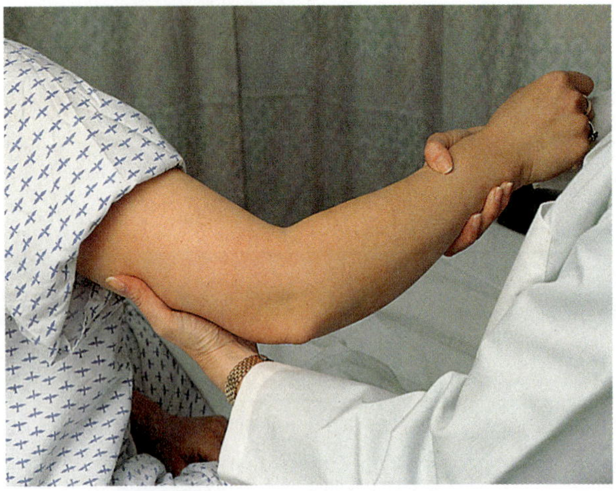

FIG. 30-73 Assessing muscle tone.

TABLE 30-34 Maneuvers to Assess Muscle Strength

MUSCLE GROUP	MANEUVER
Neck (sternocleidomastoid)	Place hand firmly against patient's upper jaw. Ask patient to turn head laterally against resistance.
Shoulder (trapezius)	Place hand over midline of patient's shoulder, exerting firm pressure. Have patient raise shoulders against resistance.
Elbow	
Biceps	Pull down on forearm as patient attempts to flex arm.
Triceps	As you flex patient's arm, apply pressure against forearm. Ask patient to straighten arm.
Hip	
Quadriceps	When patient is sitting, apply downward pressure to thigh. Ask patient to raise leg up from table.
Gastrocnemius	Patient sits while examiner holds shin of flexed leg. Ask patient to straighten leg against resistance.

TABLE 30-35 Muscle Strength

	SCALES		
MUSCLE FUNCTION LEVEL	GRADE	% NORMAL	LOVETT SCALE
No evidence of contractility	0	0	0 (zero)
Slight contractility, no movement	1	10	T (trace)
Full range of motion, gravity eliminated*	2	25	P (poor)
Full range of motion with gravity	3	50	F (fair)
Full range of motion against gravity, some resistance	4	75	G (good)
Full range of motion against gravity, full resistance	5	100	N (normal)

Modified from Walker J: The role of the nurse in the management of osteoporosis, *Br J Nurs* 19(19):1243, 2010.
*Passive movement.

Muscle Tone and Strength

Assess muscle strength and tone during ROM measurement. Integrate these findings with those from the neurological assessment. Note muscle tone, the slight muscular resistance felt as you move the relaxed extremity passively through its ROM.

Ask the patient to allow an extremity to relax or hang limp. This is often difficult, particularly if the patient feels pain in it. Support the extremity and grasp each limb, moving it through the normal ROM (Fig. 30-73). Normal tone causes a mild, even resistance to movement through the entire range.

If a muscle has increased tone, or **hypertonicity,** there is considerable resistance with any sudden passive movement of a joint. Continued movement eventually causes the muscle to relax. A muscle that has little tone **(hypotonicity)** feels flabby. The involved extremity hangs loosely in a position determined by gravity.

For assessment of muscle strength, have the patient assume a stable position. He or she performs maneuvers demonstrating strength of major muscle groups (Table 30-34). Use a grading scale of "0 to 5" to compare symmetrical muscle pairs for strength (Table 30-35). The arm on the dominant side normally is stronger than the arm on the nondominant side. In older adults a loss of muscle mass causes bilateral weakness, but muscle strength remains greater in the dominant arm or leg.

Examine each muscle group. Ask the patient to first flex the muscle you are examining and then to resist when you apply an opposing force against that flexion. It is important to not allow the patient to move the joint. Gradually increase pressure to a muscle group (e.g., elbow extension). Have the patient resist the pressure you apply by attempting to move against resistance (e.g., elbow flexion) until instructed to stop. Vary the amount of pressure applied and observe the joint move. If you identify a weakness, compare the size of the muscle with its opposite counterpart by measuring the circumference of the muscle body with a tape measure. A muscle that has **atrophied** (reduced in size) feels soft and boggy when palpated.

TABLE 30-36 Nursing History for Neurological Assessment

ASSESSMENT	RATIONALE
Determine if patient uses analgesics, alcohol, sedatives, hypnotics, antipsychotics, antidepressants, nervous system stimulants, or recreational drugs.	These medications alter level of consciousness or cause behavioral changes. Abuse sometimes causes tremors, ataxia, and changes in peripheral nerve function.
Determine if patient has recent history of seizures/convulsions: clarify sequence of events (aura, fall to ground, motor activity, loss of consciousness); character of any symptoms; and relationship of seizure to time of day, fatigue, or emotional stress.	Seizure activity often originates from central nervous system alteration. Characteristics of seizure help determine its origin.
Screen patient for symptoms of headache, tremors, dizziness, vertigo, numbness or tingling of body part, visual changes, weakness, pain, or changes in speech. Presence of any symptom requires more detailed review (onset, severity, precipitating factors or sequence of events).	These symptoms frequently originate from alterations in central or peripheral nervous system function. Identification of specific patterns aids in diagnosis of pathological condition.
Discuss with patient's family any recent changes in patient's behavior (e.g., increased irritability, mood swings, memory loss, change in energy level).	Behavioral changes sometimes result from intracranial pathological states.
Assess patient for history of change in vision, hearing, smell, taste, or touch.	Major sensory nerves originate from brainstem. These symptoms help to localize nature of problem.
If an older patient displays sudden acute confusion (delirium), review history for drug toxicity (anticholinergics, diuretics, digoxin, cimetidine, sedatives, antihypertensives, antiarrhythmics), serious infections, metabolic disturbances, heart failure, and severe anemia.	Delirium is one of the most common mental disorders in older persons. Condition is always potentially reversible (see Box 30-31).
Review past history for head or spinal cord injury, meningitis, congenital anomalies, neurological disease, or psychiatric counseling.	Factors cause neurological symptoms or behavioral changes to develop, focusing assessment on possible cause.

NEUROLOGICAL SYSTEM

The neurological system is responsible for many functions, including initiation and coordination of movement, reception and perception of sensory stimuli, organization of thought processes, control of speech, and storage of memory. A close integration exists between the neurological system and all other body systems. For example, urine production relies in part on the adequacy of blood flow to the kidneys, and the size of arterioles supplying the kidneys is under neural control.

A full assessment of neurological function requires much time and attention to detail. For efficiency, integrate neurological measurements with other parts of the physical examination. For example, test cranial nerve function while assessing the head and neck. Observe mental and emotional status during the initial interview.

Consider many variables when deciding the extent of the neurological examination. A patient's level of consciousness influences his or her ability to follow directions. General physical status influences tolerance to assessment. A patient's chief complaint also helps determine the need for a thorough neurological assessment. If a patient complains of headache or a recent loss of function in an extremity, he or she needs a complete neurological review. Table 30-36 lists the data collected in the nursing history. You will need the following items for a complete examination:

- Reading material
- Vials containing aromatic substances (e.g., vanilla extract and coffee)
- Opposite tip of cotton swab or tongue blade broken in half
- Snellen eye chart
- Penlight
- Vials containing sugar or salt
- Tongue blade
- Two test tubes, one filled with hot water and the other with cold water
- Cotton balls or cotton-tipped applicators
- Tuning fork
- Reflex hammer

Mental and Emotional Status

You learn a great deal about mental capacities and emotional state simply by interacting with a patient. Ask questions during an examination to gather data and observe the appropriateness of emotions and thoughts. Special assessment tools are designed to assess a patient's mental status. The Mini-Mental State Examination (MMSE) is an instrument developed by Folstein et al. (1975) that measures orientation and cognitive function. The questions in Box 30-30 offer examples of questions found on the MMSE. The maximum score on the MMSE is 30. Patients with scores of 21 or less generally reveal cognitive impairment requiring further evaluation.

To ensure an objective assessment, consider a patient's cultural and educational background, values, beliefs, and previous experiences. Such factors influence response to questions. An alteration in mental or emotional status reflects a disturbance in cerebral functioning. The cerebral cortex controls and integrates intellectual and emotional functioning. Primary brain disorders, medication, and metabolic changes are examples of factors that change cerebral function.

Delirium is an acute mental disorder that occurs among hospitalized patients. Obtain a thorough history of a patient's behavior before delirium develops so as to recognize the condition early. Family members are usually a good resource. Among older adults delirium most often presents within the first 48 to 72 hours of hospital admission (Rigney, 2010). It is an acute mental disorder characterized by confusion, disorientation, and restlessness. It is

BOX 30-30 MINI-MENTAL STATE EXAMINATION SAMPLE QUESTIONS

- Orientation to time
  "What is the date?"
- Registration
  "Listen carefully. I am going to say three words. Say them back after I stop. Ready? Here they are . . .
  HOUSE (pause), CAR (pause), LAKE (pause). Now repeat these words back to me."
  (Repeat up to 5 times but score only the first trial.)
- Naming
  "What is this?" (Point to a pencil or pen.)
- Reading
  "Please read this and do what it says." (Show examinee the words on the stimulus form.)
  CLOSE YOUR EYES

BOX 30-31 CLINICAL CRITERIA FOR DELIRIUM

Definition: An acute disturbance of consciousness that is accompanied by a change in cognition. It is not caused by a preexisting or evolving dementia. Delirium develops over a short period of time, usually hours to days, and tends to fluctuate during the course of the day. It is usually a direct physiological consequence of a general medical condition. It is most common in older adults but occurs occasionally in younger patients.

- There is reduced clarity of awareness of the environment.
- Ability to focus, sustain, or shift attention is impaired (questions must be repeated).
- Irrelevant stimuli easily distract the person.
- There is an accompanying change in cognition (memory impairment, disorientation, or language disturbance).
- Recent memory is commonly affected.
- Disorientation usually occurs, with patient disoriented to time, place, or person.
- Language disturbance involves impaired ability to name objects or ability to write; speech is sometimes rambling.
- Perceptual disturbances include misinterpretations, delusions, or visual and auditory hallucinations. Neurological signs include tremor, unsteady gait, asterixis, or myoclonus.

often a sign of an impending or underlying physical illness in older adults (Flood and Buckwalter, 2009). The acute condition differs from dementia, a more progressive, organic mental disorder such as Alzheimer's disease. You need to recognize the difference so you can try to learn the underlying cause of delirium. Fortunately the condition often reverses when it is correctly assessed and the underlying cause is treated (i.e., central nervous system [CNS], metabolic, and cardiopulmonary disorders; systemic illnesses; and sensory deprivation or overload). To avoid misdiagnosis you need to adequately assess mental status. Frequently patients who develop delirium are labeled with "sundown syndrome" because the delirium frequently worsens at night. Many practitioners mistake this as being common with old age. Be aware that children are vulnerable to delirium from causes such as infection, drugs, serious trauma, autoimmune disorders, general anesthesia, and after transplant (Hatherill and Fisher, 2010). Box 30-31 summarizes clinical criteria for delirium.

Level of Consciousness. A person's level of consciousness exists along a continuum from full awakening, alertness, and cooperation to unresponsiveness to any form of external stimuli. Talk with the patient, asking questions about events involving his or her concerns about any health problems. A fully conscious patient responds to questions quickly and expresses ideas logically. With a lowering of a patient's consciousness, use the Glasgow Coma Scale (GCS) for an objective measurement of consciousness on a numerical scale (Table 30-37). The patient needs to be as alert as possible before testing. Take care when using the scale if the patient has sensory losses (e.g., vision or hearing). The GCS allows evaluation of a patient's neurological status over time. The higher the score, the better the patient's neurological function. Ask short, simple questions such as "What is your name?" "Where are you?" and "What day is this?" Also ask the patient to follow simple commands such as "Move your toes."

If the patient is not conscious enough to follow commands, try to elicit the pain response. Apply firm pressure with the thumb over the root of the patient's fingernail. The normal response to the painful stimuli is withdrawal of the body part from the stimulus. A patient with serious neurological impairment exhibits abnormal posturing in response to pain. A flaccid response indicates the absence of muscle tone in the extremities and severe injury to brain tissue.

TABLE 30-37 Glasgow Coma Scale

(The total score is the sum of the scores in the three categories)

ACTION	RESPONSE	SCORE
Eyes open	Spontaneously	4
	To speech	3
	To pain	2
	None	1
Best verbal response	Oriented	5
	Confused	4
	Inappropriate words	3
	Incomprehensible sounds	2
	None	1
Best motor response	Obeys commands	6
	Localized pain	5
	Flexion withdrawal	4
	Abnormal flexion	3
	Abnormal extension	2
	Flaccid	1
	TOTAL SCORE	**3 to 15**

Behavior and Appearance. Behavior, moods, hygiene, grooming, and choice of dress reveal pertinent information about mental status. Remain perceptive of a patient's mannerisms and actions during the entire physical assessment. Note nonverbal and verbal behaviors. Does the patient respond appropriately to directions? Does his or her mood vary with no apparent cause? Does he or she show concern about appearance? Is his or her hair clean and neatly groomed, and are the nails trim and clean? The patient should behave in a manner expressing concern and interest in the examination. He or she should make eye contact with you and express appropriate feelings that correspond to the situation. Normally the patient shows some degree of personal hygiene.

Choice and fit of clothing reflect socioeconomic background or personal taste rather than deficiency in self-concept or self-care. Avoid being judgmental and focus assessment on the appropriateness of clothing for the weather. Older adults sometimes neglect their appearance because of a lack of energy, finances, or reduced vision.

Language. Normal cerebral function allows a person to understand spoken or written words and express the self through written words or gestures. Assess the patient's voice inflection, tone, and manner of speech. Normally a patient's voice has inflections, is clear and strong, and increases in volume appropriately. Speech is fluent. When communication is clearly ineffective (e.g., omission or addition of letters and words, misuse of words, or hesitations), assess for **aphasia.** Injury to the cerebral cortex results in aphasia.

The two types of aphasia are sensory (or receptive) and motor (or expressive). With receptive aphasia a person cannot understand written or verbal speech. With expressive aphasia a person understands written and verbal speech but cannot write or speak appropriately when attempting to communicate. A patient sometimes suffers a combination of receptive and expressive aphasia. Assess language capabilities when it is clear that a patient is communicating ineffectively. Some simple assessment techniques include the following:

- Point to a familiar object, and ask the patient to name it.
- Ask the patient to respond to simple verbal and written commands such as "Stand up" or "Sit down."
- Ask the patient to read simple sentences out loud.

Normally a patient names objects correctly, follows commands, and reads sentences correctly.

Intellectual Function

Intellectual function includes memory (recent, immediate, and past), knowledge, abstract thinking, association, and judgment. Testing each aspect of function involves a specific technique. However, because cultural and educational background influences the ability to respond to test questions, do not ask questions related to concepts or ideas with which a patient is unfamiliar.

Memory. Assess immediate recall and recent and remote memory. Patients demonstrate immediate recall by repeating a series of numbers (e.g., *7, 4, 1*) in the order they are presented or in reverse order. Patients normally recall a series of five to eight digits forward and four to six digits backward.

First ask to test the patient's memory. Then state clearly and slowly the name of three unrelated objects. After mentioning all three, ask the patient to repeat each. Continue until he or she is successful. Later in the assessment, ask the patient to repeat the three words again. He or she should be able to identify them. Another test for recent memory involves asking the patient to recall events occurring during the same day (e.g., what was eaten for breakfast). Validate information with a family member.

To assess past memory, ask the patient to recall his or her mother's maiden name, a birthday, or a special date in history. It is best to ask open-ended rather than simple yes/no questions. A patient usually has immediate recall of such information. With older adults do not interpret hearing loss as confusion. Good communication techniques are essential throughout the examination to ensure that a patient clearly understands all directions and testing.

Knowledge. Assess knowledge by asking how much the patient knows about his or her illness or the reason for seeking health care. A knowledge assessment allows you to determine a patient's ability to learn or understand. If there is an opportunity to teach, test a patient's mental status by asking for feedback during a follow-up visit.

Abstract Thinking. Interpreting abstract ideas or concepts reflects the capacity for abstract thinking. For an individual to explain common phrases such as "A stitch in time saves nine" or "Don't count your chickens before they're hatched" requires a higher level of intellectual function. Note whether a patient's explanations are relevant and concrete. A patient with altered mental status probably interprets the phrase literally or merely rephrases the words.

Association. Another higher level of intellectual functioning involves finding similarities or associations between concepts: a dog is to a beagle as a cat is to a Siamese. Name related concepts and ask the patient to identify their associations. Ask questions that are appropriate to the patient's level of intelligence, using simple concepts.

Judgment. Judgment requires a comparison and evaluation of facts and ideas to understand their relationships and form appropriate conclusions. Attempt to measure the patient's ability to make logical decisions with questions such as "Why did you seek health care?" or "What would you do if you became ill at home?" Normally a patient makes logical decisions.

Cranial Nerve Function

To assess cranial nerve function, you may test all 12 cranial nerves, a single nerve, or related group of nerves. A dysfunction in one nerve reflects an alteration at some point along the distribution of the cranial nerve. Measurements used to assess the integrity of organs within the head and neck also assess cranial nerve function. A complete assessment involves testing the 12 cranial nerves in their numerical order. To remember the order of the nerves, use this simple phrase, "On old Olympus' towering tops, a Finn and German viewed some hops." The first letter of each word in the phrase is the same as the first letter of the names of the cranial nerves listed in order (Table 30-38).

Sensory Function

The sensory pathways of the CNS conduct sensations of pain, temperature, position, vibration, and crude and finely localized touch. Different nerve pathways relay the sensations. Most patients require only a quick screening of sensory function unless there are symptoms of reduced sensation, motor impairment, or paralysis. The risk of skin breakdown is greater in a patient with impaired sensation. When assessing decreased sensation, complete a skin and tissue assessment of the area affected by the sensory loss. In addition, teach the patient to avoid pressure, thermal, and/or chemical trauma to the area.

Normally a patient has sensory responses to all stimuli that are tested. He or she feels sensations equally on both sides of the body in all areas. Assess the major sensory nerves by knowing the sensory dermatome zones (Fig. 30-74, *A* and *B*). Some areas of the skin are innervated by specific dorsal root cutaneous nerves. For example, if assessment reveals reduced sensation when checking for light touch along an area of the skin (e.g., the lower neck), this

TABLE 30-38 Cranial Nerve Function and Assessment

NUMBER	NAME	TYPE	FUNCTION	METHOD
I	Olfactory	Sensory	Sense of smell	Ask patient to identify different nonirritating aromas such as coffee and vanilla.
II	Optic	Sensory	Visual acuity	Use Snellen chart or ask patient to read printed material while wearing glasses.
III	Oculomotor	Motor	Extraocular eye movements: inward, up and inward, up and outward, down and outward	Assess six directions of gaze.
			Pupil constriction and dilation Opening the eye	Measure pupillary reaction to light reflex and accommodation.
IV	Trochlear	Motor	Downward, inward eye movements	Assess six directions of gaze.
V	Trigeminal	Sensory and motor	Sensory nerve to skin of face	Lightly touch cornea with wisp of cotton. Assess corneal reflex. Measure sensation of light pain and touch across skin of face.
			Motor nerve to muscles of jaw	Palpate temples as patient clenches teeth.
VI	Abducens	Motor	Lateral movement of eyeballs	Assess six directions of gaze.
VII	Facial	Sensory and motor	Facial expression	As patient smiles, frowns, puffs out cheeks, and raises and lowers eyebrows, look for asymmetry.
			Taste	Have patient identify salty or sweet taste on front of tongue.
VIII	Auditory	Sensory	Hearing	Assess ability to hear spoken word.
IX	Glossopharyngeal	Sensory and motor	Taste	Ask patient to identify sour or sweet taste on back of tongue.
			Ability to swallow	Use tongue blade to elicit gag reflex.
X	Vagus	Sensory and motor	Sensation of pharynx	Ask patient to say "ah." Observe movement of palate and pharynx.
			Movement of vocal cords	Assess speech for hoarseness.
XI	Spinal accessory	Motor	Movement of head and shoulders	Ask patient to shrug shoulders and turn head against passive resistance.
XII	Hypoglossal	Motor	Position of tongue	Ask patient to stick out tongue to midline and move it from side to side.

BOX 30-32 PATIENT TEACHING

Neurological Assessment

Objective

- Patient and family or significant others will understand relationship of patient's behavioral and mental changes to physical status.

Teaching Strategies

- Explain to family caregiver the implications of any behavioral or mental impairment shown by patient.
- If patient has sensory or motor impairments, explain measures to ensure safety (e.g., use of ambulation aids or safety bars in bathrooms or stairways).
- Teach older adult to plan enough time to complete tasks because reaction time is slow.
- Teach older adult to observe skin surfaces for areas of trauma since pain perception is reduced.

Evaluation

- Ask family member to discuss patient behaviors that result from neurological impairments.
- Have patient explain safety measures used to avoid injury from sensory and motor limitations.
- Have older patient explain reason for inspecting skin surface routinely.

determines in general where a neurological lesion exists (e.g., fourth cervical spinal cord segment).

Perform all sensory testing with the patient's eyes closed so he or she is unable to see when or where a stimulus touches the skin (Table 30-39). Then touch the patient's skin in a random, unpredictable order to maintain his or her attention and prevent detection of a predictable pattern. Ask the patient to describe when, what, and where he or she feels each stimulus. Compare symmetrical areas of the body while applying stimuli to the patient's arms, trunk, and legs.

Motor Function

An examination of motor function includes assessments made during the musculoskeletal examination. In addition, the nurse assesses cerebellar function. The cerebellum coordinates muscular activity, maintains balance and equilibrium, and controls posture.

Coordination. To avoid confusion, demonstrate each maneuver and then have the patient repeat it, observing for smoothness and balance in his or her movements (Box 30-32). In older adults normally slow reaction time causes movements to be less rhythmical.

To assess fine-motor function, have the patient extend the arms out to the sides and touch each forefinger alternately to the nose

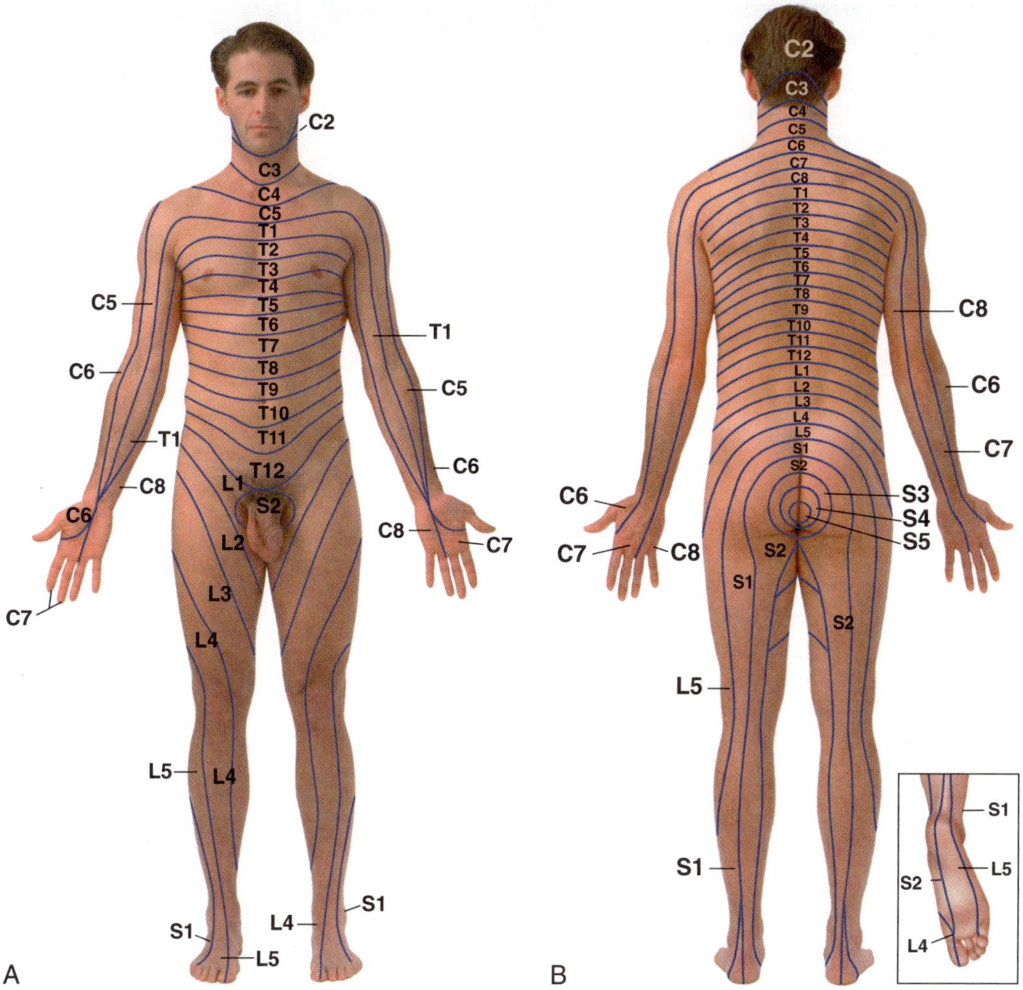

FIG. 30-74 Dermatomes of body (body surface areas innervated by particular spinal nerves); C1 usually has no cutaneous distribution. **A,** Anterior view. **B,** Posterior view. It appears that there is a distinct separation of surface area controlled by each dermatome, but there is almost always overlap between spinal nerves. (From Seidel HM et al: *Mosby's guide to physical examination,* ed 7, St Louis, 2011, Mosby.)

(first with eyes open, then with eyes closed). Normally a patient alternately touches the nose smoothly. Performing rapid, rhythmical, alternating movements demonstrates coordination in the upper extremities. While sitting, the patient begins by patting the knees with both hands. Then he or she alternately turns up the palm and back of the hands while continuously patting the knees. Normally patients perform the maneuver smoothly and regularly with increasing speed.

An additional maneuver for upper-extremity coordination involves touching each finger with the thumb of the same hand in rapid sequence. A patient moves from the index finger to the little finger and back, with one hand tested at a time. The dominant hand is slightly less awkward when performing this movement. Movement is smooth and in succession.

Test lower-extremity coordination with the patient lying supine, legs extended. Place a hand at the ball of the patient's foot. The patient taps the hand with the foot as quickly as possible. Test each foot for speed and smoothness. The feet do not move as rapidly or evenly as the hands.

Balance. Use one or two of the following tests to assess balance and gross-motor function. When examining the older adult for balance and equilibrium, be aware of the risk for falls. Some older adults need help with this portion of the examination.

Have the patient perform a Romberg's test by standing with feet together, arms at the sides, both with eyes open and eyes closed. Protect the patient's safety by standing at the side, observe for swaying. Expect slight swaying of the body in the Romberg's test. A loss of balance (positive Romberg) causes a patient to fall to the side. Normally he or she does not break the stance.

Have the patient close the eyes, with arms held straight at the sides, and stand on one foot and then the other. Normally patients are able to maintain balance for 5 seconds with slight swaying. Another test involves asking the patient to walk a straight line by placing the heel of one foot directly in front of the toes of the other foot.

Reflexes

Eliciting reflex reactions provides data about the integrity of sensory and motor pathways of the reflex arc and specific spinal cord segments. Assessment of reflexes does not determine higher neural center functioning. Fig. 30-75 traces the pathway of the reflex arc. Each muscle contains a small sensory unit called a *muscle*

TABLE 30-39 Assessment of Sensory Nerve Function

FUNCTION	EQUIPMENT	METHOD	PRECAUTIONS
Pain	Broken tongue blade or wooden end of cotton applicator	Ask patients to voice when they feel dull or sharp sensation. Alternately apply sharp and blunt ends of tongue blade to surface of skin. Note areas of numbness or increased sensitivity.	Remember that areas where skin is thick such as heel or sole of foot are less sensitive to pain.
Temperature	Two test tubes, one filled with hot water and another with cold	Touch skin with tube. Ask patient to identify hot or cold sensation.	Omit test if pain sensation is normal.
Light touch	Cotton ball or cotton-tip applicator	Apply light wisp of cotton to different points along surface of skin. Ask patients to voice when they feel a sensation.	Apply at areas where skin is thin or more sensitive (e.g., face, neck, inner aspect of arms, top of feet and hands).
Vibration	Tuning fork	Apply stem of vibrating fork to distal interphalangeal joint of fingers and interphalangeal joint of great toe, elbow, and wrist. Have patients voice when and where they feel vibration.	Be sure that patient feels vibration and not merely pressure.
Position		Grasp finger or toe, holding it by its sides with thumb and index finger. Alternate moving finger or toe up and down. Ask patient to state when finger is up or down. Repeat with toes.	Avoid rubbing adjacent appendages as you move finger or toe. Do not move joint laterally; return to neutral position before moving again.
Two-point discrimination	Two broken tongue blades	Lightly apply one or both tongue blade tips simultaneously to the surface of the skin. Ask patients whether they feel one or two pricks. Find the distance at which patient can no longer distinguish two points.	Apply blade tips to same anatomical site (e.g., fingertips, palm of hand, or upper arms). Minimum distance at which patient discriminates two points varies (2 to 8 mm on fingertips).

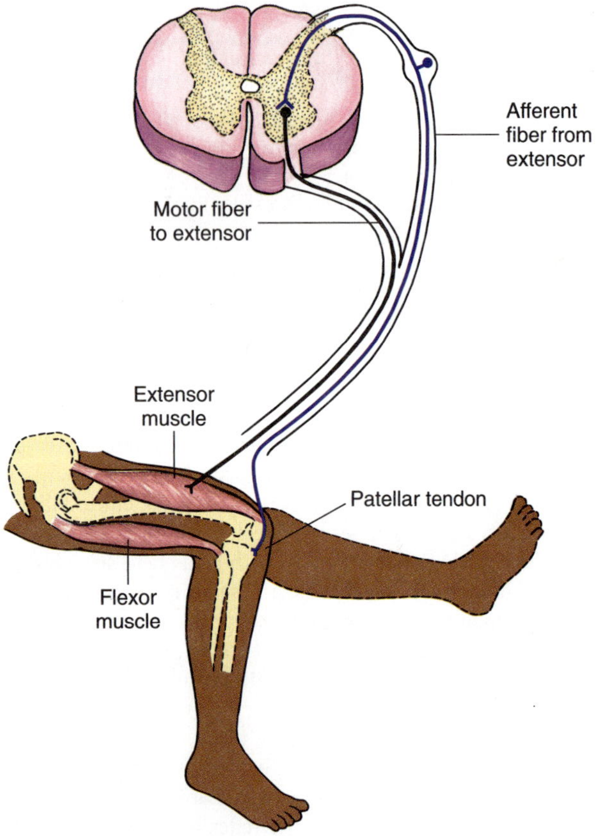

FIG. 30-75 Pathway of the reflex arc.

spindle, which controls muscle tone and detects changes in the length of muscle fibers. Tapping a tendon with a reflex hammer stretches the muscle and tendon, lengthening the spindle. The spindle sends nerve impulses along afferent nerve pathways to the dorsal horn of the spinal cord segment. Within milliseconds the impulses reach the spinal cord and synapse to travel to the efferent motor neuron in the spinal cord. A motor nerve sends the impulses back to the muscle, causing the reflex response.

The two categories of normal reflexes are deep tendon reflexes, elicited by mildly stretching a muscle and tapping a tendon, and cutaneous reflexes, elicited by stimulating the skin superficially. Grade reflexes as follows (Seidel et al., 2011):

0: No response
1+: Sluggish or diminished
2+: Active or expected response
3+: More brisk than expected, slightly hyperactive
4+: Brisk and hyperactive with intermittent or transient clonus

When assessing reflexes have the patient relax as much as possible to avoid voluntary movement or tensing of muscles. Position the limbs to slightly stretch the muscle being tested. Hold the reflex hammer loosely between the thumb and fingers so it is able to swing freely and tap the tendon briskly (Fig. 30-76). Compare the responses on corresponding sides. Normally the older adult presents with diminished reflexes. Reflexes are hyperactive in patients with alcohol, cocaine, or opioid intoxication. Table 30-40 summarizes common deep tendon and cutaneous reflexes.

AFTER THE EXAMINATION

Record findings from the physical assessment either during the examination or when it is completed. Special forms are available to record data. Review all findings before helping the patient dress

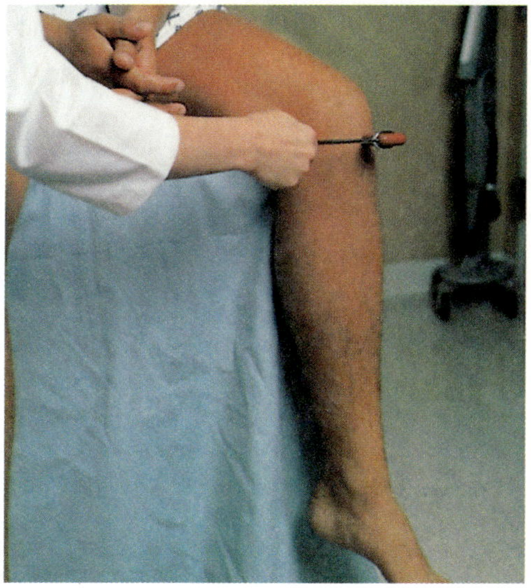

FIG. 30-76 Position for eliciting patellar tendon reflex. The lower leg normally extends.

in case it is necessary to recheck any information or gather additional data. Integrate physical assessment findings into the plan of care.

After completing the assessment give the patient time to dress. The hospitalized patient sometimes needs help with hygiene and returning to bed. When the patient is comfortable, it helps to share a summary of the assessment findings. If the findings have revealed serious abnormalities such as a mass or highly irregular heart rate, consult the patient's health care provider before revealing them. It is the health care provider's responsibility to make definitive medical diagnoses. Explain the type of abnormality found and the need for the health care provider to conduct an additional examination.

Delegate cleaning the examination area to support staff if needed. Use infection control practice to remove materials or instruments soiled with potentially infectious wastes. If the patient's bedside was the examination site, clear away soiled items from the bedside table and make sure that the bed linen is dry and clean. A patient appreciates a clean gown and the opportunity to wash the face and hands. Afterward be sure to perform hand hygiene.

Be sure to record a complete assessment. If you delayed entering any items into the assessment form, record them at this time to avoid forgetting any important information. If you made entries periodically during the examination, review them for accuracy and thoroughness. Communicate significant findings to appropriate medical and nursing personnel, either verbally or in the patient's written care plan.

TABLE 30-40 Assessment of Common Reflexes

TYPE	PROCEDURE	NORMAL REFLEX
Deep Tendon Reflexes		
Biceps	Flex patient's arm up to 45 degrees at elbow with palms down. Place your thumb in antecubital fossa at base of biceps tendon and your fingers over biceps muscle. Strike biceps tendon with reflex hammer.	Flexion of arm at elbow
Triceps	Flex patient's arm at elbow, holding arm across chest, or hold upper arm horizontally and allow lower arm to go limp. Strike triceps tendon just above elbow.	Extension at elbow
Patellar	Have patient sit with legs hanging freely over side of table or chair or have him or her lie supine and support knee in a flexed 90-degree position. Briskly tap patellar tendon just below patella.	Extension of lower leg
Achilles	Have patient assume same position as for patellar reflex. Slightly dorsiflex patient's ankle by grasping toes in palm of your hand. Strike Achilles tendon just above heel at ankle malleolus.	Plantar flexion of foot
Cutaneous Reflexes		
Plantar	Have patient lie supine with legs straight and feet relaxed. Take handle end of reflex hammer and stroke lateral aspect of sole from heel to ball of foot, curving across ball of foot toward big toe.	Plantar flexion of all toes
Abdominal	Have patient stand or lie supine. Stroke abdominal skin with base of cotton applicator over lateral borders of rectus abdominis muscle toward midline. Repeat test in each abdominal quadrant.	Contraction of rectus abdominis muscle with pulling of umbilicus toward stimulated side

KEY POINTS

- Baseline assessment findings reflect a patient's functional abilities and serve as the basis for comparison with subsequent assessment findings.
- Physical assessment of a child or infant requires the application of the principles of growth and development.
- Recognize that the normal process of aging affects physical findings collected from an older adult.
- Integrate patient teaching throughout the examination to help patients learn about health promotion, disease prevention, and skills to help with any current health issue.
- Inspection includes visual and olfaction and requires good lighting; full view of the body part; and a careful, systematic approach that compares a body part with its counterpart on the opposite side of the body.
- Palpation involves the use of parts of the hand to detect different types of physical characteristics.
- Use auscultation to assess the character of sounds created in various body organs.
- Perform a physical examination only after proper preparation of the environment and equipment and after preparing the patient physically and psychologically.
- Throughout the examination keep the patient warm, comfortable, and informed of each step of the process.
- A competent examiner is systematic while combining assessment of different body systems simultaneously.
- Information from the history helps to focus on body systems likely to be affected.

- When assessing a seriously ill patient, first concentrate on the body systems most affected.
- Creating a mental image of internal organs in relation to external anatomical landmarks enhances accuracy in assessing the thorax, heart, and abdomen.
- When assessing heart sounds, imagine events occurring during the cardiac cycle.
- Never palpate both of the carotid arteries simultaneously.
- When examining a woman's breasts, explain the techniques for breast self-examination.
- The order of the abdominal assessment is inspection, auscultation, percussion (if used), and palpation.
- During assessment of the genitalia explain the technique for genital self-examination.
- Conduct an assessment of musculoskeletal function when observing a patient ambulate or participate in other active movements.
- Assess mental and emotional status by interacting with a patient throughout the examination.
- At the end of the examination provide for the patient's comfort and then document a detailed summary of physical assessment findings.

CLINICAL APPLICATION QUESTIONS

Preparing for Clinical Practice

You receive morning report for Ms. Malone, age 63, admitted to the hospital yesterday with fatigue, a cough, and dyspnea; she is diagnosed with chronic heart failure. She states that she had increasing difficulty with shortness of breath and swelling in her legs. Pedal pulses are +1 bilaterally. On auscultation you hear bilateral crackles in the lung bases and an S_3 gallop when auscultating the heart. Respiratory rate is 18; heart rate is 84 and regular. The patient has an occasional nonproductive cough. She is receiving 2 L of oxygen by nasal cannula.

1. During the assessment Ms. Malone reports that she had difficulty breathing during the night while lying flat. Which assessment approach should the nurse take first?
   1. Raise the head of the bed up to a 45-degree angle to auscultate the lungs.
   2. Auscultate for adventitious sounds in the lung bases.
   3. Assess the patency of the nasal sinuses.
   4. Palpate legs to determine whether there is increased edema from circulating blood volume.
2. When examining Ms. Malone's lower extremities, you note bilateral pedal edema of +2. Which statement by the patient shows that she correctly understands this finding?
   1. "I ate too many fruits and vegetables with vitamin C, and that causes me to retain water."
   2. "I know that when my heart condition is not well controlled, my feet swell."
   3. "My parents both had foot swelling as they aged, and that's why my feet swell too."
   4. "When my heart isn't strong, the circulation doesn't get down to my feet."
3. After receiving medications to manage her heart failure, you return to reassess Ms. Malone's cardiac status. Select the techniques you use to correctly examine her lungs. (Select all that apply.)
   1. Listen to an entire inspiration and expiration.
   2. Place the diaphragm of the stethoscope over the ribs.
   3. Begin auscultation at the apex, moving downward, auscultating the entire right lung and then the left.
   4. If you auscultate an abnormal breath sound, check for the presence of bronchophony.

evolve *Answers to Clinical Application Questions can be found on the Evolve website.*

REVIEW QUESTIONS

Are You Ready to Test Your Nursing Knowledge?

1. The nurse prepares to conduct a general survey on an adult patient. Which assessment is performed first while the nurse initiates the nurse-patient relationship?
   1. Appearance and behavior
   2. Measurement of vital signs
   3. Observing specific body systems
   4. Conducting a detailed health history
2. The nurse is teaching a young mother to palpate her 8-year-old child to quickly evaluate if the child has a fever. Which information is important for the nurse to include?
   1. Place the palm of the hand on the child's back.
   2. Lightly touch the child's forehead with the fingertips.
   3. Place the back of your hand against the child's forehead and then on the back of the neck.
   4. Use the pads of your fingers and press against the child's neck and over the thorax.
3. While assessing the adult patient's lungs, the nurse identifies the following assessment findings. Which finding should be reported to the health care provider?
   1. Respiratory rate: 14
   2. Pain reported when palpating posterior lower thorax
   3. Thorax rising and falling symmetrically for right and left lungs
   4. Vesicular breath sounds heard with auscultation of peripheral lung fields
4. The nurse is teaching a young female patient to practice good skin health. Which information is important for the nurse to include?
   1. Avoid sunbathing between 3 PM and 7 PM.
   2. Oral contraceptives and antiinflammatories make the skin more sensitive to the sun.
   3. Call the health care provider for the presence of a mole on an arm or leg that appears uniformly brown.
   4. Wear sunscreen with an SPF of 30 or greater if using a sunlamp or tanning parlor.
5. As a nurse prepares to provide morning care and treatments, it is important to question a patient about a latex allergy before which intervention? (Select all that apply.)
   1. Applying adhesive tape to anchor a nasogastric tube
   2. Inserting a rubber Foley catheter into the patient's bladder
   3. Providing oral hygiene using a standard toothbrush and toothpaste
   4. Giving an injection using plastic syringes with rubber-coated plungers
   5. Applying a transparent wound dressing
6. The nurse is assessing a patient who returned 3 hours ago from a cardiac catheterization, during which the large catheter was inserted into the patient's femoral artery in the right groin. Which assessment finding would require immediate follow-up?
   1. Palpation of a femoral pulse with a heart rate of 76
   2. Auscultation of a heart murmur over the left thorax

3. Identification of mild bruising at the catheter insertion site
4. Palpation of a right dorsalis pedis pulse with strength of +1

7. The patient reports having a sore throat, coughing, and sneezing. While performing a focused assessment, which finding supports the patient's reported symptoms related to upper respiratory infection?
   1. Buccal mucosa is moist and dark pink.
   2. Respiratory rate is 18, rhythm is even.
   3. Retropharyngeal lymph nodes are enlarged and firm.
   4. Inspection with a tongue depressor on the posterior tongue causes gagging.
8. The nurse is teaching a patient with poor arterial circulation about checking blood flow in the legs. Which information should the nurse include? (Select all that apply.)
   1. A normal pulse on the top of the foot indicates adequate blood flow to the foot.
   2. To locate the dorsalis pedis pulse, take the fingers and palpate behind the knee
   3. When there is poor arterial blood flow, the leg is generally warm to the touch.
   4. Loss of hair on the lower leg indicates a long-term problem with arterial blood flow.
9. How should the patient be positioned to best palpate for lumps or tumors during an examination of the right breast?
   1. Supine with both arms overhead with palms upward
   2. Sitting with hands clasped just above the umbilicus
   3. Supine with the right arm abducted and hand under the head and neck
   4. Lying on the right side, adducting the right arm on the side of the body
10. The nurse is planning a staff education conference about abdominal assessment. Which point is important for the nurse to include?
    1. The aorta can be felt using deep palpation in the upper abdomen near the midline.
    2. The patient should be sitting to best determine the contour and shape of the abdomen.
    3. Always wear gloves when palpating the skin on the patient's abdomen.
    4. Avoid palpating the abdomen if the patient reports any discomfort or feelings of fullness.
11. The nurse is teaching a patient how to perform a testicular self-examination. Which statement by the nurse is correct?
    1. "The testes are normally round and feel smooth and rubbery."
    2. "The best time to do a testicular self-examination is before your bath or shower."
    3. "Perform a testicular self-examination weekly to detect signs of testicular cancer."
    4. "Since you are over 40 years old, you are in the highest risk group for testicular cancer."
12. The patient is assessed for range of joint movement. He or she is unable to move the right arm above the shoulder. How should the nurse document this finding?
    1. Patient was not able to flex arm at shoulder.
    2. Extension of right arm is limited.
    3. Patient's abduction of right arm was limited to 100 degrees.
    4. Internal rotation of right arm is limited to less than 90 degrees.
13. The nurse plans to assess the patient's abstract reasoning. Which task should the nurse ask the patient to perform?
    1. "Tell me where you are."
    2. "What can you tell me about your illness?"
    3. "Repeat these numbers back to me: 7…5…8."
    4. "What does this mean: 'A stitch in time saves nine?'"
14. The nurse teaches a patient about cranial nerves to help explain why the patient's right side of the mouth droops instead of moving up into a smile. What nerve does the nurse explain to the patient?
    1. VII—Facial
    2. V—Trigeminal
    3. XII—Hypoglossal
    4. XI—Spinal accessory
15. The nurse is planning to teach the student nurse how to assess the hydration status of an older adult. Which techniques are appropriate for this situation? (Select all that apply.)
    1. Inspect the lips and mucous membranes to determine if they are moist.
    2. Pinch the skin on the back of the hand to see if the skin tents.
    3. Check the patient's pulse and blood pressure.
    4. Weigh the patient daily.

Answers: **1.** 1; **2.** 3; **3.** 2; **4.** 2; **5.** 1, 2, 4; **6.** 4; **7.** 3; **8.** 1, 4; **9.** 3; **10.** 1; **11.** 1; **12.** 3; **13.** 4; **14.** 1; **15.** 1, 3, 4.

REFERENCES

American Cancer Society (ACS): *Cancer facts and figures 2011*, Atlanta, 2011, The Society.

American Heart Association: Know Your Fats, 2011, http://www.heart.org/HEARTORG/Conditions/Cholesterol/PreventionTreatmentofHighCholesterol/Know-Your-Fats_UCM_305628_Article.jsp. Accessed September 20, 2011.

Boyle AR, Davis H: Early screening and assessment of alcohol and substance abuse in the elderly: clinical implications, *J Addictions Nurs* 17(2):95, 2006.

Centers for Disease Control and Prevention (CDC): Vaccines and immunizations: HPV vaccine questions and answers. 2011, http://www.cdc.gov/vaccines/vpd-vac/hpv/vac-faqs.htm. Accessed September 19, 2011.

Dufault M, et al: Translating best practices in assessing capillary refill, *Worldviews Evid Based Nurs* 5(1):36, 2008.

Flood M, Buckwalter KC: Recommendations for mental health care of older adults. Part 2. An overview of dementia, delirium, and substance abuse, *J Gerontol Nurs* 35(2):35, 2009.

Frakes MA, Evans T: TB: your vigilance is vital, *RN* 67(11):31, 2004.

Hatherill S, Fisher AJ: Delirium in children and adolescents: a systematic review of the literature, *J Psychosomatic Res* 68:337, 2010.

Hockenberry MJ, Wilson P: *Wong's nursing care of infants and children*, ed 9, St Louis, 2011, Mosby.

Josephson AM, AACAP Work Group on Quality Issues: Practice parameter for the assessment of the family, *J Am Acad Child Adolesc Psych* 46(7):922, 2007.

Kresevic DM: Assessment of function. In Capezuti E, et al, editors: *Evidence-based geriatric nursing protocols for best practice*, ed 3, New York, 2008, Springer, p 23.

Marret L, et al: *Screening for skin cancer: a clinical practice guideline*, evidence-based series no. 15-11, Toronto, 2007, Cancer Care Ontario.

Meiner SE: *Gerontologic nursing*, ed 4, St Louis, 2011, Mosby.

Moore MC: *Pocket guide to nutritional assessment and care*, ed 5, St Louis, 2005, Mosby.

Nelson HD, et al: Screening for osteoporosis: an update for the US Preventive Services Task Force, *Ann Intern Med* 153(2):1, 2010, http://www.annals.org.

Oral Cancer Foundation: Oral cancer facts, 2011, http://oralcancerfoundation.org/facts/index.htm. Accessed August 28, 2011.

Ridky TW: Nonmelanoma skin cancer, *J Am Acad Dermatol* 57(3):484, 2007.

Seidel HM, et al: *Mosby's guide to physical examination*, ed 7, St Louis, 2011, Mosby.

US Department of Agriculture (USDA), US Department of Health and Human Services (USDHHS): *Dietary guidelines for Americans, 2010*, ed 7, Washington, DC, 2010, US Government Printing Office.

Walker J: The role of the nurse in the management of osteoporosis, *Br J Nurs* 19(19):1243, 2010.

Wolff T, et al: Screening for skin cancer: an update of the evidence for the US Preventive Services Task Force, *Ann Intern Med* 150(3):194, 2009.

RESEARCH REFERENCES

Bundesen I: Natural rubber latex: a matter of concern for nurses, *AORN* 88(2):197, 2008.

Chait SR, et al: Relationship of body image to breast and skin self-examination intentions and behaviors, *Body Image* 6:60, 2009.

Cohen M, et al: Elder abuse: disparities between older people's disclosure of abuse, evident signs of abuse, and high risk of abuse, *J Am Geriatr Soc* 55:1224, 2007.

Folstein MF, et al: Mini-mental state: a practical method for grading the cognitive state of patients for the clinician, *J Psychiatr Res* 12:82, 1975.

Glanz K, et al: A randomized trial of tailored skin cancer prevention messages for adults: project SCAPE, *Am J Public Health* 100(4):735, 2010.

Lecat P, et al: Ethanol-based cleanser versus isopropyl alcohol to decontaminate stethoscopes, *Am J Infect Contro* 37(3):241, 2009.

Loescher LJ, et al: Thorough skin self-examination in patients with melanoma, *Oncol Nurs Forum* 33(3):633, 2006.

Mujumdar UJ, et al: Sun protection and skin self-examination in melanoma survivors, *Psych Oncol* 18:1106, 2009.

Rigney T: Allostatic load and delirium in the hospitalized older adult, *Nurs Res* 59(5):322, 2010.

Shargorodsky J, et al: Change in prevalence of hearing loss in US adolescents, *JAMA* 304(7):772, 2010.

CHAPTER

31

Medication Administration

OBJECTIVES

- Discuss the nurse's role and responsibilities in medication administration.
- Describe the physiological mechanisms of medication action.
- Differentiate among different types of medication actions.
- Discuss developmental factors that influence pharmacokinetics.
- Discuss factors that influence medication actions.
- Discuss methods used to educate patients about prescribed medications.
- Compare and contrast the roles of the prescriber, pharmacist, and nurse in medication administration.
- Implement nursing actions to prevent medication errors.
- Describe factors to consider when choosing routes of medication administration.
- Calculate prescribed medication doses correctly.
- Discuss factors to include in assessing a patient's needs for and response to medication therapy.
- Identify the six rights of medication administration and apply them in clinical settings.
- Correctly and safely prepare and administer medications.

KEY TERMS

Absorption, p. 567
Adverse effects, p. 569
Anaphylactic reactions, p. 569
Biological half-life, p. 570
Biotransformation, p. 568
Buccal, p. 572
Detoxify, p. 568
Idiosyncratic reaction, p. 569
Infusions, p. 570
Injection, p. 567
Instillation, p. 572
Intraarticular, p. 572
Intracardiac, p. 572
Intradermal (ID), p. 572
Intramuscular (IM), p. 572
Intraocular, p. 573
Intravenous (IV), p. 572
Irrigations, p. 573
Medication allergy, p. 569
Medication error, p. 582
Medication interaction, p. 569
Medication reconciliation, p. 583
Metric system, p. 573
Nurse Practice Acts (NPAs), p. 566
Ophthalmic, p. 596
Parenteral administration, p. 572
Peak, p. 570
Pharmacokinetics, p. 567
Polypharmacy, p. 591
Prescriptions, p. 581
Pressurized metered-dose inhalers (pMDIs), p. 599
Side effects, p. 569
Solution, p. 573
Subcutaneous, p. 572
Sublingual, p. 571
Synergistic effect, p. 569
Therapeutic effect, p. 569
Toxic effects, p. 569
Transdermal disk, p. 572
Trough, p. 570
Verbal order, p. 577
Z-track method, p. 607

evolve WEBSITE

http://evolve.elsevier.com/Potter/fundamentals/

- Review Questions
- Video Clips
- Animations
- Concept Map Creator
- Case Study with Questions
- Skills Performance Checklists
- Audio Glossary
- Interactive Learning Activities
- Calculations Tutorial
- Key Term Flashcards
- Content Updates

Patients with acute or chronic health problems restore or maintain their health using a variety of strategies. One of these strategies is medication, a substance used in the diagnosis, treatment, cure, relief, or prevention of health problems. No matter where they receive their health care—hospitals, clinics, or home—nurses play an essential role in safe medication preparation, administration, and evaluation of medication effects. When patients cannot administer their own medications at home, family members, friends, or home care personnel are often responsible for medication administration. In all settings, nurses are responsible for evaluating the effects of medications on the patient's ongoing health status, teaching them about their medications and side effects, ensuring adherence to the medication regimen, and evaluating the patient's and family caregiver's ability to self-administer medications.

SCIENTIFIC KNOWLEDGE BASE

Medications are frequently used to manage diseases. Because medication administration and evaluation are a critical part of nursing practice, nurses need to have knowledge about the actions and effects of the medications taken by their patients. Administering medications safely requires an understanding of legal aspects of health care, pharmacology, pharmacokinetics, the life sciences, pathophysiology, human anatomy, and mathematics.

Medication Legislation and Standards

Federal Regulations. The U.S. government regulates the pharmaceutical industry to protect the health of the people by ensuring that medications are safe and effective. The first American law to regulate medications was the Pure Food and Drug Act. This law simply requires all medications to be free of impure products. Subsequent legislation has set standards related to safety, potency, and efficacy. Enforcement of medication laws currently rests with the Food and Drug Administration (FDA), which ensures that all medications on the market undergo vigorous testing before they are sold to the public. Federal medication law extends and refines controls on medication sales and distribution; testing, naming, and labeling; and the regulation of controlled substances. Official publications such as the *United States Pharmacopeia* (USP) and the *National Formulary* set standards for medication strength, quality, purity, packaging, safety, labeling, and dose form. In 1993 the FDA instituted the MedWatch program. This voluntary program encourages nurses and other health care professionals to report when a medication, product, or medical event causes serious harm to a patient by completing the MedWatch form. The form is available on the MedWatch website (USFDA, 2010).

State and Local Regulation of Medication. State and local medication laws must conform to federal legislation. States often have additional controls, including control of substances not regulated by the federal government. Local governmental bodies regulate the use of alcohol and tobacco.

Health Care Institutions and Medication Laws. Health care agencies establish individual policies to meet federal, state, and local regulations. The size of the agency, the types of services it provides, and the types of professional personnel it employs influence these policies. Agency policies are often more restrictive than governmental controls. For example, a common agency policy is the automatic discontinuation of narcotics after a set number of days. Although a prescriber can reorder the narcotic, this policy helps to control unnecessarily prolonged medication therapy and requires the prescriber to review the need for this class of medication on a regular basis.

Medication Regulations and Nursing Practice. State Nurse Practice Acts (NPAs) have the most influence over nursing practice by defining the scope of nurses' professional functions and responsibilities. Most NPAs are purposefully broad so nurses' professional responsibilities are not limited. Health care agencies often interpret specific actions allowed under NPAs; but they are not able to modify, expand, or restrict the intent of the act. The primary intent of NPAs is to protect the public from unskilled, undereducated, and unlicensed personnel.

The nurse is responsible for following legal provisions when administering controlled substances such as opioids, which are carefully controlled through federal and state guidelines. Violations of the Controlled Substances Act are punishable by fines, imprisonment, and loss of nurse licensure. Hospitals and other health care agencies have policies for the proper storage and distribution of narcotics (Box 31-1).

BOX 31-1 GUIDELINES FOR SAFE NARCOTIC ADMINISTRATION AND CONTROL

- Store all narcotics in a locked, secure cabinet or container. (Computerized, locked cabinets are preferred.)
- Frequently count narcotics with the opening of narcotic drawers and/or at shift change.
- Report discrepancies in narcotic counts immediately.
- Use a special inventory record each time a narcotic is dispensed. Records are often kept electronically and provide an accurate ongoing count of narcotics used, wasted, and remaining.
- Use the record to document the patient's name, date, time of medication administration, name of medication, dose, and signature of nurse dispensing the medication.
- A second nurse witnesses disposal of the unused portion if a nurse gives only part of a dose of a controlled substance. If paper records are kept, both nurses sign their names on the form. Computerized systems record the nurses' names electronically. Follow agency policy for appropriate waste of narcotics. Do not place wasted portions of medications in sharps containers.

Pharmacological Concepts

Medication Names. Some medications have as many as three different names. The chemical name of a medication provides an exact description of its composition and molecular structure. Nurses rarely use chemical names in clinical practice. An example of a chemical name is *N*-acetyl-para-aminophenol, which is commonly known as Tylenol. The manufacturer who first develops the medication gives the generic or nonproprietary name, with United States Adopted Names (USAN) Council approval (AMA, 2010). Acetaminophen is an example of a generic name. It is the generic name for Tylenol. The generic name becomes the official name listed in official publications such as the USP. The trade name, brand name, or proprietary name is the name under which a manufacturer markets a medication. The trade name has the symbol (™) at the upper right of the name, indicating that the manufacturer has trademarked the name of the medication (e.g., Panadol,™ Tempra,™ and St. Joseph Aspirin-Free Fever Reducer for Children™).

Manufacturers choose trade names that are easy to pronounce, spell, and remember. Many companies produce the same medication, and similarities in trade names are often confusing. Therefore be careful to obtain the exact name and spelling for each medication you administer to your patients. Because similarities in drug names are a common cause of medical errors, The Institute for Safe Medication Practices (ISMP) (2010a) (http://www.ismp.org/Tools/confuseddrugnames.pdf) and The Joint Commission (TJC) (2011a) (http://www.jointcommission.org/standards_information/npsgs.aspx) publish a list of medications that are frequently confused with one another. TJC's list includes recommendations to prevent mixing these medications.

Classification. Medication classification indicates the effect of the medication on a body system, the symptoms the medication relieves, or its desired effect. Usually each class contains more than one medication that is used for the same type of health problem. For example, patients who have asthma often take a variety of medications to control their illness such as $beta_2$-adrenergic agonists. The *$beta_2$-adrenergic* classification contains at least eight different medications (Lehne, 2010). Some are part of more than one class. For example, aspirin is an analgesic, an antipyretic, and an antiinflammatory medication.

Medication Forms. Medications are available in a variety of forms, or preparations. The form of the medication determines its route of administration. The composition of a medication enhances its absorption and metabolism. Many medications come in several

TABLE 31-1 Forms of Medication

FORM	DESCRIPTION
Medication Forms Commonly Prepared for Administration by Oral Route	
Solid Forms	
Caplet	Shaped like capsule and coated for ease of swallowing
Capsule	Medication encased in gelatin shell
Tablet	Powdered medication compressed into hard disk or cylinder; in addition to primary medication, contains binders (adhesive to allow powder to stick together), disintegrators (to promote tablet dissolution), lubricants (for ease of manufacturing), and fillers (for convenient tablet size)
Enteric-coated tablet	Coated tablet that does not dissolve in stomach; coatings dissolve in intestine, where medication is absorbed
Liquid Forms	
Elixir	Clear fluid containing water and/or alcohol; often sweetened
Extract	Syrup or dried form of pharmacologically active medication, usually made by evaporating solution
Aqueous solution	Substance dissolved in water and syrups
Aqueous suspension	Finely divided drug particles dispersed in liquid medium; when suspension is left standing, particles settle to bottom of container
Syrup	Medication dissolved in a concentrated sugar solution
Other Oral Forms and Terms Associated with Oral Preparations	
Troche (lozenge)	Flat, round tablets that dissolve in mouth to release medication; not meant for ingestion
Aerosol	Aqueous medication sprayed and absorbed in mouth and upper airway; not meant for ingestion
Sustained release	Tablet or capsule that contains small particles of a medication coated with material that requires a varying amount of time to dissolve
Medication Forms Commonly Prepared for Administration by Topical Route	
Ointment (salve or cream)	Semisolid, externally applied preparation, usually containing one or more medications
Liniment	Usually contains alcohol, oil, or soapy emollient applied to skin
Lotion	Liquid suspension that usually protects, cools, or cleanses skin
Paste	Thick ointment; absorbed through skin more slowly than ointment; often used for skin protection
Transdermal disk or patch	Medicated disk or patch absorbed through skin slowly over long period of time (e.g., 24 hours, 1 week)
Medication Forms Commonly Prepared for Administration by Parenteral Route	
Solution	Sterile preparation that contains water with one or more dissolved compounds
Powder	Sterile particles of medication that are dissolved in a sterile liquid (e.g., water, normal saline) before administration
Medication Forms Commonly Prepared for Instillation Into Body Cavities	
Intraocular disk	Small, flexible oval (similar to contact lens) consisting of two soft, outer layers and a middle layer containing medication; slowly releases medication when moistened by ocular fluid
Suppository	Solid dosage form mixed with gelatin and shaped in form of pellet for insertion into body cavity (rectum or vagina); melts when it reaches body temperature, releasing medication for absorption

forms such as tablets, capsules, elixirs, and suppositories. When administering a medication, be certain to use the proper form (Table 31-1).

Pharmacokinetics As the Basis of Medication Actions

For medications to be therapeutic they must be taken into a patient's body; be absorbed and distributed to cells, tissues, or a specific organ; and alter physiological functions. **Pharmacokinetics** is the study of how medications enter the body, reach their site of action, metabolize, and exit the body. Use knowledge of pharmacokinetics when timing medication administration, selecting the route of administration, considering the patient's risk for alterations in medication action, and evaluating the patient's response.

Absorption. **Absorption** is the passage of medication molecules into the blood from the site of medication administration. Factors that influence absorption are the route of administration, ability of the medication to dissolve, blood flow to the site of administration, body surface area (BSA), and lipid solubility of medication.

Route of Administration. Each route of medication administration has a different rate of absorption. When applying medications on the skin, absorption is slow because of the physical makeup of the skin. Medications placed on the mucous membranes and respiratory airways are absorbed quickly because these tissues contain many blood vessels. Because orally administered medications pass through the gastrointestinal (GI) tract, the overall rate of absorption is usually slow. Intravenous (IV) **injection** produces the most rapid absorption because medications are immediately available when they enter the systemic circulation.

Ability of the Medication to Dissolve. The ability of an oral medication to dissolve depends largely on its form or preparation. The body absorbs solutions and suspensions already in a liquid state more readily than tablets or capsules. Acidic medications pass through the gastric mucosa rapidly. Medications that are basic are not absorbed before reaching the small intestine.

Blood Flow to the Site of Administration. Medications are absorbed as blood comes in contact with the site of administration. The richer the blood supply to the site of administration, the faster the medication is absorbed.

Body Surface Area. When a medication comes in contact with a large surface area, it is absorbed at a faster rate. This helps explain why the majority of medications are absorbed in the small intestine rather than the stomach.

Lipid Solubility. Because the cell membrane has a lipid layer, highly lipid-soluble medications cross cell membranes easily and are absorbed quickly. Another factor that often affects medication absorption is whether or not food is in the stomach. Some oral medications are absorbed more easily when administered between meals because food changes the structure of a medication and sometimes impairs its absorption. When some medications are administered together, they interfere with one another, which impairs the absorption of both medications.

Safe medication administration requires knowledge of factors that alter or impair absorption of prescribed medications. You need an understanding of medication pharmacokinetics, the patient's health history, the physical examination, and knowledge gained through daily interactions with patients. Use this knowledge to ensure that you administer medications at the correct time for best absorption. When medications interact with food, know which medications must be administered before or between meals or on an empty stomach. When medications interact with one another, ensure that they are not given at the same time. Consult and collaborate with the patient's prescribers to ensure that the patient achieves the therapeutic effect of all medications. Before administering any medication, check pharmacology books, drug references, or package inserts or consult with pharmacists to identify medication-medication or medication-food interactions.

Distribution. After a medication is absorbed, it is distributed within the body to tissues and organs and ultimately to its specific site of action. The rate and extent of distribution depend on the physical and chemical properties of the medication and the physiology of the person taking it.

Circulation. Once a medication enters the bloodstream, it is carried throughout the tissues and organs. How fast it reaches the site depends on the vascularity of the various tissues and organs. Conditions that limit blood flow or blood perfusion inhibit the distribution of a medication. For example, patients with heart failure have impaired circulation, which slows medication delivery to the intended site of action. Therefore the efficacy of medications in these patients is often delayed or altered.

Membrane Permeability. Membrane permeability refers to the ability of the medication to pass through tissues and membranes to enter target cells. To be distributed to an organ, a medication has to pass through all of the tissues and biological membranes of the organ. Some membranes serve as barriers to the passage of medications. For example, the blood-brain barrier allows only fat-soluble medications to pass into the brain and cerebral spinal fluid. Therefore central nervous system infections often require treatment with antibiotics injected directly into the subarachnoid space in the spinal cord. Some older patients experience adverse effects (e.g., confusion) as a result of the change in the permeability of the blood-brain barrier, with easier passage of fat-soluble medications. The placental membrane also has a nonselective barrier to medications. Fat-soluble and nonfat-soluble agents often cross the placenta and produce fetal deformities. After birth neonates often experience respiratory depression and withdrawal symptoms when their mothers use or abuse narcotics.

Protein Binding. The degree to which medications bind to serum proteins such as albumin affects their distribution. Most medications partially bind to albumin. Medications bound to albumin cannot exert pharmacological activity. The unbound or "free" medication is its active form. Older adults have a decrease in albumin, probably caused by a change in liver function. The same is true for patients with liver disease or malnutrition. In both examples patients are at risk for an increase in medication activity, toxicity, or both.

Metabolism. After a medication reaches its site of action, it becomes metabolized into a less active or inactive form that is easier to excrete. **Biotransformation** occurs under the influence of enzymes that **detoxify,** break down, and remove biologically active chemicals. Most biotransformation occurs within the liver, although the lungs, kidneys, blood, and intestines also metabolize medications. The liver is especially important because its specialized structure oxidizes and transforms many toxic substances. The liver degrades many harmful chemicals before they become distributed to the tissues. If a decrease in liver function occurs such as with aging or liver disease, a medication is usually eliminated more slowly, resulting in its accumulation. Patients are at risk for medication toxicity if organs that metabolize medications are not functioning correctly. For example, a small sedative dose of a barbiturate sometimes causes a patient with liver disease to lapse into a coma.

Excretion. After medications are metabolized, they exit the body through the kidneys, liver, bowel, lungs, and exocrine glands. The chemical makeup of a medication determines the organ of excretion. Gaseous and volatile compounds such as nitrous oxide and alcohol exit through the lungs. Deep breathing and coughing (see Chapter 40) help patients eliminate anesthetic gases more rapidly after surgery. The exocrine glands excrete lipid-soluble medications. When medications exit through sweat glands, the skin often becomes irritated, requiring you to instruct patients in good hygiene practices (see Chapter 39). If a medication is excreted through the mammary glands, there is a risk that a nursing infant will ingest the chemicals. Check the safety of any medication used in breastfeeding women.

The GI tract is another route for medication excretion. Medications that enter the hepatic circulation are broken down by the liver and excreted into the bile. After chemicals enter the intestines through the biliary tract, the intestines resorb them. Factors that increase peristalsis (e.g., laxatives and enemas) accelerate medication excretion through the feces, whereas factors that slow peristalsis (e.g., inactivity and improper diet) often prolong the effects of a medication.

The kidneys are the main organs for medication excretion. Some medications escape extensive metabolism and exit unchanged in the urine. Others undergo biotransformation in the liver before the kidneys excrete them. If renal function declines, a patient is at risk for medication toxicity. When the kidney cannot adequately excrete a medication, it is necessary to reduce the dose. Maintenance of an adequate fluid intake (8 to 9 cups, or about 2 L of water/day) promotes proper elimination of medications for the average adult.

Types of Medication Action

Medications vary considerably in the way they act and their types of action. Patients do not always respond in the same way to each successive dose of a medication. Sometimes the same medication causes very different responses in different patients. Therefore it is essential to understand all the effects that medications have on patients.

Therapeutic Effects. The **therapeutic effect** is the expected or predicted physiological response that a medication causes. Each medication has a desired therapeutic effect. For example, nitroglycerin reduces cardiac workload and increases myocardial oxygen supply. Some medications have more than one therapeutic effect. For example, prednisone, a steroid, decreases swelling, inhibits inflammation, reduces allergic responses, and prevents rejection of transplanted organs. Knowing the desired therapeutic effect for each medication allows you to provide patient education and accurately evaluate its desired effect.

Side Effects/Adverse Effects. Every medication has a potential to harm a patient. **Side effects** are predictable and often unavoidable secondary effects produced at a usual therapeutic dose. They are either harmless or cause injury. For example, some antihypertensive medications cause impotence in men. If the side effects are serious enough to negate the beneficial effects of the therapeutic action of the medication, the prescriber discontinues the medication. Patients often stop taking medications because of side effects. **Adverse effects** are unintended, undesirable, and often unpredictable severe responses to medication. Some adverse effects are immediate, whereas others take weeks or months to develop. Early recognition is important. When adverse responses to medications occur, the prescriber discontinues the medication immediately. Health care providers report adverse effects to the FDA using the MedWatch program (USFDA, 2010).

Toxic Effects. **Toxic effects** develop after prolonged intake of a medication or when a medication accumulates in the blood because of impaired metabolism or excretion. Excess amounts of a medication within the body sometimes have lethal effects, depending on its action. For example, toxic levels of morphine, an opioid, cause severe respiratory depression and death. Antidotes are available to treat specific types of medication toxicity. For example, naloxone (Narcan), an opioid antagonist, reverses the effects of opioid toxicity.

Idiosyncratic Reactions. Medications sometimes cause unpredictable effects such as an **idiosyncratic reaction,** in which a patient overreacts or underreacts to a medication or has a reaction different from normal. For example, a child who receives diphenhydramine (Benadryl), an antihistamine, becomes extremely agitated or excited instead of drowsy. It is not always possible to predict if a patient will have an idiosyncratic response to a medication.

Allergic Reactions. Allergic reactions also are unpredictable responses to a medication. Some patients become immunologically sensitized to the initial dose of a medication. With repeated administration the patient develops an allergic response to it, its chemical preservatives, or a metabolite. The medication or chemical acts as an antigen, triggering the release of the antibodies in the body. A patient's **medication allergy** symptoms vary, depending on the individual and the medication (Table 31-2). Among the different classes of medications, antibiotics cause a high incidence of allergic reactions. Severe or **anaphylactic reactions,** which are life threatening, are characterized by sudden constriction of bronchiolar muscles, edema of the pharynx and larynx, and severe wheezing and shortness of breath. Immediate medical attention is required to treat anaphylactic reactions. A patient with a known history of an allergy to a medication needs to avoid exposure to that medication in the future and wear an identification bracelet or medal (Fig. 31-1), which alerts nurses and physicians to the allergy if the patient is unconscious when receiving medical care.

TABLE 31-2 Mild Allergic Reactions

SYMPTOM	DESCRIPTION
Urticaria	Raised, irregularly shaped skin eruptions with varying sizes and shapes; eruptions have reddened margins and pale centers
Rash	Small, raised vesicles that are usually reddened; often distributed over entire body
Pruritus	Itching of skin; accompanies most rashes
Rhinitis	Inflammation of mucous membranes lining nose; causes swelling and clear, watery discharge

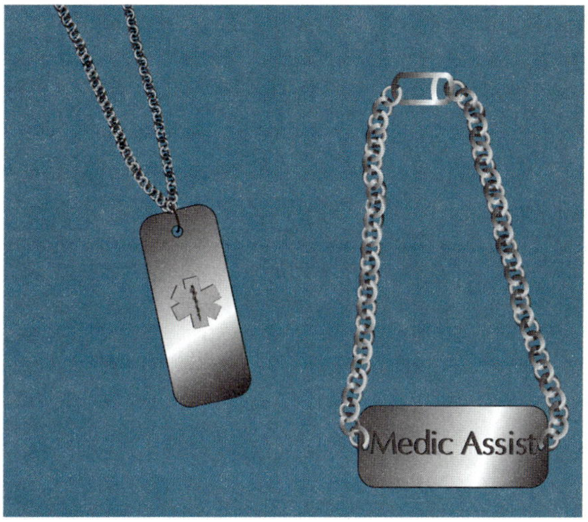

FIG. 31-1 Allergy identification bracelet and medal.

Medication Interactions

When one medication modifies the action of another, a **medication interaction** occurs. Medication interactions are common in individuals taking several medications. Some medications increase or diminish the action of others and may alter the way another medication is absorbed, metabolized, or eliminated from the body. When two medications have a **synergistic effect,** their combined effect is greater than the effect of the medications when given separately. For example, alcohol is a central nervous system depressant that has a synergistic effect on antihistamines, antidepressants, barbiturates, and narcotic analgesics. Sometimes a medication interaction is desired. Prescribers often combine medications to create an interaction that has a beneficial effect. For example, a patient with high blood pressure takes several medications such as diuretics and vasodilators that act together to control the blood pressure when one medication is not effective on its own.

Timing of Medication Dose Responses

Medications administered intravenously enter the bloodstream and act immediately, whereas medications given in other routes take time to enter the bloodstream and have an effect. The quantity and distribution of a medication in different body compartments change constantly. Medications are ordered at various times, depending on when their response begins, becomes most intense, and ceases.

The minimum effective concentration (MEC) is the plasma level of a medication below which the effect of the medication does

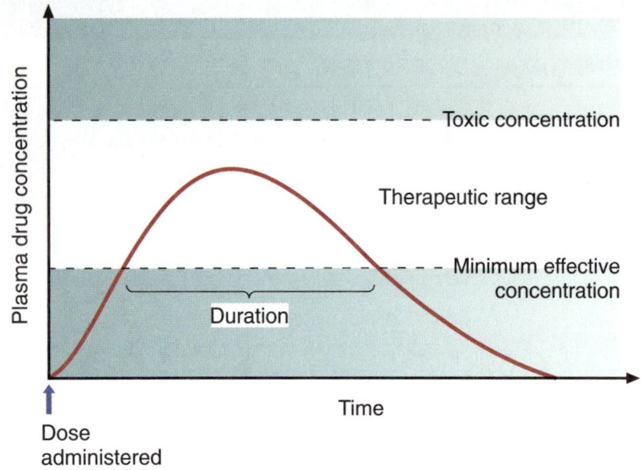

FIG. 31-2 The therapeutic range of a medication occurs between the minimum effective concentration and the toxic concentration. (From Lehne RA: *Pharmacology for nursing care*, ed 7, St Louis, 2010, Saunders.)

TABLE 31-3 Common Dosage Administration Schedules

DOSAGE SCHEDULE	ABBREVIATION
Before meals	AC, ac
As desired	ad lib
At bedtime	"nightly" or "at bedtime"
After meals	PC, pc
Whenever there is a need	prn
Every morning, every AM	qAM
Every day	Daily
Give immediately	STAT, stat

TABLE 31-4 Terms Associated with Medication Actions

TERM	MEANING
Onset	Time it takes after a medication is administered for it to produce a response
Peak	Time it takes for a medication to reach its highest effective concentration
Trough	Minimum blood serum concentration of medication reached just before the next scheduled dose
Duration	Time during which the medication is present in concentration great enough to produce a response
Plateau	Blood serum concentration of a medication reached and maintained after repeated fixed doses

not occur. The toxic concentration is the level at which toxic effects occur. When a medication is prescribed, the goal is to achieve a constant blood level within a safe therapeutic range, which falls between the MEC and the toxic concentration (Fig. 31-2). When a medication is administered repeatedly, its serum level fluctuates between doses. The highest level is called the **peak** concentration, and the lowest level is called the **trough** concentration. After reaching its peak, the serum concentration of the medication falls progressively. With IV **infusions** the peak concentration occurs quickly, but the serum level also begins to fall immediately. Some medication doses (e.g., vancomycin) are based on peak and trough serum levels. The trough level is generally drawn 30 minutes before administering the drug, and the peak level is drawn whenever the drug is expected to reach its peak concentration. The time it takes for a drug to reach its peak concentration varies, depending on the pharmacokinetics of the medication.

All medications have a **biological half-life,** which is the time it takes for excretion processes to lower the amount of unchanged medication by half. A medication with a short half-life needs to be given more frequently than a medication with a longer half-life. The half-life does not change, no matter how much medication is given. For example, if the nurse gives 1 g of a medication that has a half-life of 8 hours, the patient excretes 500 mg of the medication in 8 hours. In the next 8 hours the patient excretes 250 mg. This process continues until the medication is totally eliminated from the body.

To maintain a therapeutic plateau the patient must receive regular fixed doses. For example, current evidence shows that pain medications are most effective when they are given around the clock (ATC) rather than when the patient intermittently complains of pain because ATC allows the body to maintain an almost constant level of pain medication. After an initial medication dose, the patient receives each successive dose when the previous dose reaches its half-life.

Safe drug administration involves adherence to prescribed doses and dosage schedules (Table 31-3). Some agencies set schedules for medication administration. However, nurses are able to alter this schedule based on knowledge about a medication. For example, at some agencies medications that are to be taken once a day are given at 9:00 AM. However, if a medication works best when given before bedtime, the nurse administers it before the patient goes to sleep. In addition, acute care agencies use guidelines from the Institute for Safe Medication Practices (CMS, 2011; ISMP, 2011) to determine safe, effective, and timely administration of scheduled medications. According to the ISMP guidelines, hospitals need to determine which medications are time-critical and which are non–time-critical. Time-critical medications are medications in which early or delayed administration of maintenance doses (more than 30 minutes before or after the scheduled dose) will most likely cause harm or result in subtherapeutic responses in a patient. Non–time-critical medications include medications in which the timing of administration will most likely not affect the desired effect of the medication if given 1 to 2 hours before or after its scheduled time. You need to administer time-critical medications at a precise time or within 30 minutes before or after the scheduled time. You administer medications identified as non–time-critical within 1 to 2 hours of their scheduled time. Follow your agency's medication administration policies about the timing of medications to ensure you administer medications at the right time (CMS, 2011; ISMP, 2011).

When teaching patients about dosage schedules, use language that is familiar to the patient. For example, when teaching a patient about medication dosing twice a day, instruct him or her to take it in the morning and again in the evening. Use knowledge about the time intervals and terms used to describe medication actions to anticipate the effect of a medication and educate the patient about when to expect a response (Table 31-4).

TABLE 31-5 Factors Influencing Choice of Administration Routes

ADVANTAGES	DISADVANTAGES OR CONTRAINDICATIONS
Oral, Buccal, Sublingual Routes	
Convenient and comfortable for patient Economical Easy to administer Often produce local or systemic effects Rarely cause anxiety for patient.	Oral route is avoided when patient has alterations in gastrointestinal function (e.g., nausea, vomiting), reduced motility (after general anesthesia or bowel inflammation), and surgical resection of gastrointestinal tract. Oral administration is contraindicated in patients unable to swallow (e.g., patients with neuromuscular disorders, esophageal strictures, mouth lesions). Oral administration is contraindicated in unconscious or confused patient who is unable or unwilling to swallow or hold medication under tongue. Oral medications cannot be administered when patients have gastric suction; are contraindicated before some tests or surgery. Oral medications sometimes irritate lining of gastrointestinal tract, discolor teeth, or have unpleasant taste. Gastric secretions destroy some medications.
Subcutaneous, Intramuscular (IM), Intravenous (IV), Intradermal (ID) Routes	
Provide means of administration when oral medications are contraindicated More rapid absorption than with topical or oral routes IV infusion provides medication delivery when patient is critically ill or long-term therapy is necessary; if peripheral perfusion is poor, IV route preferred over injections	There is risk of introducing infection, and some medications are expensive. Some patients experience pain from repeated needlesticks. Subcutaneous, IM, and ID routes are avoided in patients with bleeding tendencies. There is risk of tissue damage. IM and IV routes have higher absorption rates, thus placing patient at higher risk for reactions. They often cause considerable anxiety in many patients, especially children.
Skin	
Primarily provides local effect Painless Limited side effects	Patients with skin abrasions are at risk for rapid medication absorption and systemic effects. Medications are absorbed through skin slowly.
Transdermal	
Prolonged systemic effects with limited side effects	Medication leaves oily or pasty substance on skin and sometimes soils clothing.
Mucous Membranes*	
Therapeutic effects provided by local application to involved sites Aqueous solutions readily absorbed and capable of causing systemic effects Potential route of administration when oral medications are contraindicated	Mucous membranes are highly sensitive to some medication concentrations. Patient with ruptured eardrum cannot receive ear irrigations. Insertion of rectal and vaginal medication often causes embarrassment. Rectal suppositories contraindicated if patient has had rectal surgery or if active rectal bleeding is present.
Inhalation	
Provides rapid relief for local respiratory problems Used for introduction of general anesthetic gases	Some local agents cause serious systemic effects.

*Includes eyes, ears, nose, vagina, rectum, and ostomy.

Routes of Administration

The route prescribed for administering a medication depends on the properties and desired effect of the medication and the patient's physical and mental condition (Table 31-5). Work with the prescriber in determining the best route for a patient's medication.

Oral Routes. The oral route is the easiest and the most commonly used route. Medications are given by mouth and swallowed with fluid. Oral medications have a slower onset of action and a more prolonged effect than parenteral medications. Patients generally prefer the oral route.

Sublingual Administration. Some medications are readily absorbed after being placed under the tongue to dissolve (Fig. 31-3). A medication given by the **sublingual** route should not be swallowed because the medication does not have the desired effect. Nurses often give nitroglycerin by the sublingual route. Tell the patient not to drink anything until the medication is completely dissolved.

Building Competency in Patient-Centered Care Mr. Koop is recovering from abdominal surgery 2 days ago for removal of a tumor in his colon and is feeling progressively worse. His temperature was 37° C (98.6° F) 4 hours ago and is now 39.2° C (102.6° F). He is no longer able to tolerate oral fluids and states that he is nauseated. You check his order, which reads, "Acetaminophen 650 mg orally for temperature above 38.4° C (101.2° F)." On the basis of the assessment, you believe that, because Mr. Koop is nauseated, he will not be able to tolerate an oral dose of acetaminophen. Thus you decide that you need to call Mr. Koop's health care provider to see if the medication route can be changed to a rectal suppository. Using SBAR (Situation-Background-Assessment-Recommendation) as your guide, create a report that you will use when calling his health care provider.

Answers to questions can be found on the Evolve website.

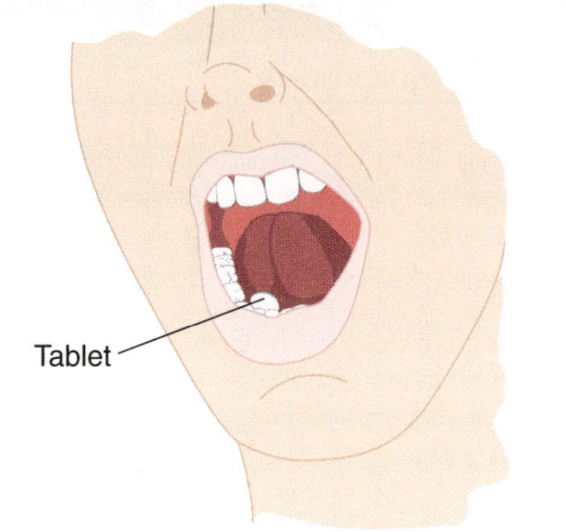

FIG. 31-3 Sublingual administration of a tablet.

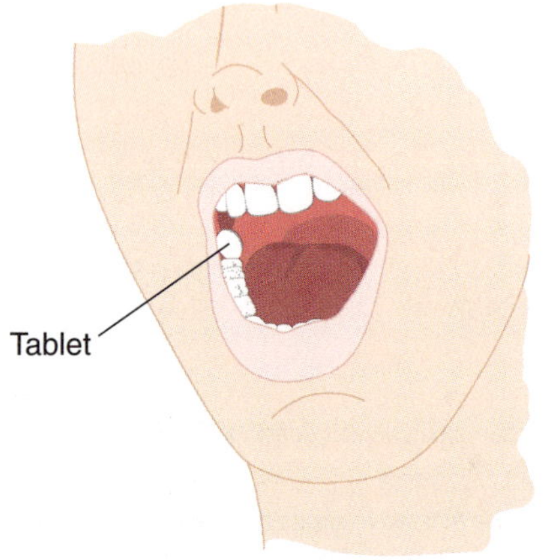

FIG. 31-4 Buccal administration of a tablet.

Buccal Administration. Administration of a medication by the **buccal** route involves placing the solid medication in the mouth against the mucous membranes of the cheek until it dissolves (Fig. 31-4). Teach patients to alternate cheeks with each subsequent dose to avoid mucosal irritation. Warn patients not to chew or swallow the medication or to take any liquids with it. A buccal medication acts locally on the mucosa or systemically as it is swallowed in a person's saliva.

Parenteral Routes. **Parenteral administration** involves injecting a medication into body tissues. The following are the four major sites of injection:

1. **Intradermal (ID):** Injection into the dermis just under the epidermis
2. **Subcutaneous:** Injection into tissues just below the dermis of the skin
3. **Intramuscular (IM):** Injection into a muscle
4. **Intravenous (IV):** Injection into a vein

Some medications are administered into body cavities other than the four types listed here. These additional routes include epidural, intrathecal, intraosseous, intraperitoneal, intrapleural, and intraarterial. Nurses usually are not responsible for the administration of medications through these advanced techniques. Whether or not you actually administer the medication, you remain responsible for monitoring the integrity of the medication delivery system, understanding the therapeutic value of the medication, and evaluating the patient's response to the therapy.

Epidural. Epidural medications are administered in the epidural space via a catheter, which is placed by a nurse anesthetist or an anesthesiologist. This route is used for the administration of regional analgesia for surgical procedures (see Chapter 43). Nurses who have advanced education in the epidural route can administer medications by continuous infusion or by a bolus dose.

Intrathecal. Physicians and specially educated nurses administer intrathecal medications through a catheter placed in the subarachnoid space or one of the ventricles of the brain. Intrathecal administration is often associated with long-term medication administration through surgically implanted catheters.

Intraosseous. This method of medication administration involves the infusion of medication directly into the bone marrow. It is most commonly used in infants and toddlers who have poor access to their intravascular space and when an emergency arises and IV access is impossible.

Intraperitoneal. Medications administered into the peritoneal cavity are absorbed into the circulation. Chemotherapeutic agents, insulin, and antibiotics are administered in this fashion.

Intrapleural. A syringe and needle or a chest tube is used to administer intrapleural medications directly into the pleural space. Chemotherapeutic agents are the most common medications administered via this method. Physicians also instill medications that help resolve persistent pleural effusion. This is called *pleurodesis,* which promotes adhesion between the visceral and parietal pleura.

Intraarterial. Intraarterial medications are administered directly into the arteries. Intraarterial infusions are common in patients who have arterial clots. The nurse manages a continuous infusion of clot-dissolving agents and carefully monitors the integrity of the infusion to prevent inadvertent disconnection of the system and subsequent bleeding.

Other methods of medication administration that are usually limited to physician administration are **intracardiac,** an injection of a medication directly into cardiac tissue, and **intraarticular,** an injection of a medication into a joint.

Topical Administration. Medications applied to the skin and mucous membranes generally have local effects. You apply topical medications to the skin by painting or spreading the medication over an area, applying moist dressings, soaking body parts in a solution, or giving medicated baths. Systemic effects often occur if a patient's skin is thin or broken down, the medication concentration is high, or contact with the skin is prolonged. A **transdermal disk** or patch (e.g., nitroglycerin, scopolamine, and estrogens) has systemic effects. The disk secures the medicated ointment to the skin. These topical applications are left in place for as little as 12 hours or as long as 7 days.

Nurses administer medications to mucous membranes in a variety of ways, including the following, by:

1. Directly applying a liquid or ointment (e.g., eyedrops, gargling, or swabbing the throat).
2. Inserting a medication into a body cavity (e.g., placing a suppository in rectum or vagina or inserting medicated packing into vagina).
3. Instilling fluid into a body cavity (e.g., eardrops, nose drops, or bladder and rectal **instillation** [fluid is retained]).
4. Irrigating a body cavity (e.g., flushing eye, ear, vagina, bladder, or rectum with medicated fluid [fluid is not retained]).
5. Spraying a medication into a body cavity (e.g., instillation into nose and throat).

Inhalation Route. The deeper passages of the respiratory tract provide a large surface area for medication absorption. Nurses

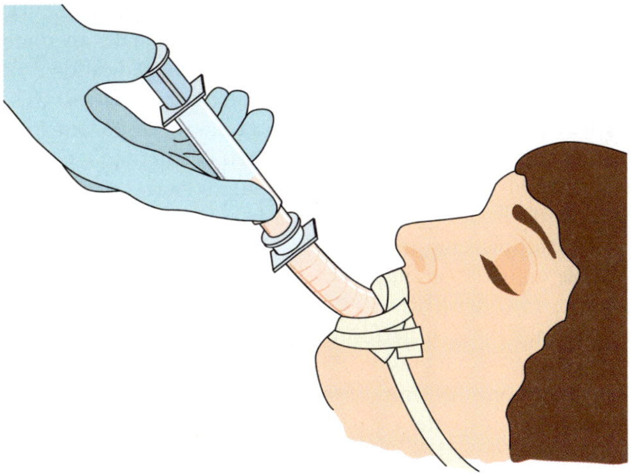

FIG. 31-5 Medication instilled through an endotracheal tube.

TABLE 31-6 Equivalents of Measurement		
METRIC	**APOTHECARY**	**HOUSEHOLD**
1 mL	15-16 minims*	15 drops (gtt)
5 mL	1 dram*	1 teaspoon (tsp)
15 mL	4 drams*	1 tablespoon (tbsp)
30 mL	1 fluid ounce	2 tablespoons (tbsp)
240 mL	8 fluid ounces	1 cup (c)
480 mL (approximately 500 mL)	1 pint (pt)	1 pint (pt)
960 mL (approximately 1 L)	1 quart (qt)	1 quart (qt)
3840 mL (approximately 4 L)	1 gallon (gal)	1 gallon (gal)

*Minums and drams are no longer acceptable units of measure for medication administration although some medication cups and syringes still have them listed. Use mL for safe medication preparation (Morris, 2010).

administer inhaled medications through the nasal and oral passages or endotracheal or tracheostomy tubes. Endotracheal tubes enter the patient's mouth and end in the trachea (Fig. 31-5), whereas tracheostomy tubes enter the trachea directly through an incision made in the neck. Inhaled medications are readily absorbed and work rapidly because of the rich vascular alveolar capillary network present in the pulmonary tissue. Many inhaled medications have local or systemic effects.

Intraocular Route. **Intraocular** medication delivery involves inserting a medication similar to a contact lens into the patient's eye. The eye medication disk has two soft outer layers that have medication enclosed in them. The nurse inserts the disk into the patient's eye, much like a contact lens, and it can remain there for up to 1 week.

Systems of Medication Measurement

The proper administration of a medication depends on your ability to compute medication doses accurately and measure medications correctly. Mistakes in calculating or measuring medications correctly often lead to fatal errors. As a nurse you are responsible for checking calculations carefully before giving a medication.

Medication therapy uses the metric, apothecary, and household systems of measurement. The apothecary system is used infrequently today. Although the U.S. Congress has not officially adopted the metric system, most health professionals in the United States use it. Health care providers usually write prescriptions to be self-administered in household measures for patients.

Metric System. As a decimal system, the **metric system** is the most logically organized. Metric units are easy to convert and compute through simple multiplication and division. Each basic unit of measurement is organized into units of 10. Multiplying or dividing by 10 forms secondary units. In multiplication the decimal point moves to the right; in division the decimal moves to the left. For example:

$$10 \text{ mg} \times 10 = 100 \text{ mg}$$

$$10 \text{ mg} \div 10 = 1 \text{ mg}$$

The basic units of measurement in the metric system are the meter (length), the liter (volume), and the gram (weight). For medication calculations only use the volume and weight units. In the metric system use lowercase or capital letters to designate basic units:

Gram = g or Gm

Liter = l or L

Use lowercase letters for abbreviations for other units:

Milligram = mg

Milliliter = mL

A system of Latin prefixes designates subdivision of the basic units: *deci-* ($\frac{1}{10}$ or 0.1), *centi-* ($\frac{1}{100}$ or 0.01), and *milli-* ($\frac{1}{1000}$ or 0.001). Greek prefixes designate multiples of the basic units: *deka-* (10), *hecto-* (100), and *kilo-* (1000). When writing medication doses in metric units, prescribers and nurses use fractions or multiples of a unit. Convert fractions to decimals.

500 mg or 0.5 g, *not* $\frac{1}{2}$ g

10 mL or 0.01 L, *not* $\frac{1}{100}$ L

Many actual and potential medication errors happen with the use of fractions and decimal points. Follow practice standards when medications are ordered in fractions to prevent medication errors. For example, to make the decimal point more visible, a leading zero is *always* placed in front of a decimal (e.g., use 0.25 *not* .25). *Never* use a trailing zero (i.e., a zero after a decimal point) because, if a health care worker does not see the decimal point, the patient may receive 10 times more medication than that prescribed (e.g., use 5 *not* 5.0) (ISMP, 2010b; TJC, 2011).

Household Measurements. Household units of measure are familiar to most people. Their disadvantage is their inaccuracy. Household utensils such as teaspoons and cups vary in size. Scales to measure pints or quarts are not well calibrated. Household measures include drops, teaspoons, tablespoons, and cups for volume and pints and quarts for weight. The advantage of household measurements is their convenience and familiarity. When the accuracy of a medication dose is not critical (e.g., [OTC medications]), it is safe to use household measures. To calculate medications accurately, you need to know common equivalents of metric and household units (Table 31-6).

Solutions. The nurse uses solutions of various concentrations for injections, **irrigations,** and infusions. A **solution** is a given mass of solid substance dissolved in a known volume of fluid or a given volume of liquid dissolved in a known volume of another fluid. When a solid is dissolved in a fluid, the concentration is in units of mass per units of volume (e.g., g/L, mg/mL). A concentration of a solution can also be expressed as a percentage. For example, a 10% solution is 10 g of solid dissolved in 100 mL of solution. A proportion also expresses concentrations. A $\frac{1}{1000}$ solution represents a solution containing 1 g of solid in 1000 mL of liquid or 1 mL of liquid mixed with 1000 mL of another liquid.

NURSING KNOWLEDGE BASE

The IOM (2003) published the book *To Err Is Human: Building a Safer Health System*. This book created a new national awareness of problems within the health care system. It estimated that up to 98,000 people die in any given year from medical errors that occur in hospitals. This means that more people die from medical errors than from motor vehicle accidents, breast cancer, acquired immunodeficiency syndrome (AIDS), and workplace injuries. Health care experts estimate that medication-related errors for hospitalized patients cost more than $3.5 billion annually (IOM, 2007).

Nurses play an important role in patient safety, especially in the area of medication administration. The safe administration of medications is also an important topic for current nursing researchers (Box 31-2). Nurses need to know how to calculate medication doses accurately and understand the different roles that members of the health care team play in prescribing and administering medications. All of the nurse's previous learning is important and is often applied to ensure safe medication administration.

BOX 31-2 EVIDENCE-BASED PRACTICE

Reducing Errors During Medication Administration

PICO Question: In hospitals does the use of bar-code scanning and an electronic medication administration record (eMAR) during medication administration decrease the incidence of medication errors made by nurses when compared with nurses who do not use bar-code scanning and eMAR?

Evidence Summary

Medication administration is a highly complex process. Errors often result from problems within one or more parts of the process. Many errors occur either when a medication is ordered or when it is administered. Research shows the combined use of bar-code technology and eMAR decreases most medication errors in various hospital settings (Foote and Coleman, 2008; Fowler, Sohler, and Zarillo, 2009; Green, 2008; Helmons, Wargel, and Daniels, 2009; Poon et al., 2010). However, sometimes these systems uncover increases in certain types of errors. For example, errors of omission (e.g., a patient not receiving a medication on time because he or she is off the nursing unit at a procedure) may become more apparent (Fowler, Sohler, and Zarillo, 2009; Helmons, Wargel, and Daniels, 2009).

Application to Nursing Practice

- The process of implementing bar-code and eMAR technology is complex and needs to be well planned and involve nursing staff to ensure successful implementation (Foote and Coleman, 2008).
- Even though the use of bar code scanning and eMAR reduces many errors, it does not eliminate all of them (Poon et al., 2010). Therefore nurses need to remain vigilant and consistently follow medication administration policies and protocols to ensure safe medication administration.
- Nurses need to analyze data collected from computerized systems about medication errors to identify ways to improve the medication administration process and enhance patient safety (Helmons, Wargel, and Daniels, 2009).

Clinical Calculations

To administer medications safely, you need to have an understanding of basic mathematics skills to calculate medication doses, mix solutions, and perform a variety of other activities. This is important because medications are not always dispensed in the unit of measure in which they are ordered. Medication companies package and bottle medications in standard dosages. For example, the patient's health care provider orders 20 mg of a medication that is available only in 40-mg vials. Nurses frequently convert available units of volume and weight to desired doses. Therefore be aware of equivalents in all major measurement systems. You use equivalents when performing other nursing actions such as when calculating patients' intake and output and IV flow rates.

Conversions Within One System. Converting measurements within one system is relatively easy; simply divide or multiply in the metric system. To change milligrams to grams, divide by 1000, moving the decimal 3 points to the left.

$$1000 \text{ mg} = 1 \text{ g}$$
$$350 \text{ mg} = 0.35 \text{ g}$$

To convert liters to milliliters, multiply by 1000 or move the decimal 3 points to the right.

$$1 \text{ L} = 1000 \text{ mL}$$
$$0.25 \text{ L} = 250 \text{ mL}$$

To convert units of measurement within the household system, consult an equivalent table. For example, when converting fluid ounces to quarts, you first need to know that 32 ounces is the equivalent of 1 quart. To convert 8 ounces to a quart measurement, divide 8 by 32 to get the equivalent, $\frac{1}{4}$ or 0.25 quart.

Conversion Between Systems. Nurses frequently determine the proper dose of a medication by converting weights or volumes from one system of measurement to another. Thus sometimes you convert metric units to equivalent household measures for use at home. To calculate medications it is necessary to work with units in the same measurement system. Tables of equivalent measurements are available in all health care institutions. The pharmacist is also a good resource.

Before converting, compare the measurement system available with that ordered. For example, the prescriber orders Robitussin 30 mL, but the patient only has tablespoons at home. To properly instruct the patient, you convert mL to tablespoons, which requires you to know the equivalent or refer to a table such as Table 31-6.

Dose Calculations. Methods used to calculate medication doses include the ratio and proportion method, the formula method, and dimensional analysis. Before completing any calculation, make a mental estimate of the approximate and reasonable dosage. If the estimate does not match the calculated solution, recheck the calculation before preparing and administering the medication. Many nursing students are anxious when calculating medication doses. To enhance accuracy and reduce anxiety, think critically about the processes used during the calculation and practice doing calculations until you feel confident about your mathematics skills (Walsh, 2008). In addition, choose the method of calculation with which you are most comfortable and use it consistently (Morris, 2010). Most health care agencies require a nurse to double-check calculations with another nurse before giving medications, especially when the risk for giving the wrong medication is high (e.g., heparin, insulin). *Always* have another nurse double-check your work if you are unsure about the answer or if the answer to a medication calculation seems unreasonable or inappropriate.

The Ratio and Proportion Method. A ratio indicates the relationship between two numbers separated by a colon (:). The colon in the ratio indicates the need to use division. Think of a ratio as a fraction; the number to the left is the numerator, and the number to the right is the denominator. For example, the ratio 1:2 is the same as ½. Write a proportion in one of three ways:

Example 1:	1:2 = 4:8
Example 2:	1:2 :: 4:8
Example 3:	1/2 = 4/8

In a proportion the first and last numbers are called the *extremes,* and the second and third numbers are called the *means.* When multiplying the extremes, the answer is the same when multiplying the means. For example, in the previous proportions, multiplying the extremes (1 × 8 = 8) is the same result as multiplying the means (2 × 4 = 8). Because of this relationship, if you know three of the numbers in the proportion, calculating the unknown fourth number is easy. The numbers need to all be in the same unit and system of measurement. To solve a calculation using the ratio and proportion method, first estimate the answer in your mind. Then set up the proportion, labeling all the terms. Put the terms of the ratio in the same sequence (e.g., mg : mL = mg : mL). Cross multiply the means and the extremes and divide both sides by the number before the *x* to obtain the dosage. *Always* label the answer; if the answer is not close to the estimate, recheck the calculation.

Example: The prescriber orders 500 mg of amoxicillin to be administered in a gastric tube every 8 hours. The bottle of amoxicillin is labeled 400 mg/5 mL. Use the following steps to calculate how much amoxicillin to give:

1. **Estimate the answer:** The amount to be given is a little more than the amount that is provided in the solution; therefore the answer is a little more than 5 mL.
2. **Set up the proportion:**

$$\frac{400\text{ mg}}{5\text{ mL}} = \frac{500\text{ mg}}{x\text{ mL}}$$

3. **Cross multiply the means and the extremes:**

$$400x = 500 \times 5$$

$$400x = 2500$$

4. **Divide both sides by the number before** ***x*****:**

$$\frac{400x}{400} = \frac{2500}{400}$$

$$x = \frac{2500}{400}$$

$$x = 6.25\text{ mL}$$

5. **Compare the estimate in Step 1 with the answer in Step 4:** The answer (6.25 mL) is close to the estimated amount (a little more than 5 mL). Therefore the answer is correct; prepare and administer 6.25 mL in the patient's gastric tube.

The Formula Method. Using this method requires you to first memorize the formula. Estimate the answer and then place all the information from the medication order into the formula. Label all the parts of the formula and ensure that all measures in the formula are in the same units and system of measurement before calculating the dosage. If the measures are not in the same measurement system, convert the numbers to the same system before calculating the dose. Calculate and label the answer and compare the answer with the estimated answer. If the estimate is not similar to the answer, recheck the calculation. Use the following basic formula when using the formula method:

$$\frac{\text{Dose ordered}}{\text{Dose on hand}} \times \text{Amount on hand} = \text{Amount to administer}$$

The dose ordered is the amount of medication prescribed. The dose on hand is the dose (e.g., mg, units) of medication supplied by the pharmacy. The amount on hand is the basic unit or quantity of the medication that contains the dose on hand. For solid medications the amount on hand is often one capsule; the amount of liquid on hand is sometimes 1 mL or 1 L, depending on the container. For example, a liquid medication comes in the strength of 125 mg per 5 mL. In this case 125 mg is the dose on hand, and 5 mL is the amount on hand. The amount to administer is the actual amount of medication the nurse administers. Always express the amount to administer in the same unit as the amount on hand.

Example: The prescriber orders morphine sulfate 2 mg IV. The medication is available in a vial containing 10 mg/mL. The formula is applied as follows:

1. **Estimate the answer:** The medication is a liquid; thus the answer will be in milliliters (mL). The amount to be given is less than ½ of the dose; thus the answer will be less than ½ mL.
2. **Set up the formula:**

$$\frac{\text{Dose ordered}}{\text{Dose on hand}} \times \text{Amount on hand} = \text{Amount to administer}$$

$$\frac{2\text{ mg}}{10\text{ mg}} \times 1\text{ mL} = \text{Amount to administer}$$

3. **Calculate the answer:**

$$\frac{2\text{ mg}}{10\text{ mg}} \times 1\text{ mL} = 0.2\text{ mL}$$

4. **Compare the estimate in Step 1 with the answer in Step 3:** The answer is less than ½ mL; thus it is close to the estimated answer. Prepare 0.2 mL of the medication in a syringe and administer it to the patient.

Dimensional Analysis. Dimensional analysis is the factor-label or the unit factor method. There is no need to memorize a formula since only one equation is needed and the same steps are used in solving every medication calculation. One research study shows that nursing students who use dimensional analysis often calculate medications more accurately than when they use the formula method (Greenfield, Whelan, and Cohn, 2006). Use the following steps to calculate medication doses by dimensional analysis:

1. Identify the unit of measure that you need to administer. For example, if you are giving a pill, you usually give a tablet or a capsule; for parenteral or liquid oral medications, the unit is milliliters.
2. Estimate the answer.
3. Place the name or appropriate abbreviation for *x* on the left side of the equation (e.g., *x* tab, *x* mL).
4. Place available information from the problem in a fraction format on the right side of the equation. Place the abbreviation or unit that matches what you are going to administer (determined in Step 1) in the numerator.

5. Look at the medication order and add other factors into the problem. Set up the numerator so it matches the unit in the previous denominator.
6. Cancel out like units of measurement on the right side of the equation. You should end up with only one unit left in the equation, and it should match the unit on the left side of the equation.
7. Reduce to the lowest terms if possible, and solve the problem or solve for *x*. Label your answer.
8. Compare your estimate from Step 1 with your answer in Step 2.

Example: The prescriber orders 0.45 g penicillin V potassium through a gastric tube. The bottle says: penicillin V potassium 125 mg/5 mL.

1. **Identify the unit of measure that you need to administer.** This medication is given in a gastric tube, which is a liquid medication; therefore the answer will be in milliliters (mL).
2. **Estimate the answer.** The medication order is more than three times but less than four times is the amount in the vial; thus the answer is more than 15 mL but less than 20 mL.
3. **Place the name or appropriate abbreviation for *x* on the left side of the equation.**

$$x\ \text{mL} =$$

4. **Place available information from the problem in a fraction format on the right side of the equation.** Since the medication will be administered in milliliters, place mL in the numerator.

$$x\ \text{mL} = \frac{5\ \text{mL}}{125\ \text{mg}}$$

5. **Look at the medication order and add other factors into the problem.** Set up the numerator so it matches the unit in the previous denominator. The order is for 0.45 g, and the medication is available in 125-mg bottles. Knowing that 1 g = 1000 mg, add this conversion to the calculation.

$$x\ \text{mL} = \frac{5\ \text{mL}}{125\ \text{mg}} \times \frac{1000\ \text{mg}}{1\text{g}} \times \frac{0.45\ \text{g}}{1}$$

6. **Cancel out like units of measurement on the right side of the equation.**

$$x\ \text{mL} = \frac{5\ \text{mL}}{125\ \cancel{\text{mg}}} \times \frac{1000\ \cancel{\text{mg}}}{1\ \cancel{\text{g}}} \times \frac{0.45\ \cancel{\text{g}}}{1}$$

7. **Reduce to the lowest terms if possible and solve the problem or solve for *x*.** Label your answer.

$$x = \frac{5 \times 1000 \times 0.45}{125}$$

$$x = \frac{2250}{125}$$

$$x = 18\ \text{mL}$$

8. **Compare the estimate from Step 2 with the answer in Step 7.** The calculated answer is 18 mL, which is between 15 mL and 20 mL. This matches the estimate made in Step 2. Prepare and administer 18 mL of medication as ordered.

Pediatric Doses. Current evidence shows that children are three times more at risk for experiencing a medication error than adults (TJC, 2008). Medication errors involving children frequently happen for the following reasons (Morris, 2010):

- Confusion between formulations for adults and children
- Availability of multiple pediatric concentrations of oral liquid medications
- Inaccurate preparation of medications that need to be diluted
- Similar packaging of medications and names of medications that look alike and sound alike
- Parents who do not understand how to correctly prepare and administer medications
- Errors in calculation and use of inaccurate measuring devices (e.g., household teaspoons and tablespoons) as opposed to devices made to measure small volume doses

Calculating children's medication doses requires caution (Hockenberry and Wilson, 2009). Even small errors or discrepancies in medication amounts can negatively affect a child's health (Morris, 2010). The child's age, weight, and maturity of body systems affect the ability to metabolize and excrete medications. Nurses sometimes have difficulties evaluating the child's response to a medication, especially when he or she cannot communicate verbally. For example, a side effect of vancomycin is ototoxicity. If a child cannot talk yet, it is challenging to assess for ototoxicity.

Use the following guidelines when calculating pediatric doses:

1. Most pediatric medications are ordered in milligrams per kilogram (mg/kg). Therefore ensure that the patient's weight is expressed in kilograms. Avoid converting the patient's weight whenever possible. If you have to convert pounds to kilograms, remember that 1 kg = 2.2 lb and convert the patient's weight before calculating the medication dosage.
2. Pediatric doses are usually a lot smaller than adult doses for the same medication. You frequently use micrograms and small syringes (e.g., tuberculin or 1 mL).
3. IM doses are very small and usually do not exceed 1 mL in small children or 0.5 mL in infants.
4. Subcutaneous dosages are also very small and do not usually exceed 0.5 mL.
5. Most medications are not rounded off to the nearest tenth. Instead they are rounded to the nearest thousandth.
6. Measure dosages that are less than 1 mL in syringes that are marked in tenths of a milliliter if the dosage calculation comes out even and does not need to be rounded. Use a tuberculin syringe for medication preparation when the medication needs to be rounded to the nearest thousandth.
7. Estimate the patient's dose before beginning the calculation; label and compare the answer with the estimate before preparing the medication.
8. To determine if a dose is safe before giving the medication, compare and evaluate the amount of medication ordered over 24 hours with the recommended dosage.

Different formulas and methods are used to calculate drug dosages in children. The two most common methods of calculating pediatric dosages are based on a child's weight or BSA. BSA is used in rare situations (e.g., determining chemotherapy doses). To estimate a child's BSA, use Mosteller's formula or the standard nomogram (e.g., the West nomogram). Refer to a pediatric or pharmacology resource and consult with the patient's health care provider or the pharmacist if you have to calculate a medication based on BSA.

Most of the time you calculate medications based on a child's weight. You can use the ratio and proportion method, the formula method, or dimensional analysis to calculate a pediatric dose using body weight. The example that follows explains how to use dimensional analysis to calculate pediatric doses. Refer to the previous sections on ratio and proportion and the formula method if you decide that they are easier for you to use.

Example: You receive an order to give ticarcillin/clavulanate 50 mg/kg q4h for a 5-year-old child who weighs 18 kg. The medication label says that there is 200 mg of ticarcillin/clavulanate in 1 mL of normal saline. How much ticarcillin/clavulanate do you give?

1. **Identify the unit of measure that you need to administer.** This medication is given IV piggyback, which is a parenteral medication. Therefore your answer will be in milliliters.
2. **Estimate the answer.** The medication is ordered 50 mg/kg. Round the child's weight up to 20 kg and multiply it by 50 mg to estimate the total amount of mg to be given. In your estimate the patient needs about 1000 mg. Because the medication comes in a vial of 200 mg in 1 mL and 1000 mg is 5 times larger than the dose of the medication and because you rounded the patient's weight up to 20 kg, you need to give a little less than 5 mL.
3. **Place the name or appropriate abbreviation for x on the left side of the equation.**

$$x \text{ mL} =$$

4. **Place available information from the problem in a fraction format on the right side of the equation.** Set up the numerator so it matches the unit in the previous denominator: You are going to administer the medication in milliliters; therefore place the mL in the numerator.

$$x \text{ mL} = \frac{1 \text{ mL}}{200 \text{ mg}}$$

5. **Look at the medication order and add other factors into the problem. Set up the numerator so that it matches the unit in the previous denominator.** You know that you need to give 50 mg/kg and that your patient weighs 18 kg.

$$x \text{ mL} = \frac{1 \text{ mL}}{200 \text{ mg}} \times \frac{50 \text{ mg}}{1 \text{ kg}} \times \frac{18 \text{ kg}}{1}$$

6. **Cancel out like units of measurement on the right side of the equation.**

$$x \text{ mL} = \frac{1 \text{ mL}}{200 \cancel{\text{mg}}} \times \frac{50 \cancel{\text{mg}}}{1 \cancel{\text{kg}}} \times \frac{18 \cancel{\text{kg}}}{1}$$

7. **Reduce to the lowest terms if possible and solve the problem or solve for *x*. Label your answer.**

$$x = \frac{50 \times 18}{200}$$

$$x = \frac{900}{200}$$

$$x = 4.5 \text{ mL}$$

8. **Compare the estimate from Step 2 with the answer in Step 7.** The answer is 4.5 mL, which is a little less than 5 mL. Since this is close to the estimate you made in Step 2, the calculation is correct, and you can continue with medication preparation at this time.

Prescriber's Role

The physician, nurse practitioner, or physician's assistant prescribes medications by writing an order on a form in the patient's medical record, in an order book, or on a legal prescription pad. Some prescribers use a desktop, laptop, or handheld electronic device to enter medication orders. Many hospitals are implementing computerized physician order entry (CPOE) to handle medication orders to decrease medication errors. In these systems the prescriber completes all computerized fields before the order for the medication is filled, thus avoiding incomplete or illegible orders.

Sometimes a prescriber orders a medication by talking directly to the nurse or by telephone. An order for a medication or medical treatment made over the telephone is called a telephone order. If the order is given verbally to the nurse, it is called a **verbal order.** When a verbal or telephone order is received, the nurse who took the order writes the complete order or enters it into a computer, reads it back, and receives confirmation from the prescriber to confirm accuracy. The nurse indicates the time and name of the prescriber who gave the order, signs it, and follows agency policy to indicate that it was read back. The prescriber countersigns the order at a later time, usually within 24 hours after giving it. Follow guidelines for taking verbal or telephone orders for medications safely (Box 31-3). Institutional policies vary regarding personnel who can take verbal or telephone orders. Nursing students cannot take them. They only give newly ordered medications after a registered nurse has written and verified the order.

Common abbreviations are often used when writing orders. Abbreviations indicate dosage frequencies or times, routes of administration, and special information for giving the medication (see Table 31-3). Medication errors frequently involve the use of abbreviations. Table 31-7 lists abbreviations that are associated with a high incidence of medication errors. Do ***not*** use these abbreviations when documenting medication orders or other information about medications (ISMP, 2010b; TJC, 2011b). Sometimes abbreviations used in different agencies vary. Check agency policy to determine which abbreviations are acceptable to use and their meaning.

Building Competency in Safety Your patient's health care provider has written the following orders. Which orders do you need to clarify before administering the medication? Provide rationale for your answers and rewrite the order so it follows the ISMP current medication order safety guidelines.

Lanoxin .25 mg QOD
Heparin 5,000 u SC twice a day
Aspirin 325 mg PO daily
Enalapril 10 mg PO twice a day
Lasix 40 mg IVP q day, hold for systolic blood pressure <100

Answers to questions can be found on the Evolve website.

Types of Orders in Acute Care Agencies

You must have a medication order before giving a medicine to a patient. Five common types of medication orders are based on the frequency and/or urgency of medication administration. Some conditions change the status of a patient's medication orders. For example, in some agencies the patient's preoperative medications are automatically discontinued, and the health care provider writes new medication orders after surgery (see Chapter 50). Agency policies that surround medication orders often vary. Nurses need to be aware of and follow these policies.

Standing Orders or Routine Medication Orders. A standing order is carried out until the prescriber cancels it by another order or a prescribed number of days elapse. A standing order often indicates a final date or number of treatments or doses. Many agencies have policies for automatically discontinuing standing orders. The following are examples of standing orders:

Tetracycline 500 mg PO q6h
Decadron 10 mg daily × 5 days

BOX 31-3 RECOMMENDATIONS TO REDUCE MEDICATION ERRORS ASSOCIATED WITH VERBAL MEDICATION ORDERS AND PRESCRIPTIONS (NCCMERP, 2006)*

Council Recommendations

Recommendations to Reduce Medication Errors Associated with Verbal Medication Orders and Prescriptions

Adopted February 20, 2001

Revised February 24, 2006

Preamble

Confusion over the similarity of drug names accounts for approximately 25% of all reports to the USP Medication Errors Reporting (MER) Program. To reduce confusion pertaining to verbal orders and to further support the Council's mission to minimize medication errors, the following recommendations have been developed.

In these recommendations verbal orders are prescriptions or medication orders that are communicated as oral, spoken communications between senders and receivers face to face, by telephone, or by other auditory device.

Recommendations

1. Verbal communication of prescription or medication orders should be limited to urgent situations where immediate written or electronic communication is not feasible.
2. Health care organizations† should establish policies and procedures that:
   - Describe limitations or prohibitions on use of verbal orders.
   - Provide a mechanism to ensure validity/authenticity of the prescriber.
   - List the elements required for inclusion in a complete verbal order.
   - Describe situations in which verbal orders may be used.
   - List and define the individuals who may send and receive verbal orders.
   - Provide guidelines for clear and effective communication of verbal orders.
3. Leaders of health care organizations should promote a culture in which it is acceptable, and strongly encouraged, for staff to question prescribers when there are any questions or disagreements about verbal orders. Questions about verbal orders should be resolved prior to the preparation, dispensing, or administration the medication.
4. Verbal orders for antineoplastic agents should ***NOT*** be permitted under any circumstances. These medications are not administered in emergency or urgent situations, and they have a narrow margin of safety.
5. Elements that should be included in a verbal order include:
   - Name of patient.
   - Age and weight of patient, when appropriate.
   - Drug name.
   - Dosage form (e.g., tablets, capsules, inhalants).
   - Exact strength or concentration.
   - Dose, frequency, and route.
   - Quantity and/or duration.
   - Purpose or indication (unless disclosure is considered inappropriate by the prescriber).
   - Specific instructions for use.
   - Name of prescriber and telephone number when appropriate.
   - Name of individual transmitting the order if different from the prescriber.
6. The content of verbal orders should be clearly communicated:
   - The name of the drug should be confirmed by any of the following:
     - Spelling
     - Providing both the brand and generic names of the medication
     - Providing the indication for use
   - In order to avoid confusion with spoken numbers, a dose such as 50 mg should be dictated as "fifty milligrams . . . five zero milligrams" to distinguish from "fifteen milligrams . . . one five milligrams."
   - In order to avoid confusion with drug name modifiers, such as prefixes and suffixes, additional spelling-assistance methods should be used (i.e., S as in Sam, X as in x-ray).
   - Instructions for use should be provided without abbreviations. For example, "1 tab tid" should be communicated as "Take/give one tablet three times daily."
   - Whenever possible, the receiver of the order should ***write*** down the complete order to enter it into a computer, then ***read*** it back, and receive confirmation from the individual who gave the order or test result.
7. All verbal orders should be reduced immediately to writing and signed by the individual receiving the order.
8. Verbal orders should be documented in the patient's medical record, reviewed, and countersigned by the prescriber as soon as possible.

†Health care organizations include community pharmacies, physicians' offices, hospitals, nursing homes, and home care agencies.

prn Orders. Sometimes the prescriber orders a medication to be given only when a patient requires it. This is a prn order. Use objective and subjective assessment and discretion in determining whether or not the patient needs the medication. An example of a prn order is:

Morphine sulfate 2 mg IV q2h prn for incisional pain

This order indicates that the patient needs to wait at least 2 hours between doses and can take the medication if experiencing pain at the incision. When administering medications, document the assessment findings that show why the patient needs the medication and the time of administration. Frequently evaluate the effectiveness of the medication and record findings in the appropriate record. Orders for prn medications that include a range (e.g., morphine sulfate IM 5-10 mg every 4-6 hours) are unclear and a source of medication errors. If a range order is written, ensure that the order follows agency policy for these types of orders. An example of a safer range order is to increase morphine dosage 50% to 100% if pain is moderate to severe.

Single (One-Time) Orders. Sometimes a prescriber orders a medication to be given only once at a specified time. This is common for preoperative medications or medications given before diagnostic examinations, for example:

Ativan 1 mg IV on call to MRI

STAT Orders. A STAT order signifies that a single dose of a medication is to be given immediately and only once. STAT orders are often written for emergencies when a patient's condition changes suddenly. For example:

Apresoline 10 mg IV STAT

Now Orders. A now order is more specific than a one-time order and is used when a patient needs a medication quickly but not right away, as in a STAT order. When receiving a now order,

TABLE 31-7 ISMP List of Error-Prone Abbreviations, Symbols, and Dose Designations

The abbreviations, symbols, and dose designations found in this table have been reported to ISMP through the USP-ISMP Medication Error Reporting Program as being frequently misinterpreted and involved in harmful medication errors. They should NEVER be used when communicating medical information. This includes internal communications, telephone/verbal prescriptions, computer-generated labels, labels for drug storage bins, medication administration records, as well as pharmacy and prescriber computer order entry screens. The Joint Commission (TJC) has established a National Patient Safety Goal that specifies that certain abbreviations must appear on the accredited organization's do-not-use list; we have highlighted these items with a double asterisk (**). However, we hope that you will consider others beyond the minimum TJC requirements. By using and promoting safe practices and educating one another about hazards, we can better protect our patients.

ABBREVIATIONS	INTENDED MEANING	MISINTERPRETATION	CORRECTION
µg	Microgram	Mistaken as "mg"	Use "mcg"
AD, AS, AU	Right ear, left ear, each ear	Mistaken as OD, OS, OU (right eye, left eye, each eye)	Use "right ear," "left ear," or "each ear"
BT	Bedtime	Mistaken as "BID" (twice daily)	Use "bedtime"
cc	Cubic centimeters	Mistaken as "u" (units)	Use "mL"
D/C	Discharge or discontinue	Premature discontinuation of medications if D/C (intended to mean "discharge") has been misinterpreted as "discontinued" when followed by a list of discharge medications	Use "discharge" and "discontinue"
IJ	Injection	Mistaken as "IV" or "intrajugular"	Use "injection"
IN	Intranasal	Mistaken as "IM" or "IV"	Use "intranasal" or "NAS"
HS	Half-strength	Mistaken as bedtime	Use "half-strength" or "bedtime"
hs	At bedtime, hours of sleep	Mistaken as half-strength	Use "bedtime" or "half-strength"
IU**	International unit	Mistaken as IV (intravenous) or 10 (ten)	Use "units"
o.d. or OD	Once daily	Mistaken as "right eye" (OD—oculus dexter), leading to oral liquid medications administered in the eye	Use "daily"
OJ	Orange juice	Mistaken as OD or OS (right or left eye); drugs meant to be diluted in orange juice may be given in the eye	Use "orange juice"
Per os	By mouth, orally	The "os" can be mistaken as "left eye" (OS—oculus sinister)	Use "PO," "by mouth," or "orally"
q.d. or QD**	Every day	Mistaken as q.i.d., especially if the period after the "q" or the tail of the "q" is misunderstood as an "I"	Use "daily"
qhs	Nightly at bedtime	Mistaken as "qhr" or every hour	Use "nightly"
qn	Nightly or at bedtime	Mistaken as "qh" (every hour)	Use "nightly" or "at bedtime"
q.o.d. or QOD**	Every other day	Mistaken as "q.d." (daily) or "q.i.d. (four times daily) if the "o" is poorly written	Use "every other day"
q1d	Daily	Mistaken as q.i.d. (four times daily)	Use "daily"
q6PM, etc.	Every evening at 6 PM	Mistaken as every 6 hours	Use "6 PM nightly" or "6 PM daily"
SC, SQ, sub q	Subcutaneous	SC mistaken as SL (sublingual); SQ mistaken as "5 every"; the "q" in "sub q" has been mistaken as "every" (e.g., a heparin dose ordered "sub q 2 hours before surgery" misunderstood as every 2 hours before surgery)	Use "subcut" or "subcutaneously"
ss	Sliding scale (insulin) or ½ (apothecary)	Mistaken as "55"	Spell out "sliding scale;" use "one-half" or "½"
SSRI	Sliding scale regular insulin	Mistaken as selective-serotonin reuptake inhibitor	Spell out "sliding scale (insulin)"
SSI	Sliding scale insulin	Mistaken as Strong Sol of Iodine (Lugol's)	

Continued

TABLE 31-7 ISMP List of Error-Prone Abbreviations, Symbols, and Dose Designations—cont'd

ABBREVIATIONS	INTENDED MEANING	MISINTERPRETATION	CORRECTION
i- /d	One daily	Mistaken as "tid"	Use "1 daily"
TIW or tiw	3 times a week	Mistaken as "3 times a day" or "twice in a week"	Use "3 times weekly"
U or u**	Unit	Mistaken as the number 0 or 4, causing a 10-fold overdose or greater (e.g., 4 U seen as "40" or 4 u seen as "44"); mistaken as "cc" so dose given in volume instead of units (e.g., 4 u seen as 4 cc)	Use "unit"
DOSE DESIGNATIONS AND OTHER INFORMATION	**INTENDED MEANING**	**MISINTERPRETATION**	**CORRECTION**
Trailing zero after decimal point (e.g., 1.0 mg)**	1 mg	Mistaken as 10 mg if the decimal point is not seen	Do not use trailing zeros for doses expressed in whole numbers
"Naked" decimal point (e.g., .5 mg)**	0.5 mg	Mistaken as 5 mg if the decimal point is not seen	Use zero before a decimal point when the dose is less than a whole unit
Drug name and dose run together (especially problematic for drug names that end in "l" such as Inderal40 mg; Tegretol300 mg)	Inderal 40 mg Tegretol 300 mg	Mistaken as Inderal 140 mg Mistaken as Tegretol 1300 mg	Place adequate space between the drug name, dose, and unit of measure
Numerical dose and unit of measure run together (e.g., 10mg, 100mL)	10 mg 100 mL	The "m" is sometimes mistaken as a zero or two zeros, risking a 10- to 100-fold overdose	Place adequate space between the dose and unit of measure
Abbreviations such as mg. or mL. with a period following the abbreviation	mg mL	The period is unnecessary and could be mistaken as the number 1 if written poorly	Use mg, mL, etc. without a terminal period
Large doses without properly placed commas (e.g., 100000 units; 1000000 units)	100,000 units 1,000,000 units	100000 has been mistaken as 10,000 or 1,000,000; 1000000 has been mistaken as 100,000	Use commas for dosing units at or above 1,000, or use words such as 100 "thousand" or 1 "million" to improve readability
DRUG NAME ABBREVIATIONS	**INTENDED MEANING**	**MISINTERPRETATION**	**CORRECTION**
ARA A	vidarabine	Mistaken as cytarabine (ARA C)	Use complete drug name
AZT	zidovudine (Retrovir)	Mistaken as azathioprine or aztreonam	Use complete drug name
CPZ	Compazine (prochlorperazine)	Mistaken as chlorpromazine	Use complete drug name
DPT	Demerol-Phenergan-Thorazine	Mistaken as diphtheria-pertussis-tetanus (vaccine)	Use complete drug name
DTO	Diluted tincture of opium, or deodorized tincture of opium (Paregoric)	Mistaken as tincture of opium	Use complete drug name
HCl	hydrochloric acid or hydrochloride	Mistaken as potassium chloride (The "H" is misinterpreted as "K")	Use complete drug name unless expressed as a salt of a drug
HCT	hydrocortisone	Mistaken as hydrochlorothiazide	Use complete drug name
HCTZ	hydrochlorothiazide	Mistaken as hydrocortisone (seen as HCT250 mg)	Use complete drug name
MgSO4**	magnesium sulfate	Mistaken as morphine sulphate	Use complete drug name
MS, MSO4**	morphine sulfate	Mistaken as magnesium sulphate	Use complete drug name
MTX	methotrexate	Mistaken as mitoxantrone	Use complete drug name
PCA	procainamide	Mistaken as patient-controlled analgesia	Use complete drug name
PTU	propylthiouracil	Mistaken as mercaptopurine	Use complete drug name
T3	Tylenol with codeine No. 3	Mistaken as liothyronine	Use complete drug name

TABLE 31-7 ISMP List of Error-Prone Abbreviations, Symbols, and Dose Designations—cont'd

DRUG NAME ABBREVIATIONS	INTENDED MEANING	MISINTERPRETATION	CORRECTION
TAC	triamcinolone	Mistaken as tetracaine, Adrenalin, cocaine	Use complete drug name
TNK	TNKase	Mistaken as "TPA"	Use complete drug name
ZnSO4	zinc sulfate	Mistaken as morphine sulphate	Use complete drug name
STEMMED DRUG NAMES	**INTENDED MEANING**	**MISINTERPRETATION**	**CORRECTION**
"Nitro" drip	nitroglycerin infusion	Mistaken as sodium nitroprusside infusion	Use complete drug name
"Norflox"	norfloxacin	Mistaken as Norflex	Use complete drug name
"IV Vanc"	intravenous vancomycin	Mistaken as Invanz	Use complete drug name
SYMBOLS	**INTENDED MEANING**	**MISINTERPRETATION**	**CORRECTION**
ʒ	Dram	Symbol for dram mistaken as "3"	Use the metric system
♍	Minim	Symbol for minim mistaken as "mL"	
×3d	For three days	Mistaken as "3 doses"	Use "for three days"
> and <	Greater than and less than	Mistaken as opposite of intended; mistakenly use incorrect symbol; "<10" mistaken as "40"	Use "greater than" or "less than"
/ (slash mark)	Separates two doses or indicates "per"	Mistaken as the number 1 (e.g., "25 units/10 units" misread as "25 units and 110" units)	Use "per" rather than a slash mark to separate doses
@	At	Mistaken as "2"	Use "at"
&	And	Mistaken as "2"	Use "and"
+	Plus or and	Mistaken as "4"	Use "and"
°	Hour	Mistaken as a zero (e.g., q2° seen as q20)	Use "hr," "h," or "hour"

ISMP, Institute for Safe Medication Practices.
**These abbreviations are included on TJC's "minimum list" of dangerous abbreviations, acronyms and symbols that must be included on an organization's "Do Not Use" list, effective January 1, 2004. Visit www.jointcommission.org for more information about this TJC requirement.

the nurse has up to 90 minutes to administer the medication. Only administer now medications one time. For example:

Vancomycin 1 g IV piggyback now

Prescriptions. The prescriber writes **prescriptions** for patients who are to take medications outside the hospital. The prescription includes more detailed information than a regular order because the patient needs to understand how to take the medication and when to refill the prescription if necessary. Some agencies require prescribers to write prescriptions for controlled substances on a special prescription pad that is different (e.g., a different color) than the prescription pad used for other medications. Fig. 31-6 illustrates the parts of a prescription.

Pharmacist's Role

The pharmacist prepares and distributes prescribed medications. Pharmacists work with nurses, physicians, and other health care providers to evaluate the efficacy of patients' medications. They are responsible for filling prescriptions accurately and being sure that prescriptions are valid. Pharmacists in health care agencies rarely mix compounds or solutions, except in the case of IV solutions. Most medication companies deliver medications in a form ready for use. Dispensing the correct medication, in the proper dosage and amount, with an accurate label is the pharmacist's main task. He or she also provides information about medication side effects, toxicity, interactions, and incompatibilities.

Distribution Systems

Systems for storing and distributing medications vary. Pharmacists provide the medications, but nurses distribute them to patients. Institutions providing nursing care have a special area for stocking and dispensing medications. Special medication rooms, portable locked carts, computerized medication cabinets, and individual storage units next to patients' rooms are examples of storage areas used. Medication storage areas need to be locked when unattended.

Unit Dose. The unit-dose system uses carts containing a drawer with a 24-hour supply of medications for each patient. Each drawer is labeled with the name of the patient in his or her designated room. The unit dose is the ordered dose of medication that the patient receives at one time. Each tablet or capsule is wrapped in a foil or paper container. At a designated time each day the pharmacist or a pharmacy technician refills the drawers in the cart with a fresh supply. The cart also contains limited amounts of prn and stock medications for special situations. Controlled substances are not kept in the individual patient drawer. Instead they are kept

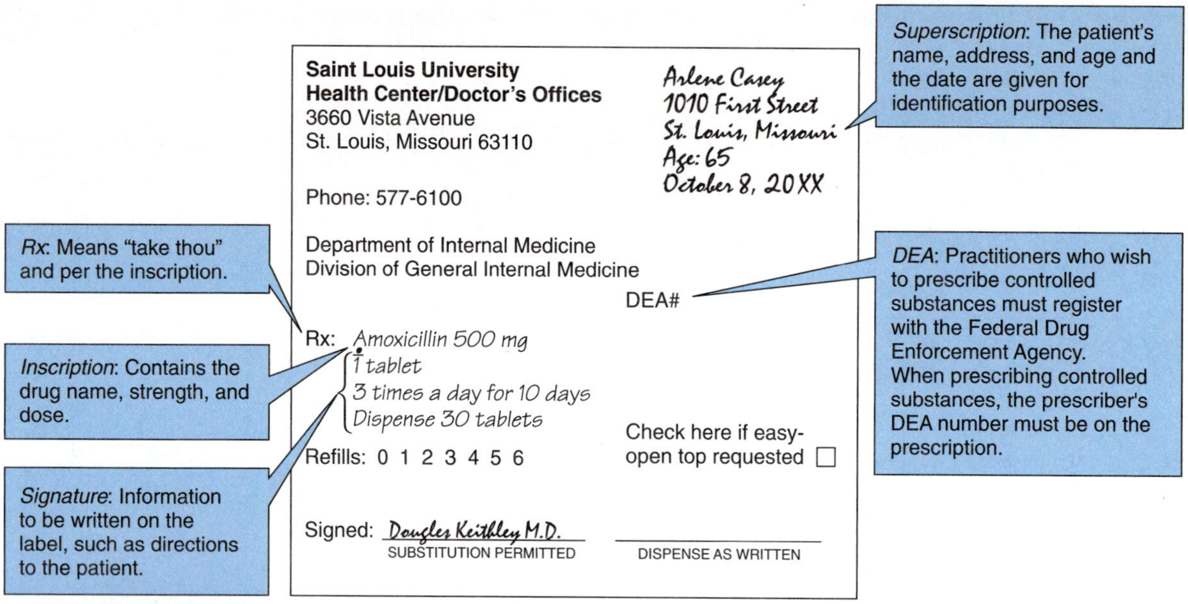

Saint Louis University
Health Center/Doctor's Offices
3660 Vista Avenue
St. Louis, Missouri 63110
Phone: 577-6100
Arlene Casey
1010 First Street
St. Louis, Missouri
Age: 65
October 8, 20XX
Superscription: The patient's name, address, and age and the date are given for identification purposes.
Department of Internal Medicine
Division of General Internal Medicine
DEA#
DEA: Practitioners who wish to prescribe controlled substances must register with the Federal Drug Enforcement Agency.
When prescribing controlled substances, the prescriber's DEA number must be on the prescription.
Rx: Means "take thou" and per the inscription.
Rx: Amoxicillin 500 mg
1 tablet
3 times a day for 10 days
Dispense 30 tablets
Inscription: Contains the drug name, strength, and dose.
Refills: 0 1 2 3 4 5 6
Check here if easy-open top requested
Signature: Information to be written on the label, such as directions to the patient.
Signed: Douglas Keithley M.D.
SUBSTITUTION PERMITTED
DISPENSE AS WRITTEN

FIG. 31-6 Example of a medication prescription. (Courtesy Saint Louis University Medical Center, St Louis, Mo.)

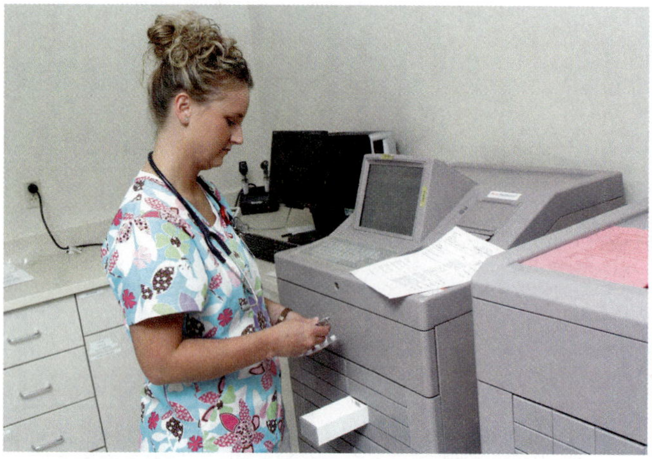

FIG. 31-7 Automated medication dispensing system.

in a larger locked drawer to keep them secure. The unit-dose system reduces the number of medication errors and saves steps in dispensing medications.

Automated Medication Dispensing Systems. Automated medication dispensing systems (AMDSs) are used throughout the country (Fig. 31-7). The systems within an agency are networked with one another and with other agency computer systems (e.g., computerized medical record). AMDSs control the dispensing of all medications, including narcotics. Each nurse accesses the system by entering a security code. Some systems require bioidentification as well. In these systems you place your finger on a screen to access the computer. You select the patient's name and his or her drug profile before the AMDS dispenses a medication. In these systems you are allowed to select the desired medication, dosage, and route from a list displayed on the computer screen. The system causes the drawer containing medication to open, records it, and charges it to the patient. Systems that are connected to the patient's computerized medical record then record information about the medication (e.g., medication name, dose, time) and the nurse's name in the patient's medical record. Some systems require nurses to scan bar codes to identify the patient, the medication, and the nurse administering the medication before recording this information in the patient's computerized medical record. Agencies that implement AMDS with bar-code scanning often reduce the incidence of medication errors (see Box 31-2).

Nurse's Role

Administering medications to patients requires knowledge and a set of skills that are unique to a nurse. You first assess that the medication ordered is the correct medication. Do not assume that all medications that are in the patient's "drawer" or pillbox are to be given to him or her. Assess the patient's ability to self-administer medications, determine whether a patient should receive a medication at a given time, administer medications correctly, and closely monitor their effects. Patient and family education about proper medication administration and monitoring is an integral part of your role. Do not delegate any part of the medication administration process to nursing assistive personnel (NAP) and use the nursing process to integrate medication therapy into care.

Medication Errors

A **medication error** can cause or lead to inappropriate medication use or patient harm. Medication errors include inaccurate prescribing, administering the wrong medication, giving the medication using the wrong route or time interval, and administering extra doses or failing to administer a medication. Preventing medication errors is essential. The process of administering medications has many steps and involves many members of the health care team. Because nurses play an essential role in preparing and administering medications, they need to be vigilant in preventing errors (Box 31-4). Advances in technology have helped to decrease the occurrence of medication errors (Box 31-5).

Medication errors are related to practice patterns, health care product design, or procedures and systems such as product labeling

BOX 31-4 STEPS TO TAKE TO PREVENT MEDICATION ERRORS

- Prepare medications for one person at a time.
- Follow the six rights of medication administration.
- Be sure to read labels at least three times (comparing medication administration record [MAR] with label) before administering the medication.
- Use at least two patient identifiers and review the patient's allergies whenever administering a medication.
- Do not allow any other activity to interrupt administration of medication to a patient (e.g., phone call, pager, discussion with other staff).
- Double-check all calculations and other high-risk medication administration processes (e.g., patient-controlled analgesia) and verify with another nurse.
- Do not interpret illegible handwriting; clarify with prescriber.
- Question unusually large or small doses.
- Document all medications as soon as they are given.
- When you have made an error, reflect on what went wrong and ask how you could have prevented the error.
- Evaluate the context or situation in which a medication error occurred. This helps to determine if nurses have the necessary resources for safe medication administration.
- Attend in-service programs that focus on the medications commonly administered.
- Ensure that you are well rested when caring for patients. Nurses make more errors when they are fatigued.
- Involve and educate the patient when administering medications. Address patients' concerns about medications before administering them (e.g., concerns about their appearance or side effects).
- Follow established policies and procedures when using technology to administer medications (e.g., automated medication dispensing systems [AMDSs] and bar-code scanning). Medication errors occur when nurses "work around" the technology (e.g., override alerts without thinking about them).

Data from Koppel et al: Workarounds to barcode medication administration systems: their occurrences, causes, and threats to patient safety, *J Am Med Inform Assoc* 15(4):408, 2008; Lockley SW et al: Effects of health care provider work hours and sleep deprivation on safety and performance, *Joint Comm J Qual Patient Safety* 33(11):7, 2007; National Coordinating Council for Medication Error Reporting and Prevention (NCCMERP): Reducing medication errors associated with at-risk behaviors, 2007, http://www.nccmerp.org/council/council2007-06-08.html.

BOX 31-5 INFORMATICS AND MEDICATION SAFETY

Many medication errors occur when the nurse incorrectly administers medications at the patient's bedside. The following innovations and advances in technology have helped reduce the number of medication errors in nursing practice:

- Networked computers allow all the patient's health care providers to see a current list of ordered and discontinued medications.
- Internet and intranet access allows nurses and other health care providers to access current information about medications (e.g., indications, desired effects, adverse effects) and specific agency policies that address medication administration (e.g., how fast to administer an intravenous [IV] push medication, how to administer medications through a nasogastric tube).
- In some agencies prescribers enter medication orders directly into a networked computer system or a personal handheld computer.
- Automated medication dispensing systems and electronic medication administration records (MARs) help with medication reconciliation, administration, and documentation.
- Bar-coding technology requires nurses to scan the medication, the patient's identification bracelet, and the nurse's identification badge before administering the medication, which helps ensure the six rights of medication administration.

Application to Nursing Practice

- Actively participate in selecting and evaluating advanced technologies and creating nursing policies and protocols used for medication administration.
- Always follow agency policies when administering medications.
- Implement agency policies when the technology cannot be used (e.g., during down time or power outages).
- Follow manufacturer guidelines for care of electronic equipment and report problems with technology immediately.

and distribution. When an error occurs, the patient's safety and well-being become the top priority. The nurse first assesses and examines the patient's condition and notifies the health care provider of the incident as soon as possible. Once the patient is stable, the nurse reports the incident to the appropriate person in the institution (e.g., manager or supervisor). The nurse is responsible for preparing a written occurrence or incident report that usually needs to be filed within 24 hours of the error. The report includes patient identification information; the location and time of the incident; an accurate, factual description of what occurred and what was done; and the signature of the nurse involved. The occurrence report is not a permanent part of the medical record and is not referred to anywhere in the record (see Chapters 23 and 26). This legally protects the nurse and institution. Agencies use occurrence reports to track incident patterns and initiate quality improvement programs as needed.

Report all medication errors, including those that do not cause obvious or immediate harm or near misses. It is important to feel comfortable in reporting an error and not fear repercussions from managerial staff. Even when a patient suffers no harm from a medication error, the institution can still learn why the mistake occurred and what can be done to avoid similar errors in the future.

Medication errors often happen when patients experience changes in the health care setting, level of care, or health care provider (e.g., goes to a health care provider's office, transfers from one patient care unit to another, is discharged from a health care setting). Reconciling the list of a patient's medications is essential to medication safety (TJC, 2011a). Nurses play an essential role in **medication reconciliation** (Box 31-6). Whenever a nurse admits a patient to a health care setting, he or she compares the medications that the patient took in the previous setting (e.g., home or another nursing unit) with his or her current medication orders (Mayhew, 2010). When the patient leaves that setting for another setting (e.g., skilled care facility or intensive care unit), the nurse communicates the patient's current medications with the health care providers in the new setting. The nurse also reconciles the patient's medications when he or she is discharged from an agency or is seen in an outpatient setting. Many agencies have computerized or written forms to facilitate the process of medication reconciliation. The process is challenging and takes a lot of time and concentration. Eliminate distractions and go slowly when reconciling patients' medications. Always clarify information when needed. Nurses need to consult with the patient, caregivers, family members, pharmacists, and other members of the health care team when reconciling medications.

BOX 31-6 PROCESS FOR MEDICATION RECONCILIATION

1. **Verify:** Obtain a comprehensive and current list of the patient's medications. Be sure to ask about vitamins, herbal and nutritional supplements, over-the-counter medications, insulin pens, transdermal patches, inhalers, and other medications that people do not typically consider to be medications (Razzi, 2009).
2. **Clarify:** Make sure that the list of medications, dosages, and frequencies is accurate; clarify the list with as many people as necessary (e.g., patient, caregiver, health care providers, pharmacists) to ensure accuracy.
3. **Reconcile:** Compare new medication orders with the current list; investigate any discrepancies with the patient's health care provider. Use computerized medical records and computerized prescriber order entry when possible to help with this process (Razzi, 2009).
4. **Transmit:** Communicate the updated and verified list to caregivers and the patient as appropriate. Teach patients to carry list of current medications and share with all health care providers (Razzi, 2009).

CRITICAL THINKING

Knowledge

You will use knowledge from many disciplines when administering medications to understand why a particular medication is prescribed for a patient and how the medication will alter the patient's physiology to have a therapeutic effect. For example, in physiology you learn that potassium is a major intracellular ion. When patients do not have enough potassium in their body (hypokalemia), they experience signs and symptoms such as muscle fatigue or weakness. In some cases severe hypokalemia is fatal as a result of associated cardiac dysrhythmias. Prescribed medications help to restore the patient's potassium level to normal, which then relieves the signs and symptoms of hypokalemia. In another example knowledge about child development indicates that children often associate medication administration with a negative experience. Use principles from child development to ensure that the child cooperates with the medication experience.

Nurses administer a variety of medications, and new medications are constantly approved. As a result, they do not always have knowledge about the medications they are asked to administer. Critical thinkers admit what they do not know and acquire the knowledge needed to safely administer unfamiliar medications. This means consulting more expert nurses, a pharmacist, the prescriber, or a medication book.

Experience

Nursing students have limited experience with medication administration as it applies to professional practice. Clinical experiences provide you with opportunities to use the nursing process as it applies to medication administration. As you gain experience in medication administration, your psychomotor skills ("the how-to") become more refined. However, psychomotor skills represent a small part of medication administration. Patient attitudes, knowledge, physical and mental status, and responses make medication administration a complex experience.

Attitudes

To administer medications safely, many critical thinking skills are essential. For example, be disciplined and take adequate time to prepare and administer medications. Take the time to read your patient's medical record before administering medications and carefully review his or her history, physical examination, and orders. Look up medications that you do not know in a medication reference and determine why each patient is taking each of his or her prescribed medications. Every step of safe medication administration requires a disciplined attitude and a comprehensive, systematic approach. Following the same procedure each time medications are administered ensures safe administration.

Responsibility and accountability are other critical thinking attitudes essential to safe medication administration. Accept full accountability and responsibility for all actions surrounding the administration of medications. Do not assume that a medication that is ordered for a patient is the correct medication or the correct dose. Be responsible for knowing that the medications and doses ordered are correct and appropriate. You are accountable if you give an ordered medication that is knowingly inappropriate for the patient. Therefore be familiar with each therapeutic effect, usual dosage, anticipated changes in laboratory data, and side effects of a drug. You are also responsible for ensuring that patients or caregivers who self-administer medications have been properly informed about all aspects of self-administration (TJC, 2010). If it is determined that a patient cannot safely self-administer medications, design interventions such as involving family caregivers to ensure safe self-administration of medications.

Standards

Standards are actions that ensure safe nursing practice. Standards for medication administration are set by individual health care agencies and the nursing profession. Agency policy usually sets limits on the nurse's ability to administer medications in certain units of the acute care setting. Sometimes nurses are limited by certain medication routes or dosages. Most institutions have nursing procedure manuals that contain policies that define the types of medications nurses can and cannot administer. The types and dosages of medications that nurses deliver often vary from unit to unit within the same facility. For example, phenytoin (Dilantin), a powerful medication for treating seizures, may be administered by mouth or IV push. In large dosages phenytoin affects heart rhythm. Therefore some agencies place limits on how much nurses can give to a patient on a nursing unit that does not have the ability to monitor the patient's heart rate and rhythm. Not all prescribers are aware of all of the limitations and sometimes prescribe medications that nurses cannot give in a particular health care setting. Recognize these limitations and inform the prescriber accordingly. Take appropriate actions to ensure that patients receive medications as prescribed and within the time prescribed in the appropriate environment.

Professional standards such as *Nursing: Scope and Standards of Practice* (American Nurses Association [ANA], 2010) (see Chapters 1 and 23) apply to the activity of medication administration. To prevent medication errors, follow the six rights of medication administration consistently every time you administer medications. Many medication errors can be linked, in some way, to an inconsistency in adhering to these six rights:

1. The right medication
2. The right dose
3. The right patient
4. The right route
5. The right time
6. The right documentation

Right Medication. A medication order is required for every medication that you administer to a patient. Sometimes prescribers write orders by hand in the patient's medical record. However, many agencies use CPOE. CPOE allows prescribers to electronically order medications, eliminating the need for written orders and enhancing medication safety (Sowan et al., 2010). Regardless of how the nurse receives a medication order, he or she compares the prescriber's written orders with the medication administration record (MAR) or electronic medication administration record (eMAR) when it is initially ordered. Nurses verify medication information whenever new MARs are created or distributed or when patients transfer from one nursing unit or health care setting to another (TJC, 2011a).

Once you determine that information on the patient's MAR is accurate, use it to prepare and administer medications. When preparing medications from bottles or containers, compare the label of the medication container with the MAR three times: (1) before removing the container from the drawer or shelf, (2) as the amount of medication ordered is removed from the container, and (3) at the patient's bedside before administering the medication to the patient. Never prepare medications from unmarked containers or containers with illegible labels (TJC, 2010). With unit-dose prepackaged medications, check the label with the MAR when taking medications out of the medication dispensing system. Finally verify all medications at the patient's bedside with the patient's MAR and use at least two identifiers before giving the patient any medications (TJC, 2011a).

Patients who self-administer medications need to keep them in their original labeled containers, separate from other medications, to avoid confusion. Many hospitals request that all medication administration in the hospital setting be completed through nurses rather than letting patients self-administer to ensure that patients are not receiving double doses. Because the nurse who administers the medication is responsible for any errors related to it, nurses administer only the medications they prepare. You cannot delegate preparation of medication to another person and then administer the medication to the patient. If a patient questions the medication, do not ignore these concerns. An alert patient or a family caregiver familiar with a patient's medications knows whether a medication is different from those received before. In most cases the patient's medication order has changed; however, some patient questions reveal an error. When this occurs, withhold the medication and recheck it against the prescriber's orders. If a patient refuses a medication, discard it rather than returning it to the original container. Unit-dose medications can be saved if they are not opened. If a patient refuses narcotics, follow proper hospital procedure by having someone else witness the "wasted" medication.

Right Dose. The unit-dose system is designed to minimize errors. When preparing a medication from a larger volume or strength than needed or when the prescriber orders a system of measurement different from that which the pharmacy supplies, the chance of error increases. When performing medication calculations or conversions, have another qualified nurse check the calculated doses. After calculating doses, prepare the medication using standard measurement devices. Use graduated cups, syringes, and scaled droppers to measure medications accurately. At home have patients use kitchen measuring spoons rather than household teaspoons and tablespoons, which vary in volume.

Medication errors often occur when pills need to be split. To promote patient safety in inpatient settings, pharmacists split the medications, label and package them, and then send them to the nurse for administration. Because pill splitting is particularly problematic in the home care setting, the Institute for Safe Medication Practices (ISMP) (2006) developed suggestions to help with this process. Determine if the patient has the motor dexterity or visual acuity to split tablets. If at all possible, prescribers need to avoid ordering medications that require splitting.

Tablets are sometimes crushed and mixed with food. Be sure to completely clean a crushing device before crushing the tablet. Remnants of previously crushed medications increase the concentration of a medication or result in the patient receiving a portion of a medication that was not prescribed. Mix crushed medications with very small amounts of food or liquid (e.g., a single tablespoon). Do not use the patient's favorite foods or liquids because medications alter their taste and decrease the patient's desire for them. This is especially a concern for pediatric patients.

Not all medications are suitable for crushing. Some medications (e.g., extended-release capsules) have special coatings to prevent them from being absorbed too quickly. These medications should not be crushed. Refer to the "Do Not Crush List" (ISMP, 2010d, http://www.ismp.org/Tools/DoNotCrush.pdf) to ensure that a medication is safe to crush.

Right Patient. Medication errors often occur because one patient gets a drug intended for another patient. Therefore an important step in safe medication administration is being sure that you give the right medication to the right patient. It is difficult to remember every patient's name and face. Before administering a medication, use at least two patient identifiers (TJC, 2010). Acceptable patient identifiers include the patient's name, an identification number assigned by a health care agency, or a telephone number. Do not use the patient's room number as an identifier. To identify a patient correctly in an acute care setting, compare the patient identifiers on the MAR with the patient's identification bracelet while at the patient's bedside. If an identification bracelet becomes smudged or illegible or is missing, obtain a new one. In health care settings that are not acute care settings, TJC (2008) does not require the use of armbands for identification. However, nurses still need to use a system that verifies the patient's identification with at least two identifiers before administering medications.

Patients do not need to state their names and other identifiers when administering medications. Collect patient identifiers reliably when the patient is admitted to a health care setting. Once the identifiers are assigned to the patient (e.g., putting identifiers on an armband and placing the armband on the patient), the nurse uses the identifiers to match the patient with the MAR, which lists the correct medications. Asking patients to state their full names and identification information provides a third way to verify that the nurse is giving medications to the right patient.

In addition to using two identifiers, some agencies use a wireless bar-code scanner to help identify the right patient (Fig. 31-8). This system requires the nurse to scan a personal bar code that is commonly placed on the nurse's name tag first. Then he or she scans a bar code on the single-dose medication package. Finally the nurse scans the patient's armband. All this information is then stored in a computer for documentation purposes. This system helps eliminate medication errors because it provides another step to ensure that the right patient receives the right medication.

Right Route. Always consult the prescriber if an order does not designate a route of administration. Likewise, if the specified route is not the recommended route, alert the prescriber immediately. Recent evidence shows that medication errors involving the wrong route are common. For example, enteral and parenteral medications are at risk for confusion in the pediatric population because liquid medications are frequently given orally. When oral medications are prepared in parenteral syringes, there is a high risk for giving an oral medication through the parenteral route (ISMP,

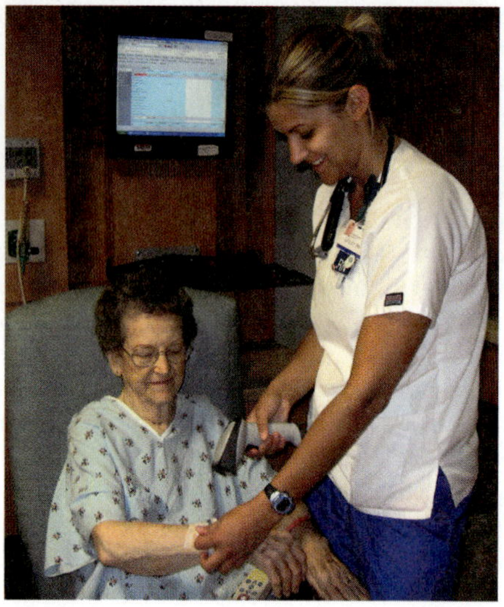

FIG. 31-8 Nurse using bar-code scanner to identify patient during medication administration.

2010c; Paparella, 2008). The injection of a liquid designed for oral use produces local complications such as sterile abscess or fatal systemic effects. Prepare injections from preparations designed for parenteral use only. Medication companies label parenteral medications "for injectable use only." Label the syringe after preparing the medication and always use different syringes for enteral and parenteral medication administration (ISMP, 2010c). The enteral syringes are often a different color than the parenteral syringes and are clearly labeled for oral or enteral use. The syringe tips of enteral syringes are incompatible with parenteral medication administration systems. Needles do not attach to the syringes, and the syringes cannot be inserted into any type of IV line. In addition, be sure to remove any caps from the tip of an oral syringe before administering the medication. Failure to remove the cap can result in the patient aspirating it, thus blocking his or her trachea (Guenter, 2010; Paparella, 2008).

Right Time. In addition, you need to know why a medication is ordered for certain times of the day and whether you are able to alter the time schedule. For example, two medications are ordered, one q8h (every 8 hours) and the other 3 times a day. Both medications are scheduled for 3 times within a 24-hour period. The prescriber intends the q8h medication to be given around-the-clock to maintain therapeutic blood levels of the medication. In contrast, the nurse needs to give the 3-times-a-day medication during the waking hours. Each agency has a recommended time schedule for medications ordered at frequent intervals. You can alter these recommended times if necessary or appropriate.

The prescriber often gives specific instructions about when to administer a medication. A preoperative medication to be given "on call" means that the nurse gives the medication when the operating room staff members notify him or her that they are coming to get the patient for surgery. Give a medication ordered PC (after meals) within half an hour after a meal, when the patient has a full stomach. Give a STAT medication immediately.

Give priority to time-critical medications that must act and therefore be given at certain times. Hospitals designate which medications are time-critical and which are non–time-critical (CMS, 2011; ISMP, 2011). You administer time-critical medications within 30 minutes before or after their scheduled time. For example, give insulin (a time-critical medication) at a precise interval before a meal. Give antibiotics 30 minutes before or after they are scheduled, around-the-clock to maintain therapeutic blood levels. Give all routinely ordered non–time-critical medications within 1 to 2 hours before or after the scheduled time or per agency policy (CMS, 2011; ISMP, 2011).

Some medications require the nurse's clinical judgment in deciding the proper time for administration. Administer a prn sleeping medication when the patient is prepared for bed. In addition, use judgment when administering prn analgesics. For example, the nurse sometimes needs to obtain a STAT order from the prescriber if the patient requires a medication before the prn interval has elapsed. Nurses always document whenever they call the patient's health care provider to obtain a change in a medication order.

Before discharge from the hospital setting, evaluate a patient's need for home care, especially if he or she was admitted to the hospital because of a problem with medication self-administration. Patients often leave the hospital with a basic knowledge of their medications but are unable to remember or implement this knowledge once back home. Before patients are discharged from the hospital, evaluate whether the medications are adequate or prescribed at therapeutic levels for them.

At home some patients take several medications throughout the day. Help to plan schedules based on preferred medication intervals, the pharmacokinetics of the medications, and the patient's daily schedule. For patients who have difficulty remembering when to take medications, make a chart that lists the times to take each medication or prepare a special container to hold each timed dose.

Right Documentation. Nurses and other health care providers use accurate documentation to communicate with one another. Many medication errors result from inaccurate documentation. Therefore always document medications accurately at the time of administration and verify any inaccurate documentation before giving medications.

Before administering a medication, ensure that the MAR clearly reflects the patient's full name; the name of the ordered medication written out in full (no medication name abbreviations); the time the medication is to be administered; and the dosage, route, and frequency. Common problems with medication orders include incomplete information; inaccurate dosage form or strength; illegible order or signature; incorrect placement of decimals, leading to the wrong dosage; and nonstandard terminology. If there is any question about a medication order because it is incomplete, illegible, vague, or not understood, contact the prescribing health care provider before administering the medication. The prescribing health care provider is responsible to provide accurate, complete, and understandable medication orders. If health care providers are unable to do this, nurses implement agency policy (usually a "chain of command" policy) to determine who to contact until they resolve issues related to patients' medications. You are responsible to begin this chain of command to ensure that patients receive the correct medication. You are also responsible for documenting any preassessment data required of certain medications such as a blood pressure measurement for antihypertensive medications or laboratory values, as in the case of phenytoin, before giving the drug.

After administering a medication, indicate which medication was given on the patient's MAR per agency policy to verify that it was given as ordered. Record each medication on the patient's MAR as soon as you give medications to a patient. Inaccurate documentation such as failing to document giving a medication or documenting an incorrect dose leads to errors in subsequent decisions about patient care. For example, errors in documentation about insulin often result in negative patient outcomes. Consider the following

BOX 31-7 NURSES' SIX RIGHTS FOR SAFE MEDICATION ADMINISTRATION

1. The right to a complete and clearly written order
2. The right to have the correct drug route and dose dispensed
3. The right to have access to information
4. The right to have policies on medication administration
5. The right to administer medications safely and identify problems in the system
6. The right to stop, think, and be vigilant when administering medications

From Cook MC: Nurses' six rights for safe medication administration, *Mass Nurse* 69(6):8, 1999.

situation: a patient receives insulin before breakfast, but the nurse who gave the insulin forgot to document it. The nurse caring for the patient goes home, and the patient has a new nurse for the day. The new nurse notices that the insulin is not documented and assumes that the previous nurse did not give the insulin. Therefore the new nurse gives the patient another dose of insulin. Approximately 2 hours later, the patient experiences a low blood glucose level, which causes him or her to have seizures. Accurate documentation would have prevented this situation from happening.

Never document that you have given a medication until you have actually given it. The name of the medication, the dose, the time of administration, and the route all need to be documented on the MAR. Also document the site of any injections and the patient's responses to medications, either positive or negative. Nurses notify the patient's health care provider of any negative responses to medications and document the time, date, and name of the health care provider that was notified in the patient's medical record. The efforts you make in ensuring proper documentation help provide safe care (Box 31-7).

Maintaining Patients' Rights. In accordance with *The Patient Care Partnership* (American Hospital Association, 2003) and because of the potential risks related to medication administration, a patient has the following rights:

- To be informed of the name, purpose, action, and potential undesired effects of a medication
- To refuse a medication regardless of the consequences
- To have qualified nurses or physicians assess a medication history, including allergies and use of herbals
- To be properly advised of the experimental nature of medication therapy and give written consent for its use
- To receive labeled medications safely without discomfort in accordance with the six rights of medication administration
- To receive appropriate supportive therapy in relation to medication therapy
- To not receive unnecessary medications
- To be informed if medications are a part of a research study

Know these rights and handle all inquiries by patients and families courteously and professionally. Do not become defensive if a patient refuses medication therapy, recognizing that every person of consenting age has a right to refusal.

NURSING PROCESS

Apply the nursing process and use a critical thinking approach in your care of patients. The nursing process provides a clinical decision-making approach for you to develop and implement an individualized plan of care.

BOX 31-8 NURSING ASSESSMENT QUESTIONS

- Which prescription and nonprescription medications and herbal and nutritional supplements do you take, when do you take them, and how do you take them? Do you have a list of medications from your pharmacy or health care provider's office?
- Why do you take the medications?
- Which side effects have you experienced?
- What have you been told to do if a side effect develops?
- Have you ever stopped taking your medications? If so, why?
- What do you do to help you remember to take your medications?
- Do you have any allergies to medications or foods? If so, describe what happens when you take the medication or eat the food.
- Describe your normal eating patterns. Which foods and at what times do you normally eat?
- How do your religious or cultural beliefs influence your beliefs about your medications?
- How do you pay for your medications? Do you sometimes have to stretch your budget to afford them or space them out to save money?
- What questions do you have about your medications?

ASSESSMENT

During the assessment process, thoroughly assess each patient and critically analyze findings to ensure that you make patient-centered clinical decisions required for safe nursing care.

Through the Patient's Eyes. Use professional knowledge, skills, and attitudes to provide compassionate and coordinated care. This requires you to take the patient's preferences, values, and needs into consideration while determining his or her need for and potential response to medication therapy. Assess patients' experiences and encourage them to express their beliefs, feelings, and concerns about their medications. Putting patients in the center of their care helps you to see the situation through their eyes and contributes to safe medication administration. Begin your assessment by asking a variety of questions that help you better understand your patients' current medication management routine, the ability to afford medications, and beliefs and expectations about medications (Box 31-8).

History. Before administering medications, obtain or review the patient's medical history. A patient's medical history provides indications or contraindications for medication therapy. Disease or illness places patients at risk for adverse medication effects. For example, if a patient has a gastric ulcer, medications containing aspirin increase the likelihood of bleeding. Long-term health problems (e.g., diabetes or arthritis) require specific medications. This knowledge helps the nurse anticipate the type of medications that a patient requires. A patient's surgical history indicates use of medications. For example, after a thyroidectomy a patient requires thyroid hormone replacement.

Allergies. Inform the other members of the health care team if the patient has a history of allergies to medications and foods. Many medications have ingredients also found in food sources. For example, propofol (Diprivan), which is used for anesthesia and sedation, includes egg lecithin and soybean oil as inactive ingredients. Therefore patients who have an egg or soy allergy should not receive propofol (Skidmore-Roth, 2011). In some health care settings patients wear identification bands listing medication and food allergies. Ensuring that all allergies and the patient's reactions are noted on the patient's admission notes, medication records, and history and physical examination facilitates communication of this essential information to members of the health care team.

Medications. Assess information about each medication that the patient takes, including length of time the medication has been taken, the current dosage, and whether or not the patient experiences side effects or has had adverse effects from the medication. In addition, review the action, purpose, normal dosage, routes, side effects, and nursing implications for administering and monitoring each medication. Often you need to consult several resources to gather necessary information. Pharmacology textbooks and handbooks; electronic medication manuals available on a computer, handheld computer, or AMDS; nursing journals; the *Physician's Desk Reference* (PDR); medication package inserts; and pharmacists are valuable resources. Nurses are responsible for knowing as much as possible about each medication given.

Diet History. A diet history reveals a patient's normal eating patterns and food preferences. An effective dosage schedule is planned around them. Teach the patient to avoid foods that interact with medications. In addition, some medications are more effective when taken with meals; teach patients about specific medications that must be taken with food.

Patient's Perceptual or Coordination Problems. A patient with perceptual fine-motor or coordination limitations has difficulty self-administering medication. For example, a patient who takes insulin to manage blood glucose and has arthritis has difficulty manipulating a syringe. Assess the patient's ability to prepare doses and take medications correctly. If the patient is unable to self-administer medications, assess if family or friends are available to assist or make a home care referral.

Patient's Current Condition. The ongoing physical or mental status of a patient affects whether a medication is given or how it is administered. *Assess a patient carefully before giving any medication.* For example, check the patient's blood pressure before giving an antihypertensive. A patient who is nauseated is probably unable to swallow a tablet. Notify the patient's health care provider if he or she is unable to take a medication. Assessment findings serve as a baseline in evaluating the effects of medication therapy.

Patient's Attitude About Medication Use. The patient's attitude about medications sometimes reveals a level of medication dependence or drug avoidance. Some patients do not express their feelings about taking a particular medication, particularly if dependence is a problem. Observe the patient's behavior for evidence of dependence or avoidance. Also be aware that his or her cultural beliefs about Western medicine sometimes interfere with medication compliance (Box 31-9; see Chapter 9).

Patient's Understanding of and Adherence to Medication Therapy. The patient's knowledge and understanding of medication therapy influence the willingness or ability to follow a medication regimen. If the patient has a history of poor adherence (e.g., frequently missed doses or failure to fill prescriptions), investigate if he or she can afford prescribed medications and review resources available for purchase of medications if indicated. Also determine if the patient understands the purpose of the medication, the importance of regular dosage schedules, proper administration methods, and the possible side effects. Without adequate knowledge and motivation, adherence to medication schedules is unlikely.

Patient's Learning Needs. Health-related information is difficult to understand because of the use of technical terminology. Serious errors can occur when patients do not understand information about their medications. Assess patients' health literacy regarding medication administration to determine their need for instruction (Cornett, 2009) (see Chapter 25). Consider patient responses to assessment questions that you ask about medications such as those listed in Box 31-8. When a patient is unable to answer questions about medications appropriately, assess him or her for challenges in health literacy.

BOX 31-9 CULTURAL ASPECTS OF CARE

Influences in Medication Administration

Health beliefs vary by culture and often influence how patients manage and respond to drug therapy. Significant differences in values, beliefs, and attitudes affect a patient's adherence to drug therapy. For example, cultures attach different symbolic meanings to medications and drug therapy. Herbal remedies and alternative therapies are common in various cultures and ethnic groups and interfere with prescribed medications. People from some cultures stop taking medications when their symptoms are resolved, even if the medications are still needed for management of a chronic illness (Krueger, 2009; Qureshi, 2010). In addition, health beliefs often differ markedly between health providers and patients, which further affects a patient's compliance with medical therapy (Krueger, 2009). Demographic changes in both age and race are factors that affect nursing practice in medication administration. In addition to the psychosocial aspect of medication therapy, pharmacological research has shown that different ethnic and racial groups experience differences in drug response, metabolism, and side effects.

Implications for Practice

- Assess cultural beliefs, attitudes, and values when administering and teaching patients about their medications.
- Resolve conflicts between medications and cultural beliefs to achieve optimal patient outcomes.
- Investigate if the patient practices any alternative therapies or is taking any herbal preparations.
- Consider cultural influences on drug response, metabolism, and side effects if a patient is not responding to drug therapy as expected. A change in the patient's medication is sometimes necessary.
- Assess food preferences that may interfere with patients' medication therapy (Giger and Davidhizar, 2008).

NURSING DIAGNOSIS

Assessment provides data about the patient's condition, ability to self-administer medications, and medication adherence, which determine actual or potential problems with medication therapy. Certain data are defining characteristics that, when clustered together, reveal nursing diagnoses. For example, *ineffective self-health management related to complexity of medical regimen* is indicated when patients do not respond as expected to their medications and admit to having difficulty in managing them. This list of nursing diagnoses may apply to patients during the administration of medications:

- Anxiety
- Ineffective health maintenance
- Readiness for enhanced immunization status
- Deficient knowledge (medications)
- Noncompliance (medications)
- Disturbed visual sensory perception
- Impaired swallowing
- Effective therapeutic regimen management

After selecting the diagnosis, identify the related factor, which drives the selection of nursing interventions. In the example of *ineffective self-health management,* the related factor of inadequate resources versus lack of knowledge requires different interventions. If the patient's nursing diagnosis is related to inadequate finances, collaborate with family members, social workers, or community agencies to help him or her receive necessary medications. If the related factor is lack of knowledge, implement a teaching plan with appropriate follow-up.

PLANNING

Always organize your care activities to ensure the safe administration of medications. Hurrying to give patients medications leads to errors. It is important to minimize distractions or interruptions when preparing and administering medications (Brady, Malone, and Fleming, 2009).

Goals and Outcomes. Setting goals and related outcomes contributes to patient safety and allows for wise use of time during medication administration. For example, the nurse establishes the following goal and related outcomes for a patient with newly diagnosed type 2 diabetes:

Goal: The patient will safely administer all ordered medications before discharge.

Outcomes:

- The patient will verbalize understanding of desired and adverse effects of medications.
- The patient will state signs, symptoms, and treatment of hypoglycemia.
- The patient will be able to monitor blood glucose levels to determine if medication is appropriate to take or if a low blood glucose level should be treated.
- The patient will establish a daily routine that will coordinate timing of medication with mealtimes.

Setting Priorities. Prioritize care when administering medications. Use information gathered from the patient's assessment in determining which medications to give first and if it is appropriate to administer prn medications. For example, if a patient is in pain, it is important to provide pain medication as soon as possible. If the patient's blood pressure is elevated, administer the blood pressure medications before other medications. Nurses also prioritize when providing patient education about medications. Provide the most important information about the medications first. For example, hypoglycemia is a serious side effect of insulin. The patient taking insulin needs to be able to identify and treat hypoglycemia immediately; thus first teach him or her about the recognition and treatment of hypoglycemia before teaching about how to administer the injection.

Teamwork and Collaboration. Collaborate with a variety of health care providers when administering medications. First it is important to collaborate with the patient's family or friends whenever possible. Family members often reinforce the importance of medication regimens in the home setting. Nurses often collaborate with the prescriber, the pharmacist, and case managers to ensure that patients are able to afford their medications. On discharge ensure that patients know where and how to obtain medications. Be sure that patients are able to read medication labels and printed medication teaching sheets. Some patients also need to understand how to calculate dosages and prepare complex medication regimens. Collaborate with community resources (e.g., agency on aging, public health department, medical interpreters) when patients are illiterate or have difficulty understanding medication instructions (see Chapter 25).

IMPLEMENTATION

Health Promotion. In promoting or maintaining a patient's health, the nurse identifies factors that improve or diminish well-being. Health beliefs, personal motivations, socioeconomic factors, and habits (e.g., excessive alcohol intake) influence the patient's adherence with medications. Several nursing interventions promote adherence to the medication regimen and foster independence. Teach the patient and family about the benefit of a medication and the knowledge needed to take it correctly and integrate the patient's health beliefs and cultural practices into the treatment plan. Help the patient and family establish a medication routine that fits into the patient's normal schedule. Make referrals to community resources if the patient is unable to afford or cannot arrange transportation to obtain necessary medications.

Patient and Family Teaching. Patients may take medications incorrectly or not at all unless they are properly informed about them. Follow principles of patient education (see Chapter 25). Provide information about the purpose of medications and their actions and effects in a way that patients can understand. Many health care agencies offer easy-to-read teaching sheets about specific types of medications. Patients need to know how to take medications properly and the risks associated with failing to do so. For example, after receiving a prescription for an antibiotic, a patient needs to understand the importance of taking the full prescription. Failure to do this can lead to a worsening of the condition and the development of bacteria resistant to the medication.

Nurses teach patients how to correctly administer their medications. For example, teach a patient how to accurately measure a liquid medication. Provide special education to patients who depend on daily injections (Box 31-10). The patient learns to prepare and administer an injection correctly using aseptic technique. Teach family members or friends how to give injections in case the patient becomes ill or physically unable to handle a syringe. Provide specially designed equipment such as syringes with enlarged calibrated scales or medications with labels in Braille when patients have visual alterations.

Patients need to know the symptoms of medication side effects or toxicity. For example, patients taking anticoagulants learn to notify their health care providers immediately when signs of bleeding or bruising develop. Inform family members or friends of medication side effects such as changes in behavior because they are often the first persons to recognize such effects. Patients cope better with problems caused by medications if they understand how and when to act. All patients need to learn the basic guidelines for medication safety, which ensure the proper use and storage of medications in the home.

Acute Care. Patients are often hospitalized to receive expert nursing observation and documentation of responses to medications. When a nurse receives a medication order, several nursing interventions are essential for safe and effective medication administration.

Receiving, Transcribing, and Communicating Medication Orders. An order is required to administer any medication. Many health care agencies use CPOE. In these systems health care providers directly enter orders for their patients into the computer. Current evidence shows that CPOE helps to reduce medication errors and mortality rates (Longhurst et al., 2010). In the absence of CPOE, the health care provider handwrites orders onto an order sheet in the patient's chart. If orders are handwritten, be sure that medication names, dosages, and symbols are legible. Rewrite any unclear or illegible transcribed orders.

BOX 31-10 PATIENT TEACHING

Safe Insulin Administration

Objective

- Patient will correctly self-administer subcutaneous insulin.

Teaching Strategies

- Teach patient how to determine if insulin is expired.
- Instruct patient to keep medication in its original labeled container and refrigerated if needed.
- Demonstrate how to prepare a single insulin preparation.
- Assess visual acuity to ensure that patient is able to draw up the appropriate amount of insulin. Coach patient through the steps of administering subcutaneous insulin injection.
- Demonstrate how to rotate insulin injection sites.
- Help patient determine the amount of insulin required based on the results of home capillary glucose monitoring as ordered by the health care provider.
- Show patient how to keep a daily logbook for insulin injections, including results of home capillary glucose monitoring, type and amount of insulin given, expiration date on insulin vial, time of insulin injection, and injection site used.

Evaluation

- Ask patient to describe procedure used at home for determining the correct dose of insulin needed and injection site.
- Watch patient prepare insulin dose based on results of capillary glucose monitoring, select injection site, and self-administer injection.
- Review information recorded in patient logbook for completeness.
- If patient is unable to prepare the correct amount of insulin or self-administer safely, instruct a family caregiver and notify the health care provider.

The process of verifying medical orders varies among health care agencies. Nurses follow agency policy and current national patient safety standards when receiving, transcribing, and communicating medication orders. *Nursing students are prohibited from receiving verbal and telephone orders.*

Medication orders need to contain all of the elements in Box 31-11. If the medication order is incomplete, inform the prescriber and ensure completeness before carrying it out. Nurses read back verbal or telephone orders to the prescriber to ensure that the correct order is obtained. The registered nurse follows institutional policy regarding receiving, recording, and transcribing verbal and telephone orders. Generally the prescriber must sign them within 24 hours.

Nurses and pharmacists check all medication orders for accuracy and thoroughness several times during the transcription process. They also take patients' current problems, treatments, laboratory values, and other prescribed medications into consideration to determine if the ordered medication is safe and appropriate. Once the nurse and pharmacist determine that a medication order is safe and appropriate, it is placed on the appropriate medication form, usually called the *MAR*. The MAR is either printed out on paper or is available electronically. An electronic version of the MAR is called an *eMAR*. Whether it is handwritten, printed out from a computer, or in an electronic version, it includes the patient's name, room, and bed number, medical record number, medical and food allergies, other patient identifiers (e.g., birth date); and medication name, dose, frequency, and route and time of administration. Each time a medication dose is prepared, the nurse refers to the MAR.

BOX 31-11 COMPONENTS OF MEDICATION ORDERS

A medication order is incomplete unless it has the following parts:

Patient's full name: The patient's full name distinguishes the patient from other persons with the same last name. In the acute care setting patients are sometimes assigned special identification numbers (e.g., medical record number) to help distinguish patients with the same names. This number is often included on the order form.

Date and time that the order is written: The day, month, year, and time need to be included. Designating the time that an order is written helps clarify when certain orders are to start and stop. If an incident occurs involving a medication error, it is easier to document what happened when this information is available.

Medication name: The health care provider orders a medication by its generic or trade name. Correct spelling is essential in preventing confusion with medications with similar spelling.

Dose: The amount or strength of the medication is included.

Route of administration: The health care provider uses accepted abbreviations for medication routes. Accuracy is important to ensure that patients receive medications by the intended route.

Time and frequency of administration: The nurse needs to know what time and how frequently to administer medications. Orders for multiple doses establish a routine schedule for medication administration.

Signature of health care provider: The signature makes an order a legal request.

It is essential to verify the accuracy of every medication you give to your patients with the patients' orders. If the medication order is incomplete, incorrect, or inappropriate or if there is a discrepancy between the original order and the information on the MAR, consult with the prescriber. Do not give the medication until you are certain that you can follow the six rights of medication administration. When you give the wrong medication or an incorrect dose, *you* are legally responsible for the error.

Accurate Dose Calculation and Measurement. When measuring liquid medications, use standard measuring containers. The procedure for medication measurement is systematic to lessen the chance of error. Calculate each dose when preparing the medication, pay close attention to the process of calculation, and avoid interruptions from other people or nursing activities. Ask another nurse to double-check your calculations against the original medication order if you are *ever* in doubt about the accuracy of your calculation or if you are calculating a new or unusual dose.

Correct Administration. For safe administration follow the six rights of medication administration. Verify the patient's identity by using at least two patient identifiers (TJC, 2011a). In the acute care setting identifiers are usually on a patient's armband. Carefully compare the patient identifiers with the MAR to ensure that you are giving the medication to the right patient. When they are able, you can also ask patients to state their name as a third identifier. Use aseptic technique and proper procedures when handling and giving medications and perform necessary assessments (e.g., assess heart rate before giving antidysrhythmic medications) before administering a medication to a patient. Carefully monitor the patient's response to the medication, especially when he or she receives the first dose of a new medication.

Recording Medication Administration. Follow all agency policies when documenting medication administration. After administering a medication, record the name of the medication, dose, route, and exact time of administration immediately on the appropriate record form. Include the site of any injections per agency policy.

If a patient refuses a medication or is undergoing tests or procedures that result in a missed dose, explain the reason that the medication was not given in the nurses' notes. Some agencies require the nurse to circle the prescribed administration time on the medication record or to notify the health care provider when a patient misses a dose. Be aware of the effects that missing doses have on a patient (e.g., with hypertension or diabetes). Coordinating care with health care providers and other services when testing or diagnostic procedures are being completed helps to ensure patient safety and therapeutic control of the disease.

Restorative Care. Because of the numerous types of restorative care settings, medication administration activities vary. Patients with functional limitations often require a nurse to fully administer all medications. In the home care setting patients usually administer their own medications or receive assistance from family caregivers. Regardless of the type of medication activity, the nurse remains responsible for instructing patients and families in medication action, administration, and side effects. The nurse is also responsible for monitoring compliance with medication and determining the effectiveness of medications that have been prescribed.

Special Considerations for Administering Medications to Specific Age-Groups. A patient's developmental level is a factor for nurses to consider when administering medications. Knowledge of developmental needs helps you anticipate responses to medication therapy.

Infants and Children. Children vary in age; weight; surface area; and the ability to absorb, metabolize, and excrete medications. Children's doses are lower than those of adults; thus special caution is necessary when preparing medications for them. Medications are usually not prepared and packaged in standardized dose ranges for children. Preparing an ordered dose from an available amount requires careful calculation. In many pediatric settings the standard of practice is to have another nurse verify all pediatric dose calculations prior to administration.

All children require special psychological preparation before receiving medications. The child's parents are often valuable resources for determining the best way to give the child medication. Sometimes it is less traumatic for the child if a parent gives the medication and the nurse supervises. Supportive care is necessary if a child is expected to cooperate. Explain the procedure to a child, using words appropriate to his or her level of comprehension. Long explanations increase a child's anxiety, especially for painful procedures such as an injection. Involving the child in choices when possible usually results in greater success. For example, saying "It's time to take your tablet now. Do you want it with water or juice?" allows a child to make a choice. Do not give the child the option of not taking a medication. After giving a medication, praise him or her and even offer a simple reward such as a star or token. Tips for administering medication to children are in Box 31-12.

Older Adults. Older adults also require special consideration during medication administration (Box 31-13). In addition to physiological changes of aging (Fig. 31-9), behavioral and economic factors influence an older person's use of medications.

Polypharmacy. Polypharmacy happens when a patient takes two or more medications to treat the same illness, takes two or more medications from the same chemical class, uses two or more medications with the same or similar actions to treat several

BOX 31-12 TIPS FOR ADMINISTERING MEDICATIONS TO CHILDREN

Oral Medications

- Liquid forms are safer to swallow to avoid aspiration.
- Use droppers for administering liquids to infants; straws often help older children swallow pills.
- When mixing medications in other foods, use only a small amount. The child may refuse to take all of a larger mixture.
- Avoid mixing a medication with foods or liquids that the child is taking well because the child may in turn refuse them.
- A plastic, disposable oral syringe is the most accurate device for preparing liquid doses, especially those less than 10 mL. (Cups, teaspoons, and droppers are inaccurate.)
- When administering liquid medications, a spoon, plastic cup, or oral syringe (without needle) is useful.

Injections

- Use caution when selecting intramuscular (IM) injection sites. Infants and small children have underdeveloped muscles. Follow agency policy.
- Children are sometimes unpredictable and uncooperative. Make sure that someone (preferably another nurse) is available to restrain a child if needed. Have the parent act as a comforter, not restrainer, if restraint is necessary.
- Always awaken a sleeping child before giving an injection.
- Distracting the child with conversation, bubbles, or a toy reduces pain perception.
- If time allows, apply a lidocaine ointment to an injection site before the injection to reduce pain perception during the injection.

BOX 31-13 FOCUS ON OLDER ADULTS

Safety in Medication Administration

- Consult with prescriber to simplify the drug therapy plan whenever possible (Lehne, 2010).
- Keep instructions clear and simple and provide written material in large print (Lehne, 2010).
- Assess functional status to determine if patient will require assistance in taking medications (Ebersole et al., 2008).
- Provide memory aids (e.g., calendar, medication schedule) and written information about medications in print large enough for the patient to see (Ebersole et al., 2008).
- Some older adults have a greater sensitivity to drugs, especially those that act on the central nervous system. Therefore carefully monitor patients' responses to medications and anticipate dosage adjustments as needed (Ebersole et al., 2008).
- If patient has difficulty swallowing a capsule or tablet (Ebersole et al., 2008):
  - Ask the physician to substitute a liquid medication if possible.
  - Instruct patient to place medication on the front of the tongue and then swallow fluid to help wash it to the back of the throat; if patient continues to have problems, have him or her try taking medication with a small amount of semisolid food (e.g., applesauce).
- Teach alternatives to medications such as proper diet instead of vitamins and exercise instead of laxatives (Ebersole et al., 2008).
- Frequently review medication history, including over-the-counter medications (Ebersole et al., 2008).

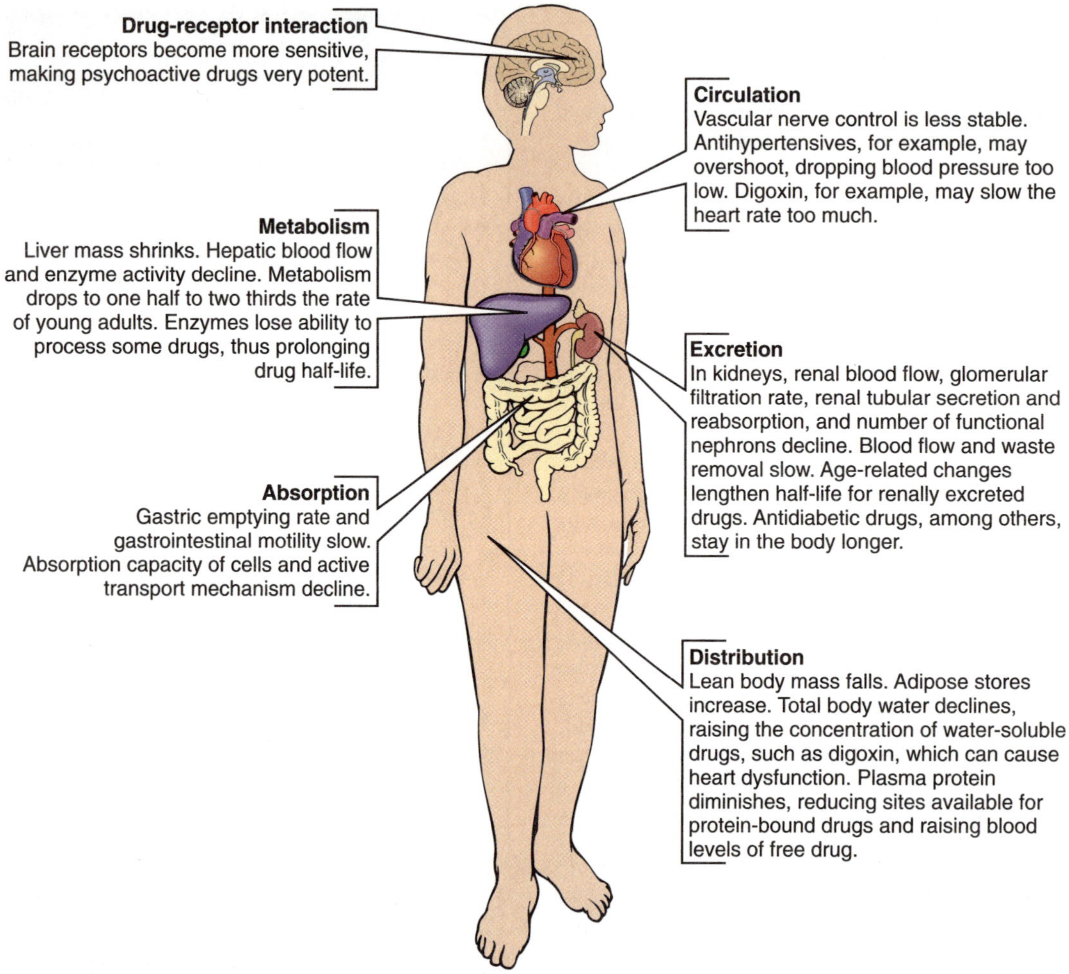
Drug-receptor interaction
Brain receptors become more sensitive, making psychoactive drugs very potent.
Circulation
Vascular nerve control is less stable. Antihypertensives, for example, may overshoot, dropping blood pressure too low. Digoxin, for example, may slow the heart rate too much.
Metabolism
Liver mass shrinks. Hepatic blood flow and enzyme activity decline. Metabolism drops to one half to two thirds the rate of young adults. Enzymes lose ability to process some drugs, thus prolonging drug half-life.
Excretion
In kidneys, renal blood flow, glomerular filtration rate, renal tubular secretion and reabsorption, and number of functional nephrons decline. Blood flow and waste removal slow. Age-related changes lengthen half-life for renally excreted drugs. Antidiabetic drugs, among others, stay in the body longer.
Absorption
Gastric emptying rate and gastrointestinal motility slow. Absorption capacity of cells and active transport mechanism decline.
Distribution
Lean body mass falls. Adipose stores increase. Total body water declines, raising the concentration of water-soluble drugs, such as digoxin, which can cause heart dysfunction. Plasma protein diminishes, reducing sites available for protein-bound drugs and raising blood levels of free drug.

FIG. 31-9 Effects of aging on medication metabolism. (From Lewis SM et al: *Medical-surgical nursing,* ed 7, St Louis, 2007, Mosby.)

disorders simultaneously, or mixes nutritional supplements or herbal products with medications (Ebersole et al., 2008; Maggiore, Gross, and Hurria, 2010). Older adults also often experience polypharmacy when they seek relief from a variety of symptoms (e.g., pain, constipation, insomnia, and indigestion) by using OTC preparations. Sometimes polypharmacy is unavoidable. For example, some patients need to take more than one medication to control their high blood pressure. When the patient experiences polypharmacy, the risk of adverse reactions and medication interactions with other medications and food is increased.

Because many older adults suffer chronic health problems, polypharmacy is common. However, it is also becoming more common in children and patients with mental illnesses. Taking OTC medications frequently, lack of knowledge about medications, incorrect beliefs about medications, and visiting several health care providers to treat different illnesses increase the risk for polypharmacy. To minimize risks associated with polypharmacy, frequent communication among health care providers is essential to make sure that the patients' medication regimen is as simple as possible.

EVALUATION

Evaluation of medication administration is an essential role of professional nursing that requires assessment skills; critical thinking; analysis; and knowledge of medications, physiology, and pathophysiology. Nurses thoroughly and accurately gather data and complete a holistic evaluation of their patients. The goal of safe and effective medication administration involves the patient's response to therapy and ability to assume responsibility for self-care. When patients do not experience expected outcomes of medication therapy, investigate possible reasons and determine appropriate revisions to the patient's plan of care.

Through the Patient's Eyes. Evaluation is more effective when you value your patients' participation. Therefore partner with your patients and include them in the evaluation process. Ensure that they understand and are able to safely administer their medications. For example, if you are caring for a child who needs an inhaler, be sure to watch the patient use the inhaler. To determine if patients understand their medication schedules, ask them to explain when they take their medications and if they are able to take them as prescribed. When patients struggle with their medication schedule, determine barriers to medication adherence (e.g., cost, lack of knowledge) and remove these barriers if possible. Also remember that patients have different values and define health differently. These values and beliefs influence their perception of the effectiveness of their medications. Therefore ask patients to describe this effectiveness. Ask if they are satisfied with their medications and how they make them feel. Use patients' statements and

TABLE 31-8 Example Evaluation for Patient Goals

GOAL	EXPECTED OUTCOMES	EVALUATIVE MEASURE WITH EXAMPLE
Patient and family will understand medication therapy.	Patient and family will describe information about medication, dosage, schedule, purpose, and adverse effects.	*Written measurement:* Have patient write out medication schedule for a 24-hour period. *Oral questioning:* Ask patient to describe purpose, dosage, and adverse effects of each prescribed medication.
	Patient and family will identify situations that require medical intervention.	*Oral questioning:* Have family describe what to do when a patient has adverse effects from a medication.
	Patient and family demonstrate appropriate administration technique.	*Direct observation:* Have patient demonstrate filling of an insulin syringe and self-injection.
Patient will safely self-administer medications.	Patient follows prescribed treatment regimen.	*Anecdotal notes:* Have family keep log of patient's adherence to therapy for 1 week.
	Patient performs administration techniques correctly.	*Direct observation:* Observe patient instill eyedrops.
	Patient identifies available resources for obtaining necessary medication.	*Oral questioning:* Ask family to identify how to contact local pharmacy or community clinic for necessary medications.

responses to questions (e.g., "I feel less anxious now") when determining the effectiveness of medications. Including patients in the evaluation process empowers them and helps them become more actively involved in their care.

Patient Outcomes. A patient's clinical condition can change minute by minute. Use knowledge of the desired effect and common side effects of each medication to compare expected outcomes with actual findings. A change in a patient's condition is often physiologically related to health status or results from medications or both. Be alert for reactions in a patient taking several medications. Nurses use a variety of measures to evaluate patient responses to medications such as direct observation of physiological measures (e.g., blood pressure or laboratory values), behavioral responses (e.g., agitation), and rating scales (e.g., rating on a pain scale). The type of measurement used varies with the action being evaluated, the reading skill and knowledge level of the patient, and the patient's cognitive and psychomotor ability. The most common type of measurement that the nurse uses is a physiological measure. Examples of physiological measures are blood pressure, heart rate, and visual acuity. Nurses also use patient statements as evaluative measures. Table 31-8 contains examples of goals, expected outcomes, and corresponding evaluative measures.

BOX 31-14 PROTECTING THE PATIENT FROM ASPIRATION

- Assess patient's ability to swallow and cough and check for presence of gag reflex.
- Prepare oral medications in the form that is easiest to swallow.
- Allow patient to self-administer medications if possible.
- If patient has unilateral weakness, place the medication in the stronger side of the mouth.
- Administer pills one at a time, ensuring that each medication is properly swallowed before the next one is introduced.
- Thicken regular liquids or offer fruit nectars if patient cannot tolerate thin liquids.
- Avoid straws because they decrease the control patient has over volume intake, which increases the risk of aspiration.
- Have patient hold and drink from a cup if possible.
- Time medications to coincide with mealtimes or when patient is well rested and awake if possible.
- Administer medications using another route if risk of aspiration is severe.

MEDICATION ADMINISTRATION

A sound knowledge base is required for medications to be administered safely. Nurses need to be prepared to administer medications using a variety of routes. The following sections explain the steps involved in administering medications using various routes.

Oral Administration

The easiest and most desirable way to administer medications is by mouth (Skill 31-1 on pp. 612-615). Patients usually are able to ingest or self-administer oral medications with a minimum of problems. Food delays stomach emptying, which may decrease the therapeutic effects of oral medications. Therefore most oral medications reach their therapeutic action best if given 30 minutes to 1 hour before meals. In addition, some medications must be taken with food. Some situations contraindicate the patient's receiving medications by mouth (see Table 31-5). Many medications interact with nutritional and herbal supplements. You need to be knowledgeable about these interactions to determine the best time to give oral medications.

An important precaution to take when administering any oral preparation is to protect patients from aspiration. Aspiration occurs when food, fluid, or medication intended for GI administration inadvertently enters the respiratory tract. Protect the patient from aspiration by assessing his or her ability to swallow. Box 31-14 provides techniques that protect patients from aspirating. Proper positioning is essential in preventing aspiration. Position a patient in a seated position at a 90-degree angle when administering oral medications if not contraindicated by his or her condition. Usually having the patient slightly flex the head in a chin-down position reduces aspiration. Use a multidisciplinary approach (e.g., speech therapist, dietitian, and occupational therapist) with patients who have difficulty swallowing (Eisenstadt, 2010).

Special consideration is needed when administering medications to patients with enteral or small-bore feeding tubes (Box 31-15). Failing to follow current evidence-based recommendations from the American Society for Parenteral and Enteral Nutrition (ASPEN) can result in tube obstruction, reduced medication effectiveness, and increased risk of medication toxicity (Boullata, 2009). Before giving a medication by this route, verify that the location of the tube (e.g., stomach or jejunum) is compatible with medication absorption. For example, iron dissolves in the stomach and is mostly absorbed in the duodenum. If iron is administered through a jejunal tube, it has poor bioavailability. Use liquid medications when possible. When liquid medications are not available, crush simple tablets or open gelatin capsules and dilute them in sterile water. Do not use tap water (Bankhead et al., 2009). Tap water often contains contaminants (e.g., pathogens, heavy metals) that can interact with a medication and affect its bioavailability (Boullata, 2009). Only use oral syringes when preparing medications for this route to prevent accidental parenteral administration. Flush tubes with at least 15 mL of sterile water before and after giving medications. When administering more than one medication at a time, give each separately and flush between medications with at least 15 mL of sterile water (Bankhead et al., 2009). Determine if medications need to be given on an empty stomach or if they are compatible with the patient's enteral feeding. If a medication needs to be given on an empty stomach or is not compatible with the feeding (e.g., phenytoin, carbamazepine [Tegretol], warfarin [Coumadin], fluoroquinolones, proton pump inhibitors), the feeding

BOX 31-15 PROCEDURAL GUIDELINES

View Video!

Giving Medications Through an Enteral Tube (Nasogastric Tube, G-tube, J-Tube, or Small-Bore Feeding Tube)

Delegation Considerations

The skill of giving medications through an enteral tube cannot be delegated to nursing assistive personnel (NAP). Instruct the NAP about:

- Potential side effects of medications and reporting their occurrence to the nurse.

Equipment

60-mL Oral syringe, gastric pH test strips (scale of 1.0 to 11.0 or greater), graduated container, sterile water, medication to be administered, pill crusher if medication in tablet form, medication administration record (MAR) (electronic or printed), clean gloves

1. Check accuracy and completeness of each MAR with prescriber's medication order. Check patient's name and medication name, dosage, and route and time of administration. Recopy or reprint any portion of printed MAR that is difficult to read.
2. Assess patient's knowledge about medication. Also assess medical history and for history or allergies to medications and foods. Make sure that patient's food and drug allergies are listed on the MAR and are prominently displayed on the patient's medical record per agency policy.
3. Avoid complicated medication regimens that frequently interrupt enteral feedings. Investigate and use alternative routes of medication administration if possible (e.g., intravenous, transdermal, rectal).
   a. Evaluate where medication is absorbed and ensure that point of absorption is not bypassed by feeding tube. For example, some medications (e.g., antacids) are absorbed in the stomach. If the patient's tube is placed in the intestines, these medications are not absorbed because the stomach is bypassed by the tube (Williams, 2008).
   b. Determine if medication interacts with enteral feeding. If interaction occurs, hold the feeding for at least 30 minutes before giving the medication (see agency policy or consult with pharmacist or drug reference).
4. Perform hand hygiene and prepare medication (see Skill 31-1, Steps 1a to 1g). Check label of medication with MAR two times for accuracy. *This is the first and second accuracy check.*
   a. Prepare medications in a liquid form (suspension, elixir, or solution) when possible to prevent tube obstruction (Bankhead et al., 2009).
   b. Before crushing tablets, be sure that they are crushable. Buccal, sublingual, enteric-coated or sustained-release medications cannot be crushed (Williams, 2008).
5. *Never* add medications directly to a tube feeding (Bankhead et al., 2009). Sometimes the tube feeding needs to be held. Verify this and the amount of time that you hold a feeding with agency policy, a pharmacist, or a medication reference before administering the medication to maximize the therapeutic effect of the medication (Bankhead et al., 2009; Williams, 2008).
6. Take medications to patient at correct time (see agency policy). Give time-critical, STAT, and single-order medications at the time ordered. Perform hand hygiene.
7. Identify the patient using at least two patient identifiers (e.g., name and birth date or name and account number) according to facility policy. Compare identifiers with information on the patient's medical record.
8. Compare label of medications against MAR one more time at patient's bedside. *This is the third accuracy check.*
9. Explain procedure and medications to patient.
10. Grind simple compressed tablets to a fine powder. Open hard gelatin capsules and pour powder into a medication cup. Dissolve crushed tablets, contents of capsules, and powders in 15 to 30 mL of sterile water. Dissolve each medication separately (Bankhead et al., 2009).
11. Do not give whole or undissolved medications through the feeding tube (Williams, 2008).
12. Put on clean gloves. NOTE: If patient has a latex allergy, use latex-free gloves.
13. Stop feeding if applicable and verify placement of any feeding tube that enters the mouth or nose using pH testing (see Chapter 44).
14. Assess gastric residual (see Chapter 44).
15. Flush tube with at least 15 mL of sterile water.
16. Draw up medication in syringe. Do ***not*** mix medications together (Bankhead et al., 2009).
17. Connect syringe with medication to nasogastric tube, G-tube, J-tube, or small-bore feeding tube. Do not use pigtail vent.
18. Administer medication by either pushing the medication through the tube with the syringe or allowing it to flow into the body freely using gravity. Administer each medication separately. If resistance is felt when pushing medication through the tube, stop administration and contact the patient's health care provider.
19. Flush tube with at least 15 mL of sterile water between each medication (Bankhead et al., 2009).
20. After giving all the medications, flush tube with at least 15 mL of sterile water (Bankhead et al., 2009).
21. Restart tube feeding if appropriate; hold feeding for 30 minutes or longer if needed to avoid alterations in medication bioavailability (Bankhead et al., 2009).
22. Clean area and put supplies away. Remove gloves and perform hand hygiene.
23. Document administration of medications, dose, route, and time on MAR.
24. Evaluate patient's response to the medication at times that correspond with onset, peak and duration of the medication. If the desired effect is not achieved, a different medication or route of administration is probably indicated because of problems with the drug bioavailability when given the enteral route. If patient self-administers medications, evaluate his or her ability to give them and technique used. Provide and reinforce medication as needed.

needs to be held at least 30 minutes before or 30 minutes after medication administration (Boullata, 2009). Verify the time with a drug reference or consult with a pharmacist. Monitor the patient closely for adverse reactions. The risk for drug-drug interactions is high when two or more medications are given in this route because they can interact together as soon as they are administered.

Topical Medication Applications

Topical medications are medications that are applied locally, most often to intact skin. They come in many forms (see Table 31-1). They are also applied to mucous membranes.

Skin Applications. Because many locally applied medications such as lotions, pastes, and ointments create systemic and local effects, apply these medications using gloves and applicators. Use sterile technique if the patient has an open wound. Skin encrustation and dead tissues harbor microorganisms and block contact of medications with the tissues to be treated. Before applying medications, clean the skin thoroughly by washing the area gently with soap and water, soaking an involved site, or locally debriding tissue.

Apply each type of medication according to directions to ensure proper penetration and absorption. When applying ointments or pastes, spread the medication evenly over the involved surface and cover the area well without applying an overly thick layer. Prescribers sometimes order a gauze dressing to be applied over the medication to prevent soiling clothes and wiping away the medication. Lightly spread lotions and creams onto the surface of the skin; rubbing often causes irritation. Apply a liniment by rubbing it gently but firmly into the skin. Dust a powder lightly to cover the affected area with a thin layer.

Some topical medications are applied in the form of a transdermal patch that remains in place for an extended amount of time (e.g., 12 hours or 7 days). Before applying a new patch, remove the old one. Medication remains on the patch even after its recommended duration of use. Nurses and patients have inadvertently left old transdermal patches in place, resulting in the patient receiving an overdose of the medication. For example, patients who use fentanyl transdermal patches for pain management can experience respiratory depression, coma, and death when the patches are not removed. Many patches are clear, which makes them difficult to see. Therefore carefully assess the patient's skin and be sure to remove the existing patch before applying a new patch. Follow these guidelines to ensure safe administration of transdermal or topical medications (ISMP, 2007b):

- Document the location on the patient's body where the medication was placed on the MAR.
- When applying a transdermal patch, ask the patient if he or she has an existing patch.
- When taking a medication history or reconciling medications, specifically ask the patient if he or she takes any medications in the forms of patches, topical creams, or any route other than the oral route.
- If the dressing or patch is difficult to see (e.g., clear), apply a noticeable label to the patch.
- Document removal of the patch or medication on the MAR.

Nasal Instillation. Patients with nasal sinus alterations sometimes receive medications by spray, drops, or tampons (Box 31-16). The most commonly administered form of nasal instillation is decongestant spray or drops, used to relieve symptoms of sinus congestion and colds. Caution patients to avoid abuse of medications because overuse leads to a rebound effect in which the nasal congestion worsens. When excess decongestant solution is swallowed, serious systemic effects also develop, especially in children.

BOX 31-16 PROCEDURAL GUIDELINES

Administering Nasal Instillations

Delegation Considerations

The skill of administering nasal instillations cannot be delegated to nursing assistive personnel (NAP). Instruct the NAP about:

- Potential side effects of medications and reporting their occurrence.

Equipment

Prepared medication with clean dropper or spray container, facial tissue, small pillow (optional), washcloth (optional), clean gloves (if patient has extensive nasal drainage), medication administration record (MAR) (electronic or printed), penlight

1. Check accuracy and completeness of each MAR with prescriber's medication order. Check patient's name and medication name, dosage, and route and time of administration. Recopy or reprint any portion of printed MAR that is difficult to read.
2. Refer to the medical record to determine which sinus is affected if giving nasal drops.
3. Assess patient's medical history (e.g., history of hypertension, heart disease, diabetes mellitus, hyperthyroidism) and for history or allergies to medications and foods. Make sure that patient's food and drug allergies are listed on the MAR and prominently displayed on his or her medical record per agency policy.
4. Perform hand hygiene. Using a penlight, inspect condition of nose and sinuses. Palpate sinuses for tenderness (see Chapter 30).
5. Assess patient's knowledge regarding use of nasal instillation, technique for instillation, and willingness to learn self-administration.
6. Review pertinent information related to medication: action, purpose, normal dose and route, side effects, time of onset and peak action, and nursing implications.
7. Perform hand hygiene and prepare medication (see Skill 31-1, Steps 1a to 1g). Compare medication label against MAR at least two times while preparing medication. *This is the first and second accuracy check.*
8. Take medication to patient at correct time (see agency policy). Perform hand hygiene.
9. Identify the patient using two patient identifiers (e.g., name and birth date or name and account number) according to facility policy. Compare identifiers with information on the patient's medical record.
10. Compare names of medication on label with MAR one more time at patient's bedside. *This is the third accuracy check.*
11. Explain procedure to patient regarding positioning and sensations to expect such as burning or stinging of mucosa or choking sensation as medication trickles into throat.
12. Arrange supplies and medications at bedside. Apply clean gloves if patient has nasal drainage. NOTE: If patient has a latex allergy, use latex-free gloves.
13. Gently roll or shake container.
14. Instruct patient to clear or blow nose gently unless contraindicated (e.g., risk of increased intracranial pressure or nosebleeds).
15. *Administer nasal drops:*

Continued

BOX 31-16 **PROCEDURAL GUIDELINES**

***Administering Nasal Instillations*—cont'd**

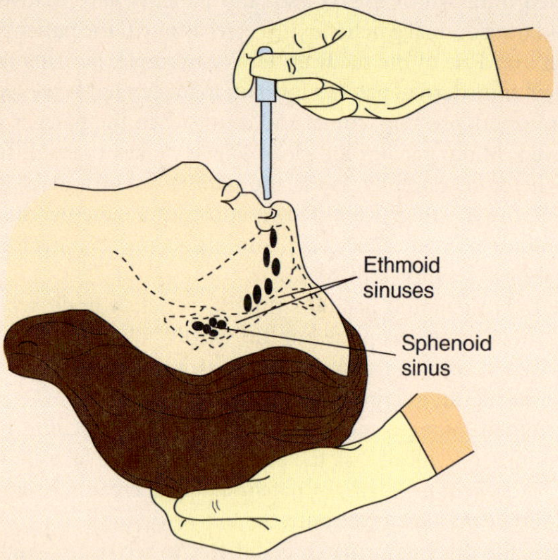

STEP 15a(2) Position for instilling nose drops into ethmoid or sphenoid sinus.

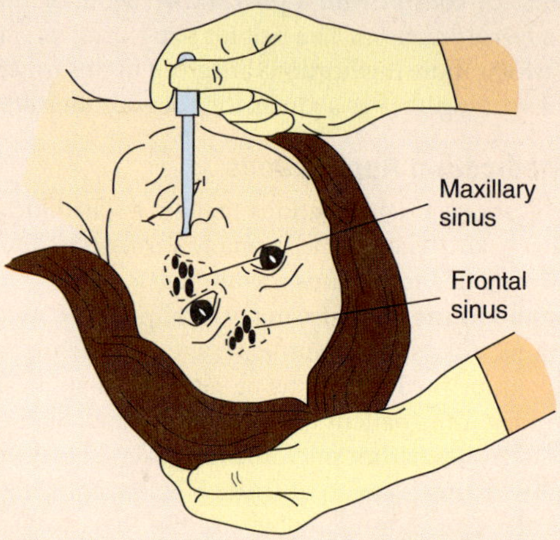

STEP 15a(3) Position for instilling nose drops into frontal and maxillary sinus.

a. Help patient to supine position and position head properly.
 (1) For access to posterior pharynx, tilt patient's head backward.
 (2) For access to ethmoid or sphenoid sinus, tilt head back over edge of bed or place small pillow under patient's shoulder and tilt head back (see illustration).
 (3) For access to frontal and maxillary sinus, tilt head back over edge of bed or pillow with head turned toward side to be treated (see illustration).
b. Support patient's head with nondominant hand.
c. Instruct patient to breathe through mouth.
d. Hold dropper 1 cm (½ inch) above nares and instill prescribed number of drops toward midline of ethmoid bone.
e. Have patient remain in supine position 5 minutes.
f. Offer facial tissue to blot runny nose but caution patient against blowing nose for several minutes.

16. *Administer nasal spray:*
 a. Help patient to supine position and position head slightly tilted forward.
 b. Help patient place spray nozzle into appropriate nares, pointing the nozzle to the side and away from the center of the nose.
 c. Have patient spray medication into the nose while inhaling.
 d. Help patient take nozzle out of nose and instruct him or her to breathe out through the mouth.
 e. Offer facial tissue but caution patient against blowing nose for several minutes.
17. Assist patient to a comfortable position after medication is absorbed.
18. Dispose of soiled supplies in proper container and perform hand hygiene.
19. Document name of medication, dose, route, and time of administration on MAR.
20. Observe patient for onset of side effects 15 to 30 minutes after administration. Ask if he or she is able to breathe through nose after decongestant administration. It may be necessary to have patient occlude one nostril at a time and breathe deeply.
21. Evaluate patient's response to medications at times that correlate with the onset, peak, and duration of the medication. Evaluate patient for both desired effect and adverse effects. Reinspect condition of nasal passages between instillations.
22. Ask patient to review risks of overuse of decongestants and methods for administration.
23. Have patient demonstrate self-medication.

Saline drops are safer than nasal preparations that contain sympathomimetics (e.g., Afrin or Neo-Synephrine) as a decongestant for children.

It is easier to have the patient self-administer sprays because he or she is able to control the spray and inhale as it enters the nasal passages. For patients who use nasal sprays repeatedly, check the nares for irritation. Nasal drops are effective in treating sinus infections. Position patients to permit the medication to reach the affected sinus. Severe nosebleeds are usually treated with packing or nasal tampons, which are treated with epinephrine, to reduce blood flow. Usually a physician or advanced practice clinician places nasal tampons.

Eye Instillation. Common medications used by patients are eyedrops and ointments, including OTC preparations such as artificial tears and vasoconstrictors (e.g., Visine and Murine). Many patients, especially older adults, receive prescribed **ophthalmic** medications for eye conditions such as glaucoma or after cataract extraction. Age-related problems, including poor vision, hand tremors, and difficulty grasping or manipulating containers, affect the older adult's ability to self-administer eye medications. Instruct patients and family members about the proper techniques for administering them (Skill 31-2 on pp. 616-619). Determine the patient's and family's ability to self-administer through a return demonstration of the procedure. Showing patients each step of the procedure for instilling eyedrops can improve adherence. Follow these principles when administering eye medications:

- Avoid instilling any form of eye medications directly onto the cornea. The cornea of the eye has many pain fibers and thus is very sensitive to anything applied to it.
- Avoid touching the eyelids or other eye structures with eyedroppers or ointment tubes. The risk of transmitting infection from one eye to the other is high.
- Use eye medication only for the patient's affected eye.
- Never allow a patient to use another patient's eye medications.

BOX 31-17 PROCEDURAL GUIDELINES

View Video!

Administering Ear Medications

Delegation Considerations

The skill of administering ear medications cannot be delegated to nursing assistive personnel (NAP). Instruct the NAP about:

- Potential side effects and the need to report their occurrence.

Equipment

Medication administration record (MAR) (electronic or printed), clean gloves, and washcloth if patient has drainage from the ear; *for drops:* medication bottle with dropper, cotton-tipped applicator, cotton ball (optional); *for irrigation:* irrigating syringe, kidney-shaped basin, towel

1. Check accuracy and completeness of each MAR with prescriber's medication order. Check patient's name and medication name, dosage, and route and time of administration. Recopy or reprint any portion of printed MAR that is difficult to read.
2. Assess patient's medical history (e.g., history of dizziness, hearing loss) and allergies to medications, food, and latex.
3. Perform hand hygiene. Prepare medication (see Skill 31-1, Steps 1a to 1g). Check label of medication with MAR two times for accuracy. *This is the first and second accuracy check.*
4. Take medication to patient at correct time (see agency policy). Perform hand hygiene.
5. Identify the patient using two identifiers (e.g., name and birth date or name and account number) according to facility policy. Compare identifiers with information on the patient's medical record.
6. Compare names of medications on label with the MAR one more time at the patient's bedside. *This is the third accuracy check.* Hold medication container in hands for a few minutes to bring medication to body temperature.
7. Explain procedure to patient regarding positioning and sensations to expect such as hearing bubbling or feeling water in ear as medication trickles into ear.
8. Teach patient about medication.
9. Administer eardrops:
   a. Apply clean gloves and gently clean outer ear with washcloth if drainage is present. NOTE: If patient has a latex allergy, use latex-free gloves.
   b. Place patient in side-lying position (if not contraindicated by his or her condition) with ear to be treated facing up or have him or her sit in chair or at the bedside. If eardrops are a cloudy suspension, shake them for about 10 seconds.
   c. Straighten ear canal by pulling auricle down and back (children younger than 3 years) or upward and outward (children 4 years of age and older and adults).
   d. Instill prescribed drops holding dropper 1 cm (½ inch) above ear canal (see illustration).

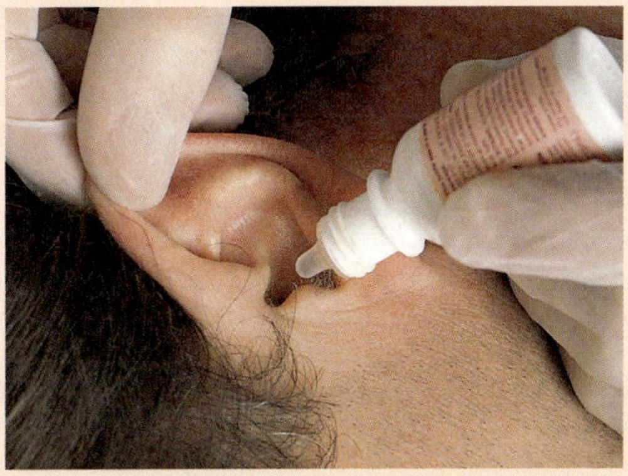

STEP 9d Placing eardrop in ear.

   e. Ask patient to remain in side-lying position 2 to 3 minutes. Apply gentle massage or pressure to tragus of ear with finger unless contraindicated because of pain.
   f. If cotton ball is needed, place it into outermost part of canal. Do not press cotton deep into canal. Remove it after 15 minutes.
10. Clean the area and put supplies away.
11. Remove gloves and perform hand hygiene.
12. Document medication administration on MAR.
13. Evaluate patient's response to the medication at times that correspond with its onset, peak, and duration.

Intraocular Administration. The nurse administers some medications intraocularly (see Skill 31-2). Medications delivered this way resemble a contact lens. Place the medication into the conjunctival sac where it remains in place for up to 1 week. Medications such as pilocarpine are administered this way. Patients require teaching about monitoring for adverse reactions to the disk. They also need to know how to insert and remove the disk.

Ear Instillation. Internal ear structures are very sensitive to temperature extremes. Instill eardrops at room temperature to prevent vertigo, dizziness, or nausea. Although the structures of the outer ear are not sterile, sterile solutions are used in case the eardrum is ruptured. The entrance of nonsterile solutions into middle ear structures can result in infection. If a patient has ear drainage, be sure that the eardrum has not ruptured. Never occlude or block the ear canal with the dropper or irrigating syringe. Forcing medication into an occluded ear canal creates pressure that injures the eardrum. Box 31-17 provides guidelines for administering eardrops.

Vaginal Instillation. Vaginal medications are available as suppositories, foam, jellies, or creams. Solid, oval-shaped suppositories come individually packaged in foil wrappers and are sometimes stored in the refrigerator to prevent them from melting. After a suppository is inserted into the vaginal cavity, body temperature causes it to melt and be distributed and absorbed. Foam, jellies, and creams are administered with an applicator inserter (Box 31-18). Give a suppository with a gloved hand in accordance with standard precautions (see Chapter 28). Patients often prefer administering their own vaginal medications and need privacy. Because vaginal medications are often given to treat infection, discharge is usually foul smelling. Follow aseptic technique and offer the patient frequent opportunities to maintain perineal hygiene (see Chapter 39).

Rectal Instillation. Rectal suppositories are thinner and more bullet-shaped than vaginal suppositories. The rounded end prevents anal trauma during insertion. Rectal suppositories contain medications that exert local effects such as promoting defecation or systemic effects such as reducing nausea. Rectal suppositories are often stored in the refrigerator until administered. Sometimes it is necessary to clear the rectum with a small cleansing enema before inserting a suppository (Box 31-19).

BOX 31-18 PROCEDURAL GUIDELINES

Administering Vaginal Medications

Delegation Considerations

The skill of administering vaginal medications cannot be delegated to nursing assistive personnel (NAP). Instruct the NAP to:

- Report new or increased vaginal discharge or bleeding and occurrence of potential side effects of medications.

Equipment

Vaginal cream, foam, jelly, or suppository with applicator (if required); clean gloves; towels and/or washcloth; perineal pad; drape or sheet; water-soluble lubricating jelly; medication administration record (MAR) (electronic or printed)

1. Check accuracy and completeness of each MAR with prescriber's medication order. Check patient's name and medication name, form (cream or suppository), dosage, and route and time of administration. Recopy or reprint any portion of printed MAR that is difficult to read.
2. Assess patient's medical history (e.g., history of vaginal drainage) and allergies to medications, food, and latex.
3. Perform hand hygiene. Prepare medication (see Skill 31-1, Steps 1a to 1g). Check name of medication on label with MAR two times for accuracy. *This is the first and second accuracy check.*
4. Take medication to patient at the correct time (see agency policy). Perform hand hygiene.
5. Identify patient using two patient identifiers (e.g., name and birth date or name and account number) according to facility policy. Compare identifiers with information on patient's medical record.
6. Compare names of medication on label with the MAR one more time at patient's bedside. *This is the third accuracy check.*
7. Teach patient about the medication. Explain procedure regarding positioning and sensations to expect such as feelings of moisture or wetness in the vaginal area. Assess patient's ability to manipulate applicator or suppository and position self to insert medication. Be sure that patient understands the procedure if she plans to self-administer the medication.
8. Close room door or pull curtain to provide privacy.
9. Put on clean gloves. NOTE: If patient has a latex allergy, use latex-free gloves.
10. Be sure that lighting is adequate to visualize vaginal opening. Inspect condition of external genitalia and vaginal canal (see Chapter 30), noting appearance of any discharge. Clean area with towel or washcloth if necessary (see Chapter 39).
11. Help patient into dorsal recumbent position and keep abdomen and lower extremities draped.
12. Administer vaginal suppository:
    a. Remove suppository from foil wrapper and apply liberal amount of sterile, water-based lubricating jelly to the smooth or rounded end. Lubricate gloved index finger of dominant hand.
    b. With nondominant gloved hand expose vaginal orifice by gently retracting labial folds.
    c. With dominant gloved hand gently insert rounded end of suppository along posterior wall of vaginal canal entire length of finger (7.5 to 10 cm [3 to 4 inches]) to ensure equal distribution of medication along walls of vaginal cavity (see illustration).
    d. Withdraw finger and wipe away remaining lubricant from around orifice and labia.
13. Administer cream or foam:
    a. Fill cream or foam applicator following package directions.
    b. With nondominant gloved hand, expose vaginal orifice by gently retracting labial folds.
    c. With dominant gloved hand, insert applicator approximately 5 to 7.5 cm (2 to 3 inches). Push applicator plunger to deposit medication into vagina to allow equal distribution of medication (see illustration).

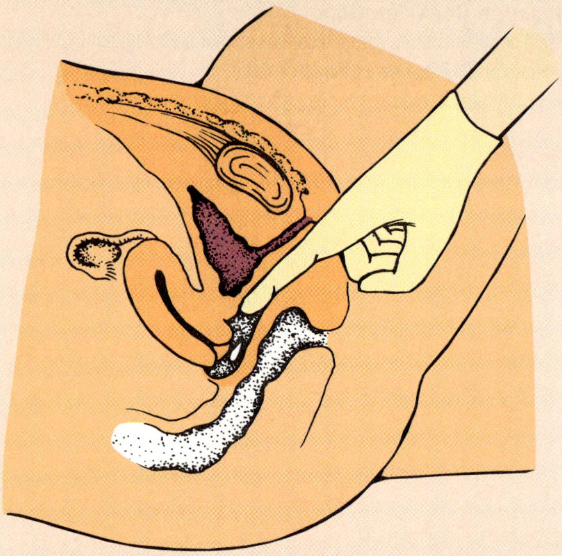

STEP 12c Insertion of suppository into vaginal canal.

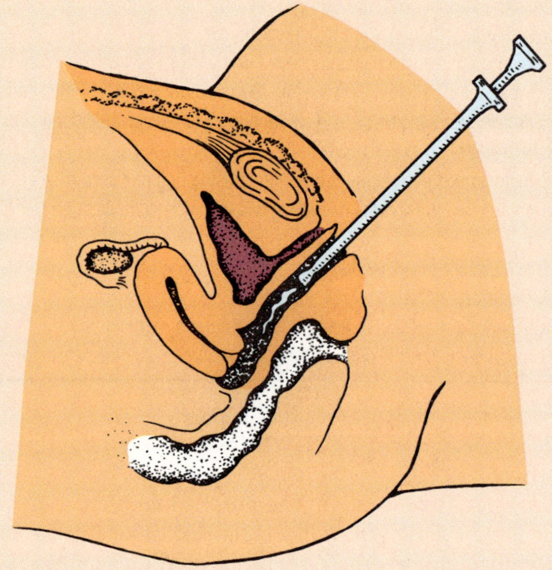

STEP 13c Instillation of medication in vaginal canal.

    d. Withdraw applicator and place on paper towel. Wipe off residual cream from labia or vaginal orifice.
14. Dispose of supplies, remove gloves, and perform hand hygiene.
15. Instruct patient to remain on back for at least 10 minutes to allow medication to be distributed and absorbed evenly throughout vaginal cavity and not lost through orifice.
16. Document medication administration on MAR.
17. If using an applicator, wearing gloves, wash with soap and warm water, rinse, and store for future use.
18. Offer patient perineal pad when she resumes ambulation.
19. Evaluate patient's response to medication at times that correspond with the onset, peak, and duration of the medication. Inspect appearance of discharge of vaginal canal and condition of external genitalia between applications.

BOX 31-19 PROCEDURAL GUIDELINES

Administering Rectal Suppositories

Delegation Considerations

The skill of administering rectal suppositories cannot be delegated to nursing assistive personnel (NAP). Instruct NAP to:

- Expect and report fecal discharge or bowel movement.
- Report occurrence of potential side effects of medications.

Equipment

Rectal suppository, water-soluble lubricating jelly, clean gloves, drape or sheet, tissue, medication administration record (MAR) (electronic or printed)

1. Check accuracy and completeness of each MAR with prescriber's medication order. Check patient's name and medication name, dosage, and route and time of administration. Recopy or reprint any portion of printed MAR that is difficult to read.
2. Review medical history (e.g., hemorrhoids, anal fissures, rectal surgery, or bleeding) and allergies to medications, food, and latex.
3. Perform hand hygiene and prepare medication (see Skill 31-1, Steps 1a to 1g). Compare names of medication on label with the MAR two times for accuracy. *This is the first and second accuracy check.*
4. Take medication to patient at the correct time and perform hand hygiene.
5. Identify patient using two patient identifiers (e.g., name and birth date or name and account number) according to facility policy. Compare identifiers with information on patient's medical record.
6. Compare names of medication on label with the MAR one more time at patient's bedside. *This is the third accuracy check.*
7. Teach patient about the medication. Explain procedure regarding positioning and sensations to expect such as feelings of needing to defecate. Be sure that patient understands the procedure if he or she is going to self-administer the medication.
8. Close room door or pull curtain to ensure privacy.
9. Put on clean gloves. NOTE: If patient has a latex allergy, use latex-free gloves.
10. Help patient to the Sims' position. Keep him or her draped with only anal area exposed.
11. Be sure that there is adequate lighting to visualize anus. Examine condition of anus externally and palpate rectal walls as needed (see Chapter 30). Dispose of gloves in proper receptacle if soiled.
12. Apply new pair of clean gloves (if previous gloves were soiled). NOTE: If patient has a latex allergy, use latex-free gloves.
13. Remove suppository from wrapper and lubricate rounded end (see illustration) with sterile water-soluble lubricating jelly. Lubricate index finger of dominant hand with a water-soluble lubricant.
14. Ask patient to take slow deep breaths through mouth and relax anal sphincter.
15. Retract buttocks with nondominant hand. Insert suppository gently through anus, past internal sphincter and against rectal wall, 10 cm (4 inches) in adults, 5 cm (2 inches) in children and infants (see illustration). Apply gentle pressure to hold buttocks together momentarily if needed to keep medication in place.

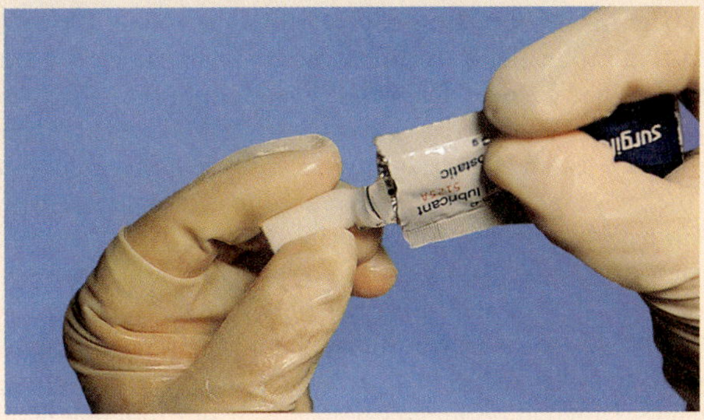

STEP 13 Remove suppository from wrapper.

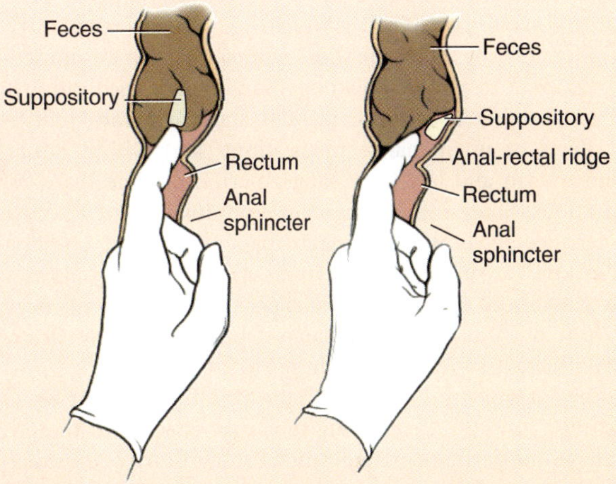

STEP 15 Inserting rectal suppository. (From deWit S: *Fundamental concepts and skills for nursing,* ed 3, Philadelphia, 2009, Saunders.)

16. Withdraw finger and wipe anal area with tissue.
17. Dispose of supplies, remove gloves, and perform hand hygiene.
18. Ask patient to remain flat or on side for at least 5 minutes to prevent expulsion of suppository.
19. Place call light within patient's reach.
20. Document medication administration on MAR.
21. Observe for effects of suppository (e.g., bowel movement, relief of nausea) at times that correlate with the onset, peak, and duration of the medication.

Administering Medications by Inhalation

Medications administered with handheld inhalers are dispersed through an aerosol spray, mist, or powder that penetrates lung airways. The alveolar-capillary network absorbs medications rapidly.

Pressurized metered-dose inhalers (pMDIs), breath-actuated metered dose inhalers (BAIs), and dry powder inhalers (DPIs) deliver medications that produce local effects such as bronchodilation. Some medications create serious systemic side effects. pMDIs use a chemical propellant to push the medication out of the inhaler and require the patient to apply approximately 5 to 10 pounds of pressure to the top of the canister to administer the medication. Children or older adults with chronic respiratory diseases often use pMDIs. These two populations have diminished hand strength. Therefore it is essential to assess if patients in these groups have enough strength to use the pMDI.

BAIs release medication when a patient raises a lever and inhales. Release of the medication depends on the strength of the patient's breath on inspiration and is a good choice for patients who have difficulty using pMDIs (Restrepo and Gardner, 2010).

DPIs hold dry powdered medication and create an aerosol when the patient inhales through a reservoir that contains a dose of the medication. Some DPIs are unit dosed. These inhalers require patients to load a single dose of medication into the inhaler with each use. Other DPIs hold enough medication to be used in 1 month. DPIs require less manual dexterity. Because the device is activated with the patient's breath, there is no need to coordinate puffs with inhalation. However, the medication inside the DPI can clump if the patient is in a humid climate, and some patients cannot inspire fast enough to administer the entire dose of the medication.

Patients who receive medications by inhalation frequently suffer chronic respiratory disease such as chronic asthma, emphysema, or bronchitis. Different respiratory problems require different inhaled medication. For example, patients with asthma usually receive antiinflammatory medications because asthma is primarily an inflammatory disease, whereas patients with chronic obstructive pulmonary disease (COPD) receive bronchodilators because they usually have problems with bronchoconstriction. Inhaled medications are also often described as "rescue" or "maintenance" medications. Rescue medications are short acting and taken for immediate relief of acute respiratory distress. Maintenance medications are used on a daily schedule to prevent acute respiratory distress. The effects of maintenance medications start within hours of administration and last for a longer period of time than rescue medications. Some inhalers contain combinations of rescue and maintenance medications. Because patients depend on inhaled medications for disease control and current evidence shows that many patients do not use their inhalers correctly, patients need to learn how to self-administer inhalers safely and effectively (Restrepo and Gardner, 2010) (Skill 31-3 on pp. 619-622).

Some patients use a spacer with the pMDI. The spacer is a 4- to 8-inch (10.16 to 20.32 cm) long tube that attaches to the pMDI and allows the particles of medication to slow down and break into smaller pieces, which improves drug absorption in the patient's airway. Spacers have a face mask for infants and children less than 4 years of age. They are especially helpful when the patient has difficulty coordinating the steps involved in self-administering inhaled medications. When patients do not use their inhalers and spacers correctly, they do not receive the full effect of the medication. Therefore patient education is essential. BAIs and DPIs do not use spacers.

One important aspect of patient teaching is to help the patient determine when the MDI, BAI, or DPI is empty and needs to be replaced. Floating the MDI in water to determine how much medication is left is no longer recommended because extra propellant causes the container to float even if no medication remains in the inhaler. Furthermore, non–ozone-depleting MDIs with hydrofluoroalkanes (HFAs) should never be immersed (Hess, 2008). Devices that count down the number of remaining doses are available for MDIs. Some DPIs have mechanisms that indicate how many doses are left. However, these mechanisms are not always accurate. Therefore, to calculate how long medication in an inhaler will last, divide the number of doses in the container by the number of doses the patient takes per day. For example, a patient is to take albuterol. The ordered dose is 2 puffs 4 times a day. The canister has a total of 200 puffs. Complete the following calculations to determine how long the MDI will last:

$$2 \text{ puffs} \times 4 \text{ times a day} = 8 \text{ puffs per day}$$
$$200 \text{ puffs} \div 8 \text{ puffs per day} = 25 \text{ days}$$

The canister in this example will last 25 days. To ensure that the patient does not run out of medication, teach him or her to refill it at least 7 to 10 days before it runs out.

BOX 31-20 PREVENTING INFECTION DURING AN INJECTION

- To prevent contamination of solution, draw medication from ampule quickly. Do not allow it to stand open.
- To prevent needle contamination, avoid letting needle touch contaminated surface (e.g., outer edges of ampule or vial, outer surface of needle cap, nurse's hands, countertop, table surface).
- To prevent syringe contamination, avoid touching length of plunger or inner part of barrel. Keep tip of syringe covered with cap or needle.
- To prepare skin, wash with soap and water if soiled with dirt, drainage, or feces and dry. Use friction and a circular motion while cleaning with an antiseptic swab. Swab from center of site and move outward in a 2-inch (5 cm) radius.

Administering Medications by Irrigations

Some medications irrigate or wash out a body cavity and are delivered through a stream of solution. Irrigations most commonly use sterile water, saline, or antiseptic solutions on the eye, ear, throat, vagina, and urinary tract. Use aseptic technique if there is a break in the skin or mucosa. Use clean technique when the cavity to be irrigated is not sterile, as in the case of the ear canal or vagina. Irrigations cleanse an area, instill a medication, or apply hot or cold to injured tissue (see Chapter 48).

Parenteral Administration of Medications

Parenteral administration of medications is the administration of medications by injection into body tissues. When medications are administered this way, it is an invasive procedure that is performed using aseptic techniques (Box 31-20). After a needle pierces the skin, there is risk of infection. Each type of injection requires certain skills to ensure that the medication reaches the proper location. The effects of a parenterally administered medication develop rapidly, depending on the rate of medication absorption. The nurse closely observes the patient's response.

Equipment. A variety of syringes and needles are available, each designed to deliver a certain volume of a medication to a specific type of tissue. Use nursing judgment when determining the syringe or needle that will be most effective.

Syringes. Syringes consist of a cylindrical barrel with a tip designed to fit the hub of a hypodermic needle and a close-fitting plunger. In general syringes are classified as being Luer-Lok or non–Luer-Lok. This nomenclature is based on the design of the tip of the syringe. Luer-Lok syringes have needles that are twisted onto the tip and lock themselves in place (Fig. 31-10, *A* and *B*). This design prevents the inadvertent removal of the needle. Non–Luer-Lok syringes (Fig. 31-10, C and *D*) have needles that slip onto the tip. Syringes have safety devices to prevent needlestick injury.

Syringes come in a number of sizes, from 0.5 to 60 mL. It is unusual to use a syringe larger than 5 mL for an injection. A 1- to 3-mL syringe is usually adequate for a subcutaneous or IM injection. A larger volume creates discomfort. Use larger syringes to administer certain IV medications and irrigate wounds or drainage tubes. Syringes often come prepackaged with a needle attached. However, you sometimes change a needle based on the route of administration and size of the patient.

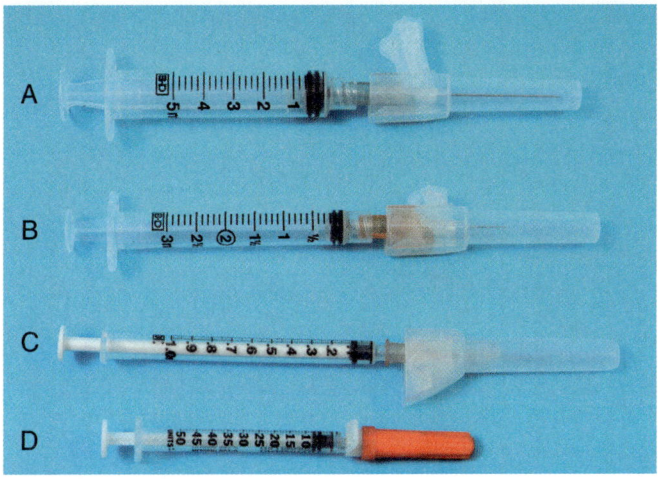

FIG. 31-10 Types of syringes. **A,** 5-mL syringe. **B,** 3-mL syringe. **C,** Tuberculin syringe marked in 0.01 (hundredths) for doses less than 1 mL. **D,** Insulin syringe marked in units (50).

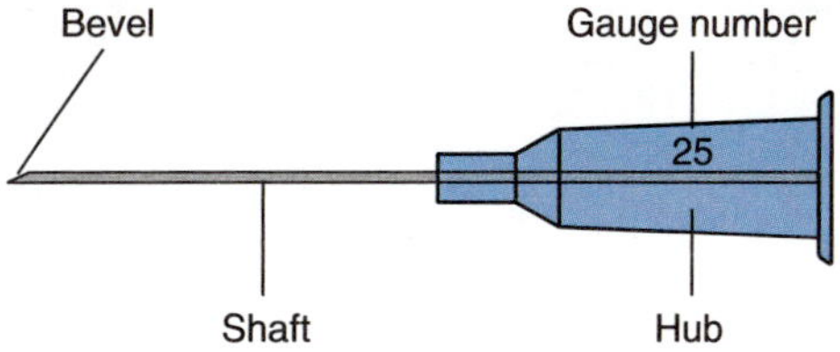

FIG. 31-12 Parts of the needle.

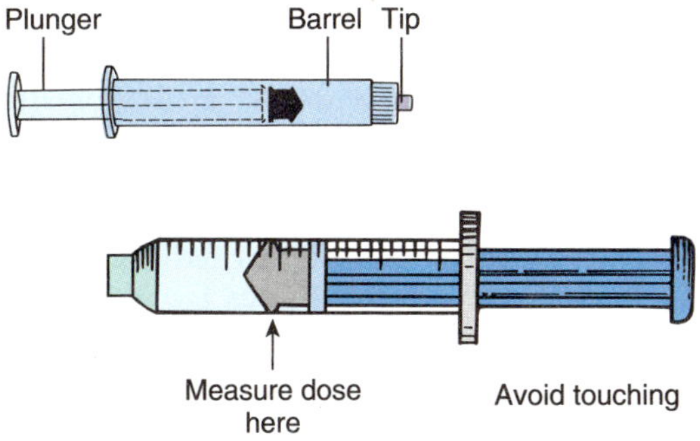

FIG. 31-11 Parts of a syringe.

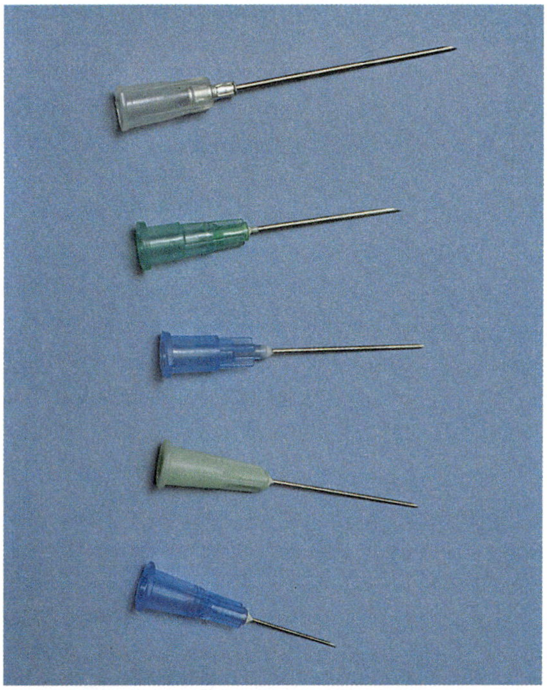

FIG. 31-13 Needles. Top to bottom: 19 gauge, 1½-inch length; 20 gauge, 1-inch length; 21 gauge, 1-inch length; 23 gauge, 1-inch length; and 25 gauge, ⅝-inch length.

The tuberculin syringe (Fig. 31-10, *C*) is calibrated in sixteenths of a minim and hundredths of a milliliter and has a capacity of 1 mL. Use a tuberculin syringe to prepare small amounts of medications (e.g., intradermal or subcutaneous injections). A tuberculin syringe is also useful when preparing small, precise doses for infants or young children.

Insulin syringes (Fig. 31-10, *D*) are available in sizes that hold 0.3 to 1 mL and are calibrated in units. Most insulin syringes are U-100s, designed to be used with U-100 strength insulin. Each milliliter of U-100 insulin contains 100 units of insulin.

Fill a syringe by pulling the plunger outward while the needle tip remains immersed in the prepared solution. Only touch the outside of the syringe barrel and the handle of the plunger to maintain sterility. Avoid letting any unsterile object touch the tip or inside of the barrel, the hub, the shaft of the plunger, or the needle (Fig. 31-11).

Needles. Some needles come packaged in individual sheaths to allow flexibility in choosing the right needle for a patient, whereas others are preattached to standard-size syringes. Most needles are made of stainless steel, and all are disposable. A needle has three parts: the hub, which fits onto the tip of a syringe; the shaft, which connects to the hub; and the bevel, or slanted tip (Fig. 31-12). The tip of a needle, or the bevel, is always slanted. The bevel creates a narrow slit when injected into tissue that quickly closes when the needle is removed to prevent leakage of medication, blood, or serum. Long beveled tips are sharper and narrower, minimizing discomfort when entering tissue used for subcutaneous or IM injections.

Most needles vary in length from ¼ to 3 inches (Fig. 31-13). Choose the needle length according to the patient's size and weight and the type of tissue into which the medication is to be injected. A child or slender adult generally requires a shorter needle. Use longer needles (1 to 1½ inches) for IM injections and a shorter needle (⅜ to ⅝ inch) for subcutaneous injections. As the needle gauge becomes smaller, the needle diameter becomes larger. The selection of a gauge depends on the viscosity of fluid to be injected or infused.

Disposable Injection Units. Disposable, single-dose, prefilled syringes are available for some medications. Be careful to check the medication and concentration because all prefilled syringes appear very similar. With these syringes you do not have to prepare

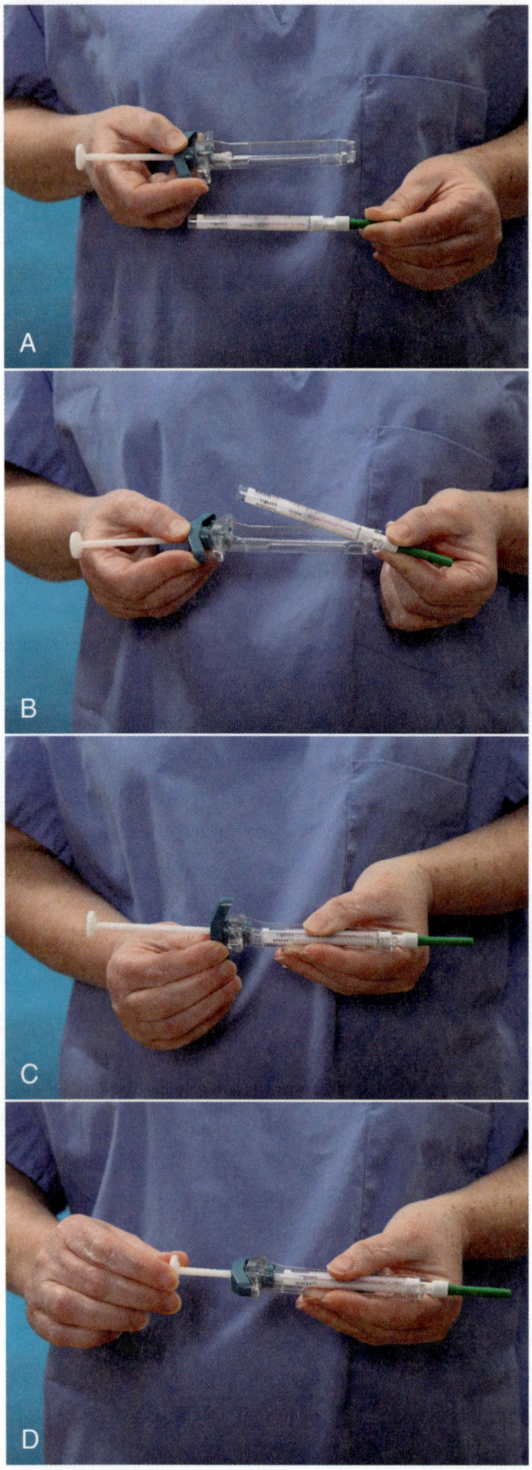

FIG. 31-14 **A,** Carpuject syringe and prefilled sterile cartridge with needle. **B,** Assembling the Carpuject. **C,** The cartridge slides into the syringe barrel. Turn and lock the syringe into the cartridge. **D,** Screw the plunger into the end of the cartridge. Expel excess medication to obtain accurate dose *(not pictured).*

medication doses, except perhaps to expel portions of unneeded medications.

The Tubex and Carpuject injection systems include reusable plastic mechanisms that hold prefilled, disposable, sterile cartridge-needle units (Fig. 31-14). Load the cartridge Luer tip first into the plastic syringe holder, secure it (following package directions), and check for air bubbles in the syringe. Advance the plunger to expel air and excess medication as in a regular syringe. The glass cartridge can be used with needleless systems or safety needles. After giving the medication, safely dispose of the glass cartridge in a puncture-proof and leak-proof receptacle.

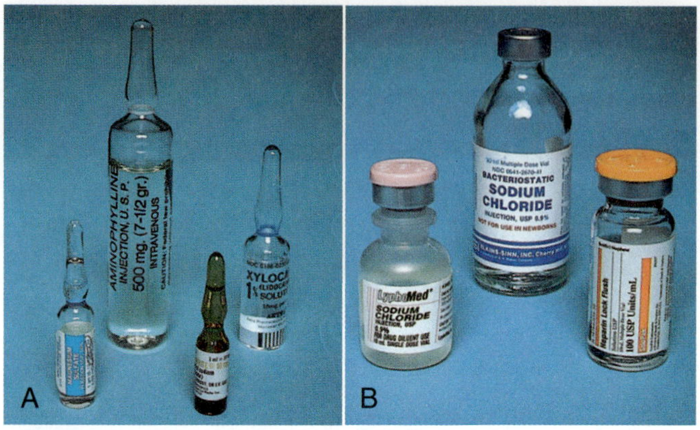

FIG. 31-15 **A,** Medication in ampules. **B,** Medication in vials.

Preparing an Injection From an Ampule. Ampules contain single doses of medication in a liquid. Ampules are available in several sizes, from 1 mL to 10 mL or more (Fig. 31-15, *A*). An ampule is made of glass with a constricted neck that must be snapped off to allow access to the medication. A colored ring around the neck indicates where the ampule is prescored so you can break it easily. Carefully aspirate the medication into a syringe (Skill 31-4 on pp. 622-626) with a filter needle. The use of a filter needle prevents particulate matter such as small glass fragments from entering the syringe (Cocoman and Murray, 2008; Nicoll and Hesby, 2002). Replace the filter needle with an appropriate-size needle or a needleless access device before administering the injection.

Preparing an Injection From a Vial. A vial is a single-dose or multidose container with a rubber seal at the top (see Fig. 31-15, *B*). A metal cap protects the seal until it is ready for use. Vials contain liquid or dry forms of medications. Medications that are unstable in solution are packaged dry. The vial label specifies the solvent or diluent used to dissolve the medication and the amount of diluent needed to prepare a desired medication concentration. Normal saline and sterile distilled water are commonly used to dissolve medications.

Unlike the ampule, the vial is a closed system, and air needs to be injected into it to permit easy withdrawal of the solution. Failure to inject air when withdrawing creates a vacuum within the vial that makes withdrawal difficult. If concerned about drawing up parts of the rubber stopper or other particles into the syringe, use a filter needle when preparing medications from vials (Cocoman and Murray, 2008; Nicoll and Hesby, 2002). Some vials contain powder, which is mixed with a diluent during preparation and before injection (see Skill 31-4). After mixing multidose vials, make a label that includes the date and time of mixing and the concentration of medication per milliliter. Some multidose vials require refrigeration after the contents are reconstituted.

Mixing Medications. If two medications are compatible, it is possible to mix them in one injection if the total dose is within accepted limits so a patient does not have to receive more than one injection at a time. Most nursing units have charts that list common compatible medications. If there is any uncertainty about

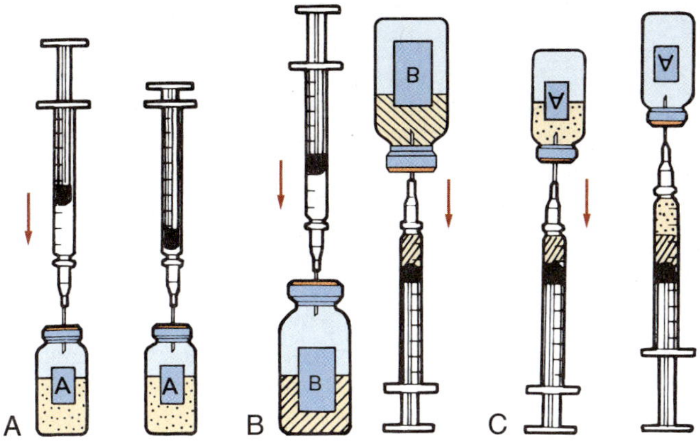

FIG. 31-16 **A,** Injecting air into vial A. **B,** Injecting air into vial B and withdrawing dose. **C,** Withdrawing medication from vial A; medications are now mixed.

medication compatibilities, consult a pharmacist or a medication reference.

Mixing Medications From a Vial and an Ampule. When mixing medication from both a vial and ampule, prepare medication from the vial first. Using the same syringe and filter needle, next withdraw medication from the ampule. Nurses prepare the combination in this order because it is not necessary to add air to withdraw medication from an ampule.

Mixing Medications From Two Vials. Apply these principles when mixing medications from two vials:

1. Do not contaminate one medication with another.
2. Ensure that the final dose is accurate.
3. Maintain aseptic technique.

Use only one syringe with a needle or needleless access device attached to mix medications from two vials (Fig. 31-16). Aspirate the volume of air equivalent to the dose of the first medication (vial A) (Fig. 31-16, *A*). Inject the air into vial A, making sure that the needle does not touch the solution. Withdraw the needle and aspirate air equivalent to the dose of the second medication (vial B). Inject the volume of air into vial B (Fig. 31-16, *B*). Immediately withdraw the medication from vial B into the syringe and insert the needle back into vial A, being careful not to push the plunger and expel the medication within the syringe into the vial. Withdraw the desired amount of medication from vial A into the syringe (Fig. 31-16, *C*). After withdrawing the necessary amount, withdraw the needle and apply a new safety needle or needleless access device suitable for injection.

Insulin Preparation. Insulin is the hormone used to treat diabetes. It is administered by injection because the GI tract breaks down and destroys an oral form of insulin. Most patients with diabetes who take insulin injections learn to administer their own injections. In the United States and Canada health care providers usually prescribe insulin in concentrations of 100 units per milliliter of solution. This is called *U-100 insulin*. Insulin is also commercially available in concentrations of 500 units per milliliter of solution; it is called *U-500 insulin*. U-500 insulin is 5 times as strong as U-100 insulin and is used only in rare cases when patients are very resistant to insulin (Davidson et al., 2010).

Use the correct syringe when preparing insulin. Use a 100-unit insulin syringe or an insulin pen to prepare U-100 insulin. Because there is no syringe currently designed to prepare U-500 insulin, many medication errors result with this kind of insulin. When ordering U-500 insulin, ensure that prescribers specify units and volume (e.g., 150 units, 0.3 mL of U-500 insulin) and use tuberculin syringes to draw up the doses. Verify dose with another nurse or pharmacist before administering it to the patient. Additional safety measures common with U-500 insulin include having the insulin listed as being concentrated in computerized medication dispensing systems, making prescribers and pharmacists verify that the patients is to receive U-500 insulin when it is ordered, and only stocking U-500 insulin on patient care units when it is ordered for a specific patient (ISMP, 2007a).

BOX 31-21 EXAMPLE OF CORRECTION INSULIN ORDER

Give regular insulin subcutaneously:
- 2 units for glucose 150 to 200 mg/dL
- 4 units for glucose 201 to 275 mg/dL
- Call for glucose greater than 275 mg/dL

Clinical scenario: Before lunch patient's blood glucose level is 201. After referring to patient's correction insulin dose, the nurse administers 4 units of insulin to patient.

Insulin is classified by rate of action, including rapid, short, intermediate, and long acting. To provide safe and effective care, you need to know the onset, peak, and duration for each of your patients' ordered insulin doses. Refer to a medication reference or consult with a pharmacist if you are unsure of this information. Only regular insulin can be given intravenously. Orders for insulin injections attempt to imitate the normal pattern of a patient's insulin release from the pancreas. Some insulins come in a stable premixed solution (e.g., 70/30 insulin is 70% NPH [intermediate] and 30% regular), eliminating the need to mix the insulins in a syringe. Other patients use an insulin pen. The insulin pen provides multiple doses and allows the patient or nurse to dial in the dose, avoiding the need to use a syringe for insulin preparation. A patient with diabetes sometimes requires more than one type of insulin. For example, by receiving a short-acting (regular) and an intermediate-acting (NPH) insulin, a patient receives more sustained control of blood glucose levels over 24 hours.

Insulin is ordered by a specific dose at select times. Correction insulin, also known as sliding-scale insulin, provides a dose of insulin based on the patient's blood glucose level (Box 31-21). The term *correction insulin* is preferred because it indicates that small doses of rapid- or short-acting insulins are needed to correct a patient's elevated blood sugar. Reliance on correction insulin is unlikely to achieve long-term glucose control; therefore it should only be ordered on a temporary basis (ADA, 2010).

Before drawing up insulin doses, gently roll all cloudy insulin preparations between the palms of the hands to resuspend the insulin (ADA, 2004). Do not shake insulin vials; shaking causes bubbles to form. Bubbles take up space in the syringe and alter the dose.

If more than one type of insulin is required to manage the patient's diabetes, the nurse can mix two different types of insulin into one syringe *if* they are compatible (Box 31-22). If regular and intermediate-acting insulin is ordered, prepare the regular insulin first to prevent the regular insulin from becoming contaminated with the intermediate-acting insulin (ADA, 2004). Use the following principles when mixing insulins (ADA, 2004; Novo Nordisk, 2010):

- Patients whose blood glucose levels are well controlled on a mixed-insulin dose need to maintain their individual routine when preparing and administering their insulin.

BOX 31-22 PROCEDURAL GUIDELINES

Mixing Two Types of Insulin in One Syringe

Delegation Considerations

The skill of mixing two types of insulin in one syringe cannot be delegated to nursing assistive personnel (NAP).

Equipment

Insulin vials, insulin syringe, alcohol swabs, medication administration (MAR) (electronic or printed)

1. Check accuracy and completeness of each MAR with prescriber's medication order. Check patient's name and medication name, dosage, and route and time of administration.
2. Review medical history (e.g., type of diabetes, reason for elevated blood sugars) and allergies to medications, food, and latex.
3. Carefully verify insulin labels; compare labels against the MAR before preparing the dose to ensure that the correct type of insulin is prepared. *This is the first accuracy check.*
4. Perform hand hygiene.
5. If patient takes insulin that is cloudy, roll the bottle of insulin between the hands to resuspend the preparation.
6. Wipe off tops of both insulin vials with alcohol swabs.
7. Verify insulin dosages against MAR a second time. *This is the second accuracy check.*
8. If mixing rapid- or short-acting insulin with intermediate-acting insulin, take insulin syringe and aspirate volume of air equivalent to the dose of insulin to be withdrawn from intermediate-acting insulin first. If two intermediate-acting insulins are mixed, it makes no difference which vial you prepare first.
9. Insert needle and inject air into vial of intermediate-acting insulin. Do not let the tip of the needle touch the insulin.
10. Remove the syringe from the vial of intermediate-acting insulin without aspirating the insulin.
11. With the same syringe, inject air equal to the dose of insulin to be withdrawn into the vial of rapid- or short-acting insulin. Then withdraw the correct dose into the syringe.
12. Remove the syringe from the rapid- or short-acting insulin vial after carefully removing air bubbles in the syringe to ensure correct dose.
13. After verifying insulin dosages with MAR a third time, show insulin prepared in syringe to another nurse to verify that correct dosage of insulin was prepared. *This is the third accuracy check.* Determine which point on the syringe scale combined the units of insulin measured by adding the number of units of both insulins together (e.g., 3 units regular + 10 units NPH = 13 units total).
14. Place the needle of the syringe back into the vial of intermediate-acting insulin. Be careful not to push the plunger and inject insulin in syringe into the vial.
15. Invert vial and carefully withdraw the desired amount of insulin into the syringe.
16. Withdraw needle and check the fluid level in syringe. Keep needle of prepared syringe sheathed or capped until ready to administer medication. Show another nurse the syringe to verify that the correct dose was prepared.
17. Dispose of soiled supplies in proper receptacle. Place used vials in puncture-proof and leak-proof container and perform hand hygiene.
18. Because rapid- or short-acting insulin binds with intermediate-acting insulin, which reduces the action of the faster-acting insulin, administer mixture within 5 minutes of preparing it.

Modified from American Diabetes Association: Insulin administration: position statement, *Diabetes Care* 27(1S):S106, 2004.

- Do not mix insulin with any other medications or diluents unless approved by the prescriber.
- Never mix insulin glargine (Lantus) or insulin detemir (Levemir) with other types of insulin.
- Inject rapid-acting insulins mixed with NPH insulin within 15 minutes before a meal.
- Verify insulin doses with another nurse while preparing them if required by agency policy.

Administering Injections

Each injection route differs based on the type of tissues the medication enters. The characteristics of the tissues influence the rate of medication absorption and thus the onset of medication action. Before injecting a medication, know the volume of the medication to administer, the characteristics and viscosity of the medication, and the location of anatomical structures underlying injection sites (Skill 31-5 on pp. 626-631).

If a nurse does not administer injections correctly, negative patient outcomes result. Failure to select an injection site in relation to anatomical landmarks results in nerve or bone damage during needle insertion. Inability to maintain stability of the needle and syringe unit can result in pain and tissue damage. If you fail to aspirate the syringe before injecting an IM medication, the medication may accidentally be injected directly into an artery or vein. Injecting too large a volume of medication for the site selected causes extreme pain and results in local tissue damage.

Many patients, particularly children, fear injections. Patients with serious or chronic illness often are given several injections daily. Minimize the patient's discomfort in the following ways:

- Use a sharp-beveled needle in the smallest suitable length and gauge.
- Position the patient as comfortably as possible to reduce muscular tension.
- Select the proper injection site, using anatomical landmarks.
- Apply a vapocoolant spray (e.g., Fluori-Methane spray or ethyl chloride) or topical anesthetic (e.g., EMLA cream) to the injection site before giving the medication when possible.
- Divert the patient's attention from the injection through conversation using open-ended questioning.
- Insert the needle quickly and smoothly to minimize tissue pulling.
- Hold the syringe steady while the needle remains in tissues.
- Inject the medication slowly and steadily.

Subcutaneous Injections. Subcutaneous injections involve placing medications into the loose connective tissue under the dermis (see Skill 31-5). Because subcutaneous tissue is not as richly supplied with blood as the muscles, medication absorption is somewhat slower than with IM injections. However, medications are absorbed completely if the patient's circulatory status is normal. Because subcutaneous tissue contains pain receptors, the patient often experiences slight discomfort.

The best subcutaneous injection sites include the outer posterior aspect of the upper arms, the abdomen from below the costal margins to the iliac crests, and the anterior aspects of the thighs (Fig. 31-17). The site most frequently recommended for heparin injections is the abdomen (Fig. 31-18). Alternative subcutaneous sites for other medications include the scapular areas of the upper back and the upper ventral or dorsal gluteal areas. The injection site chosen needs to be free of skin lesions, bony prominences, and large underlying muscles or nerves.

The administration of low-molecular-weight heparin (LMWH) (e.g., enoxaparin) requires special considerations. When injecting the medication, use the right or left side of the abdomen at least 2 inches from the umbilicus (the patient's "love handles") and pinch the injection site as you insert the needle. Administer LMWH in its prefilled syringe with the attached needle and do not expel the air bubble in the syringe before giving the medication (Sanofi-Aventis, 2010).

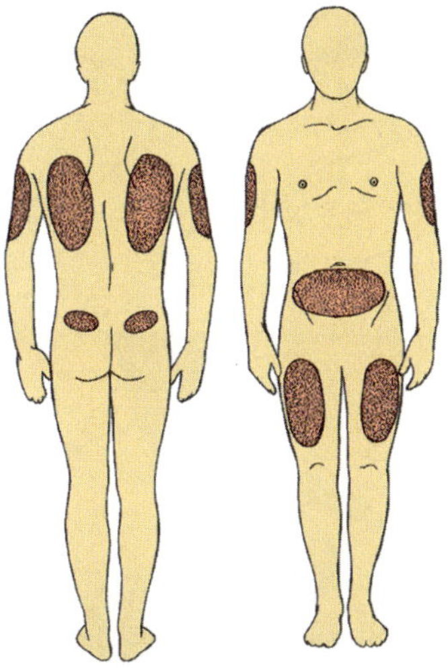

FIG. 31-17 Sites recommended for subcutaneous injections.

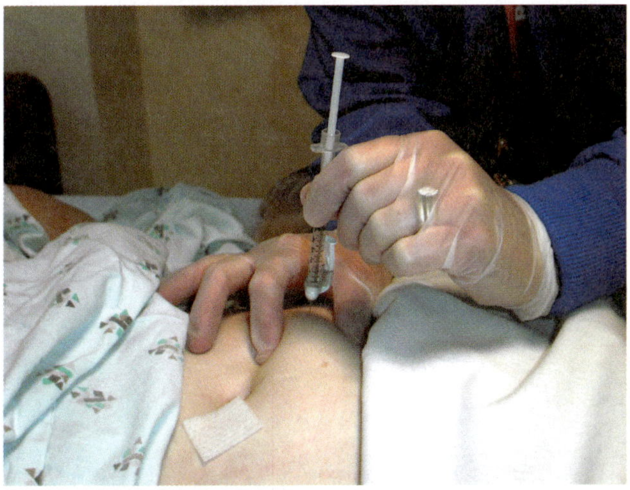

FIG. 31-18 Giving subcutaneous heparin in abdomen.

Use U-100 insulin syringes with preattached 25- to 31-gauge needles when giving U-100 insulin and 1-mL tuberculin syringes when giving U-500 insulin (ADA, n.d.; ISMP, 2002). Recommended sites for insulin injections include the upper arm and the anterior and lateral portions of the thigh, buttocks, and abdomen. Rotating injections within the same body part (intrasite rotation) provides more consistency in the absorption of the insulin. For example, if the patient receives the morning insulin in the right arm, give the next injection in a different place in the same arm. The injections are to be given at least an inch (2.5 cm) away from the previous site. No injection site should be used again for at least 1 month. The rate of insulin absorption varies based on the site; the abdomen has the quickest absorption, followed by the arms, thighs, and buttocks (ADA, 2004).

Only small volumes (0.5 to 1.5 mL) of water-soluble medications are given subcutaneously because the tissue is sensitive to irritating solutions and large volumes of medications. In children smaller volumes up to 0.5 mL are given (Hockenberry and Wilson, 2009). Collection of medications within the tissues causes sterile abscesses, which appear as hardened, painful lumps under the skin.

A patient's body weight indicates the depth of the subcutaneous layer. Therefore choose the needle length and angle of insertion based on the patient's weight and an estimation of the amount of subcutaneous tissue (Annersten and Willman, 2005). Generally a 25-gauge, ⅝-inch needle inserted at a 45-degree angle (Fig. 31-19) or a ½-inch needle inserted at a 90-degree angle deposits medications into the subcutaneous tissue of a normal-size patient. Some children require only a ½-inch needle. If the patient is obese, pinch the tissue and use a needle long enough to insert through fatty tissue at the base of the skinfold. Thin patients often do not have sufficient tissue for subcutaneous injections; the upper abdomen is usually the best site in this case. To ensure that a subcutaneous medication reaches the subcutaneous tissue, follow this rule: If you can grasp 2 inches (5 cm) of tissue, insert the needle at a 90-degree angle; if you can grasp 1 inch (2.5 cm) of tissue, insert the needle at a 45-degree angle (Rushing, 2004).

Intramuscular Injections. The IM route provides faster medication absorption than the subcutaneous route because of the greater vascularity of the muscle. However, IM injections are associated with many risks. Therefore, whenever administering a medication by the IM route, first verify that the injection is justified (Nicoll and Hesby, 2002; WHO, 2006). In many cases such as

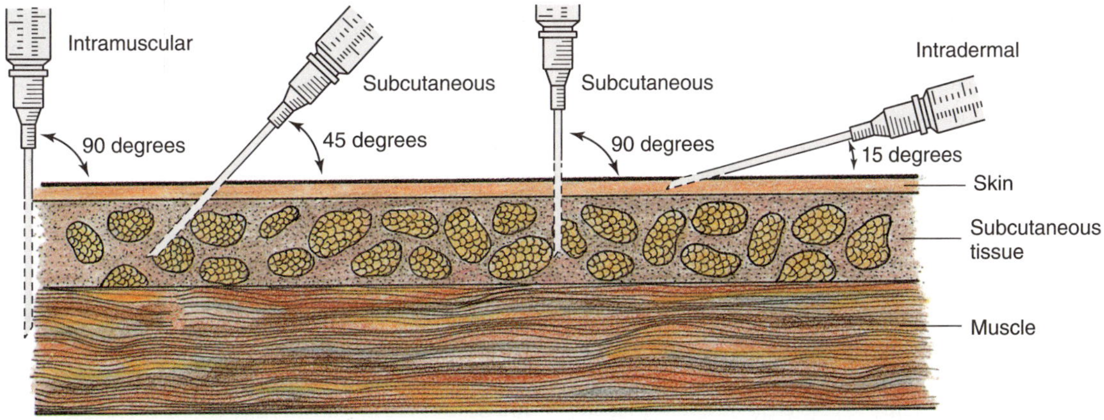

FIG. 31-19 Comparison of angles of insertion for intramuscular (90 degrees), subcutaneous (45 to 90 degrees), and intradermal (15 degrees) injections.

influenza and pneumonia shots, no alternative sites are available to give the medication.

Use a longer and heavier-gauge needle to pass through subcutaneous tissue and penetrate deep muscle tissue (see Skill 31-5). Weight and the amount of adipose tissue influence needle size selection. For example, a very obese patient often requires a needle 3 inches long, whereas a thin patient only requires a ½- to 1-inch needle (Koster et al., 2009; Zaybak et al., 2007). Because most agencies have needles that range in length from only ⅜ to 1½ inches, investigate different medication routes when IM injections are ordered for patients who are obese (TCHP Education Consortium, 2005).

The angle of insertion for an IM injection is 90 degrees (see Fig. 31-19). Muscle is less sensitive to irritating and viscous medications. A normal, well-developed adult patient tolerates 2 to 5 mL of medication into a larger muscle without severe muscle discomfort (Nicoll and Hesby, 2002; Prettyman, 2005). However, larger volumes of medication (4 to 5 mL) are unlikely to be absorbed properly. Children, older adults, and thin patients tolerate only 2 mL of an IM injection. Do not give more than 1 mL to small children and older infants, and do not give more than 0.5 mL to smaller infants (Hockenberry and Wilson, 2009).

Assess the muscle before giving an injection. Properly identify the site for the IM injection by palpating bony landmarks, and be aware of the potential complications associated with each site (Nicoll and Hesby, 2002). It needs to be free of tenderness. Repeated injections in the same muscle cause severe discomfort. With the patient relaxed, palpate the muscle to rule out any hardened lesions. Minimize discomfort during an injection by helping the patient assume a position that helps to reduce muscle strain. Other interventions such as distraction and applying pressure to the IM site decrease pain during an IM injection.

Sites. When selecting an IM site, consider the following: Is the area free of infection or necrosis? Are there local areas of bruising or abrasions? What is the location of underlying bones, nerves, and major blood vessels? What volume of medication is to be administered? Each site has different advantages and disadvantages.

Ventrogluteal. The ventrogluteal muscle involves the gluteus medius; it is situated deep and away from major nerves and blood vessels. This site is the preferred and safest site for all adults, children, and infants, especially for medications that have larger volumes and are more viscous and irritating (Hockenberry and Wilson, 2009; Nicoll and Hesby, 2002). The ventrogluteal site is recommended for volumes greater than 2 mL (Nicoll and Hesby, 2002). Research shows that injuries such as fibrosis, nerve damage, abscess, tissue necrosis, muscle contraction, gangrene, and pain are associated with all the common IM sites *except* the ventrogluteal site. Actually the only published case study of a complication at the ventrogluteal site reported a local reaction to the medication, which is not a complication associated with the site itself (Nicoll and Hesby, 2002).

Locate the ventrogluteal muscle by positioning the patient in a supine or lateral position. Flexing the knee and hip helps to relax this muscle. Place the palm of your hand over the greater trochanter of the patient's hip with the wrist perpendicular to the femur. Use the right hand for the left hip and use the left hand for the right hip. Point the thumb toward the patient's groin and the index finger toward the anterior superior iliac spine; extend the middle finger back along the iliac crest toward the buttock. The index finger, the middle finger, and the iliac crest form a V-shaped triangle; the injection site is the center of the triangle (Fig. 31-20, *A* to *C*).

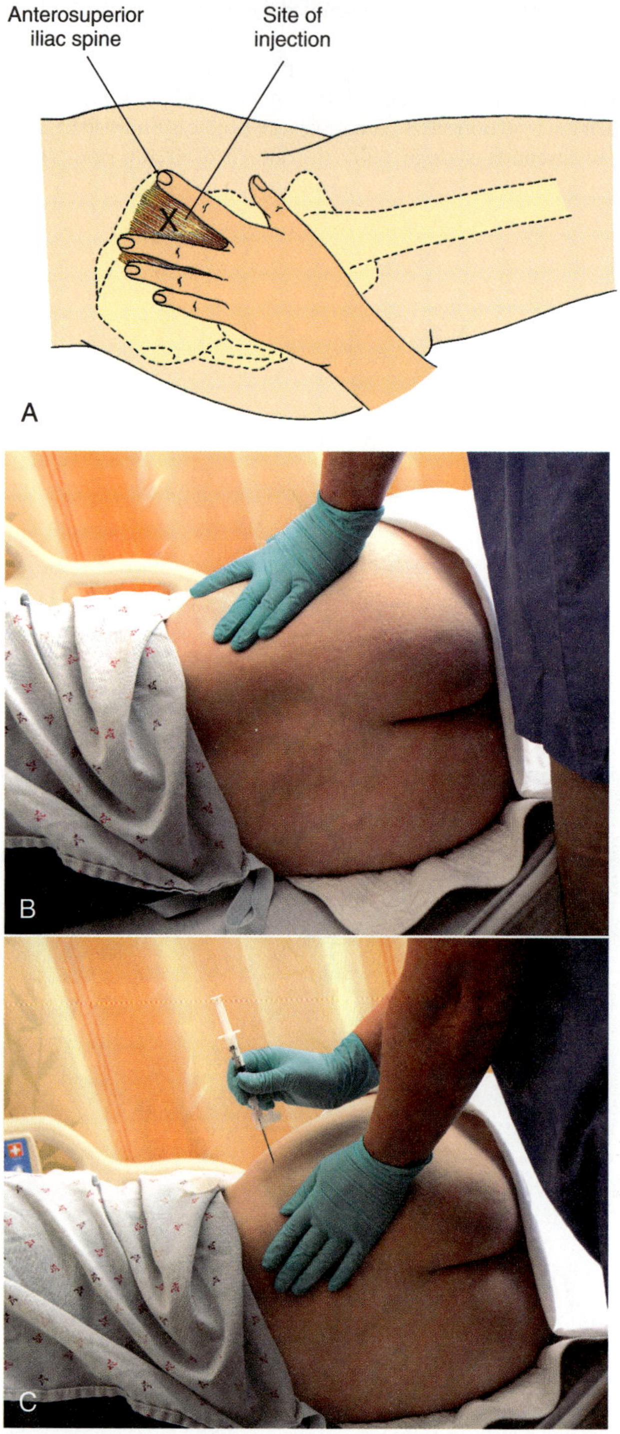

FIG. 31-20 **A,** Landmarks for ventrogluteal site. **B,** Locating ventrogluteal site in patient. **C,** Giving intramuscular injection in ventrogluteal muscle using the Z-track method.

Vastus Lateralis. The vastus lateralis muscle is another injection site for adults and children. The muscle is thick and well developed, is located on the anterior lateral aspect of the thigh, and extends in an adult from a hand breadth above the knee to a hand breadth below the greater trochanter of the femur (Fig. 31-21, *A* and *B*). Use the middle third of the muscle for injection. The width of the muscle usually extends from the midline of the thigh to the midline of the outer side of the thigh. With young children or

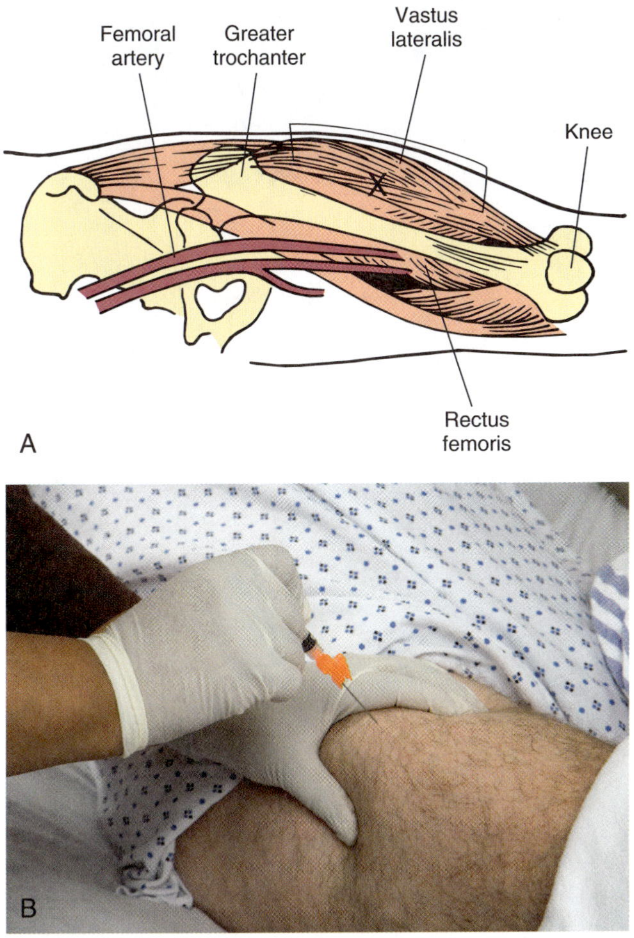

FIG. 31-21 **A,** Landmarks for vastus lateralis site. **B,** Giving intramuscular injection in vastus lateralis muscle.

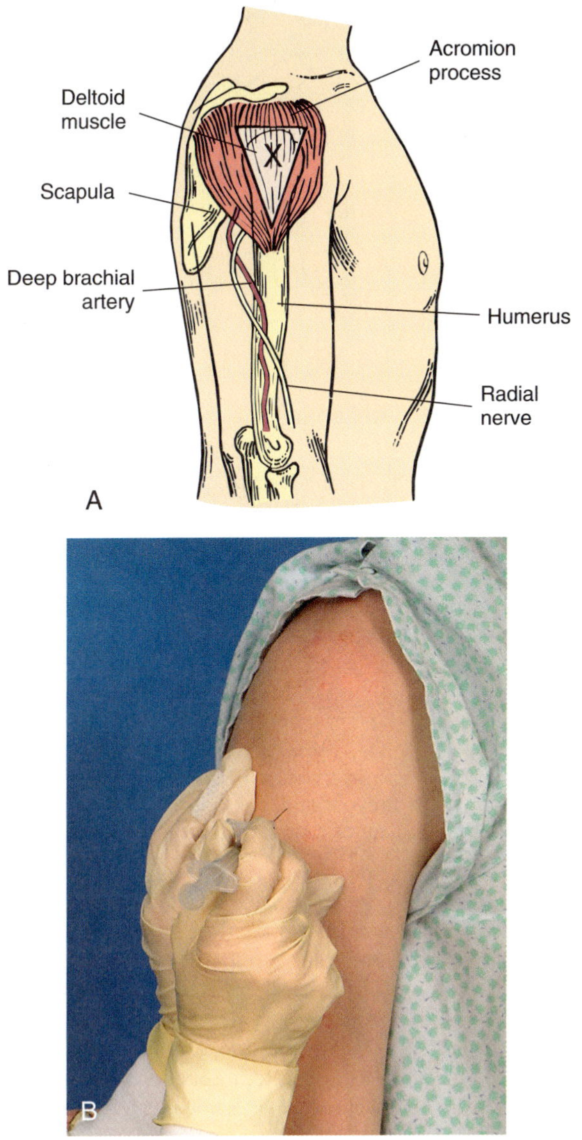

FIG. 31-22 **A,** Landmarks for deltoid site. **B,** Giving intramuscular injection in deltoid muscle.

cachectic patients, it helps to grasp the body of the muscle during injection to be sure that the medication is deposited in muscle tissue. To help relax the muscle, ask the patient to lie flat with the knee slightly flexed or in a sitting position. The vastus lateralis site is often used for infants, toddlers, and children receiving biologicals (e.g., immunoglobulins, vaccines, or toxoids) (Nicoll and Hesby, 2002).

Deltoid. Although the deltoid site is easily accessible, this muscle is not well developed in many adults. There is a potential for injury because the axillary, radial, brachial, and ulnar nerves, as well as the brachial artery, lie within the upper arm under the triceps and along the humerus. Use this site for small medication volumes (2 mL or less) (Nicoll and Hesby, 2002). Carefully assess the condition of the deltoid muscle, consult medication references for suitability of the medication, and carefully locate the injection site using anatomical landmarks (Fig 31-22, *A*). Use this site only for small medication volumes, when giving immunizations (e.g., hepatitis B, flu shots), or when other sites are inaccessible because of dressings or casts (Nicoll and Hesby, 2002). To locate the muscle, fully expose the patient's upper arm and shoulder. Do not roll up a tight-fitting sleeve. Have the patient relax the arm at the side and flex the elbow. The patient may sit, stand, or lie down (Fig. 31-22, *B*). Palpate the lower edge of the acromion process, which forms the base of a triangle in line with the midpoint of the lateral aspect of the upper arm. The injection site is in the center of the triangle, about 3 to 5 cm (1 to 2 inches) below the acromion process. You can also locate the site by placing four fingers across the deltoid muscle, with the top finger along the acromion process. The injection site is then three finger widths below the acromion process.

Use of the Z-Track Method in Intramuscular Injections. It is recommended that, when administering IM injections, the **Z-track method** be used to minimize local skin irritation by sealing the medication in muscle tissue (Nicoll and Hesby, 2002). To use the Z-track method, put a new needle on the syringe after preparing the medication so no solution remains on the outside needle shaft. Then select an IM site, preferably in a large, deep muscle such as the ventrogluteal muscle. Place the ulnar side of the nondominant hand just below the site and pull the overlying skin and subcutaneous tissues approximately 2.5 to 3.5 cm (1 to 1½ inches) laterally or downward (Nicoll and Hesby, 2002). Hold the skin in this position until you administer the injection. After preparing the site with an antiseptic swab, inject the needle deep into the muscle. Grasp the barrel of the syringe with the thumb and index finger of the nondominant hand and slowly inject the medication at a rate of 10 seconds per mL if there is no blood return on aspiration (Nicoll

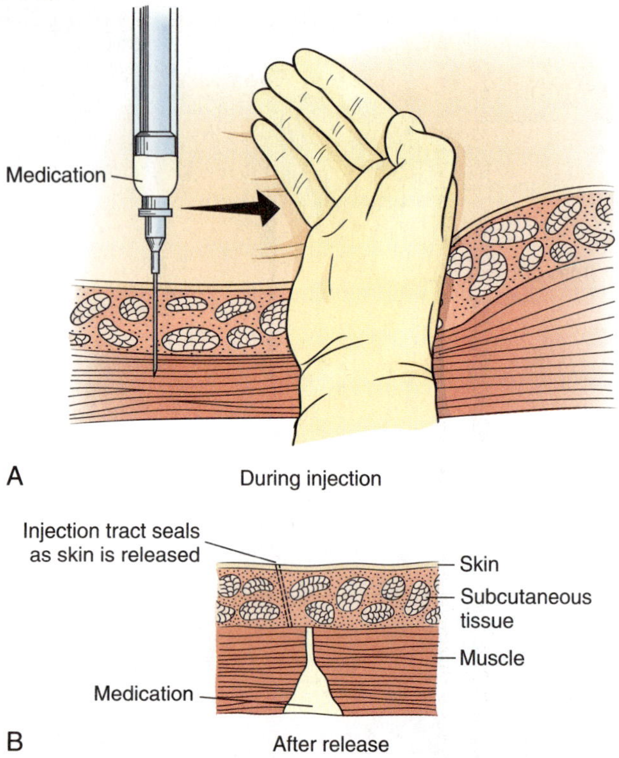

FIG. 31-23 **A,** Pulling on overlying skin during intramuscular injection moves tissue to prevent later tracking. **B,** Z-track method of injection prevents deposit of medication into sensitive tissue.

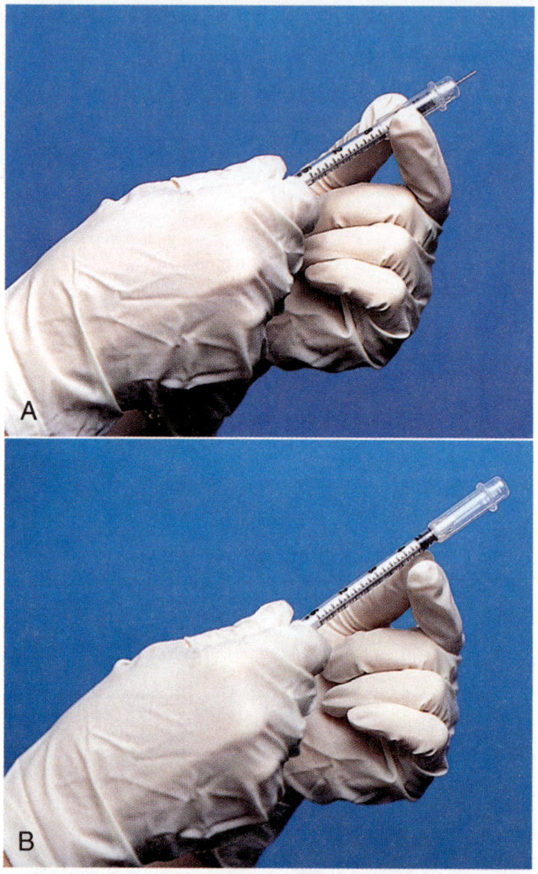

FIG. 31-24 Needle with plastic guard to prevent needlesticks. **A,** Position of guard before injection. **B,** After injection the guard locks in place, covering the needle.

and Hesby, 2002). The needle remains inserted for 10 seconds to allow the medication to disperse evenly rather than channeling back up the track of the needle (Nicoll and Hesby, 2002). Release the skin after withdrawing the needle. This leaves a zigzag path that seals the needle track where tissue planes slide across one another (Fig. 31-23, *A* and *B*). The medication cannot escape from the muscle tissue. Injections using this technique result in less discomfort and decrease the occurrence of lesions at the injection site (Nicoll and Hesby, 2002).

Intradermal Injections. Intradermal injections typically are used for skin testing (e.g., tuberculin screening and allergy tests). Because these medications are potent, they are injected into the dermis, where blood supply is reduced and medication absorption occurs slowly. Sometimes patients have a severe anaphylactic reaction if the medications enter the circulation too rapidly. Skin testing requires that the nurse be able to clearly see the injection sites for changes in color and tissue integrity. Intradermal sites need to be lightly pigmented, free of lesions, and relatively hairless. The inner forearm and upper back are ideal locations.

Use a tuberculin or small hypodermic syringe for skin testing. The angle of insertion for an intradermal injection is 5 to 15 degrees (see Fig. 31-19), and the bevel of the needle is pointed up. As you inject the medication, a small bleb resembling a mosquito bite appears on the surface of the skin. If a bleb does not appear or if the site bleeds after needle withdrawal, there is a good chance that the medication entered subcutaneous tissues. In this case test results will not be valid.

Safety in Administering Medications by Injection

Needleless Devices. Between 600,000 and 1 million accidental needlesticks and sharps injuries occur annually in health care settings (OSHA, 2009). Needlestick injuries commonly occur when health care workers recap needles, mishandle IV lines and needles, or leave needles at a patient's bedside. Exposure to bloodborne pathogens is one of the deadliest hazards to which nurses are exposed on a daily basis. Most needlestick injuries are preventable with the implementation of safe needle devices. The Needlestick Safety and Prevention Act mandates the use of special needle safety devices to reduce the frequency of needlestick injuries.

Safety syringes have a sheath or guard that covers a needle after it is withdrawn from the skin (Fig. 31-24, *A* and *B*). The needle is immediately covered, eliminating the chance for a needlestick injury. The syringe and sheath are disposed of together in a receptacle. Use needleless devices whenever possible to reduce the risk of needlestick and sharps injuries (OSHA, 2009). Always dispose of needles and other instruments considered sharps into clearly marked, appropriate containers (Fig. 31-25). Containers need to be puncture proof and leak proof. Never force a needle into a full needle disposal receptacle. Never place used needles and syringes in a wastebasket, in your pocket, on a patient's meal tray, or at the patient's bedside. Box 31-23 summarizes the recommendations for the prevention of needlestick injuries.

Intravenous Administration. The nurse administers medications intravenously by the following methods:

1. As mixtures within large volumes of IV fluids
2. By injection of a bolus or small volume of medication through an existing IV infusion line or intermittent venous access (heparin or saline lock)
3. By "piggyback" infusion of a solution containing the prescribed medication and a small volume of IV fluid through an existing IV line

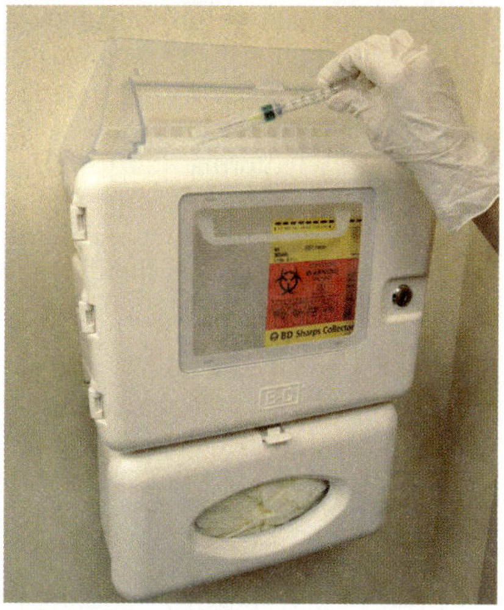

FIG. 31-25 Sharps disposal using only one hand.

BOX 31-23 RECOMMENDATIONS FOR PREVENTION OF NEEDLESTICK INJURIES

- Avoid using needles when effective needleless systems or sharps with engineered sharps injury protection (SESIP) safety devices are available.
- Do not recap any needle.
- Plan safe handling and disposal of needles before beginning the procedure.
- Immediately dispose of needles, needleless systems, and SESIP into puncture-proof and leak-proof sharps disposal containers.
- Maintain a sharps injury log that includes the following: type and brand of device involved in the incident; location of the incident (e.g., department or work area); description of the incident; privacy of the employees who have had sharps injuries.

Data from Occupational Safety and Health Administration: Toxic and hazardous substances: bloodborne pathogens, *Fed Reg* CFR 29, part 1910.1030, April 3, 2006, http://www.osha.gov/SLTC/bloodbornepathogens/index.html. Accessed on September 18, 2011.

In all three methods the patient has either an existing IV infusion running continuously or an IV access site for intermittent infusions. In most agencies policies and procedures list persons who are able to give IV medications and the situations in which they may be given. These policies are based on the medication, capability, and availability of staff, and the type of monitoring equipment available.

Chapter 41 describes the technique for performing venipuncture and establishing continuous IV fluid infusions. Medication administration is only one reason for supplying IV fluids. IV fluid therapy is used primarily for fluid replacement in patients unable to take oral fluids and as a means of supplying electrolytes and nutrients.

When using any method of IV medication administration, observe patients closely for symptoms of adverse reactions. After a medication enters the bloodstream, it begins to act immediately, and there is no way to stop its action. Thus take special care to avoid errors in dose calculation and preparation. Carefully follow the six rights of safe medication administration, double-check medication calculations with another nurse, and know the desired action and side effects of every medication you give. If the medication has an antidote, make sure that it is available during administration. When administering potent medications, assess vital signs before, during, and after infusion.

Administering medications by the IV route has advantages. Often the nurse uses this route in emergencies when a fast-acting medication must be delivered quickly. The IV route is also best when it is necessary to give medications to establish constant therapeutic blood levels. Some medications are highly alkaline and irritating to muscle and subcutaneous tissue. These medications cause less discomfort when given intravenously. Because IV medications are immediately available to the bloodstream once they are administered, verify the prescribed rate of administration with a medication reference or a pharmacist before giving them to ensure that the medication is given safely over the appropriate amount of time. Patients experience severe adverse reactions if IV medications are administered too quickly.

Large-Volume Infusions. Of the three methods of administering IV medications, mixing them in large volumes of fluids is the safest and easiest. Because the medication is not in a concentrated form, the risk of side effects or fatal reactions is minimal when infused over the prescribed time frame. Medications are diluted in large volumes (500 or 1000 mL) of compatible IV fluids such as normal saline or lactated Ringer's solution. Vitamins and potassium chloride are two types of medications commonly added to IV fluids. There is a danger with continuous infusion: if the IV fluid is infused too rapidly, the patient is at risk for medication overdose and circulatory fluid overload.

In the past nurses often mixed medications into IV fluids. However, standards developed by the U.S. Pharmacopeia and other health care professional organizations no longer support this practice on a routine basis (ASHP, n.d.b). Many patient safety risks such as incorrect calculation, nonaseptic preparation, and incorrect labeling occur when nurses have to prepare medications in IV containers on patient care units. Current best practices include use of IV medications that come in standardized concentrations and dosages; standardized procedures for ordering, preparing, and administering IV medications; and ready-to-administer doses when possible (ASHP, 2008). Nurses only mix medications into IV fluids in emergency situations. The nurse *never* prepares high-alert medications (e.g., heparin, dopamine, dobutamine, nitroglycerin, potassium, antibiotics, or magnesium) on a patient care unit. Check with a pharmacist before mixing a medication in an IV container. If the pharmacist confirms that you need to prepare the medication, ask another nurse to verify your medication calculations and have that nurse watch you during the entire procedure to ensure that you prepare the medication safely. First ensure that the IV fluid and medication are compatible. Then prepare the medication in a syringe (see Skill 31-4) using strict aseptic technique. Clean the injection port of the IV bag with an alcohol swab, remove the cap from the needle, and stick the needle into the IV fluid. Push the medication into the IV fluid and mix the solution by turning the IV bag gently end to end. Finally attach a medication label following ISMP safe label guidelines (2010e). Administer the medication to the patient at the prescribed rate (see Chapter 41). ***Do not*** add medications to IV bags that are already hanging because there is no way to tell the exact concentration of the medication. Add medications ***only*** to new IV bags.

When administering medications in large IV infusions, regulate the IV rate according to the health care provider's order. Monitor patients closely for adverse reactions to the medication and fluid volume overload. Also check the site frequently for infiltration and phlebitis (see Chapter 41).

Intravenous Bolus. An IV bolus involves introducing a concentrated dose of a medication directly into the systemic circulation (Skill 31-6 on pp. 631-635). Because a bolus requires only a small amount of fluid to deliver the medication, it is an advantage when the amount of fluid that the patient can take is restricted. The IV bolus, or "push," is the most dangerous method for administering medications because there is no time to correct errors. In addition, a bolus may cause direct irritation to the lining of blood vessels. Before administering a bolus confirm placement of the IV line. Never give a medication intravenously if the insertion site appears puffy or edematous or the IV fluid cannot flow at the proper rate. Accidental injection of a medication into the tissues around a vein causes pain, sloughing of tissues, and abscesses, depending on the composition of the medication.

Determine the rate of administration of an IV bolus medication by the amount of medication that can be given each minute. For example, if a patient is to receive 4 mL of a medication over 2 minutes, give 2 mL of the IV bolus medication every minute. Look up each medication to determine the recommended concentration and rate of administration. Consider the purpose for which an IV medication is prescribed and any potential adverse effects related to the rate or route of administration.

Volume-Controlled Infusions. Another way of administering IV medications is through small amounts (50 to 100 mL) of compatible IV fluids. The fluid is within a secondary fluid container separate from the primary fluid bag. The container connects directly to the primary IV line or to separate tubing that inserts into the primary line (Skill 31-7 on pp. 635-639). Three types of containers are volume-control administration sets (e.g., Volutrol or Pediatrol), piggyback sets, and mini-infusers. Using volume-controlled infusions has several advantages:

- It reduces risk of rapid-dose infusion by IV push. Medications are diluted and infused over longer time intervals (e.g., 30 to 60 minutes).
- It allows for administration of medications (e.g., antibiotics) that are stable for a limited time in solution.
- It allows for control of IV fluid intake.

Piggyback. A piggyback is a small (25 to 250 mL) IV bag or bottle connected to a short tubing line that connects to the *upper* Y-port of a primary infusion line or to an intermittent venous access (Fig. 31-26). The label on the medication follows the ISMP IV piggyback medication label format (2010e) (Fig. 31-27). The piggyback tubing is a microdrip or macrodrip system (see Chapter 41). The set is called a piggyback because the small bag or bottle is higher than the primary infusion bag or bottle. In the piggyback

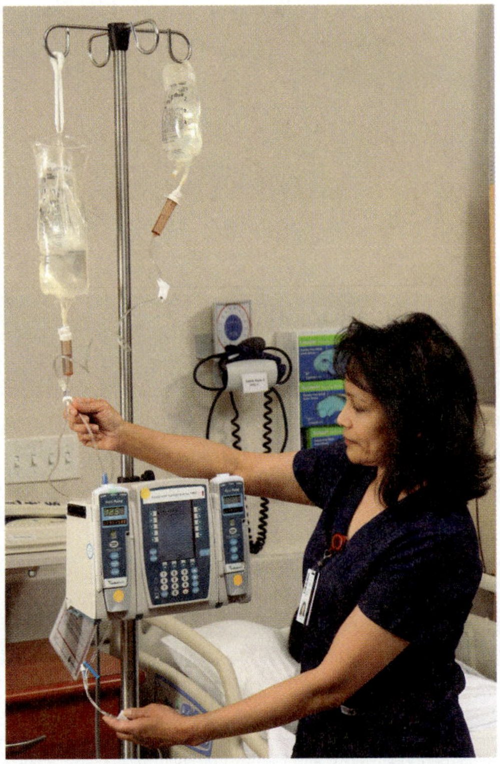

FIG. 31-26 Piggyback setup.

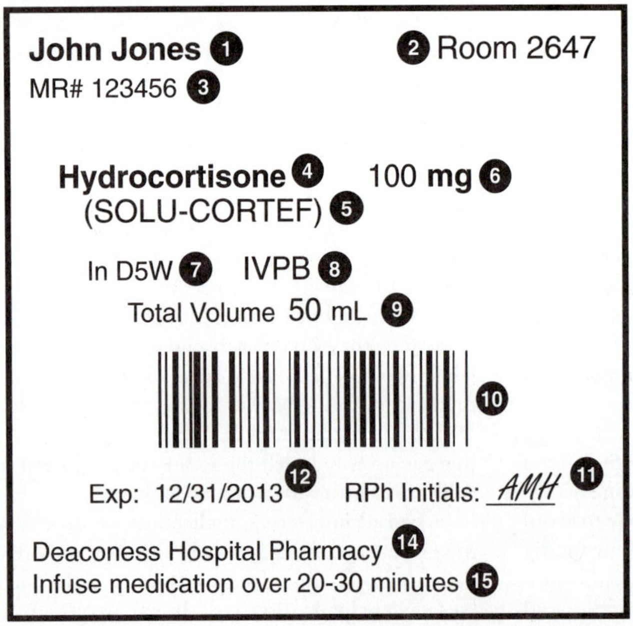
John Jones 1
2 Room 2647
MR# 123456 3
Hydrocortisone 4
100 mg 6
(SOLU-CORTEF) 5
In D5W 7
IVPB 8
Total Volume 50 mL 9
10
Exp: 12/31/2013 12
RPh Initials: AMH 11
Deaconess Hospital Pharmacy 14
Infuse medication over 20-30 minutes 15

1. **Patient name**
2. Location
3. Second identifier (Date of birth, financial #, Encounter #, Medical Record #)
4. **Generic name**
5. BRAND name
6. **Patient dose**
7. Diluent
8. Route
9. Total volume
10. Bar code
11. Initials as needed
12. Expiration Date as needed in a MM/DD/YYYY format
13. Other information as required by state or federal law
14. Pharmacy information if required
15. Comments

FIG. 31-27 IV piggyback medication with label following ISMP safe-labeling guidelines.

setup the main line does not infuse when the piggybacked medication is infusing. The port of the primary IV line contains a back-check valve that automatically stops flow of the primary infusion once the piggyback infusion flows. After the piggyback solution infuses and the solution within the tubing falls below the level of the primary infusion drip chamber, the back-check valve opens, and the primary infusion again flows.

Volume-Control Administration. Volume-control administration (e.g., Buretrol) sets are small (150-mL) containers that attach just below the primary infusion bag or bottle. The set is attached and filled in a manner similar to that used with a regular IV infusion. Follow package directions for priming sets (see Chapter 41).

Mini-Infusion Pump. The mini-infusion pump is battery operated and allows medications to be given in very small amounts of fluid (5 to 60 mL) within controlled infusion times using standard syringes.

Intermittent Venous Access. An intermittent venous access (commonly called a *saline lock)* is an IV catheter capped off on the end with a small chamber covered by a rubber diaphragm or a specially designed cap. Special rubber-seal injection caps usually accept needle safety devices (see Chapter 41). Advantages to intermittent venous access include the following:

- Cost savings resulting from the omission of continuous IV therapy
- Effectiveness of nurse's time enhanced by eliminating constant monitoring of flow rates
- Increased mobility, safety, and comfort for the patient

Before administering an IV bolus or piggyback medication, assess the patency and placement of the IV site. After the medication has been administered through an intermittent venous access, the access must be flushed with a solution to keep it patent. Generally normal saline is an effective flush solution for peripheral catheters. Some agencies require the use of heparin. Nurses need to verify and follow institution policies regarding the care and maintenance of the IV site.

Administration of Intravenous Therapy in the Home. Sometimes patients are discharged from an acute care setting and continue to receive IV therapy in the home. Medications such as antibiotics, chemotherapy, total parenteral nutrition, analgesics, and blood transfusions are given in the home. Most patients who have home IV therapy have a central venous catheter inserted before discharge (see Chapter 41). In addition, patients who need to receive IV therapy in the home have home care nurses to assist with maintenance and monitoring.

Carefully assess patients and their families to determine their ability to manage this therapy at home. Begin instruction on IV care management while the patient is still in the hospital. Patients and families need to learn how to recognize problems and what to do when these problems occur. It is important for the family to recognize signs of infection and complications and know when to notify the home care nurse or health care provider when these occur. In addition, patients and their families need information regarding maintenance of IV administration equipment, including the infusion pump.

SAFETY GUIDELINES FOR NURSING SKILLS

Ensuring patient safety is an essential role of the professional nurse. To ensure patient safety, communicate clearly with members of the health care team, assess and incorporate the patient's priorities of care and preferences, and use the best evidence when making decisions about your patient's care. When performing the skills in this chapter, remember the following points to ensure safe, individualized patient care.

- Be vigilant during the entire process of medication administration. Ensure that your patients receive the appropriate medications. Know why each medication is ordered for your patient. Understand what you need to do before, during, and after medication administration. Evaluate the effectiveness and assess for adverse effects after your patients take their medications.
- Take care of yourself. You think as clearly and critically as possible if you are healthy. Healthy behaviors such as getting adequate sleep, making healthy food choices, and relaxing pelvic floor muscles during stress are positive ways to help you better process information and make safe decisions during medication administration.
- Set up and prepare medications in distraction-free areas.
- Verify expiration date of medications during preparation. Do not administer expired medications.
- Identify each patient using at least two identifiers before administering medications.
- Clarify all unclear orders and ask for help whenever you are uncertain about a medication order or calculation. Consult with your peers, pharmacists, and other health care providers. Resolve all your concerns related to medication administration before preparing and giving medications.
- Use technology (e.g., bar-code scanning, electronic MARs) that is available to you when preparing and administering medications. Follow all policies related to the safe use of technology and do not use "work-arounds." Nurses who use "work-arounds" fail to follow agency protocols, policies, or procedures during medication administration in an attempt to administer medications to patients in a timelier manner. Failure to follow the standard of care greatly increases the risk for making a medication error, impairs patient safety, and places the nurse at risk for malpractice and disciplinary action (see Chapter 23).
- Educate patients about their medications during medication administration. Patients are often able to identify inappropriate medications. Answer all patient questions and resolve their concerns before giving medications. Include family caregivers in medication education when appropriate.
- In most circumstances you cannot delegate medication administration. Ensure that you follow standards set by your state Nurse Practice Act and guidelines established by the health care agency. Licensed practical nurses (LPNs) or licensed vocational nurses (LVNs) can usually administer medications given PO, subcutaneously, intramuscularly, and intradermally. In some cases they can give medications intravenously if they have had special training and if the medications are not high alert. Some states also allow certified medical assistants (CMAs) to administer some types of medications (e.g., PO medications) in some health care settings (e.g., long-term care facilities). The skills in this chapter assume that you are not in a setting where you can delegate medication administration to nursing assistive personnel (NAP). If you are practicing in a state and a health care setting that allow you to delegate medication administration, follow the guidelines for safe delegation (see Chapter 21), agency policies, and the standards outlined in the Nurse Practice Act in your state.

SKILL 31-1 ADMINISTERING ORAL MEDICATIONS

View Video!

Delegation Considerations

The skill of administering oral medications cannot be delegated to nursing assistive personnel (NAP). Instruct the NAP about:

- Potential side effects of medications that you summarize, and reporting their occurrence.

Equipment

- Disposable medication cups
- Glass of water, juice, or preferred liquid
- Drinking straw
- Device for crushing or splitting tablets (optional)
- Clean gloves (if handling a medication)
- MAR (electronic or printed)

STEP	RATIONALE
ASSESSMENT	
1 Check accuracy and completeness of each medication administration record (MAR) with prescriber's medication order. Check patient's name and medication name, dosage, and route and time of administration. Recopy or reprint any portion of printed MAR that is difficult to read.	The order sheet is the most reliable source and only legal record of medications that patient is to receive. Ensures that patient receives the correct medications. Illegible MARs are a source of medication errors (Poon et al., 2010).
2 Review pertinent information related to medication: action, purpose, normal dose and route, side effects, time of onset and peak action, and nursing implications.	Allows you to anticipate effects of drug and observe patient's response.
3 Assess for any contraindications to patient receiving oral medication, including being NPO, inability to swallow, nausea/vomiting, bowel inflammation or reduced peristalsis, recent gastrointestinal (GI) surgery, gastric suction, and decreased level of consciousness. Check patient's swallow, cough, and gag reflexes.	Alterations in GI function interfere with medication distribution, absorption, and excretion. Patients with GI suction do not receive benefit from oral medications because they are suctioned from the GI tract before they can be absorbed. Patients with impaired swallowing are at a risk for aspiration (Edmiaston et al., 2010).

CLINICAL DECISION: *If there are any contraindications to the patient receiving oral medications or if in doubt of the patient's ability to swallow oral medications, temporarily withhold medication and inform prescriber.*

STEP	RATIONALE
4 Assess patient's medical, medication, and diet history and history of allergies. List patient's food and drug allergies on *each* page of the MAR and prominently display it on the patient's medical record per agency policy. When patient has allergy, provide allergy bracelet.	Information reflects patient's need for and potential responses to medications. Information also indicates potential food and drug interactions. Communication of allergies is essential for safe, effective care.
5 Gather physical examination and laboratory data that influence medication administration (e.g., vital signs, renal and liver function, laboratory findings).	Data sometimes reveal need to hold medication or that medication is contraindicated. Poor liver and kidney function affects metabolism and excretion of medications (Lehne, 2010).
6 Assess patient's knowledge regarding health and medication use.	Determines patient's need for medication education and guidance needed to achieve drug adherence. Assessment often reveals problems such as medication tolerance, nonadherence, abuse, addiction, or dependence.
7 Assess patient's preferences for fluids. Maintain fluid restrictions when applicable. Determine if medication can be given with preferred fluid.	Fluids ease swallowing and facilitate absorption from the GI tract. They are necessary to maintain fluid restrictions. Some fluids interfere with absorption of medications.
PLANNING	
1 Collect appropriate equipment (e.g., disposable medication cup) and MAR.	Enhances time management and efficiency.
2 Plan preparation to avoid interruptions. Do not take phone calls or talk with others. Follow agency policy.	Interruption contributes to medication errors (Biron, Lavoie-Tremblay, and Loiselle, 2009).
IMPLEMENTATION	
1 Prepare medications:	
a. Perform hand hygiene.	Reduces transfer of microorganisms.
b. If using a medication cart, move it outside patient's room.	Organization of equipment saves time and reduces error.
c. Access automated dispensing system (ADS) or unlock medicine drawer or cart.	Medications are safeguarded when locked in cabinet, cart, or computerized medication dispensing system.
d. Prepare medication for *one patient at a time.* Follow the six rights of medication administration. Keep all pages of MARs for one patient together or look at only one patient's medication administration computer screen.	Preventing distractions limits preparation errors (Brady, Malone, and Fleming, 2009).
e. Select correct medication from stock supply, unit-dose drawer, or ADS. Compare name of medication on the label with MAR (see illustration). Exit ADS after removing drug(s).	Reading labels and comparing them with the transcribed order reduces error. *This is the first accuracy check.*
f. Check expiration date on each medication, one at a time. Return outdated drug to pharmacy.	

STEP	RATIONALE
g. Check or calculate medication dose as necessary. Double-check calculation. If needed, have another nurse verify calculations.	Double-checking reduces risk of error (Dickinson et al., 2010).
h. If preparing a controlled substance, check record for previous medication count and compare current count with supply available.	Controlled substance laws require nurses to carefully monitor and count dispensed narcotics.

CLINICAL DECISION: *Splitting tablets in half, even if they are prescored with a line down the middle, leads to medication errors. Medications need to be provided in the correct dose whenever possible. If a pill must be split within inpatient settings, the pharmacist splits the pill, repackages and labels it, and sends it to the nurse for administration. Nurses* ***should not*** *split pills (ISMP, 2006).*

STEP	RATIONALE
i. Prepare solid forms of oral medications:	
(1) To prepare tablets or capsules from a floor stock bottle, pour required number into bottle cap and transfer medication to medication cup. Do not touch medication with fingers. Return extra tablets or capsules to bottle.	Avoids contamination of medications and avoids waste.
(2) To prepare unit-dose tablets or capsules, place packaged tablet or capsule directly into medicine cup. Do not remove wrapper (see illustration).	Wrapper maintains cleanliness of medications and allows you to identify medication name and dose at patient's bedside.
(3) When using a blister pack, "pop" medications through foil or paper backing into a medication cup.	Packs provide a 1-month supply, with each "blister" usually containing a single dose.
(4) Place all tablets or capsules for patient in one medicine cup, except for those requiring preadministration assessments (e.g., pulse rate or blood pressure); keep medications in their wrappers.	Keeping medications that require preadministration assessments separate from others makes it easier to withhold medications as necessary.
(5) If the patient has difficulty swallowing and liquid medications are not an option, use pill-crushing device (see illustration). Clean crushing device before using it. If a pill-crushing device is not available, place tablet between two medication cups and grind with a blunt instrument. Mix ground tablet in small amount (e.g., teaspoon) of soft food (custard or applesauce).	Large tablets are often difficult to swallow. Ground tablet mixed with palatable soft food is usually easier to swallow. Cleaning pill-crushing device ensures that contamination of medications does not occur.

STEP 1e The nurse verifies each medication with the medication administration record.

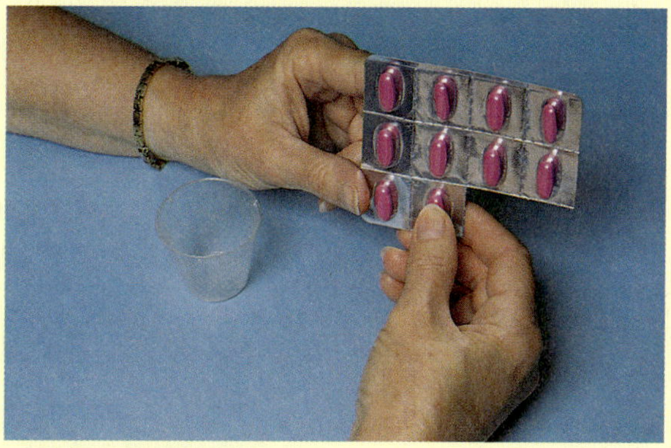

STEP 1i(2) Place tablet into medicine cup without removing wrapper.

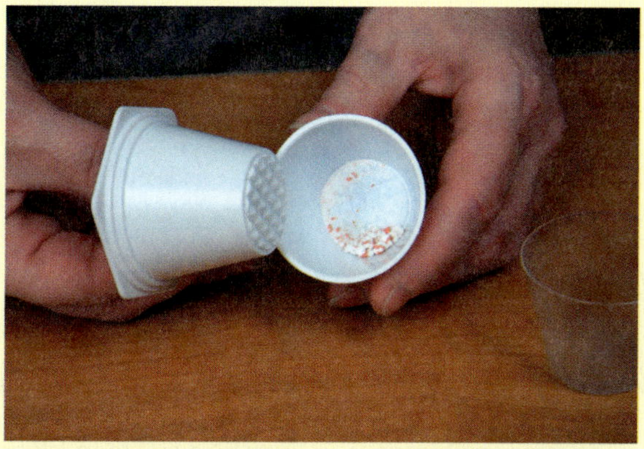

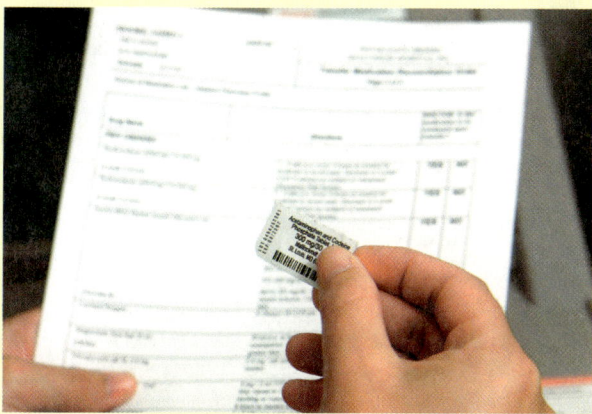

STEP 1i(5) Pill-crushing device used to crush pills when necessary.

SKILL 31-1 ADMINISTERING ORAL MEDICATIONS—cont'd

STEP	RATIONALE
CLINICAL DECISION: *Not all medications can be crushed (e.g., capsules, enteric-coated drugs). Consult with pharmacist and/or the "Do Not Crush List" when in doubt (ISMP, 2010d).*	
j. Prepare liquids:	
(1) Gently shake container. If medication is in a unit-dose container with correct amount to administer, no further preparation is necessary. If medication is in a multidose bottle, remove bottle cap from container and place cap upside down.	Shaking container ensures that medication is mixed before administration. Placing cap of bottle upside down prevents contamination of inside of cap.
(2) Hold multidose bottle with label against palm of hand while pouring.	Spilled liquid does not soil or fade label.
(3) Place medication cup at eye level on hard surface (e.g., countertop). Fill to desired level on scale (see illustration A). Make sure that scale is even with fluid level at its surface or base of meniscus, not edges. Draw up volumes of less than 10 mL in syringe designed for oral medication use without needle (see illustration B). *Do not* use parenteral syringe to draw up oral medications.	Ensures accuracy of measurement. Use of special oral syringe for oral medications prevents accidental parenteral administration of oral medication and is more accurate for small doses of medication (ISMP, 2010c).

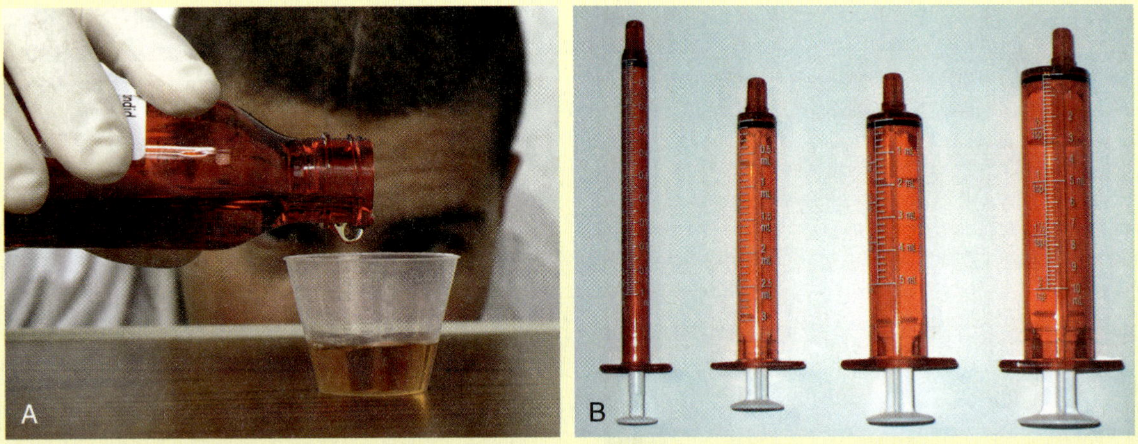

STEP 1j(3) A, Pour desired volume of liquid so base of meniscus is level with line on scale. **B,** Use special oral medication syringes to prepare small amounts of liquid medications.

STEP	RATIONALE
(4) Discard any excess liquid into sink or a place specially designated for wasting of medications. Wipe lip and neck of bottle with paper towel.	Prevents contamination of contents of bottle and prevents bottle cap from sticking.
(5) Administer liquid medication packaged in single-dose cup directly from the single-dose cup. Do not pour into medicine cup.	Avoids unnecessary manipulation of dose.
k. Before going to patient's room, compare patient's name and name of medication on label of prepared drugs with MAR.	Reading labels a second time reduces error. *This is the second accuracy check.*
l. Return stock containers or unused unit-dose medications to shelf or drawer and read label again.	Reading the label of medications in multiple-dose containers reduces administration errors.
m. Do not leave medications unattended.	Nurse is responsible for safekeeping of drugs.
2 Administer medications:	
a. Take medications to patient at correct time (see agency policy). Give time-critical, STAT, and single-order medications at time ordered. Perform hand hygiene.	Ensures intended therapeutic effect and complies with professional standards. Hospitals need to adopt a medication administration policy and procedure for the timing of medication administration that considers the patient needs, the prescribed medication, and the specific clinical indications (CMS, 2011; ISMP, 2011). Hand hygiene decreases transfer of microorganisms.
b. Identify patient using at least two patient identifiers (e.g., name and birth date or name and account number) according to facility policy. Compare identifiers with information on patient's MAR or medical record.	Ensures correct patient. Complies with a recommended National Patient Safety Goal (TJC, 2011a).
CLINICAL DECISION: *Replace patient identification bracelets that are missing, illegible, or faded.*	
c. Compare names of medications on labels with MAR at patient's bedside.	Final check of medication labels against MAR at patient's bedside reduces medication administration errors. *This is the third check for accuracy.*
d. Explain purpose of each medication, its action, and possible adverse effects to patient. Allow patient to ask any questions about drugs.	Patient has right to be informed; questions often indicate need for teaching, nonadherence to therapy, or potential medication error.

STEP	RATIONALE
e. Perform necessary preadministration assessments (e.g., blood pressure, pulse).	Determines whether specific medications should be withheld at that time.
f. Assist patient to sitting or Fowler's position. Use side-lying position if sitting is contraindicated. Have patient stay in this position for 30 minutes after administration.	Sitting position prevents aspiration during swallowing (Eisenstadt, 2010; Palmer and Metheny, 2008).
g. Administer medications	
(1) **For tablets:** Some patients want to hold solid medications in hand or cup before placing in mouth. Offer water or juice to help patient swallow.	Patient becomes familiar with medications by seeing each drug. Choice of fluid can improve fluid intake.
(2) **For sublingual-administered medications:** Have patient place medication under tongue and allow it to dissolve completely (see Fig. 31-3, p. 572). Caution patient against swallowing tablet.	Medication is absorbed through blood vessels of undersurface of tongue. If swallowed, gastric juices destroy medication, or the liver detoxifies it so rapidly that therapeutic blood levels are not attained.
(3) **For buccal medications:** Have patient place medication in mouth against mucous membranes of the cheek until it dissolves (see Fig. 31-4, p. 572). Avoid administering liquids until buccal medication has dissolved.	Buccal medications act locally on mucosa or systemically as they are swallowed in saliva.
(4) **For powdered medications:** Mix with liquids at bedside and give to patient to drink.	When prepared in advance, powdered medications often thicken and even harden, making swallowing difficult.
(5) **For crushed medications mixed in food:** Give each medication separately in teaspoon of food.	Ensures that patient swallows all of medicine.
(6) Caution patient against chewing or swallowing lozenges.	Medication acts through slow absorption through oral mucosa, not gastric mucosa.
(7) Give effervescent powders and tablets immediately after dissolving.	Effervescence improves unpleasant taste and often relieves GI problems.
h. If patient is unable to hold medications, place medication cup to lips and gently introduce each drug into the mouth, one at a time. Do not rush.	Administering single tablet or capsule eases swallowing and decreases risk of aspiration.

CLINICAL DECISION: *If tablet or capsule falls to the floor, discard it and repeat preparation.*

i. Stay until patient has completely swallowed each medication. Ask patient to open mouth if uncertain whether medication has been swallowed.	You are responsible for ensuring that patient receives ordered dosage. If left unattended, some patients do not take dose or save medications, causing risk to health.
j. For highly acidic medications (e.g., aspirin), offer patient nonfat snack (e.g., crackers) if not contraindicated by patient's condition.	Reduces gastric irritation.
k. Help patient return to comfortable position.	Maintains patient's comfort.
l. Dispose of soiled supplies and perform hand hygiene.	Reduces transmission of microorganisms.
m. Replenish stock such as cups and straws, return cart to medication room if used, and clean work area.	Clean and organized work space helps other staff complete duties efficiently.

EVALUATION

1 Evaluate patient's response to medications at times that correlate with onset, peak, and duration of the medication.	Evaluates therapeutic benefit of medication and detects onset of side effects or allergic reactions.
2 Ask patient or family member to identify medication name and explain purpose, action, dosage schedule, and potential side effects of drug.	Determines level of knowledge gained by patient and family.

UNEXPECTED OUTCOMES AND RELATED INTERVENTIONS

1 Patient exhibits adverse effects (side effect, toxic effect, allergic reaction) such as urticaria, rash, wheezing.
- *Always* notify prescriber and pharmacy when patient exhibits adverse effects.
- Withhold further doses and add allergy information to patient's medical record.

2 Patient refuses medication.
- Explore reasons why patient does not want medication.
- Educate if misunderstandings of medication therapy are apparent.
- Do not force patient to take medication; patients have the right to refuse treatment. If patient continues to refuse medication despite educational attempts, record why the drug was withheld on patient's chart and notify prescriber.

RECORDING AND REPORTING

- Chart medication dose, route, time and date given on MAR immediately after administering.
- Record the reason that any drug is withheld and follow agency policy for proper recording.
- Record and report evaluation of medication effect to prescriber if required (e.g., report urine output following administration of diuretic if ordered by prescriber).

HOME CARE CONSIDERATIONS

- Instruct patients and family caregivers about all aspects of medication administration, including dosage, desired effect, when to take medications, proper storage of medications, anticipated side effects, and whether to take medication with or without food, to ensure safe medication administration at home.
- Evaluate patient's ability to safely self-administer medications. If unable to safely self-administer, attempt nursing interventions such as a chart or pillbox to assist in self-administration. If interventions fail and patient still is unable to administer medications safely, notify the prescriber.

SKILL 31-2 ADMINISTERING OPHTHALMIC MEDICATIONS

View Video!

Delegation Considerations

The skill of administering ophthalmic medications cannot be delegated to nursing assistive personnel (NAP). Instruct NAP about:

- Potential side effects of medications and to report their occurrence, including the potential for visual changes.

Equipment

- Medication bottle with sterile eyedropper or ointment tube or medicated intraocular disk
- Cotton ball or tissue
- Washbasin filled with warm water and washcloth if eyes have crust or drainage
- Eye patch and tape (optional)
- Clean gloves
- MAR

STEP	RATIONALE
ASSESSMENT	
1 Check accuracy and completeness of each medication administration record (MAR) with prescriber's medication order. Check patient's name and medication name and dosage (e.g., number of drops [if a liquid] and eye [right, left, or both eyes]), and route and time of administration. Recopy or reprint any portion of MAR that is difficult to read.	The order sheet is the most reliable source and only legal record of medications that patient is to receive. Ensures that patient receives the correct medications. Illegible MARs are a source of medication errors (Poon et al., 2010).
2 Review pertinent information related to medication: action, purpose, normal dose and route, side effects, time of onset and peak action, and nursing implications.	Allows you to anticipate effects of drug and observe patient's response.
3 Assess condition of external eye structures (see Chapter 30). (You may also do this just before medication administration.)	Provides baseline to later determine if local response to medication occurs. Also indicates need to clean eye before medication application.
4 Assess patient's medical history, history of allergies (including latex), and medication history. If patient has latex allergy, use nonlatex gloves.	Factors in history influence how certain drugs act. Protects patient from risk of allergic medication response.
5 Determine whether patient has any symptoms of visual alterations.	Certain eye medications act to either lessen or increase these symptoms. Provides baseline assessment for recognizing change in patient's condition.
6 Assess patient's level of consciousness and ability to follow directions.	If patient becomes restless or combative during procedure, a greater risk of accidental eye injury exists.
7 Assess patient's knowledge regarding medication therapy and desire to self-administer medication.	Patient's level of understanding indicates need for health teaching. Motivation influences teaching approach.
8 Assess patient's ability to manipulate and hold dropper.	Reflects patient's ability to learn to self-administer medication.
PLANNING	
1 Collect appropriate equipment (e.g., tissue, clean gloves) and MAR.	Enhances time management and efficiency.
2 Plan preparation to avoid interruptions. Do not take phone calls. Follow agency policy.	Interruption contributes to medication errors (Biron, Lavoie-Tremblay, and Loiselle, 2009).
IMPLEMENTATION	
1 Perform hand hygiene and prepare medication (see Skill 31-1, Steps 1a to 1g). Be sure to check the label two times while preparing medication.	Hand hygiene reduces transmission of microorganisms. Ensures that patient receives correct medication. *This is the first and second accuracy check.*
2 Take medication to patient at correct time (see agency policy). Give time-critical, STAT, and single-order medications at time ordered. Perform hand hygiene.	Ensures intended therapeutic effect and complies with professional standards. Hospitals need to adopt a medication administration policy and procedure for the timing of medication administration that considers the patient needs, the prescribed medication, and the specific clinical indications (CMS, 2011; ISMP, 2011). Hand hygiene decreases transfer of microorganisms.
3 Identify patient using at least two patient identifiers (e.g., name and birth date or name and account number) according to facility policy. Compare identifiers with information on patient's MAR or medical record.	Ensures correct patient. Complies with a recommended National Patient Safety Goal (TJC, 2011a).
4 Compare names of medications on labels with MAR at patient's bedside.	*Third check for accuracy ensures that right medication is administered.*
5 Explain procedure to patient; describe positioning and sensations to expect such as burning or eye irritation. Ask if patient has any questions.	Relieves anxiety about medication being instilled into eye.
6 Arrange supplies at bedside; apply clean gloves. If eyedrops are stored in refrigerator, allow them to come to room temperature before giving them.	Reduces transmission of microorganisms and follows standards to prevent accidental exposure to body fluids. Warming eyedrops reduces irritation to eye.

STEP	RATIONALE
7 Gently roll eyedrop container between your hands.	Ensures that medication is mixed before administration. Shaking bottle causes bubbles, which makes medication administration difficult.
8 Ask patient to lie supine or sit back in chair with head slightly hyperextended.	Position provides easy access to eye for medication instillation and minimizes drainage of medication through tear duct.

CLINICAL DECISION: *Do not hyperextend the neck of a patient with cervical spine injury.*

STEP	RATIONALE
9 If crusts or drainage is present along eyelid margins or inner canthus, gently wash away. Soak any crusts that are dried and difficult to remove by applying damp washcloth or cotton ball over eye for a few minutes. Always wipe clean from inner to outer canthus.	Crusts or drainage harbors microorganisms. Soaking allows easy removal and prevents pressure from being applied directly over eye. Cleaning from inner to outer canthus avoids entrance of microorganism into lacrimal duct.
10 Hold cotton ball or clean tissue in nondominant hand on patient's cheekbone just below lower eyelid.	Cotton or tissue absorbs medication that escapes eye.
11 With tissue or cotton resting below lower lid, gently press downward with thumb or forefinger against bony orbit.	Technique exposes lower conjunctival sac. Retraction against bony orbit prevents pressure and trauma to eyeball and fingers from touching eye.
12 Ask patient to look at ceiling.	Action retracts sensitive cornea up and away from conjunctival sac and reduces stimulation of blink reflex.
13 **Instill ophthalmic drops:**	
a. With dominant hand resting on patient's forehead, hold filled medication eyedropper or ophthalmic solution approximately 1 to 2 cm (½ to ¾ inches) above conjunctival sac (see illustration).	Helps prevent accidental contact of eyedropper with eye structures, thus reducing risk of injury to eye and transfer of infection to dropper. Ophthalmic medications are sterile.
b. Drop prescribed number of medication drops into conjunctival sac.	Conjunctival sac normally holds 1 or 2 drops. Provides even distribution of medication across eye.
c. If patient blinks or closes eye or if drops land on outer lid margins, repeat instillation.	Patient obtains therapeutic effect of drug only when drops enter conjunctival sac.
d. After instilling drops, ask patient to close eye gently.	Helps to distribute medication. Squinting or squeezing of eyelids forces medication from conjunctival sac (ASHP, n.d.a).
e. When administering medications that cause systemic effects, apply gentle pressure with your finger and clean tissue on the patient's nasolacrimal duct for 30 to 60 seconds.	Prevents overflow of medication into nasal and pharyngeal passages. Prevents absorption into systemic circulation (ASHP, n.d.a).
f. If patient receives more than one eye medication to the same eye at the same time, wait at least 5 minutes before administering the next medication and use a different cotton ball or tissue with each medication.	Avoids interaction between medications (ASHP, n.d.a).
14 **Instill ophthalmic ointment:**	
a. Holding ointment applicator above lower lid margin, apply thin stream of ointment evenly along inner edge of lower eyelid on conjunctiva (see illustration) from the inner canthus to outer canthus.	Distributes medication evenly across eye and lid margin.
b. Have patient close eye and rub lid lightly in circular motion with cotton ball if rubbing is not contraindicated.	Distributes medication evenly across eye and lid margin.

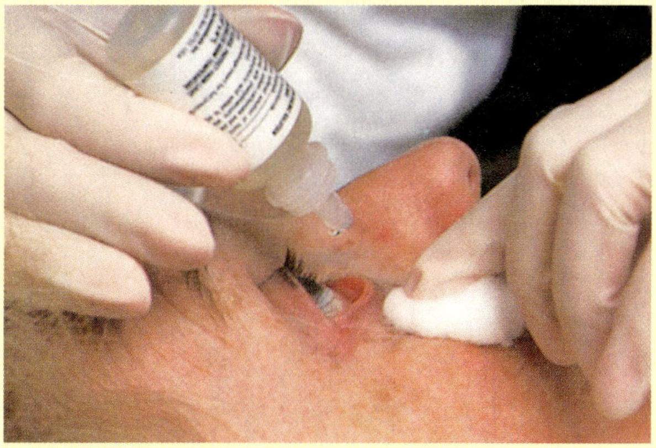

STEP 13a Hold eyedropper above conjunctival sac.

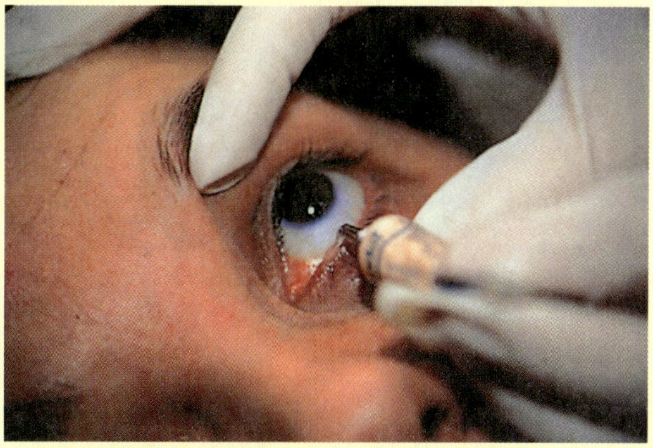

STEP 14a Apply ointment along lower eyelid.

SKILL 31-2 ADMINISTERING OPHTHALMIC MEDICATIONS—cont'd

STEP	RATIONALE
15 Administer intraocular disk:	
a. Open package containing disk. Gently press fingertip against disk so it adheres to finger. Position convex side of disk on fingertip (see illustration).	Allows you to inspect disk for damage or deformity.
b. With other hand gently pull patient's lower eyelid away from the eye. Ask patient to look up.	Prepares conjunctival sac for receiving medicated disk.
c. Place disk in conjunctival sac so it floats on the sclera between the iris and lower eyelid (see illustration).	Ensures delivery of medication (Alvarez-Lorenzo et al., 2006).
d. Pull patient's lower eyelid out and over disk (see illustration). You should not be able to see the disk at this time. Repeat Step 15 if you can see the disk.	Ensures accurate medication delivery.
16 Removal of intraocular disk	
a. Perform hand hygiene and apply gloves.	Prevents transfer of microorganisms.
b. Explain procedure to patient.	Relieves anxiety about manipulation of disk in eye.
c. Gently pull on patient's lower eyelid using nondominant hand.	Exposes intraocular disk.
d. Using forefinger and thumb of opposite hand, pinch disk and lift it out of patient's eye (see illustration).	
17 If excess medication is on eyelid, gently wipe it from inner to outer canthus.	Promotes comfort and prevents trauma to eye (ASHP, n.d.a).
18 If patient had eye patch, apply clean one by placing it over affected eye so entire eye is covered. Tape securely without applying pressure to eye.	Clean eye patch reduces chance of infection.
19 Remove gloves, dispose of soiled supplies in proper receptacle, and perform hand hygiene.	Maintains neat environment at bedside and reduces transmission of microorganisms.

EVALUATION

STEP	RATIONALE
1 Note patient's immediate response to instillation; ask if patient felt any discomfort.	Determines if procedure performed correctly and safely.
2 Observe response to medication by assessing visual changes and noting any side effects.	Evaluates effects of medication.
3 Ask patient to discuss purpose, action, side effects, and technique of administration of medication.	Determines patient's level of understanding.
4 Have patient demonstrate self-administration of next dose.	Provides feedback regarding competency with skill.

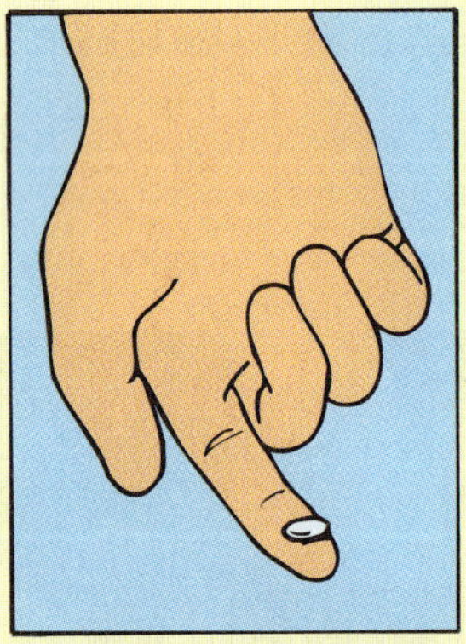
STEP 15a Gently position convex side of disk against fingertips.

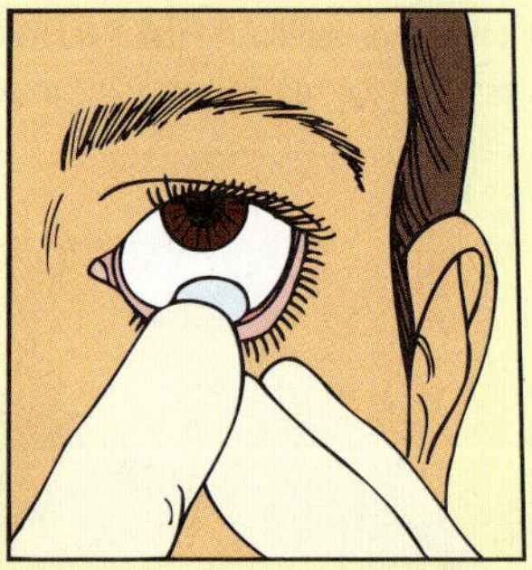
STEP 15c Place disk in conjunctival sac between the iris and lower eyelid.

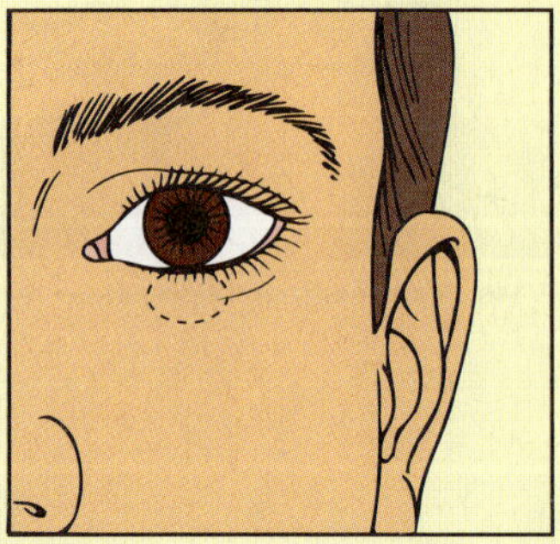
STEP 15d Gently pull lower eyelid over the disk.

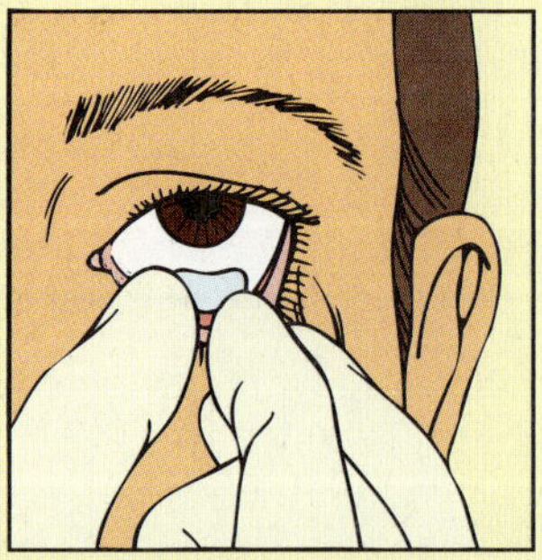
STEP 16d Carefully pinch disk to remove it from patient's eye.

UNEXPECTED OUTCOMES AND RELATED INTERVENTIONS

1 Patient cannot instill drops without supervision.
   - Reinforce teaching and allow patient to self-administer drops as much as possible to enhance confidence.
   - If patient cannot self-administer drops, teach family caregivers to instill them into patient's eye.
2 Patient displays signs of allergic reaction (e.g., tearing, reddened sclera) or systemic response (e.g., bradycardia) to medication.
   - Hold medication and speak with prescriber.
   - Follow institutional policy or guidelines for reporting adverse or allergic reaction to medications.
   - Add information about allergy to medical record per agency policy.

RECORDING AND REPORTING

- Record medication, concentration, number of drops, time and date of administration, and eye (left, right, or both) that received medication on MAR.
- Record appearance of eye in nurses' notes.

HOME CARE CONSIDERATIONS

- Have patients with chronic health care problems consult with their health care provider before using over-the-counter eye medication.
- When using eyedrops at home, patients should not share medications with other family members because risk of infection transmission is high.

SKILL 31-3 USING METERED-DOSE OR DRY POWDER INHALERS

Delegation Considerations

The skill of administering metered-dose inhalers (MDIs) or dry powder inhalers (DPIs) and supervision of patients who self-administer them cannot be delegated to nursing assistive personnel (NAP). Instruct NAP about:

- Potential side effects of medications and changes in the patient's respiratory status (e.g., increased coughing) and reporting their occurrence.

Equipment

- MDI or DPI
- Spacer (optional with MDI)
- Facial tissues (optional)
- Washbasin or sink with warm water
- Paper towel
- MAR (electronic or printed)

STEP	RATIONALE
ASSESSMENT	
1 Check accuracy and completeness of each medication administration record (MAR) with prescriber's medication order. Check patient's name and medication name, dosage (e.g., number of puffs), route, and time for administration. Recopy or reprint any portion of MAR that is difficult to read.	The order sheet is the most reliable source and only legal record of medications that patient is to receive. Ensures that patient receives the correct medications. Illegible MARs are a source of medication errors (Poon et al., 2010).
2 Review pertinent information related to medication: action, purpose, normal dose and route, side effects, time of onset and peak action, and nursing implications.	Allows you to anticipate effects of drug and observe patient's response.
3 Assess patient's medical history, history of allergies, and medication history.	Factors influence how drugs act. Reveals patient's risk for allergic response.
4 Assess patient's respiratory pattern and auscultate breath sounds.	Establishes baseline of airway status for comparison during and after treatment.
5 If previously instructed in self-administration, assess patient's ability to use inhaler (e.g., hold, manipulate, and depress canister; strength of inhalation).	Instruction sometimes only requires reinforcement of previous learning. Any impairment in ability to grasp container, breathe, or coordinate hand movement interferes with patient's ability to use MDI or DPI correctly.
6 Assess patient's *readiness* and *ability* to learn: patient asks questions about medication, disease, or complications; requests education in use of inhaler; is mentally alert, not fatigued or in pain, or in respiratory distress; and participates in own care.	Readiness affects patient's ability to understand explanations and actively participate in instruction. Mental or physical limitations affect patient's ability to learn and methods nurse uses for instruction (Bastable, 2008).
7 Assess patient's knowledge and understanding of disease and purpose and action of prescribed medications.	Knowledge of disease is essential for patient to realistically understand use of inhaler.
8 Determine medication schedule and number of inhalations prescribed for each dose.	Influences explanations nurse provides for use of inhaler.
PLANNING	
1 Collect appropriate equipment (e.g., spacer) and MAR.	Enhances time management and efficiency.
2 Provide adequate time for teaching session.	Prevents interruptions and enhances learning (Bastable, 2008).

SKILL 31-3 USING METERED-DOSE OR DRY POWDER INHALERS—cont'd

STEP	RATIONALE
IMPLEMENTATION	
1 Perform hand hygiene and prepare medication (see Skill 31-1, Steps 1a to 1g). Be sure to compare the label of the medication with the MAR two times while preparing the medication.	Following the same routine when preparing medications, eliminating distractions, and checking the label of the medication with transcribed order reduce error (Brady, Malone, and Fleming, 2009). *First and second check ensures that right medication is administered.*
2 Take medications to patient at correct time (see agency policy). Give time-critical, STAT, and single-order medications at time ordered. Perform hand hygiene.	Ensures intended therapeutic effect and complies with professional standards. Hospitals need to adopt a medication administration policy and procedure for the timing of medication administration that considers the patient needs, the prescribed medication, and the specific clinical indications (CMS, 2011; ISMP, 2011). Hand hygiene decreases transfer of microorganisms.
3 Identify patient using at least two patient identifiers (e.g., name and birth date or name and account number) according to facility policy. Compare identifiers with information on patient's MAR or medical record.	Ensures correct patient. Complies with a recommended National Patient Safety Goal (TJC, 2011a).
4 Compare names of medications on labels with MAR at patient's bedside.	*Third check for accuracy ensures that right medication is administered.*
5 Instruct patient in comfortable environment by sitting in chair in hospital room or at kitchen table in home.	Patient is more likely to remain receptive of nurse's explanations if in a comfortable environment (Bastable, 2008).
6 Allow patient opportunity to manipulate inhaler, canister, and spacer device. Explain and demonstrate how canister fits into inhaler.	Patient needs to be familiar with how to use equipment.

CLINICAL DECISION: *If patient is using an MDI with or without a spacer and the inhaler is new or has not been used for several days, push a "test spray" into the air. You do not need to do this for a DPI.*

STEP	RATIONALE
7 Explain what metered dose is, and warn patient about overuse of inhaler, including medication side effects.	Patient must not administer excessive inhalations because of risk of serious side effects. If medication is given in recommended doses, side effects are uncommon.
8 Explain steps for administering squeeze-and-breathe MDI (demonstrate steps when possible):	Use of simple, step-by-step explanations allows patient to ask questions at any point during procedure (Bastable, 2008).
a. Insert MDI canister into the holder.	
b. Remove mouthpiece cover from inhaler.	

CLINICAL DECISION: *Clean dirt or foreign objects from mouthpiece before using inhaler to avoid inhalation of unwanted material.*

STEP	RATIONALE
c. Shake inhaler vigorously five or six times. Hold inhaler in dominant hand.	Ensures that fine particle are aerosolized.
d. Have patient sit up or stand and take a deep breath and exhale.	Empties lungs and prepares the patient's airway to receive the medication.
e. Instruct the patient to position the inhaler in one of two ways.	Proper positioning of inhaler is essential to administering medication correctly.
(1) Close mouth around mouthpiece with opening toward back of throat (see illustration) and lips held tight around it.	Position directs aerosol toward airways.
(2) Position mouthpiece 2 to 4 cm (1 to 2 inches) in front of the mouth (see illustration).	
f. With inhaler properly positioned, have patient hold it with thumb at mouthpiece and index and middle fingers at the top. This is called a *three-point* or *lateral hand position.*	MDIs work best when patients use a three-point or lateral hand position to activate canisters (Lilley et al., 2007).

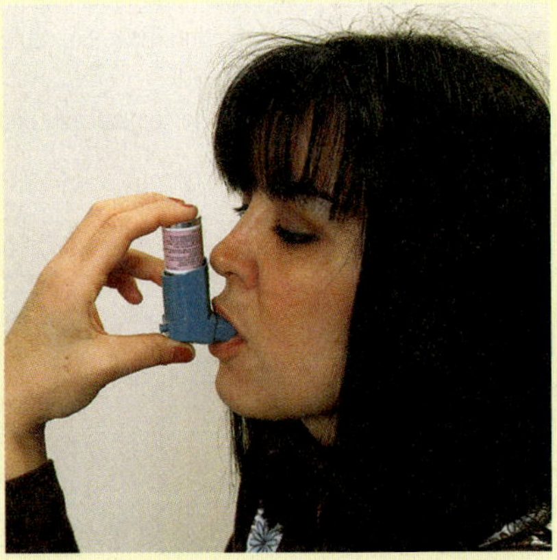

STEP 8e(1) Patient opens lips and places inhaler in mouth with opening toward back of throat.

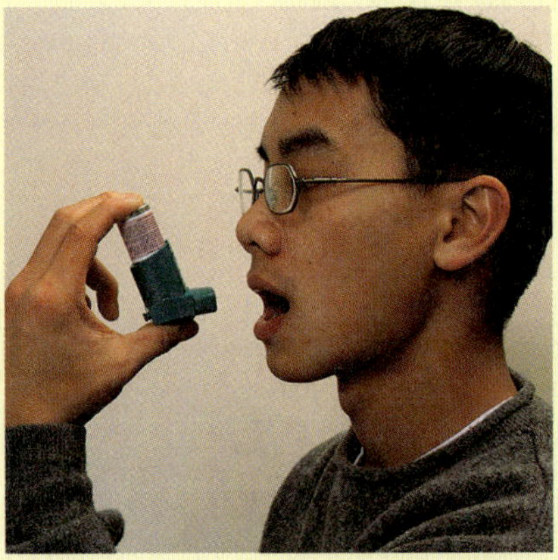

STEP 8e(2) Patient positions mouthpiece 1 to 2 inches away from mouth.

STEP	RATIONALE
g. Instruct patient to tilt head back slightly and inhale slowly and deeply through mouth for 3 to 5 seconds while depressing canister fully.	Distributes medication to airways during inhalation. Inhalation through mouth rather than nose draws medication more effectively into airways.
h. Have patient hold breath for about 10 seconds.	Allows tiny drops of aerosol spray to reach deeper branches of airways (MayoClinic.com, 2009b).
i. Remove MDI from mouth and exhale through pursed lips.	Keeps small airways open during exhalation.
9 Explain steps to administer MDI using a spacer such as an Aerochamber (demonstrate when possible):	Use of simple, step-by-step explanations allows patient to ask questions at any point during instruction.
a. Insert canister into holder. Remove mouthpiece cover from MDI and mouthpiece of spacer. Inspect spacer for foreign objects and ensure that valve is intact if spacer has one.	Inhaler fits into end of spacer.
b. Shake MDI inhaler vigorously five or six times.	Ensures that fine particles are aerosolized.
c. Insert MDI into end of spacer.	Spacer traps medication released from MDI; patient then inhales the drug from the device. These devices break up and slow down the medication particles, increasing the amount of medication that goes into the patient's lungs (MayoClinic.com, 2009a).
d. Instruct patient to place spacer mouthpiece into mouth and close lips. Do not insert beyond raised lip on mouthpiece. Avoid covering small exhalation slots with lips (see illustration).	Medication should not escape through the mouth.
e. Have patient breathe in and exhale completely and then breathe normally through spacer mouthpiece.	Empties lungs and prepares for medication.
f. Have patient depress medication canister, spraying one puff into spacer.	Emits spray that allows finer particles to be inhaled. Large droplets are retained in spacer.
g. Instruct patient to inhale deeply and slowly through mouth for 3 to 5 seconds.	Maximizes amount of medication that enters the lung.
h. Have patient hold breath for 10 seconds.	Ensures full medication distribution.
i. Remove MDI and spacer before exhaling.	Allows patient to exhale normally.
10 Explain steps to administer DPI or breath-activated MDI (demonstrate when possible):	
a. Remove cover from mouthpiece. **Do not shake** inhaler.	
b. Prepare medication as directed by manufacturer (e.g., hold inhaler upright and turn wheel to right and then to left until a click is heard, load medication pellet).	Primes inhaler, ensuring that medication is delivered to patient (MayoClinic.com, 2009a).
c. Exhale away from inhaler before inhalation.	Prevents loss of powder.
d. Position mouthpiece between lips (see illustration).	Prevents medication from escaping through mouth.
e. Inhale deeply and forcefully through mouth.	Creates aerosol.
f. Hold breath for 5 to 10 seconds.	Ensures full medication distribution.
11 Instruct patient to wait at least 20 to 30 seconds between inhalations of the same medication and 2 to 5 minutes between inhalations of different medications or as ordered by prescriber.	Medications must be inhaled sequentially. Always give bronchodilators before steroids. First inhalation opens airways. Second or third inhalation reduces inflammation and/or penetrates deeper airways.

CLINICAL DECISION: *If patient uses a corticosteroid, have him or her rinse mouth out with water or salt water or brush teeth after inhalation to reduce risk of fungal infection. Also teach patient to inspect oral cavity daily for redness, sores, or white patches. Report abnormal assessment findings to the patient's health care provider (MayoClinic.com, 2009a).*

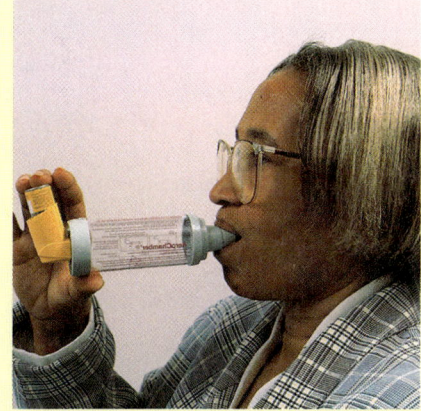

STEP 9d Have patient place mouthpiece in mouth and close lips, being careful to keep exhalation slots exposed.

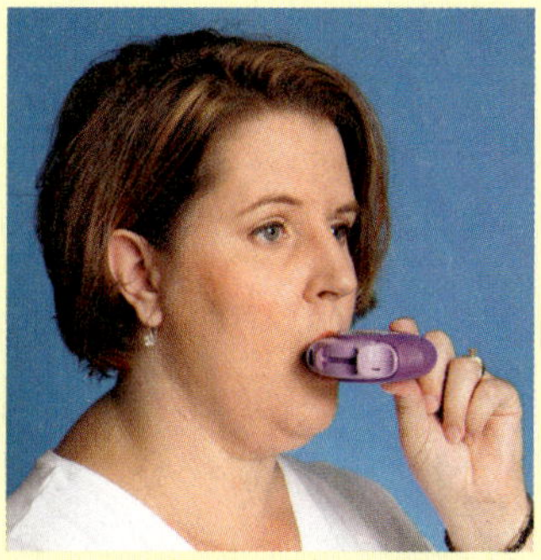

STEP 10d Have patient place mouthpiece of dry powdered inhaler between lips.

SKILL 31-3 USING METERED-DOSE OR DRY POWDER INHALERS—cont'd

STEP	RATIONALE
12 Instruct patient against repeating inhalations before next scheduled dose.	Medications are prescribed at intervals during day to provide constant drug levels and minimize side effects.
13 Explain that patient may feel gagging sensation in throat caused by droplets of medication on pharynx or tongue. Approximately 2 minutes after dose have patient rinse mouth out with warm water.	Results when inhalant is sprayed and inhaled incorrectly.
14 Instruct patient how to clean inhaler:	
a. Once a day remove canister from inhaler. Inhaler and cap need to be rinsed in warm running water. Inhaler needs to be completely dry before using.	Accumulation of spray around mouthpiece interferes with proper distribution during use.
b. Twice a week, the L-shaped plastic mouthpiece needs to be washed with mild dishwashing soap and warm water. Rinse and dry well before putting canister back inside mouthpiece.	Removes residual medication. Do not place inhalers holding cromolyn, nedocromil, or hydrofluoroalkanes (HFAs) in water.
EVALUATION	
1 Ask if patient has any questions.	Clarifies misconceptions or misunderstanding.
2 Have patient explain and demonstrate steps in use of inhaler.	Return demonstration provides feedback for measuring patient's learning.
3 Ask patient to explain medication schedule, side effects, and when to call health care provider.	Improves likelihood of adherence to therapy.
4 Ask patient to calculate how many days the inhaler will last.	Helps patient determine when to reorder prescription.
5 Assess patient's respiratory status: ease of respirations, auscultation of lungs, and use of pulse oximetry (see Chapter 30).	Determines status of breathing pattern and adequacy of ventilation.

UNEXPECTED OUTCOMES AND RELATED INTERVENTIONS

1 Patient needs a bronchodilator more than every 4 hours.
- Indicates respiratory problems; reassessment of type of medication and delivery methods is needed.
- Notify health care provider if respiratory status does not improve.

2 Patient experiences cardiac dysrhythmias, light-headedness, and/or syncope, especially if receiving beta-adrenergics.
- Withhold all further doses of medication.
- Consult with health care provider.

3 Patient is not able to self-administer medication properly.
- Explore alternative delivery routes or methods of medication administration.

4 Patient experiences paroxysms of coughing caused by irritation of posterior pharynx.
- Consult with health care provider to reassess type of medication or delivery method.

RECORDING AND REPORTING

- Document skills taught and patient's ability to perform skills.
- Record medication, time and date of administration, route, and number of puffs on the MAR.
- Document patient's response to medication in nurses' notes.
- Report any undesirable effects from medication.

HOME CARE CONSIDERATIONS

- Remind patients to carry their prescribed inhalers to use emergently in case of an acute asthma attack.

SKILL 31-4 PREPARING INJECTIONS

Delegation Considerations

The skill of preparing injections cannot be delegated to nursing assistive personnel (NAP).

Equipment

- Small gauze pad or unopened alcohol swab
- MAR (electronic or printed)
- Medication in an ampule
  - Safety syringe, needle, and filter needle
- Medication in a vial
  - Safety syringe
  - Needles:
    - — Blunt tip vial access cannula (if needleless system used)
    - — Filter needle (if indicated)
    - — Needle for drawing up medication (if needed)
    - — Safety needle for injection
- Diluent (e.g., normal saline or sterile water) (if indicated)

STEP	RATIONALE
ASSESSMENT	
1 Check accuracy and completeness of each medication administration record (MAR) with prescriber's medication order. Check patient's name and medication name, dosage, and route and time for administration. Recopy or reprint any portion of MAR that is difficult to read.	The order sheet is the most reliable source and only legal record of medications that patient is to receive. Ensures that patient receives the correct medications. Illegible MARs are a source of medication errors (Poon et al., 2010).
2 Review pertinent information related to medication, including action, purpose, dose and route, side effects, and nursing implications.	Allows nurse to administer medication properly and monitor patient's response.
3 Assess patient's body build, muscle size, and weight.	Determines type and size of syringe and needles for injection.
PLANNING	
1 Collect appropriate equipment (e.g., disposable medication cup) and MAR.	Enhances time management and efficiency.
2 Plan preparation to avoid interruptions. Do not take phone calls or talk with others. Follow agency policy.	Interruption contributes to medication errors (Biron, Lavoie-Tremblay, and Loiselle, 2009).
IMPLEMENTATION	
1 Perform hand hygiene.	Reduces transmission of microorganisms.
2 Prepare medication (see Skill 31-1, Steps 1a to 1h). Be sure to check the label two times while preparing medication.	Following the same routine when preparing medications, eliminating distractions, and checking the label of the medication with transcribed order reduces error (Brady et al., 2009). *First and second check ensures that right medication is administered.*
a. **Ampule preparation**	
(1) Tap top of ampule lightly and quickly with finger until fluid moves from neck of ampule (see illustration).	Dislodges any fluid that collects above neck of ampule. All solution moves into lower chamber.
(2) Place small gauze pad or unopened alcohol swab just above neck of ampule (see illustration).	Placing pad around neck of ampule protects nurse's fingers from trauma as glass tip is broken off.
(3) Snap neck of ampule quickly and firmly away from hands (see illustration).	Protects nurse's fingers and face from shattering glass.
(4) Draw up medication quickly, using filter needle long enough to reach bottom of ampule.	System is open to airborne contaminants. Needle needs to be long enough to access medication for preparation. Filter needles filter out any fragments of glass (Nicoll and Hesby, 2002).
(5) Hold ampule upside down or set it on a flat surface with filter needle in center of ampule opening. Do not allow needle tip or shaft to touch rim of ampule.	Broken rim of ampule is considered contaminated. When ampule is inverted, solution comes out if needle tip or shaft touches rim of ampule.

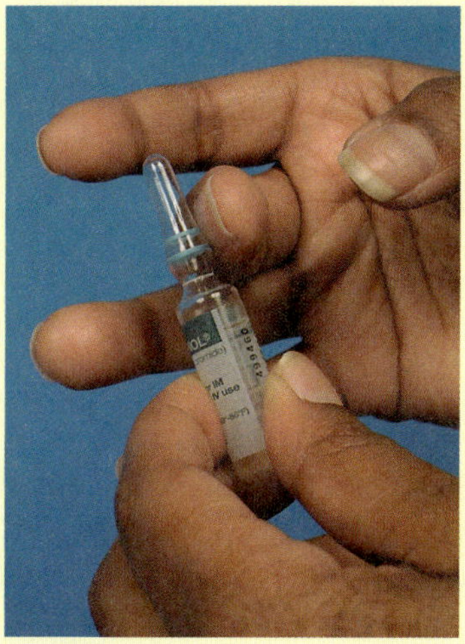

STEP 2a(1) Tapping ampule moves fluid down neck.

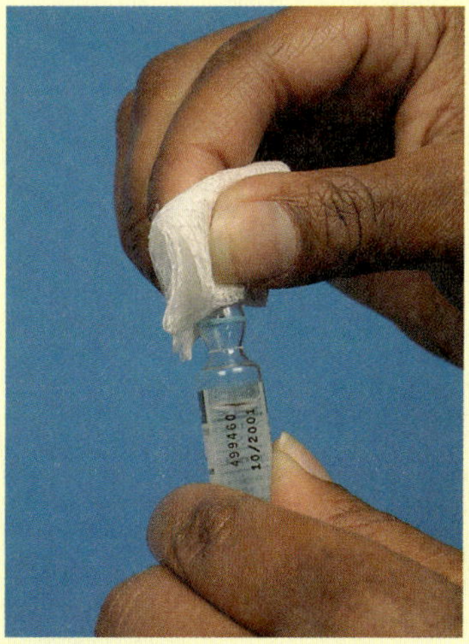

STEP 2a(2) Gauze pad placed just above neck of ampule.

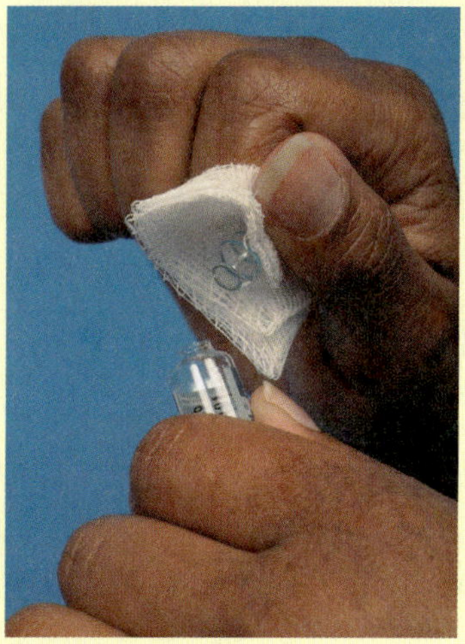

STEP 2a(3) Snapping neck away from hands.

SKILL 31-4 PREPARING INJECTIONS—cont'd

STEP	RATIONALE
(6) Aspirate medication into syringe by gently pulling back on plunger (see illustrations).	Withdrawal of plunger creates negative pressure within syringe barrel, which pulls fluid into syringe.
(7) Keep needle tip under surface of liquid. Tip ampule to bring all fluid within reach of needle.	Prevents aspiration of air bubbles.
(8) If air bubbles are aspirated, do not expel air into ampule.	Air pressure forces liquid out of ampule and medication is lost.
(9) To expel excess air bubbles, remove needle from ampule. Hold syringe with needle pointing up. Tap side of syringe to cause bubbles to rise toward needle. Draw back slightly on plunger and push plunger upward to eject air. Do not eject fluid.	Withdrawing plunger too far removes it from barrel. Holding syringe vertically allows fluid to settle in bottom of barrel. Pulling back on plunger allows fluid within needle to enter barrel so it is not expelled. Air at top of barrel and within needle is then expelled.
(10) If syringe contains excess fluid, use sink or other specially designated area for medication disposal. Hold syringe vertically with needle tip up and slanted slightly toward sink. Slowly eject excess fluid into sink. Recheck fluid level in syringe by holding it vertically.	Medication dose prepared accurately. Position of needle allows medication to be expelled without flowing down needle shaft. Rechecking fluid level ensures proper dose.
(11) Cover needle with its safety sheath or scoop needle to recap. Replace filter needle with safety needle or needleless access device for injection.	Prevents contamination of needle. Filter needles cannot be used for injection. Scooping technique prevents needlestick injury.
b. Vial containing a solution	
(1) Remove cap covering top of unused vial to expose sterile rubber seal, keeping rubber seal sterile. If a multidose vial has been used before, cap is already removed. Firmly and briskly wipe surface of rubber seal with alcohol swab and allow it to dry.	Vial comes packaged with seal that cannot be replaced after cap removal. Not all drug manufacturers guarantee that caps of unused vials are sterile. Therefore swab seals with alcohol before preparing medication. Allowing alcohol to dry prevents needle from being coated with alcohol and mixing with medication.
(2) Pick up syringe and remove needle cap or cap covering needleless vial access device (see illustration). Pull back on plunger to draw amount of air into syringe equal to volume of medication to be aspirated from vial.	Inject air first into vial to prevent buildup of negative pressure in vial when aspirating medication.

CLINICAL DECISION: *Some medications and agencies require use of a filter needle when preparing medications from a vial. See agency policy (Nicoll and Hesby, 2002). If using a filter needle to aspirate the medication, it is changed to a regular needle of suitable size to administer the medication.*

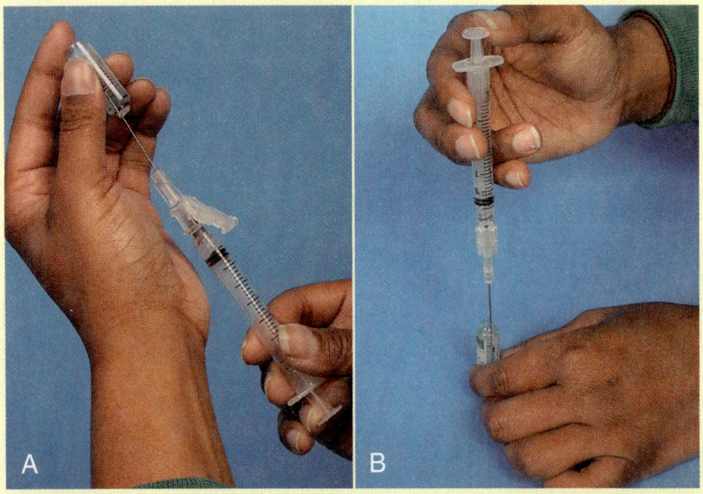

STEP 2a(6) A, Medication aspirated with ampule inverted. **B,** Medication aspirated with ampule on flat surface.

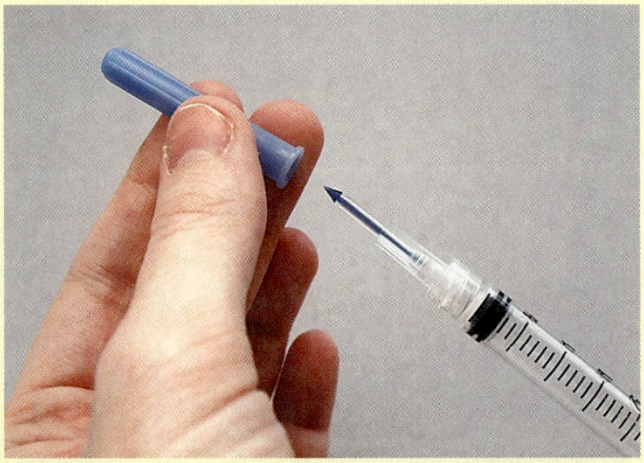

STEP 2b(2) Syringe with needleless adapter.

STEP	RATIONALE
(3) With vial on flat surface, insert tip of needle with beveled tip entering first or needleless access device through center of rubber seal (see illustration). Apply pressure to tip of needle during insertion.	Center of seal is thinner and easier to penetrate. Injecting beveled tip first and using firm pressure prevent coring of rubber seal, which could enter vial or needle.
(4) Inject air into the airspace of the vial, holding on to plunger. Hold plunger with firm pressure; air pressure within the vial sometimes forces the plunger backward.	Injecting air before aspirating fluid creates vacuum needed to get medication to flow into syringe. Injecting into airspace of vial prevents formation of bubbles and inaccuracy in dose.
(5) Invert vial while keeping firm hold on syringe and plunger (see illustration). Hold vial between thumb and middle fingers of nondominant hand. Grasp end of syringe barrel and plunger with thumb and forefinger of dominant hand to counteract pressure in vial.	Inverting vial allows fluid to settle in lower half of container. Position of hands prevents forceful movement of plunger and permits easy manipulation of syringe.
(6) Keep tip of needle below fluid level.	Prevents aspiration of air.
(7) Allow air pressure from vial to fill syringe gradually with medication. If necessary, pull back slightly on plunger to obtain correct amount of solution.	Positive pressure within vial forces fluid into syringe.
(8) When desired volume is obtained, position needle into airspace of vial; tap side of syringe barrel carefully to dislodge any air bubbles. Eject any air remaining at top of syringe into vial.	Forcefully striking barrel while needle is inserted in vial bends needle. Accumulation of air displaces medication and causes dose errors.
(9) Remove needle from vial by pulling back on barrel of syringe.	Accidentally pulling plunger rather than barrel causes plunger to separate from barrel, resulting in loss of medication.
(10) Hold syringe at eye level at 90-degree angle to ensure correct volume and absence of air bubbles. Remove any remaining air by tapping barrel to dislodge air bubbles (see illustration). Draw back slightly on plunger; push plunger upward to eject air. Do not eject fluid. Recheck volume of medication.	Holding syringe vertically allows fluid to settle in bottom of barrel. Pulling back on plunger allows fluid within needle to enter barrel so it is not expelled. Air at top of barrel and within needle is then expelled.

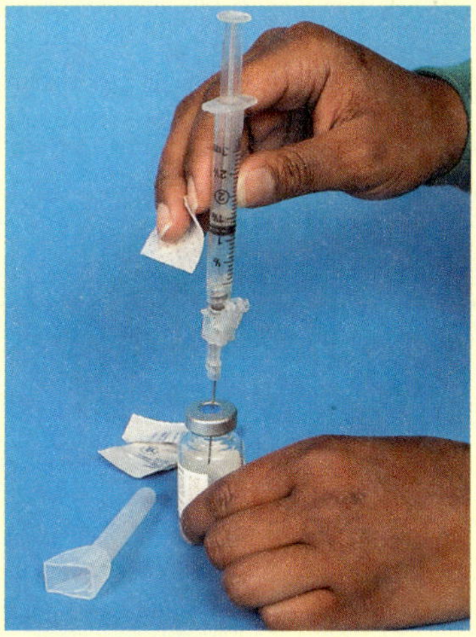

STEP 2b(3) Insert safety needle through center of vial diaphragm (with vial flat on table).

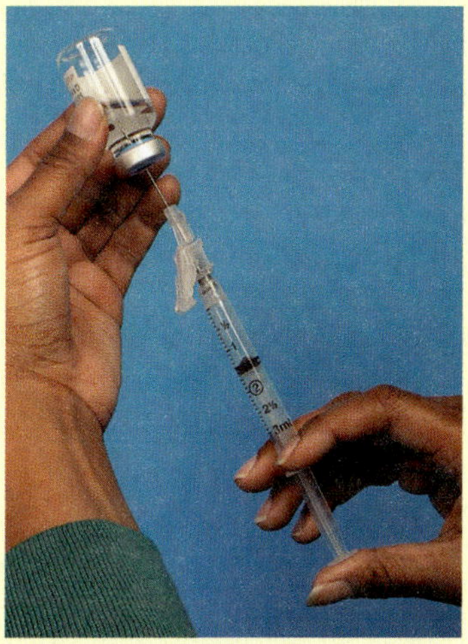

STEP 2b(5) Withdraw fluid with vial inverted.

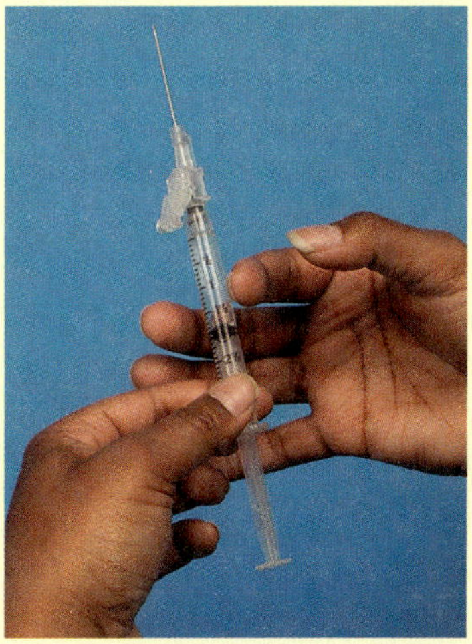

STEP 2b(10) Hold syringe upright; tap barrel to dislodge air bubbles.

SKILL 31-4 PREPARING INJECTIONS—cont'd

STEP	RATIONALE
(11) If medication will be injected into patient's tissue, change needle to appropriate gauge and length according to route of medication.	Inserting needle through a rubber stopper dulls beveled tip. New needle is sharper. Because no fluid is along shaft, needle does not track medication through tissues.
(12) For multidose vial make label that includes date of mixing, concentration of medication per milliliter, and your initials.	Ensures that future doses will be prepared correctly. Some medications need to be discarded a certain number of days after mixing of vial.
c. **Vial containing a powder (reconstituting medications)**	
(1) Remove cap covering vial of powdered medication and cap covering vial of proper diluent. Firmly swab both seals with alcohol swab and allow to dry.	Not all drug manufacturers guarantee that caps of unused vials are sterile. Therefore seals must be swabbed with alcohol before preparing medication. Allowing alcohol to dry prevents needle from being coated with alcohol and mixing with medication.
(2) Draw up diluent into syringe following Steps 2b(2)-(10).	Prepares diluent for injection into vial containing powdered medication.
(3) Insert tip of safety needle or needleless access device through center of rubber seal of vial of powdered medication. Inject diluent into vial. Remove needle.	Diluent begins to dissolve and reconstitute medication.
(4) Mix medication thoroughly. Roll in palms. **Do not shake.**	Ensures proper dispersal of medication throughout solution. Shaking produces bubbles.
(5) Reconstituted medication in vial is ready to be drawn into new syringe. Read label carefully to determine dose after reconstitution.	Once diluent is added, concentration of medication (mg/mL) determines dose to be given. Read medication label carefully to avoid medication errors.
(6) Prepare medication in syringe following Steps 2b(2)-(12).	

CLINICAL DECISION: *Some agencies require prepared parenteral medications to be verified for accuracy by another nurse. Check policies before administering medication.*

3 Compare label of medication with MAR for the final time at the patient's bedside before administering medication.	*Third check for accuracy ensures that right medication is administered.*
4 Dispose of soiled supplies. Place broken ampule and/or used vials and used needle in puncture-proof and leak-proof container. Clean work area and perform hand hygiene.	Proper disposal of glass and needle prevents accidental injury to staff. Controls transmission of infection.

EVALUATION

1 Compare dose in syringe with desired dose.	Determines that dose is accurate.

UNEXPECTED OUTCOMES AND RELATED INTERVENTIONS

1 Air bubbles remain in syringe.
- Expel air from syringe and add medication to syringe until correct dose is prepared.

2 Incorrect dose is prepared.
- Discard prepared dose and prepare corrected new dose.

SKILL 31-5 ADMINISTERING INJECTIONS

View Video!

Delegation Considerations

The skill of administering injections cannot be delegated to nursing assistive personnel (NAP). Instruct the NAP about:

- Potential medication side effects and to report their occurrence along with any changes in a patient's vital signs or level of consciousness (e.g., sedation).

Equipment

- Proper size safety syringe and needle:
  - *Subcutaneous:* Syringe (1 to 3 mL) and needle (27 to 25 gauge, 3/8 to 5/8 inch)
  - *Subcutaneous U-100 insulin:* Insulin syringe (0.3, 0.5, or 1 mL) with preattached needle (28 to 31 gauge, 5/16 to 1/2 inch)
  - *Subcutaneous U-500 insulin:* 1-mL tuberculin syringe with needle (25 to 27 gauge, 1/2 to 5/8 inch)
  - *Intramuscular (IM):* Syringe 2 to 3 mL for adult, 0.5 to 1 mL for infants and small children
  - Needle, length corresponding to site of injection and age of patient. Refer to following guidelines; length needed may vary outside of these guidelines for patients who are smaller or larger than average.

Site	Child (Hockenberry and Wilson, 2009)	Adult (Nicoll and Hesby, 2002)
Ventrogluteal	1/2 to 1 inch	1 1/2 inch
Vastus lateralis	5/8 to 1 inch	5/8 to 1 inch
Deltoid	1/2 to 1 inch	1 to 1 1/2 inch

Equipment—cont'd
- Needle gauge often depends on length of needle. Administer most biologicals and medications in aqueous solutions with 20- to 25-gauge needle. Use 18- to 25-gauge needles for medications in oil-based solutions (Nicoll and Hesby, 2002).
  - *Intradermal (ID):* 1-mL tuberculin syringe with needle (25 to 27 gauge, ½ to ⅝ inch)
- Small gauze pad
- Alcohol swab
- Vial or ampule of medication or skin test solution
- Clean gloves
- MAR (electronic or printed)

STEP	RATIONALE
ASSESSMENT	
1 Check accuracy and completeness of each medication administration record (MAR) with prescriber's medication order. Check patient's name and medication name, dosage, and route and time for administration. Recopy or reprint any portion of MAR that is difficult to read.	The order sheet is the most reliable source and only legal record of medications patient is to receive. Ensures that patient receives the correct medications. Illegible MARs are a source of medication errors (Poon et al., 2010).
2 Review pertinent information related to medication: action, purpose, normal dose and route, side effects, time of onset and peak action, nursing implications.	Allows you to anticipate effects of drug and observe patient's response.
3 Assess patient's medical and medication history and history of allergies. Know his or her normal response to an allergy.	Reveals need for medication. Allows for early identification of patient risk for allergic response. May require different medication prescription. Do not administer medication to which patient is allergic.
4 Check date of expiration for medication.	Drug potency increases or decreases when outdated.
5 Observe verbal and nonverbal responses toward receiving injection.	Injections are often painful. Some patients have anxiety, which increases pain.
6 Assess for contraindications.	
a. **For subcutaneous injections**	
(1) Assess for factors such as circulatory shock or reduced local tissue perfusion. Assess adequacy of patient's adipose tissue.	Reduced tissue perfusion interferes with medication absorption and distribution. Physiological changes of aging or patient illness often influence the amount of subcutaneous tissue that a patient possesses. This influences methods for administering injections.
b. **For IM injections**	
(1) Assess for factors such as muscle atrophy, reduced blood flow, or circulatory shock.	Atrophied muscle absorbs medication poorly. Factors interfering with blood flow to muscles impair medication absorption.
7 Assess patient symptoms or condition for which medication has been prescribed.	Provides baseline to determine response to therapy.

CLINICAL DECISION: *Because of documented adverse effects of IM injections, other routes of medication administration are safer. Verify that IM injection is necessary and explore alternative medication routes if possible (Nicoll and Hesby, 2002; World Health Organization [WHO], 2006).*

STEP	RATIONALE
PLANNING	
1 Collect appropriate equipment (e.g., safety syringe, needles) and MAR.	Enhances time management and efficiency.
2 Plan preparation to avoid interruptions. Do not take phone calls or talk with others. Follow agency policy.	Interruption contributes to medication errors (Biron, Lavoie-Tremblay, and Loiselle, 2009).
IMPLEMENTATION	
1 Perform hand hygiene. Aseptically prepare correct medication dose from ampule or vial (see Skill 31-4). Check label of medication with MAR two times while preparing medication.	Ensures that medication is sterile. Preparation techniques differ for ampule and vial. *First and second checks ensure that right medication is administered.*
2 Take medication to patient at the correct time (see agency policy). Give time-critical, STAT, and single-order medications at time ordered. Perform hand hygiene.	Ensures intended therapeutic effect and complies with professional standards. Hospitals need to adopt a medication administration policy and procedure for the timing of medication administration that considers the patient needs, the prescribed medication, and the specific clinical indications (CMS, 2011; ISMP, 2011). Hand hygiene decreases transfer of microorganisms.
3 Close room curtain or door.	Provides privacy.
4 Identify patient using two identifiers (e.g., name and birth date or name and account number) according to facility policy. Compare identifiers with information on patient's MAR or medical record.	Ensures correct patient. Complies with a recommended National Patient Safety Goal (TJC, 2011a).
5 Compare name of medication on label with MAR one more time at patient's bedside.	Third check for accuracy ensures that right medication is administered.
6 Explain steps of procedure and tell patient that injection will cause a slight burning or sting.	Helps minimize patient's anxiety.

SKILL 31-5 ADMINISTERING INJECTIONS—cont'd

STEP	RATIONALE
7 Apply clean gloves. NOTE: If patient has latex allergy, use latex-free gloves.	Reduces transfer of microorganisms.
8 Keep sheet or gown draped over body parts not requiring exposure.	Respects dignity of patient while area to be injected is exposed.
9 Select appropriate injection site. Inspect skin surface over sites for bruises, inflammation, or edema.	Injection sites need to be free of abnormalities that interfere with medication absorption. Sites used repeatedly become hardened from lipohypertrophy (increased growth in fatty tissue). Do not use an area that is bruised or has signs associated with infection.
a. *Subcutaneous:* Palpate sites for masses or tenderness. Avoid these areas. For daily insulin, rotate site within anatomical area. Be sure that needle is correct size by grasping skinfold at site with thumb and forefinger. Measure fold from top to bottom. Needle should be one-half length.	Subcutaneous injections are sometimes mistakenly given in the muscle, especially in abdomen and thigh sites. Appropriate size of needle and angle of injection ensures that medication is injected in the subcutaneous tissue (Birkebaek et al., 2008).
b. *IM:* Note integrity and size of muscle and palpate for tenderness or hardness. Avoid these areas. If injections are given frequently, rotate sites. Use ventrogluteal site if possible.	The ventrogluteal site is the preferred site for adults. This site is also preferred for children who are receiving viscous or irritating solutions (Hockenberry and Wilson, 2009; Nicoll and Hesby, 2002).
c. *ID:* Note lesions or discolorations of skin. If possible, select site three to four finger widths below antecubital space and a hand width above wrist. If you cannot use forearm, inspect upper back. If necessary, use sites for subcutaneous injections.	An ID site needs to be clear so you can see results of skin test and interpret them correctly (CDC, 2010).
10 Help patient to comfortable position:	
a. *Subcutaneous:* Have patient relax arm, leg, or abdomen, depending on site chosen for injection.	Relaxation of site minimizes discomfort.
b. *IM:* Position patient depending on site chosen (e.g., sit or lie flat, on side, or prone).	Reduces strain on muscle and minimizes discomfort of injections.
c. *ID:* Have patient extend elbow and support it and forearm on flat surface.	Stabilizes injection site for easiest accessibility.
d. Have patient talk about subject of interest. Ask open-ended questions.	Distraction reduces anxiety.

CLINICAL DECISION: *Ensure that patient's position is not contraindicated by medical condition.*

STEP	RATIONALE
11 Relocate site using anatomical landmarks.	Injection into correct anatomical site prevents injury to nerves, bones, and blood vessels (Nicoll and Hesby, 2002).
12 Clean site with an antiseptic swab. Apply swab at center of site and rotate outward in circular direction for approximately 5 cm (2 inches) (see illustration).	Mechanical action of swab removes secretions containing microorganisms.
13 Hold swab or gauze between third and fourth fingers of nondominant hand.	Gauze or swab remains readily accessible when needle is withdrawn.
14 Remove needle cap or sheath from needle by pulling it straight off.	Preventing needle from touching sides of cap prevents contamination.
15 Hold syringe between thumb and forefinger of dominant hand.	
a. *Subcutaneous:* Hold as dart, palm down (see illustration).	Quick, smooth injection requires proper manipulation of syringe parts.
b. *IM:* Hold as dart, palm down.	
c. *ID:* Hold bevel of needle pointing up.	With bevel up, medication is less likely to be deposited into tissues below dermis.

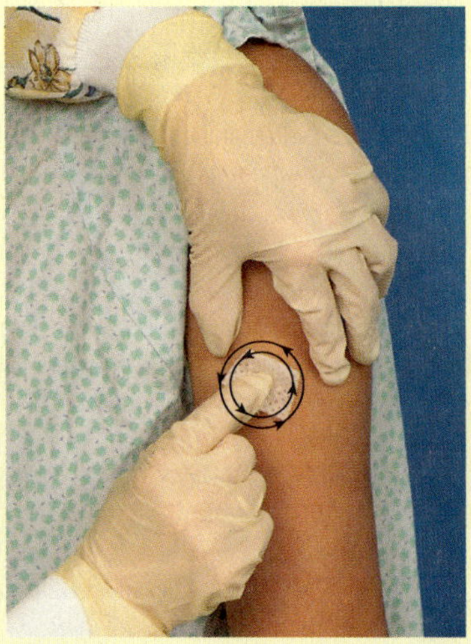

STEP 12 Clean site with circular motion.

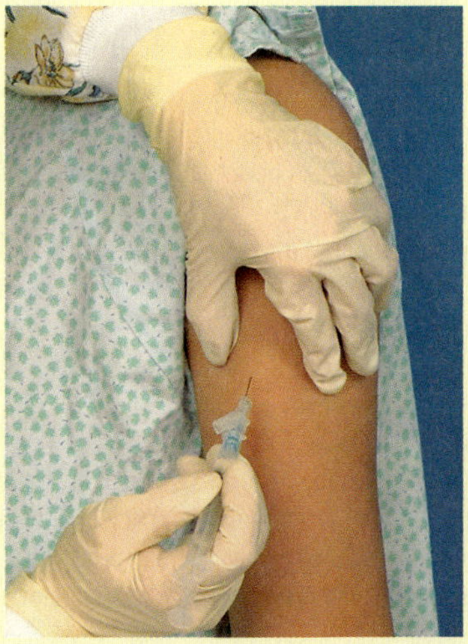

STEP 15a Hold syringe as if grasping a dart.

STEP	RATIONALE
16 Administer injection:	
a. **Subcutaneous**	
(1) For average-size patient, pinch skin with nondominant hand.	Pinching skin elevates subcutaneous tissue and desensitizes area.
(2) Inject needle quickly and firmly at 45- to 90-degree angle. Release skin. *Option:* Continue to pinch skin and release after injecting medications.	Quick, firm insertion minimizes discomfort. (Injecting medication into compressed tissue irritates nerve fibers.) Correct angle prevents accidental injection into muscle.
(3) For obese patient pinch skin at site and inject needle at 90-degree angle below tissue fold.	Obese patients have fatty layer of tissue above subcutaneous layer.

CLINICAL DECISION: *Piercing a blood vessel during a subcutaneous injection is very rare. Therefore aspiration is not necessary when administering subcutaneous injections.*

STEP	RATIONALE
(4) Inject medication slowly (see illustration).	Minimizes discomfort.

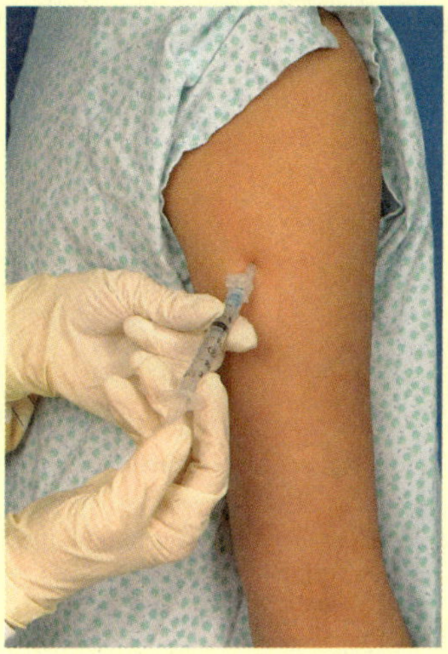

STEP 16a(4) Inject medication slowly.

STEP	RATIONALE
b. **Intramuscular**	
(1) Position ulnar aspect of your nondominant hand just below site and pull skin approximately 2.5 to 3.5 cm (1.5 inches) down or laterally to administer in a Z-track. Hold position until medication is injected (see Fig. 31-23, p. 608). With dominant hand inject needle quickly at 90-degree angle into muscle.	Z-track creates zigzag path through tissues that seals needle track to avoid tracking of medication. Use Z-track for all IM injections (Nicoll and Hesby, 2002). A quick, dartlike injection reduces discomfort.
(2) *Option:* If patient's muscle mass is small, grasp body of muscle between thumb and fingers.	Ensures that medication reaches muscle mass (Hockenberry and Wilson, 2009).
(3) Insert needle into the muscle using a smooth, steady motion. After needle pierces skin, grasp lower end of syringe barrel with nondominant hand to stabilize syringe. Continue to hold skin tightly with nondominant hand. Move dominant hand to end of plunger. Do not move syringe.	A smooth, steady motion reduces pain at the moment of injection (Nicoll and Hesby, 2002). Smooth manipulation of syringe reduces discomfort from needle movement. Skin needs to remain pulled until after injecting medication to ensure Z-track administration.
(4) Pull back on plunger 5 to 10 seconds. If no blood appears, inject medicine slowly, at a rate of 1 mL/10 seconds.	This time is necessary to ensure that the needle in not in a low-flow blood vessel (Nicoll and Hesby, 2002). Aspiration of blood into syringe indicates intravenous (IV) placement of needle. Slow injection rate reduces pain and tissue trauma, and reduces chance of leakage of medication back through the needle track (Hockenberry and Wilson, 2009; Nicoll and Hesby, 2002).

CLINICAL DECISION: *If blood appears in syringe, remove needle and dispose of medication and syringe properly. Prepare another dose of medication for injection.*

STEP	RATIONALE
(5) Wait 10 seconds. Then smoothly and steadily withdraw needle and release skin.	Allows for medication to absorb into muscle before removing syringe rather than leaking back out through the track that the needle created (Nicoll and Hesby, 2002).
c. **Intradermal**	
(1) With nondominant hand stretch skin over site with forefinger or thumb.	Needle pierces tight skin more easily.
(2) With needle almost against patient's skin, insert it slowly with bevel up at a 5- to 15-degree angle until resistance is felt. Advance it through epidermis to approximately 3 mm (⅛ inch) below skin surface. You will see needle tip through skin.	Ensures that needle tip is in dermis. You obtain inaccurate results if you do not inject needle at correct angle and depth (CDC, 2010).

SKILL 31-5 ADMINISTERING INJECTIONS—cont'd

STEP	RATIONALE
(3) Inject medication slowly. Normally you feel resistance. If not, needle is too deep; remove and begin again. Nondominant hand can stabilize needle during the injection.	Slow injection minimizes discomfort at site. Dermal layer is tight and does not expand easily when solution is injected. Stabilizing needle prevents unnecessary movements and decreases patient discomfort.
(4) While injecting medication, notice that small bleb approximately 6 mm (¼ inch) in diameter (resembling mosquito bite) appears on surface of skin (see illustration). Instruct patient that this is a normal finding.	Bleb indicates that medication is deposited in dermis.

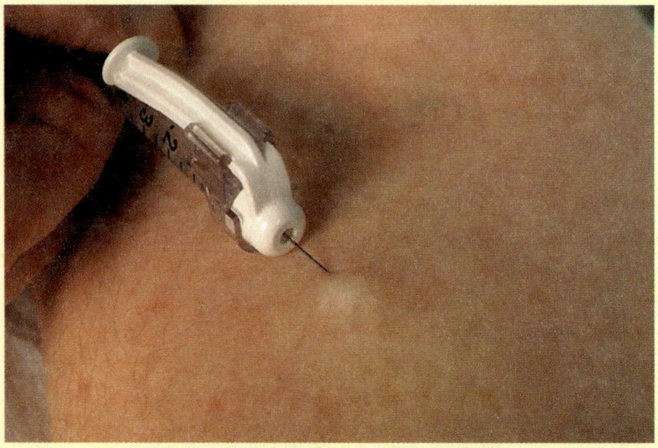

STEP 16c(4) Injection creates a small bleb.

STEP	RATIONALE
17 Withdraw needle while applying alcohol swab or gauze gently over site.	Support of tissue around injection site minimizes discomfort during needle withdrawal. Dry gauze minimizes patient discomfort associated with alcohol on nonintact skin.
18 Apply gentle pressure. *Do not massage site.* Apply bandage if needed.	Massage causes underlying tissue damage. Massaging ID site disperses medication into underlying tissue layers and alters test results.
19 Help patient to comfortable position.	Gives patient sense of well-being.
20 Discard uncapped needle or needle enclosed in safety shield and attached syringe into puncture-proof and leak-proof receptacle.	Prevents injury to patient and health care personnel. Recapping needles increases risk of needlestick injury (OSHA, 2009).
21 Remove gloves and perform hand hygiene.	Reduces transmission of microorganisms.
22 Stay with patient and observe for allergic reactions.	Dyspnea, wheezing, and circulatory collapse are signs of severe anaphylactic reaction, which is a life-threatening emergency.

EVALUATION

STEP	RATIONALE
1 Return to room and ask if patient feels any acute pain, burning, numbness, or tingling at injection site.	Continued discomfort often indicates injury to underlying bones or nerves.
2 Inspect site, noting any bruising or induration. Document bruising or induration if present. Notify health care provider and provide warm compress to site.	Bruising or induration indicates complication associated with injection.
3 Observe patient's response to medication at times that correlate with onset, peak, and duration of medication.	IM medications are rapidly absorbed. Adverse effects of parenteral medications develop rapidly. Nurse's observations determine efficacy of medication action.
4 Ask patient to explain purpose and effects of medication.	Evaluates patient's understanding of information taught.
5 *For ID injections:* Use skin pencil and draw circle around perimeter of injection site. Read site within appropriate amount of time, designated by type of medication or skin test administered.	Pencil mark makes site easy to find. Results of skin testing are read at various times, based on type of medication used or type of skin testing completed. Refer to manufacturer directions to determine when to read results of test.

CLINICAL DECISION: *Read tuberculin test at 48 to 72 hours. Induration (hard, dense, raised area) of skin around injection site indicates positive reaction, as follows:*

- *15 mm or more in patients with no known risk factors for tuberculosis (TB)*
- *10 mm or more in patients who are recent immigrants; injection drug users; residents and employees of high-risk settings; mycobacteriology laboratory personnel; patients with clinical conditions placing them at high risk; children less than 4 years of age; and infants, children, and adolescents exposed to high-risk adults*
- *5 mm or more in patients who are human immunodeficiency virus (HIV) positive, have fibrotic changes on chest x-ray film consistent with previous TB infection, have had organ transplants, or are immunosuppressed (CDC, 2010).*

UNEXPECTED OUTCOMES AND RELATED INTERVENTIONS

1 Raised, reddened, or hard zone (induration) forms around ID test site.
- Notify patient's health care provider.
- Document sensitivity to injected allergen or positive test if tuberculin skin testing was completed.

2 Hypertrophy of skin develops from repeated subcutaneous injections.
- Do not use this site for future injections.
- Instruct patient not to use site for 6 months.

3 Patient develops signs and symptoms of allergy or side effects.
- Follow agency policy or guidelines for appropriate response to adverse drug reactions.
- Notify patient's health care provider immediately.
- Add allergy information to patient's medical record.

4 Patient complains of localized pain, numbness, tingling, or burning at injection site, indicating possible injury to nerve or tissues.
- Assess injection site.
- Document findings.
- Notify patient's health care provider.

RECORDING AND REPORTING

- Chart medication dose, route, site, time, and date given on MAR immediately after giving medication per agency policy.
- Document if scheduled medication is withheld and record the reason per agency policy.
- Report any undesirable effects from medication to prescriber.
- Record patient's response to medications in nurses' notes and report to prescriber if required.

HOME CARE CONSIDERATIONS

- Assess patient's readiness to learn before instructing in self-injections. Some patients are hesitant to administer injections to themselves; thus relieve any anxiety before teaching this skill to a patient.
- Some patients prefer to reuse their syringes to save costs. This practice is safe and practical if the needle is not contaminated during the preparation and administration of the injection. Teach patients to immediately recap needles after use.
- Patients can often purchase or obtain sharps boxes for home use. If this is not possible, they can use a hard plastic bottle that they cannot see through (e.g., a fabric softener bottle or detergent bottle) to safely store syringes after use. Disposal of needles used in the home varies among communities. Check with local authorities to verify how to dispose of needles.

SKILL 31-6 ADMINISTERING MEDICATIONS BY INTRAVENOUS BOLUS

Delegation Considerations

The skill of administering medications by intravenous (IV) bolus cannot be delegated to nursing assistive personnel (NAP). Inform NAP about:
- Potential side effects of medications and need to report their occurrence.
- The need to report discomfort at infusion site as soon as possible.
- Obtaining any required vital signs and reporting these findings to the nurse.

Equipment

- Watch with second hand
- MAR (electronic or printed)
- Clean gloves
- Antiseptic swab
- Medication in vial or ampule
- Safety syringe for medication preparation
- Needleless device or sterile safety needle (21 to 25 gauge)
- IV lock: vial of appropriate flush solution (saline most common, heparinized flush is sometimes used; if using heparin, most common concentration is 10 to 100 units/mL; see agency policy)

STEP	RATIONALE
ASSESSMENT	
1 Check accuracy and completeness of each medication administration record (MAR) with prescriber's medication order. Check patient's name and medication name, dosage, route, and time for administration. Recopy or reprint any portion of MAR that is difficult to read.	The order sheet is the most reliable source and only legal record of medications that patient is to receive. Ensures that patient receives the correct medications. Illegible MARs are a source of medication errors (Poon et al., 2010).

SKILL 31-6 ADMINISTERING MEDICATIONS BY INTRAVENOUS BOLUS—cont'd

STEP	RATIONALE
CLINICAL DECISION: *Some IV medications can only be pushed safely when a patient is being continuously monitored for dysrhythmias, blood pressure changes, or other adverse effects. Therefore some medications can only be pushed in specific areas within a health care agency. See agency policy for special monitoring requirements before giving medication (Lehne, 2010).*	
2 Review pertinent information related to medication: action, purpose, normal dose and route, side effects, time of onset and peak action, how slowly to give medication, compatibility with IV fluids, and nursing implications.	Allows you to give medication safely and monitor patient's response to therapy (Lehne, 2010). Prevents incompatible drug reaction.
3 If pushing medication into an IV line, determine compatibility of medication with IV fluids and any additives within IV solution.	IV medications are not always compatible with IV solution and/or additives.
4 Perform hand hygiene. Assess IV or saline lock insertion site for signs of infiltration or phlebitis (see Chapter 41).	Confirming placement of IV catheter and integrity of surrounding tissue ensures that medication is administered safely. Do not administer medication if site is inflamed or edematous.
5 Check patient's medical history and history of drug or latex allergies.	IV bolus delivers medication rapidly. Allergic reactions can be fatal.
6 Assess patient's understanding of purpose of medication therapy.	Reveals need for patient education.
PLANNING	
1 Collect appropriate equipment (e.g., syringe, medication) and MAR.	Enhances time management and efficiency.
CLINICAL DECISION: *Some IV medications require dilution before administration. Verify with agency policy. If a small amount of medication is given (e.g., less than 1 mL), dilute medication in 5 to 10 mL of normal saline or sterile water so medication does not collect in "dead spaces" (e.g., Y-site injection port, IV cap) of the IV delivery system. Verify that medication can be diluted by consulting medication reference or checking with pharmacist first.*	
2 Plan preparation to avoid interruptions. Do not take phone calls or talk with others. Follow agency policy.	Interruption contributes to medication errors (Biron, Lavoie-Tremblay, and Loiselle, 2009).
IMPLEMENTATION	
1 Perform hand hygiene. Prepare ordered medication from vial or ampule using aseptic technique (see Skill 31-4). Check label of medication carefully with MAR two times.	Ensures that medication is sterile. Preparation techniques differ for ampule and vial. *First and second checks ensure that right medication is administered.*
2 Take medication to patient at correct time (see agency policy). Give time-critical, STAT, and single-order medications at time ordered. Perform hand hygiene.	Ensures intended therapeutic effect and complies with professional standards. Hospitals need to adopt a medication administration policy and procedure for the timing of medication administration that considers the patient needs, the prescribed medication, and the specific clinical indications (CMS, 2011; ISMP, 2011). Hand hygiene decreases transfer of microorganisms.
3 Identify patient using at least two patient identifiers (e.g., name and birth date or name and account number) according to facility policy. Compare identifiers with information on patient's MAR or medical record.	Ensures correct patient. Complies with a recommended National Patient Safety Goal (TJC, 2011a).
4 Compare names of medications on labels with MAR one more time at patient's bedside.	*Third check for accuracy ensures that right medication is administered.*
5 Explain procedure to patient. Encourage patient to report symptoms of discomfort at IV site.	Keeps patient informed and ensures patient-centered care. Helps identify possible infiltration early.
6 Put on clean gloves. NOTE: If patient has latex allergy, use latex-free gloves.	Reduces transmission of microorganisms. During IV bolus administration there is a risk of blood exposure.
7 **IV push (existing line):**	
a. Select injection port of IV tubing closest to patient. Whenever possible, injection port should accept a needleless syringe. Use IV filter if required by medication reference or agency policy.	Follows provisions of the Needle Safety and Prevention Act of 2001 (OSHA, 2009).
CLINICAL DECISION: *Never administer IV medications through tubing that is infusing blood, blood products, or parenteral nutrition solutions.*	
b. Clean injection port with antiseptic swab. Allow to dry.	Prevents introduction of microorganisms during needle insertion.
c. Connect syringe to port of IV line. Insert needleless tip or small-gauge needle of syringe containing prepared drug through center of injection port (see illustration).	Prevents damage to diaphragm of port and subsequent leakage.

STEP	RATIONALE
d. Occlude IV line by pinching tubing just above injection port (see illustration). Pull back gently on syringe plunger to aspirate blood return.	Final check that medication is being delivered into bloodstream.

CLINICAL DECISION: *In some cases, especially with a smaller-gauge IV needle, blood return is not always aspirated, even if IV is patent. If IV site shows no signs of infiltration and IV fluid is infusing without difficulty, proceed with IV push.*

STEP	RATIONALE
e. Release tubing and inject medication within amount of time recommended by institutional policy, pharmacist, or medication reference manual. Use watch to time administration (see illustration). You can pinch the IV line while pushing medication and release when not pushing it. Allow IV fluids to infuse when not pushing medication.	Ensures safe medication infusion. Rapid injection of IV medication can be fatal (Lehne, 2010). Allowing IV fluids to infuse while pushing IV drug enables medications to be delivered to patient at prescribed rate.

CLINICAL DECISION: *When IV medication is incompatible with IV fluids, stop the IV fluids, clamp the IV line above the injection site, flush with 10 mL of normal saline or sterile water, give the IV bolus over the appropriate amount of time, flush with another 10 mL of normal saline or sterile water at the same rate as the medication was administered, and restart the IV fluids at the prescribed rate. If IV line that is currently hanging contains a medication (e.g., ranitidine), disconnect IV line and administer IV push as outlined in Step 8 to avoid giving a sudden bolus of the medication in existing IV line. Some IV medications and fluids cannot be stopped. Verify agency policy regarding temporarily stopping IV fluids or continuous IV medications. If unable to stop IV infusion, start a new IV site (see Chapter 41) and administer medication using the IV lock method.*

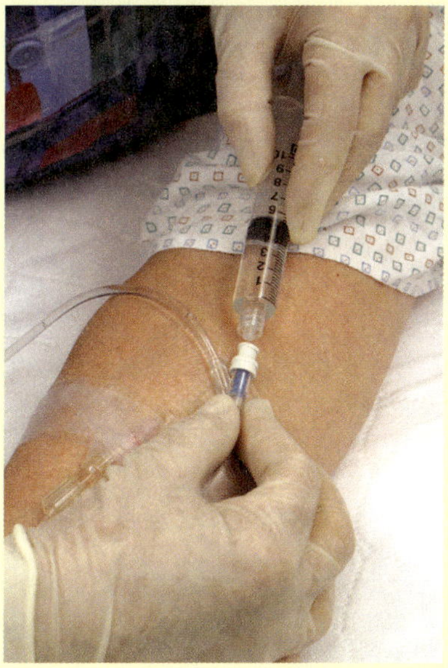

STEP 7c Connecting syringe to IV line with blunt needleless cannula tip.

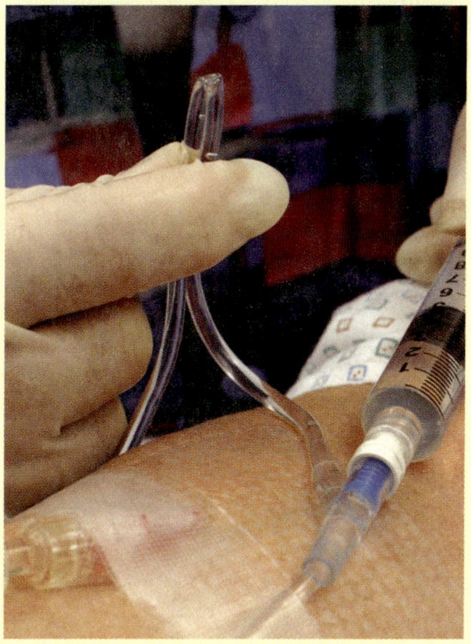

STEP 7d Intravenous line pinched above injection port to aspirate for blood return.

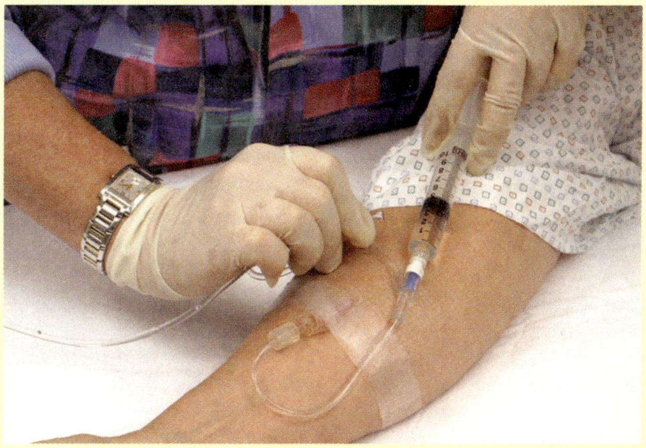

STEP 7e Using watch to time an IV push medication.

SKILL 31-6 ADMINISTERING MEDICATIONS BY INTRAVENOUS BOLUS—cont'd

STEP	RATIONALE
f. After injecting medication, release tubing, withdraw syringe, and recheck fluid infusion rate.	Injection of bolus alters rate of fluid infusion. Rapid fluid infusion causes circulatory overload.
8 **IV push (IV lock)**	
a. Prepare two syringes with 2 to 3 mL of normal saline (0.9%) in syringe.	

CLINICAL DECISION: *Current evidence reflects that saline flushes are effective in maintaining patency of IV lines and do not carry risk of thrombocytopenia associated with heparin flushes.*

STEP	RATIONALE
b. Administer medication:	
(1) Clean injection port of lock with antiseptic swab.	Prevents introduction of microorganisms during needle insertion.
(2) Insert syringe containing normal saline (0.9%) into injection port of IV lock (see illustration).	

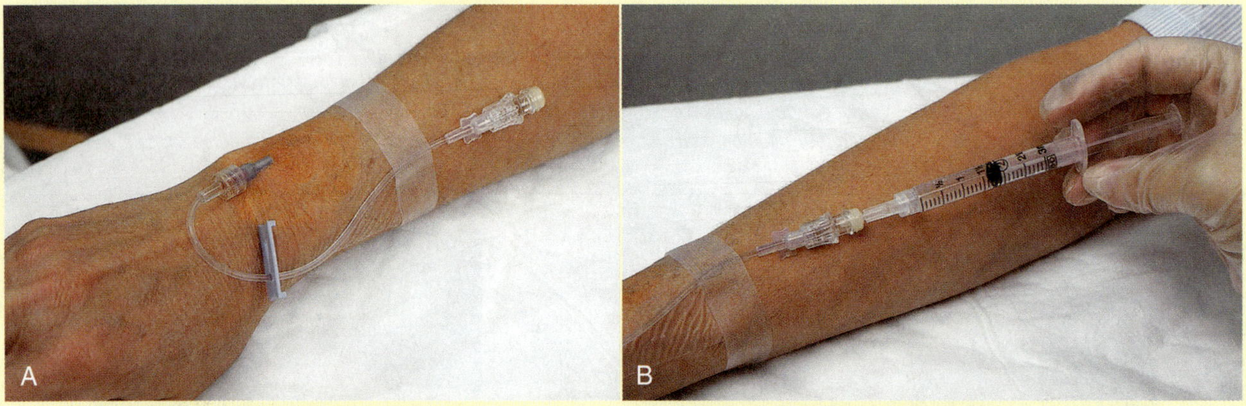

STEP 8b(2) A, IV catheter with saline lock adapter. **B,** Syringe inserted into injection port.

STEP	RATIONALE
(3) Pull back gently on syringe plunger and look for blood return.	Determines whether IV needle or catheter is positioned in vein.

CLINICAL DECISION: *At times a blood return is not aspirated even though lock is patent. If IV site does not show signs of infiltration and IV site flushes without difficulty, proceed with IV push.*

STEP	RATIONALE
(4) Flush IV lock with normal saline by pushing slowly on plunger.	Clears IV lock of blood.

CLINICAL DECISION: *Observe closely area of skin above IV catheter. Note any puffiness or swelling as IV lock is flushed, which indicates infiltration into vein, requiring removal of catheter.*

STEP	RATIONALE
(5) Remove saline flush syringe.	
(6) Clean injection port of lock with antiseptic swab.	Prevents transmission of infection.
(7) Insert syringe containing prepared medication into injection port of IV lock.	
(8) Inject medication within amount of time recommended by institutional policy, pharmacist, or medication reference manual. Use watch to time administration.	Rapid injection of IV medication can result in death. Following guidelines for IV push rates promotes patient safety (Lehne, 2010).
(9) After administering bolus, withdraw syringe.	
(10) Clean injection port of lock with antiseptic swab.	Prevents transmission of microorganisms.
(11) Flush injection port by attaching syringe with normal saline. Inject normal saline flush at same rate medication was delivered.	Irrigation with saline prevents occlusion of IV access device and ensures that all medication is delivered. Flushing IV site at same rate as medication ensures that any medication remaining within IV needle is delivered at correct rate.
9 Dispose of uncapped needles and syringes in puncture-proof and leak-proof container.	Reduces accidental needlesticks (OSHA, 2009).
10 Remove and dispose of gloves. Perform hand hygiene.	Reduces transmission of microorganisms.

STEP	RATIONALE
EVALUATION	
1 Observe patient closely for adverse reaction as drug is administered and for several minutes thereafter.	IV medications act rapidly.
2 Observe IV site during injection for sudden swelling.	Swelling indicates infiltration into tissues surrounding vein.
3 Assess patient's status after giving medication to evaluate its effectiveness.	IV bolus medications often cause rapid changes in patient's physiological status. Some medications require careful monitoring and possibly laboratory testing (e.g., vasopressors require monitoring of blood pressure and heart rate; dilantin requires laboratory studies to determine if it is in a therapeutic level).
4 Ask patient to explain purposes and side effects of medication.	Evaluates learning.

UNEXPECTED OUTCOMES AND RELATED INTERVENTIONS

1 Patient develops adverse reaction to medication.
- Stop delivering medication immediately and follow institution policy or guidelines for appropriate response and reporting of adverse drug reactions.
- Add allergy information to patient's medical record.

2 IV site shows symptoms of infiltration or phlebitis (see Chapter 41).
- Stop infusing medication.
- Treat IV site as indicated by agency policy.
- Insert new IV site if continuing IV therapy.

3 Patient is unable to explain medication information.
- Patient requires reinstruction or is unable to learn at this time.

RECORDING AND REPORTING

- Record medication, dose, time and date, and route of administration.
- Report any adverse reactions immediately to health care provider. Patient's response may indicate need for additional medical therapy.
- Record patient's response to medication in nurses' notes.

SKILL 31-7 ADMINISTERING INTRAVENOUS MEDICATIONS BY PIGGYBACK, INTERMITTENT INTRAVENOUS INFUSION SETS, AND MINI-INFUSION PUMPS

Delegation Considerations

The skill of administering intravenous (IV) medications by piggyback, intermittent IV infusion sets, and mini-infusion pumps cannot be delegated to nursing assistive personnel (NAP). Instruct NAP about:
- Potential side effects of medications and to report their occurrence to the nurse immediately.
- Reporting patient's verbalization of discomfort at infusion site.
- Reporting changes in patient's condition or vital signs.

Equipment

- Adhesive tape (optional)
- Antiseptic swab
- IV pole
- MAR (electronic or printed)
- Clean gloves
- Piggyback or mini-infusion pump
  - Medication prepared in 5- to 250-mL labeled infusion bag or syringe
  - Short microdrip, macrodrip or mini-infusion tubing set for piggyback with needleless system attachment
    - —Needleless device or stopcocks
    - —Mini-infusion pump if needed
- Volume-control administration set
  - Buretrol
  - Infusion tubing with needleless system attachment
  - Syringe (1 to 20 mL)
  - Vial or ampule of ordered medication

STEP	RATIONALE
ASSESSMENT	
1 Check accuracy and completeness of each medication administration record (MAR) with prescriber's medication order. Check patient's name and medication name, dosage, and route and time of administration. Recopy or reprint any portion of MAR that is difficult to read.	The order sheet is the most reliable source and only legal record of medications that patient is to receive. Ensures that patient receives the correct medications. Illegible MARs are a source of medication errors (Poon et al., 2010).
2 Review patient's medical history and history of allergies.	Helps you anticipate therapeutic effect of medication. Intravenous bolus delivers medication rapidly. Allergic reactions can be fatal.

SKILL 31-7 ADMINISTERING INTRAVENOUS MEDICATIONS BY PIGGYBACK, INTERMITTENT INTRAVENOUS INFUSION SETS, AND MINI-INFUSION PUMPS—cont'd

STEP	RATIONALE
3 Review pertinent information related to medication: action, purpose, normal dose and route, side effects, time of onset and peak action, compatibility with existing IV fluids, and nursing implications.	Allows you to give medication safely and to monitor patient's response to therapy.
4 Assess patency of patient's existing IV infusion line by noting infusion rate of main IV line (see Chapter 41).	IV line must be patent, and fluids need to infuse easily for medication to reach venous circulation effectively.

CLINICAL DECISION: *If the patient's IV site is saline locked, clean the port with alcohol and assess the patency of the IV line by flushing it with 2 to 3 mL of sterile normal saline. Attach appropriate IV tubing to the saline lock and administer the medication via piggyback, tandem, mini-infusion, or volume-control administration set. When the infusion is completed, disconnect the tubing, clean the port with alcohol, and flush the IV line with 2 to 3 mL of sterile normal saline. Maintain sterility of IV tubing between intermittent infusions.*

STEP	RATIONALE
5 Perform hand hygiene. Assess IV insertion site for signs of infiltration or phlebitis: redness, pallor, swelling, and tenderness on palpation.	Confirmation of placement of IV needle or catheter and integrity of surrounding tissues ensures safe medication administration.
6 Assess patient's understanding of purpose of medication therapy.	Reveals need for education.
PLANNING	
1 Collect appropriate equipment (e.g., medication, tubing) and MAR.	Enhances time management and efficiency.
2 Plan preparation to avoid interruptions. Do not take phone calls or speak with others. Follow agency policy.	Interruption contributes to medication errors (Biron, Lavoie-Tremblay, and Loiselle, 2009).
IMPLEMENTATION	
1 Perform hand hygiene. Prepare medication from an ampule or vial (see Skill 31-4). Be sure to compare the label of the medication with the MAR two times while preparing the medication.	Ensures that medication is sterile. Preparation techniques differ for ampule and vial. *First and second checks ensure that right medication is administered.*
2 Take medication to patient at correct time (see agency policy). Give time-critical, STAT, and single-order medications at time ordered. Perform hand hygiene.	Ensures intended therapeutic effect and complies with professional standards. Hospitals need to adopt a medication administration policy and procedure for the timing of medication administration that considers the patient needs, the prescribed medication, and the specific clinical indications (CMS, 2011; ISMP, 2011). Hand hygiene decreases transfer of microorganisms.
3 Identify patient using at least two patient identifiers (e.g., name and birth date or name and account number) according to facility policy. Compare identifiers with information on patient's MAR or medical record.	Ensures correct patient. Complies with a recommended National Patient Safety Goal (TJC, 2011a).
4 Explain purpose of medication and side effects to patient. Explain that you will give medication through existing IV line. Encourage patient to report symptoms of discomfort at site immediately.	
5 Compare names of medications on labels with MAR one more time at patient's bedside.	*Third check for accuracy ensures that right medication is administered.*
6 Put on clean gloves. NOTE: If patient has a latex allergy, use latex-free gloves.	Reduces transmission of microorganisms. During IV administration there is a risk of blood exposure.
7 Administer medications	
a. Piggyback infusion	

CLINICAL DECISION: *Never administer IV medications through tubing that is infusing blood, blood products, or parenteral nutrition solutions.*

STEP	RATIONALE
(1) Connect infusion tubing to medication bag (see Chapter 41). Allow solution to fill tubing by opening regulator flow clamp. Once tubing is full, close clamp and cap end of tubing.	Infusion tubing needs to be filled with solution and free of air bubbles to prevent air embolus.
(2) Hang piggyback medication bag above level of primary fluid bag (use hook to lower main bag) (see Fig. 31-26, p. 610).	Height of fluid bag affects rate of flow to patient.
(3) Connect tubing of piggyback infusion to appropriate connector on primary infusion line.	

STEP	RATIONALE
(a) *Needleless system:* Wipe off needleless port of main IV line and insert tip of piggyback infusion tubing (see illustration).	Use needleless connections to prevent accidental needlestick injuries (OSHA, 2009). Establishes route for IV medication to enter main IV line.
(b) *Stopcock:* Wipe off stopcock port with alcohol swab and connect tubing. Turn stopcock to open position.	Stopcock eliminates need for needle.
(4) Regulate flow rate of medication solution by adjusting regulator clamp or IV pump infusion rate (see Chapter 41). Infusion times vary. Refer to medication reference or agency policy for safe flow rate.	Provides slow, intermittent infusion of medication and maintains therapeutic blood levels.
(5) After medication has infused, check flow regulator on primary infusion. Primary infusion automatically begins to flow after piggyback solution is empty. If stopcock is used, turn it to off position.	Back-check valve on piggyback stops flow of the primary infusion until second medication infuses. Checking flow rate ensures proper administration of IV fluids.
(6) Regulate main infusion line to desired rate if necessary.	Infusion of piggyback sometimes interferes with main line infusion rate.
(7) Leave IV piggyback bag and tubing in place for future medication administration or discard in appropriate containers.	Establishment of secondary line produces route for microorganisms to enter main line. Repeated changes in tubing increase risk of infection transmission (see agency policy).
b. Mini-infusion administration	
(1) Connect prefilled syringe to mini-infusion tubing.	Special tubing designed to fit syringe delivers medication to main IV line.
(2) Carefully apply pressure to syringe plunger, allowing tubing to fill with medication.	Ensures that tubing is free of air bubbles to prevent air embolus.
(3) Place syringe into mini-infusion pump (follow product directions). Be sure that syringe is secured (see illustration).	
(4) Connect mini-infusion tubing to main IV line.	
(a) *Needleless system:* Wipe off needleless port and insert tip of mini-infusion tubing.	Needleless system reduces risk of needlestick injuries (OSHA, 2009).
(b) *Stopcock:* Wipe off stopcock port with alcohol swab and connect tubing. Turn stopcock to open position.	Stopcock reduces risk of needlestick injuries.
(5) Hang infusion pump with syringe on IV pole alongside main IV bag. Set pump to deliver medication within time recommended by institutional policy, pharmacist, or medication reference manual. Use alarm if medication is delivered into heparin/saline lock. Press button on pump to begin infusion.	Pump automatically delivers medication at safe, constant rate based on volume in syringe.
(6) After medication has infused, check flow rate on primary infusion. The infusion automatically begins to flow once the pump stops. Regulate main infusion line to desired rate as needed. (NOTE: If stopcock is used, turn off mini-infusion line.)	Maintains patency of primary IV line.

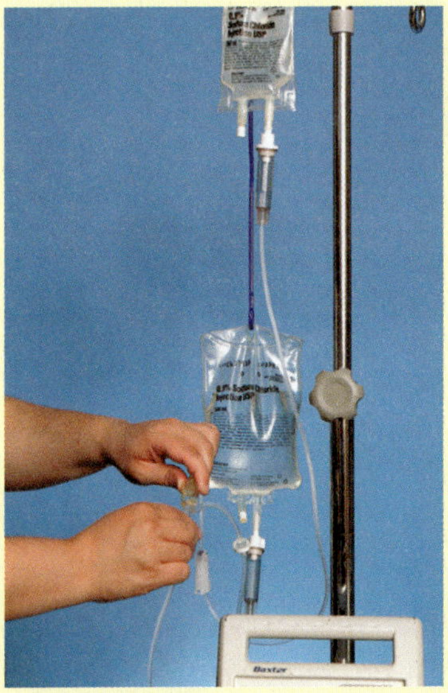

STEP 7a(3)(a) For needleless system insert tip of piggyback infusion tubing into port.

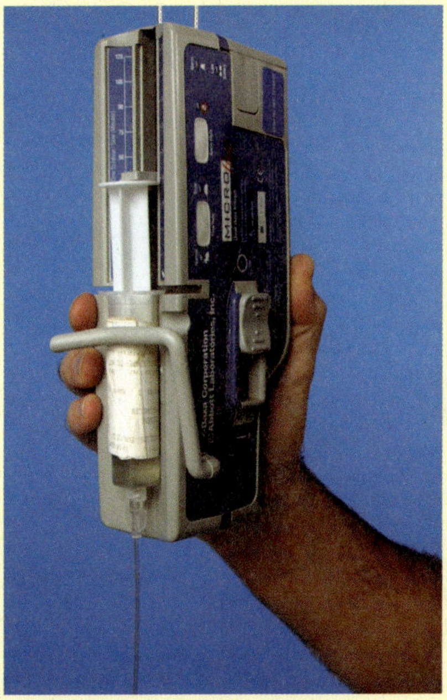

STEP 7b(3) Ensure that syringe is secure after placing it into mini-infusor pump.

SKILL 31-7 ADMINISTERING INTRAVENOUS MEDICATIONS BY PIGGYBACK, INTERMITTENT INTRAVENOUS INFUSION SETS, AND MINI-INFUSION PUMPS—cont'd

STEP	RATIONALE
c. **Volume-control administration set (e.g., Buretrol)**	
(1) Fill Buretrol with desired amount of fluid (50 to 100 mL) by opening clamp between Buretrol and main IV bag (see illustration).	Small volume of fluid dilutes IV medication and reduces risk of too-rapid infusion.
(2) Close clamp and check to be sure that clamp on air vent of Buretrol chamber is open.	Prevents additional leakage of fluid into Buretrol. Air vent allows fluid in Buretrol to exit at regulated rate.
(3) Clean injection port on top of Buretrol with antiseptic swab.	Prevents introduction of microorganisms during needle insertion.
(4) Remove needle cap or sheath, insert syringe needle through port, and inject medication (see illustrations). Gently rotate Buretrol between hands.	Rotating mixes medication with solution in Buretrol to ensure equal distribution.
(5) Regulate IV infusion rate to allow medication to infuse in time recommended by agency policy, a pharmacist, or a medication reference manual.	For optimal therapeutic effect, medication needs to infuse in prescribed time interval.
(6) Label Buretrol with name of medication, dosage, and total volume, including diluent and time of administration following ISMP (2010e) safe medication label format (see Fig. 31-27, p. 610).	Alerts nurses to medication being infused. Prevents other medications from being added to Buretrol.
(7) If patient is receiving a continuous IV infusion, check continuous infusion rate after Buretrol infusion is complete to ensure the appropriate rate of IV fluid administration.	Ensures appropriate fluid balance.
8 Dispose of uncapped needle or needle enclosed in safety shield and syringe in proper container.	Prevents accidental needlesticks (OSHA, 2009).
9 Discard supplies in appropriate container and perform hand hygiene.	Reduces transmission of microorganisms.
EVALUATION	
1 Assess patient's status after administering medication.	Evaluates effect of medication.
2 Observe patient for signs of adverse reactions.	IV medications act rapidly.
3 During infusion periodically check infusion rate and condition of IV site.	IV line needs to remain patent for proper medication administration. Development of infiltration necessitates discontinuing infusion.
4 Ask patient to explain purpose and side effects of medication.	Evaluates patient's understanding of instruction.

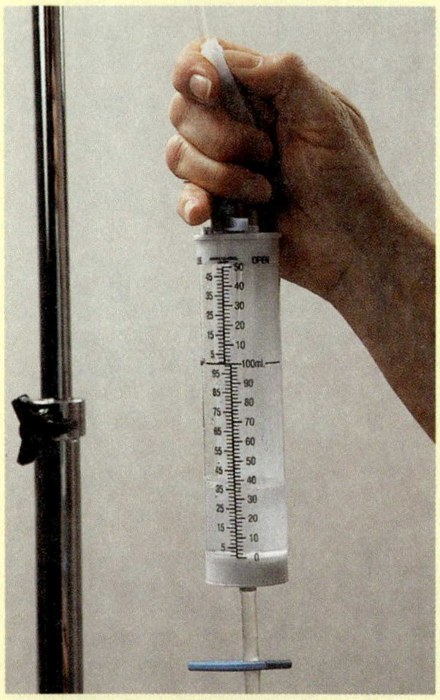

STEP 7c(1) Filling volume-control administration device.

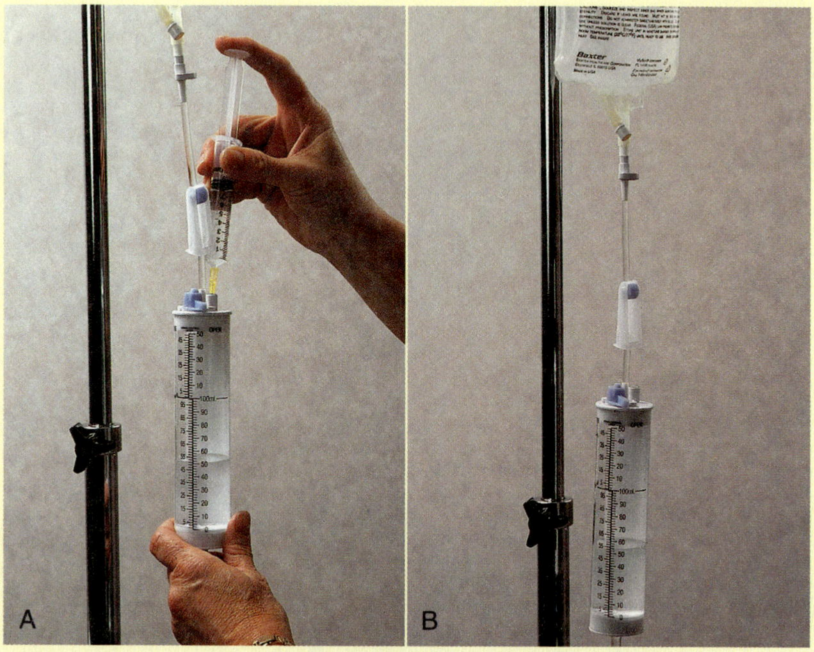

STEP 7c(4) **A,** Medication injected into device. **B,** Prepared device.

UNEXPECTED OUTCOMES AND RELATED INTERVENTIONS

1 Patient develops adverse drug reaction.
- Stop medication infusion immediately.
- Follow institutional policy or guidelines for appropriate response and reporting of adverse drug reactions.
- Document allergy in patient's medical record.

2 Medication does not infuse over desired period.
- Determine reason (e.g., improper calculation of flow rate, malpositioning of IV needle at insertion site, or infiltration).
- Take corrective action as indicated.

3 IV site shows signs of phlebitis or infiltration (see Chapter 41).
- See related interventions in Skill 31-6.

RECORDING AND REPORTING

- Record medication, dose, route, time and date administered on MAR.
- Record volume of fluid in medication bag or Buretrol on intake and output form.
- Report adverse reactions to patient's health care provider.

HOME CARE CONSIDERATIONS

- Teach patient and family caregiver to dispose of needles and contaminated equipment in puncture-proof containers (e.g., coffee can).
- Instruct family about community resources to obtain supplies.

KEY POINTS

- Learning medication classifications improves understanding of nursing implications for administering medications with similar characteristics.
- All controlled substances are handled according to strict procedures that account for each medication.
- The nurse applies understanding of the physiology of medication action when timing administration, selecting routes, initiating actions to promote medication efficacy, and observing responses to medications.
- The older adult's body undergoes structural and functional changes that alter medication actions and influence the manner in which nurses provide medication therapy.
- Verify medication calculations with another nurse to ensure accuracy.
- Medications given parenterally are absorbed more quickly than those administered by other routes.
- Each medication order needs to include the patient's name, order date, medication name, dosage, route, time of administration, drug indication, and prescriber's signature.
- A medication history reveals allergies, medications a patient is taking, and the patient's adherence to therapy.
- The six rights of medication administration contribute to accurate preparation and administration of medication doses.
- The six rights of medication administration are the right medication, right dose, right patient, right route, right time, and right documentation.
- Nurses need to avoid distractions and follow the same routine when preparing medications to reduce medication errors.
- Nurses administer only medications they prepare, and prepared medications are never left unattended.
- Document medications immediately after administration.
- A nurse uses clinical judgment in determining the best time to administer prn medications.
- The nurse reports a medication error immediately.
- When preparing medications, the nurse checks the medication container label against the MAR three times.
- The Z-track method for IM injections protects subcutaneous tissues from irritating parenteral fluids.
- Failure to select injection sites by anatomical landmarks leads to tissue, bone, or nerve damage.

CLINICAL APPLICATION QUESTIONS

Preparing for Clinical Practice

Janice, a nursing student, is caring for Esteban, a 48-year-old Latino who had diabetes and hypertension. Esteban's health care provider writes a new medication order for furosemide 30 mg IVP STAT and then q8h.

1. What does Janice need to know about furosemide before administering it?
2. Three vials of furosemide arrive on the patient care unit. The labels on the vials say: "40 mg furosemide/4 mL." How much medication does Janice prepare in the syringe?
3. Janice collects the appropriate equipment to administer the medication, performs hand hygiene, prepares the medication in the syringe, and takes it to Esteban at the correct time. Which step does she need to take next in administering the medication?

evolve *Answers to Clinical Application Questions can be found on the Evolve website.*

REVIEW QUESTIONS

Are You Ready to Test Your Nursing Knowledge?

1. The nurse is having difficulty reading a physician's order for a medication. He or she knows that the physician is very busy and does not like to be called. What is the most appropriate next step for the nurse to take?
   1. Call a pharmacist to interpret the order
   2. Call the physician to have the order clarified
   3. Consult the unit manager to help interpret the order
   4. Ask the unit secretary to interpret the physician's handwriting

2. The patient has an order for 2 tablespoons of Milk of Magnesia. How much medication does the nurse give him or her?
   1. 2 mL
   2. 5 mL
   3. 16 mL
   4. 30 mL
3. A nurse is administering eardrops to an 8-year-old patient with an ear infection. How does the nurse pull the patient's ear when administering the medication?
   1. Outward
   2. Back
   3. Upward and back
   4. Upward and outward
4. A patient is to receive cephalexin (Keflex) 500 mg PO. The pharmacy has sent 250-mg tablets. How many tablets does the nurse administer?
   1. ½ tablet
   2. 1 tablet
   3. 1½ tablets
   4. 2 tablets
5. A nurse is administering medications to a 4-year-old patient. After he or she explains which medications are being given, the mother states, "I don't remember my child having that medication before." What is the nurse's next action?
   1. Give the medications
   2. Identify the patient using two patient identifiers
   3. Withhold the medications and verify the medication orders
   4. Provide medication education to the mother to help her better understand her child's medications
6. A patient is transitioning from the hospital to the home environment. A home care referral is obtained. What is a priority in relation to safe medication administration for the discharge nurse?
   1. Set up the follow-up appointments with the physician for the patient.
   2. Ensure that someone will provide housekeeping for the patient at home.
   3. Ensure that the home care agency is aware of medication and health teaching needs.
   4. Make sure that the patient's family knows how to safely bathe him or her and provide mouth care.
7. A nursing student takes a patient's antibiotic to his room. The patient asks the nursing student what it is and why he should take it. Which information does the nursing student include when replying to the patient?
   1. Only the patient's physician can give this information.
   2. The student provides the name of the medication and a description of its desired effect.
   3. Information about medications is confidential and cannot be shared.
   4. He has to speak with his assigned nurse about this.
8. The nurse is administering a sustained-release capsule to a new patient. The patient insists that he cannot swallow pills. What is the nurse's next best course of action?
   1. Ask the prescriber to change the order
   2. Crush the pill with a mortar and pestle
   3. Hide the capsule in a piece of solid food
   4. Open the capsule and sprinkle it over pudding
9. The nurse takes a medication to a patient, and the patient tells him or her to take it away because she is not going to take it. What is the nurse's next action?
   1. Ask the patient's reason for refusal
   2. Explain that she must take the medication
   3. Take the medication away and chart the patient's refusal
   4. Tell the patient that her physician knows what is best for her
10. The nurse receives an order to start giving a loop diuretic to a patient to help lower his or her blood pressure. The nurse determines the appropriate route for administering the diuretic according to:
    1. Hospital policy.
    2. The prescriber's orders.
    3. The type of medication ordered.
    4. The patient's size and muscle mass.
11. A patient is receiving an intravenous (IV) push medication. If the drug infiltrates into the outer tissues, the nurse:
    1. Continues to let the IV run.
    2. Applies a warm compress to the infiltrated site.
    3. Stops the administration of the medication and follows agency policy.
    4. Should not worry about this because vesicant filtration is not a problem.
12. If a patient who is receiving intravenous (IV) fluids develops tenderness, warmth, erythema, and pain at the site, the nurse suspects:
    1. Sepsis.
    2. Phlebitis.
    3. Infiltration.
    4. Fluid overload.
13. After seeing a patient, the physician gives a nursing student a verbal order for a new medication. The nursing student first needs to:
    1. Follow ISMP guidelines for safe medication abbreviations.
    2. Explain to the physician that the order needs to be given to a registered nurse.
    3. Write down the order on the patient's order sheet and read it back to the physician.
    4. Ensure that the six rights of medication administration are followed when giving the medication.
14. A nurse accidently gives a patient a medication at the wrong time. The nurse's first priority is to:
    1. Complete an occurrence report.
    2. Notify the health care provider.
    3. Inform the charge nurse of the error.
    4. Assess the patient for adverse effects.
15. A patient is taking albuterol through a pressurized metered-dose inhaler (pMDI) that contains a total of 200 puffs. The patient takes 2 puffs every 4 hours. How many days will the pMDI last?

    ________ days

Answers: 1. 2; 2. 4; 3. 4; 4. 4; 5. 3; 6. 3; 7. 2; 8. 1; 9. 1; 10. 2; 11. 3; 12. 2; 13. 2; 14. 4; 15. 16.

REFERENCES

Alvarez-Lorenzo C, et al: Contact lenses for drug delivery: achieving sustained release with novel systems, *Am J Drug Deliv* 4(3):131, 2006.

American Diabetes Association (ADA): Insulin administration: position statement, *Diabetes Care* 27(1S):S106, 2004.

American Diabetes Association (ADA): Standards of medical care in diabetes—2010: position statement, *Diabetes Care* 33(1):S11, 2010, http://care.diabetesjournals.org/content/33/Supplement_1/S11.full.pdf+html. Accessed September 3, 2011.

American Diabetes Association (ADA): Syringes (U-100), n.d., http://forecast.diabetes.org/files/images/issues/SyringesChart.pdf. Accessed September 3, 2011.

American Hospital Association: *The patient care partnership*, 2003, http://www.aha.org/aha/issues/Communicating-With-Patients/pt-care-partnership.html. Accessed September 3, 2011.

American Medical Association (AMA): *United States Adopted Name Council,* 2010, http://www.ama-assn.org/ama/pub/about-ama/our-people/coalitions-consortiums/united-states-adopted-names-council.shtml. Accessed September 3, 2011.

American Nurses Association: *Nursing: scope and standards of practice*, ed 2, Silver Spring, Md, 2010, The Association.

American Society of Health-System Pharmacists (ASHP): *Healthcare leaders vow to stop intravenous medication errors,* 2008, http://www.ashp.org/menu/AboutUs/ForPress/PressReleases/PressRelease.aspx?id=511. Accessed September 18, 2011.

American Society of Health-System Pharmacists (ASHP): *How to use eye drops properly,* n.d.a, http://www.safemedication.com/safemed/MedicationTipsTools/HowtoAdminister/HowtoUseEyeDropsProperly.aspx. Accessed September 3, 2011.

American Society of Health-System Pharmacists [ASHP]: *The ASHP discussion guide for compounding sterile preparations: summary and implementation of USP chapter <797>*, n.d.b, http://www.ashp.org/s_ashp/docs/files/HACC_797guide.pdf. Accessed September 3, 2011.

Bankhead R, et al: Enteral nutrition practice recommendations, *JPEN J Parenter Enteral Nutr* 33:1, 2009.

Bastable S: *Nurse as educator: principles of teaching and learning for nursing practice*, ed 3, Sudbury, Mass, 2008, Jones & Bartlett.

Biron AD, Lavoie-Tremblay M, Loiselle CG: Characteristics of work interruptions during medication administration, *J Nurs Scholarship* 41(4):330, 2009.

Boullata JI: Drug administration through an enteral feeding tube: the rationale behind the guidelines, *Am J Nurs* 109(10):34, 2009.

Centers for Disease Control and Prevention (CDC): *Tuberculosis (TB),* 2010, http://www.cdc.gov/tb/. Accessed September 18, 2011.

Centers for Medicare and Medicaid Services, 2011, http://www.ismp.org/download/files/Updated_IGs_Medication_Adminis_Nov-18-11.pdf. Accessed January 3, 2012.

Cornett S: Assessing and addressing health literacy, *Online J Issues Nurs* 14(3), 2009.

Ebersole P, et al: *Toward healthy aging: human needs and nursing response*, ed 7, St Louis, 2008, Mosby.

Eisenstadt ES: Dysphagia and aspiration pneumonia in older adults, *J Am Acad Nurse Pract* 22(1):17, 2010.

Giger JL, Davidhizar RE: *Transcultural nursing: assessment and intervention*, ed 5, St Louis, 2008, Mosby.

Guenter P: Safe practices for enteral nutrition in critically ill patients, *Crit Care Nurs Clin North Am* 22(2):197, 2010.

Hess DR: Aerosol delivery devices in the treatment of asthma, *Respir Care* 53(6):699, 2008.

Hockenberry MJ, Wilson D: *Wong's essentials of pediatric nursing*, ed 8, St Louis, 2009, Mosby.

Institute for Safe Medication Practices (ISMP): *ISMP medication safety alert!* 2002, http://www.ismp.org/Newsletters/acutecare/articles/A1Q02Action.asp. Accessed September 3, 2011.

Institute for Safe Medication Practices (ISMP): *ISMP Acute Care Guidelines for Timely Administration of Scheduled Medications,* 2011, http://www.ismp.org/Tools/guidelines/acutecare/tasm.pdf. Accessed September 1, 2011.

Institute for Safe Medication Practices (ISMP): *Preventing errors with tablet splitting,* 2006, http://www.accessdata.fda.gov/scripts/cdrh/cfdocs/psn/transcript.cfm?show=54#7. Accessed September 3, 2011.

Institute for Safe Medication Practices (ISMP): *Humulin R concentrate U-500,* 2007a, http://www.ismp.org/Newsletters/ambulatory/archives/200708_2.asp. Accessed September 3, 2011.

Institute for Safe Medication Practices (ISMP): Patches: what you can't see can harm patients, *Nurse Advise-ERR* 5(4):1, 2007b.

Institute for Safe Medication Practices (ISMP): *ISMP's list of confused drug names,* 2010a, http://www.ismp.org/Tools/confuseddrugnames.pdf. Accessed September 3, 2011.

Institute for Safe Medication Practices (ISMP): *ISMP's list of error-prone abbreviations, symbols, and dose designations,* 2010b, http://www.ismp.org/Tools/errorproneabbreviations.pdf. Accessed September 3, 2011.

Institute for Safe Medication Practices (ISMP): *Never use parenteral syringes for oral medications,* 2010c, http://www.accessdata.fda.gov/psn/transcript.cfm?show=94#9. Accessed September 3, 2011.

Institute for Safe Medication Practices (ISMP): *Oral dosage forms that should not be crushed,* 2010d, http://www.ismp.org/Tools/DoNotCrush.pdf. Accessed September 3, 2011.

Institute for Safe Medication Practices (ISMP): *Principles of designing a medication label for intravenous piggyback medication for patient specific, inpatient use,* 2010e, http://www.ismp.org/tools/guidelines/labelFormats/IVPB.asp. Accessed September 3, 2011.

Institute of Medicine (IOM): *Preventing medication errors,* 2007, http://books.nap.edu/openbook.php?record_id=11623. Accessed September 3, 2011.

Institute of Medicine (IOM): *Report brief, to err is human: building a safer health system,* 2003, http://iom.edu/CMS/8089/5575/4117.aspx. Accessed September 3 2011.

Lehne RA: *Pharmacology for nursing care,* ed 7, St Louis, 2010, Saunders.

Lilley LL, et al: *Pharmacology and the nursing process,* ed 5, St Louis, 2007, Mosby.

Maggiore RJ, Gross CP, Hurria A: Polypharmacy in older adults with cancer, *Oncologist* 15(5):507, 2010.

Mayhew MS: Medication reconciliation and discontinuity of care, *J Nurse Pract* 6(1):61, 2010.

MayoClinic.com: *Asthma inhalers: which one's right for you?* 2009a, http://www.mayoclinic.com/health/asthma-inhalers/HQ01081. Accessed September 7, 2011.

MayoClinic.com: Using a metered-dose asthma inhaler and spacer, 2009b, http://www.mayoclinic.com/health/asthma/MM00608. Accessed September 7, 2011.

Morris DG: *Calculate with confidence*, ed 5, St Louis, 2010, Mosby.

Novo Nordisk: *Levimir,* 2010, http://www.novomedlink.com/products/Levemir/levemir-home.aspx. Accessed November 13, 2011.

Occupational Safety and Health Administration (OSHA): *Bloodborne pathogens and needlestick prevention,* 2009, http://osha.gov/SLTC/bloodbornepathogens/index.html. Accessed September 7, 2011.

Palmer J, Metheny NA: Preventing aspiration in older adults with dysphagia, *Am J Nurs* 108(2):40, 2008.

Paparella S: Death by syringe: a call to action, *J Emerg Nurs* 34(1):49, 2008.

Prettyman J: Subcutaneous or intramuscular? Confronting a parenteral administration dilemma, *MedSurg Nurs* 14(2):93 2005.

Qureshi B: Cultural, religious and ethnic issues in prescribing, *Practice Nurse* 39(5):35, 2010.

Razzi CC: Incorporating the BEERS criteria may reduce ED visits in elderly patients, *J Emerg Nurs* 35(5):453, 2009.

Restrepo RD, Gardner DD: Selecting the best inhaler device: not always an easy task, *J Respir Care Pract* 23(6):8, 2010.

Rushing J: How to administer a subcutaneous injection, *Nursing* 34(6):32, 2004.

Sanofi-Aventis: Lovenox® injections at home, 2010, http://www.lovenox.com/consumer/prescribed-lovenox/lovenox-at-home.aspx. Accessed September 7, 2011.

Skidmore-Roth L: *Mosby's drug guide for nurses,* ed 9, St Louis, 2011, Mosby.

The Joint Commission (TJC): *Joint Commission alert: prevent pediatric medication errors children are three times more at risk than adults,* 2008, http://www.jointcommission.org/NewsRoom/NewsReleases/nr_04_11_08.htm.

The Joint Commission (TJC): Comprehensive accreditation manual for hospitals: the official handbook (E-dition), 2010, TJC.

The Joint Commission (TJC): *2011 National patient safety goals (NPGs),* 2011a, http://www.jointcommission.org/hap_2011_npsgs/. Accessed September 18, 2011.

The Joint Commission (TJC): *Official do not use list,* 2011b, http://www.jointcommission.org/facts_about_the_official_/. Accessed September 18, 2011.

Twin Cities Health Professionals (TCHP) Education Consortium: Management of the obese patient, 2005, http://tchpeducation.com/homestudies/generalinterest/obesity/obesitybook_2011_final.pdf. Accessed September 18, 2011.

US Food and Drug Administration (USFDA): *MedWatch: the FDA safety information and adverse event reporting program,* 2010, http://www.fda.gov/Safety/MedWatch/default.htm. Accessed September 7, 2011.

Williams NT: Medication administration through enteral feeding tubes, *Am J Health-System Pharm* 65(24):2347, 2008.

World Health Organization (WHO): *Injection safety: misuse and overuse of injection worldwide,* 2006, http://www.who.int/mediacentre/factsheets/fs231/en/index.html. Accessed September 7, 2011.

RESEARCH REFERENCES

Annersten M, Willman A: Performing subcutaneous injections; a literature review, *Worldviews Evid Based Nurs* 2(3):122, 2005.

Birkebaek NH, et al: A 4-mm needle reduces the risk of intramuscular injections without increasing backflow to skin surface in lean diabetic children and adults, *Diabetes Care* 31(9):e65, 2008.

Brady A, Malone A, Fleming S: A literature review of the individual and systems factors that contribute to medication errors in nursing practice, *J Nurs Manage* 17(6): 679, 2009.

Cocoman A, Murray J: Intramuscular injections: a review of best practice for mental health nurses, *J Psych Mental Health Nurs* 15(5):424, 2008.

Davidson MB, et al: U-500 regular insulin: clinical experience and pharmacokinetics in obese, severely insulin-resistant type 2 diabetic patients, *Diabetes Care* 33(2):281, 2010.

Dickinson A, et al: Paediatric nurses' understanding of the process and procedure of double-checking medications, *J Clin Nurs* 19(5-6):728, 2010.

Edmiaston J, et al: Validation of a dysphagia screening tool in acute stroke patients, *Am J Crit Care* 19(4):357, 2010.

Foote SO, Coleman JR: Medication administration: the implementation process of bar-coding for medication administration to enhance medication safety, *Nurs Econ* 26(3):207, 2008.

Fowler SB, Sohler P, Zarillo DF: Bar-code technology for medication administration: medication errors and nurse satisfaction, *MedSurg Nurs* 18(2):103, 2009.

Green R: A descriptive correlation study of medication error and nursing, *South Online J Nurs Res* 8(2), 2008.

Greenfield S, Whelan B, Cohn E: Use of dimensional analysis to reduce medication errors, *J Nurs Educ* 45(2):91, 2006.

Helmons PJ, Wargel LN, Daniels CE: Effect of bar-code-assisted medication administration on medication administration errors and accuracy in multiple patient care areas, *Am J Health-Syst Pharm* 66:1202, 2009.

Koster MP, et al: Needle length for immunization of early adolescents as determined by ultrasound, *Pediatrics* 124(2):667, 2009.

Krueger L: Experiences of Hmong patients on hemodialysis and the nurses working with them, *Nephrol Nurs J* 36(4):379, 2009.

Longhurst CA, et al: Decrease in hospital-wide mortality rate after implementation of a commercially sold computerized physician order entry system, *Pediatrics* 126(1):14, 2010.

Nicoll LH, Hesby A: Intramuscular injection: an integrative research review and guideline for evidence-based practice, *Appl Nurs Res* 16(2):149, 2002.

Poon EG, et al: Effect of bar-code technology on the safety of medication administration, *N Engl J Med* 362(18):1698, 2010.

Sowan AK, et al: Impact of computerized orders for pediatric continuous drug infusions on detecting infusion pump programming errors: a simulated study, *J Pediatr Nurs* 25(2):108, 2010.

Walsh KA: The relationship among mathematics anxiety, beliefs about mathematics, mathematics self-efficacy, and mathematics performance in associate degree nursing students, *Nurs Educ Perspect* 29(4):226, 2008.

Zaybak A, et al: Does obesity prevent the needle from reaching muscle in intramuscular injections? *J Adv Nurs* 58(6):552, 2007.

CHAPTER

32

Complementary and Alternative Therapies

OBJECTIVES

- Differentiate between complementary and alternative therapies.
- Describe the clinical applications of relaxation therapies.
- Discuss the relaxation response and its effect on somatic ailments.
- Identify the principles and effectiveness of imagery, meditation, and breathwork.
- Describe the purpose and principles of biofeedback.
- Describe the methods of and the psychophysiological responses to therapeutic touch.
- Explain the scope of practice of chiropractic therapy.
- Discuss the principles and applications of acupuncture.
- Describe safe and unsafe herbal therapies.

KEY TERMS

Acupoints, p. 650
Acupuncture, p. 649
Allopathic medicine, p. 643
Alternative therapies, p. 644
Biofeedback, p. 649
Chiropractic therapy, p. 650
Complementary therapies, p. 643
Creative visualization, p. 648
Cupping, p. 652
Imagery, p. 648
Integrative health care, p. 644
Integrative health care programs, p. 644
Meditation, p. 648
Meridians, p. 649
Moxibustion, p. 652
Passive relaxation, p. 647
Progressive relaxation, p. 647
***Qi gong*, p. 652**
Relaxation response, p. 646
Stress response, p. 644
Tai chi, p. 652
Therapeutic touch (TT), p. 650
Traditional Chinese medicine (TCM), p. 651
Vital energy *(qi)*, p. 649
Whole medical systems, p. 644
Yin and yang, p. 651

evolve WEBSITE

http://evolve.elsevier.com/Potter/fundamentals/

- Review Questions
- Case Study with Questions
- Audio Glossary
- Interactive Learning Activities
- Key Term Flashcards
- Content Updates

The general health of North American people has steadily improved over the course of the last century as evidenced by lower mortality rates and increased life expectancies. Changes in science and medicine have provided the knowledge and technology to successfully alter the course of many illnesses. Despite the success of **allopathic medicine** (conventional western medicine), many conditions such as chronic back and neck pain, arthritis, gastrointestinal problems, allergies, headache, and anxiety are sometimes difficult to treat. As a result, more patients are exploring alternative methods to relieve their symptoms. Researchers estimate that up to 75% of patients seek care from their primary care practitioners for stress, pain, and health conditions for which there are no known causes or cures (Rakel and Faass, 2006). Although allopathic medicine is quite effective in treating numerous physical ailments (e.g., bacterial infections, structural abnormalities, and acute emergencies), it is generally less effective in decreasing stress-induced illnesses, managing chronic disease, caring for the emotional and spiritual needs of individuals, and improving quality of life and general well-being.

The number of patients seeking unconventional treatments has risen considerably over the past decade. The most recent comprehensive national survey estimates that between 38.3% and 62.1% of the U.S. population uses complementary and alternative medicine (CAM) (Barnes et al., 2008). In part this increase is caused by (1) a desire for less invasive, less toxic, "more natural" treatments; (2) lack of satisfaction with allopathic treatments; (3) an increasing desire by patients to take a more active role in their treatment process; (4) beliefs that a combination of treatments (allopathic and complementary) result in better overall results; (5) the increased number of research articles in journals such as *Journal of Alternative and Complementary Medicine* and the *Journal of Holistic Nursing;* and (6) beliefs and values that are consistent with an approach to health that incorporates the mind, body, and spirit or a holistic approach (Koithan, 2009).

COMPLEMENTARY AND ALTERNATIVE APPROACHES TO HEALTH

The National Institutes of Health/National Center for Complementary and Alternative Medicine (NIH/NCCAM, 2010b) defines CAM as "a group of diverse medical and health care systems, practices, and products that are not presently considered to be part of conventional medicine." **Complementary therapies** are therapies used in addition to conventional treatment recommended by the person's health care provider. As the name implies, complementary therapies complement conventional treatments. Many of them such as therapeutic touch contain diagnostic and therapeutic methods that require special training. Others such as guided imagery and breathwork are easily learned and applied. Complementary therapies also include relaxation; exercise; massage; reflexology; prayer; biofeedback; hypnotherapy; creative therapies, including art, music, or dance therapy; meditation; chiropractic therapy; and herbs/supplements (Fontaine, 2005). Another term that is used to describe interventions used in this fashion, particularly by licensed health care providers, is *integrative therapies* (Kreitzer et al., 2009).

Alternative therapies may include the same interventions as complementary therapies; but they become the primary treatment, replacing allopathic medical care. For example, a person with chronic pain uses yoga to encourage flexibility and relaxation at the same time that nonsteroidal antiinflammatory or opioid medications are prescribed. Both sets of interventions are based on conventional pathophysiology and anatomy while acknowledging the mind-body connection that contributes to the physiological pain response. In this case yoga is used as a complementary intervention. However, another patient decides a meditative practice that includes yoga and other lifestyle changes is more helpful than an allopathic approach to chronic pain. This patient studies these practices more deeply, adhering to one of the many schools or traditions, and decides to use these practices as the primary approach to manage chronic pain. In this case yoga is an alternative treatment. Several therapies are always considered alternative because they are based on completely different philosophies and life systems than those used by allopathic medicine. These are identified by NIH/NCCAM as **whole medical systems** such as traditional Chinese medicine (TCM), Ayurveda, and various forms of traditional or folk medicine. Table 32-1 presents types of complementary and alternative therapies.

Because of the increased interest in complementary therapies, many institutions, including medical and nursing schools, have training programs that incorporate complementary and alternative therapy content into the curriculum. Some schools have **integrative health care programs** that allow health care consumers the opportunity to be treated by a team of providers consisting of both allopathic and complementary practitioners. More fully defined, **integrative health care** emphasizes the importance of the relationship between practitioner and patient; focuses on the whole person; is informed by evidence; and makes use of appropriate therapeutic approaches, health care professionals, and disciplines to achieve optimal health (Kreitzer et al., 2009).

Nurses have historically practiced in an integrative fashion; a review of nursing theory (see Chapter 4) reveals the values of holism, relational care, and informed practice. However, nursing has identified its practice as holistic rather than integrated. Holistic nursing regards and treats the mind-body-spirit of the patient. Nurses use holistic nursing interventions such as relaxation therapy, music therapy, touch therapies, and guided imagery. Such interventions affect the whole person (mind-body-spirit) and are effective, economical, noninvasive, nonpharmacological complements to medical care. Nurses use holistic interventions to augment standard treatments, replace interventions that are ineffective or debilitating, and promote or maintain health (Dossey and Keegan, 2009). The American Holistic Nurses Association maintains Standards of Holistic Nursing Practice, which defines and establishes the scope of holistic practice and describes the level of care expected from a holistic nurse (AHNA/ANA, 2007).

Increasing interest in CAM is evident in the increased number of publications on CAM topics in respected health care journals and the development of new journals that specifically focus on complementary and alternative therapies (e.g., *Evidence-Based Complementary and Alternative Medicine* and *Integrative Cancer Therapies*). The ongoing mission of the National Institutes of Health/National Center for Complementary and Alternative Medicine (NCCAM) supports the investigation of the benefits and safety of CAM interventions. Although the body of evidence about CAM is growing, limited data make it difficult to establish the specific benefits of complementary therapies. Reasons are varied but reflect the growing and developing nature of the science. Therefore nurses should weigh the risk and benefits of each intervention and consider the following when recommending complementary therapies: (1) the history of each therapy (many have been used by cultures for thousands of years to support health and ameliorate suffering); (2) nursing's history and experience with a particular therapy; (3) other forms of evidence reporting outcomes and safety data, including case study and qualitative research; and (4) the cultural influences and context for certain patient populations.

This chapter discusses several types of complementary and alternative therapies, including a description, the clinical applications, and the limitations of each therapy. The therapies are organized into two categories. The first are nursing-accessible therapies that you can begin to learn and apply in patient care. The second category includes training-specific therapies such as chiropractic therapy or acupressure that a nurse cannot perform without additional training and/or certification.

NURSING-ACCESSIBLE THERAPIES

Some complementary therapies and techniques are general in nature and use natural processes (e.g., breathing, thinking and concentration, presence, movement) to help people feel better and cope with both acute and chronic conditions (Box 32-1). You need to learn about these techniques and incorporate them as a part of your independent nursing practice with patients (AHNA/ANA, 2007). Assess your patients and obtain their permission before using complementary therapies. In addition, conduct ongoing outcomes assessment and evaluation of your patients' responses to the interventions. Sometimes changes to physician-prescribed therapies, such as medication doses, are needed when complementary therapies alter physiological responses and lead to therapeutic responses.

Complementary therapies teach individuals ways in which to change their behavior to alter physical responses to stress and improve symptoms such as muscle tension, gastrointestinal discomfort, pain, or sleep disturbances. Active involvement is a primary principle for these therapies; individuals achieve better responses if they commit to practice the techniques or exercises daily. Therefore to achieve effective outcomes, therapeutic strategies need to be matched with an individual's lifestyle, his or her beliefs and values, and his or her treatment preferences.

Relaxation Therapy

People face stressful situations in everyday life that evoke the **stress response** (see Chapter 37). The mind varies the biochemical functions of the major organ systems in response to feedback. Thoughts and feelings influence the production of chemicals (i.e., neurotransmitters, neurohormones, and peptides) that circulate throughout the body and convey messages via cells to various

TABLE 32-1 **Complementary and Alternative Therapies**

TYPES	DEFINITIONS
Biologically Based Therapies (Natural products)	
Dietary supplements	Defined by the Dietary Supplement Health and Education Act of 1994 and used to supplement dietary/nutritional intake by mouth; contain one or more dietary ingredients, including vitamins, minerals, herbs or other botanical products
Herbal medicines	Plant-based therapies used in whole systems of medicine or as individual preparations by allopathic providers and consumers for specific symptoms or issues
Macrobiotic diet	Predominantly a vegan diet (no animal products except fish); initially used in the management of a variety of cancers; emphasis placed on whole cereal grains, vegetables, and unprocessed foods
Mycotherapies	Fungi-based (mushroom) products
Orthomolecular medicine (megavitamin)	Increased intake of nutrients such as vitamin C and beta-carotene; treats cancer, schizophrenia, autism, and certain chronic diseases such as hypercholesterolemia and coronary artery disease
Probiotics	Live microorganisms (in most cases, bacteria) that are similar to beneficial microorganisms found in the human gastrointestinal system; also called *good bacteria*
The "Zone"	Dietary program that requires eating protein, carbohydrate, and fat in a 30 : 40 : 30 ratio: 30% of calories from protein, 40% from carbohydrate, and 30% from fat; used to balance insulin and other hormones for optimal health
Energy Therapies (Use or manipulation of energy fields)	
Healing touch	Biofield therapy; uses gentle touch directly on or close to body to influence and support the human energy system and bring balance to the whole body (physical, spiritual, emotional, and mental); a formal educational and certification system provides credentials for practitioners
Reiki therapy	Biofield therapy derived from ancient Buddhist rituals; practitioner places hands on or above a body area and transfers "universal life energy," providing strength, harmony, and balance to treat a patient's health disturbances
Therapeutic touch	Biofield therapy involving direction of a practitioner's balanced energies in an intentional manner toward those of a patient; practitioner's hands lay on or close to a patient's body
Magnet therapy	Bioelectromagnetic therapy; devices (magnets) applied to the body surface, producing a measurable magnetic field; used primarily to alleviate pain associated with musculoskeletal injuries or disorders
Manipulative and Body-Based Methods (Involve movement of body with focus on body structures and systems)	
Acupressure	Applying digital pressure in a specified way on designated points on the body to relieve pain, produce analgesia, or regulate a body function
Chiropractic medicine	Manipulating the spinal column; includes physiotherapy and diet therapy
Craniosacral therapy	Assessing the craniosacral motion for rate, amplitude, symmetry, and quality and attuning/aligning the spinal column, cerebrospinal fluid, and rhythmic processes releasing restrictions or abnormal barriers to motion
Massage therapy	Manipulating soft tissue through stroking, rubbing, or kneading to increase circulation, improve muscle tone, and provide relaxation
Simple touch	Touching the patient in appropriate and gentle ways to make connection, display acceptance, and give appreciation
Mind-Body Interventions (Honor connections between thoughts and physiological functioning using emotion to influence health and well-being)	
Acupuncture	Traditional Chinese method of producing analgesia or altering the function of a body system by inserting thin needles along a series of lines or channels, called *meridians;* direct needle manipulation of energetic meridians influences deeper internal organs by redirecting *qi*
Art therapy	Use of art to reconcile emotional conflicts, foster self-awareness, and express patients' unspoken and frequently unconscious concerns about their disease
Biofeedback	Process providing a person with visual or auditory information about autonomic physiological functions of the body such as muscle tension, skin temperature, and brain wave activity through the use of instruments
Breathwork	Using a variety of breathing patterns to relax, invigorate, or open emotional channels
Guided imagery	Concentrating on an image or series of images to treat pathological conditions
Healing intention (prayer)	Variety of techniques used in multiple cultures that incorporate caring, compassion, love, or empathy with the target of prayer
Meditation	Self-directed practice for relaxing the body and calming the mind using focused rhythmic breathing

Continued

TABLE 32-1 Complementary and Alternative Therapies—cont'd

TYPES	DEFINITIONS
Music therapy	Using music to address physical, psychological, cognitive, and social needs of individuals with disabilities and illnesses; improves physical movement and/or communication, develops emotional expression, evokes memories, and distracts people who are in pain
Psychotherapy	Treatment of emotional and mental disorders by psychological techniques
Tai chi	Incorporating breath, movement, and meditation to cleanse, strengthen, and circulate vital life energy and blood; stimulate the immune system and maintain external and internal balance
Yoga	Focuses on body musculature, posture, breathing mechanisms, and consciousness; goal is attainment of physical and mental well-being through mastery of body achieved through exercise, holding of postures, proper breathing, and meditation
Movement Therapies **(Eastern or Western approaches to promote well-being)**	
Dance therapy	Intimate and powerful medium because it is a direct expression of the mind and body; treats persons with social, emotional, cognitive, or physical problems
Feldenkrais method	Alternative therapy based on establishment of good self-image through awareness and correction of body movements; integrates the understanding of the physics of body movement patterns with an awareness of the way people learn to move, behave, and interact
Pilates	Method of body movement used to strengthen, lengthen, and improve the voluntary control of muscles and muscle groups, especially those used for posture and core strengthening; awareness of breathing and precise movements are integral components
Whole Medical Systems **(Complete systems of theory and practice that have evolved independently from or parallel to allopathic [conventional] medicine)**	
Ayurvedic medicine	One of the oldest systems of medicine practiced in India since the first century AD. Ancient Sanscrit books are considered the main texts on Ayurveda medicine—*Caraka Samhita* and *Sushruta Samhita*. There are eight branches of Ayurvedic medicine, including internal medicine; surgery; treatment of head and neck disease; gynecology, obstetrics, and pediatrics; toxicology; psychiatry; elder care and rejuvenation; and sexual vitality. Treatments balance the doshas using a combination of dietary and lifestyle changes, herbal remedies and purgatives, massage, meditation, and exercise.
Homeopathic medicine	Developed in Germany and practiced in the United States since the mid-1800s. It is a system of medical treatments based on the theory that certain diseases can be cured by giving small, highly diluted doses of substances that in a healthy person would produce symptoms like those of the disease. Prescribed substances called *remedies* are made from naturally occurring plant, animal, or mineral substances and are used to stimulate the vital force of the body so it can heal itself.
Latin American traditional healing	*Curanderismo* is a Latin American traditional healing system that includes a humoral model for classifying food, activity, drugs, and illnesses and a series of folk illnesses. The goal is to create a balance between the patient and his or her environment, thereby sustaining health.
Native American traditional healing	Tribal traditions are individualistic, but similarities across traditions include the use of sweating and purging, herbal remedies, and ceremonies in which a shaman (a spiritual healer) makes contact with spirits to ask their direction in bringing healing to people to promote wholeness and healing.
Naturopathic medicine	A system of therapeutics focused on treating the whole person and promoting health and well-being rather than an individual disease. Therapeutics include herbal medicine, nutritional supplementation, physical medicine, homeopathy, lifestyle counseling, and mind-body therapies with an orientation toward assisting the person's internal capacity for self-healing (vitalism).
Traditional Chinese medicine	An ancient healing tradition identified in the first century AD focused on balancing yin/yang energies. It is a set of systematic techniques and methods, including acupuncture, herbal medicines, massage, acupressure, moxibustion (use of heat from burning herbs), Qi gong (balancing energy flow through body movement), cupping, and massage. Fundamental concepts are from Taoism, Confucianism, and Buddhism.

systems within the body. The stress response is a good example of the way in which systems cooperate to protect an individual from harm. Physiologically the cascade of changes associated with the stress response causes increased heart and respiratory rates; tightened muscles; increased metabolic rate; and a general sense of foreboding, fear, nervousness, irritability, and negative mood. Other physiological responses include elevated blood pressure; dilated pupils; stronger cardiac contractions; and increased levels of blood glucose, serum cholesterol, circulating free fatty acids, and triglycerides. Although these responses prepare a person for short-term stress, the effects on the body of long-term stress sometimes include structural damage and chronic illness such as angina, tension headaches, cardiac arrhythmias, pain, ulcers, and atrophy of the immune system organs (Dossey and Keegan, 2009).

The **relaxation response** is the state of generalized decreased cognitive, physiological, and/or behavioral arousal. Relaxation also involves arousal reduction. The process of relaxation elongates the muscle fibers, reduces the neural impulses sent to the brain, and

BOX 32-1 EVIDENCE-BASED PRACTICE

Pain in Hospitalized Children

PICO Question: Do complementary therapies safely and effectively reduce pain and discomfort in hospitalized children?

Evidence Summary

Pain is a complex phenomenon for children, involving psychological, biological, and sociological factors. Hospitalization and pain are often linked in the minds of children. Despite advances in pediatric pain management, recent studies demonstrate that many children continue to have uncontrolled moderate-to-severe pain when they are in the hospital. Several systematic analyses focusing on the use of alternative therapies to control pain show that many complementary and nonpharmacological therapies, such as relaxation, distraction, focused breathing, imagery, art therapy and humor, are effective in reducing discomfort in children who are hospitalized (Chambers et al., 2009; Lasseter, 2006; Rheingans, 2007). Barriers to the use of alternative and complementary therapies included nurses' heavy workloads and the need for further education about how to use these techniques.

Application to Nursing Practice

- Children who are hospitalized often respond positively to complementary therapies, experience reduced pain, and need fewer medications to control their pain.
- Instructing parents on specific complimentary therapies used for their child's pain control (e.g., breathing techniques, art therapy) allows the parents to use these techniques.
- Nurses need to learn about and use complementary therapies such as breathing techniques and distraction to alleviate the pain associated with painful and stressful procedures, especially among children.

thus decreases the activity of the brain and other body systems. Decreased heart and respiratory rates, blood pressure, and oxygen consumption and increased alpha brain activity and peripheral skin temperature characterize the relaxation response. The relaxation response occurs through a variety of techniques that incorporate a repetitive mental focus and the adoption of a calm, peaceful attitude (Snyder and Lindquist, 2010).

Relaxation helps individuals develop cognitive skills to reduce the negative ways in which they respond to situations within their environment. Cognitive skills include the following:

- Focusing (the ability to identify, differentiate, maintain attention on, and return attention to simple stimuli for an extended period)
- Passivity (the ability to stop unnecessary goal-directed and analytic activity)
- Receptivity (the ability to tolerate and accept experiences that are uncertain, unfamiliar, or paradoxical).

The long-term goal of relaxation therapy is for people to continually monitor themselves for indicators of tension and consciously let go and release the tension contained in various body parts.

Progressive relaxation training teaches the individual how to effectively rest and reduces tension in the body. The person learns to detect subtle localized muscle tension sequentially, one muscle group at a time (e.g., the upper arm muscles, the forearm muscles). In doing so the individual learns to differentiate between high-intensity tension (strong fist clenching), very subtle tension, and relaxation (Dossey and Keegan, 2009). He or she practices this activity using different muscle groups. One active progressive relaxation technique involves the use of slow, deep abdominal breathing while tightening and relaxing an ordered succession of muscle groups, focusing on the associated bodily sensations while letting go of extraneous thoughts. When guiding a patient, you may decide to begin with the muscles in the face, followed by those in the arms, hands, abdomen, legs, and feet. Conversely you may also guide a patient to tense and relax muscles, beginning with the feet and working up the body.

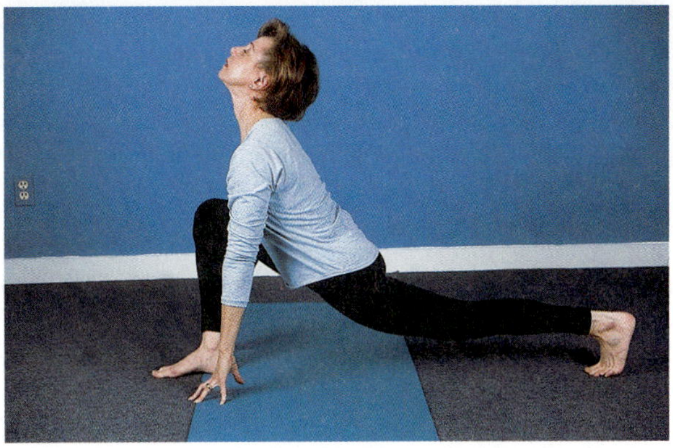

FIG. 32-1 Yoga is a discipline that focuses on muscles, posture, breathing, and consciousness.

The goal of **passive relaxation** is to still the mind and body intentionally without the need to tighten and relax any particular body part. One effective passive relaxation technique incorporates slow, abdominal breathing exercises while imagining warmth and relaxation flowing through specific body parts such as the lungs or hands. Passive relaxation is useful for persons for whom the effort and energy expenditure of active muscle contracting leads to discomfort or exhaustion.

Clinical Applications of Relaxation Therapy. Research shows relaxation techniques effectively lower blood pressure and heart rate, decrease muscle tension, improve well-being, and reduce symptom distress in persons experiencing a variety of situations (e.g., complications from medical treatments, chronic illness, or loss of a significant other) (Bloch et al., 2010; Kwekkeboom et al., 2008). Research also indicates that relaxation, alone or in combination with imagery, yoga (Fig. 32-1), and music, reduces pain and anxiety while improving well-being (Schmidt et al., 2008; Weeks and Nilsson, 2010). Other benefits of relaxation include the reduction of hypertension (Dickinson et al., 2008), depression (Jorm et al., 2008), and menopausal symptoms, including vasomotor responses, insomnia, mood, and musculoskeletal pain (Innes et al., 2010).

Relaxation enables individuals to exert control over their lives. Some experience a decreased feeling of helplessness and a more positive psychological state overall. Relaxation also reduces workplace stress on nursing units. For example, deep-breathing exercises, centering, and focusing attention often lead to improved staff satisfaction, staff relationships and communication, and workload perceptions (Clarke et al., 2009). Nursing units that incorporate relaxation activities into daily routines experience reduced turnover and improved patient satisfaction scores (Zborowsky and Kreitzer, 2009).

Limitations of Relaxation Therapy. During relaxation training individuals learn to differentiate between low and high levels of muscle tension. During the first months of training sessions, when the person is learning how to focus on body sensations and tensions, there are reports of increased sensitivity in detecting muscle tension. Usually these feelings are minor and resolve as the person continues with the training. However, be aware that on occasion some relaxation techniques result in continued intensification of symptoms or the development of altogether new symptoms (Dossey and Keegan, 2009).

An important consideration when choosing any type of relaxation technique is the physiological and psychological status of the individual. Some patients with advanced disease such as cancer or acquired immunodeficiency syndrome (AIDS) seek relaxation training to reduce their stress response. However, techniques such as active progressive relaxation training require a moderate expenditure of energy, which often increases fatigue and limits an individual's ability to complete relaxation sessions and practice. Therefore active progressive relaxation is not appropriate for patients with advanced disease or those who have decreased energy reserves. Passive relaxation or guided imagery is more appropriate for these individuals.

Meditation and Breathing

Meditation is any activity that limits stimulus input by directing attention to a single unchanging or repetitive stimulus so the person is able to become more aware of self (Snyder and Lindquist, 2010). It is a general term for a wide range of practices that involve relaxing the body and stilling the mind. The root word, *meditari,* means to consider or pay attention to something. Although the meditation has its roots in eastern religious practices (Hindu, Buddhism, and Taoism), conventional health care practitioners began to recognize its healing potential in the early 1970s (Snyder and Lindquist, 2010). According to Benson (1975), the four components of meditation are (1) a quiet space, (2) a comfortable position, (3) a receptive attitude, and (4) a focus of attention. He described meditation as a process that anyone can use to calm down; cope with stress; and, for those with spiritual inclinations, feel one with God or the universe.

Meditation is different from relaxation; the purpose of meditation is to become "mindful," increasing our ability to live freely and escape destructive patterns of negativity. Meditation is self-directed; it does not necessarily require a teacher and can be learned from books or audiotapes (Kabat-Zinn, 2005). Most meditation techniques involve slow, relaxed, deep, abdominal breathing that evokes a restful state, lowers oxygen consumption, reduces respiratory and heart rates, and reduces anxiety (Chiesa and Serretti, 2010).

Clinical Applications of Meditation. Several recent studies support the clinical benefits of meditation. For example, meditation reduces overall systolic and diastolic blood pressures and significantly reduces hypertensive risk (Nidich et al., 2009). It also successfully reduces relapses in alcohol treatment programs (Garland et al., 2010). Patients with cancer who use mindfulness-based cognitive therapies often experience less depression, anxiety, and distress and report an improved quality of life (Foley et al., 2010). Patients suffering from posttraumatic stress disorders and chronic pain also benefit from mindfulness meditation (Kimbrough et al., 2010). In addition, meditation increases productivity, improves mood, increases sense of identity, and lowers irritability (Dossey and Keegan, 2009).

Considerations for the appropriateness of meditation include the person's degree of self-discipline; it requires ongoing practice to achieve lasting results. Most meditation activities are easy to learn and do not require memorization or particular procedures. Patients typically find mindfulness and meditation self-reinforcing. The peaceful, positive mental state is usually pleasurable and provides an incentive for individuals to continue meditating.

Limitations of Meditation. Although meditation contributes to improvement in a variety of physiological and psychological ailments, it is contraindicated for some people. For example, a person who has a strong fear of losing control will possibly perceive it as a form of mind control and thus will be resistant to learning the technique. Some individuals also become hypertensive during meditation and require a much shorter session than the average 15- to 20-minute session.

Meditation may also increase the effects of certain drugs. Therefore monitor individuals learning meditation closely for physiological changes with respect to their medications. Prolonged practice of meditation techniques sometimes reduces the need for antihypertensive, thyroid-regulating, and psychotropic medications (e.g., antidepressants and anti-anxiety agents). In these cases, adjustment of the medication is necessary.

Imagery

Imagery or visualization is a mind-body therapy that uses the conscious mind to create mental images to stimulate physical changes in the body, improve perceived well-being, and/or enhance self-awareness. Frequently imagery, combined with some form of relaxation training, facilitates the effect of the relaxation technique. Imagery is self-directed, in which individuals create their mental images, or guided, during which a practitioner leads an individual through a particular scenario (Dossey and Keegan, 2009). When guiding an imagery exercise, direct the patient to begin slow abdominal breathing while focusing on the rhythm of breathing. Then direct the patient to visualize a specific image such as ocean waves coming to shore with each inspiration and receding with each exhalation. Next instruct the patient to take notice of the smells, sounds, and temperatures that he or she is experiencing. As the imagery session progresses, instruct the patient to visualize warmth entering the body during inspiration and tension leaving the body during exhalation. Individualize imagery scenarios for each patient to ensure that the image does not evoke negative memories or feelings.

Imagery often evokes powerful psychophysiological responses such as alterations in gastric secretions, body chemistry, internal and superficial blood flow, wound healing, and heart rate/heart rate variability (Pincus and Sheikh, 2009). Although most imagery techniques involve visual images, they also include the auditory, proprioceptive, gustatory, and olfactory senses. An example of this involves visualizing a lemon being sliced in half and squeezing the lemon juice on the tongue. This visualization produces increased salivation as effectively as the actual event. People typically respond to their environment according to the way they perceive it and by their own visualizations and expectancies. Therefore you need to individualize imagery for each patient (Snyder and Lindquist, 2010).

Creative visualization is one form of self-directed imagery that is based on the principle of mind-body connectivity (i.e., every mental image leads to physical or emotional changes) (Gawain, 2008). Box 32-2 lists patient teaching strategies for creative visualization.

Clinical Applications of Imagery. Imagery has applications in a number of pediatric and adult patient populations. For example, it helps control or relieve pain, decrease nightmares, and improve sleep (Pincus and Sheikh, 2009). It also aids in the treatment of chronic conditions such as asthma, cancer, sickle cell anemia, migraines, autoimmune disorders, atrial fibrillation, functional urinary disorders, menstrual and premenstrual syndromes, gastrointestinal disorders such as irritable bowel syndrome and ulcerative colitis, and rheumatoid arthritis (Snyder and Lindquist, 2010).

BOX 32-2 PATIENT TEACHING

Creative Visualization

Objective

- The patient will demonstrate skills in creative visualization.

Teaching Strategies

- Set goals the patient can meet. Success achieves confidence and increased self-esteem.
- Create a clear image. Although it is sometimes difficult to develop a visual image, if the patient views the goals of the imagery with clear thoughts and in the present tense, the patient will be more successful in creating an effective image.
- Have the patient frequently visualize the image. Have him or her perform this visualization during relaxing states and throughout the day but particularly before bedtime or on wakening, when his or her mind usually is more relaxed.
- Have the patient repeat encouraging statements while focusing on the image. This alleviates any doubts about his or her ability to achieve established goals.

Evaluation

- Observe patient behaviors for presence of anxiety or increased discomfort.
- Ask patient to describe the helpfulness of the visualization experience.
- Have patient describe use of positive self-dialogue and images of desired health habits, feelings, and desires for healing.
- Ask how the patient is coping with daily stressors.

Limitations of Imagery. Imagery is a behavioral intervention that has relatively few side effects (Roffe, Schmidt, and Ernst, 2005). Yet increased anxiety and fear sometimes occur when imagery is used to treat posttraumatic stress disorders and social anxiety disorders (Cook et al., 2010). Some patients with chronic obstructive pulmonary disease (COPD) and asthma experience increased airway constriction when using guided imagery (Reed, 2007). Thus you need to closely monitor patients when beginning this therapy.

TRAINING-SPECIFIC THERAPIES

Training-specific therapies are CAM treatments that nurses administer only after completing a specific course of study and training. These therapies require postgraduate certificates or degrees indicating completion of additional education and training, national certification, or additional licensure beyond the registered nurse (RN) to practice and administer them. Several training-specific therapies (e.g., biofeedback and acupuncture) are very effective and often recommended by western health care practitioners (Trigkilidas, 2010; Wheat and Larkin, 2010). However, others (e.g., homeopathy and naturopathy) have not been adequately studied, and their effectiveness in many conditions has been questioned (Borelli and Ernst, 2010). Although many of these complementary therapies elicit positive effects, all therapies carry some risk, particularly when used in conjunction with conventional medical therapies. Therefore you need advanced knowledge to effectively talk about them with patients and provide education about their safe use.

Biofeedback

Biofeedback is a mind-body technique that uses instruments to teach self-regulation and voluntary self-control over specific physiological responses. Electronic or electromechanical instruments measure, process, and provide information to patients about their muscle tension, cardiac activity, respiratory rates, brain-wave patterns, and autonomic nervous system activity. This information, or feedback, is given in physical, physiological, auditory, and/or visual feedback signals that increase a person's awareness of internal processes that are linked to illness and distress. Biofeedback therapies are used to change thinking, emotions, and behaviors, which in turn support beneficial physiological changes, resulting in improved health and well-being. For example, patients connected to a biofeedback device sometimes hear a sound if their pulse rate or blood pressure increases out of their therapeutic zone. Practitioners then help patients interpret these sounds and use a variety of breathing, relaxation, and imaging exercises to gain voluntary control over their racing heart or their increasing systolic blood pressure (Applied Psychophysiology and Biofeedback Association, 2008).

Biofeedback is an effective addition to more traditional relaxation programs because it immediately demonstrates to patients their ability to control some physiological responses and the relationship among thoughts, feelings, and physiological responses. It helps individuals focus on and monitor specific body parts. Biofeedback helps patients control the physiological functions that are most difficult to control by providing immediate feedback about which stress relaxation behaviors work most effectively. Eventually patients notice positive physiological changes without the need for instrument feedback.

Clinical Applications of Biofeedback. Biofeedback in a variety of forms has application in numerous situations, with evidence supporting its effectiveness dating back to the 1980s. Recent systematic literature reviews suggest that it is helpful in stroke recovery, smoking cessation, attention deficit hyperactivity disorder (ADHD), epilepsy, headache disorders, and a variety of gastrointestinal and urinary tract disorders (Arns et al., 2009; Hollands et al., 2010). One of the most critical components of any behavioral program is adherence to the treatment regimen. Patients who are compliant have more positive results.

Limitations of Biofeedback. Although biofeedback produces effective outcomes in many patients, there are several precautions, particularly in those with psychological or neurological conditions. During biofeedback sessions repressed emotions or feelings for which coping is difficult sometimes surface. For this reason practitioners who offer biofeedback need to be trained in more traditional psychological methods or have qualified professionals available for referral. In addition, long-term use of biofeedback sometimes lowers blood pressure, heart rates, and other physiological parameters. As with other biobehavioral interventions, monitor patients closely to determine the need for medication adjustments.

Acupuncture

As a key component of TCM, **acupuncture** is one of the oldest practices in the world. In TCM, acupuncture is only one intervention used. When applied outside the whole system practice of TCM, acupuncture is viewed as a mind-body therapy and is called medical acupuncture. In the United States medical acupuncture is often provided as an individual treatment by conventionally trained physicians, nurses, chiropractors, dentists, and acupuncturists for many chronic conditions. Many states now have regulations and licensure requirements to practice as an acupuncturist.

Acupuncture regulates or realigns the **vital energy *(qi)***, which flows like a river through the body in channels that form a system of pathways called **meridians.** Twelve primary and eight secondary meridians are used by medical acupuncturists. An obstruction in

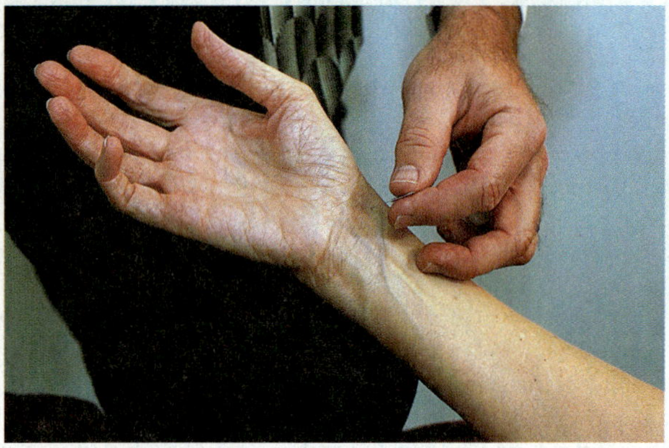

FIG. 32-2 Acupuncture accesses the *qi* through specific points along the energy meridians of the body.

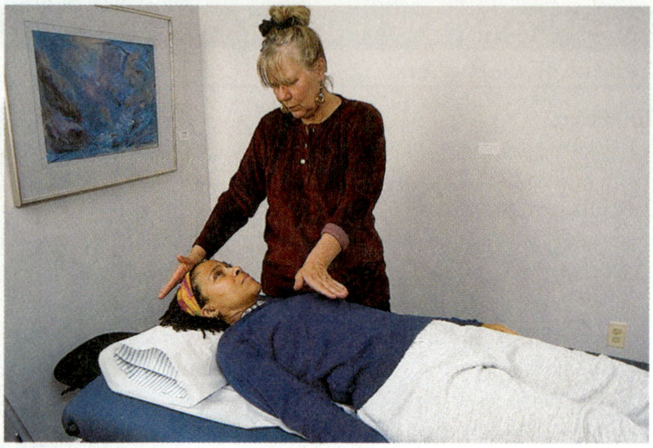

FIG. 32-3 The practitioner intentionally directs interpersonal energy to facilitate the patient's healing process during a therapeutic touch session.

these channels blocks energy flow in other parts of the body. Acupuncturists insert needles in specific areas along the channels called **acupoints,** through which the *qi* can be influenced and flow reestablished (Fig. 32-2). Application of heat or weak electrical currents enhances the effects of the needles (Fontaine, 2005).

Clinical Applications of Acupuncture. Current evidence shows that acupuncture modifies the body's response to pain and how pain is processed by central neural pathways and cerebral function (NIH/NCCAM, 2010a). Acupuncture is effective for low back pain, myofascial pain (e.g., temporomandibular joint disorder and trigeminal neuralgia), simple and migraine headaches, osteoarthritis, plantar heel pain, and chronic shoulder pain (Lee et al., 2010; Molsberger et al., 2010). It is also used to treat other problems such as sinusitis, gastrointestinal disorders, chronic pruritus, perimenstrual symptoms, menopausal symptoms, clinical depression, smoking, and other addictions with varying effectiveness (Scheid et al., 2010).

Limitations of Acupuncture. Acupuncture is a safe therapy when the practitioner has the appropriate training and uses sterilized needles. Although needle complications occur, they are rare if the practitioner takes appropriate steps to ensure the safety of the equipment and the patient. Reported complications include infections resulting from inadequately sterilized needles or those that are left in place for an extended length of time, broken needles, puncture of an internal organ, bleeding, fainting, seizures, and posttreatment drowsiness.

Caution is necessary when using acupuncture with pregnant patients and those who have a history of seizures, are carriers of hepatitis, or are infected with human immunodeficiency virus (HIV). Treatment is contraindicated in persons who have bleeding disorders and skin infections. Further, semipermanent needles should not be used with patients who have valvular heart disease because of the increased risk of infection. Electroacupuncture is not recommended for persons with a pacemaker and those who have cardiac arrhythmias or epilepsy or are pregnant (Fontaine, 2005).

Therapeutic Touch

Therapeutic touch (TT), developed in the 1970s, is one of the "touch therapies" identified by NCCAM. It affects the energy fields that surround and penetrate the human body with the conscious intent to help or heal (Dossey and Keegan, 2009). Other touch therapies include acupressure, healing touch (HT), reiki, and the M technique. Blending ancient eastern traditions with modern nursing theory, TT uses the energy of the provider to positively influence the patient's energy field.

TT consists of placing the practitioner's open palms either on or close to the body of a person (Fig. 32-3). It occurs in five phases: centering, assessing, unruffling, treating, and evaluating. To begin the practitioner centers physically and psychologically, becoming fully present in the moment and quieting outside distractions. Then the practitioner scans the body of the patient with the palms (roughly 2 to 6 inches [5 to 15 cm] from the body) from head to toe. While assessing the energetic biofield of the patient, the practitioner focuses on the quality of the *qi,* identifying areas of accumulated energetic tensions, uneasiness, sluggishness, or congestion that manifest as sensations of congestion, pressure, warmth, coolness, blockage, pulling or drawing, or static or tingling. The practitioner then redirects these energetic patterns to harmonize distressed areas or to stimulate movement of *qi* in areas that are stuck and congested. Using long downward strokes over the energy fields of the body, the practitioner touches the body or maintains the hands in a position a few inches away from the body. The final phase consists of evaluating the patient, reassessing the energy field to ensure that energy is flowing freely, and determining additional outcomes and responses to the treatment (Krieger, 1975, 1979).

Clinical Applications of Therapeutic Touch. The evidence supporting the effectiveness of TT is inconclusive, although it may be effective in treating pain in adults and children, dementia, trauma, and anxiety during acute and chronic illnesses (Jain and Mills, 2010). Box 32-3 summarizes the importance of touch in older adults.

Limitations of Therapeutic Touch. Although the use of TT causes very few complications or side effects, it is contraindicated in certain patient populations. For example, people who are sensitive to human interaction and touch (e.g., those who have been physically abused or have psychiatric disorders) often misinterpret the intent of the treatment and feel threatened and anxious by it. Other patients, including pregnant women, neonates, patients with cardiovascular and neurological instabilities, or patients who are dying, sometimes are sensitive to energy repatterning. Sessions with these populations need to be time limited and particularly gentle (Snyder and Lindquist, 2010).

Chiropractic Therapy

Chiropractic therapy, a manipulative or body-based therapy, was developed in 1895 in Iowa. Chiropractors graduate from well-established postbaccalaureate educational programs similar to medical schools. The central belief of the chiropractic profession

BOX 32-3 FOCUS ON OLDER ADULTS

The Importance of Touch

- Touch is a primal need, as necessary as food, growth, or shelter. Touch is like a nutrient transmitted through the skin, and "skin hunger" is like a form of malnutrition that has reached epidemic proportions in the United States, especially among older adults (Fontaine, 2005).
- Older adults need touch as much as or more than any other age-group. However, the elderly often experience "skin hunger." Older adults often have fewer family members or friends to touch them at a time when simple touch may enhance communication, especially when other senses are reduced (Dossey and Keegan, 2009).
- Simple touch helps older adults feel more connected to and accepted by those around them and more in tune with their environment. Touch enhances self-esteem and sense of worth.
- Nurses who react adversely to skin changes caused by aging often find it difficult to touch older adults. This reluctance communicates a negative message to the older adult (Dossey and Keegan, 2009). Therefore be aware of your own reactions to touch when caring for older adults to ensure a therapeutic approach to patient-centered care.

is that body structure (primarily that of the spine and spinal cord) and the ability of the body to function normally are closely related. When the spine is misaligned, energy flow is impeded, and the innate healing abilities of the body are impaired. Chiropractic therapy aims to normalize the relationship between structure and function by a series of manipulations. Practitioners use their hands or a device to provide manipulation, which is the application of a controlled, sudden forceful movement to a joint, moving it beyond its passive range of motion. Often manipulations are combined with additional therapeutic modalities, including ice and heat, electrical stimulation, deep tissue massage, joint immobilization, lifestyle counseling, and medications.

Chiropractic care is a popular form of complementary therapy in the United States; 8.6% of the adult and 3% of the pediatric population visit chiropractors each year, representing almost 20 million health care visits (Barnes et al., 2008). Compared to other forms of complementary therapies, chiropractic care is often covered by insurance plans, including Medicare, Medicaid, state workers' compensation plans, health maintenance organizations (HMOs), and private insurance plans. Licensure is regulated by individual state governments, and scopes of practice and prescriptive authority vary from state to state.

Clinical Applications of Chiropractic Therapy. The basic goals of chiropractic therapy focus on restoring structural and functional imbalances. Chiropractors believe that structure and function coexist with one another and that alterations or distortions in structure ultimately lead to abnormalities in function. A major structural problem that chiropractors treat is vertebral (neck/back) subluxation with its accompanying symptom of pain.

Chiropractic therapy improves acute pain and disability in some patients. This therapy is also sometimes effective over longer periods to reduce pain caused by acute and subacute low back pain and joint pain caused by osteoarthritis (Walker et al., 2010). Chiropractic care may also enhance the effects of conventional treatments in pediatric asthma (Kaminskyj et al., 2010). Chiropractic interventions are also used to treat headaches, dysmenorrhea, vertigo, tinnitus, and visual disorders (Hawk et al., 2010).

Limitations of Chiropractic Therapy. Although chiropractic therapies are safe for a variety of conditions, chiropractors do not treat several diseases or conditions with manipulation. Bone and joint infections require pharmaceutical or surgical intervention because the structural integrity of the bone is compromised if excessive force is used. Other contraindications include acute myelopathy, fractures, dislocations, rheumatoid arthritis, and osteoporosis.

Some risks are associated with chiropractic therapy. A variety of injuries, ranging in severity from mild adverse responses (e.g., mild transient headache, increased pain and stiffness) to more serious injuries (e.g., vertebral artery dissection), sometimes happen (Ernst, 2007). Degree and risk of injury depend on the type of manipulation performed, location of the manipulation (cervical spine is more susceptible to serious injury), overall health of the patient, and expertise of the provider. When educating patients about chiropractic care, you need to include educational and licensure credentials of qualified chiropractors, typical treatments, and possible complications.

TABLE 32-2 Three Causes of Disease According to Traditional Chinese Medicine

CAUSE OF DISEASE	INFLUENCES
Internal causes	Internal causes originate in emotions and affect different organs: anger (liver), joy (heart), fear (kidney), grief/sadness (lung), pensiveness/worry (spleen), and shock (heart/kidney).
External causes	Six "evils" primarily linked to weather and climate (wind, cold, fire, damp, summer heat, and dryness) are manifested as linked patterns such as wind-cold, wind-heat, fire-toxin.
Nonexternal, noninternal causes	Additional causes of disharmony include congenital weak constitutions (birth defects), trauma, overexertion, excessive sexual activity, poor quality diet, and parasites and poisons.

Traditional Chinese Medicine

Traditional Chinese medicine (TCM) is a whole system of medicine that began as a primitive ethnic healing system approximately 3600 years ago. Chinese medicine views health as "life in balance," which manifests as lustrous hair, a radiant complexion, engaged interactions, a body that functions without limitations, and emotional balance. Health promotion encourages healthy diet, moderate regular exercise, regular meditation/introspection, healthy family and social relationships, and avoidance of environmental toxins such as cigarette smoke.

Several concepts and principles guide the TCM system of assessment, diagnosis, and intervention. The most important of these is the concept of yin and yang, which represent opposing yet complementary phenomena that exist in a state of dynamic equilibrium. Examples are night/day, hot/cold, and shady/sunny. Yin represents shade, cold, and inhibition; whereas yang represents fire, light, and excitement. Yin also represents the inner part of the body, specifically the viscera, liver, heart, spleen, lung, and kidney; whereas yang represents the outer part, specifically the bowels, stomach, and bladder. Harmony and balance in every aspect of life are the keys to health, including yin/yang balance. Practitioners believe that disease occurs when there is an imbalance in these two paired opposites (Maciocia, 1989). Imbalance occurs as excess or deficiencies in three areas: external, internal, or neither internal nor external (Table 32-2). It ultimately leads to disruption of vital energy, *qi*, which then compromises the body-mind-spirit of the person, causing "*disease*." Disruptions in *qi* along the meridians can be systematically evaluated and treated by TCM practitioners.

TCM is an individualized treatment system based on a very specific assessment process. Practitioners use four methods to evaluate a patient's condition: observing, hearing/smelling, asking/interviewing, and touching/palpating. In Chinese medicine outward manifestations reflect the internal environment. For example, the color, shape, and coating of the tongue reflect the general condition of the internal organs. The pulses provide information about the condition and balance of *qi*, blood, ying and yang, and internal organs. Therapeutic modalities include acupuncture, Chinese herbs, tui na massage, **moxibustion** (burning moxa, a cone or stick of dried herbs that have healing properties on or near the skin) **cupping** (placing a heated cup on the skin to create a slight suction), **tai chi** (originally a martial art that is now viewed as a moving meditation in which patients move their bodies slowly, gently, and with awareness while breathing deeply), ***qi gong*** (originally a martial art, now viewed as a series of carefully choreographed movements or gestures that are designed to promote and manipulate the flow of *qi* within the body), lifestyle modifications, and dietary changes.

Clinical Applications of Traditional Chinese Medicine. In spite of widespread use of TCM in Asia, evidence about its effectiveness is limited. Most research in this field focuses on the study of individual treatment components of TCM such as acupuncture and herbal therapies. However, some evidence shows that TCM is helpful in treating fibromyalgia (Cao et al., 2010) and in reducing pain and spasticity in children with cerebral palsy (Zhang et al., 2010).

Limitations of Traditional Chinese Medicine. TCM is not currently regulated in most states, although acupuncture is. The federal government recognizes the Accreditation Commission for Acupuncture and Oriental Medicine (ACAOM) as responsible for accrediting schools that teach acupuncture and TCM, and approximately one third of the states that license acupuncture require graduation from an ACAOM-accredited school. The National Certification Commission for Acupuncture and Oriental Medicine (NCCAOM) offers a certification examination for acupuncture and Chinese herbal and manipulative therapies. Refer patients requesting TCM to a qualified practitioner found at http://www.nccaom.org/find/index.html.

There is some concern about the safety of Chinese herbal treatments that are used in teas, remedies, and supplements. The U.S. Food and Drug Administration (FDA) does not regulate, inspect, or ensure that the ingredients of these herbs are safe and without toxins. Recent reports about these products suggest that many Chinese herbs are contaminated with drugs, toxins, or heavy metals or that many ingredients may not be clearly listed or labeled. Further, these herbs can be very powerful, interacting with drugs and causing serious complications. When assessing a person using TCM, you always need to ask about the full complement of therapies, including the types of herbs that the patient is using. Some patients consider these as teas or dietary additives, powders, or supplements and not as over-the-counter medications.

Natural Products and Herbal Therapies

Researchers estimate that approximately 25,000 plant species are used medicinally throughout the world. It is the oldest form of medicine known to man, and archeological evidence suggests that herbal remedies have been used for over 60,000 years. Herbal medicines are a prominent part of health care among indigenous populations worldwide. In addition, interest in countries in which health care is primarily conventional allopathic medicine is also increasing (Snyder and Lindquist, 2010).

Nonvitamin, nonmineral natural products are used by almost 20% of the U.S. population to prevent disease and illness and to promote health and well-being (Barnes et al., 2008). A natural product is a chemical compound or substance produced by a living organism and includes herbal medicines (also known as botanicals), dietary supplements, vitamins, minerals, mycotherapies (fungi-based products), essential oils (aromatherapy), and probiotics. Many are sold over the counter as dietary supplements. The most frequently used products are garlic, Echinacea, saw palmetto, ginkgo biloba, cranberry, soy, ginseng, black cohosh, St. John's wort, glucosamine, peppermint, fish oil/omega 3, soy, and milk thistle (Blumenthal et al., 2006).

Herbal medicines are not approved for use as drugs and are not regulated by the FDA. For this reason many are sold as foods or food supplements. The Dietary Supplement Health and Education Act (1994) allows companies to sell herbs as dietary supplements as long as there are no health claims written on their labels. Natural products in the United States are prepared primarily from plant materials. They are provided as tinctures or extracts, elixirs, syrups, capsules, pills, tablets, lozenges, powders, ointments or creams, drops, and suppositories.

Clinical Applications of Herbal Therapy. A number of herbs are safe and effective for a variety of conditions (Table 32-3). Nurses have used cranberry juice to treat urinary tract infections for decades. Research now supports the use of cranberry supplements to prevent urinary tract infections because cranberry molecules bind with the iron that bacteria need to grow and reproduce and substances in cranberry block adherence of bacteria to the walls of the bladder (Rossi et al., 2010). Chamomile is a plant substance that has been widely used in teas to promote sleep and relaxation and treat mild gastrointestinal disturbances and premenstrual symptoms. Clinical trials have recently found that chamomile may have modest benefits for people with mild-to-moderate generalized anxiety disorder (Amsterdam et al., 2009).

Limitations of Herbal Therapy. Simply because a product is "natural" does not make it "safe." Although herbal medicines provide beneficial effects for a variety of conditions, a number of problems exist. Because they are not regulated, concentrations of the active ingredients vary considerably. Contamination with other herbs or chemicals, including pesticides and heavy metals, is also problematic. Not all companies follow strict quality control and manufacturing guidelines that set standards for acceptable levels of pesticides, residual solvents, bacterial levels, and heavy metals. For this reason, teach patients to purchase herbal medicines only from reputable manufacturers. Labels on herbal products need to contain the scientific name of the botanical, the name and address of the actual manufacturer, a batch or lot number, the date of manufacture, and the expiration date. Using natural products that have been verified by the U.S. Pharmacopeia (USP) is another way to ensure product safety, quality, and purity. Look for the USP Verified Dietary Supplement mark on product labels when buying or recommending natural products.

Some herbs also contain toxic products that have been linked to cancer. Table 32-4 lists several unsafe herbs. Some herbal substances contain powerful chemicals. As with any other medication, examine herbs for interaction and compatibility with other prescribed or over-the-counter substances that are being used simultaneously.

TABLE 32-3 Safe or Effective Herbs Determined by Non-U.S. Regulatory Authorities

COMMON NAME AND USES	EFFECTS	POTENTIAL DRUG INTERACTIONS
Aloe		
Skin disorders, including inflammation and acute injuries (used topically)	Acceleration of wound healing	Furosemide (Lasix) and loop diuretics
GI ulcerations, including Crohn's disease and ulcerative colitis (taken orally)	Unknown mechanism, although there is a known laxative effect	May enhance the effects of laxatives when taken orally
Chamomile		
Inflammatory diseases of GI and upper respiratory tracts	Antiinflammatory	Drugs that cause drowsiness (alcohol, barbiturates, benzodiazepines, narcotics, antidepressants)
Generalized anxiety disorder	Calming agent	
Echinacea		
Upper respiratory tract infections	Stimulant of immune system	Antirejection and other drugs that weaken immune system May interact with antiretrovirals and other drugs used in the treatment of HIV/AIDS
Feverfew		
Wound healing	Antiinflammatory	Warfarin (Coumadin) and blood thinners
Arthritis	Inhibition of serotonin and prostaglandins	Aspirin and ibuprofen
Garlic		
Elevated cholesterol levels	Inhibition of platelet aggregation	Warfarin and blood thinners
Hypertension		Saquinavir (Fortovase) and other anti-HIV drugs
Ginger		
Nausea and vomiting	Antiemetic	Warfarin and blood thinners Aspirin and NSAIDs
Gingko biloba		
Alzheimer's disease and dementia	Memory improvement, although these effects are now in question given results in two recent clinical trials	Warfarin and anticoagulants Aspirin and NSAIDs
Ginseng		
Age-related diseases	Increased physical endurance, improved immune function	Warfarin and anticoagulants Aspirin and NSAIDs MAO inhibitors
Licorice		
GI disorders, including gastric ulcers and hepatitis C	Unknown	Corticosteroids and other immunosuppressive drugs Digoxin Antihypertensive drugs
Saw palmetto		
Benign prostatic hyperplasia	Prevention of conversion of testosterone to dihydrotestosterone (needed for prostate cell multiplication)	Finasteride (Propecia) and antiandrogen drugs
Chronic pelvic pain	Unknown mechanism	None known
Valerian		
Sleep disorders, mild anxiety and restlessness	Central nervous system depression	Barbiturates and other sleep medications Alcohol Antihistamines

Data from National Institutes of Health/National Center for Complementary and Alternative Medicine: *Herbs at a glance,* 2010, accessed September 10, 2010, from http://nccam.nih.gov/health/herbsataglance.htm.

AIDS, Acquired immunodeficiency disease; *GI,* gastrointestinal; *HIV,* human immunodeficiency virus; *MAO,* monoamine oxidase; *NSAIDs,* nonsteroidal antiinflammatory drugs.

TABLE 32-4 **Unsafe Herbs**

COMMON NAME	EFFECTS	COMMENTS
Calamus (Indian type most toxic)	Fever Digestive aid	Contains varying amounts of carcinogenic *cis*-isoasarone Documented cases of kidney damage and seizures with oral preparations
Chaparral	Anticancer Used for bronchitis in traditional healing systems (Native American and Hispanic folk medicine) Found in "natural" weight-loss products	No proven efficacy Induces severe liver toxicity in some cases Severe uterine contractions
Coltsfoot	Antitussive	Contains carcinogenic pyrrolizidine alkaloids Hepatotoxic
Comfrey	Wound healing and acute injuries Used for antiinflammatory effects in osteoarthritis and rheumatoid arthritis	Contains carcinogenic pyrrolizidine alkaloids May induce venoocclusive disease Hepatotoxic
Ephedra (ma huang)	Central nervous system stimulant Bronchodilator Cardiac stimulation Weight loss	Unsafe for people with hypertension, diabetes, or thyroid disease Avoid consumption with caffeine
Life root	Menstrual flow stimulant	Hepatotoxic
Pokeweed	Antirheumatic Anticancer	Do not use with children, but many websites state that it is safe with observation and monitoring and proper dosing; often used with folk remedies and in native American healing

Data from National Institutes of Health/National Center for Complementary and Alternative Medicine: *Herbs at a glance,* 2010, accessed September 10, 2010, from http://nccam.nih.gov/health/herbsataglance.htm; Natural Standard, 2011, accessed April 2, 2011, from http://naturalstandard.com/; US Pharmacopeia, 2011, accessed March 29, 2011 from http://www.usp.org/.

NURSING ROLE IN COMPLEMENTARY AND ALTERNATIVE THERAPIES

The interest in complementary and alternative therapies continues to increase. Most people using and seeking information about these therapies are well educated and have a strong desire to actively participate in decision making about their health care. This increased interest comes not only from health care consumers but also from allopathic physicians who have increasing concerns that current conventional medicine is not meeting the needs of their patients. Many allopathic physicians do not refer their patients for complementary therapies because they are not familiar with them and have had little, if any, education and training about integrating these traditions with their practice. Many physicians have reservations about complementary therapies because they have not been tested appropriately in clinical trials in which other factors that influence the outcomes are strictly controlled.

In North America and Europe many professional groups are exploring the use of complementary and alternative therapies and facilitating and monitoring research in this area. Proposals put forth by several of the these groups include assessing the public use of complementary and alternative therapies, integrating CAM educational components in the curriculum for all health care programs, providing appropriate information to the public, and encouraging and facilitating communication between CAM and conventional care providers to improve public health and ensure the quality and safety of health care. For example, if health care providers want to recommend the best treatment option for each health condition, allopathic providers need to be aware of the evidence supporting complementary therapies and how to safely refer patients to complementary therapy providers. Contrastingly, complementary therapy providers need to participate in the research process, working with scientists to demonstrate the effectiveness of these therapies on patient outcomes within the more rigorous framework of western science. All providers, including nurses, need to encourage open, honest dialogue about the use of complementary and alternative therapies by patients and better understand the benefits of therapies that encourage active participation by their patients in preventing or managing illness rather than relying solely on surgery or drugs.

Integrative health care, a strategy that is gaining popularity, involves a multiple-practitioner group practice in which a patient seeks care simultaneously from more than one type of practitioner. Patients have the option to choose the type of practitioner that they believe is beneficial for their particular health problem. Patients who benefit from these groups are those who have chronic health problems that have historically been difficult to treat using traditional allopathic approaches such as fibromyalgia, chronic fatigue syndrome, or chronic pain syndromes. A multiple-practitioner group practice represents a pluralistic and truly complementary health care system in which both alternative and allopathic practitioners work side-by-side to improve the well-being of their patients. The integrative approach is consistent with the holistic approach that nurses learn to practice. Nurses have the potential for becoming essential participants in this type of health care philosophy. Many nurses already practice the use of touch, relaxation techniques, imagery, and breathwork. Familiarize yourself with the evidence in each modality that you incorporate into your practice. Know which patient is most likely to benefit from each therapy, which complications might occur, and which precautions are needed when using these therapies.

In addition, you need enough knowledge to discuss complementary and alternative therapies with patients and help them make health care decisions. Always ask patients directly about their use of complementary therapies, including self-care activities such as yoga, meditation, or dietary supplements. Be knowledgeable about the evidence for different complementary therapies so you can make appropriate recommendations about which therapies are possibly useful for patients. Know about the different credentialing processes and how to refer patients to competent providers. Understand thoroughly the potential benefits and risks so information is clearly and fully disclosed. Be knowledgeable so you can give advice to patients about when to seek conventional care and when it is safe to consider complementary care services. For example, if a patient complains of right lower abdominal pain, nausea, and vomiting, be suspicious of appendicitis and recommend assessment by an allopathic physician. However, if the patient has a chronic gastrointestinal disorder and has a diagnosis of irritable bowel syndrome, the patient may benefit from relaxation and herbal therapy. Be aware of the safety precautions for each complementary therapy and incorporate these in your teaching plans. Finally understand your state Nurse Practice Act with regard to complementary therapies and practice only within the scope of these laws.

Nurses work very closely with their patients and are in the unique position of becoming familiar with the patient's spiritual and cultural viewpoints. They are often able to determine which complementary therapies are more appropriately aligned with these beliefs and offer recommendations accordingly. Being knowledgeable about CAM therapies will help you provide accurate information to patients and other health care professionals.

KEY POINTS

- Integrative health care programs use a multidisciplinary (both allopathic and complementary) treatment approach that provides holistic care to patients.
- The stress response is an adaptive response that allows individuals to respond to stressful situations.
- A chronic stress response is often maladaptive, leading to chronic muscle tension, mood changes, and immune changes.
- Complementary therapies require commitment and regular involvement by the patient to be most effective and have prolonged beneficial outcomes.
- Choose complementary therapies appropriately according to the patient's functional status, belief or religious perspectives, access to health care, and insurance coverage.
- Medication doses need to be changed when complementary therapies significantly and consistently alter physiological responses.
- Complementary therapies accessible to nursing include relaxation, meditation and mindfulness techniques, and imagery. Evidence supports their use to decrease the effects of stress and improve overall patient well-being.
- Many complementary therapies require additional education and certification, including biofeedback, touch therapies (TT, Reiki, and HT), and acupuncture.
- Although increasing evidence supports the use of complementary therapies, many complementary and alternative therapies still lack a scientific basis but are effective based on observed positive outcomes in a number of patients.

CLINICAL APPLICATION QUESTIONS

Preparing for Clinical Practice

1. Margaret Thompson is a 76-year-old Catholic woman who has been diagnosed with a slow-growing renal tumor. She is scheduled for surgery. You are responsible for the admission assessment and initial care for this patient. What assessment questions about complementary and alternative therapies are important to include during this preoperative period?
2. During the initial assessment Ms. Thompson asks many questions. "Is it cancer? Will the surgery result in a disability? What can I expect? Will I have to be in intensive care unit (ICU)?" You conclude that she is afraid of both the surgical procedure and the outcome. What types of specific nursing-accessible complementary therapies will you offer her during the preoperative period to reduce her anxiety and help her prepare for surgery?
3. In the days following surgery you are assigned to care for Ms. Thompson. Although physically she is recovering quite well from the procedure, you note that she is becoming more despondent and depressed. Preparing for discharge, what complementary and alternative medicine (CAM) therapies do you recommend to help her deal with her depression and cancer diagnosis?

evolve *Answers to Clinical Application Questions can be found on the Evolve website.*

REVIEW QUESTIONS

Are You Ready to Test Your Nursing Knowledge?

1. When planning patient education, it is important to remember that patients with which of the following often find relief in complementary therapies?
   1. Lupus and diabetes
   2. Ulcers and hepatitis
   3. Heart disease and pancreatitis
   4. Chronic back pain and arthritis
2. Which complementary therapies are most easily learned and applied by the nurse? (Select all that apply.)
   1. Massage therapy
   2. Traditional Chinese medicine
   3. Progressive relaxation
   4. Breathwork and imagery
   5. Therapeutic touch
3. Which statement best describes the evidence associated with complementary therapies as a whole?
   1. Many clinical trials in complementary therapies support their effectiveness in a wide range of clinical problems.
   2. It is difficult to find funding for studies about complementary therapies. Therefore we should not expect to find evidence supporting its use.
   3. The science supporting the effectiveness of complementary therapies is early in its development. Systematic reviews of the evidence often indicate beginning support for therapies, but there is a lack of strong evidence supporting their widespread use.
   4. Most of the research examining complementary and alternative therapies has found little evidence, suggesting that although people like them, they are not effective.
4. The nurse understands that providing holistic care includes treating which of the following?

1. Disease, spirit, and family interactions
2. Desires and emotions of the patient
3. Mind-body-spirit of the patient and their families
4. Muscles, nerves, and spine disorders

5. In addition to an adequate patient assessment, when the nurse uses one of the nursing-accessible complementary therapies, he or she must ensure that which of the following has occurred?
   1. The family has provided permission.
   2. The patient has provided permission and consent.
   3. The health care provider has given approval or provided orders for the therapy.
   4. He or she has documented that the patient has a complete understanding of complementary and alternative medicine.
6. Which role do patients have in complementary and alternative medicine therapy?
   1. Submissive to the practitioner
   2. Actively involved in the treatment
   3. An educator for other health care professionals
   4. A total believer in what is being taught
7. The nurse is caring for a patient experiencing a stress response. The nurse plans care with the knowledge that systems respond to stress in what manner?
   1. Always fail and cause illness and disease
   2. Cause structural damage to the body
   3. React the same way for all individuals
   4. Protect an individual from harm in the short term but cause negative responses over time
8. When meditation therapy is used, nurses need to monitor patients' medications carefully because meditation may augment the effects of certain drugs such as:
   1. Prednisone and antibiotics.
   2. Insulin and vitamins.
   3. Cough syrups and aspirin.
   4. Antihypertensive and thyroid-regulating medications.
9. A patient who has been using relaxation wants a better response. The nurse recommends the addition of biofeedback. What is the expected outcome related to using this additional modality?
   1. To eat less food
   2. To control diabetes
   3. To live longer with acquired immunodeficiency syndrome (AIDS)
   4. To learn how to control some autonomic nervous system responses
10. A patient asks a nurse about therapeutic touch (TT). Which of the following does the nurse include when providing patient education about TT? Therapeutic touch:
    1. Intentionally mobilizes energy to balance, harmonize, and repattern the recipient's biofield
    2. Intentionally heals specific diseases or corrects certain symptoms
    3. Is overwhelmingly effective in many conditions
    4. Is completely safe and does not warrant any special precautions
11. A nurse provides care for a diverse group of patients, including many immigrants. To better understand various types of health care, the nurse learns the traditional Chinese medicine system:
    1. Uses acupuncture as its primary intervention modality
    2. Uses many modalities that are based on the individual and include herbal therapies, moxibustion, and acupuncture
    3. Uses primarily herbal remedies (that are known to have high levels of lead products) and exercise
    4. Is the equivalent of medical acupuncture
12. The nurse is planning care for a group of patients who have requested the use of complementary health modalities. Which patient is not a good candidate for imagery?
    1. Pregnant patient
    2. Hypertensive patient
    3. Patient with posttraumatic stress disorder (PTSD)
    4. A pediatric patient
13. Several nurses on a busy unit are using relaxation strategies while at work. What is the desired workplace outcome from this intervention? (Select all that apply.)
    1. Improved health among the staff
    2. Increased patient safety
    3. Improved staff satisfaction
    4. Increased staff retention
    5. Fewer overtime assignments
14. The nurse is caring for a patient who uses several herbal preparations in addition to prescribed medications. What does the nurse need to understand about herbal preparations?
    1. They are regulated by the Food and Drug Administration (FDA); therefore patients and providers should feel confident that they are completely safe.
    2. They are natural products and therefore are safe as long as you use them cautiously and prudently for the conditions that are indicated.
    3. They are covered by insurance, including Medicare, Medicaid, and private payers.
    4. They should be treated as though they were "drugs" of sorts because many have active ingredients that can interact with other medications and change physiological responses.
15. The nurse manager of a community clinic arranges for staff in-services about various complementary therapies available in the community. What is the purpose of this training? (Select all that apply.)
    1. Nurses have a long history of providing some of these therapies and need to be knowledgeable about their positive outcomes.
    2. Nurses are often asked for recommendations and strategies that promote well-being and quality of life.
    3. Nurses play an essential role in patient education to provide information about the safe use of these healing strategies.
    4. Nurses appreciate the cultural aspects of care and recognize that many of these complementary strategies are part of a patient's life.
    5. Nurses play an essential role in the safe use of complementary therapies.
    6. Nurses learn how to provide all of the complementary modalities during their basic education.

Answers: 1. 4; 2. 3, 4; 3. 3; 4. 3; 5. 2; 6. 2; 7. 4; 8. 4; 9. 4; 10. 1; 11. 2; 12. 3; 13. 3, 4; 14. 4; 15. 1, 2, 3, 4, 5.

REFERENCES

American Holistic Nursing Association/American Nurses Association (AHNA/ANA): *Holistic nursing: scope and standards of practice*, Silver Spring, Md, 2007, American Nurses Publishing.

Applied Psychophysiology and Biofeedback Association: *Biofeedback position statement*, 2008, http://www.aapb.org/. Accessed September 2, 2010.

Benson H: *The relaxation response*, New York, 1975, Avon.

Dossey B, Keegan L: *Holistic nursing: a handbook for practice*, ed 5, Boston, Mass, 2009, Jones & Bartlett.

Fontaine K: *Healing practices: alternative therapies for nursing*, ed 2, Upper Saddle River, NJ, 2005, Prentice Hall.

Gawain S: *Creative visualization: use the power of your imagination to create what you want in your life*, Novato, Calif, 2008, New World Library.

Kabat-Zinn J: *Coming to our senses: healing ourselves and the world through mindfulness*, New York, 2005, Hyperion.

Koithan M: Let's talk about complementary and alternative therapies, *J Nurse Pract* 5(3):214, 2009.

Kreiger D: Therapeutic touch: the imprimatur of nursing, *Am J Nurs* 25:784, 1975.

Kreiger D: Searching for evidence of physiological change, *Am J Nurs* 79:660, 1979.

Kreitzer MJ, et al:Health professions education and integrative healthcare, *Explore J Sci Healing* 5(4):2127, 2009.

Maciocia G: *The foundations of Chinese medicine: a comprehensive text for acupuncturists and herbalists*, London, England, 1989, Churchill Livingstone.

National Institutes of Health/National Center for Complementary and Alternative Medicine (NIH/NCCAM): *Acupuncture and pain: applying modern science to an ancient practice. Complementary and alternative medicine: focus on research and care*, online newsletter, February 2010a, from http://nccam.nih.gov/news/newsletter/2010_february/2010february.pdf. Accessed September 14, 2010.

National Institutes of Health/National Center for Complementary and Alternative Medicine (NIH/NCCAM): *What is CAM and CAM basics*, 2010b, accessed September 1, 2010, from http://nccam.nih.gov/health/whatiscam/.

Pincus D, Sheikh AA: *Imagery for pain relief: A scientifically grounded guidebook for clinicians*, New York, 2009, Routledge, Taylor & Francis Group.

Rakel DP, Faass N: *Complementary medicine in clinical practice*, Sudbury, Mass, 2006, Jones & Bartlett.

Snyder M, Lindquist R: *Complementary and alternative therapies in nursing*, New York, 2010, Springer.

RESEARCH REFERENCES

Amsterdam JD, et al: A randomized, double-blind, placebo-controlled trial of oral *Matricaria recutita* (chamomile) extract therapy for generalized anxiety disorder, *J Clin Psychopharmacol* 29(4):378, 2009.

Arns M, et al: Efficacy of neurofeedback treatment in ADHD: the effects on inattention, impulsivity and hyperactivity: a meta-analysis, *Clin EEG Neurosci* 40(3): 180, 2009.

Barnes PM, et al: Complementary and alternative medicine use among adults and children: United States, 2007, *National Health Statistics Rep* 12:1, 2008.

Bloch B, et al: The effects of music relaxation on sleep quality and emotional measures in people living with schizophrenia, *J Music Ther* 47(1):27, 2010.

Blumenthal M, et al: Total sales of herbal supplements in US, *Herbalgram: Am Botanical Council* 71:64, 2006.

Borrelli F, Ernst E: Alternative and complementary therapies for the menopause, *Maturitas* 66(4):3333, 2010.

Cao H, et al: Traditional Chinese medicine for treatment of fibromyalgia: a systematic review of randomized controlled trials, *J Altern Complement Med* 16(4):397, 2010.

Chambers CT, et al: Psychological interventions for reducing pain and distress during routine childhood immunizations: a systematic review, *Clin Ther* 31(suppl 2):S77, 2009.

Chiesa A, Serretti A: A systematic review of neurobiological and clinical features of mindfulness meditations, *Psychol Med* 40(8):1239, 2010.

Clarke PN, et al: From theory to practice: caring science according to Watson and Brewer, *Nurs Sci Q* 22(4):339, 2009.

Cook JM, et al: Imagery rehearsal for posttraumatic nightmares: a randomized controlled trial, *Trauma stress* [Epub ahead of print], September 2010.

Dickinson HO, et al: Relaxation therapies for the management of primary hypertension in adults, *Cochrane Database Syst Rev* 2008,1(2):CD004935, DOI:10.1002/14651858.CD004935.pub2.

Ernst E: Adverse effects of spinal manipulation: a systematic review, *J Royal Soc Med* 100(7):330, 2007.

Foley E, et al: Mindfulness-based cognitive therapy for individuals whose lives have been affected by cancer: a randomized controlled trial, *J Consult Clin Psychol* 78(1):72, 2010.

Garland EL, et al: Mindfulness training modifies cognitive, affective, and physiological mechanisms implicated in alcohol dependence: results of a randomized controlled pilot trial, *J Psychoactive Drugs* 42(2):177, 2010.

Hawk C, et al: Best practices recommendations for chiropractic care for older adults: results of a consensus process, *J Manipulative Physiological Ther* 33(6):464, 2010.

Hollands GJ, et al: Visual feedback of individuals' medical imaging results for changing health behavior, *Cochrane Database Syst Rev* 20:1, 2010.

Innes KE, et al: Mind-body therapies for menopausal symptoms: a systematic review, *Maturitas* 66(2):135, 2010.

Jain S, Mills PJ: Biofield therapies: helpful or full of hype? A best evidence synthesis, *Int J Behav Med* 17(1):1, 2010.

Jorm AF, et al: Relaxation for depression. *Cochrane Database Syst Rev* 2008, 4(2):CD007142, DOI:10.1002/14651858.CD007142.pub2.

Kaminskyj A, et al: Chiropractic care for patients with asthma: a systematic review of the literature, *J Can Chiropr Assoc* 54(1):24, 2010.

Kimbrough E, et al: Mindfulness intervention for child abuse survivors, *J Clin Psychol* 66(1):17, 2010.

Kwekkeboom K, et al: Patients' perceptions of the effectiveness of guided imagery and progressive muscle relaxation interventions used in chronic cancer pain, *Complement Ther Clin Pract* 14:185, 2008.

Lasseter JH: The effectiveness of complementary therapies on the pain experience of hospitalized children, *J Holistic Nurs* 24:196, 2006.

Lee JH, et al: Acupuncture for chronic low back pain: protocol for a multicenter, randomized, sham-controlled trial, *BMC Musculoskelet Disord* 14(11):118, 2010.

Molsberger AF, et al: German Randomized Acupuncture Trial for chronic shoulder pain (GRASP)—a pragmatic, controlled, patient-blinded, multi-centre trial in an outpatient care environment, *Pain* 151(1):146, 2010.

Nidich SI, et al: A randomized controlled trial on effects of the transcendental meditation program on blood pressure, psychological distress, and coping in young adults, *Am J Hypertens* 22(12):1326, 2009.

Reed T: Imagery in the clinical setting: a tool for healing, *Nurs Clin North Am* 42(2):261, 2007.

Rheingans JI: A systematic review of nonpharmacologic adjunctive therapies for symptom management in children with cancer, *J Pediatr Oncol Nurs* 24(2):81, 2007.

Roffe L, Schmidt K, Ernst E: A systematic review of guided imagery as an adjuvant cancer therapy, *Psycho-Oncol* 14(8):607, 2005.

Rossi R, et al: Overview on cranberry and urinary tract infections in females, *J Clin Gastroenterol* 44(suppl 1): S61, 2010.

Scheid V, et al: The treatment of menopausal symptoms by traditional East Asian medicines: review and perspectives, *Maturitas* 66(2):111, 2010.

Schmidt J, et al: Psychological and physiological correlates of a brief intervention to enhance self-regulation in chronic pain, *J Pain* 9(4):55, 2008.

Trigkilidas D: Acupuncture therapy for chronic lower back pain: a systematic review, *Ann Royal Coll Surg Engl* 92(7): 595, 2010.

Walker BF, et al: Combined chiropractic interventions for low-back pain, *Cochrane Database Syst Rev* 4, 2010.

Weeks BP, Nilsson U: Music interventions in patients during coronary angiographic procedures: a randomized controlled study of the effect on patients' anxiety and well-being, *Eur J Cardiovasc Nurs* [Epub ahead of print], August 2010.

Wheat AL, Larkin KT: Biofeedback of heart rate variability and related physiology: a critical review, *Appl Psychophysiol Biofeedback* 35(3):229, 2010.

Zborowsky T, Kreitzer MJ: People, place, and process: the role of place in creating optimal healing environments, *Creative Nurs* 15(4):1860, 2009.

Zhang Y, et al: Traditional Chinese medicine for treatment of cerebral palsy in children: a systematic review of randomized clinical trials, *J Altern Complement Med* 16(4): 375, 2010.

CHAPTER 33

Self-Concept

OBJECTIVES

- Discuss factors that influence the components of self-concept.
- Identify stressors that affect self-concept and self-esteem.
- Describe the components of self-concept as related to psychosocial and cognitive developmental stages.
- Explore ways in which a nurse's self-concept and nursing actions affect a patient's self-concept and self-esteem.
- Discuss evidence-based practice applicable for identity confusion, disturbed body image, low self-esteem, and role conflict.
- Examine cultural considerations that affect self-concept.
- Apply the nursing process to promote a patient's self-concept.

KEY TERMS

Body image, p. 658
Identity, p. 660
Identity confusion, p. 662
Role ambiguity, p. 663
Role conflict, p. 663
Role overload, p. 663
Role performance, p. 661
Role strain, p. 663
Self-concept, p. 658
Self-esteem, p. 661
Sick role, p. 663

evolve WEBSITE

http://evolve.elsevier.com/Potter/fundamentals/

- Review Questions
- Concept Map Creator
- Case Study with Questions
- Audio Glossary
- Interactive Learning Activities
- Key Term Flashcards
- Content Updates

Self-concept is an individual's view of self. It is a subjective view and a complex mixture of unconscious and conscious thoughts, attitudes, and perceptions. Self-concept, or how a person *thinks* about oneself, directly affects self-esteem, or how one *feels* about oneself. Although these two terms are often used interchangeably, nurses need to differentiate the two so they correctly and completely assess patients and develop an individualized plan of care based on the patient's needs.

Nurses care for patients who face a variety of health problems that threaten their self-concept and self-esteem. The loss of bodily function, decline in activity tolerance, and difficulty in managing a chronic illness are examples of situations that change a patient's self-concept. As a nurse, you will help patients adjust to alterations in self-concept and support components of self-concept to promote successful coping and positive health outcomes.

SCIENTIFIC KNOWLEDGE BASE

The development and maintenance of self-concept and self-esteem begin at a young age and continue across the life span with a general tendency for boys to report higher self-esteem than girls. However, the exact amount of this gender difference and the way it varies across the life span remain unclear. Parents and other primary caregivers influence the development of a child's self-concept and self-esteem. In addition, individuals learn and internalize cultural influences on self-concept and self-esteem in childhood and adolescence (Guilamo-Ramos, 2009). There is a significant amount of emphasis on fostering a school-age child's self-concept. In general, young children tend to rate themselves higher than they rate other children, suggesting that their view of themselves is positively inflated. Adolescence is a particularly critical time when many variables, including school, family, and friends, affect self-concept and self-esteem (Martyn-Nemeth et al., 2009). The adolescent experience can adversely affect self-esteem, often more strongly for girls than for boys. For example, some adolescent girls are more sensitive about their appearance and how others view them. Thus it is important to assess changes in self-esteem among early, middle, and late adolescence because changes in self-concept occur over time (Fig. 33-1).

Job satisfaction and overall performance in adulthood are also linked to self-esteem. Sometimes when individuals lose a job, their sense of self diminishes, they lose motivation to be socially active, or they even become depressed. They lose their job identity, and this alters their self-perceptions. Establishing a stable sense of self that transcends relationships and situations is a developmental goal of adulthood.

Evidence suggests that sense of self is often negatively affected in older adulthood because of the intensity of emotional and physical changes associated with aging (Ebersole et al., 2008; Price, 2010). For example, when an older adult loses a partner or experiences a change in health, sometimes there is a change in social interaction or even self-care practices.

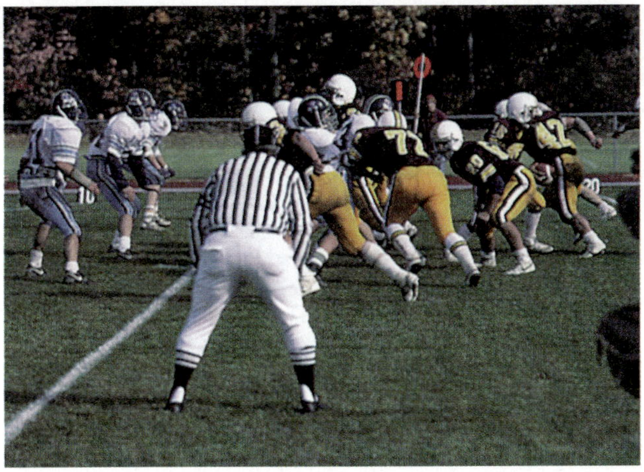

FIG. 33-1 Adolescents' participation in group activities can foster self-esteem. (From Hockenberry MJ, Wilson D: *Wong's essentials of pediatric nursing,* ed 8, St Louis, 2009, Mosby.)

Researchers also found ethnic and cultural differences in self-concept and self-esteem across the life span that impact health behaviors. In Latino youth, ethnic pride and self-esteem serve as protective factors against risk behaviors, including intentions to smoke cigarettes and to have sexual intercourse (Guilamo-Ramos, 2009). Cultural identity of older adults is one of the major elements of self-concept and a key aspect of self-esteem (Ebersole et al., 2008). Considering aging from a cultural perspective provides the context for providing the highest-quality nursing care. Sensitivity to factors that affect self-concept and self-esteem in diverse cultures is essential to ensure an individualized approach to health care.

How individuals view themselves and their perception of their health are closely related. Lower self-esteem is a risk factor that leaves one vulnerable to health problems, whereas higher self-esteem and strong social relationships support good health (Stinson et al., 2008). A patient's belief in personal health often enhances his or her self-concept. Statements such as "I can get through anything" or "I've never been sick a day in my life" indicate that a person's thoughts about personal health are positive. Illness, hospitalization, and surgery also affect self-concept. Chronic illness often affects the ability to provide financial support and maintain relationships, which then affects an individual's self-esteem and perceived roles within the family. Negative perceptions regarding health status are reflected in such statements as "It's not worth it anymore" or "I'm a burden to my family." Further, chronic illness affects identity and body image as reflected by verbalizations such as "I'll never get any better" or "I can't stand to look at myself anymore."

What individuals think and how they feel about themselves affect the way in which they care for themselves physically and emotionally and how they care for others. Further, a person's behaviors are generally consistent with both self-concept and self-esteem. Individuals who have a poor self-concept often do not feel in control of situations and worthy of care, which influences decisions regarding health care. Patients often have difficulty making even simple decisions, such as what to eat. Knowledge of variables that affect self-concept and self-esteem is critical to provide effective treatment.

BOX 33-1 SELF-CONCEPT: DEVELOPMENTAL TASKS

Trust versus Mistrust (Birth to 1 Year)
- Develops trust following consistency in caregiving and nurturing interactions
- Distinguishes self from environment

Autonomy versus Shame and Doubt (1 to 3 Years)
- Begins to communicate likes and dislikes
- Increasingly independent in thoughts and actions
- Appreciates body appearance and function (e.g., dressing, feeding, talking, and walking)

Initiative versus Guilt (3 to 6 Years)
- Identifies with a gender
- Enhances self-awareness
- Increases language skills, including identification of feelings

Industry versus Inferiority (6 to 12 Years)
- Incorporates feedback from peers and teachers
- Increases self-esteem with new skill mastery (e.g., reading, mathematics, sports, music)
- Aware of strengths and limitations

Identity versus Role Confusion (12 to 20 Years)
- Accepts body changes/maturation
- Examines attitudes, values, and beliefs; establishes goals for the future
- Feels positive about expanded sense of self

Intimacy versus Isolation (Mid-20s to Mid-40s)
- Has stable, positive feelings about self
- Experiences successful role transitions and increased responsibilities

Generativity versus Self-Absorption (Mid-40s to Mid-60s)
- Able to accept changes in appearance and physical endurance
- Reassesses life goals
- Shows contentment with aging

Ego Integrity versus Despair (Late 60s to Death)
- Feels positive about life and its meaning
- Interested in providing a legacy for the next generation

NURSING KNOWLEDGE BASE

In providing evidence-based practice to patients, incorporate professional nursing knowledge developed from the humanities, sciences, nursing research, and clinical practice. A broad knowledge base allows nurses to have a holistic view of patients, thus promoting quality patient care that best meets the self-concept needs of each patient and family. Understanding a patient's self-concept is a necessary part of all nursing care (Stuart, 2009).

Development of Self-Concept

The development of self-concept is a complex lifelong process that involves many factors. Erikson's psychosocial theory of development (1963) remains beneficial in understanding key tasks that individuals face at various stages of development. Each stage builds on the tasks of the previous stage. Successful mastery of each stage leads to a solid sense of self (Box 33-1).

Learn to recognize an individual's failure to achieve an age-appropriate developmental stage or his or her regression to an earlier stage in a period of crisis. This understanding allows you to individualize care and determine appropriate nursing interventions. Self-concept is always changing and is based on the following:

- Sense of competency
- Perceived reactions of others to one's body
- Ongoing perceptions and interpretations of the thoughts and feelings of others
- Personal and professional relationships
- Academic and employment-related identity
- Personality characteristics that affect self-expectations
- Perceptions of events that have an impact on the self
- Mastery of prior and new experiences
- Ethnic, cultural, racial, and spiritual identity

Self-esteem is usually highest in childhood, declines during adolescence, gradually rises throughout adulthood, and diminishes again in old age (Stuart, 2009). Although this pattern varies, in general it holds true across gender, socioeconomic status, and ethnicity. Children often report high self-esteem because their sense of self is inflated by a variety of extremely positive sources, and the subsequent decline is from time to time associated with a shift to more realistic information about the self.

Erikson's (1963) emphasis on the generativity stage (see Chapter 11) explains the rise in self-esteem and self-concept in adulthood. The individual focuses on being increasingly productive and creative at work, while at the same time promoting and guiding the next generation. Several individuals report a decline in self-esteem in later adulthood (Ebersole et al., 2008). Based on Erikson's stages of development, a decline in self-concept in later adulthood reflects a diminished need for self-promotion and a shift in self-concept to a more modest and balanced view of self. Identifying specific nursing interventions to address the unique needs of patients at various life stages is essential.

BOX 33-2 CULTURAL ASPECTS OF CARE

Promoting Self-Concept and Self-Esteem in Culturally Diverse Patients

Racial and cultural identity is an important component of a person's self-concept and self-esteem. Early in growth and development an individual develops this identity within the context of family. As an individual grows, the cultural aspects of his or her self-concept are reinforced through social, family, or cultural experiences. In addition, a person's self-concept is strengthened or questioned through political, social, or cultural influences experienced in the home, school, and workplace environments. Positive or negative cultural role modeling, ethnic identity, and past experiences influence self-concept.

Implications for Practice

- Develop an open, nonrestrictive attitude for assessing and encouraging cultural practices to improve patients' self-concept.
- Understand that the relationship among self-esteem, stress, and social support can facilitate the development of nursing strategies to promote effective coping in ethnically diverse adolescents (Martyn-Nemeth et al., 2009).
- Ask patients what they think is important to help them feel better or gain a stronger sense of self.
- Encourage cultural identity and ethnic pride by individualizing self-care practices and offering treatment choices to meet patients' self-concept needs.
- Facilitate culturally sensitive health promotion activities that address at-risk behaviors identified through evidence-based practice (e.g., smoking, weight and shape issues, premature sexual experiences, excessive and violent video gaming (Guilamo-Ramos, 2009; Jackson et al., 2009).

Components and Interrelated Terms of Self-Concept

A positive self-concept gives a sense of meaning, wholeness, and consistency to a person. A healthy self-concept has a high degree of stability, which generates positive feelings toward self. The components of self-concept are identity, body image, and role performance. Because how one thinks about oneself (self-concept) affects how one feels about oneself (self-esteem), both concepts need to be evaluated.

Identity. Identity involves the internal sense of individuality, wholeness, and consistency of a person over time and in different situations. It implies being distinct and separate from others. Being "oneself" or living an authentic life is the basis of true identity. Children learn culturally accepted values, behaviors, and roles through identification and modeling. They often gain an identity from self-observations and from what individuals tell them. An individual first identifies with parenting figures and later with other role models such as teachers or peers. To form an identity, the child must be able to bring together learned behaviors and expectations into a coherent, consistent, and unique whole (Erikson, 1963).

The achievement of identity is necessary for intimate relationships because individuals express identity in relationships with others (Stuart, 2009). Sexuality is a part of identity, and its focus differs across the life span. For example, as an adult ages, the focus shifts from procreation to companionship, physical and emotional intimacy, and pleasure-seeking (Ebersole et al., 2008). Gender identity is a person's private view of maleness or femaleness; gender role is the masculine or feminine behavior exhibited. This image and its meaning depend on culturally determined values (see Chapters 9 and 22).

Cultural differences in identity exist (Box 33-2). Racial or cultural identity develops from identification and socialization within an established group and through the experience of integrating the response of individuals outside the cultural or racial group into one's self-concept. Differences in ethnic identity (e.g., Mexican American or Cuban American) exist through identification with traditions, customs, and rituals within one's race/ethnic group (e.g., Hispanic/Latino). In general, the more a person identifies with social groups, the greater his or her self-esteem. In addition, when ethnic identity is central to self-concept and is positive, ethnic pride and self-esteem tend to be high (Guilamo-Ramos, 2009). An individual who experiences discrimination, prejudice, or environmental stressors such as low-income or high-crime neighborhoods often conceptualizes himself or herself differently than an individual who experiences better living conditions.

Body Image. Body image involves attitudes related to the body, including physical appearance, structure, or function. Feelings about body image include those related to sexuality, femininity and masculinity, youthfulness, health, and strength. These mental images are not always consistent with a person's actual physical structure or appearance. Some body image distortions have deep psychological origins, such as the eating disorder anorexia nervosa. Other alterations occur as a result of situational events, such as the loss or change in a body part. Be aware that most men and women experience some degree of dissatisfaction with their bodies, which affects body image and overall self-concept. Individuals often

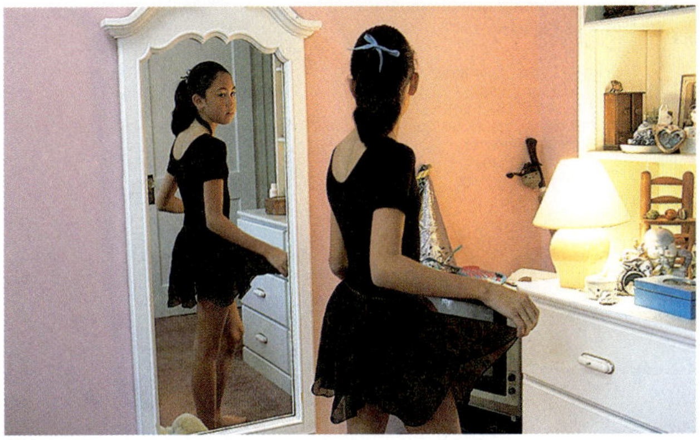

FIG. 33-2 An individual's appearance influences self-concept. (From Sorrentino SA, Remmert LN: *Mosby's textbook for nursing assistants,* ed 8, St Louis, 2012, Mosby.)

exaggerate disturbances in body image when a change in health status occurs. The way others view a person's body and the feedback offered are also influential. For example, a controlling, violent husband tells his wife that she is ugly and that no one else would want her. Over the years of marriage she incorporates this devaluation into her self-concept.

Cognitive growth and physical development also affect body image. Normal developmental changes such as puberty and aging have a more apparent effect on body image than on other aspects of self-concept. Hormonal changes during adolescence and menopause influence body image. The development of secondary sex characteristics and the changes in body fat distribution have a tremendous impact on an adolescent's self-concept. Early maturation is associated with lower psychological well-being and lower enjoyment of physical activity, which in turn could negatively impact body image (Davison et al., 2007). For both male and female adolescents, negative body image is a risk factor for suicidal thoughts (Brausch and Muehlenkamp, 2007). A threat to body image and overall self-concept can affect adherence to recommended health regimens, including diet and taking medications as prescribed (Thomas, 2007). Changes associated with aging (e.g., wrinkles; graying hair; and decrease in visual acuity, hearing, and mobility) also affect body image in an older adult.

Cultural and societal attitudes and values influence body image. Culture and society dictate the accepted norms of body image and influence one's attitudes (Fig. 33-2). Racial and ethnic background plays an integral role in body satisfaction in adolescent girls and is reflected in differences in body satisfaction among groups. Further, body image is more favorable in cultures in which girls describe more reasonable views about physical appearance, report less social pressure for thinness, and have less tendency to base self-esteem on body image. Values such as ideal body weight and shape and attitudes toward piercing and tattoos are culturally based. American society emphasizes youth, beauty, and wholeness. Western cultures have been socialized to dread the normal aging process, whereas eastern cultures view aging very positively and respect older adults. Body image issues are often associated with impaired self-concept and self-esteem.

Role Performance. Role performance is the way in which individuals perceive their ability to carry out significant roles (e.g., parent, supervisor, or close friend). Normal changes associated with maturation result in changes in role performance. For example, when a man has a child, he becomes a father. The new role of father involves many changes in behavior if the man is going to be successful. Group interventions aimed at improving fathering experiences have led to significant improvements in the father's participation in the family, including role performance, involvement, communication, self-esteem, a sense of increased competence, and decreased stress in parenting (Gearing et al., 2008). Roles that individuals follow in given situations involve socialization, expectations, or standards of behavior. The patterns are stable and change only minimally during adulthood.

Ideal societal role behaviors are often hard to achieve in real life. Individuals have multiple roles and personal needs that sometimes conflict. Successful adults learn to distinguish between ideal role expectations and realistic possibilities. To function effectively in multiple roles, a person must know the expected behavior and values, desire to conform to them, and be able to meet the role requirements. Fulfillment of role expectations leads to an enhanced sense of self. Difficulty or failure in meeting role expectations leads to deficits and often contributes to decreased self-esteem or altered self-concept.

Self-Esteem. Self-esteem is an individual's overall feeling of self-worth or the emotional appraisal of self-concept. It is the most fundamental self-evaluation because it represents the overall judgment of personal worth or value. Self-esteem is positive when one feels capable, worthwhile, and competent (Rosenberg, 1965). A person's self-esteem is related to his or her evaluation of his or her effectiveness at school, within the family, and in social settings. The evaluation of others also is likely to have a profound influence on a person's self-esteem. For example, college athletes report greater levels of self-esteem and social connectedness and lower levels of depression than nonathletes. The positive influence of team support can protect college athletes from disturbances of self-esteem and depression symptoms (Armstrong and Oomen-Early, 2009).

Considering the relationship between a person's actual self-concept and his or her ideal self enhances understanding of that person's self-esteem. The ideal self consists of the aspirations, goals, values, and standards of behavior that a person considers ideal and strives to attain. In general, a person whose self-concept comes close to matching the ideal self has high self-esteem, whereas a person whose self-concept varies widely from the ideal self suffers from low self-esteem (Stuart, 2009). Once established, basic feelings about the self tend to be constant, even though a situational crisis can temporarily affect self-esteem.

Factors Influencing Self-Concept

A self-concept stressor is any real or perceived change that threatens identity, body image, or role performance (Fig. 33-3). An individual's perception of the stressor is the most important factor in determining his or her response. The ability to reestablish balance following a stressor is related to numerous factors, including the number of stressors, duration of the stressor, and health status (see Chapter 37). Stressors challenge a person's adaptive capacities. Changes that occur in physical, spiritual, emotional, sexual, familial, and sociocultural health affect self-concept. Being able to adapt to stressors is likely to lead to a positive sense of self, whereas failure to adapt often leads to a negative self-concept.

Any change in health is a stressor that potentially affects self-concept. A physical change in the body sometimes leads to an altered body image, affecting identity and self-esteem. Chronic illnesses often alter role performance, which change an individual's identity and self-esteem. Further, an essential process in the adjustment to loss is the development of a new self-concept. A loss of a partner can lead to a loss of identity and a lower self-esteem. Unlike

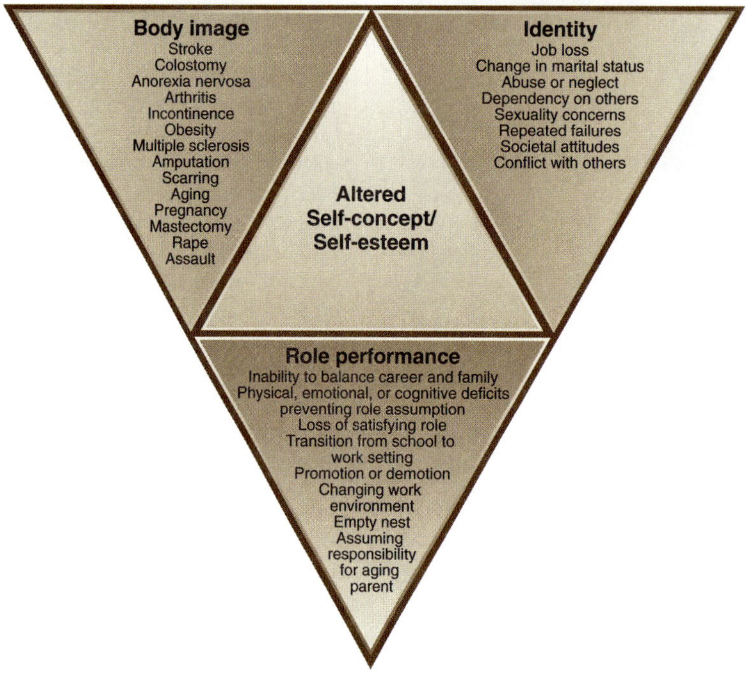

FIG. 33-3 Common stressors that influence self-concept.

the loss in self-esteem shown in vulnerable older adults, the resiliency demonstrated in some older adults may reflect more sophisticated cognitive strategies to manage losses.

The stressors created as a result of a crisis also affect a person's health. If the resulting identity confusion, disturbed body image, low self-esteem, or role conflict is not relieved, illness can result. For example, the diagnosis of cancer places additional demands on a person's established living pattern. It changes his or her appraisal of and satisfaction with the current level of physical, emotional, and social functioning. In this case assess self-esteem, effectiveness of coping strategies, and social support. During self-concept crises, supportive and educative resources are valuable in helping a person learn new ways of coping with and responding to the stressful event or situation to maintain or enhance self-concept.

Identity Stressors. Stressors affect an individual's identity throughout life, but individuals are particularly vulnerable during adolescence. Adolescents are trying to adjust to the physical, emotional, and mental changes of increasing maturity, which results in insecurity and anxiety. It is also a time when the adolescent is developing psychosocial competence, including coping strategies (see Chapter 37).

An adult generally has a more stable identity and thus a more firmly developed self-concept than an adolescent. Cultural and social stressors rather than personal stressors have more impact on an adult's identity. For example, an adult has to balance career and family or make choices regarding honoring religious traditions from one's family of origin. **Identity confusion** results when people do not maintain a clear, consistent, and continuous consciousness of personal identity. It occurs at any stage of life if a person is unable to adapt to identity stressors.

Body Image Stressors. A change in the appearance, structure, or function of a body part requires an adjustment in body image. An individual's perception of the change and the relative importance placed on body image affects the significance of a loss of function or change in appearance. For example, if a woman's body image incorporates reproductive organs as the ideal, a hysterectomy needed because of a diagnosis of uterine cancer is a significant alteration and can result in a perceived loss of femininity or wholeness. Changes in the appearance of the body such as an amputation, facial disfigurement, or scars from burns are obvious stressors affecting body image. Mastectomy and colostomy are surgical procedures that alter the appearance and function of the body, yet the changes are not apparent to others when the individual is dressed. Although potentially undetected by others, these bodily changes significantly impact the individual. Even some elective changes such as breast augmentation or reduction affect body image. Chronic illnesses such as heart and renal disease affect body image because the body no longer functions at an optimal level. The patient has to adjust to a decrease in activity tolerance that impacts his or her ability to perform normal activities of daily living. In addition, pregnancy, significant weight gain or loss, pharmacological management of illness, or radiation therapy changes body image. Negative body image often leads to adverse health outcomes.

The response of society to physical changes in an individual often depends on the conditions surrounding the alteration. Some social changes have allowed the public to respond more favorably to illness and altered body image. For example, the media frequently presents positive stories about persons adjusting in a healthy manner following serious disabilities (e.g., Christopher Reeve's spinal cord injury) or adapting to a debilitating illness (e.g., Michael J. Fox's Parkinson's disease). These stories change public awareness and the perception of what constitutes a disability and provide positive role models for individuals undergoing self-concept stressors and their families, friends, and society as a whole. In view of the growing epidemic of obesity in western cultures, parents and health care providers need to address weight management issues without causing further injury to body image. Providing a social environment that focuses on health and fitness rather than a drive for thinness for girls or muscularity for boys can potentially increase adolescent satisfaction with their bodies (Brunet et al., 2010).

Role Performance Stressors. Throughout life a person undergoes numerous role changes. Situational transitions occur when parents, spouses, children, or close friends die or people move, marry, divorce, or change jobs. It is important to recognize that a shift along the continuum from illness to wellness is as stressful as a shift from wellness to illness. Any of these transitions may lead to role conflict, role ambiguity, role strain, or role overload.

Role conflict results when a person has to simultaneously assume two or more roles that are inconsistent, contradictory, or mutually exclusive. For example, when a middle-age woman with teenage children assumes responsibility for the care of her older parents, conflicts occur in relation to being both a parent to her children and the child of her parents. Negotiating a balance of time and energy between her children and parents creates role conflicts. The perceived importance of each conflicting role influences the degree of conflict experienced. The **sick role** involves the expectations of others and society regarding how an individual behaves when sick. Role conflict occurs when general societal expectations (take care of yourself, and you will get better) and the expectations of co-workers (need to get the job done) collide. The conflict of taking care of oneself while getting everything done is often a major challenge.

Role ambiguity involves unclear role expectations, which makes people unsure about what to do or how to do it, creating stress and confusion. Role ambiguity is common in the adolescent years. Parents, peers, and the media pressure adolescents to assume adultlike roles, yet many lack the resources to move beyond the role of a dependent child. Role ambiguity is also common in employment situations. In complex, rapidly changing, or highly specialized organizations, employees often become unsure about job expectations.

Role strain combines role conflict and role ambiguity. Some express role strain as a feeling of frustration when a person feels inadequate or unsuited to a role such as providing care for a family member with Alzheimer's disease.

Role overload involves having more roles or responsibilities within a role than are manageable. This is common in an individual who unsuccessfully attempts to meet the demands of work and family while carving out some personal time. Often during periods of illness or change, those involved either as the one who is ill or as a significant other find themselves in role overload.

Self-Esteem Stressors. Individuals with high self-esteem are generally more resilient and better able to cope with demands and stressors than those with low self-esteem. Low self-worth contributes to feeling unfulfilled and disconnected from others. Decreased self-worth can potentially result in depression and unremitting uneasiness or anxiety. Illness, surgery, or accidents that change life patterns also influence feelings of self-worth. Chronic illnesses such as diabetes, arthritis, and cardiac dysfunction require changes in accepted and long-assumed behavioral patterns. The more the chronic illness interferes with the ability to engage in activities contributing to feelings of worth or success, the more it affects self-esteem.

Self-esteem stressors vary with developmental stages. Perceived inability to meet parental expectations, harsh criticism, inconsistent discipline, and unresolved sibling rivalry reduce the level of self-worth of children. A developmental milestone such as pregnancy introduces unique self-concept stressors and has significant health care implications. For some economically disadvantaged youth, safe sex behaviors are not always valued, and pregnancy is an affirmation of ethnic identity. Low self-esteem during adolescence also has significant real-world consequences in adulthood, including poor health, criminal behavior, and limited economic prospects compared to adolescents with high self-esteem. Self-esteem and health behaviors are intertwined. Stressors affecting the self-esteem of an adult include failure in work and unsuccessful relationships. Self-concept stressors in older adults include health problems, declining socioeconomic status, spousal loss or bereavement, loss of social support, and decline in achievement experiences following retirement (Box 33-3).

BOX 33-3 FOCUS ON OLDER ADULTS

Enhancing Self-Concept in Older Adults

Self-concept is sometimes negatively affected in older adulthood because of a number of life changes. However, in some individuals, aging promotes improved coping strategies that protect against the declining feelings of self-esteem, despite the physical and emotional changes associated with aging (Ebersole et al., 2008). Gender differences in the last decades of life exist as men become more negative about appearance and function of their bodies than do women (Kaminski and Hayslip, 2006). Nursing interventions aimed at enhancing self-concept and self-esteem in older adults is essential, particularly during illness, injury, or disability.

Implications for Practice

- Clarify what the life changes mean and the effect on self-concept. Discuss health problems, declining socioeconomic status, spousal loss or bereavement, and loss of social support following retirement.
- Conduct supportive conversations to understand challenges to the patient's perceptions of body image adjustments as part of aging and changes associated with illness, injury, or disability (Price, 2010).
- Be alert to preoccupation with physical complaints. Assess complaints thoroughly and, if no physical explanation exists, encourage older adult to verbalize needs (fear, insecurity, loneliness) in a nonphysical way (Stuart, 2009).
- Identify positive and negative coping mechanisms. Support effective strategies.
- Encourage the use of storytelling and review of old photographs.
- Communicate that the older adult is worthwhile by actively listening to and accepting the person's feelings, being respectful, and praising healthy behaviors.
- Allow additional time to complete tasks. Reinforce the older adult's efforts at independence (Ebersole et al., 2008).

Building Competency in Safety You are caring for Paul Taylor, a 69-year-old man, who suffered a debilitating stroke. The stroke was unexpected and sudden. Mr. Taylor did not know that he had hypertension because he had not been getting annual checkups. His body image has dramatically changed from that of a man of strength to that of a helpless individual. Mr. Taylor worries about being a burden to his family. He and his wife, Meredith, are terrified. His self-concept has changed from that of a strong laborer, one who did his own plumbing and car repairs, to a man who must completely rely on others. Mr. Taylor's identity is not clear to him anymore. He has no clear role within the family, his body image has been drastically altered, his sexual health has suffered, and his self-esteem has never been lower. He says, "My family would be better off if I were dead." What is your priority nursing intervention to ensure Mr. Taylor's safety?

Answers to questions can be found on the Evolve website.

Family Effect on Self-Concept Development

The family plays a key role in creating and maintaining the self-concepts of its members. Children develop a basic sense of who they are from their family caregivers. A child also gains accepted norms for thinking, feeling, and behaving from family members. Sometimes well-meaning parents cultivate negative self-concepts in children. Some literature suggests that parents are the most important influences on a child's development, yet variations in parenting approach depend on the culture. Specifically a child's positive self-esteem and school achievement are fostered by parents who respond in a firm, consistent, and warm manner. High parental support and parental monitoring are related to greater self-esteem and lower risk behaviors. For example, in Mexican American adolescents perceived parental educational involvement combined with their perceived acculturation and self-esteem significantly affect their aspirations and achievement (Carranza et al., 2009). Parents who are harsh, inconsistent, or have low self-esteem themselves often behave in ways that foster negative self-concepts in their children. Positive communication and social support foster self-esteem and well-being in adolescence. To reverse a patient's negative self-concept, first assess the family's style of relating (see Chapter 10). Family and cultural factors sometimes influence negative health practices such as cigarette smoking (Box 33-4). Self-concept change demands an evidence-based practice approach supported by the entire health care team.

Nurse's Effect on Patient's Self-Concept

A nurse's acceptance of a patient with an altered self-concept promotes positive change. Often this simply involves sitting with a patient and forming a therapeutic relationship. When a patient's physical appearance has changed, it is likely that both the patient and the family look to nurses and observe their verbal and nonverbal responses and reactions to the changed appearance. You need to remain aware of your own feelings, ideas, values, expectations, and judgments. Self-awareness is critical in understanding and accepting others. Nurses need to assess and clarify the following self-concept issues about themselves:

- Thoughts and feelings about lifestyle, health, and illness
- Awareness of how their own nonverbal communication affects patients and families
- Personal values and expectations and how these affect patients
- Ability to convey a nonjudgmental attitude toward patients
- Preconceived attitudes toward cultural differences in self-concept and self-esteem

Some patients with a change in body appearance or function are extremely sensitive to the verbal and nonverbal responses of the health care team. A positive, matter-of-fact approach to care provides a model for the patient and family to follow. For example, when you observe a positive change in a patient's behavior, note it and allow the patient to establish its meaning. Nurses have a significant effect on patients by conveying genuine interest and acceptance. Including self-concept issues in the planning and delivery of care can positively influence patient outcomes. Building a trusting nurse-patient relationship that incorporates both the patient and family in the decision-making process enhances self-concept. Nurses individualize their approach by highlighting a patient's unique needs and incorporating alternative health care practices or methods of spiritual expression into the plan of care. It is important that health care providers understand the degree to which self-esteem and sexuality affect patient outcomes (Figueroa-Hass, 2007).

BOX 33-4 EVIDENCE-BASED PRACTICE

Self-Concept and the Impact of Body Image, Self-Esteem, and Stress on Adolescent Smoking Behaviors

PICO Question: How does self-concept influence smoking behaviors in adolescents?

Evidence Summary

The prevalence of tobacco use in the United States is highest between ages 18 and 24 (24%), with college students representing the highest portion of smokers (CDC, 2006). In 2009, 19% of high school students reported current cigarette use, while 9% of high school students reported current smokeless tobacco use (CDC, 2010). The prevalence of current cigarette use was higher among ninth-grade female than same-grade male students and higher among 12th-grade male than same-grade female students. Overall the prevalence of current cigarette use in both males and females was higher among white, followed by Hispanic, and then black students. Previous studies have shown that weight concerns, especially in women, motivate users to continue smoking and predict smoking relapse. Smokers were more likely to perceive higher amounts of stress and lower self-esteem (Croghan et al., 2006; Nelson and Gordon-Larsen, 2006). The majority of smokers, regardless of gender, consider tobacco use to be an important stress-management practice. Identifying risk and protective factors is important for smoking prevention programs (Greene and Banerjee, 2008). Enhancing opportunities to learn communication skills and engage in alternative behaviors, including physical activity, may reduce smoking as an adolescent risk behavior (Croghan et al., 2006; Nelson and Gordon-Larsen, 2006).

Application to Nursing Practice

- Smoking cessation efforts should include stress management and self-esteem and body image improvement (Croghan et al., 2006).
- A priority nursing action is the assessment of child and adolescent coping strategies. Appropriate techniques include effective communication, conflict resolution, and stress.
- Families, peers, teachers, and health care providers should instill students' ethnic pride, which promotes self-concept and the use of protective factors against risk behaviors, such as smoking (Guilamo-Ramos, 2009).
- Body-weight concerns and family, social environment, and behavioral factors are important issues to address during preadolescence and adolescence.
- Implement effective, healthy, and realistic weight management methods for adolescents. Techniques include promoting fun, family-oriented activities such as television viewing and gaming and eliminating dieting (Nelson and Gordon-Larsen, 2006).
- Identifying risk factors for early drug and alcohol use, including genetic predisposition, family environment, ethnic identity, and sedentary behaviors needs to be a priority for health care providers (Croghan et al., 2006; Guilamo-Ramos, 2009).

Your nursing care significantly affects a patient's body image. For example, the body image of a woman following a mastectomy is positively influenced by a nurse showing acceptance of the mastectomy scar. On the other hand, a nurse who has a shocked or disgusted facial expression contributes to the woman developing a negative body image. Patients closely watch the reactions of others to their wounds and scars, and it is very important to be aware of your responses toward the patient. Statements such as "This wound is healing nicely" or "This tissue looks healthy" are affirmations for the body image of the patient. Nonverbal behaviors convey the level of caring that exists for a patient and affect self-esteem. Anticipate personal reactions, acknowledge them, and focus on the patient instead of the unpleasant task or situation. Nurses who put themselves in the patient's situation incorporate measures to ease embarrassment, frustration, anger, and denial.

Preventive measures, early identification, and appropriate treatment minimize the intensity of self-esteem stressors and the potential effects for a patient and his or her family. Learn to design specific self-concept interventions to fit a patient's profile of risk factors. It is essential to assess a patient's perception of a problem and work collaboratively to resolve self-concept issues. For example, incorporating self-esteem activities into regular school health and physical education curriculum can result in a positive change in students' physical self-esteem and family self-esteem (Lai et al., 2009). Interventions designed to promote active living and healthy eating may be beneficial for preventing childhood obesity, improving self-esteem, preventing chronic diseases, and improving mental health in adulthood (Wang et al., 2009).

Building Competency in Patient-Centered Care You are a third-year nursing student who feels insecure in the clinical setting. You hope that your clinical instructor won't ask you questions about your patient because you "forget" everything when your assigned faculty approaches; you feel embarrassed that you sometimes "hide" or "look busy" to avoid interacting with your instructor. You wonder, "How can I attend to my patient's self-concept and self-esteem issues when I can't even deal with my own?" What actions must you take to improve your self-esteem and self-concept as a student nurse?

Answers to questions can be found on the Evolve website.

CRITICAL THINKING

Successful critical thinking requires synthesis of knowledge, experience, information gathered from patients and families, critical thinking attitudes, and ethical and professional standards. Solid clinical judgment requires anticipating and securing the necessary information, analyzing the data, and making appropriate decisions regarding patient care.

In the case of self-concept, it is essential to integrate knowledge from nursing and other disciplines, including self-concept theory, communication principles, and a consideration of cultural and developmental factors. Previous experience in caring for patients with self-concept alterations helps to individualize care. Self-concept profoundly influences a person's response to illness. A critical thinking approach to care is essential.

NURSING PROCESS

Apply the nursing process and use a critical thinking approach in your care of patients. The nursing process provides a clinical decision-making approach for you to develop and implement an individualized plan of care. The nursing process is continuous until the patient's self-concept is improved, restored, or maintained.

ASSESSMENT

During the assessment process, thoroughly assess each patient and critically analyze findings to ensure that you make patient-centered clinical decisions required for safe nursing care. In assessing self-concept and self-esteem, first focus on each component of self-concept (identity, body image, and role performance). Assessment needs to include looking for the range of behaviors suggestive of an altered self-concept or self-esteem (Box 33-5), actual and potential self-concept stressors (see Fig. 33-3), and coping patterns. Gathering comprehensive assessment data requires the critical synthesis of information from multiple sources (Fig. 33-4). In addition to direct questioning (Box 33-6), nurses gather much of the data regarding self-concept through observation of the patient's nonverbal behavior and by paying attention to the content of the patient's conversations. Take note of the manner in which patients talk about the people in their lives because this provides clues to both stressful and supportive relationships and key roles the patient assumes. Using knowledge of developmental stages to determine which areas are likely to be important to the patient, inquire about these aspects of the person's life. For example, ask a 70-year-old patient about his life and what has been important to him. The individual's conversation likely provides data relating to role performance, identity, self-esteem, stressors, and coping patterns.

Through the Patient's Eyes. An important factor in assessing self-concept is the person's viewpoint of his or her health condition and its influence on self-concept. Give patients the opportunity to tell their stories of how they perceive their illness or condition affecting their identity, their image of themselves, and their ability to lead a normal lifestyle. Also assess patients' expectations of health care by asking them how interventions will make a difference. This is also an opportunity to discuss the patient's goals. For example, a nurse working with a patient who is experiencing anxiety related to an upcoming diagnostic study asks the patient

BOX 33-5 BEHAVIORS SUGGESTIVE OF ALTERED SELF-CONCEPT

- Avoidance of eye contact
- Slumped posture
- Unkempt appearance
- Overly apologetic
- Hesitant speech
- Overly critical or angry
- Frequent or inappropriate crying
- Negative self-evaluation
- Excessively dependent
- Hesitant to express views or opinions
- Lack of interest in what is happening
- Passive attitude
- Difficulty in making decisions

BOX 33-6 NURSING ASSESSMENT QUESTIONS

Nature of the Problem
- How would you describe yourself?
- What aspects of your appearance do you like?
- Tell me about the things you do that make you feel good about yourself.
- Tell me about your primary roles. How effective are you at carrying out each of these roles?

Onset and Duration
- When did you start to think or feel differently about yourself?
- How long have you struggled with _____ (specify identity, body image, role performance, or self-esteem)?
- Can you remember a time when you felt good about yourself?

Effect on Patient
- Tell me how your self-concept affects your ability to take care of yourself.
- What impact does your self-esteem have on relationships?
- How does your self-esteem affect other areas of your life?

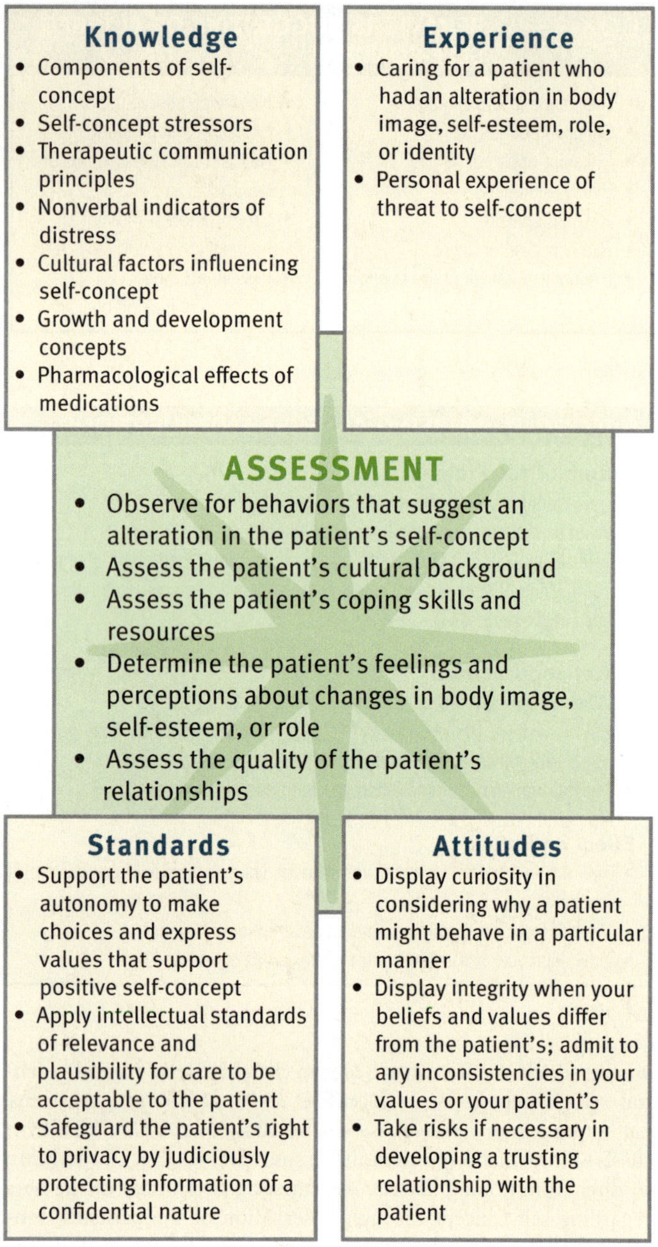
Knowledge
• Components of self-concept
• Self-concept stressors
• Therapeutic communication principles
• Nonverbal indicators of distress
• Cultural factors influencing self-concept
• Growth and development concepts
• Pharmacological effects of medications
Experience
• Caring for a patient who had an alteration in body image, self-esteem, role, or identity
• Personal experience of threat to self-concept
ASSESSMENT
• Observe for behaviors that suggest an alteration in the patient's self-concept
• Assess the patient's cultural background
• Assess the patient's coping skills and resources
• Determine the patient's feelings and perceptions about changes in body image, self-esteem, or role
• Assess the quality of the patient's relationships
Standards
• Support the patient's autonomy to make choices and express values that support positive self-concept
• Apply intellectual standards of relevance and plausibility for care to be acceptable to the patient
• Safeguard the patient's right to privacy by judiciously protecting information of a confidential nature
Attitudes
• Display curiosity in considering why a patient might behave in a particular manner
• Display integrity when your beliefs and values differ from the patient's; admit to any inconsistencies in your values or your patient's
• Take risks if necessary in developing a trusting relationship with the patient

FIG. 33-4 Critical thinking model for self-concept assessment.

about his expectations of the relaxation exercise that they have been practicing together. The patient's response gives the nurse valuable information about the patient's beliefs and attitudes regarding the efficacy of the interventions and the potential need to modify the nursing approach.

Coping Behaviors. The nursing assessment also includes consideration of previous coping behaviors; the nature, number, and intensity of the stressors; and the patient's internal and external resources. Knowledge of how a patient has dealt with stressors in the past provides insight into his or her style of coping. Patients do not address all issues in the same way, but they often use a familiar coping pattern for newly encountered stressors. Identify previous coping strategies to determine whether these patterns have contributed to healthy functioning or created more problems. For example, the use of drugs or alcohol during times of stress often creates additional stressors (see Chapter 37).

BOX 33-7 NURSING DIAGNOSTIC PROCESS

Situational Low Self-Esteem

ASSESSMENT ACTIVITIES	DEFINING CHARACTERISTICS
Ask patient to explain thoughts and feelings about self.	Patient is tearful and reports negative thoughts about self. She reports not wanting to have any visitors.
Observe patient's behavior and ask family if she is experiencing emotional or behavior changes.	Spouse describes withdrawal and avoidance of intimacy. Spouse states that wife is unable to make decisions.
Determine if patient has had issues with self-esteem in the past and her plans to improve her self-esteem.	Patient denies any self-esteem issues since adolescence. She describes a willingness to bring her husband to a counselor to discuss ways that he can support her return to high self-esteem.

Significant Others. Exploring resources and strengths such as availability of significant others or prior use of community resources is important in formulating a realistic and effective plan of care. Valuable information comes from conversations with family and significant others. Significant others sometimes have insights into the person's way of dealing with stressors. They also have knowledge about what is important to the person's self-concept. The way in which a significant other talks about the patient and the significant other's nonverbal behaviors provide information about what kind of support is available for the patient.

NURSING DIAGNOSIS

Carefully consider the assessment data to identify a patient's actual or potential problem areas. Rely on knowledge and experience, apply appropriate professional standards, and look for clusters of defining characteristics that indicate a nursing diagnosis. Although there are four nursing diagnostic labels for altered self-concept, the following list (NANDA International, 2009) also provides examples of self-concept–related nursing diagnoses:

- Disturbed body image
- Caregiver role strain
- Disturbed personal identity
- Ineffective role performance
- Readiness for enhanced self-concept
- Chronic low self-esteem
- Situational low self-esteem
- Risk for situational low self-esteem

Making nursing diagnoses about self-concept is complex. Often isolated data are defining characteristics for more than one nursing diagnosis (Box 33-7). For example, a patient expresses feelings of uncertainty and inadequacy. These are defining characteristics for both *anxiety* and *situational low self-esteem.* Realizing that the patient is demonstrating defining characteristics of more than one nursing diagnosis guides you to gather specific data to validate and differentiate the underlying problem. To further assess the possibility of *anxiety* as the nursing diagnosis, consider whether the person has any of the following defining characteristics: Is the person experiencing increased muscle tension, shakiness, a sense of being "rattled," or restlessness? These symptoms suggest *anxiety* as the more appropriate diagnosis. On the other hand, if the person expresses a predominantly negative self-appraisal, including inability to handle situations or events and difficulty making decisions, these characteristics suggest that *situational low self-esteem* is more appropriate. To further aid in differentiating between the two demonstrated diagnoses, information regarding recent events in the person's life and how the person has viewed himself or herself in the past provide insight into the most appropriate nursing diagnosis. As you gather additional data, usually the priority nursing diagnosis becomes evident.

To validate critical thinking regarding a nursing diagnosis, share observations with the patient and allow him or her to verify perceptions. This approach often results in the patient providing additional data, which further clarifies the situation. For example, "I noticed that you jumped when I touched your arm. Are you feeling uneasy today?" allows the patient to verify whether he or she is in fact anxious and describe his or her concerns.

PLANNING

During planning synthesize knowledge, experience, critical thinking attitudes, and standards (Fig. 33-5). Critical thinking ensures that a patient's plan of care integrates information known about the individual and key critical thinking elements (see the Nursing Care Plan). Professional standards are especially important to consider when developing a plan of care. These standards often establish ethical or evidence-based practice guidelines for selecting effective nursing interventions.

Another method to assist in planning care is a concept map. An example of an illustrative concept map (Fig. 33-6) shows the relationship of a primary health problem (postoperative bilateral radical mastectomy) and four nursing diagnoses and several interventions. The concept map shows how the nursing diagnoses are interrelated. It also assists in showing the interrelationships among nursing interventions. A single nursing intervention can be effective for more than one diagnosis.

Goals and Outcomes. Develop an individualized plan of care for each nursing diagnosis. Work collaboratively with the patient to set realistic expectations for care. Make sure that goals are individualized and realistic with measurable outcomes. In establishing goals, consult with the patient about whether they are achievable. Consultation with significant others, mental health clinicians, and community resources results in a more comprehensive and workable plan. When you set goals, consider the data necessary to demonstrate that the patient's problem would change if the nursing diagnosis were managed. The outcome criteria should reflect these changes. For example, a patient is diagnosed with *situational low self-esteem related to a recent job layoff.* Establish a goal: "Patient's self-esteem and self-concept will improve in 1 week." Examples of expected outcomes directed toward that goal include the following:

- The patient will discuss a minimum of three areas of her life where she is functioning well.
- The patient will be able to voice the recognition that losing her job is not reflective of her worth as a person.
- The patient will attend a support group for out-of-work professionals.

Setting Priorities. The care plan presents the goals, expected outcomes, and interventions for a patient with an alteration in self-concept. Interventions help the patient adapt to the stressors that led to the self-concept disturbance and support and reinforce the development of coping methods. Often a patient perceives a situation as overwhelming and feels hopeless about returning to the level of previous functioning. The patient often needs time to adapt to physical changes but can work toward progressive improvement in self-concept and self-esteem.

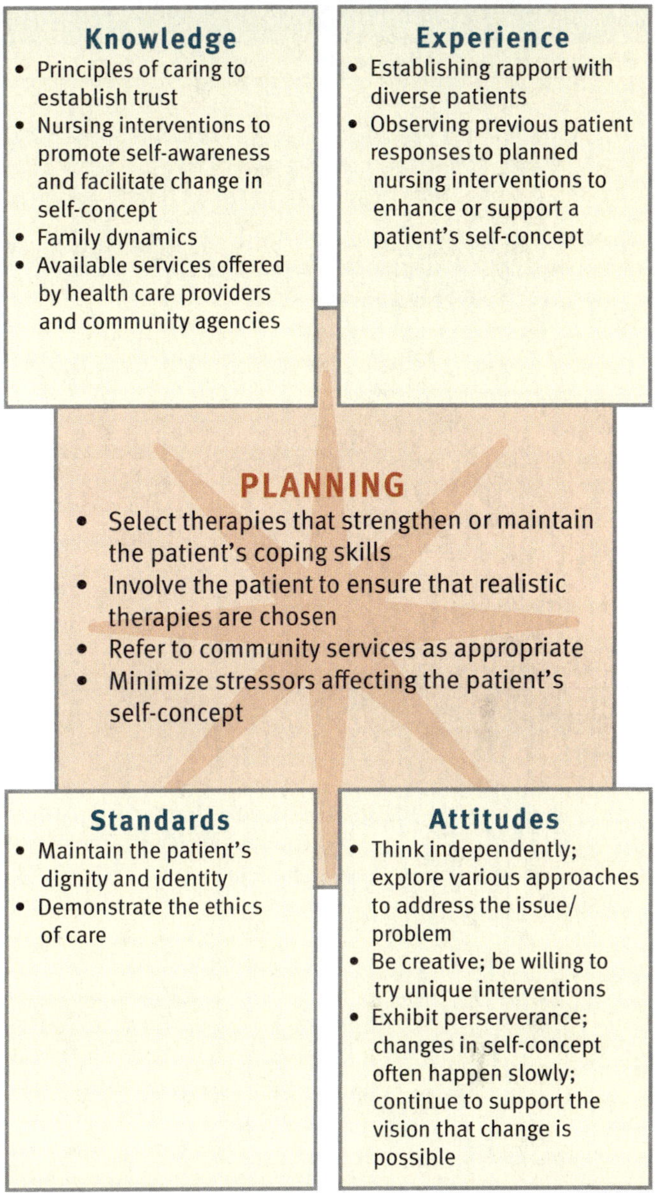
Knowledge
• Principles of caring to establish trust
• Nursing interventions to promote self-awareness and facilitate change in self-concept
• Family dynamics
• Available services offered by health care providers and community agencies
Experience
• Establishing rapport with diverse patients
• Observing previous patient responses to planned nursing interventions to enhance or support a patient's self-concept
PLANNING
• Select therapies that strengthen or maintain the patient's coping skills
• Involve the patient to ensure that realistic therapies are chosen
• Refer to community services as appropriate
• Minimize stressors affecting the patient's self-concept
Standards
• Maintain the patient's dignity and identity
• Demonstrate the ethics of care
Attitudes
• Think independently; explore various approaches to address the issue/problem
• Be creative; be willing to try unique interventions
• Exhibit perserverance; changes in self-concept often happen slowly; continue to support the vision that change is possible

FIG. 33-5 Critical thinking model for self-concept planning.

Establishing priorities includes using therapeutic communication to address self-concept issues, which ensures that the patient's ability to address physical needs is maximized. Look for strengths in both the individual and the family and provide resources and education to turn limitations into strengths. Patient teaching creates understanding of the normalcy of certain situations (e.g., nature of a chronic disease, change in relationships, or effect of a loss). Often, once patients understand their situations, their sense of hopelessness and helplessness is lessened.

Teamwork and Collaboration. A patient's perceptions of significant others are important to incorporate into the plan of care. Individuals who have experienced deficits in self-concept before the current episode of treatment have often established a system of support that includes mental health clinicians, clergy, and other community resources. Before including family members,

NURSING CARE PLAN

Situational Low Self-Esteem

ASSESSMENT

Mrs. Johnson, a 45-year-old married woman who had a bilateral radical mastectomy resulting from malignant breast cancer, has been assigned to Susan Carr, nursing student. Susan completed Mrs. Johnson's physical assessment. She has been adequately medicated for pain. Ms. Carr sits down to discuss how the mastectomy has affected Mrs. Johnson's self-concept and self-esteem.

Assessment Activities	*Findings/Defining Characteristics**
Assess identity concerns (e.g., sexual role, femininity). Ask how the loss of breasts has affected her sense of self.	Mrs. Johnson **looks away, shakes her head,** and states, **"I feel like less of a woman.** My husband says I'm still attractive, but I don't believe him."
Observe Mrs. Johnson's mood and affect and her nonverbal communication and interactions with others.	Mrs. Johnson demonstrates **intermittent eye contact, frequent crying when alone, pulling hospital gown tightly across chest,** and **superficial conversations** with family members.
Assess Mrs. Johnson's involvement in self-care activities.	Mrs. Johnson is **unable to decide when to bathe, comb hair, or apply typical makeup.** Avoids looking in a mirror.
Offer opportunities to participate in treatment and provide supportive-educative nursing care.	**Mrs. Johnson avoids** looking at or touching her chest and **does not ask questions** about her condition.

***Defining characteristics** are shown in bold type.

NURSING DIAGNOSIS: Situational low self-esteem related to negative view of self

PLANNING

Goals	*Expected Outcomes (NOC)†*
	Self-Esteem
Mrs. Johnson's perceived self-concept will improve in 1 week	Mrs. Johnson will verbalize feelings of self-acceptance and self-worth within 4 days.
Mrs. Johnson will regain sense of her ability to achieve role performance before discharge.	Mrs. Johnson will demonstrate maintenance of basic grooming and hygiene needs within 2 days.
	Role Performance
	Mrs. Johnson will describe role changes associated with mastectomy and will verbalize commitment to accessing community resources by day of discharge.
	Body Image
	Mrs. Johnson will demonstrate adjustment to changes in body appearance within 1 week.

†Outcome classification labels from Moorhead S et al: *Nursing outcomes classification (NOC),* ed 4, St Louis, 2008, Mosby.

INTERVENTIONS (NIC)‡	RATIONALE
Self-Esteem Enhancement	
Use communication techniques to facilitate an environment and activities that will increase self-esteem.	A therapeutic nurse-patient relationship promotes positive patient outcome, including the patient's assuming responsibility for her own care (Stuart, 2009).
Monitor Mrs. Johnson's statements of self-worth.	Self-esteem and body image are strong predictors of depression (MacPhee and Andrews, 2006). The nurse must assess thoughts and feelings, including depression and risk for suicide, to ensure the patient's safety and make appropriate referrals (Folse and Hahn, 2009).
Encourage increased responsibility for self and assist patient with accepting dependence on others, as appropriate.	Promoting self-care enhances self-concept, including improving role performance (Stuart, 2009).
Role Enhancement	
Assist Mrs. Johnson with identifying specific role changes brought on by mastectomy.	Only after the problem is accurately defined can alternative choices be proposed (Stuart, 2009).
Body Image Enhancement	A threat to body image and overall self-concept often influences adherence to recommended health regimens (Thomas, 2007).

‡Intervention classification labels from Bulechek GM, Butcher HK, and Dochterman JM: *Nursing interventions classification (NIC),* ed 5, St Louis, 2008, Mosby.

NURSING CARE PLAN

***Situational Low Self-Esteem*—cont'd**

EVALUATION

Nursing Actions	*Patient Response/Finding*	*Achievement of Outcome*
Ask Mrs. Johnson how effective she feels in her ability to identify and express feelings verbally and nonverbally.	Mrs. Johnson reports, "I've been able to talk with my husband, even about my concerns that he won't find me attractive anymore."	Improved verbal and nonverbal communication noted
Monitor changes in Mrs. Johnson's statements about herself.	Mrs. Johnson is making fewer negative comments and is evaluating body image more realistically but remains dissatisfied with appearance.	Small improvement in self-esteem; body image more realistic, but remains negative Discusses body image with husband and nursing student
Observe Mrs. Johnson's participation in self-care related to mastectomy.	Mrs. Johnson is more assertive in completing basic hygiene; has used a mirror to examine mastectomy scar.	Meeting self-care needs
Ask Mrs. Johnson to identify resources outside the hospital.	Mrs. Johnson has expressed interest in attending local breast cancer survivors' support group.	Scheduled to attend mastectomy support group 2 days after scheduled discharge

CONCEPT MAP

Nursing diagnosis: Disturbed body image
- Does not touch her chest
- Unable to look in mirror
- Avoids new social interactions
- Fears husband's response to loss of breasts

Interventions
- Assist patient to develop a realistic perception of her body image
- Tell patient that her feelings are similar to feelings of other people in the same situation
- Show acceptance of mastectomy when providing care

Nursing diagnosis: Acute pain
- Rates postoperative pain as a 9 on a scale of 0 to 10
- States "no relief from pain" with PCA
- Has poor sleeping patterns
- Has a lack of appetite
- Has decreased nutritional intake

Interventions
- Ask patient to describe past methods used to control pain
- Explore the need for opioid and nonnarcotic analgesics
- Discuss patient's fears of undertreated pain and addiction

Primary health problem: Postoperative bilateral radical mastectomy
Priority assessments: Self-esteem, effects of scars on body image, pain level, and feelings of fear and anxiety

Nursing diagnosis: Situational low self-esteem
- States she is unable to "cope"
- Has difficulty making decisions
- Has feelings of uselessness

Interventions
- Assess patient for signs and symptoms of depression and potential for suicide
- Actively listen to and demonstrate respect for patient
- Ask patient to identify personal strengths and talents

Nursing diagnosis: Fear
- Has decreased self-confidence
- Reports being unable to solve personal problems
- Panics when people ask about the cancer
- Experiences daily fatigue
- Worries that reconstruction "won't work"

Interventions
- Help patient distinguish between real and imagined threats
- Encourage patient to write about fears in a journal
- Explore feelings that contribute to fear

——— Link between medical diagnosis and nursing diagnosis
- - - - - Link between nursing diagnoses

FIG. 33-6 Concept map for Mrs. Johnson. *PCA,* Patient-controlled analgesia.

consider the patient's desires for their involvement and cultural norms regarding who most frequently makes decisions in the family. Patients who are experiencing threats to or alterations in self-concept often benefit from collaboration with mental health and community resources to promote increased awareness. Additional resources include physical therapy, occupational therapy, behavioral health, social services, and pastoral care. Knowledge of available resources allows appropriate referrals.

IMPLEMENTATION

As with all the steps of the nursing process, a therapeutic nurse-patient relationship is central to the implementation phase. You develop the goals and outcome criteria and then consider nursing interventions for promoting a healthy self-concept and helping the patient move toward his or her goals. To develop effective nursing interventions, consider each nursing diagnosis and individualize interventions that address the diagnosis. Collaborating with members of the health care team maximizes the comprehensiveness of the approach to self-concept issues. Regardless of the health care setting, it is important to work with patients and their families or significant others to promote a healthy self-concept. For example, select nursing interventions that help patients regain or restore the elements that contribute to a strong and secure sense of self. The approaches chosen vary according to the level of care required.

Health Promotion. Work with patients to help them develop healthy lifestyle behaviors that contribute to a positive self-concept. Measures that support adaptation to stress such as proper nutrition, regular exercise within the patient's capabilities, adequate sleep and rest, and stress-reducing practices contribute to a healthy self-concept. Nurses are in a unique position to identify lifestyle practices that put a person's self-concept at risk or are suggestive of altered self-concepts. For example, a young teacher visits a clinic with complaints of being unable to sleep and experiencing anxiety attacks. In gathering the nursing history, lifestyle practices such as too little rest, a large number of life changes occurring simultaneously, and excessive use of alcohol emerge. These data, when taken together, are suggestive of actual or potential self-concept disturbances. Determine how the patient views the various lifestyle elements to facilitate his or her insight into behaviors and make referrals or provide needed health teaching.

Acute Care. In the acute care setting some patients experience potential threats to their self-concept because of the nature of the treatment and diagnostic procedures. Threats to a person's self-concept often result in anxiety and/or fear. As a nurse, you need to address the patient's numerous stressors, including fear of unknown diagnoses (prior to diagnostic tests), the need to modify lifestyle, and anticipated changes in functioning. In the acute care setting there is often more than one stressor, thus increasing the overall stress level for the patient and family.

Nurses in the acute care setting encounter patients who face the need to adapt to an altered body image as a result of surgery or other physical change. With shortened lengths of stay, addressing these needs is difficult to do while in an acute care setting; thus appropriate follow-up and referrals, including home care, are essential. Remain sensitive to the patient's level of acceptance of any changes. Forcing confrontation with a change before the patient is ready likely delays the person's acceptance. Signs that a person is receptive to accepting a change include asking questions related to how to manage a particular aspect of what has happened or looking at the changed body area. As the patient expresses readiness to integrate the body change into his or her self-concept, let him or her know about support groups that are available and offer to make the initial contact.

BOX 33-8 PATIENT TEACHING

Alterations in Self-Concept

Objective

- Situational low self-esteem will be reduced in the home care setting.

Teaching Strategies

- Encourage opportunities for patient to care for self (Stuart, 2009).
- Elicit patient's perceptions of strengths and weaknesses.
- Express verbally and behaviorally that patient is responsible for behavior.
- Identify relevant stressors with patient and ask for appraisal of them.
- Explore patient's adaptive and maladaptive coping responses to problems.
- Incorporate psychiatric co-morbidities (e.g., depression, somatoform disorders) and alterations to self-esteem and body image when planning treatment approaches (Sertoz et al., 2009).
- Collaboratively identify alternative solutions; encourage alternatives not previously tried.
- Continue to reinforce strengths and successes.

Evaluation

- Confirm perception and actual use of improved communication skills.
- Observe level of participation in decisions that affect care.
- Observe patient's establishment of a simple routine.
- Observe patient taking necessary action to change maladaptive coping responses and maintain adaptive ones (Stuart, 2009).
- Confirm with patient and family how to apply new coping resources to continued change.

Restorative and Continuing Care. Often in a home care environment a nurse has more of an opportunity to work with a patient to reach the goal of attaining a more positive self-concept. Interventions designed to help a patient reach the goal of adapting to changes in self-concept or attaining a positive self-concept are based on the premise that the patient first develops insight and self-awareness concerning problems and stressors and then acts to solve the problems and cope with the stressors. One way to achieve this is by reframing the patient's thoughts and feelings in a more positive way. Incorporate this approach into patient teaching for alterations in self-concept, including situational low self-esteem, that sometimes are present in the home care setting (Box 33-8).

Increase the patient's self-awareness by allowing him or her to openly explore thoughts and feelings. A priority nursing intervention is the expert use of therapeutic communication skills to clarify the expectations of a patient and family. Open exploration makes the situation less threatening for a patient and encourages behaviors that expand self-awareness. Accept the patient's thoughts and feelings nonjudgmentally, help the patient clarify interactions with others, and be empathic. Support self-expression and stress the patient's self-responsibility.

Help the patient define problems clearly and identify positive and negative coping mechanisms. Work closely with him or her to analyze adaptive and maladaptive responses, contrast different alternatives, devise a plan, and discuss outcomes. Collaborate with the patient to identify alternative solutions and develop realistic goals to facilitate real change and encourage further goal-setting behaviors. Design opportunities that result in success, reinforce the patient's skills and strengths, and help him or her find needed assistance. Encourage the patient to commit to decisions and

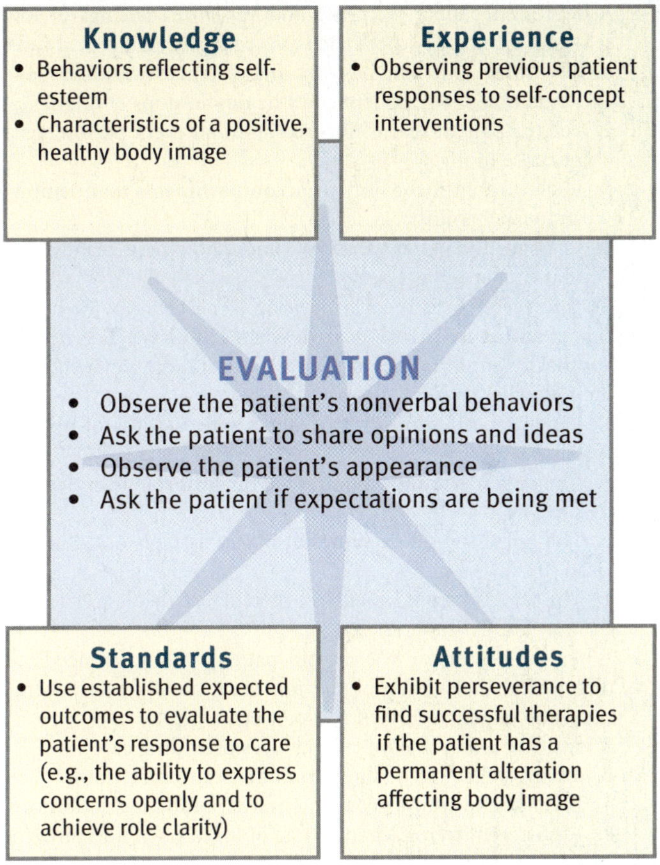

Knowledge
• Behaviors reflecting self-esteem
• Characteristics of a positive, healthy body image
Experience
• Observing previous patient responses to self-concept interventions
EVALUATION
• Observe the patient's nonverbal behaviors
• Ask the patient to share opinions and ideas
• Observe the patient's appearance
• Ask the patient if expectations are being met
Standards
• Use established expected outcomes to evaluate the patient's response to care (e.g., the ability to express concerns openly and to achieve role clarity)
Attitudes
• Exhibit perseverance to find successful therapies if the patient has a permanent alteration affecting body image

FIG. 33-7 Critical thinking model for self-concept evaluation.

actions to achieve goals by teaching him or her to move away from ineffective coping mechanisms and develop successful coping strategies. Supporting attempts that are helpful is essential because with each success a patient is able to make another attempt.

EVALUATION

Through the Patient's Eyes. Use critical thinking to evaluate the patient's perceived success in meeting each goal and the established expected outcomes (Fig. 33-7). Frequent evaluation of patient progress is necessary. Apply knowledge of behaviors and characteristics of a healthy self-concept when reviewing the actual behaviors that patients display. This determines whether outcomes have been met.

Patient Outcomes. Expected outcomes for a patient with a self-concept disturbance include nonverbal behaviors indicating a positive self-concept, statements of self-acceptance, and acceptance of change in appearance or function. Key indicators of a patient's self-concept are nonverbal behaviors. For example, a patient who has had difficulty making eye contact demonstrates a more positive self-concept by making more frequent eye contact during conversation. Social interaction, adequate self-care, acceptance of the use of prosthetic devices, and statements indicating understanding of teaching all indicate progress. Investing in satisfying activities, exerting choices in daily life, understanding own needs during transitions, and adapting to life circumstances are evidence of self-esteem and self-efficacy in older adults (Ebersole et al., 2008). A positive attitude toward rehabilitation and increased movement toward independence facilitate a return to preexisting roles at work or at home. Patterns of interacting also reflect changes in self-concept. For example, a patient who has been hesitant to express personal views more readily offers opinions and ideas as self-esteem increases.

The goals of care sometimes become unrealistic or inappropriate as a patient's condition changes. Revise the plan if needed, reflecting on successful experiences with other patients. Patient adaptation to major changes takes a year or longer, but the fact that this period is long does not suggest problems with adaptation. Look for signs that the patient has reduced some stressors and that some behaviors have become more adaptive. If initial outcomes regarding self-concept are not met, individualize the following questions:

- Tell me what you will do if you are not able to return to work (may substitute school or home) as planned.
- Who will you contact if you are not feeling any better about yourself in 2 weeks?
- What are you doing to actively promote improvement in your self-concept and self-esteem?
- How will you know that your self-concept and self-esteem are improving?

Changes in self-concept take time. Although change is often slow, care of a patient with a self-concept disturbance is rewarding.

KEY POINTS

- Self-concept is an integrated set of conscious and unconscious attitudes and perceptions about self.
- Components of self-concept are identity, body image, and role performance.
- Each developmental stage involves factors that are important to the development of a healthy, positive self-concept.
- Identity is particularly vulnerable during adolescence.
- Body image is the mental picture of one's body and is not necessarily consistent with a person's actual body structure or physical appearance.
- Body image stressors include changes in physical appearance, structure, or functioning caused by normal developmental changes or illness.
- Self-esteem stressors include developmental and relationship changes, illness, surgery, accidents, and the responses of other individuals to changes resulting from these events.
- Role stressors, including role conflict, role ambiguity, and role strain, originate in unclear or conflicting role expectations; the effects of illness often aggravate this.
- A nurse's self-concept and nursing actions have an effect on a patient's self-concept.
- Planning and implementing nursing interventions for self-concept disturbance involve expanding a patient's self-awareness, encouraging self-exploration, aiding in self-evaluation, helping formulate goals in regard to adaptation, and assisting a patient in achieving these goals.

CLINICAL APPLICATION QUESTIONS

Preparing for Clinical Practice

1. On the second postoperative day you enter the room and find Mrs. Johnson crying. She states that she has just gotten off the phone with her 23-year-old daughter and has agreed to care for her 3-month-old granddaughter while the daughter returns to work. You were informed in shift report that Mrs. Johnson had a restless night and has not taken pain medication since 2030.

You assess that she is in moderate pain, which you immediately treat with morphine. Within 40 minutes Mrs. Johnson reports that the morphine has decreased her pain rating from a 6 to a 3 on a scale of 0 to 10 but has left her somewhat drowsy. Mrs. Johnson has shared with you some of her concerns about whether or not she can actually provide child care for her granddaughter but states, "Maybe it will make me feel worthwhile and will take my mind off of how disgusting I look." She continues, "I just want to be normal again." How would you address her comment regarding "being normal again" and her lack of understanding of her physical condition, including pain management, increased fatigue, and limitations regarding lifting?

2. As a part of your home care experience, you are assigned to visit Mrs. Johnson who, in addition to caring for her infant granddaughter, is also caring for her mother, who is increasingly agitated and aggressive secondary to Alzheimer's disease. When you go to the home, you find Mrs. Johnson tearful. She says, "I can't do this anymore. She doesn't like anything I cook. She calls me two or three times during the night to sit with her; sometimes she doesn't even recognize me. The baby is constantly crying; I think she senses my stress. I feel so overwhelmed." What additional assessment data would be important to gather? What priority nursing diagnosis could be made for Mrs. Johnson?
3. You suspect that Mrs. Johnson's depressed mood and loss of interest in usual activities exceeds your previous diagnosis of situational low self-esteem. Describe which assessment data are needed to modify your plan of care. Identify your priority actions.

evolve *Answers to Clinical Application Questions can be found on the Evolve website.*

REVIEW QUESTIONS

Are You Ready to Test Your Nursing Knowledge?

1. Following a bilateral mastectomy, a 50-year-old patient refuses to eat, discourages visitors, and pays little attention to her appearance. One morning the nurse enters the room to see the patient with her hair combed and makeup applied. Which of the following is the best response from the nurse?
   1. "What's the special occasion?"
   2. "You must be feeling better today."
   3. "This is the first time I have seen you look this good."
   4. "I see that you've combed your hair and put on makeup."
2. A patient diagnosed with major depressive disorder has a nursing diagnosis of chronic low self-esteem related to negative view of self. Which of the following would be the most appropriate cognitive intervention by the nurse?
   1. Promote active socialization with other patients
   2. Role play to increase assertiveness skills
   3. Focus on identifying strengths and accomplishments
   4. Encourage journaling of underlying feelings
3. Several staff members complain about a patient's constant questions such as "Should I have a cup of coffee or a cup of tea?" and "Should I take a shower now or wait until later?" Which interpretation of the patient's behavior helps the nurses provide optimal care?
   1. Asking questions is attention-seeking behavior.
   2. Inability to make decisions reflects a self-concept issue.
   3. Dependence on staff must be stopped immediately.
   4. Indecisiveness is aimed at testing how the staff reacts.
4. A depressed patient is crying and verbalizes feelings of low self-esteem and self-worth such as "I'm such a failure ... I can't do anything right." The best nursing response would be to:
   1. Remain with the patient until he or she stops crying.
   2. Tell the patient that is not true and that every person has a purpose in life.
   3. Review recent behaviors or accomplishments that demonstrate skill ability.
   4. Reassure the patient that you know how he is feeling and that things will get better.
5. An adult woman is recovering from a mastectomy for breast cancer and is frequently tearful when left alone. The nurse's approach should be based on an understanding of which of the following:
   1. Patients need support in dealing with the loss of a body part.
   2. The patient's family should take the lead role in providing support.
   3. The nurse should explain that breast tissue is not essential to life.
   4. The patient should focus on the cure of the cancer rather than loss of the breast.
6. When caring for an 87-year-old patient, the nurse needs to understand that which of the following most directly influences the patient's current self-concept:
   1. Attitude and behaviors of relatives providing care
   2. Caring behaviors of the nurse and health care team
   3. Level of education, economic status, and living conditions
   4. Adjustment to role change, loss of loved ones, and physical energy
7. A 20-year-old patient diagnosed with an eating disorder has a nursing diagnosis of situational low self-esteem. Which of the following nursing interventions would be best to address self-esteem?
   1. Offer independent decision-making opportunities
   2. Review previously successful coping strategies
   3. Provide a quiet environment with minimal stimuli
   4. Support a dependent role throughout treatment
8. The nurse asks the patient, "How do you feel about yourself?" The nurse is assessing the patient's:
   1. Identity.
   2. Self-esteem.
   3. Body image.
   4. Role performance.
9. The nurse can increase a patient's self-awareness through which of the following actions? (Select all that apply.)
   1. Helping the patient define her problems clearly
   2. Allowing the patient to openly explore thoughts and feelings
   3. Reframing the patient's thoughts and feelings in a more positive way
   4. Have family members assume more responsibility during times of stress
10. When developing an appropriate outcome for a 15-year-old girl, the nurse considers that a primary developmental task of adolescence is to:
    1. Form a sense of identity.
    2. Create intimate relationships.
    3. Separate from parents and live independently.
    4. Achieve positive self-esteem through experimentation.
11. An appropriate nursing diagnosis for an individual who experiences confusion in the mental picture of his physical appearance is:

1. Acute confusion.
2. Disturbed body image.
3. Chronic low self-esteem.
4. Situational low self-esteem.

12. In planning nursing care for an 85-year-old male, the most important basic need that must be met is:
    1. Assurance of sexual intimacy.
    2. Preservation of self-esteem.
    3. Expanded socialization.
    4. Increase in monthly income.
13. Based on knowledge of Erikson's stages of growth and development, the nurse plans her nursing care with the knowledge that old age is primarily focused on:
    1. Intimacy versus Isolation.
    2. Autonomy versus Shame and Doubt.
    3. Generativity versus Self-Absorption.
    4. Ego Integrity versus Despair.
14. The home health nurse is visiting a 90-year-old man who lives with his 89-year-old wife. He is legally blind and is 3 weeks' post right hip replacement. He ambulates with difficulty with a walker. He comments that he is saddened now that his wife has to do more for him and he is doing less for her. Which of the following is the priority nursing diagnosis?
    1. Self-care deficit, toileting
    2. Deficient knowledge regarding resources for the visually impaired
    3. Disturbed body image
    4. Risk for situational low self-esteem
15. Based on knowledge of the developmental tasks of Erikson's Industry versus Inferiority, the nurse emphasizes proper technique for use of an inhaler with a 10-year-old boy so he will:
    1. Increase his self-esteem with mastery of a new skill.
    2. Accept changes in his appearance and physical endurance.
    3. Experience success in role transitions and increased responsibilities.
    4. Appreciate his body appearance and function.

Answers: **1.** 4; **2.** 3; **3.** 2; **4.** 1; **5.** 1; **6.** 4; **7.** 1; **8.** 2; **9.** 1, 2, 3; **10.** 1; **11.** 2; **12.** 2; **13.** 4; **14.** 4; **15.** 1.

REFERENCES

Centers for Disease Control and Prevention (CDC): Tobacco use among adults—United States, 2005, *MMWR* 55(42):1145, 2006.

Centers for Disease Control and Prevention (CDC): Youth risk behavior surveillance—United States, 2009, *MMWR* 59(SS-5):1, 2010.

Ebersole P, et al: *Toward healthy aging: human needs and nursing response*, ed 7, St Louis, 2008, Mosby.

Erikson E: *Childhood and society*, ed 2, New York, 1963, WW Norton.

NANDA International: *NANDA International nursing diagnoses: definitions and classifications, 2009-2011*, Oxford, UK, 2009, Wiley-Blackwell.

Rosenberg M: *Society and the adolescent self-image*, Princeton, NJ, 1965, Princeton University Press.

Stuart GW: *Principles and practice of psychiatric nursing*, ed 9, St Louis, 2009, Mosby.

RESEARCH REFERENCES

Armstrong S, Oomen-Early J: Social connectedness, self-esteem, and depression symptomology among collegiate athletes versus nonathletes, *J Am College Health* 57(5): 521, 2009.

Brausch AM, Muehlenkamp JJ: Body image and suicidal ideation in adolescents, *Body Image* 4(2):207, 2007.

Brunet J, et al: Exploring a model linking social physique anxiety, drive for muscularity, drive for thinness and self-esteem among adolescent boys and girls, *Body Image* 7(2):137, 2010.

Carranza FD, et al: Mexican American adolescents' academic achievement and aspirations: the role of perceived parental educational involvement, acculturation, and self-esteem, *Adolescence* 44(174):313, 2009.

Croghan IT et al: Is smoking related to body image satisfaction, stress, and self-esteem in young girls? *Am J Health Behav* 30(3):322, 2006.

Davison KK, et al: Why are early maturing girls less active: links between pubertal development, psychological well-being, and physical activity among girls ages 11 and 13, *Social Sci Med* 64(12):2391, 2007.

Figueroa-Hass CL: Effect of breast augmentation mammoplasty on self-esteem and sexuality: a quantitative analysis, *Plastic Surg Nurs* 27(1):16, 2007.

Folse VN, Hahn RL: Suicide risk screening in an emergency department: engaging staff nurses in continued testing of a brief instrument, *Clin Nurs Res* 18(3):253, 2009.

Gearing RE, et al: Remembering fatherhood: evaluating the impact of a group intervention on fathering, *J Specialists Group Work* 33(1):22, 2008.

Greene K, Banerjee SC: Adolescents' responses to peer smoking offers: the role of sensation seeking and self-esteem, *J Health Commun* 13(3):267, 2008.

Guilamo-Ramos V: Maternal influence on adolescent self-esteem, ethnic pride and intentions to engage in risk behavior in Latino youth, *Prev Sci* 10(4):366, 2009.

Jackson LA, et al: Self-concept, self-esteem, gender, race, and information technology use, *Cyberpsychol Behav* 12(4): 437, 2009.

Kaminski PL, Hayslip B: Gender differences in body esteem among older adults, *J Women Aging* 18(3):19, 2006.

Lai HR, et al: The effects of a self-esteem program incorporated into health and physical education classes, *J Nurs Res* 17(4):233, 2009.

MacPhee AR, Andrews J: Risk factors for depression in early adolescence, *Adolescence* 41(163):435, 2006.

Martyn-Nemeth P, et al: The relationships among self-esteem, stress, coping, eating behavior, and depressive mood in adolescents, *Res Nurs Health* 32(1):96, 2009.

Nelson MC, Gordon-Larsen P: Physical activity and sedentary behavior patterns are associated with selected adolescent risk behaviors, *Pediatrics* 117(4):1281, 2006.

Price B: The older woman's body image, *Nurs Older People* 22(1):31, 2010.

Sertoz OO, et al: Body image and self-esteem in somatizing patients, *Psych Clin Neurosci* 63(4):508, 2009.

Stinson DA, et al: The cost of lower self-esteem: testing a self- and social-bonds model of health, *J Personality Social-Psychol* 94(3):412, 2008.

Thomas CM: The influence of self-concept on adherence to recommended health regimens in adults with heart failure, *J Cardiovasc Nurs* 22(5):405, 2007.

Wang F, et al: The influence of childhood obesity on the development of self-esteem, *Health Rep* 20(2):21, 2009.

CHAPTER

34

Sexuality

OBJECTIVES

- Identify personal attitudes, beliefs, and biases related to sexuality.
- Discuss the nurse's role in maintaining or enhancing a patient's sexual health.
- Describe key concepts of sexual development across the life span.
- Identify causes of sexual dysfunction.
- Assess a patient's sexuality.
- Formulate appropriate nursing diagnoses for patients with alterations in sexuality.
- Identify patient risk factors in the area of sexual health.
- Identify and describe nursing interventions to promote sexual health.
- Evaluate patient outcomes related to sexual health needs.
- Identify other health care providers and community resources available to help patients resolve sexual concerns that are outside the nurse's level of expertise.
- Use critical thinking skills when helping patients meet their sexual needs.

KEY TERMS

Bisexual, p. 675
Climacteric, p. 685
Condom, p. 676
Contraception, p. 674
Diaphragm, p. 676
Dyspareunia, p. 675
Gay, p. 675
Gender identity, p. 674
Gender roles, p. 674
Hypoactive sexual desire disorder, p. 679
Infertility, p. 677
Lesbian, p. 675
Perimenopausal, p. 675
Sexual dysfunction, p. 679
Sexual health, p. 674
Sexual orientation, p. 674
Sexuality, p. 674
Sexually transmitted infection (STI), p. 674
Sterilization, p. 676
Transgender, p. 675
Tubal ligation, p. 677
Vasectomy, p. 677

evolve WEBSITE

http://evolve.elsevier.com/Potter/fundamentals/

- Review Questions
- Concept Map Creator
- Case Study with Questions
- Audio Glossary
- Interactive Learning Activities
- Key Term Flashcards
- Content Updates

Sexuality is part of a person's personality and is important for overall health. Even though discussion of sexual topics has increased over the years, many adults lack knowledge regarding **sexuality.** Although patients may be hesitant to bring up their concerns, they often share their feelings when the nurse addresses sexuality in a relaxed, matter-of-fact manner. To feel comfortable addressing sexuality, nurses need therapeutic communication skills and to be knowledgeable about sexual functioning, issues, and assessment. Many values and issues surround sexuality. Religious teachings, cultural influences on **gender roles,** beliefs about **sexual orientation,** and social and environmental climates influence the values systems for both patients and health care providers.

Sexuality has many definitions. Expression of an individual's sexuality is influenced by interaction among biological, sociological, psychological, spiritual, economic, political, religious, and cultural factors (Gorman and Sultan, 2008; World Health Organization [WHO], 2010). In addition, values, attitudes, behaviors, relationships with others, and the need to establish emotional closeness with others influence sexuality.

Sexuality differs from *sexual health.* According to WHO (2010), **sexual health** is "a state of physical, emotional, mental and social well-being in relation to sexuality; it is not merely the absence of disease, dysfunction or infirmity." People who are sexually healthy have a positive and respectful approach to sexuality and sexual relationships. They also have a potential for having pleasurable and safe sexual experiences that are free from coercion, discrimination, and violence.

SCIENTIFIC KNOWLEDGE BASE

Nurses help patients achieve sexual health by having a sound scientific knowledge base regarding sexuality. A basic understanding of sexual development, sexual orientation, **contraception,** abortion, and **sexually transmitted infections (STIs)** is necessary.

Sexual Development

Sexuality changes as a person grows and develops. Each stage of development brings changes in sexual functioning and the role of sexuality in relationships.

Infancy and Early Childhood. The first 3 years of life are crucial in the development of **gender identity** (Edelman and

Mandle, 2010). The child identifies with the parent of the same sex and develops a complementary relationship with the parent of the opposite sex. Children become aware of differences between the sexes, begin to perceive that they are either male or female, and interpret the behaviors of others as behavior appropriate for a female or a male.

School-Age Years. During the school years parents, educators, and peer groups serve as role models and teachers about how men and women act with and relate to one another. School-age children generally have questions regarding the physical and emotional aspects of sex. They need accurate information from home and school about changes in their bodies and emotions during this period and what to expect as they move into puberty (Edelman and Mandle, 2010). Knowledge about normal emotional and physical changes associated with puberty decreases anxiety as these changes begin to happen. Menstruation or nocturnal emission is sometimes frightening for uninformed children, and some view them as evidence of a dreadful disease.

Puberty/Adolescence. The emotional changes during puberty and adolescence are as dramatic as the physical ones. The adolescent functions within a powerful peer group, with the almost constant anxiety of "Am I normal?" and "Will I be accepted?" (Fig. 34-1). They face many decisions and need accurate information on topics such as body changes, sexual activity, emotional responses within intimate sexual relationships, STIs, contraception, and pregnancy.

In the United States approximately 46% of high school students report that they have had sexual intercourse at least one time and 14% of high school students had had four or more sexual partners (CDC, 2010a). One reason why adolescents are sexually active is because many believe that sexual intercourse helps them achieve goals of intimacy, relationships, and pleasure (Fantasia, 2009). A substantial number of sexually active teenagers do not protect themselves from pregnancy or STIs. The dynamics of sexual risk taking are not fully understood, but studies have found correlations among drug/alcohol use, sexual abuse, and unsafe sex (Elkington, Bauermeister, and Zimmerman, 2010; Fantasia, 2009). Adolescents tend to think that unwanted pregnancy, STIs, and other negative outcomes of sexual behavior are not likely to happen to them. Parents need to understand the importance of providing factual information, sharing their values, and promoting sound decision-making skills. They need to know that, even with the best guidance and information, adolescents make their own decisions and need to be held accountable for them.

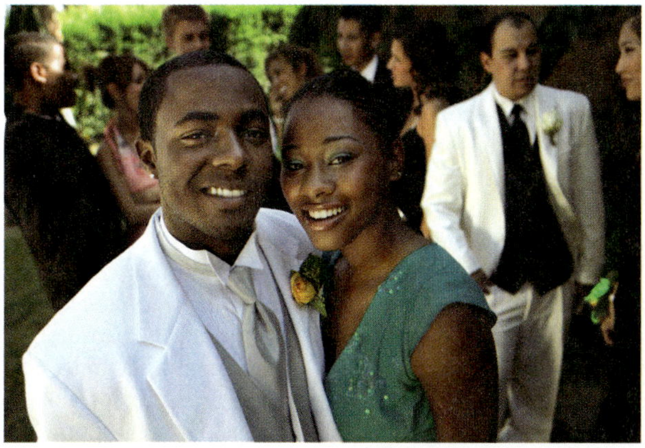

FIG. 34-1 Adolescents function within a powerful network of peers as they explore their sexual identity. (© bikeriderlondon.)

Adolescence is often a time when individuals explore their primary sexual orientation (Bowder and Greenberg, 2010). They may identify with a sexual minority group such as **lesbian, gay, bisexual,** or **transgender** (LGBT) (Young-Bruehl, 2010). Adolescents often face significant stress related to these choices and benefit from education about sexuality issues (Doty et al., 2010). Support from peers, family, school counselors, clergy, nurses, and other health professionals is important during this time.

> **Building Competency in Patient-Centered Care** A 15-year-old girl tells the nurse at a family planning clinic that she is sexually active but does not use birth control. She states that her boyfriend won't use condoms and she is concerned about pregnancy. In addition, she lives at home with her parents, and she doesn't want them to know that she is using contraception. What assessment and teaching strategies would you use to address these patient concerns?
>
> Answers to questions can be found on the Evolve website.

Young Adulthood. Although young adults have matured physically, they continue to explore and mature emotionally in relationships. Intimacy and sexuality are issues for all young adults whether they are in a sexual relationship, choose to abstain from sex, remain single by choice, are homosexual, or are widowed. People are sexually healthy in numerous ways. Sexual activity is often defined as a basic need, and healthy sexual desire is channeled into forms of intimacy throughout a lifetime.

As sexually active adults develop intimate relationships, they learn techniques of stimulation that are satisfying to both themselves and their sexual partners. Some adults need permission or affirmation that alternative ways of sexual expression other than penile-vaginal intercourse are normal. Other individuals require significant education or therapy to achieve mutually satisfying sexual relationships.

Middle Adulthood. Changes in physical appearance in middle adulthood sometimes lead to concerns about sexual attractiveness. In addition, actual physical changes related to aging affect sexual functioning. Decreasing levels of estrogen in **perimenopausal** woman lead to diminished vaginal lubrication and decreased vaginal elasticity. Both of these changes often lead to **dyspareunia,** or the occurrence of pain during intercourse. Decreasing levels of estrogen may also result in a decreased desire for sexual activity. As men age, they are likely to experience changes such as an increase in the postejaculatory refractory period and delayed ejaculation. Anticipatory guidance regarding these normal changes, using vaginal lubrication, and creating time for caressing and tenderness ease concerns regarding sexual functioning. Some aging adults also need to adjust to the impact of chronic illness, medications, aches, pains, and other health concerns about sexuality.

Later in the adult years some individuals have to adjust to the social and emotional changes associated with children moving away from home. This results in either a time of renewed intimacy between partners or a time when formerly intimate partners realize that they no longer care for one another or have common interests. In either case, when children leave home, intimate relationships usually change.

Older Adulthood. Sexuality in older adults is an important aspect of health that is often overlooked by health care providers. Studies show a positive correlation between sexual activity and physical health in older adults (Lindau and Gavrilova, 2010; Lindau et al., 2007). Many studies suggest that older adults retain

BOX 34-1 FOCUS ON OLDER ADULTS

Sexuality in Older Adults

- Sexuality and continued interest in sex throughout middle and late life is usually associated with good physical health (Lindau and Gavrilova, 2010).
- Pathological problems with the aging sexual response are often related to illnesses and side effects from medications (Hillman, 2008).
- Older adults are often reluctant to discuss sexual problems with health care providers (Green and Kodish, 2009; Lindau et al., 2007).
- Older adults who live in assisted-living or extended care facilities lose their privacy and experience a decline in physical and cognitive abilities that affects their sexual expression (Frankowski and Clark, 2009).
- The number of older lesbian, gay, bisexual, and transgendered (LGBT) population is increasing as the general population ages (Fredriksen-Goldsen and Muraco, 2010)
- Many older adults are unfamiliar with the use of condoms and other health promotion activities (e.g., having protected sex with a limited number of sexual partners) related to prevention of sexually transmitted infection (Smith and Christakis, 2009).

an interest in sexual function and are sexually active. Other studies conclude that there is a decline of sexual interest and behavior among older adults, especially in women (Box 34-1). Factors that determine sexual activity in older adults include present health status, past and present life satisfaction, and the status of marital or intimate relationships. For example, many older women are widowed or divorced and lack available sexual partners, which accounts for their decline in sexual activity. Nurses working with older adults need to be aware of the sexuality of their patients, assess interest and functioning, and plan accordingly (Wallace, 2008). It is essential to maintain a nonjudgmental attitude and convey that sexual activity is normal in later years. Emphasize that sexual activity is not essential to maintaining quality of life, especially when patients have decided not to remain sexually active.

To be effective in promoting sexual health, nurses need to understand the normal sexual changes that occur as people age. The excitement phase prolongs in both men and women, and it usually takes longer for them to reach orgasm. The refractory time following orgasm is also longer. Both genders experience a reduced availability of sex hormones. Men often have erections that are less firm and shorter acting. Women usually do not have difficulty maintaining sexual function unless they have a medical condition that impairs their sexual activity. Typically the infrequency of sex in older women is related to the age, health, and sexual function of their partner. Women continue to experience changes related to menopause, and those with problems related to urinary incontinence often experience embarrassment during intercourse. Couples who have physically disabling conditions often need information about which positions are more comfortable when having sexual intercourse.

Sexual Orientation

Sexual orientation describes the predominant pattern of a person's sexual attraction over time. Many stereotypical myths remain about people who are LGBT. Current evidence indicates that they experience decreased access to health care and do not readily seek preventive care (Brown, 2009; Williamson, 2010). Nonjudgmental nurses who have a solid knowledge base help to discourage these myths and provide nursing care that includes attention to the person's sexual orientation.

Contraception

Numerous contraceptive options are available to sexually active couples today. They provide varying levels of protection against unwanted pregnancies. Some methods do not require a prescription, whereas others require a prescription or some other type of intervention from a health care provider. Methods that are effective for contraception do not always reduce the risk of STIs. For example, the pill and intrauterine device (IUD) are effective as birth control but not for protection from STIs. Effectiveness varies with each contraceptive method and the consistency of use. Unplanned pregnancies occur because contraceptives are not used, are used inconsistently, or are used improperly (Gabelnick et al., 2009).

Nonprescription Contraceptive Methods. Nonprescription methods for contraception include abstinence, barrier methods, and timing of intercourse with regard to the woman's ovulation cycle. Although abstinence from sexual intercourse is 100% effective, it is often difficult for both men and women to use consistently. Any act of unprotected intercourse potentially results in pregnancy and exposure to STIs.

Barrier methods include over-the-counter spermicidal products and condoms. Spermicidal products (e.g., creams, jellies, foams, and sponges) are put into the vagina before intercourse to create a spermicidal barrier between the uterus and ejaculated sperm. A **condom** is a thin rubber sheath that fits over the penis to prevent entrance of sperm into the vagina. A diaphragm is a barrier method, which must be used with a spermacide with each sexual encounter. Vaginal spermicides and condoms are most effective when instructions are followed carefully; their combined use is more effective in preventing pregnancy than the use of either one alone (Warner and Steiner, 2009).

Nonprescription methods of contraception based on the physiological changes of the menstrual cycle include the rhythm, basal body temperature, cervical mucus, and fertility-awareness methods. Couples who use these methods need to understand the reproductive cycle of the woman's body and the subtle signs and signals that her body gives during the cycle. To prevent pregnancy couples abstain from sexual intercourse during designated fertile periods.

Methods That Require a Health Care Provider's Intervention. Contraceptive methods that require the intervention of a health care provider include hormonal contraception, IUDs, the diaphragm, the cervical cap, and **sterilization.** Hormonal contraception is available in several forms: oral contraceptive pills, vaginal contraceptive rings, hormonal injections, subdermal implant, transdermal skin patches, and IUDs. Hormonal contraception alters the hormonal environment to prevent ovulation, thicken cervical mucus, and thin the lining of the uterus.

An IUD is a plastic device inserted by a health care provider into the uterus through the cervical opening. IUDs contain either copper or progesterone. The primary mechanism by which both types of IUDs prevent pregnancy is to stop the sperm from fertilizing an egg (Grimes, 2009; Murphy, 2011; Ortiz and Croxatto, 2007). The release of progesterone may also increase cervical mucus thickness and alter the lining of the uterus.

The **diaphragm** is a round, rubber dome that has a flexible spring around the edge. It is used with a contraceptive cream or jelly and is inserted in the vagina so it provides a contraceptive barrier over the cervical opening. The woman needs to be refitted after a significant change in weight (10-lb gain or loss) or pregnancy. The cervical cap functions like the diaphragm; however, it covers only the cervix. It may be left in place longer, and some perceive it as more comfortable than the diaphragm.

Sterilization is the most effective contraception method other than abstinence. Female sterilization, or **tubal ligation,** involves cutting, tying, or otherwise ligating the fallopian tubes. In male sterilization, or **vasectomy,** the vas deferens, which carries the sperm away from the testicles, is cut and tied. Both a tubal ligation and a vasectomy are usually considered permanent surgical procedures.

Sexually Transmitted Infections

The incidence of STIs continues to increase. About 19 million people in the United States are diagnosed with an STI each year; almost half of them are 15 to 24 years of age (CDC, 2009). The prevalence of STIs is a major health concern for several reasons. Black and Hispanic populations are diagnosed with STIs more frequently than whites, and women have more complications associated with STIs than men. In addition, social factors such as poverty, low literacy, discrimination, use of illegal drugs (e.g., crack cocaine, methamphetamine), incarceration, sexual abuse, and racial segregation contribute to racial disparities in the STI rates (Hogben and Leichliter, 2008). Treatment of STIs in America costs about $16 million annually (CDC, 2009). Commonly diagnosed STIs include syphilis, gonorrhea, chlamydia, trichomoniasis, and infection with the human papillomavirus (HPV) and herpes simplex virus (HSV) type II (genital warts and genital herpes, respectively).

As the name implies, STIs are transmitted from infected individuals to partners during intimate sexual contact. The site of transmission is usually genital, but sometimes it is oral-genital or anal-genital. People most likely to be infected share one key characteristic: unprotected sex with multiple partners. Gonorrhea, chlamydia, syphilis, and pelvic inflammatory disease (PID) are caused by bacteria and are usually curable with antibiotics. Patients need to take antibiotics for the full course of treatment. However, an emerging concern is that some of these bacterial infections (e.g., gonorrhea and syphilis) are now developing antibiotic-resistant strains. Infections such as genital herpes, HPV, and human immunodeficiency virus (HIV) are caused by viruses and cannot be cured.

A major problem in dealing with STIs is finding and treating the people who have them. Some people do not know that they are infected because symptoms are sometimes absent or go unnoticed (CDC, 2009). Common symptoms of an STI include discharge from the vagina, penis, or anus; pain during sex or when urinating; blisters or sores in the genital area; and fever (Marrazzo et al., 2009). Because sexual behavior often includes the whole body rather than just the genitalia, many parts of the body are potential sites for an STI. The ears, mouth, throat, tongue, nose, and eyelids are sometimes used for sexual pleasure. The perineum, anus, and rectum are also frequently included in sexual activity. Furthermore, any contact with another person's body fluids around the head or an open lesion on the skin, anus, or genitalia can transmit an STI.

Sometimes people do not seek treatment because they are embarrassed to discuss sexual symptoms or concerns. They are also often hesitant to talk about their sexual behavior if they believe that it is not "normal." Any sexual behavior that embarrasses the patient often hinders the detection of an STI. Develop communication skills and a nonjudgmental attitude to provide effective care for those diagnosed with one. Detect valuable clues about an STI by establishing trust, talking with patients, and asking questions in a caring manner. Assess attitudes toward sexuality and adjust the intervention to make it acceptable to the patient's sexual value system.

Human Immunodeficiency Virus Infection. HIV infection is sometimes spread through sexual contact. Although HIV is present in most body fluids, it is a bloodborne pathogen. Transmission occurs when there is an exchange of body fluid. Primary routes of transmission include contaminated intravenous (IV) needles, anal intercourse, vaginal intercourse, oral-genital sex, and transfusion of blood and blood products. Populations that are at risk for HIV include people who use illicit IV drugs and share needles, individuals with hemophilia, and people who have unprotected sexual contact.

The natural history of HIV is composed of three stages. The primary infection stage lasts for about a month after contracting the virus. During this time the person often experiences flulike symptoms. Then he or she enters the clinical latency phase; at this time there are no symptoms of infection. HIV antibodies appear in the blood about 6 weeks to 3 months after infection. If left untreated, people who are infected with HIV live about 10 years. The last stage, acquired immunodeficiency syndrome (AIDS), happens when the person begins to show symptoms of the disease. AIDS is a serious, debilitating, and eventually fatal disease. Highly active antiretroviral therapy (HAART) greatly increases the survival time of persons who live with HIV/AIDS (Marrazzo et al., 2009).

Human Papillomavirus Infection. HPV is the most common STI in the United States, with approximately 6 million new infections every year (CDC, 2010b). Most HPV infections are asymptomatic and self-limiting. However, certain types of HPV can cause cervical cancer in women and anogenital cancers and genital warts in both men and women (CDC, 2010b; Palefsky, 2010). HPV is spread through direct contact with warts, semen, and other body fluids from others who have the disease. The textured warts often have a cauliflower appearance and are most common on the penis and scrotum in men and the vagina and cervix in women. An HPV vaccine that protects both men and woman against the types of HPV that most commonly cause health concerns is available (CDC, 2010b).

Chlamydia. An infection of the bacteria *Chlamydia trachomatis* causes chlamydia. It is the most commonly reported bacterial STI in the United States, affecting about 2.8 million Americans each year (CDC, 2009). Chlamydia infects the genitourinary tract and rectum in adults, and it causes conjunctivitis and pneumonia in newborn babies. Transmission occurs when the person comes in contact with fluids from infected sites (e.g., cervix or urethra). It is a major health issue because, if it is not treated, it causes PID, ectopic pregnancy, **infertility,** and neonatal complications. The risk of infection is higher in people who are less than 25 years old and who do not consistently use barrier contraceptives. It is also common in people who have multiple sex partners and who are infected with other STIs (Marrazzo et al., 2009). Most chlamydia infections go undiagnosed and untreated because 75% of women and 50% of men experience no symptoms (Grimshaw-Mulcahy, 2008). Symptoms that women often experience include dysuria, urinary frequency, and purulent vaginal discharge. In men it usually infects the urethra and causes nongonococcal urethritis (NGU). Dysuria and urethral discharge are common symptoms of NGU (Marrazzo et al., 2009).

NURSING KNOWLEDGE BASE

Factors Influencing Sexuality

Use critical thinking skills and basic nursing knowledge when addressing patients' sexual health needs. Draw from the following areas of nursing knowledge: sociocultural dimensions of sexuality, decisional issues, and alterations in sexual health.

BOX 34-2 CULTURAL ASPECTS OF CARE

Latinos and HIV/AIDS Risk Factors

Latinos are less likely to use condoms, less likely to seek human immunodeficiency virus/acquired immunodeficiency syndrome (HIV/AIDS) testing and have a higher incidence of HIV/AIDS than other ethnic groups in the United States. Latinos with HIV are diagnosed later in the disease process and often in the acute care setting with symptoms and complications associated with AIDS. Sociocultural factors such as gender roles, lack of knowledge, language, younger age at onset of sexual activity, and limited communication between parents and children about use of contraceptives contribute to this discrepancy (Wohl et al., 2009). Traditional Latino culture supports beliefs in abstinence until marriage, and many believe that teaching children about sex promotes sexual activity. Parents are not comfortable teaching their children, especially their daughters, about sex (Lescano et al., 2009).

Implications for Practice

- Direct interventions toward the family versus the individual since collectivism and family are fundamental to Latino culture.
- Whenever possible, first establish a strong therapeutic relationship with the patient and family before discussing sexual health.
- Design culturally sensitive and specific nursing interventions for Latino patients and families.
- Provide written and verbal information (in English and Spanish) about sex education, assertive communication, power in relationships, and negotiation skills.
- Encourage community resources such as churches and schools to improve sex education in Latino families and communities.
- Promote community and multimedia education campaigns in Spanish and English languages.
- Increase HIV testing offered at community and public clinics and consider combining HIV testing with other laboratories to promote acceptance by Latinos.

Sociocultural Dimensions of Sexuality

Cultural rules and norms regarding acceptable behavior within the culture influence sexuality. People assign different meanings to sexuality based on their culture, gender, education, socioeconomic status, and religion (Giger and Davidhizar, 2008; Stilos et al., 2008). Society plays a powerful role in shaping sexual values and attitudes and supporting specific expression of sexuality in its members.

Each cultural and social group has its own set of rules and norms that guide sexual behavior, sexual health, and the willingness to discuss this private part of life. For example, cultural norms influence how people find partners, whom they choose as partners, how they relate to one another, how often they have sex, and what they do when they have sex. Personal beliefs enable certain practices and prohibit others (Box 34-2).

Impact of Pregnancy and Menstruation on Sexuality. Sexual interest and activity of women and their partners vary during pregnancy and menstruation. Some cultures encourage sexual intercourse or male-female contact during menstruation and pregnancy, but other cultures strictly forbid it. For example, in the Hindu culture a woman avoids worship, cooking, and other members of the family during menstruation. Research has found no physiological contraindication to intercourse during menstruation or during most pregnancies. Female sexual interest tends to fluctuate during pregnancy, with increased interest during the second trimester and often decreased interest during the first and third trimesters. There is often a decrease in libido during the first trimester because of nausea, fatigue, and breast tenderness. During the second trimester blood flow to the pelvic area increases to supply the placenta, resulting in increased sexual enjoyment and libido. During the third trimester the increased abdominal size often makes finding a comfortable position difficult (Lowdermilk et al., 2010).

Discussing Sexual Issues. Sexuality is a significant part of each person's being, yet sexual assessment and interventions are not always included in health care (Lindau et al., 2007; Stilos et al., 2008). The area of sexuality is often emotionally charged for nurses and patients. Sometimes nurses avoid discussing sexual issues with patients because they lack information or have different values than their patients. Nurses who have difficulty discussing topics related to sexuality need to explore their discomfort and develop a plan to address it. If you are uncomfortable with topics related to sexuality, the patient is unlikely to share sexual concerns with you.

Decisional Issues

Individuals make many decisions about their sexuality. Some nurses help patients make decisions about contraception and abortion.

Contraception. Decisions patients make regarding contraception have far-reaching effects on their lives. Pregnancy, whether planned or unplanned, significantly affects the life of the mother and father and often their support network. Effects are physical, interpersonal, social, financial, and societal. The choice to use contraception is multifaceted and not completely understood. Factors that affect the effectiveness of contraception include the method of contraception, the couple's understanding of the contraceptive method, the consistency of use, and compliance with the requirements of the chosen method. Choice of contraception method varies in relation to the age, marital status, income, education, and previous pregnancies of the woman (Mosher and Jones, 2010).

Abortion. Half of all pregnancies in the United States are unplanned; the majority of unplanned pregnancies occur in teenagers, women over 40 years of age, and low-income nonwhite women (Paul and Stewart, 2009). Almost half of unintended pregnancies end in abortion (Mosher and Jones, 2010). Abortions have been performed since ancient times. The safety and availability of abortions in the United States improved after the 1973 Supreme Court decision *Roe v Wade,* which established the right of every woman to have an abortion. Abortions are safer and less costly when performed in the early weeks of pregnancy.

Abortion is a hotly debated issue. Women and their partners who face an unwanted pregnancy may consider it. If caring for a patient contemplating abortion, provide an environment in which the patient is able to discuss the issue openly, allowing exploration of various options with an unwanted pregnancy. Discuss religious, social, and personal issues in a nonjudgmental manner with patients. Reasons for choosing an abortion vary and include terminating an unwanted pregnancy or aborting a fetus known to have birth defects. When a woman chooses abortion as a way of dealing with an unwanted pregnancy, the woman and often her partner experience a sense of loss, grief, and/or guilt.

Be aware of personal values related to abortion. Nurses are entitled to their personal views and should not be forced to participate in counseling or procedures contrary to beliefs and values. It is essential to choose specialties or places of employment where personal values are not compromised and the care of a patient in need of health care is not jeopardized.

Prevention of Sexually Transmitted Infections. Abstinence is the only practice that is considered to be 100% effective in preventing transmission of STIs. Responsible sexual behavior includes knowing one's sexual partner, being able to openly discuss sexual and drug-use history with the partner, not allowing drugs or alcohol to influence decision making, and using protective devices.

Alterations in Sexual Health

Infertility. Infertility is the inability to conceive after 1 year of unprotected intercourse. A couple who wants to conceive and cannot has special needs. Some experience a sense of failure and feel that their bodies are defective. Sometimes the desire to become pregnant grows until it permeates most waking moments. Some individuals become preoccupied with creating just the right circumstances for conception. With advances in reproductive technology, infertile couples face many choices that involve religious and ethical values and financial limitations.

Choices for the infertile couple include pursuit of adoption, medical assistance with fertilization, or adapting to the probability of remaining childless. Organizations such as RESOLVE: The National Organization of Infertility, a national support group for couples with infertility, or international adoption groups provide couples with support and offer referral sources.

Sexual Abuse. Sexual abuse is a widespread health problem. Abuse crosses all gender, socioeconomic, age, and ethnic groups. Most often it is at the hands of a former intimate partner or family member. Sexual abuse has far-ranging effects on physical and psychological functioning (Edelman and Mandle, 2010). Sometimes sexual abuse begins, continues, or even intensifies during pregnancy. Cues that raise a question of possible sexual abuse include extreme jealousy and refusal to leave a woman's presence. The overall appearance is sometimes that of a very concerned and caring husband or boyfriend, when the underlying reason for this behavior is very different.

When you recognize abuse, mobilize support for the victim and the family. All family members usually require therapy to promote healthy interactions and relationships. Rape victims often need to work through the crisis before feeling comfortable with intimate expressions of affection. The partner needs to know how to help and support the victim. Children who have been sexually molested need to understand that they are not at fault for the incident. The parents need to understand that their response is critical to how the child reacts and adapts. Nurses are in an ideal position to assess occurrences of sexual violence, help patients confront these stressors, and educate individuals regarding community services. Nurses must also report suspected abuse to the proper authorities.

Personal and Emotional Conflicts. Ideally sex is a natural, spontaneous act that passes easily through a number of recognizable physiological stages and ends in one or more orgasms. In reality this sequence of events is more the exception than the rule. Nurses meet patients who have problems with one or more of the stages of sexual activity, including the feeling of wanting sex, the physiological processes and emotions of having sex, and the feelings experienced after sex. For example, some women and men who are taking antidepressants report that their ability to reach orgasm is negatively affected.

Sexual Dysfunction. **Sexual dysfunction,** the absence of complete sexual functioning, is common. The incidence of sexual dysfunction in the general population is estimated to be as high as 40% in men and 45% in women (Gorman and Sultan, 2008; Murtagh, 2010; Shifren et al., 2008). It is more prevalent in men and women with poor emotional and physical health (Box 34-3). Sometimes the exact cause cannot be determined.

BOX 34-3 ILLNESSES AND MEDICATIONS THAT AFFECT SEXUAL FUNCTIONING OF MEN AND WOMEN

Illnesses
- Diabetes mellitus
- Cancer (e.g., prostate, breast, colon, ovarian, testicular, rectal)
- Neuropathy
- Spina bifida
- Spinal cord injury
- Unstable angina
- Uncontrolled hypertension
- Chronic obstructive pulmonary disease
- Human immunodeficiency virus (HIV) infection
- Substance abuse
- Depression

Medications
- Antihypertensives
- Antipsychotics
- Antidepressants
- Antianxiety
- Diuretics
- Oncological agents
- Recreational or illicit drugs

Data from Chapleau C et al: Antidepressant-induced sexual dysfunction, *Consultant* 50(7):282, 2010; Harzichristou DG et al: Recommendations for the clinical evaluation of men and women with sexual dysfunction, *J Sex Med* 7:337, 2010; Gorman LM and Sultan DF: The patient with sexual dysfunction. In Gorman L, editor: *Psychosocial nursing for general patient care,* ed 3, Philadelphia, 2008, FA Davis; Lilley LL et al: *Pharmacology and the nursing process,* ed 6, St Louis, 2011, Mosby.

Erectile dysfunction (ED) affects as many as 40% of men between 40 and 70 years of age in the United States and is often unreported (Green and Kodish, 2009; Hillman, 2008). It occurs more frequently in older men, but it occurs in younger men as well (Lindau et al., 2007). Risk factors are similar to those for heart disease (i.e., diabetes mellitus, hyperlipidemia, hypertension, hypothyroidism, chronic renal failure, smoking, obesity, alcohol abuse, and lack of exercise). The etiology of ED is often multifactorial. Neurogenic problems, medications, or endocrine or psychogenic factors can cause it. An age-related decrease in testosterone often results in decreased tone of the erectile tissues.

One of the most common problems affecting women of all ages is **hypoactive sexual desire disorder** (HSDD) (Kingsberg, 2011; West et al., 2008). Biological, organic, or psychosocial factors can contribute to the incidence of HSDD. Chronic medical conditions such as breast or gynecological cancers and hormonal fluctuations, pain, or depression and anxiety can contribute to a decreased interest in sexual intimacy.

CRITICAL THINKING

Successful critical thinking requires synthesis of knowledge, experience, information gathered from patients, critical thinking attitudes, and intellectual and professional standards. Nurses use clinical judgment to anticipate information needs, analyze assessment data, and make appropriate decisions regarding patient care. Fig. 34-2 shows how to use elements of critical thinking and patient assessment data to develop appropriate nursing diagnoses.

In the case of sexuality, integrate knowledge from nursing and other disciplines. Have a thorough understanding of safe sex practices and the risks and behaviors associated with sexual problems to anticipate how to assess a patient and interpret findings. Use previous experiences to provide care for patients with sexual issues in a more reflective and helpful way. Patients have different customs and values from those of the nurse. Professional standards require respect for each patient as an individual. Critical thinking attitudes

Knowledge
- Ways to phrase questions about sexuality
- Sexual development and human sexual response patterns
- Impact of self-concept on sexuality
- Sexual orientation
- Effective contraceptive methods
- STIs and associated risk factors
- Safe sex practices
- Behaviors suggestive of current or past sexual abuse
- Diseases and/or medications that affect sexual function
- Interpersonal relationship factors and sexual functioning

Experience
- Communicating with patients and developing rapport
- Working with patients and exploring sexual concerns (e.g., working in OB-GYN setting)
- Personal sexual experience and response

ASSESSMENT
- Assess the patient's developmental stage with regard to sexuality
- Perform physical assessment of urogenital area
- Determine the patient's sexual concerns
- Assess the presence of high-risk behaviors, use of safe sex practices and contraception
- Assess medical conditions and medications that might affect sexual functioning

Standards
- Apply intellectual standards of relevance and plausibility for care to be acceptable to the patient
- Safeguard the patient's right to privacy by judiciously protecting information of a confidential nature
- Demonstrate ethics of care

Attitudes
- Display curiosity; consider why a patient might behave or respond in a particular manner
- Display integrity; your beliefs and values differ from patient's; admit to any inconsistencies in your values and in the patient's
- Take risks if necessary to explore both personal sexual issues and concerns and those of the patient

FIG. 34-2 Critical thinking model for sexuality assessment. *OB-GYN,* Obstetric-gynecological; *STI,* sexually transmitted infection.

such as integrity require you to recognize when personal opinions and values are in conflict with those of the patient and to consider how to proceed in a way that is mutually beneficial.

NURSING PROCESS

Apply the nursing process and use a critical thinking approach in your care of patients. The nursing process provides a clinical decision-making approach to help you develop and implement an individualized plan of care. Assess all relevant factors, including physical, psychological, social, and cultural, to determine a patient's sexual well-being. The nursing role in addressing sexual concerns ranges from ongoing assessment to providing information, counseling, and referral. Keep in mind that nurses are not expected to have answers to all sexual issues and concerns identified.

ASSESSMENT

During the assessment process, thoroughly assess each patient and critically analyze findings to ensure that you make patient-centered clinical decisions required for safe nursing care.

Through the Patient's Eyes. As in any patient assessment, it is important to understand the patient's expectations regarding care. Questions such as "What would you like to have happen in regard to your sexual health problems?" and "What initial steps might you take?" help the patient identify desired outcomes. It is important to set aside personal views and consider the patient's needs and preferences for care.

Factors Affecting Sexuality. In gathering a sexual history consider physical, functional, relationship, lifestyle, developmental, and self-esteem factors that influence sexual functioning. Sexual desire varies among individuals; some people want and enjoy sex every day, whereas others want sex only once a month, and still others have no sexual desire and are quite comfortable with that fact. Sexual desire becomes an issue if the person wants to satisfy sexual desire more often, if he or she believes that it is necessary to measure up to some cultural norm, or if there is a discrepancy between the sexual desires of the partners in a relationship.

Ask patients to describe factors that typically influence their sexual desire. Knowing the patients' medical history and probing for information is helpful. For example, minor illness, medications, and fatigue often decrease sexual desire. Lifestyle factors such as the use or abuse of alcohol, lack of sleep, lack of time, or the demands of caring for a new baby are other influencing factors. For example, working parents sometimes feel so overburdened that they perceive sexual advances from a partner as an additional demand on them. Confirm factors that potentially affect sexual desire and determine with the patient the extent to which sexual function is impaired.

Self-concept issues (see Chapter 33), including identity, body image, role performance, and self-esteem, affect a patient's sexuality. Consider how these factors relate to the patient's condition. For example, poor body image associated with chronic disease magnifies feelings of rejection. This often results in diminished or absent sexual desire. Problems with a person's self-esteem frequently lead to conflicts involving sexuality. Patients who experience negative feelings often suppress sexual feelings when they have not developed a healthy sense of a sexual self. Low sexual self-esteem negatively affects a person's self-concept.

Issues in a relationship often affect sexual desire. After the initial glow of a new relationship has faded, some couples find that they have major differences in their values or lifestyles. Ask couples to

TABLE 34-1 Signs and Symptoms That Indicate Possible Current Sexual Abuse or a History of Sexual Abuse

TYPES OF FINDINGS	SYMPTOMS OFTEN FOUND IN CHILDREN	SYMPTOMS OFTEN FOUND IN ADULTS
Injuries and/or physical signs	• Bruises, bleeding, soreness, or irritation of external genitalia, anus, mouth, or throat • Sexually transmitted infections • Recurrent urinary tract infections • Unintended pregnancy • Chronic pain • Difficulty walking or sitting • Unusual odor in genital area • Penile discharge • Torn, stained, or bloody underclothing	• Welts, bruising, swelling, scars, burns, or lacerations on arms, legs, breasts, or abdomen • Wounds that do not match the patient's "story" • Multiple bruises in various stages of healing • Vaginal or rectal bleeding • Fractures of face, nose, ribs, or arms • Trauma to labia, vagina, cervix, or anus • Vomiting or abdominal tenderness
Behavior, nonverbal and/or vague somatic complaints	• Physical aggression • Sexual acting out • Excessive masturbation • Expressions of low self-esteem • Poor school performance • Poor peer relationships • Sleep disturbances • Social withdrawal and excessive daydreaming • Running away from home • Substance abuse or suicide attempts	• Facial grimacing • Absence of facial response or flat affect • Anxiety • Depression • Panic attacks • Difficulty sleeping • Anorexia • Slow, unsteady gait

Data from Hockenberry MJ, Wilson D: *Wong's essentials of pediatric nursing,* ed 8, St Louis, 2009, Elsevier; Davidson MR, London ML, Ladewig PA: *Olds' Maternal-newborn nursing & women's health across the lifespan,* ed 8, Upper Saddle River, NJ, 2008, Pearson Prentice Hall; Ball JW, Bindler RC: *Pediatric nursing caring for children,* ed 4, Upper Saddle River, NJ, 2008, Pearson Prentice Hall.

BOX 34-4 PLISSIT ASSESSMENT OF SEXUALITY

Permission to discuss sexuality issues
Limited **I**nformation related to sexual health problems being experienced
Specific **S**uggestions—only when the nurse is clear about the problem
Intensive **T**herapy—referral to professional with advanced training if necessary

Modified from Annon JS: The PLISSIT model: a proposed conceptual scheme for the behavioral treatment of sexual problems, *J Sex Educ Ther* 2(2):1, 1976.

describe how close they feel to each other and how often they interact on an intimate level. Assess communication patterns between sexual partners to determine sexual satisfaction within a relationship.

Sexual Health History. Most patients want to know how medications, treatments, and surgical procedures influence their sexual relationship even though they often do not ask questions. With experience nurses recognize that most patients welcome the opportunity to talk about their sexuality, especially when they are experiencing difficulties. The PLISSIT assessment model helps nurses discuss sexuality with patients in a relaxed, matter-of-fact manner (Wallace, 2008) (Box 34-4).

Incorporate assessment questions related to sexuality in the nursing history (Box 34-5). Using an opening statement puts the patient at ease when introducing these questions (e.g., "Sex is an important part of life, and a person's health status often affects sexuality. Many people have questions and concerns about their sexual health. What questions or concerns do you have now?"). Use knowledge of developmental stages to determine which areas are likely to be important for the patient. For example, when gathering a sexual history from an older adult, it is important to keep in mind that some have difficulty discussing intimate details with health care providers.

BOX 34-5 NURSING ASSESSMENT QUESTIONS

- Are you sexually active?
- With whom do you have sex: men, women, or both?
- How many sexual partners do you have (or have you ever had)?
- How do you feel about the sexual aspects of your life?
- Have you noticed any changes in the way you feel about yourself?
- How has your illness, medication, or surgery affected your sex life?
- It is not unusual for people with your condition to be experiencing some sexual changes. Have you noticed any changes or do you have any concerns?
- Are you in a relationship in which someone is hurting you?
- Has anyone ever forced you to have sex against your will?
- Tell me what you know about safe sex practices, use of contraceptives, or prevention of sexually transmitted infections.

Nurses who conduct sexual assessments of children and adolescents face special challenges. Use language that is accurate and that the child or adolescent understands. Also promote normal development, avoid minimizing problems, and screen for sexual concerns while making the child or adolescent feel at ease. The sexual counseling of minors raises ethical and legal issues regarding the patient's rights to health care and education on the one hand and the parents' or guardian's right to supervise information on the other. Children and adolescents frequently respond when they know that having questions related to sexuality is normal. Being open, positive, and interested when introducing sexual questions is helpful.

In light of the prevalence of domestic violence and sexual abuse, questions relating to abusive relationships are important. Address these questions in private. Recognizing both subjective and objective signs and symptoms of abuse in children and adults aids in identification of this too-common problem (Table 34-1).

Some individuals are too embarrassed or do not know how to ask sexual questions directly. Look for clues that a person has questions. For example, a patient expresses concern about how his or her partner will respond now or makes a sexual comment or joke. Observing for and listening to concerns about sexuality take practice. With experience a nurse develops skill in clarifying and paraphrasing to help individuals express sexual concerns. By including sexuality in the nursing history, the nurse acknowledges that sexuality is an important component of health and creates an opportunity for the person to discuss sexual concerns.

Sexual Dysfunction. Many illnesses, injuries, medications, and aging changes have a negative effect on sexual health. Sexual dysfunction is either temporary or permanent. Apply knowledge about conditions that frequently cause sexual dysfunction while assessing a patient's risks (see Box 34-3). Awareness of the possible effects of physical problems, altered self-concept, medications, and the factors addressed thus far on sexual functioning helps in conducting a thorough assessment. Some patients bring up the topic of sexual dysfunction. Other times issues become evident as the patient answers other nursing history questions.

Physical Assessment. The physical examination is important in evaluating the cause of sexual concerns or problems and usually provides the best opportunity to teach an individual about sexuality. In examining a woman's breasts and the external and internal genitalia, a nurse has the opportunity to assess the woman's reaction, answer questions, and provide information about the examination of anatomical and physiological structures. For example, a nurse teaches a woman how to perform breast self-examination during physical assessment (see Chapter 30). During physical assessment of the genitalia, he or she teaches men how to perform testicular self-examination (see Chapter 30). Knowledge of normal scrotal anatomical structures helps men detect signs of testicular cancer. Instruct both men and women on signs and symptoms of STIs during the examination when patients' histories suggest risks for STIs.

NURSING DIAGNOSIS

After completing an assessment and applying critical thought to the diagnostic process, select diagnoses applicable to the patient's needs. Possible nursing diagnoses related to sexual functioning are listed here:

- Anxiety
- Ineffective coping
- Interrupted family processes
- Deficient knowledge (contraception/STIs)
- Sexual dysfunction
- Ineffective sexuality pattern
- Social isolation
- Risk for other-directed violence
- Risk for self-directed violence

Assessment data that signal a nursing diagnosis related to sexuality often include history of surgery of reproductive organs, changes in appearance or body image, a history of or current physical or sexual abuse, chronic illness, or developmental milestones such as puberty or menopause. To make a nursing diagnosis related to sexual dysfunction, consider anatomical, physiological, sociocultural, ethical, and situational issues thoroughly.

As with making any nursing diagnosis, clarify that the defining characteristics exist and that the patient perceives a problem or difficulty with regard to sexuality (Box 34-6). Determining the etiological or contributing factors helps in planning effectively and selecting the appropriate nursing interventions. For example, the nursing interventions appropriate for the nursing diagnosis of *sexual dysfunction* are different for different etiological factors. *Sexual dysfunction related to misinformation about the risk of sexually transmitted infections* requires counseling and education on how to maintain safe sexual practices. In contrast, patients who experience *sexual dysfunction related to physical abuse* need counseling and referral to community resources (e.g., crisis services and physical abuse support group).

BOX 34-6 NURSING DIAGNOSTIC PROCESS

Sexual Dysfunction

ASSESSMENT ACTIVITIES	DEFINING CHARACTERISTICS
Review medical and medication history	History of hypertension History of uncomplicated MI Takes propranolol (Inderal)
Have patient describe sexual problems	Less interested in having intercourse with wife since taking propranolol (Inderal) Rarely has sexual intercourse with wife Sometimes has trouble having an erection
Patient's fears and concerns	Fearful will have chest pain or another MI while having intercourse

PLANNING

Goals and Outcomes. Synthesize information from multiple resources to develop an individualized plan of care (Fig. 34-3). Critical thinking ensures that the patient's plan of care integrates all that a nurse knows about the individual and critical thinking elements as they pertain to sexuality. Professional standards are especially important to consider when developing a plan of care. Maintain a patient's dignity and identity at all times. For example, to convey respect for the patient's gender preferences, include a lesbian or gay partner in the plan to the degree that the patient wishes.

Develop an individualized plan of care for each nursing diagnosis (see the Nursing Care Plan). Set realistic goals and measurable outcomes with the patient. For example, a patient who has dyspareunia has a nursing diagnosis of *sexual dysfunction related to decreased sexual desire*. The nurse and patient develop a goal to report decreased anxiety and greater satisfaction with sexual activity within 1 month. Expected outcomes include that the patient will do the following:

- Consistently use a water-soluble lubricant before sexual intercourse within 1 week
- Discuss stressors that contribute to sexual dysfunction with partner within 2 weeks
- Identify alternative, satisfying, and acceptable sexual practices for self and partner within 4 weeks

A concept map is another method that is useful in organizing patient care (Fig. 34-4). The concept map shows the relationship of a medical diagnosis (decreased libido and depression) to the four nursing diagnoses identified from the patient assessment data. It also shows the links and relationship to the nursing diagnosis and interventions appropriate for each diagnosis. For example, *ineffective coping* affects and contributes to social isolation; and as long as the patient has ineffective coping, the social isolation continues or perhaps worsens.

NURSING CARE PLAN

Sexual Dysfunction

ASSESSMENT

Mr. Clements is a 65-year-old African American patient who had an uncomplicated myocardial infarction (MI) 3 days ago. He is stable and experienced no complications following his MI. He currently is on a cardiac telemetry nursing unit. According to Mr. Clements' medical record, he last visited his advanced practice nurse in the office 2 months ago and was diagnosed with hypertension. He was given a prescription for propranolol (Inderal). Mr. Clements is married and lives with his wife.

His blood pressure today is 122/82 mm Hg. Mr. Clements reports that he has been taking his medication regularly. The nurse knows that patients who have had MIs and are taking antihypertensive medications often experience sexual problems. When assessed by the nurse, Mrs. Clements expresses that she is still interested in having a sexual relationship with her spouse.

Assessment Activities	*Findings/Defining Characteristics**
Ask Mr. Clements if his interest in sex has changed since he started taking propranolol.	He responds that he has been **less interested in having sexual intercourse with his wife** since he started taking propranolol.
Ask Mr. Clements to compare his sexual relationship with his wife before and after taking propranolol.	He states they used to have intercourse 1 to 3 times per week, and since he started taking propranolol **they rarely have intercourse.**
Ask Mr. Clements if he has noticed any changes in his erect penis.	He states that he **sometimes has trouble having an erection.**
Ask Mr. Clements what concerns or fears he has about resuming his sexual relationship with his wife now that he has had an MI.	He states that **he is afraid that after discharge he will have chest pain or another heart attack if he has sexual intercourse** with his wife.

***Defining characteristics** are shown in bold type.

NURSING DIAGNOSIS: Sexual dysfunction related to altered body function (side effects of propranolol) and lack of knowledge.

PLANNING

Goal	*Expected Outcomes (NOC)*†
	Sexual Functioning
Patient will express satisfaction with sexual relationship with wife within 1 month.	Patient will express renewed sexual interest within 2 weeks. Patient will sustain arousal through orgasm within 3 weeks.

†Outcome classification labels from Moorhead S et al: *Nursing outcomes classification (NOC),* ed 4, St Louis, 2008, Mosby.

INTERVENTIONS (NIC)‡	RATIONALE
Sexual Counseling	
Establish trust and respect with Mr. Clements. Offer privacy during conversations.	Establishing trust and offering privacy express sense of caring, increasing likelihood of patient's ability to express concerns (Wallace, 2008). Advancing age and fear of embarrassment are major barriers to discussing erectile dysfunction (Green and Kodish, 2009).
Discuss possible effects of MI and propranolol on sexual functioning and when it is safe to resume sexual intercourse (within 7-10 days after an uncomplicated MI) (Steinke and Jaarsma, 2008).	Discussion enhances understanding about reasons for sexual difficulties and provides safe guidelines for resumption of sexual intercourse following MI (Adams and Holland, 2011).
Include Mrs. Clements in discussions about sexual issues as frequently as possible and when appropriate.	Including partner in the plan of care helps patients cope better with problems (Wallace, 2008).
Anxiety Reduction	
Encourage Mr. Clements to express fears about resuming sexual activity and assure him that others who have had MIs experience similar fears.	Knowing that feelings and fears are normal helps decrease anxiety and encourages return of sexual activity (Wallace, 2008).

‡Intervention classification labels from Bulechek GM, Butcher HK, Dochterman JM: *Nursing interventions classification (NIC),* ed 5, St Louis, 2008, Mosby.

EVALUATION

Nursing Actions	*Patient Response/Finding*	*Achievement of Outcome*
Ask Mr. Clements if he and his wife are satisfied with their sexual relationship during return office visit.	Mr. Clements reports that his interest in sex is back to normal and he is able to have an erection.	Mr. Clements reports sexual interest and function; he and his wife are satisfied with their relationship.

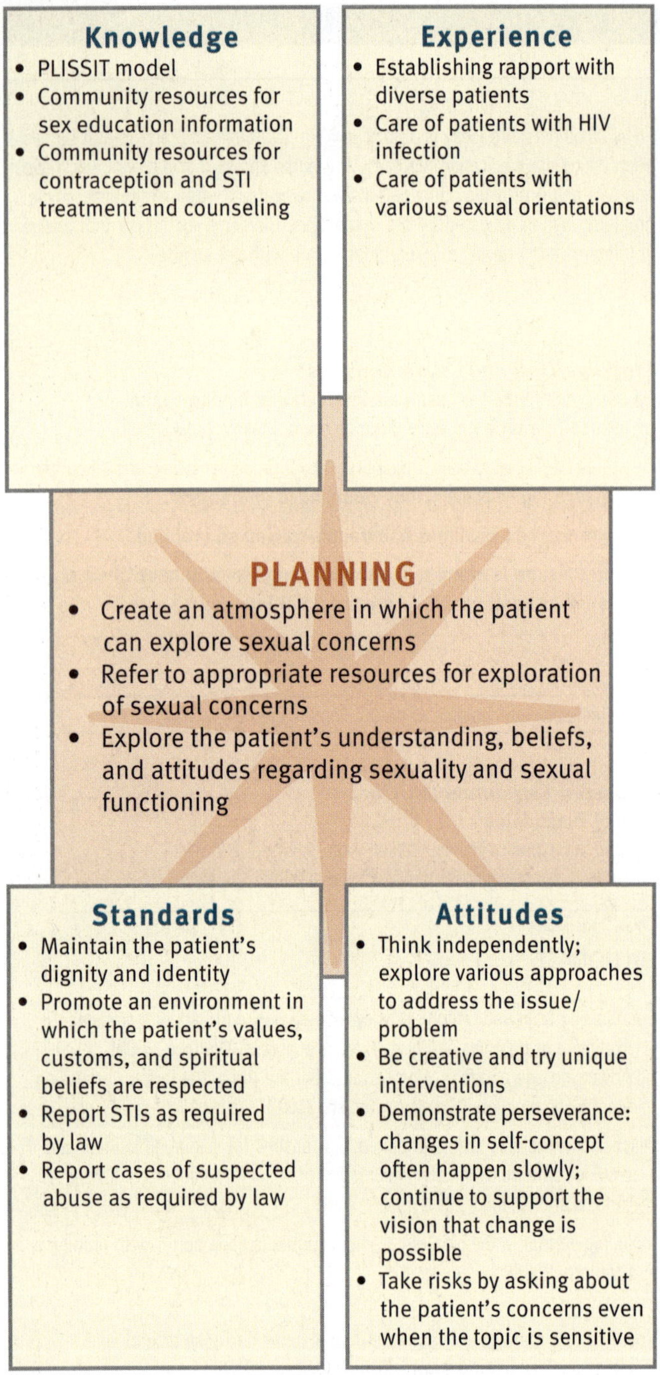
Knowledge
• PLISSIT model
• Community resources for sex education information
• Community resources for contraception and STI treatment and counseling
Experience
• Establishing rapport with diverse patients
• Care of patients with HIV infection
• Care of patients with various sexual orientations
PLANNING
• Create an atmosphere in which the patient can explore sexual concerns
• Refer to appropriate resources for exploration of sexual concerns
• Explore the patient's understanding, beliefs, and attitudes regarding sexuality and sexual functioning
Standards
• Maintain the patient's dignity and identity
• Promote an environment in which the patient's values, customs, and spiritual beliefs are respected
• Report STIs as required by law
• Report cases of suspected abuse as required by law
Attitudes
• Think independently; explore various approaches to address the issue/problem
• Be creative and try unique interventions
• Demonstrate perseverance: changes in self-concept often happen slowly; continue to support the vision that change is possible
• Take risks by asking about the patient's concerns even when the topic is sensitive

FIG. 34-3 Critical thinking model for sexuality planning. *HIV,* Human immunodeficiency virus; *STI,* sexually transmitted infection.

Setting Priorities. The care plan shows the goals, expected outcomes, and interventions for a patient experiencing sexual dysfunction. Nursing interventions for patients with sexual concerns focus on supporting the patient's need for intimacy and sexual activity. Patients often feel overwhelmed and hopeless about returning to the level of previous sexual functioning. They usually need time to adapt to physical and psychosocial changes that affect their sexuality and sexual health.

The priority in addressing needs related to sexuality includes establishing a therapeutic relationship so the patient feels comfortable in discussing issues related to sexuality. Look for strengths in both the patient and the family while providing education and access to resources to turn limitations into strengths. Patient teaching communicates the normalcy of feelings following certain situations (e.g., the diagnosis of a chronic illness or the loss of a body part). The nurse determines the patient's needs and plans accordingly.

The patient's current problems and needs help the nurse determine the priorities related to the patient's sexual health. Priorities for sexual health often include resuming sexual activities. For example, if the patient is recovering from a mastectomy and is having problems resuming an intimate relationship with her spouse because of problems related to body image, the nurse helps her adapt to and cope with the changes in her body image associated with the mastectomy. Once the patient's issues related to body image are resolved, she is able to restore intimacy with her spouse and address her sexual health needs.

BOX 34-7 EXAMPLES OF COMMUNITY RESOURCES RELATING TO SEXUALITY

- Planned Parenthood
- Health department (often for both family planning and sexually transmitted infections)
- Groups that provide education/services for those with particular conditions include the following:
  - American Diabetes Association
  - American Heart Association
  - Muscular Dystrophy Association
  - Muscular Sclerosis Society
- Sexual abuse support groups and hot lines
- Women's shelters (for those who have been physically and/or sexually abused)
- Resolve: The National Infertility Association (http://www.resolve.org)
- North America Menopause Society (http://www.menopause.org)

Teamwork and Collaboration. Planning in the area of sexuality often includes collaboration with other health care providers and referrals to community resources (Box 34-7). Nurses generally raise awareness of sexual issues, help to clarifying concerns, and/or provide information. Nurses who have specialized education in sexual functioning and counseling provide more intensive sex therapy. It is necessary to understand the limits of your knowledge base and include other health care providers such as sex therapists, clinical psychologists, and social workers as appropriate to meet patients' needs for sexual health. For example, conflicts in marriage usually require intensive treatment with a mental health professional or certified sex therapist. For the woman who is currently in an abusive relationship, the nurse collaborates with special women's shelters that provide counseling and serve as a safe place for her while further plans are made.

IMPLEMENTATION

As a nurse, promote sexual health as a component of overall wellness by identifying patients at increased risk (Box 34-8), providing appropriate information, helping individuals gain insight into their problems, and exploring methods to deal with them effectively.

Health Promotion. Helping patients maintain or gain sexual health involves consideration of factors that influence sexual satisfaction. Educate patients about sexual health, including measures for contraception, safe sex practices, and prevention of STIs.

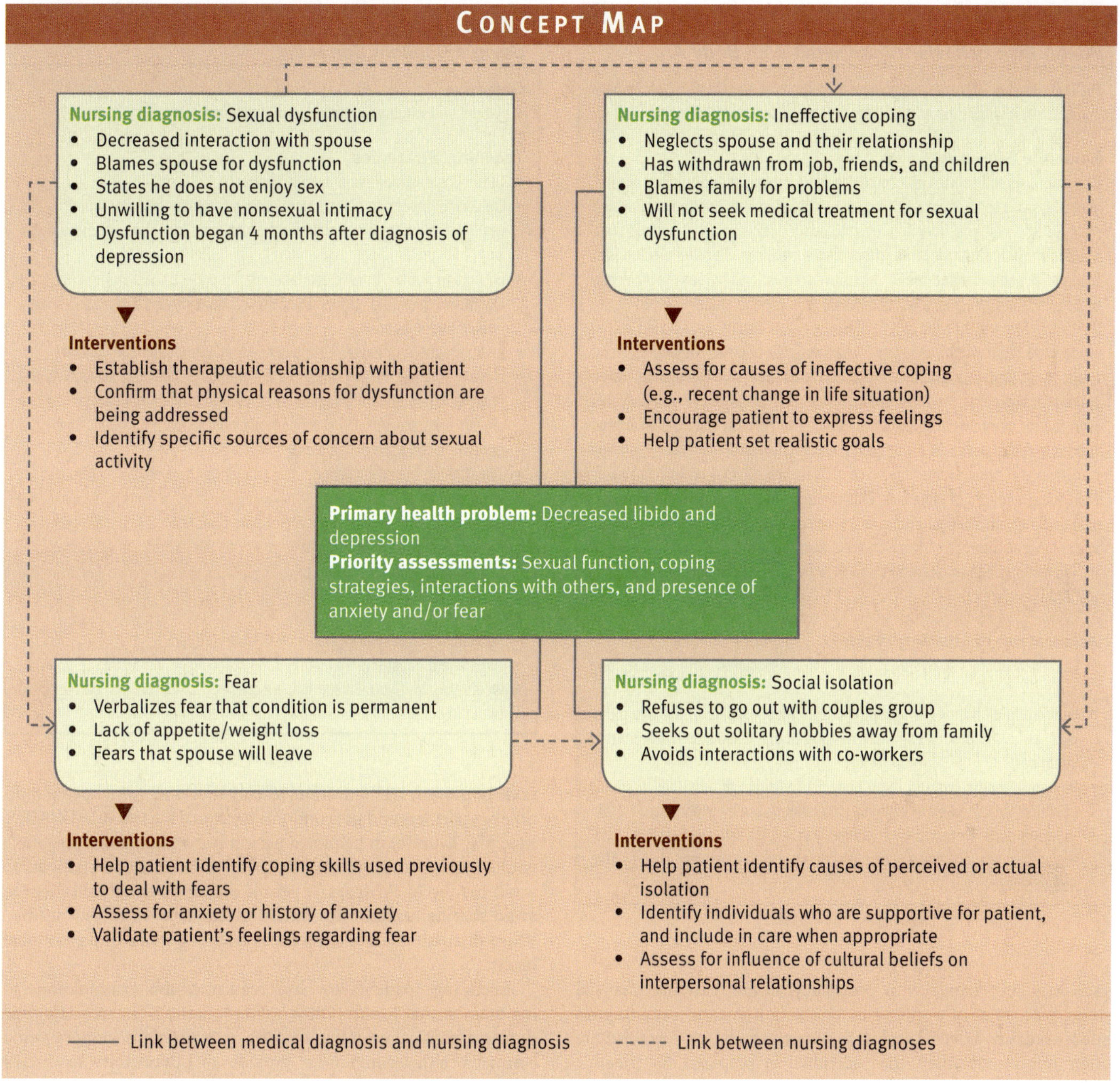
CONCEPT MAP
Nursing diagnosis: Sexual dysfunction
• Decreased interaction with spouse
• Blames spouse for dysfunction
• States he does not enjoy sex
• Unwilling to have nonsexual intimacy
• Dysfunction began 4 months after diagnosis of depression
Interventions
• Establish therapeutic relationship with patient
• Confirm that physical reasons for dysfunction are being addressed
• Identify specific sources of concern about sexual activity
Nursing diagnosis: Ineffective coping
• Neglects spouse and their relationship
• Has withdrawn from job, friends, and children
• Blames family for problems
• Will not seek medical treatment for sexual dysfunction
Interventions
• Assess for causes of ineffective coping (e.g., recent change in life situation)
• Encourage patient to express feelings
• Help patient set realistic goals
Primary health problem: Decreased libido and depression
Priority assessments: Sexual function, coping strategies, interactions with others, and presence of anxiety and/or fear
Nursing diagnosis: Fear
• Verbalizes fear that condition is permanent
• Lack of appetite/weight loss
• Fears that spouse will leave
Interventions
• Help patient identify coping skills used previously to deal with fears
• Assess for anxiety or history of anxiety
• Validate patient's feelings regarding fear
Nursing diagnosis: Social isolation
• Refuses to go out with couples group
• Seeks out solitary hobbies away from family
• Avoids interactions with co-workers
Interventions
• Help patient identify causes of perceived or actual isolation
• Identify individuals who are supportive for patient, and include in care when appropriate
• Assess for influence of cultural beliefs on interpersonal relationships
Link between medical diagnosis and nursing diagnosis
Link between nursing diagnoses

FIG. 34-4 Concept map for Mr. Clements.

Regular breast self-examinations, mammograms, and Papanicolaou (Pap) smears are important sexual health measures for women; testicular self-examinations are important for men. Offer the HPV vaccine to males and females who are between 9 and 26 years of age. The vaccine is safe for girls as young as 9 years old and is recommended for females ages 13 to 26 if they have not already completed the three required injections. Booster doses currently are not recommended. The vaccine is most effective if administered before sexual activity or exposure (CDC, 2010b; Palefsky, 2010).

Exploring an individual's values, discussing levels of satisfaction, and providing sex education require therapeutic communication skills. Structure the environment and timing to provide privacy, comfort, and uninterrupted time (Wallace, 2008). For example, when discussing methods of contraception with a woman, provide education in a private area with the patient fully dressed rather than in the examination room when the patient is only partially clothed.

Topics of education vary and often are related to the patient's developmental level. For example, a nurse talks to school-age children regarding the appearance of breast buds or pubic hair. When discussing sexual health with patients of childbearing age, always consider the patient's cultural and religious beliefs regarding contraception. The discussion includes the desire for children, usual sexual practices, and acceptable methods of contraception. Nurses review all methods of contraception to allow patients to make informed decisions.

Major developmental crises (e.g., puberty, climacteric, or menopause) prompt education about sexuality. Situational crises

BOX 34-8 EVIDENCE-BASED PRACTICE

Health Risk Behaviors Associated with Body Art

PICO Question: Do American college students who have body art participate in high-risk behaviors more frequently than college students without body art?

Evidence Summary

Body piercing and tattoos are becoming more prevalent and socially acceptable across all ages of society. They are associated with health risks ranging from local or systemic infection, even to death (Hayward and Tindale, 2008). Studies show that adolescents with multiple piercings are more predisposed to high-risk behaviors and confirm a positive correlation between the incidence of body art (tattoos, piercings) and deviance in college students (Koch et al., 2010; Rivardo and Keelan, 2010). Illegal deviant behaviors included in the study were regular marijuana use, occasional use of other illegal drugs, and a history of arrest for crimes. Legal deviant behaviors involved cheating on college assignments, multiple sex partners, and binge drinking. Individuals with four or more tattoos were 2 to 10 times more likely than those with no tattoos to report deviance. Participants reporting seven or more body piercings or piercings located in the nipples or genitals were 2 to 4 times more likely than those without intimate piercings to report regular marijuana use, occasional use of other illegal drugs, and a history of arrest for crimes. Students with higher occurrence of body art were also more likely to cheat on college assignments, binge drink, report sexual activity at a younger age, and have multiple sex partners.

Application to Nursing Practice

- Nurses need to be aware of health risks associated with piercing and tattoos.
- Individuals with multiple tattoos and piercings, especially intimate piercings, are often at increased risk for drug abuse and sexually transmitted infections.
- Routinely assess patients with body art for signs of local and systemic infection; educate about common symptoms they may experience.
- Provide education to patients with body art about safe sex practices, contraception, sexually transmitted infections, and the importance of related health screenings.

BOX 34-9 PATIENT TEACHING

Using a Condom Correctly

Objective

- Patient will verbalize correct use of a condom.

Teaching Strategies

- Develop a trusting relationship with patient.
- Explain to patient to always use a latex or rubber condom when having vaginal, oral, or anal sex and to store condoms in a cool, dry place away from sunlight.
- Encourage patient to read the label on the condom package to check the expiration date and ensure that the condom protects against sexually transmitted infections.
- Instruct patient to never reuse a condom or use a damaged condom.
- Explain how to correctly apply the condom (e.g., put it on as soon as the penis is hard and before vaginal, anal, or oral contact; gently squeeze any air out from the tip of the condom, leaving space for semen; unroll the condom to the base of the penis).
- Teach patient to pull out right after ejaculating and hold onto the condom when pulling out.
- Instruct patient to only use water-based lubricants (e.g., K-Y jelly) to prevent the condom from breaking; do not use petroleum jelly, massage oils, body lotions, or cooking oil.

Evaluation

- Ask patient to describe where condoms are stored.
- Ask patient questions that verify understanding of instruction (e.g., What would you do if you noticed that a condom you just opened had an open slit in it?).

such as a life change with pregnancy, illness, extreme financial stress, placement of a spouse in a nursing home, or loss and grief affect sexuality. Effects can last for days, months, or years and are often minimized when the individual is prepared for possible changes in sexual functioning.

Demonstrate recognition, acceptance, and respect for an older adult's sexuality by displaying a willingness to openly discuss sex and sexuality-related concerns. Strategies that enhance sexual functioning include the following (Kautz and Upadhyaya, 2010):

- Avoid alcohol and tobacco.
- Eat well-balanced meals.
- Plan sexual activity for times when the couple feels rested.
- Take pain medication if needed before sexual intercourse.
- Use pillows and alternate positioning to enhance comfort.
- Encourage touch, kissing, hugging, and other tactile stimulation.
- Communicate concerns and fears with partner and health care provider.

Individuals who have more than one sex partner or whose partner has other sexual experiences need to learn about safe sex practices. Provide information about STI symptoms and transmission, use of condoms, and risky sexual activities (e.g., trauma from penile-anal sex). To prevent HIV infection, teach patients to avoid having multiple sex partners and use condoms to reduce the risk of HIV/AIDS. Role play is useful in helping a person learn to say no or negotiate with a partner to use a condom (Box 34-9). Also teach patients to avoid the use of IV drugs. If people do use IV drugs, tell them to avoid sharing needles with others and to always use new needles. When discussing safe sex, consider patients' physical and emotional health.

Encourage patients to have regular health examinations to maintain sexual health. Often asymptomatic STIs are diagnosed during a physical examination with appropriate laboratory work. Annual health examinations provide an opportunity to discuss contraception and safe sex practices. However, some people do not routinely seek annual health examinations. Barriers to health screenings include cultural beliefs, low socioeconomic status, and low health literacy (Hogben and Leichliter, 2008; Shaw et al., 2009). Consider cultural implications as well. For example, Arab women frequently do not have breast examinations, mammograms, and cervical cancer screening because of religious and cultural beliefs about modesty (Cohen and Azaiza, 2010). Develop a therapeutic relationship with patients and provide culturally sensitive education that is written at an appropriate reading level (see Chapter 25). Encourage patients to find health care providers that they can trust and help patients who are uninsured or underinsured locate resources that can help them pay for important sexual health screenings (Hogben and Leichliter, 2008).

Acute Care. Illness and surgery create situational stressors that often affect a person's sexuality. During periods of illness individuals experience major physical changes, the effects of drugs or treatments, the emotional stress of a prognosis, concern about future functioning, and separation from significant others. Never assume that sexual functioning is not a concern merely because of an individual's age or severity of prognosis. After identifying concerns, address them in the context of his or her value system.

When a patient identifies sexual concerns, initiate discussion and education appropriately. Help patients to anticipate how their illness or disease will change over time and the adjustments that will be necessary to achieve sexual fulfillment.

Restorative and Continuing Care. Frequently nurses establish relationships with couples that encourage honest and open discussions about sexual health during restorative or continuing care. Address needs by taking a sexual health history and implementing a basic model such as PLISSIT to provide options for patients (see Box 34-4). Assessment and management of sexual concerns are important when promoting sexual intimacy and providing closeness and closure between partners at the end of life.

In the home environment it is important to provide information on how an illness limits sexual activity and give ideas for adapting or facilitating sexual activity. Interventions range from giving permission for a partner to lie in bed and hold a patient to coordinating nursing care and medications to provide opportunity for privacy and intimacy. Often nurses help individuals create an environment that is comfortable for sexual activity in the home. This sometimes involves making recommendations for ways to arrange the bedroom to accommodate physical limitations. For example, some individuals who are in a wheelchair prefer being able to move the chair close to the side of the bed at an angle that allows for more ease in touching and caressing. Suggestions regarding how to accommodate barriers such as Foley catheters or drainage tubes contribute to sexual activity.

In the long-term care setting facilities need to make proper arrangements for privacy during residents' sexual experiences (Frankowski and Clark, 2009). The ideal situation is to set up a pleasant room that is used for a variety of activities that the resident is able to reserve for private visits with a spouse or partner. If this is not possible, make arrangements for the roommate of a patient to be somewhere else to allow a couple time alone. Never leave patients alone in a situation in which they can injure themselves.

EVALUATION

Through the Patient's Eyes. Evaluate patient responses to nursing interventions to determine if goals and outcome criteria have been met (Fig. 34-5). Critical thinking ensures that the nurse applies what is known about sexuality and the patient's unique situation.

Have follow-up discussions with the patient or partner to determine whether goals and outcomes have been achieved. Sexuality is felt more than observed, and sexual expression requires an intimacy that is not amenable to observation. Therefore ask patients questions about risk factors, sexual concerns, and their level of satisfaction. Observe behavioral cues such as eye contact, posture, and extraneous hand movements that indicate comfort or suggest continued anxiety or concern as topics are addressed. Anticipate the need to modify expectations with the individual and partner when evaluating outcomes. Sometimes a nurse needs to establish more appropriate time frames in which to achieve the target goals. Ask patients to define what is acceptable and satisfying while considering the partner's level of sexual satisfaction.

Patient Outcomes. When outcomes are not met, begin to ask questions to determine appropriate changes in interventions. Examples of questions include the following:

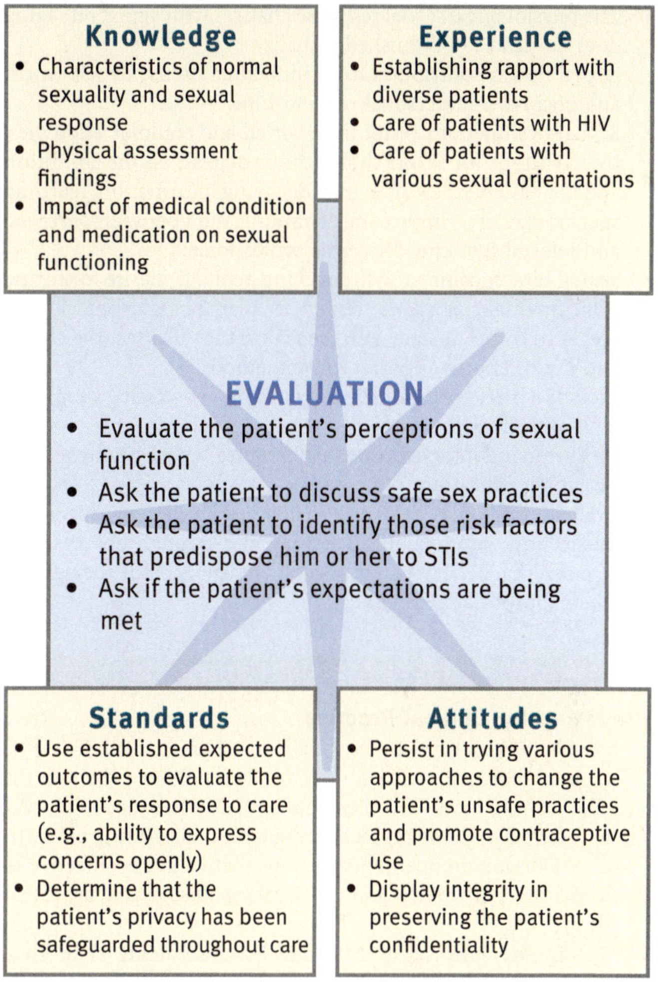
Knowledge
• Characteristics of normal sexuality and sexual response
• Physical assessment findings
• Impact of medical condition and medication on sexual functioning
Experience
• Establishing rapport with diverse patients
• Care of patients with HIV
• Care of patients with various sexual orientations
EVALUATION
• Evaluate the patient's perceptions of sexual function
• Ask the patient to discuss safe sex practices
• Ask the patient to identify those risk factors that predispose him or her to STIs
• Ask if the patient's expectations are being met
Standards
• Use established expected outcomes to evaluate the patient's response to care (e.g., ability to express concerns openly)
• Determine that the patient's privacy has been safeguarded throughout care
Attitudes
• Persist in trying various approaches to change the patient's unsafe practices and promote contraceptive use
• Display integrity in preserving the patient's confidentiality

FIG. 34-5 Critical thinking model for sexuality evaluation. *HIV,* Human immunodeficiency virus; *STI,* sexually transmitted infection.

- What other questions do you have about your sexual health?
- Did you experience less pain during sexual intercourse after taking your pain medication?
- Which positions did you find most comfortable when you had sexual intercourse? Which positions were most awkward?
- What barriers are preventing you from discussing your feelings and fears with your partner?

KEY POINTS

- Sexuality is related to all dimensions of health; therefore address sexual concerns or problems while providing routine nursing care.
- Sexuality is a part of each individual's identity and includes biological sex, gender identity, gender role, and sexual partner preference.
- Attitudes toward sexuality vary widely. Religious beliefs, values of society, the media, the family, and other factors all influence it.
- Nurses' attitudes toward sexuality vary and often differ from those of patients; be sensitive to patients' sexual preferences and needs.
- Sexual development begins in infancy and involves some level of sexual behavior or growth in all developmental stages.

- The physiological sexual response changes with aging, but aging does not lead to diminished sexuality.
- Sexual health contributes to an individual's sense of self-worth and positive interpersonal relationships.
- Sexual dysfunctions result from varied and complex etiologies.
- Interventions for sexual dysfunctions depend on the condition and the patient; they often include giving information, teaching specific exercises, improving communication between partners, and referral to a knowledgeable professional.
- Sexual biases, comfort with touching genitalia, desire for future fertility, financial status, ability to plan sexual contact, and ability to communicate with the sex partner all affect the choice and use of effective contraceptive methods.
- Include a brief review of sexuality whenever assessing a patient's level of wellness.
- Most nursing interventions that enhance sexual health require providing education.
- Evaluate outcomes of care by talking with patients regarding satisfaction with sexual functioning and through observations of nonverbal behaviors that suggest anxiety. Include the partner when appropriate.

CLINICAL APPLICATION QUESTIONS

Preparing for Clinical Practice

1. Mr. Clements returns to see the advanced practice nurse (APN) in his cardiologist's office for a routine visit. During the visit the APN plans to assess Mr. Clements' sexuality. What can the APN do to help Mr. Clements feel comfortable in discussing his sexuality? Develop an opening statement that would be effective in decreasing his anxiety about discussing this private aspect of his life.
2. During the office visit Mr. and Mrs. Clements state that, although they are able to engage in sexual intercourse, it is taking both of them longer to reach orgasm. Explain why they are experiencing this change and describe at least three strategies that they could use to enhance their sexual functioning.
3. Mrs. Clements vocalizes concern about continuing sexual activity because Mr. Clements sometimes becomes short of breath during intercourse. She also says he seems to have less energy by the end of the day than before the MI. Using the PLISSIT model, give two examples of specific suggestions that the APN might give to the couple.

evolve *Answers to Clinical Application Questions can be found on the Evolve website.*

REVIEW QUESTIONS

Are You Ready to Test Your Nursing Knowledge?

1. The nurse is providing education on sexually transmitted infections (STIs) to a group of adolescents. The nurse knows that further teaching is needed when one of the adolescents states:
   1. "A vaccine is available to reduce infection from certain types of human papillomavirus."
   2. "I should be screened for an STI after I am with a new partner."
   3. "I know I'm not infected if I don't have any symptoms such as discharge or sores."
   4. "A viral infection such as herpes or human papillomavirus cannot be treated with antibiotics."
2. A 25-year-old patient is in the emergency department and states that she has had a cough and fever for the past 3 days. While performing a physical assessment, the nurse finds several bruises that are in various stages of healing and suspects that the patient possibly is a victim of sexual abuse. Which of the following is the nurse's first action?
   1. Refer the patient to a sexual counselor
   2. Tell the patient about the safe house for women
   3. Ask the patient to describe how she got the bruises
   4. Report the abuse immediately to the proper authorities
3. A 26-year-old married woman recently discovered that she is pregnant and is at her first prenatal visit. While assessing the patient, the woman's health nurse practitioner discovers that she has purulent vaginal discharge. The patient states, "It burns when I urinate, and I seem to have to go to the bathroom frequently." Based on these symptoms, the nurse practitioner determines that further follow-up is needed because the patient:
   1. Should be tested for human immunodeficiency virus (HIV).
   2. May have a sexually transmitted infection (STI) such as chlamydia.
   3. Is experiencing normal signs of pregnancy.
   4. Needs education on proper perineal hygiene.
4. A new graduate nurse is working in a rehabilitation center that specializes in the care of patients with spinal cord injuries (SCIs). The new graduate knows that sexual issues are common among patients with SCIs. Which of the following actions enhances the nurse's comfort in discussing sexual issues with the patients? (Select all that apply.)
   1. Clarifying personal values related to sexuality
   2. Role playing discussion of sexual concerns with another nurse
   3. Attending a conference to enhance knowledge about sexuality
   4. Avoiding a discussion of sexual concerns until after completing new nurse orientation
5. The nurse is gathering a sexual history from a 68-year-old man in a nursing home. It is important for the nurse to keep in mind that:
   1. Older adults are usually not part of a sexual minority group.
   2. Older adults sometimes do not reveal intimate details.
   3. Older men and women lose their interest in sex.
   4. Older adults in nursing homes do not usually participate in sexual activity.
6. Certain cultural groups in the United States are disproportionately affected by diseases such as human immunodeficiency virus (HIV) and acquired immunodeficiency syndrome (AIDS). The nurse understands that this is most likely caused by: (Select all that apply.)
   1. Expectations about behavior by men or women in the culture.
   2. Higher percentages of lesbian, gay, bisexual, or transgender individuals in the culture.
   3. Genetic predisposition to the disease in the culture
   4. Communication patterns and language practiced by the culture.
7. Since the majority of sexually transmitted infections (STIs) have few if any symptoms, it is important for the nurse to:
   1. Encourage regular screenings in all sexually active individuals.
   2. Provide information about contraception options.

3. Administer prescribed antibiotics for human papillomavirus (HPV) or genital herpes outbreaks.
4. Ask all patients if they are experiencing any symptoms.

8. Establishing trust and encouraging disclosure about sexuality are often facilitated if the nurse begins by asking the patient:
   1. How often he or she has sexual intercourse.
   2. To disrobe in preparation for the physical assessment.
   3. For permission to discuss sexual issues.
   4. For specific examples of sexual practices and problems.
9. A 15-year-old girl states that she is having unprotected intercourse with her boyfriend. She asks for more information about birth control methods. The nurse informs the patient that: (Select all that apply.)
   1. Condoms or diaphragms must be used with each sexual encounter.
   2. Hormonal methods offer little protection against sexually transmitted infections (STIs).
   3. Barrier methods offer some protection against STIs.
   4. Sterilization is an effective option that she should consider.
10. The nurse reviews the health history of a 24-year-old woman who indicates that she has had three new sexual partners since her previous examination 2 years ago. The nurse discusses the need for sexually transmitted infection (STI) screening with the patient even though she denies symptoms or discomfort. The nurse realizes that the most serious complication from untreated STIs in females is:
    1. Genital discharge and dyspareunia.
    2. Painful menstrual cycles.
    3. Infertility and pelvic inflammatory disease.
    4. Genital warts.
11. The nurse is providing education about condom use at a community clinic for older adults. Which of following statements demonstrates that the adults understand correct use of condoms? (Select all that apply.)
    1. "I can use any kind of lubricant such as lotions or baby oil."
    2. "Before using the condom, I should check the package for damage or expiration."
    3. "I need to use a condom to help reduce the risk of sexually transmitted infections."
    4. "A good place to store condoms is in the bathroom so they don't dry out."
12. Which of the following represents a nonjudgmental approach when gathering a sexual health history?
    1. How do you and your wife/husband feel about intimacy?
    2. Do you have sex with men, women, or both?
    3. Are you heterosexual or homosexual?
    4. What is your sexual orientation?
13. A 54-year-old male patient who is being seen for an annual physical tells the nurse that he is having difficulty sustaining an erection. The nurse reviews his health history and notes no current health problems except medical treatment for depression. The nurse understands that:
    1. A personal issue such as this is best addressed by the male physician during the examination.
    2. Erectile dysfunction affects most men over the age of 50.
    3. The patient needs to be screened for sexually transmitted infections (STIs).
    4. Antidepressant medication may be affecting his sexual functioning.
14. The nurse at a community health center is teaching a group of menopausal women about normal changes in the female sexual response that occur with aging. The nurse knows that the information is understood when one of the women states that:
    1. It's normal for me to take longer to reach an orgasm.
    2. I might experience chest pain or shortness of breath during intercourse.
    3. It's normal for me to lose interest in sexual relationships.
    4. I won't need to be concerned about contraception or sexually transmitted infections because of my age.
15. A school nurse is completing a health history on an adolescent female and notices several body piercings and tattoos. The student tells the nurse that she is planning to get more tattoos and piercings over the summer break. The nurse tells the student piercing and tattoos can:
    1. Prevent you from being involved in contact sports.
    2. Only create health problems if they are located in the nipples or genital area.
    3. Increase your risk for infection at the site and in the body.
    4. Be a safe and important way of establishing your personality.

Answers: 1. 3; 2. 2; 3. 2; 4. 1, 2, 3; 5. 2; 6. 1, 4; 7. 1; 8. 3; 9. 2, 3; 10. 3; 11. 2, 3; 12. 2; 13. 4; 14. 1; 15. 3.

REFERENCES

Adams MP, Holland LN Jr: *Pharmacology for nurses: a pathophysiological approach*, ed 3, Upper Saddle River, NJ, 2011, Pearson Prentice Hall.

Bowder VR, Greenberg CS: *Children and their families*, ed 2, Philadelphia, 2010, Lippincott Williams & Wilkins.

Brown MT: LGBT aging and rhetorical silence, *Sexuality Res Social Policy: J NSRC* 6(4):65, 2009.

Centers for Disease Control and Prevention, United States Department of Health and Human Services (CDC/USDHHS): *Sexually transmitted disease surveillance, 2008*. Atlanta, Ga, November 2009, accessed from http://www.cdc.gov/std/stats08/trends.htm. Accessed September 12, 2011.

Centers for Disease Control and Prevention (CDC): *Youth risk behavior surveillance—United States, 2009. MMWR* 59(SS-5):1, 2010a, accessed from http://www.cdc.gov/mmwr/pdf/ss/ss5905.pdf. Accessed September 12, 2011.

Centers for Disease Control and Prevention, United States Department of Health and Human Services (CDC/USDHHS): *Vaccine information statement (interim) human papilloma virus (HPV) Gardasil, 3/30/2010*, 2010b, accessed from http://www.cdc.gov/vaccines/pubs/vis/downloads/vis-hpv-gardasil.pdf. Accessed September 12, 2011.

Edelman CL, Mandle CL: *Health promotion throughout the life span*, ed 7, St Louis, 2010, Mosby.

Frankowski AC, Clark LJ: Sexuality and intimacy in assisted living: residents' perceptions and experiences, *Sexuality Res Social Policy NRSC* 6(4):25, 2009.

Gabelnick HL, et al: Contraceptive research and development. In Hatcher RA, et al, editors: *Contraceptive technology*, ed 19, New York, 2009, Ardent Media.

Giger JN, Davidhizer RE: *Transcultural Nursing*, ed 5, St Louis, 2008, Mosby.

Gorman LM, Sultan DF: The patient with sexual dysfunction. In Gorman L, editor: *Psychosocial nursing for general patient care*, ed 3, Philadelphia, 2008, FA Davis.

Grimes DA: Intrauterine devices. In Hatcher RA, et al, editors: *Contraceptive technology*, ed 19, New York, 2009, Ardent Media.

Grimshaw-Mulcahy LJ: Now I know my STDs. Part II: Bacterial and protozoal, *J Nurse Pract* 4(4):271, April, 2008.

Hayward M, Tindale R: Knowing your dydoe from your madonna: an emergency nurse guide to body piercing, *Emerg Nurse* 15(10):26, 2008.

Hillman J: Sexual issues and aging within the context of work with older adult patients, *Prof Psychol Res Pract* 39(3):290, 2008.

Hogben M, Leichliter JS: Social determinants and sexually transmitted disease disparities, *Sexually Transmitted*

Dis 35(suppl 12):S13, 2008, DOI:10.1097/OLQ.0b013e31818d3cad.

Kautz DD, Upadhyaya RC: Enhancing sexual intimacy. In Mauk KL, editor: *Gerontological nursing: competencies for care*, Sudbury, Mass, 2010, Jones & Bartlett, p 602.

Kingsberg SA: Hypoactive sexual desire disorder: understanding the impact on midlife women, *Female Patient* 36(3):39, 2011.

Lowdermilk DL, et al: *Maternity nursing*, ed 8, St Louis, 2010, Mosby, p 190.

Marrazzo JM, et al: Reproductive tract infections, including HIV and other sexually transmitted infections. In Hatcher RA, et al, editor: *Contraceptive technology*, ed 19, New York, 2009, Ardent Media.

Mosher WD, Jones J: Use of contraception in the United States: 1982-2008, National Center for Health Statistics, *Vital Health Stat* 23(29), 2010, DOI: 0.1016/j.jmwh.2009.12.006.

Murphy PA: Contraception and reproductive health. In King TL, Brucker MC: *Pharmacology for women's health*, Sudbury, Mass, 2011, Jones & Bartlett.

Palefsky JM: Human papillomavirus-related disease in men: not just a women's issue, *J Adolesc Health* 46:S12, 2010.

Paul M, Stewart FH: Abortion. In Hatcher RA, et al, editor: *Contraceptive technology*, ed 19, New York, 2009, Ardent Media.

Shaw SJ, et al: The role of culture in health literacy and chronic disease screening and management, *J Immmigr Minor Health* 11(6):460, 2009.

Steinke EE, Jaarsma T: Impact of cardiovascular disease on sexuality. In Moser D, Riegel B, editors: *Cardiac nursing: a companion to Braunwald's heart disease*, St Louis, 2008, Saunders, p 241.

Stilos K, et al: Addressing the sexual health needs of patients with gynecologic cancers, *Clin J Oncol Nurs* 12(3):457, 2008, DOI:10.1188/08.CJON.457-463.

Wallace MA: Assessment of sexual health in older adults, *Am J Nurs* 108(7):52, 2008.

Warner L, Steiner MJ: In Hatcher RA, et al, editor: *Contraceptive technology*, ed 19, New York, 2009, Ardent Media.

Williamson C: Providing care to transgender persons: a clinical approach to primary care, hormones, and HIV management, *J Nurses AIDS Care* 21(3):221, 2010.

World Health Organization: *Gender and human rights: sexual health*, 2010, accessed from http://www.who.int/reproductivehealth/topics/gender_rights/sexual_health/en/. Accessed September 12, 2012.

Young-Bruehl E: Sexual diversity in cosmopolitan perspective, *Studies Gender Sexuality* 11:1, 2010.

RESEARCH REFERENCES

Cohen M, Azaiza F: Increasing breast examinations among Arab women using a tailored culture-based intervention, *Behav Med* 36:92, 2010.

Doty ND, et al: Sexuality-related social support among lesbian, gay, and bisexual youth, *J Youth Adolesc* 39:1134, 2010, DOI:10.1007/s10964-010-9566-x.

Elkington KS, Bauermeister JA, Zimmerman, MA: Psychological distress, substance abuse, and HIV/STI risk behaviors among youth, *J Youth Adolesc* 39:514, 2010, DOI:10.1007/s10964-010-9524-7.

Fantasia HC: Adolescent sexual decision making: a review of the literature, *Am J Nurse Pract* 13(11/12):22, 2009.

Fredriksen-Goldsen KI, Muraco A: Aging and sexual orientation: a 25-year review of the literature, *Res Aging* 32(2):372, 2010, DOI:10.1177/0164027509360355.

Green R, Kodish S: Discussing a sensitive topic: nurse practitioners' and physician assistants' communication strategies in managing patients with erectile dysfunction, *J Am Acad Nurse Pract* 21:698, 2009.

Koch JR, et al: Body art, deviance, and American college students, *Social Sci J* 47:151, 2010.

Lescano CM, et al: Cultural factors and family-based HIV prevention intervention for Latino youth, *J Pediatr Psychol* 34(10):1041, 2009.

Lindau ST, Gavrilova N: Sex, health and years of sexually active life gained due to good health: evidence from two US population-based cross-sectional surveys of aging, *Br Med J* 340:c810, 2010, DOI:10.1136/bmj.c810.

Lindau ST, et al: A study of sexuality and health among older adults in the United States, *N Engl J Med* 357:762, 2007.

Murtagh J: Female sexual function, dysfunction, and pregnancy: implications for practice, *Am College Nurse-Midwives* 55(5):438, 2010.

Ortiz ME, Croxatto HB: Copper-T intrauterine device and levonorgestrel intrauterine system: biological basis of their mechanism of action, *Contraception* 75(suppl):16, 2007.

Rivardo MG, Keelan CM: Body modifications, sexual activity, and religious practices, *Psychol Rep* 106(2):467, 2010.

Shifren JL, et al: Sexual problems and distress in United States women: prevalence and correlates, *Obstet Gynecol* 112:970, 2008.

Smith KP, Christakis NA: Association between widowhood and risk of diagnosis with a sexually transmitted infection in older adults, *Am J Public Health* 99(11):2055, 2009.

West SL, et al: Prevalence of low sexual desire and hypoactive sexual desire disorder in a nationally representation sample of US women, *Arch Intern Med* 168(13):1441, 2008.

Wohl AR, et al: Factors associated with late HIV testing for Latinos diagnosed with AIDS in Los Angeles, *AIDS Care* 21(9):1203, 2009.

CHAPTER 35

Spiritual Health

OBJECTIVES

- Discuss the influence of spiritual practices on the health status of patients.
- Describe the relationship among faith, hope, and spiritual well-being.
- Compare and contrast the concepts of religion and spirituality.
- Perform an assessment of a patient's spirituality.
- Explain the importance of establishing a caring relationship with patients to gain spiritual insight.
- Discuss nursing interventions designed to promote spiritual health.
- Establish presence with patients.
- Evaluate how patients attain spiritual health.

KEY TERMS

Agnostic, p. 692
Atheist, p. 692
Connectedness, p. 692
Faith, p. 693
Holistic, p. 702
Hope, p. 693
Self-transcendence, p. 692
Spiritual distress, p. 693
Spirituality, p. 691
Spiritual well-being, p. 692
Transcendence, p. 692

evolve WEBSITE

http://evolve.elsevier.com/Potter/fundamentals/

- Review Questions
- Concept Map Creator
- Case Study with Questions
- Audio Glossary
- Interactive Learning Activities
- Key Term Flashcards
- Content Updates

The word *spirituality* derives from the Latin word *spiritus*, which refers to breath or wind. The spirit gives life to a person. It signifies whatever is at the center of all aspects of a person's life (Smith, 2008). Florence Nightingale believed that spirituality was a force that provided energy needed to promote a healthy hospital environment and that caring for a person's spiritual needs was just as essential as caring for his or her physical needs (Dolamo, 2010). Today **spirituality** is often defined as an awareness of one's inner self and a sense of connection to a higher being, nature, or some purpose greater than oneself (Smith, 2008; Vachon, Fillion, and Achille, 2009). A person's health depends on a balance of physical, psychological, sociological, cultural, developmental, and spiritual factors. Spirituality is important in helping individuals achieve the balance needed to maintain health and well-being and cope with illness. Research shows that spirituality positively affects and enhances health, quality of life, health promotion behaviors, and disease prevention activities (Jurkowski, Kurlanska, and Ramos, 2010; Lee, 2009).

Too often nurses and other health care providers fail to recognize the spiritual dimension of their patients because spirituality is not scientific enough, it has many definitions, and it is difficult to measure. In addition, some nurses and health care providers do not believe in God or an ultimate being, some are not comfortable with discussing the topic, and others claim that they do not have time to address spiritual needs (Tanyi, McKenzie, and Chapek, 2009). The concepts of spirituality and religion are often interchanged, but spirituality is a much broader and more unifying concept than religion (Vachon, Fillion, and Achille, 2009).

The human spirit is powerful, and spirituality has different meanings for different people (Pesut et al., 2008). Therefore nurses need to be aware of their own spirituality to provide appropriate and relevant spiritual care to others. They need to care for the whole person and accept a patient's beliefs and experiences when providing spiritual care (Ellis and Narayanasamy, 2009; Mueller, 2010). Being able to determine the importance that spirituality holds for patients depends on a nurse's ability to develop a caring relationship (see Chapter 7). Nursing care involves helping patients use their spiritual resources as they identify and explore what is meaningful in their lives and find ways to cope with the impact of illness and the ongoing stressors of life.

SCIENTIFIC KNOWLEDGE BASE

The relationship between spirituality and healing is not completely understood. However, the individual's intrinsic spirit seems to be an important factor in healing. Healing often takes place because of believing. Current evidence shows a link between mind, body, and spirit. An individual's beliefs and expectations often have effects on his or her physical and psychological well-being (Burris et al., 2009). Many of these effects are tied to hormonal and neurological function. For example, relaxation exercises and guided imagery improve immune function in certain situations (Lahmann et al., 2010; Weigensberg et al., 2009) and reduce perceptions of pain and anxiety (Casida and Lemanski, 2010). Laughter raises pain thresholds, boosts the immune system, reduces stress and anxiety, relieves tension, and elevates mood (Harkins 2009; Swetz et al., 2009). A person's inner beliefs and convictions are powerful resources for healing. Nurses who support the spirituality of patients and their families are successful in helping patients achieve desirable health outcomes.

NURSING KNOWLEDGE BASE

Nursing research shows the association between spirituality and health. For example, Pierce et al. (2008) found that caregivers used spirituality to cope with the daily aspects of providing care to family members who have had strokes. Hollywell and Walker (2009) found that prayer often helps those who attend church or who are older, female, or less educated cope with chronic illnesses and maintain feelings of well-being. The increased interest in studying the relationship between spirituality and health has greatly contributed to nursing science.

Current Concepts in Spiritual Health

A variety of concepts describe spiritual health. To provide meaningful and supportive spiritual care, it is important to understand the concepts of spirituality, spiritual well-being, faith, religion, and hope. Each concept offers direction in understanding the views that individuals have of life and its value.

Spirituality. Spirituality is a complex concept that is unique to each individual; it depends on a person's culture, development, life experiences, beliefs, and ideas about life (McSherry, 2007). Furthermore, spirituality is an inherent human characteristic that exists in all people, regardless of their religious beliefs. It gives individuals the *energy* needed to discover themselves, cope with difficult situations, and maintain health (Villagomeza, 2006). Energy generated by spirituality helps patients feel well and guides choices made throughout life. Spirituality enables a person to love, have faith and hope, seek meaning in life, and nurture relationships with others. Because it is subjective, multidimensional, and personal, researchers and scholars cannot agree on a universal definition of spirituality (Tanyi, McKenzie, and Chapek, 2009). However, five distinct but overlapping constructs are frequently found in definitions of spirituality (Fig. 35-1).

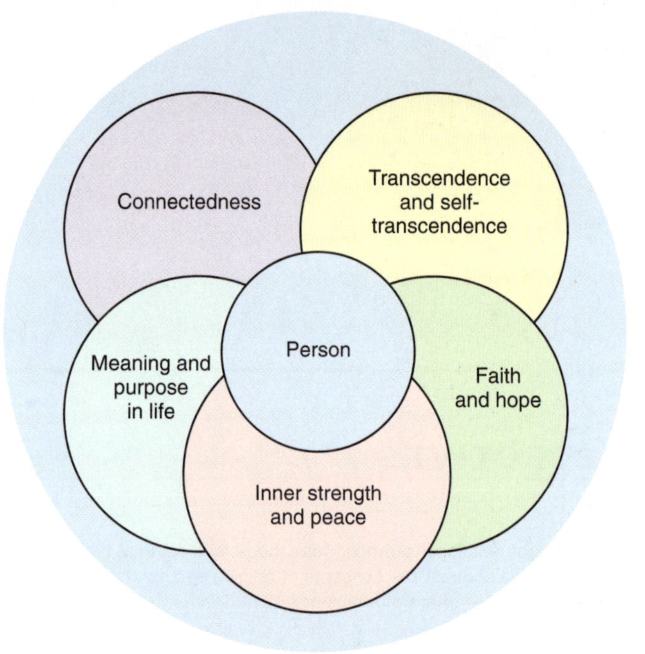

FIG. 35-1 The concept of spirituality has five distinct but overlapping constructs.

Self-transcendence is a sense of authentically connecting to one's inner self (Vachon, Fillion, and Achille, 2009), whereas **transcendence** is the belief that a force outside of and greater than the person exists beyond the material world (Bailey et al., 2009). Individuals usually see this force as positive, and it allows people to have new experiences and develop new perspectives that are beyond ordinary physical boundaries. Examples of transcendent moments include the feeling of awe when holding a new baby or looking at a beautiful sunset. Spirituality offers a sense of **connectedness** intrapersonally (connected within oneself), interpersonally (connected with others and the environment), and transpersonally (connected with the unseen, God, or a higher power). Through connectedness patients are able to move beyond the stressors of everyday life and find comfort, faith, hope, peace, and empowerment (Nelson-Becker, Nakashima, and Canda, 2007). *Faith* allows people to have firm beliefs despite lack of physical evidence. It enables them to believe in and establish transpersonal connections. Although many people associate faith with religious beliefs, it exists without religious beliefs (Villagomeza, 2006). *Hope* has several meanings that vary on the basis of how it is being experienced; it usually refers to an energizing source that has an orientation to future goals and outcomes (Phillips-Salimi et al., 2007; Vachon, Fillion, and Achille, 2009).

Spirituality gives people the ability to find a dynamic and creative sense of *inner strength* that is often used when making difficult decisions. Inner strength is a source of energy that instills hope, provides motivation, and promotes a positive outlook on life (Lundman et al., 2010). *Inner peace* fosters calm, positive, and peaceful feelings despite life experiences of chaos, fear, and uncertainty. These feelings help people feel comforted even in times of great distress (Hanson et al., 2008). Spirituality also helps people find *meaning and purpose in life* in both positive and negative life events (Bailey et al., 2009; Vachon, Fillion, and Achille, 2009).

Some people do not believe in the existence of God **(atheist)** or they believe that there is no known ultimate reality **(agnostic).** This does not mean that spirituality is not an important concept for the atheist or agnostic (Smith-Stoner, 2007). Atheists search for meaning in life through their work and their relationships with others. Agnostics discover meaning in what they do or how they live because they find no ultimate meaning for the way things are. They believe that people bring meaning to what they do.

Spirituality is an integrating theme. A person's concept of spirituality begins in childhood and continues to grow throughout adulthood (Narayanasamy et al., 2004; Smith and McSherry, 2004). It represents the totality of one's being, serving as the overriding perspective that unifies the various aspects of an individual. It spreads through all dimensions of a person's life, whether or not the person acknowledges or develops it.

Spiritual Well-Being. The concept of **spiritual well-being** is often described as having two dimensions. The vertical dimension supports the transcendent relationship between a person and God or some other higher power. The horizontal dimension describes positive relationships and connections that people have with others (Gray, 2006; Smith, 2006). Spiritual well-being has a positive effect on health. Those who experience spiritual well-being feel connected to others and are able to find meaning or purpose in their lives. Spiritual well-being leads to spiritual health. Those who are spiritually healthy experience joy, are able to forgive themselves and others, accept hardship and mortality, report an enhanced quality of life, and have a positive sense of physical and emotional well-being (Whelan-Gales et al., 2009; Yampolsky et al., 2008).

Faith. In addition to being a part of the definition of spirituality, the concept of **faith** has other common definitions. Faith is a cultural or institutional religion such as Judaism, Buddhism, Islam, or Christianity. It is also a relationship with a divinity, higher power, authority, or spirit that incorporates a reasoning faith (belief) and a trusting faith (action). Reasoning faith provides confidence in something for which there is no proof. It is an acceptance of what reasoning cannot explain. Sometimes faith involves a belief in a higher power, spirit guide, God, or Allah. Faith is also the manner in which a person chooses to live. It gives purpose and meaning to an individual's life, allowing for action. Many times patients who are ill have a positive outlook on life and continue to pursue daily activities rather than resign themselves to the symptoms of the disease. Their faith often becomes stronger because they view their illness as an opportunity for personal growth (Alcorn et al., 2010; Ford et al., 2010).

Religion. Religion is associated with the "state of doing," or a specific system of practices associated with a particular denomination, sect, or form of worship. Religion refers to the system of organized beliefs and worship that a person practices to outwardly express spirituality. Many people practice a faith or belief in the doctrines and expressions of a specific religion or sect such as the Lutheran church or Orthodox Judaism. People from different religions view spirituality differently. For example, a Buddhist believes in Four Noble Truths: life is suffering; suffering is caused by clinging; suffering can be eliminated by eliminating clinging; and to eliminate clinging and suffering, one follows an eightfold path. The path includes right understanding, intention, speech, action, livelihood, effort, mindfulness, and concentration. It promotes wisdom, moral behavior, and meditation (Wilkins, Mailoo, and Kularatne, 2010). A Buddhist turns inward, valuing self-control, whereas a Christian looks to the love of God to provide enlightenment and direction in life.

When providing spiritual care to a patient, it is important to understand the differences between religion and spirituality. Many people tend to use the terms *spirituality* and *religion* interchangeably. Although closely associated, these terms are not synonymous. Religious practices encompass spirituality, but spirituality does not need to include religious practice. Religious care helps patients maintain their faithfulness to their belief systems and worship practices. Spiritual care helps people identify meaning and purpose in life, look beyond the present, and maintain personal relationships and a relationship with a higher being or life force.

Hope. Spirituality and faith bring **hope.** When a person has the attitude of something to live for and look forward to, hope is present. It is a multidimensional concept that provides comfort while people endure life-threatening situations, hardships, and other personal challenges. It is closely associated with faith and is energizing, giving individuals a motivation to achieve and the resources to use toward that achievement. People express hope in all aspects of their lives to help them deal with life stressors. Hope is a valuable personal resource whenever someone is facing a loss (see Chapter 36) or a difficult challenge (Duggleby, Cooper, and Penz, 2009).

Spiritual Health

People gain spiritual health by finding a balance between their values, goals, and beliefs and their relationships within themselves and others. Throughout life a person often grows more spiritual, becoming increasingly aware of the meaning, purpose, and values of life. In times of stress, illness, loss, or recovery, a person often uses previous ways of responding or adjusting to a situation. Often these coping styles lie within the person's spiritual beliefs.

Spiritual beliefs change as patients grow and develop. Spirituality begins as children learn about themselves and their relationships with others. Nurses who understand a child's spiritual beliefs are able to care for and comfort the child (Mueller, 2010). As children mature into adulthood, they experience spiritual growth by entering into lifelong relationships. An ability to care meaningfully for others and self is evidence of a healthy spirituality.

Beliefs among older people vary based on many factors such as gender, past experience, religion, economic status, and ethnic background. Healthy spirituality in older adults is one that gives peace and acceptance of the self. It is often based on a lifelong relationship with a Supreme Being. Illness and loss sometimes threaten and challenge the spiritual developmental process. Older adults often express their spirituality by turning to important relationships and giving of themselves to others (Edelman and Mandle, 2010).

Factors Influencing Spirituality

When illness, loss, grief, or a major life change occurs, either people use spiritual resources to help them cope or spiritual needs and concerns develop. **Spiritual distress** is the "impaired ability to experience and integrate meaning and purpose in life through connectedness with self, others, art, music, literature, nature, and/or a power greater than oneself" (NANDA International, 2011). Spiritual distress causes a person to feel doubt, loss of faith, and a sense of being alone or abandoned. Individuals often question their spiritual values, raising questions about their way of life, purpose for living, and source of meaning. Spiritual distress also occurs when there is conflict between a person's beliefs and prescribed health regimens or the inability to practice usual rituals.

Acute Illness. Sudden, unexpected illness frequently creates significant spiritual distress. For example, both the 50-year-old patient who has a heart attack and the 20-year-old patient who is in a motor vehicle accident face crises that threaten their spiritual health. The illness or injury creates an unanticipated scramble to integrate and cope with new realities (e.g., disability). People often look for ways to remain faithful to their beliefs and value systems. Some pray, attend religious services more often, or spend time reflecting on the positive aspects of their lives. Often conflicts develop around a person's beliefs and the meaning of life. Anger is common; and patients sometimes express it against God, their families, themselves, or the nurse. The strength of a patient's spirituality influences how he or she copes with sudden illness and how quickly he or she moves to recovery. Nurses use knowledge of a person's spiritual well-being and implement spiritual interventions to maximize inner peace and healing (Yeager et al., 2010).

Chronic Illness. Many chronic illnesses threaten the person's independence, causing fear, anxiety, and spiritual distress. Dependence on others for routine self-care needs often creates feelings of powerlessness. Powerlessness and the loss of a sense of purpose in life impair the ability to cope with alterations in functioning. Spirituality significantly helps patients and their family caregivers adapt to the changes that result from chronic illness (Box 35-1). Successful adaptation often provides spiritual growth. Patients who have a sense of spiritual well-being, feel connected with a higher power and others, and are able to find meaning and purpose in life are better able to cope with and accept their chronic illness (Daaleman and Dobbs, 2010; Ebadi et al., 2009).

BOX 35-1 EVIDENCE-BASED PRACTICE

Spirituality and Caregiver Well-Being

PICO Question: What is the effect of spirituality on the well-being of adults who care for family members with chronic illnesses?

Evidence Summary

The CDC (2010) estimates that 133 million Americans have at least one chronic illness. Most people with chronic illnesses live and are cared for at home. Family caregivers of individuals with chronic illnesses often experience stress, depression, burden, and changes to their physical health (Herrera et al., 2009; Sanders et al., 2008). As the population continues to age, the number of family caregivers will continue to climb (Choi, Tirrito, and Mills, 2008). Therefore it is essential to explore ways to enhance their well-being.

Research supports a positive correlation between spirituality and family caregiver well-being. Church-based emotional support, faith in God or a higher being, and prayer help to reduce caregiver burden and stressors, especially in culturally diverse populations (Sanders et al., 2008; Strudwick and Morris, 2010). Family caregivers who are able to attend religious services and receive support from members of their congregation experience less mental distress and caregiver burden (Herrera et al., 2009). Spirituality helps caregivers find meaning during times of hardship, which enhances life satisfaction (Roscoe, 2009). Family caregivers who interpret their caregiving experience positively experience less depression and better health (Roscoe, 2009). However, caregivers still often experience grief and loss and have to work hard to obtain support from different health care agencies (Sanders et al., 2008; Strudwick and Morris, 2010). Frequently assessing family caregiver needs and providing spiritual care enhance the caregiving experience.

Application to Nursing Practice

- Use assessment data about the spirituality and spiritual behaviors or practices from caregivers of family members with chronic illnesses to identify areas of strength and support.
- When appropriate, encourage family caregivers to participate in spiritual behaviors or practices and encourage members from the caregivers' congregations to visit to enhance social support and reduce caregiver burden.
- Consider cultural differences and explore personal preferences when determining nursing interventions to enhance spiritual well-being.
- Inform caregivers of spiritual resources available in the community (e.g., parish nurses, community- or faith-based support groups, clergy, social services).
- Arrange for respite care to allow caregivers to attend religious services if desired to enhance social support and reduce caregiver burden.

Terminal Illness. Terminal illness commonly causes fears of physical pain, isolation, the unknown, and dying. It creates an uncertainty about what death means, making patients susceptible to spiritual distress. However, some patients have a spiritual sense of peace that enables them to face death without fear. Spirituality helps these patients find peace in themselves and their death. Individuals experiencing a terminal illness often find themselves reviewing their life and questioning its meaning. Common questions they ask include "Why is this happening to me?" or "What have I done?" Terminal illness often affects family and friends just as much as the patient. It causes members of the family to ask important questions about its meaning and how it will affect their relationship with the patient (see Chapter 36). In addition to managing patients' physical and psychosocial symptoms experienced at the end of life, empower them to have a greater sense of control over their disease, regardless of whether they receive care in a hospital or at home. Providing holistic care is essential because dying is a part of life that encompasses the patient's physical, social, psychological, and spiritual health (Wasserman, 2008).

Near-Death Experience. Some nurses care for patients who have had a near-death experience (NDE). An NDE is a psychological phenomenon of people who either have been close to clinical death or have recovered after being declared dead. It is not associated with a mental disorder. Persons who experience an NDE often tell the same story of feeling themselves rising above their bodies and watching caregivers initiate lifesaving measures. Most individuals describe passing through a tunnel to a bright light, encountering people who had preceded them in death, and feeling an inner tranquility and peace. Instead of moving toward the light, they learn that it is not time for them to die, and they return to life (Rominger, 2010).

Patients who have an NDE are often reluctant to discuss it, thinking that others will not understand. However, individuals experiencing an NDE who discuss it with family or caregivers find acceptance and meaning from this powerful experience. They are often no longer afraid of death. After a patient has survived an NDE, it is important to remain open and give him or her a chance to explore what happened. Provide support if the patient decides to share the experience with significant others (Duffy, 2007).

CRITICAL THINKING

The helping role is important in nursing practice (Benner, 1984). Patients look to nurses for help that is different than the help they seek from other health care professionals. Expert nurses acquire the ability to anticipate personal issues affecting patients and their spiritual well-being. Critical thinking, knowledge, and skills help nurses enhance patients' spiritual well-being and health. While using the nursing process, apply knowledge, experience, attitudes, and standards in providing appropriate spiritual care (Fig. 35-2). Nurses who are comfortable with their own spirituality often are more likely to care for their patients' spiritual needs. Nurses who foster their own personal, emotional, and spiritual health become resources for their patients and use their own spirituality as a tool when caring for themselves and their patients (Chism and Magnan, 2009; Ellis and Narayanasamy, 2009).

Taking a faith history reveals patient's beliefs about life, health, and a Supreme Being. Knowing patients' cultural preferences provides additional insight into their spiritual practices. Applying knowledge of spiritual concepts, principles of caring (see Chapter 7), and therapeutic communication skills (see Chapter 24) helps nurses readily recognize and understand patients' spiritual needs. Convey caring and openness to successfully promote honest discussion about patients' spiritual beliefs.

A sound understanding of ethics and values (see Chapter 22) is essential when providing spiritual care. A person's values or beliefs about the worth of a given idea, attitude, or custom are linked to his or her spiritual well-being. Application of ethical principles ensures respect for a patient's spiritual and religious convictions.

Personal experience in caring for patients in spiritual distress is valuable when helping patients select coping options. You need to determine if your spirituality is beneficial in assisting patients. Nurses who sense a personal faith and hope regarding life are usually better able to help their patients. Previous personal and professional experiences with dying patients, patients with chronic disease, or those who have experienced significant losses provide lessons in how to help patients face difficult challenges and how to offer support to family and friends.

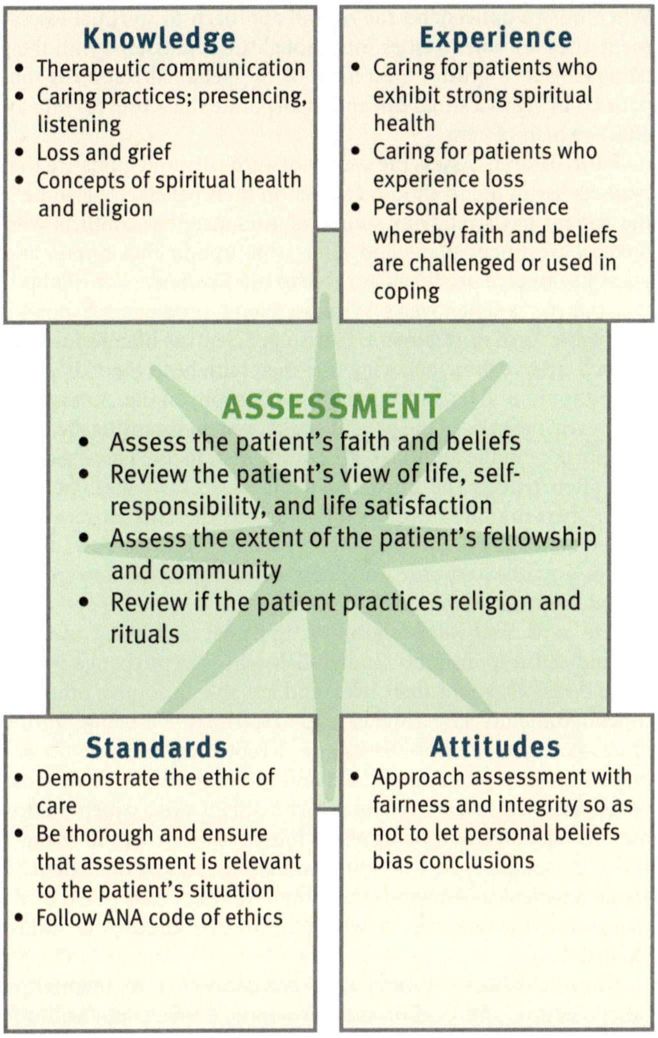

Knowledge
• Therapeutic communication
• Caring practices; presencing, listening
• Loss and grief
• Concepts of spiritual health and religion
Experience
• Caring for patients who exhibit strong spiritual health
• Caring for patients who experience loss
• Personal experience whereby faith and beliefs are challenged or used in coping
ASSESSMENT
• Assess the patient's faith and beliefs
• Review the patient's view of life, self-responsibility, and life satisfaction
• Assess the extent of the patient's fellowship and community
• Review if the patient practices religion and rituals
Standards
• Demonstrate the ethic of care
• Be thorough and ensure that assessment is relevant to the patient's situation
• Follow ANA code of ethics
Attitudes
• Approach assessment with fairness and integrity so as not to let personal beliefs bias conclusions

FIG. 35-2 Critical thinking model for spiritual health assessment. *ANA,* American Nurses Association.

Because each person has a unique spirituality, you need to know your own beliefs so you are able to care for each patient without bias (Tiew and Creedy, 2010). Use critical thinking when assessing each patient's reaction to illness and loss and when determining if spiritual intervention is necessary. Humility is essential, especially when caring for patients from diverse cultural and/or religious backgrounds. Recognize personal limitations in knowledge about patients' spiritual beliefs and religious practices. Effective nurses show genuine concern as they assess their patients' beliefs and determine how spirituality influences their patients' health. You demonstrate integrity by refraining from voicing your opinions about religion or spirituality when your beliefs conflict with those of your patients.

The application of intellectual standards helps you make accurate clinical decisions and helps patients find meaningful and logical ways to acquire spiritual healing. Critical thinking ensures that you obtain significant and relevant information when making decisions about patients' spiritual needs. The nature of a person's spirituality is complex and highly individualized. Therefore avoid making assumptions about his or her religion and beliefs. Significance and relevance are standards of critical thinking that ensure that you explore the issues that are most meaningful to patients and most likely to affect spiritual well-being.

In setting standards for quality health care, The Joint Commission (2010) requires health care organizations to assess patients' denomination, beliefs, and spiritual practices and acknowledge their rights to spiritual care. Health care organizations also need to provide for patients' spiritual needs through pastoral care or others who are certified, ordained, or lay individuals.

The American Nurses Association Code of Ethics for Nurses (Fowler, 2010) requires nurses to practice nursing with compassion and respect for the inherent dignity, worth, and uniqueness of each patient despite socioeconomic status, personal characteristics, or type of health problem. It is essential to promote an environment that respects patients' values, customs, and spiritual beliefs. Routinely implementing nursing interventions such as prayer or meditation is coercive and/or unethical. Therefore determine which interventions are compatible with the patient's beliefs and values before selecting them. An ethic of caring (see Chapter 22) provides a framework for decision making and places the nurse as the patient's advocate.

NURSING PROCESS

Apply the nursing process and use a critical thinking approach in your care of patients. The nursing process provides a clinical decision-making approach for you to use to develop and implement an individualized plan of care. The core of nursing includes a commitment to caring and respect for an individual's uniqueness. Application of the nursing process from the perspective of a patient's spiritual needs is not simple. It goes beyond assessing his or her religious practices. Understanding a patient's spirituality and then appropriately identifying the level of support and resources needed require a compassionate perspective. Remove any personal biases or misconceptions from patient assessments and be willing to share and discover another person's meaning and purpose in life, illness, and health. Love, trust, hope, forgiveness, meaning, and community are universal spiritual needs. Learning to share these needs helps you find a way to give patients spiritual care and support. Patients bring certain spiritual resources that help them assume healthier lives, recover from illness, or face impending death. Supporting and recognizing the positive side of a patient's spirituality goes a long way toward delivering effective, individualized nursing care.

ASSESSMENT

During the assessment process thoroughly assess each patient and critically analyze findings to ensure that you make patient-centered clinical decisions required for safe nursing care. Because spirituality is deeply subjective, it means different things to different people (Bailey et al., 2009).

Through the Patient's Eyes. It is essential to take the time to assess the patient's viewpoints and establish a trusting relationship with him or her. Focus nursing assessment on aspects of spirituality that life experiences and events most likely influence. As you and your patients reach a point of learning together, spiritual caring occurs.

Spiritual assessment is therapeutic because it expresses a level of caring and support. It is also a fundamental part of the nursing assessment. Because completing a spiritual assessment takes time, conduct an ongoing assessment over the course of the patient's stay in the health care setting if possible. Establish trust and rapport and make the opportunity to conduct meaningful discussions with patients a priority.

BOX 35-2 NURSING ASSESSMENT QUESTIONS

Spirituality and Spiritual Health
- What gives you energy during difficult times?
- Which aspects of your spirituality have been most helpful to you?
- Which aspects of your spirituality would you like to discuss?

Faith, Belief, Fellowship, and Community
- To what or whom do you look as a source of strength, hope, or faith in times of difficulty?
- How does your faith help you cope?
- Do you use prayer?
- What can I do to support your religious beliefs or faith commitment?
- What gives your life meaning?

Life and Self-Responsibility
- How do you feel about the changes this illness has caused?
- How do these changes affect what you now need to do?

Life Satisfaction
- How happy or satisfied are you with your life?
- What accomplishments help you feel satisfied with your life?

Connectedness
- What feelings do you have after you pray?
- Who do you feel is the most important person in your life?

Vocation
- How has your illness affected the way you live your life spiritually at home or where you work?
- In what way has your illness affected your ability to express what is important in life to you?

You can assess a patient's spiritual health in several different ways. One way is to ask direct questions (Box 35-2). This approach requires you to feel comfortable asking others about their spirituality. Several assessment tools are available to help nurses clarify values and assess spirituality. For example, the spiritual well-being (SWB) scale has 20 items that assess the individual's view of life and relationship with a higher power (Gray, 2006). The B-E-L-I-E-F assessment tool helps nurses evaluate a child's and family's spiritual and religious needs (McEvoy, 2003). The acronym stands for the following:

B—Belief system
E—Ethics or values
L—Lifestyle
I—Involvement in a spiritual community
E—Education
F—Future events

Effective spiritual assessment tools such as the SWB and B-E-L-I-E-F help nurses remember important areas to assess. A patient's response to items on assessment tools often indicates areas that need further investigation. For example, if after using an assessment tool, a nurse finds that a patient has difficulty accepting change, the nurse needs to spend time understanding how the patient is accepting and managing the new illness. Whether you use an assessment tool or direct an assessment with questions that are based on principles of spirituality, it is important not to impose your personal value systems on the patient. This is particularly true when the patient's values and beliefs are similar to those of your own because it then becomes very easy to make false assumptions. When nurses understand the overall approach to spiritual assessment, they are able to enter into thoughtful discussions with their patients, gain a greater awareness of the personal resources that patients bring to a situation, and incorporate the resources into an effective plan of care.

Faith/Belief. Assess the source of authority and guidance that patients use in life to choose and act on their beliefs. Determine if the patient has a religious source of guidance that conflicts with medical treatment plans and affects the option that nurses and other health care providers are able to offer patients. For example, if a patient is a Jehovah's Witness, blood products are not an acceptable form of treatment. Christian Scientists often refuse any medical intervention, believing that their faith heals them. It is also important to understand a patient's philosophy of life. Assessment data reveal the basis of the patient's belief system regarding meaning and purpose in life and the patient's spiritual focus. This information often reflects the impact that illness, loss, or disability has on the person's life. Considerable religious diversity exists in the United States. A patient's religious faith and practices, views about health, and the response to illness often influence how nurses provide support (Table 35-1).

Life and Self-Responsibility. Spiritual well-being includes life and self-responsibility. Individuals who accept change in life, make decisions about their lives, and are able to forgive others in times of difficulty have a higher level of spiritual well-being. During illness patients often are unable to accept limitations or do not know how to regain a functional and meaningful life. Their sense of helplessness reflects spiritual distress. However, patients often use their spiritual well-being as a resource as they adapt to changes and seek solutions to deal with limitations. Assess the extent to which a patient understands the limitations or threats posed by an illness and the manner in which he or she chooses to adjust to them.

Connectedness. People who are connected to themselves, others, nature, and God or another Supreme Being cope with the stress brought on by crisis and chronic illness. Patients remain connected with God by praying (Fig. 35-3). Prayer is personal communication with one's god. It provides a sense of hope, strength, security, and well-being; and it is a part of faith (Hollywell and Walker, 2009; Krause and Bastida, 2009). Help patients become or remain connected by respecting each patient's unique sense of spirituality. Assess whether the patient loses the ability to express a sense of relatedness to something greater than the self.

Life Satisfaction. Spiritual well-being is tied to a person's satisfaction with life and what he or she has accomplished (Katerndahl, 2008). Assessing a person's satisfaction with life often provides insight to appropriate nursing care. When people are satisfied with life, more energy is available to deal with new difficulties and resolve problems.

Culture. Spirituality is a personal experience within a cultural context. It is important to know a patient's culture of origin and assess his or her values (Tiew and Creedy, 2010). It is common in many cultures for individuals to believe that they have led a worthwhile and purposeful life. Remaining connected with their cultural heritage often helps patients define their place in the world and express their spirituality. Asking them about their faith and belief systems is a good beginning for understanding the relationship between culture and spirituality (Box 35-3).

Fellowship and Community. Fellowship is a type of relationship that an individual has with other persons (e.g., family, close friends, fellow members of a church, or neighbors). Explore the extent and nature of the patient's support networks. It is unwise

TABLE 35-1 Religious Beliefs About Health

RELIGIOUS OR CULTURAL GROUP	HEALTH CARE BELIEFS	RESPONSE TO ILLNESS	IMPLICATIONS FOR HEALTH AND NURSING
Hinduism	Accepts modern medical science	Past sins cause illness. Prolonging life is discouraged.	Allow time for prayer and purity rituals. Allow use of amulets, rituals, and symbols.
Sikhism	Accepts modern medical science	Females are to be examined by females. Removing undergarments causes great distress.	Provide time for devotional prayer. Allow use of religious symbols.
Buddhism	Accepts modern medical science	Followers sometimes refuse treatment on Holy Days. Nonhuman spirits invading the body cause illness. Sometimes followers want a Buddhist priest. They usually accept death as last stage of life and usually permit withdrawal of life support. Followers do not practice euthanasia. They often do not take time off from work or family responsibilities when sick.	Health is an important part of life. Good health is maintained by caring for self and others. Medications are not always accepted because of belief that chemical substances in the body are harmful.
Islam	Must be able to practice the Five Pillars of Islam Sometimes has a fatalistic view of health	Muslims use faith healing. Family members are a comfort. Group prayer is strengthening. They often permit withdrawal of life support. They do not practice euthanasia. They believe that time of death is predetermined and cannot be changed. They maintain a sense of hope and often avoid discussions of death.	Women prefer female health care providers. During month of Ramadan Muslims do not eat until after the sun goes down. Health and spirituality are connected. Family and friends visit during time of illness. They usually do not consider organ transplantation or donation and postmortem examinations.
Judaism	Believes in the sanctity of life Balance between God and medicine Observance of the Sabbath important Treatments sometimes refused on the Sabbath	Visiting the sick is an obligation. There is an obligation to seek care, exercise, sleep, eat well, and avoid drug and alcohol abuse. Euthanasia is forbidden. Life support is discouraged.	Jews believe that it is important to stay healthy. They expect the nurse to provide competent health care. Allow patients to express their feelings. Allow family to stay with dying patient.
Christianity	Accepts modern medical science Complementary or alternative medicine often followed (see Chapter 32)	Followers use prayer, faith healing. They appreciate visits from clergy. Some use laying on of hands. Holy Communion is sometimes practiced. Anointing of the sick is given when patient is ill or near death (Catholic).	Christians are usually in favor of organ donation. Health is important to maintain. Allow time for patients to pray by themselves, with family or friends.
Navajos	Concepts of health have a fundamental place in their concept of humans and their place in the universe	Blessingway is a practice that attempts to remove ill health by means of stories, songs, rituals, prayers, symbols, and sand paintings.	Navajos prefer holistic approach to health care. They often are not on time for appointments. Promote physical, mental, spiritual, and social health of persons, families, and communities. Allow family members to visit. Provide teaching about wellness, not disease prevention, when possible.
Appalachians	External locus of control Nature controls life and health Accept folk healers Good Christian members of community are called as servants to minister to disabled	They dislike hospitals. They tend not to follow medical regimens but expect to be helped directly when seeking episodic treatment.	They become anxious in unfamiliar settings. Encourage communication with family and friends when ill.

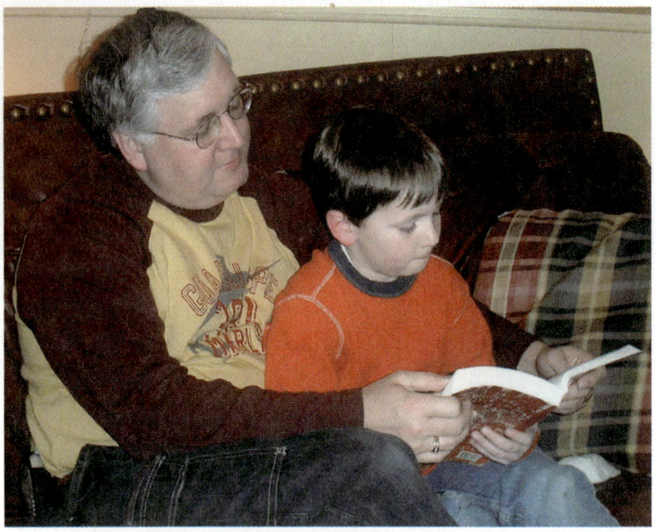

FIG. 35-3 Praying or reading a bible together enhances the connectedness between parents and their children.

BOX 35-3 CULTURAL ASPECTS OF CARE

Spirituality and Culture

Spirituality and spiritual health vary among cultures. Therefore nurses need to assess how their patients' culture affects spirituality. For example, spiritual aspects of life are frequently important to Latinos. *Personalismo* is a cultural value that indicates warmth, closeness, and empathy in relationships with other people and a universal being. *Familismo*, another Latino cultural value, indicates commitment and loyalty to immediate and extended family (Campesino et al., 2009). For African Americans spirituality is associated with guidance, coping, strength, and peace. It is often a catalyst for recovery, and community- and faith-based programs are effective in promoting health (Gallia and Pines, 2009). Although people who practice Buddhism believe that suffering is a part of life, they try to avoid it when possible (Wilkins, Mailoo, and Kularatne, 2010). At the end of life they prepare for "a good death," which requires quiet time for meditation and prayer.

Implications for Practice

- Explore the spirituality of patients from different cultures by assessing the meaning of health and how patients achieve balance, stability, peace, or comfort in their lives.
- Offer a universal and holistic approach to assessing patients' needs by demonstrating caring and using therapeutic communication techniques.
- Promote an environment during assessment that respects human rights, values, customs, and spiritual beliefs.
- Include appropriate pastoral care professionals in the assessment process.
- Avoid use of language that alienates or discriminates among different religions.

to assume that a given network offers the kind of support that a patient desires. For example, calling the patient's clergy to request a visit is inappropriate if the patient finds little fellowship with that individual.

Ritual and Practice. Assessing the use of rituals and practices helps nurses understand a patient's spirituality. Rituals include participation in worship, prayer, sacraments (e.g., baptism, Holy Eucharist), fasting, singing, meditating, scripture reading, and making offerings or sacrifices. Different religions have different rituals for life events. For example, Buddhists practice baptism later in life and find burial or cremation acceptable at death. Muslims wash the body of a dead family member and wrap it in white cloth with the head turned toward the right shoulder. Orthodox and Conservative Jews circumcise their newborn sons 8 days after birth. Determine whether illness or hospitalization has interrupted a patient's usual rituals or practices. A ritual often provides the patient with structure and support during difficult times. If rituals are important to the patient, use them as part of nursing intervention.

Vocation. Individuals express their spirituality on a daily basis in life routines, work, play, and relationships. Spirituality is often a part of a person's identity and vocation in life. Determine if illness or hospitalization alters the ability to express some aspect of spirituality as it relates to the person's work or daily activities. Expression of spirituality is highly individual and includes showing an appreciation for life in the variety of things people do, living in the moment and not worrying about tomorrow, appreciating nature, expressing love toward others, and being productive. When illness or loss prevents patients from expressing their spirituality, understand the psychological, social, and spiritual implications and provide appropriate guidance and support.

Building Competency in Patient-Centered Care You are caring for Grace, a 52-year-old who experienced multiple fractures following a motor vehicle crash. Grace is experiencing difficulties with mobility and she is not going to be able to go back to work for at least 6 months. She is currently having extensive rehabilitation to help her complete activities of daily living. When you walk into Grace's room, she will not look at you. You can tell that she has been crying. She has a flat affect and states, "I just don't know why God did this to me. How am I going to go on from here?"

Identify at least three questions you will ask Grace to assess her spiritual well-being and plan effective, evidence-based care.

Answers to questions can be found on the Evolve website.

NURSING DIAGNOSIS

A spiritual assessment allows a nurse to learn a great deal about the patient and the extent that spirituality plays in his or her life. Exploring the patient's spirituality sometimes reveals responses to health problems that require nursing intervention or the existence of a strong set of resources that allow the patient to cope effectively. Analyze data to find patterns of defining characteristics and select appropriate nursing diagnoses (Box 35-4). In identifying diagnoses, recognize the significance that spirituality has for all types of health problems. Be sure that each diagnosis has an accurate related factor to guide the selection of individualized, purposeful, and goal-directed interventions. Potential nursing diagnoses for spiritual health include the following:

- Anxiety
- Ineffective coping
- Fear
- Complicated grieving
- Hopelessness
- Powerlessness
- Readiness for enhanced spiritual well-being
- Spiritual distress
- Risk for spiritual distress

Three nursing diagnoses accepted by NANDA International (2011) pertain specifically to spirituality. *Readiness for enhanced spiritual*

BOX 35-4 NURSING DIAGNOSTIC PROCESS

Readiness for Enhanced Spiritual Well-Being

ASSESSMENT ACTIVITIES	DEFINING CHARACTERISTICS
Ask patient to describe personal source of faith and hope.	Patient expresses an inner strength and source of guidance.
Have patient describe level of satisfaction with life.	Life has purpose and meaning; patient finds satisfaction while providing community service as a volunteer.
Determine who provides the greatest source of strength and support to the patient during times of difficulty.	Patient pursues interactions with friends and family.

well-being is based on defining characteristics that show a person's ability to experience and integrate meaning and purpose in life through connectedness with self and others. A patient with this nursing diagnosis has potential resources on which to draw when faced with illness or a threat to well-being. If the patient does not know how to engage personal resources to cope with health problems, offer support in exploring options.

The nursing diagnoses of *spiritual distress* and *risk for spiritual distress* create different clinical pictures. Defining characteristics from a nurse's assessment reveal patterns that reflect a person's actual or potential dispiritedness (e.g., expressing lack of hope, meaning, or purpose in life; anger toward God; or verbalizing conflicts about personal beliefs). Patients likely to be at risk for spiritual distress include those who have poor relationships, have experienced a recent loss, or are suffering some form of mental or physical illness.

Accurate selection of diagnoses requires critical thinking. Review all concrete data (e.g., religious rituals and sources of fellowship), your assessment of previous patient experiences, your own spirituality, and your appraisal of the patient's spiritual well-being. Validate and clarify defining characteristics with the patient before making a diagnosis and plan of care. Commonly patients have multiple nursing diagnoses.

PLANNING

During the planning step of the nursing process, develop a plan of care for each of the patient's nursing diagnoses. Critical thinking at this step is important because you reflect on previous experiences and apply knowledge and critical thinking attitudes and standards in selecting the most appropriate nursing interventions (Fig. 35-4). Prior experience with other patients is valuable when selecting interventions to support spiritual well-being. Integrate assessment data with knowledge about resources and therapies available for spiritual care to develop an individualized plan of care (see the Nursing Care Plan). Match the patient's needs with evidence-based interventions that are supported and recommended in the clinical and research literature. Use a concept map (Fig. 35-5) to organize patient care and show how the patient's medical diagnosis, assessment data, and nursing diagnoses are interrelated.

Confidence, an important critical thinking attitude, builds trust, enabling you and a patient to enter into a healing relationship together. Attempting to meet or support patients' spiritual needs is not simple; frequently you need additional resources. For example,

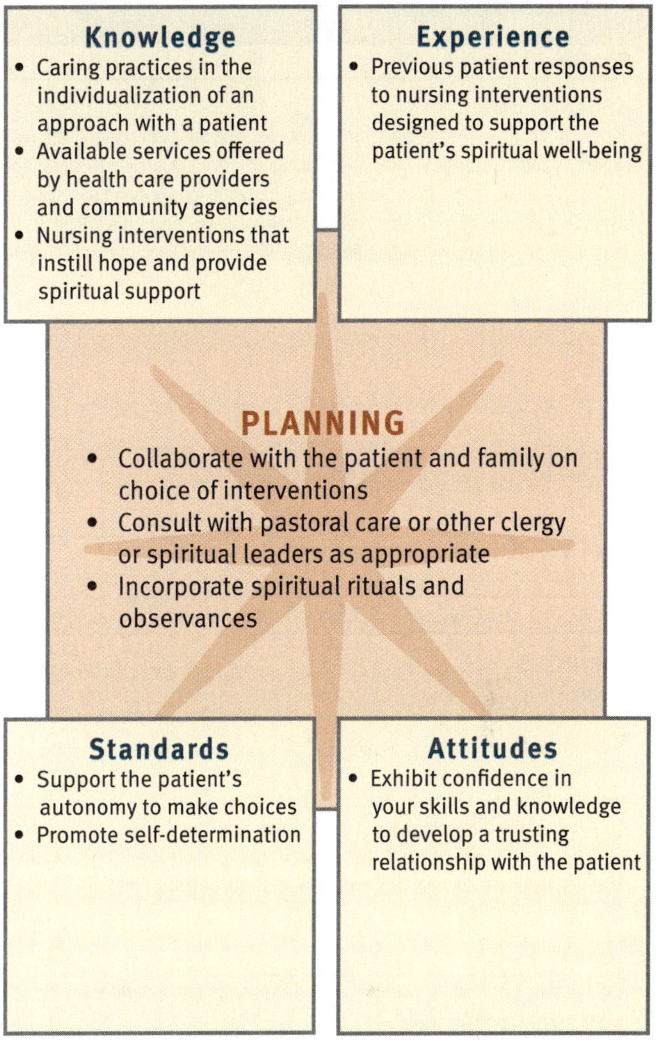

Knowledge
• Caring practices in the individualization of an approach with a patient
• Available services offered by health care providers and community agencies
• Nursing interventions that instill hope and provide spiritual support
Experience
• Previous patient responses to nursing interventions designed to support the patient's spiritual well-being
PLANNING
• Collaborate with the patient and family on choice of interventions
• Consult with pastoral care or other clergy or spiritual leaders as appropriate
• Incorporate spiritual rituals and observances
Standards
• Support the patient's autonomy to make choices
• Promote self-determination
Attitudes
• Exhibit confidence in your skills and knowledge to develop a trusting relationship with the patient

FIG. 35-4 Critical thinking model for spiritual health planning.

sometimes a nurse's skills in helping patients interpret and understand the meaning of illness and loss are limited. Because spiritual care is so personal, standards of autonomy and self-determination are critical in supporting the patient's decisions about the plan of care.

Goals and Outcomes. A spiritual care plan includes realistic and individualized goals along with relevant outcomes. It is important to collaborate closely with patients when setting goals and choosing related interventions. Setting realistic goals requires you to know a patient well. When spiritual care requires helping patients adjust to loss or stressful life situations, goals are long term. However, short-term outcomes such as renewing participation in religious practices help the patient progressively reach a more spiritually healthy situation. In establishing a plan of care, an example of a goal and associated outcomes follows:

The patient will improve personal harmony and connections with members of his or her support system.

- The patient will express an acceptance of illness.
- The patient will report the ability to rely on family members for support.
- The patient will initiate social interactions with family and friends.

Setting Priorities. Spiritual care is very personalized. Your relationship with a patient allows you to understand the patient's

NURSING CARE PLAN

Spiritual Distress

ASSESSMENT

Jose Gomez is a 24-year-old Latino who has recently been diagnosed with human immunodeficiency virus (HIV)/acquired immunodeficiency syndrome (AIDS). The clinic nurse, Leah, has been talking with Jose during his last three visits. During clinic visits Jose expresses a fear of dying. His partner, Will, visits Jose at home periodically, but he has been visiting much less often than before the diagnosis. Jose states that he "used to go to a Catholic church" when he was younger and explains that he currently has a poor relationship with his mother and his brother. The nurse practitioner recently told Jose that he is in the end stage of his illness and suggested that he consider hospice care. Leah now talks with Jose in a private conference area.

Assessment Activities	*Findings/Defining Characteristics**
Ask Jose how his illness affects his source of strength or hope.	Jose responds, "**How can God do this to me?** There are moments when I just **feel so angry**. What is going to happen to me?"
Ask Jose who provides the greatest source of support to him in his life.	He begins to cry and admits, "**I feel so alone. Will has not been there** when I need him."
Ask Jose how his illness affected his faith and beliefs.	Jose responds, "My church does not accept homosexuality, so **I don't feel like I fit in** there. I have always had faith in God."

***Defining characteristics** are shown in bold type.

NURSING DIAGNOSIS: Spiritual distress related to terminal illness.

PLANNING

Goals	*Expected Outcomes (NOC)†*
	Dignified Life Closure
Jose will maintain feelings of control as he approaches the end of his life.	Jose will share feelings about dying in 1 week. Jose will initiate contact and begin to heal relationships with his family within 3 weeks.
	Spiritual Health
Jose will establish connections with self, significant others, and God.	Jose will visit with Will in the next 2 weeks to share his thoughts, feelings, and beliefs. Jose will identify and participate in spiritual activities in 1 month.

†Outcome classification labels from Moorhead S et al: *Nursing outcomes classification (NOC),* ed 4, St Louis, 2008, Mosby.

INTERVENTIONS (NIC)‡	RATIONALE
Spiritual Growth Facilitation	
Ask Jose to identify activities that will help heal his body, mind, and spirit.	Spirituality and religious activities often help men who are HIV positive cope with their illness (Hampton, Halkitis, and Mattis, 2010).
Encourage Jose to pray; offer to pray with him.	People who are Latino sometimes pray more frequently than they attend church; prayer often provides spiritual strength (Campesino et al., 2009).
Spiritual Support	
Use therapeutic communication to establish trust and a caring presence.	Providing spiritual care requires caring, compassion, and respect (Tiew and Creedy, 2010).
Encourage Jose to renew his relationships with Will, his mother, and his brother.	The Latino cultural values of *personalismo* and *simpático* (close, personal relationships with others) enhance connection with God (Campesino et al., 2009).
Teach Jose methods of relaxation, meditation, and guided imagery.	Relaxation methods such as relaxation, meditation, and guided imagery help promote quality of life and enhance serenity and dignity in Latino patients who are dying (Elias, Giglio, and Pimenta, 2008) and in patients with HIV (Horowitz, 2010).

‡Intervention classification labels from Bulechek GM, Butcher HK, Dochterman JM: *Nursing interventions classification (NIC),* ed 5, St Louis, 2008, Mosby.

priorities. When establishing a mutually agreed-on plan with the patient, he or she is able to identify what is most important. Spiritual priorities do not need to be sacrificed for physical care priorities. For example, when a patient is in acute distress, focus care to provide the patient a sense of control. When a patient is terminally ill, spiritual care often is the most important nursing intervention.

Teamwork and Collaboration. If the patient participates in a formal religion, involve members of the clergy or members of the church, temple, mosque, or synagogue in the plan of care. In a

NURSING CARE PLAN

***Spiritual Distress*—cont'd**

EVALUATION

Nursing Actions	*Patient Response/Finding*	*Achievement of Outcome*
Ask Jose how he currently feels about having end-stage AIDS.	"I am not quite as frightened as I was a few weeks ago."	Jose reports an improved outlook. Expect continued fears about dying.
Ask Jose about his relationships with Will, his mother, and his brother.	"It meant a great deal to tell Will and my family how I feel. They did not know how to help me. We now talk on the phone almost every day."	Jose successfully increased connection with significant others.
Ask Jose which spiritual activities he finds helpful.	"I have been praying and have been using the breathing techniques you taught me every day. They have helped me feel better about myself and my situation. I don't feel so angry anymore."	Prayer and relaxation activities have enhanced positive feelings about self and reduced feelings of anger.

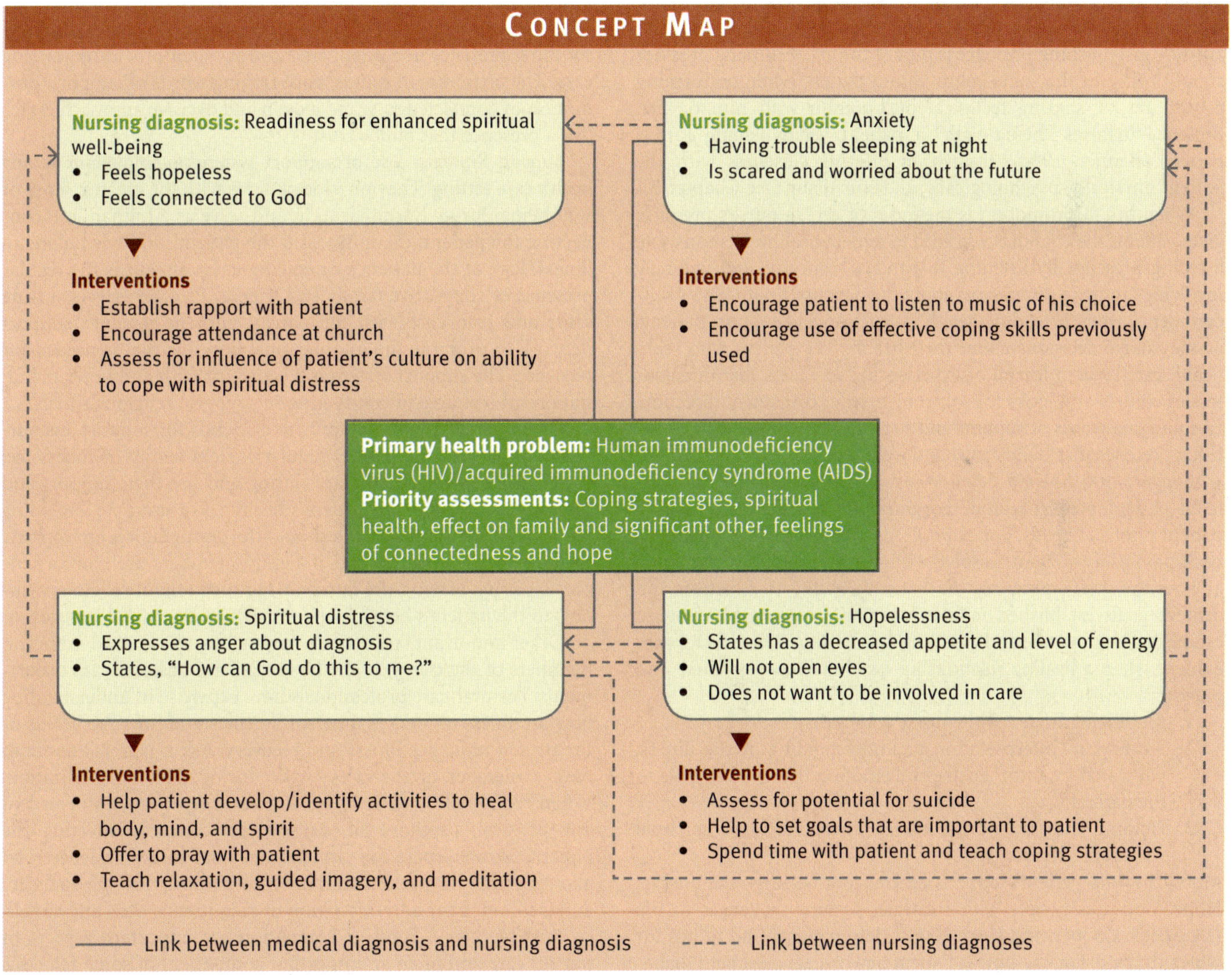

FIG. 35-5 Concept map for Jose Gomez.

hospital setting the pastoral-care department is a valuable resource. These professionals provide insight about how and when to best support patients and their families. In addition, significant others such as spouses, siblings, parents, and friends need to be involved in the patient's care as appropriate. This means that the nurse learns from the assessment which individuals or groups have formed a relationship with the patient. These individuals sometimes become involved in all levels of the nurse's plan. They often assist in giving physical care, providing emotional comfort, and sharing spiritual support.

IMPLEMENTATION

Establish caring relationships with patients to discover their beliefs about the meaning of illness or loss and the effect they have on the meaning and purpose of life. Achieving this level of understanding with patients enables you to deliver care in a sensitive, creative, and appropriate manner.

Health Promotion. Spiritual care needs to be a central theme in promoting an individual's overall well-being (Lopez et al., 2009). Spirituality is one personal resource that affects the balance between health and illness. In settings where health promotion activities occur, patients often need information, counseling, and guidance to make the necessary choices to remain healthy.

Establishing Presence. Nurses contribute to a sense of well-being and provide hope for recovery when they spend time with their patients (Tiew and Creedy, 2010). Behaviors that establish the nurse's presence include paying attention, answering questions, listening, and having a positive and encouraging (but realistic) attitude. Establishing presence is part of the art of nursing. It is not simply being in the same room with a patient while performing procedures or sharing technical information with him or her. Presence involves "being with" a patient versus "doing for" a patient (Benner, 1984). It involves offering closeness with the patient physically, psychologically, and spiritually (see Chapter 7).

When health promotion is the focus of care, a nurse's presence gives patients the confidence needed to remain healthy. Demonstrate a caring presence by listening to patients' concerns and willingly involving family in discussions about the patients' health. Show self-confidence when providing health instruction and support patients as they make decisions about their health. The patient who seeks health care is often fearful of experiencing an illness that threatens loss of control and looks for someone to offer competent direction. Encouraging words of support and a calm, decisive approach establish a presence that builds trust and well-being.

Supporting a Healing Relationship. Learn to look beyond isolated patient problems and recognize the broader picture of a patient's holistic needs. For example, do not just look at a patient's back pain as a problem to solve with quick remedies; rather look at how the pain influences the patient's ability to function and achieve goals established in life. A **holistic** view enables you to establish a helping role and a healing relationship. Three factors are evident when a healing relationship develops between nurse and patient:

1. Mobilizing hope for the nurse and patient
2. Finding an interpretation or understanding of the illness, pain, anxiety, or other stressful emotion that is acceptable to the patient
3. Helping the patient use social, emotional, and spiritual resources (Benner, 1984)

Mobilizing the patient's hope is central to a healing relationship. Hope motivates people with strategies to face challenges in life (Duggleby, Cooper, and Penz, 2009). Help patients find things for which to hope. For example, a patient newly diagnosed with diabetes wants to learn how to manage the disease to continue a productive and satisfying way of life. An adult daughter who has decided to become caregiver to her older adult parent hopes to be able to protect the parent from injury or worsening disability. Hope helps a patient work toward recovery. To help patients achieve hope, work together to find an explanation of the situation that is acceptable to the patient. Help the patient realistically exercise hope by supporting a positive attitude toward life or a desire to be informed and make decisions.

To further support a healing relationship, remain aware of the patient's spiritual resources and needs. It is always important for patients to be able to express and exercise their beliefs and find spiritual comfort. When life stressors or illness create confusion or uncertainty, recognize the possible effect on a patient's well-being. How does the nurse use and strengthen spiritual resources? Begin by encouraging a patient to discuss the effect that illness has had on personal beliefs and faith, thus giving the chance to clarify any misconceptions or inaccuracies in information. Having a clear sense of what illness will be like for an individual helps the person to apply all resources toward recovery.

Acute Care. Within acute care settings patients experience multiple stressors that threaten their sense of control. Ongoing assessment of spiritual needs is essential because the patient's needs often change rapidly (Smith, 2006). Support and enhancement of a patient's spiritual well-being are challenges when the focus of health care seems to be on treatment and cure rather than care (Tiew and Creedy, 2010). To overcome these challenges display a soothing presence and supportive touch when providing nursing care. The artful use of hands, encouraging words of support, promotion of connectedness, and a calm and decisive approach establish a presence that builds trust.

Support Systems. Use of support systems is important in any health care setting. They provide patients with the greatest sense of well-being during hospitalization and serve as a human link connecting the patient, the nurse, and the patient's lifestyle before an illness. Part of the patient's caregiving environment is the regular presence of supportive family and friends. Provide privacy during visits and plan care with the patient and the patient's support network to promote the interpersonal bonding that is needed for recovery. The support system is a source of faith and hope and an important resource in conducting meaningful religious rituals.

When patients look to family and friends for support, encourage them to visit the patient regularly. Help family members feel comfortable in the health care setting and use their support and presence to promote the patient's healing. For example, including family members in prayer is a thoughtful gesture if it is appropriate to the patient's religion and if family members are comfortable participating. Having the family bring meaningful religious symbols to the patient's bedside offers significant spiritual support.

Other important resources to patients are spiritual advisors and members of the clergy. Many hospitals have pastoral-care departments. Pastoral-care professionals have expertise in understanding how an illness influences a person's beliefs and how the beliefs of the person influence illness and recovery. Ask if patients desire to have a member of the clergy visit during their hospitalization. When requested by patients or families, keep clergy informed of any physical, psychosocial, or spiritual concerns affecting the patient. Show respect for patients' spiritual values and needs by allowing time for pastoral-care members to provide spiritual care and facilitating the administration of sacraments, rites, and rituals.

Diet Therapies. Food and nutrition are important aspects of patient care and often an important component of some religious observances (Table 35-2). Food and the rituals surrounding the preparation and serving of food are sometimes important to a person's spirituality. Consult with a dietitian to integrate patients' dietary preferences into daily care. In the event that a hospital or other health care agency cannot prepare food in the preferred way, ask the family to bring meals that fit into dietary restrictions posed by the patient's condition.

Supporting Rituals. Nurses provide spiritual care by supporting patients' participation in spiritual rituals and activities. Plan care

TABLE 35-2 **Religious Dietary Regulations Affecting Health Care**

RELIGION	DIETARY PRACTICES
Hinduism	Some sects are vegetarians. The belief is not to kill *any* living creature.
Buddhism	Some are vegetarians and do not use alcohol. Many fast on Holy Days.
Islam	Consumption of pork and alcohol is prohibited. Followers fast during the month of Ramadan.
Judaism	Some observe the kosher dietary restrictions (e.g., avoid pork and shellfish, do not prepare and eat milk and meat at the same time).
Christianity	Some Baptists, Evangelicals, and Pentecostals discourage the use of alcohol and caffeine. Some Roman Catholics fast on Ash Wednesday and Good Friday. Some do not eat meat on Fridays during Lent.
Jehovah's Witnesses	Members avoid food prepared with or containing blood.
Mormonism	Members abstain from alcohol and caffeine.
Russian Orthodox Church	Followers observe fast days and a "no meat" rule on Wednesdays and Fridays. During Lent all animal products, including dairy products and butter, are forbidden.
Native Americans	Individual tribal beliefs influence food practices.

to allow time for religious readings, spiritual visitations, or attendance at religious services. Allow family members to plan a prayer session or an organized reading of scriptures on a regular basis. Make arrangements with pastoral-care staff for the patient and family to participate in religious practices (e.g., receiving sacraments). Clergy often visit people who are unable to attend religious services. Taped meditations, classical or religious music, and televised religious services provide other effective options. The nurse respects icons, medals, prayer rugs, or crosses that patients bring to a health setting and ensures they are not accidentally lost, damaged, or misplaced. Supporting spiritual rituals is especially important for older adults (Box 35-5).

Restorative and Continuing Care. For patients who are recovering from a long-term illness or disability or who suffer chronic or terminal disease, spiritual care becomes especially important. Many of the nursing interventions applicable in health promotion and acute care apply to this level of health care as well.

Prayer. Prayer offers an opportunity to renew personal faith and belief in a higher being in a specific, focused way that is either highly ritualized and formal or quite spontaneous and informal. It is an effective coping resource for physical and psychological symptoms (Hollywell and Walker, 2009). Patients pray in private or pursue opportunities for group prayer with family, friends, or clergy. Nurses are supportive of prayer by giving patients privacy, suggesting prayer when they know that patients use it as a coping resource, and participating in prayer with patients. If prayer is not suitable for a patient, alternatives include listening to music or reading a book, poetry, or other inspirational texts selected by the patient.

Meditation. Meditation effectively creates a relaxation response that reduces daily stress. It reduces blood pressure, reduces stress and pain, and enhances the function of the immune system (Horowitz, 2009). Nurses often use guided imagery to help patients learn meditation (see Chapter 32). When patients use meditation in conjunction with their spiritual beliefs, they often report an increased spirituality that they commonly describe as experiencing the presence of a power, force, or energy or what was perceived as God (Box 35-6).

Supporting Grief Work. Patients who experience terminal illness or who have suffered permanent loss in body function because of a disabling disease or injury require the nurse's support in grieving

BOX 35-5 **FOCUS ON OLDER ADULTS**

Spirituality and Spiritual Health

- There is an association between an older adult's spirituality and his or her ability to adjust or cope with illness (Ebersole et al., 2008).
- Religious activities and spiritual experiences are very common among older adults. Those who experience spiritual well-being have strong social support and better physical and psychological health (Stranahan, 2008).
- Respecting privacy and dignity is an essential part of nursing care, especially when meeting spiritual needs of the older adult (Ellis and Narayanasamy, 2009).
- Many patients use a variety of strategies such as spiritual rituals, exercise, and complementary medicine to cope with pain and chronic illness. Including religious activities and meditation positively enhances coping and feelings of peace (Narayansamy, 2007).
- Feelings of connectedness are important for the older adult (Anderberg and Berglund, 2010). Enhance connectedness by helping older patients find meaning and purpose in life, listening actively to concerns, and being present.
- Beliefs in the afterlife increase as adults grow older. Make visits from clergy, social workers, lawyers, and financial advisors available so patients feel as though they have completed all unfinished business. Leaving a legacy to loved ones prepares the older adult to leave the world with a sense of meaning (Ebersole et al., 2008). Legacies include oral histories, works of art, publications, photographs, or other objects of significance.
- Older-adult caregivers often use their spirituality and spiritual behaviors or practices to help them deal with crisis and conflict (Strudwick, 2010).

BOX 35-6 **PATIENT TEACHING**

Meditation Techniques

Objective

- The patient will verbalize feelings of relaxation and self-transcendence after meditation.

Teaching Strategies

- Provide patient a brief description of information and a printed teaching guide that describes how to meditate.
- Help patient identify a quiet room in the home that has minimal interruptions.
- Explain that peaceful music or the quiet whirring of a fan blocks out distractions.
- Teach steps of meditation—sit in a comfortable position with the back straight; breathe slowly; and focus on a sound, prayer, or image.
- Encourage patient to meditate for 10 to 20 minutes twice a day.
- Answer questions and reinforce information as needed.

Evaluation

- Have patient describe feelings following meditation.

over and coping with their loss. Chapter 36 summarizes interventions to use in grief work. Your ability to enter into a therapeutic and spiritual relationship with patients supports them during times of grief.

EVALUATION

Through the Patient's Eyes. The evaluation of a patient's spiritual care requires you to think critically in determining if efforts at restoring or maintaining the patient's spiritual health were successful (Fig. 35-6). Include the patient in your evaluation of care. Outcomes established during the planning phase serve as the standards to evaluate the patient's progress. Ask him or her if you and the health care team met their expectations and if there is anything else you can do to enhance their spiritual well-being. In addition, evaluate ethical concerns that arise in the course of the patient's spiritual care and support. Apply critical thinking attitudes and use therapeutic communication techniques to ensure sound nursing judgments.

Patient Outcomes. Attaining spiritual health is a lifelong goal. In evaluating outcomes, compare the patient's level of spiritual health with the behaviors and perceptions noted in the nursing assessment. Evaluation data related to spiritual health are usually subjective. For example, if a nurse's assessment finds the patient losing hope, the follow-up evaluation involves asking the patient if feelings of hope have been restored. Include family and friends when gathering evaluative information. Successful outcomes reveal the patient developing an increased or restored sense of connectedness with family; maintaining, renewing, or reforming a sense of purpose in life; and for some a confidence and trust in a Supreme Being or power. When outcomes are not met, ask questions to determine appropriate continuing care. Examples of questions to ask include the following:

- Do you feel the need to forgive someone or to be forgiven by someone?
- What spiritual activities such as prayer or meditation were helpful in the past?
- Would you like for me to ask a friend, family member, or someone from pastoral care to talk with you?
- What can I do to help you feel more at peace?
- Sometimes people need to give themselves permission to feel hope when they experience difficult events. What can you do to allow yourself to feel hope again?

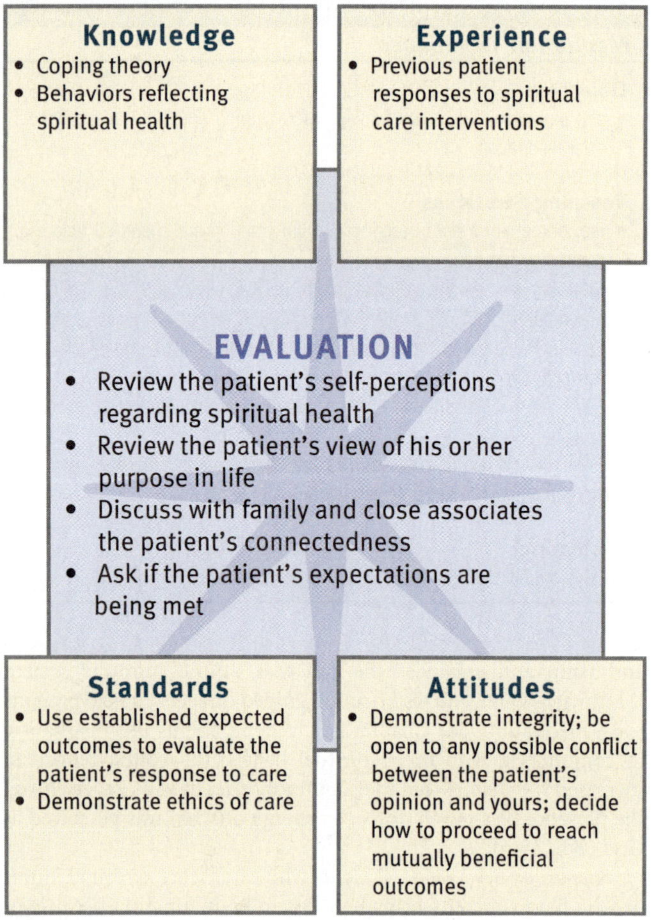

Knowledge
• Coping theory
• Behaviors reflecting spiritual health
Experience
• Previous patient responses to spiritual care interventions
EVALUATION
• Review the patient's self-perceptions regarding spiritual health
• Review the patient's view of his or her purpose in life
• Discuss with family and close associates the patient's connectedness
• Ask if the patient's expectations are being met
Standards
• Use established expected outcomes to evaluate the patient's response to care
• Demonstrate ethics of care
Attitudes
• Demonstrate integrity; be open to any possible conflict between the patient's opinion and yours; decide how to proceed to reach mutually beneficial outcomes

FIG. 35-6 Critical thinking model for spiritual health evaluation.

KEY POINTS

- Attending to a patient's spirituality ensures a holistic focus to nursing practice.
- Beneficial health outcomes occur when individuals are able to exercise their spiritual beliefs.
- Frequently spirituality and religion are interchanged, but spirituality is a much broader and more unifying concept than religion.
- Spirituality is highly personal and unique to each individual.
- Faith and hope are closely linked to a person's spiritual well-being, providing an inner strength for dealing with illness and disability.
- When patients experience acute or chronic illness or a terminal disease, spiritual resources either help them move to recovery, or spiritual distress develops.
- A spiritual assessment is most successful when the nurse applies knowledge that is relevant to therapeutic communication, principles of loss and grief, and knowledge of caring practices.
- The personal nature of spirituality requires open communication and the establishment of trust between nurse and patient.
- Nurses need to determine if a patient's religious beliefs conflict with medical treatment.
- An important part of spiritual assessment is learning who makes up the patient's community of faith.
- Establishing presence involves giving attention, answering questions, having an encouraging attitude, and expressing a sense of trust.
- Connectedness and fellowship with other persons are a source of hope for a patient.
- Part of a patient's caregiving environment is the regular presence of family, friends, and spiritual advisors.
- Prayer is an effective coping resource for physical and psychological symptoms.
- When evaluating spiritual care, successful outcomes reveal the patient developing an increased or restored sense of connectedness with family and maintaining, renewing, or reforming a sense of purpose in life.

CLINICAL APPLICATION QUESTIONS

Preparing for Clinical Practice

1. Jose continues to regularly visit the human immunodeficiency virus (HIV)/acquired immunodeficiency syndrome (AIDS) clinic. The nurse wants to incorporate a spiritual assessment

with the physical assessment. During the assessment the nurse asks Jose if he has any questions. Jose asks her about a Buddhist ritual that he heard about from a friend. The nurse has not heard about that ritual before and states, "I'm not sure what you're asking about. After we're finished here, I'll try to get some information for you." In this interaction the nurse is exhibiting the attitude for critical thinking known as ________.

2. Jose's mother comes with Jose to a clinic visit. During the visit the nurse asks Jose's mother, "Which spiritual activities are part of your life?" Jose's mother responds that she goes to daily Mass, listens to religious music, and spends time praying while she sits in her garden. When asked if there is anything the nurse can do for Jose's mother, she responds that she would like to meet with a priest while she is visiting Jose. She then states, "My biggest concern is remaining strong for Jose. It is so hard to watch your child die." Which nursing diagnosis is appropriate for Jose's mother at this time?
3. Jose is too ill to come to the clinic. He now is being seen every other day by the hospice team. Jose's family and his partner, Will, are at his side. Describe two nursing interventions the hospice nurse could implement to enhance the family's connectedness.

evolve *Answers to Clinical Application Questions can be found on the Evolve website.*

REVIEW QUESTIONS

Are You Ready to Test Your Nursing Knowledge?

1. An emergency department nurse is caring for a patient who was severely injured in a car accident. The patient's family is in the waiting room. They are crying softly. The nurse sits down next to the family, takes the mother's hand, and says, "I can only imagine how you're feeling. What can I do to help you feel more at peace right now?" In this example the nurse is demonstrating:
   1. Prayer.
   2. Presence.
   3. Coaching.
   4. Instilling hope.
2. A patient states that he does not believe in the existence of God. This patient most likely is an:
   1. Academic.
   2. Atheist.
   3. Agnostic.
   4. Anarchist.
3. As the nurse cares for a patient in an outpatient clinic, the patient states that he recently lost his position as a volunteer coordinator at a local community center. He expresses that he is angry with his former boss and with God. The nurse knows that the priority at this time is to assess the patient's spirituality in relation to his:
   1. Vocation.
   2. Life satisfaction.
   3. Fellowship and community.
   4. Connectedness with his family and co-workers.
4. A patient who is hospitalized with heart failure states that she sees her illness as an opportunity and a challenge. Despite her illness, she is still able to see that life is worth living. This is an example of:
   1. Hope.
   2. Faith.
   3. Values.
   4. Connectedness.
5. Which of the following statements made by an older adult whose husband recently died most indicates the need for follow-up by the nurse?
   1. "I planted a tree at church in my husband's honor."
   2. "I have been unable to talk with my children lately."
   3. "My friends think that I need to go to a grief support group."
   4. "I believe that someday I'll meet my husband in heaven."
6. Which of the following nursing interventions support(s) a healing relationship with a patient? (Select all that apply):
   1. Praying with the patient
   2. Giving pain medications before a painful procedure
   3. Telling a patient that it is time to take a bath before family arrive to visit
   4. Making the patient's bed following hospital protocol
   5. Helping a patient see positive aspects related to a chronic illness
7. A patient expresses the desire to learn how to meditate. What does the nurse need to do first?
   1. Answer the patient's questions
   2. Help the patient get into a comfortable position
   3. Select a teaching environment that is free from distractions
   4. Encourage the patient to meditate for 10 to 20 minutes 2 times a day
8. An older adult is receiving hospice care. Which nursing intervention(s) help the patient cope with feelings related to death and dying? (Select all that apply.)
   1. Teaching the patient how to use guided imagery
   2. Encouraging the family to visit the patient frequently
   3. Taking the patient's vital signs every time the nurse visits
   4. Teaching the patient how to manage pain and take pain medications
   5. Helping the patient put significant photographs in a scrap-book for the family
9. Which of the following questions would best assess a patient's level of connectedness?
   1. What gives your life meaning?
   2. Which aspects of your spirituality would you like to discuss right now?
   3. Who do you consider to be the most important person in your life at this time?
   4. How do you feel about the accomplishments you've made in your life so far?
10. A nurse is using the B-E-L-I-E-F tool to complete a spiritual assessment on a 12-year-old male who has recently been diagnosed with acute lymphocytic leukemia. Which of the following questions would the nurse use to assess the child's involvement in the spiritual community?
    1. Which church do you attend?
    2. Which sports do you like to play?
    3. Are there any foods you cannot eat?
    4. In which church activities do you participate?
11. A nurse is caring for a patient who refuses to eat until after the sun sets. Which religion does this patient most likely practice?
    1. Islam
    2. Sikhism
    3. Hinduism
    4. Catholicism

12. A Catholic patient with diabetes receives the following items on his meal tray on the Friday before Easter. For which of the foods does the nurse offer to substitute?
    1. Apple sauce
    2. Cheese and crackers
    3. Spaghetti with meat sauce
    4. Tossed salad with ranch dressing
13. A nurse is working in a health clinic on a Navajo reservation. He or she plans care for the patients knowing which of the following is true?
    1. The patients may not be on time for their appointments.
    2. The patients most likely do not trust the doctors and nurses.
    3. The patients probably are not comfortable if they have to remove their undergarments.
    4. Terminally ill patients probably want to receive the sacrament, the anointing of the sick.
14. A 62-year-old male patient has just been told he has a terminal illness. Which of the following statements supports a nursing diagnosis of *spiritual distress related to diagnosis of terminal illness?*
    1. "I have nothing to live for now."
    2. "What will happen to my wife when I die?"
    3. "How much longer do I have to live?"
    4. "I need to go to church and pray for a miracle."
15. Which of the following would be the most appropriate outcome for a patient who has a nursing diagnosis of *spiritual distress related to loneliness?*
    1. Encourage the patient to meditate 2 to 3 times a week.
    2. The patient will set up a time to speak to a close friend in 1 week.
    3. Encourage the patient to phone his brother and set up a time to go out for dinner.
    4. The patient will experience greater connections with family members in 2 months.

Answers: **1.** 2; **2.** 2; **3.** 1; **4.** 1; **5.** 2; **6.** 1, 5; **7.** 3; **8.** 1, 2, 5; **9.** 3; **10.** 4; **11.** 1; **12.** 3; **13.** 1; **14.** 1; **15.** 2.

REFERENCES

Alcorn SR, et al: "If God wanted me yesterday, I wouldn't be here today": religious and spiritual themes in patients' experiences of advanced cancer, *J Palliat Med* 13(5):581, 2010.

Benner P: *From novice to expert*, Menlo Park, Calif, 1984, Addison-Wesley.

Centers for Disease Control and Prevention (CDC): *Chronic diseases and health promotion*, 2010, www.cdc.gov/chronicdisease/overview/index.htm. Accessed August 21, 2011.

Dolamo BL: Spiritual nursing, *Nurs Update* 34(4):22, 2010.

Duffy N: Supporting a patient after a near-death experience, *Nursing* 37(4):46, 2007.

Ebersole P, et al: *Toward healthy aging: human needs and nursing response*, ed 7, St Louis, 2008, Mosby.

Edelman CL, Mandle CL: *Health promotion throughout the life span*, ed 7, St Louis, 2010, Mosby.

Fowler MDM: *Guide to the code of ethics for nurses: interpretation and application*, Silver Spring, Md, 2010, American Nurses Association.

Gray J: Measuring spirituality: conceptual and methodological considerations, *J Theory Construction Testing* 10(2):58, 2006.

Horowitz S: Health benefits of meditation: what the newest research shows, *Altern Complement Ther* 16(4):223, 2010.

Lundman B, et al: Inner strength: a theoretical analysis of salutogenic concepts, *Int J Nurs Stud* 47(2):251, 2010.

McEvoy M: Culture and spirituality as an integrated concept in pediatric care, *MCN Am J Matern Child Nurs* 28(1):39, 2003.

McSherry W: *The meaning of spirituality and spiritual care within nursing and health care practice*, London, 2007, Quay Books.

Mueller CR: Spirituality in children: understanding and developing interventions, *Pediatr Nurs* 36(4):197, 2010.

NANDA International: *NANDA-I nursing diagnoses: definitions and classification 2012-2014*, Philadelphia, 2012, The Association.

Narayanasamy A: Palliative care and spirituality, *Indian J Palliat Care* 13(2):32, 2007.

Nelson-Becker H, Nakashima M, Canda ER: Spiritual assessment in aging: a framework for clinicians, *J Gerontol Soc Work* 48(3/4):331, 2007.

Pesut B, et al: Conceptualising spirituality and religion for healthcare, *J Clin Nurs* 17:2803, 2008.

Smith AR: Using the synergy model to provide spiritual nursing care in critical care settings, *Crit Care Nurse* 26(4):41, 2006.

Smith S: Toward a flexible framework for understanding spirituality, *Occupational Ther Health Care* 22(1):39, 2008.

Smith J, McSherry W: Spirituality and child development: a concept analysis, *J Adv Nurs* 45(3):307, 2004.

The Joint Commission (TJC): *Standards FAQ details*, 2010, http://www.jointcommission.org/standards_information/jcfaqdetails.aspx?StandardsFaqId=290&ProgramId=1. Accessed August 21, 2011.

Vachon M, Fillion L, Achille M: A conceptual analysis of spirituality at the end of life, *J Palliat Med* 21(1):53, 2009.

Wasserman LS: Respectful death: a model for end-of-life care, *Clin J Oncol Nurs* 12(4):621, 2008.

Wilkins A, Mailoo VJ, Kularatne U: Care of the older person: a Buddhist perspective, *Nurs Residential Care* 12(6):295, 2010.

Yeager S et al: Embrace hope: an end-of-life intervention to support neurological critical care patients and their families, *Crit Care Nurs* 30(1):47, 2010.

RESEARCH REFERENCES

Anderberg P, Berglund A: Elderly persons' experiences of striving to receive care on their own terms in nursing homes, *Int J Nurs Pract* 16(1):64, 2010.

Bailey ME, et al: Creating a spiritual tapestry: nurses' experiences of delivering spiritual care to patients in an Irish hospice, *Int J Palliat Nurs* 15(9):42, 2009.

Burris JL, et al: Factors associated with the psychological well-being and distress of university students, *J Am Coll Health* 57(5):536, 2009.

Campesino M, et al: Spirituality and cultural identification among Latino and non-Latino college students, *Hispanic Health Care Int* 7(2):72, 2009.

Casida J, Lemanski SA: An evidence-based review on guided imagery utilization in adult cardiac surgery, *Clin Scholars Rev* 3(1):22, 2010.

Chism LA, Magnan MA: The relationship of nursing students' spiritual care perspectives to their expressions of spiritual empathy, *J Nurs Educ* 48(11):597, 2009.

Choi G, Tirrito T, Mills F: Caregiver's spirituality and its influence on maintaining the elderly and disabled in a home environment, *J Gerontol Soc Work* 51(3-4):247, 2008.

Daaleman TP, Dobbs D: Religiosity, spirituality, and death attitudes in chronically ill older adults, *Res Aging* 32(2):224, 2010.

Duggleby W, Cooper D, Penz K: Hope, self-efficacy, spiritual well-being and job satisfaction, *J Adv Nurs* 65(11):2376, 2009.

Ebadi A, et al: Spirituality: a key factor in coping among Iranians chronically affected by mustard gas in the disaster of war, *Nurs Health Sci* 11(4):344, 2009.

Elias ACA, Giglio JS, Pimenta CAM: Analysis of the nature of spiritual pain in terminal patients and the process through the resignification relaxation, mental images and spirituality (RIME) intervention, *Rev Lat Am Enfermagem* 16(6):959, 2008.

Ellis HK, Narayanasamy A: An investigation into the role of spirituality in nursing, *Br J Nurs* 18(14):886, 2009.

Ford D, et al: Factors associated with illness perception among critically ill patients and surrogates, *CHEST* 138(1):59, 2010.

Gallia KS, Pines EW: Narrative identity and spirituality of African American churchwomen surviving breast cancer survivors, *J Cult Diversity* 16(2):50, 2009.

Hampton MC, Halkitis PN, Mattis JS: Coping, drug use, and religiosity/spirituality in relation to HIV serostatus among gay and bisexual men, *AIDS Educ Prev* 22(5):417, 2010.

Hanson LC, et al: Providers and types of spiritual care during serious illness, *J Palliat Med* 11(6):907, 2008.

Harkins LE: Literature analysis of humor therapy research. *Am J Recreation Ther* 8(4):35, 2009.

Herrera AP, et al: Religious coping and caregiver well-being in Mexican-American families, *Aging Ment Health* 13(1):84, 2009.

Hollywell C, Walker J: Private prayer as a suitable intervention for hospitalised patients: a critical review of the literature, *J Clin Nurs* 18(5):637, 2009.

Horowitz S: Effect of positive emotions on health: hope and humor, *Altern Complement Ther* 15(4):196, 2009.

Jurkowski JM, Kurlanska C, Ramos BM: Latino women's spiritual beliefs related to health, *Am J Health Promotion* 25(1):19, 2010.

Katerndahl DA: Impact of spiritual symptoms and their interactions on health services and life satisfaction, *Ann Fam Med* 6(5):412, 2008.

Krause N, Bastida E: Core religious beliefs and providing support to others in late life, *Ment Health Religion Cult* 12(1):75, 2009.

Lahmann C, et al: Effects of functional relaxation and guided imagery on IgE in dust-mite allergic adult asthmatics: a randomized, controlled clinical trial, *J Nerv Ment Dis* 198(2):125, 2010.

Lee CJ: A comparison of health promotion behaviors in rural and urban community-dwelling spousal caregivers, *J Gerontol Nurs* 35(5):34, 2009.

Lopez AJ, et al: Spiritual well-being and practices among women with gynecologic cancer, *Oncol Nurs Forum* 36(3):300, 2009.

Narayanasamy A, et al: Responses to the spiritual needs of older people, *J Adv Nurs* 48(1):6, 2004.

Phillips-Salimi CR, et al: Psychometric properties of the Herth Hope Index in adolescents and young adults with cancer, *J Nurs Measurement* 15(1):3, 2007.

Pierce LL, et al: Spirituality expressed by caregivers of stroke survivors, *West J Nurs Res* 30(5):606, 2008.

Rominger R: Postcards from heaven and hell: understanding the near-death experience through art, *Art Ther* 27(1):18, 2010.

Roscoe LA: Well-being of family caregivers of persons with late-stage Huntington's disease: lessons in stress and coping, *Health Commun* 24(3):239, 2009.

Sanders S, et al: The experience of high levels of grief in caregivers of persons with Alzheimer's disease and related dementia, *Death Studies* 32(6):495, 2008.

Smith-Stoner M: End-of-life preferences for atheists, *J Palliat Med* 10(4):923, 2007.

Stranahan S: A spiritual screening tool for older adults, *J Relig Health* 47:491, 2008.

Strudwick A, Morris R: A qualitative study exploring the experiences of African-Caribbean informal stroke carers in the UK, *Clin Rehabil* 24(2):159, 2010.

Swetz KM, et al: Strategies for avoiding burnout in hospice and palliative medicine: peer advice for physicians on achieving longevity and fulfillment, *J Palliat Med* 12(9):773, 2009.

Tanyi RA, McKenzie M, Chapek C: How family practice physicians, nurse practitioners, and physician assistants incorporate spiritual care in practice, *J Am Acad Nurse Pract* 21(12):690, 2009.

Tiew LH, Creedy DK: Integration of spirituality in nursing practice: a literature review, *Singapore Nurs J* 37(1):15, 2010.

Villagomeza LR: Mending broken hearts: the role of spirituality in cardiac illness: a research synthesis, 1991-2004, *Holist Nurs Pract* 20(4):169, 2006.

Weigensberg MJ, et al: Acute effects of stress-reduction interactive guided imagery (SM) on salivary cortisol in overweight Latino adolescents, *J Altern Complement Med* 15(3):297, 2009.

Whelan-Gales MA, et al: Spiritual well-being, spiritual practices, and depressive symptoms among elderly patients hospitalized with acute heart failure, *Geriatr Nurs* 30(5):312, 2009.

Yampolsky MA, et al: The role of spirituality in coping with visual impairments, *J Vis Impair Blind* 102(1):28, 2008.

CHAPTER

36

The Experience of Loss, Death, and Grief

OBJECTIVES

- Identify the nurse's role when caring for patients who are experiencing loss, grief, or death.
- Describe the types of loss experienced throughout life.
- Discuss grief theories.
- Identify types of grief.
- Describe characteristics of a person experiencing grief.
- Discuss variables that influence a person's response to grief.
- Develop a nursing care plan for a patient and family experiencing loss and grief.
- Identify ways to collaborate with family members and the interdisciplinary team to provide palliative care.
- Describe interventions for symptom management in patients at the end of life.
- Discuss the criteria for hospice care.
- Describe care of the body after death.
- Discuss the nurse's own grief experience when caring for dying patients.
- Identify methods for nurse self-care in grief and loss.

KEY TERMS

Actual loss, p. 709
Ambiguous loss, p. 710
Anticipatory grief, p. 710
Autopsy, p. 724
Bereavement, p. 709
Compassion fatigue, p. 726
Complicated grief, p. 710
Disenfranchised grief, p. 710
Disorganization and despair, p. 710
Grief, p. 709
Hope, p. 712
Hospice, p. 719
Maturational loss, p. 709
Mourning, p. 709
Necessary loss, p. 709
Normal (uncomplicated) grief, p. 709
Numbing, p. 710
Organ and tissue donation, p. 724
Palliative care, p. 719
Postmortem care, p. 724
Perceived loss, p. 709
Reminiscence, p. 711
Reorganization, p. 710
Situational loss, p. 709
Yearning and searching (separation anxiety), p. 710

evolve WEBSITE

http://evolve.elsevier.com/Potter/fundamentals/

- Review Questions
- Concept Map Creator
- Case Study with Questions
- Audio Glossary
- Interactive Learning Activities
- Key Term Flashcards
- Content Updates

Nurses have a primary duty to prevent illness and injury and help patients return to health. They also play a vital role in helping patients and families cope with things that cannot be changed and facilitate a peaceful death. Patients and families need expert nursing care through grief and death, perhaps more than at any other time. Caring for patients at the end of life requires knowledge and caring to bring comfort, even when the hope for cure or continued life is not possible. Although specialized roles and a sophisticated knowledge base for palliative and hospice care nurses have expanded greatly in the last two decades, nurses in all settings (i.e., residential facilities, hospitals, nursing homes, critical care units, and home health) provide most of the care for the seriously ill and dying.

Despite the pervasiveness of serious chronic illness and the high incidence of death in health care settings, many health care professionals feel apprehensive about providing end-of-life care (Weigel et al., 2007). Talking openly about death is discouraged in American society (i.e., in our everyday lives, our language, and even our thinking) (Matzo and Sherman, 2010). Terminal illness reminds friends and family members of their own mortality, which often causes them, sometimes unconsciously, to withdraw from the dying person. Nurses also grieve when witnessing the suffering of others.

You need to know that you are capable of providing the asset most valued by patients and family members at the end of life: a compassionate, attentive, and patient-centered approach to care. With each experience of caring for people at the end of life, you gain more confidence, courage, and compassion to accompany patients and family members through this intimate and meaningful phase of human transition. Your skills and knowledge base develop quickly if you have the desire and willingness to learn, be present, and seek the help needed to learn how to give excellent care at the end of life.

SCIENTIFIC KNOWLEDGE BASE

Loss

Throughout a lifetime people grieve the loss of multiple things: body parts or function, self-esteem, friendships, confidence, or income. Children develop independence from the adults who raise them, begin and leave school, change friends, begin careers, and form new relationships. From birth to death people form attachments and suffer losses. Illness also changes or threatens a person's identity, and at some point everyone dies. People experience loss when another person, possession, body part, familiar environment, or sense of self changes or is no longer present (Table 36-1). The values learned in one's family, religious community, society, and culture shape what a person regards as loss and how to grieve (Walter and McCoyd, 2009).

Life changes are natural and often positive. As people move forward in life, they learn that change always involves a **necessary loss,** which is a part of life. They learn to expect that most necessary losses are eventually replaced by something different or better. However, some losses cause them to undergo permanent changes in their lives and threaten their sense of belonging and security. The death of a loved one, divorce, or loss of independence changes life forever and often significantly disrupts a person's physical, psychological, and spiritual health. A **maturational loss** is a form of necessary loss and includes all normally expected life changes across the life span. A mother feels loss when her child leaves home for the first day of school. A grade school child does not want to lose her favorite teacher and classroom. Maturational losses associated with normal life transitions help people develop coping skills to use when they experience unplanned, unwanted, or unexpected loss. Some losses seem unnecessary and are not part of expected maturation experiences. Sudden, unpredictable external events bring about **situational loss.** For example, a person in an automobile accident sustains an injury with physical changes that make it impossible to return to work or school, leading to loss of function, income, life goals, and self-esteem.

TABLE 36-1 Types of Loss

DEFINITION	IMPLICATIONS OF LOSS
Loss of possessions or objects (e.g., theft, deterioration, misplacement, or destruction)	Extent of grieving depends on value of object, sentiment attached to it, or its usefulness.
Loss of known environment (e.g., leaving home, hospitalization, new job, moving out of a rehabilitation unit)	Loss occurs through maturational or situational events or by injury/illness. Loneliness in an unfamiliar setting threatens self-esteem, hopefulness, or belonging.
Loss of a significant other (e.g., divorce, loss of friend, trusted caregiver, or pet)	Close friends, family members, and pets fulfill psychological, safety, love, belonging, and self-esteem needs.
Loss of an aspect of self (e.g., body part, job, psychological or physiological function)	Illness, injury, or developmental changes result in loss of a valued aspect of self, altering personal identity and self-concept.
Loss of life (e.g., death of family member, friend, co-worker, or one's own death)	Loss of life grieves those left behind. Dying persons also feel sadness or fear pain, loss of control, and dependency on others.

Losses may be actual or perceived. An **actual loss** occurs when a person can no longer feel, hear, see, or know a person or object. Examples include the loss of a body part, death of a family member, or loss of a job. Lost valued objects include those that wear out or are misplaced, stolen, or ruined by disaster. A child grieves the loss of a favorite toy washed away in a flood. A **perceived loss** is uniquely defined by the person experiencing the loss and is less obvious to other people. For example, some people perceive rejection by a friend to be a loss, which creates a loss of confidence or changes their status in a group. How an individual interprets the meaning of the perceived loss affects the intensity of the grief response. Perceived losses are easy to overlook because they are experienced so internally and individually, but they are grieved in the same way as an actual loss.

Each person responds to loss differently. The type of loss and the person's perception of it influence the depth and duration of the grief response. For some individuals the loss of an object (e.g., home or treasured inherited gift) generates the same level of distress as the loss of a person, depending on the value the person places on the object. Chronic illnesses, disabilities, and hospitalization produce multiple losses. When entering an institution for care, patients lose access to familiar people and environments, privacy, and control over body functions and daily routines. A chronic illness or disability adds financial hardships for most people and often brings about changes in lifestyle and dependence on others. Even brief illnesses or hospitalizations cause temporary changes in family role functioning, daily activities, and relationships.

Death is the ultimate loss. Although it is a necessary part of the continuum of life and of being human, death represents the unknown and generates anxiety, fear, and uncertainty for many people. Death permanently separates people physically from important persons in their lives and causes fear, sadness, and regret for the dying person, family members, friends, and caregivers. A person's culture, spirituality, personal beliefs and values, previous experiences with death, and degree of social support influence the way he or she approaches death.

Grief

Grief is the emotional response to a loss, manifested in ways unique to an individual and based on personal experiences, cultural expectations, and spiritual beliefs (Walter and McCoyd, 2009) (see Chapters 9 and 35). Coping with grief involves a period of **mourning,** the outward, social expressions of grief and the behavior associated with loss. Most mourning rituals are culturally influenced, learned behaviors. For example, the Jewish mourning ritual of *Shivah* incorporates the helping behaviors of the community toward those experiencing death, sets expectations for survivor behavior, and sustains the community with tradition and rituals (Bauer-Wu et al., 2007). The term **bereavement** encompasses both grief and mourning and includes the emotional responses and outward behaviors of a person experiencing loss (AACN, 2008). Recognizing that there are different types of grief can help nurses plan and implement appropriate care.

Normal Grief. **Normal (uncomplicated) grief** is a common, universal reaction characterized by complex emotional, cognitive, social, physical, behavioral, and spiritual responses to loss and death. Feelings of acceptance, disbelief, yearning, anger, and depression are displayed in normal bereavement grief. Although manner of death (violent, unexpected, or traumatic) poses greater risk to survivors, it does not always determine how an individual will grieve. Helpful coping mechanisms for grieving people include hardiness and resilience, a personal sense of control, and the ability to make sense of and identify positive possibilities after a loss.

Anticipatory Grief. A person experiences **anticipatory grief,** the unconscious process of disengaging or "letting go" before the actual loss or death occurs, especially in situations of prolonged or predicted loss (Simon, 2008). When grief extends over a long period of time, people absorb loss gradually and begin to prepare for its inevitability. They experience intense responses to grief (e.g., shock, denial, and tearfulness) before the actual death occurs and often feel relief when it finally happens. The idea that people actually grieve in anticipation (rather than following a loss) is debated by researchers. Another way to think about anticipatory grief is that it is a forewarning or cushion that gives people time to prepare or complete the tasks related to the impending death. However, this idea may not apply in every situation. Although forewarning is a buffer for some individuals, it increases stress for others, creating an emotional roller coaster of highs and lows.

Disenfranchised Grief. People experience **disenfranchised grief,** also known as *marginal* or *unsupported grief,* when their relationship to the deceased person is not socially sanctioned, cannot be openly shared, or seems of lesser significance. The person's loss and grief do not meet the norms of grief acknowledged by his or her culture, cutting the grieving person off from social support and the sympathy given to persons with "legitimate" losses. The grieving person often wonders if he or she should call the experience a loss. Examples include the death an ex-spouse, a gay partner, or a pet or death from a stigmatized illness such as alcoholism or during the commission of a crime (Hooyman and Kramer, 2008; Walter and McCoyd, 2009).

Ambiguous Loss. Sometimes people experience losses that are marked by uncertainty. **Ambiguous loss,** a type of disenfranchised grief, occurs when the lost person is physically present but not psychologically available, as in cases of severe dementia or severe brain injury. Other times the person is gone (e.g., after a kidnapping or as a prisoner of war); but the grieving person maintains an ongoing, intense psychological attachment, never sure of the reality of the situation. Ambiguous losses are particularly difficult to process because of the lack of finality and unknown outcomes (Walter and McCoyd, 2009).

Complicated Grief. Some people do not experience a normal grief process. In **complicated grief** a person has a prolonged or significantly difficult time moving forward after a loss. He or she experiences a chronic and disruptive yearning for the deceased; has trouble accepting the death and trusting others; and/or feels excessively bitter, emotionally numb, or anxious about the future. Complicated grief occurs more often when a person had a conflicted relationship with the deceased, prior or multiple losses or stressors, mental health issues, or lack of social support. Loss associated with homicide, suicide, sudden accidents, or the death of a child has the potential to become complicated. Specific types of complicated grief include exaggerated, delayed, and masked grief.

Exaggerated Grief. A person with an exaggerated grief response often exhibits self-destructive or maladaptive behavior, obsessions, or psychiatric disorders. Suicide is a risk for these people.

Delayed Grief. A person's grief response is unusually delayed or postponed, often because the loss is so overwhelming that the person must avoid the full realization of the loss. A delayed grief response is frequently triggered by a second loss, sometimes seemingly not as significant as the first loss.

Masked Grief. Sometimes a grieving person behaves in ways that interfere with normal functioning but is unaware that the disruptive behavior is a result of the loss and ineffective grief resolution (AACN, 2008).

Theories of Grief and Mourning

Knowledge of grief theories and normal responses to loss and bereavement will help you better understand these complex experiences and how to help a grieving person. Grief theorists describe the physical, psychological, and social reactions to loss. Remember that people who vary from expected norms of grief or theoretical descriptions are not abnormal. The variety of theories supports the complexity and individuality of grief responses. Although most grief theories describe how people cope with death, they also help to understand responses to other significant losses. A review of some classic grief theories follows.

Stages of Dying. Basing her research on interviews with dying people, Kübler-Ross (1969) describes five stages of dying in her classic behavioral theory: denial, anger, bargaining, depression, and acceptance. A person in the denial stage cannot accept the fact of the loss, which often provides psychological protection from a loss that the person cannot yet bear. When experiencing the anger stage of adjustment to loss, a person expresses resistance and sometimes feels intense anger at God, other people, or the situation. Bargaining cushions and postpones awareness of the loss by trying to prevent it from happening. Grieving or dying people make promises to self, God, or loved ones that they will live or believe differently if they can be spared death. When a person realizes the full impact of the loss, depression occurs. Some individuals feel overwhelmingly sad, hopeless, and lonely. In acceptance the person incorporates the loss into life; develops the capacity to have a breadth of emotions, even positive ones; and finds ways to move forward. The stages of dying are not linear. Patients will move back and forth through the stages.

Attachment Theory. Bowlby's (1980) attachment theory, also a stage theory, describes the experience of mourning based on his studies of children separated from their parents during World War II. Attachment, an instinctive behavior, leads to the development of bonds between children and their primary caregivers. Relational bonds are present and active throughout the life cycle, and individuals later generalize them to persons in other relationships. Attachment behavior ensures survival because it keeps people close to those who offer love, protection, and support.

Bowlby describes four stages of mourning: numbing, yearning and searching, disorganization and despair, and reorganization. **Numbing,** the shortest stage of mourning, may last from a few hours to a week or more. The grieving person describes this stage as feeling "stunned" or "unreal." Numbing protects the person from the full impact of the loss. Emotional outbursts of tearful sobbing and acute distress characterize the second bereavement stage, **yearning and searching (separation anxiety).** Common physical symptoms in this stage include tightness in the chest and throat, shortness of breath, a feeling of lethargy, insomnia, and loss of appetite. A person also experiences an inner, intense yearning for the lost person or object. This stage lasts for months or considerably longer. During the stage of **disorganization and despair,** a person endlessly examines how and why the loss occurred or expresses anger at anyone who seems responsible for the loss. The grieving person retells the loss story again and again and gradually realizes that the loss is permanent. With **reorganization,** which usually takes a year or more, the person begins to accept change, assume unfamiliar roles, acquire new skills, and build new relationships. Persons who are reorganizing begin to separate themselves from their lost relationship without feeling that they are lessening its importance.

Grief Tasks Model. Worden (1982) proposes a task-based grief theory. He describes how individuals actively engage in behaviors by responding to outside interventions to help themselves. Working through the grief tasks typically requires a minimum of a full year, although the time varies from person to person.

- *Task I: Accept the reality of the loss.* Even when a death is expected, survivors register some disbelief and surprise that it has really happened. Task I involves the process of accepting that the person or object is gone and will not return.
- *Task II: Experience the pain of grief.* Even though people respond to loss differently, it is impossible to experience a significant loss without some emotional pain. People react with sadness, loneliness, despair, or regret and work through painful feelings using the coping mechanisms most familiar and comfortable to them.
- *Task III: Adjust to a world in which the deceased is missing.* A person does not realize the full impact of a loss for at least 3 months. Family members or friends pay less attention to the bereaved person at about the same time, just as the finality of the loss becomes real. People completing this task begin to take on roles formerly filled by the deceased, including some jobs they do not want.
- *Task IV: Emotionally relocate the deceased and move on with life.* The deceased person is not forgotten but rather takes a different and less prominent place in the survivor's emotional life. People often fear that in making new attachments they will forget their loved one or seem disloyal, making this a potentially difficult task to complete. Realizing that it is possible to love other people without betraying the deceased, the person moves forward.

Rando's "R" Process Model. Rando (1993) describes grief as a series of processes instead of stages or tasks. However, her processes are similar to the stages and tasks already described. Rando's processes include recognizing the loss, reacting to the pain of separation, reminiscing, relinquishing old attachments, and readjusting to life after loss. **Reminiscence** is an important activity in grief and mourning. A person recollects and reexperiences the deceased and the relationship by mentally or verbally anecdotally reliving and remembering the person and past experiences.

Dual Process Model. Newer theories account for gender and cultural variations and address the limitations of theories focused mainly on internal, emotional responses to grief. The dual process model describes the everyday life experiences of grief as moving back and forth between loss-oriented and restoration-oriented activities (Wright and Hogan, 2008). Loss-oriented behaviors include grief work, dwelling on the loss, breaking connections with the deceased person, and resisting activities to move past the grief. Restoration-oriented activities such as attending to life changes, finding new roles or relationships, coping with finances, and participating in distractions provide balance to the loss-oriented state. The extent to which an individual engages in loss or restoration-oriented processes depends on factors such as personality, coping styles, or cultural practices.

Post Modern Grief Theories. Some experts believe the stage and task theories described previously lack empirical evidence, do not allow for cultural differences, and assume there is an end point in grieving (Walter and McCoyd, 2009). More recent grief theories take into consideration that human beings construct their own experiences and truths differently and make their own meanings when confronted with loss and death. Differences in social and historical context, family structure, and cognitive capacities shape an individual's truths and grief experiences. No one's grief follows a predetermined path.

NURSING KNOWLEDGE BASE

Nurses develop plans of care to help patients and family members who are undergoing loss, grief, or death experiences. Based on nursing research, practice evidence, nursing experience, and patient and family preferences, nurses implement plans of care in acute care, nursing home, hospice, home care, and community settings. Extensive nursing education programs support the improvement of end-of-life care at every level of practice. The End-of-Life Nursing Education Consortium (ELNEC) provides nurses with basic and advanced curricula to care for patients and families experiencing loss, grief, death, and bereavement (AACN, 2008); and nursing textbooks provide advanced discussions on multiple dimensions of palliative and end-of-life care (Ferrell and Coyle, 2010; Matzo and Sherman, 2010). In conjunction with the Hospice and Palliative Care Nurses Association, the American Nurses Association has developed the Scope and Standards of Hospice and Palliative Nursing Practice (2007). Professional nursing organizations such as the American Society of Pain Management Nurses and the American Association of Critical Care Nurses offer evidence-based practice guidelines for managing clinical and ethical issues at the end of life in many health care settings.

Factors Influencing Loss and Grief

Multiple factors influence the way a person perceives and responds to loss. They include developmental factors, personal relationships, the nature of the loss, coping strategies, socioeconomic status, and cultural and spiritual influences and beliefs.

Human Development. Patient age and stage of development affect the grief response. For example, toddlers cannot understand loss or death but often feel anxiety over the loss of objects and separation from parents. They sometimes express the sense of absence they feel with changes in eating and sleeping patterns, fussiness, or bowel and bladder disturbances. School-age children understand the concepts of permanence and irreversibility but do not always understand the causes of a loss. Some have intense periods of emotional expression. Young adults undergo many necessary developmental losses related to their evolving future. They leave home, begin school or a work life, or form significant relationships. Illness or death disrupts the young adult's future and establishment of an autonomous sense of self. Midlife adults also experience major life transitions such as caring for aging parents, dealing with changes in marital status, and adapting to new family roles (Walter and McCoyd, 2009). For older adults the aging process leads to necessary and developmental losses. Some older adults experience age discrimination, especially when they become dependent or are near death; but they show resilience after a loss as a result of their prior experiences and developed coping skills (Box 36-1).

Personal Relationships. When loss involves another person, the quality and meaning of the lost relationship influence the grief response. When a relationship between two people was very rewarding and well connected, the survivor often finds it difficult to move forward. Grief resolution is hampered by regret and a sense of unfinished business, especially when people are closely related but did not have a good relationship at the time of death. Social support and the ability to accept help from others are critical variables in recovery from loss and grief. When patients do not receive supportive understanding and compassion from

BOX 36-1 FOCUS ON OLDER ADULTS

Grief Considerations in Older Adults

- There is little evidence that grief experiences differ because of age alone. Responses to loss are more likely related to the nature of the specific loss experience and individual differences.
- Increased age increases the likelihood that older adults have faced multiple losses—loved ones, friends, valued objects, a child, or declining health. Older adults residing in communal living situations experience many losses as friends die.
- Many older adults exhibit resilience. Others around them can learn from their courage and ability to respond to life challenges graciously, accepting life with integrity and wholeness (Walter and McCoyd, 2009).
- Older adults are at risk for complicated grieving as a result of multiple losses, potential for cognitive impairment, or decreased physical resources. The risks include depression, loneliness, and accompanying functional decline.
- Physical decline caused by chronic illness sometimes leads to grief over lost health, function, and roles.
- Pain is often undertreated in older adults, particularly in people with dementia or cognitive impairments. Side effects of pain medications are usually more pronounced in older adults (Matzo and Sherman, 2010).
- Older adults benefit from the same therapeutic techniques as persons in other age-groups. Evidence indicates that positive reappraisal (cognitive restructuring) helps older adults adapt to significant losses. Older adults have opportunities for growth and development through their loss experiences (Hooyman and Kramer, 2008).
- Relieving depression and maintaining physical function are therapeutic goals for grieving older adults.

others, grief becomes complicated or prolonged (Hooyman and Kramer, 2008).

Nature of the Loss. Exploring the meaning a loss has for your patient helps you better understand the effect of the loss on the patient's behavior, health, and well-being. Highly visible losses generally stimulate a helping response from others. For example, the loss of one's home from a tornado often brings community and governmental support. A more private loss such as a miscarriage brings less support from others. A sudden and unexpected death poses different challenges than those in a debilitating chronic illness. When the death is sudden and unexpected, the survivors do not have time to let go. In chronic illness survivors have memories of prolonged suffering, pain, and loss of function. Death by violence or suicide or multiple losses by their very nature complicate the grieving process in unique ways (Walter and McCoyd, 2009).

Coping Strategies. Life experiences shape the coping strategies that a person uses to deal with the stress of loss. Patients rely first on familiar coping strategies. When the usual coping strategies do not work, they need new ones. Emotional disclosure (i.e., venting, talking about one's feelings, or expressing anger or other negative feelings) is one way to cope with loss. Negative themes that are present when people talk about grief sometimes predict more distressful reactions (Maciejewski, 2007). However, some individuals cope better in situations of loss when they instead focus on positive emotions and optimistic feelings. Emotional disclosure is often accomplished by having people write about their feelings in letters to lost loved ones or personal journals.

Socioeconomic Status. Socioeconomic status influences a person's ability to access support and resources for coping with loss and physical responses to stress (Cohen et al., 2006). When people lack financial, educational, or occupational resources, the burdens of loss multiply. For example, a patient with limited finances is not able to replace a car demolished in an accident and pay for the associated medical expenses.

Culture and Ethnicity. Culture and family or religious affiliation influences interpretations of loss and the ability to establish acceptable expressions of grief, which affects the ability to provide stability and structure in the midst of chaos and loss. Expressions of grief in one culture do not always make sense to people from a different culture (see Chapter 9). Try to understand and appreciate each patient's cultural values related to loss, death, and grieving. Grief theories commonly used to understand loss and death have cultural limitations. For example, some theorists describe grief as a process of "work" or "tasks" that occurs in stages or on projected timelines. North Americans may better understand work, tasks, and time expectations for grief compared to other cultural groups not as defined by work achievements or with a different sense of time. Some cultural groups experience grief as a timeless, communal expression or state of being. Many people in Western European and American cultures hold back their public displays of emotion. In other cultures behaviors such as public wailing and physical demonstrations of grief, including survivor body mutilation, show respect for the dead. Core American cultural values of individualism and self-determination stand in contrast with communal, family, or tribal ways of life. Americans value and expect honesty and truth telling in end-of-life situations, but some cultures have strict taboos surrounding what should be discussed regarding the diagnosis and prognosis in serious illness (Erichsen et al., 2010; Johnstone and Kanitsaki, 2009). Cultural differences influence processes such as obtaining informed consent or making life-support decisions. Research has shown that ethnicity is strongly related to attitudes toward life-sustaining treatments during terminal illness and the use of hospice services (Rosenfeld et al., 2007).

Spiritual and Religious Beliefs. The care of seriously ill patients usually involves medical interventions to restore or maintain health. A contrasting set of practices (i.e., transformative strategies) acknowledge life limits and help dying people find meaning in suffering so they are able to transcend (go beyond) their personal existence. Transformative practices are associated with healing and spiritual or religious beliefs. Spiritual resources include faith in a higher power, communities of support, friends, a sense of hope and meaning in life, and religious practices. Spirituality affects the patient's and family members' ability to cope with loss. Positive correlations show that spiritual well-being, peacefulness, comfort, and serenity are all important aspects of a peaceful death (Kruse et al., 2007). Findings in the literature verify that religious beliefs provide a sense of structure in end-of-life situations and are linked to more positive attitudes toward death (Ladd, 2007).

Hope, a multidimensional concept considered to be a component of spirituality, energizes and provides comfort to individuals experiencing personal challenges. Hopefulness gives a person the ability to see life as enduring or having meaning or purpose. As a future-shaping, motivating force, hope helps patients maintain anticipation of a continued good, an improvement in their circumstances, or a lessening of something unpleasant (Clayton et al., 2008). With hope a patient moves from feelings of weakness and vulnerability to living as fully as possible. Maintaining a sense of hope depends in part on a person having strong relationships and emotional connectedness to others. On the other hand, spiritual distress often arises from a patient's inability to feel hopeful or foresee any favorable outcomes. Spirituality and hope play a vital role in a patient's adjustment to loss and death (see Chapter 35).

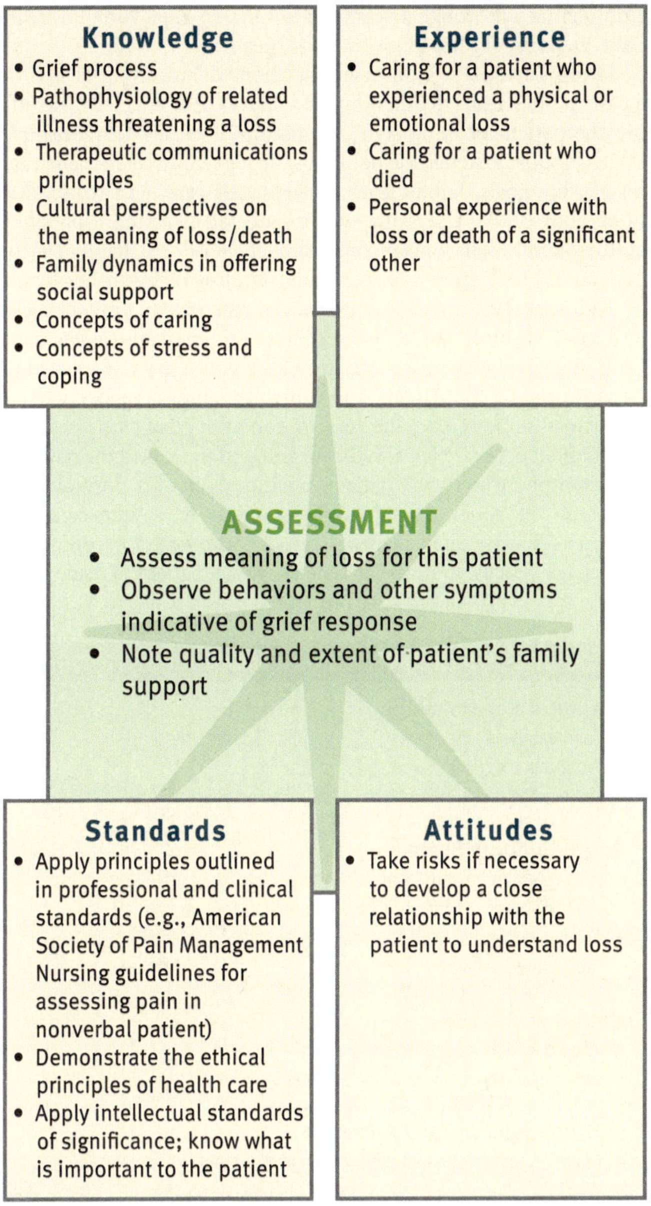
Knowledge
• Grief process
• Pathophysiology of related illness threatening a loss
• Therapeutic communications principles
• Cultural perspectives on the meaning of loss/death
• Family dynamics in offering social support
• Concepts of caring
• Concepts of stress and coping
Experience
• Caring for a patient who experienced a physical or emotional loss
• Caring for a patient who died
• Personal experience with loss or death of a significant other
ASSESSMENT
• Assess meaning of loss for this patient
• Observe behaviors and other symptoms indicative of grief response
• Note quality and extent of patient's family support
Standards
• Apply principles outlined in professional and clinical standards (e.g., American Society of Pain Management Nursing guidelines for assessing pain in nonverbal patient)
• Demonstrate the ethical principles of health care
• Apply intellectual standards of significance; know what is important to the patient
Attitudes
• Take risks if necessary to develop a close relationship with the patient to understand loss

FIG. 36-1 Critical thinking model for loss, death, and grieving assessment.

CRITICAL THINKING

To provide appropriate and responsive care for the grieving patient and family, use critical thinking skills to synthesize scientific knowledge from nursing and nonnursing disciplines, professional standards, evidence-based practice, patient assessments, previous caregiving experiences, and self-knowledge. Critical thinking informs all steps of the nursing process (see Chapter 15).

During the assessment phase use critical thinking to gather and analyze the data that lead to the selection of appropriate nursing diagnoses (Fig. 36-1). To understand a patient's subjective experiences of loss, form assessment questions based on your theoretical and professional knowledge of grief and loss but then listen carefully to the patient's perceptions. A culturally competent nurse also uses culture-specific understanding of grief to explore the meaning of loss with a patient.

BOX 36-2 A DYING PERSON'S BILL OF RIGHTS

I have the right to be treated as a living human being until I die.
I have the right to be in control.
I have the right to maintain a sense of hopefulness, however changing its focus may be.
I have the right to be cared for by those who can maintain a sense of hopefulness, however changing this may be.
I have the right to have a sense of purpose.
I have the right to express my feelings and emotions about my approaching death in my own way.
I have the right to participate in decisions about my care.
I have the right to expect continuing medical and nursing attention even though "cure" goals must be changed to "comfort" goals.
I have the right not to die alone.
I have the right to be free of pain.
I have the right to have a respected spirituality.
I have the right to have my questions answered honestly.
I have the right not to be deceived.
I have the right to have help from and for my family in accepting my death.
I have the right to die in peace and dignity.
I have the right to retain my individuality and not be judged for my decisions that may be contrary to beliefs of others.
I have the right to discuss and enlarge my religious and/or spiritual experiences, whatever these may mean to others.
I have a right to expect that the sanctity of my human body will be respected after death.
I have the right to be cared for by caring, sensitive, knowledgeable people who will try to understand my needs and will be able to gain some satisfaction in helping me face my death.

Modified from Barbus AJ: The dying person's bill of rights, *Am J Nurs* 75:99, 1975; and Dying person's bill of rights, www.kingston.gov.uk/dyingbillofrightsp.pdf. Accessed November 10, 2011.

Being familiar with commonly experienced responses to loss enables you to better understand a patient's emotions and behaviors. Some patients ignore, lash out, plead with, or withdraw from other people as part of a normal response to loss. Instead of "taking things personally," a critically thinking nurse integrates theory, prior experience, appreciation of subjective experiences, and self-knowledge to respond to the patient's emotions with patience and understanding. In designing plans of care, use professional standards, including the Nursing Code of Ethics (see Chapter 22), the dying person's bill of rights (Box 36-2), the American Nurses Association Scope and Standards of Hospice and Palliative Nursing Practice (2007), and clinical standards such as the American Society of Pain Management Nurses' guidelines for pain assessment in the nonverbal patient (Herr et al., 2006).

NURSING PROCESS

Apply the nursing process and use a critical thinking approach in your care of patients. The nursing process provides a clinical decision-making approach for you to develop and implement an individualized plan of care.

ASSESSMENT

During the assessment process, thoroughly assess each patient and critically analyze findings to ensure that you make patient-centered clinical decisions required for safe nursing care. A trusting, helping relationship with grieving patients and family members is essential to the assessment process. A caring nurse encourages a patient to tell his or her story, which then becomes a primary source of assessment data (Betcher, 2010). Look for opportunities to invite patients to share their experiences, being aware that attitudes about self-disclosure; sharing emotions; or talking about illness, fears, and death are shaped by an individual's personality, coping style, and culture.

Through the Patient's Eyes. Explore with patients their unique responses to grief or their preferences for end-of-life care, which may include advance directives. Patient perceptions and expectations influence how you prioritize your nursing diagnoses. To assess patient perceptions, you ask, "What is the most important thing I can do for you right now?" You usually gather information from patients first, but with advanced illness and as death approaches, patients often rely on family members to communicate for them. Encourage family members to share their goals and perceptions with you. Whether or not they accurately represent a patient's viewpoints or wishes has been the topic of extensive research (Gardner and Kramer, 2010). Most often they provide valuable information about patient preferences and clarify misunderstandings or identify overlooked information. Assess patients' and family members' understanding of treatment options to implement a mutually developed care plan. Assessment of grief responses extends throughout the course of an illness into the bereavement period following a death. Patients with advanced chronic illness and their families eventually face end-of-life care decisions and should discuss the content of any advance directives together. Because most deaths are now "negotiated" among patients, family members, and the health care team, discuss end-of-life care preferences early in the assessment phase of the nursing process. If you feel uncomfortable in assessing a patient's wishes for end-of-life care by yourself, ask a health care provider experienced in discussing these issues to help you. Communicate what you have learned about patient preferences during any RN hand-off, at health care team conferences, in written care plans, and through ongoing consultation (see Chapter 26).

Speak to patients and family members using honest and open communication, remembering that cultural practices influence how much information the patient shares. Keep an open mind, listen carefully, and observe the patient's verbal and nonverbal responses. Facial expressions, voice tones, and avoided topics often disclose more than words. Anticipate common grief responses, but allow patients to describe their experiences in their own words. Open-ended questions such as "What do you understand about your diagnosis?" or "You seem sad today. Can you tell me more?" may open the door to a patient-centered discussion. Many people find it difficult to talk about loss, fear, death, or grief. The use of pauses, gentle questioning, and silence honors the patient's privacy and readiness to talk. Talk to patients and family members in a private, quiet setting. Many times a patient wants to have family members present so everyone hears the same thing and has an opportunity to add to the conversation. However, some people want their concerns and questions addressed privately. Ask patients and family members about their preferences. As you gather assessment data, summarize and validate your impressions with the patient or family member. Information from the medical record and other members of the health care team, physicians, social workers, and spiritual care providers contributes to your assessment data.

Because of the importance of symptom management and priority of comfort in end-of-life care, prioritize your initial assessment to encourage patients to identify any distressing symptoms. Completing a thorough assessment is difficult when patients are in pain, anxious, depressed, or short of breath.

Grief Variables. Conversations about the meaning of loss to a patient often leads to other important areas of assessment, including the patient's coping style, the nature of family relationships, social support systems, the nature of the loss, cultural and spiritual beliefs, life goals, family grief patterns, self-care, and sources of hope (Box 36-3). Use skills appropriate for assessing a patient's culture, family, self-concept, or spiritual beliefs (see Chapters 9, 10, 33, and 35) to acquire a deeper understanding of his or her loss.

Knowing the commonly experienced reactions to grief and loss and grief theories guides your critical thinking and assessment skills. A single behavior can occur in all types of grief. If a grieving patient describes loneliness and difficulty falling asleep, consider all factors surrounding the loss in context. What was the loss? When did it occur? What was the meaning of the loss to the patient? For example, when your patient exhibits signs of a normal grief reaction, but you learn that the loss occurred 2 years ago, the patient's response most likely indicates a complicated, chronic grief experience. Focus your assessment on how a patient is reacting to

BOX 36-3 NURSING ASSESSMENT QUESTIONS

Nature of Relationships
- How long have you known _______ (the deceased person)?
- What role did (name person) play in your life?
- Tell me about your relationship with (name person).

Social Support Systems
- Who is "there for you?" Absent? Who provides support?
- What do others do for you that is most meaningful or helpful?
- Are family/friends available when needed? Which friends or relatives do you wish were here?

Nature of the Loss
- What does this loss mean to you?
- What other losses have you experienced?

Cultural and Spiritual Beliefs
- What is your belief about death? Meaning of life?
- Which rituals are important to you at the end of life?
- How do members of your culture or religious group respond to this loss?

Life Goals
- What are your life goals at this time?
- How have your goals changed because of this experience?
- Are you able to envision what you will do in the future?

Family Grief Patterns
- How have you/your family dealt with loss in the past?
- What are your family's strengths?
- How have family relationships changed as a result of your loss?
- What role do you assume in your family during stressful situations?

Self-Care
- Tell me how you are feeling.
- What are you doing to take care of yourself now?
- What helps you when you feel this sad? What doesn't help?

Hope
- What do you hope for right now?
- What helps you to remain hopeful? What causes you to lose hope?

loss or grief and not on how *you* believe that patient should be reacting.

Grief Reactions. Use psychological and physical assessment skills to assess a patient's unique grief responses. Most grieving people show some common outward signs and symptoms (Box 36-4). Analyze assessment data and identify possible related causes for the signs and symptoms that you observe. For example, after a significant loss a person has a sad affect, withdrawn behaviors, headaches, upset stomach, and decreased ability to concentrate. You associate these symptoms with several potential causes, including anxiety, gastrointestinal disturbances, medication side effects, or impaired memory. Careful analysis of the symptoms in context leads you to an accurate nursing diagnosis. Ask: How are the symptoms related to one another when they occur? When did they begin? Were they present before the loss? To what does the person attribute them?

Loss takes place in a social context; thus family assessment is a vital part of your data gathering. If a father of a young family is dying, he will not be able to fulfill certain roles, causing a change in family structure. When a person develops a disability, the patient and family members realign their roles and responsibilities to meet new demands. Family members also experience a variety of physical and psychological symptoms. Assess the family's response to loss and recognize that sometimes they are dealing with their grief at a different pace.

BOX 36-4 SYMPTOMS OF NORMAL GRIEF

Feelings
- Sorrow
- Fear
- Anger
- Guilt or self-reproach
- Anxiety
- Loneliness
- Fatigue
- Helplessness/hopelessness
- Yearning
- Relief

Cognitions (Thought Patterns)
- Disbelief
- Confusion or memory problems
- Problems with decision making
- Inability to concentrate
- Feeling the presence of the deceased

Physical Sensations
- Headaches
- Nausea and appetite disturbances
- Tightness in the chest and throat
- Insomnia
- Oversensitivity to noise
- Sense of depersonalization ("Nothing seems real")
- Feeling short of breath, choking sensation
- Muscle weakness
- Lack of energy
- Dry mouth

Behaviors
- Crying and frequent sighing
- Distancing from people
- Absentmindedness
- Dreams of the deceased
- Keeping the deceased's room intact
- Loss of interest in regular life events
- Wearing objects that belonged to the deceased

NURSING DIAGNOSIS

Use critical thinking to cluster assessment data cues, identify defining characteristics, draw conclusions regarding the patient's actual or potential needs or resources, and identify nursing diagnoses applicable to the patient's situation (Box 36-5). In addition to numerous diagnoses related to physical symptoms at the end of life, additional nursing diagnoses relevant for patients experiencing grief, loss, or death include:

- Compromised family coping
- Death anxiety
- Fear
- Impaired comfort
- Ineffective denial
- Grieving
- Complicated grieving
- Risk for complicated grieving
- Hopelessness
- Pain (Acute or Chronic)
- Risk for loneliness
- Spiritual distress
- Readiness for enhanced spiritual well-being

You cannot make accurate nursing diagnoses on the basis of just one or two defining characteristics. Carefully review the data to consider if more than one diagnosis applies. For example, a dying patient who cries often, has angry outbursts, and reports nightmares gives evidence of several possible nursing diagnoses: *pain (acute or chronic), ineffective coping, grieving,* or *spiritual distress.* Examine the available data, validate assumptions with the patient, and look for other validating behaviors and symptoms before making a diagnosis.

BOX 36-5 NURSING DIAGNOSTIC PROCESS

Hopelessness Related to Deteriorating Physical Condition

ASSESSMENT ACTIVITIES	DEFINING CHARACTERISTICS
Ask patient to discuss her understanding of her health situation.	Patient sighs and offers a negative view of her future. She is ready to give up and join her deceased husband.
Observe patient's nonverbal behavior.	Patient keeps eyes closed and has sad facial and voice expressions.
Observe patient's responses to care options.	Patient does not want scheduled test. "There is nothing they can do."
Assess activity level.	Patient states that she has no energy and reports pain; wants to stay in bed.
Observe patient's interactions with others.	Patient shows lack of interest, communicates minimally, and does not want to contact daughter yet.

As part of the diagnostic process, identify the appropriate "related to" factor for each diagnosis. Clarification of the related factors ensures that you select appropriate interventions. For example, a nursing diagnosis of *complicated grieving related to the permanent loss of mobility* requires different interventions than a diagnosis of *complicated grieving related to infertility after an ectopic pregnancy.*

When identifying nursing diagnoses related to a patient's grief or loss, you sometimes identify other related diagnoses. Some patients experiencing grief or impending death have nursing diagnoses such as *disturbed body image* or *impaired physical mobility.* A patient entering the phase of active dying often has diagnoses related to physical changes, including *impaired urinary elimination, bowel incontinence, acute pain, nausea, disturbed sensory perception,* and *ineffective breathing pattern.*

PLANNING

Nurses provide holistic, physical, emotional, social, and spiritual care to patients experiencing grief, death, or loss. Fig. 36-2 illustrates the interrelatedness of critical thinking factors during the planning phase of the nursing process. The use of critical thinking ensures a well-designed care plan that supports a patient's self-esteem and autonomy by including him or her in the planning process. A care plan for the dying patient focuses on comfort; preserving dignity and quality of life; and providing family members with emotional, social, and spiritual support (see the Nursing Care Plan).

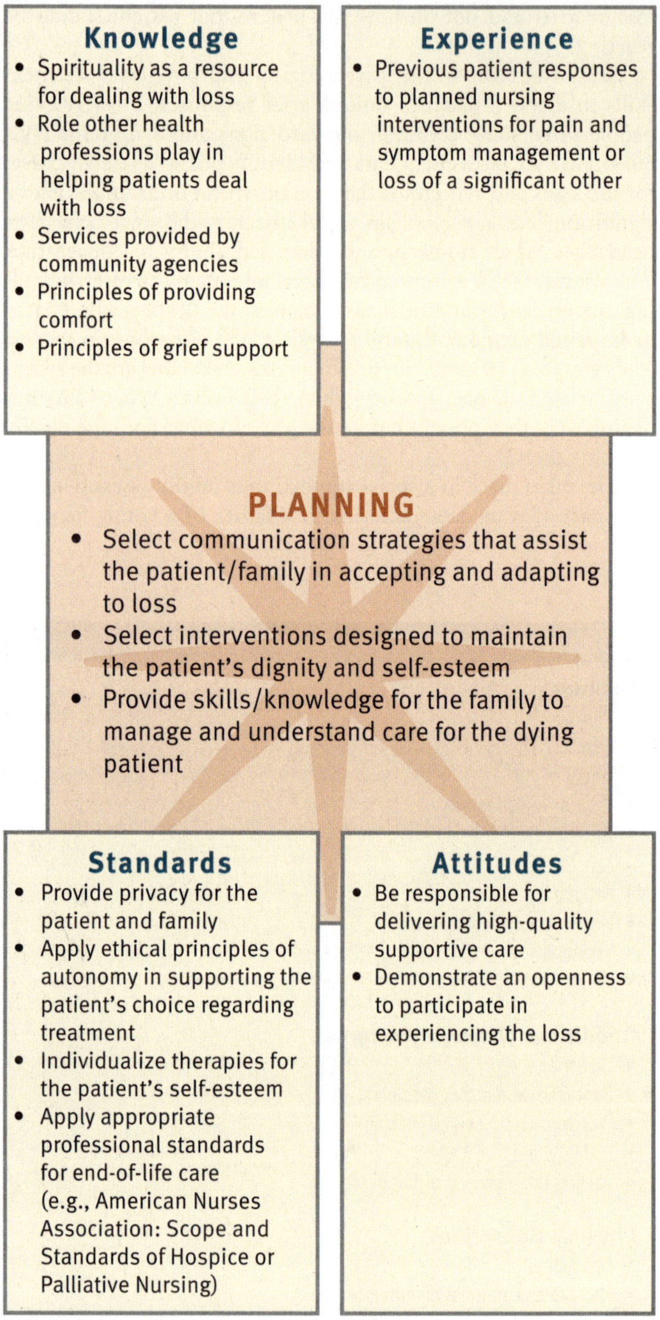

Knowledge
• Spirituality as a resource for dealing with loss
• Role other health professions play in helping patients deal with loss
• Services provided by community agencies
• Principles of providing comfort
• Principles of grief support
Experience
• Previous patient responses to planned nursing interventions for pain and symptom management or loss of a significant other
PLANNING
• Select communication strategies that assist the patient/family in accepting and adapting to loss
• Select interventions designed to maintain the patient's dignity and self-esteem
• Provide skills/knowledge for the family to manage and understand care for the dying patient
Standards
• Provide privacy for the patient and family
• Apply ethical principles of autonomy in supporting the patient's choice regarding treatment
• Individualize therapies for the patient's self-esteem
• Apply appropriate professional standards for end-of-life care (e.g., American Nurses Association: Scope and Standards of Hospice or Palliative Nursing)
Attitudes
• Be responsible for delivering high-quality supportive care
• Demonstrate an openness to participate in experiencing the loss

FIG. 36-2 Critical thinking model for loss, death, and grief planning.

Goals and Outcomes. During planning establish realistic goals and expected outcomes based on the nursing diagnoses. Consider a patient's own resources such as physical energy and activity tolerance, family support, and coping style. A nursing diagnosis of *powerlessness related to experimental cancer therapy* with a goal of "Patient will be able to describe the expected course of disease" is realistic for a patient who frequently asks for clarification about the treatment plan and participates in educational discussions. In contrast, an expected outcome of "Patient will identify a minimum of three effective coping skills" is appropriate for a patient with the same nursing diagnosis who is experiencing depression from feeling powerless about having experimental cancer treatment.

The goals of care for a patient experiencing loss are either short or long term, depending on the nature of the loss and the patient's condition. Some nursing care goals for patients facing loss or death include accommodating grief, accepting the reality of a loss, or maintaining meaningful relationships. A possible goal for a young woman with advanced breast cancer is "Maintain a sense of control," with the following potential expected outcomes:

- Patient will participate in all treatment decisions.
- Patient will identify a minimum of three ways to maintain a parental role in the care of her young child.
- Patient will communicate a minimum of three treatment side effects or concerns to the health care team.

Setting Priorities. Encourage patients and family members to share their priorities for care at the end of life. Patients at the end of life or with advanced chronic illness are more likely to want their comfort, social, or spiritual needs met rather than pursuing medical cures. Give priority to a patient's most urgent physical or psychological needs while also considering his or her expectations and priorities. If a terminally ill patient's goals include pain control and promoting self-esteem, pain control takes priority when the patient experiences acute physical discomfort. When comfort needs have been met, then you address other issues important to the patient and family. When it is realistic for the patient to remain independent, strategies that foster his or her sense of autonomy and ability to function independently take priority. A patient's condition at the end of life often changes quickly; therefore maintain an ongoing assessment to revise the plan of care according to patient needs and preferences.

When a patient has multiple nursing diagnoses, it is not possible to address them all simultaneously. Fig. 36-3 illustrates a concept map developed for Mrs. Allison, an elderly patient with a medical diagnosis of advanced cancer (leukemia). In conjunction with her recent medical diagnosis, she experiences associated health problems identified in the nursing diagnoses *chronic pain, imbalanced nutrition: less than body requirements, fatigue, and hopelessness.* In

NURSING CARE PLAN

Hopelessness

ASSESSMENT

Mrs. Allison, an 80-year-old woman, was brought to the hospital after a neighbor found her lying on the floor. She was unable to get up after falling down 4 hours earlier. She was admitted to the hospital with low blood pressure, dehydration, and weakness. She reports having severe pain in her back and toes, making it difficult for her to walk. She has also lost weight, has a poor appetite, and is too tired to cook or enjoy activities. Blood tests and physical examination reveal that she has a more serious health problem, likely a form of leukemia, for which she needs a bone marrow biopsy to make a medical diagnosis. Mrs. Allison lives alone since her husband's death 2 years earlier. She has the support of her neighbors and church community and one daughter who lives out of town. On entering the room the nurse notes that Mrs. Allison appears withdrawn and tearful. The nurse talks to her to gather more information.

Assessment Activities	*Findings/Defining Characteristics**
Ask open-ended questions. "It looks like you're having a difficult time. What do you understand about your situation right now?"	"The doctors say that **I might have cancer. Shrugging her shoulders** she states, **"There's nothing they can do. I don't want the test."**
Observe Mrs. Allison's behaviors and nonverbal communication.	Mrs. Allison **appears sad and keeps her eyes closed.** She **cries and sighs frequently.**
Assess Mrs. Allison's pain and energy level.	Mrs. Allison's **great toes are swollen and red.** Reports **constant back pain.** She has **"no energy for anything."**
Observe Mrs. Allison's interactions and interest in others.	Mrs. Allison **does not look at people and does not want to talk to her daughter yet.**
Assess meaning of recent events with Mrs. Allison and invite her to talk about her situation.	Mrs. Allison states that **"It's time to quit on life and be with my late husband."**

***Defining characteristics** are shown in bold type.

NURSING DIAGNOSIS: Hopelessness related to declining physical condition.

PLANNING

Goals	*Expected Outcomes (NOC)†*
Mrs. Allison will discuss care priorities and preferences within 1 day.	Mrs. Allison identifies the concerns causing the greatest amount of suffering or distress.
Mrs. Allison will communicate with support persons within next 12 hours.	Daughter, church community, and neighbors provide supportive care.
Mrs. Allison will identify what help she needs to live at home by discharge from the hospital.	Mrs. Allison identifies ways she can live at home with the help of others.

†Outcome classification labels from Moorhead S et al: *Nursing outcomes classification (NOC),* ed 4, St Louis, 2008, Mosby.

INTERVENTIONS (NIC)‡	RATIONALE
Presence	
Develop an open and caring relationship through active listening and emotional support.	Active listening provides opportunity for patients to find new coping strategies (Benzein and Saveman, 2008).
Establish trust and positive regard for patient in her grief and suffering.	A trusting relationship decreases feelings of abandonment. Believing that others are present gives hope in suffering (Ferrell and Coyle, 2008).
Symptom Management	
Provide pharmacological and nonpharmacological relief for chronic back and foot pain.	When people feel relaxed and obtain relief from discomfort, they are able to communicate their spiritual needs and resources (Bephage, 2009).
Grief Work Facilitation	
Help Mrs. Allison identify her personal goals, desires, and priorities. Evaluate effectiveness and promote goal achievement as appropriate.	Having a future orientation and a degree of normalcy fosters hope and sense of control over circumstances (Innes and Payne, 2009).
Assist Mrs. Allison in identifying available resources. Initiate discussions with interdisciplinary team as appropriate.	Hope is strengthened when one finds realistic possibilities and can adapt to life challenges (McDonald and McCallin, 2010).
Discuss Mrs. Allison's spiritual beliefs, practices, needs, and resources.	Spiritual and religious practices provide structure, a sense of belonging, and a more positive outlook in negative events (Ladd, 2007).

‡Intervention classification labels from Bulechek GM, Butcher HK, and Dochterman JM: *Nursing interventions classification (NIC),* ed 5, St Louis, 2008, Mosby.

Continued

NURSING CARE PLAN

***Hopelessness*—cont'd**

EVALUATION

Nursing Actions	*Patient Response/Finding*	*Achievement of Outcome*
Validate Mrs. Allison's experience: "It must be difficult to face such a big life change."	Mrs. Allison responds, "My life has changed, but I have good friends and a good daughter."	Mrs. Allison shows beginning acceptance of her changed health condition.
Use open-ended question: "Tell me how you're feeling now."	Mrs. Allison explains, "I'm not sure what will happen. I may not be able to take care of myself much longer, but I'll try."	She is able to express normal grieving behaviors and feelings of uncertainty resulting from loss of her life as she knew it.
Observe Mrs. Allison's planning activities and behavior with her daughter and friends.	Mrs. Allison and daughter discuss what they can do so she can stay at home longer.	She indicates ability to make plans for a change of care location. Daughter supports revised plans.

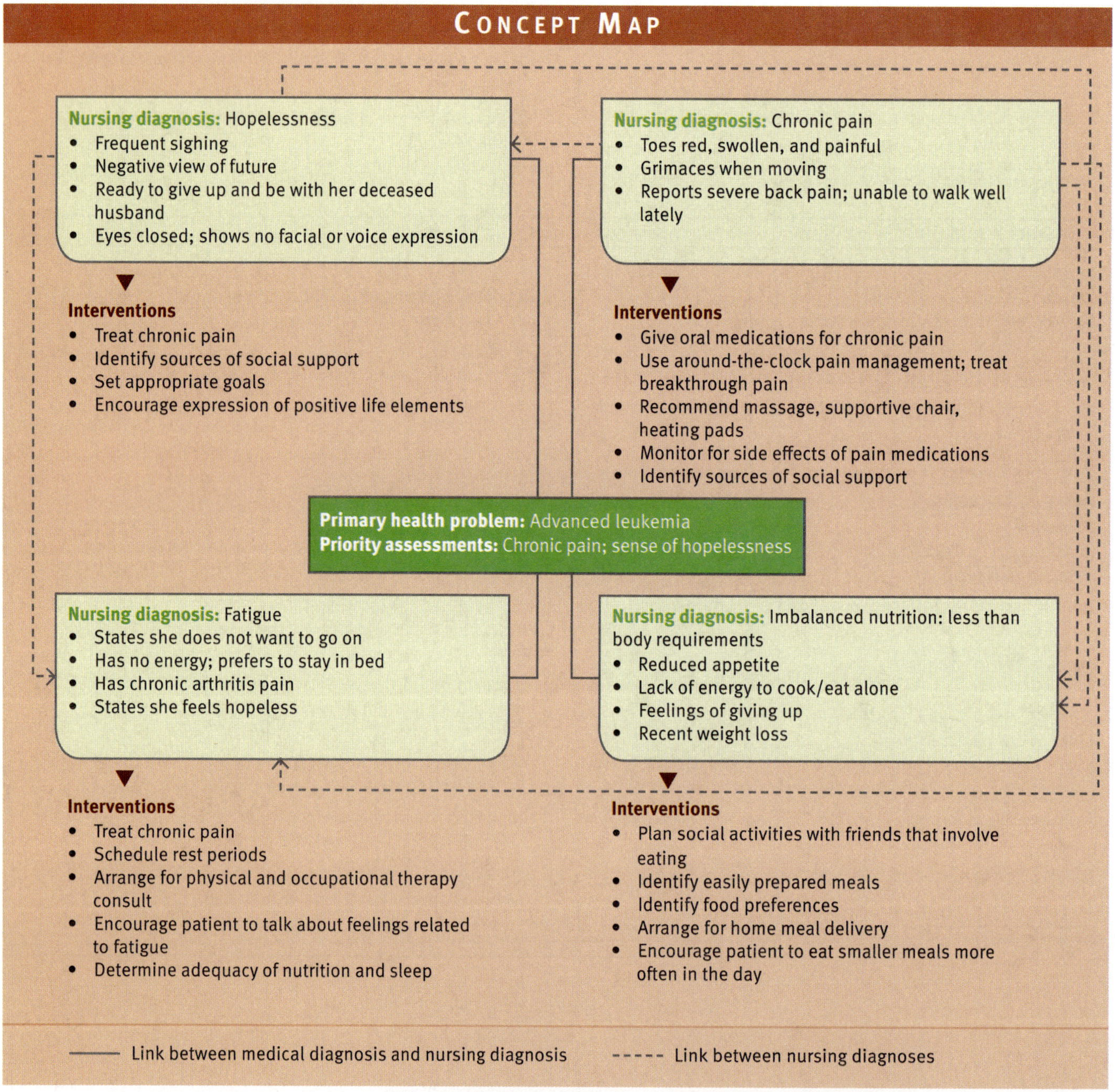
CONCEPT MAP
Nursing diagnosis: Hopelessness
• Frequent sighing
• Negative view of future
• Ready to give up and be with her deceased husband
• Eyes closed; shows no facial or voice expression
Interventions
• Treat chronic pain
• Identify sources of social support
• Set appropriate goals
• Encourage expression of positive life elements
Nursing diagnosis: Chronic pain
• Toes red, swollen, and painful
• Grimaces when moving
• Reports severe back pain; unable to walk well lately
Interventions
• Give oral medications for chronic pain
• Use around-the-clock pain management; treat breakthrough pain
• Recommend massage, supportive chair, heating pads
• Monitor for side effects of pain medications
• Identify sources of social support
Primary health problem: Advanced leukemia
Priority assessments: Chronic pain; sense of hopelessness
Nursing diagnosis: Fatigue
• States she does not want to go on
• Has no energy; prefers to stay in bed
• Has chronic arthritis pain
• States she feels hopeless
Interventions
• Treat chronic pain
• Schedule rest periods
• Arrange for physical and occupational therapy consult
• Encourage patient to talk about feelings related to fatigue
• Determine adequacy of nutrition and sleep
Nursing diagnosis: Imbalanced nutrition: less than body requirements
• Reduced appetite
• Lack of energy to cook/eat alone
• Feelings of giving up
• Recent weight loss
Interventions
• Plan social activities with friends that involve eating
• Identify easily prepared meals
• Identify food preferences
• Arrange for home meal delivery
• Encourage patient to eat smaller meals more often in the day
Link between medical diagnosis and nursing diagnosis
Link between nursing diagnoses

FIG. 36-3 Concept map for Mrs. Allison.

such a situation determine which of the four diagnoses should take priority. The chronic pain experienced by the patient is often the first focus. Until the patient's pain is under control, it will not be possible for her to feel more energized, eat well, or regain her sense of hopefulness.

Teamwork and Collaboration. As described previously, grief, loss, and death affect people physically, emotionally, spiritually, and culturally. No one is able to address all of these dimensions alone. A team of nurses, physicians, social workers, spiritual care providers, nutritionists, pharmacists, physical and occupational therapists, patients, and family members works together to provide palliative care, grief care, and care at the end of life. Massage or music/art therapists who provide alternative therapies are sometimes part of the team (see Chapter 32). As a patient's care needs change, team members take a more or less active role, depending on the patient's shifting priorities. Team members communicate with one another on a regular basis to ensure coordination and effectiveness of care.

Building Competency in Teamwork and Collaboration You are caring for Ms. Allison, an older patient who has recently been diagnosed with a terminal illness. She wants to go home again for as long as possible but lives alone. She has lost strength as a result of decreased activity, depression, and back pain. She has a decreased appetite and has had little desire or energy to prepare meals. How can you help Mrs. Allison achieve her goal of returning home by addressing her multiple health concerns through interdisciplinary collaboration?

Answers to questions can be found on the Evolve website.

BOX 36-6 PATIENT TEACHING

Maintaining Self-Care

Objective

- The patient will participate in activities to manage symptoms and prepare for death.

Teaching Strategies

- Encourage patient to set realistic goals and help him or her identify ways to achieve them.
- Identify ways patient can maintain usual daily routines that provide comfort and sense of normalcy.
- Demonstrate forms of complementary therapy that patient can use for symptom management.
- Discuss ways that patient can prepare for death to enhance his or her sense of control over end-of-life planning and maintain a realistic outlook (advance directives, funeral planning, and preferred location of death).
- Discuss patient's needs for presence of particular support people or for solitude.
- Identify methods to facilitate safety and ease in managing activities of daily living as patient's abilities change (assistive devices, in-home caregivers).
- Provide patient with information about who to call for questions or emergencies so he or she knows that constant support exists in difficult times.

Evaluation

- Ask patient to describe symptom management methods used and rate their effectiveness.
- Have patient describe wishes related to end-of-life planning.

IMPLEMENTATION

Health Promotion. Health promotion in serious chronic illness or death focuses on facilitating successful coping and optimizing physical, emotional, and spiritual health. Many people continue to look for and find meaning even in difficult life circumstances. They often find personal growth and spiritual insights they have not previously experienced and need family and nurse support as they strive to maintain a degree of normalcy; live with loss; make health care decisions; prepare for death; and adjust to disappointments, frustration, and anxieties along the way (Box 36-6).

Palliative Care in Acute and Restorative Settings. Interventions for people who face chronic life-threatening illnesses or who are at the end of life need palliative care. **Palliative care** focuses on the prevention, relief, reduction, or soothing of symptoms of disease or disorders throughout the entire course of an illness, including care of the dying and bereavement follow-up for the family. The primary goal of palliative care is to help patients and families achieve the best possible quality of life. Although it is especially important in advanced or chronic illness, it is appropriate for patients of any age, with any diagnosis, at any time, or in any setting.

Patients who have complex serious illnesses often benefit from palliative care throughout the course of their illness, even while seeking treatment for their disease. As the goals of care change and cure for illnesses becomes less likely, the focus shifts to more palliative care strategies. Palliative care interventions are not only appropriate at the end of life. Making this distinction is important because some patients, family members, or health care professionals refuse helpful palliative care interventions, believing that palliative care is only for the dying.

Hospice Care. **Hospice** care is a philosophy and a model for the care of terminally ill patients and their families. Hospice is not a place but rather a patient- and family-centered approach to care. It gives priority to managing a patient's pain and other symptoms; comfort; quality of life; and attention to physical, psychological, social, and spiritual needs and resources. Patients accepted into a hospice program usually have less than 6 to 12 months to live. Hospice services are available in home, hospital, extended care, or nursing home settings.

Many patients prefer to die at home in a familiar setting, whereas others fear burdening their families or prefer to die in a hospital or nursing home. It is important that the hospice team knows the patient's preference. When family issues complicate the options, hospice caregivers try to support the patient's wishes but also consider what is best for everyone. Sometimes the complexity and severity of patients' symptoms prevent them from being cared for at home, despite the willingness of family and friends to provide care. Patients receiving hospice care are active participants in all aspects of care, and caregivers prioritize care according to patient wishes. Patient care goals are mutually set, and all participants fully understand the patient's care preferences and try to honor them. Hospice services provide bereavement visits made by the staff after the death of the patient to help the family move through the grieving process.

To be eligible for home hospice services, a patient must have a family caregiver to provide care when the patient is no longer able to function alone. Home care aides offer help with hygienic needs, and a nurse is available to coordinate and manage symptom relief. Nurses providing hospice care use therapeutic communication, offer psychosocial care and expert symptom management, promote patient dignity and self-esteem, maintain a comfortable and peaceful environment, provide spiritual comfort and hope, protect against abandonment or isolation, offer family support, assist with ethical decision making, and facilitate mourning. Hospice team members offer 24-hour accessibility and coordinate care between the home and inpatient setting. A patient receiving home hospice care may enter the hospital for stabilization of symptoms or for caregiver respite. As a patient's death comes closer, the hospice team provides intensive support to the patient and family (Hospice Foundation of America, 2010).

Use Therapeutic Communication. Establish a caring, trusting relationship with a patient and family by using an "open hearted," nonassuming communication style (Galvin and Todres, 2009; Wright et al., 2009). Open-ended questions invite patients to expand on their thoughts and tell their stories. Patients usually give short answers (yes or no) when you use closed-ended questions, which limits what you can learn about a patient's situation. Use active listening, learn to be comfortable with silence, and use prompts (e.g., "go on," "tell me more") to encourage continued conversation (Fig. 36-4). Empathize with the patient's grief; offer your caring, transformative presence and use intentional, meaningful touch (Newman, 2008).

Feelings of sadness, numbing, denial, or anger make talking about these situations especially difficult. For example, a grieving patient experiences anger and becomes hostile with family members or caregivers. Some patients become demanding and accusing. Remain supportive by letting patients and family members know that feelings such as anger are normal by saying, "You are understandably upset right now. I just want you to know I'm here to talk with you if you want." Invite patients to reveal the emotions and concerns of greatest importance to them and acknowledge their feelings and concerns in a nonjudgmental manner. If a patient chooses not to share feelings or concerns, express a willingness to be available at any time. Some patients do not discuss emotions for personal or cultural reasons, and other patients hesitate to express their emotions for fear that others will abandon them. If you are reassuring and respectful of a patient's privacy, a therapeutic relationship likely develops. Sometimes patients need to begin resolving their grief privately before they discuss their loss with others, especially strangers.

Avoid communication barriers such as denying a patient's grief, providing false reassurance, or avoiding discussion of sensitive issues (see Chapter 24). When you sense that a patient wants to talk about something, make time immediately if at all possible. This is very challenging if you have limited experience with dying patients or are in a busy acute care setting. Above all, remember that a patient's emotions are not something you can "fix." Instead view emotional expression as a necessary part of the patient's adjustment to significant life changes and development of effective coping skills. Help family members access other professional resources. For example, call on a spiritual care provider to help patients and family members discuss difficult issues related to personal meanings, faith beliefs, and values.

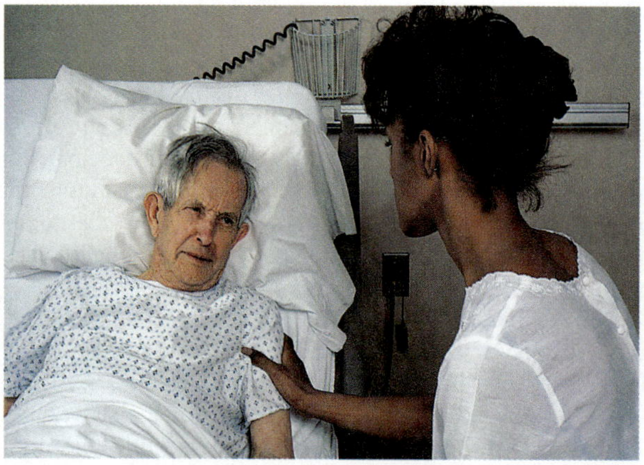

FIG. 36-4 A nurse's presence and active listening affirm the patient's dignity and worth.

Provide Psychosocial Care. Patients at the end of life experience a range of psychological symptoms, including anxiety, depression, altered body image, denial, powerlessness, uncertainty, and isolation (Taylor and Ashelford, 2008). Patients experience anguish from not knowing or being unaware of aspects of their health status or treatment. Worry or fear is common in many patients and often heightens their perception of discomfort and suffering. Providing information helps patients understand their condition, the course of their disease, and the benefits and burdens of treatment options. Suffering, a complex social and psychological response to illness, loss, and death, goes beyond psychological diagnoses. Nurses validate and support those who suffer (Ferrell and Coyle, 2008).

Manage Symptoms. Managing the multiple symptoms commonly experienced by chronically ill or dying patients remains a primary goal of palliative care nursing. Symptom distress, discomfort, and anguish often complicate a patient's dying experience. Despite the availability of effective treatment options for pain, many patients suffer with avoidable pain at the end of life. Maintain an ongoing assessment by reassessing pain and medication side effects, using pain management expertise, and advocating for change if the patient does not obtain relief from the prescribed regimen. Implement evidence-based pain management protocols (Paice, 2010) (see Chapter 43). It is essential for you to learn how to assess patients who are debilitated or dying because they often lose their ability to communicate or self-advocate (Herr et al., 2006). During the dying process, patients' renal and liver function decline, decreasing metabolism and rate of drug clearance and leading to a need for decreased medication dosages to avoid toxicities. Also be aware that advancing disease pathology, anxiety, or delirium sometimes requires the use of higher doses or different drug therapies.

Remain alert to the potential side effects of opioid administration: constipation, nausea, sedation, respiratory depression, or myoclonus. Family members often worry about potential addiction to opioid medications. Not only is the incidence of true addiction very low, but a patient's need for pain relief at the end of life takes priority. Table 36-2 provides a basic overview of nursing care for common symptoms experienced at the end of life.

Promote Dignity and Self-Esteem. A sense of dignity includes a person's positive self-regard, an ability to invest in and gain strength from one's own meaning in life, feeling valued by others, and how one is treated by caregivers. Nurses promote patients' self-esteem and dignity by respecting them as a whole (i.e., as people with feelings, accomplishments, and passions independent of the illness experience). Giving importance to the things that a patient cares about validates the person, at the same time strengthening communication among the patient, family members, and the nurse. Spending time with patients as they share their life stories helps you know him or her better and facilitates the development of individualized interventions. Show respect for older patients by calling them by surnames and titles and obtaining their permission to include others in private conversations.

Attending to the patient's physical appearance promotes dignity and self-esteem. Cleanliness, absence of body odors, and attractive clothing give patients a sense of worth. When caring for a patient's bodily functions, show patience and respect, especially after the patient becomes dependent. Allow patients to make decisions such as how and when to administer personal hygiene, diet preferences, and timing of nursing interventions. Keep the patient and family members informed about daily activities, tests, or therapies; their purposes; and anticipated effects. Provide privacy during nursing care procedures and be sensitive to when the patient and family need time alone together.

Maintain a Comfortable and Peaceful Environment. A comfortable, clean, pleasant environment helps patients relax, promotes good sleep patterns, and minimizes symptom severity. Keep a patient comfortable through frequent repositioning, making sure that bed linens are dry and controlling extraneous environmental noise and offensive odors. Pictures, cherished objects, and cards or letters from family members and friends create a familiar and

TABLE 36-2 Promoting Comfort in the Terminally Ill Patient

SYMPTOMS	CHARACTERISTICS OR CAUSES	NURSING IMPLICATIONS
Pain	Multiple causes, depending on patient diagnosis.	See Chapter 43 for a full discussion of pain management.
Skin and mucous membrane discomfort	Any source of skin irritation increases discomfort.	Provide skin care as needed based on patient comfort or preference. Apply lotion to skin; dry, clean bed linens to reduce irritants (see Chapter 39).
Mucous membrane discomfort	Mouth breathing or dehydration leads to dry mucous membranes; tongue and lips become dry or chapped.	Provide oral care, including tongue, every 2 to 4 hours with soft toothbrushes or foam swabs and using nonabrasive toothpaste or water. Apply a light film of lip balm for dryness. Apply topical analgesics to oral lesions (see Chapter 39).
Corneal irritation	Blinking reflexes diminish near death, causing drying of cornea.	Optical lubricants or artificial tears reduce corneal drying. Eye care with warm water removes crusts from eyelid margins.
Fatigue	Metabolic demands, stress, disease states, decreased oral intake, and heart function cause weakness and fatigue.	Balance activity and rest periods according to patient's priorities and preferred time of day. Conserve patient energy by modifying environment (Kehl, 2008).
Anxiety	Physical, social, or spiritual distress causes anxiety; causes may be situational or event specific.	Address underlying cause; provide calm, supportive environment, active listening; use benzodiazepines for acute anxiety (Pasacreta et al., 2010).
Nausea	Medications, pain, or decreased intestinal blood flow with impending death	Administer antiemetics or promotility agents; discontinue medications or foods that cause nausea; provide oral care at least every 2 to 4 hours; offer clear liquid diet and ice chips; avoid liquids that increase stomach acidity (Acreman, 2009).
Constipation	Opioids, medications, and immobility slow peristalsis. Lack of bulk in diet or reduced fluid.	Use a stimulant laxative with opioids. Make dietary alterations as preferred or tolerated; increase fluid intake if tolerated (Enck, 2009).
Diarrhea	Disease processes, treatment or medications, and gastrointestinal (GI) infections.	Assess for fecal impaction. Confer with health care provider to change medication if identified as the cause. Protect skin with moisture barrier (Kyle, 2010).
Urinary incontinence	Progressive disease and decreased level of consciousness.	Protect skin from irritation or breakdown by maintaining dry linens and clothing. Use indwelling urinary catheter or condom catheters for comfort or prevention of skin problems (Kyle, 2010).
Altered nutrition	Medications, depression, decreased activity, and decreased blood flow to the GI tract; nausea produces anorexia.	Offer smaller portions of patient-preferred foods. Treat underlying cause of anorexia if patient still wants to eat. Do not force food on patients (Acreman, 2009).
Dehydration	Patient is less willing or able to maintain oral fluid intake; has fever.	Reduce discomfort from dehydration; give mouth care at least every 2 to 4 hours; offer ice chips or moist cloth to lips. Keep lips and tongue moist.
Ineffective breathing patterns (e.g., dyspnea, shortness of breath)	Anxiety; fever; pain; increased oxygen demand; disease processes; and anemia, which reduces oxygen-carrying capacity.	Treat or control underlying cause. Position for comfort and maximal respiratory excursion, provide supplemental oxygen if comforting; reduce anxiety or fever; and provide effective pain management. Use fan for air movement, stimulating trigeminal nerve in cheek, which decreases dyspneic sensation. Administer anxiolytics, bronchodilators, inhaled steroids, or opioids to suppress cough and ease breathing and apprehension (Balkstra, 2010).
Noisy breathing ("death rattle")	Noisy breathing is the sound of secretions moving in the airway during inspiratory and expiratory phases caused by thick secretions, decreased muscle tone, swallow, and cough.	Elevate head to facilitate postural drainage. Turn from side to side to mobilize and drain secretions. Stop oral intake; avoid suctioning because of discomfort and ineffectiveness. Anticholinergic medications are sometimes helpful (Hipp and Letizia, 2009).

comforting environment for the patient dying in an institutional setting. Consider nonpharmacological interventions to increase patient comfort (Running et al., 2008). Family members are often able to provide these interventions, increasing their sense that they are making a positive contribution. Research supports the use of soft massage and brief hand massages for reducing stress (Osaka et al., 2009). Use patient-preferred music in the background, provide guided-imagery exercises, and dim the lights to provide a soothing environment for the patient and family. Patient-preferred forms of complementary therapies offer noninvasive methods to increase comfort and well-being at the end of life (Mariano, 2010) (see Chapter 32).

Promote Spiritual Comfort and Hope. Help patients make connections to their spiritual practice or cultural community. Patients are comforted when they have assurance that some aspect of their lives will transcend death. Draw on the resources of spiritual care providers in an institutional setting or collaborate with the patient's own spiritual or religious leaders and communities. Making an audiotape or videotape for the family, writing letters, or keeping a journal assures patients that something of their essence will survive past their death.

The spiritual concept of hope takes on special significance near the end of life. Nursing strategies that promote hope are often quite simple: be present and provide holistic care that affirms a patient's life and maintains dignity (Daaleman et al., 2008). Patients perceive the love of family and friends, faith, goal setting, positive relationships with professional caregivers, humor, and uplifting memories as hope promoting. Circumstances that hinder the preservation of hope include abandonment or isolation, uncontrolled symptoms, or being devalued as a person. Patients and their families hope for different things over the course of their experience with illness and death. Some hope to live for an anniversary, sit outdoors for a meal, see an important person one last time, gain pain relief, or have a peaceful death. Listen for shifts in patients' hopes and find ways to help them meet their desired goals.

Protect Against Abandonment and Isolation. Many patients with terminal illness fear dying alone. Patients feel more hopeful when others are near to help them. Nurses in institutional settings need to answer call lights promptly and check on patients often to reassure them that someone is close at hand. Consider carefully whether or not to place a patient who is actively dying in a private room. If family members plan to stay with the patient at all times or if you have assessed high privacy needs for the patient and family, a private room is best. On the other hand, many patients appreciate being able to stay involved and interact with others, which is possible when sharing a room.

Some family members who have a difficult time accepting a patient's impending death cope by making fewer visits. When family members do visit, inform them of the patient's status and share meaningful insights or encounters that you have had with the patient. Find simple and appropriate care activities for the family to perform such as offering food, cooling the patient's face, combing hair, or filling out a menu. Nighttime can be particularly lonely. Suggest that a family member stay through the night if possible. Make exceptions to visiting policies, allowing family members to remain with patients who are dying at any time. Family members appreciate having open access or closeness to their loved one through their experiences at the end of life. Record contact information for them so you can reach them at any time.

Support the Grieving Family. In palliative care patients and family members constitute the unit of care. When a patient becomes debilitated or approaches the end of life, family members also suffer. They describe caregiving at the end of life as unpredictable, frightening, and anguishing. On the other hand, they report being deeply moved by their experiences and describe their activities as affirming (Phillips, 2009). In these extremely intimate and emotionally challenging times, offer holistic, family-centered support, compassion, and education that incorporates the uniqueness of each patient. Often family members face challenging and complex situations long before their loved one is actively dying. Family members caring for people with serious life-limiting illness need attention and support early and consistently throughout the experience of illness and death (Box 36-7).

Families report that they especially value having access to the information they need to make important decisions (Spichiger, 2008). Educate family members in all settings about the symptoms that the patient will likely experience and the implications for care. For example, patients in the last days of life often develop anorexia or feel nauseated by food. Illness, decreased activity, treatments, and fatigue decrease a patient's caloric needs and appetite. Family members, distressed with the decline, often believe that they need to encourage the patient to eat. Forcing food or fluids stresses the patient's compromised gastrointestinal and cardiovascular systems, potentially creating increased discomfort (Acreman, 2009). Help families shift their focus to other helping activities during this time.

BOX 36-7 EVIDENCE-BASED PRACTICE

Patient and Family Member Satisfaction with End-of-Life Care

PICO Question: For patients who are dying and their family members, which nursing interventions are most successful in enhancing satisfaction with end-of-life care?

Evidence Summary

Above all nurses strive for positive patient-centered outcomes at the end of life. A growing body of research literature reveals what patients and family members perceive to be important at the end of life (i.e., helping caregivers focus on behaviors that bring about the highest degree of patient and family satisfaction). A systematic review of research literature included 21 qualitative studies that focused on caregiver interventions that patients and family members described as satisfying care. The dominant themes of satisfaction that surfaced in the research studies include accessibility, coordination of care, competence, communication and relationships, education, emotional support, personalization of care, and support for patient decision making (Dy et al., 2008). Other important nursing interventions include symptom management and providing comfort care and emotional support. Patients and family members are most satisfied when they receive attentive, compassionate care. Novice nurses who are grounded in authentic, open-hearted, holistic nursing care practices are capable of providing valuable care to patients at the end of life.

Application to Nursing Practice

- Individualize your plan of care. Discuss priorities and preferences for care with patients and family members frequently.
- Give as much time as needed to discuss a sensitive topic, maintain contact, and respond to requests promptly.
- Coordinate care by maintaining effective interdisciplinary communication.
- Support patient's decision making and provide assistance with end of life to maintain a sense of control.
- Provide information about what to expect at a level understandable to the patient.

BOX 36-8 PHYSICAL CHANGES HOURS OR DAYS BEFORE DEATH

- Increased periods of sleeping/unresponsiveness
- Coolness and color changes in extremities, nose, fingers
- Bowel or bladder incontinence
- Decreased urine output; dark-colored urine
- Restlessness or disorientation
- Decreased intake of food or fluids; inability to swallow
- Congestion/increased pulmonary secretions; noisy respirations (death rattle)
- Altered breathing (apnea, labored or irregular breathing, Cheyne-Stokes pattern)
- Decreased muscle tone, relaxed jaw muscles, sagging mouth
- Weakness and fatigue

Family members who have limited prior experience with death do not know what to expect. They may need personal time with the nurse to share their concerns, ask about treatment options, validate perceived changes in the patient's status, or explore the possible meaning of patient behaviors. Whenever possible, communicate news of a patient's declining condition or impending death when family members are together so they can support each other. Provide information privately and stay with the family as long as needed or desired. Reduce family member anxiety, stress, or fear by describing what to expect as death approaches. Become familiar with common manifestations of impending death (Box 36-8), remembering that patients usually experience some but not all of these changes. Do not try to predict the time of death; instead use your assessments to help family members anticipate what is happening. Share your observations and through your role modeling encourage a sense of patience, compassion, and comfort throughout the dying process.

After death assist the family with decision making such as notification of a funeral home, transportation of family members, and collection of the patient's belongings. Nurses are a primary source of family support. Remember that, because of differing responses to grief, some family members prefer to be alone at the time of a death, whereas others want to be surrounded by a support community. When uncertain about what a family member prefers for support, pose simple questions and offer suggestions for assistance.

With the death of a patient, family members benefit from the many resources of the health care team. When the patient chooses to die at home, family members provide direct care, which is often emotionally stressful and physically exhausting. In the home setting fatigued family caregivers benefit from respite care. During respite care, a patient temporarily receives care from others so family members are able to get away to rest and relax. Hospice program benefits include some days of respite care. Inform family members of home care, hospice, and community service options so they can access the best resources for their situation.

Assist with End-of-Life Decision Making. Patients and family members often face complex treatment decisions at the end of life. Decisions the family often need to make include: Which medical interventions would the patient want to use? Should life-extending treatments be stopped if there appears to be little chance of recovery? Should artificial nutrition and hydration be provided when a patient is near death and no longer able to eat? (Wainwright and Gallagher, 2007). They need time and careful explanations by nurses and other health care providers to make decisions (Mahon, 2010).

Difficult ethical decisions at the end of life complicate a survivor's grief, create family divisions, or increase family uncertainty at the time of death (see Chapter 22). When ethical decisions are handled well, survivors achieve a sense of control and experience a meaningful conclusion to their loved one's death. Suggest to patients that they clearly communicate their wishes for end-of-life care so family members are able to act as faithful surrogates when the patient can no longer speak for himself or herself. Advance directives often decrease the stress of family members when end-of-life decisions must be made (see Chapter 23) (Tilden et al., 2001). Some patients and family members rely on the nurse and other members of the health care team to initiate discussions regarding end-of-life care. Nurses often provide options that family members do not know are available and are advocates for patients and family members making decisions at the end of life.

Facilitate Mourning. Nurses who work with grieving family members often provide bereavement care after the patient's death. Helpful strategies for assisting grieving persons include the following:

- Help the survivor accept that the loss is real. Discuss how the loss or illness occurred or was discovered, when, under what circumstances, who told him or her about it, and other factual topics to reinforce the reality of the event and put it in perspective.
- Support efforts to adjust to the loss. Use a problem-solving approach. Have survivors make a list of their concerns or needs, help them prioritize, and lead them step-by-step through a discussion of how to proceed. Encourage survivors to ask for help.
- Encourage establishment of new relationships. Reassure people that new relationships do not mean that they are replacing the person who has died. Encourage involvement in nonthreatening group social activities (e.g., volunteer activities or church events).
- Allow time to grieve. "Anniversary reactions" (i.e., renewed grief around the time of the loss in subsequent years) are common. A return to sadness or the pain of grief is often worrisome. Openly acknowledge the loss, provide reassurance that the reaction is normal, and encourage the survivor to reminisce.
- Interpret "normal" behavior. Being distractible, having difficulty sleeping or eating, and thinking that they have heard the deceased's voice are common behaviors following loss. These symptoms do not mean that an individual has an emotional problem or is becoming ill. Reinforce that these behaviors are normal and will resolve over time.
- Provide continuing support. Survivors need the support of a nurse with whom they have bonded for a time following a loss, especially in home care or hospice nursing. The nurse has become an important "actor" in the drama of the deceased's life and death and has helped them through some very intimate and memorable times. Attachment for awhile after the death is appropriate and healing for both the survivor and the nurse.
- Be alert for signs of ineffective, potentially harmful coping mechanisms such as alcohol and substance abuse or excessive use of over-the-counter analgesics or sleep aids.

Care After Death. Federal and state laws require institutions to develop policies and procedures for certain events that occur after death: requesting organ or tissue donation, performing an autopsy, certifying and documenting the occurrence of a death, and providing safe and appropriate postmortem care. In accordance with federal law, a specially trained professional (e.g., transplant coordinator or social worker) makes requests for **organ and tissue donation** at the time of every death. The person requesting organ or tissue donation provides information about who can legally give consent, which organs or tissues can be donated, associated costs, and how donation affects burial or cremation.

In extremely stressful circumstances created by the loss of a loved one, grieving survivors usually cannot remember all they were told. Nurses provide support and reinforce and clarify explanations given to them during the request process. In addition, understanding the physiology of organ donation is often difficult for family members. Even though a patient who is brain dead is legally declared dead, he or she remains on life support to provide the vital organs with blood and oxygen before transplant. The appearance of a live-looking body confuses the family, and they need help to understand that the life support is only preserving the vital organs. Nonvital tissues such as corneas, skin, long bones, and middle ear bones are taken at the time of death without artificially maintaining vital functions. If the deceased has not left behind instructions concerning organ and tissue donation, the family gives or denies consent at the time of death. Review your state organ retrieval laws and institutional policy and procedure regarding the formal consent process. Be aware that the laws governing who to approach for organ donation may not be acceptable in other cultures.

Family members give consent for an **autopsy** (i.e., the surgical dissection of a body after death) to determine the exact cause and circumstances of death or discover the pathway of a disease (see Chapter 23). In most cases a coroner or medical examiner determines the need to perform an autopsy. Law sometimes requires that an autopsy be performed when death is the result of foul play; homicide; suicide; or accidental causes such as motor vehicle crashes, falls, the ingestion of drugs, or deaths within 24 hours of hospital admission. Unattended deaths or those that occur in the workplace or during incarceration also usually require an autopsy (AMA, 2004).

Usually the physician or other designated health care provider asks for autopsy permission while the nurse answers questions and supports the family's choices. Inform family members that an autopsy does not deform the body and that all organs are replaced in the body. Family members are often comforted to know that others may be helped by either the gift of organ and tissue donation or through autopsy. Respect and honor family wishes and final decisions.

Documentation of a death provides a legal record of the event. Follow agency policies and procedures carefully to provide an accurate and reliable medical record of all assessments and activities surrounding a death. Physicians or coroners sign some medical forms such as a request for autopsy, but the registered nurse gathers and records much of the remaining information surrounding a death. Nurses also usually witness or delegate the signing of forms (e.g., release of body or personal belongings forms). Nursing documentation becomes relevant in risk management or legal investigations into a death, underscoring the importance of accurate, legal reporting. Documentation also validates success in meeting patient goals or provides justification for changes in treatment or expected outcomes. Box 36-9 lists important documentation elements for end-of-life care.

Family members deserve and expect a clear description of what happened to their loved one, especially in cases of sudden, unusual, or unexpected circumstances. Give only factual information in a nonjudgmental, objective manner and avoid sharing your opinions. State law and agency policy govern the sharing of the written medical record information, which usually involves a written request. Follow legal guidelines for documentation and sharing of medical records (see Chapter 23).

BOX 36-9 DOCUMENTATION OF END-OF-LIFE CARE

- Time and date of death and all actions taken to respond to the impending death
- Name of health care provider certifying the death
- Persons notified of the death (e.g., health care providers, family members, organ request team, morgue, funeral home, spiritual care providers) and person who comes to declare time of death
- Name of person making request for organ or tissue donation
- Special preparations of the body (e.g., desired or required religious/cultural rituals)
- Medical tubes, devices, or lines left in or on the body
- Personal articles left on and secured to the body
- Personal items given to the family with description, date, time, to whom given
- Location of body identification tags
- Time of body transfer and destination
- Any other relevant information or family requests that help clarify special circumstances

When a patient dies in an institutional or home care setting, nurses provide or delegate **postmortem care,** the care of a body after death. Above all, a human body deserves the same respect and dignity as a living person and needs to be prepared in a manner consistent with the patient's cultural and religious beliefs. Death produces physical changes in the body quite quickly; thus you need to perform postmortem care as soon as possible to prevent discoloration, tissue damage, or deformities.

Maintaining the integrity of cultural and religious rituals and mourning practices at the time of death gives survivors a sense of fulfilled obligations and promotes acceptance of the patient's death (Box 36-10). The ability of families to mourn in a manner consistent with cultural values helps survivors experience some predictability and control in an otherwise uncertain and confusing time. Some cultures consider "family" as more than a nuclear biological unit. Health care providers need to understand the makeup of a family network and know which individuals to involve in end-of-life decisions and care.

The nurse coordinates patient and family care during and after a death. Become familiar with applicable policies and procedures for postmortem care because they vary across settings or institutions. See the procedural guideline (Box 36-11) for standard activities for care of the body after death.

EVALUATION

Through the Patient's Eyes. The success of the evaluation process depends partially on the bond that you have formed with the patient. Patients are more likely to share personal expectations or their wishes if you form a trusting relationship with them. Refer back to the goals and expected outcomes established during the planning phase to determine the effectiveness of nursing interventions. A patient's responses and perceptions of the effectiveness of the interventions determine if the existing plan of care is effective or if different strategies are necessary. For example, if the goal

BOX 36-10 CULTURAL ASPECTS OF CARE

Care of the Body After Death

There are culturally specific rituals and mourning practices that loved ones use to achieve a sense of acceptance and inner peace and participate in socially accepted expressions of grief. One's culture greatly influences what behaviors and rituals are expected at the time of death. Institutional guidelines and end-of-life care procedures for patients from all cultures provide standards based on compassion, maintaining privacy and dignity, and respect for patients' and family members' cultural beliefs and practices. Expert end-of-life care allows time for patients and their families to make private and public preparations and complete unfinished communication. Understanding the uniqueness of cultural expectations at the end of life helps a nurse know what questions to ask. The cultural or religious practices described below are not necessarily exclusive to the culture named but are offered to give you an idea of some culturally specific concerns you may encounter in end-of-life care.

Implications for Practice

- **African American:** Care of the body after death depends on the African American's country of origin and degree of American acculturation. The presence of large extended family groups, including the church family, is common at time of death. The mourning period is relatively short, with a memorial service and a public viewing of the body or a wake before burial. Organ donation and autopsy are allowable.
- **Chinese:** Death is regarded as a negative life event, and there is no concept of an afterlife. The dead are treated with the same respect as the living and may be buried with food and other artifacts. Members of an extended family usually stay with the deceased for up to 8 hours after death. The oldest son or daughter bathes the body under direction from an older relative or a temple priest. They often believe the body should remain intact; thus organ donation and autopsy are uncommon (Xu Y, 2007).
- **Hispanic or Latino:** Honoring family values and roles is essential in providing care and making decisions at the end of life. People in Hispanic and Mexican-American cultures often use special objects such as amulets or rosary beads, alternative healing practices (folk medicine), and prayer. Grief is expressed openly. Religious and spiritual rituals (predominantly Catholic) are essential at the end of life. Death is often believed to be the will of God (Gonzales et al., 2008; Taxis et al., 2008).
- **Native American:** Native Americans encompass diverse tribal groups with differing practices, traditions, and ceremonies. Traditional Navajos do not touch the body after death. Care of the body in the large Navajo tribe includes cleansing the body, painting the deceased's face, dressing in clothing, and attaching an eagle feather to symbolize a return home. Mourners also have a ritual cleansing of their bodies. The dead are buried on the deceased's homeland (Hanley, 2008).
- **Islamic:** The deceased's body is ritualistically washed, wrapped, cried over, prayed for, and buried as soon as possible after death. The eyes and mouth are closed, and the face of the deceased is turned toward Mecca. Muslims of the same gender prepare the body for burial. Bodies are buried, not cremated. Autopsies interfere with a quick burial; make autopsy requests with sensitivity and only if necessary. The proximity of loved ones after death is important since it is believed that the soul stays with the body until it is buried. Organ donation is permissible by some Qur'an interpretations (Gatrad and Sheikh, 2008).
- **Buddhist:** Buddhists believe in an afterlife in which humans manifest in different forms. Death is preferred at home, and a person's state at the time of death is important. Individuals usually minimize emotional expressions and maintain a peaceful, compassionate atmosphere. Male family members prepare the body. Buddhists recommend not touching the body after death to give the deceased a smoother transition to the afterlife. People often say prayers while touching and standing at the head of the deceased. The body is not left alone after death. Family and friends pay respects after death and before cremation of the body (Bauer-Wu et al., 2007).
- **Hindu:** The body is placed on the floor with the head facing north. Persons of the same gender handle the body after death. There are no general prohibitions against autopsy. Bodies are cremated after death to purify by fire (Gatrad et al., 2008).
- **Jewish:** If the family practices Orthodox Judaism, determine if members from the Jewish Burial Society are coming to the facility before preparing the body. A family member often stays with the body until burial. Usually the burial occurs within 24 hours but not on the Sabbath. Some but not all types of Judaism avoid cremation, autopsy, and embalming (Bauer-Wu et al., 2007).

is to have the patient communicate a sense of hope to family members, evaluate verbal and nonverbal communication and behaviors for cues related to expressions of hope. Continue to evaluate the patient's progress, the effectiveness of the interventions, and patient and family interactions. Even when a patient is not seeking care specifically related to a loss, be alert for signs and symptoms of grief. They provide the criteria for evaluating whether a patient is coping with a loss and how he or she is moving through the grief process. Critical thinking ensures that the evaluation process accurately reflects the patient's situation and desired outcomes (Fig. 36-5).

Patient Outcomes. The following questions help you validate achievement of patient goals and expectations:

- What is the most important thing I can do for you at this time?
- Are your needs being addressed in a timely manner?
- Are you getting the care for which you hoped?
- Would you like me to help you in a different way?
- Do you have a specific request that I have not met?

Especially in home care settings, you include family members in the evaluation process. The short- and long-term outcomes that signal a family's recovery from a loss guide your evaluation. Short-term outcomes indicating effectiveness of grief interventions include talking about the loss without feeling overwhelmed, improved energy level, normalized sleep and dietary patterns, reorganization of life patterns, improved ability to make decisions, and finding it easier to be around other people. Long-term achievements include the return of a sense of humor and normal life patterns, renewed or new personal relationships, and decrease of inner pain.

Importance of Nurses' Self-Care

You cannot give fully engaged, compassionate care to others when you feel depleted or do not feel cared for yourself. Nurses experience grief and loss too. Many times, even before a nurse has a chance to recover from an emotionally draining situation, he or she encounters another difficult human story. Nurses in acute care settings often witness prolonged, concentrated suffering on a daily basis, leading to feelings of frustration, anger, guilt, sadness, or anxiety. Nursing students report initially feeling hesitant and uncomfortable with their first encounters with a dying patient and identify feelings of sadness, anxiety, and discomfort (Allchin, 2006).

BOX 36-11 PROCEDURAL GUIDELINES

Care of the Body After Death

Delegation Considerations

The skill of care of the body after death can be delegated to nursing assistive personnel (NAP). Nurses often find it meaningful to help care for a patient after death and assist the NAP whenever possible. Instruct the NAP to:

- Contact the nurse for all questions and procedures related to organ/tissue donation and autopsy requests.
- Alert nurse to family members' questions related to manner of death or after-death activities.

Equipment

Bath towels, washcloths, washbasin, scissors, shroud kit with name tags, bed linen, documentation forms.

1. Confirm the health care provider certified the death and documented the time of death and actions taken.
2. Determine if the health care provider requested an autopsy. An autopsy is required for deaths that occur under certain circumstances.
3. Validate the status of request for organ or tissue donation. Given the complex and sensitive nature of such requests, only specially trained personnel make the requests. Maintain sensitivity to personal, religious, and cultural beliefs in this process.
4. Identify the patient using two identifiers (e.g., name and birth date or name and account number) according to facility policy. Compare identifiers with information on the patient's medical record.
5. Provide sensitive and dignified nursing care to the patient and family.
   a. Elevate the head of the bed as soon as possible after death to prevent discoloration of the face.
   b. Collect ordered specimens.
   c. Ask if the family wishes to participate in preparation of the body. Offer to make arrangements for supportive company for the family (patient/family religious leader, spiritual care personnel, or bereavement specialist) during body preparation.
   d. Ask about family requests for body preparation such as wearing special clothing or religious artifacts. Be aware that personal, religious, or cultural practices determine whether or not to shave male facial hair. Get permission before shaving a beard.
   e. Remove all equipment, tubes, and indwelling lines. Note that autopsy or organ donation often poses exceptions to removal; thus consult agency policy in these situations.
   f. Cleanse the body thoroughly, maintaining safety standards for body fluids and contamination when indicated. Comb patient's hair or apply personal hairpieces.
   g. Cover body with a clean sheet, place head on a pillow, and leave arms outside covers if possible. Close eyes by gently holding them shut; leave dentures in the mouth to maintain facial shape; cover any signs of body trauma.
   h. Prepare and clean the environment, deodorize room if needed, and lower the lights.
   i. Offer family members the option to view the body and ask if they want you or other support persons to accompany them. Honor and respect individual choices.
   j. Encourage grievers to say good-bye in their own way: words, touch, singing, religious rituals, or prayers.
   k. Provide privacy and an unrushed atmosphere. Assess family members' need or desire for your presence at this time. If you leave, tell them how to reach you.
   l. Determine which personal belongings stay with the body (e.g., wedding ring or religious symbol) and give other personal items to family members. Document time, date, description of the items taken, and who received them. Save any items that are accidentally left behind and contact family for further instructions.
   m. Apply identifying name tags and shroud according to agency policy before transporting the body. Follow safety procedures for body fluid precautions or contamination concerns.
   n. Complete documentation in the narrative notes section (see Box 36-9).
   o. Maintain privacy and dignity when transporting the body to another location; cover the body or stretcher with a clean sheet.

Frequent, intense, or prolonged exposure to grief and loss places nurses at risk for developing **compassion fatigue.** Compassion fatigue, described as physical, emotional, and spiritual exhaustion resulting from seeing patients suffer, leads to a decreased capacity to show compassion or empathize with suffering people (Bush, 2009).

To avoid the extremes of either becoming overly involved in patients' suffering or detaching from them, nurses develop self-care strategies to maintain balance. Self-reflection, an element of critical thinking, serves as a useful tool when you feel overwhelmed. For example, ask yourself if your sadness is related to caring for a patient or to an unresolved, disruptive experience in your personal life. Talking with friends, a spiritual care provider, or a close colleague helps you recognize your own grief and reflect on the meaning of caring for dying patients. Creative strategies help you cope with the loss of a patient to whom you have become attached. You sometimes gain closure by attending a mortuary viewing or a funeral or writing a sympathy letter to the family. Stress management techniques (see Chapter 37) help restore your energy and enjoyment in caring for patients. In some instances nurses choose to work temporarily in less emotionally stressful settings.

Nurses who practice self-care are more likely to experience professional and personal growth and find meaning in their work. Care for your physical health by eating well, exercising, engaging in relaxing activities, laughing, and getting enough sleep. To promote emotional health, participate in calming activities such as meditation, daily gratitude reflections, deep breathing, walking, or listening to music (Showalter, 2010). Activities for self-transcendence (spiritual awareness) include journal writing, sharing stories, recognizing one's own positive contributions and unique gifts, and connecting with one's self (Hunnibell et al., 2008). Because of the ongoing demands of professional caregiving, set limits on the how much you do and spend time enjoying your favorite activities (Fig. 36-6). Pay attention to the people who nurture you.

Research indicates that nurses maintain hope and a positive outlook when they have adequate resources to care for patients, believe they are making a difference, and feel supported by team members (Duggleby and Wright, 2007). Receiving recognition for the many ways in which nurses make valuable contributions to the quality of patients' lives contributes greatly to job satisfaction (Perry, 2009). Nurture your work relationships and learn to ask for and accept help. Creative workplace strategies and educational offerings provide nurses with opportunities for healing, restoration of balance, and personal recognition (Parsons, 2009).

Remember that caring for seriously ill and dying people gives you opportunities to find meaning and importance in being a

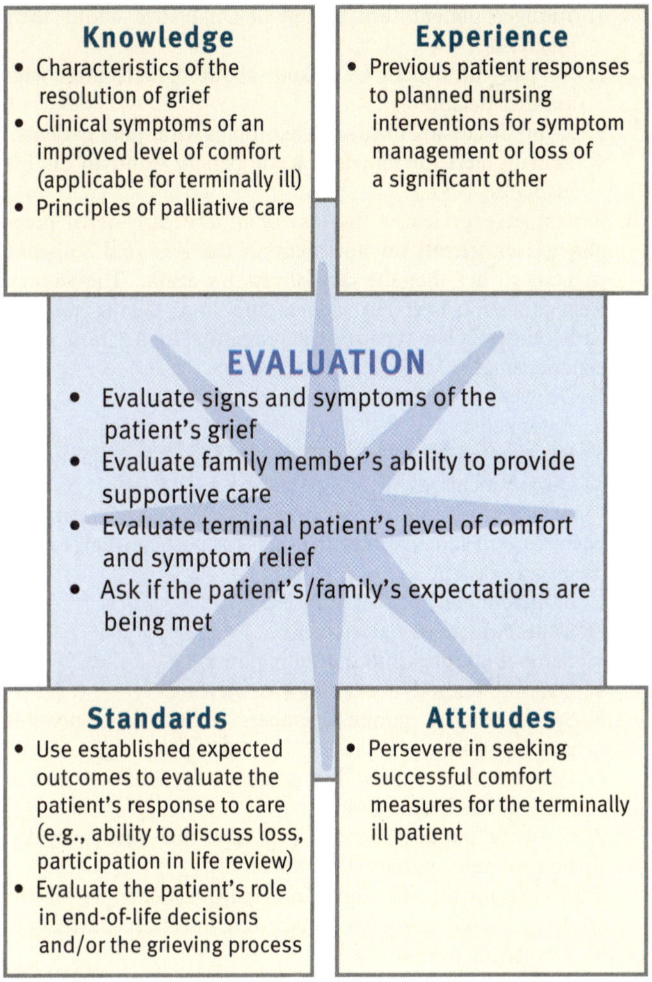
Knowledge
• Characteristics of the resolution of grief
• Clinical symptoms of an improved level of comfort (applicable for terminally ill)
• Principles of palliative care
Experience
• Previous patient responses to planned nursing interventions for symptom management or loss of a significant other
EVALUATION
• Evaluate signs and symptoms of the patient's grief
• Evaluate family member's ability to provide supportive care
• Evaluate terminal patient's level of comfort and symptom relief
• Ask if the patient's/family's expectations are being met
Standards
• Use established expected outcomes to evaluate the patient's response to care (e.g., ability to discuss loss, participation in life review)
• Evaluate the patient's role in end-of-life decisions and/or the grieving process
Attitudes
• Persevere in seeking successful comfort measures for the terminally ill patient

FIG. 36-5 Critical thinking model for loss, death, and grief evaluation.

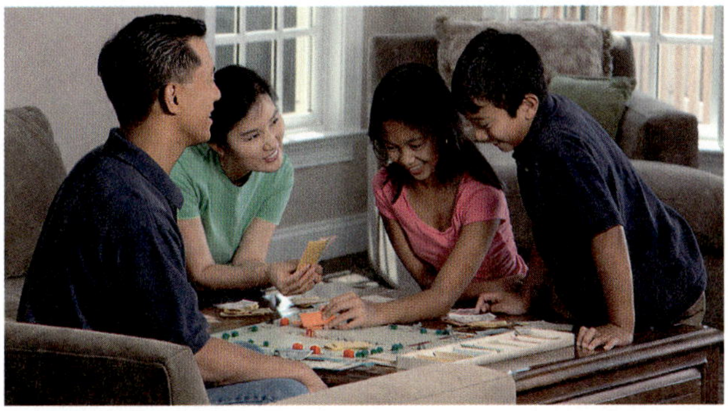

FIG. 36-6 Nurses participate in self-care to maintain balance needed for compassionate caregiving. (Courtesy Bill Branson, National Cancer Institute.)

nurse. You learn from the courage of your patients, find joy and beauty in life, and become more open to others. The same nursing students who experience discomfort in their first experiences with death also note that they reflect on those experiences well beyond their clinical time and are able to identify personal and professional benefits to their experience (Allchin, 2006).

KEY POINTS

- When caring for patients who have experienced a loss, facilitate the grief process by helping survivors feel the loss, express it, and move through their grief.
- Loss comes in many forms, based on the values and priorities learned within a person's sphere of influence (i.e., family, friends, religion, society, and culture).
- The type and perception of the loss influence how a person experiences grief.
- Death is difficult for the dying person and the person's family, friends, and caregivers.
- Theorists describe grief as stages, tasks, and processes undertaken by survivors to successfully complete their bereavement and adapt to life with a loss.
- Survivors move back and forth through a series of stages and/or tasks many times, possibly extending over a long period of time.
- Grieving people use their own unique history, context, and resources to make meaning out of their loss experiences. Listen as patients share the experience in their own way.
- Knowledge of the types of grief helps nurses identify appropriate interventions.
- A person's development, coping strategies, socioeconomic status, personal relationships, nature of loss, and cultural and spiritual beliefs influence the way he or she perceives and responds to grief.
- Nursing interventions involve reinforcing patients' successful coping mechanisms and introducing new coping approaches when needed.
- Assess the terminally ill patient and family wishes for end-of-life care, including the preferred place for death, desired level of intervention, and expectations for pain and symptom management.
- Establish a caring presence and use effective communication strategies to encourage patients to share to the degree they are comfortable.
- Palliative care allows patients to make more informed choices, achieve better alleviation of symptoms, and experience a higher quality of life through an illness or death experience.
- Hospice is not a place but rather a philosophy of family-centered, whole-person care at the end of life.
- Practice self-care, ask for and accept help, and reflect on the meaning of nursing experiences of caring for the dying patient and family.

CLINICAL APPLICATION QUESTIONS

Preparing for Clinical Practice

1. Mrs. Allison feels hopeless and uncertain about her future. As noted in the concept map, her chronic pain and associated hopelessness contribute to other health problems. She has lost her desire to eat or see other people and has difficulty walking. As a result her activity and balance are also decreased. Describe how you plan to communicate with Mrs. Allison, who is having intense emotional reactions to loss and grief.
2. Mrs. Allison's family members express concern about how they can best offer support when she goes home. What do you include in a family teaching plan?
3. Mrs. Allison wants to go home to live independently as long as she is able. Her daughter arrives to help make decisions for her

mother's care. Mrs. Allison and her daughter do not understand hospice care and want you to tell them about it to see if it might be a good care option for them. What major points do you plan to include in a conversation with the patient and family related to hospice philosophy, services, and impact on the family?

evolve *Answers to Clinical Application Questions can be found on the Evolve website.*

REVIEW QUESTIONS

Are You Ready to Test Your Nursing Knowledge?

1. Regarding the request for organ and tissue donation at the time of death, the nurse needs to be aware that:
   1. Specially educated personnel make requests.
   2. Requests are usually made by the nurse caring for the patient at the time of death.
   3. Only patients who have given prior instruction regarding donation become donors.
   4. Professionals need to be very selective in whom they ask for organ and tissue donation.
2. The nurse notes that a woman who recently began cancer treatment appears quiet and withdrawn, states that she does not believe the treatments will make any difference, does not ask about her progress, and missed two chemotherapy sessions. Based on the above assessment data, the nurse gathers more information to consider making which of the following nursing diagnoses?
   1. Anxiety
   2. Hopelessness
   3. Spiritual distress
   4. Complicated grieving
3. A family member asks a home care nurse what he should do if the patient's serious chronic illness worsens even with increased medical interventions. How does the nurse best begin a conversation about the goals of care at the end of life?
   1. Encourage the family member to think more positively about the patient's new therapy
   2. Avoid the discussion because it has to do with medical, not nursing, diagnoses
   3. Initiate a discussion about advance directives with the patient, family, and health care team
   4. Begin the discussion by asking the patient to identify his or her beliefs about the goals of care while the family member is present
4. Which of the following nursing actions best reflects sensitivity to cultural differences related to end-of-life care?
   1. Practice honesty with everyone, telling patients about their illness, even if the news is not good.
   2. Ask family members if they prefer to help with the care of the body after death.
   3. Provide postmortem care at the time of death to relieve family members of this difficult job.
   4. Value patient self-determination, understanding that each person makes his or her own decisions.
5. A young man is diagnosed with a serious, life-changing illness. His conversations during his first 2 days of hospitalization are abrupt, superficial, and unrelated to his illness. What understanding about communication enhances your therapeutic communication with this patient?
   1. Younger patients are usually less talkative about their diagnosis.
   2. All patients benefit by talking about their feelings with another person.
   3. Avoid discussing illness-related topics with quiet patients.
   4. Remain alert for signals that the patient wants to discuss his illness.
6. A woman experiences the loss of a very early–term pregnancy. Her friends do not mention the loss, and someone suggests to her that she can "always try again." The woman feels confusion over her sadness and stops talking about it with others. What type of grief response is she most likely experiencing?
   1. Delayed
   2. Anticipated
   3. Exaggerated
   4. Disenfranchised
7. A nurse has the responsibility of managing a deceased patient's post-mortem care. Arrange the steps for post-mortem care in the proper order.
   1. Bathe the body of the deceased.
   2. Collect any needed specimens.
   3. Remove all tubes and indwelling lines.
   4. Position the body for family visit/viewing.
   5. Speak to the family members about their possible participation.
   6. Confirm that request for organ/tissue donation and/or autopsy has been made.
   7. Notify a support person (e.g., spiritual care provider, bereavement specialist) for the family.
   8. Accurately tag the body, indicating the identity of the deceased and safety issues regarding infection control.
   9. Elevate the head of the bed.
8. A family member of a recently deceased patient talks casually with the nurse at the time of the patient's death and expresses relief that she will not have to visit at the hospital anymore. What theoretical description of grief best applies to this family member?
   1. Denial
   2. Anticipatory grief
   3. Dysfunctional grief
   4. Yearning and searching
9. A self-care goal you set when caring for dying and grieving patients includes:
   1. Learning not to take losses so seriously.
   2. Limiting involvement with patients who are grieving.
   3. Maintaining life balance and reflecting on the meaning of your work.
   4. Admitting that you are not well suited to care for people who are grieving and asking the charge nurse not to assign you to care for these patients.
10. A nurse is providing postmortem care. Which action is the priority?
    1. Locating the patient's clothing
    2. Providing culturally and religiously sensitive care in body preparation
    3. Transporting the body to the morgue as soon as possible to prevent body decomposition
    4. Providing all postmortem care to protect the family of the deceased from having to see the body
11. Which approach to helping grieving people is most consistent with postmodern grief theories?

1. Help the patient identify the tasks to be accomplished during his or her grief.
2. Encourage people to recognize stages of grieving in anticipation of what is to come.
3. Listen carefully to a person's story of how his or her grief experience is unfolding.
4. Offer general grief timelines to help the person know when a phase will pass.

12. A patient who has a serious, life-limiting chronic illness wants to continue to engage in self-care and live as normally as possible. Which of the following nursing responses reflect a helpful understanding of patient self-care at the end of life?
    1. "Learning to accept that you can't perform some activities anymore will bring you more acceptance and peace."
    2. "Which activities are most important to you, and how can you continue to do them?"
    3. "People in your life want to help you with things; allow them to do what they want for you."
    4. "Spending more of your time resting or reading will conserve your energy."
13. The nurse suggests that a patient receive a palliative care consultation for symptom management related to anxiety and increasing pain. A family member asks the nurse if this means that the patient is dying and is now "in hospice." What does the nurse tell the family member about palliative care? (Select all that apply.)
    1. Hospice and palliative care are the same thing.
    2. Palliative care is for any patient, any time, any disease, in any setting.
    3. Palliative care strategies are primarily designed to treat the patient's illness.
    4. Palliative care interventions relieve the symptoms of illness and treatment.
14. You have identified three nursing diagnoses for a patient who is having anxiety and hopelessness as a result of a loss. Which general approach do you take to prioritize the nursing diagnoses? (Select all that apply.)
    1. Use family members and physician orders as primary resources for prioritizing your actions.
    2. Address the nursing diagnosis that most affects the medical diagnosis.
    3. Ask the patient to identify the most distressing symptom and first address that diagnosis.
    4. Use nursing knowledge to address the problem that is the underlying cause of other diagnoses.
15. Regarding grief in older adults, which understanding helps guide your relationship with an elderly patient?
    1. Older adults have usually sustained many losses in life, which influence the current loss.
    2. Older adults with a poor memory experience grief less intensely.
    3. Older adults generally handle loss better because they have more experience with it.
    4. Social support is less important because an older adult's circle of friends has become smaller.

Answers: **1.** 1; **2.** 2; **3.** 4; **4.** 2; **5.** 4; **6.** 4; **7.** 6, 9, 2, 5, 7, 3, 1, 4, 8; **8.** 2; **9.** 3; **10.** 2; **11.** 3; **12.** 2; **13.** 2, 4; **14.** 3, 4; **15.** 1.

REFERENCES

Acreman S: Nutrition in palliative care, *Br J Commun Nurs* 14(10):127, 2009.

American Association of Colleges of Nursing (AACN) and City of Hope National Medical Center: *End-of-Life Nursing Education Consortium (ELNEC)-Core*, Duarte, Calif, 2008, The Associations.

American Medical Association (AMA): *Autopsy: life's final chapter*, 2004, http://ukhealthcare.uky.edu/publications/healthsmart/healthsmart_autopsy.pdf. Accessed November 6, 2011.

American Nurses Association (ANA): *Scope and standards of hospice and palliative nursing practice*, Atlanta, 2007, ANA.

Balkstra C: Dyspnea. In Matzo M, Sherman D, editors: *Palliative care nursing: quality care at the end of life*, ed 3, New York, 2010, Springer Publishing Co.

Bauer-Wu S, et al: Spiritual perspectives and practices at the end of life: a review of the major world religions and application to palliative care, *Indian J Palliat Care* 13(2): 53, 2007.

Bephage G: Promoting spiritual comfort in palliative care settings, *Nurs Residential Care* 11(9):463, 2009.

Betcher D: Elephant in the room project: improving caring efficacy through effective and compassionate communication with palliative care patients, *Medsurg Nurs* 19(2): 101, 2010.

Bowlby J: *Attachment and loss:* vol 3, *Loss, sadness, and depression*, New York, 1980, Basic Books.

Bush N: Compassion fatigue: are you at risk? *Oncol Nurs Forum* 26(1):24, 2009.

Enck R: An overview of constipation and newer therapies, *Am J Hospice Palliat Med* 26(3):157, 2009.

Ferrell B, Coyle N, editors: *Textbook of palliative nursing*, ed 3, New York, 2010, Oxford University Press.

Ferrell B, Coyle N: The nature of suffering and the goals of nursing, *Oncol Nurs Forum* 35(2):241, 2008.

Galvin K, Todres L: Embodying nursing open-heartedness, *J Holistic Nurs* 27(2):141, 2009.

Gatrad R, Sheikh A: Palliative care for Muslims. In Gatrad R, Sheikh A, Brown E, editors: *Palliative care for South Asians: Muslims, Hindus, & Sikhs*, London, 2008, Quay Books.

Gatrad R, et al: Palliative care for Hindus. In Gatrad R, Sheikh R, Brown E, editors: *Palliative care for South Asians: Muslims, Hindus, & Sikhs*, London, 2008, Quay Books.

Gonzales E, et al: Mexican Americans. In Giger JN, Davidhizar RN, editors: *Transcultural nursing: assessment and intervention*, ed 5, St Louis, 2008, Mosby.

Hanley K. Navajos. In Giger JN, Davidhizar RN, editors: *Transcultural nursing: assessment and intervention*, ed 5, St Louis, 2008, Mosby.

Herr K, et al: Pain assessment in the nonverbal patient: position statement with clinical practice recommendations, *J Pain Symptom Manage* 31(2):170, 2006.

Hipp B, Letizia M: Understanding and responding to the death rattle in dying patients, *Medsurg Nurs* 18(1):17, 2009.

Hooyman N, Kramer B: *Living through loss: interventions across the lifespan*, New York, 2008, Columbia University Press.

Hospice Foundation of America: *Services*, 2010, http://www.hospicefoundation.org/pages/page.asp?page_id=47055. Accessed November 10, 2011.

Johnstone L, Kanitsaki O: Ethics and advance care planning in a culturally diverse society, *J Transcult Nurs* 20(4):405, 2009.

Kehl K: Caring for the patient and the family in the last hours of life, *Home Health Care Mange Pract* 20(5):408, 2008.

Kübler-Ross E: *On death and dying*, New York, 1969, Macmillan.

Kyle B: Bowel and bladder care at the end of life, *Br J Nurs* 19(7):408, 2010.

Mahon M: Advanced care decision making: asking the right people the right questions, *J Psychosocial Nurs* 48(7):13, 2010.

Mariano C: Holistic integrative therapies in palliative care. In Matzo M, Sherman D, editors, *Palliative care nursing: quality care to the end-of-life*, ed 3, New York, 2010, Springer.

Matzo M, Sherman D: *Palliative care nursing: quality care to the end of life*, ed 3, New York, 2010, Springer.

McDonald C, McCallin A: Interprofessional collaboration in palliative nursing: what is the patient-family role? *Internat J Palliat Nurs* 16(6):285, 2010.

Newman M: *Transforming presence*, Philadelphia, 2008, Davis.

Paice J: Pain at the end of life. In Ferrell B, Coyle N, editors, *Textbook of palliative nursing*, ed 3, New York, 2010, Oxford University Press.

Pasacreta JV, Minarik PA, Nield-Anderson L: Anxiety and depression. In Ferrell B, Coyle N, editors: *Textbook of palliative nursing*, ed 3, New York, 2010, Oxford University Press.

Parsons S: The meaning of Friday afternoon tea for informal caregivers on a palliative care unit, *Internat J Palliat Nurs* 15(2):74, 2009.

Rando T: *Treatment of complicated mourning*, Champaign, Ill, 1993, Research Press.

Showalter S: Compassion fatigue: what is it? Why does it matter? Recognizing the symptoms, acknowledging the impact, developing the tools to prevent compassion fatigue, and strengthen the professional already suffering from the effects, *Am J Hosp Palliat Med* 27(4):239, 2010.

Simon J: Anticipatory grief: recognition and coping, *J Palliat Med* 11(9):1280, 2008.

Taxis JC, et al: Mexican Americans and hospice care: culture, control and communication, *J Hospice Palliat Nurs* 10(3):133, 2008.
Taylor V, Ashelford S: Understanding depression in palliative and end-of-life care, *Nurs Standard* 23(12):48, 2008.
Tilden VP, et al: Family decision-making to withdraw life-sustaining treatments from hospitalized patients, *Nurs Res* 50:105, 2001.
Wainwright P, Gallagher A: Ethical aspects of withdrawing and withholding treatment, *Nurs Standard* 21(33):46, 2007.
Walter C, McCoyd J: *Grief and loss across the lifespan: a biopsychosocial perspective*, New York, 2009, Springer.
Worden JW: *Grief counseling and grief therapy*, New York, 1982, Springer.
Wright P, Hogan N: Grief theories and models: applications to hospice nursing practice, *J Hospice and Palliat Nurs* 10(6):350, 2008.
Wright D, et al: Human relationships at the end of life, *J Hosp Palliat Nurs* 11(4):219, 2009.
Xu Y: Death and dying in the Chinese culture: implications for health care practice, *Home Health Care Manage Pract* 19:412, 2007.

RESEARCH REFERENCES

Allchin L: Caring for the dying: nursing student perspectives, *J Hosp Palliat Nurs* 8(2):112, 2006.
Benzein G, Saveman B: Health-promoting conversations about hope and suffering with couples in palliative care, *Internat J Palliat Nurs* 14(9):439, 2008.
Clayton J, et al: Sustaining hope when communicating with terminally ill patients and their families: a systematic review, *Psych Oncol* 17:641, 2008.
Cohen S, et al: Socioeconomic status is associated with stress hormones, *Psychosom Med* 68:414, 2006.
Daaleman T, et al: An exploratory study of spiritual care at the end of life, *Ann Fam Med* 6(5):406, 2008.
Duggleby W, Wright K: The hope of professional caregivers caring for persons at the end of life, *J Hosp Palliat Nurs* 9(1):42, 2007.
Dy S, et al: A systematic review of satisfaction with care at the end of life, *J Am Geriatric Soc* 56(1):124, 2008.
Erichsen E, et al: A phenomenological study of nurses' understanding of honesty in palliative care, *Nurs Ethics* 17(1):39, 2010.
Gardner D, Kramer B: End-of-life concerns and care preferences: congruence among terminally ill elders and their family caregivers, *Omega* 60(3):273, 2010.
Hunnibell L, et al: Self-transcendence and burnout in hospice and oncology nurses, *J Hosp Palliat Nurs* 10(3):172, 2008.
Innes P, Payne S: Advanced cancer patients' prognostic information preferences: a review, *Pall Med* 23(1):29, 2009.
Kruse B, et al: Spirituality and coping at the end of life, *J Hospice Palliat Nurs* 9(6):296, 2007.
Ladd K: Religiosity, the need for structure, death attitudes, and funeral preferences, *Mental Health Religion Cult* 10(5):451, 2007.
Maciejewski PK, et al: An empirical examination of the stage theory of grief, *JAMA* 297:716, 2007.
Osaka I, et al: Endocrinological evaluations of brief hand massage in palliative care, *J Altern Complement Med* 15(9):981, 2009.
Perry B: Achieving professional fulfillment as a palliative care nurse, *J Hosp Palliat Nurs* 11(2):109, 2009.
Phillips L: Into the abyss of someone else's dying, *Clin Nurs Res* 18(1):80, 2009.
Rosenfeld P, et al: Are there racial differences in attitudes toward hospice care? A study of hospice-eligible patients at the visiting nurse service of New York, *Am J Hosp Palliat Med* 24(5):408, 2007.
Running A, et al: A survey of hospices' use of complementary therapy, *J Hospice Palliat Nurs* 10(5):304, 2008.
Spichiger E: Living with terminal illness: patient and family experiences of hospital end-of-life care, *Internat J Palliat Nurs* 14(5):220, 2008.
Weigel C, et al: Apprehension among hospital nurses providing end-of-life care, *J Hospice Palliat Nurs* 9(2):86, 2007.

CHAPTER 37

Stress and Coping

OBJECTIVES

- Describe the three stages of the general adaptation syndrome.
- Describe characteristics of posttraumatic stress disorder.
- Discuss the integration of stress theory with nursing theories.
- Describe stress management techniques beneficial for coping with stress.
- Discuss the process of crisis intervention.
- Develop a care plan for patients who are experiencing stress.
- Discuss how stress in the workplace affects the nurse.

KEY TERMS

Adventitious crises, p. 734
Alarm reaction, p. 732
Allostatic load, p. 732
Appraisal, p. 731
Burnout, p. 741
Coping, p. 732
Crisis, p. 731
Crisis intervention, p. 742
Developmental crises, p. 734
Ego-defense mechanisms, p. 733
Exhaustion stage, p. 732
Fight-or-flight response, p. 731
Flashback, p. 734
General adaptation syndrome (GAS), p. 732
Posttraumatic stress disorder (PTSD), p. 733
Primary appraisal, p. 732
Resistance stage, p. 732
Secondary appraisal, p. 732
Situational crises, p. 734
Stress, p. 731
Stressors, p. 731
Trauma, p. 731

evolve WEBSITE

http://evolve.elsevier.com/Potter/fundamentals/

- Review Questions
- Concept Map Creator
- Case Study with Questions
- Audio Glossary
- Interactive Learning Activities
- Key Term Flashcards
- Content Updates

Health care professionals need to know about stress so they are able to recognize it in patients and families and intervene effectively. Caregiver stress frequently affects family members of patients and must be considered in patient care. Equally important, health care professionals also experience stressful events that occur in the course of clinical practice and in their own lives. Nurses need to recognize the signs and symptoms of stress and understand stress management techniques to aid personal coping and design stress management interventions for their patients and families.

People use the term **stress** in many ways. It is an experience to which a person is exposed through a stimulus or stressor. **Stressors** are tension-producing stimuli operating within or on any system (Neuman and Fawcett, 2011). It is also the appraisal, or perception, of a stressor. **Appraisal** is how people interpret the impact of the stressor on themselves or on what is happening and what they are able to do about it (Lazarus, 2007). Finally stress is a physical, emotional, or psychological demand that often leads to growth or overwhelms a person and leads to illness (Varcarolis and Halter, 2010). Stress refers to the consequences of the stressor and the person's appraisal of it.

People experience stress as a consequence of daily life events and experiences. It stimulates thinking processes and helps people stay alert to their environment. It results in personal growth and facilitates development. How people react to stress depends on how they view and evaluate the impact of the stressor, its effect on their situation and support at the time of the stress, and their usual coping mechanisms. When stress overwhelms existing coping mechanisms, patients lose emotional balance, and a **crisis** results. If symptoms of stress persist beyond the duration of the stressor, a person has experienced a **trauma.**

SCIENTIFIC KNOWLEDGE BASE

The **fight-or-flight response** to stress, which is arousal of the sympathetic nervous system, prepares a person for action (Fig. 37-1). Neurophysiological responses to stress function through negative feedback. The process of negative feedback senses an abnormal state such as lowered body temperature and makes an adaptive response such as initiating shivering to generate body heat. Three structures, the medulla oblongata, the reticular formation, and the pituitary gland, control the response of the body to a stressor.

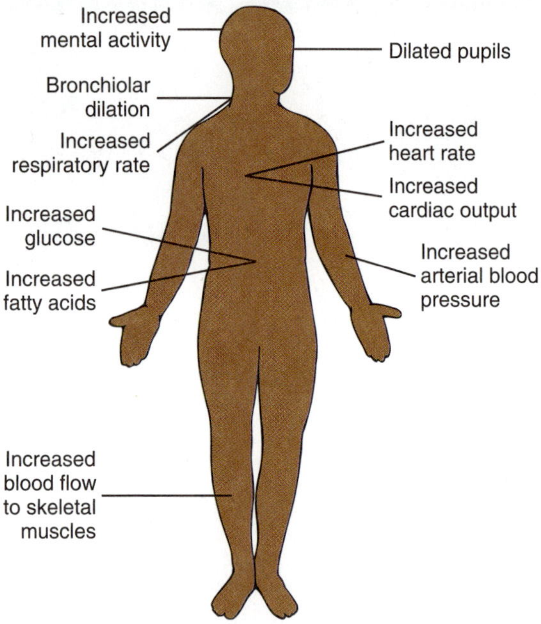

FIG. 37-1 Fight-or-flight response.

Medulla Oblongata

The medulla oblongata, located in the lower portion of the brainstem, controls heart rate, blood pressure, and respirations. Impulses traveling to and from the medulla oblongata increase or decrease these vital functions. For example, sympathetic or parasympathetic nervous system impulses traveling from the medulla oblongata to the heart control regulation of the heartbeat. The heart rate increases in response to impulses from sympathetic fibers and decreases with impulses from parasympathetic fibers.

Reticular Formation

The reticular formation, a small cluster of neurons in the brainstem and spinal cord, continuously monitors the physiological status of the body through connections with sensory and motor tracts. For example, certain cells within the reticular formation cause a sleeping person to regain consciousness or increase the level of consciousness when a need arises.

Pituitary Gland

The pituitary gland is a small gland immediately beneath the hypothalamus. It produces hormones necessary for adaptation to stress such as adrenocorticotropic hormone, which in turn produces cortisol. In addition, the pituitary gland regulates the secretion of thyroid, gonadal, and parathyroid hormones. A feedback mechanism continuously monitors hormone levels in the blood and regulates hormone secretion. When hormone levels drop, the pituitary gland receives a message to increase hormone secretion. When they rise, it decreases hormone production.

General Adaptation Syndrome

The **general adaptation syndrome (GAS),** a three-stage reaction to stress, describes how the body responds to stressors through the alarm reaction, the resistance stage, and the exhaustion stage. The GAS is triggered either directly by a physical event or indirectly by a psychological event. It involves several body systems, especially the autonomic nervous and endocrine systems, and responds immediately to stress (Fig. 37-2). When the body encounters a physical demand such as an injury, the pituitary gland initiates the GAS.

During the **alarm reaction** rising hormone levels result in increased blood volume, blood glucose levels, epinephrine and norepinephrine amounts, heart rate, blood flow to muscles, oxygen intake, and mental alertness. In addition, the pupils of the eyes dilate to produce a greater visual field. If the stressor poses an extreme threat to life or remains for a long time, the person progresses to the second stage, resistance.

During the **resistance stage** the body stabilizes and responds in a manner opposite to that of the alarm reaction. Hormone levels, heart rate, blood pressure, and cardiac output return to normal; and the body repairs any damage that has occurred. However, if the stress response is chronically activated, a state of allostasis occurs. This chronic arousal with the presence of powerful hormones causes excessive wear and tear on the person and is called **allostatic load.** An increased allostatic load leads to chronic illness (Diamond, 2009/2010). A persistent allopathic load can cause long-term physiological problems such as chronic hypertension, depression, sleep deprivation, chronic fatigue syndrome, and autoimmune disorders (McEwen, 2005).

The **exhaustion stage** occurs when the body is no longer able to resist the effects of the stressor and has depleted the energy necessary to maintain adaptation. The physiological response has intensified; but with a compromised energy level, the person's adaptation to the stressor diminishes.

Reaction to Psychological Stress. The GAS is activated indirectly for psychological threats, which are different for each person and produce differing reactions. The intensity and duration of the psychological threat and the number of other stressors that occur at the same time affect the person's response to the threat. In addition, whether or not the person anticipated the stressor influences its effect. It is often more difficult to cope with an unexpected stressor. Personal characteristics that influence the response to a stressor include the level of personal control, presence of a social support system, and feelings of competence.

A person experiences stress only if the event or circumstance is personally significant. Evaluating an event for its personal meaning is **primary appraisal.** Appraisal of an event or circumstance is an ongoing perceptual process. If primary appraisal results in the person identifying the event or circumstance as a harm, loss, threat, or challenge, the person experiences stress. If stress is present, **secondary appraisal** focuses on possible coping strategies. Balancing factors contribute to restoring equilibrium. According to crisis theory, feedback cues lead to reappraisals of the original perception. Therefore coping behaviors constantly change as individuals perceive new information.

Coping is the person's effort to manage psychological stress. Effectiveness of coping strategies depends on the individual's needs. A person's age and cultural background influence these needs. For this reason no single coping strategy works for everyone or for every stressor. The same person may cope differently from one time to another. In stressful situations most people use a combination of problem- and emotion-focused coping strategies. In other words, when under stress a person obtains information, takes action to change the situation, and regulates emotions tied to the stress. In some cases people avoid thinking about the situation or change the way they think about it without changing the actual situation itself. The type of stress, people's goals, their beliefs about themselves and the world, and personal resources determine how people cope with stress. Resources include intelligence, money, social skills, supportive family and friends, physical attractiveness,

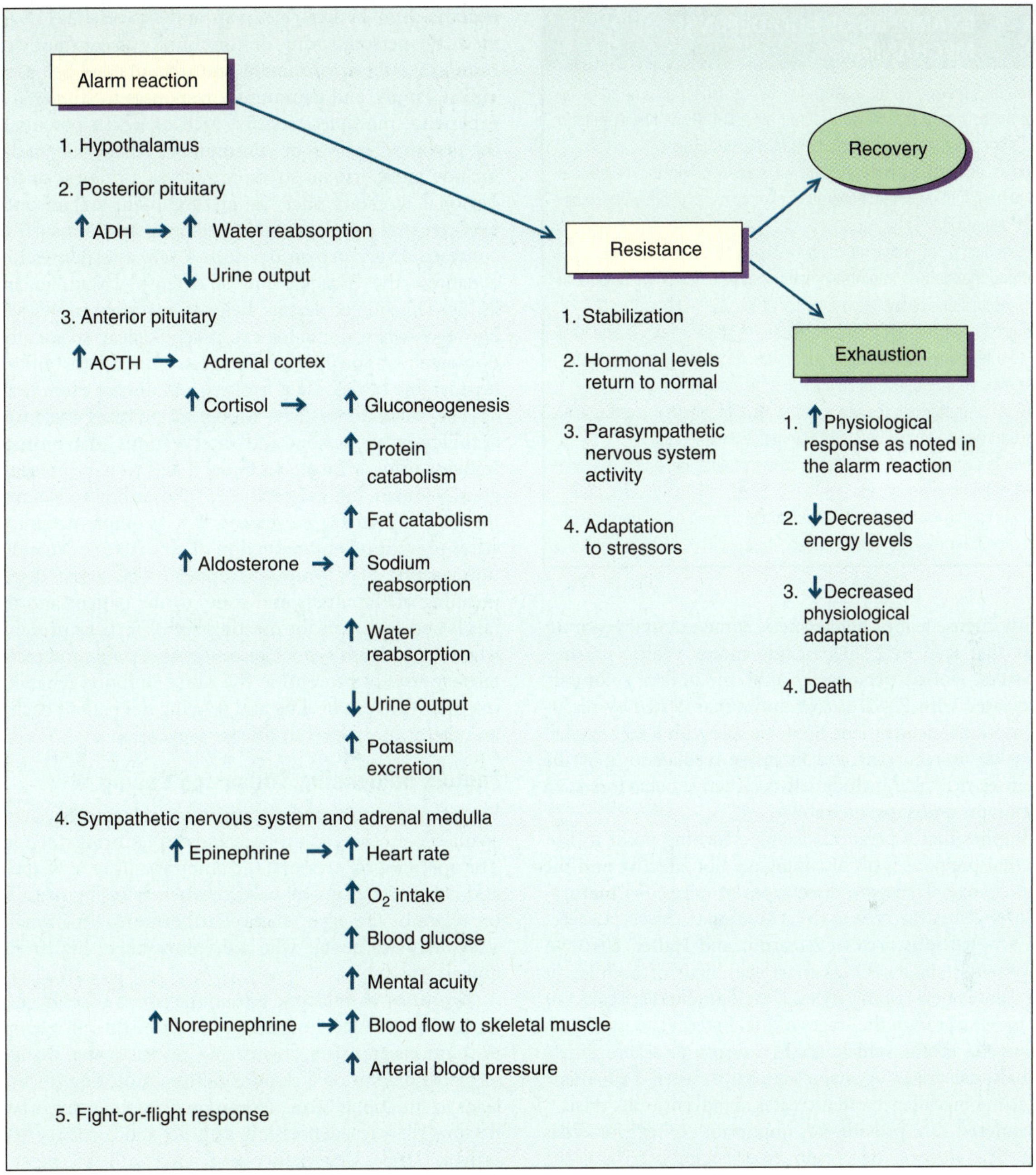

FIG. 37-2 General adaptation syndrome (GAS).

health and energy, and ways of thinking such as optimism (Lazarus, 2007).

Coping mechanisms include psychological adaptive behaviors. Such behaviors are often task oriented, involving the use of direct problem-solving techniques to cope with threats. **Ego-defense mechanisms** regulate emotional distress and thus give a person protection from anxiety and stress. Ego-defense mechanisms help a person cope with stress indirectly and offer psychological protection from a stressful event. Everyone uses them unconsciously to protect against feelings of worthlessness and anxiety. Occasionally a defense mechanism becomes distorted and no longer helps the person adapt to a stressor. However, people generally find them very helpful in coping and use them spontaneously (Box 37-1). Frequently short-term stressors activate ego-defense mechanisms. These usually do not result in psychiatric disorders.

Types of Stress

Stress includes work, family, chronic, and acute stress; daily hassles; trauma; and crisis. One person looks at a stimulus and sees it as a challenge, leading to mastery and growth. Another sees the same stimulus as a threat, leading to stagnation and loss. The individual with family responsibilities and a full-time job outside the home can experience chronic stress. It occurs in stable conditions and from stressful roles. Living with a long-term illness produces chronic stress. Conversely, time-limited events that threaten a person for a relatively brief period provoke acute stress. Recurrent daily hassles such as commuting to work, maintaining a house, dealing with difficult people, and managing money further complicate chronic or acute stress.

Posttraumatic stress disorder (PTSD) begins when a person experiences, witnesses, or is confronted with a traumatic event and

BOX 37-1 EXAMPLES OF EGO-DEFENSE MECHANISMS

- Compensation is making up for a deficiency in one aspect of self-image by strongly emphasizing a feature considered an asset. (Example: A person who is a poor communicator relies on organizational skills.)
- Conversion is unconsciously repressing an anxiety-producing emotional conflict and transforming it into nonorganic symptoms (e.g., difficulty sleeping, loss of appetite).
- Denial is avoiding emotional conflicts by refusing to consciously acknowledge anything that causes intolerable emotional pain. (Example: A person refuses to discuss or acknowledge a personal loss.)
- Displacement is transferring emotions, ideas, or wishes from a stressful situation to a less anxiety-producing substitute. (Example: A person transfers anger over an interpersonal conflict to a malfunctioning computer.)
- Identification is patterning behavior after that of another person and assuming that person's qualities, characteristics, and actions.
- Dissociation is experiencing a subjective sense of numbing and a reduced awareness of one's surroundings.
- Regression is coping with a stressor through actions and behaviors associated with an earlier developmental period.

responds with intense fear or helplessness. Some examples of traumatic events that lead to PTSD include motor vehicle crashes, natural disasters, violent personal assault, and military combat. Anxiety associated with PTSD is sometimes manifested by nightmares and emotional detachment. Some people with PTSD experience **flashbacks,** or recurrent and intrusive recollections of the event. Responses may also include self-destructive behaviors such as suicide attempts and substance abuse.

A crisis implies that a person is facing a turning point in life. This means that previous ways of coping are not effective and the person must change. There are three types of crises: (a) maturational or **developmental crises,** (b) **situational crises,** and (c) disasters or **adventitious crises** (Varcarolis and Halter, 2010). A new developmental stage such as marriage, birth of a child, or retirement requires new coping styles. Developmental crises occur as a person moves through the stages of life. External sources such as a job change, a motor vehicle crash, a death, or severe illness provoke situational crises. A major natural disaster, man-made disaster, or crime of violence often creates an adventitious crisis.

Patient-centered care provides an important context for crisis intervention. The view of the person experiencing a crisis is the frame of reference for the crisis. The vital questions for a person in crisis are, "What does this mean to you; how is it going to affect your life?" What causes extreme stress for one person is not always stressful to another. The perception of the event, situational supports, and coping mechanisms all influence return of equilibrium or homeostasis. A person either advances or regresses as a result of a crisis, depending on how he or she manages the crisis (Lazarus, 2007).

NURSING KNOWLEDGE BASE

Nurses have proposed theories related to stress and coping. Because stress plays a central role in vulnerability to disease, symptoms of stress often require nursing intervention.

Nursing Theory and the Role of Stress

The Neuman Systems Model is based on the concepts of stress and reaction to it. Nurses are responsible for developing interventions to prevent or reduce stressors on the patient or make them more bearable him or her (Neuman and Fawcett, 2011). This model views the person, family, or community as constantly changing in response to the environment and stressors and helps explain individual, family, and community responses to stressors. All systems experience multiple stressors, each of which potentially disturbs the person's, family's, or community's balance. Examples of stress include intrapersonal stressors such as an illness or injury, interpersonal stressors such as an argument or misunderstanding between two people, or extrapersonal stressors such as financial concerns. Every person develops a set of responses to stress that constitute the "normal line of defense" (Neuman and Fawcett, 2011). This line of defense helps to maintain health and wellness. However, when physiological, psychological, sociocultural, developmental, or spiritual resources are unable to buffer stress, the normal line of defense is broken, and disease often results.

The Neuman Systems Model emphasizes the importance of accuracy in assessment and interventions that promote optimal wellness using primary, secondary, and tertiary prevention strategies (Neuman and Fawcett, 2011). According to Neuman's theory, the goal of primary prevention is to promote patient wellness by stress prevention and reduction of risk factors. Secondary prevention occurs after symptoms appear. The nurse determines the meaning of the illness and stress to the patient and the patient's needs and resources for meeting them. Tertiary prevention begins when the patient's system becomes more stable and recovers. At the tertiary level of prevention the nurse supports rehabilitation processes involved in healing and moving the patient back to wellness and the primary level of disease prevention.

Factors Influencing Stress and Coping

Potential stressors and coping mechanisms vary across the life span. Adolescence, adulthood, and old age bring different stressors. The appraisal of stressors, the amount and type of social support, and coping strategies all balance when assessing stress and depend on previous life experiences. Furthermore, situational and social stressors place people who are vulnerable at higher risk for prolonged stress.

Situational Factors. Situational stress arises from personal or family job changes or relocation. Stressful job changes include promotions, transfers, downsizing, restructuring, changes in supervisors, and additional responsibilities. Adjusting to chronic illness leads to situational stress. Common diseases such as obesity, hypertension, diabetes, depression, asthma, and coronary artery disease provoke stress. Uncertainty associated with treatment and illness triggers stress in patients of all ages. Paying for treatment and limited access to providers also create stress. Although being a family caregiver for someone with a chronic illness such as Alzheimer's disease is associated with stress, the actions of competent health care providers often minimize the stress for caregivers (Box 37-2).

Maturational Factors. Stressors vary with life stage. Children identify stressors related to their physical appearance, their families, their friends, and school. Preadolescents experience stress related to self-esteem issues, changing family structure as a result of divorce or death of a parent, or hospitalizations. As adolescents search for their identity with peer groups and separate from their families, they experience stress. In addition, they face stressful questions about using mind-altering substances, sex, jobs, school, and career choices. Stress for adults centers around major changes in life circumstances. These include the many milestones of beginning a family and a career, losing parents, seeing children leave home, and accepting physical aging. In old age stressors include the loss of

BOX 37-2 EVIDENCE-BASED PRACTICE

Recognizing Sources of Caregiver Stress

PICO Question: How do family caregivers of patients with chronic illness perceive caregiving?

Evidence Summary

Research about effects of family caregiving on caregivers typically focuses on multiple stressors experienced by family caregivers and the personal benefits of caregiving. A common stressor for family caregivers is dealing with the patient's emotional well-being and mood. For example, when caring for a family member with heart failure, the most difficult tasks for family caregivers often include dealing with behavior problems (e.g., moodiness), providing emotional support, and managing dietary needs (Pressler et al., 2009). Similarly, when caring for a family member who has had a stroke, the most stressful caregiving tasks for family caregivers often include managing problems with mood (depression, loneliness, and anxiety), memory, and physical care (bowel control) (Haley et al., 2009).

Family caregivers also experience positive aspects of caregiving. For example, family members who care for patients who have had strokes often appreciate life more, feel needed, experience stronger relationships with others, and develop a more positive attitude toward life (Haley et al., 2009).

Attitude toward caregiving is sometimes a good predictor of stress in both Japanese American and American cultures (Anngela-Cole and Hilton, 2009). Caregivers who believe that their job is important and who want to provide care may experience lower levels of depression and greater life satisfaction than those who see caregiving as a burden.

Two psychosocial themes emerge from the findings of these studies: the urgent desire to deal with mood problems of the patient and the benefit of the caregiver having a positive attitude toward being a caregiver.

Application to Nursing Practice

- Focus education for family caregivers on behavior management strategies, communication skills (including therapeutic silence), and assessment tools that family caregivers can use to anticipate and reduce behavior problems.
- Engage family caregivers in discussions to help them identify benefits of caregiving (Haley et al., 2009).
- Develop supportive interventions to help family caregivers reframe their caregiving as loving and generous while recognizing the impact of stressors on them (Anngela-Cole and Hilton, 2009).

autonomy and mastery resulting from general frailty or health problems that limit stamina, strength, and cognition (Box 37-3).

Sociocultural Factors. Environmental and social stressors often lead to developmental problems. Potential stressors that affect any age-group but are especially stressful for young people include prolonged poverty and physical handicap. Children become vulnerable when they lose parents and caregivers through divorce, imprisonment, or death or when parents have mental illness or substance abuse disorders. Living under conditions of continuing violence, disintegrated neighborhoods, or homelessness affects people of any age, especially young people (Pender et al., 2011). A person's culture also influences stress and coping (Box 37-4).

BOX 37-3 FOCUS ON OLDER ADULTS

Understanding Differences in Stress and Coping Among Older Adults

- Ordinary hassles of day-to-day living are a source of stress; older people have more hassles with home maintenance and health than do younger people (Folkman et al., 1987).
- Older adults use more passive, intrapersonal, emotion-focused forms of coping such as distancing, humor, accepting responsibility, and reappraising the stressor in a positive way (Folkman et al., 1987).
- Life experiences and perspectives of older adults make most problems seem insignificant, and many older adults have acquired appropriate stress-management techniques (Folkman et al., 1987).
- Older adults' coping improves based on earlier experience with coping with traumatic situations (Yancura and Aldwin, 2008).
- Coping affects health in older adults more than in younger adults (Yancura and Aldwin, 2008).
- Because of the high incidence of depression in older adults, you need to assess for suicidal thoughts and intent.
- Conditions such as hypoxia and thyroid dysfunction are common in older adults and initially present symptoms that mimic the consequences of stress and anxiety.
- Differentiate signs of stress and crisis in older adults from dementia and acute confusion.

BOX 37-4 CULTURAL ASPECTS OF CARE

Cultural Variations in Stress Appraisal and Coping Strategies

A patient's culture defines what is stressful to the person and ways of coping with stress (Aldwin, 2007). Cultural context shapes the types of environmental stimuli that produce stress. For example, diverse cultures address developmental transitions and turning points in life differently. Culture affects how a person leaves the parental home, experiences health crises or chronic illness, cares for the family, or becomes disabled or dependent. Furthermore, how a person appraises stress also depends on his or her culture. What is perceived as a major stressor in one culture might be viewed as a minor problem in another. A person's response to the stress of pain is an example of a culture-based response to stress. In some cultures patients maintain personal control, whereas others become emotionally expressive. Coping strategies are also influenced by one's cultural background. Cultures vary in their emotion- and problem-focused coping strategies. Some cultures stress that emotions should be controlled, whereas others believe in expressing emotions. Problem-focused coping refers to controlling or managing stress. Different cultures control stress in different ways. Cultures provide different resources for coping with stress. These include the legal system for conflict resolution, advice givers or support groups, and rituals.

Implications for Practice

- Realize that stressors and coping styles vary with different cultures.
- Reflect on your own perceptions of stress and coping in a cultural context.
- Assess the influence of culture on a patient's appraisal of stress.
- Determine resources in a patient's culture that facilitate coping.

CRITICAL THINKING

When caring for a patient experiencing stress, use critical thinking skills to understand the patient's stressor and the stress response. Integrate knowledge from nursing and other disciplines, previous experiences, and information gathered from patients to understand stress and its impact on the patient and family. Know the neurophysiological changes that occur in the patient experiencing the alarm reaction, resistance stage, and exhaustion stage of the general adaptation syndrome. In addition, know communication principles that contribute to assessing patient's behaviors. Give utmost attention to determining the patient's perception of the situation and his or her ability to cope with the stress. If the patient's usual coping skills have not helped or his or her support systems have failed, use crisis intervention counseling.

Experience teaches you to understand the patient's unique perspective and view each person as an individual, recognizing that no two people are exactly alike. Experience with patients also helps you to recognize responses to stress. In addition, personal experiences with stress and coping increase your ability to empathize with a patient temporarily immobilized by stress.

Be confident in the belief that you and your patients can effectively manage stress. Patients who feel overwhelmed and perceive events as being beyond their capacity to cope rely on you as an expert. Patients respect your advice and counsel and gain confidence from your belief in their ability to move past the stressful event or illness. Patients overwhelmed by life events are often unable, at least initially, to act on their own behalf and require either direct intervention or guidance. Integrity is an essential attitude through which you respect the patient's perception of the stressor. Make the effort to have the patient explain his or her unique viewpoint and situation.

The practice standards for psychiatric mental health nursing (ANA, 2007) guide assessment of a patient's stress, coping mechanisms, and support system before intervening. Use linguistic and culturally effective communication skills to clearly and precisely understand a patient's perception of stress. Focus on factors relevant to his or her well-being. In addition, the patient expects you to exhibit confidence and integrity when he or she feels vulnerable. Be especially aware of the ethical responsibility in caring for someone who has diminished autonomy as a result of stress.

NURSING PROCESS

Apply the nursing process and use a critical thinking approach in your care of patients. The nursing process provides a clinical decision-making approach for you to develop and implement an individualized plan of care.

ASSESSMENT

During the assessment process thoroughly assess each patient and critically analyze findings to ensure that you make patient-centered clinical decisions required for safe nursing care.

Through the Patient's Eyes. Assessment of a patient's stress level and coping resources requires that you first establish a trusting nurse-patient relationship because you are asking a patient to share personal and sensitive information. Learn from the patient both by asking questions and by making observations of nonverbal behavior and the patient's environment. Synthesize the information and adopt a critical thinking attitude while observing and analyzing patient behavior (Fig. 37-3). Often the patient has difficulty expressing exactly what is most bothersome about the situation until there is an opportunity to discuss it with someone who has time to listen.

Begin your assessment with an open-ended question such as, "What is happening in your life that caused you to come today?" or "What happened in your life that is *different?*" This requires some focusing by the patient. Next assess the patient's perception of the event, available situational supports, and what he or she usually does when there is a problem that he or she cannot solve. Determine if a person is suicidal or homicidal by asking directly. For example, ask, "Are you thinking of killing yourself or someone else?" If so, determine in a caring and concerned manner if the person has a plan and determine how lethal the means are.

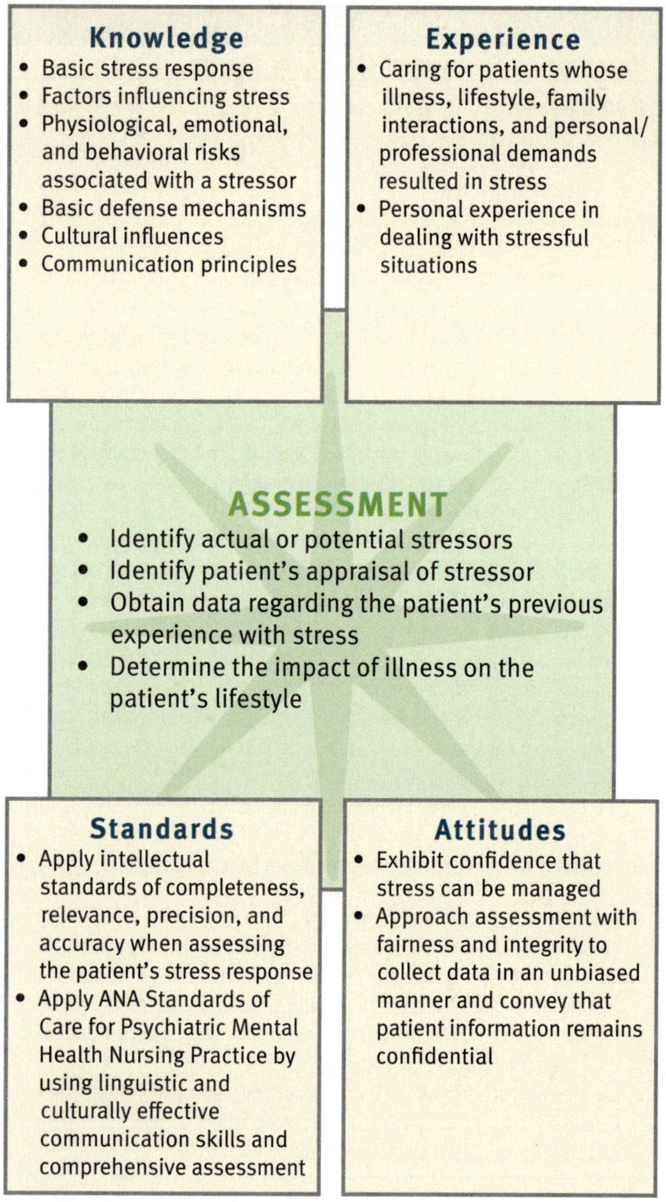

Knowledge
• Basic stress response
• Factors influencing stress
• Physiological, emotional, and behavioral risks associated with a stressor
• Basic defense mechanisms
• Cultural influences
• Communication principles
Experience
• Caring for patients whose illness, lifestyle, family interactions, and personal/professional demands resulted in stress
• Personal experience in dealing with stressful situations
ASSESSMENT
• Identify actual or potential stressors
• Identify patient's appraisal of stressor
• Obtain data regarding the patient's previous experience with stress
• Determine the impact of illness on the patient's lifestyle
Standards
• Apply intellectual standards of completeness, relevance, precision, and accuracy when assessing the patient's stress response
• Apply ANA Standards of Care for Psychiatric Mental Health Nursing Practice by using linguistic and culturally effective communication skills and comprehensive assessment
Attitudes
• Exhibit confidence that stress can be managed
• Approach assessment with fairness and integrity to collect data in an unbiased manner and convey that patient information remains confidential

FIG. 37-3 Critical thinking model for stress and coping assessment. *ANA,* American Nurses Association.

Take time to understand a patient's meaning of the precipitating event and the ways in which stress is affecting his or her life. Allow time for him or her to express priorities for coping with stress. For example, in the case of a woman who has just been told that a breast mass was identified on a routine mammogram, it is important to know what the patient wants and needs most from the nurse. Although some women in this situation identify their need for information about biopsy or mastectomy as their personal priority, others need guidance and support in discussing how to share the news with family members. In some cases, when there is nothing that will change or improve the situation, allowing the patient to use denial as a coping mechanism is helpful. Gaining an understanding of patient expectations does not mean excluding certain types of care that are important simply because a patient does not identify them as needs. However, by inquiring about patient expectations and priorities, you are better able to ensure that you address *all* of the patient's needs in some way.

BOX 37-5 NURSING ASSESSMENT QUESTIONS

Perception of Stressor
- What is bothering you most right now?
- What do you think about when you're lying awake?

Maladaptive Coping Used
- Do you live alone or with others?
- Who helps you?
- Have you started drinking or smoking?
- Has your caffeine intake increased?

Adherence to Healthy Practices
- Do you have high blood pressure?
- Have you noticed an increase or decrease in weight?
- Are you taking your prescribed medications?
- Have you increased any medications?

Stress also occurs in a family or a community. Stress in a family is sometimes from a critically ill family member, the sudden loss of a job, a move, or becoming homeless. An example of stress in a community is a natural disaster such as a major flood or the sudden, unexpected death of a beloved teacher or teenager. To develop appropriate and safe nursing care when caring for families or communities, ensure that you understand the meaning that the stress has for that group.

Subjective Findings. When assessing a patient's level of stress and coping resources, create a nonthreatening physical environment for the interaction. Assume the same height as the patient, arranging the interview environment so you can maintain or avoid eye contact comfortably. You do this by placing chairs at a 90-degree angle or side by side to reduce the intensity of the interaction (Varcarolis and Halter, 2010). Gather information about the health status of the patient from his or her perspective and begin the process of developing a trusting relationship with him or her. Use the interview to determine the patient's view of the stress, coping resources, any possible maladaptive coping, and adherence to prescribed medical recommendations such as medication or diet (Box 37-5). If the patient is using denial as a coping mechanism, be alert to whether he or she is overlooking necessary information. As in all interactions with the patient, respect the confidentiality and sensitivity of the information shared.

Objective Findings. Obtain objective findings related to stress and coping through observation of the appearance and nonverbal behavior of a patient. Observe grooming and hygiene, gait, characteristics of the handshake, actions while sitting, quality of speech, eye contact, and the attitude of the patient during the interview. Before the interview begins or at the end of the interview, depending on the anxiety level of the patient, obtain basic vital signs to assess for physiological signs of stress such as elevated blood pressure, heart rate, or respiratory rate. Make certain to incorporate cultural components of interpreting the patient's nonverbal communication behaviors.

Building Competency in Safety You are caring for Lois, an 80-year-old woman who appears highly anxious and distressed about the health of her dog. Her concerns seem rather unspecific to you, yet Lois is having insomnia and anorexia. She's lost 5 pounds since you last visited her home. What conditions do you need to consider in addition to her apparent stress and anxiety?

Answers to questions can be found on the Evolve website.

BOX 37-6 NURSING DIAGNOSTIC PROCESS

Ineffective Coping

ASSESSMENT ACTIVITIES	DEFINING CHARACTERISTICS
Ask patient about change in sleeping patterns.	Sleep disturbance Difficulty falling asleep at nights Sighing
Ask patient to complete a sleep diary for 2 weeks.	Excessive sleeping
Observe patient's behavior and response to questions during assessment.	Fatigue Inability to concentrate Inaccurate response to questions Inappropriate laugh or crying
Observe patient's appearance.	Poor grooming Self-harm
Ask patient about changes in eating patterns.	Weight gain or loss Lack of interest in food

NURSING DIAGNOSIS

A review of assessment data leads the nurse to cluster data that indicate a potential or actual stressor and the patient's response. Clustering data, along with the application of the nurse's knowledge and experiences with patients in stress, leads to individualized nursing diagnoses (Box 37-6).

Nursing diagnoses for people experiencing stress generally focus on coping. Specifically major defining characteristics of *ineffective coping* include verbalization of an inability to cope and an inability to ask for help. To identify defining characteristics, ask the patient what is of most concern at the time of the interview. It is important to allow him or her sufficient time to answer. Observe for nonverbal signs of anxiety, fear, anger, irritability, and tension in a patient who is experiencing ineffective coping. Other defining characteristics include the presence of life stress, an inability to meet role expectations and basic needs, alteration in societal participation, self-destructive behavior, change in usual communication patterns, high rate of accidents, excessive food intake, drinking, smoking, and sleep disturbances. Stress often results in multiple nursing diagnoses. Examples of these diagnoses include but are not limited to the following:

- Anxiety
- Caregiver role strain
- Ineffective coping
- Fear
- Risk for post-trauma syndrome
- Insomnia
- Situational low self-esteem
- Stress overload

PLANNING

Goals and Outcomes. Desirable outcomes for persons experiencing stress frequently include effective coping, family coping, caregiver emotional health, and psychosocial adjustment: life change. The nurse often selects interventions for stress and improved coping such as coping enhancement and crisis intervention in addition to individualized interventions after considering

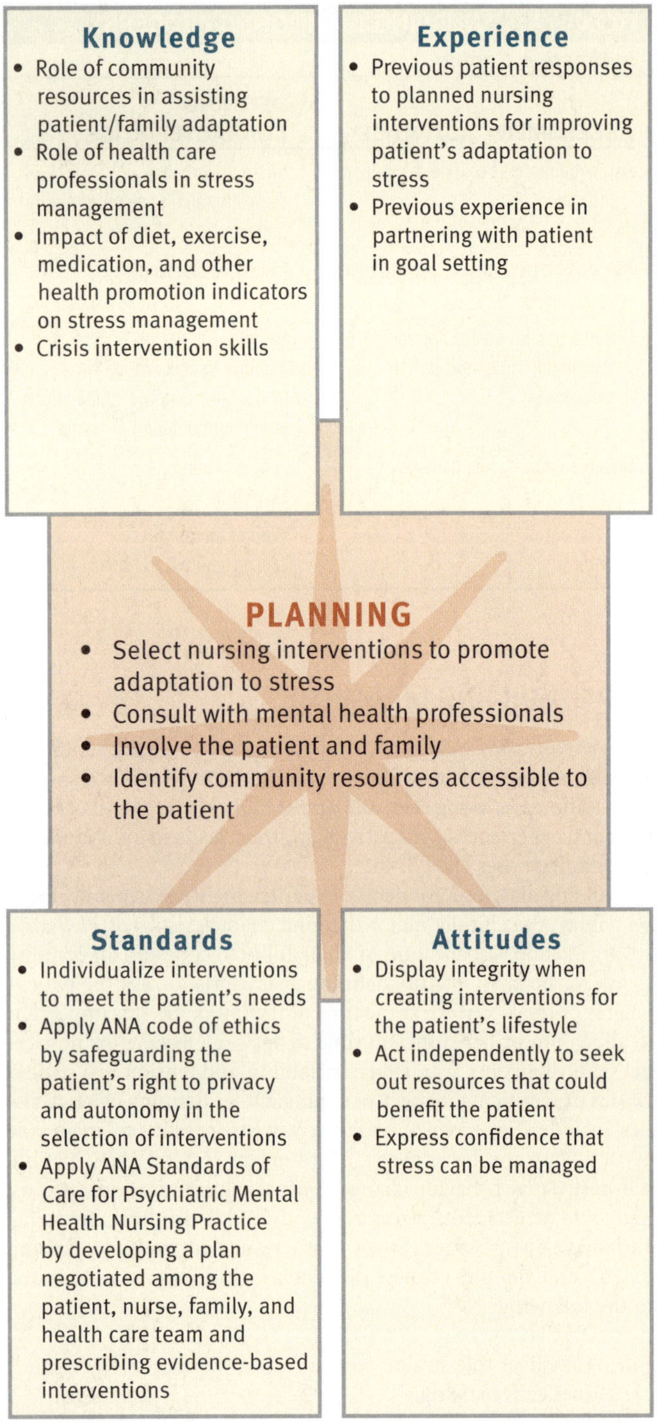
Knowledge
• Role of community resources in assisting patient/family adaptation
• Role of health care professionals in stress management
• Impact of diet, exercise, medication, and other health promotion indicators on stress management
• Crisis intervention skills
Experience
• Previous patient responses to planned nursing interventions for improving patient's adaptation to stress
• Previous experience in partnering with patient in goal setting
PLANNING
• Select nursing interventions to promote adaptation to stress
• Consult with mental health professionals
• Involve the patient and family
• Identify community resources accessible to the patient
Standards
• Individualize interventions to meet the patient's needs
• Apply ANA code of ethics by safeguarding the patient's right to privacy and autonomy in the selection of interventions
• Apply ANA Standards of Care for Psychiatric Mental Health Nursing Practice by developing a plan negotiated among the patient, nurse, family, and health care team and prescribing evidence-based interventions
Attitudes
• Display integrity when creating interventions for the patient's lifestyle
• Act independently to seek out resources that could benefit the patient
• Express confidence that stress can be managed

FIG. 37-4 Critical thinking model for stress and coping planning. *ANA,* American Nurses Association.

the nursing diagnosis, the resources available to the patient, and the goals identified by the patient and nurse (Fig. 37-4).

Nursing interventions are designed within the framework of primary, secondary, and tertiary prevention. At the primary level of prevention you direct nursing activities to identifying individuals and populations who are possibly at risk for stress. Nursing interventions at the secondary level include actions directed at symptoms such as protecting the patient from self-harm. Tertiary-level interventions assist the patient in readapting and can include relaxation training and time-management training. The nurse and the patient assess the level and source of the existing stress and determine the appropriate points for intervention to reduce it (Pender et al., 2011) (see the Nursing Care Plan).

Another method of planning care is through the use of a concept map (Fig. 37-5 on p. 740). Concept maps identify multiple nursing diagnoses from the assessment database and show how they are related. In this example the nursing diagnoses are linked to the patient's medical diagnosis of depression. In addition, the concept map shows the relationship among the nursing diagnoses *chronic low self-esteem, ineffective coping, anxiety, and caregiver role strain.* Use of a concept map requires critical thinking skills to organize patient data and assists in planning for patient-centered care.

Just as the nursing assessment of the patient's stress and coping depends on the patient's perception of the problem and coping resources, the interventions focus on a partnership with the patient and support system, usually the family. In the case of a family or community stressor and impaired family or community coping, the view of the situation and resources is broader.

Setting Priorities. Consider the patient's perspective and responses to assessment questions when setting priorities for care (see the Nursing Care Plan). The patient's clinical condition and perception of stress determine which nursing diagnosis has the greatest priority. As in all areas of nursing, safety of the patient and others in his or her environment is the first priority.

> **Building Competency in Safety** You are interviewing Dave, a 60-year-old man who has recently lost his job and whose wife has terminal cancer. He says, "I don't see how I can go on." This raises a warning flag for you. How would you determine if Bob is suicidal?
>
> Answers to questions can be found on the Evolve website.

If suicide or homicide is not an issue, examine other potential threats to the safety of vulnerable people who are under the care of the patient. Provide for their temporary care or supervision if necessary. Other potential threats to safety include nutritional deficits; insomnia; self-care deficits; and poor judgment and impulsiveness that possibly lead to unsafe decisions about sex, drugs, money, or damage to personal relationships that the person might later regret. Determine the degree of work, school, home, and family disruption in the person's life. When you have completed immediate assessment and ensured safety, begin the problem-solving process.

Teamwork and Collaboration. Collaborate with occupational therapists, dietitians, pastoral care professionals, and health care professionals from other clinical specialties, depending on the patient's situation. The scope of your nursing practice cannot meet all of the patient's needs. Patients experiencing stress from medical conditions or psychiatric disorders present needs that make it necessary for you to consult with advanced practice mental health nurses, psychiatrists, psychologists, or psychiatric social workers. A multidisciplinary approach addresses the holistic needs of the patient. Recognize the need for collaboration and consultation; inform the patient about potential resources; and make arrangements for interventions such as consultations, group sessions, or therapy as needed. A hospital social worker shares ideas for available resources both within the hospital and in the community. A home care nurse knows community services, groups, and appropriate contacts.

In addition to maximizing use of available resources for the patient, collaborative care also benefits the nurse. While working

NURSING CARE PLAN
Caregiver Role Strain

ASSESSMENT

Evelyn was recently diagnosed with Alzheimer's dementia. Carl, her husband, is her main caregiver. When the home health nurse first goes to Evelyn and Carl's house, she finds the home in slight disarray. The lawn is overgrown, there are dirty dishes in the sink, and an empty can of soup is sitting on the kitchen counter. Carl is standing in the living room folding clothes from a laundry basket, and Evelyn is watching television. Carl looks tired and states, "I'm just worn out." The home health nurse knows that a new diagnosis of dementia often creates stress, especially for the caregiver.

Assessment Activities	*Findings/Defining Characteristics**
Ask Carl about his recent stressors and coping strategies.	Carl states, **"There's so much to do that I don't even know where to begin."** He **awakens 3 to 4 times per night** to find Evelyn wandering about.
Observe Carl's grooming and hygiene.	Carl is **unshaven and appears disheveled.**
Ask Carl about his sleep and nutrition patterns.	Carl states that he has **lost 20 pounds in the past 6 months** and that his **appetite has been poor.**
Assess Carl's mood and affect by asking how he is feeling.	Carl states, **"I feel very tired. Everything feels overwhelming."**
Assess Carl's suicide potential.	Carl denies being suicidal.
Assess health status and health care status.	Carl **has not seen a health care provider for his own health in over a year.**

*Defining characteristics are shown in **bold type.**

NURSING DIAGNOSIS: Caregiver role strain related to recent diagnosis of wife's Alzheimer's dementia

PLANNING

Goals	*Expected Outcomes (NOC)†*
Carl will appear rested in 1 month.	**Caregiver Physical Health** Carl will verbalize approaches used to involve others in Evelyn's caregiving activities within 2 weeks.
Carl will state that he has resumed one outside activity within 1 month.	**Caregiver Lifestyle Disruption** Carl will report a balanced routine that incorporates time for own rest or relaxation within 1 week.

†Outcome classification labels from Moorhead S et al: Nursing outcomes classification (NOC), ed 4, St Louis, 2008, Mosby.

INTERVENTIONS (NIC)‡	RATIONALE
Caregiver Support	
Help Carl locate an Internet video support group.	An Internet video support group helps lower stress related to the care recipient's cognitive impairment and decline in function (Marziali and Garcia, 2011).
Identify sources of respite care in the form of adult day care programs.	Adult day programs reduce caregiver burden much more successfully than in-home services (Sussman and Regehr, 2009).
Explore community resources for a short-term education group for Carl that teaches self-care tools to reduce stress.	Education groups help caregivers develop self-care tools to reduce stress, change negative self-talk, communicate more effectively, and make difficult decisions (Oken et al., 2010).
Teach Carl mindfulness meditation strategies.	Mindfulness meditation, a form of cognitive therapy, reduces stress in caregivers (Oken et al, 2010).

‡Intervention classification labels from Bulechek GM, Butcher HK, Dochterman JM: *Nursing interventions classification (NIC),* ed 5, St Louis, 2008, Mosby.

EVALUATION

Nursing Actions	*Patient Response/Finding*	*Achievement of Outcome*
Ask Carl if his fatigue and stress level have decreased.	Carl states that he feels more rested and less depressed.	Carl sleeps for 6 hours at night and takes a 30-minute nap in the afternoon.
Ask Carl to describe modifications that he has made in his daily routine.	Carl uses mindfulness meditation several times a week and states that he is feeling much more relaxed.	Meditation is reducing stress and allowing Carl to care for his own needs.

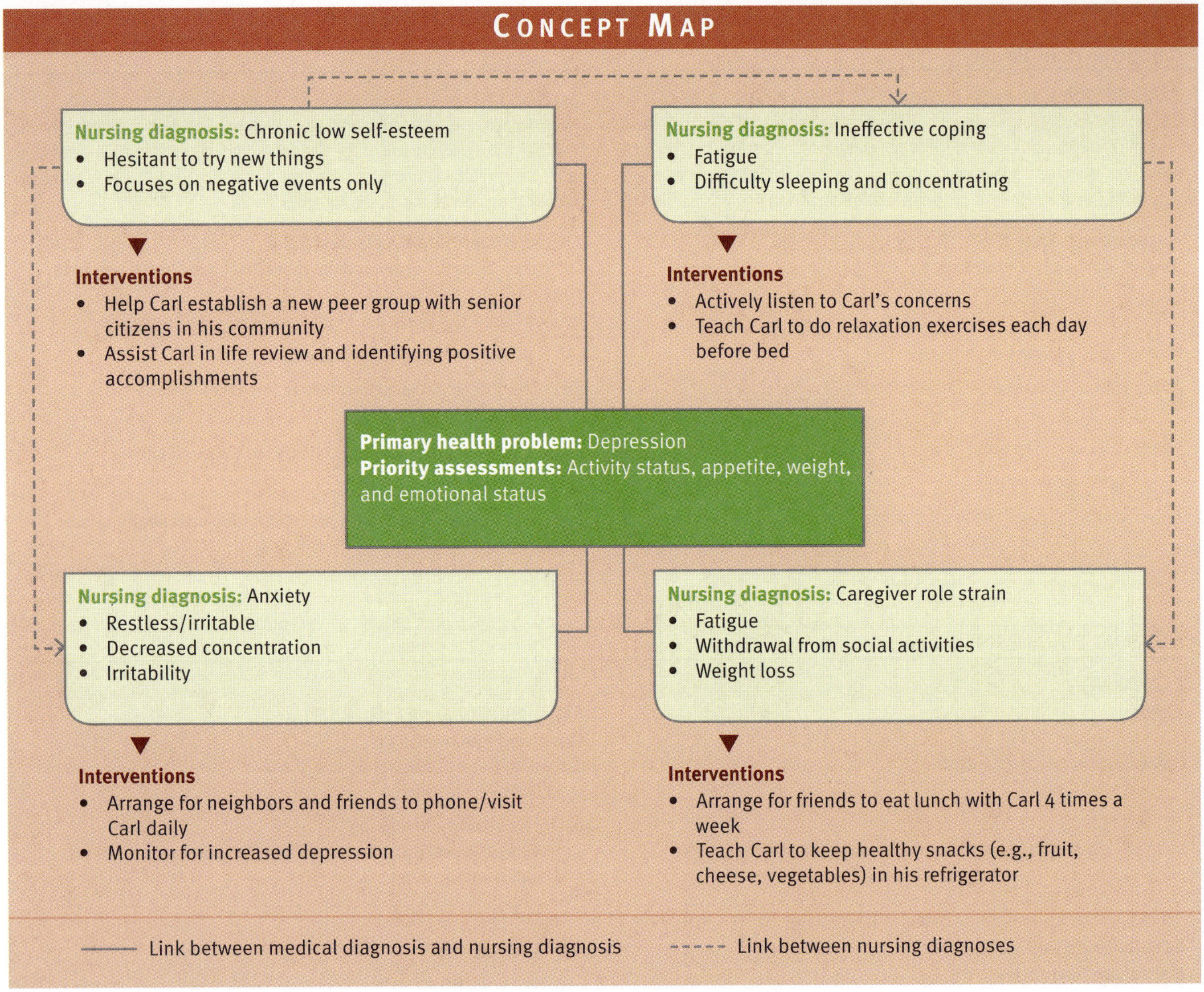
CONCEPT MAP
Nursing diagnosis: Chronic low self-esteem
• Hesitant to try new things
• Focuses on negative events only
Interventions
• Help Carl establish a new peer group with senior citizens in his community
• Assist Carl in life review and identifying positive accomplishments
Nursing diagnosis: Ineffective coping
• Fatigue
• Difficulty sleeping and concentrating
Interventions
• Actively listen to Carl's concerns
• Teach Carl to do relaxation exercises each day before bed
Primary health problem: Depression
Priority assessments: Activity status, appetite, weight, and emotional status
Nursing diagnosis: Anxiety
• Restless/irritable
• Decreased concentration
• Irritability
Interventions
• Arrange for neighbors and friends to phone/visit Carl daily
• Monitor for increased depression
Nursing diagnosis: Caregiver role strain
• Fatigue
• Withdrawal from social activities
• Weight loss
Interventions
• Arrange for friends to eat lunch with Carl 4 times a week
• Teach Carl to keep healthy snacks (e.g., fruit, cheese, vegetables) in his refrigerator
Link between medical diagnosis and nursing diagnosis
Link between nursing diagnoses

FIG. 37-5 Concept map for Carl.

with patients experiencing stress, you gain a broad understanding of the multitude of health care disciplines. Work becomes more satisfying. Contacts with other members of the multidisciplinary team and the community provide a feeling of contributing to the teamwork of providing holistic care.

IMPLEMENTATION

Health Promotion. Three primary modes of intervention for stress are to decrease stress-producing situations, increase resistance to stress, and learn skills that reduce physiological response to stress (Pender et al., 2011). Educate patients and families about the importance of health promotion (Box 37-7).

Regular Exercise. A regular exercise program improves muscle tone and posture, controls weight, reduces tension, and promotes relaxation. In addition, exercise reduces the risk of cardiovascular disease and improves cardiopulmonary functioning. Patients who have a history of a chronic illness, are at risk for developing an illness, or are older than 35 years of age should begin a physical exercise program only after discussing the plan with a health care provider (Fig. 37-6).

Building Competency in Evidence-Based Practice You are a nurse educator for a diabetes rehabilitation program. You recognize the value of exercise for these patients, yet you are not sure about the best way to persuade the patients to increase their exercise. You've located a current systematic review (which represents the highest quality of research evidence) that found three types of interventions to be most effective in promoting physical activity among chronically ill adults. These are to (1) target physical activity exclusively, (2) use behavioral (as opposed to cognitive) strategies, and (3) encourage self-monitoring (Ruppar and Conn, 2010). On the basis of the evidence, which of the following interventions is (are) most likely to be successful? (Select all that apply.)

1. Develop a program that focuses on multiple behaviors, including diet, exercise, and medication compliance.
2. Develop a program that teaches tai chi.
3. Ask patients to keep a written log of the amount of physical activity they have each day.
4. Ask patients to list the ways that exercise helps them.
5. Provide patients with pedometers to record their daily steps.
6. Ask patients to set goals for exercise every day.

Answers to questions can be found on the Evolve website.

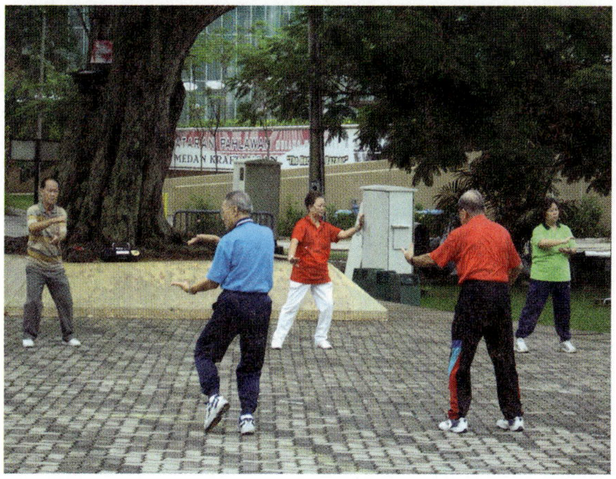

FIG. 37-6 Regular exercise assists in coping with stress. (Courtesy Rudolph A. Furtado.)

BOX 37-7 PATIENT TEACHING

Stress Management

Objective

- Patient will report less anxiety, depression, and pain related to chronic health problems.

Teaching Strategies

- Familiarize patient with one or more of the following mind-body therapies, referring to a group or specialized practitioner when necessary (Bertisch et al., 2009):
  - Meditation
  - Deep breathing
  - Progressive muscle relaxation
  - Guided imagery
  - Hypnosis
  - Biofeedback
  - Yoga
  - Tai Chi
  - Qigong
- Teach patient to exercise for at least 15-30 minutes every day.
- Encourage patient to lower or stop caffeine intake (i.e., in coffee, tea, and soda).
- Instruct patient to do the following:
  - Listen to music that you enjoy.
  - Keep a journal of your thoughts and feelings.
  - Replace unnecessary time-consuming activities with activities that are pleasurable or interesting.
  - Look for humor in stressful situations.

Evaluation

- Ask the patient to report effects of the alternative therapy(ies) on pain, anxiety, and depression.
- Observe the patient for signs of stress.

Support Systems. A support system of family, friends, and colleagues who listen, offer advice, and provide emotional support benefits a patient experiencing stress. Many support groups are available to individuals (e.g., those sponsored by the American Heart Association and the American Cancer Society, local hospitals and churches, and mental health organizations).

Time Management. Time management techniques include developing lists of prioritized tasks. For example, help patients list tasks that require immediate attention, those that are important and can be delayed, and those that are routine and can be accomplished when time becomes available. In many cases setting priorities helps individuals identify tasks that are not necessary or can be delegated to someone else.

Guided Imagery and Visualization. Guided imagery is based on the belief that a person significantly reduces stress with imagination. It is a relaxed state in which a person actively uses imagination in a way that allows visualization of a soothing, peaceful setting. Typically the image created or suggested uses many sensory words to engage the mind and offer distraction and relaxation.

Progressive Muscle Relaxation. In the presence of anxiety-provoking thoughts and events, a common physiological symptom is muscle tension. Diminish physiological tension through a systematic approach to releasing tension in major muscle groups. Typically an individual achieves a relaxed state through deep chest breathing. Once the patient is breathing deeply, direct him or her to alternately tighten and relax muscles in specific groupings.

Assertiveness Training. Assertiveness includes skills for helping individuals communicate effectively regarding their needs and desires. The ability to resolve conflict with others through assertiveness training is important for reducing stress. Teaching assertiveness in a group setting increases the benefits of the experience.

Journal Writing. For many people keeping a private, personal journal provides a therapeutic outlet for stress. Suggest that patients keep journals, especially during difficult situations. In a private journal patients are able to express a full range of emotion and vent their honest feelings without hurting anyone else's feelings and without concern for how they appear to others.

Stress Management in the Workplace. Stressors such as rapid changes in health care technology, diversity in the workforce, organizational restructuring, and changing work systems place stress on employees. **Burnout** occurs as a result of chronic stress. In nursing burnout frequently results from intense caregiving and manifests as emotional exhaustion, loss of a sense of personal identity, and feelings of failure.

If you or your patients experience burnout, it helps to make changes in behavior to cope with workplace stress. An important step is identifying the limits and scope of responsibilities at work. Recognizing the areas over which you have control and can change and those for which you do not have responsibility is a vital insight. Making a clear separation between work and home life is also crucial. Strengthening friendships outside of the workplace, arranging for temporary social isolation for personal "recharging" of emotional energy, and spending off-duty hours in interesting activities all help reduce burnout.

Acute Care

Crisis Intervention. When stress overwhelms a person's usual coping mechanisms and demands mobilization of all available resources, it becomes a crisis. A crisis creates a turning point in a person's life because it changes the direction of his or her life in some way. The precipitating event usually occurs approximately 1 to 2 weeks before the individual seeks help, but sometimes it has occurred within the past 24 hours. Generally a person resolves the crisis in some way within approximately 6 weeks. Crisis intervention aims to return the person to a precrisis level of functioning and promote growth (Fig. 37-7).

Because an individual's or family's usual coping strategies are ineffective in managing the stress of the precipitating event, the use of new coping mechanisms is necessary. This experience forces the use of unfamiliar strategies and results in either a heightened awareness of previously unrecognized strengths and resources or deterioration in functioning. Thus a crisis is often referred to as a situation of both danger and opportunity. Some individuals or families emerge from a crisis state functioning more effectively, whereas others find themselves weakened, and still others are completely dysfunctional.

Crisis intervention is a specific type of brief psychotherapy with prescribed steps. It is more directive than traditional psychotherapy or counseling, and any member of the health care team who has been trained in its techniques can use it. The basic approach is problem solving, and it focuses only on the problem presented by the crisis.

When using a crisis intervention approach, you help the patient make the mental connection between the stressful event and his or her reaction to it. This is crucial because he or she is sometimes unable to see the whole situation clearly. You also help the person become aware of present feelings such as anger, grief, or guilt to help him or her reduce feelings of tension. In addition, you help the patient explore coping mechanisms, perhaps identifying new methods of coping. Finally you help the person increase social contacts if he or she has been isolated and overly self-focused.

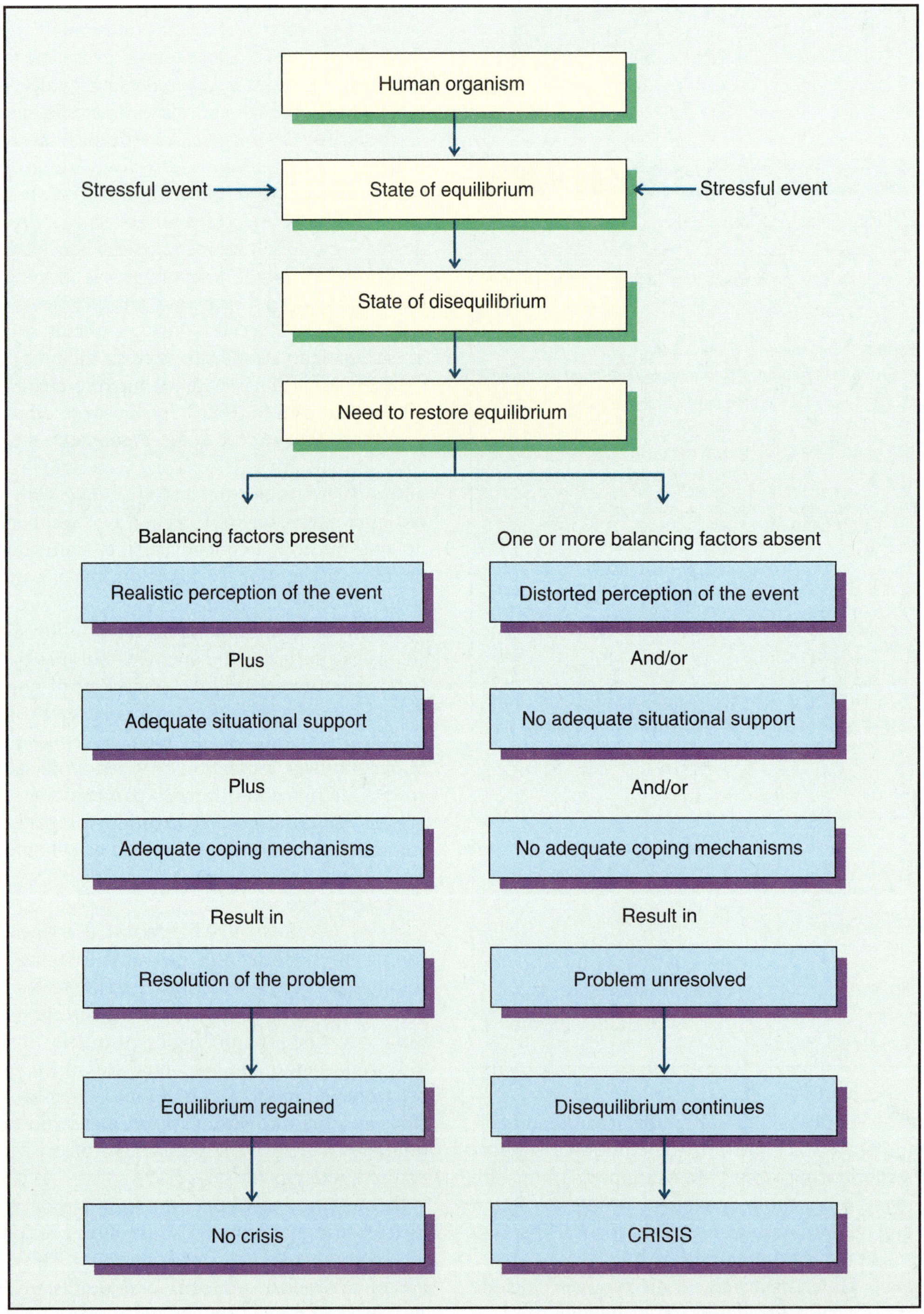

FIG. 37-7 Crisis intervention model. (Redrawn from Aguilera DC: *Crisis intervention: theory and methodology,* ed 8, St Louis, 1998, Mosby.)

Restorative and Continuing Care. A person under stress recovers when the stress is removed or coping strategies are successful; however, a person who has experienced a crisis has changed, and the effects often last for years or for the rest of the person's life. The final stage of adapting to a crisis is acknowledgment of the long-term implications of the crisis. If a person has successfully coped with a crisis and its consequences, he or she becomes more mature and healthy. When a person recovers from a stressful situation, the time is right for introducing stress management skills to reduce the number and intensity of stressful situations in the future.

EVALUATION

Through the Patient's Eyes. A patient recovering from acute stress often spontaneously reports feeling better when the stressor is gone. The recovery from chronic stress occurs more gradually as the patient emerges from the strain. In either situation reassess the patient for the presence of new or recurring stress-related symptoms (Fig. 37-8). Observe patient behaviors and talk with the patient and family if appropriate. Ask the patient about sleep patterns, appetite, and ability to concentrate. Ask about coping strategies that the patient uses and determine their effectiveness. Ask patients to compare current feelings and behaviors with feelings and behaviors 6 months ago. If desired outcomes have been met, the patient reports feeling better now than 6 months ago.

Patient Outcomes. Remember that coping with stress takes time. Maintain ongoing communication with patients regarding their coping. Patients under severe stress, or trauma, often experience feelings of powerlessness, vulnerability, and loss of control. The nurse addresses these feelings by actively involving patients and families in the processes of problem identification (assessment), prioritizing, goal setting, and evaluation. Involving patients in these processes gives them an opportunity to direct their energy in a positive way and moves them toward taking greater responsibility for health maintenance and promotion.

Engaging the patient as a partner in health care sets the stage for open communication. In such an environment the patient feels freer to give important feedback about interventions that are successful and helps the nurse better understand why some interventions fail to meet the established goals. If he or she reports continued acute stress, assess for safety by asking about whether or not there have been any recent accidents at home, in the car, or at work. Ask about coping strategies to determine if the patient is using unsafe, maladaptive strategies. If the patient reports continued chronic stress, ask about his or her perception of the stressor and coping behaviors used. Discuss the stressor with the patient to determine if it needs to be redefined. If contact with a patient ends before you have achieved the resolution of goals, it is important to refer him or her to appropriate resources so progress is not delayed or interrupted.

An essential part of the evaluation process is collaborating with patients to determine if their own expectations from nursing have been met. Any revision in the plan of care includes steps to address patient expectations.

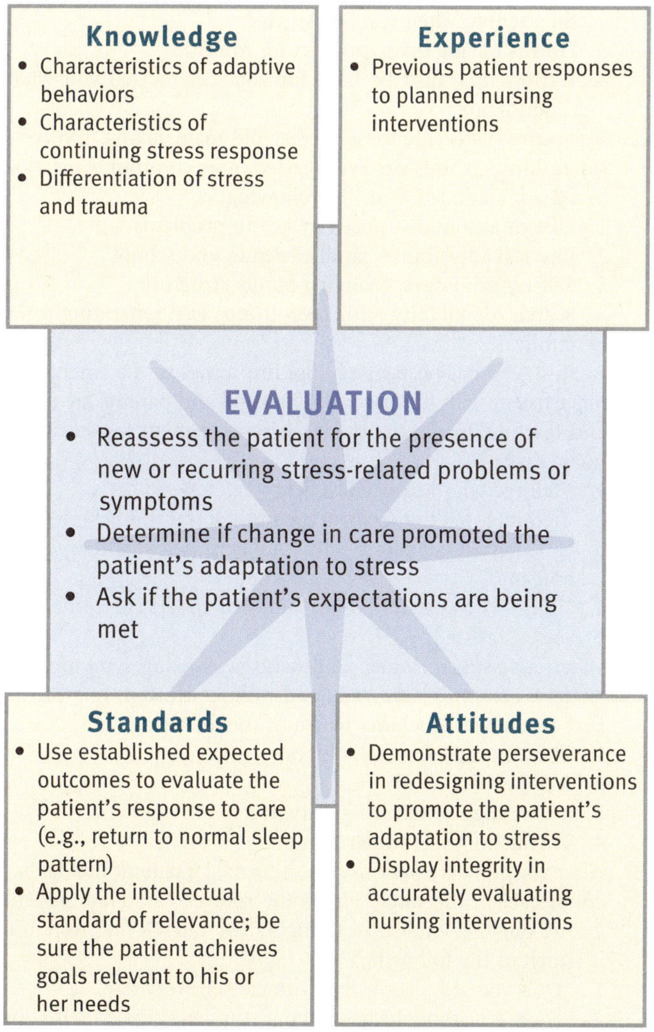

Knowledge
• Characteristics of adaptive behaviors
• Characteristics of continuing stress response
• Differentiation of stress and trauma
Experience
• Previous patient responses to planned nursing interventions
EVALUATION
• Reassess the patient for the presence of new or recurring stress-related problems or symptoms
• Determine if change in care promoted the patient's adaptation to stress
• Ask if the patient's expectations are being met
Standards
• Use established expected outcomes to evaluate the patient's response to care (e.g., return to normal sleep pattern)
• Apply the intellectual standard of relevance; be sure the patient achieves goals relevant to his or her needs
Attitudes
• Demonstrate perseverance in redesigning interventions to promote the patient's adaptation to stress
• Display integrity in accurately evaluating nursing interventions

FIG. 37-8 Critical thinking model for stress and coping evaluation.

KEY POINTS

- The general adaptation syndrome is an immediate physiological response of the whole body to stress and involves several body systems, especially the autonomic nervous and endocrine systems. Physiological responses to stress also include immunological changes.
- Stress can make people ill as a result of increased levels of powerful hormones that change bodily processes.
- A person is under psychological stress only if he or she evaluates the event or circumstance as personally significant. Such an evaluation of an event for its personal meaning is called *primary appraisal.*
- There are several types of stress, including work, family, chronic, and acute stress; daily hassles; trauma; and crisis.
- Nurses recognize and respond to caregiver stress of family members of patients.
- Rapid changes in health care technology, diversity in the workforce, organizational redesign, and changing work systems place stress on employees, including nurses.
- Potential stressors and coping mechanisms vary across the life span.
- Coping means making an effort to manage psychological stress.
- Coping is a process that constantly changes to manage demands on a person's resources.
- Three primary modes for stress intervention are to decrease stress-producing situations, increase resistance to stress, and learn skills that reduce physiological response to stress.
- A patient whose stress is so severe that he or she is unable to cope using any of the means that have worked before is experiencing a crisis.

- A crisis is a turning point in life and is developmental, situational, or adventitious.
- Generally a crisis is resolved in some way within approximately 6 weeks. Crisis intervention aims to return the person to a pre-crisis level of functioning and to promote growth.

CLINICAL APPLICATION QUESTIONS

Preparing for Clinical Practice

1. You are making a home visit to see 80-year-old Carl and 81-year-old Evelyn because Evelyn has Alzheimer's dementia and her health care provider is concerned about her nutrition. He also wants to know if she is taking her medications. Carl has been providing Evelyn's care, and he is also worried about his own health. Discuss the various stressors that need to be considered when assessing their situation.
2. Carl reports dizziness; however, based on your thorough assessment, you do not identify any physical findings that would account for this. As you talk with Carl, he tells you that his life is very stressful and he is barely coping. He is the sole caregiver for his wife, Evelyn, who has dementia. He is worried about what might happen to her if his health failed. He has not been able to play golf with his friends or go to church in months. His only social activity is a trip to the grocery store while his neighbor stays with Evelyn. He is worried that they will spend all their life savings if she needs to go to a nursing home, and he loses his patience with her. Develop nursing diagnoses related to this situation.
3. Carl is admitted to the hospital with a fractured hip sustained from a fall when he got up during the night to check on Evelyn who was wandering in the house. Before his injury he cared for Evelyn, who suffers from advancing Alzheimer's disease. While he is hospitalized, Evelyn stays with a niece who lives 100 miles away, but this cannot be a permanent situation because their niece is also in frail health. Carl and Evelyn's children live across the country and are very involved in their careers. He is concerned about who will care for Evelyn and how he will manage when he is discharged. What approach would be the best to take in planning Carl's care?

evolve *Answers to Clinical Application Questions can be found on the Evolve website.*

REVIEW QUESTIONS

Are You Ready to Test Your Nursing Knowledge?

1. When teaching a patient about the negative feedback response to stress, the nurse includes which of the following to describe the benefits of this stress response?
   1. Results in neurophysiological response.
   2. Reduces body temperature
   3. Causes a person to be hypervigilant
   4. Reduces level of consciousness to conserve energy.
2. A nurse observes that a patient whose home life is chaotic with intermittent homelessness, a child with spina bifida, and an abusive spouse appears to be experiencing an allostatic load. As a result, the nurse expects to detect which of the following while assessing the patient?
   1. Posttraumatic stress disorder
   2. Rising hormone levels
   3. Chronic illness
   4. Return of vital signs to normal
3. A patient who is having difficulty managing his diabetes mellitus responds to the news that his hemoglobin A1C, a measure of blood sugar control over the past 90 days, has increased by saying, "The hemoglobin A1C is wrong. My blood sugar levels have been excellent for the last 6 months." The patient is using the defense mechanism:
   1. Denial.
   2. Conversion.
   3. Dissociation.
   4. Displacement.
4. When doing an assessment of a young woman who was in an automobile accident 6 months before, the nurse learns that the woman has vivid images of the crash whenever she hears a loud, sudden noise. The nurse recognizes this as ____________.
5. A grandfather living in Japan worries about his two young grandsons who disappeared after a tsunami. This is an example of:
   1. A situational crisis.
   2. A maturational crisis.
   3. An adventitious crisis.
   4. A developmental crisis.
6. During the assessment interview of an older woman experiencing a developmental crisis, the nurse asks which of the following questions?
   1. How is this flood affecting your life?
   2. Since your husband has died, what have you been doing in the evening when you feel lonely?
   3. How is having diabetes affecting your life?
   4. I know this must be hard for you. Let me tell you what might help.
7. The nurse plans care for a 16-year-old male, taking into consideration that stressors experienced most commonly by adolescents include which of the following?
   1. Loss of autonomy caused by health problems
   2. Physical appearance, family, friends, and school
   3. Self-esteem issues, changing family structure
   4. Search for identity with peer groups and separating from family
8. A child who has been in a house fire comes to the emergency department with her parents. The child and parents are upset and tearful. During the nurse's first assessment for stress the nurse says:
   1. "Tell me who I can call to help you."
   2. "Tell me what bothers you the most about this experience."
   3. "I'll contact someone who can help get you temporary housing."
   4. "I'll sit with you until other family members can come help you get settled."
9. When assessing an older adult who is showing symptoms of anxiety, insomnia, anorexia, and mild confusion, one of the first assessments includes which of the following?
   1. The amount of family support
   2. A 3-day diet recall
   3. A thorough physical assessment
   4. Threats to safety in her home
10. After a health care provider has informed a patient that he has colon cancer, the nurse enters the room to find the patient gazing out the window in thought. The nurse's first response is which of the following?
    1. "Don't be sad. People live with cancer every day."
    2. "Have you thought about how you are going to tell your family?"

3. "Would you like for me to sit down with you for a few minutes so you can talk about this?"
4. "I know another patient whose colon cancer was cured by surgery."

11. A 34-year-old man who is anxious, tearful, and tired from caring for his three young children tells you that he feels depressed and doesn't see how he can go on much longer. Your best response would be which of the following?
    1. "Are you thinking of suicide?"
    2. "You've been doing a good job raising your children. You can do it!"
    3. "Is there someone who can help you?"
    4. "You have so much to live for."
12. The nurse is evaluating the coping success of a patient experiencing stress from being newly diagnosed with multiple sclerosis and psychomotor impairment. The nurse realizes that the patient is coping successfully when the patient says:
    1. "I'm going to learn to drive a car so I can be more independent."
    2. "My sister says she feels better when she goes shopping, so I'll go shopping."
    3. "I've always felt better when I go for a long walk. I'll do that when I get home."
    4. "I'm going to attend a support group to learn more about multiple sclerosis."
13. A patient newly diagnosed with type 2 diabetes says, "My blood sugar was just a little high. I don't have diabetes." The nurse responds:
    1. "Let's talk about something cheerful."
    2. "Do other members of your family have diabetes?"
    3. "I can tell that you feel stressed to learn that you have diabetes."
    4. With silence.
14. A staff nurse is talking with the nursing supervisor about the stress that she feels on the job. The supervising nurse recognizes that:
    1. Nurses who feel stress usually pass the stress along to their patients.
    2. A nurse who feels stress is ineffective as a nurse and should not be working.
    3. Nurses who talk about feeling stress are unprofessional and should calm down.
    4. Nurses frequently experience stress with the rapid changes in health care technology and organizational restructuring.
15. A crisis intervention nurse working with a mother whose Down syndrome child has been hospitalized with pneumonia and who has lost her entitlement check while the child is hospitalized can expect the mother to regain stability after how long?
    1. After 2 weeks when the child's pneumonia begins to improve
    2. After 6 weeks when she adjusts to the child's respiratory status and reestablishes the entitlement checks
    3. After 1 month when the child goes home and the mother gets help from a food pantry
    4. After 6 months when the child is back in school

Answers: 1. 1; 2. 3; 3. 1; 4. Posttraumatic stress disorder (PTSD); 5. 3; 6. 2; 7. 4; 8. 2; 9. 3; 10. 3; 11. 1; 12. 4; 13. 4; 14. 4; 15. 2.

REFERENCES

Aldwin CM: *Stress, coping and development: an integrative perspective*, ed 2, New York, 2007, Guilford Press.

American Nurses Association (ANA): *Psychiatric–mental health nursing: scope and standards of practice*, Silver Spring, Md, 2007, ANA.

Diamond JW: Allostatic medicine: bringing stress, coping, and chronic disease into focus. Part 1, *Integrat Med* 8(6):40, Dec 2009/Jan 2010.

Lazarus RS: Stress and emotion: a new synthesis. In Monat A, Lazarus RS, Reevy G: *The Praeger handbook on stress and coping*, Westport, Conn, 2007, Praeger.

McEwen BS: Stressed or stressed out: what is the difference, *J Psychiatry Neurosci* 50(5):315, 2005.

Neuman B, Fawcett J, editors: *The Neuman Systems Model*, ed 5, Upper Saddle River, NJ, 2011, Pearson.

Pender NJ, Murdaugh C, Parsons MA: *Health promotion in nursing practice*, ed 6, Upper Saddle River, NJ, 2011, Howorth Press.

Varcarolis EM, Halter MJ: *Foundations of psychiatric mental health nursing: a clinical approach*, ed 6, St Louis, 2010, Saunders.

RESEARCH REFERENCES

Anngela-Cole L, Hilton JM: The role of attitudes and culture in family caregiving for older adults, *Home Health Care Services Q* 28:59, 2009.

Bertisch SM, Wee CC, Phillips RS, McCarthy EP: Alternative mind-body therapies used by adults with medical conditions, *J Psychosom Res* 66(6):511, 2009.

Folkman S, et al: Age differences in stress and coping, *Psychol Aging* 2(2):171, 1987.

Haley WE, et al: Problems and benefits reported by stroke family caregivers: results from a prospective epidemiological study, *Stroke J Am Heart Assoc* 40:2129, 2009.

Marziali E, Garcia LJ: Dementia caregivers' responses to 2 internet-based intervention programs, *Am J Alzheimers Dis Other Dementias* 26(1):36, 2011.

Oken BS, et al: Pilot controlled trial of mindfulness meditation and education for dementia caregivers, *J Altern Complement Med* 16:1031, 2010.

Pressler SJ, et al: Family caregiver outcomes in heart failure, *Fam Crit Care* 18:149, 2009.

Ruppar TM, Conn VS: Interventions to promote physical activity in chronically ill adults, *Am J Nurs* 110(7):30, 2010.

Sussman T, Regehr C: The influence of community-based services on the burden of spouses caring for their partners with dementia, *Health Social Work* 34(1):29, 2009.

Yancura LA, Aldwin CM: Coping and health in older adults, *Curr Psych Rep* 10:10, 2008.

CHAPTER

38

Activity and Exercise

OBJECTIVES

- Describe the role of the musculoskeletal and nervous systems in the regulation of movement.
- Discuss physiological and pathological influences on body alignment and joint mobility.
- Describe how to maintain and use proper body mechanics.
- Describe how exercise and activity benefit physiological and psychological functioning.
- Describe the benefits of implementing an exercise program for the purpose of health promotion.
- Describe important factors to consider when planning an exercise program for patients across the life span and for those with specific chronic illnesses.
- Assess patients for impaired mobility and activity intolerance.
- Formulate nursing diagnoses for patients experiencing problems with impaired mobility and activity intolerance.
- Write a nursing care plan for a patient with impaired mobility and activity intolerance.
- Describe interventions for maintaining activity tolerance and mobility.
- Evaluate the nursing care plan for maintaining activity and exercise for patients across the life span and with specific chronic illnesses.

KEY TERMS

Activities of daily living (ADLs), p. 746
Activity tolerance, p. 747
Antagonistic muscles, p. 748
Antigravity muscles, p. 748
Cartilage, p. 748
Cartilaginous joints, p. 747
Center of gravity, p. 747
Crutch gait, p. 761
Exercise, p. 746
Fibrous joints, p. 747
Footboards, p. 747
Friction, p. 747
Gait, p. 753
Hemiparesis, p. 752
Hemiplegia, p. 749
Isometric contraction, p. 747
Isotonic contraction, p. 747
Joint, p. 747
Ligaments, p. 747
Mobility, p. 752
Muscle tone, p. 746
Posture, p. 746
Proprioception, p. 748
Range of motion (ROM), p. 751
Synergistic muscles, p. 748
Synovial joints, p. 747
Tendons, p. 748

evolve WEBSITE

http://evolve.elsevier.com/Potter/fundamentals/

- Review Questions
- Video Clips
- Concept Map Creator
- Case Study with Questions
- Audio Glossary
- Interactive Learning Activities
- Key Term Flashcards
- Content Updates

A program of regular physical activity and **exercise** has the potential to enhance all aspects of a patient's biopsychosocial and spiritual model of health. This chapter provides you with knowledge of exercise and activity as they relate to health promotion, the acute phase of illness, and the restorative and continuing care of patients, as well as nursing strategies to help plan an individualized exercise and activity program for a variety of patients with specific disease entities and needs.

SCIENTIFIC KNOWLEDGE BASE

Regular physical activity and exercise contribute to both physical and emotional well-being (Edelman and Mandle, 2010; Ferrand et al., 2008). Knowing the physiology and regulation of body mechanics, exercise, and activity helps provide individualized care.

Overview of Exercise and Activity

The coordinated efforts of the musculoskeletal and nervous systems maintain balance, **posture,** and body alignment during lifting, bending, moving, and performing **activities of daily living (ADLs).** Proper balance, posture, and body alignment reduce the risk of injury to the musculoskeletal system and facilitate body movements, allowing physical mobility without muscle strain and excessive use of muscle energy.

Body Alignment. Body alignment refers to the relationship of one body part to another along a horizontal or vertical line. Correct alignment involves positioning so no excessive strain is placed on a person's joints, tendons, ligaments, or muscles, thereby maintaining adequate **muscle tone** and contributing to balance.

Body Balance. Body balance occurs when a relatively low center of gravity is balanced over a wide, stable base of support and a vertical line falls from the center of gravity through the base of support. When the vertical line from the center of gravity does not fall through the base of support, the body loses balance. Proper posture or a body position that most favors function, requires the least muscular work to maintain, and places the least strain on muscles, ligaments, and bones enhances body balance (Patton and Thibodeau, 2010). Nurses use balance to maintain proper body alignment and posture through two simple techniques. First widen the base of support by separating the feet to a comfortable distance. Second, increase balance by bringing the center of gravity closer to the base of support. For example, you raise the height of the bed when performing a procedure such as changing a dressing to prevent bending too far at the waist and shifting the base of support.

Coordinated Body Movement. Coordinated body movement is a result of weight, center of gravity, and balance. Weight is the force exerted on a body by gravity. When an object is lifted, the lifter must overcome the weight of the object and be aware of the center of gravity of the object. In symmetrical objects the center of gravity is located at the exact center of the object. The force of weight is always directed downward. An unbalanced object has its center of gravity away from the midline and falls without support. Because people are not geometrically perfect, their centers of gravity are usually midline, at 55% to 57% of standing height. Like unbalanced objects, patients who are unsteady do not maintain a balance with their center of gravity, which places them at risk for falling. You need to be able to identify these patients and intervene to maintain their safety.

Friction. Friction is a force that occurs in a direction to oppose movement. Reduce friction by following some basic principles. When you move objects, those with a greater surface area create more friction. To reduce friction, you need to decrease the object's surface area. For example, when helping patients move up in bed, place their arms across the chest. This decreases surface area and reduces friction.

A patient who is passive or immobilized produces greater friction to movement (see Chapter 47). When possible, use some of your patients' strength and mobility when positioning and transferring them. Explain the procedure and tell your patients when to move. You decrease friction when your patients bend their knees as you help them move up in the bed.

You can also reduce friction by using an air-assisted device when performing lateral patient transfers (Baptiste et al., 2006). Air-assisted devices are commercially available transfer devices that are effective solutions to reducing injury to health care employees and patients.

Exercise and Activity. Exercise is physical activity used to condition the body, improve health, and maintain fitness. Sometimes exercise is also a therapeutic measure. A patient's individualized exercise program depends on the patient's activity tolerance or the type and amount of exercise or activity that the patient is able to perform. Physiological, emotional, and developmental factors influence the patient's activity tolerance.

An active lifestyle is important for maintaining and promoting health; it is also an essential treatment for chronic illnesses (Perez et al., 2009). Regular physical activity and exercise enhance functioning of all body systems, including cardiopulmonary functioning (endurance), musculoskeletal fitness (flexibility and bone integrity), weight control and maintenance (body image), and psychological well-being (ACSM, 2007; Edelman and Mandle, 2010).

The best program of physical activity includes a combination of exercises that produces different physiological and psychological benefits. Three categories of exercise are isotonic, isometric, and resistive isometric. The type of muscle contraction involved determines the classification of the exercise. Isotonic exercises cause muscle contraction and change in muscle length (isotonic contraction). Examples are walking, swimming, dance aerobics, jogging, bicycling, and moving arms and legs with light resistance. Isotonic exercises enhance circulatory and respiratory functioning; increase muscle mass, tone, and strength; and promote osteoblastic activity (activity by bone-forming cells), thus combating osteoporosis.

Isometric exercises involve tightening or tensing muscles without moving body parts (isometric contraction). Examples are quadriceps set exercises and contraction of the gluteal muscles. This form of exercise is ideal for patients who do not tolerate increased activity. A patient who is immobilized in bed can perform isometric exercises. The benefits are increased muscle mass, tone, and strength, thus decreasing the potential for muscle wasting; increased circulation to the involved body part; and increased osteoblastic activity.

Resistive isometric exercises are those in which the individual contracts the muscle while pushing against a stationary object or resisting the movement of an object (Hoeman, 2006). A gradual increase in the amount of resistance and length of time that the muscle contraction is held increases muscle strength and endurance. Examples of resistive isometric exercises are push-ups and hip lifting, in which a patient in a sitting position pushes with the hands against a surface such as a chair seat and raises the hips. In some long-term care settings, footboards are placed on the end of beds; patients push against them to move up in bed. Resistive isometric exercises help promote muscle strength and provide sufficient stress against bone to promote osteoblastic activity.

Regulation of Movement

Coordinated body movement involves the integrated functioning of the skeletal, muscular, and nervous systems. Because these three systems cooperate so closely in mechanical support of the body, they are often considered as a single functional unit.

Skeletal System. Bones perform five functions in the body: support, protection, movement, mineral storage, and hematopoiesis (blood cell formation). In the discussion of body mechanics, two of these functions (i.e., support and movement) are most important (see Chapter 47). Bones serve as support by providing the framework and contributing to the shape, alignment, and positioning of the body parts. Bones, together with their joints, constitute levers for muscle attachment to provide movement. As muscles contract and shorten, they pull on bones, producing joint movement (Patton and Thibodeau, 2010).

Joints. An articulation, or joint, is the connection between bones. Each joint is classified according to its structure and degree of mobility. On the basis of connective structures, joints are classified as fibrous, cartilaginous, or synovial (Huether and McCance, 2008). Fibrous joints fit closely together and are fixed, permitting little, if any, movement such as the syndesmosis between the tibia and fibula. Cartilaginous joints have little movement but are elastic and use cartilage to unite separate body surfaces such as the synchondrosis that attaches the ribs to the costal cartilage. Synovial joints, or true joints, such as the hinge type at the elbow, are freely movable and the most mobile, numerous, and anatomically complex body joints.

Ligaments, Tendons, and Cartilage. Ligaments, tendons, and cartilage support the skeletal system (see Chapter 47). Ligaments are white, shiny, flexible bands of fibrous tissue that bind joints and connect bones and cartilage. They are elastic and aid joint flexibility and support. **Tendons** are white, glistening, fibrous bands of tissue that connect muscle to bone. **Cartilage** is nonvascular, supporting connective tissue with the flexibility of a firm, plastic material. Because of its gristle-like nature, cartilage sustains weight and serves as a shock absorber between articulating bones.

Skeletal Muscle. Contraction of skeletal muscles allows people to walk, talk, run, breathe, or participate in physical activity. There are more than 600 skeletal muscles in the body. In addition to facilitating movement, these muscles determine the form and contour of our bodies. Most of our muscles span at least one joint and attach to both articulating bones. When contraction occurs, one bone is fixed while the other moves. The origin is the point of attachment that remains still; the insertion is the point that moves when the muscle contracts (Patton and Thibodeau, 2010).

Muscles Concerned with Movement. The muscles of movement are located near the skeletal region, where a lever system causes movement (Patton and Thibodeau, 2010). The lever system makes the work of moving a weight or load easier. It occurs when specific bones such as the humerus, ulna, and radius and the associated joints such as the elbow act as a lever. Thus the force applied to one end of the bone to lift a weight at another point tends to rotate the bone in the direction opposite that of the applied force. Muscles that attach to bones of leverage provide the necessary strength to move the object.

Muscles Concerned with Posture. Gravity continually pulls on parts of the body; the only way the body is held in position is for muscles to pull on bones in the opposite direction. Muscles accomplish this counterforce by maintaining a low level of sustained contraction. Poor posture places more work on muscles to counteract the force of gravity. This leads to fatigue and eventually interferes with bodily functions and causes deformities.

Muscle Groups. The nervous system coordinates the antagonistic, synergistic, and antigravity muscle groups that are responsible for maintaining posture and initiating movement. **Antagonistic muscles** cause movement at the joint. During movement the active mover muscle contracts while its antagonist relaxes. For example, during flexion of the arm the active mover, the biceps brachii, contracts; and its antagonist, the triceps brachii, relaxes. During extension of the arm the active mover, now the triceps brachii, contracts; and the new antagonist, the biceps brachii, relaxes.

Synergistic muscles contract to accomplish the same movement. When the arm is flexed, the strength of the contraction of the biceps brachii is increased by contraction of the synergistic muscle, the brachialis. Thus with synergistic muscle activity there are now two active movers (i.e., the biceps brachii and the brachialis), which contract while the antagonistic muscle, the triceps brachii, relaxes.

Antigravity muscles stabilize joints. These muscles continuously oppose the effect of gravity on the body and permit a person to maintain an upright or sitting posture. In an adult the antigravity muscles are the extensors of the leg, the gluteus maximus, the quadriceps femoris, the soleus muscles, and the muscles of the back.

Skeletal muscles support posture and carry out voluntary movement. The muscles are attached to the skeleton by tendons, which provide strength and permit motion. The movement of the extremities is voluntary and requires coordination from the nervous system.

Nervous System. The nervous system regulates movement and posture. The major voluntary motor area, located in the cerebral cortex, is the precentral gyrus, or motor strip. A majority of motor fibers descend from the motor strip and cross at the level of the medulla. Thus the motor fibers from the right motor strip initiate voluntary movement for the left side of the body, and motor fibers from the left motor strip initiate voluntary movement for the right side of the body.

Transmission of the impulse from the nervous system to the musculoskeletal system is an electrochemical event and requires a neurotransmitter. Basically neurotransmitters are chemicals (e.g., acetylcholine) that transfer the electrical impulse from the nerve across the myoneural junction to stimulate the muscle, causing movement. Several disorders impair movement. For example, Parkinson's disease alters neurotransmitter production, myasthenia gravis disrupts transfer from the neurotransmitter to the muscle, and multiple sclerosis impairs muscle activity (Huether and McCance, 2008).

Proprioception. **Proprioception** is the awareness of the position of the body and its parts (Huether and McCance, 2008). Proprioceptors located on nerve endings in muscles, tendons, and joints monitor proprioception. The nervous system regulates posture, which requires coordination of proprioception and balance. As a person carries out ADLs, proprioceptors monitor muscle activity and body position. For example, the proprioceptors on the soles of the feet contribute to correct posture while standing or walking. In standing, pressure is continuous on the bottom of the feet. The proprioceptors monitor the pressure, communicating this information through the nervous system to the antigravity muscles. The standing person remains upright until deciding to change position. As a person walks, the proprioceptors on the bottom of the feet monitor pressure changes. Thus, when the bottom of the moving foot comes in contact with the walking surface, the individual automatically moves the stationary foot forward.

Balance. A person needs adequate balance to stand, run, lift, or perform ADLs. The nervous system controls balance specifically through the cerebellum and the inner ear. The cerebellum coordinates all voluntary movement, particularly highly skilled movements such as those required in skiing.

Within the inner ear are the semicircular canals, three fluid-filled structures that help maintain balance. Fluid within the canals has a certain inertia; when the head is suddenly rotated in one direction, the fluid remains stationary for a moment, but the canal turns with the head. This allows a person to change position suddenly without losing balance.

Principles of Transfer and Positioning Techniques

Using principles of safe patient transfer and positioning during routine activities decreases work effort (Box 38-1). Teach colleagues and patients' families how to transfer or position patients properly. Teaching a patient's family to transfer the patient from bed to chair increases and reinforces the family's knowledge about proper transfer and position techniques.

Whether you are moving a patient who is immobile, assisting a patient from the bed to the chair, or teaching a patient to carry out ADLs efficiently, knowledge of safe patient transfer and positioning is crucial. You also incorporate knowledge of physiological and pathological influences on body alignment and mobility.

Pathological Influences on Body Alignment and Mobility. Many pathological conditions affect body alignment and mobility. These conditions include congenital defects; disorders of bones, joints, and muscles; central nervous system damage; and musculoskeletal trauma.

BOX 38-1 PRINCIPLES OF SAFE PATIENT TRANSFER AND POSITIONING

- Mechanical lifts and lift teams are essential when the patient is unable to assist.
- When a patient is able to assist, remember the following principles:
  - The wider the base of support, the greater the stability of the nurse.
  - The lower the center of gravity, the greater the stability of the nurse.
  - The equilibrium of an object is maintained as long as the line of gravity passes through its base of support.
  - Facing the direction of movement prevents abnormal twisting of the spine.
  - Dividing balanced activity between arms and legs reduces the risk of back injury.
  - Leverage, rolling, turning, or pivoting requires less work than lifting.
  - When friction is reduced between the object to be moved and the surface on which it is moved, less force is required to move it.

Congenital Defects. Congenital abnormalities affect the efficiency of the musculoskeletal system in regard to alignment, balance, and appearance. Osteogenesis imperfecta is an inherited disorder that affects bone. Bones are porous, short, bowed, and deformed; as a result, children experience curvature of the spine and shortness of stature. Scoliosis is a structural curvature of the spine associated with vertebral rotation. Muscles, ligaments, and other soft tissues become shortened. Balance and mobility are affected in proportion to the severity of abnormal spinal curvatures (Hockenberry and Wilson, 2011).

Disorders of Bones, Joints, and Muscles. Osteoporosis, a well-known and well-publicized disorder of aging, results in the reduction of bone density or mass. The bone remains biochemically normal but has difficulty maintaining integrity and support. The cause is uncertain, and theories vary from hormonal imbalances to insufficient intake of nutrients (Huether and McCance, 2008).

Osteomalacia is an uncommon metabolic disease characterized by inadequate and delayed mineralization, resulting in compact and spongy bone (Lewis et al., 2011). Mineral calcification and deposition do not occur. Replaced bone consists of soft material rather than rigid bone.

Joint mobility is altered by inflammatory and noninflammatory joint diseases and articular disruption. Inflammatory joint disease (e.g., arthritis) is characterized by inflammation or destruction of the synovial membrane and articular cartilage and by systemic signs of inflammation. Noninflammatory diseases have none of these characteristics, and the synovial fluid is normal (Huether and McCance, 2008). Joint degeneration, which can occur with inflammatory and noninflammatory disease, is marked by changes in articular cartilage combined with overgrowth of bone at the articular ends. Degenerative changes commonly affect weight-bearing joints.

Articular disruption involves trauma to the articular capsules and ranges from mild, such as a tear resulting in a sprain, to severe, such as a separation leading to dislocation. Articular disruption usually results from trauma but sometimes is congenital, as with developmental dysplasia of the hip (Hockenberry and Wilson, 2011).

Central Nervous System Damage. Damage to any part of the central nervous system that regulates voluntary movement causes impaired body alignment and immobility. For example, a patient with a traumatic head injury experiences damage in the motor strip in the cerebrum. The amount of voluntary motor impairment is directly related to the amount of destruction of the motor strip. For example, a patient with a right-sided cerebral hemorrhage and permanent damage to the right motor strip has left-sided **hemiplegia,** whereas a patient with a right-sided head injury experiences cerebral edema around (but not destruction of) the motor strip. The patient with hemiplegia does not regain movement, whereas the second patient's voluntary movement gradually returns to the left side following extensive physical therapy.

Musculoskeletal Trauma. Musculoskeletal trauma often results in bruises, contusions, sprains, and fractures. A fracture is a disruption of bone tissue continuity. Fractures most commonly result from direct external trauma. They also occur because of some deformity of the bone (e.g., with pathological fractures of osteoporosis) (see Chapter 47).

NURSING KNOWLEDGE BASE

Application of nursing knowledge allows you to think critically about the holistic needs of patients. Nursing knowledge as it pertains to activity and exercise helps you assess, identify, and intervene when patients have decreased activity tolerance or physical limitation that affects their ability to exercise.

Factors Influencing Activity and Exercise

Factors influencing activity and exercise include developmental changes, behavioral aspects, family and social support, cultural and ethnic origin, and environmental issues. Consider these areas of knowledge and incorporate into the plan of care whether the patient is seeking health promotion, acute care, or restorative and continuing care.

Developmental Changes. Throughout the life span the appearance and functioning of the body undergo change. The greatest change and effect on the maturational process occurs in childhood and old age.

Infants Through School-Age Children. The newborn infant's spine is flexed and lacks the anteroposterior curves of the adult. The first spinal curve occurs when the infant extends the neck from the prone position. As growth and stability increase, the thoracic spine straightens, and the lumbar spinal curve appears, which allows sitting and standing.

The toddler's posture is awkward because of the slight swayback and protruding abdomen. As the child walks, the legs and feet are usually far apart, and the feet are slightly everted (turned outward). Toward the end of toddlerhood, posture appears less awkward, curves in the cervical and lumbar vertebrae are accentuated, and foot eversion disappears.

By the third year the body is slimmer, taller, and better balanced. Abdominal protrusion decreases, the feet are not as far apart, and the arms and legs have increased in length. The child appears more coordinated. From the third year through the beginning of adolescence, the musculoskeletal system continues to grow and develop (see Chapter 12).

Adolescence. The period of adolescence usually begins with a tremendous growth spurt. Growth is frequently uneven. As a result, the adolescent appears awkward and uncoordinated. Adolescent girls usually grow and develop earlier than boys. Hips widen; and fat deposits in the upper arms, thighs, and buttocks. The adolescent boy's changes in shape are usually a result of long-bone growth and increased muscle mass (see Chapter 12).

Young to Middle Adults. An adult with correct posture and body alignment feels good, looks good, and generally appears self-confident. The healthy adult also has the necessary musculoskeletal development and coordination to carry out ADLs (see Chapter 13). Normal changes in posture and body alignment in adulthood occur mainly in pregnant women. These changes result from the adaptive response of the body to weight gain and the growing fetus. The center of gravity shifts toward the anterior. The pregnant woman leans back and is slightly swaybacked; as a result, pregnant women often complain of back pain.

Older Adults. A progressive loss of total bone mass occurs with the older adult. Some of the possible causes of this loss include physical inactivity, hormonal changes, and increased osteoclastic activity (i.e., activity by cells responsible for bone tissue absorption). The effect of bone loss is weaker bones, causing vertebrae to be softer and long shaft bones to be less resistant to bending.

In addition, older adults may walk more slowly and appear less coordinated. They often take smaller steps and keep their feet closer together, which decreases the base of support. Thus body balance is unstable, and they are at greater risk for falls and injuries (see Chapter 14).

Behavioral Aspects. Patients are more likely to incorporate an exercise program into their daily lives if supported by family, friends, nurses, health care providers, and other members of the health care team. The nurse takes into consideration the patient's knowledge of exercise and activity, barriers to a program of exercise and physical activity, and current exercise habits. Patients are more open to developing an exercise program when they are at a stage of readiness to change their behavior (Prochaska, Norcross, and DiClemente, 1994). Information about the benefits of regular exercise is often helpful to the patient who is not at the stage of readiness to act. Patients' decisions to change behavior and include a daily exercise routine in their lives sometimes occur gradually with repeated information individualized to patients' needs and lifestyle (Box 38-2). Once the patient is at the stage of readiness, collaborate with him or her to develop an exercise program that fits his or her needs and provide continued follow-up support and assistance until the exercise program becomes a daily routine.

Environmental Issues

Work Site. A common barrier for many patients is the lack of time needed to engage in a daily exercise program. Some work sites help their employees overcome the obstacle of time constraints by offering opportunities, reminders, and rewards for those committed to physical fitness (Kuoppala, Lamminpää, and Husman, 2008). Reminders such as signs that encourage employees to use the stairs instead of elevators are useful. Rewards such as free parking or discounted parking fees are also effective for employees who park in distant lots and walk.

Schools. Children today are less active, resulting in an increase in childhood obesity (Harper, 2006; Ward et al., 2010). Schools are excellent facilitators of physical fitness and exercise. Strategies for physical activity incorporated early into a child's daily routine often provide a foundation for lifetime commitment to exercise and physical fitness.

Community. Community support of physical fitness is instrumental in promoting the health of its members (e.g., providing walking trails and track facilities in parks and physical fitness classes). Success in implementing physical fitness programs depends on a collaborative effort from public health agencies, parks and recreational associations, state and local government agencies, health care agencies, and the members of the community (Bors et al., 2009; Harper, 2006).

Cultural and Ethnic Influences. Exercise and physical fitness are beneficial to all people. When developing a physical fitness program for culturally diverse populations, consider what motivates them and what they see as appropriate and enjoyable. It is also important to know which specific disease entities are associated with different cultural and ethnic origins (Box 38-3).

BOX 38-2 GENERAL GUIDELINES FOR INITIATING AN EXERCISE PROGRAM

Five steps to beginning an exercise program:

Step 1: Assess fitness level.
- Seek approval from a health care provider to begin. Are there any limitations to consider before determining the exercises in the fitness program?
- Record baseline fitness scores such as pulse rate, how long it takes to walk 1 mile, waist circumference, and body mass index.

Step 2: Design the fitness program.
- Consider fitness goals. Make goals attainable.
- Plan a logical progression of activities (e.g., walk a mile and gradually increase the pace).
- Build the program into a daily routine.
- Plan the fitness program with creativity and different activities.

Step 3: Assemble equipment.
- Choose athletic shoes designed for the chosen exercise.
- Try equipment at a fitness center before purchasing to make sure it fits into the fitness program.
- Buy used fitness equipment.
- Try homemade equipment (e.g., half-gallon milk jugs filled with sand for weights).

Step 4: Get started.
- Start slowly, including a warm-up and cool-down period.
- Divide exercise time throughout day if time or fatigue is a barrier. Ten minutes of exercise 3 times a day instead of a single 30-minute workout may be better for some patients' schedules and medical conditions.

Step 5: Monitor progress.
- Retake fitness assessment at 6 weeks and then every 3 to 6 months.
- If losing motivation: set new goals, exercise with a friend, or incorporate new activities

Modified from American College of Sports Medicine: *Position stand on fitness: the recommended quantity and quality of exercise for developing and maintaining cardiorespiratory and muscular fitness and flexibility in healthy adults,* 2007, accessed August 2010 from http://www.50plus.org/Libraryitems/1_5positionstandonfitness.htm; and Mayo Clinic Tools for Healthier Lives: *Fitness programs: 5 steps to getting started,* 2008, accessed August 2010 from http://www.mayoclinic.com/health/fitness/HQ00171/NSECTIONGROUP=2.

Family and Social Support. Social support is one motivational tool to encourage and promote exercise and physical fitness. For example, a patient engages a friend or significant other to participate in a "buddy system" where they walk together each day at a specified time. This companionship provides for socialization, increases the enjoyment, and develops a lifelong commitment to physical fitness. Parents support their children in sports and physical activity by providing encouragement, praise, and transportation (Davison and Jago, 2010; Dunton, 2010). Other parents support physical activity by including their children in family outings such as bicycling or a basketball game in the neighborhood schoolyard.

CRITICAL THINKING

Successful critical thinking requires a synthesis of knowledge, experience, information gathered from patients, critical thinking attitudes, and intellectual and professional standards. Patients' conditions are always changing. Clinical judgments require you to

BOX 38-3 CULTURAL ASPECTS OF CARE

Incidence and Challenges of Type 2 Diabetes Among Ethnic Groups in the United States

Studies of ethnic groups indicate that physical inactivity is one of the risk factors associated with type 2 diabetes. In the United States type 2 diabetes is more prevalent in blacks and Native Americans. Physical activity plays an important role in the prevention and treatment of type 2. However, the black and Native American populations have a disproportionate number of individuals who are poor, unemployed, and disadvantaged and who lack access to the health care system (Huang et al., 2009; Maskarinec et al., 2009).

Implications for Practice

- Physical inactivity is a modifiable risk factor for the development of type 2. Prevention and treatment programs need to focus on exercise and be tailored to the activity tolerance and interests of each patient.
- Support promotion of physical activity through formal programs in schools, churches, and government agencies within black and Native American communities.
- Incorporate motivational factors into the exercise program such as providing a healthy snack or meal for the participants and furnishing each patient with a log to monitor weight loss and blood glucose levels.
- Exercise and diabetes prevention programs need to remove potential barriers such as transportation and cost to facilitate commitment to the program.

anticipate the necessary information, analyze the data, and make decisions regarding patient care.

To understand activity tolerance, physical fitness, and the effect on the patient, you integrate knowledge from nursing and other disciplines, previous experiences, and information gathered from patients. As you plan patient care, consider the relationship among a variety of concepts to provide the best outcome for the patient. For example, you lay the foundation for planning and decision making by understanding the relationship between the musculoskeletal system and health alterations that create problems with activity and exercise, positioning, and transferring. Professional standards such as those developed by the American College of Sports Medicine (ACSM) (2007) and the American Diabetes Association (ADA) (2007) provide valuable guidelines for exercise and physical fitness. In addition, using the recommendations from the American Nurses Association (ANA) (2008) reduces the risk for work-related musculoskeletal disorders.

Any acquired or congenital condition that affects the structure of the musculoskeletal or nervous system impairs activity, body alignment, or joint mobility to some degree. The impairment is sometimes temporary, such as casting of an extremity, or is permanent, such as a contracture. For patients with limited **range of motion (ROM)** or mobility, the nursing care plan needs to include interventions that maintain the present level of alignment and joint mobility and increase the level of motor function.

Your experiences and critical thinking attitude affect the problem-solving approach with patients and are evaluated with each new patient. Remember that some patients have the capacity for recovery in spite of the loss of some physical function. Restoration of function begins early in the care of patients whose ability to perform self-care is disrupted. Encouragement, support, commitment, and perseverance are important attitudes in critical thinking for these patients.

Perseverance is necessary when caring for patients who depend on you for assistance with positioning, turning, or ambulation. Hourly responsibility for turning often becomes repetitive, and some nurses lose sight of its importance. Perseverance is especially important in delegating these activities to other personnel. Making certain that the task is performed correctly is an essential nursing function. Problems with activity and mobility are often prolonged; creativity is necessary when designing interventions for improving activity tolerance and mobility skills.

NURSING PROCESS

Apply the nursing process and use a critical thinking approach in your care of patients. The nursing process provides a clinical decision-making approach for you to develop and implement an individualized plan of care.

ASSESSMENT

During the assessment process, you thoroughly assess each patient and critically analyze findings to ensure that you make patient-centered clinical decisions required for safe nursing care. Complete the assessment of body alignment and posture with the patient standing, sitting, or lying down. Use assessment to determine normal physiological changes in growth and development; deviations related to poor posture, trauma, muscle damage, or nerve dysfunction; and any learning needs of patients. In addition, provide opportunities for patients to observe their posture and obtain important information about other factors that contribute to poor alignment such as inactivity, fatigue, malnutrition, and psychological problems. Ask questions related to the patient's exercise and activity tolerance to gather important information (Box 38-4). During assessment (Fig. 38-1) consider all of the elements that help you make appropriate nursing diagnoses. The first step in assessing body alignment is to put the patient at ease so he or she does not assume unnatural or rigid positions. When assessing body alignment of a patient who is immobilized or unconscious, remove pillows from the bed if not contraindicated and place the patient in the supine position.

Through the Patient's Eyes. In patient-centered care, assessing the patient's expectations concerning activity and exercise and determining individual perceptions of what is normal or acceptable is of utmost importance in developing a plan of care. For example, one of the factors affecting physical activity is freedom from pain. When patients experience pain or fatigue following exercise, they often lack commitment to desired interventions. When patients are content with their present physical activity and fitness, they do not perceive a need for improvement.

Standing. Assessment of the standing patient includes the following: the head is erect and midline, body parts are symmetrical, the spine is straight with normal curvatures (cervical concave, thoracic convex, lumbar concave), the abdomen is comfortably tucked, the knees are in a straight line between the hips and ankles and slightly flexed, the feet are flat on the floor and pointed directly forward and slightly apart to maintain a wide base of support, and the arms hang comfortably at the sides (Fig. 38-2). The patient's center of gravity is in the midline, and the line of gravity is from the middle of the forehead to a midpoint between the feet. Laterally the line of gravity runs vertically from the middle of the skull to the posterior third of the foot (Wilson and Giddens, 2009).

Sitting. Assessment of the patient in the sitting position includes the following: the head is erect, and the neck and vertebral column are in straight alignment; the body weight is distributed on the buttocks and thighs; the thighs are parallel and in a

BOX 38-4 NURSING ASSESSMENT QUESTIONS

Nature of the Problem
- Which types of problems are you having with activities and exercise?
- What makes you think your exercise and activity are inadequate?
- Describe for me your typical daily exercise routine and activity.
- Which type of exercise do you prefer?
- How long do you exercise at any given time?

Signs and Symptoms
- Do you experience muscular or joint pain during or after exercise?
- Do you experience shortness of breath during activity?
- Do you experience chest discomfort or pain during exercise or activity?

Onset and Duration
- Which activities cause you to become short of breath?
- How long does it take to resume normal breathing after exercise or an activity?

Severity
- How far do you walk before the pain in your legs begins?
- On a scale of 0 to 10 (10 being the worse discomfort), rate your leg pain.
- Do you describe your shortness of breath as minimal, moderate, or severe after activities and/or exercise?

Barriers to Exercise and Activity
- Do you have any chronic illnesses that affect your ability to carry out activities of daily living or exercise?
- Do you have any physical limitations that prevent you from exercising on a daily basis?
- Do you have access to a community walking path and exercise equipment?
- What prevents you from exercising 30 minutes each day?

Effect on Patient
- How has the lack of an exercise routine affected your weight?
- Do you feel more fatigued since you have not been able to exercise routinely?
- Have you noticed any increase in shortness of breath when performing activities that require little exertion?

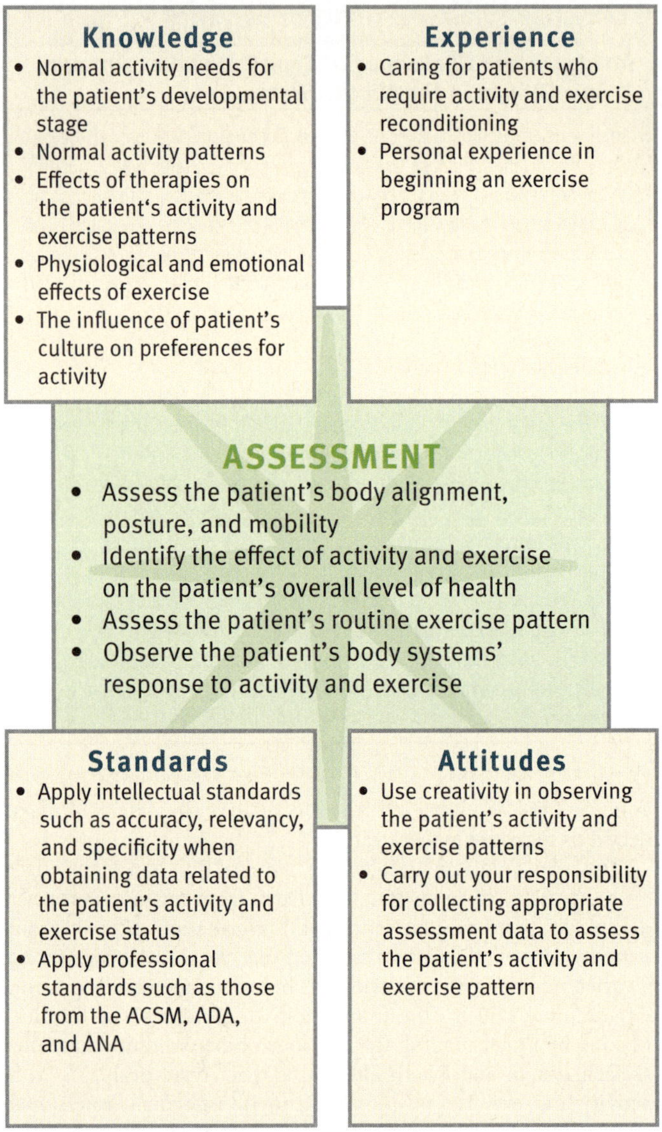
Knowledge
• Normal activity needs for the patient's developmental stage
• Normal activity patterns
• Effects of therapies on the patient's activity and exercise patterns
• Physiological and emotional effects of exercise
• The influence of patient's culture on preferences for activity
Experience
• Caring for patients who require activity and exercise reconditioning
• Personal experience in beginning an exercise program
ASSESSMENT
• Assess the patient's body alignment, posture, and mobility
• Identify the effect of activity and exercise on the patient's overall level of health
• Assess the patient's routine exercise pattern
• Observe the patient's body systems' response to activity and exercise
Standards
• Apply intellectual standards such as accuracy, relevancy, and specificity when obtaining data related to the patient's activity and exercise status
• Apply professional standards such as those from the ACSM, ADA, and ANA
Attitudes
• Use creativity in observing the patient's activity and exercise patterns
• Carry out your responsibility for collecting appropriate assessment data to assess the patient's activity and exercise pattern

FIG. 38-1 Critical thinking model for activity and exercise assessment. *ACSM,* American College of Sports Medicine; *ADA,* American Diabetes Association; *ANA,* American Nurses Association.

horizontal plane (be careful to avoid pressure on the popliteal nerve and blood supply); the feet are supported on the floor; and the forearms are supported on the armrest, in the lap, or on a table in front of the chair.

Assessment of alignment in the sitting position is particularly important for the patient with muscle weakness, muscle paralysis, or nerve damage. A patient with these alterations has diminished sensation in affected areas and is unable to perceive pressure or decreased circulation. Proper sitting alignment reduces the risk of musculoskeletal system damage.

Recumbent Position. When assessing the patient in the recumbent position, you place the patient in the lateral position, removing all positioning supports and all but one pillow. The vertebrae are in straight alignment without observable curves. This assessment provides baseline data concerning the patient's body alignment.

Conditions that create a risk of damage to the musculoskeletal system when lying down include impaired mobility (e.g., traction), decreased sensation (e.g., hemiparesis from a stroke), impaired circulation (e.g., diabetes), and lack of voluntary muscle control (e.g., spinal cord injuries).

When a patient is unable to change position voluntarily, assess the position of body parts while the patient is lying down. Make sure that the vertebrae are in straight alignment without any observable curves. Also check that the extremities are in alignment and not crossed over one another. The head and neck need to be aligned without excessive flexion or extension.

Mobility. Assessment of mobility helps to determine the patient's coordination and balance while walking, the ability to carry out ADLs, and the ability to participate in an exercise program. The assessment of mobility has three components: ROM, gait, and exercise.

Range of Motion. Assessing ROM is one assessment technique used to determine the degree of damage or injury to a joint (see Chapter 47). By measuring the ROM of a joint you are able to answer questions about joint stiffness, swelling, pain, limited movement, and unequal movement. Limited ROM often indicates inflammation such as arthritis, fluid in the joint, altered nerve supply, or contractures. Increased mobility (beyond normal) of a

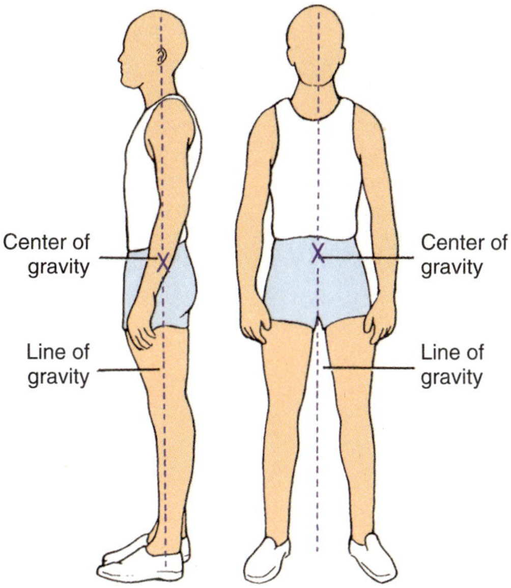

FIG. 38-2 Correct body alignment when standing.

joint sometimes indicates connective tissue disorders, ligament tears, or possible joint fractures.

Gait. Gait is the manner or style of walking, including rhythm, cadence, and speed. Assessing gait allows you to draw conclusions about balance, posture, and the ability to walk without assistance. Assessment findings in patients with normal gait include a regular, smooth rhythm; symmetry in the length of leg swing; smooth swaying related to the gait phase; and a smooth, symmetrical arm swing (Wilson and Giddens, 2009).

Exercise. Exercise conditions the body, improves health, maintains fitness, and provides therapy for correcting a deformity or restoring the overall body to a maximal state of health. When a person engages in physical activity, physiological changes occur in body systems (Box 38-5). Determine how much the patient exercises regularly.

Activity Tolerance. Activity tolerance is the kind and amount of exercise or activity that a person is able to perform. Assessment of activity tolerance is necessary when planning physical activity for health promotion and for patients with acute or chronic illness. This assessment provides baseline data about the patient's activity patterns and helps determine which factors (physical, psychological, or motivational) affect activity tolerance (Box 38-6).

NURSING DIAGNOSIS

Assessment of the patient's activity tolerance, physical fitness, body alignment, and joint mobility provides clusters of data or defining characteristics to support a nursing diagnosis. You need to be accurate when identifying diagnoses. For example, you consider nursing diagnoses of *activity intolerance* or *fatigue* in a patient who reports being tired and weak. Further review of assessed defining characteristics (e.g., abnormal heart rate and dyspnea) leads to the definitive diagnosis *(activity intolerance)*.

When patients have problems with activity and exercise, nursing diagnoses often focus on the ability to move. The diagnostic label and related factors direct nursing interventions. This requires the correct selection of the related factors. For example, *activity intolerance related to excess weight gain* requires very different interventions than if the related factor is prolonged bed rest. Box 38-7 provides an example of how the diagnostic process leads to accurate diagnosis selection. The following are examples of nursing diagnoses related to activity and exercise:

- Activity intolerance
- Ineffective coping
- Impaired gas exchange
- Risk for injury
- Impaired physical mobility
- Imbalanced nutrition: more than body requirements
- Acute or chronic pain

BOX 38-5 EFFECTS OF EXERCISE

Cardiovascular System
- Increased cardiac output
- Improved myocardial contraction, thereby strengthening cardiac muscle
- Decreased resting heart rate
- Improved venous return

Pulmonary System
- Increased respiratory rate and depth followed by a quicker return to resting state
- Improved alveolar ventilation
- Decreased work of breathing
- Improved diaphragmatic excursion

Metabolic System
- Increased basal metabolic rate
- Increased use of glucose and fatty acids
- Increased triglyceride breakdown
- Increased gastric motility
- Increased production of body heat

Musculoskeletal System
- Improved muscle tone
- Increased joint mobility
- Improved muscle tolerance to physical exercise
- Possible increase in muscle mass
- Reduced bone loss

Activity Tolerance
- Improved tolerance
- Decreased fatigue

Psychosocial Factors
- Improved tolerance to stress
- Reports of "feeling better"
- Reports of decrease in illness (e.g., colds, influenza)

Data from Huether SE, McCance KL: *Understanding pathophysiology,* ed 4, St Louis, 2008, Mosby.

PLANNING

During planning synthesize information from multiple resources (Fig. 38-3). Critical thinking ensures that the patient's plan of care integrates all patient information. Professional standards are especially important to consider when developing a plan of care. These standards often establish scientifically proven guidelines for selecting effective nursing interventions.

Concept maps are a tool to assist in the planning of care. Fig. 38-4 shows the relationship between a patient's medical diagnosis of heart failure and the identified nursing diagnosis.

Goals and Outcomes. Once you identify the nursing diagnoses, you and the patient set goals and expected outcomes to direct

BOX 38-6 FACTORS INFLUENCING ACTIVITY TOLERANCE

Physiological Factors
- Skeletal abnormalities
- Muscular impairments
- Endocrine or metabolic illnesses (e.g., diabetes mellitus, thyroid disease)
- Hypoxemia
- Decreased cardiac function
- Decreased endurance
- Impaired physical stability
- Pain
- Sleep pattern disturbance
- Prior exercise patterns
- Infectious processes and fever

Emotional Factors
- Anxiety
- Depression
- Chemical addictions
- Motivation

Developmental Factors
- Age
- Sex

Pregnancy
- Physical growth and development of muscle and skeletal support

Modified from Monahan FD et al: *Phipps' medical-surgical nursing: health and illness perspectives,* ed 8, St Louis, 2007, Mosby.

BOX 38-7 NURSING DIAGNOSTIC PROCESS

Impaired Physical Mobility

ASSESSMENT ACTIVITIES	DEFINING CHARACTERISTICS
Observe patient's gait.	Shuffled gait Uncoordinated gait Patient reports slower walking speed
Observe patient performing tasks such as feeding, dressing, or recreational activities.	Uncoordinated movements Limited fine-motor coordination
Measure range of joint motion.	Reduced joint motion in lower and/or upper extremities Stiffness in joints

interventions. The plan includes consideration of any risks for injury to the patient and preexisting health concerns. It is especially important to have knowledge of the patient's home environment when planning therapies to maintain or improve activity, body alignment, and mobility. Include the patient's family in the care plan. For some patients with alterations in joint mobility, family members may be caregivers. The general goal related to exercise and activity is to improve or maintain the patient's motor function and independence. The following are examples of outcomes for patients with deficits in activity and exercise (Ackley and Ladwig, 2008):

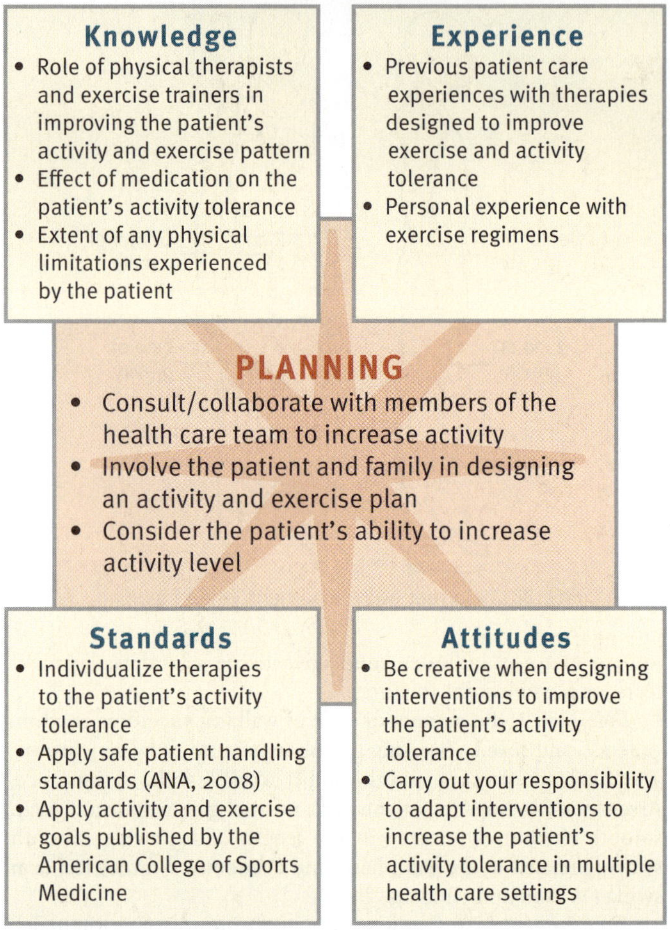

Knowledge
• Role of physical therapists and exercise trainers in improving the patient's activity and exercise pattern
• Effect of medication on the patient's activity tolerance
• Extent of any physical limitations experienced by the patient
Experience
• Previous patient care experiences with therapies designed to improve exercise and activity tolerance
• Personal experience with exercise regimens
PLANNING
• Consult/collaborate with members of the health care team to increase activity
• Involve the patient and family in designing an activity and exercise plan
• Consider the patient's ability to increase activity level
Standards
• Individualize therapies to the patient's activity tolerance
• Apply safe patient handling standards (ANA, 2008)
• Apply activity and exercise goals published by the American College of Sports Medicine
Attitudes
• Be creative when designing interventions to improve the patient's activity tolerance
• Carry out your responsibility to adapt interventions to increase the patient's activity tolerance in multiple health care settings

FIG. 38-3 Critical thinking model for activity and exercise planning.

- Participates in prescribed physical activity while maintaining appropriate heart rate, blood pressure, and breathing rate
- Verbalizes an understanding of the need to gradually increase activity based on tolerance and symptoms
- Expresses understanding of balancing rest and activity

Setting Priorities. Care planning is patient centered, taking into consideration the patient's most immediate needs. You determine the immediacy of any problem by the effect of the problem on the patient's mental and physical health. Because of the many skills associated with the care of patients with activity intolerance; improper body mechanics; and/or impaired mobility such as turning, transferring, and positioning, it is easy to overlook the complications associated with these health alterations. Therefore be vigilant in monitoring the patient and supervising assistive personnel in carrying out activities to prevent complications and potential injury.

Teamwork and Collaboration. Planning involves understanding the patient's need to maintain function and independence. For example, it is important to collaborate with physical and occupational therapists. Sometimes long-term rehabilitation is necessary. Discharge planning begins when a patient enters the health care system. In addition, always individualize a plan of care directed at meeting the actual or potential needs of the patient (see the Nursing Care Plan).

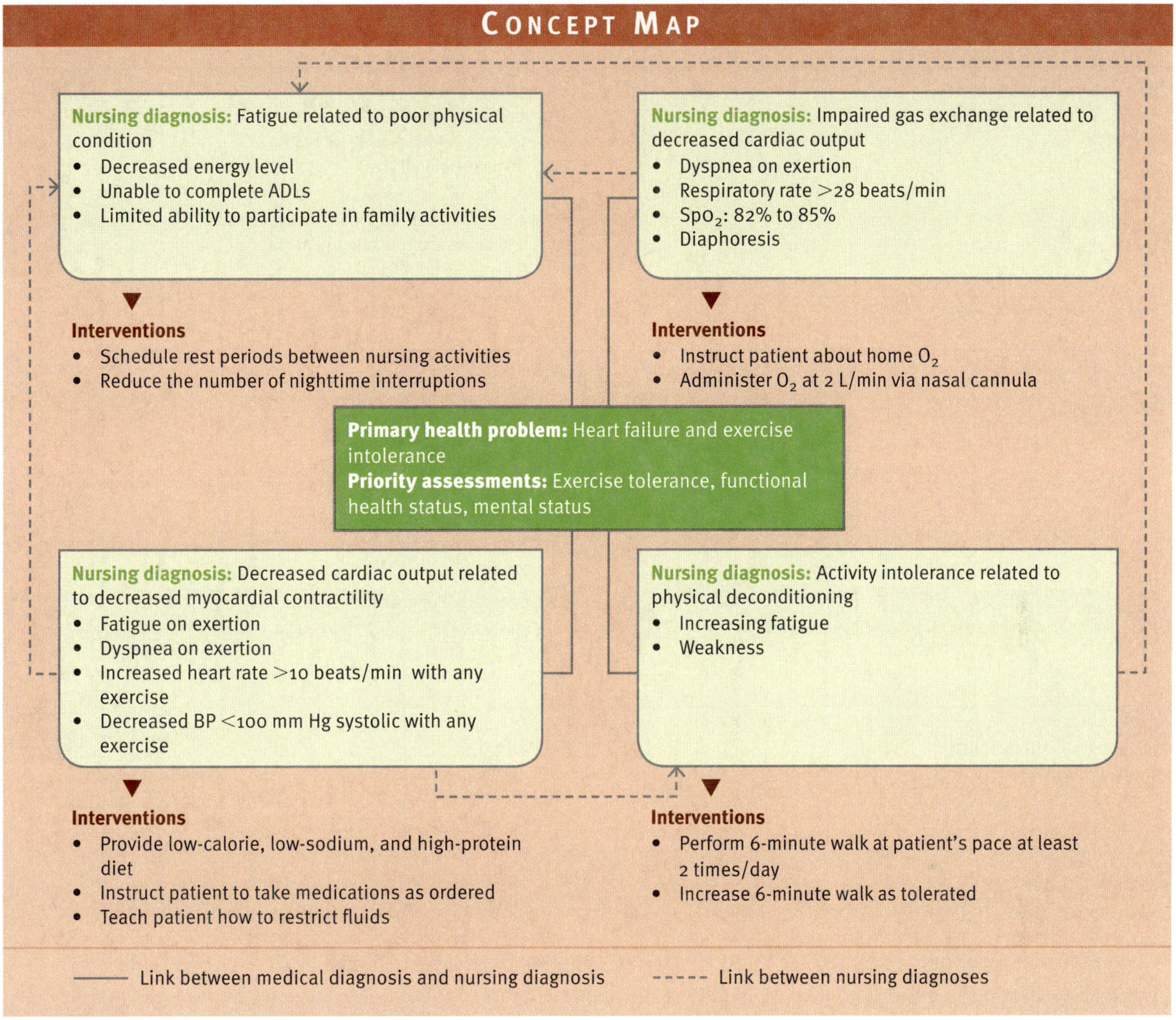

FIG. 38-4 Concept map for Mrs. Smith. *ADLs,* Activities of daily living.

NURSING CARE PLAN

Activity Intolerance

ASSESSMENT

Mrs. Smith is a 45-year-old housewife. She is in a cardiovascular rehabilitation program prescribed by her health care provider and conducted by Erich Sieple, a registered nurse. Mrs. Smith has a history of cardiovascular disease with mild heart failure. She expresses feelings of stress caused by excessive demands on her time. Erich's assessment includes a discussion of Mrs. Smith's current health problem and a pertinent physical examination.

Assessment Activities	*Findings/Defining Characteristics**
Ask Mrs. Smith what prompted her health care provider to recommend a cardiovascular rehabilitation program.	She responds, "I **gained 50 pounds** over the past year. I become easily **fatigued** and lack the energy to keep up with even simple household chores. I don't want to leave the house anymore. I don't have extra money to join one of those fancy gyms."
Ask Mrs. Smith about her exercise and eating habits.	She responds, "I want to exercise, but with the demands of child care and taking care of my aging parents, I just don't feel like it. I feel pulled in every direction; that increases my **stress**, and then I want to eat, eat, and eat!"

Continued

NURSING CARE PLAN

***Activity Intolerance*—cont'd**

Perform baseline assessment.	Height: 5 feet 3 inches Weight: **225 pounds** (102 kg) Blood pressure: **152/90 mm Hg (at rest)** Pulse: **96 beats/min (at rest)** Breathing rate: 20 breaths/min (at rest) Blood pressure: **164/96 mm Hg (climbing 10 steps)** Pulse: **120 beats/min (climbing 10 steps)** Breathing rate: **36 breaths/min (climbing 10 steps)**

*__Defining characteristics__ are shown in bold type.

NURSING DIAGNOSIS: Activity intolerance related to inactivity and lack of cardiovascular fitness

PLANNING

Goals	*Expected Outcomes (NOC)*†
	Activity Tolerance
Mrs. Smith's activity tolerance will improve above baseline.	Mrs. Smith will perform and record exercise patterns 3 to 4 times over the next 2 weeks. Mrs. Smith's level of fatigue associated with exercise will remain the same or decrease.
	Cardiovascular Pump Effectiveness
Mrs. Smith's cardiopulmonary response to exercise will improve.	Mrs. Smith's resting diastolic blood pressure will remain below 80 mm Hg. Her systolic blood pressure will be below 140 mm Hg. Mrs. Smith's resting heart rate will range between 75 and 85 beats/min.

†Outcome classification labels from Moorhead S, et al: *Nursing outcomes classification (NOC),* ed 4, St Louis, 2008, Mosby.

INTERVENTIONS (NIC)‡	RATIONALE
Exercise Promotion	
Instruct Mrs. Smith about the physiological benefits of a regular exercise program.	Physical activity and exercise protect against the further development of cardiovascular disease (CVD) and decrease other risk factors associated with CVD such as obesity, hypertension, and hyperlipidemia (Donges et al., 2010; Hamer and Stamatakis, 2009; Mandic et al., 2009).
Develop a progressive plan of exercise with Mrs. Smith, such as 2 to 3 miles of brisk walking and quadriceps, bicep, and gluteal muscle isometric exercises 3 to 4 times per week.	Cross-training (combination of exercise activities) provides variety to combat boredom and increases potential for total-body conditioning (Edelman and Mandle, 2010).
Instruct Mrs. Smith to use an exercise log and record the day, time, duration, and responses (pulse, feelings, shortness of breath, daily weight).	Keeping a log may increase adherence to exercise prescription.
Schedule routine visits with Mrs. Smith for follow-up and review of exercise log, progress, and barriers.	Patients are more likely to increase physical activity and remain compliant with an exercise program if they are counseled by a health care professional (Edelman and Mandle, 2010).

‡Intervention classification labels from Bulechek GM, Butcher HK, Dochterman JM: *Nursing interventions classification (NIC),* ed 5, St Louis, 2008, Mosby.

EVALUATION

Nursing Actions	*Patient Response/Finding*	*Achievement of Outcome*
Record weight, blood pressure, and pulse.	Weight, 210 pounds. Resting heart rate remains between 80 and 85 beats/min. Blood pressure, 146/86 mm Hg.	Improved cardiovascular effects of exercise: • Heart rate is within normal range. • Blood pressure is lower but not at expected range. Monitor blood pressure as patient continues to lose weight.
Ask Mrs. Smith if exercise is helping to lower fatigue level.	"At first, finding time to exercise was hard, but once I started feeling less tired and even less stressed, it was easy to integrate exercise into my daily activities."	Activity tolerance improved with exercise.

BOX 38-8 PROCEDURAL GUIDELINES

Helping Patients to Exercise

Delegation Considerations

The skill of helping patients to exercise can be delegated to nursing assistive personnel (NAP). However, the nurse first must assess the patient's ability and tolerance to exercise. The nurse also teaches patients and their families how to implement exercise programs. NAP can prepare patients for exercise (e.g., putting on shoes and clothing, providing hygiene needs and obtaining preexercise and postexercise vital signs). Instruct NAP to do the following:

- Notify nurse if patient reports pain before, during, or after exercise.
- Notify nurse if patient complains of increased fatigue, dizziness, or lightheadedness when obtaining preexercise and/or postexercise vital signs.
- Notify nurse of vital sign values.

1. Identify patient using two identifiers (i.e., name and birth date or name and account number) according to facility policy.
2. Assess for any medical limitations (e.g., weight-bearing status, untreated fracture, cardiovascular disease).
3. Know patient's mobility level before hospitalization.
4. Teach patient breathing skills to help reduce anxiety and fully oxygenate tissues and expand lungs.
5. Assess for patient's physiological and psychological limitations for learning and implementing an exercise program.
6. Assess for joint limitations and do not force a muscle or a joint during exercise.
7. Teach patient to wear comfortable shoes and clothing for exercise.
8. Let each patient move at his or her own pace.
9. Observe for proper posture, body alignment, and proper body mechanics during exercise.
10. Monitor vital signs before, during, and after exercise.
11. Assess for pain, shortness of breath, or a change in vital signs. If present, stop exercise.
12. Document patient's progress and provide feedback as patient exercises.

Data from Edelman CL, Mandle CL, editors: *Health promotion throughout the life span,* ed 7, St Louis, 2010, Mosby; and Monahan FD, et al: *Phipps' medical-surgical nursing: health and illness perspectives,* ed 8, St Louis, 2007, Mosby.

IMPLEMENTATION

Health Promotion. A sedentary lifestyle contributes to the development of health-related problems. You promote health by encouraging patients to engage in a regular exercise program (Box 38-8). Take a holistic approach to develop and implement a plan that enhances the patient's overall physical fitness. Discuss recommendations for physical activity and fitness and collaborate with the patient to design a program of exercise.

Before starting an exercise program, teach patients to calculate their maximum heart rate by subtracting their current age in years from 220 and then obtaining their target heart rate by taking 60% to 90% of the maximum, depending on their health care provider's recommendation. No matter which exercise prescription is implemented for the patient, a warm-up and cool-down period needs to be included in the program (Edelman and Mandle, 2010). The warm-up period usually lasts about 5 to 10 minutes and frequently includes stretching, calisthenics, and/or the aerobic activity performed at a lower intensity. It prepares the body and decreases the potential for injury. The cool-down period follows the exercise routine and usually lasts about 5 to 10 minutes. It allows the body to readjust gradually to baseline functioning and provides an opportunity to combine movement such as stretching with relaxation-enhancing mind-body awareness.

BOX 38-9 INCORPORATING ACTIVE EXERCISE INTO ACTIVITIES OF DAILY LIVING (ADLs)

Lower-Intensity ADLs

- Doing laundry
- Making the bed
- Ironing
- Washing dishes

Moderate-Intensity ADLs

- Sweeping the kitchen or sidewalk
- Washing windows
- Folding clothes
- Vacuuming

High-Intensity ADLs

- Moving furniture
- Carrying boxes or heavier items up and down stairs

Hints to a Good Workout While Doing Housework

- To make housework more aerobic, work faster, scrub harder
- Bend your legs rather than your back
- Start daily household chores with gentle stretches
- Alternate cleaning activities to prevent overworking the same muscle groups

From Collins A: *Getting fit: unstructured exercise,* http://www.suite101.com/lesson.cfm/18274/1552). Accessed August 2010.

Building Competency in Safety In order for patients to exercise safely, you need to be able to calculate their maximum heart rate. Determine the range of maximum heart rate for the patient in the nursing care plan, 45-year-old Mary Smith.

Answers to questions can be found on the Evolve website.

Many patients find it difficult to incorporate an exercise program into their daily lives because of time constraints. For these patients it is beneficial to reinforce that they can use ADLs to accumulate the recommended 30 minutes or more per day of moderate-intensity physical activity (Box 38-9).

Other patients benefit from a prescribed exercise and physical fitness program carefully designed to meet their needs and expectations. An exercise prescription usually includes a combination of aerobic exercises, stretching and flexibility exercises, and resistance training. Aerobic exercise includes walking, running, bicycling, aerobic dance, jumping rope, and cross-country skiing. Recommended frequency of aerobic exercise is 3 to 5 times per week or every other day for approximately 30 minutes. Cross-training is recommended for the patient who prefers to exercise every day. For example, the patient runs one day and does yoga the next day.

Stretching and flexibility exercises include active ROM and stretch all muscle groups and joints. This form of exercise is ideal for warm-up and cool-down periods. Benefits include increased flexibility, improved circulation and posture, and an opportunity for relaxation.

Resistance training increases muscle strength and endurance and is associated with improved performance of daily activities and avoidance of injuries and disability. Formal resistance training includes weight training; but patients can obtain the same benefits by performing ADLs such as pushing a vacuum cleaner, raking leaves, shoveling snow, and kneading bread. Some patients use

TABLE 38-1 **PREVENTING LIFT INJURIES IN HEALTH CARE WORKERS**

ACTION	RATIONALE
When planning to move a patient, arrange for adequate help. If your institution has a lift team, use it as a resource.	A lift team is properly educated in techniques to prevent musculoskeletal injuries.
Use patient-handling equipment and devices such as height-adjustable beds, ceiling-mounted lifts, friction-reducing slide sheets, and air-assisted devices (Nelson and Baptiste, 2004; Nelson and Hughes, 2009; Tullar et al., 2010).	These devices reduce the caregiver's muscular strain during patient handling.
Encourage patient to assist as much as possible.	This promotes patient's independence and strength while minimizing workload.
Keep back, neck, pelvis, and feet aligned. Avoid twisting.	Reduces risk of injury to lumbar vertebrae and muscle groups. Twisting increases risk of injury.
Flex knees; keep feet wide apart.	A broad base of support increases stability.
Position self close to patient (or object being lifted).	Reduces horizontal reach and stress on caregiver's back.
Use arms and legs (not back).	The leg muscles are stronger, larger muscles capable of greater work without injury.
Slide patient toward your body using a pull sheet or slide board. When transferring a patient onto a stretcher or bed, a slide board is more appropriate.	Sliding requires less effort than lifting. Pull sheet minimizes shearing forces, which can damage patient's skin.
Person with the heaviest load coordinates efforts of team involved by counting to three.	Simultaneous lifting minimizes the load for any one lifter.
Perform manual lifting as last resort and only if it does not involve lifting most or all of patient's weight (Nelson and Baptiste, 2004; Nelson and Hughes, 2009; Tullar, 2010).	Lifting is a high-risk activity that causes significant biochemical and postural stressors.

weight training to bulk up their muscles. However, the purpose of weight training from a health perspective is to develop tone and strength and stimulate and maintain healthy bone (O'Donovan et al., 2010).

Body Mechanics. The U.S. Occupational Safety and Health Administration released federal ergonomic guidelines to prevent musculoskeletal injuries in the workplace (OSHA, 2009). Half of all back pain is associated with manual lifting tasks (Box 38-10). Coordinated musculoskeletal activity is necessary when positioning and transferring patients. The most common back injury is strain on the lumbar muscle group, which includes the muscles around the lumbar vertebrae. Injury to these areas affects the ability to bend forward, backward, and from side to side. The ability to rotate the hips and lower back is also decreased (Nelson and Hughes, 2009). Body mechanics alone are not sufficient to prevent musculoskeletal injuries when positioning or transferring patients (Table 38-1).

Before lifting, assess the weight to be lifted, determine the assistance needed, and evaluate available resources. Use safe patient-handling equipment when the patient is unable to assist in transfer. Lift teams, consisting of two physically fit people competent in lifting techniques, reduce the risk of injury to the patient and members of the health care team (Baptiste et al., 2006; Pelczarski, 2007). Use manual lifting only as a last resort when you need to lift a small portion of the patient's weight (Nelson and Baptiste, 2004; Nelson et al., 2008; Tullar et al., 2010). Teaching health care workers about patient-handling equipment, proper body mechanics, and the use of lift teams is most effective in preventing injury (Nelson and Baptiste, 2004; Nelson et al., 2008).

Acute Care. Encourage patients who are hospitalized to do stretching and isometric exercises, active ROM exercises, and low-intensity walking, depending on their condition. When patients cannot participate in active ROM, maintain joint mobility and prevent contractures by implementing passive ROM into the plan of care. If needed, medicate patients for pain 30 minutes before exercise.

BOX 38-10 **EVIDENCE-BASED PRACTICE**

Promoting Safe Handling of Patients and Prevention of Injury to Nurses and Their Patients

PICO Question: What is the effect on patient and nurse safety in health care agencies that have safe patient handling policies when compared with agencies that do not have these policies?

Evidence Summary

Musculoskeletal disorders are the most prevalent and debilitating occupational health hazards for nurses. Preventive interventions are needed to avoid the hazards and economic burdens associated with patient-handling tasks. The American Nurses Association (ANA, 2008) position statements call for the use of assistive equipment and devices to promote a safe health care environment for nurses and their patients. The use of assistive equipment and continued use of proper body mechanics significantly reduces the risk of musculoskeletal injuries. In addition, the Occupational Safety and Health Administration (OSHA, 2009) recommends minimizing or eliminating manual lifting of patients. Current evidence supports the benefits of instituting safe patient handling (SPH) programs in health care organizations. The U.S. Bureau of Labor Statistics (2007) reported a reduction in workers' compensation claims and costs associated with absenteeism because of SPH programs. As a result, many facilities are moving toward limited lift policies to minimize patient handling by nurses and using lift devices. Research shows these policies effectively reduce on-the-job injuries (Nelson and Baptiste, 2004; Nelson and Hughes, 2009; Tullar et al., 2010).

Application to Nursing Practice

- Be familiar with health care facility safety information and training concerning the transfer, positioning, and lifting of patients.
- Use recommended back safety guidelines to prevent musculoskeletal injuries.
- Use current research, standards, and guidelines regarding safe positioning and transferring of patients.
- Use "lift teams" and patient-handling equipment such as mechanical lifts to prevent injury to yourself and the patient.

Musculoskeletal System. Help maintain the musculoskeletal system during acute care by encouraging the use of stretching and isometric exercises. Review the patient's chart and collaborate with the health care provider to identify possible contraindications before initiating isometric exercises. You design an isometric exercise program for the specific needs of a patient. For example, an exercise program includes isometric exercises of the biceps and triceps to prepare your patient for crutch walking. Instruct the patient to stop the activity if pain, fatigue, or discomfort is experienced.

Generally the muscle group is tightened (contracted) for 10 seconds and then completely relaxed for several seconds (Hoeman, 2006). Repetitions are gradually increased for each muscle group until the isometric exercise is repeated 8 to 10 times. Instruct patients to perform the exercises slowly and increase repetitions as their physical condition improves. Patients need to isometrically exercise muscle groups (quadriceps and gluteal) used for walking 4 times per day until they are ambulatory.

Joint Mobility. The easiest intervention to maintain or improve joint mobility for patients and one that can be coordinated with other activities is the use of ROM exercises (see Chapter 47). In active ROM exercises patients are able to move their joints independently. With passive ROM exercises you move each joint in patients who are unable to perform these exercises themselves. The use of ROM exercises provides data to systematically assess and improve the patient's joint mobility.

Joints that are not moved periodically are at risk for contractures, a permanent shortening of a muscle followed by the eventual shortening of associated ligaments and tendons. Over time the joint becomes fixed in one position, and the patient loses normal use of it. Passive ROM exercises are the exercises of choice for patients who do not have voluntary motor control.

Older adults experiencing a decline in physical activity and changes in joints often have limited mobility and joint flexibility. Use a variety of recommended approaches to help older adults use proper body mechanics and prevent injury (Box 38-11).

Mechanical devices place specific joints through continuous passive motion (CPM). You will use CPM machines most commonly after joint replacement surgery to place joints through a selective repetitive ROM. You set the machine to certain degrees of joint mobility, with increasing joint mobility or flexion as the goal. Unless contraindicated, the nursing care plan includes exercising each joint through as nearly a full ROM as possible. Initiate passive ROM exercises as soon as the patient loses the ability to move the extremity or joint. Chapter 47 details ROM exercises for each area and illustrates the motion of each joint.

Walking. Walking increases joint mobility. Measure distances walked in feet or yards instead of charting "ambulated to nurses' station and back." Illness or trauma usually reduces activity tolerance, resulting in the need for assistance with walking or the use of mechanical devices such as crutches, canes, or walkers.

Helping a Patient to Walk. Helping a patient to walk requires preparation. Assess the patient's activity tolerance, strength, coordination, baseline vital signs, and balance to determine the type of assistance needed. Also assess the patient's orientation and determine if there are any signs of distress. Postpone walking if you determine the patient cannot safely walk. Evaluate the environment for safety before ambulation; this includes the removal of obstacles, a clean and dry floor, and the identification of rest points in case the patient's activity tolerance becomes less than expected or if the patient becomes dizzy. Also have the patient wear supportive, nonskid shoes.

BOX 38-11 FOCUS ON OLDER ADULTS

Helping the Older Adult Initiate and Maintain an Exercise Program

- Encourage older adults to avoid prolonged sitting and get up and stretch. Frequent stretching decreases the risk of developing joint contractures.
- Be sure that the older patient maintains proper body alignment when sitting to minimize joint and muscle stress.
- Teach patients how to use stronger joints or larger muscle groups. Efficient distribution of the workload decreases joint stress and pain.
- Provide resources for planned exercise programs. Weight-bearing and resistance exercise slows bone loss and prevents fractures in older adults with osteoporosis (De Kam et al., 2009; Monahan et al., 2007).
- Recommend resistance- and agility-training programs. These forms of exercise reduce fear of falling and increase sense of well-being in older adults (De Kam et al., 2009; Sherrington et al., 2008).
- Teach older adults that it is never too late to begin an exercise program (Chodzko-Zajko et al., 2009; Edelman and Mandle, 2010). Consult a health care provider before beginning an exercise program, particularly in the presence of heart or lung disease and other chronic illnesses.
- Use assessment data to determine when you need to make adjustments to exercise programs for those in advanced age.
- When developing an exercise program for older adults, consider current activity level, range of motion, muscle strength and tone, response to physical activity, and personal interests, capacities, and limitations.
- Encourage older adults who are unable to participate in a formal exercise program to improve joint mobility and enhance circulation by simply stretching and exaggerating movements during the performance of routine activities of daily living.

Help the patient to a position of sitting at the side of the bed and dangling the legs over the side of the bed for 1 to 2 minutes before standing. Some patients experience orthostatic hypotension, a drop in blood pressure that occurs when they change from a horizontal to a vertical position (Capan and Lynch, 2007; Monahan et al., 2007). Those at higher risk are patients who are immobilized, patients who are on prolonged bed rest, older adults, and patients with chronic illnesses such as diabetes mellitus and cardiovascular disease (Capan and Lynch, 2007). Signs and symptoms of orthostatic hypotension include dizziness, light-headedness, nausea, tachycardia, pallor, and even fainting. Dangling a patient's legs before standing is an intermediate step that allows assessment of the patient before changing positions to maintain safety and prevent injury to the patient. In some instances you will need to obtain the patient's blood pressure while he or she is sitting on the side of the bed.

Several methods are used to assist a patient with ambulation. Provide support at the waist so the patient's center of gravity remains midline. This is achieved with the use of a gait belt. A gait belt encircles the patient's waist and may have handles attached for the nurse to hold while the patient ambulates.

If the patient has a fainting (syncope) episode or begins to fall, assume a wide base of support with one foot in front of the other, thus supporting the patient's body weight (Fig. 38-5, *A*). Extend one leg, let the patient slide against the leg, and gently lower the patient to the floor, protecting the head (Fig. 38-5, *B* and *C*). Practice this technique with a friend or classmate before attempting it in a clinical setting. When the patient attempts to ambulate again, proceed more slowly, monitoring for reports of dizziness, and take the patient's blood pressure before, during, and after ambulation.

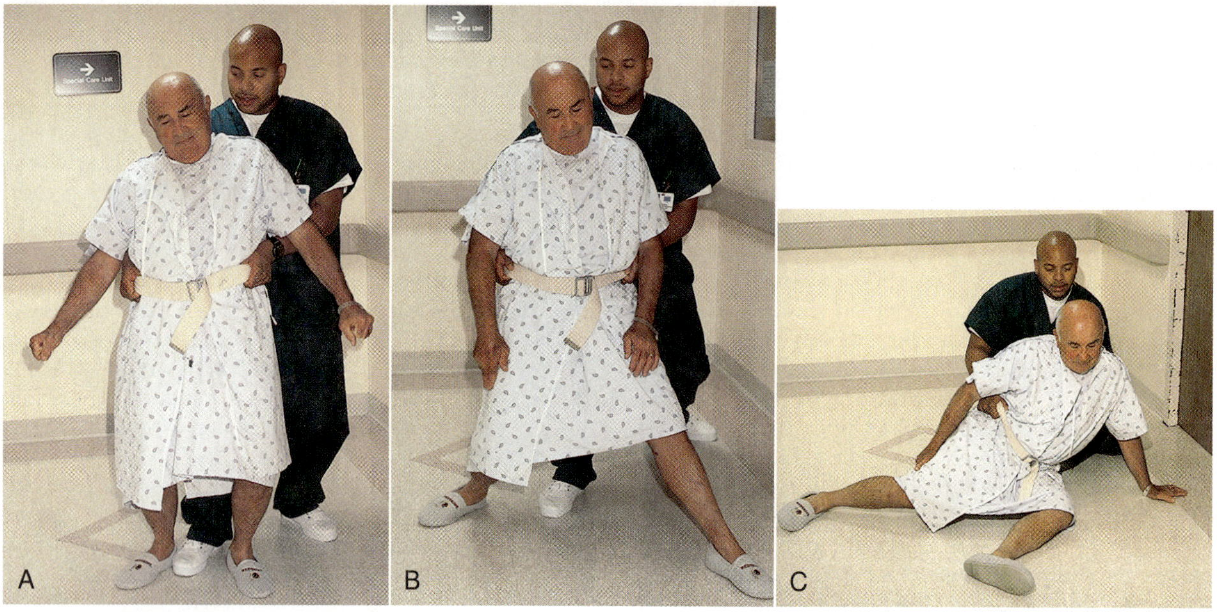

FIG. 38-5 A, Stand with feet apart to provide a broad base of support. **B,** Extend one leg and let patient slide against it to the floor. **C,** Bend knees to lower body as patient slides to the floor.

Restorative and Continuing Care. Restorative and continuing care involves implementing activity and exercise strategies to assist the patient with ADLs after acute care is no longer needed. Restorative and continuing care also includes activities and exercises that restore and promote optimal functioning in patients with specific chronic illnesses such as coronary heart disease (CHD), hypertension, chronic obstructive pulmonary disease (COPD), and diabetes mellitus.

Assistive Devices for Walking. In collaboration with other health care professionals such as physical therapists, promote activity and exercise by teaching the proper use of canes, walkers, or crutches, depending on the assistive device most appropriate for the patient's condition.

Walkers. Walkers are extremely light, movable devices that are about waist high and made of metal tubing (Fig. 38-6). They have four widely placed, sturdy legs. The patient holds the handgrips on the upper bars, takes a step, moves the walker forward, and takes another step. A walker requires a patient to lift the device up and forward. In the home many patients prefer walkers with wheels or short runners on the legs that allow them to push the walker. Instruct patients on how to use walkers safely and avoid risk of falling.

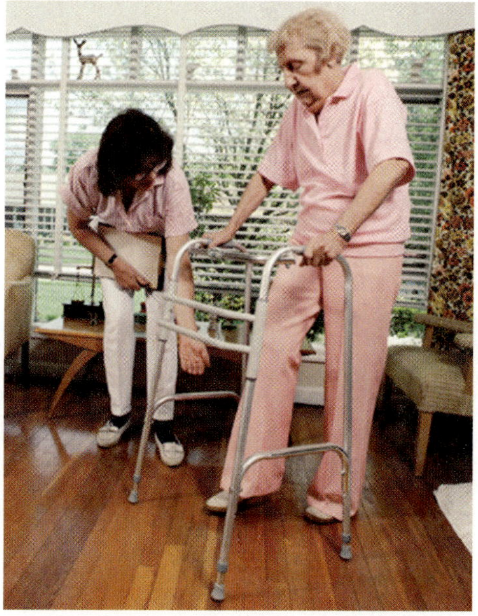

FIG. 38-6 Patient using a walker.

Canes. Canes are lightweight, easily movable devices made of wood or metal. They provide less support than a walker and are less stable. A person's cane length is equal to the distance between the greater trochanter and the floor (Pierson and Fairchild, 2008). Two common types of canes are the single straight-legged cane and the quad cane. The single straight-legged cane is more common and is used to support and balance a patient with decreased leg strength. Have the patient keep the cane on the stronger side of the body. For maximum support when walking, the patient places the cane forward 15 to 25 cm (6 to 10 inches), keeping body weight on both legs. The weaker leg is moved forward to the cane so body weight is divided between the cane and the stronger leg. The stronger leg is then advanced past the cane so the weaker leg and the body weight are supported by the cane and weaker leg. During walking the patient continually repeats these three steps. The patient needs to learn that two points of support such as both feet or one foot and the cane are on the floor at all times.

The quad cane provides the most support and is used when there is partial or complete leg paralysis or some hemiplegia (Fig. 38-7). You teach the patient the same three steps that are used with the straight-legged cane.

Crutches. Crutches are often needed to increase mobility. Begin crutch instruction with guidelines for safe use (Box 38-12). The use of crutches is often temporary (e.g., after ligament damage to the knee). However, some patients with paralysis of the lower extremities need them permanently. A crutch is a wooden or metal staff. The two types of crutches are the double adjustable Lofstrand or forearm crutch and the axillary wooden or metal crutch. The

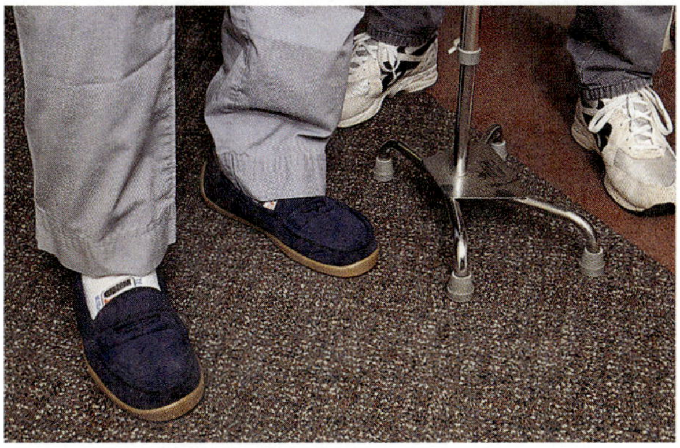

FIG. 38-7 Bottom of quad cane.

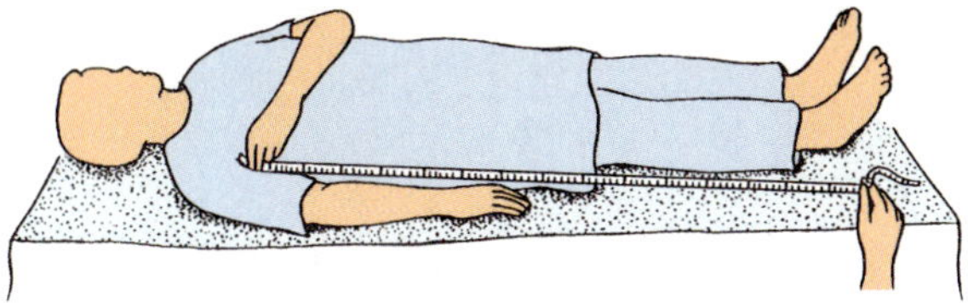

FIG. 38-8 Measuring crutch length.

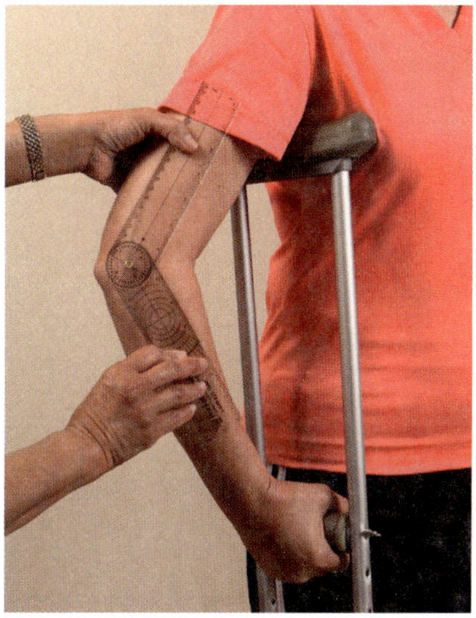

FIG. 38-9 Using the goniometer to verify correct degree of elbow flexion for crutch use.

BOX 38-12 PATIENT TEACHING

Crutch Safety

Objective
- Patient will state and demonstrate safe crutch walking.

Teaching Strategies
- Teach patient not to lean on crutches to support body weight.
- Teach patient with axillary crutches about the dangers of pressure on the axillae, which occurs when leaning on the crutches to support body weight.
- Explain why patient needs to use crutches that were measured for him or her.
- Show patient how to routinely inspect crutch tips. Securely attach rubber tips to the crutches. Replace worn tips. Rubber crutch tips increase surface friction and help prevent slipping.
- Explain that the crutch tips need to remain dry. Water decreases surface friction and increases the risk of slipping. Show patient how to dry the crutch tips if they become wet; patient may use paper or cloth towels.
- Show patient how to inspect the structure of the crutches. Cracks in a wooden crutch decrease its ability to support weight. Bends in aluminum crutches alter body alignment.
- Provide patient with a list of medical supply companies in the community for obtaining repairs, new rubber tips, handgrips, and crutch pads.
- Instruct patient to have spare crutches and tips readily available.

Evaluation
- Patient states principles of crutch safety.
- Patient correctly demonstrates proper use of crutches.
- Axilla is free of pressure.

forearm crutch has a handgrip and a metal band that fits around the patient's forearm. The metal band and the handgrip are adjusted to fit the patient's height. The axillary crutch has a padded curved surface at the top, which fits under the axilla. A handgrip in the form of a crossbar is held at the level of the palms to support the body. It is important to measure crutches for the appropriate length and to teach patients how to use their crutches safely to achieve a stable gait, ascend and descend stairs, and rise from a sitting position.

Measuring for Crutches. The axillary crutch is the more common crutch used. Measurements include the patient's height, the angle of elbow flexion, and the distance between the crutch pad and the axilla. When crutches are fitted, ensure the length of the crutch is three to four finger widths from the axilla to a point 15 cm (6 inches) lateral to the patient's heel (Pierson and Fairchild, 2008) (Fig. 38-8).

Position the handgrips so the axillae are not supporting the patient's body weight. Pressure on the axillae increases risk to underlying nerves, which sometimes results in partial paralysis of the arm. Determine correct position of the handgrips with the patient upright, supporting weight by the handgrips with the elbows slightly flexed at 30 degrees (Pierson and Fairchild, 2008). Elbow flexion may be verified with a goniometer (Fig. 38-9). When you determine the height and placement of the handgrips, verify that the distance between the crutch pad and the patient's axilla is three to four finger widths (Fig. 38-10).

Crutch Gait. Patients assume a crutch gait by alternately bearing weight on one or both legs and on the crutches. Determine the gait by assessing the patient's physical and functional abilities and the disease or injury that resulted in the need for crutches. This section summarizes the basic crutch stance and the four standard gaits: four-point alternating gait, three-point alternating gait, two-point gait, and swing-through gait.

The basic crutch stance is the tripod position, formed when the crutches are placed 15 cm (6 inches) in front of and 15 cm (6 inches) to the side of each foot (Fig. 38-11). This position improves the patient's balance by providing a wider base of support. The body alignment of the patient in the tripod position includes an erect head and neck, straight vertebrae, and extended hips and knees. The axillae should not bear any weight. The patient assumes the tripod position before crutch walking.

Four-point alternating, or four-point, gait gives stability to the patient but requires weight bearing on both legs. Each leg is moved alternately with each opposing crutch so three points of support are on the floor at all times (Fig. 38-12, *A*).

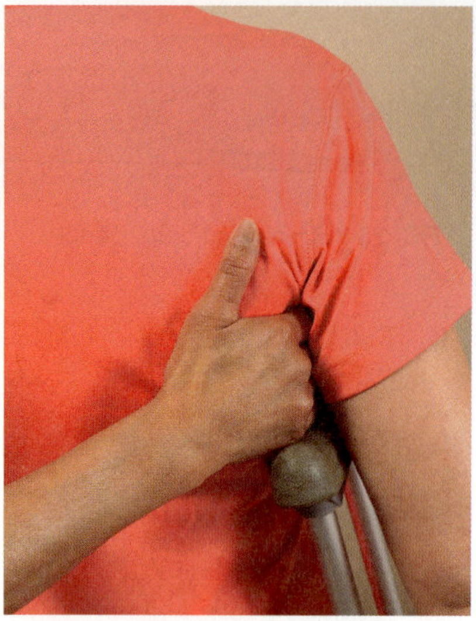

FIG. 38-10 Verifying correct distance between crutch pads and axilla.

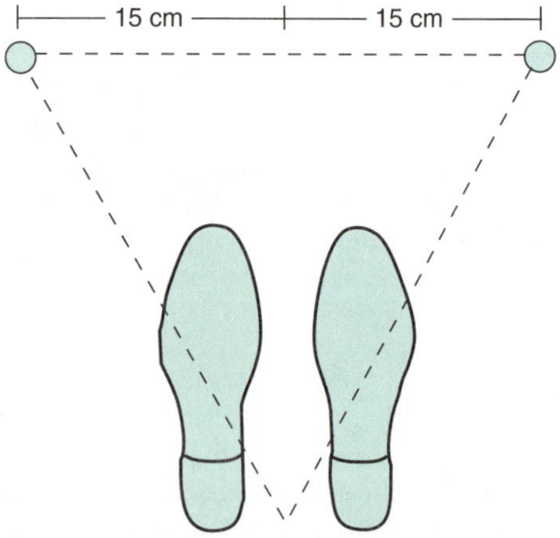

FIG. 38-11 Tripod position, basic crutch stance.

Three-point alternating, or three-point, gait requires the patient to bear all of the weight on one foot. In a three-point gait the patient bears weight on both crutches and then on the uninvolved leg, repeating the sequence (Fig. 38-12, *B*). The affected leg does not touch the ground during the early phase of the three-point gait. Gradually the patient progresses to touchdown and full weight bearing on the affected leg.

The two-point gait requires at least partial weight bearing on each foot (Fig. 38-12, *C*). The patient moves a crutch at the same time as the opposing leg so the crutch movements are similar to arm motion during normal walking.

Individuals with paraplegia who wear weight-supporting braces on their legs frequently use the swing-through gait. With weight placed on the supported legs, the patient places the crutches one stride in front and then swings to or through them while they support his or her weight.

Crutch Walking on Stairs. When ascending stairs on crutches, the patient usually uses a modified three-point gait (Fig. 38-13). He or she stands at the bottom of the stairs and transfers body weight to the crutches. The unaffected leg is advanced between the crutches to the stairs. The patient then shifts weight from the crutches to the unaffected leg. Finally he or she aligns both crutches on the stairs. The patient repeats this sequence until he or she reaches the top of the stairs.

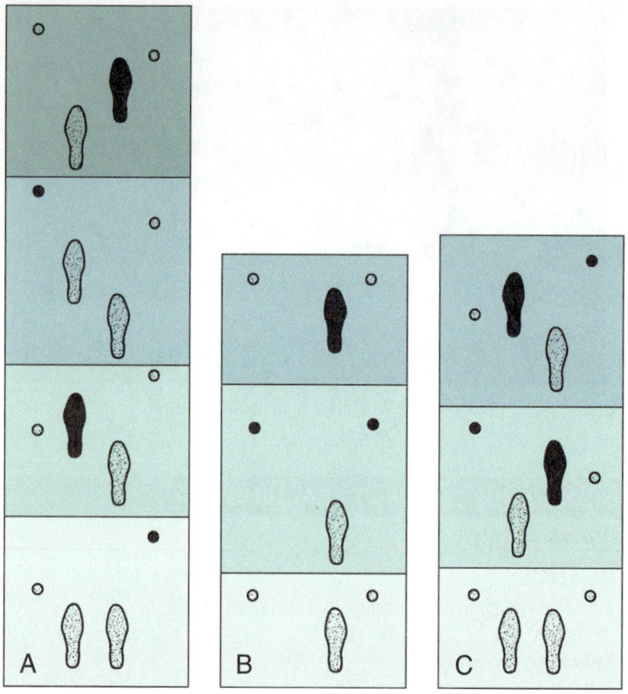

FIG. 38-12 **A,** Four-point alternating gait. Solid feet and crutch tips show the order of foot and crutch tip movement in each of the four phases. (Read from bottom to top.) **B,** Three-point gait with weight borne on unaffected leg. Solid foot and crutch tips show weight bearing in each phase. (Read from bottom to top.) **C,** Two-point gait with weight borne partially on each foot and each crutch advancing with opposing leg. Solid areas indicate leg and crutch tips bearing weight. (Read from bottom to top.)

A three-phase sequence is also used to descend the stairs (Fig. 38-14). The patient transfers body weight to the unaffected leg. The crutches are placed on the stairs, and the patient begins to transfer body weight to the crutches, moving the affected leg forward. Finally the unaffected leg is moved to the stairs with the crutches. The patient repeats the sequence until reaching the bottom of the stairs.

Because in most cases patients need to use crutches for some time, they need to be taught to use them on stairs before discharge. This instruction applies to all patients who are dependent on crutches, not only those who have stairs in their homes. You will frequently collaborate with physical therapists to provide instruction about crutch walking.

Building Competency in Patient-Centered Care You are caring for Mr. Slane, a 72-year-old patient who has undergone a left total knee replacement. His orders are that he is allowed no weight bearing on the left leg, and he has been fitted with crutches. As you prepare for his discharge he states, "I'm not sure how I'm going to get up and down the stairs to go to bed and down the basement stairs to do my laundry. I can't read these silly directions on how to use my crutches on the stairs; the print is so small." Which assessment questions and teaching strategies, approaches, and tools do you use to enhance Mr. Slane's learning and ability to safely use his crutches when ascending and descending stairs?

Answers to questions can be found on the Evolve website.

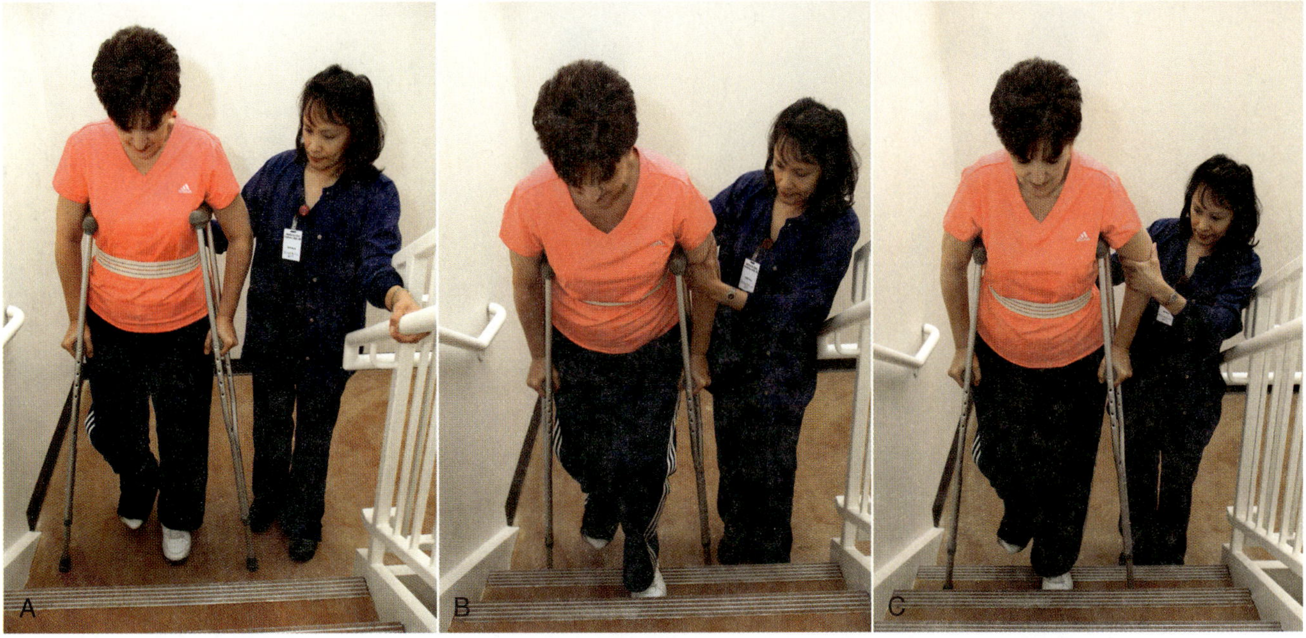

FIG. 38-13 Ascending stairs. **A,** Weight is placed on crutch. **B,** Weight is transferred from crutches to unaffected leg on stairs. **C,** Crutches are aligned with unaffected leg on stairs.

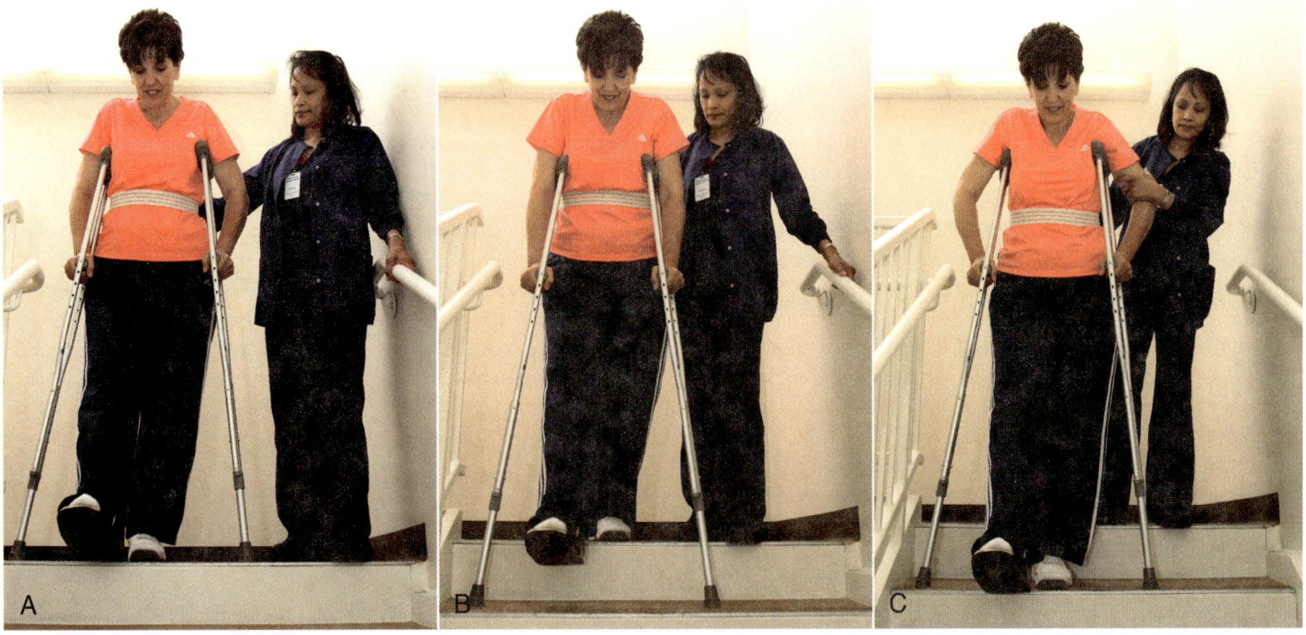

FIG. 38-14 Descending stairs. **A,** Body weight is on unaffected leg. **B,** Body weight is transferred to crutches. **C,** Unaffected leg is aligned on stairs with crutches.

Sitting in a Chair with Crutches. As with crutch walking and crutch walking up and down stairs, the procedure for sitting in a chair involves phases and requires the patient to transfer weight (Fig. 38-15). First the patient positions himself or herself at the center front of the chair with the posterior aspect of the legs touching the chair. Then the patient holds both crutches in the hand opposite the affected leg. If both legs are affected, as with a person with paraplegia who wears weight-supporting braces, the crutches are held in the hand on the patient's stronger side. With both crutches in one hand, the patient supports body weight on the unaffected leg and the crutches. While still holding the crutches, the patient grasps the arm of the chair with the remaining hand and lowers his or her body into it. To stand the procedure is reversed; and the patient, when fully erect, assumes the tripod position before beginning to walk.

Restoration of Activity and Chronic Illness. Nurses design care plans to increase activity and exercise in patients with specific disease conditions and chronic illnesses such as CHD, hypertension, COPD, and diabetes mellitus.

Coronary Heart Disease. Research shows activity and exercise play a role in secondary prevention or recurrence of CHD. Cardiac rehabilitation is an integral part of comprehensive care of patients

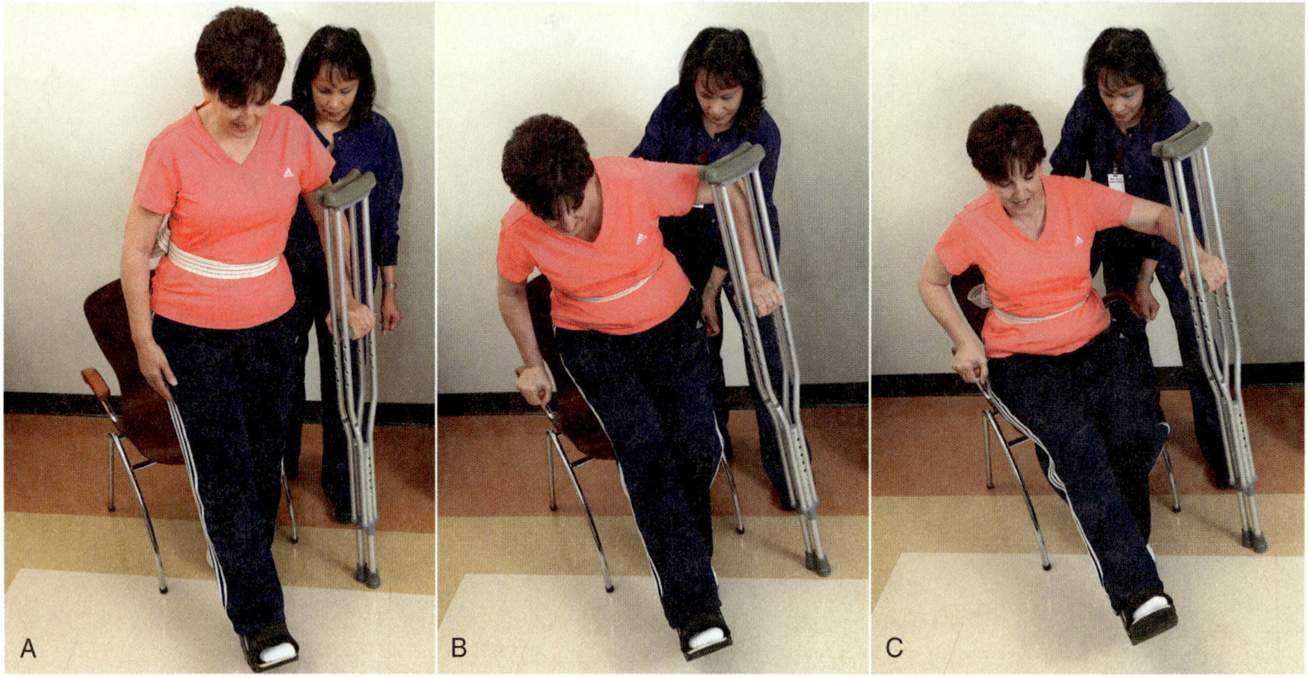

FIG. 38-15 Sitting in a chair. **A,** Both crutches are held in one hand. Patient transfers weight to crutches and unaffected leg. **B,** Patient grasps arm of chair with free hand and begins to lower herself into chair. **C,** Patient completely lowers herself into chair.

diagnosed with CHD. Nurses are involved in many aspects of cardiac rehabilitation and assist patients to develop a program of exercise that fits their needs and level of functioning. Increased physical activity benefits individuals with myocardial infarction (MI), angina pectoris, or heart failure and patients who have had a coronary artery bypass graft (CABG) or percutaneous transluminal coronary angioplasty (PTCA). Patients with CHD benefit from exercise and activity in terms of reduced mortality and morbidity, improved quality of life, improved left ventricular function, increased functional capacity, decreased blood lipids and apolipoproteins (protein components of lipoprotein complexes), and psychological well-being (Donges et al., 2010; Hamer and Stamatakis, 2009; Mandic et al., 2009).

Hypertension. Exercise reduces systolic and diastolic blood pressure readings. Low- to moderate-intensity aerobic exercise (brisk walking or bicycling) is the most effective in lowering blood pressure, whereas weight training and high-intensity aerobics have minimal benefits (Balady et al., 2010; Ciolac et al., 2009; Edelman and Mandle, 2010).

Chronic Obstructive Pulmonary Disease. Pulmonary rehabilitation helps patients reach an optimal level of functioning. Some patients are fearful of participating in exercise because of the potential of worsening dyspnea (difficulty breathing). This aversion to physical activity sets up a progressive deconditioning in which minimal physical exertion results in dyspnea. Pulmonary rehabilitation provides a safe environment for monitoring patients' progress. In addition, they receive encouragement and support to increase activity and exercise (Berry et al., 2010; Salhi et al., 2010).

Diabetes Mellitus. Along with diet, glucose monitoring, and medication, exercise is an important component in the care of patients with diabetes mellitus. Individuals with type 1 diabetes need to exercise because it leads to improved glucose control, cardiovascular fitness, and psychological well-being. Exercise lowers blood sugar levels, and the effects of exercise on blood sugar levels often last for at least 24 hours. Instruct the patient with type 1 diabetes about the risks and precautions regarding exercise. Instruction includes the need for a physical examination before beginning an exercise program and precautions to monitor blood glucose level immediately before and after exercise. Also instruct patients to perform low- to moderate-intensity exercises, carry a concentrated form of carbohydrates (sugar packets or hard candy), and wear a medical alert bracelet. The patient with type 2 diabetes who decides to participate in a regular program of exercise needs to include low-intensity warm-up and cool-down exercises, aerobic exercise at 50% to 75% of maximal oxygen uptake, and exercise for 20 to 45 minutes 3 days per week (ADA, 2007; Morrato et al., 2006).

EVALUATION

Through the Patient's Eyes. For activity and exercise you measure the effectiveness of nursing interventions by the success of meeting the patient's expected outcomes and goals of care. The patient is the only one who knows the effectiveness and benefits of activity and exercise (Fig. 38-16). Continuous evaluation helps to determine whether new or revised therapies are needed and if new nursing diagnoses have developed.

Patient Outcomes. To evaluate the effectiveness of nursing interventions to enhance activity and exercise, make comparisons with baseline measures that include pulse, blood pressure, strength, endurance, and psychological well-being. Compare actual outcomes with expected outcomes to determine the patient's health status and progression. The following is an example of questions you ask when your patients do not meet their expected outcomes:

- The last time we met, you planned to walk outside for 20 minutes three days a week. However, you report that you are only able to walk twice a week right now. What do you think is preventing you from meeting your goal?
- Your weight is the same this month as it was last month. We were hoping that increasing your activity would lead to a

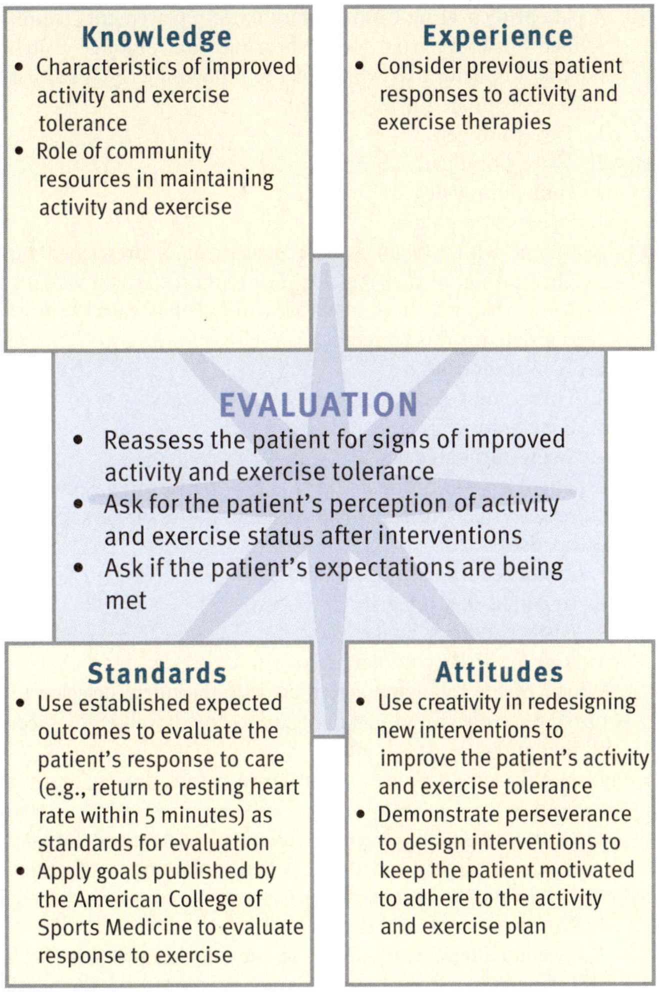
Knowledge
• Characteristics of improved activity and exercise tolerance
• Role of community resources in maintaining activity and exercise
Experience
• Consider previous patient responses to activity and exercise therapies
EVALUATION
• Reassess the patient for signs of improved activity and exercise tolerance
• Ask for the patient's perception of activity and exercise status after interventions
• Ask if the patient's expectations are being met
Standards
• Use established expected outcomes to evaluate the patient's response to care (e.g., return to resting heart rate within 5 minutes) as standards for evaluation
• Apply goals published by the American College of Sports Medicine to evaluate response to exercise
Attitudes
• Use creativity in redesigning new interventions to improve the patient's activity and exercise tolerance
• Demonstrate perseverance to design interventions to keep the patient motivated to adhere to the activity and exercise plan

FIG. 38-16 Critical thinking model for activity and exercise evaluation.

decrease in your weight. Help me understand the factors you believe are preventing you from losing weight right now.
- You state that you experience leg pain after walking short distances. Describe your pain. What pain-relieving measures have you tried?

KEY POINTS

- Exercise is physical activity for the purpose of conditioning the body, improving health, and maintaining fitness; it also is a therapeutic measure.
- Activity tolerance is the kind and amount of exercise or work that a person is able to perform. Physiological, emotional, and developmental factors influence the patient's activity tolerance.
- The best program of physical activity includes a combination of exercises that produces different physiological and psychological benefits.
- Body mechanics are the coordinated efforts of the musculoskeletal and nervous systems as the person moves, lifts, bends, stands, sits, lies down, and completes daily activities.
- Coordinated body movement requires integrated functioning of the skeletal system, skeletal muscles, and nervous system.
- Muscles primarily associated with movement are located near the skeletal region, where movement results from leverage, which is characteristic of movements of the upper extremities.
- Coordination and regulation of muscle groups depend on muscle tone and activity of antagonistic, synergistic, and antigravity muscles.
- The nervous system controls balance through the functions of the cerebellum and inner ear.
- You achieve body balance when there is a wide base of support, the center of gravity falls within the base of support, and a vertical line falls from the center of gravity through the base of support.
- Developmental changes, behavioral aspects, environmental issues, cultural and ethnic origin, and family and social support influence the patient's perception and motivation to engage in physical activity and exercise.
- Ability to engage in normal physical activity and exercise depends on intact and functioning nervous and musculoskeletal systems.
- Use the nursing process to provide care for patients who are experiencing or are at risk for activity intolerance and impaired physical mobility.
- After identifying nursing diagnoses, plan and implement interventions to increase activity and exercise in collaboration with the patient when possible.
- Range-of-motion exercises incorporated into daily activities include one or all of the body joints.
- Mechanical devices to promote walking include canes, walkers, and crutches.

CLINICAL APPLICATION QUESTIONS

Preparing for Clinical Practice

Mrs. Smith has experienced some success in initiating an exercise program. However, maintaining her exercise plan is becoming challenging, and she is not seeing the improvements that she expects. She states, "I feel like I'm doing everything right, but I'm getting few results for my efforts."

1. Mrs. Smith states, "I don't want to leave the house anymore." She also expresses feelings of overwhelming stress and excessive demands on her time. What interventions do you suggest to Mrs. Smith to help overcome this barrier to exercise?
2. Mrs. Smith has several challenges to initiating and maintaining an exercise program. Develop a stepwise approach for Mrs. Smith that helps her initiate and maintain an exercise program, keeping in mind the challenges that she faces.
3. Develop an educational component to Mrs. Smith's care plan, emphasizing the benefits of exercise.

evolve *Answers to Clinical Application Questions can be found on the Evolve website.*

REVIEW QUESTIONS

Are You Ready to Test Your Nursing Knowledge?

1. A patient on bed rest for several days attempts to walk with assistance. He becomes dizzy and nauseated. His pulse rate jumps from 85 to 110 beats/min. These are most likely symptoms of which of the following?
   1. Rebound hypertension
   2. Orthostatic hypotension
   3. Dysfunctional proprioception.
   4. Central nervous system rebound hypotension
2. Which action(s) are appropriate for the nurse to implement when a patient experiences orthostatic hypotension? (Select all that apply.)

1. Call for assistance.
2. Allow patient to sit down.
3. Take patient's blood pressure and pulse.
4. Continue to ambulate patient to build endurance.
5. If patient begins to faint, allow him to slide against the nurse's leg to the floor.

3. Which of the following *best* motivates a patient to participate in an exercise program?
   1. Giving a patient information on exercise
   2. Providing information to the patient when the patient is ready to change behavior
   3. Explaining the importance of exercise when a patient is diagnosed with a chronic disease such as diabetes
   4. Following up with instructions after the health care provider tells a patient to begin an exercise program
4. Which of the following is a principle of proper body mechanics when lifting or carrying objects?
   1. Keep the knees in a locked position.
   2. Bend at the waist to maintain a center of gravity.
   3. Maintain a wide base of support.
   4. Hold objects away from the body for improved leverage.
5. Which group of patients is at most risk for severe injuries related to falls?
   1. Adolescents
   2. Older adults
   3. Toddlers
   4. Young children
6. A nurse plans to provide education to the parents of school-aged children and includes which of the following result of children being less physically active outside of school?
   1. An increase in obesity
   2. An increase in heart disease
   3. Higher computer literacy
   4. Improved school attendance and grades
7. A nursing assistive personnel asks for help to transfer a patient who is 125 pounds (56.8 kg) from the bed to a wheelchair. The patient is unable to assist. What is the nurse's best response?
   1. "As long as we use proper body mechanics, no one will get hurt."
   2. "The patient only weighs 125 lb. You don't need my assistance."
   3. "Call the lift-team for additional assistance."
   4. "The two of us can easily lift the patient."
8. You are transferring a patient who weighs 320 lb (145.5 kg) from his bed to a chair. The patient has an order for partial weight bearing as a result of bilateral reconstructive knee surgery. Which of the following is the best technique for transfer?
   1. Use a transfer board.
   2. Obtain a stand assist device.
   3. Implement a three-person carry.
   4. Use the ceiling-mounted lift.
9. Which is the correct gait when a patient is ascending stairs on crutches?
   1. A modified two-point gait. The affected leg is advanced between the crutches to the stairs.
   2. A modified three-point gait. The unaffected leg is advanced between the crutches to the stairs.
   3. A swing-through gait.
   4. A modified four-point gait. Both legs advance between the crutches to the stairs.
10. A patient recovering from bilateral knee replacements is prescribed bilateral partial weight bearing. You reinforce crutch walking knowing that which of the following crutch gaits is most appropriate for this patient?
    1. Two-point gait
    2. Three-point gait
    3. Four-point gait
    4. Swing-through gait
11. A patient with a right knee replacement is prescribed no weight bearing on the right leg. You reinforce crutch walking knowing that which of the following crutch gaits is most appropriate for this patient?
    1. Two-point gait
    2. Three-point gait
    3. Four-point gait
    4. Swing-through gait
12. A patient on week-long bed rest is now performing isometric exercises. Which nursing diagnosis best addresses the safety of this patient?
    1. Disturbed thought processes
    2. Impaired skin integrity
    3. Disturbed body image
    4. Risk for activity intolerance
13. Which of the following activities does the nurse delegate to nursing assistive personnel in regard to crutch walking? (Select all that apply.)
    1. Notify nurse if patient reports pain before, during, or after exercise.
    2. Notify nurse of patient complaints of increased fatigue, dizziness, light-headedness when obtaining vital signs before and/or after exercise.
    3. Notify nurse of vital sign values.
    4. Evaluate the patient's ability to use crutches properly.
    5. Prepare the patient for exercise by assisting in dressing and putting on shoes.
14. Select statements that apply to the proper use of a cane. (Select all that apply.)
    1. For maximum support when walking, the patient places the cane forward 15 to 25 cm (6 to 10 inches), keeping body weight on both legs. The weaker leg is moved forward to the cane so body weight is divided between the cane and the stronger leg.
    2. A person's cane length is equal to the distance between the elbow and the floor.
    3. Canes provide less support than a walker and are less stable.
    4. The patient needs to learn that two points of support such as both feet or one foot and the cane need to be present at all times.
15. A patient is discharged after an exacerbation of chronic obstructive pulmonary disease (COPD). She states, "I'm afraid to go to pulmonary rehabilitation." What is your best response?
    1. Pulmonary rehabilitation provides a safe environment for monitoring your progress.
    2. You have to participate or you will be back in the hospital.
    3. Tell me more about your concerns with going to pulmonary rehabilitation.
    4. The staff at our pulmonary rehabilitation facility are professionals and will not cause you any harm.

Answers: **1.** 2; **2.** 1, 2, 3, 5; **3.** 2; **4.** 3; **5.** 2; **6.** 1; **7.** 3; **8.** 4; **9.** 2; **10.** 1; **11.** 2; **12.** 4; **13.** 1, 2, 3, 5; **14.** 1, 3, 4; **15.** 1.

REFERENCES

Ackley BJ, Ladwig GB: *Nursing diagnosis handbook: an evidence-based guide to planning care*, ed 8, St Louis, 2008, Mosby.

American College of Sports Medicine (ACSM): *Position stand on fitness: the recommended quantity and quality of exercise for developing and maintaining cardiorespiratory and muscular fitness and flexibility in healthy adults*, 2007, http://www.50plus.org/Libraryitems/1_5positionstandonfitness.htm. Accessed August 2010.

American Diabetes Association (ADA): Diabetes and exercise: position statement, *Diabetes Care* S58, 2007.

American Nurses Association (ANA): *Position statement on elimination of manual patient handling to prevent work-related musculoskeletal disorders*, 2008, http://www.nursingworld.org/readroom/postion/workplace/pathand.htm. Accessed August 2010.

Balady GJ, et al: Clinician's guide to cardiopulmonary exercise testing in adults: a scientific statement from the American Heart Association, *Circulation* 122(2):191, 2010.

Chodzko-Zajko WJ, et al: Exercise and physical activity for older adults, *Med Sci Sports Exercise* 41(7):1510, 2009.

Edelman CL, Mandle CL, editors: *Health promotion throughout the life span*, ed 7, St Louis, 2010, Mosby.

Harper MG: Childhood obesity: strategies for prevention, *Fam Commun Health* 29(4):288, 2006.

Hockenberry M, Wilson D: *Nursing care of infants and children*, ed 9, St Louis, 2011, Mosby.

Hoeman SP: *Rehabilitation nursing: process, application, and outcomes*, ed 4, St Louis, 2006, Mosby.

Huether SE, McCance KL: *Understanding pathophysiology*, ed 4, St Louis, 2008, Mosby.

Lewis SL, et al: *Medical-surgical nursing assessment and management of clinical problems*, ed 8, St Louis, 2011, Mosby.

Monahan FD, et al: *Phipps' medical-surgical nursing: health and illness perspectives*, ed 8, St Louis, 2007, Mosby.

Morrato E, et al: Are health care professionals advising patients with diabetes or at risk for developing diabetes to exercise more? *Diabetes Care* 29(3):543, 2006.

Nelson A, Baptiste A: Evidence-based practices for safe patient handling and movement, *Online J Issues Nurs* 9(3), 2004.

Nelson A, et al: Myths and facts about safe patient handling in rehabilitation, *Rehabil Nurs* 33(1):10, 2008.

Occupational Safety and Health Administration (OSHA): *Guidelines for nursing homes: ergonomics for the prevention of musculoskeletal disorders*, 2009, http://www.osha.gov/ergonomics/guidelines/nursinghome/final_nh_guidelines.pdf. Accessed November 6, 2011.

O'Donovan G, et al: The ABCs of physical activity for health: a consensus statement from the British association of sport and exercise sciences, *J Sports Sci* 28(6):573, 2010.

Patton KT, Thibodeau GA: *Anatomy and physiology*, ed 7, St Louis, 2010, Mosby.

Pelczarski K: Take a proactive approach to bariatric patient needs, *Material Manage* 16(6):24, 2007.

Pierson F, Fairchild S: *Principles & techniques of patient care*, ed 4, St Louis, 2008, Saunders.

Prochaska JO, Norcross JC, DiClemente CC: *Changing for good*, New York, 1994, William Morrow.

United States Department of Labor: Bureau of Labor Statistics 2007, http://www.dol.gov/dol/topic/statistics/index.htm. Accessed November 6, 2011.

Wilson SF, Giddens JF: *Health assessment for nursing practice*, ed 4, St Louis, 2009, Mosby.

RESEARCH REFERENCES

Baptiste A, et al: Friction-reducing devices for lateral patient transfers: a clinical evaluation, *AAOHN J* 54(4):173, 2006.

Berry MJ, et al: A lifestyle activity intervention in patients with chronic obstructive pulmonary disease, *Respir Med* 104(6):829, 2010.

Bors P, et al: The active living by design national program: community initiatives and lessons learned, *Am J Prevent Med* 37(6 suppl 2):S313, 2009.

Capan K, Lynch B: A hospital fall assessment and intervention project, *J Clin Outcomes Manage* 14(3):155, 2007.

Ciolac EG, et al: Acute effects of continuous and interval aerobic exercise on 24-hour ambulatory blood pressure in long-term treated hypertensive patients, *Int J Cardiol* 133(3):381, 2009.

Davison KK, Jago R: Change in parent and peer support across ages 9 to 15 years and adolescent girls' physical activity, *Med Sci Sports Exercise* 41(9):1816, 2010.

De Kam D, et al: Exercise interventions to reduce fall-related fractures and their risk factors in individuals with low bone density: a systematic review of randomized controlled trials, *Osteoporosis Int* 20(12):2111, 2009.

Donges CE, et al: Effects of resistance or aerobic exercise training on interleukin-6, C-reactive protein, and body composition, *Med Sci Sports Exercise* 42(2):304, 2010.

Dunton GF: Adolescents' sports and exercise environments in the US time use survey, *Am J Prevent Med* 39(2):122, 2010.

Ferrand C, et al: Motives for regular physical activity in women and men: a qualitative study in French adults with type 2 diabetes, *Health Social Care Commun* 16(5):511, 2008.

Hamer M, Stamatakis E: Physical activity and risk of cardiovascular disease events: inflammatory and metabolic mechanisms, *Med Sci Sports Exercise* 41(6):1206, 2009.

Huang ES, et al: Racial/ethnic differences in concerns about current and future medications among patients with type 2 diabetes, *Diabetes Care* 32(2):311, 2009.

Kuoppala J, Lamminpää A, Husman P: Workplace health promotion, job well-being, and sickness absences—a systematic review and meta-analysis, *J Occupational Environmental Med* 50(11):1216, 2008.

Mandic S, et al: Characterizing differences in mortality at the low end of the fitness spectrum, *Med Sci Sports Exercise* 41(8):1573, 2009.

Maskarinec G, et al: Diabetes prevalence and body mass index differ by ethnicity: the multiethnic cohort, *Ethnicity Dis* 19(1):49, 2009.

Nelson NA, Hughes RE: Quantifying relationships between selected work-related risk factors and back pain: a systematic review of object biomechanical measures and cost-related health outcomes, *Int J Industrial Ergonomics* 39(1):202, 2009.

Perez AP, et al: Promoting dietary change among state health employees in Arkansas through a worksite wellness program, *Preventing Chronic Dis* 6(4):A123, 2009.

Salhi B, et al: Effects of pulmonary rehabilitation in patients with restrictive lung diseases, *Chest* 137(2):273, 2010.

Sherrington D, et al: Effective exercise for the prevention of falls: a systematic review and meta-analysis, *J Am Geriatr Soc* 56(12):2234, 2008.

Tullar JM, et al: Occupational safety and health interventions, *J Occupational Rehabil* 20(2):199, 2010.

Ward DS, et al: Interventions for increasing physical activity at child care, *Med Sci Sports Exercise* 42(3):526, 2010.

CHAPTER 39

Hygiene

OBJECTIVES

- Describe factors that influence personal hygiene practices.
- Discuss the role that critical thinking plays in providing hygiene.
- Conduct a comprehensive assessment of a patient's total hygiene needs.
- Discuss conditions that place patients at risk for impaired skin integrity.
- Discuss factors that influence the condition of the nails and feet.
- Explain the importance of foot care for the patient with diabetes.
- Discuss conditions that place patients at risk for impaired oral mucous membranes.
- List common hair and scalp problems and their related interventions.
- Describe how hygiene care for the older adult differs from that for the younger patient.
- Discuss different approaches used in maintaining a patient's comfort and safety during hygiene care.
- Successfully perform hygiene procedures for the care of the skin, perineum, feet and nails, mouth, eyes, ears, and nose.
- Adapt hygiene care for a patient who is cognitively impaired.

KEY TERMS

Acne, p. 771
Alopecia, p. 776
Caries, p. 772
Cerumen, p. 776
Complete bed bath, p. 783
Cuticle, p. 769
Dental caries, p. 770
Edentulous, p. 772
Effleurage, p. 785
Enucleation, p. 790
Epidermis, p. 769
Gingivitis, p. 770
Glossitis, p. 775
Halitosis, p. 775
Mucositis, p. 779
Partial bed bath, p. 783
Pediculosis capitis, p. 776
Perineal care, p. 784
Stomatitis, p. 786
Xerostomia, p. 770

evolve WEBSITE

http://evolve.elsevier.com/Potter/fundamentals/

- Review Questions
- Video Clips
- Concept Map Creator
- Case Study with Questions
- Skills Performance Checklists
- Audio Glossary
- Interactive Learning Activities
- Key Term Flashcards
- Content Updates

Personal hygiene affects patients' comfort, safety, and well-being. Hygiene care includes cleaning and grooming activities that maintain personal body cleanliness and appearance. Personal hygiene activities such as taking a bath or shower, brushing and flossing the teeth, washing and grooming the hair, and performing nail care promote comfort and relaxation, foster a positive self-image, promote healthy skin, and help prevent infection and disease. Healthy people fulfill their own hygiene needs; but when ill or physically or emotionally challenged, people often require some degree of assistance with hygiene care. A variety of personal, social, and cultural factors influence hygiene practices.

In both agency and home care settings, determine a patient's ability to perform self-care and provide hygiene care according to individual needs and preferences. In addition, in the home setting help the patient and family adapt hygiene techniques and approaches. Use the close contact required for hygiene care to promote a caring therapeutic relationship and provide needed patient teaching and counseling. Integrate other nursing activities during hygiene care, including assessment and interventions such as range-of-motion (ROM) exercises, application of dressings, or inspection and care of intravenous (IV) sites. During hygiene care preserve as much of the patient's independence as possible, assess his or her ability to perform hygiene care, ensure privacy, convey respect, and foster his or her physical comfort.

SCIENTIFIC KNOWLEDGE BASE

Proper hygiene care requires an understanding of the anatomy and physiology of the skin, nails, oral cavity, eyes, ears, and nose. The skin and mucosal cells exchange oxygen, nutrients, and fluids with underlying blood vessels. The cells require adequate nutrition, hydration, and circulation to resist injury and disease. Good hygiene techniques promote the normal structure and function of these tissues.

Apply knowledge of pathophysiology to provide preventive hygiene care. Recognize disease states that create changes in the integument, oral cavity, and sensory organs. For example, diabetes mellitus often results in chronic vascular changes that impair healing of the skin and mucosa. In the early stages of acquired

TABLE 39-1 Function of the Skin and Implications for Care

FUNCTION/DESCRIPTION	IMPLICATIONS FOR CARE
Protection	
Epidermis is relatively impermeable layer that prevents entrance of microorganisms. Although microorganisms reside on skin surface and in hair follicles, relative dryness of surface of skin inhibits bacterial growth. Sebum removes bacteria from hair follicles. Acidic pH of skin further retards bacterial growth.	Weakening of epidermis occurs by scraping or stripping its surface (e.g., use of dry razors, tape removal, improper turning or positioning techniques). Excessive dryness causes cracks and breaks in skin and mucosa that allow bacteria to enter. Emollients soften skin and prevent moisture loss, soaking skin improves moisture retention, and hydrating mucosa prevents dryness. However, constant exposure of skin to moisture causes maceration or softening, interrupting dermal integrity and promoting ulcer formation and bacterial growth. Keep bed linen and clothing dry. Misuse of soap, detergents, cosmetics, deodorant, and depilatories cause chemical irritation. Alkaline soaps neutralize the protective acid condition of skin. Cleaning skin removes excess oil, sweat, dead skin cells, and dirt, which promote bacterial growth.
Sensation	
Skin contains sensory organs for touch, pain, heat, cold, and pressure.	Minimize friction to avoid loss of stratum corneum, which results in development of pressure ulcers. Smoothing linen removes sources of mechanical irritation. Remove rings from fingers to prevent accidentally injuring patient's skin. Make sure that bath water is not excessively hot or cold.
Temperature Regulation	
Radiation, evaporation, conduction, and convection control body temperature.	Factors that interfere with heat loss alter temperature control. Wet bed linen or gowns interfere with convection and conduction. Excess blankets or bed coverings interfere with heat loss through radiation and conduction. Coverings promote heat conservation.
Excretion and Secretion	
Sweat promotes heat loss by evaporation. Sebum lubricates skin and hair.	Perspiration and oil harbor microorganisms. Bathing removes excess body secretions; although, if excessive, it causes dry skin.

immunodeficiency syndrome (AIDS), fungal infections of the oral cavity are common. Paralysis of the trigeminal nerve (cranial nerve V) eliminates the blink reflex, causing risk of corneal drying. In the presence of conditions such as these, adapt hygiene practices to minimize injury. Use time spent providing hygiene care to identify abnormalities and initiate appropriate actions to prevent further injury to sensitive tissues.

The Skin

The skin serves several functions, including protection, secretion, excretion, body temperature regulation, and cutaneous sensation (Table 39-1). It consists of two primary layers: the epidermis and the dermis. Just beneath the skin lies the subcutaneous tissue (also known as the hypodermis), which shares some of the protective functions of the skin.

Several thin layers of epithelial cells comprise the outer layer, or **epidermis;** these cells shield underlying tissue against water loss and injury and prevent entry of disease-producing microorganisms. The innermost layer of the epidermis generates new cells to replace the dead cells that the outer surface of the skin continuously sheds. Bacteria commonly reside on the outer epidermis. These resident bacteria are normal flora (see Chapter 28) that do not cause disease but instead inhibit the multiplication of disease-causing microorganisms.

Bundles of collagen and elastic fibers form the thicker dermis that underlies and supports the epidermis. Nerve fibers, blood vessels, sweat glands, sebaceous glands, and hair follicles run through the dermal layers. Sebaceous glands secrete sebum, an oily, odorous fluid, into the hair follicles. Sebum softens and lubricates the skin and slows water loss from the skin when the humidity is low. More important, sebum has bactericidal action.

The subcutaneous tissue layer contains blood vessels, nerves, lymph, and loose connective tissue filled with fat cells. The fatty tissue functions as a heat insulator for the body. Subcutaneous tissue also supports upper skin layers to withstand stresses and pressure without injury and anchors the skin loosely to underlying structures such as muscle. Very little subcutaneous tissue underlies the oral mucosa.

The skin often reflects a change in physical condition by alterations in color, thickness, texture, turgor, temperature, and hydration (see Chapter 30). As long as the skin remains intact and healthy, its physiological function remains optimal. Hygiene practices frequently influence skin status and can have both beneficial and negative effects on the skin. For example, too-frequent bathing and use of hot water frequently leads to dry, flaky skin and loss of protective oils.

The Feet, Hands, and Nails

The feet, hands, and nails often require special attention to prevent infection, odor, and injury. The condition of a patient's hands and feet influences the ability to perform hygiene care. Without the ability to bear weight, ambulate, or manipulate the hands, the patient is at risk for losing self-care ability.

A wide range of dexterity exists in the hand because of the movement between the thumb and fingers. Any condition that interferes with movement of the hand (e.g., superficial or deep pain or joint inflammation) impairs a patient's self-care abilities. Foot pain often changes the patient's gait, causing strain on different joints and muscle groups. Discomfort while standing or walking limits self-care abilities.

The nails grow from the root of the nail bed, which is located in the skin at the nail groove, hidden by the fold of skin called the **cuticle.** A scalelike modification of the epidermis forms the visible part of the nail (nail body), which has a crescent-shaped white area known as the lunula. Under the nail lies a layer of epithelium called the nail bed. A normal healthy nail appears transparent, smooth, and convex, with a pink nail bed and translucent white tip. Disease causes changes in the shape, thickness, and curvature of the nail (see Chapter 30).

The Oral Cavity

The oral cavity consists of the lips surrounding the opening of the mouth, the cheeks running along the sidewalls of the cavity, the tongue and its muscles, and the hard and soft palate. The mucous membrane, continuous with the skin, lines the oral cavity. The floor of the mouth and the undersurface of the tongue are richly supplied with blood vessels. Normal oral mucosa glistens and is pink, soft, moist, smooth, and without lesions. Ulcerations or trauma frequently result in significant bleeding. Several glands within and outside the oral cavity secrete saliva. Saliva cleanses the mouth, dissolves food chemicals to promote taste, moistens food to facilitate bolus formation, and contains enzymes that start breakdown of starchy foods. The effects of medications, exposure to radiation, dehydration, and mouth breathing impair salivary secretion in the mouth. Strong sympathetic nervous system stimulation almost completely inhibits the release of saliva and results in **xerostomia** or dry mouth.

The teeth lie in sockets in the gum-covered mandible and maxilla; they tear and grind ingested food so it can be mixed with saliva and swallowed for digestion. A normal tooth consists of the crown, neck, and root. The enamel-covered crown extends above the gingiva or gum, which normally surrounds the tooth like a tight collar. A constricted portion of the tooth called the *neck* connects the crown and the root; the root is embedded in the jawbone. The periodontal membrane lies just below the gum margins, surrounds a tooth, and holds it firmly in place. Healthy teeth appear white, smooth, shiny, and properly aligned.

Difficulty in chewing develops when surrounding gum tissues become inflamed or infected or when teeth are lost or become loosened. Regular oral hygiene helps to prevent **gingivitis** (i.e., inflammation of the gums) and **dental caries** (i.e., tooth decay produced by interaction of food with bacteria).

The Hair

Hair growth, distribution, and pattern indicate a person's general health status. Hormonal changes, nutrition, emotional and physical stress, aging, infection, and some illnesses affect hair characteristics. The hair shaft itself is lifeless, and physiological factors do not directly affect it. However, hormonal and nutrient deficiencies of the hair follicle cause changes in hair color or condition.

The Eyes, Ears, and Nose

When providing hygiene care, the eyes, ears, and nose require careful attention. Chapter 30 describes the structure and function of these organs. Clean the sensitive sensory tissues in a way that prevents injury and discomfort for a patient, such as using care not to get soap in his or her eyes. In addition, the time you spend with your patient during hygiene provides an excellent opportunity to ask if there are any changes in vision, hearing, or sense of smell.

NURSING KNOWLEDGE BASE

A number of factors influence personal preferences for hygiene and the ability to maintain hygiene practices. Since no two individuals perform hygiene care in the same manner, you individualize patient care based on learning about his or her unique hygiene practices and preferences. Individualized hygiene care requires use of therapeutic communication skills to promote the therapeutic relationship. In addition, use the opportunity provided during hygiene care to assess a patient's health promotion practices, emotional status, and health care education needs. Be aware that developmental changes influence the need and preferences for type of hygiene care.

Factors Influencing Hygiene

Social Practices. Social groups influence hygiene preferences and practices, including the type of hygiene products used and the nature and frequency of personal care practices. Parents and caregivers perform hygiene care for infants and young children. Family customs play a major role during childhood in determining hygiene practices such as the frequency of bathing, the time of day bathing is performed, and even whether certain hygiene practices such as brushing of the teeth or flossing are performed. As children enter adolescence, peer groups and media often influence hygiene practices. For example, some young girls become more interested in their personal appearance and begin to wear makeup. During the adult years involvement with friends and work groups shape the expectations that people have about personal appearance. Some older adults' hygiene practices change because of changes in living conditions and available resources.

Personal Preferences. Patients have individual desires and preferences about when to perform hygiene and grooming care. Some patients prefer to shower, whereas others prefer to bathe. Patients select different hygiene and grooming products according to personal preferences. Knowing patients' personal preferences promotes individualized care. Help the patient develop new hygiene practices when indicated by an illness or condition. For example, you need to teach a patient with diabetes proper foot hygiene. Safe and effective patient-centered nursing care elicits individual preferences, allows patients to make personal choices whenever possible, and promotes patient involvement and independence (Cronenwett et al., 2007).

Body Image. Body image is a person's subjective concept of his or her body, including physical appearance, structure, or function (see Chapter 33). Body image affects the way in which individuals maintain personal hygiene. If a patient maintains a neatly groomed appearance, be sure to consider the details of grooming when planning care and consult with the patient before making decisions about how to provide hygiene care. Patients who appear unkempt or uninterested in hygiene sometimes need education about its importance or further assessment regarding their ability to participate with daily hygiene.

Surgery, illness, or a change in emotional or functional status often affects a patient's body image. Discomfort and pain, emotional stress, or fatigue diminish the ability or desire to perform hygiene self-care and require extra effort to promote hygiene and grooming.

Socioeconomic Status. A person's economic resources influence the type and extent of hygiene practices used. Be sensitive in considering that the patient's economic status influences the ability to regularly maintain hygiene. He or she may not be able to afford desired basic supplies such as deodorant, shampoo, and toothpaste. A patient may need to modify the home environment by adding safety devices such as nonskid surfaces and grab bars in the bath to perform hygiene self-care safely. When he or she lacks socioeconomic resources, it becomes difficult to participate and take a responsible role in health promotion activities such as basic hygiene.

Health Beliefs and Motivation. Knowledge about the importance of hygiene and its implications for well-being influences hygiene practices. However, knowledge alone is not enough. Motivation also plays a key role in a patient's hygiene practices. Patient teaching is often needed to foster hygiene self-care. Provide information that focuses on a patient's health-related issues relevant to the desired hygiene care behaviors. Patient perceptions of the benefits of hygiene care and the susceptibility to and

BOX 39-1 CULTURAL ASPECTS OF CARE

Hygiene Practices

Patients deserve a culturally congruent plan for hygiene care. For many patients culture influences hygiene practices, and hygiene care becomes a potential source of conflict and stress in the caregiving environment. Patient-centered care mandates that care be based on respect for the individual patient's cultural background (Cronenwett et al., 2007).

Implications for Practice

- Maintain privacy, especially for women from cultures that value female modesty (e.g., Muslim, Hispanic, Nigerian) (Galanti, 2008).
- Avoid uncovering the lower torso and exposing the arms of Middle Eastern and East Asian Women.
- Allow family members to participate in care if desired by adapting the schedule of hygiene activities.
- Provide gender-congruent caregivers as needed or requested.
- Recognize that some cultures prohibit or restrict touching. For some patients from Arab and Hispanic cultures touching between unrelated males and females is forbidden (Maier-Lorentz, 2008).
- Incorporate awareness that people from various cultures have differing preferences regarding personal space. Hispanics, Asians, and Middle Easterners often feel very comfortable in closer proximity than people of European and North American descent (Maier-Lorentz, 2008).
- Do not cut or shave hair without prior discussion with patient or family (Galanti, 2008).
- Be aware that toileting practices vary by culture (e.g., Asians may prefer squatting for toileting) (Galanti, 2008).
- Recognize that people from the Japanese culture often prefer to cleanse while sitting before getting into a bath tub. Immersion in a tub occurs after cleansing because the bath represents spiritual cleansing. Japanese people prefer that the water be deeper (submerged to the neck) and hotter than the typical western bath (McGraw and Drennan, 2009).

seriousness of developing a problem affect the motivation to change behavior (Pender, Murdaugh, and Parsons, 2011). For example, do patients perceive that they are at risk for dental disease, that dental disease is serious, and that brushing and flossing are effective in reducing risk? When they recognize that there is a risk and that they can take reasonable action without negative consequences, they are more likely to be receptive to nurses' counseling and teaching efforts.

Cultural Variables. Cultural beliefs and personal values influence hygiene care (Box 39-1). People from diverse cultural backgrounds frequently follow different self-care practices (see Chapter 9). Maintaining cleanliness does not hold the same importance for some ethnic or social groups as it does for others (Galanti, 2008). In North America it is common to bathe or shower daily and use deodorant to prevent body odors. However, people from some cultures are not sensitive to body odors, prefer to bathe less frequently, and do not use deodorant. Some homeless people believe that a layer of dirt helps protect them from becoming sick (Galanti, 2008). Do not express disapproval when caring for patients whose hygiene practices differ from yours. Avoid forcing changes in hygiene practices unless the practices affect the patient's health. In these situations use tact, provide information, and allow choices. Religious beliefs associated with culture sometimes influence hygiene practices. Facilitate a patient's religious practices whenever possible. For example, Muslim patients often remove their shoes and assume different positions for prayer. This increases the risk of developing foot pathology such as calluses on the toes and lateral ankles. When caring for Muslim patients who have diabetes mellitus, you need to be supportive of religious practices while also stressing the need to be diligent in inspecting the feet after prayer sessions for any blisters or calluses.

Developmental Stage. The normal process of aging influences the condition of body tissues and structures. A patient's developmental stage affects the ability of the patient to perform hygiene care and the type of care needed. Apply knowledge of developmental changes as you assess your patients and plan, implement, and evaluate hygiene care.

Skin. The neonate's skin is relatively immature at birth. The epidermis and dermis are loosely bound together, and the skin is very thin. Friction against the skin layers causes bruising. Handle the neonate carefully during bathing. Any break in the skin easily results in an infection.

A toddler's skin layers become more tightly bound together. Thus the child has a greater resistance to infection and skin irritation. However, because of his or her more active play and the absence of established hygiene habits, parents and caregivers need to provide thorough hygiene and teach good hygiene habits.

During adolescence the growth and maturation of the integument increases. In girls estrogen secretion causes the skin to become soft, smooth, and thicker with increased vascularity. In boys male hormones produce an increased thickness of the skin with some darkening in color. Sebaceous glands become more active, predisposing adolescents to acne (i.e., active inflammation of the sebaceous glands accompanied by pimples). Sweat glands become fully functional during puberty. Adolescents usually begin to use antiperspirants. More frequent bathing and shampooing also become necessary to reduce body odors and eliminate oily hair.

The condition of the adult's skin depends on hygiene practices and exposure to environmental irritants. Normally the skin is elastic, well hydrated, firm, and smooth. When an adult bathes frequently or is exposed to an environment with low humidity, it becomes dry and flaky. With aging the rate of epidermal cell replacement slows, and the skin thins and loses resiliency. Moisture leaves the skin, increasing the risk for bruising and other types of injury. As the production of lubricating substances from skin glands decreases, the skin becomes dry and itchy (Meiner, 2011). These changes warrant caution when turning and repositioning older adults and when bathing. Too-frequent bathing and bathing with hot water or harsh soap cause the skin to become excessively dry (American Academy of Dermatology, 2009).

Feet and Nails. With aging and continued exposure the patient is more likely to develop chronic foot problems as a result of poor foot care, improper fit of footwear, and systemic disease. Older adults do not always have the strength, flexibility, visual acuity, or manual dexterity to care for their feet and nails. Long or roughened nails lead to traumatic nail avulsions in which the nail plate is torn from the nail bed (Berridge, 2009).

Older adults often have dry feet because of a decrease in sebaceous gland secretion and dehydration of epidermal cells. Common problems of the feet affecting older adults include corns, calluses, bunions, hammertoe, and fungal infections (Wright, 2009). Older adults frequently complain of foot pain (Meiner, 2011). Painful feet result from a variety of congenital deformities, weak structure, injuries, and diseases such as diabetes and rheumatoid arthritis.

The Mouth. At approximately 6 to 8 months of age, infants begin teething. The first permanent (secondary) teeth erupt at about 6 years of age (Hockenberry and Wilson, 2011). From adolescence, when all of the permanent teeth are in place, through middle adulthood, the teeth and gums remain healthy if a person follows healthy eating patterns and dental care. Avoiding fermentable carbohydrates and sticky sweets helps to keep the teeth free of **caries.** In addition, regular brushing and flossing help to prevent caries and periodontal disease.

As a person ages, numerous factors result in poor oral health. These include age-related changes of the mouth, chronic disease such as diabetes, physical disabilities involving hand grasp or strength affecting the ability to perform oral care, lack of attention to oral care, and prescribed medications that have oral side effects. Gums lose vascularity and tissue elasticity, which causes dentures to fit poorly. If the older adult becomes **edentulous** (i.e., without teeth) and wears complete or partial dentures, include assessment of underlying gums and palate.

Hair. Throughout life changes in the growth, distribution, and condition of the hair influence hair hygiene. As males reach adolescence, shaving becomes a part of routine grooming. Young girls who reach puberty often begin to shave their legs and axillae. With aging, as scalp hair becomes thinner and drier, shampooing is usually performed less frequently.

Eyes, Ears, and Nose. Chapter 49 addresses changes in hearing, vision, and olfaction across the life span as a result of growth and development. Alterations in sensory function often require modifications in hygiene care. Use your knowledge of developmental changes when planning hygienic care.

Physical Condition. Patients with certain types of physical limitations or disabilities associated with disease and injury lack the physical energy and dexterity to perform hygiene self-care safely. A patient whose arm is in a cast or who has an IV line needs help with hygiene care. A weakened grasp resulting from arthritis, stroke, or muscular disorders makes using a toothbrush, washcloth, or hairbrush difficult or ineffective. Sensory deficits not only alter a patient's ability to perform care but also place the patient at risk for injury. Safety is a priority for a patient with a sensory deficit. For example, the inability to feel that the water is too hot can lead to a burn injury during bathing.

Chronic illnesses such as cardiac disease, cancer, neurological disorders, and some mental health illnesses often exhaust or incapacitate patients. Patients who become fatigued frequently need to have complete hygiene care provided. Include periods of rest during care to allow patients who are fatigued the opportunity to participate in their care. Pain often accompanies illness and injury, limiting a patient's ability to tolerate hygiene and grooming activities or perform self-care. Pain frequently limits ROM, resulting in impaired use of the arms or hands or limited ability to move about in the environment, impairing the ability to perform hygiene self-care. Sedation and drowsiness associated with analgesics used for pain management also limit a patient's ability to safely participate in care.

Limited mobility caused by a variety of factors (e.g., physical injury, weakness, surgery, pain, prolonged inactivity, medication effect, and presence of indwelling catheter or IV line) decreases a patient's ability to perform hygiene self-care activities safely. Individualized care considers a patient's ability to perform care, the amount of assistance needed, and the need for assistive and safety devices to facilitate safe hygiene care.

Acute and chronic cognitive impairments such as stroke, brain injury, psychoses, and dementia often result in the inability to perform self-care independently. When people with cognitive impairments are unaware of their hygiene and grooming needs, they become fearful and agitated during hygiene care, resulting in aggressive behavior (Hoeffer et al., 2006). Safe, effective patient care takes the effect of cognitive impairment on hygiene care into consideration and allows for appropriate modifications.

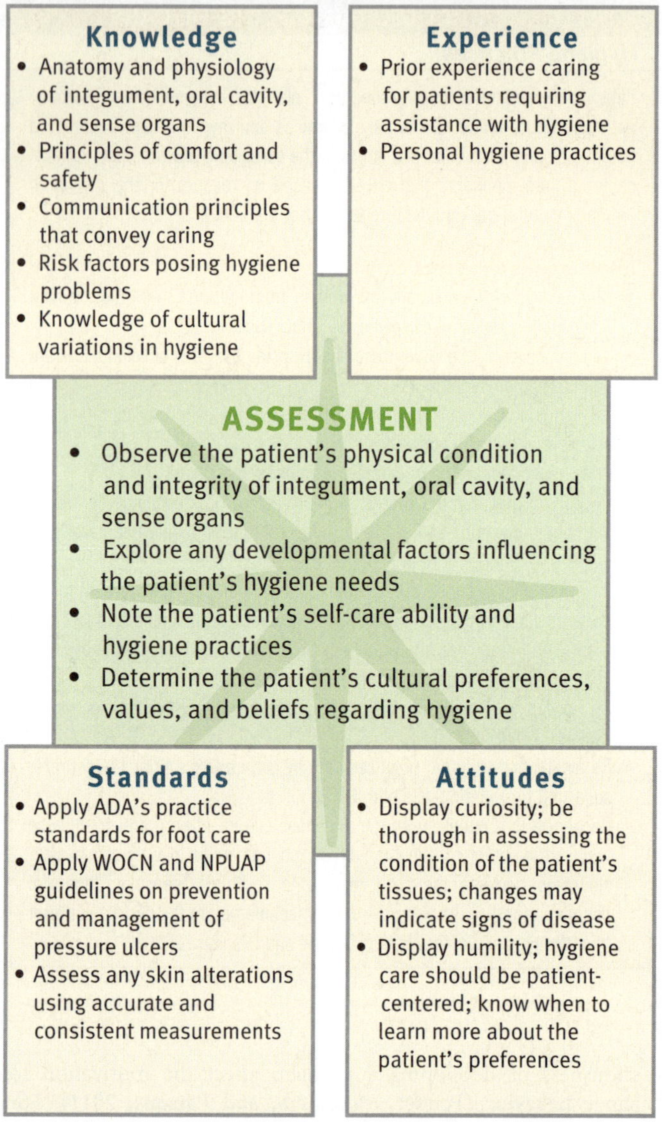

Knowledge
• Anatomy and physiology of integument, oral cavity, and sense organs
• Principles of comfort and safety
• Communication principles that convey caring
• Risk factors posing hygiene problems
• Knowledge of cultural variations in hygiene
Experience
• Prior experience caring for patients requiring assistance with hygiene
• Personal hygiene practices
ASSESSMENT
• Observe the patient's physical condition and integrity of integument, oral cavity, and sense organs
• Explore any developmental factors influencing the patient's hygiene needs
• Note the patient's self-care ability and hygiene practices
• Determine the patient's cultural preferences, values, and beliefs regarding hygiene
Standards
• Apply ADA's practice standards for foot care
• Apply WOCN and NPUAP guidelines on prevention and management of pressure ulcers
• Assess any skin alterations using accurate and consistent measurements
Attitudes
• Display curiosity; be thorough in assessing the condition of the patient's tissues; changes may indicate signs of disease
• Display humility; hygiene care should be patient-centered; know when to learn more about the patient's preferences

FIG. 39-1 Critical thinking model for hygiene assessment. *ADA,* American Diabetes Association; *NPUAP,* National Pressure Ulcer Advisory Panel; *WOCN,* Wound Ostomy Continence Nurses.

CRITICAL THINKING

Effective critical thinking requires synthesis of knowledge, experience, information gathered from patients, critical thinking attitudes, and intellectual and professional standards. Clinical judgments require you to anticipate the information necessary to analyze data and make decisions regarding care. A patient's condition is always changing, requiring ongoing critical thinking. During assessment consider all elements that build toward making appropriate nursing diagnoses (Fig. 39-1). Apply the elements of critical thinking as you use the nursing process to meet patients' hygiene needs.

Integrate nursing knowledge with knowledge from other disciplines. For example, the patient with diabetes mellitus has special needs for nail and foot care. Knowledge about the pathophysiology of diabetes and its potential effects on his or her peripheral circulation and sensory status provides the scientific knowledge base needed to implement safe and effective foot care. In addition, integrate knowledge about developmental and cultural influences as you identify and meet hygiene needs.

Be aware of the impact of critical thinking attitudes as you plan and implement care. For example, think creatively to help patients adapt existing hygiene practices or develop new hygiene practices when illness or loss of function impairs self-care abilities. Be nonjudgmental and confident when providing care. Because of variations in individual patients' physical status and hygiene practices, you need to approach care with an attitude of flexibility. For example, when caring for a patient who is fatigued, you pace activities and plan rest periods during hygiene care to prevent exhaustion.

Draw on your own experiences as you assist with your patients' hygiene care. Reflect on times when you helped family members or others close to you with their hygiene. Usually an early clinical experience involves providing or assisting with hygiene care for a patient. Finally rely on professional standards such as those for skin and foot care from the American Diabetes Association (ADA) and specialty nursing groups such as Wound Ostomy Continency Nurses (WOCN) when planning care to meet a patient's hygiene needs. As your experience and knowledge grow, your comfort and expertise in meeting the individualized hygiene needs of your patients increase.

NURSING PROCESS

Apply the nursing process and use a critical thinking approach in your care of patients. The nursing process provides a clinical decision-making approach for you to develop and implement an individualized plan of care.

ASSESSMENT

During the assessment process thoroughly assess each patient and critically analyze findings to ensure that you make patient-centered clinical decisions required for safe nursing care. Assessment of a patient's hygiene status and self-care abilities requires you to complete a nursing history and perform a physical assessment. You do not routinely assess all body regions before providing hygiene. However, you need to conduct a brief history to determine priority areas and help you plan individualized hygiene care. Assessment of a patient's ability to provide hygiene self-care helps you make decisions about the kind and amount of hygiene care to provide and how much the patient can be encouraged to participate in care.

Through the Patient's Eyes. Providing safe, quality hygiene care requires a complete awareness of the patient's perspective. Because patients have varying expectations, you need to avoid making personal hygiene care a simple routine. Complete a nursing history that not only elicits personal preferences but also addresses the patient's cultural or religious customs and beliefs.

Explore the patient's viewpoint regarding hygiene care by asking him or her about preferred personal hygiene and grooming practices. Ask about personal care products desired and preferences such as frequency, time of day, and amount of assistance needed. Also ask questions such as "To make you most comfortable and feel at home, how can I best perform your bath and personal care?" Determine the patient's awareness of any hygiene-related problems and his or her knowledge and ability to perform hygiene care measures (Box 39-2). Learning a patient's expectations and applying them in practice fosters a caring relationship. Fully individualizing hygiene care shows the nurse's respect for the patient's needs.

> **BOX 39-2 NURSING ASSESSMENT QUESTIONS**
>
> **Cultural and/or Religious Practices**
> - Do any cultural or religious practices affect your personal hygiene care?
> - How can I include these in your care?
>
> **Tolerance of Hygiene Activities**
> - Do hygiene activities cause any symptoms such as shortness of breath, pain, or fatigue?
> - What can I do to minimize these symptoms?
> - Which aspects of hygiene care worsen your discomfort or make you fatigued?
>
> **Assistance with Hygiene**
> - Do you use any aids to help you with your bath such as grab bars in your tub or shower?
> - Do you prefer someone of the same gender to assist in your hygiene care?
> - Which parts of personal hygiene can you do for yourself? With which parts of hygiene care do you need help?
>
> **Skin Care**
> - Which type of bath do you prefer?
> - How often and when do you usually bathe?
> - What kind of soap and lotion do you use?
> - Have you noticed any skin changes or irritation?
> - Do you have any known allergies or reactions to soaps, cosmetics, or skin care products?
>
> **Mouth Care**
> - Do you have any mouth pain or toothaches, or have you noticed any sores in your mouth?
> - Do you wear dentures or a partial plate?
>
> **Foot and Nail Care**
> - How do you usually care for your feet and nails? Do you soak your feet?
> - Do you file or trim your own fingernails and toenails?
>
> **Hair and Scalp Care**
> - Have you recently experienced itching of the scalp or noticed flaking or dandruff?
> - Have you noticed any changes in the texture or thickness of your hair?

As you learn what the patient expects, you incorporate this information into a plan of care.

Assessment of Self-Care Ability. Assess a patient's physical status as it relates to ability to perform or assist with hygiene care safely and efficiently; include assessment of the patient's muscle strength, flexibility, balance, visual acuity, and ability to detect thermal and tactile stimuli. Determine your patient's mental status, including orientation and cognitive function (see Chapter 30). The patient with impaired cognitive function may be unaware of hygiene care needs or less able to follow instructions and assist with care. Observe the patient performing hygiene care, noting complaints or physical manifestations that suggest activity intolerance. Assess respiratory rate and effort, skin color, and pulse rate. Ask questions to assess the patient for dizziness, weakness, or fatigue. To determine the amount of assistance the patient needs, observe him or her performing care activities such as brushing teeth or combing hair (Fig. 39-2). Patients who have limited upper-extremity mobility, reduced vision, fatigue, or inability to grasp small objects require assistance. For example, current evidence

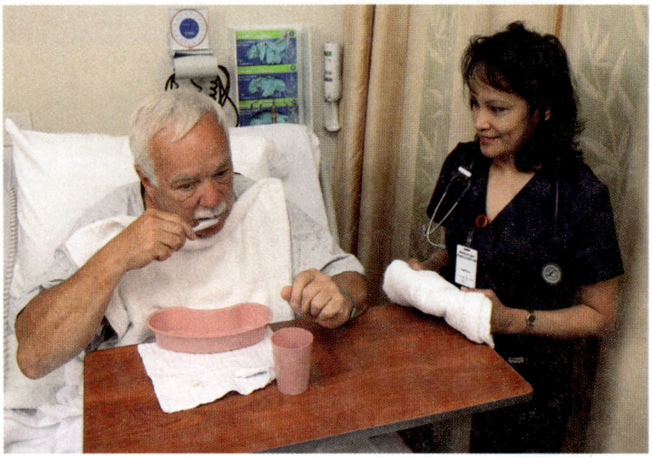

FIG. 39-2 The nurse observes the patient brushing teeth. During such observations the nurse can determine how much assistance the patient may need.

shows that older adults who have poor hand function have more dental plaque when they perform their own oral care (Padilha et al., 2007). Also note the presence of equipment such as IV lines or urinary catheters. When patients have self-care limitations, family may assist with care. Determine how the family can help the patient, how often they can provide this assistance, and what their feelings are about being caregivers. In addition, assess the home environment and its influence on the patient's hygiene practices. Are there barriers in the home that affect his or her self-care abilities? Water faucets that are too tight to adjust easily, bathtubs with high sides, and a bathroom too small to fit a chair in front of a sink are a few examples.

Assessment of the Skin. Perform an assessment of the skin (see Chapter 30), noting color, texture, thickness, turgor, temperature, and hydration. In the healthy person the skin is smooth, warm, and supple with good turgor. Pay special attention to the presence and condition of any lesions. Note dryness of the skin indicated by flaking, redness, scaling, and cracking. Discovering manifestations of common skin problems influences how you administer hygiene care (Table 39-2).

TABLE 39-2 Common Skin Problems

CHARACTERISTICS	IMPLICATIONS	INTERVENTIONS
Dry Skin		
Flaky, rough texture on exposed areas such as hands, arms, legs, or face	Skin becomes infected if epidermal layer cracks.	Bathe less frequently and rinse body of all soap because residue left on skin can cause irritation and breakdown. Add moisture to air with use of humidifier. Increase fluid intake when skin is dry. Use moisturizing cream to aid healing. (Cream forms protective barrier and helps maintain fluid within skin.) Use creams to clean skin that is dry or allergic to soaps and detergents.
Acne		
Inflammatory, papulopustular skin eruption, usually involving bacterial breakdown of sebum; appears on face, neck, shoulders, and back	Infected material within pustule spreads if area is squeezed or picked. Permanent scarring can result.	Wash hair and skin thoroughly each day with warm water and soap to remove oil. Use cosmetics sparingly because oily cosmetics or creams accumulate in pores and tend to make condition worse. Implement dietary restrictions if necessary. (Eliminate foods that aggravate condition from diet.) Use prescribed topical antibiotics for severe forms of acne.
Skin Rashes		
Skin eruptions that result from overexposure to sun or moisture or from allergic reaction (flat or raised, localized or systemic, pruritic or nonpruritic)	If skin is continually scratched, inflammation and infection may occur. Rashes also cause discomfort.	Wash area thoroughly and apply antiseptic spray or lotion to prevent further itching and aid in healing process. Apply warm or cold soaks to relieve inflammation if indicated.
Contact Dermatitis		
Inflammation of skin characterized by abrupt onset with erythema; pruritus; pain; and appearance of scaly, oozing lesions (seen on face, neck, hands, forearms, and genitalia)	Dermatitis is often difficult to eliminate because person is usually in continual contact with substance causing skin reaction. Substance is often hard to identify.	Avoid causative agents (e.g., cleansers and soaps).
Abrasion		
Scraping or rubbing away of epidermis that results in localized bleeding and later weeping of serous fluid	Infection occurs easily because of loss of protective skin layer.	Be careful not to scratch patient with jewelry or fingernails. Wash abrasions with mild soap and water; dry thoroughly and gently. Observe dressing or bandage for retained moisture because it increases risk of infection.

Determine the degree of cleanliness by observing the appearance of the skin and detecting body odors that possibly indicate inadequate cleansing or excessive perspiration caused by fever or pain. Inspect less obvious or difficult-to-reach skin surfaces such as under the breasts or scrotum, around the female patient's perineum, or in the groin for redness, excessive moisture, and soiling or debris. Separate skinfolds for observation and palpation.

Be attentive to characteristics of skin problems most influenced by hygiene measures. Is the skin dry from too much bathing or from use of hot water or irritating soap? Does the patient have a rash caused by an allergic reaction to a skin care product? Certain conditions place patients at risk for impaired skin integrity (Box 39-3). Because of increased risk be particularly alert when assessing patients with reduced sensation, impaired circulation, nutrition or hydration alterations, body secretions, incontinence, altered cognition, external devices, and decreased mobility. Patients may be unaware of skin problems because they are unable to feel pain or pressure or see their skin in some places (e.g., the back or the feet). Carefully assess the skin under orthopedic devices (braces, splints, casts) and beneath items such as antiembolic stockings and tape. Assess the condition and cleanliness of the perineal and anal areas during hygiene care and when the patient requires toileting assistance. When prolonged contact of urine or feces occurs such as with diarrhea or incontinence, skin breakdown often results. Most people consider these areas to be private. Use sensitivity in your approach.

When caring for patients with dark skin pigmentation, be aware of assessment techniques and skin characteristics unique to highly pigmented skin (see Chapter 30). Carefully assess the skin in dark-skinned patients at risk for pressure ulcers (see Chapter 48).

Assessment of the Feet and Nails. A variety of common foot and nail problems can be caused by inadequate hygiene and are actually detected during hygiene care. Problems sometimes result from abuse or poor care of the feet and hands such as nail biting or trimming nails improperly, exposure to harsh chemicals, and wearing poorly fitting shoes. Question the patient to determine type of footwear and usual foot and nail care practices.

Examine all skin surfaces of the feet, including the areas between the toes and over the entire sole of the foot. Poorly fitting shoes often irritate the heels, soles, and sides of the feet. Inspection of the feet for lesions includes noting areas of dryness, inflammation, or cracking. Chronic foot problems are common in older adults who often experience dry feet because of a decrease in sebaceous gland secretion, dehydration, or poor condition of footwear.

People are often unaware of foot or nail problems until pain or discomfort occurs. Assess patients with diseases that affect peripheral circulation and sensation for the adequacy of circulation and sensation of the feet. Foot ulceration is the most common single precursor to lower-extremity amputations among people with diabetes (Frykberg et al., 2006). Daily inspection and preventive foot care help maintain ulcer-free feet. Palpate the dorsalis pedis and posterior tibial pulses and assess for intact sensation to light touch, pinprick, and temperature (see Chapter 30).

Observe the patient's gait. Painful foot disorders or decreased sensation cause limping or an unnatural gait. Ask whether the patient has foot discomfort and determine factors that aggravate the pain. Foot problems sometimes result from bone or muscular alterations or wearing poorly fitting footwear.

Inspect the condition of the fingernails and toenails, looking for lesions, dryness, inflammation, or cracking, which are often associated with a variety of common nail problems (Table 39-3). The cuticle that surrounds the nail can grow over it and become inflamed if nail care is not performed correctly and periodically. Ask women whether they frequently polish their nails and use polish remover because chemicals in these products cause excessive nail dryness. Disease changes the shape and curvature of the nails (see Chapter 30). Inflammatory lesions and fungus of the nail bed cause thickened, horny nails that separate from the nail bed.

Assessment of the Oral Cavity. The condition of the oral cavity reflects overall health and also indicates oral hygiene needs. Inspect all areas of the mouth carefully for color, hydration, texture, and lesions (see Chapter 30). Patients frequently develop common oral problems as a result of inadequate oral care or consequence of disease (e.g., oral malignancy) or as a side effect of treatments such as radiation and chemotherapy. These problems include receding gum tissue, inflamed gums (gingivitis), a coated tongue, **glossitis** (inflamed tongue), discolored teeth (particularly along gum margins), dental caries, missing teeth, and **halitosis** (foul-smelling breath). Localized pain and infection commonly accompany oral problems. Apply clean gloves to palpate any tender areas or lesions. Observe for cleanliness and use olfaction to detect halitosis. If you

BOX 39-3 RISK FACTORS FOR SKIN IMPAIRMENT

Immobilization

When restricted from moving freely, dependent body parts are exposed to pressure that reduces circulation to affected tissues. Know which patients require help to turn and change positions.

Reduced Sensation

Patients with paralysis, circulatory insufficiency, or local nerve damage are unable to sense an injury to the skin. During a bath assess the status of sensory nerve function by checking for pain, tactile sensation, and temperature sensation.

Nutrition and Hydration Alterations

Patients with limited caloric and protein intake develop thinner, less elastic skin with loss of subcutaneous tissue, which results in impaired or delayed wound healing.

Secretions and Excretions on the Skin

Moisture on the surface of the skin serves as a medium for bacterial growth and causes irritation, softens epidermal cells, and leads to skin maceration. Presence of perspiration, urine, watery fecal material, and wound drainage on the skin results in breakdown and infection.

Vascular Insufficiency

Inadequate arterial supply to tissues and impaired venous return decrease circulation to the extremities. Inadequate blood flow causes ischemia and breakdown. Risk of infection also exists because delivery of nutrients, oxygen, and white blood cells to injured tissues is inadequate.

External Devices

An external device applied to or around the skin exerts pressure or friction on the skin. Assess all surfaces exposed to casts, cloth restraints, bandages and dressings, tubing, or orthopedic braces.

Altered Cognition

Patients who have decreased level of awareness as a result of altered thought processes may be unaware of or unable to verbalize their skin care needs. They may not realize the effect of pressure or prolonged contact with secretions or excretions. Be extra vigilant for warning signs of skin breakdown and provide preventive hygiene care.

TABLE 39-3 Common Foot and Nail Problems

CHARACTERISTICS	IMPLICATIONS	INTERVENTIONS
Callus		
Thickened portion of epidermis consists of mass of horny, keratotic cells. Callus is usually flat, painless, and found on undersurface of foot or palm of hand.	Local friction or pressure causes callus formation, which causes discomfort when wearing tight shoes.	Soft-sole shoes with insoles are recommended. Advise patient to wear gloves when using tools or objects that create friction on palmar surfaces. Advise patients, especially with callus formation, not to self-treat but seek interventions from a podiatrist.
Corns		
Friction and pressure from ill-fitting or loose shoes causes keratosis. It is seen mainly on or between toes, over bony prominence. Corn is usually cone shaped, round, and raised. Soft corns are macerated.	Compresses the underlying dermis, making it thin and tender. Pain is aggravated when wearing tight shoes. Tissue becomes attached to bone if allowed to grow. Patient suffers alteration in gait resulting from pain.	Surgical removal is necessary, depending on severity of pain and size of corn. Avoid use of oval corn pads, which increase pressure on toes and reduce circulation. Warm water soaks soften corns before gentle rubbing with a callus file or pumice stone (consult with health care provider). Wider and softer shoes, especially shoes with a wider toe box, are helpful.
Plantar Warts		
Fungating lesion appears on sole of foot and is caused by the papilloma virus.	Some warts are contagious. They are painful and make walking difficult.	Treatment ordered by health care provider often includes applications of salicylic acid, electrodessication (burning with electrical spark), or freezing with solid carbon dioxide.
Athlete's Foot (Tinea Pedis)		
Athlete's foot is fungal infection of foot; scaling and cracking of skin occurs between toes and on soles of feet. Small blisters containing fluid appear.	Athlete's foot spreads to other body parts, especially hands. It is contagious and frequently recurs.	Make sure that feet are well ventilated. Drying feet well after bathing and applying powder help prevent infection. Wearing clean socks or stockings reduces incidence. Health care provider orders application of griseofulvin, miconazole, or tolnaftate.
Ingrown Nails		
Toenail or fingernail grows inward into soft tissue around nail. Ingrown nail often results from improper nail trimming.	Ingrown nails cause localized pain when pressure is applied.	Treatment is frequent hot soaks in antiseptic solution and removal of part of nail that has grown into skin. Instruct patient in proper nail-trimming techniques and refer to podiatrist.
Foot Odors		
Foot odors are result of excess perspiration, promoting microorganism growth.	Condition causes discomfort because of excess perspiration.	Frequent washing, use of foot deodorants and powders, and wearing clean footwear prevent or reduce problem.

identify any oral problems, notify the patient's health care provider. Early identification of poor oral hygiene practices and common oral problems reduces the risk for gum disease and dental caries.

Assessment of the Hair and Hair Care. Before performing hair care, assess the condition of the patient's hair and scalp. Findings help determine the frequency and type of care needed. Normally the hair is clean, shiny, and untangled; and the scalp is clear of lesions. Table 39-4 summarizes hair and scalp problems with implications and interventions.

Observe the patient's ability to perform hair care. A person's appearance and feeling of well-being often are related to the way the hair looks and feels. Illness, disability, and conditions such as arthritis, fatigue, and the presence of physical barriers (e.g., cast or IV access) alter a patient's ability to maintain daily hair care.

In community health and home care settings it is particularly important to inspect the hair for lice so you can provide appropriate hygienic treatment. If you suspect **pediculosis capitis** (head lice), guard against self-infestations by handwashing and using gloves or tongue blades to inspect the patient's hair.

The loss of hair **(alopecia)** results from the effects of chemotherapy medications, hormonal changes, or improper hair care practices. Alopecia often appears as brittle and broken hair in the hair line that progresses to bald patches. If noted, be sure to question the patient about specific hair care practices, especially the use of chemicals and heat application during hair care.

Assessment of the Eyes, Ears, and Nose. Examine the condition and function of the eyes, ears, and nose (see Chapter 30). The healthy eye is not inflamed and is without drainage. The presence of redness indicates allergic or infectious conjunctivitis, which can be highly contagious. The crusty drainage associated with conjunctivitis easily spreads from one eye to the other. Wear clean gloves to examine the eyes and perform proper hand hygiene before and after the examination. Determine if a patient wears contact lenses, especially when he or she enters the health care agency in an unresponsive or confused state. To determine if a contact lens is present, stand to the side of the patient's eyes and observe the corneas for the presence of a soft or rigid lens. Also observe the sclera because the lens may have shifted off the cornea. An undetected contact lens causes corneal injury when left in place too long.

Assessment of the external ear structures includes inspection of the auricle and external ear canal (see Chapter 30). Observe for the presence of accumulated **cerumen** (earwax) or drainage in the ear

TABLE 39-4 Hair and Scalp Problems

CHARACTERISTICS	IMPLICATIONS	INTERVENTIONS
Dandruff		
Scaling of scalp is accompanied by itching. In severe cases dandruff is on eyebrows.	Dandruff causes person embarrassment. If it enters eyes, conjunctivitis often develops.	Shampoo regularly with medicated shampoo. In severe cases obtain health care provider's advice.
Ticks		
Small, gray-brown parasites burrow into skin and suck blood.	Ticks transmit several diseases to people. Most common are Rocky Mountain spotted fever, tularemia, and Lyme disease.	Using blunt tweezers, grasp tick as close to the head as possible and pull upward with even, steady pressure. Hold until tick pulls out, usually for about 3-4 minutes. Save tick in plastic bag and put in freezer if it is necessary to identify type of tick.
Pediculosis (Lice)		
Pediculosis Capitis (Head Lice)		
Parasite resides on scalp attached to hair strands. Eggs look like oval particles, similar to dandruff. Bites or pustules may be observed behind ears and at hairline.	Head lice are difficult to remove and spread to furniture and other people if not treated. They do not carry disease, cannot fly or jump, and are carried by animals.	Wearing gloves, check entire scalp by using a tongue depressor or special lice comb. Use medicated shampoo for eliminating lice. *Caution against use of products containing lindane because the ingredient is toxic and known to cause adverse reactions* (CDC, 2008). Manual removal is best option when treatment has failed. Vacuum infested areas of home.
Pediculosis Corporis (Body Lice)		
Parasites tend to cling to clothing; thus they are not always easy to see. Body lice suck blood and lay eggs on clothing and furniture.	Patient itches constantly. Scratches seen on skin become infected. Hemorrhagic spots appear on skin where lice are sucking blood.	Bathe or shower thoroughly. After skin is dried, apply recommended pediculicide lotion. After 12 to 24 hours take another bath or shower. Bag infested clothing or linen until laundered in hot water. Vacuum rooms thoroughly and throw away bag after completion.
Pediculosis Pubis (Crab Lice)		
Parasites are in pubic hair. Crab lice are gray-white with red legs.	Lice spread through bed linen, clothing, or furniture or between people via sexual contact.	Shave hair off affected area. Clean as for body lice. If lice were sexually transmitted, notify partner.
Hair Loss (Alopecia)		
Alopecia occurs in all races. Balding patches are in periphery of hair line. Hair becomes brittle and broken.	Patches of uneven hair growth and loss alter patient's appearance.	Stop hair care practices that damage hair. The use of hair curlers, hair picks, tight braiding, and hot comb contributes to hair-loss condition.

canal and local inflammation. Question patients about tenderness on palpation or the presence of pain and ask how they usually clean their ears.

Inspect the nares for signs of inflammation, discharge, lesions, edema, and deformity (see Chapter 30). The nasal mucosa is normally pink and clear and has little or no discharge. Allergies cause a clear, watery discharge. If patients have any form of tubing exiting the nose (e.g., nasogastric), observe for tissue damage, localized tenderness, inflammation, drainage, and bleeding where the tubing comes in contact with the nares..

Use of Sensory Aids. For patients who wear eyeglasses, contact lenses, artificial eyes, or hearing aids, assess their knowledge and methods used for care and have them describe the typical approach used in routine care. When possible observe the patient performing care. Compare information gathered from him or her with the proper care technique for these devices. Any difference between patient and standard practice provides an opportunity for patient education.

Assessment of Hygiene Care Practices. Assessment of hygiene practices reveals the patient's preferences for grooming. For example, a patient chooses to groom the hair in a certain style or trim nails in a certain way. When a patient has a physical disability, special precautions may be necessary to perform grooming without injury. For example, teach patients with loss of sensation to file nails instead of clipping. By observing the patient perform hygiene care, you can detect any needed areas of teaching or assistance while maintaining the patient's maximal level of independence.

Assessment of Cultural Influences. A patient's cultural background influences hygiene needs. Culture plays a role not only in hygiene practices and preferences but also in sensitivity to personal space and gender sensitivity (see Box 39-1 and Chapter 9). Ask what makes the patient feel most comfortable during a bath. Perhaps he or she prefers a partial instead of a full bath from the nurse, with a family member completing the bathing of more private body parts. Some patients also defer part of hygiene. If you believe that hygiene is critical to prevent developing or worsening problems such as skin breakdown, take the time to understand the patient's concerns and then offer an explanation that helps him or her accept your intervention.

Patients at Risk for Hygiene Problems. Some patients present risks that require more attentive and rigorous hygiene care (Table 39-5). These risks result from side effects of medications or other medical therapy; a lack of knowledge; immobilization; an inability to perform hygiene; or a physical condition that potentially injures the skin, mouth, feet and nails, or hair. Anticipate whether a patient is predisposed to risks and follow through with a complete assessment. For example, if a patient is receiving cancer chemotherapy, there is a risk of the medication producing ulcerations of the mouth, which are painful and create a risk for infection and impaired nutrition because of reluctance to eat and drink.

TABLE 39-5 Risk Factors for Hygiene Problems

RISKS	HYGIENE IMPLICATIONS
Oral Problems	
Patients who are unable to use upper extremities because of paralysis, weakness, or restriction (e.g., cast, dressing)	Patient lacks upper-extremity strength or dexterity needed to brush teeth (Lewis et al., 2011).
Dehydration, inability to take fluids or food by mouth (NPO)	Dehydration causes excess drying and fragility of mucosa; increases accumulation of secretions on tongue and gums.
Presence of nasogastric or oxygen tubes; mouth breathers	Tubes cause drying of mucosa and lips.
Chemotherapeutic drugs	Drugs kill rapidly multiplying cells, including normal cells lining oral cavity. Ulcers and inflammation develop.
Lozenges, cough drops, antacids, and chewable over-the-counter vitamins	Medications contain large amounts of sugar. Repeated use increases sugar or acid content in mouth, causing dental caries.
Radiation therapy to head and neck	Radiation therapy reduces salivary flow and lowers pH of saliva; leads to stomatitis and tooth decay (Lewis et al., 2011).
Oral surgery, trauma to mouth, placement of oral airway	These cause trauma to oral cavity with swelling, ulcerations, inflammation, and bleeding.
Immunosuppression; altered blood clotting	These predispose to inflammation and bleeding gums.
Diabetes mellitus	Patients are prone to dryness of mouth, gingivitis, periodontal disease, and loss of teeth.
Endotracheal intubation with mechanical ventilation	Potential for ventilator-associated pneumonia (VAP) exists. Use of chlorhexidine reduces risk of VAP. Chlorhexidine is an inexpensive effective agent for reducing VAP, especially in patients who have heart surgery (Berry et al., 2007).
Dialysis	Oral problems commonly found in these patients include halitosis, xerostomia (dry mouth), gingivitis, stomatitis, tooth decay, tooth loss, and jaw problems. Causes include decreased saliva production, uremia, and inattention to care (Gonyea, 2009).
Skin Problems	
Immobilization	Dependent body parts are exposed to pressure from underlying surfaces. The inability to turn or change position increases risk for pressure ulcers.
Reduced sensation caused by stroke, spinal cord injury, diabetes, local nerve damage	Patient does not receive normal transmission of nerve impulses when applying excessive heat or cold, pressure, friction, or chemical irritants to skin.
Limited protein or caloric intake and reduced hydration (e.g., fever, burns, gastrointestinal alterations, poorly fitting dentures)	Limited caloric and protein intake predispose to impaired tissue synthesis. Skin becomes thinner, less elastic, and smoother with a loss of subcutaneous tissue. Poor wound healing results. Reduced hydration impairs skin turgor.
Excessive secretions or excretions on skin from perspiration, urine, watery fecal material, and wound drainage	Moisture is a medium for bacterial growth and causes local skin irritation, softening of epidermal cells, and skin maceration.
Presence of external devices (e.g., cast, restraint, bandage, dressing)	Device exerts pressure or friction against surface of skin.
Vascular insufficiency	Arterial blood supply to tissues is inadequate, or venous return is impaired, causing decreased circulation to extremities. Tissue ischemia and breakdown often occur. Risk for infection is high.
Foot Problems	
Patient unable to bend over or has reduced visual acuity	Patient is unable to fully visualize entire surface of each foot, impairing ability to adequately assess condition of skin and nails.
Eye Care Problems	
Reduced dexterity and hand coordination	Physical limitations create inability to safely insert or remove contact lenses.

A patient who receives broad-spectrum antibiotics develops an opportunistic infection when the normal flora of the mouth is disrupted by the antibiotic. These examples demonstrate the need to identify patients at risk and be thorough and detailed during the oral examination, checking all surfaces of the tongue and mucosa. For a patient who is diaphoretic, provide special attention to body areas such as beneath the woman's breasts and in the groin and perineal area, where moisture collects and irritates skin surfaces. Anticipate problems created by these risks to provide preventive care. Assessment includes a review of the patient's medical and surgical history, medications, and the specific risk factors that the patient presents.

NURSING DIAGNOSIS

Thorough assessment of a patient's hygiene status and self-care abilities identifies clusters of data or defining characteristics that support actual or at-risk hygiene-related diagnoses. Identification of the defining characteristics leads you to select the NANDA International diagnostic label that best communicates the individual

BOX 39-4 NURSING DIAGNOSTIC PROCESS

Bathing Self-Care Deficit

ASSESSMENT ACTIVITIES	FINDINGS/DEFINING CHARACTERISTICS
Observe patient attempt to bathe self.	Patient is unable to wash lower body, back, or perineal area.
Assess patient's upper-extremity strength and range of motion.	Patient has restricted upper-extremity range of motion and weakness and is unable to turn water faucets on and off.
Observe patient's ability to move from bed to bathroom and to maneuver in bathroom.	Patient cannot transfer from bed to chair without assistance, cannot ambulate, relies on wheelchair to move around, is unable to maneuver the wheelchair in the bathroom without help or transfer to shower seat unassisted.

patient's situation. For example, when caring for an older adult with degenerative arthritis you observe swollen joints, weakness, and limited ROM in the dominant hand along with a generally unkempt appearance. Closer review of data reveals defining characteristics of an inability to wash body parts and difficulty turning and regulating a water faucet. The nursing diagnosis of *bathing self-care deficit* becomes part of the plan of care. Accurate selection of nursing diagnoses requires critical thinking to identify actual or potential problems. Be thorough in assessment to reveal all appropriate defining characteristics so you can make an accurate diagnosis (Box 39-4).

Use a patient's actual alteration (e.g., *impaired tissue integrity)* or the alteration for which the patient is at risk (e.g., *risk for infection)* to determine the focus of nursing interventions. The patient with an actual alteration requires extensive hygiene care, often more thorough than routine hygiene. For example, if a patient has skin breakdown, initiate care more frequently to keep skin surfaces clean and dry and eliminate factors such as moisture or drainage that worsen skin condition. Also provide care to promote healing of injured skin surfaces (see Chapter 48). If the patient is at risk for a problem, take preventive measures. For example, if a patient is at risk for developing an infection in his or her mouth and has the nursing diagnosis *risk for infection,* keep the mucosa well hydrated, minimize foods irritating to tissues, and provide cleaning that soothes and reduces tissue inflammation.

Completing a nursing diagnosis requires identification of the related factor, which will guide your selection of nursing interventions. A diagnosis of *impaired oral mucous membrane related to malnutrition* and a diagnosis of *impaired oral mucous membrane related to chemical trauma* require different interventions. When poor nutrition is a causal factor, you need to consult with a dietitian for appropriate dietary supplements and incorporate patient education into the plan. When chemotherapy injures the oral mucosa, you follow cancer nursing guidelines regarding care for oral **mucositis** (i.e., painful inflammation of oral mucous membranes), including frequent gentle brushing with soft toothbrush, flossing, rinsing with bland rinse, limiting diet to soft foods, and applying water-based moisturizer to lips (Harris et al., 2008). Although many possible nursing diagnoses apply to patients in need of supportive hygiene care, the following list represents examples of diagnoses commonly associated with hygiene problems:

- Activity intolerance
- Bathing self-care deficit

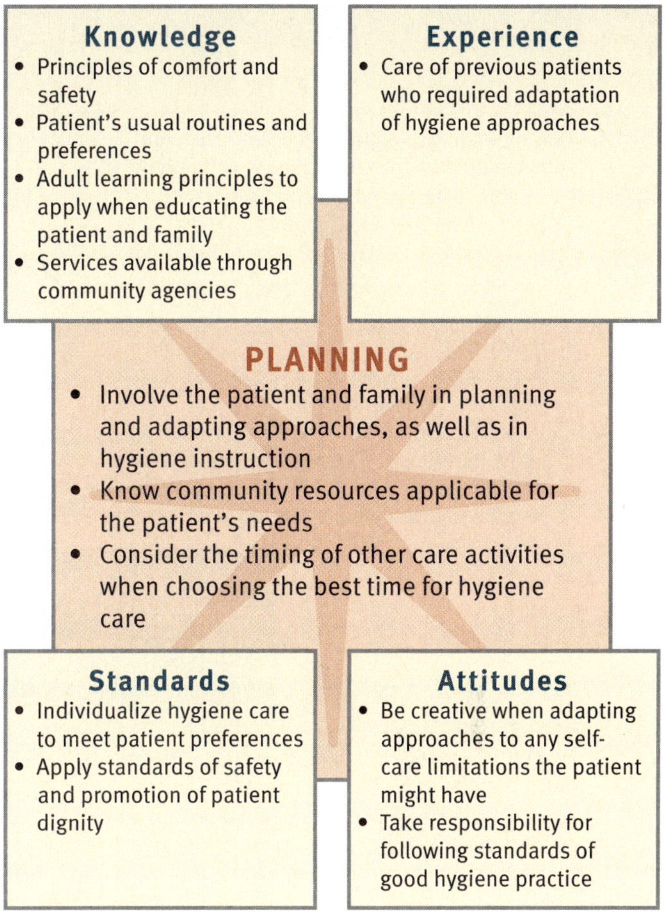

Knowledge
• Principles of comfort and safety
• Patient's usual routines and preferences
• Adult learning principles to apply when educating the patient and family
• Services available through community agencies
Experience
• Care of previous patients who required adaptation of hygiene approaches
PLANNING
• Involve the patient and family in planning and adapting approaches, as well as in hygiene instruction
• Know community resources applicable for the patient's needs
• Consider the timing of other care activities when choosing the best time for hygiene care
Standards
• Individualize hygiene care to meet patient preferences
• Apply standards of safety and promotion of patient dignity
Attitudes
• Be creative when adapting approaches to any self-care limitations the patient might have
• Take responsibility for following standards of good hygiene practice

FIG. 39-3 Critical thinking model for hygiene planning.

- Dressing self-care deficit
- Impaired physical mobility
- Impaired oral mucous membrane
- Ineffective health maintenance
- Risk for infection

PLANNING

During planning synthesize information from multiple resources (Fig. 39-3). Critical thinking ensures that a patient's plan of care integrates all that is known about the individual patient and key critical thinking elements. In many situations patients present with multiple nursing diagnoses. Use a concept map (Fig. 39-4) to visualize how nursing diagnoses interrelate. Rely on knowledge, experience, and established standards of care when developing the care plan. Remember critical thinking attitudes such as creativity when developing a patient-centered plan for hygiene care. Consciously include the patient in this important step of the nursing process. Identify patient goals and outcomes, set priorities for care, and select evidence-based interventions. Consider continuity of care and involve other health care team members (e.g., occupational or physical therapy) when developing the plan.

Previous experience with other patients is useful in knowing how to adapt hygiene techniques for special needs. Professional standards guide selection of the most effective nursing interventions. These standards often establish evidence-based guidelines for care.

Goals and Outcomes. Partner with the patient and family to identify goals and expected outcomes and develop an

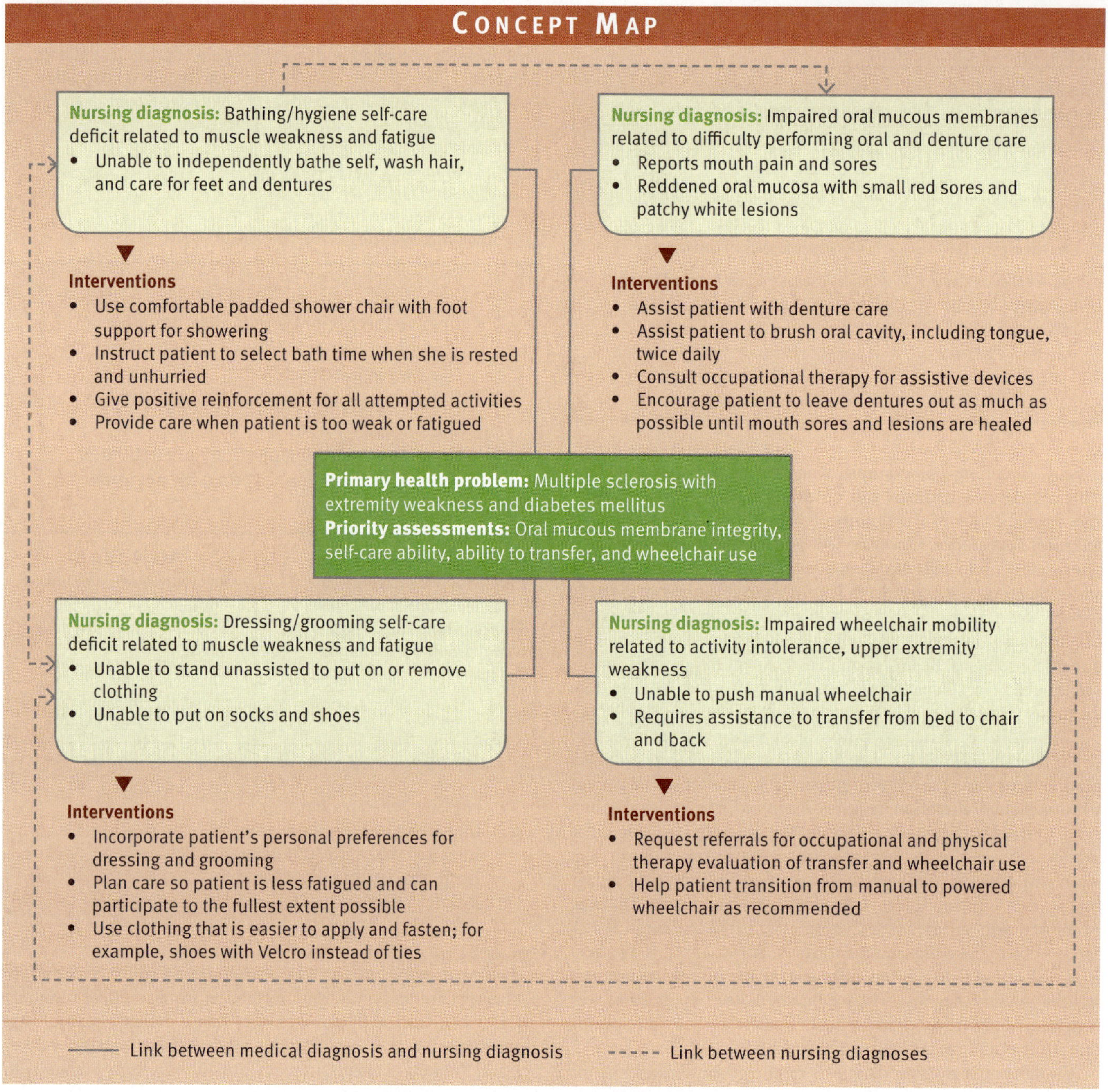
CONCEPT MAP
Nursing diagnosis: Bathing/hygiene self-care deficit related to muscle weakness and fatigue
• Unable to independently bathe self, wash hair, and care for feet and dentures
Interventions
• Use comfortable padded shower chair with foot support for showering
• Instruct patient to select bath time when she is rested and unhurried
• Give positive reinforcement for all attempted activities
• Provide care when patient is too weak or fatigued
Nursing diagnosis: Impaired oral mucous membranes related to difficulty performing oral and denture care
• Reports mouth pain and sores
• Reddened oral mucosa with small red sores and patchy white lesions
Interventions
• Assist patient with denture care
• Assist patient to brush oral cavity, including tongue, twice daily
• Consult occupational therapy for assistive devices
• Encourage patient to leave dentures out as much as possible until mouth sores and lesions are healed
Primary health problem: Multiple sclerosis with extremity weakness and diabetes mellitus
Priority assessments: Oral mucous membrane integrity, self-care ability, ability to transfer, and wheelchair use
Nursing diagnosis: Dressing/grooming self-care deficit related to muscle weakness and fatigue
• Unable to stand unassisted to put on or remove clothing
• Unable to put on socks and shoes
Interventions
• Incorporate patient's personal preferences for dressing and grooming
• Plan care so patient is less fatigued and can participate to the fullest extent possible
• Use clothing that is easier to apply and fasten; for example, shoes with Velcro instead of ties
Nursing diagnosis: Impaired wheelchair mobility related to activity intolerance, upper extremity weakness
• Unable to push manual wheelchair
• Requires assistance to transfer from bed to chair and back
Interventions
• Request referrals for occupational and physical therapy evaluation of transfer and wheelchair use
• Help patient transition from manual to powered wheelchair as recommended
Link between medical diagnosis and nursing diagnosis
Link between nursing diagnoses

FIG. 39-4 Concept map for Mrs. Winkler.

individualized plan of care based on the patient's nursing diagnoses (see the Nursing Care Plan). For example, establish goals with the patient's self-care abilities and resources in mind and focus on maintaining or improving the condition of the skin and oral cavity. Make outcomes measurable and achievable within patient limitations. In addition, work with the patient to select individualized hygiene measures.

When providing for patient hygiene, you care for a variety of patients with different self-care abilities and needs. For example, the nurse and a patient who has one-sided paralysis following a cerebral vascular accident develop the following goal: "Patient's skin remains free of breakdown." Then the nurse establishes a series of realistic, individualized expected outcomes to measure the patient's progress toward meeting this goal. These outcomes may include the following:

- Patient's skin is clean, dry, and intact without signs of inflammation.
- Patients' skin remains elastic and well hydrated.
- Patient's skin is free from areas of pressure.

Setting Priorities. The patient's condition influences your priorities for hygiene care. Set priorities based on the necessary assistance required by the patient, the extent of the hygiene-related problems, and the nature of the patient's nursing diagnoses. For example, a seriously ill patient usually needs a daily bath because body secretions accumulate and the patient is unable to independently maintain cleanliness. Some older patients at home require

NURSING CARE PLAN

Impaired Oral Mucous Membrane

ASSESSMENT

Mrs. Winkler is a 58-year-old woman admitted recently to an extended care nursing facility with a medical history of multiple sclerosis and diabetes mellitus. She uses a wheelchair for mobility. She recently became weaker, is now unable to push the chair herself, and requires assistance with transferring to and from the chair. She has both upper- and lower-extremity weakness. She wears full dentures. Jamie Johnson is a nursing student assigned to care for Mrs. Winkler today. As Jamie is talking with Mrs. Winkler before breakfast is served, she learns that Mrs. Winkler likes to wash her face and hands and then put in her dentures. Mrs. Winkler states, "I want to stay in bed today because I'm tired and I don't feel well. I just get so weak when I do anything. Also, I think I have sores on the roof of my mouth. They really hurt."

Assessment Activities	*Findings/Defining Characteristics**
Ask Mrs. Winkler what care is important this morning.	Mrs. Winkler says, "I want to be able to wear my teeth and feel clean and look nice."
Assess the condition of Mrs. Winkler's oral cavity.	Mrs. Winkler **reports mouth pain and sores.** On visual inspection, Jamie observes generalized **reddened oral mucosa** with small **red sores** and **patchy white lesions** most notable on the roof of the mouth; thick secretions **coating** the gums, cheeks, and tongue; and some **bleeding** from the **inflamed, swollen tissues.** Jamie detects **halitosis.**
Assess Mrs. Winkler's ability to bathe and perform oral hygiene care, including an assessment of her range of motion and upper-extremity strength.	Mrs. Winkler states, "I have trouble holding my arms up above my waist, and I have trouble holding my brush or small things. My muscles are just so weak. I get so tired doing anything." Unable to raise arms over head with restricted shoulder range of motion to flexion of 90 degrees and upper extremity muscle strength 2/5.

*__Defining characteristics__ are shown in bold type.

NURSING DIAGNOSIS: Impaired oral mucous membrane related to difficulty performing oral and denture care associated with upper-extremity weakness

PLANNING

Goals	*Expected Outcomes (NOC)*†
	Knowledge: Illness Care
Mrs. Winkler will verbalize preventive and routine oral and denture care by discharge.	Mrs. Winkler will state importance of reporting signs and symptoms, including mouth tenderness and discomfort, sores, dry mouth, and presence of coating, within 2 days. Mrs. Winkler will describe correct preventive oral hygiene care practices within 1 week.
	Oral Hygiene
Mrs. Winkler will have return of intact oral mucosa within 1 week.	Mrs. Winkler's oral mucosa will be moist and free of thick coating and sores within 1 week. Mrs. Winkler's oral cavity will be odor free within 2 days. Mrs. Winkler will report mouth feels clean within 1 day.

†Outcome classification labels from Moorhead S, et al: *Nursing outcomes classification (NOC),* ed 4, St Louis, 2008, Mosby.

INTERVENTIONS (NIC)‡	RATIONALE
Oral Health Restoration	
Provide oral care at least twice a day, cleaning for a minimum of 90 seconds with a soft-bristled toothbrush or toothette. Explain importance of oral care and problems to report to health care provider during care.	Stimulates gums and cleans oral cavity. Recommended oral care protocol for mucositis (Harris et al., 2008). Provides patient education during routine care to enhance learning.
Assist Mrs. Winkler with rinsing mouth 4 times a day with a bland rinse (normal saline, sodium bicarbonate, or mixture of saline and sodium bicarbonate).	Rinses remove loose debris and aid in oral hydration. Sodium bicarbonate reduces acidity of oral fluids, dilutes accumulating mucus, and discourages yeast colonization (Harris et al., 2008).
Remove, clean, and do not replace dentures except for meals (if desired).	Promotes healing during cases of mild-to-moderate stomatitis (Sciubba, 2009).
Refer for dental appointment to check fit of dentures and possibility of denture-induced stomatitis.	Denture-induced stomatitis is related in part to dentures that fit poorly, especially if worn while sleeping (Sciubba, 2009).
Carefully observe oral mucosa at least twice daily, noting worsening of manifestations.	Monitor effectiveness of treatment and patient progress toward goal.

‡Intervention classification labels from Bulechek GM, Butcher HK, and Dochterman JM: *Nursing interventions classification (NIC),* ed 5, St Louis, 2008, Mosby.

Continued

NURSING CARE PLAN

Impaired Oral Mucous Membrane—cont'd

EVALUATION

Nursing Actions	Patient Response/Finding	Achievement of Outcome
Ask Mrs. Winkler about importance of reporting signs and symptoms.	Mrs. Winkler states that she now realizes that her oral discomfort and sores may be related to how she cares for her dentures and that she will report these if they recur.	Able to participate in prevention of oral problems by reporting signs and symptoms indicating a problem.
Ask Mrs. Winkler about preventive oral care.	Mrs. Winkler lists the steps that she needs to take to prevent the recurrence of oral problems. She states, "I will now always take my teeth out at night so they can soak and clean. Until my mouth sores are gone I will only wear my dentures when eating."	Although Mrs. Winkler does not currently have the ability to perform her own care, she is involved in care by requesting oral and denture care.
Assess Mrs. Winkler's oral cavity.	Mrs. Winkler's oral cavity mucosa is pink, moist, and not swollen; no lesions or sores are present. No odor is detected. No coating is observed.	Inflammation and infection in the mouth are resolved.

a visit from a home care aide to help with a tub bath or shower. Patients who are normally inactive during the day and have skin that tends to be dry may need to bathe only twice a week, whereas a patient with urinary and bowel incontinence needs perineal cleaning with each episode of soiling. Plan for necessary assistance for patients who are weakened or possess poor coordination. For example, a patient who is partially paralyzed and has difficulty getting out of a tub needs a tub chair, handrails, or extra personnel available for help.

Timing is also important in planning hygiene care. Being interrupted in the middle of a bath often frustrates and embarrasses the patient.

Teamwork and Collaboration. Plan for care throughout the stay in a hospital, including discharge to a rehabilitation facility or home. In hospital or extended care settings, work closely with nursing assistive personnel who often provide hygiene care. Provide them with the necessary information and equipment so they can provide safe, effective hygiene care. Collaborate with other health team members as indicated (e.g., work with physical therapy and occupational therapy to enhance the patient's independence with self-care activities).

When a patient needs assistance as a result of a self-care limitation, the family often becomes a valuable resource to the nurse and helps with hygiene measures. In these cases family members often need guidance in adapting techniques to fit patient limitations. Be aware of equipment and procedures used in the agency so the patient and family are knowledgeable about the care, have the skills needed to provide it, and have access to necessary equipment. Depending on the patient's limitations, some insurance plans provide staff to assist with basic hygiene needs. Explore this option with the patient and family members.

Collaborate with community agencies as needed. For example, the nurse involved in the care of a homeless patient needs to be aware of the location of clothing distribution centers for basic hygiene supplies, a shelter where bathing facilities are available, and any organization that offers free health care or reduced fees. Partner with social workers or staff in local area churches, not-for-profit organizations, and schools to be sure that patients have the resources they need to maintain hygiene.

IMPLEMENTATION

Hygiene is a part of basic patient care. Use caring practices when performing hygiene measures to reduce patient anxiety and promote comfort and relaxation. For example, while giving a patient a bath and changing a gown, use a gentle approach as you turn and reposition him or her. A soft, gentle voice while conversing with the patient helps to relieve fears or concerns. For patients suffering symptoms such as pain or nausea, administering medications to relieve the symptoms before providing hygiene interventions helps to maintain patient comfort during hygiene care. Consider the stress that hygiene care invokes and be alert for any cues of anxiety or fear. Some patients fear pain or are frightened about falling or sustaining injury associated with hygiene care.

Implementation also focuses on assisting and preparing patients to be able to perform as much of their hygiene care as they can independently. Teach patients proper hygiene techniques and signs and symptoms of hygiene problems. Inform patients about available resources in the community for dealing with these problems if they arise.

Health Promotion. In primary health care situations educate and counsel patients and caregivers on proper hygiene techniques. For example, a new mother needs to learn how to bathe her newborn, whereas an older adult needs information on the importance of regular ear care to avoid accumulated cerumen and hearing impairment. The hygiene skills described throughout this chapter provide standards for excellent physical care. When caring for patients in primary health care settings, maintain these standards and incorporate adaptations as needed to meet the patient's lifestyle, functional status, living arrangements, and preferences. Key points when teaching patients about hygiene include the following:

- Make any instruction relevant based on your assessment of the patient's knowledge, motivation, preferences, and health beliefs. For example, when teaching the patient with diabetes, include how circulation to the feet is impaired and how this causes poor healing and infection, especially when the skin is injured or broken.
- Adapt instruction to the patient's personal bathing facilities and resources. Not all patients have the ideal situation that exists in a health care setting (e.g., easily accessible shower or a bedside table to place over a bed). Adapt available resources so the patient can comfortably and safely reach and use needed items. For example, a young mother has more room and believes that bathing her infant is safer if she uses her kitchen sink and counter rather than her bathroom sink.

- Teach the patient ways to avoid injury. Almost any hygiene procedure poses risks (e.g., cutting a nail too close to the skin or failing to adjust the water temperature of the bath). Include safety risks and tips with all instructions.
- Reinforce infection control practices. Damage to the skin, mucosa, eyes, or other tissues creates an immediate risk for infection. Determine that the patient understands the relationship among healthy and intact skin and tissues, hand hygiene practices, and the prevention of infection.

Acute, Restorative, and Continuing Care. Nursing knowledge and skills needed for performing hygiene care are consistent across all health care settings where acute care, restorative care, and continuing care are provided. In addition, some of the skills in this section are applicable in areas of health promotion.

The variety and timing of hygiene measures vary across health care settings and according to individual patient needs. In the acute care setting factors such as more frequent diagnostic and treatment plans and the need for more extensive hygiene care resulting from acute illness or injury affect scheduling. In extended care facilities and nursing homes, bathing may be scheduled less frequently.

Bathing and Skin Care. Consider a patient's normal grooming routines, including type of hygiene products used and the time of day when hygiene is routinely performed. Individualize your care based on the patient's preferences. The extent, type, and timing or frequency of bathing and the methods used depend on a patient's physical abilities, health problems, and the degree of hygiene required (Boxes 39-5 and 39-6). In addition to cleansing baths, the health care provider may prescribe therapeutic baths, including sitz baths or medicated baths (e.g., oatmeal, cornstarch, or Aveeno). A sitz bath cleans and reduces pain and inflammation of perineal and anal areas. Medicated baths relieve skin irritation and create an antibacterial and drying effect.

If a patient is physically dependent or cognitively impaired, increase the frequency of skin assessment and provide skin care directed toward reducing the risk for skin breakdown. When bathing patients with cognitive impairments, consider special needs and challenges (Box 39-7). These patients easily become afraid and use physical and verbal aggressive behaviors to express their needs. Apply available evidence to your care of the patient who is cognitively impaired. When family members assist in bathing cognitively impaired patients, you need to provide them with coaching, practice, and support (Mahoney et al., 2006).

Building Competency in Patient-Centered Care You are a home health nurse and visit the home of your patient, Anna, a 74-year-old female with Alzheimer's disease. Anna lives with her daughter Rose. You notice that Anna appears unkempt and her gown is soiled with food and urine. Rose tearfully tells you, "I just don't know what we are going to do. It's such a battle to clean Mom. She yells and hits me when I try to wash her." Which assessments do you make and which teaching do you implement to help Rose provide the necessary hygiene care in a caring manner?

Answers to questions can be found on the Evolve website.

BOX 39-5 HYGIENE CARE SCHEDULE IN ACUTE AND LONG-TERM CARE SETTINGS

Early Morning Care

Nursing personnel on the night shift provide basic hygiene to patients getting ready for breakfast, scheduled tests, or early morning surgery. "AM care" includes offering a bedpan or urinal if the patient is not ambulatory, washing the patient's hands and face, and assisting with oral care.

Routine Morning Care

After breakfast assist by offering a bedpan or urinal to patients confined to bed; provide a bath or shower, including perineal care and oral, foot, nail, and hair care; give a back rub; change the patient's gown or pajamas; change the bed linens; and straighten the patient's bedside unit and room. This is often referred to as "complete AM care."

Afternoon Care

Hospitalized patients often undergo many exhausting diagnostic tests or procedures in the morning. In rehabilitation centers patients participate in physical therapy in the morning. Afternoon hygiene care includes washing the hands and face, assisting with oral care, offering a bedpan or urinal, and straightening bed linen.

Evening, or Hour-Before-Sleep, Care

Before bedtime offer personal hygiene care that helps patients relax and promotes sleep. "PM care" often includes changing soiled bed linens, gowns, or pajamas; helping patients wash the face and hands; providing oral hygiene; giving a back massage; and offering the bedpan or urinal to nonambulatory patients. Some patients enjoy a beverage such as juice; check diet to determine which beverages are allowed.

BOX 39-6 TYPES OF BATHS

Complete bed bath: Bath administered to totally dependent patient in bed (see Skill 39-1).

Partial bed bath: Bed bath that consists of bathing only body parts that would cause discomfort if left unbathed such as the hands, face, axillae, and perineal area. Partial bath may also include washing back and providing back rub. Provide a partial bath to dependent patients in need of partial hygiene or self-sufficient bedridden patients who are unable to reach all body parts.

Sponge bath at the sink: Involves bathing from a bath basin or sink with patient sitting in a chair. Patient is able to perform part of the bath independently. Assistance is needed for hard-to-reach areas.

Tub bath: Involves immersion in a tub of water that allows more thorough washing and rinsing than a bed bath. Patient may still require the nurse's assistance. Some institutions have tubs equipped with lifting devices that facilitate positioning dependent patients in the tub.

Shower: Patient sits or stands under a continuous stream of water. The shower provides more thorough cleaning than a bed bath but can cause fatigue.

Bag bath/travel bath: Contains several soft, nonwoven cotton cloths that are premoistened in a solution of no-rinse surfactant cleanser and emollient. The bag bath offers an alternative because of the ease of use, reduced time bathing, and patient comfort.

A **complete bed bath** (Skill 39-1 on pp. 797-805) often exhausts a patient. Turning during a complete bed bath and receiving back care increase oxygen consumption and demand. Anticipate and assess whether patients are physically able to tolerate a complete bath. Assessing heart rate before, during, and after the bath provides a measure of their physical tolerance. Provide a **partial bed bath** (see Skill 39-1) to patients who are aging, dependent, in need of only partial hygiene, or bedridden and unable to reach all body parts. Wear gloves when there is a risk of contacting body fluids. Control environmental factors that alter skin integrity,

BOX 39-7 EVIDENCE-BASED PRACTICE

Making Bathing Better for Patients with Cognitive Impairment

PICO Question: Do patients who are cognitively impaired have fewer negative behaviors when nurses and other caregivers use person-centered care techniques during bathing than patients who do not receive patient-centered care during bathing?

Evidence Summary

For patients with Alzheimer's disease and related dementia, bathing frequently creates high levels of discomfort. Confusion causes these patients to feel vulnerable or as if they are being attacked during bathing, resulting in screaming, crying, and even aggressively lashing out at caregivers. Bathing leaves both the patient and caregiver feeling unsatisfied. Research shows that using nontraditional bathing techniques and educating caregivers to provide person-centered care ease the conflict and reduce aggressive, negative behaviors associated with bathing activities (Hoeffer et al., 2006). Caregivers need to recognize and eliminate triggers that cause negative behaviors during bathing. Use of patient-centered showering techniques and the in-bed towel bath with no-rinse soap results in a reduction of discomfort and aggressive incidents compared with traditional methods (Rader et al., 2006). Evidence disputes the need to force people against their wishes to bathe at routine intervals and in traditional ways (Rader et al., 2006).

Application to Nursing Practice

- Use person-centered care techniques when bathing patients with cognitive impairments. Develop a therapeutic relationship with the patient. Include him or her in planning care as much as possible, especially in regard to comfort and personal preferences. For example, let the patient select whether to shower or take a towel bath. Show respect in all interactions and communication. Use a gentle approach and avoid rushing. Approach the situation focusing on the person instead of on the task (Rader et al., 2006).
- Address factors that contribute to bathing difficulties, including pain; fatigue and weakness; fear and misunderstanding; anxiety and apprehension associated with fear of falling, noisy bathing areas, and being naked in front of strangers; triggers specific to the patient; and discomfort associated with cold, drafty air or cold water spray (Rader et al., 2006). Provide privacy and promote comfort. Close the door and pull room curtains around the bathing area. Control drafts and keep the patient covered, exposing only the body part being washed. For showering, consider leaving a light gown on during the shower. Change the bathing environment to be more inviting and calming. Avoid common triggers such as starting the bath by washing the face or forcing the patient to bathe.
- Support caregivers by providing education and materials needed for person-centered care. Empower staff as caregivers to recognize that agitation and aggressive behaviors are used by patients to communicate their needs (Hoeffer et al., 2006).

including moisture, heat, and external sources of pressure such as wrinkled bed linen and improperly placed drainage tubing.

When administering either a complete or partial bath, assess the condition of the skin to determine if soap is necessary or if the patient requires daily bathing. Patients with excessively dry skin are predisposed to skin impairment. Use soaps that contain emollients to hydrate dry skin. Avoid overly hot water because it can dry the skin by removing natural oils. Lubricate the skin with emollient lotions to reduce dryness.

Use the tub bath or shower (see Skill 39-1) to give a more thorough bath than a bed bath. Implement safety measures to prevent fall injuries because the surface of the tub or shower stall is slippery. In some settings a health care provider's order for a shower or tub bath is necessary. Place a chair in the shower for patients with weakness or poor balance. Both tubs and showers need to have grab bars for patients to hold during entry and exit and maneuvering during the bath or shower. Patients vary in how much help they need.

Regardless of the type of bath the patient receives, use the following guidelines:

- *Provide privacy.* Close the door and/or pull room curtains around the bathing area. While bathing the patient, expose only the areas being bathed by using proper draping.
- *Maintain safety.* Keep side rails up when away from the patient's bedside when patients are dependent or unconscious. NOTE: When side rails serve as a restraint, you need a health care provider's order (see agency-specific policy for restraint usage) (see Chapter 27). Place the call light in the patient's reach if leaving the bedside even temporarily.
- *Maintain warmth.* Keep the room warm because the patient is partially uncovered and easily chilled. Wet skin causes an excess loss of heat through evaporation. Control drafts and keep windows closed. Keep patient covered, only exposing the body part being washed during the bath.
- *Promote independence.* Encourage the patient to participate in as much of the bathing activities as possible. Offer assistance when needed.
- *Anticipate needs.* Bring a new set of clothing and hygiene products to the bedside or bathroom.

Teach patients to follow a few general rules for skin health. Encourage them to routinely inspect their skin for changes in color or texture and report abnormalities to their health care provider. Instruct patients to handle the skin gently, avoiding excessive rubbing. Also encourage them to eat nutritious foods from all food groups, including those rich in vitamins and minerals, and to consume adequate fluids. Stress safety concerns such as failing to adjust or check the water temperature, cutting nails too close to the skin, and slipping on wet surfaces. Ensure that patients understand that healthy and intact skin and tissues protect them from infection. Reinforce infection control practice, including proper hand hygiene.

Bag Baths. This innovative approach to the traditional bed bath was developed because of nurses' concern for patients who are predisposed to dry skin and the risk for infection (see Skill 39-1). Not cleaning and drying washbasins completely after use provides a risk for contamination by disease-producing gram-negative organisms. Based on their study in intensive care units, Johnson, Lineweaver, and Maze (2009) concluded that bath basins provide a reservoir for bacteria and are a possible source of transmission of hospital-acquired infections. The bag bath contains a no-rinse surfactant, a humectant to trap moisture, and an emollient. Nurses in another study expressed a significant overall preference for the disposable bag bath versus the traditional basin bath, especially for patients who are unable to bathe themselves in critical and long-term care settings (Larson et al., 2004). Some facilities have switched from the traditional bath in favor of the bag bath because of concerns related to infection control.

Perineal Care. Cleansing patients' genital and anal areas is called **perineal care.** It usually occurs as part of a complete bed bath (see Skill 39-1). Patients most in need of perineal care include those at greatest risk for acquiring an infection (e.g., uncircumcised males, patients who have indwelling urinary catheters, or those who are recovering from rectal or genital surgery or childbirth). In addition, women who are having a menstrual period require perineal care. Encourage patients to perform their own perineal care. Sometimes you are embarrassed about providing perineal care, particularly to patients of the opposite sex. Similarly the patient may feel embarrassed. Do not let embarrassment cause you to overlook the patient's hygiene needs. When staffing levels permit, use a gender-congruent caregiver. A professional, dignified, and sensitive approach reduces embarrassment and helps put the patient at ease.

If a patient performs self-care, various problems such as vaginal and urethral discharge, skin irritation, and unpleasant odors often go unnoticed. Stress the importance of perineal care in preventing skin breakdown and infection. Be alert for complaints of burning during urination or localized soreness, excoriation, or pain in the perineum. Inspect vaginal and perineal areas and the patient's bed linen for signs of discharge and use your sense of smell to detect abnormal odors. Risk factors for skin breakdown in the perineal area include urinary or fecal incontinence, rectal and perineal surgical dressings, indwelling urinary catheters, and morbid obesity.

Back Rub. A back rub or back massage usually follows the patient's bath. It promotes relaxation, relieves muscular tension, and decreases perception of pain. **Effleurage** (i.e., long, slow, gliding strokes of a massage) is associated with reduced measured anxiety, heart rate, and respiratory rate. Studies show that slow-stroke back massages of 3 minutes and hand massages of 10 minutes significantly improve both physiological and psychological indicators of relaxation in older people (Harris and Richards, 2010).

When providing a back rub, enhance relaxation by reducing noise and ensuring that the patient is comfortable. It is important to ask whether a patient would like a back rub or if he or she prefers gentle instead of deep massage, because some individuals dislike physical contact. Consult the medical record for any contraindications to a massage (e.g., fractured ribs, burns, and heart surgery).

Foot and Nail Care. Incorporate foot and nail care into a person's regular hygiene routine. Routine care involves soaking to soften cuticles and layers of horny cells, thorough cleaning, drying, and proper nail trimming. Patients with diabetes mellitus should not soak their nails because of the risk of overdrying the feet and developing breaks in the skin with resulting infection. When providing nail care, the patient remains in bed or sits in a chair (Skill 39-2 on pp. 805-808). In some settings or with specific patients such as a person with diabetes mellitus, you need a health care provider's order to trim toenails. Before implementing this procedure, check agency policy to determine if the order is necessary.

Take time during the procedure to teach the patient and family proper techniques for cleaning and nail trimming. You need to stress measures to prevent infection and promote good circulation. Patients learn to protect the feet from injury, keep them clean and dry, and wear footwear that fits properly. Instruct patients in the proper way to inspect all surfaces of the feet and hands for redness, lesions, dryness, or signs of infection. Teach foot care to family members or caregivers for patients who need regular foot care and have peripheral vascular disease, visual difficulties, physical constraints preventing movement, or cognitive problems.

Certain conditions place patients with diabetes at increased risk for amputation (American Diabetes Association, 2007). These factors include peripheral neuropathy, limited joint mobility, bony deformity, peripheral vascular disease, and a history of skin ulcers or previous amputation. Observe for changes that indicate peripheral neuropathy or vascular insufficiency (Box 39-8). Advise patients to use the following guidelines in a routine foot and nail care program (American Diabetes Association, 2010):

BOX 39-8 SIGNS OF PERIPHERAL NEUROPATHY OR VASCULAR INSUFFICIENCY

Peripheral Neuropathy

- Muscle wasting of lower extremities
- Absence of deep tendon reflexes
- Foot deformities
- Infections
- Abnormal gait
- Decreased or absent vibratory sensation

Vascular Insufficiency

- Decreased hair growth on legs and feet
- Absent or decreased pulses
- Infection in the foot
- Poor wound healing
- Thickened nails
- Shiny appearance of the skin
- Blanching of the skin on elevation

Data from American Diabetes Association: Position statement on standards of medical care in diabetes 2007, *Diabetes Care* 30:S4, 2007.

- Receive a thorough foot examination at least once a year. People with one or more high-risk foot conditions need an evaluation more frequently.
- Inspect the feet daily, including the bottoms and tops, heels, and areas between the toes. Use a mirror to help inspect the feet thoroughly or ask a family member to check daily.
- Wash feet daily in lukewarm water. Dry thoroughly, especially between the toes.
- Wear shoes and clean, dry socks at all times; never go barefoot. Check inside shoes before wearing them for rough areas or objects that may rub against the foot.
- Keep skin soft and smooth by applying an emollient lotion over all surfaces of the feet but not between the toes.
- If you can see and reach your toenails, trim them straight across and square file the edges smooth.
- Keep the blood flowing to your feet by putting them up when sitting and wiggling your toes and moving your ankles up and down for 5 minutes 2 or 3 times a day. Do not cross your legs for long periods and don't smoke.
- Protect the feet from hot and cold. Do not use heating pads or electric blankets and always wear shoes at the beach or on hot pavement.

Oral Hygiene. Regular oral hygiene, including brushing, flossing, and rinsing, prevents and controls plaque-associated oral diseases. Evidence relates poor oral health to risk of impaired nutrition, stroke, poor blood sugar control in diabetes, and nursing home–acquired pneumonia (Jablonski, 2009). Inadequate oral care and some medications diminish salivary production, which in turn reduces the ability of the oral environment to help fight effects of pathogens (Box 39-9).

Brushing cleans the teeth of food particles, plaque, and bacteria. It also massages the gums and relieves discomfort resulting from unpleasant odors and tastes. Flossing removes tartar that collects at the gum line. Rinsing removes dislodged food particles and excess toothpaste. Complete oral hygiene enhances well-being and comfort and stimulates the appetite.

When patients become ill, many factors influence their need for oral hygiene. Patients in hospitals or long-term care facilities do

BOX 39-9 FOCUS ON OLDER ADULTS

Oral Health

- Many older adults are edentulous (without teeth), and the teeth that are present are often diseased or decayed (Meiner, 2011).
- The periodontal membrane weakens with aging, making it more prone to infection. Periodontal disease predisposes the older adult to systemic infection.
- Dentures or partial plates do not always fit properly, causing pain and discomfort, which in turn affect digestive processes, enjoyment of food, and nutritional status.
- An age-related decline in saliva secretion and some medications (e.g., antihypertensives, diuretics, antiinflammatories, antidepressants) cause dry mouth (Meiner, 2011).
- Financial limitations and the belief that dentures eliminate the need for routine dental care are reasons why older adults do not seek dental care (Meiner, 2011).

not always receive the aggressive oral care they need. Base the frequency of care on the condition of the oral cavity and the patient's level of comfort. Some patients require oral care as often as every 1 to 2 hours.

Acidic fruits in the patient's diet reduce plaque formation. A well-balanced diet contributes to the integrity of oral tissues. To prevent tooth decay, patients sometimes need to change eating habits (e.g., reducing intake of carbohydrates, especially sweet snacks between meals). Advise patients of all ages to visit a dentist regularly for checkups. Education about common gum and tooth disorders and methods of prevention may motivate patients to follow good oral hygiene practices.

Brushing. The American Dental Association (2010) guidelines for effective oral hygiene include brushing the teeth at least twice a day with American Dental Association–approved fluoride toothpaste. Fluoride and antimicrobial mouth rinses also help prevent tooth decay. Do not use fluoride rinse in children ages 6 or under because of the risk of swallowing the rinse. Use antimicrobial toothpastes and 0.12% chlorhexidine oral rinses for patients at increased risk for poor oral hygiene (e.g., older adults and patients with cognitive impairments and who are immunocompromised) (Garcia and Caple, 2011). The toothbrush needs to have a straight handle and a brush small enough to reach all areas of the mouth. Rounded soft bristles stimulate the gums without causing abrasion and bleeding. Any patient who experiences decreased dexterity as a result of a medical condition or the aging process requires an enlarged handle with an easier grip.

Brush all tooth surfaces thoroughly (Skill 39-3 on pp. 808-811). Commercially made foam swabs are ineffective in removing plaque (Garcia and Caple, 2011). Electric or powered toothbrushes improve the quality of cleaning and may be easier to use than manual brushes when nurses provide care for dependent patients. Do not use lemon-glycerin sponges because they dry mucous membranes and erode tooth enamel.

To prevent cross-contamination, teach patients to avoid sharing toothbrushes with family members or drinking directly from a bottle of mouthwash. The use of disclosure tablets or drops to stain the plaque that collects at the gum line is useful for showing patients how effectively they brush. Instruct patients to obtain a new toothbrush every 3 months or following a cold or upper respiratory infection to minimize growth of microorganisms on the brush surfaces (American Dental Association, 2010).

Flossing. Dental flossing removes plaque and tartar between teeth. Flossing involves inserting waxed or unwaxed dental floss between all tooth surfaces, one at a time. The seesaw motion used to pull floss between teeth removes plaque and tartar from tooth enamel. Use unwaxed floss and avoid vigorous flossing near the gum line on patients who are receiving chemotherapy, radiation, or anticoagulant therapy to prevent bleeding. If toothpaste is applied to the teeth before flossing, fluoride comes in direct contact with tooth surfaces, aiding in cavity prevention. According to American Dental Association (2010) recommendations, flossing once a day is sufficient. Because it is important to clean all teeth surfaces thoroughly, do not rush to complete flossing. Placing a mirror in front of the patient helps you demonstrate the proper method for holding the floss and cleaning between the teeth. Flossing a patient's teeth is not realistic or appropriate in all care settings.

Patients with Special Needs. Some patients require special oral hygiene methods. For example, patients with diabetes mellitus frequently experience periodontal disease. Therefore they need to visit the dentist every 3 to 4 months, clean their teeth up to 4 times a day, and handle oral tissues gently with a minimum of trauma. Other patients depend on their caregivers for oral care. Being unconscious or having an artificial airway (e.g., endotracheal or tracheal tubes) increases the susceptibility for patients to have drying of salivary secretions because they are unable to eat or drink, frequently breathe through the mouth, and often receive oxygen therapy. Unconscious patients cannot swallow salivary secretions that accumulate in the mouth. These secretions often contain gram-negative bacteria that cause pneumonia if aspirated into the lungs. While providing hygiene, protect the patient from choking and aspiration and use topical chlorhexidine, especially in ventilated patients. Current evidence shows that use of chlorhexidine with oral hygiene reduces the risk for ventilator-associated pneumonia (Munro et al., 2009).

Patients with decreased levels of consciousness need special attention because they often do not have a gag reflex. Proper oral hygiene requires keeping the mucosa moist and removing secretions that contribute to infection. When providing oral hygiene to an unconscious patient, you need to protect him or her from choking and aspiration. Have two nurses provide the care; turn the patient's head toward you, and place the bed in semi-Fowler's position. You can delegate nursing assistive personnel to participate. One nurse does the actual cleaning, and the other caregiver removes secretions with suction equipment. Some agencies use equipment that combines a mouth swab with the suction device; you can use this equipment safely by yourself. While cleansing the oral cavity, use a small oral airway or a padded tongue blade to hold the mouth open. Never use your fingers to hold the patient's mouth open. A human bite contains multiple pathogenic microorganisms. Even though the patient is not awake or alert, explain the steps of mouth care and the sensations that he or she will feel. Also tell the patient when the procedure is completed (Skill 39-4 on pp. 811-813).

Some treatments such as chemotherapy, immunosuppressive agents, head and neck radiation, and nasogastric intubation place patients at higher risk of experiencing stomatitis or inflammation of the oral mucosa. **Stomatitis** causes burning, pain, and change in food and fluid tolerance. When caring for patients with stomatitis, brush with a soft toothbrush and floss gently to prevent bleeding of the gums. In some cases flossing needs to be temporarily omitted from oral care. Advise patients to avoid alcohol and commercial mouthwash and stop smoking. Normal saline rinses (approximately 30 mL) on awaking in the morning, after each meal, and at bedtime help clean the oral cavity. Patients can increase the rinses to every 2 hours if necessary. Consult with the health care provider to obtain topical or oral analgesics for pain control.

Denture Care. Encourage patients to clean their dentures on a regular basis to avoid gingival infection and irritation. When patients become disabled, someone else assumes responsibility for denture care (Box 39-10). Dentures are the patient's personal property and must be handled with care because they break easily. They must be removed at night to rest the gums and prevent bacterial buildup. To prevent warping, keep dentures covered in water when they are not worn and always store them in an enclosed, labeled cup with the cup placed in the patient's bedside stand. Discourage patients from removing their dentures and placing them on a napkin or tissue because they could easily be thrown away.

Implement measures to prevent denture-induced stomatitis when caring for patients who wear dentures. Poorly fitting dentures, wearing dentures while sleeping, and poor dental hygiene habits contribute to denture-induced stomatitis (Sciubba, 2009). Signs and symptoms range from redness and swelling under the dentures to painful red sores on the roof of the mouth and infection with the yeast *Candida albicans*. Some patients deny pain, and others complain of pain worsened by wearing dentures. To prevent denture-induced stomatitis, rinse the mouth and dentures after meals, clean them carefully and regularly, remove and soak them overnight, brush and floss any remaining teeth, and visit a dentist regularly for examination (Sciubba, 2009).

Hair and Scalp Care. A person's appearance and feeling of well-being often depend on the way the hair looks and feels. Illness or disability often prevents a patient from maintaining daily hair care. When patients are immobilized, their hair soon becomes tangled. Some dressings or diagnostic procedures leave sticky residue on the hair. Basic hair and scalp care includes brushing, combing, and shampooing.

Brushing and Combing. Frequent brushing helps keep hair clean and distributes oil evenly along hair shafts. Combing prevents hair from tangling. Encourage patients to maintain routine hair care and provide help for patients with limited mobility or weakness and those who are confused or weakened by illness. Patients in a hospital or extended care facility appreciate the opportunity to have their hair brushed and combed before being seen by others.

When caring for patients from different cultures, learn as much as possible from them or their family about preferred hair care practices. For example, the hair of African Americans tends to be quite dry. Use special lanolin conditioners for conditioning. Cultural preferences also affect how hair is combed and styled and whether it can be cut.

Long hair easily becomes matted when a patient is confined to bed, even for a short period. When lacerations or incisions involve the scalp, blood and topical medications also cause tangling. Frequent brushing and combing keep long hair neatly groomed. Braiding helps to avoid repeated tangles; however, patients need to unbraid hair periodically and comb it to ensure good hygiene. Braids that are too tight lead to bald patches. Obtain permission from the patient before braiding the hair.

To brush hair part it into two sections and separate each section into two more sections. Brushing from the scalp toward the hair ends minimizes pulling. Moistening the hair with water or an alcohol-free detangle product makes it easier to comb. Never cut a patient's hair without consent.

Patients who develop head lice require special considerations in the way combing is performed. The lice are small, about the size of a sesame seed; thus you need bright light or natural sunlight to see

BOX 39-10 PROCEDURAL GUIDELINES

View Video!

Care of Dentures

Delegation Considerations

The skill of denture care can be delegated to nursing assistive personnel (NAP). Instruct the NAP to:

- Inform the nurse if there are cracks in dentures.
- Inform the nurse if the patient complains of oral discomfort.
- Inform the nurse of any lesions in the mouth.

Equipment

Soft-bristle toothbrush or denture toothbrush, denture-cleaning agent or toothpaste, denture adhesive *(optional)*, glass of water, emesis basin or sink, washcloth, clean gloves, denture cup (if dentures are to be stored after cleaning)

1. Identify the patient using two identifiers (i.e., name and birth date or name and account number) according to facility policy.
2. Ask patient if dentures fit and if there is any gum or mucous membrane tenderness or irritation.
3. Ask patient about preferences for denture care and products used. If patient is unable to care for own dentures, provide this care. Clean dentures for patient during routine mouth care.
4. Fill emesis basin with tepid water; or, if using sink, place washcloth in bottom of sink and fill sink with an inch (2.5 cm) of water.
5. Remove dentures: If patient is unable to do this independently, perform hand hygiene and apply gloves, grasp upper plate at front with thumb and index finger wrapped in gauze, and pull downward. To remove lower denture, gently lift it from the jaw and rotate one side downward. Place dentures in emesis basin or sink.
6. Apply cleaning agent to brush and brush surfaces of dentures (see illustration). Hold dentures close to water. Hold brush horizontally and use back-and-forth motion to clean biting surfaces. Use short strokes from top of denture to biting surfaces to clean outer and inner teeth surfaces. Hold brush vertically and use short strokes to clean inner tooth surfaces. Hold brush horizontally and use back-and-forth motion to clean undersurface of dentures.

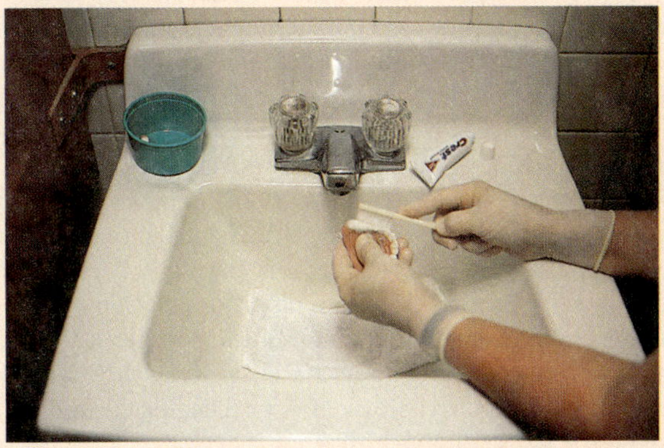

STEP 6 Brushing dentures.

7. Some patients use an adhesive to seal dentures in place. Apply a thin layer to undersurface before inserting.
8. If patient needs help inserting dentures, moisten upper denture and press firmly to seal it in place. Insert moistened lower denture. Ask if dentures feel comfortable.
9. Some patients prefer to have their dentures stored to rest the gums and reduce risk of infection. Keeping dentures moist prevents warping and facilitates easier insertion. Store in a secure place to prevent loss.
10. Remove and discard gloves and perform hand hygiene.

them. Thorough combing is more effective than use of pediculicidal shampoos, which are often toxic and ineffective against resistant lice. Follow these steps:

- Apply disposable gown and gloves.
- Use a grooming comb or hairbrush to remove tangles.
- Divide the patient's hair in sections and fasten off hair that is not being combed.
- Comb out from the scalp to the end of the hair (special combs are available in drug stores).
- Dip the comb in a cup of water or use a paper towel to remove lice between each passing.
- After combing look through the hair carefully for attached lice.
- You can catch live lice with a tweezers or comb.
- After combing thoroughly, move to next section.
- Instruct family to clean the comb with an old toothbrush and dental floss and boil the comb. The ideal is to discard the comb after each use, but some patient's financial situations prevent the purchase of multiple combs.
- Instruct family to comb and screen for lice daily.
- Instruct family to contain patient's clothes and wash them in hot water.
- Instruct family to vacuum the home and patient's room and immediately empty vacuum bag or bagless collection device.
- Instruct caregivers in how to prevent transmission of lice:
  - Do not share bed linens or hair care products.
  - Avoid placing bare hand on patient's head.
  - Immediately wash hands after providing hair care.

If a pediculicidal shampoo is ordered, instruct the patient and caregiver in its proper use. These shampoos have neurological side effects. The very young and very old have increased susceptibility to the toxic effects of seizure, dizziness, headache, paresthesia, and death. Never use organochloride lindane to treat people with seizure disorders, pregnant or breastfeeding women, people with irritated skin or sores where lindane will be applied, people who weigh less than 110 pounds, and older adults (CDC, 2008). As with any medication preparation, it is important to review and understand pertinent information. Most side effects associated with pediculicidal shampoos occur as a result of applying too much medicated shampoo, leaving the shampoo in place too long, or repeating a shampoo too soon. To avoid overtreatment, teach patients that itching is a common side effect (Grose, 2011).

Shampooing. Frequency of shampooing depends on a person's daily routines and the condition of the hair. Remind patients in hospitals or extended care facilities that staying in bed, excess perspiration, or treatments that leave blood or solutions in the hair require more frequent shampooing. In some agencies you need a health care provider's order to shampoo a patient who is dependent or has limited mobility because it is challenging to find ways to shampoo the hair without causing injury.

The patient who can shower or tub bathe usually shampoos the hair without difficulty. A shower or tub chair facilitates shampooing for patients who are ambulatory and weight bearing and become tired or faint. Handheld shower nozzles allow patients to easily wash the hair in the tub or shower. Some patients allowed to sit in a chair choose to be shampooed in front of a sink or over a washbasin; however, certain conditions (e.g., eye surgery or neck injury) limit bending. In these situations teach the patient and family the degree of bending allowed.

If a patient is unable to sit but can be moved, transfer him or her to a stretcher for transportation to a sink or shower equipped with a handheld nozzle. Use caution when positioning the patient's head and neck, particularly in patients with any form of head or neck injury.

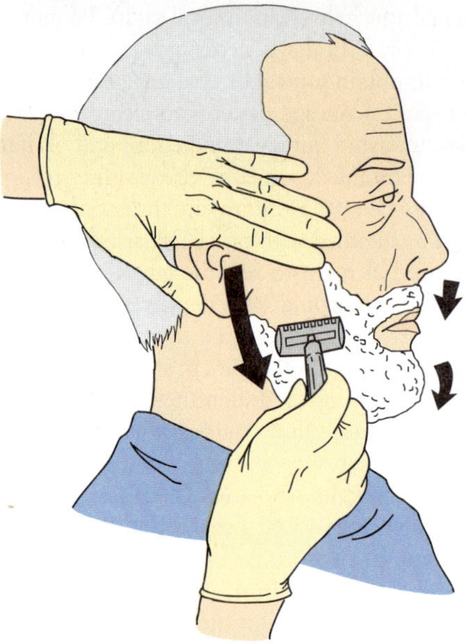

FIG. 39-5 Shave in the direction of hair growth. Use longer strokes on the larger areas of the face. Use short strokes around the chin and lips. (From Sorrentino SA, Remmert LN: *Mosby's textbook for nursing assistants*, ed 8, St Louis, 2012, Mosby.)

If a patient is unable to sit in a chair or be transferred to a stretcher, shampoo the hair with the patient in bed (Box 39-11). Position a special shampoo trough under his or her head to catch water and suds. After shampooing, patients like having their hair styled and dried. Most health care centers have portable hair dryers. Dry shampoos that reduce the need to wet the patient's hair are also available but are not highly effective. Dry shampoo preparations vary; therefore follow the application procedures listed on the container.

Shaving. Shave facial hair after the bath or shampoo. Some women prefer to shave their legs or axillae while bathing. When assisting a patient, take care to avoid cutting him or her with the razor blade. Patients prone to bleeding (e.g., those receiving anticoagulants or high doses of aspirin or those with low platelet counts) need to use an electric razor. Before using an electric razor, check for frayed cords or other electrical hazards. Use razor blades and electric razors on only one patient because of infection control considerations.

When using a razor blade for shaving, the skin must be softened to prevent pulling, scraping, or cuts. Moisten the skin with lukewarm water and apply shaving cream. Avoid use of bar soap, which leaves a film on the blade, resulting in a poorer-quality shave (Draelos, 2010). You need to shave patients when they are unable to shave themselves independently. To avoid causing discomfort or razor cuts, gently pull the skin taut and use long, firm razor strokes in the direction the hair grows (Fig. 39-5). Short downward strokes work best to remove hair over the upper lip or chin. The patient usually explains the best way to move the razor across the skin. Facial hair of African Americans tends to be curly and becomes ingrown unless shaved close to the skin.

Mustache and Beard Care. Mustaches or beards require daily grooming. Grooming keeps food particles and mucus from collecting in the hair. If a patient is unable to carry out self-care, do so

BOX 39-11 PROCEDURAL GUIDELINES

View Video!

Shampooing Hair of Patient Who Is Bed-Bound

Delegation Considerations

The skill of shampooing hair can be delegated to nursing assistive personnel (NAP). Instruct the NAP:

- About any precautions needed in positioning the patient.
- To inform the nurse if the patient reports neck pain.
- To inform the nurse of any new skin lesions.

Equipment

Brush, comb, shampoo board, shampoo, conditioner *(optional)*, hydrogen peroxide *(optional)*, towels (three or more), waterproof pad, hair dryer, basin of very warm water, clean gloves (if needed)

1. Identify patient using two identifiers (i.e., name and birth date or name and account number) according to facility policy.
2. Before washing patient's hair, determine that there are no contraindications to procedure.
3. Perform hand hygiene and apply gloves if needed. Inspect the hair and scalp before initiating the procedure to determine the presence of any conditions that require the use of special shampoos or treatments (e.g., for dandruff or the removal of dried blood).
4. Place waterproof pad under patient's shoulders, neck, and head. Position patient supine, with head and shoulders at top edge of bed. Place plastic trough under patient's head and washbasin at end of trough. Be sure that trough spout extends beyond edge of mattress.
5. Place rolled towel under patient's neck and bath towel over patient's shoulders (see illustration).
6. Brush and comb patient's hair.
7. Obtain warm water.
8. Offer patient the option of holding face towel or washcloth over eyes.
9. Slowly pour water from water pitcher over hair until it is completely wet (see illustration). If hair contains matted blood, put on gloves, apply peroxide to dissolve clots, and rinse hair with saline. Apply small amount of shampoo.
10. Work up lather with both hands. Start at hairline and work toward back of neck. Lift head slightly with one hand to wash back of head. Shampoo sides of head. Massage scalp by applying pressure with fingertips.
11. Rinse hair with water. Make sure that water drains into basin. Repeat rinsing until hair is free of soap.
12. Apply conditioner or cream rinse if requested and rinse hair thoroughly.
13. Wrap patient's head in bath towel. Dry patient's face with cloth used to protect eyes. Dry off any moisture along neck or shoulders.
14. Dry patient's hair and scalp. Use second towel if first becomes saturated.
15. Comb hair to remove tangles and dry with dryer if desired.
16. Apply oil preparation or conditioning product to hair if desired by patient.
17. Assist patient to comfortable position and complete styling of hair.

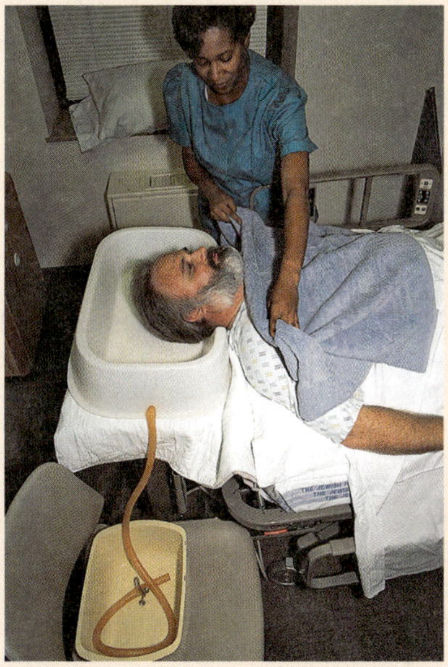

STEP 5 Placing bath towel over patient's shoulders.

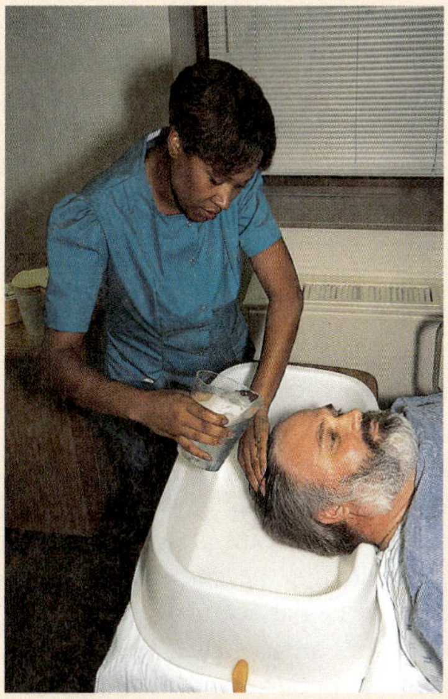

STEP 9 Pouring water over hair.

at his or her request. Comb out beards gently and obtain the patient's permission before trimming or shaving off a mustache or beard.

Care of the Eyes, Ears, and Nose. Give special attention to cleaning the eyes, ears, and nose during a routine bath and when drainage or discharge accumulates. This aspect of hygiene not only makes a patient more comfortable but also improves sensory reception (see Chapter 49). Care focuses on preventing infection and maintaining normal sensory function. In addition, care of the eyes, ears, and nose requires approaches that consider the patient's special needs.

Basic Eye Care. Cleaning the eyes involves simply washing with a clean washcloth moistened in water (see Skill 39-1). Soap causes burning and irritation. Never apply direct pressure over the eyeball because it causes serious injury. When cleaning a patient's eyes, obtain a clean washcloth and clean from inner to outer canthus. Use a different section of the washcloth for each eye.

Unconscious patients often require more frequent eye care. Secretions collect along the lid margins and inner canthus when the blink reflex is absent or when the eye does not close completely. When an eye does not close completely, you may need to place an eye patch over the involved eye to prevent corneal drying and irritation. Apply lubricating eyedrops according to the health care provider's orders.

Eyeglasses. Glasses are made of hardened glass or plastic that is impact resistant to prevent shattering. Nevertheless, because of

BOX 39-12 PATIENT TEACHING

Contact Lens Care

Objective

- Patient verbalizes and/or demonstrates proper care for contact lenses and common warning signs of problems associated with contact lens wear.

Teaching Strategies

- Instruct patients on the following:
  - Do not use fingernail on lens to remove dirt or debris.
  - Do not use tap water to clean soft lenses.
  - Follow recommendations of lens manufacturer or eye care practitioner when inserting, cleaning, and disinfecting lenses.
  - Keep lenses moist or wet when not worn.
  - Use fresh solution daily when storing and disinfecting lenses.
  - Thoroughly wash and rinse lens storage case on a daily basis. Clean periodically with soap or liquid detergent, rinse thoroughly with warm water, and air dry.
  - If lens is dropped, moisten finger with cleaning or wetting solution and gently touch it to pick it up. Then clean, rinse, and disinfect lens.
- To avoid mix-up, always start with the same lens when removing or inserting lenses.
- Throw away disposable or planned replacement lenses after prescribed wearing period.
- Encourage patient to remember the acronym RSVP: *R*edness, *S*ensitivity, *V*ision problems, and *P*ain. If one of these problems occurs, remove contact lenses immediately. If problems continue, contact a vision care specialist (Lewis et al., 2011).

Evaluation

- Ask patient to state warning signs of corneal irritation and eye infection.
- Ask patient to describe methods of contact lens care that lead to infection.
- Ask patient to demonstrate cleaning and storing contact lenses.

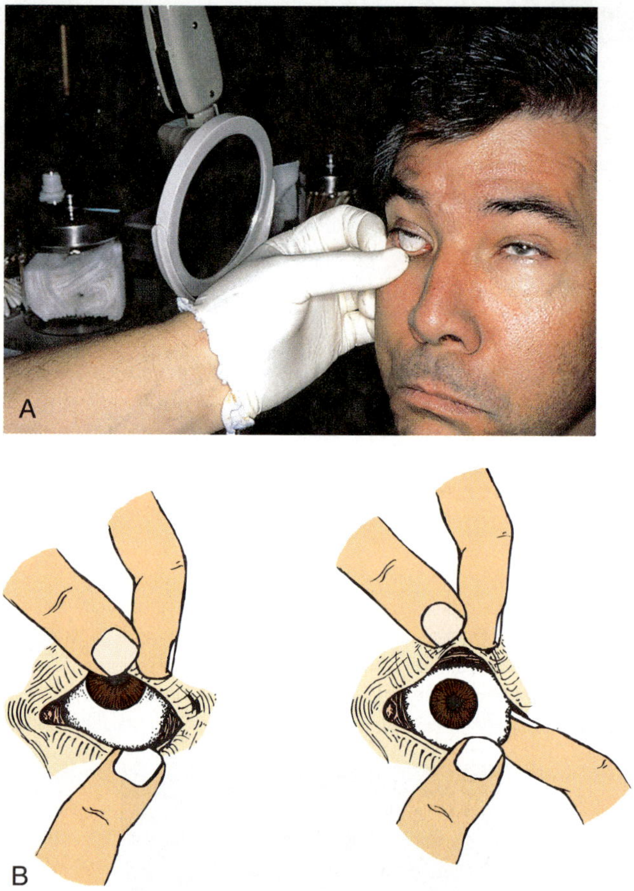

FIG. 39-6 Removal of prosthetic eye.

the cost, be careful when cleaning glasses and protect them from breakage or other damage when they are not worn. Put glasses in a case in a drawer of the bedside table when not in use.

Cool water sufficiently cleans glass lenses. Use a soft cloth for drying to prevent scratching the lens since paper towels can scratch it. Plastic lenses in particular scratch easily; special cleaning solutions and drying tissues are available.

Contact Lenses. A contact lens is a thin, transparent, circular disk that fits directly over the cornea of the eye. Contact lenses correct refractive errors of the eye or abnormalities in the shape of the cornea. Daily-wear lenses are removed nightly for cleansing and disinfection, whereas extended-wear lenses may be worn overnight and removed at least weekly for cleaning and disinfection. Remove disposable-wear lenses nightly and replace when indicated (e.g., daily, weekly, monthly). All contact lenses must be removed periodically to prevent ocular infection and corneal ulcers or abrasions. Common infectious agents are *Pseudomonas aeruginosa* and staphylococci. Patient education includes a discussion of proper lens care techniques (Box 39-12). Pain, tearing, discomfort, and redness of the conjunctivae indicate lens overwear. Report persistence of these symptoms even after lens removal to the patient's vision health care provider.

Care of contact lenses includes proper cleaning and disinfection, insertion and removal, and storage. When patients require help to clean their contact lenses, first perform hand hygiene and then clean and disinfect the lenses with appropriate contact lens solution. Before reinsertion rinse the lenses with an appropriate solution such as sterile saline. Caution patients to never use saliva or homemade saline when cleaning lenses because these solutions contain microorganisms that can cause serious infection. Instruct the patient to clean the contact lens case frequently with warm water and allow it to air dry.

When patients are admitted to the hospital or agency in an unresponsive or confused state, determine if they normally wear contact lenses and if the lenses are in place. If a patient wears contact lenses and no one detects this, severe corneal injury can result. If you find that your patient is wearing contact lenses and the patient cannot remove them, seek assistance. Once the lenses are removed, document the removal, the condition of the patient's eyes following removal, and the storage of the lenses.

Artificial Eyes. Patients with artificial eyes have had an **enucleation** (i.e., removal) of an entire eyeball as a result of tumor growth, severe infection, or eye trauma. Some artificial eyes are permanently implanted, whereas others must be removed for cleaning. Patients with artificial eyes usually prefer to care for their own eyes. Respect the patient's wishes and help by assembling needed equipment.

At times patients require assistance in prosthesis removal and cleaning. To remove an artificial eye, retract the lower eyelid and exert slight pressure just below the eye (Fig. 39-6). This action causes the artificial eye to rise from the socket because the suction holding the eye in place has been broken. You can also use a small, rubber bulb syringe or medicine-dropper bulb to create a suction effect. Place the bulb tip directly over the eye and squeeze it to create suction needed to lift the eye from the socket.

The artificial eye is usually made of glass or plastic. Warm normal saline cleans the prosthesis effectively. Also clean the edges of the eye socket and surrounding tissues with soft gauze moistened in saline or clean tap water. Report signs of infection immediately because bacteria can spread to the neighboring eye, underlying sinuses, or even underlying brain tissue. To reinsert the eye, retract the upper and lower lids and gently slip the eye into the socket, fitting it neatly under the upper eyelid. Store an artificial eye in a labeled container filled with tap water or saline.

Ear Care. Routine ear care involves cleaning the ear with the end of a moistened washcloth, rotated gently into the ear canal. Gentle, downward retraction at the entrance of the ear canal usually causes visible cerumen to loosen and slip out. Instruct patients never to use objects such as bobby pins, toothpicks, paper clips, or cotton-tipped applicators to remove earwax. These objects can injure the ear canal and rupture the tympanic membrane. They may also cause cerumen to become impacted within the ear canal.

Children and older adults commonly have impacted cerumen. You can usually remove excessive or impacted cerumen by irrigation, which requires a health care provider's order. Review the order for type of solution and ear(s) to receive the irrigation. Before irrigation question the patient for history of perforated eardrum and inspect his or her tympanic membrane to be sure that it is intact; a perforated tympanic membrane contradicts performing irrigation. Visually inspect the pinna and external meatus for redness, swelling, drainage, and presence of foreign objects. Also determine the patient's ability to hear in the affected ear before irrigation.

To irrigate the ear, have the patient sit or lie on the side with the affected ear up. For adults and children over 3 years of age, gently pull the pinna up and back. In children 3 years of age or younger, the pinna should be pulled down and back. Using a bulb-irrigating syringe or a Water Pik set on No. 2 setting; gently wash the ear canal with warm solution (37° C or 98.6° F), being careful to not occlude the canal, which results in pressure on the tympanic membrane. Direct the fluid slowly and gently toward the superior aspect of the ear canal, maintaining the flow in a steady stream. Periodically during the irrigation ask if the patient is experiencing pain, nausea, or vertigo. These symptoms indicate that the solution is too hot or too cold or is being instilled with too much pressure. After the canal is clear, wipe off any moisture from the ear with cotton balls and inspect the canal for remaining earwax.

Hearing Aid Care. A hearing aid amplifies sounds in a controlled manner; the aid receives normal low-intensity sound inputs and delivers them to the patient's ear as louder output. Hearing aids come in a variety of types. The new class of hearing aids reduces background noise interference. Computer chips placed in the aids allow for fine adjustments to the specific patient's hearing needs. People who are hard of hearing (slight or moderate hearing loss) or deaf (severe or profound hearing loss) use hearing aids.

There are three popular types of hearing aids. An in-the-canal (ITC) aid (Fig. 39-7, *A*) is the newest, smallest, and least visible and fits entirely in the ear canal. It has cosmetic appeal, is easy to manipulate and place in the ear, and does not interfere with wearing eyeglasses or using the telephone; and the patient can wear it during most physical exercise. However, it requires adequate ear diameter and depth for proper fit. It does not accommodate progressive hearing loss; and it requires manual dexterity to operate, insert, remove, and change batteries. In addition, cerumen tends to plug this model more than the others.

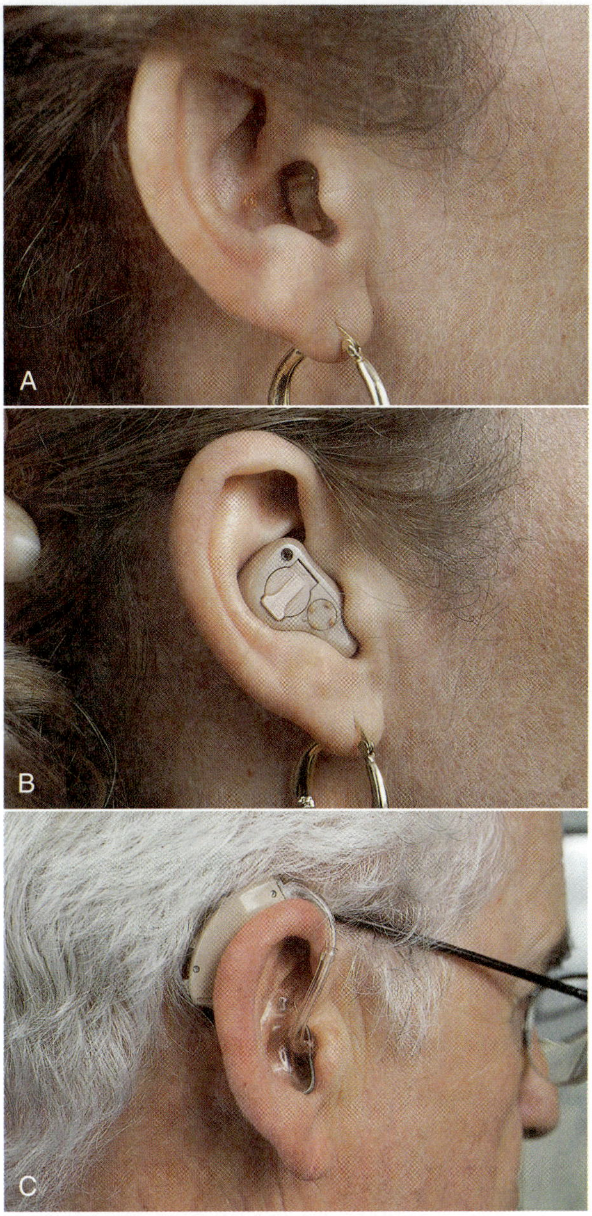

FIG. 39-7 Three common types of hearing aids. **A,** In the canal (ITC). **B,** In the ear (ITE). **C,** Behind the ear (BTE).

An in-the-ear (ITE, or intraaural) aid (Fig. 39-7, *B*) fits into the external auditory canal and allows for more fine tuning. It is more powerful and stronger and therefore is useful for a wider range of hearing loss than the ITC aid. It is easy to position and adjust and does not interfere with eyeglass wearing. However, it is more noticeable than the ITC aid and is not for people with moisture or skin problems in the ear canal.

A behind-the-ear (BTE, or postaural) aid (Fig. 39-7, *C*) hooks around and behind the ear and is connected by a short, clear, hollow plastic tube to an ear mold inserted into the external auditory canal. It allows for fine tuning. It is the largest of the three aids and is useful for patients with rapidly progressing hearing loss or manual dexterity difficulties or those who find partial ear occlusion

BOX 39-13 CARE AND USE OF HEARING AIDS

- Initially wear a hearing aid 15 to 20 minutes; gradually increase time to 10 to 12 hours.
- Once inserted, turn the aid slowly to one-third to one-half volume.
- A whistling sound indicates incorrect ear mold insertion, improper fit of aid, or buildup of earwax or fluid.
- Adjust volume to a comfortable level for talking at a distance of 1 yard.
- Do not wear aid under heat lamps or a hair dryer or in very wet, cold weather.
- Batteries last 1 week with daily wearing of 10 to 12 hours.
- Remove or disconnect battery when not in use.
- Replace ear molds every 2 or 3 years.
- Routinely check battery compartment: Is it clean? Are batteries inserted properly? Is compartment shut all the way?
- Make sure that dials on hearing aid are clean and easy to rotate, creating no static during adjusting.
- Keep aid clean. See manufacturer instructions. Aids are usually cleaned with a soft cloth.
- Avoid use of hairspray and perfume while wearing hearing aids, the residue from the spray causes aid to become oily and greasy.
- Do not submerse in water.
- Routinely check cord or tubing (depending on type of aid) for cracking, fraying, and poor connections.
- Routine follow-up with audiologist is recommended to evaluate effectiveness of current aid.

Data from Ebersole P, et al: *Toward healthy aging,* ed 7, St Louis, 2008, Mosby.

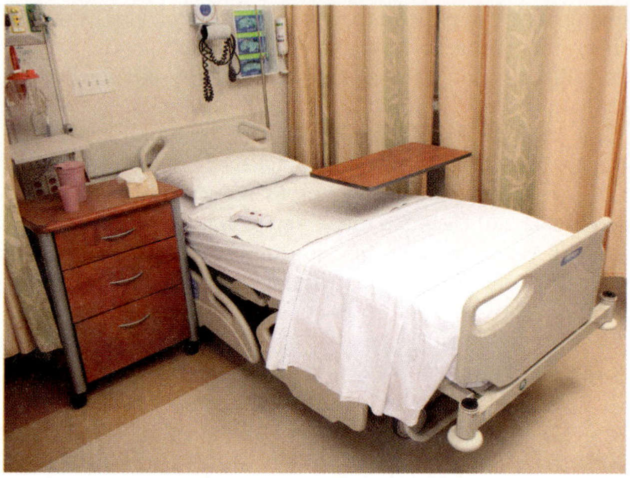

FIG. 39-8 Typical hospital room.

intolerable. The larger size of this type of aid can make use of eyeglasses and phones difficult; it is more difficult to keep in place during physical exercise. Box 39-13 reviews guidelines for the care and cleaning of hearing aids.

Nasal Care. The patient usually removes secretions from the nose by gently blowing into a soft tissue. Caution the patient against harsh blowing that creates pressure capable of injuring the eardrum, nasal mucosa, and even sensitive eye structures. Bleeding from the nares is a sign of harsh blowing.

If the patient is unable to remove nasal secretions, help by using a wet washcloth or a cotton-tipped applicator moistened in water or saline. Never insert the applicator beyond the length of the cotton tip. You can remove excessive nasal secretions by gentle suctioning.

When nasogastric, feeding, or endotracheal tubes are inserted through a patient's nose, change the tape anchoring the tube at least once a day. When tape becomes moist from nasal secretions, the skin and mucosa easily become macerated. Friction from a tube causes tissue sloughing. After carefully removing the tape, maintain hold of the tubing and thoroughly clean and dry the nasal surface.

Patient's Room Environment. Attempt to make a patient's room as comfortable as the home. It needs to be safe and large enough to allow the patient and visitors to move about freely. Control room temperature, ventilation, noise, and odors. Keeping the room neat and orderly also contributes to the patient's sense of well-being.

Maintaining Comfort. What makes a comfortable environment depends on a patient's age, severity of illness, and level of normal daily activity. Depending on age and physical condition, maintain the room temperature between 20° and 23° C (68° and 73.4° F). Infants, older adults, and the acutely ill often need a warmer room. However, certain ill patients benefit from cooler room temperatures to lower the metabolic demands of the body.

An effective ventilation system keeps stale air and odors from lingering in the room. Protect the acutely ill, infants, and older adults from drafts by ensuring that they are adequately dressed and covered with a lightweight blanket. Always empty and rinse commodes, bedpans, and urinals promptly. Room deodorizers help remove many unpleasant odors. Before using room deodorizers determine that the patient is not allergic or sensitive to the deodorizer itself. Thorough hygiene measures provide the best control of body or breath odors.

Ill patients seem to be more sensitive to noises and lighting commonly found in health care. Try to control the noise level, especially when the patient is trying to sleep. Explain the source of unfamiliar noises such as an IV pump or pulse oximeter alarm. Proper lighting provides for safety and comfort. A brightly lit room usually stimulates, whereas a darkened room promotes rest and sleep. Adjust room lighting by closing or opening drapes, regulating over-bed and floor lights, and closing or opening room doors. When entering a patient's room at night, refrain from abruptly turning on an overhead light unless necessary.

Room Equipment. Although there are variations across health care settings, a typical hospital room contains the following basic pieces of furniture: over-bed table, bedside stand, chairs, and bed (Fig. 39-8). Long-term care and rehabilitation facilities often have similar equipment. You can adjust the over-bed table, which rolls on wheels, to various heights over the bed or a chair. The table provides ideal working space for performing procedures. It also provides a surface on which to place meal trays, toiletry items, and objects frequently used by the patient. Clean the top of the over-bed table with an antiseptic cleaner before using it for meals. Do not place the bed pan or urinal on the over-bed table. The bedside stand is for storing the patient's personal possessions and hygiene equipment. The telephone, water pitcher, and drinking cup are usually on top of the bedside stand.

Most hospital rooms contain an armless straight-backed chair or an upholstered lounge chair with arms. Straight-backed chairs

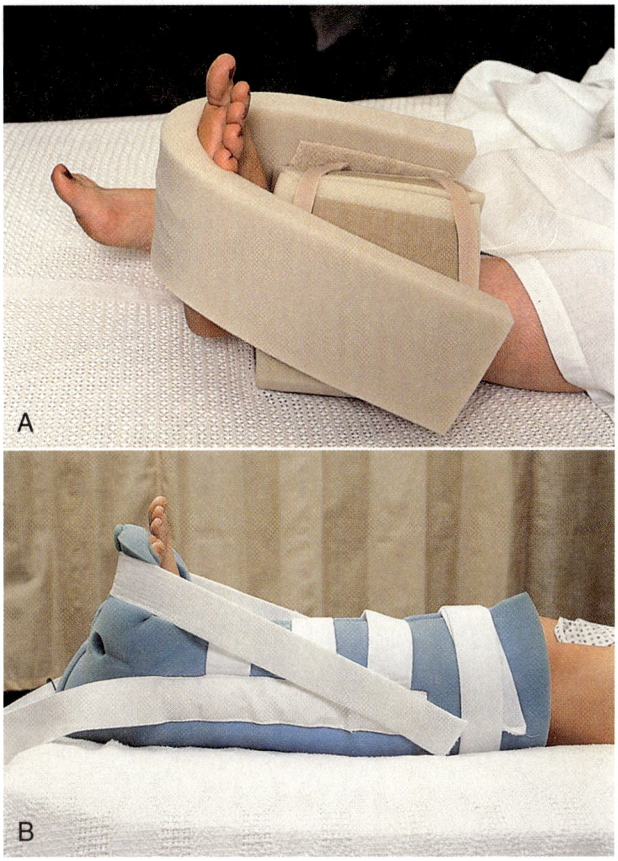

FIG. 39-9 **A,** Foot boot. **B,** Foot boot with lower leg extension.

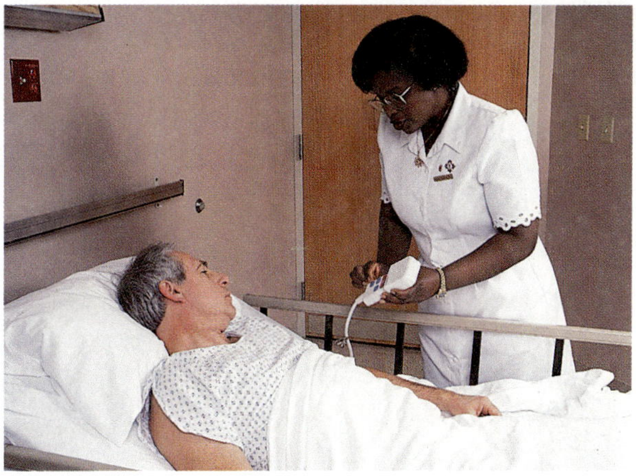

FIG. 39-10 Nurse instructing patient in use of call light and bed controls.

are convenient when temporarily transferring the patient from the bed such as during bed making. Lounge chairs tend to be more comfortable when a patient is willing and able to sit for an extended period.

Each room usually has an over-bed light and floor level night lighting. Position movable lights that extend over the bed from the wall for easy reach, but move them aside when not in use. Additional portable lighting provides extra light during bedside procedures. Some facilities have permanent examination lights mounted in the ceiling or wall.

Other equipment usually found in a patient's room includes a call light, a television set, a wall-mounted blood pressure gauge, oxygen and vacuum wall outlets, and personal care items. Special equipment designed for comfort or positioning patients includes foot boots (Fig. 39-9), special mattresses (see Chapter 48), and bed boards. Whenever you use comfort and positioning equipment, check agency policy and manufacturer directions before application.

Beds. Seriously ill patients often remain in bed for a long time. Because a bed is the piece of equipment used most by a hospitalized patient, it is designed for comfort, safety, and adaptability for changing positions.

The typical hospital bed has a firm mattress on a metal frame that you can raise and lower horizontally. More and more hospitals are converting the standard hospital bed to one in which the mattress surface can be electronically adjusted for patient safety and comfort. Different bed positions promote patient comfort, minimize symptoms, promote lung expansion, and improve access during certain procedures (Table 39-6).

You change the position of a bed usually by using electrical controls incorporated into the patient's call light and in a panel on the side or foot of the bed (Fig. 39-10). Be familiar with use of the bed controls. Ease in raising and lowering a bed and changing position of the head and foot eliminates undue musculoskeletal strain on a nurse. Instruct patients in the proper use of controls and caution them against raising the bed to a position that causes harm. Maintain the bed height at the lowest horizontal position when the patient is unattended.

Beds contain safety features such as locks on the wheels or casters. Lock wheels when the bed is stationary to prevent accidental movement. Side rails allow patients to move more easily in bed and prevent accidents. Do not use side rails to restrict a patient from moving in bed. When using side rails as a restraint, you need a health care provider's order (see Chapter 27). You can remove the headboard and footboard from most beds. This is important when the medical team needs to have easy access to the patient such as during cardiopulmonary resuscitation.

Bed Making. Keep a patient's bed clean and comfortable. This requires frequent inspection to be sure that linen is clean, dry, and free of wrinkles. When patients are diaphoretic, have draining wounds, or are incontinent, check more frequently for wet or soiled linen.

Usually you make the bed in the morning after the patient's bath or while he or she is bathing, in a shower, sitting in a chair eating, or out of the room for procedures or tests. Throughout the day straighten linen that is loose or wrinkled. Also check the bed linen for food particles after meals and for wetness or soiling. Change any linen that becomes soiled or wet.

When changing bed linen, follow principles of medical asepsis by keeping soiled linen away from the uniform (Fig. 39-11). Place soiled linen in special linen bags before placing in a hamper. To avoid air currents that spread microorganisms, never shake the linen. To avoid transmitting infection, do not place soiled linen on the floor. If clean linen touches the floor or any unclean surface, immediately place it in the dirty linen container.

During bed making use safe patient handling procedures and proper body mechanics (see Chapter 47). Always raise the bed to the appropriate height before changing linen so you do not have

TABLE 39-6 Common Bed Positions

POSITION	DESCRIPTION	USES
Fowler's 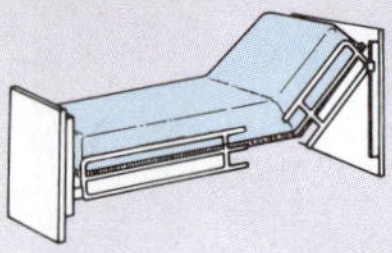	Head of bed raised to angle of 45 degrees or more; semi-sitting position; foot of bed may also be raised at knee	While patient is eating During nasogastric tube insertion and nasotracheal suction Promotes lung expansion Eases difficult breathing
Semi-Fowler's 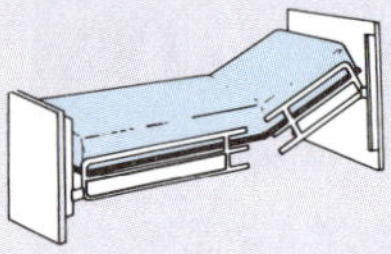	Head of bed raised approximately 30 degrees; inclination less than Fowler's position; foot of bed may also be raised at knee	Promotes lung expansion, especially with ventilator-assisted patients Used when patients receive gastric feedings to reduce regurgitation and risk of aspiration
Trendelenburg's 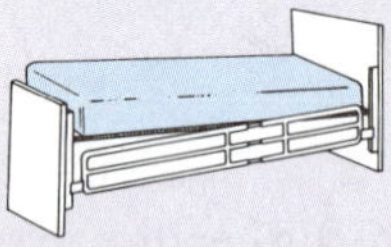	Entire bed frame tilted with head of bed down	Used for postural drainage Facilitates venous return in patients with poor peripheral perfusion
Reverse Trendelenburg's 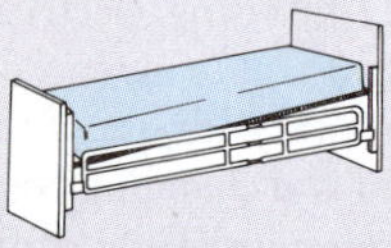	Entire bed frame tilted with foot of bed down	Used infrequently Promotes gastric emptying Prevents esophageal reflux
Flat 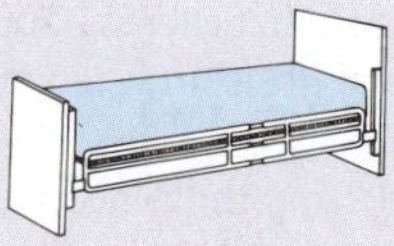	Entire bed frame horizontally parallel with floor	Used for patients with vertebral injuries and in cervical traction Used for patients who are hypotensive Patients usually prefer for sleeping

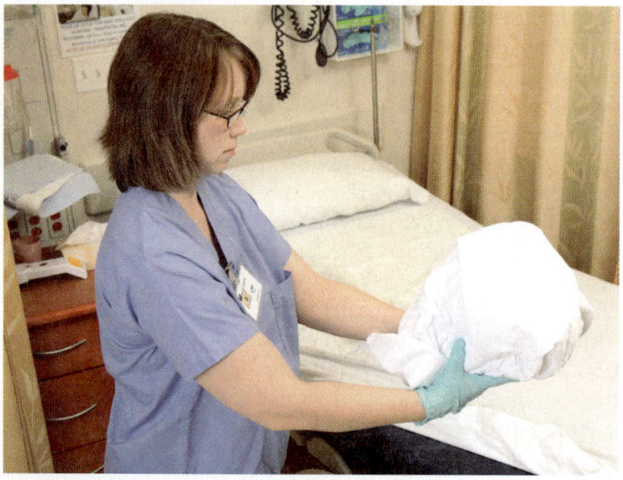

FIG. 39-11 Holding linen away from the uniform prevents contact with microorganisms.

to bend or stretch over the mattress. You move back and forth to opposite sides of the bed while applying new linen. Body mechanics and safe handling are important when turning or repositioning the patient in bed.

When patients are confined to bed, organize bed-making activities to conserve time and energy (Skill 39-5 on pp. 813-817). The patient's privacy, comfort, and safety are all important when making a bed. Using side rails to aid positioning and turning, keeping call lights within the patient's reach and maintaining the proper bed position help promote comfort and safety. After making a bed, return it to the lowest horizontal position and verify that the wheels are locked to prevent accidental falls when the patient gets in and out alone.

When possible, make the bed while it is unoccupied (Box 39-14). Use judgment to determine the best time for the patient to sit up in a chair so you can make the bed. When making an unoccupied bed, follow the same basic principles as for occupied bed making.

An unoccupied bed can be made as an open or closed bed. In an open bed the top covers are folded back so it is easy for a patient to get into bed. In a closed bed the top sheet, blanket, and bedspread are drawn up to the head of the mattress and under the pillows. A closed bed is prepared in a hospital room before a new patient is admitted to that room. A surgical, recovery, or postoperative bed is a modified version of the open bed. The top bed linen is arranged for easy transfer of the patient from a stretcher to the bed. The top sheets and spread are not tucked or mitered at the corners. Instead they are folded to one side or to the bottom third of the bed (Fig. 39-12). This makes patient transfer into the bed easier.

Linens. Many agencies have "nurse servers" either within or just outside a patient's room where a daily supply of linen is stored. Because of the importance of cost control in health care, avoid bringing excess linen into a patient's room. Once you bring the

BOX 39-14 PROCEDURAL GUIDELINES

Making an Unoccupied Bed

Delegation Considerations

The skill of making an unoccupied bed can be delegated to nursing assistive personnel (NAP).

Equipment

Linen bag, mattress pad (change only when soiled), bottom sheet (flat or fitted), drawsheet *(optional)*, top sheet, blanket, bedspread, waterproof pads *(optional)*, pillowcases, bedside chair or table, clean gloves (if linen is soiled), washcloth, and antiseptic cleanser

1. If patient has been incontinent or if excess drainage is on linen, gloves are necessary.
2. Assess activity orders or restrictions in mobility in planning if patient can get out of bed for procedure. Assist to bedside chair or recliner.
3. Lower side rails on both sides of bed and raise bed to comfortable working position.
4. Remove soiled linen and place in laundry bag. Avoid shaking or fanning linen.
5. Reposition mattress and wipe off any moisture using a washcloth moistened in antiseptic solution. Dry thoroughly.
6. Apply all bottom linen on one side of bed before moving to opposite side.
7. Be sure that fitted sheet is placed smoothly over mattress. To apply a flat unfitted sheet, allow about 25 cm (10 inches) to hang over mattress edge. Make sure that lower hem of sheet lies seam down, even with bottom edge of mattress. Pull remaining top portion of sheet over top edge of mattress.
8. While standing at head of bed, miter top corner of bottom sheet (see Skill 39-5, Step 14).
9. Tuck remaining portion of unfitted sheet under mattress from head to foot of bed.
10. *Optional:* Apply drawsheet, laying centerfold along middle of bed lengthwise. Smooth drawsheet over mattress and tuck excess edge under mattress, keeping palms down.
11. Move to opposite side of bed and spread bottom sheet smoothly over edge of mattress from head to foot of bed.
12. Apply fitted sheet smoothly over each mattress corner. For an unfitted sheet, miter top corner of bottom sheet (see Step 8), making sure that corner is taut.
13. Grasp remaining edge of unfitted bottom sheet and tuck tightly under mattress while moving from head to foot of bed. Smooth folded drawsheet over bottom sheet and tuck under mattress, first at middle, then at top, and then at bottom.
14. If needed, apply waterproof pad over bottom sheet or drawsheet.
15. Place top sheet over bed with vertical centerfold lengthwise down middle of bed. Open sheet out from head to foot, being sure that top edge of sheet is even with top edge of mattress.
16. Make horizontal toe pleat: stand at foot of bed and make fanfold in sheet 5 to 10 cm (2 to 4 inches) across bed. Pull sheet up from bottom to make fold approximately 15 cm (6 inches) from bottom edge of mattress (see illustration, Skill 39-5, Step 31).
17. Tuck in remaining portion of sheet under foot of mattress. Then place blanket over bed with top edge parallel to top edge of sheet and 15 to 20 cm (6 to 8 inches) down from edge of sheet. (*Optional:* Apply additional spread over bed.)
18. Make cuff by turning edge of top sheet down over top edge of blanket and spread.
19. Standing on one side at foot of bed, lift mattress corner slightly with one hand; with other hand tuck top sheet, blanket, and spread under mattress. Be sure that toe pleats are not pulled out.
20. Make modified mitered corner with top sheet, blanket, and spread. After making triangular fold, do not tuck tip of triangle (see illustration).

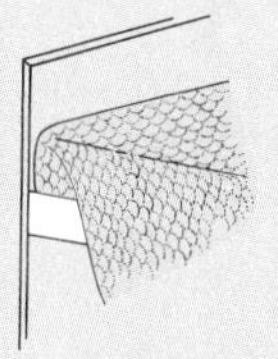

STEP 20 Modified mitered corner.

21. Go to other side of bed. Spread sheet, blanket, and spread out evenly. Make cuff with top sheet and blanket. Make modified corner at foot of bed.
22. Apply clean pillowcase.
23. Place call light within patient's reach on bed rail or pillow and return bed to height allowing for patient transfer. Assist patient to bed.
24. Arrange patient's room. Remove and discard supplies. Perform hand hygiene.

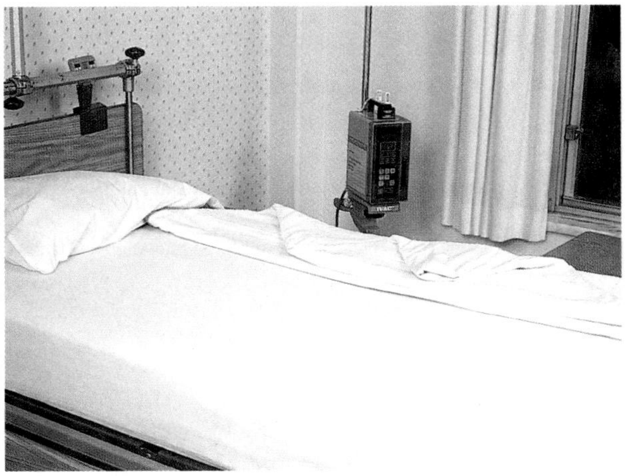

FIG. 39-12 Surgical or recovery bed.

linen into a patient's room, if unused, it must be laundered before being used. This increases agency costs. Excess linen lying around a patient's room creates clutter and obstacles for patient care activities.

Before making a bed collect necessary bed linens and the patient's personal items. In this way all equipment is accessible to prepare the bed and room. When fitted sheets are not available, flat sheets usually are pressed with a center crease to be placed down the center of the bed. The linens unfold easily to the sides, with creases often fitting over the mattress edge. Apply clean linens whenever there is soiling.

Handle linen properly to minimize the spread of infection (see Chapter 28). Agency policies provide guidelines for the proper way to bag and dispose of soiled linen. After a patient is discharged, all bed linen goes to the laundry, and housekeeping cleans the mattress and bed before clean linen is applied.

EVALUATION

Through the Patient's Eyes. Evaluate patient responses to nursing interventions to determine if goals and outcome criteria have been met. A critical thinking approach considers all factors when evaluating the patient's care (Fig. 39-13). Critical thinking ensures that the nurse considers the patient's perspectives and applies what is known about hygiene to the patient's unique situation.

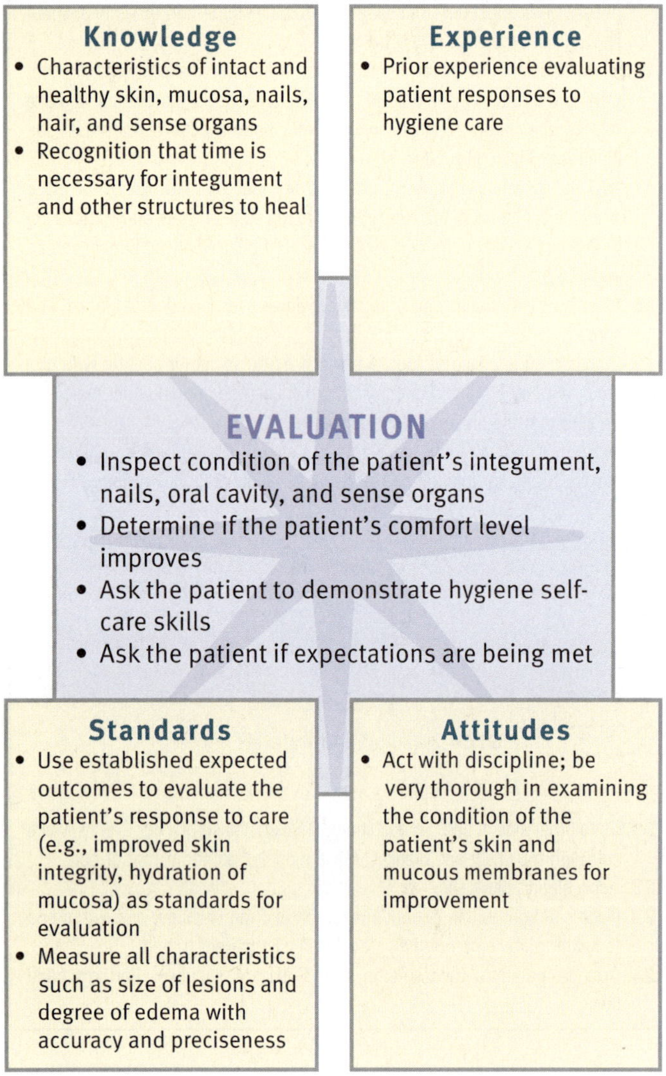
Knowledge
• Characteristics of intact and healthy skin, mucosa, nails, hair, and sense organs
• Recognition that time is necessary for integument and other structures to heal
Experience
• Prior experience evaluating patient responses to hygiene care
EVALUATION
• Inspect condition of the patient's integument, nails, oral cavity, and sense organs
• Determine if the patient's comfort level improves
• Ask the patient to demonstrate hygiene self-care skills
• Ask the patient if expectations are being met
Standards
• Use established expected outcomes to evaluate the patient's response to care (e.g., improved skin integrity, hydration of mucosa) as standards for evaluation
• Measure all characteristics such as size of lesions and degree of edema with accuracy and preciseness
Attitudes
• Act with discipline; be very thorough in examining the condition of the patient's skin and mucous membranes for improvement

FIG. 39-13 Critical thinking model for hygiene evaluation.

The patient's expectations are important guidelines in determining patient satisfaction. You need to feel comfortable in addressing his or her concerns and expectations. A caring approach facilitates discussion of these issues. Evaluate patient responses to hygiene measures both during and after each particular hygiene intervention. For example, when the bath is completed, ask if the patient's comfort and relaxation have improved. When evaluating for the effectiveness of hygiene measures, observe for changes in his or her behavior. Does the patient assume a more relaxed position? Is he or she free of body odor? Is he or she able to fall asleep? Does his or her facial expression convey a sense of comfort?

Patient Outcomes. Frequently it takes time for hygiene care to result in an improvement in the patient's condition. The presence of oral lesions, a scalp infestation, or skin excoriation often requires repeated measures and a combination of nursing interventions. The nurse's knowledge base and experience provide important perspectives when analyzing assessment data about a patient. For example, frequent observation of the oral mucosa helps to determine the effectiveness of oral hygiene practices. Are previously inflamed mucosa improving? The standards for evaluation are the expected outcomes established in the planning stage of the patient's care. If outcomes are not met, you need to revise the care plan. Continue to apply critical thinking attitudes when considering all evaluation findings.

The final aspect of evaluation determines whether or not the patient's expectations for hygiene were met.

When outcomes are not met, ask questions to determine appropriate changes in interventions. Examples of questions include:

- Did your bath and back rub help make you comfortable?
- Are there ways we can do a better job with your foot care?
- What is preventing you from being able to perform your foot care at home?
- Which further measures do you think are necessary to keep your mouth clean and refreshed?
- What other questions do you have about helping your father with his bath?
- What do you think would help you be more independent with your hygiene care?

SAFETY GUIDELINES FOR NURSING SKILLS

Ensuring patient safety is an essential role of the professional nurse. To ensure patient safety, communicate clearly with members of the health care team, assess and incorporate the patient's priorities of care and preferences, and use the best evidence when making decisions about your patient's care. When performing the skills in this chapter, remember the following points to ensure safe, individualized patient care.

- Always perform hygiene measures moving from the cleanest to less clean or dirty areas. This often requires you to change gloves and perform hand hygiene during care activities.
- Use clean gloves when you anticipate contact with nonintact skin or mucous membranes or when there will likely be contact with drainage, secretions, excretions, or blood during hygiene care.
- When using water or solutions for hygiene care, be sure to test the temperature to prevent burn injury.
- To avoid injury when performing hygiene care, use principles of body mechanics and safe patient handling.
- When giving or assisting with hygiene care, be sensitive to the invasion of privacy and possible loss of self-esteem associated with these procedures. Foster acceptance and comfort by using therapeutic communication techniques, draping and providing privacy, and informing the patient before touching sensitive or private body parts.
- Remember that you are responsible and accountable for assessing the patient both before and after care to detect unexpected outcomes and give proper direction to nursing assistive personnel when delegating hygiene care.

SKILL 39-1 BATHING AND PERINEAL CARE

Delegation Considerations

The skill of bathing and perineal care can be delegated to nursing assistive personnel (NAP). Direct the NAP to:

- Avoid massaging reddened skin areas.
- Report early signs of impaired skin integrity, including redness or pale skin, to the nurse.
- Properly position patients with musculoskeletal limitations and indwelling catheters or intravenous (IV) lines.
- Report patient fatigue, shortness of breath, or pain during hygiene care.
- Report changes in patient's skin to the nurse.

Equipment

- Washcloths and bath towels (optional disposable cloths)
- Bath blanket
- Soap and soap dish or liquid soap (optional no rinse solution)
- Toiletry items (deodorant, powder, lotion, cologne)
- Toilet tissue or wipes
- Warm water
- Clean hospital gown or patient's own pajamas or gown
- Laundry bag
- Clean gloves (when risk for contacting body fluids)
- Washbasin

STEP	RATIONALE
ASSESSMENT	
1 Assess patient's tolerance for bathing: activity tolerance, comfort level during movement, cognitive ability, musculoskeletal function, and the presence of shortness of breath.	Determines patient's ability to perform or tolerate bathing and level of assistance required (e.g., tub bath, partial bed bath).
CLINICAL DECISION: *Patients with dementia may become agitated and aggressive during bathing activities. Consider using alternative bathing procedures with these patients (see Box 39-7).*	
2 Assess patient's visual status, ability to sit without support, hand grasp, range of motion (ROM) of extremities.	Determines degree of assistance patient needs for bathing.
3 Assess for presence of equipment (e.g., IV line, oxygen tubing, Foley catheter)	Affects how you plan bathing activities and positioning. Helps determine how to set up supplies.
4 Assess patient's bathing preferences: frequency and time of day preferred, type of hygiene products used, and other factors related to patient preferences.	Patient participates in plan of care. Promotes patient's comfort and willingness to cooperate. Includes cultural or personal hygiene preferences into care.
5 Ask if patient has noticed any problems related to condition of skin and genitalia: excess moisture, inflammation, drainage or excretions from lesions or body cavities, rashes or other skin lesions.	Provides you with information to direct physical assessment of skin and genitalia during bathing. Also influences selection of skin care products.
6 Before or during bath, assess condition of patient's skin. Note presence of dryness, indicated by flaking, redness, scaling, and cracking.	Provides a baseline for comparison over time in determining if bathing improves condition of skin.
7 Assess patient's knowledge of skin hygiene in terms of its importance, preventive measures to take, and common problems.	Determines patient's learning needs.
PLANNING	
1 Review orders for specific precautions concerning patient's movement or positioning.	Prevents injury to patient during bathing activities. Determines level of assistance required by patient.
2 Check for a health care provider's therapeutic bath order; if there is an order, note type of solution, length of time for bath, body part to be attended.	Therapeutic baths are ordered for specific physical effect, which usually includes promotion of healing or soothing effects.
3 Identify the patient using two identifiers (i.e., name and birth date or name and account number) according to facility policy.	Ensures correct patient. Complies with recommended National Patient Safety Goal (TJC, 2011).
4 Explain procedure and ask patient for suggestions on how to prepare supplies. If partial bath, ask how much of bath patient wishes to complete.	Promotes patient's cooperation and participation.
5 Prepare equipment and supplies. If it is necessary to leave room, be sure that call light is within patient's reach.	Avoids interrupting procedure or leaving patient unattended to retrieve missing equipment.
IMPLEMENTATION	
1 **Complete or partial bed bath**	
a. Offer patient bedpan or urinal. Provide toilet tissue.	Patient feels more comfortable after voiding. Prevents interruption of bath.
b. Perform hand hygiene. If patient has nonintact skin or skin is soiled with drainage, excretions, or body secretions, apply clean gloves. Ensure that patient is not allergic to latex.	Reduces transmission of microorganisms. Prevents allergic reaction if latex gloves are used.
c. Verify that bed is in locked position and raise bed to a comfortable working height. Lower side rail closest to you and assist patient into comfortable supine position, maintaining body alignment. Bring patient toward side closest to you.	Prevents bed from moving. Helps you reach patient without stretching and reaching across bed, thus minimizing strain on back muscles.

SKILL 39-1 BATHING AND PERINEAL CARE—cont'd

STEP	RATIONALE
d. Place bath blanket over patient and loosen and remove top covers without exposing him or her. If possible, have patient hold top of bath blanket. Place soiled linen in laundry bag. Take care to not allow linen to touch your uniform. *Optional:* Use top sheet when bath blanket is not available or patient prefers.	Bath blanket provides warmth and privacy during bath.
e. Remove patient's gown or pajamas.	Provides full exposure of body parts during bathing.
(1) If available, use gown with ties or snaps on sleeves for patient with IV line, upper-extremity injury, or limited ROM.	
(2) If snap-on gown or gown with ties on arms is not used and patient has limited upper-extremity ROM or an IV access, remove gown from *unaffected side first.*	Undressing unaffected side first allows easier manipulation of gown over body part with reduced ROM.
(3) Remove gown from arm without IV line first. Then remove gown from arm with IV line (see illustrations). Remove IV tubing from pole and slide IV container and tubing through arm of patient's gown. Rehang IV container and check flow rate. Regulate if necessary.	Manipulation of IV tubing and container may disrupt flow rate. Do **not** delegate regulation of IV flow rate to NAP.

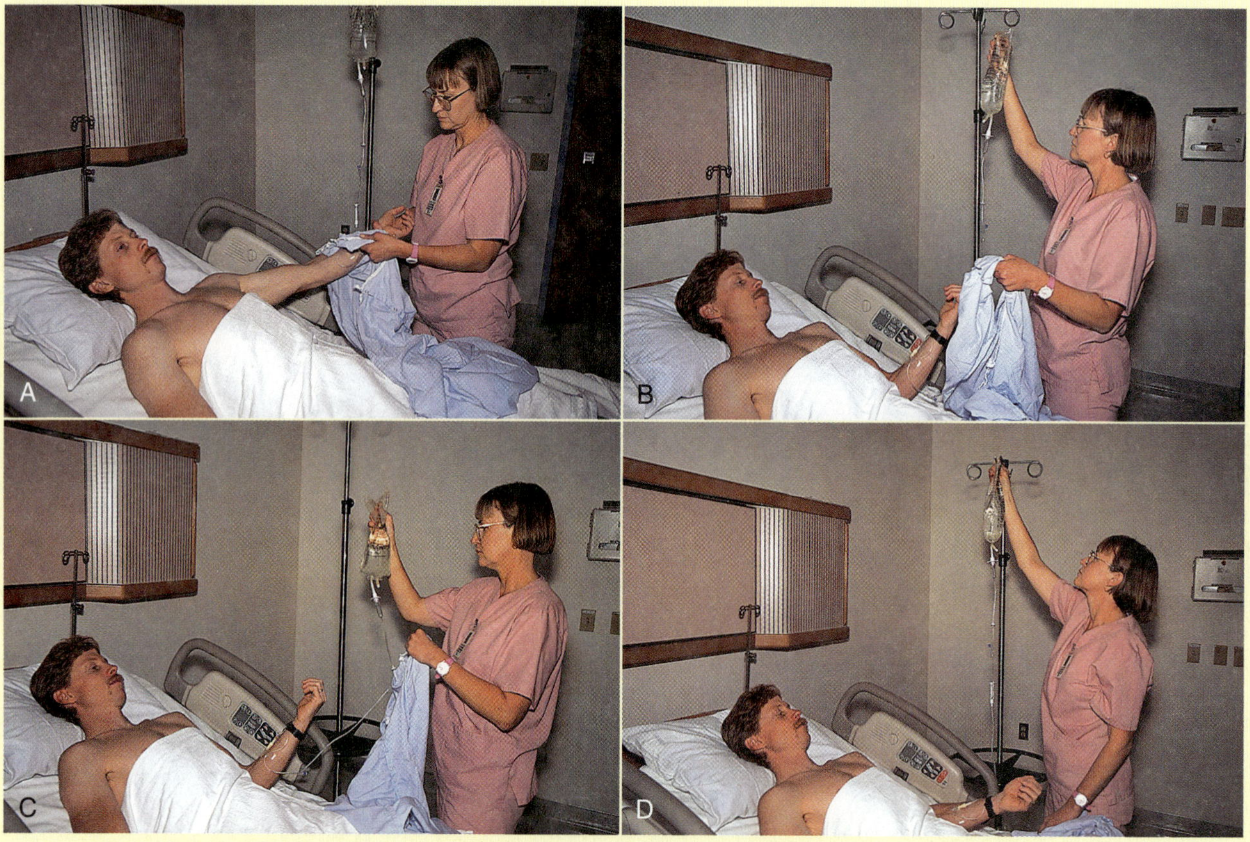

STEP 1e(3) A, Remove patient's gown. **B,** Remove IV tubing from pole. **C,** Slide IV tubing through arm of patient's gown. **D,** Rehang IV bag.

STEP	RATIONALE
(4) If IV pump is in use, turn pump off, clamp tubing, remove tubing from pump, and proceed as in Step (3). Reinsert tubing into pump, unclamp tubing, and turn pump on at correct rate. Observe flow rate and regulate if necessary. *Do not disconnect tubing.*	Regulation is necessary to prevent improper infusion of fluids. Do **not** delegate regulation of IV pump to NAP. Disconnecting IV tubing places patient at risk of introduction of microorganisms into the IV line.
f. Pull side rail up. Lower bed temporarily to lowest position and raise to comfortable working height on return after filling washbasin two-thirds full with warm water. Place basin and supplies on over-bed table. Check water temperature and also have patient place fingers in water to test temperature tolerance. Place plastic container of bath lotion in bath water to warm if desired.	Raising side rail and lowering bed position maintain patient's safety while you leave bedside. Keeping bed at working height during bath prevents back strain. Warm water promotes comfort, relaxes muscles, and prevents unnecessary chilling. Testing temperature prevents accidental burns. Bath water warms lotion for application to patient's skin.

STEP	RATIONALE
g. Lower side rail, remove pillow if tolerated, and raise head of bed 30 to 45 degrees if allowed. Place bath towel under patient's head. Place second bath towel over patient's chest.	Aids your access to patient. You do not have to reach across bed, thus minimizing strain on back muscles. Removal of pillow makes it easier to wash patient's ears and neck. Placing towels prevents bed linen and bath blanket from getting soiled or wet.
h. Wash face.	
(1) Ask if patient is wearing contact lenses.	Prevents accidental injury to eyes.
(2) Fold washcloth around fingers of your hand to form a mitt (see illustration). Immerse mitt in water and wring thoroughly.	Mitt retains water and heat better than loosely held washcloth; keeps cold edges from brushing against patient and prevents splashing.
(3) Wash patient's eyes with plain warm water. Use different section of mitt for each eye. Move mitt from inner to outer canthus (see illustration). Soak any crusts on eyelid for 2 to 3 minutes with damp cloth before attempting removal. Dry eyes thoroughly but gently.	Soap irritates eyes. Use of separate sections of mitt reduces infection transmission. Bathing eye from inner to outer canthus prevents secretions from entering nasolacrimal duct. Pressure can cause internal injury.
(4) Ask if patient prefers to use soap on face. Otherwise wash, rinse, and dry forehead, cheeks, nose, neck, and ears without using soap. (Men may wish to shave at this point or wait until after bath.)	Soap tends to dry face, which is exposed to air more than other body parts.
i. Wash trunk and upper extremities.	
(1) Remove bath blanket from patient's arm that is closest to you. Place bath towel lengthwise under arm. Bathe arm with soap and water using long, firm strokes from distal to proximal areas (fingers to axilla).	Towel prevents soiling of bed. Soap lowers surface tension and facilitates removal of debris and bacteria when friction is applied during washing. Long, firm strokes stimulate circulation; moving distal to proximal promotes venous return.
(2) Raise and support arm above head (if possible) to wash, rinse, and dry axilla thoroughly (see illustration). Apply deodorant or powder to underarms if desired or needed.	Movement of arm exposes axilla and exercises normal ROM of joint. Alkaline residue from soap discourages growth of normal skin bacteria. Drying prevents excess moisture, which can cause skin maceration or softening. Respect patient's preference for use of hygiene products.

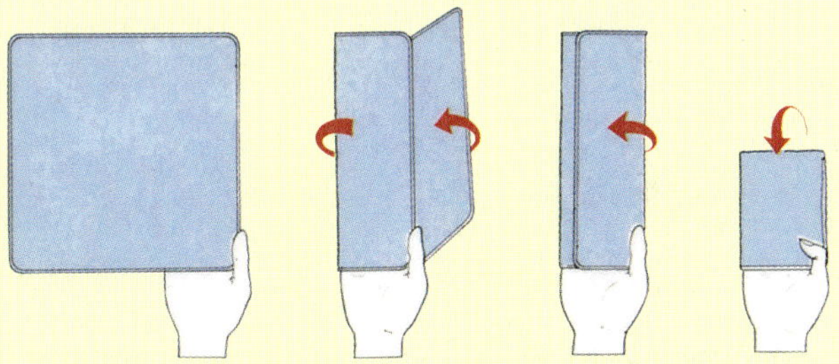

STEP 1h(2) Steps for folding washcloth to form a mitt.

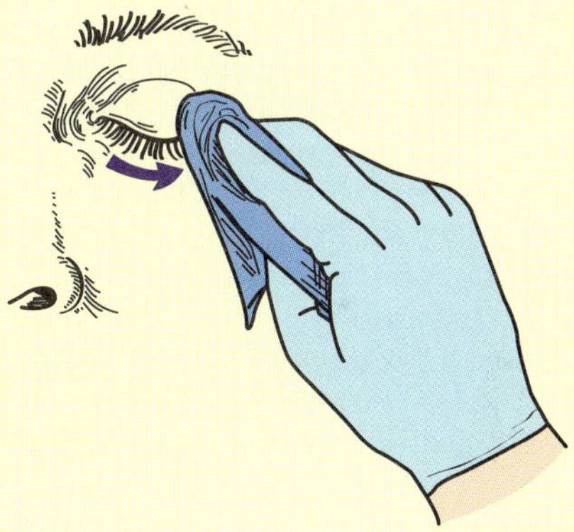

STEP 1h(3) Wash eye from inner to outer canthus.

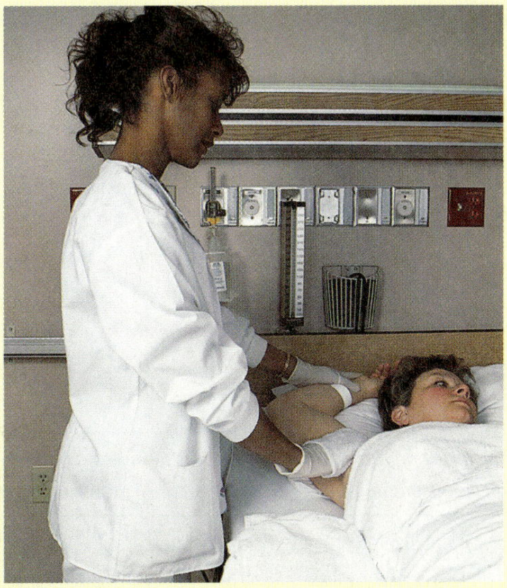

STEP 1i(2) Positioning arm to wash axilla.

SKILL 39-1 BATHING AND PERINEAL CARE—cont'd

STEP	RATIONALE
(3) Move to other side of bed and repeat Steps (1) and (2) with other arm.	Provides for better access to patient and helps prevents back strain.
(4) Place bath towel across patient's chest so it covers chest and arms and fold bath blanket down to umbilicus. While lifting edge of towel away from chest with one hand, bathe chest with mitted washcloth on other hand using long, firm strokes. Take special care to wash skinfolds under female's breasts. It is often necessary to lift breast upward while bathing underneath it. Keep patient's chest covered between wash and rinse periods. Rinse and dry well.	Draping prevents unnecessary exposure of body parts. Towel maintains warmth and privacy. Secretions and dirt collect easily in areas of tight skinfolds. Skin under breasts is vulnerable to excoriation if not kept clean and dry.
j. Wash hands and nails.	
(1) Fold bath towel in half and lay it on bed beside patient. Place basin on towel. Immerse patient's hand in water. Allow hand to soak for 2 to 3 minutes before washing hand and fingernails. Remove basin and dry hand well. Repeat for other hand.	Soaking softens cuticles and calluses of hand, loosens debris beneath nails, and enhances feeling of cleanliness. Thorough drying removes moisture between fingers.
k. Check temperature of bath water and change water when cool or soapy.	Warm water maintains patient's comfort. Alkaline soap residue is irritating to skin and can decrease the normal protectiveness of acid ph.

CLINICAL DECISION: *If patient is at risk for falling, be sure that two side rails are up before obtaining fresh water. In addition, lower bed when it is necessary to leave bedside. Note: Having all side rails raised is considered a restraint. Check agency policy.*

STEP	RATIONALE
l. Wash the abdomen.	
(1) Place bath towel lengthwise over chest and abdomen. (Two towels may be needed.) Fold bath blanket down to just above pubic region. With one hand lift bath towel. With mitted hand bathe and rinse abdomen, giving special attention to umbilicus and skinfolds of abdomen and groin. Stroke from side to side. Keep abdomen covered between washing and rinsing. Rinse and dry well.	Draping prevents unnecessary exposure of body parts. Towel maintains warmth and privacy. Keeping skinfolds clean and dry helps prevent odor and skin irritation. Moisture and sediment that collect in skinfolds predispose skin to maceration.
(2) Apply clean gown or pajama top. If an extremity is injured or immobilized, dress affected side first. (This step may be omitted until completion of bath; gown should not become soiled during remainder of bath.)	Maintains patient's warmth and comfort. Dressing affected side first allows easier manipulation of gown over body part with reduced ROM.
m. Wash the lower extremities.	
(1) Cover chest and abdomen with top of bath blanket. Cover legs with bottom of blanket. Expose near leg by folding blanket toward midline. Be sure to keep other leg and perineum draped.	Prevents unnecessary exposure.
(2) Place bath towel under leg, supporting leg at knee and ankle. If appropriate, place patient's foot in bath basin to soak while washing and rinsing. (Bend patient's leg at knee; and, while grasping patient's heel, elevate leg from mattress slightly and place bath basin on towel.) If patient is unable to support leg, cleaning can be done by washing feet thoroughly with washcloth.	Towel prevents soiling of bed linen. Support of joint and extremity during lifting prevents strain on musculoskeletal structures. Sudden movement by patient could spill bath water. Soaking softens calluses and rough skin.

CLINICAL DECISION: *If patient has diabetes or peripheral vascular disease with impaired circulation and/or sensation, do not soak feet.*

STEP	RATIONALE
(3) Wash leg using long, firm strokes from ankle to knee and from knee to thigh (see illustration). Do not rub or massage the back of the calf. Rinse and dry well. Clean foot, making sure to bathe between toes. Rinse and dry toes and feet completely. Clean and clip nails as needed (see Skill 39-2). Remove and discard towel.	Promotes circulation and venous return. Excess massage of calf could loosen deep vein thrombus. Secretions and moisture may be present between toes, predisposing patient to maceration and breakdown.
(4) Raise side rail, move to opposite side of bed, lower side rail, and repeat Steps (2) and (3) for other leg and foot. If skin is dry, apply moisturizer. When finished, cover patient with bath blanket.	

CLINICAL DECISION: *Do not use long, firm strokes to wash the lower extremities of patients with history of deep vein thromboses or blood-clotting disorders. Use short, light strokes instead.*

STEP	RATIONALE
n. Cover patient with bath blanket, raise side rail for patient's safety, remove soiled gloves, and/or perform hand hygiene. Change bath water.	Decreased bath water temperature causes chilling. Clean water reduces microorganism transmission to perineal structures.

STEP	RATIONALE
o. Provide perineal hygiene.	
(1) If patient is able to maneuver and handle washcloth, allow him or her to clean perineum on own.	Maintains patient's dignity and self-care ability.
(2) Female patient	
(a) Apply pair of clean gloves. Lower side rail. Assist patient into dorsal recumbent position. Note restrictions or limitations in patient's positioning. Place waterproof pad under patient's buttocks. Drape patient with bath blanket placed in the shape of a diamond. Lift lower edge of bath blanket to expose perineum (see illustration).	Provides full exposure of female genitalia. If patient is totally dependent, provide assistance to support patient in side-lying position and raise leg as perineum is bathed. If position causes patient discomfort, reduce degree of abduction in female's hips.
(b) Fold lower corner of bath blanket up between patient's legs onto abdomen. Wash and dry patient's upper thighs.	Keeping patient draped until procedure begins minimizes anxiety. Buildup of perineal secretions soils surrounding skin surfaces.
(c) Wash labia majora. Use nondominant hand to gently retract labia from thigh: with dominant hand, wash carefully in skinfolds. Wipe in direction from perineum to rectum. Repeat on opposite side using separate section of washcloth. Rinse and dry area thoroughly.	Perineal care involves thorough cleaning of the patient's external genitalia and surrounding skin. Skinfolds may contain body secretions that harbor microorganisms. Wiping front to back reduces chance of transmitting fecal organisms to urinary meatus.
(d) Gently separate labia with nondominant hand to expose urethral meatus and vaginal orifice. With dominant hand, wash downward from pubic area toward rectum in one smooth stroke (see illustration). Wash middle and both sides of the perineum. Use separate section of cloth for each stroke. Clean thoroughly around labia minora, clitoris, and vaginal orifice. Avoid placing tension on indwelling catheter if present and clean area around it thoroughly.	Cleansing method reduces transfer of microorganisms to urinary meatus. (For menstruating women or patients with indwelling catheters, clean with cotton balls.)
(e) Provide catheter care as needed (see Chapter 45).	Cleaning along catheter from exit site reduces incidence of health care–associated urinary infection.
(f) Rinse area thoroughly. May use bedpan and pour warm water over perineal area. Dry thoroughly from front to back.	Rinsing removes soap and microorganisms more effectively than wiping. Retained moisture harbors microorganisms.

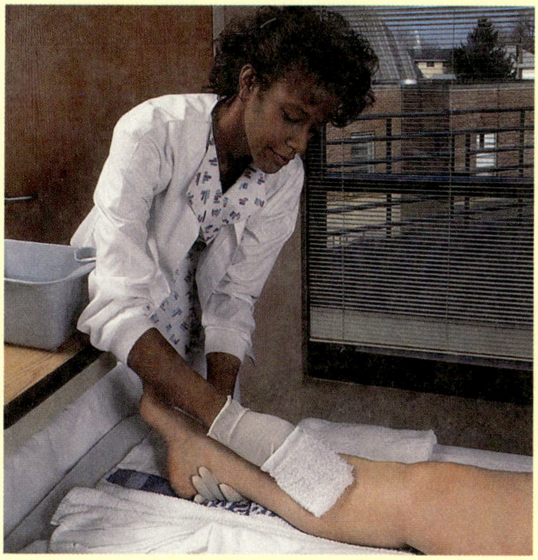

STEP 1m(3) Washing leg.

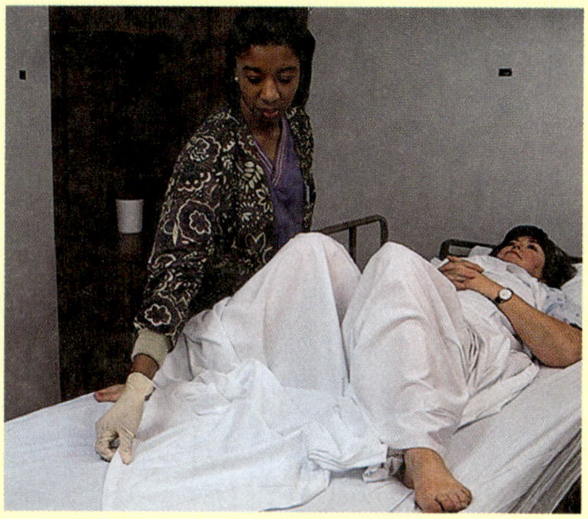

STEP 1o(2)(a) Drape patient for perineal care.

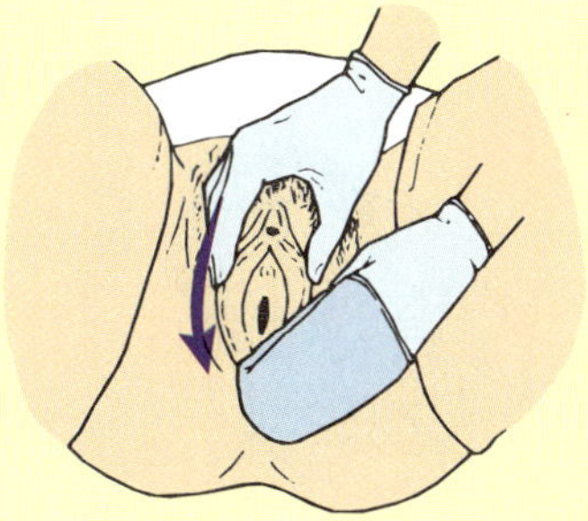

STEP 1o(2)(d) Cleanse from perineum to rectum.

SKILL 39-1 BATHING AND PERINEAL CARE—cont'd

STEP	RATIONALE
(g) Fold lower corner of bath blanket back between patient's legs and over perineum. Ask patient to lower legs and assume comfortable position.	
(3) Male patient	
(a) Apply pair of clean gloves. Lower side rail. Assist patient to supine position. Note any restriction in mobility.	Provides full exposure of male genitalia. Position patients who are unable to lie supine on their side.
(b) Fold lower half of bath blanket up to expose upper thighs. Wash and dry thighs.	Buildup of perineal secretions soils surrounding skin surfaces.
(c) Cover thighs with bath towels. Raise bath blanket up to expose genitalia. Gently raise penis and place bath towel underneath. Gently grasp shaft of penis. If patient is uncircumcised, retract foreskin (see illustration). If patient has an erection, defer procedure until later.	Draping minimizes patient anxiety. Towel prevents moisture from collecting in inguinal area. Gentle but firm handling of penis reduces chance of an erection. Secretions capable of harboring microorganisms collect underneath foreskin.
(d) Wash tip of penis at urethral meatus first. Using circular motion, clean from meatus outward (see illustration). Discard washcloth and repeat with a clean cloth until penis is clean. Rinse and dry gently.	Direction of cleaning moves from area of least contamination to area of most contamination, preventing microorganisms from entering urethra.
(e) Return foreskin to its natural position. This is extremely important in patients with decreased sensation in their lower extremities.	Tightening of foreskin around shaft of penis causes local edema and discomfort. Patients with reduced sensation do not feel tightening of foreskin.
(f) Gently clean shaft of penis and scrotum by having patient abduct legs. Pay special attention to underlying surface of penis. Lift scrotum carefully and wash underlying skinfolds. Rinse and dry thoroughly.	Vigorous massage of penis may cause an erection. Underlying surface of penis is an area where secretions accumulate. Abduction of legs provides easier access to scrotal tissues. Secretions easily collect between skinfolds.
(g) Avoid placing tension on indwelling catheter if present and clean area around it thoroughly. Provide catheter care (see Chapter 45).	Cleaning along catheter from exit site reduces incidence of nosocomial urinary infection.
p. Remove soiled gloves and discard in trash; raise side rail before leaving bedside to dispose of water and obtain fresh water.	Prevents transmission of infection. Protects patient from injury.
q. Wash back. (This follows both female and male perineal care.)	
(1) Perform hand hygiene and apply clean pair of gloves if indicated. Lower side rail. Assist patient into prone or side-lying position (as applicable). Place towel lengthwise along patient's side and keep him or her covered with bath blanket.	Exposes back and buttocks for bathing while limiting exposure.
(2) Keep patient draped by sliding bath blanket over shoulders and thighs during bathing. Wash, rinse, and dry back from neck to buttocks using long, firm strokes. Move from back to buttocks and anus. Pay special attention to folds of buttocks and anus.	Cleaning buttocks and anus after back prevents contamination of water.
(3) Perform hand hygiene and apply clean pair of gloves. Lower side rail. Assist patient into prone or side-lying position (as applicable). Place towel lengthwise along patient's side and keep him or her covered with bath blanket.	Exposes back and buttocks for bathing while limiting exposure.
(4) If fecal material is present, enclose in a fold of underpad or toilet tissue and remove with disposable wipes.	Skinfolds near buttocks and anus may contain fecal secretions that harbor microorganisms.
(5) Clean buttocks and anus, washing front to back (see illustration). Clean, rinse, and dry area thoroughly. If needed, place a clean absorbent pad under patient's buttocks. Remove contaminated gloves. Raise side rail and perform hand hygiene.	Cleaning motion prevents contaminating perineal area with fecal material or microorganisms.

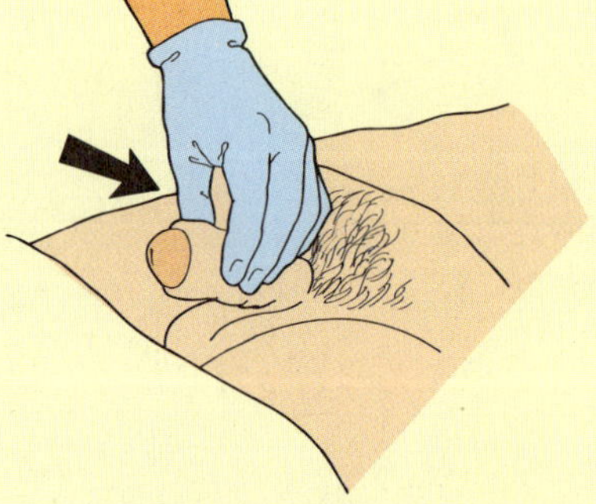

STEP 1o(3)(c) Retract foreskin.

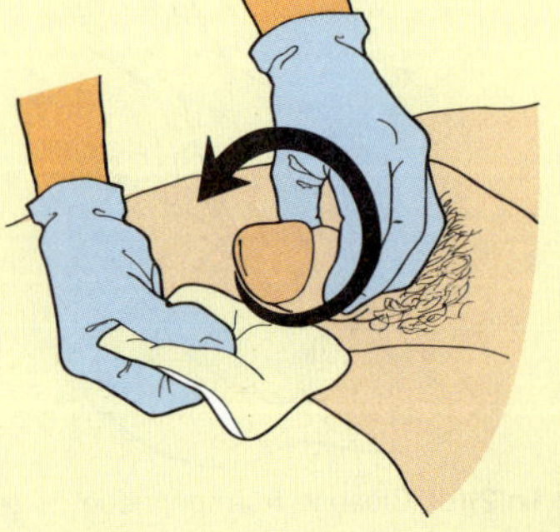

STEP 1o(3)(d) Use circular motion to cleanse tip of penis.

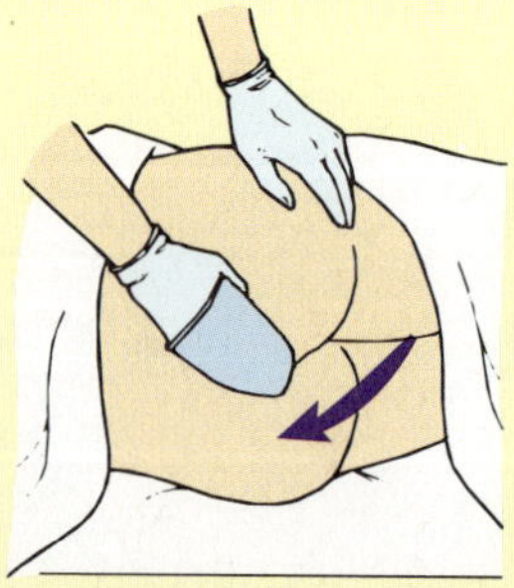

STEP 1q(5) Cleanse buttocks from front to back.

STEP	RATIONALE
(6) Return to bed and lower side rail; give a back rub.	Promotes patient relaxation. Make sure that a back rub is appropriate for your patient. Back rubs are contraindicated in some cardiac patients.
r. Apply additional body lotion or oil to patient's skin as needed.	Moisturizing lotion prevents dry, chapped skin.
s. Remove soiled linen and place in dirty-linen bag. Clean and replace bathing equipment. Wash hands.	Reduces transmission of microorganisms.
t. Assist patient in dressing. Comb patient's hair. Women may want to apply makeup. Help as needed.	Promotes patient's body image.
u. Make patient's bed (see Skill 39-5 and Box 39-14).	Provides clean, comfortable environment.
v. Check the function and position of external devices (e.g., indwelling urethral catheters, nasogastric tubes, IV lines).	Ensures that systems remain functional after bathing activities.
w. Place bed in lowest position.	Maintains patient's safety by decreasing height of bed frame from floor.
x. Replace call light and personal possessions. Leave room as clean and comfortable as possible.	Prevents transmission of infection. Clean environment promotes patient's comfort. Keeping call light and articles of care within reach promotes patient's safety.
y. Perform hand hygiene.	Reduces transmission of microorganisms.
2 Commercial bag bath or cleansing pack	
a. The cleansing pack contains 8 to 10 premoistened towels for cleaning (see illustrations). Warm package contents in microwave following package directions.	Provides warm soothing heat.

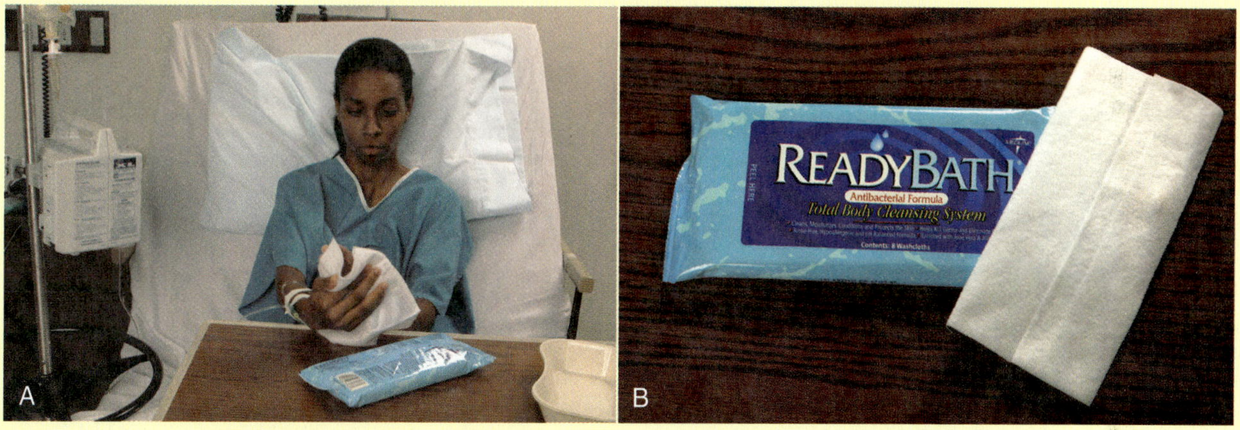

STEP 2a A, Patient uses individual towels to bathe. **B,** Commercial bath cleansing pack.

STEP	RATIONALE
b. Use a single towel for each general body part cleaned. Follow the same order of cleaning as the total or partial bed bath.	Reduces transmission of microorganisms.
c. Allow the skin to air dry for 30 seconds. It is permissible to lightly cover patient with a bath towel to prevent chilling.	Drying the skin with a towel removes the emollient that is left behind after the water/cleaner solution evaporates.
d. Note: If there is excessive soiling (e.g., in the perineal region), use an extra bag bath or conventional washcloths, soap, water, and towels.	
3 Tub Bath or Shower	
a. Consider patient's condition and review orders for precautions concerning his or her movement or positioning.	Prevents accidental injury to patient during bathing.
b. Schedule use of shower or tub.	Prevents unnecessary waiting, which causes fatigue.
c. Check tub or shower for cleanliness. Use cleaning techniques outlined in agency policy. Place rubber mat on tub or shower bottom. Place disposable bath mat or towel on floor in front of tub or shower.	Cleaning prevents transmission of microorganisms. Mats prevent slipping and falling.
d. Collect all hygienic aids, toiletry items, and linens requested by patient. Place within easy reach of tub or shower.	Placing items close at hand prevents possible falls when patient reaches for equipment.
e. Assist patient to bathroom if necessary. Have him or her wear robe and slippers.	Assistance prevents accidental falls. Wearing robe and slippers prevents chilling.
f. Demonstrate how to use call signal for assistance.	Bathrooms are equipped with signaling devices in case patient feels faint or weak or needs immediate assistance. Patients prefer privacy during bath if safety is not jeopardized.

SKILL 39-1 BATHING AND PERINEAL CARE—cont'd

STEP	RATIONALE
g. Place "occupied" sign on bathroom door.	Maintains patient's privacy.
h. Fill bath tub halfway with warm water. Check temperature of bath water, have patient test water, and adjust temperature if water is too warm. Explain which faucet controls hot water. If patient is taking shower, turn shower on and adjust water temperature before patient enters shower stall. Use shower seat or tub chair if needed (see illustration).	Adjusting water temperature prevents accidental burns. Older adults and patients with neurological alterations (e.g., diabetes, spinal cord injury) are at high risk for burn as a result of reduced sensation. Use of assistive devices facilitates bathing and minimizes physical exertion.

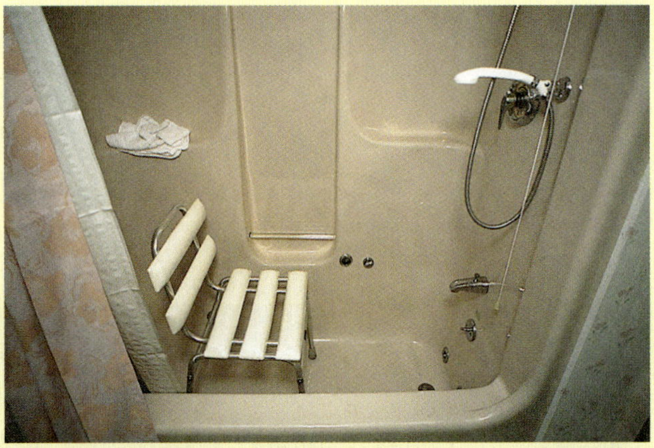

STEP 3h Shower seat for patient safety.

STEP	RATIONALE
i. Instruct patient to use safety bars when getting in and out of tub or shower. Also instruct to pull cord to summon assistance (if available). Caution patient against use of bath oil in tub water.	Prevents slipping and falling. Oil causes tub surfaces to become slippery.
j. Instruct patient not to remain in tub longer than 10 to 15 minutes. Check on him or her every 5 minutes.	Prolonged exposure to warm water causes vasodilation and pooling of blood in some patients, leading to light-headedness or dizziness.
k. Return to bathroom when patient signals and knock before entering.	Provides privacy.
l. For patient who is unsteady, drain tub of water before he or she attempts to get out. Place bath towel over patient's shoulders. Assist patient out of tub as needed and help with drying.	Prevents accidental falls. Patient may become chilled as water drains.

CLINICAL DECISION: *Weak or unstable patients need extra assistance in getting out of a tub. Planning for additional personnel is essential before attempting to help the patient.*

STEP	RATIONALE
m. Help patient as needed with getting dressed in a clean gown or pajamas, slippers, and robe. (In home setting patient may put on regular clothing.)	Maintains warmth to prevent chilling.
n. Assist patient to room and comfortable position in bed or chair.	Maintains relaxation gained from bathing.
o. Clean tub or shower according to agency policy. Remove soiled linen and place in dirty-linen bag. Discard disposable equipment in proper receptacle. Place "unoccupied" sign on bathroom door. Return supplies to storage area.	Prevents transmission of infection through soiled linen and moisture.
p. Perform hand hygiene.	Reduces transfer of microorganisms.

EVALUATION

STEP	RATIONALE
1 Observe skin, paying particular attention to areas previously soiled, reddened, dry, or showing early signs of breakdown.	Techniques used during bathing leave skin clean and clear. Over time dry skin diminishes. If patient shows areas of redness, use Braden scale to measure risk for pressure ulcers (see Chapter 48).
2 Observe ROM during bath.	Measures joint mobility.
3 Ask patient to rate level of comfort.	Determines patient's tolerance of bathing activities.
4 Ask patient to rate level of fatigue.	Determines patient's tolerance of bathing activities.

STEP	RATIONALE

UNEXPECTED OUTCOMES AND RELATED INTERVENTIONS

1. Areas of excessive dryness, rashes, or pressure ulcers appear on skin.
   - Complete pressure ulcer assessment (see Chapter 48).
   - Apply moisturizing lotions or topical skin applications per agency policy.
   - Limit frequency of complete baths.
   - Obtain special bed surface if patient is at risk for skin breakdown.
2. Patient becomes excessively fatigued or unable to cooperate or participate in bathing.
   - Reschedule bathing to a time when patient is more rested.
   - Provide pillow or elevate head of bed during bath for patient with breathing difficulties.
   - Notify health care provider if this is a change in patient's fatigue level.
   - Perform hygiene measures in stages between scheduled rest periods.
3. The rectum, perineum, or genital area is inflamed or swollen or has foul-smelling odor.
   - Bathe perineal area frequently enough to keep clean and dry.
   - Obtain an order for a sitz bath.
   - Apply protective barrier ointment or antiinflammatory cream.
   - Report findings to health care provider.

RECORDING AND REPORTING

- Report any breaks in skin or ulcerations to nurse in charge or health care provider. These are serious in patients with altered circulation to the lower extremities.
- Report intolerance of activity to patient's nurse.
- Record procedure, amount of assistance provided, patient's participation in care, condition of skin, and any significant findings (e.g., reddened areas, breaks in skin, inflammation, ulcerations).

HOME CARE CONSIDERATIONS

- Assess patient's tub and shower area for need for safety devices (e.g., grab bars).
- Assess patient for the need for assistive bathing devices (e.g., shower chair, handheld shower).

SKILL 39-2 PERFORMING NAIL AND FOOT CARE

Delegation Considerations

The skill of nail and foot care of patients *without* circulatory problems or diabetes can be delegated to nursing assistive personnel (NAP). Instruct the NAP to:

- Not clip patient's toenails.
- Use warm, not hot, water for soaking nails.
- Not soak feet of patients who have diabetes or peripheral vascular disease.
- Report any changes that may indicate inflammation or injury to tissue.

Equipment

- Washbasin
- Emesis basin
- Washcloth
- Bath or face towel
- Nail clippers
- Soft cuticle or nail brush
- Orangewood stick
- Emery board or nail file
- Body lotion
- Disposable bath mat (optional)
- Paper towels
- Clean gloves (if drainage is present)
- Linen bag or hamper

STEP	RATIONALE
ASSESSMENT	
1 Inspect all surfaces of fingers, toes, feet, and nails. Pay particular attention to areas of dryness, inflammation, or cracking. Also inspect areas between toes, heels, and soles of feet.	Integrity of feet and nails determines frequency and level of hygiene required. Heels, soles, and sides of feet are prone to irritation from ill-fitting shoes.

CLINICAL DECISION: *Patients with peripheral vascular diseases or diabetes mellitus, older adults, and patients whose immune system is suppressed often require nail care from a specialist to reduce the risk of tissue injury and infection. Defer care other than washing the feet in these cases until patient has been evaluated.*

STEP	RATIONALE
2 Assess color and temperature of toes, feet, and fingers. Assess capillary refill of nails. Palpate radial and ulnar pulse of each hand and dorsalis pedis pulse of foot; note character of pulses (see Chapter 30).	Assesses adequacy of blood flow to extremities. Circulatory alterations often change integrity of nails and increase patient's chance of localized infection when break in skin integrity occurs.

SKILL 39-2 PERFORMING NAIL AND FOOT CARE—cont'd

STEP	RATIONALE
3 Ask female patients about whether they use nail polish and polish remover frequently.	Chemicals in these products cause excessive dryness.
4 Assess type of footwear worn by patient: Does patient wear socks? Are shoes tight or ill fitting? Does patient wear garters or knee-high nylons? Is footwear clean?	Types of shoes and footwear predispose patient to foot and nail problems (e.g., infection, areas of friction, ulcerations). These conditions decrease mobility and increase the risk for amputation in the patient with diabetes.
5 Identify patient's risk for foot or nail problems:	Certain conditions increase likelihood of foot or nail problems.
a. Older adult	Poor vision, lack of coordination, or inability to bend over contributes to difficulty in performing foot and nail care. Normal physiological changes of aging also result in nail and foot problems (Meiner, 2011).
b. Diabetes mellitus, peripheral vascular disease	Vascular changes associated with diabetes mellitus reduce blood flow to peripheral tissues. Break in skin integrity places patient with diabetes at high risk for skin infection.
c. Heart failure, renal disease	Both conditions increase tissue edema, particularly in dependent areas (e.g., feet). Edema reduces blood flow to neighboring tissues.
d. Cerebrovascular accident (stroke)	Presence of residual foot or leg weakness or paralysis results in altered walking patterns. Altered gait pattern causes increased friction and pressure on feet.
6 Assess type of home remedies that patient uses for existing foot problems:	Certain preparations or applications cause more injury to soft tissue than initial foot problem.
a. Over-the-counter liquid preparations to remove corns	Liquid preparations cause burns and ulcerations.
b. Cutting corns or calluses with razor blade or scissors	Cutting corns or calluses sometimes results in infection caused by break in skin integrity. The patient with diabetes or any patient with decreased peripheral circulation has an increased risk for infection secondary to a break in skin integrity.
c. Use of oval corn pads	Oval pads exert pressure on toes, thereby decreasing circulation to surrounding tissues.
d. Application of adhesive tape	Skin of older adult is thin and delicate and prone to tearing when adhesive tape is removed.
7 Assess patient's ability to care for nails or feet: visual alterations, fatigue, and musculoskeletal weakness.	Determines patient's ability to perform self-care and degree of assistance required from nurse.
8 Assess patient's knowledge of foot and nail care practices.	Determines patient's need for health teaching.
PLANNING	
1 Obtain health care provider's order for cutting nails if agency policy requires it.	Patients with reduced circulation are more at risk for infection. Accidental cutting of skin increases risk for infection for them.
2 Identify the patient using two identifiers (i.e., name and birth date or name and account number) according to facility policy.	Patient needs to be able to place fingers and feet in basin for 10 to 20 minutes. Some patients may become fatigued.
3 Explain procedure. Include proper soaking; requires several minutes.	
4 Collect appropriate equipment.	Ensures correct patient. Complies with recommended National Patient Safety Goal (TJC, 2011).
IMPLEMENTATION	
1 Perform hand hygiene. Apply gloves if lesions or drainage present or anticipated.	Reduces transmission of microorganisms.
2 Arrange equipment on over-bed table.	Easy access to equipment prevents delays.
3 Provide privacy by closing curtains around bed or closing door.	Maintaining privacy reduces embarrassment and anxiety.
4 Assist ambulatory patient to sit in bedside chair. Help bed-bound patient to supine position with head of bed elevated. Place disposable bath mat or towel on floor under patient's feet or place towel on bed.	Sitting in chair facilitates immersing feet in basin. Bath mat or towel protects feet from exposure to soil or microorganisms on floor; towel lessens chance of splashing water on floor or bed.
5 Fill wash basin with warm water. Test water temperature.	Warm water softens nails and thickened epidermal cells, reduces inflammation of skin, and promotes local circulation. Proper water temperature prevents burns.
6 Place basin on bath mat or towel and help patient place feet in basin. Place call light within patient's reach.	Patients with muscular weakness or tremors often have difficulty positioning feet. Maintains patient's safety.

CLINICAL DECISION: *Soaking the feet of patients with diabetes mellitus or peripheral vascular disease is not recommended. Soaking may lead to maceration (excessive softening of the skin) and drying of the skin (ADA, 2010) leading to tissue breakdown and infection.*

STEP	RATIONALE
7 Adjust over-bed table to low position and place it over patient's lap. (Patient sits in chair or lies in bed).	Easy access prevents accidental spills.
8 Fill emesis basin with warm water and place basin on paper towels on over-bed table.	Warm water softens nails and thickened epidermal cells.
9 Instruct patient to place fingers in emesis basin and arms in comfortable position.	Prolonged positioning causes discomfort unless normal anatomical alignment is maintained.
10 Allow patient's feet and fingernails to soak for 10 to 20 minutes. Rewarm water after 10 minutes.	Softening of corns, calluses, and cuticles ensures easy removal of dead cells and easy manipulation of cuticle.
11 Clean gently under fingernails with orangewood stick while fingers are immersed (see illustration). Remove emesis basin and dry fingers thoroughly.	Orangewood stick removes debris under nails that harbors microorganisms. Thorough drying impedes fungal growth and prevents maceration of tissues.
12 Using nail clippers, clip fingernails straight across and even with tops of fingers; check agency policy regarding clipping of nails (see illustration). Using a file, shape nails straight across. If patient has circulatory problems, do not cut nail; file the nail only.	Cutting straight across prevents splitting of nail margins and formation of sharp nail spikes that irritate lateral nail margins. Filing prevents cutting nail too close to nail bed.
13 Use a soft cuticle brush or nail brush around cuticles. Do not push cuticles back roughly or cut cuticles.	Reduces incidence of inflamed cuticles.
14 Move over-bed table away from patient.	Provides easier access to feet.
15 Put on clean gloves and scrub callused areas of feet with washcloth.	Gloves prevent transmission of fungal infection. Friction removes dead skin layers.
16 Clean gently under nails with orangewood stick. Remove feet from basin and dry thoroughly.	Nails harbor debris and dirt and are a source of potential infection (Berridge, 2009).
17 Clean and trim toenails using procedures in Steps 11 and 12. Do not file corners of toenails. Check agency policy for trimming patient's nails.	Shaping corners of toenails damages tissues.
18 Apply lotion to feet and hands and assist patient back to bed and into comfortable position.	Lotion lubricates dry skin by helping to retain moisture.
19 Remove clean gloves and place in receptacle. Clean and return equipment and supplies to proper place. Dispose of soiled linen in hamper. Perform hand hygiene.	Reduces transmission of infection.

EVALUATION

1 Inspect nails and surrounding skin surfaces after soaking and nail trimming.	Evaluates condition of skin and nails. Allows nurse to note any remaining rough nail edges.
2 Ask patient to explain or demonstrate nail care.	Evaluates patient's level of learning foot and nail care techniques.
3 Observe patient's walk after toenail care.	Evaluates level of comfort and mobility achieved.

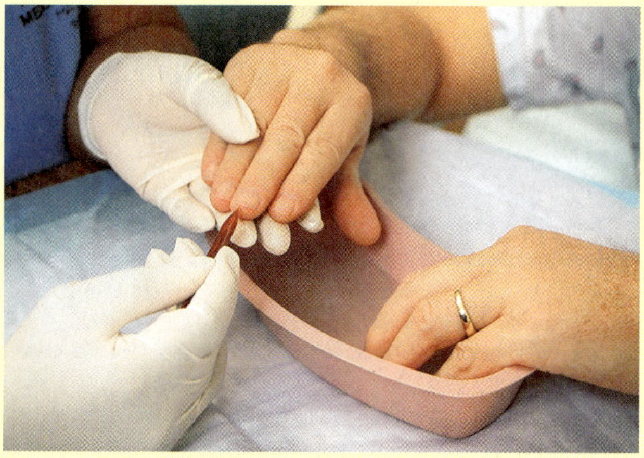

STEP 11 Clean under fingernails.

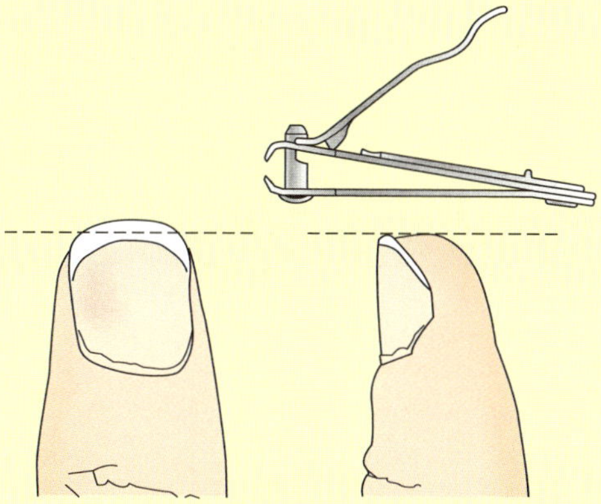

STEP 12 Use nail clippers to clip nails straight across.

SKILL 39-2 PERFORMING NAIL AND FOOT CARE—cont'd

STEP | **RATIONALE**

UNEXPECTED OUTCOMES AND RELATED INTERVENTIONS

1 Cuticles and surrounding tissues are inflamed and tender to touch.
- Repeated soakings are necessary to relieve inflammation and loosen layers of cells from calluses or corns.
- Patients with peripheral vascular disease or diabetes often require referral to a podiatrist.
- Evaluate need for antifungal cream.

2 Localized areas of tenderness occur on feet with calluses or corns at point of friction.
- Change in footwear is necessary.
- Refer to a podiatrist or nurse in charge.

3 Ulcer appears between toes or other pressure areas in foot.
- Notify physician or nurse in charge.
- Refer to a podiatrist or nurse certified in foot care.
- Increase frequency of foot assessment and hygiene.

RECORDING AND REPORTING

- Record procedure and observations (e.g., breaks in skin, inflammation, ulcerations).
- Report any breaks in skin or ulcerations to nurse in charge or physician. These are serious in patients with peripheral vascular disease and illnesses in which the patient's circulation is impaired. Special foot care treatments are often necessary.
- Record procedure and observations (e.g., breaks in skin, inflammation, ulcerations).

HOME CARE CONSIDERATIONS

- If the patient has diabetes or decreased peripheral circulation, perform procedure only after consulting with a health care provider.
- Alternative therapies: moleskin applied to areas of feet that are under friction is less likely to cause pressure than corn pads; spot adhesive bandages guard against friction, but they do not have padding to protect against pressure; wrapping small pieces of lamb's wool around toes reduces irritation of soft corns between toes.
- If patient is ambulatory, instruct to soak feet in bathtub. When patient's mobility is limited, use a large basin or pan.

SKILL 39-3 PROVIDING ORAL HYGIENE

View Video!

Delegation Considerations

The skill of performing oral hygiene can be delegated to nursing assistive personnel (NAP). However, the nurse is responsible for assessing the risk for aspiration. Direct the NAP to:
- Position the patient to avoid aspiration.
- Immediately report to the nurse excessive patient coughing or choking during or after oral hygiene.
- Report bleeding of oral mucosa or gums, patient report of pain, or lesions.

Equipment

- Soft-bristle toothbrush (hard toothbrushes damage enamel and gums)
- Nonabrasive fluoride toothpaste or dentifrice
- Dental floss
- Tongue depressor
- Water glass with cool water
- Normal saline or an essential-oil antiseptic mouthwash (optional; follow patient's preference)
- Emesis basin
- Face towel
- Paper towels
- Clean gloves

STEP	RATIONALE
ASSESSMENT	
1 Perform hand hygiene and apply clean gloves.	Reduces transmission of microorganisms.
2 Instruct patient to not bite down. Inspect integrity of lips, teeth, buccal mucosa, gums, palate, and tongue (see Chapter 30).	Determines status of patient's oral cavity and extent of need for oral hygiene.
3 Identify presence of common oral problems:	Helps determine type of hygiene patient requires and information that he or she needs for self-care.
a. Dental caries—Chalky white discoloration of tooth or presence of brown or black discoloration	
b. Gingivitis—Inflammation of gums	
c. Periodontitis—Receding gum lines, inflammation, gaps between teeth	Receding gums occur with aging; as a result older patients require meticulous oral hygiene.
d. Halitosis—Bad breath	
e. Cheilitis—Cracked lips	
f. Stomatitis—Inflammation of the mouth	Patients receiving immunosuppressive chemotherapy (e.g., cancer chemotherapy, antirejection medication after organ transplant) or patients with suppressed immune function are at risk for stomatitis.

STEP	RATIONALE
4 Assess patient's risk for aspiration: impaired swallowing, reduced gag reflex.	Accumulation of secretions and dentifrice increase patient's risk for aspiration because of reduced ability to control oral secretions.
5 Remove gloves and perform hand hygiene.	Prevents spread of microorganisms.
6 Assess risk for oral hygiene problems (see Table 39-5).	Certain conditions increase likelihood of impaired oral cavity integrity and need for preventive care.
7 Determine patient's oral hygiene practices; question him or her and observe patient performing care if possible.	Allows you to identify errors in technique, deficiencies in preventive oral hygiene, and patient's level of knowledge regarding dental care.
a. Frequency of toothbrushing and flossing	The American Dental Association (2010) recommends at least twice-a-day brushing and once-daily flossing as part of routine oral care.
b. Type of toothpaste or dentifrice used	The American Dental Association (2010) recommends the use of an ADA-approved fluoride toothpaste.
c. Last dental visit and frequency of dental visits	The American Dental Association (2010) recommends regular visits to the dentist for professional cleanings and oral examinations.
d. Type of mouthwash or moistening preparation	Lemon-glycerin preparations are harmful. Glycerin is an astringent that dries and shrinks mucous membranes and gums. Lemon exhausts salivary reflex and erodes tooth enamel. Mouthwash provides pleasant aftertaste but dries mucosa after extended use if it has an alcohol base. Mouthwashes are not a replacement for flossing (American Dental Association, 2010).
8 Assess patient's ability to grasp and manipulate toothbrush.	Toothbrush test assesses dexterity and strength. Determines level of assistance required. Older adults or people with musculoskeletal or nervous system alterations are sometimes unable to hold toothbrush with firm grip or manipulate brush.
PLANNING	
1 Identify the patient using two identifiers (i.e., name and birth date or name and account number) according to facility policy.	Ensures correct patient. Complies with recommended National Patient Safety Goal (TJC, 2011).
2 Explain procedure to patient and discuss preferences regarding use of hygiene aids.	Some patients feel uncomfortable about having the nurse care for their basic needs. Patient involvement with procedure minimizes anxiety.
3 Place paper towels on over-bed table and arrange other equipment within easy reach.	Creates organized work space.
IMPLEMENTATION	
1 Raise bed to comfortable working position. Raise head of bed (if allowed) and lower side rail. Move patient or help patient move closer. Use side-lying position if needed.	Raising bed and positioning patient prevent nurse from straining muscles. Semi-Fowler's position helps prevent patient from choking or aspirating. Side-lying position facilitates drainage of secretions.
2 Place towel over patient's chest.	Prevents soiling of patient's gown.
3 Apply clean gloves.	Prevents contact with microorganisms or blood in saliva.
4 Apply toothpaste to brush. Holding brush over emesis basin, pour small amount of water over toothpaste.	Moisture aids in distribution of toothpaste over tooth surfaces.
5 Patient may assist with brushing. Hold toothbrush bristles at 45-degree angle to gum line. Be sure that tips of bristles rest against and penetrate under gum line. Brush inner and outer surfaces of upper and lower teeth by brushing from gum to crown of each tooth. Clean biting surfaces of teeth by holding top of bristles parallel with teeth and brushing gently back and forth. Brush sides of teeth by moving bristles back and forth (see illustration).	Angle allows brush to reach all tooth surfaces and clean under gum line where plaque and tartar accumulate. Back-and-forth motion dislodges food particles caught between teeth and along chewing surfaces.

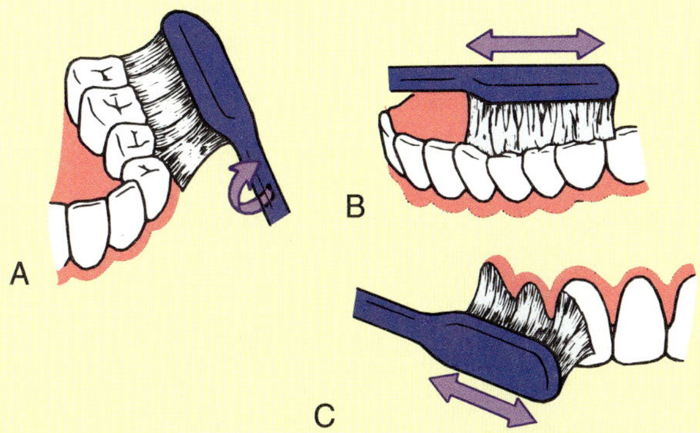

STEP 5 Direction for toothbrush placement. **A,** A 45-degree angle brushes gum line. **B,** Parallel position brushes biting surfaces. **C,** Lateral position brushes sides of teeth.

SKILL 39-3 PROVIDING ORAL HYGIENE—cont'd

STEP	RATIONALE
6 Have patient hold brush at 45-degree angle and lightly brush over surface and sides of tongue (see illustration). Avoid initiating gag reflex.	Microorganisms collect and grow on surface of tongue and contribute to bad breath. Gagging can cause aspiration of toothpaste.

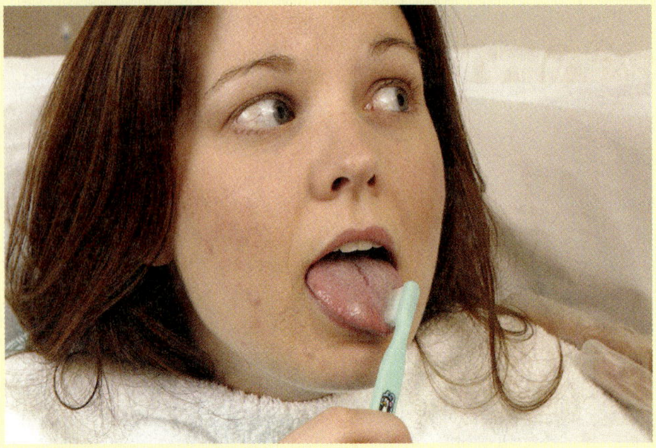

STEP 6 Assisting patient with brushing tongue.

STEP	RATIONALE
7 Allow patient to rinse mouth thoroughly by taking several sips of water, swishing water across all tooth surfaces and spitting into emesis basin.	Irrigation removes food particles.
8 Allow patient to gargle to rinse mouth with mouthwash as desired.	Mouthwash leaves a pleasant taste in mouth but dries mucosa after extended use if it has an alcohol base.
9 Assist in wiping patient's mouth.	Promotes sense of comfort.
10 Allow patient to floss. Floss between all teeth. Hold floss against tooth while moving it up and down sides of teeth and under gum line.	Reduces tartar on tooth surfaces and prevents gum disease. The American Dental Association (2010) recommends flossing once daily.
11 Allow patient to rinse mouth thoroughly with cool water and spit into emesis basin. Help to wipe patient's mouth.	Irrigation removes plaque and tartar from oral cavity.
12 Remove one soiled glove before raising side rail and lowering bed to original position. Remove second soiled glove and perform hand hygiene.	Reduces transmission of microorganisms to environmental surfaces and provides for patient safety.
13 Assist patient to comfortable position, raising bed as needed to working height and lowering when finished.	Provides for patient comfort and safety; prevents straining for nurse when helping patient to move.
14 Apply clean gloves. Wipe off over-bed table, cleanse and dry emesis basin, discard paper towels in trash. Remove gloves and perform hand hygiene. Return equipment to proper place. Gather soiled linen bag and paper towels in appropriate containers.	Reduces transmission of microorganisms. Preventing areas of residual moisture decreases microorganism reservoir. Proper disposal of soiled equipment prevents spread of Infection.
15 Perform hand hygiene.	Reduces transmission of microorganisms.

EVALUATION

1 Ask patient if any area of oral cavity feels uncomfortable or irritated.	Pain indicates an oral cavity problem.
2 Apply gloves and inspect condition of oral cavity.	Determines effectiveness of hygiene and rinsing.
3 Ask patient to describe proper hygiene techniques.	Evaluates patient's learning.
4 Observe patient brushing and flossing.	Evaluates patient's ability to use correct technique.

UNEXPECTED OUTCOMES AND RELATED INTERVENTIONS

1 Oral mucosa is dry and inflamed.
- Increase frequency of oral hygiene.
- Increase patient's hydration.
- Apply protectant to patient's lips.

2 Gum margins are retracted from teeth, with localized areas of inflammation. Bleeding occurs around gum margins.
- Determine if patient has underlying bleeding tendency (e.g., anticoagulant therapy).
- Report findings to health care provider.
- Use soft-bristle toothbrush.
- Increase frequency of oral hygiene.

3 Teeth show signs of dental caries.
- Refer patient to dentist on order from health care provider.
- Review patient's hygiene routine.
- Teach patient oral hygiene.

STEP	RATIONALE

RECORDING AND REPORTING

- Record procedure on flow sheet. Note condition of oral cavity in nurses' notes.
- Report bleeding or presence of lesions to nurse in charge or health care provider.

HOME CARE CONSIDERATIONS

- Teach patient and caregiver to assess oral cavity daily to determine any effects of medications on it (e.g., reddened, inflamed gums) and to detect oral cavity problems.

SKILL 39-4 PERFORMING MOUTH CARE FOR AN UNCONSCIOUS OR DEBILITATED PATIENT

Delegation Considerations

The skill of performing mouth care for an unconscious or debilitated patient can be delegated to nursing assistive personnel (NAP). However, the nurse assesses the patient's risk for aspiration before care, including determining presence of the gag reflex. Instruct the NAP about:

- Proper positioning of patient to lessen chance of aspiration.
- The safe use of an oral suction catheter for clearing oral secretions (see Skill 40-1),
- Signs of impaired integrity of oral mucosa to report to the nurse.
- Reporting any bleeding of mucosa or gums, painful reaction by patient, or excessive coughing or choking to the nurse.

Equipment

- Antibacterial solution (e.g., 0.12% chlorhexidine rinse and paste) (requires a health care provider's order) (IHI, 2011)
- Small pediatric soft-bristle toothbrush, sponge toothettes or swabs
- Tongue blade
- Face towel
- Small oral airway
- Paper towels
- Emesis basin
- Water glass with cool water
- Water-soluble lip lubricant
- Small-bulb syringe or suction machine equipment (required for patients with poor or absent gag reflex)
- Clean gloves

STEP	RATIONALE
ASSESSMENT	
1 Identify the patient using two identifiers (i.e., name and birth date or name and account number) according to facility policy.	Ensures correct patient. Complies with recommended National Patient Safety Goal (TJC, 2011).
2 Perform hand hygiene. Apply clean gloves.	Reduces transmission of microorganisms. Gloves prevent contact with microorganisms in blood or saliva.
3 Assess patient's risk for oral hygiene problems (see Table 39-5).	Impaired level of consciousness increases the likelihood of alterations in integrity of oral cavity structures and requires more frequent care. Proper oral care reduces the risk of pneumonia (Bassim et al., 2008).
4 Test for presence of gag reflex by placing tongue blade on back half of patient's tongue.	Reveals whether patient is at risk for aspiration. Helps determine need for and type of suction apparatus to have available.
5 Inspect condition of oral cavity (see Chapter 30).	Determines integrity of gums, teeth, mucosa, and tongue and need for hygiene.
6 Remove gloves. Perform hand hygiene.	Prevents spread of infection.
PLANNING	
1 Explain procedure to patient even if patient is unconscious.	Allows debilitated patient to anticipate procedure without anxiety. Unconscious patient may retain ability to hear.
2 Collect appropriate equipment.	Prevents interruptions during procedure.
3 Place paper towels on over-bed table and arrange equipment. If needed, turn on suction machine and connect tubing to suction catheter.	Prevents soiling of table top. Equipment prepared in advance ensures smooth, safe procedure.
IMPLEMENTATION	
1 Unless contraindicated (e.g., head injury, neck trauma), raise bed, lower side rail, and position patient close to side of bed with head of bed raised up to 30 degrees; turn patient's head toward mattress. Patient can also be placed on side (Sims' position). Raise side rail.	Turning patient's head to the side allows secretions to drain from mouth instead of collecting in back of pharynx. Prevents aspiration, which could cause lower respiratory tract infection (pneumonia). Moving patient close to side of bed and raising bed facilitate proper body mechanics during the skill and reduce risk for injury to the nurse. Proper use of side rail protects caregiver from straining and provides for patient safety.
2 Pull curtain around bed or close room door.	Provides privacy.
3 Lower side rail.	Prevents straining to reach.

SKILL 39-4 PERFORMING MOUTH CARE FOR AN UNCONSCIOUS OR DEBILITATED PATIENT—cont'd

STEP	RATIONALE
4 Apply clean gloves.	Reduces transfer of microorganisms.
5 Place towel under patient's head and emesis basin under chin.	Prevents soiling of bed linen.
6 Remove partial plate or dentures if present (see Box 39-10)	Allows for thorough cleaning of prosthetics later. Provides clearer access to oral cavity.
7 If patient is unconscious, uncooperative, or having difficulty keeping mouth open, insert an oral airway. Insert upside down and turn the airway sideways and then over tongue to keep teeth apart. Do not use force.	Prevents patient from biting down on nurse's fingers and provides access to oral cavity.

CLINICAL DECISION: *Never place fingers into the mouth of an unconscious or debilitated patient. The normal response of the patient is to bite down.*

STEP	RATIONALE
8 Clean mouth using brush moistened with water or a cleaning agent such as chlorhexidine paste if prescribed. Clean chewing and inner tooth surfaces first. Clean outer tooth surfaces. Moisten brush with chlorhexidine rinse to rinse. Use swab or toothette to clean roof of mouth, gums, and inside cheeks (see illustration). Gently swab or brush tongue but avoid stimulating gag reflex. Moisten clean swab or toothette with chlorhexidine to rinse. Use bulb syringe as needed to remove excess rinse.	Brushing action removes food particles between teeth and along chewing surfaces. Chlorhexidine 0.12% is an antimicrobial agent effective against dental plaque biofilms (IHI, 2011). Swabbing helps remove secretions and crusts from mucosa and moistens mucosa. Repeated rinsing removes peroxide, which is irritating to mucosa, and debris.
9 For patients without teeth, use a toothette moistened in chlorhexidine rinse to clean oral cavity.	This is less traumatic to mucosa of gums.
10 Suction oral secretions as they accumulate if needed.	Suction removes secretions and fluid that collect in posterior pharynx.
11 Apply thin layer of water-soluble jelly to lips (see illustration).	Water-soluble jelly lubricates lips to prevent drying and cracking.
12 Inform patient that procedure is completed.	Provides meaningful stimulation to patient.
13 Remove gloves and dispose in proper receptacle. Raise side rail. Perform hand hygiene.	Prevents transmission of microorganisms to environmental surfaces (e.g., side rails, patient's linens). Reduces risk for patient injury.
14 Reposition patient comfortably, raise side rail, and return bed to original position.	Maintains patient's comfort and safety.
15 Apply clean gloves to clean equipment. Return supplies to proper place. Place soiled linen in proper receptacle.	Proper disposal of soiled equipment and handling of soiled linens prevent spread of infection.
16 Remove and discard soiled gloves. Perform hand hygiene.	Reduces transmission of microorganisms.

EVALUATION

STEP	RATIONALE
1 Apply clean gloves and inspect oral cavity.	Determines efficacy of cleaning. Once you have removed thick secretions, this reveals any underlying inflammation or lesions.
2 Remove gloves and dispose in proper receptacle. Perform hand hygiene.	Reduces transmission of microorganisms.
3 Ask patient if mouth feels clean.	Evaluates level of comfort.
4 Assess patient's respirations and auscultate lung sounds on an ongoing basis.	Ensures early recognition of aspiration.

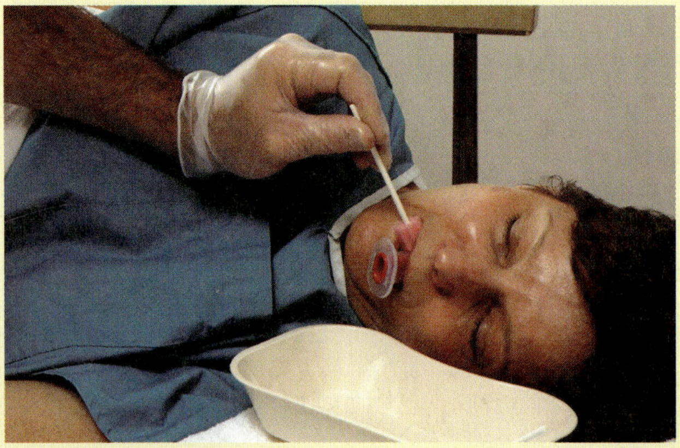

STEP 8 Using moistened toothette to rinse teeth in patient with oral airway inserted.

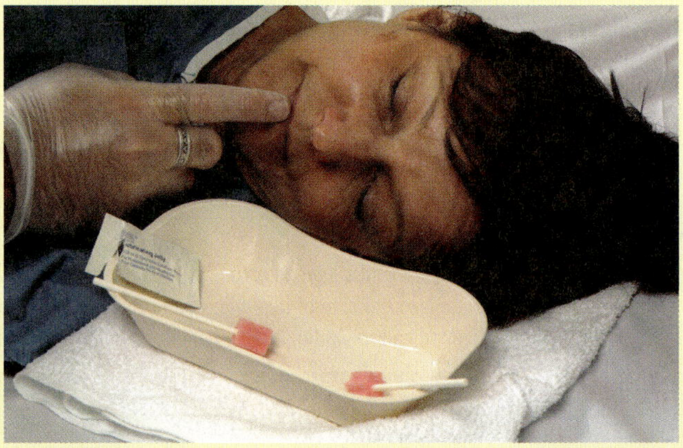

STEP 11 Application of water-soluble moisturizer to lips.

UNEXPECTED OUTCOMES AND RELATED INTERVENTIONS

1 Secretions or crusts remain on oral mucosa, tongue, or gums.
  - Increase frequency of oral hygiene.
  - Use a pediatric-size toothbrush to provide better hygiene.

2 Localized inflammation of gums or mucosa is present, or lips are cracked and inflamed.
  - Increase frequency of oral hygiene with a soft-bristle toothbrush.
  - Apply water-soluble moisturizing gel on oral mucosa and massage.
  - Apply water-soluble moisturizing gel or lubricant to lips.

3 Patient aspirates secretions.
  - Suction oral airway as secretions accumulate to maintain patent airway.
  - Perform tracheal bronchial suctioning.
  - Notify health care provider immediately.
  - Elevate patient's head of bed to facilitate breathing.
  - Be prepared to have chest x-ray film examination ordered by health care provider.

RECORDING AND REPORTING

- Record procedure, including pertinent observations (e.g., presence of bleeding gums, dry mucosa, ulcerations, crusts on tongue).
- Report any unusual findings to nurse in charge or health care provider.

HOME CARE CONSIDERATIONS

- Irrigate oral cavity with bulb syringe; patient can use a gravy baster to remove secretions.
- Give mouth care at least twice a day.
- Have caregivers demonstrate positioning patient to prevent aspiration.

SKILL 39-5 MAKING AN OCCUPIED BED

Delegation Considerations

The skill of making an occupied bed can be delegated to nursing assistive personnel (NAP). The nurse reviews any precautions or activity restrictions. Instruct the NAP about:

- Any activity or positioning restrictions for the patient.
- Looking for wound drainage, dressing materials, drainage tubes, or intravenous (IV) tubing that becomes dislodged or is found in the linens.
- What to do if patient becomes fatigued.

Equipment (Fig. 39-14)

- Linen bag(s)
- Mattress pad (optional depending on facility practice; needs to be changed only when soiled)
- Bottom sheet (flat or fitted)
- Drawsheet
- Top sheet
- Blanket (optional depending on patient preference)
- Bedspread
- Waterproof pads and/or bath blankets (optional)
- Pillowcases
- Bedside chair or table
- Clean gloves (optional)
- Towel
- Disinfectant

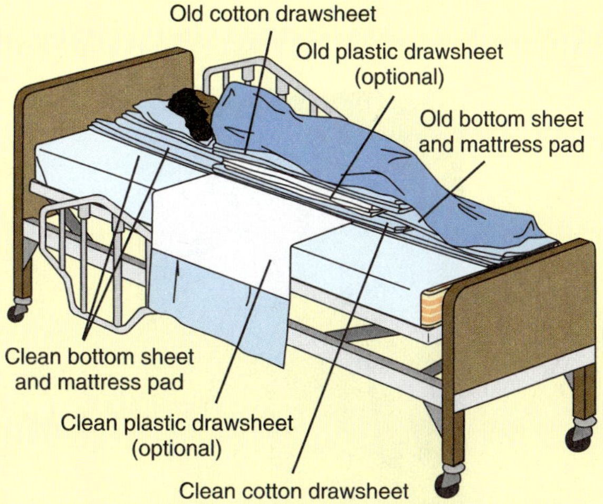

FIG. 39-14 Equipment for making occupied bed.

SKILL 39-5 MAKING AN OCCUPIED BED—cont'd

STEP	RATIONALE
ASSESSMENT	
1 Assess potential for patient incontinence or excess drainage on bed linen.	Determines need for protective waterproof pads or extra bath blankets on bed and whether gloves are likely needed for procedure.
2 Check chart for orders or specific precautions concerning movement and positioning.	Ensures patient safety and use of proper body mechanics.
PLANNING	
1 Explain procedure to patient, including that he or she will be asked to turn on side and roll over linen.	Minimizes anxiety and promotes cooperation.
2 Gather needed supplies, being sure to not let clean linen touch your uniform.	Securing needed supplies ensures that procedure can be implemented without interruption. Uniform is less clean than the clean linen.
IMPLEMENTATION	
1 Perform hand hygiene and apply clean gloves (wear gloves only if old linen is soiled or there is risk for contact with body secretions).	Reduces transmission of microorganisms.
2 Arrange equipment on bedside chair or over-bed table. Remove unnecessary equipment such as a dietary tray or items used for hygiene.	Organizing equipment provides for smooth procedure and assists in increasing patient's comfort. Placing linen on clean surface minimizes spread of infection.
3 Pull room curtain around bed and/or close door.	Maintains patient's privacy.
4 Adjust bed height to comfortable working position with bed flat if patient can tolerate. Lower raised side rail on one side of bed. Remove call light.	Minimizes strain on back. It is easier to remove and apply linen evenly to bed in flat position. Provides easy access to bed and linen. If patient has trouble breathing, leave head of bed elevated to comfort level.
5 Loosen top linen at foot of bed.	Makes linen easier to remove.
6 Remove bedspread and blanket separately. If spread and blanket are soiled, place them in linen bag. Keep soiled linen away from uniform.	Reduces transmission of microorganisms.
7 If blanket and spread are to be reused, fold them by bringing the top and bottom edges together. Fold farthest side over onto nearer bottom edge. Bring top and bottom edges together again. Place folded linen over back of chair.	Folding method facilitates replacement and minimizes wrinkles.
8 Cover patient with bath blanket in the following manner: unfold bath blanket over top sheet. Ask patient to hold top edge of bath blanket. If patient is unable to help, tuck top of bath blanket under shoulders. Grasp top sheet under bath blanket at patient's shoulders and bring sheet down to foot of bed. Remove sheet and discard in linen bag.	Bath blanket provides warmth and keeps body parts covered during linen removal.
9 With assistance from 1 or 2 other care providers, slide mattress toward head of bed if needed.	If mattress slides toward foot of bed when head of bed is raised, it is difficult to tuck in linen. In addition, it is uncomfortable for the patient because his or her feet may be pressed against or hang over the foot of the bed.
10 Position patient on far side of bed, turned onto side and facing away from you. Be sure that side rail in front of patient is up. Adjust pillow under patient's head.	Turning patient onto side provides space for placement of clean linen. Side rail ensures patient's safety from forward falls from bed surface and helps patient in moving.
11 Loosen bottom linens, moving from head to foot. With seam side down (facing the mattress), fanfold bottom sheet and drawsheet toward patient—first drawsheet, then bottom sheet. Tuck edges of linen just under buttocks, back, and shoulders. Do not fanfold mattress pad if it is to be reused (see illustration).	Prepares for removal of all bottom linen simultaneously. Provides maximum work space for placing clean linen. Later, when patient turns to other side, you can remove soiled linen easily.

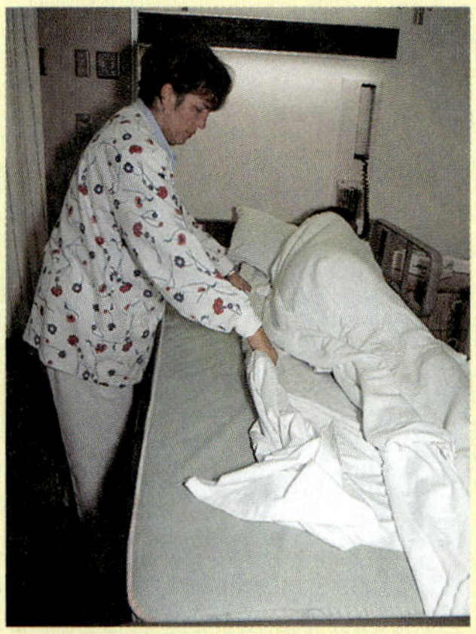

STEP 11 Old linen tucked under patient.

STEP	RATIONALE
12 Wipe off any moisture on exposed mattress with towel and appropriate disinfectant. Make sure that mattress surface is dry before applying linens.	Reduces transmission of microorganisms.
13 Apply clean linen to exposed half of bed:	
a. Place clean mattress pad on bed (if used) by folding it lengthwise with center crease in middle of bed. Fanfold top layer over mattress. (If pad is reused, simply smooth out any wrinkles.)	Applying linen over bed in successive layers minimizes energy and time used in bed making.
b. If using flat sheet for bottom sheet, unfold sheet lengthwise so center crease is situated lengthwise along center of bed. Fanfold top layer of sheet toward center of bed alongside the patient. Smooth bottom layer of sheet over mattress and bring edge over closest side of mattress. If using a fitted sheet, pull sheet smoothly over mattress ends. Allow edge of flat unfitted sheet to hang about 25 cm (10 inches) over mattress edge. Make sure that lower hem of bottom flat sheet lies seam down and even with bottom edge of mattress (see illustration).	Proper positioning of linen on one side ensures that adequate linen is available to cover opposite side of bed. Keeping seam edges down eliminates irritation to patient's skin.
14 If flat sheet is used for bottom sheet, miter bottom flat sheet at head of bed:	Ensures that secure flat sheet does not loosen easily.
a. Face head of bed diagonally. Place hand away from head of bed under top corner of mattress, near mattress edge, and lift.	
b. With other hand tuck top edge of bottom sheet smoothly under mattress so side edges of sheet above and below mattress meet when brought together.	
c. Face side of bed and pick up top edge of sheet at approximately 45 cm (18 inches) from top of mattress (see illustration).	
d. Lift sheet and lay it on top of mattress to form a neat triangular fold, with lower base of triangle even with mattress side edge (see illustration).	
e. Tuck lower edge of sheet, which is hanging free below the mattress, under mattress. Tuck with palms down without pulling triangular fold (see illustration).	
f. Hold portion of sheet covering side of mattress in place with one hand. With the other hand, pick up top of triangular linen fold and bring it down over side of mattress. Tuck this portion under mattress (see illustrations).	Mitered corner cannot be loosened easily even if patient frequently moves in bed.

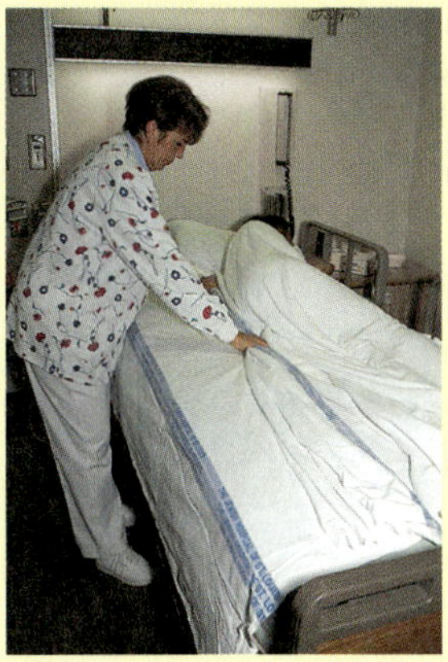

STEP 13b Clean linen applied to bed.

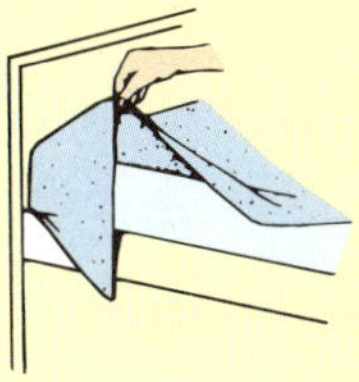

STEP 14c Top edge of sheet picked up.

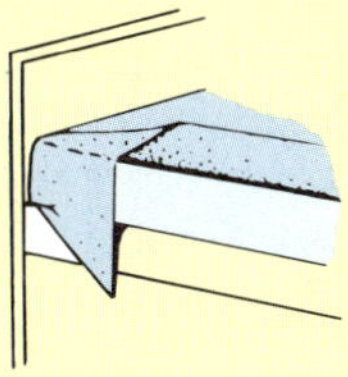

STEP 14d Sheet on top of mattress in a triangular fold

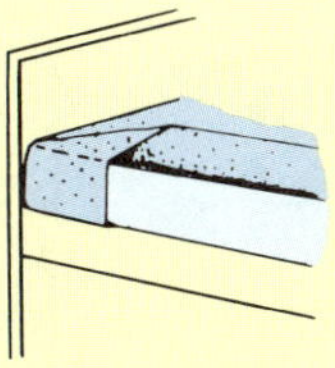

STEP 14e Lower edge of sheet tucked under mattress.

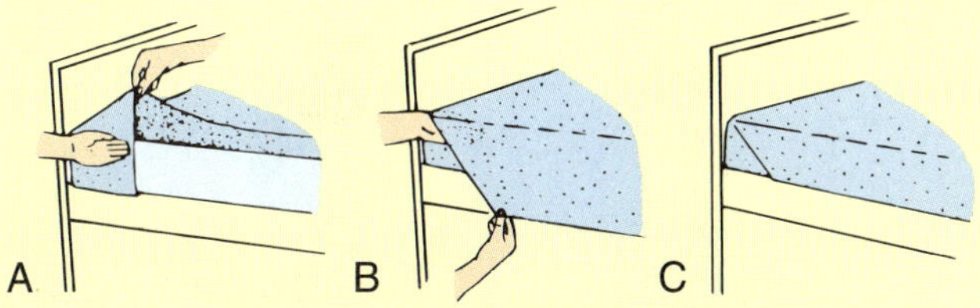

STEP 14f A and **B,** Triangular fold placed over side of mattress. **C,** Linen tucked under mattress.

SKILL 39-5 MAKING AN OCCUPIED BED—cont'd

STEP	RATIONALE
15 Tuck remaining portion of sheet under mattress, moving toward foot of bed. Keep linen smooth.	Folds of linen are source of irritation.
16 *(Optional)* Open clean drawsheet so it unfolds in half. Lay centerfold along middle of bed lengthwise and position sheet so it is under patient's buttocks and torso (see illustration). Fanfold top layer toward patient with edge along patient's back. Smooth bottom layer out over mattress and tuck excess edge under mattress (keep palms down).	Drawsheet is used to lift and reposition patient. Placement under patient's torso distributes most of patient's body weight over sheet.
17 Place waterproof pad over drawsheet, *(optional)* with centerfold against patient's side. Fanfold top layer toward patient.	Protects bed linen from being soiled.
18 Advise patient that rolling over thick layer of linens is necessary and that he or she will feel a lump. Have patient roll slowly toward you over the layers of linen. Raise side rail on working side before going to other side of bed.	Positions patient for removal and placement of linens. Maintains patient's safety.
19 Lower side rail. Assist patient in positioning on other side as needed. Loosen edges of soiled linen from under mattress (see illustration).	Ensures patient comfort. Exposes opposite side of bed for removal of soiled linen and placement of clean linen. Makes linen easier to remove.
20 Remove soiled linen by folding it into a bundle or square with soiled side turned in. Discard in linen bag. If necessary, wipe mattress with antiseptic solution and dry mattress surface before applying new linen.	Reduces transmission of microorganisms.
21 Pull clean, fanfolded linen smoothly over edge of mattress from head to foot of bed.	Smooth linen does not irritate patient's skin.
22 Help patient roll back into supine position. Reposition pillow.	Maintains patient's comfort.
23 Pull fitted sheet smoothly over mattress ends. Miter top corner of bottom sheet (see Step 14). When tucking corner, be sure that sheet is smooth and free of wrinkles.	Wrinkles and folds cause irritation to skin.
24 Facing side of bed, grasp remaining edge of bottom flat sheet. Lean back, keep back straight, and pull while tucking excess linen under mattress. Proceed from head to foot of bed. (Avoid lifting mattress during tucking to ensure fit.)	Proper use of body mechanics while tucking linen prevents injury.
25 Smooth fanfolded drawsheet out over bottom sheet. Grasp edge of sheet with palms down, lean back, and tuck sheet under mattress. Tuck from middle to top and then to bottom.	Tucking first at top or bottom pulls sheet sideways, causing poor fit.
26 Place top sheet over patient with centerfold lengthwise down middle of bed. Open sheet from head to foot and unfold over patient.	Correctly positioning centerfold ensures that sheet is equally distributed over bed.
27 Ask patient to hold clean top sheet or tuck sheet around his or her shoulders. Remove bath blanket and discard in linen bag.	Sheet prevents exposure of body parts. Having patient hold sheet encourages patient participation in care.
28 Place blanket on bed, unfolding it so crease runs lengthwise along middle of bed. Unfold blanket to cover patient. Make sure that top edge is parallel with edge of top sheet and 15 to 20 cm (6 to 8 inches) from edge of top sheet.	Blanket covers patient completely and provides adequate warmth.
29 Place spread over bed according to Step 28. Be sure that top edge of spread extends about 2.5 cm (1 inch) above edge of blanket. Tuck top edge of spread over and under top edge of blanket.	Gives bed neat appearance and provides extra warmth.
30 Make cuff by turning edge of top sheet down over top edge of blanket and spread.	Protects patient's face from rubbing against blanket or spread.

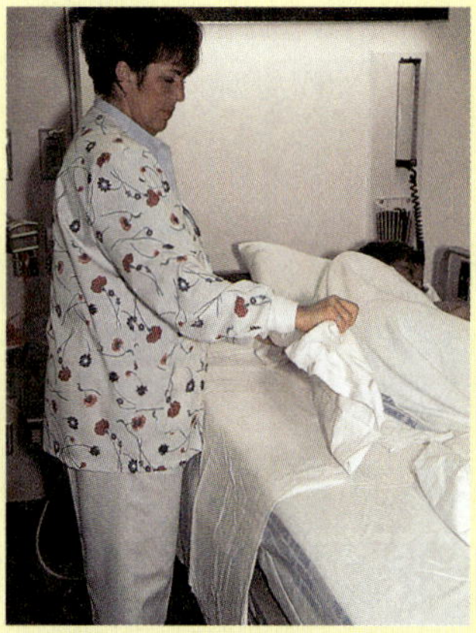

STEP 16 Optional drawsheet.

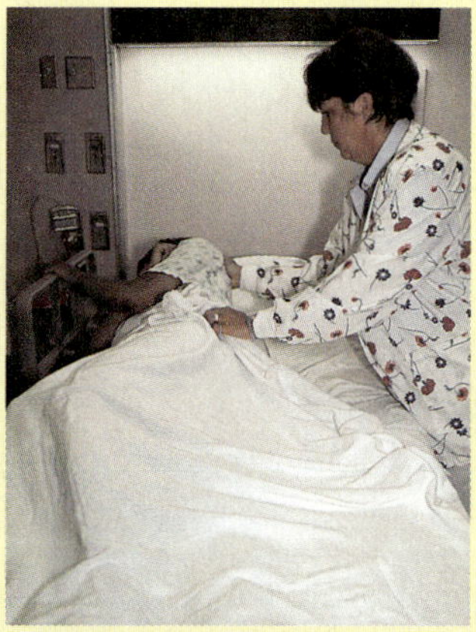

STEP 19 Assisting patient to position after rolling over folds of linen.

STEP	RATIONALE
31 Standing on one side at foot of bed, lift mattress corner slightly with one hand and tuck linens under mattress. Top sheet and blanket are tucked under together. Be sure that linens are loose enough to allow movement of patient's feet. Making a horizontal toe pleat is an option (see illustration).	Makes neat-appearing bed. Pressure ulcers develop on patient's toes and heels from feet rubbing against tight-fitting bed sheets.

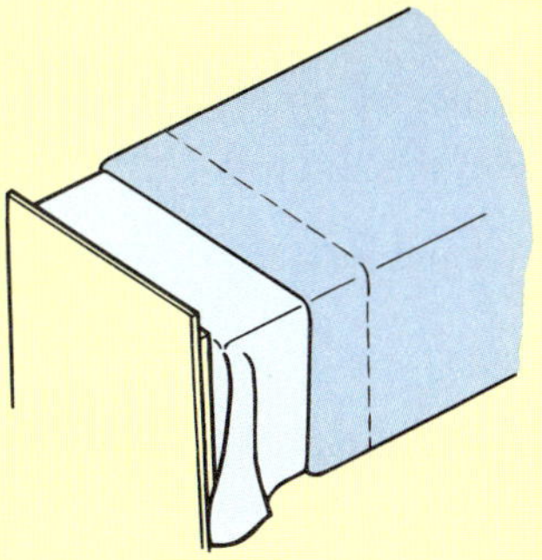

STEP 31 Optional toe pleat.

STEP	RATIONALE
32 Make modified mitered corner with top sheet, blanket, and spread (see illustration in Box 39-14, Step 20).	Ensures that top covers do not loosen easily.
a. Pick up side edge of top sheet, blanket, and spread approximately 45 cm (18 inches) from foot of mattress. Lift linen to form triangular fold and lay it on bed.	
b. Tuck lower edge of sheet, which is hanging free below mattress, under mattress. Do not pull triangular fold.	
c. Pick up triangular fold and bring it down over mattress while holding linen in place alongside of mattress. Do not tuck tip of triangle.	Secures top linen but keeps even edge of blanket and top sheet draped over mattress.
33 Raise side rail. Make other side of bed; spread sheet, blanket, and bedspread out evenly. Fold top edge of spread over blanket and make cuff with top sheet (see Step 30); make modified mitered corner at foot of bed (see Step 32).	Correct use of side rails aids patient's movement in bed.
34 Change pillowcase:	
a. Have patient raise head. While supporting neck with one hand, remove pillow. Allow patient to lower head.	Support of neck muscles prevents injury during flexion and extension of neck.
b. Remove soiled case by grasping pillow at open end with one hand and pulling case back over pillow with other hand. Discard case in linen bag.	Pillows slide out easily, thus minimizing contact with soiled linen.
c. Grasp clean pillowcase at center of closed end. Gather case, turning it inside out over the hand holding it. With same hand pick up middle of one end of pillow. Pull pillowcase down over pillow with other hand.	Eases sliding of pillowcase over pillow.
d. Be sure that pillow corners fit evenly into corners of pillowcase. Place pillow under patient's head.	Poorly fitting case constricts fluffing and expansion of pillow and interferes with patient comfort.
35 Place call light within patient's reach and return bed to comfortable position and height.	Ensures patient safety and comfort.
36 Open room curtains and rearrange furniture. Place personal items within easy reach on over-bed table or bedside stand.	Promotes sense of well-being.
37 Place dirty linen in hamper or chute. Remove gloves (if worn); dispose and perform hand hygiene.	Prevents transmission of microorganisms.

EVALUATION

1 Ask if patient feels comfortable.	Ensures that bed linens are smooth and patient is positioned comfortably.
2 Inspect skin for areas of irritation.	Folds or creases in linen cause pressure on skin.
3 Assess patient for signs and symptoms of fatigue, dyspnea, pain, or discomfort.	Provides you with data about patient's level of activity tolerance and ability to participate in other procedures.

UNEXPECTED OUTCOMES AND RELATED INTERVENTIONS

1 Patient feels discomfort from linen fold.
- Tighten sheets.
- Change patient's position frequently.

2 Patient's skin shows signs of breakdown.
- Institute skin care measures to reduce risk of pressure ulcer (see Chapter 48).
- Change patient's position more frequently.

RECORDING AND REPORTING

- Making an occupied bed does not need to be recorded.

KEY POINTS

- Assess a patient's physical and cognitive ability to perform basic hygiene measures.
- Provide hygiene care according to a patient's needs and preference.
- During hygiene integrate other activities such as physical assessment, wound care, and ROM exercises.
- While providing daily hygiene needs, use teaching and communication skills to develop a caring relationship with the patient.
- Various personal, sociocultural, economic, and developmental factors influence patients' hygiene practices.
- Patients' health beliefs predict the likelihood of assuming health promotion behavior such as maintaining good hygiene.
- Reduced sensation, vascular insufficiency, and immobility place a patient at greater risk for impaired skin integrity.
- Administering symptom relief therapies before hygiene to patients suffering symptoms such as pain or nausea better prepares them for any procedure.
- When administering oral care to unconscious patients, take measures to prevent aspiration.
- A patient's room needs to be comfortable, safe, and large enough to allow the patient and visitors to move about freely.
- Evaluation of hygiene care is based on a patient's sense of comfort, relaxation, well-being, and understanding of hygiene techniques.

CLINICAL APPLICATION QUESTIONS

Preparing for Clinical Practice

Mrs. Winkler is an 87-year-old resident of an extended care facility who has diabetes mellitus. When Jamie, the nursing student, enters the room, she finds Mrs. Winkler's daughter, Carol, preparing a basin of hot water. Carol tells Jamie, "Mom needs a good pedicure. I'm going to soak her feet in hot sudsy water, clip her toenails, and then put on her favorite polish." Jamie notices that Mrs. Winkler's nails are thick, long, and curved.

1. Which response or action by Jamie is the appropriate initial response to the daughter's statement?
   a. Sits down and helps pick out a nail polish color
   b. "Oh my gosh! You shouldn't soak her feet."
   c. Explains why not to soak the feet.
   d. Checks with Mrs. Winkler's nurse to see if it is okay to soak her feet
2. Which assessment does Jamie need to complete before helping Mrs. Winkler and Carol continue with foot care?
   a. Measuring blood glucose at the bedside
   b. Observing condition of the feet and nails
   c. Asking Mrs. Winkler about her last bowel movement
   d. Observing condition of the skin
3. Jamie helps wash Mrs. Winkler's feet and applies a lanolin cream. Which approach should Jamie take regarding trimming Mrs. Winkler's toenails?
   a. Collaborate with Mrs. Winkler's nurse to obtain a podiatrist consult order
   b. Carefully cut the nails using nail scissors
   c. File the long curving nails
   d. Ask Carol to trim the nails

evolve *Answers to Clinical Application Questions can be found on the Evolve website.*

REVIEW QUESTIONS

Are You Ready to Test Your Nursing Knowledge?

1. The nurse is assisting a patient with rheumatoid arthritis to bathe at the sink. During the bath the patient states that she is tired. The nurse notices the patient is breathing rapidly and the pulse is rapid. What is the nurse's best response?
   1. Finish the bath quickly
   2. Help the patient return to bed
   3. Leave the patient alone to rest in the chair at the sink for a few minutes
   4. Instruct the patient to take deep breaths and try to relax
2. A patient who is cognitively impaired and has dementia requires hygiene care. The patient often displays aggressive behavior such as screaming and hitting during the bath. Which techniques make the bathing experience less stressful for both the nurse and the patient? (Select all that apply.)
   1. Allow the patient to perform as much of the care as possible.
   2. Start by washing the face.
   3. Try an alternative to traditional bathing such as the "bag bath."
   4. Use restraints to prevent the patient from injuring self or the nurse.
3. What is the priority concern when providing oral hygiene for a patient who is unconscious?
   1. Thoroughly brushing all tooth and oral surfaces
   2. Preventing aspiration
   3. Controlling mouth odor
   4. Applying local antiseptic such as chlorhexidine
4. A male nurse is caring for a 32-year-old female Muslim patient who has an indwelling Foley catheter. After introducing himself to the patient, the nurse learns that the patient does not want him to help her with personal hygiene care. Which of the following is(are) appropriate actions? (Select all that apply.)
   1. Finding a female nurse to help the patient
   2. Convincing the patient that he will work quickly and provide as much privacy as possible
   3. Skipping hygiene care for the day except for the parts that the patient can complete independently
   4. Asking the patient if she prefers a family member assist with the care
5. You are helping a female patient bathe. As you are about to perform perineal care, the patient says, "I can finish my bath." The patient has discomfort and burning in the perineal area. What action do you need to take initially?
   1. Explain to the patient that, because of her symptoms, you need to observe the perineal area.
   2. Insist that you are supposed to complete the care.
   3. Honor the patient's request to complete her own perineal care to avoid any embarrassment.
   4. Ask the patient if a family member can complete the care instead.
6. Your patient wears full dentures. His usual denture care includes taking the teeth out once a day to brush. He wears the dentures overnight. You are concerned that he might be at risk for developing denture-induced stomatitis. Which points do you include in a teaching plan for denture care? (Select all that apply.)
   1. Remove dentures overnight once a week while they soak in a cleansing bath.
   2. Do not wear damaged or poorly fitting dentures.

3. Observe mouth for reddened areas under the dentures and small red sores on the roof of the mouth.
4. See dentist regularly.
5. Rinse dentures after meals.
6. Clean dentures every night with cleanser, rinsing well before replacing in mouth at bedtime.

7. A patient who is receiving chemotherapy has inflamed gums and oral mucosa and painful sores in the mouth. Which of the following oral care actions are appropriate? (Select all that apply.)
   1. Decreasing frequency of oral hygiene
   2. Applying water-soluble moisturizing gel on the oral mucosa
   3. Encouraging intake of soft foods
   4. Using commercial mouthwash
8. While planning morning care, which of the following patients would receive the highest priority to receive his or her bath first?
   1. A patient who just returned to the nursing unit from surgery and is experiencing pain at a level of 7 on a scale of 0 to 10
   2. A patient who prefers a bath in the evening when his wife visits and can help him
   3. A patient who is experiencing frequent incontinent diarrheal stools
   4. A patient who has just returned from diagnostic testing and complains of being very fatigued
9. During bathing your patient experiences shortness of breath and labored breathing with a respiratory rate of 30. The bed is in a flat position. You change the bed position to:
   1. Trendelenburg's.
   2. Reverse Trendelenburg's.
   3. Fowler's.
   4. Semi-Fowler's.
10. A nurse caring for a male patient observes the nursing assistive personnel (NAP) performing perineal care. Which of the following observed actions indicates a need for further teaching for the NAP? The NAP:
    1. Used clean gloves.
    2. Did not retract the foreskin before cleansing.
    3. Used the clean portion of washcloth for each cleansing wipe.
    4. Used a circular motion to cleanse from urinary meatus outward.
11. A nurse teaching a family member caregiver how to bathe the patient explains the importance of using long strokes on the patient's extremities, moving from distal to proximal. Which explanation does the nurse include? Long strokes moving from distal to proximal are used to:
    1. Decrease the chance of infection.
    2. Help remove dry, flaky skin.
    3. Prevent skin trauma.
    4. Stimulate venous return.
12. Which of the following actions would best help prevent skin breakdown in a patient who is incontinent of stools and very weak and drowsy?
    1. Checking frequently for soiling
    2. Washing the perineal area with strong soap and water
    3. Placing the call light within easy reach
    4. Keeping a pad under the patient
13. The nurse is caring for a patient who has reduced sensation in both feet. Which of the following should the nurse do? (Select all that apply.)
    1. Avoid cleaning the feet until an order from the health care provider is received.
    2. Wash the feet with lukewarm water and then dry well.
    3. Apply moisturizing lotion to the feet, especially between the toes.
    4. File the toenails straight across.
14. The nurse recognizes that her older-adult patient needs additional teaching about skin care when the older adult says, "I should:
    1. Bathe twice a week.
    2. Rinse well after using soap.
    3. Use hot water for bathing.
    4. Drink plenty of fluids.
15. You ask the nursing assistive personnel (NAP) to clean a patient who has been incontinent of urine. Several minutes later you pass the open door of the room and see the NAP changing the patient's gown and linen. Which of the following requires your immediate attention?
    1. Room temperature is overly warm.
    2. Room door is open to the hallway.
    3. Television volume is too loud.
    4. Strong odor of urine is detected.

Answers: **1.** 2; **2.** 1, 3; **3.** 2; **4.** 1, 4; **5.** 1; **6.** 2, 3, 4, 5; **7.** 2, 3; **8.** 3; **9.** 3; **10.** 2; **11.** 4; **12.** 1; **13.** 2, 4; **14.** 3; **15.** 2.

REFERENCES

American Academy of Dermatology: *Dry skin & keratosis pilaris,* 2009, http://www.aad.org/public/publications/pamphlets/skin_dry.html. Accessed October 3, 2011.

American Dental Association: *Oral health topics : cleaning your teeth and gums (oral hygiene),* 2010, http://www.ada.org/2624.aspx. Accessed September 29, 2011.

American Diabetes Association (ADA): Position statement on standards of medical care in diabetes 2007, *Diabetes Care* 30:S4, 2007.

American Diabetes Association (ADA): *Foot care,* 2010, accessed Sept. 20, 2010, from http://www/diabetes.org/living-with-diabetes/complications/foot-care.html.

Berridge M: Guidance on maintaining personal hygiene in nail care, *Nurs Standard* 23(41):35, 2009.

Berry AM, et al: Systematic literature review of oral hygiene practices for intensive care patients receiving mechanical ventilation, *Am J Crit Care* 16(6):552, 2007.

Centers for Disease Control and Prevention (CDC): *Head lice: treatment,* 2008, www.cdc.gov/lice/head/treatment.html. Accessed October 3, 2011.

Cronenwett L, et al: Quality and safety education for nurses, *Nurs Outlook* 55:122, 2007.

Draelos Z: Smooth approach, *Dermatol Times* 31(2):58, 2010.

Galanti GA: *Caring for patients from different cultures,* ed 4, Philadelphia, 2008, University of Pennsylvania Press.

Garcia M, Caple C: Evidence-based care sheet: oral care of the hospitalized patient, 2011, *Cumulative Index to Nursing and Allied Health Literature (CINAHL),* January 11, 2011.

Gonyea J: Oral health care for patients on dialysis, *Nephrol Nurs J* 36(3):327, 2009.

Grose S: Evidence-based care sheet—bites: head lice, 2011, *Cumulative Index to Nursing and Allied Health Literature (CINAHL),* July 1, 2011.

Harris DJ, et al: Putting evidence into practice: evidence-based interventions for the management of oral mucositis, *Clin J Oncol Nurs* 12(1):141, 2008.

Hockenberry ML, Wilson D: *Wong's nursing care of infants and children,* ed 8, St Louis, 2011, Mosby.

Institute for Healthcare Improvement (IHI): *Ventilator bundle: daily oral care with chlorhexidine,* 2011, http://www.ihi.org. Accessed December 11, 2011.

Jablonski RA: Mouth care in nursing homes: knowledge, beliefs, and practices of nursing assistants, *Geriatr Nurs* 30(2):99, 2009.

Lewis SL, et al: *Medical-surgical nursing: assessment and management of clinical problems,* ed 8, St Louis, 2011, Mosby.

Maier-Lorentz M: Transcultural nursing: its importance in nursing practice, *J Cult Divers* 15(1):37, 2008.

McGraw C, Drennan V: Assisting older people with bathing, *J Commun Nurs* 23(9):12, 2009.

Meiner S: *Gerontologic nursing*, ed 4, St Louis, 2011, Mosby.

Pender N, Murdaugh C, Parsons M: *Health promotion in nursing practice*, Upper Saddle River, NJ, 2011, Pearson Education.

Sciubba JJ: Denture stomatitis, 2009, http://www.emedicine.com/derm/topic642.htm. Accessed October 3, 2011.

The Joint Commission: *2011 National Patient Safety Goals (NPGs)*, 2011, TJC, http://www.jointcommission.org/standards_information/npsgs.aspx. Accessed October 3, 2011.

Wright K: A practical guide to foot care for older adults, *Nurs Residential Care* 11(10):496, 2009.

RESEARCH REFERENCES

Bassim CW, et al: Modification of the risk of mortality from pneumonia with oral hygiene care, *J Amer Geriatr Soc* 56(9):1601, 2008.

Frykberg R, et al: Diabetic foot disorders: a clinical practice guideline, *J Foot Ankle Surg* 45(5):S2, 2006.

Harris M, Richards KC: The physiological and psychological effects of slow-stroke back massage and hand massage on relaxation in older people, *J Clin Nurs* 19(7-8):917, 2010.

Hoeffer B, et al: Assisting cognitively impaired nursing home residents with bathing: effects of two bathing interventions on caregiving, *Gerontologist* 46(4):524, 2006.

Johnson D, Lineweaver L, Maze L: Patients' bath basins as potential sources of infection: a multicenter sampling study, *Am J Crit Care* 18(1):31, 2009.

Larson E, et al: Comparison of traditional and disposable bed baths in critically ill patients, *Am J Crit Care* 13(3): 235, 2004.

Mahoney EK, et al: Challenges to intervention implementation lessons learned in the Bathing Persons With Alzheimer's Disease at Home Study, *Nurs Res* 55(2 suppl): S10, 2006.

Munro CL, et al: Chlorhexidine, toothbrushing, and preventing ventilator-associated pneumonia in critically ill adults, *Am J Crit Care* 18(5):428, 2009.

Padilha DM, et al: Hand function and oral hygiene in older institutionalized Brazilians, *J Am Geriatr Soc* 55(9):1333, 2007.

Rader J, et al: The bathing of older adults with dementia, *Am J Nurs* 106(4):40, 2006.

CHAPTER

40

Oxygenation

OBJECTIVES

- Describe the structure and function of the cardiopulmonary system.
- Describe the physiological processes of ventilation, perfusion, and exchange of respiratory gases.
- State the process of the neural and chemical regulation of respiration.
- Differentiate among the physiological processes of cardiac output, myocardial blood flow, and coronary artery circulation.
- Describe the relationship of cardiac output, preload, afterload, contractility, and heart rate to the process of oxygenation.
- Identify the clinical outcomes occurring as a result of hyperventilation, hypoventilation, and hypoxemia.
- Identify the clinical outcomes occurring as a result of disturbances in conduction, altered cardiac output, impaired valvular function, myocardial ischemia, and impaired tissue perfusion.
- Discuss the effect of a patient's level of health, age, lifestyle, and environment on oxygenation.
- Assess for the risk factors affecting a patient's oxygenation.
- Assess for the physical manifestations that occur with alterations in oxygenation.
- Develop a plan of care for a patient with altered need for oxygenation.
- Describe nursing care interventions used to promote oxygenation in the primary care, acute care, and restorative and continuing care settings.

KEY TERMS

Acute coronary syndrome (ACS), p. 828
Afterload, p. 824
Angina pectoris, p. 828
Apnea, p. 834
Atelectasis, p. 822
Bilevel positive airway pressure (BiPAP), p. 848
Bronchoscopy, p. 832
Cardiac output, p. 824
Cardiopulmonary rehabilitation, p. 854
Cardiopulmonary resuscitation (CPR), p. 853
Chest physiotherapy (CPT), p. 842
Chest tube, p. 849
Cheyne-Stokes respiration, p. 834
Continuous positive airway pressure (CPAP), p. 848
Diaphragmatic breathing, p. 854
Dyspnea, p. 831
Dysrhythmias, p. 827
Electrocardiogram (ECG), p. 825
Endotracheal (ET) tube, p. 846
Expiration, p. 822
Hematemesis, p. 832
Hemoptysis, p. 832
Hemothorax, p. 849
Humidification, p. 842
Hyperventilation, p. 827
Hypoventilation, p. 827
Hypovolemia, p. 826
Hypoxia, p. 827
Incentive spirometry, p. 848
Inspiration, p. 822
Kussmaul respiration, p. 834
Myocardial infarction (MI), p. 828
Myocardial ischemia, p. 828
Nasal cannula, p. 851
Nebulization, p. 842
Noninvasive positive-pressure ventilation (NPPV), p. 848
Normal sinus rhythm (NSR), p. 825
Orthopnea, p. 832
Perfusion, p. 822
Pneumothorax, p. 849
Postural drainage, p. 843
Preload, p. 824
Pursed-lip breathing, p. 854
Stroke volume, p. 823
Surfactant, p. 822
Tracheostomy, p. 847
Ventilation, p. 822
Ventricular tachycardia/fibrillation, p. 827
Wheezing, p. 832

evolve WEBSITE

http://evolve.elsevier.com/Potter/fundamentals/

- Review Questions
- Video Clips
- Animations
- Concept Map Creator
- Case Study with Questions
- Skills Performance Checklists
- Audio Glossary
- Interactive Learning Activities
- Key Term Flashcards
- Content Updates

SCIENTIFIC KNOWLEDGE BASE

Oxygen is necessary to sustain life. The cardiac and respiratory systems supply the oxygen demands of the body. Blood is oxygenated through the mechanisms of ventilation, perfusion, and transport of respiratory gases. Neural and chemical regulators control the rate and depth of respiration in response to changing tissue oxygen demands. The cardiovascular system provides the transport mechanisms to distribute oxygen to cells and tissues of the body.

Respiratory Physiology

The exchange of respiratory gases occurs between the environment and the blood. Respiration is the exchange of oxygen and

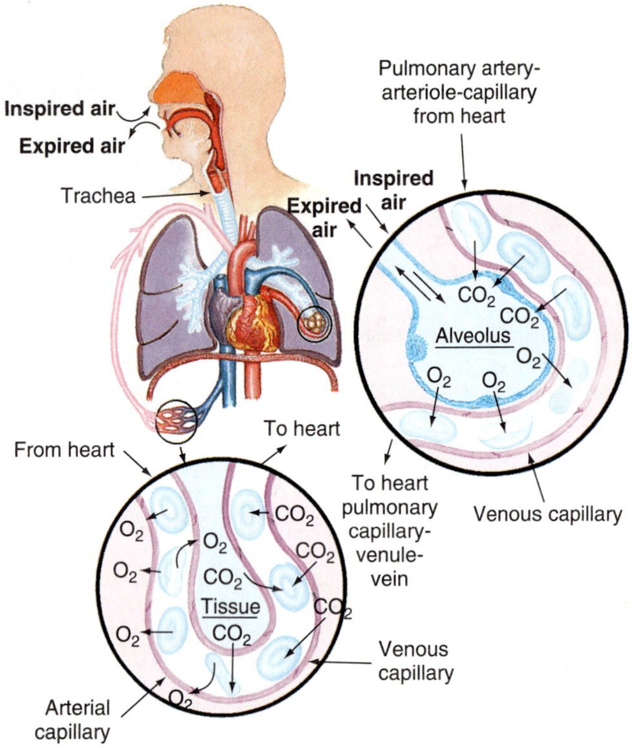

FIG. 40-1 Structures of pulmonary system. (From Thompson J et al: *Mosby's manual of clinical nursing,* ed 3, St Louis, 1993, Mosby.)

carbon dioxide during cellular metabolism. The airways of the lung transfer oxygen from the atmosphere to the alveoli, where the oxygen is exchanged for carbon dioxide. Through the alveolar capillary membrane, oxygen transfers to the blood, and carbon dioxide transfers from the blood to the alveoli. There are three steps in the process of oxygenation: ventilation, perfusion, and diffusion.

Structure and Function. Conditions or diseases that change the structure and function of the pulmonary system alter respiration. The respiratory muscles, pleural space, lungs, and alveoli (Fig. 40-1) are essential for ventilation, perfusion, and exchange of respiratory gases. Gases move into and out of the lungs through pressure changes. Intrapleural pressure is negative, or less than atmospheric pressure, which is 760 mm Hg at sea level. For air to flow into the lungs, intrapleural pressure becomes more negative, setting up a pressure gradient between the atmosphere and the alveoli. The diaphragm and external intercostal muscles contract to create a negative pleural pressure and increase the size of the thorax for inspiration. Relaxation of the diaphragm and contraction of the internal intercostal muscles allow air to escape from the lungs.

Ventilation is the process of moving gases into and out of the lungs. It requires coordination of the muscular and elastic properties of the lung and thorax. The major inspiratory muscle of respiration is the diaphragm. It is innervated by the phrenic nerve, which exits the spinal cord at the fourth cervical vertebra. **Perfusion** relates to the ability of the cardiovascular system to pump oxygenated blood to the tissues and return deoxygenated blood to the lungs. Finally, diffusion is responsible for moving the respiratory gases from one area to another by concentration gradients. For the exchange of respiratory gases to occur, the organs, nerves, and muscles of respiration need to be intact; and the central nervous system needs to be able to regulate the respiratory cycle.

Work of Breathing. Work of breathing (WOB) is the effort required to expand and contract the lungs. In the healthy individual breathing is quiet and accomplished with minimal effort. The amount of energy expended on breathing depends on the rate and depth of breathing, the ease in which the lungs can be expanded (compliance), and airway resistance.

Inspiration is an active process, stimulated by chemical receptors in the aorta. **Expiration** is a passive process that depends on the elastic recoil properties of the lungs, requiring little or no muscle work. **Surfactant** is a chemical produced in the lungs to maintain the surface tension of the alveoli and keep them from collapsing. Patients with advanced chronic obstructive pulmonary disease (COPD) lose the elastic recoil of the lungs and thorax. As a result, the patient's work of breathing increases. In addition, patients with certain pulmonary diseases have decreased surfactant production and sometimes develop atelectasis. **Atelectasis** is a collapse of the alveoli that prevents normal exchange of oxygen and carbon dioxide.

Accessory muscles of respiration can increase lung volume during inspiration. Patients with COPD, especially emphysema, frequently use these muscles to increase lung volume. Prolonged use of the accessory muscles does not promote effective ventilation and causes fatigue. During assessment observe for elevation of the patient's clavicles during inspiration, which can indicate ventilatory fatigue, air hunger, or decreased lung expansion.

Compliance is the ability of the lungs to distend or expand in response to increased intraalveolar pressure. Compliance decreases in diseases such as pulmonary edema, interstitial and pleural fibrosis, and congenital or traumatic structural abnormalities such as kyphosis or fractured ribs.

Airway resistance is the increase in pressure that occurs as the diameter of the airways decreases from mouth/nose to alveoli. Any further decrease in airway diameter by bronchoconstriction can increase airway resistance. Diseases causing airway obstruction such as asthma and tracheal edema increase airway resistance. When airway resistance increases, the amount of oxygen delivered to the alveoli decreases.

Decreased lung compliance, increased airway resistance, and the increased use of accessory muscles increase the WOB, resulting in increased energy expenditure. Therefore the body increases its metabolic rate and the need for more oxygen. The need for elimination of carbon dioxide also increases. This sequence is a vicious cycle for a patient with impaired ventilation, causing further deterioration of respiratory status and the ability to oxygenate adequately.

Lung Volumes. The normal lung values are determined by age, gender, and height. Tidal volume is the amount of air exhaled after normal inspiration. Residual volume is the amount of air left in the alveoli after a full expiration. Forced vital capacity is the maximum amount of air that can be removed from the lungs during forced expiration (McCance and Huether, 2010). Variations in tidal volume and other lung volumes are associated with alterations in patients' health status or activity, such as pregnancy, exercise, obesity, or obstructive and restrictive conditions of the lungs.

Pulmonary Circulation. The primary function of pulmonary circulation is to move blood to and from the alveolar capillary membrane for gas exchange. Pulmonary circulation begins at the pulmonary artery, which receives poorly oxygenated mixed venous blood from the right ventricle. Blood flow through this system depends on the pumping ability of the right ventricle. The flow continues from the pulmonary artery through the pulmonary

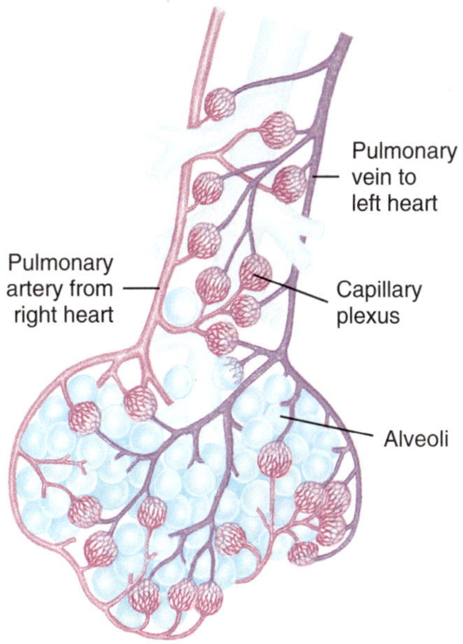

FIG. 40-2 Alveoli at terminal end of lower airway. (From Thompson J et al: *Mosby's manual of clinical nursing,* ed 3, St Louis, 1993, Mosby.)

arterioles to the pulmonary capillaries, where blood comes in contact with the alveolar capillary membrane and the exchange of respiratory gases occurs. The oxygen-rich blood then circulates through the pulmonary venules and pulmonary veins, returning to the left atrium.

Respiratory Gas Exchange. Diffusion is the process for the exchange of respiratory gases in the alveoli and the capillaries of the body tissues. Diffusion of respiratory gases occurs at the alveolar capillary membrane (Fig. 40-2). The thickness of the membrane affects the rate of diffusion. Increased thickness of the membrane impedes diffusion because gases take longer to transfer across the membrane. Patients with pulmonary edema, pulmonary infiltrates, or pulmonary effusion have a thickened membrane, resulting in slow diffusion, slow exchange of respiratory gases, and decreased delivery of oxygen to tissues. Chronic diseases (e.g., emphysema), acute diseases (e.g., pneumothorax), and surgical processes (e.g., lobectomy) often alter the amount of alveolar capillary membrane surface area.

Oxygen Transport. The oxygen-transport system consists of the lungs and cardiovascular system. Delivery depends on the amount of oxygen entering the lungs (ventilation), blood flow to the lungs and tissues (perfusion), rate of diffusion, and oxygen-carrying capacity. Three things influence the capacity of the blood to carry oxygen: the amount of dissolved oxygen in the plasma, the amount of hemoglobin, and the tendency of hemoglobin to bind with oxygen. Hemoglobin, which is a carrier for oxygen and carbon dioxide, transports most oxygen (approximately 97%). The hemoglobin molecule combines with oxygen to form oxyhemoglobin. The formation of oxyhemoglobin is easily reversible, allowing hemoglobin and oxygen to dissociate (deoxyhemoglobin), which frees oxygen to enter tissues.

Carbon Dioxide Transport. Carbon dioxide, a product of cellular metabolism, diffuses into red blood cells and is rapidly hydrated into carbonic acid (H_2CO_3). The carbonic acid then dissociates into hydrogen (H) and bicarbonate (HCO_3^-) ions. Hemoglobin buffers the hydrogen ion, and the (HCO_3^-) diffuses into the plasma (see Chapter 41). Reduced hemoglobin (deoxyhemoglobin) combines with carbon dioxide, and the venous blood transports the majority of carbon dioxide back to the lungs to be exhaled.

Regulation of Respiration. Regulation of respiration is necessary to ensure sufficient oxygen intake and carbon dioxide elimination to meet the demands of the body (e.g., during exercise, infection, or pregnancy). Neural and chemical regulators control the process of respiration. Neural regulation includes the central nervous system control of respiratory rate, depth, and rhythm. The cerebral cortex regulates the voluntary control of respiration by delivering impulses to the respiratory motor neurons by way of the spinal cord. Chemical regulation maintains the appropriate rate and depth of respirations based on changes in the carbon dioxide (CO_2), oxygen (O_2), and hydrogen ion (H^+) concentration (pH) in the blood. Changes in chemical content of O_2, CO_2, and H (pH) stimulate the chemoreceptors located in the medulla, aortic body, and carotid body, which in turn stimulate neural regulators to adjust the rate and depth of ventilation to maintain normal arterial blood gas levels.

Cardiovascular Physiology

Cardiopulmonary physiology involves delivery of deoxygenated blood (blood high in carbon dioxide and low in oxygen) to the right side of the heart and then to the lungs, where it is oxygenated. Oxygenated blood (blood high in oxygen and low in carbon dioxide) then travels from the lungs to the left side of the heart and the tissues. The cardiac system delivers oxygen, nutrients, and other substances to the tissues and facilitates the removal of cellular metabolism waste products by way of blood flow through other body systems such as respiratory, digestive, and renal (McCance and Huether, 2010).

Structure and Function. The right ventricle pumps deoxygenated blood through the pulmonary circulation (Fig. 40-3). The left ventricle pumps oxygenated blood through the systemic circulation. As blood passes through the circulatory system, there is an exchange of respiratory gases, nutrients, and waste products between the blood and the tissues.

Myocardial Pump. The pumping action of the heart is essential to oxygen delivery. There are four cardiac chambers, two atria and two ventricles. The ventricles fill with blood during diastole and empty during systole. The volume of blood ejected from the ventricles during systole is the **stroke volume.** Hemorrhage and dehydration cause a decrease in circulating blood volume and a decrease in stroke volume.

Myocardial fibers have contractile properties that allow them to stretch during filling. In a healthy heart this stretch is proportionally related to the strength of contraction. As the myocardium stretches, the strength of the subsequent contraction increases; this is known as the *Frank-Starling (Starling's) law of the heart.* In the diseased heart (cardiomyopathy or myocardial infarction [MI]) Starling's law does not apply because the increased stretch of the myocardium is beyond the physiological limits of the heart. The subsequent contractile response results in insufficient stroke volume, and blood begins to "back up" in the pulmonary (left heart failure) or systemic (right heart failure) circulation.

Myocardial Blood Flow. To maintain adequate blood flow to the pulmonary and systemic circulation, myocardial blood flow must supply sufficient oxygen and nutrients to the myocardium itself. Blood flow through the heart is unidirectional. The four heart valves ensure this forward blood flow (see Fig. 40-3). During ventricular diastole the atrioventricular (mitral and tricuspid) valves open, and blood flows from the higher-pressure atria into the relaxed ventricles. As systole begins, ventricular pressure rises and

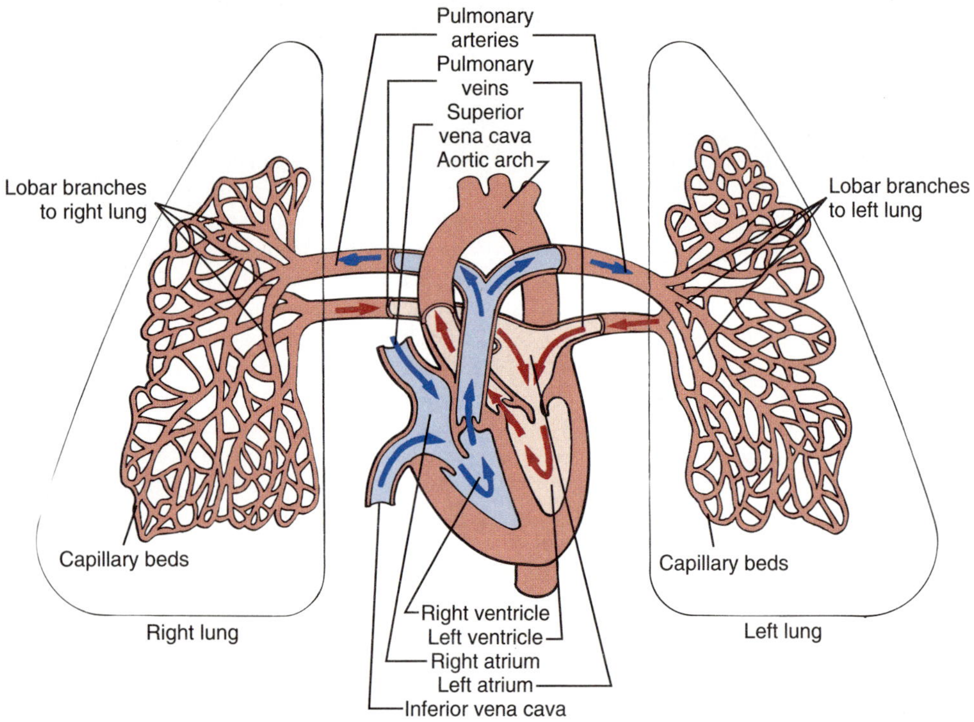

FIG. 40-3 Schematic representation of blood flow through the heart. *Arrows* indicate direction of flow and pulmonary circulation. (From McCance KL, Huether SE: *Pathophysiology: the biologic basis for disease in adults and children,* ed 6, St Louis, 2010, Mosby.)

closes the mitral and tricuspid valves. Valve closure causes the first heart sound (S_1).

During the systolic phase the semilunar (aortic and pulmonic) valves open, and blood flows from the ventricles into the aorta and pulmonary artery. The mitral and tricuspid valves stay closed during systole so all of the blood is moved forward into the pulmonary artery and aorta. As the ventricles empty, the ventricular pressures decrease, allowing closure of the aortic and pulmonic valves, which causes the second heart sound (S2). Some patients with valvular disease have backflow or regurgitation of blood through the incompetent valve, causing a murmur that you can hear on auscultation (see Chapter 30).

Coronary Artery Circulation. The coronary circulation is the branch of the systemic circulation that supplies the myocardium with oxygen and nutrients and removes waste. The coronary arteries fill during ventricular diastole (McCance and Huether, 2010). The left coronary artery has the most abundant blood supply and feeds the more muscular left ventricular myocardium, which does most of the work of the heart.

Systemic Circulation. The arteries of the systemic circulation deliver nutrients and oxygen to tissues, and the veins remove waste from tissues. Oxygenated blood flows from the left ventricle through the aorta and into large systemic arteries. These arteries branch into smaller arteries; then arterioles; and finally the smallest vessels, the capillaries. The exchange of respiratory gases occurs at the capillary level, where the tissues are oxygenated. The waste products exit the capillary network through venules that join to form veins. These veins become larger and form the vena cava, which carry deoxygenated blood to the right side of the heart, where it then returns to the pulmonary circulation.

Blood Flow Regulation. The amount of blood ejected from the left ventricle each minute is the **cardiac output.** The normal cardiac output is 4 to 6 L/min in the healthy adult at rest. The circulating volume of blood changes according to the oxygen and metabolic needs of the body. For example, cardiac output increases during exercise, pregnancy, and fever but decreases during sleep. The following formula represents cardiac output:

$$\text{Cardiac output (CO)} = \text{Stroke volume (SV)} \times \text{Heart rate (HR)}$$

The amount of blood in the left ventricle at the end of diastole (preload), the resistance to left ventricular ejection (afterload), and myocardial contractility all affect stroke volume.

Preload is the end-diastolic volume. The ventricles stretch when filling with blood. The more stretch on the ventricular muscle, the greater the contraction and the greater the stroke volume (Starling's law). In clinical situations, medical treatment can alter the preload and subsequent stroke volumes by changing the amount of circulating blood volume. For example, during treatment of a patient who is hemorrhaging, increased fluid therapy and replacement of blood increase circulating volume, thus increasing the preload and stroke volume, which increases cardiac output. If volume is not replaced, preload, stroke volume and the subsequent cardiac output decreases.

Afterload is the resistance to left ventricular ejection. The heart works harder to overcome the resistance so blood can be fully ejected from the left ventricle. The diastolic aortic pressure is a good clinical measure of afterload. In hypertension the afterload increases, making cardiac workload also increase.

Myocardial contractility also affects stroke volume and cardiac output. Poor ventricular contraction decreases the amount of blood ejected. Injury to the myocardial muscle such as an acute MI causes a decrease in myocardial contractility. The myocardium of the older adult is stiffer with a slower ventricular filling rate and prolonged contraction time (Linton and Lach, 2007).

Heart rate affects blood flow because of the relationship between rate and diastolic filling time. With a sustained heart rate greater

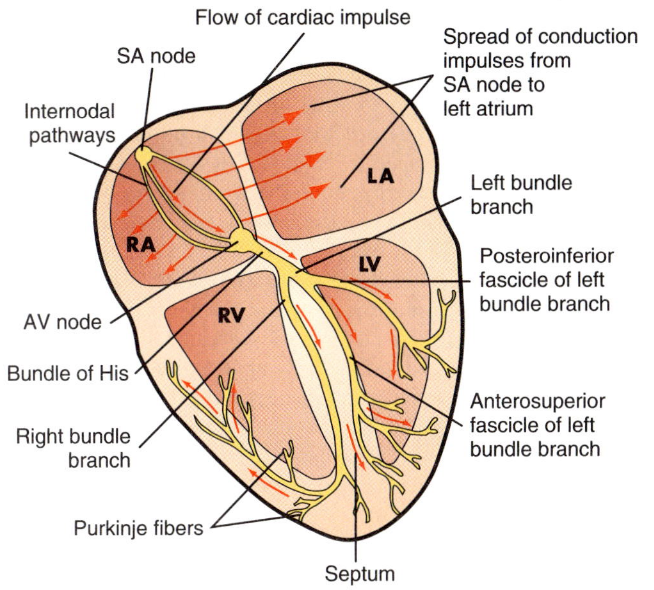

FIG. 40-4 Conduction system of the heart. *AV,* Atrioventricular; *LA,* Left atrium; *LV,* left ventricle; *RA,* right atrium; *RV,* right ventricle; *SA,* sinoatrial. (From Lewis SM et al: *Medical-surgical nursing: assessment and management of clinical problems,* ed 7, St Louis, 2007, Mosby.)

than 160 beats/min, diastolic filling time decreases, decreasing stroke volume and cardiac output. The heart rate of the older adult is slow to increase under stress, but studies have found that this may be caused more by lack of conditioning than age. Exercise is beneficial in maintaining function at any age (Linton and Lach, 2007).

Conduction System. The rhythmic relaxation and contraction of the atria and ventricles depend on continuous, organized transmission of electrical impulses. The cardiac conduction system generates and transmits these impulses (Fig. 40-4).

The conduction system of the heart generates the impulses needed to initiate the electrical chain of events for a normal heartbeat. The autonomic nervous system influences the rate of impulse generation and the speed of transmission through the conductive pathway and the strength of atrial and ventricular contractions. Sympathetic and parasympathetic nerve fibers innervate all parts of the atria and ventricles and the sinoatrial (SA) and atrioventricular (AV) nodes. Sympathetic fibers increase the rate of impulse generation and speed of transmission. The parasympathetic fibers originating from the vagus nerve decrease the rate.

The conduction system originates with the SA node, the "pacemaker" of the heart. The SA node is in the right atrium next to the entrance of the superior vena cava. Impulses are initiated at the SA node at an intrinsic rate of 75 cardiac action potentials per minute in an adult at rest (McCance and Huether, 2010).

The electrical impulses are transmitted through the atria along intraatrial pathways to the AV node. The AV node mediates impulses between the atria and the ventricles. It assists atrial emptying by delaying the impulse before transmitting it through the bundle of His and the ventricular Purkinje network.

An **electrocardiogram (ECG)** reflects the electrical activity of the conduction system. An ECG monitors the regularity and path of the electrical impulse through the conduction system; however, it does not reflect the muscular work of the heart. The normal sequence on the ECG is called the **normal sinus rhythm (NSR)** (Fig. 40-5).

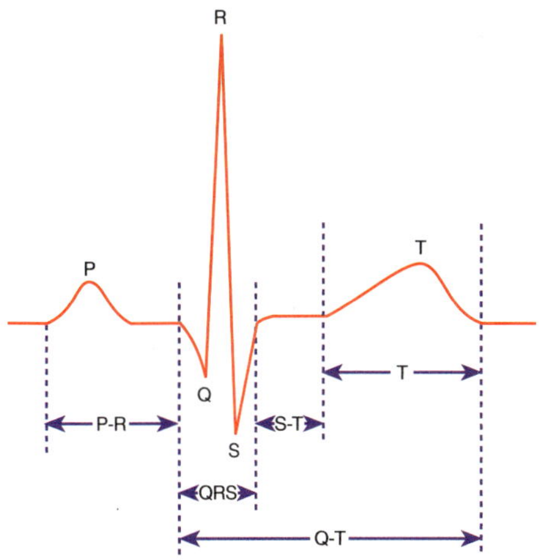

FIG. 40-5 Normal electrocardiogram waveform.

NSR implies that the impulse originates at the SA node and follows the normal sequence through the conduction system. The P wave represents the electrical conduction through both atria. Atrial contraction follows the P wave. The PR interval represents the impulse travel time from the SA node through the AV node, through the bundle of His, and to the Purkinje fibers. The normal length for the PR interval is 0.12 to 0.2 second. An increase in the time greater than 0.2 second indicates a block in the impulse transmission through the AV node; whereas a decrease, less than 0.12 second, indicates the initiation of the electrical impulse from a source other than the SA node.

The QRS complex indicates that the electrical impulse traveled through the ventricles. Normal QRS duration is 0.06 to 0.1 second. An increase in QRS duration indicates a delay in conduction time through the ventricles. Ventricular contraction usually follows the QRS complex.

The QT interval represents the time needed for ventricular depolarization and repolarization. The normal QT interval is 0.12 to 0.42 second. This interval varies inversely with changes in heart rate (McCance and Huether, 2010). Changes in electrolyte values such as hypocalcemia or therapy with drugs such as disopyramide (Norpace) or amiodarone (Cordarone) increase the QT interval. Shortening of the QT interval occurs with digitalis therapy, hyperkalemia, and hypercalcemia.

Factors Affecting Oxygenation

Four factors influence adequacy of circulation, ventilation, perfusion, and transport of respiratory gases to the tissues: (1) physiological, (2) developmental, (3) lifestyle, and (4) environmental. The physiological factors are discussed here, and the others are discussed in the Nursing Knowledge Base section that follows.

Physiological Factors. Any condition affecting cardiopulmonary functioning directly affects the ability of the body to meet oxygen demands. Respiratory disorders include hyperventilation, hypoventilation, and hypoxia. Cardiac disorders include disturbances in conduction, impaired valvular function, myocardial hypoxia, cardiomyopathic conditions, and peripheral tissue hypoxia. Other physiological processes affecting a patient's oxygenation include alterations affecting the oxygen-carrying capacity of blood, decreased inspired oxygen concentration, increases in the metabolic demand of the body, and alterations affecting chest wall movement caused by musculoskeletal abnormalities or neuromuscular alterations.

Decreased Oxygen-Carrying Capacity. Hemoglobin carries the majority of oxygen to tissues. Anemia and inhalation of toxic substances decrease the oxygen-carrying capacity of blood by reducing the amount of available hemoglobin to transport oxygen. Anemia (i.e., a lower-than-normal hemoglobin level) is a result of decreased hemoglobin production, increased red blood cell destruction, and/or blood loss. Patients have fatigue, decreased activity tolerance, increased breathlessness, increased heart rate, and pallor (especially seen in the conjunctiva of the eye). Oxygenation decreases as a secondary effect with anemia. The physiological response to chronic hypoxemia is the development of increased red blood cells (polycythemia). This is the adaptive response of the body to increase the amount of hemoglobin and the available oxygen-binding sites.

Carbon monoxide (CO) is the most common toxic inhalant decreasing the oxygen-carrying capacity of blood. In CO toxicity hemoglobin strongly binds with CO, creating a functional anemia. Because of the strength of the bond, CO does not easily dissociate from hemoglobin, making hemoglobin unavailable for oxygen transport.

Hypovolemia. Conditions such as shock and severe dehydration cause extracellular fluid loss and reduced circulating blood volume, or **hypovolemia.** Decreased circulating blood volume results in hypoxia to body tissues. With significant fluid loss, the body tries to adapt by peripheral vasoconstriction and increasing the heart rate to increase the volume of blood returned to the heart, thus increasing the cardiac output.

Decreased Inspired Oxygen Concentration. With the decline of the concentration of inspired oxygen, the oxygen-carrying capacity of the blood decreases. Decreases in the fraction of inspired oxygen concentration (FiO_2) are caused by upper or lower airway obstruction, which limits delivery of inspired oxygen to alveoli; decreased environmental oxygen (at high altitudes); or hypoventilation (occurs in drug overdoses).

Increased Metabolic Rate. Increased metabolic activity increases oxygen demand. The level of oxygenation declines when body systems are unable to meet this demand. An increased metabolic rate is normal in pregnancy, wound healing, and exercise because the body is using energy or building tissue. Most people are able to meet the increased oxygen demand and do not display signs of oxygen deprivation. Fever increases the need of tissues for oxygen; as a result carbon dioxide production increases. When fever persists, the metabolic rate remains high, and the body begins to break down protein stores. This causes muscle wasting and decreased muscle mass, including respiratory muscles such as the diaphragm and intercostal muscles.

The body attempts to adapt to the increased carbon dioxide levels by increasing the rate and depth of respiration. The patient's WOB increases, and the patient eventually displays signs and symptoms of hypoxemia. Patients with pulmonary diseases are at greater risk for hypoxemia.

Conditions Affecting Chest Wall Movement. Any condition reducing chest wall movement results in decreased ventilation. If the diaphragm does not fully descend with breathing, the volume of inspired air decreases, delivering less oxygen to the alveoli and tissues.

Pregnancy. As the fetus grows during pregnancy, the enlarging uterus pushes abdominal contents upward against the diaphragm. In the last trimester of pregnancy, the inspiratory capacity declines, resulting in dyspnea on exertion and increased fatigue.

Obesity. Patients who are morbidly obese have reduced lung volumes from the heavy lower thorax and abdomen, particularly when in the recumbent and supine positions. Many morbidly obese patients suffer from obstructive sleep apnea. Morbidly obese patients have a reduction in lung and chest wall compliance as a result of encroachment of the abdomen into the chest, increased WOB, and decreased lung volumes. In some patients an obesity-hypoventilation syndrome develops in which oxygenation is decreased and carbon dioxide is retained. The obese patient is also susceptible to atelectasis or pneumonia after surgery because the lungs do not expand fully and the lower lobes retain pulmonary secretions.

Musculoskeletal Abnormalities. Musculoskeletal impairments in the thoracic region reduce oxygenation. Such impairments result from abnormal structural configurations, trauma, muscular diseases, and diseases of the central nervous system. Abnormal structural configurations impairing oxygenation include those affecting the rib cage such as pectus excavatum and the vertebral column such as kyphosis, lordosis, or scoliosis.

Trauma. Flail chest is a condition in which multiple rib fractures cause instability in part of the chest wall. The unstable chest wall allows the lung underlying the injured area to contract on inspiration and bulge on expiration, resulting in hypoxia. Patients with thoracic or upper abdominal surgical incisions use shallow respirations to avoid pain, which also decreases chest wall movement. Opioids used to treat pain depress the respiratory center, further decreasing respiratory rate and chest wall expansion.

Neuromuscular Diseases. Neuromuscular diseases affect tissue oxygenation by decreasing the patient's ability to expand and contract the chest wall. Ventilation is impaired, resulting in atelectasis, hypercapnia, and hypoxemia. Examples of conditions causing hypoventilation include myasthenia gravis, Guillain-Barré syndrome, and poliomyelitis.

Central Nervous System Alterations. Diseases or trauma of the medulla oblongata and/or spinal cord result in impaired respiration. When the medulla oblongata is affected, neural regulation of respiration is impaired, and abnormal breathing patterns develop. Cervical trauma at C3 to C5 usually results in paralysis of the phrenic nerve. When the phrenic nerve is damaged, the diaphragm does not descend properly, thus reducing inspiratory lung volumes and causing hypoxemia. Spinal cord trauma below the C5 vertebra usually leaves the phrenic nerve intact but damages nerves that innervate the intercostal muscles, preventing anteroposterior chest expansion.

Influences of Chronic Disease. Oxygenation decreases as a direct consequence of chronic lung disease. Changes in the anteroposterior diameter of the chest wall (barrel chest) occur because of overuse of accessory muscles and air trapping in emphysema. The diaphragm is flattened, and the lung fields are overdistended, resulting in varying degrees of hypoxemia and/or hypercapnia (McCance and Huether, 2010).

Alterations in Respiratory Functioning

Illnesses and conditions affecting ventilation or oxygen transport cause alterations in respiratory functioning. The three primary alterations are hypoventilation, hyperventilation, and hypoxia.

The goal of ventilation is to produce a normal arterial carbon dioxide tension ($PaCO_2$) between 35 and 45 mm Hg and a normal arterial oxygen tension (PaO_2) between 80 and 100 mm Hg. Hypoventilation and hyperventilation are often determined by arterial blood gas analysis (McCance and Huether, 2010). Hypoxemia refers to a decrease in the amount of arterial oxygen. Nurses monitor arterial oxygen saturation (SpO_2) using a noninvasive oxygen saturation monitor pulse oximeter. Normally SpO_2 is greater than or equal to 95% (see Chapter 41).

Hypoventilation. Hypoventilation occurs when alveolar ventilation is inadequate to meet the oxygen demand of the body or eliminate sufficient carbon dioxide. As alveolar ventilation decreases, the body retains carbon dioxide. For example, atelectasis, a collapse of the alveoli, prevents normal exchange of oxygen and carbon dioxide. As more alveoli collapse, less of the lung is ventilated, and hypoventilation occurs.

In patients with COPD, the administration of excessive oxygen results in hypoventilation. These patients have adapted to a high carbon dioxide level so their carbon dioxide–sensitive chemoreceptors are essentially not functioning. Their peripheral chemoreceptors of the aortic arch and carotid bodies are primarily sensitive to lower oxygen levels, causing increased ventilation. Because the stimulus to breathe is a decreased arterial oxygen (PaO_2) level, administration of oxygen greater than 24% to 28% (1 to 3 L/min) prevents the PaO_2 from falling to a level (60 mm Hg) that stimulates the peripheral receptors, thus destroying the stimulus to breathe (McCance and Huether, 2010). The resulting hypoventilation causes excessive retention of carbon dioxide, which can lead to respiratory acidosis and respiratory arrest.

Signs and symptoms of hypoventilation include mental status changes, dysrhythmias, and potential cardiac arrest. If untreated, the patient's status rapidly declines, leading to convulsions, unconsciousness, and death.

Hyperventilation. Hyperventilation is a state of ventilation in which the lungs remove carbon dioxide faster than it is produced by cellular metabolism. Severe anxiety, infection, drugs, or an acid-base imbalance induces hyperventilation. Acute anxiety leads to hyperventilation and exhalation of excessive amounts of carbon dioxide. Increased body temperature (fever) increases the metabolic rate, thereby increasing carbon dioxide production. The increased carbon dioxide level stimulates an increase in the patient's rate and depth of respiration, causing hyperventilation.

Hyperventilation is sometimes chemically induced. Salicylate (aspirin) poisoning and amphetamine use result in excess carbon dioxide production, stimulating the respiratory center to compensate by increasing the rate and depth of respiration. It also occurs as the body tries to compensate for metabolic acidosis. For example, the patient with diabetes in ketoacidosis produces large amounts of metabolic acids. The respiratory system tries to correct the acid-base balance by overbreathing. Ventilation increases to reduce the amount of carbon dioxide available to form carbonic acid (see Chapter 41). This can also result in the patient developing respiratory alkalosis. Signs and symptoms of hyperventilation include rapid respirations, sighing breaths, numbness and tingling of hands/feet, light-headedness, and loss of consciousness (Ackley and Ladwig, 2011).

Hypoxia. Hypoxia is inadequate tissue oxygenation at the cellular level. It results from a deficiency in oxygen delivery or oxygen use at the cellular level. It is a life-threatening condition. Untreated it produces possibly fatal cardiac dysrhythmias.

Causes of hypoxia include (1) a decreased hemoglobin level and lowered oxygen-carrying capacity of the blood; (2) a diminished concentration of inspired oxygen, which occurs at high altitudes; (3) the inability of the tissues to extract oxygen from the blood, as with cyanide poisoning; (4) decreased diffusion of oxygen from the alveoli to the blood, as in pneumonia; (5) poor tissue perfusion with oxygenated blood, as with shock; and (6) impaired ventilation, as with multiple rib fractures or chest trauma.

The clinical signs and symptoms of hypoxia include apprehension, restlessness, inability to concentrate, decreased level of consciousness, dizziness, and behavioral changes. The patient with hypoxia is unable to lie flat and appears both fatigued and agitated. Vital sign changes include an increased pulse rate and rate and depth of respiration. During early stages of hypoxia the blood pressure is elevated unless the condition is caused by shock. As the hypoxia worsens, the respiratory rate declines as a result of respiratory muscle fatigue.

Cyanosis, blue discoloration of the skin and mucous membranes caused by the presence of desaturated hemoglobin in capillaries, is a late sign of hypoxia. The presence or absence of cyanosis is not a reliable measure of oxygen status. Central cyanosis, observed in the tongue, soft palate, and conjunctiva of the eye where blood flow is high, indicates hypoxemia. Peripheral cyanosis, seen in the extremities, nail beds, and earlobes, is often a result of vasoconstriction and stagnant blood flow.

Alterations in Cardiac Functioning

Illnesses and conditions affecting cardiac rhythm, strength of contraction, blood flow through the heart or to the heart muscle, and decreased peripheral circulation cause alterations in cardiac functioning. Older adults experience alterations in cardiac function as a result of calcification of the conduction pathways, thicker and stiffer heart valves caused by lipid accumulation and fibrosis, and a decrease in the number of pacemaker cells in the SA node (Linton and Lach, 2007; Meiner, 2011).

Disturbances in Conduction. Electrical impulses that do not originate from the SA node cause conduction disturbances. These rhythm disturbances are called dysrhythmias, meaning a deviation from the normal sinus heart rhythm. Dysrhythmias occur as a primary conduction disturbance such as in response to ischemia; valvular abnormality; anxiety; drug toxicity; caffeine, alcohol, or tobacco use; or as a complication of acid-base or electrolyte imbalance (see Chapter 41).

Dysrhythmias are classified by cardiac response and site of impulse origin. Cardiac response is tachycardia (greater than 100 beats/min), bradycardia (less than 60 beats/min), a premature (early) beat, or a blocked (delayed or absent) beat. Tachydysrhythmias and bradydysrhythmias lower cardiac output and blood pressure. Tachydysrhythmias reduce cardiac output by decreasing diastolic filling time. Bradydysrhythmias lower cardiac output because of the decreased heart rate.

Atrial fibrillation is a common dysrhythmia frequently seen in older adults. The electrical impulse in the atria is chaotic and originates from multiple sites. The rhythm is irregular because of the multiple pacemaker sites and the unpredictable conduction to the ventricles. The QRS complex is normal; however, it occurs at irregular intervals. Atrial fibrillation is often described as an irregularly irregular rhythm.

Abnormal impulses originating above the ventricles are supraventricular dysrhythmias. The abnormality on the waveform is the configuration and placement of the P wave. Ventricular conduction usually remains normal, and there is a normal QRS complex.

Paroxysmal supraventricular tachycardia is a sudden, rapid onset of tachycardia originating above the AV node. It often begins and ends spontaneously. Sometimes excitement, fatigue, caffeine, smoking, or alcohol use precipitates paroxysmal supraventricular tachycardia.

Ventricular dysrhythmias represent an ectopic site of impulse formation within the ventricles. It is ectopic in that the impulse originates in the ventricle, not the SA node. The configuration of the QRS complex is usually widened and bizarre. P waves are not always present; often they are buried in the QRS complex. Ventricular tachycardia and ventricular fibrillation are life-threatening rhythms that require immediate intervention. Ventricular tachycardia is a life-threatening dysrhythmia because of the decreased cardiac output and the potential to deteriorate into ventricular fibrillation or sudden cardiac death (AHA, 2010b).

Altered Cardiac Output. Failure of the myocardium to eject sufficient volume to the systemic and pulmonary circulations occurs in heart failure. Primary coronary artery disease, cardiomyopathy, valvular disorders, and pulmonary disease lead to myocardial pump failure.

Left-Sided Heart Failure. Left-sided heart failure is an abnormal condition characterized by decreased functioning of the left ventricle. If left ventricular failure is significant, the amount of blood ejected from the left ventricle drops greatly, resulting in decreased cardiac output. Signs and symptoms include fatigue, breathlessness, dizziness, and confusion as a result of tissue hypoxia from the diminished cardiac output. As the left ventricle continues to fail, blood begins to pool in the pulmonary circulation, causing pulmonary congestion. Clinical findings include crackles in the bases of the lungs on auscultation, hypoxia, shortness of breath on exertion, cough, and paroxysmal nocturnal dyspnea.

Right-Sided Heart Failure. Right-sided heart failure results from impaired functioning of the right ventricle. It more commonly results from pulmonary disease or as a result of long-term left-sided failure. The primary pathological factor in right-sided failure is elevated pulmonary vascular resistance (PVR). As the PVR continues to rise, the right ventricle works harder, and the oxygen demand of the heart increases. As the failure continues, the amount of blood ejected from the right ventricle declines, and blood begins to "back up" in the systemic circulation. Clinically the patient has weight gain, distended neck veins, hepatomegaly and splenomegaly, and dependent peripheral edema.

Impaired Valvular Function. Valvular heart disease is an acquired or congenital disorder of a cardiac valve that causes either hardening (stenosis) or impaired closure (regurgitation) of the valves. When stenosis occurs, the flow of blood through the valves is obstructed. For example, when stenosis occurs in the semilunar valves (aortic and pulmonic valves), the adjacent ventricles have to work harder to move the ventricular blood volume beyond the stenotic valve. Over time the stenosis causes the ventricle to hypertrophy (enlarge); and, if the condition is untreated, left- or right-sided heart failure occurs. When regurgitation occurs, there is a backflow of blood into an adjacent chamber. For example, in mitral regurgitation the mitral leaflets do not close completely. When the ventricles contract, blood escapes back into the atria, causing a murmur, or "whooshing" sound (see Chapter 30).

Myocardial Ischemia. Myocardial ischemia results when the supply of blood to the myocardium from the coronary arteries is insufficient to meet myocardial oxygen demands. Two common outcomes of this ischemia are angina pectoris and MI.

Angina. Angina pectoris is a transient imbalance between myocardial oxygen supply and demand. The condition results in chest pain that is aching, sharp, tingling, or burning or that feels like pressure. Typically chest pain is left sided or substernal and often radiates to the left or both arms, the jaw, neck, and back. In some patients angina pain does not radiate. It usually lasts from 3 to 5 minutes (McCance and Huether, 2010). Patients report that it is often precipitated by activities that increase myocardial oxygen demand (e.g., eating heavy meals, exercise, or stress). It is usually relieved with rest and coronary vasodilators, the most common being a nitroglycerin preparation.

Myocardial Infarction. Myocardial infarction (MI) or acute coronary syndrome (ACS) results from sudden decreases in coronary blood flow or an increase in myocardial oxygen demand without adequate coronary perfusion. Infarction occurs because ischemia is not reversed. Cellular death occurs after 20 minutes of myocardial ischemia (McCance and Huether, 2010).

Chest pain associated with MI in men is usually described as crushing, squeezing, or stabbing. The pain is often in the left chest and sternal area; may be felt in the back; and radiates down the left arm to the neck, jaws, teeth, epigastric area, and back. It occurs at rest or exertion and lasts more than 20 minutes. Rest, position change, or sublingual nitroglycerin administration does not relieve the pain.

There is a significant difference between men and women in relation to coronary artery disease. As women get older, their risk of heart disease begins to rise (AHA, 2010a). Women on average have greater blood cholesterol and triglyceride levels than men. Obesity in women is more prevalent, which also increases risk for diabetes and cardiac disease (Shaw et al., 2009). Women's symptoms differ from those of men. The most common initial symptom in women is angina, but they also present with atypical symptoms such as fatigue, indigestion, shortness of breath, and back or jaw pain. Women have twice the risk of dying within the first year after a heart attack than men.

NURSING KNOWLEDGE BASE

Factors Influencing Oxygenation

In addition to physiological factors, multiple developmental, lifestyle, and environmental factors affect patients' oxygenation status. It is important to recognize these as possible risks or factors that impact their health care goals.

Developmental Factors. The developmental stage of a patient and the normal aging process affect tissue oxygenation.

Infants and Toddlers. Infants and toddlers are at risk for upper respiratory tract infections as a result of frequent exposure to other children, an immature immune system, and exposure to secondhand smoke. In addition, during the teething process some infants develop nasal congestion, which encourages bacterial growth and increases the potential for respiratory tract infection. Upper respiratory tract infections are usually not dangerous, and infants or toddlers recover with little difficulty.

School-Age Children and Adolescents. School-age children and adolescents are exposed to respiratory infections and respiratory risk factors such as cigarette smoking or secondhand smoke. A healthy child usually does not have adverse pulmonary effects from respiratory infections. The American Lung Association (2008) reported a study showing that cigarette smoking in college students (19.2%) had declined in 2006 compared to those smoking in 1999 (30.6%). Although this is still higher than the national goal set by the U.S. Department of Health and Human Services (12%), there is hope that the decline will continue. The biggest risk factor for those still smoking in college was if they started smoking in high school (American Lung Association, 2008). A person who starts smoking in adolescence and continues to smoke into middle age has an increased risk for cardiopulmonary disease and lung cancer.

Young and Middle-Age Adults. Young and middle-age adults are exposed to multiple cardiopulmonary risk factors: an unhealthy diet, lack of exercise, stress, over-the-counter and prescription drugs not used as intended, illegal substances, and smoking. Reducing these modifiable factors decreases a patient's risk for cardiac or pulmonary diseases. This is also the time when individuals

BOX 40-1 FOCUS ON OLDER ADULTS

Oxygenation Changes in Older Adults

- The tuberculin skin test is an unreliable indicator of tuberculosis in older patients. They frequently display false-positive or false-negative skin test reactions.
  - Older patients are at an increased risk for reactivation of dormant organisms that were present for decades as a result of age-related changes in the immune system.
  - The standard 5-TU Mantoux test is given and repeated or repeated with the 250-TU strength to create a booster effect.
  - If the older patient has a positive reaction, a complete history is necessary to determine any risk factors.
- Older adults have more atypical signs and symptoms of coronary artery disease (Meiner, 2011).
- The incidence of atrial fibrillation increases with age and is the leading contributing factor for stroke in the older adult (Meiner, 2011).
- Mental status changes are often the first signs of respiratory problems and often include forgetfulness and irritability.
- Older adults do not always complain of dyspnea until it affects the activities of daily living that are important to them.
- Changes in the older adult's cough mechanism lead to retention of pulmonary secretions, airway plugging, and atelectasis if patients do not use cough suppressants with caution.
- Age-related changes in the immune system lead to a decline of both cell-mediated and humoral immunity, resulting in an increased risk of respiratory infections (McCance and Huether, 2010).
- Changes in the thorax that occur from ossification of costal cartilage, decreased space between vertebrae, and diminished respiratory muscle strength lead to problems with chest expansion and oxygenation (Linton and Lach, 2007).

establish lifelong habits and lifestyles. In 2007 20.6% of adults were smokers (LungUSA, 2010). It is important to help your patients make good choices and informed decisions about their health care practices. The increased cost of cigarettes plus the state smoke-free air policies and laws that reduce smoking in public places have proven to be helpful in smoking cessation (American Lung Association, 2008).

Older Adults. The cardiac and respiratory systems undergo changes throughout the aging process (Box 40-1). The changes are associated with calcification of the heart valves, SA node, and costal cartilages. The arterial system develops atherosclerotic plaques.

Osteoporosis leads to changes in the size and shape of the thorax. The trachea and large bronchi become enlarged from calcification of the airways. The alveoli enlarge, decreasing the surface area available for gas exchange. The number of functional cilia is reduced, causing a decrease in the effectiveness of the cough mechanism, putting the older adult at increased risk for respiratory infections (Meiner, 2011).

Lifestyle Factors. Lifestyle modifications are difficult for patients because they often have to change an enjoyable habit such as cigarette smoking or eating certain foods. Risk-factor modification is important and includes smoking cessation, weight reduction, a low-cholesterol and low-sodium diet, management of hypertension, and moderate exercise (see Chapter 6). Although it is difficult to change long-term behavior, helping patients acquire healthy behaviors reduces the risk for or slows or halts the progression of cardiopulmonary diseases (Meiner, 2011).

Nutrition. Nutrition affects cardiopulmonary function in several ways. Severe obesity decreases lung expansion, and increased body weight increases tissue oxygen demands. The malnourished patient experiences respiratory muscle wasting, resulting in decreased muscle strength and respiratory excursion. Cough efficiency is reduced secondary to respiratory muscle weakness, putting the patient at risk for retention of pulmonary secretions.

Patients who are morbidly obese and/or malnourished are at risk for anemia. Diets high in carbohydrates play a role in increasing the carbon dioxide load for patients with carbon dioxide retention. As carbohydrates are metabolized, an increased load of carbon dioxide is created and excreted via the lungs.

Dietary practices also influence the prevalence of cardiovascular diseases. Cardioprotective nutrition includes diets rich in fiber; whole grains; fresh fruits and vegetables; nuts; antioxidants; lean meats, fish, and chicken; and omega-3 fatty acids. The latest update by the Joint National Committee (JNC, 2003) recommended that dietary restriction of sodium is beneficial in reducing antihypertensive medication requirements; in some cases it causes left ventricular hypertrophy to regress. Diets high in potassium prevent hypertension and help improve control in patients with hypertension. A 2000-calorie diet of fruits; vegetables; and low-fat dairy foods that are high in fiber, potassium, calcium, and magnesium and low in saturated and total fat helps prevent and reduce the effects of hypertension.

Exercise. Exercise increases the metabolic activity and oxygen demand of the body. The rate and depth of respiration increase, enabling the person to inhale more oxygen and exhale excess carbon dioxide. A physical exercise program has many benefits (see Chapter 38). People who exercise for 30 to 60 minutes daily have a lower pulse rate and blood pressure, decreased cholesterol level, increased blood flow, and greater oxygen extraction by working muscles. Fully conditioned people increase oxygen consumption by 10% to 20% because of increased cardiac output and increased efficiency of the myocardial muscle (JNC, 2003).

Smoking. Cigarette smoking and secondhand smoke are associated with a number of diseases, including heart disease, COPD, and lung cancer. Cigarette smoking worsens peripheral vascular and coronary artery diseases (McCance and Huether, 2010). Inhaled nicotine causes vasoconstriction of peripheral and coronary blood vessels, increasing blood pressure and decreasing blood flow to peripheral vessels.

Women who take birth control pills and smoke cigarettes have an increased risk for thrombophlebitis and pulmonary emboli. Smoking during pregnancy can result in low-birth-weight babies, preterm delivery, and babies with reduced lung function (LungUSA, 2010). Even exposure to secondhand smoke can be a risk for low-birth-weight babies, preterm delivery, and miscarriages (ACS, 2010).

The risk of lung cancer is 10 times greater for a person who smokes than for a nonsmoker. In the United States the use of tobacco accounts for 30% of all cancer deaths. This includes 87% of the deaths from lung cancer and cancer of the larynx, mouth, pharynx, esophagus, and bladder. Smoking has been linked to the development of other cancers, including kidney, cervix, and leukemia (ACS, 2010). Nicotine patches, gum, and lozenges are available over the counter, and nicotine nasal spray and inhalers can be obtained by prescription. Prescription drugs such as bupropion (Zyban) and varenicline (Chantix) are also available to help people quit smoking (LungUSA, 2010).

Exposure to environmental tobacco smoke (secondhand smoke) increases the risk of lung cancer and cardiovascular disease in the nonsmoker. Children with parents who smoke have a higher incidence of asthma, pneumonia, and ear infections. Babies exposed to secondhand smoke are at higher risk for sudden infant death syndrome (ACS, 2010).

Substance Abuse. Excessive use of alcohol and other drugs impairs tissue oxygenation in two ways. First, the person who chronically abuses substances often has a poor nutritional intake. With the resultant decrease in intake of iron-rich foods, hemoglobin production declines. Second, excessive use of alcohol and certain other drugs depresses the respiratory center, reducing the rate and depth of respiration and the amount of inhaled oxygen. Substance abuse by either smoking or inhaling substances such as crack cocaine or fumes from paint or glue cans causes direct injury to lung tissue that leads to permanent lung damage. The report on inhalant abuse (huffing) by teenagers to get a euphoric effect includes use of a wide variety of substances such as paint thinner, nail polish remover, glue, spray paint, nitrous oxide, and other common household products. Sudden death can occur from cardiac arrhythmias; or chronic abuse can cause damage to heart, lungs, and kidneys (Stoppler, 2005).

Stress. A continuous state of stress or severe anxiety increases the metabolic rate and oxygen demand of the body. The body responds to anxiety and other stresses with an increased rate and depth of respiration. Most people adapt; but some, particularly those with chronic illnesses or acute life-threatening illnesses such as an MI, cannot tolerate the oxygen demands associated with anxiety (see Chapter 37).

Environmental Factors. The environment also influences oxygenation. The incidence of pulmonary disease is higher in smoggy, urban areas than in rural areas. In addition, a patient's workplace sometimes increases the risk for pulmonary disease. Occupational pollutants include asbestos, talcum powder, dust, and airborne fibers. For example, farm workers in dry regions of the southwestern United States are at risk for coccidioidomycosis, a fungal disease caused by inhalation of spores of the airborne bacterium *Coccidioides immitis.* Asbestosis is an occupational lung disease that develops after exposure to asbestos. The lung with asbestosis often has diffuse interstitial fibrosis, creating a restrictive lung disease. Patients exposed to asbestos are at risk for developing lung cancer, and this risk increases with exposure to tobacco smoke.

CRITICAL THINKING

Successful critical thinking requires a synthesis of knowledge, experience, information gathered from patients, critical thinking attitudes, and intellectual and professional standards. Clinical judgments require you to anticipate information, analyze the data, and make decisions regarding your patient's care. During assessment consider all elements that build toward making an appropriate nursing diagnosis (Fig. 40-6).

To understand how alterations in oxygenation affect patients and the interventions necessary, you need to integrate knowledge from nursing and other disciplines and information gathered from patients. Critical thinking attitudes ensure that you approach patient care in a methodical and logical way. The use of professional standards such as those developed by the Agency for Healthcare Research and Quality (AHRQ), the American Cancer Society (ACS), the American Heart Association (AHA), the American Lung Association (ALA), the American Thoracic Society (ATS), and the American Nurses Association (ANA) provide valuable guidelines for care and management of patients.

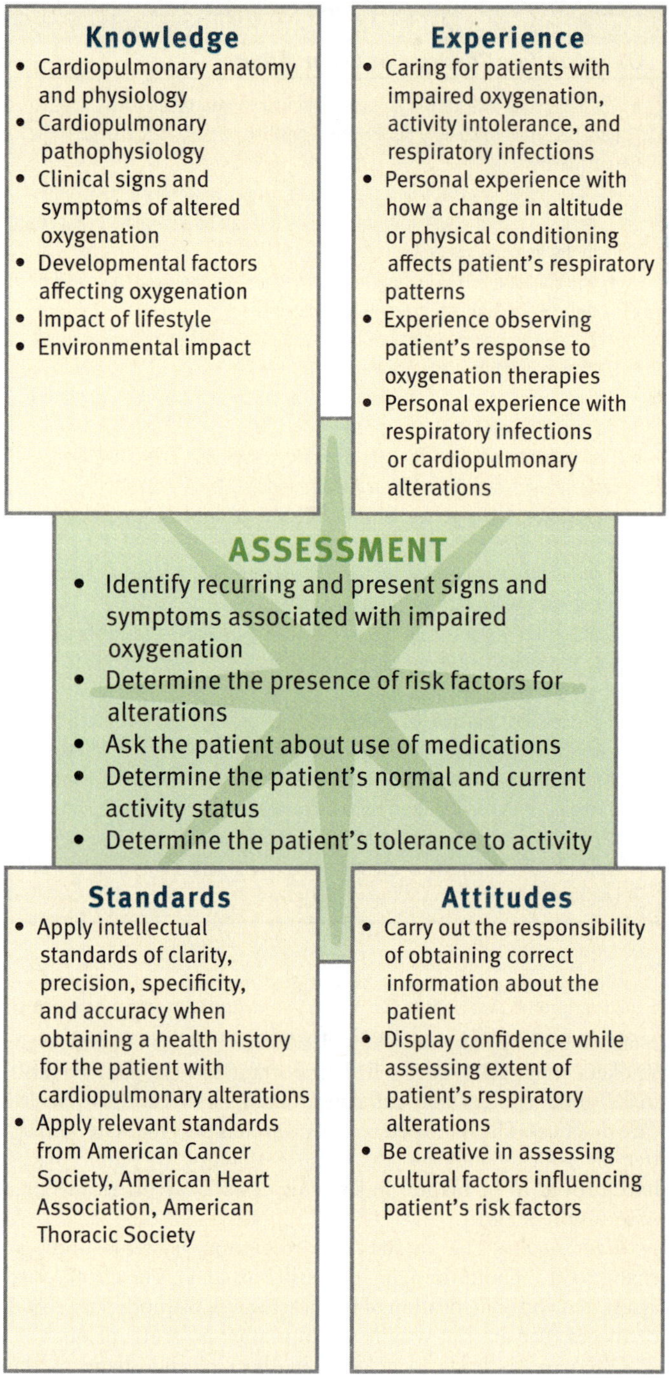

Knowledge
• Cardiopulmonary anatomy and physiology
• Cardiopulmonary pathophysiology
• Clinical signs and symptoms of altered oxygenation
• Developmental factors affecting oxygenation
• Impact of lifestyle
• Environmental impact
Experience
• Caring for patients with impaired oxygenation, activity intolerance, and respiratory infections
• Personal experience with how a change in altitude or physical conditioning affects patient's respiratory patterns
• Experience observing patient's response to oxygenation therapies
• Personal experience with respiratory infections or cardiopulmonary alterations
ASSESSMENT
• Identify recurring and present signs and symptoms associated with impaired oxygenation
• Determine the presence of risk factors for alterations
• Ask the patient about use of medications
• Determine the patient's normal and current activity status
• Determine the patient's tolerance to activity
Standards
• Apply intellectual standards of clarity, precision, specificity, and accuracy when obtaining a health history for the patient with cardiopulmonary alterations
• Apply relevant standards from American Cancer Society, American Heart Association, American Thoracic Society
Attitudes
• Carry out the responsibility of obtaining correct information about the patient
• Display confidence while assessing extent of patient's respiratory alterations
• Be creative in assessing cultural factors influencing patient's risk factors

FIG. 40-6 Critical thinking model for oxygenation assessment.

NURSING PROCESS

Apply the nursing process and use a critical thinking approach in your care of patients. The nursing process provides a clinical decision-making approach for you to develop and implement an individualized plan of care.

ASSESSMENT

During the assessment process, thoroughly assess each patient and critically analyze findings to ensure that you make patient-centered clinical decisions required for safe nursing care. Nursing assessment of cardiopulmonary functioning includes an in-depth history of a patient's normal and present cardiopulmonary function, past impairments in circulatory or respiratory functioning, and methods that a patient uses to optimize oxygenation. The nursing history includes a review of drug, food, and other allergies. Physical examination of a patient's cardiopulmonary status reveals the extent of existing signs and symptoms. Finally, a review of laboratory and diagnostic test results provides valuable assessment data.

Through the Patient's Eyes. Ask patients about their priorities and what they expect from their health care visit. Identifying their expectations involves patients in the decision-making process and helps them participate in their care. For example, planning a smoking cessation program for a patient who is not ready for the change is frustrating for both the patient and the nurse. Establish realistic, short-term outcomes that build to a larger goal. For example, tobacco cessation treatments are effective, but the patient needs to be willing to participate in the program and may need to use several strategies to be successful. Educating the patient on the opportunities for individual, group, or telephone counseling and identifying a social support system give more individual choices when developing the cessation plan. After this is determined, the various nicotine and nonnicotine medications for treatment of tobacco dependence can be discussed to find one that may fit the patient's lifestyle. A combination of counseling and medication is more effective than either one alone (CDC, 2008).

Remember that your goals and expectations do not always coincide with those of your patient. By addressing a patient's concerns and expectations, you establish a relationship that addresses other health care goals and expected outcomes. Knowing your patients' mindsets and respecting their wishes goes a long way in helping them make significant beneficial lifestyle changes.

Nursing History. The nursing history focuses on the patient's ability to meet oxygen needs. The nursing history for respiratory function includes the presence of a cough, shortness of breath, dyspnea, wheezing, pain, environmental exposures, frequency of respiratory tract infections, pulmonary risk factors, past respiratory problems, current medication use, and smoking history or secondhand smoke exposure. The nursing history for cardiac function includes pain and characteristics of pain, fatigue, peripheral circulation, cardiac risk factors, and the presence of past or concurrent cardiac conditions. Ask specific questions related to cardiopulmonary disease (Box 40-2).

Pain. The presence of chest pain requires an immediate thorough evaluation, including location, duration, radiation, and frequency. Cardiac pain does not occur with respiratory variations. Chest pain in men is most often on the left side of the chest and radiates to the left arm. Chest pain in women is much less definitive and is often a sensation of breathlessness, jaw or back pain, nausea, and fatigue (AHA, 2006a). Pericardial pain results from inflammation of the pericardial sac, occurs on inspiration, and does not usually radiate.

Pleuritic chest pain is peripheral and radiates to the scapular regions. Inspiratory maneuvers such as coughing, yawning, and sighing worsen pleuritic chest pain. An inflammation or infection in the pleural space often causes this; and patients usually describe it as knifelike, lasting from a minute to hours and always in association with inspiration.

Musculoskeletal pain is often present following exercise, rib trauma, and prolonged coughing episodes. Inspiration worsens this pain, and patients often confuse it with pleuritic chest pain.

BOX 40-2 NURSING ASSESSMENT QUESTIONS

Nature of the Cardiopulmonary Problem
- What types of breathing problems are you having?
- Describe the problem that you're having with your heart.
- Does the problem (e.g., chest pain, rapid heart rate) occur at a specific time of the day, during or after exercise, or all the time?

Signs and Symptoms
- How has your breathing pattern changed?
- Do you have sputum with coughing? Is this different?
- Is your sputum a different color?
- Are you having any chest pain? Does the pain occur with breathing?

Onset and Duration
- If you are having chest pain, what causes the pain and how long does it last? Is this a different type of pain?
- When did you notice your sputum change in color and amount?
- When did your coughing increase? How does this differ from your usual pattern of coughing?

Severity
- On a scale of 0 to 10, with 10 being the most severe, rate your shortness of breath.
- What helps relieve your shortness of breath?
- On a scale of 0 to 10, with 0 being no pain and 10 the most severe pain, rate your chest pain. Is the severity of your pain different today?
- What do you do for this pain?

Predisposing Factors
- Have you been exposed to a cold or flu?
- Are you taking your prescribed medications?
- Do you smoke? Have you been exposed to secondhand smoke?
- Have you been doing any unusual exercises?

Effect of Symptoms on Patient
- Do these symptoms affect your daily activities? If so how?
- What impact do these symptoms have on your appetite, sleeping habits, activity status?

Fatigue. Fatigue is a subjective sensation in which the patient reports a loss of endurance. Fatigue in the patient with cardiopulmonary alterations is often an early sign of a worsening of the chronic underlying process. To provide an objective measure of fatigue, ask the patient to rate it on a scale of 0 to 10, with 10 being the worst level and 0 representing no fatigue.

Dyspnea. Dyspnea is a clinical sign of hypoxia. It is the subjective sensation of difficult or uncomfortable breathing. Dyspnea is shortness of breath usually associated with exercise or excitement, but in some patients it is present without any relation to activity or exercise. It is associated with many conditions such as pulmonary diseases, cardiovascular diseases, neuromuscular conditions, and anemia. In addition, it occurs in the pregnant woman in the final months of pregnancy. Finally, environmental factors such as pollution, cold air, and smoking also cause or worsen dyspnea.

Dyspnea is associated with exaggerated respiratory effort, use of the accessory muscles of respiration, nasal flaring, and marked increases in the rate and depth of respirations. The use of a Visual Analogue Scale (VAS) helps patients objectively assess their dyspnea. The VAS is a 100-mm vertical line. Have patients rate their dyspnea on a scale of 0 to 10, with 0 equated with no dyspnea and

10 equated with the worst breathlessness a patient has experienced. The use of the VAS to assess the level of a patient's dyspnea is helpful in later evaluating nursing interventions designed to reduce dyspnea (Meek and Lareau, 2003).

When conducting a nursing history on a patient with dyspnea, ask when it occurs (such as with exertion, stress, or respiratory tract infection). Determine whether the patient's dyspnea affects the ability to lie flat. **Orthopnea** is an abnormal condition in which a patient uses multiple pillows when reclining to breathe easier or sits leaning forward with arms elevated. The number of pillows used usually helps to quantify the orthopnea (e.g., two or three-pillow orthopnea). Also ask if the patient must sleep in a recliner chair to breathe easier.

Cough. Cough is a sudden, audible expulsion of air from the lungs. The person breathes in, the glottis is partially closed, and the accessory muscles of expiration contract to expel the air forcibly. Coughing is a protective reflex to clear the trachea, bronchi, and lungs of irritants and secretions. A cough is difficult to evaluate, and almost everyone has periods of coughing. Patients with a chronic cough tend to deny, underestimate, or minimize their coughing, often because they are so accustomed to it that they are unaware of how frequently it occurs.

Patients with chronic sinusitis usually cough only in the early morning or immediately after rising from sleep. This clears the airway of mucus resulting from sinus drainage. Patients with chronic bronchitis generally cough and produce sputum all day, although greater amounts are produced after rising from a semirecumbent or flat position. This is a result of the dependent accumulation of sputum in the airways and is associated with reduced mobility (see Chapter 38).

If the patient has a cough, determine how frequently it occurs and whether it is productive or nonproductive. A productive cough results in sputum production (i.e., material coughed up from the lungs that a patient swallows or expectorates). Sputum contains mucus, cellular debris, microorganisms, and sometimes pus or blood. Collect data about the type and quantity of sputum. Instruct the patient to try to cough up some sputum and not to simply clear the throat, which produces only saliva. Inspect the sputum for color such as green or blood tinged, consistency such as thin or thick, odor such as none or foul, and amount such as increased or decreased.

If **hemoptysis** (bloody sputum) is present, determine if it is associated with coughing and bleeding from the upper respiratory tract, sinus drainage, or the gastrointestinal tract **(hematemesis).** Hemoptysis has an alkaline pH, and hematemesis has an acidic pH; thus pH testing of the specimen may help to determine the source (McCance and Huether, 2010). Describe hemoptysis according to amount and color and whether it is mixed with sputum. When there is bloody or blood-tinged sputum, health care providers frequently perform diagnostic tests such as examination of sputum specimens, chest x-ray examinations, **bronchoscopy,** and other x-ray film studies.

Wheezing. **Wheezing** is a high-pitched musical sound caused by high-velocity movement of air through a narrowed airway. It is associated with asthma, acute bronchitis, or pneumonia. It occurs during inspiration, expiration, or both. Determine if there are any precipitating factors such as respiratory infection, allergens, exercise, or stress.

Environmental or Geographical Exposures. Environmental exposure to inhaled substances is closely linked with respiratory disease. Investigate exposures in the patient's home and workplace. The most common environmental exposures in the home are cigarette smoke, CO, and radon. In addition, determine whether a patient who is a nonsmoker is exposed to secondhand smoke.

CO poisoning often results from a blocked furnace flue or fireplace. The patient will have vague complaints of general malaise, flulike symptoms, and excessive sleepiness. Patients are particularly at risk in the late fall when they turn the furnace on or begin to use the fireplace again. Radon gas is a radioactive substance from the breakdown of uranium in soil, rock, and water that enters homes through the ground or well water. When homes are poorly ventilated, this gas is unable to escape and becomes trapped. If a patient who smokes also lives in a home with a high radon level, the risk for lung cancer is very high (EPA, 2010). Ask if there are any CO or radon detectors in the home.

Smoking. It is important to determine patients' direct and secondary exposure to tobacco. Ask about any history of smoking; include the number of years smoked and the number of packages smoked per day. This is recorded as pack-year history. For example, if a patient smoked two packs a day for 20 years, the patient has a 40 pack-year history (packages per day × years smoked). Determine exposure to secondhand smoke because any form of tobacco exposure increases a patient's risk for cardiopulmonary diseases.

Respiratory Infections. Obtain information about the patient's frequency and duration of respiratory tract infections. Although everyone occasionally has a cold, for some people it results in bronchitis or pneumonia. On average patients have four colds per year. Determine if and when the patient has had a pneumococcal or influenza (flu) vaccine. This is especially important when assessing older adults because of their increased risk for respiratory disease (Linton and Lach, 2007). Ask about any known exposure to tuberculosis (TB) and the date and results of the last tuberculin skin test.

Determine the patient's risk for human immunodeficiency virus (HIV) infection. Patients with a history of intravenous (IV) drug use and multiple unprotected sexual partners are at risk of developing HIV infection. Patients do not always display symptoms of HIV infection until they present with *Pneumocystis carinii* pneumonia (PCP) or *Mycoplasma* pneumonia. Presentation with PCP or *Mycoplasma* pneumonia indicates a significant depression of a patient's immune system and progression to acquired immunodeficiency syndrome (AIDS).

Allergies. Inquire about your patient's exposure to airborne allergens (e.g., pet dander or mold). The allergic response is often watery eyes, sneezing, runny nose, or respiratory symptoms such as cough or wheezing. When obtaining information, ask specific questions about the type of allergens, response to these allergens, and successful and unsuccessful relief measures. In addition, determine the effect of environmental air quality and secondhand smoke exposure on the patient's allergy and symptoms.

Safe nursing practice also includes obtaining information about food, drug, or insect sting allergies on the initial history and physical. However, always double-check this information with the patient on any subsequent assessment, especially concerning respiratory allergens.

Health Risks. Determine familial risk factors such as a family history of lung cancer or cardiovascular disease. Documentation includes blood relatives who had the disease and their present level of health or age at time of death. Other family risk factors include the presence of infectious diseases, particularly TB.

Medications. Another component of the nursing history describes medications that a patient is using. These include prescribed medications, over-the-counter medications, folk medicine, herbal medicines, alternative therapies, and illicit drugs and

TABLE 40-1 Assessment Findings in the Aging Cardiopulmonary System

FUNCTION	PATHOPHYSIOLOGICAL CHANGE	KEY CLINICAL FINDINGS
Heart		
Muscle contraction	Thickening of the ventricular wall, increased collagen and decreased elastin in the heart muscle	Decreased cardiac output Diminished cardiac reserve
Blood flow	Heart valves become thicker and stiffer, more often in the mitral and aortic valves	Systolic ejection murmur
Conduction system	SA node becomes fibrotic from calcification; decrease of number of pacemaker cells in SA node	Increased PR, QRS, and Q-T intervals, decreased amplitude of QRS complex Irregular heart rhythm
Arterial vessel compliance	Calcified vessels, loss of arterial distensibility, decreased elastin in vessel walls, more tortuous vessels	Hypertension with an increase in systolic blood pressure.
Lungs		
Breathing mechanics	Decreased chest wall compliance, loss of elastic recoil Decreased respiratory muscle mass/strength	Prolonged exhalation phase Decreased vital capacity
Oxygenation	Increased ventilation/perfusion mismatch Decreased alveolar surface area Decreased carbon dioxide diffusion capacity	Decreased PaO_2 Decreased cardiac output Slightly increased $PaCO_2$
Breathing control/breathing pattern	Decreased responsiveness of central and peripheral chemoreceptors to hypoxemia and hypercapnia	Increased respiratory rate Decreased tidal volume
Lung defense mechanisms	Decreased number of cilia Decreased IgA production and humoral and cellular immunity	Decreased airway clearance Diminished cough reflex Increased risk for infection
Sleep and breathing	Decreased respiratory drive Decreased tone of upper airway muscles	Increased risk of aspiration and respiratory infection Decreased PaO_2 Snoring, obstructive sleep apnea

IgA, Immunoglobulin A; *$PaCO_2$,* arterial carbon dioxide tension; *PaO_2,* arterial oxygen tension; *SA,* sinoatrial.

substances. Some of these preparations have adverse effects by themselves or because of interactions with other drugs. For example, a person using a prescribed bronchodilator drug decides to use an over-the-counter inhalant as well. Many of these contain ephedrine or *ma huang,* a natural ephedrine, which acts like epinephrine. This product reacts with the prescribed medication by potentiating or decreasing the effect of the prescribed medication. Patients taking warfarin (Coumadin) for blood thinning prolong the prothrombin time (PT)/international normalized ratio (INR) results if they are taking gingko biloba, garlic, or ginseng with the anticoagulant. The drug interaction can precipitate a life-threatening bleed.

It is important to determine if a patient uses illicit drugs. Illicit drugs, particularly inhaled opioids, which are often diluted with talcum powder, cause pulmonary disorders resulting from the irritant effect of the powder on lung tissues. Marijuana is usually smoked in the form of a joint or pipe. Marijuana smoke contains carcinogens and is an irritant to the lungs, putting users at higher risk for lung cancer and respiratory illnesses (NIDA, 2009). Cocaine is snorted through the nose, smoked, or injected. Cocaine abusers can have acute changes such as constricted blood vessels and increased heart rate and blood pressure, which result in heart attack or stroke. Cocaine deaths are caused by cardiac arrest and respiratory failure (NIDA, 2010).

As with all medications, assess the patient's knowledge and ability to self-administer medications correctly (see Chapter 31). Of particular importance is the assessment that the patient understands the potential side effects of medications. Patients need to recognize adverse reactions and be aware of the dangers in combining prescribed medications with over-the-counter drugs.

Building Competency in Safety You are caring for Mary, an 87-year-old patient with diabetes, hypertension, and heart failure. She has recently developed an increase in shortness of breath, weakness, and fatigue. Her daughter brings in a paper bag containing all the medications found in Mary's medicine cabinet. Which of the following medications would put Mary at increased risk of further cardiopulmonary or other problems caused by drug interactions?

- Glucotrol 5 mg 30 minutes before breakfast for diabetes
- Enalapril (Vasotec) 10 mg morning and evening for heart failure and elevated blood pressure
- Furosemide (Lasix) 20 mg every morning as a diuretic for heart failure and to lower blood pressure
- Warfarin (Coumadin) 5 mg every afternoon as a blood thinner to prevent clot formation
- Melatonin 50 mg at bedtime for sleep
- Ginseng 200 mg at bedtime to reduce cholesterol and blood sugar

Answers to questions can be found on the Evolve website.

Physical Examination. The physical examination includes assessment of the cardiopulmonary system (see Chapter 30). Give special consideration when assessing an older adult patient of changes that occur with the aging process (Table 40-1). These changes affect the patient's activity tolerance and level of fatigue or cause transient changes in vital signs and are not always associated with a specific cardiopulmonary disease.

Inspection. Using inspection techniques, perform a head-to-toe observation of the patient for skin and mucous membrane color, general appearance, level of consciousness, adequacy of systemic circulation, breathing patterns, and chest wall movement (Table 40-2). Investigate any abnormalities further during palpation, percussion, and auscultation.

Inspection includes observations of the nails for clubbing (see Chapter 29). Clubbed nails often occur in patients with prolonged oxygen deficiency, endocarditis, and congenital heart defects.

Observe chest wall movement for retraction (i.e., sinking in of soft tissues of the chest between the intercostal spaces) and use of accessory muscles. Also observe the patient's breathing pattern and assess for paradoxical breathing (the chest wall contracts during inspiration and expands during exhalation) or asynchronous breathing. At rest the normal adult rate is 12 to 20 regular breaths/min. Bradypnea is less than 12 breaths/min, and tachypnea is greater than 20 breaths/min (see Chapter 29). In some conditions, such as metabolic acidosis, the acidic pH stimulates an increase in both rate and depth of respirations (**Kussmaul respiration**) to compensate by decreasing carbon dioxide levels. **Apnea** is the absence of respirations for a period of time. **Cheyne-Stokes respiration** occurs when there is decreased blood flow or injury to the brainstem. This respiratory pattern has periods of apnea followed by periods of deep breathing and then shallow breathing followed by more apnea. The apnea periods can last 15 to 60 seconds (McCance and Huether, 2010). Also note the shape of the chest wall. Conditions such as emphysema, advancing age, and COPD cause the chest to assume a rounded "barrel" shape.

TABLE 40-2 Inspection of Cardiopulmonary Status

ABNORMALITY	CAUSE
Eyes	
Xanthelasma (yellow lipid lesions on eyelids)	Hyperlipidemia
Corneal arcus (whitish opaque ring around junction of cornea and sclera)	Abnormal finding in young to middle-age adults with hyperlipidemia (normal finding in older adults with arcus senilis)
Pale conjunctivae	Anemia
Cyanotic conjunctivae	Hypoxemia
Petechiae on conjunctivae	Fat embolus or bacterial endocarditis
Mouth and Lips	
Cyanotic mucous membranes	Decreased oxygenation (hypoxia)
Pursed-lip breathing	Associated with chronic lung disease
Neck Veins	
Distention	Associated with right-sided heart failure
Nose	
Flaring nares	Air hunger, dyspnea
Chest	
Retractions	Increased work of breathing, dyspnea
Asymmetry	Chest wall injury
Skin	
Peripheral cyanosis	Vasoconstriction and diminished blood flow
Central cyanosis	Hypoxemia
Decreased skin turgor	Dehydration (normal finding in older adults as a result of decreased skin elasticity)
Dependent edema	Associated with right- and left-sided heart failure
Periorbital edema	Associated with kidney disease
Fingertips and Nail Beds	
Cyanosis	Decreased cardiac output or hypoxia
Splinter hemorrhages	Bacterial endocarditis
Clubbing	Chronic hypoxemia

From Potter PA, Weilitz PB: *Health assessment, pocket guide series,* ed 6, St Louis, 2007, Mosby.

Palpation. Palpation of the chest provides assessment data in several areas. It documents the type and amount of thoracic excursion; elicits any areas of tenderness; and helps to identify tactile fremitus, thrills, heaves, and the cardiac point of maximal impulse (PMI). Palpation of the extremities provides data about the peripheral circulation (i.e., the presence and quality of peripheral pulses, skin temperature, color, and capillary refill) (see Chapter 30).

Palpation of the feet and legs determines the presence or absence of peripheral edema. Patients with alterations in cardiac function such as those with heart failure or hypertension often have pedal or lower-extremity edema. Edema is graded from +1 to +4 depending on the depth of visible indentation after firm finger pressure (see Chapter 30).

Palpate the pulses in the neck and extremities to assess arterial blood flow (see Chapter 30). Use a scale of 0 (absent pulse) to +4 (full, bounding pulse) to describe what you feel. The normal pulse is +2; and a weak, thready pulse is +1.

Percussion. Percussion detects the presence of abnormal fluid or air in the lungs. It also determines diaphragmatic excursion (see Chapter 30).

Auscultation. Auscultation helps identify normal and abnormal heart and lung sounds (see Chapter 30). Auscultation of the cardiovascular system includes assessment for normal S_1 and S_2 sounds and the presence of abnormal S_3 and S_4 sounds (gallops), murmurs, or rubs. Identify the location, radiation, intensity, pitch, and quality of a murmur. Auscultation also identifies any bruit over the carotid, abdominal aorta, and femoral arteries.

Auscultation of lung sounds involves listening for movement of air throughout all lung fields: anterior, posterior, and lateral. Adventitious, or abnormal, breath sounds occur with collapse of a lung segment, fluid in a lung segment, or narrowing or obstruction of an airway.

Diagnostic Tests. A variety of diagnostic tests monitor cardiopulmonary functioning. Some of these screening tests involve simple blood specimens, x-rays, or other noninvasive means. One screening mechanism is TB skin testing (Box 40-3). This is a simple test and is required for health care workers; restaurant employees; students on entry to school, teachers, and other school employees; prisoners and correctional facility employees; and residents of long-term care facilities (CDC, 2010a, 2010b).

Diagnostic testing used in the assessment and evaluation of the patient with cardiopulmonary alterations are summarized in Tables 40-3 through 40-5. When reviewing results of pulmonary function studies, be aware of expected variations in patients from different cultures. These changes are caused by structural variations in chest wall size (Box 40-4).

Invasive diagnostic tests such as a thoracentesis are painful. How painful a diagnostic procedure is depends on the patient's tolerance for pain (see Chapter 43). Reduce the patient's anxiety by explaining the thoracentesis procedure and telling him or her what to expect. Be sure that he or she understands the importance of following instructions such as taking a deep breath and holding it when requested and not coughing during the procedure. Provide appropriate pain management before the procedure to reduce the perception of pain. After any procedure monitor the patient for signs of changes in cardiopulmonary functioning such as sudden shortness of breath, pain, oxygen desaturation, and anxiety.

BOX 40-3 TUBERCULOSIS SKIN TESTING

- Skin testing determines whether a person is infected with *Mycobacterium tuberculosis.*
- Tuberculosis (TB) skin testing (TST) is performed by an intradermal injection of 0.1 mL of tuberculin purified protein derivative (PPD) on the inner surface of the forearm (see Chapter 31). The injection produces a pale elevation of the skin (a wheal) 6 to 10 mm in diameter. Afterward the injection site is circled, and the patient is instructed not to wash the circle off.
- Read tuberculin skin tests between 48 to 72 hours after the test. If the site is not read within 72 hours, a patient must have another skin test.
- *Positive results:* A palpable, elevated, hardened area around the injection site, caused by edema and inflammation from the antigen-antibody reaction, measured in millimeters. (See Chapter 31 for evaluation of positive results by millimeters.) People born outside the United States may have had bacille Calmette Guérin (BCG) vaccine for TB disease, which results in a positive reaction to the TST and may complicate the treatment plan. The positive skin reaction does not indicate that the BCG vaccine provided protection against the disease (CDC, 2010b).
- Reddened flat areas are *not* positive reactions and are not measured.
- TST is less reliable in older adults (see Box 40-1) and those with an altered immune function such as a human immunodeficiency virus (HIV)–positive patient or someone receiving chemotherapy.

NURSING DIAGNOSIS

Based upon your assessment, you develop nursing diagnoses for patients with oxygenation alterations by clustering specific defining characteristics and identifying the related etiology (Box 40-5). The defining characteristics for diagnoses related to oxygenation can be similar. For example, both *impaired gas exchange* and *ineffective*

BOX 40-5 NURSING DIAGNOSTIC PROCESS

Impaired Gas Exchange Related to Decreased Lung Expansion

ASSESSMENT ACTIVITIES	DEFINING CHARACTERISTICS
Ask patient or family about patient's mood, attentiveness, memory, and activity level.	Confusion Decreased activity Fatigue Irritability Restlessness Sleepiness
Observe patient's respirations for rate, rhythm, depth.	Dyspnea Nasal flaring Tachypnea Use of accessory muscles
Inspect skin and mucous membranes.	Diaphoresis Pallor Cyanosis
Auscultate chest.	Decreased respiratory excursion Abnormal, distant lung sounds

BOX 40-4 CULTURAL ASPECTS OF CARE

Cultural Impact on Pulmonary Diseases

The impact of pulmonary diseases on the patient and family varies among cultures. It is important to understand these variations in terms of assessing for and providing care in patients with lung diseases.

- Differences occur as a result of the variation in chest size. Caucasians have the largest chest volumes, followed by African Americans, Asian Americans, and Native Americans. The variations in the chest size affect the forced expiratory volume (FEV_1), forced vital capacity (FVC), and the FEV_1/FVC ratio (Meiner, 2011).
- In 2008 Asian Americans had the highest incidence rate of tuberculosis (TB), followed by native Hawaiians and Pacific Islanders. Asian Americans had 23.3 times the incidence rate of Caucasians. United States–born Asian Americans only make up 3% of TB cases compared to 43% of foreign-born Asian Americans. Major countries of origin for foreign-born TB cases are the Philippines, Vietnam, India, and China (American Lung Association, 2010b). Ask if they have had the bacille Calmette-Guérin (BCG) vaccine, which can cause a positive reaction to the TB skin test.
- The cigarette smoking prevalence rate in America's youth is highest in Alaskan Natives (23.1%), followed by Caucasians (14.9%), Hispanics (9.3%), African Americans (6.5%), and Asian Americans (4.3%). This puts them at risk for lung cancer, chronic obstructive pulmonary disease (COPD), and heart disease (American Lung Association, 2010a).
- African Americans have higher mortality rates from lung cancer despite the lower smoking prevalence. African American men are 37% more likely to get lung cancer, and 22.5% are more likely to die of the disease compared to Caucasian men (American Lung Association, 2010a).
- Air pollution has also been linked to cancer, asthma, and heart disease, which puts both African Americans and Hispanics at increased risk since they are more likely to live in areas with high levels of air toxins and heavy vehicle traffic (American Lung Association, 2010b). Female African Americans have the highest mortality rates from asthma among all ethnic/gender groups (Lewis et al., 2007).
- Caucasians have the highest incidences of COPD and cystic fibrosis, which is uncommon among African Americans, Hispanics, and Asian Americans (Lewis et al., 2007). They are more likely to die from COPD than any other racial group (American Lung Association, 2010b).
- African Americans and Hispanics are less likely to get flu or pneumonia vaccines than Caucasians. A recent report on health care disparities found that Asian Americans over the age of 65 had the highest rates of never having received a pneumococcal vaccine, which explains why influenza and pneumonia are the fourth leading cause of death in this group (American Lung Association, 2010b). Community Health Departments need to target these groups during education programs for their flu and pneumonia vaccine clinics.

Implications for Practice

- Public health programs for those at highest risk for pulmonary diseases should focus on pollution prevention and smoking cessation programs.
- Immunization clinics should concentrate on the underserved urban communities, especially those with large numbers of older adults.

TABLE 40-3 Cardiopulmonary Diagnostic Blood Studies

TEST AND NORMAL VALUES	INTERPRETATION
Complete Blood Count	
Normal values for a complete blood count (CBC) vary with age and gender	A CBC determines the number and type of red and white blood cells per cubic millimeter of blood.
Cardiac Enzymes	
Creatine kinase (CK): A serial CK with 50% increase between two samples 3-6 hours apart, peaking 12-24 hours after chest pain or a single CK elevation twofold is diagnostic for an acute myocardial infarction. Male normal: 55-170 units/L; female normal: 30-135 units/L	Providers use cardiac enzymes to diagnose acute myocardial infarcts.
Cardiac Troponins	
Plasma cardiac troponin I <0.03 ng/mL	Value elevates as early as 3 hours after myocardial injury. Value often remains elevated for 7-10 days.
Plasma cardiac troponin T <0.1 ng/mL	Value often remains elevated for 10-14 days.
Myoglobin	
<90 mcg/L	Early index of damage to myocardium in myocardial infarction or reinfarction. Increases within 3 hours.
Serum Electrolytes	
Potassium (K+) 3.5-5 mEq/L or 3.5-5 mmol/L	Patients on diuretic therapy are at risk for hypokalemia (low potassium). Patients receiving angiotensin-converting enzyme (ACE) inhibitors are at risk for hyperkalemia (elevated potassium).
Cholesterol	
Fasting cholesterol less than 200 mg/dL or less than 5.2 mmol/L (SI units)	Contributing factors include sedentary lifestyle with intake of saturated fatty acids, familial hypercholesterolemia.
Low-density lipoproteins (LDLs) (bad cholesterol) <130 mg/dL Very low–density lipoproteins (VLDLs) 7-32 mg/dl	High LDL cholesterol (hypercholesterolemia) is caused by excessive intake of saturated fatty acids, dietary cholesterol intake, and obesity. Familial hypercholesterolemia and hyperlipidemia, hypothyroidism, nephrotic syndrome, and diabetes mellitus are also contributing factors. VLDLs are predominant carriers of triglycerides and can be converted to LDL by lipoprotein lipase. Levels in excess of 25%-50% indicate increased risk of cardiac disease.
High-density lipoproteins (HDLs) (good cholesterol) Male: >45 mg/dL; female: >55 mg/dL	Factors such as cigarette smoking, obesity, lack of regular exercise, beta-adrenergic blocking agents, genetic disorders of HDL metabolism, hypertriglyceridemia, and type 2 diabetes cause low HDL cholesterol.
Triglycerides Male: 40-160 mg/dL; female: 35-135 mg/dL	Obesity, excessive alcohol intake, diabetes mellitus, beta-adrenergic blocking agents, and familial hypertriglyceridemia cause hypertriglyceridemia.

Data from Pagana KD, Pagana TJ: *Mosby's diagnostic and laboratory test reference,* ed 10, St Louis, 2011, Mosby.

TABLE 40-4 Cardiac Function Diagnostic Tests

TEST	SIGNIFICANCE
Holter monitor	Portable ECG worn by a patient. The test produces a continuous ECG tracing over a period of time. Patients keep a diary of activity, noting when they experience rapid heartbeats or dizziness. Evaluation of the ECG recording along with the diary provides information about the electrical activity of the heart during activities of daily living.
ECG exercise stress test	ECG is monitored while a patient walks on a treadmill at a specified speed and duration of time. Test evaluates the cardiac response to physical stress. It is not a valuable tool for evaluation of cardiac response in women because of an increased false-positive finding.
Thallium stress test	ECG stress test with the addition of thallium-201 injected intravenously. It determines coronary blood flow changes with increased activity.
Electrophysiological study (EPS)	EPS is an invasive measure of intracardiac electrical pathways. It provides more specific information about difficult-to-treat dysrhythmias and assesses adequacy of antidysrhythmic medication.
Echocardiography	This is a noninvasive measure of heart structure and heart wall motion. It graphically demonstrates overall cardiac performance.
Scintigraphy	Scintigraphy is radionuclide angiography; used to evaluate cardiac structure, myocardial perfusion, and contractility.
Cardiac catheterization and angiography	These are used to visualize cardiac chambers, valves, the great vessels, and coronary arteries. Pressures and volumes within the four chambers of the heart are also measured.

ECG, Electrocardiogram.

TABLE 40-5 Ventilation and Oxygenation Diagnostic Studies

MEASUREMENT AND NORMAL VALUES	INTERPRETATION
Arterial Blood Gases	
pH 7.35-7.45 PCO_2 35-45 mm Hg HCO_3 21-28 mEq/L PO_2 80-100 mm Hg SaO_2 saturation >95% Base excess 0 ± 2 mEq/L	Provide important information for assessment of patient's respiratory and metabolic acid/base balance and adequacy of oxygenation (see Chapter 41)
Pulmonary Function Tests	
Basic ventilation studies (Pulmonary functions vary by ethnic group.)	Determines ability of the lungs to efficiently exchange oxygen and carbon dioxide Used to differentiate pulmonary obstructive from restrictive disease
Peak Expiratory Flow Rate (PEFR)	
The point of highest flow during maximal expiration (Normal is based on age and body weight.)	Reflects changes in large airway sizes; an excellent predictor of overall airway resistance in a patient with asthma Daily measurement for early detection of asthma exacerbations
Bronchoscopy	
Normal airways without masses, pus, or foreign bodies	Visual examination of the tracheobronchial tree through a narrow, flexible fiberoptic bronchoscope Performed to obtain fluid, sputum, or biopsy samples; remove mucus plugs or foreign bodies
Lung Scan	
Normal lung structure without masses	Nuclear scanning test used to identify abnormal masses by size and location Identification of masses used in planning therapy and treatments Also used to find a blood clot preventing normal perfusion or ventilation ($\dot{V}/\dot{Q}$ scan)
Thoracentesis	
Surgical perforation of chest wall and pleural space with a needle to aspirate fluid for diagnostic or therapeutic purposes or to remove a specimen for biopsy; performed using aseptic technique and local anesthetic (Patient usually sits upright with the anterior thorax supported by pillows or an over-bed table.)	Specimen of plural fluid obtained for cytological examination Results may indicate an infection or neoplastic disease Identification of infection or a type of cancer important in determining a plan of care
Sputum Specimens	
Normal: negative	
Sputum culture and sensitivity	Obtained to identify a specific microorganism or organism growing in sputum Identifies drug resistance and sensitivities to determine appropriate antibiotic therapy
Sputum for acid-fast bacillus (AFB)	Screens for presence of AFB for detection of tuberculosis by early-morning specimens on 3 consecutive days
Sputum for cytology	Obtained to identify lung cancer Differentiates type of cancer cells (small cell, oat cell, large cell)

breathing pattern have the defining characteristics of dyspnea and nasal flaring. A closer review of assessment findings as well as an analysis of the patient's history will help you clarify and select the correct diagnosis. For example, a patient who is a victim of trauma and has rib pain and is showing an increased respiratory rate is more likely to be suffering *ineffective breathing pattern*. The clustered defining characteristics and related factor must support the nursing diagnosis.

These nursing diagnosis examples are appropriate for the patient with alterations in oxygenation (Ackley and Ladwig, 2011):

- Activity intolerance
- Decreased cardiac output
- Fatigue
- Impaired gas exchange
- Impaired spontaneous ventilation
- Impaired verbal communication
- Ineffective airway clearance
- Ineffective breathing pattern
- Ineffective health maintenance
- Risk for aspiration
- Risk for imbalanced fluid volume
- Risk for infection
- Risk for suffocation

PLANNING

During planning, use critical thinking skills to synthesize information from multiple sources (Fig. 40-7). Critical thinking ensures that your plan of care integrates individualized patient needs. Professional standards are especially important to consider when developing a plan of care. These standards often establish scientifically proven guidelines for selecting effective nursing interventions.

Goals and Outcomes. Develop an individualized plan of care for each nursing diagnosis (see the Nursing Care Plan). Together with your patient set realistic expectations, goals, and measurable outcomes of care.

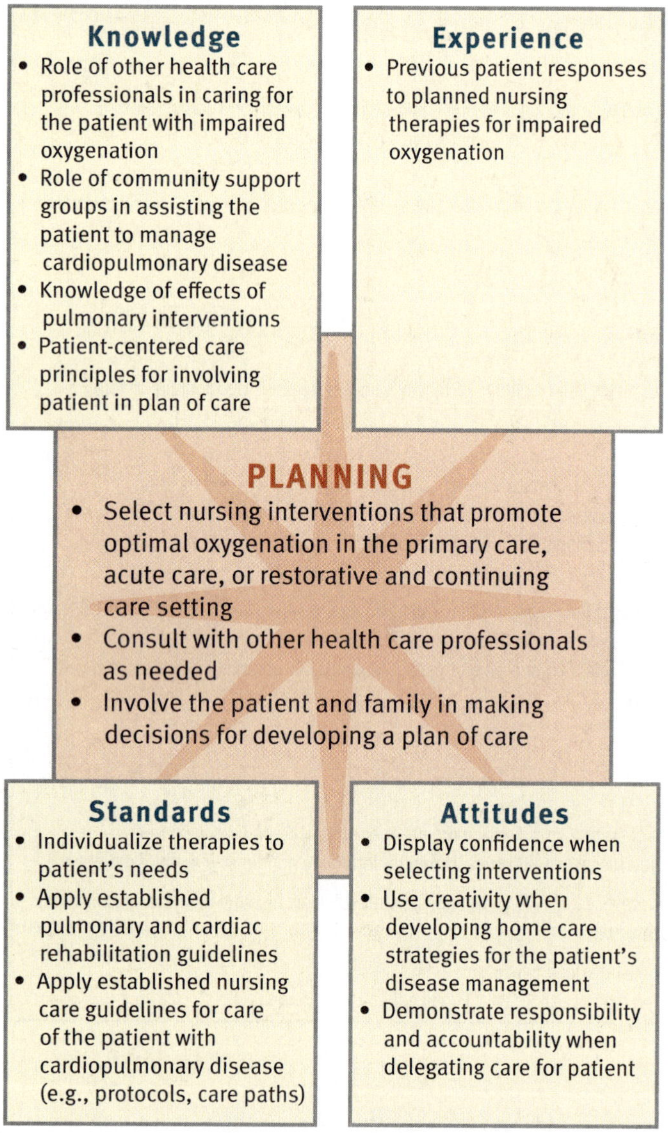

Knowledge
• Role of other health care professionals in caring for the patient with impaired oxygenation
• Role of community support groups in assisting the patient to manage cardiopulmonary disease
• Knowledge of effects of pulmonary interventions
• Patient-centered care principles for involving patient in plan of care
Experience
• Previous patient responses to planned nursing therapies for impaired oxygenation
PLANNING
• Select nursing interventions that promote optimal oxygenation in the primary care, acute care, or restorative and continuing care setting
• Consult with other health care professionals as needed
• Involve the patient and family in making decisions for developing a plan of care
Standards
• Individualize therapies to patient's needs
• Apply established pulmonary and cardiac rehabilitation guidelines
• Apply established nursing care guidelines for care of the patient with cardiopulmonary disease (e.g., protocols, care paths)
Attitudes
• Display confidence when selecting interventions
• Use creativity when developing home care strategies for the patient's disease management
• Demonstrate responsibility and accountability when delegating care for patient

FIG. 40-7 Critical thinking model for oxygenation planning.

Patients with impaired oxygenation require a nursing care plan directed toward meeting actual or potential oxygenation needs. Allow patients to collaborate in setting relevant goals of care. Develop individual outcomes based on patient-centered goals. For example, for the goal of maintaining a patent airway, select specific expected outcomes for the patient, such as the following:

- Patient's lungs are clear to auscultation.
- Patient achieves bilateral lung expansion.
- Patient coughs productively.
- Pulse oximetry (SpO_2) is maintained or improved.

Often a patient with cardiopulmonary disease has multiple nursing diagnoses (Fig. 40-8). In this case identify when goals or outcomes apply to more than one diagnosis. The presence of multiple diagnoses also makes priority setting a critical activity.

Setting Priorities. A patient's level of health, age, lifestyle, and environmental risks affect the level of tissue oxygenation. Patients with severe impairments in oxygenation frequently require nursing interventions in multiple areas. Consider which goal is the most important to achieve while the patient is in the hospital or primary care setting. For example, in an acute care setting maintaining a patent airway has a higher priority than improving the patient's exercise tolerance. The need for a patent airway is immediate; and, as the patient's level of oxygen improves, activity tolerance increases. In a second example, when caring for a patient who has an abdominal incision, pain control is a priority. In this situation controlling the patient's pain facilitates coughing and deep breathing.

However, in a community-based or primary care setting, priorities often focus on smoking cessation, exercise, and/or diet modifications. Both you and the patient need to focus on the same goal and expected outcomes. In addition to individualizing each goal, be sure that the goals are realistic, have a reasonable time frame, and are attainable for the patient. In addition, be sure to respect the patient's preferences for his or her degree of active engagement in the care process. Some will choose to be very active and desire to make day-to-day decisions. Others may choose to assume a more passive role, preferring you to choose a course of action while keeping them informed.

Teamwork and Collaboration. The time spent with a patient in any setting is limited. Therefore collaborate with family members, colleagues, and other specialists to achieve the established goals and expected outcomes. Some patients need to improve their exercise and activity tolerance; for other patients continuing care involves participating in a community-based cardiopulmonary rehabilitation program. Finally, some patients need home physical therapy.

Collaboration with physical therapists, nutritionists, and community-based nurses is valuable for patients with heart failure or chronic lung conditions. These professionals work with patients and use resources in the community to assist them

NURSING CARE PLAN

Ineffective Airway Clearance

ASSESSMENT

Mr. Edwards is a 75-year-old Caucasian male who is currently lying in a semi-Fowler's position in bed talking with his wife. Kathy Allen is a nursing student completing a respiratory assessment. Mr. Edwards has a history of chronic obstructive pulmonary disease for 2 years. He continues to smoke ½ pack of cigarettes a day and does not participate in any exercise. He does not "see any reason" to increase his fluid intake. His SpO_2 ranges from 78% to 84%. He must do his self-care activities slowly because of fatigue. Presently he is admitted for right upper lobe pneumonia. He reports having an intermittent productive cough that occasionally produces thick, yellow sputum. He has more episodes of coughing when lying flat. His vital signs are temperature, 101.4° F (38.5° C); pulse, 102 beats/min; respirations, 30 breaths/min; blood pressure, 130/90 mm Hg; and SpO_2, 84%. He has episodes of chilling and diaphoresis. His health care provider has told him that, if he gradually increases his exercise, drinks more fluids, and stops smoking, his respiratory status will improve.

NURSING CARE PLAN

***Ineffective Airway Clearance*—cont'd**

Assessment Activities	*Findings/Defining Characteristics**
Ask Mr. Edwards how long he has had this cough.	He replies, "I have a morning **cough** every day, but this cough is different. It started about a week ago. It is worse when I lie flat."
Ask Mr. Edwards what is different about this cough.	He replies, "My ribs are getting sore. It is difficult to cough up anything, my **mouth** is **dry**, and I have become more **fatigued**."
Observe Mr. Edwards' skin and mucous membranes.	**Skin and mucous membranes** are **dry.**
Auscultate lung fields.	**Abnormal lung sounds** (crackles) are heard in lower lobes bilaterally.
Ask Mr. Edwards to produce a sputum sample.	Sputum is **thick** and **discolored** yellow to yellow-green.

***Defining characteristics** are shown in bold type.

NURSING DIAGNOSIS: Ineffective airway clearance related to retained thick pulmonary secretions

PLANNING

Goals	*Expected Outcomes (NOC)*†
	Respiratory Status: Airway Patency
Mr. Edwards will be able to effectively clear secretions by discharge.	Lung sounds will be clear in 48 hours. Mr. Edwards will notice increased ease in coughing within 48 hours. Sputum will be thin and white within 3 days. Respiratory rate will be within 12 to 20 breaths/min in 48 hours.
Mr. Edwards will increase oral hydration within 48 hours.	Mr. Edwards will drink 2500 mL of water or preferred liquids every 24 hours starting today. Mr. Edwards will verbalize that his mouth is not dry in 48 hours.

†Outcome classification labels from Moorhead S et al.: *Nursing outcomes classification (NOC),* ed 4, St Louis, 2008, Mosby.

INTERVENTIONS (NIC)‡	RATIONALE
Airway Management	
Position Mr. Edwards with head elevated 30-45 degrees.	An upright angle allows for thoracic expansion; lying flat allows abdominal organs to push up against the diaphragm, compromising inspiration. This allows for a more normal respiratory rate (Lawrence et al., 2006).
Ambulate in room or hall as tolerated at least 2 times a day. If unable to ambulate, reposition from side to side every 2 hours or more.	Body movement helps mobilize secretions (Perme and Chandrashekar, 2009).
Have Mr. Edwards deep breathe and cough every 2 hours. Teach him to take a deep breath, hold it for several seconds, open his mouth, tighten his abdominal muscles, and cough 2 to 3 times with his mouth open.	Retained secretions predispose patient to atelectasis and pneumonia. Controlled coughing that uses the diaphragmatic muscles make the cough more effective in removing mucus (AARC, 1993).
Administer 2 L/min of oxygen as ordered per nasal cannula if SpO_2 less than 90%.	This dependent nursing intervention will relieve hypoxia.
Increase fluids to 2500 mL in 24 hours if not contraindicated by cardiac or renal status. Offer fluids Mr. Edwards prefers.	Fluids help to liquefy secretions and promote ease of removal. Fluids relieve oral mucosa and skin dryness.

‡Intervention classification labels from Bulechek GM, Butcher HK, and Dochterman JM: *Nursing interventions classification (NIC),* ed 5, St Louis, 2008, Mosby.

EVALUATION

Nursing Actions	*Patient Response/Finding*	*Achievement of Outcome*
Auscultate the chest.	Mr. Edwards reports that he has not heard any rattling in his chest.	Lung sounds are normal.
Ask Mr. Edwards if he can deep breathe and cough and measure SpO_2.	Mr. Edwards reports that it is easier to cough up his secretions. SpO_2 is 95%.	Airway clears with coughing. SpO_2 is within normal levels.
Observe sputum.	Mr. Edwards states, "My sputum is thinner and white now."	Sputum is thin and white.
Monitor respiratory rate.	Mr. Edwards says that it is easier to breathe.	Rate is between 12 and 20 breaths/min.
Assess Mr. Edwards' level of hydration (skin turgor, condition of mucosa).	Mucous membranes are moist. Fluid intake in previous 24 hours was 2600 mL.	Oral membranes are pink and moist. Minimum fluid intake of 2500 mL was achieved.

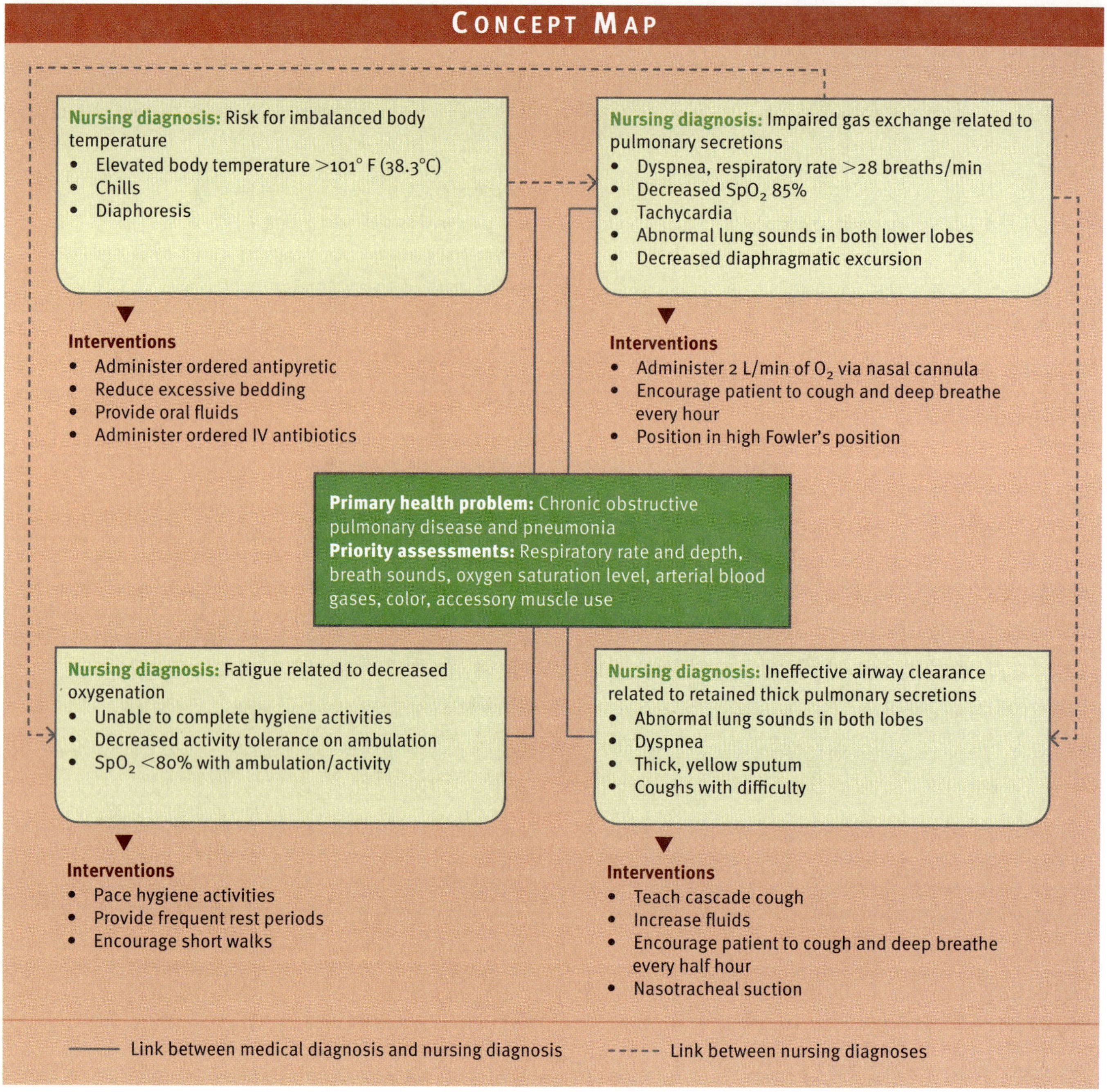
CONCEPT MAP
Nursing diagnosis: Risk for imbalanced body temperature
• Elevated body temperature >101° F (38.3°C)
• Chills
• Diaphoresis
Interventions
• Administer ordered antipyretic
• Reduce excessive bedding
• Provide oral fluids
• Administer ordered IV antibiotics
Nursing diagnosis: Impaired gas exchange related to pulmonary secretions
• Dyspnea, respiratory rate >28 breaths/min
• Decreased SpO2 85%
• Tachycardia
• Abnormal lung sounds in both lower lobes
• Decreased diaphragmatic excursion
Interventions
• Administer 2 L/min of O2 via nasal cannula
• Encourage patient to cough and deep breathe every hour
• Position in high Fowler's position
Primary health problem: Chronic obstructive pulmonary disease and pneumonia
Priority assessments: Respiratory rate and depth, breath sounds, oxygen saturation level, arterial blood gases, color, accessory muscle use
Nursing diagnosis: Fatigue related to decreased oxygenation
• Unable to complete hygiene activities
• Decreased activity tolerance on ambulation
• SpO2 <80% with ambulation/activity
Interventions
• Pace hygiene activities
• Provide frequent rest periods
• Encourage short walks
Nursing diagnosis: Ineffective airway clearance related to retained thick pulmonary secretions
• Abnormal lung sounds in both lobes
• Dyspnea
• Thick, yellow sputum
• Coughs with difficulty
Interventions
• Teach cascade cough
• Increase fluids
• Encourage patient to cough and deep breathe every half hour
• Nasotracheal suction
Link between medical diagnosis and nursing diagnosis
Link between nursing diagnoses

FIG. 40-8 Concept map for Mr. Edwards. *IV,* Intravenous.

in attaining and maintaining the highest possible level of wellness. In addition, professionals identify community resources and support systems for both the patient and family in preventing and managing symptoms related to cardiopulmonary diseases. Communicating among everyone on the patient's health care team and recognizing everyone's contributions in achieving the health care goals for the patient are imperative.

IMPLEMENTATION

There are interventions for promoting and maintaining adequate oxygenation across the continuum of care. As a nurse, you will be responsible for independent interventions such as positioning, coughing techniques, and health education for disease prevention. In addition, you will provide physician-initiated interventions such as oxygen therapy, lung inflation techniques, and chest physiotherapy.

Health Promotion. Maintaining the patient's optimal level of health is important in reducing the number and/or severity of respiratory symptoms. Prevention of respiratory infections is foremost in maintaining optimal health. Providing cardiopulmonary-related health information (Box 40-6) is an important nursing responsibility.

Vaccinations. Annual flu vaccines are recommended for all people 6 months and older. Patients with chronic illnesses (heart, lung, kidney, or immunocompromised), infants, older adults, and pregnant women can get very sick; thus they should be immunized. Close contacts of infants under 6 months should also be

BOX 40-6 PATIENT TEACHING

Prevention of Respiratory Infections

Objective

- The patient will be able to verbalize the methods to reduce the risk factors for respiratory infection and the steps needed to adopt health promotion behaviors.

Teaching Strategies

- Establish rapport with the patient and maintain eye contact as long as it is culturally acceptable.
- Teach the importance of not smoking. Refer to smoking cessation programs and discuss appropriate medication to support smoking cessation from the primary health provider.
- If a patient does not smoke, teach the importance of avoiding secondhand smoke and areas of high air pollution.
- Inform patient about other risk factors for pulmonary disease such as diabetes, obesity, and lack of physical inactivity.
- Teach how to implement a balanced diet low in fat, sodium, and carbohydrates. Provide sample menus.
- Discuss the benefits of exercising 30 to 60 minutes a day and help patient develop an exercise program suited to lifestyle.
- Teach patient about the importance of getting annual influenza vaccines and the pneumovax vaccine. If younger than 65 at the time of the primary vaccination, a one-time revaccination is recommended within 5 years (CDC, 2011).
- Teach the importance of handwashing during flu and cold season.
- Inform patient of signs of respiratory infection that should be reported to health care provider such as increased coughing, shortness of breath, change of color of sputum, fever, and fatigue.

Evaluation

- Ask patient to verbalize what they learned about smoking cessation, secondhand smoke, diet and exercise.
- Ask patient to describe in simple terms the symptoms of respiratory infection and when to call the health care provider.
- Have patient tell you how he or she plans to prevent exposure to respiratory infections.
- Ask if patient has any other questions or need for additional information or referrals.

immunized. Anyone who had the 2009 H1N1 (pandemic) vaccine or who actually had the pandemic flu in 2009 should get the 2010-2011 vaccine because it provides protection against A/H1N1 and two other flu viruses. The vaccine is also recommended for people in close or frequent contact with anyone in the high-risk groups. It is effective in reducing the severity of illness and the risk of serious complications and death (CDC, 2010c).

Researchers do not fully understand the value of vaccination in immune-compromised patients. HIV-positive patients receive the flu vaccine; however, they often require a second vaccine to gain protection. People with a known hypersensitivity to eggs or other components of the vaccine should not be vaccinated. Adults with an acute febrile illness should schedule the vaccination after they have recovered. The vaccines are formulated annually based on worldwide surveillance data. The live, attenuated nasal spray vaccine is given to people from 2 through 49 years of age if they are not pregnant or do not have certain long-term health problems such as asthma; heart, lung or kidney disease; diabetes; or anemia. The inactivated flu shot should be given to these individuals and those 50 and older (CDC, 2010c).

Pneumococcal vaccine (PCV13) is routinely given to infants in a series of four doses and is recommended for patients at increased risk of developing pneumonia. This includes all adults over 65 years of age, those with chronic illnesses or who are immunocompromised (such as HIV/AIDS), any adult who smokes or has asthma, and those living in special environments such as nursing homes or long-term care facilities (CDC, 2010d, 2011).

Healthy Lifestyle. Identification and elimination of risk factors for cardiopulmonary disease are important parts of primary care. Encourage patients to eat a healthy low-fat, high-fiber diet; monitor their cholesterol, triglyceride, high-density lipoprotein (HDL), and low-density lipoprotein (LDL) levels; reduce stress; exercise; and maintain a body weight in proportion to their height. Eliminating cigarettes and other tobacco, reducing pollutants, monitoring air quality, and adequately hydrating are additional healthy behaviors. Encourage patients to examine their habits and make appropriate changes.

Exercise is a key factor in promoting and maintaining a healthy heart and lungs. Encourage patients to exercise at least 3 to 4 times a week for 30 to 60 minutes. Aerobic exercise is necessary to improve lung and heart function and strengthen muscles. Walking is an efficient way to achieve a good aerobic workout. Many shopping malls have programs allowing people to walk in the enclosed mall before the shops open. During the hot summer months teach patients to limit activities to early in the day or late in the evening, when temperatures are lower. Teach patients how to maintain adequate hydration and sodium intake, especially if they are taking diuretics.

Patients with cardiopulmonary alterations need to minimize their risk for infection, especially during the winter months. Teach them to avoid large, crowded places; keep their mouth and nose covered; and be sure to dress warmly, including a scarf, hat, and gloves. This is especially important during the peak of the flu season.

Patients with known cardiac disease and those with multiple risk factors are cautioned to avoid exertion in cold weather. Shoveling snow is especially risky and often precipitates a cardiac event. Other activities such as hanging holiday lights and decorations in the extreme cold can precipitate chest pain and bronchospasm.

Environmental Pollutants. Avoiding exposure to secondhand smoke is essential to maintaining optimal cardiopulmonary function. Most businesses and restaurants now ban smoking or have separate areas designated as smoking areas. If patients are exposed to secondhand smoke in their home environments, counseling and support for all family members are necessary to assist the smoker in successful smoking cessation or alterations in behavior patterns such as smoking outside.

Consider if a patient is exposed to chemicals and pollutants in the work environment. Farmers, painters, carpenters, and others benefit from the use of particulate filter masks to reduce the inhalation of particles.

Acute Care. Patients with acute pulmonary illnesses require nursing interventions directed toward halting the pathological process (e.g., respiratory tract infection); shortening the duration and severity of the illness (e.g., hospitalization with pneumonia); and preventing complications from the illness or treatments (e.g., hospital-acquired infection resulting from invasive procedures).

Dyspnea Management. Dyspnea is difficult to measure and treat. Health care providers will individualize treatments for each patient and usually implement more than one therapy. Treatment of the underlying process causing dyspnea is then followed with other therapies (e.g., pharmacological measures, oxygen therapy, physical techniques, and psychosocial techniques). Pharmacological agents include bronchodilators, inhaled steroids, mucolytics, and low-dose antianxiety medications. Oxygen therapy reduces dyspnea associated with exercise and hypoxemia. Physical techniques such as cardiopulmonary reconditioning (e.g., exercise, breathing techniques, and cough control), relaxation techniques, biofeedback, and meditation are also beneficial.

Airway Maintenance. The airway is patent when the trachea, bronchi, and large airways are free from obstructions. Airway maintenance requires adequate hydration to prevent thick, tenacious secretions. Proper coughing techniques remove secretions and keep the airway open. A variety of interventions such as suctioning, chest physiotherapy, and nebulizer therapy assist patients in managing alterations in airway clearance.

Mobilization of Pulmonary Secretions. The ability of a patient to mobilize pulmonary secretions makes the difference between a short-term illness and a long recovery involving complications. Nursing interventions promoting removal of pulmonary secretions assist in achieving and maintaining a clear airway and help to promote lung expansion and gas exchange.

Hydration. Maintenance of adequate systemic hydration keeps mucociliary clearance normal. In patients with adequate hydration, pulmonary secretions are thin, white, watery, and easily removable with minimal coughing. Excessive coughing to clear thick, tenacious secretions is fatiguing and energy depleting. The best way to maintain thin secretions is to provide a fluid intake of 1500 to 2500 mL/day unless contraindicated by cardiac or renal status. The color, consistency, and ease of mucus expectoration determine adequacy of hydration.

Humidification. **Humidification** is the process of adding water to gas. Temperature is the most important factor affecting the amount of water vapor a gas can hold. Relative humidity is the percentage of water in the gas. Air or oxygen with a high relative humidity keeps the airways moist and loosens and mobilizes pulmonary secretions. Humidification is necessary for patients receiving oxygen therapy at greater than 4 L/min (check agency protocol). It might be necessary to add humidification at lower oxygen concentrations if the environment is dry and arid. Bubbling oxygen through water adds humidity to the oxygen delivered to the upper airways (see Skill 40-4).

An oxygen hood is used for infants, and a humidity tent is used for children with illnesses such as croup and tracheitis to liquefy secretions and help reduce fever (Hockenberry and Wilson, 2011). The nebulizer at the top of the humidity tent remains filled with water to prevent nonhumidified air or oxygen from entering the tent. Air in the humidity tent sometimes becomes cool and falls below 20° C (68° F), causing the child to become chilled. Children in humidity tents require frequent changes of clothing and bed linen to remain warm and dry.

Nebulization. **Nebulization** adds moisture or medications to inspired air by mixing particles of varying sizes with the air. Aerosolization suspends the maximum number of water drops or particles of the desired size in inspired air. The moisture added through nebulization improves clearance of pulmonary secretions. Nebulization is used for administration of bronchodilators and mucolytic agents.

When the thin layer of fluid supporting the mucous layer over the cilia dries, the cilia are damaged and unable to adequately clear the airway. Humidification through nebulization enhances mucociliary clearance, the natural mechanism of the body for removing mucus and cellular debris from the respiratory tract.

Coughing and Deep-Breathing Techniques. Coughing is effective for maintaining a patent airway. Directed coughing is a deliberate maneuver that is effective when spontaneous coughing is not adequate (AARC, 1993). Directed coughing permits a patient to remove secretions from both the upper and lower airways. The normal series of events in the cough mechanism are deep inhalation, closure of the glottis, active contraction of the expiratory muscles, and glottis opening. Deep inhalation increases the lung volume and airway diameter, allowing the air to pass through partially obstructing mucus plugs or other foreign matter. Contraction of the expiratory muscles against the closed glottis causes a high intrathoracic pressure to develop. When the glottis opens, a large flow of air is expelled at a high speed, providing momentum for mucus to move to the upper airways where the patient can expectorate or swallow it.

Diaphragmatic breathing/belly breathing is a technique that encourages deep breathing to increase air to the lower lungs. The belly moves out when breathing in and sinks in when breathing out (CFF, 2005). Deep breathing also opens the pores of Kohn between alveoli to allow sharing of oxygen between alveoli. This is especially important if the airway of the alveoli is plugged with mucus. The neighboring alveoli can share the air distribution through the pores of Kohn (McCance and Huether, 2010).

Evaluate the effectiveness of coughing by sputum expectoration, the patient's report of swallowed sputum, or clearing of adventitious sounds by auscultation. Encourage patients with chronic pulmonary diseases, upper respiratory tract infections, and lower respiratory tract infections to deep breathe and cough at least every 2 hours while awake. Encourage patients with a large amount of sputum to cough every hour while awake and then awaken them at night in order to cough every 2 to 3 hours. This is necessary until the acute phase of mucus production has ended. After surgery it is recommended that directed cough be performed every 2 to 4 hours while awake to prevent accumulation of secretions. Offer postoperative patients support devices (folded blanket, pillow, or palmed hands) to splint an abdominal or thoracic incision to minimize pain during directed coughing. Cough is a source of droplet transmission of pulmonary pathogens; thus the health care provider should follow Standard Precautions. Coughing techniques include deep breathing and coughing for the postoperative patient, cascade, huff, and quad coughing (AARC, 1993).

With the *cascade cough* the patient takes a slow, deep breath and holds it for 2 seconds while contracting expiratory muscles. Then he or she opens the mouth and performs a series of coughs throughout exhalation, thereby coughing at progressively lowered lung volumes. This technique promotes airway clearance and a patent airway in patients with large volumes of sputum.

The *huff cough* stimulates a natural cough reflex and is generally effective only for clearing central airways. While exhaling, the patient opens the glottis by saying the word *huff.* With practice he or she inhales more air and is able to progress to the cascade cough.

The *quad cough* technique is for patients without abdominal muscle control such as those with spinal cord injuries. While the patient breathes out with a maximal expiratory effort, the patient or nurse pushes inward and upward on the abdominal muscles toward the diaphragm, causing the cough.

Chest Physiotherapy. **Chest physiotherapy (CPT)** is a group of therapies for mobilizing pulmonary secretions. These therapies include postural drainage, chest percussion, and vibration. CPT is followed by productive coughing or suctioning of a patient who has a decreased ability to cough. It is recommended for patients who produce greater than 30 mL of sputum per day or have evidence of atelectasis on chest x-ray examination. The procedure is safe for infants and young children; however, at times conditions and diseases unique to children contraindicate it. CPT is for a select group of patients. Box 40-7 describes the guidelines to determine if CPT is indicated.

Postural drainage is a component of pulmonary hygiene; it consists of drainage, positioning, and turning and is sometimes accompanied by chest percussion and vibration (CFF, 2005). It improves secretion clearance and oxygenation. Positioning includes most lung segments (Table 40-6) and helps to drain secretions from specific segments of the lungs and bronchi into the trachea. Some patients do not require postural drainage of all lung segments, and clinical assessment is crucial in identifying specific lung segments requiring it. For example, patients with left lower lobe atelectasis require postural drainage of only the affected region, whereas a child with cystic fibrosis often requires postural drainage of all lung segments.

Chest percussion involves rhythmically clapping on the chest wall over the area being drained to force secretions into larger airways for expectoration. Position the hand so the fingers and thumb touch and the hands are cupped. The cupping makes the hand conform to the chest wall while trapping a cushion of air to soften the intensity of the clapping. The procedure should produce a hollow sound and should not be painful (CFF, 2005). Perform chest percussion by vigorously striking the chest wall alternately with cupped hands (Fig. 40-9). Perform percussion over a single layer of clothing, not over buttons, snaps, or zippers. The single layer of clothing prevents slapping the patient's skin. Thicker or multiple layers of material dampen the vibrations.

Percussion is contraindicated in patients with bleeding disorders, osteoporosis, or fractured ribs. Avoid percussion over burns,

BOX 40-7 GUIDELINES FOR CHEST PHYSIOTHERAPY

Nursing and respiratory therapy collaborate with the health care provider to determine if chest physiotherapy (CPT) is best for the patient. The following guidelines help in physical assessment and subsequent decision making:

- Know a patient's normal range of vital signs. Conditions requiring CPT such as atelectasis and pneumonia affect vital signs. The degree of change is related to the level of hypoxia, overall cardiopulmonary status, and tolerance to activity.
- Conduct a respiratory assessment to confirm need for CPT, including sputum production, effectiveness of cough, history of pulmonary problems successfully relieved with CPT, abnormal lung sounds, documented conditions such as atelectasis, pneumonia, and changes in oxygenation status.
- Know the patient's medications. Certain medications, particularly diuretics and antihypertensives, cause fluid and hemodynamic changes. These decrease a patient's tolerance to positional changes and postural drainage. Long-term steroid use increases a patient's risk of pathological rib fractures and often contraindicates vibration.
- Know the patient's medical history. Certain conditions such as increased intracranial pressure, spinal cord injuries, and abdominal aneurysm resection contraindicate the positional changes of postural drainage. Thoracic trauma or surgery contraindicates percussion and vibration.
- Know the patient's level of cognitive function. Participation in controlled coughing techniques requires him or her to follow instructions. Congenital or acquired cognitive limitations alter a patient's ability to learn and participate in these techniques.
- Be aware of the patient's exercise tolerance. CPT maneuvers are fatiguing. When a patient is not used to physical activity, initial tolerance to the maneuvers is often decreased. However, with gradual increases in activity and planned CPT, patient tolerance for the procedure improves.

TABLE 40-6 Positions for Postural Drainage

LUNG SEGMENT	POSITION OF PATIENT	LUNG SEGMENT	POSITION OF PATIENT
Adult			
Bilateral 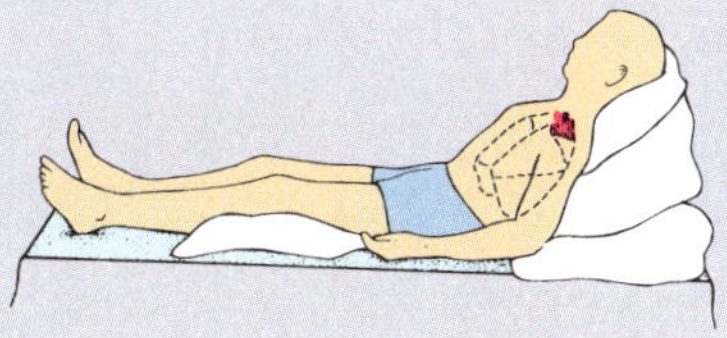	High-Fowler's	Left lower lobe—lateral segment 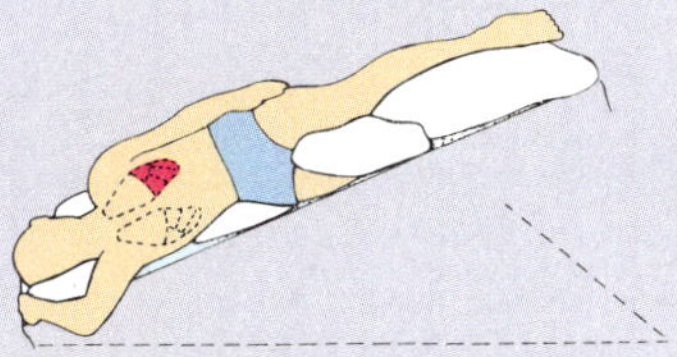	Right side-lying in Trendelenburg's position
Apical segments	Sitting on side of bed	Right lower lobe—lateral segment 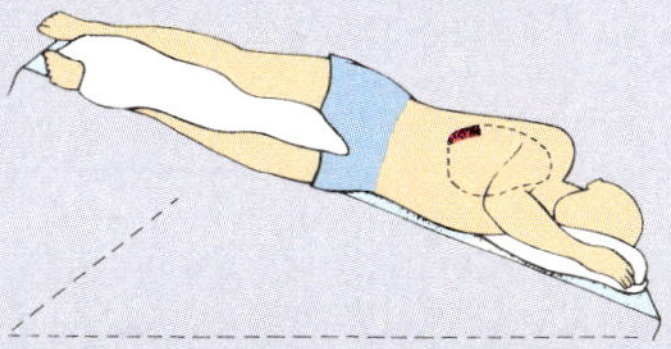	Left side-lying in Trendelenburg's position
Right upper lobe—anterior segment 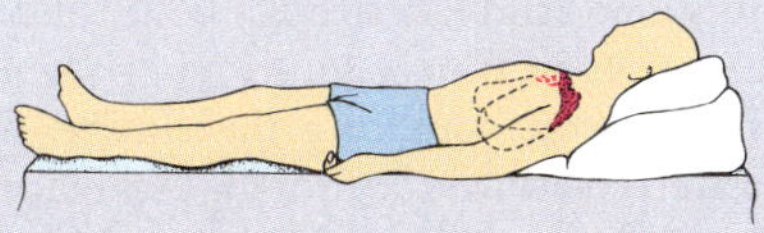	Supine with head elevated	Right lower lobe—posterior segment 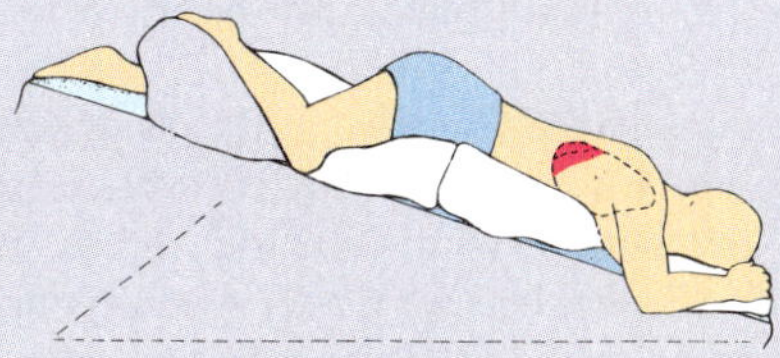	Prone with right side of chest elevated in Trendelenburg's position

Continued

TABLE 40-6 Positions for Postural Drainage—cont'd

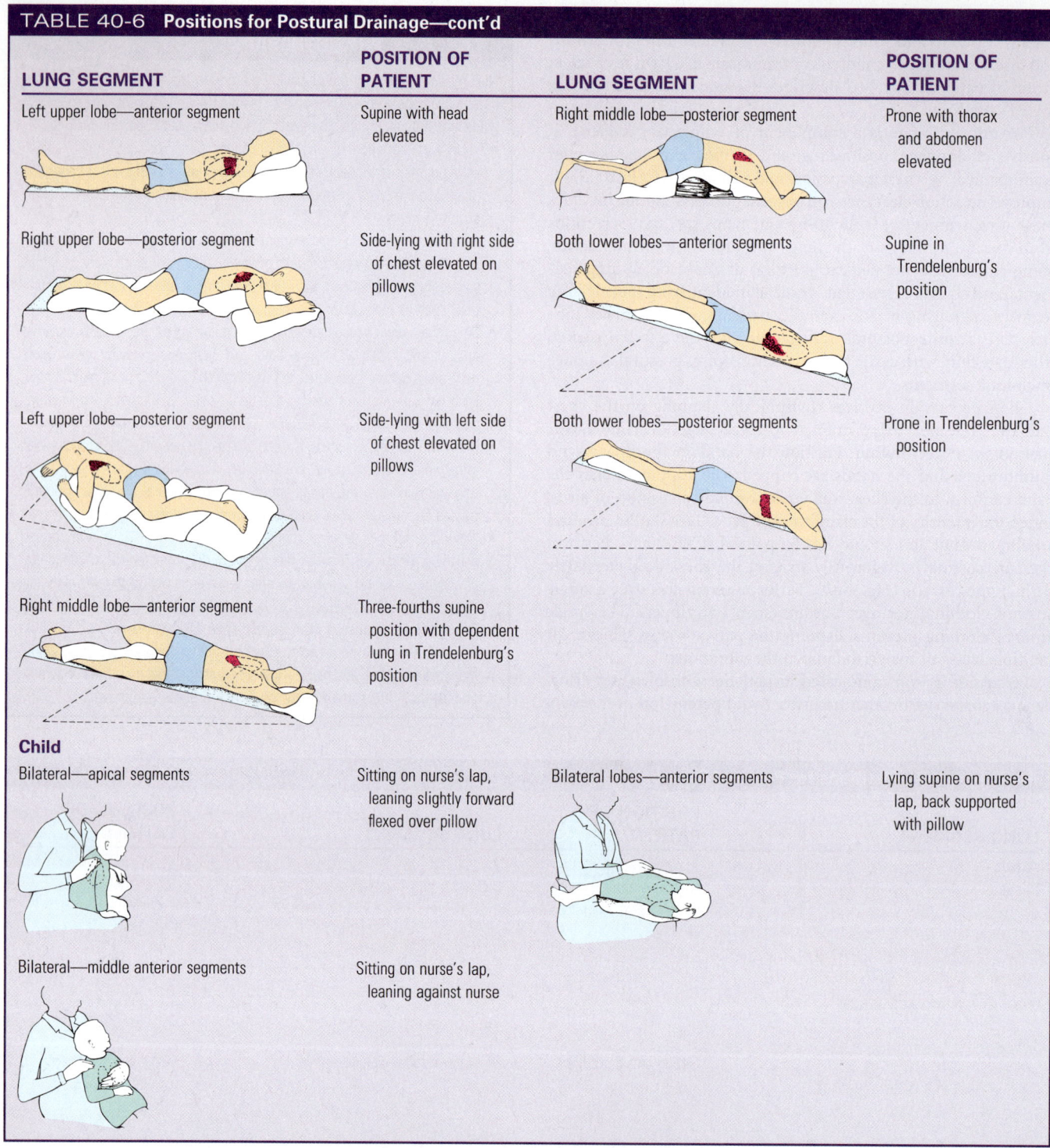

LUNG SEGMENT	POSITION OF PATIENT	LUNG SEGMENT	POSITION OF PATIENT
Left upper lobe—anterior segment 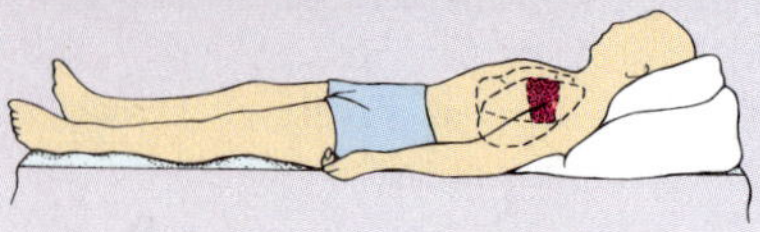	Supine with head elevated	Right middle lobe—posterior segment 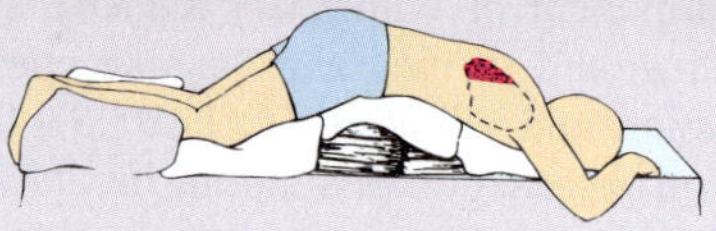	Prone with thorax and abdomen elevated
Right upper lobe—posterior segment 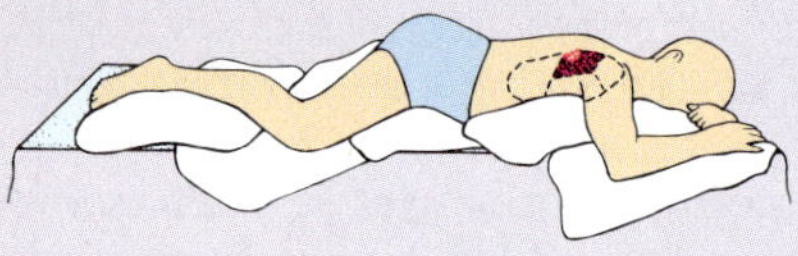	Side-lying with right side of chest elevated on pillows	Both lower lobes—anterior segments 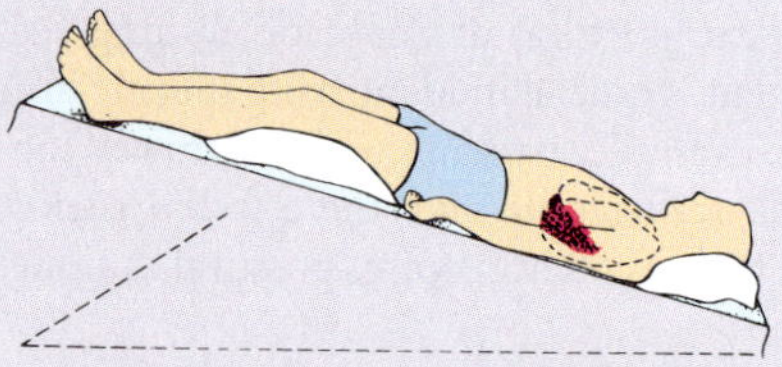	Supine in Trendelenburg's position
Left upper lobe—posterior segment 	Side-lying with left side of chest elevated on pillows	Both lower lobes—posterior segments 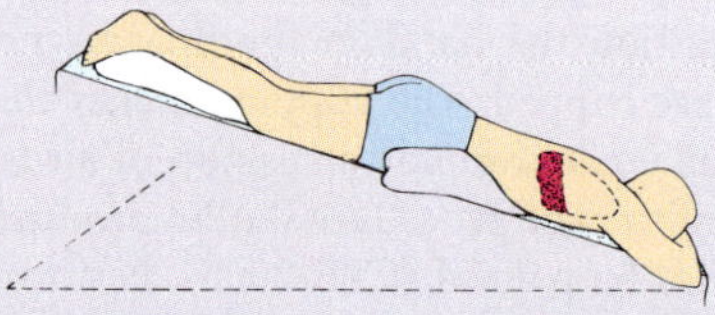	Prone in Trendelenburg's position
Right middle lobe—anterior segment 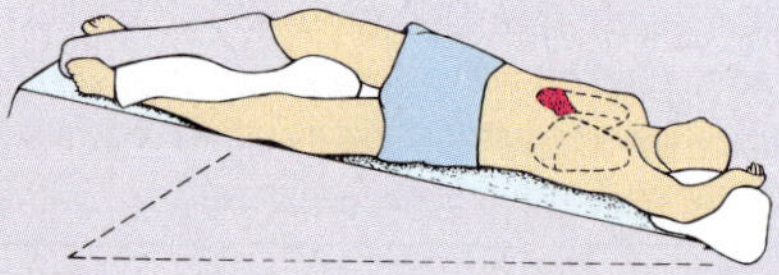	Three-fourths supine position with dependent lung in Trendelenburg's position		
Child			
Bilateral—apical segments 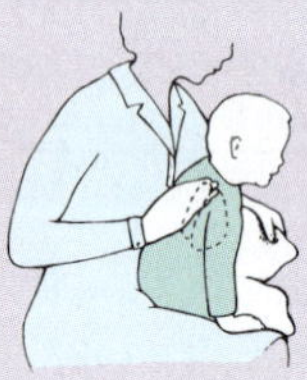	Sitting on nurse's lap, leaning slightly forward flexed over pillow	Bilateral lobes—anterior segments 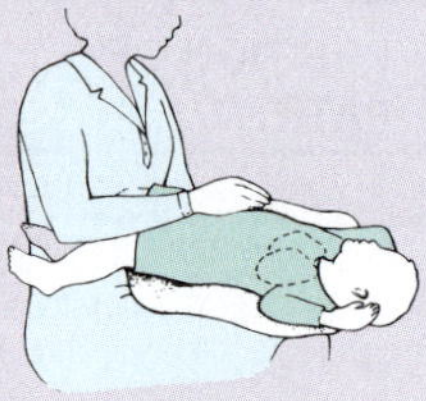	Lying supine on nurse's lap, back supported with pillow
Bilateral—middle anterior segments 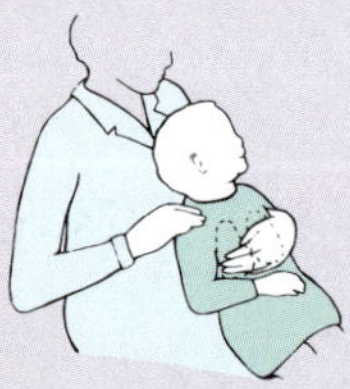	Sitting on nurse's lap, leaning against nurse		

open wounds, or skin infections of the thorax. Take caution to percuss the lung fields under the ribs and not the over the spine, breastbone, stomach or lower back or trauma can occur to the spleen, liver, or kidneys (CFF, 2005).

Vibration is a gentle, shaking pressure applied to the chest wall to shake secretions into larger airways. Place a flattened hand or two hands (pressing top and bottom hand into each other to vibrate) firmly on the chest wall over the appropriate segment and tense the muscles of the arm to provide a shaking motion. Have the patient exhale as slowly as possible during the vibration. This technique increases the velocity and turbulence of exhaled air, facilitating secretion removal. Vibration increases the exhalation of trapped air, shakes mucus loose, and induces a cough (CFF, 2005).

Suctioning Techniques. Suctioning is necessary when patients are unable to clear respiratory secretions from the airways by coughing or other less invasive procedures. Suctioning techniques include oropharyngeal and nasopharyngeal suctioning, orotracheal and nasotracheal suctioning, and suctioning an artificial airway.

In most cases use sterile technique for suctioning because the oropharynx and trachea are considered sterile. The mouth is

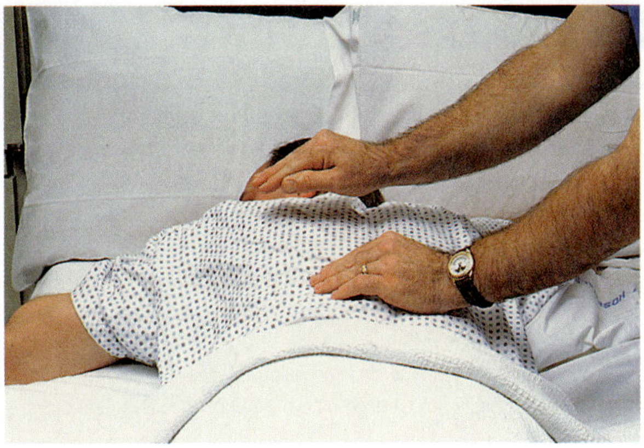

FIG. 40-9 Chest wall percussion, alternating hand clapping against patient's chest wall.

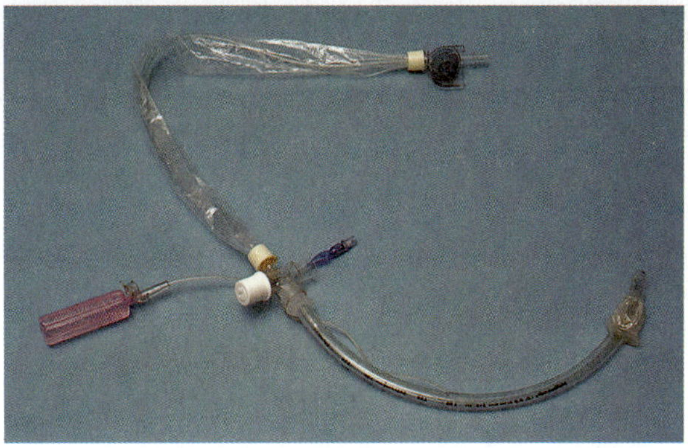

FIG. 40-10 Ballard tracheal care, closed suction catheter.

considered clean; therefore you suction oral secretions after suctioning the oropharynx and trachea. In the home setting a "clean" versus "sterile" technique is used because the patient is not exposed to pathogens common to health care settings; however, appropriate measures for disinfecting equipment should be taught (AARC, 2004).

Each type of suctioning requires the use of a round-tipped, flexible catheter with holes on the sides and end of the catheter. When suctioning, you apply negative pressures (not greater than 150 mm Hg) during withdrawal of the catheter, never on insertion. Patient assessment determines the frequency of suctioning. It is indicated when audible on auscultation (rhonchi, gurgling breath sounds, diminished breath sounds) or visible secretions are present after other methods to remove airway secretions have failed. You may also use suctioning to obtain a sputum specimen for culture or cytology if the patient is not able to cough productively. Too-frequent suctioning puts patients at risk for development of hypoxemia, hypotension, arrhythmias, and possible trauma to the mucosa of the lungs (AARC, 2004).

Oropharyngeal and Nasopharyngeal Suctioning. Oropharyngeal or nasopharyngeal suctioning is used when the patient is able to cough effectively but unable to clear secretions by expectorating. Apply suction after a patient has coughed (Skill 40-1 on pp. 855-861). Once the pulmonary secretions decrease and a patient is less fatigued, he or she is then able to expectorate or swallow the mucus, and suctioning is no longer necessary.

Orotracheal and Nasotracheal Suctioning. Orotracheal or nasotracheal suctioning is necessary when a patient with pulmonary secretions is unable to manage secretions by coughing and does not have an artificial airway present (see Skill 40-1). You pass a sterile catheter through the mouth or nose into the trachea. The nose is the preferred route because stimulation of the gag reflex is minimal. The procedure is similar to nasopharyngeal suctioning, but you advance the catheter tip farther into the patient's trachea. The entire procedure from catheter passage to its removal is done quickly, lasting no longer than 15 seconds (AARC, 2004). Unless in respiratory distress, allow the patient to rest between passes of the catheter. If the patient is using supplemental oxygen, replace the oxygen cannula or mask during rest periods.

Tracheal Suctioning. You perform tracheal suctioning through an artificial airway such as an endotracheal (ET) or tracheostomy tube. The size of a catheter should be as small as possible but large enough to remove secretions. Recommendation is about half the internal diameter of the ET tube (Pedersen et al., 2009). Never apply suction pressure while inserting the catheter to avoid traumatizing the lung mucosa. Once you insert a catheter the necessary distance, maintain suction pressure between 120 and 150 mm Hg (AARC, 2004) as you withdraw. Apply suction intermittently ***only*** while withdrawing the catheter. Rotating the catheter enhances removal of secretions that have adhered to the sides of the ET tube.

The practice of normal saline instillation (NSI) into artificial airways to improve secretion removal is inconclusive. Clinical studies comparing the results of suctioning following NSI with standard suctioning have not shown any clinical or significant results (Box 40-8). There are anecdotal results supporting the theory that NSI stimulates patients to cough and as a result the airway secretions are loosened and dislodged. However, the practice of NSI has the potential of causing detrimental effects such as increased heart rate and blood pressure and an increased risk of respiratory infection (Kuriakose, 2008).

The two current methods of suctioning are the open and closed methods. Open suctioning involves using a new sterile catheter for each suction session (Pedersen et al., 2009). Wear sterile gloves and follow Standard Precautions during the suction procedure. Closed suctioning involves using a reusable sterile suction catheter that is encased in a plastic sheath to protect it between suction sessions (Fig. 40-10). Closed suctioning is most often used on patients who require mechanical ventilation to support their respiratory efforts because it permits continuous delivery of oxygen while suction is performed and reduces the risk of oxygen desaturation. Although sterile gloves are not used in this procedure, nonsterile gloves are recommended to prevent contact with splashes from body fluids (Box 40-9).

Artificial Airways. An artificial airway is for a patient with a decreased level of consciousness or airway obstruction and aids in removal of tracheobronchial secretions. The presence of an artificial airway places a patient at high risk for infection and airway injury. Use clean technique for oral airways, but use sterile technique in caring for and maintaining endotracheal and tracheal airways to prevent health care–associated infections (HAIs). Artificial airways need to stay in the correct position to prevent airway damage (Skill 40-2 on pp. 861-869).

Oral Airway. The oral airway, the simplest type of artificial airway, prevents obstruction of the trachea by displacement of the tongue into the oropharynx (Fig. 40-11). The oral airway extends from the teeth to the oropharynx, maintaining the tongue in the normal position. Use the correct-size airway. Determine the proper oral airway size by measuring the distance from the corner of the mouth to the angle of the jaw just below the ear. The length is equal

BOX 40-8 EVIDENCE-BASED PRACTICE

The Effectiveness of Instilling Normal Saline into Artificial Airways Before Suctioning

PICO Question: In patients with artificial airways, does instilling normal saline into artificial airways before suctioning increase the output of mucus?

Evidence Summary

The practice of instilling normal saline before suctioning artificial airways to dilute and loosen secretions has been questioned by researchers. Several meta-analysis studies report more harmful effects from normal saline instillation than benefits. One of the complications found was significant decreased oxygenation saturation in patients receiving normal saline instillation compared to patients who did not. The saline group actually took 5 minutes to return to baseline SaO_2 after suctioning (Halm and Krisko-Hagel, 2008; Kuriakose, 2008; Rauen et al., 2008).

Another complication reported was increased dyspnea in people over 60 years if they had saline instilled (Kuriakose, 2008; Pedersen et al., 2009). Along with dyspnea, patients reported anxiety, dread, and increased pain when saline was used (Halm and Krisko-Hagel, 2008).

Increased colonization of the lower respiratory tract after 48 hours was found to be five times higher in patients receiving saline. It was thought that the saline actually dislodged colonies and dispersed them to the lower airways (Halm and Krisko-Hagel, 2008; Kuriakose, 2008).

Studies looking at the amount of sputum yield after suctioning following saline instillation showed that the amount obtained was not clinically important. It was even found that the saline was rapidly absorbed and did not really mix with the secretions (Halm and Krisko-Hagel, 2008). The problem with the yield studies was how to quantify the amount removed (Rauen et al., 2008).

The evidence of adverse effects of instilling saline both physically and psychologically supports not using saline instillation before suctioning. However, change in practice is a challenge since surveys have found that 2 to 3 times as many respiratory therapists report that they continue to use saline before suctioning compared to nurses (Halm and Krisko-Hagel, 2008; Rauen et al., 2008). However, surveys of nursing practice report that 24% to 33% of nurses still use saline (Rauen et al., 2008). What may help change practice is the American Association of Respiratory Care guideline for endotracheal suctioning of mechanically ventilated patients with artificial airways (2010a), which states that normal saline should not be used before suctioning on a routine basis.

Application to Nursing Practice

- Normal saline and mucus do not appear to mix so it does not thin or mobilize secretions. It would be better to increase humidification by improving systemic hydration either orally or by intravenous infusion.
- Use humidification with oxygen and refer to respiratory therapy for appropriate nebulizer treatments to disperse the humidification more uniformly.
- Increase ambulation and mobility even in intensive care units to help mobilize secretions.
- Use chest physiotherapy to help mobilize secretions.
- Use positioning such as "good lung down" to facilitate oxygenation and elevation of head of bed to at least 45 degrees. Turn critically ill patients more frequently than every 2 hours.

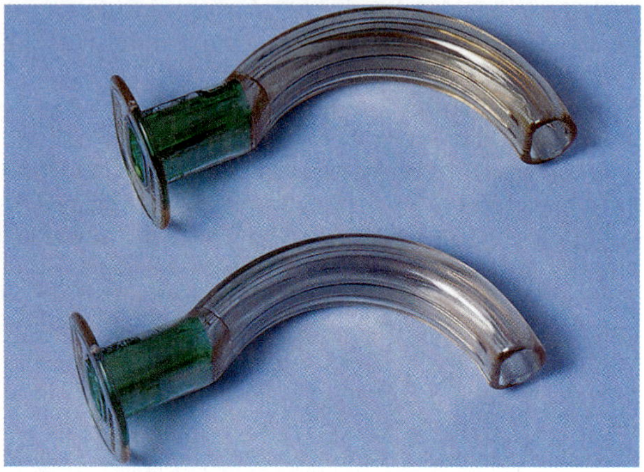

FIG. 40-11 Artificial oral airways.

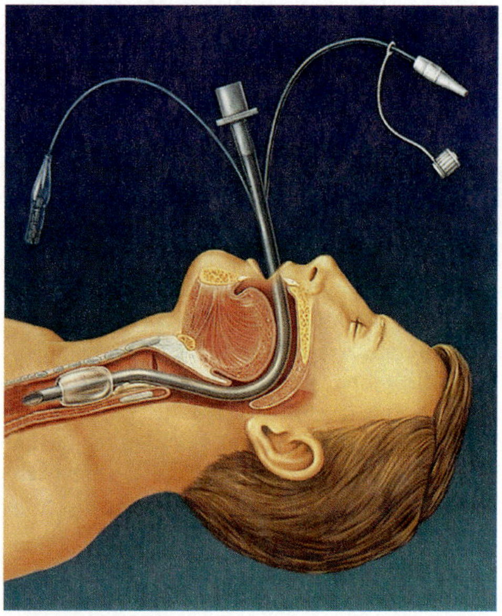

FIG. 40-12 Endotracheal tube inserted into trachea. Cuff inflated to maintain position. (From Nellcor Puritan Bennett: *Hi-Lo Evac endotracheal tube with evacuation lumen,* http://www.nellcor.com/_Catalog/PDF/Product/Hi-LoEvac.pdf. Accessed August 2, 2011).

to the distance from the flange of the airway to the tip. If the airway is too small, the tongue does not stay in the anterior portion of the mouth; if the airway is too large, it forces the tongue toward the epiglottis and obstructs the airway.

Insert the airway by turning the curve of the airway toward the cheek and placing it over the tongue. When the airway is in the oropharynx, turn it so the opening points downward. Correctly placed, the airway moves the tongue forward away from the oropharynx, and the flange (i.e., the flat portion of the airway) rests against the patient's teeth. Incorrect insertion merely forces the tongue back into the oropharynx.

Endotracheal and Tracheal Airway. An **endotracheal (ET) tube** is a short-term artificial airway to administer mechanical ventilation, relieve upper airway obstruction, protect against aspiration, or clear secretions. A physician or specially trained clinician inserts the ET tube. The tube is passed through the patient's mouth, past the pharynx, and into the trachea (Fig. 40-12). It is generally removed within 14 days; however, it is sometimes used for a longer period of time if the patient is still showing progress toward weaning from mechanical ventilation and extubation.

BOX 40-9 PROCEDURAL GUIDELINES

Closed (In-Line) Suction Catheter

Delegation Considerations

Airway suctioning with a closed (in-line) suction catheter cannot be routinely delegated to nursing assistive personnel (NAP). This procedure may be delegated when suctioning a patient with a permanent tracheostomy is necessary (follow agency policy). The nurse is responsible for the patient's cardiopulmonary assessment and evaluation. The nurse informs the NAP about:

- Any individualized aspects of patient care that pertain to suctioning (e.g., position, duration of suction, pressure settings).
- The expected quality, quantity, and color of secretions and to immediately report any changes to the nurse.
- Patient's anticipated response to suction and to immediately report to the nurse changes in vital signs, complaints of pain, changes in respiratory status, mental status, or increased restlessness

Equipment

Closed system or in-line suction catheter; suction machine, 6 feet of connecting tubing, clean gloves (optional), face shield, goggles (optional) or mask (optional), saline vial or syringe (for rinsing tubing), clean towel, pulse oximeter and stethoscope

1. Identify the patient using two identifiers (e.g., name and birth date or name and account number) according to facility policy. Compare identifiers with information on the patient's medical record.
2. Perform assessment as in Skill 40-1.
3. Explain the procedure to patient and the importance of coughing during the suctioning procedure.
4. Assist patient with assuming a position of comfort usually semi-or high-Fowler's position. Place towel across patient's chest.
5. Perform hand hygiene, apply face shield and clean gloves, and attach suction. NOTE: If risk for splash is present or patient is on respiratory precautions, mask and goggles may be needed.
   a. In some settings a respiratory therapist attaches the catheter to the closed ventilator circuit. If catheter is not already in place, open closed-suction catheter package using aseptic technique, attach catheter to ventilator circuit by removing swivel adapter, and place catheter apparatus on endotracheal or tracheostomy tube. Connect Y on mechanical ventilator circuit to closed-suction catheter with flex tubing (see Fig. 40-10).
   b. Connect one end of connecting tubing to suction machine and the other to the end of a closed system or in-line suction catheter, if not already done. Turn suction device on and set vacuum regulator to appropriate negative pressure (see manufacturer directions). Many closed-system suction catheters require slightly higher suction; consult manufacturer guidelines.
6. Hyperinflate and/or hyperoxygenate patient with bag-valve mask or manual breathing mechanism on mechanical ventilator according to institution protocol and clinical status (usually 100% oxygen).
7. Unlock suction-control mechanism if required by manufacturer. Open saline port and attach saline syringe or vial.
8. Pick up suction catheter enclosed in plastic sleeve with dominant hand.

   CLINICAL DECISION: The instillation of normal saline into the airway before closed in-line suctioning may not be appropriate for all patients and needs further investigation. Normal saline instillation in conjunction with artificial airway suctioning may lead to the dispersion of microorganisms into the lower respiratory tract (Kuriakose, 2008).

9. Insert catheter; use a repeating maneuver of pushing catheter and sliding (or pulling) plastic sleeve back between thumb and forefinger until you feel resistance or patient coughs.
10. Encourage patient to cough and apply suction by squeezing on suction-control mechanism while withdrawing catheter. It is difficult to apply intermittent pulses of suction and nearly impossible to rotate the catheter compared with a standard catheter. Be sure to withdraw catheter completely into plastic sheath so it does not obstruct airflow (AARC, 2004).
11. Reassess cardiopulmonary status, including pulse oximetry, to determine need for subsequent suctioning or complications. Repeat Steps 5 through 9 one to two more times to clear secretions. Allow adequate time (at least 1 full minute) between suction passes for ventilation and reoxygenation (AARC, 2004).
12. When airway is clear, withdraw catheter completely into sheath. Be sure that colored indicator line on catheter is visible in the sheath. Squeeze vial or push syringe while applying suction to rinse the inner lumen of catheter. Use at least 5 to 10 mL of saline to rinse the catheter until it is clear of retained secretions, which cause bacterial growth and increase the risk of infection (AARC, 2004). Lock suction mechanism, if applicable, and turn off suction.
13. If patient requires oral or nasal suctioning, perform Skill 40-1 with separate standard suction catheter.
14. Reposition patient.
15. Remove gloves and face shield, discard into appropriate receptacle, and perform hand hygiene.
16. Compare patient's respiratory assessment with evaluation findings after suctioning and observe airway secretions.

If a patient requires long-term assistance from an artificial airway, a **tracheostomy** is considered. A surgical incision is made into the trachea, and a short artificial airway (a tracheostomy tube) is inserted. Most tracheostomies have a small plastic inner tube that fits inside a larger one (the inner cannula). The most common complication of a tracheostomy tube is partial or total airway obstruction caused by buildup of respiratory secretions. If this occurs, the inner tube can be removed and cleaned or replaced with a temporary spare inner tube that should be kept at the patient's bedside. Keep tracheal dilators at the bedside to have available for emergency tube replacement or reinsertion. Humidification from air humidifiers or humidified oxygen tracheostomy collars can help prevent drying of secretions that cause occlusion. Tracheostomy suctioning should be done as often as necessary to clear secretions. The majority of patients with a tracheostomy tube cannot speak because the tube is inserted below the vocal cords. It is important to use written or nonverbal communication (lip reading) strategies to help patients communicate. Be sure to assess patients for anxiety caused by the inability to speak (Higgins, 2009). Care and cleaning of the tracheostomy tube is discussed in Skill 40-2.

Maintenance and Promotion of Lung Expansion. Nursing interventions to maintain or promote lung expansion include noninvasive techniques such as ambulation, positioning, incentive spirometry, and noninvasive ventilation. Invasive medical interventions such as chest tube insertion and management assist in restoring lung expansion.

Ambulation. Immobility is a major factor in developing atelectasis, ventilator-associated pneumonia (VAP), and functional limitations. The research has shown that, after 1 week of bed rest, muscle strength declines by as much as 20%, which results in an increased oxygen demand, weakened respiratory muscles, and a decline of functional status. Early ambulation studies indicate that the therapeutic benefits of activity include an increase in general strength and lung expansion. Even the patient who requires mechanical ventilation benefits by an early mobility program. Such mobility programs should include input from both respiratory and physical therapists in the treatment plan (Perme and Chandrashekar, 2009). Progressive mobilization from dangling the legs to standing and then walking is safe for intubated patients (Rauen et al., 2008).

Positioning. The healthy, completely mobile person maintains adequate ventilation and oxygenation by frequent position changes during daily activities. However, when a person's illness or injury restricts mobility, the risk for respiratory impairment is increased. Frequent changes of position are simple and cost-effective methods for reducing stasis of pulmonary secretions and decreased chest wall expansion, both of which increase the risk of pneumonia. Research has shown that turning critically ill patients every 2 hours is not often enough to prevent pneumonia (Rauen et al., 2008).

The 45-degree semi-Fowler's is the most effective position to promote lung expansion and reduce pressure from the abdomen on the diaphragm. When a patient is in this position, be sure that he or she does not slide down in bed, which can reduce lung expansion. A patient with unilateral lung disease such as pneumothorax, atelectasis, pneumonia, thoracotomy, and trauma of one lung should be positioned in a manner to promote perfusion of the healthy lung and improve oxygenation. In most cases, position the patient with the good lung down (Rauen et al., 2008). In the presence of pulmonary abscess or hemorrhage, position the patient with the affected lung down to prevent drainage toward the healthy lung. For bilateral lung disease the best position depends on the severity of the disease.

Incentive Spirometry. **Incentive spirometry** encourages voluntary deep breathing by providing visual feedback to patients about inspiratory volume. It promotes deep breathing and prevents or treats atelectasis in the postoperative patient. There is solid evidence to support the use of lung expansion with incentive spirometry in preventing postoperative pulmonary complications following abdominal surgery (Lawrence et al., 2006).

Flow-oriented incentive spirometers consist of one or more plastic chambers that contain freely moving colored balls. A patient inhales slowly and with an even flow to elevate the balls and keep them floating as long as possible to ensure a maximally sustained inhalation.

Volume-oriented incentive spirometry devices have a bellows that is raised to a predetermined volume by an inhaled breath (Fig. 40-13). An achievement light or counter is used to provide feedback. Some devices are constructed so the light does not turn on unless the bellows is held at a minimum desired volume for a specified period to enhance lung expansion (see Chapter 50).

Incentive spirometry encourages patients to use visual feedback to maximally inflate their lungs and sustain that inflation (Basoglu et al., 2005). A postoperative inspiratory capacity one half to three fourths of the preoperative volume is acceptable because of postoperative pain. The AARC guidelines (2011) recommend 5 to 10 breaths per session every hour while awake. Administration of pain medications before incentive spirometry helps a patient achieve deep breathing by reducing pain and splinting.

Noninvasive Ventilation. **Noninvasive positive-pressure ventilation (NPPV)** is used to prevent using invasive artificial airways (ET tube or tracheostomy) in patients with acute respiratory failure, cardiogenic pulmonary edema, or exacerbation of COPD. It has also been used following extubation of an ET tube (Agarwal et al., 2007). The purpose of NPPV is to maintain a positive airway pressure and improve alveolar ventilation. This prevents or treats atelectasis by inflating the alveoli, reducing pulmonary edema by forcing fluid out of the lungs back into circulation, and improving oxygenation in those with sleep apnea. Ventilatory support is achieved using a variety of modes, including **continuous positive airway pressure (CPAP)** and **bilevel positive airway pressure (BiPAP).**

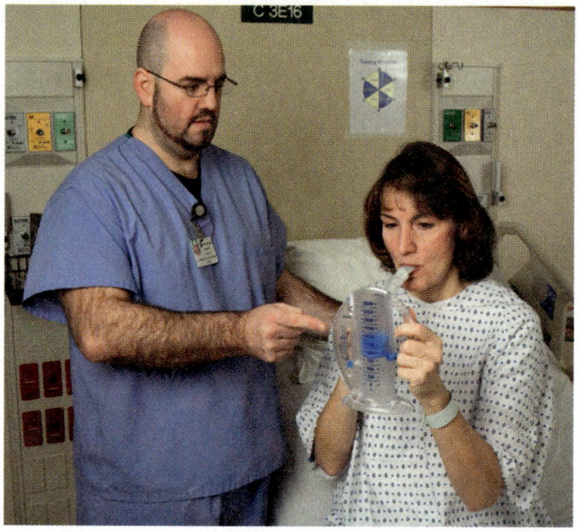

FIG. 40-13 Volume-oriented incentive spirometer.

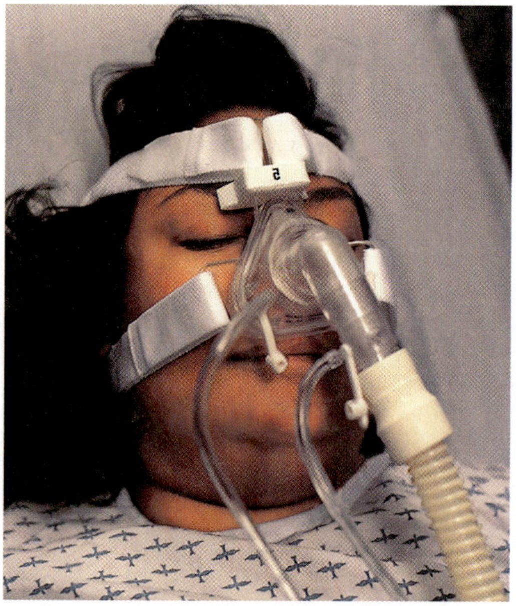

FIG. 40-14 CPAP mask.

CPAP treats patients with obstructive sleep apnea, patients with heart failure, and preterm infants with underdeveloped lungs. In obstructive sleep apnea, airways collapse, causing shallow or absent breathing. Any air moving past the obstruction results in loud snoring. An overnight sleep study may be needed to determine the correct settings for a CPAP machine (see Chapter 42). Equipment includes a mask (Fig. 40-14) that fits over the nose or both nose and mouth and a CPAP machine that delivers air to the mask (National Heart Lung and Blood Institute, 2010). The smallest mask with the proper fit is the most effective. Because straps hold the mask in place, it is important to assess for excess pressure on the patient's face or nose that could cause skin breakdown or necrosis. The mask should have enough slack to allow one to two fingers between the straps and the face (Soo Hoo, 2010). However, it must also be tight enough to form a tight seal on the face so the air does not escape. With higher pressures escape of some air may be avoidable.

The most common mode of support is BiPAP that provides both inspiratory positive airway pressure (IPAP) and expiratory airway pressure (EPAP), also known as *positive end-expiratory pressure (PEEP)*. The difference between these two pressures indicates the amount of pressure support a patient needs (Soo Hoo, 2010). During inhalation the positive pressure increases the patient's tidal volume and alveolar ventilation. The pressure support decreases when the patient exhales, allowing for easier exhalation.

Complications of noninvasive ventilation include facial and nasal injury and skin breakdown, dry mucous membranes and thick secretions, and aspiration of gastric contents if vomiting occurs during ventilation. Complications avoided by noninvasive ventilation are VAP, sinusitis, and effects of large-dose sedative agents. Use of noninvasive ventilation results in shorter intensive care unit (ICU) and hospital stays (Soo Hoo, 2010). Perform good oral hygiene every few hours while a patient is on BiPAP to relieve dryness.

Chest Tubes. A **chest tube** (Fig. 40-15) is a catheter inserted through the thorax to remove air and fluids from the pleural space, to prevent air or fluid from reentering the pleural space, or to reestablish normal intrapleural and intrapulmonic pressures (Roman and Mercado, 2006). Chest tubes are common after chest surgery and chest trauma and are used for treatment of pneumothorax or hemothorax to promote lung reexpansion (Skill 40-3 on pp. 869-873).

A **pneumothorax** is a collection of air in the pleural space. The loss of negative intrapleural pressure causes the lung to collapse. There are a variety of causes for a pneumothorax. A secondary pneumothorax can occur as a result of chest trauma (e.g., stabbing, gunshot wound, or rib fracture from striking the chest against the steering wheel in an automobile accident). Other causes of secondary pneumothorax are the rupture of an emphysematous bleb on the surface of the lung (the destruction caused by emphysema), tearing of the pleura from an invasive procedure such as surgery, insertion of a subclavian IV line, and mechanical ventilation, including PEEP. Spontaneous (primary) pneumothorax is a genetic condition that occurs unexpectedly in healthy individuals who develop blisterlike formations (blebs) on the visceral pleura, usually on the apex of the lungs. The blebs can rupture during sleep or exercise (McCance and Huether, 2010). A patient with a pneumothorax usually feels pain as atmospheric air irritates the parietal pleura. The pain is sharp and pleuritic and worsens on inspiration. Dyspnea is common and worsens as the size of the pneumothorax increases.

A **hemothorax** is an accumulation of blood and fluid in the pleural cavity between the parietal and visceral pleura, usually as a result of trauma. It produces a counter pressure and prevents the lung from full expansion. A rupture of small blood vessels from inflammatory processes such as pneumonia or TB can cause a hemothorax. In addition to pain and dyspnea, signs and symptoms of shock develop if blood loss is severe.

A variety of chest tubes are available to drain air or excess fluid from the pleural space to relieve respiratory distress. A small-bore chest tube (12 to 20 Fr) is used to remove a small amount of air, and a larger-bore chest tube is used to remove large amounts of fluid or blood and large amounts of air (Coughlin and Parchinsky, 2006).

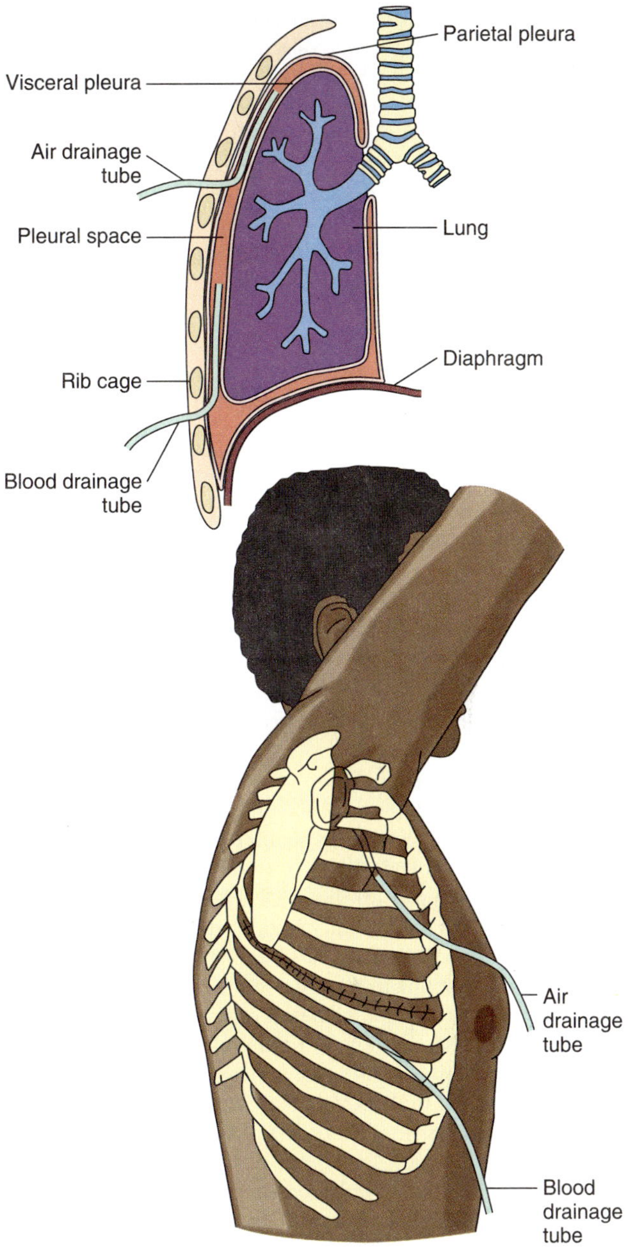

FIG. 40-15 Chest tube placement.

After a chest tube is inserted, it is attached to a drainage system. A traditional chest drainage unit (CDU) has three chambers for collection, water seal, and suction control. This unit can drain a large amount of both fluid and air (Coughlin and Parchinsky, 2006). Mobile systems rely on gravity, not suction, for drainage. In selected patients these mobile drains reduce the length of time needed for the chest tube, improve ambulation, and decrease the length of time in the hospital (Carroll, 2005). Nonventilated patients and patients who had thoracoscopic lung surgery or minimally invasive cardiac surgery do well with these mobile chest drains. They are lighter and smaller; thus patients are able to move more easily. As a result this reduces the risks of deep vein thrombosis and pulmonary embolism.

The simplest closed drainage system is the single chamber unit. The chamber serves as a fluid collector and a water seal. During normal respiration the fluid in the chamber ascends with inspiration and descends with expiration. A single chamber is used for smaller amounts of drainage such as an empyema (i.e., a collection of infected fluid or pus in the pleural space).

The use of two chambers permits any fluid to flow into the collection chamber as air flows into the water-seal chamber. Fluctuations in the water-seal tube are still anticipated. Two chambers allow for more accurate measurement of chest drainage and are used when larger amounts of drainage are expected.

When a volume of air or fluid needs to be evacuated with controlled suction, all three chambers are used. Mark the suction control with centimeter readings to adjust the amount of suction. Usually 15 to 20 cm of water is used for adults (Roman and Mercado, 2006). This means that the chamber is filled with sterile water to the 15- or 20-cm water level.

There is a new dry chest drainage system that does not use water in the suction chamber. An automatic control valve (ACV) is located inside the regulator and continuously balances the force of the suction with the atmospheres. As a result, the ACV responds and adjusts to changes in patient air leaks and fluctuations in suction source vacuum to deliver accurate suction. Set the pressure between −10 cm H_2O and −40 cm H_2O (Roman and Mercado, 2006). Regardless of the system used, the principles of patient management are the same.

Special Considerations. Keep a chest tube system closed and below the chest (see Skill 40-3). The tube should be secured to the chest wall. Watch for slow, steady bubbling in the suction-control chamber and keep it filled with sterile water at the prescribed level. Make sure that the water-seal chamber is filled to the manufacturer-specified level and watch for fluctuation (tidaling) of the fluid level to ensure that the chest tube and system are working. A constant or intermittent bubbling in the water-seal chamber indicates a leak in the drainage system, and the health care provider must be notified immediately. Mark the level on the outside of the collection chambers every shift. Report any unexpected cloudy or bloody drainage. Do not let the tubing kink or loop, and ideally it should lie horizontally across the bed or chair before dropping vertically into the drainage device. Encourage your patient to cough, deep breath, and use the incentive spirometer. Make sure that he or she is frequently repositioned and ambulated if not contraindicated. Routinely assess respiratory rate, breath sounds, SpO_2 levels, and the insertion site for subcutaneous emphysema (Rushing, 2007).

Clamping a chest tube is contraindicated when ambulating or transporting a patient. Clamping can result in a tension pneumothorax. Air pressure builds in the pleural space, collapsing the lung and creating a life-threatening event. A chest tube is only clamped when replacing the chest drainage system, assessing for an air leak, or during removal (Rushing, 2007).

Chest tubes are not routinely stripped or milked to move clots or increase chest tube drainage (Rushing, 2007). Stripping or milking chest tubes is based on nursing assessment (see Skill 40-3). Stripping is when the thumb and forefinger are used to compress the chest tube and the other hand is used to pull the tube away from the chest wall. Milking is squeezing, twisting, or kneading the tube to create a burst of suction to move clots. The excessive pressure caused by milking can lead to damaged tissue being trapped in the eyelets of the chest tube, resulting in increased bleeding (Halm, 2007).

Handle the chest drainage unit carefully and maintain the drainage device below the patient's chest. If the tubing disconnects from the drainage unit, instruct the patient to exhale as much as possible and to cough. This maneuver rids the pleural space of as much air as possible. Temporarily reestablish a water seal by immersing the open end of the chest tube into a container of sterile water (Roman and Mercado, 2006).

Removal of chest tubes requires patient preparation. The most frequent sensations reported by patients during chest tube removal include burning, pain, and a pulling sensation. Make sure that the patient is given pain medication at least 30 minutes before removal. The nurse assists the health care provider in removing the chest tube and monitors the dressing placed over the insertion site and the patient's respiratory status after tube removal.

Maintenance and Promotion of Oxygenation. Promotion of lung expansion, mobilization of secretions, and maintenance of a patent airway assist patients in meeting their oxygenation needs. However, some patients also require oxygen therapy to keep a healthy level of tissue oxygenation.

Oxygen Therapy. Oxygen therapy is widely available and used in a variety of settings to relieve or prevent tissue hypoxia. The goal of oxygen therapy (AARC, 2007) is to prevent or relieve hypoxia by delivering oxygen at concentrations greater than ambient air (21%). Oxygen is a medical gas and should be used in accordance with federal, state, and local regulations. It has dangerous side effects such as oxygen toxicity. The dosage or concentration of oxygen is monitored continuously. Routinely check the health care provider's orders to verify that the patient is receiving the prescribed oxygen concentration. The six rights of medication administration also pertain to oxygen administration (see Chapter 31).

Safety Precautions. Oxygen is a highly combustible gas. Although it does not burn spontaneously or cause an explosion, it can easily cause a fire in a patient's room if it contacts a spark from an open flame or electrical equipment. With increasing use of home oxygen therapy, patients and health care professionals need to be aware of the dangers of combustion. Chapter 27 describes steps to take in case of fire.

Promote oxygen safety by the following measures:

- Oxygen is a therapeutic gas and must be prescribed and adjusted only with a health care provider's order. Distribution must be in accordance with federal, state, and local regulations (AARC, 2007).
- Place an "Oxygen in Use" sign on the patient's door and in the patient's room. If using oxygen at home, place a sign on the door of the house. No smoking should be allowed on the premises.
- Keep oxygen-delivery systems 10 feet from any open flames.
- Determine that all electrical equipment in the room is functioning correctly and properly grounded (see Chapter 27). An electrical spark in the presence of oxygen can result in a serious fire.
- When using oxygen cylinders, secure them so they do not fall over. Store them upright and either chained or secured in appropriate holders.
- Check the oxygen level of portable tanks before transporting a patient to ensure that there is enough oxygen in the tank.

Supply of Oxygen. Oxygen is supplied to a patient's bedside either by oxygen tanks or through a permanent wall-piped system. Oxygen tanks are transported on wide-based carriers that allow the tank to be placed upright at the bedside. Regulators control the amount of oxygen delivered. One common type is an upright flowmeter with a flow adjustment valve at the top. A second type is a cylinder indicator with a flow adjustment handle. In the home setting oxygen therapy is also supplied in a variety of

TABLE 40-7 Approximate FIO_2 with Different Oxygen-Delivery Devices

OXYGEN-DELIVERY DEVICE	FIO_2 DELIVERED	ADVANTAGES	DISADVANTAGES
Nasal cannula	1 L/min: 24% 2 L/min: 28% 3 L/min: 32% 4 L/min: 36% 5 L/min: 40% 6 L/min: 44%	Safe and simple Easily tolerated Delivers low concentrations while allowing patients to eat, speak, and drink Does not impede eating or talking Disposable	Unable to use with nasal obstruction Drying to mucous membranes, so flow greater than 4 L/min needs to be humidified Can dislodge from nares easily Causes skin irritation or breakdown over ears or at nares Not good for mouth breathers Patient's breathing pattern affects exact FIO_2
Transtracheal oxygen cannula	Flow rates range from ¼ to 4 L/min and range from 22%-45% (AARC, 2007).	Small intravenous-size catheter inserted directly into trachea that provides individualized delivery for patients with chronic lung disease More comfortable and cosmetic than nasal cannula Provides adequate oxygen at lower flow rates; thus less expensive	Requires more monitoring and has more complications Patient needs to be educated on cleaning of catheter to prevent infection
Simple face mask	5-6 L/min: 40% 6-7 L/min: 50% 7-8 L/min: 60% >8 L/min: 60%	Assists in providing humidified oxygen	Exact FIO_2 level is difficult to estimate Requires high FIO_2 levels at 5 L/min or more to prevent rebreathing of carbon dioxide Patient inhales room air through the side holes in the mask Possible pressure areas and skin irritation with long-term use More difficult to eat, speak, or drink when in place
Partial nonrebreather mask with a reservoir bag	Delivers high concentrations of oxygen at 6-10 L/min to provide 40%-70% FIO_2.	Oxygen flow supplied to maintain the reservoir bag at least ⅓ to ½ full on inspiration (AARC, 2002).	Possible pressure areas and skin irritation with long-term use More difficult to eat, speak, or drink when in place Need to check frequently to make sure that bag is inflated
Nonrebreather mask with reservoir bag	Minimum flow of 10 L/min and delivers FIO_2 of 60%-80%	Similar to partial nonrebreather with reservoir bag but has valve between bag and mask to prevent exhaled air from returning to bag	Possible pressure areas and skin irritation with long-term use More difficult to eat, speak, or drink when in place
Venturi mask	4 L/min: 24%-28% 8 L/min: 35%-40% 12 L/min: 50%-60%	Controls amount of specified oxygen concentration; delivers percentage of FIO_2 from 24% to 60% Does not dry mucous membranes Delivers humidity with oxygen concentration	Hot and confining, increased levels of humidification irritate skin Specific flow rate necessary to deliver a specific FIO_2; possible decrease in FIO_2 if mask does not fit properly Interferes with eating and talking

FIO_2, Fraction of inspired oxygen concentration.

methods, including oxygen concentrators and refillable cylinders (AARC, 2007).

In the hospital or home oxygen tanks are delivered with the regulator in place. In the hospital the respiratory care department usually connects the regulator to the oxygen source. Home care vendors are usually responsible for connecting the oxygen tank to the regulator for home use.

Methods of Oxygen Delivery. The nasal cannula and oxygen masks are the most common devices to deliver oxygen to patients.

Nasal Cannula. A nasal cannula is a simple, comfortable device used for precise oxygen delivery (Skill 40-4 on pp. 873-875). The two nasal prongs are slightly curved and inserted in a patient's nostrils. To keep the nasal prongs in place, fit the attached tubing over the patient's ears and secure it under the chin using the sliding connector. Be alert for skin breakdown over the ears and in the nostrils from too tight an application. Attach the nasal cannula to a humidified oxygen source with a flow rate up to 6 L/min (24% to 40% oxygen). Flow rates equal to or greater than 4 L/min have a drying effect on the mucosa and thus need to be humidified (AARC, 2007). Know which flow rate produces a given percentage of inspired oxygen concentration (FIO_2) (Table 40-7).

Oxygen Masks. An oxygen mask is a plastic device that fits snugly over the mouth and nose and is secured in place with a strap. It delivers oxygen as the patient breathes through either the mouth or nose by way of a plastic tubing at the base of the mask that is attached to an oxygen source. An adjustable elastic band is attached to either side of the mask that slides over the head to above the ears to hold the mask in place. There are two primary types of oxygen masks: those delivering low concentrations of oxygen and those delivering high concentrations.

The simple face mask (Fig. 40-16) is used for short-term oxygen therapy. It fits loosely and delivers oxygen concentrations from

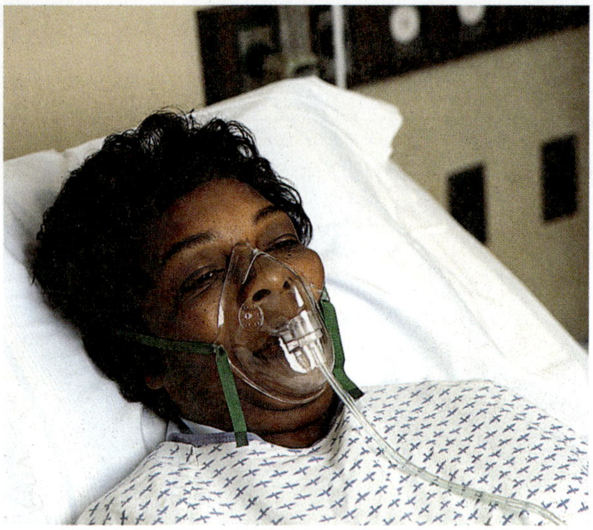

FIG. 40-16 Simple face mask.

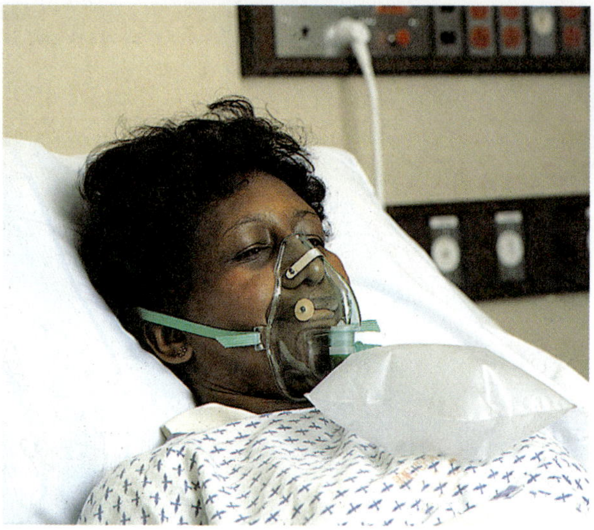

FIG. 40-17 Plastic face mask with reservoir bag.

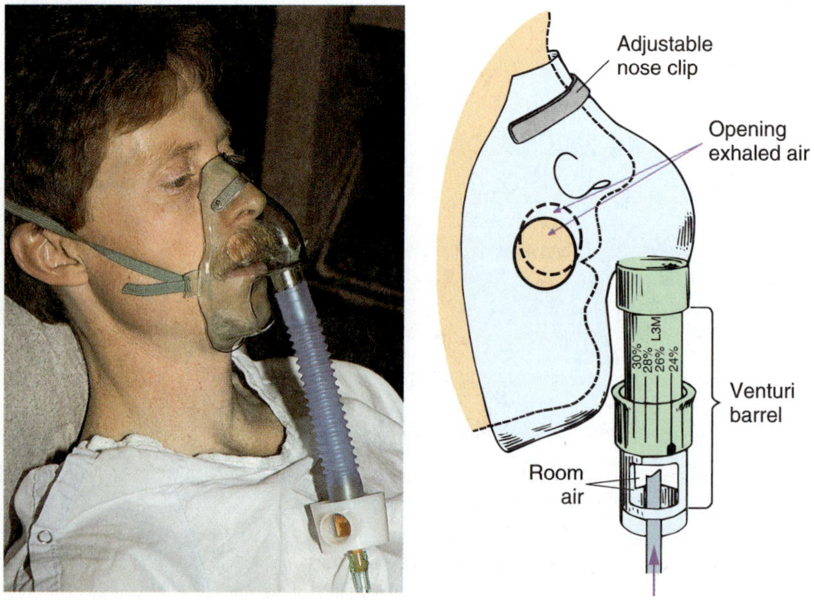

FIG. 40-18 Venturi mask.

35% to 50% FIO_2. The mask is contraindicated for patients with carbon dioxide retention because retention can be worsened. Flow rates should be 5 L or more to avoid rebreathing exhaled carbon dioxide retained in the mask. Be alert to skin breakdown under the mask with long-term use (AARC, 2002).

A plastic face mask with a reservoir bag (Fig. 40-17) is capable of delivering higher concentrations of oxygen. A partial rebreather mask is a simple mask with a reservoir bag that should be at least one third to one half full on inspiration and delivers from 40% to 70% FIO_2 with a flow rate of 6 to 10 L/min. When used as a nonrebreather mask, a similar face mask has one-way valves that prevent exhaled air from returning to the reservoir bag. The flow rate should be a minimum of 10 L/min and deliver FIO_2 of 60% to 80% (AARC, 2002). Frequently inspect the reservoir bag to make sure that it is inflated. If it is deflated, the patient is breathing large amounts of exhaled carbon dioxide. High-flow oxygen systems should be humidified (AARC, 2007).

The Venturi mask (Fig. 40-18) delivers higher oxygen concentrations of 24% to 60% with oxygen flow rates of 4 to 12 L/min, depending on the flow-control meter selected.

Home Oxygen Therapy. Indications for home oxygen therapy include an arterial partial pressure (PaO_2) of 55 mm Hg or less or an arterial oxygen saturation (SaO_2) of 88% or less on room air at rest, on exertion, or with exercise. Home oxygen therapy is administered via nasal cannula or face mask. Patients with permanent tracheostomies use either a T tube or tracheostomy collar (AARC, 2007). Home oxygen therapy has beneficial effects for patients with chronic cardiopulmonary diseases. This therapy improves patients' exercise tolerance and fatigue levels and in some situations assists in the management of dyspnea.

There are three types of oxygen delivery systems: compressed gas cylinders, liquid oxygen, and oxygen concentrators. Before placing a certain delivery system in a home, assess the advantages and disadvantages (Table 40-8) of each type, along with the

TABLE 40-8 **Home Oxygen Systems**

PRIMARY USE	ADVANTAGES	DISADVANTAGES
Compressed Gas Cylinders		
Intermittent therapy such as for exercise or sleep only	100% oxygen stored in steel or aluminum cylinders; relatively inexpensive, no loss of gas during storage, relatively portable, delivery of up to 15 L/min; does not require electrical source; smaller tanks available	Bulky and heavy; frequent refilling necessary with continuous use; patient must know how to read regulator and understand when to call supplier; portable cylinders weigh 15 lbs
Liquid Oxygen Systems		
System of choice for high-volume users and active patients	100% oxygen; more oxygen occupies a smaller space; patient carries convenient ambulatory units refilled at home as shoulder bag, backpack, or wheeled luggage cart; delivery of up to 6 L/min; patient can safely refill ambulatory units from larger reservoir; quiet and easy operation; does not require electricity for operation; requires relatively fewer deliveries of oxygen	Evaporates, especially in warmer temperatures and when not in use; potential for connections to freeze together or form frost at connections if tight connection not maintained during filling; costly setup and delivery fees
Oxygen Concentrators		
Cost-effective for patients requiring low-flow continuous oxygen and patients with limited mobility inside or outside the home	Inexpensive, fixed monthly costs; most units with delivery of 1 to 5 L/min; good choice for people who do not leave their homes frequently; no cylinders or tanks to refill; delivery up to 10 L/min with specific makes and models	Oxygen concentration decreases as liter flow increases (usually 85% or greater 90%); power supply needed; increased electric costs; is not an ambulatory unit, therefore requires second system for portability; requires regular maintenance and backup system

Data from AARC: *Clinical practice guideline—2007 revision and update,* Cleveland Clinic Foundation: *Home oxygen therapy,* 2010b, from http://www.cchs.net/health/health-info/docs/2400/2412.asp?index=8707. Accessed September 14, 2010.

patient's needs and community resources. In the home the major consideration is the oxygen-delivery source.

Patients and their family caregivers need extensive teaching to be able to manage oxygen therapy efficiently and safely (Skill 40-5 on pp. 875-878). Teach the patient and family about home oxygen delivery (i.e., oxygen safety, regulation of the amount of oxygen, and how to use the prescribed home oxygen-delivery system) to ensure their ability to maintain the oxygen-delivery system. The home health nurse coordinates the efforts of the patient and family, home respiratory therapist, and home oxygen equipment vendor. The social worker usually assists initially with arranging for the home care nurse and oxygen vendor.

Restoration of Cardiopulmonary Functioning. If a patient's hypoxia is severe and prolonged, cardiac arrest results. A cardiac arrest is a sudden cessation of cardiac output and circulation. When this occurs, oxygen is not delivered to tissues, carbon dioxide is not transported from tissues, tissue metabolism becomes anaerobic, and metabolic and respiratory acidosis occurs. Permanent heart, brain, and other tissue damage occur within 4 to 6 minutes.

Cardiopulmonary Resuscitation. During cardiac arrest there is an absence of pulse and respiration. The American Heart Association continues to research cardiac arrest treatment and outcomes. The 2010 Consensus Conference reviewed the most current and comprehensive resuscitation literature/research to develop the *2010 AHA Guidelines for Cardiopulmonary Resuscitation (CPR) and Emergency Cardiac Care (ECC),* thus simplifying the basic life support (BLS) steps (AHA, 2010b).

The previous ABC (establish an ***A***irway, initiate ***B***reathing, and maintain ***C***irculation) of **cardiopulmonary resuscitation (CPR)** is changed to CAB (***C***hest compression, ***A***irway, ***B***reathing) for adults and pediatric patients (excluding newborns). In adults (the majority of cardiac arrests) the critical initial elements found to be essential for survival were chest compressions and early defibrillation. In the previous ABC sequence, establishing an airway first delays chest compressions. Now ventilation is done after the first cycle of 30 chest compressions. Another issue is that bystander CPR may increase if those not comfortable with doing ventilations would at least perform chest compression. For most adults with out-of-the-hospital arrest, hands-only CPR by bystanders has had similar outcomes to conventional CPR. A lone health care provider who sees an adult in cardiac arrest should activate the emergency response system, get and use an automatic external defibrillator (AED) if available, and give CPR. Defibrillation by AED (Box 40-10) is needed to stop an abnormal heart rhythm, and AEDs are now available in public places such as schools, airports, and workplaces (AHA, 2006a, 2010b).

BOX 40-10 **AUTOMATED EXTERNAL DEFIBRILLATOR**

- An automated external defibrillator (AED) is a device used to administer an electrical shock through the chest wall to the heart to stop the abnormal rhythm and restore a normal heart rhythm.
- Built-in computers assess patient's heart rhythm and determine if defibrillation is necessary. New technology has made them user friendly with audio and visual cues telling users what to do when using them (AHA, 2010b).
- The AED analyzes the patient's heart rhythm and determines if a shock is needed. It delivers a shock to the patient after announcing, "Everyone stand clear of patient." A shock is only delivered if the patient needs it.
- Lay rescuer AED programs train lay personnel (security guards, police, and firefighters) on the use of the AED (AHA, 2006b, 2010b).
- The AED is used to strengthen the chain of survival. Every minute of a sudden cardiac arrest without defibrillation decreases the survival rate by 7% to 10% (AHA, 2010b).
- For witnessed ventricular fibrillation, early cardiopulmonary resuscitation with defibrillation within the first 3 to 5 minutes can result in greater than 50% long-term survival (AHA, 2010a).

Restorative and Continuing Care. Restorative and continuing care emphasizes cardiopulmonary reconditioning as a structured rehabilitation program. **Cardiopulmonary rehabilitation** helps patients achieve and maintain an optimal level of health through controlled physical exercise, nutrition counseling, relaxation and stress-management techniques, and prescribed medications and oxygen. As physical reconditioning occurs, a patient's complaints of dyspnea, chest pain, fatigue, and activity intolerance decrease. In addition, the patient's anxiety, depression, or somatic concerns often decrease. The patient and the rehabilitation team define the goals of rehabilitation.

Respiratory Muscle Training. Respiratory muscle training improves muscle strength and endurance, resulting in improved activity tolerance. Respiratory muscle training prevents respiratory failure in patients with COPD. One method for respiratory muscle training is the incentive spirometer resistive breathing device (ISRBD). Patients achieve resistive breathing by placing a resistive breathing device into a volume-dependent incentive spirometer. Patients achieve muscle training when they use the ISRBD on a scheduled routine (e.g., twice a day for 15 minutes or 4 times a day for 15 minutes).

Breathing Exercises. Breathing exercises include techniques to improve ventilation and oxygenation. The three basic techniques are deep-breathing and coughing exercises, pursed-lip breathing, and diaphragmatic breathing. Deep-breathing and coughing exercises, previously discussed, are routine interventions used by postoperative patients (see Chapter 50).

Pursed-Lip Breathing. **Pursed-lip breathing** involves deep inspiration and prolonged expiration through pursed lips to prevent alveolar collapse. While sitting up, instruct the patient to take a deep breath and exhale slowly through pursed lips as if blowing through a straw. Have him or her blow through a straw into a glass of water to learn the technique. Patients need to gain control of the exhalation phase so it is longer than inhalation. The patient is usually able to perfect this technique by counting the inhalation time and gradually increasing the count during exhalation. In studies using pulse oximetry as a feedback tool, patients are able to demonstrate an increase in their arterial oxygen saturation during pursed-lip breathing (AARC, 1993).

Diaphragmatic Breathing. **Diaphragmatic breathing** is useful for patients with pulmonary disease, postoperative patients, and women in labor to promote relaxation and provide pain control. The exercise improves efficiency of breathing by decreasing air trapping and reducing the WOB.

Diaphragmatic breathing is more difficult than other breathing methods because it requires a patient to relax intercostal and accessory respiratory muscles while taking deep inspirations, which takes practice. The patient places one hand flat below the breastbone (upper hand) and the other hand (lower hand) flat on the abdomen. Ask him or her to inhale slowly, making the abdomen push out (as the diaphragm flattens, the abdomen should extend out) and moving the lower hand outward. When the patient exhales, the abdomen goes in (the diaphragm ascends and pushes on lungs to help expel trapped air). The patient practices these exercises initially in the supine position and then while sitting and standing. The exercise is often used with the pursed-lip breathing technique.

EVALUATION

Evaluate nursing interventions and therapies by comparing the patient's progress with the goals and expected outcomes of the nursing care plan (Fig. 40-19). Patient expectations evaluate the care from the patient's perspective.

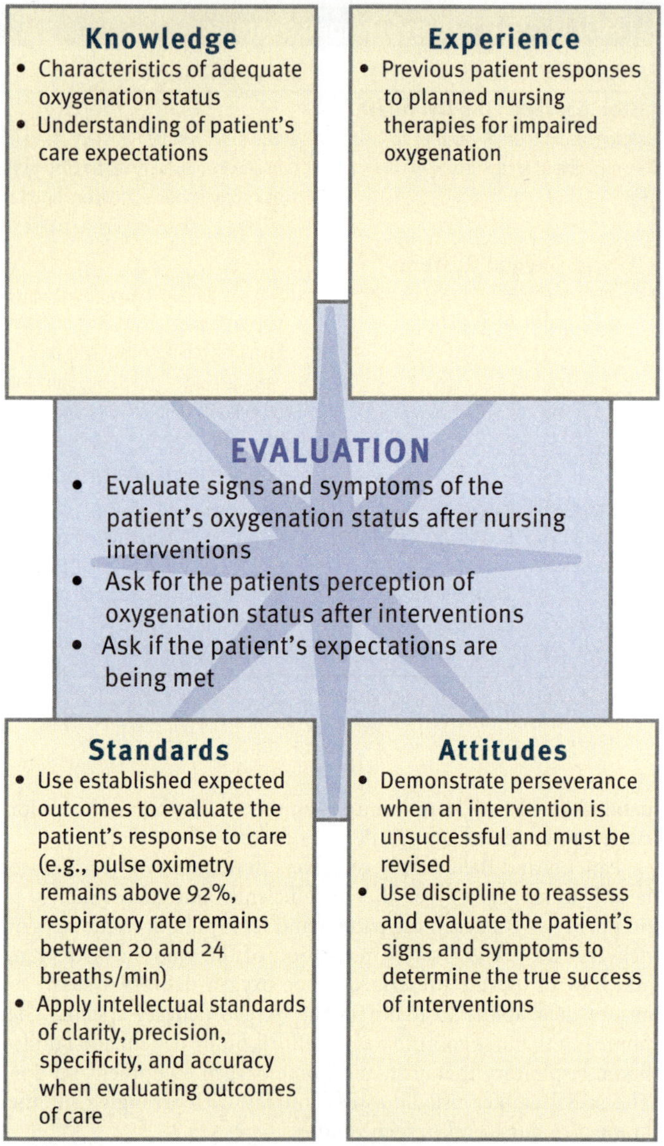

Knowledge
• Characteristics of adequate oxygenation status
• Understanding of patient's care expectations
Experience
• Previous patient responses to planned nursing therapies for impaired oxygenation
EVALUATION
• Evaluate signs and symptoms of the patient's oxygenation status after nursing interventions
• Ask for the patients perception of oxygenation status after interventions
• Ask if the patient's expectations are being met
Standards
• Use established expected outcomes to evaluate the patient's response to care (e.g., pulse oximetry remains above 92%, respiratory rate remains between 20 and 24 breaths/min)
• Apply intellectual standards of clarity, precision, specificity, and accuracy when evaluating outcomes of care
Attitudes
• Demonstrate perseverance when an intervention is unsuccessful and must be revised
• Use discipline to reassess and evaluate the patient's signs and symptoms to determine the true success of interventions

FIG. 40-19 Critical thinking model for oxygenation evaluation.

Through the Patient's Eyes. It is important to determine a patient's perceptions of how the disease affecting his or her need for oxygenation is also affecting his or her lifestyle. Focus on evaluating how the disease is affecting day-to-day activities and how the patient believes he or she is responding to treatment. Patients who have chronic lung problems often must be motivated to participate in necessary therapies. Evaluate the patient's motivation and emotional readiness to adhere to treatments provided. Be aware of the need to change a treatment plan to be culturally sensitive to improve adherence to it. Determine if the patient or family/caregiver feels more in control of the health situation after you have provided instruction. Consider the use of survey tools such as COPD Self Efficacy Scale, Chronic Respiratory Disease Questionnaire, and Pulmonary-Specific Quality of Life for COPD Scale (AARC, 2010b) to evaluate a patient's perception of his or her quality of life.

Patient Outcomes. Compare the patient's actual progress to the goals and expected outcomes of the nursing care plan to determine his or her health status. If the nursing measures used are not successful in improving oxygenation, modify the care plan and reevaluate. Continuous evaluation helps to determine whether new or revised therapies are required and if new nursing diagnoses have developed and require a new plan of care. Do not hesitate to notify the health care provider about a patient's deteriorating oxygenation status. Prompt notification helps avoid an emergency situation or even the need for CPR.

- Ask the patient about his or her degree of breathlessness. Observe respiratory rate before, during, and after any activity or procedure.
- Ask the patient if the distance ambulated without fatigue has increased.
- Ask the patient to rate breathlessness on a scale of 0 to 10, with 0 being no shortness of breath and 10 being severe shortness of breath.
- Ask the patient which interventions help reduce dyspnea.
- Ask the patient about frequency of cough and sputum production and assess any sputum produced.
- Auscultate lung sounds for improvement in adventitious sounds.
- Evaluate pulse oximetry changes to decreases in oxygen delivery.
- Monitor arterial blood gas levels, pulmonary function tests, chest x-ray films, ECG tracings, and physical assessment data to provide objective measurement of the success of therapies and treatments.

SAFETY GUIDELINES FOR NURSING SKILLS

Ensuring patient safety is an essential role of the professional nurse. To ensure patient safety, communicate clearly with members of the health care team, assess and incorporate the patient's priorities of care and preferences, and use the best evidence when making decisions about your patient's care. When performing the skills in this chapter, remember the following points to ensure safe, individualized patient care.

- Patients with sudden changes in their vital signs, level of consciousness, or behavior are possibly experiencing profound hypoxia (McCance and Huether, 2010).
- Perform tracheal suctioning before pharyngeal suctioning whenever possible. The mouth and pharynx contain more bacteria than the trachea. If a large amount of oral secretions is present before beginning the procedure, suction mouth with separate oral suction device.
- Use caution when suctioning patients with a head injury. The suction procedure causes elevations in intracranial pressure (ICP). Reduce this risk by presuctioning hyperventilation, which results in hypocarbia, which in turn induces vasoconstriction, thereby reducing the risk of increased ICP. It is recommended that you limit the introduction of the catheter to 2 times with each suctioning procedure (Gholamzadeh and Javadi, 2009).
- The routine use of NSI into the airway before ET and tracheostomy suctioning is not recommended. Normal saline is not effective in thinning secretions or improving removal. Use of NSI is associated with the adverse effects of excessive coughing, bronchospasm, spread of organisms to the lower respiratory tract, and decreased oxygen saturation (AARC, 2010b).
- Check your institutional policy before stripping or milking chest tubes. Nursing assessment determines if these procedures are necessary. These procedures can cause excessive pressure that has the potential to damage tissue trapped in the eyelets of the chest tube and cause increased bleeding.
- The most serious tracheostomy complication is airway obstruction, which can result in cardiac arrest. Most tracheostomy tubes are designed with a small plastic inner tube that sits inside the larger one. If the airway becomes occluded, the smaller one can be removed and replaced with a temporary spare. It is important to always have a spare at the bedside for emergency replacement (Higgins, 2009).
- Patients with COPD who are breathing spontaneously should never receive high levels of oxygen therapy because it results in a decreased stimulus to breathe. Do not administer oxygen more than 2 L/min unless a health care provider's order is obtained (AARC, 2007).

SKILL 40-1 SUCTIONING

View Video!

Delegation Considerations

The skill of nasotracheal suctioning and suctioning a new artificial airway cannot be delegated to nursing assistive personnel (NAP). However, when a patient has been assessed by the nurse to be stable, oropharyngeal and permanent tracheostomy tube suctioning can be delegated to NAP. Instruct NAP about:

- Unique modifications of the skill such as the need to reapply any supplemental oxygen equipment following the procedure.
- Reporting to the nurse any change in patient's respiratory status, level of consciousness, secretion color or volume, or unresolved coughing or gagging.
- Reporting to the nurse any change in patient's color, vital signs, or complaints of pain.

Equipment

- Appropriate-size suction catheter (smallest diameter that removes secretions effectively) or Yankauer catheter (oral suction). Outer diameter of catheter should not exceed half of internal diameter of an artificial airway (AARC, 2010a)
- Nasal or oral airway (if indicated)
- Two sterile gloves (open suction) or clean gloves (closed or oropharyngeal suction)
- Clean towel or paper drape
- Portable or wall suction as vacuum source
- Mask, goggles, or face shield
- Connecting tube (6 feet) and collection bottle
- Oxygen source and/or manual resuscitation bag equipped with oxygen-enrichment device
- Pulse oximeter
- Stethoscope

If not using closed-suction catheter

- Water-soluble lubricant
- Small Y adapter if catheter does not have a suction port
- Sterile basin
- Sterile normal saline solution or water (about 100 mL)

SKILL 40-1 SUCTIONING—cont'd

STEP	RATIONALE
ASSESSMENT	
1 Identify the patient using two identifiers (i.e., name and birth date or name and account number) according to facility policy. Compare identifiers with information on the patient's medical record.	Ensures correct patient. Complies with a recommended National Patient Safety Goal (TJC, 2011).
2 Assess for signs and symptoms of upper and lower airway obstruction requiring suctioning: abnormal respiratory rate, adventitious sounds on inspiration or expiration, nasal secretions, gurgling, drooling, restlessness, gastric secretions or vomitus in mouth, and coughing without clearing secretions from airway.	Physical signs and symptoms result from decreased oxygen to tissues and pooling of secretions in upper and lower airways. Complete assessment measures before and after suction procedure (AARC, 2004).
3 Assess signs and symptoms associated with hypoxia and hypercapnia: decreased SpO_2, increased pulse and blood pressure, increased respiratory rate, apprehension, anxiety, decreased ability to concentrate, lethargy, decreased level of consciousness (especially acute), increased fatigue, dizziness, behavioral changes (especially irritability), dysrhythmias, pallor, and cyanosis.	Physical signs and symptoms resulting from decreased oxygen to tissues indicate need for suctioning (AARC, 2004).
4 Assess for risk factors for upper or lower airway obstruction, including chronic obstructive pulmonary disease, pulmonary infection, fluid imbalance, lack of humidity, impaired mobility, decreased level of consciousness, decreased gag or cough reflex, dysphagia, presence of feeding tube.	The presence of these risk factors impairs a patient's ability to clear secretions from the airway, thickens secretions, or increases risk for retaining secretions and thus requires suctioning.
5 Assess for anatomic factors that influence upper or lower airway function, such as recent surgery; head, chest, or neck trauma; tumors; neuromuscular disease.	Abnormal anatomy or head and neck trauma impairs normal drainage of secretions. Tumors in or around the lower airway impair secretion removal by occluding or externally compressing lumen of airway.
6 Identify **contraindications to nasotracheal suctioning** (AARC, 2004): occluded nasal passages; nasal bleeding, epiglottitis, or croup; acute head, facial, or neck injury or surgery, coagulopathy or bleeding disorder; irritable airway; laryngospasm or bronchospasm; gastric surgery with high anastomosis; myocardial infarction.	These conditions are **contraindicated because the passage of a catheter through the nasal route** causes trauma to existing facial trauma or surgery, increases nasal bleeding, or causes severe bleeding in the presence of bleeding disorders. In the presence of epiglottitis, croup, laryngospasm, or irritable airway, the entrance of a suction catheter via the nasal route causes intractable coughing, hypoxemia, and severe bronchospasm, necessitating emergency intubation or tracheostomy. Hypoxemia could worsen cardiac damage in myocardial infarction (AARC, 2004).
7 Review sputum microbiology data.	Certain bacteria are easier to transmit or require isolation because of virulence or antibiotic resistance.
8 Assess patient's understanding of procedure.	Reveals need for patient instruction and encourages cooperation.
PLANNING	
1 Explain to patient how procedure will help clear airway and relieve breathing problems and that temporary coughing, sneezing, gagging, or shortness of breath is normal. Encourage patient to cough out secretions.	Encourages cooperation and minimizes risks, anxiety, and pain.
2 Explain importance of and encourage coughing during procedure. Practice coughing if able. Splint surgical incisions if necessary.	Facilitates secretion removal and reduces frequency and duration of future suctioning.
3 Assist patient with assuming comfortable position (usually semi-Fowler's or sitting upright with head hyperextended, unless contraindicated). Nurse should stand on patient's right if nurse is right-handed or on patient's left if nurse is left-handed.	Reduces stimulation of gag reflex, promotes patient comfort and secretion drainage, and prevents aspiration. Hyperextension facilitates insertion of catheter into trachea.
4 Place pulse oximeter on patient's finger. Take reading and leave pulse oximeter in place.	Provides baseline SpO_2 to determine patient's response to suctioning.
5 Place towel across patient's chest.	Reduces transmission of microorganisms by protecting gown from secretions.
IMPLEMENTATION	
1 Perform hand hygiene. Apply mask, goggles, or face shield if splashing is likely.	Reduces transmission of microorganisms.
2 Connect one end of connecting tubing to suction machine and place other end in convenient location near patient. Turn suction device on and set vacuum regulator to appropriate negative pressure (120 to 150 mm Hg) (AARC, 2004).	Excessive negative pressure damages nasal, pharyngeal, and tracheal mucosa and induces greater hypoxia. Negative pressures should not exceed 150 mm Hg because higher pressure increases risk for airway trauma, hypoxemia, and atelectasis (AARC, 2004).
3 If indicated, increase supplemental oxygen therapy to 100% or as ordered by health care provider. Encourage patient to deep breathe.	Hyperoxygenation provides some protection from suction-induced decline in oxygenation. It is most effective in the presence of hyperinflation such as encouraging the patient to deep breathe or increase ventilator tidal volume settings (Bourgault et al., 2006; Pedersen et al., 2009).

STEP	RATIONALE
4 Preparation for all types of suctioning	
a. Open appropriate suction kit or catheter, using aseptic technique. If sterile drape is available, place it across patient's chest or on the over-bed table. Do not allow the suction catheter to touch any nonsterile surfaces.	Prepares catheter and prevents transmission of microorganisms. Provides sterile surface on which to lay suction catheter between passes, if needed.
b. Unwrap or open sterile basin and place on bedside table. Fill basin or cup with approximately 100 mL of sterile normal saline solution or water (see illustration).	Solution is used to flush catheter after each suction pass.
c. Open lubricant. Squeeze small amount onto open sterile catheter package without touching package. NOTE: Lubricant is not necessary for oropharyngeal or artificial airway suctioning.	Prepares lubricant while maintaining sterility. Use water-soluble lubricant to avoid lipoid aspiration pneumonia. Excessive lubricant application can occlude the catheter.
5 Apply gloves:	
a. Apply clean glove to each hand or dominant hand for oropharyngeal suctioning.	Suction of oral cavity does not require sterile glove use.
b. Apply sterile glove to each hand or nonsterile glove to nondominant hand and sterile glove to dominant hand for nasopharyngeal, nasotracheal, and artificial airway suctioning.	Reduces transmission of microorganisms and allows nurse to maintain sterility of suction catheter.
c. For artificial airway, see Step 8c.	Personal protective equipment is applied before gloving.
6 Pick up suction catheter with dominant hand without touching nonsterile surface. Pick up connecting tubing with nondominant hand. Secure catheter to tubing (see illustration)	
7 Place tip of catheter into sterile basin and suction a small amount of normal saline by occluding suction vent.	Ensures suction is functioning. Lubricates internal catheter and tubing.
8 Suction airway.	
a. Oropharyngeal suctioning	
(1) Remove oxygen mask if present. Keep oxygen mask near patient's face. If patient has a nasal cannula, it may remain in place.	Allows access to patient's mouth while having access to oxygen-delivery system.

CLINICAL DECISION: *Be prepared to quickly reapply oxygen mask if SpO_2 falls or respiratory distress develops during or at the end of suctioning.*

STEP	RATIONALE
(2) Insert Yankauer catheter into patient's mouth. With suction applied intermittently, move catheter around mouth, including pharynx and gum line, until secretions are cleared.	If catheter does not have a suction control to apply intermittent suction, take care not to allow suction tip to irritate oral mucosal surfaces with continuous suction.
(3) Encourage patient to cough and repeat suctioning if needed. Replace oxygen mask if used.	Coughing moves secretions from lower to upper airways into mouth.
(4) Rinse catheter with saline or water from basin with suction on continuously until catheter is cleared of secretions.	Clearing secretions before they dry reduces probability of transmission of microorganisms and enhances delivery of preset suction pressures.
b. Nasopharyngeal and nasotracheal suctioning	
(1) Lightly coat distal 6-8 cm (2-3 inches) of catheter tip with water-soluble lubricant.	Lubricates catheter for easier insertion.
(2) Remove oxygen-delivery device, if applicable, with nondominant hand. Without applying suction and using dominant thumb and forefinger, gently insert catheter into naris during inhalation.	Application of suction pressure while introducing catheter into nasopharyngeal tissues increases risk of damage to mucosa. When advanced into trachea, suction could damage mucosa and increase risk of hypoxia.

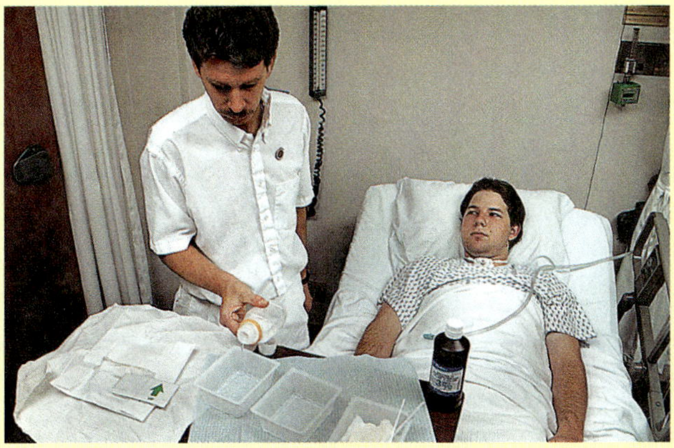

STEP 4b Pouring saline into basin.

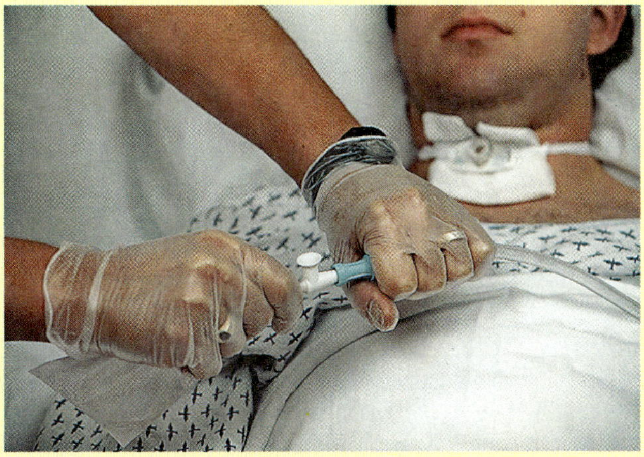

STEP 6 Attaching catheter to suction.

SKILL 40-1 SUCTIONING—cont'd

STEP	RATIONALE

CLINICAL DECISION: *Be sure to insert catheter during patient inhalation, especially if inserting into trachea because epiglottis is open. Do not insert during swallowing, or catheter will most likely enter the esophagus. If patient gags or becomes nauseated, the catheter is most likely in the esophagus and must be removed.* ***Never apply suction during insertion.***

STEP	RATIONALE
(3) *Nasopharyngeal:* Have patient take a deep breath and insert catheter, following natural course of naris; slightly slant catheter downward and advance to back of pharynx. Do not force through naris. In adults insert catheter about 16 cm (6 inches); in older children, 8 to 12 cm (3 to 5 inches); in infants and young children, 4 to 8 cm (2 to 3 inches). Rule of thumb is to insert catheter distance from tip of nose (or mouth) to angle of mandible.	Proper placement ensures removal of pharyngeal secretions.
(a) Apply intermittent suction for no more than 15 seconds by placing and releasing nondominant thumb over catheter vent. Slowly withdraw catheter while rotating it back and forth between thumb and forefinger.	Intermittent suction up to 15 seconds safely removes pharyngeal secretions. Suction time greater than 15 seconds increases risk for suction-induced hypoxemia (AARC, 2004).
(4) *Nasotracheal:* Follow natural course of naris and advance catheter slightly slanted and downward to just above entrance into trachea. While patient takes a deep breath, quickly insert catheter about 15 to 20 cm (6 to 8 inches in adult) into trachea (see illustration). Patient will begin to cough. **NOTE:** In older children advance the catheter 16 to 20 cm (6 to 8 inches), and in young children and infants, 8 to 14 cm (3 to 5½ inches).	Ensures that catheter is inserted into trachea with minimum stress to patient. In young children and infants, shallow suctioning is recommended instead of deep tracheal suctioning, which increases the risk of tracheal edema and inflammation (AARC, 2010a). Premeasured suction catheters are used in some pediatric settings to avoid deep suctioning (Hockenberry and Wilson, 2011).

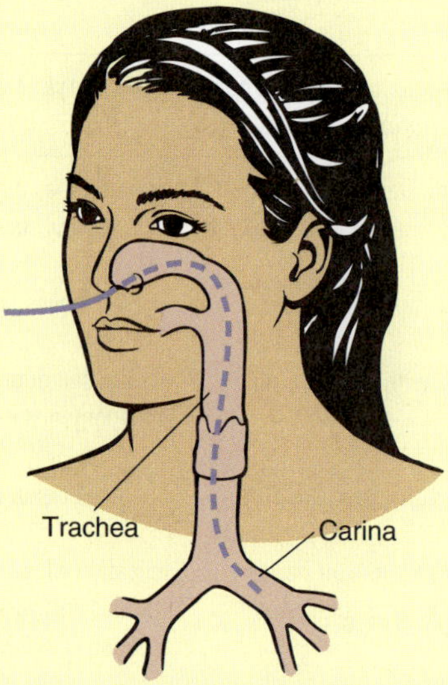

STEP 8b(4) Distance of insertion of nasotracheal catheter.

CLINICAL DECISION: *When there is difficulty passing the catheter, ask patient to cough or say "ahh" or try to advance during inspiration. Both these measures assist in opening the glottis to permit passage of the catheter into the trachea.*

STEP	RATIONALE
(a) *Positioning option:* In some instances turning patient's head to right helps suction the left mainstem bronchus; turning head to left helps suction the right mainstem bronchus. If you feel resistance after insertion of catheter to maximum recommended distance, catheter has probably hit carina. Pull it back 1 to 2 cm (½ inch) before applying suction.	Turning patient's head to the side elevates the bronchial passage on the opposite side and facilitates passage of the catheter.

CLINICAL DECISION: *Use nasotracheal suctioning before pharyngeal suctioning whenever possible. The mouth and pharynx contain more bacteria than the trachea. If copious oral secretions are present before beginning the procedure, suction mouth with oral suction device.*

STEP	RATIONALE
(b) Apply intermittent suction for no more than 15 seconds by placing and releasing nondominant thumb over vent of catheter. Slowly withdraw catheter while rotating it back and forth between the dominant thumb and forefinger. Encourage patient to cough. Replace oxygen device if applicable.	Intermittent suction and rotation of catheter prevent injury to mucosa. If catheter "grabs" mucosa, remove thumb to release suction. Suctioning longer than 15 seconds causes cardiopulmonary compromise, usually from hypoxemia or vagal overload.

CLINICAL DECISION: *Monitor patient's vital signs and oxygen saturation during procedure; note whether there is a change of 20 beats/min (either increase or decrease) or if pulse oximetry falls below 90% or 5% from baseline. If this occurs, stop suctioning.*

(5) Rinse catheter and connecting tubing with normal saline or water until cleared.	Removes secretions from catheter. Secretions that remain in suction catheter or connecting tubing decrease suctioning efficiency.
(6) Assess for need to repeat suctioning procedure. Do not perform more than two passes with catheter. Allow at least 1 minute between passes for ventilation and oxygenation (AARC, 2004). Ask patient to deep breathe and cough.	Observe for alterations in cardiopulmonary status. Suctioning induces hypoxemia, dysrhythmias, laryngospasm, and bronchospasm (AARC, 2004). Deep breathing hyperventilates and reoxygenates alveoli and reduces the risk for suction-induced hypoxemia (Bourgault et al., 2006). Repeated passes clear the airway of excessive secretions but also remove oxygen and can induce laryngospasm.
c. Artificial airway (tracheostomy or endotracheal [ET] tube) suctioning	
(1) Apply mask, goggles, or face shield.	Reduces transmission of microorganisms.
(2) Apply one sterile glove to each hand or nonsterile glove to nondominant hand and sterile glove to dominant hand.	Reduces transmission of microorganisms and allows nurse to maintain sterility of suction catheter.
(3) Pick up suction catheter with dominant hand without touching nonsterile surfaces. Pick up connecting tubing with nondominant hand. Secure catheter to tubing.	Maintains catheter sterility. Establishes suction.
(4) Check that equipment is functioning properly by placing tip of catheter into basin and suctioning small amount of saline.	Ensures equipment function; lubricates catheter and tubing.
(5) Hyperinflate and/or hyperoxygenate patient before suctioning, using manual resuscitation AMBU-bag connected to oxygen source or sigh mechanism on mechanical ventilator. Some mechanical ventilators have a button that, when pushed, delivers 100% oxygen for a few minutes and then resets to the previous value.	Hyperinflation along with hyperoxygenation decreases the risk for a decrease in oxygenation saturation. Routine use of hyperinflation is not recommended because of the possibility of trauma resulting from large volumes and high peak pressures (Pedersen et al., 2009).
(6) If patient is receiving mechanical ventilation, open swivel adapter or, if necessary, remove oxygen- or humidity-delivery device with nondominant hand.	Exposes artificial airway.
(7) Without applying suction gently but quickly insert catheter using dominant thumb and forefinger into artificial airway (see illustration) (best to time catheter insertion with inspiration) until you meet resistance or patient coughs; then pull back 1 cm (½ inch).	Application of suction pressure while introducing catheter into trachea increases risk of damage to tracheal mucosa and increased hypoxia related to removal of entrained oxygen present in airways. Pulling back stimulates cough and removes catheter from mucosal wall so catheter is not resting against tracheal mucosa during suctioning.

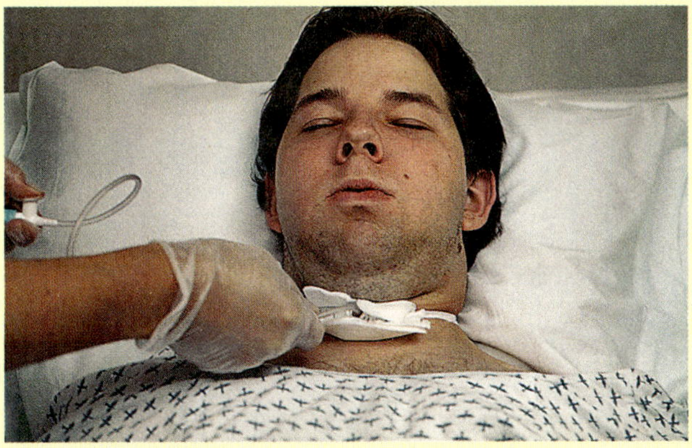

STEP 8c(7) Suctioning tracheostomy.

CLINICAL DECISION: *If unable to insert catheter past the end of the ET tube, it is probably caught in the Murphy eye (i.e., side hole at the distal end of the ET tube that allows for collateral airflow in the event of mainstem intubation). If this happens, rotate the catheter to reposition it away from the Murphy eye or withdraw it slightly and reinsert with the next inhalation. Usually the catheter meets resistance at the carina. One indication that the catheter is at the carina is acute onset of coughing because the carina contains many cough receptors. Pull the catheter back 1 cm (½ inch).*

SKILL 40-1 SUCTIONING—cont'd

STEP	RATIONALE
(8) Apply intermittent suction by placing and releasing nondominant thumb over vent of catheter; slowly withdraw catheter while rotating it back and forth between dominant thumb and forefinger. Encourage patient to cough. Watch for respiratory distress.	Intermittent suction and rotation of catheter prevent injury to tracheal mucosal lining. If catheter "grabs" mucosa, remove thumb to release suction.

CLINICAL DECISION: *If patient develops respiratory distress, immediately withdraw catheter and supply additional oxygen and breaths as needed. In an emergency administer oxygen directly through the catheter. Disconnect suction and give 100% oxygen through the catheter.*

STEP	RATIONALE
(9) If patient is receiving mechanical ventilation, close swivel adapter or replace oxygen-delivery device.	Reestablishes the artificial airway.
(10) Encourage patient to deep breathe if able. Some patients respond well to several manual breaths from the mechanical ventilator or bag-valve mask.	Reoxygenates and expands alveoli. Suctioning sometimes causes hypoxemia and atelectasis.
(11) Rinse catheter and connecting tubing with normal saline until clear. Use continuous suction.	Removes catheter secretions. Secretions left in tubing decrease suction and provide environment for microorganism growth. Secretions left in connecting tube decrease suctioning efficiency.
(12) Assess patient's cardiopulmonary status for secretion clearance and complications. Repeat Steps (5) through (8) once or twice more to clear secretions. Allow adequate time (at least 1 full minute) between suction passes for ventilation and hyperoxygenation. Do not perform more than two passes with the catheter (AARC, 2010a).	Suctioning sometimes induces dysrhythmias, hypoxia, and bronchospasm and impairs cerebral circulation or adversely affects hemodynamics (AARC, 2010a). Repeated passes with suction catheter clear airway of excessive secretions and promote improved oxygenation.
(13) Perform nasopharyngeal and oropharyngeal suctioning if necessary. After performing nasopharyngeal and oropharyngeal suctioning, catheter is contaminated; do not reinsert into ET or tracheostomy tube.	Upper airway is "clean," and lower airway is "sterile." Therefore you can use the same catheter to suction from sterile to clean areas but not from clean to sterile areas.
9 Complete procedure.	
a. Place Yankauer catheter in a clean, dry area for reuse with suction turned off or within patient's reach with suction on if patient is capable of suctioning self.	Facilitates prompt removal of airway secretions when suctioning is necessary in the future.
b. Disconnect nasal and artifical airway catheters from connecting tubing. Turn off suction. Roll catheter around fingers of dominant hand. Pull glove off inside out so catheter remains in glove. Pull off other glove over first glove in same way to contain contaminants. Discard into appropriate receptacle. Turn off suction device.	Reduces transmission of microorganisms. Do not touch clean equipment with contaminated gloves.
c. Remove towel and place in laundry or remove drape and discard in appropriate receptacle.	Reduces transmission of organisms.
d. Reposition patient as indicated by condition. Reapply clean gloves for patient's personal care (e.g., oral hygiene).	Proper positioning based on patient's condition promotes comfort, encourages secretion drainage, and reduces risk of aspiration.
e. If indicated, readjust oxygen to original level.	Helps patient's blood oxygen level return to baseline.

CLINICAL DECISION: *If patient develops respiratory distress during the suctioning procedure, immediately withdraw catheter and supply additional oxygen and breaths as needed. In an emergency administer oxygen directly through the catheter. Disconnect suction and attach oxygen at prescribed flow rate through the catheter.*

STEP	RATIONALE
f. Discard remainder of normal saline into appropriate receptacle. If basin is disposable, discard into appropriate receptacle. If basin is reusable, rinse and place in soiled utility room.	Solution is contaminated; this reduces transmission of microorganisms.
g. Remove and discard goggles, mask, or face shield and perform hand hygiene.	Reduces transmission of microorganisms.
h. Place unopened suction kit on suction machine table or at head of bed according to institution preference.	Provides for immediate access of suction catheter and equipment in event of an emergency or for next suctioning procedure.

EVALUATION

STEP	RATIONALE
1 Compare patient's vital signs and SpO_2 saturation before and after suctioning.	Provides objective data about any physiological effects of suctioning.
2 Ask patient if breathing is easier and congestion is decreased.	Provides subjective confirmation that airway obstruction is relieved with suctioning procedure.
3 Auscultate lungs for change in adventitious lung sounds.	Provides objective information about any improvement in lung sounds.
4 Observe airway secretions.	Provides data to document presence or absence of respiratory tract infection.

UNEXPECTED OUTCOMES AND RELATED INTERVENTIONS

1 Worsening cardiopulmonary status
- Limit length of suctioning.
- Determine need for presuctioning hyperoxygenation and hyperinflation.
- Determine need for more frequent suctioning, possibly shorter duration.
- Notify health care provider of changes.

2 Return of bloody secretions
- Determine amount of suction pressure used and adjust accordingly.
- Evaluate suctioning frequency and reduce if appropriate.
- Determine other factors that lead to bloody secretions (e.g., prolonged bleeding time).
- Provide more frequent oral hygiene.

3 Unable to pass suction catheter through first naris attempted
- Try other naris or oral route.
- Insert nasal airway, especially if suctioning through patient naris frequently.
- Guide catheter along naris floor to avoid turbinates.
- If obstruction is mucus, apply suction to relieve obstruction but do not apply suction to mucosa. If you think obstruction is a blood clot, consult health care provider.
- Increase lubrication of catheter.

RECORDING AND REPORTING

- Record amount, consistency, color, and odor of secretions.
- Record patient's response to procedure.
- Record and report patient's presuctioning and postsuctioning cardiopulmonary status.

HOME CARE CONSIDERATIONS

- Adhere to best practices for infection control while weighing cost-effectiveness in the presence of a chronic situation. If a patient has an established tracheostomy or requires long-term nasotracheal suctioning and infection is not present, clean suction technique is appropriate.
- Although most patients with airway clearance problems at home have a tracheostomy, some also require nasal pharyngeal suctioning. Catheters are often used for a 24-hour period and then cleaned and disinfected; or they are cleaned with soapy water after each use and discarded after 24 hours.
- Stress to family caregivers the importance of brief intervals of applying suction pressure. Instruct those performing suction to hold their breath during the application of negative suction pressure to help them remember to not suction too long.
- Instruct patient to clean and disinfect or change the secretion collection container every 24 hours according to home care or institutional protocol.
- Teach patient and family how to practice infection-control measures when emptying the suction container jar. These secretions are emptied in the toilet but have a splash risk. Instruct caregiver to apply mask (shield if available) and gloves and bring the jar as close to the toilet bowel as possible to decrease the risk of splash.

SKILL 40-2 CARE OF AN ARTIFICIAL AIRWAY

View Video!

Delegation Considerations

The skill of performing artificial airway care cannot be delegated to nursing assistive personnel (NAP). In some settings patients who have well-established tracheostomy tubes may have their care delegated to the NAP. Instruct the NAP to:
- Immediately report to the nurse changes in patient's respiratory status, change in level of consciousness, confusion, restlessness or irritability, change in vital signs (range to report), decreased pulse oximetry level (values to report), or change in level of comfort.
- Immediately report to the nurse if the endotracheal (ET) tube or tracheostomy tube appears to have becomes dislodged, obstructed, or moved.
- Immediately report to the nurse any unexpected drainage or secretions from tracheostomy or change in color of stoma.

Equipment

- Stethoscope
- ET tube care
  - Towel
  - ET and oropharyngeal suction equipment
  - 1- to 1½-inch (2.5- to 4-cm) adhesive or waterproof tape (not paper or silk tape) or commercial ET holder and mouth guard (follow manufacturer instructions for securing)
  - Clean gloves (two pairs)
  - Adhesive remover swab
  - Mouth care supplies
  - Powdered toothbrush or brush with non-foaming paste (sodium monoflurophosphate 0.7% [Sona et al., 2009])
  - 0.12% to 0.20% Chlorhexidine mouthwash, rinse, or gel
  - Tap water
  - Clean toothette
  - Face cleaner (e.g., wet washcloth, towel, soap, shaving supplies)
  - Clean 2 × 2 gauze
  - Tincture of benzoin, liquid adhesive, or skin preparation pad

SKILL 40-2 CARE OF AN ARTIFICIAL AIRWAY—cont'd

Equipment—cont'd

- Face shield, mask, goggles (if indicated)
- Tongue blade (optional)
- Oral airway

- Tracheostomy care
  - Towel
  - Tracheostomy suction supplies
  - Sterile tracheostomy care kit, if available, or two sterile 4 × 4 gauze pads
  - Sterile cotton-tipped applicators
  - Sterile tracheostomy dressing (precut and sewn surgical dressing)
  - Sterile basin
  - Small sterile brush (or disposable inner cannula)
  - Tracheostomy ties (e.g., twill tape, manufactured tracheostomy ties, Velcro tracheostomy ties)
  - Normal saline (NS)
  - Scissors
  - Clean gloves (two)
  - Face shield, mask, or goggle if indicated

STEP	RATIONALE
ASSESSMENT	
1 Identify the patient using two identifiers (i.e., name and birth date or name and account number) according to facility policy. Compare identifiers with information on the patient's medical record.	Ensures correct patient. Complies with a recommended National Patient Safety Goal (TJC, 2011).
2 Auscultate lung sounds and observe respiratory rate and depth.	Provides baseline measure of ventilation and ease of breathing.
3 Assess condition of surrounding tissues (soiled or loose tape, ties, or dressing; pressure sores on nares, lips, or corner of mouth; excess nasal, oral, or peristomal secretions; patient moving endotracheal tube with tongue; biting tube or tongue; or foul-smelling mouth).	Determines need for airway care and identifies potential pressure sites from airway devices.
4 Observe patency of airway. Excess intratracheal or endotracheal secretions, diminished airflow through airway, signs and symptoms of airway obstruction.	Buildup of secretions in airways impair oxygenation.
5 Observe for factors that increase risk for complications from ET tube: type and size of tube, movement of tube up and down trachea, cuff size and overinflation or underinflation, duration of tube placement, facial trauma, malnutrition, and neck or thoracic radiation.	Movement of tube predisposes patient to tracheal trauma or tube dislodgment and indicates the need for another size airway. Cuff size indicates the amount of air needed to properly inflate cuff. An underinflated cuff increases patient's risk for aspiration. Cuff overly inflated may cause ischemia or necrosis of tracheal tissue. Longer duration of intubation increases risk for lower airway complications (Hess, 2005). Tissue is prone to breakdown in the presence of malnutrition and radiation.
6 Determine proper ET tube depth, noted by centimeters at lip or gum line. Line is marked on tube and recorded in medical record at time of intubation.	
7 Assess patient's knowledge of procedure and ability to perform trach care at home, and answer any questions of family.	Reinforces information given to patient and family and provides opportunity to ask additional questions. Encourages cooperation and minimizes anxiety.
PLANNING	
1 Obtain assistance from available staff for this procedure.	Reduces risk for accidental extubation of artificial airway.
2 Assist patient with assuming comfortable position for both patient and nurse (usually supine or semi-Fowlers).	Provides access to site and facilitates completion of procedure without causing the nurse muscle strain or patient discomfort.
3 Place towel across patient's chest.	Reduces transmission of microorganisms to linens and bedclothes.
4 Explain importance of patient's participation, including importance of not biting or moving ET tube with tongue, trying not to cough when tape is temporarily removed from the airway, not pulling on tube with hand.	Reduces anxiety, encourages cooperation, and reduces risks. Removal of tape can be uncomfortable.
IMPLEMENTATION	
1 Perform hand hygiene. Apply mask, goggles, or face shield if indicated.	Reduces transmission of microorganisms.
2 Perform tracheal (tracheostomy), endotracheal (endotracheal tube), nasopharyngeal, or oropharyngeal suction (see Skill 40-1). (When suctioning tracheostomy, remove soiled dressing and discard in glove with coiled catheter.)	Removes secretions and diminishes patient's need to cough during procedure.
3 Connect Yankauer suction catheter to suction source.	Prepares for oropharyngeal suctioning.

STEP	RATIONALE
4 Care of artificial airways	
a. Endotracheal (ET) tube care	
(1) Prepare method to secure ET tube (check agency policy).	
(a) Tape method: Cut piece of tape long enough to go completely around patient's head from naris to naris plus 15 cm (6 inches): adult, about 30 to 60 cm (1 to 2 feet). Lay adhesive side up on bedside table. Cut and lay 8 to 15 cm (3 to 6 inches) of tape, adhesive sides together, in center of long strip to prevent tape from sticking to hair. Smaller strip of tape covers area between ears around back of head.	Preparing tape ahead will allow you to have one hand positioned on ET tube throughout the procedure. Adhesive tape needs to be placed around head from cheek to cheek below ears. Avoid over ears because this results in a pressure sore.
(b) Commercially available ET tube holder: Open package per manufacturer instructions. Set device aside with head guard in place and Velcro strips open.	Commercial devices are latex free, fast, and convenient. These devices avoid need for tape and resultant skin breakdown and are easily applied in presence of facial hair.
(2) Apply clean gloves and instruct NAP or another RN to apply gloves and hold ET tube firmly at patients' lips or naris throughout the procedure. Note the number marking on ET tube at gum line or lips.	Reduces transmission of microorganisms. Maintains proper tube position and prevents accidental extubation.
(3) Remove old tape or device.	Provides access to underlying skin for assessment and hygiene. Reduces transmission of microorganisms.
(a) Tape: Carefully remove tape from ET tube and patient's face. If tape is difficult to remove, moisten with soapy water or adhesive tape remover. Discard tape in appropriate receptacle if nearby.	Limits tape burns around face and neck.
(b) Commercially available device: Remove Velcro strips from ET tube and remove ET tube holder from patient.	Velcro strips secure ET tube in place and provide a marker to measure distance to patient's lips or gums. These devices all permit access to patient's mouth and lips for ease in oropharyngeal suctioning and oral hygiene.

CLINICAL DECISION: *Do not allow helper to hold the tube away from the lips or naris. Doing so allows too much "play" in the tube and increases the risk for tube movement and accidental extubation. Never let go of the ET tube because it could become dislodged.*

STEP	RATIONALE
(4) Remove excess secretions or adhesive left on patient's face. Use adhesive remover swab to remove excess adhesive left on face after tape removal. Wash adhesive remover from face.	Promotes hygiene. Retained adhesive causes damage to skin and makes it difficult for new tape to adhere.
(5) Remove oral airway or bite block if present and place on towel.	Provides access and complete observation of patient's oral cavity.

CLINICAL DECISION: *Do not remove oral airway if patient is actively biting. Wait until tape or device is partially or completely secured to ET tube.*

STEP	RATIONALE
(6) Provide oral care. (Have Yankauer suction catheter on and at hand.) Brush oral mucosa, gums, and teeth with powdered toothbrush, or brush with nonfoaming antiseptic paste for 2 minutes (Sona et al., 2009; Needleman et al., 2011). Rinse carefully using tap water. Suction orally as needed during brushing and rinsing. Moisten brush with water to rinse, then use brush or a clean toothette to apply chlorhexidine rinse or gel (Sona et al., 2009; Morris et al., 2011; Labeau et al., 2011). Perform oral care twice daily at 12-hour intervals (Sona et al., 2009).	The use of an oral antiseptic for oral care of intubated patients has a beneficial effect in preventing ventilator-associated pneumonia (Labeau et al., 2011; Sona et al., 2009; Morris et al., 2011).
(7) Oral ET tube only: Note "cm" ET tube marking at lips or gums. With help of assistant, move ET tube to opposite side or center of mouth. Do not change tube depth.	Prevents pressure sore formation at sides of patient's mouth. Ensures correct position of tube and allows for quick visual of displaced tube. Measuring tube at lip line can be distorted because of edema, trauma, or disease process (Vollman, 2006).
(8) Repeat oral cleaning as in Step (6) on opposite side of mouth.	Cleanses oral cavity and removes secretions from mouth and oropharynx.
(9) Clean face and neck with soapy washcloth; rinse and dry. Shave male patient as necessary.	Moisture and beard growth prevent adhesive tape adherence.
(10) Use small amount of skin protectant or liquid adhesive on clean 2×2 gauze and dot on upper lip (oral ET tube) or across nose (nasal ET tube) and cheeks to ear. Allow tincture to dry completely.	Protects and makes skin more receptive to tape.
(11) Secure ET tube.	
(a) Tape method	
[1] Slip tape under patient's head and neck, adhesive side up. Take care not to twist tape or catch hair. Do not allow tape to stick to itself. It helps to stick tape gently to a tongue blade, which serves as a guide as tape is passed behind patient's head. Center tape so double-faced tape extends around back of neck from ear to ear.	Positions tape to secure ET tube in proper position.

SKILL 40-2 CARE OF AN ARTIFICIAL AIRWAY—cont'd

STEP	RATIONALE
[2] On one side of face, secure tape from ear to naris (nasal ET tube) or over lip to edge of mouth (oral ET tube). Tear remaining tape in half lengthwise, forming two pieces that are $\frac{1}{2}$- to $\frac{3}{4}$-inch (1 to 1.5 cm) wide. Secure bottom half of tape across upper lip (oral ET tube) or across top of nose (nasal ET tube) to opposite ear (see illustration, *A*). Wrap top half of tape around tube (see illustration, *B*). Tape should encircle main part of tube at least 2 times for security.	Secures tape to face. Using top tape to wrap prevents downward drag on ET tube.
[3] Gently pull other side of tape firmly to pick up slack and secure to remaining side of face (see illustration). Have assistant release hold when tube is secure.	Secures tape to face and tube. ET tube should be at same depth as the lips. Check earlier assessment for verification of tube depth in centimeters.
(b) Commercially available device	
[1] Thread ET tube through opening designed to secure it. Be sure that pilot balloon to ET tube is accessible.	Commercially available holders have a slit in front of holder designed to secure the ET tube.
[2] Place Velcro strips of ET holder under patient at occipital region of the head.	
[3] Verify that ET tube is at established depth, using lip or gum line marker as guide.	Ensures that ET tube remains at correct depth as determined during assessment.
[4] Secure Velcro strips at base of patient's head. Leave 1 cm ($\frac{1}{2}$ inch) slack in strips.	
[5] Verify that tube is secure, it does not move forward from patient's mouth or backward down into patient's throat, and there are no pressure areas on the oral mucosa or the occipital region of the head (see illustration).	The tube needs to be secure so its position remains at correct depth. It can be secured without being tight and causing pressure.

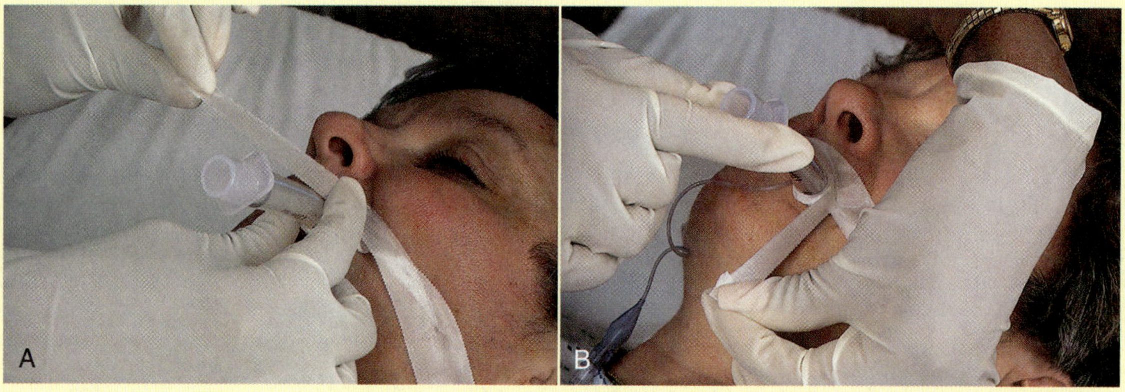

STEP 4a(11)(a)[2] A, Securing bottom half of tape across patient's upper lip. **B,** Securing top half of tape around tube.

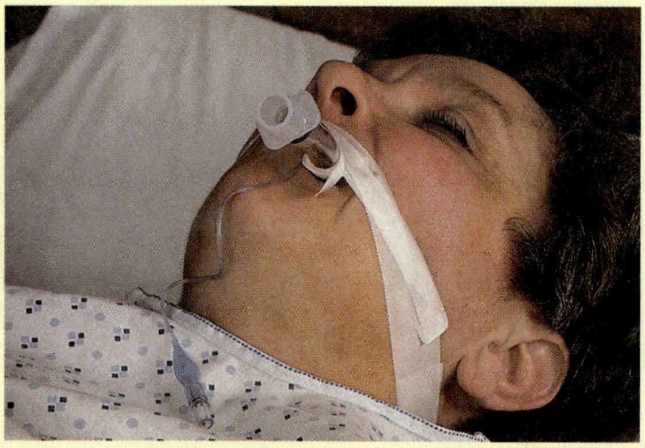

STEP 4a(11)(a)[3] Tape securing ET tube.

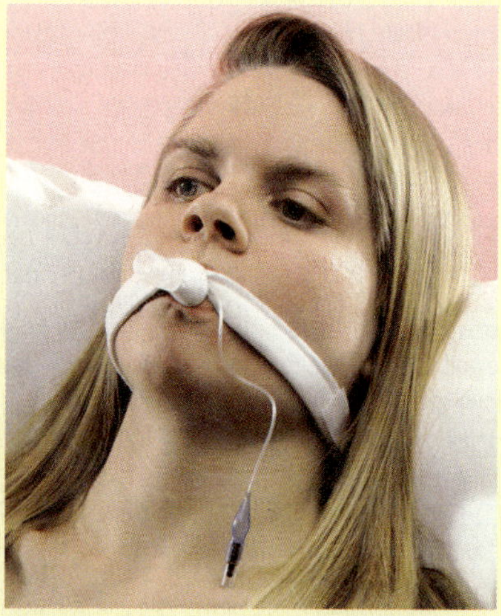

STEP 4a(11)(b)[5] ET holder in place. (Courtesy Dale Medical Products, Plainesville, Mass.)

STEP	RATIONALE
(12) Remove and clean oral airway in warm soapy water and rinse well. Then rinse in chlorhexidine rinse. Shake excess solution from oral airway. **Option:** Insert new oral airway if secretions are difficult to remove.	Promotes hygiene. Reduces transmission of microorganisms.
(13) For unconscious patient reinsert oral airway without pushing tongue into oropharynx and secure with tape.	Prevents patient from biting ET tube and allows access for oropharyngeal suctioning. An oral airway in a conscious, cooperative patient causes excessive gagging and pressure ulcers to mouth and tongue.
b. Tracheostomy care	
(1) While patient is replenishing oxygen stores following suctioning, prepare equipment on bedside table.	Preparation and organization of equipment allows completion of tracheostomy care procedure efficiently and reconnection of patient to oxygen source in timely manner.
(a) Open two packages of cotton-tipped swabs. Keeping contents sterile, pour NS onto one of the packages.	
(b) Open tracheostomy kit. Open two 4 × 4 gauze packages using aseptic technique and pour saline on one package. Leave second package dry. Do not recap NS.	A tracheostomy tube has multiple components (see illustration). Some of these components might be used during tracheostomy care.

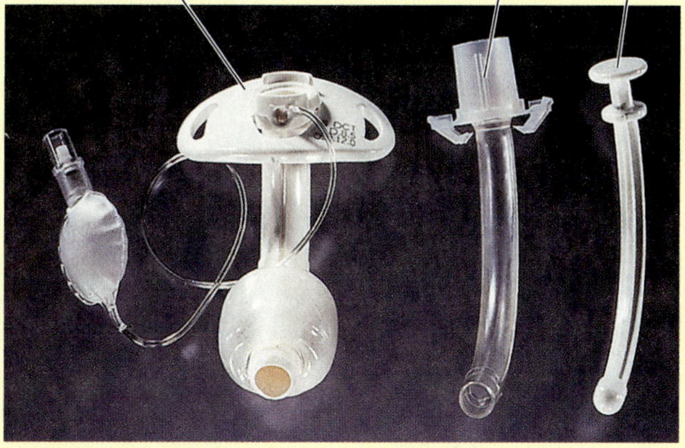

STEP 4b(1)(b) Tracheostomy tube. (Courtesy Mallinckrodt Inc. Shiley Tracheostomy Products, St Louis, Mo.)

STEP	RATIONALE
(c) Unwrap sterile basin and pour about 2 cm (1 inch) of NS into it.	
(d) Open small sterile brush package and place aseptically into sterile basin.	
(e) Open sterile tracheostomy dressing package.	
(f) Prepare length of twill tape long enough to go around patient's neck two times, about 60 to 75 cm (25 to 30 inches) for an adult. Cut ends on the diagonal. Lay aside in dry area.	Cutting ends of tie on a diagonal aids in inserting tie through eyelet.
(g) If using commercial tracheostomy tube holder, open package according to manufacturer's directions.	
(2) Apply sterile gloves. Keep dominant hand sterile throughout procedure.	Reduces transmission of microorganisms.
(3) Hyperoxygenate patient if oxygen saturation levels are below 92% (Demir and Dramali, 2005). Apply oxygen source loosely over tracheostomy if patient desaturates during procedure.	Helps reduce amount of desaturation.

CLINICAL DECISION: *It is important to stabilize the tracheostomy tube at all times during tracheostomy care to prevent injury and unnecessary discomfort. Have another nurse or NAP assist during procedure if necessary.*

CLINICAL DECISION: *For tracheostomy tube with no inner cannula or Kistner button, continue with Step (6).*

STEP	RATIONALE
(4) Tracheostomy with **inner cannula** care.	
(a) While touching only the outer aspect of tube, unlock and remove inner cannula with nondominant hand. Drop inner cannula into NS basin.	Removes inner cannula for cleaning. Hydrogen peroxide loosens secretions from inner cannula; but, if it is too irritating, use NS only (Johns Hopkins, 2010).

SKILL 40-2 CARE OF AN ARTIFICIAL AIRWAY—cont'd

STEP	RATIONALE
(b) Place tracheostomy collar or T tube and ventilator oxygen source over or near outer cannula. (NOTE: T tube and ventilator oxygen devices cannot be attached to all outer cannulas when inner cannula is removed.)	Maintains supply of oxygen to patient.
(c) To prevent oxygen desaturation in affected patients, quickly pick up inner cannula and use small brush to remove secretions inside and outside cannula (see illustration).	Tracheostomy brush provides mechanical force to remove thick or dried secretions.
(d) Hold inner cannula over basin and rinse with NS, using nondominant hand to pour.	Removes secretions from inner cannula (Cleveland Clinic, 2010a).
(e) Replace inner cannula (see illustration) and secure "locking" mechanism. Hyperventilate patient if needed. Reapply ventilator or oxygen sources.	Secures inner cannula and reestablishes oxygen supply.
(5) Disposable inner cannula care	
(a) Remove cannula from manufacturer packaging.	
(b) While touching only the outer aspect of tube, withdraw inner cannula and replace with new cannula. Lock into position.	Reestablishes airway quickly.
(c) Dispose of contaminated cannula in appropriate receptacle and apply oxygen source or ventilator.	Prevents unnecessary oxygen desaturation.
(6) Using NS-saturated cotton-tipped sterile swabs and 4 × 4 gauze, clean exposed outer cannula surfaces and stoma under faceplate, extending 5 to 10 cm (2 to 4 inches) in all directions from stoma (see illustration). Clean in circular motion from stoma site outward using dominant hand to handle sterile supplies.	Aseptically removes secretions from stoma site. Moving in outward circle pulls mucus and other contaminants from stoma to periphery.

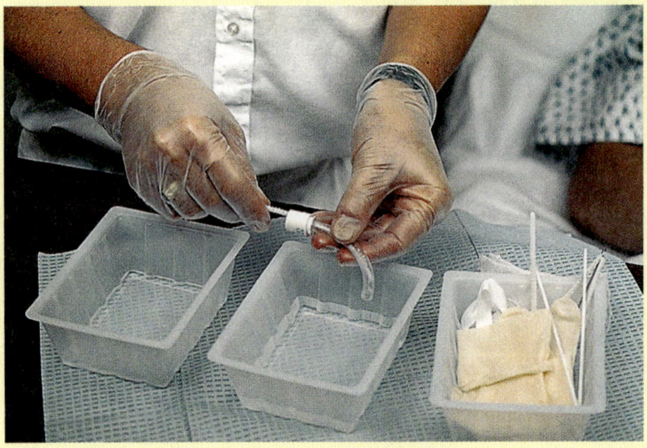

STEP 4b(4)(c) Cleaning tracheostomy inner cannula.

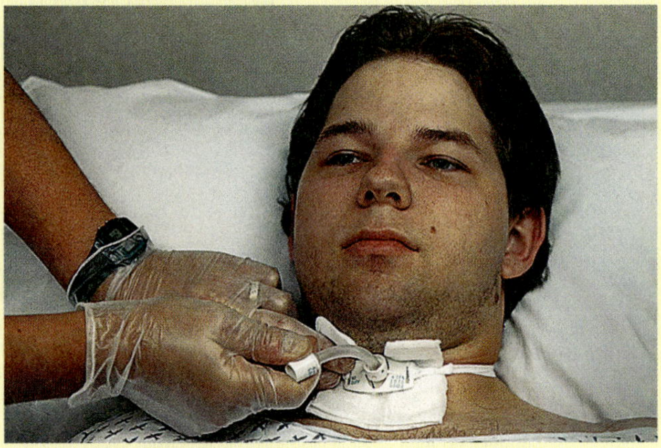

STEP 4b(4)(e) Reinserting inner cannula.

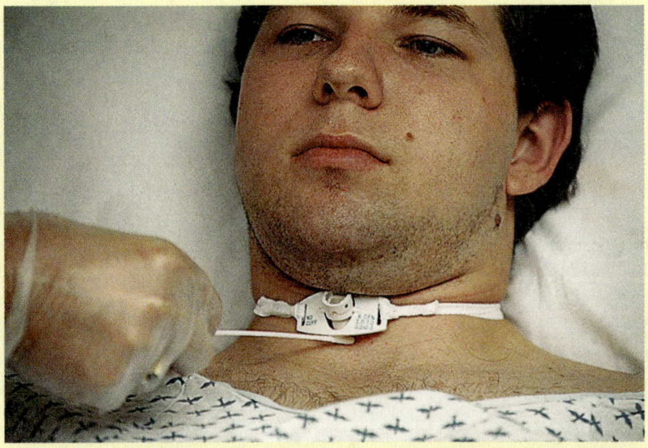

STEP 4b(6) Cleaning around stoma.

STEP	RATIONALE
(7) Using NS-prepared cotton-tipped swabs and 4 × 4 gauze, clean outer tracheostomy tube flange and skin surfaces.	Removes secretions that can be source of infection.
(8) Using dry 4 × 4 gauze, pat lightly at skin and exposed outer cannula surfaces.	Dry surfaces prohibit formation of moist environment for microorganism growth and skin excoriation.
(9) Securing tracheostomy	
(a) Tracheostomy tie method	
[1] Instruct assistant, if available, to apply clean gloves and securely hold tracheostomy tube securely in place, then cut old ties.	Promotes hygiene, reduces transmission of microorganisms. Secures tracheostomy tube to prevent incidental extubation.

CLINICAL DECISION: *Assistant must not release hold on tracheostomy tube until new ties are firmly tied to reduce risk of accidental extubation. If no assistant is present, do not cut old ties until new ties are in place and securely tied.*

STEP	RATIONALE
[2] Take prepared twill tape, insert one end of tie through faceplate eyelet, and pull ends even (see illustration).	
[3] Slide both ends of ties behind head and around neck to other eyelet and insert one tie through second eyelet.	
[4] Pull snugly.	Secures tracheostomy tube in place.
[5] Tie ends securely in double square knot, allowing space for only one loose or two snug finger widths in tie.	One-finger slack prevents ties from being too tight when tracheostomy dressing is in place and also prevents movement of tracheostomy into lower airway.
(b) Tracheostomy tube holder method (see illustration)	
[1] While wearing gloves, maintain secure hold on tracheostomy tube. This can be done with an assistant or, when an assistant is not available, leave old tracheostomy tube holder in place until new device is secure.	Prevents incidental displacement of tube.
[2] Align strap under patient's neck. Be sure that Velcro attachments are positioned on either side of tracheostomy tube.	
[3] Place narrow end of ties under and through faceplate eyelets. Pull ends even and secure with Velcro closures.	
[4] Verify that there is space for only one loose or two snug finger width(s) under neck strap.	Prevents skin necrosis.

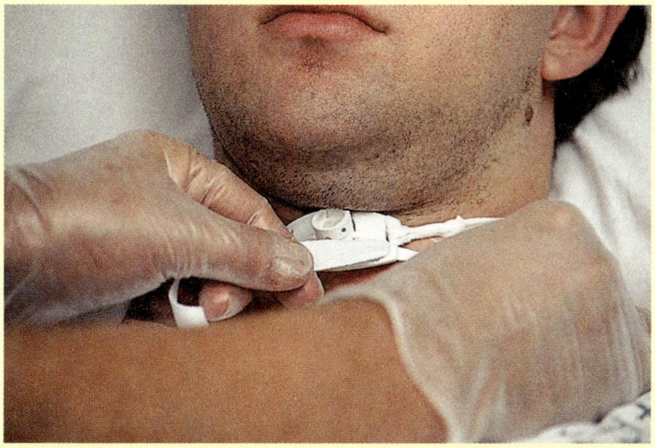

STEP 4b(9)(a)[2] Replacing tracheostomy ties when an assistant is not available. Do not remove old tracheostomy ties until new ones are secure.

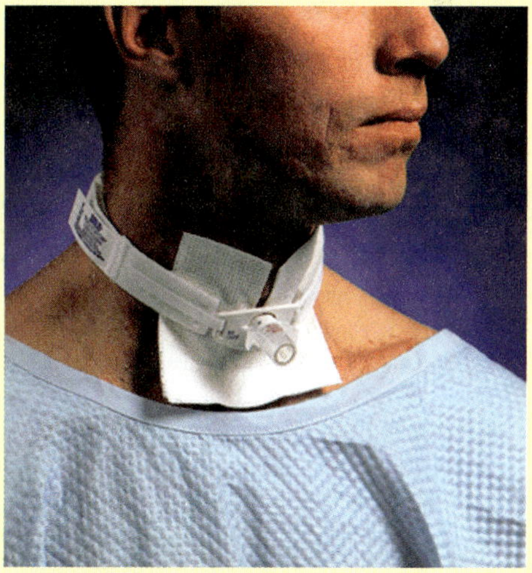

STEP 4b(9)(b) Tracheostomy tube holder in place. (Courtesy Dale Medical Products, Plainesville, Mass.)

SKILL 40-2 CARE OF AN ARTIFICIAL AIRWAY—cont'd

STEP	RATIONALE
(10) Insert fresh tracheostomy dressing under clean ties/holder and faceplate (see illustration).	Absorbs drainage. Dressing prevents pressure on clavicle heads.

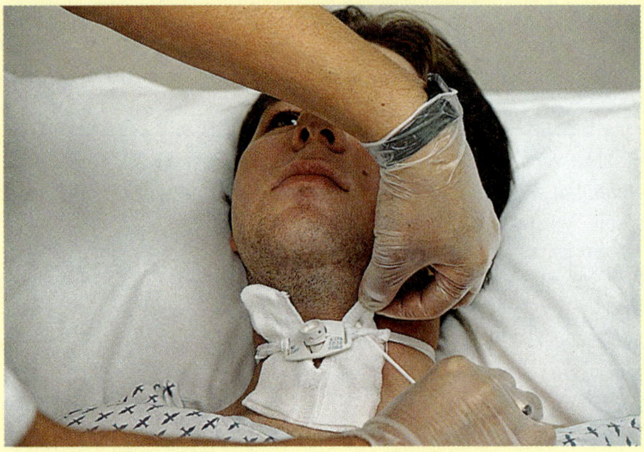

STEP 4b(10) Applying tracheostomy dressing.

STEP	RATIONALE
5 Position patient comfortably and evaluate respiratory status.	Promotes comfort. Some patients require posttracheostomy care suctioning.
6 Replace any oxygen-delivery devices.	Maintains oxygen therapy.
7 Remove and discard gloves. Perform hand hygiene.	Prevents transmission of microorganisms.

CLINICAL DECISION: *Keep tracheostomy obturator at bedside with a fresh tracheostomy to facilitate reinsertion of the outer cannula if dislodged. Keep an additional tracheostomy tube of the same size and shape on hand for emergency replacement (Higgins, 2009).*

EVALUATON

STEP	RATIONALE
1 Compare respiratory assessments before and after procedure.	Identifies any changes in presence and quality of breath sounds after procedure. Determines effectiveness of artificial airway care.
2 Observe depth and position of ET tubes according to health care provider's recommendation.	Verifies that position of tube is correct and not altered.
3 Assess security of tape/holder securing ET tube by gently tugging at tube.	Artificial airway (ET tube) should not move. Patient may cough.
4 Assess fit of new tracheostomy ties and ask patient if tube feels comfortable.	If tracheostomy ties are uncomfortable, ties that are too loose or tight place patient at risk for injury.
5 Assess skin around mouth, oral mucosa (ET tube), and tracheostomy stoma for drainage, pressure, irritation, or signs of infection.	Skin breakdown and/or irritation should not be present. Broken skin places patient at risk for infection.

UNEXPECTED OUTCOMES AND RELATED INTERVENTIONS

1 Unexpected extubation of ET tube
- Call for assistance while remaining with patient.
- Assist respirations with bag-valve mask as needed.
- Assess patient for airway patency, spontaneous breathing, and vital signs.
- Prepare for reintubation.

2 Accidental decannulation of tracheostomy tube
- Call for assistance while remaining with patient.
- Replace old tracheostomy tube with new spare tube of same size and kind kept at the bedside. Some experienced nurses or respiratory therapists may be able to quickly reinsert tracheostomy tube (Higgins, 2009).
- Same-size ET tube can be inserted in stoma in an emergency.
- Be prepared to manually ventilate patient who develops respiratory distress.

3 Movement of ET tube
- Repeat taping or securing procedure.
- In very active patients without facial injury who are at risk for self-extubation, consider applying a second piece of tape around back of head.

4 Pressure area around tracheostomy tube
- Increase frequency of tracheostomy care. Keep dressing under faceplate at all times.
- Consider using double dressing or applying hydrocolloid or stoma adhesive dressing around stoma.

RECORDING AND REPORTING

- Record respiratory assessment measures before and after care.
- Record ET tube care: depth of ET tube, frequency and extent of care, patient tolerance of procedure, and special care of any unexpected outcomes related to presence of the tube.
- Record tracheostomy care: type and size of tracheostomy tube, frequency and extent of care, patient tolerance of procedure, and special care of any unexpected outcomes related to presence of the tube.

HOME CARE CONSIDERATIONS TRACHEOSTOMY ONLY (CLEVELAND CLINIC, 2010A).

- Instruct family caregivers in how to obtain supplies. Routine tracheostomy care should be done at least once a day after discharge from hospital. At home clean technique is used with nonsterile gloves.
- Immediately after tracheostomy insertion, patients must communicate with others by writing or use of computer.
- Instruct caregivers in signs and symptoms of respiratory distress, tube dysfunction, and respiratory and stoma infections. Call health care provider if patient feels pain or discomfort longer than a week after insertion, if breathing does not improve after usual method of clearing secretions, or if secretions become thick or mucus plugs are present.
- When outside, use tracheostomy covers to protect from dust or cold air.
- Never remove the outer cannula unless instructed by health care provider to do so.

SKILL 40-3 CARE OF PATIENTS WITH CHEST TUBES

Delegation Considerations

The skill of care of patients with chest tubes cannot be delegated to nursing assistive personnel (NAP). Instruct the NAP about:

- Proper positioning of patient with chest tubes to facilitate chest tube drainage and optimal function of the system.
- How to safely ambulate and transfer patient with chest drainage.
- The appropriate setup of drainage equipment for the type of system to be used.
- Reporting to the nurse any changes in vital signs or SpO_2, chest pain, sudden shortness of breath, or excessive bubbling in water-seal chamber.
- Immediately notifying the nurse if there is disconnection of system, change in type and amount of drainage, sudden bleeding, or sudden cessation of bubbling in water-seal chamber.

Equipment

- Stethoscope
- Pulse oximeter
- Clean gloves
- Two rubber-tipped (also called *shodded*) hemostats for each tube
- 2-inch (5-cm) adhesive tape for taping connections
- Sterile gauze sponges
- Suction source and setup (wall canister or portable) if physician is inserting chest tube
- Water suction system: Add sterile water or normal saline (NS) solution to cover the lower 2.5 cm (1 inch) of water-seal U tube, sterile water or NS solution to put into the suction-control chamber if suction is to be used (see manufacturer directions)
- Waterless system: Add vial of 30 mL injectable sodium chloride or water, 20-mL syringe, 21-gauge needle, and antiseptic swab

STEP	RATIONALE
ASSESSMENT	
1 Identify the patient using two identifiers (i.e., name and birthday or name and account number) according to facility policy. Compare identifiers with information on the patient's medical record.	Ensures correct patient. Complies with recommended National Patient Safety Goal (TJC, 2011).
2 Assess pulmonary status,	
a. Signs and symptoms of increased respiratory distress (displaced trachea, decreased breath sounds over affected and nonaffected lungs, marked cyanosis, asymmetrical chest movements).	Baseline measures allow you to determine if signs and symptoms of respiratory distress improve after insertion of chest tube. If respiratory distress is not relieved or worsens or if there is sharp stabbing chest pain with or without decreased blood pressure and increased heart rate, notify health care provider immediately. These symptoms indicate a pneumothorax.
b. Assess for sharp, stabbing chest pain or chest pain on inspiration; hypotension; and tachycardia. Ask patient to rate level of comfort on a scale of 0 to 10.	Symptoms may indicate a tension pneumothorax. Presence of a pneumothorax or hemothorax is painful, often causing sharp inspiratory pain.
3 Obtain baseline and serial vital signs, level of cognition, and SpO_2.	Changes in pulse, SpO_2, and blood pressure often indicate infection, respiratory distress, or pain. Cognitive changes indicate hypoxia.
4 Assess patient's current hemoglobin and hematocrit levels	Provides measure reflecting blood loss and subsequent levels of oxygenation.
5 Observe chest tube status:	
a. Chest tube dressing and site surrounding tube insertion. Apply clean gloves if drainage is present.	Ensures that dressing is intact, without air or fluid leaks, and that area surrounding insertion site is free of drainage or skin irritation.

SKILL 40-3 CARE OF PATIENTS WITH CHEST TUBES—cont'd

STEP	RATIONALE
b. Tubing for kinks, dependent loops, or clots.	Maintains patent, freely draining system, preventing fluid accumulation in chest cavity. Presence of kinks, dependent loops, or clotted drainage increases patient's risk for infection, atelectasis, and tension pneumothorax (Centre for Reviews and Dissemination, 2008).
c. Check existing drainage system to ensure that it is upright and below level of tube insertion. Note amount of drainage in system (see illustration).	Facilitates drainage. Ensures that system is in this position to function properly.

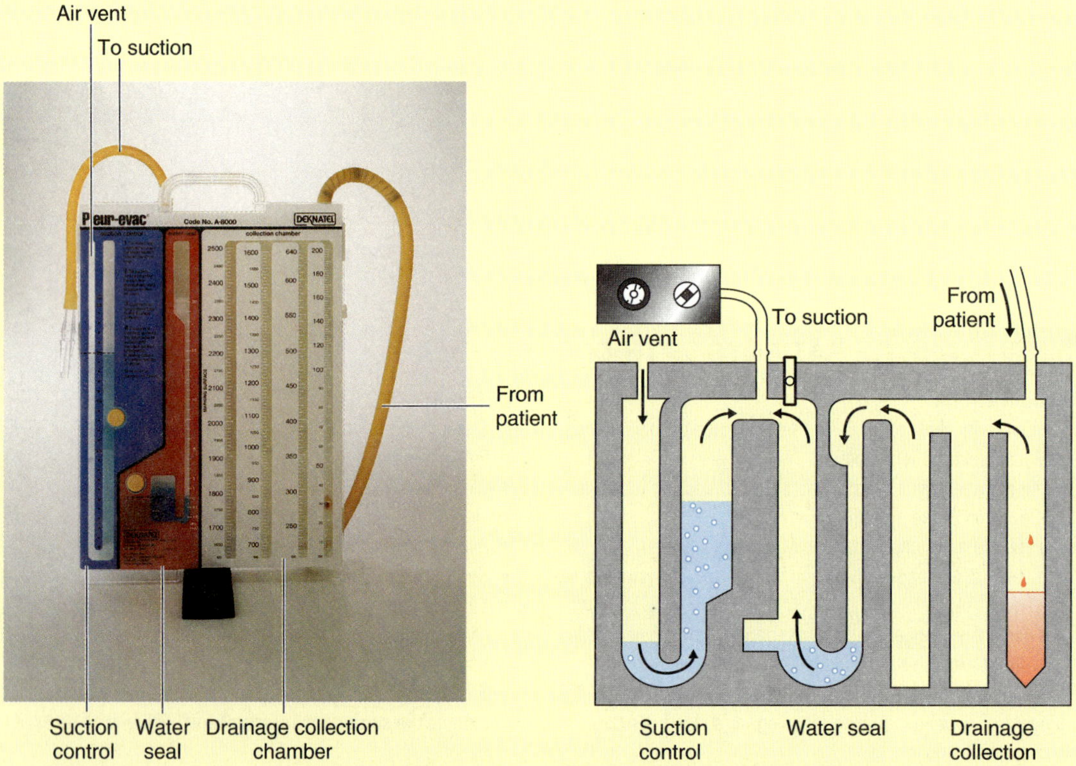

STEP 5c *Left,* Pleur-Evac drainage system, a commercial three-bottle chest drainage device. *Right,* Schematic of drainage device.

PLANNING

STEP	RATIONALE
1 Provide two rubber-tipped hemostats or approved clamps for each chest tube, attached to top of patient's bed with adhesive tape. Chest tubes are only clamped under specific circumstances per health care provider's order or nursing policy and procedure:	Hemostat has a covering to prevent it from penetrating chest tube. Use of these rubber-tipped hemostats or other clamps prevents air from reentering pleural space in emergencies (Rushing, 2007).
a. To assess air leak.	
b. To quickly empty or change disposable systems; performed by a nurse who has received education in the procedure.	
c. To assess if patient is ready to have chest tube removed (which is done by health care provider's order); monitor patient for recurrent pneumothorax (see illustration).	
2 Position patient.	Permits optimal drainage of fluid and/or air.
a. Semi-Fowler's position to evacuate air (pneumothorax)	Air rises to highest point in chest. Pneumothorax tubes are usually placed on anterior aspect at midclavicular line, second or third intercostal space.
b. High-Fowler's position to drain fluid (hemothorax, effusion)	Permits optimal drainage of fluid. Posterior tubes are placed on midaxillary line, eighth or ninth intercostal space.

IMPLEMENTATION

STEP	RATIONALE
1 Be sure that tube connection between chest and drainage tube is intact and taped.	Secures chest tube to drainage system and reduces risk of air leak causing breaks in airtight system.
a. Make sure that water-seal vent on drainage system is not occluded.	Permits displaced air to pass into atmosphere.
b. Make sure that suction-control chamber vent is not occluded when using suction. Waterless systems have relief valves without caps.	Provides safety factor of releasing excess negative pressure into atmosphere.

STEP	RATIONALE

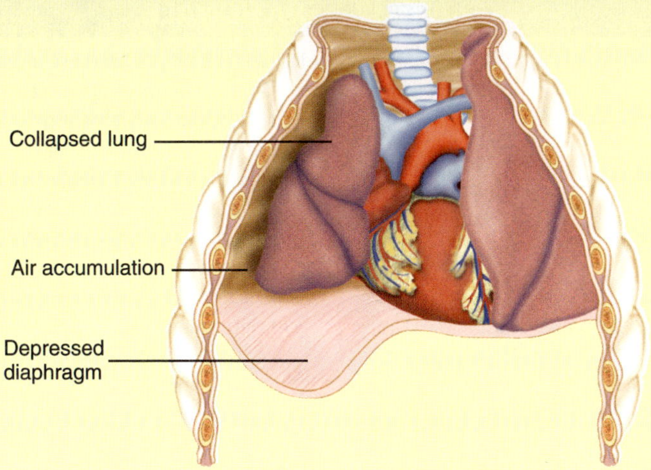

STEP 1c Pneumothorax. (From Seidel HM et al: *Mosby's guide to physical examination*, ed 7, St Louis, 2011, Mosby.)

STEP	RATIONALE
2 Coil excess drainage tubing on mattress next to patient. Secure with rubber band, safety pin, or plastic clamp. Allow enough room for patient to reposition.	Prevents excess tubing from hanging over edge of mattress in dependent loop. It is possible for drainage to collect in loop and occlude drainage system (Centre for Reviews and Dissemination, 2008).
3 Adjust tubing to hang in straight line from top of mattress to drainage chamber.	Promotes drainage and prevents fluid or blood from accumulating in pleural cavity (Halm, 2007).
4 If chest tube is draining fluid, indicate time (e.g., 0900) that you began measuring drainage on adhesive tape on drainage bottle or on write-on surface of disposable commercial system.	Provides a baseline for continuous assessment of type and quality of drainage.
5 Strip or milk chest tube only if indicated (this means compressing along tube to encourage clots to pass through the tube) (See agency policy.) Stripping is compression along length of tubing beginning at patient and continuing until reaching drainage unit. Milking is compressing and releasing tube sequentially.	Stripping may cause complications because it can create excessive negative intrapleural pressure (over 100 cm H_2O). Milking causes less of a pressure change and is recommended (Halm, 2007).
a. Manipulate postoperative mediastinal chest tubes if assessment indicates an obstruction or decreased drainage from clots or debris in tubing.	Stripping is performed only if hospital policy permits and there is a health care provider's order. There is no evidence that stripping or milking increases output or causes significant complications (Centre for Reviews and Dissemination, 2008).
6 Perform hand hygiene.	Reduces transmission of infection.

EVALUATION

STEP	RATIONALE
1 Monitor vital signs and pulse oximetry as ordered or if patient's condition changes.	Provides ongoing data about patient's level of oxygenation.
Evaluate patient for decreased respiratory distress and chest pain, auscultate lung sounds over affected lung area, and monitor SpO_2.	Increasing respiratory distress, decreased breath sounds, marked cyanosis, asymmetrical chest wall movements, presence of subcutaneous emphysema around insertion site or neck, hypotension, tachycardia, and/or mediastinal shift are critical and indicate a severe change in patient status such as excessive blood loss or tension pneumothorax. Notify health care provider immediately.
2 Observe:	
a. Appearance of chest tube dressing.	Drainage is often caused by tube occlusion, causing drainage to exit around tube.

CLINICAL DECISION: *Check the dressing carefully because it needs to remain occlusive. It can come loose from the skin, although this is not readily apparent. Assess for drainage and reinforce to maintain seal. Follow hospital policy as needed.*

STEP	RATIONALE
b. Make sure that tubing is free of kinks and dependent loops.	Straight and coiled drainage tube positions are optimal for pleural drainage. However, when a dependent loop is unavoidable, periodic lifting and draining the tube promote pleural drainage.
c. Make sure that chest drainage system is upright and below level of tube insertion. Note presence of clots or debris in tubing. Monitor position of system relative to chest tube carefully, especially during patient transport.	System must be in the upright position to function and facilitate proper drainage.

SKILL 40-3 CARE OF PATIENTS WITH CHEST TUBES—cont'd

STEP	RATIONALE
d. Observe water seal for fluctuations with patient's inspiration and expiration.	Indicates appropriate function of negative pressure system.
(1) *Waterless system:* Diagnostic indicator for fluctuations with patient's inspirations and expirations	In nonmechanically ventilated patient, fluid rises in water seal or diagnostic indicator with inspiration and falls with expiration. Opposite occurs in patient who is mechanically ventilated. This indicates that system is functioning properly (Lewis et al., 2007).
(2) *Water-seal system:* Bubbling in water-seal chamber	When system is initially connected to patient, expect bubbles from the chamber. These are from air present in system and from patient's intrapleural space. After a short time bubbling stops. Fluid continues to fluctuate in water seal on inspiration and expiration until lung reexpands or system is occluded.
(3) *Water-seal system:* Bubbling in suction-control chamber (when using suction)	Suction-control chamber has constant gentle bubbling. Tubing remains free of obstruction, and suction source is turned to appropriate setting.
e. Observe type and amount of fluid drainage: note color of drainage and skin color. Look at fluid in drainage tubing and not just in collection chamber. What is the normal amount of drainage? Is it bright red, dark red, or pink? Is it opaque, or can you see through it?	Character of drainage indicated if it is as expected or if infection or hemorrhage is developing.
(1) *In adult:* less than 50 to 200 mL/hr immediately after surgery in a mediastinal chest tube; approximately 500 mL in first 24 hours.	Dark-red drainage is normal only in postoperative period, turning serous with time.
(2) Between 100 and 300 mL of fluid drains in a pleural chest tube in an adult during first 3 hours after insertion. Rate decreases after 2 hours; expect 500 to 1000 mL in first 24 hours. Drainage is grossly bloody during first several hours after surgery and then changes to serous. Sudden gush of drainage is often retained blood and not active bleeding and is usually the result of patient repositioning (Lewis et al., 2007).	Reexpansion of lungs forces drainage into tube. Coughing also causes large gushes of drainage or air. Report excessive amounts and/or continued presence of frank, bloody drainage the first several hours after surgery to health care provider, along with patient's vital signs and respiratory status.

CLINICAL DECISION: *If drainage increases suddenly or is bright red or if there is more than 100 mL/hr of bloody drainage (except for the first 3 hours after surgery), notify the health care provider, remain with the patient, and assess vital signs and cardiopulmonary status. This may indicate hemorrhage or perforation of the lung.*

STEP	RATIONALE
f. *Waterless system:* The suction control (float ball) indicates the amount of suction that patient's intrapleural space is receiving.	Suction float ball dictates amount of suction in system. Float ball allows no more suction than dictated by its setting. If suction source is set too low, suction float ball cannot reach prescribed setting. In this case increase suction for float ball to reach the prescribed setting.
g. Ask patient to rate level of comfort on a scale of 0 to 10.	Indicates need for analgesia. Patient with chest tube discomfort hesitates to take deep breaths and as a result is at risk for pneumonia and atelectasis.

UNEXPECTED OUTCOMES AND RELATED INTERVENTIONS

1 Air leak unrelated to patient respirations
- Assess all connections between patient and drainage system to find source and tighten any loose connections (Coughlin and Parchinsky, 2006).
- If air leak persists, notify health care provider to change drainage system.

2 Tension pneumothorax present
- Determine that chest tubes are not clamped, kinked, or occluded. Obstructed chest tubes trap air in intrapleural space when air leak originates within patient and can cause a tension pneumothorax.
- Notify patient's health care provider immediately.
- Prepare immediately for another chest tube insertion; obtain a flutter (Heimlich) valve or large-gauge needle for short-term emergency release of air in intrapleural space; have emergency equipment (e.g., oxygen, code cart) near patient.

3 Continuous bubbling in water-seal chamber, indicating that leak is between patient and water seal
- Tighten loose connections between patient and water-seal system.
- Check agency policy and, if instructed, cross-clamp chest tube closer to patient's chest using hemostat clamps. If bubbling stops, the air leak is inside patient's thorax or at chest tube insertion site.
- Unclamp chest tube.
- Reinforce dressing.
- Notify health care provider.

RECORDING AND REPORTING

- Record and report patency of chest tube; presence, type, and amount of drainage; presence of fluctuations; patient's vital signs; chest dressing status; amount of suction and/or water seal; and patient's level of comfort.

HOME CARE CONSIDERATIONS

- Patients with chronic conditions (e.g., uncomplicated pneumothorax, effusions, empyema) that require long-term chest tube may be discharged with smaller mobile drains. These systems do not have a suction-control chamber and use a mechanical one-way valve instead of a water-seal chamber.
- Instruct patient in how to ambulate and remain active with a mobile chest tube drainage system.
- Provide patient with information as to when to contact health care professionals regarding changes in health status or drainage system (e.g., chest pain, breathlessness, change in drainage).

SKILL 40-4 APPLYING A NASAL CANNULA OR OXYGEN MASK

View Video!

Delegation Considerations

The skill of applying (not adjusting oxygen flow) a nasal cannula or oxygen mask can be delegated to nursing assistive personnel (NAP). The nurse is responsible for assessing patient's respiratory system; response to oxygen therapy; and setup of oxygen therapy, including adjustment of oxygen flow rate. Direct the NAP by:

- Informing how to safely position and adjust the device (e.g., loosening the strap on oxygen mask) and clarifying its correct placement and positioning.
- Instructing to inform the nurse immediately about any vital sign changes; skin irritation from the cannula, mask, or straps; if patient reports pain or breathlessness; or if patient presents with decreased level of consciousness or increased confusion.
- Having personnel provide skin care around patient's ears and nose.

Equipment

- Oxygen-delivery device as ordered by patient's health care provider
- Oxygen tubing (consider extension tubing)
- Humidifier if indicated
- Sterile water for humidifier
- Oxygen source
- Oxygen flowmeter
- Stethoscope, pulse oximeter
- Appropriate room signs

STEP	RATIONALE
ASSESSMENT	
1 Identify the patient using two identifiers (i.e., name and birth date or name and account number) according to facility policy. Compare identifiers with information on the patient's medical record.	Ensures correct patient. Complies with recommended National Patient Safety Goal (TJC, 2011).
2 Assess patient's respiratory status, including symmetry of chest wall expansion, chest wall abnormalities (e.g., kyphosis), temporary conditions (e.g., pregnancy, trauma) affecting ventilation, respiratory rate and depth, sputum production, and lung sounds.	Decreased chest wall movement, crackles or decreased lung sounds, increased respiratory rate, increased sputum production, and/or hypoxia indicate need for noninvasive ventilation to improve oxygenation.
3 Observe for patent airway and remove secretions by having patient cough and expectorate mucus or by suctioning.	Presence of airway secretions decreases effectiveness of oxygen delivery by plugging airway.

CLINICAL DECISION: *Patients with sudden changes in their vital signs, level of consciousness, or behavior are often experiencing profound hypoxia. Patients who demonstrate subtle changes over time have worsening of a chronic or existing condition or a new medical condition (Jarvis, 2006).*

STEP	RATIONALE
4 Obtain patient's most recent SpO_2 or arterial blood gas (ABG) values if available.	Provides objective baseline data to use to compare outcome of oxygen therapy.
5 Review patient's medical record for medical order for oxygen, noting delivery method, flow rate, and duration of oxygen therapy.	Ensures safe and accurate oxygen administration. Safe oxygen delivery includes the six rights of medication administration.
PLANNING	
1 Explain to patient and family what happens during procedure and the purpose of oxygen therapy.	Decreases patient's anxiety, which reduces oxygen consumption and increases patient/family adherence and cooperation.
IMPLEMENTATION	
1 Perform hand hygiene.	Reduces transmission of infection.
2 Attach oxygen-delivery device (e.g., nasal cannula or mask) to oxygen tubing and attach to humidified oxygen source adjusted to prescribed flow rate (see illustration).	Humidity prevents drying of nasal and oral mucous membranes and airway secretions. Ensures correct oxygen delivery.
3 Position tips of nasal cannula properly in patient's nares and adjust elastic headband or plastic slide on cannula so it is snug and comfortable (see illustration). Position face mask so it is snug and comfortable. If using an oxygen mask, adjust elastic headband until mask fits comfortably over patient's face and mouth.	Directs flow of oxygen into patient's upper respiratory tract. Patient is more likely to keep cannula or face mask in place if it fits comfortably.

SKILL 40-4 APPLYING A NASAL CANNULA OR OXYGEN MASK—cont'd

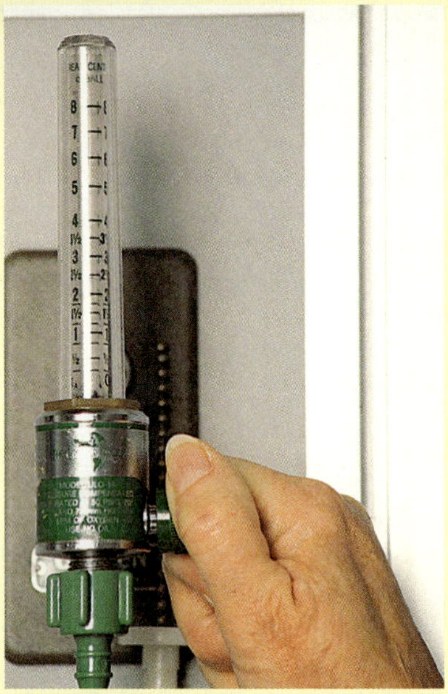

STEP 2 Adjusting flowmeter to prescribed oxygen flow rate.

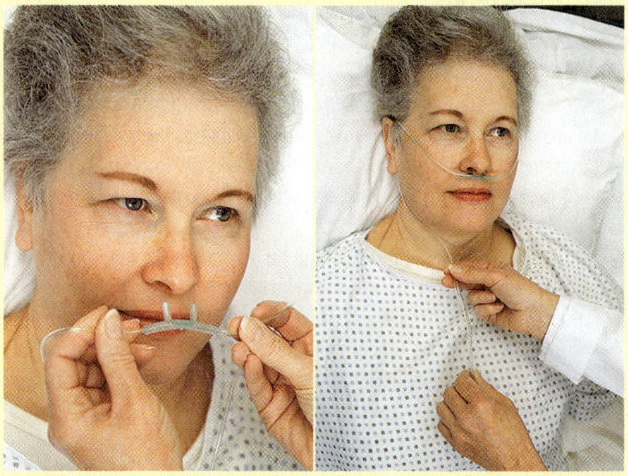

STEP 3 Applying nasal cannula and adjusting fit to patient comfort.

STEP	RATIONALE
4 Maintain sufficient slack on oxygen tubing and secure to patient's clothes.	Allows patient to turn head without removing oxygen mask or dislodging cannula and reduces pressure on tips of nares.
5 Observe for proper functioning of oxygen-delivery device:	Ensures patency of delivery device and proper oxygen flow.
a. *Nasal cannula:* Cannula is positioned properly in nares with humidification functioning.	Oxygen therapy causes drying of nasal mucosa. Oxygen delivered at flow rates greater than 4 L/min must be humidified (AARC, 2002).
b. *Reservoir nasal cannula Oxymizer:* Fit as for nasal cannula. Reservoir is positioned under patient's nose or worn as a pendant.	Delivers higher flow of oxygen than cannula without changing to a mask, which is claustrophobic for some patients. Delivers a 2:1 ratio (e.g., 6 L/min nasal cannula is approximately equivalent to 3.5 L/min with Oxymizer device).
c. *Nonrebreathing mask:* Apply mask over patient's mouth and nose to form tight seal. Valves on mask close so exhaled air does not enter reservoir bag.	Does not allow exhaled air to be rebreathed. Valves on mask side ports permit exhalation but close during inhalation to prevent inhaling room air.
d. *Partial rebreathing mask:* Apply mask over patient's mouth and nose to form tight seal. Ensure that bag remains partially inflated.	Allow exhaled air to mix with inhaled air. Port on side of mask permits most of expired air to escape; however, the bag remains partially inflated.
e. *Venturi mask:* Apply mask over patient's mouth and nose to form a tight seal. Select appropriate flow rate.	Reduces carbon dioxide buildup.
f. *Face tent:* Apply tent under patient's chin and over mouth and nose. It will be loose, and a mist is always present.	Excellent source of humidification; however, you cannot control oxygen concentrations.
6 Verify setting on flowmeter and oxygen source for proper setup and prescribed flow rate.	Ensures delivery of prescribed oxygen therapy in conjunction with the specific cannula/mask.
7 Check cannula/mask every 8 hours. Keep humidification container filled at all times.	Ensures patency of cannula and oxygen flow. Oxygen is a dry gas: when it is administered via any route, you must add humidification so the patient inhales humidified oxygen (Woodrow, 2007).
8 Perform hand hygiene.	Reduces transmission of microorganisms.

EVALUATION

1 Monitor patient's response to changes in oxygen flow rate with pulse oximetry. Note: Monitor ABGs when ordered; however, obtaining ABG measurement is an invasive procedure, and ABGs are not measured frequently.	Continual monitoring with pulse oximetry is required for patients on oxygen therapy. Base changes in supplemental oxygen on individual patient's oxygen saturation levels.
2 Observe for decreased anxiety, improved level of consciousness and cognitive abilities, decreased fatigue, absence of dizziness, decreased respiratory rate, improved color, improved oxygen saturation, and return to patient's baseline vital signs.	Evaluates patient's response to supplemental oxygen. As patient's oxygen level improves, physical signs and symptoms improve.
3 Check adequacy of oxygen flow each shift.	Ensures patency of oxygen-delivery device.
4 Observe patient's external ears, bridge of nose, nares, and nasal mucous membranes for evidence of skin breakdown.	Oxygen therapy sometimes causes drying of nasal mucosa. The delivery device can cause skin breakdown where it comes in contact with face, neck, and ears.

UNEXPECTED OUTCOMES AND RELATED INTERVENTIONS

1 Patient experiences continued hypoxia.
- Check that oxygen-delivery device is patent, not kinked, and attached to oxygen flowmeter.
- Check oxygen level set on flowmeter; determine if delivered amount is consistent with health care provider's order.
- Obtain orders for follow-up pulse oximetry monitoring or ABG assessment.
- Consider measures to improve airway patency, coughing techniques, and oropharyngeal suctioning.
- Notify health care provider.

2 Dry nasal and upper airway mucosa or epistaxis.
- If oxygen flow rate is greater than 4 L/min, determine need for humidification.
- Assess patient's fluid status and increase fluids if appropriate.
- Provide frequent oral care.
- Obtain health care provider's order for use of sterile nasal saline intermittently.

3 Skin irritation or breakdown (e.g., at ears, bridge of nose, nares, other pressure areas).
- Adjust tightness of elastic strap to looser level.
- Provide good hygiene and skin care around the ears.
- Use soft, woven 4 × 4s as nonabrasive pad between elastic and ears.
- Reposition elastic strap frequently.

RECORDING AND REPORTING

- Record and report type of oxygen-delivery device and liter flow in medical record; document patient and family education.
- Record respiratory assessment findings; patient response to oxygen therapy, and any adverse reactions or side effects.
- Report any unexpected outcomes to health care provider or nurse in charge.

SKILL 40-5 USING HOME OXYGEN EQUIPMENT

Delegation Considerations

The skill of administering home oxygen equipment cannot be delegated to nursing assistive personnel (NAP). Instruct the NAP about:
- The unique needs of patient (e.g., amount of assistance in applying nasal cannula or mask) and any assistance needed in filling liquid canisters.
- The type of equipment patient should have in the home and the oxygen flow rate.
- Immediately reporting to the nurse increased rate of breathing, decreased level of consciousness, increased confusion, and pain.

Equipment
- Nasal cannula equipment (see Skill 40-4)
- Humidification device if oxygen delivery greater than 4 L/min
- Oxygen tubing available in lengths of 50 feet
- Home low-flow oxygen-delivery system with appropriate equipment

STEP	RATIONALE
ASSESSMENT	
1 While patient is still in the hospital, determine patient's or family caregiver's ability to use oxygen equipment correctly. In home setting reassess for appropriate use of equipment.	Physical or cognitive impairments necessitate instructing family member or significant other how to operate home oxygen equipment. Ongoing assessment enables nurse to determine specific components of skill that patient or family can complete easily.
2 Assess home environment for adequate electrical service if oxygen concentrator is ordered.	Oxygen concentrators require electricity to work. Continuous oxygen therapy must not be interrupted.
3 Assess patient's and family's ability to observe for signs and symptoms of hypoxia: apprehension, anxiety, decreased ability to concentrate, decreased level of consciousness, increased fatigue, dizziness, behavioral changes, increased pulse, increased respiratory rate, pallor, or cyanosis of the mucous membranes.	Hypoxia occurs at home despite use of oxygen therapy. Worsening of patient's physical condition or another underlying condition such as change in the respiratory status can cause hypoxia.
PLANNING	
1 Identify the patient using two identifiers (i.e., name and birth date or name and account number) according to facility policy. Compare identifiers with information on the patient's medical record.	Ensures correct patient. Complies with recommended National Patient Safety Goal (TJC, 2011).
2 Determine appropriate resources in community for equipment and assistance, including maintenance and repair services and medical equipment supplier.	Ensures readily available assistance for patients with home oxygen systems. Delivery and setup with basic instruction on how to use and maintain the home oxygen equipment must be in accordance with federal, state, and local laws (AARC, 2007).

SKILL 40-5 USING HOME OXYGEN EQUIPMENT—cont'd

STEP	RATIONALE
3 In case of power failure, determine appropriate backup systems when using compressor. Have spare oxygen tank available.	Many municipalities require that patients with home oxygen equipment notify emergency medical service (EMS) before bringing the equipment home. When there is a power outage, EMS calls the home, and in some cases the home is on a priority list for power restoration.
4 Obtain appropriate referrals to determine if patient meets standards for third-party reimbursement.	Indications include (1) a PaO_2 less than or equal to 55 mm Hg or SaO_2 less than or equal to 88% breathing room air; (2) PaO_2 less than or equal to 56-59 mm Hg or SaO_2 less than or equal to 89% with conditions such as cor pulmonale, heart failure, or hematocrit greater than 56%; (3) oxygen therapy is needed during activities that cause hypoxia such as ambulation, sleep, or exercise causing an SaO_2 of less than or equal to 88% (AARC, 2007).

IMPLEMENTATION

STEP	RATIONALE
1 Perform hand hygiene.	Reduces transmission of infection.
2 Place oxygen-delivery system in clutter-free environment that is well ventilated; away from walls, drapes, bedding, and combustible materials; and at least 8 feet from heat source.	Prevents injury from improper placement of oxygen equipment.
3 Demonstrate each step for preparation and completion of oxygen therapy.	Teaches psychomotor skills and enables patient to ask questions.
a. **Compressed oxygen system**—available in large cylinders as stationary units or smaller, lightweight cylinders in carrying bags and/or wheel carts.	Smaller units are used for ambulation and as a backup of stationary unit if there is power failure or equipment malfunction (AARC, 2007).
(1) Turn cylinder valve counterclockwise two or three turns with wrench. Store wrench with oxygen tank.	Turns on oxygen. Keeps wrench available.
(2) Check cylinders by reading amount on pressure gauge (see illustration).	Verifies adequate oxygen supply for patient use.

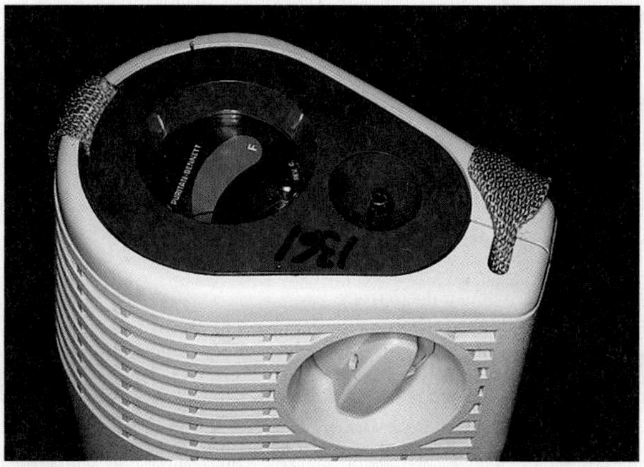

STEP 3a(2) Verify oxygen level by reading gauge on top of canister.

STEP	RATIONALE
b. **Oxygen concentrator system**—available as stationary unit or portable device.	Extracts oxygen from other gases in atmospheric air (AARC, 2007).
(1) Plug concentrator into appropriate outlet.	Provides power source. Make sure that it is in an open area and never in a closet or other closed space (Cleveland Clinic, 2010b).
(2) Turn on power switch.	Starts concentrator motor.
(3) Alarm sounds for a few seconds.	Alarm turns off when desired pressure inside concentrator is reached.
c. **Liquid oxygen systems**—available in large-reservoir canisters that can be used to refill a smaller portable unit (AARC, 2007). Portable unit weighs 5 to 13 lbs and can be carried with a shoulder strap or pulled on a cart.	When liquid oxygen is warmed, it goes from liquid to gas. More oxygen can be stored as a liquid than gas.
d. Refill oxygen tank	
(1) Check for amount of oxygen in tank	If not in use, evaporation empties portable canister; thus always check it before use (Cleveland Clinic, 2001b).
(2) Wipe both filling connectors with clean, dry, lint-free cloth.	Removes dust and moisture from system.
(3) Turn off flow selector of ambulatory unit.	
(4) Attach ambulatory unit to stationary reservoir by inserting adapter from ambulatory tank into adapter of stationary reservoir.	

STEP	RATIONALE
(5) Open fill valve on ambulatory tank and apply firm pressure to top of stationary reservoir (see illustration). Stay with unit while it is filling. You will hear a loud hissing noise. Tank fills in about 2 minutes.	Prevents leaking of oxygen during filling process. If oxygen leaks during filling process, connection between ambulatory tank and reservoir ices up and valves stick together.

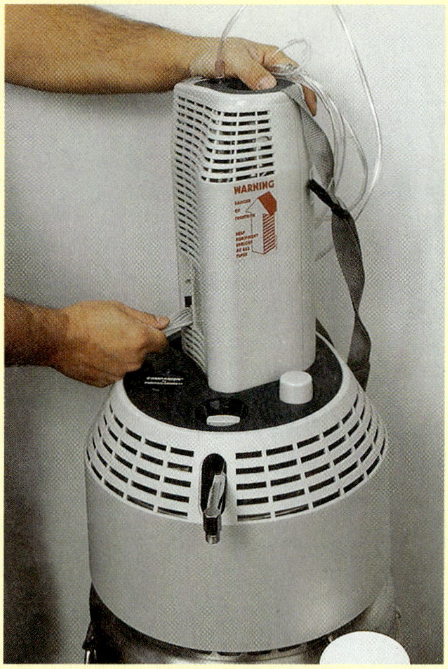

STEP 3d(5) Open fill valve on ambulatory tank while applying firm pressure to top of ambulatory unit.

(6) Disengage ambulatory unit from stationary reservoir when hissing noise changes and vapor cloud begins to form from stationary unit.	Overfilling causes ambulatory unit to malfunction caused by high pressure in tank.
(7) Wipe both filling connectors with clean, dry, lint-free cloth.	Ice sometimes forms during filling. Removes moisture from oxygen system.

CLINICAL DECISION: *If ambulatory unit does not separate easily, valves from reservoir and ambulatory unit may be frozen together. Wait until valves warm to disengage (about 5 to 10 minutes). Do not touch any frosted areas because contact with skin causes skin damage from frostbite.*

4 Connect oxygen-delivery device to oxygen system.	Connects oxygen source to delivery system.
5 Adjust to prescribed flow rate (L/min).	Ensures appropriate oxygen prescription.
6 Place oxygen-delivery device on patient.	Delivers oxygen to patient.
7 Perform hand hygiene.	Reduces transmission of microorganisms.
8 Instruct patient and family not to change oxygen flow rate.	
9 Guide patient and family caregiver as they perform each step. Provide written material for reinforcement and review.	Allows nurse to correct for errors in technique and discuss their implications.
10 Instruct patient and family caregiver to notify health care provider if signs or symptoms of hypoxia or respiratory tract infection (e.g., fever, increased sputum, change in color of sputum, or odor) occur.	Respiratory tract infections increase oxygen demand and affect oxygen transfer from lungs to blood. Can create severe exacerbation of patient's pulmonary disease.
11 Discuss emergency plan for power loss, natural disaster, and acute respiratory distress. Have patient or family/caregiver call 911 and notify health care provider and home care agency.	Ensures appropriate response and prevents worsening of patient's condition.
12 Instruct patient and family caregiver in safe home oxygen practices, including not allowing smoking in the house, keeping oxygen tanks away from open flame, and storing tanks upright.	Ensures safe use of oxygen in the home and prevents injury to patient and family.
13 Monitor oxygen-delivery rate. All oxygen-delivery equipment should be checked at least daily by patient or caregiver.	Determines if patient is using oxygen at prescribed rate.
14 Oxygen-delivery equipment must be maintained and serviced routinely according to manufacturer's guidelines (AARC, 2007).	Routine maintenance ensures proper function of equipment.

SKILL 40-5 USING HOME OXYGEN EQUIPMENT—cont'd

STEP	RATIONALE
EVALUATION	
1 Ask patient and family caregiver about ease of administering or problems associated with home oxygen.	Determines ability of patient and family to deal with stressors associated with home oxygen use.
2 Ask patient and family caregiver to state safety guidelines, emergency precautions, and emergency plan.	Determines patient's knowledge of what to do if power fails, there is a failure in equipment, or patient's status worsens.

UNEXPECTED OUTCOMES AND RELATED INTERVENTIONS

1 Patient reports no oxygen flow.
- Check tank pressure gauge. If level of oxygen is low, refill tank if portable or provide alternate source of oxygen such as concentrator.
- Notify home oxygen supplier of need for refill.
- Reassure patient and family.

2 Patient or family caregiver is unable to fill portable liquid oxygen from main source.
- Check to see that portable tank is connected correctly.
- Determine if valve is frozen.
- Contact home oxygen supplier for service visit.
- Provide alternate oxygen source if necessary.

RECORDING AND REPORTING

- Record teaching plan and patient's and family caregiver's ability to safely use home oxygen equipment; report type of home oxygen equipment to be used, patient's and family's understanding of how to use equipment, knowledge of safety guidelines and unexpected outcomes, and ability to return demonstrate proper use of oxygen-delivery device.

KEY POINTS

- The primary function of the lungs is to transfer oxygen from the atmosphere into the alveoli and carbon dioxide out of the body as a waste product.
- Changes in intrapleural and intraalveolar pressures and lung volumes cause the process of inspiration (active process) and expiration (passive process).
- Decreased hemoglobin levels alter the patient's ability to transport oxygen.
- Impaired chest wall movement reduces the level of tissue oxygenation.
- Hyperventilation is a respiratory rate greater than that required to maintain normal levels of carbon dioxide.
- Hypoventilation causes carbon dioxide retention.
- Hypoxia occurs if the amount of oxygen delivered to tissues is too low.
- The primary functions of the heart are to deliver deoxygenated blood to the lungs for oxygenation and oxygen and nutrients to the tissues.
- The nursing history includes information about the patient's cough, dyspnea, fatigue, wheezing, chest pain, environmental exposures, respiratory infection, cardiopulmonary risk factors, and use of medications.
- Nursing assessment includes respiratory pattern, thoracic inspection, palpation, and auscultation for deviations from normal.
- Diagnostic and laboratory tests complete the database for a patient with decreased oxygenation.
- Health promotion includes vaccinations against flu and pneumonia, exercise programs, nutrition support, smoking cessation, and environmental assessment for pollutants and air quality.
- Airway maintenance requires mobilization of secretions by increased fluid intake, humidification, or nebulization.
- Breathing exercises improve ventilation, oxygenation, and sensations of dyspnea.
- Chest physiotherapy includes postural drainage, percussion, and vibration to mobilize pulmonary secretions.
- Airway maintenance may require use of artificial airways and suctioning.
- Promotion of lung expansion can be achieved by mobility, positioning, incentive spirometry, and chest tube insertion.
- Nasal cannulas and oxygen masks deliver oxygen therapy, which improves the levels of tissue oxygenation.
- Learning breathing exercises, including pursed-lip breathing and diaphragmatic breathing, benefits patients with chronic pulmonary diseases.

CLINICAL APPLICATION QUESTIONS

Preparing for Clinical Practice

Forty-eight hours after admission to the hospital, Mr. Edwards had abnormal lung sounds (crackles) in the left base and both upper lobes. His vital signs were as follows: temperature, 102.4° F (39.1° C); blood pressure, 140/92 mm Hg; pulse, 110 beats/min; respirations, 32 breaths/min; and SpO_2, 82%. He could not lie flat, and it was difficult for him to speak because of dyspnea. He was placed on a nonrebreather mask at an oxygen concentration of 60%. He was also unable to cough up any sputum.

Mr. Edwards's health care provider determined his pneumonia had worsened. A chest x-ray film and arterial blood gas levels were obtained. His chest x-ray film indicated that both upper lobes and the left lower lobe had infiltrates. The arterial blood gas levels indicated respiratory acidosis (see Chapter 41). His PaO_2 was 55 mm Hg, $PaCO_2$ was 65 mm Hg, pH was 7.30, and SpO_2 was

80%. He spent 5 days in an intensive care unit (ICU) and 2 weeks in a transitional care unit. He is being discharged on home oxygen therapy. His discharge plan includes an outpatient rehabilitation program to begin 1 month after discharge.

1. When Mr. Edwards was hypoxic (PaO_2 55 mm Hg, SpO_2 80%), which additional assessment findings would you expect to find?
2. Based on the case scenario and information in Question 1, determine the two priority nursing diagnoses for Mr. Edwards and list the appropriate interventions or nursing activities that you must implement.
3. What do you need to do to prepare Mr. and Mrs. Edwards for home oxygen therapy?

evolve *Answers to Clinical Application Questions can be found on the Evolve website.*

REVIEW QUESTIONS

Are You Ready to Test Your Nursing Knowledge?

1. A patient who started smoking in adolescence and continues to smoke 40 years later comes to the clinic. The nurse understands that this patient has an increased risk for being diagnosed with which disorder:
   1. Alcoholism and hypertension
   2. Obesity and diabetes
   3. Stress-related illnesses
   4. Cardiopulmonary disease and lung cancer
2. A patient has been diagnosed with severe iron deficiency anemia. During physical assessment for which of the following symptoms would the nurse assess to determine the patient's oxygen status?
   1. Increased breathlessness but increased activity tolerance
   2. Decreased breathlessness and decreased activity tolerance
   3. Increased activity tolerance and decreased breathlessness
   4. Decreased activity tolerance and increased breathlessness
3. A patient is admitted to the emergency department with suspected carbon monoxide poisoning. Even though the patient's color is ruddy, not cyanotic, the nurse understands that the patient is at a risk for decreased oxygen-carrying capacity of blood because carbon monoxide does which of the following:
   1. Stimulates hyperventilation, causing respiratory alkalosis
   2. Forms a strong bond with hemoglobin, creating a functional anemia.
   3. Stimulates hypoventilation, causing respiratory acidosis
   4. Causes alveoli to overinflate, leading to atelectasis
4. A 6-year-old boy is admitted to the pediatric unit with chills and a fever of 104° F (40° C). What physiological process explains why the child is at risk for developing dyspnea?
   1. Fever increases metabolic demands, requiring increased oxygen need.
   2. Blood glucose stores are depleted, and the cells do not have energy to use oxygen.
   3. Carbon dioxide production increases as result of hyperventilation.
   4. Carbon dioxide production decreases as a result of hypoventilation.
5. A patient is admitted with the diagnosis of severe left-sided heart failure. The nurse expects to auscultate which adventitious lung sounds?
   1. Sonorous wheezes in the left lower lung
   2. Rhonchi midsternum
   3. Crackles only in apex of lungs
   4. Inspiratory crackles in lung bases
6. The nurse is caring for a patient who has decreased mobility. Which intervention is a simple and cost-effective method for reducing the risks of stasis of pulmonary secretions and decreased chest wall expansion?
   1. Antibiotics
   2. Frequent change of position
   3. Oxygen humidification
   4. Chest physiotherapy
7. A patient is admitted with severe lobar pneumonia. Which of the following assessment findings would indicate that the patient needs airway suctioning?
   1. Coughing up thick sputum only occasionally
   2. Coughing up thin, watery sputum easily after nebulization
   3. Decreased independent ability to cough
   4. Lung sounds clear only after coughing
8. A patient was admitted after a motor vehicle accident with multiple fractured ribs. Respiratory assessment includes signs/symptoms of secondary pneumothorax, which includes which of the following?
   1. Sharp pleuritic pain that worsens on inspiration
   2. Crackles over lung bases of affected lung
   3. Tracheal deviation toward the affected lung
   4. Increased diaphragmatic excursion on side of rib fractures
9. A patient has been newly diagnosed with emphysema. In discussing his condition with the nurse, which of his statements would indicate a need for further education?
   1. "I'll make sure that I rest between activities so I don't get so short of breath."
   2. "I'll rest for 30 minutes before I eat my meal."
   3. "If I have trouble breathing at night, I'll use two to three pillows to prop up."
   4. "If I get short of breath, I'll turn up my oxygen level to 6 L/min."
10. The nurse goes to assess a new patient and finds him lying supine in bed. The patient tells the nurse that he feels short of breath. Which nursing action should the nurse perform first?
    1. Raise the head of the bed to 45 degrees.
    2. Take his oxygen saturation with a pulse oximeter.
    3. Take his blood pressure and respiratory rate.
    4. Notify the health care provider of his shortness of breath.
11. The nurse is caring for a patient who exhibits labored breathing and uses accessory muscles. The patient has crackles in both lung bases and diminished breath sounds. Which would be priority assessments for the nurse to perform? (Select all that apply.)
    1. SpO_2 levels
    2. Amount of sputum production
    3. Change in respiratory rate and pattern
    4. Pain in lower calf area
12. Which of the following statements made by a student nurse indicates the need for further teaching about suctioning a patient with an endotracheal tube?
    1. "Suctioning the patient requires sterile technique."
    2. "I'll apply suction while rotating and withdrawing the suction catheter."
    3. "I'll suction the mouth after I suction the endotracheal tube."
    4. "I'll instill 5 mL of normal saline into the tube before hyperoxygenating the patient."
13. Two hours after surgery the nurse assesses a patient who had a chest tube inserted during surgery. There is 200 mL of

dark-red drainage in the chest tube at this time. What is the appropriate action for the nurse to perform?
1. Record the amount and continue to monitor drainage
2. Notify the health care provider
3. Strip the chest tube starting at the chest
4. Increase the suction by 10 mm Hg

14. Which nursing intervention is appropriate for preventing atelectasis in the postoperative patient?
1. Postural drainage
2. Chest percussion
3. Incentive spirometer
4. Suctioning

15. The nurse needs to apply oxygen to a patient who has a precise oxygen level prescribed. Which of the following oxygen-delivery systems should the nurse select to administer the oxygen to the patient?
1. Nasal cannula
2. Venturi mask
3. Simple face mask without inflated reservoir bag
4. Plastic face mask with inflated reservoir bag

Answers: 1. 4; 2. 4; 3. 2; 4. 1; 5. 4; 6. 2; 7. 3; 8. 1; 9. 4; 10. 1; 11. 1, 2, 3; 12. 4; 13. 1; 14. 3; 15. 1.

REFERENCES

Ackley BJ, Ladwig, GB: *Nursing diagnosis handbook: an evidence-based guide to planning care*, ed 9, St Louis, 2011, Mosby.

American Association of Respiratory Care (AARC): Clinical practice guideline: Incentive spirometry, *Respir Care* 56(10):1600, 2011.

American Association of Respiratory Care (AARC): AARC clinical practice guideline, directed cough, *Respir Care* 38(5):495, 1993, http://www.rcjournal.com/cpgs/dccpg.html.

American Association of Respiratory Care (AARC): AARC clinical practice guideline, oxygen therapy for adults in the acute care facility—2002 revision and update, *Respir Care* 47:717, 2002.

American Association of Respiratory Care (AARC): AARC clinical practice guideline, nasotracheal suction—2004 revision and update, *Respir Care* 49:1080, 2004.

American Association of Respiratory Care (AARC): AARC clinical practice guideline, oxygen therapy in the home or alternate site health care facility—2007 revision and update, *Respir Care* 52:1063, 2007.

American Association of Respiratory Care (AARC): AARC clinical practice guideline, endotracheal suctioning of mechanically ventilated patients with artificial airways—2010 update, *Respir Care* 55(60):758, 2010a.

American Association of Respiratory Care (AARC): AARC clinical practice guideline, providing patient and caregiver training—2010, *Respir Care* 55:765, 2010b.

American Cancer Society (ACS): *Questions about smoking, tobacco, and health, 2010,* http://www.cancer.org/Cancer/CancerCauses/QuestionsaboutSmokingTob. Accessed August 18, 2010.

American Heart Association (AHA): *Women and coronary heart disease,* 2006a, http://www.americanheart.org/presenter.jhtml?identifier=2859. Accessed June 29, 2007.

American Heart Association (AHA): Community lay rescuer automated external defibrillator programs, *Circulation* 113:1260, 2006b.

American Heart Association (AHA): *Cardiopulmonary resuscitation (CPR) statistics,* 2010a, http://www.americanheart.org/print_presenter.jhtml;jsessionid=GZVUF13G0X1LACQFCX. Accessed September 1, 2010.

American Heart Association (AHA): Part 1: Executive Summary: 2010 American Heart Association guidelines for cardiopulmonary resuscitation and emergency cardiovascular care, *Circulation* 122(suppl):S640-S656, 2010b.

American Lung Association: *Big tobacco on campus: ending the addiction,* 2008, http://www.lungusa.org/stop-smoking/tobacco-control-advocacy/reports-resources/tobacco-policy-trend-reports/college-report.pdf. Accessed September 27, 2011.

American Lung Association: *Many lung diseases more prevalent in diverse populations,* 2010a, from http://www.lungusa.org/press-room/press-releases/many-lung-diseases-more.html. Accessed July 16, 2010.

American Lung Association: *State of the lung disease in diverse communities 2010,* 2010b, http://www.lungusa.org/assets/documents/publications/lung-disease-data/solddc_2010.pdf. Accessed September 27, 2011.

Carroll P: Keeping up with mobile chest drains, *RN* 68(10):26, 2005.

Centers for Disease Control and Prevention (CDC): *2008 Smoking cessation clinical practice guideline,* 2008, http://www.cdc.gov/tobacco/quit_smoking/cessation/index.htm. Accessed August 18, 2010.

Centers for Disease Control and Prevention (CDC): *Testing for TB infection*, Atlanta, 2010a, Centers for Disease Control and Prevention, http://www.cdc.gov/tb/topic/testing/default.htm .

Centers for Disease Control and Prevention (CDC): *Tuberculin testing and diagnosis,* Atlanta, 2010b, http:www.cdc.gov/tb/topic/testing/default.htm. Accessed September 8, 2010.

Centers for Disease Control and Prevention (CDC): *Adult immunization schedule 2010–11, National immunization program*, Atlanta, 2010c, Centers for Disease Control and Prevention, http://www.cdc.gov/vaccines/pubs/vis/default.htm.

Centers for Disease Control and Prevention (CDC): *Vaccines & immunizations: pneumococcal disease in short*, Atlanta, 2010d, Centers for Disease Control and Prevention, Vaccines and Preventable Diseases. http://www.cdc.gov/vaccines/vpd-vac/pneumo/in-short-both.htm.

Centers for Disease Control and Prevention (CDC): *Recommended adult immunization schedule—United States*, Atlanta, 2011, Centers for Disease Control and Prevention, Morbidity and Mortality Weekly, http://www.cdc.gov/mmwr/preview/mmwrhtml/mm604a10.htm?s_cid=mm6004a10_e.

Cleveland Clinic: *Information for patients: tracheostomy care*, Cleveland Clinic Head and Neck Institute, 2010a, http://my.clevelandclinic.org/head_neck/patients/head_neck_cancer/tracheostomy_care.aspx. Accessed July 14, 2010.

Cleveland Clinic: *Home oxygen therapy*, Cleveland Clinic Foundation, 2010b, http://www.cchs.net/health/health-info/docs/2400/2413.asp?index=8707. Accessed September 14, 2010.

Coughlin AM, Parchinsky C: Go with the flow of chest tube therapy, *Nursing 2006* 36(3):36, 2006.

Cystic Fibrosis Foundation (CFF): *An introduction to postural drainage & percussion—consumer fact sheet*, Bethesda, Md, 2005, Cystic Fibrosis Foundation.

Demir F, Dramali A: Requirement for 100% oxygen before and after closed suction. *J Adv Nurs* 51(3):245, 2005.

Environmental Protection Agency (EPA): *A citizen's guide to radon*, 2010, http://www.epa.gov/radon/pubs/citguide.html. Accessed August 18, 2010.

Hess DR: Tracheostomy tubes and related appliances, *Respir Care* 50:497, 2005.

Higgins D: Basic principles of caring for patients with a tracheostomy, *Nurs Times* 105(3):14, 2009

Hockenberry MJ, Wilson D: *Wong's nursing care of infants and children*, ed 9, St Louis, 2011, Mosby.

Johns Hopkins Medicine: *Stoma care,* 2010, http://www.hopkinsmedicine.org/se/util/display_mod.cfm?MODULE=se_server/mod/mod. Accessed July 14, 2010.

The Joint National Committee (JNC): The Seventh Report of the Joint National Committee on Prevention, Detection, Evaluation, and Treatment of High Blood Pressure—Complete Report, *Hypertension* 42:1206, 2003.

Lewis SL, et al: *Medical-surgical nursing: assessment and management of clinical problems*, ed 7, St Louis, 2007, Mosby.

Linton AD, Lach HW: *Matteson & McConnell's Gerontological nursing: concepts and practice*, ed 3, Philadelphia, 2007, Saunders Elsevier.

LungUSA: Facts about secondhand smoke: American Lung Association, 2010, http://www.lungusa.org/stop-smoking/health-effects/secondhand-smoke.html. Accessed July 16, 2010.

McCance KL, Huether SE: *Pathophysiology: the biologic basis for disease in adults and children*, ed 6, St Louis, 2010, Mosby Elsevier.

Meiner S: *Gerontologic nursing*, ed 4, St Louis, 2011, Mosby.

National Heart Lung and Blood Institute: *What is CPAP?* National Institutes of Health, 2010, http://www.nhlbi.nih.gov/health/dci/Diseases/cpap/cpap_what.html. Accessed August 25, 2010.

National Institute on Drug Abuse (NIDA): *NIDA InfoFacts: marijuana*, National Institutes of Health, 2009, http://drugabuse.gov/infofacts/marijuana.html. Accessed August 18, 2010.

National Institute on Drug Abuse (NIDA): *InfoFacts: cocaine*, National Institutes of Health, 2010, http://www.drugabuse.gov/infofacts/cocaine.html. Accessed August 18, 2010.

Roman M, Mercado D: Review of chest tube use, *Medsurg Nurs* 15(1):41, 2006.

Rushing J: Managing a water-seal chest drainage unit, *Nursing* 379(12):12, 2007.

Stoppler MC: *Is your child or teen "huffing"*, MedicineNet.com, 2005, http://www.medicinenet.com/script/main/art.asp?articlekey=47975. Accessed September 8, 2010.

Soo Hoo GW: Ventilation, noninvasive, http://emedicine.medscape.com/article/304235. Accessed August 25, 2010.

The Joint Commission: *2011 National Patient Safety Goals (NPGs)*, 2011, TJC; available at http://www.jointcommission.org/standards_information/npsgs.aspx.

Vollman K: Ask the experts, *Crit Care Nurs* 26(4):53, 2006.

Woodrow MA: Caring for patients receiving oxygen therapy, *Nurs Older Adults* 19(1):31, 2007.

RESEARCH REFERENCES

Agarwal R, et al: Role of noninvasive positive-pressure ventilation in postextubation respiratory failure: a meta-analysis, *Respir Care* 52(11):1472, 2007.

Basoglu O, et al: The efficacy of incentive spirometry in patients with COPD, *Respirology* 10:349, 2005.

Bourgault AM et al: Effects of endotracheal tube suctioning on arterial oxygen tension and heart rate variability, *Biol Res Nurs* 7:268, 2006.

Centre for Reviews and Dissemination: The nursing management of chest drains; a systematic review, *Joanna Briggs Institute for Evidence-Based Nursing and Midwifery* 3:5, 2008.

Gholamzadeh S, Javadi M: Effect of endotracheal suctioning on intracranial pressure in severe head-injured patients, *Crit Care* 13(suppl 1):80, 2009.

Halm MA: To strip or not to strip? Physiological effects of chest tube manipulation, *Am J Crit Care* 16:609, 2007.

Halm M, Krisko-Hagel K: Instilling normal saline with suctioning: beneficial technique or potentially harmful sacred cow, *Am J Crit Care* 17(5):469, 2008.

Jarvis H: Exploring the evidence base of the use of non-invasive ventilation, *Br J Nurs* 15:756, 2006.

Kuriakose A: Using the synergy model as best practice in endotracheal tube suctions of critically ill patients, *Dimens Crit Care Nurs* 27:10, 2008.

Labeau SO, et al: Prevention of ventilator-associated pneumonia with oral antiseptics: a systematic review and meta-analysis, *Lancet Infect Dis* 2011, Jul 25 [Epub ahead of print]; http://www.thelancet.com/journals/laninf/article/PIIS1473–3099%2811%2970127-X/abstract.

Lawrence VA, et al: Strategies to reduce postoperative pulmonary complications after noncardiothoracic surgery: systematic review for the American College of Physicians, *Ann Intern Med* 144:596, 2006.

Meek PM, Lareau SC: Critical outcomes in pulmonary rehabilitation: assessment and evaluation of dyspnea and fatigue, *J Rehabil Res Dev* 40(5):13, 2003, http://www.rehab.research.va.gov/jour/03/40/5Sup2/Meek.html.

Morris AC, et al: Reducing ventilator-associated pneumonia in intensive care: impact of implementing a care bundle. *Crit Care Med* 39(10):2218, 2011.

Needleman M, et al: Randomized controlled trial of toothbrushing to reduce ventilator-associated pneumonia pathogens and dental plaque in a critical care unit. *J Clin Periodont* 38(3):246, 2011.

Pederson CM, et al: Endotracheal suctioning of the adult intubated patient—what is the evidence? *Intensive Crit Care Nurs* 25:21, 2009.

Perme C, Chandrashekar R: Early mobility and walking program for patients in intensive care units: creating a standard of care, *Am J Crit Care* 18(3):212, 2009.

Rauen CA, et al: Seven evidenced-based practice habits: putting some sacred cows out to pasture, *Crit Care Nurs* 28(2):98, 2008.

Shaw LJ, et al: Women and ischemic heart disease: evolving knowledge, *J Am Coll Cardiol* 54(17):1561, 2009.

Sona CS, et al. The impact of a simple, low-cost oral care protocol on ventilator-associated pneumonia rates in a surgical intensive care unit. *J Intens Care Med* 24(1):54, 2009.

The Joint National Committee on Prevention, Detection, Evaluation and Treatment of High Blood Pressure (JNC): *The sixth report of the Joint National Committee on Prevention, Detection, Evaluation and Treatment of High Blood Pressure (JNC VII)*, Bethesda, Md, 2003, US Department of Health and Human Services, National Heart, Lung, and Blood Institute, http://www.nhlbi.nih.gov/guidelines/hypertension/express.pdf.

CHAPTER

41

Fluid, Electrolyte, and Acid-Base Balance

OBJECTIVES

- Describe the processes involved in regulating extracellular fluid volume, body fluid osmolality, and fluid distribution.
- Describe the processes involved in regulating plasma concentrations of potassium, calcium, magnesium, and phosphate ions.
- Describe the processes involved in regulating acid-base balance.
- Describe common fluid, electrolyte, and acid-base imbalances.
- Identify risk factors for fluid, electrolyte, and acid-base imbalances.
- Choose appropriate clinical assessments for specific fluid, electrolyte, and acid-base imbalances.
- Interpret basic fluid, electrolyte, and acid-base laboratory values.
- Apply the nursing process when caring for patients with fluid, electrolyte, and acid-base imbalances.
- Discuss purpose and procedure for initiation and maintenance of intravenous therapy.
- Calculate an intravenous flow rate.
- Describe how to measure and record fluid intake and output.
- Explain how to change intravenous solutions and tubing and discontinue an infusion.
- Describe potential complications of intravenous therapy and what to do if they occur.
- Discuss the procedure for initiating a blood transfusion and interventions to manage a transfusion reaction.

KEY TERMS

Acidosis, p. 893
Active transport, p. 884
Alkalosis, p. 893
Anion gap, p. 893
Anions, p. 883
Arterial blood gases (ABGs), p. 891
Autologous transfusion, p. 911
Buffers, p. 891
Cations, p. 883
Colloid osmotic pressure, p. 885
Colloids, p. 885
Crystalloids, p. 904
Dehydration, p. 887
Electrolytes, p. 883
Electronic infusion devices (EIDs), p. 907
Extracellular fluid (ECF), p. 883
Extracellular fluid volume deficit (ECV deficit), p. 887
Extracellular fluid volume excess (ECV excess), p. 887
Extravasation, p. 909
Filtration, p. 884
Fluid, p. 883
Hydrostatic pressure, p. 885
Hypercalcemia, p. 890
Hyperkalemia, p. 889
Hypermagnesemia, p. 891
Hypernatremia, p. 887
Hypertonic, p. 884
Hypocalcemia, p. 889
Hypokalemia, p. 889
Hypomagnesemia, p. 890
Hyponatremia, p. 887
Hypotonic, p. 884
Hypovolemia, p. 887
Infiltration, p. 909
Interstitial fluid, p. 883
Intracellular fluid (ICF), p. 883
Intravascular fluid, p. 883
Ions, p. 883
Isotonic, p. 884
Metabolic acidosis, p. 893
Metabolic alkalosis, p. 893
Oncotic pressure, p. 885
Osmolality, p. 883
Osmosis, p. 884
Osmotic pressure, p. 884
Phlebitis, p. 909
Respiratory acidosis, p. 893
Respiratory alkalosis, p. 893
Transcellular fluids, p. 883
Transfusion reaction, p. 909
Vascular access devices (VADs), p. 906
Venipuncture, p. 906

evolve WEBSITE

http://evolve.elsevier.com/Potter/fundamentals/

- Review Questions
- Video Clips
- Case Study with Questions
- Skills Performance Checklists
- Audio Glossary
- Interactive Learning Activities
- Calculations Tutorial
- Key Term Flashcards
- Butterfield's Fluids and Electrolytes Tutorial
- Content Updates

Fluid surrounds all the cells in the body and is also inside cells. Body fluids contain electrolytes such as sodium and potassium; they also have a certain degree of acidity. Fluid, electrolyte, and acid-base balances within the body maintain the health and function of all body systems. The characteristics of body fluids influence body system function because of their effects on cell function. These characteristics include the fluid amount (volume), concentration (osmolality), composition (electrolyte concentration), and degree of acidity (pH). All of these characteristics have regulatory mechanisms, which keeps them in balance for normal function. In this chapter you learn how the body normally maintains fluid, electrolyte, and acid-base balance. You also learn how imbalances develop; how various fluid, electrolyte, and acid-base imbalances affect patients; and ways to help patients maintain or restore balance safely.

SCIENTIFIC KNOWLEDGE BASE

This section provides the foundation for your critical thinking regarding patients who have or are at risk of having, fluid, electrolyte, or acid-base imbalances.

Location and Movement of Water and Electrolytes

Water makes up a substantial proportion of body weight. In fact, about 60% of the body weight of an adult man is water. This proportion decreases with age; approximately 50% of an older man's weight is water. Women typically have less water content than men. Obese people have less water in their bodies than lean people because fat contains less water than muscle. The term **fluid** means water that contains dissolved or suspended substances such as glucose, mineral salts, and proteins.

Fluid Compartments. Body fluids are located in two distinct compartments: **extracellular fluid (ECF)** outside the cells, and **intracellular fluid (ICF)** inside the cells (Fig. 41-1). In adults ICF is approximately two thirds of total body water. ECF is approximately one third of total body water. ECF has two major divisions (**intravascular fluid** and **interstitial fluid**) and a minor division (**transcellular fluids**). Intravascular fluid is the liquid portion of the blood (i.e., the plasma). Interstitial fluid is located between the cells and outside the blood vessels. Transcellular fluids such as cerebrospinal, pleural, peritoneal, and synovial fluids are secreted by epithelial cells (Hall, 2011).

Fluid in the body compartments contains mineral salts known technically as **electrolytes.** An electrolyte is a compound that separates into **ions** (charged particles) when it dissolves in water. Ions that are positively charged are called **cations;** ions that are negatively charged are called **anions.** Cations in body fluids are sodium (Na^+), potassium (K^+), calcium (Ca^{2+}), and magnesium ions (Mg^{2+}). Anions in body fluids are chloride (Cl^-) and bicarbonate (HCO_3^-). Anions and cations combine to make salts. If you put table salt (NaCl) in water, it separates into Na^+ and Cl^-. Other combinations of anions and cations do the same. Clinical laboratories usually report electrolyte measurements in milliequivalents per liter (mEq/L) or millimoles per liter (mmol/L), two different units of concentration (Table 41-1). Millimoles per liter represent the number of milligrams of the electrolyte divided by its molecular weight that are contained in a liter of the fluid being measured (usually blood plasma or serum). Milliequivalents per liter is the millimoles per liter multiplied by the electrolyte charge (e.g., 1 for Na^+, 2 for Ca^{2+}). A milliequivalent of one electrolyte can combine with a milliequivalent of another electrolyte, which is why this measurement unit is used (Rose, 2011).

Fluid that contains a large number of dissolved particles is more concentrated than the same amount of fluid that contains only a few particles. **Osmolality** of a fluid is a measure of the number of particles per kilogram of water. Some particles (e.g., urea) pass easily through cell membranes; others such as Na^+ cannot cross easily. The particles that cannot cross cell membranes easily (nonpermeant particles) determine tonicity of a fluid (Caon, 2008). A fluid with the same concentration of nonpermeant particles as

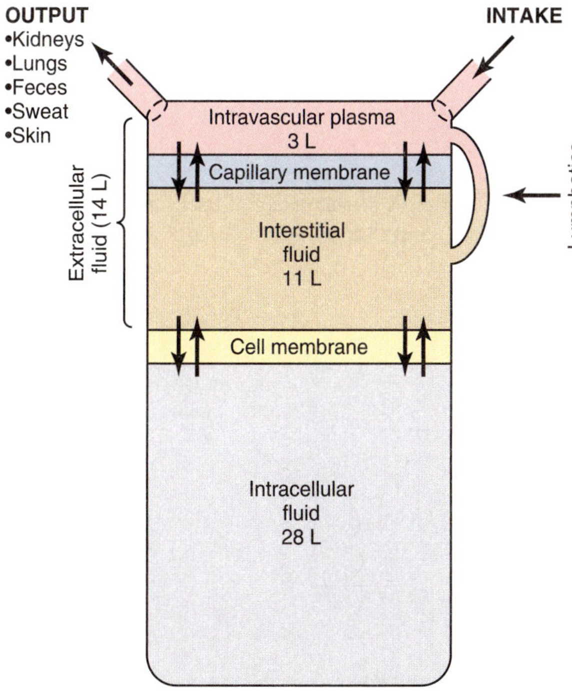

FIG. 41-1 Body fluid compartments. (From Hall JE: *Guyton and Hall textbook of medical physiology*, ed 12, Philadelphia, 2011, Saunders.)

TABLE 41-1 Laboratory Normal Values for Adults

ITEM MEASURED	NORMAL VALUE IN SERUM OR BLOOD
Osmolality	280-300 mOsm/kg H_2O (280-300 mmol/kg H_2O)
Electrolytes	
Sodium (Na^+)	136-145 mEq/L (136-145 mmol/L)
Potassium (K^+)	3.5-5.0 mEq/L (3.5-5 mmol/L)
Chloride (Cl^-)	98-106 mEq/L (98-106 mmol/L)
Total CO_2 (CO_2 total content)	22-30 mEq/L (22-30 mmol/L)
Bicarbonate (HCO_3^-)	Arterial 22-26 mEq/L (22-26 mmol/L) Venous 24-30 mEq/L (24-30 mmol/L)
Total calcium (Ca^{2+})	8.4-10.5 mg/dL (2.1-2.6 mmol/L)
Ionized calcium (Ca^{2+})	4.5-5.3 mg/dL (1.1-1.3 mmol/L)
Magnesium (Mg^{2+})	1.5-2.5 mEq/L (0.75-1.25 mmol/L)
Phosphate (PO_4^{3-})	2.7-4.5 mg/dL (0.87-1.45 mmol/L)
Anion gap	5-11 mEq/L (5-11 mmol/L)
Arterial Blood Gases	
pH	7.35-7.45
$PaCO_2$	35-45 mm Hg (4.7-6 kPa)
PaO_2	80-100 mm Hg (10.7-13.3 kPa)
O_2 saturation	95%-100% (0.95-1.00)
Base excess	−2 to +2 mmol/L

normal blood is called **isotonic.** A **hypotonic** solution is more dilute than the blood, and a **hypertonic** solution is more concentrated than normal blood (Fig. 41-2).

Movement of Water and Electrolytes. Active transport, diffusion, osmosis, and filtration are processes that move water and electrolytes between body compartments. These processes maintain equal osmolality in all compartments while allowing for different electrolyte concentrations.

Active Transport. Fluids in different body compartments have different concentrations of electrolytes that are necessary for normal function. For example, concentrations of Na^+, Cl^-, and HCO_3^- are higher in the ECF than in the ICF, whereas the concentrations of K^+, Mg^{2+}, and PO_4^{3-} are higher in the ICF than in the ECF. Cells maintain their high intracellular electrolyte concentration by **active transport.** Active transport requires energy in the form of adenosine triphosphate (ATP) to move electrolytes across cell membranes against the concentration gradient (from areas of lower concentration to areas of higher concentration). One example of active transport is the sodium-potassium pump, which moves Na^+ out of a cell and K^+ into it, keeping ICF lower in Na^+ and higher in K^+ than the ECF.

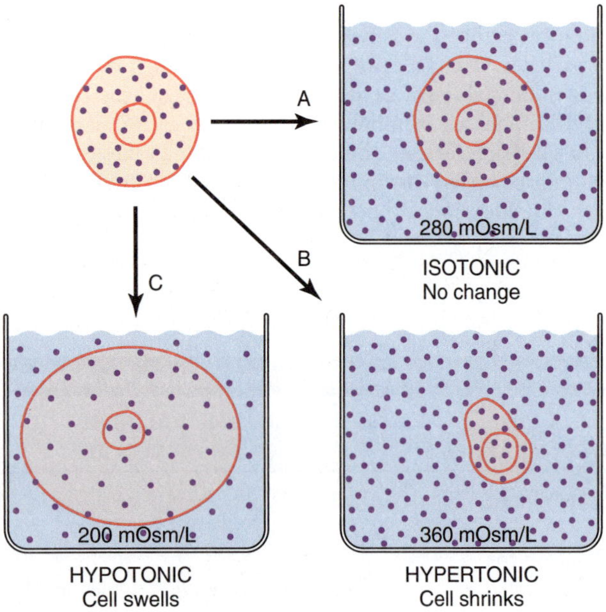

FIG. 41-2 Effects of isotonic, hypotonic, and hypertonic solutions. (From Hall JE: *Guyton and Hall textbook of medical physiology*, ed 12, Philadelphia, 2011, Saunders.)

Diffusion. Diffusion is passive movement of electrolytes or other particles down the concentration gradient (from areas of higher concentration to areas of lower concentration). Within a body compartment electrolytes diffuse easily by random movements until the concentration is the same in all areas. However, diffusion of electrolytes across cell membranes requires proteins that serve as ion channels. For example, when a sodium channel in a cell membrane is open, Na^+ diffuses passively across the cell membrane into the ICF because concentration is lower in the ICF. Opening of ion channels is tightly controlled and plays an important part in muscle and nerve function.

Osmosis. Water moves across cell membranes by **osmosis,** a process by which water moves through a membrane that separates fluids with different particle concentrations (Fig. 41-3). Cell membranes are semipermeable, which means that water crosses them easily but they are not freely permeable to many types of particles, including electrolytes such as sodium and potassium. These semipermeable cell membranes separate interstitial fluid from ICF. The fluid in each of these compartments exerts **osmotic pressure,** an inward-pulling force caused by particles in the fluid. The particles already inside the cell exert ICF osmotic pressure, which tends to pull water into the cell. The particles in the interstitial fluid exert interstitial fluid osmotic pressure, which tends to pull water out of the cell. Water moves into the compartment that has a higher osmotic pressure (inward-pulling force) until the particle concentration is equal in the two compartments.

If the particle concentration in the interstitial compartment changes, osmosis occurs rapidly and moves water into or out of cells to equalize the osmotic pressures. For example, when a hypotonic solution (more dilute than normal body fluids) is administered intravenously, it dilutes the interstitial fluid, decreasing its osmotic pressure below intracellular osmotic pressure. Water moves rapidly into cells until the two osmotic pressures are equal again. On the other hand, infusion of a hypertonic intravenous (IV) solution (more concentrated than normal body fluids) causes water to leave cells by osmosis to equalize the osmolality between interstitial and intracellular compartments.

Filtration. Fluid moves into and out of capillaries (between the vascular and interstitial compartments) by the process of **filtration** (Fig. 41-4). Filtration is the net effect of four forces, two that tend to move fluid out of capillaries and small venules and two that tend

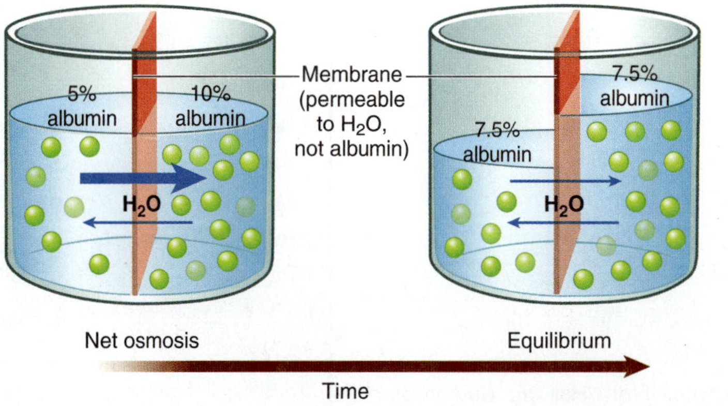

FIG. 41-3 Osmosis moves water through semipermeable membrane. (From Patton KT, Thibodeau GA: *Anatomy and physiology*, ed 7, St Louis, 2010, Mosby.)

to move fluid back into them (Rose, 2011). **Hydrostatic pressure** is the force of the fluid pressing outward against a surface. Similarly, capillary hydrostatic pressure is a relatively strong outward-pushing force that helps move fluid from capillaries into the interstitial area. Interstitial fluid hydrostatic pressure is a weaker opposing force that tends to push fluid back into capillaries.

Blood contains albumin and other proteins known as **colloids.** These proteins are much larger than electrolytes, glucose, and other molecules that dissolve easily. Most colloids are too large to leave capillaries in the fluid that is filtered, so they remain in the blood. Because they are particles, colloids exert osmotic pressure. Blood **colloid osmotic pressure,** also called **oncotic pressure,** is an inward-pulling force caused by blood proteins that helps move fluid from the interstitial area back into capillaries. Interstitial fluid colloid osmotic pressure normally is a very small opposing force.

At the arterial end of a normal capillary, capillary hydrostatic pressure is strongest, and fluid moves from the capillary into the interstitial area, bringing nutrients to cells. At the venous end capillary hydrostatic pressure is weaker, and the colloid osmotic pressure of the blood is stronger. Thus fluid moves into the capillary at the venous end, removing waste products from cellular metabolism. Lymph vessels remove any extra fluid and proteins that have leaked into the interstitial fluid.

Disease processes and other factors that alter these forces may cause accumulation of excess fluid in the interstitial space, known as *edema*. For example, people with heart failure develop edema. In this situation, venous congestion from a weakened heart, which no longer pumps effectively, increases capillary hydrostatic pressure, causing edema by moving excessive fluid into the interstitial space. Inflammation is another cause of edema. It increases capillary blood flow and allows capillaries to leak colloids into the interstitial space. The resulting increased capillary hydrostatic pressure and increased interstitial colloid osmotic pressure produce localized edema in the inflamed tissues.

Fluid Balance

Fluid homeostasis is the dynamic interplay of three processes: fluid intake and absorption, fluid distribution, and fluid output (Felver, 2010b). Human total daily fluid output consists of hypotonic sodium-containing fluid. People must have intake of an equivalent amount of hypotonic sodium-containing fluid (or water plus foods with some salt) to maintain fluid balance.

Fluid Intake. Fluid intake occurs orally through drinking but also through eating because most foods contain some water. Food metabolism creates additional water. Average fluid intake from these routes for healthy adults is about 2300 mL, although it varies widely (Table 41-2). Other routes of fluid intake include IV, rectal (e.g., enemas), and irrigation of body cavities that can absorb fluid.

Although you might think that the major regulator of oral fluid intake is thirst, habit and social reasons actually account for most fluid intake (Johnson, 2007). Thirst, the conscious desire for water, is an important regulator of fluid intake when plasma osmolality increases (osmoreceptor-mediated thirst) or the blood volume decreases (baroreceptor-mediated thirst and angiotensin II– and III–mediated thirst). The thirst-control mechanism is located within the hypothalamus in the brain (Fig. 41-5). Osmoreceptors continually monitor plasma osmolality; when it increases, they cause thirst by stimulating neurons in the hypothalamus. Dry oral mucous membranes also cause thirst. People who are alert can obtain fluid or communicate their thirst to others, and fluid intake restores fluid balance. Infants, patients with neurological or psychological problems, and some older adults who are unable to perceive or communicate their thirst are at risk for dehydration.

Fluid Distribution. The term *fluid distribution* means the movement of fluid among its various compartments. Fluid

TABLE 41-2 Healthy Adult Average Daily Fluid Intake and Output

FLUID INTAKE	NORMAL	PROLONGED HEAVY EXERCISE
Fluids ingested:		
Oral	1100-1400 mL	?
Foods	800-1000 mL	?
Metabolism	300 mL	200 mL
TOTAL	**2200-2700 mL**	**?**
FLUID OUTPUT		
Skin (insensible and sweat)	500-600 mL	5350 mL
Insensible-lungs	400 mL	650 mL
GI	100-200 mL	100 mL
Urine	1200-1500 mL	500 mL
TOTAL	**2200-2700 mL**	**6600 mL**

Data from Heitz UE, Horne MM: *Mosby's pocket guide series: Fluid, electrolyte and acid base balance,* ed 5, St Louis, 2005, Mosby; Hall JE: *Guyton and Hall textbook of medical physiology,* ed 12, Philadelphia, 2011, Saunders.

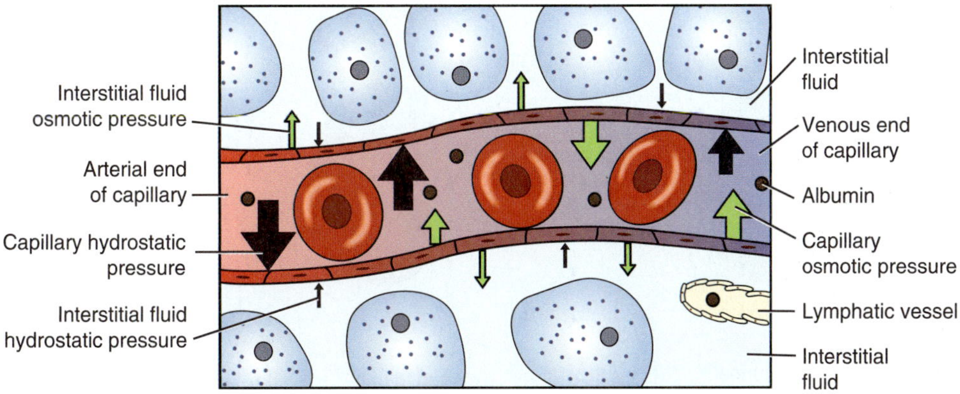

FIG. 41-4 Capillary filtration moves fluid between vascular and interstitial compartments. (From Copstead LC, Banasik JL: *Pathophysiology,* ed 4, St Louis, 2010, Saunders.)

distribution between the extracellular and intracellular compartments occurs by osmosis. Fluid distribution between the vascular and interstitial portions of the ECF occurs by filtration.

Fluid Output. Fluid output normally occurs through four organs: the skin, lungs, gastrointestinal (GI) tract, and kidneys. Examples of abnormal fluid output include vomiting, wound drainage, or hemorrhage (Felver, 2010b). Table 41-2 shows average amounts of fluid excretion for healthy adults, although urine output varies greatly, depending on fluid intake. Insensible (not visible) water loss through the skin and lungs is continuous. It increases when a person has a fever or a recent burn to the skin (Metheny, 2010). Sweat, which is visible and contains sodium, occurs intermittently and increases fluid output substantially. The GI tract plays a vital role in fluid balance. Approximately 3 to 6 L of fluid moves into the GI tract daily and then returns again to the ECF. The average adult normally excretes only 100 mL of fluid each day through feces. However, diarrhea causes a large fluid output from the GI tract.

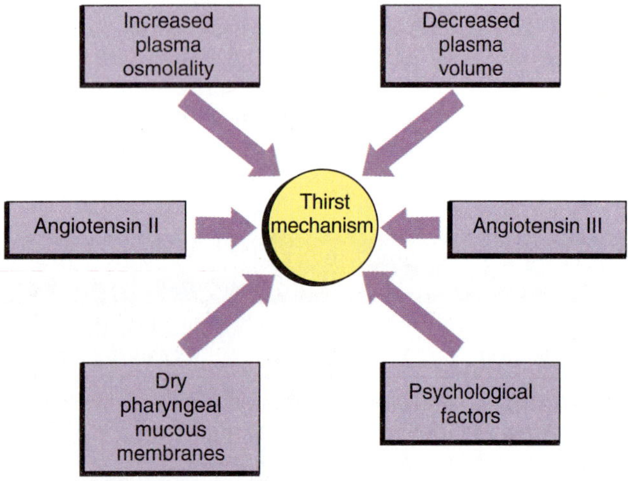

FIG. 41-5 Stimuli affecting thirst mechanism.

The kidneys are the major regulator of fluid output because they respond to hormones that influence urine production. When healthy adults drink more water, they increase urine production to maintain fluid balance. If they drink less water, sweat a lot, or lose fluid by vomiting, their urine volume decreases to maintain fluid balance. These adjustments primarily are caused by the actions of antidiuretic hormone (ADH), the renin-angiotensin-aldosterone system (RAAS), and atrial natriuretic peptides (ANPs) (Goldstein et al., 2010) (Fig. 41-6).

Antidiuretic Hormone. ADH regulates the osmolality of the body fluids by influencing how much water is excreted in urine. It is synthesized by neurons in the hypothalamus that release it from the posterior pituitary gland. ADH circulates in the blood to the kidneys, where it acts on the collecting ducts (Koeppen and Stanton, 2008). Its name—antidiuretic hormone—tells you what it does. It causes renal cells to resorb water, taking water from the renal tubular fluid and putting it back in the blood. This action decreases urine volume, concentrating the urine while diluting the blood by adding water to it (see Fig. 41-6, *A*).

People normally have some ADH release to maintain fluid balance. More ADH is released if body fluids become more concentrated. Factors that increase ADH levels include severely decreased blood volume (e.g., dehydration, hemorrhage), pain, stressors, and some medications.

ADH levels decrease if body fluids become too dilute. This allows more water to be excreted in urine, creating a larger volume of dilute urine and concentrating the body fluids back to normal osmolality. For example, ethyl alcohol decreases ADH release,

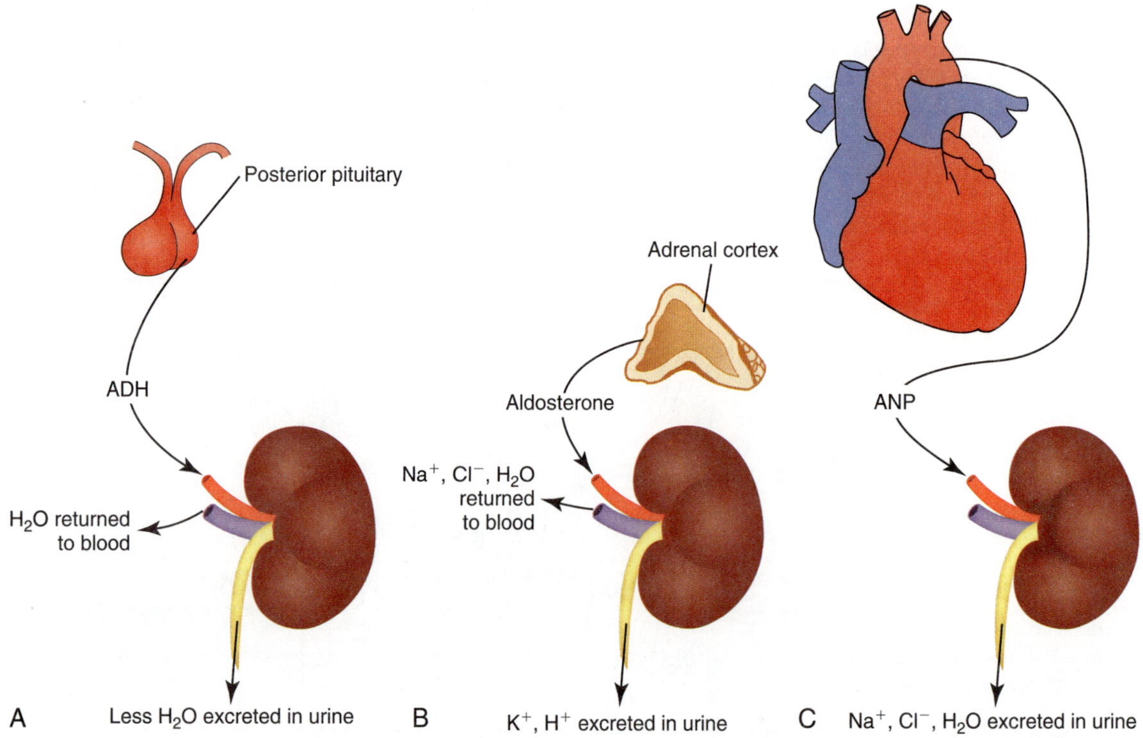

FIG. 41-6 Major hormones that influence renal fluid excretion. **A,** Antidiuretic hormone (ADH). **B,** Aldosterone. **C,** Atrial natriuretic peptide (ANP).

which causes people to urinate frequently when they drink alcoholic beverages.

Renin-Angiotensin-Aldosterone System. The renin-angiotensin-aldosterone system (RAAS) regulates ECF volume by influencing how much sodium and water are excreted in urine. It also contributes to regulation of blood pressure. Specialized cells in the kidneys release the enzyme renin, which acts on angiotensinogen, an inactive protein secreted by the liver that circulates in the blood. Renin converts angiotensinogen to angiotensin I, which other enzymes in the lung capillaries convert to angiotensin II (Koeppen and Stanton, 2008). Angiotensin II has several functions, one of which is vasoconstriction in some vascular beds. The important fluid homeostasis functions of angiotensin II include stimulation of aldosterone release from the adrenal cortex.

Aldosterone circulates to the kidneys, where it causes resorption of sodium and water in isotonic proportion in the distal renal tubules. Removing sodium and water from the renal tubules and returning it to the blood increases the volume of the ECF (see Fig. 41-6, *B*). Aldosterone also contributes to electrolyte and acid-base balance by increasing urinary excretion of potassium and hydrogen ions.

To maintain fluid balance, normally some action of the RAAS occurs. Certain stimuli increase or decrease the activity of this system to restore fluid balance. For example, if hemorrhage or vomiting decreases the extracellular fluid volume (ECV), blood flow decreases through the renal arteries, and more renin is released. This increased RAAS activity causes more sodium and water retention, helping to restore ECV.

Atrial Natriuretic Peptide. Atrial natriuretic peptide (ANP) also regulates ECV by influencing how much sodium and water are excreted in urine. Cells in the atria of the heart release ANP when they are stretched (e.g., by an increased ECV). ANP is a weak hormone that inhibits ADH by increasing the loss of sodium and water in the urine (see Fig. 41-6, *C*). Thus ANP opposes the effect of aldosterone (Koeppen and Stanton, 2008).

Fluid Imbalances

If disease processes, medications, or other factors disrupt fluid intake or output, imbalances sometimes occur (Felver, 2010b). For example, with diarrhea there is an increase in fluid output, and a fluid imbalance (dehydration) occurs if fluid intake does not increase appropriately. There are two major types of fluid imbalances: volume imbalances and osmolality imbalances (Fig. 41-7). Volume imbalances are disturbances of the *amount of fluid in the extracellular compartment.* Osmolality imbalances are disturbances of the *concentration of body fluids.* Volume and osmolality imbalances occur separately or in combination.

Extracellular Fluid Volume Imbalances. In an ECV imbalance there is either too little (ECV deficit) or too much (ECV excess) isotonic fluid. **ECV deficit** is present when there is insufficient isotonic fluid in the extracellular compartment. Remember that there is a lot of sodium in normal ECF. With ECV deficit, output of isotonic fluid exceeds intake of sodium-containing fluid. Because ECF is both vascular and interstitial, signs and symptoms arise from lack of volume in both of these compartments. Table 41-3 lists specific causes and signs and symptoms of ECV deficit. The term **hypovolemia** means decreased vascular volume and often is used when discussing ECV deficit (Metheny, 2010).

ECV excess occurs when there is too much isotonic fluid in the extracellular compartment. Intake of sodium-containing isotonic fluid has exceeded fluid output. For example, when you eat more salty foods than usual and drink water, you may notice that your ankles swell or rings on your fingers feel tight and you gain 2 lbs (1 kg) or more overnight. These are manifestations of mild ECV excess. See Table 41-3 for other specific causes and signs and symptoms.

Osmolality Imbalances. In an osmolality imbalance body fluids become hypertonic or hypotonic, which causes osmotic shifts of water across cell membranes. The osmolality imbalances are called *hypernatremia* and *hyponatremia.*

Hypernatremia, also called *water deficit,* is a hypertonic condition. Two general causes make body fluids too concentrated: loss of relatively more water than salt or gain of relatively more salt than water (Felver, 2010b). Table 41-3 lists specific causes under these categories. When the interstitial fluid becomes hypertonic, water leaves cells by osmosis, and they shrivel. Signs and symptoms of hypernatremia are those of cerebral dysfunction, which arise when brain cells shrivel. Hypernatremia may occur in combination with ECV deficit; this combined disorder is called clinical **dehydration.**

Hyponatremia, also called *water excess* or *water intoxication,* is a hypotonic condition. It arises from gain of relatively more water than salt or loss of relatively more salt than water (Felver, 2010b) (see Table 41-3). The excessively dilute condition of interstitial fluid causes water to enter cells by osmosis, causing the cells to swell. Signs and symptoms of cerebral dysfunction occur when brain cells swell.

Clinical Dehydration. ECV deficit and hypernatremia often occur at the same time; this combination is called *clinical dehydration* (Bryant, 2007). The ECV is too low, and the body fluids are too concentrated. Clinical dehydration is common with gastroenteritis or other causes of severe vomiting and diarrhea when people are not able to replace their fluid output with enough intake of dilute sodium-containing fluids. Signs and symptoms of clinical dehydration are those of both ECV deficit and hypernatremia (see Table 41-3).

Electrolyte Balance

You can best understand electrolyte balance by considering the three processes involved in electrolyte homeostasis: electrolyte intake and absorption, electrolyte distribution, and electrolyte

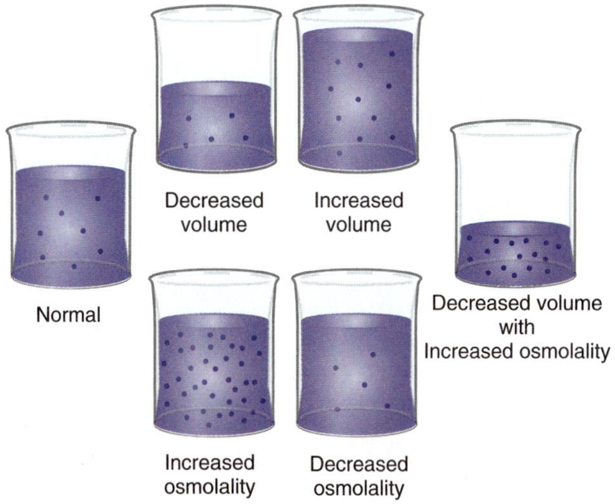

FIG. 41-7 Fluid volume and osmolality imbalances. (From Copstead LC, Banasik JL: *Pathophysiology online for pathophysiology,* ed 4, St Louis, 2010, Mosby.)

TABLE 41-3 Fluid Imbalances

IMBALANCE AND RELATED CAUSES	SIGNS AND SYMPTOMS
Volume Imbalances	
Extracellular Fluid Volume Deficit—Body Fluids Have Decreased Volume but Normal Tonicity	
Sodium and water intake less than output, causing isotonic loss: Severely decreased oral intake of water and salt *Increased GI output:* Diarrhea, vomiting, laxative overuse, or drainage from fistulas or tubes *Increased renal output:* Use of diuretics, adrenal insufficiency, salt-wasting renal disorders *Loss of blood or plasma:* Hemorrhage, burns Massive sweating without water and salt replacement	*Physical examination:* Sudden weight loss (e.g., overnight), postural hypotension, tachycardia, thready pulse, neck veins flat or collapsing with inhalation when supine, slow vein filling, oliguria (<30 mL/hr), dark yellow urine, dry mucous membranes, inelastic skin turgor, absence of tears and sweat, longitudinal furrows in tongue, thirst, restlessness, confusion, cold clammy skin, hypotension, ***hypovolemic shock.*** *Laboratory findings:* Increased hematocrit; BUN greater than 25 mg/dL (8.9 mmol/L) caused by hemoconcentration; urine specific gravity greater than 1.030
Extracellular Fluid Volume Excess—Body Fluids Have Increased Volume but Normal Tonicity	
Sodium and water intake greater than output, causing isotonic gain: Excessive administration of sodium-containing isotonic parenteral fluids Excessive oral intake of salty foods and water *Decreased renal output caused by elevated aldosterone:* Chronic heart failure, cirrhosis, aldosterone-secreting tumor *Decreased renal output from other causes:* Oliguric acute kidney disease, end-stage chronic renal disease, glucocorticoid excess	*Physical examination:* Sudden weight gain (e.g., overnight), edema (especially in dependent areas), neck veins full when upright or semi-upright, crackles in dependent portion of lungs, ***pulmonary edema*** *Laboratory findings:* Decreased hematocrit; BUN less than 10 mg/dL (3.6 mmol/L) caused by hemodilution
Osmolality Imbalances	
Hypernatremia (Water Deficit; Hyperosmolar Imbalance)—Hypertonic Body Fluids	
Loss of relatively more water than salt: Diabetes insipidus (ADH deficiency) Osmotic diuresis Greatly increased insensible perspiration and respiratory water output without increased water intake Gain of relatively more salt than water: Overuse of salt tablets Administration of tube feedings or hypertonic parenteral fluids Difficulty swallowing fluids, as in Parkinson's disease Lack of access to water or deliberate water deprivation Inability to respond to thirst (immobility, aphasia) Dysfunction of osmoreceptor-driven thirst drive	*Physical examination:* Extreme thirst, dry and flushed skin, postural hypotension, fever, restlessness, confusion, agitation, ***coma***, ***seizures*** if develops rapidly or is very severe *Laboratory findings:* Serum Na^+ level greater than 145 mEq/L (145 mmol/L) and serum osmolality greater than 295 mOsm/kg (295 mmol/kg), urine specific gravity 1.030
Hyponatremia (Water Excess; Water Intoxication; Hypoosmolar Imbalance)—Hypotonic Body Fluids	
Gain of relatively more water than salt: Excessive ADH (SIADH) Psychogenic polydipsia or forced excessive water drinking Excessive IV administration of 5% dextrose in water (D_5W) Use of hypotonic irrigating solutions Tap-water enemas Loss of relatively more salt than water: Renal salt-wasting disease Replacement of large body fluid output (diarrhea, vomiting, gastric suction) with water but not salt	*Physical examination:* Apprehension, nausea and vomiting, headaches, decreased level of consciousness (confusion, lethargy, muscle weakness, ***coma***); ***seizures*** if develops rapidly or is very severe *Laboratory findings:* Serum Na^+ level less than 135 mEq/L (135 mmol/L) and serum osmolality 280 mOsm/kg (280 mmol/kg) or less, urine specific gravity below 1.010 (if not SIADH)
Combined Volume and Osmolality Imbalance	
Clinical Dehydration (Extracellular Fluid Volume Deficit plus Hypernatremia)—Body Fluids Have Decreased Volume and Are Hypertonic	
Sodium and water intake less than output, with loss of relatively more water than salt: Most of the causes of ECV deficit (see previous causes) with no water intake, often with increased insensible water output through skin with fever	*Physical examination and laboratory findings:* Combination of those for ECV deficit plus those for hypernatremia (see previous signs)

ADH, Antidiuretic hormone; *BUN*, blood urea nitrogen; *ECV*, extracellular fluid volume; *GI*, gastrointestinal; *IV*, intravenous; *SIADH*, syndrome of inappropriate secretion of antidiuretic hormone.

Text in bold italics denotes potentially life-threatening manifestations.

TABLE 41-4 **Electrolyte Intake and Absorption, Distribution, and Output**

ELECTROLYTE	INTAKE AND ABSORPTION	DISTRIBUTION	OUTPUT/LOSS	IMPORTANT FUNCTION
Potassium (K^+)	Fruits Potatoes Instant coffee Molasses Brazil nuts Absorbs easily	Low in ECF, high in ICF. Insulin, epinephrine, and alkalosis shift K^+ into cells. Some types of acidosis shift K^+ out of cells.	Aldosterone, black licorice, hypomagnesemia, and polyuria increase renal excretion; oliguria decreases renal excretion. Acute or chronic diarrhea increases fecal excretion.	Maintains resting membrane potential of skeletal, smooth, and cardiac muscle, allowing for normal muscle function
Calcium (Ca^{2+})	Dairy products Canned fish with bones Broccoli Oranges Requires vitamin D for best absorption Undigested fat prevents absorption	Ca^{2+} is low in ECF, mostly in bones and intracellular. Some Ca^{2+} in blood is bound and inactive; only ionized Ca^{2+} is active. Parathyroid hormone shifts Ca^{2+} out of bone; calcitonin shifts Ca^{2+} into bone. Ca^{2+} decreases in blood if phosphate rises and vice versa.	Thiazide diuretics decrease renal excretion. Chronic diarrhea and undigested fat increase fecal excretion.	Influences excitability of nerve and muscle cells; necessary for muscle contraction
Magnesium (Mg^{2+})	Dark green leafy vegetables Whole grains Mg^{2+}-containing laxatives and antacids Undigested fat prevents absorption	Mg^{2+} is low in ECF, mostly in bones and intracellular. Some Mg^{2+} in blood is bound and not active; only free Mg^{2+} is active.	Rising blood ethanol increases renal excretion; oliguria decreases renal excretion. Chronic diarrhea and undigested fat increase fecal excretion.	Influences function of neuromuscular junctions and is a cofactor for numerous enzymes
Phosphate (PO_4)	Milk Processed foods Aluminum antacids prevent absorption	PO_4 is low in ECF; it is higher in ICF and in bones. Insulin and epinephrine shift phosphate into cells. Decreases in blood if calcium rises and vice versa.	Oliguria decreases renal excretion.	Necessary for production of ATP, the energy source for cellular metabolism

ATP, Adenosine triphosphate; *ECF,* extracellular fluid; *ICF,* intracellular fluid.

output (Table 41-4) (Felver, 2010b). Although sodium is an electrolyte, it is not included here because serum sodium imbalances are the osmolality imbalances discussed previously.

Electrolyte distribution is an important issue. Plasma concentrations of K^+, Ca^{2+}, Mg^{2+}, and phosphate are very low compared with their concentrations in cells and bone (Metheny, 2010). These concentration differences are necessary for normal muscle and nerve function. The electrolyte values that you review from laboratory reports are measured in blood serum and do not measure intracellular levels.

Electrolyte output occurs through normal excretion in urine, feces, and sweat. Output also occurs through vomiting, drainage tubes or fistulas. When electrolyte output increases, electrolyte intake must increase to maintain electrolyte balance. Similarly, if electrolyte output decreases such as with oliguria, electrolyte intake must also decrease to maintain balance (Felver, 2010b).

Electrolyte Imbalances

Factors such as diarrhea, endocrine disorders, and medications that disrupt electrolyte homeostasis cause electrolyte imbalances. Electrolyte intake greater than electrolyte output or a shift of electrolytes from cells or bone into the ECF causes plasma electrolyte excess. Electrolyte intake less than electrolyte output or shift of electrolyte from the ECF into cells or bone causes plasma electrolyte deficit (Felver, 2010b).

Potassium Imbalances. Hypokalemia is abnormally low potassium concentration in the blood. Hypokalemia results from decreased potassium intake and absorption, a shift of potassium from the ECF into cells, and an increased potassium output (Table 41-5). Common causes of hypokalemia from increased potassium output include diarrhea, repeated vomiting, and use of potassium-wasting diuretics. People who have these conditions need to increase their potassium intake to reduce their risk of hypokalemia. Hypokalemia causes muscle weakness, which becomes life threatening if it includes respiratory muscles and potentially life-threatening cardiac dysrhythmias.

Hyperkalemia is abnormally high potassium ion concentration in the blood. Its general causes are increased potassium intake and absorption, shift of potassium from cells into the ECF, and decreased potassium output (see Table 41-5). People who have oliguria (decreased urine output) are at high risk of hyperkalemia from the resultant decreased potassium output unless their potassium intake also decreases substantially. Understanding this principle helps you remember to check urine output before you administer IV solutions containing potassium. Hyperkalemia can cause muscle weakness, potentially life-threatening cardiac dysrhythmias, and cardiac arrest.

Calcium Imbalances. Hypocalcemia is abnormally low calcium concentration in the blood. The physiologically active form of calcium in the blood is ionized calcium. Total blood

TABLE 41-5 Electrolyte Imbalances

IMBALANCE AND RELATED CAUSES	SIGNS AND SYMPTOMS
Hypokalemia—Low Serum Potassium (K^+) Level	
Decreased K^+ intake and absorption: Excessive use of potassium-free IV solutions Shift of K^+ from ECF into cells: Alkalosis Treatment of diabetic ketoacidosis with insulin Increased K^+ output: Aldosterone excess Polyuria Use of potassium-wasting diuretics Glucocorticoid therapy Acute or chronic diarrhea, vomiting, or other GI losses	*Physical examination:* Bilateral muscle weakness that begins in quadriceps and may ascend to respiratory muscles, abdominal distention, decreased bowel sounds, constipation, ***cardiac dysrhythmias;*** signs of digoxin toxicity at normal digoxin levels *Laboratory findings:* Serum K^+ level less than 3.5 mEq/L (3.5 mmol/L); possible ECG abnormalities
Hyperkalemia—High Serum Potassium (K^+) Level	
Increased K^+ intake and absorption: Iatrogenic administration of large amounts of IV potassium Rapid infusion of stored blood Excessive ingestion of K^+ salt substitutes Shift of K^+ from cells into ECF: Massive cellular damage such as from crushing trauma or cytotoxic chemotherapy Insufficient insulin (e.g., diabetic ketoacidosis) Some types of acidosis Decreased K^+ output: Acute or chronic oliguria (e.g., severe ECV deficit, end-stage renal disease) Adrenal insufficiency Use of potassium-sparing diuretics	*Physical examination:* Bilateral muscle weakness in quadriceps, transient abdominal cramps and diarrhea, ***cardiac dysrhythmias, cardiac arrest*** *Laboratory findings:* serum K^+ level greater than 5 mEq/L (5 mmol/L); possible ECG abnormalities
Hypocalcemia—Low Serum Calcium (Ca^{2+}) Level	
Decreased Ca^{2+} intake and absorption: Calcium-deficient diet Vitamin D deficiency (includes end-stage renal disease) Chronic diarrhea, laxative misuse Steatorrhea (e.g., pancreatitis) Shift of Ca^{2+} from ECF into bone or inactive form: Hypoparathyroidism Rapid administration of citrated blood Hypoalbuminemia Alkalosis Hyperphosphatemia (includes end-stage renal disease) Increased Ca^{2+} output: Steatorrhea Chronic diarrhea	*Physical examination:* Positive Chvostek's sign (contraction of facial muscles when facial nerve is tapped), positive Trousseau's sign (carpal spasm with hypoxia), numbness and tingling of fingers and circumoral (around mouth) region, hyperactive reflexes, muscle twitching and cramping, tetany, seizures, ***laryngospasm, cardiac dysrhythmias*** *Laboratory findings:* Total serum Ca^{2+} less than 8.4 mg/dL (2.1 mmol/L) or serum ionized Ca^{2+} level less than 4.5 mg/dL (1.1 mmol/L); ECG abnormalities possible

calcium also contains inactive forms that are bound to plasma proteins and small anions such as citrate. Factors that cause too much ionized calcium to shift to the bound forms cause symptomatic *ionized hypocalcemia*. Table 41-5 summarizes general causes. People who have acute pancreatitis frequently develop hypocalcemia because calcium binds to undigested fat in their feces and is excreted. This process decreases absorption of dietary calcium and also increases calcium output by preventing resorption of calcium contained in GI fluids. Hypocalcemia increases neuromuscular excitability, the basis for its signs and symptoms.

Hypercalcemia is abnormally high calcium concentration in the blood. Hypercalcemia results from increased calcium intake and absorption, shift of calcium from bones into the ECF, and decreased calcium output (see Table 41-5). Patients with cancer often develop hypercalcemia because some cancer cells secrete chemicals into the blood that are related to parathyroid hormone. When these chemicals reach the bones, they cause shift of calcium from bones into the ECF. This weakens bones, and the person sometimes develops pathological fractures (i.e., bone breakage caused by forces that would not break a healthy bone). Hypercalcemia decreases neuromuscular excitability, the basis for its other signs and symptoms, the most common of which is lethargy.

Magnesium Imbalances. Hypomagnesemia is abnormally low magnesium concentration in the blood. Its general causes are decreased magnesium intake and absorption, shift of plasma magnesium to its inactive bound form, and increased magnesium output (see Table 41-5). Signs and symptoms are similar to those of hypocalcemia because hypomagnesemia also increases neuromuscular excitability.

TABLE 41-5 Electrolyte Imbalances—cont'd

IMBALANCE AND RELATED CAUSES	SIGNS AND SYMPTOMS
Hypercalcemia—High Serum Calcium (Ca^{2+}) Level	
Increased Ca^{2+} intake and absorption: Milk-alkali syndrome Shift of Ca^{2+} from bone into ECF: Prolonged immobilization Hyperparathyroidism Bone tumors Nonosseous cancers that secrete bone-resorbing factors Decreased Ca^{2+} output: Use of thiazide diuretics	*Physical examination:* Anorexia, nausea and vomiting, constipation, fatigue, diminished reflexes, lethargy, decreased level of consciousness, confusion, personality change, ***cardiac dysrhythmias;*** possible flank pain from renal calculi; with hypercalcemia caused by shift of calcium from bone: pathological fractures; signs of digoxin toxicity at normal digoxin levels *Laboratory findings:* Total serum Ca^{2+} greater than 10.5 mg/dL (2.6 mmol/L) or serum ionized Ca^{2+} greater than 5.3 mg/dL (1.3 mmol/L); possible ECG abnormalities
Hypomagnesemia—Low Serum Magnesium (Mg^{2+}) Level	
Decreased Mg^{2+} intake and absorption: Malnutrition Chronic alcoholism Chronic diarrhea, laxative misuse Steatorrhea (e.g., pancreatitis) Shift of Mg^{2+} into inactive form: Rapid administration of citrated blood Increased Mg^{2+} output: Aldosterone excess Use of thiazide or loop diuretics Steatorrhea, chronic diarrhea or other GI losses	*Physical examination:* Positive Chvostek's and Trousseau's signs, hyperactive deep tendon reflexes, insomnia, muscle cramps and twitching, grimacing, dysphagia, tachycardia, hypertension, tetany, seizures, ***cardiac dysrhythmias;*** signs of digoxin toxicity at normal digoxin levels *Laboratory findings:* Serum Mg^{2+} level less than 1.5 mEq/L (0.75 mmol/L)
Hypermagnesemia—High Serum Magnesium (Mg^{2+}) Level	
Increased Mg^{2+} intake and absorption: Excessive use of Mg^{2+}-containing laxatives and antacids Parenteral overload of magnesium Decreased Mg^{2+} output: End-stage renal disease Adrenal insufficiency	*Physical examination:* Lethargy, hypoactive deep tendon reflexes, bradycardia, hypotension; acute elevation in magnesium levels: flushing, sensation of warmth; severe hypermagnesemia: flaccid muscle paralysis, ***decreased rate and depth of respirations, cardiac dysrhythmias, cardiac arrest*** *Laboratory findings:* Serum Mg^{2+} level greater than 2.5 mEq/L (1.25 mmol/L); possible ECG abnormalities

Data from Felver L: Fluid and electrolyte homeostasis and imbalances. In Copstead LC, Banasik JL: *Pathophysiology,* ed 4, St Louis, 2010b, Saunders; Goldstein MB et al: *Fluid, electrolyte and acid-base physiology: a problem-based approach,* ed 4, St Louis, 2010, Saunders; and Rose BD: *Clinical physiology of acid-base disorders,* ed 6, New York, 2011, McGraw-Hill.

ECF, Extracellular fluid, *ECG,* electrocardiogram, *ECV,* extracellular fluid volume, *GI,* gastrointestinal, *IV,* intravenous. ***Text in bold italics denotes potentially life-threatening manifestations.***

Hypermagnesemia is abnormally high magnesium concentration in the blood (see Table 41-5). End-stage renal disease causes hypermagnesemia unless the person decreases magnesium intake to match the decreased output. Signs and symptoms are caused by decreased neuromuscular excitability, with lethargy and decreased deep tendon reflexes being most common.

Acid-Base Balance

For optimal cell function the body maintains a balance between acids and bases. Acid-base homeostasis is the dynamic interplay of three processes: acid production, acid buffering, and acid excretion (Felver, 2010a). Normal acid-base balance is maintained with acid excretion equal to acid production. Acids release hydrogen (H^+) ions; bases (alkaline substances) take up H^+ ions. The more H^+ ions that are present, the more acidic is the solution.

The degree of acidity in blood and other body fluids is reported from the clinical laboratory as pH. The pH scale goes from 1.0 (very acid) to 14.0 (very alkaline; basic). A pH of 7.0 is considered neutral. The normal pH range of adult arterial blood is 7.35 to 7.45. Maintaining pH within this normal range is very important for optimal cell function. If the pH goes outside the normal range, enzymes within cells do not function properly; hemoglobin does not manage oxygen properly; and serious physiological problems occur, including death. Laboratory tests of a sample of arterial blood called **arterial blood gases (ABGs)** are used to monitor a patient's acid-base balance (Kramer and Raymond, 2009) (Table 41-6).

Acid Production. Cellular metabolism constantly creates two types of acids: carbonic acid and metabolic acids (Fig. 41-8). Cells produce carbon dioxide (CO_2), which acts like an acid in the body by converting to carbonic acid (H_2CO_3):

$$CO_2 + H_2O \leftrightarrow H_2CO_3 \leftrightarrow H^+ + HCO_3^-$$

$$\text{Carbon dioxide} + \text{Water} \leftrightarrow \text{Carbonic acid} \leftrightarrow \text{Hydrogen ion} + \text{Bicarbonate}$$

Metabolic acids are any acids that are not carbonic acid. They include citric acid, lactic acid, and many others.

Acid Buffering. **Buffers** are pairs of chemicals that work together to maintain normal pH of body fluids. If there are too many free H^+ ions, a buffer takes them up so they no longer are free. If there are too few, a buffer can release H^+ ions to prevent an acid-base imbalance. Buffers work rapidly, within seconds.

TABLE 41-6 Arterial Blood Gas Measures

LABORATORY MEASURE	NORMAL RANGE IN ADULT ARTERIAL BLOOD	DEFINITION AND INTERPRETATION
pH	7.35-7.45	pH is a negative logarithm of the free H^+ concentration, a measure of how acid or alkaline the blood is. Values below 7.35 indicate abnormally acid, and above 7.45 indicate abnormally alkaline. Small changes in pH denote large changes in H^+ concentration and are clinically important.
$PaCO_2$	35-45 mm Hg (4.7-6 kPa)	$PaCO_2$ is partial pressure of carbon dioxide (CO_2), a measure of how well the lungs are excreting CO_2 produced by cells. Increased $PaCO_2$ indicates CO_2 accumulation in blood (more carbonic acid) caused by hypoventilation; decreased $PaCO_2$ indicates excessive CO_2 excretion (less carbonic acid) through hyperventilation.
HCO_3^-	22-26 mEq/L (22-26 mmol/L)	HCO_3^- is concentration of the base (alkaline substance) bicarbonate, a measure of how well the kidneys are excreting metabolic acids. Increased HCO_3^- indicates that the blood has too few metabolic acids; decreased HCO_3^- indicates that the blood has too many metabolic acids.
PaO_2	80-100 mm Hg (10.7-13.3 kPa)	PaO_2 is partial pressure of oxygen (O_2), a measure of how well gas exchange is occurring in the alveoli of the lungs. Values below normal indicate poor oxygenation of the blood.
SaO_2	95%-100%	SaO_2 is oxygen saturation, the percentage of hemoglobin that is carrying as much O_2 as possible. It is influenced by pH, $PaCO_2$, and body temperature. It drops rapidly when PaO_2 falls below 60 mm Hg (8 kPa).
Base excess	−2 to +2 mmol/L	Base excess is observed buffering capacity minus the normal buffering capacity, a measure of how well the blood buffers are managing metabolic acids. Values below −2 (negative base excess) indicate excessive metabolic acids; values above +2 indicate excessive amounts of bicarbonate.

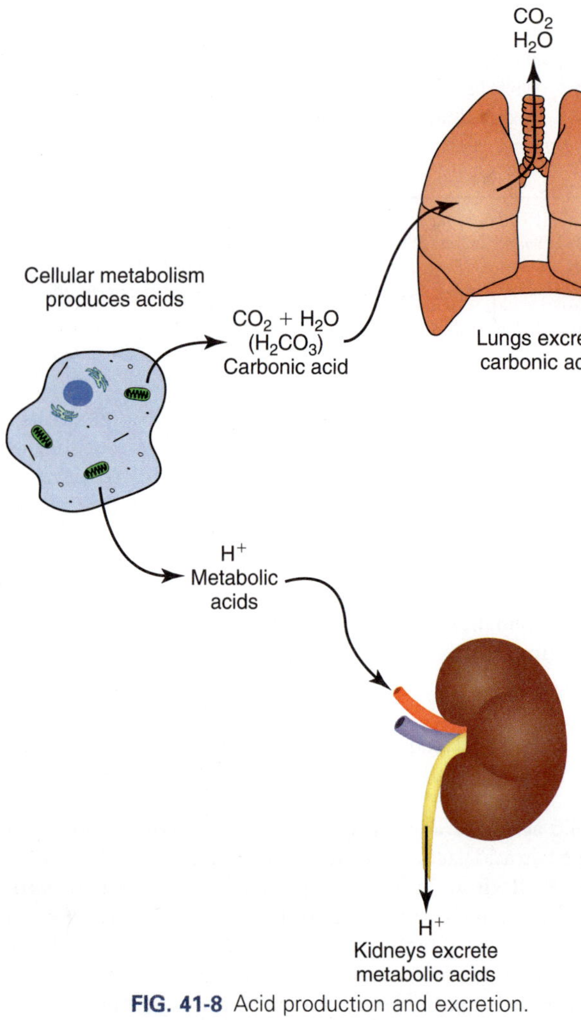

FIG. 41-8 Acid production and excretion.

All body fluids contain buffers. The major buffer in the ECF is the bicarbonate (HCO_3^-) buffer system, which buffers metabolic acids. It consists of a lot of bicarbonate and a small amount of carbonic acid (normally a 20 to 1 ratio). Addition of H^+ released by a metabolic acid to a bicarbonate ion makes more carbonic acid. Now the H^+ is no longer free and will not decrease the blood pH:

$$HCO_3^- + H^+ \leftrightarrow H_2CO_3$$

$$\text{Bicarbonate ion} + \text{Hydrogen ion} \leftrightarrow \text{Carbonic acid}$$

If there are too few H^+ ions, the carbonic acid portion of the buffer pair will release some, increasing the bicarbonate, again returning pH to normal.

$$H_2CO_3 \leftrightarrow HCO_3^- + H^+$$

$$\text{Carbonic acid} \leftrightarrow \text{Bicarbonate ion} + \text{Hydrogen ion}$$

Other buffers include hemoglobin, protein buffers, and phosphate buffers. Cellular and bone buffers also contribute. Buffers normally keep the blood from becoming too acid when acids that are produced by cells circulate to the lungs and kidneys for excretion.

Acid Excretion. The body has two acid-excretion systems: lungs and kidneys. The lungs excrete carbonic acid; the kidneys excrete metabolic acids (see Fig. 41-8).

Excretion of Carbonic Acid. When you exhale, you excrete carbonic acid in the form of CO_2 and water. If the $PaCO_2$ (i.e., level of CO_2 in the blood) rises, the chemoreceptors trigger faster and deeper respirations to excrete the excess. If the $PaCO_2$ falls, the chemoreceptors trigger slower and shallower respirations so more of the CO_2 produced by cells remains in the blood and makes up the deficit. These alterations in respiratory rate and depth maintain the carbonic acid portion of acid-base balance (Coggon, 2008a). Sometimes people who have lung disease have difficulty with normal excretion of carbonic acid, which causes it to accumulate and make the blood more acid.

Excretion of Metabolic Acids. The kidneys excrete all acids except carbonic acid. They secrete H^+ into the renal tubular fluid, putting HCO_3^- back into the blood at the same time. If there are too many H^+ ions in the blood, renal cells move more H^+ ions into the renal tubules for excretion, retaining more HCO_3^- in the process. If there are too few H^+ ions in the blood, renal cells secrete fewer H^+ ions.

Phosphate buffers in the renal tubular fluid keep the urine from becoming too acidic when the kidneys excrete H^+ ions. If the kidneys need to excrete a lot of H^+, renal tubular cells secrete ammonia, which combines with the H^+ ions in the tubules to make NH_4^+, ammonium ions. Buffering by phosphate and the creation of NH_4^+ turn free H^+ ions into other molecules in the renal tubular fluid (Rose, 2011). This process enables metabolic acid excretion in urine without making urine too acidic. People who have kidney disease often have difficulty with normal excretion of metabolic acids.

Acid-Base Imbalances

People develop acid-base imbalances when their normal homeostatic mechanisms are dysfunctional or overwhelmed. The term **acidosis** describes a condition that tends to make the blood relatively too acidic. Because our cells produce two types of acid, there are two different types of acidosis: respiratory acidosis and metabolic acidosis. The term **alkalosis** describes a condition that tends to make the blood relatively too basic (alkaline). There are two types of alkalosis: respiratory alkalosis and metabolic alkalosis.

The body has compensatory mechanisms that limit the extent of pH change with acid-base imbalances (Coggon, 2008b; Rose, 2011). It is important to remember that the kidney or lung cannot compensate for itself. Therefore the kidneys compensate for respiratory acid-base imbalances; the respiratory system compensates for metabolic acid-base imbalances. These compensatory mechanisms do not correct the problem, but they assist the body to adapt. However, if the underlying condition is not corrected, these compensatory mechanisms will fail.

Respiratory Acidosis. **Respiratory acidosis** arises from alveolar hypoventilation; the lungs are unable to excrete enough CO_2. The $PaCO_2$ rises, creating an excess of carbonic acid in the blood, which decreases pH (Table 41-7). The kidneys compensate by increasing excretion of metabolic acids in the urine, which increases blood bicarbonate. This compensatory process is slow, often taking 24 hours to show clinical effect and 3 to 5 days to reach steady state. Decreased cerebrospinal fluid (CSF) pH and intracellular pH of brain cells cause decreased level of consciousness.

Respiratory Alkalosis. **Respiratory alkalosis** arises from alveolar hyperventilation; the lungs excrete too much carbonic acid (CO_2 and water). The $PaCO_2$ falls, creating a deficit of carbonic acid in the blood, which increases pH (see Table 41-7). Respiratory alkalosis usually is short lived; thus the kidneys do not have time to compensate. When the pH of blood, CSF, and ICF increases acutely, cell membrane excitability also increases, giving rise to neurological symptoms such as excitement, confusion, and paresthesias. If the pH rises high enough, central nervous system (CNS) depression can occur.

Metabolic Acidosis. **Metabolic acidosis** occurs from an increase of metabolic acid or a decrease of base (bicarbonate). The kidneys are unable to excrete enough metabolic acids, which accumulate in the blood, or bicarbonate is removed from the body directly as with diarrhea (see Table 41-7). In either case the blood HCO_3^- decreases, and the pH falls. With an increase of metabolic acids, blood HCO_3^- decreases because it is used to buffer metabolic acids. Similarly, when patients have conditions that cause the removal of HCO_3^-, the amount of HCO_3^- in the blood decreases. To help identify the specific cause, health care providers and the laboratory calculate the **anion gap,** a reflection of unmeasured anions in plasma. You calculate anion gap by subtracting the sum of plasma concentrations of the anions Cl^- and HCO_3^- from the plasma concentration of the cation Na^+ (Rose, 2011). When reviewing laboratory reports, check the reference values from the laboratory that measured the electrolyte concentrations (Table 41-8).

The abnormally low pH in metabolic acidosis stimulates the chemoreceptors so the respiratory system compensates for the acidosis by hyperventilation. Compensatory hyperventilation begins in a few minutes and removes carbonic acid from the body. This process does not correct the problem, but it helps limit the pH decrease. Metabolic acidosis decreases one's level of consciousness (see Table 41-7).

Metabolic Alkalosis. **Metabolic alkalosis** occurs from a direct increase of base (HCO_3^-) or a decrease of metabolic acid, which increases blood HCO_3^- by releasing it from its buffering function. Common causes include vomiting and gastric suction (see Table 41-7). The respiratory compensation for metabolic alkalosis is hypoventilation. The decreased rate and depth of respiration allow carbonic acid to increase in the blood, as seen by an increased $PaCO_2$. The need for oxygen may limit the degree of respiratory compensation for metabolic alkalosis. Because HCO_3^- crosses the blood-brain barrier with difficulty, neurological signs and symptoms are less severe or even absent with metabolic alkalosis (Rose, 2011).

NURSING KNOWLEDGE BASE

You will apply knowledge about fluid, electrolyte, and acid-base imbalance in many clinical settings. Use the scientific knowledge base in clinical decision making to provide safe, optimal fluid therapy. For example, apply knowledge of risk factors for fluid imbalances and physiology of normal aging when assessing older adults, knowing that this age-group has high risk of fluid imbalances (Bryant, 2007). Nursing knowledge includes questions to ask to elicit risk factors for fluid, electrolyte, and acid-base imbalance; specific clinical assessments for signs and symptoms of these imbalances; and nursing and collaborative interventions to maintain or restore fluid and electrolyte balance (Metheny, 2010). Skills and techniques for safe IV therapy, are a vital area of the nursing knowledge base and the focus of much nursing research to support evidence-based practice.

CRITICAL THINKING

Successful critical thinking requires a synthesis of knowledge, experience, information gathered from patients, critical thinking attitudes, and intellectual and professional standards. Clinical judgments require you to anticipate the information necessary to analyze the data and make decisions regarding patient care. Patients' conditions are always changing. During assessment, consider all critical thinking elements and data about the specific patient to develop appropriate nursing diagnoses.

In the case of fluid, electrolyte, and acid-base balance, you integrate knowledge of physiology, pathophysiology, and pharmacology and previous experiences and information gathered from patients. Critical analysis of data enables an understanding of how fluid, electrolyte, and acid-base imbalances affect a specific patient and his or her family. In addition, critical thinking attitudes such

TABLE 41-7 Acid-Base Imbalances

IMBALANCE AND RELATED CAUSES	SIGNS AND SYMPTOMS
Respiratory Acidosis—Excessive Carbonic Acid Caused by Alveolar Hypoventilation	
Impaired gas exchange: Type B COPD (chronic bronchitis) or end-stage type A COPD (emphysema) Pneumonia Severe acute asthma episode Airway obstruction Extensive atelectasis Obstructive sleep apnea Impaired neuromuscular function: Respiratory muscle weakness or paralysis from hypokalemia or neurological dysfunction Respiratory muscle fatigue, respiratory failure Chest injury or surgery causing pain with respiration Dysfunction of brainstem respiratory control: Drug overdose with a respiratory depressant Central sleep apnea	*Physical examination:* Headache, light-headedness, decreased level of consciousness (confusion, lethargy, ***coma***), ***cardiac dysrhythmia***, warm and flushed skin, muscular twitching Laboratory findings in blood: pH less than 7.35 $PaCO_2$ greater than 45 mm Hg (6 kPa) HCO_3^- level normal if uncompensated or greater than 26 mEq/L (26 mmol/L) if compensated
Respiratory Alkalosis—Deficient Carbonic Acid Caused by Alveolar Hyperventilation	
Hypoxemia Acute pain Anxiety, psychological distress, prolonged sobbing Inappropriate mechanical ventilator settings Stimulation of brainstem respiratory control: head injuries, meningitis, gram-negative sepsis, salicylate overdose	*Physical examination:* Increased rate and depth of respirations (hyperventilation), light-headedness, numbness and tingling of extremities and circumoral region (paresthesias), excitement and confusion possibly followed by decreased level of consciousness, ***cardiac dysrhythmias*** Laboratory findings in blood: pH greater than 7.45 $PaCO_2$ less than 35 mm Hg (4.7 kPa) HCO_3^- level normal if short lived or uncompensated or less than 22 mEq/L (22 mmol/L) if compensated K^+ level may be decreased (less than 3.5 mEq/L) Ionized Ca^{2+} level may be decreased (below 4.5 mg/dL)
Metabolic Acidosis—Excessive Metabolic Acids	
Increase of metabolic acid: Ketoacidosis (diabetes, starvation, alcoholism) Hypermetabolic state (severe hyperthyroidism, burns, severe infection) Oliguric renal disease (acute kidney injury, end-stage renal disease) Circulatory shock (lactic acidosis) Ingestion of acid or acid precursors (e.g., methanol, ethylene glycol, boric acid, salicylate overdose) Decrease of base (bicarbonate): Diarrhea Pancreatic fistula or intestinal decompression Renal tubular acidosis	*Physical examination:* Decreased level of consciousness (lethargy, confusion, ***coma***), abdominal pain, ***cardiac dysrhythmias,*** increased rate and depth of respirations (compensatory hyperventilation) Laboratory findings in blood: pH less than 7.35 $PaCO_2$ normal if uncompensated or less than 35 mm Hg (4.7 kPa) if compensated HCO_3^- level less than 22 mEq/L (22 mmol/L) Anion gap normal or high, depending on cause K^+ level may be elevated (greater than 5 mEq/L), depending on cause
Metabolic Alkalosis—Deficient Metabolic Acids	
Increase of base (bicarbonate): Excessive administration of $NaHCO_3$ Massive blood transfusion (liver converts citrate to HCO_3^-) Mild or moderate ECV deficit (contraction alkalosis) Decrease of metabolic acid: Excessive or prolonged vomiting Prolonged gastric suctioning Hypokalemia Excess aldosterone	*Physical examination:* Light-headedness, numbness and tingling of fingers, toes, and circumoral region (paresthesias); possible excitement and confusion followed by decreased level of consciousness, ***cardiac dysrhythmias*** (may be caused by hypokalemia) Laboratory findings in blood: pH greater than 7.45 $PaCO_2$ normal if uncompensated or greater than 45 mm Hg (6.0 kPa) if compensated HCO_3^- greater than 26 mEq/L (26 mmol/L) K^+ level often decreased (less than 3.5 mEq/L) Ionized Ca^{2+} level may be decreased (less than 4.5 mg/dL)

COPD, Chronic obstructive pulmonary disease, *ECV,* extracellular fluid volume. ***Text in bold italics denotes potentially life-threatening manifestations.***

TABLE 41-8 Anion Gap in Metabolic Acidosis

ANION GAP TYPE	VALUES (WITHOUT K^+)	CAUSES
Normal anion gap	5-11 mEq/L (5-11 mmol/L) Varies, depending on laboratory	*Excess output of bicarbonate:* Diarrhea, pancreatic fistula, intestinal decompression, renal tubular acidosis Increase of chloride-containing acid: Parenteral HCl therapy
High anion gap	Greater than 11 mEq/L (11 mmol/L) Varies, depending on laboratory	*Increase of any acid except HCl:* Ketoacids (DKA, starvation, alcoholism), lactic acid (circulatory shock, extreme exercise), excessive normal metabolic acids (oliguric acute kidney injury, end-stage renal disease, severe hyperthyroidism, burns, severe infection), unusual organic acids (salicylate overdose, acids metabolized from methanol, ethylene glycol, paraldehyde)

Data from Rose BD: *Clinical physiology of acid-base disorders*, ed 6, New York, 2011, McGraw-Hill.
DKA, Diabetic ketoacidosis.

as accountability, discipline, and integrity assist you in identifying appropriate nursing diagnoses and planning successful interventions. Professional standards such as the Infusion Nurses Society (INS) standards of practice (INS, 2011) provide valuable guidance for appropriate assessment.

NURSING PROCESS

Apply the nursing process and use a critical thinking approach in your care of patients. The nursing process provides a clinical decision-making approach for you to develop and implement an individualized plan of care. For patients at high risk for fluid, electrolyte, and/or acid-base imbalances or those who already have these imbalances, an individualized approach is the foundation for safe and effective patient-centered nursing care.

ASSESSMENT

During the assessment process, thoroughly assess each patient and critically analyze findings to ensure you make patient-centered clinical decisions required for safe nursing care. Using a systematic approach in assessment enables you to help patients maintain or restore fluid, electrolyte, and acid-base balances safely (Fig. 41-9).

Through the Patient's Eyes. A patient's fluid, electrolyte, or acid-base imbalance is sometimes so severe that it prevents initial discussion of his or her expressed needs, values, and preferences. However, when a patient is alert enough to discuss care, you need to elicit this information. Focus on the patient's experience with fluid, electrolyte, or acid-base alterations and his or her perceptions of the illness. For example, for a patient who is hospitalized for clinical dehydration from diarrhea, ask if he or she has experienced dehydration previously, and assess his or her interpretation of the signs and symptoms experienced and possible causes. For example, ask how the person manages diarrhea at home to assess

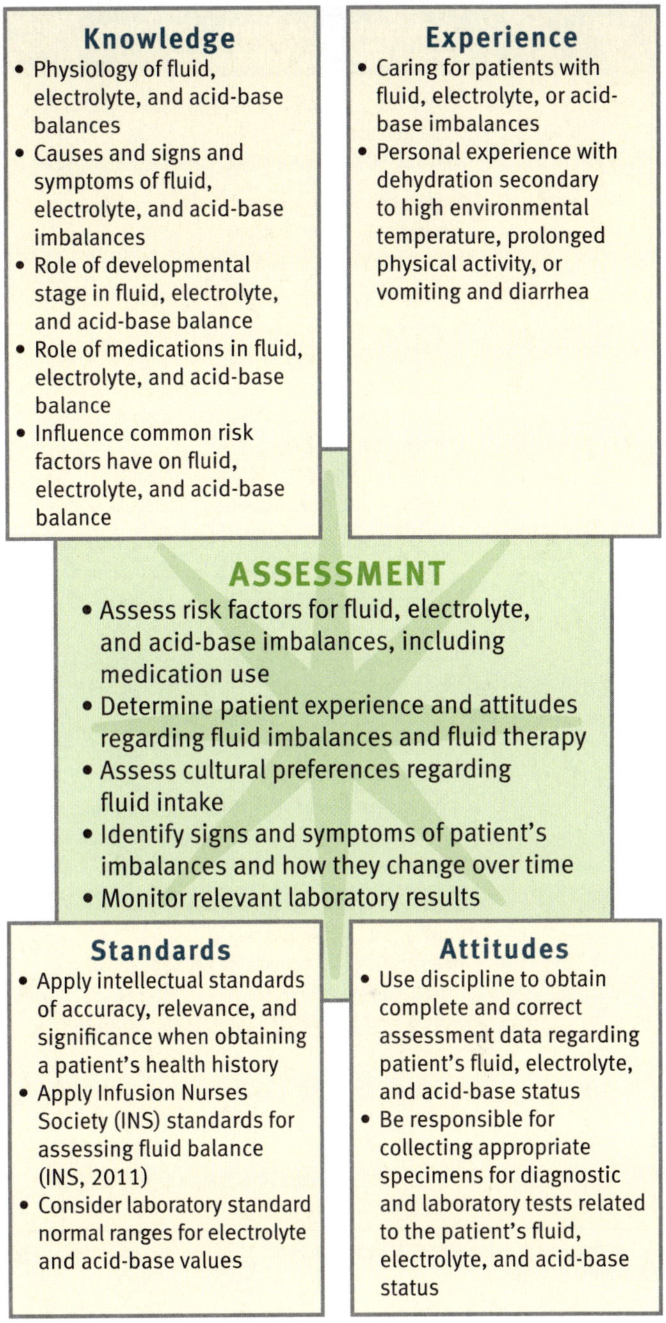
Knowledge
• Physiology of fluid, electrolyte, and acid-base balances
• Causes and signs and symptoms of fluid, electrolyte, and acid-base imbalances
• Role of developmental stage in fluid, electrolyte, and acid-base balance
• Role of medications in fluid, electrolyte, and acid-base balance
• Influence common risk factors have on fluid, electrolyte, and acid-base balance
Experience
• Caring for patients with fluid, electrolyte, or acid-base imbalances
• Personal experience with dehydration secondary to high environmental temperature, prolonged physical activity, or vomiting and diarrhea
ASSESSMENT
• Assess risk factors for fluid, electrolyte, and acid-base imbalances, including medication use
• Determine patient experience and attitudes regarding fluid imbalances and fluid therapy
• Assess cultural preferences regarding fluid intake
• Identify signs and symptoms of patient's imbalances and how they change over time
• Monitor relevant laboratory results
Standards
• Apply intellectual standards of accuracy, relevance, and significance when obtaining a patient's health history
• Apply Infusion Nurses Society (INS) standards for assessing fluid balance (INS, 2011)
• Consider laboratory standard normal ranges for electrolyte and acid-base values
Attitudes
• Use discipline to obtain complete and correct assessment data regarding patient's fluid, electrolyte, and acid-base status
• Be responsible for collecting appropriate specimens for diagnostic and laboratory tests related to the patient's fluid, electrolyte, and acid-base status

FIG. 41-9 Critical thinking model for fluid, electrolyte, and acid-base balances assessment.

the patient's understanding of how to prevent the imbalances from occurring in the future. Assess potential barriers to rehydration, such as concerns regarding IV therapy or lack of availability of favorite fluids at the preferred fluid temperature. Ask about the patient's greatest concerns regarding fluid status to build the basis for active partnership in planning, implementing, and evaluating patient-centered care.

Nursing History

Clinical assessment begins with a patient history designed to reveal risk factors that cause or contribute to fluid, electrolyte, and acid-base imbalances (Table 41-9). Ask specific, focused questions to

TABLE 41-9 Risk Factors for Fluid, Electrolyte, and Acid-Base Imbalances

Age	*Very young:* ECV deficit, osmolality imbalances, clinical dehydration *Very old:* ECV excess or deficit, osmolality imbalances
Environment	Sodium-rich diet: ECV excess Electrolyte-poor diet: Electrolyte deficits *Hot weather:* Clinical dehydration
Gastrointestinal output	*Diarrhea:* ECV deficit, clinical dehydration, hypokalemia, hypocalcemia (if chronic), hypomagnesemia (if chronic), metabolic acidosis *Drainage (e.g., nasogastric suctioning, fistulas):* ECV deficit, hypokalemia; metabolic acidosis if intestinal or pancreatic drainage *Vomiting:* ECV deficit, clinical dehydration, hypokalemia, hypomagnesemia, metabolic alkalosis
Chronic diseases	*Cancer:* Hypercalcemia; with tumor lysis syndrome: hyperkalemia, hypocalcemia, hyperphosphatemia; other imbalances, depending on side effects of therapy Chronic obstructive pulmonary disease: Respiratory acidosis *Cirrhosis:* ECV excess, hypokalemia *Heart failure:* ECV excess; other imbalances, depending on therapy *Oliguric renal disease:* ECV excess, hyperkalemia, hypermagnesemia, hyperphosphatemia, metabolic acidosis
Trauma	*Burns:* ECV deficit, metabolic acidosis Crush injuries: Hyperkalemia *Head injuries:* Hyponatremia or hypernatremia, depending on ADH response *Hemorrhage:* ECV deficit; hyperkalemia if circulatory shock
Therapies	Diuretics and other medications (see Box 41-3) *IV therapy:* ECV excess, osmolality imbalances, electrolyte excesses *PN:* Any fluid or electrolyte imbalance, depending on components of solution

ADH, Antidiuretic hormone; *ECV,* extracellular fluid volume; *IV,* intravenous; *PN,* parenteral nutrition.

identify factors that contribute to a patient's potential imbalances (Box 41-1).

Age. First assess a patient's age. An infant's proportion of total body water (70% to 80% total body weight) is greater than that of children or adults. Infants and young children have greater water needs and immature kidneys (Hockenberry and Wilson, 2011). They are at greater risk for ECV deficit and hypernatremia because body water loss is proportionately greater per kilogram of weight.

Children who are between the ages of 2 and 12 frequently respond to illnesses with fevers of higher temperatures and longer duration than those of adults (Hockenberry and Wilson, 2011). At any age fever increases the rate of insensible water loss. Adolescents have increased metabolism and increased water production because of their rapid growth changes. Fluctuations in fluid balance are greater in adolescent girls because of hormonal changes associated with the menstrual cycle.

Older adults experience a number of age-related changes that potentially affect fluid, electrolyte, and acid-base balances (Box 41-2). They often have more difficulty recovering from imbalances resulting from the combined effect of normal aging, various disease conditions, and multiple medications.

Environment. Hot environments increase fluid output through sweating. Sweat is a hypotonic sodium-containing fluid.

BOX 41-1 NURSING ASSESSMENT QUESTIONS

Environment
- Do you work or exercise in a hot environment?
- If so, which type of fluid do you drink during that time?

Dietary Intake
- How much do you usually drink every day? Which type of fluids do you drink?
- Tell me what you eat in a typical day.
- Which snacks do you usually eat?
- Are you on a special diet because of a medical problem? How does that work for you?
- Are you following any weight loss program?
- Do you use a salt substitute?
- Do you take calcium, magnesium, or potassium supplements? If so, how often?
- Do you have any difficulties chewing or swallowing?

Lifestyle
- How much alcohol do you drink in a typical week?

Gastrointestinal Output
- Have you had recent vomiting or diarrhea? If so, for how long? How many times per day?

Medications and Other Therapies
- Which medications/herbal remedies do you use regularly? Occasionally?
- Do you take diuretics? Drugs for high blood pressure?
- Do you use antacids? If so, which ones? How often? Do you ever use baking soda as an antacid? Do you use fizzy (effervescent) medications for colds?
- Do you use laxatives? If so, how often? Which type of stool do you get when you use them?
- What do you use for an upset stomach?

Signs and Symptoms
- If you weigh yourself every day, how has your weight changed over the past few days?
- Do you get light-headed when you stand up?
- Do you feel thirsty, have a dry mouth, or notice a lack of tears?
- Have you noticed a change in your urine output: decreased volume, dark color, or concentrated appearance?
- Are you experiencing swelling of your fingers, feet, or ankles?
- Do you have difficulty breathing when you lie down at night?
- Are you having difficulty concentrating, or do you feel confused? What is normal for you?
- Are you having more difficulty than usual standing up from a sofa or soft chair? Do your legs feel unusually heavy when you climb stairs? Do you have muscle weakness that is unusual for you?
- Have you noticed any muscle cramps or unusual sensations such as numbness or tingling fingers?

BOX 41-2 FOCUS ON OLDER ADULTS

Factors Affecting Fluid, Electrolyte, and Acid-Base Balance

- Body composition changes, causing a decreased percentage of body weight as water (50%), which increases risk of extracellular fluid volume (ECV) deficit and dehydration (Felver, 2010b).
- Some older adults restrict fluid intake because of impaired mobility or concerns about bladder control; this increases their risk of hypernatremia and ECV deficit.
- Decreased elasticity of skin alters skin turgor even with normal fluid balance; do not rely on skin turgor to assess ECV deficit or dehydration in older adults.
- Decreased thirst sensation increases risk of hypernatremia and dehydration; do not rely on thirst to assess hypernatremia, ECV deficit, or dehydration in older adults (Wotton, Crannitch, and Munt, 2008).
- Baroreceptors become sluggish with age, often causing brief postural hypotension; have older adults arise slowly when you take orthostatic blood pressure measurements.
- Cardiovascular changes with aging often decrease the ability to adapt to a sudden increase in vascular volume, increasing risk of pulmonary edema with rapid infusion of isotonic intravenous fluids.
- Older-adult kidneys are less able to concentrate urine, making them less able to conserve fluid when needed; this increases the risk of hypernatremia, ECV deficit, and dehydration (Meiner, 2010).
- Kidney changes of normal aging make it more difficult to excrete a large acid load, increasing the risk of metabolic acidosis.
- Increased sensitivity to anticholinergic effects of medications causes dry mouth; use several different assessments for ECV deficit and dehydration rather than relying solely on dry mouth (Lehne, 2010).
- The combined effects of normal aging, chronic diseases, and multiple medications often pose challenges to maintaining fluid and electrolyte balance.

Excessive sweating without adequate replacement of salt and water can lead to ECV deficit, hypernatremia, or clinical dehydration. Ask patients about their normal level of physical work and whether they engage in vigorous exercise in hot environments. Do the patients have fluid replacements containing salt available during exercise and activity?

Dietary Intake. Assess dietary intake of fluids; salt; and foods rich in potassium, calcium, and magnesium (see Table 41-4). Ask patients if they follow weight-loss diets. Starvation diets or those with high fat and no carbohydrate content often lead to metabolic acidosis (see Table 41-7). In addition, assess the patient's ability to chew and swallow, which, if altered, interferes with adequate intake of electrolyte-rich foods and fluids.

Lifestyle. Take an alcohol intake history. Chronic alcohol abuse commonly causes hypomagnesemia, in part because it increases renal magnesium excretion.

Medications. Obtain a complete list of your patient's current medications, including over-the-counter (OTC) and herbal preparations, to assess the risk for fluid, electrolyte, and acid-base imbalances (Box 41-3). Use a drug reference book or reputable online database to check the potential effects of other medications. Ask specifically about the use of baking soda as an antacid, which can cause ECV excess because of its high sodium content that holds water in the extracellular compartments. For an individual who uses laxatives, ask about the consistency and frequency of stools. Multiple loose stools remove fluid and electrolytes from the body, thus causing numerous imbalances.

BOX 41-3 COMMONLY USED MEDICATIONS THAT CAUSE FLUID, ELECTROLYTE, AND ACID-BASE IMBALANCES

- *ACE inhibitors (e.g., captopril [Capoten]) and angiotensin II receptor blockers (e.g., Losartan [Cozaar]):* Hyperkalemia
- *Antidepressants, SSRI (e.g., fluoxetine [Prozac]):* Hyponatremia
- *Calcium carbonate antacids:* Hypercalcemia, mild metabolic alkalosis
- *Corticosteroids (e.g., prednisone):* Hypokalemia, metabolic alkalosis
- *Diuretics, potassium-wasting (e.g., furosemide [Lasix], thiazides):* ECV deficit, hyponatremia (thiazides), hypokalemia, hypomagnesemia, mild metabolic alkalosis
- *Diuretics, potassium-sparing (e.g., spironolactone [Aldactone]):* Hyperkalemia, mild metabolic acidosis
- *Effervescent (fizzy) antacids and cold medications (high Na^+ content):* ECV excess
- *Laxatives:* ECV deficit, hypokalemia, hypocalcemia, hypomagnesemia, metabolic acidosis
- *Magnesium hydroxide (e.g., Milk of Magnesia):* Hypermagnesemia
- *Nonsteroidal antiinflammatory drugs (e.g., ibuprofen [Advil]):* Mild ECV excess, hyponatremia
- *Penicillins, high-dose (e.g., carbenicillin):* Hypokalemia, metabolic alkalosis; hyperkalemia with penicillin G (contains K^+)

Data from Haskal R: Current issues for nurse practitioners: hyponatremia, *J Am Acad Nurs Practitioners* 19(11):563, 2007; Lehne, RA: *Pharmacology for nursing care*, ed 7, Philadelphia, 2010, Saunders; Metheny NM: *Fluids and electrolytes balance: nursing applications*, ed 5, Sudbury, Mass, 2010, Jones & Bartlett Learning.

ACE, Angiotensin-converting enzyme; *ECV*, extracellular fluid volume; *SSRI*, selective serotonin reuptake inhibitor.

Medical History

Recent Surgery. Surgery causes a physiological stress response, which increases with extensive surgery and blood loss. In the second to fifth postoperative day, increased secretion of aldosterone, glucocorticoids, and ADH cause increased ECV, decreased osmolality, and increased potassium excretion (Monahan et al., 2007). In otherwise healthy patients these imbalances resolve without difficulty, but patients who have preexisting illnesses or additional risk factors often need treatment during this time period.

Gastrointestinal Output. Increased output of fluid through the GI tract is a common and important cause of fluid, electrolyte, and acid-base imbalances that requires careful assessment. Vomiting and diarrhea, either acute or chronic, can cause ECV deficit, hypernatremia, clinical dehydration, and hypokalemia by increasing the output of fluid, Na^+, and K^+. In addition, chronic diarrhea can cause hypocalcemia and hypomagnesemia by decreasing electrolyte absorption. Removal of gastric acid from the body through vomiting or nasogastric suction can cause metabolic alkalosis. In contrast, removal of the bicarbonate-rich intestinal or pancreatic fluids through diarrhea, intestinal suction, or fistula can cause metabolic acidosis.

Acute Illness or Trauma. Acute conditions that place patients at high risk for fluid, electrolyte, and acid-base alterations include respiratory diseases, burns, trauma, GI alterations, and acute oliguric renal disease.

Respiratory Disorders. Many acute respiratory disorders predispose patients to respiratory acidosis. For example, bacterial pneumonia causes alveoli to fill with exudate that impairs gas exchange, causing the patient to retain carbon dioxide, which leads to increased $PaCO_2$ and respiratory acidosis.

Burns. Burns place patients at high risk for ECV deficit from numerous mechanisms, including plasma-to-interstitial fluid shift and increased evaporative and exudate output. The greater the body surface burned, the greater is the fluid loss (Copstead and Banasik, 2010). Patients with burns often develop metabolic acidosis because of greatly increased cellular metabolism, which produces more metabolic acids than their kidneys are able to excrete.

Trauma. Hemorrhage from any type of trauma causes ECV deficit from blood loss. Some types of trauma create additional risks. For example, crush injuries cause hyperkalemia. The trauma from the crush injury destroys the cellular structure, resulting in a massive release of intracellular K^+ into the blood.

Head injury typically alters ADH secretion. It may cause diabetes insipidus (secretion of too little ADH), in which patients excrete large volumes of very dilute urine and develop hypernatremia. In contrast, head injury may cause the syndrome of inappropriate antidiuretic hormone (SIADH), in which excess secretion of ADH causes hyponatremia by retaining too much water and concentrating the urine (Copstead and Banasik, 2010).

Chronic Illness. Many chronic diseases create ongoing risk of fluid, electrolyte, and acid-base imbalances. In addition, the treatment regimens for chronic disease often cause imbalances. Assess patients for the presence of these conditions.

Cancer. The types of fluid and electrolyte imbalances that occur with cancer depend on the type and progression of the cancer and treatment regimen. Many patients with cancer develop hypercalcemia when their cancer cells secrete chemicals that circulate into bones and cause calcium to enter the blood. Other fluid and electrolyte imbalances occur in cancer because some types of tumors cause metabolic and endocrine abnormalities. In addition, patients with cancer are at risk for fluid and electrolyte imbalances as a result of the side effects (e.g., anorexia, diarrhea) of chemotherapy, biological response modifiers, or radiation (Copstead and Banasik, 2010).

Heart Failure. Patients who have chronic heart failure have diminished cardiac output, which reduces kidney perfusion and activates the RAAS. The action of aldosterone on the kidneys causes ECV excess and risk of hypokalemia. Most diuretics used to treat heart failure increase the risk of hypokalemia while reducing the ECV excess. Dietary sodium restriction is important with heart failure because Na^+ holds water in the ECF, making the ECV excess worse. In severe heart failure restriction of both fluid and sodium is prescribed to decrease the workload of the heart by reducing excess circulating fluid volume (Copstead and Banasik, 2010).

Oliguric Renal Disease. Oliguria occurs when the kidneys have a reduced capacity to make urine. Some conditions, such as acute rephritis, cause a sudden onset of oliguria, whereas other problems, such as chronic kidney disease, lead to chronic oliguria. Oliguric renal disease prevents normal excretion of fluid, electrolytes, and metabolic acids, resulting in ECV excess, hyperkalemia, hypermagnesemia, hyperphosphatemia, and metabolic acidosis. The severity of these imbalances is proportional to the degree of renal failure. Although chronic kidney disease is progressive, successful management of imbalances is possible with dietary restriction of sodium and other electrolytes, fluid restriction in severe cases, and eventually dialysis or renal transplant (Copstead and Banasik, 2010).

Physical Assessment

Data gathered through a focused physical assessment validates and extends the information collected in the patient history. Table 41-10 summarizes focused assessments for patients with fluid, electrolyte, and acid-base imbalances. Focus your assessment on the areas pertinent to each patient situation. For example, for patients at risk of fluid imbalances, focus your assessment on body weight changes, clinical markers of vascular and interstitial volume, thirst, behavior changes, and level of consciousness. Additional focused assessments for patients at high risk of electrolyte and acid-base imbalances include specific cardiac, respiratory, neuromuscular, and GI markers. Grouping your assessments under these categories helps you know which assessments to prioritize and enables you to assess effectively.

Daily Weights and Fluid Intake and Output Measurement. Daily weights are an important indicator of fluid status (Metheny, 2010). Each kilogram (2.2 lbs) of weight gained or lost overnight is equal to 1 L of fluid retained or lost. These fluid gains or losses indicate changes in the amount of total body fluid, usually ECF, but do not indicate shift between body compartments. Weigh patients with heart failure and those who are at high risk for or actually have ECV excess daily. Daily weights are also useful for patients with clinical dehydration or other causes or risks for ECV deficit. Weigh the patient at the same time each day with the same scale after a patient voids. Calibrate the scale each day or routinely. The patient needs to wear the same clothes or clothes that weigh the same; if using a bed scale, use the same number of sheets on the scale with each weighing. Compare the weight of each day with that of the previous day to determine fluid gains or losses. Look at the weights over several days to recognize trends. Interpretation of daily weights guides medical therapy and nursing care. Teach patients with heart failure to take and record their daily weights at home and to contact their health care provider if their weight increases suddenly by a set amount (obtain parameters from their health care providers). Recognizing trends in daily weights taken at home is important. Research shows that patients who are hospitalized for decompensated heart failure often experience steady increases in daily weights during the week before hospitalization. A weight gain of more than 2.2 lbs (1 kg) was associated with increased risk of hospitalization because of heart failure (Chaudry et al., 2007).

Measuring and recording all liquid intake and output (I&O) during a 24-hour period is an important aspect of fluid balance assessment. Compare a patient's 24-hour intake with his or her 24-hour output. The two measures should be approximately equal if the person has normal fluid balance. To interpret situations in which I&O are substantially different, consider the individual patient. For example, if intake is substantially greater than output, there are two possibilities: the patient may be gaining excessive fluid or may be returning to normal fluid status by replacing fluid lost previously from the body. Similarly, if intake is substantially smaller than output, there are also two possibilities: The patient may be losing needed fluid from the body and developing ECV deficit and/or hypernatremia or may be returning to normal fluid status by excreting excessive fluid gained previously.

In most health care settings I&O measurement is a nursing assessment. Some agencies require a health care provider's order for I&O. If you want to measure I&O for a patient with compromised fluid status, check your agency policies to determine whether you can institute it or if you need a health care provider's order.

Fluid intake includes all liquids that a person eats (e.g., gelatin, ice cream, soup), drinks, (e.g., water, coffee, juice), or receives through nasogastric or jejunostomy feeding tubes (see Chapter 44). IV fluids (continuous infusions and intermittent IV piggybacks) and blood components are also sources of intake. Water swallowed while taking pills and liquid medications also counts as intake. A patient receiving tube feedings often receives numerous liquid medications, and water is used to flush the tube before and/or after medications. Over a 24-hour period these liquids amount to significant intake and always are recorded on the I&O record.

TABLE 41-10 Focused Nursing Assessments for Patients with Fluid, Electrolyte, and Acid-Base Imbalances

ASSESSMENT	IMBALANCES
Body Weight Changes from Previous Day	
Loss of 2.2 lbs (1 kg) or more in 24 hours for adults	ECV deficit
Gain of 2.2 lbs (1 kg) or more in 24 hours for adults	ECV excess
Clinical Markers of Vascular Volume	
Blood pressure:	
Hypotension or orthostatic hypotension	ECV deficit
Light-headedness on sitting upright or standing	ECV deficit
Pulse rate and character:	
Rapid, thready	ECV deficit
Bounding	ECV excess
Fullness of neck veins:	
Flat or collapsing with inhalation when supine	ECV deficit
Full or distended when upright or semi-upright	ECV excess
Capillary refill: Sluggish	ECV deficit
Lung auscultation, dependent portions: Crackles or rhonchi with progressive dyspnea	ECV excess
Urine output: Small volume of dark yellow urine	ECV deficit
Clinical Markers of Interstitial Volume	
Presence of edema: Present in dependent areas (ankles or sacrum) and possibly fingers or around eyes	ECV excess
Mucous membranes: Dry between cheek and gum, decreased or absent tearing	ECV deficit
Skin turgor: Pinched skin fails to return to normal position within 3 seconds	ECV deficit
Presence of thirst: Thirst present	Hypernatremia, severe ECV deficit
Behavior and Level of Consciousness	
Restlessness and mild confusion	Severe ECV deficit
Decreased level of consciousness (lethargy, confusion, coma)	Hyponatremia, hypernatremia, hypercalcemia, acid-base imbalances
Cardiac and Respiratory Signs of Electrolyte or Acid-Base Imbalances	
Pulse rhythm and ECG: Irregular pulse and ECG changes	K^+, Ca^{2+}, Mg^{2+}, and/or acid-base imbalances
Rate and depth of respirations:	
Increased rate and depth	Metabolic acidosis (compensatory mechanism); respiratory alkalosis (cause)
Decreased rate and depth	Metabolic alkalosis (compensatory mechanism); respiratory acidosis (cause)
Neuromuscular Markers of Electrolyte or Acid-Base Imbalances	
Muscle strength bilaterally, especially quadriceps muscles:	
Muscle weakness	Hypokalemia, hyperkalemia
Reflexes and sensations:	
Decreased deep tendon reflexes	Hypercalcemia, hypermagnesemia
Hyperactive reflexes, muscle twitching and cramps, tetany	Hypocalcemia, hypomagnesemia
Numbness, tingling in fingertips, around mouth	Hypocalcemia, hypomagnesemia, respiratory alkalosis
Muscle cramps, tetany	Hypocalcemia, hypomagnesemia, respiratory alkalosis
Tremors	Hypomagnesemia
Gastrointestinal Signs of Electrolyte Imbalances	
Inspection and auscultation:	
Abdominal distention	Hypokalemia, third-spacing of fluid
Decreased bowel sounds	Hypokalemia
Motility: Constipation	Hypokalemia, hypercalcemia

ECG, Electrocardiogram; *ECV,* extracellular fluid volume.

Ask patients who are alert and oriented to assist with measuring their oral intake and explain to families why they should not drink or eat from the patient's meal trays or water pitcher.

Fluid output includes urine, diarrhea, vomitus, gastric suction, and drainage from postsurgical wounds or other tubes (see Chapter 50). Record a patient's urinary output after each voiding. Instruct patients who are alert, oriented, and ambulatory to save their urine in a calibrated insert, which attaches to the rim of the toilet bowl (Fig. 41-10). Teach patients and families the purpose of I&O measurements. Teach them to notify the nurse or nursing assistive personnel (NAP) to empty any container with voided fluid or how to measure and empty the container themselves and report the result appropriately. Patients need to have good vision and motor skills to perform these measurements. Active involvement of patient and family is an aspect of patient-centered care that is essential to maintaining accurate I&O measurements. When a patient has an indwelling urinary catheter, drainage tube, or suction, record output (e.g., at the end of each nursing shift or every hour) as the patient's condition requires.

You can delegate portions of I&O measurement and recording to NAP with competent skills in measurement. Research shows that visual estimates of fluid volumes often are unreliable; actual measurement is preferable (McConnell et al., 2007). In many institutions NAP record oral intake but not intake through feeding or IV tubes, which are nursing responsibilities. Similarly NAP often record urine, diarrhea, and vomitus output but not drainage through tubes. The responsible registered nurse (RN) or licensed practical nurse/licensed vocational nurse (LPN/LVN) and the NAP work as a team to record measurements in the designated location in the electronic health record (EHR), often on a flow sheet with other information. The EHR program usually calculates the 24-hour totals. If an EHR is not used, record I&O on paper forms attached to the bedside chart or room door. You or the NAP calculate the 24-hour totals (see agency policy). Accurate I&O facilitates ongoing evaluation of a patient's hydration status.

Laboratory Values

Review the patient's laboratory test results and compare them with the normal ranges to obtain further objective data about fluid, electrolyte, and acid-base balances. Normal and abnormal test results are summarized in Tables 41-1, 41-3, 41-5, 41-6, and 41-7. The frequency of electrolyte level measurements depends on the severity of the patient's illness. Analysis of laboratory results requires a good medical clinician, especially if a person develops an acute imbalance while also having a chronic disease. Serum electrolyte tests usually are performed routinely on any patient entering a hospital to screen for imbalances and serve as a baseline for future comparisons.

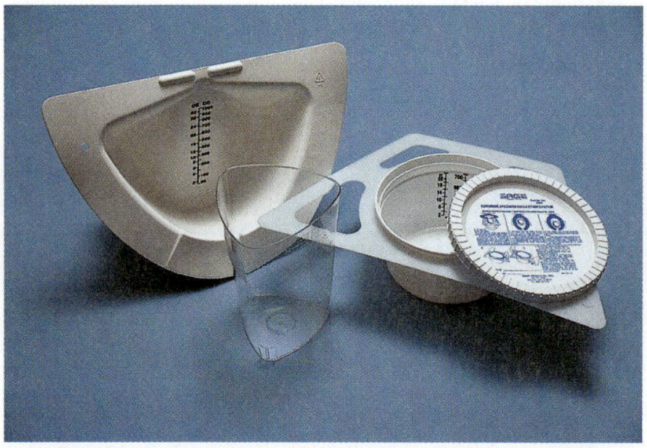

FIG. 41-10 Containers for measuring urine output.

NURSING DIAGNOSIS

When caring for patients with suspected fluid, electrolyte, and acid-base imbalances, it is particularly important to use critical thinking to formulate nursing diagnoses. The assessment data that establish the risk for or the actual presence of a nursing diagnosis in these areas are often subtle, and patterns and trends emerge only when there has been astute assessment. Multiple body systems are often involved; careful clustering of defining characteristics leads to selection of the appropriate diagnoses (Box 41-4).

In addition to the accurate clustering of assessment data, an important part of formulating nursing diagnoses is identifying the relevant causative or related factor. You choose interventions that treat or modify the related factor for the diagnosis to be resolved. For example, *deficient fluid volume related to loss of GI fluids from vomiting* requires therapies that manage the patients' emesis and restore fluid volume with IV therapy. In contrast, the diagnosis of *deficient fluid volume related to elevated body temperature* requires therapies to lower the patient's body temperature and replace lost body fluids through oral fluid replacement or possibly IV therapy. Possible nursing diagnoses for patients with fluid, electrolyte, and acid-base alterations include the following:

- Decreased cardiac output
- Acute confusion
- Risk for electrolyte imbalance
- Deficient fluid volume
- Excess fluid volume
- Impaired gas exchange
- Risk for injury
- Deficient knowledge regarding disease management
- Impaired oral mucous membrane
- Impaired skin integrity
- Ineffective tissue perfusion

PLANNING

During the planning process use critical thinking to synthesize information from multiple resources (Fig. 41-11). Ensure that

BOX 41-4 NURSING DIAGNOSTIC PROCESS

Deficient Fluid Volume Related to Loss of Gastrointestinal Fluids via Vomiting

ASSESSMENT ACTIVITIES	DEFINING CHARACTERISTICS
Assess postural blood pressure and pulse.	Patient has postural hypotension with increased heart rate; pulse is weak.
Inspect oral mucous membranes for degree of moisture.	Oral mucous membranes between cheek and gum are dry.
Obtain daily weight measurements.	Adult patient loses 2.2 lbs (1 kg) or more in 24 hours.
Measure urine output and observe color; if available, measure specific gravity of urine.	Patient produces small volume of dark yellow urine; urine specific gravity is increased.
Test skin turgor (not reliable for older adults).	Decreased skin turgor noted.

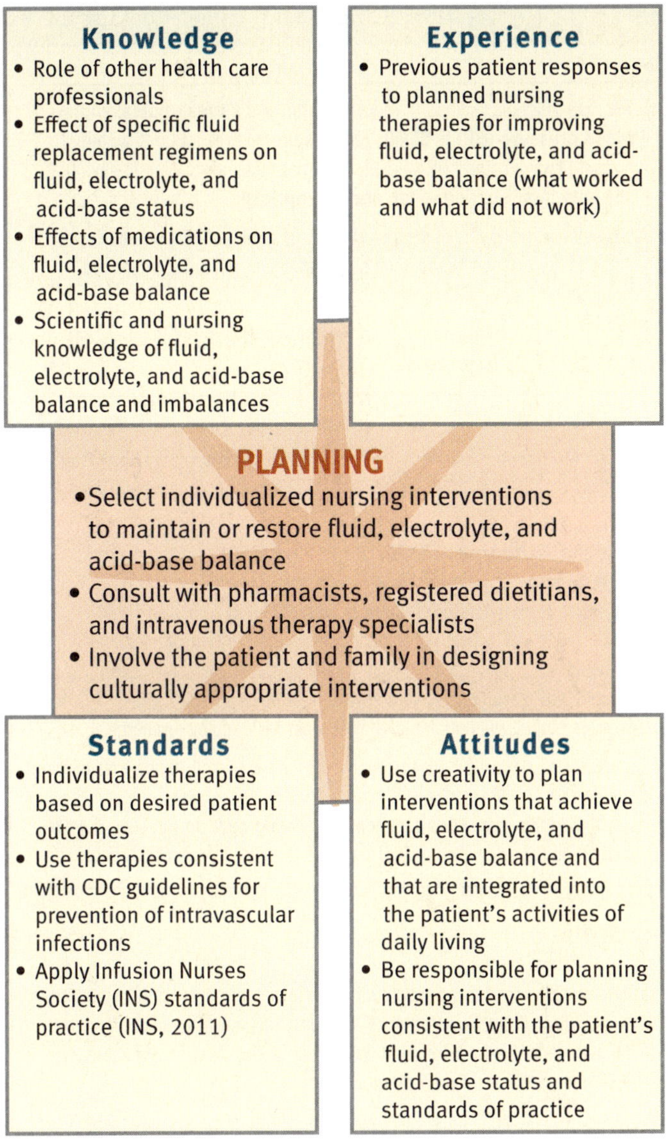
Knowledge
• Role of other health care professionals
• Effect of specific fluid replacement regimens on fluid, electrolyte, and acid-base status
• Effects of medications on fluid, electrolyte, and acid-base balance
• Scientific and nursing knowledge of fluid, electrolyte, and acid-base balance and imbalances
Experience
• Previous patient responses to planned nursing therapies for improving fluid, electrolyte, and acid-base balance (what worked and what did not work)
PLANNING
• Select individualized nursing interventions to maintain or restore fluid, electrolyte, and acid-base balance
• Consult with pharmacists, registered dietitians, and intravenous therapy specialists
• Involve the patient and family in designing culturally appropriate interventions
Standards
• Individualize therapies based on desired patient outcomes
• Use therapies consistent with CDC guidelines for prevention of intravascular infections
• Apply Infusion Nurses Society (INS) standards of practice (INS, 2011)
Attitudes
• Use creativity to plan interventions that achieve fluid, electrolyte, and acid-base balance and that are integrated into the patient's activities of daily living
• Be responsible for planning nursing interventions consistent with the patient's fluid, electrolyte, and acid-base status and standards of practice

FIG. 41-11 Critical thinking model for fluid, electrolyte, and acid-base balances planning. *CDC,* Centers for Disease Control and Prevention.

the patient's plan of care integrates both scientific and nursing knowledge and all of the information that you collected about the individual patient.

Goals and Outcomes. Establish an individual patient plan of care for each nursing diagnosis (see the Nursing Care Plan) that includes mutually established patient goals for each diagnosis. Goals need to be individualized and realistic with measurable outcomes. For example, with a nursing diagnosis of *deficient fluid volume,* the following related outcomes may be established for the goal, "The patient will achieve normal hydration status at discharge":

- The patient will be free of complications associated with the IV device throughout the duration of IV therapy.
- The patient will demonstrate balanced I&O measurements within 48 hours.
- The patient will have serum electrolytes within the normal range within 48 hours.

Setting Priorities. The patient's clinical condition determines which of the nursing diagnoses takes the greatest priority. Many nursing diagnoses in the area of fluid, electrolyte, and acid-base balances are of highest priority because the consequences for the patient can be serious or even life threatening. For example, in the concept map (Fig. 41-12 on p. 903) for Mrs. Beck, the occurrence of vomiting and diarrhea created a high-priority nursing diagnosis of *fluid volume deficit.* In this situation intervention is necessary to help resolve her vomiting and diarrhea and replace her deficient fluid volume. If these priorities are unmet, Mrs. Beck's fluid imbalance likely will worsen.

Teamwork and Collaboration. Consultation with a patient's health care provider helps to set realistic time frames for the goals of care, particularly when the patient's physiological status is unstable. Ongoing communication and consultation are important because the patient's condition can change quickly. Collaboration with the patient and family and other members of the interdisciplinary health care team such as IV therapy and pharmacy assists in achieving patient outcomes. Patient and family are very helpful in identifying approaches for successful therapies, such as ways to increase fluid intake. Incorporate patient preferences and resources into the plan of care. Do **not** delegate administration of IV fluid and hemodynamic assessment to NAP. When the patient is stable, you can delegate daily weights, I&O, and direct physical care to NAP.

NURSING CARE PLAN

Deficient Fluid Volume

ASSESSMENT

Mrs. Hilda Beck is a 72-year-old seen by her health care provider this morning after falling at home and telephoning a neighbor for assistance. She lives alone in an apartment and has no chronic disease except for osteoarthritis of her hands. She has had diarrhea and vomiting for over 24 hours and has not eaten anything. Despite feeling slightly nauseated, she tried to drink a little water, because she knew she needed it. Mrs. Beck is admitted for intravenous (IV) fluid therapy. X-ray films indicate that she has no broken bones. Mrs. Beck voids a small amount of dark yellow urine. Review of laboratory findings: hematocrit 55% (hemoconcentration caused by hypovolemia); sodium 148 mEq/L, and potassium 3 mEq/L. (Note: Mrs. Beck has hypokalemia in addition to extracellular fluid volume [ECV] deficit and hypernatremia [clinical dehydration].)

Assessment Activities	*Findings/Defining Characteristics**
Ask Mrs. Beck to describe when her vomiting and diarrhea began and any accompanying signs and symptoms.	She states that her gastrointestinal (GI) problems began suddenly yesterday and that she **gets weak and light-headed when she stands or sits upright,** which is why she fell. She feels **weak** and has a **dry mouth.**
Ask her about current status of vomiting and diarrhea.	Says she still was vomiting earlier this morning. Has not done so for the past 3 hours. Feels slightly nauseated. Had three episodes of watery diarrhea this morning and more than six yesterday.

NURSING CARE PLAN

Deficient Fluid Volume—cont'd

Assess Mrs. Beck's vital signs.	**Heart rate 102** beats/min with regular rhythm and a **weak pulse; supine blood pressure (BP) is 90/58.** Temperature and respirations within normal limits. Postural BP measurement not taken since patient says that she **gets light-headed when she sits upright.**
Evaluate physical signs of ECV.	Neck veins flat when she is supine; **100 mL of dark yellow urine** in past 4 hours; dry mucous membranes between cheek and gum; prolonged capillary refill time of 5 seconds.
Weigh Mrs. Beck using a bed scale.	Weight 120 lb (54.5 kg). States usual weight at home is 127 lb (46.27 kg) **(7 lb [3.17 kg] weight loss).**

*__Defining characteristics__ are shown in bold type.

NURSING DIAGNOSIS: Deficient fluid volume related to increased output of GI fluids from vomiting and diarrhea

PLANNING

Goals	*Expected Outcomes (NOC)*†
	Fluid Balance
Mrs. Beck's fluid volume will return to normal by hospital discharge.	Heart rate and BP will return to normal within 24 hours. Mrs. Beck will not report light-headedness when sitting or standing within 24 hours. Urine color will become light yellow within 24 hours. Daily urine output will equal intake of at least 1500 mL by discharge.
Mrs. Beck will describe how to manage fluid balance at home before hospital discharge.	Mrs. Beck will describe how to replace GI fluid loss with fluids that contain sodium. She will describe signs and symptoms indicating need to increase fluid and sodium intake.

†Outcome classification labels from Moorhead S et al: *Nursing outcomes classification (NOC)*, ed 4, St Louis, 2008, Mosby.

INTERVENTIONS‡ (NIC)	RATIONALE
Fluid/Electrolyte Management	
Provide Mrs. Beck her favorite noncaffeinated fluids at her preferred temperature.	Patient-centered care takes individual preferences into account (Cronenwett et al., 2007). Cultural preferences regarding temperature of oral fluid influence fluid intake (Giger and Davidhizar, 2008). Avoid caffeinated beverages because of their diuretic effect.
Provide a pitcher and glass of water at Mrs. Beck's preferred temperature at her bedside; ensure that she can access and pour from it easily; provide a straw if she wishes.	Weakness or chronic disease such as osteoarthritis of hands may make it difficult to manipulate a full water pitcher. Make fluid available in a form that is easy for a patient to access.
Administer IV therapy as prescribed, monitoring closely for early side effects of complications.	IV fluid replacement augments oral replacement when ECV deficit exists. Age-appropriate care is needed because of older adult's anatomical and physiological changes that effect volume delivery (INS, 2011).
Discuss different ways to prevent and treat dehydration at home. Provide written handout of information.	Patient education is enhanced in older adults when you use multiple senses during teaching sessions (Meiner, 2011).

‡Intervention classification labels from Bulechek GM, Butcher HK, and Dochterman JM: *Nursing interventions classification (NIC)*, ed 5, St Louis, 2008, Mosby.

EVALUATION

Nursing Actions	*Patient Response/Finding*	*Achievement of Outcome*
Monitor vital signs, intake and output (I&O), daily weight, and postural BP when no longer light-headed.	T 37° C (98.6° F), RR 10, HR 72 bpm, BP 120/78 sitting, 122/78 standing, denies light-headedness Intake 2000 mL, output 2000 mL of light yellow urine Today's weight 129 lb (58.5 kg)	Vital signs returned to normal range. No postural hypotension. I&O measurements are balanced, urine is light yellow. Daily weight returned to Mrs. Beck's normal.
Assess neck vein fullness when supine, mucous membranes.	Neck veins full when supine; mucous membranes moist	Additional markers of ECV are normal.
Evaluate effectiveness of teaching regarding maintaining fluid balance at home.	Mrs. Beck identified salty broth and commercial electrolyte replacement fluids for replacing GI fluid loss and indicated need to increase her intake if her urine becomes dark yellow or she becomes light-headed when sitting upright.	Mrs. Beck describes effective home management of fluid balance.

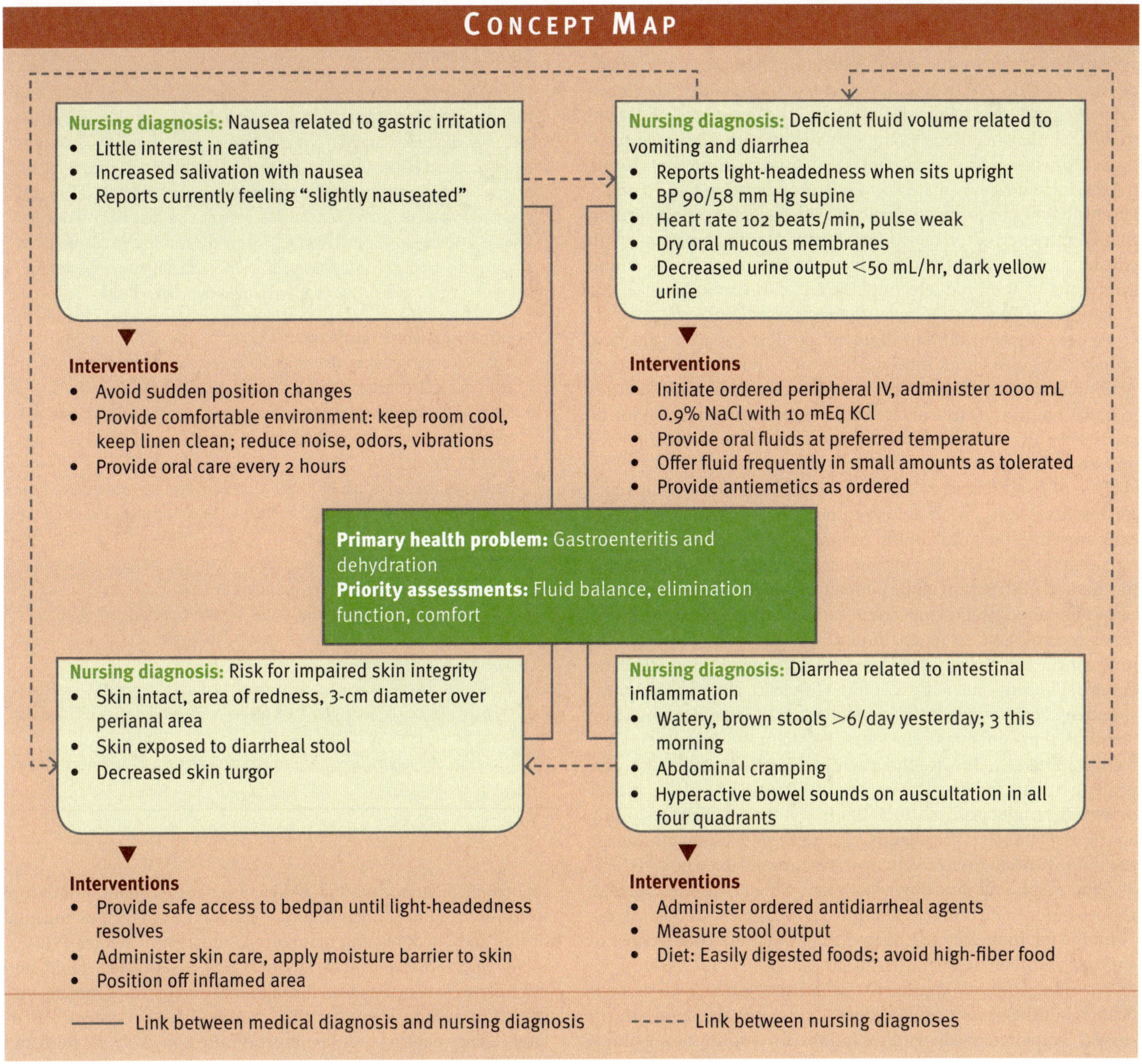
CONCEPT MAP
Nursing diagnosis: Nausea related to gastric irritation
• Little interest in eating
• Increased salivation with nausea
• Reports currently feeling "slightly nauseated"
Interventions
• Avoid sudden position changes
• Provide comfortable environment: keep room cool, keep linen clean; reduce noise, odors, vibrations
• Provide oral care every 2 hours
Nursing diagnosis: Deficient fluid volume related to vomiting and diarrhea
• Reports light-headedness when sits upright
• BP 90/58 mm Hg supine
• Heart rate 102 beats/min, pulse weak
• Dry oral mucous membranes
• Decreased urine output <50 mL/hr, dark yellow urine
Interventions
• Initiate ordered peripheral IV, administer 1000 mL 0.9% NaCl with 10 mEq KCl
• Provide oral fluids at preferred temperature
• Offer fluid frequently in small amounts as tolerated
• Provide antiemetics as ordered
Primary health problem: Gastroenteritis and dehydration
Priority assessments: Fluid balance, elimination function, comfort
Nursing diagnosis: Risk for impaired skin integrity
• Skin intact, area of redness, 3-cm diameter over perianal area
• Skin exposed to diarrheal stool
• Decreased skin turgor
Interventions
• Provide safe access to bedpan until light-headedness resolves
• Administer skin care, apply moisture barrier to skin
• Position off inflamed area
Nursing diagnosis: Diarrhea related to intestinal inflammation
• Watery, brown stools >6/day yesterday; 3 this morning
• Abdominal cramping
• Hyperactive bowel sounds on auscultation in all four quadrants
Interventions
• Administer ordered antidiarrheal agents
• Measure stool output
• Diet: Easily digested foods; avoid high-fiber food
Link between medical diagnosis and nursing diagnosis
Link between nursing diagnoses

FIG. 41-12 Concept map for Mrs. Beck.

Begin discharge planning early for patients with acute or chronic fluid and electrolyte disturbances by anticipating the needs of the patient and family as they transition to another setting. In the hospital, collaboration with other members of the health care team ensures that care will continue in the home or long-term care setting with few disruptions. You ensure that therapeutic regimens established in one setting continue through completion at the next setting. For example, for a patient who is discharged on IV therapy, you assess the knowledge and skills of the family member or friend who is to assume caregiving responsibilities and initiate a referral to home IV therapy as soon as possible. Close collaboration with members of the health care team such as the patient's health care provider, dietitian, and pharmacist is essential to ensure positive patient outcomes. A dietitian is a valuable resource in recommending food sources to increase or reduce intake of specific electrolytes (see Chapter 44). A pharmacist helps identify medications or combinations of medications likely to cause electrolyte or acid-base disturbances and offer information regarding patient education about side effects to anticipate for prescribed drugs. The patient's health care provider directs the treatment of fluid, electrolyte, or acid-base imbalances.

IMPLEMENTATION

Health Promotion. Health promotion activities focus primarily on patient education. Teach patients and caregivers to recognize risk factors for developing imbalances and implement appropriate preventive measures. For example, parents of infants need to understand that GI losses lead quickly to serious imbalances; therefore, when vomiting or diarrhea occurs in an infant, they need to promptly rehydrate with sodium-containing fluid or seek health care to restore normal balance. People of any age need to learn to replace body fluid losses with sodium-containing fluid and water.

Patients with chronic health alterations often are at risk for developing fluid, electrolyte, and acid-base imbalances. They need to understand their own risk factors and the measures to be taken to avoid imbalances. For example, patients with end-stage renal disease often need to restrict intake of fluid, sodium, potassium, magnesium, and phosphate. Through diet education these patients learn the types of foods to avoid and the suitable volume of fluid that they are permitted daily (see Chapter 44). Teach patients with chronic diseases and their family caregivers the early signs and symptoms of the fluid, electrolyte, and acid-base imbalances for which they are at risk and what to do if these occur.

Acute Care. Although fluid, electrolyte, and/or acid-base imbalances occur in all settings, they are common in acute care. Acute care nurses administer medications and oral and IV fluids to replace fluid and electrolyte deficits or maintain normal homeostasis; they also assist with restricting intake as part of therapy for excesses.

Enteral Replacement of Fluids. Oral replacement of fluids and electrolytes is appropriate as long as the patient is not so physiologically unstable that oral fluids cannot be replaced rapidly. Oral replacement of fluids is contraindicated when the patient has a mechanical obstruction of the GI tract, is at high risk for aspiration, or has impaired swallowing. Some patients unable to tolerate solid foods are still able to ingest fluids. Strategies to encourage fluid intake include offering small sips of fluid frequently, popsicles, and ice chips. Record one half the volume of the ice chips in I&O measurement. For example, if a patient ingests 240 mL of ice chips, you record 120 mL of intake. Encourage patients to keep their own record of intake to involve them actively. Family members who are properly instructed can also assist. Pay attention to each patient's preferred temperature of oral fluids. Cultural beliefs regarding appropriate fluid temperature may interfere with fluid intake unless the fluid with the preferred temperature is available (Box 41-5).

BOX 41-5 CULTURAL ASPECTS OF CARE

Fluid Therapy

Cultural and religious beliefs influence how you manage fluid therapy and how patients communicate their needs. For example, the family elder may be the person who receives explanations and makes health care decisions rather than the patient. A person's cultural and religious beliefs may cause refusal of therapies. For example, hot-cold beliefs often cause patients to refuse cold oral fluids when they have certain illnesses because they believe that hot fluids are needed to restore balance (Giger and Davidhizar, 2008). Religious practices may require modifications of intravenous (IV) tubing length (e.g., patients need to kneel on the floor and pray several times daily).

Implications for Practice

- Establish communication. If appropriate, determine who the family elder is and explain fluid restriction or IV therapy procedures.
- Elicit patient/family values and preferences in your clinical interview. Ask specifically about preferred temperature of oral fluids and provide (if oral intake is allowed).
- Determine needed length of IV tubing and incorporate one or more segments of long extension tubing into the IV setup if patient kneels on the floor to pray.
- Determine acceptance of or abstinence from therapeutic regimens and respect patients/family choices regarding therapy.
- Although some patients refuse whole blood or packed red blood cells because of religious or personal beliefs, they may accept other blood products or alternatives.
- When the natural skin color is dark, assess carefully for subtle color changes at vascular access device site that might indicate phlebitis, which may be more difficult to recognize.
- Communicate patient/family values and choices to other members of the health care team.

When replacing fluids by mouth in a patient with ECV deficit, choose fluids that contain sodium (e.g., Pedialyte and Gastrolyte). Liquids containing lactose, caffeine, or low-sodium content are not appropriate when a patient has diarrhea.

A feeding tube is appropriate when the patient's GI tract is healthy but the patient cannot ingest fluids (e.g., after oral surgery or with impaired swallowing). Options for administering fluids include gastrostomy or jejunostomy instillations or infusions through small-bore nasogastric feeding tubes (see Chapter 44).

Restriction of Fluids. Patients who have hyponatremia usually require restricted water intake. Patients who have very severe ECV excess sometimes have both sodium and fluid restrictions. Fluid restriction often is difficult for patients, particularly if they take medications that dry the oral mucous membranes or if they are mouth breathers. Explain the reason that fluids are restricted and ensure that the patient and family visitors know the amount of fluid permitted orally and understand that ice chips, gelatin, and ice cream are fluids. Help the patient decide the amount of fluid to drink with each meal, between meals, before bed, and with medications. It is important to allow patients to choose preferred fluids unless contraindicated. Frequently patients on fluid restriction can swallow a number of pills with as little as 1 oz (30 mL) of liquid.

In acute care settings fluid restrictions usually allot half the total oral fluids between 7 AM and 3 PM, the period when patients are more active, receive two meals, and take most of their oral medications. Offer the remainder of the fluids during the evening and night shifts. Patients on fluid restriction need frequent mouth care to moisten mucous membranes, decrease the chance of mucosal drying and cracking, and maintain comfort (see Chapter 39).

Parenteral Replacement of Fluids and Electrolytes. Fluid and electrolytes may be replaced through infusion of fluids directly into veins (intravenously) rather than via the digestive system. Parenteral replacement includes parenteral nutrition (PN), IV fluid and electrolyte therapy **(crystalloids),** and blood and blood component (colloids) administration. IV devices are called *peripheral IVs* when the catheter tip lies in a vein in one of the extremities; they are called *central venous IVs* when the catheter tip lies in the central circulatory system (e.g., in the vena cava close to the right atrium of the heart) (Fig. 41-13).

Practice standard body fluid precautions when administering parenteral fluids (see Chapter 28) to minimize your own risk for exposure to bloodborne pathogens. Read and understand the policy and procedures for parenteral infusions at the institution for which you work.

Parenteral Nutrition. PN, also called *total parenteral nutrition (TPN),* is IV administration of a complex, highly concentrated solution containing nutrients and electrolytes that is formulated to meet a patient's needs. Depending on their osmolality, PN solutions are administered through a central IV catheter (high osmolality) or peripherally (lower osmolality). Chapter 44 reviews principles and guidelines for PN administration, which is used when patients are unable to receive enough nutrition orally or through enteral feeding.

TABLE 41-11 Intravenous Solutions

SOLUTION	CONCENTRATION	COMMENTS
Dextrose in Water Solutions		Dextrose is another name for glucose.
Dextrose 5% in water (D_5W)	Isotonic	Isotonic when first enters vein. Dextrose enters cells rapidly, leaving free water, which dilutes ECF; most of the water then enters cells by osmosis.
Dextrose 10% in water ($D_{10}W$)	Hypertonic	Dextrose enters cells rapidly, leaving free water, which dilutes ECF; most of the water then enters cells by osmosis.
Saline Solutions		Saline is sodium chloride in water.
0.225% sodium chloride (quarter normal saline; ¼ NS; 0.225% NaCl)	Hypotonic	Expands ECV (vascular and interstitial) and rehydrates cells
0.45% sodium chloride (half normal saline; ½ NS; 0.45% NaCl)	Hypotonic	Expands ECV (vascular and interstitial) and rehydrates cells
0.9% sodium chloride (normal saline; NS; 0.9% NaCl)	Isotonic	Expands ECV (vascular and interstitial); does not enter cells
3% or 5% sodium chloride (hypertonic saline; 3% or 5% NaCl)	Hypertonic	Draws water from cells into ECF by osmosis
Dextrose in Saline Solutions		
Dextrose 5% in 0.45% NaCl sodium chloride (D_5½NS; $D_5$0.45% NaCl)	Hypertonic	Dextrose enters cells rapidly, leaving 0.45% sodium chloride.
Dextrose 5% in 0.9% sodium chloride (D_5NS; $D_5$0.9% NaCl)	Hypertonic	Dextrose enters cells rapidly, leaving 0.9% sodium chloride.
Balanced Electrolyte Solutions		
Lactated Ringer's (LR)	Isotonic	Contains Na^+, K^+, Ca^{2+}, Cl^-, and lactate, which the liver metabolizes to HCO_3^-. Expands ECV (vascular and interstitial); does not enter cells.
Dextrose 5% in lactated Ringer's (D_5LR)	Hypertonic	Dextrose enters cells rapidly, leaving lactated Ringer's.

ECF, Extracellular fluid; *ECV,* extracellular fluid volume.

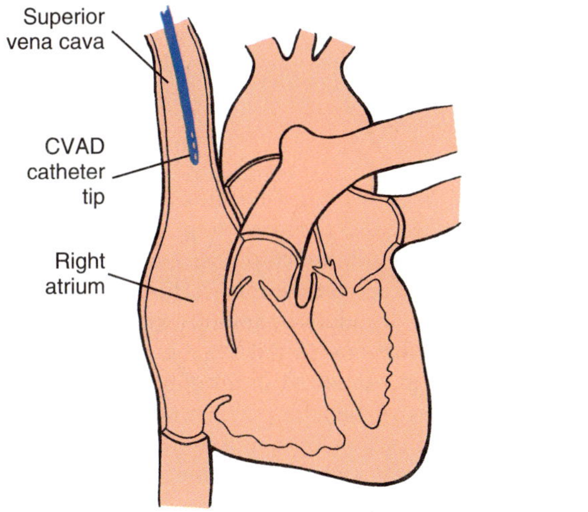

FIG. 41-13 Central venous lines deliver intravenous fluid into superior vena cava near heart. *CVAD,* Central venous access device.

Intravenous Therapy (Crystalloids). The goal of IV fluid administration is to correct or prevent fluid and electrolyte disturbances. It allows for direct access to the vascular system, permitting the continuous infusion of fluids over a period of time. You regulate IV fluid therapy continuously because of ongoing changes in a patient's fluid and electrolyte balance. To provide safe and appropriate therapy to patients who require IV fluids, you need knowledge of the correct ordered solution, the reason the solution was ordered, the equipment needed, the procedures required to initiate an infusion, how to regulate the infusion rate and maintain the system, how to identify and correct problems, and how to discontinue the infusion.

Types of Solutions. Many prepared IV solutions are available for use (Table 41-11). An IV solution is isotonic, hypotonic, or hypertonic. Isotonic solutions have the same effective osmolality as body fluids. Sodium-containing isotonic solutions such as normal saline are indicated for ECV replacement to prevent or treat ECV deficit. Hypotonic solutions have an effective osmolality less than body fluids, thus decreasing osmolality by diluting body fluids and moving water into cells. Hypertonic solutions have an effective osmolality greater than body fluids. If they are hypertonic sodium-containing solutions, they increase osmolality rapidly and pull water out of cells, causing them to shrivel (David, 2007). The decision to use a hypotonic or hypertonic solution is based on the patient's specific fluid and electrolyte imbalance. For example, a patient with hypernatremia that cannot be treated with oral water generally receives a hypotonic IV solution to dilute the ECF and rehydrate cells. Too rapid or excessive infusion of any IV fluid has the potential to cause serious patient problems.

Additives such as potassium chloride (KCl) are common in IV solutions. A health care provider's order is necessary if an IV is to have additives added (e.g., 1000 mL D_5½NS with 20 mEq KCl at 125 mL/hr). Administer KCl carefully because hyperkalemia can cause fatal cardiac dysrhythmias. Under no circumstances should it be administered by IV push (directly through a port in IV tubing). Verify that a patient has adequate kidney function and urine output before administering an IV solution containing potassium. Patients with normal renal function who are receiving nothing by mouth should have potassium added to IV solutions. The body cannot conserve potassium, and the kidneys continue to excrete potassium even when the plasma level falls. Without potassium intake, hypokalemia develops quickly.

Vascular Access Devices. Vascular access devices (VADs) are catheters or infusion ports designed for repeated access to the vascular system. Peripheral catheters are for short-term use (e.g., fluid restoration after surgery and short-term antibiotic administration). Devices for long-term use include central catheters and implanted ports, which empty into a central vein. Remember that the term *central* applies to the location of the catheter tip, not to the insertion site. Peripherally inserted central catheters (PICC lines) enter a peripheral arm vein and extend through the venous system to the superior vena cava where they terminate. Other central lines enter a central vein such as the subclavian or jugular vein or are tunneled through subcutaneous tissue before entering a central vein. Central lines are more effective than peripheral catheters for administering large volumes of fluid, PN, and medications or fluids that irritate veins. Proper care of central line insertion sites is critical for the prevention of catheter-related bloodstream infections (CRBSI). The National Quality Forum (NQF) (2010) identified CRBSIs as one of their endorsed patient safety measures that health care institutions are encouraged to report. *Beginning in October of 2008, the Centers for Medicare and Medicaid Services (CMS) no longer reimburses* over and above the typical inpatient prospective payment system rate for care required to manage and correct a CRBSI. This means that a hospital is not paid for the added costs and hospital days needed to treat it. Nurses require specialized education regarding care of central venous catheters and implanted infusion ports. Nursing responsibilities for central lines include careful monitoring, flushing to keep the line patent, and site care and dressing changes to prevent CRBSIs.

Equipment. Correct selection and preparation of IV equipment assists in safe and quick placement of an IV line. Because fluids infuse directly into the bloodstream, sterile technique is necessary. Organize all equipment at the bedside for an efficient insertion. IV equipment includes VADs, tourniquet, clean gloves, dressings, IV fluid containers, various types of tubing, and electronic infusion devices (EIDs), also called *infusion pumps.* VADs that are short, peripheral IV catheters are available in a variety of gauges such as the commonly used 20 and 22 gauges. A larger gauge indicates a smaller-diameter catheter. A peripheral VAD is called an over-the-needle catheter; it consists of a small plastic tube or catheter threaded over a sharp stylet (needle). Once you insert the stylet and advance the catheter into the vein, you withdraw the stylet, leaving the catheter in place. These devices have a safety mechanism that covers the sharp stylet when withdrawing it to reduce the risk of needlestick injury (Fig. 41-14). Needleless systems allow you to make connections without using needles, which reduces needlestick injuries (Hadaway and Richardson, 2010).

The main IV fluid used in a continuous infusion flows through tubing called the *primary line.* The primary line connects to the IV catheter. Injectable medications such as antibiotics are usually added to a small IV solution bag and "piggybacked" as a secondary set into the primary line or as a primary intermittent infusion to be administered over a 30- to 60-minute period (see Chapter 31). The type and amount of solution are prescribed by the patient's health care provider and depend on the medication added and the patient's physiological status. If an IV infusion is connected to an EID, use the tubing designated for that EID. For gravity-flow IVs (not using an EID), select tubing as described in the equipment list of Skill 41-1 on pp. 916-925. Add IV extension tubing to increase the length of the primary line, which reduces pulling of the tubing and increases a patient's mobility in changing position.

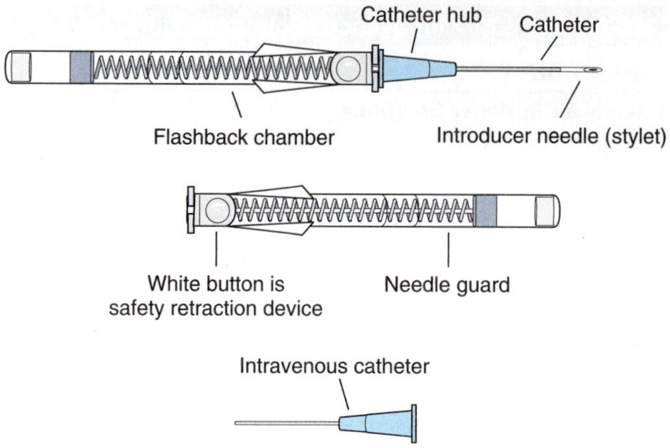

FIG. 41-14 Over-the-needle catheter for venipuncture.

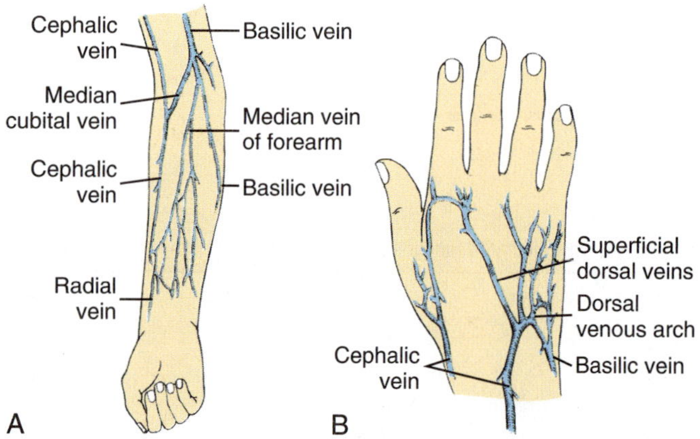

FIG. 41-15 Common IV sites. **A,** Inner arm. **B,** Dorsal surface of hand.

Initiating the Intravenous Line. After you collect the equipment at the patient's bedside, prepare to insert the IV line by assessing the patient for a venipuncture site (see Skill 41-1). The most common IV sites are on the inner arm (Fig. 41-15). Do not use hand veins on older adults or ambulatory patients. IV insertion in a foot vein is common with children, but avoid these sites in adults because of the increased risk of thrombophlebitis (INS, 2011).

As you assess a patient for potential venipuncture sites, consider conditions that exclude certain sites. Venipuncture is contraindicated in a site that has signs of infection, infiltration, or thrombosis. An infected site is red, tender, swollen, and possibly warm to the touch. Exudate may be present. Do not use an infected site because of the danger of introducing bacteria from the skin surface into the bloodstream. Avoid using an extremity with a vascular (dialysis) graft/fistula or on the same side as a mastectomy. Avoid areas of flexion if possible (INS, 2011). Choose the most distal appropriate site (INS, 2011). Using a distal site first allows for the use of proximal sites later if the patient needs a venipuncture site change.

Venipuncture is a technique in which a vein is punctured through the skin by a sharp rigid stylet (e.g., metal needle). The stylet is partially covered either with a plastic catheter or a needle attached to a syringe. General purposes of venipuncture are to collect a blood specimen, start an IV infusion, provide vascular access for later use, instill a medication, or inject a radiopaque or other tracer for special diagnostic examinations. Skill 41-1 describes

BOX 41-6 FOCUS ON OLDER ADULTS

Protection of Skin and Veins During Intravenous Therapy

- Use the smallest-gauge catheter or needle possible (e.g., 22 to 24 gauge). Veins are very fragile, and a smaller gauge allows better blood flow to provide increased hemodilution of the intravenous (IV) fluids or medications (Fabian, 2010).
- Avoid the back of the hand, which may compromise the patient's need for independence and mobility (O'Halloran, El-Masri, and Fox-Wasylyshyn, 2008).
- Avoid placement of IV line in veins that are easily bumped because older adults have less subcutaneous support tissue.
- Avoid vigorous friction while cleaning the site to prevent tearing fragile skin.
- If the patient has fragile skin and veins, use minimal or no tourniquet pressure.
- If using a tourniquet, place it over the patient's sleeve or use a blood pressure cuff.
- With loss of supportive tissue, veins tend to lie more superficially; lower the insertion angle for venipuncture to 10 to 15 degrees after penetrating the skin (Fabian, 2010).
- Veins roll away from the needle easily because of loss of subcutaneous tissue. To stabilize the vein, apply traction to the skin below the projected insertion site (Fabian, 2010).
- Secure IV site with a catheter stabilization device and perhaps a mesh dressing for protection, avoiding excessive use of tape on fragile skin (Fabian, 2010).
- Numerous medications and supplements (e.g., anticoagulants, antibiotics, glucocorticoids, and garlic) increase the likelihood of bruising and bleeding.

venipuncture for peripheral IV fluid infusion, incorporating INS (2011) standards of practice. It takes practice to become proficient in venipuncture. Only experienced practitioners perform it for patients whose veins are fragile or collapse easily, such as older adults. Box 41-6 describes principles to follow for venipuncture in older adults.

Nurses require specialized knowledge and education to place PICCs. Some central lines and implanted ports require insertion by physicians or advanced practice nurses. Both types of central catheters require close monitoring and maintenance. This chapter focuses on peripheral catheters.

Regulating the Infusion Flow Rate. After initiating a peripheral IV infusion and checking it for patency, regulate the rate of infusion according to the health care provider's orders (Skill 41-2 on pp. 925-929). For patient safety avoid uncontrolled flow of IV fluid into a patient. You are responsible for calculating the flow rate per hour that delivers the IV fluid in the prescribed time frame. The correct IV infusion rate ensures patient safety by preventing too-slow or too-rapid administration of IV fluids. An infusion rate that is too slow often leads to further physiological compromise in a patient who is dehydrated, in circulatory shock, or critically ill. An infusion rate that is too rapid overloads the patient with IV fluid, causing fluid and electrolyte imbalances and cardiac complications in vulnerable patients (e.g., older adults or patients with preexisting heart disease).

Electronic infusion devices (EIDs), also called *IV pumps* or *infusion pumps,* deliver an accurate hourly IV infusion rate. EIDs use positive pressure to deliver a measured amount of fluid during a specified unit of time (e.g., 125 mL/hr). Familiarize yourself with the brand of EID in use at your agency so you are able to accurately set the flow rate. Many EIDs have capabilities that allow for single- and multiple-solution infusions at different rates. A variety of electronic detectors and alarms respond to air in IV lines, occlusion, completion of infusion, high and low pressure, and low battery power.

When you open a roller clamp or other type of clamp on an infusion tubing that is not yet properly inserted in an EID or on a gravity-flow IV system, the IV fluid infuses very rapidly. Nonelectronic volume control devices are used occasionally with an IV solution infused by gravity to prevent accidental infusion of a large fluid volume. These devices hang between the IV bag and the patient and hold only a small volume of fluid that can infuse into the patient. Regardless of the device in use, monitor the patient regularly to verify correct infusion of IV fluids. Patency of an IV catheter means that IV fluid flows easily through it. For patency there must be no clots at the tip of the catheter, and the catheter tip must not be against the vein wall. A blocked catheter slows or stops the rate of infusion of the IV fluids. IV flow rate also can be slowed by infiltration, vasospasm, a knot or kink in the tubing, external pressure on the tubing, and position changes of the patient's extremity. If the flow decreases or stops and the EID is working correctly, inspect the tubing. Sometimes the patient is lying or sitting on it. Also inspect the area around the insertion site for anything that obstructs the flow of IV fluids. For gravity flow, the height of the container influences flow rate. Raising the container usually increases the rate because of increased driving pressure.

Flexion of an extremity, particularly at the wrist or elbow, can decrease IV flow rate by compressing the vein. Although VAD placement in areas of flexion is discouraged, occasionally it becomes necessary. In that case INS standards specify use of an arm board or other joint stabilization device to protect the IV site by keeping the joint extended (INS, 2011). Use padding with arm boards because they may cause skin or nerve damage from pressure. Starting an infusion in a new location rather than relying on a site that causes problems may be more comfortable for a patient. Before discontinuing the current infusion, choose another site and start the infusion to verify that the patient has other accessible veins.

Maintaining the System. After placing an IV line and regulating the flow rate, maintain the IV system. Line maintenance involves (1) keeping the system sterile and intact; (2) changing IV fluid containers, tubing, and contaminated site dressings; (3) assisting a patient with self-care activities so as not to disrupt the system; and (4) monitoring for complications of IV therapy. The frequency and options for maintaining the system are identified in agency policies.

An important component of patient care is maintaining the integrity of an IV line to prevent infection. Potential sites for contamination of a VAD are shown in Fig. 41-16. Inserting an IV line under appropriate aseptic technique reduces the chances of contamination from the patient's skin microflora. After insertion the conscientious use of infection control principles, including thorough hand hygiene before and after handling any part of the IV system and maintaining sterility of the system during tubing and fluid container changes, prevents infection.

Always maintain the integrity of an IV system. Never disconnect tubing because it becomes tangled or it might seem more convenient for positioning or moving a patient or applying a gown. If a patient needs more room to maneuver, use aseptic technique to add extension tubing to an IV line. However, keep the use of extension tubing to a minimum, because each connection of tubing

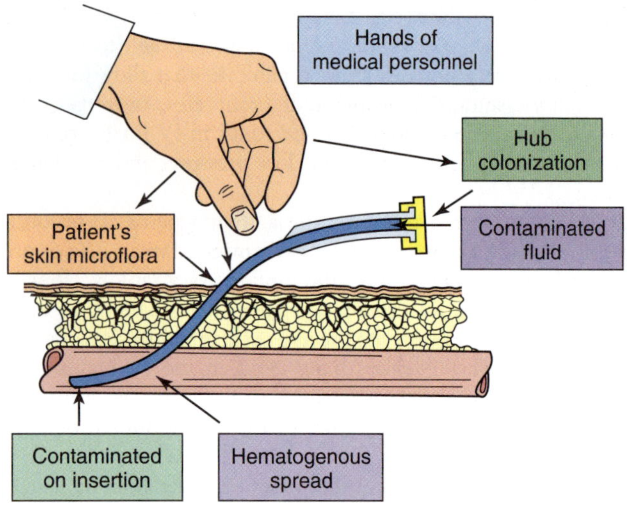

FIG. 41-16 Potential sites for contamination of vascular access device.

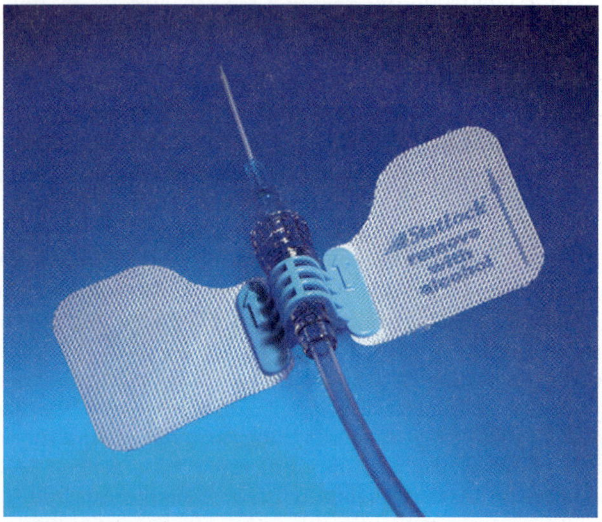

FIG. 41-17 Catheter stabilization device. (Copyright © C.R. Bard, Inc. Used with permission.)

BOX 41-7 EVIDENCE-BASED PRACTICE

Preventing Complications at Peripheral Intravenous Sites

PICO Question: Does use of standard taping compared with a catheter stabilization device prevent phlebitis and other complications of peripheral intravenous (IV) catheters in adult patients?

Evidence Summary

Phlebitis and infiltration are the most frequent complications of peripheral IV therapy. To prevent these and other complications such as catheter dislodgement, nurses traditionally stabilized the catheter by taping the hub to the skin, often with a chevron taping method. Commercially manufactured catheter stabilization devices are now available. Research shows that catheter stabilization devices extend the time that a catheter remains in a vein without complications. One study used a protocol requiring routine IV catheter removal and reinsertion every 96 hours unless complications occurred. The study found that only 8% of taped peripheral IV sites survived 96 hours compared to 52% of sites that used a specific brand of catheter stabilization device (Smith, 2006). Pooled data from over 10,000 patients in 83 hospitals showed a 67% reduction in total complications and a 76% reduction in unscheduled peripheral IV starts with the use of manufactured catheter stabilization devices (Schears, 2006). Substantial cost savings were achieved as well. Infusion Nurses Society standards of practice indicate that a catheter stabilization device is preferred over tape (INS, 2011).

Application to Nursing Practice

- If available, use a manufactured catheter stabilization device when you initiate IV therapy or change a peripheral IV site to reduce the incidence of phlebitis, infiltration, and infection.
- Work with an IV therapy team or other knowledgeable nurses to develop your skills in applying manufactured catheter stabilization devices if you are not familiar with them.
- If manufactured catheter stabilization devices are available at your agency but not widely used, consider educational offerings and other techniques to increase their use.
- If manufactured catheter stabilization devices are not available at your agency, review the research on these devices in a nursing practice committee or with your IV therapy team to influence policy and procedures and request their purchase.

provides opportunity for contamination. *Never let IV tubing touch the floor.* You do not use stopcocks for connecting more than one solution to a single IV site because they are sources of contamination (CDC, 2002; INS, 2011). IV tubing contains needleless injection ports through which syringes or other adaptors can be inserted for medication administration. Clean an injection port thoroughly with 2% chlorhexidine (preferred), 70% alcohol, or povidone-iodine solution and let it dry before accessing the system (INS, 2011).

Protective devices designed to prevent movement or accidental dislodgment of a VAD are called *catheter stabilization devices* (Fig. 41-17). These devices are available in many hospitals, and nurses decide whether or not to use them when starting an IV line (Box 41-7). This is a patient safety issue. INS standards indicate that use of these devices is preferable over taping when feasible (INS, 2011).

Changing Intravenous Fluid Containers, Tubing, and Dressings. Patients receiving IV therapy over several days require periodic changes of IV fluid containers (Skill 41-3 on pp. 929-934). It is important to organize tasks so you can change containers rapidly before a thrombus forms in the catheter.

Recommended frequency of IV tubing change depends on whether it is used for continuous or intermittent infusion. INS (2011) standards specify that continuous infusion tubing changes occur *no more frequently* than every 96 hours unless the tubing has been compromised or has become contaminated, which requires immediate tubing change. In contrast, change tubing for *intermittent* infusion every 24 hours because of the increased risk of contamination from opening the IV system (INS, 2011). Blood, blood components, and lipids are likely to promote bacterial growth in tubing. INS standards (2011) specify tubing changes every 4 hours for blood and blood components and every 24 hours for continuous IV lipids. For lipids use tubing that is free of diethylhexylphthalate (DEHP), a toxin that leaches into lipid solutions (INS, 2011). Whenever possible, schedule tubing changes when it is time to hang a new IV container to decrease risk of infection (INS, 2011). To prevent entry of bacteria into the bloodstream, maintain sterility during tubing and IV fluid container changes (INS, 2011).

A sterile dressing over an IV site reduces the entrance of bacteria into the insertion site. Transparent dressings, the most common type, help secure the VAD, allow continuous visual inspection of the IV site, and become less easily soiled or moistened than gauze dressings. You leave transparent dressings in place until the IV tubing is replaced (INS, 2011). If a gauze dressing is used, change it every 48 hours (INS, 2011). Both types of dressings must be changed when the IV device is removed or replaced or when the dressing becomes damp, loosened, or soiled (INS, 2011) (Skill 41-4 on pp. 934-936).

Assisting Patients to Protect Intravenous Integrity. To prevent the accidental disruption of an IV system, a patient often needs assistance with hygiene, comfort measures, meals, and ambulation. Changing gowns is difficult for a patient with an IV in the arm. Teach nursing assistive personnel (NAP) and patients that they must not break the integrity of an IV line to change a gown because it leads to contamination. It helps to use a gown with snaps along the top sleeve seam to facilitate changing the gown without disturbing the venipuncture site. Change regular gowns by following these steps for maximum speed and arm mobility:

1. *To remove a gown,* remove the sleeve of the gown from the arm without the IV line, maintaining the patient's privacy.
2. Remove the sleeve of the gown from the arm with the IV line.
3. Remove the IV solution container from its stand and pass it and the tubing through the sleeve. (If this involves removing the tubing from an EID, use the roller clamp to slow the infusion to prevent the accidental infusion of a large volume of solution or medication).
4. *To apply a gown,* place the IV solution container and tubing through the sleeve of the clean gown and hang it on its stand. (If the IV line is controlled by an EID, reassemble, turn on the pump, and open the roller clamp.)
5. Place the arm with the IV line through the gown sleeve.
6. Place the arm without the IV line through the gown sleeve.

A patient with an arm or a hand infusion is able to walk unless contraindicated. Offer a rolling IV pole on wheels. Help the patient to get out of bed and place the IV pole next to the involved arm. Teach the patient to hold on to the pole with the involved hand and to push it while walking. Check that the IV container is at the proper height, there is no tension on the tubing, and the flow rate is correct. Instruct the patient to report any blood in the tubing, a stoppage in the flow, or increased discomfort.

Complications of Intravenous Therapy. Table 41-12 presents complications of IV therapy, with assessments and nursing interventions. A potentially dangerous complication of IV therapy is circulatory overload with IV solution, which occurs when a patient receives too-rapid administration or an excessive amount of fluids. Assessment findings depend on the type of IV solution that infuses in excess (see Table 41-12). The signs and symptoms often arise rapidly, which highlights the importance of frequent assessment of patients receiving IV therapy.

> **Building Competency in Safety** You have an order to change an IV fluid container for Mrs. Jamison, age 48, who has no oral intake. The new IV fluid is 1000 mL NS with 20 mEq KCl; the previous IV fluid was 1000 mL NS and did not contain KCl. Which nursing assessments related to fluid and electrolyte imbalances do you need to make before you hang the new IV fluid container? Why?
>
> Answers to questions can be found on the Evolve website.

Infiltration occurs when an IV catheter becomes dislodged or a vein ruptures and IV fluids inadvertently enter subcutaneous tissue around the venipuncture site. When the IV fluid contains additives that damage tissue, **extravasation** occurs (Hadaway, 2007). Infiltration or extravasation causes coolness, paleness, and swelling of the area. When infiltration occurs, immediately assess for any additives in the infiltrated fluid to determine what type of action is necessary to prevent local tissue damage and sloughing. Vasoconstrictors, high-dose potassium, and other IV additives in subcutaneous tissue need different treatments from those needed for an infiltrated additive-free IV (Doellman et al., 2009) (see Table 41-12). Although the INS removed their previous infiltration scale from their 2011 standards because of insufficient research validation, the society does recommend use of an infiltration scale to provide objectivity in infiltration measurement (Table 41-13).

Phlebitis (i.e., inflammation of a vein) results from chemical, mechanical, or bacterial causes. Risk factors for phlebitis include acidic or hypertonic IV solutions; rapid IV rate; IV drugs such as KCl, vancomycin, and penicillin; VAD inserted in area of flexion, poorly secured catheter; poor hand hygiene; and lack of aseptic technique (Roszell and Jones, 2010). The typical signs of inflammation (i.e., heat, erythema [redness], tenderness) occur along the course of the vein (Table 41-14). Phlebitis can be dangerous because blood clots (thrombophlebitis) form along the vein and in some cases cause emboli. This may cause permanent damage to veins. Although some agencies require routine removal of VADs and site rotation to help prevent phlebitis and other complications, the INS Standards of Practice (2011) recommend replacement of a peripheral IV catheter only if clinically indicated in adults (Webster et al., 2010). Avoid routine replacement of peripheral IV catheters in infants and children (INS, 2011).

In the absence of phlebitis, local infection at the venipuncture site is usually caused by poor aseptic technique during catheter insertion, daily monitoring, or catheter removal. Early recognition of local infection and treatment are important to prevent bacteria from entering the bloodstream (see Table 41-12).

Bleeding can occur around the venipuncture site during the infusion or through the catheter or tubing if these become disconnected inadvertently (see Table 41-12). Bleeding is more common in patients who receive heparin or other anticoagulants or who have a bleeding disorder (e.g., hemophilia or thrombocytopenia).

Discontinuing Peripheral Intravenous Access. Discontinue IV access after infusion of the prescribed amount of fluid; when infiltration, phlebitis, or local infection occurs; or if the IV catheter develops a thrombus at its tip. Skill 41-3 presents the steps for discontinuing peripheral IV access. You help patients and families understand that moving from IV infusion to oral fluid intake is a sign of progress toward recovery.

Blood Transfusion. Blood transfusion, or blood component therapy, is the IV administration of whole blood or a blood component such as packed red blood cells (RBCs), platelets, or plasma. Objectives for administering blood transfusions include (1) increasing circulating blood volume after surgery, trauma, or hemorrhage; (2) increasing the number of RBCs and maintaining hemoglobin levels in patients with severe anemia; and (3) providing selected cellular components as replacement therapy (e.g., clotting factors, platelets, albumin).

Blood Groups and Types. Blood transfusions must be matched to each patient to avoid incompatibility. RBCs have antigens in their membranes; the plasma contains antibodies against specific RBC antigens. If incompatible blood is transfused (i.e., a patient's RBC antigens differ from those transfused), the patient's antibodies trigger RBC destruction in a potentially dangerous **transfusion reaction** (i.e., an immune response to the transfused blood components).

TABLE 41-12 Complications of Intravenous Therapy with Nursing Interventions

COMPLICATION	DESCRIPTION	ASSESSMENT FINDINGS	NURSING INTERVENTIONS
Circulatory overload of IV solution	IV solution infused too rapidly or in too great an amount	Depends on type of solution ECV excess with Na^+ containing isotonic fluid (crackles in dependent portions of lungs, shortness of breath, dependent edema) Hyponatremia with hypotonic fluid (confusion, seizures) Hypernatremia with Na^+ containing hypertonic fluid (confusion, seizures) Hyperkalemia from K^+ containing fluid (cardiac dysrhythmias, muscle weakness, abdominal distention)	If symptoms appear, reduce IV flow rate and notify patient's health care provider. With ECV excess raise head of bed; administer oxygen and diuretics if ordered. Monitor vital signs and laboratory reports of serum levels. Health care provider may adjust additives in IV solution or type of IV fluid; watch for and implement order.
Infiltration or extravasation	IV fluid entering subcutaneous tissue around venipuncture site Extravasation: technical term used when a vesicant (tissue-damaging) drug enters tissues	Skin around catheter site taut, blanched, cool to touch, edematous; may be painful as infiltration or extravasation increases; infusion may slow or stop	Stop infusion. Discontinue IV infusion if no vesicant drug (see Skill 41-3). If vesicant drug, disconnect IV tubing and aspirate drug from catheter (Doellman et al., 2009). Agency policy and procedures may require delivery of antidote through catheter before removal. Elevate extremity. Contact health care provider if solution contained KCl, a vasoconstrictor, or other potential vesicant. Apply warm moist or cold compress according to procedure for type of solution infiltrated. Start new IV line in other extremity.
Phlebitis	Inflammation of inner layer of a vein	Redness, tenderness, pain, warmth along course of vein starting at access site; possible red streak and/or palpable cord along vein	Stop infusion and discontinue IV line (see Skill 41-3). Start new IV line in other extremity or proximal to previous insertion site if continued IV therapy is necessary. Apply warm moist compress or contact IV therapy team or health care provider if area needs additional treatment.
Local infection	Infection at catheter-skin entry point, during infusion or after removal of IV catheter	Redness, heat, swelling at catheter-skin entry point; possible purulent drainage	Culture any drainage (if ordered). Clean skin with alcohol; remove catheter and save for culture; apply sterile dressing. Notify health care provider. Start new IV line in other extremity. Initiate appropriate wound care (see Chapter 48) if needed.
Bleeding at venipuncture site	Oozing or slow, continuous seepage of blood from venipuncture site	Fresh blood evident at venipuncture site, sometimes pooling under extremity	Assess if IV system is intact. If catheter is within vein, apply pressure dressing over site or change dressing. Start new IV line in other extremity or proximal to previous insertion site if VAD is dislodged, IV is disconnected, or bleeding from site does not stop.

ECV, Extracellular volume; *IV,* intravenous; *VAD,* vascular access device.

The most important grouping for transfusion purposes is the ABO system, which identifies A, B, O, and AB blood types. Determination of blood type is based on the presence or absence of A and B red blood cell (RBC) antigens. Individuals with type A blood have A antigens on their RBCs and anti-B antibodies in their plasma. Individuals with type B blood have B antigens on their RBCs and anti-A antibodies in their plasma. A person who has type AB blood has both A and B antigens on the RBCs and no antibodies against either antigen in the plasma. A type O individual has neither A nor B antigens on RBCs but has both anti-A and anti-B antibodies in the plasma (Trick, 2010). Table 41-15 shows the compatibilities between blood types of donors and recipients. People with type O blood are considered universal blood donors because they can donate packed RBCs and platelets to people with any ABO blood type. People with type AB blood are called *universal blood recipients* because they can receive packed RBCs and platelets of any ABO type.

Another consideration when matching blood components for transfusions is the Rh factor, which refers to another antigen in RBC membranes. Most people have this antigen and are Rh

TABLE 41-13 Infiltration Scale

GRADE	CLINICAL CRITERIA
0	No symptoms
1	Skin blanched Edema <2.54 cm (1 inch) in any direction Cool to touch With or without pain
2	Skin blanched Edema 2.54-15.2 cm (1-6 inches) in any direction Cool to touch With or without pain
3	Skin blanched, translucent Gross edema >15.2 cm (6 inches) in any direction Cool to touch Mild-moderate pain Possible numbness
4	Skin blanched, translucent Skin tight, leaking Skin discolored, bruised, swollen Gross edema >15.2 cm (6 inches) in any direction Deep pitting tissue edema Circulatory impairment Moderate-to-severe pain Infiltration of any amount of blood product, irritant, or vesicant

From Groll D et al: Evaluation of the psychometric properties of the phlebitis and infiltration scales for the assessment of complications of peripheral vascular access devices, *J Infus Nurs* 33(6):385, 2010.

TABLE 41-14 Phlebitis Scale

GRADE	CLINICAL CRITERIA
0	No symptoms
1	Erythema at access site with or without pain
2	Pain at access site with erythema and/or edema
3	Pain at access site with erythema and/or edema; streak formation; palpable venous cord
4	Pain at access site with erythema and/or edema; streak formation; palpable venous cord >2.54 cm (1 inch) in length; purulent drainage

From Infusion Nurses Society: Infusion nursing standards of practice, *J Intraven Nurs* 29(15), 2006.

positive; a person without it is Rh negative. People who are Rh negative receive only Rh-negative blood components.

Autologous Transfusion. Autologous transfusion (autotransfusion) is the collection and reinfusion of a patient's own blood. Blood for an autologous transfusion most commonly is obtained by preoperative donation up to 6 weeks before a scheduled surgery (e.g., heart, orthopedic, plastic, or gynecological). A patient can donate several units of blood, depending on the type of surgery and his or her ability to maintain an acceptable hematocrit. Blood for autologous transfusion is also obtained at the time of surgery by normovolemic hemodilution or through blood salvage (e.g., during surgery for liver transplantation, trauma, or vascular and

TABLE 41-15 ABO Compatibilities for Transfusion Therapy

COMPONENT	COMPATIBILITIES	
Whole blood	Give type-specific blood only	
Packed red cells (stored, washed, or frozen/washed)	**Donor**	**Recipient**
	O	O, A, B, AB
	A	A, AB
	B	B, AB
	AB	AB
Fresh-frozen plasma	**Donor**	**Recipient**
	O	O
	A	A, O
	B	B, O
	AB	AB, B, A, O
Platelets	RBC: ABO and Rh compatible *preferred*	
	Donor	**Recipient**
	O	O, A, B, AB
	A	A, AB
	B	B, AB
	AB	AB

From Alexander M et al: *Infusion nursing: an evidence-based approach,* ed 3, St Louis, 2010, Saunders.
ABO, Blood group consisting of groups A, AB, B, and O.

orthopedic conditions). After surgery blood is salvaged from drainage from chest tubes or joint cavities. Autologous transfusions are safer for patients because they decrease the risk of mismatched blood and exposure to bloodborne infectious agents (Trick, 2010).

Transfusing Blood. Transfusion of blood or blood components is a nursing procedure that requires an order from a health care provider. A blood transfusion reaction is one of the National Quality Forum's patient safety measures that should be included in a health care institution's public reporting of safety events (NQF, 2010). Patient safety is a nursing priority, and patient assessment, verification of health care provider's order, and verification of correct blood products for the correct patient are imperative.

Perform a thorough patient assessment before initiating a transfusion and monitor carefully during and after the transfusion. Assessment is critical because of the risk of transfusion reactions. Pretransfusion assessment includes establishing whether the patient knows the reason for the blood transfusion and whether he or she has ever had a previous transfusion or transfusion reaction. A patient who has had a transfusion reaction is usually at no greater risk for a reaction with a subsequent transfusion. However, he or she may be anxious about the transfusion, requiring nursing intervention. Before beginning a transfusion, explain the procedure and instruct the patient to report any side effects (e.g., chills, dizziness, or fever) once the transfusion begins. Ensure that he or she has signed an informed consent. Patients with certain cultural backgrounds may refuse blood transfusions (see Box 41-5).

Because of the danger of transfusion reactions, your pretransfusion assessment always includes the patient's baseline vital signs. These data allow you to identify when vital sign changes occur as a result of a transfusion reaction.

For patient safety always verify three things: that blood components delivered are the ones that were ordered; that blood delivered to the patient is compatible with the blood type listed in the medical record; and that the right patient receives the blood.

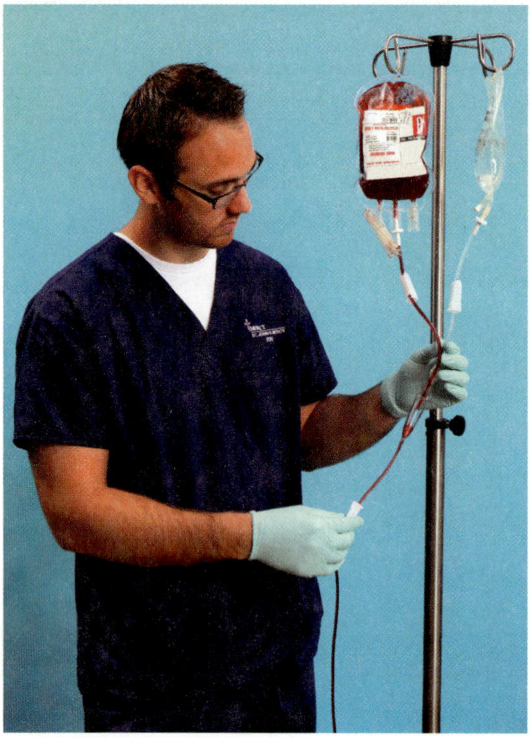

FIG. 41-18 Filling tubing for blood administration.

Together two RNs or one RN and an LPN (check agency policy and procedures) must check the label on the blood product against the medical record and against the patient's identification number, blood group, and complete name. If even a minor discrepancy exists, **do not** give the blood; notify the blood bank immediately to prevent infusion errors.

When administering a transfusion you need an appropriate-size IV catheter and blood administration tubing that has a special in-line filter (Fig. 41-18). Adults require a large catheter (e.g., 18- or 20-gauge) because blood is more viscous than crystalloid IV fluids. Children with small veins use a smaller catheter. Prime the tubing with 0.9% sodium chloride (normal saline) to prevent hemolysis or breakdown of RBCs. Initiate a transfusion slowly to allow for the early detection of a transfusion reaction. Maintain the ordered infusion rate, monitor for side effects, assess vital signs, and promptly record all findings. It is important to stay with the patient during the first 15 minutes, the time when a reaction is most likely to occur. After the initial time period, continue to monitor the patient and obtain vital signs periodically during the transfusion as directed by agency policy. If a transfusion reaction is anticipated or suspected, obtain vital signs more frequently (Table 41-16).

The transfusion rate usually is specified in the health care provider's orders. Ideally a unit of whole blood or packed RBCs is transfused in 2 hours. This time can be lengthened to 4 hours if the patient is at risk for ECV excess. Beyond 4 hours there is a risk for bacterial contamination of the blood.

When patients have a severe blood loss such as with hemorrhage, they often receive rapid transfusions through a central venous catheter. A blood-warming device often is necessary because the tip of the central venous catheter lies in the superior vena cava, above the right atrium. Rapid administration of cold blood can cause cardiac dysrhythmias. Patients who receive large-volume transfusion of citrated blood have high risk of hyperkalemia, hypocalcemia, hypomagnesemia, and metabolic alkalosis.

Transfusion Reactions and Other Adverse Effects. A transfusion reaction is an immune system reaction to the transfusion that ranges from a mild response to severe anaphylactic shock or acute intravascular hemolysis, both of which are life threatening. Table 41-16 presents the causes, manifestations, management, and prevention of transfusion reactions. Prompt intervention when a transfusion reaction occurs maintains or restores the patient's physiological stability. When you suspect acute intravascular hemolysis, do the following (Trick, 2010):

- Stop the transfusion immediately.
- Keep the IV line open by replacing the IV tubing down to the catheter hub with new tubing and running 0.9% sodium chloride (normal saline).
- *Do not* turn off the blood and simply turn on the 0.9% sodium chloride (normal saline) that is connected to the Y-tubing infusion set. This would cause blood remaining in the IV tubing to infuse into the patient. Even a small amount of mismatched blood can cause a major reaction.
- Immediately notify the health care provider or emergency response team.
- Remain with the patient, observing signs and symptoms and monitoring vital signs as often as every 5 minutes.
- Prepare to administer emergency drugs such as antihistamines, vasopressors, fluids, and corticosteroids per health care provider order or protocol.
- Prepare to perform cardiopulmonary resuscitation.
- Save the blood container, tubing, attached labels, and transfusion record for return to the blood bank.
- Obtain blood and urine specimens per health care provider order or protocol.

Acute adverse effects that do not involve an immune response to the blood components also can occur during a transfusion (see Table 41-16). Circulatory overload is a risk when a patient receives massive whole blood or packed RBC transfusions for massive hemorrhagic shock or when a patient with normal blood volume receives blood. Patients particularly at risk for circulatory overload are older adults and those with cardiopulmonary diseases. Transfusion of blood components that are contaminated with bacteria, especially gram-negative bacteria, can cause sepsis.

Another category of adverse transfusion effects is diseases transmitted by blood from infected donors who are asymptomatic. Symptoms of these conditions may arise long after the transfusion. Diseases transmitted through transfusions include hepatitis B and C, human immunodeficiency virus (HIV) infection and acquired immunodeficiency syndrome (AIDS), and cytomegalovirus infection (CDC, 2010). In the United States all units of blood for blood banks undergo screening for HIV, hepatitis B virus (HBV), hepatitis C virus (HCV), and syphilis, which reduces the risk of acquiring these bloodborne infections.

Interventions for Electrolyte Imbalances. In addition to the administration of prescribed medical therapies, there are nursing interventions for preserving or restoring electrolyte imbalance. For example, people who have hypokalemia or hypercalcemia often need bowel management for constipation. Patient safety interventions to prevent falls (see Chapter 27) are vital for patients who become lethargic from hypercalcemia and those with muscle weakness. Patients who have hypercalcemia need an increased fluid intake to prevent renal damage; nurses can help them meet the oral fluid intake goals. Teach patients the reasons for their therapies and the importance of balancing electrolyte I&O to prevent imbalances in the future.

TABLE 41-16 Acute Adverse Effects of Transfusions

ADVERSE EFFECT	CAUSE	CLINICAL MANIFESTATIONS	MANAGEMENT	PREVENTION
Transfusion Reactions—Caused by Immune Response to Blood Components				
Acute intravascular hemolytic	Infusion of ABO-incompatible whole blood, RBCs, or components containing 10 mL or more of RBCs Antibodies in recipient's plasma attach to antigens on transfused RBCs, causing RBC destruction	Chills, fever, low back pain, flushing, tachycardia, tachypnea, hypotension, hemoglobinuria, hemoglobinemia, sudden oliguria (acute kidney injury), circulatory shock, cardiac arrest, death	Stop transfusion and save blood bag and administration set for follow-up. Keep IV site open with normal saline infused through new tubing. Maintain BP and treat shock as ordered, if present. Obtain blood samples slowly to avoid hemolysis; then send for serological testing. Send urine specimen to laboratory. Give diuretics as prescribed to maintain urine flow. Insert indwelling urinary catheter or measure each voiding to monitor hourly urine output. Dialysis may be required if acute kidney injury occurs. ***Patient safety alert:*** Do not transfuse additional RBC-containing components until transfusion service provides newly cross-matched units.	Meticulously verify and document patient identification from sample collection to component infusion.
Febrile nonhemolytic (most common)	Antibodies against donor white blood cells	Sudden shaking chills (rigors), fever (rise in temperature 1° F [0.5° C] or more from start), headache, flushing, anxiety, muscle pain	Stop transfusion. Give antipyretics as prescribed; avoid aspirin in thrombocytopenic patients. ***Patient safety alert:*** Do not restart transfusion.	Consider leukocyte-poor blood products (filtered, washed, or frozen). Pretreat with antipyretics if prior history.
Mild allergic	Antibodies against donor plasma proteins	Flushing, itching, urticaria (hives)	Stop transfusion temporarily. Give antihistamine as directed. If symptoms are mild and transient, restart transfusion slowly. ***Patient safety alert:*** Do not restart transfusion if fever, pulmonary symptoms, or hypotension develop.	Treat prophylactically with antihistamines.
Anaphylactic	Antibodies to donor plasma, especially anti-IgA	Anxiety, urticaria, dyspnea, wheezing, progressing to cyanosis, severe hypotension, circulatory shock, possible cardiac arrest	Stop transfusion. Have epinephrine ready for injection (0.4 mL of 1:1000 solution subcutaneously or 0.1 mL of 1:1000 solution diluted to 10 mL with saline for IV use). Provide blood pressure support as ordered. Initiate CPR if indicated. ***Patient safety alert:*** Do not restart transfusion.	Transfuse extensively washed RBC products from which all plasma has been removed. Alternately use blood from IgA-deficient donor.
Other Acute Adverse Effects				
Circulatory overload	Blood administered faster than circulation can accommodate	Dyspnea, cough, crackles, or rales in dependent portions of lungs; distended neck veins when upright	Turn down transfusion rate or stop transfusion. Place patient upright with feet in dependent position. Administer prescribed diuretics, oxygen, morphine. Phlebotomy may be indicated.	Adjust transfusion volume and flow rate based on patient size and clinical status. Have transfusion service divide unit into smaller aliquots for better spacing of fluid input.
Sepsis	Bacterial contamination of transfused blood components	Rapid onset of chills, high fever, severe hypotension, and circulatory shock *May occur:* Vomiting, diarrhea, sudden oliguria (acute kidney injury), DIC	Stop transfusion. Obtain culture of patient's blood and send bag with remaining blood to transfusion service for further study. Treatment as ordered: antibiotics, IV fluids, vasopressors, glucocorticoids.	Collect, process, store, and transfuse blood products according to blood-banking standards and infuse within 4 hours of starting time.

Data from Roback J et al., editors: *Technical manual,* ed 16, Bethesda, Md, 2008, American Association of Blood Banks; and Trick NL: Blood component therapy. In Alexander M et al: *Infusion nursing: an evidence-based approach,* ed 3, St Louis, 2010, Saunders.

ABO, Blood group consisting of groups A, AB, B, and O; *BP,* blood pressure; *CPR,* cardiopulmonary resuscitation; *DIC,* disseminated intravascular coagulation; *IgA,* immunoglobulin A; *IV,* intravenous; *RBC,* red blood cell.

Interventions for Acid-Base Imbalances. Nursing interventions to promote acid-base balance support prescribed medical therapies and aim at reversing the existing acid-base imbalance while providing for patient safety. When imbalances are life threatening, they require rapid treatment. Maintain a functional IV line and check the health care provider's orders frequently for new medications or fluids. Give fluid and electrolyte replacement and prescribed drugs such as insulin promptly. In addition, monitor patients closely for changes in their status. Use protective measures such as side rails for patients with decreased level of consciousness. Support compensatory hyperventilation for patients with metabolic acidosis by keeping their oral mucous membranes moist and positioning them to facilitate chest expansion. Chapter 40 reviews appropriate therapies for patients with respiratory acidosis. Patients with acid-base imbalances often require repeated ABG analysis.

Arterial Blood Gases. Determination of a patient's acid-base status requires obtaining a sample of arterial blood for laboratory testing. An ABG reveals acid-base status and the adequacy of ventilation and oxygenation. A qualified RN or other health care provider draws arterial blood from a peripheral artery (usually the radial) or from an existing arterial line (see agency policy and procedures). Before an arterial blood draw ensure that the patient has an ulnar pulse to prevent loss of blood flow to the hand if the radial artery is damaged. After the ABG puncture apply pressure to the puncture site for at least 5 minutes to reduce the risk of hematoma formation. A longer time is necessary if the patient takes anticoagulant medications. Reassess the radial pulse after removing the pressure. After obtaining the specimen, take care to prevent air from entering the syringe because this alters the blood gas values. To reduce oxygen usage by blood cells, submerge the syringe in crushed ice and transport it immediately to the laboratory.

Restorative Care. After experiencing acute alterations in fluid, electrolyte, or acid-base balance, patients often require ongoing maintenance to prevent a recurrence of health alterations. Older adults require special considerations to prevent complications from developing (see Box 41-2).

Home Intravenous Therapy. IV therapy often continues in the home setting for patients requiring long-term hydration, PN, or long-term medication administration. A home IV therapy nurse works closely with the patient to ensure that a sterile IV system is maintained and complications can be avoided or recognized promptly. Box 41-8 summarizes patient education guidelines for home IV therapy.

Nutritional Support. Most patients who have had electrolyte disorders or metabolic acid-base imbalances require ongoing nutritional support. Depending on the type of disorder, fluid or food intake may be encouraged or restricted (see Chapter 44). Patients or family members who are responsible for meal preparation need to learn to understand nutritional content of foods and read the labels of commercially prepared foods.

Medication Safety. Numerous medications, OTC drugs, and herbal preparations contain components or create potential side effects that can alter fluid and electrolyte balance. Patients with chronic disease who are receiving multiple medications and those with renal disorders are at significant risk for alterations. Once patients return to a restorative care setting, whether in the home, long-term care, or other setting, drug safety is very important. Patient and family education regarding potential side effects and drug interactions that can alter fluid, electrolyte, or acid-base balance is essential. Review all medications with patients, and encourage them to consult with their local pharmacist, especially if they wish to try a new OTC drug or herbal preparation.

BOX 41-8 PATIENT TEACHING

Home Intravenous Therapy

Objective
- The patient and/or family caregiver will demonstrate competence with administering intravenous (IV) therapy safely in the home.

Teaching Strategies
- Explain the importance of IV therapy in maintaining hydration and access for the delivery of medications.
- Emphasize the risks involved when the IV system is not kept sterile.
- Be sure that the patient and/or caregiver is able to manipulate the required equipment.
- Instruct in aseptic technique and hand hygiene in the handling of all IV equipment.
- Instruct in how to change IV solutions, tubing, and dressing when they become soiled or dislodged. (NOTE: The home care nurse may be able to visit frequently enough to perform scheduled tubing changes.)
- Instruct in procedures for safe disposal in appropriate containers of all sharps and IV materials exposed to blood. Keep sharps containers away from children.
- Instruct to apply pressure with sterile gauze if catheter falls out and, if patient is on anticoagulants, to tape pieces of sterile gauze in place for at least 20 minutes with pressure or until bleeding stops.
- Instruct about signs and symptoms of infiltration, phlebitis, and infection and reporting symptoms immediately.
- Instruct patient and/or caregiver to report if the infusion slows or stops or if blood is seen in the tubing.
- Teach patient with family caregiver's assistance how to ambulate, perform hygiene, and participate in other activities of daily living without dislodging or disconnecting catheter and tubing:
  - For showering, protect the IV site and dressing from getting wet by covering it completely with plastic. If using an EID, unplug around water.
  - Wear clothes that avoid pressure on the IV site and avoid trauma to the site when changing clothes.
  - Have patient avoid strenuous exercise of the arm with the IV line.

Evaluation
- Ask patient and family caregiver why it is necessary to maintain hydration and IV access for the delivery of medications.
- Ask what to do if the IV infusion stops.
- Ask patient and caregiver to describe signs and symptoms of complications and the action they should take.
- Observe the patient or caregiver changing the IV container, tubing, and dressing.
- Observe the patient ambulating and participating in activities of daily living to see how he or she protects and manipulates the IV catheter and apparatus.

EVALUATION

Through the Patient's Eyes. Review with patients how well their major concerns regarding fluid, electrolyte, or acid-base situations were alleviated or addressed. For example, ask a person admitted with dehydration who was concerned about falling due to light-headedness, "How confident are you in your ability to stand without getting light-headed now?" If the patient's concern was feeling uncomfortable with very dry mouth, ask, "How does your mouth feel now?" If the patient's concerns involved having a better understanding of a chronic problem, focus the evaluation on the patient's view of the patient education provided. A patient's perspectives regarding care often depend in part on involvement of family and friends. If patients have concerns about returning home or to a different care setting, it is important to evaluate how well prepared they feel for the transition from acute care.

Patient Outcomes. Evaluate the effectiveness of interventions using the goals and outcomes established for the patient's nursing diagnoses. Evaluation of a patient's clinical status is especially important if acute fluid, electrolyte, and/or acid-base imbalances exist. A patient's condition can change very quickly, and it is important to recognize impending problems by integrating information about his or her presenting risk factors, clinical status, effects of the present treatment regimen, and potential causative agent. Knowledge of how various pathophysiological conditions affect fluid, electrolyte, and acid-base balance; the effects of medications and fluids; and the patient's presenting clinical status aid in evaluation (Fig. 41-19).

Compare your current assessment findings with the previous patient assessment. For example, a patient's hypokalemia demonstrates improvement when the serum potassium is increasing toward normal and the physical signs and symptoms of hypokalemia begin to disappear or lessen in intensity. Specifically the patient's heart rhythm becomes more regular, and normal bowel function returns.

For patients with less acute alterations, evaluation likely occurs over a longer period of time. In this situation evaluation may be more focused on behavioral changes (e.g., the patient's adherence to dietary restrictions and medication schedules). Another important element of evaluation is the family's ability to anticipate alterations and prevent problems from recurring.

The patient's level of progress determines whether the plan of care needs to continue or be revised. If goals are not met, you may need to consult a health care provider to discuss additional methods such as increasing the frequency of an intervention (e.g., providing more fluids to a dehydrated patient), introducing a new therapy (e.g., initiating insertion of an IV line), or discontinuing a particular therapy. Once outcomes are met, the nursing diagnosis is resolved, and you are able to focus on other priorities, including maintaining normal fluid, electrolyte, and acid-base balance. If established outcomes are not achieved, explore factors that contributed to why the planned outcomes were not met. Modification of the care plan occurs after this evaluation. Questions asked if outcomes are not achieved may include the following:

- "What difficulties are you having with measuring your I&O daily and keeping a record?"
- "What barriers are you experiencing to obtaining the potassium-rich foods you need?"
- "Are you continuing to have frequent loose stools or diarrhea?"
- "Have you purchased an antacid, or are you still using baking soda as an antacid?"

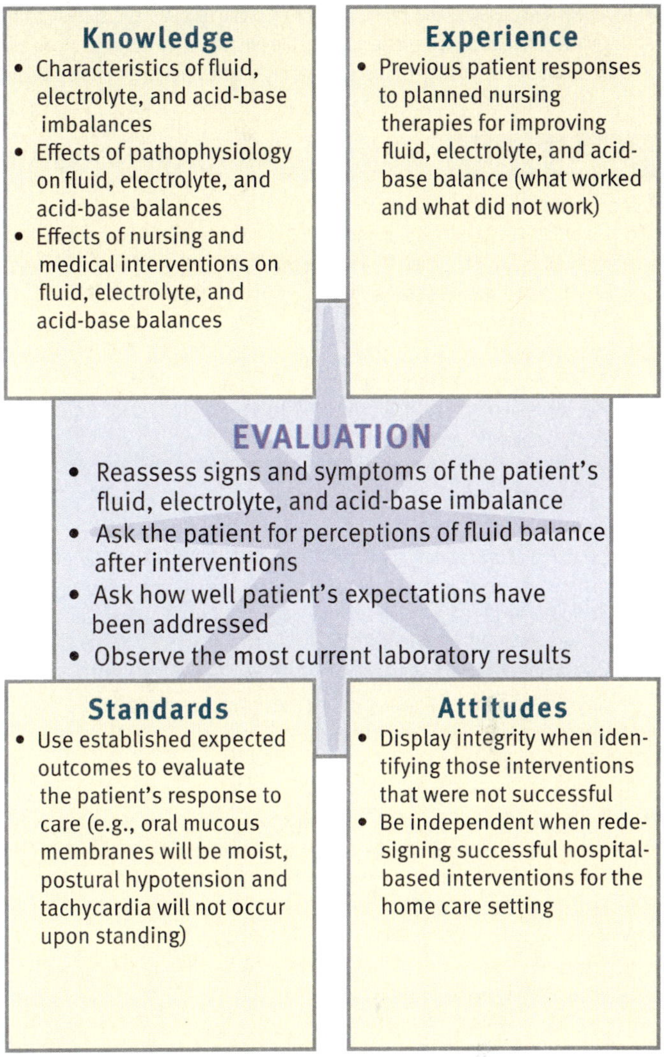
Knowledge
• Characteristics of fluid, electrolyte, and acid-base imbalances
• Effects of pathophysiology on fluid, electrolyte, and acid-base balances
• Effects of nursing and medical interventions on fluid, electrolyte, and acid-base balances
Experience
• Previous patient responses to planned nursing therapies for improving fluid, electrolyte, and acid-base balance (what worked and what did not work)
EVALUATION
• Reassess signs and symptoms of the patient's fluid, electrolyte, and acid-base imbalance
• Ask the patient for perceptions of fluid balance after interventions
• Ask how well patient's expectations have been addressed
• Observe the most current laboratory results
Standards
• Use established expected outcomes to evaluate the patient's response to care (e.g., oral mucous membranes will be moist, postural hypotension and tachycardia will not occur upon standing)
Attitudes
• Display integrity when identifying those interventions that were not successful
• Be independent when redesigning successful hospital-based interventions for the home care setting

FIG. 41-19 Critical thinking model for fluid, electrolyte, and acid-base balances evaluation.

SAFETY GUIDELINES FOR NURSING SKILLS

Ensuring patient safety is an essential role of the professional nurse. To ensure patient safety, communicate clearly with members of the health care team, assess and incorporate the patient's priorities of care and preferences, and use the best evidence when making decisions about your patient's care. When performing the skills in this chapter, remember the following points to ensure safe, individualized patient care:

- Check that you have the necessary information, a health care provider's order if required, and equipment available for the procedure before beginning.
- Before initiation of therapy, check patient identification using two patient identifiers, and assess the appropriate route and rate of infusion and potential incompatibilities between infusing fluids and medications (INS, 2011).
- Determine if the patient has a latex allergy and use nonlatex items if allergy is present (INS, 2011).
- Use special designated tubing for the brand of EID and for blood transfusions and some medications.
- Review the steps of the procedure mentally before entering a patient's room (i.e., consider modifications that you may need to make for this specific patient and verify that the type of IV solution is appropriate for this patient).

- Maintain strict aseptic and sterile techniques when required and sterility and integrity of the IV system to prevent bloodstream infections (INS, 2011).
- If you contaminate a sterile object during the procedure, do not use it. Use a new sterile one.
- Use standard body fluid precautions during procedures and place all disposable blood-contaminated items and sharp items in designated puncture-resistant biohazard containers (INS, 2011).

SKILL 41-1 INITIATING INTRAVENOUS THERAPY

View Video!

Delegation Considerations

The skill of initiating peripheral intravenous (IV) therapy cannot be delegated to nursing assistive personnel (NAP). Delegation to licensed practical nurses (LPNs) varies by state Nurse Practice Act. Instruct the NAP to inform you if:

- Patient indicates burning, bleeding, swelling, or coolness at the catheter insertion site.
- An IV dressing becomes wet or loose.
- Electronic infusion device (EID) alarm signals.
- Fluid container is almost empty.

Equipment

- Proper vascular access device (VAD) for venipuncture such as an over-the-needle catheter of appropriate gauge, depending on vein size; for continuous fluid infusions: peripheral 20-gauge catheter for an adult, 22-gauge for older adults and children (Perucca, 2010)
- IV start kit (available in some agencies)—contains a sterile drape to place under patient's arm, tourniquet, cleaning and antiseptic preparations, dressings, and a small roll of sterile tape
- If IV kit not available:
  - Disposable drape or towel
  - Tourniquet (Determine type of tourniquet based on patient assessment [e.g., blood pressure [BP] cuff—older adult, rubber band—infants]. Use single-use tourniquets to prevent transfer of microorganisms between patients.) (Perucca, 2010)
  - Antiseptic swabs (2% chlorhexidine preferred) (INS, 2011)]
  - Transparent dressing or, less commonly, 2 × 2 or 4 × 4 gauze sponge
  - Nonallergenic tape and sterile tape
- Local anesthetic (e.g., intradermal lidocaine, topical transdermal anesthetic, vapocoolant) (optional)
- Short extension tubing with fused or separate needleless connector (also called *saline lock, heparin lock, IV plug, injection cap, PRN adapter, buff cap,* or *buffalo cap)*
- Syringe containing 1 to 3 mL of preservative-free sterile 0.9% sodium chloride (normal saline) for adults, children, and neonates (INS, 2011; Mok, Kwong, and Chan, 2007); less frequently for neonates, heparin lock solution (10 units/mL or per agency protocol)
- Manufactured catheter stabilization device (e.g., STATLOCK), if available (see Fig. 41-17).
- Clean gloves
- Protective equipment: goggles, mask (optional, check agency policy)
- Patient gown with snaps at shoulder seams if available
- Needle disposal container (sharps container)
- For continuous IV fluid infusion, in addition to the above:
  - Correct type and amount of IV fluid
  - IV tubing administration set with tubing specific for the type of EID (If using gravity-flow, use microdrip tubing for small or very precise volumes and macrodrip tubing to infuse fluid more rapidly.)
  - In-line filter if particulate matter is likely, long-term or high-volume IV therapy is expected, or required by agency policy; size appropriate to type of solution (e.g., 0.22 micron for nonlipid solution, 1.2 microns for lipid solution)
  - Long extension tubing if desired for patient mobility
  - EID
  - IV pole, rolling, ceiling mounted, or attached to bed
  - Handheld bar code scanner, if using bar code system

STEP	RATIONALE
ASSESSMENT	
1 Review accuracy and completeness of health care provider's order for patient name, type and amount of IV fluid, medication additives, infusion time, and purpose of infusion. Follow six rights of medication administration (see Chapter 31).	Ensures that correct IV fluid is administered.

CLINICAL DECISION: *In most institutions health care providers do not write orders to "initiate peripheral access" or "perform venipuncture." The statement "Start IV" usually is written followed by the exact IV therapy order. The order to perform the venipuncture is implied. If the order is confusing or in question, clarify with the health care provider before proceeding.*

STEP	RATIONALE
2 Assess for clinical variables that respond to or are affected by IV fluid administration:	Provides baseline to determine effect that IV fluids have on patient's fluid and electrolyte balance.
a. Body weight	Daily weights reflect fluid retention or loss. One liter of fluid weighs 2.2 lb (1 kg). Compare with previous day's weight if available. Gain or loss of 2 lbs (1 kg) in 24 hours indicates gain or loss of 1 L of fluid. Body fat gain or loss takes longer.
b. Clinical markers of vascular volume:	Assess signs and symptoms as a group to interpret them accurately. Infusion of Na^+-containing IV fluid expands extracellular fluid volume (ECV) (vascular and interstitial).
(1) BP	Decreased BP or orthostatic hypotension may indicate ECV deficit caused by decreased stroke volume. Increased BP may indicate ECV excess.
(2) Pulse	Baroreceptor response causes rapid, thready pulse with ECV deficit; bounding, full pulse with ECV excess.
(3) Fullness of neck veins (normally neck veins are full when person is supine and flat when person is upright or semi-upright)	Indicator of fluid volume status: flat or collapsing with inhalation when supine with ECV deficit; full or distended when upright or semi-upright with ECV excess.

STEP	RATIONALE
(4) Capillary refill	Provides an indirect measure of tissue perfusion. Can indicate poor tissue perfusion (sluggish with ECV deficit).
(5) Auscultation of lungs	Crackles or rhonchi in dependent portions of lung may signal fluid buildup in lungs caused by ECV excess.
(6) Urine output (decreased; dark yellow with ECV deficit)	Kidneys respond to ECV deficit by reducing urine production and concentrating the urine. Average daily adult urine output is 1500 mL; oliguria is urine output of less than 400 mL/24 hr. Kidney disease and SIADH also can cause oliguria. Dark yellow indicates concentrated urine (Scales and Pilsworth, 2008)
c. Clinical markers of interstitial volume:	Assess signs and symptoms as a group to interpret them accurately. Infusion of Na^+-containing IV fluid expands ECV (vascular and interstitial).
(1) Dependent edema (rate severity by assessing pitting over bony prominences; 1+ indicates barely detectable edema to 4+ indicates deep persistent pitting (see Chapter 30)	Edema, indicating expanded interstitial fluid volume, is most evident in dependent areas bilaterally (i.e., feet and ankles if sitting) or sacrum if bedfast.
(2) Oral mucous membranes between cheek and gum.	More reliable indicator than dry lips or skin. Dry between cheek and gums indicates ECV deficit.
(3) Skin turgor (pinch skin over sternum or inside of forearm). Failure of skin to return to normal position within 3 seconds indicates ECV deficit.	Pinched skin that stays elevated for several seconds is called *poor skin turgor* or *"tenting."* May occur from ECV deficit, rapid weight loss, or normal aging.
d. Thirst	Occurs with hypernatremia and severe ECV deficit. Not a reliable indicator for older adults because thirst sensation decreases with age (Meiner, 2010).
e. Behavior and level of consciousness	
(1) Restlessness and mild confusion	Occurs with severe ECV deficit caused by lack of blood flow to brain.
(2) Decreased level of consciousness (lethargy, confusion, coma)	May occur with osmolality imbalances (hyponatremia and hypernatremia) and acid-base imbalances.
f. Cardiac signs of electrolyte or acid-base imbalances (e.g., irregular pulse and electrocardiogram [ECG] changes)	Rhythm and ECG changes may occur with K^+, Ca^{2+}, Mg^{2+}, and/or acid-base imbalances. Should improve as IV fluid replaces deficient electrolytes or occur if electrolyte infusion is excessive.
3 Assess patient's previous experience with and perceptions of IV therapy, understanding of purpose of IV therapy, and arm placement preference.	Provides patient-centered care by determining level of emotional support and instruction necessary. If patient is apprehensive about venipuncture, use a local anesthetic.
4 Obtain information from approved online database, drug reference book, or pharmacist about composition of IV fluids, purposes of administration, potential incompatibilities, side effects, monitoring guidelines, and need for special catheter or tubing for administration.	Allows detection of an inadvisable IV fluid order and helps to determine priority assessments.
5 Determine if patient is to undergo any planned surgeries or procedures.	Allows anticipation and placement of appropriate VAD and gauge for fluid infusion and avoids placement in an area that will interfere with medical procedures.
6 Assess for following risk factors: child or older adult; presence of heart failure or oliguric renal disease; skin lesions or infection near potential venipuncture sites; low platelet count or patient receiving anticoagulants	Older adults have proportionately less body water; persons with heart failure cannot adapt to sudden increases in vascular volume; and persons with oliguria cannot eliminate excess extracellular fluid, K^+, or Mg^{2+}. Skin lesions or infection influence choice of access site. Low platelet count or anticoagulant use increases patient's risk for bleeding from VAD site and seepage of blood from puncture site during venipuncture.
7 Assess laboratory data.	Helps determine priority assessments, establishes baseline for determining if therapy is effective, and may allow detection of an inadvisable fluid order.

CLINICAL DECISION: *If the current K^+, Ca^{2+}, or Mg^{2+} serum values are high, clarify order with health care provider before administering an IV solution containing the elevated electrolyte to avoid worsening the electrolyte excess.*

STEP	RATIONALE
8 Assess patient's history of allergies, especially to iodine, adhesive, or latex.	Equipment used during insertion of VAD may contain substances to which patient is allergic. Use alternatives if patient has allergy.

PLANNING

STEP	RATIONALE
1 Collect appropriate equipment. Be sure that you have the correct infusion set for the EID that will be used. If the IV container is rigid rather than collapsible, you need a vented spike on the IV tubing.	Provides patient safety.
2 Identify the patient using two identifiers (e.g., name and birth date or name and account number) according to facility policy. Compare identifiers with information on patient's medication administration record (MAR) or medical record.	Ensures correct patient. Complies with a recommended National Patient Safety Goal (TJC, 2011).

SKILL 41-1 INITIATING INTRAVENOUS THERAPY—cont'd

STEP	RATIONALE
3 Explain to patient and family the rationale for IV fluids and medications, procedure for initiating an IV infusion, signs and symptoms of complications, what is expected of patient, and which sensations patient should expect.	Cognitive and sensory information decreases anxiety and helps promote cooperation.
4 Assist patient to comfortable sitting or supine position. Position a chair so you are level with patient. Provide adequate lighting.	Promotes comfort and relaxation for patient. Provides proper body mechanics for nurse. Aids in successful vein location.
IMPLEMENTATION	
1 Perform hand hygiene. Organize equipment on clean, clutter-free bedside stand or over-bed table.	Reduces transmission of infection and risk of accidents.
2 Change patient's gown to more easily removable gown with snaps at shoulder if available.	Use of a special IV gown makes gown removal easier and protects VAD site from trauma during gown changes.
3 Open sterile packages using sterile aseptic technique (see Chapter 28).	Maintains sterility of equipment and reduces spread of microorganisms.
4 Prepare short extension tubing with needleless connector or stand-alone saline lock (check agency policy and procedures) to attach to VAD catheter hub.	Short extension tubing prevents traction on VAD. Many facilities use short extension tubing for continuous infusions and stand-alone saline locks (capped catheters). Continuous infusion attaches to needleless connector on short extension tubing. Saline locks provide IV access when continuous IV infusions are not needed.
a. Remove protective cap from needleless connector and attach syringe with 1 to 3 mL 0.9% sodium chloride (normal saline), maintaining sterility. Slowly inject enough saline to prime (fill) short extension tubing and connector, removing all air. Leave syringe attached to tubing (see illustration).	Replaces air with normal saline, preventing air from entering patient's vein during VAD insertion.

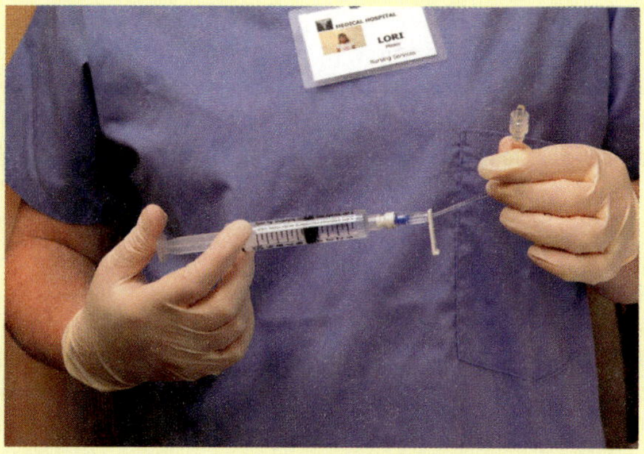

STEP 4a Prime short extension tubing, leaving syringe attached.

STEP	RATIONALE
b. Maintain sterility of end of connector and set aside for attaching to catheter hub after successful venipuncture.	Prevents touch contamination, which allows microorganisms to enter infusion equipment and bloodstream.
5 ***For continuous infusion:*** Prepare IV tubing and solution	
a. Check IV solution, using six rights of medication administration (see Chapter 31). If using bar-code system, scan bar code on patient's wristband and then on IV fluid container. Be sure prescribed additives such as potassium or vitamins are included and noted on bag label. Check solution for color, clarity, and expiration date. Check bag for leaks.	IV solutions are medications and need to be checked carefully to reduce risk of error. Bar-code systems reduce medication errors by verifying right patient, medication, dose, route, and time with EHR (Poon et al., 2010). Do not use solutions that are discolored, contain particles, or are expired. Do not use leaky bags because they present an opportunity for infection.
b. Open infusion set, maintaining sterility of both ends of tubing.	Prevents touch contamination, which allows microorganisms to enter infusion equipment and bloodstream.
c. Removing appropriate end caps, attach extension tubing with injection port to distal end of infusion set, maintaining sterility of the connection. Do not touch point of entry of connection. Leave end cap on distal end of extension tubing.	Distal end of extension tubing with injection port attaches to IV catheter hub after venipuncture, providing greater ease of access and ability to change easily between continuous and intermittent IV infusion. Prevents touch contamination, which allows microorganisms to enter infusion equipment and bloodstream.

STEP	RATIONALE
d. Place roller clamp of IV tubing approximately 2 to 5 cm (1 to 2 inches) below drip chamber and move it to closed position (see illustrations).	Close proximity of roller clamp to drip chamber allows more accurate regulation of flow rate. Closing clamp prevents accidental spillage of IV fluid on patient, nurse, bed, or floor.
e. Remove protective sheath from IV tubing port on plastic IV solution bag or top of bottle while maintaining sterility (see illustration).	Provides access for insertion of infusion tubing into solution while preventing touch contamination.
f. *Insert infusion set into fluid bag or bottle:* Remove protective cap from tubing insertion spike, not touching spike, and insert it into port of IV container, using a twisting motion (see illustration). Clean rubber stopper on glass-bottled solution with single-use antiseptic and insert spike into rubber stopper of IV bottle.	Prevents contamination of IV solution during insertion of spike. Flat surface on top of bottled solution may contain contaminants, whereas opening to plastic bag is recessed.

CLINICAL DECISION: *Do not touch spike (it is sterile). If contamination occurs (e.g., you accidentally touch outside of bag with the spike or drop spike), discard that IV tubing and obtain a new one.*

STEP	RATIONALE
g. Compress drip chamber and release, allowing it to fill one-half full with infusion fluid (see illustration).	Creates suction effect; fluid enters drip chamber, which prevents air from entering tubing.
h. Prime tubing by filling with IV solution: Remove protector cap on end of tubing if necessary (you can prime some tubing without removing cap) and slowly open roller clamp to allow fluid to travel from drip chamber through tubing to distal end. Maintain sterility of the end. Return roller clamp to closed position after tubing is filled with IV fluid. Replace protective cap on end of tubing if you removed it.	Priming replaces air in tubing with IV solution so air does not enter patient's vein. Slow fill of tubing decreases turbulence and chance of bubble formation. Closing clamp prevents continued flow of IV fluid. Cap on end of tubing maintains system sterility.

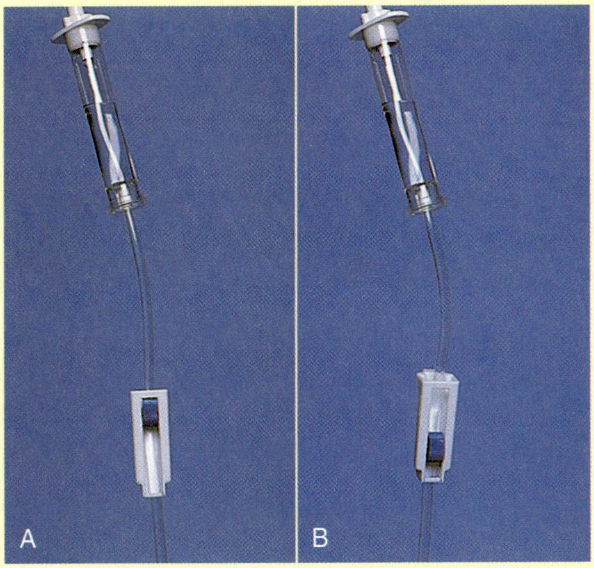

STEP 5d A, Roller clamp in open position. **B,** Roller clamp in off or closed position.

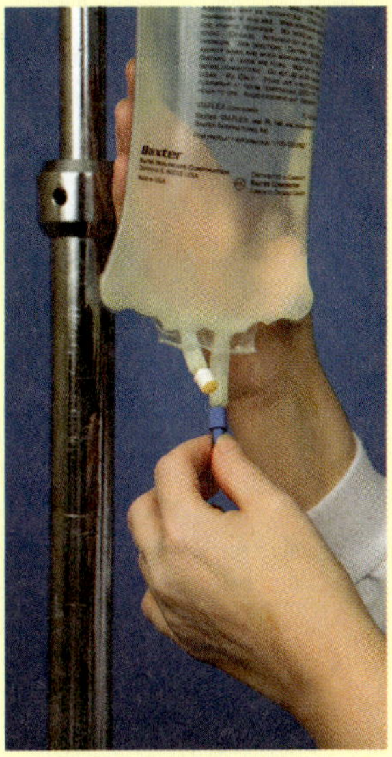

STEP 5e Remove protective covering from IV solution tubing port.

SKILL 41-1 INITIATING INTRAVENOUS THERAPY—cont'd

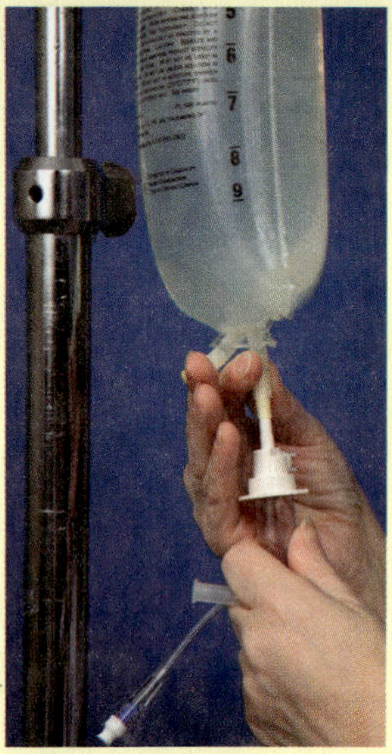

STEP 5f Insert tubing spike into IV container.

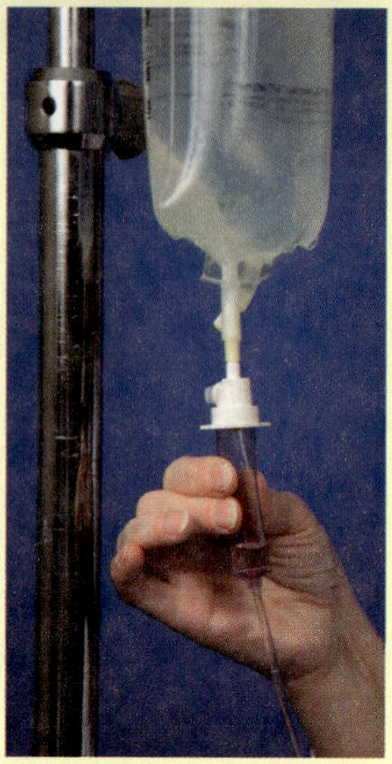

STEP 5g Squeeze drip chamber to fill with fluid.

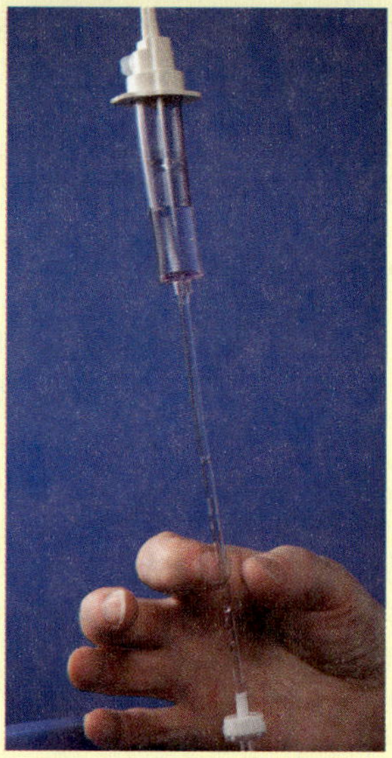

STEP 5i Removing air bubbles from tubing.

STEP	RATIONALE
i. Be certain that tubing is clear of air and air bubbles. To remove small air bubbles, firmly tap tubing where they are located (see illustration). Check entire length of tubing to ensure that all air bubbles are removed. If using multiple-port tubing, turn ports upside down and tap to fill and remove air.	Tapping causes air bubbles to rise up to drip chamber. Large air bubbles may act as emboli.
CLINICAL DECISION: *Add a long extension tubing to IV tubing to provide more length, which enables patient to move much more freely while still keeping IV line stable.*	
j. If using optional long extension tubing (not short extension tubing in Step 4), remove protective cap and attach it to distal end of IV tubing, maintaining sterility. Then prime the long extension tubing.	Priming replaces air in tubing with IV solution so air does not enter patient's vascular system.
k. Insert primed tubing into EID, with power off.	Facilitates starting infusion as soon as IV site is ready.
6 Apply clean gloves. Wear eye protection and mask (check agency policy) if splash or spray of blood is possible.	Reduces transmission of microorganisms. Prevents spraying of blood on nurse's mucous membranes.
CLINICAL DECISION: *You can apply gloves before or after assessing veins. You must apply them before VAD insertion.*	
7 Apply tourniquet to begin vein selection around arm above antecubital fossa or 10 to 15 cm (4 to 6 inches) above proposed insertion site. Do not apply tourniquet too tightly to avoid injury, bruising the skin, or occluding arterial flow. Check for presence of radial pulse.	Tourniquet slows venous return but should not occlude arterial flow. If you cannot find a vein in hand or lower arm, move up to antecubital fossa. Use antecubital fossa primarily for blood draws because a VAD there limits mobility.
Option a: You may apply tourniquet on top of a thin layer of clothing such as a gown sleeve to protect fragile or hairy skin.	
Option b: Use BP cuff instead of tourniquet. Inflate it to a level just below patient's normal diastolic pressure (less than 50 mm Hg).	Use of BP cuff reduces trauma to skin and underlying tissues.
8 Select vein for VAD insertion. Veins on dorsal and ventral surfaces of upper extremities (e.g., cephalic, basilic, and median veins) are preferred in adults (see Fig. 41-15).	Ensures adequate vein that is easy to puncture and less likely to rupture.
a. Use most distal site in nondominant arm, if possible.	Patients with VAD placement in their dominant hand have decreased ability to perform activities of daily living (O'Halloran, El-Masri, and Fox-Wasylyshyn, 2008). Performing venipuncture distal to proximal increases availability of other sites for future IV therapy (INS, 2011).

STEP	RATIONALE
b. Select a well-dilated vein. Methods to foster venous distention include:	Increased volume of blood in vein at venipuncture site makes vein more visible.
(1) Stroking extremity from distal to proximal below proposed venipuncture site.	Promotes venous filling.
(2) Applying warmth to extremity for several minutes (e.g., with a warm washcloth).	Increases blood in vein by causing dilation.
(3) If possible, placing extremity in dependent position.	Gravity promotes venous dilation.

CLINICAL DECISION: *Vigorous friction and multiple tapping of a vein, especially in older adults, causes hematoma and/or venous constriction. Choose appropriate dilation method.*

STEP	RATIONALE
c. Select vein large enough for a VAD.	Prevents interruption of venous flow while allowing adequate blood flow around catheter.
d. With your index finger, palpate vein by pressing downward. Note resilient, soft, bouncy feeling while releasing pressure (see illustration).	Fingertip is more sensitive and better for assessing vein location and condition.
e. Avoid vein selection in:	
(1) Area with tenderness, pain, infection, or wound.	May indicate inflamed vein or increase risk of infection.
(2) Extremity affected by previous stroke (cerebrovascular accident [CVA]), paralysis, mastectomy, or dialysis graft.	Increases risk of complications such as lymphedema or vessel damage.
(3) Site distal to previous venipuncture site, sclerosed or hardened veins, infiltrate site or phlebotic vessels, bruised areas, or areas of venous valves.	Such sites cause infiltration around newly placed VAD site and excessive vessel damage.
(4) Fragile dorsal veins in older adult patients and vessels in an extremity with compromised circulation.	Small, fragile veins have increased risk of infiltration, hematoma from vessel rupture, and phlebitis from vessel damage.
f. Choose a site that does not interfere with patient's activities of daily living (ADLs), use of mobility aids such as a cane, or planned procedures. Clip arm hair with scissors if necessary (explain to patient).	Keeps patient as mobile and independent as possible. Hair impedes venipuncture or adherence of dressing.

CLINICAL DECISION: *If hair removal is needed, do not shave area with a razor. Shaving may cause microabrasions that increase risk of infection (INS, 2011).*

STEP	RATIONALE
9 Release tourniquet temporarily and carefully. *Option:* At this point in procedure you may apply a local anesthetic to site; wait several minutes for it to take effect (see product directions). Monitor for allergic reaction.	Restores blood flow and prevents venospasm while preparing for venipuncture. Local anesthetic reduces insertion pain (Anderson et al., 2010).
10 Apply clean gloves, if not done in Step 6.	Reduces transmission of microorganisms.
11 Place distal end of short infusion tubing (prepared in Step 4) or adaptor end of saline lock nearby on sterile gauze, avoiding touch contamination.	Permits smooth, quick connection to VAD after accessing vein. Prevents microorganisms from entering infusion equipment and bloodstream.
12 If area of insertion appears to need cleaning, use soap and water first and dry. Use antiseptic swab or applicator to clean insertion site, using friction in a horizontal plane with first swab, in a vertical plane with second swab, and in a circular motion moving outward with third swab (see illustration). Allow to dry completely. Refrain from touching clean site unless using sterile technique.	Mechanical friction penetrates antiseptic solution into cracks and fissures of the skin. Allowing antiseptic solution to air-dry completely reduces microbial counts and risk of phlebitis. Chlorhexidine 2% preparation is preferred (CDC, 2002; INS, 2011). If your fingers touch clean area, you have introduced microorganisms from your gloves and you must clean it again.
13 Reapply tourniquet or BP cuff 10 to 12 cm (4 to 6 inches) above anticipated insertion site or keep BP cuff inflated <50 mm Hg until venipuncture completed. Check presence of distal pulse.	Diminished arterial flow prevents venous filling. The pressure of the tourniquet cause vein to fill and dilate.

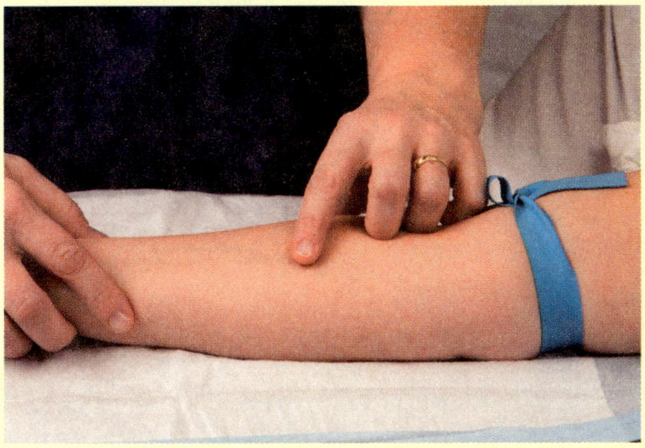

STEP 8d Palpate vein for resilience.

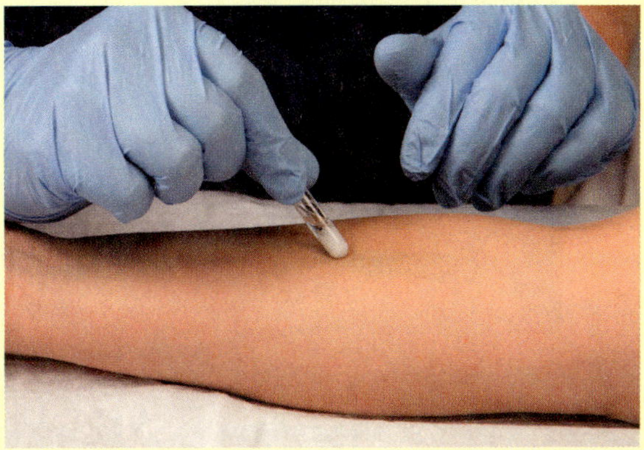

STEP 12 Clean site with chlorhexidine.

SKILL 41-1 INITIATING INTRAVENOUS THERAPY—cont'd

STEP	RATIONALE
14 Perform venipuncture. Anchor vein by placing thumb over it and stretching skin against direction of insertion 4 to 5 cm ($1\frac{1}{2}$ to 2 inches) distal to the site (see illustration).	Stabilizes vein for needle insertion. Places VAD parallel to vein.
a. Warn patient of sharp, quick stick.	Prepares patient to avoid movement of extremity during venipuncture.
b. Insert VAD with bevel up at 10- to 30-degree angle slightly distal to actual site of venipuncture in direction of vein (see illustration).	Places needle at optimal angle to vein to reduce risk of puncturing posterior vein wall when entering vein. Superficial veins require smaller insertion angle. Deeper veins require greater angle.

CLINICAL DECISION: *Use each VAD only once for each insertion attempt. If you need to try again, use a new VAD for patient safety and protection from infection.*

STEP	RATIONALE
15 Observe for blood return in flashback chamber of catheter, indicating that needle has entered vein (see illustration). Lower catheter until almost flush with skin. Advance catheter approximately $\frac{1}{4}$ inch into vein and loosen stylet. Continue to hold skin taut and advance catheter into vein until hub is near venipuncture site (see illustration). *Do not reinsert stylet once it is loosened.* Advance catheter while safety device automatically retracts stylet. (Techniques for retracting stylet vary with different VADs.) Follow manufacturer guidelines for specific safety catheter use. Place stylet directly into sharps container.	Increased venous pressure caused by tourniquet increases backflow of blood into catheter or tubing. Allows for full penetration of vein wall, placement of catheter in vein lumen, and advancement of catheter off stylet. Reduces risk of introduction of infectious microorganisms along catheter. Advancing entire stylet into vein may penetrate posterior vein wall, causing a hematoma. Reinsertion of stylet can cause catheter shearing and potential catheter embolization. Proper sharps disposal prevents needlestick injury (OSHA, 2011).

CLINICAL DECISION: *Each nurse should make no more than two attempts at initiating IV access (INS, 2011). If you are not successful with two attempts, have another nurse attempt the insertion.*

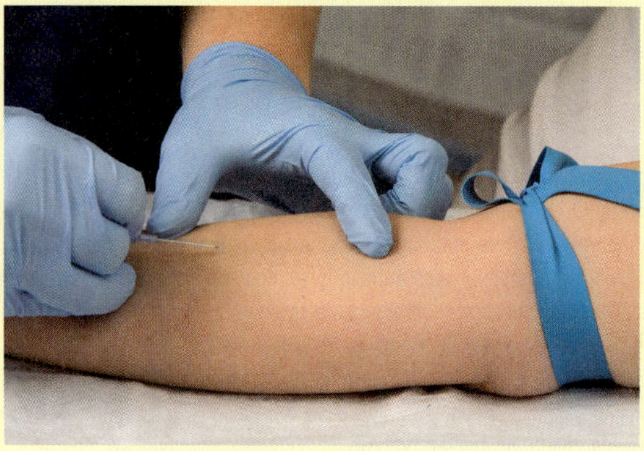

STEP 14 Stabilize vein below insertion site.

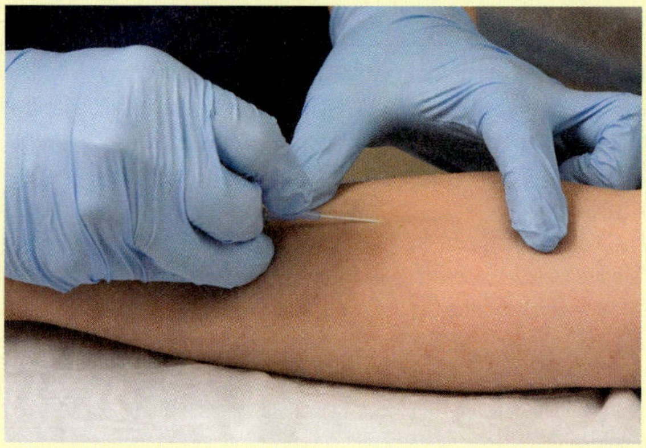

STEP 14b Puncture vein with catheter at a 10- to 30-degree angle. Catheter enters vein.

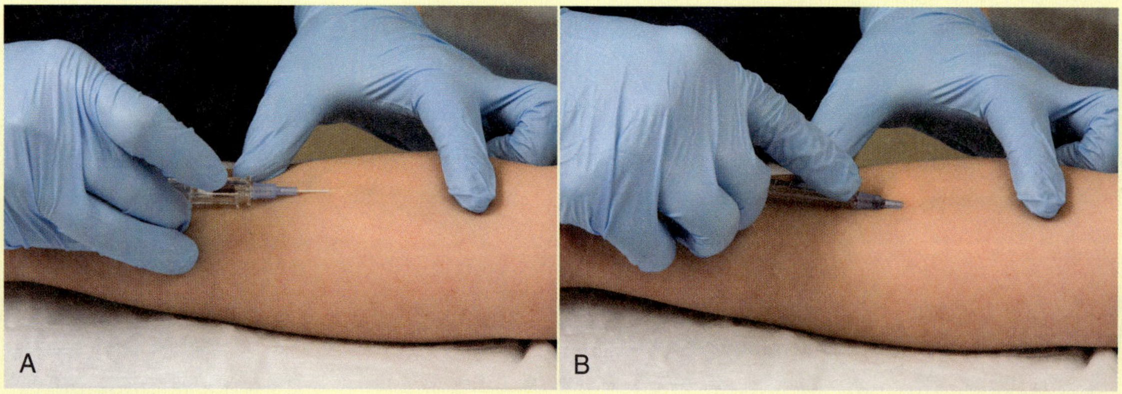

STEP 15 **A,** Look for blood return in flashback chamber. **B,** Advance catheter into vein until hub is near insertion site.

STEP	RATIONALE
16 Stabilize catheter with nondominant hand and release tourniquet or BP cuff with other. Apply gentle but firm pressure with middle finger of nondominant hand 3 cm (1¼ inches) above insertion site. Keep catheter stable with index finger.	Tourniquet release permits venous flow. Pressure with finger on vein reduces backflow of blood and allows connection with short extension tubing or saline lock with minimal blood loss.
17 Quickly connect distal end of primed short extension tubing from Step 11 or end of a prepared saline lock to catheter. Do not touch point of entry of connection. Secure connection.	Prompt connection of infusion set maintains patency of vein and prevents risk for exposure to blood. Maintains sterility.
18 Gently flush catheter using attached saline syringe to ensure that site is patent (see illustration). Observe for swelling at site while flushing.	Provides patient safety by not beginning infusion if site is not patent. Swelling during flush indicates infiltration, and site must be discontinued.
19 Remove syringe. For continuous infusion, attach distal end of IV tubing to needleless connector on short extension tubing that is attached to catheter (see illustration). Turn on EID, program it, and begin infusion at correct rate (see Skill 41-2). If using gravity flow instead of EID, begin infusion by slowly opening roller clamp to regulate rate.	Initiates flow of fluid through IV catheter, preventing clotting of device.

CLINICAL DECISION: *Be sure to calculate rate (see Skill 41-2) and set EID correctly to infuse IV solution at prescribed rate.*

STEP	RATIONALE
20 Observe insertion site for swelling.	Swelling indicates infiltration, which requires catheter removal.
21 Secure catheter and apply sterile dressing over site (procedures differ; follow agency policy).	Prevents accidental dislodgement of catheter and protects site from infection.
a. *Manufactured catheter stabilization device:* Wipe selected area with single-use skin protectant and allow to dry completely (10-15 seconds). Apply sterile adhesive strip over catheter hub. Place retainer over tubing end just behind spin nut. Peel off half of liner; press to adhere to skin. Repeat on other side (see Fig. 41-17). Then apply dressing.	A manufactured catheter stabilization device holds the catheter in place, improving patient outcomes by reducing risk of catheter dislodgement, phlebitis, and other complications (Harnage, 2007; INS, 2011).
b. *Transparent dressing:* Continue to secure catheter with nondominant hand.	Prevents accidental dislodgement of catheter.
(1) Remove adherent backing. Apply one edge of dressing and gently smooth remaining dressing over IV site, leaving connection between IV tubing and catheter hub uncovered. Remove outer covering and smooth dressing gently over site (see illustration).	Occlusive dressing protects site from bacterial contamination. Connection between administration set and hub needs to be uncovered to facilitate changing tubing if necessary.

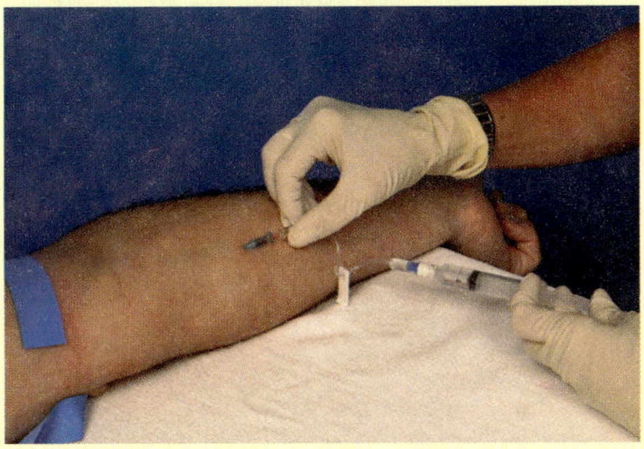

STEP 18 Flush catheter gently to ensure patency.

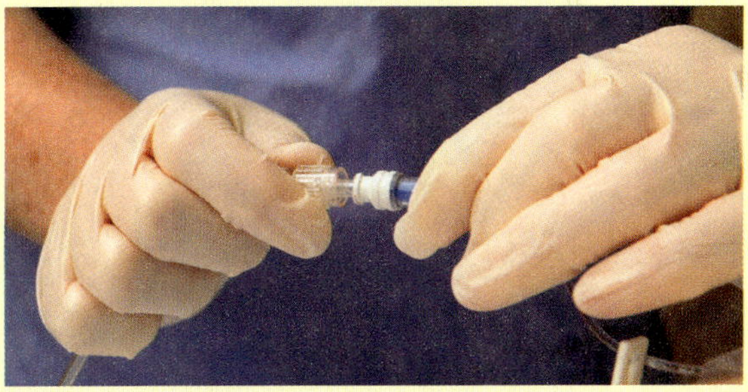

STEP 19 Connect IV tubing to the short extension set that is attached to catheter.

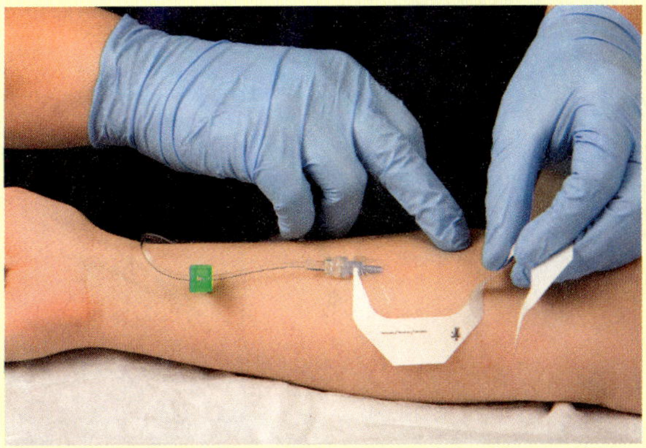

STEP 21b(1) Apply transparent dressing.

SKILL 41-1 INITIATING INTRAVENOUS THERAPY—cont'd

STEP	RATIONALE
(2) If manufactured catheter stabilization device is not used, secure catheter by placing a 2.5-cm (1-inch) piece of transparent tape over extension tubing or administration set. Do not apply tape on top of transparent dressing.	Removal of tape from transparent dressing might cause accidental dislodgement of catheter. Tape on top of a transparent dressing prevents moisture from being carried away from skin.
c. *Sterile gauze dressing:* If manufactured catheter stabilization device is not used, secure catheter by placing a narrow piece (½ inch) of sterile tape over catheter hub (see illustration). Place sterile tape only on hub, *never* over insertion site. Secure site for easy visualization. Avoid applying tape or gauze around arm.	Less frequently used than transparent dressing. Prevents accidental removal of catheter from vein. Prevents back-and-forth motion, which can irritate vein and introduce microorganisms on skin into vein. Sterile tape prevents site contamination. Wrapping anything around arm compresses veins or prevents visualization of insertion site.
(1) Place 2 × 2 gauze pad over insertion site and catheter hub. Secure all edges with tape (see illustration). Do not cover connection between IV tubing and catheter hub.	Secure dressing is less likely to allow entrance of microorganisms.
(2) *Option:* Fold 2 × 2 gauze pad in half and cover with a 2.5 cm (1 inch)–wide tape extending about an inch from each side. Place under tubing/catheter hub junction.	Tape on top of gauze makes it easier to access hub/tubing junction. Gauze pad elevates hub off skin to prevent pressure area.

CLINICAL DECISION: *Think carefully about where you place tape. Do not apply it over the catheter insertion site, over the connection between the tubing or port and the IV catheter hub, or on top of the transparent dressing.*

STEP	RATIONALE
22 Curl loop of tubing alongside arm and place second piece of tape directly over tubing to secure it (see illustration).	Securing loop of tubing reduces risk of dislodging catheter if IV tubing is pulled (i.e., loop comes apart before catheter dislodges).
23 For gravity-flow IV fluid administration, recheck flow rate to correct drops per minute (see Skill 41-2).	Manipulation of catheter during dressing application may alter flow rate. Check flow rate to maintain accurate administration of IV fluids. Flow can fluctuate; thus it must be checked at intervals for accuracy.
24 Label dressing per agency policy. Include date and time of IV insertion, VAD gauge and length, and your initials (see illustration).	Provides immediate access to data regarding when IV was inserted and when to rotate site.

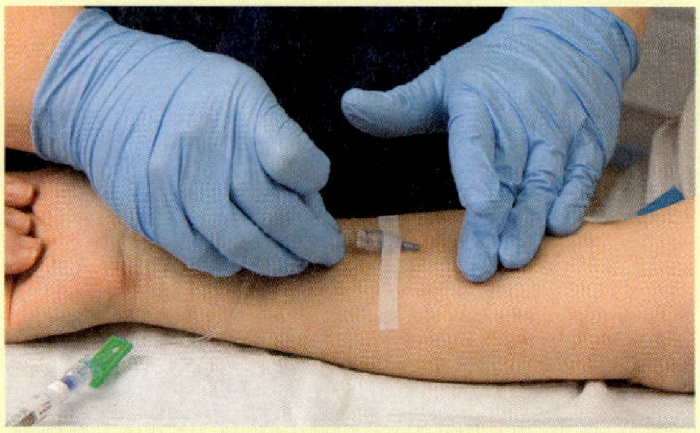

STEP 21c Apply tape over catheter hub.

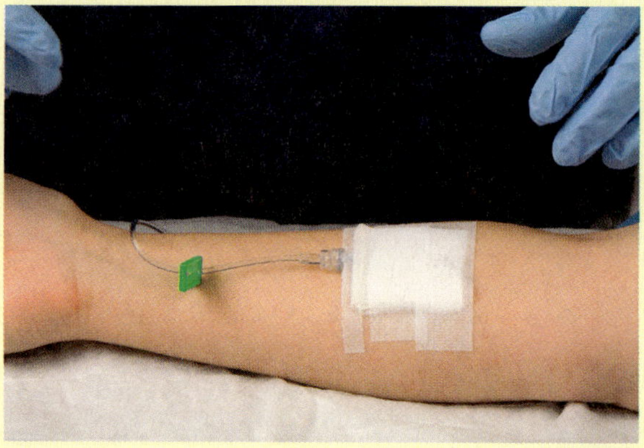

STEP 21c(1) Place 2 × 2 inch gauze over insertion site and catheter hub.

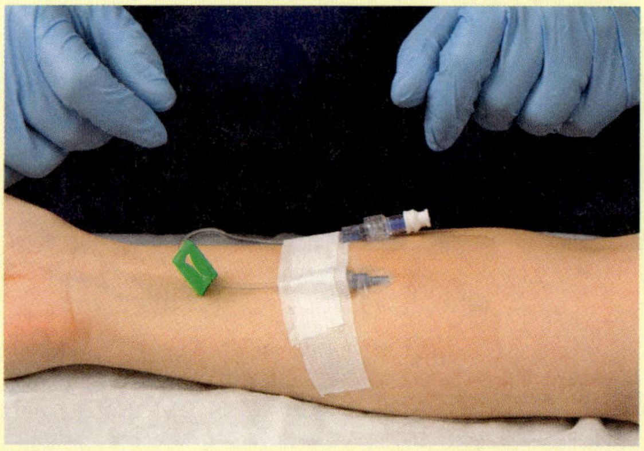

STEP 22 Curl a loop of the short or long intravenous tubing alongside the arm. Secure tubing.

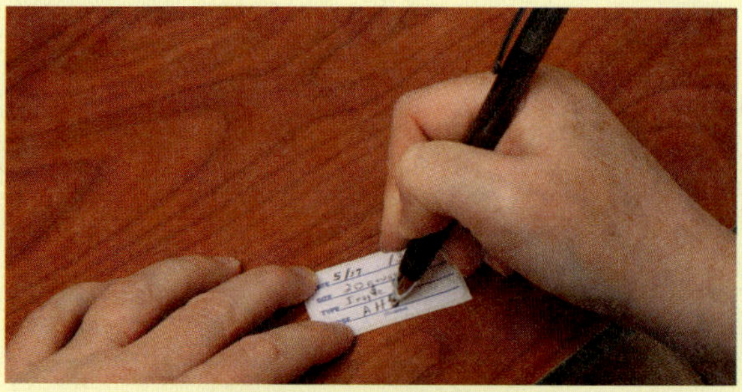

STEP 24 Label IV dressing.

STEP	RATIONALE
25 Dispose of used stylet or other sharps in appropriate sharps container if not done previously. Discard supplies. Remove gloves and perform hand hygiene.	Reduces transmission of microorganisms, prevents accidental needlestick injuries, and follows guidelines for disposal of sharps (OSHA, 2011).
26 Teach patient how to move or turn without dislodging VAD.	Prevents accidental dislodgement of catheter.

EVALUATION

1 Observe patient every 1 to 2 hours.	
a. Check that correct amount of IV fluid has infused by observing fluid level in IV container.	Administration of prescribed amount of fluid maintains or restores fluid balance.
b. Check rate on EID or count drip rate (if gravity drip).	Accurate monitoring of rate further ensures administration of correct amount of fluid.
c. Check patency of VAD.	Flow rate slows or stops if catheter becomes partially occluded or obstructed.

CLINICAL DECISION: *If IV line is positional, fluid runs quickly, slowly, or stops, depending on position of patient's arm. Instruct patient to position arm to maintain flow; if this continues, consider restarting IV in another site.*

d. Observe patient during palpation of vessel for signs of discomfort.	Tenderness is an early sign of phlebitis.
e. Inspect insertion site, note skin color (e.g., redness, pallor). Inspect for presence of swelling, infiltration (see Table 41-13), and phlebitis (see Table 41-14). Palpate temperature of skin above dressing.	Redness, tenderness, and warmth indicate vein inflammation or phlebitis. Swelling above insertion site and cool temperature often indicate infiltration of fluid into tissues.
2 Change peripheral IV access per agency policy, per health care provider's orders, or immediately on suspected contamination or complication.	INS standards recommend VAD replacement and site rotation when clinically indicated rather than at set intervals (INS, 2011). A retrospective review showed that it was possible to have long catheter indwell times without complications in some patients (Powell et al., 2008).
3 Observe patient to determine response to therapy (e.g., measure intake and output [I&O], daily weights, vital signs).	IV fluids and additives are administered to maintain or restore fluid and electrolyte balance. Early recognition of complications leads to prompt treatment.

UNEXPECTED OUTCOMES AND RELATED INTERVENTIONS

1. Overload of IV solution, infiltration, phlebitis, local infection, and bleeding at venipuncture site
   - See Table 41-12.
2. Lack of effectiveness of IV therapy for ECV
   - Notify patient's health care provider, providing baseline and current heart rate and BP and length of time IV has been infusing; adjust infusion rate or type of IV solution as ordered.
   - Be prepared to draw blood for laboratory testing.

RECORDING AND REPORTING

- Document in nurses' notes or other designated location in an electronic health record (EHR) date and time of insertion; number and sites of attempts, precise description of insertion site (e.g., cephalic vein on dorsal surface of right lower arm, 2.5 cm above wrist); catheter gauge, type, length, and brand; type of dressing and catheter stabilization; flow rate; type of infusion, EID use, and your identity (INS, 2011). If using bar-code system, fluid type and time record automatically.
- Record patient's status, IV fluid, amount infused, and integrity and patency of system according to agency policy.
- Report to oncoming nursing staff: type of fluid, flow rate, status of VAD, amount of fluid remaining in present container, expected time to hang subsequent IV container, and patient condition.
- Report to health care provider: any adverse reactions.

HOME CARE CONSIDERATIONS

- Ensure that patient is able and willing to self-administer IV therapy or that a reliable family caregiver will provide IV therapy at home.
- Teach patient and caregiver information needed to administer IV therapy safely (see Box 41-8).

SKILL 41-2 REGULATING INTRAVENOUS FLOW RATE

View Video!

Delegation Considerations

The skill of regulating intravenous (IV) flow rate cannot be delegated to nursing assistive personnel (NAP). Delegation to licensed practical nurses (LPNs) varies by state Nurse Practice Act. Instruct the NAP to inform you if:

- Patient indicates burning, bleeding, swelling, or coolness at catheter insertion site.
- Electronic infusion device (EID) alarm signals.
- Fluid container is almost empty.

Equipment

- Electronic infusion device (EID, IV pump) or for gravity infusion: volume control device and watch with second hand
- Calculator or paper and pen/pencil
- Tape
- Label

SKILL 41-2 REGULATING INTRAVENOUS FLOW RATE—cont'd

STEP	RATIONALE
ASSESSMENT	
1 Review accuracy and completeness of health care provider's order for patient name, type, and amount of IV fluid, medication additives, infusion time, and purpose of infusion. Follow six rights of medication administration (see Chapter 31).	Ensures administration of correct IV fluid at proper rate. IV fluids are medications. The six rights prevent medication administration error.
2 Perform hand hygiene.	Prevents transmission of microorganisms.
3 Observe for patency of IV tubing and vascular access device (VAD).	For fluid to infuse at proper rate, IV line and VAD must be free of kinks, knots, and clots.
4 Inspect IV site and verify with patient how existing IV site feels (e.g., determine if any tenderness, pain, or burning).	Tenderness, pain, or burning may be early indication of phlebitis. Includes patient in own care.
5 Assess patient's knowledge of how positioning of IV site affects flow rate.	Fosters patient participation in maintaining most effective position of arm with IV equipment.
6 Assess patient risk for fluid and electrolyte imbalance, given type of IV fluid (e.g., neonate, cardiac or kidney disease)	Helps prioritize nursing assessments.
PLANNING	
1 Gather paper and pencil or calculator to calculate flow rate.	Use accurate mathematical calculations to obtain correct rate for patient safety.
2 Check order to see how long each liter of fluid should infuse. If hourly rate (mL/hr) is not provided in order, calculate it by dividing volume by hours. For example:	Provides even infusion of fluid over prescribed hourly rate. A volume of 1 L = 1000 mL.

$$\text{mL/hr} = \frac{\text{Total infusion volume (mL)}}{\text{Hours of infusion}}$$

1000 mL/8 hr = 125 mL/hr
or if 3 L is ordered for 24 hours,
3000 mL/24 hr = 125 mL/hr

CLINICAL DECISION: *It is common for health care providers to write an abbreviated IV order such as "D_5W with 20 mEq KCl 125 mL/hr continuous." This order implies that IV infusion should be maintained at this rate until an order has been written for IV infusion to be discontinued. Occasionally an IV order calls for 1 L "TKO" or "KVO," either of which means at a slow rate to keep vein open. Clarify with the provider if any part of the order is unclear.*

STEP	RATIONALE
3 If KVO (or TKO) rate is ordered, check agency policy regarding flow rate. KVO often falls in the range of 10 to 25 mL/hr.	KVO rate prevents catheter clotting, thus preserving venous access while infusing a minimal amount of fluid.
4 Use hourly rate to program EID (see Implementation) or, if gravity-flow infusion, use to calculate minute flow rate (gtt/min).	EID automatically delivers correct minute flow rate. Gravity infusion requires nurse calculation.
5 Calculate minute flow rate for gravity-flow infusion:	Use microdrip tubing when infusing small or very precise volumes. Use macrodrip tubing to infuse fluid more rapidly.
a. Determine drop factor (calibration) in drops per milliliter (gtt/mL) of infusion set currently in use: *Microdrip:* 60 gtt/mL *Macrodrip:* 10 or 15 gtt/mL; see label on administration set packaging.	Drop factor for macrodrip tubing varies with manufacturer.
b. Select one of the following formulas to calculate minute flow rate (drops/min) based on drop factor of infusion set: **(1)** mL/hr/60 min = mL/min Drop factor × mL/min = gtt/min *Or* **(2)** mL/hr × drop factor/60 min = gtt/min Using formula (2) above, calculate minute flow rate for an IV solution that should infuse at 125 mL/hr:	Formulas compute correct flow rate over a minute.
Microdrip: 125 mL/hr × 60 gtt/mL = 7500 gtt/hr 7500 gtt ÷ 60 minutes = 125 gtt/min	When using microdrip, mL/hr always equals gtt/min.
Macrodrip: 125 mL/hr × 15 gtt/mL = 1875 gtt/hr 1875 gtt ÷ 60 minutes = 31-32 gtt/min	Multiple hourly rate (mL/hr) by drop factor and divide product by 60 to convert hours to minutes.
(3) Option—use dimensional analysis (see Chapter 31)	

STEP	RATIONALE
IMPLEMENTATION	
1 Identify the patient using two identifiers (e.g., name and birth date or name and account number) according to facility policy. Compare identifiers with information on patient's medication administration record (MAR) or medical record.	Ensures correct patient. Complies with a recommended National Patient Safety Goal (TJC, 2011).
2 Using an EID (infusion pump or smart pump):	Smart pumps with medication safety software are designed for administration of IV fluid that contains medications.
a. Consult manufacturer directions for setup of infusion. Use tubing compatible with EID.	Special infusion tubing is required for most EIDs. It is designed to prevent free flow of fluid when tubing is removed from device. Check agency equipment and associated policies and procedures.
b. Close roller clamp on primed IV tubing and insert tubing into chamber of EID control mechanism or pump module per manufacturer directions (see illustration). Roller clamp on IV tubing goes between EID and patient.	Most electronic infusion pumps use positive pressure to infuse. They move fluid through IV tubing by compressing and milking tubing.
c. Turn on EID power; test alarm; select required volume per hour, volume to be infused (VTBI), and any other information required. Close control chamber door if not already done and press run/start button. If smart pump alarms immediately and shuts down, your settings were outside unit parameters. Recalculate infusion rate and set EID again.	Program EID per manufacturer instructions for patient safety. Smart pumps require additional information such as patient unit and medication. They contain a computer that matches pump setting against a drug dose database (Hertzel and Sousa, 2009). If your setting does not match the database, the pump alarms and automatically shuts down for patient safety.
d. Open roller clamp completely while EID is in use.	Ensures that EID regulates infusion rate.
e. Check intermittently to see that correct amount of IV fluid has infused by observing fluid level in IV container.	EIDs do not replace frequent, accurate nursing evaluation. They may continue to infuse IV fluids even after an infiltration or other complication.
f. Assess patency of system if EID alarm signals.	Alarm indicates problem in system. Empty solution container, kinked tubing, air in tubing, closed clamp, infiltration, clotted catheter, and/or low battery all trigger EID alarm.
3 Using gravity flow:	
a. Ensure that IV container is 36 inches above IV site for adults.	Pressure caused by gravity is necessary to overcome venous pressure and resistance from tubing and catheter.
b. Slowly open roller clamp on tubing until you can see drops in drip chamber. Hold a watch with second hand at same level as drip chamber and count drip rate for 1 minute (see illustration). Adjust roller clamp to increase or decrease drip rate until you obtain desired number of drops per minute.	Regulate to prescribed rate of fluid infusion.
c. Monitor drip rate at least hourly.	Many factors influence drip rate; frequent monitoring ensures IV fluid administration as prescribed.
4 Using a volume-control device with gravity flow:	Device is a graduated chamber with tubing inserted in an IV line just below IV container. It is used in pediatric units if an EID is not used.
a. Insert volume-control device spike into IV container and insert spike of infusion set into bottom end of volume controller tubing using aseptic technique.	Delivers small volume of fluid to prevent bolus administration in case of equipment malfunction; especially important in pediatric units. You refill it as it becomes low.

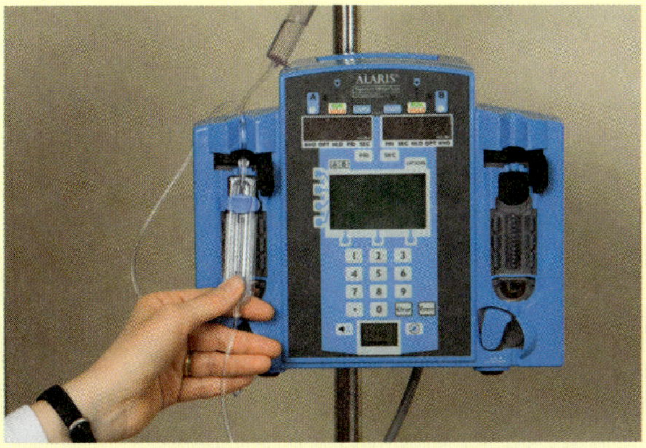

STEP 2b Insert IV tubing into chamber of control mechanism of EID.

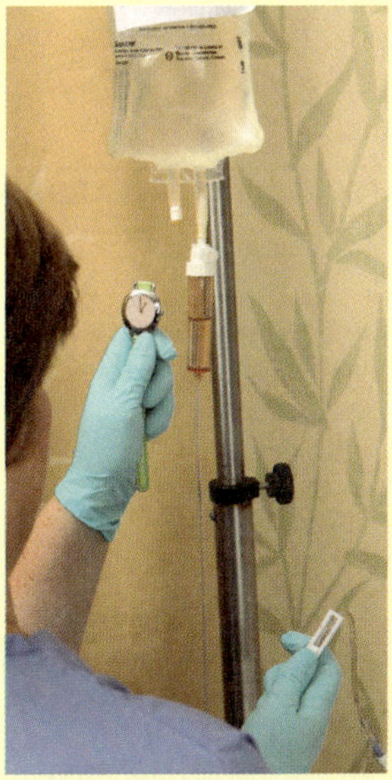
STEP 3b Nurse counting drip rate on gravity-flow infusion.

SKILL 41-2 REGULATING INTRAVENOUS FLOW RATE—cont'd

STEP	RATIONALE
b. Place no more than 2 hours' allotment of fluid into device by opening clamp between IV fluid container and device (see illustration).	Allows for continuous fluid infusion if you do not return in exactly 60 minutes to refill volume controller. If infusion rate accidentally increases, patient receives only a 2-hour allotment of fluid.

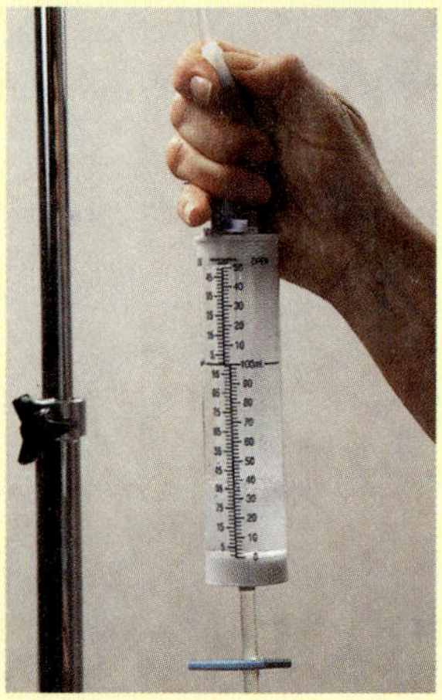

STEP 4b Open regulator clamp to fill volume control device.

STEP	RATIONALE
c. Regulate flow rate manually with roller clamp by counting drops in drip chamber for 1 minute by watch and adjusting roller clamp to increase or decrease rate of infusion.	Regulate to prescribed rate of fluid infusion.
d. Assess system at least hourly; add fluid to volume-control device. Regulate flow rate.	Maintains patency of system and patient monitoring.
5 Attach piece of tape or label to IV fluid container with date and time of container change (check agency policy). If using polyvinylchloride (PVC) container, mark only on label and not container.	Provides reference to determine next time for container change, especially with KVO rate. Ink may leak into IV fluid through PVC container.
6 Instruct patient to avoid raising arm with IV line because it can affect flow rate; to avoid touching control clamp or other equipment; and about purpose of EID alarms.	Provides information so patient does not alter infusion rate. Ask patient to instruct family if appropriate.

EVALUATION

1 Monitor IV infusion at least every hour, noting volume of IV fluid infused and rate.	Ensures that correct volume infuses over prescribed time period.
2 Observe patient for signs of overhydration or dehydration to determine response to therapy and restoration of fluid balance.	Signs and symptoms of new overhydration or continued dehydration warrant changing rate of fluid infused. Contact health care provider for new infusion rate order.
3 Evaluate for signs of infiltration, inflammation at site, kink or knot in infusion tubing, or occluded VAD.	Prevents or identifies conditions that decrease or stop flow rate.

UNEXPECTED OUTCOMES AND RELATED INTERVENTIONS

1. Circulatory overload of IV solution occurs.
   - See Table 41-12.
2. IV fluid container empties with subsequent loss of VAD patency.
   - Discontinue present IV infusion and start new IV line in other extremity or proximal to previous insertion site.
3. IV fluid infuses more slowly than ordered.
   - Check for positional change that might affect rate, EID malfunction (or insufficient height of IV fluid container with gravity flow), kinking or obstruction of tubing, infiltration or other complications at VAD site.
   - Consult health care provider for new order to provide necessary fluid volume.

RECORDING AND REPORTING

- Record rate of infusion in milliliters per hour (or drops per minute with gravity flow) in designated location in the patient's medical record.
- Document use of EID or volume-control device.
- Immediately record any new IV fluid rate.
- At change of shift or when leaving on break, report rate and volume left of infusion to nurse in charge or next nurse assigned to care for patient.

HOME CARE CONSIDERATIONS

- Ensure that patient is able and willing to operate infusion pump and administer IV therapy. If he or she is unable to provide self-care, be sure that a reliable family caregiver is available in the home.
- Ensure that EID functions properly before use and that patient's electrical outlets are properly grounded.
- Teach patient and caregiver what EID alarms mean, methods to troubleshoot them, and how to disconnect the tubing from the EID pump in case of pump failure. Provide a 24-hour access telephone number for patient to call for assistance.
- If using gravity administration, teach patient and family caregiver how to time drops per minute using watch with second hand.

SKILL 41-3 MAINTENANCE OF INTRAVENOUS SYSTEM

Delegation Considerations

The skills of changing an intravenous (IV) fluid container and tubing cannot be delegated to nursing assistive personnel (NAP). Some states allow NAP to discontinue peripheral IV access. Delegation to licensed practical nurses (LPNs) varies by state Nurse Practice Act. Instruct the NAP to inform you if:

- The IV fluid container is nearly empty.
- Any bleeding occurs after you remove the vascular access device (VAD).

Equipment

- Changing an IV fluid container and tubing (continuous infusion)
  - Correct type and volume of IV solution
  - Infusion tubing
  - Tape or tubing label
  - Filter (size appropriate to solution) and extension tubing (if necessary)
  - Handheld bar-code scanner if using bar-code system
- Changing an IV fluid container and tubing (intermittent infusion or saline lock)
  - Syringe containing 1 to 3 mL of preservative-free sterile 0.9% sodium chloride (normal saline) for adults, children, and neonates (INS, 2011; Mok, Kwong, and Chan 2007) (less frequently for neonates), heparin lock solution (10 units/mL or per agency protocol)
  - 2 × 2 gauze pads (optional)
  - Tape or label
  - Clean gloves
  - Antiseptic swab (chlorhexidine 2% preferred [INS, 2011])
- Discontinuing peripheral IV access
  - Clean gloves
  - Sterile 2 × 2 or 4 × 4 gauze sponge
  - Antiseptic swab
  - Tape

STEP	RATIONALE
ASSESSMENT	
1 Changing IV fluid container:	
a. Review accuracy and completeness of health care provider's order for patient name, type and amount of IV fluid, medication additives, infusion time, and purpose of infusion. Follow six rights of medication administration (see Chapter 31). If order is written for KVO (keep vein open) or TKO (to keep open), note date and time of last fluid container change and refer to agency policy to determine need for IV fluid container change.	Provides patient safety by preventing medication errors. Agency policy determines how often IV fluid container change is required for KVO infusion rate.
b. Determine compatibility of all IV fluids and additives by consulting approved online database, drug reference book, or pharmacist.	Incompatibilities cause physical and chemical changes with adverse patient outcomes.
2 Changing IV tubing:	
a. Assess current tubing for puncture, contamination, or occlusion, which requires immediate tubing change.	Compromised tubing allows fluid leakage, bacterial contamination, and entry of pathogens into patient's bloodstream. Whole blood, blood component products, or incompatible mixtures can occlude or partially occlude tubing because viscous solutions adhere to walls of tubing, decreasing size of lumen.
b. Note date and time of last IV tubing change. Agency policy indicates frequency of routine change for IV administration sets and saline/heparin locks.	INS (2011) recommends changing continuous IV tubing no more often than 96-hour intervals unless tubing becomes compromised. Change primary intermittent tubing set every 24 hours (INS, 2011).
3 Discontinuing peripheral IV access: Review accuracy and completeness of health care provider's order for discontinuing IV therapy.	Order required for discontinuing IV therapy.
4 Determine patient's/family member's understanding of need for IV therapy or reason for discontinuing it.	Reveals need for patient teaching.

SKILL 41-3 MAINTENANCE OF INTRAVENOUS SYSTEM—cont'd

STEP	RATIONALE
PLANNING	
1 Collect appropriate equipment at patient's bedside.	Keeps procedure organized and provides patient safety.
For changing IV fluid container: Have next solution prepared at least 1 hour before needed. If prepared in pharmacy, ensure that it has been delivered to patient care unit. Check that solution is correct and properly labeled. Allow solution to warm to room temperature if refrigerated. Check solution expiration date. Observe for precipitate, discoloration, and leakage.	Adequate planning for changing solution reduces risk of clot formation at catheter tip caused by lack of flow from an empty IV container. Checking that solution is correct prevents medication error.
2 Coordinate tubing changes with IV fluid container changes if possible.	Promotes patient safety by reducing number of times IV system is open.
3 Identify the patient using two identifiers (e.g., name and birth date or name and account number) according to facility policy. Compare identifiers with information on patient's medication administration record (MAR) or medical record. If using bar-code system, scan bar code on patient's wristband and then on IV fluid container.	Ensures correct patient. Complies with a recommended National Patient Safety Goal (TJC, 2011). Bar-code systems reduce medication errors by verifying right patient, medication, dose, and time with EHR (Poon et al., 2010).
4 Explain to patient/family member procedure, its purpose, and what is expected of patient.	Promotes patient cooperation and decreases anxiety.
For discontinuing peripheral IV access: Explain that patient must hold extremity still, that he or she may feel burning sensation when you remove catheter, and that procedure will take about 5 minutes.	
IMPLEMENTATION	
1 Perform hand hygiene.	Reduces transmission of microorganisms.
2 Changing IV fluid container:	
a. Determine patency of current VAD site: Look for swelling, coolness to touch, or tenderness around VAD site. With EID use VAD should be patent if site is not infiltrated and EID functions without alarm signals. If not using EID, carefully adjust roller clamp to see an increase in flow rate and then regulate back to prescribed rate.	New IV access site is necessary if infiltration or phlebitis is present, IV tubing is compromised, or VAD site is not patent. EID alarm signals when system is occluded. In absence of EID, adjusting roller clamp increases flow rate if there is no obstruction.

CLINICAL DECISION: *Lowering IV container below level of IV site for presence of blood return (retrograde) is an unreliable indicator of patency.*

STEP	RATIONALE
b. Prepare to change solution when about 50 mL of fluid remains in container. Be sure that drip chamber is at least half full.	Prevents air from entering tubing and vein from clotting from lack of flow.
c. Prepare new IV fluid container for changing. If using plastic bag, hang on IV pole and remove protective cover from IV tubing port. If using glass bottle, remove metal cap and disks.	Permits quick, smooth, and organized change from old to new IV fluid container.
d. Close roller clamp to stop flow of existing infusion. Remove tubing from EID. Then remove old IV fluid container from IV pole and hold it with tubing port pointing upward.	Prevents solution remaining in drip chamber from emptying while changing IV fluid container. Port held upward prevents IV fluid from spilling.
e. Quickly remove spike from old solution container (see illustration) and, without touching tip, insert it into new container (see illustration).	Reduces risk of solution in drip chamber running dry and maintains sterility.

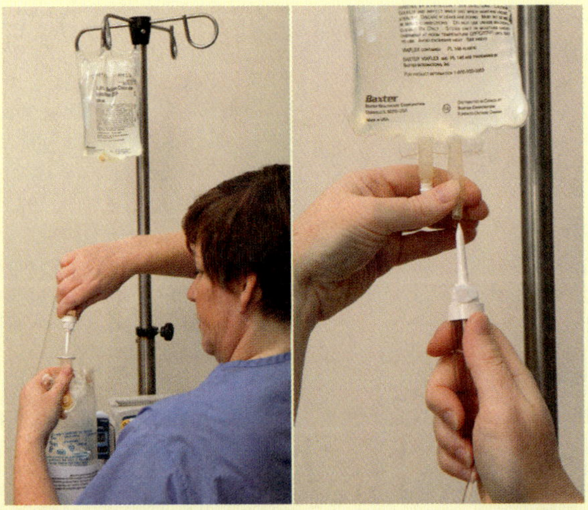

STEP 2e A, Quickly remove spike from old solution container. **B,** Without touching tip, insert spike into new container.

STEP	RATIONALE
CLINICAL DECISION: *If you contaminate the spike, discard that IV tubing and use a new one.*	
f. Hang new fluid container on IV pole.	Gravity assists delivery of fluid into drip chamber.
g. Check for air in tubing. If bubbles form, remove them by closing roller clamp below them, stretching tubing downward, and tapping tubing with finger (bubbles rise in fluid to drip chamber) (see illustration). For larger amount of air, swab port below air with alcohol and allow to dry; insert needleless syringe into port and aspirate air into the syringe.	Reduces risk of air descending the tubing. Use of air-eliminating filter also reduces this risk.
h. Make sure that drip chamber is one-third to one-half full. If it is too full, pinch off tubing below it, invert container, squeeze drip chamber (see illustration) to push fluid into container, release tubing, and hang container.	Reduces risk of air entering tubing. If chamber is completely filled, you cannot observe drips.
i. Insert tubing into EID and restart pump. If no EID, regulate flow to prescribed rate with roller clamp.	Delivers IV fluid as ordered.
j. Attach piece of tape or label to IV fluid container with date and time of container change (check agency policy). If using polyvinylchloride (PVC) container, mark only on label and not container.	Provides reference to determine next time for container change, especially with KVO rate. Ink may leak into IV fluid through PVC container.
3 Changing IV tubing:	
a. Open new infusion set and connect add-on pieces (e.g., filter, extension tubing). Keep protective coverings over infusion spike and distal connector for VAD. Secure all connections.	Protective covers maintain sterility of IV system. Securing connections reduces risk of contamination, infection, and hemorrhage.
b. Apply clean gloves.	Reduces transmission of microorganisms (OSHA, 2011).
c. If catheter hub is not accessible, remove IV dressing as directed in Skill 41-4. Do not remove tape or catheter securement device that secures catheter to skin.	Catheter hub must be accessible to provide smooth transition when removing old and inserting new tubing.
d. *Prepare tubing, using existing continuous IV infusion:*	
(1) Close roller clamp on new IV tubing.	Prevents spillage of fluid after spiking container.
(2) Slow rate of infusion through old tubing to KVO rate, using EID or roller clamp if no EID.	Prevents complete infusion of fluid remaining in tubing, thus decreasing risk of VAD clotting.
(3) Compress and fill drip chamber of old tubing.	Ensures that drip chamber contains enough fluid to maintain IV patency while changing tubing.

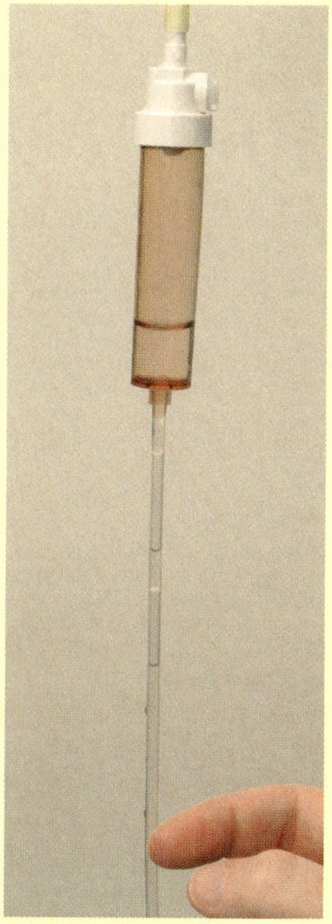

STEP 2g Nurse taps tubing to cause air bubbles to rise up to drip chamber.

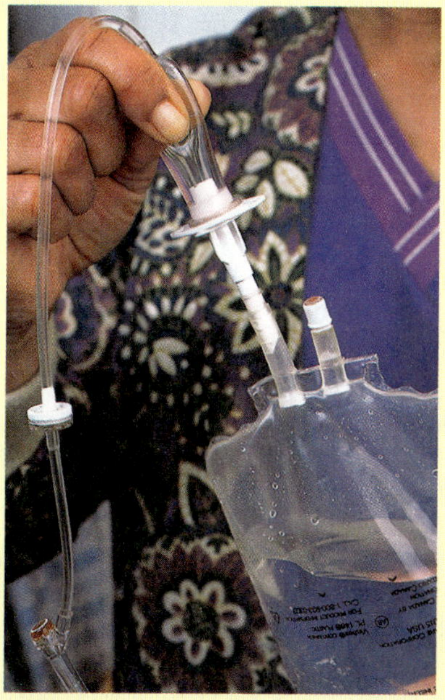

STEP 2h Remove excess fluid from drip chamber.

SKILL 41-3 MAINTENANCE OF INTRAVENOUS SYSTEM—cont'd

STEP	RATIONALE
(4) Invert IV fluid container and remove old tubing. Keep spike sterile and upright. *Optional:* Tape old drip chamber to IV pole without contaminating spike.	Allows fluid to continue to flow through IV catheter while new tubing is prepared.
(5) Place insertion spike of new tubing into IV fluid container. Hang container on IV pole, compress and release drip chamber on new tubing, and fill drip chamber one-third to one-half full.	Permits flow of fluid from solution into new infusion tubing.

CLINICAL DECISION: *If you contaminate the spike, discard that IV tubing and use a new one.*

STEP	RATIONALE
(6) Slowly open roller clamp, remove protective cap from adapter (if necessary), and flush new tubing with solution. Close roller clamp when full. Replace cap. Place capped end of adapter near patient's IV site.	Priming slowly instead of allowing a wide-open flow reduces formation of air in tubing. Removes air from tubing and replaces it with fluid. Positions equipment for quick smooth connection of new tubing.
(7) Stop EID if used and close roller clamp on old tubing.	Prevents spillage of fluid as tubing is removed from catheter.
e. *Prepare tubing, using existing saline lock:*	
(1) If loop or short extension tubing is needed, use sterile technique to connect new injection cap to new loop or tubing.	Sterile technique prevents transmission of infection.
(2) Swab injection cap with antiseptic swab and let dry. Insert syringe with 1 to 3 mL saline solution and inject through injection cap into loop of extension tubing (see illustration). Place capped end of tubing near patient's IV site.	Maintains patency of VAD.

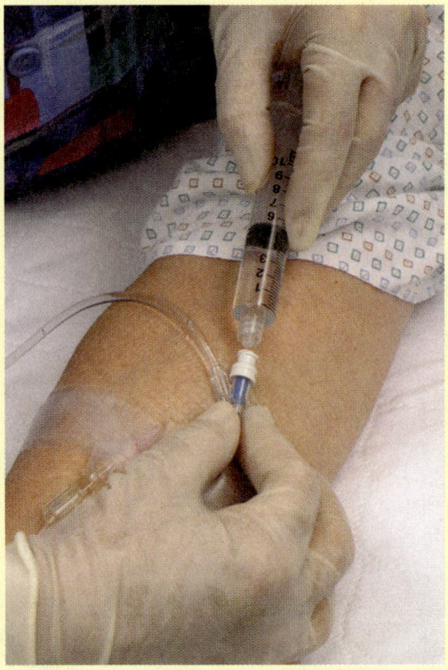

STEP 3e(2) Flush injection port slowly.

STEP	RATIONALE
f. *Reestablish infusion:*	
(1) Remove manufactured catheter stabilization device or tape from tubing. Gently disconnect old tubing from catheter hub (see illustration A) and quickly insert adapter of new tubing into catheter hub, being sure that it is secure, thus maintaining sterility of point of entry of connection (see illustration B).	Allows smooth transition from old to new tubing, minimizing time that system is open to infection. Careful technique prevents VAD dislodgement or vein trauma during tubing change and transmission of microorganisms.
(2) *For continuous infusion:* Open roller clamp on new tubing, allowing solution to run rapidly for 30 to 60 seconds, and then regulate drip rate using EID or roller clamp if gravity drip.	Brief rapid flow ensures catheter patency and prevents occlusion. Regulation restores infusion rate to deliver IV fluid as prescribed.

STEP	RATIONALE

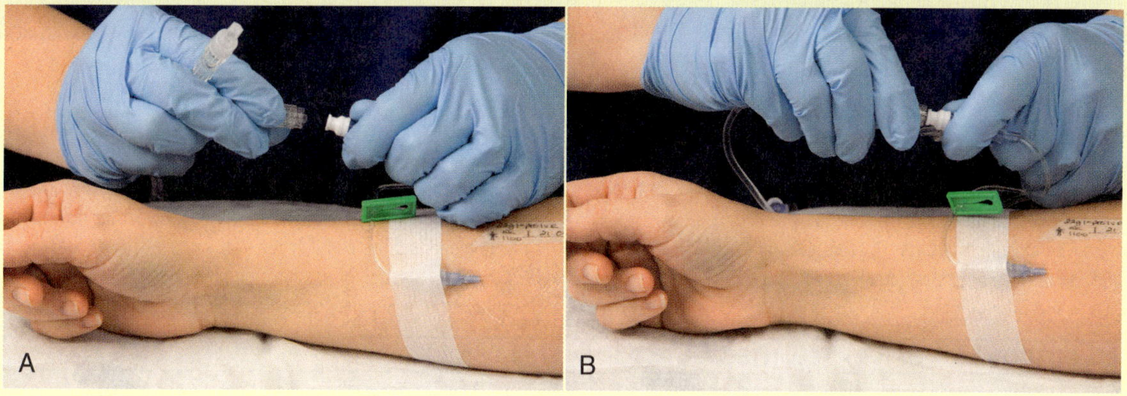

STEP 3f(1) A, Disconnect old intravenous tubing. **B,** Connect Luer-Lok adapter of new intravenous tubing.

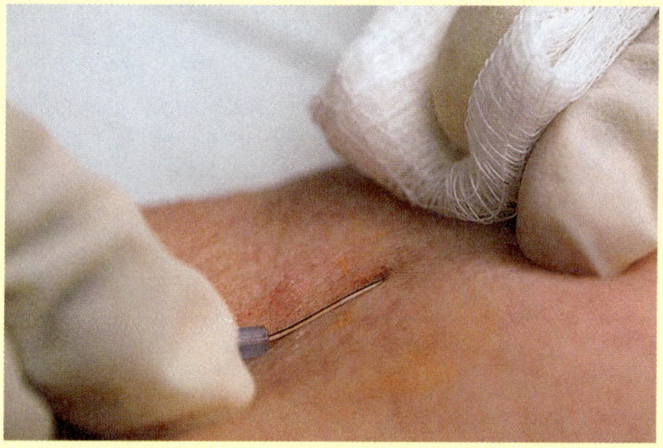

STEP 4e IV catheter is removed slowly, keeping catheter parallel to vein.

STEP	RATIONALE
(3) Attach piece of tape or label with date and time of tubing change onto tubing below drip chamber.	Provides reference to determine next time for tubing change.
(4) Apply new manufactured catheter stabilization device or tape if used. Form loop of tubing and secure it to patient's arm with strip of tape.	Avoids accidental pulling against site and stabilizes catheter.
g. Remove and discard old IV tubing. If necessary, apply new dressing (see Skill 41-4). Remove and dispose of gloves. Perform hand hygiene.	Reduces transmission of microorganisms.
4 Discontinuing peripheral IV access	
a. Perform hand hygiene. Apply clean gloves.	Reduces transmission of microorganisms.
b. Turn off EID and close roller clamp or, if no EID, close roller clamp that controls rate.	Prevents spillage of IV fluid.
c. Remove IV site dressing and manufactured catheter stabilization device (see Skill 41-4). Remove any tape that secures catheter. Do not use scissors.	Exposes catheter with minimal discomfort. Scissors might accidentally damage catheter or injure patient (INS, 2011).
d. Hold catheter hub and clean site with antiseptic swab. Allow to dry completely.	Removes secretions around skin puncture site.
e. Place sterile gauze over venipuncture site and apply light pressure while withdrawing catheter, using slow, steady motion. Keep hub parallel to skin (see illustration). Do not raise or lift catheter before it is completely out of vein. Inspect end of catheter for intactness after removal.	Dry pad causes less irritation to puncture site. Removal technique avoids trauma to vein or hematoma formation. Inspection determines if catheter tip is intact. Tip of catheter can break off and embolize, an emergency situation.
f. Keep gauze in place and apply continuous pressure to site for 2 to 3 minutes and assess bleeding.	Controls bleeding and hematoma formation. Pressure should be applied until hemostasis occurs (INS, 2011).

CLINICAL DECISION: *If patient receives anticoagulants or platelet inhibitors (e.g., low-dose aspirin, warfarin sodium [Coumadin], heparin) or has a low platelet count, apply steady pressure longer (for 5 to 10 minutes) and assess bleeding.*

STEP	RATIONALE
g. Apply sterile folded gauze dressing over insertion site and secure with tape.	Maintains pressure to prevent bleeding and reduces bacterial entry into puncture site.
h. Discard used supplies, remove gloves, and perform hand hygiene.	Reduces transmission of microorganisms.

SKILL 41-3 MAINTENANCE OF INTRAVENOUS SYSTEM—cont'd

STEP	RATIONALE
EVALUATION	
1 *For changing IV fluid container and/or tubing:*	
a. Evaluate IV flow rate hourly; observe connections for leaking and patency of system.	Ensures proper fluid administration.
b. Observe patient for signs of overhydration or dehydration to determine response to therapy and restoration of fluid balance.	Signs and symptoms of overhydration or continued dehydration warrant changing rate of fluid infused. Contact health care provider for new infusion rate order.
2 *For discontinuing peripheral IV access:* Observe site for bleeding soon after procedure and redness, tenderness, drainage, or swelling during a later evaluation.	Detects bleeding after catheter removal. Detects local infection or postinfusion phlebitis (INS, 2011). Postinfusion phlebitis may occur 48 to 96 hours after catheter removal.

UNEXPECTED OUTCOMES AND RELATED INTERVENTIONS

1. Flow rate is incorrect; patient receives too little or too much fluid.
   - Readjust infusion rate to ordered rate.
   - Evaluate patient for adverse effects; notify health care provider if apparent.
   - Determine and correct cause of incorrect flow rate (e.g., positional change that might affect rate, EID malfunction (or poor height of IV container with gravity flow), kinking or obstruction of tubing, infiltration or other complications of VAD site).
   - Notify health care provider if patient's anticipated infusion is 100 to 200 mL less than or greater than expected (check agency policy).
2. Catheter tip is missing after withdrawal.
   - Apply tourniquet high on extremity to restrict mobility of catheter embolus.
   - Immediately notify health care provider.
3. See Table 41-12 for infiltration, phlebitis, and local infection.

RECORDING AND REPORTING

- Record amount and type of fluid infused, amount and type of fluid started, and tubing change on patient's medical record according to agency policy. If using bar-code system, fluid type and time record automatically in an EHR.
- Record time that peripheral IV access was discontinued on patient's record according to agency policy. Include site assessment information and status of catheter, including gauge, length, and catheter tip integrity.

HOME CARE CONSIDERATIONS

- Ensure that patient is able and willing to self-manage IV therapy (including changing IV containers) or that reliable family caregiver is at home to provide IV care.
- Instruct patient or caregiver in procedure for performing an IV solution and tubing change.
- Instruct patient or caregiver to notify health care provider if bleeding or drainage is noted at insertion site or if pain or tenderness occurs up to 4 days after catheter removal.

SKILL 41-4 CHANGING A PERIPHERAL INTRAVENOUS DRESSING

Delegation Considerations

The skill of changing a peripheral intravenous (IV) dressing cannot be delegated to nursing assistive personnel (NAP). Delegation to licensed practical nurses (LPNs) varies by state Nurse Practice Act. Instruct the NAP to inform you if:

- Patient indicates moistness or loosening of an IV dressing.

Equipment

- Antiseptic swabs (chlorhexidine 2% preferred [INS, 2011])
- Adhesive remover *(optional)*
- Skin protectant swab
- Clean gloves
- Strips of nonallergenic tape
- Manufactured catheter stabilization device, if available
- Dressing: Sterile transparent dressing (preferred) or sterile 2 × 2 or 4 × 4 inch gauze pad

STEP	RATIONALE
ASSESSMENT	
1 Determine agency policy regarding peripheral IV dressing changes. Transparent dressings usually remain in place until IV site is changed unless dressing becomes wet, soiled, or loose.	Dressing change increases risk of catheter displacement and is performed only if dressing is compromised.
2 Perform hand hygiene. Observe present dressing for moisture and intactness. Determine whether moisture is from site leakage or external source.	Moisture is a medium for bacterial growth and renders dressing contaminated. Loose dressing increases risk for bacterial contamination of venipuncture site or displacement of vascular access device (VAD).

STEP	RATIONALE
3 Observe IV system for proper functioning or complications. Apply clean gloves if dressing is moist. Palpate VAD site through intact dressing, assessing for pain or burning.	Unexplained decrease in flow rate requires investigating VAD placement and patency. Pain is associated with both phlebitis and infiltration.
4 Assess patient's understanding of need for continued IV infusion.	Determines need for patient teaching.
PLANNING	
1 Identify the patient using two identifiers (e.g., name and birthday or name and account number) according to facility policy. Compare identifiers with information on patient's medication administration record (MAR) or medical record.	Ensures correct patient. Complies with a recommended National Patient Safety Goal (TJC, 2011).
2 Explain procedure and purpose to patient and family. Explain that patient must hold affected extremity still and how long procedure will take.	Decreases anxiety, promotes cooperation, and gives patient time frame around which to plan personal activities.
IMPLEMENTATION	
1 Perform hand hygiene. Collect equipment. Apply clean gloves.	Reduces transmission of microorganisms.
2 Remove transparent dressing by pulling up one corner and pulling dressing laterally while holding catheter hub and tubing with nondominant hand (see illustration). Leave tape or catheter stabilization device that secures IV catheter in place. *For gauze dressing:* Stabilize catheter hub while removing old dressing one layer at a time. Be cautious if catheter tubing becomes tangled between two layers of dressing.	Prevents accidental displacement of VAD.
3 Observe insertion site for signs and symptoms of infiltration, phlebitis (see Tables 41-12 to 41-14), and local infection (inflammation and exudate). Discontinue infusion if complication exists (see Skill 41-3).	Presence of infiltration, phlebitis, or local infection requires removal of VAD and new IV start in other extremity or proximal to previous insertion site if continued therapy is necessary.
4 If IV is infusing properly, gently remove any tape or stabilization device that secures catheter. Stabilize catheter with one hand. Use adhesive remover to clean skin and remove adhesive residue if needed.	Exposes venipuncture site. Stabilization prevents accidental displacement of catheter. Adhesive residue decreases ability of new tape to adhere securely to skin.

CLINICAL DECISION: *Keep one finger stabilizing VAD at all times until dressing is applied. This requires careful advance planning regarding placing and opening supplies and how to work with one hand. If patient is restless or uncooperative, ask another nurse to assist with dressing change.*

STEP	RATIONALE
5 While stabilizing VAD, clean insertion site with antiseptic swab using friction in a horizontal plane and then a vertical plane, followed by a circular motion moving from insertion site outward (see illustration). Allow antiseptic to dry completely.	Mechanical friction in this pattern allows penetration of antiseptic solution into cracks and fissures of epidermal layer of skin.
6 *Optional:* Apply skin protectant solution (e.g., Skin Prep, No Sting Barrier Film) to area where you will apply tape or dressing. Allow to dry.	Coats skin with protective solution to maintain skin integrity, prevents irritation from adhesive, and promotes adherence of dressing.
7 Secure catheter with stabilization device or tape (see Skill 41-1) and apply sterile dressing over site (procedures differ; follow agency policy).	Prevents accidental dislodgement of catheter and protects site from infection.
a. *Transparent dressing:* Apply as directed in Skill 41-1, Step 21b.	Occlusive dressing protects site from bacterial contamination.
b. *Gauze dressing:* Apply as directed in Skill 41-1, Step 21c.	Less frequently used than transparent dressing.

CLINICAL DECISION: *Think carefully about where you place tape. Do not apply it over catheter insertion site, over connection between tubing or port and IV catheter hub, or on top of transparent dressing.*

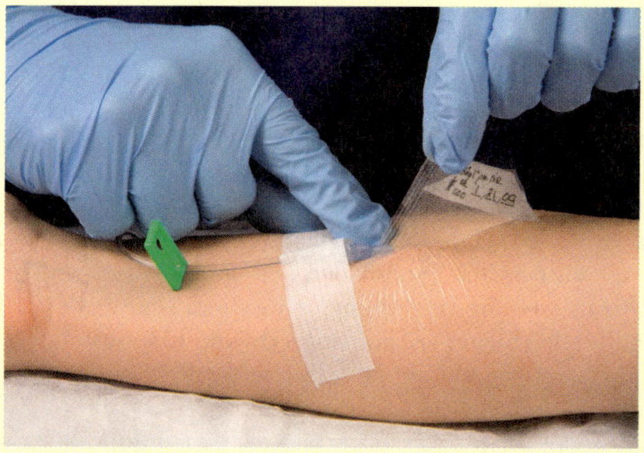

STEP 2 Remove transparent dressing while pulling it laterally.

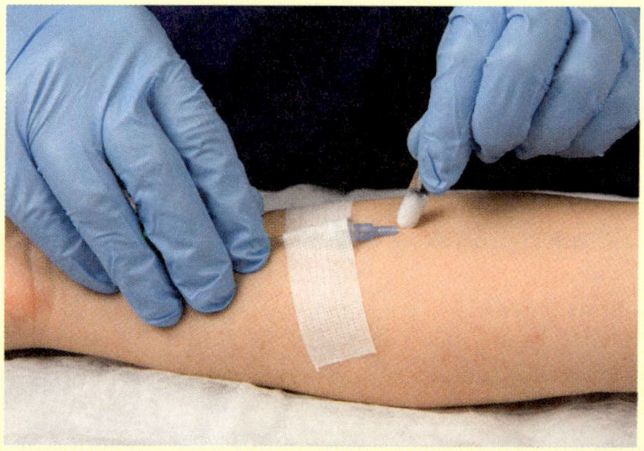

STEP 5 Cleanse peripheral insertion site with antiseptic swab.

SKILL 41-4 CHANGING A PERIPHERAL INTRAVENOUS DRESSING—cont'd

STEP	RATIONALE
8 Remove and discard gloves.	Reduces transmission of microorganisms.
9 *Optional:* Apply protective device over area if patient may pick at or bump dressing (see illustration).	Site protection devices include vented plastic or stretch netting coverings and mitts for hands. Designed to reduce risk of phlebitis, infiltration, or catheter displacement from mechanical motion.

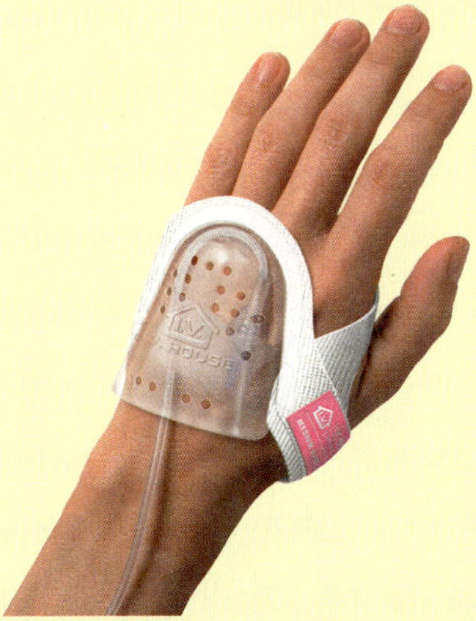

STEP 9 IV House protective device. (Courtesy IV House, St Louis, Mo.)

STEP	RATIONALE
10 Anchor IV tubing with additional pieces of tape if necessary.	Prevents accidental displacement of IV catheter.
11 Label dressing per agency policy. Label information should include date and time of original IV insertion and VAD gauge and length.	Labeling with IV insertion date and VAD length facilitates appropriate site rotation and safe discontinuation of IV access.
12 Discard equipment and perform hand hygiene.	Reduces transmission of microorganisms.
13 Ensure that flow rate is accurate.	Validates that IV line is patent and functioning correctly. Manipulation of catheter and tubing may affect rate of infusion.

UNEXPECTED OUTCOMES AND RELATED INTERVENTIONS

1 VAD is accidentally dislodged or removed.
- Start new IV line in other extremity or proximal to previous insertion site if continued therapy is necessary.

2 IV site develops infiltration, phlebitis, and local infection.
- See Table 41-12.

RECORDING AND REPORTING

- Record time that peripheral dressing was changed, reason for change, type of dressing material used, patency of system, and description of venipuncture site.
- Report to charge nurse or oncoming nursing shift that dressing was changed and any significant information about integrity of system.
- Report any complications to health care provider and document them.

KEY POINTS

- Body fluids containing water, Na^+, and other electrolytes are distributed between ECF and ICF compartments.
- A dynamic interplay of fluid intake and absorption, fluid distribution, and fluid output determines fluid balance.
- Fluid moves between blood vessels and interstitial fluid by filtration; water moves between ECF and ICF by osmosis.
- ECV deficit and excess are abnormal volumes of isotonic fluid, manifested as sudden changes in body weight and changes in markers of vascular and interstitial volume.
- Osmolality imbalances are abnormal concentrations of body fluids, manifested as altered serum Na^+ levels and decreased level of consciousness.
- Interplay of electrolyte intake and absorption, electrolyte distribution, and electrolyte output determines balance of K^+, Ca^{2+}, Mg^{2+}, and phosphate.
- Interplay of acid production, acid buffering, and acid excretion determines acid-base balance.
- Acid-base imbalances are caused by excesses or deficits of carbonic or metabolic acids, manifested as changes in level of consciousness and abnormalities of $PaCO_2$, HCO_3^-, and pH.
- Patients who are very young or very old, whose I&O of fluid and/or electrolytes are not equal, or who have various chronic diseases or trauma are at high risk for fluid, electrolyte, and acid-base imbalances.
- Treatment for ECV excess is Na^+ restriction and fluid restriction if severe; treatment for hyponatremia usually is water restriction.

- Prevention and treatment of ECV deficit, hypernatremia, and electrolyte deficits are accomplished with enteral or parenteral administration of appropriate fluid.
- Initiation and maintenance of IV therapy require clinical decision making, skill, and organized procedures to maintain sterility and patency of the system.
- Good IV practice requires periodic updating of procedures based on current research evidence.
- Nurses monitor vigilantly for complications of IV therapy, which include fluid overload, infiltration, phlebitis, local infection, and bleeding at the infusion site.
- Administration of blood or blood products requires a specific procedure for correctly identifying patient and blood product and responding to transfusion reactions quickly.
- Patient and family teaching is important for preventing fluid, electrolyte, and acid-base imbalances and effective restorative care.

CLINICAL APPLICATION QUESTIONS

Preparing for Clinical Practice

Mrs. Hilda Beck is a 72-year-old seen by her health care provider this morning after falling at home because she became light-headed after vomiting and having diarrhea that has lasted over 24 hours. She was admitted for oral and intravenous (IV) fluid therapy.

1. Why is Mrs. Beck likely becoming light-headed? When should you expect this to resolve?
2. Mrs. Beck's IV fluid order is 1000 mL 0.9% sodium chloride to run over 8 hours. Calculate the milliliters per hour that you should program into her infusion pump.
3. You auscultate crackles in Mrs. Beck's lung bases while her IV is infusing. What is your next action?

evolve *Answers to Clinical Application Questions can be found on the Evolve website.*

REVIEW QUESTIONS

Are You Ready to Test Your Nursing Knowledge?

1. A patient who is comatose is admitted to the hospital with an unknown history. Respirations are deep and rapid. Arterial blood gas levels on admission are pH, 7.20; $PaCO_2$, 21 mm Hg; PaO_2, 92 mm Hg; and HCO_3^-, 8. You interpret these laboratory values to indicate:
   1. Metabolic acidosis
   2. Metabolic alkalosis
   3. Respiratory acidosis
   4. Respiratory alkalosis
2. A patient with a cardiac history is taking the diuretic furosemide (Lasix) and is seen in the emergency department for muscle weakness. Which laboratory value do you assess first?
   1. Serum albumin
   2. Serum sodium
   3. Hematocrit
   4. Serum potassium
3. Which of these patients do you expect will need teaching regarding dietary sodium restriction?
   1. An 88-year-old with a fractured femur scheduled for surgery
   2. A 65-year-old recently diagnosed with heart failure
   3. A 50-year-old recently diagnosed with asthma and diabetes
   4. A 20-year-old with vomiting and diarrhea from gastroenteritis
4. You teach patients to replace sweat, vomiting, or diarrhea fluid losses with which type of fluid?
   1. Tap water or bottled water
   2. Fluid that has sodium (salt) in it
   3. Fluid that has K^+ and HCO_3^- in it
   4. Coffee or tea, whichever they prefer
5. You assess four patients. Which patient is at greatest risk for the development of hypocalcemia?
   1. 56-year-old with acute kidney renal failure
   2. 40-year-old with appendicitis
   3. 28-year-old who has acute pancreatitis
   4. 65-year-old with hypertension and asthma
6. Which of the following activities can you delegate to nursing assistive personnel (NAP)? (Select all that apply.)
   1. Measuring oral intake and urine output
   2. Preparing intravenous (IV) tubing for routine change
   3. Reporting an IV container that is low in fluid
   4. Changing an IV fluid container
7. Place the following steps for intravenous (IV) catheter insertion in the correct order:
   1. Perform hand hygiene.
   2. Open and prepare infusion set.
   3. Select appropriate vein and insert catheter.
   4. Use two identifiers to ensure correct patient.
   5. Assess for risk factors such as age or platelet count.
   6. Carefully check the health care provider's order for the IV therapy.
8. Assessment findings consistent with intravenous (IV) fluid infiltration include: (Select all that apply.)
   1. Edema and pain
   2. Streak formation
   3. Pain and erythema
   4. Pallor and coolness
   5. Numbness and pain
9. Which of the following defining characteristics is consistent with *fluid volume deficit?*
   1. A 1-lb (0.5 kg) weight loss, pale yellow urine
   2. Engorged neck veins when upright, bradycardia
   3. Dry mucous membranes, thready pulse, tachycardia
   4. Bounding radial pulse, flat neck veins when supine
10. Which of the following assessments do you perform routinely when an older adult patient is receiving intravenous 0.9% NaCl?
    1. Auscultate dependent portions of lungs
    2. Check color of urine
    3. Assess muscle strength
    4. Check skin turgor over sternum or shin
11. While receiving a blood transfusion, your patient develops chills, tachycardia, and flushing. What is your priority action?
    1. Notify a health care provider
    2. Insert an indwelling catheter
    3. Alert the blood bank
    4. Stop the transfusion
12. The health care provider's order is 1000 mL 0.9% NaCl with 20 mEq K^+ intravenously over 8 hours. Which assessment finding causes you to clarify the order with the health care provider before hanging this fluid?
    1. Flat neck veins
    2. Tachycardia
    3. Hypotension
    4. Oliguria
13. Your patient who has diabetic ketoacidosis is breathing rapidly and deeply. Intravenous (IV) fluids and other treatments have

just been started. What should you do about this patient's breathing?
1. Notify her health care provider that she is hyperventilating
2. Provide frequent oral care to keep her mucous membranes moist
3. Ask her to breathe slower and help her to calm down and relax
4. Assess her for pain and request an order for a sedative

14. Your patient had 200 mL of ice chips and 900 mL intravenous (IV) fluid during your shift. Which total intake should you record?
1. 700 mL
2. 900 mL
3. 1000 mL
4. 1100 mL

15. The health care provider's order is 1000 mL 0.9% NaCl IV over 6 hours. Which rate do you program into the infusion pump?
1. 125 mL/hr
2. 167 mL/hr
3. 200 mL/hr
4. 1000 mL/hr

Answers: 1. 1; 2. 4; 3. 2; 4. 2; 5. 3; 6. 1, 3; 7. 6, 5, 4, 1, 2, 3; 8. 1, 4; 9. 3; 10. 1; 11. 4; 12. 4; 13. 2; 14. 3; 15. 2.

REFERENCES

Bryant H: Dehydration in older people: assessment and management, *Emerg Nurs* 15(4):22, 2007.

Caon M: Osmoles, osmolality and osmotic pressure: clarifying the puzzle of solution concentration, *Contemp Nurs* 29(1):92, 2008.

Centers for Disease Control and Prevention (CDC): Guidelines for the prevention of intravascular catheter-related infections, *MMWR Morb Mortal Wkly Rep* 51(RR-10), 2002.

Centers for Disease Control and Prevention (CDC): HIV transmission through transfusion—Missouri and Colorado, 2008, *MMWR Morb Mortal Wkly Rep* 59(41), 2010.

Coggon JM: Arterial blood gas analysis 1: understanding ABG reports, *Nurs Times* 104(18):18, 2008a.

Coggon JM: Arterial blood gas analysis 2: compensatory mechanisms, *Nurs Times* 104(19):24, 2008b.

Copstead LC, Banasik JL: *Pathophysiology online for pathophysiology*, ed 4, St Louis, 2010, Mosby.

Cronenwett L, et al: Quality and safety education for nurses, *Nurs Outlook* 55(3):122, 2007.

David K: IV fluids: do you know what's hanging and why? *RN* 70(10):35, 2007.

Doellman D, et al: Infiltration and extravasation: update on prevention and management, *J Infus Nurs* 32(4):203, 2009.

Fabian B: Infusion therapy in the older adult. In Alexander M, et al, editors: *Infusion nursing an evidence-based approach*, ed 3, St Louis, 2010, Saunders.

Felver L: Acid-base homeostasis and imbalances. In Copstead LC, Banasik JL, editors: *Pathophysiology*, ed 4, St. Louis, 2010a, Saunders.

Felver L: Fluid and electrolyte homeostasis and imbalances. In Copstead LC, Banasik JL, editors: *Pathophysiology*, ed 4, St Louis, 2010b, Saunders.

Giger JN, Davidhizar RE: *Transcultural nursing: assessment and intervention*, ed 4, St Louis, 2008, Mosby.

Goldstein MB, et al: *Fluid, electrolyte and acid-base physiology: a problem-based approach*, ed 4, St Louis, 2010, Saunders.

Hadaway L: Infiltration and extravasation: preventing a complication of IV catheterization, *Am J Nurs* 107(8):64, 2007.

Hadaway L, Richardson D: Needleless connectors: a primer on terminology, *J Infus Nurs* 33(1):22, 2010.

Hall JE: *Guyton and Hall textbook of medical physiology*, ed 12, Philadelphia, 2011, Saunders.

Hockenberry MJ, Wilson D: *Wong's nursing care of infants and children*, ed 9, St Louis, 2011, Mosby.

Infusion Nurses Society (INS): Infusion nursing standards of practice, *J Infus Nurs* 34(1S):S1, 2011.

Johnson A: Psychobiology of thirst and salt appetite, *Med Sci Sports Exercise* 39(8):1388, 2007.

Koeppen BM, Stanton BA: *Berne & Levy physiology*, ed 6, St Louis, 2008, Mosby.

Kramer BJ, Raymond MK: Arterial blood gases, *RN* 72(4):22, 2009.

Lehne RA: *Pharmacology for nursing care*, ed 7, Philadelphia, 2010, Saunders.

Meiner SE: *Gerontologic nursing*, ed 4, St Louis, 2011, Mosby.

Metheny NM: *Fluids and electrolytes balance: nursing applications*, ed 5, Sudbury, Mass, 2010, Jones & Bartlett Learning.

Monahan F, et al: *Phipps' medical-surgical nursing: health and illness perspectives*, ed 8, St Louis, 2007, Mosby.

National Quality Forum (NQF): *National Voluntary Consensus Standards for Public Reporting of Patient Safety Event Information: a consensus report*, Washington, DC, 2010, NQF.

Occupational Safety and Health Administration [OSHA]: *Bloodborne pathogen and needlestick prevention*, United States Department of Labor, last updated July 11, 2011, http://www.osha.gov/SLTC/bloodbornepathogens/index.html. Accessed October 9, 2011.

Perucca R: Peripheral venous access devices. In Alexander M, et al, editors: *Infusion nursing an evidence-based approach*, ed 3, St Louis, 2010, Saunders.

Rose BD: *Clinical physiology of acid-base disorders*, ed 6, New York, 2011, McGraw-Hill.

Scales K, Pilsworth J: The importance of fluid balance in clinical practice, *Nurs Standard* 22(4):50, 2008.

The Joint Commission (TJC): *2011 National patient safety goals (NPGs)*, 2011, TJC; http://jointcommission.org/standards_information/npsgs.aspx. Last accessed October 10, 2011.

Trick NL: Blood component therapy. In Alexander M, et al, editors: *Infusion nursing an evidence-based approach*, ed 3, St Louis, 2010, Saunders.

Wotton K, Crannitch K, Munt R: Prevalence, risk factors and strategies to prevent dehydration in older adults, *Contemp Nurs* 31(1):44, 2008.

RESEARCH REFERENCES

Anderson S, et al: Administration of local anesthetic agents to decrease pain associated with peripheral vascular access, *J Infus Nurs* 33(6):353, 2010.

Chaudry SI, et al: Patterns of weight change preceding hospitalization for heart failure, *Circulation* 116(14):1549, 2007.

Harnage SA: Achieving zero catheter related bloodstream infections: 15 months success in a community based medical center. *J Assoc Vasc Access* 12(4):218, 2007.

Hertzel C, Sousa VD: The use of smart pumps for preventing medication errors, *J Infus Nurs* 32(5):257, 2009.

McConnell JS, et al: "About a cupful"—a prospective study into accuracy of volume estimation by medical and nursing staff, *Accident Emerg Nurs* 15(2):101, 2007.

Mok E, Kwong TK, Chan MF: A randomized controlled trial for maintaining peripheral intravenous lock in children, *Int J Nurs Pract* 13(1):33, 2007.

O'Halloran L, El-Masri MM, Fox-Wasylyshyn SM: Home intravenous therapy and the ability to perform self-care activities of daily living, *J Infus Nurs* 31(6):367, 2008.

Poon EG, et al: Effect of bar-code technology on the safety of medication administration, *New Engl J Med* 362(18):1698, 2010.

Powell J, Tarnow KG, Perucca R: The relationship between peripheral intravenous catheter indwell time and the incidence of phlebitis, *J Infus Nurs* 31(1):39, 2008.

Roszell S, Jones C: Intravenous administration issues: a comparison of intravenous insertions and complications in vancomycin versus other antibiotics, *J Infus Nurs* 33(2):112, 2010.

Schears GJ: Summary of product trials for 10,164 patients: comparing an intravenous stabilizing device to tape, *J Infus Nurs* 29(4):225, 2006.

Smith B: Peripheral intravenous catheter dwell times: a comparison of three securement methods for implementation of a 96-hour scheduled change protocol, *J Infus Nurs* 29(1):17, 2006.

Webster J, et al: Clinically indicated replacement versus routine replacement of peripheral venous catheters, *Cochrane Database Syst Rev* 3:CD007798, 2010.

CHAPTER 42

Sleep

OBJECTIVES

- Explain the effect that the 24-hour sleep-wake cycle has on biological function.
- Discuss mechanisms that regulate sleep.
- Describe the stages of a normal sleep cycle.
- Explain the functions of sleep.
- Compare and contrast the sleep requirements of different age-groups.
- Identify factors that normally promote and disrupt sleep.
- Discuss characteristics of common sleep disorders.
- Conduct a sleep history for a patient.
- Identify nursing diagnoses appropriate for patients with sleep alterations.
- Identify nursing interventions designed to promote normal sleep cycles for patients of all ages.
- Describe ways to evaluate sleep therapies.

KEY TERMS

Biological clocks, p. 940
Cataplexy, p. 944
Circadian rhythm, p. 939
Excessive daytime sleepiness (EDS), p. 943
Hypersomnolence, p. 942
Hypnotics, p. 957
Insomnia, p. 942
Narcolepsy, p. 944
Nocturia, p. 942
Nonrapid eye movement (NREM) sleep, p. 940
Polysomnogram, p. 942
Rapid eye movement (REM) sleep, p. 940
Rest, p. 944
Sedatives, p. 957
Sleep, p. 939
Sleep apnea, p. 943
Sleep deprivation, p. 944
Sleep hygiene, p. 942

evolve WEBSITE

http://evolve.elsevier.com/Potter/fundamentals/

- Review Questions
- Concept Map Creator
- Case Study with Questions
- Audio Glossary
- Interactive Learning Activities
- Key Term Flashcards
- Content Updates

Proper rest and sleep are as important to health as good nutrition and adequate exercise. Physical and emotional health depends on the ability to fulfill these basic human needs. Individuals need different amounts of sleep and rest. Without proper amounts, the ability to concentrate, make judgments, and participate in daily activities decreases; and irritability increases.

Identifying and treating patients' sleep pattern disturbances are important goals. To help patients you need to understand the nature of sleep, the factors influencing it, and patients' sleep habits. Patients require individualized approaches based on their personal habits, patterns of sleep, and the particular problem influencing sleep. Nursing interventions are often effective in resolving short- and long-term sleep disturbances.

Sleep provides healing and restoration (McCance et al., 2010). Achieving the best possible sleep quality is important for the promotion of good health and recovery from illness. Ill patients often require more sleep and rest than healthy patients. However, the nature of illness often prevents some patients from getting adequate rest and sleep. The environment of a hospital or long-term care facility and the activities of health care personnel make sleep difficult. Some patients have preexisting sleep disturbances; other patients develop sleep problems as a result of illness or hospitalization.

SCIENTIFIC KNOWLEDGE BASE

Physiology of Sleep

Sleep is a cyclical physiological process that alternates with longer periods of wakefulness. The sleep-wake cycle influences and regulates physiological function and behavioral responses.

Circadian Rhythms. People experience cyclical rhythms as part of their everyday lives. The most familiar rhythm is the 24-hour, day-night cycle known as the diurnal or **circadian rhythm** (derived from Latin: *circa,* "about," and *dies,* "day"). The suprachiasmatic nucleus (SCN) nerve cells in the hypothalamus control the rhythm of the sleep-wake cycle and coordinate this cycle with other circadian rhythms (McCance et al., 2010). Circadian rhythms influence the pattern of major biological and behavioral functions. The predictable changing of body temperature, heart rate, blood pressure, hormone secretion, sensory acuity, and mood depend on the maintenance of the 24-hour circadian cycle (Van der Zee et al., 2009).

Factors such as light, temperature, social activities, and work routines affect circadian rhythms and daily sleep-wake cycles. All

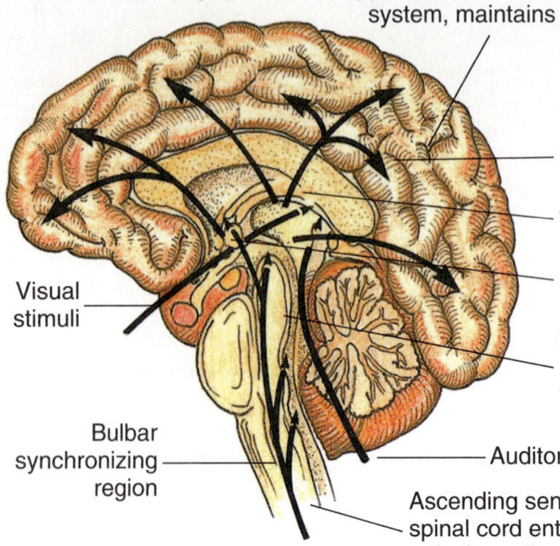

FIG. 42-1 Reticular activating system (RAS) and bulbar synchronizing region (BSR) control sensory input, intermittently activating and suppressing the higher centers of the brain to control sleep and wakefulness.

persons have **biological clocks** that synchronize their sleep cycles. This explains why some people fall asleep at 8 PM, whereas others go to bed at midnight or early in the morning. Different people also function best at different times of the day.

Hospitals or extended care facilities usually do not adapt care to an individual's sleep-wake cycle preferences. Typical hospital routines interrupt sleep or prevent patients from falling asleep at their usual time. Poor quality of sleep results when a person's sleep-wake cycle changes. Reversals in the sleep-wake cycle, such as when a person who is normally awake during the day falls asleep during the day, often indicate a serious illness.

The biological rhythm of sleep frequently becomes synchronized with other body functions. For example, changes in body temperature correlate with sleep patterns. Normally body temperature peaks in the afternoon, decreases gradually, and then drops sharply after a person falls asleep. When the sleep-wake cycle becomes disrupted (e.g., by working rotating shifts), other physiological functions usually change as well. For example, a new nurse who starts working the night shift experiences a decreased appetite and loses weight. Anxiety, restlessness, irritability, and impaired judgment are other common symptoms of sleep cycle disturbances. Failure to maintain an individual's usual sleep-wake cycle negatively influences the patient's overall health.

Sleep Regulation. Sleep involves a sequence of physiological states maintained by highly integrated central nervous system (CNS) activity. It is associated with changes in the peripheral nervous, endocrine, cardiovascular, respiratory, and muscular systems (McCance et al., 2010). Specific physiological responses and patterns of brain activity identify each sequence. Instruments such as the electroencephalogram (EEG), which measures electrical activity in the cerebral cortex; the electromyogram (EMG), which measures muscle tone; and the electrooculogram (EOG), which measures eye movements provide information about some structural physiological aspects of sleep.

The major sleep center in the body is the hypothalamus. It secretes hypocreatins (orexins) that promote wakefulness and rapid eye movement sleep. Prostaglandin D_2, L-tryptophan, and growth factors control sleep (McCance et al., 2010).

Researchers believe that the ascending reticular activating system (RAS) located in the upper brainstem contains special cells that maintain alertness and wakefulness. The RAS receives visual, auditory, pain, and tactile sensory stimuli. Activity from the cerebral cortex (e.g., emotions or thought processes) also stimulates the RAS. Arousal, wakefulness, and maintenance of consciousness result from neurons in the RAS releasing catecholamines such as norepinephrine (Izac, 2006).

Researchers hypothesize that the release of serotonin from specialized cells in the raphe nuclei sleep system of the pons and medulla produces sleep. This area of the brain is also called the *bulbar synchronizing region (BSR)*. Whether a person remains awake or falls asleep depends on a balance of impulses received from higher centers (e.g., thoughts), peripheral sensory receptors (e.g., sound or light stimuli), and the limbic system (emotions) (Fig. 42-1). As people try to fall asleep, they close their eyes and assume relaxed positions. Stimuli to the RAS decline. If the room is dark and quiet, activation of the RAS further declines. At some point the BSR takes over, causing sleep.

Stages of Sleep. Current theory suggests that sleep is an active multiphase process. Different brain-wave, muscle, and eye activity is associated with different stages of sleep (Izac, 2006). Normal sleep involves two phases: **nonrapid eye movement (NREM) sleep** and **rapid eye movement (REM) sleep** (Box 42-1). During NREM a sleeper progresses through four stages during a typical 90-minute sleep cycle. The quality of sleep from stage 1 through stage 4 becomes increasingly deep. Lighter sleep is characteristic of stages 1 and 2, during which a person is more easily aroused. Stages 3 and 4 involve a deeper sleep, called *slow-wave sleep*. REM sleep is the phase at the end of each sleep cycle. Different factors promote or interfere with various stages of the sleep cycle.

Sleep Cycle. The normal sleep pattern for an adult begins with a presleep period during which the person is aware only of a gradually developing sleepiness. This period normally lasts 10 to 30 minutes; however, if a person has difficulty falling asleep, it lasts an hour or more.

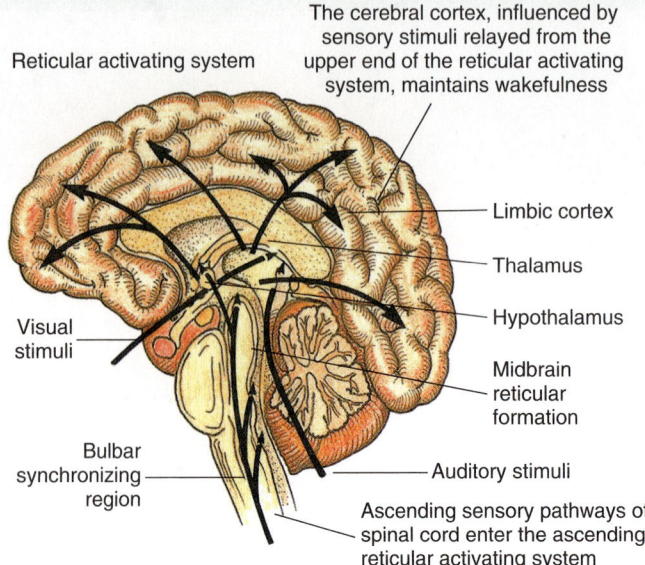

Once asleep, the person usually passes through four or five complete sleep cycles per night, each consisting of four stages of

BOX 42-1 STAGES OF THE SLEEP CYCLE

Stage 1: NREM

- Stage lasts a few minutes.
- It includes lightest level of sleep.
- Decreased physiological activity begins with gradual fall in vital signs and metabolism.
- Sensory stimuli such as noise easily arouses person.
- Awakened, person feels as though daydreaming has occurred.

Stage 2: NREM

- Stage lasts 10 to 20 minutes.
- It is a period of sound sleep.
- Relaxation progresses.
- Body functions continue to slow.
- Arousal remains relatively easy.

Stage 3: NREM

- Stage lasts 15 to 30 minutes.
- It involves initial stages of deep sleep.
- Muscles are completely relaxed.
- Vital signs decline but remain regular.
- Sleeper is difficult to arouse and rarely moves.

Stage 4: NREM

- Stage lasts approximately 15 to 30 minutes.
- It is the deepest stage of sleep.
- If sleep loss has occurred, sleeper spends considerable portion of night in this stage.
- Vital signs are significantly lower than during waking hours.
- Sleepwalking and enuresis (bed-wetting) sometimes occur.
- It is very difficult to arouse sleeper.

REM Sleep

- Stage usually begins about 90 minutes after sleep has begun.
- Duration increases with each sleep cycle and averages 20 minutes.
- Vivid, full-color dreaming occurs; less vivid dreaming occurs in other stages.
- Stage is typified by rapidly moving eyes, fluctuating heart and respiratory rates, increased or fluctuating blood pressure, loss of skeletal muscle tone, and increase of gastric secretions.
- It is very difficult to arouse sleeper.

NREM, Nonrapid eye movement; *REM,* rapid eye movement.

NREM sleep and a period of REM sleep (McCance et al., 2010). Each cycle lasts approximately 90 to 100 minutes. The cyclical pattern usually progresses from stage 1 through stage 4 of NREM, followed by a reversal from stages 4 to 3 to 2, ending with a period of REM sleep (Fig. 42-2). A person usually reaches REM sleep about 90 minutes into the sleep cycle. Seventy-five to eighty percent of sleep time is spent in NREM sleep.

With each successive cycle stages 3 and 4 shorten, and the period of REM lengthens. REM sleep lasts up to 60 minutes during the last sleep cycle. Not all people progress consistently through the stages of sleep. For example, a sleeper moves back and forth for short intervals between NREM stages 2, 3, and 4 before entering REM stage. The amount of time spent in each stage varies over the life span. Newborns and children spend more time in deep sleep. Sleep becomes more fragmented with aging, and a person spends more time in lighter stages (National Sleep Foundation, 2009). Shifts from stage to stage of sleep tend to accompany body movements. Shifts to light sleep or wakefulness tend to occur suddenly,

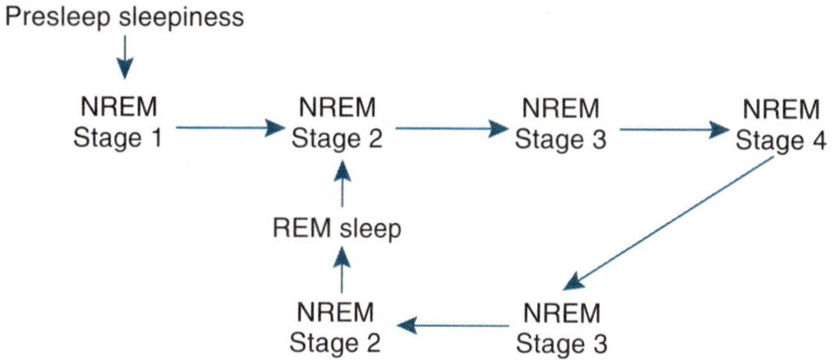

FIG. 42-2 Stages of adult sleep cycle.

whereas shifts to deep sleep tend to be gradual (Izac, 2006). The number of sleep cycles depends on the total amount of time that the person spends sleeping.

Functions of Sleep

The purpose of sleep remains unclear. It contributes to physiological and psychological restoration. NREM sleep contributes to body tissue restoration (McCance et al., 2010). During NREM sleep biological functions slow. A healthy adult's normal heart rate throughout the day averages 70 to 80 beats/min or less if the individual is in excellent physical condition. However, during sleep the heart rate falls to 60 beats/min or less, which benefits cardiac function. Other biological functions decreased during sleep are respirations, blood pressure, and muscle tone (McCance et al., 2010).

The body needs sleep to routinely restore biological processes. During deep slow-wave (NREM stage 4) sleep, the body releases human growth hormone for the repair and renewal of epithelial and specialized cells such as brain cells (McCance et al., 2010). Protein synthesis and cell division for renewal of tissues such as the skin, bone marrow, gastric mucosa, or brain occur during rest and sleep. NREM sleep is especially important in children, who experience more stage 4 sleep.

Another theory about the purpose of sleep is that the body conserves energy during sleep. The skeletal muscles relax progressively, and the absence of muscular contraction preserves chemical energy for cellular processes. Lowering of the basal metabolic rate further conserves body energy supply (Izac, 2006).

REM sleep is necessary for brain tissue restoration and appears to be important for cognitive restoration. It is associated with changes in cerebral blood flow, increased cortical activity, increased oxygen consumption, and epinephrine release. This association assists with memory storage and learning (McCance et al., 2010).

The benefits of sleep on behavior often go unnoticed until a person develops a problem resulting from sleep deprivation. A loss of REM sleep leads to feelings of confusion and suspicion. Various body functions (e.g., mood, motor performance, memory, and equilibrium) are altered when prolonged sleep loss occurs (National Sleep Foundation, 2010a). Changes in the natural and cellular immune function also occur with moderate-to-severe sleep deprivation. Traffic, home, and work-related accidents caused by falling asleep cost billions of dollars a year in the United States because of lost productivity, health care costs, and accidents (Irwin et al., 2006).

Dreams. Although dreams occur during both NREM and REM sleep, the dreams of REM sleep are more vivid and elaborate; and some believe that they are functionally important to learning, memory processing, and adaptation to stress (Kryger et al., 2011). REM dreams progress in content throughout the night from dreams about current events to emotional dreams of childhood or the past. Personality influences the quality of dreams (e.g., a creative person has elaborate and complex dreams, whereas a depressed person dreams of helplessness).

Most people dream about immediate concerns such as an argument with a spouse or worries over work. Sometimes a person is unaware of fears represented in bizarre dreams. Clinical psychologists try to analyze the symbolic nature of dreams as part of a patient's psychotherapy. The ability to describe a dream and interpret its significance sometimes helps resolve personal concerns or fears.

Another theory suggests that dreams erase certain fantasies or nonsensical memories. Because most people forget their dreams, few have dream recall or do not believe they dream at all. To remember a dream, a person has to consciously think about it on awakening. People who recall dreams vividly usually awake just after a period of REM sleep.

Physical Illness

Any illness that causes pain, physical discomfort, or mood problems such as anxiety or depression often results in sleep problems. People with such alterations frequently have trouble falling or staying asleep. Illnesses also force patients to sleep in unfamiliar positions. For example, it is difficult for a patient with an arm or leg in traction to rest comfortably.

Respiratory disease often interferes with sleep. Patients with chronic lung disease such as emphysema are short of breath and frequently cannot sleep without two or three pillows to raise their heads. Asthma, bronchitis, and allergic rhinitis alter the rhythm of breathing and disturb sleep. A person with a common cold has nasal congestion, sinus drainage, and a sore throat, which impair breathing and the ability to relax.

Connections between heart disease, sleep, and sleep disorders exist (Redeker, 2008). Sleep-related breathing disorders are linked to increased incidence of nocturnal angina (chest pain), increased heart rate, electrocardiogram changes, high blood pressure, and risk of heart diseases and stroke (McCance et al., 2010). Hypertension often causes early-morning awakening and fatigue. Hypothyroidism decreases stage 4 sleep, whereas hyperthyroidism causes persons to take more time to fall asleep. Research also identifies an increased risk of sudden cardiac death in the first hours after awakening.

Nocturia, or urination during the night, disrupts sleep and the sleep cycle. After repeated awakenings to urinate, returning to sleep is difficult, and the sleep cycle is not complete. This condition is most common in older people with reduced bladder tone or people with cardiac disease, diabetes, urethritis, or prostatic disease.

Many people experience restless legs syndrome (RLS), which occurs before sleep onset. More common in women, older people, and those with iron deficiency anemia, RLS symptoms include recurrent, rhythmical movements of the feet and legs. Patients feel an itching sensation deep in the muscles. Relief comes only from moving the legs, which prevents relaxation and subsequent sleep. RLS is sometimes a relatively benign condition, depending on how severely sleep is disrupted. Primary RLS is a CNS disorder. Researchers associate secondary RLS with lower levels of iron, pregnancy, and renal failure (Natarajan, 2010).

People with peptic ulcer disease often awaken in the middle of the night. Studies showing a relationship between gastric acid secretion and stages of sleep are conflicting. One consistent finding is that people with duodenal ulcers fail to suppress acid secretion in the first 2 hours of sleep (Kryger et al., 2011).

Sleep Disorders

Sleep disorders are conditions that, if untreated, generally cause disturbed nighttime sleep that results in one of three problems: insomnia, abnormal movements or sensation during sleep or when awakening at night, or excessive daytime sleepiness (Kryger et al., 2011). Many adults in the United States have significant sleep problems from inadequacies in either the quantity or quality of their nighttime sleep and experience **hypersomnolence** on a daily basis (National Sleep Foundation, 2010a). The American Academy of Sleep Medicine developed the International Classification of Sleep Disorders version 2 (ICSD-2), which classifies sleep disorders into eight major categories (Box 42-2).

The insomnias are disorders related to difficulty falling asleep. Individuals with sleep-related breathing disorders have disordered respirations during sleep. Hypersomnia not caused by sleep-related breathing disorders is a group of disorders that is not caused by disturbed circadian rhythms or nocturnal sleep. The circadian rhythm sleep disorders are caused by a misalignment between the timing of sleep and individual desires or the societal norm. The parasomnias are undesirable behaviors that occur usually during sleep. Sleep and wake disturbances are associated with many medical and psychiatric sleep disorders, including psychiatric, neurological, or other medical disorders. In sleep-related movement disorders the person experiences simple stereotyped movements that disturb sleep. The category of isolated symptoms, apparently normal variants, and unresolved issues includes sleep-related symptoms that fall between normal and abnormal sleep. The other sleep disorders category contains sleep problems that do not fit into other categories.

Sleep laboratory studies diagnose a sleep disorder. A **polysomnogram** involves the use of EEG, EMG, and EOG to monitor stages of sleep and wakefulness during nighttime sleep. The Multiple Sleep Latency Test (MSLT) provides objective information about sleepiness and selected aspects of sleep structure by measuring eye movements, muscle-tone changes, and brain electrical activity during at least four napping opportunities spread throughout the day. The MSLT takes 8 to 10 hours to complete. Patients wear an Actigraph device on the wrist to measure sleep-wake patterns over an extended period of time. Actigraphy data provide information about sleep time, sleep efficiency, number and duration of awakenings, and levels of activity and rest (Natale et al., 2009).

Insomnia. **Insomnia** is a symptom that patients experience when they have chronic difficulty falling asleep, frequent awakenings from sleep, and/or a short sleep or nonrestorative sleep (Kryger et al., 2011). It is the most common sleep-related complaint. People with insomnia experience excessive daytime sleepiness and insufficient sleep quantity and quality. However, frequently a patient gets more sleep than he or she realizes. Insomnia often signals an underlying physical or psychological disorder. It occurs more frequently in and is the most common sleep problem for women.

People experience transient insomnia as a result of situational stresses such as family, work, or school problems; jet lag; illness; or loss of a loved one. Insomnia sometimes recurs, but between episodes a patient is able to sleep well. However, a temporary case of insomnia caused by a stressful situation can lead to chronic difficulty in getting enough sleep, perhaps because of the worry and anxiety that develop about getting it.

Insomnia is often associated with poor **sleep hygiene,** or practices that a patient associates with sleep. If the condition continues, the fear of not being able to sleep is enough to cause wakefulness. During the day people with chronic insomnia feel sleepy, fatigued, depressed, and anxious. Treatment is symptomatic, including

BOX 42-2 CLASSIFICATION OF SELECT SLEEP DISORDERS

Insomnias
- Adjustment sleep disorder (acute insomnia)
- Inadequate sleep hygiene
- Behavioral insomnia of childhood
- Insomnia caused by medical condition

Sleep-Related Breathing Disorder
Central Sleep Apnea Syndromes
- Primary central sleep apnea
- Central sleep apnea caused by medical condition
- Obstructive sleep apnea syndromes

Hypersomnias Not Caused by a Sleep-Related Breathing Disorder
- Narcolepsy (four specified types)
- Menstrual-related hypersomnia
- Hypersomnia caused by a medical condition

Parasomnias
Disorders of Arousal
- Sleepwalking
- Sleep terrors

Parasomnias Usually Associated with REM Sleep
- Nightmare disorder
- REM sleep behavior disorder

Other Parasomnias
- Sleep-related hallucinations
- Sleep-related eating disorder
- Sleep-related enuresis (bed-wetting)

Circadian Rhythm Sleep Disorders
Primary Circadian Rhythm Sleep Disorders
- Delayed sleep phase type
- Advanced sleep phase type

Behaviorally Induced Circadian Rhythm Sleep Disorders
- Jet lag type
- Shift work type
- Drug or substance use

Sleep-Related Movement Disorders
- Restless legs syndrome
- Periodic limb movements
- Sleep-related bruxism (teeth grinding)

Isolated Symptoms, Apparently Normal Variants, and Unresolved Issues
- Long sleeper
- Short sleeper
- Sleep talking

Other Sleep Disorders
- Physiological (organic) sleep disorders
- Environmental sleep disorder

Data from American Academy of Sleep Medicine: International classes of diseases and international classification of sleep disorders. In Kryger HM et al: *Principles and practice of sleep medicine,* ed 5, St Louis, 2011, Saunders. *REM,* Rapid eye movement.

improved sleep hygiene measures, biofeedback, cognitive techniques, and relaxation techniques. Behavioral and cognitive therapies have few adverse effects and show evidence of sustained improvement in sleep over time (Babson et al., 2010).

Sleep Apnea. Sleep apnea is a disorder characterized by the lack of airflow through the nose and mouth for periods of 10 seconds or longer during sleep. There are three types of sleep apnea: central, obstructive, and mixed apnea. The most common form is obstructive sleep apnea (OSA). Research estimates that 2% to 4% of the adults in the United States meet the diagnostic criteria for OSA (Adult Obstructive Sleep Apnea Task Force, 2009). The two major risk factors for OSA are obesity and hypertension (Sheldon et al., 2009). Smoking, heart failure, type II diabetes, alcohol, and a positive family history of OSA also greatly increase the risk of developing the problem (Adult Obstructive Sleep Apnea Task Force, 2009). It occurs in up to 2% of middle-age women and up to 4% of middle-age men, with occurrence higher in the older-adult population and African Americans (Malhotra and Desai, 2010).

OSA occurs when muscles or structures of the oral cavity or throat relax during sleep. The upper airway becomes partially or completely blocked, diminishing nasal airflow (hypopnea) or stopping it (apnea) for as long as 30 seconds (Kryger et al., 2011). The person still attempts to breathe because chest and abdominal movement continue, which often results in loud snoring and snorting sounds. When breathing is partially or completely diminished, each successive diaphragmatic movement becomes stronger until the obstruction is relieved. Structural abnormalities such as a deviated septum, nasal polyps, certain jaw configurations, larger neck circumference, or enlarged tonsils predispose a patient to OSA (Pinto and Caple, 2010). The effort to breathe during sleep results in arousals from deep sleep often to the stage 2 cycle. In severe cases hundreds of hypopnea/apnea episodes occur every hour, resulting in severe interference with deep sleep.

Excessive daytime sleepiness (EDS) and fatigue are the most common complaints of people with OSA. Persons with severe OSA often report taking daytime naps and experience a disruption in their daily activities because of sleepiness (Adult Obstructive Sleep Apnea Task Force, 2009). Feelings of sleepiness are usually most intense on awakening, right before going to sleep, and about 12 hours after the midsleep period. EDS often results in impaired waking function, poor work or school performance, accidents while driving or using equipment, and behavioral or emotional problems.

Obstructive apnea causes a serious decline in arterial oxygen saturation level. Patients are at risk for cardiac dysrhythmias, right heart failure, pulmonary hypertension, angina attacks, stroke, and hypertension. Sleep apnea contributes to high blood pressure and increased risk for heart attack and stroke (National Sleep Foundation, 2010b).

Central sleep apnea (CSA) involves dysfunction in the respiratory control center of the brain. The impulse to breathe fails temporarily, and nasal airflow and chest wall movement cease. The oxygen saturation of the blood falls. The condition is common in patients with brainstem injury, muscular dystrophy, and encephalitis. Less than 10% of sleep apnea is predominantly central in origin. People with CSA tend to awaken during sleep and therefore complain of insomnia and EDS. Mild and intermittent snoring is also present.

Patients with sleep apnea rarely achieve deep sleep. In addition to complaints of EDS, sleep attacks, fatigue, morning headaches, irritability, depression, difficulty concentrating, and decreased sex drive are common (Kryger et al., 2011). OSA affects quality of life issues such as marital relationships and interactions within and outside the family and often is an embarrassment to a patient (Adult Obstructive Sleep Apnea Task Force, 2009). Treatment includes therapy for underlying cardiac or respiratory complications and emotional problems that occur as a result of the symptoms of this disorder.

Narcolepsy. Narcolepsy is a dysfunction of mechanisms that regulate sleep and wake states. Excessive daytime sleepiness is the most common complaint associated with this disorder. During the day a person suddenly feels an overwhelming wave of sleepiness and falls asleep; REM sleep occurs within 15 minutes of falling asleep. Cataplexy, or sudden muscle weakness during intense emotions such as anger, sadness, or laughter, occurs at any time during the day. If the cataplectic attack is severe, a patient loses voluntary muscle control and falls to the floor. A person with narcolepsy often has vivid dreams that occur as he or she is falling asleep. These dreams are difficult to distinguish from reality. Sleep paralysis, or the feeling of being unable to move or talk just before waking or falling asleep, is another symptom. Some studies show a genetic link for narcolepsy (Ahmed and Thorpy, 2010).

A person with narcolepsy falls asleep uncontrollably at inappropriate times. When individuals do not understand this disorder, a sleep attack is easily mistaken for laziness, lack of interest in activities, or drunkenness. Typically the symptoms first begin to appear in adolescence and are often confused with the EDS that commonly occurs in teens. Narcoleptic patients are treated with stimulants or wakefulness-promoting agents such as sodium oxybate, modafinil (Provigil) or armodafinil (Nuvigil) that only partially increase wakefulness and reduce sleep attacks. Patients also receive antidepressant medications that suppress cataplexy and the other REM-related symptoms. Brief daytime naps no longer than 20 minutes help reduce subjective feelings of sleepiness. Other management methods that help are following a regular exercise program, practicing good sleep habits, avoiding shifts in sleep, strategically timed daytime naps if possible, eating light meals high in protein, practicing deep breathing, chewing gum, and taking vitamins (Kryger et al., 2011). Patients with narcolepsy need to avoid factors that increase drowsiness (e.g., alcohol; heavy meals; exhausting activities; long-distance driving; and long periods of sitting in hot, stuffy rooms).

Sleep Deprivation. Sleep deprivation is a problem many patients experience as a result of dyssomnia. Causes include symptoms (e.g., fever, difficulty breathing, or pain) caused by illnesses, emotional stress, medications, environmental disturbances (e.g., frequent nursing care), and variability in the timing of sleep because of shift work. Physicians and nurses are particularly prone to sleep deprivation as a result of long work schedules and rotating shifts. Chronic sleep deprivation is associated with development of cardiovascular disease, weight gain, type II diabetes, poor memory, depression, and digestive problems (Ohlmann and O'Sullivan, 2009).

Hospitalization, especially in intensive care units (ICUs), makes patients particularly vulnerable to the extrinsic and circadian sleep disorders that cause the "ICU syndrome of sleep deprivation" (Fontana and Pittiglio, 2010). Constant environmental stimuli within the ICU such as strange noises from equipment, the frequent monitoring and care given by nurses, and ever-present lights confuse patients. Repeated environmental stimuli and the patient's poor physical status lead to sleep deprivation (Fontana and Pittiglio, 2010).

A person's response to sleep deprivation is highly variable. Patients experience a variety of physiological and psychological symptoms (Box 42-3). The severity of symptoms is often related to the duration of sleep deprivation.

BOX 42-3 SLEEP DEPRIVATION SYMPTOMS

Physiological Symptoms
- Ptosis, blurred vision
- Fine-motor clumsiness
- Decreased reflexes
- Slowed response time
- Decreased reasoning and judgment
- Decreased auditory and visual alertness
- Cardiac arrhythmias

Psychological Symptoms
- Confused and disoriented
- Increased sensitivity to pain
- Irritable, withdrawn, apathetic
- Agitated
- Hyperactive
- Decreased motivation
- Excessive sleepiness

Parasomnias. The parasomnias are sleep problems that are more common in children than adults. Some have hypothesized that sudden infant death syndrome (SIDS) is thought to be related to apnea, hypoxia, and cardiac arrhythmias caused by abnormalities in the autonomic nervous system that are manifested during sleep (Kryger et al., 2011). Because of an association between the prone position and the occurrence of SIDS, the American Academy of Pediatrics recommends that parents place apparently healthy infants in the supine position during sleep (Koren et al., 2010).

Parasomnias that occur among older children include somnambulism (sleepwalking), night terrors, nightmares, nocturnal enuresis (bed-wetting), body rocking, and bruxism (teeth grinding). When adults have these problems, it often indicates more serious disorders. Specific treatment varies. However, in all cases it is important to support patients and maintain their safety.

NURSING KNOWLEDGE BASE

Sleep and Rest

When people are at rest, they usually feel mentally relaxed, free from anxiety, and physically calm. Rest does not imply inactivity, although everyone often thinks of it as settling down in a comfortable chair or lying in bed. When people are at rest, they are in a state of mental, physical, and spiritual activity that leaves them feeling refreshed, rejuvenated, and ready to resume the activities of the day. People have their own habits for obtaining rest and can find ways to adjust to new environments or conditions that affect the ability to rest. They rest by reading a book, practicing a relaxation exercise, listening to music, taking a long walk, or sitting quietly.

Illness and unfamiliar health care routines easily affect the usual rest and sleep patterns of people entering a hospital or other health care facility. Nurses frequently care for patients who are on bed rest to reduce physical and psychological demands on the body in a variety of health care settings. However, these people do not necessarily feel rested. Some still have emotional worries that prevent complete relaxation. For example, concern over physical limitations or a fear of being unable to return to their usual lifestyle causes such patients to feel stressed and unable to relax. You must always be aware of a patient's need for rest. A lack of rest for long periods causes illness or worsening of existing illness.

Normal Sleep Requirements and Patterns

Sleep duration and quality vary among people of all age-groups. For example, one person feels adequately rested with 4 hours of sleep, whereas another requires 10 hours. Nurses play an important role in identifying treatable sleep-deprivation problems.

Neonates. The neonate up to the age of 3 months averages about 16 hours of sleep a day, sleeping almost constantly during the first week. The sleep cycle is generally 40 to 50 minutes with wakening occurring after one to two sleep cycles. Approximately 50% of this sleep is REM sleep, which stimulates the higher brain centers. This is essential for development because the neonate is not awake long enough for significant external stimulation.

Infants. Infants usually develop a nighttime pattern of sleep by 3 months of age. The infant normally takes several naps during the day but usually sleeps an average of 8 to 10 hours during the night for a total daily sleep time of 15 hours. About 30% of sleep time is in the REM cycle. Awakening commonly occurs early in the morning, although it is not unusual for an infant to awaken during the night.

Toddlers. By the age of 2 children usually sleep through the night and take daily naps. Total sleep averages 12 hours a day. After 3 years of age children often give up daytime naps (Hockenberry and Wilson, 2011). It is common for toddlers to awaken during the night. The percentage of REM sleep continues to fall. During this period toddlers may be unwilling to go to bed at night because they need autonomy or fear separation from their parents.

Preschoolers. On average a preschooler sleeps about 12 hours a night (about 20% is REM). By the age of 5 he or she rarely takes daytime naps except in cultures in which a siesta is the custom (Hockenberry and Wilson, 2011). The preschooler usually has difficulty relaxing or quieting down after long, active days and has bedtime fears, awakens during the night, or has nightmares. Partial awakening followed by normal return to sleep is frequent (Hockenberry and Wilson, 2011). In the awake period the child exhibits brief crying, walking around, unintelligible speech, sleepwalking, or bed-wetting.

School-Age Children. The amount of sleep needed varies during the school years. A 6-year-old averages 11 to 12 hours of sleep nightly, whereas an 11-year-old sleeps about 9 to 10 hours (Hockenberry and Wilson, 2011). The 6- or 7-year-old usually goes to bed with some encouragement or by doing quiet activities. The older child often resists sleeping because he or she is unaware of fatigue or has a need to be independent.

Adolescents. On average teenagers get about 7½ hours of sleep per night. The typical adolescent is subject to a number of changes such as school demands, after-school social activities, and part-time jobs, which reduce the time spent sleeping (Noland et al., 2009). Shortened sleep time often results in EDS, which frequently leads to reduced performance in school, vulnerability to accidents, behavior and mood problems, and increased use of alcohol (Noland et al., 2009; Vallido et al., 2009).

Young Adults. Most young adults average 6 to 8½ hours of sleep a night. Approximately 20% of sleep time is REM sleep, which remains consistent throughout life. It is common for the stresses of jobs, family relationships, and social activities to frequently lead to insomnia and the use of sleep medication. Daytime sleepiness contributes to an increased number of accidents, decreased productivity, and interpersonal problems in this age-group. Pregnancy increases the need for sleep and rest. Insomnia, periodic limb movements, RLS, and sleep-disordered breathing are common problems during the third trimester of pregnancy (Kryger et al., 2011).

Middle Adults. During middle adulthood the total time spent sleeping at night begins to decline. The amount of stage 4 sleep begins to fall, a decline that continues with advancing age. Insomnia is particularly common, probably because of the changes and stresses of middle age. Anxiety, depression, or certain physical illnesses cause sleep disturbances. Women experiencing menopausal symptoms often experience insomnia.

Older Adults. Complaints of sleeping difficulties increase with age. More than 50% of older adults report sleep problems (Neikrug and Ancoli-Israel, 2010). Older adults experience weakening, desynchronized circadian rhythms that alter the sleep-wake cycle (Neikrug and Ancoli-Israel, 2010). Episodes of REM sleep tend to shorten. There is a progressive decrease in stages 3 and 4 NREM sleep; some older adults have almost no stage 4, or deep sleep. An older adult awakens more often during the night, and it takes more time for him or her to fall asleep. The tendency to nap seems to increase progressively with age because of the frequent awakenings experienced at night.

The presence of chronic illness often results in sleep disturbances for the older adult. For example, an older adult with arthritis frequently has difficulty sleeping because of painful joints. Changes in sleep pattern are often caused by changes in the CNS that affect the regulation of sleep. Sensory impairment reduces an older person's sensitivity to time cues that maintain circadian rhythms.

Factors Influencing Sleep

A number of factors affect the quantity and quality of sleep. Often a single factor is not the only cause for a sleep problem. Physiological, psychological, and environmental factors frequently alter the quality and quantity of sleep.

Drugs and Substances. Sleepiness, insomnia, and fatigue often result as a direct effect of commonly prescribed medications (Box 42-4). These medications alter sleep and weaken daytime alertness, which is problematic (Kryger et al., 2011). Medications prescribed for sleep often cause more problems than benefits. Older adults take a variety of drugs to control or treat chronic illness, and the combined effects of their drugs often seriously disrupt sleep. Some substances such as L-tryptophan, a natural protein found in foods such as milk, cheese, and meats, promote sleep.

Lifestyle. A person's daily routine influences sleep patterns. An individual working a rotating shift (e.g., 2 weeks of days followed by a week of nights) often has difficulty adjusting to the altered sleep schedule. For example, the body's internal clock is set at 11 PM, but the work schedule forces sleep at 9 AM instead. The individual is able to sleep only 3 or 4 hours because his or her body clock perceives that it is time to be awake and active. Difficulties maintaining alertness during work time result in decreased and even hazardous performance. After several weeks of working a night shift, a person's biological clock usually does adjust. Other alterations in routines that disrupt sleep patterns include performing unaccustomed heavy work, engaging in late-night social activities, and changing evening mealtime.

Usual Sleep Patterns. In the past century the amount of sleep obtained nightly by U.S. citizens has decreased to about 6.7 hours per night, causing many Americans to be sleep deprived and experience excessive sleepiness during the day (Ohlmann and O'Sullivan, 2009). Sleepiness becomes pathological when it occurs at times when individuals need or want to be awake. People who experience temporary sleep deprivation as a result of an active social evening or lengthened work schedule usually feel sleepy the next day. However, they are able to overcome these feelings even though they have difficulty performing tasks and remaining attentive. Chronic lack of sleep is much more serious and causes serious alterations in the ability to perform daily functions. Sleepiness

BOX 42-4 DRUGS AND THEIR EFFECTS ON SLEEP

Hypnotics
- Interfere with reaching deeper sleep stages
- Provide only temporary (1 week) increase in quantity of sleep
- Eventually cause "hangover" during day; excess drowsiness, confusion, decreased energy
- Sometimes worsen sleep apnea in older adults

Antidepressants and Stimulants
- Suppress REM sleep
- Decrease total sleep time

Alcohol
- Speeds onset of sleep
- Reduces REM sleep
- Awakens person during night and causes difficulty returning to sleep

Caffeine
- Prevents person from falling asleep
- Causes person to awaken during night
- Interferes with REM sleep

Diuretics
- Nighttime awakenings caused by nocturia

Beta-Adrenergic Blockers
- Cause nightmares
- Cause insomnia
- Cause awakening from sleep

Benzodiazepines
- Alter REM sleep
- Increase sleep time
- Increase daytime sleepiness

Nicotine
- Decreases total sleep time
- Decreases REM sleep time
- Causes awakening from sleep
- Causes difficulty staying asleep

Narcotics
- Suppress REM sleep
- Cause increased daytime drowsiness

Anticonvulsants
- Decrease REM sleep time
- Cause daytime drowsiness

REM, Rapid eye movement.

tends to be most difficult to overcome during sedentary (inactive) tasks such as driving. There is an increased risk of motor vehicle accidents if an individual drives after less than 7 hours of sleep (Heaton et al., 2009).

Emotional Stress. Worry over personal problems or a situation frequently disrupts sleep. Emotional stress causes a person to be tense and often leads to frustration when sleep does not occur. Stress also causes a person to try too hard to fall asleep, to awaken frequently during the sleep cycle, or to oversleep. Continued stress causes poor sleep habits.

Older patients frequently experience losses that lead to emotional stress such as retirement, physical impairment, or the death of a loved one. Older adults and other individuals who experience depressive mood problems experience delays in falling asleep, earlier appearance of REM sleep, frequent or early awakening, feelings of sleeping poorly, and daytime sleepiness (National Sleep Foundation, 2010c).

Environment. The physical environment in which a person sleeps significantly influences the ability to fall and remain sleep. Good ventilation is essential for restful sleep. The size, firmness, and position of the bed affect the quality of sleep. If a person usually sleeps with another individual, sleeping alone often causes wakefulness. On the other hand, sleeping with a restless or snoring bed partner disrupts sleep.

In hospitals and other inpatient facilities noise creates a problem for patients. Noise in hospitals is usually new or strange and often loud. Thus patients wake easily. This problem is greatest the first night of hospitalization, when patients often experience increased total wake time, increased awakenings, and decreased REM sleep and total sleep time. People-induced noises (e.g., nursing activities) are sources of increased sound levels. ICUs are sources of high noise levels because of staff, monitor alarms, and equipment. Close proximity of patients, noise from confused and ill patients, ringing alarm systems and telephones, and disturbances caused by emergencies make the environment unpleasant. Noise causes increased agitation; delayed healing; impaired immune function; and increased blood pressure, heart rate, and stress (Dennis et al., 2010).

Light levels affect the ability to fall asleep. Some patients prefer a dark room, whereas others such as children or older adults prefer keeping a soft light on during sleep. Patients also have trouble sleeping because of the room temperature. A room that is too warm or too cold often causes a patient to become restless.

Exercise and Fatigue. A person who is moderately fatigued usually achieves restful sleep, especially if the fatigue is the result of enjoyable work or exercise. Exercising 2 hours or more before bedtime allows the body to cool down and maintain a state of fatigue that promotes relaxation. However, excess fatigue resulting from exhausting or stressful work makes falling asleep difficult. This is often seen in grade-school children and adolescents who keep stressful, long schedules because of school, social activities, and work.

Food and Caloric Intake. Following good eating habits is important for proper sleep. Eating a large, heavy, and/or spicy meal at night often results in indigestion that interferes with sleep. Caffeine, alcohol, and nicotine consumed in the evening produce insomnia. Coffee, tea, cola, and chocolate contain caffeine and xanthines that cause sleeplessness. Thus drastically reducing or avoiding these substances can improve sleep. Some food allergies cause insomnia. A milk allergy sometimes causes nighttime waking and crying or colic in infants.

Weight loss or gain influences sleep patterns. Weight gain contributes to OSA because of increased size of the soft tissue structures in the upper airway (Kryger et al., 2011). Weight loss causes insomnia and decreased amounts of sleep (Benca and Schneck, 2005). Certain sleep disorders are the result of the semi-starvation diets popular in a weight-conscious society.

CRITICAL THINKING

Successful critical thinking requires a synthesis of knowledge, including information gathered from patients, experience, critical thinking attitudes, and intellectual and professional standards.

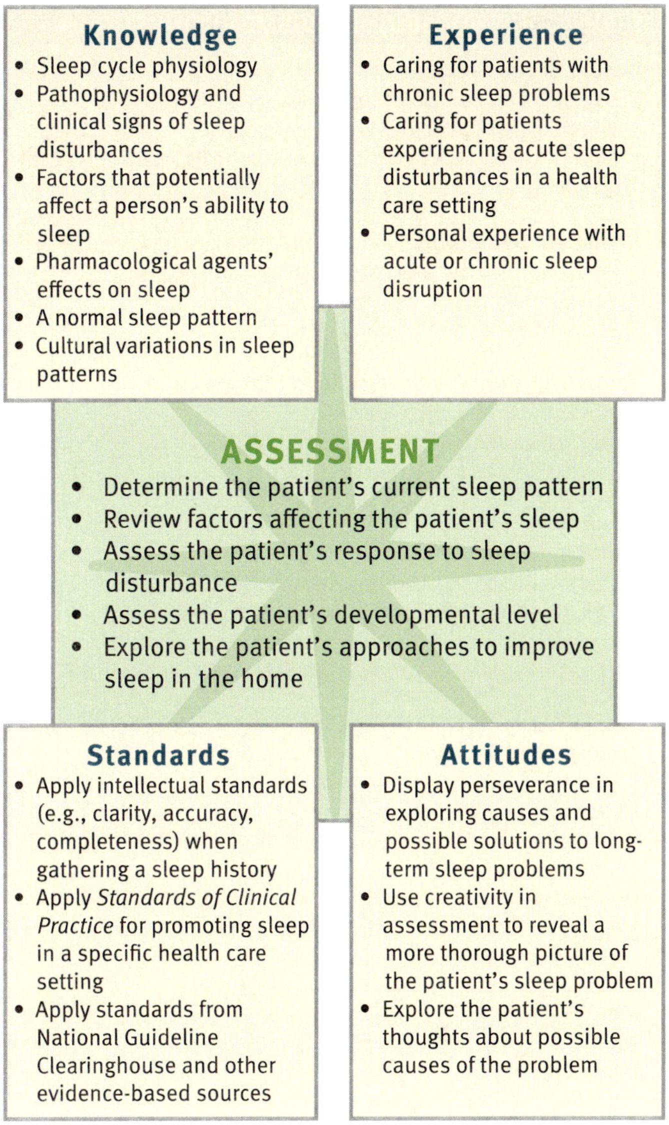

Knowledge
• Sleep cycle physiology
• Pathophysiology and clinical signs of sleep disturbances
• Factors that potentially affect a person's ability to sleep
• Pharmacological agents' effects on sleep
• A normal sleep pattern
• Cultural variations in sleep patterns
Experience
• Caring for patients with chronic sleep problems
• Caring for patients experiencing acute sleep disturbances in a health care setting
• Personal experience with acute or chronic sleep disruption
ASSESSMENT
• Determine the patient's current sleep pattern
• Review factors affecting the patient's sleep
• Assess the patient's response to sleep disturbance
• Assess the patient's developmental level
• Explore the patient's approaches to improve sleep in the home
Standards
• Apply intellectual standards (e.g., clarity, accuracy, completeness) when gathering a sleep history
• Apply Standards of Clinical Practice for promoting sleep in a specific health care setting
• Apply standards from National Guideline Clearinghouse and other evidence-based sources
Attitudes
• Display perseverance in exploring causes and possible solutions to long-term sleep problems
• Use creativity in assessment to reveal a more thorough picture of the patient's sleep problem
• Explore the patient's thoughts about possible causes of the problem

FIG. 42-3 Critical thinking model for sleep assessment.

Clinical judgments require you to anticipate the information necessary, analyze the data, and make decisions regarding patient care. You adapt critical thinking to the changing needs of the patient. During assessment (Fig. 42-3) consider all elements to make appropriate nursing diagnoses.

In the case of sleep, integrate knowledge from nursing and disciplines such as pharmacology and psychology. Personal experience with a sleep problem and experience with patients prepares you to know effective forms of sleep therapies. You use critical thinking attitudes such as perseverance, confidence, and discipline to complete a comprehensive assessment and develop a plan of care to provide successful management of the sleep problem. Professional standards such as the *Nursing Scope and Standards of Practice* (American Nurses Association, 2010), *Clinical Guidelines for the Evaluation and Management of Chronic Insomnia* (National Guideline Clearinghouse, 2008) and "Excessive Sleepiness" in *Evidence-based Geriatrics Nursing Protocols for Best Practice* (Chasens et al., 2008) provide valuable guidelines to assess and address the needs of patients with sleep disorders.

NURSING PROCESS

Apply the nursing process and use a critical thinking approach in the care of patients. The nursing process provides a clinical decision-making approach for you to develop and implement an individualized plan of care.

ASSESSMENT

During the assessment process, thoroughly assess each patient and critically analyze findings to ensure that you make patient-centered clinical decisions required for safe nursing care.

Through the Patient's Eyes. Assess patients' sleep patterns by using a nursing history to gather information about factors that usually influence sleep. Sleep is a subjective experience. Only the patient is able to report whether or not it is sufficient and restful. If the patient is satisfied with the quantity and quality of sleep received, you consider it normal, and the nursing history is brief. If a patient admits to or suspects a sleep problem, you need a detailed history and assessment. If a patient has an obvious sleep problem, consider asking if his or her sleep partner can be approached for further assessment data.

A poor night's sleep for a patient often starts a vicious cycle of anticipatory anxiety. The patient fears that sleep will again be disturbed while trying harder and harder to sleep. Use a skilled and caring approach to assess the patient's sleep needs. A caring nurse individualizes care for each patient. Always ask patients what they expect regarding sleep. This includes asking about the interventions that they currently use and how successful they are. It is important to understand patients' expectations regarding their sleep pattern. When patients ask for assistance because of sleep disturbances, they typically expect a nurse to respond promptly to help them improve the quantity and quality of their sleep.

Sleep Assessment. Most persons are able to provide a reasonably accurate estimate of their sleep patterns, particularly if any changes have occurred. Aim your assessment at understanding the characteristics of the patient's sleep problem and usual sleep habits so you incorporate ways for promoting sleep into nursing care. For example, if the nursing history reveals that a patient always reads before falling asleep, it makes sense to offer reading material at bedtime.

Sources for Sleep Assessment. Usually patients are the best resource for describing sleep problems and how they are a change from their usual sleep and waking patterns. Often the patient knows the cause for sleep problems such as a noisy environment or worry over a relationship.

In addition, bed partners are able to provide information about patients' sleep patterns that help reveal the nature of certain sleep disorders. For example, partners of patients with sleep apnea often complain that the patient's snoring disturbs their sleep. Often the partners must sleep in different beds or rooms to obtain adequate sleep. Ask bed partners (if the patient agrees) whether patients have breathing pauses during sleep and how frequently the apneic attacks occur. Some partners mention becoming fearful when patients apparently stop breathing for periods.

When caring for children, seek information about sleep patterns from parents or guardians because they are usually a reliable source of information. Hunger, excessive warmth, and separation anxiety often contribute to an infant's difficulty going to sleep or frequent awakenings during the night. Parents of infants need to keep a 24-hour log of their infant's waking and sleeping behavior for several days to determine the cause of the problem. They also need to describe the infant's eating pattern and sleeping environment because these influence sleeping behavior. Older children often are able to relate fears or worries that inhibit their ability to fall asleep. If children frequently awaken in the middle of bad dreams, parents are able to identify the problem but perhaps do not understand the meaning of the dreams. Ask parents to describe the typical behavior patterns that foster or impair sleep. For example, excessive stimulation from active play or visiting friends predictably impairs sleep. With chronic sleep problems, parents need to relate the duration of the problem, its progression, and children's responses.

Tools for Sleep Assessment. Two effective subjective measures of sleep are the Epworth Sleepiness Scale and the Pittsburgh Sleep Quality Index. The Epworth Sleepiness Scale evaluates the severity of EDS (Chasens et al., 2008). The Pittsburgh Sleep Quality Index assesses sleep quality and sleep patterns (Smyth, 2008). Another effective, brief method for assessing sleep quality is the use of a visual analogue scale (Lashley, 2004). Draw a straight horizontal line 100 mm (4 inches) long. Opposing statements such as "best night's sleep" and "worst night's sleep" are at opposite ends of the line. Ask patients to place a mark on the horizontal line at the point corresponding to their perceptions of the previous night's sleep. Measuring the distances of the mark along the line in millimeters offers a numerical value for satisfaction with sleep. Use the scale repeatedly to show change over time. Such a scale is useful to assess an individual patient, not to compare patients.

Another brief subjective method to assess sleep is a numeric scale with a 0-to-10 sleep rating (Lashley, 2004). Ask individuals to separately rate the quantity and quality of their sleep on the scale. Instruct them to indicate with a number between 0 and 10 their sleep quantity and then their quality of sleep, with 0 being the worst sleep and 10 being the best.

Sleep History. When a patient reports having adequate sleep, a sleep history is usually brief. A determination of usual bedtime, normal bedtime rituals, preferred environment for sleeping, and what time the patient usually rises gives you information for planning care conducive to sleep. When suspecting a sleep problem, assess the quality and characteristics of sleep in greater depth by asking the patient to describe the problem. This includes recent changes in sleep pattern, sleep symptoms experienced during waking hours, use of sleep and other prescribed or over-the-counter medications, diet and intake of substances such as caffeine or alcohol that influence sleep, and recent life events that have affected the patient's mental and emotional status.

Description of Sleeping Problems. Conduct a more detailed history when a patient has a sleep problem. This ensures that you provide appropriate therapeutic care. Open-ended questions help a patient describe a problem more fully. A general description of the problem followed by more focused questions usually reveals specific characteristics that are useful in planning therapies. To begin, you need to understand the nature of the sleep problem, its signs and symptoms, its onset and duration, its severity, any predisposing factors or causes, and the overall effect on the patient. Ask specific questions related to the sleep problem (Box 42-5).

Proper questioning helps to determine the type of sleep disturbance and the nature of the problem. Box 42-6 gives examples of additional questions for you to ask a patient when you suspect specific sleep disorders. The questions assist in selecting specific sleep therapies and the best time for implementation.

As an adjunct to the sleep history, have the patient and bed partner keep a sleep-wake log for 1 to 4 weeks (Cuellar et al., 2007). The patient completes the sleep-wake log daily to provide information on day-to-day variations in sleep-wake patterns over extended periods. Entries in the log often include 24-hour information about various waking and sleeping health behaviors such as physical activities, mealtimes, type and amount of intake (alcohol and caffeine), time and length of daytime naps, evening and bedtime routines, the time the patient tries to fall asleep, nighttime awakenings, and the time of morning awakening. A partner helps record the estimated times the patient falls asleep or awakens. Although the log is helpful, the patient needs to be motivated to participate in its completion.

Usual Sleep Pattern. Normal sleep is difficult to define because individuals vary in their perception of adequate quantity and quality of sleep. However, it is important to have patients describe their usual sleep pattern to determine the significance of the changes caused by a sleep disorder. Knowing a patient's usual, preferred sleep pattern allows you to try to match sleeping conditions in a health care setting with those in the home. Ask the following questions to determine a patient's sleep pattern:

BOX 42-5 NURSING ASSESSMENT QUESTIONS

Nature of the Problem
- Describe for me the type of sleep problem you are having.
- Why do you think you are not getting enough sleep?
- Describe a recent night's sleep. How is this sleep different from your usual sleep?

Signs and Symptoms
- Do you have difficulty falling asleep, staying asleep, or waking up?
- Have you been told that you snore loudly?
- Do you have headaches when awakening?

Onset and Duration of Signs and Symptoms
- When did you notice the problem?
- What do you do to relieve the symptom?
- How long has this problem lasted?

Severity
- How long does it take you to fall asleep?
- How often during the week do you have trouble falling asleep?
- How many hours of sleep a night did you get this week?
- How does this compare to your usual amount of sleep?
- What do you do when you awaken during the night or too early in the morning?

Predisposing Factors
- What do you do just before you go to bed?
- Have you recently had any changes at work or at home?
- How is your mood? Have you noticed any changes recently?
- Which medications or recreational drugs do you take on a regular basis
- Are you taking any new prescriptions or over-the-counter medications?
- Do you eat food (spicy or greasy foods) or drink substances (alcohol or caffeinated beverages) that affect your sleep?
- Do you have a physical illness that affects your sleep?
- Does anyone in your family have a history of sleep problems?

Effect on Patient
- How has the loss of sleep affected you?
- Do you feel excessively sleepy or irritable or have trouble concentrating during waking hours?
- Do you have trouble staying awake? Have you fallen asleep at the wrong times (e.g., while driving, sitting quietly in a meeting)?

BOX 42-6 QUESTIONS TO ASK TO ASSESS FOR SPECIFIC SLEEP DISORDERS

Insomnia
- How easily do you fall asleep?
- Do you fall asleep and have difficulty staying asleep? How many times do you awaken?
- What time do you awaken in the morning? What causes you to awaken early?
- What do you do to prepare for sleep? To improve your sleep?
- What do you think about as you try to fall asleep?
- How often do you have trouble sleeping?

Sleep Apnea
- Do you snore loudly? Does anyone else in your family snore loudly?
- Has anyone ever told you that you often stop breathing for short periods during sleep? (Spouse or bed partner/roommate may report this.)
- Do you experience headaches after awakening?
- Do you have difficulty staying awake during the day?

Narcolepsy
- Do you fall asleep at the wrong times? (Friends or relatives may report this.)
- Do you have episodes of losing muscle control or falling to the floor?
- Have you ever had the feeling of being unable to move or talk just before waking or falling asleep?
- Do you have vivid, lifelike dreams when going to sleep or awakening?

1. What time do you usually get in bed each night?
2. How much time does it usually take to fall asleep? Do you do anything special to help you fall asleep?
3. How many times do you awaken during the night? Why?
4. What time do you typically wake up in the morning?
5. On average, how many hours do you sleep each night?

Compare patient data with their pattern before the sleep problem or with the predominant pattern usually found for other patients of the same age. On the basis of this comparison, you begin to assess for identifiable patterns such as insomnia.

Patients with sleep problems frequently show patterns drastically different from their usual one, or sometimes the change is relatively minor. Hospitalized patients usually need or want more sleep as a result of illness. However, some require less sleep because they are less active. Some patients who are ill think that it is important to try to sleep more than usual, eventually making sleeping difficult.

Physical and Psychological Illness. Determine whether the patient has any preexisting health problems that interfere with sleep. A history of psychiatric problems also makes a difference. For example, a patient who is living with bipolar disorder sleeps more when depressed than when manic. A patient who is depressed often experiences an inadequate amount of fragmented sleep. Chronic diseases such as chronic obstructive pulmonary disease and painful disorders such as arthritis interfere with sleep. Also assess the patient's medication history, including a description of over-the-counter and prescribed drugs. If a patient takes medications to aid sleep, gather information about the type and amount of medication and frequency used. Also assess the patient's daily caffeine intake.

If the patient has recently had surgery, expect him or her to experience some sleep disturbance. Patients usually awaken frequently during the first night after surgery and receive little deep or REM sleep. Depending on the type of surgery, it takes several days to months for a normal sleep cycle to return.

Current Life Events. In your assessment learn if the patient is experiencing any changes in lifestyle that disrupt sleep. A person's occupation often offers a clue to the nature of the sleep problem. Changes in job responsibilities, rotating shifts, or long hours contribute to a sleep disturbance. Questions about social activities, recent travel, or mealtime schedules help clarify the assessment.

Emotional and Mental Status. A patient's emotions and mental status affect the ability to sleep. For example, if a patient is experiencing anxiety, emotional stress related to illness, or situational crises such as loss of job or a loved one, he or she often experiences insomnia. When a sleep disturbance is related to an emotional problem, the key is to treat the primary problem; its resolution often improves sleep (Ramakrishnan and Scheid, 2007). Patients with mental illnesses may need mild sedation for adequate rest. Assess the effectiveness of any medication and its effect on daytime function.

Bedtime Routines. Ask patients what they do to prepare for sleep. For example, some patients drink a glass of milk, take a sleeping pill, eat a snack, or watch television. Assess habits that are beneficial compared with those that disturb sleep. For example, watching television promotes sleep for one person, whereas it stimulates another to stay awake. Sometimes pointing out that a particular habit is interfering with sleep helps patients find ways to change or eliminate habits that are disrupting sleep.

Pay special attention to a child's bedtime rituals. For example, the parents need to report whether it is necessary to read a bedtime story, rock the child to sleep, or engage in quiet play. Some young children need a special blanket or stuffed animal when going to sleep.

Bedtime Environment. During assessment ask the patient to describe preferred bedroom conditions, including preferences for lighting in the room, music or television in the background, or needing to have the door open versus closed. In addition, some children need the company of a parent to fall asleep. In a health care environment environmental distractions such as a roommate's television, an electronic monitor in the hallway, a noisy nurses' station, or another patient who cries out at night often interfere with sleep. Identify factors to reduce or control the environment.

Behaviors of Sleep Deprivation. Some patients are unaware of how their sleep problems are affecting their behavior. Observe for behaviors such as irritability, disorientation (similar to a drunken state), frequent yawning, and slurred speech. If sleep deprivation has lasted a long time, psychotic behavior such as delusions and paranoia sometimes develop. For example, a patient reports seeing strange objects or colors in the room, or he or she acts afraid when the nurse enters the room.

NURSING DIAGNOSIS

Review your assessment data, looking for clusters of data that include defining characteristics for a sleep pattern disturbance or other health problem. If you identify a sleep problem, specify the condition, such as insomnia or sleep deprivation. By specifying the sleep disturbance diagnosis, you are able to design more effective interventions. For example, you choose different therapies for patients with insomnia who are unable to fall asleep than for those with sleep deprivation. Box 42-7 demonstrates how to use nursing assessment activities to identify and cluster defining characteristics to make an accurate nursing diagnosis.

Assessment also identifies the related factor or probable cause of a sleep disturbance such as a noisy environment or a high intake of caffeinated beverages in the evening. These causes become the

BOX 42-7 NURSING DIAGNOSTIC PROCESS

Insomnia

ASSESSMENT ACTIVITIES	DEFINING CHARACTERISTICS
Ask patient to explain nature of sleep problem.	Patient reports difficulty falling asleep, taking up to 1 hour. Patient reports awakening two to three times nightly with difficulty returning to sleep.
Observe patient's behavior and ask spouse if patient is experiencing behavior changes.	Patient admits to not feeling well rested. Spouse describes times when patient was lethargic and irritable.
Determine if patient has had recent lifestyle changes.	Spouse reports that patient recently lost job and is concerned about finding new position.

focus of interventions for minimizing or eliminating the problem. For example, if a patient is experiencing insomnia as a result of a noisy health care environment, offer some basic recommendations for helping sleep such as controlling the noise of hospital equipment, reducing interruptions, or keeping doors closed. If the insomnia is related to worry over a threatened marital separation, introduce coping strategies and create an environment for sleep. If you incorrectly define the probable cause or related factors, the patient does not benefit from care.

Sleep problems affect patients in other ways. For example, you find that a patient with sleep apnea has problems with a spouse who is tired and frustrated over the patient's snoring. In addition, the spouse is concerned that the patient is breathing improperly and thus is in danger. The nursing diagnosis of *compromised family coping* indicates that you need to provide support to the patient and spouse so they understand sleep apnea and obtain the medical treatment needed. Examples of nursing diagnoses for patients with sleep problems include the following:

- Anxiety
- Ineffective breathing pattern
- Acute confusion
- Compromised family coping
- Ineffective coping
- Insomnia
- Fatigue
- Sleep deprivation
- Readiness for enhanced sleep

PLANNING

Goals and Outcomes. During planning you again synthesize information from multiple resources to develop an individualized plan of care (Fig. 42-4) (see the Nursing Care Plan). Professional standards are especially important to consider in developing a care plan. These standards often offer evidence-based guidelines for effective nursing interventions. For example, *the Evidence-based Geriatrics Protocol for Best Practice* (Chasens et al., 2008) titled "Excessive Sleepiness" recommends individualized nursing interventions that maintain and support an older adult's normal sleep pattern and bedtime ritual. It is important for a plan of care for sleep promotion to include strategies appropriate to the patient's sleep routines, living environment, and lifestyle.

As you plan care for a patient with sleep disturbances, creation of a concept map is another method for developing holistic

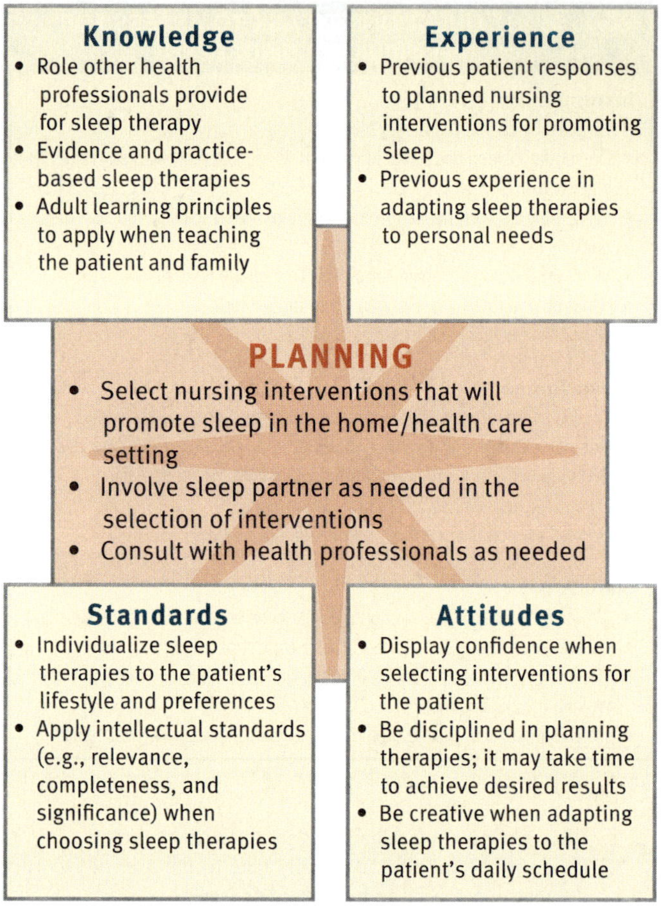

Knowledge
• Role other health professionals provide for sleep therapy
• Evidence and practice-based sleep therapies
• Adult learning principles to apply when teaching the patient and family
Experience
• Previous patient responses to planned nursing interventions for promoting sleep
• Previous experience in adapting sleep therapies to personal needs
PLANNING
• Select nursing interventions that will promote sleep in the home/health care setting
• Involve sleep partner as needed in the selection of interventions
• Consult with health professionals as needed
Standards
• Individualize sleep therapies to the patient's lifestyle and preferences
• Apply intellectual standards (e.g., relevance, completeness, and significance) when choosing sleep therapies
Attitudes
• Display confidence when selecting interventions for the patient
• Be disciplined in planning therapies; it may take time to achieve desired results
• Be creative when adapting sleep therapies to the patient's daily schedule

FIG. 42-4 Critical thinking model for sleep planning.

patient-centered care (Fig. 42-5 on p. 953). Create the map after identifying relevant nursing diagnoses from the assessment database. In this example the nursing diagnoses are linked to the patient's medical diagnosis of depression and situational stress. The concept map shows the relationships among the nursing diagnoses *insomnia, stress overload, sedentary lifestyle,* and *readiness for enhanced sleep.* This approach to planning care helps the nurse recognize relationships among planned interventions. For this patient, interventions and successful outcomes for one nursing diagnosis affect the resolution of another nursing diagnosis.

When developing goals and outcomes, it is important for a nurse and patient to collaborate. As a result, you are more likely to set realistic goals and measurable outcomes with your patients. An effective plan includes outcomes established over a realistic time frame that focus on the goal of improving the quantity and quality of sleep in the home. Often family members are very helpful in contributing to the plan. A sleep-promotion plan frequently requires many weeks to accomplish. The following is an example of a goal with patient outcomes:

Goal: The patient will control environmental sources disrupting sleep within 1 month.

Outcomes:

- Patient will identify factors in the immediate home environment that disrupt sleep in 2 weeks.
- Patient will report having a discussion with family members about environmental barriers to sleep in 2 weeks.
- Patient will report changes made in the bedroom to promote sleep within 4 weeks.

NURSING CARE PLAN

Insomnia

ASSESSMENT

Julie Arnold, a 42-year-old attorney, is the first patient of the morning at the neighborhood health clinic where you work. When you ask her how she is doing, she tells you that she is having difficulty sleeping. Her physician has diagnosed that she is suffering from depression. Julie is married and has two school-age children. She also tells you that she is caring for her mother, who is currently staying with them after she was discharged from the hospital following an exacerbation of her heart failure. Julie's assessment includes a thorough sleep history and a discussion of how the sleep problem has affected her life. You also conduct a physical examination.

Assessment Activities	*Findings/Defining Characteristics**
Ask Julie to explain the nature of her sleep problem.	Julie explains that she wakes up once or twice a night. She states, "I feel tired when I wake up, and I have trouble concentrating at work in the afternoon." She also reports that she has less patience with her children at home and no energy in the evenings.
Ask Julie if there have been any recent changes in her life.	Julie says that she is feeling pressured at work to complete an important case that she started on 2 weeks ago and because of this she is working longer hours. She also reports that, because of her heavy work schedule, she has **stopped** her **routine of walking 1 to 2 miles daily.** She reports that she **has no time for any exercise** when she gets home because **she needs to take care of her mother and the children.**
Ask Julie to describe her bedtime routine.	Julie responds that she is going to bed between 12 AM and 1 AM, which is 2 hours later than her usual bedtime. **It takes her an hour to fall asleep.** She says that she used to get 7 to 8 hours of sleep a night and now **it is more like 5 to 6 hours.** She drinks two to three cups of coffee after dinner while she is working on her case before bedtime. Julie reports drinking a glass of wine just before bedtime to help relax because she has been having trouble falling asleep.
Assess Julie for physical signs of sleep problems.	During the examination you note that Julie has dark circles under her eyes; she shifts her position in the chair multiple times and yawns frequently.

***Defining characteristics** are shown in bold type.

NURSING DIAGNOSIS: Insomnia related to psychological stress from job pressures.

PLANNING

Goals	*Expected Outcomes (NOC)†*
	Sleep
Patient will achieve an improved sense of adequate sleep within 4 weeks.	Patient will report waking up less frequently during the night and feeling rested within 4 weeks. Patient will verbalize adherence to a regular bedtime routine within 4 weeks.
Patient will achieve a more normal sleep pattern within 4 weeks.	Patient will fall asleep within 30 minutes of going to bed within 4 weeks. Patient will report sleeping 7 hours nightly within 4 weeks.

†Outcome classification labels from Moorhead S et al: *Nursing outcomes classification (NOC),* ed 4, St Louis, 2008, Mosby.

INTERVENTIONS (NIC)‡	RATIONALE
Sleep Enhancement	
Encourage patient to establish a bedtime routine and a regular sleep pattern.	Maintaining a consistent schedule helps induce sleep (National Guideline Clearinghouse, 2008).
Instruct patient to avoid caffeine, nicotine, and alcohol before bedtime.	Caffeine and nicotine are stimulants and cause difficulty in falling asleep. Alcohol lightens and fragments sleep (Reeve and Bailes, 2010).
Help patient identify ways to eliminate stressful concerns about work before bedtime (e.g., taking time before actual sleep time to read a light novel).	Excess worry and intense activities before bedtime stimulate patient and prevent sleep (Reeve and Bailes, 2010).
Adjust environment; have patient control noise, temperature, and light in the bedroom.	Develop an environment conducive to sleep (Wickwire and Collop, 2010).
Exercise Promotion	
Encourage patient to begin walking routinely during the day but not 2 to 3 hours before bedtime.	Regular exercise increases activity levels and improves sleep quality. Exercise just before bedtime is a stimulant that prevents sleep (Reeve and Bailes, 2010).

Continued

NURSING CARE PLAN

***Insomnia*—cont'd**

Relaxation Therapy	
Instruct patient in how to perform muscle relaxation before bedtime; include demonstration.	Relaxation therapy helps reduce anxiety, which interferes with sleep (National Guideline Clearinghouse, 2008).

‡Intervention classification labels from Bulechek GM, Butcher HK, and Dochterman JM: *Nursing interventions classification (NIC)*, ed 5, St Louis, 2008, Mosby.

EVALUATION

Nursing Actions	*Patient Response/Finding*	*Achievement of Outcome*
Ask Julie if she is able to fall asleep and stay asleep.	Julie responds, "It usually takes 15 to 20 minutes to fall asleep, and I woke up once for only two nights last week."	Julie reports that she falls asleep within 30 minutes and wakes up less frequently during the night.
Ask Julie to describe her waking behaviors at work and home during the day.	Julie responds that she has completed her case at work and feels less pressure. She has restarted her walking routine and is better able to cope with her children. She is able to concentrate at work more.	Julie reports feeling more rested.
Observe Julie's waking nonverbal expressions and behavior.	Julie sits in the chair without shifting position. She does not yawn during the conversation. The dark circles under her eyes are almost gone.	Julie reports that she is sleeping an average of 7 hours a night.

- Patient will report having fewer than two awakenings per night within 4 weeks.

Setting Priorities. Work with patients to establish priority outcomes and interventions. Frequently sleep disturbances are the result of other health problems. For example, when physical symptoms are interfering with sleep, managing the symptoms is your first priority. After symptoms are relieved, focus on sleep therapies. Patients are a helpful resource in determining which interventions hold priority. For example, once patients understand the factors that disrupt sleep, they make choices about the types of changes they would like to make in their lifestyle or sleeping environment.

Teamwork and Collaboration. Partner closely with the patient and sleep partner to ensure that any therapies such as a change in the sleep schedule or changes to the bedroom environment are realistic and achievable. In a health care setting plan treatments or routines so the patient is able to rest. For example, in the ICU use available electronic monitors to track trends in vital signs without awakening a patient each hour. Other staff members need to be aware of the care plan so they can cluster activities at certain times to reduce awakenings. In a nursing home the focus of the plan involves better planning of rest periods around the activities of the other residents. Roommates often have very different schedules.

When patients have chronic sleep problems, the initial referral for a patient is often to a comprehensive sleep center for assessment of the problem. The nature of the sleep disturbance then determines whether referrals to additional health care providers are necessary. For example, if a sleep problem is related to a situational crisis or emotional problem, refer the patient to a mental health clinical nurse specialist or clinical psychologist for counseling. If the nurse works in an inpatient setting and the patient needs a referral for continued care after discharge, offering information about the sleep problem is useful to the home care nurse. The success of sleep therapy depends on an approach that fits the patient's lifestyle and the nature of the sleep disorder.

IMPLEMENTATION

Nursing interventions designed to improve the quality of a person's rest and sleep are largely focused on health promotion. Patients need adequate sleep and rest to maintain active and productive lifestyles. During times of illness, rest and sleep promotion are important for recovery. Nursing care in an acute, restorative, or continuing care setting differs from that provided in a patient's home. The primary differences are in the environment and the nurse's ability to support normal rest and sleep habits. A patient's age also influences the types of therapies that are most effective. Box 42-8 provides principles for promoting sleep in older patients.

Health Promotion. In community health and home settings help patients develop behaviors conducive to rest and relaxation. To develop good sleep habits at home, patients and their bed partners need to learn techniques that promote sleep and conditions that interfere with it (Kryger et al., 2011) (Box 42-9 on p. 954). Parents also learn how to promote good sleep habits for their children. Patients benefit most from instructions based on information about their homes and lifestyles such as which type of activities promotes sleep in a night-shift worker or how to make the home environment more conducive to sleep. They will more likely apply information that is useful and valued.

Environmental Controls. All patients require a sleeping environment with a comfortable room temperature and proper ventilation, minimal sources of noise, a comfortable bed, and proper lighting (National Heart, Lung, and Blood Institute, 2009). Children and adults vary more in regard to comfortable room temperature. Instruct parents to position cribs away from open windows or drafts and to cover the infant with a light, warm blanket. Older adults often require extra blankets or covers.

Eliminate distracting noise so the bedroom is as quiet as possible. In the home the television, telephone, or the intermittent chiming of a clock often disrupts a patient's sleep. Involve the family in identifying approaches for reducing noise in the home, especially if there are several family members, all with different sleep schedules. It is also important to remember that some patients sleep with familiar inside noises such as the hum of a fan. Commercial products that produce a soothing noise such as ocean waves or rainfall create a soothing environment for sleep.

A bed and mattress need to provide support and comfortable firmness. Bed boards placed under mattresses add support.

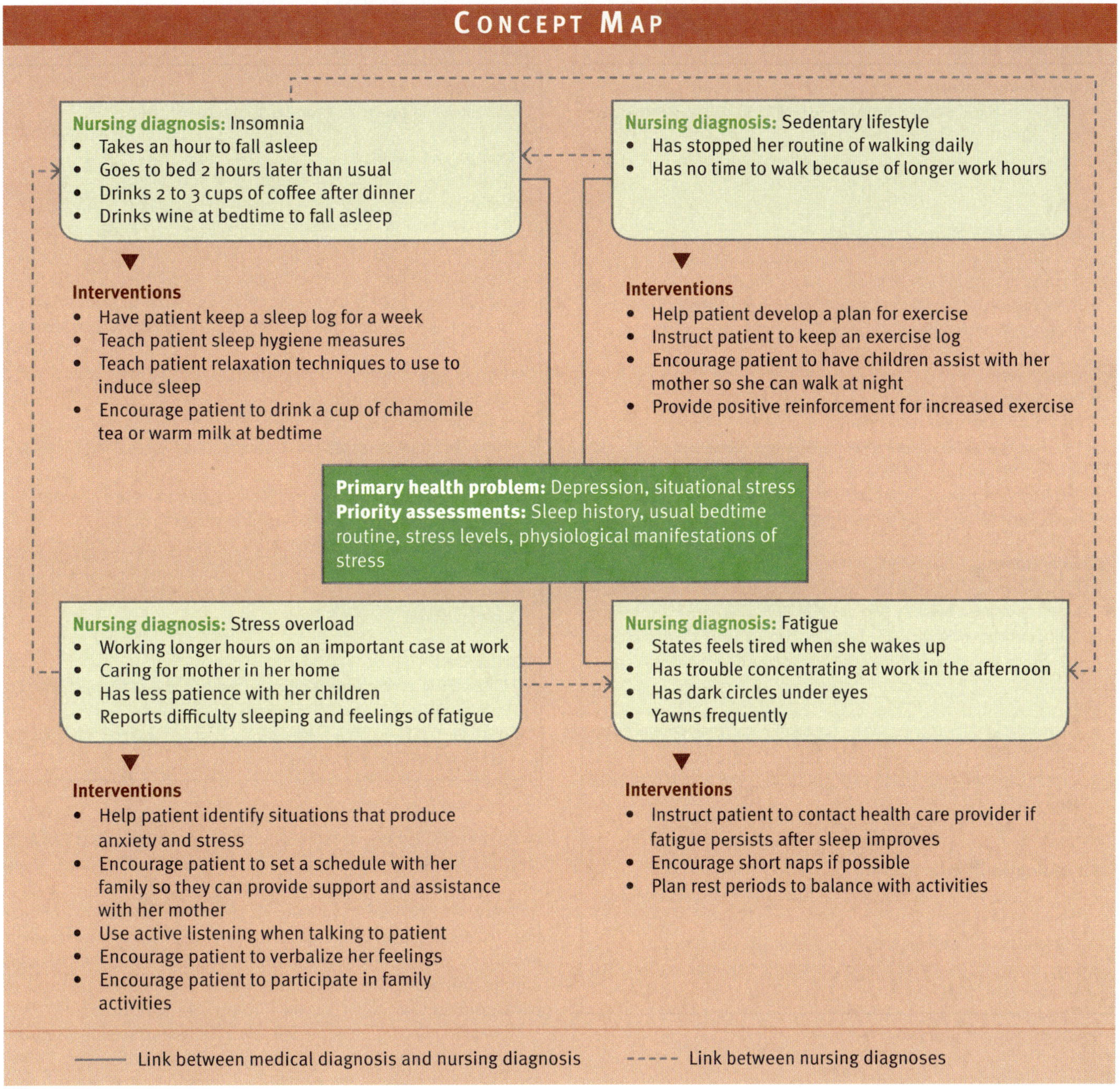
CONCEPT MAP
Nursing diagnosis: Insomnia
• Takes an hour to fall asleep
• Goes to bed 2 hours later than usual
• Drinks 2 to 3 cups of coffee after dinner
• Drinks wine at bedtime to fall asleep
Interventions
• Have patient keep a sleep log for a week
• Teach patient sleep hygiene measures
• Teach patient relaxation techniques to use to induce sleep
• Encourage patient to drink a cup of chamomile tea or warm milk at bedtime
Nursing diagnosis: Sedentary lifestyle
• Has stopped her routine of walking daily
• Has no time to walk because of longer work hours
Interventions
• Help patient develop a plan for exercise
• Instruct patient to keep an exercise log
• Encourage patient to have children assist with her mother so she can walk at night
• Provide positive reinforcement for increased exercise
Primary health problem: Depression, situational stress
Priority assessments: Sleep history, usual bedtime routine, stress levels, physiological manifestations of stress
Nursing diagnosis: Stress overload
• Working longer hours on an important case at work
• Caring for mother in her home
• Has less patience with her children
• Reports difficulty sleeping and feelings of fatigue
Interventions
• Help patient identify situations that produce anxiety and stress
• Encourage patient to set a schedule with her family so they can provide support and assistance with her mother
• Use active listening when talking to patient
• Encourage patient to verbalize her feelings
• Encourage patient to participate in family activities
Nursing diagnosis: Fatigue
• States feels tired when she wakes up
• Has trouble concentrating at work in the afternoon
• Has dark circles under eyes
• Yawns frequently
Interventions
• Instruct patient to contact health care provider if fatigue persists after sleep improves
• Encourage short naps if possible
• Plan rest periods to balance with activities
Link between medical diagnosis and nursing diagnosis
Link between nursing diagnoses

FIG. 42-5 Concept map for Julie Arnold.

Sometimes extra pillows are important to help a person position comfortably in bed. The position of the bed in the room also makes a difference for some patients.

Patients vary in regard to the amount of light that they prefer at night. Infants and older adults sleep best in softly lit rooms. Light should not shine directly on their eyes. Small table lamps prevent total darkness. For older adults light reduces the chance of confusion and prevents falls when walking to the bathroom. If streetlights shine through windows or when patients nap during the day, heavy shades, drapes, or slatted blinds are helpful.

Promoting Bedtime Routines. Bedtime routines relax patients in preparation for sleep (Bulechek, Butcher, and Dochterman, 2008). It is always important for persons to go to sleep when they feel fatigued or sleepy. Going to bed while fully awake and thinking about other things often causes insomnia and interferes with the bed as a stimulus for sleep. Newborns and infants sleep through so much of the day that a specific routine is hardly necessary. However, quiet activities such as holding them snugly in blankets, singing or talking softly, and gentle rocking help infants fall asleep.

A bedtime routine (e.g., same hour for bedtime, snack, or quiet activity) used consistently helps young children avoid delaying sleep. Parents need to reinforce patterns of preparing for bedtime. Quiet activities such as reading stories, coloring, allowing children to sit in a parent's lap while listening to music or listening to a prayer are routines that are often associated with preparing for bed.

Adults need to avoid excessive mental stimulation just before bedtime. Reading a light novel, watching an enjoyable television

BOX 42-8 FOCUS ON OLDER ADULTS

Promoting Sleep

Sleep-Wake Pattern

- Maintain a regular bedtime and wake-up schedule (Townsend-Roccichelli et al., 2010).
- Eliminate naps unless they are a routine part of the schedule.
- If naps are taken, limit to 20 minutes or less twice a day (Touhy and Jett, 2010).
- Go to bed when sleepy.
- Use warm bath and relaxation techniques (Ebersole et al., 2008).
- If unable to sleep in 15 to 30 minutes, get out of bed.
- Avoid stimulating activities before bedtime such as exercise or watching television (Townsend-Roccichelli et al., 2010).

Environment

- Sleep where you sleep best.
- Keep noise to minimum; use soft music to mask it if necessary.
- Use night-light and keep path to bathroom free of obstacles.
- Set room temperature to preference; use socks to promote warmth.
- Listen to relaxing music (Touhy and Jett, 2010).
- Increase exposure to bright light during the day (Neubauer, 2009).

Medications

- Use sedatives and hypnotics with caution as last resort and then only short term if absolutely necessary (Neubauer, 2009).
- Adjust medications being taken for other conditions and assess for drug interactions that may cause insomnia or excessive daytime sleepiness.

Diet

- Limit alcohol, caffeine, and nicotine in late afternoon and evening (Touhy and Jett, 2010).
- Consume carbohydrates or milk as a light snack before bedtime (Ebersole et al., 2008).
- Decrease fluids 2 to 4 hours before sleep (Ebersole et al., 2008).

Physiological/Illness Factors

- Elevate head of bed and provide extra pillows as preferred (Townsend-Roccichelli et al., 2010).
- Use analgesics 30 minutes before bed to ease aches and pains.
- Use therapeutics to control symptoms of chronic conditions as prescribed (Chasens et al., 2008).

BOX 42-9 PATIENT TEACHING

Sleep Hygiene Habits

Objective

- Patient will follow proper sleep hygiene habits at home.

Teaching Strategies

- Instruct patient to try to exercise daily, preferably in the morning or afternoon, and to avoid vigorous exercise in the evening within 2 hours of bedtime.
- Caution patient against sleeping long hours during weekends or holidays to prevent disturbance of normal sleep-wake cycle.
- Explain that, if possible, patients should not use the bedroom for intensive studying, snacking, television watching, or other nonsleep activity besides sex.
- Encourage patients to try to avoid worrisome thinking when going to bed and to use relaxation exercises.
- If patient does not fall asleep within 30 minutes of going to bed, advise him or her to get out of bed and do some quiet activity until feeling sleepy enough to go back to bed.
- Recommend that patient limit caffeine to morning coffee and limit alcohol intake (more than 1 to 2 drinks a day interrupts sleep cycle).
- Ask patient to examine environment. Instruct that use of earplugs and eyeshades may be helpful.
- Instruct patient to avoid heavy meals for 3 hours before bedtime; a light snack may help.

Evaluation

- Have patient complete sleep-wake log for 1 week and compare it with previous sleep-wake log.
- Ask patient to periodically complete visual analogue or sleep-rating scale for perceptions of quality of sleep.

program, or listening to music helps a person relax. Relaxation exercises such as slow, deep breathing for 1 or 2 minutes relieve tension and prepare the body for rest (see Chapter 43). Guided imagery and praying also promote sleep for some patients.

At home discourage patients from trying to finish office work or resolve family problems before bedtime. The bedroom is not a place to work, and patients need to always associate it with sleep. Working toward a consistent time for sleep and awakening helps most patients gain a healthy sleep pattern and strengthens the rhythm of the sleep-wake cycle.

Promoting Safety. For any patient prone to confusion or falls, safety is critical. A small night-light helps a patient orient to the room environment before going to the bathroom. Beds set lower to the floor lessen the chance of a person falling when first standing. Instruct patients to remove clutter and throw rugs from the path used to walk from the bed to the bathroom. If a patient needs assistance in ambulating from a bed to the bathroom, place a small bell at the bedside to call family members. Sleepwalkers are unaware of their surroundings and are slow to react, increasing the risk of falls. Do not startle sleepwalkers but instead gently awaken them and lead them back to bed.

Infants' beds need to be safe. To reduce the chance of suffocation, do not place pillows, stuffed toys, or the ends of loose blankets in cribs. Loose-fitting plastic mattress covers are dangerous because infants pull them over their faces and suffocate. Parents need to place an infant on his or her back to prevent suffocation.

Promoting Comfort. People fall asleep only after feeling comfortable and relaxed (Bulechek, Butcher, and Dochterman, 2008). Minor irritants often keep patients awake. Soft cotton nightclothes keep infants or small children warm and comfortable. Instruct patients to wear loose-fitting nightwear. An extra blanket is sometimes all that is necessary to prevent a person from feeling chilled and being unable to fall asleep. Patients need to void before retiring so they are not kept awake by a full bladder.

Establishing Periods of Rest and Sleep. In the home it helps to encourage patients to stay physically active during the day so they are more likely to sleep at night. Increasing daytime activity lessens problems with falling asleep. In a home setting you will frequently care for patients with chronic debilitating disease. The nursing care plan includes having patients set aside afternoons for rest to promote optimal health. Help adjust medication schedules, instruct patients to regularly void before rest periods, and suggest silencing the telephone ringer so rest periods are uninterrupted.

Stress Reduction. The inability to sleep because of emotional stress also makes a person feel irritable and tense. When patients are emotionally upset, encourage them to try not to force sleep.

Otherwise insomnia frequently develops, and soon bedtime is associated with the inability to relax. Encourage a patient who has difficulty falling asleep to get up and pursue a relaxing activity such as sewing or reading rather than staying in bed and thinking about sleep.

Preschoolers have bedtime fears (fear of the dark or strange noises), awaken during the night, or have nightmares. After nightmares the parent enters the child's room immediately and talks to him or her briefly about fears to provide a cooling-down period. One approach is to comfort children and leave them in their own beds so their fears are not used as excuses to delay bedtime. Keeping a light on in the room also helps some children. Cultural tradition causes families to approach sleep practices differently (Box 42-10). Always respect those that differ from traditional recommendations.

Bedtime Snacks. Some people enjoy bedtime snacks, whereas others cannot sleep after eating. A dairy product such as warm milk or cocoa that contains L-tryptophan is often helpful in promoting sleep. A full meal before bedtime often causes gastrointestinal upset and interferes with the ability to fall asleep.

Warn patients against drinking or eating foods with caffeine before bedtime. Coffee, tea, colas, and chocolate act as stimulants, causing a person to stay awake or to awaken throughout the night. Caffeinated foods and liquids and alcohol act as diuretics and cause a person to awaken in the night to void (National Heart, Lung, & Blood Institute, 2009).

Infants require special measures to minimize nighttime awakenings for feeding. It is common for children to need middle-of-the-night bottle-feeding or breastfeeding. Hockenberry and Wilson (2011) recommend offering the last feeding as late as possible. Tell parents not to give infants bottles in bed.

Pharmacological Approaches. Melatonin is a neurohormone produced in the brain that helps control circadian rhythms and promote sleep (Kryger et al., 2011). It is a popular nutritional supplement that is found to be helpful in improving sleep efficiency and decreasing nighttime awakenings (Pandi-Perumal et al., 2007). The recommended dose is 0.3 to 1 mg taken 2 hours before bedtime. Older adults who have decreased levels of melatonin find it beneficial as a sleep aid (Kryger et al., 2011). Short-term use of melatonin has been found to be safe, with mild side effects of nausea, headache, and dizziness being infrequent (Larzelere et al., 2010). Ramelton (Rozerem), a melatonin receptor agonist, is well tolerated and appears to be effective in improving sleep (Morin et al., 2007).

Several other herbal products assist in sleep. Valerian is effective in mild insomnia and RLS. It effects release of neurotransmitters and produces very mild sedation (Cuellar and Ratcliffe, 2009). Kava helps promote sleep in patients with anxiety. It needs to be used cautiously because of its potential toxic effects on the liver (Larzelere et al., 2010). Chamomile, an herbal tea, has a mild sedative effect that may be beneficial in promoting sleep (Moquin et al., 2009). Caution patients about the dosage and use of herbal compounds because the U.S. Food and Drug Administration (FDA) does not regulate them. Herbal compounds may interact with prescribed medication, and patients need to avoid using these together (Meiner, 2011).

Building Competency in Evidence-Based Practice Julie Arnold tells you that her mother used melatonin to help her sleep before her fall at home. She asks you if she should start taking melatonin to help her sleep. Based on the evidence, what is your best response to Julie?

Answers to questions can be found on the Evolve website.

BOX 42-10 CULTURAL ASPECTS OF CARE

Co-sleeping

Practices and patterns of sleep and rest vary among cultures. Culture and biology influence the development of sleep problems in children. Sleep patterns, bedtime routines, sleep aids, and sleep arrangements are components of cultural practices related to the use of space and interaction distances (Giger and Davidhizer, 2008). Traditionally experts recommend having infants and children sleep in their own beds. Co-sleeping, in which infants and children sleep with their parents, is a culturally preferred habit; and the practice of co-sleeping varies between cultures (AABMPC, 2008). It is more common in nonindustrialized countries. In some parts of the world co-sleeping practices are seen as part of the bonding process and warmth and protection for an infant (i.e., against the cold) (Sobralske and Gruber, 2009). This practice is also common in the United States with Asian, Hispanic, and African American families (AABMPC, 2008; Lahr et al., 2007). Health care providers in the United States discourage this practice because of safety issues, even though research does not show that the practice is unsafe. American culture promotes independence in childhood. One belief is that co-sleeping does not promote this independence; thus health care providers discourage it (Getter and McKenna, 2010). Research results related to co-sleeping and the incidence of sudden infant death syndrome (SIDS) are mixed (Getter and McKenna, 2010). As a nurse, be culturally sensitive when discussing co-sleeping practices with parents and developing sleeping plans for children. The type of bed for a child also varies. Some Native American tribes use a cradle board for infants, whereas American Samoan infants sleep on a pandanus mat covered with a blanket. These approaches lessen the child's anxiety and create a strong sense of security (Andrews and Boyle, 2008).

Implications for Practice

- Complete a thorough sleep assessment of the child and family.
- Discuss the risks of co-sleeping with parents. During the discussion remain culturally sensitive and respectful of the parents' views (Sobralske and Gruber, 2009).
- Co-sleeping has been linked to increased risk of SIDS under certain conditions such as parental smoking and alcohol or drug use (Getter and McKenna, 2010).
- Instruct parents that practice co-sleeping to avoid using alcohol or drugs that impair arousal. Decreased arousal prevents the parents from awakening if the child is having problems (Sobralske and Gruber, 2009).
- Co-sleeping should occur only with parents and not another adult or child (AABMPC, 2008).
- Co-sleeping should occur on a firm mattress (never on a water bed, sofa or couch) (AABMPC, 2008; Sobralske and Gruber, 2009).
- Encourage parents to use light sleeping clothes, keep room temperature comfortable, and not bundle the child tightly or in too many clothes.
- Avoid using heavy quilts, comforters, pillows, and stuffed animals in the bed (AABMPC, 2008).

The use of nonprescription sleeping medications is not advisable. Patients need to learn the risks of such drugs. Over the long term these drugs lead to further sleep disruption, even when they initially seemed to be effective. Caution older adults about using over-the-counter antihistamines because of their long duration of action, which can cause confusion, constipation, urinary retention, and increased risk of falls (Passarella and Duong, 2008). Help patients use behavioral and proper sleep hygiene measures to establish sleep patterns that do not require the use of drugs.

Acute Care. Patients in acute care settings have their normal rest and sleep routine disrupted, which generally leads to sleep

BOX 42-11 EVIDENCE-BASED PRACTICE

Creating a Sleep Environment in the Hospital

PICO Question: What are best practices for a sleep hygiene protocol to create an environment conducive to sleep for adult patients in a hospital?

Evidence Summary

Hospitalization causes a disruption in normal sleep habits for patients. Sleep in hospitalized patients is disrupted by noise, lighting, and patient-care activities. Sleep is needed for healing and recovery (Richardson et al., 2009). Implementing a specific sleep protocol that includes sleep hygiene measures is an effective strategy to improve sleep quality and ability to stay asleep in hospitalized patients (LaReau et al., 2008). A specified daytime quiet-time intervention that includes limiting treatment activities, use of positioning and pain-relief methods, and reduction of environmental stressors such as lighting and noise significantly improves patient sleep. There is a direct relationship between noise levels and number of patients sleeping (Gardner et al., 2009; Richardson et al., 2009). Raising staff awareness of noise levels and harmful effects of noise and providing education about strategies to reduce noise are effective in removing barriers to patient sleep (Richardson et al., 2009).

Application to Nursing Practice

- Cluster nursing activities to provide uninterrupted periods of sleep (LaReau et al., 2008).
- Provide programs for staff on the effects of noise and noise-reduction strategies (Richardson et al., 2009).
- Develop a designated quiet time period during the day that incorporates rest and reduction of noise on the unit (Gardner et al., 2009).
- Reduce lighting, telephone volumes, and staff conversations in the halls during quiet time and nighttime (Gardner et al., 2009)
- Use sleep hygiene measures with patients such as personal hygiene, adjusting room temperature, and relaxation methods (LaReau et al., 2008).

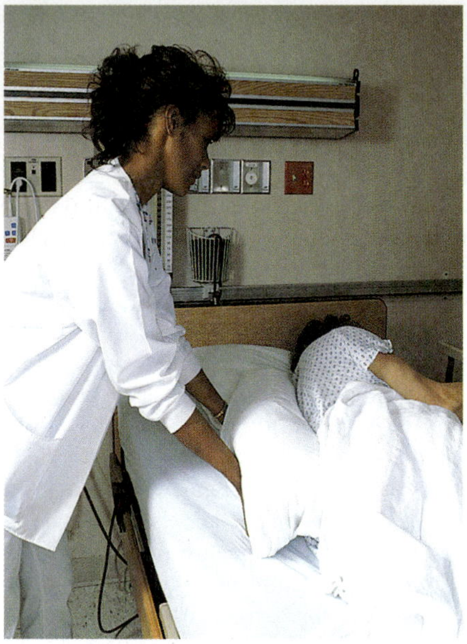

FIG. 42-6 Positioning patient for sleep.

BOX 42-12 CONTROL OF NOISE IN THE HOSPITAL

- Close doors to patients' room when possible.
- Keep doors to work areas on unit closed when in use.
- Reduce volume of nearby telephone and paging equipment.
- Wear rubber-soled shoes. Avoid clogs.
- Turn off bedside oxygen and other equipment that is not in use.
- Turn down alarms and beeps on bedside monitoring equipment.
- Turn off room television and radio unless patient prefers soft music.
- Avoid abrupt loud noise such as flushing a toilet or moving a bed.
- Keep necessary conversations at low levels, particularly at night.
- Conduct conversations and reports in a private area away from patient rooms.

problems. In this setting nursing interventions focus on controlling factors in the environment that disrupt sleep, relieving physiological or psychological disruptions to sleep, and providing for uninterrupted rest and sleep periods for the patient. "Excessive Sleepiness" in the *Evidence-based Geriatric Nursing Protocols for Best Practice* is based on the principle that nurses need to individualize an effective strategy based on patient needs and that sleep medications are a last-resort intervention (Chasens et al., 2008).

Environmental Controls. In a hospital the nurse controls the environment in several ways (Box 42-11). Close the curtains between patients in semiprivate rooms. Dim lights on a hospital nursing unit at night. One of the biggest problems for patients in the hospital is noise. Important ways to reduce noise are to conduct conversations and reports in a private area away from patient rooms and keep necessary conversations to a minimum, especially at night (Gardner et al., 2009). Additional ways to control noise in the hospital are listed in Box 42-12.

Promoting Comfort. Compared with beds at home, hospital beds are often harder and of a different height, length, or width. Keeping them clean and dry and in a comfortable position helps patients relax. Some patients suffer painful illnesses requiring special comfort measures such as application of dry or moist heat, use of supportive dressings or splints, and proper positioning before retiring (Fig. 42-6).

Establishing Periods of Rest and Sleep. In a hospital or extended care setting it is difficult to provide patients with the time needed to rest and sleep. The most effective treatment for sleep disturbances is elimination or correction of factors that disrupt the sleep pattern. You need to plan care to avoid awakening patients for nonessential tasks. Do this by scheduling assessments, treatments, procedures, and routines for times when patients are awake. For example, if a patient's physical condition has been stable, avoid awakening him or her to check vital signs. Allowing patients to determine the timing and methods of delivery of basic care measures promotes rest. Do not give baths and routine hygiene measures during the night for nursing convenience. Draw blood samples at a time when the patient is awake. Unless maintaining the therapeutic blood level of a drug is essential, give medications during waking hours. Work with the radiology department and other support services to schedule diagnostic studies and therapies at intervals that allow patients time for rest. Always try to provide the patient with 2 to 3 hours of uninterrupted sleep during the night.

When the patient's condition demands more frequent monitoring, plan activities to allow extended rest periods. A nurse instructs assistive personnel in the coordination of patient care to reduce patient disturbances. This means planning activities so the patient has as long as an hour or more to rest quietly rather than having a nurse or other personnel return to the room every few minutes.

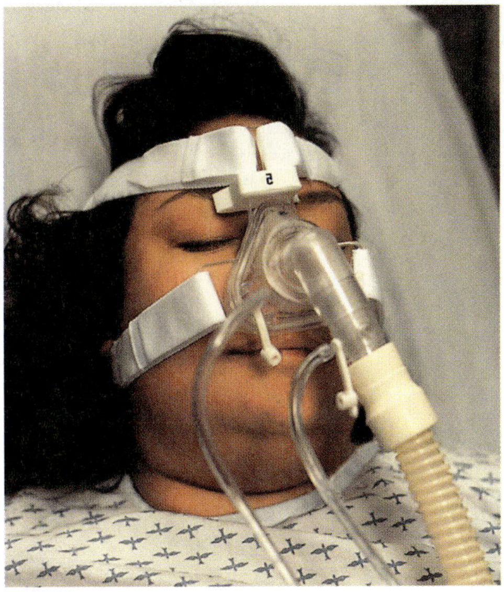

FIG. 42-7 Mask suitable for continuous positive airway pressure (CPAP).

For example, if a patient needs frequent dressing changes, is receiving intravenous therapy, and has drainage tubes from several sites, do not make a separate trip into the room to check each problem. Instead use a single visit to perform all three tasks. Become the patient's advocate for promoting optimal sleep. This means becoming a gatekeeper by postponing or rescheduling visits by family, asking consultants to reschedule visits, or questioning the frequency of certain procedures.

Promoting Safety. Patients with OSA are at risk for complications while in the hospital. Surgery and anesthesia disrupt normal sleep patterns. After surgery patients reach deep levels of REM sleep. This deep sleep causes muscle relaxation that leads to OSA (Hwang et al., 2008). Patients with OSA who are given opioid analgesics after surgery have an increased risk of developing airway obstruction because the medications suppress normal arousal mechanisms (Hwang et al., 2008). These patients often need ventilator support in the postoperative period because of the increased risk of respiratory complications. Monitor the patient's airway, respiratory rate, depth, and breath sounds frequently after surgery.

Recommend lifestyle changes to patients with OSA that include sleep hygiene, alcohol moderation, smoking cessation, and a weight-loss program (Freedman, 2010). Teach the patient to elevate the head of the bed and use a side or prone position for sleep. Use pillows to prevent a supine position (Lamm et al., 2008; Pinto and Caple, 2010).

One of the most effective therapies is use of a nasal continuous positive airway pressure (CPAP) device at night, which requires a patient to wear a mask over the nose. A mask delivers room air at a high pressure (Fig. 42-7). The air pressure prevents airway collapse. The CPAP device is portable and effective particularly for obstructive apnea. Another treatment option is the use of an oral appliance. These appliances advance the mandible or tongue to relieve pharyngeal obstruction (Wickwire and Collop, 2010). In cases of severe sleep apnea the tonsils, uvula, or portions of the soft palate are surgically removed. The success of surgical procedures to correct OSA varies.

Stress Reduction. Patients who are hospitalized for extensive diagnostic testing often have difficulty resting or sleeping because of uncertainty about the state of their health. Giving patients control over their health care minimizes uncertainty and anxiety. Providing information about the purpose of procedures and routines and answering questions give patients the peace of mind needed to rest or fall asleep. A nurse on the night shift needs to take time to sit and talk with patients unable to sleep. This helps to determine the factors keeping patients awake. Back rubs also help patients relax more thoroughly. If a sedative is indicated, confer with the patient's health care provider to be sure that the lowest dose is used initially. Discontinuing a sedative as soon as possible prevents a dependence that seriously disrupts the normal sleep cycle. Older adults' metabolism of drugs is slow, making them more vulnerable to the side effects of sedatives, hypnotics, antianxiety drugs, or analgesics.

Restorative or Continuing Care. The nursing interventions implemented in the acute care setting are also used in the restorative or continuing care environment. Controlling the environment, especially noise; establishing periods of rest and sleep; and promoting comfort are important considerations. Nursing interventions related to stress reduction and controlling physiological disturbances are also implemented in these settings. Helping a patient achieve restful sleep in this environment sometimes takes time.

Promoting Comfort. Providing for personal hygiene improves a patient's sense of comfort. A warm bath or shower before bedtime is relaxing. Offer patients restricted to bed the opportunity to void and wash their face and hands. Toothbrushing and care of dentures also help to prepare patients for sleep. Position patients to support their dependent body parts and protect pressure points. Offer a back or hand massage to aid in muscle relaxation just before a patient goes to sleep (Harris and Richards, 2010) (see Chapter 43).

Controlling Physiological Disturbances. As a nurse you will learn to control symptoms of physical illness that disrupt sleep. For example, a patient with respiratory abnormalities sleeps with two pillows or in a semi-sitting position to ease the effort to breathe. He or she benefits from taking prescribed bronchodilators before sleep to prevent airway obstruction. A patient with a hiatal hernia also needs special care. After meals he or she often experiences a burning sensation as a result of gastric reflux. To prevent sleep disturbances have the patient eat a small meal several hours before bedtime and sleep in a semi-sitting position. Patients with pain, nausea, or other recurrent symptoms receive any symptom-relieving medication timed so the drug takes effect at bedtime. Remove or change any irritants against the patient's skin such as moist dressings or drainage tubes.

Pharmacological Approaches. The liberal use of drugs to manage insomnia is quite common in American culture. CNS stimulants such as amphetamines, caffeine, nicotine, terbutaline, theophylline, and modafinil need to be used sparingly and under medical management (Lehne, 2010). In addition, withdrawal from CNS depressants such as alcohol, barbiturates, tricyclic antidepressants (amitriptyline, imipramine, and doxepin), and triazolam causes insomnia. You need to manage these carefully.

Medications that induce sleep are called **hypnotics. Sedatives** are medications that produce a calming or soothing effect (Lehne, 2010). A patient who takes sleep medications needs to know about their proper use and their risks and possible side effects. Long-term use of antianxiety, sedative, or hypnotic agents disrupts sleep and leads to more serious problems. The FDA requires that the product labels of all sleep medications contain safety information related to the potential adverse effects of severe allergic reactions; severe facial swelling; and complex sleep behaviors such as sleep-driving, making phone calls, and preparing and eating food while asleep (USFDA, 2010).

Benzodiazepines and nonbenzodiazepines are common classifications of drugs used to treat sleep problems. The nonbenzodiazepines have become the treatment of choice for insomnia because of improved efficacy and safety of use (Neubauer, 2009). Experts recommend a low dose of a short-acting medication such as zolpidem (Ambien) for short-term use (no longer than 2 to 3 weeks) (Cramwell-Bruce, 2007). These drugs cause fewer problems with dependence and abuse and fewer rebound insomnia and hangover effects than benzodiazepines (Passarella and Duong, 2008).

The benzodiazepines cause relaxation, antianxiety, and hypnotic effects by facilitating the action of neurons in the CNS that suppress responsiveness to stimulation, thereby decreasing levels of arousal (Lehne, 2010). Short-acting benzodiazepines (e.g. oxazepam, lorazepam, or temazepam) at the lowest possible dose are recommended. Initial doses are small; and increments are added gradually, based on patient response, for a limited time. Warn patients not to take more than the prescribed dose, especially if the medication seems to become less effective after initial use. The use of benzodiazepines in older adults is potentially dangerous because of the tendency of the drugs to remain active in the body for a longer time. As a result, they also cause respiratory depression; next-day sedation; amnesia; rebound insomnia; and impaired motor functioning and coordination, which leads to increased risk of falls (Cramwell-Bruce, 2007; Neubauer, 2009). If older patients who were recently continent, ambulatory, and alert become incontinent or confused and/or demonstrate impaired mobility, the use of benzodiazepines needs to be considered as a possible cause.

Use benzodiazepines cautiously with children under 12 years of age. These medications are contraindicated in infants less than 6 months. Pregnant patients need to avoid them because their use is associated with risk of congenital anomalies. Nursing mothers do not receive the drugs because they are excreted in breast milk.

Regular use of any sleep medication often leads to tolerance and withdrawal. Rebound insomnia is a problem after stopping the medication. Immediately administering a sleeping medication when a hospitalized patient complains of being unable to sleep does the patient more harm than good. Consider alternative approaches to promote sleep. Routine monitoring of patient response to sleeping medications is important.

EVALUATION

Through the Patient's Eyes. With regard to problems with sleep, the patient is the source for evaluating outcomes. Each patient has a unique need for sleep and rest. The patient is the only one who knows if sleep problems are improved and which interventions or therapies are most successful in promoting sleep (Fig. 42-8). To evaluate the effectiveness of nursing interventions, make comparisons with baseline assessment data to evaluate if sleep has improved. It is important to ask the patient if his or her sleep needs have been met. For example, ask the patient, "Are you feeling more rested?"; "Can you tell me if you feel we have done all we can to help improve your sleep?"; or "What interventions have been most effective in helping you sleep?" If expectations have not been met, you need to spend more time trying to understand the patient's needs and preferences. Working closely with the patient and bed partner enables you to redefine expectations that can be met realistically within the limits of the patient's condition and treatment.

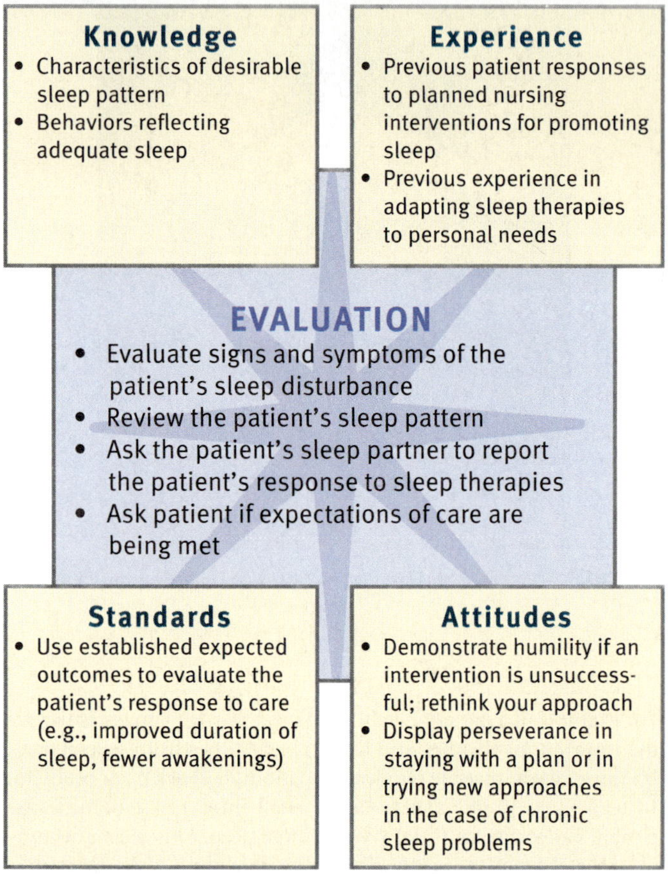

Knowledge
• Characteristics of desirable sleep pattern
• Behaviors reflecting adequate sleep
Experience
• Previous patient responses to planned nursing interventions for promoting sleep
• Previous experience in adapting sleep therapies to personal needs
EVALUATION
• Evaluate signs and symptoms of the patient's sleep disturbance
• Review the patient's sleep pattern
• Ask the patient's sleep partner to report the patient's response to sleep therapies
• Ask patient if expectations of care are being met
Standards
• Use established expected outcomes to evaluate the patient's response to care (e.g., improved duration of sleep, fewer awakenings)
Attitudes
• Demonstrate humility if an intervention is unsuccessful; rethink your approach
• Display perseverance in staying with a plan or in trying new approaches in the case of chronic sleep problems

FIG. 42-8 Critical thinking model for sleep evaluation.

Patient Outcomes. Determine whether expected outcomes have been met. Use evaluative measures shortly after a therapy has been tried (e.g., observing whether a patient falls asleep after reducing noise and darkening a room). Use other evaluative measures after a patient awakens from sleep (e.g., asking a patient to describe the number of awakenings during the previous night). The patient and bed partner usually provide accurate evaluative information. Over longer periods use assessment tools such as the visual analogue or sleep-rating scale to determine whether sleep has progressively improved or changed.

Also evaluate the level of understanding that patients or family members gain after receiving instruction in sleep habits. You measure compliance with these practices during a home visit, when you are able to observe the environment. When expected outcomes are not met, revise the nursing measures or expected outcomes based on the patient's needs or preferences. When outcomes are not met, ask questions such as:

- Are you able to fall asleep within 20 minutes of getting in bed?
- Describe how well you sleep when you exercise.
- Does the use of quiet music at bedtime help you to relax?
- Do you feel rested when you wake up?

If a nurse has successfully developed a good relationship with a patient and a therapeutic plan of care, subtle behaviors often indicate the level of the patient's satisfaction. Note the absence of signs of sleep problems such as lethargy or frequent yawning or position changes in the patient. You are effective in promoting rest and sleep if the patient's goals and expectations are met.

KEY POINTS

- Sleep provides physiological and psychological restoration.
- The 24-hour sleep-wake cycle is a circadian rhythm that influences physiological function and behavior.
- The control and regulation of sleep depends on a balance among regulators within the CNS.
- During a typical night's sleep a person passes through four to five complete sleep cycles. Each sleep cycle contains three NREM stages of sleep and a period of REM sleep.
- The most common type of sleep disorder is insomnia.
- The hectic pace of a person's lifestyle, emotional and psychological stress, and alcohol ingestion frequently disrupt the sleep pattern.
- If a patient's sleep is adequate, assess his or her usual bedtime, normal bedtime ritual, preferred environment for sleeping, and usual preferred rising time.
- When a patient has a sleep problem, conduct a complete sleep history. Diagnosing sleep problems depends on identifying factors that impair sleep.
- When planning interventions to promote sleep, considers the usual characteristics of the patient's home environment and normal lifestyle.
- A regular bedtime routine of relaxing activities prepares a person physically and mentally for sleep.
- An environment with a darkened room, reduced noise, comfortable bed, and good ventilation promotes sleep.
- Important nursing interventions for promoting sleep in the hospitalized patient are establishing periods for uninterrupted sleep and rest and controlling noise levels.
- Pain or other disease symptom control is essential to promoting the ability to sleep.
- Long-term use of sleeping pills often leads to difficulty initiating and maintaining sleep.

CLINICAL APPLICATION QUESTIONS

Preparing for Clinical Practice

Julie returns to the neighborhood health clinic with her husband, David, for a follow-up visit. She tells you that since she started her sleep hygiene plan she feels more rested but is still having some problems sleeping because of her husband's loud snoring. Besides Julie's report of David's snoring, you note that he is overweight.

1. Based on Julie's report of David's snoring, which additional assessment data should you gather from David?
2. Based on David's reported symptoms, what problem do you suspect he might have? What recommendations do you give David to improve his sleeping?
3. Julie and David tell you that they are concerned about their 6-year-old daughter. She just started school and is having sleep problems. List at least four interventions for Julie and David to use to improve their daughter's sleep patterns.

evolve *Answers to Clinical Application Questions can be found on the Evolve website.*

REVIEW QUESTIONS

Are You Ready to Test Your Nursing Knowledge?

1. The nurse is gathering a sleep history from a patient who is being evaluated for obstructive sleep apnea. Which common symptoms does the patient most likely report? (Select all that apply.)
   1. Headache
   2. Early wakening
   3. Excessive daytime sleepiness
   4. Difficulty falling asleep
   5. Snoring
2. The nurse incorporates which priority nursing intervention into a plan of care to promote sleep for a hospitalized patient?
   1. Have patient follow hospital routines
   2. Avoid awakening patient for nonessential tasks
   3. Give prescribed sleeping medications at dinner
   4. Turn television on low to late-night programming.
3. Older adults are cautioned about the long-term use of sedatives and hypnotics because these medications can:
   1. Cause headaches and nausea.
   2. Be expensive and difficult to obtain.
   3. Cause severe depression and anxiety.
   4. Lead to sleep disruption.
4. The nurse is providing health teaching for a patient using herbal compounds such as melatonin for sleep. Which points need to be included? (Select all that apply.)
   1. Can cause urinary retention
   2. Should not be used indefinitely
   3. May cause diarrhea and anxiety
   4. May interfere with prescribed medications
   5. Can lead to further sleep problems over time
   6. Are not regulated by the U.S. Food and Drug Administration (FDA)
5. The patient reports vivid dreaming to the nurse. Through understanding of the sleep cycle, the nurse recognizes that vivid dreaming occurs during which sleep phase?
   1. REM sleep
   2. Stage 1 NREM sleep
   3. Stage 4 NREM sleep
   4. Transition period from NREM to REM sleep
6. The nurse teaches a patient taking a benzodiazepine that this group of medications causes which symptom of a sleep problem?
   1. Nocturia
   2. Hyperactivity
   3. Grogginess and feeling hung over
   4. Increased sleep time
7. Which intervention is appropriate to include on a care plan for improving sleep in the older adult?
   1. Decrease fluids 2 to 4 hours before sleep
   2. Exercise in the evening to increase fatigue
   3. Allow the patient to sleep as late as possible
   4. Take a nap during the day to make up for lost sleep
8. Which statement made by a mother being discharged to home with her newborn infant indicates a need for further teaching?
   1. "I won't put the baby to bed with a bottle."
   2. "For the first few weeks we're putting the cradle in our room."
   3. "My grandmother told me that babies sleep better on their stomachs."
   4. "I know I'll have to get up during the night to feed the baby when he wakes up."
9. The nurse is developing a plan of care for a patient experiencing narcolepsy. Which intervention is appropriate to include on the plan?

1. Instruct the patient to increase carbohydrates in the diet
2. Have patient limit fluid intake 2 hours before bedtime
3. Preserve energy by limiting exercise to morning hours
4. Encourage patient to take one or two 20-minute naps during the day

10. Which nursing measure best promotes sleep in a school-age child?
    1. Encourage evening exercise
    2. Offer a glass of hot chocolate before bedtime
    3. Make sure that the room is dark and quiet
    4. Use quiet activities consistently before bedtime
11. Which action by the nursing assistant at bedtime requires the nurse to intervene?
    1. Giving the patient a back rub
    2. Turning on quiet music
    3. Dimming the lights in the patient's room
    4. Giving a patient a cup of coffee
12. Which statement made by the patient indicates a need for further teaching on sleep hygiene?
    1. "I'm going to do my exercises before I eat dinner."
    2. "I'll have a glass of wine at bedtime to relax."
    3. "I set my alarm to get up at the same time every morning."
    4. "I moved my computer to the den to do my work."
13. Which statement made by an older adult best demonstrates understanding of taking a sleep medication?
    1. "I'll take the sleep medicine for 4 or 5 weeks until my sleep problems disappear."
    2. "Sleep medicines won't cause any sleep problems once I stop taking them."
    3. "I'll talk to my health care provider before I use an over-the-counter sleep medication."
    4. "I'll contact my health care provider if I feel extreme sleepy in the mornings."
14. The school nurse is teaching health-promoting behaviors that improve sleep to a group of high school students. Which points should be included in the education? (Select all that apply.)
    1. Do not study in your bed.
    2. Go to sleep each night whenever you feel tired.
    3. Turn off your cell phone at bedtime.
    4. Avoid drinking coffee or soda before bedtime.
    5. Turn on the television to help you fall asleep.
15. The nurse is taking a sleep history from a patient. Which statement made by the patient needs further follow-up?
    1. I always feel tired when I wake up in the morning.
    2. I go to bed at the same time each night.
    3. It takes me about 15 minutes to fall asleep.
    4. Sometimes I have to get up during the night to urinate.

Answers: **1.** 1, 3, 5; **2.** 2; **3.** 4; **4.** 2, 4, 6; **5.** 1; **6.** 3; **7.** 1; **8.** 3; **9.** 4; **10.** 4; **11.** 4; **12.** 2; **13.** 3; **14.** 1, 3, 4; **15.** 1.

REFERENCES

Adult Obstructive Sleep Apnea Task Force of the American Academy of Sleep Medicine: Clinical guideline for the evaluation, management and long-term care of obstructive sleep apnea in adults, *J Clin Sleep Med* 5(3):263, 2009.

Ahmed I, Thorpy M: Clinical features, diagnosis and treatment of narcolepsy, *Clin Chest Med* 31(2):371, 2010.

American Academy of Breastfeeding Medical Protocol Committee (AABMPC): ABM clinical protocol #6: guideline on co-sleeping and breastfeeding, *Breastfeeding Med* 3(1):38, 2008.

American Nurses Association: *Nursing scope and standards of practice*, Washington, DC, 2010, The Association.

Andrews MM, Boyle JS: *Transcultural concepts in nursing care*, ed 5, Philadelphia, 2008, Lippincott.

Babson KA, et al: Cognitive behavioral therapy for sleep disorders, *Psych Clin North Am* 33(3):629, 2010.

Benca RM, Schneck CH: Sleep and eating disorders. In Kruger MH et al, editors: *Principles and practice of sleep medicine*, ed 4, St Louis, 2005, Saunders.

Bulechek GM, Butcher HK, Dochterman JM: *Nursing interventions classification (NIC)*, ed 5, St Louis, 2008, Mosby.

Chasens ER, et al: Excessive sleepiness. In Capezuti E et al, editors: *Evidence-based geriatric nursing protocols for best practice*, ed 3, New York, 2008, Springer.

Cramwell-Bruce LA: Hypnotic sedative drugs, *Medsurg Nurs* 16(3):198, 2007.

Cuellar NG, et al: Assessment and treatment of sleep disorders in the elderly, *Geriatr Nurs* 28(4):254, 2007.

Ebersole P, et al: *Toward healthy aging: human needs and nursing response*, ed 7, St Louis, 2008, Mosby.

Freedman N: Treatment of obstructive sleep apnea, *Clin Chest Med* 31:187, 2010.

Getter LT, McKenna JJ: Never sleep with baby? Or keep me close but keep me safe; eliminating inappropriate "safe infant sleep" rhetoric in the United States, *Curr Pediatr Rev* 6(1):71, 2010.

Giger JN, Davidhizar RE: *Transcultural nursing: assessment and intervention*, ed 5, St Louis, 2008, Mosby.

Heaton K, et al: Sleep and motor vehicle crashes, *J Emerg Nurs* 35(4):363, 2009.

Hockenberry MJ, Wilson D: *Wong's nursing care of infants and children*, ed 9, St Louis, 2011, Mosby.

Hwang D, et al: Association of sleep-disordered breathing with post-operative complications, *CHEST* 133(5):1128, 2008.

Izac SM: Basic anatomy and physiology of sleep, *Am J Electroneurodiagnostic Technol* 46:18, 2006.

Kryger MH, et al: *Principles and practice of sleep medicine*, ed 5, St Louis, 2011, Saunders.

Lamm J, et al: Obtaining a thorough sleep history and routinely screening for obstructive sleep apnea, *J Am Acad Nurs Pract* 20:225, 2008.

Larzelere MM, et al: Complementary and alternative medicine usage for behavioral health indicators, *Prim Care Clin Office Pract* 37(2):213, 2010.

Lashley F: Measuring sleep. In Frank-Stromborg M, Olsen SJ, editors: *Instruments for clinical-healthcare research*, ed 3, Boston, 2004, Jones & Bartlett.

Lehne RA: *Pharmacology for nurses*, ed 7, St Louis, 2010, Mosby.

Malhotra RK, Desai AK: Healthy brain aging: what has sleep got to do with it? *Clin Geriatr Med* 26:45, 2010.

McCance KL et al, editors: *Pathophysiology: the biologic basis for disease in adults and children*, ed 6, St Louis, 2010, Mosby.

Meiner SE: *Gerontologic nursing*, ed 4, St Louis, 2011, Mosby.

Moquin B, et al: Complementary and alternative medicine, *Geriatr Nurs* 30(3):196, 2009.

Morin AK, et al: Therapeutic options for sleep-maintenance and sleep-onset insomnia, *Pharmacotherapy* 27(1):89, 2007.

Natarajan R: Review of periodic limb movement and restless leg syndrome, *J Postgrad Med* 56(2):157, 2010.

National Guideline Clearinghouse: *Clinical guideline for the evaluation and management of chronic insomnia in adults*, NCG7396, 2008, http://www.guideline.gov/content.aspx?id=15089. Accessed October 10, 2011.

National Heart, Lung, and Blood Institute: *How is insomnia treated?* 2009, http://www.nhlbi.nih.gov/health/health-topics/topics/inso/treatment.html. Accessed December 10, 2011.

National Sleep Foundation: *Aging and sleep*, Washington, DC, 2009, http://www.sleepfoundation.org/article/sleep-topics/aging-and-sleep. Accessed October 10, 2011.

National Sleep Foundation: *The ABCs of ZZZs* [Brochure], Washington, DC, 2010a, The Foundation.

National Sleep Foundation: *Apnea and sleep*, Washington, DC, 2010b, http://www.sleepfoundation.org/article/sleep-topics/sleep-apnea-and-sleep. Accessed October 10, 2011.

National Sleep Foundation: *Depression and sleep*, 2010c, http://www.sleepfoundation.org/article/sleep-topics/depression-and-sleep. Accessed October 10, 2011.

Neikrug AB, Ancoli-Israel S: Sleep disorders in the older adult—a mini review, *Gerontology* 56:181, 2010.

Neubauer DN: Current and new thinking in the management of comorbid insomnia, *Am J Manag Care* 15(1):S24, 2009.

Ohlmann KK, O'Sullivan MI: The costs of short sleep, *AAOHN J* 57(9):381, 2009.

Pandi-Perumal SR, et al: Role of melatonin system in the control of sleep, *CNS Drugs 2007* 21(12):995, 2007.

Passarella S, Duong M: Diagnosis and treatment of insomnia, *Am J Health Syst Pharmacol* 65:927, 2008.

Pinto S, Caple C: Obstructive sleep apnea in adults, *CINAHL Information Systems*, April 23, 2010.

Ramakrishnan K, Scheid DC: Treatment options for insomnia, *Am Fam Physician* 76(4):517, 2007.

Redeker N: Sleep disturbance in people with heart failure: implications for self-care, *J Cardiovasc Nurs* 23(3):231, 2008.

Reeve K, Bailes B: Insomnia in adults: etiology and management, *J Nurs Pract* 6(1):53, 2010.

Smyth CA: Evaluating sleep quality in older adult, *Am J Nurs* 108(5):42, 2008.

Touhy TA, Jett KF: *Ebersole and Hess' gerontological nursing healthy aging*, ed 3, St Louis, 2010, Mosby.

Townsend-Roccichelli J, et al: Managing sleep disorders in the elderly, *Nurse Pract* 35(5):30, 2010.

US Food and Drug Administration: *Side effects of sleep drugs*, 2010, http://www.fda.gov/ForConsumers/ConsumerUpdates/ucm107757.htm. Accessed October 10, 2011.

Van der Zee EA, et al: The neurobiology of circadian rhythms, *Curr Opinion Pulmonary Med* 15:534, 2009.

Wickwire EM, Collop NA: Insomnia and sleep-related breathing disorders, *CHEST* 137(6):1449, 2010.

RESEARCH REFERENCES

Cuellar NG, Ratcliffe SJ: Does valerian improve sleepiness and symptom severity in people with restless legs syndrome? *Alt Ther Health Med* 15(2):22, 2009.

Dennis CM, et al: Benefits of quiet time for neurointensive care patients, *J Neurosci Nurs* 42(4):217, 2010.

Fontana CJ, Pittiglio LI: Sleep deprivation among critical care patients, *Crit Care Nurs Q* 33(1):75, 2010.

Gardner G, et al: Creating a therapeutic environment: a non-randomized controlled trial of a quiet time intervention for patients in acute care, *Int J Nurs Stud* 46:778, 2009.

Harris M, Richards KC: The physiological and psychological effect of slow-stroke back massage and hand massage on relaxation in older people, *J Clin Nurs* 19:197, 2010.

Irwin MR, et al: Comparative meta-analysis of behavioral interventions for insomnia and their efficacy in middle-aged adults and in older adults 55+ years of age, *Health Psych* 25(1):3, 2006.

Koren A, et al: Parental information and behaviors and provider practices related to tummy time and back to sleep, *J Pediatr Health Care* 24(4):222, 2010.

Lahr MAB, et al: Maternal-infant bed sharing: risk factors for bedsharing in a population-based survey of new mothers and implications for SIDS risk reduction, *Matern Chld Health J* 11(3):277, 2007.

LaReau R, et al: Examining the feasibility of implementing specific nursing interventions to promote sleep in hospitalized elderly patients, *Geriatr Nurs* 29(3):197, 2008.

Natale V, et al: Actigraphy in the assessment of insomnia: a quantitative approach, *Sleep* 32(6):767, 2009.

Noland H, et al: Adolescents' sleep behaviors and perceptions of sleep, *J School Health* 79(5):224, 2009.

Richardson A, et al: Development and implementation of a noise reduction intervention programme: a pre- and postaudit of three hospital wards, *J Clin Nurs* 18:3316, 2009.

Sheldon A, et al: Nursing assessment of obstructive sleep apnea in hospitalized adults: a review of risk factors and screening tools, *Contemp Nurse* 34(1):19, 2009.

Sobralske MC, Gruber ME: Risks and benefits of parent/child bed sharing, *J Am Acad Nurs Pract* 21:474, 2009.

Vallido T, et al: Sleep in adolescence: a review of issues for nursing practice, *J Clin Nurs* 18:1819, 2009.

CHAPTER

43

Pain Management

OBJECTIVES

- Discuss common misconceptions about pain.
- Describe the physiology of pain.
- Identify components of the pain experience.
- Explain how the physiology of pain relates to selecting interventions for pain relief.
- Describe the components of pain assessment.
- Be able to perform an assessment of a patient experiencing pain.
- Explain how cultural factors influence the pain experience.
- Describe guidelines for selecting and individualizing pain interventions.
- Explain various pharmacological approaches to treating pain.
- Describe applications for use of nonpharmacological pain interventions.
- Discuss nursing implications for administering analgesics.
- Identify barriers to effective pain management.
- Evaluate a patient's response to pain interventions.

KEY TERMS

Acupressure, p. 980
Acute pain, p. 965
Addiction, p. 988
Adjuvants, p. 981
Analgesics, p. 981
Biofeedback, p. 978
Breakthrough pain, p. 986
Chronic pain, p. 965
Cutaneous stimulation, p. 978
Drug tolerance, p. 988
Epidural analgesia, p. 985
Guided imagery, p. 978
Idiopathic pain, p. 966
Local anesthesia, p. 985
Modulation, p. 964
Neurotransmitters, p. 963
Nociceptor, p. 963
Opioids, p. 981
Pain threshold, p. 964
Pain tolerance, p. 964
Patient-controlled analgesia (PCA), p. 983
Perception, p. 963
Perineural infusion, p. 984
Physical dependence, p. 988
Placebos, p. 989
Prostaglandins, p. 963
Pseudoaddiction, p. 965
Regional anesthesia, p. 985
Relaxation, p. 978
Transcutaneous electrical nerve stimulation (TENS), p. 981
Transduction, p. 963
Transmission, p. 963

evolve WEBSITE

http://evolve.elsevier.com/Potter/fundamentals/

- Review Questions
- Video Clips
- Concept Map Creator
- Case Study with Questions
- Skills Performance Checklists
- Audio Glossary
- Interactive Learning Activities
- Key Term Flashcards
- Content Updates

Everyone eventually experiences some type or degree of pain. Although it is the most common reason that people seek health care, pain is not well understood. A person in pain feels distress or suffering and seeks relief. As the nurse you cannot see or feel the patient's pain. It is purely subjective. No two people experience pain in the same way, and no two painful events create identical responses or feelings in a person. The International Association for the Study of Pain (IASP) defines pain as "an unpleasant, subjective sensory *and* emotional experience associated with actual or potential tissue damage, or described in terms of such damage" (IASP, 2010).

Congress declared 2000 to 2010 the Decade of Pain Control and Research, yet pain continues to be a leading public health problem in the United States. Providing pain relief is a basic human right and is in the Pain Care Bill of Rights (APF, 2007). According to the American Bar Association (2009), pain management is a basic right of people who are seriously ill. Nurses are legally and ethically responsible for managing pain and relieving suffering.

When caring for patients in pain, consider the nurse-patient relationship, patient advocacy, patient empowerment, compassion, and respect (Vaartio et al., 2009). Caring for patients in pain requires recognition that pain can and should be relieved. Effective communication among the patient, family, and professional caregivers is essential to achieve adequate pain management. You show respect for a patient in pain when you accept McCaffery's classic definition: "Pain is whatever the experiencing person says it is, existing whenever he says it does" (Pasero and McCaffery, 2011). Effective pain management improves quality of life; reduces physical discomfort; promotes earlier mobilization and return to previous activity levels; results in fewer hospital and clinic visits; and decreases hospital lengths of stay, resulting in lower health care costs.

SCIENTIFIC KNOWLEDGE BASE

Nature of Pain

The pain experience is complex, involving physical, emotional, and cognitive components. Pain is subjective and highly individualized. Its stimulus is physical and/or mental in nature. Pain uses a person's energy. It interferes with personal relationships and influences the meaning of life. You cannot measure it objectively. Only the patient knows whether pain is present and how the experience feels. It is not the responsibility of patients to prove that they are in pain; it is a nurse's responsibility to accept their report (APS, 2003).

Physiology of Pain

There are four physiological processes of nociceptive (normal) pain: transduction, transmission, perception, and modulation (Pasero and McCaffery, 2011). A patient in pain cannot discriminate among the processes. Understanding each process helps you recognize factors that cause pain, symptoms that accompany it, and the rationale for selected therapies.

Thermal, chemical, or mechanical stimuli usually cause pain. **Transduction** converts energy produced by these stimuli into electrical energy Transduction begins in the periphery when a pain-producing stimulus sends an impulse across a sensory peripheral pain nerve fiber **(nociceptor),** initiating an action potential. Once transduction is complete, **transmission** of the pain impulse begins.

Cellular damage caused by thermal, mechanical, or chemical stimuli results in the release of excitatory **neurotransmitters** such as **prostaglandins,** bradykinin, substance P, and histamine (Box 43-1). These pain-sensitizing substances surround the pain fibers in the extracellular fluid, creating an "inflammatory soup," spreading the pain message and causing an inflammatory response (Pasero and McCaffery, 2011). The pain stimulus enters the spinal cord via the dorsal horn and travels one of several routes until ending within the gray matter of the spinal cord. At the dorsal horn substance P is released, causing a synaptic transmission from the afferent (sensory) peripheral nerve to spinothalamic tract nerves, which cross to the opposite side (Pasero and McCaffery, 2011) (Fig. 43-1).

Nerve impulses resulting from the painful stimulus travel along afferent (sensory) peripheral nerve fibers. Two types of peripheral nerve fibers conduct painful stimuli: the fast, myelinated A-delta fibers and the very small, slow, unmyelinated C fibers. The A fibers send sharp, localized, and distinct sensations that specify the source of the pain and detect its intensity. The C fibers relay impulses that are poorly localized, burning, and persistent. For example, after stepping on a nail, a person initially feels a sharp, localized pain, which is a result of A-fiber transmission. Within a few seconds the pain becomes more diffuse and widespread, until the whole foot hurts because of C-fiber innervations (Pasero and McCaffery, 2011).

Along the spinothalamic tract, pain impulses travel up the spinal cord (Fig. 43-2). After the pain impulse ascends the spinal cord, the thalamus transmits information to higher centers in the brain, including the reticular formation, limbic system, somatosensory cortex, and association cortex. Once a pain stimulus reaches the cerebral cortex, the brain interprets the quality of the pain and processes information from past experience, knowledge, and cultural associations in the perception of the pain (Pasero and McCaffery, 2011). **Perception** is the point at which a person is aware of pain. The somatosensory cortex identifies the location and intensity of pain, whereas the association cortex, primarily

BOX 43-1 NEUROPHYSIOLOGY OF PAIN: NEUROREGULATORS

Neurotransmitters (Excitatory)

Prostaglandins

- Generated from the breakdown of phospholipids in cell membranes
- Thought to increase sensitivity to pain

Bradykinin

- Released from plasma that leaks from surrounding blood vessels at the site of tissue injury
- Binds to receptors on peripheral nerves, increasing pain stimuli
- Binds to cells that cause the chain reaction producing prostaglandins

Substance P

- Found in the pain neurons of the dorsal horn (excitatory peptide)
- Needed to transmit pain impulses from the periphery to higher brain centers
- Causes vasodilation and edema

Histamine

- Produced by mast cells causing capillary dilation and increases capillary permeability

Serotonin

- Released from the brainstem and dorsal horn to inhibit pain transmission

Neuromodulators (Inhibitory)

- Are natural supply of morphine-like substances in the body
- Activated by stress and pain
- Located within the brain, spinal cord, and gastrointestinal tract
- Cause analgesia when they attach to opiate receptors in the brain
- Present in higher levels in people who have less pain than others with a similar injury

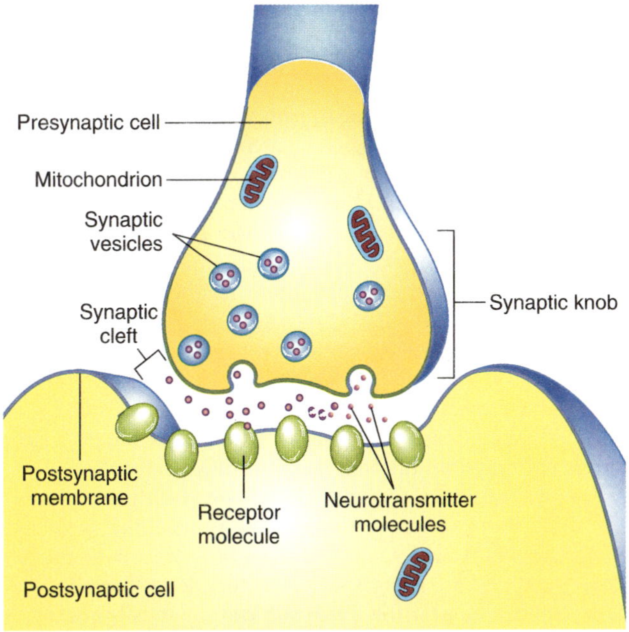

FIG. 43-1 Chemical synapses involve transmitter chemicals (neurotransmitters) that signal postsynaptic cells. (From Patton KT, Thibodeau GA: *Anatomy & physiology*, ed 7, St Louis, 2010, Mosby.)

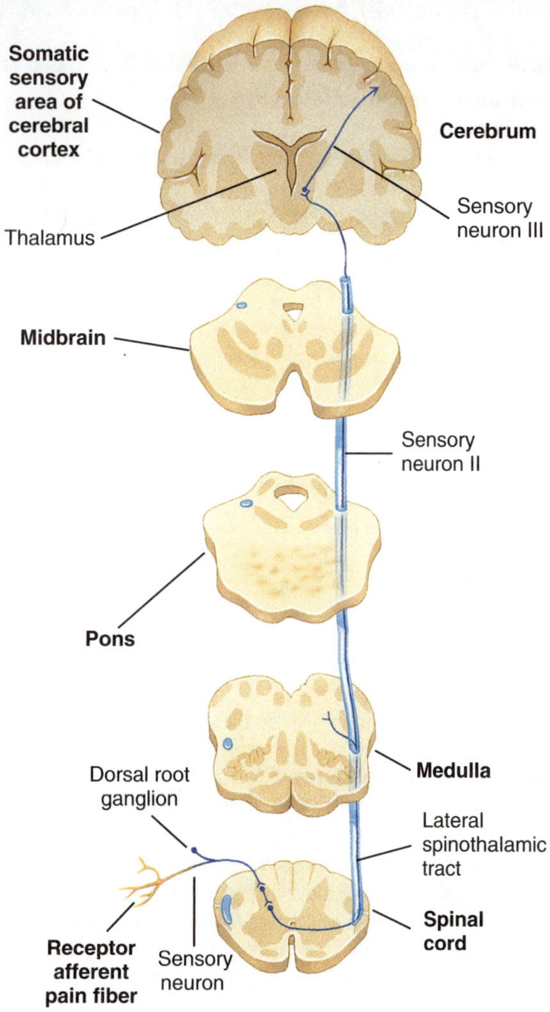

FIG. 43-2 Spinothalamic pathway that conducts pain stimuli to the brain.

the limbic system, determines how a person feels about it. There is no single pain center.

As a person becomes aware of pain, a complex reaction occurs. Psychological and cognitive factors interact with neurophysiological ones in the perception of pain. Perception gives awareness and meaning to pain, resulting in a reaction. The reaction to pain includes the physiological and behavioral responses that occur after an individual perceives pain (Pasero and McCaffery, 2011).

Once the brain perceives pain, there is a release of inhibitory neurotransmitters (see Box 43-1) such as endogenous opioids, serotonin, norepinephrine, and gamma aminobutyric acid (GABA), which work to hinder the transmission of pain and help produce an analgesic effect (Pasero and McCaffery, 2011). This inhibition of the pain impulse is the fourth and last phase of the nociceptive process known as **modulation** (Pasero and McCaffery, 2011).

A protective reflex response also occurs with pain reception (Fig. 43-3). A-delta fibers send sensory impulses to the spinal cord, where they synapse with spinal motor neurons. The motor impulses travel via a reflex arc along efferent (motor) nerve fibers back to a peripheral muscle near the site of stimulation, thus bypassing the brain. Contraction of the muscle leads to a protective withdrawal from the source of pain. For example, when you accidentally touch a hot iron, you feel a burning sensation, but your hand also reflexively withdraws from the surface of the iron.

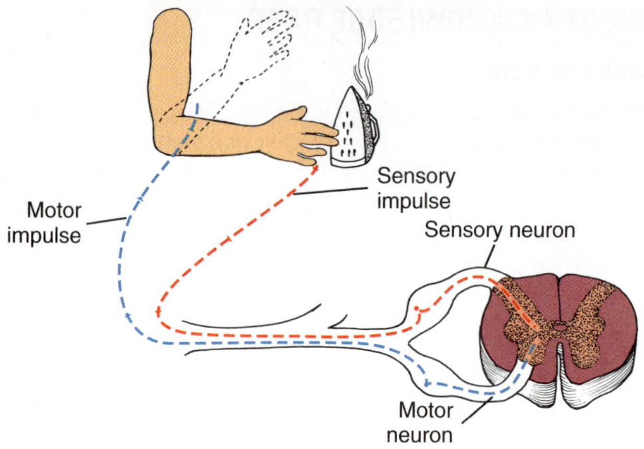

FIG. 43-3 Protective reflex to pain stimulus.

Gate-Control Theory of Pain. Melzack and Wall's gate-control theory (1965) first suggested that pain has emotional and cognitive components in addition to a physical sensation. According to this theory, gating mechanisms located along the central nervous system regulate or even block pain impulses. Pain impulses pass through when a gate is open and are blocked when a gate is closed. Closing the gate is the basis for nonpharmacological pain-relief interventions. You gain a useful conceptual framework for pain management by understanding the physiological, emotional, and cognitive influences on the gates. For example, factors such as stress and exercise increase the release of endorphins, often raising an individual's **pain threshold** (the point at which a person feels pain). Because the amount of circulating substances varies with every individual, the response to pain varies.

Physiological Responses. As pain impulses ascend the spinal cord toward the brainstem and thalamus, the stress response stimulates the autonomic nervous system. Pain of low to moderate intensity and superficial pain elicit the fight-or-flight reaction of the general adaptation syndrome (see Chapter 37). Stimulation of the sympathetic branch of the autonomic nervous system results in physiological responses (Table 43-1). Continuous, severe, or deep pain typically involving the visceral organs (e.g., with a myocardial infarction or colic from gallbladder or renal stones) activates the parasympathetic nervous system. Sustained physiological responses to pain sometimes seriously harm individuals. Except in cases of severe traumatic pain, which causes a person to go into shock, most people adapt to their pain, and their physical signs return to normal. Thus patients in pain do *not* always have changes in their vital signs. Changes in vital signs more often indicate problems other than pain.

Behavioral Responses. If left untreated or unrelieved, pain significantly alters quality of life. It usually interferes with every aspect of a person's life, which supports why effective pain management is essential. It threatens physical and psychological well-being. Some patients choose not to report pain if they believe that it inconveniences others or if it signals loss of self-control, and some endure severe pain without assistance. Encourage your patients to accept pain-relieving measures so they remain active and continue to maintain daily activities. In contrast, other patients seek relief before pain occurs, having learned that prevention is easier than treatment. A patient's ability to tolerate pain significantly influences your perceptions of the degree of the patient's discomfort. Patients who have a low **pain tolerance** (level of pain a person is willing to accept) are sometimes inaccurately perceived

TABLE 43-1 Physiological Reactions to Pain

RESPONSE	CAUSE OR EFFECT
Sympathetic Stimulation*	
Dilation of bronchial tubes and increased respiratory rate	Provides increased oxygen intake
Increased heart rate	Provides increased oxygen transport
Peripheral vasoconstriction (pallor, elevation in blood pressure)	Elevates blood pressure with shift of blood supply from periphery and viscera to skeletal muscles and brain
Increased blood glucose level	Provides additional energy
Diaphoresis	Controls body temperature during stress
Increased muscle tension	Prepares muscles for action
Dilation of pupils	Affords better vision
Decreased gastrointestinal motility	Frees energy for more immediate activity
Parasympathetic Stimulation†	
Pallor	Causes blood supply to shift away from periphery
Muscle tension	Results from fatigue
Decreased heart rate and blood pressure	Results from vagal stimulation
Rapid, irregular breathing	Causes body defenses to fail under prolonged stress of pain

*Pain of low-to-moderate intensity and superficial pain.
†Severe or deep pain.

as complainers. Teach patients the importance of reporting their pain sooner rather than later.

Body movements and facial expressions indicating pain include clenched teeth, holding the painful area, bent posture, and grimacing. Some patients cry or moan, are restless, or make frequent requests of a nurse. You soon learn to recognize patterns of behavior that reflect pain. This becomes especially important in patients who are unable to report their pain such as the cognitively impaired. However, lack of pain expression does not indicate that the patient is not experiencing pain (Pasero and McCaffery, 2011).

Types of Pain

Pain is categorized by duration (acute or chronic) or pathological condition (e.g., cancer or neuropathic).

Acute/Transient Pain. Acute pain is protective, has an identifiable cause, is of short duration, and has limited tissue damage and emotional response. It eventually resolves, with or without treatment, after an injured area heals. Because acute pain has a predictable ending (healing) and an identifiable cause, health team members are usually willing to treat it aggressively. Unrelieved acute pain can progress to chronic pain (Kehlet et al., 2006).

Acute pain seriously threatens a patient's recovery by resulting in prolonged hospitalization, increased risks of complications from immobility (see Chapter 47), and delayed rehabilitation. Physical and psychological progress is delayed as long as acute pain persists because a patient focuses all energy on pain relief. Efforts aimed at teaching and motivating the patient toward self-care are often hampered until the pain is successfully managed. Complete pain relief is not always achievable, but reducing pain to a tolerable level is realistic. Thus a primary nursing goal is to provide pain relief that allows patients to participate in their recovery.

Chronic/Persistent Noncancer Pain. Unlike acute pain, chronic pain is not protective and thus serves no purpose. Chronic pain lasts longer than 6 months and is constant or recurring with a mild-to-severe intensity (Ackley and Ladwig, 2011). It does *not* always have an identifiable cause and leads to great personal suffering. Examples of chronic noncancer pain include arthritis, low back pain, myofascial pain, headache, and peripheral neuropathy. Chronic pain is usually non–life threatening. Sometimes an injured area healed long ago, yet the pain is ongoing and does not respond to treatment.

The possible unknown cause of chronic pain, combined with the unrelenting nature and uncertainty of its duration, frustrates a patient, frequently leading to psychological depression and even suicide. Chronic pain is a major cause of psychological and physical disability, leading to problems such as job loss, inability to perform simple daily activities, sexual dysfunction, and social isolation.

The person with chronic noncancer pain often does not show obvious symptoms and does not adapt to the pain. Rather, he or she seems to suffer more with time because of physical and mental exhaustion. Associated symptoms of chronic pain include fatigue, insomnia, anorexia, weight loss, apathy, hopelessness, and anger. Chronic pain creates the uncertainty of how one will feel from day to day. If there is no objective evidence to confirm the existence of pain, the "burden of proof" lies with the patient (Shaw, 2006). Health care workers are usually less willing to treat chronic noncancer pain with opioids, although a policy statement supports the use of opioids for it (Chou et al., 2009). In addition, the American Society of Anesthesiologists (2010) developed "Practice Guidelines for Chronic Pain Management," which includes the use of opioids. Often a person with chronic pain who consults with numerous health care providers is labeled a drug seeker, when he or she is actually seeking adequate pain relief. This situation is called pseudoaddiction. Nurses need to discourage patients from having multiple health care providers for treating pain and refer them to pain specialists. Pain centers offer a holistic approach to chronic pain using both nonpharmacological and pharmacological strategies for pain management (Pasero and McCaffery, 2011).

Chronic Episodic Pain. Pain that occurs sporadically over an extended period of time is episodic pain. Pain episodes last for hours, days, or weeks. Examples are migraine headaches and pain related to sickle cell disease (Gruener and Lande, 2006).

Cancer Pain. Not all patients with cancer experience pain. For those who do, as many as 90% are able to have their pain managed with relatively simple means (Lehne, 2010). Some patients with cancer experience acute and/or chronic pain. The pain is nociceptive and/or neuropathic. Cancer pain is usually caused by tumor progression and related pathological processes, invasive procedures, toxicities of treatment, infection, and physical limitations. A patient senses pain at the actual site of the tumor or distant to the site, called *referred pain*. Assess reports of new pain by a patient with existing pain. Although the treatment of cancer pain has improved, undertreatment of cancer pain continues. Approximately 70% to 90% of patients with advanced cancer experience pain. Sixty percent of them report moderate-to-severe pain (Maxwell et al., 2005).

Pain by Inferred Pathological Process. Identifying the cause of pain is the first step in successful treatment. Nociceptive pain includes somatic (musculoskeletal) and visceral (internal organ) pain. Neuropathic pain arises from abnormal or damaged

TABLE 43-2 **Classification of Pain by Inferred Pathology**

NOCICEPTIVE PAIN	NEUROPATHIC PAIN
I. *Nociceptive pain:* Normal processing of stimuli that damages normal tissues or has the potential to do so if prolonged; usually responsive to nonopioids and/or opioids A. *Somatic pain:* Comes from bone, joint, muscle, skin, or connective tissue; is usually aching or throbbing in quality and well localized B. *Visceral pain:* Arises from visceral organs such as the gastrointestinal tract and pancreas; is sometimes subdivided: 1. Tumor involvement of organ capsule that causes aching and fairly well–localized pain 2. Obstruction of hollow viscus, which causes intermittent cramping and poorly localized pain	II. *Neuropathic pain:* Abnormal processing of sensory input by the peripheral or central nervous system; treatment usually includes adjuvant analgesics A. Centrally generated pain 1. *Deafferentation pain:* Injury to either the peripheral or central nervous system *Examples:* Phantom pain indicates injury to the peripheral nervous system; burning pain below the level of a spinal cord lesion reflects injury to the central nervous system. 2. *Sympathetically maintained pain:* Associated with impaired regulation of the autonomic nervous system *Examples:* Pain associated with complex regional pain syndrome, type I, type II B. Peripherally generated pain 1. *Painful polyneuropathies:* Pain felt along the distribution of many peripheral nerves. *Examples:* Diabetic neuropathy, alcohol-nutritional neuropathy, and Guillain-Barré syndrome. 2. *Painful mononeuropathies:* Usually associated with a known peripheral nerve injury; pain felt at least partly along the distribution of the damaged nerve *Examples:* Nerve root compression, nerve entrapment, trigeminal neuralgia

From Pasero C, McCaffery M: *Pain assessment and pharmacologic management*, St Louis, 2011, Mosby.

pain nerves (Table 43-2). Each of these pathological processes has distinct pain characteristics. The pain assessment section discusses these further.

Idiopathic Pain. **Idiopathic pain** is chronic pain in the absence of an identifiable physical or psychological cause or pain perceived as excessive for the extent of an organic pathological condition. An example of idiopathic pain is complex regional pain syndrome (CRPS). Research is needed to better identify the causes of idiopathic pain, thus leading to a more effective treatment (Pasero and McCaffery, 2011).

NURSING KNOWLEDGE BASE

Nursing knowledge of pain mechanisms and interventions continues to grow through nursing research. This section explores factors that influence the pain experience.

Knowledge, Attitudes, and Beliefs

Attitudes of nurses and other health care providers affect pain management. The traditional medical model of illness generates attitudes about pain. This model suggests that physical problems result from physical causes. Thus pain is a physical response to organic dysfunction. When there is no obvious source of pain (e.g., the patient with chronic low back pain or neuropathies), health care providers sometimes stereotype pain sufferers as malingerers, complainers, or difficult patients.

Studies of nurses' attitudes regarding pain management show that a nurse's personal opinion about a patient's report of pain affects pain assessment and titration of opioid doses. The amount of analgesia administered varies based on whether a patient is grimacing or smiling during the nurse's assessment (Pasero and McCaffery, 2011). Nurses with more than 6 years of work experience, higher job motivation, and perceived higher levels of pain-care skills in themselves often use more patient advocacy skills in providing pain management for patients (Vaartio et al., 2009).

Nurses' assumptions about patients in pain seriously limit their ability to offer pain relief. Biases based on culture, education, and experience influence everyone. Too often nurses allow misconceptions about pain (Box 43-2) to affect their willingness to intervene. Some nurses avoid acknowledging a patient's pain because of their own fear and denial. They do not believe a patient's report of pain if he or she does not look in pain. You are entitled to your personal beliefs; however, you must *accept* a patient's report of pain and act according to professional guidelines, standards, position statements, policies and procedures, and evidence-based research findings (Pasero and McCaffery, 2011).

BOX 43-2 **COMMON BIASES AND MISCONCEPTIONS ABOUT PAIN**

The following statements are *false:*
- Patients who abuse substances (e.g., use drugs or alcohol) overreact to discomforts.
- Patients with minor illnesses have less pain than those with severe physical alteration.
- Administering analgesics regularly leads to drug addiction.
- The amount of tissue damage in an injury accurately indicates pain intensity.
- Health care personnel are the best authorities on the nature of a patient's pain.
- Psychogenic pain is not real.
- Chronic pain is psychological.
- Patients who are hospitalized will experience pain.
- Patients who cannot speak do not feel pain.

To help a patient gain pain relief, view the experience through the patient's eyes. Acknowledging personal prejudices or misconceptions helps you address patient problems more professionally. When you become an active, knowledgeable observer of a patient in pain, you more objectively analyze the pain experience. The patient makes the diagnosis that pain is present, and you apply interventions that ultimately give relief.

Factors Influencing Pain

Pain is a complex process, involving physiological, social, spiritual, psychological, and cultural influences. Thus each individual's pain experience is different. Consider all factors that affect the patient in pain to ensure a holistic approach to the assessment and care of the patient.

BOX 43-3 FOCUS ON OLDER ADULTS

Factors Influencing Pain in Older Adults

- With aging, muscle mass decreases, body fat increases, and percentage of body water decreases. This increases concentration of water-soluble drugs such as morphine, and the volume of distribution for fat-soluble drugs such as fentanyl increases (Lehne, 2010).
- Older adults frequently eat poorly, resulting in low serum albumin levels. Many drugs are highly protein bound. In the presence of low serum albumin, more free drug (active form) is available, thus increasing the risk for side and/or toxic effects (Lehne, 2010).
- A decline of liver and renal function naturally occurs with aging. This results in reduced metabolism and excretion of drugs. Thus older adults often experience a greater peak effect and longer duration of analgesics (Arnstein, 2010).
- Age-related changes in the skin such as thinning and loss of elasticity affect the absorption rate of topical analgesics.

TABLE 43-3 Pain in Infants

MISCONCEPTION	CORRECTION
Infants cannot feel pain.	Infants have the anatomical and functional requirements for pain processing by mid-to-late gestation.
Infants are less sensitive to pain than older children and adults.	Term neonates have the same sensitivity to pain as older infants and children. Preterm neonates have a greater sensitivity to pain than term neonates or older children.
Infants cannot express pain.	Although infants cannot verbalize pain, they respond with behavioral cues and physiological indicators that are observable.
Infants must learn about pain from previous painful experiences.	Pain requires no prior experience; infants do not need to learn it from earlier painful experience. It occurs with the first insult.
You cannot accurately assess pain in infants.	You use behavioral cues (e.g., facial expressions, cry, body movements) and physiological indicators of pain (e.g., changes in vital signs) to reliably and validly assess pain in infants.
You cannot safely give analgesics and anesthetics to infants and neonates because of their immature capacity to metabolize and eliminate drugs and their sensitivity to opioid-induced respiratory depression.	Infants are very sensitive to drugs. Response to drugs is often intense and prolonged. Absorption is faster than expected. Dosages of drugs excreted by the kidneys need to be reduced (Lehne, 2010). Prescribers carefully select the medication, dosage, administration route, and time. Nurses monitor frequently for desired and undesired effects. Nurses also follow medication orders to titrate and wean medications to minimize adverse effects.

Physiological Factors

Age. Age influences pain, particularly in infants and older adults. Developmental differences found between these age-groups influence how children and older adults react to pain. Young children have trouble understanding pain and the procedures that cause it. If they have not developed full vocabularies, they have difficulty verbally describing and expressing pain to parents or caregivers. Toddlers and preschoolers are unable to recall explanations about pain or associate it with experiences that occur in various situations. With these developmental considerations in mind, you need to adapt approaches for assessing a child's pain, including what to ask and the behaviors to observe, and how to prepare a child for a painful medical procedure.

Pain is not an inevitable part of aging. However, older adults have a greater likelihood of developing pathological conditions, which are accompanied by pain. Serious impairment of functional status often accompanies pain in older patients. Pain potentially reduces mobility, activities of daily living (ADLs), social activities, and activity tolerance. The presence of pain in an older adult requires aggressive assessment, diagnosis, and management (Box 43-3).

The ability of older patients to interpret pain is complicated. They often suffer from multiple diseases with vague symptoms that affect similar parts of the body. You need to make detailed assessments when there is more than one source of pain. Different diseases sometimes cause similar symptoms. For example, chest pain does not always indicate a heart attack; it also is a symptom of arthritis of the spine or an abdominal disorder. When older adults experience cognitive impairment and confusion, they have difficulty recalling pain experiences and providing detailed explanations of their pain (Pasero and McCaffery, 2011). You need to address misconceptions about pain management in the very young and in older adults before intervening for a patient (Tables 43-3 and 43-4).

Fatigue. Fatigue heightens the perception of pain and decreases coping abilities. If it occurs along with sleeplessness, the perception of pain is even greater. Pain is often experienced less after a restful sleep than at the end of a long day.

Genes. Research on healthy human subjects suggests that genetic information passed on by parents possibly increases or decreases the person's sensitivity to pain and determines pain threshold or pain tolerance. A study of twins by Kato et al. (2006) suggested modest genetic influence in the development of chronic widespread pain without significant differences experienced between men and women.

Neurological Function. A patient's neurological function influences the pain experience. Any factor that interrupts or influences normal pain reception or perception (e.g., spinal cord injury, peripheral neuropathy, or neurological disease) affects the patient's awareness of and response to pain. Some pharmacological agents (analgesics, sedatives, and anesthetics) influence pain perception and response and thus require close monitoring.

Social Factors

Attention. The degree to which a patient focuses attention on pain influences pain perception. Increased attention is associated with increased pain, whereas distraction is associated with a diminished pain response. This concept is one that nurses apply in various pain-relief interventions such as relaxation, guided imagery, and massage. By focusing patients' attention and concentration on other stimuli, their perception of pain declines (see Chapter 32).

Previous Experience. Each person learns from painful experiences. Prior experience does not mean that a person accepts pain more easily in the future. Previous frequent episodes of pain without relief or bouts of severe pain cause anxiety or fear. In contrast, if a person repeatedly experiences the same type of pain that was relieved successfully in the past, the patient finds it easier to interpret the pain sensation. As a result, the patient is better prepared to take necessary actions to relieve the pain.

TABLE 43-4 Misconceptions About Pain in Older Adults

MISCONCEPTION	CORRECTION
Pain is a natural outcome of growing old.	Older adults are at greater risk (as much as twofold) than younger adults for many painful conditions; however, pain is not an inevitable result of aging.
Pain perception, or sensitivity, decreases with age.	This assumption is unsafe. Although there is evidence that emotional suffering specifically related to pain is possibly less in older than in younger patients, no scientific basis exists for the claim that a decrease in perception of pain occurs with age or that age dulls sensitivity to pain.
If the older patient does not report pain, he or she does not have pain.	Older patients commonly underreport pain. Reasons include expecting to have pain with increasing age; not wanting to alarm loved ones; being fearful of losing their independence; not wanting to distract, anger, or bother caregivers; and believing that caregivers know they have pain and are doing all they can to relieve it. The absence of a report of pain does not mean the absence of pain.
If an older patient appears to be occupied, asleep, or otherwise distracted from pain, he or she does not have pain.	Older patients often believe that it is unacceptable to show pain and have learned to use a variety of ways to cope with it (e.g., many patients use distraction successfully for short periods of time). Sleeping is sometimes a coping strategy; alternately, it indicates exhaustion, not pain relief. Do not make assumptions about the presence or absence of pain solely on the basis of a patient's behavior.
The potential side effects of opioids make them too dangerous to use to relieve pain in older adults.	Opioids are safe to use in older adults with moderate-to-severe pain (Arnstein, 2010). Although the opioid-naive older adult is usually more sensitive to opioids, this does not justify withholding their use in pain management. Slow titration prevents potentially dangerous opioid-induced side effects. Regular, frequent monitoring and assessment of a patient's response are necessary. Adjust dose and interval between doses when you detect side effects. If necessary, administer an opioid antagonist drug to reverse clinically significant respiratory depression.
Patients with Alzheimer's disease and other cognitive impairments do not feel pain, and their reports of pain are most likely invalid.	No evidence exists that cognitively impaired older adults experience less pain or that their reports of pain are less valid than those of individuals with intact cognitive function (Herr, 2010). Patients with dementia or other deficits of cognition most likely suffer significant unrelieved pain and discomfort. Assessment of pain in these patients is challenging but possible. The best approach is to accept a patient's report of pain and treat it as you would treat it in an individual with intact cognitive function.
Older patients report more pain as they age.	Even though older patients experience a higher incidence of painful conditions such as arthritis, osteoporosis, peripheral vascular disease, and cancer than younger patients, studies show that they underreport pain. Many older adults grew up valuing the ability to "grin and bear it" (Pasero and McCaffery, 2011).

When a patient has no experience with a painful condition, the first perception of it often impairs the ability to cope. For example, after abdominal surgery it is common for patients to experience severe incisional pain for several days. Unless a patient knows this is a common occurrence following surgery, the onset of pain seems like a serious complication. Rather than participate actively in postoperative breathing exercises (see Chapter 50), the patient lies immobile in bed and breathes shallowly because of fear that something is not right. In the anticipatory phase of the pain experience, you need to prepare a patient with a clear explanation of the type of pain to expect and methods to reduce it. This usually results in a reduced perception of pain.

Family and Social Support. People in pain often depend on family members or close friends for support, assistance, or protection. Although pain still exists, the presence of family or friends can often make the pain experience less stressful. The presence of parents is especially important for children experiencing pain.

Spiritual Factors. Spirituality stretches beyond religion and includes an active searching for meaning to situations in which one finds oneself. Spiritual questions include "Why has this happened to me?" "Why am I suffering?" Spiritual pain goes beyond what we can see. "Why has God done this to me?" "Is this suffering teaching me something?" Other spiritual concerns include loss of independence and becoming a burden to family (Otis-Green et al., 2002). Consider making a referral to pastoral care for patients in pain. Recall that pain is an experience that has physical *and* emotional components. Thus providing interventions designed to treat both aspects is essential for the best possible pain management (see Chapter 35).

Psychological Factors

Anxiety. A person perceives pain differently if it suggests a threat, loss, punishment, or challenge. For example, a woman in labor perceives pain differently than a woman with a history of cancer who is experiencing a new pain and fearing recurrence. In addition, the degree and quality of pain perceived by a patient influences the meaning of pain. The relationship between pain and anxiety is complex. Anxiety often increases the perception of pain, and pain causes feelings of anxiety. It is difficult to separate the two sensations.

Critically ill or injured patients who perceive a lack of control over their environment and care have high anxiety levels. This anxiety leads to serious pain-management problems. Pharmacological and nonpharmacological approaches to the management of anxiety are appropriate; however, anxiolytic medications are not a substitute for analgesia (Pasero and McCaffery, 2011).

Coping Style. Coping style influences the ability to deal with pain. Persons with internal loci of control perceive themselves as having control over events in their life and the outcomes such as pain. In contrast, persons with external loci of control perceive that other factors in their life such as nurses are responsible for the outcome of events. Patient-controlled analgesia (PCA) uses this concept. Patients who self-administer small doses of intravenous (IV) pain medication using PCA during an acute episode successfully achieve pain control more quickly than those who rely on nurses to administer intermittent doses of pain medications.

BOX 43-4 CULTURAL ASPECTS OF CARE

Assessing Pain in Culturally Diverse Patients

Pain is a biopsychosocial phenomenon. Culture shapes the experience of pain, its expression, its behaviors, or coping responses. Culture also affects lay remedies, help-seeking activities, and receptivity to medical treatment. Some health care providers undertreat pain because they do not understand the cultural effects on the perception of pain intensity. Differences exist both within cultural and ethnic groups and among them. Nurses care for patients with pain from a variety of cultures; thus you need to develop strategies to assess and manage pain in culturally diverse patients.

Implications for Practice

- Use culturally appropriate assessment tools to assess pain such as tools written in the patient's native language (Pasero and McCaffery, 2011).
- Recognize variations in subjective responses to pain. Some patients are stoic and less expressive, whereas others are emotive and more likely to verbalize pain.
- Be sensitive to variations in communication styles. Some cultures believe that nonverbal expression of pain is sufficient to describe the pain experience; whereas others assume that, if pain medication is appropriate, the nurse will bring it; thus asking is inappropriate.
- Understand that expression of pain is unacceptable within certain cultures. Some patients believe asking for help indicates a lack of respect, whereas others believe acknowledging pain is a sign of weakness.
- The meaning of pain varies among cultures. Pain is personal and related to religious beliefs. Some cultures consider suffering a part of life to be endured to enter heaven.
- Use knowledge of biological variations of pain. Significant differences in drug metabolism, dosing requirements, therapeutic response, and adverse effects occur in racial and ethnic groups. A wide range of responses is also possible within a cultural group. Therefore assess each patient's response to pain medication carefully.
- Develop a personal awareness of your own values and beliefs that affect your responses to patients' reports of pain.

You need to understand patients' coping resources during painful experiences. Use resources such as communicating with a supportive family, being active, or praying, in your plan of care to support patients and offer a degree of pain relief (see Chapter 37).

Cultural Factors. The meaning that a person associates with pain affects the experience of pain and how one adapts to it. This is often closely associated with a person's cultural background. Cultural beliefs and values affect how individuals cope with pain. Individuals learn what is expected and accepted by their culture, including how to react to pain. Health care providers often mistakenly assume that everyone responds to pain in the same way. Different meanings and attitudes are associated with pain across various cultural groups. An understanding of the cultural meaning of pain helps you design culturally sensitive care for people with pain (Pasero and McCaffery, 2011).

Culture affects pain expression. Some cultures believe that it is natural to be demonstrative about pain. Others tend to be more introverted. In addition, it is also important to know to what extent a member of a particular culture has assimilated into American society. For example, if several generations of a Hispanic patient's family have lived in the United States, the influence of the Spanish culture may be limited, whereas newly immigrated patients still embrace their cultural norms.

As a nurse, explore the impact of cultural differences on a patient's pain experience and make adjustments to the plan of care (Box 43-4). Work with the patient and family to facilitate communication about the assessment and management of pain. Find a culturally appropriate assessment tool and communicate use of that tool to other health care providers.

CRITICAL THINKING

Successful critical thinking requires a synthesis of knowledge, experience, information gathered from patients, critical thinking attitudes, and intellectual and professional standards. To make clinical judgments, you anticipate the information you need, analyze the data, and make decisions regarding patient care. A patient's condition or situation is always changing. During assessment consider all critical thinking elements that lead to appropriate nursing diagnoses.

Knowledge of pain physiology and the many factors that influence pain help you manage a patient's pain. Previous experience in caring for patients with pain sharpens your assessment skills and ability to choose effective therapies. Critical thinking attitudes and intellectual standards ensure the aggressive assessment, creative planning, and thorough evaluation needed to obtain an acceptable level of patient pain relief. Successful pain management does not necessarily mean pain elimination but rather attainment of a mutually agreed-on pain-relief goal that allows patients to control their pain instead of the pain controlling them.

NURSING PROCESS

Apply the nursing process and use a critical thinking approach in your care of patients. The nursing process provides a clinical decision-making approach for you to develop and implement an individualized plan of care.

Nurses approach pain management systematically to understand and treat a patient's pain. Successful management of pain depends on establishing a relationship of trust among health care providers, patient, and family. Pain management extends beyond pain relief, encompassing the patient's quality of life and ability to work productively, enjoy recreation, and function normally in the family and society.

The American Nurses Association (ANA) (2005) upholds that pain assessment and management is within the scope of every nurse's practice. Thus the ANA offers a certification examination in pain management to staff nurses (http://www.aspmn.org/certification). Several clinical guidelines are available for managing pain in specific disorders. Guidelines are available through the American Pain Society (APS) on the management of pain in the primary care setting; sickle cell pain; cancer pain in adults and children; and pain in osteoarthritis, rheumatoid arthritis, and juvenile chronic arthritis. Sigma Theta Tau International offers guidelines for the older adult on their website (www.geriatricpain.org). In addition, the National Guidelines Clearinghouse (www.guideline.gov) posts a variety of pain-management guidelines, including ones on acute, chronic, spinal, chest, low back, cancer, and pancreatic pain.

ASSESSMENT

During the assessment process, thoroughly assess each patient and critically analyze findings to ensure that you make patient-centered clinical decisions required for safe nursing care.

Through the Patient's Eyes. Many people view pain as a part of life. Some patients experience it for hours or days before seeking health care assistance. They often expect and even accept a

BOX 43-5 NURSING ASSESSMENT QUESTIONS

Current Pain

- *P*alliative or *P*rovocative factors: What makes your pain worse? What makes it better?
- *Q*uality: How do you describe your pain?
- *R*egion or *R*adiation: Show me where you hurt. Does it stay there or does it spread somewhere else?
- *S*everity: On a scale of 0 to 10, how bad is your pain now?
- What is the worst pain you have had in the past 24 hours?
- What is the average pain you have had in the past 24 hours?
- *T*iming: Is your pain constant, intermittent, or both?
- *U:* Effect of pain: What does your pain prevent you from doing that you would like to do?

Allergies

- Do you have any allergies to medications?
- What type of problems have these allergies caused?
- How are these allergies treated?

Current Medications

- What medications are you taking now?
- Are you taking any herbs?
- Are these medications and herbs effective in relieving the pain?
- Which nonpharmacological treatments have you tried to relieve the pain?
- Which medications have you tried in the past that worked to stop your pain?
- Have you ever used recreational drugs or alcohol to alleviate pain?
- Have you ever been diagnosed with a gastrointestinal bleed or a kidney or liver disorder?
- Are you being treated for any other medical conditions?
- With whom do you live, and how do they help you when you have pain?

BOX 43-6 ROUTINE CLINICAL APPROACH TO PAIN ASSESSMENT AND MANAGEMENT: ABCDE

A: ***Ask*** about pain regularly. Assess pain systematically.
B: ***Believe*** the patient and family in their report of pain and what relieves it.
C: ***Choose*** pain control options appropriate for the patient, family, and setting.
D: ***Deliver*** interventions in a timely, logical, and coordinated fashion.
E: ***Empower*** patients and their families. Enable them to control their course to the greatest extent possible.

From Jacox A et al.: *Management of cancer pain,* Clinical Practice Guideline No. 9, AHCPR Publication No. 94-0592, Rockville, Md, 1994, Agency for Health Care Policy and Research, Public Health Service, US Department of Health and Human Services.

BOX 43-7 POSSIBLE SOURCES FOR ERROR IN PAIN ASSESSMENT

- Bias, which causes nurses to consistently overestimate or underestimate the pain that patients experience
- Vague or unclear assessment questions, which lead to unreliable assessment data
- Use of pain assessment tools that are not evidence based
- Patients who do not always provide complete, relevant, and accurate pain information
- Patients who are cognitively impaired and unable to use pain scales

certain amount of pain while being hospitalized. Asking patients about their tolerable pain level is the first step in helping them regain control. Assessing previous pain experiences and effective home interventions provides a foundation on which you can build. Patients expect nurses to accept their reports of pain and be prompt in meeting their pain needs.

When assessing pain, be sensitive to the level of discomfort and determine what level will allow your patient to function. For example, when caring for a patient with pain, you ask, "What level of pain will allow you to walk down the hall?" The patient answers that walking is possible when pain is at a level of 2 on a scale of 0 to 10, with 0 being no pain and 10 being worst pain imaginable. You then focus efforts on decreasing the pain to that level. If pain is acute or severe, it is unlikely that the patient is able to provide a detailed description of the entire experience. During an episode of acute pain you primarily assess its location, severity, and quality. Collect a more detailed acute pain assessment when the patient is more comfortable (Box 43-5). For patients with chronic pain, a thorough pain assessment includes affective, cognitive, behavioral, spiritual, and social dimensions. In the home care setting family members assess pain. Using the ABCs of pain management is an effective way to manage pain (Box 43-6).

Because pain is not static but dynamic, you monitor it on a regular basis along with other vital signs. Some institutions treat pain as the fifth vital sign. Pain assessment is *not* simply a number. Relying solely on a number is unsafe (Vila et al., 2005). Although pain assessment is a nursing function, nursing assistive personnel (NAP) also screen for pain (Schulman-Green et al., 2005). NAP have the responsibility to inform the nurse immediately when a patient is having pain so the nurse is able to confirm the assessment and begin appropriate treatment.

The ability to establish a nursing diagnosis, decide on appropriate interventions, and evaluate the patient's response (outcomes) to interventions depends on the fundamental activity of a factual, timely, accurate pain assessment (Fig. 43-4). The core of this complex activity is the exploration of the pain experience through the eyes of the patient. Nurses use a variety of tools to assess nociceptive pain and neuropathic pain (Jensen et al., 2006). The goal in using these tools is to identify how much pain exists without interfering with patient function, not to identify how much pain the patient tolerates.

The Agency for Healthcare Research and Quality (AHRQ) established specific guidelines for assessing patients with acute and cancer pain. The focus is on planning successful pain-management interventions before a patient has pain. Because it involves a collaborative approach, the AHRQ pain treatment flow chart (Fig. 43-5) offers a useful conceptual approach to the control of acute pain. Patients need to understand that informed reporting of pain is valuable and necessary if the health care team is to manage it effectively.

Always be aware of possible errors in pain assessment (Box 43-7). Using the right tools and methods helps you avoid errors and ensures that you choose the right pain interventions. Failure of clinicians to assess a patient's pain, accept the findings, and treat the report of pain is a common cause of unrelieved pain and suffering (Hughes, 2008).

Patient's Expression of Pain. A patient's self-report of pain is the single most reliable indicator of its existence and intensity (APS, 2003; Pasero and McCaffery, 2011). Pain is individualistic. Many patients fail to report or discuss discomfort. At the same time

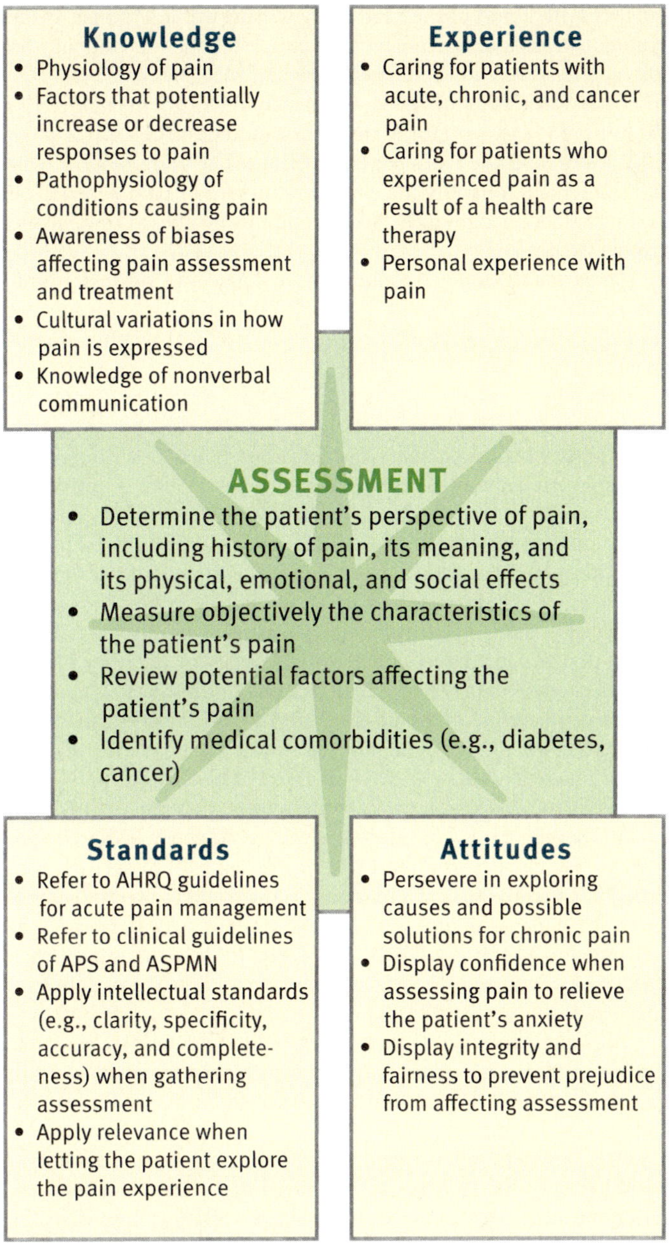
Knowledge
• Physiology of pain
• Factors that potentially increase or decrease responses to pain
• Pathophysiology of conditions causing pain
• Awareness of biases affecting pain assessment and treatment
• Cultural variations in how pain is expressed
• Knowledge of nonverbal communication
Experience
• Caring for patients with acute, chronic, and cancer pain
• Caring for patients who experienced pain as a result of a health care therapy
• Personal experience with pain
ASSESSMENT
• Determine the patient's perspective of pain, including history of pain, its meaning, and its physical, emotional, and social effects
• Measure objectively the characteristics of the patient's pain
• Review potential factors affecting the patient's pain
• Identify medical comorbidities (e.g., diabetes, cancer)
Standards
• Refer to AHRQ guidelines for acute pain management
• Refer to clinical guidelines of APS and ASPMN
• Apply intellectual standards (e.g., clarity, specificity, accuracy, and completeness) when gathering assessment
• Apply relevance when letting the patient explore the pain experience
Attitudes
• Persevere in exploring causes and possible solutions for chronic pain
• Display confidence when assessing pain to relieve the patient's anxiety
• Display integrity and fairness to prevent prejudice from affecting assessment

FIG. 43-4 Critical thinking model for pain assessment. *AHRQ,* Agency for Healthcare Research and Quality; *ANA,* American Nurses Association; *ASPMN,* American Society for Pain Management Nursing.

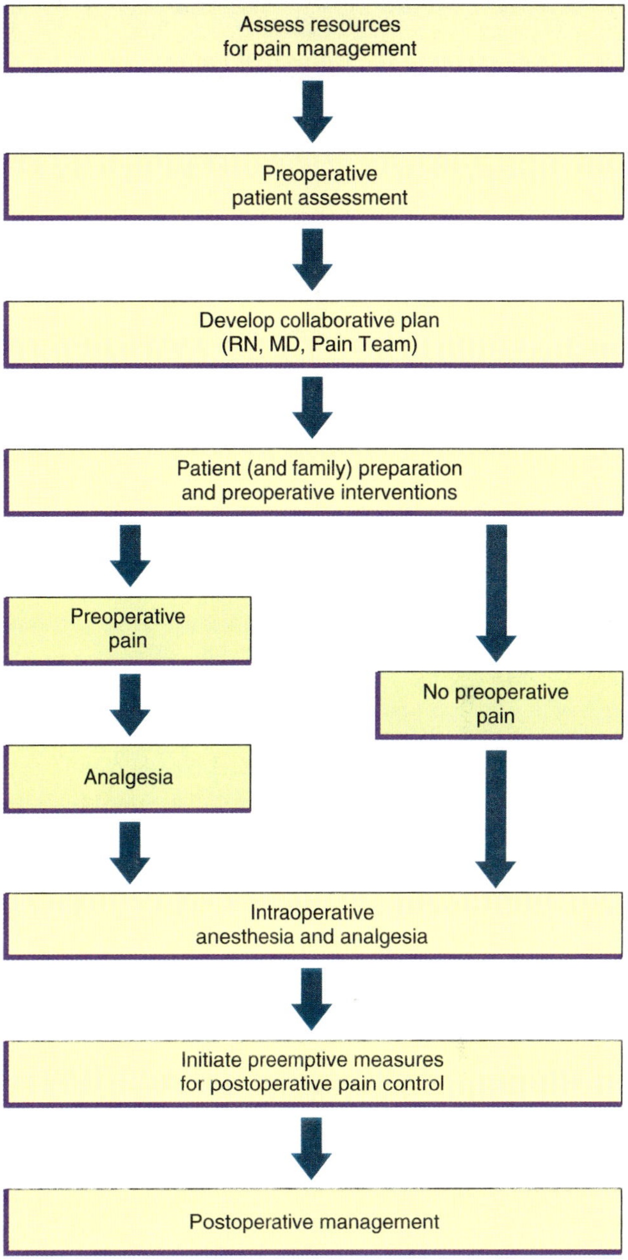

FIG. 43-5 Pain treatment flow chart: preoperative and intraoperative phases. *MD,* Medical doctor, *RN,* registered nurse. (From Agency for Health Care Policy and Research, Acute Pain Management Guideline Panel: *Acute pain management: operative or medical procedures and trauma,* Clinical Practice Guideline, AHCPR Pub No. 92-0032, Rockville, Md, 1992, Agency for Health Care Policy and Research, Public Health Service, US Department of Health and Human Services; and Jacox A et al: *Management of cancer pain,* Clinical Practice Guideline No. 9, AHCPR Pub No. 94-0592, Rockville, Md, 1994, Agency for Health Care Policy and Research, Public Health Service, US Department of Health and Human Services.)

many nurses believe that patients report pain if they have it. If patients sense that you doubt that pain exists, they share little information about their pain experience or minimize their report. You need to establish a caring therapeutic relationship that allows for open communication. Simple measures such as sitting when talking to patients about pain lets them know that you are sincerely concerned about their pain.

Patients unable to communicate effectively often require special attention during assessment. Children, people who are developmentally delayed, patients who are psychotic, the critically ill, patients with dementia, and patients who do not speak English all require different approaches. Herr et al. (2006a, 2006b) examined various pain behavior assessment tools used with patients who were cognitively impaired. Although no one tool had sufficient reliability and validity, there are clinical practice recommendations (Box 43-8). However, you need to understand that "the number obtained when using a pain-behavior scale is a pain-behavior score, not a pain-intensity rating" (Pasero and McCaffery, 2005). These tools identify the presence of pain but do not determine its intensity.

BOX 43-8 **EVIDENCE-BASED PRACTICE**

Pain Assessment in the Nonverbal Patient

PICO Question: In patients who are nonverbal, which method of pain assessment is the most effective?

Evidence Summary

A common misconception is that individuals who are nonverbal as a result of dementia or cognitive impairments do not experience pain (Herr, 2010). Patients who are nonverbal often present with atypical manifestations of pain caused by pathophysiological changes in the brain. Manifestations often include hitting, fearful expressions, combativeness, and resistance to care (Herr, 2010). An appointed task force of the American Society for Pain Management Nursing developed an evidence-based position statement and clinical practice recommendations for pain assessment in the nonverbal patient (Herr et al., 2006a). No single assessment strategy such as interpretation of behaviors, pathology, or estimates of pain by others is sufficient by itself in determining the presence of pain in a nonverbal patient.

Application to Nursing Practice

- Recommended assessment considerations:
  - Attempt a self-report of pain using simple yes/no responses or vocalizations or a numerical rating scale (Herr and Titler, 2009).
  - Search for potential causes of pain (Herr, 2010).
  - Assume that pain is present (APP) after ruling out other problems (infection, constipation) that cause pain.
  - Identify pathological conditions or procedures that cause pain.
  - Observe patient behaviors and list behaviors (e.g., facial expressions, vocalizations, body movements, changes in interactions or mental status) that indicate pain. These vary, depending on patient's developmental level (Herr, 2010).
  - Ask family members, parents, or caregivers for a surrogate report.
- Use behavioral pain assessment tools.
  - Use evidence-based tools to ensure appropriate pain assessment (Herr, 2010).
  - Evidence supports use of the Behavioral Pain Scale and the Nonverbal Pain Scale for patients who are mechanically ventilated (Juarez et al., 2010).
- Determine the appropriate scale based on individual patient needs; no one scale measures pain accurately for all groups of patients.
- Vital signs are not sensitive indicators for the presence of pain.
- For severe pain, consider starting the analgesic trial with an opioid. (Herr et al., 2006a).
- Choose analgesic, dose, and titration based on estimated intensity of pain.
- For mild-to-moderate pain, give nonopioid analgesics around the clock.
- After 24 hours reassess. If behaviors improve, assume that pain was the cause.
- If behaviors persist, consider giving a single, low-dose short-acting opioid (e.g., morphine). Observe effect.
- If behaviors continue, titrate dose upward by 25% to 50% and observe effect.
- Continue to titrate up until a therapeutic effect or bothersome adverse effects occur or if there is no benefit.
- If behaviors continue after a reasonable analgesic trial, explore other potential causes.

Patients with cognitive impairments often require simple assessment approaches involving close observation of behavior changes, especially with movement. Patients who are critically ill and have a clouded sensorium or the presence of nasogastric tubes or artificial airways require you to ask specific questions that they can answer with a nod of the head or by writing out a response. If the patient speaks a different language, pain assessment is difficult. An interpreter is often necessary (Pasero and McCaffery, 2011).

Characteristics of Pain. Assessment of common characteristics of pain helps you form an understanding of the type of pain, its pattern, and the types of interventions that bring relief. Use of instruments to quantify the extent and degree of pain depends on a patient being cognitively alert enough to be able to understand your instructions.

Onset and Duration. Ask questions to determine the onset, duration, and sequence of pain. When did it begin? How long has it lasted? Does it occur at the same time each day? How often does it recur?

Location. To assess pain location, ask the patient to describe or point to all areas of discomfort. Do not assume that your patient's pain always occurs in the same location. When describing pain location, use anatomical landmarks and descriptive terminology. The statement "Pain is localized in the upper right abdominal quadrant" is more specific than "The patient states the pain is in the abdomen." Pain classified by location is superficial or cutaneous, deep or visceral, referred, or radiating (Table 43-5).

Intensity. One of the most subjective and therefore most useful characteristics for reporting pain is its severity or intensity. Nurses use a variety of pain scales to help patients communicate their pain intensity. Examples of pain intensity scales include the verbal descriptor scale (VDS), the numerical rating scale (NRS), and the visual analogue scale (VAS) (Fig. 43-6). When using the NRS, a report of 0 to 3 indicates mild pain; 4 to 6, moderate pain; and 7 to 10, severe pain, considered a pain emergency (Miaskowski, 2005). These scales work best when assessing pain intensity before and after therapeutic interventions. Many of them are available in several languages to aid nurses when an interpreter is not present (Pasero and McCaffery, 2011). In addition to the current pain level, also ask patients to rate their average pain and the worst pain they have had over the past 24 hours.

Although different patients prefer different pain scales, it is important for you to select and consistently use the same scale with a specific patient. Do not use a pain scale to compare the pain of one patient to that of another.

Assessing pain intensity in children requires special techniques. Children's verbal statements are most important (Hockenberry and Wilson, 2011). Young children do not always know what the word *pain* means; therefore assessment requires you to use words such as *owie, boo-boo,* or *hurt.* Some unique tools are available to measure pain intensity in children. The "Oucher" (Beyer et al., 1992) uses photographs of the face of a child (in increasing levels of discomfort) to cue children into understanding pain and its severity. A child points to a face on the tool, thus simplifying the task of describing the pain. There are ethnic versions of the tool (Fig. 43-7). The FACES scale (Wong and Baker, 1988) assesses pain in verbal children (Fig. 43-8). The scale consists of six cartoon faces ranging from a smiling face ("no hurt") to increasingly less happy faces; to a final sad, tearful face ("hurts worst"). Children as young as 3 years of age use the scale. Nurses use a variety of other tools to assess pain in neonates, infants, nonverbal toddlers, and children with cognitive impairments.

Quality. Because there is no common or specific pain vocabulary in general use, the words patients choose to describe pain vary. Patients of American descent often use *hurt* and *ache* to describe their pain, reserving the word *pain* for severe discomfort. Always use words other than *pain* to obtain an accurate report. For example, you say, "Tell me what your discomfort feels like." The

TABLE 43-5 Classification of Pain by Location

LOCATION	CHARACTERISTICS	EXAMPLES OF CAUSES
Superficial or Cutaneous		
Pain resulting from stimulation of skin	Pain is of short duration and localized. It usually is a sharp sensation.	Needlestick; small cut or laceration
Deep or Visceral		
Pain resulting from stimulation of internal organs	Pain is diffuse and radiates in several directions. Duration varies, but it usually lasts longer than superficial pain. Pain is sharp, dull, or unique to organ involved.	Crushing sensation (e.g., angina pectoris); burning sensation (e.g., gastric ulcer)
Referred		
Common phenomenon in visceral pain because many organs themselves have no pain receptors; entrance of sensory neurons from affected organ into same spinal cord segment as neurons from areas where individual feels pain; perception of pain in unaffected areas	Pain is in part of body separate from source of pain and assumes any characteristic.	Myocardial infarction, which causes referred pain to the jaw, left arm, and left shoulder; kidney stones, which refer pain to groin
Radiating		
Sensation of pain extending from initial site of injury to another body part	Pain feels as though it travels down or along body part. It is intermittent or constant.	Low back pain from ruptured intravertebral disk accompanied by pain radiating down leg from sciatic nerve irritation

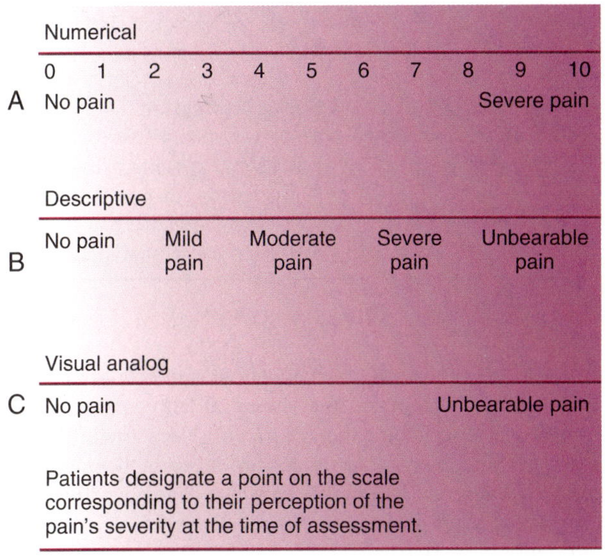

FIG. 43-6 Sample pain scales. **A,** Numerical. **B,** Verbal descriptive. **C,** Visual analogue.

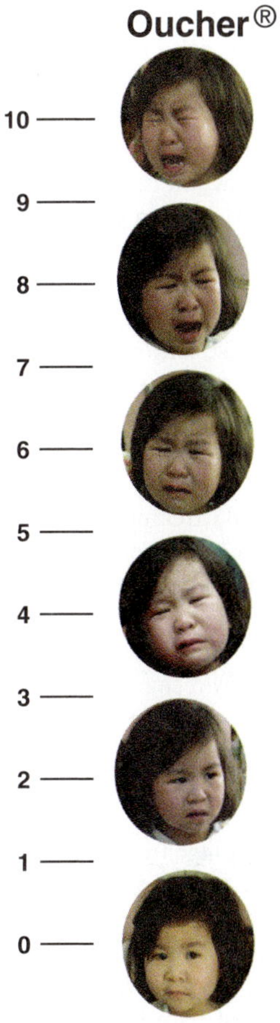

FIG. 43-7 Asian girl version of the Oucher pain scale. (The Asian versions of the Oucher [male and female] were developed and copyrighted in 2003 by CH Yeh [University of Pittsburgh] and CH Wang, Taiwan.)

patient likely describes the pain as crushing, throbbing, sharp, or dull. Although a list of descriptive terms is available, it is more accurate to have patients describe the pain in their own words whenever possible.

There is some consistency in the way people describe certain types of pain. The pain associated with a myocardial infarction is often described as crushing or viselike; whereas the pain of a surgical incision is often described as dull, aching, and throbbing, indicating nociceptive pain. Neuropathic pain is usually burning, shooting, or electric-like (Williams, 2006). When a patient's descriptions fit the pattern forming in the assessment, you then make a clearer analysis of the nature and type of pain. This leads to more appropriate pain management because you treat nociceptive and neuropathic pain differently.

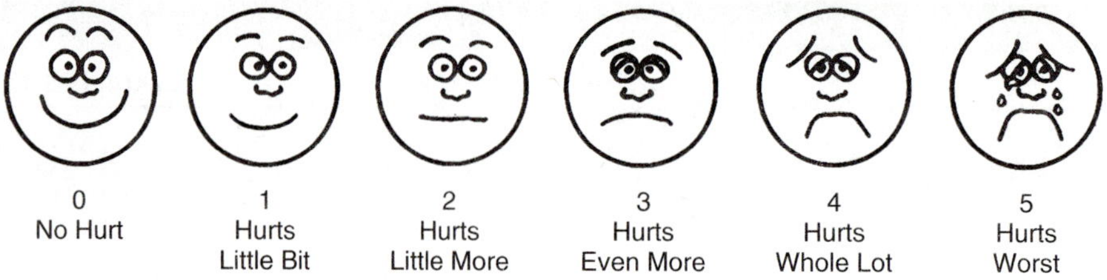
0
No Hurt
1
Hurts
Little Bit
2
Hurts
Little More
3
Hurts
Even More
4
Hurts
Whole Lot
5
Hurts
Worst
Brief word instructions: Point to each face using the words to describe the pain intensity. Ask the child to choose face that best describes own pain and record the appropriate number.

FIG. 43-8 Wong-Baker FACES pain-rating scale. (From Hockenberry MJ, Wilson D: *Wong's nursing care of infants and children,* ed 9, St Louis, 2011, Mosby.)

Pain Pattern. Various factors affect the pattern of pain. It helps to assess specific events or conditions that precipitate or aggravate pain. Ask the patient to describe activities that cause pain such as physical movement or food. Also ask him or her to demonstrate actions that cause a painful response such as coughing or turning a certain way. For example, with a ruptured intravertebral disk the low back pain usually radiates down the leg to the foot, and bending over or lifting objects aggravates it. Asking the patient if there is a particular time of day that the pain is worse or if the pain is intermittent, constant, or a combination helps you plan interventions to prevent it from occurring or worsening.

Relief Measures. It is useful to know whether a patient has an effective way of relieving pain such as changing position, using ritualistic behavior (pacing, rocking, or rubbing), eating, meditating, praying, or applying heat or cold to the painful site. The patient's methods are ones you can use for treatment. Patients gain trust when they know you are willing to try their relief measures. They also gain a sense of control over the pain instead of the pain controlling them. Assessment of relieving factors includes identification of all the patient's health care providers (e.g., internist, orthopedist, acupuncturist, chiropractor, or dentist).

Contributing Symptoms. Some symptoms (depression, anxiety, fatigue, sedation, anorexia, sleep disruption, spiritual distress, and guilt) cause worsening of pain. You need to assess for these associated symptoms and evaluate their effects on the patient's pain perception. Reporting and treating associated symptoms contributes to successful pain management.

Effects of Pain on the Patient. Pain alters a person's lifestyle and affects psychological well-being. Chronic/persistent pain causes suffering, loss of control, loneliness, disabilities, exhaustion, and impaired quality of life. By recognizing the effects that pain has on patients, you better understand the patient's experience and provide the best pain management. When a patient is in pain, you need to conduct a focused physical and neurological examination and observe for nonverbal responses to pain (e.g., "grimacing, rigid body posture, limping, frowning, or crying") (Pasero and McCaffery, 2011). Examine the painful area to see if palpation or manipulation of the site increases pain.

Behavioral Effects. When a patient has pain, assess verbalization, vocal response, facial and body movements, and social interaction. A verbal report of pain is a vital part of assessment. You need to be willing to listen and understand. Many patients are unable to communicate their pain. An infant or a patient who is unconscious, disoriented or confused, aphasic or who speaks a foreign language is unable to explain the pain experience. In these cases it is especially important for you to be alert for behaviors that indicate pain (Box 43-9).

BOX 43-9 BEHAVIORAL INDICATORS OF EFFECTS OF PAIN

Vocalizations
- Moaning
- Crying
- Gasping
- Grunting

Facial Expressions
- Grimace
- Clenched teeth
- Wrinkled forehead
- Tightly closed or widely opened eyes or mouth
- Lip biting

Body Movement
- Restlessness
- Immobilization
- Muscle tension
- Increased hand and finger movements
- Pacing activities
- Rhythmic or rubbing motions
- Protective movement of body parts
- Grabbing or holding a body part

Social Interaction
- Avoidance of conversation
- Focus only on activities for pain relief
- Avoidance of social contacts
- Reduced attention span
- Reduced interaction with environment

The nonverbal expression of pain either supports or contradicts other information about it. If a woman in labor reports that her labor pains are occurring more frequently and if she begins to massage her abdomen more often, this confirms her report. If a patient reports severe abdominal pain but continues to grasp the chest, a more detailed assessment is necessary.

Influence on Activities of Daily Living. Patients who live with daily pain are less able to participate in routine activities, which results in physical deconditioning. Assessment of these changes reveals the extent of the patient's disability and adjustments necessary to help patients participate in self-care. Your primary goal as a nurse is to improve patient function.

Ask the patient whether pain interferes with sleep. Some patients experience difficulty in falling asleep and/or staying asleep. The pain awakens the patient during the night and makes it hard to fall back to sleep. Consider giving medications or trying nonpharmacological interventions to promote sleep (see Chapter 42). Do not use medications that promote sleep as a substitute for pain relief.

Depending on the location of the pain, some patients have difficulty independently performing ADLs. For example, some pain restricts mobility to the point at which the patient is no longer able to bathe in a bathtub. Patients with severe arthritis find it painful to grasp eating utensils or lower themselves to a toilet seat. Assess the patient's need for assistance with self-care activities and collaborate with members of the health care team (e.g., physical and

BOX 43-10 NURSING DIAGNOSTIC PROCESS

Chronic Pain

ASSESSMENT ACTIVITIES	DEFINING CHARACTERISTICS
Have patient describe pain intensity.	Pain constant; patient verbally reports 5 on a scale of 0 to 10
Assess onset and location of pain.	Present for 7 months in lower lumbar area
Observe patient behaviors.	Grimaces and grunts with movement, rubs flanks frequently; reduced movement
Assess effect of pain on activities of daily living (ADLs).	Appetite poor; gets little sleep; difficulty dressing
Review medical history.	Previous trauma; effectiveness of past pain control measures

occupational therapy). Also consider the need for family members or friends to assist patients with basic hygiene.

Pain sometimes impairs the ability to maintain normal sexual relations. Include in your assessment the extent to which pain affects the patient's sexual activity. It also helps to learn whether a patient is physically unable to participate or if pain reduces the desire for sexual intercourse.

Pain threatens a person's ability to work. The more physical activity required in a job, the greater the risk of discomfort when the pain is associated with movement. Pain related to emotional stress increases in individuals whose jobs involve stressful decision making. Assess the work that patients do and their abilities to function in their jobs. Assess the daily chores of homemakers in the same manner as the duties involved in jobs outside the home. Also assess whether it is necessary for patients to stop activity occasionally because of pain, and then help them select ways to minimize or control it so they are able to remain productive.

Include an assessment of the effect of pain on social activities. Some pain is so debilitating that the patient becomes too exhausted to socialize. Identify the patient's normal social activities, the extent to which activities have been disrupted, and the desire to participate in these activities.

NURSING DIAGNOSIS

You make an accurate diagnosis only after you have performed a complete assessment. The development of an accurate nursing diagnosis for a patient in pain results from thorough data collection and analysis (Box 43-10). Careful assessment reveals the presence or potential for pain. In addition, examine the patient's history for recent procedures or preexisting painful conditions.

The nursing diagnosis focuses on the specific nature of the pain to identify the most useful types of interventions for alleviating it and improving the patient's function. *Acute pain related to physical trauma* and *acute pain related to natural childbirth processes* require very different nursing interventions. Accurate identification of related factors is necessary in choosing appropriate nursing interventions. For example, interventions for *acute pain related to physical trauma* require pharmacological intervention, whereas *acute pain related to natural childbirth processes* is sometimes managed more appropriately with nonpharmacological interventions such as controlled breathing techniques.

Your assessment often directs you to diagnoses other than that of *acute* or *chronic pain*. The extent to which pain affects a patient's function and general state of health determines whether other nursing diagnoses are relevant. For example, your assessment reveals that a patient has pain of the hands and shoulders as a result of crippling arthritis for over 3 years. As a result the patient is unable to remove or fasten necessary items of clothing. The nursing diagnoses for this patient are *dressing/grooming self-care deficit* and *chronic pain*. The diagnosis of *self-care deficit* requires involvement by members of the interdisciplinary health care team to provide the patient with assistive devices for performing self-care. Examples of other diagnoses that are applicable to patients experiencing pain include the following:

- Activity intolerance
- Anxiety
- Ineffective coping
- Fatigue
- Fear
- Hopelessness
- Impaired physical mobility
- Imbalanced nutrition: less than body requirements
- Insomnia
- Powerlessness
- Chronic low self-esteem
- Impaired social interaction
- Spiritual distress

PLANNING

During the planning step of the nursing process, you synthesize information from multiple resources. Critical thinking ensures that the patient's plan of care (see the Nursing Care Plan) integrates all that you know about the individual patient and key critical thinking elements (Fig. 43-9, p. 978). Professional standards are especially important to consider when you develop a plan of care. These standards establish evidence-based guidelines for selecting effective nursing interventions. Professional standards of care regarding pain management are available as agency policies or through professional organizations such as the American Society for Pain Management Nursing (ASPMN).

Another effective method for planning care is a concept map. Patients who are in pain frequently have interrelated problems. As one problem gets worse, other aspects of a patient's level of health also change. The concept map helps you determine how the nursing diagnoses are interrelated with one another and linked to the patient's medical diagnosis. Using the example here, as you plan care for the patient with rheumatoid arthritis, note the relationships among *acute pain, impaired physical mobility, dressing and feeding self-care deficit,* and *fatigue* (Fig. 43-10). Identifying these relationships helps you develop a holistic and patient-centered plan of care.

Goals and Outcomes. When managing pain, goals of care promote a patient's optimal function. Determine, along with the patient, what the pain has prevented the patient from doing. Then decide on a mutually acceptable level of pain that allows return of function. An indication of the success of the plan is determined through attainment of goals and outcomes. For example, for the goal "the patient will achieve a satisfactory level of pain relief within 24 hours," the following are possible outcomes:

- Reports that pain is a 3 or less on a scale of 0 to 10
- Identifies factors that intensify pain
- Uses pain-relief measures safely
- Level of discomfort does not interfere with ADLs

NURSING CARE PLAN

Acute Pain

ASSESSMENT

Mrs. Mays, 75 years old, was diagnosed with a cancerous tumor in her left lung 2 months ago. She also has a history of osteoarthritis. After chemotherapy and radiation therapy, she took ibuprofen (Advil) 200 mg on an as-needed (prn) basis. Until today she was able to clean her home and climb the stairs to her bedroom without difficulty. She also maintained her body weight and slept well through the night. However, she is now admitted to the hospital with uncontrollable chest pain and possible pneumonia. Her husband is with her. The nurse begins a patient-controlled analgesia (PCA) of morphine 0.5 mg demand dose with a 10-minute lockout.

Assessment Activities	*Findings/Defining Characteristics**
Ask Mrs. Mays what she did at home to control her pain.	Her **pain escalated** from a 3 to a 10 on a scale of 0 to 10, so she doubled her medication and went to bed; but this did not help.
Ask Mrs. Mays what her pain intensity is now.	On a scale of 0 to 10, **she reports a 9.**
Ask Mrs. Mays what her pain has prevented her from doing.	She responds that she is **unable to complete her own hygiene activities, sleep, or eat well.**
Observe Mrs. Mays's nonverbal behavior.	She is **restless,** is **unable to stay focused,** her **muscles tense, and** she is **frowning** during the history taking.
Ask Mrs. Mays her pain-intensity goal (on a scale of 0 to 10).	She says that a pain intensity of 5 on a scale of 10 helps her function better right now. A goal of 3 is preferable.

***Defining characteristics** are shown in bold type.

NURSING DIAGNOSIS: Acute pain related to abrupt onset of inflammation

PLANNING

Goals	*Expected Outcomes (NOC)†*
	Pain Control
Mrs. Mays will reach a tolerable level of pain before discharge.	Mrs. Mays will report pain at target goal of 3 or below. Mrs. Mays uses PCA device appropriately.
	Pain: Disruptive Effects
Mrs. Mays will actively participate in activities of daily living (ADLs).	Mrs. Mays will report sleeping for 5 to 6 hours without interruption from pain. Mrs. Mays will complete her own hygiene with minimal assistance. Mrs. Mays will walk the hallway with her husband every 4 hours for 15 minutes.
	Medication Response
Mrs. Mays will not experience unmanageable opioid side effects.	Mrs. Mays will report having a normal bowel movement every other day.

†Outcome classification labels from Moorhead S et al: *Nursing outcomes classification (NOC),* ed 4, St Louis, 2008, Mosby.

INTERVENTIONS (NIC)‡	**RATIONALE**
Pain Management	
Begin PCA at ordered dose. Explain to patient and spouse how to use the PCA. Emphasize the importance of only the patient pushing the button, not the husband.	Acute cancer pain rated a 7 (or more) on a scale of 0 to 10 requires immediate-release opioid. Discouraging the husband from pushing the button prevents unnecessary doses and reduces potential toxic effects of the opioid. Patient needs to be awake to perceive the pain and push the button (Pasero and McCaffery, 2011).
Monitor IV PCA morphine use. Explain to patient and spouse the action of the medication, potential side effects, and the importance of reporting unrelieved pain.	Pain is easier to prevent than to treat. Side effects are usually transient, except for constipation. Calculating 24-hour dosage of opioid helps determine appropriate oral dose (Pasero and McCaffery, 2011).
Have patients select nonpharmacological interventions that have relieved pain in the past (e.g., distraction, music, simple relaxation therapy) or that are acceptable to them.	Nonpharmacological approaches augment pharmacological therapy and help patients improve quality of life and decrease anxiety and depression (Chen and Francis, 2010).
Teach spouse how to perform slow-stroke back massage.	Slow-stroke back massage is easy to do, takes a brief time, and induces relaxation (Walters, 2010).

‡Intervention classification labels from Bulechek GM, Butcher HK, and Dochterman JM: *Nursing interventions classification (NIC),* ed 5, St Louis, 2008, Mosby.

NURSING CARE PLAN

***Acute Pain*—cont'd**

EVALUATION

Nursing Actions	*Patient Response/Finding*	*Achievement of Outcome*
Ask Mrs. Mays if she attained her pain relief goal most of the time.	She responds, "My pain usually runs around a 3, except when I start walking."	Mrs. Mays reports an acceptable level of pain. Instruct her to push her button before ambulating.
Observe Mrs. Mays performing ADLs, walking, and during sleep.	Mrs. Mays is dressed for breakfast, walking the hallway every 4 hours with her husband. The night nurse's notes indicate that she slept through the night.	Ability to perform ADLs and sleep has improved. Continue to monitor.
Observe Mrs. Mays as she ambulates in the hallway.	Mrs. Mays successfully ambulated in the hallway with her husband twice during the shift with minimal increase in pain intensity.	Improved pain control increased her activity, a nonverbal indicator of pain. Continue to monitor.
Ask Mr. Mays if he was able to give his wife a back rub.	Mr. Mays reported that she did not want a back rub but preferred to have her feet rubbed, which he was happy to do. "She said it made her feel more relaxed."	Nonpharmacological intervention was successful but needs to be changed from back rub to foot rub in the nursing care plan.
Ask Mrs. Mays when she last had a bowel movement and its consistency.	She has not had a bowel movement in 3 days (since starting the morphine PCA).	Assess her abdomen for bowel sounds and distention and return of flatus. Consult with health care provider about starting a stimulant laxative once intestinal obstruction is ruled out (Pasero and McCaffery, 2011).
Observe Mrs. Mays for excessive drowsiness.	Mrs. Mays is awake and alert during conversations and interacts frequently with her husband.	Sedation, an indicator of too much opioid, is not identified. Continue to monitor.

Setting Priorities. When setting priorities in pain management, consider the type of pain the patient is experiencing and the effect that it has on various body functions. Work with the patient to select interventions that are appropriate. For example, if an analgesic relieves acute pain, center your attention on how the pain is affecting your patient's activity, appetite, and sleep. In contrast, when a patient's pain continues to be severe, preventing you from implementing other interventions, immediate pain relief is the obvious priority. Your priorities change as a patient's pain experience changes.

Teamwork and Collaboration. A comprehensive plan includes a variety of resources for pain control. Resources available include advanced practice nurses, doctors of pharmacology (PharmDs), physical therapists, occupational therapists, and clergy. An oncology or pain clinical nurse specialist is very familiar with pharmacological and nonpharmacological interventions that are most effective for chronic/persistent pain. PharmDs are knowledgeable about pharmacological treatments of pain. Physical therapists plan exercises that strengthen muscle groups and lessen pain in affected areas. Occupational therapists devise splints to support painful body parts. Clergy members help patients focus on spiritual health. It is important to involve the family in the plan of care because they often administer care in the home after discharge. If the pain-management plan is not successful in achieving the identified pain relief goal, talk with the patient's health care provider about revising it. Consultation with a pain expert is sometimes necessary.

IMPLEMENTATION

Pain therapy requires an individualized approach, perhaps more so than any other patient problem. The nurse, patient, and frequently the family are partners in pain management. Nurses administer and monitor interventions ordered by health care providers for pain relief in addition to complementary pain-relief measures. Usually you try the least invasive or safest therapy first along with previously used successful patient remedies. If there is a question about a medical therapy, consult with the health care provider.

Health Promotion. Patients are better prepared to handle almost any situation when they understand it. The experience of pain is no exception. However, patients with moderate-to-severe pain are not always able to participate in the decision-making process until the pain is controlled at an acceptable level. Once you accomplish this, you are able to begin teaching.

Because pain affects physical and mental functioning, holistic health approaches are important interventions for maintaining wellness. Holistic health is an ongoing state of wellness that involves taking care of the physical self, expressing emotions appropriately and effectively, using the mind constructively, being creatively involved with others, and becoming aware of higher levels of consciousness (American Holistic Health Association, 2007). The concept of holistic health parallels the values of nursing in maintaining the integrity of the whole person.

Patients actively participate in their own well-being whenever possible. Common holistic health approaches include wellness education, regular exercise, rest, attention to good hygiene practices and nutrition, and management of interpersonal relationships. When a person develops pain, you can offer nonpharmacological and pharmacological strategies. Several of the nonpharmacological interventions are nurse initiated.

Nonpharmacological Pain-Relief Interventions. A number of nonpharmacological interventions lessen pain; however, they are to be used *with,* and not in place of, pharmacological measures (Gruener and Lande, 2006; Hughes, 2008). Nonpharmacological interventions include cognitive-behavioral and physical approaches. Cognitive-behavioral interventions change patients' perceptions of

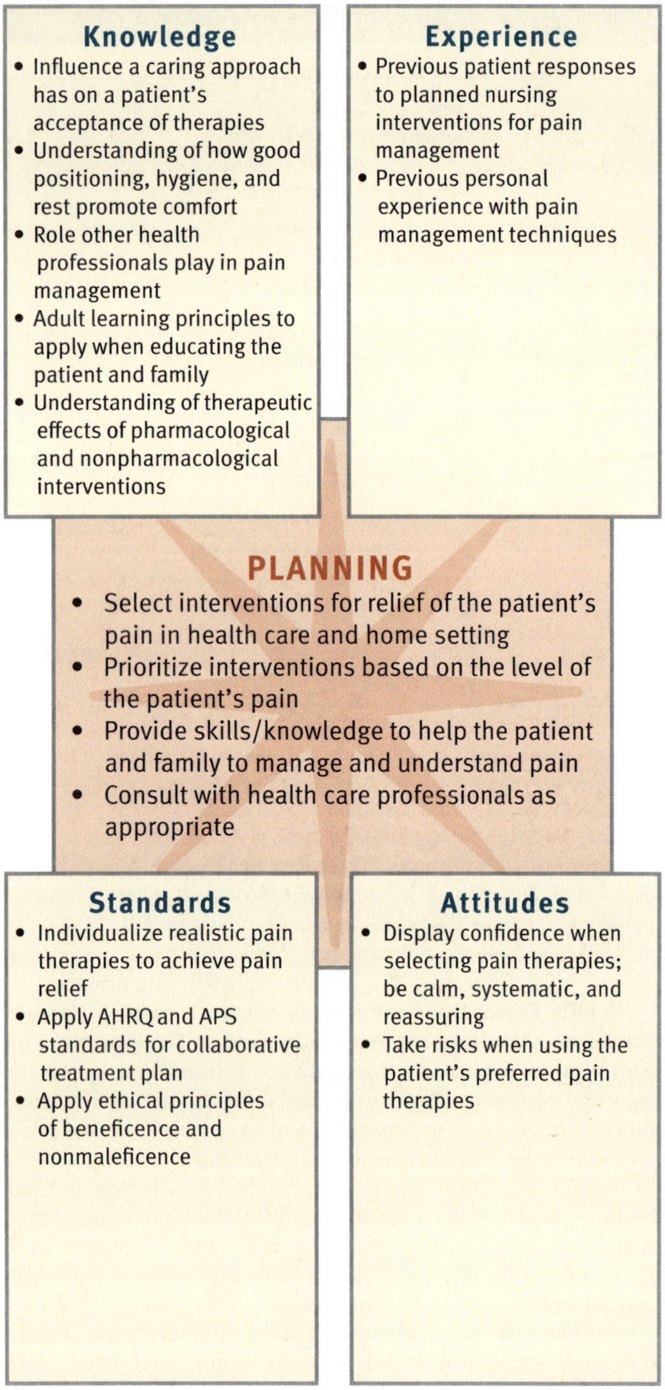
Knowledge
• Influence a caring approach has on a patient's acceptance of therapies
• Understanding of how good positioning, hygiene, and rest promote comfort
• Role other health professionals play in pain management
• Adult learning principles to apply when educating the patient and family
• Understanding of therapeutic effects of pharmacological and nonpharmacological interventions
Experience
• Previous patient responses to planned nursing interventions for pain management
• Previous personal experience with pain management techniques
PLANNING
• Select interventions for relief of the patient's pain in health care and home setting
• Prioritize interventions based on the level of the patient's pain
• Provide skills/knowledge to help the patient and family to manage and understand pain
• Consult with health care professionals as appropriate
Standards
• Individualize realistic pain therapies to achieve pain relief
• Apply AHRQ and APS standards for collaborative treatment plan
• Apply ethical principles of beneficence and nonmaleficence
Attitudes
• Display confidence when selecting pain therapies; be calm, systematic, and reassuring
• Take risks when using the patient's preferred pain therapies

FIG. 43-9 Critical thinking model for pain management planning. *AHRQ,* Agency for Healthcare Research and Quality; *APS,* American Pain Society.

pain, alter pain behavior, and provide patients with a greater sense of control. Distraction, prayer, relaxation, guided imagery, music, and **biofeedback** are examples. Physical approaches aim to provide pain relief, correct physical dysfunction, alter physiological responses, and reduce fears associated with pain-related immobility. Chiropractic therapy and acupuncture/acupressure therapy are examples (see Chapter 32). Complementary and alternative medicine (CAM) therapies such as therapeutic touch also help to alleviate pain in some patients. The Agency for Health Care Policy and Research guidelines for acute pain management (AHCPR, 1992) cite nonpharmacological interventions to be appropriate for patients who meet the following criteria:

- Find such interventions appealing
- Express anxiety or fear
- Possibly benefit from avoiding or reducing drug therapy
- Are likely to experience and need to cope with a prolonged interval of postoperative pain
- Have incomplete pain relief after use of pharmacological interventions

Relaxation and Guided Imagery. Relaxation and **guided imagery** allow patients to alter affective-motivational and cognitive pain perception. **Relaxation** is mental and physical freedom from tension or stress that provides individuals a sense of self-control. You use relaxation techniques at any phase of health or illness. Physiological and behavioral changes associated with relaxation include the following: decreased pulse, blood pressure, and respirations; heightened awareness; decreased oxygen consumption; a sense of peace; and decreased muscle tension and metabolic rate. Relaxation techniques include meditation, yoga, Zen, guided imagery, and progressive relaxation exercises (see Chapter 32). For effective relaxation, teach techniques only when a patient is not distracted by acute discomfort. Sometimes you need to use a combination of these techniques to achieve optimal pain relief. With practice the patient performs relaxation exercises independently.

Distraction. The reticular activating system inhibits painful stimuli if a person receives sufficient or excessive sensory input. With sufficient sensory stimuli, a person ignores or becomes unaware of pain. Persons who are bored or in isolation have only their pain to think about and thus perceive it more acutely. Distraction directs a patient's attention to something other than pain and thus reduces awareness of it. One disadvantage of distraction is that, if it works, health care providers or family members question the existence or severity of the pain. Distraction works best for short, intense pain lasting a few minutes such as during an invasive procedure or while waiting for an analgesic to work. Use activities enjoyed by the patient as distractions (e.g., singing, praying, listening to music, humor or laughter therapy, playing games).

Music. Music treats acute or chronic pain, stress, anxiety, and depression (Allred et al., 2010). It diverts a person's attention away from the pain and creates a relaxation response. Music therapy uses all kinds of music. It is important to let patients select the type of music they prefer. Music produces an altered state of consciousness through sound, silence, space, and time. Therapeutic sessions usually last 20 to 30 minutes (Hughes, 2008). Patients use earphones to enhance their concentration on the music. This allows patients to adjust the volume of the music without interrupting other patients or staff. Evidence shows that music decreases the use of analgesics in some postoperative patients (Engwall and Duppils, 2009).

Cutaneous Stimulation. Stimulation of the skin helps relieve pain. A massage, warm bath, ice bag, and transcutaneous electrical nerve stimulation (TENS) stimulate the skin to reduce pain perception (Pain Management Center Staff, 2002). How **cutaneous stimulation** works is unclear. One suggestion is that it causes release of endorphins, thus blocking the transmission of painful stimuli. The gate-control theory suggests that cutaneous stimulation activates larger, faster-transmitting A-beta sensory nerve fibers. This closes the gate, thus decreasing pain transmission through small-diameter C fibers (Melzack and Wall, 1965).

Cutaneous stimulation gives patients and families some control over pain symptoms and treatment in the home. Using it properly helps to reduce muscle tension, resulting in less pain. When using

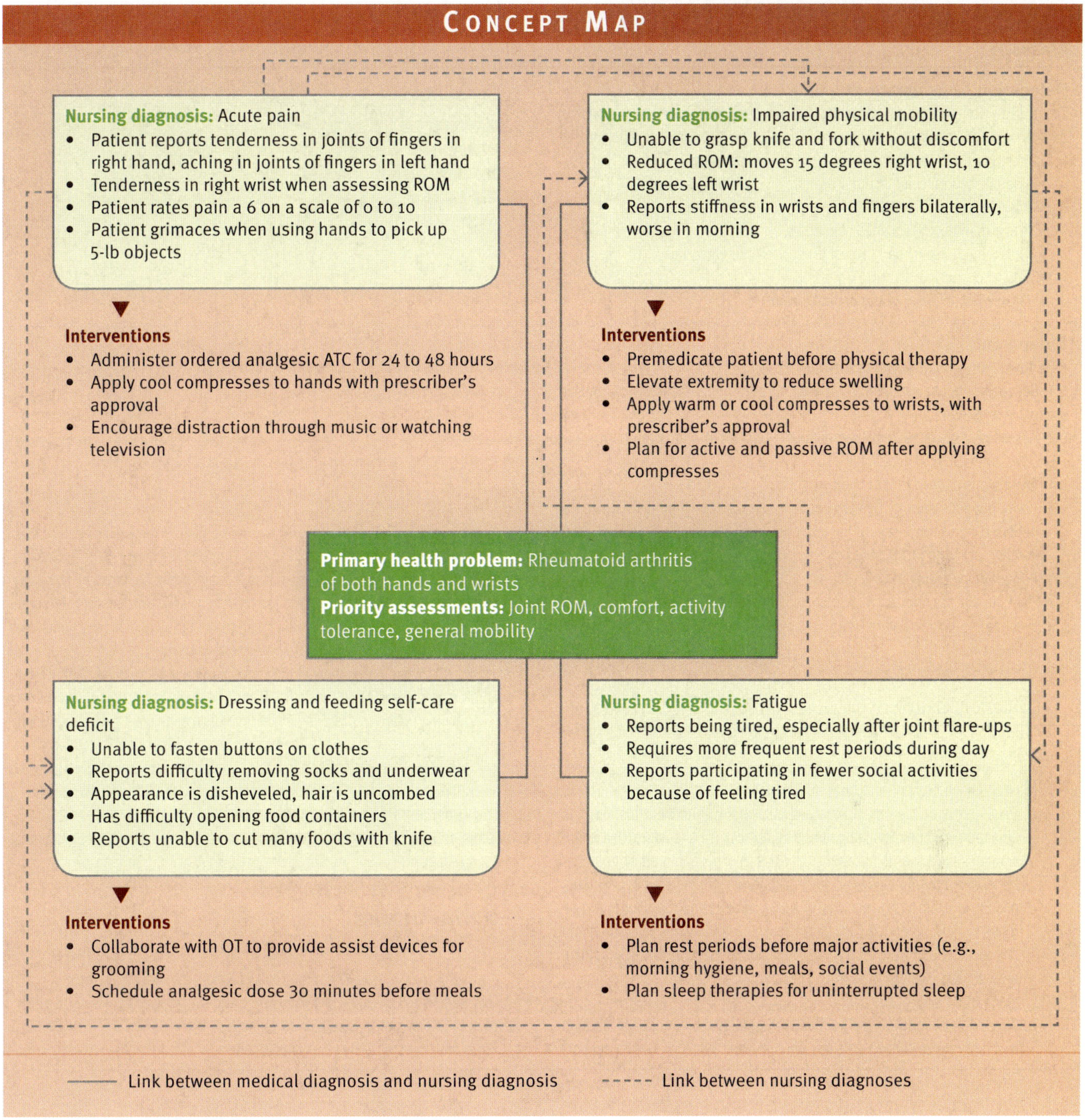
CONCEPT MAP
Nursing diagnosis: Acute pain
• Patient reports tenderness in joints of fingers in right hand, aching in joints of fingers in left hand
• Tenderness in right wrist when assessing ROM
• Patient rates pain a 6 on a scale of 0 to 10
• Patient grimaces when using hands to pick up 5-lb objects
Interventions
• Administer ordered analgesic ATC for 24 to 48 hours
• Apply cool compresses to hands with prescriber's approval
• Encourage distraction through music or watching television
Nursing diagnosis: Impaired physical mobility
• Unable to grasp knife and fork without discomfort
• Reduced ROM: moves 15 degrees right wrist, 10 degrees left wrist
• Reports stiffness in wrists and fingers bilaterally, worse in morning
Interventions
• Premedicate patient before physical therapy
• Elevate extremity to reduce swelling
• Apply warm or cool compresses to wrists, with prescriber's approval
• Plan for active and passive ROM after applying compresses
Primary health problem: Rheumatoid arthritis of both hands and wrists
Priority assessments: Joint ROM, comfort, activity tolerance, general mobility
Nursing diagnosis: Dressing and feeding self-care deficit
• Unable to fasten buttons on clothes
• Reports difficulty removing socks and underwear
• Appearance is disheveled, hair is uncombed
• Has difficulty opening food containers
• Reports unable to cut many foods with knife
Interventions
• Collaborate with OT to provide assist devices for grooming
• Schedule analgesic dose 30 minutes before meals
Nursing diagnosis: Fatigue
• Reports being tired, especially after joint flare-ups
• Requires more frequent rest periods during day
• Reports participating in fewer social activities because of feeling tired
Interventions
• Plan rest periods before major activities (e.g., morning hygiene, meals, social events)
• Plan sleep therapies for uninterrupted sleep
Link between medical diagnosis and nursing diagnosis
Link between nursing diagnoses

FIG. 43-10 Concept map for Mrs. Mays. *ATC,* Around the clock; *OT,* occupational therapist; *ROM,* range of motion.

cutaneous stimulation, eliminate sources of environmental noise, help the patient to assume a comfortable position, and explain the purpose of the therapy. Do not use it directly on sensitive skin areas (e.g., burns, bruises, skin rashes, inflammation, and underlying bone fractures).

Massage is effective for producing physical and mental relaxation, reducing pain, and enhancing the effectiveness of pain medication. Massaging the back, shoulders, hands, and/or feet for 3 to 5 minutes relaxes muscles and promotes sleep and comfort. Cutshall et al. (2010) reported a significant decrease in pain, anxiety, and tension in patients with cardiac problems who received a 20-minute massage. In older adults slow back massage and a 20-minute hand massage improved pain, anxiety, tension, and insomnia (Harris and Richards, 2010). Massages communicate caring and are easy for family members or other health care personnel to learn (Box 43-11).

Cold and heat applications (see Chapter 48) relieve pain and promote healing. The selection of heat versus cold interventions varies with patients' conditions (McCarberg and O'Connor, 2004). For example, moist heat helps to relieve the pain from a tension headache, and cold applications reduce the acute pain from inflamed joints. When using any form of heat or cold application,

BOX 43-11 PROCEDURAL GUIDELINES

Massage

Delegation Considerations

The skill of administering a massage may be delegated to nursing assistive personnel (NAP). However, the nurse must first assess for any possible contraindication and evaluate the patient's response to massage. Direct the NAP to:

- Use massage techniques that are effective with the patient.
- Massage specific body parts.
- Avoid massaging reddened skin areas.
- Notify the nurse of early signs of impaired skin integrity.
- Report changes in the skin appearance.
- Report a worsening in the patient's pain.

Equipment

Bath towel, lotion, bath towel or blanket.

1. Based on patient assessment, decide on performing massage on one or more body parts.
2. Assess skin areas for reddened areas or impaired skin integrity.
3. Collect appropriate equipment.
4. Explain procedure to the patient.
5. Verify patient's identity by using at least two patient identifiers. Compare patient's name and one other identifier such as hospital identification number, according to facility policy.
6. Perform hand hygiene.
7. Help patient assume a comfortable lying or sitting position.
8. Dim room lights and/or turn on soft music according to patient preference.
9. Use warm body lotion as lubricant.

CLINICAL DECISION: *Do not give back or neck massages to patients who have had neck or spinal trauma and/or surgery without an order from their health care provider.*

10. Massage each body part at least 10 minutes.
    a. *Back:* Begin at the sacral area and massage in a circular motion (see illustration) while moving upward from buttocks to shoulders. Use a firm smooth stroke over the scapula. Continue in one smooth stroke to upper arms and laterally along sides of back down to iliac crests. Use long, gliding strokes along muscles of spine. Knead any muscles that feel tense or tight. Knead skin by gently grasping tissue between thumb and fingers. Knead upward along one side of spine from buttocks to shoulders around nape of neck. Knead or stroke downward toward sacrum. Repeat along other side of the back.
    b. *Neck:* Support neck at the hairline with one hand and massage up with a gliding stroke. Knead muscles on one side. Switch hands to support neck and knead other side. Stretch neck slightly, with one hand at top and the other at bottom.
    c. *Arms:* Use gliding stroke to massage from patient's wrist or forearm. With thumb and forefinger of both hands, knead muscles from forearm to shoulder. Continue kneading biceps, deltoid, and triceps muscles. Finish with gliding strokes from wrists to shoulder.
    d. *Hands:* Using both hands, slowly open patient's palm; glide fingers over palmar surface. While supporting the patient's hand, use both thumbs to apply friction to palm and move thumbs in a circular motion to stretch palm outward. Massage each finger using a corkscrew-like motion from base of finger to tip. With thumb and forefinger gently knead each muscle in the patient's fingers. Glide hands smoothly from fingertips to wrists. Repeat for other hand.
    e. *Feet:* Gently massage top and bottom of each foot. Using gliding motion, massage from heel to toe. Gently massage dorsal surface of foot and each toe. Repeat for other foot.

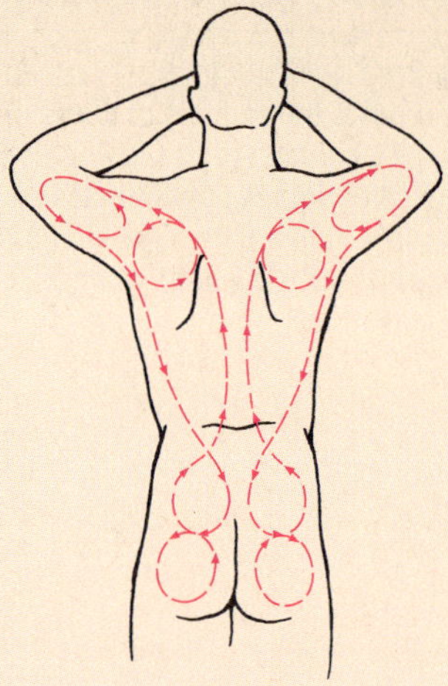

STEP 10a Back massage pattern.

CLINICAL DECISION: *Do not massage patient's legs or calf muscles because there is a risk of dislodging a vascular clot.*

11. At end of massage have patient relax, taking slow, deep breaths.
12. Ask patient to rate level of pain.
13. Note any areas of muscle pain or tension.
14. Note any areas of redness or impairment.

instruct the patient to avoid injury to the skin by checking the temperature and not applying cold or heat directly to the skin. Especially at risk are patients with spinal cord or other neurological disorders, older adults, and patients who are confused.

Cold therapies are particularly effective for pain relief. Ice massage involves the use of a large ice cube or a small paper cup filled with water and frozen (water rises out of the cup as it freezes to create a smooth surface of ice for massage). A nurse or the patient applies the ice with firm pressure to the skin, which is covered with a lightweight cloth. Then you use a slow, steady, circular massage over the area. You apply cold near the pain site, on the opposite side of the body corresponding to the pain site, or on a site located between the brain and the pain site. Each patient responds differently to the site of application. Application near the actual site of pain tends to work best. A patient feels cold, burning, and aching sensations and numbness. When numbness occurs, remove the ice for usually 5 to 10 minutes. Cold is effective for tooth or mouth pain when you place the ice on the web of the hand between the thumb and index finger. This point on the hand is an **acupressure** point that influences nerve pathways to the face and head. Cold applications are also effective before invasive needle punctures.

Heat application is more effective for some patients. You use heating pads, warm compresses, or commercial pillows that are warmed in the microwave. Teach patients to check the temperature of the compress and not to lie on the heating element, because burning can occur.

BOX 43-12 CONTROLLING PAINFUL STIMULI IN THE PATIENT'S ENVIRONMENT

- Tighten and smooth wrinkled bed linen.
- Reposition patient to avoid lying on tubing (e.g., IV tubing, chest tubes).
- Loosen constricting bandages (unless specifically applied as a pressure dressing).
- Change wet dressings and linens.
- Position patient in anatomical alignment according to individual preference or requirements.
- Check temperature of hot or cold applications, including bath water.
- Lift patient in bed—do not pull.
- Position patient correctly on bedpan.
- Avoid exposing skin or mucous membranes to irritants (e.g., urine, stool, wound drainage).
- Keep patients clean, dry, and turned if needed. Use urinary incontinence pads if indicated.
- Prevent urinary retention by keeping Foley catheters patent and free flowing while also monitoring urinary output.
- Prevent constipation with fluids, diet, exercise, and stimulant laxatives if needed.

Another form of cutaneous stimulation is **transcutaneous electrical nerve stimulation (TENS),** involving stimulation of the skin with a mild electrical current passed through external electrodes (Melzack and Wall, 2003). The therapy requires an order from a health care provider. The TENS unit consists of a battery-powered transmitter, lead wires, and electrodes. Place the electrodes directly over or near the site of pain. Remove any hair or skin preparations before attaching the electrodes. The patient turns the transmitter on when feeling pain. This creates a buzzing or tingling sensation. The patient adjusts the intensity and quality of skin stimulation and applies the tingling sensation until pain relief occurs. TENS is effective for postsurgical and procedural pain control.

Herbals. Many patients use herbals such as echinacea, ginseng, ginkgo biloba, and garlic supplements despite a lack of evidence supporting their use in pain relief (Wirth et al., 2005). Herbals often interact with prescribed analgesics; thus ask patients to report all substances they take to relieve pain (Yoon and Schaffer, 2006) (see Chapter 32).

Reducing Pain Perception. One simple way to promote comfort is to remove or prevent painful stimuli (Box 43-12). This is especially important for patients who are immobilized or have difficulty expressing themselves. For example, your patient becomes constipated and has abdominal distention and cramping. As the nurse you intervene to ensure that the normal elimination process continues: increasing fluids, ambulating the patient, and/or requesting stool softeners or laxatives. Another example involves reducing pain perception in the way you perform procedures. Always consider the patient's condition, aspects of the procedure that are uncomfortable, and techniques to avoid causing pain. In a patient with severe arthritic knee pain who has severe discomfort during any extreme flexion of the knee, take precautions before walking the patient to the bathroom. Use an elevated toilet seat to allow the patient to sit and rise with minimal discomfort.

Acute Care

Acute Pain Management. Nurses often care for patients who have acute pain resulting from invasive procedures (e.g., surgery) or trauma. The AHCPR established a pain treatment flow chart in 1992 that is still used today (Fig. 43-11) for treatment of postoperative pain and pain from medical procedures and trauma. This systematic approach ensures quick caregiver response to patient discomfort. The key to success is ongoing evaluation of interventions: Does the patient feel relief? Are there any unacceptable side effects from the medications? It is the responsibility of the health care team to collaborate to find the combination of therapy that works best for a patient.

Pharmacological Pain-Relief Interventions. Many pharmacological agents are available to provide pain relief. A nurse's judgment in the use and management of analgesics helps ensure the best pain relief possible. Unfortunately the ideal analgesic has yet to be developed.

Analgesics. **Analgesics** are the most common and effective method of pain relief. However, health care providers and nurses still tend to undertreat patients because of incorrect drug information, concerns about addiction, anxiety over errors in using opioid analgesics, and administration of excessive medication. You need to understand the drugs available for pain relief and their pharmacological effects.

There are three types of analgesics: (1) nonopioids, including acetaminophen and nonsteroidal antiinflammatory drugs (NSAIDs); (2) **opioids** (traditionally called *narcotics);* and (3) **adjuvants,** a variety of medications that enhance analgesics or have analgesic properties that were originally unknown (Pasero and McCaffery, 2011).

Acetaminophen (Tylenol) is considered one of the most tolerated and safest analgesics available. It has no antiinflammatory effects, and its action is unknown. Its major adverse effect is hepatotoxicity. It is in a variety of over-the-counter (OTC) cold, flu, and allergy remedies. The maximum 24-hour dose is 4 g (the same dose limitation for aspirin). It is often combined with opioids (e.g., Percocet [oxycodone], Vicodin [hydrocodone], Lortab [hydrocodone], and Ultracet [tramadol]) because it reduces the dose of opioid needed to achieve successful pain control. You treat overdoses of acetaminophen with acetylcysteine (Mucomyst) (Pasero and McCaffery, 2011).

Nonselective NSAIDs such as aspirin and ibuprofen provide relief for mild-to-moderate acute intermittent pain such as the pain associated with a headache or muscle strain. Treatment of mild-to-moderate postoperative pain begins with an NSAID unless contraindicated (Pasero and McCaffery, 2011). NSAIDs most likely inhibit the synthesis of prostaglandins (Lehne, 2010) and thus inhibit cellular responses to inflammation. Most NSAIDs act on peripheral nerve receptors to reduce transmission of pain stimuli and inflammation. Unlike opioids, NSAIDs do not depress the central nervous system, nor do they interfere with bowel or bladder function (Pasero and McCaffery, 2011). However, chronic NSAID use in the older patient is not recommended because it is associated with more frequent adverse effects (gastrointestinal bleeding and renal insufficiency). Mild-to-moderate musculoskeletal pain in older adults is effectively managed with the acetaminophen (AGS, 2002; Pasero and McCaffery, 2011). Some patients with asthma or an allergy to aspirin are also allergic to other NSAIDs (Kaufman, 2010). Some NSAIDs are available over-the-counter (OTC); thus advise patients to discuss the use of OTC NSAIDs to manage pain with their health care provider (D'Arcy, 2006).

Current evidence shows nonselective NSAIDs are safe when taken for short periods. Some patients who took selective COX-2 inhibitors for longer periods experienced heart attacks and strokes; thus Celebrex is the only selective COX-2 inhibitor currently available. The rest are no longer available on the market. Celebrex is not to be used in patients with a sulfa allergy.

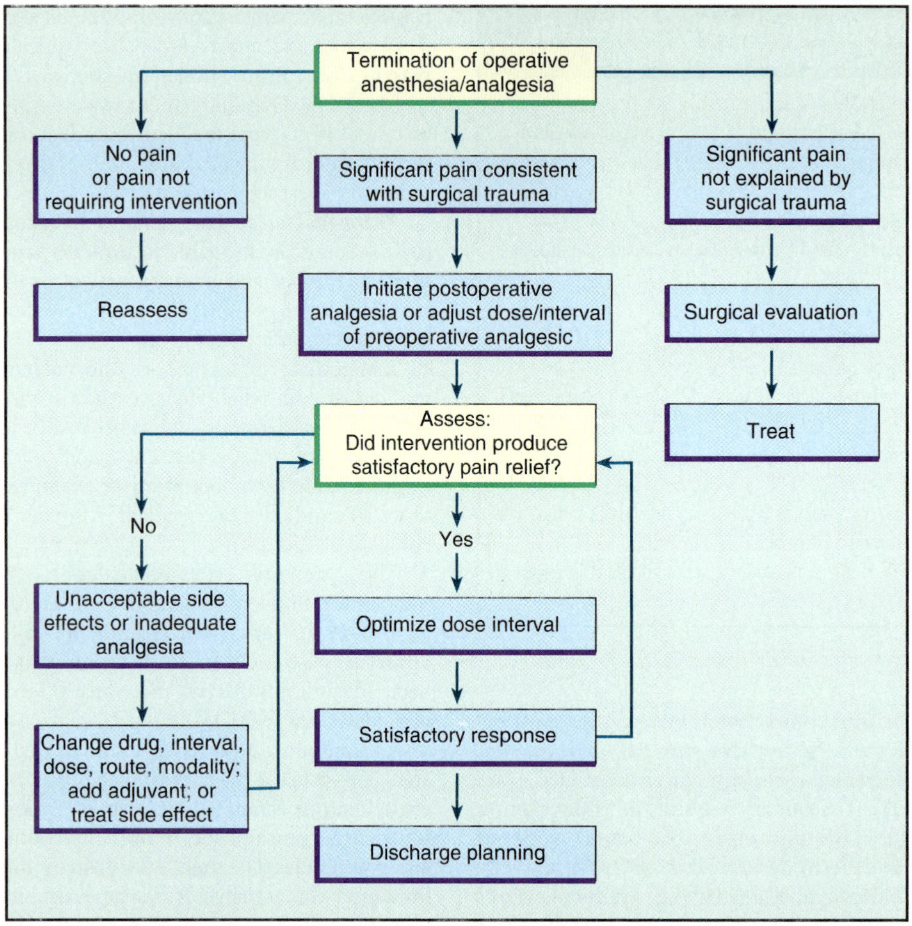

FIG. 43-11 Pain treatment flow chart: postoperative phase. (From Agency for Health Care Policy and Research, Acute Pain Management Guideline Panel: *Acute pain management: operative or medical procedures and trauma,* Clinical Practice Guideline, AHCPR Pub No. 92-0032, Rockville, Md, 1992, Agency for Health Care Policy and Research, Public Health Service, US Department of Health and Human Services.)

Opioid or opioid-like analgesics are generally prescribed for moderate-to-severe pain. These analgesics act on higher centers of the brain and spinal cord by binding with opiate receptors to modify perceptions of pain. A rare adverse effect of opioids in opioid-naive patients is respiratory depression. Respiratory depression is only clinically significant if there is a decrease in the rate *and* depth of respirations from the patient's baseline assessment (Pasero and McCaffery, 2011). Patients who are breathing deeply rarely have clinical respiratory depression. Sedation, another adverse effect of opioids, *always* occurs before respiratory depression. Thus closely monitor for sedation in opioid-naive patients (Pasero and McCaffery, 2011).

If a patient experiences respiratory depression, administer naloxone (Narcan) (0.4 mg diluted with 9 mL saline) intravenous push (IVP) at a rate of 0.5 mL every 2 minutes until the respiratory rate is greater than 8 breaths/min with good depth. Administering naloxone faster than recommended possibly causes severe pain and serious complications (Pasero and McCaffery, 2011). Reassess patients who receive naloxone every 15 minutes for 2 hours following drug administration because its duration is less than that of the opioid and respiratory depression sometimes returns.

Additional adverse effects of opioids include nausea, vomiting, constipation, itching, urinary retention, myoclonus, and altered mental processes (Ersek et al., 2004). Except for constipation, these side effects usually stop once a patient receives an opioid around the clock (ATC) for 4 to 10 days. Consider patients to be opioid naive until this point and opioid tolerant after about a week of ATC opioid dosing.

One way to maximize pain relief while potentially decreasing drug use is to administer analgesics on an ATC rather than a prn basis. The American Pain Society (APS, 2003) supports ATC administration if pain is anticipated for the majority of the day.

According to the American Geriatrics Society (AGS, 2002), opioids are probably not used enough with older persons. The AGS suggests a "start-low" (dose) and "go-slow" (upward dose titration) philosophy. Furthermore, do not use meperidine in older adults (AGS, 2002; Pasero and McCaffery, 2011). Meperidine (Demerol) is not recommended as an analgesic at any age because of its toxic metabolite, normeperidine, which causes seizures (APS, 2003; Pasero and McCaffery, 2011).

The proper use of analgesics requires careful assessment and critical thinking in the application of pharmacological principles and logic (Box 43-13). A person's response to an analgesic is highly individualized. If the pain is caused by inflammation, an NSAID is sometimes as effective as, or more effective than, an opioid. An orally administered analgesic usually has a longer onset

BOX 43-13 NURSING PRINCIPLES FOR ADMINISTERING ANALGESICS

Know Patient's Previous Response to Analgesics

- Determine whether patient has allergies.
- Know whether patient is at risk for using NSAIDs (e.g., history of GI bleeding or renal insufficiency) or opioids (e.g., history of obstructive or central sleep apnea).
- Identify previous doses and routes of analgesic administration to avoid undertreatment.
- Determine whether patient obtained relief.
- Ask whether a nonopioid was as effective as an opioid.

Select Proper Medications When More Than One Is Ordered

- Use nonopioid analgesics or opioid combination drugs for mild-to-moderate pain.
- You can give opioids with nonopioids.
- In older adults avoid combinations of opioids.
- Fentanyl patches, morphine, or hydromorphone are opioids of choice for long-term management of severe pain.
- Intravenous medications act more quickly and usually relieve severe, acute pain within 1 hour; whereas oral medications take as long as 2 hours to relieve pain.
- Avoid intramuscular analgesics, especially in older adults.
- Use an opioid with a nonopioid analgesic for severe pain because such combinations treat pain peripherally and centrally.
- For chronic pain give sustained-release oral formulations ATC.

Know Accurate Dosage

- Recall that 4 g is considered the maximum 24-hour dosage for acetaminophen and acetylsalicylic acid (ASA); 3200 mg for ibuprofen.
- Adjust doses as appropriate for children and older patients.
- Large doses of opioids are acceptable in opioid-tolerant patients, but not opioid-naive patients.
- When titrating opioids it is important to titrate to effect or to uncontrollable side effects.

Assess Right Time and Interval for Administration

- Administer analgesics as soon as pain occurs and before it increases in severity.
- An ATC administration schedule is usually best.
- Give analgesics before pain-producing procedures or activities.
- Know the average duration of action for a drug and the time of administration so the peak effect occurs when the pain is most intense.
- Use extended-release opioid formulations to treat chronic pain.
- Avoid abruptly stopping opioids in patients who are opioid tolerant.

Modified from Pasero, C. McCaffery M: *Pain assessment and pharmacological management,* St Louis, 2011, Mosby.
ATC, Around the clock; *GI,* gastrointestinal; *NSAIDs,* nonsteroidal antiinflammatory drugs.

and duration of action than an injectable form. In addition, controlled- or extended-release opioid formulations (morphine [MS Contin, Kadian, Avinza], oxycodone [OxyContin], and methadone) are available for administration every 8 to 12 hours ATC; they are not ordered prn.

You need to know the comparative potencies of analgesics in oral and injectable form. In addition, know the route of administration most effective for a patient so controlled, sustained pain relief is achieved. If nurses on succeeding shifts choose different routes for the same dose, the patient does not receive the same level of analgesia; and pain control will be poor. Equianalgesic charts (i.e., charts converting one opioid to another or parenteral forms of opioids [e.g., morphine to hydromorphone] to oral forms ([or vice versa]) are available on most nursing units or by contacting pharmacy staff.

Before administering opioids, it is important to consider a patient's situation, including current treatments, diseases/conditions, and/or organ (kidneys/liver) function. Opioid doses often need to be adjusted up or down according to patient circumstances. Situations requiring special considerations include breast-feeding mothers, patients on dialysis, those with neurological or respiratory conditions, and patients with recent abdominal surgery.

The Joint Commission requires health care agencies to have range-order policies in place to guide nurses in selecting the most appropriate dose of a medication. "Range orders are medication orders in which the dose varies over a prescribed range depending on the situation or the patient's status" (Manworren, 2006). An example is "Administer 5 to 10 mg morphine sulfate IVP for acute pain." Such an order is dangerous when there are no clinical guidelines to use for selecting the exact dose. Range orders give nurses the flexibility needed to treat patients' pain in a timely way while allowing for differences in patient response to pain and analgesia. Safe and effective range orders consider the patient's age, pain intensity, and co-morbidities; avoid frequency ranges; and prescribe a maximum dose that is at least two times but not more than four times the minimum dose in the range (Pasero et al., 2007; ASPMN, 2004).

Adjuvants are drugs originally developed to treat conditions other than pain but also have analgesic properties. For example, tricyclic antidepressants (e.g., nortriptyline [Pamelor]), anticonvulsants (e.g., gabapentin [Neurontin]), and infusional lidocaine successfully treat neuropathic pain. Corticosteroids relieve pain associated with inflammation and bone metastasis. Other examples of adjuvants are bisphosphonates and calcitonin given for bone pain (Pasero and McCaffery, 2011).

Sedatives, antianxiety agents, and muscle relaxants have *no* analgesic effect; however, they often cause drowsiness and impaired coordination, judgment, and mental alertness and contribute to respiratory depression. It is important to avoid attributing these adverse effects solely to opioids.

Patient-Controlled Analgesia. When patients depend on nurses for prn analgesia, an erratic cycle of alternating pain and analgesia often occurs. The patient feels pain and asks for medication, but you must first assess the patient and then prepare the medication. Under this circumstance analgesia finally occurs in about an hour, but pain relief may last only 30 minutes. Gradually the patient again feels discomfort, and the cycle begins again. The patient is constantly going in and out of analgesic therapeutic range.

A drug delivery system called **patient-controlled analgesia (PCA)** is a safe method for pain management that many patients prefer (Skill 43-1 on pp. 990-992). It is a drug delivery system that allows patients to self-administer opioids (morphine, hydromorphone, and fentanyl) with minimal risk of overdose. The goal is to maintain a constant plasma level of analgesic to avoid the problems of prn dosing. Systemic PCA traditionally involves IV or subcutaneous drug administration; however, a controlled analgesia device for oral medications, Medication on Demand (MOD), is now available. This device allows patients access to their own oral prn mediations, including opioids and other analgesics, antiemetics, and anxiolytics, at the bedside (Avancen, 2006).

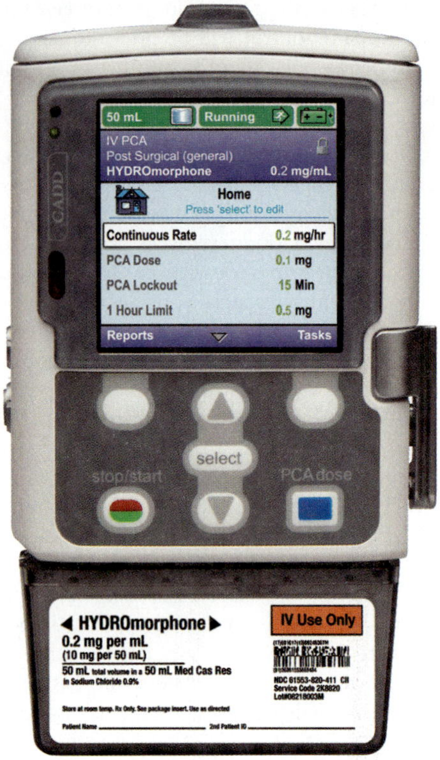

FIG. 43-12 Patient-controlled analgesia pump with cassette. (Courtesy of Smiths Medical ASD, Inc, St Paul, Minn.)

PCA infusion pumps are portable and computerized and contain a chamber for a syringe or bag that delivers a small, preset dose of opioid (Fig. 43-12). To receive a demand dose, the patient pushes a button attached to the PCA device. Systems are designed to deliver a specified number of doses every 1 to 4 hours (depending on the pump settings) given every 5 to 15 minutes (programmable) to avoid overdoses (APS, 2003). Most pumps have locked safety systems that prevent tampering by patients or family members and are generally safe to be managed in the home. For patients with cancer pain, a low-dose continuous infusion (basal rate) of 0.5 to 1 mg/hr is sometimes programmed to deliver a steady dose of continuous medication (Pasero and McCaffery, 2011).

There are many benefits to PCA use. The patient gains control over pain, and pain relief does not depend on nurse availability. Patients also have access to medication when they need it. This decreases anxiety and leads to decreased medication use. Small doses of medications are delivered at short intervals, stabilizing serum drug concentrations for sustained pain relief.

Patient preparation and teaching is critical to the safe and effective use of PCA devices (Box 43-14). Patients need to understand PCA and be physically able to locate and press the button to deliver the dose. Be sure to instruct family members not to "push the button" for the patient. Use Authorized Agent Controlled Analgesia (AACA) guidelines to *authorize* a family member or nurse to administer the analgesic, when appropriate (Wuhrman et al., 2006).

Check the IV line and PCA device per institutional policy to ensure proper functioning. Even though patients control administration of analgesics, diligence of the nurse is needed to prevent errors related to programmable PCA devices. In opioid-naive patients, do not increase demand or basal dose *and* shorten the interval time simultaneously because this increases the risk for oversedation and respiratory depression. Document drug dosages and track medication wastes according to agency policy (Pasero and McCaffery, 2011). PCA basal doses are *not* recommended for opioid-naive patients following surgery because of the possibility for respiratory depression.

BOX 43-14 PATIENT TEACHING

Patient-Controlled Analgesia

Objective

- Patient achieves pain control with proper use of the patient-controlled analgesia (PCA) device.

Teaching Strategies

- Teach the use of PCA before procedures so patient understands how to use it after awakening from anesthesia or sedation. Reinforce as needed.
- Instruct patient in the purpose of PCA, emphasizing that patient controls medication delivery.
- Explain that the pump prevents the risk of overdose.
- Tell family members or friends not to operate the PCA device for patient.

Evaluation

- Ask patient to tell you the purpose of the PCA device.
- Observe patient administering a dose.
- Evaluate the severity of patient's pain while using the PCA device.

Building Competency in Patient-Centered Care You are caring for Mrs. Gonzales, a 62-year-old patient who had surgery earlier today for a total knee replacement. Her husband is at her side and very concerned about her condition. Mrs. Gonzales had preoperative instruction on use of PCA, and you are reinforcing that education with her and her husband. She states she does not want to become addicted to the pain medication and is hesitant to push the button to administer it. Mr. Gonzales tells her that he will push the button for her when she needs pain medication. What knowledge, skills and attitudes will best help you provide patient-centered care to Mrs. Gonzales?

Answers to questions can be found on the Evolve website.

Perineural Local Anesthetic Infusion. You are able to manage pain for a variety of inpatient and outpatient adult and pediatric surgical procedures with **perineural infusion** pumps (e.g., Breg and On-Q). An unsutured catheter from a surgical wound placed near a nerve or groups of nerves connects to a pump containing a local anesthetic (bupivacaine or ropivacaine). You set the pump on demand or continuous mode, and it is usually left in place for 48 hours. Patients learn how to discontinue the pump at home and bring the catheter to their next health care provider visit. Some patients still need oral analgesics, but perineural infusions often reduce the total dosage (Pasero, 2004).

Topical Analgesics. Topical analgesics such as ELA-Max/LMX and eutectic mixture of local anesthetics (EMLA) are available for children. Apply EMLA via a disk or thick cream to the skin 30 to 60 minutes before minor procedures (e.g., IV start, IM injection) or anesthetic infiltration of soft tissue. Do not place EMLA around the eyes, the tympanic membrane, or over large skin surfaces.

The Lidoderm patch is a topical analgesic effective for cutaneous neuropathic pain in adults. You place three patches, cut to size, on and around the pain site using a 12-hour on, 12-hour

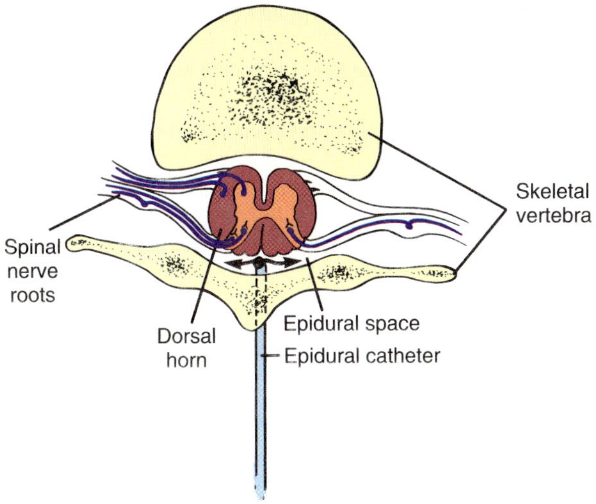

FIG. 43-13 Anatomical drawing of epidural space.

off schedule to avoid lidocaine toxicity. Other topical analgesics include ketoprofen patch and capsaicin lotion (Pasero and McCaffery, 2011).

Local and Regional Anesthetics. Local anesthesia is the local infiltration of an anesthetic medication to induce loss of sensation to a body part. Health care providers often use local anesthesia during brief surgical procedures such as removal of a skin lesion or suturing a wound by applying local anesthetics topically on skin and mucous membranes or by injecting them subcutaneously or intradermally to anesthetize a body part. The drugs produce temporary loss of sensation by inhibiting nerve conduction. Local anesthetics also block motor and autonomic functions, depending on the amount used and the location and depth of an injection. Smaller sensory nerve fibers are more sensitive to local anesthetics than are large motor fibers. As a result, the patient loses sensation before losing motor function, and conversely, motor activity returns before sensation.

Local anesthetics cause side effects, depending on their absorption into the circulation. Itching or burning of the skin or a localized rash is common after topical applications. Application to vascular mucous membranes increases the chance of systemic effects such as a change in heart rate.

Regional anesthesia is the injection of a local anesthetic to block a group of sensory nerve fibers. Tissues are anesthetized layer by layer as the surgeon or anesthesia provider introduces the agent into deeper structures of the body. Kinds of regional anesthesia include epidural anesthesia, pudendal blocks, and spinal anesthesia. Epidural analgesia is common for the treatment of acute postoperative pain, labor and delivery pain, and chronic cancer pain (Chumbley and Thomas, 2010). It permits control or reduction of severe pain and reduces the patient's overall opioid requirement, thus minimizing adverse effects. Epidural analgesia is short or long term, depending on a patient's condition and life expectancy.

The health care provider administers epidural analgesia into the spinal epidural space (Fig. 43-13) by inserting a blunt-tip needle into the level of the vertebral interspace nearest to the area requiring analgesia. The health care provider advances the catheter into the epidural space, removes the needle, and secures the remainder of the catheter with a dressing. Ensure the catheter is taped securely along the back of the patient. If the catheter is temporary, it is connected to tubing positioned along the spine and over the patient's shoulder. The end of the catheter is then placed on the patient's chest for the nurse's access. Nurse anesthetists, anesthesiologists, and nurses control epidural analgesia, depending on agency policy. Some patients control their demand dose, known as *patient-controlled epidural analgesia (PCEA)* (Pasero and McCaffery, 2011).

Nursing Implications. You maintain responsibility for providing emotional support to patients receiving local or regional anesthesia by explaining the insertion technique and warning patients that they will temporarily lose sensory function within minutes of injection. In the case of regional anesthesia, motor and autonomic (bowel and bladder control) function are also quickly lost. It is common for patients to fear paralysis because epidural and spinal injections come close to the spinal cord. To reassure the patient, explain that numbness, tingling, and coldness are common. Catheter insertion is painful unless the health care provider numbs the injection site. Prepare patients for such discomfort. Before a patient receives an analgesic, check for allergies. Also check to be sure that the drugs (morphine [Duramorph] and fentanyl [Sublimaze]) administered via the epidural catheter are free of potentially neurotoxic substances such as preservatives and additives. Assess vital signs to monitor systemic effects.

After administration of a local anesthetic, protect the patient from injury until full sensory and motor function return. Patients are at risk for injuring the anesthetized body part without knowing it. For example, after an injection into a joint, warn the patient to avoid using the joint until function returns. For patients with topical anesthesia, avoid applying heat or cold to numb areas. After spinal anesthesia the patient stays in bed until sensory and motor function return. Assist the patient the first time he or she tries to get out of bed.

When managing epidural infusions, connect the catheter to an infusion pump, a port, or reservoir or cap it off for bolus injections. To reduce the risk of accidental epidural injection of drugs intended for IV use, clearly label the catheter *epidural catheter*. Always administer continuous infusions through electronic infusion devices for proper control. Because of the catheter location, use surgical asepsis to prevent a serious and potentially fatal infection. Notify a patient's health care provider immediately of any signs or symptoms of infection or pain at the insertion site. Thorough hygiene is necessary during nursing procedures to keep the catheter system clean and dry.

Nursing implications for managing epidural analgesia are numerous (Table 43-6). Do not administer supplemental doses of opioids or sedative/hypnotics because of possible additive central nervous system adverse effects. Monitoring for effects of medications differs, depending on whether infusions are intermittent or continuous. Complications of epidural opioid use include nausea and vomiting, urinary retention, constipation, respiratory depression, and pruritus (Lehne, 2010). When patients receive epidural analgesia, you monitor them as often as every 15 minutes, including assessment of vital signs, respiratory effort, and skin color. Once stabilized, monitoring occurs every hour (refer to agency policy).

The patient needs to receive thorough education about epidural analgesia in terms of the action of the medication and its advantages and disadvantages. Instruct patients about the potential for side effects and to notify you or their health care provider if side effects develop. If the patient requires long-term epidural use, the health care provider tunnels a permanent catheter through the skin. The catheter exits at the patient's side. Teach a patient on long-term therapy how to safely administer home infusions with minimal ongoing nursing intervention.

TABLE 43-6 Nursing Care for Patients with Epidural Infusions

GOAL	ACTIONS
Prevent catheter displacement.	Secure catheter (if not connected to implanted reservoir) carefully to outside skin.
Maintain catheter function.	Check external dressing around catheter site for dampness or discharge. (Leak of cerebrospinal fluid may develop.) Use transparent dressing to secure catheter and aid inspection. Inspect catheter for breaks.
Prevent infection.	Use strict aseptic technique when caring for catheter (see Chapter 28). Do not routinely change dressing over site. Change infusion tubing every 24 hours.
Monitor for respiratory depression.	Monitor vital signs, especially respirations, per policy. Use pulse oximetry and apnea monitoring.
Prevent undesirable complications.	Assess for pruritus (itching) and nausea and vomiting. Administer antiemetics as ordered.
Maintain urinary and bowel function.	Monitor intake and output. Assess for bladder and bowel distention. Assess for discomfort, frequency, and urgency.

Invasive Interventions for Pain Relief. When severe pain persists despite medical treatment, invasive interventions available for consideration include intrathecal implantable pumps or injections, spinal cord stimulators, deep brain stimulation, neuroablative procedures (cordotomy, rhizotomy, thalamotomy), trigger point injections, radiofrequency ablation, cryoablation, intradiscal electrothermal (IDET) annuloplasty, vertebroplasty, and intraspinal medications (opioids, steroids, local anesthetics, alpha agonists). It is not acceptable to tell a patient with severe unrelieved pain that there is "nothing more we can do for you." Refer patients with pain unresponsive to medications to a pain expert.

Procedure Pain Management. The Thunder Project II (Puntillo et al., 2001) identified several procedures causing pain in critical care patients: turning, wound drain removal, tracheal suctioning, femoral catheter removal, placement of a central line, and changing of nonburn wound dressings.

Premedicating patients before painful procedures allows patients to cooperate more fully and reduces the experience of pain. The American Society of Anesthesiologists practice guidelines (2004) recommend premedicating patients before surgery as part of a multimodal analgesic pain management program.

Chronic Noncancer and Cancer Pain Management. Cancer pain is either chronic or acute. The AHCPR published clinical practice guidelines for cancer pain management in 1994 that continue to be a reference today (Lehne, 2010). The guidelines support comprehensive and aggressive treatment of cancer pain, including many options for pain relief (Fig. 43-14). The best choice of treatment often changes as the patient's condition and the characteristics of pain change. You can use nonpharmacological interventions with pharmacological interventions.

Various medications and routes of administration provide relief for patients with cancer pain. Long-acting or controlled-release medications are very successful in managing all types of chronic pain. These controlled-released medications (e.g., morphine [MS Contin, Roxanol SR], and oxycodone [OxyContin]) relieve pain for 8 to 12 hours. A 72-hour fentanyl patch is also available. You can manage most chronic pain by using oral or patch medications. Do not use the intramuscular route for controlling pain because the injection is painful and there is inconsistent, erratic drug absorption (Pasero and McCaffery, 2011).

BOX 43-15 TYPES OF BREAKTHROUGH PAIN

Incident pain: Pain that is predictable and elicited by specific behaviors such as physical therapy or wound dressing changes

End-of-dose failure pain: Pain that occurs toward the end of the usual dosing interval of a regularly scheduled analgesic

Spontaneous pain: Pain that is unpredictable and not associated with any activity or event

Data from Gruener D, Lande S: *Pain control in the primary care setting,* Glenview, Ill, 2006, American Pain Society.

Estimates of addiction in patients with persistent pain range from 6% to 10% (Pasero and McCaffery, 2011). Patients with persistent pain requiring prolonged opioid administration sometimes develop an opioid tolerance. As a result, patients require higher doses of opioids to attain pain relief. The higher opioid dose is not lethal because patients also develop a tolerance to respiratory depression.

It is necessary to give patients with chronic pain required analgesics on a regular basis. Prescribing analgesics on a prn basis for chronic pain is ineffective and causes more suffering. The patient with chronic pain needs to take an analgesic ATC, even when the pain subsides. Regular administration maintains therapeutic drug blood levels for ongoing pain control.

Administering analgesics to treat chronic pain requires applying principles different from those used to treat acute pain. The World Health Organization (Pasero and McCaffery, 2011) recommends a three-step approach to managing cancer pain (Fig. 43-15). Therapy begins with using NSAIDs and/or adjuvants and progresses to strong opioids if pain persists. Side effects of opioids such as nausea and constipation are treated aggressively so patients are able to continue using them. Patients usually become tolerant to their side effects, with the exception of constipation. Routinely administer stimulant laxatives, not simple stool softeners, to prevent and treat constipation.

Transdermal fentanyl, which is 100 times more potent than morphine, is available at predetermined doses that provide analgesia for 48 to 72 hours. The transdermal route is useful when patients are unable to take drugs orally. Fentanyl patches are only used with patients who are opioid tolerant. Patients find this system easy to use because it allows for continuous opioid administration without needles or pumps. Self-adhesive patches release the medication slowly over time, achieving effective analgesia. Transdermal fentanyl is not for adult patients who weigh less than 100 pounds (too little subcutaneous tissue for absorption) or who are hyperthermic (increases drug absorption). Do not place heating pads over the patch and never cut it. To dispose of the patch, fold in half, adhesive side onto itself, and flush down the toilet (Pasero and McCaffery, 2011).

A transmucosal fentanyl "unit" now exists to treat **breakthrough pain** (Box 43-15) in opioid-tolerant patients. Breakthrough pain is a transient flare of moderate-to-severe pain superimposed on continuous or persistent pain. Swab the fentanyl unit in the mouth over the buccal mucosa and gums. The unit remains intact to

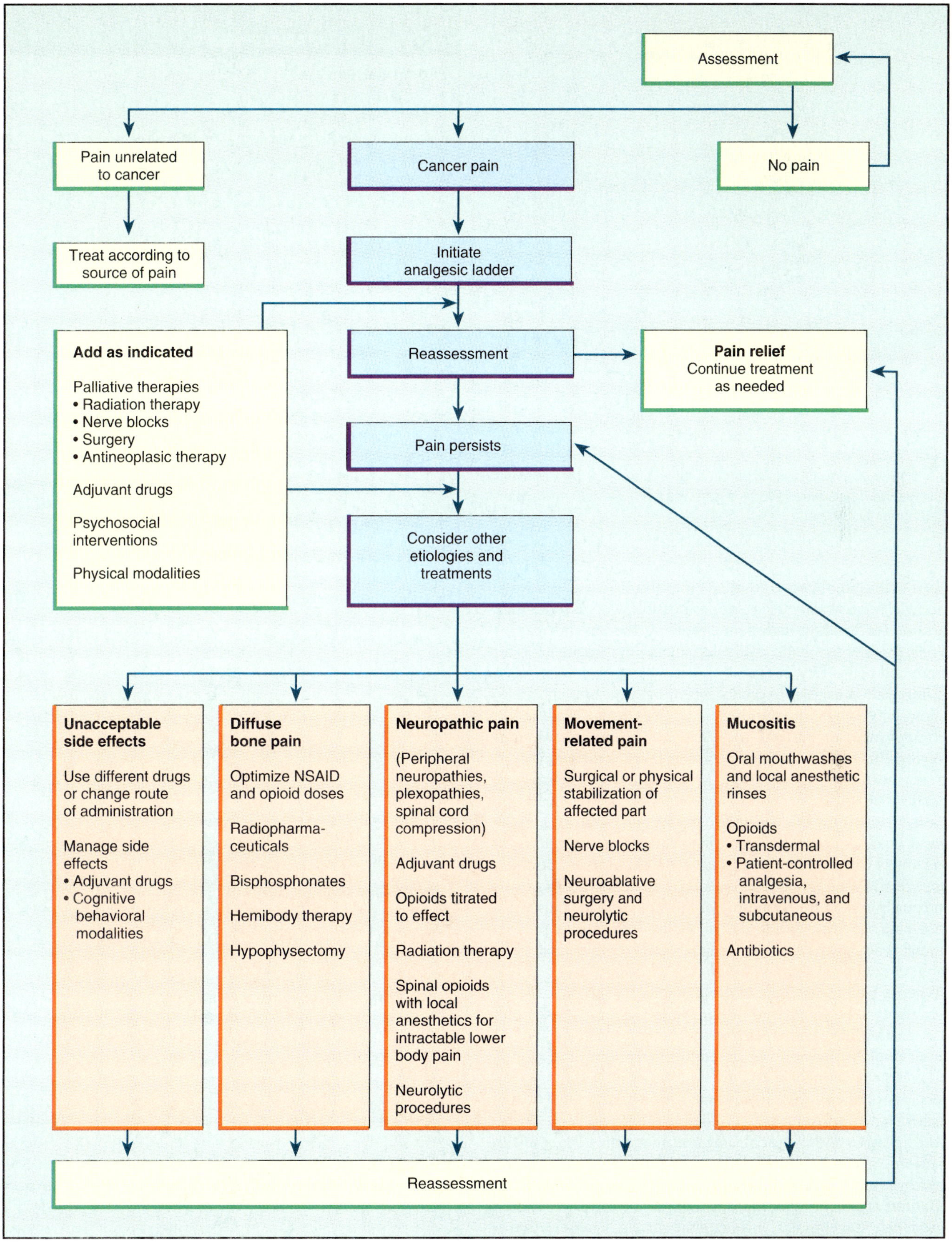

FIG. 43-14 Flow chart: continuing pain management in patients with cancer. *NSAID,* Nonsteroidal antiinflammatory drug. (From Jacox A et al: *Management of cancer pain,* Clinical Practice Guideline No. 9, AHCPR Pub No. 94-0592, Rockville, Md, 1994, Agency for Health Care Policy and Research, Public Health Service, US Department of Health and Human Services.)

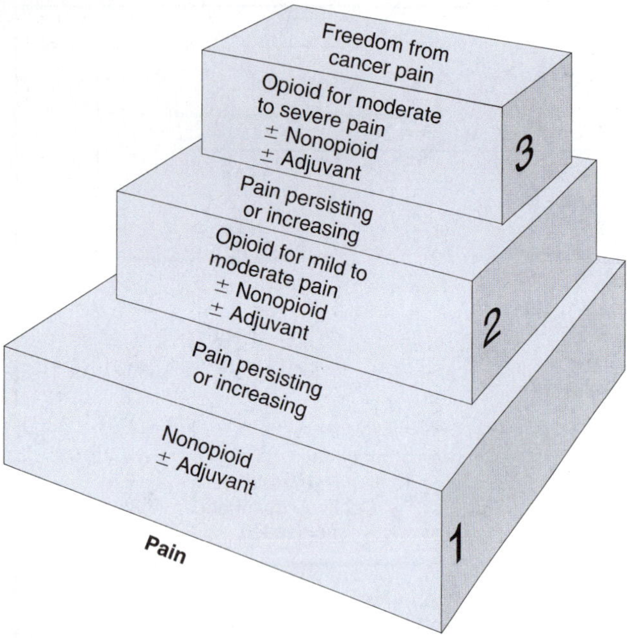

FIG. 43-15 WHO analgesic ladder is a three-step approach in treating cancer pain, accessed 9/27/10 from http://www.who.int/cancer/palliative/painladder/en/.

dissolve in the mouth, not chewed. Allow to absorb over a 15-minute period, delaying swallowing as long as possible. Use no more than two units per breakthrough pain episode. If the patient's pain is not relieved after two units, notify the patient's health care provider (Pasero and McCaffery, 2011).

Administer analgesics rectally when patients are unable to swallow, have nausea or vomiting, or are near death. This route is contraindicated for patients with diarrhea or cancerous lesions involving the anus or rectum. Morphine, hydromorphone, and oxymorphone are available in suppositories (Pasero and McCaffery, 2011).

Some patients use PCA devices to treat severe cancer pain in the home or acute care setting. PCA devices provide improved, uniform pain control with fewer peaks and valleys in plasma concentration, more effective drug action, and lower drug dosages overall. Patients who usually benefit from continuous infusions include those with severe pain for whom oral and injectable medications provide minimal relief, those with severe nausea and vomiting, and those unable to swallow oral medications.

When a patient first receives continuous-drip opioids, the IV access needs to be patent and without complications (see Chapter 41). A central-line catheter such as a Groshong or Hickman catheter, an implanted venous access port, or a peripherally inserted central catheter is usually best for long-term IV infusion. When IV access is poor, the subcutaneous route with a concentrated dose is possible. When infusions begin, monitor the patient very closely for the first hour and then according to agency policy. Patients who are placed on continuous analgesic infusions are opioid tolerant; thus respiratory depression is rare.

Barriers to Effective Pain Management. Barriers to effective pain management are complex, involving the patient, health care provider, and health care system (Box 43-16). Some health care providers require opioid agreements and random urine testing from patients who need long-term opioid therapy. However, evidence of the effectiveness of agreements is lacking, and there are ethical concerns about using them for all patients who require long-term opioid therapy (Arnold et al., 2006). This raises the question as to whether agreements protect patients or health care providers.

Patients and health care providers often do not understand the differences between **physical dependence, addiction,** and **drug tolerance** (Box 43-17). Experiencing a physical dependency does not imply addiction, and drug tolerance in and of itself is not the same as addiction. That is not to say that addiction does not occur

BOX 43-16 BARRIERS TO EFFECTIVE PAIN MANAGEMENT

Patient Barriers
- Fear of addiction
- Worry about side effects
- Fear of tolerance (won't be there when I need it)
- Takes too many pills already
- Fear of injections
- Concern about not being a "good" patient
- Doesn't want to worry family and friends
- May need more tests
- Needs to suffer to be cured
- Pain necessary for past indiscretions
- Inadequate education
- Reluctance to discuss pain
- Pain inevitable
- Pain part of aging
- Fear of disease progression
- Believes health care providers and nurses are doing all they can
- Just forgets to take analgesics
- Fear of distracting health care providers from treating illness
- Believes health care providers have more important or sicker patients to see
- Suffering in silence noble and expected

Health Care Provider Barriers
- Inadequate pain assessment skills
- Concern with addiction
- Opiophobia, fear of opioids
- Fear of legal repercussions
- No visible cause of pain
- Belief that patients need to learn to live with pain
- Reluctance to deal with side effects of analgesics
- Not believing patient's report of pain
- Fear that giving a dose will kill the patient
- Health care provider time constraints
- Inadequate reimbursement
- Belief that opioids "mask" symptoms
- Belief that pain is part of aging
- Overestimation of rates of respiratory depression

Health Care System Barriers
- Concern with creating "addicts"
- Difficulty in filling prescriptions
- Absolute dollar restriction on amount reimbursed for prescriptions
- Mail-order pharmacy restrictions
- Advanced practice nurses not used efficiently
- Extensive documentation requirements
- Poor pain policies and procedures regarding pain management
- Lack of money
- Inadequate access to pain clinics
- Poor understanding of economic impact of unrelieved pain

BOX 43-17 DEFINITIONS RELATED TO THE USE OF OPIOIDS IN PAIN TREATMENT*

Physical Dependence
A state of adaptation that is manifested by a drug class specific withdrawal syndrome produced by abrupt cessation, rapid dose reduction, decreasing blood level of the drug, and/or administration of an antagonist.

Addiction
A primary, chronic, neurobiological disease with genetic, psychosocial, and environmental factors influencing its development and manifestations. Addictive behaviors include one or more of the following: impaired control over drug use, compulsive use, continued use despite harm, and craving.

Drug Tolerance
A state of adaptation in which exposure to a drug induces changes that result in a diminution of one or more effects of the drug over time.

*Approved by the Boards of Directors of the American Academy of Pain Medicine, the American Pain Society, and the American Society of Addiction Medicine, February 2001 (American Pain Society, 2011).

or that true addicts should not be treated for pain. "Patients with addictive disease and pain have the right to be treated with dignity, respect, and the same quality of pain assessment and management as all other patients" (ASPMN Position Statement, 2002). Nurses and health care providers need to avoid labeling patients as *drug seeking* because this term is poorly defined and can cause bias and prejudice. If you are concerned that a patient is abusing opioids, voice your concerns to the patient and notify the patient's health care provider, explaining the reasons for your concern.

Follow recommendations for the management of acute pain in patients dependent on opioids who are not necessarily addicted (Mehta and Langford, 2006). A study of patients who had addictions and pain revealed that they did not feel respected by nurses who cared for them (Morgan, 2006). These patients used presentation (try to be nice and thank the nurse) and self-management strategies (do not get angry or make waves) to obtain pain relief.

Placebos. Placebos are medications or procedures that produce positive or negative effects in patients. These effects are not related to the specific physical or chemical properties of the placebo. Professional organizations discourage their use to treat pain. It is considered unethical and deceitful to administer them. Placebo use jeopardizes the trust between patients and their caregivers. If a placebo is ordered, you must question the order. Many health care agencies have policies that limit the use of placebos to research only (Pasero and McCaffery, 2011).

Restorative and Continuing Care

Pain Clinics, Palliative Care, and Hospices. Health professionals recognize pain as a significant health problem. Growth of pain centers, palliative care departments, and hospices designed to manage pain and suffering has increased. The Commission on Accreditation of Rehabilitation Facilities (CARF) accredits chronic pain treatment programs and sets standards for chronic pain management. A comprehensive pain center treats persons on an inpatient or outpatient basis. Staff members representing all health care disciplines (e.g., nursing, medicine, physical therapy, pastoral care, and dietetics) work with patients to find the most effective pain-relief measures. A comprehensive clinic provides not only diverse therapy but also research into new treatments and training for professionals.

Many hospitals have palliative-care departments to help patients and their family members successfully manage their diseases (Morrison et al., 2005). The goal of palliative care is to learn to live life fully with an incurable condition (see Chapter 36). Patients and their family members need ongoing assistance in managing their pain at home. A National Patient Safety Goal (TJC, 2011) recommends standardizing communication when a patient transfers into, out of, and within the medical system. Teaching pain management during discharge and ensuring continuation of pain management after discharge is essential.

Hospices are programs that care for patients at the end of life (see Chapter 36). The emphasis is on quality of life over quantity (Douglass et al., 2004). Hospice helps terminally ill patients continue to live at home or in a health care setting in comfort and privacy. Pain control is a priority for hospices. Under the guidance of hospice nurses, families learn to monitor patients' symptoms and become the primary caregivers. Some hospice patients become hospitalized, such as in the event of a brief acute care crisis or family problem.

Hospice programs help nurses overcome their fears of contributing to a patient's death when administering large doses of opioids. The American Nurses Association supports aggressive treatment of pain and suffering even if it hastens a patient's death (Fowler, 2010). Recent research suggests that moderate opioid dose increases in patients who are terminally ill do not hasten death (Bengoechea et al., 2010). The disease, not the opioid, is killing the patient.

EVALUATION

Through the Patient's Eyes. Evaluate patients' perceptions of the effectiveness of interventions used to relieve pain. Patients help decide the best times to attempt pain treatments. Essentially they are the best judge of whether a pain-relief intervention works. Often the family is another valuable resource, particularly in the case of a patient with pain who is not able to express discomfort. Also ask patients about tolerance to therapy and the overall amount of relief obtained. If patients state that an intervention is not helpful or even aggravates the discomfort, stop it immediately and seek an alternative. Time and patience are necessary to maximize the effectiveness of pain management. Educate the patient about what to expect. Reassure the patient that you will check back frequently to assess for changes in pain level. Continually assess whether the character of the patient's pain changes and whether individual interventions are effective.

Patient Outcomes. Evaluation of pain is one of many nursing responsibilities that require effective critical thinking (Fig. 43-16). A patient's behavioral responses to pain-relief interventions are not always obvious. Evaluating the effectiveness of a pain intervention requires you to evaluate the patient's pain after an appropriate period of time. For instance, oral medications usually peak in about 1 hour; whereas IVP medications peak in 15 to 30 minutes. Ask the patient if the medication alleviated the pain when it was peaking. Do not expect the patient to volunteer the information. Evaluate psychological and physiological responses to pain (e.g., "Does your pain ever cause you to get depressed or angry?").

If you evaluate that a patient continues to have discomfort after an intervention, try a different approach. For example, if an analgesic provides only partial relief, add relaxation exercises or guided-imagery exercises. You also consult with the patient's health care provider about increasing the dose, decreasing the interval between doses, or trying different analgesics. If patient outcomes are not met, ask the patient:

- What is your current pain level?
- How far away is your pain level from your goal?

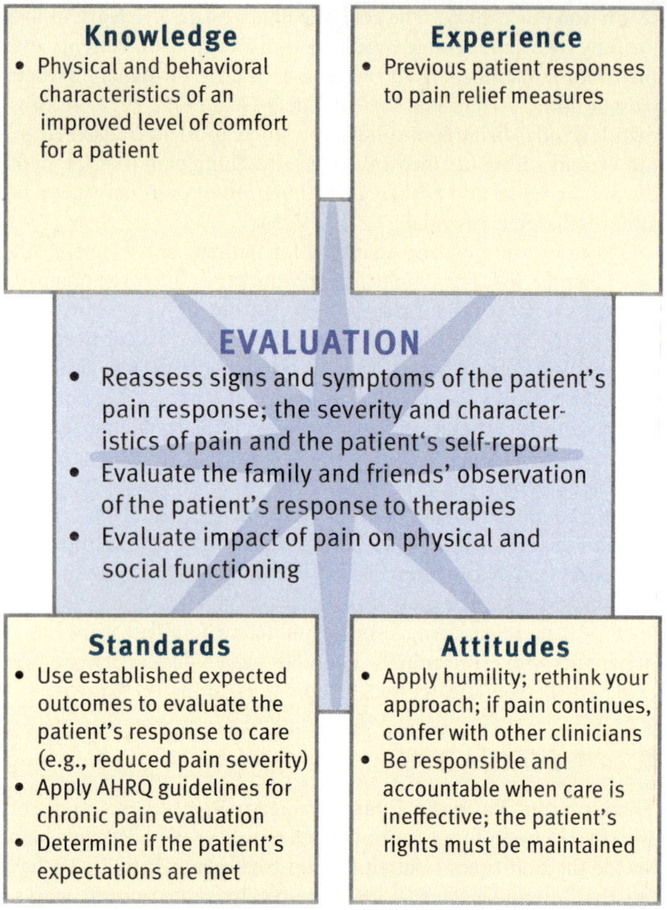
Knowledge
• Physical and behavioral characteristics of an improved level of comfort for a patient
Experience
• Previous patient responses to pain relief measures
EVALUATION
• Reassess signs and symptoms of the patient's pain response; the severity and characteristics of pain and the patient's self-report
• Evaluate the family and friends' observation of the patient's response to therapies
• Evaluate impact of pain on physical and social functioning
Standards
• Use established expected outcomes to evaluate the patient's response to care (e.g., reduced pain severity)
• Apply AHRQ guidelines for chronic pain evaluation
• Determine if the patient's expectations are met
Attitudes
• Apply humility; rethink your approach; if pain continues, confer with other clinicians
• Be responsible and accountable when care is ineffective; the patient's rights must be maintained

FIG. 43-16 Critical thinking model for pain-management evaluation. *AHRQ*, Agency for Healthcare Research and Quality.

BOX 43-18 CHECKLIST FOR COMMUNICATING PATIENTS' UNRELIEVED PAIN TO COLLEAGUES

- What is the pain rating now? Over the past period of time?
- Which pain rating is acceptable to the patient?
- How do you recommend that the patient's treatment be changed to reduce the pain rating?
- Which professional reference can be used, if needed, to support this recommendation?

From Pasero C, McCaffery M: *Pain assessment and pharmacologic management*, St Louis, 2011, Mosby.

- What side effects are you experiencing from your pain medication?
- Describe limitations in function you are experiencing related to uncontrolled pain.
- How is your pain limiting or altering your rest and sleep?

Effective communication of your assessment of a patient's pain and the response to intervention is facilitated by accurate and thorough documentation. This communication needs to happen from nurse to nurse, shift to shift, and nurse to other health care providers. It is your professional responsibility as the nurse caring for the patient to report the effectiveness of interventions for managing the patient's pain and evaluation of patient care goals and outcomes. A variety of tools such as a pain flow sheet or diary help centralize information about pain management. The patient expects you to be sensitive to his or her pain and to be attentive in attempts to manage that pain. Effectively communicating with colleagues (Box 43-18) helps you achieve optimal pain relief for patients.

SAFETY GUIDELINES FOR NURSING SKILLS

Ensuring patient safety is an essential role of the professional nurse. To ensure patient safety, communicate clearly with members of the health care team, assess and incorporate the patient's priorities of care and preferences, and use the best evidence when making decisions about your patient's care. When performing the skills in this chapter, remember the following points to ensure safe, individualized patient care.

- The patient is the only person who should press the button to administer the pain medication when using PCA.
- Monitor the patient for signs and symptoms of oversedation and respiratory depression.

SKILL 43-1 PATIENT-CONTROLLED ANALGESIA

View Video!

Delegation Considerations

The skill of administration of patient-controlled analgesia (PCA) cannot be delegated to nursing assistive personnel (NAP). Instruct the NAP to:

- Notify the nurse if the patient complains of pain or has signs of becoming oversedated.
- Notify the nurse if the patient has questions about the PCA process or equipment.
- Never administer a PCA dose for the patient.

Equipment

- PCA system
- Identification label and time tape (may already be attached and completed by pharmacy)
- Alcohol swab
- Adhesive tape
- Clean gloves, when applicable
- Equipment for vital signs and pulse oximeter

STEP	RATIONALE
ASSESSMENT	
1 Assess patient's cognitive ability.	Determines if patient is able to use PCA for pain management.
2 Assess for physical, behavioral, and emotional signs and symptoms of pain or discomfort.	Combination of signs and symptoms reveals source and nature of pain.
3 Assess characteristics of patient's pain.	Reveals source and nature of pain and factors that may increase pain.
4 Assess patency of intravenous (IV) access and surrounding tissue for inflammation or swelling.	IV line needs to be patent for safe administration of pain medication. Confirmation of placement of IV catheter and integrity of surrounding tissues ensures that medication is administered safely.
5 Check accuracy and completeness of each MAR or computer printout with health care provider's order for patient's name, name of medication, dose, frequency of medication (continuous or demand or both), and lockout period.	Health care provider order required for administration of opioid medication. Ensures patient receives right medications.
6 Have a second registered nurse (RN) confirm health care provider's order and correct setup of PCA. The second RN **independently checks** health care provider's order and the machine, not simply look at the first RN's setup.	Prevents medication errors.
7 Check patient's history for drug allergies. Be aware that nausea is not an allergic reaction and it can be treated; itching alone is not an allergic reaction and is common to opioid use. Itching is also treatable and does not rule out the use of PCA.	Avoids placing patient at risk for allergic reaction.
PLANNING	
1 Collect appropriate equipment.	
2 Review medication information in drug reference manual or consult with pharmacist if uncertain about any medications to be administered.	Understanding medications before administering them prevents medication errors (Brady, Malone, and Fleming, 2009).
3 Explain purpose and demonstrate function of PCA to patient and family (see Box 43-14).	Allows patient participation in care and independence in pain control. Preoperative education about PCA therapy improves postoperative pain relief (ASPMN, 2006).
4 Check infuser and patient-controlled module for accurate labeling or evidence of leaking.	Avoids medication error. Damage to system can occur in shipping and handling; inspect to avoid injury or harm to patient, self, or others.
5 Program computerized PCA pump to deliver prescribed medication dose and lockout interval.	Ensures safe, therapeutic drug administration.
6 Draw curtains around patient's bed or close door to room.	Maintains patient's privacy.
7 Position patient comfortably for procedure. Maintain any position restrictions. Venipuncture or central line site needs to be accessible.	Comfortable position enhances effectiveness of analgesia.
IMPLEMENTATION	
1 Perform hand hygiene.	Reduces transmission of infection.
2 Follow the six rights to be sure of correct medication. Identify the patient using two identifiers (i.e., name and birth date or name and account number) according to facility policy. Compare identifiers with information on patient's medication administration record (MAR) or medical record (see Chapter 31).	Minimizes risk for medication error and harm to patient. Ensures correct patient. Complies with recommended National Patient Safety Goal (TJC, 2011).
3 Attach drug reservoir to infusion device and prime tubing.	Locks system and prevents air from infusing into IV tubing.
4 Apply clean gloves.	Reduces potential contact with blood when working with IV line.
5 Attach needleless adapter to tubing adapter of patient-controlled module.	Needed to connect with IV line.
6 Wipe injection port of maintenance IV line with alcohol if using a closed port.	Alcohol is a topical antiseptic that minimizes entry of surface microorganisms during needle insertion.
7 Insert and secure needleless adapter into injection port nearest patient.	Establishes route for medication to enter main IV line. Prevents delay of medication delivery to patient. Needleless systems prevent needlestick injuries.
8 Administer loading dose of analgesia as prescribed.	Give one-time doses manually or program into PCA pump.
9 Discard gloves and supplies in appropriate containers.	Reduces transmission of microorganisms.
10 If experiencing pain, have patient demonstrate use of PCA system; if not, have patient repeat instructions given earlier by nurse.	Repeating instructions reinforces learning. Checking patient's understanding through return demonstration helps nurse determine patient's level of understanding and ability to manipulate device.
11 Dispose of empty cassette or syringe in compliance with institutional policy.	The federal Controlled Substances Act regulates the control and dispensation of opioids for all institutions.
12 If PCA is discontinued before device is completely empty, record drug wastage on PCA medication administration record (MAR) per institutional policy. Note date, time, amount of drug wasted, and reason for wastage.	Two RNs must witness wastage of opioids (narcotics) and sign the record to meet requirements of the Controlled Substances Act for scheduled drugs.
13 Most PCA systems need a secondary IV infusion running at TKO (to keep open rate). Be sure that infusion is running properly (see Chapter 41).	To maintain patency of vein between PCA intermittent (bolus) doses.

SKILL 43-1 PATIENT-CONTROLLED ANALGESIA—cont'd

STEP	RATIONALE
EVALUATION	
1 Use pain-rating scale to evaluate patient's pain intensity according to agency policy.	Determines response to PCA dosing. Documenting "PCA in use" or "PCA effective" is not an adequate record of the patient's pain level.
2 Observe patient for nausea or itching.	Common side effects of opioid.
3 Observe for signs of adverse reactions, especially excessive sedation. Monitor level of sedation, vital signs, and pulse oximetry every 2 hours for the first 12 hours (APS, 2003).	Patient is at highest risk the first 12 hours of use. Excess sedation precedes respiratory depression.
4 Have patient demonstrate dose delivery.	Evaluates skill in use of PCA.
5 According to agency policy, evaluate number of attempts (number of times patient pushed the button), delivery of demand doses (number of times drug actually given), and basal dose if ordered.	Assists in evaluating effectiveness of PCA dose and frequency in relieving pain. Maintains compliance with Controlled Substances Act.

UNEXPECTED OUTCOMES AND RELATED INTERVENTIONS

1 Patient verbalizes continued or worsening discomfort or displays nonverbal behaviors indicative of pain, suggesting that underlying condition has changed or patient is undermedicated.
- Perform complete pain assessment.
- Inspect IV site for possible catheter occlusion or infiltration.
- Consult with health care provider.

2 Patient is not readily arousable.
- Stop PCA, elevate head of bed unless contraindicated, and assess vital signs. **Do not** leave the patient's bedside.
- Notify health care provider and/or call for help.
- Prepare to administer an opioid-reversing agent.

3 Patient unable to manipulate PCA device to maintain pain control.
- Consult with health care provider regarding alternative medication route.
- Discuss with health care provider possible basal (continuous) dose.
- Assess patient support system for significant other who can responsibly manipulate PCA device (ASPMN, 2006).

RECORDING AND REPORTING

- Record drug, dose, and time begun on MAR. Note lockout time, demand, and basal dose.
- Record regular assessments of patient pain, vital signs, and oxygen saturation.
- Record amount of drug delivered and amount wasted.

KEY POINTS

- Pain is a purely subjective physical and psychosocial experience.
- Misconceptions about pain often result in doubt about the degree of the patient's suffering and unwillingness to provide relief.
- Knowledge of the nociceptive pain processes of the pain experience—transmission, transduction, perception, and modulation—provides guidelines for selecting pain-relief measures.
- An interaction of psychological and cognitive factors affects pain perception.
- A person's cultural background influences the meaning of pain and how it is expressed.
- It is common for older patients not to report pain.
- Patients who are in chronic pain are unlikely to show behavioral changes.
- The difference between acute and chronic pain involves the concept of harm. Acute pain is protective, thus preventing harm; chronic pain is no longer protective.
- Do not collect an in-depth pain history when the patient is experiencing severe discomfort.
- Pain causes physical signs and symptoms similar to those of other diseases.
- Individualize pain interventions by collaborating closely with the patient, using assessment findings, and trying a variety of interventions.
- Eliminating sources of painful stimuli is a basic nursing measure for promoting comfort.
- Using a regular schedule around-the-clock (ATC) for analgesic administration is more effective than an as-needed schedule in pain control.
- Sedation is an adverse effect of opioids that always precedes respiratory depression (which is rare).
- A PCA device gives patients pain control with low risk of overdose.
- While caring for a patient who receives local anesthesia, protect him or her from injury.
- Nursing implications for administering epidural analgesia include preventing infection and monitoring closely for respiratory depression.
- Addiction rarely occurs in patients who take opioids to relieve pain.
- The goal of pain management is to anticipate and prevent pain rather than treat it.

- Pain evaluation includes measuring the changing character of pain, the patient's response to interventions, and the patient's perceptions of the effectiveness of a therapy.

CLINICAL APPLICATION QUESTIONS

Preparing for Clinical Practice

After three doses (0.5 mg each) of morphine from the patient-controlled analgesia (PCA) device, Mrs. Mays started vomiting and stated that she was feeling "out of her head." She rated her chest pain as 3 on a scale of 0 to 10. She is breathing comfortably on 2 L of nasal cannula oxygen, and her lung sounds are clear to auscultation. Her husband is very concerned and anxious about his wife and wants the morphine stopped so she will not become "addicted."

1. Do you think Mrs. Mays is allergic to morphine? Support your answer.
2. What do you need to tell Mr. and Mrs. Mays about the adverse effects of morphine?
3. Which interventions do you need to complete before consulting the health care provider?

evolve *Answers to Clinical Application Questions can be found on the Evolve website.*

REVIEW QUESTIONS

Are You Ready to Test Your Nursing Knowledge?

1. Which of the following signs or symptoms in an opioid-naive patient is of greatest concern to the nurse when assessing the patient 1 hour after administering an opioid?
   1. Oxygen saturation of 95%
   2. Difficulty arousing the patient
   3. Respiratory rate of 10 breaths/min
   4. Pain intensity rating of 5 on a scale of 0 to 10
2. A health care provider writes the following order for an opioid-naive patient who returned from the operating room following a total hip replacement. "Fentanyl patch 100 mcg, change every 3 days." Based on this order, the nurse takes the following action:
   1. Calls the health care provider, and questions the order
   2. Applies the patch the third postoperative day
   3. Applies the patch as soon as the patient reports pain
   4. Places the patch as close to the hip dressing as possible
3. A patient is being discharged home on an around-the-clock (ATC) opioid for chronic back pain. Because of this order, the nurse anticipates an order for which class of medication?
   1. Stool softener
   2. Stimulant laxative
   3. H_2 receptor blocker
   4. Proton pump inhibitor
4. A new medical resident writes an order for OxyContin SR 10 mg PO q12 hours prn. Which part of the order does the nurse question?
   1. The drug
   2. The time interval
   3. The dose
   4. The route
5. The nurse notices that a patient has received oxycodone/acetaminophen (Percocet) (5/325), two tablets PO every 3 hours for the past 3 days. What concerns the nurse the most?
   1. The patient's level of pain
   2. The potential for addiction
   3. The amount of daily acetaminophen
   4. The risk for gastrointestinal bleeding
6. A patient with chronic low back pain who took an opioid around-the-clock (ATC) for the past year decided to abruptly stop the medication for fear of addiction. He is now experiencing shaking chills, abdominal cramps, and joint pain. The nurse recognizes that this patient is experiencing symptoms of:
   1. Addiction.
   2. Tolerance.
   3. Pseudoaddiction.
   4. Physical dependence.
7. After having received 0.2 mg of naloxone (Narcan) intravenous push (IVP), a patient's respiratory rate and depth are within normal limits. The nurse now plans to implement the following action:
   1. Discontinue all ordered opioids
   2. Close the room door to allow the patient to recover
   3. Administer the remaining naloxone over 4 minutes
   4. Assess patient's vital signs every 15 minutes for 2 hours
8. Which one of the following instructions is crucial for the nurse to give to both family members and the patient who is about to be started on a patient-controlled analgesia (PCA) of morphine?
   1. Only the patient should push the button.
   2. Do not use the PCA until the pain is severe.
   3. The PCA prevents overdoses from occurring.
   4. Notify the nurse when the button is pushed.
9. A patient with a history of a stroke that left her confused and unable to communicate returns from interventional radiology following placement of a gastrostomy tube. The health care provider's order reads as follows: "Vicodin 1 tab, per tube, q4 hours, prn." Which action by the nurse is most appropriate?
   1. No action is required by the nurse because the order is appropriate.
   2. Request to have the ordered changed to ATC for the first 48 hours.
   3. Ask for a change of medication to meperidine (Demerol) 50 mg IVP, q3 hours, prn.
   4. Begin the Vicodin when the patient shows nonverbal symptoms of pain.
10. A patient returning to the nursing unit after knee surgery is verbalizing pain at the surgical site. The nurse's first action is to:
    1. Call the patient's health care provider.
    2. Administer pain medication as ordered.
    3. Check the patient's vital signs.
    4. Assess the characteristics of the pain.
11. The patient rates his pain as a 6 on a scale of 0 to 10, with 0 being no pain and 10 being the worst pain. The patient's wife says that he can't be in that much pain since he has been sleeping for 30 minutes. Which is the most accurate resource for assessing the pain?
    1. The patient's wife is the best resource for determining the level of pain since she has been with him continually for the entire day.
    2. The patient's report of pain is the best method for assessing the pain.
    3. The patient's health care provider has the best knowledge of the level of pain that the patient that should be experiencing.
    4. The nurse is the most experienced at assessing pain.

12. When using ice massage for pain relief, which of the following are correct? (Select all that apply.)
    1. Apply ice using firm pressure over skin.
    2. Apply ice until numbness occurs and remove the ice for 5 to 10 minutes.
    3. Apply ice until numbness occurs and discontinue application.
    4. Apply ice for no longer than 10 minutes.
13. When teaching a patient about transcutaneous electrical nerve stimulation (TENS), which information do you include?
    1. TENS works by causing distraction.
    2. TENS therapy does not require a health care provider's order.
    3. TENS requires an electrical source for use.
    4. TENS electrodes are applied near or directly on the site of pain.
14. While caring for a patient with cancer pain, the nurse knows that the World Health Organization (WHO) analgesic ladder recommends:
    1. Transitioning use of adjuvants with nonsteroidal antiinflammatory drugs (NSAIDs) to opioids.
    2. Using acetaminophen for refractory pain.
    3. Limiting the use of opioids because of the likelihood of side effects.
    4. Avoiding total sedation, regardless of how severe the pain is.
15. A postoperative patient is currently asleep. Therefore the nurse knows that:
    1. The sedative administered may have helped him sleep, but assessment of pain is still needed.
    2. The intravenous (IV) pain medication is effectively relieving his pain.
    3. Pain assessment is not necessary.
    4. The patient can be switched to the same amount of medication by the oral route.

Answers: **1.** 2; **2.** 1; **3.** 2; **4.** 2; **5.** 3; **6.** 4; **7.** 4; **8.** 1; **9.** 2; **10.** 4; **11.** 2; **12.** 1, 2; **13.** 4; **14.** 1; **15.** 1.

REFERENCES

Ackley B, Ladwig G: *Nursing diagnosis handbook*, ed 9, St Louis, 2011, Mosby.

Agency for Health Care Policy and Research, Acute Pain Management Guideline Panel (AHCPR): *Acute pain management: operative or medical procedures and trauma*, Clinical Practice Guideline, AHCPR Pub No. 92-0032, Rockville, Md, 1992, Agency for Health Care Policy and Research, Public Health Service, US Department of Health and Human Services.

American Bar Association: *Legal guide for the seriously ill*, 2009, http://apps.americanbar.org/abanet/media/release/news_release.cfm?releaseid=849. Accessed October 10, 2011.

American Geriatrics Society (AGS): The management of persistent pain in older persons, *J Am Geriatr Soc* 50(S6):205, 2002.

American Holistic Health Association: *Wellness from within: the first step*, Anaheim, Calif, 2007, The Association.

American Nurses Association (ANA): *Pain management nursing: scope and standards of practice*, Silver Spring, Md, 2005, The Association.

American Pain Foundation (APF): *Pain care bill of rights*, 2007, http://www.painfoundation.org/. Accessed September 25, 2010.

American Pain Society (APS): *Principles of analgesic use in the treatment of acute and cancer pain*, ed 5, Glenview, Ill, 2003, The Society.

American Pain Society (APS): *Definitions related to the use of opioids for the treatment of pain*, Glenview, Ill, 2011, The Society, www.ampainsoc.org/advocacy/opioids2.htm.

American Society of Anesthesiologists (ASA): Practice guidelines for acute pain management in the perioperative setting, *Anesthesiology* 100:1573, 2004.

American Society of Anesthesiologists (ASA): Practice guidelines for chronic pain management, *Anesthesiology* 112:1, 2010.

American Society for Pain Management Nursing (ASPMN): *Position statement on pain management in patients with addictive disease*, Pensacola, Fla, 2002, http://www.asmpn.org/Organization/documents/AddictiveDisease.pdf.

American Society for Pain Management Nursing (ASPMN): *Position statement on the use of "as needed" range orders for opioid analgesics in the management of acute pain*, Pensacola, Fla, 2004, http://www.asmpn.org/pdfs/As%20Needed%20Range%20Orders.pdf/.

American Society for Pain Management Nursing (ASPMN): Patient-controlled analgesia: authorized agent controlled analgesia, a position statement, *Pain Manag Nurs* 7(4):134, 2006.

Arnold R, et al: Opioid contracts in chronic nonmalignant pain management: objectives and uncertainties, *Am J Med* 119(4):292, 2006.

Arnstein P: Balancing analgesic efficacy with safety concerns in the older adult, *Pain Manage Nurs* 11(2):S11, 2010.

Avancen: *Medication on demand*, 2006, http://www.avancen.com. Accessed November 26, 2011.

Chou R, et al: Clinical guidelines for the use of chronic opioid therapy in chronic noncancer pain, *J Pain* 10(2):113, 2009.

Chumbley G, Thomas S: Care of the patient receiving epidural analgesia, *Nurs Standard* 25(9):35, 2010.

D'Arcy Y: Hot topics in pain management: using NSAIDs safely, *Nursing* 35(2):22, 2006.

Douglass AB, et al: Principles of palliative care medicine. I. Patient assessment, *Adv Stud Med* 4(1):15, 2004.

Ersek M, et al: The cognitive effects of opioids, *Pain Manag Nurs* 5(2):75, 2004.

Fowler MDM: *Guide to the code of ethics for nurses*, Silver Spring, Md, 2010, American Nurses Association.

Gruener D, Lande S: *Pain control in the primary care setting*, Glenview, Ill, 2006, American Pain Society.

Herr K, et al: Pain assessment in the nonverbal patient: position statement with clinical practice recommendations, *Pain Manag Nurs* 7(2):44, 2006a.

Herr K, et al: Tools for assessment of pain in nonverbal older adults with dementia: a state-of-the-science review, *J Pain Symptom Manage* 31(2):170, 2006b.

Herr K: Pain in the older adult: an imperative across all health care settings, *Pain Manage Nurs* 11(2):S1, 2010.

Hockenberry MJ, Wilson D: *Wong's nursing care of infants and children*, ed 9, St Louis, 2011, Mosby.

Hughes RG, editor: *Patient safety and quality: an evidence-based handbook for nurses*, prepared with support from the Robert Wood Johnson Foundation. AHRQ Publication No. 08-0043, Rockville, Md, March 2008, Agency for Healthcare Research and Quality.

International Association for the Study of Pain (IASP): *Pain terms*, 2010, http://www.iasp-pain.org/AM/Template.cfm?Section=Pain_Definitions&Template=/CM/HTMLDisplay.cfm&ContentID=1728#Pain. Accessed September 10, 2010.

Kaufman G: Basic pharmacology of nonopioid analgesics, *Nurs Standard* 24(30):55, 2010.

Kehlet H, et al: Persistent postsurgical pain: risk factors and prevention, *Lancet* 367(9522):1618, 2006.

Lehne R: *Pharmacology for nursing care*, ed 7, Philadelphia, 2010, Saunders.

Manworren R: A call to action to protect range orders, *Am J Nurs* 106(7):65, 2006.

Maxwell T, et al: *Palliative and end-of-life pain management: self-directed learning module*, Pensacola, Fla, 2005, American Society for Pain Management Nursing.

McCarberg B, O'Connor A: A new look at heat treatment for pain disorders, part I, *APS Bulletin* 14(6):4, 2004.

Mehta V, Langford R: Acute pain management for opioid dependent patients, *Anaesthesia* 61(3):269, 2006.

Melzack R, Wall PD: Pain mechanisms: a new theory, *Science* 150:971, 1965.

Melzack R, Wall D: *Handbook of pain management*, London, 2003, Churchill Livingstone.

Miaskowski C: The next step to improving cancer pain management, *Pain Manag Nurs* 6(1):1, 2005.

Morrison R, et al: The growth of palliative care programs in United States hospitals, *J Palliat Med* 8(6):1127, 2005.

Otis-Green S, et al: An integrated psychosocial model for cancer pain management, *Cancer Pract* 10(S1):58, 2002.

Pain Management Center Staff: *When your pain flares up: easy, proven techniques for managing chronic pain*, Minneapolis, 2002, Fairview Press.

Pasero C: Perineural local anesthetic infusion, *Am J Nurs* 104(7):89, 2004.

Pasero C, McCaffery M: No self-report means no pain-intensity rating, *Am J Nurs* 205(10):50, 2005.

Pasero C, McCaffery M: *Pain assessment and pharmacologic management*, St Louis, 2011, Mosby.

Pasero C, et al: Pain control: IV opioid range orders for acute pain management, *Am J Nurs* 107(2):52, 2007.

Schulman-Green D, et al: Unlicensed staff members' experiences with patients' pain on an inpatient oncology unit: implications for redesigning the care delivery system, *Cancer Nurs* 28(5):340, 2005.

Shaw S: Nursing and supporting patients with chronic pain, *Nurs Stand* 20(19):60, 2006.

The Joint Commission (TJC): *2011 National Patient Safety Goals (NPSG)*, 2011, http://jointcommission.org/Patient/Safety/NationalPatient/SafetyGoals/. Accessed January 31, 2011.

Vila H, et al: The efficacy and safety of pain management before and after implementation of hospital-wide pain management standards: is patient safety compromised

by treatment based solely on numerical pain ratings? *Anesth Analg* 101(2):474, 2005.
Williams H: Assessing, diagnosing and managing neuropathic pain, *Nurs Times* 102(16):22, 2006.
Wirth J, et al: Use of herbal therapies to relieve pain: a review of efficacy and adverse effects, *Pain Manag Nurs* 6(4):145, 2005.
Wong DL, Baker CM: Pain in children: comparison of assessment scales, *Oklahoma Nurse* 33(1):8, 1988.
Wuhrman E, et al: *Authorized and unauthorized ("PCA by PROXY") dosing of analgesic infusion pumps*, 2006, http://www.aspmn.org/organization/documents/PCAbyProxy-final-ew_004.pdf. Accessed October 10, 2011.
Yoon S, Schaffer S: Herbal, prescribed, and over-the-counter drug use in older women: prevalence of drug interactions, *Geriatr Nurs* 27(2):118, 2006.

RESEARCH REFERENCES

Allred K, et al: The effect of music on postoperative pain and anxiety, *Pain Manage Nurs* 11(1):15, 2010.
Bengoechea I, et al: Opioid use at the end of life and survival in a hospital at home unit, *J Palliat Med* 13(9):1079, 2010.
Beyer JE, et al: The creation, validation, and continuing development of the Oucher: a measure of pain intensity in children, *J Pediatr Nurs* 7(5):335, 1992.
Brady A, Malone A, Fleming S: A literature review of the individual and systems factors that contribute to medication errors in nursing practice, *J Nurs Manage* 17(6): 679, 2009.
Chen Y, Francis A: Relaxation and imagery for chronic, nonmalignant pain: effects on pain symptoms, quality of life, and mental health, *Pain Manage Nurs* 11(3):159, 2010.
Cutshall SM, et al: Effect of massage therapy on pain, anxiety, and tension in cardiac surgical patients: a pilot study, *Complement Ther Clin Pract* 16(2):92, 2010.
Engwall M, Duppils GS: Music as a nursing intervention for postoperative pain: a systematic review, *J PeriAnesth Nurs* 24(6):370, 2009.
Harris M, Richards KC: The physiological and psychological effects of slow-stroke back massage and hand massage on relaxation in older people, *J Clin Nurs* 19(7-8):917, 2010.
Herr K, Titler M: Acute pain assessment and pharmacological management practices for the older adult with a hip fracture: review of ED trends, *J Emerg Nurs* 35(4):312, 2009.
Jensen M, et al: The validity of the neuropathic pain scale for assessing diabetic neuropathic pain in a clinical trial, *Clin J Pain* 22(1):97, 2006.
Juarez P, et al: Comparison of two pain scales for the assessment of pain in the ventilated adult patient, *Dimens Crit Care Nurs* 29 (6):307, 2010.
Kato K, et al: Importance of genetic influences on chronic widespread pain, *Arthritis Rheum* 54:1682, 2006.
Morgan B: Knowing how to play the game: hospitalized substance abusers' strategies for obtaining pain relief, *Pain Manag Nurs* 7(1):31, 2006.
Puntillo K, et al: Patients' perceptions and responses to procedural pain: results from Thunder Project II, *Am J Crit Care* 10(4):238, 2001.
Vaartio H, et al: Nursing advocacy in procedural pain care, *Nurs Ethics* 16(3):340, 2009.
Walters SJ: Massage and cancer: practice guidelines, *J Aust Traditional Med Soc* 16(3): 141, 2010.

CHAPTER

44

Nutrition

OBJECTIVES

- Explain the importance of a balance between energy intake and energy requirements.
- List the end products of carbohydrate, protein, and fat metabolism.
- Explain the significance of saturated, unsaturated, and polyunsaturated fats.
- Describe food guidelines and discuss their value in planning meals for good nutrition.
- List the current dietary guidelines for the general population.
- Explain the variance in nutritional requirements throughout growth and development.
- Discuss the major methods of nutritional assessment.
- Identify three major nutritional problems and describe patients at risk.
- Establish a plan of care to meet the nutritional needs of a patient.
- Describe the procedure for initiating and maintaining enteral feedings.
- Describe the methods to avoid complications of enteral feedings.
- Describe the methods for avoiding complications of parenteral nutrition.
- Discuss medical nutrition therapy in relation to three medical conditions.
- Discuss diet counseling and patient teaching in relation to patient expectations.

KEY TERMS

Amino acid, p. 997
Anabolism, p. 1000
Anorexia, p. 1015
Anorexia nervosa, p. 1003
Anthropometry, p. 1009
Basal metabolic rate (BMR), p. 997
Body mass index (BMI), p. 1009
Bulimia nervosa, p. 1003
Carbohydrates, p. 997
Catabolism, p. 1000
Chyme, p. 1000
Daily values, p. 1001
Dietary reference intakes (DRIs), p. 1001
Dispensable amino acids, p. 997
Dysphagia, p. 1010
Enteral nutrition (EN), p. 1018
Enzymes, p. 998
Fat-soluble vitamins, p. 998
Fatty acids, p. 998
Fiber, p. 997
Food security, p. 996
Gluconeogenesis, p. 1000
Glycogenesis, p. 1000
Glycogenolysis, p. 1000
Hypervitaminosis, p. 998
Ideal body weight (IBW), p. 1009
Indispensable amino acids, p. 997
Intravenous fat emulsions, p. 1021
Ketones, p. 1000
Kilocalorie (kcal), p. 997
Lipids, p. 998
Macrominerals, p. 998
Malabsorption, p. 1024
Malnutrition, p. 1007
Medical nutrition therapy (MNT), p. 1024
Metabolism, p. 1000
Minerals, p. 998
Monounsaturated fatty acids, p. 998
Nitrogen balance, p. 998
Nutrient density, p. 997
Nutrients, p. 997
Parenteral nutrition (PN), p. 1021
Peristalsis, p. 999
Polyunsaturated fatty acids, p. 998
Resting energy expenditure (REE), p. 997
Saccharides, p. 997
Saturated fatty acids, p. 998
Simple carbohydrates, p. 997
Trace elements, p. 998
Triglycerides, p. 998
Unsaturated fatty acids, p. 998
Vegetarianism, p. 1006
Vitamins, p. 998
Water-soluble vitamins, p. 998

evolve WEBSITE

http://evolve.elsevier.com/Potter/fundamentals/

- Review Questions
- Video Clips
- Animations
- Concept Map Creator
- Case Study with Questions
- Skills Performance Checklists
- Audio Glossary
- Interactive Learning Activities
- Key Term Flashcards
- Content Updates

Nutrition is a basic component of health and is essential for normal growth and development, tissue maintenance and repair, cellular metabolism, and organ function. The human body needs an adequate supply of nutrients for essential functions of cells. **Food security** is critical for all members of a household. This means that all household members have access to sufficient, safe, and nutritious food to maintain a healthy lifestyle; sufficient food is available on a consistent basis; and the household has resources to obtain appropriate food for a nutritious diet. Food also holds symbolic meaning. Giving or taking food is part of ceremonies, social gatherings, holiday traditions, religious events, the celebration of birth, and the mourning of death. The difficulty of the decision to withdraw food in a terminal illness, even in the form of intravenous (IV) nutrients, is a testament to the symbolic power of food and feeding.

Florence Nightingale understood the importance of nutrition, stressing a nurse's role in the science and art of feeding during the mid-1800s (Dossey, 1999). Since then the nurse's role in nutrition and diet therapy has changed. Medical nutrition therapy

BOX 44-1 EXAMPLES OF NUTRITION OBJECTIVES FOR *HEALTHY PEOPLE 2020*

Weight and Growth

- Increase proportion of adults who are at a healthy weight (body mass index [BMI] 18.5 to 24.9).
- Reduce the proportion of adults who are obese.
- Reduce the proportion of children (2 to 11 years) who are overweight or obese.

Food and Nutrient Consumption

- Decrease saturated fat intake in population 2 years and older.
- Increase the variety of vegetables and fruit intake in the population 2 years and older.
- Increase grain product intake and consumption of calcium in the population 2 years and older.
- Reduce sodium daily intake in the population 2 years and older.

Iron Deficiency and Anemia

- Reduce prevalence of iron deficiency in children and childbearing women.
- Reduce prevalence of anemia in pregnant women in third trimester to 20%.

Schools, Work Sites, and Nutrition Counseling

- Increase work-site nutrition-education and weight-management program offerings.
- Offer nutrition assessment and individualized planning at primary care sites.
- Increase the percentage of schools that offer nutritious foods and beverages outside of school meals.
- Increase the number of states with nutrition standards for food and beverages provided to preschool-age children in child care.

Food Security

- Increase food security to 94% of households.

Data from U.S. Department of Health and Human Services: *Healthy people 2020,* 2010, http://www.healthypeople.gov/hp2020/objectives.

(MNT) uses nutrition therapy and counseling to manage diseases (American Dietetic Association, 2010b). In some illnesses such as type 1 diabetes mellitus (DM) or mild hypertension, diet therapy is often the major treatment for disease control (ADA, 2008; American Heart Association, 2010). Other conditions such as severe inflammatory bowel disease require specialized nutrition support such as enteral nutrition (EN) or parenteral nutrition (PN). Current standards of care promote optimal nutrition in all patients (American Heart Association, 2010; ACS, 2011).

The U.S. Department of Health and Human Services (USDHHS) and the Public Health Service established nutritional goals and objectives for *Healthy People 2020* (USDHHS, 2010). *Healthy People 2020* is the United States' contribution to the "Health for All" strategy of the World Health Organization (WHO, 2010). *Healthy People 2020* (Box 44-1) continues the objectives initiated in *Healthy People 2000* and *Healthy People 2010,* with overall goals of promoting health and reducing chronic disease. All nutrition-related objectives include baseline data from which progress is measured. The challenge remains to motivate consumers to put these dietary recommendations into practice.

SCIENTIFIC KNOWLEDGE BASE

Nutrients: The Biochemical Units of Nutrition

The body requires fuel to provide energy for cellular metabolism and repair, organ function, growth, and body movement. The **basal metabolic rate (BMR)** is the energy needed to maintain life-sustaining activities (breathing, circulation, heart rate, and temperature) for a specific period of time at rest. Factors such as age, body mass, gender, fever, starvation, menstruation, illness, injury, infection, activity level, or thyroid function affect energy requirements. The **resting energy expenditure (REE),** or resting metabolic rate, is the amount of energy that an individual needs to consume over a 24-hour period for the body to maintain all of its internal working activities while at rest. Factors that affect metabolism include illness, pregnancy, lactation, and activity level.

In general, when energy requirements are completely met by **kilocalorie (kcal)** intake in food, weight does not change. When the kilocalories ingested exceed a person's energy demands, the individual gains weight. If the kilocalories ingested fail to meet a person's energy requirements, the individual loses weight.

Nutrients are the elements necessary for the normal function of numerous body processes. Energy needs are met from a variety of nutrients: carbohydrates, proteins, fats, water, vitamins, and minerals. Food is sometimes described according to its **nutrient density** (i.e., the proportion of essential nutrients to the number of kilocalories). High–nutrient dense foods such as fruits and vegetables provide a large number of nutrients in relationship to kilocalories. Low–nutrient dense foods such as alcohol or sugar are high in kilocalories but nutrient poor.

Carbohydrates. **Carbohydrates,** composed of carbon, hydrogen, and oxygen, are the main source of energy in the diet. Each gram of carbohydrate produces 4 kcal/g and serves as the main source of fuel (glucose) for the brain, skeletal muscles during exercise, erythrocyte and leukocyte production, and cell function of the renal medulla. People obtain carbohydrates primarily from plant foods, except for lactose (milk sugar). They are classified according to their carbohydrate units, or **saccharides.**

Monosaccharides such as glucose (dextrose) or fructose cannot be broken down into a more basic carbohydrate unit. Disaccharides such as sucrose, lactose, and maltose are composed of two monosaccharides and water. Both monosaccharides and disaccharides are classified as **simple carbohydrates** and are found primarily in sugars. Polysaccharides such as glycogen are made up of many carbohydrate units (i.e., complex carbohydrates). They are insoluble in water and digested to varying degrees. Starches are polysaccharides.

The body is unable to digest some polysaccharides because humans do not have enzymes capable of breaking them down. **Fiber** is a polysaccharide that is the structural part of plants that is not broken down by the human digestive enzymes. Because fiber is not broken down, it does not contribute calories to the diet. Insoluble fibers are not digestible and include cellulose, hemicellulose, and lignin. Soluble fibers dissolve in water and include barley, cereal grains, cornmeal, and oats.

Proteins. Proteins provide a source of energy (4 kcal/g), and they are essential for synthesis (building) of body tissue in growth, maintenance, and repair. Collagen, hormones, enzymes, immune cells, deoxyribonucleic acid (DNA), and ribonucleic acid (RNA) are all made of protein. In addition, blood clotting, fluid regulation, and acid-base balance require proteins. These proteins transport nutrients and many drugs in the blood. Ingestion of proteins maintains nitrogen balance.

The simplest form of protein is the **amino acid,** which is made up of hydrogen, oxygen, carbon, and nitrogen. The body does not synthesize **indispensable amino acids;** thus these need to be provided in the diet. Examples of indispensable amino acids are histidine, lysine, and phenylalanine. The body synthesizes **dispensable amino acids.** Examples of amino acids synthesized in the body are alanine, asparagine, and glutamic acid. Amino acids can link together. Albumin and insulin are simple proteins because they contain only amino acids or their derivatives. The combination of a simple protein with a nonprotein substance produces a complex protein such as lipoprotein, formed by a combination of a lipid and a simple protein.

A complete protein, also called a *high-quality protein,* contains all essential amino acids in sufficient quantity to support growth and maintain nitrogen balance. Examples of foods that contain complete proteins are fish, chicken, soybeans, turkey, and cheese. Incomplete proteins are missing one or more of the nine indispensable amino acids and include cereals, legumes (beans, peas), and vegetables. Complementary proteins are pairs of incomplete proteins that, when combined, supply the total amount of protein provided by complete protein sources.

Nitrogen balance is achieved when the intake and output of nitrogen are equal. When the intake of nitrogen is greater than the output, the body is in positive nitrogen balance. Positive nitrogen balance is required for growth, normal pregnancy, maintenance of lean muscle mass and vital organs, and wound healing. The body uses nitrogen to build, repair, and replace body tissues. Negative nitrogen balance occurs when the body loses more nitrogen than it gains (e.g., with infection, burns, fever, starvation, head injury, and trauma). The increased nitrogen loss is the result of body tissue destruction or loss of nitrogen-containing body fluids. Nutrition during this period needs to provide nutrients to put patients into positive balance for healing.

Protein provides energy; however, because of the essential role of protein in growth, maintenance, and repair, a diet needs to provide adequate kilocalories from nonprotein sources. When there is sufficient carbohydrate in the diet to meet the energy needs of the body, protein is spared as an energy source.

Fats. Fats **(lipids)** are the most calorie-dense nutrient, providing 9 kcal/g. Fats are composed of triglycerides and fatty acids. **Triglycerides** circulate in the blood and are composed of three fatty acids attached to a glycerol. **Fatty acids** are composed of chains of carbon and hydrogen atoms with an acid group on one end of the chain and a methyl group at the other. Fatty acids can be **saturated,** in which each carbon in the chain has two attached hydrogen atoms; or **unsaturated,** in which an unequal number of hydrogen atoms are attached and the carbon atoms attach to each other with a double bond. **Monounsaturated** fatty acids have one double bond, whereas **polyunsaturated** fatty acids have two or more double carbon bonds. The various types of fatty acids have significance for health and the incidence of disease and are referred to in dietary guidelines.

Fatty acids are also classified as essential or nonessential. Linoleic acid, an unsaturated fatty acid, is the only essential fatty acid in humans. Linolenic acid and arachidonic acid (also unsaturated fatty acids) are important for metabolic processes but are manufactured by the body when linoleic acid is available. Deficiency occurs when fat intake falls below 10% of daily nutrition. Most animal fats have high proportions of saturated fatty acids, whereas vegetable fats have higher amounts of unsaturated and polyunsaturated fatty acids.

Water. Water is critical because cell function depends on a fluid environment. Water makes up 60% to 70% of total body weight. The percent of total body water is greater for lean people than obese people because muscle contains more water than any other tissue except blood. Infants have the greatest percentage of total body water, and older people have the least. When deprived of water, a person cannot survive for more than a few days.

An individual meets fluid needs by drinking liquids and eating solid foods high in water content such as fresh fruits and vegetables. Water is also produced during digestion when food is oxidized. In a healthy individual fluid intake from all sources equals fluid output through elimination, respiration, and sweating (see Chapters 41 and 45). An ill person has an increased need for fluid (e.g., with fever or gastrointestinal [GI] losses). By contrast, he or she also has a decreased ability to excrete fluid (e.g., with cardiopulmonary or renal disease), which often leads to the need for fluid restriction.

Vitamins. **Vitamins** are organic substances present in small amounts in foods that are essential to normal metabolism. They are chemicals that act as catalysts in biochemical reactions. When there is enough of any specific vitamin to meet the body's catalytic demands, the rest of the vitamin supply acts as a free chemical and is often toxic to the body. Certain vitamins are currently of interest in their role as antioxidants. These vitamins neutralize substances called *free radicals,* which produce oxidative damage to body cells and tissues. Researchers think that oxidative damage increases a person's risk for various cancers. These vitamins include betacarotene and vitamins A, C, and E (Nix, 2009).

The body is unable to synthesize vitamins in the required amounts and depends on dietary intake. Vitamin content is usually highest in fresh foods that are used quickly after minimal exposure to heat, air, or water. Vitamins are classified as fat soluble and water soluble.

Fat-Soluble Vitamins. The **fat-soluble vitamins** (A, D, E, and K) are stored in the fatty compartments of the body. With the exception of vitamin D, people acquire vitamins through dietary intake. **Hypervitaminosis** of fat-soluble vitamins results from megadoses (intentional or unintentional) of supplemental vitamins, excessive amounts in fortified food, and large intake of fish oils.

Water-Soluble Vitamins. The **water-soluble vitamins** are vitamin C and the B complex (which is eight vitamins). The body does not store water-soluble vitamins; thus they need to be provided in daily food intake. Water-soluble vitamins absorb easily from the GI tract. Although they are not stored, toxicity can still occur.

Minerals. **Minerals** are inorganic elements essential to the body as catalysts in biochemical reactions. They are classified as **macrominerals** when the daily requirement is 100 mg or more and microminerals or **trace elements** when less than 100 mg is needed daily. Macrominerals help to balance the pH of the body, and specific amounts are necessary in the blood and cells to promote acid-base balance. Interactions occur among trace minerals. For example, excess of one trace mineral sometimes causes deficiency of another. Selenium is a trace element that also has antioxidant properties. Silicon, vanadium, nickel, tin, cadmium, arsenic, aluminum, and boron play an unidentified role in nutrition. Arsenic, aluminum, and cadmium have toxic effects.

Anatomy and Physiology of the Digestive System

Digestion. Digestion of food is the mechanical breakdown that results from chewing, churning, and mixing with fluid and chemical reactions in which food is reduced to its simplest form. Each part of the GI system has an important digestive or absorptive function (Fig. 44-1). **Enzymes** are the proteinlike substances that act as catalysts to speed up chemical reactions. They are an essential part of the chemistry of digestion.

Most enzymes have one specific function. Each enzyme works best at a specific pH. For example, the enzyme amylase in the saliva breaks down starches into sugars. The secretions of the GI tract have very different pH levels. For example, saliva is relatively

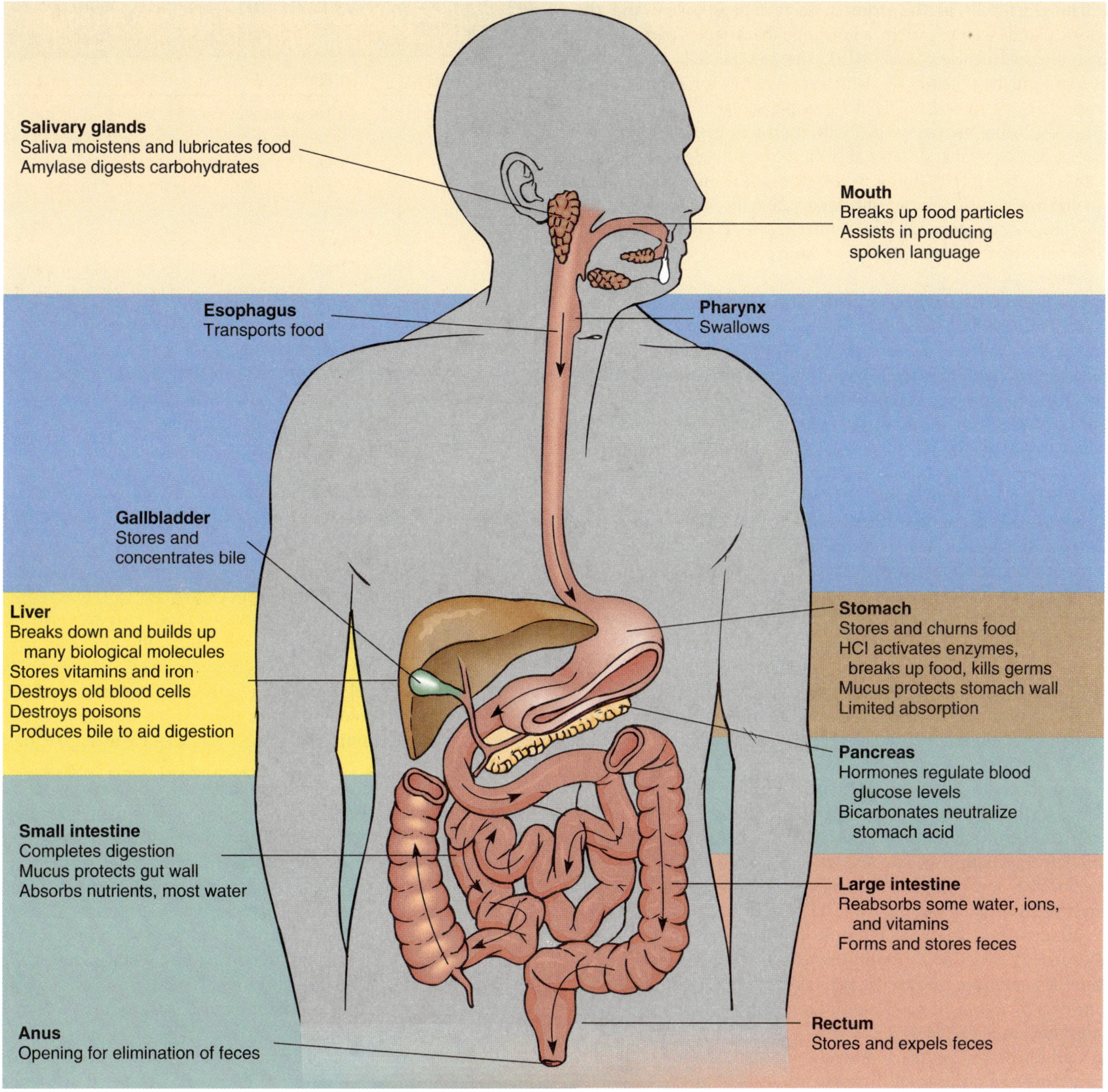
Salivary glands
Saliva moistens and lubricates food
Amylase digests carbohydrates
Mouth
Breaks up food particles
Assists in producing spoken language
Esophagus
Transports food
Pharynx
Swallows
Gallbladder
Stores and concentrates bile
Liver
Breaks down and builds up many biological molecules
Stores vitamins and iron
Destroys old blood cells
Destroys poisons
Produces bile to aid digestion
Stomach
Stores and churns food
HCl activates enzymes, breaks up food, kills germs
Mucus protects stomach wall
Limited absorption
Pancreas
Hormones regulate blood glucose levels
Bicarbonates neutralize stomach acid
Small intestine
Completes digestion
Mucus protects gut wall
Absorbs nutrients, most water
Large intestine
Reabsorbs some water, ions, and vitamins
Forms and stores feces
Anus
Opening for elimination of feces
Rectum
Stores and expels feces

FIG. 44-1 Summary of digestive system anatomy/organ function. *HCl,* Hydrochloric acid. (From Rolin Graphics.)

neutral, gastric juice is highly acidic, and the secretions of the small intestine are alkaline.

The mechanical, chemical, and hormonal activities of digestion are interdependent. Enzyme activity depends on the mechanical breakdown of food to increase its surface area for chemical action. Hormones regulate the flow of digestive secretions needed for enzyme supply. Physical, chemical, and hormonal factors regulate the secretion of digestive juices and the motility of the GI tract. Nerve stimulation from the parasympathetic nervous system (e.g., the vagus nerve) increases GI tract action.

Digestion begins in the mouth, where chewing mechanically breaks down food. The food mixes with saliva, which contains ptyalin (salivary amylase), an enzyme that acts on cooked starch to begin its conversion to maltose. The longer an individual chews food, the more starch digestion occurs in the mouth. Proteins and fats are broken down physically but remain unchanged chemically because enzymes in the mouth do not react with these nutrients. Chewing reduces food particles to a size suitable for swallowing, and saliva provides lubrication to further ease swallowing of the food. The epiglottis is a flap of skin that closes over the trachea as a person swallows to prevent aspiration. Swallowed food enters the esophagus, and wavelike muscular contractions **(peristalsis)** move the food to the base of the esophagus, above the cardiac sphincter. Pressure from a bolus of food at the cardiac sphincter causes it to relax, allowing the food to enter the fundus, or uppermost portion, of the stomach.

The chief cells in the stomach secrete pepsinogen; and the pyloric glands secrete gastrin, a hormone that triggers parietal cells to secrete hydrochloric acid (HCl). The parietal cells also secrete HCl and intrinsic factor (IF), which is necessary for absorption of vitamin B_{12} in the ileum. HCl turns pepsinogen into pepsin, a protein-splitting enzyme. The body produces gastric lipase and amylase to begin fat and starch digestion, respectively. A thick layer of mucus protects the lining of the stomach from autodigestion. Alcohol and aspirin are two substances directly absorbed through the lining of the stomach. The stomach acts as a reservoir where food remains for approximately 3 hours, with a range of 1 to 7 hours.

Food leaves the antrum, or distal stomach, through the pyloric sphincter and enters the duodenum. Food is now an acidic, liquefied mass called **chyme.** Chyme flows into the duodenum and quickly mixes with bile, intestinal juices, and pancreatic secretions. The small intestine secretes the hormones secretin and cholecystokinin (CCK). Secretin activates release of bicarbonate from the pancreas, raising the pH of chyme. CCK inhibits further gastrin secretion and initiates release of additional digestive enzymes from the pancreas and gallbladder.

Bile is manufactured in the liver and concentrated and stored in the gallbladder. It acts as a detergent because it emulsifies fat to permit enzyme action while suspending fatty acids in solution. Pancreatic secretions contain six enzymes: amylase to digest starch; lipase to break down emulsified fats; and trypsin, elastase, chymotrypsin, and carboxypeptidase to break down proteins.

Peristalsis continues in the small intestine, mixing the secretions with chyme. The mixture becomes increasingly alkaline, inhibiting the action of the gastric enzymes and promoting the action of the duodenal secretions. Epithelial cells in the small intestinal villi secrete enzymes (e.g., sucrase, lactase, maltase, lipase, and peptidase) to facilitate digestion. The major portion of digestion occurs in the small intestine, producing glucose, fructose, and galactose from carbohydrates; amino acids and dipeptides from proteins; and fatty acids, glycerides, and glycerol from lipids. Peristalsis usually takes approximately 5 hours to pass food through the small intestine.

Absorption. The small intestine is the primary absorption site for nutrients. It is lined with fingerlike projections called *villi.* Villi increase the surface area available for absorption. The body absorbs nutrients by means of passive diffusion, osmosis, active transport, and pinocytosis (Table 44-1).

TABLE 44-1 Mechanisms for Intestinal Absorption of Nutrients

MECHANISM	DEFINITION
Active transport	An energy-dependent process whereby particles move from an area of greater concentration to an area of lesser concentration. A special "carrier" moves the particle across the cell membrane.
Passive diffusion	The force by which particles move outward from an area of greater concentration to lesser concentration. The particles do not need a special "carrier" to move outward in all directions.
Osmosis	Movement of water through a membrane that separates solutions of different concentrations. Water moves to equalize the concentration pressures on both sides of the membrane.
Pinocytosis	Engulfing of large molecules of nutrients by the absorbing cell when the molecule attaches to the absorbing cell membrane.

Data from Nix S: *Williams' basic nutrition and diet therapy*, ed 13, St Louis, 2009, Mosby.

Carbohydrates, protein, minerals, and water-soluble vitamins are absorbed by the small intestine, processed in the liver, and released into the portal vein circulation. Fatty acids are absorbed in the lymphatic circulatory systems through lacteal ducts at the center of each microvilli in the small intestine.

Approximately 85% to 90% of water is absorbed in the small intestine (Huether et al., 2008). Approximately 8.5 L of GI secretions and 1.5 L of oral intake are managed daily within the GI tract. The small intestine resorbs 9.5 L, and the colon absorbs approximately 0.4 L. The remaining 0.1 L is eliminated in feces. In addition, electrolytes and minerals are absorbed in the colon, and bacteria synthesize vitamin K and some B-complex vitamins. Finally, feces are formed for elimination.

Metabolism and Storage of Nutrients. **Metabolism** refers to all of the biochemical reactions within the cells of the body. Metabolic processes are anabolic (building) or catabolic (breaking down). **Anabolism** is the building of more complex biochemical substances by synthesis of nutrients. Anabolism occurs when an individual adds lean muscle through diet and exercise. Amino acids are anabolized into tissues, hormones, and enzymes. Normal metabolism and anabolism are physiologically possible when the body is in positive nitrogen balance. **Catabolism** is the breakdown of biochemical substances into simpler substances and occurs during physiological states of negative nitrogen balance. Starvation is an example of catabolism when wasting of body tissues occurs.

Nutrients absorbed in the intestines, including water, are transported through the circulatory system to the body tissues. Through the chemical changes of metabolism, the body converts nutrients into a number of required substances. Carbohydrates, protein, and fat are metabolized to produce chemical energy and maintain a balance between anabolism and catabolism. To carry out the work of the body, the chemical energy produced by metabolism converts to other types of energy by different tissues. Muscle contraction involves mechanical energy, nervous system function involves electrical energy, and the mechanisms of heat production involve thermal energy.

Some of the nutrients required by the body are stored in tissues. The major form of body reserve energy is fat, stored as adipose tissue. Protein is stored in muscle mass. When the energy requirements of the body exceed the energy supplied by ingested nutrients, stored energy is used. Monoglycerides from the digested portion of fats are converted to glucose by gluconeogenesis. Amino acids are also converted to fat and stored or catabolized into energy through gluconeogenesis. All body cells except red blood cells and neurons oxidize fatty acids into **ketones** for energy when dietary carbohydrates (glucose) are not adequate. Glycogen, synthesized from glucose, provides energy during brief periods of fasting (e.g., during sleep). It is stored in small reserves in liver and muscle tissue. Nutrient metabolism consists of three main processes:

1. Catabolism of glycogen into glucose, carbon dioxide, and water **(glycogenolysis)**
2. Anabolism of glucose into glycogen for storage **(glycogenesis)**
3. Catabolism of amino acids and glycerol into glucose for energy **(gluconeogenesis)**

Elimination. Chyme moves by peristaltic action through the ileocecal valve into the large intestine, where it becomes feces (see Chapter 46). Water absorbs in the mucosa as feces move toward the rectum. The longer the material stays in the large intestine, the more water is absorbed, causing the feces to become firmer. Exercise and fiber stimulate peristalsis, and water maintains consistency. Feces contain cellulose and similar indigestible substances, sloughed epithelial cells from the GI tract, digestive secretions, water, and microbes.

Dietary Guidelines

Dietary Reference Intakes. Dietary reference intakes (DRIs) present evidence-based criteria for an acceptable range of amounts of vitamins and nutrients for each gender and age-group (Institute of Medicine, 2006). There are four components to the DRIs. The estimated average requirement (EAR) is the recommended amount of a nutrient that appears sufficient to maintain a specific body function for 50% of the population based on age and gender. The recommended dietary allowance (RDA) is the average needs of 98% of the population, not the exact needs of the individual. The adequate intake (AI) is the suggested intake for individuals based on observed or experimentally determined estimates of nutrient intakes and is used when there is not enough evidence to set the RDA. The tolerable upper intake level (UL) is the highest level that likely poses no risk of adverse health events. It is not a recommended level of intake (Tolerable upper level intake, 2010).

Food Guidelines. The U.S. Department of Agriculture (USDA) and the U.S. Department of Health and Human Services (USDHHS) published the *Dietary Guidelines for Americans 2010* and provide average daily consumption guidelines for the five food groups: grains, vegetables, fruits, dairy products, and meats (Box 44-2). These guidelines are for Americans over the age of 2 years. As a nurse, consider the food preferences of patients from different racial and ethnic groups, vegetarians, and others when planning diets. The *ChooseMyPlate* program was developed by the U.S. Department of Agriculture to replace the *My Food Pyramid* program. *ChooseMyPlate* provides a basic guide for making food choices for a healthy lifestyle (Fig. 44-2). The *ChooseMyPlate* program includes guidelines for balancing calories; decreasing portion size; increasing healthy foods; increasing water consumption; and decreasing fats, sodium, and sugars (USDA, 2011a).

Daily Values. The Food and Drug Administration (FDA) created daily values for food labels in response to the 1990 Nutrition Labeling and Education Act (NLEA). The FDA first established two sets of reference values. The referenced daily intakes (RDIs) are the first set, comprising protein, vitamins, and minerals based on the RDA. The daily reference values (DRVs) make up the second set and consist of nutrients such as total fat, saturated fat, cholesterol, carbohydrates, fiber, sodium, and potassium. Combined, both sets make up the daily values used on food labels (USFDA, 2008). Daily values did not replace RDAs but provided a separate, more understandable format for the public. Daily values are based on percentages of a diet consisting of 2000 kcal/day for adults and children 4 years or older.

BOX 44-2 2010 DIETARY GUIDELINES FOR AMERICANS: KEY RECOMMENDATIONS FOR THE GENERAL POPULATION

- Adopt a balanced eating pattern with a variety of nutrient-dense food and beverages among the basic food groups.
- Maintain body weight in a healthy range.
- Encourage physical activity and decrease sedentary activities.
- Encourage fruits, vegetables, whole-grain products, seafood, and fat-free or low-fat milk.
- Reduce amount of foods containing sugars.
- Eat moderate amount of lean meats, poultry, and eggs.
- Keep total fat intake between 20% and 35% of total calories, with most fats coming from polyunsaturated or monounsaturated fatty acids.
- Choose and prepare foods and beverages with little added sugar or sweeteners.
- Choose and prepare foods with little salt and eat potassium-rich foods.
- Limit intake of alcohol to moderate use (i.e., one drink daily for women and two drinks daily for men).
- Practice food safety to prevent bacterial foodborne illness. Use food safety principles of Clean, Separate, Cook, and Chill.

Data from US Department of Agriculture and US Department of Health and Human Services: Dietary Guidelines for Americans, 2010. *Report of Dietary Guidelines Advisory Committee on the dietary guidelines for Americans 2010,* http://www.cnpp.usda.gov/dietaryguidelines.htm. Accessed October 29, 2011.

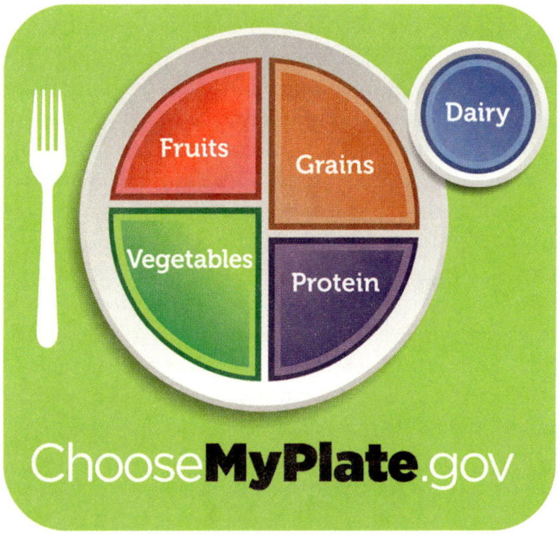

FIG. 44-2 ChooseMyPlate. (From US Department of Agriculture: ChooseMyPlate, 2011, http://www.choosemyplate.gov).

NURSING KNOWLEDGE BASE

Sociological, cultural, psychological, and emotional factors are associated with eating and drinking in all societies. Holidays and events are celebrated with food, food is brought to those who are grieving, and food is used for medicinal purposes. It is incorporated into family traditions and rituals and is often associated with eating behaviors. You need to understand patients' values, beliefs, and attitudes about food and how these values affect food purchase, preparation, and intake to affect eating patterns.

Nutritional requirements depend on many factors. Individual caloric and nutrient requirements vary by stage of development, body composition, activity levels, pregnancy and lactation, and the presence of disease. Registered dietitians (RDs) use predictive equations that take into account some of these factors to estimate patients' nutritional requirements.

Factors Influencing Nutrition

Environmental Factors. Environmental factors beyond the control of individuals contribute to the development of obesity. Obesity is an epidemic in the United States. The prevalence of obesity in adults has doubled since 1980, with 33% of adults in the United States overweight, 34% obese, and 6 % extremely obese (body mass index [BMI] ≥40) (Khan et al., 2009). Proposed contributing factors are sedentary lifestyle, work schedules, and poor meal choices often related to the increasing frequency of eating away from home and eating fast food (Kruskall, 2006). The likelihood of healthy eating and participation in exercise or other activities of healthy living is limited by environmental factors. Lack of access to full-service grocery stores, high cost of healthy food, widespread availability of less healthy foods in fast-food restaurants, widespread advertising of less healthy food, and lack of access to safe places to play and exercise are environmental factors that contribute to obesity (Khan et al., 2009).

Developmental Needs

Infants Through School-Age. Rapid growth and high protein, vitamin, mineral, and energy requirements mark the developmental stage of infancy. The average birth weight of an American baby is 3.2 to 3.4 kg (7 to 7½ pounds). An infant usually doubles birth weight at 4 to 5 months and triples it at 1 year. Infants need an energy intake of approximately 90 to 110 kcal/kg of body weight, with premature infants needing 105 to 130 kcal/kg per day (Nix, 2009). Commercial formulas and human breast milk both provide approximately 20 kcal/oz. A full-term newborn is able to digest and absorb simple carbohydrates, proteins, and a moderate amount of emulsified fat. Infants need about 100 to 120 mL/kg/day of fluid because a large portion of total body weight is water.

Breastfeeding. The American Dietetic Association strongly supports exclusive breastfeeding for the first 6 months of life and breastfeeding with complementary foods from 6 to 12 months (American Dietetic Association, 2009). Breastfeeding has multiple benefits for both infant and mother, including fewer food allergies and intolerances; fewer infant infections; easier digestion; convenience, availability, and freshness; temperature always correct; economical because it is less expensive than formula; and increased time for mother and infant interaction.

Formula. Infant formulas contain the approximate nutrient composition of human milk. Protein in the formula is typically whey, soy, cow's milk base, casein hydrolysate, or elemental amino acids. The American Academy of Pediatrics sets standards for the level of nutrients in infant formulas. Soy protein–based formulas are used for infants allergic or intolerant to cow's milk (Nix, 2009).

Infants should not have regular cow's milk during the first year of life. It is too concentrated for an infant's kidneys to manage, increases the risk of milk product allergies, and is a poor source of iron and vitamins C and E (Nix, 2009). Honey and corn syrup are potential sources of botulism toxin and should not be used in an infant's diet. This toxin is potentially fatal in children under 1 year of age (Nix, 2009).

Introduction to Solid Food. Breast milk or formula provides sufficient nutrition for the first 4 to 6 months of life. The development of fine-motor skills of the hand and fingers parallels an infant's interest in food and self-feeding. Iron-fortified cereals are typically the first semisolid food to be introduced. For infants 4 to 11 months, cereals are the most important nonmilk source of protein (Fox et al., 2006).

The addition of foods to an infant's diet is governed by an infant's nutrient needs, physical readiness to handle different forms of foods, and the need to detect and control allergic reactions. Foods such as wheat, egg white, nuts, citrus juice, and chocolate have a high incidence of allergies and should be added late (Nix, 2009). Caregivers should introduce new foods one at a time, approximately 4 to 7 days apart to identify allergies. It is best to introduce new foods before milk or other foods to avoid satiety (Hockenberry and Wilson, 2011).

The growth rate slows during toddler years (1 to 3 years). A toddler needs fewer kilocalories but an increased amount of protein in relation to body weight; consequently appetite often decreases at 18 months of age. Toddlers exhibit strong food preferences and become picky eaters. Small frequent meals consisting of breakfast, lunch, and dinner with three interspersed high nutrient–dense snacks help improve nutritional intake (Hockenberry and Wilson, 2011). Calcium and phosphorus are important for healthy bone growth.

Toddlers who consume more than 24 ounces of milk daily in place of other foods sometimes develop milk anemia because milk is a poor source of iron. Toddlers need to drink whole milk until the age of 2 years to make sure that there is adequate intake of fatty acids necessary for brain and neurological development. Certain foods such as hot dogs, candy, nuts, grapes, raw vegetables, and popcorn have been implicated in choking deaths and need to be avoided. Dietary requirements for preschoolers (3 to 5 years) are similar to those for toddlers. They consume slightly more than toddlers, and nutrient density is more important than quantity.

School-age children, 6 to 12 years old, grow at a slower and steadier rate, with a gradual decline in energy requirements per unit of body weight. Despite better appetites and more varied food intake, you need to assess school-age children's diets carefully for adequate protein and vitamins A and C. They often fail to eat a proper breakfast and have unsupervised intake at school. High fat, sugar, and salt result from too-liberal intake of snack foods. Physical activity level decreases consistently, and high-calorie, readily available food increases in consumption, leading to an increase in childhood obesity (Budd and Hayman, 2008).

In the last 20 years the prevalence of overweight children has risen. The percent of obesity in children ages 6 to 11 years has doubled to 17%, and the percent of overweight adolescents has more than tripled to 17.6% (Li and Hooker, 2010). A combination of factors contributes to the problem, including a diet rich in high-calorie foods, food advertising targeting children, inactivity, genetic predisposition, use of food as a coping mechanism for stress or boredom or as a reward or celebration, and family and social factors (Budd and Hayman, 2008). Childhood obesity contributes to medical problems related to the cardiovascular system, endocrine system, and mental health (Budd and Hayman, 2008). As a result of the obesity, the incidence of type II diabetes in children is also increasing. Prevention of childhood obesity is critical because of the long-term effects. Family education is an important component in decreasing the prevalence of this problem. Promote healthy food choices and eating in moderation along with increased physical activity.

Adolescents. During adolescence physiological age is a better guide to nutritional needs than chronological age. Energy needs increase to meet greater metabolic demands of growth. Daily requirement of protein also increases. Calcium is essential for the rapid bone growth of adolescence, and girls need a continuous source of iron to replace menstrual losses. Boys also need adequate iron for muscle development. Iodine supports increased thyroid activity, and use of iodized table salt ensures availability. B-complex vitamins are necessary to support heightened metabolic activity.

Many factors other than nutritional needs influence the adolescent's diet, including concern about body image and appearance, desire for independence, eating at fast-food restaurants, peer pressure, and fad diets. Nutritional deficiencies often occur in adolescent girls as a result of dieting and use of oral contraceptives. An adolescent boy's diet is often inadequate in total kilocalories, protein, iron, folic acid, B vitamins, and iodine. Snacks provide approximately 25% of a teenager's total dietary intake. Fast food, particularly value-size or super-size meals, is common and adds extra salt, fat, and kilocalories (Budd and Hayman, 2008). Skipping meals or eating meals with unhealthy choices of snacks contributes to nutrient deficiency and obesity (Hockenberry and Wilson, 2011).

Fortified foods (nutrients added) are important sources of vitamins and minerals. Snack food from the dairy and fruit and vegetable groups are good choices. To counter obesity, increasing physical activity is often more important than curbing intake. The onset of eating disorders such as **anorexia nervosa** or **bulimia nervosa** often occurs during adolescence. Recognition of eating disorders is essential for early intervention (Box 44-3).

Sports and regular moderate-to-intense exercise necessitate dietary modification to meet increased energy needs for adolescents. Carbohydrates, both simple and complex, are the main source of energy, providing 55% to 60% of total daily kilocalories. Protein needs increase to 1 to 1.5 g/kg/day. Fat needs do not increase. Adequate hydration is very important. Adolescents need to ingest water before and after exercise to prevent dehydration, especially in hot, humid environments. Vitamin and mineral supplements are not required, but intake of iron-rich foods is required to prevent anemia.

Parents have more influence on adolescents' diets than they believe. Effective strategies include limiting the amount of unhealthy food choices kept at home, encouraging smart snacks such as fruit vegetables or string cheese, and enhancing the appearance and taste of healthy foods (Mayo Clinic Staff, 2009). Making healthy food choices more convenient at home and at fast-food restaurants and discouraging adolescents from eating while watching television are ways to promote healthy eating (Befort et al., 2006).

Pregnancy occurring within 4 years of menarche places a mother and fetus at risk because of anatomical and physiological immaturity. Malnutrition at the time of conception increases risk to the adolescent and her fetus. Most teenage girls do not want to gain weight. Counseling related to nutritional needs of pregnancy is often difficult, and teens tolerate suggestions better than rigid directions. The diet of pregnant adolescents is often deficient in calcium, iron, and vitamins A and C. Prenatal vitamin and mineral supplements are recommended.

Young and Middle Adults. There is a reduction in nutrient demands as the growth period ends. Mature adults need nutrients for energy, maintenance, and repair. Energy needs usually decline over the years. Obesity becomes a problem because of decreased physical exercise, dining out more often, and increased ability to afford more luxury foods. Adult women who use oral contraceptives often need extra vitamins. Iron and calcium intake continues to be important.

Pregnancy. Poor nutrition during pregnancy causes low birth weight in infants and decreases chances of survival. Generally the needs of a fetus are met at the expense of the mother. However, if nutrient sources are not available, both suffer. The nutritional status of the mother at the time of conception is important. Significant aspects of fetal growth and development often occur before the mother suspects the pregnancy. The energy requirements of pregnancy are related to the mother's body weight and activity. The quality of nutrition during pregnancy is important, and food intake in the first trimester includes balanced portions of essential nutrients with emphasis on quality. Protein intake throughout pregnancy needs to increase to 60 g daily. Calcium intake is especially critical in the third trimester, when fetal bones are mineralized. Iron needs to be supplemented to provide for increased maternal blood volume, fetal blood storage, and blood loss during delivery.

Folic acid intake is particularly important for deoxyribonucleic acid (DNA) synthesis and the growth of red blood cells. Inadequate intake can lead to fetal neural tube defects, anencephaly, or maternal megaloblastic anemia (Nix, 2009). Women of childbearing age need to consume 400 mcg of folic acid daily, increasing to 600 mcg daily during pregnancy. Prenatal care usually includes vitamin and mineral supplementation to ensure daily intakes; however, pregnant women should not take additional supplements beyond prescribed amounts.

Lactation. The lactating woman needs 500 kcal/day above the usual allowance because the production of milk increases energy requirements. Protein requirements during lactation are greater than those required during pregnancy. The need for calcium remains the same as during pregnancy. There is an increased need for vitamins A and C. Daily intake of water-soluble vitamins (B and C) is necessary to ensure adequate levels in breast milk. Fluid intake needs to be adequate but not excessive. Caffeine, alcohol, and drugs are excreted in breast milk and should be avoided.

Older Adults. Adults 65 years and older have a decreased need for energy because their metabolic rate slows with age. However, vitamin and mineral requirements remain unchanged from middle adulthood. Numerous factors influence the nutritional status of the older adult (Box 44-4). Age-related changes in appetite, taste, smell, and the digestive system affect nutrition (Touhy and Jett, 2010). For example, older adults often experience a decrease in taste cells that alters food flavor and may decrease intake. Multiple factors

BOX 44-3 POTENTIAL ASSESSMENT FOR EATING DISORDERS

Anorexia Nervosa

- Refusal to maintain body weight over a minimal normal weight for age and height (e.g., weight loss leading to maintenance of body weight less than 85% of ideal body weight) or failure to make expected weight gain during period of growth, leading to body weight less than 85% of that expected
- Intense fear of gaining weight or becoming fat, although underweight
- Disturbance in the way in which one's body weight, size, or shape is experienced (e.g., the person claims to "feel fat" even when emaciated; believes that one area of the body is "too fat" even when obviously underweight)
- In females absence of at least three consecutive menstrual cycles when otherwise expected to occur (primary or secondary amenorrhea). (A woman is considered to have amenorrhea if her periods occur only following hormone [e.g., estrogen] administration.)

Bulimia Nervosa

- Recurrent episodes of binge eating (rapid consumption of a large amount of food in a discrete period of time)
- A feeling of lack of control over eating behavior during eating binges
- Regularly engages in self-induced vomiting, use of laxatives or diuretics, strict dieting or fasting, or vigorous exercise to prevent weight gain
- Minimum average of two binge-eating episodes a week for at least 3 months

TABLE 44-2 Sample of Drug-Nutrient Interactions*

DRUG	EFFECT
Analgesic	
Acetaminophen	Decreased drug absorption with food; overdose associated with liver failure
Aspirin	Absorbed directly through stomach; decreased drug absorption with food; decreased folic acid, vitamins C and K, and iron absorption
Antacid	
Aluminum hydroxide	Decreased phosphate absorption
Sodium bicarbonate	Decreased folic acid absorption
Antiarrhythmic	
Amiodarone (Codarone)	Taste alteration
Digitalis	Anorexia, decreased renal clearance in older people
Antibiotic	
Penicillin	Decreased drug absorption with food, taste alteration
Cephalosporin	Decreased vitamin K
Rifampin (Rifadin)	Decreased vitamin B_6, niacin, vitamin D
Tetracycline	Decreased drug absorption with milk and antacids; decreased nutrient absorption of calcium, riboflavin, vitamin C caused by binding
Trimethoprim/sulfamethoxazole	Decreased folic acid

BOX 44-4 FOCUS ON OLDER ADULTS

Factors Affecting Nutritional Status

- Age-related gastrointestinal changes that affect digestion of food and maintenance of nutrition include changes in the teeth and gums, reduced saliva production, atrophy of oral mucosal epithelial cells, increased taste threshold, decreased thirst sensation, reduced gag reflex, and decreased esophageal and colonic peristalsis (Touhy and Jett, 2010).
- The presence of chronic illnesses (e.g., diabetes mellitus, end-stage renal disease, cancer) often affects nutrition intake (Ebersole et al., 2008).
- Adequate nutrition in older adults is affected by multiple causes such as lifelong eating habits, ethnicity, socialization, income, educational level, physical functional level to meet activities of daily living (ADLs), loss, dentition, and transportation (Touhy and Jett, 2010).
- Adverse effects of medications cause problems such as anorexia, gastrointestinal bleeding, xerostomia, early satiety, and impaired smell and taste perception (Lehne, 2010).
- Cognitive impairments such as delirium, dementia, and depression affect ability to obtain, prepare, and eat healthy foods (Chang and Roberts, 2008; Ebersole et al., 2008).

contribute to the risk of food insecurity in the older adult. Income is significant because living on a fixed income often reduces the amount of money available to buy food. Health is another important influence that affects a person's desire and ability to eat. Lack of transportation or ability to get to the grocery store because of mobility problems contributes to inability to purchase adequate and nutritious food. Often availability of nutritionally adequate and safe foods is limited or uncertain.

Maintaining good oral health is significant throughout adulthood, particularly as an individual ages. Difficulty chewing, missing teeth, having teeth in poor condition, and oral pain result from poor oral health. These often contribute to malnutrition and dehydration in older adults (Touhy and Jett, 2010). Poor oral hygiene and periodontal disease are potential risk factors for systemic diseases such as joint infections, ischemic stroke, cardiovascular disease, DM, and aspiration pneumonia (O'Connor, 2008).

The older adult is often on a therapeutic diet or has difficulty eating because of physical symptoms, lack of teeth, or dentures or is at risk for drug-nutrient interactions (Table 44-2). Caution older adults to avoid grapefruit and grapefruit juice because they alter absorption of many drugs. Thirst sensation diminishes, leading to inadequate fluid intake or dehydration (see Chapter 41). Symptoms of dehydration in older adults include confusion; weakness; hot, dry skin; furrowed tongue; rapid pulse; and high urinary sodium. Some older adults avoid meats because of cost or because they are difficult to chew. Cream soups and meat-based vegetable soups are nutrient-dense sources of protein. Cheese, eggs, and peanut butter are also useful high-protein alternatives. Milk continues to be an important food for older women and men who need adequate calcium to protect against osteoporosis (a decrease of bone mass density). Screening and treatment are necessary for both older men and women. Vitamin D supplements are important for improving strength and balance, strengthening bone health, and preventing bone fractures and falls (Park et al., 2008). The diet of older adults needs to contain choices from all food groups and often requires a vitamin and mineral supplement. MyPlate for Older Adults addresses the specific nutritional needs for older adults and encourages physical activity (Tufts University, 2011).

The USDHHS Administration on Aging (AOA) requires states to provide nutrition screening services to older adults who benefit from home-delivered or congregate meal services. This program requires meals to provide at least one third of the DRI for an older adult and meet the Dietary Guidelines for Americans (American Dietetic Association, 2010a). Homebound older adults with chronic illnesses have additional nutritional risks. They frequently live alone with little or no social or financial resources to assist in obtaining or preparing nutritionally sound meals, contributing to

TABLE 44-2 **Sample of Drug-Nutrient Interactions*—cont'd**

DRUG	EFFECT
Anticoagulant	
Warfarin (Coumadin)	Acts as antagonist to vitamin K
Anticonvulsant	
Carbamazepine (Tegretol)	Increased drug absorption with food
Phenytoin (Dilantin)	Decreased calcium absorption; decreased vitamins D and K and folic acid; taste alteration; decreased drug absorption with food
Antidepressant	
Amitriptyline	Appetite stimulant
Clomipramine (Anafranil)	Taste alteration, appetite stimulant
Fluoxetine (Prozac) (selective serotonin reuptake inhibitors [SSRIs])	Taste alteration, anorexia
Antihypertensive	
Captopril (Capoten)	Taste alteration, anorexia
Hydralazine	Enhanced drug absorption with food, decreased vitamin B_6
Labetalol (Normodyne)	Taste alteration (weight gain for all beta-blockers)
Methyldopa	Decreased vitamin B_{12}, folic acid, iron
Antiinflammatory	
All steroids	Increased appetite and weight, increased folic acid, decreased calcium (osteoporosis with long-term use), promotes gluconeogenesis of protein
Antiparkinson	
Levodopa (Dopar)	Taste alteration, decreased vitamin B_6 and drug absorption with food
Antipsychotic	
Chlorpromazine	Increased appetite
Thiothixene	Decreased riboflavin, increased need
Bronchodilator	
Albuterol sulfate	Appetite stimulant
Theophylline	Anorexia
Cholesterol Lowering	
Cholestyramine (Prevalite)	Decreased fat-soluble vitamins (A, D, E, K); vitamin B_{12}; iron
Diuretic	
Furosemide (Lasix)	Decreased drug absorption with food
Spironolactone (Aldactone)	Increased drug absorption with food
Thiazides	Decreased magnesium, zinc, and potassium
Laxative	
Mineral oil	Decreased absorption of fat-soluble vitamins (A, D, E, K), carotene
Platelet Aggregate Inhibitor	
Dipyridamole (Persantine)	Decreased drug absorption with food
Potassium Replacement	
Potassium chloride	Decreased vitamin B_{12}
Tranquilizer	
Benzodiazepines	Increased appetite

Data from Hermann J: *Nutrient and drug interactions,* http://pods.dasnr.okstate.edu/docushare/dsweb/Get/Document-2458/T-3120web.pdf; accessed October 31, 2010; Lehne RA: *Pharmacology for nursing care,* ed 7, St Louis, 2010, Saunders.

*Not intended to be an exhaustive or all-inclusive list. Always check pharmacology references before administering medications.

the risk for food insecurity. Approximately 19% of older adults experience some degree of food insecurity as a result of low income or poverty (American Dietetic Association, 2010a). Increased nutrition screening by the nurse results in early recognition and treatment of nutritional deficiencies. Undernourishment of older adults often results in health problems that lead to admission to acute care hospitals or long-term care facilities.

Alternative Food Patterns

Long before the FDA issued recommended allowances and guidelines, many people followed special patterns of food intake based on religion (Table 44-3), cultural background (Box 44-5), ethics, health beliefs, personal preference, or concern for the efficient use of land to produce food. Such special diets are not necessarily more or less nutritious than diets based on the MyPlate or other

TABLE 44-3 Religious Dietary Restrictions

MUSLIM	CHRISTIANITY	HINDUISM	JUDAISM	CHURCH OF JESUS CHRIST OF LATTER-DAY SAINTS (MORMONS)	SEVENTH-DAY ADVENTISTS CHURCH
Pork Alcohol Caffeine Ramadan fasting sunrise to sunset for month Ritualized methods of animal slaughter required for meat ingestion	Some faiths, such as Baptists, have minimal or no alcohol Some meatless days may be observed during the calendar year, commonly during Lent	All meats Fish, shellfish with some restrictions Alcohol	Pork Predatory fowl Shellfish (eat only fish with scales) Rare meats Blood (e.g., blood sausage) Mixing of milk or dairy products with meat dishes Must adhere to kosher food preparation methods 24 hr of fasting on Yom Kippur, a day of atonement No leavened bread eaten during Passover (8 days) No cooking on the Sabbath from sundown Friday to sundown Saturday	Alcohol Tobacco Caffeine, such as teas, coffees, and sodas	Pork Shellfish Fish Alcohol Caffeine Vegetarian or ovolactovegetarian diets encouraged

BOX 44-5 CULTURAL ASPECTS OF CARE

Nutrition

Food patterns developed as a child, habits, and culture interact to influence food intake. Culture also influences the meaning of food not related to nutrition. Eating is associated with sentiments and feelings such as "good" and "bad." For example, children are often rewarded for "being good" with a treat such as candy. They then associate candy with "being good." Food frequently enhances interpersonal relationships and demonstrates love and caring (Andrews and Boyle, 2008).

The incidence of lactose intolerance around the world occurs in the following ethnic or racial groups: Asian-Pacific, African and African American, Native American, Mexican American, Middle Eastern, and Caucasians. The incidence is highest in Asian-Pacific populations and lowest in Caucasians. It affects nutrient absorption. Calcium deficiency often results, causing decreased bone mass density.

The theory of hot and cold foods predominates in many cultures. The origin appears to be from Hippocratic beliefs concerning health and the four humors. Arabs were keepers of this knowledge during the Dark Ages and later influenced the Spanish to adopt this belief system in the later Middle Ages. The foundation of the theory is keeping harmony with nature by balancing "cold," "hot," "wet," and "dry." Some cultures believe that hot is warmth, strength, and reassurance; whereas cold is menacing and weak. Classification has nothing to do with spiciness but is a symbolic representation of temperature (Giger and Davidhizar, 2008). Different cultures also have beliefs about food and special dishes that should be eaten when sick (e.g., chicken soup during illness).

Implications for Practice

- Identify the meaning that types of food have for each patient.
- Lactose and other food intolerances unique to specific cultures require diet adaptation to meet nutrient, mineral, and vitamin daily intake requirements.
- When patients use hot and cold foods as part of their cultural health practices, dietary modifications are necessary. Hot foods include rice, grain cereals, alcohol, beef, lamb, chili peppers, chocolate, cheese, temperate zone fruits, eggs, peas, goat's milk, cornhusks, oils, onions, pork, radishes, and tamales. By contrast, cold foods are beans, citrus fruits, tropical fruits, dairy products, most vegetables, honey, raisins, chicken, fish, and goat.
- In some cultures specific conditions require hot foods. Menstruation, cancer, pneumonia, earache, colds, paralysis, headache, and rheumatism are cold illnesses requiring hot foods.
- Other conditions such as pregnancy, fever, infections, diarrhea, rashes, ulcers, liver problems, constipation, kidney problems, and sore throats are hot conditions requiring cold foods.

nutritional guidelines because good nutrition depends on a balanced intake of all required nutrients.

Vegetarian Diet. A common alternative dietary pattern is the vegetarian diet. **Vegetarianism** is the consumption of a diet consisting predominantly of plant foods. Some vegetarians are ovolactovegetarian (avoid meat, fish, and poultry but eat eggs and milk), lactovegetarians (drink milk but avoid eggs), or vegans (consume only plant foods). Through careful selection of foods, individuals following a vegetarian diet can meet recommendations for proteins and essential nutrients (Nix, 2009). Zen macrobiotic (primarily brown rice, other grains, and herb teas) and fruitarian (only fruit, nuts, honey, and olive oil) diets are nutrient poor and frequently result in malnutrition. Knowledge related to complementary use of high and low biological value proteins is necessary. Children who follow a vegetarian diet are especially at risk for protein and vitamin deficiencies such as vitamin B_{12}. Careful planning helps to ensure a balanced, healthy diet.

CRITICAL THINKING

Effective critical thinking requires a synthesis of knowledge, experience, information collected from patients, critical thinking

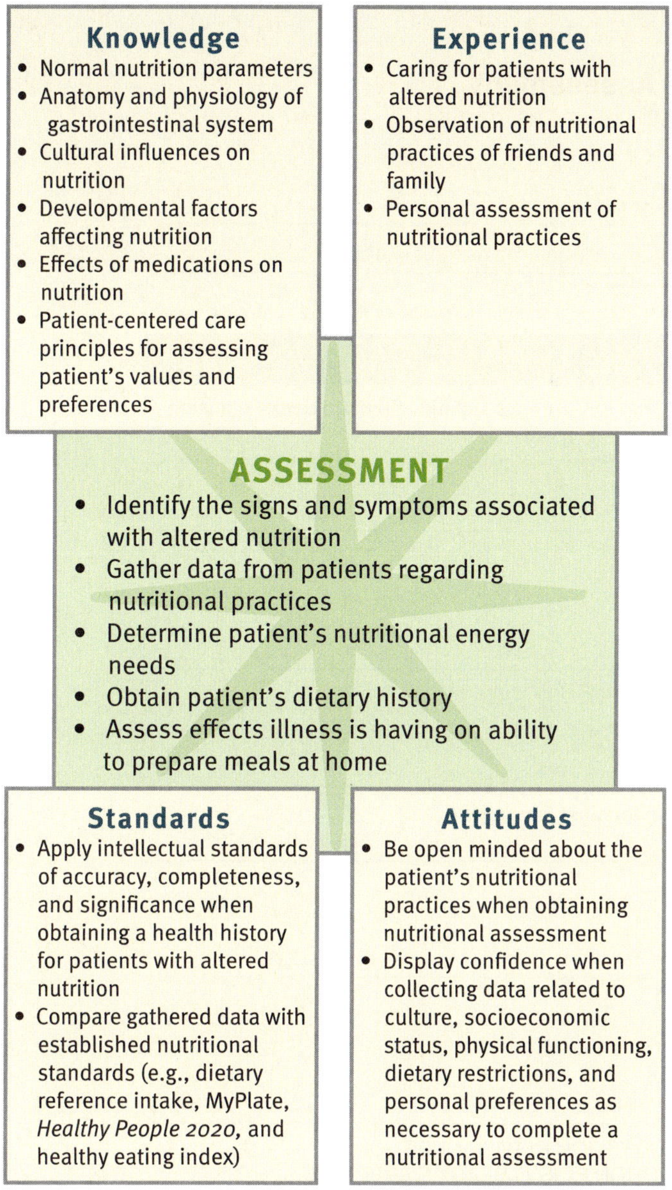
Knowledge
• Normal nutrition parameters
• Anatomy and physiology of gastrointestinal system
• Cultural influences on nutrition
• Developmental factors affecting nutrition
• Effects of medications on nutrition
• Patient-centered care principles for assessing patient's values and preferences
Experience
• Caring for patients with altered nutrition
• Observation of nutritional practices of friends and family
• Personal assessment of nutritional practices
ASSESSMENT
• Identify the signs and symptoms associated with altered nutrition
• Gather data from patients regarding nutritional practices
• Determine patient's nutritional energy needs
• Obtain patient's dietary history
• Assess effects illness is having on ability to prepare meals at home
Standards
• Apply intellectual standards of accuracy, completeness, and significance when obtaining a health history for patients with altered nutrition
• Compare gathered data with established nutritional standards (e.g., dietary reference intake, MyPlate, Healthy People 2020, and healthy eating index)
Attitudes
• Be open minded about the patient's nutritional practices when obtaining nutritional assessment
• Display confidence when collecting data related to culture, socioeconomic status, physical functioning, dietary restrictions, and personal preferences as necessary to complete a nutritional assessment
FIG. 44-3 Critical thinking model for nutrition assessment.

attitudes, and intellectual and professional standards. Clinical judgments require you to anticipate the required information, analyze the data, and make decisions regarding patient care. Critical thinking is a dynamic process. During assessment (Fig. 44-3) consider all elements that build toward making appropriate nursing diagnoses.

Integrate knowledge from nursing and other disciplines, previous experiences, and information gathered from patients and families regarding customary food preferences and recent diet history. Use of professional standards such as the DRIs, the USDA MyPlate dietary guidelines, and *Healthy People 2020* objectives provide guidelines to assess and maintain patients' nutritional status. Other professional standards by the American Heart Association (AHA, 2010), the American Diabetes Association (ADA, 2008), The American Cancer Society (ACS, 2011), and the American Society for Parenteral and Enteral Nutrition (ASPEN) (Bankhead et al., 2009) are available. These standards are evidence based and regularly updated for optimal patient care.

NURSING PROCESS

Apply the nursing process and use a critical thinking approach in your care of patients. The nursing process provides a clinical decision-making approach for you to develop and implement an individualized plan of care.

ASSESSMENT

During the assessment process, thoroughly assess each patient and critically analyze findings to ensure that you make patient-centered clinical decisions required for safe nursing care. Early recognition of malnourished or at-risk patients has a strong positive influence on both short- and long-term health outcomes. Studies indicate that 40% to 55% of adult hospitalized patients are either malnourished or at risk for malnutrition (Mason, 2006). Patients who are malnourished on admission are at greater risk of life-threatening complications such as arrhythmia, sepsis, or hemorrhage during hospitalization.

Through the Patient's Eyes. Assess patients' nutritional status by using the nursing history to gather information about factors that usually influence nutrition. As the nurse you are in an excellent position to recognize signs of poor nutrition and take steps to initiate change. Close contact with patients and their families enables you to make observations about physical status, food intake, food preferences, weight changes, and response to therapy. Always ask patients about their food preferences, their values regarding nutrition, and what they expect from nutritional therapy. In attempting to affect eating patterns, you need to understand patient's values, beliefs, and attitudes about food. Also assess family traditions and rituals related to food, cultural values and beliefs, and nutritional needs. Determine how these factors affect food purchase, preparation, and intake.

Screening. Nutrition screening is an essential part of an initial assessment. Screening a patient is a quick method of identifying **malnutrition** or risk of malnutrition using sample tools (Charney, 2008). Nutrition screening tools need to gather data on the current condition, stability of the condition, assessment of whether it will worsen, and if the disease process accelerates. These tools typically include objective measures such as height, weight, weight change, primary diagnosis, and the presence of other co-morbidities (Charney, 2008). Combine multiple objective measures with subjective measures related to nutrition to adequately screen for nutritional problems. Identification of risk factors such as unintentional weight loss, presence of a modified diet, or the presence of altered nutritional symptoms (i.e., nausea, vomiting, diarrhea, and constipation) requires nutritional consultation.

Several standardized nutrition screening tools are available for use in the outpatient setting. The Subjective Global Assessment (SGA) uses the patient history, weight, and physical assessment data to evaluate nutritional status (Charney, 2008). SGA is a simple, inexpensive technique that is able to predict nutrition-related complications. The Mini Nutritional Assessment (MNA) (Fig. 44-4) was developed to use for screening older adults in home care programs, nursing homes, and hospitals. The tool has 18 items that are divided into screening and assessment. If a patient scores 11 or less on the screening portion, the health care provider completes the assessment portion (Kondrup et al., 2003). A total score of less than 17 indicates protein-energy malnutrition (Guigoz et al., 1996; Guigoz and Vellas, 1999). The Malnutrition Screening Tool (MST) is an effective measure of nutritional problems for patients in a variety of health care settings (Charney, 2008).

Nestlé Nutrition Institute

Mini Nutritional Assessment MNA®

Last name: First name:

Sex: Age: Weight, kg: Height, cm: Date:

Complete the screen by filling in the boxes with the appropriate numbers. Total the numbers for the final screening score.

Screening

A Has food intake declined over the past 3 months due to loss of appetite, digestive problems, chewing or swallowing difficulties?
0 = severe decrease in food intake
1 = moderate decrease in food intake
2 = no decrease in food intake ☐

B Weight loss during the last 3 months
0 = weight loss greater than 3 kg (6.6 lbs)
1 = does not know
2 = weight loss between 1 and 3 kg (2.2 and 6.6 lbs)
3 = no weight loss ☐

C Mobility
0 = bed or chair bound
1 = able to get out of bed / chair but does not go out
2 = goes out ☐

D Has suffered psychological stress or acute disease in the past 3 months?
0 = yes 2 = no ☐

E Neuropsychological problems
0 = severe dementia or depression
1 = mild dementia
2 = no psychological problems ☐

F1 Body Mass Index (BMI) (weight in kg) / (height in m^2)
0 = BMI less than 19
1 = BMI 19 to less than 21
2 = BMI 21 to less than 23
3 = BMI 23 or greater ☐

IF BMI IS NOT AVAILABLE, REPLACE QUESTION F1 WITH QUESTION F2.
DO NOT ANSWER QUESTION F2 IF QUESTION F1 IS ALREADY COMPLETED.

F2 Calf circumference (CC) in cm
0 = CC less than 31
3 = CC 31 or greater ☐

Screening score
(max. 14 points) ☐☐

12-14 points:	Normal nutritional status
8-11 points:	At risk of malnutrition
0-7 points:	Malnourished

Ref. Vellas B, Villars H, Abellan G, et al. *Overview of the MNA® - Its History and Challenges.* J Nutr Health Aging 2006;10:456-465.
Rubenstein LZ, Harker JO, Salva A, Guigoz Y, Vellas B. *Screening for Undernutrition in Geriatric Practice: Developing the Short-Form Mini Nutritional Assessment (MNA-SF).* J. Geront 2001;56A: M366-377.
Guigoz Y. *The Mini-Nutritional Assessment (MNA®) Review of the Literature - What does it tell us?* J Nutr Health Aging 2006; 10:466-487.
Kaiser MJ, Bauer JM, Ramsch C, et al. *Validation of the Mini Nutritional Assessment Short-Form (MNA®-SF): A practical tool for identification of nutritional status.* J Nutr Health Aging 2009; 13:782-788.

For more information: www.mna-elderly.com

FIG. 44-4 Mini Nutritional Assessment (MNA). (Copyright © Nestlé, 1994, Revision 2009. N67200 12/99 10M.)

Assess patients for malnutrition when they have conditions that interfere with their ability to ingest, digest, or absorb adequate nutrients. Use standardized tools to assess nutrition risks when possible. Congenital anomalies and surgical revisions of the GI tract interfere with normal function. Patients fed only by IV infusion of 5% or 10% dextrose are at risk for nutritional deficiencies. Chronic diseases or increased metabolic requirements are risk factors for development of nutritional problems. Infants and older adults are at greatest risk.

Anthropometry. Anthropometry is a measurement system of the size and makeup of the body. Nurses obtain height and weight for each patient on hospital admission or entry into any health care setting. If you are not able to measure height with the patient standing, position him or her lying flat in bed as straight as possible with arms folded on the chest and measure him or her lengthwise. Serial measures of weight over time provide more useful information than one measurement. The patient needs to be weighed at the same time each day, on the same scale, and with the same clothing or linen. Document his or her weight and compare height and weight to standards for height-weight relationships. An ideal body weight (IBW) provides an estimate of what a person should weigh. Rapid weight gain or loss is important to note because it usually reflects fluid shifts. One pint or 500 mL of fluid equals 1 lb (0.45 kg). For example, for a patient with renal failure, a weight increase of 2 lbs (0.90 kg) in 24 hours is significant because it usually indicates that the patient has retained a liter (1000 mL) of fluid.

Other anthropometric measurements often obtained by dietitians help identify nutritional problems. These include the ratio of height-to-wrist circumference, midupper arm circumference (MAC), triceps skinfold (TSF), and midupper arm muscle circumference (MAMC). A dietitian will compare values for MAC, TSF, and MAMC to standards and calculate them as a percentage of the standard. Changes in values for an individual over time are of greater significance than isolated measurements (Nix, 2009).

Body mass index (BMI) measures weight corrected for height and serves as an alternative to traditional height-weight relationships. Calculate BMI by dividing the patient's weight in kilograms by height in meters squared: Weight (kg) divided by height^2 (m^2). For example, a patient who weighs 165 lbs (75 kg) and is 1.8 m (5 feet 9 inches) tall has a BMI of 23.15 ($75 \div 1.8^2 = 23.15$). The website for the National Heart Lung and Blood Institute (http://www.nhlbisupport.com/bmi/) provides an easy way to calculate BMI. A patient is overweight if his or her BMI is 25 to 30. A BMI of greater than 30 is defined as obesity and places a patient at higher medical risk of coronary heart disease, some cancers, DM, and hypertension.

Laboratory and Biochemical Tests. No single laboratory or biochemical test is diagnostic for malnutrition. Factors that frequently alter test results include fluid balance, liver function, kidney function, and the presence of disease. Common laboratory tests used to study nutritional status include measures of plasma proteins such as albumin, transferrin, prealbumin, retinol binding protein, total iron-binding capacity, and hemoglobin. After feeding, the response time for changes in these proteins ranges from hours to weeks. The metabolic half-life of albumin is 21 days, transferrin is 8 days, prealbumin is 2 days, and retinol binding protein is 12 hours. Use this information to determine the most effective measure of plasma proteins for your patients. Factors that affect serum albumin levels include hydration; hemorrhage; renal or hepatic disease; large amounts of drainage from wounds, drains, burns, or the GI tract; steroid administration; exogenous albumin infusions; age; and trauma, burns, stress, or surgery. Albumin level is a better indicator for chronic illnesses, whereas prealbumin level is preferred for acute conditions (Pagana and Pagana, 2009).

Nitrogen balance is important to determining serum protein status (see discussion of protein in this chapter). Calculate nitrogen balance by dividing 6.25 into the total grams of protein ingested in a day (24 hours). Use laboratory analysis of a 24-hour urinary urea nitrogen (UUN) to determine nitrogen output. For patients with diarrhea or fistula drainage, estimate a further addition of 2 to 4 g of nitrogen output. Calculate nitrogen balance by subtracting the nitrogen output from the nitrogen intake. A positive 2- to 3-g nitrogen balance is necessary for anabolism. By contrast, negative nitrogen balance is present when catabolic states exist.

Diet History and Health History. In addition to the general nursing history, use data from a more specific diet history to assess a patient's actual or potential needs. Box 44-6 lists some specific assessment questions to ask in the diet history. The diet history focuses on a patient's habitual intake of foods and liquids and includes information about preferences, allergies, and other relevant areas such as the patient's ability to obtain food. Gather information about the patient's illness/activity level to determine

BOX 44-6 NURSING ASSESSMENT QUESTIONS

Dietary Intake and Food Preferences
- What type of food do you like?
- How many meals a day do you eat?
- What times do you normally eat meals and snacks?
- What portion sizes do you eat at each meal?
- Are you on a special diet because of a medical problem?
- Do you have any diet preferences because of your religion or culture?
- Who prepares the food at home?
- Who purchases the food?
- How do you cook your food (e.g., fried, broiled, baked, grilled)?

Unpleasant Symptoms
- Which foods cause indigestion, gas, or heartburn?
- Does this occur each time you have the food?
- What relieves the symptoms?

Allergies
- Are you allergic to any foods?
- Which types of problems do you have with these foods?
- How are these food allergies treated (e.g., EpiPen, oral antihistamines)?

Taste, Chewing, and Swallowing
- Have you noticed any changes in taste?
- Did these changes occur with medications or following an illness?
- Do you wear dentures? Are the dentures comfortable?
- Do you have any mouth pain or sores (e.g., cold sore, canker sores)?
- Do you have difficulty swallowing?
- Do you cough or gag when you swallow?

Appetite and Weight
- Have you had a change in appetite?
- Have you noticed a change in your weight?
- Was this change anticipated (e.g., were you on a weight-reduction diet)?

Use of Medications
- Which medications do you take?
- Do you take any over-the-counter medications that your doctor does not prescribe?
- Do you take any nutritional or herbal supplements?

BOX 44-7 CAUSES OF DYSPHAGIA

Myogenic
- Myasthenia gravis
- Aging
- Muscular dystrophy
- Polymyositis

Neurogenic
- Stroke
- Cerebral palsy
- Guillain-Barré syndrome
- Multiple sclerosis
- Amyotrophic lateral sclerosis (Lou Gehrig disease)
- Diabetic neuropathy
- Parkinson's disease

Obstructive
- Benign peptic stricture
- Lower esophageal ring
- Candidiasis
- Head and neck cancer
- Inflammatory masses
- Trauma/surgical resection
- Anterior mediastinal masses
- Cervical spondylosis

Other
- Gastrointestinal or esophageal resection
- Rheumatological disorders
- Connective tissue disorders
- Vagotomy

energy needs and compare food intake. Your nursing assessment of nutrition includes health status; age; cultural background (see Box 44-5); religious food patterns (see Table 44-3); socioeconomic status; personal food preferences; psychological factors; use of alcohol or illegal drugs; use of vitamin, mineral, or herbal supplements; prescription or over-the-counter (OTC) drugs (see Table 44-2); and the patient's general nutrition knowledge.

In outpatient settings the patient keeps a 3- to 7-day food diary. This allows you to calculate nutritional intake and to compare it with DRI to see if the patient's dietary habits are adequate. Use food questionnaires to establish patterns over time (Bankhead et al., 2009). In health care settings nurses collaborate with RDs to complete calorie counts for patients.

Physical Examination. The physical examination is one of the most important aspects of a nutritional assessment. Because improper nutrition affects all body systems, observe for malnutrition during physical assessment (see Chapter 30). Complete the general physical assessment of body systems and recheck relevant areas to evaluate a patient's nutritional status. The clinical signs of nutritional status (Table 44-4) serve as guidelines for observation during physical assessment.

Dysphagia. Dysphagia refers to difficulty swallowing. The causes (Box 44-7) and complications of dysphagia vary. Complications include aspiration pneumonia, dehydration, decreased nutritional status, and weight loss. Dysphagia leads to disability or decreased functional status, increased length of stay and cost of care, increased likelihood of discharge to institutionalized care, and increased mortality (Ashley et al., 2006).

Be aware of warning signs for dysphagia. They include cough during eating; change in voice tone or quality after swallowing; abnormal movements of the mouth, tongue, or lips; and slow, weak, imprecise, or uncoordinated speech. Abnormal gag, delayed swallowing, incomplete oral clearance or pocketing, regurgitation, pharyngeal pooling, delayed or absent trigger of swallow, and inability to speak consistently are other signs of dysphagia. Patients with dysphagia often do not show overt signs such as coughing when food enters the airway. *Silent aspiration* is aspiration that occurs in patients with neurological problems that lead to decreased sensation. It often occurs without a cough, and symptoms usually do not appear for 24 hours (Palmer and Metheny, 2008). Silent aspiration accounts for most of the 40% to 70% of aspiration in patients with dysphagia following stroke (Kwon et al., 2006).

BOX 44-8 NURSING DIAGNOSTIC PROCESS

Imbalanced Nutrition: Less Than Body Requirements

ASSESSMENT ACTIVITIES	DEFINING CHARACTERISTICS
Body mass index (BMI)	BMI = 17
Obtain weight	68-year-old woman 24-lb (10.8-kg) weight loss Weight is 20% below her ideal body weight
Obtain 24-hour food and fluid history	Lack of satiety Lack of interest in food Fluid intake is juice and coffee Eats sandwich in afternoon
Physical assessment	Poor muscle tone Fatigue Hair loss Dry scaly skin Pale conjunctiva and mucous membranes
Medication	Takes sertraline for depression
Social	Husband died 6 months ago Has quit attending monthly quilting club Started counseling 3 months ago

Dysphagia often leads to an inadequate amount of food intake, which often results in malnutrition. Frequently patients with dysphagia become frustrated with eating and show changes in skinfold thickness and albumin. Adjustment to new dietary restrictions during the rehabilitation period affects intake for long periods of time. Malnutrition significantly slows swallowing recovery and may increase mortality (Robbins et al., 2007).

Dysphagia screening quickly identifies problems with swallowing and helps nurses initiate referrals for more in-depth assessment by a speech pathologist (Skill 44-1 on pp. 1026-1027). Early and ongoing assessment of patients with swallowing difficulties and use of a valid dysphagia screening tool increase quality of care and decrease incidence of aspiration pneumonia (AY Cichero et al., 2009). Dysphagia screening includes medical record review; observation of a patient at a meal for change in voice quality, posture, and head control; percentage of meal consumed; eating time; drooling or leakage of liquids and solids; cough during/after a swallow; facial or tongue weakness; palatal movement; difficulty with secretions; pocketing; choking; and presence of voluntary and dry cough. A number of validated screening tools are available, such as the Bedside Swallowing Assessment, Burke Dysphagia Screening Test, Acute Stroke Dysphagia Screen, and Standardized Swallowing Assessment (Edmiaston et al., 2010). The Acute Stroke Dysphagia screen is an easily administered and reliable tool for health care professionals who are not speech-language pathologists. Screening for and treatment of dysphagia requires a multidisciplinary team approach of nurses, RDs, health care providers, and speech language pathologists (SLPs) (Robbins et al., 2007).

NURSING DIAGNOSIS

Cluster all assessment data to identify actual or at-risk nursing diagnoses (Box 44-8). A nutritional problem often occurs when overall intake is significantly decreased or increased or when one or more nutrients are not ingested, completely digested, or completely absorbed. Nursing diagnoses are related to either the actual

TABLE 44-4 **Physical Signs of Nutritional Status**

BODY AREA	SIGNS OF GOOD NUTRITION	SIGNS OF POOR NUTRITION
General appearance	Alert: responsive	Listless, apathetic, cachectic
Weight	Weight normal for height, age, body build	Obesity (usually 10% above ideal body weight [IBW]) or underweight (special concern for underweight)
Posture	Erect posture; straight arms and legs	Sagging shoulders; sunken chest; humped back
Muscles	Well-developed, firm; good tone; some fat under skin	Flaccid, poor tone, underdeveloped tone; "wasted" appearance; impaired ability to walk properly
Nervous system control	Good attention span; not irritable or restless; normal reflexes; psychological stability	Inattention; irritability; confusion; burning and tingling of hands and feet (paresthesia); loss of position and vibratory sense; weakness and tenderness of muscles (may result in inability to walk); decrease or loss of ankle and knee reflexes; absent vibratory sense
Gastrointestinal function	Good appetite and digestion; normal regular elimination; no palpable organs or masses	Anorexia; indigestion; constipation or diarrhea; liver or spleen enlargement
Cardiovascular function	Normal heart rate and rhythm; lack of murmurs; normal blood pressure for age	Rapid heart rate (above 100 beats/min), enlarged heart; abnormal rhythm; elevated blood pressure
General vitality	Endurance; energy; sleeps well; vigorous	Easily fatigued; no energy; falls asleep easily; tired and apathetic
Hair	Shiny, lustrous; firm; not easily plucked; healthy scalp	Stringy, dull, brittle, dry, thin, and sparse, depigmented; easily plucked
Skin (general)	Smooth and slightly moist skin with good color	Rough, dry, scaly, pale, pigmented, irritated; bruises; petechiae; subcutaneous fat loss
Face and neck	Uniform color; smooth, pink, healthy appearance; not swollen	Greasy, discolored, scaly, swollen; dark skin over cheeks and under eyes; lumpiness or flakiness of skin around nose and mouth
Lips	Smooth; good color; moist; not chapped or swollen	Dry, scaly, swollen; redness and swelling (cheilosis); angular lesions at corners of mouth; fissures or scars (stomatitis)
Mouth, oral membranes	Reddish-pink mucous membranes in oral cavity	Swollen, boggy oral mucous membranes
Gums	Good pink color; healthy and red; no swelling or bleeding	Spongy gums that bleed easily; marginal redness, inflammation; receding
Tongue	Good pink or deep reddish color; no swelling; smooth, presence of surface papillae; lack of lesions	Swelling, scarlet and raw; magenta, beefiness (glossitis); hyperemic and hypertrophic papillae; atrophic papillae
Teeth	No cavities; no pain; bright, straight; no crowding; well-shaped jaw; clean with no discoloration	Unfilled caries; missing teeth; worn surfaces; mottled (fluorosis), malpositioned
Eyes	Bright, clear, shiny; no sores at corner of eyelids; moist and healthy pink conjunctivae; prominent blood vessels; no fatigue circles beneath eyes	Eye membranes pale (pale conjunctivas); redness of membrane (conjunctival injection); dryness; signs of infection; Bitot's spots; redness and fissuring of eyelid corners (angular palpebritis); dryness of eye membrane (conjunctival xerosis); dull appearance of cornea (corneal xerosis); soft cornea (keratomalacia)
Neck (glands)	No enlargement	Thyroid or lymph node enlargement
Nails	Firm, pink	Spoon shape (koilonychia); brittleness; ridges
Legs, feet	No tenderness, weakness, or swelling; good color	Edema; tender calf; tingling; weakness
Skeleton	No malformations	Bowlegs; knock-knees; chest deformity at diaphragm; prominent scapulae and ribs

From Nix S: *Williams' basic nutrition and diet therapy,* ed 13, St Louis, 2009, Mosby.

nutrition problems (e.g., inadequate intake) or problems that place the patient at risk for nutritional deficiencies such as oral trauma, severe burns, or infections.

Select a nursing diagnostic statement based on defining characteristics in the assessment database. Make sure the nursing diagnosis is as precise as possible. The following are examples of nursing diagnoses that apply to nutritional problems:

- Risk for aspiration
- Diarrhea
- Deficient knowledge
- Imbalanced nutrition: less than body requirements
- Imbalanced nutrition: more than body requirements
- Risk for imbalanced nutrition: more than body requirements
- Readiness for enhanced nutrition
- Feeding self-care deficit
- Impaired swallowing

Be sure to select the appropriate related factor for a nursing diagnosis. Related factors need to be accurate so you select the appropriate interventions. In addition, there are also clinical situations in which patients have multiple related problems. The concept map in Fig. 44-5 shows the relationship of nursing diagnoses for Mrs. Cooper.

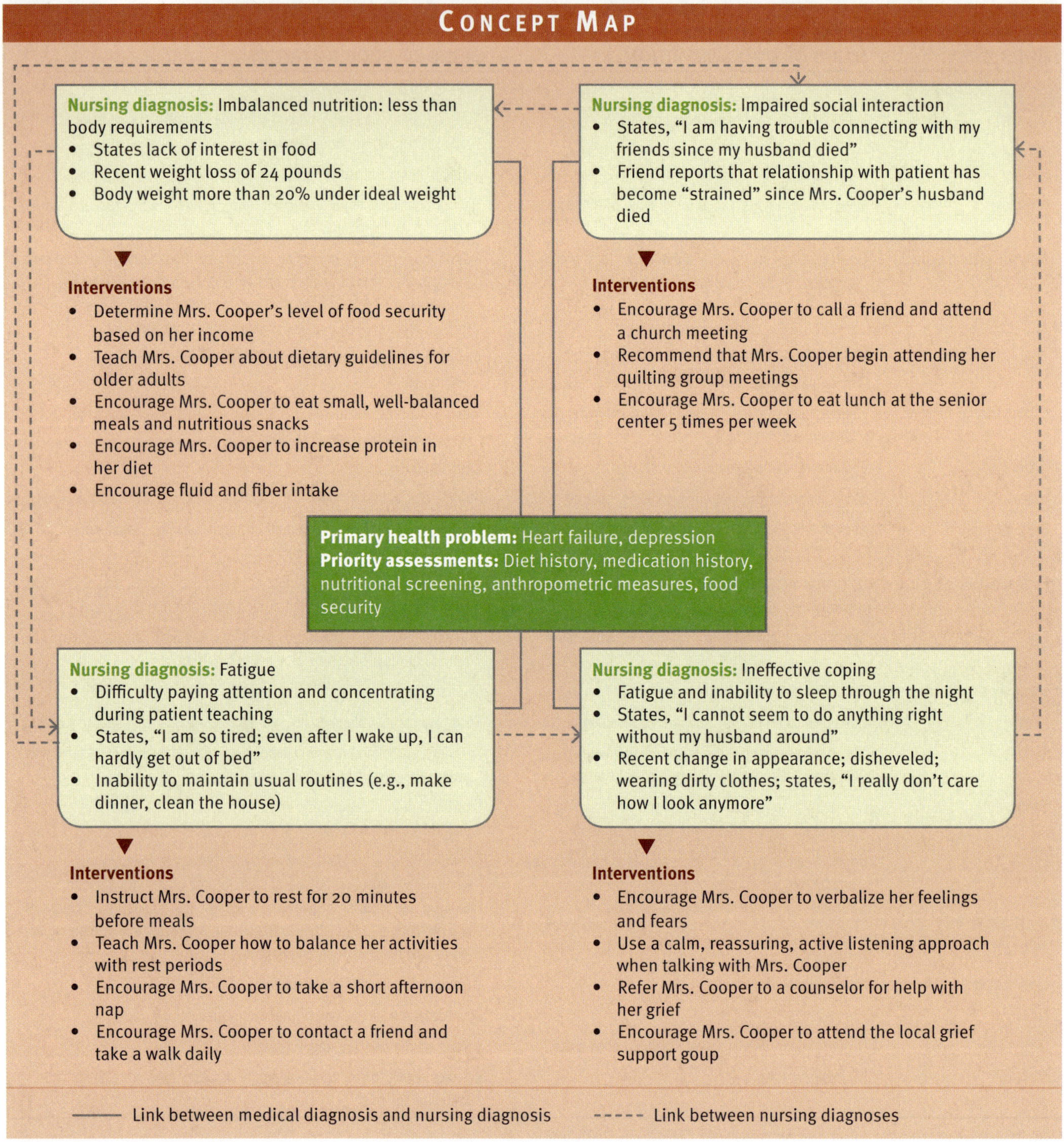

CONCEPT MAP
Nursing diagnosis: Imbalanced nutrition: less than body requirements
• States lack of interest in food
• Recent weight loss of 24 pounds
• Body weight more than 20% under ideal weight
Interventions
• Determine Mrs. Cooper's level of food security based on her income
• Teach Mrs. Cooper about dietary guidelines for older adults
• Encourage Mrs. Cooper to eat small, well-balanced meals and nutritious snacks
• Encourage Mrs. Cooper to increase protein in her diet
• Encourage fluid and fiber intake
Nursing diagnosis: Impaired social interaction
• States, "I am having trouble connecting with my friends since my husband died"
• Friend reports that relationship with patient has become "strained" since Mrs. Cooper's husband died
Interventions
• Encourage Mrs. Cooper to call a friend and attend a church meeting
• Recommend that Mrs. Cooper begin attending her quilting group meetings
• Encourage Mrs. Cooper to eat lunch at the senior center 5 times per week
Primary health problem: Heart failure, depression
Priority assessments: Diet history, medication history, nutritional screening, anthropometric measures, food security
Nursing diagnosis: Fatigue
• Difficulty paying attention and concentrating during patient teaching
• States, "I am so tired; even after I wake up, I can hardly get out of bed"
• Inability to maintain usual routines (e.g., make dinner, clean the house)
Interventions
• Instruct Mrs. Cooper to rest for 20 minutes before meals
• Teach Mrs. Cooper how to balance her activities with rest periods
• Encourage Mrs. Cooper to take a short afternoon nap
• Encourage Mrs. Cooper to contact a friend and take a walk daily
Nursing diagnosis: Ineffective coping
• Fatigue and inability to sleep through the night
• States, "I cannot seem to do anything right without my husband around"
• Recent change in appearance; disheveled; wearing dirty clothes; states, "I really don't care how I look anymore"
Interventions
• Encourage Mrs. Cooper to verbalize her feelings and fears
• Use a calm, reassuring, active listening approach when talking with Mrs. Cooper
• Refer Mrs. Cooper to a counselor for help with her grief
• Encourage Mrs. Cooper to attend the local grief support goup
—— Link between medical diagnosis and nursing diagnosis
----- Link between nursing diagnoses

FIG. 44-5 Concept map for Mrs. Cooper.

PLANNING

Planning to maintain patients' optimal nutritional status requires a higher level of care than simply correcting nutritional problems. Often there is a need for patients to make long-term changes for nutrition to improve. Synthesis of patient information from multiple sources is necessary to create an individualized approach of care that is relevant to a patient's needs and situation (Fig. 44-6). Apply critical thinking to ensure that you consider all data sources in developing a patient's plan of care. The accurate identification of nursing diagnoses related to patients' nutritional problems results in a care plan that is relevant and appropriate (see the Nursing Care Plan). Referring to professional standards for nutrition is especially important during this step, because published standards are based on scientific findings.

Goals and Outcomes. Goals and outcomes of care reflect a patient's physiological, therapeutic, and individualized needs. Nutrition education and counseling are important to prevent disease and promote health. Patients on therapeutic diets need to understand the implications of their diets and how prescribed diets

NURSING CARE PLAN

Imbalanced Nutrition: Less Than Body Requirements

ASSESSMENT

Maria Steiner, a nurse practitioner in a senior citizens' center, is seeing Mrs. Cooper, who is 68 years old and has a history of heart failure. Recently Mrs. Cooper experienced an unexpected 15% weight loss. Three months have passed since she started taking sertraline (Zoloft) for depression related to the loss of her husband 6 months ago. She no longer participates in her monthly quilting club. She was also referred for counseling 3 months ago for help with grief and depression through a local senior service agency. When Maria inquired about her financial situation, Mrs. Cooper responded that it was tight living on a small pension and Social Security but she was able to manage.

Assessment Activities	*Findings/Defining Characteristics**
Ask Mrs. Cooper about her food intake during the last 2 days.	She responds that she drinks some juice in the morning and two or three cups of coffee. In addition, she often has a sandwich in the late afternoon. **"I'm just not interested in food. It has no taste."**
Ask Mrs. Cooper about social interaction.	Mrs. Cooper complains of loneliness and says that she does not get out much, although her psychologist recommended more socializing. Her friends at church call her to come back to meetings, but she is just not ready. She says that she tires easily and no longer attends the monthly meetings of her quilt club.
Weigh patient and assess posture.	Her **weight is 20% below her IBW** and her **BMI is 17.** This weight loss has happened over the past 6 months, and she has **lost 24 pounds.** **Stooped posture**
Observe Mrs. Cooper for signs of poor nutrition.	**Hair loss** **Sore oral mucous membranes** **Pale conjunctivae** and mucous membranes
Palpate muscles	**Generalized poor muscle tone**

***Defining characteristics** are shown in bold type.
BMI, Body mass index; *IBW,* ideal body weight.

NURSING DIAGNOSIS: Imbalanced nutrition: less than body requirements related to a decreased ability to ingest food as a result of depression

PLANNING

Goals	*Expected Outcomes (NOC)†*
	Weight Gain Behavior
Mrs. Cooper will progressively gain weight.	Mrs. Cooper will gain 1 to 2 pounds per month until goal of 130 pounds is reached.
	Nutritional Status
Mrs. Cooper will consume adequate nourishment each day.	Mrs. Cooper will ingest 1900 kcal/day, including 50 g of protein per day.
	Nutritional Status: Biochemical Measures
Mrs. Cooper will exhibit no signs of malnutrition.	Physical assessment findings will be within normal limits. Laboratory values will be within normal limits.

†Outcome classification labels from Moorhead S et al: *Nursing outcomes classification (NOC),* ed 4, St Louis, 2008, Mosby.

INTERVENTIONS (NIC)‡	RATIONALE
Nutritional Counseling	
Coordinate plan of care with health care provider, psychologist, Mrs. Cooper, and registered dietitian.	Successful nutrition care planning is a multidisciplinary approach throughout the continuum of care (DiMaria-Ghalili, 2008).
Individualize menu plans according to Mrs. Cooper's preferences.	Encourages patient to eat by incorporating her food preferences into the meal plans (DiMaria-Ghalili, 2008).
Teach Mrs. Cooper about MyPlate for Older Adults.	MyPlate for Older Adults is adapted to meet the nutritional requirements for older adults (Shelnutt et al., 2009).

‡Intervention classification labels from Bulechek GM, Butcher HK, and Dochterman JM: *Nursing interventions classification (NIC),* ed 5, St Louis, 2008, Mosby.

Continued

NURSING CARE PLAN

Imbalanced Nutrition: Less Than Body Requirements—cont'd

Nutritional Management

Encourage Mrs. Cooper to eat small nutritious meals and snacks and increase dietary intake to help offset anorexia secondary to sertraline.	Sertraline is a selective serotonin reuptake inhibitor (SSRI) antidepressant medication, which causes diminished taste and anorexia. Frequent small nutritious meals and snacks help to reduce anorexia-associated weight loss.
Encourage fluid intake.	Older adults need eight 8-oz (240 mL) glasses per day of fluid from beverage and food sources. Concentrating intake in morning and early afternoon is acceptable to prevent nocturia (Meiner, 2011).
Encourage fiber intake.	Deters constipation, enhancing appetite.
Encourage Mrs. Cooper to eat lunch at the senior center 5 times per week.	Eating with others encourages good nutrition and promotes socialization with peers (Krondl et al., 2008; Nix, 2009).

EVALUATION

Nursing Actions	*Patient Response/Finding*	*Achievement of Outcome*
Monitor Mrs. Cooper monthly for weight gain, anemia, serum albumin level, and transferrin levels.	After 2 weeks Mrs. Cooper has gained 3 lbs, and her Hgb level is 12.	Mrs. Cooper is making progress with weight gain; her hemoglobin level still reflects mild anemia.
Ask Mrs. Cooper to keep a food diary for 3 days.	Food diary reflects that she ate her main meal at the senior center, has fruit and bran flakes for breakfast, and in the evening either has soup or a sandwich with fruit.	Mrs. Cooper is selecting more nutritionally rich foods, consistent with current guidelines.
Observe Mrs. Cooper's physical appearance.	At 2 weeks, her skin is less pale, and her hair appears to be in better condition and styled.	Mrs. Cooper has improved physical parameters of nutrition; still needs follow-up.
Ask Mrs. Cooper about appetite and energy level.	Mrs. Cooper responds that on days that she eats at the senior center her appetite seems better and she "wants to do more things." She notes that weekends are very lonely.	Weekday support for nutritional status appears effective; needs to increase patient's activity status and nutritional intake during weekends.

help to control their illnesses. When planning care, be aware of all factors that influence a patient's food intake. In one study patients with heart failure identified that decreased hunger, diet restrictions, fatigue, shortness of breath, anxiety, and sadness influenced their food intake (Lennie et al., 2006).

Individualized planning is essential. Explore patients' feelings about their weight and diet and help them set realistic and achievable goals (Daniels, 2006). Mutually planned goals negotiated among the patient, RD, and nurse ensure success. For the patient with heart failure described previously, an overall goal is "Patient will achieve appropriate BMI height-weight range or be within 10% of IBW." The following outcomes assist in achievement of this goal:

- Patient's daily nutritional intake meets the minimal DRIs.
- Patient's daily nutritional fat intake is less than 30%.
- Patient removes sugared beverages from diet.
- Patient refrains from eating unhealthy foods between meals and after dinner.
- Patient loses at least ½ to 1 lb (0.2 to 0.45 kg) per week.

Meeting nutritional goals requires input from the patient and the multidisciplinary team. Knowledge of the role of each discipline in providing nutrition support is necessary to maximize nutritional outcomes. For example, collaboration with an RD helps develop appropriate nutrition treatment plans. Calorie counts are frequently ordered, and assistance is necessary in obtaining accurate data. An effective plan of care requires accurate exchange of information among disciplines.

Setting Priorities. After identifying patients' nursing diagnoses, you determine priorities in order to plan timely and successful interventions. For example, managing a patient's oral pain will be a priority over the diagnosis of *imbalanced nutrition: less than body requirements* if the patient is unable to swallow and maintain adequate food intake. *Deficient knowledge* regarding diet therapy will be a priority if it is necessary to promote long-term and effective weight loss.

During acute illness or surgery the intake of food is often altered in the perioperative period. The priority of care is to provide optimal preoperative nutrition support in patients with malnutrition. The priority for the resumption of food intake after surgery depends on the return of bowel function, the extent of the surgical procedure, and the presence of any complications (see Chapter 50). For example, when patients have oral and throat surgery, they chew and swallow food in the presence of excision sites, sutures, or tissue manipulated during surgery. The priority of care is to first provide comfort and pain control. Then address nutritional priorities and plan care to maintain nutrition that does not cause pain or injury to the healing tissues.

The patient and family must collaborate with the nurse in planning care and setting priorities. This is important because food preferences, food purchases, and preparation involve the entire family. The plan of care cannot succeed without their commitment to, involvement in, and understanding of the nutritional priorities.

Teamwork and Collaboration. The care of the patient often extends beyond the acute hospital setting, requiring continued collaboration among members of the health care team. It is important that discharge planning include nutritional interventions as patients return to their homes or extended care facilities.

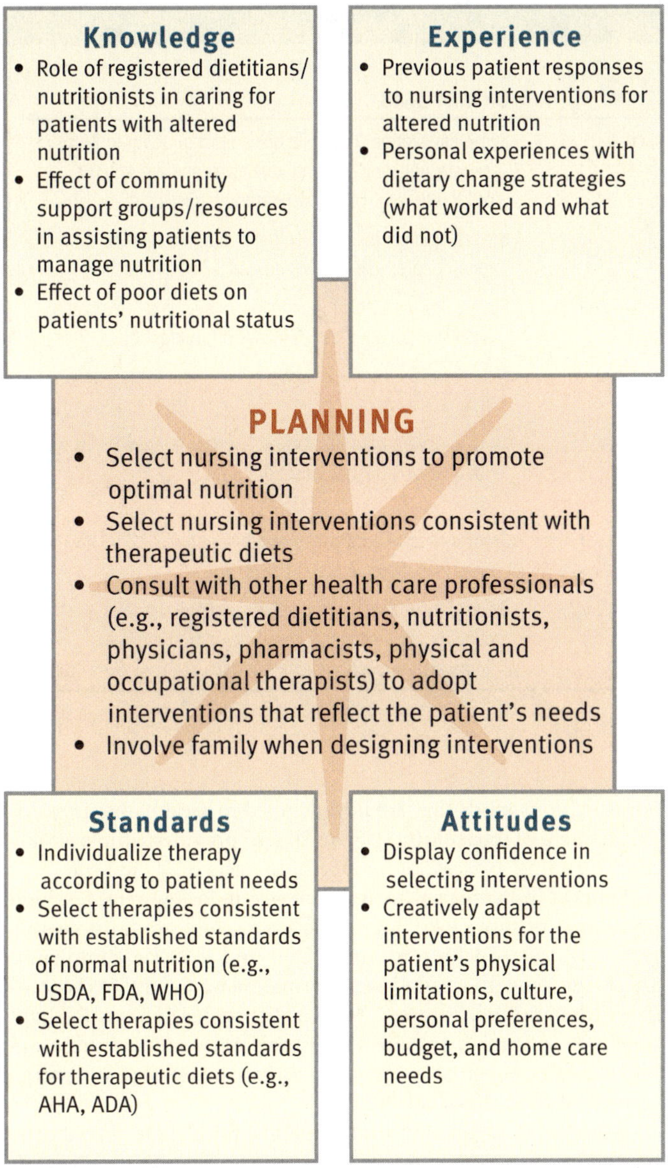

Knowledge
• Role of registered dietitians/nutritionists in caring for patients with altered nutrition
• Effect of community support groups/resources in assisting patients to manage nutrition
• Effect of poor diets on patients' nutritional status
Experience
• Previous patient responses to nursing interventions for altered nutrition
• Personal experiences with dietary change strategies (what worked and what did not)
PLANNING
• Select nursing interventions to promote optimal nutrition
• Select nursing interventions consistent with therapeutic diets
• Consult with other health care professionals (e.g., registered dietitians, nutritionists, physicians, pharmacists, physical and occupational therapists) to adopt interventions that reflect the patient's needs
• Involve family when designing interventions
Standards
• Individualize therapy according to patient needs
• Select therapies consistent with established standards of normal nutrition (e.g., USDA, FDA, WHO)
• Select therapies consistent with established standards for therapeutic diets (e.g., AHA, ADA)
Attitudes
• Display confidence in selecting interventions
• Creatively adapt interventions for the patient's physical limitations, culture, personal preferences, budget, and home care needs

FIG. 44-6 Critical thinking model for nutrition planning. *ADA,* American Diabetes Association; *AHA,* American Heart Association; *FDA,* Food and Drug Administration; *USDA,* U.S. Department of Agriculture; *WHO,* World Health Organization.

Communicate patient goals and planned interventions to all team members to achieve expected patient outcomes. Consult with an SLP, RD, pharmacist, and/or occupational therapist when working with patients with dysphagia or who need ongoing nutritional assessment and interventions to meet their nutritional needs.

Enteral tube feedings are often administered into the stomach or intestines via a tube inserted through the nose or a percutaneous access (Skills 44-2 and 44-3 on pp. 1028-1035). These enteral feedings supplement a patient's oral nutritional intake in the home, acute care, extended care, or rehabilitation setting when they cannot meet their nutritional needs by mouth. Regardless of the setting, the RD assesses and monitors the patient's nutritional status and intake and makes recommendations for changes. RDs are expert in the choice of enteral formulas and dietary modifications required for specific disease states. Long-term management of nutritional problems is a challenge that requires collaboration among the patient, family, and health care team members.

Patients who cannot tolerate nutrition through the GI tract receive parenteral nutrition, a solution consisting of glucose, amino acids, lipids, minerals, electrolytes, trace elements, and vitamins, through an indwelling peripheral or central venous catheter (CVC) (see Chapter 41). The pharmacist is an expert who reviews medications to identify drug-nutrient interactions. Pharmacists are also experts in preparing mixtures of total parenteral nutrition (TPN).

When patients have difficulty feeding themselves, occupational therapists work with them and their families to identify assistive devices. Devices such as utensils with large handles and plates with elevated sides help a patient with self-feeding. An SLP helps a patient with swallowing exercises and techniques to reduce the risk of aspiration. Occupational therapists also help patients maintain function in the home setting by rearranging food preparation areas in an effort to maximize a patient's functional capacity.

IMPLEMENTATION

Diet therapies are numerous and are chosen on the basis of a patient's overall health status, ability to eat and digest normally, and long-term nutritional needs. The focus of health promotion is to educate patients and family caregivers about balanced nutrition and to assist them in obtaining resources to eat high-quality meals. In acute care, your role as a nurse is to manage acute conditions that alter patients' nutritional status and assist in ways to promote their appetite and ability to take in nutrients. Patients who are ill or debilitated often have poor appetites (anorexia). **Anorexia** has many causes (e.g., pain, fatigue, and the effects of medications). Help patients understand the factors that cause anorexia and use creative approaches to stimulate appetite. In the restorative care setting, you will assist patients in learning how to follow the therapeutic diets necessary for recovery and treatment of chronic health conditions.

Health Promotion. As a nurse you are in a key position to educate patients about healthy diet choices and good nutrition. Incorporating knowledge of nutrition into patients' lifestyles serves to prevent the development of many diseases. Outpatient and community-based settings are optimal locations for nursing assessment of nutritional practices and status. Early identification of potential or actual problems is the best way to avoid more serious problems. Similarly, in other health care settings patients with nutritional problems such as obesity often require assistance in menu planning and compliance strategies. Your role as educator includes educating families and providing information about community resources. Telephone numbers of an RD or nurse for follow-up questions are always a part of counseling.

Meal planning takes into account the family's budget and different preferences of family members. Choose specific foods on the basis of the dietary prescription and recommended food groups. For families on limited budgets use substitutes. For example, bean or cheese dishes often replace meat in a meal, and evaporated milk or dry skim milk is used for cooking. Have patients modify the method of preparation when it is necessary to minimize certain substances. Baking rather than frying reduces fat intake, and patients can use lemon juice or spices to add flavor to low-sodium diets.

Planning menus a week in advance has several benefits. It helps ensure good nutrition or compliance with a specific diet and helps a family stay within their allotted budget. Nurses or RDs need to check menus for content. Often a simple tip is helpful in meal planning such as avoiding grocery shopping when hungry, which can lead to spur-of-the-moment purchases of more expensive or

TABLE 44-5 Food Safety

FOODBORNE DISEASE	ORGANISM	FOOD SOURCE	SYMPTOMS*
Botulism	*Clostridium botulinum*	Improperly home-canned foods, smoked and salted fish, ham, sausage, shellfish	Symptoms varied from mild discomfort to death in 24 hours; initially nausea, vomiting, dizziness, and weakness progressing to motor (respiratory) paralysis
Escherichia coli	*E. coli*	Undercooked meat (ground beef)	Severe cramps, nausea, vomiting, diarrhea (may be bloody), renal failure; appears 1-8 days after eating; lasts 1-7 days
Listeriosis	*Listeria monocytogenes*	Soft cheese, meat (hot dogs, paté, lunch meats), unpasteurized milk, poultry, seafood	Severe diarrhea, fever, headache, pneumonia, meningitis, endocarditis; appears 3-21 days after infection
Perfringens enteritis	*Clostridium perfringens*	Cooked meats, meat dishes held at room or warm temperature	Mild diarrhea, vomiting; appears 8-24 hours after eating; lasts 1-2 days
Salmonellosis	*Salmonella* *S. typhi* *S. paratyphi*	Milk, custards, egg dishes, salad dressings, sandwich fillings, polluted shellfish	Mild-to-severe diarrhea, cramps, vomiting; appears up to 72 hours after ingestion; lasts 4-7 days
Shigellosis	*Shigella dysenteriae*	Milk, milk products, seafood, salads	Cramps, diarrhea to fatal dysentery; appears 12-50 hours after ingestion; lasts 3-14 days
Staphylococcus	*Staphylococcus aureus*	Custards, cream fillings, processed meats, ham, cheese, ice cream, potato salad, sauces, casseroles	Severe abdominal cramps, pain, vomiting, diarrhea, perspiration, headache, fever, prostration; appears 1-6 hours after ingestion; lasts 1-2 days

From Nix S: *Williams' basic nutrition and diet therapy,* ed 13, St Louis, 2009, Mosby.
*Symptoms are generally most severe for youngest and oldest age-groups.

BOX 44-9 PATIENT TEACHING

Food Safety

Objective

- Patient is able to verbalize measures to protect from foodborne illness.

Teaching Strategies

- Explain that food safety is an important public health issue. Populations particularly at risk are older and younger persons and immunosuppressed individuals.
- Instruct patients using the following four principles:

1. CLEAN
   - Wash hands with warm, soapy water before touching or eating food.
   - Wash fresh fruits and vegetables thoroughly.
   - Clean the inside of refrigerator and microwave regularly to prevent microbial growth.
2. SEPARATE
   - Wash cooking utensils and cutting boards with hot soapy water.
   - Wash hands after handling foods, especially meats, poultry, and eggs.
   - Clean vegetables and lettuce used in salads thoroughly.
   - Wash dishrags, towels, and sponges regularly or use paper towels
3. COOK
   - Use a food thermometer to verify that meat, poultry, and fish are cooked properly.
   - Do not eat raw meats or unpasteurized milk.
4. CHILL
   - Keep foods properly refrigerated at 40° F and frozen at 0° F.
   - Do not save leftovers for more than 2 days in refrigerator.

Evaluation

- Ask patient to verbalize measures to prevent foodborne illnesses.
- Observe the patient at home for safe practices if making home visit.

Data from US Department of Agriculture and US Department of Health and Human Services: *Report of the dietary guidelines advisory committee dietary guidelines for Americans 2010,* 2010, http://www.cnpp.usda.gov/dietaryguidelines.htm. Accessed November 23, 2011.

less nutritious foods that are not included in meal plans. The U.S. Department of Agriculture (USDA, 2011b) provides sample weekly meal-planning services for a range of budgets on its website.

Support individuals who are interested in losing weight. A high percentage of those who attempt to lose weight are unsuccessful, regaining lost weight over time. Diet and exercise compliance affects success with weight loss. Information on weight loss is available from multiple sources. Help patients develop a successful weight-loss plan that considers their preferences and resources and includes awareness of portion sizes and knowledge of energy content of food (Kruskall, 2006).

Food safety is an important public health issue. Foodborne bacteria can occur from improper food cleaning, preparation, or poor hygiene practices of food workers. Health care professionals not only need to be aware of the factors related to food safety but also should provide patient education to reduce the risks for foodborne illnesses (Table 44-5; Box 44-9).

Building Competency in Safety You are a nurse planning a community health program on food safety at the senior center. Develop an outline of key topics to present using the 2010 Dietary Guidelines for Americans food safety principles.

Answers to questions can be found on the Evolve website.

Acute Care. The nutritional care of acutely ill patients requires a nurse to consider a variety of factors that influence nutritional intake. Diagnostic testing and procedures in the acute care setting disrupt food intake. Often as preparation for or immediately following a diagnostic procedure, a patient is to receive nothing by mouth (NPO). Mealtimes in a health care setting are frequently interrupted, or patients have poor appetites. Patients often are too fatigued or uncomfortable to eat. It is important to continuously assess a patient's nutritional status and adopt interventions that

TABLE 44-6 Nutrition and the Immune System

IMMUNE/ PHYSIOLOGICAL COMPONENT	MALNUTRITION EFFECT	VITAL NUTRIENT
Antibodies	Decreased amount	Protein, vitamins A, B_6, B_{12}, C, folic acid, thiamin, biotin, riboflavin, niacin
GI tract	Systemic movement of bacteria	Arginine, glutamine, omega-3 fatty acids
Granulocytes and macrocytes	Longer time for phagocytosis kill time and lymphocyte activation	Protein, vitamins A, B_6, B_{12}, C, folic acid, thiamin, riboflavin, niacin, zinc, iron
Mucus	Flat microvilli in GI tract, decreased antibody secretion	Vitamins B_{12}, B_6, C, biotin
Skin	Integrity compromised, density reduced, wound healing slowed	Protein, vitamins A, B_{12}, C, niacin, copper, zinc
T-lymphocytes	Depressed T-cell distribution	Protein, arginine, iron, zinc, omega-3 fatty acids, vitamins A, B_6, B_{12}, folic acid, thiamin, riboflavin, niacin, pantothenic acid

Modified from Grodner M, Long S, DeYoung S: *Foundations and clinical applications of nutrition: a nursing approach,* ed 5, St Louis, 2012, Mosby.
GI, Gastrointestinal.

promote normal intake, digestion, and metabolism of nutrients. Patients who are NPO and receive only standard IV fluids for more than 4 to 7 days are at nutritional risk.

Advancing Diets. Acute and chronic conditions affect a patient's immune system and nutritional status. Patients with decreased immune function (e.g., from cancer, chemotherapy, human immunodeficiency virus/acquired immunodeficiency syndrome [HIV/AIDS], or organ transplants) require special diets that decrease their exposure to microorganisms and are higher in selected nutrients. Table 44-6 gives an overview of the immune system, the malnutrition impact, and which nutrients are beneficial. In addition, patients who are ill, who have had surgical procedures, or who were NPO for a period of time have specialized dietary needs. Health care providers order a gradual progression of dietary intake or therapeutic diet to manage patients' illness (Box 44-10).

Promoting Appetite. Providing an environment that promotes nutritional intake includes keeping a patient's environment free of odors, providing oral hygiene as needed to remove unpleasant tastes, and maintaining patient comfort. Offering smaller, more frequent meals often helps. In addition, certain medications affect dietary intake and nutrient use. For example, medications such as insulin, glucocorticoids, and thyroid hormones affect metabolism. Other medications such as antifungal agents frequently affect taste. Some of the psychotropic medications affect appetite, cause nausea, and also alter taste. The nurse and RD help patients to select foods that reduce the altered taste sensations or nausea. Consult with an RD regarding seasonings that may be used to improve food taste.

BOX 44-10 DIET PROGRESSION AND THERAPEUTIC DIETS

Clear Liquid
Clear fat-free broth, bouillon, coffee, tea, carbonated beverages, clear fruit juices, gelatin, fruit ices, popsicles

Full Liquid
As for clear liquid, with addition of smooth-textured dairy products (e.g., ice cream), strained or blended cream soups, custards, refined cooked cereals, vegetable juice, pureed vegetables, all fruit juices, sherbets, puddings, frozen yogurt

Pureed
As for clear and full liquid, with addition of scrambled eggs; pureed meats, vegetables, and fruits; mashed potatoes and gravy

Mechanical Soft
As for clear and full liquid and pureed, with addition of all cream soups, ground or finely diced meats, flaked fish, cottage cheese, cheese, rice, potatoes, pancakes, light breads, cooked vegetables, cooked or canned fruits, bananas, soups, peanut butter, eggs (not fried)

Soft/Low Residue
Addition of low-fiber, easily digested foods such as pastas, casseroles, moist tender meats, and canned cooked fruits and vegetables; desserts, cakes, and cookies without nuts or coconut

High Fiber
Addition of fresh uncooked fruits, steamed vegetables, bran, oatmeal, and dried fruits

Low Sodium
4-g (no added salt), 2-g, 1-g, or 500-mg sodium diets; vary from no added salt to severe sodium restriction (500-mg sodium diet), which requires selective food purchases

Low Cholesterol
300 mg/day cholesterol, in keeping with American Heart Association guidelines for serum lipid reduction

Diabetic
Nutrition recommendations by the American Diabetes Association: focus on total energy, nutrient and food distribution; include a balanced intake of carbohydrates, fats, and proteins; varied caloric recommendations to accommodate patient's metabolic demands

Regular
No restrictions, unless specified

In other situations medications need to be changed. Assessing patients for the need for pharmacological agents to stimulate appetite such as cyproheptadine (Periactin), megestrol (Megace), or dronabinol (Marinol) or to manage symptoms that interfere with nutrition requires health care provider consultation.

Mealtime is usually a social activity. If appropriate, encourage visitors to eat with the patient. When patients experience anorexia, encourage other nurses or care providers to converse and engage them in conversation. Mealtime is also an excellent opportunity for patient education. Instruct a patient about any therapeutic diets, medications, energy conservation measures, or adaptive devices to assist with independent feeding.

Assisting Patients with Oral Feeding. When a patient needs help with eating, it is important to protect his or her safety, independence, and dignity. Clear the table or over-bed tray of clutter. Assess his or her risk of aspiration (see Skill 44-1). Patients at high risk for aspiration have decreased level of alertness, decreased gag and/or cough reflexes, and difficulty managing saliva (see Assessment section of this chapter).

Patients with dysphagia are at risk for aspiration and need more assistance with feeding and swallowing. An SLP identifies patients at risk and provides recommendations for therapy (Nowlin, 2006). Provide a 30-minute rest period before eating (Palmer and Metheny, 2008). Position the patient in an upright, seated position in a chair or raise the head of the bed to 90 degrees. Have the patient flex the head slightly to a chin-down position to help prevent aspiration. If the patient has unilateral weakness, teach him or her and the caregiver to place food in the stronger side of the mouth. With the help of an SLP, determine the viscosity of foods that the patient tolerates best through the use of trials of different consistencies of foods and fluids. Thicker fluids are generally easier to swallow. The American Dietetic Association published the National Dysphagia Diet Task Force National Dysphagia Diet in 2002 to provide uniformity of diets provided to patients with dysphagia (NDDTF, 2002). There are four levels of diet: dysphagia puree, dysphagia mechanically altered, dysphagia advanced, and regular. The four levels of liquid include thin liquids (low viscosity), nectar-like liquids (medium viscosity), honey-like liquids (viscosity of honey), and spoon-thick liquids (viscosity of pudding) (NDDTF, 2002).

Feed a patient with dysphagia slowly, providing smaller-size bites. Allow him or her to chew thoroughly and swallow the bite before taking another. More frequent chewing and swallowing assessments throughout the meal are necessary. Allow the patient time to empty the mouth after each spoonful, matching the speed of feeding to the patient's readiness (see Skill 44-1). If the patient begins to cough or choke, remove the food immediately (Nowlin, 2006). Sometimes it is necessary to have oral suction equipment available at the patient's bedside.

Provide opportunities for patients to direct the order in which they want to eat the food items and how fast they wish to eat. Determine the patient's food preferences; and, unless contraindicated, try to have these items included on his or her dietary tray. Ask the patient if the food is the right temperature. These seem like small acts, but they go a long way in maintaining the patient's sense of independence.

Patients with visual deficits also need special assistance. Patients with decreased vision are able to independently feed themselves when they are given adequate information. Identify the food location on a meal plate as if it were a clock (e.g., meat at 9 o'clock and vegetable at 3 o'clock). Tell the patient where the beverages are located in relation to the plate. Be sure that other care providers set the meal tray and plate in the same manner. Patients with impaired vision and those with decreased motor skills are more independent during mealtimes with the use of large-handled adaptive utensils (Fig. 44-7). These are easier to grip and manipulate.

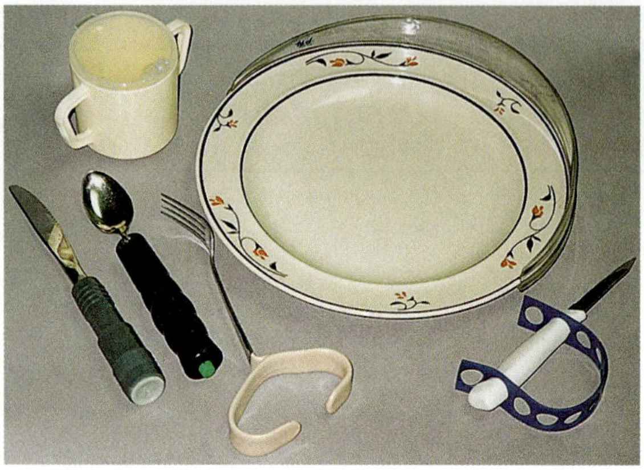

FIG. 44-7 Adaptive equipment. Clockwise from upper left: Two-handled cup with lid, plate with plate guard, utensils with splints, and utensils with enlarged handles.

Enteral Tube Feeding. Enteral nutrition (EN) provides nutrients into the GI tract. It is the preferred method of meeting nutritional needs if a patient is unable to swallow or take in nutrients orally yet has a functioning GI tract. Enteral nutrition provides physiological, safe, and economical nutritional support. Patients with enteral feedings receive formula via nasogastric, jejunal, or gastric tubes. Patients with a low risk of gastric reflux receive gastric feedings; however, if there is a risk of gastric reflux, which leads to aspiration, jejunal feeding is preferred. Box 44-11 lists indications for tube feeding. Enteral tube feedings can easily be given in the home setting by either the nurse or a family caregiver. After an enteral tube is inserted, verification of tube placement by x-ray film examination needs to occur before the patient receives the first enteral feeding (see Skill 44-2).

An enteral formula is usually one of four types. Polymeric (1 to 2 kcal/mL) includes milk-based blenderized foods prepared by hospital dietary staff or in a patient's home. The polymeric classification also includes commercially prepared whole-nutrient formulas. For this type of formula to be effective, the patient's GI tract needs to be able to absorb whole nutrients. The second type, modular formulas (3.8 to 4 kcal/mL), are single macronutrient (e.g., protein, glucose, polymers, or lipids) preparations and are not nutritionally complete. This type of formula is added to other foods to meet a patient's individual nutritional needs. The third type, elemental formulas (1 to 3 kcal/mL), contain predigested nutrients that are easier for a partially dysfunctional GI tract to absorb. Finally, specialty formulas (1 to 2 kcal/mL) are designed to meet specific nutritional needs in certain illness (e.g., liver failure, pulmonary disease, or HIV infection).

Tube feedings are typically started at full strength at slow rates (see Skill 44-3 and Box 44-12). Increase the hourly rate every 8 to 12 hours per health care provider's order if no signs of intolerance appear (high gastric residuals, nausea, cramping, vomiting, and diarrhea). Studies have demonstrated a beneficial effect of enteral feedings compared with PN. Feeding by the enteral route reduces sepsis, minimizes the hypermetabolic response to trauma, decreases hospital mortality, and maintains intestinal structure and function (Khalid et al., 2010). Enteral nutrition is successful within 24 to 48 hours after surgery or trauma to provide fluids, electrolytes, and nutritional support. Gastric ileus prevents nasogastric feedings from being given. Nasointestinal or jejunal tubes allow successful postpyloric feeding because formula is placed directly into the small intestine or jejunum or beyond the pyloric sphincter of the stomach (Bankhead et al., 2009).

A serious complication associated with enteral feedings is aspiration of formula into the tracheobronchial tree. Aspiration of enteral formula into the lungs irritates the bronchial mucosa, resulting in decreased blood supply to affected pulmonary tissue (McCance et al., 2010). This leads to necrotizing infection,

BOX 44-11 INDICATIONS FOR ENTERAL AND PARENTERAL NUTRITION

Enteral Nutrition

Cancer
- Head and neck
- Upper GI

Critical illness/trauma

Neurological and muscular disorders
- Brain neoplasm
- Cerebrovascular accident
- Dementia
- Myopathy
- Parkinson's disease

Gastrointestinal disorders
- Enterocutaneous fistula
- Inflammatory bowel disease
- Mild pancreatitis

Respiratory failure with prolonged intubation

Inadequate oral intake
- Anorexia nervosa
- Difficulty chewing, swallowing
- Severe depression

Parenteral Nutrition

Nonfunctional gastrointestinal tract
- Massive small bowel resection/GI surgery/massive GI bleed
- Paralytic ileus
- Intestinal obstruction
- Trauma to abdomen, head, or neck
- Severe malabsorption
- Intolerance to enteral feeding (established by trial)
- Chemotherapy, radiation therapy, bone marrow transplantation

Extended bowel rest
- Enterocutaneous fistula
- Inflammatory bowel disease exacerbation
- Severe diarrhea
- Moderate-to-severe pancreatitis

Preoperative total parenteral nutrition
- Preoperative bowel rest
- Treatment for co-morbid severe malnutrition in patients with nonfunctional GI tracts
- Severely catabolic patients when GI tract nonusable for more than 4 to 5 days

GI, Gastrointestinal.

pneumonia, and potential abscess formation. The high glucose content of a feeding serves as a bacterial medium for growth, promoting infection. Acute respiratory distress syndrome (ARDS) is also an outcome frequently associated with pulmonary aspiration. Some of the common conditions that increase the risk of aspiration include coughing, gastroesophageal reflux disease (GERD), nasotracheal suctioning, an artificial airway, decreased level of consciousness, and lying flat. Prokinetic medications such as metoclopramide, erythromycin, or cisapride promote gastric emptying and decrease the risk of aspiration (Bourgault et al., 2007; Metheny, 2006). Keep the head of the bed elevated a minimum of 30 degrees, preferably 45 degrees, unless medically contraindicated (Bankhead et al., 2009). Measure gastric residual volumes (GRVs) every 4 to 6 hours in patients receiving continuous feedings and immediately before the feeding in patients receiving

BOX 44-12 ADVANCING THE RATE OF TUBE FEEDING

Protocols for advancing tube feedings are commonly institution specific. Most of these protocols are untested for validity. There does not appear to be a benefit to slow initiation of enteral nutrition over days. Most patients are able to tolerate feeding 24 to 48 hours after initiation. Do not dilute formulas with water; this increases the risk of bacterial contamination (Bankhead et al., 2009).

Intermittent

1. Start formula at full strength for isotonic formulas (300 to 400 mOsm) or at ordered concentration.
2. Infuse bolus of formula over at least 20 to 30 minutes via syringe or feeding container.
3. Begin feedings with a volume of 2.5-5 mL/kg 5 to 8 times per day. Increase by 60-120 mL per feeding every 8-12 hours to achieve needed volume and calories in four to six feedings (Bankhead et al., 2009).

Continuous

1. Start formula at full strength for isotonic formulas (300 to 400 mOsm) or at ordered concentration.
2. Begin infusion rate at designated rate typically at 10 to 40 mL/hr (Bankhead et al., 2009).
3. Advance rate slowly (e.g., 10 to 20 mL/hr every 8 to 12 hours) to target rate if tolerated (tolerance indicated by absence of nausea and diarrhea and low gastric residuals) (Bankhead et al., 2009).

intermittent feedings (Metheny et al., 2006). Delayed gastric emptying is a concern if 250 mL or more remains in a patient's stomach on two consecutive assessments (1 hour apart) or if a single GRV measurement exceeds 500 mL (Bankhead et al., 2009). There is a lack of consensus for recommendations for stopping feedings; decisions to stop feedings must include assessment of patient's condition (Metheny et al., 2008). The North American Summit on Aspiration in the Critically Ill Patient recommends the following: (1) stop feedings immediately if aspiration occurs; (2) withhold feedings and reassess patient tolerance to feedings if GRV is over 500 mL; (3) routinely evaluate the patient for aspiration; and (4) use nursing measures to reduce the risk of aspiration if GRV is between 250 and 500 mL (Bankhead et al., 2009).

Enteral Access Tubes. When patients are unable to ingest food but are still able to digest and absorb nutrients, enteral tube feeding is indicated. Feeding tubes are inserted through the nose (nasogastric or nasointestinal), surgically (gastrostomy or jejunostomy), or endoscopically (percutaneous endoscopic gastrostomy or jejunostomy [PEG or PEJ]). If EN therapy is for less than 4 weeks, total, nasogastric, or nasojejunal feeding tubes may be used. Surgical or endoscopically placed tubes are preferred for long-term feeding (more than 4 weeks) to reduce the discomfort of a nasal tube and provide a more secure, reliable access (Rolandelli et al., 2005). Some patients such as those with gastroparesis (decreased or absent innervation to the stomach that results in delayed gastric emptying) or esophageal reflux or with a history of aspiration pneumonia require placement of tubes beyond the stomach into the intestine (Cirgin Ellett, 2006; Metheny et al., 2007).

Most health care settings use small-bore feeding tubes because they create less discomfort for a patient (Fig. 44-8). For the adult most of these tubes are 8- to 12-Fr and 36 to 44 inches (90 to 110 cm) long. A stylet is often used during insertion of a small-bore tube to stiffen it. The stylet is removed when the correct position

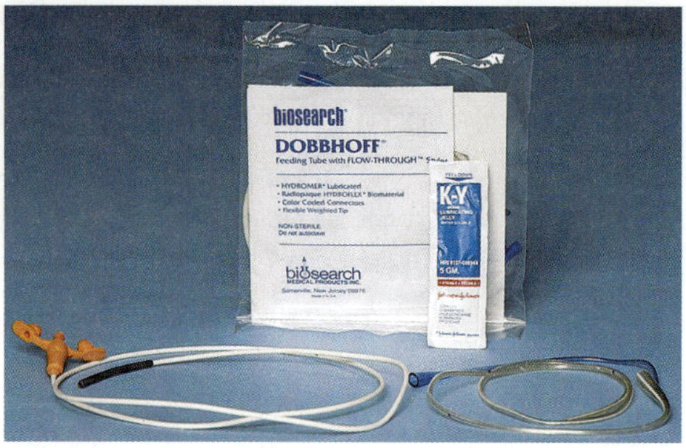

FIG. 44-8 Enteral tubes, small-bore.

of the feeding tube is confirmed. Skill 44-3 describes the procedure for initiating beginning nasogastric, gastrostomy, and jejunostomy enteral feedings.

Historically nurses verified feeding tube placement by injecting air through the tube while auscultating the stomach for a gurgling or bubbling sound or asking the patient to speak. Auscultation has repeatedly been shown to be ineffective in detecting tubes accidentally placed in the lung (Bourgault et al., 2007). Some patients are able to speak despite placement of feeding tubes in the lung (Rolandelli et al., 2005). Furthermore, auscultation is not effective in distinguishing between gastric and intestinal placement for feeding tubes (Rauen et al., 2008). The measurement of pH of secretions withdrawn from the feeding tube helps to differentiate the location of the tube (Box 44-13). At present the most reliable

BOX 44-13 PROCEDURAL GUIDELINES

Obtaining Gastrointestinal Aspirate for pH Measurement, Large-Bore, and Small-Bore Feeding Tubes: Intermittent and Continuous Feeding

Delegation Considerations

The skill of measuring pH in gastrointestinal (GI) aspirate is not delegated to nursing assistive personnel.

Equipment

Cone-tipped or Asepto syringe, pH test paper (scale of 1.0 to 11.0 or greater), paper towel, small medication cup, clean gloves

1. Perform measures to verify placement of tube:
   a. For intermittently fed patients, test placement immediately before feeding (usually a period of at least 4 hours has elapsed since previous feeding). More frequent checking has been associated with increased clogging of small-bore tubes. To avoid clogging, flush tube with 30 mL water after aspirating for the gastric residual volume (Bourgault et al., 2007).
   b. For continuously tube-fed patients, test placement every 4 to 6 hours (Metheny, 2006). If patient is tolerating the feedings without incident and other indicators of correct location are present (i.e., the mark on the tube at the exit site has remained in its original position, and the most recent x-ray films confirm correct position of tube), it is reasonable to continue feedings. If risk of tube displacement is high, and the tube has moved, consider the need for an x-ray film to verify placement (Bankhead et al., 2009). Plan pH testing at times when feeding may be withheld (e.g., during diagnostic testing or chest physiotherapy or to avoid medication interaction).
   c. Wait at least 1 hour after medication administration by tube or mouth.
2. Perform hand hygiene and apply clean gloves.
3. Draw up 30 mL of air into syringe and attach to end of feeding tube. Flush tube with 30 mL of air before attempting to aspirate fluid. It is likely to be more difficult to aspirate fluid from the small intestine than from the stomach. Repositioning patient from side to side is helpful. More than one bolus of air through the tube is necessary in some cases. Burst of air aids in aspirating fluid more easily.
4. Draw back on syringe and obtain 5 to 10 mL of gastric aspirate. Observe appearance of aspirate (see illustration). Gently mix aspirate in syringe. Expel a few drops into a clean medicine cup. Dip the pH strip into the fluid or apply a few drops of the fluid to the strip (see illustration). Compare the color of the strip with the color on the chart provided by the manufacturer (Metheny, 2006).
   a. Gastric fluid from patient who has fasted for at least 4 hours usually has pH range of 1 to 4.
   b. Fluid from nasointestinal tube of fasting patient usually has pH greater than or equal to 6.0 (Bankhead et al., 2009).
   c. Patient with continuous tube feeding often has pH of 5.0 or higher.
   d. pH of pleural fluid from tracheobronchial tree is generally greater than 6.0.
5. Remove gloves and discard supplies. Perform hand hygiene.

CLINICAL DECISION: If after repeated attempts it is not possible to aspirate fluid from a tube that was originally established by x-ray film examination to be in desired position and (a) there are no risk factors for tube dislocation, (b) there is no change in external marked tube length, and (c) patient is not experiencing difficulty, assume that tube is correctly placed (Roberts et al., 2007).

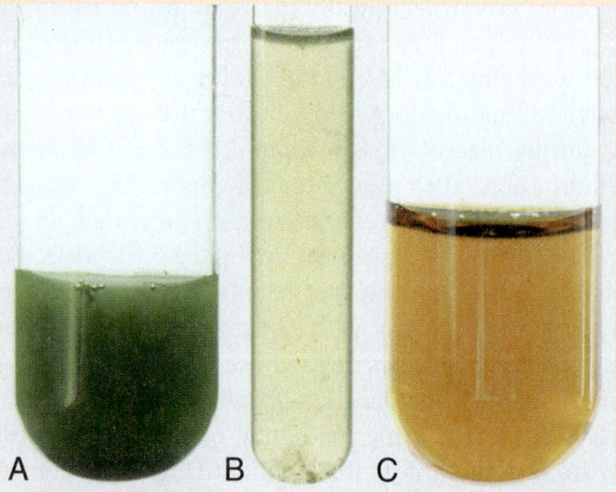

STEP 4a Gastrointestinal contents. **A,** Stomach. **B,** Stomach. **C,** Intestinal. (Courtesy Dr. Norma Metheny, Professor, St Louis University School of Nursing.)

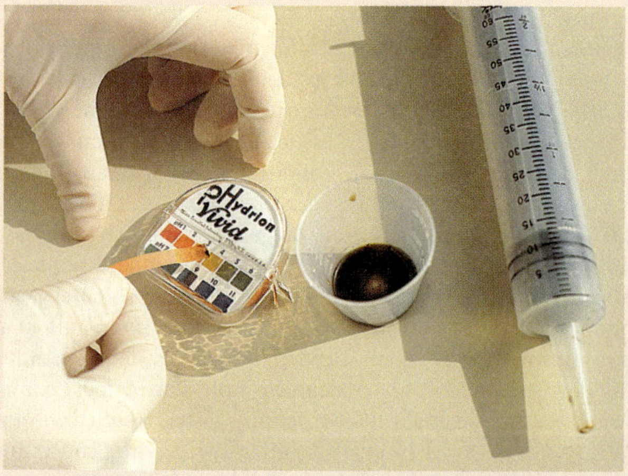

STEP 4b Comparing pH strip with color chart.

method for verification of placement of small-bore feeding tubes is x-ray film examination (Box 44-14).

The addition of blue food coloring to enteral formula to assist with the detection of formula aspirated into the lung, presumably by staining the tracheobronchial secretions, is no longer used. The FDA issued a public health advisory reporting an association between use of Blue No. 1 food coloring and patient deaths (McClave et al., 2009).

BOX 44-14 EVIDENCE-BASED PRACTICE

Accuracy in Determining Placement of Feeding Tubes

PICO Question: In adult patients, what method determines stomach placement of enteral feeding tubes for preventing aspiration?

Evidence Summary

Two of the most frequent complications associated with tube feedings are pulmonary aspiration, potentially leading to pneumonia, and accidental placement of a nasoenteric feeding tube into the lung. Patients at highest risk for aspiration have decreased level of consciousness, confusion, uncooperativeness, agitation, presence of an endotracheal tube and absent or poor gag reflex (Metheny, 2006). Gastric residual volume has not been found to be consistently related to aspiration (Bankhead et al., 2009). A traditional bedside method used to assess for pulmonary aspiration of enteral feeding into the respiratory tract was the glucose method. The premise of the glucose method was that normal tracheal secretions contain minimal levels of glucose. Therefore, if glucose-rich enteral formula is aspirated into the airway, glucose levels of tracheal secretions increase. However, researchers have shown that the glucose levels of tracheal secretions vary widely and this method is not sufficiently sensitive or specific to be useful to detect aspiration (Metheny et al., 2007). Researchers are currently trying to develop new bedside methods for assessing for pulmonary aspiration such as using electromagnetic tracking devices and assessing for the presence of pepsin, a substance produced in the stomach in tracheal secretions (Bankhead et al., 2009).

Traditionally nurses have used the auscultatory method of assessing placement. This method has been shown to be unreliable. Auscultation does not detect when a feeding tube has inadvertently been placed into the respiratory tract and does not distinguish between placement in the stomach versus the intestine. The most accurate method for checking feeding tube placement is x-ray film examination (Bankhead et al., 2009; Kenny and Goodman, 2010). The most effective nonradiological methods include aspirating fluid from the feeding tube, measuring its pH, and describing its appearance (Bourgault et al., 2007; Bankhead et al., 2009).

Application to Nursing Practice

- X-ray film verification of feeding tube placement is the most reliable method available to confirm correct tube location. It is required in most acute care facilities after insertion of a small-bore tube.
- Verify the placement of the feeding tube every 4 to 6 hours by aspirating gastric contents, observing its appearance, and testing pH. A properly obtained pH of 0 to 4.0 is a good indication of gastric placement. A pH of 6.0 or higher likely indicates placement in the lung, intestine, or even the stomach when gastric pH is unusually high. Intestinal fluid is usually bile stained (dark golden yellow). Gastric fluid is usually grassy green, off-white to tan, or clear and colorless (Bankhead et al., 2009).
- Do not use the auscultatory method to determine tube location.
- Do not use the glucose detection method to determine if aspiration has occurred.
- Check gastric residual volumes every 4 hours in patients at high risk for aspiration (Bankhead et al., 2009).

Table 44-7 outlines major complications of EN. Of special note, patients who are severely malnourished are at risk for electrolyte disturbances from re-feeding syndrome during EN or PN therapy. In re-feeding syndrome potassium, magnesium, and phosphate move intracellularly, resulting in low serum (extracellular) levels and edema. These changes cause cardiac dysrhythmias, heart failure, respiratory distress, convulsions, coma, or death.

Parenteral Nutrition. **Parenteral nutrition (PN)** is a form of specialized nutrition support in which nutrients are provided intravenously. A basic PN formula is a combination of crystalline amino acids, hypertonic dextrose, electrolytes, vitamins, and trace elements. TPN, administered through a central line, is a 2-in-1 formula in which fat emulsions are administered separately from the protein and dextrose solution (Krzywda and Meyer, 2010). Safe administration depends on appropriate assessment of nutrition needs, meticulous management of the central venous catheter (CVC), and careful monitoring to prevent or treat metabolic complications. PN is administered in a variety of settings, including a patient's home. Regardless of the setting, adhere to principles of asepsis and infusion management to ensure safe nutrition support.

Patients who are unable to digest or absorb EN benefit from PN. Patients in highly stressed physiological states such as sepsis, head injury, or burns are candidates for PN therapy (see Box 44-11).

Clinical and laboratory monitoring by a multidisciplinary team is required throughout PN therapy. The need for continued PN is consistently reevaluated. The goal to move toward use of the GI tract is constant (McClave et al., 2009). Disuse of the GI tract has been associated with villus atrophy and generalized cell shrinkage. As a result of disuse of the GI tract, bacteria may move from the unused gut into the bloodstream, resulting in gram-negative septicemia.

Intravenous fat emulsions are sometimes added to PN to provide supplemental kilocalories, prevent essential fatty acid deficiencies, and help control hyperglycemia during periods of stress (Phillips, 2010). Administer these emulsions through a separate peripheral line, through the central line by using Y-connector tubing (see Chapter 41), or as an admixture to the PN solution. The addition of fat emulsion to a PN solution is called a *3-in-1 admixture* or *total nutrient admixture*. The patient receives it over a 24-hour period. Do not use the admixture if you observe oil droplets or an oily or creamy layer on the surface of the admixture. This observation indicates that the emulsion has broken into large lipid droplets that cause fat emboli if administered. IV fat emulsions are white and opaque. Take care to avoid confusing enteral formula with parenteral lipids.

Initiating Parenteral Nutrition. Patients with short-term nutritional needs often receive IV solutions of less than 10% dextrose via a peripheral vein in combination with amino acids and lipids. Peripheral solutions are not as calorically dense as TPN solutions and therefore are usually temporary. PN with greater than 10% dextrose requires a CVC that a health care provider places into a high-flow central vein such as the superior vena cava under sterile conditions (see Chapter 41). If you are using a CVC that has multiple lumens, use a port that is exclusively dedicated for the TPN. Label the port for TPN and do not infuse other solutions or medications through it (Krzywda and Meyer, 2010). Nurses with special training insert peripherally inserted central catheters (PICCs) that are started in a vein of the arm and threaded into the subclavian or superior vena cava vein.

TABLE 44-7 Enteral Tube Feeding Complications

PROBLEM	POSSIBLE CAUSE	INTERVENTION*
Pulmonary aspiration	Regurgitation of formula	Verify tube placement. Place patient in high Fowler's position or elevate head of bed a minimum of 30 (preferably 45) degrees during feedings and for 2 hours afterward.
	Feeding tube displaced	Reposition tube and verify tube placement.
	Deficient gag reflex	Reassess for return of normal gag reflex; until then place patient on aspiration precautions and in semi-Fowler's position.
	Delayed gastric emptying	See delayed gastric emptying that follows.
Diarrhea	Hyperosmolar formula or medications	Deliver formula continuously, lower rate, dilute, or change to isotonic enteral nutrition.
	Antibiotic therapy	Antibiotics destroy normal intestinal flora; consult with health care provider to consider changing medication; treat symptoms with antidiarrheal agents; culture stool for *Clostridium difficile*.
	Bacterial contamination	Do not hang formula longer than 4-8 hours in bag, wash bag out well when refilling, change tube feeding bags and tubing q24h and use aseptic practices. Check expiration dates.
	Malabsorption	Check for pancreatic insufficiency; use low-fat, lactose-free formula and continuous feedings.
Constipation	Lack of fiber	Consult with a dietitian to select a formula containing fiber.
	Lack of free water	Add water as needed as flushes.*
	Inactivity	Monitor patient's ability to ambulate; collaborate with health care provider and/or physical therapist for activity order.
Tube occlusion	Pulverized medications given per tube	Irrigate with 30 mL water before and after each medication per tube.* Use liquid medications when available. Completely dissolve crushed medications in liquid if liquid medication is not available.
	Sedimentation of formula	Shake cans well before administering (read label).
	Reaction of incompatible medications or formula	Read pharmacological information on compatibility of drugs and formula.
Tube displacement	Coughing, vomiting	Replace tube and confirm placement before restarting tube feeding.
	Not taped securely	With placement verification check that tape is secure (nasoenteric).
Abdominal cramping, nausea/vomiting	High osmolality of formula	Suggest an isotonic formula or dilution of current formula to health care provider.
	Rapid increase in rate/volume	Lower rate of delivery to increase tolerance. Maintain head of bed at least 30 degrees.
	Lactose intolerance	Suggest use of lactose-free formula.
	Intestinal obstruction	Stop feeding with GI obstruction.
	High-fat formula used	Use greater proportion of carbohydrate.
	Cold formula used	Warm formula to room temperature.
Delayed gastric emptying	Diabetic gastroparesis	Consult with health care provider regarding prokinetic medication for increasing gastric motility.
	Serious illnesses	Consult health care provider regarding advancing tube to intestinal placement.
	Inactivity	Monitor medications and pathological conditions that affect GI motility.
Serum electrolyte imbalance	Excess GI losses Dehydration Presence of disease states such as cirrhosis, renal insufficiency, heart failure, or diabetes mellitus	Monitor serum electrolyte levels daily. Provide free water per registered dietitian recommendation.
Fluid overload	Refeeding syndrome in malnutrition	Restrict fluids if necessary and use either a specialized formula or a diluted enteral formula at first.
	Excess free water or diluted (hypotonic) formula	Monitor levels of serum proteins and electrolytes. Use a more concentrated formula with fluid volume excess without risk of refeeding syndrome.
Hyperosmolar dehydration	Hypertonic formula with insufficient free water	Slow rate of delivery, dilute, or change to isotonic formula.

*Check first for fluid-restricted conditions that affect volume of water that can be safely given.
GI, Gastrointestinal.

TABLE 44-8 **Metabolic Complications of Parenteral Nutrition**

PROBLEM	SIGNS/SYMPTOMS	INTERVENTION
Electrolyte imbalance	See Chapter 41 for signs of deficiency/toxicity	Check TPN for supplemental electrolyte levels. Notify health care provider of imbalances. Maintain steady rate of infusion. Monitor intake and output.
Hypercapnia	Increased oxygen consumption, CO_2, respiratory quotient (>1), and minute ventilation	Ventilator-dependent patients are at risk; provide 30% to 60% of energy requirements per health care provider's order.
Hypoglycemia	Diaphoresis, shakiness, confusion, loss of consciousness	To prevent hypoglycemia, do not abruptly discontinue TPN but taper rate down to within 10% of infusion rate 1 to 2 hours before stopping. If you suspect hypoglycemia, test blood glucose and administer IV bolus of 50% dextrose or glucagon per order or protocol if necessary.
Hyperglycemia	Thirst, headache, lethargy, increased urination	Monitor blood glucose level every 6 hours. Initiate TPN slowly and taper up to maximal infusion rate to prevent hyperglycemia. Additional insulin may be required during therapy if problem persists or patient has diabetes mellitus.
Hyperglycemic hyperosmolar nonketotic coma (HHNKC) or hyperosmolar hyperglycemic nonketotic syndrome (HHNS)	Hyperglycemia (>500 mg/dl), glycosuria, serum osmolarity >350 mOsm/L, confusion, azotemia, headache, severe signs of dehydration (see Chapter 41), hypernatremia, metabolic acidosis, convulsions, coma	Monitor blood glucose, BUN, serum osmolarity, glucose in urine, and fluid losses; administer insulin as ordered; replace fluids as ordered; maintain constant infusion rate; and provide 30% of daily energy needs as fat. Patients at risk are those receiving steroids; older adults diagnosed with diabetes, who have impaired renal or pancreatic function or increased metabolism, or who are septic.

BUN, Blood urea nitrogen; *IV,* intravenous; *TPN,* total parenteral nutrition.

After catheter placement, wait to flush and use the catheter until the position is radiographically confirmed. The health care provider secures the CVC with a securement device and covers the site with a sterile dressing. A PICC is usually stabilized with sterile strips of tape and a sterile dressing. A chest x-ray film examination verifies catheter tip placement for a CVC or PICC before starting a PN infusion (DeChicco et al., 2007).

Before beginning any PN infusion, verify the health care provider's order and inspect the solution for particulate matter or a break in the fat emulsion. Always use an infusion pump to deliver a constant rate. The initial rate delivers no more than 50% of estimated needs for the first 24 to 48 hours. The rate is gradually increased until a patient's complete nutrition needs are supplied (National Guideline Clearinghouse, 2008). Patients receiving PN at home frequently administer the entire daily solution over 12 hours at night. This allows the patient to disconnect from the infusion each morning, flush the central line, and have independent mobility during the day. Home PN therapy often interferes with patients' normal activities, causing a poorer quality of life (Siepler, 2007).

Preventing Complications. Complications of PN include catheter-related problems and metabolic alterations (Table 44-8). Pneumothorax results from a puncture insult to the pulmonary system and involves the accumulation of air in the pleural cavity with subsequent collapse of the lung and impaired breathing. Pneumothorax is usually accompanied by symptoms of sudden sharp chest pain, dyspnea, and coughing. In relation to PN, pneumothorax most often occurs during CVC placement. Monitor a patient with a CVC for the first 24 hours for signs and symptoms of pulmonary distress.

An air embolus possibly occurs during insertion of the catheter or when changing the tubing or cap. Turn the patient into a left lateral decubitus position, and have the patient perform a Valsalva maneuver (holding the breath and "bearing down") during catheter insertion to help prevent air embolus. The increased venous pressure created by the maneuver prevents air from entering the bloodstream. Maintaining integrity of the closed IV system also helps prevent air embolus.

Catheter occlusion is present when there is sluggish or no flow through the catheter. Temporarily stop the infusion and flush with saline or heparin per protocol or orders. If this is unsuccessful, attempt to aspirate a clot. If still unsuccessful, follow institution protocol for use of a thrombolytic agent (e.g., urokinase).

Suspect catheter sepsis if a patient develops fever, chills, or glucose intolerance and has a positive blood culture. To prevent infection, change the TPN infusion tubing every 24 hours. Do not hang a single container of PN for more than 24 hours or lipids more than 12 hours. Change the administration system every 72 hours when infusing a 2-in-1 solution and every 24 hours for a 3-in-1 solution (Phillips, 2010). During CVC dressing changes, always use a sterile mask and gloves and assess insertion sites for signs and symptoms of infection (see Chapter 41). Change the CVC dressing per institution policy and anytime it becomes wet or contaminated. Use either alcohol or an alcoholic solution of chlorhexidine gluconate to clean the injection port or catheter hub 15 seconds before and after each time it is used (National Guideline Clearinghouse, 2008). Use a 1.2-micron filter for 3-in-1 formulas and an inline 0.22-micron filter for PN solutions that do not include IV fat emulsions (Task Force for the Revision of Safe Practices for Parenteral Nutrition, 2004).

PN solutions contain most of the major electrolytes, vitamins, and minerals. Patients also need supplemental vitamin K as ordered throughout therapy. Vitamin K is synthesized by microflora found in the jejunum and ileum with normal use of the GI tract; however, because PN circumvents GI use, patients need to receive exogenous vitamin K.

Electrolyte and mineral imbalances often occur. Administration of concentrated glucose is accompanied by increases in endogenous insulin production, which causes cations (potassium, magnesium, and phosphorus) to move intracellularly. Monitor blood glucose levels every 6 hours to assess for hyperglycemia and administer supplemental insulin as needed (Phillips, 2010) (Skill 44-4 on pp. 1035-1039).

Too-rapid administration of hypertonic dextrose can result in an osmotic diuresis and dehydration (see Chapter 41). If an infusion falls behind schedule, do not increase the rate in an attempt to catch up. Sudden discontinuation of a solution can cause hypoglycemia. Usually 10% dextrose is infused when PN solution is suddenly discontinued. Patients with diabetes are more at risk.

The goal is to move patients from PN to EN and/or oral feeding. Once patients are meeting one third to one half of their kilocalorie needs per day, PN is usually decreased to half the original volume. EN feedings are then increased to meet needs. Patients who make the transition from PN to oral feedings typically have early satiety and decreased appetite. PN is gradually decreased in response to increased oral intake. If oral intake is inadequate, small frequent meals are helpful. Calorie/protein counts are recommended when patients begin taking soft foods. When 75% of needs are being met by enteral feedings or reliable dietary intake, PN therapy is usually discontinued. PN may also be discontinued if complications occur or the health care provider determines that it is not benefiting the patient (Krzywda and Meyer, 2010).

Restorative and Continuing Care. Patients discharged from a hospital with diet prescriptions often need dietary education to plan meals that meet specific therapeutic requirements. Restorative care includes both immediate postsurgical care and routine medical care and therefore includes patients in the hospital and at home. The following sections address nutritional interventions for some common disease states.

Medical Nutrition Therapy. Optimal nutrition is important in health and illness, but the specific dietary intake pattern that results in optimal nutrition is modified for patients with particular diseases. Medical nutrition therapy (MNT) is the use of specific nutritional therapies to treat an illness, injury, or condition. MNT is necessary to help the body metabolize certain nutrients, correct nutritional deficiencies related to the disease, and eliminate foods that may exacerbate disease symptoms. It is most effective using a team approach that promotes collaboration between the health care team and an RD (American Dietetic Association, 2010b).

Gastrointestinal Diseases. Peptic ulcers are controlled with regular meals and medications such as histamine receptor antagonists that block secretion of HCl or proton pump inhibitors. Marshall and Warren first identified *Helicobacter pylori* in 1984. *H. pylori* is a bacterium that causes up to 85% of peptic ulcers and is confirmed by laboratory tests or a biopsy during endoscopy (Nix, 2009). It is treated with antibiotics that control the bacterial infection. Stress and overproduction of gastric HCl also irritate a preexisting ulcer. Encourage patients to avoid foods that increase stomach acidity and pain such as caffeine, decaffeinated coffee, frequent milk intake, citric acid juices, and certain seasonings (hot chili peppers, chili powder, black pepper). Discourage smoking, alcohol, aspirin, and nonsteroidal antiinflammatory drugs (NSAIDs). Teach patients to eat a well-balanced, healthy diet; avoid eating large meals; and eat three regular meals (or several small meals) without snacks, especially at bedtime (Nix, 2009). Family members of the patient with a *H. pylori* infection also need to be tested and treated if indicated.

Inflammatory bowel disease includes Crohn's disease and idiopathic ulcerative colitis. Treatment of acute inflammatory bowel disease includes elemental diets (formula with the nutrients in their simplest form ready for absorption) or PN when symptoms such as diarrhea and weight loss are prevalent. In the chronic stage of the disease a regular highly-nourishing diet is appropriate. Vitamins and iron supplements are often required to correct or prevent anemia. Patients manage irritable bowel syndrome by increasing fiber, reducing fat, avoiding large meals, and avoiding lactose or sorbitol-containing foods for susceptible individuals.

The treatment of malabsorption syndromes such as celiac disease includes a gluten-free diet. Gluten is present in wheat, rye, barley, and oats. Short-bowel syndrome results from extensive resection of bowel, after which patients suffer from malabsorption caused by lack of intestinal surface area. These patients require lifetime feeding with either elemental enteral formulas or PN.

Diverticulitis is a condition that results from an inflammation of diverticula, which are abnormal but common pouchlike herniations that occur in the bowel lining. This condition is nutritionally treated with a moderate- or low-residue diet until the infection subsides. Afterward a high-fiber diet is generally prescribed for chronic diverticula problems.

Diabetes Mellitus. Type 1 diabetes mellitus (DM) requires both insulin and dietary restrictions for optimal control, with treatment beginning at diagnosis (ADA, 2008). By contrast, patients often control type 2 DM initially with exercise and diet therapy. If these measures prove ineffective, it is common to add oral medications. Insulin injections often follow if type 2 diabetes worsens or fails to respond to these initial interventions.

Individualize the diet according to a patient's age, build, weight, and activity level. Maintaining a prescribed carbohydrate intake is the key in diabetes management. A diet that includes carbohydrates from fruits, vegetables, whole grains, legumes, and low-fat milk is recommended (American Dietetic Association, 2010b). Monitoring carbohydrate consumption is a key strategy in achieving glycemic control (ADA, 2008). Limit saturated fat to less than 7% of the total calories and cholesterol intake to less than 200 mg/day. Also recommended are a variety of foods containing fiber. Patients are able to substitute sucrose-containing foods for carbohydrates but need to make sure to avoid excess energy intake. Sugar alcohols and non-nutritive sweeteners are able to be eaten as long as the recommended daily intake levels are followed (ADA, 2008). Patients with diabetes and normal renal function should continue to consume usual amounts of protein (15% to 20% of energy) (ADA, 2008).

The goal of MNT treatment is to have glycemic levels that are normal or as close to normal as safely possible; lipid and lipoprotein profiles that decrease the risk of microvascular (e.g., renal and eye disease), cardiovascular, neurological, and peripheral vascular complications; and blood pressure in the normal or near-normal range (ADA, 2008). Be aware of signs and symptoms of hypoglycemia and hyperglycemia.

Cardiovascular Diseases. The American Heart Association (AHA) dietary guidelines (AHA, 2010) are intended to reduce risk factors for the development of hypertension and coronary artery disease. Diet therapy for reducing the risk of cardiovascular disease includes balancing calorie intake with exercise to maintain a healthy body weight; eating a diet high in fruits, vegetables, and whole-grain high-fiber foods; eating fish at least 2 times per week; and limiting food and beverages that are high in added sugar and salt. The AHA guidelines also recommend limiting saturated fat to less than 7%, trans-fat to less than 1%, and cholesterol to less than 300 mg/day. To accomplish this goal, patients choose lean meats and vegetables, use fat-free dairy products, and limit intake of fats and sodium (Nix, 2009).

Cancer and Cancer Treatment. Malignant cells compete with normal cells for nutrients, increasing a patient's metabolic needs. Most cancer treatments cause nutritional problems. Patients with cancer often experience anorexia, nausea, vomiting, and taste distortions. The goal of nutrition therapy is to meet the increased metabolic needs of a patient (Nix, 2009). Malnutrition in cancer is associated with increased morbidity and mortality. Enhanced nutritional status often improves a patient's quality of life.

Radiation therapy destroys rapidly dividing malignant cells; however, other normal rapidly dividing cells such as the epithelial lining of the GI tract are often affected. Radiation therapy causes anorexia, stomatitis, severe diarrhea, strictures of the intestine, and pain. Radiation treatment of the head and neck region causes taste and smell disturbances, decreased salivation, and dysphagia. Nutrition management of a patient with cancer focuses on maximizing intake of nutrients and fluids. Individualize diet choices to a patient's needs, symptoms, and situation (Nix, 2009). Use creative approaches to manage alterations in taste and smell. For example, patients with altered taste often prefer chilled foods or foods that are spicy. Encourage patients to eat small frequent meals and snacks that are nutritious and easy to digest.

Human Immunodeficiency Virus/Acquired Immunodeficiency Syndrome. Patients with HIV/AIDS typically experience body wasting and severe weight loss. The wasting is related to anorexia, stomatitis, oral thrush infection, nausea, or recurrent vomiting, all resulting in inadequate intake. Factors associated with weight loss and malnutrition include severe diarrhea, GI malabsorption, and altered metabolism of nutrients. Systemic infection results in hypermetabolism from cytokine elevation. Often the medications taken to treat HIV infection cause side effects that alter nutritional status.

Restorative care of malnutrition resulting from AIDS focuses on maximizing kilocalories and nutrients. Diagnose and address each cause of nutritional depletion in the care plan. Individually tailored nutrition support progresses in stages from oral, to enteral, and finally to parenteral. Good hand hygiene and food safety are essential because of a patient's reduced resistance to infection. For example, minimization of exposure to *Cryptosporidium* in drinking water, lakes, or swimming pools is important. Small, frequent, nutrient-dense meals that limit fatty and overly sweet foods are easier to tolerate. Patients benefit from eating cold foods and drier or saltier foods with fluid in between (Nix, 2009).

EVALUATION

Through the Patient's Eyes. Patients expect competent and accurate care. If ongoing nutrition therapies do not result in successful outcomes, patients expect nurses to recognize this and alter the plan of care accordingly. Expectations and health care values held by nurses frequently differ from those held by patients. Successful interventions and outcomes require nurses to know what patients expect in addition to nursing knowledge and skill. Work closely with patients to define their expectations, and talk with them about their concerns if their expectations are not realistic. Consider the limits of their conditions and treatment, their dietary preferences, and their cultural beliefs when evaluating outcomes.

Patient Outcomes. Care plans need to reflect achievable goals and outcomes. Evaluate the actual outcomes of nursing actions and compare with expected outcomes to determine if the goals are met (Fig. 44-9). Multidisciplinary collaboration remains essential in providing nutritional support. Nutrition therapy does not always produce rapid results. Ongoing comparisons need to be made with baseline measures of weight, serum albumin or prealbumin, and protein and kilocalorie intake. If you do not observe gradual weight gain or if weight loss continues, evaluate the dietary EN prescription and determine if the patient is experiencing any adverse effects from medications that are affecting his or her nutritional status. Changes in condition also indicate a need to change the nutritional plan of care. Consult multidisciplinary members of the health care team in an effort to better individualize this plan. The patient is an active participant whenever possible. In the end, a patient's ability to incorporate dietary changes into his or her lifestyle with the least amount of stress or disruption facilitates attainment of outcome measures. When expected outcomes are not met, revise the nursing interventions or expected outcomes based on the patient's needs or preferences. When outcomes are not met, ask questions such as "How has your appetite been?" "Have you noticed a change in your weight?" "How much would you like to weigh?" or "Have you changed your exercise pattern?"

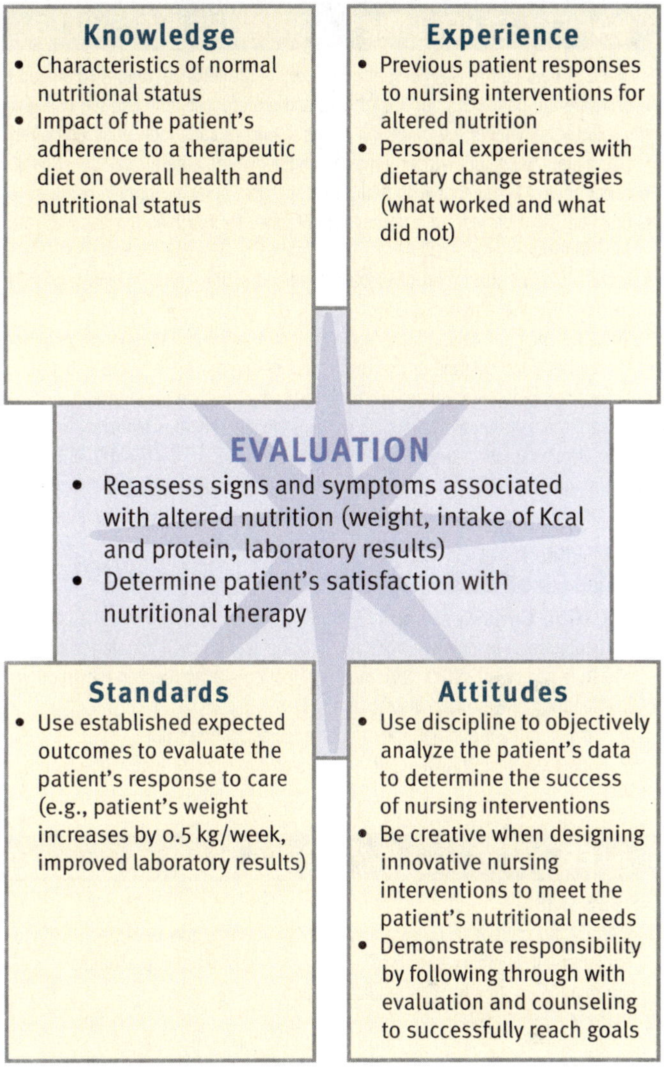
Knowledge
• Characteristics of normal nutritional status
• Impact of the patient's adherence to a therapeutic diet on overall health and nutritional status
Experience
• Previous patient responses to nursing interventions for altered nutrition
• Personal experiences with dietary change strategies (what worked and what did not)
EVALUATION
• Reassess signs and symptoms associated with altered nutrition (weight, intake of Kcal and protein, laboratory results)
• Determine patient's satisfaction with nutritional therapy
Standards
• Use established expected outcomes to evaluate the patient's response to care (e.g., patient's weight increases by 0.5 kg/week, improved laboratory results)
Attitudes
• Use discipline to objectively analyze the patient's data to determine the success of nursing interventions
• Be creative when designing innovative nursing interventions to meet the patient's nutritional needs
• Demonstrate responsibility by following through with evaluation and counseling to successfully reach goals
FIG. 44-9 Critical thinking model for nutrition evaluation.

SAFETY GUIDELINES FOR NURSING SKILLS

Ensuring patient safety is an essential role of the professional nurse. To ensure patient safety, communicate clearly with members of the health care team, assess and incorporate the patient's priorities of care and preferences, and use the best evidence when making decisions about your patient's care. When performing the skills in this chapter, remember the following points to ensure safe, individualized patient care.

- Use aseptic technique when preparing and delivering enteral feedings. Check agency policy for wearing gloves when handling feedings (Bankhead et al., 2009).
- Label enteral equipment with patient name, room number, formula name, rate, date and time of initiation, and nurse initials (Bankhead et al., 2009).
- Practice "right patient, right formula, right tube" by matching formula and rate to feeding order and verifying that an enteral tubing set connects formula to a feeding tube (Bankhead et al., 2009).
- Have a patient sit upright or elevate the head of the bed a minimum of 30 (preferably 45) degrees unless medically contraindicated for patients receiving enteral feedings (Bankhead et al., 2009).
- Trace all lines and tubing back to the patient to ensure that you have only enteral-to-enteral connections (Bankhead et al., 2009).
- Do not add food coloring or dye to EN. Use of dye has been linked to hypotension, metabolic acidosis, and death (Metheny et al., 2007).
- Refer to manufacturer guidelines to determine hang time for enteral feedings. Maximum hang time for formula is 8 hours in an open system and 24 to 48 hours in a closed, ready-to-hang system (if it remains closed). There is increased risk of bacterial growth in feedings that exceed the recommended hang time.
- Auscultation is not a reliable method for verification of nasogastric or nasointestinal tube placement because a tube inadvertently placed in the lungs, pharynx, or esophagus also transmits a sound similar to that of air entering the stomach (Metheny et al., 2007; Serna and McCarthy, 2006).
- Continuous enteral feedings and PN are always administered using an infusion pump.

SKILL 44-1 ASPIRATION PRECAUTIONS

View Video!

Delegation Considerations

The skill of assessing a patient's risk for aspiration cannot be delegated to nursing assistive personnel (NAP). NAP may feed patients after receiving instructions in aspiration precautions. Instruct NAP to:

- Position patient appropriately to decrease aspiration risk.
- Report any onset of coughing, gagging, or pocketing of food in the mouth.

Equipment

- Chair or electric bed (to allow patient to sit upright)
- Thickening agents as needed (rice, cereal, yogurt, gelatin, commercial thickening agent)
- Tongue blade
- Oral hygiene supplies (see Chapter 39)
- Penlight

STEP	RATIONALE
ASSESSMENT	
1 Identify the patient using two identifiers (i.e., name and birth date or name and account number) according to facility policy. Compare identifiers with information on the patient's medical record.	Ensures correct patient. Complies with a recommended National Patient Safety Goal (TJC, 2011).
2 Perform nutrition screening.	Patients at risk for aspiration from dysphagia often alter their eating patterns or choose foods that do not provide adequate nutrition (White et al., 2008).
3 Perform dysphagia screening. Note symptoms such as cough, pharyngeal pooling, change in voice after swallowing. Use a validated screening tool (when available).	Patients at risk for dysphagia include those who have neurological or neuromuscular diseases and those who have had trauma to or surgical procedures of the oral cavity or throat.
4 Observe patient during mealtime for signs of dysphagia and allow him or her to attempt to feed self. Observe patient eat various consistencies of foods and liquids. Note at end of meal if patient becomes tired.	Helps detect abnormal eating patterns such as frequent clearing of throat or prolonged eating time. Fatigue increases risk of aspiration.
5 Ask patient and or family caregiver about any difficulties with chewing or swallowing various textures of food.	Certain types of food are more easily aspirated than others.
PLANNING	
1 Report signs and symptoms of dysphagia to the health care provider.	Signs or symptoms associated with aspiration indicate the need for further evaluation of swallowing by a radiologist or speech language pathologist such as a fluoroscopic swallow study (Ashley et al., 2006).
2 Place information on patient's medical record indicating that dysphagia is present.	Alerts the health care team to the patient's problem to help the team develop and implement an individualized plan of care (Nowlin, 2006).
3 Explain to patient why you are observing him or her while he or she eats.	Increases patient cooperation.
4 Provide a 30-minute rest period before meals.	Swallowing difficulty is less likely in a well-rested patient (Palmer and Metheny, 2008).

STEP	RATIONALE
IMPLEMENTATION	
1 Perform hand hygiene.	Reduces transmission of microorganisms.
2 Perform oral hygiene, including brushing of tongue, before meals.	Risk of aspiration pneumonia is associated with poor oral hygiene (Palmer and Metheny, 2008).
3 Using penlight and tongue blade, gently inspect mouth for pockets of food.	Pockets of food in the mouth often indicate difficulty swallowing.
4 Have patient sit upright, or elevate head of patient's bed so hips are flexed at a 90-degree angle and head is flexed slightly forward or help patient to same position in a chair. Have him or her assume chin tuck position.	Chin-tuck or chin-down position helps reduce aspiration (Huang et al., 2006). A supine position increases the probability of aspiration (Palmer and Metheny, 2008).
5 Observe patient consume various consistencies of foods and liquids.	Referral to a dietitian is appropriate if a patient has difficulty with a particular consistency.
6 Add thickener to thin liquids to create the consistency of mashed potatoes or serve patient pureed foods.	Thin liquids such as water and fruit juice are difficult to control in the mouth and are more easily aspirated (White et al., 2008).
7 Place ½ to 1 teaspoon of food on unaffected side of the mouth, allowing utensil to touch the mouth or tongue.	Placement of food in the mouth varies based on the type of deficit (Palmer and Metheny, 2008).
8 Place hand on throat to gently palpate swallowing event as it occurs. Swallowing twice is often necessary to clear the pharynx.	Helps evaluate swallowing effort.
9 Provide verbal coaching while feeding patient and give positive reinforcement, as follows: **a.** Open your mouth. **b.** Feel the food in your mouth. **c.** Chew and taste the food. **d.** Raise your tongue to the roof of your mouth. **e.** Think about swallowing. **f.** Close your mouth and swallow. **g.** Swallow again. **h.** Cough to clear airway.	Verbal cueing keeps patient focused on swallowing. Positive reinforcement enhances patient's confidence in ability to swallow (Palmer and Metheny, 2008).
10 Observe for coughing, choking, gagging, and drooling food; suction airway as necessary.	These are indications that suggest dysphagia and risk for aspiration (Ashley et al., 2006).
11 Provide rest periods as necessary during meal to avoid rushed or forced feeding.	Avoiding fatigue decreases the risk of aspiration (Palmer and Metheny, 2008).
12 Ask patient to remain sitting upright for at least 30 to 60 minutes after the meal.	Requiring patients to remain upright after meals or snacks reduces the chance of aspiration by allowing food particles remaining in the pharynx to clear (Frey and Ramsberger, 2011).
13 Help patient perform hand hygiene and mouth care.	Mouth care after meals helps prevent dental caries and reduces colonization of bacteria, which reduces the risk of pneumonia (Palmer and Metheny, 2008).
14 Return patient's tray to appropriate place and perform hand hygiene.	Reduces spread of microorganisms.
EVALUATION	
1 Observe patient's ability to ingest foods of various textures and thickness.	Indicates whether aspiration risk is increased with thin liquids.
2 Monitor patient's food and fluid intake.	Patient needs to avoid certain types and textures of food that are difficult to swallow.
3 Weigh patient weekly at the same time on the same scale.	Determines if weight is stable and reflects adequate caloric level.
4 Observe patient's oral cavity after meal to detect pockets of food.	Determines patient's ability to swallow.

UNEXPECTED OUTCOMES AND RELATED INTERVENTIONS

1 Patient coughs, gags, complains of food "stuck in throat," or has pockets of food in mouth.
- Patient may require a swallowing evaluation.
- Initiate consultation with a speech-language pathologist (SLP) for swallowing exercises and techniques to improve swallowing and reduce risk of aspiration.
- Notify health care provider and SLP of any symptoms that occurred during meal and which foods caused the symptoms.

2 Patient avoids certain textures of food.
- Change consistency and texture of food.

3 Patient experiences weight loss.
- Discuss findings with health care provider, SLP, and/or RD.

RECORDING AND REPORTING

- Document the following in the patient's medical record: patient's tolerance of various food textures, amount of assistance required, position during meal, absence or presence of any symptoms of dysphagia, and amount eaten.
- Report any coughing, gagging, choking, or swallowing difficulties to nurse in charge or health care provider.

SKILL 44-2 INSERTING A SMALL-BORE NASOENTERIC TUBE FOR ENTERAL FEEDINGS

Delegation Considerations

The skill of inserting a small-bore nasoenteric tube cannot be delegated to nursing assistive personnel (NAP). The nurse guides the NAP to assist with patient positioning during tube insertion.

Equipment

- Nasogastric or nasointestinal tube (8- to 12-Fr) with guidewire or stylet
- Stethoscope
- Water-soluble lubricant
- 60-mL or larger Luer-Lok or catheter-tip syringe
- Hypoallergenic tape and tincture of benzoin or tube fixation device
- pH indicator strip (scale 1.0 to 11.0 or greater)
- Glass of water and straw
- Emesis basin
- Towel
- Facial tissues
- Clean gloves
- Suction equipment in case of aspiration
- Penlight to check placement in nasopharynx
- Tongue blade

STEP	RATIONALE
ASSESSMENT	
1 Assess patient for the need for enteral tube feeding: NPO or insufficient intake for more than 5 days, functional gastrointestinal (GI) tract, unable to ingest sufficient nutrients.	Identifying patients who need tube feedings before they become nutritionally depleted helps to prevent complications related to malnutrition.
2 Review patient's medical history for nasal problems (e.g., nosebleeds, oral facial surgery, facial trauma, past history of aspiration, anticoagulation therapy or coagulopathy).	A history of these problems may contraindicate tube placement and require you to consult with health care provider to change route of nutrition support.
3 Assess patient's mental status.	Alert patient is better able to cooperate with tube insertion. If vomiting occurs, an alert patient usually expectorates vomitus, which helps reduce the risk of aspiration.
4 Review health care provider's order for type of tube and enteral feeding schedule.	Procedure and tube feedings require a health care provider's order.
5 Perform hand hygiene. Assess patency of nares. Have patient close each nostril alternately and breathe. Examine each naris for patency and skin breakdown.	Evaluates nares for patency. Nares are often obstructed or irritated, or septal defect is present.
6 Assess for gag reflex. Place tongue blade in patient's mouth, touching uvula to induce a gag response.	Identifies ability to swallow and determines if there is a risk for aspiration.
7 Determine if health care provider wants a prokinetic agent administered before tube placement.	Prokinetic agents such as metoclopramide given before tube placement help advance the tube into the intestine (Metheny, 2006).

CLINICAL DECISION: *Patients with impaired level of consciousness often have impaired gag reflex; their risk of aspiration is increased during insertion of feeding tubes and subsequent tube feedings (Roberts et al., 2007).*

STEP	RATIONALE
8 Auscultate abdomen for bowel sounds.	Absence of bowel sounds indicates decreased or absent peristalsis and increased risk for aspiration and/or abdominal distention.
PLANNING	
1 Identify the patient using two identifiers (i.e., name and birth date or name and account number) according to facility policy. Compare identifiers with information on the patient's medical record.	Ensures correct patient. Complies with a recommended National Patient Safety Goal (TJC, 2011).
2 Explain procedure to patient, including sensations that will be felt during insertion (burning in nasal passages) and how to communicate during intubation by raising index finger to indicate gagging or discomfort.	Reduces anxiety and helps patient assist in insertion.
3 Stand on same side of bed as naris chosen for insertion and assist patient to high-Fowler's position unless contraindicated. Place pillow behind head and shoulders.	Allows easier manipulation of tube. Fowler's position reduces risk of aspiration and promotes effective swallowing.
4 Place bath towel over chest. Keep facial tissues within reach.	Prevents soiling of gown. Insertion of tube frequently produces tearing.

STEP	RATIONALE
5 Determine length of tube to be inserted and mark with tape:	
a. *Traditional method:* Measure distance from tip of nose to earlobe to xiphoid process of sternum (see illustration).	Length approximates distance from nose to stomach in 98% of patients. For duodenal or jejunal placement, an additional 20 to 30 cm (8 to 12 inches) is required.
6 Prepare nasogastric or nasointestinal tube for intubation: NOTE: Do not ice plastic tubes.	Tubes becomes stiff and inflexible, causing trauma to mucous membranes.
a. Inject 10 mL of water from 30-mL or larger Luer-Lok or catheter-tip syringe into tube.	Aids in guidewire or stylet insertion.
b. Make certain that guidewire is securely positioned against weighted tip and that both Luer-Lok connections are snugly fitted together.	Promotes smooth passage of tube into GI tract. Improperly positioned stylet induces serious trauma.
7 Cut tape 10 cm (4 inches) long, or prepare tube fixation device.	Anchors tubing following insertion.

IMPLEMENTATION

1 Perform hand hygiene. Apply clean gloves.	Reduces transmission of microorganisms.
2 Dip tube with surface lubricant into glass of water.	Activates lubricant to facilitate passage of tube into naris to GI tract.
3 Insert tube through nostril to back of throat (posterior nasopharynx). Aim back and down toward ear (see illustration).	Natural contour facilitates passage of tube into GI tract and reduces gagging by patient.
4 Have patient flex head toward chest after tube has passed through nasopharynx.	Closes off glottis and reduces risk of tube entering trachea.
5 Encourage patient to swallow by giving small sips of water or ice chips when possible. Advance tube as patient swallows.	Swallowing facilitates passage of tube past oropharynx.
6 Emphasize need to mouth breathe and swallow during procedure.	Helps facilitate passage of tube and alleviates patient's fears during procedure.
7 When tip of tube reaches carina (about 25 cm [10 inches] in an adult), stop, hold end of tube near ear, and listen for air exchange from distal portion of tube.	If you hear air, tube is possibly in respiratory tract; remove tube and start over. *Never* use this step for tube verification (Baskin, 2006).
8 Advance tube each time patient swallows until desired length has been passed.	Reduces discomfort and trauma to patient.

CLINICAL DECISION: *Do not force the tube. If you meet resistance or patient starts to cough, choke, or become cyanotic, stop advancing the tube and pull it back.*

9 Check for position of tube in the back of throat with penlight and tongue blade.	Tube may be coiled, kinked, or entering trachea.
10 Keep tube secure as you measure gastric pH to verify placement of tube (see Box 44-13) by obtaining gastric aspirate.	Properly obtained pH of 0 to 4 is a good indication of gastric placement (Metheny, 2006).

CLINICAL DECISION: *Auscultation is not a reliable method for verification of tube placement because a tube inadvertently placed in the lungs, pharynx, or esophagus also transmits a sound similar to that of air entering the stomach (Bankhead et al., 2009; Kenny and Goodman, 2010).*

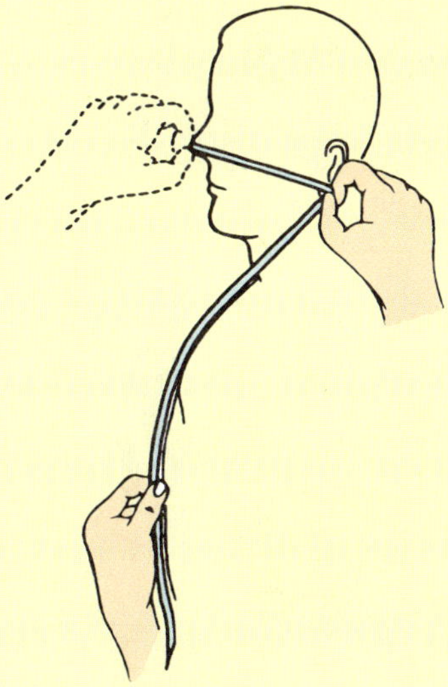

STEP 5a Determine length of tube to be inserted.

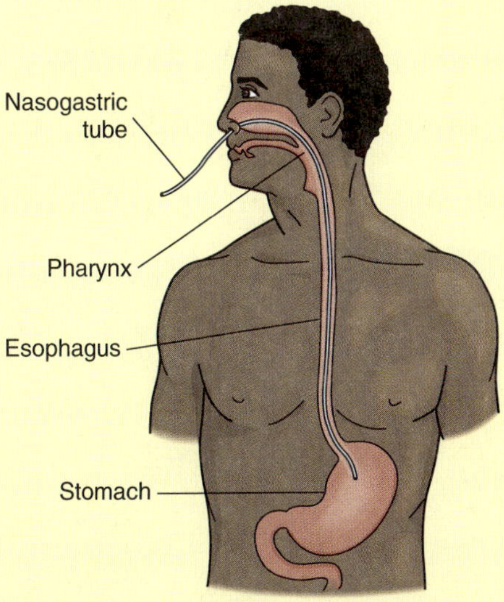

STEP 3 NG tube inserted through nose and esophagus into stomach.

SKILL 44-2 INSERTING A SMALL-BORE NASOENTERIC TUBE FOR ENTERAL FEEDINGS—cont'd

STEP	RATIONALE
11 After gastric aspirates are obtained, anchor tube to nose and avoid pressure on nares. Mark exit site with indelible ink. Select one of the following options.	Properly secured tube allows patient more mobility and prevents trauma to nasal mucosa.
a. Apply tape	
(1) Apply tincture of benzoin or other skin adhesive on tip of patient's nose and tube and allow it to become "tacky."	Helps tape adhere better. Protects skin.
(2) Remove gloves and split one end of tape lengthwise 5 cm (2 inches).	
(3) Place intact end of tape over bridge of patient's nose. Wrap each of the 5-cm (2-inch) strips around tube as it exits nose (see illustration).	Securing tape to nares prevents tissue necrosis.
b. Apply tube fixation device using shaped adhesive patch.	Secures tube and reduces friction on naris.
(1) Apply wide end of patch to bridge of nose (see illustration).	
(2) Slip connector around tube as it exits nose (see illustration).	
12 Fasten end of nasogastric tube to patient's gown using piece of tape (see illustration). Do not use safety pins to fasten tube to gown.	Reduces traction on naris if tube moves. Safety pins become unfastened and possibly cause injury to patient.
13 For intestinal placement, position patient on right side when possible until radiological confirmation of correct placement has been verified.	Promotes passage of tube into small intestine (duodenum or jejunum).
14 Remove gloves, perform hand hygiene, and assist patient to a comfortable position.	Prevents transmission of infection.

CLINICAL DECISION: *Leave guidewire or stylet in place until a radiologist verifies correct position by x-ray film. Never attempt to reinsert partially or fully removed guidewire or stylet while feeding tube is in place.*

STEP	RATIONALE
15 Obtain x-ray film of chest/abdomen.	X-ray film examination is the gold standard for verifying tube placement (Bankhead et al., 2009).
16 Apply clean gloves and administer oral hygiene (see Chapter 39). Clean tubing at nostril.	Promotes patient comfort and integrity of oral mucous membranes.
17 Remove gloves, dispose of equipment, and perform hand hygiene.	Reduces transmission of microorganisms.

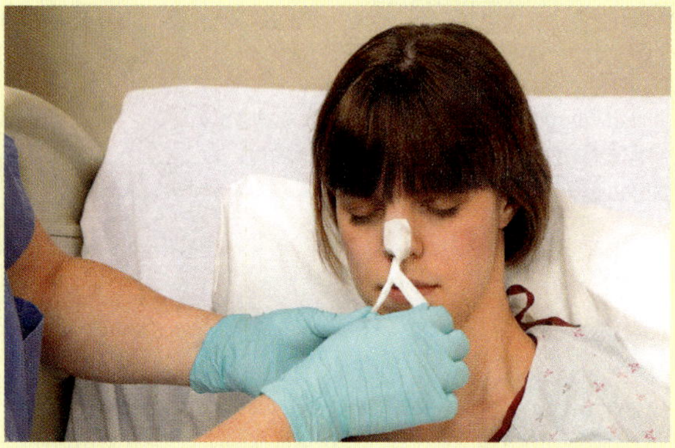

STEP 11a(3) Wrapping tape to anchor nasoenteral tube.

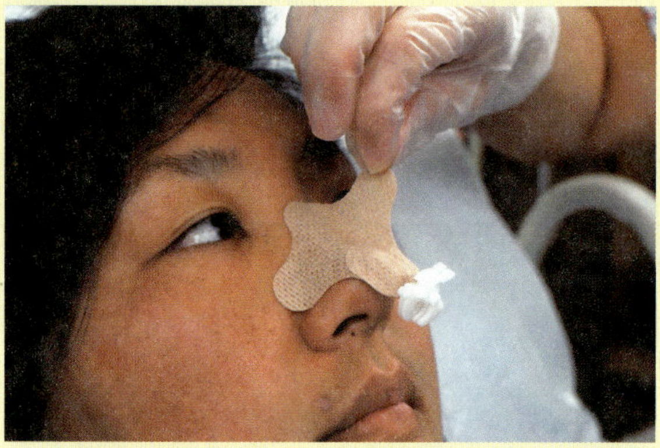

STEP 11b(1) Applying patch to bridge of nose.

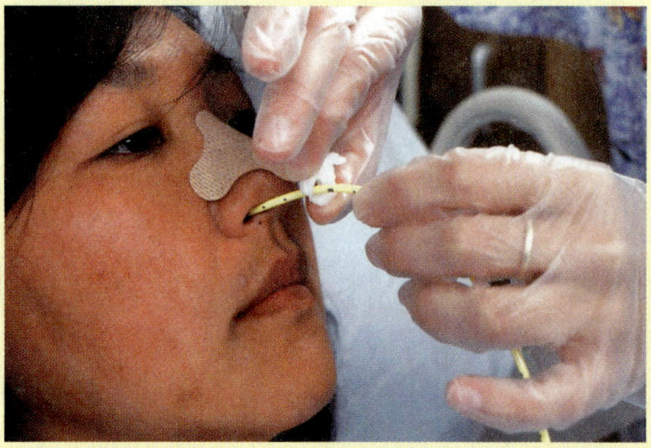

STEP 11b(2) Slip connector around feeding tube.

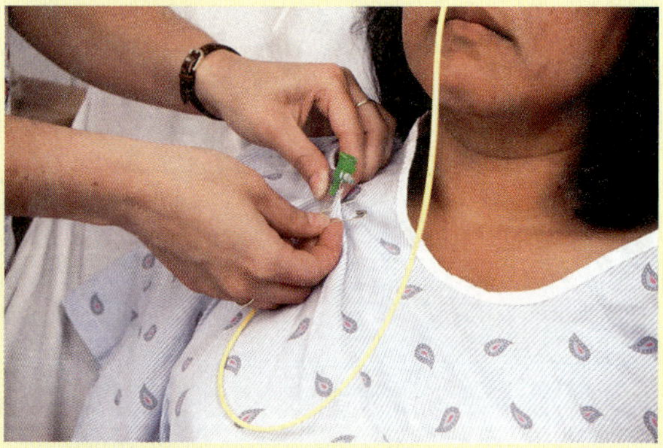

STEP 12 Fastening feeding tube to patient's gown.

STEP	RATIONALE
EVALUATION	
1 Inspect naris and oropharynx for any irritation after insertion.	If insertion was difficult, irritation of naris or oropharynx possibly occurred.
2 Ask if patient feels comfortable.	Evaluates patient's level of comfort.
3 Observe patient for any difficulty breathing, coughing, or gagging.	Malposition of tube causes these symptoms.
4 Auscultate lung sounds.	Abnormal lung sounds are early sign of aspiration.
5 Confirm x-ray film results.	Verifies position of tube before initiating enteral feeding.

UNEXPECTED OUTCOMES AND RELATED INTERVENTIONS

1 Aspiration of stomach contents into the respiratory tract
- Position patient on side.
- Suction nasotracheally and orotracheally.
- Consult health care provider immediately to order chest x-ray film examination.
- Prepare for possible initiation of antibiotics.

2 Displacement of feeding tube to another site (e.g., from duodenum to stomach, mark at exit site if tube is moved); possibly occurs when patient coughs or vomits
- Aspirate GI contents and measure pH.
- Remove displaced tube and insert and verify placement of new tube.
- If there is a question of aspiration, obtain chest x-ray film.

RECORDING AND REPORTING

- Record and report type and size of tube placed, location of distal tip of tube, patient's tolerance of procedure, pH value, and confirmation of tube position by x-ray film examination.
- If patient develops signs of aspiration, notify health care provider immediately.

SKILL 44-3 ADMINISTERING ENTERAL FEEDINGS VIA NASOENTERIC, GASTROSTOMY, OR JEJUNOSTOMY TUBES

View Video!

Delegation Considerations

The skill of administering enteral tube feeding via a nasoenteric, gastrostomy, or jejunostomy can be delegated to nursing assistive personnel (NAP) after the tube placement is verified by the nurse (refer to agency policy). The nurse is responsible for patient assessment and verification of tube placement and patency. The nurse directs the NAP to:

- Have the patient sit upright in bed/chair or elevate the head of the patient's bed at least 30 (preferably 45) degrees.
- Infuse the feeding slowly.
- Report any difficulty infusing the feeding or any discomfort voiced by the patient.
- Report any gagging, paroxysms of coughing, or choking.

Equipment

- Disposable feeding bag and tubing or ready-to-hang system
- 30-mL or larger Luer-Lok or catheter-tip syringe
- Stethoscope
- pH indicator strip (scale 1.0 to 11.0 or greater)
- Infusion pump (required for continuous or intestinal feedings): use pump designed for tube feedings
- Prescribed enteral feedings
- Clean gloves
- Equipment to obtain blood glucose by fingerstick

STEP	RATIONALE
ASSESSMENT	
1 Assess patient's need for enteral tube feedings: impaired swallowing, decreased level of consciousness, head or neck surgery, facial trauma, surgeries of upper alimentary canal.	Identify patients who need tube feedings before they become nutritionally depleted.
2 Evaluate patient's nutritional status (see Table 44-4). Obtain baseline weight and laboratory values. Assess patient for fluid volume excess or deficit, electrolyte abnormalities, and metabolic abnormalities such as hyperglycemia.	Enteral feedings are to restore or maintain a patient's nutritional status. Provides objective data to measure effectiveness of feedings.
3 Verify health care provider's order for formula, rate, route, and frequency. Laboratory data and bedside assessments such as fingerstick blood glucose measurement are also ordered by health care provider.	Tube feedings, laboratory tests, and bedside tests must be ordered by health care provider.
4 For feedings administered through tubes placed through abdominal wall, assess tube site for breakdown, irritation, or drainage.	Infection, pressure from tube, or drainage of gastric secretions causes skin breakdown.
5 Auscultate for bowel sounds before feeding.	Absent bowel sounds indicate decreased ability of gastrointestinal (GI) tract to digest or absorb nutrients. May require holding of feeding (see agency policy).

SKILL 44-3 ADMINISTERING ENTERAL FEEDINGS VIA NASOENTERIC, GASTROSTOMY, OR JEJUNOSTOMY TUBES—cont'd

STEP	RATIONALE
PLANNING	
1 Identify the patient using two identifiers (i.e., name and birth date or name and account number) according to facility policy. Compare identifiers with information on the patient's medical record.	Ensures correct patient. Complies with a recommended National Patient Safety Goal (TJC, 2011).
2 Explain procedure to patient.	Well-informed patient is more cooperative and at ease.
3 Perform hand hygiene and apply clean gloves.	Reduces transmission of microorganisms.
4 Prepare feeding container and formula:	
a. Check expiration date on formula and integrity of container.	Tube feedings administered within designated shelf life from container without cracks or breaks reduces patient's risk of obtaining tube feeding–borne GI infections. In addition, a container without cracks or breaks prevents leakage of tube feeding.
b. Have tube feeding at room temperature.	Cold formula causes gastric cramping and discomfort because mouth and esophagus do not warm liquid.
c. Connect tubing to container as needed or prepare ready-to-hang container. Use aseptic technique and avoid handling feeding system or touching can tops, container openings, spike, and spike port.	Ensures that feeding system, including bag, connections, and tubing, is free of contamination to prevent bacterial growth (Bankhead et al., 2009; Matlow et al., 2006).
d. Shake formula container well. Cleanse the top of canned formula with an alcohol swab before opening it. Fill container with formula (see illustration). Open roller clamp on tubing and fill with formula to remove air. Reclamp tubing. Hang on intravenous (IV) pole.	Filling tubing with formula prevents excess air from entering GI tract.

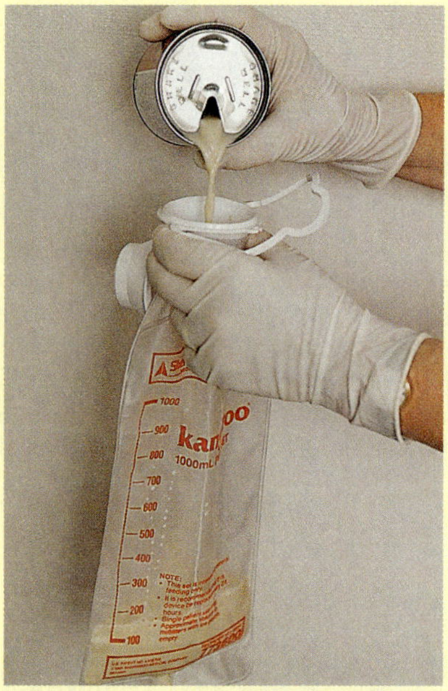

STEP 4d Pour formula into feeding container.

STEP	RATIONALE
5 For intermittent feeding have syringe ready and be sure that formula is at room temperature.	Cold formula causes gastric cramping.
IMPLEMENTATION	
1 Place patient in high-Fowler's position or elevate head of bed at least 30 (preferably 45) degrees. For patients forced to remain supine, place in reverse Trendelenburg's position.	Elevated head helps prevent aspiration (Kenny and Goodman, 2010).
2 Verify tube placement:	
a. Nasoenteric (see Box 44-14.)	
b. *Gastrostomy tube:* Attach syringe and aspirate 5 to 10 mL of gastric secretions; observe their appearance and check pH.	Gastric fluid of patient who has fasted for at least 4 hours usually has a pH of 1 to 4, especially when patient is not receiving gastric-acid inhibitor. Continuous administration of tube feedings elevates pH (Bankhead et al., 2009).
c. *Jejunostomy tube:* Aspirate intestinal secretions, observe their appearance, and check pH.	Presence of intestinal fluid indicates that end of tube is in small intestine. If fluid tests acidic on pH test, if it looks like gastric fluid, or if residual volume is large (>10 mL), displacement of tube into stomach has possibly occurred.

STEP	RATIONALE
CLINICAL DECISION: *Auscultation is not a reliable method for verification of placement of a tube because a tube inadvertently placed in lungs, pharynx, or esophagus transmits sound similar to that of air entering the stomach (Bankhead et al., 2009; Kenny and Goodman, 2010).*	
3 Check for gastric residual volume (GRV) before each feeding for bolus and intermittent feedings and every 4 hours in critically ill patients and every 4 to 6 hours in non–critically ill patients for continuous feedings (Metheny, 2006; Bankhead et al., 2009).	Gastric residual volume (GRV) indicates if gastric emptying is delayed.
a. Draw up 10 to 30 mL of air into syringe. Connect to end of feeding tube. Flush tube with air. Pull back slowly to aspirate total amount of gastric contents (see illustration).	
b. Return aspirated contents to stomach unless volume exceeds 250 mL, then check agency policy. Some questions exist regarding the safety of returning high volumes of fluid into the stomach (Bankhead et al., 2009; Delegge, 2011).	Return of aspirate prevents fluid and electrolyte imbalance (Bankhead et al., 2009).
c. Do not administer feeding when a single GRV exceeds 500 mL or when two consecutive measurements (taken 1 hour apart) each exceed 250 mL (Metheny, 2006; Bankhead et al., 2009) (check agency policy).	Some controversy exists regarding the ability of elevated GRVs to identify risk for pulmonary aspiration. However, frequent interruptions of feeding based on GRV levels is a well-recognized reason for failure to meet nutritional goals (Metheny et al., 2008; Bankhead et al., 2009; Delegge, 2011).
4 Flush tubing with 30 mL water. Before attaching feeding administration set to feeding tube, trace tube to origin and label "Tube feeding only."	Ensures that tube is clear and patent (Bourgault et al., 2007). Usually patients receive enteral feedings continuously. Avoids misconnections (Bankhead et al., 2009). However, they often receive initial feedings by bolus to assess formula tolerance. See Box 44-12 for guidelines to advance enteral feedings.
5 Initiate feeding:	
a. Syringe for intermittent feeding	
(1) Pinch proximal end of feeding tube.	Prevents excessive air from entering patient's stomach/intestine or leaking of contents.
(2) Remove plunger from syringe and attach barrel of syringe to end of tube.	
(3) Fill syringe with measured amount of formula (see illustration). Release tube, elevate syringe to no more than 45 cm (18 inches) above insertion site, and allow it to empty gradually by gravity. Repeat Steps (1) to (3) until you have delivered prescribed amount to patient.	Height of syringe allows for safe, slow, gravity drainage of formula. This gradual emptying of tube feeding by gravity reduces risk of abdominal discomfort, vomiting, or diarrhea induced by bolus or too-rapid infusion of tube feedings.
b. Feeding bag for intermittent feeding	
CLINICAL DECISION: *Before attaching feeding administration set to a feeding tube, trace the tube to its point of origin. Label the administration set "Tube Feeding Only." This prevents misconnections between feeding set and intravenous systems or other medical tubing or devices (Bankhead et al., 2009).*	

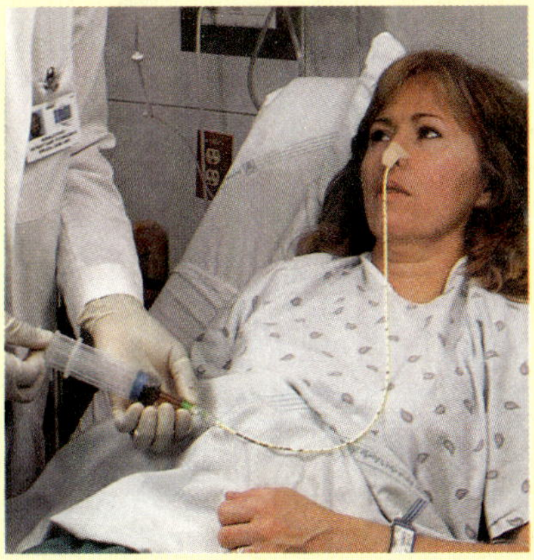

STEP 3a Check for gastric residual (small-bore tube).

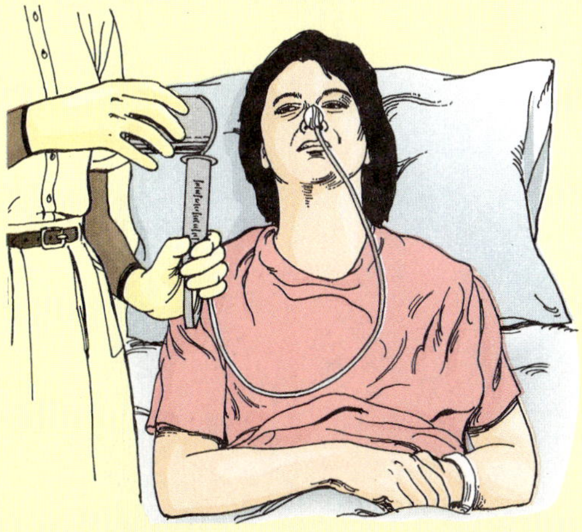

STEP 5a(3) Fill syringe with formula.

SKILL 44-3 ADMINISTERING ENTERAL FEEDINGS VIA NASOENTERIC, GASTROSTOMY, OR JEJUNOSTOMY TUBES—cont'd

STEP	RATIONALE
(1) Attach feeding bag tubing to end of feeding tube. Set rate by adjusting roller clamp on tubing or placing on feeding pump.	Reduces air introduced to stomach.
(2) Allow bag to empty gradually over 30 to 45 minutes (see illustration). Label bag with tube-feeding type, strength, and amount (include date, time, and initials). Change bag every 24 hours.	Gradual emptying of tube feeding by gravity reduces risk for abdominal discomfort, vomiting, or diarrhea induced by bolus or too-rapid infusion of tube feedings. Helps decrease bacterial colonization.
c. Continuous-drip method	
(1) Attach administration set tubing to end of feeding tube.	Continuous feeding method is designed to deliver prescribed hourly rate of feeding. This method reduces risk of abdominal discomfort.
(2) Insert tubing through infusion pump and set rate (see illustration). Use a pump designated for tube feeding and not one for intravenous fluids.	Use of an infusion pump delivers continuous feeding at a steady rate and pressure. Pump alarms for increased resistance.
6 Advance rate of tube feeding gradually as ordered (see Box 44-12).	Tube feedings are advanced gradually to prevent diarrhea and gastric intolerance to formula.

CLINICAL DECISION: *Use pump designated for tube feeding and not for intravenous fluids.*

STEP	RATIONALE
7 Flush with 30 mL water every 4 hours during continuous feeding, before and after an intermittent feeding. Have registered dietitian recommend total free water requirement per day and obtain a health care provider's order.	Clears tubing of formula and prevents clogging of tube (Bankhead et al., 2009). Provides patient with source of water to help maintain fluid and electrolyte balance.

CLINICAL DECISION: *Flush tube with 30 mL sterile water in immunocompromised or critically ill patients (Bankhead et al., 2009).*

STEP	RATIONALE
8 When tube feedings are not being administered, cap or clamp proximal end of feeding tube.	Prevents air from entering stomach between feedings.
9 Rinse bag and tubing with warm water whenever feedings are interrupted.	Clears old tube feedings and reduces bacterial growth.
10 Change bag and use a new administration set every 24 hours.	Reduces patient's exposure to bacterial growth occurring in bag and tubing.
11 Dispose of supplies, and perform hand hygiene.	Reduces transmission of microorganisms.

EVALUATION

STEP	RATIONALE
1 Measure amount of aspirated GRV every 4 to 6 hours.	Evaluates tolerance of tube feeding.
2 Monitor fingerstick blood glucose every 6 hours until maximum administration rate is reached and maintained for 24 hours (see Skill 44-4).	Alerts nurse to patient's tolerance of glucose. Glucose testing is often continued if blood glucose levels are elevated.

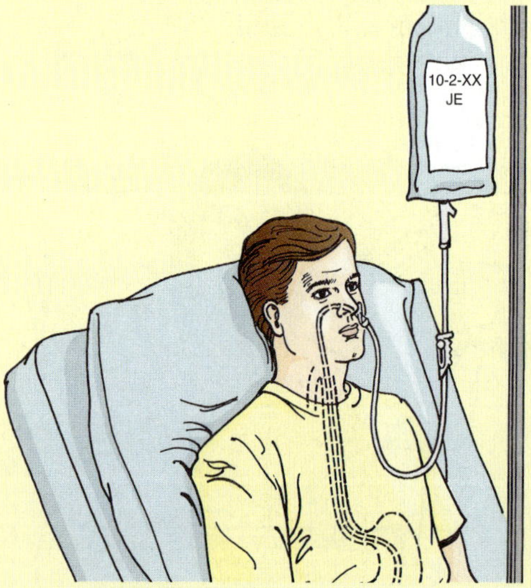

STEP 5b(2) Administer feeding.

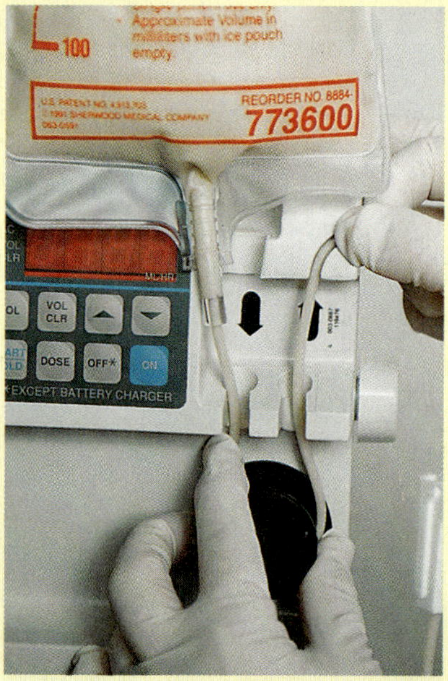

STEP 5c(2) Connect tubing through infusion pump.

STEP	RATIONALE
3 Monitor intake and output every 8 hours and calculate daily totals every 24 hours.	Intake and output are indications of fluid balance, fluid volume excess or deficit.
4 Weigh patient daily until maximum administration rate is reached and maintained for 24 hours; then weigh patient 3 times per week at same time using same scale.	Weight gain is indicator of improved nutritional status; however, sudden gain of more than 2 pounds in 24 hours usually indicates fluid retention.
5 Monitor laboratory values.	Improving laboratory values (e.g., albumin, transferrin, and prealbumin) indicate an improved nutritional status (Bankhead et al., 2009).
6 Observe patient's respiratory status.	Change in respiratory status (e.g., increased rate, declining SpO_2) may indicate aspiration of tube feeding.
7 Auscultate bowel sounds.	Assesses gastric peristalsis.
8 For tubes placed through abdominal wall, inspect insertion site for signs of impaired skin integrity.	Enteral tubes often cause pressure and excoriation at insertion site. Gastric secretions also cause irritation to skin.

UNEXPECTED OUTCOMES AND RELATED INTERVENTIONS (IN ADDITION TO THOSE IN SKILL 44-1)

1 GRV exceeds 250 mL for each of two consecutive assessments (see agency policy).
- Hold feeding and notify health care provider..
- Maintain patient in upright position in chair/bed or elevate HOB at least 30 (preferably 45) degrees.
- Recheck residual in 1 hour.

2 Patient develops diarrhea 3 times or more in 24 hours.
- Notify health care provider.
- Confer with dietitian.
- Institute skin care measures.
- Consider change in antibiotics, only for patients receiving antibiotics.

3 Patient develops nausea, vomits, and aspirates formula when gastric emptying is delayed or formula is administered too rapidly and produces vomiting.
- Position patient in side-lying position.
- Suction airway.
- Notify health care provider.
- Obtain chest x-ray film.
- Check patency of tube.
- Aspirate for GRV.

RECORDING AND REPORTING

- Record amount and type of feeding instilled. Record patient's response to tube feeding, patency of tube, condition of naris or skin at tube site for tubes placed in abdominal wall, and any side effects.
- Report patient's tolerance and adverse effects.

HOME CARE CONSIDERATIONS

- Teach patient or family caregiver how to determine correct placement of feeding tube.
- Inform patient or family caregiver of signs associated with pulmonary aspiration, delayed gastric emptying.
- Reinforce signs and symptoms associated with feeding tube complications and when to call health care provider.
- Explain and demonstrate how to do skin care around gastrostomy or jejunostomy tube and explain signs and symptoms of infection at the insertion site.

SKILL 44-4 BLOOD GLUCOSE MONITORING

Delegation Considerations

The skill of measuring blood glucose level after skin puncture (capillary puncture) can be delegated to properly trained nursing assistive personnel (NAP). You must first assess the patient to determine that serum glucose monitoring is appropriate for delegation. When the patient's condition changes frequently, you should not delegate this skill to NAP. The nurse directs the NAP by:
- Explaining appropriate sites to use for puncture and when to obtain glucose levels.
- Reviewing expected levels and when to report unexpected glucose levels to the nurse.

Equipment

- Antiseptic swab
- Cotton ball
- Sterile lancet or blood-letting device
- Heel-warming device *(optional)*
- Paper towel
- Blood glucose meter (e.g., OneTouch) (Fig. 44-10)
- Blood glucose reagent strips (brand determined by meter used)
- Clean gloves

SKILL 44-4 BLOOD GLUCOSE MONITORING—cont'd

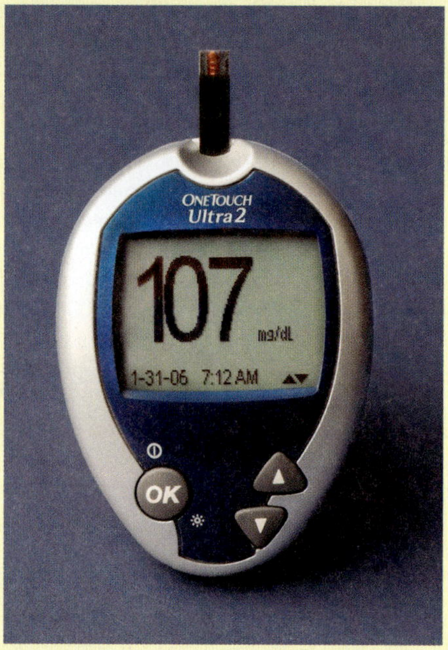

FIG. 44-10 Blood glucose monitor. (Courtesy LifeScan, Inc., Milpitas, Calif.)

STEP	RATIONALE
ASSESSMENT	
1 Assess patient's understanding of procedure and purpose of glucose monitoring. Determine if patient with diabetes mellitus performs test at home and, if so, confirm his or her competency.	Data set guidelines for nurse to develop teaching plan.
2 Determine if specific conditions need to be met before or after sample collection (e.g., with fasting, after meals, after certain medications, before insulin doses).	Dietary intake of carbohydrates and ingestion of concentrated glucose preparations alter blood glucose levels.
3 Determine if risks exist for performing skin puncture (e.g., low platelet count, anticoagulant therapy, bleeding disorders).	Abnormal clotting mechanisms increase risk for local ecchymosis and bleeding.
4 Assess area of skin that you will use as puncture site (e.g., fingers or heel). Alternative sites are palm, arm, or thigh. Avoid areas of bruising and open lesions.	Sides of fingers and heels are commonly selected because they have fewer nerve endings. Measurements from alternative sites are meter specific and may be different than those from traditional sites (Corbett, 2008). Puncture site should not be edematous, inflamed, or recently punctured because these factors cause increased interstitial fluid and blood to mix and also increase risk for infection.
5 Review health care provider's order for time of frequency of measurement.	Health care provider determines test schedule on basis of patient's physiological status and risk for glucose imbalance.
6 For patient with diabetes who performs test at home, assess ability to handle skin-puncturing device. If patient chooses, he or she may wish to continue self-testing while in hospital.	Patient's physical health may change (e.g., vision disturbance, fatigue, pain, disease process), preventing him or her from performing test.
PLANNING	
1 Identify the patient using two identifiers (i.e., name and birth date or name and account number) according to facility policy. Compare identifiers with information on the patient's medical record.	Ensures correct patient. Complies with a recommended National Patient Safety Goal (TJC, 2011).
2 Explain procedure and purpose to patient and/or family. Offer patient and family opportunity to practice testing procedures. Provide resources/teaching aids for patient.	Promotes understanding and cooperation.
IMPLEMENTATION	
1 Perform hand hygiene.	Reduces transfer of microorganisms.
2 Instruct adult to perform hand hygiene with soap and warm water if able.	Promotes skin cleaning and vasodilation at selected puncture site. Handwashing establishes practice for patient when test is performed at home.
3 Position patient comfortably in chair or in semi-Fowler's position in bed.	Ensures easy accessibility to puncture site. Patient assumes position when self-testing.

STEP	RATIONALE
4 Remove reagent strip from container; tightly seal cap. Check code on test strip vial.	Protects strips from accidental discoloration caused by exposure to air or light. Code on test strip vial must match code entered into glucose meter.
5 Turn on glucose meter if necessary.	Activates meter.
CLINICAL DECISION: *Some monitors are activated when the reagent strip is inserted and therefore do not have a specific on/off switch.*	
6 Insert strip into glucose meter (refer to manufacturer directions) and make necessary adjustments (see illustration).	Some machines must be calibrated; others require zeroing of timer. Each meter is adjusted differently.
7 Remove unused reagent strip from meter and place on paper towel or clean, dry surface with test pad facing up (see manufacturer directions). (Note that for some models of meters, strip remains in device as you apply blood to tip of strip.)	Moisture on strip can alter accuracy of final test results.
8 Apply clean gloves.	Reduces risk for contamination by blood.
9 Choose puncture site. Puncture site should be vascular. In adult select lateral side of finger; be sure to avoid central tip of finger, which has more dense nerve supply.	Ensures free flow of blood following puncture.
10 Hold finger that you will puncture in dependent position while gently massaging it toward puncture site.	Increases blood flow to area before puncture.
11 Clean site with antiseptic swab and *allow it to dry completely.*	Alcohol can cause blood to hemolyze.
12 Remove cover of lancet or blood-letting device. Hold lancet perpendicular to puncture site and pierce finger or heel quickly in one continuous motion (do not force lancet).	Cover keeps tip of lancet/needle sterile.
13 Some agencies use lancet devices with an automatic blade retraction system. This reduces the possibility of self-sticks, preventing exposure to bloodborne pathogens. Place blood-letting device firmly against side of finger and push release button, causing needle to pierce skin (see illustration).	Blood-letting devices are designed to pierce skin for specific depth, ensuring adequate blood flow. Perpendicular position ensures proper skin penetration.
14 Wipe away first droplet of blood with cotton ball. (See manufacturer directions for meter used.)	First drop of blood may contain more serous fluid than blood cells.
15 Lightly squeeze puncture site (without touching) until large droplet of blood has formed (see illustration). Repuncturing is necessary if large-enough drop does not form to ensure accurate test results. (See manufacturer directions regarding how blood is applied.)	Adequate-size droplet is needed to activate monitor and obtain accurate results. Excessive squeezing of tissues during blood sample collection may contribute to pain, bruising, scarring, and hematoma formation (Pagana and Pagana, 2009).

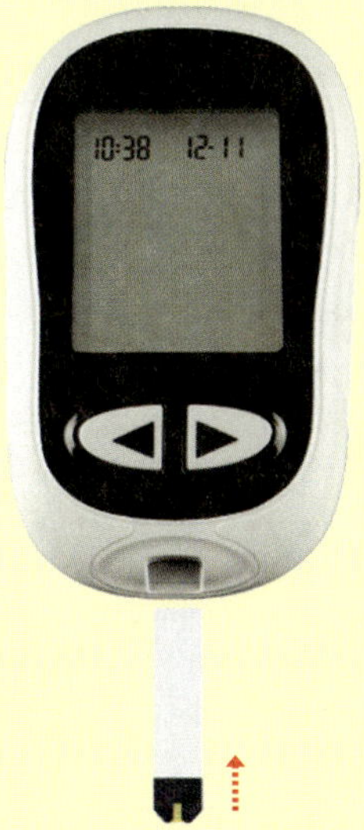

STEP 6 Load test strip into meter. (Courtesy of the manufacturer.)

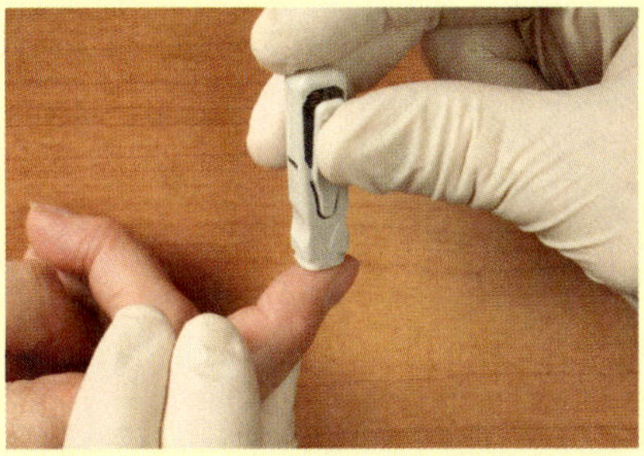

STEP 13 Prick side of finger with lancet.

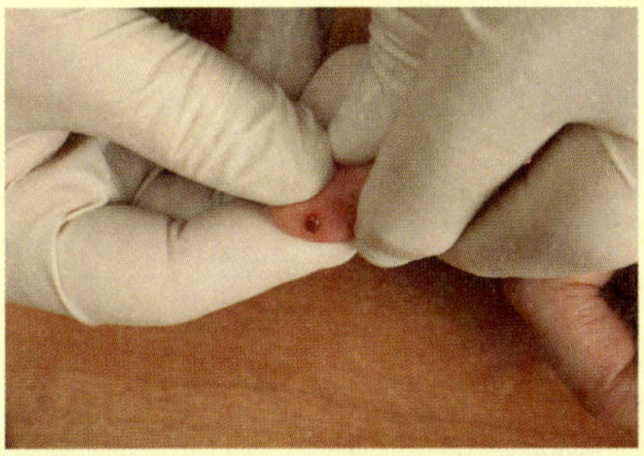

STEP 15 Squeeze puncture site until large droplet of blood is formed.

SKILL 44-4 BLOOD GLUCOSE MONITORING—cont'd

STEP	RATIONALE
CLINICAL DECISION: *Patients with diabetes frequently have peripheral vascular disease, making it difficult to produce a large drop of blood after a fingerstick. Be sure to hold finger in dependent position before puncturing to improve blood flow.*	
16 Obtain test results.	Exposure of blood to test strip for prescribed time ensures proper results.
CLINICAL DECISION: *Some meters (e.g., OneTouch [LifeScan]) require blood sample to be applied to test strip already in the meter. Once the drop of blood is applied, the meter automatically calculates the reading.*	
a. Be sure that meter is still on. Bring test strip in meter to drop of blood. The blood is wicked onto the test strip (see manufacturer's instructions).	Blood enters strip, and glucose device shows message on screen to signal that enough blood is obtained.
CLINICAL DECISION: *Do not scrape blood onto the test strips or apply it to the wrong side of the test strip. This prevents accurate glucose measurement.*	
b. Blood glucose test result appears on screen (see illustration). Some devices "beep" when completed.	

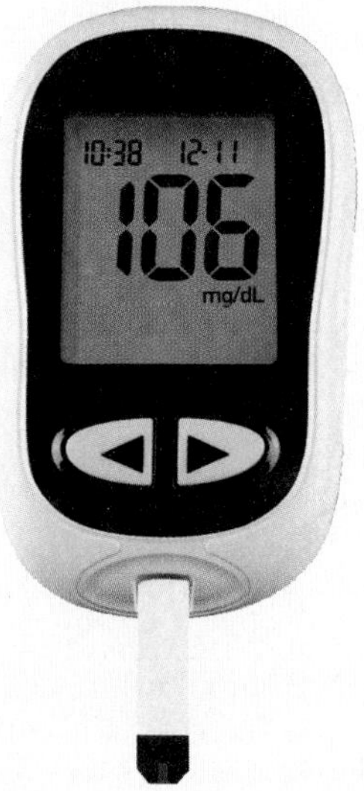

STEP 16b Results appear on meter screen. (Courtesy of the manufacturer.)

STEP	RATIONALE
17 Turn meter off. Dispose of test strip, lancet, and gloves in proper receptacles.	Meter is battery powered. Proper disposal reduces risk for needlestick injury and spread of infection.
18 Discuss test results with patient.	Promotes participation and compliance with therapy.

EVALUATION

1 Reinspect puncture site for bleeding or tissue injury.	Site is a possible source of discomfort and infection.
2 Compare glucose meter reading with normal blood glucose levels and previous test results.	Determines if glucose level is normal.
3 Ask patient to discuss procedure.	Validates level of learning.
4 Ask patient to explain test and results.	Results of test may cause anxiety. Patient may misunderstand specific step of procedure.

UNEXPECTED OUTCOMES AND RELATED INTERVENTIONS

1 Puncture site continues to bleed or is bruised.
- Apply pressure to site.
- Notify health care provider if bleeding lasts more than 5 minutes.

2 Glucose meter malfunctions.
- Repeat test, following directions.
- Follow manufacturer directions for malfunctions.

3 Blood glucose level is above or below target range.
- Continue to monitor patient.
- Follow agency protocol for laboratory confirmation testing of very high or very low results. Laboratory testing is generally considered more accurate.
- Check medical record to see if there is a medication order for deviations in glucose level; if not, notify health care provider.
- Administer insulin or carbohydrate source as ordered (depending on glucose level).
- Notify health care provider of patient's response.

RECORDING AND REPORTING

- Record glucose results on appropriate flow sheet and describe response, including presence or absence of pain or excessive oozing of blood at puncture site.
- Describe explanations or teaching provided in medical record.
- Report blood glucose levels out of target range and take appropriate action for hypoglycemia or hyperglycemia.

KEY POINTS

- Ingestion of a diet balanced with carbohydrates, fats, proteins, vitamin, and minerals provides the essential nutrients to carry out the normal physiological functioning of the body throughout the life span.
- Through digestion food is broken down into its simplest form for absorption. Digestion and absorption occur mainly in the small intestine.
- Guidelines for dietary change recommend reduced fat, saturated fat, sodium, refined sugar, and cholesterol and increased intake of complex carbohydrates and fiber.
- Because improper nutrition affects all body systems, nutritional assessment includes a review of total physical assessment.
- Enteral feedings are for patients who are unable to ingest food but are able to digest and absorb food in the gastrointestinal tract.
- EN protects intestinal structure and function and enhances immunity.
- TPN supplies essential nutrients in appropriate amounts to support life through the administration of a concentrated nutrient solution into the superior vena cava near the right atrium of the heart.
- MNT is a recognized treatment modality for both acute and chronic disease states.
- One of the most important responsibilities of a nurse administering enteral feedings is to take precautions to prevent patients from aspirating feeding formula.
- Special diets alter the composition, texture, digestibility, and residue of foods to suit the patient's particular needs.

CLINICAL APPLICATION QUESTIONS

Preparing for Clinical Practice

1. As part of your next visit to the senior citizens' center where Mrs. Cooper lives, you plan to present a program to the residents to help decrease their risk of cardiovascular disease. Using your knowledge of medical nutrition therapy (MNT), summarize five points that you will include in the program for the residents.
2. Six months later, Mrs. Cooper is admitted to the hospital for a viral infection. She had a recent weight loss of 6 pounds in the week before admission and lost an additional 4 pounds during the week of hospitalization. Her appetite is poor; she has frequent nausea and vomiting. Her abdomen is soft and nontender, and bowel sounds are present. The health care provider orders enteral feedings to be started.
   a. What type of tube should be selected?
   b. How is the tube placement verified?
   c. Describe the type of feeding and initiation of feedings.
   d. Which complications of tube feeding should be assessed?
3. Two years after her husband died, Mrs. Cooper suffered a stroke and developed dysphagia. Develop a plan of care for assisting Mrs. Cooper with meals to reduce the risk of aspiration.

evolve *Answers to Clinical Application Questions can be found on the Evolve website.*

REVIEW QUESTIONS

Are You Ready to Test Your Nursing Knowledge?

1. Which statement made by an adult patient demonstrates understanding of healthy nutrition teaching?
   1. I need to stop eating red meat.
   2. I will increase the servings of fruit juice to four a day.
   3. I will make sure that I eat a balanced diet and exercise regularly.
   4. I will not eat so many dark green vegetables and eat more yellow vegetables.
2. The nurse teaches a patient who has had surgery to increase which nutrient to help with tissue repair?
   1. Fat
   2. Protein
   3. Vitamin
   4. Carbohydrate
3. The nurse is caring for a patient experiencing dysphagia. Which interventions help decrease the risk of aspiration during feeding? (Select all that apply.)
   1. Sit the patient upright in a chair.
   2. Give liquids at the end of the meal.
   3. Place food in the strong side of the mouth.
   4. Provide thin foods to make it easier to swallow.
   5. Feed the patient slowly, allowing time to chew and swallow.
   6. Encourage patient to lie down to rest for 30 minutes after eating.
4. The nurse suspects that the patient receiving parenteral nutrition (PN) through a central venous catheter (CVC) has an air embolus. What action does the nurse need to take first?
   1. Raise head of bed to 90 degrees
   2. Turn patient to left lateral decubitus position
   3. Notify health care provider immediately
   4. Have patient perform the Valsalva maneuver
5. Which action is initially taken by the nurse to verify correct position of a newly placed small-bore feeding tube?

1. Placing an order for x-ray film examination to check position
2. Confirming the distal mark on the feeding tube after taping
3. Testing the pH of the gastric contents and observing the color
4. Auscultating over the gastric area as air is injected into the tube

6. The catheter of the patient receiving parenteral nutrition (PN) becomes occluded. Place the steps for caring for the occluded catheter in the order in which the nurse would perform them.
   1. Attempt to aspirate a clot.
   2. Temporarily stop the infusion.
   3. Flush the line with saline or heparin.
   4. Use a thrombolytic agent if ordered or per protocol.
7. Based on knowledge of peptic ulcer disease (PUD), the nurse anticipates the presence of which bacteria when reviewing the laboratory data for a patient suspected of having PUD?
   1. *Micrococcus*
   2. *Staphylococcus*
   3. *Corynebacterium*
   4. *Helicobacter pylori*
8. The nurse is assessing a patient receiving enteral feedings via a small-bore nasogastric tube. Which assessment findings need further intervention?
   1. Gastric pH of 4.0 during placement check
   2. Weight gain of 1 pound over the course of a week
   3. Active bowel sounds in the four abdominal quadrants
   4. Gastric residual aspirate of 350 mL for the second consecutive time
9. The home care nurse is seeing the following patients. Which patient is at greatest risk for experiencing inadequate nutrition?
   1. A 55-year-old obese man recently diagnosed with diabetes mellitus
   2. A recently widowed 76-year-old woman recovering from a mild stroke
   3. A 22-year-old mother with a 3-year-old toddler who had tonsillectomy surgery
   4. A 46-year-old man recovering at home following coronary artery bypass surgery
10. The nurse is checking feeding tube placement. Place the steps in the proper sequence.
    1. Draw 5 to 10 mL gastric aspirate into syringe.
    2. Flush tube with 30 mL air.
    3. Mix aspirate in syringe and place in medicine cup.
    4. Observe color of gastric aspirate.
    5. Perform hand hygiene and put on clean gloves.
    6. Dip pH strip into gastric aspirate.
    7. Compare strip with color chart from manufacturer.
11. Which statement made by a patient of a 2-month-old infant requires further education?
    1. I'll continue to use formula for the baby until he is a least a year old.
    2. I'll make sure that I purchase iron-fortified formula.
    3. I'll start feeding the baby cereal at 4 months.
    4. I'm going to alternate formula with whole milk starting next month.
12. The nurse is teaching a program on healthy nutrition at the senior community center. Which points should be included in the program for older adults? (Select all that apply.)
    1. Avoid grapefruit and grapefruit juice, which impair drug absorption.
    2. Increase the amount of carbohydrates for energy.
    3. Take a multivitamin that includes vitamin D for bone health.
    4. Cheese and eggs are good sources of protein.
    5. Limit fluids to decrease the risk of edema.
13. The nurse sees the nursing assistive personnel (NAP) perform the following for a patient receiving continuous enteral feedings. What intervention does the nurse need to address immediately with the NAP? The NAP:
    1. Fastens the tube to the gown with tape.
    2. Places the patient supine while giving a bath.
    3. Performs oral care for the patient.
    4. Elevates the head of the bed 45 degrees.
14. The patient receiving total parenteral nutrition (TPN) asks the nurse why his blood glucose is being checked since he does not have diabetes. What is the best response by the nurse?
    1. TPN can cause hyperglycemia, and it is important to keep your blood glucose level in an acceptable range.
    2. The high concentration of dextrose in the TPN can give you diabetes; thus you need to be monitored closely.
    3. Monitoring your blood glucose level helps to determine the dose of insulin that you need to absorb the TPN.
    4. Checking your blood glucose level regularly helps to determine if the TPN is effective as a nutrition intervention.
15. The nurse is performing blood glucose monitoring for a patient receiving parenteral nutrition. Place the steps of the procedure in the correct sequence.
    1. Clean puncture site with antiseptic solution.
    2. Identify patient using two identifiers.
    3. Check code on test strip vial.
    4. Wick blood drop into test strip.
    5. Gently squeeze fingertip until drop of blood appears.
    6. Assess area of skin to be used as puncture site.
    7. Read results and document in medical record.

Answers: **1.** 3; **2.** 2; **3.** 1, 3, 5; **4.** 2; **5.** 1; **6.** 2, 3, 1, 4; **7.** 4; **8.** 4; **9.** 2; **10.** 5, 2, 1, 4, 3, 6, 7; **11.** 4; **12.** 1, 3, 4; **13.** 2; **14.** 1; **15.** 6, 2, 3, 1, 5, 4, 7.

REFERENCES

American Cancer Society (ACS): *American Cancer Society guidelines on nutrition and physical activity for cancer prevention*, 2011, http://www.cancer.org/acs/groups/cid/documents/webcontent/002577-pdf.pdf. Accessed October 17, 2011.

American Diabetes Association (ADA): Position statement: nutrition recommendations and interventions for diabetes, *Diabetes Care* 31(suppl 1):561, 2008.

American Dietetic Association: Position of the American Dietetic Association: Promoting and supporting breastfeeding, *J Am Diet Assoc* 109:1926, 2009.

American Dietetic Association: Position of the American Dietetic Association, American Society for Nutrition, and Society for Nutrition Education: Food and nutrition programs for community-residing older adults, *J Am Diet Assoc* 110(3):463, 2010a.

American Dietetic Association: Position of the American Dietetic Association: Integration of medical nutrition therapy and pharmacotherapy, *J Am Diet Assoc* 110(6):950, 2010b.

American Heart Association: *Diet and lifestyle recommendations revision*, 2010, http://www.heart.org/HEARTORG/GettingHealthy/Diet-and-Lifestyle-Recommendations_UCM_305855_Article.jsp. Accessed October 17, 2011.

Andrews MM, Boyle JS: *Transcultural concepts in nursing care*, ed 5, Philadelphia, 2008, Lippincott Williams & Wilkins.

Ashley J, et al: Speech, language, and swallowing disorders in the older adult, *Clin Geriatr Med* 22:291, 2006.

Baskin WN: Acute complications associated with bedside placement of feeding tubes, *Nutr Clin Pract* 21:40, 2006.

Budd GM, Hayman LL: Addressing the childhood obesity crisis: a call to action, *Matern Child Nurs* 33(2):111, 2008.

Charney P: Nutrition screening vs nutrition assessment: how do they differ? *Nutr Clin Pract* 23(4):366, 2008.

Corbett JV: *Laboratory tests and diagnostic procedures with nursing diagnoses*, ed 7, Upper Saddle River, NJ, 2008, Prentice-Hall.

Daniels J: Obesity: America's epidemic, *Am J Nurs* 106(1):40, 2006.

Delegge DH: Managing gastric residual volumes in the critically ill patient: An update, *Curr Opin Nutr Metab Care* 14:193, 2011.

DiMaria-Ghalili RA: *Nutrition in the elderly: nursing standard of practice protocol: nutrition in aging*, 2008, http://consultgerirn.org/topics/nutrition_in_the_elderly/want_to_know_more. Accessed October 17, 2011.

Dossey B: *Florence Nightingale: mystic, visionary, and healer*, Philadelphia, 1999, Springhouse.

Ebersole P, et al: *Toward healthy aging: human needs and nursing response*, ed 7, St Louis, 2008, Mosby.

Giger JN, Davidhizar RE: *Transcultural nursing: assessment and intervention*, ed 5, St Louis, 2008, Mosby.

Hockenberry MJ, Wilson D: *Wong's nursing care of infants and children*, ed 9, St Louis, 2011, Mosby.

Huether SE, et al: *Understanding pathophysiology*, ed 4, St Louis, 2008, Mosby.

Institute of Medicine: *Dietary reference intakes: essential nutrient guide*, 2006, http://iom.edu/Reports/2006/Dietary-Reference-Intakes-Essential-Guide-Nutrient-Requirements.aspx. Accessed October 31, 2010.

Khan LK, et al: Recommended community strategies and measurements to prevent obesity in the United States, *MMWR Morb Mortal Wkly Rep* 58(RR-7):1, 2009.

Kondrup J, et al: ESPEN guidelines for nutrition screening 2002, *Clin Nutr* 22(4):415, 2003.

Krondl M, et al: Helping older adults meet nutritional challenges, *J Nutr Elderly* 27(3/4):2005, 2008.

Kruskall LJ: Portion distortion: sizing up food servings, *ACSM Health Fitness J* 10(3):8, 2006.

Krzywda EA, Meyer D: Parenteral nutrition. In Alexander M, et al, editors: *Infusion nursing society infusion nursing: an evidence-based approach*, ed 3, St Louis, 2010, Saunders.

Lehne RA: *Pharmacology for nursing care*, ed 7, St Louis, 2010, Saunders.

Li J, Hooker NH: Childhood obesity and schools: evidence from the national survey of children's health, *J School Health* 80(2):96, 2010.

Mason P: Undernutrition in hospital: causes and consequences, *Hosp Pharm* 13:353, 2006.

Mayo Clinic Staff: *Teen weight loss: healthy habits count*, 2009, http://www.mayoclinic.com/health/teen-weight-loss/WT00012. Accessed October 17, 2011.

McCance KL, et al: *Pathophysiology: the biologic basis for disease in adults and children*, ed 6, St Louis, 2010, Mosby.

McClave SA, et al: Guidelines for the provision and assessment of nutrition support therapy in the adult critically ill patient, *J Parenter Enter Nutr* 33(3):277, 2009.

Meiner SE: *Gerontologic nursing*, ed 4, St Louis, 2011, Mosby.

Metheny NA, et al: Tracheobronchial aspiration of gastric contents in critically ill tube-fed patients: frequency, outcomes, and risk factors, *Crit Care Med* 34(4):1007, 2006.

Metheny NA, et al: Gastric residual volume and aspiration in critically ill patients receiving gastric feedings, *Am J Crit Care* 17(6):512, 2008.

National Dysphagia Diet Task Force (NDDTF): *National Dysphagia Diet: standardization for optimal care*, Chicago, 2002, American Dietetic Association.

National Guideline Clearinghouse: *Strategies to prevent central-line associated bloodstream infections in acute care hospitals*, 2008, http://www.guideline.gov/content.aspx?id=13395&search=prevention+of+healthcare+associated+infection. Accessed October 17, 2011.

Nix S: *Williams' basic nutrition and diet therapy*, ed 13, St Louis, 2009, Mosby.

Nowlin A: The dysphagia dilemma: how you can help, *RN* 69(6):44, 2006.

O'Connor L: Oral health care. In Capezuti E et al, editors: *Evidence-based geriatric nursing protocols for best practice*, ed 3, New York, 2008, Springer.

Pagana KD, Pagana TJ: *Mosby's diagnostic and laboratory test reference*, ed 9, St Louis, 2009, Mosby.

Palmer JL, Metheny NA: Preventing aspiration in older adults with dysphagia, *Am J Nurs* 108(2):40, 2008.

Park S, et al: Vitamin and mineral supplements: barriers and challenges for older adults, *J Nutr Elderly* 27(3/4):297, 2008.

Phillips LD: *Manual of IV therapeutics: evidence-based practice for infusion therapy*, ed 5, Philadelphia, 2010, FA Davis.

Rauen CA, et al: Seven evidence-based practice habits: putting some sacred cows to pasture, *Crit Care Nurs* 28(2):98, 2008.

Robbins J, et al: Team management of dysphagia in the institutional setting, *J Nutr Elderly* 26(3/4):59, 2007.

Roberts S, et al: Devices and techniques for bedside enteral feeding tube placement, *Nutr Clin Pract* 22:412, 2007.

Rolandelli RH, et al: *Clinical nutrition: enteral feeding and tube feeding*, Philadelphia, 2005, Saunders.

Serna ED, McCarthy MS: Heads up to prevent aspiration during enteral feeding, *Nursing* 36(1):76, 2006.

Siepler J: Principles and strategies for monitoring home parenteral nutrition, *Nutr Clin Pract* 22(3):340, 2007.

Task Force for the Revision of Safe Practices for Parenteral Nutrition: Safe practices for parenteral nutrition, *J Parenter Enter Nutr* 28(6):S39, 2004.

The Joint Commission (TJC): *2011 National patient safety goals (NPGs)*, 2011, http://www.jointcommission.org/standards_information/npsgs.aspx.

Tolerable upper level intake, 2010, National Institutes of Health http://ods.od.nih.gov/pubs/conferences/tolerable_upper_intake.pdf. Accessed October 19, 2010.

Touhy TA, Jett KF: *Ebersole and Hess' gerontological nursing healthy aging*, St Louis, 2010, Mosby.

Tufts University: *MyPlate for Older Adults*, 2011, http://nutrition.tufts.edu/research/myplate-older-adults. Accessed February 7, 2012.

US Department of Agriculture (USDA): *Choose MyPlate*, 2011a, http://www.choosemyplate.gov. Accessed October 17, 2011.

US Department of Agriculture (USDA): *Shopping, cooking, and meal planning*, 2011b, http://www.nutrition.gov/nal_display/index.php?info_center=11&tax_level=2&tax_subject=391&level3_id=0&level4_id=0&level5_id=0&topic_id=1756&&placement_default=0. Accessed October 17, 2011.

US Department of Health and Human Services (USDHHS): *Healthy people 2020*, 2010, http://www.healthypeople.gov/hp2020/objectives. Accessed October 17, 2011.

US Food and Drug Administration (USFDA): Appendix F. Calculate the percent daily value for the appropriate nutrients, 2008, http://www.fda.gov/Food/GuidanceComplianceRegulatoryInformation/GuidanceDocuments/FoodLabelingNutrition/FoodLabelingGuide/ucm064928.htm. Accessed October 17, 2011.

White G, et al: Dysphagia: cause, assessment, and management, *Geriatrics* 3(5):15, 2008.

World Health Organization (WHO): Food security, 2010, http://www.who.int/trade/glossary/story028/en. Accessed October 17, 2011.

RESEARCH REFERENCES

AY Cichero J, et al: Triaging dysphagia: nurse screening for dysphagia in an acute hospital, *J Clin Nurs* 18:1649, 2009.

Bankhead R, et al: Enteral nutrition practice recommendations, *JPEN J Parenter Enteral Nutr* 33:122, 2009.

Befort C, et al: Fruit, vegetable and fat intake among non-Hispanic black and non-Hispanic white adolescents: associations with home availability and food consumption settings, *J Am Diet Assoc* 106(3):367, 2006.

Bourgault AN, et al: Development of evidence-based guidelines and critical care nurses' knowledge of enteral feedings, *Crit Care Nurse* 27(4):17, 2007.

Chang C, Roberts B: Feeding difficulty in older adults with dementia, *J Clin Nurs* 17:2266, 2008.

Cirgin Ellett ML: Important facts about intestinal feeding tube placement, *Gastroenterol Nurs* 29(2):112, 2006.

DeChicco R, et al: Tip position of long-term central venous access devices used for parenteral nutrition, *J Parenter Enter Nutr* 31(5):382, 2007.

Edmiaston J, et al: Validation of a dysphagia screening tool in acute stroke patients, *Am J Crit Care* 19(4):357, 2010.

Fox MK, et al: Sources of energy and nutrients in the diets of infants and toddlers, *J Am Diet Assoc* 106(suppl 1): S28e1, 2006.

Frey K, Ramsberger G: Comparison of outcomes before and after implementation of a water protocol for patients with cerebrovascular accident and dysphagia, *J Neurosci Nurs* 43(3): 165-170, 2011.

Guigoz Y, Vellas B: The Mini Nutritional Assessment (MNA) for grading the nutritional state of elderly patients: presentation of the MNA, history and validation, *Nestle Nutr Workshop Ser Clin Perform Programme* 1:3, 1999.

Guigoz YB, et al: Assessing the nutritional status of the elderly: the Mini Nutritional Assessment as part of the geriatric evaluation, *Nutr Rev* 54(1 pt 2):S59, 1996.

Huang G, et al: Training in swallowing prevents aspiration pneumonia in stroke patients with dysphagia, *J Int Med Res* 34(3):303, 2006.

Kenny DJ, Goodman P: Care of the patient with enteral tube feeding: an evidence-based practice protocol, *Nurs Res* 59(1S):S22, 2010.

Khalid I, et al: early enteral nutrition and outcomes of critically ill patients treated with vasopressors and mechanical ventilation, *Am J Crit Care* 19(3):261, 2010.

Kwon HM, et al: The pneumonia score: a simple grading scale for prediction of pneumonia after acute stroke, *Am J Infect Control* 34(2):64, 2006.

Lennie TA, et al: Factors influencing food intake in patients with heart failure: a comparison with healthy elders, *J Cardiovasc Nurs* 21(2):123, 2006.

Matlow A, et al: Enteral tube hub as a reservoir for the transmissible enteric bacteria, *Am J Infect Control* 34(3): 131, 2006.

Metheny NA: Preventing respiratory complications of tube feedings: evidence-based practice, *Am J Crit Care* 15(4): 360, 2006.

Metheny NA, et al: Complications related to feeding tube placement, *Curr Opin Gastroenterol* 23:178, 2007.

CHAPTER 45

Urinary Elimination

OBJECTIVES

- Describe the process of urination.
- Identify factors that commonly influence urinary elimination.
- Compare and contrast common alterations in urinary elimination.
- Obtain a nursing history for a patient with urinary elimination problems.
- Identify nursing diagnoses appropriate for patients with alterations in urinary elimination.
- Obtain urine specimens correctly.
- Describe characteristics of normal and abnormal urine.
- Describe the nursing implications of common diagnostic tests of the urinary system.
- Discuss nursing measures to promote normal micturition and reduce episodes of incontinence.
- Insert a urinary catheter correctly.
- Discuss nursing measures to reduce urinary tract infection.
- Irrigate a urinary catheter correctly.
- Identify two modalities of renal replacement therapy.

KEY TERMS

Anuria, p. 1045
Bacteremia, p. 1046
Bacteriuria, p. 1046
Catheterization, p. 1061
Cystitis, p. 1047
Diuresis, p. 1045
Dysuria, p. 1047
Erythropoietin, p. 1043
Hematuria, p. 1047
Hyperactive/overactive bladder, p. 1047
Meatus, p. 1051
Micturition, p. 1044
Nephron, p. 1043
Nephrostomy, p. 1047
Nocturia, p. 1045
Nocturnal enuresis, p. 1049
Oliguria, p. 1045
Overflow incontinence, p. 1044
Pelvic floor exercises (Kegel exercises), p. 1066
Polyuria, p. 1045
Proteinuria, p. 1043
Pyelonephritis, p. 1047
Reflex incontinence, p. 1044
Renal calculus, p. 1044
Renal replacement therapy, p. 1045
Renin, p. 1043
Residual urine, p. 1046
Specific gravity, p. 1053
Stoma, p. 1046
Uremic syndrome, p. 1045
Urge incontinence, p. 1047
Urinalysis, p. 1053
Urinary diversion, p. 1046
Urinary frequency, p. 1049
Urinary incontinence, p. 1047
Urinary retention, p. 1046
Urosepsis, p. 1046

evolve WEBSITE

http://evolve.elsevier.com/Potter/fundamentals/

- Review Questions
- Video Clips
- Concept Map Creator
- Case Study with Questions
- Skills Performance Checklists
- Audio Glossary
- Interactive Learning Activities
- Key Term Flashcards
- Content Updates

Normal elimination of urinary wastes is a basic function that most people take for granted. When the urinary system fails to function properly, eventually all organ systems are affected. Patients with alterations in urinary elimination often suffer emotionally from body image changes. It is important to know the reasons for urinary elimination problems, find acceptable solutions, and provide understanding and sensitivity to all patients' needs.

SCIENTIFIC KNOWLEDGE BASE

Urinary elimination depends on the function of the kidneys, ureters, bladder, and urethra. Kidneys remove wastes from the blood to form urine. Ureters transport urine from the kidneys to the bladder. The bladder holds urine until the urge to urinate develops. Urine leaves the body through the urethra. All organs of the urinary system must be intact and functional for successful removal of urinary wastes. Intact efferent and afferent nerves from the bladder to the spinal cord and brain must be present (Fig. 45-1).

Kidneys

The kidneys lie on either side of the vertebral column behind the peritoneum and against the deep muscles of the back. Normally the left kidney is higher than the right because of the anatomical position of the liver.

Kidneys filter waste products of metabolism that collect in the blood. The blood reaches each kidney by a renal (kidney) artery that branches from the abdominal aorta. Approximately 20% to 25% of the cardiac output circulates each minute through the

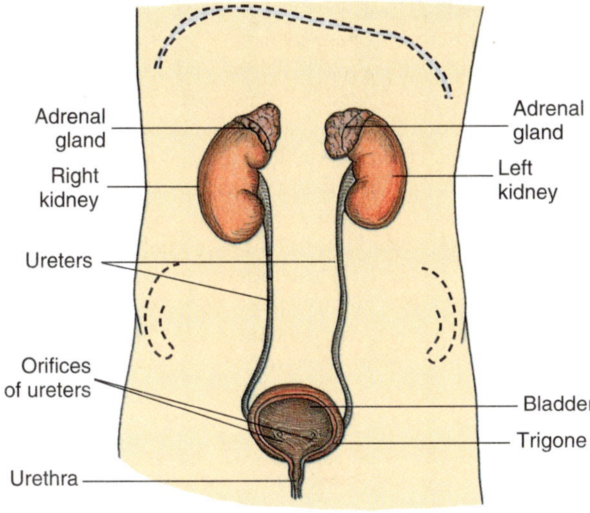

FIG. 45-1 Organs of urinary system.

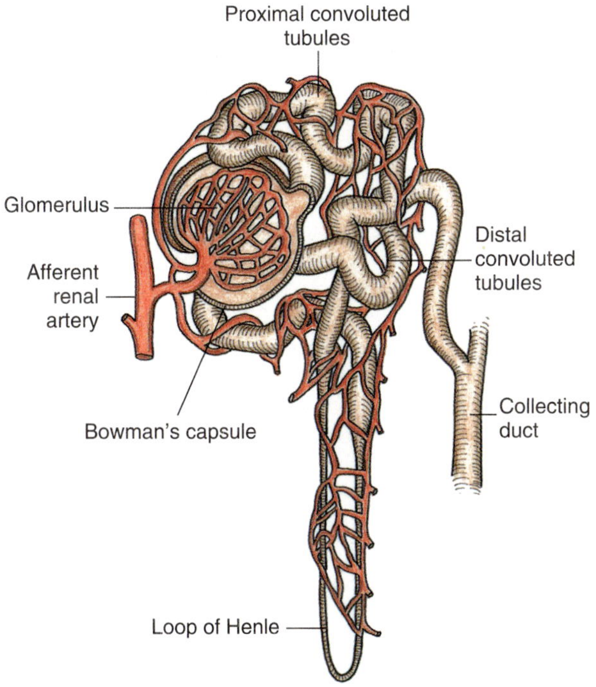

FIG. 45-2 Renal nephron.

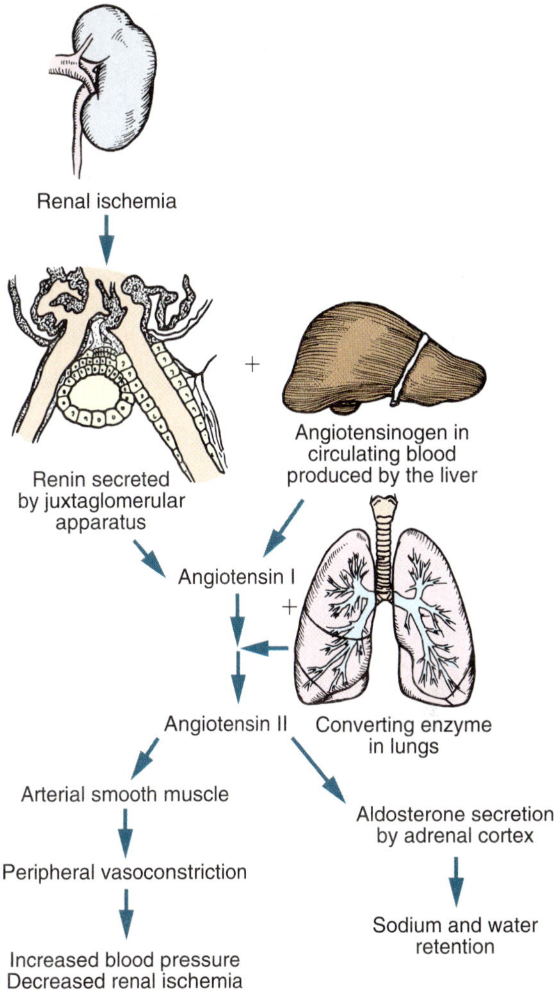

FIG. 45-3 Physiological effects of renin-angiotensin mechanism.

kidneys. The **nephron,** the functional unit of the kidney, forms the urine. It is composed of the glomerulus, Bowman's capsule, proximal convoluted tubule, loop of Henle, distal tubule, and collecting duct (Fig. 45-2).

A cluster of blood vessels forms the capillary network of the glomerulus, which is the initial site of filtration of the blood and the beginning of urine formation. The glomerular capillaries permit filtration of water, glucose, amino acids, urea, creatinine, and major electrolytes into Bowman's capsule. Large proteins and blood cells do not normally filter through the glomerulus. The presence of large proteins in the urine **(proteinuria)** is a sign of glomerular injury. The glomerulus filters approximately 125 mL of filtrate per minute.

Not all of the glomerular filtrate is excreted as urine. Approximately 99% is resorbed into the plasma, with the remaining 1% excreted as urine (Huether et al., 2008). The kidneys play a key role in fluid and electrolyte balance (see Chapter 41). Although output does depend on intake, the normal adult urine output averages 1200 to 1500 mL/day. An output of less than 30 mL/hr indicates possible circulatory, blood volume, or renal alterations.

The kidneys produce several substances vital to red blood cell (RBC) production, blood pressure, and bone mineralization. They are responsible for maintaining a normal RBC volume by producing **erythropoietin.** Erythropoietin functions within the bone marrow to stimulate RBC production and maturation and prolongs the life of mature RBCs (Huether et al., 2008). Patients with chronic kidney conditions cannot produce sufficient quantities of this hormone; therefore they are prone to anemia.

Renal hormones affect blood pressure regulation in several ways. In times of renal ischemia (decreased blood supply), **renin** is released from juxtaglomerular cells (Fig. 45-3). Renin functions as an enzyme to convert angiotensinogen (a substance synthesized by the liver) into angiotensin I. Angiotensin I is converted to angiotensin II in the lungs. Angiotensin II causes vasoconstriction and stimulates aldosterone release from the adrenal cortex. Aldosterone causes retention of water, which increases blood volume. The kidneys also produce prostaglandin E_2 and prostacyclin, which help maintain renal blood flow through vasodilation. These mechanisms increase arterial blood pressure and renal blood flow (Huether et al., 2008).

The kidneys affect calcium and phosphate regulation by producing a substance that converts vitamin D into its active form. Patients with chronic alterations in kidney function do not make sufficient amounts of the active vitamin D. They are prone to develop renal bone disease resulting from the demineralization of bone caused by impaired calcium absorption.

Ureters

The ureters are tubular structures that enter the urinary bladder. Urine draining from the ureters to the bladder is usually sterile.

Peristaltic waves cause the urine to enter the bladder in spurts. The ureters enter obliquely through the posterior bladder wall. This arrangement prevents the reflux of urine from the bladder into the ureters during the act of **micturition** by the compression of the ureter at the ureterovesical junction (the juncture of the ureters with the bladder). An obstruction within a ureter such as a kidney stone **(renal calculus)** results in strong peristaltic waves that attempt to move the obstruction into the bladder. These waves result in pain often referred to as *renal colic*.

Bladder

The urinary bladder is a hollow, distensible, muscular organ (detrusor muscle) that stores and excretes urine. When empty, the bladder lies in the pelvic cavity behind the symphysis pubis. In men the bladder lies against the anterior wall of the rectum, and in women it rests against the anterior walls of the uterus and vagina.

The bladder expands as it becomes filled with urine. Pressure within it is usually low even when partly full, a factor that protects against infection. When the bladder is full, it expands and extends above the symphysis pubis. A greatly distended bladder may reach the level of the umbilicus. In a pregnant woman the developing fetus pushes against the bladder, reducing the capacity of the bladder and causing a feeling of fullness. This effect is more likely to occur in the first and third trimesters.

The trigone (a smooth triangular area on the inner surface of the bladder) is at the base of the bladder. An opening exists at each of the three angles of the trigone. Two are for the ureters, and one is for the urethra.

Urethra

Urine exits the bladder through the urethra and passes out of the body through the urethral meatus. Normally the turbulent flow of urine through the urethra washes it free of bacteria. Mucous membrane lines the urethra, and urethral glands secrete mucus into the urethral canal. Thick layers of smooth muscle surround the urethra. In addition, it descends through a layer of skeletal muscles called the *pelvic floor muscles*. When these muscles are contracted, it is possible to prevent urine flow through the urethra (Huether et al., 2008).

In women the urethra is approximately 4 to 6.5 cm (1½ to 2½ inches) long. The external urethral sphincter, which is composed of skeletal muscle located about halfway down the urethra, permits voluntary flow of urine. However, the internal sphincter muscle is composed of smooth muscle and therefore is not under voluntary control. The short length of the urethra predisposes women and girls to infection. It is easy for bacteria to enter the urethra from the perineal area.

In men the urethra, which is both a urinary canal and a passageway for cells and secretions from reproductive organs, is about 20 cm (8 inches) long. The male urethra has three sections: prostatic, membranous, and penile.

Act of Urination

Several brain structures influence bladder function, including the cerebral cortex, thalamus, hypothalamus, and brainstem. Together they inhibit the urge to void or allow voiding. Normal voiding involves contraction of the bladder and coordinated relaxation of the urethral sphincter and pelvic floor muscles.

Bladder capacity varies with the individual but generally ranges from 600 to 1000 mL of urine (Lewis et al., 2011), and an adult normally voids every 2 to 4 hours. However, individuals are able to sense the desire to urinate when the bladder contains a smaller amount of urine (150 to 200 mL in an adult and 50 to 100 mL in a child). It is important to teach parents that children do not have enough neurological development to be toilet trained until after 24 months and some are not developed enough until 36 months. As the volume increases, the bladder walls stretch, sending sensory impulses to the micturition center in the sacral spinal cord. Impulses from the micturition center respond to or ignore this urge, thus making urination under voluntary control. If the person chooses not to void, the external urinary sphincter remains contracted, inhibiting the micturition reflex. However, when a person is ready to void, the external sphincter relaxes, the micturition reflex stimulates the detrusor muscle to contract, and efficient emptying of the bladder occurs. It is vital that nurses understand this process to be able to assess and determine which form of incontinence or bladder problem may be occurring.

Damage to the spinal cord above the sacral region causes **reflex incontinence.** This condition causes loss of voluntary control of urination; but the micturition reflex pathway often remains intact, allowing urination to occur without sensation of the need to void. If a chronic obstruction caused by neurological damage such as prostate enlargement hinders bladder emptying, over time the micturition reflex changes, causing bladder overactivity and possibly causing the bladder to not empty completely. **Overflow incontinence** occurs when a bladder is overly full and bladder pressure exceeds sphincter pressure, resulting in involuntary leakage of urine. Causes often include head injury; spinal injury; multiple sclerosis; diabetes; trauma to the urinary system; and postanesthesia sedatives/hypnotics, tricyclics, and analgesia (Lewis et al., 2011). Hyperreflexia, a life-threatening problem affecting heart rate and blood pressure, is caused by an overly full bladder. It is usually neurogenic in nature; however, it can be caused functionally by blockage.

Factors Influencing Urination. Many factors influence the volume and quality of urine and the patient's ability to urinate. Some pathophysiological conditions are acute and reversible (urinary tract infection [UTI]), whereas others are chronic and irreversible (slow, progressive development of renal dysfunction). Sociocultural factors, psychological factors, fluid balance, and surgical and diagnostic procedures affect urine and urination in several ways. In addition, medications, including anesthesia, interfere with both the production and characteristics of urine, affect the act of urination, and affect the ability to completely empty or control voiding.

Disease Conditions. Disease processes that affect urine elimination affect renal function (changes in urine volume or quality), the act of urine elimination, or both. Conditions that affect urine volume and quality are generally categorized as prerenal, renal, or postrenal in origin.

Decreased blood flow to and through the kidney (prerenal), disease conditions of the renal tissue (renal) and obstruction in the lower urinary tract that prevents urine flow from the kidneys (postrenal) sometimes alter renal function. Conditions of the lower urinary tract, including narrowing of the urethra, altered innervation of the bladder, or weakened pelvic and/or perineal muscles, affect urinary elimination.

Diabetes mellitus and neuromuscular diseases such as multiple sclerosis cause changes in nerve functions that can lead to possible loss of bladder tone, reduced sensation of bladder fullness, or inability to inhibit bladder contractions. Older men often suffer from benign prostatic hyperplasia (BPH), which makes them prone to urinary retention and incontinence. Some patients with cognitive impairments, such as Alzheimer's disease, lose the ability to sense a full bladder or are unable to recall the procedure for voiding. Diseases that slow or hinder physical activity interfere with the ability to void. Degenerative joint disease and Parkinsonism are examples of conditions that make it difficult to reach and use toilet facilities.

Diseases that cause irreversible damage to kidney tissue result in end-stage renal disease (ESRD). Eventually the patient has symptoms resulting from **uremic syndrome.** An increase in nitrogenous wastes in the blood, marked fluid and electrolyte abnormalities, nausea, vomiting, headache, coma, and convulsions characterize this syndrome. As the uremic symptoms worsen, aggressive treatment is indicated for survival (Box 45-1). These treatments are **renal replacement therapies.**

Dialysis and organ transplantation are two methods of renal replacement. Dialysis takes one of two forms, peritoneal dialysis or hemodialysis. Patients can use both dialysis modalities for a short or long term, but they require specialized equipment and nurses with specialized education.

Peritoneal dialysis is an indirect method of cleaning the blood of waste products using osmosis and diffusion, with the peritoneum functioning as a semipermeable membrane. This method removes excess fluid and waste products from the bloodstream when a sterile electrolyte solution (dialysate) is instilled into the peritoneal cavity by gravity via a surgically placed catheter. The dialysate remains in the cavity for a prescribed time interval and then is drained out by gravity, taking accumulated wastes and excess fluid and electrolytes with it.

Hemodialysis requires a machine equipped with a semipermeable filtering membrane (artificial kidney) that removes accumulated waste products and excess fluids from the blood. In the dialysis machine dialysate fluid is pumped through one side of the filter membrane (artificial kidney) while a patient's blood passes through the other side. The processes of diffusion, osmosis, and ultrafiltration clean the patient's blood. Then the blood returns through a specially placed vascular access device (Gore-Tex graft, arteriovenous fistula, or hemodialysis catheter).

Organ transplantation is the replacement of a patient's diseased kidney with a healthy one from a living or cadaver donor of compatible blood and tissue type. The new organ is surgically implanted into the abdomen. Special medications (immunosuppressives) are administered, often for life, to prevent the body from rejecting the transplanted organ. Unlike the other treatments, successful organ transplantation offers patients the potential for restoration of normal kidney function.

BOX 45-1 INDICATIONS FOR DIALYSIS

- Renal failure that can no longer be controlled by conservative management (i.e., dietary modifications and administration of medications to correct electrolyte abnormalities)
- Worsening of uremic syndrome associated with ESRD (i.e., nausea, vomiting, neurological changes, pericarditis)
- Severe electrolyte and/or fluid abnormalities that cannot be controlled by simpler measures (e.g., hyperkalemia, pulmonary edema)

ESRD, End-stage renal disease.

Sociocultural Factors. The degree of privacy needed for urination varies with cultural norms. North Americans expect toilet facilities to be private, whereas some European cultures accept communal toilet facilities. Social expectations (e.g., school recesses) influence the time of urination.

Psychological Factors. Anxiety and emotional stress cause a sense of urgency and increased frequency of urination. Anxiety often prevents a person from being able to urinate completely; as a result, the urge to void returns shortly after voiding. Emotional tension makes it difficult to relax abdominal and perineal muscles. Attempting to void in a public restroom sometimes results in a temporary inability to void. Privacy and adequate time to urinate are usually important to most people.

Fluid Balance. The kidneys primarily maintain the balance between retention and excretion of fluids (see Chapter 41). If fluids and the concentration of electrolytes and solutes are in equilibrium, an increase in fluid intake causes an increase in urine production. This amount varies with food and fluid intake. The volume of urine formed at night is about half of the volume formed during the day because both intake and metabolism decline. **Nocturia** (awakening to void one or more times at night) is often a sign of renal alteration. In a healthy person the intake of water in food and fluids balances the output of water in urine, feces, and insensible losses in perspiration and respiration. An excessive output of urine is **polyuria.** A urine output that is decreased despite normal intake is called **oliguria.** Oliguria often occurs when fluid loss through other means (e.g., perspiration, diarrhea, or vomiting) increases. It also occurs in early kidney disease. Often in severe kidney disease no urine is produced **(anuria).**

Ingestion of certain fluids directly affects urine production and excretion. Coffee, tea, cocoa, and cola drinks that contain caffeine promote increased urine formation **(diuresis).** Alcohol inhibits the release of antidiuretic hormone (ADH), also resulting in increased water loss in urine.

Febrile conditions affect urine production. A patient with excessive perspiration loses a large amount of fluids through insensible water loss, which decreases urine production. Fever causes an increase in body metabolism and accumulation of body wastes. Although urine volume is reduced, it is highly concentrated.

Surgical Procedures. The stress of surgery initially triggers the general adaptation syndrome (see Chapter 37). Preoperative orders of nothing-by-mouth or an underlying disease condition affect fluid balance before surgery, which reduces urine output. In addition, the stress response releases an increased amount of ADH, which increases water resorption. Stress also elevates the level of aldosterone, causing retention of sodium and water. Both of these substances reduce urine output in an effort to maintain circulatory fluid volume.

Anesthetics and narcotic analgesics slow the glomerular filtration rate, reducing urine output. These pharmacological agents also impair sensory and motor impulses traveling among the bladder, spinal cord, and brain. Patients are often unable to sense bladder fullness and initiate or inhibit micturition. Spinal anesthetics, in particular, create the risk of urinary retention because of an inability to sense the need to void and a possible inability of the bladder muscles and urethral sphincters to respond (Lewis et al., 2011).

Surgery of lower abdominal and pelvic structures sometimes impairs urination because of local trauma to surrounding tissues. After returning from surgery involving the ureters, bladder, and urethra, patients routinely have urinary catheters.

Medications. Many medications directly or indirectly contribute to urinary dysfunction. Antipsychotics, antidepressants, alpha-adrenergic agonists, and calcium channel blockers can cause urinary retention and overflow incontinence. Alpha-antagonists, diuretics, sedative hypnotics, opioid analgesics, angiotensin-converting enzyme (ACE) inhibitors, and antihistamines can cause urinary incontinence. Antiparkinson medications may cause urinary urgency and subsequent incontinence. Always consider these medications as the cause of new-onset urinary incontinence, especially in older adults.

Some medications change the color of urine. For example, phenazopyridine (Pyridium) colors the urine a bright orange to rust; amitriptyline causes a green or blue discoloration, whereas levodopa discolors the urine to brown or black. Cancer chemotherapy drugs also color the urine and are often toxic to the bladder and/or kidneys. Patients with impaired kidney function require dosage adjustments in medications excreted by the kidneys.

Diagnostic Examination. Examination of the urinary system influences micturition. Some procedures such as an intravenous pyelogram (IVP) require patients to limit fluids before the test. A restriction in fluid intake commonly lowers urine output. Diagnostic examinations (e.g., cystoscopy) involving direct visualization of urinary structures cause localized edema of the urethral passageway and spasm of the bladder sphincter. After the procedure, a patient may have difficulty voiding or have red or pink urine because of trauma to the urethral or bladder mucosa.

Alterations in Urinary Elimination. Most patients with urinary problems are unable to store urine or fully empty the bladder. These disturbances result from impaired bladder function, obstruction to urine outflow, or inability to voluntarily control micturition.

Some patients may have permanent or temporary changes in the normal pathway of urinary excretion. The surgical formation of a **urinary diversion** temporarily or permanently bypasses the bladder and urethra as the exit routes for urine. Permanent urinary diversions are often necessary in the patient with cancer of the bladder. The patient with a urinary diversion has a **stoma** (artificial opening) on the abdomen to drain urine. He or she has many special needs because urine drains to the outside through a stoma.

Urinary Retention. **Urinary retention** is an accumulation of urine resulting from an inability of the bladder to empty properly. Normally urine production slowly fills the bladder and prevents activation of stretch receptors until it distends to a certain level of stretch. The micturition reflex occurs, and the bladder empties. In urinary retention the bladder is unable to respond to the micturition reflex and thus is unable to empty. Urine continues to collect in the bladder, stretching its walls and causing feelings of pressure, discomfort, tenderness over the symphysis pubis, restlessness, and diaphoresis (sweating).

As retention progresses, retention with overflow develops. Pressure in the bladder builds to a point at which the external urethral sphincter is unable to hold back urine. The sphincter temporarily opens to allow a small volume of urine (25 to 60 mL) to escape. As urine exits, the bladder pressure falls enough to allow the sphincter to regain control and close. With retention a patient may void small amounts of urine 2 or 3 times an hour with no real relief of discomfort or may continually dribble urine. Be aware of the volume and frequency of voiding to assess for urinary retention. Assess the abdomen for evidence of bladder distention and tenderness.

In acute retention key signs are bladder distention and absence of urine output over several hours. A patient under the influence of anesthetics or analgesics often feels only pressure, but the alert patient has severe pain as the bladder distends beyond its normal capacity. In severe urinary retention the bladder holds as much as 2000 to 3000 mL of urine. Retention occurs as a result of urethral obstruction, surgical or childbirth trauma, and alterations in motor and sensory innervation of the bladder such as occurs with neuropathy secondary to diabetes. It may occur after removal of an indwelling catheter. Medication side effects or anxiety may also result in urinary retention. If a patient cannot void or completely empty the bladder, he or she must be catheterized because a UTI, kidney stones, and hyperreflexia can occur.

Retained or **residual urine,** also referred to as *postvoid residual (PVR),* occurs if a patient has urinary retention or cannot empty the bladder completely. You can use a portable noninvasive bladder ultrasound device (bladder scanner) or the technique of straight/intermittent catheterization to assess for PVR. Bladder scanners are often not readily available for nurses to use in all clinical settings, and straight/intermittent catheterization may be the only means to determine bladder urine volume. Regardless of the method used to determine PVR, assess the amount of urine left in the bladder within 10 to 15 minutes after a patient voids (Altschuler and Diaz, 2006). Instruct the patient not to void again before measurement. At least two residuals should be obtained since a patient may empty well one time and not the next. Spastic bladders and some medications and problems such as using a bedpan or not sitting upright to void cause inconsistent emptying. In normal micturition or in a normal void the bladder should empty completely.

Urinary Tract Infections. UTI is the most common health care–acquired infection; 80% of these infections result from the use of an indwelling urethral catheter (Lo et al., 2009). Catheterization results in over 1 million UTIs each year in the United States (Matteucci and Walsh, 2011). Infection frequently occurs after placement of urinary catheters, and each day a catheter is in place there is a 5% increase in bacteria in the urine (Saint et al., 2009). Catheter-associated UTIs (CAUTIs) are associated with increased hospitalizations, increased morbidity and mortality, longer hospital stay, and increased hospital costs (Newman, 2007). Each episode of CAUTI and ensuing complications are estimated to cost between $600 and $2800 (Saint et al., 2009). Because a CAUTI is common, costly, and believed to be reasonably preventable, as of October 1, 2008, the Centers for Medicare and Medicaid Services (CMS) chose it as one of the complications for which hospitals no longer receive additional payment to compensate for the extra cost of treatment (Saint et al., 2009). Consequently there has been a shift in reimbursement practices from its traditional focus on early recognition and prompt treatment to one of prevention (Wilson et al., 2009).

Although several different microorganisms cause CAUTIs, the patient's own colonic flora, including *Escherichia coli,* remains the most common causative pathogen (Ksycki and Namias, 2009). **Bacteriuria** (bacteria in the urine) leads to the spread of organisms into the kidneys and possibly to **bacteremia** or **urosepsis** (bacteria in the bloodstream) (Lewis et al., 2011). Microorganisms commonly enter the urinary tract through the ascending urethral route. Bacteria inhabit the distal urethra and external genitalia in men and women and the vagina in women. Organisms enter the urethral meatus easily and travel up the inner mucosal lining to the bladder. Women are more susceptible to infection because of a short urethra and the proximity of the anus to the urethral meatus.

In men prostatic secretions containing an antibacterial substance and the length of the urethra reduce the susceptibility to UTIs. However, men are at increased risk for infection-related renal disease. Older adults and patients with progressive underlying disease or decreased immunity are also at increased risk.

In a healthy person with good bladder function, organisms are flushed out during voiding. Residual (retained) urine in the bladder becomes more alkaline and is an ideal site for microorganism growth. Any condition resulting in urinary retention such as a kinked, obstructed, or clamped catheter increases the risk of a UTI.

Poor perineal hygiene is another cause of UTIs in women. Inadequate handwashing, failure to wipe from front to back after voiding or defecating, and frequent sexual intercourse predispose women to infection.

Patients with lower UTIs have pain or burning during urination **(dysuria)** as urine flows over inflamed tissues. Fever, chills, nausea, vomiting, and malaise develop as an infection worsens. An irritated bladder **(cystitis)** causes a frequent and urgent sensation of the need to void. Irritation to bladder and urethral mucosa results in blood-tinged urine **(hematuria)**. The urine appears concentrated and cloudy because of the presence of white blood cells (WBCs) or bacteria. If infection spreads to the upper urinary tract (kidneys—**pyelonephritis**), flank pain, tenderness, fever, and chills are common.

Another common cause of infection is the introduction of instruments into the urinary tract. For example, the introduction of a catheter through the urethra provides a direct route for microorganisms (Nazarko, 2008). With an indwelling catheter bacteria ascend along the outside of the catheter on the urethral wall or travel up its lumen. Local irritation to the urethra or bladder predisposes tissues to bacterial invasion.

Urinary Incontinence. **Urinary incontinence** is the involuntary leakage of urine that is sufficient to be a problem. It can be either temporary or permanent, continuous or intermittent. Urinary incontinence related to urinary causes is called either *stress* or *urge urinary incontinence* (Palmer and Newman, 2007). Urge incontinence is more common in younger women and may be caused by local irritating factors such as UTIs (Ebersole et al., 2008). Individuals sense the urge to urinate but cannot keep from urinating long enough to reach a toilet. *Stress incontinence* occurs more often in older women when intraabdominal pressure exceeds urethral resistance. Muscles around the urethra become weak; thus even a small amount of urine may leak spontaneously (Ebersole et al., 2008). Some patients may have a mixed form of incontinence that has features of both stress and urge urinary incontinence. Table 45-5 on p. 1060 describes the types of urinary incontinence, their symptoms, and treatment interventions. **Hyperactive or overactive bladder (OAB)** is associated with individuals of all ages, but older adults are more likely to have incontinence associated with it following physical and cognitive decline associated with aging and effects of medications (Stewart, 2010). OAB results from sudden, involuntary contraction of the muscles of the urinary bladder, resulting in an urge to urinate **(urge incontinence)**. Common abnormalities of the nervous system that cause OAB include cerebrovascular accident (CVA) and other head injuries, spinal cord injury, and diabetic neuropathy. Other causes include UTI and anxiety.

Approximately 15% to 30% of adult women experience urinary incontinence. It is present in as many as 30% to 70% of nursing home residents and in 30% of adults living at home (Touhy and Jett, 2010). Incontinence can impair body image and often leads to a loss of independence. Clothing becomes wet with urine, and the accompanying odor adds to the embarrassment. As a result, patients with this problem often avoid social activities. They often fail to discuss this condition with health care providers or nurses, and as a result urinary incontinence is underreported and undertreated. Resources for information about continence care, patient education, and treatment are available at the following websites: the Society for Urological Nurses and Associates (http://www.suna.org), the National Association for Continence (http://www.nafc.org), and the Simon Foundation (http://www.simonfoundation.org).

Physical limitations and environmental barriers are risks for incontinence. People with restricted mobility have greater chances of being incontinent because of their inability to reach toilet facilities in time. Low-set chairs and beds raised well above the floor are obstacles for people who must get up to reach a toilet. Some patients often lack the energy to walk very far at one time. The toilet is sometimes too far away for patients with urge incontinence. Patients who have difficulty undoing buttons or manipulating zippers face another obstacle.

Continued episodes of incontinence is a risk for impaired skin integrity. The character of urine changes when it remains in contact with skin, causing skin breakdown. The immobilized patient with frequent incontinence is especially at risk for pressure ulcers (see Chapter 48). Additional health care and patient education resources are available at the websites for the American Geriatrics Society (http://www.americangeriatrics.org) or the American Urogynecologic Society (http://www.augs.org).

Urinary Diversions. Conditions such as bladder cancer, radiation injury to the bladder, or chronic urinary infections may necessitate a urinary diversion to drain urine from a diseased or dysfunctional bladder. There are two types of continent urinary diversions (Fig. 45-4, *A*). One is a continent urinary reservoir that is created from a distal portion of the ileum and proximal portion of the colon. The ureters are embedded in the reservoir. This reservoir is situated under the abdominal wall and has a narrow ileal segment brought out through the abdominal wall to form a small stoma. The ileocecal valve creates a one-way valve in the pouch through which a catheter is inserted to empty the urine from the pouch. Patients must be willing and able to catheterize the pouch 4 to 6 times a day for the rest of their lives.

The second continent urinary diversion is an orthotopic neobladder that also uses an ileal pouch to replace the bladder. Anatomically the pouch is in the same position where the bladder was before removal, allowing patients to void normally.

Incontinent urinary diversions are less commonly performed. The surgery involves connecting the ureters to a section of the intestinal ileum with formation of a stoma on the abdominal wall (Fig. 45-4, *B*). Urine drains continuously because a patient has no sensation or control over urinary output, requiring the application of a collection pouch at all times.

Some patients need urinary drainage directly from one or both kidneys. In this case a tube is placed directly into the renal pelvis. This procedure is called a **nephrostomy**.

Any urinary diversion poses threats to a patient's body image. The patient must learn how to manage the diversion, and those who do not have a continent urinary diversion must wear an artificial device at all times. However, most patients are able to wear normal clothing, engage in physical activity, travel, and have sexual relations. Care must be taken not to pull on tubing, especially in a nephrostomy, since it can be pulled out, causing tissue and organ damage and infection. Most nephrostomies are sutured into the kidney.

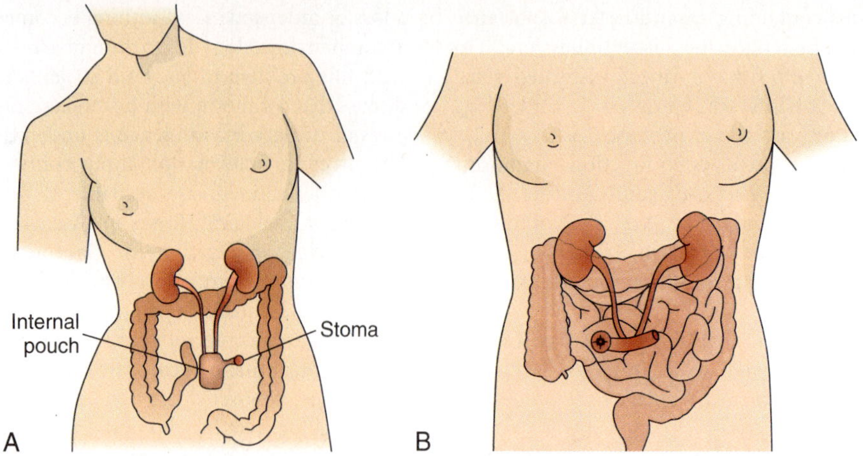

FIG. 45-4 Types of urinary diversions. **A,** Continent urinary reservoir. **B,** Urostomy (ileal conduit).

Refer patients with a urinary diversion to an ostomy nurse (a nurse with specialized education in this area). This specialist is a valuable resource for assisting a patient and family with matters pertaining to all aspects of care. The ostomy nurse often meets with the patient and family before surgery. In addition, refer the patient to the United Ostomy Associations of America (http://www.uoaa.org). This organization provides information about support groups to enhance coping and adaptation to lifestyle and body-image changes.

NURSING KNOWLEDGE BASE

Urinary elimination is a basic function and is usually a private process. Many patients need physiological and psychological assistance from the nurse. Whether a patient has an actual or potential urinary problem, be sensitive to his or her elimination needs. You need knowledge of concepts beyond the anatomy and physiology of the urinary system to give appropriate care. In addition, you need to understand and apply knowledge about infection control principles.

Infection Control and Hygiene

The urinary tract is sterile. Use infection control principles to help prevent the development and spread of UTIs and treat existing infections. *E. coli,* a common bacteria found in feces, causes many CAUTIs. Infection can occur in any location of the urinary tract. Apply knowledge of medical and surgical asepsis when providing care involving the urinary tract or external genitalia (see Chapter 28). Any invasive procedure of the urinary tract such as catheterization requires sterile technique. Procedures such as perineal care or examination of the genitalia require medical asepsis, including proper hand hygiene. Use medical asepsis by wiping off tubing with antiseptic wipes when changing from a large-volume urinary bag to a small-volume leg bag.

Factors Influencing Urination

Factors in a patient's history that normally affect urination are age, environmental factors, medication history, psychological factors, muscle tone, fluid balance, current surgical or diagnostic procedures, and presence of disease conditions. Be alert to individual needs related to normal changes of aging that predispose older adults to certain elimination problems (Box 45-2). Also assess the bowel elimination pattern because constipation often interferes with normal urine elimination (see Chapter 46). Problems with urination also stem from dehydration. Evaluate environmental barriers in the home or health care setting. Aids such as elevated toilet seats, grab bars, or a portable commode are often necessary to ensure patient safety.

BOX 45-2 FOCUS ON OLDER ADULTS

Promoting Urinary Health

- Facilitate more frequent opportunities to void. Older adults have a smaller bladder capacity than younger adults (Ebersole et al., 2008).
- Encourage older adults to empty bladder completely before and after meals and at bedtime (Touhy and Jett, 2010).
- Encourage patient to increase fluid intake to at least six to eight glasses a day unless medically contraindicated. Dilute urine discourages bacterial growth. Discourage drinking of coffee, tea, brown cola, and alcohol since these have a diuretic effect and increase urinary frequency (Touhy and Jett, 2010).
- Make fluids such as cranberry juice available as part of patient's fluid intake. Cranberry juice and vitamin C help acidify the urine to decrease bacterial infections of the bladder (Ebersole et al., 2008).
- Restricting fluid intake does not decrease urinary incontinence severity or frequency (Touhy and Jett, 2010).
- Avoid routine use of indwelling catheters. If one is necessary, use it no longer than necessary. The risk of infection increases dramatically for catheterized patients (Fernandez and Griffiths, 2006).
- Note that incontinence is not a normal part of aging and make efforts to assess incontinence and provide interventions to promote return to continence (Touhy and Jett, 2010).

Growth and Development. Growth and development factors determine a patient's ability to control the act of urination during the life span. Infants and young children cannot effectively concentrate urine. Their urine appears light yellow or clear. In relation to their small body size, infants and children excrete large volumes of urine. For example, a 6-month-old infant who weighs 13 to 18 pounds (6 to 8 kg) excretes 400 to 500 mL of urine daily.

The neurological system is not well developed until 2 to 3 years of age in a normal toddler. Until this age he or she is not able to associate the sensations of bladder filling and urination. A child must be able to recognize the feeling of bladder fullness, to hold urine for 1 to 2 hours, and to communicate the sense of urgency.

Many toddlers are then able to control the external sphincter, and toilet training begins. Daytime control of urination is easier to accomplish than nighttime control and occurs earlier in the child's development, usually by 2 to 3 years of age. Some children do not gain full control until age 4 or 5. Occasional daytime accidents or **nocturnal enuresis** (nighttime voiding without awakening) sometimes continue until age 5 (see Chapter 12).

During pregnancy urinary frequency is common, and susceptibility to UTI increases. Temporary or permanent changes resulting from repeated deliveries or hormonal changes often result in decreased perineal muscle tone, leading to urgency and stress incontinence.

Aging often impairs micturition. In men prostate enlargement usually begins during the 40s and continues throughout life, resulting in urinary frequency and possible urinary retention. In women changes in the urethral mucosa associated with loss of estrogen during and after menopause contribute to increased susceptibility to UTIs (Palmer and Newman, 2007).

Changes in kidney and bladder function also occur with aging. The ability of the kidney to concentrate urine declines. The older adult often experiences nocturia. The bladder loses muscle tone, and capacity decreases, resulting in increased **urinary frequency.** Because the bladder cannot contract effectively, an older adult often retains urine in it after voiding. These changes increase the risk for bacterial growth and development of UTIs.

Muscle Tone. Weak abdominal and pelvic floor muscles impair the ability of the urinary sphincter to maintain tone during increased abdominal pressure. Poor control of micturition or incontinence results from muscle wasting caused by prolonged immobility, muscle damage during vaginal childbirth, being overweight, caffeine use because caffeine relaxes the smooth muscle of the sphincter, muscle atrophy secondary to menopause, or other traumatic damage to pelvic nerves and muscles.

CRITICAL THINKING

Successful critical thinking requires synthesis of knowledge, experience, information gathered from patients, critical thinking attitudes, and intellectual and professional standards. Clinical judgments require you to collect necessary information, analyze the data, and anticipate and make decisions regarding patient care.

During assessment consider all elements that build toward making appropriate nursing diagnoses. In the case of urinary elimination, integrate knowledge from nursing and other disciplines, previous experiences, and information gathered from patients to understand the process of urinary elimination and the impact on a patient and family. As a result, you are able to identify the unique impact of these problems on patients and families.

In addition, use critical thinking attitudes such as perseverance to find a plan of care to provide successful management of urinary elimination problems. Professional standards provide valuable directions for management. You are in a key position to serve as a patient advocate by suggesting noninvasive alternatives to catheterization use (e.g., the use of a bladder scanner to evaluate urine volume without invasive instrumentation or implementation of a voiding schedule for the incontinent patient).

When planning and implementing care for the patient with alterations in urinary elimination, also use standards developed by professional organizations such as the American Nurses Association (ANA), the International Continence Society (ICS), and the United Ostomy Associations of America as a guide for individualized patient care.

NURSING PROCESS

Apply the nursing process and use a critical thinking approach in the care of patients. The nursing process provides a clinical decision-making approach for you to develop and implement an individualized plan of care.

ASSESSMENT

During the assessment process, thoroughly assess each patient and critically analyze findings to ensure that you make patient-centered clinical decisions required for safe nursing care.

Through the Patient's Eyes. Throughout the assessment process it is important to consider the patient's frame of reference of his or her illness experience. Also consider whether the patient understands his or her health status along with his or her self-care ability. Value the patient's expertise with his or her own health and symptoms. Consider the patient's cognitive ability to understand the signs and symptoms of the illness. Remember that you are in partnership with the patient or designated surrogates in planning, implementing, and evaluating care. Always ask what he or she expects from care. Does the patient expect that the UTI will be resolved?

Make sure that your approach to a patient's elimination needs considers personal, social, and gender habits. Be sensitive and ask questions in a straightforward manner. Gender influences positioning for urination: males stand, whereas females sit. Place patients in a position of comfort. Some men who cannot stand to urinate become overly distressed. Gender differences also affect risk factors associated with urinary alterations. If a patient prefers privacy, try to prevent interruptions as he or she voids. Treat all patients with understanding and acceptance.

Be aware of your own attitudes and values about working with patients from diverse ethnic, social, and cultural backgrounds. Know that culture influences the choice of appropriate nursing interventions. In some cultures the embarrassment related to urinary elimination problems is so great that many patients, especially women, refuse to seek treatment. In some cultures patients prefer to squat over a receptacle rather than sit on one. Culture dictates when and where it is appropriate to urinate. It also determines whether it is proper for a male to care for the urinary needs of a female or if gender-congruent care is needed (see Chapter 9).

Identifying Urinary Alterations. To identify a urinary elimination problem and gather data for a care plan, use scientific and nursing knowledge, conduct a nursing history, perform a physical assessment, assess the patient's urine, and review information from diagnostic tests and examinations. Use critical thinking to synthesize this information as assessment proceeds (Fig. 45-5). Adequate assessment results in the formulation of nursing diagnoses appropriate for alterations in urinary elimination. When assessing for problems with urinary elimination, be aware of the impact of the patient's culture and language in the assessment process (Box 45-3).

Nursing History. The nursing history includes a review of a patient's elimination patterns and symptoms of urinary alterations and an assessment of other factors that possibly affect the ability to urinate normally. Use questions to help direct the patient to focus on specific urinary problems (Box 45-4).

Pattern of Urination. Ask the patient about daily voiding patterns, including frequency and times of day, normal volume at each voiding, and any recent changes. Frequency varies among individuals and with intake and other types of fluid losses. The common times for urination are on awakening, after meals, and before

Knowledge
- Physiology of fluid balance
- Anatomy and physiology of normal urine production and urination
- Pathophysiology of selected urinary alterations
- Factors affecting urination
- Principles of communication used to address issues related to self-concept and sexuality

Experience
- Caring for patients with alterations in urinary elimination
- Caring for patients at risk for urinary infection
- Personal experience with changes in urinary elimination

ASSESSMENT
- Gather nursing history for the patient's urination pattern, symptoms, and factors affecting urination
- Conduct physical assessment of the patient's body systems potentially affected by urinary change
- Assess characteristics of urine
- Assess the patient's perception of urinary problems as it affects self-concept and sexuality
- Gather relevant laboratory and diagnostic test data

Standards
- Maintain the patient's privacy and dignity
- Apply intellectual standards to ensure patient history and assessment are complete and in depth
- Apply professional standards of care from professional organizations such as ANA, International Continence Society (ICS), United Ostomy Associations of America

Attitudes
- Display humility in recognizing limitations in knowledge
- Establish trust with the patient to reveal full picture of this potentially sensitive area of assessment

FIG. 45-5 Critical thinking model for urinary elimination assessment. *ANA,* American Nurses Association.

bedtime. Most people void an average of 5 or more times a day. Some patients who void frequently during the night may have renal disease, prostate enlargement, or cardiac disease. Information about the pattern of urination establishes a baseline for comparison.

Symptoms of Urinary Alterations. Certain symptoms specific to urinary alterations may occur in more than one type of disorder. During assessment ask the patient about any symptoms related to urination (Table 45-1). Also assess whether the patient is aware of conditions or factors that precipitate or aggravate symptoms and determine what the patient does when any of these symptoms occur.

BOX 45-3 CULTURAL ASPECTS OF CARE

Urinary Elimination

Urine elimination is a personal, private activity that individuals do not share with others. When patients have needs related to urine elimination, be aware of the intrusive nature of intervention. Because of the embarrassing nature of urinary problems such as incontinence, many women do not report symptoms (Beji et al., 2010; Gemmill and Wells, 2010). In addition, other characteristics such as a patient's culture also affect care. Although you cannot be knowledgeable about the impact of every culture on patient care, it is important to be open to and respect practices different from your own.

Implications for Practice
- When English is a second language, use simple and clear sentences in communicating with patients. Remember, speaking louder or more slowly does not always help. Learn at least a few important words in the patient's language to allow for future interchanges. In some situations an interpreter is needed (Giger and Davidhizar, 2008).
- If available, provide written materials in patient's primary language. If not, provide the English version. Some patients are able to read better than they understand the spoken word. Time to review the information also increases understanding.
- In some cultures intimate contact or discussion of urinary problems between genders is forbidden outside marriage. Urological care, whether involving questions, discussion, or contact, is usually considered intimate care. Gender-congruent caregivers are assigned to a patient from these cultures (e.g., Muslim) (Beji et al., 2010; Giger and Davidhizar, 2010).
- Cultures view disease differently. It is important to understand how the culture views the cause and treatment of the condition and how traditional Western medicine may or may not fit with that understanding. Programs to help with urinary problems need to be adapted to the cultural values of the woman seeking assistance (Bradway et al., 2010).
- Cultures allow for varied involvement of family in a patient's care. This source of strength is important to the health of the patient, and family must be included in the plan of care (Giger and Davidhizar, 2008).
- Cultural influences may affect the willingness of a patient to seek care. Be aware of topics that specific cultures may find offensive, which can make discussion of nursing interventions difficult (Giger and Davidhizar, 2008).

Note the presence of an indwelling catheter. It places a patient at risk for infection, catheter blockage, or skin-care problems. Monitor fluid balance through regular intake and output (I&O) measurements (see Chapter 41). Patients with a urinary diversion sometimes need special assistance to maintain adequate urine elimination and skin care integrity.

Physical Assessment. A physical examination (see Chapter 30) provides you with data to determine the presence and severity of urinary elimination problems. The primary structures to assess include the skin and mucosal membranes, kidneys, bladder, and urethral meatus. Fluid intake and the pattern and amounts, which are objective data, are important to assess (see Chapter 41).

Skin and Mucosal Membranes. Observe the condition of the skin and mucosal membranes. Problems with urinary elimination are frequently associated with fluid and electrolyte disturbances. By assessing skin turgor and the oral mucosa you gather data about the patient's hydration status. Urinary incontinence increases the risk for skin breakdown. Observe the perineum for rashes, blistering, irritation, and breakdown.

Kidneys. Nurses with advanced examination skills learn to palpate the kidneys during abdominal examination. The position, shape, and size of the kidneys reveal problems such as tumors;

BOX 45-4 NURSING ASSESSMENT QUESTIONS

Nature of the Problem
- What type of problems are you having with urination?
- Describe a recent day and or night when you were having urinary problems.
- Has this pattern remained constant, or do you have different patterns on different days or nights?

Signs and Symptoms
- Do you have urgency (i.e., feeling as though you have to void immediately)?
- Do you ever lose urine when you cough or sneeze?
- Does leakage occur at other times?

Onset and Duration
- When did you first notice a problem?
- How long has this problem lasted?

Severity
- How many times a day or night do you void or have leakage?
- How does this pattern compare with the pattern you last remember?
- What do you do when the symptoms occur?

Predisposing Factors
- Have you ever had a vaginal birth? More than once?
- Do you notice what you are doing at the time of urinary incidents?
- Do your symptoms increase after eating or drinking food with caffeine or alcohol?
- Which medications do you take routinely, and have any recently changed?
- Do you have a physical illness that may interfere with your usual urinary pattern?

Effect on Patient
- How have these symptoms affected your life?
- Have you had to change any of your usual activities?
- Have you sought any health care assistance with this problem?

TABLE 45-1 Common Types of Urinary Alterations

SYMPTOMS	DESCRIPTIONS	CAUSES OR ASSOCIATED FACTORS
Urgency	Feeling of need to void immediately	Full bladder, bladder irritation or inflammation from infection, overactive bladder, psychological stress
Dysuria	Painful or difficult urination	Bladder inflammation, trauma or inflammation of urethral sphincter
Frequency	Voiding at frequent intervals (less than 2 hours)	Increased fluid intake, bladder inflammation, increased pressure on bladder (pregnancy), diuretic therapy
Hesitancy	Difficulty initiating urination	Prostate enlargement, anxiety, urethral edema
Polyuria	Voiding large amounts of urine	Excess fluid intake, diabetes mellitus or insipidus, use of diuretics, postobstructive diuresis
Oliguria	Diminished urinary output relative to intake (usually 400 mL/24 hr)	Dehydration, renal failure, UTI, increased ADH secretion, heart failure
Nocturia	Voiding one or more times at night	Excessive fluid intake before bed (especially coffee or alcohol), renal disease, aging process, prostate enlargement
Dribbling	Leakage of urine despite voluntary control of urination	Stress incontinence, overflow from urinary retention (e.g., from BPH)
Incontinence	Involuntary loss of urine	Multiple factors: Unstable urethra, loss of pelvic muscle tone, fecal impaction, neurological impairment, overactive bladder
Hematuria	Blood in urine	Neoplasms of kidney or bladder, glomerular disease, infection of kidney or bladder, trauma to urinary structures, calculi, bleeding disorders
Retention	Accumulation of urine in bladder, with inability of bladder to empty fully	Urethral obstruction (stricture), decreased sensory activity, neurogenic bladder, prostate enlargement, postanesthesia effects, side effects of medications (e.g., anticholinergics, opioids)
Residual urine	Volume of urine remaining after voiding (≥100 mL)	Inflammation or irritation of bladder mucosa from infection, neurogenic bladder, prostate enlargement, trauma, or inflammation of urethra

ADH, Antidiuretic hormone; *BPH,* benign prostatic hyperplasia; *UTI,* urinary tract infection.

whereas tenderness indicates inflammation. Auscultation is sometimes performed to detect the presence of a renal artery bruit (sound resulting from turbulent blood flow through a narrowed artery).

Bladder. In adults the bladder rests below the symphysis pubis. When it is distended, it rises above the symphysis pubis at the midline of the abdomen and often extends to just below the umbilicus. On inspection you may note a swelling or convex curvature of the lower abdomen. Gently palpate the lower abdomen. The partially filled bladder normally feels smooth and rounded. Gentle palpation on a distended bladder causes the patient to feel the urge to urinate, tenderness, or even pain. Percussion of a full bladder yields a dull percussion note.

Urethral Meatus. Observe the urinary meatus for any discharge, inflammation, and lesions. To examine the female, a dorsal recumbent position provides full exposure of the genitalia. While wearing clean gloves, retract the labial folds to see the urethral meatus. Normally it is pink, it appears as a small slitlike opening below the clitoris and above the vaginal orifice, and there is no discharge; if discharge is present, obtain specimens of urethral discharge before the patient voids.

Women with vaginal infections are susceptible to UTIs because it is easy for the drainage to travel to the urethral meatus. If yeast (candidiasis) is found in urine, it is important to inspect the vagina, in the groin area, under the breasts, and in the mouth for the source. It needs to be treated to keep UTI from yeast recurring. Older women may have vaginitis as a result of estrogen deficiency. Inspect the vaginal orifice carefully for signs of inflammation and describe any drainage.

A man's urethral meatus is normally a small opening at the tip of the penis. Inspect the meatus for discharge, inflammation, and lesions. It is necessary to retract the foreskin in uncircumcised men to see the meatus. Wear clean gloves when retracting the foreskin. Be sure to replace it after the examination is complete to prevent swelling of the tissue around the glans of the penis.

Assessment of Urine. Assessment of urine involves measuring patients' fluid I&O and observing characteristics of their urine.

Intake and Output. Assess the patient's average daily fluid intake. If you need an accurate measurement of fluid intake from the patient who is at home, ask him or her to estimate his or her intake by showing a measurement on a commonly used glass or cup.

In a health care setting measure a patient's fluid intake either when the health care provider orders I&O measurements or when you judge that measurement is needed (see Chapter 41). A change in urine volume is a significant indicator of fluid alterations or kidney disease. While caring for the patient, use a graduated receptacle to measure urinary output from a bedpan or urinal after each voiding. Special receptacles (urimeters) that attach between indwelling catheters and drainage bags are a convenient means of accurately measuring urine volume. A urimeter holds 100 to 200 mL of urine. After measuring urine from a urimeter, drain the cylinder into the urinary drainage bag or into a receptacle for disposal. Use urimeters when precise hourly measurements of urine are necessary.

When you measure urine from a drainage bag, the use of a separate plastic graduated measuring receptacle obtains a more precise measurement of urine output (Fig. 45-6). Each patient needs to have a graduated receptacle for his or her exclusive use to prevent potential cross-contamination. Label each container with patient name. The container needs to be rinsed after emptying, and the tubing that drains the bag securely clamped and cleaned with alcohol before putting it back in the holder.

Report any extreme increase or decrease in urine volume. An individual's daily output generally ranges from 1200 to 1500 mL of urine (Hall, 2011). An hourly output of less than 30 mL for more than 2 consecutive hours is cause for concern. Similarly, you need to report consistently high volumes of urine (polyuria) (i.e., over 2000 to 2500 mL daily).

Characteristics of Urine. Inspect the patient's urine for color, clarity, and odor.

Color. Normal urine ranges from a pale, straw color to amber, depending on its concentration. Urine is usually more concentrated in the morning or with fluid volume deficits. As a person drinks more fluids, urine becomes less concentrated.

Bleeding from the kidneys or ureters causes dark red urine; bleeding from the bladder or urethra causes bright red urine. Various medications and foods also change urine color. For example, phenazopyridine, a urinary analgesic, colors urine bright orange. Eating beets, rhubarb, or blackberries causes red urine. Special dyes used in intravenous diagnostic studies eventually discolor urine.

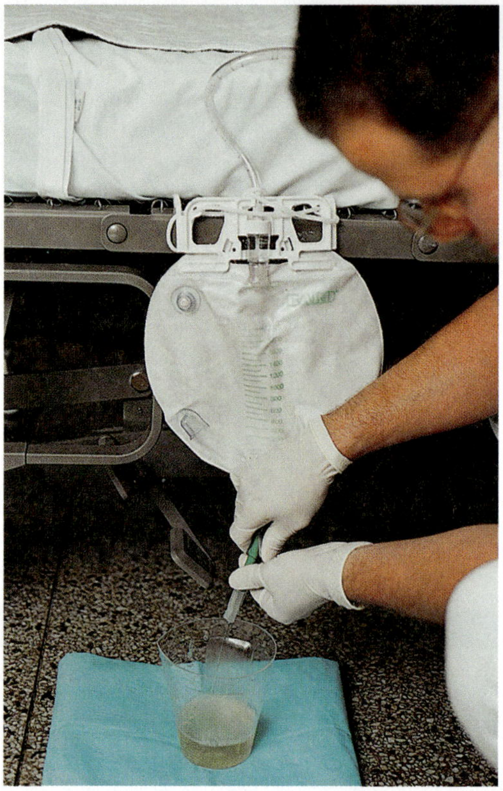

FIG. 45-6 Urine drainage bag.

Dark amber urine is the result of high concentrations of bilirubin caused by liver dysfunction. Document and report any abnormal color or sediment, especially if the cause is unknown.

Clarity. Normal urine appears transparent at voiding. Urine that stands in a container becomes cloudy. Freshly voided urine in patients with renal disease appears cloudy or foamy because of high protein concentrations. Urine may also appear thick and cloudy as a result of bacteria and WBCs.

Odor. Urine has a characteristic odor. The more concentrated the urine, the stronger the odor. Stagnant urine has an ammonia odor, which is common in patients who are repeatedly incontinent. A sweet or fruity odor occurs from acetone or acetoacetic acid (by-products of incomplete fat metabolism) seen with diabetes mellitus or starvation. Some food and medications can affect the odor of urine (e.g., asparagus and amoxicillin). A foul odor is often associated with a possible infection.

Urine Testing. Nurses often collect urine specimens for laboratory testing. The type of test determines the method of collection. Label all specimens with the patient's name, date, and time of collection. Transport specimens to the laboratory in a timely fashion to ensure accuracy of test results. Agency infection control policies require the adherence to standard precautions by all personnel during specimen handling (see Chapter 34).

Specimen Collection. The nurse collects random, clean-voided or midstream, sterile, and timed specimens (Table 45-2). The method of collection varies based on a patient's developmental level and the type of specimen ordered.

Urine Collection in Children. Specimen collection from infants and children is often difficult. Adolescents and school-age children are usually able to cooperate, although some are embarrassed. Preschool children and toddlers have difficulty voiding on request. It often helps to offer the child fluids 30 minutes before requesting a

TABLE 45-2 **Urine Testing**

COLLECTION TYPE/ USE OF SPECIMEN	NURSING CONSIDERATIONS
Random (routine urinalysis)	Collect during normal voiding or from an indwelling catheter or urinary diversion collection bag. Do not collect from an indwelling catheter drainage bag. Use a clean specimen cup.
Clean-voided or midstream (culture and sensitivity)	See Skill 45-1 on pp. 1068-1070. Use a sterile specimen cup.
Sterile specimen (culture and sensitivity)	If the patient has an indwelling catheter, collect a sterile specimen by using aseptic technique through the special sampling port (Fig. 45-7) found on the side of the catheter. Clamp the tubing below the port, allowing fresh, uncontaminated urine to collect in the tube. After wiping the port with an antimicrobial swab, insert a sterile syringe hub and withdraw at least 3 to 5 mL of urine (check agency policy). Using sterile aseptic technique, transfer the urine to a sterile container (see Chapter 28).
Timed urine specimens (for measuring levels of adrenocortical steroids or hormones, creatinine clearance, or protein quantity tests)	Time required may be 2-, 12-, or 24-hour collections. The timed period begins after the patient urinates and ends with a final voiding at the end of the time period. The patient voids into a clean receptacle, and the urine is transferred to the special collection container, which often contains special preservatives. Each specimen must be free of feces and toilet tissue. Missed specimens make the whole collection inaccurate. Check with agency policy and the laboratory for specific instructions.

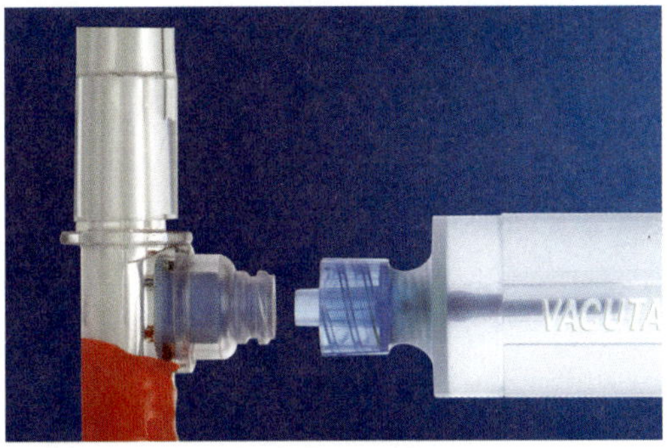

FIG. 45-7 Urine specimen collection: aspiration from a collection port in drainage tubing of indwelling catheter (needleless technique). (Courtesy and © Becton, Dickinson and Company).

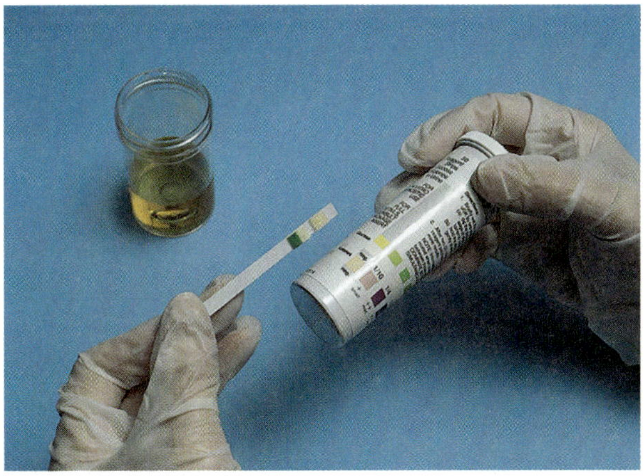

FIG. 45-8 Checking results of chemical reagent strip dipped in urine.

specimen. You need to use terms for urination that the child is able understand. A young child is often reluctant to void in unfamiliar receptacles. A potty chair or specimen hat placed under the toilet seat is usually effective. You will need to use special collection devices for infants or toddlers who are not toilet trained. You can attach clear plastic, single-use bags with self-adhering material over the child's urethral meatus. Do not obtain specimens by squeezing urine from the diaper because the results will be inaccurate.

Common Urine Tests

Urinalysis. The laboratory performs a **urinalysis** on a specimen obtained by any of the previously described methods. Table 45-3 lists normal values for a urinalysis. A lab examines specimens as soon as possible, preferably within 2 hours. Make sure that it is the first voided specimen in the morning to ensure a uniform concentration of constituents. For a quick screening perform certain portions of the urinalysis with special reagent strips. Dip the strips into the urine and observe for a color change in the time interval designated on the package (Fig. 45-8).

Specific Gravity. The **specific gravity** is the weight or degree of concentration of a substance compared with an equal volume of water. Pour a urine specimen into a special clean, dry cylinder. The weighted urinometer is suspended in the cylinder of urine. The concentration of dissolved substances in the urine aids in determination of a patient's fluid balance. This measurement is always part of a complete urinalysis. Nurses in critical care units are often responsible for doing periodic measurements of urine specific gravity (see Table 45-3).

If questions regarding the accuracy of specific gravity measurements arise, obtain a urine osmolality test. Although both tests measure urine concentration, the osmolality test is more accurate because it measures the total number of particles in a solution (see Chapter 41).

Urine Culture. A urine culture requires a sterile or clean-voided sample of urine. It takes approximately 24 to 48 hours before the laboratory can report findings of bacterial growth. While awaiting results, a broad-spectrum antibiotic is sometimes ordered as soon as a culture has been obtained. The test for sensitivity determines which specific antibiotics are effective. The results (sensitivities) of a urine culture may show that another antibiotic would be more effective. In this case a new antibiotic is ordered.

Diagnostic Examinations. The urinary system is one of the few organ systems amenable to accurate diagnostic study by several

View Video!

TABLE 45-3 Routine Urinalysis

MEASUREMENT AND NORMAL VALUE	INTERPRETATION
pH (4.6-8.0)	pH of urine indicates acid-base balance. An acid pH helps protect against bacterial growth. Urine that stands for several hours becomes alkaline.
Protein (none or up to 8 mg/100 mL)	Normally protein is not present in urine. It is common in renal disease because damage to glomeruli or tubules allows it to enter urine.
Glucose (none)	Patients with diabetes mellitus often have glucose in urine as a result of inability of tubules to resorb high glucose concentrations (>180 mg/100 mL). Ingestion of high concentrations of glucose causes some glucose to appear in urine of healthy persons.
Ketones (none)	Patients whose diabetes mellitus is poorly controlled experience breakdown of fatty acids. End products of fat metabolism are ketones. Some patients with dehydration, starvation, or excessive aspirin usage also have *ketonuria.*
Blood	A positive test for occult blood occurs when intact erythrocytes, hemoglobin, or myoglobin is present. Blood in a routine urine specimen in a woman may be a result of contamination with menstrual fluid.
Specific gravity (1.0053-1.030)	Specific gravity measures concentration of particles in urine. High specific gravity reflects concentrated urine, and low specific gravity reflects diluted urine. Dehydration, reduced renal blood flow, and increased ADH secretion elevate specific gravity. Overhydration, early renal disease, and inadequate ADH secretion reduce specific gravity.
Microscopic Examination	
RBCs (up to 2)	Damage to glomeruli or tubules allows RBCs to enter the urine. Trauma, disease, or surgery of the lower urinary tract also causes blood to be present.
WBCs (0-4 per low-power field)	Greater numbers indicate urinary tract infection.
Bacteria (none)	Bacteria indicate urinary tract infection. (Patients do not always have symptoms.)
Casts (none)	Casts are cylindrical bodies the shapes of which take on likeness of objects within the renal tubule. Types include hyaline, WBCs, RBCs, granular cells, and epithelial cells. Their increased presence is always an abnormal finding and indicates renal alterations.
Crystals (none)	Crystals are the result of food metabolism. Excess crystals such as uric acid or calcium phosphate result in renal stone formation.

Data from Pagana KD, Pagana TJ: *Mosby's diagnostic and laboratory test reference,* ed 10, St Louis, 2011, Mosby.
ADH, Antidiuretic hormone; *RBCs,* red blood cells; *WBCs,* white blood cells.

radiographic techniques. The two approaches for visualization of urinary structures, direct and indirect techniques, are either quite simple or very complex, requiring extensive nursing intervention. These procedures are further subdivided into invasive or noninvasive categories (Table 45-4).

Many of the nursing responsibilities related to diagnostic examinations of the urinary tract are common to many of the studies. The common responsibilities before the study include the following:

- Obtain a signed consent (check agency policy)
- Assess patient for history of any allergies and whether they have had a previous reaction to a contrast agent (Schabelman and Witting, 2010). Allergic individuals in general (including individuals with asthma) are at mildly increased risk for developing adverse reactions to radiocontrast media (Beaty, Lieberman, and Slavin, 2008).
- Administer bowel-cleaning medications as ordered (check agency policy)
- Ensure that patient receives appropriate pretest diet (clear liquids) or nothing by mouth (NPO) as needed

The common responsibilities following the study include the following:

- Assessing I&O
- Observing characteristics of urine (color, clarity, presence of blood)
- Encouraging fluid intake, especially if using radiopaque dye

NURSING DIAGNOSIS

A thorough assessment of a patient's urinary elimination function reveals patterns of data that allow a nurse to make relevant and accurate nursing diagnoses. Use critical thinking to reflect on knowledge of previous patients, apply knowledge of urinary function and the effects of disorders, review defining characteristics, and make a specific nursing diagnosis. Data from questions about the urinary system are important in identifying nursing diagnoses. The diagnosis focuses on a specific urinary elimination alteration or an associated problem such as *impaired skin integrity related to urinary incontinence.* Identification of defining characteristics leads to selection of an appropriate diagnosis. An important part of formulating nursing diagnoses is identifying the relevant causative or related factor. You choose interventions that treat or modify the related factor for the diagnosis to be resolved. Specifying related factors for each diagnosis allows selection of individualized nursing interventions (Ackley and Ladwig, 2011). For example, *impaired skin integrity related to incontinence* requires interventions such as a toileting schedule or assisting the patient to the toilet at frequent intervals. In contrast, *impaired skin integrity related to inability to change positions* requires interventions such as placing the patient on a turning schedule. Box 45-5 provides an example of diagnostic reasoning. Some nursing diagnoses common to patients with urine elimination alterations include the following:

TABLE 45-4 Diagnostic Examinations

NAME OF PROCEDURE	PURPOSE AND METHOD OF PROCEDURE	SPECIAL NURSING CONSIDERATIONS
Noninvasive Procedures		
Abdominal roentgenogram (plain film; kidney, ureter, bladder [KUB], or flat plate)	Determine the size, shape, symmetry, and location of the kidneys.	No special preparation or precautions are required.
Computerized axial tomography (CT) scan	Obtain detailed images of structures within a selected plane of the body. The computer reconstructs cross-sectional image and thus allows the health care provider to view pathological conditions such as tumors and obstructions.	Bowel cleaning per agency or health care provider preference. Assess for shellfish (iodine) allergy if a CT scan with contrast is ordered. Prepare patient for the procedure (e.g., patient is placed into a large machine and needs to lie still; feelings of claustrophobia in some patients).
Intravenous pyelogram (IVP)	View the collecting ducts and renal pelvis and outline the ureters, bladder, and urethra. A special intravenous injection (iodine-based) that converts to a dye in urine is injected intravenously.	Bowel cleaning is completed per agency or health care provider preference. Only clear liquids are permitted until after test is completed. Assess patient for any allergies before test. After test encourage fluid intake to dilute and flush dye from patient. Observe for late symptoms of allergy (e.g., rash).
Ultrasound		
Renal	Identify gross renal structures and structural abnormalities in the kidney using high-frequency, inaudible sound waves.	No bowel cleaning needed.
Bladder	Identify structural abnormalities of bladder or lower urinary tract. It is also used to estimate the volume of urine in the bladder.	If needed, ask patient to drink fluids before the test to cause bladder distention for better results. No special care is necessary after either study.
Urodynamic testing (uroflowmetry)	Determine bladder muscle function and evaluate causes of urinary incontinence. Generally the patient urinates into a toilet equipped with a funnel and uroflowmeter. Voiding activates the uroflowmeter, and electronic data are recorded and analyzed.	The nurse explains the procedure to the patient. After the test, provide materials for perineal hygiene.
Invasive Procedures		
Endoscopy-cystoscopy	Provide direct visualization, specimen collection, and/or treatment of the interior of the bladder and urethra. Although this procedure is usually performed using local anesthesia, general anesthesia or conscious sedation is more common to avoid unnecessary anxiety and trauma for the patient. Surgery on the male prostate is also performed using a special endoscope.	Obtain signed consent. Complete a bowel cleaning if ordered. Follow agency policy for preoperative preparation and checklist (see Chapter 50). After patient's return assess the vital signs and the characteristics of urine; monitor intake and output (I&O); encourage fluids; and observe for fever, dysuria, and pain in suprapubic region.
Arteriogram (angiography)	Visualize the renal arteries and/or their branches to detect narrowing or occlusion. A catheter is placed in one of the femoral arteries and introduced up to the level of the renal arteries. Radiopaque contrast is injected through the catheter while x-ray film images are taken in rapid succession.	Obtain signed consent. Assess for any allergy. Follow agency preprocedure checklist. After the procedure monitor vital signs frequently until stable. Patient maintains bed rest for prescribed time interval. Encourage fluids to flush the contrast from the system. Also monitor the affected extremity for neurocirculatory function (pulse, skin temperature, sensation, and movement) and observe catheter site for bleeding, swelling, increased tenderness, or hematoma formation. Notify health care provider immediately of any postprocedure abnormality.

Modified from Pagana KD, Pagana TJ: *Mosby's diagnostic and laboratory test reference,* ed 10, St Louis, 2011, Mosby.

- Social isolation
- Disturbed body image
- Urinary incontinence (functional, stress, urge, overflow)
- Pain (acute, chronic)
- Risk for infection
- Toileting self-care deficit
- Impaired skin integrity
- Impaired urinary elimination
- Constipation
- Urinary retention

BOX 45-5 NURSING DIAGNOSTIC PROCESS

Stress Urinary Incontinence Related to Weakened Pelvic Musculature

ASSESSMENT ACTIVITIES	DEFINING CHARACTERISTICS
Have patient describe situations that accompany urine leakage.	Patient states that she "loses a little urine" whenever she sneezes, coughs, or laughs. Patient states she has been having problems for the past 2 years.
Observe patient behavior.	Patient wears a menstrual minipad continuously. Patient is reluctant to interact with others and tries not to cough or laugh.
Review medical history.	Patient is postmenopausal after three vaginal births.

PLANNING

During planning integrate the knowledge from assessment and information about available resources and therapies to develop an individualized plan of care (see the Nursing Care Plan). Match the patient's needs with clinical and professional standards recommended in the literature (Fig. 45-9). Building a relationship of trust with patients is important because the implementation of care involves interaction of a very personal nature.

Goals and Outcomes. The plan of care for urinary elimination alterations must include realistic and individualized goals along with relevant outcomes. The nurse and the patient need to collaborate in setting goals and outcomes and ultimately in choosing nursing interventions. A general goal is often normal urinary elimination; but sometimes the individual goal differs, depending on the problem. The goals are short or long term. For example, urinary retention following surgery requires a short-term goal: "Patient will have normal voiding with complete bladder emptying within 24 hours." Relevant expected outcomes for this goal include the following:

- Patient will void within 4 hours.
- Urinary output of 300 mL or greater will occur with each voiding.
- Patient's bladder is not distended to palpation.

Conversely, the patient with stress incontinence often has a long-term goal that depends on weeks of pelvic floor muscle exercise to achieve urinary control: "Patient will achieve full urinary continence within 8 weeks after start of exercise program (Kegel)." Make sure that goals are reasonably achievable and relevant to the patient's situation.

Setting Priorities. Urinary elimination is a personal and intimate activity. Establish a relationship with the patient that allows discussion and intervention. While you are collaborating with the patient, his or her priorities become apparent, and he or she should develop an understanding of all the goals.

When a patient has multiple nursing diagnoses (Fig. 45-10), it is important to recognize the primary health problem and its influence on other problems. In the example of the patient with chronic confusion, the resultant incontinence creates several risks. Focusing on the management of incontinence resolves more than one nursing diagnosis. Although physical needs appear to have higher priority, the psychological needs related to self-esteem or sexuality are sometimes a higher priority for the patient. Attention

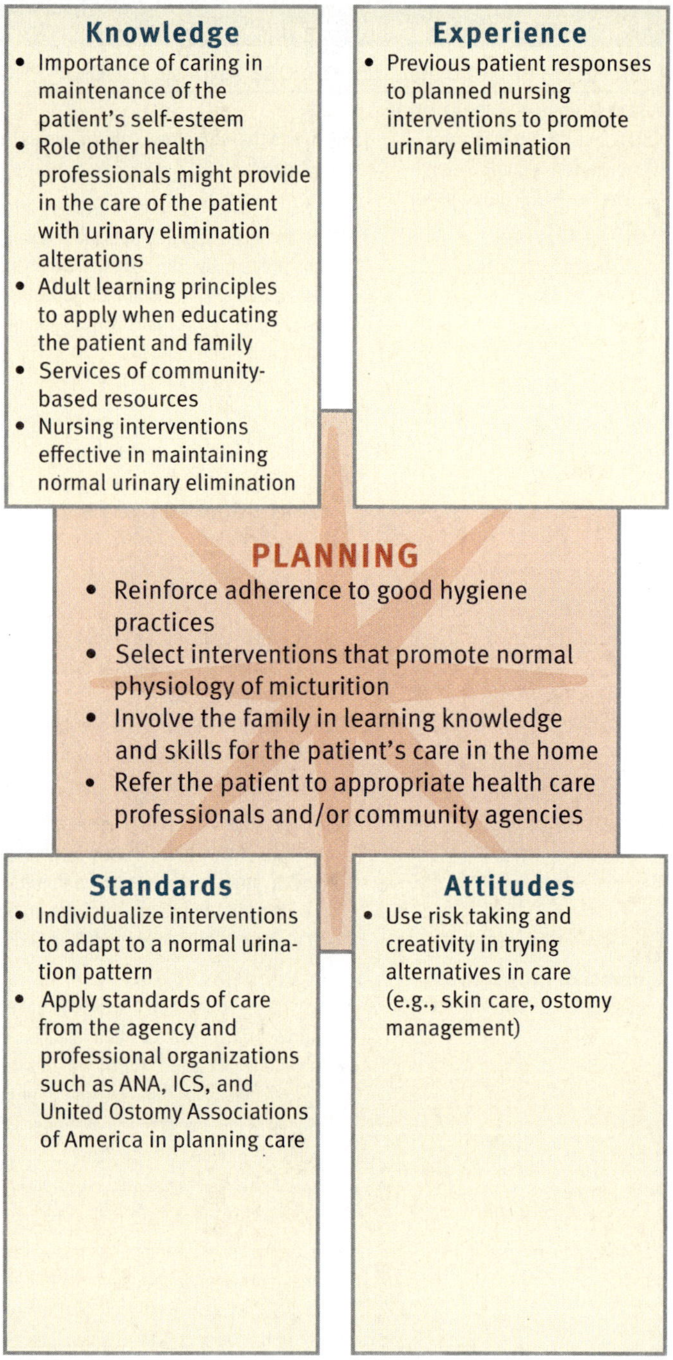

Knowledge
• Importance of caring in maintenance of the patient's self-esteem
• Role other health professionals might provide in the care of the patient with urinary elimination alterations
• Adult learning principles to apply when educating the patient and family
• Services of community-based resources
• Nursing interventions effective in maintaining normal urinary elimination
Experience
• Previous patient responses to planned nursing interventions to promote urinary elimination
PLANNING
• Reinforce adherence to good hygiene practices
• Select interventions that promote normal physiology of micturition
• Involve the family in learning knowledge and skills for the patient's care in the home
• Refer the patient to appropriate health care professionals and/or community agencies
Standards
• Individualize interventions to adapt to a normal urination pattern
• Apply standards of care from the agency and professional organizations such as ANA, ICS, and United Ostomy Associations of America in planning care
Attitudes
• Use risk taking and creativity in trying alternatives in care (e.g., skin care, ostomy management)

FIG. 45-9 Critical thinking model for urinary elimination planning. *ANA,* American Nurses Association; *ICS,* International Continence Society.

to the patient's perceived needs is the most satisfactory and successful approach to accomplishing all the goals. Reinforcement of good health habits that are already followed improves compliance with the care plan.

Teamwork and Collaboration. Incorporate individualized health promotion activities and therapeutic interventions to meet the patient's needs. Consider the patient's home environment and normal elimination routines when planning therapies. Collaborate with several health care disciplines, the patient, and the patient's family. For example, a nurse specialist in urinary continence teaches pelvic floor exercises, whereas a physical therapist designs an

NURSING CARE PLAN

Stress Urinary Incontinence

ASSESSMENT

Mrs. Kay, the nurse, is seeing Mrs. Grayson, a 55-year-old woman, for symptoms of urinary incontinence. Mrs. Grayson is postmenopausal, has a history of three vaginal births, and is "overweight." She lives with her husband, and her three grown children live nearby. Mrs. Grayson works as a secretary for a local social service agency. She confided to her gynecological practitioner that uncontrollable urine leakage has affected her life. Mrs. Kay's assessment includes a discussion of Mrs. Grayson's current health status with emphasis on her urinary concerns.

Assessment Activities	*Findings/Defining Characteristics**
Ask Mrs. Grayson about the effects of her urinary symptoms on her daily life.	She responds, "I find myself being embarrassed and frustrated for **losing control.** If my bladder is a little full, I **dribble** easily just picking something up or when I'm on my way to the bathroom. I'm afraid to laugh anymore because I **leak urine.** At work I try to avoid being close to my co-workers because I'm afraid I might have an odor."
Ask her what she has been doing about her condition.	She states that she has been wearing "one of those little pads" all the time now.
Ask Mrs. Grayson about any other effects caused by her leakage.	She begins to cry and states, "You know, I don't even like to go out to the movies or a party anymore. It's safer to stay home. I have problems being intimate with my husband because of leaking. We used to go dancing occasionally, but we don't do that anymore."
Observe Mrs. Grayson's behavior.	She appears anxious and is slowly pacing the floor.
Take a focused nursing history addressing urinary leakage and other lower urinary tract symptoms.	Mrs. Grayson's report of **urine leakage on physical exertion, sneezing, and laughing** increases the likelihood of a diagnosis of stress incontinence. Her risk factors for this condition include a **history of three pregnancies,** being **postmenopausal,** and being **overweight.** The history helps to define the proper interventions.
Have Mrs. Grayson complete a 3-day 24-hour log of urination.	The bladder log provides objective verification of urine elimination pattern and patterns of urine leakage and baseline for evaluation of effectiveness. It also demonstrates pattern of voiding that indicates more serious urinary problems related to urinary tract infections or other renal diseases (Lewis et al., 2011).

***Defining characteristics** are shown in bold type.

NURSING DIAGNOSIS: Stress urinary incontinence related to weakened pelvic musculature

PLANNING

Goals	*Expected Outcomes (NOC)†*
	Urinary Continence
Mrs. Grayson will have reduced episodes of urine leakage (incontinence) between voidings within 1 month.	Patient will report less than two episodes of incontinence following initiation of a pattern of pelvic muscle strengthening exercises (Kegel). Patient will state increased comfort between voidings.
	Urinary Elimination
Mrs. Grayson will achieve and maintain an optimum urinary elimination pattern within 2 months.	Patient will remain free of urinary tract infection. Patient will demonstrate ability to start and stop urinary stream with no leaking between voidings. Patient will void more than 150 mL each time.

†Outcome classification labels from Moorhead S et al: *Nursing outcomes classification (NOC),* ed 4, St Louis, 2008, Mosby.

INTERVENTIONS (NIC)‡	RATIONALE
Urinary Incontinence Care	
Assist Mrs. Grayson with supportive measures to reduce intraabdominal pressure by • Losing weight. • Avoiding heavy lifting. • Referring to urinary continence specialist if needed.	These measures reduce intraabdominal and bladder pressure, which increase leakage.

‡Intervention classification labels from Bulechek GM, Butcher HK, Dochterman JM: *Nursing interventions classifications (NIC),* ed 5, St Louis, 2008, Mosby.

Continued

NURSING CARE PLAN

Stress Urinary Incontinence—cont'd

Pelvic Muscle Exercise

Work with Mrs. Grayson to establish a program of pelvic muscle exercises that increase bladder control. Instruct her to tighten and then relax the ring of muscle around the urethra and anus, as if trying to prevent urination. Instruct her to work up to a total of 15 (3 sets of 5) contractions a day, ultimately holding the contraction for 10 seconds each, resting 10 seconds between each contraction, and resting 30 seconds between sets (Doughty, 2006).

Pelvic muscle rehabilitation alleviates or even cures stress incontinence for many women. Noticeable change will probably take 4 weeks, and maximum effect may take 6 weeks (Touhy and Jett, 2010).

EVALUATION

Nursing Actions	*Patient Response/Finding*	*Achievement of Outcomes*
Ask Mrs. Grayson about frequency of incontinence since starting pelvic muscle exercises.	She responds, "I'm dry most of the time now; and, when I do leak, it's only a few drops."	Mrs. Grayson reports increasing success with bladder control. She is satisfied that with time her success will be complete. Mrs. Grayson has had no symptoms of a urinary tract infection and states that she is voiding larger amounts.
Perform an ultrasound of Mrs. Grayson's bladder after voiding.	Residual volume is less than 30 mL.	Mrs. Grayson achieves improved bladder emptying.

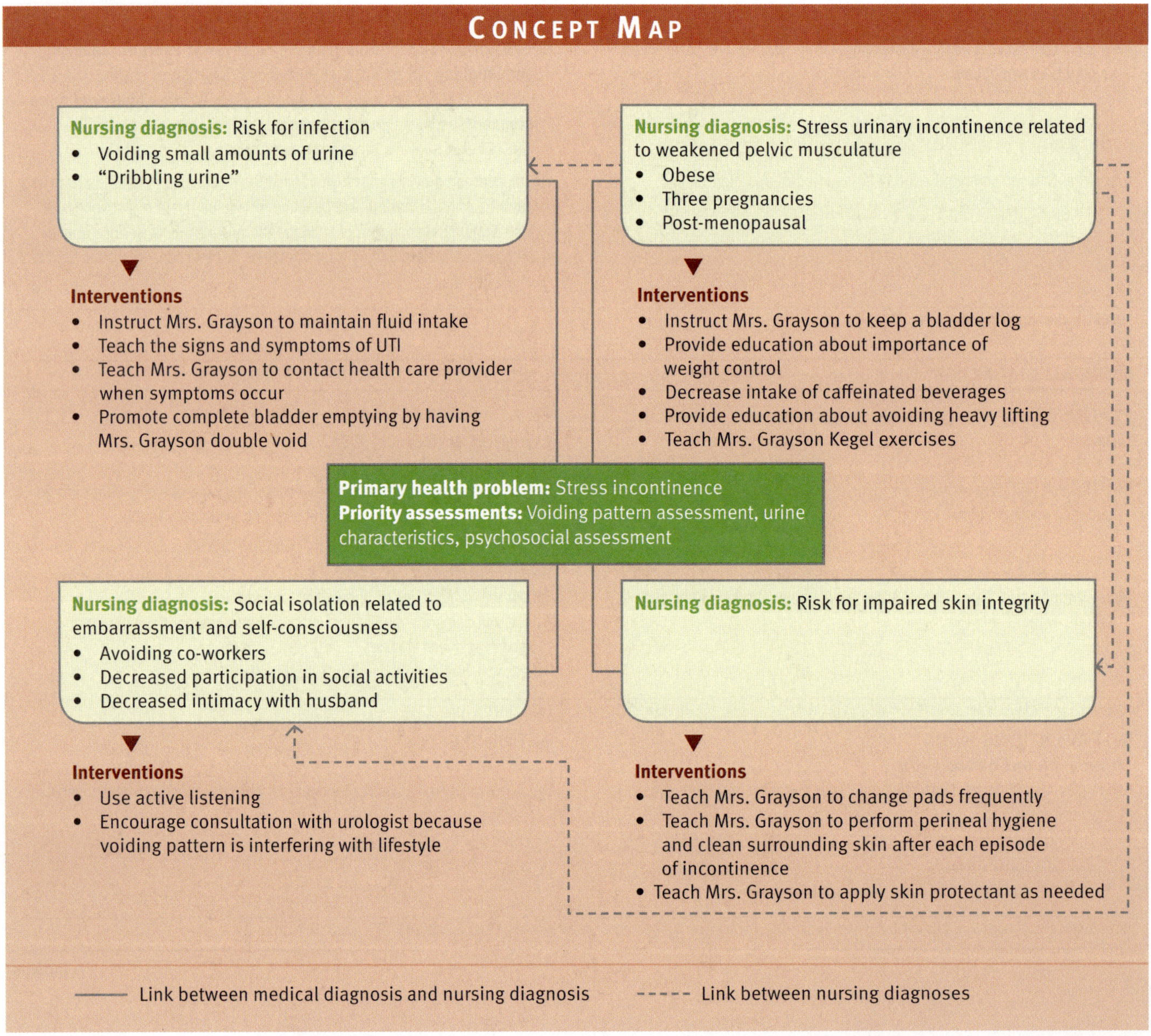
Concept Map
Nursing diagnosis: Risk for infection
• Voiding small amounts of urine
• "Dribbling urine"
Interventions
• Instruct Mrs. Grayson to maintain fluid intake
• Teach the signs and symptoms of UTI
• Teach Mrs. Grayson to contact health care provider when symptoms occur
• Promote complete bladder emptying by having Mrs. Grayson double void
Nursing diagnosis: Stress urinary incontinence related to weakened pelvic musculature
• Obese
• Three pregnancies
• Post-menopausal
Interventions
• Instruct Mrs. Grayson to keep a bladder log
• Provide education about importance of weight control
• Decrease intake of caffeinated beverages
• Provide education about avoiding heavy lifting
• Teach Mrs. Grayson Kegel exercises
Primary health problem: Stress incontinence
Priority assessments: Voiding pattern assessment, urine characteristics, psychosocial assessment
Nursing diagnosis: Social isolation related to embarrassment and self-consciousness
• Avoiding co-workers
• Decreased participation in social activities
• Decreased intimacy with husband
Interventions
• Use active listening
• Encourage consultation with urologist because voiding pattern is interfering with lifestyle
Nursing diagnosis: Risk for impaired skin integrity
Interventions
• Teach Mrs. Grayson to change pads frequently
• Teach Mrs. Grayson to perform perineal hygiene and clean surrounding skin after each episode of incontinence
• Teach Mrs. Grayson to apply skin protectant as needed
Link between medical diagnosis and nursing diagnosis
Link between nursing diagnoses

FIG. 45-10 Concept map for Mrs. Grayson. *UTI,* Urinary tract infection.

exercise plan to increase overall strength and endurance so the patient is able to ambulate to the bathroom. In addition, a health care provider prescribes an indwelling catheter. The nurse monitors the length of time that it is in place and communicates this to the health care provider. Explore the need for home care services and make the appropriate referrals. The family may need to alter the home environment to make it easier and safer for the patient to use the bathroom. The patient's plan requires multiple interventions.

IMPLEMENTATION

Complete independent and collaborative interventions to help the patient achieve the desired outcomes and goals. The independent activities are those in which nurses use their own judgment. An example of this is teaching self-care activities to the patient. Collaborative activities are those prescribed by the health care provider and carried out by the nurse such as medication administration.

Health Promotion. Health promotion assists the patient in understanding and participating in self-care practices to preserve and protect healthy urinary system function. You can achieve this focus using several means.

Patient Education. Success of therapies aimed at eliminating or minimizing urinary elimination problems depends in part on successful patient education (Box 45-6). Although many patients need to learn about all aspects of urinary elimination, first focus the teaching on their specific elimination problems. For example, patients who practice poor hygiene benefit most from learning about normal sterility of the urinary tract and how frequent handwashing and proper perineal hygiene reduce the risks for infection. Patients also learn the significance of symptoms of urinary alterations so they can initiate early preventive health care.

You can easily incorporate teaching when giving nursing care. For example, a good time to discuss the benefits of increasing fluid intake is while giving fluids with medications or meals. Often you are more successful in teaching about perineal hygiene while giving a bath or performing catheter care.

Promoting Normal Micturition. Maintaining normal urinary elimination helps to prevent many urination problems. Many nursing measures promote normal voiding in patients at risk for urination difficulties and in those with established urination problems. Some of these measures are independent nursing interventions.

Stimulating Micturition Reflex. A patient's ability to void depends on feeling the urge to urinate, being able to control the urethral sphincter, and being able to relax during voiding. Help patients learn to relax and stimulate the reflex to void by helping them assume the normal position for voiding. A woman is better able to void in a squatting or sitting position. If the patient is unable to use toilet facilities, position him or her in a squatting position on a bedpan (see Chapter 46) or bedside commode. A man voids more easily in the standing position. If the man cannot reach toilet facilities, have him stand at the bedside and void into a urinal (a metal or plastic receptacle for urine) (Fig. 45-11). At times it is necessary for one or more nurses to help a man stand.

Other measures that promote relaxation and the ability to void include sensory stimuli. The sound of running water helps many patients void through the power of suggestion. Stroking the inner aspect of the thigh stimulates sensory nerves and promotes the micturition reflex. You can also pour warm water over the patient's perineum and create the sensation to urinate. If you need to measure urine output, first measure the volume of water that you pour over the perineal area.

Maintaining Elimination Habits. Many patients follow routines to promote normal voiding. In a hospital or long-term care facility health care routines often conflict with those of patients. Integrating patients' habits into the care plan fosters normal voiding and helps prevent problems related to urination.

Maintaining Adequate Fluid Intake. A simple method of promoting normal micturition is maintaining optimal fluid intake. A patient with normal renal function who does not have heart or

BOX 45-6 PATIENT TEACHING

Urinary Elimination Problems Related to Urinary Sphincter Dysfunction

Objective

- Patient will achieve continence through increased sphincter control.

Teaching Strategies

- Have patient attempt to tighten urinary sphincter during urination to feel the sensations associated with urinary sphincter contraction.
- Teach patient progressive use of pelvic floor exercises (Kegel exercises).
  - Provide written instructions and/or audiotape for reinforcement of technique.
  - Have patient sit or stand without tensing muscles of legs, buttocks, or abdomen.
  - Have patient contract circumvaginal muscles and urinary and anal sphincters for 10 seconds and then relax for 10 seconds.
  - Have patient repeat these cycles for 30 to 100 times per day.
  - For maintenance, have patient do 1 to 2 sets per week. Patient should contract pelvic muscles and sphincters before sneezing, coughing, or lifting.
  - Maintain optimum strength through practicing hard contractions.
- Teach and monitor use of a voiding record. Inform patient that it may take 2 to 4 weeks of exercises before improvement is seen.

Evaluation

- Ask patient and caregiver about voiding record to identify changes in patterns of urinary elimination.
- Ask patient and caregiver about degree of satisfaction related to control achieved in urinary elimination.
- Ask patient and caregiver about selection and usage of incontinence control devices.

Teaching strategies modified from Bradway C, Cacchione P: Teaching strategies for assessing and managing urinary incontinence in older adults, *J Gerontol Nurs* 36(7):18, 2010; Touhy TA, Jett KF: *Ebersole and Hess' Gerontological nursing healthy aging*, ed 3, St Louis, 2010, Mosby.

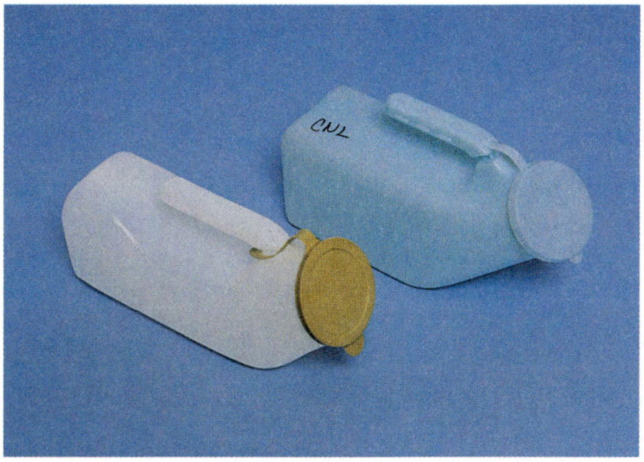

FIG. 45-11 Types of male urinals.

kidney disease needs to drink 2200 to 2700 mL of fluid daily. However, a minimal daily intake of 1200 to 1500 mL of fluids is usually adequate unless the patient has a history of UTI.

Increasing fluid intake helps flush out solutes or particles that collect in the urinary system. Because some patients are unwilling to drink 2500 mL of water daily, encourage fluids that the patient prefers. Many vegetables and fruits also have a high fluid content. At home it helps to set a schedule for drinking fluids (e.g., with meals or medications). To minimize nocturia, avoid fluids 2 hours before bedtime.

Promoting Complete Bladder Emptying. Under normal conditions a small amount of a patient's urine remains in the bladder after voiding (residual urine). Encouraging patients to wait until urine stops flowing or to attempt to void again (double voiding) can improve bladder emptying (Table 45-5). Urinary retention care includes scheduled toileting (Lewis et al., 2011). In addition, Credé's method or manual compression of the bladder walls with each attempted void may be used (Madineh, 2008). Instruct the patient to place both hands flat on the abdomen below the umbilicus and above the symphysis pubis with the fingers pointed down toward the bladder dome. Have him or her compress the hands downward against the walls of the bladder while tightening the perineum, contracting the abdominal wall, and holding the breath. The maneuver promotes bladder emptying by relaxing the urethral sphincter.

Preventing Infection. One of the most important considerations is to prevent infection of the urinary system. Good perineal hygiene that includes cleaning the urethral meatus after each voiding or bowel movement is essential. A minimal daily fluid intake of 1200 to 1500 mL dilutes urine, promotes regular micturition, and flushes

TABLE 45-5 Urinary Incontinence and Treatment Options

TYPE	SIGNS AND SYMPTOMS	INTERVENTIONS
Functional		
Loss of urine caused by factors outside the urinary tract that interfere with the ability to respond in a socially appropriate way to the urge to void Relevant factors: Environmental barriers Sensory, cognitive, and mobility issues	Urge to void that causes loss of urine before reaching appropriate receptacle	Clothing modifications Environmental alterations Scheduled toileting Absorbent products
Stress		
Involuntary leakage of urine during increased abdominal pressure in the absence of bladder muscle contraction	Loss of urine with increased intraabdominal pressure (coughing, laughing, sneezing, or lifting with a full bladder)	Pelvic floor exercises (Kegel) Surgical interventions Biofeedback Electrical stimulation Absorbent products
Urge		
Involuntary passage of urine after a strong sense of urgency to void	Urinary urgency, often with frequency (more often than every 2 hours); bladder spasm or contraction	Antimuscarinic agents Behavioral interventions Biofeedback Bladder retraining Pelvic floor exercises Lifestyle modifications (smoking cessation, weight loss and fluid modifications) Absorbent products
Mixed		
Combination of urge and stress urinary incontinence signs and symptoms	Combination of urge and stress symptoms	Main treatments usually based on symptoms that are most bothersome to patient
Overflow Incontinence		
Involuntary loss of urine at intervals without sensation of urge to void Relevant factors: Spinal cord dysfunction—loss of cerebral awareness or impairment of reflex arc	Lack of urge to void, unawareness of bladder filling, reflex emptying when certain volume reached	Intermittent catheterization Condom catheter (male) Credé's method
Hyperactive/Overactive Bladder		
Urinary urgency that is associated with urinary frequency and nocturia	Sudden compelling desire to urinate that is difficult to deter	Pelvic floor exercises (Kegel) Intake of 1.5-2 L of fluid a day Limit carbonated and caffeinated Beverages Bladder training Biofeedback

Modified from Palmer MH, Newman DK: Urinary incontinence and estrogen, *Am J Nurs* 107(3):35, 2007; Doughty DB: *Urinary and fecal incontinence: current management concepts*, ed 3, St Louis, 2006, Mosby; and McKertich K: Urinary incontinence: Assessment in women: Stress, urge or both? *Aust Fam Physician* 37(3):112, 2008.

the urethra of microorganisms. Voiding after intercourse; not using excessive soap or taking bubble baths; wearing cotton underwear; and drinking enough fluids, especially fluids high in acid ash such as apple or cranberry juice help prevent UTI.

Acute Care

Maintaining Elimination Habits. Patients usually require time to void. Requesting a urine specimen on demand does not contribute to relaxation and normal voiding habits. Give patients at least 30 minutes to provide a specimen. Patients normally void on awakening or before meals; therefore offer the opportunity to use toilet facilities then. Also important is the need to respond to and anticipate patients' urges to urinate. For example, many older-adult falls are related to the urge to urinate. Anticipate the need and provide for scheduled bathroom visits to help reduce the fall risk in these patients.

Many patients need privacy for voiding. If a patient cannot reach the bathroom and uses a bedside commode or bedpan, make sure that the bedside curtain is closed. Patients who are debilitated and live at home often prefer using a bedside commode screened by a partition or room divider. Young children are often unable to void in the presence of persons other than their parents.

When possible encourage the continued use of special measures that the patient uses to void. Some patients are able to relax and void more easily while reading or listening to music. Having a cup or glass of fluids also promotes urination.

Medications. Drug therapy given alone or with other therapies often helps problems of incontinence or retention. The bladder is innervated by the parasympathetic nervous system. Drugs that block the muscarinic receptors suppress bladder contractions and reduce incontinence caused by bladder irritation. Examples include solifenacin (VESIcare) and oxybutynin chloride (Ditropan). These medications can cause constipation, dry mouth, and skin irritation (Lehne, 2010). Irritants present in the urine such as caffeine or alcohol may cause uncontrolled bladder contractions, and thus patients should avoid them.

When the bladder empties, the detrusor muscle contracts in response to parasympathetic stimulation. Incomplete bladder emptying results from impaired innervation or weakness of the detrusor muscle. The patient experiences retention and possible overflow incontinence. Cholinergic drugs increase contraction of the bladder and improve emptying. Bethanechol (Urecholine) stimulates parasympathetic nerves to increase bladder wall contraction and relax the sphincter. You can administer bethanechol by subcutaneous or oral routes. Cholinergic drugs often cause diarrhea as a side effect (Lehne, 2010).

The dribbling or overflow incontinence seen in men with prostatic enlargement can be treated with an $alpha_1$-adrenergic blocker such as tamsulosin (Flomax). Tamsulosin is given orally and relaxes prostatic smooth muscle, thus relieving obstructive symptoms. This drug has few side effects and does not cause transient hypotension as other alpha-adrenergic blockers do (Lehne, 2010).

Catheterization. Catheterization of the bladder involves introducing a latex or plastic tube through the urethra and into the bladder. The catheter provides a continuous flow of urine in patients unable to control micturition or those with obstructions. It also provides a means of assessing urine output in hemodynamically unstable patients. Because bladder catheterization carries the risk of UTI, blockage, and trauma to the urethra, it is preferable to rely on other measures for either specimen collection or management of incontinence.

Types of Catheterization. Intermittent and indwelling retention catheterizations are the two forms of catheter insertion. With the intermittent technique you introduce a straight single-use catheter (Fig. 45-12, *A)* long enough to drain the bladder (5 to 10 minutes). When the bladder is empty, you immediately withdraw the catheter. You can repeat intermittent catheterization as necessary, but each catheter insertion increases risk of trauma and infection. It is common for people with spinal cord injury or other neurological problems such as multiple sclerosis to perform self–intermittent catheterization up to every 4 hours daily for months or years. If done correctly with use of clean technique, they frequently do not experience more UTIs; in fact, the UTI rate is lower than for patients with long-term indwelling catheters. An indwelling or Foley catheter (Fig. 45-12, *B*) remains in place for a longer period, until a patient is able to void voluntarily or continuous accurate urine measurements are no longer needed (Box 45-7).

The straight single-use catheter has a single lumen with a small opening about 1.3 cm (½ inch) from the tip. Urine drains from the tip, through the lumen, and to a receptacle. An indwelling Foley catheter has a small inflatable balloon that encircles the catheter just above the tip. When inflated the balloon rests against the bladder outlet to anchor the catheter in place. The indwelling retention catheter often has two or three lumens within the body of the catheter (see Fig. 45-12, *B*). One lumen drains urine through the catheter to a collecting tube. A second lumen carries sterile

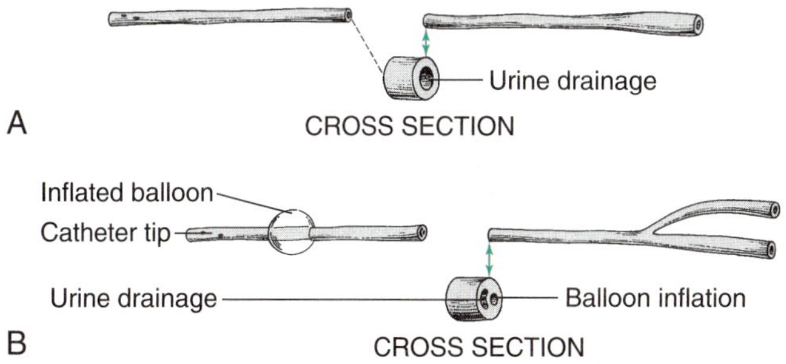

FIG. 45-12 Types of urinary catheters. **A,** Straight. **B,** Indwelling (Foley).

BOX 45-7 INDICATIONS FOR CATHETERIZATION

Intermittent Catheterization
- Relieving discomfort of bladder distention, providing decompression
- Obtaining sterile urine specimen when clean-catch specimen is unobtainable
- Assessing residual urine after urination
- Managing patients with spinal cord injuries, neuromuscular degeneration, or incompetent bladders long term

Short-Term Indwelling Catheterization
- Obstruction to urine outflow (e.g., prostate enlargement)
- Surgical repair of bladder, urethra, and surrounding structures
- Prevention of urethral obstruction from blood clots after genitourinary surgery
- Measurement of urinary output in critically ill patients
- Continuous or intermittent bladder irrigations

Long-Term Indwelling Catheterization
- Severe urinary retention with recurrent episodes of UTI
- Skin rashes, ulcers, or wounds irritated by contact with urine
- Terminal illness when bed linen changes are painful for patient

UTI, Urinary tract infection.

BOX 45-8 GUIDELINES FOR APPROPRIATE CATHETER SELECTION

- The catheter size should be determined by the size of the patient's urethral canal. When the French system is used, the larger the gauge number, the larger the catheter size. Generally children require an 8- to 10-Fr, women require a 14- to 16-Fr, and men require a 16- to 18-Fr (Gray et al., 2006). To prevent trauma, the smallest effective catheter size is preferred. Larger sizes than 18-Fr create discomfort, increase risk of blockage, and lead to urinary tract infection, urethral irritation, and erosion (Gray et al., 2006)
- The expected duration of the catheterization determines the catheter material selection.
  - Plastic catheters are suitable only for intermittent use because of their inflexibility.
  - Latex catheters are recommended for use up to 3 weeks. Be aware of allergies.
  - Pure silicon or Teflon catheters are best suited for long-term use (2 to 3 months) because of less encrustation at the urethral meatus.
- Balloon size is important in selecting an indwelling catheter. Balloon sizes range from 3 mL (pediatric) to large postoperative volumes (75 mL). In adults the 5-mL and 30-mL sizes are the most common: The 5-mL size allows for optimal drainage, whereas the 30-mL size is used after prostatectomies to provide hemostasis of the prostatic bed (Gray et al., 2006).
- Use only sterile water to inflate the balloon because saline crystallizes, resulting in incomplete deflation of the balloon at the time of removal.
- If leakage occurs around the catheter, a change in lumen size or use of antispasmodic medication is necessary.

water to and from the balloon when it is inflated or deflated. A third (optional) lumen is sometimes used to instill fluids or medications into the bladder. It is easy to determine the number of lumens by the number of drainage and injection ports at the end of the catheter.

A second type of intermittent catheter has a curved tip. A Coudé catheter is used on male patients who may have enlarged prostates that partly obstruct the urethra. It is less traumatic during insertion because it is stiffer and easier to control than the straight-tip catheter.

Catheters come in many diameters to fit the size of a patient's urethral canal. Box 45-8 provides suggestions for how to make appropriate decisions regarding catheter selection.

Catheter Insertion. Urethral catheterization requires a health care provider's order. You must use strict aseptic technique (see Chapter 28). Organizing equipment before the procedure prevents interruptions. The steps for inserting indwelling and single-use straight catheters are basically the same. The difference lies in the procedure taken to inflate the indwelling catheter balloon and secure the catheter. Skill 45-2 on pp. 1071-1079 lists steps for performing female and male urethral catheterization.

Closed Drainage Systems. After inserting an indwelling catheter, maintain a closed urinary drainage system to minimize the risk of infection. Standard urinary drainage bags are plastic and hold about 1000 to 1500 mL of urine. The bag hangs on the bed frame or wheelchair without touching the floor. Never hang the bag on the bedrail because it can accidentally be raised above the level of the bladder. In patients with indwelling catheters you can obtain specimens without opening the drainage system using a special port in the tubing (see Fig. 45-7).

An alternative to a large-volume urinary drainage bag is a small-volume leg bag. A urinary drainage bag attached to the patient's calf or thigh provides the catheterized patient with greater mobility. These drainage bags are usually worn during the day and replaced at night with a standard drainage bag.

When the patient ambulates, the nurse or patient carries the standard urinary drainage bag below the patient's waist. As with leg bags, never raise the drainage bag above the level of the patient's bladder. Urine in the bag and tubing becomes a medium for bacteria, and infection is likely to develop if urine flows back into the bladder.

Most drainage bags contain an antireflux valve to prevent urine in the bag from reentering the drainage tubing and contaminating the patient's bladder. A spigot at the base of urinary drainage bags provides a means for emptying the bag. The spigot on a leg bag is covered with a protective cap. The spigot on a standard drainage bag always needs to be clamped, except during emptying, and tucked into the protective pouch on the side of the bag (see agency policy). To keep urinary drainage systems patent so urine can flow into the drainage bag, check for kinks or bends in the tubing, avoid positioning the patient on the tubing, and observe for clots or sediment that occlude it. Patients with indwelling catheters have a number of special care needs. Direct nursing measures at preventing infection and maintaining unobstructed flow of urine through the catheter drainage system.

Perineal Hygiene. Buildup of secretions or encrustation at the catheter insertion site is a source of irritation and potential infection. Nurses provide perineal hygiene (see Chapter 39) at least 3 times daily or as needed for a patient with a retention catheter. Soap and water are effective in reducing the number of organisms around the urethra. Accidentally advancing the catheter further into the bladder during cleaning increases the risk of introducing bacteria into the bladder.

Catheter Care. In addition to routine perineal hygiene, many institutions recommend that patients with catheters receive special care 3 times a day and after defecation or bowel incontinence to help minimize discomfort and infection (Skill 45-3 on pp. 1079-1081).

Fluid Intake. All patients with catheters should have a daily intake of 2000 to 2500 mL if permitted. Patients can do this through oral intake or intravenous infusion. A high fluid intake produces a large volume of urine that flushes the bladder and keeps catheter tubing free of sediment. Cranberry, apple, and prune juices are high in acid ash and help prevent infection; conversely citrus juices such as orange, grapefruit, and pineapple should be used sparingly because they can create an environment in the bladder more prone to infection.

Preventing Infection. Maintaining a closed urinary drainage system is important in infection control. A break in the system leads to introduction of microorganisms (Box 45-9). Sites at risk are the site of catheter insertion, the drainage bag, the spigot, the tube junction, and the junction of the tube and bag (Fig. 45-13).

In addition, monitor the patency of the system to prevent pooling of urine within the tubing. Urine in the drainage bag is an excellent medium for microorganism growth. Bacteria can travel up drainage tubing to grow in pools of urine. If this urine flows back into the patient's bladder, an infection is more likely to develop. Many urine drainage systems are equipped with an antireflux valve. Suggestions for ways to prevent infections in patients with catheters are provided in Box 45-10.

Catheter Irrigations and Instillations. To maintain the patency of indwelling urinary catheters, it is sometimes necessary to irrigate or flush a catheter with sterile solution. If a catheter becomes plugged with pus or sediment, it is best to change it rather than

BOX 45-9 EVIDENCE-BASED PRACTICE

Factors to Decrease Urinary Tract Infections

PICO Question: Which factors decrease the risk of urinary tract infections (UTIs) in hospitalized patients with indwelling urinary catheters?

Evidence Summary

Urinary catheterization is a common procedure in health care settings. Nine percent of patients in hospitals acquire a health care–associated infection. UTIs account for approximately 40% of them (Parker et al., 2009). The risk of catheter-associated urinary tract infections (CAUTIs) increases by the number of days that a catheter remains in place.

Nazarko (2008) stresses that decreasing the risk for CAUTIs starts by avoiding unnecessary use of indwelling catheters and removing them as soon as medically indicated. Indications for catheterization include surgery, urinary retention, and need for accurate measurement of output (Holroyd-Leduc et al., 2007). The authors designed a study to determine the association between indwelling urinary catheterization without a specific medical indication and adverse outcomes. They found that patients older than 70 years with limited functional ability are often catheterized to facilitate their care. The results suggested that nonmedical use of indwelling catheters in older adults may result in longer hospital stays and greater risk of death resulting from the development of a UTI and subsequent development of bacteremia or urosepsis.

Urinary catheters vary in composition and design. Research related to catheter composition focuses on altering the catheter surface to slow biofilm development (adherence of microorganisms to the catheter surface). According to Parker et al. (2009), there is robust evidence supporting the insertion of a silver alloy–coated catheter to reduce the risk of CAUTIs for up to 2 weeks and an antibiotic-impregnated catheter for up to 7 days in adult patients. In addition, further research needs to be conducted on which type of catheter is effective in decreasing the risk of CAUTI for long-term use.

Many catheterizations can be avoided by using noninvasive alternatives. For example, instead of using catheterization to evaluate residual urine in the bladder, a bladder scanner can be used. When it is determined that bladder volume is normal, the invasive procedure of catheterization may not be needed (Chen et al., 2005). In addition, the incidence of CAUTI significantly decreases when nurses give the prescriber daily reminders to remove unnecessary catheters and suggest the use of alternative noninvasive treatments such as condom catheters to manage urinary elimination (Holroyd-Leduc et al., 2007; Nazarko, 2008).

Application to Nursing Practice

- Avoid the routine use of catheters; use only when clinically indicated.
- Collaborate with health care providers to remove catheters when medical indications no longer exist.
- Suggest noninvasive continent devices such as condom catheters to reduce the risk of UTI and resulting complications.
- Nurses need to be patient advocates by taking an active role in monitoring duration of treatment.

irrigate because irrigation washes the pus and sediment back into the bladder, creating a worse infection. Change the catheter as needed. It is appropriate to use irrigation after surgery for blood clots and short-term catheter use; but for long-term use irrigation can create a chronic sediment and pus problem, requiring lifelong irrigation in long-term indwelling catheters. For patients with bladder infections, a health care provider often orders antiseptic or antibiotic bladder irrigations to wash out the bladder or treat local infection. In both irrigations follow sterile aseptic technique.

BOX 45-10 TIPS FOR PREVENTING INFECTION IN PATIENTS WITH CATHETERS

- Follow good hand hygiene techniques (see Chapter 28).
- Do not allow the spigot on the drainage system to touch a contaminated surface.
- Only use sterile technique to collect specimens from a closed drainage system.
- If the drainage tube becomes disconnected, do not touch the ends of the catheter or tubing. Wipe the end of the tubing and catheter with an antimicrobial solution before reconnecting.
- Ensure that each patient has a separate receptacle for measuring urine to prevent cross-contamination.
- Prevent pooling of urine in the tubing and reflux of urine into the bladder.
- Avoid raising the drainage bag above the level of the bladder.
- If it becomes necessary to raise the bag during transfer of the patient to a bed or stretcher, clamp the tubing or empty its contents to the drainage bag first.
- Provide for drainage of urine from the tubing to the bag by positioning the tubing.
- Before exercise or ambulation drain all urine from the tubing into the drainage bag.
- Avoid prolonged kinking or clamping of the tubing.
- Empty the drainage bag at least every 8 hours. If you note large outputs, empty more frequently.
- Encourage fluid intake (if not contraindicated).
- Remove the catheter as soon as clinically necessary (Fernandez and Griffiths, 2006).
- Tape or secure the catheter appropriately for the patient (see Skill 45-2).
- Perform routine perineal hygiene per agency policy and after defecation or bowel incontinence (see Skill 45-3).

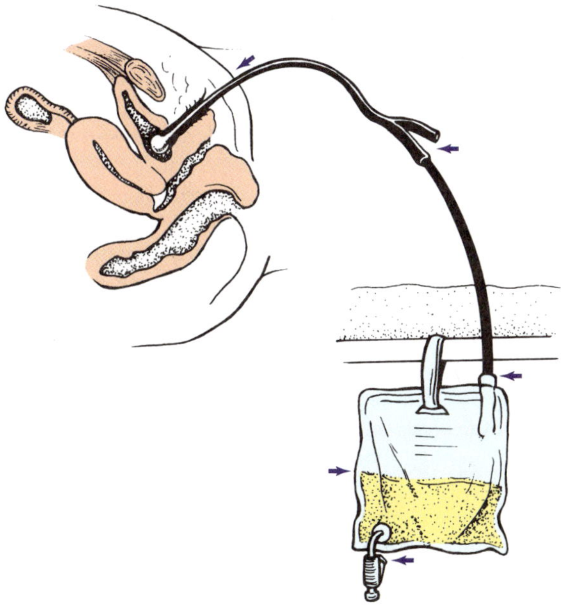

FIG. 45-13 Potential sites for introduction of infectious organisms into a urinary drainage system.

Before performing irrigation assess the catheter for blockage. If the amount of urine in the drainage bag is less than the patient's intake or output during the previous shift, expect some blockage. If urine does not drain freely, milk the tubing. Milk the tube by squeezing and then releasing it, starting at a point close to the patient and then out to the drainage bag so a clot or sediment is not forced back into the catheter. Many times this takes care of the problem without irrigation.

Maintenance of a closed system is recommended during intermittent irrigations or instillations. This technique is effective for irrigating a partially blocked catheter or for bladder instillations. One method of closed-bladder irrigation provides for frequent intermittent irrigations or continuous irrigation without disruption of the sterile catheter system through use of a three-way catheter (Skill 45-4 on pp. 1081-1084). This method is used most often in patients who have had genitourinary surgery and are at risk for blood clots and mucus fragments occluding the catheter. The other method involves accessing the closed drainage system to instill bladder irrigations (see Skill 45-4). This method is often used for unanticipated irrigation or intermittent instillations.

Removal of Indwelling Catheter. When removing an indwelling catheter, promote normal bladder function and prevent trauma to the urethra. Removing a catheter requires a clean, disposable towel; a trash receptacle; and a sterile syringe the same size as the volume of solution within the inflated balloon of the catheter. Perform hand hygiene and put on clean gloves before removing the catheter. The end of each catheter contains a label that denotes the volume of solution (5 to 30 mL) within the balloon. If a different volume was used, there should be a notation on the patient record.

Position the patient in the same position as during catheterization. Some institutions recommend collecting a sterile urine specimen at this time or sending the catheter tip for culture and sensitivity tests. After removing the tape, place the towel between a female patient's thighs or over a male patient's thighs. Insert the syringe into the balloon injection port. Most ports are self-sealing and require that only the tip of the syringe be inserted. Slowly withdraw all of the solution to deflate the balloon totally. If a portion of the solution remains, the partially inflated balloon traumatizes the urethral canal as the catheter is removed. After deflation, explain that the patient will feel a burning sensation as the catheter is withdrawn. Then pull the catheter out smoothly and slowly.

It is normal for the patient to experience some dysuria, especially if the catheter has been in place several days or weeks. Until the bladder regains full tone, some patients also experience frequency of urination or urinary retention.

Assess the patient's urinary function by noting the first voiding after catheter removal and documenting the time and amount of voiding for the next 24 hours. If amounts are small, frequent assessment of bladder for distention is necessary. If 4 hours have elapsed without voiding or the patient experiences discomfort, it often becomes necessary to reinsert the catheter.

Alternatives to Urethral Catheterization. To avoid the risks associated with urethral catheters, two alternatives are available for urinary drainage.

Suprapubic Catheterization. Suprapubic catheterization involves surgical placement of a catheter through the abdominal wall above the symphysis pubis and into the urinary bladder. A health care provider performs the procedure under local or general anesthesia. The catheter is anchored in place with sutures, a commercially prepared ring seal, or both. Urine drains into a urinary drainage bag. Maintenance of the tubing and drainage bag is the same as for an indwelling catheter. Studies comparing the use of this method of urinary drainage with indwelling catheters have shown mixed results. Infection rates may be slightly lower; however, long-term complications are similar (Doughty, 2006). Sediment, clots, or the abdominal wall itself can block the suprapubic catheter. Adequate fluid intake helps to minimize risk of blockage by increasing urine flow. The suprapubic catheter must remain patent at all times. Monitor the patient's I&O carefully, monitor the urine characteristics, and observe for signs of infection (e.g., fever and chills). Also administer skin care around the insertion site. This method may be used in men and women.

Condom Catheter. The second alternative to catheterization is the condom catheter (Box 45-11), which is suitable for incontinent or comatose men who still have complete and spontaneous bladder emptying. The condom is a soft, pliable, latex sheath that slips over the penis. Patients wear it only at night or continuously, depending on their needs. There are three general methods of securing a condom catheter. One method uses a strip of elastic tape or rubber that encircles the top of the condom to secure it in place. Another type uses a self-adhesive condom sheath. The third method uses an inflatable ring within the condom to secure placement. Take care to ensure that, whatever type or size is used, blood supply to the penis is not impaired. Never use standard adhesive tape to secure a condom catheter because it does not expand with change in penis size and is painful to remove.

The end of the condom is attached to plastic drainage tubing and a bag that you attach to the side of the bed or strap to the patient's leg. The condom catheter itself poses little risk of UTI. Infections usually result from buildup of secretions around the urethra, trauma to the urethral meatus, or buildup of pressure in the outflow tubing. If the condom catheter is made of opaque material, remove it daily to check for skin irritation. Some new condom catheters are more transparent, and you are able to observe the skin through them more easily. Change the condom catheter daily. With each catheter change clean the urethral meatus and penis thoroughly. Check the drainage tubing often for patency because twisting the condom at the drainage tube attachment irritates the skin and obstructs urine outflow. Make sure that the tip of the penis is at the end of the catheter. If there is space between the end of the penis and the catheter, urine can pool in this space and excoriate the end of the penis.

For a man with a retracted penis, maintaining a conventional condom catheter often proves difficult. Special devices are available to help alleviate this problem (Fig. 45-14). Consult manufacturer guidelines for product application.

No collection devices for women are as effective as the condom catheter is for men; thus frequently the only devices used are pads and protective clothing. To maintain dignity, do not refer to pads

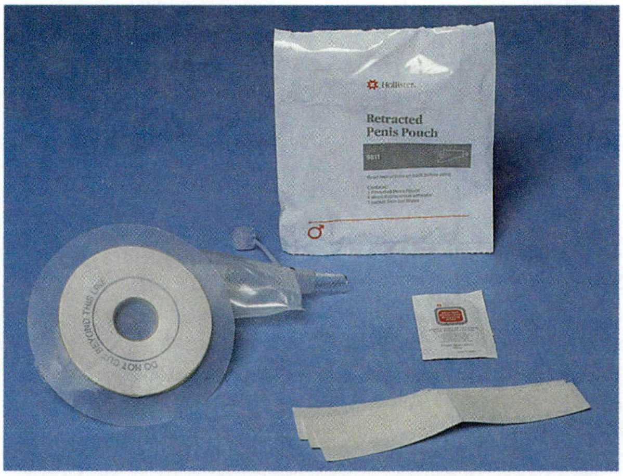

FIG. 45-14 Retracted penis pouch external urinary device.

BOX 45-11 **PROCEDURAL GUIDELINES**

Applying a Condom Catheter

Delegation Considerations

After assessing patient for latex allergy, you can delegate the skill of applying a condom catheter to nursing assistive personnel (NAP). The nurse instructs NAP to:

- Be sensitive to privacy needs of patients.
- Be sure that the skin of the penile shaft is intact and free from swelling, redness, or open lesions before applying the condom catheter.
- Ask for assistance if the NAP is uncertain how to apply the adhesive strip that secures the condom catheter.

Equipment

Condom catheter (sometimes comes with self-adhesive or an elastic adhesive), collection bag, skin preparation, basin with warm water, towel and washcloth, clean gloves, scissors or hair guard, bath blanket and sheet

1. Check health care provider's order. Identify patient using two identifiers (i.e., name and birth date or name and account number) according to facility policy.
2. Perform hand hygiene.
3. Assess urinary elimination patterns, patient's ability to urinate voluntarily, and continence.
4. Assess mental status of patient and explain procedure.
5. Provide for privacy by closing room door or bedside curtain. Raise bed to working height and lower side rail on working side.
6. Prepare condom catheter and drainage bag and tubing (see manufacturer directions).
7. Assist patient to supine or sitting position. Place bath blanket over upper torso; fold sheet over lower torso so only penis is exposed.
8. Apply clean gloves, provide perineal care (see Chapter 28), and dry thoroughly. If patient is uncircumcised, return foreskin to normal position.
9. If needed, clip hair at base of penile shaft. Do not shave the pubic area. An alternative to trimming pubic hair is placing a hair guard (see manufacturer directions) over penis before applying catheter.
10. Assess condition of penis and scrotum. Use manufacturer measuring guide to measure diameter of penis in flaccid state. Penile shaft should be at least 2 cm (approximately 1 inch) in length to ensure successful application.
11. *Option:* Apply skin-cleaning preparation to penile shaft and allow to dry.
12. Hold penis along shaft in nondominant hand. With dominant hand hold condom sheath at tip of penis and smoothly roll sheath onto penis. Allow 2.5 to 5 cm (1 to 2 inches) of space between tip of penis and end of catheter (see illustration).

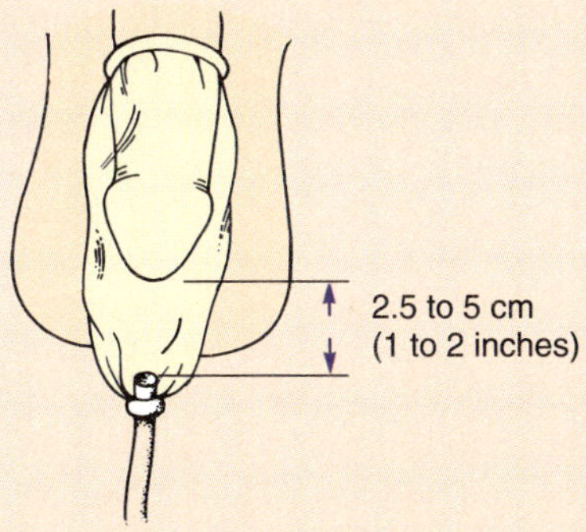

STEP 12 Distance between end of penis and tip of condom.

13. Secure condom catheter according to manufacturer directions.
    a. If using elastic adhesive, wrap strip of adhesive over condom to secure it in place by using spiral technique (see illustration). *Note: Never use adhesive tape.*
    b. For self-adhesive catheter, apply catheter as in Steps 11 and 12; then apply gentle pressure on penile shaft for 10 to 15 seconds to secure.
14. Connect drainage tubing to end of condom catheter. Be sure that condom is not twisted. Connect catheter to large-volume drainage bag or leg bag (see illustration). Attach large-volume drainage bag to lower bed frame. Coil excess tubing on bed.
15. Make patient comfortable, lower bed, and place side rails as appropriate.
16. Dispose of contaminated supplies, remove gloves, and perform hand hygiene.
17. Observe urinary drainage, drainage tube patency, condition of penis, and tape placement.

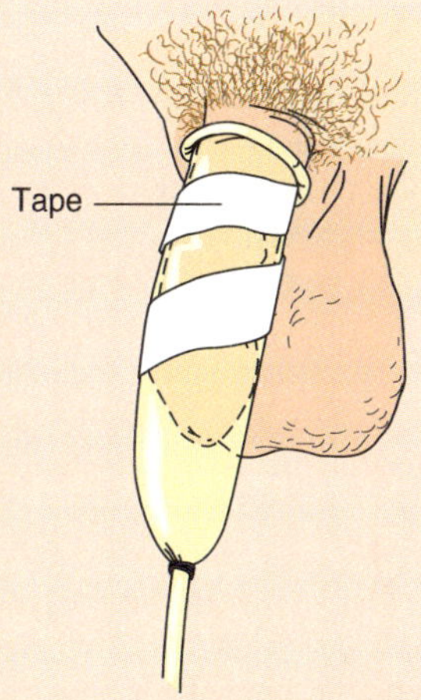

STEP 13a Apply elastic tape in spiral fashion to secure condom catheter to penis.

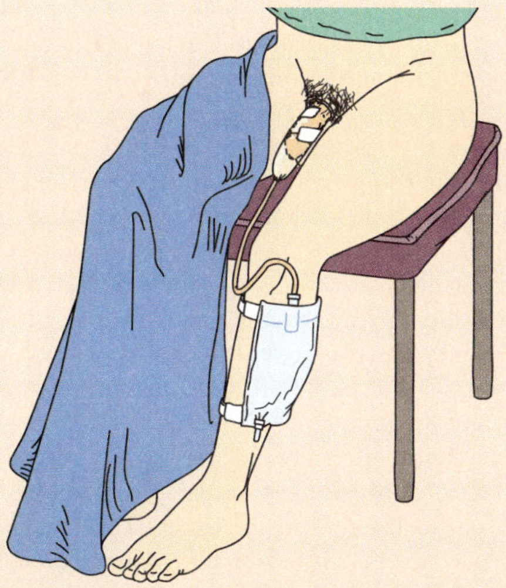

STEP 14 Attach condom catheter tubing to leg bag.

and protective clothing as adult diapers and change them frequently to control odor. Only use these products temporarily to minimize or prevent episodes of incontinence while treatment is ongoing. Monitor patients frequently and provide good skin care to prevent irritation caused by urine. Some manufacturers have developed a female urinal; however, their ease of use may be an issue.

Restorative Care. Some patients regain normal urinary voiding function through special activities such as bladder retraining, habit training, or cognitive therapy. In some cases self-catheterization may be used to restore a measure of control to the patient.

Strengthening Pelvic Floor Muscles. Patients who have stress or urge urinary incontinence and difficulty starting and stopping urination may benefit from **pelvic floor exercises.** Pelvic floor exercises, also known as **Kegel exercises,** improve the strength of pelvic floor muscles and consist of repetitive contractions of muscle groups. These exercises have demonstrated effectiveness in treating stress incontinence, OAB, and mixed cause of urinary incontinence. A patient begins these exercises during voiding to learn the technique. They are then practiced at nonvoiding times. Improvement is usually gradual. Patients need to be alert and motivated to perform the exercises. They need to continue to use them to maintain effectiveness (see Box 45-6). The exercises are noninvasive and carry a low risk of adverse effects.

Bladder Retraining. The goal of bladder retraining is to reduce the voiding frequency and perhaps the bladder capacity (Doughty, 2006). This method is a specific program for patients who have a decreased urge to void or have stress incontinence since it keeps the bladder from getting full; thus there is less dribbling. Ultimately the overall goal of this retraining is to restore a normal pattern of voiding by teaching patients to keep the patient continent. Initially patients keep a bladder diary or log noting times, volumes, fluid intake, and any other related symptoms. This provides a baseline for comparison during the retraining. For bladder retraining to be successful, patients must agree to it and be alert and physically able to follow a training program. Bladder retraining is very important in long-term care and rehabilitation facilities. Remember that keeping a patient with a severely spastic bladder from frequent toileting causes pain for the patient. Nurses should never refuse to toilet a patient. Urological consultation can be helpful; and, if treated properly, bladder capacity will increase.

Assess the patient's current pattern of urination. This information allows the nurse to plan a program that often takes 2 weeks or more to learn. Although patients may start the program in the hospital or in rehabilitation, they may need to continue it in an extended care facility or at home. Generally the patient is asked to suppress urination for each voiding and increase time by increments of 15 minutes every week. The goal is to void every 3 to 4 hours in volumes of 240 to 500 mL. If the patient has an underlying UTI, treat this at the same time.

As part of restorative and rehabilitative care, patients with different types of incontinence may benefit from specific measures that address particular continence issues. These guidelines help patients control factors that affect the number of incontinence episodes.

The following measures may help patients with stress urinary incontinence to gain control over urination:

- Learning exercises to strengthen the pelvic floor (see Box 45-6)
- Initiating a toileting schedule on awakening, at least every 2 hours during the day and evening, before getting into bed, and every 4 hours at night (individualizing time frame as needed)
- Avoiding an overfilled bladder because this increases chances of incontinence related to increased bladder pressure
- Minimizing tea, coffee, other caffeine drinks (increases urine production, frequency, and urgency) and alcohol (increases urine production)
- Taking prescribed diuretic medication early in the morning
- Following a weight-control program if obesity is a problem that is causing increased abdominal pressure

Habit Training. A patient with functional incontinence benefits from habit training, which helps patients improve voluntary control over urination. A patient establishes a flexible toileting schedule based on his or her pattern. Have the patient establish the pattern by documenting episodes of incontinence and scheduling voiding opportunities just before the urge time interval. The goal is to keep the patient dry. Help him or her to the bathroom before the urge usually occurs. Time fluids and medications to prevent interference with the toileting schedule. Patients with moderate or severe mental or physical dysfunction and those who have normal bladder function or overflow reflex incontinence benefit from habit training. When combined with positive reinforcement to reward successful voiding, this approach is also called *prompted voiding.*

Building Competency in Safety You are caring for a 70-year-old male patient who has urgency and is incontinent of urine. An indwelling catheter is prescribed for the incontinence. What is your responsibility in this situation to promote patient safety? Provide the rationales for your answer.

Answers to questions can be found on the Evolve website.

Self-Catheterization. Some patients with chronic disorders such as spinal cord injury learn to perform self-catheterization. A patient must be able to physically manipulate equipment and assume a position for successful catheterization. You teach the patient the structures of the urinary tract, clean-versus-sterile technique, the importance of adequate fluid intake, and the frequency of self-catheterization. Generally the goal is to have patients perform self-catheterization 4 to 6 times a day with volumes of 400 to 500 mL; but be sure to individualize the schedule.

Maintenance of Skin Integrity. The normal acidity of urine is irritating to skin. Urine allowed to remain in contact with the skin becomes alkaline, causing encrustations or precipitates to collect on it, fostering breakdown. Washing with mild soap and warm water is the best way to remove urine from skin. Body lotion keeps skin moisturized, and petroleum-based ointments provide a barrier to the urine. Patients who wet their clothing need to receive partial baths and dry clothing after voiding. Continuous exposure of the perineal area or skin around an ostomy leads to gradual maceration and excoriation (see Chapter 48) requiring special care.

When the skin becomes irritated or inflamed, often the health care provider prescribes a cream or spray containing steroids (e.g., Kenalog) to reduce inflammation. If fungal growth develops, the antifungal drug nystatin (Mycostatin), available in cream or powder, is effective.

Promotion of Comfort. Patients with urinary alterations become uncomfortable as a result of the symptoms of urinary problems. Frequent or unpredictable voiding, dysuria, and painful distention are sources of discomfort.

The incontinent patient gains comfort from having clean, dry clothing. When stress incontinence is the problem, a protective pad offers protection against soiling. Wet clothing adheres to the skin and can cause rubbing and irritation.

Urinary analgesics that act on the urethral and bladder mucosa (e.g., phenazopyridine) relieve dysuria. Often you combine this drug with sulfonamide antibiotics in preparations such as Azo-Gantanol and Azo-Gantrisin. Patients taking drugs with phenazopyridine need to be aware that their urine will be orange. They must drink large amounts of fluids to prevent toxicity from the sulfonamides and maintain optimal flow through the urinary system (Lehne, 2010).

If the patient has local discomfort from an inflamed urethra, an iced sitz bath provides pain relief. The patient is often relaxed after a sitz bath; thus voiding occurs easily. Patients cannot relieve pain of distention unless they are able to empty the bladder. Interventions that stimulate micturition or intermittent catheterization may be the only sources of pain relief.

EVALUATION

Through the Patient's Eyes. The patient is the best source of evaluation of outcomes and responses to nursing care (Fig. 45-15). Note his or her responses to questions about urination. Does he or she seem hesitant or embarrassed? Psychosocial factors such as culture or sexuality sometimes influence the patient's response. Because urination is often considered a private matter, some people find it difficult to talk about their voiding habits. Remember that urinary elimination problems are not just physiological in nature. Be sensitive to any changes in self-concept and sexuality. Self-concept, which includes body image, self-esteem, roles, and identity, develops over a life span. Because the penis is an organ for both urination and sex, urinary dysfunction often greatly affects a man's self concept.

Patient Outcomes. You also evaluate the effectiveness of nursing interventions through comparisons with the outcome goals. Evaluate for changes in the patient's voiding pattern and continued presence of urinary tract alteration. Actual outcomes are compared with expected outcomes to determine success or partial success in achieving those outcomes. Examples of questions to ask for evaluation include:

- "Tell me, how frequently are you voiding now?"
- "Do you continue to have the feeling of urgency every time you void?"
- "Have the symptoms of urgency decreased since you changed your caffeine intake?
- "Do you still have burning when you pass urine?
- "Do you still feel uncomfortable over your lower abdomen?"

Evaluation of an intervention that may take weeks to accomplish such as pelvic floor exercises requires follow-up beyond the hospital or rehabilitation facility. Specific information about how well an intervention has met the need determines if you need to revise the plan of care. Continuous evaluation allows you to determine whether any new symptoms or nursing diagnoses have developed. Help the patient redefine goals when impairment in function is not likely to be altered as completely as the patient might like.

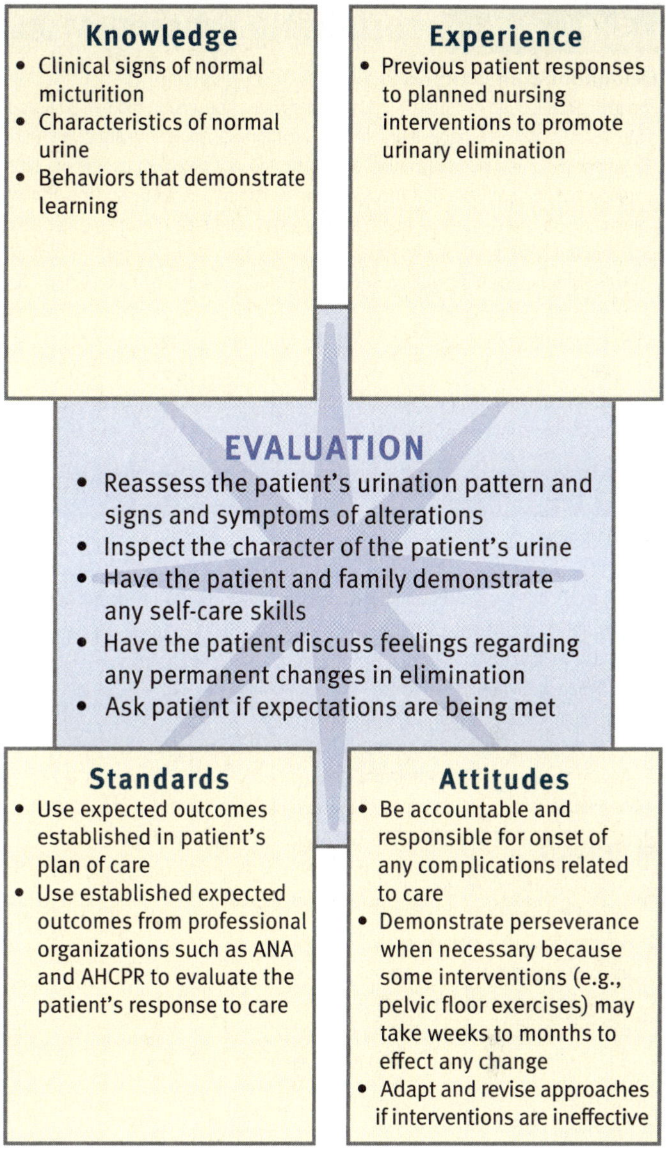
Knowledge
• Clinical signs of normal micturition
• Characteristics of normal urine
• Behaviors that demonstrate learning
Experience
• Previous patient responses to planned nursing interventions to promote urinary elimination
EVALUATION
• Reassess the patient's urination pattern and signs and symptoms of alterations
• Inspect the character of the patient's urine
• Have the patient and family demonstrate any self-care skills
• Have the patient discuss feelings regarding any permanent changes in elimination
• Ask patient if expectations are being met
Standards
• Use expected outcomes established in patient's plan of care
• Use established expected outcomes from professional organizations such as ANA and AHCPR to evaluate the patient's response to care
Attitudes
• Be accountable and responsible for onset of any complications related to care
• Demonstrate perseverance when necessary because some interventions (e.g., pelvic floor exercises) may take weeks to months to effect any change
• Adapt and revise approaches if interventions are ineffective

FIG. 45-15 Critical thinking model for urinary elimination evaluation. *AHCPR,* Agency for Health Care Policy and Research; *ANA,* American Nurses Association.

SAFETY GUIDELINES FOR NURSING SKILLS

Ensuring patient safety is an essential role of the professional nurse. To ensure patient safety, communicate clearly with members of the health care team, assess and incorporate a patient's priorities of care and preferences and use the best evidence when making decisions about your patient's care. When performing the skills in this chapter, remember the following points to ensure safe individualized patient care.

- Follow principles of surgical and medical asepsis as indicated when performing catheterizations, handling urine specimens, or helping patients with their toileting needs.
- Identify patients at risk for latex allergies (i.e., patient history of hay fever; asthma; and allergies to certain foods such as bananas, grapes, apricots, kiwi fruit, and hazelnuts).
- Identify patients with allergies to povidone-iodine (Betadine). Provide alternatives such as chlorhexidine.

SKILL 45-1 COLLECTING MIDSTREAM (CLEAN-VOIDED) URINE SPECIMEN

View Video!

Delegation Considerations

The skill of collecting midstream (clean-voided) urine specimens can be delegated to nursing assistive personnel (NAP). If appropriate, you can instruct an alert patient who is physically able to collect the specimen. It is the nurse's responsibility to ensure that this specimen is obtained correctly and in a timely manner. Be knowledgeable about agency policy regarding specimen collection. Direct the NAP to:

- Consider patient's mobility restrictions and inform the nurse when the specimen is obtained.
- Inform the nurse if patient is unable to initiate a stream or has pain or burning on urination.
- Inform the nurse if the collected specimen is dark, bloody, cloudy, or odorous or contains mucus.

Equipment

- Soap or cleaning solution, washcloth, and towel
- Commercial kit for clean-voided specimen or individual supplies as listed
  - Sterile cotton balls or sterile 2 × 2 or 4 × 4 gauze pads
  - Antiseptic solution (e.g., chlorhexidine [Hibiclens] or povidone-iodine [Betadine]); check for patient allergy to iodine (if allergic, provide alternative such as chlorhexidine)
  - Sterile water or saline
  - Sterile specimen container
- Clean gloves
- Bedpan, bedside commode, or specimen hat
- Completed specimen label with proper patient identifiers
- Completed laboratory requisition form and biohazard bag

STEP	RATIONALE
ASSESSMENT	
1 Identify the patient using two identifiers (i.e., name and birth date or name and account number) according to facility policy. Compare identifiers with information on patient's medical record.	Ensures correct patient. Complies with recommended National Patient Safety Goal (TJC, 2011).
2 Assess voiding status of patient.	
a. When patient last voided	Indicates bladder fullness.
b. Level of awareness or developmental stage	Reveals patient's ability to cooperate during procedure.
c. Mobility, balance, coordination, and physical limitations	Determines level of assistance in acquiring specimen.
3 Assess for signs and symptoms of UTI.	Indicates need to screen for bacteria in urine.
4 Assess patient's understanding of purpose of test and method of collection.	Allows you to clarify misunderstandings and promotes patient cooperation.
PLANNING	
1 Provide fluids to drink ½ hour before collection unless contraindicated (i.e., fluid restriction) if patient does not feel urge to void.	Improves likelihood of patient being able to void.
2 Explain procedure to patient:	Helps patient understand procedure.
a. Reason midstream specimen is necessary	
b. Ways for patient and family to assist	
c. Ways to obtain specimen free of feces	Feces change characteristics of urine and cause abnormal values.
d. Use visual aids (if applicable) to explain procedure	Illustrations demonstrating midstream collection techniques help to clarify a complex procedure, especially with patients for whom English is a second language.
IMPLEMENTATION	
1 Perform hand hygiene.	Decreases likelihood of transfer of microorganisms.
2 Provide privacy for patient by closing door or bed curtain.	Privacy allows patient to relax and produce specimen more quickly.
3 Give patient or family member cleaning towelette or soap, washcloth, and towel to clean perineal area or assist dependent patient (wear gloves).	Patient often prefers to wash own perineal area. Cleaning prevents contamination of specimen as urine passes from urethra.
4 Assist patient who cannot ambulate onto bedpan. Raise head of bed.	Provides easy access to perineal area to collect specimen. Semi-sitting position may ease voiding.
5 Using surgical asepsis, open sterile kit (see illustration) or prepare sterile supplies.	Sterile technique is essential to maintaining sterility of equipment and specimen.
6 Apply sterile gloves (when assisting dependent patient) after opening sterile specimen cup, placing cap with sterile inside surface up; do not touch inside of container or cap (see Chapter 28).	Sterile gloves prevent introduction of microorganisms from nurse's hands to specimen. Contaminated specimen is most frequent reason for inaccurate reporting of urine cultures and sensitivities.
7 Pour antiseptic solution over cotton balls or gauze pads unless kit contains prepared gauze pads in antiseptic solution.	Use cotton balls or gauze pads to further clean the perineum.

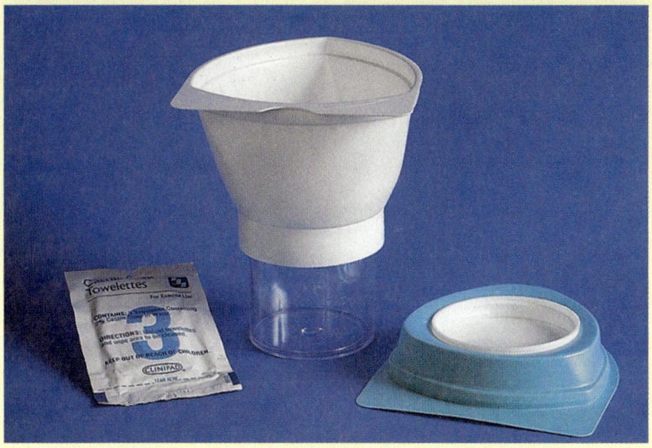

STEP 5 Commercial midstream urine collection kit.

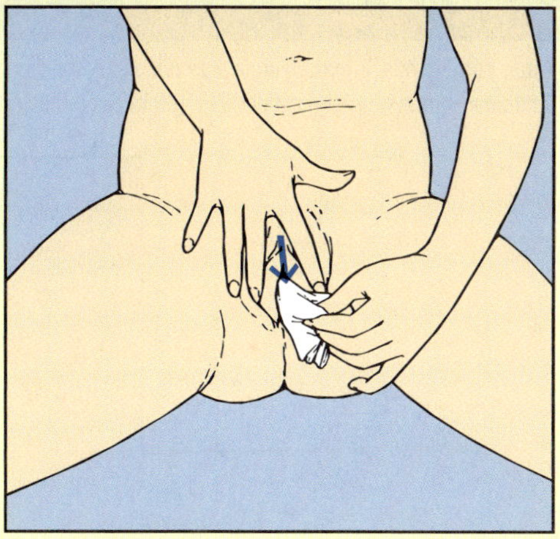

STEP 8a(2) Cleaning technique (female).

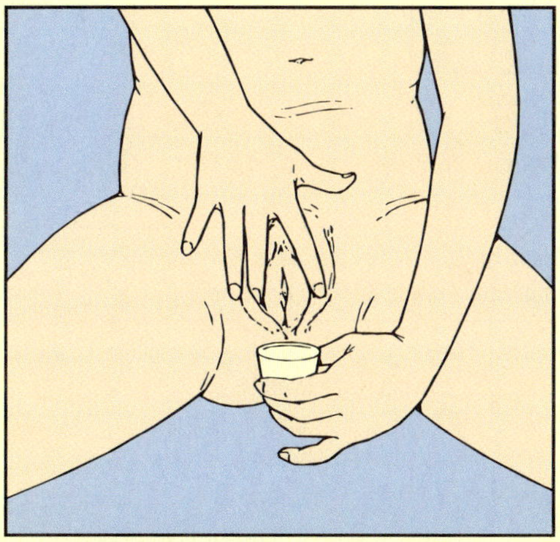

STEP 8a(4) Specimen collection (female).

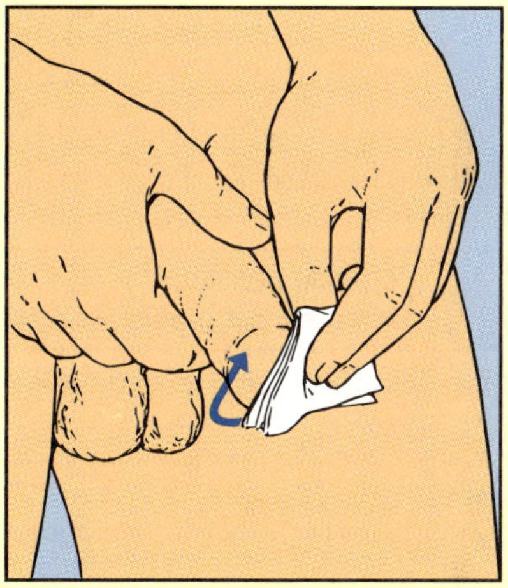

STEP 8b(1) Cleaning technique (male).

STEP	RATIONALE
8 Perform urine collection by assisting or allowing patient to independently clean perineum and collect specimen:	
a. Female	
(1) Spread labia with thumb and forefinger of nondominant hand.	Provides access to urethral meatus.
(2) Clean area with cotton ball or gauze, moving from front (above urethral orifice) to back (toward anus). Using a fresh swab each time, repeat front-to-back motion 3 times (begin with left side, then right side, then center) (see illustration).	Clean from area of least contamination to area of greatest contamination to decrease bacterial levels.
(3) If agency policy indicates, rinse area with sterile water and dry with dry cotton ball or gauze.	Prevents contamination of specimen with antiseptic solution.
(4) While continuing to hold labia apart, have patient initiate stream. After patient starts urine stream, pass container into stream and collect 30 to 60 mL (see illustration).	Initial stream flushes out microorganisms that accumulate at urethral meatus and prevents transfer into specimen.
(5) If menstruating, record this on the laboratory requisition form.	
b. Male	
(1) Hold penis with one hand and, using circular motion and antiseptic swab, clean end of penis, moving from center to outside (see illustration). In uncircumcised men retract foreskin before cleaning.	Clean from area of least contamination to area of greatest contamination to decrease bacterial levels.
(2) If agency procedure indicates, rinse area with sterile water and dry with cotton or gauze.	Prevents contamination of specimen with antiseptic solution.

SKILL 45-1 COLLECTING MIDSTREAM (CLEAN-VOIDED) URINE SPECIMEN—cont'd

STEP	RATIONALE
(3) After patient has initiated urine stream, pass specimen collection container into stream and collect 30 to 60 mL (see illustration).	Initial stream flushes out microorganisms that accumulate at urethral meatus and prevents transfer into specimen.

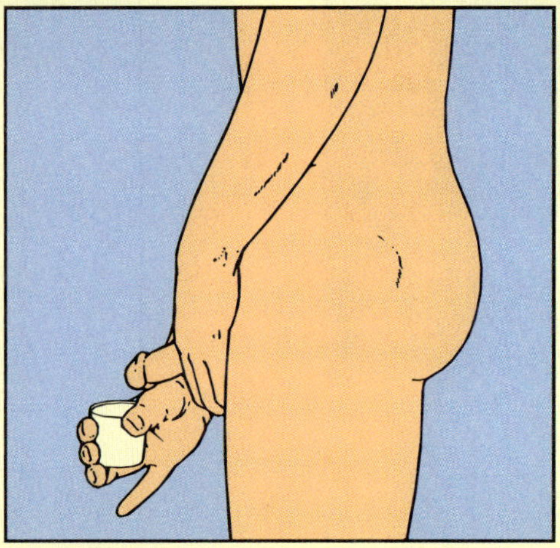

STEP 8b(3) Specimen collection (male).

STEP	RATIONALE
9 Remove specimen container before flow of urine stops and before releasing labia or penis. Patient finishes voiding in bedpan or toilet.	Prevents contamination of specimen with skin flora.

CLINICAL DECISION: *If foreskin was retracted for specimen collection, replace it over the glans. If foreskin is not replaced, swelling and constriction occur, causing pain and possible obstruction to urine flow.*

STEP	RATIONALE
10 Replace cap securely on specimen container (touch outside only).	Retains sterility of inside of container and prevents spillage of urine.
11 Clean any urine from exterior surface of container. Attach label on side of container in front of patient. Place in a plastic specimen biohazard bag as required by agency.	Prevents transfer of microorganisms to others.
12 Remove and empty bedpan (if applicable) and assist patient to comfortable position.	Promotes relaxing environment.
13 Attach laboratory requisition to specimen bag.	Prevents inaccurate identification and minimizes errors in diagnosis or treatment.
14 Remove gloves, dispose of them in proper receptacle, and perform hand hygiene.	Reduces transmission of infection.
15 Transport specimen to laboratory within 15 to 30 minutes or refrigerate immediately.	Because bacteria grow quickly in urine, urine not received by laboratory within 30 minutes should be refrigerated. However, refrigeration should not exceed 2 hours (Pagana and Pagana, 2010).

EVALUATION

1 Observe characteristics of urine and contaminants.	Contaminants prevent specimen from being used.
2 Evaluate laboratory results of urine test.	Determines presence of bacteria and kidney function.

UNEXPECTED OUTCOMES AND RELATED INTERVENTIONS

1 Urine specimen is contaminated with feces or toilet paper.
- Repeat instruction to patient or assist patient in obtaining specimen.
- Obtain a new specimen.
- Request an order for using a straight catheterization to obtain specimen.

2 Specimen is accidentally discarded.
- Repeat specimen collection.

RECORDING AND REPORTING

- Record date and time urine specimen was obtained in nurses' notes.
- Notify health care provider of any significant abnormalities.

HOME CARE CONSIDERATIONS

- If patient is to collect specimen as outpatient, a clean technique may be used. Provide instruction for collection and appropriate equipment.
- Provide information about storing specimen until time for delivery to health care provider's office or hospital laboratory.

SKILL 45-2 INSERTING A STRAIGHT OR INDWELLING CATHETER

Delegation Considerations

The skill of inserting a straight or an indwelling catheter cannot be delegated. The nurse is responsible for assessing the need for and evaluation of catheterization. The nurse directs nursing assistive personnel (NAP) to:

- Assist with positioning the patient and maintaining patient privacy and comfort, emptying urine from the collection bag, and providing perineal care.
- Report patient discomfort or fever to the nurse.
- Report abnormal color, odor, and amount of urine in drainage bag to the nurse.

Equipment

- Catheterization kit containing the following sterile items:
  - Gloves (extra pair optional)
  - Drapes, one fenestrated
  - Lubricant
  - Antiseptic cleaning solution such as povidone-iodine (Betadine) or alternative chlorhexidine (Hibiclens) if allergic to iodine
  - Cotton balls
  - Forceps
  - Prefilled syringe with sterile water to inflate balloon of indwelling catheter
  - Catheter of correct size and type for procedure (i.e., intermittent or indwelling)
  - Sterile drainage tubing with collection bag and multipurpose tube holder or tape and elastic band for securing tubing to bed if patient is bed bound (for indwelling catheter)
  - Receptacle or basin (usually bottom of catheterization tray)
  - Specimen container
- Also needed
  - Clean gloves for perineal care
  - Bath blanket
  - Appropriate light source (e.g., room lighting adapted or additional lighting such as an examination lamp)

STEP	RATIONALE
ASSESSMENT	
1 Review patient's medical record, including health care provider's order and nurses' notes. When appropriate, determine previous catheterization, including catheter size.	Determines purpose of inserting catheter: preparation for surgery, urinary irrigations, collection of sterile specimens, or measurement of residual urine.
2 Identify the patient using two identifiers (i.e., name and birth date or name and account number) according to facility policy. Compare identifiers with information on patient's medical record.	Ensures correct patient. Complies with a recommended National Patient Safety Goal (TJC, 2011).
3 Assess status of patient:	
a. Last time patient urinated from intake and output (I&O) flow sheet or palpate bladder or perform bladder scan	Determine time of last voiding or potential for bladder fullness. Scanner measures presence of urine.
b. Level of awareness or developmental stage	Reveals patient's ability to cooperate and level of explanation needed.
c. Mobility and physical limitations of patient	Affect way the nurse positions patient.
d. Patient's gender and age	Determines catheter size: 5- to 6-Fr generally for an infant; 8- to 10-Fr used for children; 14- to 16-Fr recommended for most patients. Men often need a slightly larger size (such as a 16- to 18-Fr) than women. Large catheters (greater than 16-Fr can distend the urethra, permanently damage the urethra and bladder neck, and cause bladder spasms and leaking around the catheter (Hart, 2008). Use the smallest size catheter possible to minimize trauma and promote adequate drainage of the periurethral glands. This decreases the risk for infection (Hart, 2008; Senese et al., 2006a).
e. Note any pathological condition that impairs passage of catheter (e.g., enlarged prostate in men).	Obstruction prevents passage of catheter through urethra into bladder. Often requires use of Coudé catheter.
f. Perform hand hygiene. Apply clean gloves. Inspect perineum for erythema, drainage, and odor. Remove gloves following inspection and perform hand hygiene.	Reduces infection. Determines condition of perineum.
g. Allergies.	Procedure risks exposure to allergies associated with antiseptic, tape, latex, and lubricant. Allergy to povidone-iodine is common. Alternatives to povidone-iodine include chlorhexidine or Sur-Clens (Senese et al., 2006b, 2006c).
4 Assess patient's knowledge of purpose for catheterization.	Reveals need for patient instruction.

SKILL 45-2 INSERTING A STRAIGHT OR INDWELLING CATHETER—cont'd

STEP	RATIONALE
PLANNING	
1 Explain procedure to patient.	Promotes cooperation.
2 Arrange for extra nursing personnel to assist as necessary.	Some patients are unable to assume positioning for procedure.
IMPLEMENTATION	
1 Perform hand hygiene.	Reduces transmission of microorganisms.
2 Close curtain or door.	Offers privacy, reduces embarrassment, and aids in relaxation during procedure.
3 Raise bed to appropriate working height. Facing patient, stand on left side of bed if right-handed (on right side of bed if left-handed). Clear bedside table and arrange equipment. If side rails are in use, raise side rail on opposite side of bed and put side rail down on working side.	Promotes use of proper body mechanics. Successful catheter insertion requires nurse to assume comfortable position with all equipment easily accessible. Use of side rails in this manner promotes patient safety.
4 Place waterproof pad under patient.	Prevents soiling of bed linen.
5 Position patient.	
a. Female patient	
(1) Assist to dorsal recumbent position (supine with knees flexed). Ask patient to relax thighs so you can rotate hips. Support legs with pillows to reduce muscle tension and promote comfort.	Provides good visualization of perineal structures. This position is optimal because it minimizes risk for contamination by fecal material (Cochran, 2007).
(2) Position female patient in side-lying (Sims) position with upper leg flexed at hip if unable to assume dorsal recumbent position.	This alternate position is used if patient cannot abduct leg at hip joint (e.g., if patient has an arthritic joint). It is also more comfortable for patient. Support patient with pillows if necessary to maintain position.
b. Male patient	
(1) Assist to supine position with thighs slightly abducted.	Comfortable position for patient that aids in visualization.
6 Drape patient.	
a. Female patient	
(1) Drape with bath blanket. Place blanket diamond fashion over patient, with one corner at patient's midsection, side corners over each thigh and abdomen, and last corner over perineum (see illustration).	Avoids unnecessary exposure of body parts and maintains patient's comfort.
b. Male patient	
(1) Drape upper trunk with bath blanket and cover lower extremities with bed sheets, exposing only genitalia (see illustration).	Avoids unnecessary exposure of body parts and maintains patient's comfort.

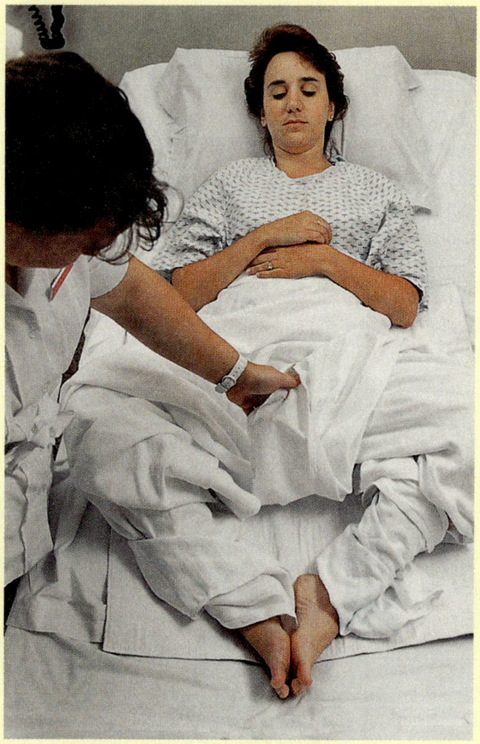

STEP 6a(1) Draping technique (female).

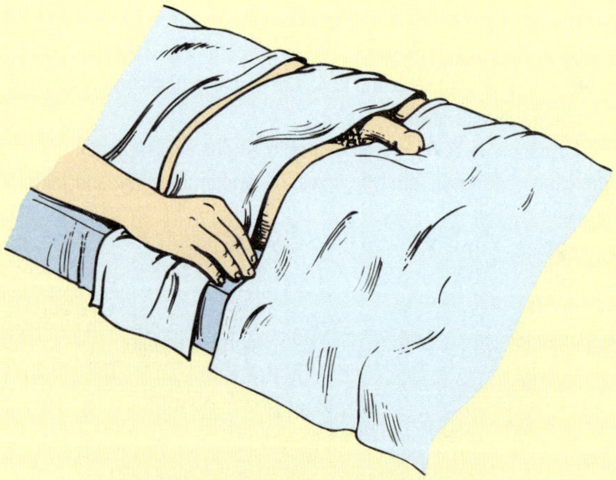

STEP 6b(1) Draping technique (male).

STEP	RATIONALE
7 Wearing clean gloves, wash perineal area with soap and water as needed; dry thoroughly. Remove and discard gloves; perform hand hygiene. Position light source to illuminate perineal area. (Have an assistant hold flashlight if necessary.)	Washing ensures that area is not contaminated before catheter insertion (Leaver, 2007). It is sometimes difficult to see urinary meatus of female patient because of individual anatomical differences (Senese et al., 2006a). Permits accurate identification and good visualization of urethral meatus.
8 Open outer wrapping of the indwelling Foley catheterization kit by tearing package on paper-lined edge of plastic wrap. Place inner wrapped box on easily accessible, clean bedside table or set between patient's legs. Patient's size and positioning dictates exact placement. Place empty package (outer plastic wrap) near end of bed and use for waste disposal.	Provides easy access to supplies during catheter insertion. Maintains aseptic technique during procedure.
9 *Open sterile wrap covering box containing catheter supplies:* Using sterile technique (see Chapter 28), fold back each flap of sterile package one at a time, with last flap opened toward patient.	The tray is now open and sitting on its own sterile field.
a. Supplies in intermittent catheterization tray are contained in sterile receptacle that can be used for urine collection.	
b. Supplies in an indwelling catheter box are arranged in sequence of use.	
10 Apply waterproof sterile drape (when packed as first item in tray). Sterile gloves may be packed as first item (see Step 11).	
a. Female patient	
(1) Remove square sterile drape from the tray, touching edges (2.5 cm [1-inch] border) only. Do not touch any other item in kit (see Chapter 28).	Keeps drape and items sterile.
(2) Maintain sterility of drape and let it unfold after removing from tray. Fold top edge of drape (2.5-5 cm [1-2 inches]) away from patient to form cuff over both hands.	
(3) Have patient lift hips (if patient is unable to lift hips, get assistance).	
(4) Place sterile drape with plastic (shiny) side down under patient's buttocks.	Creates sterile field over which you work during catheterization.
(5) Apply sterile gloves and proceed to Step 12.	
b. Male patient	Creates sterile field.
(1) Use of square sterile drape is optional; you may apply fenestrated drape instead (see Step 12). Remove and unfold as with female (see Step 10a).	
(2) Apply drape over thighs just below penis (instead of under buttocks as in female).	
11 Apply sterile gloves. (When packed as first item in tray, apply and then place square drape [see Step 10].)	Apply drapes either with or without sterile gloves, depending on sequence of packaging.
12 Apply fenestrated drape:	
a. Female patient	
(1) Pick up fenestrated drape out of tray. Allow it to unfold without touching nonsterile surface. Form cuff from edges to protect sterile gloves. Apply drape over perineum, exposing labia, and be sure not to touch contaminated surface.	Creates sterile field around perineum with opening that allows you to manipulate perineum.
b. Male patient	
(1) Apply drape over thighs and below penis without completely opening it. Use this technique when you choose not to apply square sterile drape.	Either a square or fenestrated drape may be used with male patient to create sterile field.
(2) Pick up fenestrated sterile drape and allow it to unfold without touching nonsterile surface. Form cuff from edges to protect sterile gloves; drape it over penis with fenestrated slit resting over penis (see illustration).	Maintains sterility of work surface while only exposing penis.
13 Move tray/box on sterile field closer to patient. In the case of female patient, sterile wrap under tray/box and drape form a continuous field.	Prevents you from reaching over nonsterile area when manipulating sterile catheter.
a. Organize remaining items on sterile field. *Indwelling catheter:* Take top tray out of box and place it on sterile field. (Sterile catheter and drainage bag are under top tray in box.) Make sure that clamp on drainage port of bag is closed. If drainage bag is preconnected to catheter, leave bag on sterile field until catheter is inserted. If drainage bag is not connected to catheter, open package containing sterile collection bag and drainage tubing. Keep cover on tip of drainage tubing until ready to connect to catheter.	Maintains principles of surgical asepsis and organizes work area. Keeping cover on tip of sterile drainage tubing prevents contamination.

SKILL 45-2 INSERTING A STRAIGHT OR INDWELLING CATHETER—cont'd

STEP	RATIONALE

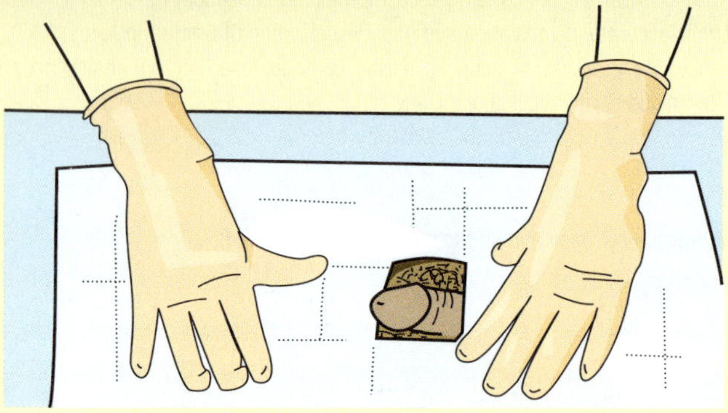

STEP 12b(2) Draping male with fenestrated drape.

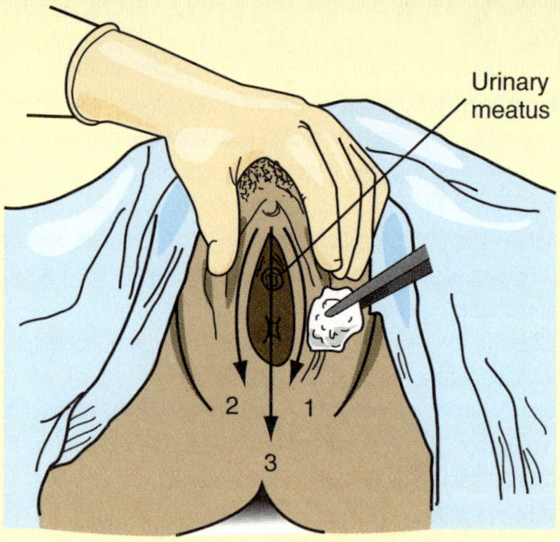

STEP 16a(2) Cleaning female perineum.

STEP	RATIONALE
b. *Intermittent catheter:* There is no drainage bag in container or specimen container.	
c. Loosen lid on sterile specimen container if urine specimen is required. Otherwise discard into waste disposal bag.	Makes container accessible to receive urine from catheter if specimen is needed.
d. Open package of sterile antiseptic solution. Pour solution over sterile cotton balls. NOTE: Sometimes there are sterile antiseptic swabs instead of solution. If swabs are available, open package with "stick" ends up.	
e. Open packet containing lubricant. NOTE: Lubricant is sometimes in prefilled syringe. If in prefilled syringe, remove protective cap. Spread lubricant into sterile tray.	Prepares lubricant for catheter.
14 Remove plastic covering from catheter (usually on indwelling catheter only). Take care to coil length of catheter in palm. Do not pretest balloon.	Prevents contamination of catheter.

CLINICAL DECISION: *Pretesting balloon by injecting fluid from the prefilled sterile water syringe into the balloon port is no longer recommended. Testing the balloon may distort and stretch it and lead to damage, causing increased trauma on insertion (Smith, 2006).*

STEP	RATIONALE
15 Place length of catheter in lubricant: Lubricate catheter 2.5-5 cm (1-2 inches) for women and 12.5-17.5 cm (5-7 inches) for men.	Lubricating catheter minimizes urethral trauma and discomfort when inserting it.
16 Clean urethral meatus:	
a. Female patient	
(1) With nondominant hand fully expose urethral meatus by spreading labia. Have NAP use flashlight if unable to visualize with available lighting. Maintain position of nondominant hand throughout procedure.	Optimal visualization of urethral meatus is possible. Fully spreading labia prevents contamination of urethral meatus during cleaning. NOTE: Closure of labia during cleaning requires that cleaning procedure be repeated.
(2) Using forceps in sterile dominant hand, pick up cotton ball saturated with antiseptic solution or antiseptic swab stick and clean perineal area, wiping from front to back from clitoris toward anus. Using a new cotton ball or swab for each area you clean, wipe far labial fold, near labial fold, and directly over center of urethral meatus (see illustration).	Cleaning reduces number of microorganisms at urethral meatus. Use of a new cotton ball for each wipe prevents transfer of microorganisms. Cleaning for each of the three areas proceeds from area of least to most contamination. Dominant hand remains sterile.

STEP	RATIONALE
b. Male patient	
(1) If patient is not circumcised, retract foreskin with nondominant hand.	Exposes urethral meatus
(a) Grasp penis at shaft just below glans.	
(b) Gently spread urethral meatus so opening is more visible. Keep nondominant hand in this position throughout procedure.	Accidental release of foreskin or dropping of penis during cleaning requires repeating process because area becomes contaminated.
(2) With dominant hand pick up antiseptic-soaked cotton ball with forceps or swab stick and clean penis. Move cotton ball or swab in circular motion from urethral meatus down to base of glans. Repeat cleaning 3 more times, using clean cotton ball/stick each time (see illustration).	Reduces number of microorganisms at urethral meatus. Follows principles of medical aseptic technique (see Chapter 28). Dominant gloved hand remains sterile.
17 Pick up catheter with gloved dominant hand 7.5-10 cm (3-4 inches) from catheter tip. Hold end of catheter loosely coiled in palm of dominant hand. Place distal end of catheter in urine tray receptacle if straight catheterization is ordered.	Prevents soiling of patient and bed with draining urine.
18 Insert catheter:	
a. Female patient	
(1) Ask patient to bear down gently as if to void and slowly insert catheter through urethral meatus (see illustration).	Relaxation of external sphincter aids in insertion of catheter.
(2) Advance catheter a total of 7.5 cm (3 inches) in adult or **until urine flows out of catheter end.** When urine appears, advance catheter another 2.5-5 cm (1-2 inches). Do not use force to insert catheter.	Female urethra is short. Appearance of urine indicates that catheter tip is in bladder or lower urethra.
(3) Release labia and hold catheter securely with nondominant hand. **Proceed to Step 20 for balloon inflation (indwelling Foley only).**	Bladder or sphincter contraction causes accidental expulsion of catheter.

CLINICAL DECISION: *If no urine appears, catheter may be in vagina. If misplaced, leave catheter in vagina as landmark indicating where not to insert and insert new sterile catheter.*

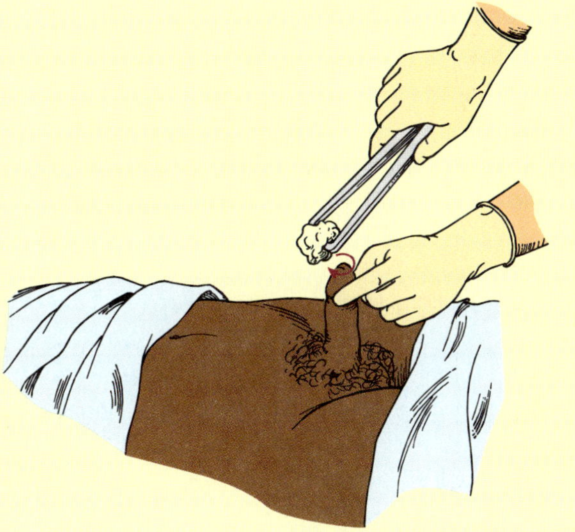

STEP 16b(2) Cleaning male urinary meatus.

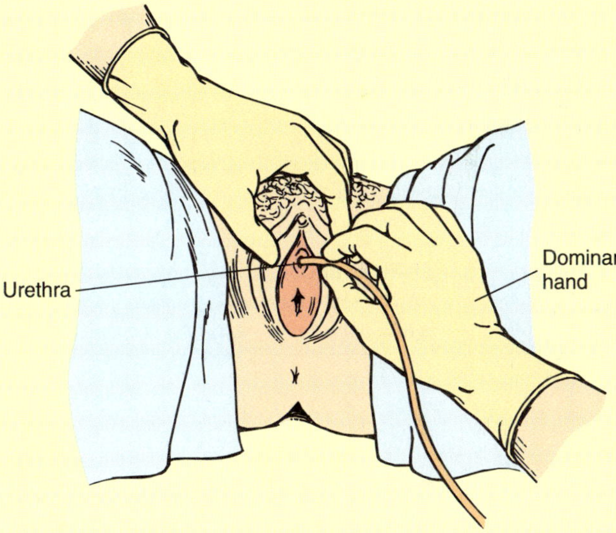

STEP 18a(1) Inserting catheter.

SKILL 45-2 INSERTING A STRAIGHT OR INDWELLING CATHETER—cont'd

STEP	RATIONALE
b. Male Patient	
(1) Lift penis to position perpendicular to patient's body and apply light traction (see illustration).	Straightens urethral canal to ease catheter insertion.
(2) Ask patient to bear down as if to void and slowly insert catheter through urethral meatus.	Relaxation of external sphincter aids in insertion of catheter.
(3) Advance catheter 17-22.5 cm (7-9 inches) in adult *or until urine flows out catheter.* If you feel resistance, withdraw catheter; do not force it through urethra. **If there is resistance to catheter insertion, have patient take slow deep breaths while you insert it slowly** (Senese et al., 2006c). When urine appears, advance catheter to bifurcation (see illustration).	The adult male urethra is long. It is normal to meet resistance at the prostatic sphincter. When resistance is met, hold catheter firmly against sphincter without forcing catheter. After a few seconds the sphincter relaxes, and you advance the catheter. Appearance of urine indicates that catheter tip is in bladder or urethra. Advancement of catheter to bifurcation of drainage and balloon inflation port ensures proper placement of catheter through longer urethra of male patients (Daneshgari et al., 2002; Senese et al., 2006c). Deep breathing during catheter insertion promotes relaxation (Senese et al., 2006c).
(4) Lower penis and hold catheter securely in nondominant hand. **Proceed to Step 20 for balloon inflation (indwelling Foley) only.**	Bladder or urethral contraction can accidentally expel catheter. Prevents accidental dislodgement of catheter.
(5) Reduce (or reposition) foreskin if necessary.	Paraphimosis (retraction and constriction of foreskin behind glans penis) secondary to catheterization occurs if foreskin is not reduced.
19 Collect urine specimen as needed. Fill specimen cup to correct level (20-30 mL).	Allows you to obtain sterile specimen for culture analysis.
20 Inflate balloon fully per manufacturer direction.	
a. While holding catheter with nondominant hand at urethral meatus, take end of catheter in dominant hand and place it between first two fingers of nondominant hand. Maintain secure hold on catheter with nondominant hand.	
b. With free dominant hand connect syringe to end of catheter at inflation valve and slowly inject total amount of solution. Follow manufacturer instructions regarding amount of fluid used for balloon inflation (see illustration).	Inflation of balloon anchors catheter tip in place above bladder outlet to prevent removal of catheter. Note size of balloon on catheter. Most commonly a 5-mL balloon is used and should be inflated with the amount (10 mL) supplied in the prefilled syringe to allow symmetrical expansion (Smith, 2006).
c. After inflating balloon, pull *gently* on catheter tubing until resistance is felt (see illustration).	Ensures that catheter tip is anchored.
d. Connect drainage tubing to retention catheter if it is not already preconnected. Place drainage bag below level of bladder (see illustration); do not place bag on side rails of bed.	Ensures proper drainage by gravity. Placement on side rails increases risk for tension applied to catheter, and bag can be raised above level of bladder.

CLINICAL DECISION: *If you notice resistance to inflation or if patient complains of pain, the balloon is not entirely in the bladder. Stop inflation, aspirate the fluid injected into the balloon, and advance the catheter a little more before attempting to inflate the balloon again.*

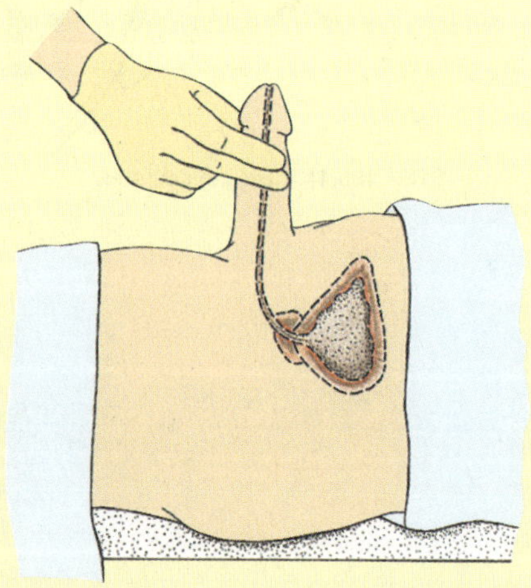

STEP 18b(1) Position penis perpendicular to body for catheter insertion.

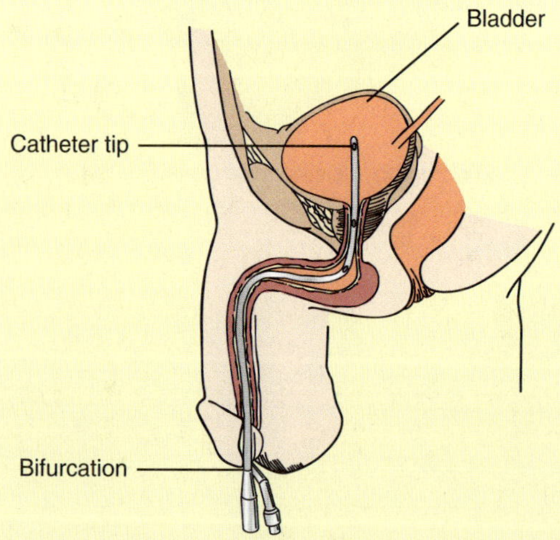

STEP 18b(3) Male anatomy with correct catheter insertion to bifurcation.

STEP	RATIONALE

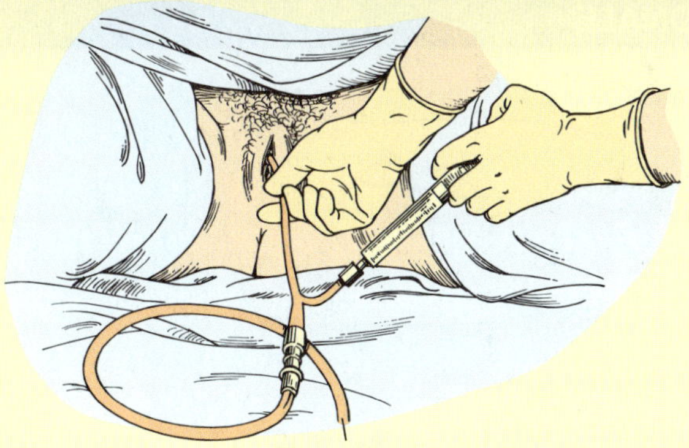

STEP 20b Inflating balloon (indwelling catheter) of drainage and balloon inflation port.

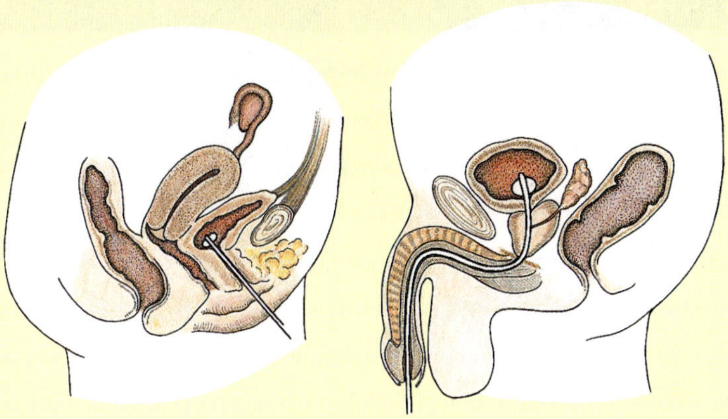

STEP 20c Placement of inflated balloon in bladder.

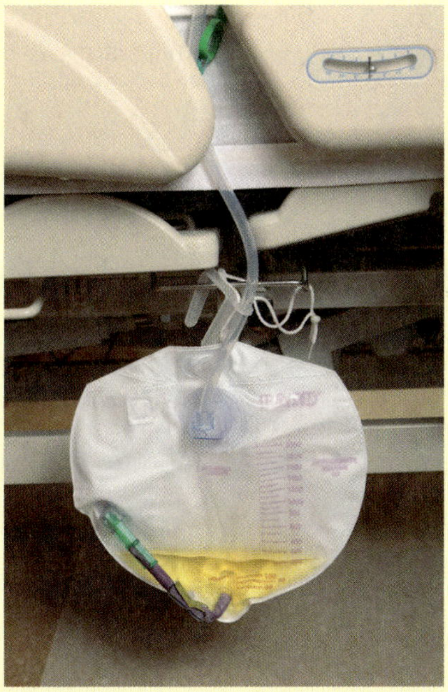

STEP 20d Attach drainage bag to lower bed frame.

STEP	RATIONALE
21 Allow bladder to empty fully unless agency policy restricts maximal volume of urine to drain with each catheterization (about 500 to 800 mL).	Relieves bladder distention. There is no definitive evidence regarding whether there is benefit in limiting maximal volume drained. Retained urine serves as a reservoir for growth of microorganisms (Smith, 2006).
22 Anchor indwelling catheter:	
a. Female patient	
(1) Secure catheter tubing to inner thigh with strip of nonallergenic tape (use paper tape if allergic to silk tape or a multipurpose tube holder with a Velcro strap). Allow for slack so movement of thigh does not create tension on catheter (see illustration).	Anchoring catheter to inner thigh reduces pressure on urethra, thus reducing possibility of tissue injury (Smith, 2006). Also minimizes risk for bleeding, trauma, meatal necrosis, and bladder spasms from pressure and traction (Senese et al., 2006a).
b. Male patient	
(1) Secure catheter tubing to top of thigh or lower abdomen (with penis directed toward chest). Allow slack in catheter so movement does not create tension on catheter (see illustration).	Anchoring catheter to lower abdomen reduces pressure on urethra at junction of penis and scrotum, thus reducing possibility of tissue injury (Senese et al., 2006a).

SKILL 45-2 INSERTING A STRAIGHT OR INDWELLING CATHETER—cont'd

STEP	RATIONALE

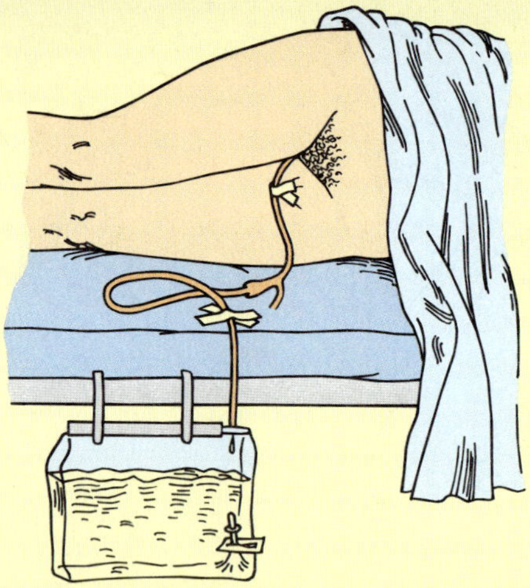

STEP 22a(1) Tape catheter to inner thigh (female) and coil excess tubing on bed and attach to sheet.

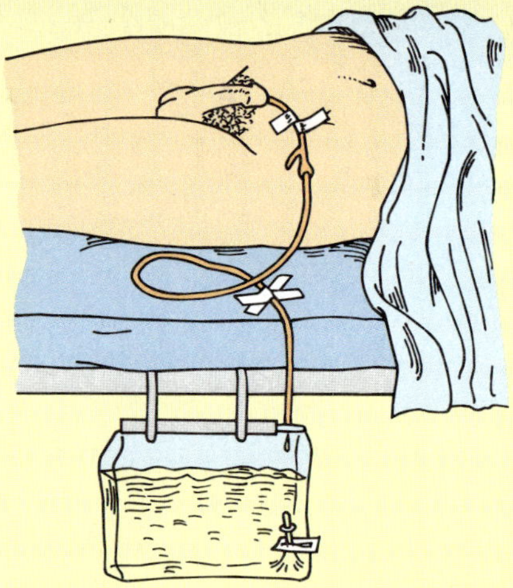

STEP 22b(1) Tape catheter to lower abdomen (male) and coil extra tubing on bed and attach to sheet.

STEP	RATIONALE
23 Be sure that there are no obstructions in tubing. Coil excess tubing on bed and fasten it to bottom sheet with clip from kit.	Obstructions prevent free flow of urine, leading to bladder retention.
24 Assist patient to comfortable position. Perform catheter care routinely and when secretions build up in perineum (see Skill 45-3).	Maintains comfort and security.
25 Dispose of equipment in proper receptacles, remove gloves, and perform hand hygiene.	Reduces transmission of microorganisms.
26 *For straight or intermittent catheter:* Follow Steps 1-18. Note differences identified between indwelling and straight catheter.	
a. Once catheter is in bladder, allow urine to drain out of end of catheter into sterile urine receptacle. Do not release hold on catheter.	Aim is to drain bladder fully without removing catheter too early.
b. Collect urine specimen if needed by placing end of catheter over specimen container. Collect 20-30 mL of urine.	Urine is used to test for microorganisms.
c. Gently withdraw catheter from bladder while palpating over the patient's bladder with nonsterile hand.	Allows for complete emptying of bladder.
d. Place urine in receptacle in graduated cylinder to measure. Remember to record amount in sterile specimen container as well.	Determines urinary output.
e. Complete Steps 24-25.	

EVALUATION

STEP	RATIONALE
1 Palpate bladder for distention or perform bladder scan.	Determines if distention is relieved.
2 Ask about patient's comfort.	Determines if patient's sensation of discomfort or fullness has been relieved.
3 Observe character and amount of urine in drainage system.	Determines if urine is flowing adequately.
4 Determine that no urine is leaking from catheter or tubing connections.	Prevents injury to patient's skin.

UNEXPECTED OUTCOMES AND RELATED INTERVENTIONS

1 Urethral or perineal irritation is present.
- Observe for catheter leaking; replace if necessary.
- Assess that indwelling catheter is anchored properly.
- Perform perineal hygiene and catheter care more frequently.

2 Patient has fever, and/or odor is present; or he or she experiences small frequent voiding, burning or bleeding on voiding.
- Obtain clean-voided urine specimen.
- Notify health care provider.

3 Patient experiences urinary retention and is unable to void after you remove the catheter.
- Provide adequate fluid intake and ensure patient privacy.
- If patient is unable to void 4 hours following catheter removal, notify health care provider.

RECORDING AND REPORTING

- Report and record type and size of catheter inserted, amount of fluid used to inflate the balloon, characteristics and amount of urine, reasons for catheterization, specimen collection if appropriate, and patient's response to procedure and teaching concepts.
- Initiate intake and output (I&O) record.
- If catheter is definitely in bladder and no urine is produced within an hour, immediately report absence of urine to health care provider.

HOME CARE CONSIDERATIONS

- Patients at home often use a leg bag during the day and switch to a large-volume bag at night so sleep is uninterrupted.
- Patients who catheterize themselves at home frequently use a clean technique.

SKILL 45-3 INDWELLING CATHETER CARE

Delegation Considerations

The skill of perineal care is often part of routine hygiene care that can be delegated to nursing assistive personnel (NAP). Proper assessment and care of the perineal area is the responsibility of the nurse. If patient has had trauma or surgical procedures that involve the perineal area, do not delegate this care.

The nurse instructs the NAP to:

- Report patient discomfort and perineal pain, discharge, perineal rash, and/or odor.
- Report condition of the catheter and drainage tubing (e.g., leaks, encrustations).
- Report any discolored or foul-smelling urine.

Equipment

- Catheter care kit or individual supplies
  - Clean gloves
  - Cotton balls or large swabs
  - Clean washcloth and towel
  - Warm water and soap
- Bath blanket
- Waterproof absorbent pad

STEP	RATIONALE
ASSESSMENT	
1 Identify the patient using two identifiers (i.e., name and birth date or name and account number) according to facility policy. Compare identifiers with information on patient's medical record.	Ensures correct patient. Complies with a recommended National Patient Safety Goal (TJC, 2011).
2 Assess for episode of bowel incontinence or patient discomfort or provide care per agency routine as part of hygiene measures (see Chapter 39).	Accumulation of secretions or feces causes irritation to perineal tissues and acts as source of bacterial growth.
3 Observe any discharge or redness around urethral meatus.	Indicates inflammatory process and possible infection.
4 Assess patient's knowledge of catheter care.	Patients who perform own catheter care may be unsure of touching catheter. Assesses patient's ability and knowledge to provide instruction as needed (Leaver, 2007).
PLANNING	
1 Explain procedure to patient. Offer opportunity to perform self-care to able patient.	Reduces anxiety and promotes cooperation. Embarrassment often motivates patient to perform own hygiene.
2 Close door or bedside curtain.	Maintains patient privacy.
IMPLEMENTATION	
1 Perform hand hygiene.	Reduces transmission of infection.
2 Position patient:	Ensures easy access and visualization of perineal tissues.
a. **Female**	
(1) Dorsal recumbent position	
b. **Male**	
(1) Supine or Fowler's position	
3 Place waterproof pad under patient.	Protects bed linens from soiling.
4 Drape bath blanket on patient so only perineal area is exposed.	Prevents unnecessary exposure of body parts.
5 Apply clean gloves.	
6 Remove anchor device to free catheter tubing.	

SKILL 45-3 INDWELLING CATHETER CARE—cont'd

STEP	RATIONALE
7 With nondominant hand:	
a. Female	
(1) Gently retract labia to fully expose urethral meatus and catheter insertion site, maintaining position of hand throughout procedure.	Provides full visualization of urethral meatus. Full retraction of labia prevents contamination of meatus during cleaning.
b. Male	
(1) Retract foreskin if not circumcised and hold penis at shaft just below glans, maintaining position throughout procedure.	Retraction of foreskin provides full visualization of urethral meatus.
8 Assess urethral meatus and surrounding tissue for inflammation, swelling, and discharge. Note amount, color, odor, and consistency of discharge. Ask patient if he or she feels any burning or discomfort.	Determines presence of local infection and status of hygiene.
9 Clean perineal tissue:	
a. Female	
(1) Use clean cloth, soap, and water. Clean around urethral meatus and catheter. Avoid getting soap into urethra. Cleaning from pubis toward anus, clean labia minora. Use clean side of cloth for each wipe. Finally clean around anus. Dry each area well.	Perineal care with soap and water is sufficient to keep area clean (Leaver, 2007). Soap entering urethra may cause urinary tract infection (UTI). Application of topical antimicrobial products is not effective in reducing meatal bacterial flora and reducing risk of UTI. Do not include them as part of routine catheter care (Leaver, 2007).
b. Male	
(1) While spreading urethral meatus, clean around catheter first and then wipe in circular motion around meatus and glans.	Cleaning moves from area of least to most contamination.
10 While stabilizing catheter with nondominant hand, clean length of catheter from meatus to tubing in circular motion. Follow agency guidelines (see illustration).	Reduces presence of secretions, drainage, and bacteria on exterior of catheter surface.

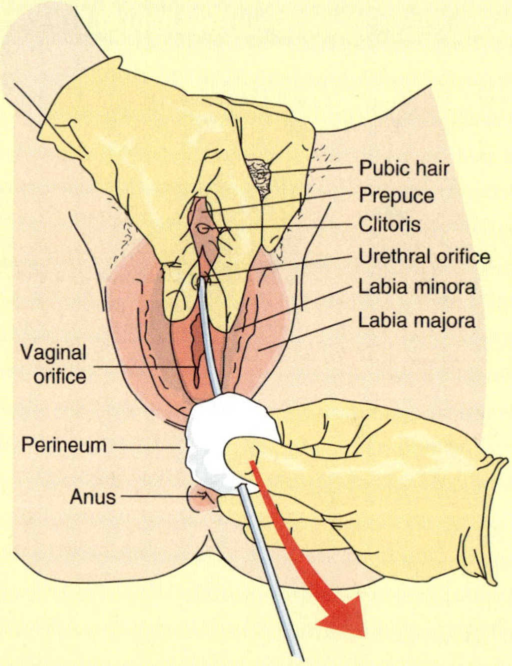

STEP 10 Cleaning catheter during catheter care. (From Sorrentino S: *Mosby's textbook for nursing assistants,* St Louis, 2007, Mosby.)

STEP	RATIONALE
11 Reduce (or reposition) foreskin after care.	
12 Reanchor catheter tubing.	
13 Place patient in safe, comfortable position.	Promotes comfort.
14 Dispose of contaminated supplies, remove gloves, and perform hand hygiene.	Prevents spread of infection.

EVALUATION

STEP	RATIONALE
1 Inspect condition of urethra and surrounding tissue and ask patient about discomfort.	Determines if area is cleaned properly and/or if patient has any irritation.

UNEXPECTED OUTCOMES AND RELATED INTERVENTIONS

1 Urethral discharge or perineal irritation present
- Observe for leaking from around catheter; catheter may need replacing.
- Increase frequency of indwelling catheter care.
- Notify health care provider.

2 Accidental catheter dislodgement
- Notify health care provider.
- Assess for urethral trauma.
- Monitor urine output.

RECORDING AND REPORTING

- Report and record presence and characteristics of drainage, condition of perineal tissue, and any discomfort reported by patient.
- If infection is suspected, report findings to health care provider.

HOME CARE CONSIDERATIONS

- If patient is discharged with indwelling catheter, teach patient and family catheter care and signs and symptoms to report to nurse or health care provider.

SKILL 45-4 CLOSED CATHETER IRRIGATION

Delegation Considerations

The skill of closed catheter irrigation or instillation cannot be delegated to nursing assistive personnel (NAP). The nurse is responsible for assessing the need for irrigation. Catheter irrigation is usually done in patients with complications such as urinary tract infections (UTIs) or after prostatectomy. The nurse directs NAP caring for the patient to:
- Report patient complaints of pain, discomfort, or fever and leakage of urine around catheter.
- Report the presence of blood clots or a change in color of the urine.
- Monitor and record intake and output (I&O); immediately report any decrease in urinary output.

Equipment

- Closed intermittent method for irrigation or instillation
  - Sterile irrigation or instillation solution at room temperature (unless otherwise ordered)
  - Sterile graduated container
  - Sterile 30- to 50-mL irrigation syringe (used to instill irrigant into catheter)
  - Luer-Lok syringe without needles if used for needleless access port (this varies depending on manufacturer)
  - Sterile 19- to 22-gauge 1-inch needle (if catheter access port is not needleless)
  - Clean gloves
  - Antiseptic swabs
  - Clamp for catheter or tubing
- Closed continuous method
  - Sterile irrigation solution at room temperature (unless otherwise ordered)
  - Irrigation tubing and clamp (with or without a Y connector) (Clamp regulates irrigation flow rate. Y connector allows intravenous [IV] or irrigant bags to be connected to tubing.)
  - IV pole
  - Antiseptic swab
  - Y connector (optional) (used to connect irrigation tubing to double-lumen catheter).
  - Bath blanket

STEP	RATIONALE
ASSESSMENT	
1 Assess patient's record to determine:	
a. Purpose of bladder irrigation.	Allows you to anticipate observations to make (e.g., blood or mucus in urine).
b. Prescriber's order for type and amount of irrigant (e.g., saline).	Order required to initiate therapy. Ensures that correct medication or solution and amount are administered. Amount of solution used to flush system may be a nursing judgment or indicated by prescriber or institution policy. Frequency of irrigation is based on patient's need (e.g., patient who has just had prostate gland surgery may require continuous irrigation for 24 hours).

SKILL 45-4 CLOSED CATHETER IRRIGATION—cont'd

STEP	RATIONALE
c. Type of irrigation: continuous or intermittent.	Allows for selection of proper equipment. In continuous irrigation clamp regulates slow, steady flow into bladder. Because outflow should correspond to regulated drip, patency of catheter must be checked frequently to prevent distention of bladder. For intermittent irrigation instill designated amount of irrigation solution into catheter and clamp catheter or tubing for no longer than 30 minutes. Intermittent irrigation requires close observation of catheter patency between irrigations.
d. Type of catheter used. (NOTE: Appropriate catheter should be inserted during original catheterization.)	Indicates if it is necessary to break into closed system for irrigation.
(1) Single lumen (single use) for open intermittent irrigation only	
(2) Double lumen (one lumen to inflate balloon, one to allow outflow of urine)	
(3) Triple lumen (one lumen to inflate balloon, one to instill irrigation solution, one to allow outflow of urine)	
2 Assess the following:	
a. Color of urine and presence of mucus, clots, or sediment	Indicates if patient is bleeding or sloughing tissue and determines necessity for increasing irrigation rates with continuous irrigations or increasing frequency with intermittent irrigations.
b. Bladder palpation	Determines if urine is draining freely from bladder.
c. Existing closed irrigation system	
(1) Note if fluid entering bladder and fluid draining from bladder are in approximate proportions.	Determines presence of bladder distention.
(2) Determine that drainage tubing is not kinked, clamped off incorrectly, or looped below bladder level.	Determines if system is obstructed. You would expect more output than fluid instilled because of urine production.
(3) Note amount of fluid remaining in existing irrigating solution container.	Allows you to anticipate hanging of new irrigation bag.
3 Review I&O record.	Determines baseline for prior urine output measures. All patients with continuous bladder irrigations should have I&O measurements (see Chapter 41).
4 Identify the patient using two identifiers (i.e., name and birth date or name and account number) according to facility policy. Compare identifiers with information on patient's medical record.	Ensures correct patient. Complies with recommended National Patient Safety Goal (TJC, 2011).
5 Assess patient's knowledge regarding purpose of performing catheter irrigations.	Reveals need for patient instruction.
PLANNING	
1 Explain procedure to patient.	Reduces anxiety and promotes cooperation.
IMPLEMENTATION	
1 Perform hand hygiene and apply clean gloves.	Prevents transmission of microorganisms.
2 Provide privacy by pulling bed curtains closed. Fold back covers so catheter is exposed. Cover patient's upper torso with bath blanket.	Promotes patient comfort and provides easy access to catheter.
3 Position patient in dorsal recumbent or supine position.	Promotes flow of irrigating solution into bladder.
4 *Closed intermittent irrigation or instillation with double-lumen catheter:*	
a. Pour prescribed sterile solution in sterile graduated cup.	Ensures that irrigation or instillation fluid remains sterile.
b. Clamp indwelling retention catheter just below specimen port.	Occlusion of catheter provides resistance against which nurse can forcefully instill irrigant into catheter.
c. Draw sterile solution into syringe using aseptic technique (usually 30 to 50 mL). Place sterile cap on tip of needleless syringe. Attach capped, sterile needle on end of syringe (if needleless system is not used).	Ensures sterility of irrigation fluid.

CLINICAL DECISION: *Avoid cold solution as irrigant or instillation because it results in bladder spasm and discomfort.*

STEP	RATIONALE
d. Using circular motion, clean injection port with antiseptic swab (same port used for specimen collection).	Reduces transmission of infection.
e. Insert tip of needleless syringe using twisting motion into irrigation port (see manufacturer instructions for possible variation). *Alternative:* Insert needle through port at 30-degree angle toward bladder.	Ensures that hub enters lumen of catheter and flow is directed into bladder.
f. Slowly inject fluid into catheter and bladder.	Slow, continuous pressure dislodges clots and sediment without traumatizing bladder wall.

STEP	RATIONALE

CLINICAL DECISION: *If catheter does not irrigate easily, the tip of the catheter is incorrectly placed in the urethra and not in the bladder. Use slow pressure when injecting fluid. Too much pressure traumatizes the urethral or bladder wall.*

g. Withdraw syringe, remove clamp, and allow solution to drain into drainage bag. If an instillation, keep catheter clamped to allow solution to remain in bladder for ordered time, especially if irrigant is medicated per prescriber's order.	Allows drainage by gravity.

CLINICAL DECISION: *If solution is to remain in bladder, do not forget to unclamp tubing at the end of the instillation period.*

5 *Closed continuous irrigation (see illustration):*

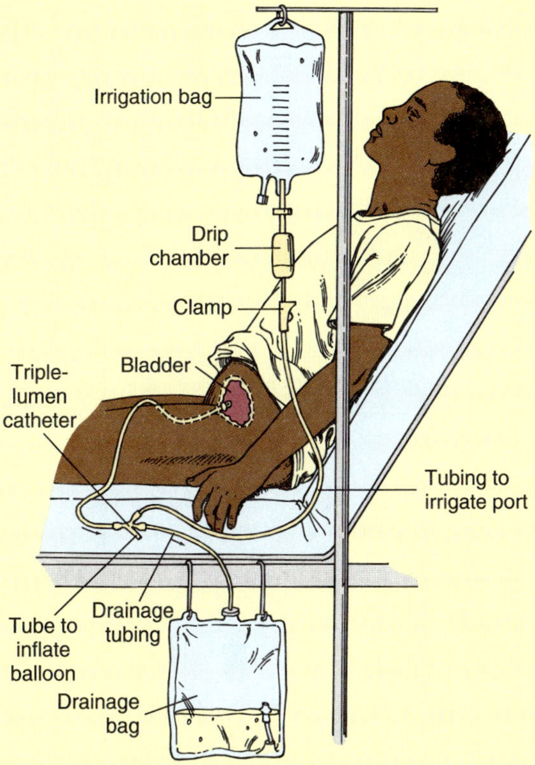

STEP 5 Closed continuous bladder irrigation.

a. Apply clean gloves.	Prevents entrance of microorganisms.
b. Close clamp on tubing and hang bag of solution on IV pole. Using aseptic technique, insert spike of sterile irrigation tubing into bag of sterile irrigating solution.	
c. Open clamp and allow solution to flow through tubing, keeping end of tubing sterile. Close clamp and recap end of tubing.	Removes air from tubing.
d. Use aseptic technique to wipe off irrigation port of triple-lumen catheter or attach sterile Y-connector to double-lumen catheter and then attach to irrigation tubing.	Third lumen or Y-connector provides means for irrigation solution to enter bladder. System must remain sterile.
e. Be sure that drainage bag and tubing are securely connected to drainage port of triple-lumen catheter or other arm of Y-connector.	Ensures that urine and irrigation solution drains from bladder without leaking.
f. For continuous drainage, calculate drip rate and adjust clamp on irrigation tubing accordingly. Be sure that clamp on drainage tubing is open and check volume of drainage in drainage bag. Make sure that drainage tubing is patent and avoid kinks.	Ensures continuous, even irrigation of catheter system. Prevents accumulation of solution in bladder, which causes bladder distention and possible injury.
g. For intermittent flow, clamp tubing on drainage system, open clamp on irrigation tubing, and allow prescribed amount of fluid to enter bladder (100 mL is normal for adults). Close irrigation clamp and then open drainage tubing clamp. *(Optional:* Leave clamp closed for 20 to 30 minutes if ordered.)	Fluid instills through catheter into bladder, flushing system. Fluid drains out after irrigation is completed. Do not clamp catheter for longer than 30 minutes because it can cause damage to bladder, backup to kidneys, and hyperreflexia if bladder gets too full.

SKILL 45-4 CLOSED CATHETER IRRIGATION—cont'd

STEP	RATIONALE
6 When procedure is completed, dispose of contaminated supplies, remove gloves, and perform hand hygiene.	Prevents spread of infection.
EVALUATION	
1 Calculate amount of irrigation or instillation fluid and subtract from total output.	Determines accurate urinary output.
2 Assess characteristics of output: viscosity, color, clarity, odor, and presence of matter (e.g., sediment, clots, blood).	Evaluates results of irrigation or instillation and provides baseline data to judge response to therapy. Determines presence of UTI.
3 Observe for catheter patency.	Ensures that bladder is emptying freely.
4 Observe patient for signs of pain and fever.	Evaluates for presence of infection.

UNEXPECTED OUTCOMES AND RELATED INTERVENTIONS

1 Irrigant or instillation solution not returning; or continuous solution not flowing at prescribed rate, which indicates possible occlusion of catheter
- Examine tubing for kinks, clots, or urine sediment.
- Notify health care provider if irrigant or instillation is retained, patient complains of pain, or bladder is distended.

2 Cloudy or foul urine, fever
- Monitor fever.
- Notify health care provider.
- Obtain sterile urine specimen if ordered by health care provider.

3 Increase in bladder spasms; indicates occlusion of catheter with foreign object (e.g., blood clot)
- Notify health care provider.
- Perform intermittent irrigations until clots clear as directed.

RECORDING AND REPORTING

- Record type and amount of irrigation solution used, amount returned as drainage, and the character of drainage.
- Record and report any findings such as complaints of bladder spasms, inability to instill fluid into bladder, and/or presence of blood clots.

HOME CARE CONSIDERATIONS

- If patient is discharged with indwelling catheter and requires bladder irrigations, instruct the patient and/or the family on proper care.
- Because irrigation or instillation carries a risk of contamination, assess the level of understanding of surgical asepsis by the patient and family and provide appropriate instruction. The patient and family need guidelines for the skill and for conditions requiring a call to the health care provider.

KEY POINTS

- Voluntary control from higher brain centers and involuntary control from the spinal cord influence the act of micturition or voiding.
- Symptoms common to urinary disturbances include frequency, urgency, dysuria, polyuria, oliguria, incontinence, and difficulty in starting the urinary stream.
- When collected properly, a clean-voided urine specimen does not contain bacteria from the urethral meatus.
- Methods of promoting the micturition reflex help patients sense the urge to urinate and control urethral sphincter relaxation.
- An increased fluid intake results in increased diluted urine formation that reduces the risk of urinary tract infections.
- An indwelling urinary catheter remains in the bladder for an extended period, making the risk of infection greater than with intermittent catheterization.
- Catheter irrigation becomes necessary when the catheter becomes occluded with sediment or blood clots.
- A catheter drainage system should be a closed system positioned to allow free drainage of urine by gravity.
- Incontinence is classified as functional, overflow, stress, urge, or total. Each type has specific nursing interventions.
- Follow specific guidelines for catheter selection so the catheter does not cause harm.

CLINICAL APPLICATION QUESTIONS

Preparing for Clinical Practice

Mrs. Grayson is a 55-year-old woman who has had problems with stress incontinence for the past 2 years. She has not spoken to anyone about her problems because she is embarrassed. She finally confides to her health care practitioner that the problem is causing her to avoid social situations and she would like help to regain urinary control. Mrs. Grayson weighs 200 pounds, and her height is 5 feet 1 inch. She has been referred to a continence specialist. A plan of care was developed after a thorough assessment of her urinary pattern and symptoms.

1. She has recently begun Kegel exercises to attempt improvement in her urinary control. She doesn't see any improvement. She has been trying to deal with the problem by using an absorbent pad in her underwear, but she feels as though everyone knows her problem. What additional teaching does Mrs. Grayson need?
2. Two months after your first encounter with Mrs. Grayson, she has been seen by her primary health care provider for burning on urination with increased frequency and urgency. She has also noted blood in her urine for a week. What is Mrs. Grayson experiencing and what can you teach her to minimize her symptoms?
3. Mrs. Grayson says she is not satisfied with her current state of urinary control and has decided on a more permanent solution

to her stress incontinence. She opts for a minimally invasive procedure that will provide support for the urethra. She will be going home with an indwelling catheter. She asks how to care for the catheter while she is home. She does not want another urinary tract infection. What do you tell her about measures at home to remain infection free?

evolve *Answers to Clinical Application Questions can be found on the Evolve website.*

REVIEW QUESTIONS

Are You Ready to Test Your Nursing Knowledge?

1. A female patient reports that she is experiencing burning on urination, frequency, and urgency. The nurse notes that a clean-voided urine specimen is markedly cloudy. The probable cause of these symptoms and findings is:
   1. Cystitis.
   2. Hematuria.
   3. Pyelonephritis.
   4. Dysuria.
2. A male patient returned from the operating room 6 hours ago with a cast on his right arm. He has not yet voided. Which action would be the most beneficial in assisting the patient to void?
   1. Suggest he stand at the bedside
   2. Stay with the patient
   3. Give him the urinal to use in bed
   4. Tell him that, if he doesn't urinate, he will be catheterized
3. Elimination changes that result from inability of the bladder to empty properly may cause which of the following? (Select all that apply.)
   1. Incontinence
   2. Frequency
   3. Urgency
   4. Urinary retention
   5. Urinary tract infection
4. An older male patient states that he is having problems starting and stopping his stream of urine and he feels the urgency to void. The best way to assist this patient is to:
   1. Help him stand to void.
   2. Place a condom catheter.
   3. Have him practice Credé's method.
   4. Initiate Kegel exercises.
5. Since removal of the patient's Foley catheter, the patient has voided 50 to 100 mL every 2 to 3 hours. Which action should the nurse take first?
   1. Check for bladder distention
   2. Encourage fluid intake
   3. Obtain an order to recatheterize the patient
   4. Document the amount of each voiding for 24 hours
6. To minimize the patient experiencing nocturia, the nurse would teach him or her to:
   1. Perform perineal hygiene after urinating.
   2. Set up a toileting schedule.
   3. Double void.
   4. Limit fluids before bedtime.
7. A patient with a Foley catheter carries the collection bag at waist level when ambulating. The nurse tells the patient that he or she is at risk for: (Select all that apply.)
   1. Infection.
   2. Retention.
   3. Stagnant urine.
   4. Reflux of urine.
8. The patient is incontinent, and a condom catheter is placed. The nurse should take which action?
   1. Secure the condom with adhesive tape
   2. Change the condom every 48 hours
   3. Assess the patient for skin irritation
   4. Use sterile technique for placement
9. After a transurethral prostatectomy a patient returns to his room with a triple-lumen indwelling catheter and continuous bladder irrigation. The irrigation is normal saline at 150 mL/hr. The nurse empties the drainage bag for a total of 2520 mL after an 8-hour period. How much of the total is urine output?

   ____
10. The nurse is planning to remove a Foley catheter at 1300. The nurse would check if the patient has voided by:
    1. 1400.
    2. 1600
    3. 1700.
    4. 2300.
11. The postoperative patient has difficulty voiding after surgery and is feeling "uncomfortable" in the lower abdomen. Which action should the nurse implement first?
    1. Encourage fluid intake
    2. Administer pain medication
    3. Catheterize the patient
    4. Turn on the bathroom faucet as he tries to void
12. The patient is to have an intravenous pyelogram (IVP). Which of the following apply to this procedure? (Select all that apply.)
    1. Note any allergies.
    2. Monitor intake and output.
    3. Provide for perineal hygiene.
    4. Assess vital signs.
    5. Encourage fluids after the procedure.
13. The nurse assesses that the patient has a full bladder, and the patient states that he or she is having difficulty voiding. The nurse would teach the patient to:
    1. Use the double-voiding technique.
    2. Perform Kegel exercises.
    3. Use Credé's method.
    4. Keep a voiding diary.
14. The patient states that she "loses urine" every time she laughs or coughs. The nurse teaches the patient measures to regain urinary control. The nurse recognizes the need for further teaching when the patient states:
    1. "I will perform my Kegel exercises every day."
    2. "I joined weight watchers."
    3. "I drink two glasses of wine with dinner."
    4. "I have tried urinating every 3 hours."
15. The nurse notes that the patient's Foley catheter bag has been empty for 4 hours. The priority action would be to:
    1. Irrigate the Foley.
    2. Check for kinks in the tubing.
    3. Notify the health care provider.
    4. Assess the patient's intake.

Answers: **1.** 1; **2.** 1; **3.** 1, 2, 3, 4, 5; **4.** 4; **5.** 1; **6.** 4; **7.** 1, 4; **8.** 3; **9.** 1320 mL; **10.** 3; **11.** 4; **12.** 1, 5; **13.** 3; **14.** 3; **15.** 2.

REFERENCES

Ackley BJ, Ladwig GB: *Nursing diagnosis handbook: a guide to planning care*, ed 7, St Louis, 2011, Mosby.

Altschuler V, Diaz L: Bladder ultrasound, *Medsurg Nurs* 15(5):317, 2006.

Beaty AD, Lieberman PL, Slavin RG: Seafood allergy and radiocontrast media: Are physicians propagating a myth? *Am J Med* 121(2):158, 2008.

Beji NK, et al: Overview of the social impact of urinary incontinence with a focus on Turkish women, *Urol Nurs* 30(6):327, 2010.

Bradway C, Cacchione P: Teaching strategies for assessing and managing urinary incontinence in older adults, *J Gerontol Nurs* 36(7):18, 2010.

Cochran S: Care of the indwelling urinary catheter: is it evidenced based? *J Wound Ostomy Cont Nurs* 34(3):282, 2007.

Daneshgari F, et al: Evidence-based multidisciplinary practice: improving the safety and standards of male bladder catheterization, *MedSurg Nurs* 11(5): 236, 2002.

Doughty DB: *Urinary and fecal incontinence: current management concepts*, ed 3, St Louis, 2006, Mosby.

Ebersole P, et al: *Toward healthy aging: human needs and nursing response*, ed 7, St Louis, 2008, Mosby.

Gemmill R, Wells A: Promotion of urinary continence worldwide, *Urol Nurs* 30(6):336, 2010.

Giger JN, Davidhizar RE: *Transcultural nursing: assessment and intervention*, ed 5, St Louis, 2008, Mosby.

Gray M, et al: *Expert review: best practices in managing the indwelling catheter*, Perspectives, special edition sponsored by Dale Medical Products, Burlington, Vt, 2006, Saxe Health.

Hall JE: *Guyton and Hall textbook of medical physiology*, ed 12, Philadelphia, 2011, Saunders.

Hart S: Urinary catheterization, *Nurs Stand* 22(27):44, 2008.

Huether SE, et al: *Understanding pathophysiology*, ed 4, St Louis, 2008, Mosby.

Ksycki MF, Namias N: Nosocomial urinary tract infection, *Surg Clin North Am* 89:475, 2009.

Leaver R: The evidence for urethral meatal cleaning, *Nurs Stand* 21(41):39, 2007.

Lehne RA: *Pharmacology for nursing care*, ed 7, St Louis, 2010, Saunders.

Lewis SM, et al: *Medical-surgical nursing: assessment and management of clinical problems*, ed 8, St Louis, 2011, Mosby.

Madineh SMA: Avicenna's cannon of medicine and modern urology, *Urol J* 5(4): 284, 2008.

Newman DK: The indwelling urinary catheter: principles for best practices, *J Wound Ostomy Cont Nurs* 34(6):655, 2007.

Pagana KD, Pagana TJ: *Mosby's diagnostic and laboratory reference*, ed 10, St Louis, 2010, Mosby.

Palmer MH, Newman DK: Urinary incontinence and estrogen, *Am J Nurs* 107(3):35, 2007.

Saint S, et al: Catheter-associated urinary tract infection and the Medicare rule change, *Ann Intern Med* 150(112):877, 2009.

Schabelman E, Witting M: The relationship of radiocontrast, iodine, and seafood allergies: A medical myth exposed, *J Emerg Med* 39(5):701, 2010.

Smith JM: Current concepts in catheter management. In Doughty DB: *Urinary and fecal incontinence: current management concepts*, ed 3, St Louis, 2006, Mosby.

Stewart E: Treating urinary incontinence in older women, *Br J Commun Nurs* 15(11):526, 2010.

The Joint Commission (TJC): *2011 National Patient Safety Goals (NPGs)*, 2011, http://www.jointcommission.org/standards_information/npsgs.aspx. Accessed November 4, 2011.

Touhy TA, Jett KF: Ebersole and Hess' gerontological nursing healthy aging, ed 3, St Louis, 2010, Mosby.

RESEARCH REFERENCES

Bradway C, et al: How women conceptualize urinary incontinence: a cultural model, *J Women's Health* 19(8):1533, 2010.

Chen L, et al: Utility of bedside bladder ultrasound before urethral catheterization in young children, *Pediatrics* 115:108, 2005.

Fernandez RS, Griffiths RD: Duration of short-term indwelling catheters: a systematic review of the evidence, *J Wound Ostomy Cont Nurs* 33(2):145, 2006.

Holroyd-Leduc JM, et al: The relationship of indwelling urinary catheters to death, length of hospital stay, functional decline and nursing home admission in the hospitalized older medical patients, *J Am Geriatr Soc* 55 (2):227, 2007.

Lo E, et al: Strategies to prevent catheter-associated urinary tract infections in acute care hospitals, *Infect Control Hosp Epidemiol* 30(4):404, 2009.

Matteucci R, Walsh K: Urinary catheter use and prevention of infection: evidenced-based care sheet, *CINAHL Information Aug* 19(2p), 2011.

Nazarko L: Reducing the risk of catheter-related urinary tract infection, *Br J Nurs* 17(16):1002, 2008.

Parker D, et al: Nursing interventions to reduce the risk of catheter-associated urinary tract infection. Part 1: Catheter selection, *J Wound Ostomy Cont Nurs* 36(1):23, 2009.

Senese V, et al: SUNA clinical practice guidelines: care of the patient with an indwelling catheter, *Urol Nurs* 26(1):80, 2006a.

Senese V, et al: SUNA clinical practice guidelines: female urethral catheterization, *Urol Nurs* 26(4):314, 2006b.

Senese V, et al: SUNA clinical practice guidelines: male urethral catheterization, *Urol Nurs* 26(4):315, 2006c.

Wilson M, et al: Nursing interventions to reduce the risk of catheter-associated urinary tract infection. Part 2: Staff education, monitoring, and care techniques, *J Wound Ostomy Cont Nurs* 36(2):137, 2009.

CHAPTER

46

Bowel Elimination

OBJECTIVES

- Discuss the role of gastrointestinal organs in digestion and elimination.
- Describe three functions of the large intestine.
- Explain the physiological aspects of normal defecation.
- Discuss psychological and physiological factors that influence the elimination process.
- Describe common physiological alterations in elimination.
- Assess a patient's elimination pattern.
- List nursing diagnoses related to alterations in elimination.
- Describe nursing implications for common diagnostic examinations of the gastrointestinal tract.
- List nursing interventions that promote normal elimination.
- List nursing interventions included in bowel training.
- Discuss nursing care measures required for patients with a bowel diversion.
- Use critical thinking in the provision of care to patients with alterations in bowel elimination.

KEY TERMS

Bowel training, p. 1110
Cathartics, p. 1091
***Clostridium difficile*, p. 1092**
Colostomy, p. 1093
Constipation, p. 1091
Diarrhea, p. 1092
Effluent, p. 1109
Endoscopy, p. 1091
Enema, p. 1107
Fecal occult blood test (FOBT), p. 1099
Flatulence, p. 1092
Hemorrhoids, p. 1092
Ileostomy, p. 1093
Impaction, p. 1091
Incontinence, p. 1092
Laxatives, p. 1091
Paralytic ileus, p. 1091
Polyps, p. 1094
Stoma, p. 1093
Valsalva maneuver, p. 1089
Wound ostomy continence nurse (WOCN), p. 1109

evolve WEBSITE

http://evolve.elsevier.com/Potter/fundamentals/

- Review Questions
- Video Clips
- Animations
- Concept Map Creator
- Case Study with Questions
- Skills Performance Checklists
- Audio Glossary
- Interactive Learning Activities
- Key Term Flashcards
- Content Updates

Regular elimination of bowel waste products is essential for normal body functioning. Alterations in bowel elimination are often early signs or symptoms of problems within either the gastrointestinal (GI) or other body systems. Because bowel function depends on the balance of several factors, elimination patterns and habits vary among individuals.

Understanding normal bowel elimination and factors that promote, impede, or cause alterations in elimination help manage patients' elimination problems. Supportive nursing care respects the patient's privacy and emotional needs. Measures designed to promote normal elimination also need to minimize discomfort for the patient.

SCIENTIFIC KNOWLEDGE BASE

The GI tract is a series of hollow mucous membrane–lined muscular organs. These organs absorb fluid and nutrients, prepare food for absorption and use by body cells, and provide for temporary storage of feces (Fig. 46-1). The GI tract absorbs high volumes of fluids, making fluid and electrolyte balance a key function of the GI system. In addition to ingested fluids and foods, the GI tract also receives secretions from the gallbladder and pancreas.

Mouth

Digestion begins in the mouth and ends in the small intestine. The mouth mechanically and chemically breaks down nutrients into a usable size and form. The teeth masticate food, breaking it down into a size suitable for swallowing. Saliva, produced by the salivary glands in the mouth, dilutes and softens the food in the mouth for easier swallowing.

Esophagus

As food enters the upper esophagus, it passes through the upper esophageal sphincter, a circular muscle that prevents air from entering the esophagus and food from refluxing into the throat. The bolus of food travels down the esophagus and is pushed along by peristalsis, which propels it through the length of the GI tract.

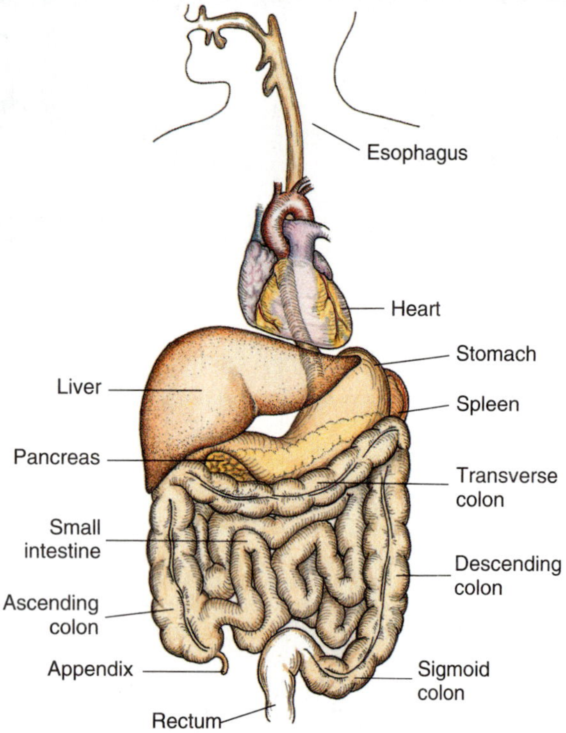

FIG. 46-1 Organs of gastrointestinal tract (with heart as reference point).

As food moves down the esophagus, it reaches the cardiac or lower esophageal sphincter, which lies between the esophagus and the upper end of the stomach. The sphincter prevents reflux of stomach contents back into the esophagus.

Stomach

The stomach performs three tasks: storing swallowed food and liquid; mixing food, liquid, and digestive juices; and emptying its contents into the small intestine. It produces and secretes hydrochloric acid (HCl), mucus, the enzyme pepsin, and the intrinsic factor. Pepsin and HCl facilitate the digestion of protein. Mucus protects the stomach mucosa from acidity and enzyme activity. The intrinsic factor is essential for the absorption of vitamin B_{12}.

Small Intestine

Segmentation and peristaltic movement in the small intestine facilitate both digestion and absorption (Fig. 46-2). Chyme mixes with digestive juices (e.g., bile and amylase). Resorption in the small intestine is so efficient that, by the time the chyme reaches the end of the small intestine, it is pastelike in consistency.

The small intestine has three sections: the duodenum, the jejunum, and the ileum. The duodenum is approximately 20 to 28 cm (8 to 11 inches) long and continues to process the chyme from the stomach. The jejunum is approximately 2.5 m (8 feet) long and absorbs carbohydrates and proteins. The ileum is approximately 3.7 m (12 feet) long and absorbs water, fats, certain vitamins, iron, and bile salts. The duodenum and jejunum absorb most of the nutrients and electrolytes. The intestinal wall also absorbs nutrients across the mucosa and into lymph fluids or blood vessels. Substances, such as plant fiber, that the small intestine cannot digest empty into the cecum at the lower right side of the abdomen. The large intestine begins at the cecum.

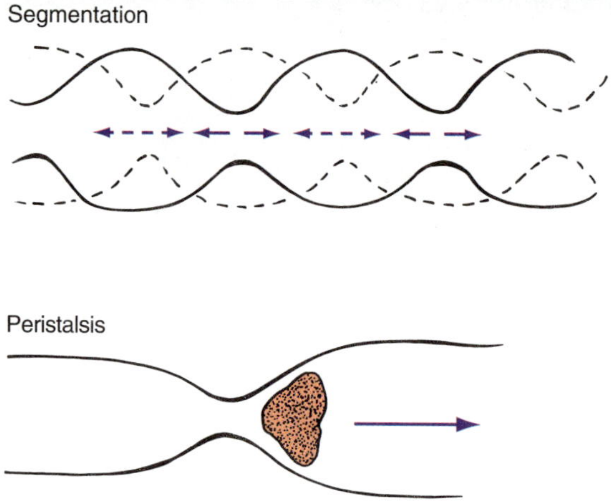

FIG. 46-2 Segmented and peristaltic waves.

Impairment of the small intestine alters the digestive process. For example, conditions such as inflammation, surgical resection, or obstruction disrupt peristalsis, reduce the area of absorption, or block the passage of chyme. Electrolyte and nutrient deficiencies then develop.

Large Intestine

The lower GI tract is called the *large intestine* (colon) because it is larger in diameter than the small intestine. The large intestine is shorter (1.5 to 1.8 m [5 to 6 feet]) but much wider than the small intestine. The large intestine is divided into the cecum, colon, and rectum (Fig. 46-3). The large intestine is the primary organ of bowel elimination. It is positioned like a question mark, partially encircling the small intestine.

Chyme enters the large intestine by waves of peristalsis through the ileocecal valve, a circular muscular layer that prevents regurgitation. The colon is divided into the ascending, transverse, descending, and sigmoid colons. The muscular tissue of the colon allows it to accommodate and eliminate large quantities of waste and gas (flatus). It has three functions: absorption, secretion, and elimination. The large intestine absorbs water, sodium, and chloride from the digested food that has passed from the small intestine. Healthy adults absorb more than a gallon of water and an ounce of salt from the colon every 4 hours. The amount of water absorbed from chyme depends on the speed at which colonic contents move. Chyme is normally a soft, formed mass. If peristalsis is abnormally fast, there is less time for water to be absorbed, and the stool is watery. If peristaltic contractions slow, water continues to be absorbed; and a hard mass of stool forms, resulting in constipation (JBI, 2008).

The secretory function of the colon aids in electrolyte balance. The colon secretes bicarbonate in exchange for chloride. The colon also excretes about 4 to 9 mEq of potassium daily. Therefore serious alterations in colon function (e.g., diarrhea) cause severe electrolyte disturbances.

Slow peristaltic contractions move contents through the colon. Intestinal content is the main stimulus for contraction. Mass peristalsis pushes undigested food toward the rectum. These mass movements occur only three or four times daily, with the strongest during the hour after mealtime.

The rectum is the final portion of the large intestine. Here bacteria convert fecal matter into its final form. Normally the rectum is empty of waste products (feces) until just before defecation. It

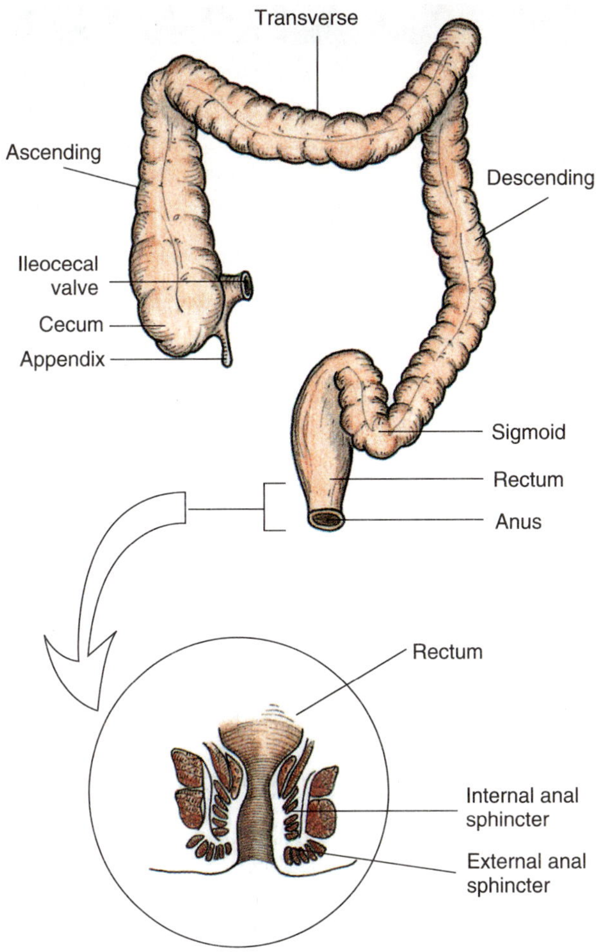

FIG. 46-3 Divisions of large intestine.

contains vertical and transverse folds of tissue that help to temporarily hold fecal contents during defecation. Each fold contains an artery and vein that can become distended from pressure during straining. This distention often results in hemorrhoid formation.

Anus

The body expels feces and flatus from the rectum through the anal canal and anus. Contraction and relaxation of the internal and external sphincters, innervated by sympathetic and parasympathetic stimuli, aid in the control of defecation. The anal canal is richly supplied with sensory nerves that help to control continence.

Defecation

The physiological factors critical to bowel function and defecation include normal GI tract function, sensory awareness of rectal distention and rectal contents, voluntary sphincter control, and adequate rectal capacity and compliance. Normal defecation begins with movement in the left colon, moving stool toward the anus. When stool reaches the rectum, the distention causes relaxation of the internal sphincter and an awareness of the need to defecate. At the time of defecation, the external sphincter relaxes, and abdominal muscles contract, increasing intrarectal pressure and forcing the stool out (Huether and McCance, 2008). Sometimes people use the **Valsalva maneuver** to assist in stool passage. The Valsalva maneuver exerts pressure to expel feces through a voluntary contraction of the abdominal muscles while maintaining forced expiration against a closed airway. Patients with cardiovascular disease, glaucoma, increased intracranial pressure, or a new surgical wound are at greater risk for cardiac dysrhythmias and elevated blood pressure with the Valsalva maneuver and need to avoid straining to pass the stool. Normal defecation is painless, resulting in passage of soft, formed stool.

NURSING KNOWLEDGE BASE

Factors Influencing Bowel Elimination

Many factors influence the process of bowel elimination. Knowledge of these factors helps to anticipate measures required to maintain a normal elimination pattern.

Age. Developmental changes affecting elimination occur throughout life. An infant has a small stomach capacity and less secretion of digestive enzymes. Food passes quickly through an infant's intestinal tract because of rapid peristalsis. The infant is unable to control defecation because of a lack of neuromuscular development. This neuromuscular development usually does not take place until 2 to 3 years of age.

Systemic changes in the function of digestion and absorption of nutrients result from changes in older patients' cardiovascular and neurological systems rather than their GI system. For example, arteriosclerosis causes decreased mesenteric blood flow, thus decreasing absorption from the small intestine (Meiner, 2011). In addition, peristalsis decreases, and esophageal emptying slows. Older adults often experience changes in the GI system that impair digestion and elimination (JBI, 2008) (Table 46-1).

Older adults also lose muscle tone in the perineal floor and anal sphincter (Holman et al., 2008). Although the integrity of the sphincter remains intact, they often have difficulty controlling bowel evacuation and are at risk for incontinence. In addition, nerve impulses to the anal region slow, causing some individuals to become less aware of the need to defecate. Older adults, especially residents in long-term care facilities, sometimes develop irregular bowel movements and an increased risk for constipation (Kyle, 2007a).

Diet. Regular daily food intake helps maintain a regular pattern of peristalsis in the colon. Fiber, the nondigestible residue in the diet, provides the bulk of fecal material. Bulk-forming foods such as whole grains, fresh fruits, and vegetables help flush the fats and waste products from the body with more efficiency (Holman et al., 2008). The bowel walls stretch, creating peristalsis and initiating the defecation reflex. With stimulation of peristalsis, bulk foods pass quickly through the intestines, keeping the stool soft. Ingestion of a high-fiber diet improves the likelihood of a normal elimination pattern if other factors are normal. Diets high in vegetables and fruits have been linked to decreased risk of colorectal cancer (ACS, 2011b).

Gas-producing foods such as onions, cauliflower, and beans also stimulate peristalsis. The gas formed distends intestinal walls and increases colon motility. Some spicy foods increase peristalsis but also cause indigestion and watery stools.

Food intolerance is not an allergy but rather a particular food that causes the body distress within a few hours of ingestion. The result is diarrhea, cramps, or flatulence. For example, people who drink cow's milk and have these symptoms are not allergic to milk but lack the enzyme needed to digest the milk sugar lactase and therefore are lactose intolerant. Another condition called *celiac disease* is a syndrome in which the patient has a hypersensitivity to protein in certain cereal grains and gluten.

TABLE 46-1 Normal Age-Related Changes in the Gastrointestinal Tract

PORTION OF GASTROINTESTINAL TRACT	FUNCTIONAL OR PHYSIOLOGICAL CHANGE	CAUSES
Mouth	Decreased chewing and salivation, including oral dryness	Degeneration of cells, medications (Gray-Vickrey, 2010; Meiner, 2011)
Esophagus	Reduced motility, especially in lower third	Degeneration of neural cells (Meiner, 2011)
Stomach	Decrease in:	
	Acid secretions	Degeneration of gastric mucosa (Banning, 2008) (Alkaline gastric medium contributes to malabsorption of iron. Although digestive enzymes are decreased, enough remain available for digestion.)
	Motor activity	Delayed gastric emptying, causing fewer hunger contractions (Gray-Vickrey, 2010)
	Mucosal thickness	Loss of parietal cells; leads to loss of intrinsic factor, which is necessary for vitamin B_{12} absorption
Small intestine	Decreased nutrient absorption	Fewer absorbing cells
Large intestine	Increase in pouches on weakened intestinal wall called *diverticulosis*	Weakened musculature Does not significantly affect absorption (Banning, 2008)
	Constipation	Decreased peristalsis (Gray-Vickrey, 2010)
	Missed defecation signal, increasing risk for fecal incontinence	Duller nerve sensations (Gray-Vickrey, 2010)
Liver	Size decreased	Reduced storage capacity and ability to synthesize protein and metabolize medications

Fluid Intake. An inadequate fluid intake or disturbances resulting in fluid loss (such as vomiting) affect the character of feces. Fluid liquefies intestinal contents, easing its passage through the colon. Reduced fluid intake slows passage of food through the intestine and results in hardening of stool contents. Unless there is a medical contraindication, an adult needs to drink at least 1100 to 1400 mL of fluid daily. An increase in fluid intake with the use of fruit juices softens stool and increases peristalsis. Poor fluid intake increases the risk of constipation because of greater resorption of fluid in the colon, resulting in hard, dry stools (Kyle, 2007a).

Physical Activity. Physical activity promotes peristalsis, whereas immobilization depresses it. Encourage early ambulation as illness begins to resolve or as soon as possible after surgery to promote maintenance of peristalsis and normal elimination. Maintaining tone of skeletal muscles used during defecation is important. Weakened abdominal and pelvic floor muscles impair the ability to increase intraabdominal pressure and control the external sphincter. Muscle tone is sometimes weakened or lost as a result of long-term illness, spinal cord injury, or neurological disease that impairs nerve transmission. As a result of these changes in the abdominal and pelvic floor muscles, there is an increased risk for constipation.

Psychological Factors. Prolonged emotional stress impairs the function of almost all body systems (see Chapter 37). During emotional stress the digestive process is accelerated, and peristalsis is increased. Side effects of increased peristalsis are diarrhea and gaseous distention. A number of diseases of the GI tract are associated with stress, including ulcerative colitis, irritable bowel syndrome, certain gastric and duodenal ulcers, and Crohn's disease. If a person becomes depressed, the autonomic nervous system slows impulses; peristalsis decreases, resulting in constipation.

Personal Habits. Personal elimination habits influence bowel function. Most people benefit from being able to use their own toilet facilities at a time that is most effective and convenient for them. A busy work schedule sometimes prevents the individual from responding appropriately to the urge to defecate, disrupting regular habits and causing possible alterations such as constipation. Individuals need to recognize the best time for elimination.

Chronically ill and hospitalized patients are not always able to maintain privacy during defecation. In a hospital or extended care setting, patients sometimes share bathroom facilities with a roommate with different hygienic habits. In addition, chronic illness limits a patient's balance, activity tolerance, or physical activity and requires the use of a bedpan or bedside commode. The sights, sounds, and odors associated with sharing toilet facilities or using bedpans are often embarrassing. This embarrassment often causes patients to ignore the urge to defecate, which begins a vicious cycle of constipation and discomfort.

Position During Defecation. Squatting is the normal position during defecation. Modern toilets facilitate this posture, allowing the person to lean forward, exert intraabdominal pressure, and contract the thigh muscles. For the patient immobilized in bed, defecation is often difficult. In a supine position it is impossible to contract the muscles used during defecation. If the patient's condition permits, raise the head of the bed to assist the patient to a more normal sitting position on a bedpan, enhancing the ability to defecate.

Pain. Normally the act of defecation is painless. However, a number of conditions such as hemorrhoids, rectal surgery, rectal fistulas, and abdominal surgery result in discomfort. In these instances the patient often suppresses the urge to defecate to avoid pain, contributing to the development of constipation.

Pregnancy. As pregnancy advances, the size of the fetus increases, and pressure is exerted on the rectum. A temporary obstruction created by the fetus impairs passage of feces. Slowing of peristalsis during the third trimester often leads to constipation. A pregnant woman's frequent straining during defecation or delivery results in formation of permanent hemorrhoids.

Surgery and Anesthesia. General anesthetic agents used during surgery cause temporary cessation of peristalsis (see Chapter 50). Inhaled anesthetic agents block parasympathetic impulses to

TABLE 46-2 Medications and the Gastrointestinal System

MEDICATIONS	ACTION
Dicyclomine HCl (Bentyl)	Suppresses peristalsis and decreases gastric emptying
Opioid analgesics	Slow peristalsis and segmental contractions, often resulting in constipation (Lehne, 2010)
Anticholinergic drugs such as atropine or glycopyrrolate (Robinul)	Inhibit gastric acid secretion and depress gastrointestinal (GI) motility (Lehne, 2010) (Although useful in treating hyperactive bowel disorders, anticholinergics cause constipation.)
Antibiotics	Produce diarrhea by disrupting the normal bacterial flora in the GI tract (An increase in the use of fluoroquinolones in recent years has provided a selective advantage for the epidemic of *Clostridium difficile*) (Vonberg et al., 2008)
Nonsteroidal antiinflammatory drugs	Cause GI irritation that increases the incidence of bleeding with serious consequences to older adults; rectal bleeding is often observed with GI irritation (Lehne, 2010)
Aspirin	Prostaglandin inhibitor; interferes with the formation and production of protective mucus and causes GI bleeding (Lehne, 2010)
Histamine$_2$ (H_2) antagonists	Suppress the secretion of hydrochloric acid and interfere with the digestion of some foods
Iron	Causes discoloration of the stool (black), nausea, vomiting, constipation (diarrhea is less commonly reported), and abdominal cramps (Lehne, 2010)

the intestinal musculature. The action of the anesthetic slows or stops peristaltic waves. The patient who receives a local or regional anesthetic is less at risk for elimination alterations because this type of anesthesia generally affects bowel activity minimally or not at all.

Any surgery that involves direct manipulation of the bowel temporarily stops peristalsis. This condition, called **paralytic ileus,** usually lasts about 24 to 48 hours. If the patient remains inactive or is unable to eat after surgery, return of normal bowel elimination is further delayed.

Medications. Some medications have certain expected actions on the bowel (e.g., there are medications to promote defecation or control diarrhea). In addition, medications prescribed for acute and chronic conditions often have secondary effects on the patient's bowel elimination patterns (Table 46-2).

Laxatives and **cathartics** soften the stool and promote peristalsis. Although similar, laxatives are milder in action than cathartics. When used correctly, laxatives and cathartics safely maintain normal elimination patterns. However, chronic use of cathartics causes the large intestine to become less responsive to stimulation by laxatives. Laxative overuse can also cause serious diarrhea, leading to dehydration and electrolyte depletion. Mineral oil, a common laxative, decreases fat-soluble vitamin absorption. Laxatives often influence the efficacy of other medications by altering the transit time (i.e., the time the medication remains in the GI tract and is available for absorption).

Diagnostic Tests. Diagnostic examinations involving visualization of GI structures often require a prescribed bowel preparation (e.g., medications, cathartics, and/or enemas) to ensure that the bowel is empty. In addition, the patient cannot eat or drink several hours before the examinations such as an **endoscopy,** colonoscopy, or other testing that requires visualization of the GI tract. Following the diagnostic procedure, changes in elimination such as increased gas or loose stools often occur until the patient resumes a normal eating pattern.

BOX 46-1 COMMON CAUSES OF CONSTIPATION

- Irregular bowel habits and ignoring the urge to defecate
- Chronic illnesses (e.g., Parkinson's disease, multiple sclerosis, rheumatoid arthritis, chronic bowel diseases, depression, diabetic neuropathy, eating disorders (McWilliams, 2010)
- Low-fiber diet high in animal fats (e.g., meats, dairy products, eggs) (McWilliams, 2010)
- Low fluid intake, which slows peristalsis (Holman et al., 2008)
- Anxiety, depression, cognitive impairment (McWilliams, 2010)
- Lengthy bed rest or lack of regular exercise (McWilliams, 2010)
- Laxative misuse (Durston, 2009)
- Slowed peristalsis, loss of abdominal muscle elasticity, and reduced intestinal mucus secretion experienced by older adults (Durston, 2009)
- Neurological conditions that block nerve impulses to the colon (e.g., spinal cord injury, tumor) (Kyle, 2007c)
- Illnesses such as hypothyroidism, hypocalcemia, or hypokalemia
- Medications such as anticholinergics, antispasmodics, anticonvulsants, antidepressants, antihistamines, antihypertensives, antiparkinsonism drugs, bile acid sequestrants, diuretics, antacids, iron supplements, calcium supplements, and opioids slow colonic action (Lehne, 2010)

Common Bowel Elimination Problems

Caring for patients who have or are at risk for elimination problems because of emotional stress (anxiety or depression), physiological changes in the GI tract such as surgical alteration of intestinal structures, inflammatory diseases, prescribed therapy, or disorders impairing defecation is common in the practice of nursing.

Constipation. **Constipation** is a symptom, not a disease (Box 46-1). Improper diet, reduced fluid intake, lack of exercise, and certain medications can cause constipation. For example, patients receiving opiates for pain after surgery often require a stool softener or laxative to prevent constipation. The signs of constipation include infrequent bowel movements (less than every 3 days), difficulty passing stools, excessive straining, inability to defecate at will, and hard feces (McWilliams, 2010). When intestinal motility slows, the fecal mass becomes exposed over time to the intestinal walls, and most of the fecal water content is absorbed. Little water is left to soften and lubricate the stool. Passage of a dry, hard stool causes rectal pain (Fig. 46-4).

Constipation is a significant health hazard. Straining during defecation causes problems for the patient with recent abdominal, gynecological, or rectal surgery. The effort to pass a stool often causes sutures to separate, reopening the wound. In addition, patients with histories of cardiovascular disease, diseases causing elevated intraocular pressure (glaucoma), and increased intracranial pressure need to prevent constipation and avoid using the Valsalva maneuver.

Impaction. Fecal **impaction** results from unrelieved constipation. It is a collection of hardened feces wedged in the rectum that a person cannot expel. In cases of severe impaction the mass extends up into the sigmoid colon. If not resolved or removed,

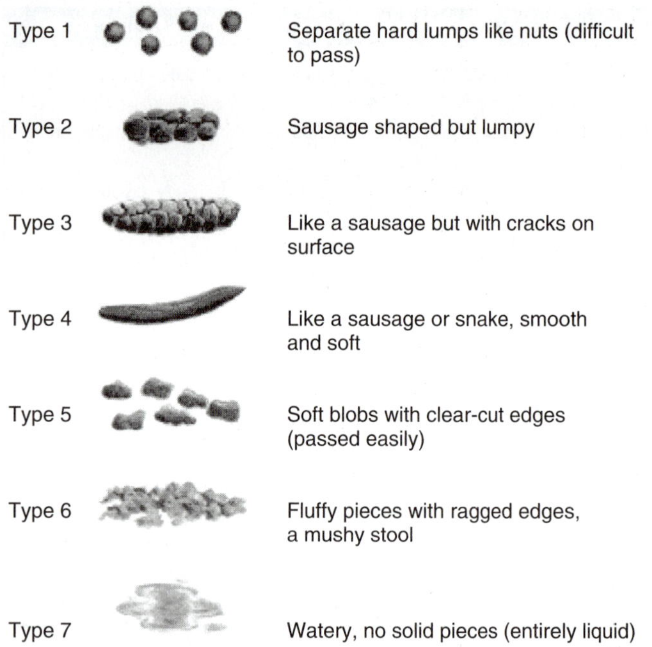
Type 1
Separate hard lumps like nuts (difficult to pass)
Type 2
Sausage shaped but lumpy
Type 3
Like a sausage but with cracks on surface
Type 4
Like a sausage or snake, smooth and soft
Type 5
Soft blobs with clear-cut edges (passed easily)
Type 6
Fluffy pieces with ragged edges, a mushy stool
Type 7
Watery, no solid pieces (entirely liquid)

FIG. 46-4 Bristol stool form scale. (Used with permission. *Bristol Stool Form Guideline,* http://www.aboutconstipation.org/bristol.html, accessed July 31, 2006.)

severe impaction often results in intestinal obstruction. Patients who are debilitated, confused, or unconscious are most at risk for impaction. They are dehydrated or too weak or unaware of the need to defecate, and the stool becomes too hard and dry to pass.

An obvious sign of impaction is the inability to pass a stool for several days, despite the repeated urge to defecate (Chien and Bradway, 2010). You suspect impaction when a continuous oozing of diarrhea stool occurs. The liquid portion of feces located higher in the colon seeps around the impacted mass. Loss of appetite (anorexia), nausea and/or vomiting, abdominal distention and cramping, and rectal pain often accompany the condition. If an impaction is suspected, gently perform a digital examination of the rectum and palpate for the impacted mass (Steggall, 2008).

Diarrhea. Diarrhea is an increase in the number of stools and the passage of liquid, unformed feces. It is associated with disorders affecting digestion, absorption, and secretion in the GI tract. Intestinal contents pass through the small and large intestine too quickly to allow for the usual absorption of fluid and nutrients. Irritation within the colon results in increased mucus secretion. As a result, feces become watery, and the patient is unable to control the urge to defecate. Normally an anal bag is safe and effective in long-term treatment of patients with fecal incontinence at home, in hospice, or in the hospital. Fecal incontinence is expensive and a potentially dangerous condition in terms of contamination and risk of skin ulceration (Gray, 2007).

Excess loss of colonic fluid results in serious fluid and electrolyte or acid-base imbalances. Infants and older adults are particularly susceptible to associated complications (see Chapter 41). Because repeated passage of diarrhea stools also exposes the skin of the perineum and buttocks to irritating intestinal contents, meticulous skin care and containment of fecal drainage is necessary to prevent skin breakdown (see Chapter 48).

Many conditions cause diarrhea. Antibiotic use via any route of administration alters the normal flora in the GI tract (Vonberg et al., 2008). Patients receiving enteral nutrition are also at risk for diarrhea. Consult a dietitian when diarrhea occurs (Tabloski, 2009). See Chapter 44 for interventions to decrease diarrhea caused by enteral feedings. Food allergies and intolerances increase peristalsis and cause diarrhea. Surgeries or diagnostic testing of the lower GI tract also cause diarrhea. The aim of treatment is to remove precipitating conditions and slow peristalsis.

Another common causative agent of diarrhea is ***Clostridium difficile*** (*C. difficile*), in which symptoms range from mild diarrhea to severe colitis. *C. difficile* infection is acquired in one of two ways: by factors that cause an overgrowth of *C. difficile,* and by contact with the *C. difficile* organism. A new strain of *C. difficile* has been identified that is more virulent with more toxic effects (Grossman, 2010). Antibiotics (cephalosporins, ampicillin, amoxicillin, and clindamycin (Calfee, 2008), chemotherapy, and invasive bowel procedures such as surgery or colonoscopy disrupt normal bowel flora and may cause an overgrowth of *C. difficile.* Some patients acquire the organism from a health care worker's hands or direct contact with the environmental surfaces contaminated with it. Only hand hygiene with soap and water is effective to physically remove *C. difficile* spores from the hands. In addition, evidence supports the use of diluted bleach (1:10) as an environmental disinfectant to decrease the incidence of *C. difficile* (Calfee, 2008; Vonberg, 2008). The most common diagnostic test for the bacteria is the enzyme-linked immunosorbent assay (ELISA) test, which detects *C. difficile* A and B in the stool.

Communicable foodborne pathogens also cause diarrhea. Hand hygiene following the use of the bathroom, before and after preparing foods, and when cleaning and storing fresh produce and meats greatly reduces the risk of foodborne illnesses. When diarrhea is the result of a foodborne virus, the goal usually is to rid the GI system of the pathogen rather than slow peristalsis.

Incontinence. Fecal incontinence is the inability to control passage of feces and gas from the anus. Incontinence harms a patient's body image (see Chapter 33). In many situations the patient is mentally alert but physically unable to avoid defecation. The embarrassment of soiling clothes often leads to social isolation. Physical conditions that impair anal sphincter function or control cause incontinence. It occurs in a variety of settings. Conditions that create frequent, loose, large-volume, watery stools also predispose to incontinence. Using an anal bag or a bowel management system helps to prevent perineal skin breakdown (Fig. 46-5).

Flatulence. As gas accumulates in the lumen of the intestines, the bowel wall stretches and distends (flatulence). It is a common cause of abdominal fullness, pain, and cramping. Normally intestinal gas escapes through the mouth (belching) or the anus (passing of flatus). However, flatulence causes abdominal distention and severe, sharp pain if intestinal motility is reduced because of opiates, general anesthetics, abdominal surgery, or immobilization.

Hemorrhoids. Hemorrhoids are dilated, engorged veins in the lining of the rectum. They are either external or internal. External hemorrhoids are clearly visible as protrusions of skin. If the underlying vein is hardened, there is usually a purplish discoloration (thrombosis). This causes increased pain and often needs to be excised. Internal hemorrhoids have an outer mucous membrane. Increased venous pressure from straining at defecation, pregnancy, heart failure, and chronic liver disease causes hemorrhoids.

Bowel Diversions

Certain diseases cause conditions that prevent normal passage of feces through the rectum. The treatment for these disorders results in the need for a temporary or permanent artificial opening

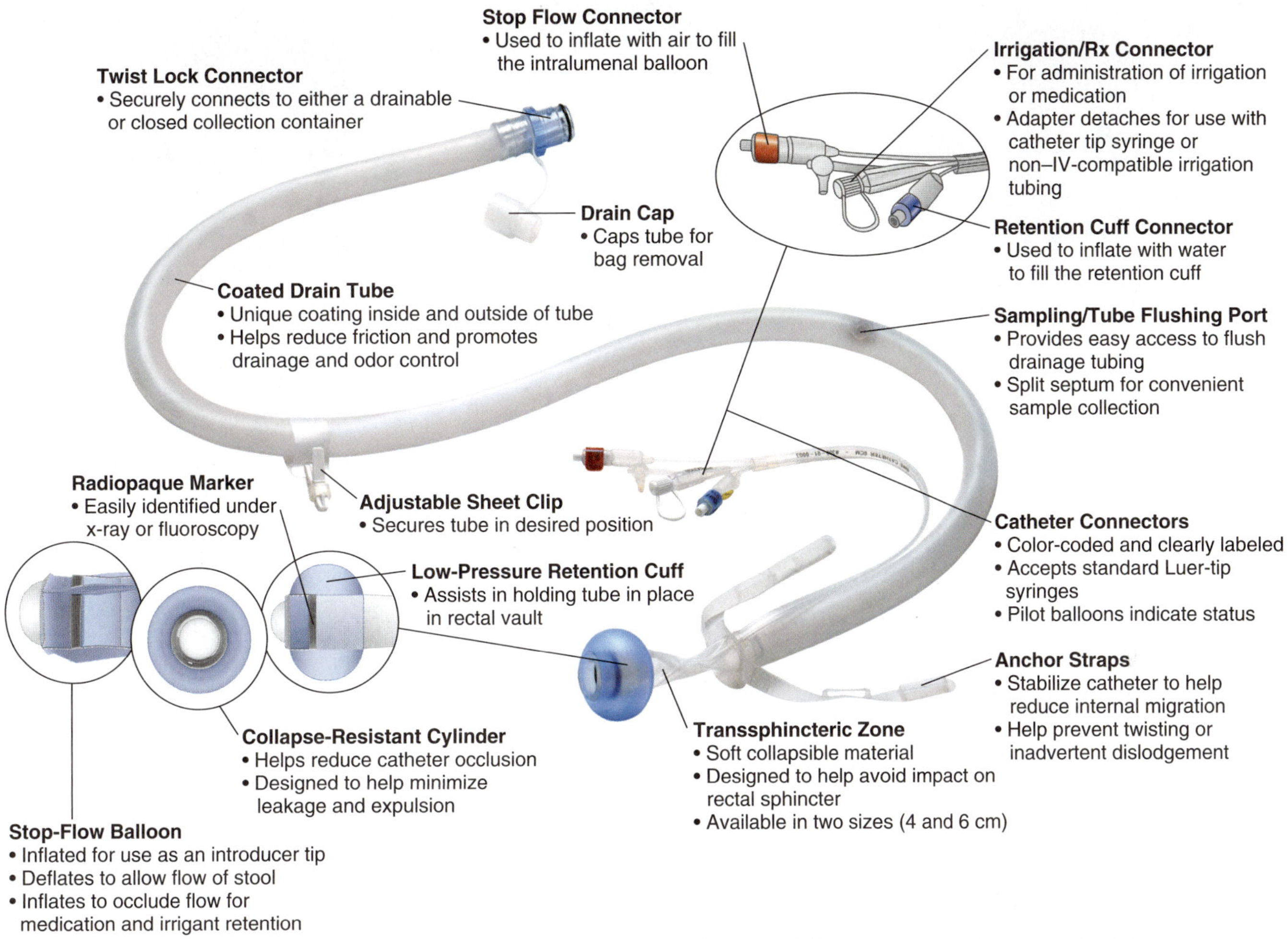
Stop Flow Connector
• Used to inflate with air to fill the intralumenal balloon
Twist Lock Connector
• Securely connects to either a drainable or closed collection container
Irrigation/Rx Connector
• For administration of irrigation or medication
• Adapter detaches for use with catheter tip syringe or non–IV-compatible irrigation tubing
Retention Cuff Connector
• Used to inflate with water to fill the retention cuff
Drain Cap
• Caps tube for bag removal
Coated Drain Tube
• Unique coating inside and outside of tube
• Helps reduce friction and promotes drainage and odor control
Sampling/Tube Flushing Port
• Provides easy access to flush drainage tubing
• Split septum for convenient sample collection
Radiopaque Marker
• Easily identified under x-ray or fluoroscopy
Adjustable Sheet Clip
• Secures tube in desired position
Catheter Connectors
• Color-coded and clearly labeled
• Accepts standard Luer-tip syringes
• Pilot balloons indicate status
Low-Pressure Retention Cuff
• Assists in holding tube in place in rectal vault
Anchor Straps
• Stabilize catheter to help reduce internal migration
• Help prevent twisting or inadvertent dislodgement
Transsphincteric Zone
• Soft collapsible material
• Designed to help avoid impact on rectal sphincter
• Available in two sizes (4 and 6 cm)
Collapse-Resistant Cylinder
• Helps reduce catheter occlusion
• Designed to help minimize leakage and expulsion
Stop-Flow Balloon
• Inflated for use as an introducer tip
• Deflates to allow flow of stool
• Inflates to occlude flow for medication and irrigant retention

FIG. 46-5 ActiFlo™ Indwelling Bowel Catheter System. (Courtesy Hollister Incorporated, Libertyville, Ill.)

(stoma) in the abdominal wall. Surgical openings are created in the ileum **(ileostomy)** or colon **(colostomy),** with the ends of the intestine brought through the abdominal wall to create the stoma (Durston, 2009).

The standard bowel diversion creates a stoma, or the patient has reconstructive bowel surgery that uses the native sphincter for bowel continence. The reconstructive surgery includes a continent stoma procedure or the ileoanal pouch anastomosis, which is described later in the chapter.

Ostomies. The location of an ostomy determines the consistency of stool. An ileostomy bypasses the entire large intestine. As a result, stools are frequent and liquid. The same is true for a colostomy of the ascending colon. A colostomy of the transverse colon generally results in a more solid, formed stool. The sigmoid colostomy releases near-normal stool. The patient's medical problem and general condition determine the location of a colostomy. There are three types of colostomy construction: loop, end, and double-barrel.

Loop Colostomy. A loop colostomy is usually performed in a medical emergency when health care providers anticipate closure of the colostomy (Fig. 46-6). It is usually a temporary large stoma constructed in the transverse colon. The surgeon pulls a loop of bowel onto the abdomen. An external supporting device such as a plastic rod, bridge, or rubber catheter is temporarily placed under the bowel loop to keep it from slipping back. The surgeon then opens the bowel and sutures it to the skin of the abdomen. A communicating wall remains between the proximal and distal bowel. The loop ostomy has two openings through one stoma. The proximal end drains stool, whereas the distal portion drains mucus. Within 7 to 10 days the surgeon removes the supporting device.

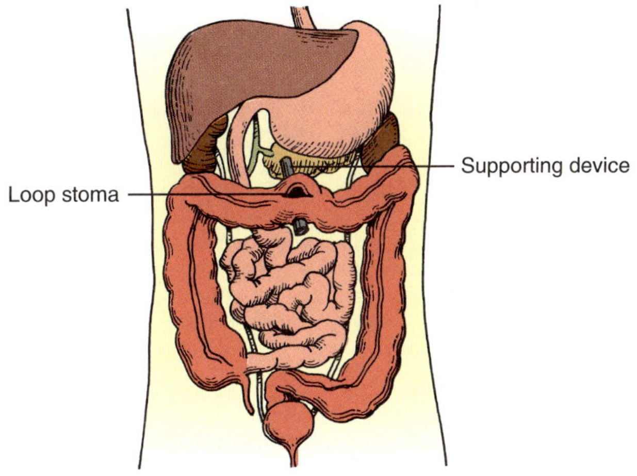
Supporting device
Loop stoma

FIG. 46-6 Loop colostomy. Loop of colon is exteriorized over plastic rod for temporary fecal diversion. (Modified from Phillips N: *Berry & Kohn's operating room technique,* ed 11, St Louis, 2007, Mosby.)

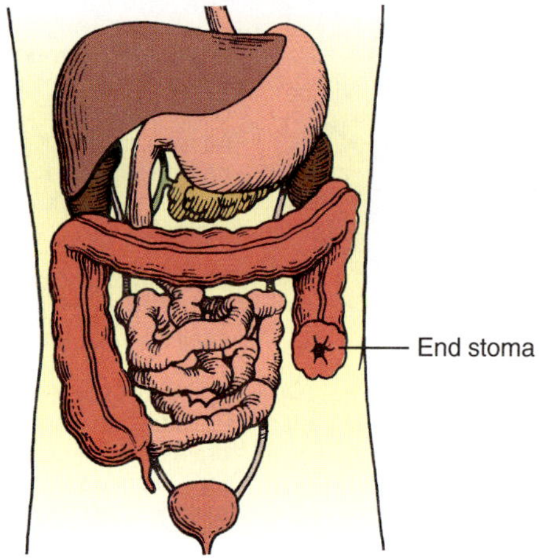

FIG. 46-7 Permanent (end) colostomy. Terminal end of descending or sigmoid colon is brought out through peritoneum and muscle and sutured to skin. (Modified from Phillips N: *Berry & Kohn's operating room technique,* ed 11, St Louis, 2007, Mosby.)

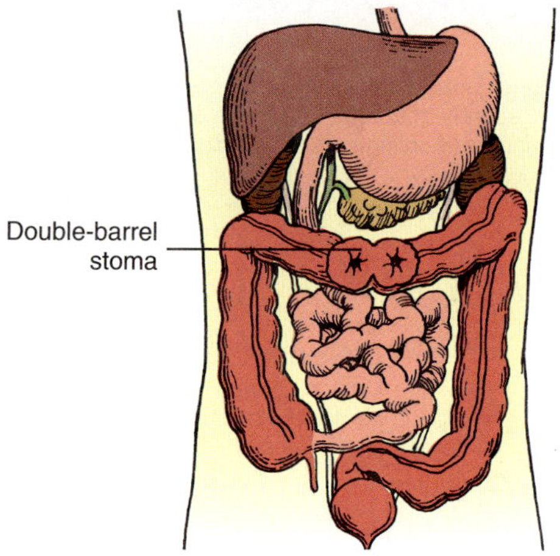

FIG. 46-8 Double-barrel colostomy. Both ends of transected colon are brought out to skin. (Modified from Phillips N: *Berry & Kohn's operating room technique,* ed 11, St Louis, 2007, Mosby.)

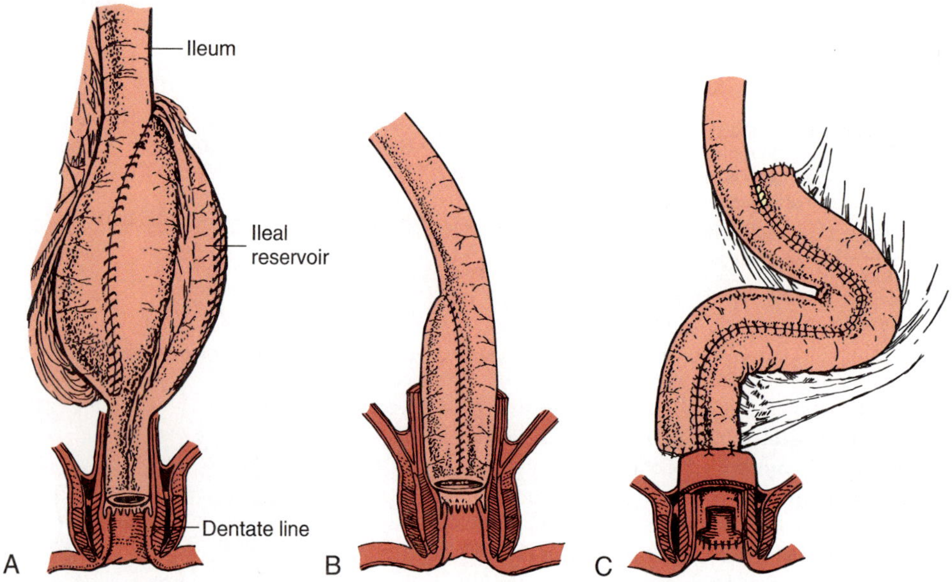

FIG. 46-9 Ileoanal reservoirs (IARs). **A,** S-shaped configuration for IAR. Three 10-cm limbs of ileum are used, antimesenteric surface of each limb is opened, and adjacent bowel walls are anastomosed. **B,** J-shaped configuration for IAR. Distal ileum is aligned in J shape, antimesenteric surface of J shape is opened, and adjacent bowel walls are anastomosed. Side-to-end anastomosis of bowel to dentate line is evident. **C,** Lateral or side-by-side ileoanal pouch configuration. (From Hampton BG, Bryant RA: *Ostomies and continent diversions: nursing management,* St Louis, 1992, Mosby.)

End Colostomy. The end colostomy consists of one stoma formed from the proximal end of the bowel, with the distal portion of the GI tract either removed or sewn closed (called *Hartmann's pouch)* and left in the abdominal cavity. For many patients end colostomies are a result of surgical treatment of colorectal cancer. In such cases the rectum is usually removed. Patients with diverticulitis who are treated surgically often have a temporary end stoma with a Hartmann's pouch (Fig. 46-7).

Double-Barrel Colostomy. Unlike the loop colostomy, the surgeon divides the intestine and brings both the proximal and distal ends through the abdominal incision to the abdominal surface when creating a double-barrel colostomy. A small incision is made in the proximal stoma for fecal drainage. The distal stoma leads to the inactive intestine and is left intact. When the intestinal injury has healed, the colostomy is reversed, and the divided ends are anastomosed to restore intestinal integrity (Fig. 46-8).

Alternative Procedures

Ileoanal Pouch Anastomosis. The ileoanal pouch anastomosis is a surgical procedure that is used in patients who need to have a colectomy for treatment of ulcerative colitis or familial polyps (Dorman, 2009). In this procedure the surgeon removes the colon, creates a pouch from the end of the small intestine, and attaches the pouch to the patient's anus (Fig. 46-9). This pouch provides for the collection of waste material, which is similar to the rectum. The patient is continent of stool because stool is evacuated via the anus.

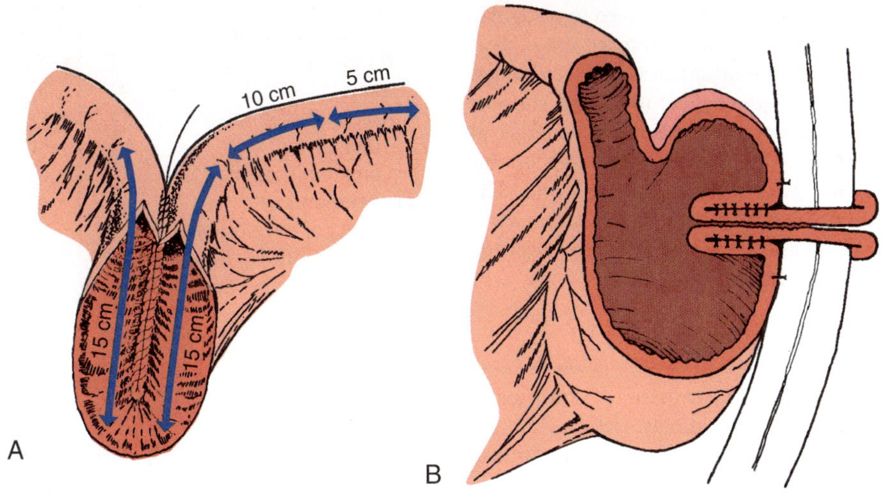

FIG. 46-10 Construction of Kock continent ileostomy—Kock pouch. **A,** Two 15-cm limbs are used to create a pouch, and one 15-cm limb is used to fashion a nipple valve and stoma. **B,** Distal limb is intussuscepted into reservoir to create one-way valve and accomplish continence. Sutures or staples, or both, are placed to stabilize and maintain intussuscepted nipple. Anterior surface of reservoir is anchored to anterior peritoneal wall. (From Hampton BG, Bryant RA: *Ostomies and continent diversions: nursing management,* St Louis, 1992, Mosby.)

When the ileal pouch is created, the patient has a temporary ileostomy to allow the anastomosis to heal.

Kock Continent Ileostomy. The Kock continent ileostomy is created using the patient's small intestine, changing its cylindrical shape into a spherical reservoir (Gordon, 2007). This procedure is occasionally used in the treatment of ulcerative colitis. The pouch has a continent stoma, a nipple type of valve that is drained with an external catheter, which the patient places intermittently in the stoma (Fig. 46-10).

Macedo-Malone Antegrade Continence Enema. The Macedo-Malone antegrade continence enema (MACE) procedure improves continence in patients with fecal soiling associated with neuropathic or structural abnormalities of the anal sphincter. This procedure isolates a 3-cm (1.2-inch) flap on the left colon. A Foley catheter placed on the surface of the flap creates a tubular passage. This produces a continence valve mechanism. The surgeon takes the distal end of the tube and makes a V shape to the skin flap (Fig. 46-11). Enema administration begins 7 to 10 days after surgery. Patients receive enemas daily. The volume of the enema varies from 250 to 800 mL and takes 45 to 60 minutes to administer. Colonic evacuation occurs within 30 to 60 minutes (Meurette et al., 2010).

Psychological Considerations. A stoma causes serious body image changes, particularly if it is permanent. After the surgery, patients face a variety of anxieties and concerns, from learning how to manage their stoma to coping with conflicts of self-esteem and body image. Provide emotional support before and after surgery (Deitz, 2010a). Patients often perceive a stoma as invasive and disfiguring. However, a well-placed stoma usually does not interfere with the patient's activities and is concealed with clothing. Nonetheless, even though clothing conceals the ostomy, the patient feels different. Many patients have difficulty maintaining or initiating normal sexual relations (see Chapter 34) (Ramirez et al., 2009). Important factors affecting reactions to the stoma include the character of fecal secretions and the ability to control them. Foul odors, spillage, or leakage of liquid stools and inability to regulate bowel movements cause the patient to lose self-esteem (Richbourg et al., 2007). The aging process often affects the ability to manage stomas,

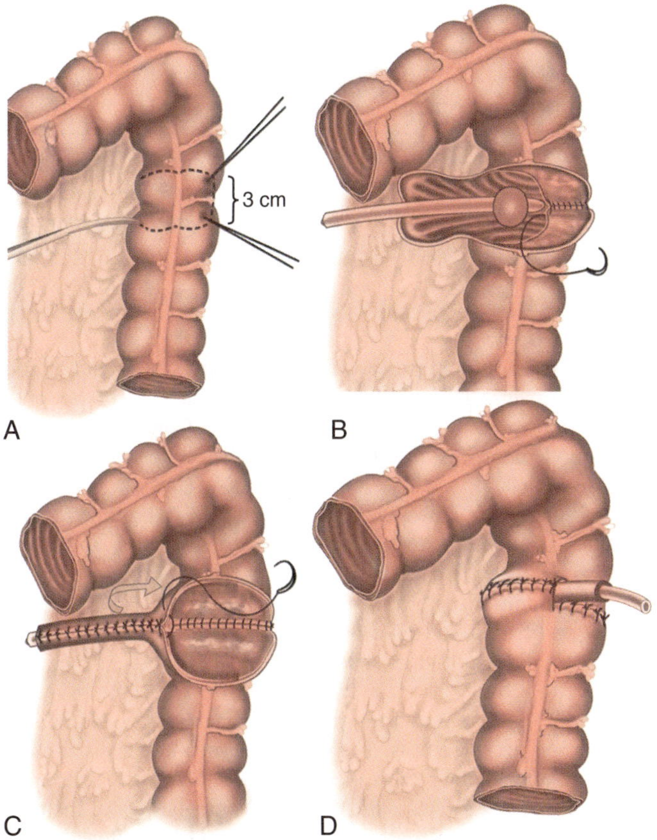

FIG. 46-11 Macedo-Malone antegrade continence enema procedure. **A,** Isolation of the flap on left colon. **B,** Foley catheters placed on mucosal surface of flap. **C,** Tubularization of plate creating efferent tubular conduit. **D,** Continence valve mechanism is created. (Used with permission. From Calado A et al: The Macedo-Malone antegrade continence enema procedure: early experience, *J Urol* 173:1340, 2005.)

even in people who have had them for years. You need to recognize and intervene when problems resulting from advanced age such as skin changes, weight loss or gain, visual impairments, or changes in diet occur (Pearson, 2010). Refer the patient to ostomy support groups such as the United Ostomy Associations of America at http://www.uoaa.org, which has discussion boards for various types of incontinent and continent diversions and networks. The Wound, Ostomy and Continence Nurses Society (http://www.wocn.org) provides information and helps patients locate a wound, ostomy continence nurse (WOCN) (Dorman, 2009).

CRITICAL THINKING

Successful critical thinking requires a synthesis of knowledge, experience, information gathered from patients, critical thinking attitudes, and intellectual and professional standards. Clinical judgments require you to anticipate the information necessary, analyze the data, and make decisions regarding patient care.

In the case of bowel elimination, integrate the knowledge from nursing and other disciplines to understand the patient's response to bowel elimination alterations. Experience in caring for patients with elimination alterations helps you provide an appropriate plan of care. Use critical thinking attitudes such as fairness, confidence, and discipline when listening to and exploring the patient's nursing history. Apply relevant standards of practice (e.g., wound care standards, quality and safety standards) when selecting nursing measures.

NURSING PROCESS

Apply the nursing process and use a critical thinking approach in your care of patients. The nursing process provides a clinical decision-making approach for you to develop and implement an individualized plan of care.

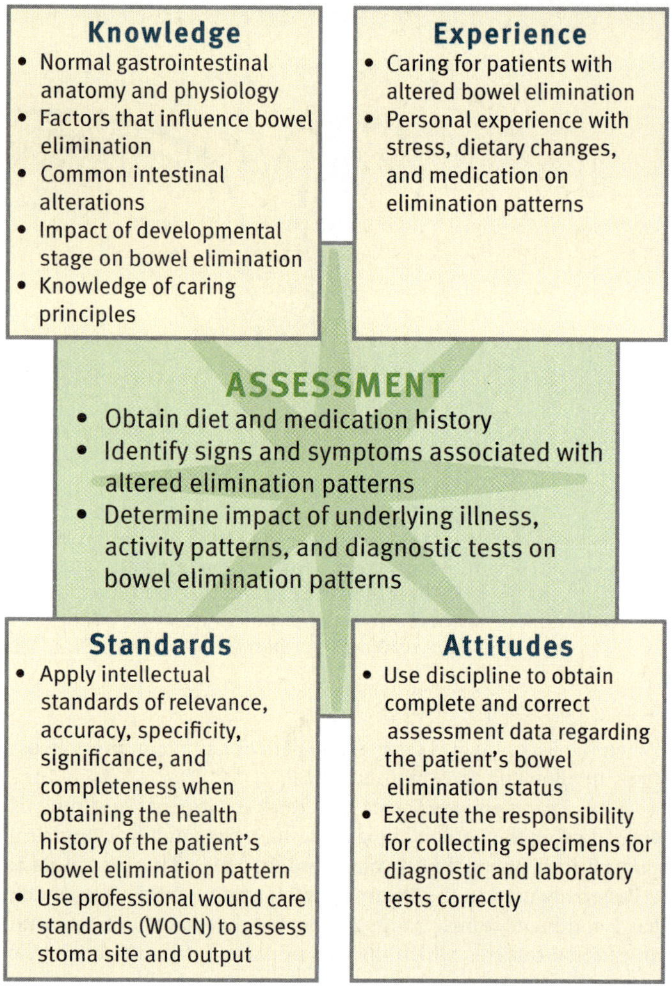

Knowledge
• Normal gastrointestinal anatomy and physiology
• Factors that influence bowel elimination
• Common intestinal alterations
• Impact of developmental stage on bowel elimination
• Knowledge of caring principles
Experience
• Caring for patients with altered bowel elimination
• Personal experience with stress, dietary changes, and medication on elimination patterns
ASSESSMENT
• Obtain diet and medication history
• Identify signs and symptoms associated with altered elimination patterns
• Determine impact of underlying illness, activity patterns, and diagnostic tests on bowel elimination patterns
Standards
• Apply intellectual standards of relevance, accuracy, specificity, significance, and completeness when obtaining the health history of the patient's bowel elimination pattern
• Use professional wound care standards (WOCN) to assess stoma site and output
Attitudes
• Use discipline to obtain complete and correct assessment data regarding the patient's bowel elimination status
• Execute the responsibility for collecting specimens for diagnostic and laboratory tests correctly

FIG. 46-12 Critical thinking model for elimination assessment. *WOCN,* Wound, Ostomy and Continence Nurses Society.

ASSESSMENT

During the assessment process, thoroughly assess each patient and critically analyze findings to ensure you make patient-centered clinical decisions required for safe nursing care. Consider all critical thinking elements that build toward making appropriate diagnoses (Fig. 46-12).

Assessment for bowel elimination patterns and abnormalities includes a nursing history, physical assessment of the abdomen, inspection of fecal characteristics, and review of relevant test results. In addition, determine the patient's medical history, pattern and types of fluid and food intake, chewing ability, medications, and recent illnesses and/or stressors.

Through the Patient's Eyes. Patients expect the nurse to answer all of their questions regarding diagnostic tests and the preparation for these tests. They are concerned about discomfort and exposure of their more personal areas. Bowel problems are often devastating for the patient and their families. Fecal incontinence in older people, most commonly caused by overflow leakage as a result of constipation, often means the breakdown of care at home, causing them to be admitted to a residential facility (Continence Care Position Statement, 2009). Some older patients who fail to recognize their elimination needs need monitoring for elimination patterns so negative consequences do not occur. Remember that each patient has a unique situation and a perception of what is "right" for him or her. Patients expect a knowledgeable nurse with the ability to teach methods of promoting and maintaining normal bowel elimination patterns. Consider the patient's cultural practices and preferences because patients of different cultures can have various expectations (Box 46-2).

Nursing History. The nursing history provides a review of the patient's usual bowel pattern and habits. What a patient describes as normal or abnormal is often different from factors and conditions that tend to promote normal elimination. Identifying normal and abnormal patterns, habits, and the patient's perception of normal and abnormal in regard to bowel elimination allows you to accurately determine a patient's problems. Organize the nursing history around factors that affect elimination (Wisniewski, 2010):

- *Determination of the usual elimination pattern:* Include frequency and time of day. Having the patient or caregiver complete a bowel elimination diary provides an accurate assessment of a patient's current bowel elimination pattern.
- *Patient's description of usual stool characteristics:* Determines whether the stool is normally watery or formed soft or hard, the typical color, and the presence of blood. Ask the patient to describe the usual shape of the stool and the number of stools per day.
- *Identification of routines followed to promote normal elimination:* Examples are drinking hot liquids, eating specific foods, or taking time to defecate during a certain part of the day.
- *Assessment of the use of artificial aids at home:* Assess whether and how often the patient uses enemas, laxatives,

BOX 46-2 CULTURAL ASPECTS OF CARE

Variables Influencing Colorectal Cancer Screening in African Americans

Biological, psychological, behavioral, and social variables influence colorectal cancer (CRC) screenings in African Americans. African Americans have a 20% higher rate of CRC and 40% higher incidence of disease-related death when compared with Caucasians (ACS, 2011b). Prevention resulting in early detection is key to finding CRC when it is often curable, but screening rates are low in African Americans.

Implications for Practice

- Lack of routine visits to a primary care provider is one of the strongest predictors for inadequate CRC screening and advanced stage at presentation (Griffin, 2009).
- Patients who do not have health insurance do not frequently seek CRC screening (Griffin, 2009).
- Patients who participate in preventive health practices (e.g., regular physical activity) often seek regular screening for CRC because these patients are often interested in promoting their own health (Griffin, 2009).
- Identification of additional social system predictors such as family support, church affiliation, and geographical access also help in receiving timely CRC screening (Griffin, 2009).
- Removing barriers of safety, quality, and cost-effectiveness improves the involvement of patients in CRC screening (Cronenwett et al., 2007).

or bulk-forming food additives before having a bowel movement.

- *Presence and status of bowel diversions:* If the patient has an ostomy, assess frequency of fecal drainage, character of feces, appearance and condition of the stoma (color, swelling, and irritation), type of fecal collection device used, and methods used to maintain the function of the ostomy.
- *Changes in appetite:* Include changes in eating patterns and a change in weight (amount of loss or gain). If a change of weight is present, ask if the patient planned it (e.g., weight loss with a diet).
- *Diet history:* Determine the patient's dietary preferences for a day. Determine the intake of fruits, vegetables, cereals, and breads and also if mealtimes are regular or irregular.
- *Description of daily fluid intake:* This includes the type and amount of fluid. The patient often estimates the amount using common household measurements.
- *History of surgery or illnesses affecting the GI tract:* This information helps explain symptoms, the potential for maintaining or restoring normal bowel elimination pattern, and whether there is a family history of GI cancer.
- *Medication history:* Ask whether the patient takes medications (e.g., laxatives, antacids, iron supplements, and analgesics) that alter defecation or fecal characteristics.
- *Emotional state:* The patient's emotions significantly alter frequency of defecation. During assessment observation of the patient's emotions, tone of voice, and mannerisms reveal significant behaviors that indicate stress.
- *History of exercise:* Ask the patient to specifically describe the type and amount of daily exercise.
- *History of pain or discomfort:* Ask the patient whether there is a history of abdominal or anal pain. The type, frequency, and location of pain help identify the source of the problem.
- *Social history:* Patients have many different living arrangements. Where patients live affects their toileting habits. If patients share living quarters, ask how many bathrooms there are. Find out if patients have their own bathroom or if they need to share bathrooms, creating a need to adjust the time they use the bathroom to accommodate others. If patients live alone, can they ambulate safely to the toilet? When patients are not independent in bowel management, determine who assists them and how.
- *Mobility and dexterity:* Evaluate patients' mobility and dexterity to determine if they need assistive devices or help from personnel.

Box 46-3 summarizes types of assessment questions to use for gathering a detailed nursing history.

Physical Assessment. Conduct a physical assessment of body systems and functions likely to be influenced by the presence of elimination problems (see Chapter 30).

Mouth. Inspect the patient's teeth, tongue, and gums. Poor dentition or poorly fitting dentures influence the ability to chew. Sores in the mouth make eating not only difficult but also painful.

Abdomen. Inspect all four abdominal quadrants for contour, shape, symmetry, and skin color. Note masses, peristaltic waves, scars, venous patterns, stomas, and lesions. Normally you do not see peristaltic waves. Observable peristalsis is often a sign of intestinal obstruction.

Abdominal distention appears as an overall outward protuberance of the abdomen. Intestinal gas, large tumors, or fluid in the peritoneal cavity cause distention. A distended abdomen feels tight like a drum; and the skin is taut and appears stretched.

Auscultate the abdomen with a stethoscope to assess bowel sounds in each quadrant (see Chapter 30). Normal bowel sounds occur every 5 to 15 seconds and last a second to several seconds. During auscultation note the character and frequency of bowel sounds. You hear an increase in pitch or a tinkling sound with abdominal distention. Absent (no auscultated bowel sounds) or hypoactive sounds (less than five sounds per minute) occur with paralytic ileus such as after abdominal surgery. High-pitched and hyperactive bowel sounds (35 or more sounds per minute) occur with small intestine obstruction and inflammatory disorders.

Percussion identifies underlying abdominal structures and detects lesions, fluid, or gas within the abdomen. Gas or flatulence creates a tympanic note. Masses, tumors, and fluid are dull to percussion (Wisniewski, 2010).

Gently palpate the abdomen for masses or areas of tenderness. It is important for the patient to relax. Tensing abdominal muscles interferes with palpating underlying organs or masses.

Rectum. Inspect the area around the anus for lesions, discoloration, inflammation, and hemorrhoids. Carefully record abnormalities.

Laboratory Tests. Laboratory and diagnostic examinations yield useful information concerning elimination problems (Table 46-3). Laboratory analysis of fecal contents detects pathological conditions such as tumors, bleeding, parasites, and infection.

Fecal Specimens. The nurse ensures that specimens are obtained accurately, labeled properly in appropriate containers, and transported to the laboratory on time. Institutions provide special containers for fecal specimens. Some tests require that specimens are placed in chemical preservatives. Use medical aseptic technique during collection of stool specimens (see Chapter 28). Because about 25% of the solid portion of a stool is bacteria from the colon, wear clean gloves when handling specimens.

Hand hygiene is necessary for anyone who comes in contact with the specimen. Often the patient is able to obtain the specimen if properly instructed. Teach the patient to avoid mixing feces with

BOX 46-3 NURSING ASSESSMENT QUESTIONS

Signs and Symptoms

Nausea or Vomiting: Onset, Duration, Associated Symptoms, Character, Exposures

- When did the nausea/vomiting start?
- Is it related to particular stimuli (odors, after eating specific food)?
- How does the emesis look (mucus type, bloody or coffee grounds, color, or undigested food)?
- Do you have other symptoms such as dizziness, headaches, abdominal pain, or weight loss?
- Do you have family members who are experiencing the same symptoms?

Indigestion: Onset, Character, Location, Associated Symptoms, Alleviating Factors

- Is the indigestion related to meals, types or quantity of food, time of day or night?
- Does the discomfort from indigestion radiate to the shoulders or arms?
- Do you feel bloated after eating?
- Do you have any other symptoms (vomiting, headaches, diarrhea, belching, flatulence, heartburn, or pain)?
- Does the indigestion respond to antacids or other self-care measures?

Diarrhea: Onset, Duration, Character, Associated Symptoms, Alleviating Factors, Exposure

- When did the diarrhea start? Was it gradual or sudden?
- How many stools do you have per day? Is it watery or explosive? What is the color and consistency?
- Have you had fever, chills, weight loss, or abdominal pain?
- Have you taken antibiotics recently?
- Have you been under stress?
- What have you used to try to alleviate the diarrhea? Was it successful?
- Have you been out of the country recently?

Constipation: Onset, Character, Symptoms, Alleviating Factors

- When was your last bowel movement? How many bowel movements do you have in a typical week?
- Is this a recent occurrence or a long-standing problem?
- Describe your bowel movements.
- Do you have to strain to have a bowel movement?
- Do you have abdominal or rectal pain when you have a bowel movement?
- Do you feel as though your bowel movements are incomplete?
- Have you recently changed your diet or fluid intake?
- Do you use stool softeners, laxatives, or enemas?
- Is it necessary to manually remove the bowel movements?

Medical History

- Do you have a previous history of gastrointestinal problems? If yes, explain.
- Have you had abdominal surgery or trauma?
- Do you have a history of major illnesses such as cancer, arthritis, respiratory disease (steroid use), kidney disease, or cardiac disease?

Effect on the Patient

- How do these symptoms affect you?
- Have you missed work or social engagements because of these symptoms?

TABLE 46-3 Laboratory and Diagnostic Tests for Bowel Function

MEASUREMENT AND NORMAL VALUES	INTERPRETATION
Laboratory Tests	
Total bilirubin: 0.3-1 mg/dL	Bilirubin is increased in hepatobiliary diseases, obstructions in bile duct, certain anemias, and following transfusion reactions (Pagana and Pagana, 2011).
Alkaline phosphatase: 30-120 units/L	Alkaline phosphatase is elevated in obstructive hepatobiliary diseases, hepatobiliary carcinomas, bone tumors, and healing fractures (Pagana and Pagana, 2011).
Amylase: 60-120 Somogyi units/dL	Amylase is elevated in abnormalities of the pancreas such as inflammation or tumors, cholecystitis, necrotic bowel, and diabetic ketoacidosis (Pagana and Pagana, 2011).
Carcinoembryonic antigen (CEA): less than 5 ng/mL	CEA is elevated in the presence of cancer or inflammation of the GI tract or hepatobiliary organs (Pagana and Pagana, 2011).
Direct Visualization	
Endoscopy, colonoscopy	Routine examination such as a colonoscopy is recommended for people after 50 years of age who have no family history of CRC. People with a personal or family history need to talk with their health care provider to determine if they need to start screening at an earlier age and recommended frequency of screening (ACS, 2011b). Normally the GI tract is free of polyps, tumors, inflammation, ulcers, hernias, obstruction, and ulcerations. If a lesion such as a polyp is identified, the health care provider removes the growth or a portion of the growth and sends it to pathology for analysis. If bleeding is present, the health care provider usually attempts to stop it at the source. In some cases the identification of an abnormality indicates the need for follow-up surgery for the patient.
Indirect Visualization	
X-ray film with contrast medium	X-ray identifies the presence of abnormalities in the GI tract. A series of x-ray films allow for indirect visualization of the entire tract (ACS, 2011b). The presence of tumors, ulcerations, inflammation, or other abnormalities indicates the need for further diagnostic testing and medical or surgical intervention.

BOX 46-4 PROCEDURAL GUIDELINES

View Video!

Performing a Guaiac Fecal Occult Blood Test

Delegation Considerations

The skill of performing a guaiac fecal occult blood test (gFOBT) can be delegated to nursing assistive personnel (NAP). However, the nurse must evaluate the significance of the findings. Instruct the NAP to

- Notify nurse immediately if frank red blood is noted or if a positive result for occult blood is found in the sample specimen.
- Have the patient void first to avoid contamination of the specimen.

Equipment

Hemoccult test paper, Hemoccult developer, and wooden applicator (Fig. 46-13)

1. Patient identification: Identify the patient using two identifiers (e.g., name and birth date or name and account number) according to facility policy. Compare identifiers with information on the patient's medical record (TJC, 2011).
2. Explain purpose of the test and ways for patient to assist. Patient can collect own specimen if possible.
3. Perform hand hygiene and apply clean disposable gloves.
4. Use tip of wooden applicator to obtain a small portion of a stool specimen. Be sure that specimen is free of tissue paper.
5. Perform Hemoccult slide test.
   a. Open flap of slide and, using the wooden applicator, thinly smear stool in the first box of the guaiac paper. Apply a second fecal specimen from a different portion of the stool to the second box of the slide (see illustration).
   b. Close slide cover and turn the packet over to the reverse side (see illustration). After waiting 3 to 5 minutes, open cardboard flap and apply 2 drops of developing solution on each smear.
   c. Interpret the color of the guaiac paper within 60 seconds. A blue color indicates a positive guaiac or presence of fecal occult blood.
   d. After determining if the patient's specimen is positive or negative, apply 1 drop of developer to the quality control section and interpret within 10 seconds.
6. Dispose of test slide in proper receptacle.
7. Wrap wooden applicator in paper towel, remove gloves, and discard in proper receptacle and perform hand hygiene.
8. Note color, changes on guaiac paper, and observe character of stool specimen.
9. Record results of test, noting any unusual fecal characteristics.

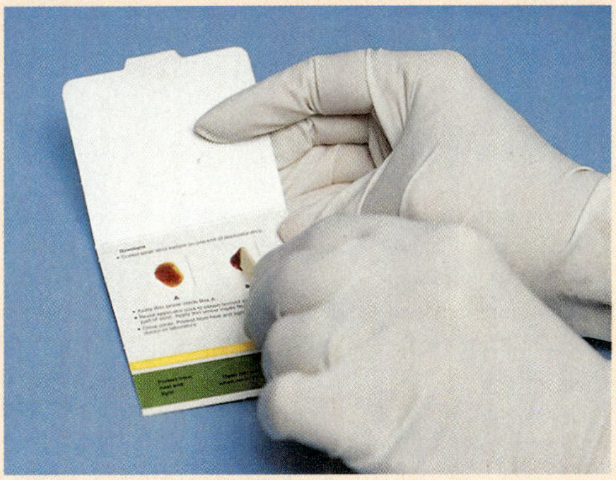

STEP 5a Application of fecal specimen on guaiac paper.

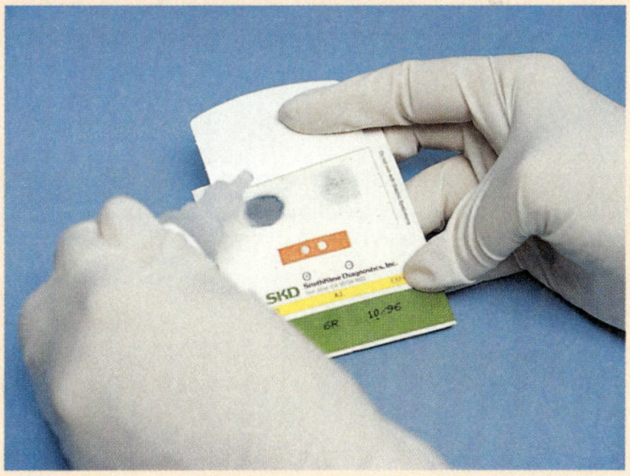

STEP 5b Application of hemoccult developing solution on guaiac paper on reverse side of test kit.

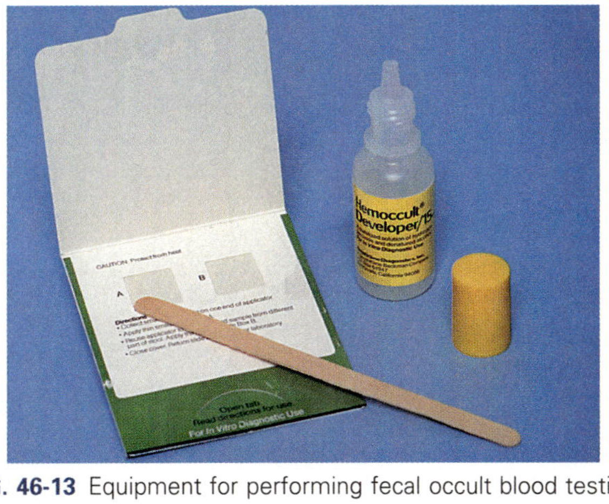

FIG. 46-13 Equipment for performing fecal occult blood testing.

urine or water. The patient defecates into a clean, dry bedpan or a special container under the toilet seat.

Tests performed by the laboratory for occult (microscopic) blood in the stool and stool cultures require only a small sample. Collect about 2.54 cm (1 inch) of formed stool or 15 to 30 mL of liquid diarrhea stool. Tests for measuring the output of fecal fat require a 3- to 5-day collection of stool. You need to save all fecal material throughout the test period.

After obtaining a specimen, label and tightly seal the container and complete all laboratory requisition forms. Record specimen collections in the patient's medical record. It is important to avoid delays in sending specimens to the laboratory. Some tests such as measurement for ova and parasites require the stool to be warm. When stool specimens remain at room temperature, bacteriological changes that alter test results occur.

A common laboratory test that patients perform at home or nurses perform at the patient's bedside is the **fecal occult blood test (FOBT),** or guaiac test, which measures microscopic amounts of blood in feces (Box 46-4). It is useful as a diagnostic screening

TABLE 46-4 Fecal Characteristics

CHARACTERISTIC	NORMAL	ABNORMAL	ABNORMAL CAUSE
Color	Infant: yellow; adult: brown	White or clay Black or tarry (melena) Red Pale with fat Translucent mucus Bloody mucus	Absence of bile Iron ingestion or upper gastrointestinal (GI) bleeding Lower GI bleeding, hemorrhoids Malabsorption of fat Spastic constipation, colitis, excessive straining Blood in feces, inflammation, infection
Odor	Pungent; affected by food type	Noxious change	Blood in feces or infection
Consistency	Soft, formed	Liquid Hard	Diarrhea, reduced absorption Constipation
Frequency	*Varies:* Infant 4-6 times daily (breastfed) or 1-3 times daily (bottle-fed); adult daily or 2-3 times a week	Infant more than 6 times daily or less than once every 1-2 days; adult more than 3 times a day or less than once a week	
Amount	150 g/day (adult)		Hypomotility or hypermotility
Shape	Resembles diameter of rectum	Narrow, pencil shaped	Obstruction, rapid peristalsis
Constituents	Undigested food, dead bacteria, fat, bile pigment, cells lining intestinal mucosa, water	Blood, pus, foreign bodies, mucus, worms Excess fat	Internal bleeding, infection, swallowed objects, irritation, inflammation Malabsorption syndrome, enteritis, pancreatic disease, surgical resection of intestine

BOX 46-5 SCREENING FOR COLON CANCER

Risk Factors

- *Age:* Over 50 years of age
- *Family history:* Colorectal cancer
- Personal history of colorectal cancer; colorectal polyps; chronic inflammatory bowel disease (IBD), including ulcerative colitis and Crohn's disease
- *Ethnic background:* Jews of Eastern European descent
- *Race:* African Americans
- *Diet:* High intake of animal fats and low in fruits and vegetables
- Obesity and inactivity
- Smoking and alcohol intake
- Diabetes

Warning Signs

- Change in bowel habits
- Rectal bleeding
- Sensation of incomplete bowel evacuation

Beginning at age 50, men and women who are at average risk for developing colorectal cancer need to have one of the following five screening options:

- A fecal occult blood test or fecal immunochemical test (also called the iFOBT)] every year *or*
- Flexible sigmoidoscopy every 5 years *or*
- A gFOBT or iFOBT every year plus flexible sigmoidoscopy every 5 years (Of these first three options, the combination of gFOBT or iFOBT every year plus flexible sigmoidoscopy every 5 years is preferable.) *or*
- Double contrast barium enema every 5 years *or*
- Colonoscopy every 10 years

Data from The American Cancer Society (ACS): *Detailed guide: colon and rectum cancer: revised 6/17/2011,* 2011b, http://www.cancer.org/Cancer/ColonandRectumCancer/DetailedGuide/index. Accessed December 3, 2011.
gFOBT, Guaiac fecal occult blood test; *iFOBT,* immunochemical fecal occult blood test.

tool for colon cancer (Box 46-5). The noninvasive FOBT is one of five colorectal cancer screening regimens recommended by the American Cancer Society (ACS, 2011a; 2011b). Three types of FOBT are available to date. They include the most commonly used guaiac fecal occult blood test (gFOBT), the immunochemical fecal occult blood test (iFOBT), and the stool deoxyribonucleic acid (DNA) test. One positive gFOBT result does not confirm GI bleeding. You need to repeat the test at least three times while the patient refrains from ingesting foods (e.g., some raw vegetables, red meat, poultry, fish) and medications (e.g., vitamin C, aspirin, nonsteroidal anti-inflammatory drugs) that cause false-positive results (Peters, 2008). Patients who take anticoagulants or who have a bleeding disorder or a GI disorder known to cause bleeding (e.g., intestinal tumors, bowel inflammation, or ulcerations) need regular screening for fecal occult blood.

Fecal Characteristics. Inspection of fecal characteristics (Table 46-4) reveals information about the nature of elimination alterations. Several factors influence each characteristic. Knowing whether there have been any recent changes is a key to assessment. The patient best provides this information during the nursing history.

Diagnostic Examinations. A variety of radiological and diagnostic tests are used with the patient experiencing altered bowel elimination (Box 46-6). Direct or indirect approaches are used to visualize GI structures. Many facilities use moderate sedation during these procedures. The most common types of drugs used to achieve moderate sedation include benzodiazepines and opiates. It is essential to understand the safety precautions involved concerning this form of anesthesia. In many institutions special training is required. A crash cart must be present at the bedside; and you must monitor the patient continuously with pulse oximetry and frequent vital signs, usually every 15 minutes

BOX 46-6 RADIOLOGICAL AND DIAGNOSTIC TESTS

Plain Film of Abdomen/Kidneys, Ureter, Bladder
- A simple x-ray film of the abdomen requires no preparation.

Upper Gastrointestinal/Barium Swallow
- An x-ray film examination using an opaque contrast medium (barium) examines the structure and motility of the upper gastrointestinal (GI) tract, including pharynx, esophagus, and stomach.
- Patient is ordered to have nothing by mouth (NPO) after midnight the night before the examination.
- Patient removes all jewelry or other metallic objects before the test.
- After the test patient needs to increase fluids to facilitate passage of barium.

Upper Endoscopy
- An endoscopic examination of the upper GI tract allows more direct visualization through a lighted fiber-optic tube that contains a lens, forceps, and brushes for biopsy.
- Preparation is similar to that for the upper GI.
- Light sedation is required (Herman, 2010).

Barium Enema with Air Contrast
- An x-ray film examination uses an opaque contrast medium and air that outlines the colon and rectum to examine the lower GI tract.
- Preparation includes NPO after midnight, a bowel preparation such as magnesium citrate, and in some instances enemas to empty out any remaining stool particles (ACS, 2011b).

Ultrasound
- This technique uses high-frequency sound waves to echo off body organs, creating a picture.
- Preparation depends on the organ to be visualized and includes NPO or no preparation.

Colonoscopy
- An endoscopic examination of the entire colon uses a colonoscope inserted into the rectum.
- Preparation is similar to that for barium enema: clear liquids the day before and then some form of bowel cleanser such as GoLytely. Enemas until clear are also common.
- Light sedation is required (Herman, 2010).

Flexible Sigmoidoscopy
- An examination of the interior of the sigmoid colon with a flexible or rigid lighted tube.
- Preparation is similar to that for a barium enema or colonoscopy.
- Light sedation is required (ACS, 2011b).

Computerized Tomography Scan
- An x-ray film examination of the body from many angles uses a scanner analyzed by a computer.
- Preparation is usually NPO.
- The patient needs to lie very still. If claustrophobia is a problem, use light sedation.

Magnetic Resonance Imaging
- A noninvasive examination uses magnet and radio waves to produce a picture of the inside of the body.
- Preparation is NPO 4 to 6 hours before examination.
- No metallic objects, including metal objects on clothes, are allowed in the room.

Enteroclysis
- Contrast material is introduced to jejunum, allowing entire small intestine to be studied.
- Preparation is 24 hours of clear liquid diet and colon cleansing such as GoLytely or enemas until clear.

during and immediately following the procedure (check agency policy).

NURSING DIAGNOSIS

The nursing assessment of the patient's bowel function reveals data that indicate an actual or potential elimination problem or a problem resulting from elimination alterations. In the examples discussed in the Nursing Care Plan, a patient has constipation as a result of pain medications and decreased fiber intake. Examples of diagnoses that apply to patients with elimination problems include the following:

- Bowel incontinence
- Constipation
- Risk for constipation
- Perceived constipation
- Diarrhea
- Toileting self-care deficit

Associated problems such as age, body-image changes, or skin breakdown require interventions unrelated to bowel function impairment. Ability to identify the correct diagnosis depends not only on the thoroughness of assessment but also on recognition of defining characteristics and factors that impair elimination (Box 46-7). Determine the patient's risk and institute measures to ensure maintenance of normal bowel function.

BOX 46-7 NURSING DIAGNOSTIC PROCESS

Constipation

ASSESSMENT ACTIVITIES	DEFINING CHARACTERISTICS
Ask patient about bowel elimination patterns.	Patient reports no bowel movement for 4 days.
Auscultate bowel sounds.	Bowel sounds are decreased in all four quadrants.
Ask patient to describe recent food and fluid intake.	Patient reports drinking six cups of coffee throughout day but no water. Eating his regular diet but no extra fiber.
Palpate abdomen.	Patient reports pain. Left lower quadrant is tender and firm.

PLANNING

When planning care, synthesize information from multiple resources (Fig. 46-14). Critical thinking ensures that the plan of care integrates everything known about the patient and the clinical problem. Rely on professional standards. The guidelines on incontinence assist in protecting the patient's skin, promoting continence, and reducing the embarrassment associated with

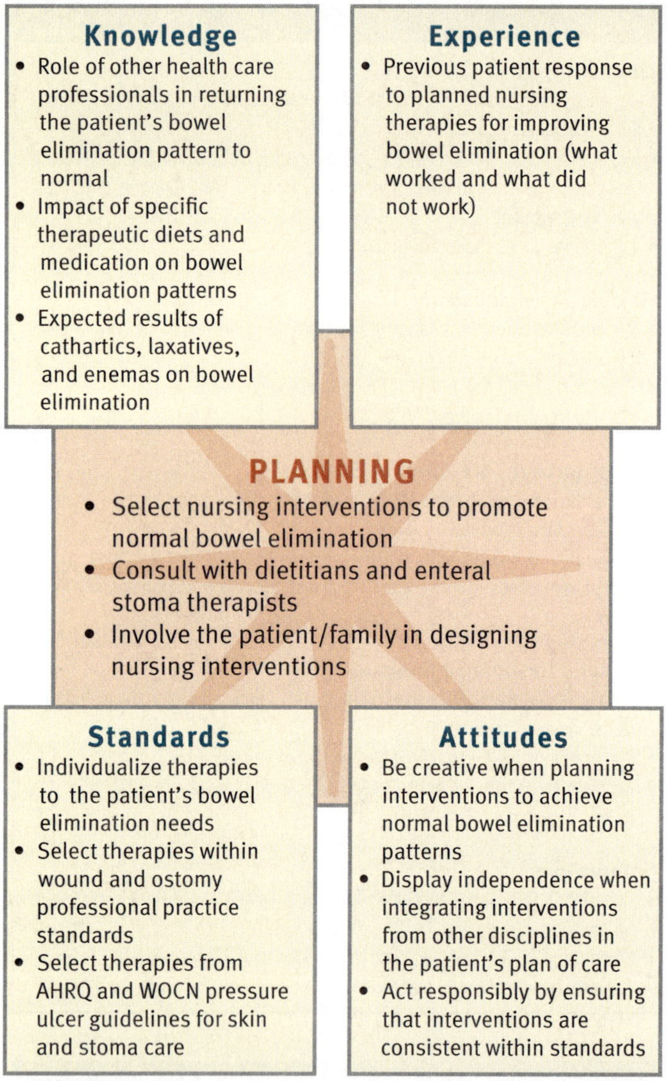
Knowledge
• Role of other health care professionals in returning the patient's bowel elimination pattern to normal
• Impact of specific therapeutic diets and medication on bowel elimination patterns
• Expected results of cathartics, laxatives, and enemas on bowel elimination
Experience
• Previous patient response to planned nursing therapies for improving bowel elimination (what worked and what did not work)
PLANNING
• Select nursing interventions to promote normal bowel elimination
• Consult with dietitians and enteral stoma therapists
• Involve the patient/family in designing nursing interventions
Standards
• Individualize therapies to the patient's bowel elimination needs
• Select therapies within wound and ostomy professional practice standards
• Select therapies from AHRQ and WOCN pressure ulcer guidelines for skin and stoma care
Attitudes
• Be creative when planning interventions to achieve normal bowel elimination patterns
• Display independence when integrating interventions from other disciplines in the patient's plan of care
• Act responsibly by ensuring that interventions are consistent within standards

FIG. 46-14 Critical thinking model for elimination planning. *AHRQ,* Agency for Healthcare Research and Quality; *WOCN,* Wound, Ostomy and Continence Nurses Society.

incontinence. In addition, the Agency for Healthcare Research and Quality (AHRQ) provides guidelines on reduction of pressure ulcers that also help you develop a plan of care for patients with bowel incontinence (see Chapter 48).

Goals and Outcomes. Help patients establish goals and outcomes by incorporating their elimination habits or routines as much as possible and reinforcing the routines that promote health (see the Nursing Care Plan). In addition, consider preexisting health concerns. For example, if a patient is at risk for worsening heart failure, you need to individualize an outcome of increased fluid intake to accommodate cardiac function and the patient's ability to safely handle the increased fluid. In another example, if a patient's bowel habits caused the elimination problem, help the patient learn new habits. The overall goal of returning the patient to a normal bowel elimination pattern includes the following outcomes:

- Patient sets regular defecation habits.
- Patient is able to list proper fluid and food intake needed to achieve bowel elimination.
- Patient implements a regular exercise program.
- Patient reports daily passage of soft, formed brown stool.
- Patient does not report discomfort associated with defecation.

Setting Priorities. Defecation patterns vary among individuals. For this reason the nurse and patient work together closely to plan effective interventions. Patients often have multiple diagnoses. The concept map (Fig. 46-15) shows an example of how the nursing diagnosis of constipation is related to three other diagnoses and their respective interventions. A realistic time frame to establish a normal defecation pattern for one patient is sometimes very different for another. In the patient with recent abdominal surgery, the priorities of pain management and the avoidance of constipation through increasing fiber in the diet and increasing activity help in the recovery process.

Teamwork and Collaboration. When patients are disabled or debilitated by illness, you need to include the family in the plan of care. In some situations family members have the same ineffective elimination habits as the patient. Thus patient and family teaching is an important part of the care plan. Other health team members such as dietitians and WOCNs are often valuable resources. You coordinate activities of the multidisciplinary health care team.

The patient with alterations in bowel elimination requires intervention from many members of the health care team. Certain tasks such as assisting patients onto the bedpan or bedside commode are appropriate to delegate to nursing assistive personnel (NAP). It is important to remind the NAP to report any abnormal findings or difficulties encountered during the elimination process. Many of the diagnostic tests for evaluation of the GI system are performed by nonnursing personnel. Maintain ongoing communication with these caregivers to ensure that you provide safe and effective patient-centered care and address the patient's needs, wants, and concerns (Cronenwett et al., 2007).

IMPLEMENTATION

Successful nursing interventions improve the patients' and family members' understanding of bowel elimination. Teach the patient and family about proper diet, adequate fluid intake, and factors that stimulate or slow peristalsis such as emotional stress. This is often best done during the patient's mealtime. Patients also need to learn the importance of establishing regular bowel routines, regular exercise, and taking appropriate measures when elimination problems develop.

Health Promotion. One of the most important habits to teach regarding bowel habits is to take time for defecation. To establish regular bowel habits, a patient needs to know when the urge to defecate normally occurs. Advise the patient to begin establishing a routine during a time when defecation is most likely to occur, usually an hour after a meal. When patients are restricted to bed or need help to ambulate, offer a bedpan or help them reach the bathroom in a timely manner.

Many patients have established routines for defecation. In a hospital or long-term care facility make certain that treatment routines do not interfere with the patient's routine. It is important to provide privacy. When patients forced to use a bedpan share rooms with other people, pull the curtain around the area so patients are able to relax, knowing that interruptions will not occur. Always place the call light and toilet tissue within the patient's reach. When patients are at risk for falls, you stand near them or leave the door partially open so you can see them at all times.

Promotion of Normal Defecation. A number of interventions stimulate the defecation reflex, affect the character of feces, or

NURSING CARE PLAN

Constipation

ASSESSMENT

Javier, a home care nurse, is visiting Larry Johnston at his home on one of the local cattle ranches. Larry lives 20 miles from town. He is 22 years old and had surgery 6 days ago for repair of a badly broken right leg, after being thrown from a horse. Larry tells Javier that he "just doesn't feel well." His past history includes pneumonia at age 12 and a recent traumatic injury to the abdomen. The injury required emergency surgery after he was struck by a bull's horns.

Assessment Activities	*Findings/Defining Characteristics**
Ask Larry about his bowel elimination patterns over the last 5 days.	Larry tells Javier that he **has not had a bowel movement since he left the hospital 4 days ago** and that his **abdomen is tight and sore.**
Review patient's medication.	Larry says he is taking one Percocet tablet for pain, up to three tablets a day.
Review dietary and fluid intake over last day.	Diet included eggs, bacon, and toast for breakfast; soup for lunch; and chicken, rice, and corn for dinner. He drinks about six cups of coffee each day, no water, but will drink a cola.
Ask about any nausea or vomiting.	**Denies any nausea or vomiting.**
Auscultate patient's abdomen.	**Decreased bowel sounds** are auscultated throughout all four abdominal quadrants.
Palpate abdomen.	While Javier is palpating Larry's abdomen, Larry tells Javier, **"It really hurts."** On palpation **left lower quadrant is tender and firm.**

***Defining characteristics** are shown in bold type.

NURSING DIAGNOSIS: Constipation related to opiate-containing pain medication and decreased fiber intake

PLANNING

Goals	*Expected Outcomes (NOC)†*
	Bowel Elimination
Larry will establish normal defecation.	Larry will report passage of soft, formed stool without straining in next 24 hours.
	Nutritional Status: Food and Fluid Intake
Larry will make changes to his diet to prevent constipation.	Larry will drink at least 1500 mL of fluid over the next 8 hours. Larry will increase the fiber content of his diet.

†Outcome classification labels from Moorhead S et al: *Nursing outcomes classification (NOC)*, ed 4, St Louis, 2008, Mosby.

INTERVENTIONS (NIC)‡ ***Constipation/Impaction Management***	**RATIONALE**
Encourage fluid intake of appropriate fluids, fruit juice, and water.	At least 1500 mL fluid intake daily is necessary to prevent hard, dry stool (JBI, 2008).
Encourage activity within patient's mobility regimen.	Minimal activity (such as leg lifts) increases peristalsis.
Instruct Larry to add 20g/day of wheat bran to diet.	Bran along with physical activity prevents constipation (JBI, 2008).
Provide laxative or stool softeners as ordered.	Medications soften the stool and prevent straining (Lehne, 2010).
Provide privacy during toileting.	Patients need to feel relaxed when moving bowels (Holman et al., 2008).

‡Intervention classification labels from Bulechek GM, Butcher HK, Dochterman JM: *Nursing interventions classification (NIC)*, ed 5, St Louis, 2008, Mosby.

EVALUATION

Nursing Actions	*Patient Response/Finding*	*Achievement of Outcomes*
Ask Larry to identify foods high in fiber.	Able to state appropriate foods.	Larry is making excellent progress in introducing high-fiber and low-fat foods into his diet.
	Review of 24-hour diet diary shows Larry is selecting high-fiber, low-fat foods.	
Ask Larry about physical activity.	Larry states that he has not changed his activity pattern.	Larry did not increase activity pattern and needs to continue to work on this intervention.
Observe Larry's subsequent stool for characteristics such as consistency and color.	Stools are now every 24 to 48 hours. Larry does not "feel regular." Abdomen is soft and nondistended. Stools are formed and hard, but Larry does report straining.	Larry did not achieve passage of regular, formed stool.

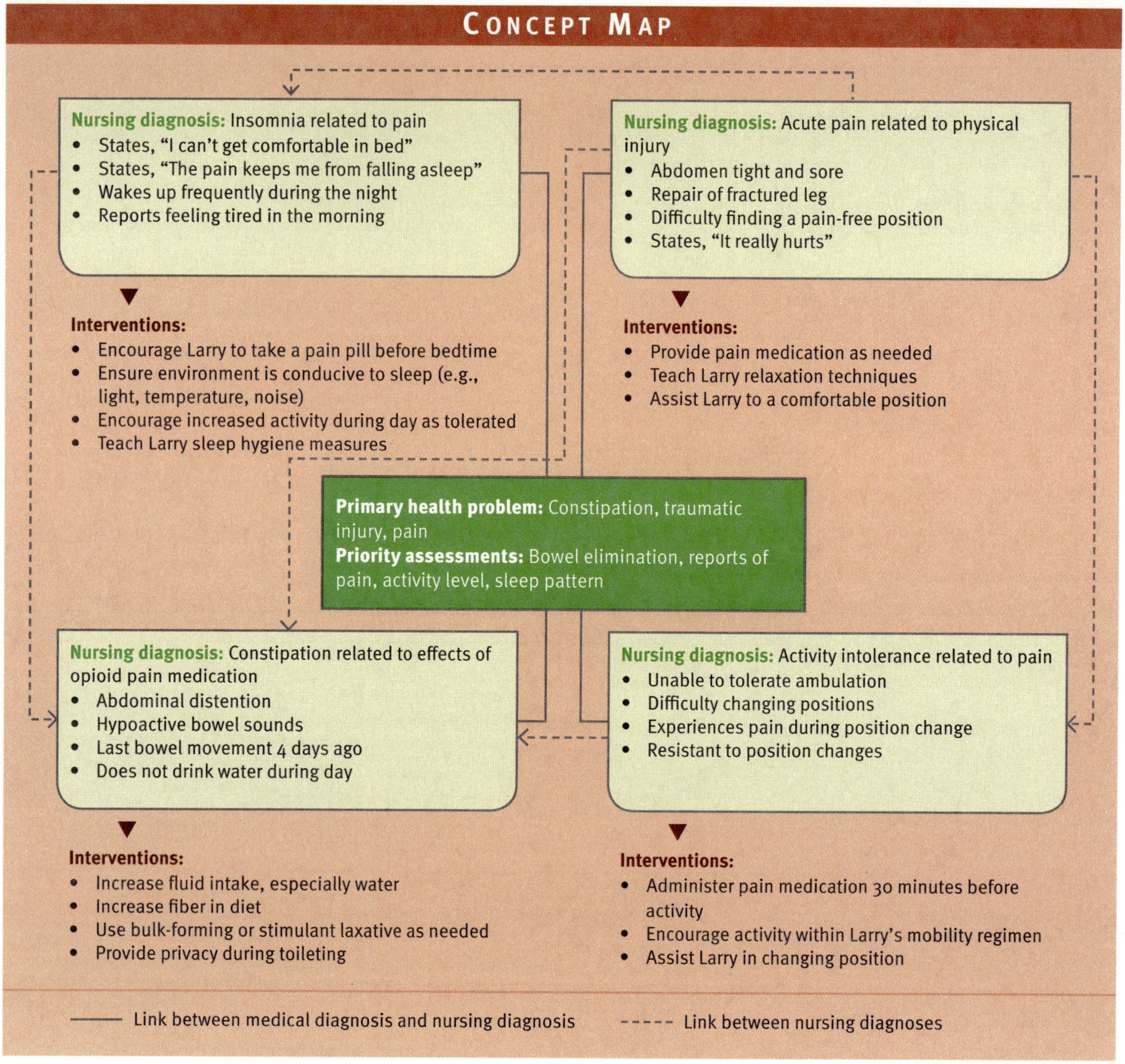
CONCEPT MAP
Nursing diagnosis: Insomnia related to pain
• States, "I can't get comfortable in bed"
• States, "The pain keeps me from falling asleep"
• Wakes up frequently during the night
• Reports feeling tired in the morning
Interventions:
• Encourage Larry to take a pain pill before bedtime
• Ensure environment is conducive to sleep (e.g., light, temperature, noise)
• Encourage increased activity during day as tolerated
• Teach Larry sleep hygiene measures
Nursing diagnosis: Acute pain related to physical injury
• Abdomen tight and sore
• Repair of fractured leg
• Difficulty finding a pain-free position
• States, "It really hurts"
Interventions:
• Provide pain medication as needed
• Teach Larry relaxation techniques
• Assist Larry to a comfortable position
Primary health problem: Constipation, traumatic injury, pain
Priority assessments: Bowel elimination, reports of pain, activity level, sleep pattern
Nursing diagnosis: Constipation related to effects of opioid pain medication
• Abdominal distention
• Hypoactive bowel sounds
• Last bowel movement 4 days ago
• Does not drink water during day
Interventions:
• Increase fluid intake, especially water
• Increase fiber in diet
• Use bulk-forming or stimulant laxative as needed
• Provide privacy during toileting
Nursing diagnosis: Activity intolerance related to pain
• Unable to tolerate ambulation
• Difficulty changing positions
• Experiences pain during position change
• Resistant to position changes
Interventions:
• Administer pain medication 30 minutes before activity
• Encourage activity within Larry's mobility regimen
• Assist Larry in changing position
Link between medical diagnosis and nursing diagnosis
Link between nursing diagnoses

FIG. 46-15 Concept map for Larry Johnston. *PCA,* Patient-controlled analgesia.

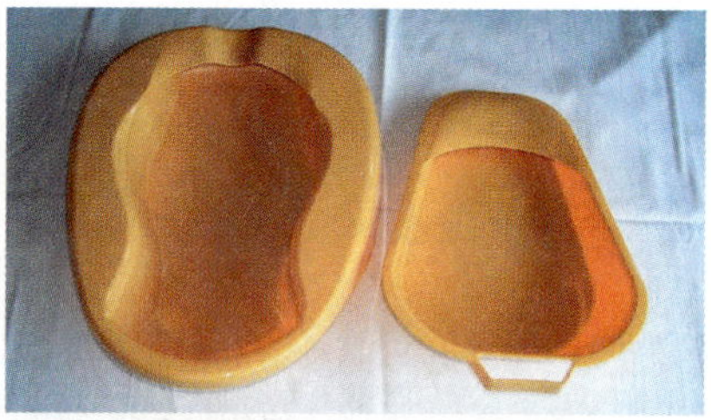

FIG. 46-16 Types of bedpans. *From left,* Regular bedpan and fracture bedpan.

increase peristalsis to help patients evacuate bowel contents normally and without discomfort.

Sitting Position. Assist patients who have difficulty sitting because of muscular weakness and mobility problems. Place an elevated seat on the toilet when patients are unable to lower themselves to a sitting position because of joint- or muscle-wasting diseases. These seats require patients to use less effort to sit or stand.

Positioning on Bedpan. Patients restricted to bed use bedpans for defecation. Women use bedpans to pass both urine and feces, whereas men use bedpans only for defecation. Sitting on a bedpan is extremely uncomfortable. Help position patients comfortably. Two types of bedpans are available (Fig. 46-16). The regular bedpan, made of plastic, has a curved smooth upper end and a sharper-edged lower end and is about 5 cm (2 inches) deep. The smaller fracture pan, designed for patients with lower-extremity fractures, has a shallow upper end about 1.3 cm (½ inch) deep. The shallow end of the pan fits under the buttocks toward the sacrum; the deeper end, which has a handle, goes just under the upper thighs. The pan needs to be high enough so feces enter it.

When positioning a patient, it is important to prevent muscle strain and discomfort. Never try to lift a patient onto a bedpan. Never place a patient on a bedpan and then leave with the bed flat unless activity restrictions demand it. If the bed is flat, the hips remain hyperextended.

Fig. 46-17 shows proper and improper positions on bedpans. The best method for bedpan placement is to first be sure that the patient is positioned high in bed. Then raise the patient's head about 30 degrees to prevent hyperextension of the back and provide support to the upper torso. The patient then raises the hips by bending the knees and lifting the hips upward. Place a hand palm up under the patient's sacrum, resting the elbow on the mattress and using it as a lever to help in lifting while slipping the pan under the patient. Patients who have had abdominal surgery are hesitant to exert strain on suture lines and often have difficulty positioning on a pan. Always wear gloves when handling a bedpan.

When patients are immobile or it is unsafe to allow them to raise their hips, they remain flat and roll onto the bedpan by using the following steps:

1. Lower the head of the bed flat and help the patient roll onto one side, backside toward the nurse.
2. Apply a small amount of powder to back and buttocks or cover bedpan edge with tissue to prevent skin from sticking to the pan.
3. Place the bedpan firmly against the buttocks, down into the mattress with the open rim toward the patient's feet (Fig. 46-18).
4. Keeping one hand against the bedpan, place the other around the patient's fore hip. Ask the patient to roll back onto the pan, flat in bed. Do not shove the pan under the patient.
5. With the patient positioned comfortably, raise the head of the bed 30 degrees.
6. Place a rolled towel or small pillow under the lumbar curve of the patient's back for added comfort.
7. Raise the knee gatch or ask the patient to bend the knees to assume a squatting position. Do not raise the knee gatch if contraindicated.

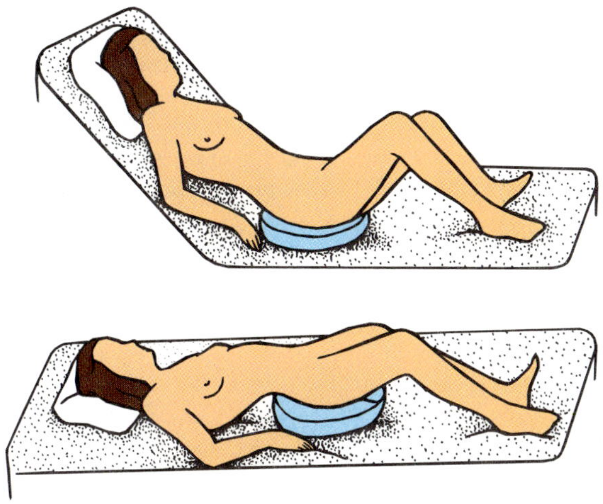

FIG. 46-17 Positions on a bedpan. *Top,* Proper position reduces patient's back strain. *Bottom,* Improper positioning of patient.

Privacy. Maintain the patient's privacy during bowel elimination. This is especially important for a patient using a bedpan. The call light and a supply of toilet paper need to be within easy reach. When the patient finishes, respond to the call signal immediately and remove the pan. The patient often requires assistance with wiping. To remove the pan, ask the patient to roll off to the side or raise the hips. While wearing gloves, hold the pan steady to avoid spilling. Avoid pulling or shoving it from under the patient's hips because this pulls the patient's skin and causes tissue injury such as shearing (see Chapter 48). Remove the pan and clean the perineum front to back.

After assessing the stool, immediately empty the contents of the bedpan into the toilet or in a special receptacle in the utility room. A spray faucet attached to most toilets allows for the ability to rinse the bedpan thoroughly. The patient uses the same bedpan each time. Finally, document the characteristics of the feces.

Offer the bedpan often. Patients will accidentally soil bedclothes if forced to wait. Many patients try to avoid using a bedpan because it is embarrassing and uncomfortable. They often try to get to the bathroom even though their conditions prohibit ambulation. Warn patients about the risk of falls or accidents.

Acute Care. With some acute illnesses the GI system becomes affected. Changes in the patient's fluid status, mobility patterns, nutrition, and sleep cycle affect regular bowel habits. Surgical interventions on the GI tract obviously affect bowel elimination. However, surgery on other systems (e.g., the musculoskeletal and cardiovascular systems) sometimes affects the patient's bowel elimination patterns. Remain sensitive to patients' elimination needs and intervene to help them maintain as normal bowel elimination habits as possible.

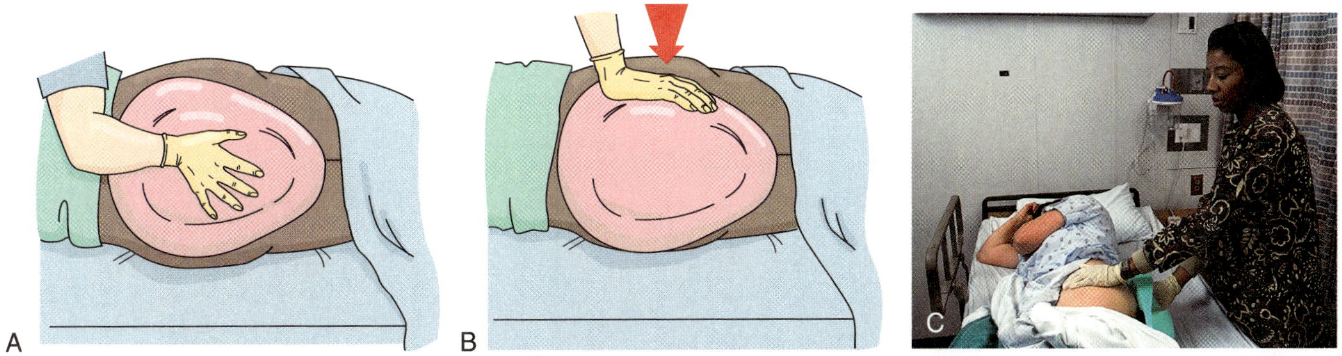

FIG. 46-18 Positioning immobilized patient on bedpan. **A,** Place bedpan firmly against buttocks. **B,** Push buttocks down into mattress with open rim toward feet. **C,** Place one hand against bedpan; place other hand around patient's fore hip.

Medications. Some medications initiate and facilitate bowel elimination. Cathartics, laxatives, and occasionally an enema are used to resolve constipation; antidiarrheal preparations help the patient to resolve diarrhea. All of these medications are available over the counter; stronger preparations are available through prescriptions. Caution patients not to use these over-the-counter medications on a prolonged basis without consulting their health care provider.

Building Competency in Patient-Centered Care You are caring for Mr. Miner, an 82-year-old male who reports experiencing constipation. He is hard of hearing and has bilateral cataracts. He admits to using laxatives and/or enemas at least on a biweekly basis. What assessment questions and teaching strategies, approaches, and tools do you use to enhance Mr. Miner's learning and ability to prevent constipation?

Answers to questions can be found on the Evolve website.

Cathartics and Laxatives. Often a patient is unable to defecate normally because of pain, constipation, or impaction. Cathartics and laxatives have the short-term action of emptying the bowel. They are prescribed for bowel evacuation for patients undergoing GI tests and abdominal surgery. Although the terms *cathartic* and *laxative* are often used interchangeably, cathartics have a stronger effect on the intestines. Five types of laxatives and cathartics are available (Table 46-5).

Cathartics and laxatives come in oral, tablet, powder, and suppository dosage forms (see Chapter 31). Although the oral route is most commonly used, suppositories are more effective because of their stimulant effect on the rectal mucosa. Cathartic suppositories such as bisacodyl (Dulcolax) act within 30 minutes. Older adults often get a strong sudden urge to defecate with Dulcolax.

Excessive use of laxatives, enemas, and/or bulk-forming agents increases the patient's risk for diarrhea and abnormal bowel elimination. It can impair the patient's normal defecation reflex. In

TABLE 46-5 Common Types of Laxatives and Cathartics

AGENT/BRAND NAME	ACTION	INDICATIONS	RISKS
Bulk Forming			
Methylcellulose (Citrucel) Psyllium (Metamucil, Naturacil) Polycarbophil (Fibercon)	High-fiber content absorbs water and increases solid intestinal bulk (JBI, 2008; Lehne, 2010). Agents stretch intestinal wall to stimulate peristalsis.	Agents are least irritating, most natural, and safest cathartics. Agents are drugs of choice for chronic constipation (e.g., pregnancy, low-residue diet). Also relieves mild diarrhea. If treating diarrhea, administer less water.	Agents that are in powder form cause obstruction if not mixed with at least 240 mL of water or juice and swallowed quickly. Caution is necessary with bulk-forming laxatives that also contain stimulants. Agents are not for patients for whom large fluid intake is contraindicated. Follow each dose with 8 oz water.
Emollient or Wetting			
Docusate sodium (Colace, Correctol, Disonate) Docusate calcium (Surfak) Docusate potassium (Dialose)	Stool softeners are detergents that lower surface tension of feces, allowing water and fat to penetrate. They increase secretion of water by intestine (Lehne, 2010).	Agents are for short-term therapy to relieve straining on defecation (e.g., hemorrhoids, perianal surgery, pregnancy, recovery from myocardial infarction).	Agents are of little value for treatment of chronic constipation.
Saline			
Magnesium citrate or citrate of magnesia Magnesium hydroxide (Milk of Magnesia) Sodium phosphate (Fleet Phospho-Soda, Fleet Enema)	Agents contain salt preparation not absorbed by intestines. Osmotic effect increases pressure in bowel to act as stimulant for peristalsis (Lehne, 2010).	Agents are only for acute emptying of bowel (e.g., endoscopic examination, suspected poisoning, acute constipation).	Agents are not for long-term management of constipation. Agents are not for patients with kidney dysfunction (toxic buildup of magnesium). Phosphate salts are not for patients on fluid restriction.
Stimulant Cathartics			
Bisacodyl (Dulcolax) Castor oil Casanthranol (Peri-Colace) Senna (Ex-Lax, Senokot)	Agents irritate intestinal mucosa to increase motility (Lehne, 2010). Agents decrease absorption in small bowel and colon (Lehne, 2010).	Agents prepare bowel for diagnostic procedures.	Agents cause severe cramping. Agents are not for long-term use. Chronic use causes fluid and electrolyte imbalances.
Lubricants			
Mineral oil (Haley's M-O, Petrogalar Plain)	Agents coat fecal contents, allowing easier passage of stool (Lehne, 2010). Agents reduce water absorption in colon.	Agents prevent straining on defecation (e.g., hemorrhoids, perianal surgery).	Agents decrease absorption of fat-soluble vitamins (A, D, E, and K). They cause dangerous form of pneumonia if aspirated into lungs. When taken with emollients, mineral oil increases risk for fat emboli.

addition, the patient develops altered absorption of nutrients, fluid and electrolyte imbalances, and generalized weakness. In chronically ill or older adult patients weakness and the frequent need to use toilet facilities result in an increased risk for falls and other injuries.

Antidiarrheal Agents. For patients with diarrhea, frequent passage of liquid stools becomes a problem. Many patients use over-the-counter agents such as Imodium to relieve common diarrhea. However, the most effective antidiarrheal agents are prescriptive opiates such as codeine phosphate, opium tincture (Paregoric), and diphenoxylate (Lomotil). Antidiarrheal opiate agents decrease intestinal muscle tone to slow passage of feces. Opiates inhibit peristaltic waves that move feces forward, but they also increase segmental contractions that mix intestinal contents. As a result, the intestinal walls absorb more water. Use antidiarrheal agents with caution because opiates are habit forming. Patients with diarrhea lasting more than 2 days need a stool culture and evaluation of diet and fluid intake for intolerances of food and fluids (e.g., excessive use of fruits, lactose).

Enemas. An enema is the instillation of a solution into the rectum and sigmoid colon. The primary reason for an enema is to promote defecation by stimulating peristalsis. The volume of fluid instilled breaks up the fecal mass, stretches the rectal wall, and initiates the defecation reflex. Enemas are also a vehicle for medications that exert a local effect on rectal mucosa. The most common use for an enema is temporary relief of constipation. Other indications include removing impacted feces, emptying the bowel before diagnostic tests or surgery, and beginning a program of bowel training.

Cleansing Enemas. Cleansing enemas promote the complete evacuation of feces from the colon. They act by stimulating peristalsis through the infusion of a large volume of solution or through local irritation of the mucosa of the colon. They include tap water, normal saline, soapsuds solution, and low-volume hypertonic saline. Each solution has a different osmotic effect, influencing the movement of fluids between the colon and interstitial spaces beyond the intestinal wall. Infants and children receive only normal saline because they are at risk for fluid imbalance.

Tap Water. Tap water is hypotonic and exerts an osmotic pressure lower than fluid in interstitial spaces. After infusion into the colon, tap water escapes from the bowel lumen into interstitial spaces. The net movement of water is low. The infused volume stimulates defecation before large amounts of water leave the bowel. Do not repeat tap-water enemas because water toxicity or circulatory overload develops if the body absorbs large amounts of water.

Normal Saline. Physiologically normal saline is the safest solution to use because it exerts the same osmotic pressure as fluids in interstitial spaces surrounding the bowel. The volume of infused saline stimulates peristalsis. Giving saline enemas does not create the danger of excess fluid absorption.

Hypertonic Solutions. Hypertonic solutions infused into the bowel exert osmotic pressure that pulls fluids out of interstitial spaces. The colon fills with fluid, and the resultant distention promotes defecation. Patients unable to tolerate large volumes of fluid benefit most from this type of enema, which is by design low volume. This type of enema is contraindicated for patients who are dehydrated and young infants. A hypertonic solution of 120 to 180 mL (4 to 6 oz) is usually effective. The commercially prepared Fleet enema is the most common.

Soapsuds. You add soapsuds to tap water or saline to create the effect of intestinal irritation to stimulate peristalsis. Use only pure castile soap that comes in a liquid form included in most soapsuds enema kits. Use soapsuds enemas with caution in pregnant women and older adults because they cause electrolyte imbalance or damage to the intestinal mucosa.

The health care provider sometimes orders a high or low cleansing enema. The terms *high* and *low* refer to the height from which, and hence the pressure with which, the fluid is delivered. High enemas cleanse the entire colon. After the enema is infused, ask the patient to turn from the left lateral to the dorsal recumbent, over to the right lateral position. The position change ensures that fluid reaches the large intestine. A low enema cleanses only the rectum and sigmoid colon.

Oil Retention. Oil-retention enemas lubricate the rectum and colon. The feces absorb the oil and become softer and easier to pass. To enhance action of the oil, the patient retains the enema for several hours if possible.

Other Types of Enemas. Carminative enemas provide relief from gaseous distention. They improve the ability to pass flatus. An example of a carminative enema is MGW solution, which contains 30 mL of magnesium, 60 mL of glycerin, and 90 mL of water.

Medicated enemas contain drugs. An example is sodium polystyrene sulfonate (Kayexalate), used to treat patients with dangerously high serum potassium levels. This drug contains a resin that exchanges sodium ions for potassium ions in the large intestine. Another medicated enema is neomycin solution, an antibiotic used to reduce bacteria in the colon before bowel surgery.

Enema Administration. Enemas are available in commercially packaged, disposable units or with reusable equipment prepared before use. Sterile technique is unnecessary because the colon normally contains bacteria. However, wear gloves to prevent the transmission of fecal microorganisms.

Explain the procedure, including the position to assume, precautions to take to avoid discomfort, and length of time necessary to retain the solution before defecation. If the patient needs to take the enema at home, explain the procedure to a family member.

Often the health care provider orders "enemas until clear." This means that the enema is repeated until the patient passes fluid that is clear and contains no fecal material. It is often necessary to give as many as three enemas, but caution the patient against using more than three. Excess enema use seriously depletes fluids and electrolytes. If the enema fails to return a clear solution after three times (check agency policy) or if the patient seems to not be tolerating the rigors of repeated enemas, notify the health care provider.

Giving an enema to a patient who is unable to contract the external sphincter poses difficulties. Give the enema with the patient positioned on the bedpan. Giving the enema with the patient sitting on the toilet is unsafe because the curved rectal tubing scrapes the rectal wall. Skill 46-1 on pp. 1112-1115 outlines the steps for an enema administration.

Digital Removal of Stool. For a patient with an impaction, the fecal mass is sometimes too large to pass voluntarily. If enemas fail, break up the fecal mass with the fingers and remove it in sections. Digital removal is a last resort in the management of severe constipation and practiced when all other methods have failed. The procedure is very uncomfortable for the patient. Excess rectal manipulation causes irritation to the mucosa; bleeding; and stimulation of the vagus nerve, which results in a reflex slowing of the heart rate. Because of the potential complications of the procedure, a health care provider's order is necessary to remove a fecal impaction (Kyle, 2007c) (Box 46-8).

BOX 46-8 PROCEDURAL GUIDELINES

Digital Removal of Stool

Delegation Considerations

The skill of digital removal of stool cannot be delegated to nursing assistive personnel (NAP).

Equipment

Clean gloves, stethoscope, water-soluble anesthetic lubricant (check agency policy on type of lubricant), towel, washcloth, soap and water, and bedpan

1. Patient identification. Identify the patient using two identifiers (e.g., name and birth date or name and account number) according to facility policy. Compare identifiers with information on the patient's medical record (TJC, 2011).
2. Explain the purpose of the procedure and ways patient can assist.
3. Verify medical history of impaction and patient's last bowel movement.
4. Observe for abdominal distention and auscultate abdomen.
5. Obtain baseline vital signs before the procedure.
6. Position patient on the left side with knees flexed and back toward you (Steggall, 2008).
7. Pull curtains around bed. Drape the trunk and lower extremities with a bath blanket and place a waterproof pad under the buttocks. Place a bedpan next to the patient.
8. Apply gloves and lubricate the index and middle fingers of your dominant hand with anesthetic lubricating jelly (Steggall, 2008).
9. Instruct patient to take slow deep breaths, gently and gradually insert the gloved index finger, and feel the anal sphincter relax around the finger. Then insert middle finger into the rectum and advance the finger slowly along the rectal wall toward the umbilicus (Kyle, 2007c; Steggall, 2008).
10. Gently loosen the fecal mass by moving fingers in a scissors motions to fragment fecal mass. Work the finger into the hardened mass.
11. Work the feces downward toward the end of the rectum. Remove small pieces at a time and discard into bedpan.
12. Periodically assess patient's vital signs and look for signs of fatigue.

    CLINICAL DECISION: Stop the procedure if the heart rate drops significantly or the rhythm changes.

13. Continue to remove feces and allow patient to rest at intervals (Chien and Bradway, 2010).
14. After completion wash and dry the buttocks and anal area.
15. Remove bedpan and dispose of feces. Remove gloves by turning them inside out and discard.
16. Assist patient to toilet or clean bedpan if urge to defecate develops.
17. Perform hand hygiene.
18. Assess patient's vital signs and determine level of comfort. Auscultate bowel sounds and gently palpate abdomen.
19. Observe for rectal bleeding, diarrhea, changes from baseline vital signs, and increasing pain or abdominal distention.
20. Record results of removal of impaction by describing fecal characteristics.

Inserting and Maintaining a Nasogastric Tube. A patient's condition or situation sometimes requires special interventions to decompress the GI tract. Such conditions include surgery (see Chapter 50), infections of the GI tract, trauma to the GI tract, and conditions in which peristalsis is absent.

A nasogastric (NG) tube is a pliable hollow tube that is inserted through the patient's nasopharynx into the stomach. NG intubation has several purposes (Table 46-6). There are two main categories of NG tubes: Fine- or small-bore tubes and large-bore tubes.

TABLE 46-6 Purposes of Nasogastric Intubation

PURPOSE	DESCRIPTION	TYPE OF TUBE
Decompression	Removal of secretions and gaseous substances from gastrointestinal (GI) tract; prevention or relief of abdominal distention (Lewis et al., 2011)	Salem sump, Levin, Miller-Abbott
Enteral feeding (see Chapter 44)	Instillation of liquid nutritional supplements or feedings into stomach for patients unable to swallow fluid (Lewis et al., 2011)	Duo, Dobhoff, Levin
Compression	Internal application of pressure by means of inflated balloon to prevent internal esophageal or GI hemorrhage (Lewis et al., 2011)	Sengstaken-Blakemore
Lavage	Irrigation of stomach in cases of active bleeding, poisoning, or gastric dilation (Lewis et al., 2011)	Levin, Ewald, Salem sump

Large-bore tubes, 12-Fr and above, are usually used for gastric decompression or removal of gastric secretions. Small-bore tubes are frequently used for medication administration and enteral feedings (see Chapter 44 for enteral feedings). The Levin and Salem sump tubes are the most common for stomach decompression. The Levin tube is a single-lumen tube with holes near the tip. You connect it to a drainage bag or to an intermittent suction device to drain stomach secretions.

The Salem sump tube is preferable for stomach decompression. The tube has two lumina: one for removal of gastric contents and one to provide an air vent. A blue "pigtail" is the air vent that connects with the second lumen. When the main lumen of the sump tube is connected to suction, the air vent permits free, continuous drainage of secretions. Never clamp off the air vent, connect it to suction, or use it for irrigation.

NG tube insertion does not require sterile technique. Simply use clean technique. The procedure is uncomfortable. The patient experiences a burning sensation as the tube passes through the sensitive nasal mucosa. When it reaches the back of the pharynx, the patient sometimes begins to gag. Help him or her relax to make tube insertion easier. Some institutions allow you to use Xylocaine jelly when inserting the tube because it increases patient comfort during the procedure (Skill 46-2 on pp. 1115-1120).

One of the greatest problems in caring for a patient with an NG tube is maintaining comfort. Because the tube constantly irritates the nasal mucosa, you assess the condition of the patient's nares and mucosa for inflammation and excoriation. The tape or fixation device used to anchor the tube often becomes soiled. Change it every day to lessen irritation. Frequent lubrication of the nares also minimizes excoriation. With one nares occluded, the patient breathes through the mouth. Frequent mouth care (at least every 2 hours) helps minimize dehydration. A glass of cool water for rinsing is useful, but the patient who is allowed nothing by mouth (NPO) should not swallow the water. The patient frequently complains of a sore throat. An ice bag applied externally to the throat helps. If ordered by the health care provider, the patient gargles with topical Xylocaine jelly and/or uses lozenges to minimize the irritation.

After you insert the tube, you need to maintain its patency. Sometimes the tip of the tubing rests against the stomach wall, or the tube becomes blocked with thick secretions. Therefore regular irrigation is necessary. Flushing the tube with normal saline by way of a catheter-tipped syringe clears blockages in the tube. If an NG tube continues to drain improperly after irrigation, reposition it by advancing or withdrawing it slightly. Any change in tube position requires you to verify its placement in the patient's GI tract.

The NG tube sometimes causes distention. Its presence causes many patients to swallow large volumes of air. Channels of gastric secretions also form along the walls of the stomach and bypass the suction holes. Turning the patient regularly helps to collapse the channels and promotes emptying of stomach contents (Durston, 2009).

Continuing and Restorative Care. Regular elimination patterns need to begin for a patient to recover and return home or to an extended care facility. When patients have a colostomy, they need to learn to care for the ostomy. Other patients require bowel retraining. It is important to remember that you initiate ostomy care and bowel retraining in acute care settings. However, because these are long-term care needs, teaching is usually completed in restorative care settings. Evidence-based interventions reduce the risk of stoma problems in the older adult population over time (Box 46-9).

Care of Ostomies. Patients with temporary or permanent bowel diversions have unique elimination needs. An individual with an ostomy wears a pouch or appliance to collect **effluent,** stool discharged from the stoma (Dorman, 2009). The patient needs to use meticulous skin care to prevent liquid stool from irritating the skin around the stoma.

Irrigating a Colostomy. Although this practice is not as common as it once was, some patients irrigate their left-sided colostomies to regulate colon emptying. Other patients do not want to spend the additional 60 to 90 minutes in the bathroom every day; thus they empty their pouch as necessary (Dorman, 2009). Only colostomies can be irrigated.

Never use an enema set to irrigate a colostomy. Instead you use specific equipment, which includes a special cone-tipped irrigator to prevent bowel penetration and backflow of the irrigating solution (Fig. 46-19). Help patients to schedule irrigations at times that fit within their daily routine. Before irrigating the stoma, patients usually sit on the toilet and place an irrigating sleeve over the stoma. The end of this sleeve extends into the bowl of the commode. The health care provider orders the amount and type of irrigation solution. For adults the amount typically ranges from 500 to 700 mL of tap water. The patient instills the solution slowly through the lubricated cone tip. Irrigation usually takes 5 to 10 minutes. The patient then removes the cone tip and waits 30 to 45 minutes for the solution and feces to drain out of the irrigation sleeve. Once the drainage stops, the patient applies a stoma cap or a pouch.

Pouching Ostomies. An ostomy requires a pouch to collect fecal material. An effective pouching system protects the skin, contains fecal material, remains odor free, and is comfortable and inconspicuous. A person wearing a pouch needs to feel secure enough to participate in any activity (Deitz, 2010b).

Many pouching systems are available. To ensure that a pouch fits well and meets the patient's needs, consider the location of the ostomy, type and size of the stoma, type and amount of ostomy drainage, size and contour of the abdomen, condition of the skin around the stoma, physical activities of the patient, patient's personal preference, age and dexterity, and cost of equipment. A **wound ostomy continence nurse (WOCN)** is a nurse specially educated to care for ostomy patients; the WOCN collaborates with staff nurses to be sure that the patient uses the correct pouching system, especially when the patient is ill or is experiencing health changes or problems with the ostomy. For example, you initiate a referral to a WOCN when planning the care of a patient who has a high-output ostomy that requires a pouch modification.

BOX 46-9 EVIDENCE-BASED PRACTICE

Recognition of Skin Problems

PICO Question: In patients with ostomies, what is the effect of patient education and knowledge on the prevention of skin breakdown around the ostomy?

Evidence Summary

Patients with an ostomy are at risk for development of peristomal skin problems. Maintenance of healthy peristomal skin, with the skin around the stoma being clean, dry, and intact is a priority following ostomy surgery (Williams et al., 2010). Persons with an ileostomy experience the highest incidence of skin problems, whereas persons with a colostomy have a lower incidence of skin problems (Herlufsen et al., 2006). The most common cause of peristomal skin disorders is effluent, which causes skin irritation, ulceration, or erosion. Reasons for effluent leakage include poor-fitting stoma appliances, poor adhesive adherence, peristomal hernia, and surgical complications (Williams et al., 2010).With shorter postoperative hospital stays, it is challenging for nurses to provide the extensive patient education on pouching systems, ostomy care, and problem-solving techniques needed to prevent peristomal skin problems (Ratliff, Scarano, and Donovan, 2005). Patients often failed to recognize early signs of skin irritation and did not report a skin problem (Herlufsen et al., 2006; Thompson et al., 2011). This lack of knowledge resulted in patients delaying to seek health care to treat the skin problem (Herlufsen et al., 2006). Patient education is an important factor in preventing complications following ostomy surgery. Nurses need to provide education to patients before discharge and follow up with patients after discharge to prevent peristomal skin problems.

Implications for Practice

- Evaluate patient's knowledge and ability to assess skin disorders for early recognition and treatment of skin disorders.
- Provide patient education on signs and symptoms of skin disorders to ensure early identification of skin problems (Herlufsen et al., 2006; Williams et al., 2010).
- Work with the patient to find the simplest ostomy appliance possible with minimal or no accessories (William et al., 2010).
- Refer patients to an ostomy specialist if assistance is needed to manage the ostomy (Thompson et al., 2011).

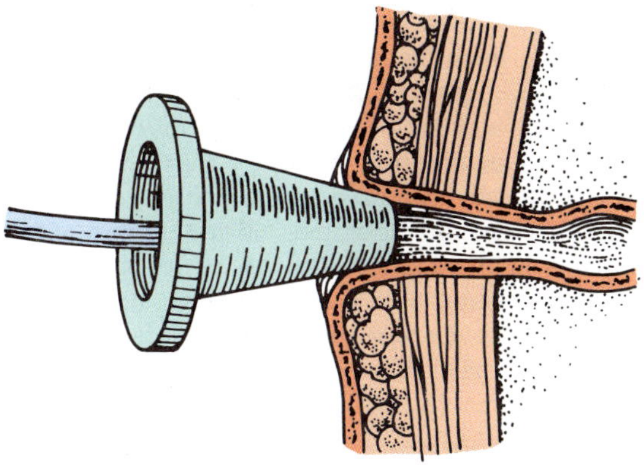

FIG. 46-19 Ostomy irrigation cone inserted into stoma.

A pouching system consists of a pouch and skin barrier. Some pouching systems such as Squibb-ConvaTec, Hollister, Coloplast, and Smith & Nephew are attached to the patient's skin from the adhesive surface of the product; whereas other pouching systems such as VIP are nonadhesive. Pouches come in one- and two-piece systems that are disposable or reusable. Some pouches have the opening precut by the manufacturer; others require the stoma opening to be custom cut to the patient's specific stoma size.

Skin barriers include wafers, pastes, powders, and liquid film applied to the skin around the stoma (Hoeflok et al., 2009). Some wafer skin barriers are permanently attached to the ostomy pouch. These are called *one-piece pouch systems*. With a two-piece system, the patient detaches the pouch from the skin barrier for emptying or changing. This allows the skin barrier to remain around the patient's stoma for several days, thus minimizing the chance of skin damage from too-frequent removal of the skin barrier from the peristomal skin. When using a two-piece pouching system, it is important to remember that the skin barrier and pouch need to be the corresponding size and from the same manufacturer. A pouch from one manufacturer does not fit correctly on a skin barrier from another manufacturer. Be sure to use an ostomy pouch made for collecting fecal matter (colostomy or ileostomy) and not one for collecting urine (urostomy).

Assess the stoma color. A normal stoma is bright pink or brick red. Notify the health care provider if the stoma is blue, brown, or black, which indicates circulation problems to the stoma (WOCN et al., 2010). You need to measure the stoma size carefully when selecting and cutting out the opening on the wafer skin barrier. Too tight of an opening constricts the stoma and causes irritation and necrosis. Subtle stoma changes occur over time. Encourage patients to visit their enterostomal nurse at least annually to ensure proper pouching and fit (see Box 46-9). A good skin barrier protects the skin, prevents irritation from repeated removal of the pouch, and is comfortable for the patient to wear (see Fig. 46-21 in Skill 46-3). Skill 46-3 on p. 1121-1124 describes steps for applying a pouching system.

Patients with new stomas often feel vulnerable when they leave the hospital. To provide a smooth transition from hospital to home, offer help for the patient and family caregivers (Richbourg et al., 2007). Effective patient teaching helps patients with a new ostomy transition smoothly to home (Dixon, 2007) (Box 46-10).

BOX 46-10 PATIENT TEACHING

Teaching the Patient How to Provide Ostomy Care

Objective

- Patient/caregiver will demonstrate how to change an ostomy pouch.

Teaching Strategies

- Provide a comprehensive list of the products needed to care for the ostomy (Durston, 2009; Rust, 2007).
- Provide patient/caregiver with supplies to last 1 to 2 weeks and the contact number and location of nearest medical supply store (Dorman, 2009).
- Show patient/caregiver the step-by-step approach for changing an ostomy pouch (Deitz, 2010b; Durston, 2009).
- Provide at least one opportunity for patient/caregiver to change the ostomy pouch while patient is in the hospital.
- Arrange visits from a community stoma care nurse or home care nurse and provide contact numbers (Deitz, 2010b; Pearson, 2010).
- Provide detailed discharge instructions for skin care, clothing, driving, lifting, resuming exercise, and when to contact the health care provider (Dixon, 2007).

Evaluation

- Observe patient/caregiver change ostomy pouch.
- Ask patient/caregiver to state signs of stoma irritation and how to relieve it.
- Ask patient/caregiver to describe expected output from stoma and when to call the health care provider.

Nutritional Considerations for Patients with Ostomies. Nutritional therapy is important for patients with ostomies. During the first weeks after surgery many health care providers recommend low-fiber diets, particularly for patients with ileostomies, because the small bowel requires time to adapt to the diversion. Low-fiber foods include bread, noodles, rice, cream cheese, eggs (not fried), strained fruit juices, lean meats, fish, and poultry. As ostomies heal, patients are able to eat almost any food. High-fiber foods such as fresh fruits and vegetables help ensure a more solid stool. Patients need to avoid blockages of the bowel. The surgical construction of the stoma affects the likelihood of blockage.

A patient with an ileostomy needs to eat slowly and chew food completely. Drinking 10 to 12 glasses of water daily (unless contraindicated) also prevents blockage. High-fiber foods that cause problems include stringy meats, mushrooms, popcorn, fruits such as cherries, and some seafood such as shrimp and crab. Patients with ostomies often benefit from avoiding foods that cause gas and odor, including broccoli, cauliflower, dried beans, and Brussels sprouts.

Bowel Training. The patient with incontinence is unable to maintain bowel control. A **bowel training** program helps some patients defecate normally, especially those who still have some neuromuscular control.

The training program involves setting up a daily routine. By attempting to defecate at the same time each day and using measures that promote defecation, the patient gains control of bowel reflexes (Mengel, 2009). The program requires time, patience, and consistency. The health care provider determines the patient's physical readiness and ability to benefit from bowel training. A successful program includes the following:

- Assessing the normal elimination pattern and recording times when the patient is incontinent
- Incorporating principles of gerontological nursing when providing bowel retraining programs for the older adult (Box 46-11)
- Choosing a time in the patient's pattern to initiate defecation-control measures
- Giving stool softeners orally every day or a cathartic suppository at least half an hour before the selected defecation time (lower colon needs to be free of stool so suppository contacts intestinal mucosa)
- Offering a hot drink (hot tea) or fruit juice (prune juice) (or whatever fluids normally stimulate peristalsis for the patient) before the defecation time
- Helping the patient to the toilet at the designated time
- Avoiding medications such as opioids that increase constipation
- Providing privacy and setting a time limit for defecation (15 to 20 minutes)
- Instructing the patient to lean forward at the hips while sitting on the toilet, apply manual pressure with the hands over the abdomen, and bear down but not strain to stimulate colon emptying
- Not criticizing or conveying frustration if the patient is unable to defecate

BOX 46-11 FOCUS ON OLDER ADULTS

Bowel Retraining

- Constipation is common in older patients (Gray-Vickrey, 2010).
- Coarse bran rather than refined fiber is more effective in increasing stool weight (Holman et al., 2008).
- A minimum of 1500 mL of fluid per day reduces the risk of constipation, with increased fluid needs during summer months and for those on diuretics with stable cardiovascular status (Holman et al., 2008; JBI, 2008).
- If holding a drinking cup is a problem, consider using a lighter plastic cup and filling half full, refilling frequently.
- Fruit juices increase fiber content and intake.
- Encourage regular exercise. Maintaining an erect posture in an immobile patient reduces the risk of constipation (Holman et al., 2008; JBI, 2008).
- Patients need to feel at ease during elimination. Lack of privacy leads the patient to ignore the urge to defecate (Pegram et al., 2008).
- Review all medications with the health care provider to provide substitute medications that are less likely to cause constipation whenever possible (Chien and Bradway, 2010).
- Behavioral interventions such as habit training provide relief of constipation. Have patients sit on the toilet about 30 minutes after a meal, whether or not they feel the urge to defecate (Chien and Bradway, 2010).

- Maintaining normal exercise within the patient's physical ability

Maintenance of Proper Fluid and Food Intake. In choosing a diet for promoting normal elimination, consider the frequency of defecation, characteristics of feces, and types of foods that impair or promote defecation. The patient with frequent constipation or impaction requires an increased intake of high-fiber foods and more fluids. However, he or she needs to realize that diet therapy provides only long-term relief of elimination problems and does not give immediate relief from problems such as constipation.

When diarrhea is a problem, recommend foods with low-fiber content and discourage foods that typically cause gastric upset or abdominal cramping. Diarrhea caused by illness is sometimes debilitating. If the patient cannot tolerate foods or liquids orally, intravenous therapy (with potassium supplements) is necessary. The patient returns to a normal diet slowly, often beginning with fluids. Excessively hot or cold fluids stimulate peristalsis, causing abdominal cramps and further diarrhea. As tolerance to liquids improves, the patient eats solid foods.

Promotion of Regular Exercise. A daily exercise program helps prevent elimination problems. Walking, riding a stationary bicycle, or swimming stimulates peristalsis. Patients who are sedentary at work are most in need of regular exercise.

For a patient temporarily immobilized, attempt ambulation as soon as possible. If the condition permits, help the patient walk to a chair on the evening of the day of surgery. Have him or her walk farther each day.

Some patients have difficulty passing stool because of weak abdominal and pelvic floor muscles. Exercises help patients who are confined to bed use a bedpan. The patient practices the exercises as follows:

- Lie supine; tighten the abdominal muscles as though pushing them to the floor. Hold the muscles tight to the count of three; relax. Repeat 5 to 10 times as tolerated.
- Flex and contract the thigh muscles by raising one knee slowly toward the chest. Repeat for each leg at least 5 times and increase frequency as tolerated.

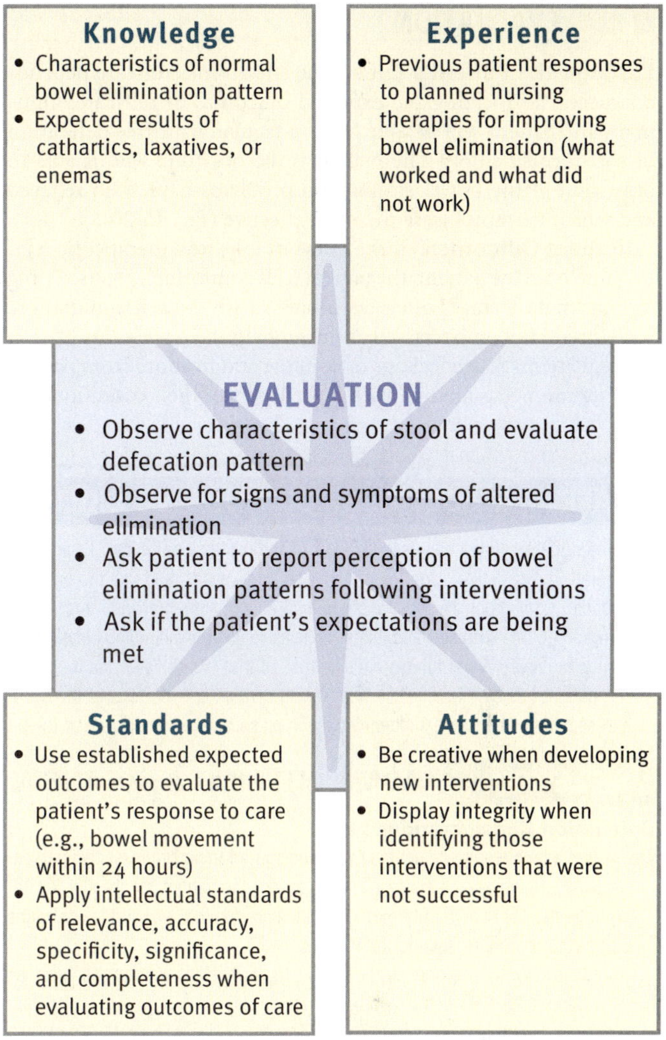

Knowledge
• Characteristics of normal bowel elimination pattern
• Expected results of cathartics, laxatives, or enemas
Experience
• Previous patient responses to planned nursing therapies for improving bowel elimination (what worked and what did not work)
EVALUATION
• Observe characteristics of stool and evaluate defecation pattern
• Observe for signs and symptoms of altered elimination
• Ask patient to report perception of bowel elimination patterns following interventions
• Ask if the patient's expectations are being met
Standards
• Use established expected outcomes to evaluate the patient's response to care (e.g., bowel movement within 24 hours)
• Apply intellectual standards of relevance, accuracy, specificity, significance, and completeness when evaluating outcomes of care
Attitudes
• Be creative when developing new interventions
• Display integrity when identifying those interventions that were not successful

FIG. 46-20 Critical thinking model for elimination evaluation.

Hemorrhoids. Pain results when hemorrhoid tissues are irritated directly. The primary goal for the patient with hemorrhoids is to have soft-formed, painless bowel movements. Proper diet, fluids, and regular exercise improve the likelihood of stools being soft. If the patient becomes constipated, passage of hard stools causes bleeding and irritation. An ice pack or a warm sitz bath (see Chapter 48) provides temporary relief of swollen hemorrhoids.

Maintenance of Skin Integrity. The patient with diarrhea or fecal incontinence is at risk for skin breakdown when fecal contents remain on the skin. The same problem exists for the patient with an ostomy that drains liquid stool. Liquid stool is usually acidic and contains digestive enzymes. Irritation from repeated wiping with toilet tissue aggravates skin breakdown. Bathing the skin after soiling helps, but sometimes it results in more breakdown unless the patient dries the skin thoroughly.

When caring for a patient who is debilitated, incontinent, and unable to ask for assistance, check often for defecation. You can protect the anal areas with petrolatum, zinc oxide, or another ointment that holds moisture in the skin, preventing drying and cracking. Yeast infections of the skin often develop easily. Several powdered antifungal agents are effective against yeast. Do not use baby powder or cornstarch because they have no medical properties, often cake on the skin, are difficult to remove, and enhance fungal infections of the skin.

EVALUATION

Through the Patient's Eyes. The effectiveness of care depends on success in meeting the expected outcomes of self-care. Optimally the patient will be able to have regular, pain-free defecation of soft-formed stools. The patient is the only one who is able to determine if the bowel elimination problems have been relieved and which therapies were the most effective (Fig. 46-20).

Patient Outcomes. If the nurse establishes a therapeutic relationship with the patient, the patient feels comfortable in discussing the intimate details often associated with bowel elimination. Patients are not embarrassed as nurses help them with elimination needs. Patients relate feelings of comfort and freedom from pain as elimination needs are met within the limits of their condition and treatment. Evaluate a patient's level of knowledge regarding establishing a normal elimination pattern, caring for an ostomy, and promoting skin integrity. Also determine the extent to which the patient accomplishes normal defection. Ask the patient to describe changes in diet, fluid intake, and activity to promote bowel health. You ask the following questions when a patient's outcomes are not met:

- Do you use medications such as laxatives or enemas to help you defecate?
- What barriers are preventing you from eating a diet high in fiber and participating in regular exercise?
- How much fluid do you drink in a typical day? What types of fluids do you normally drink?
- What challenges do you encounter when you change your ostomy pouch?

SAFETY GUIDELINES FOR NURSING SKILLS

Ensuring patient safety is an essential role of the professional nurse. To ensure patient safety, communicate clearly with members of the health care team, assess and incorporate the patient's priorities of care and preferences, and use the best evidence when making decisions about your patient's care. When performing the skills in this chapter, remember the following points to ensure safe, individualized, patient care.

- Instruct patients who self-administer enemas to use the side-lying position. Tell them not to self-administer an enema while sitting on the toilet because this position results in curved rectal tubing, causing friction that wears down the rectal wall.
- If a patient has cardiac disease or is taking cardiac or hypertensive medication, obtain pulse rate because manipulation of rectal tissue stimulates the vagus nerve and sometimes causes a sudden decline in pulse rate, which increases the patient's risk of fainting while on the bedpan, bedside commode, or toilet.

SKILL 46-1 ADMINISTERING A CLEANSING ENEMA

View Video!

Delegation Considerations

The skill of administering an enema can be delegated to nursing assistive personnel (NAP). However, the nurse must first assess the patient for specific considerations such as need for alternative positioning, comfort, and stable vital signs before the procedure. Instruct NAP about:

- Proper way to position patients who have mobility restrictions such as patients with arthritis or severe fatigue.
- How to position patients who also have therapeutic equipment present such as drains, intravenous (IV) catheters, or traction.
- Specific signs and symptoms of patient's intolerance to the procedure and when to stop it such as abdominal pain more than a pressure sensation, abdominal cramping, abdominal distention, or rectal bleeding.

Equipment

- Clean gloves
- Water-soluble lubricant
- Waterproof, absorbent pads
- Bath blanket
- Toilet tissue
- Bedpan, bedside commode, or access to toilet
- Washbasin, washcloths, towel, and soap
- IV pole
- Enema kit with
  - Enema container
  - Tubing and clamp (if not already attached to container)
  - Appropriate-size rectal tube
    - *Adult:* 22- to 30-Fr
    - *Child:* 12- to 18-Fr
  - Correct volume of warmed solution:
    - *Adult:* 750 to 1000 mL
    - *Child:*
      - 150 to 250 mL, infant
      - 250 to 350 mL, toddler
      - 300 to 500 mL, school-age child
      - 500 to 750 mL, adolescent

or

- Prepackaged enema container with rectal tip

STEP	RATIONALE
ASSESSMENT	
1 Assess status of patient: last bowel movement, normal bowel patterns, hemorrhoids, mobility, external sphincter control, and abdominal pain.	Determines factors indicating need for enema and influencing type of enema used.
2 Assess for presence of increased intracranial pressure, glaucoma, or recent rectal or prostate surgery.	Conditions contraindicate use of enemas (Pegram et al., 2008).
3 Check patient's medical record to clarify rationale for the enema.	Determines purpose of enema administration: preparation for special procedure or relief of constipation.

STEP	RATIONALE
4 Review health care provider's order for enema.	Order by health care provider is required. Determines number and type of enema to give.
5 Identify patient using two identifiers (e.g., name and birth date or name and account number) according to facility policy. Compare identifiers with information on the patient's medical record.	Ensures correct patient. Complies with a recommended National Patient Safety Goal (TJC, 2011).
6 Inspect for abdominal distention and auscultate for bowel sounds.	Establishes baseline for determining effectiveness of enema.
PLANNING	
1 Explain purpose of enema and determine patient's level of understanding.	Allows time to plan for appropriate teaching measures.
2 Collect appropriate equipment and arrange at beside.	Ensures smooth procedure.
IMPLEMENTATION	
1 Assemble enema bag with appropriate solution and rectal tube.	
2 Perform hand hygiene and apply gloves.	Reduces transmission of microorganisms.
3 Provide privacy by closing curtains around bed or closing door.	Reduces embarrassment for patient.
4 Raise bed to appropriate working height and raise side rail on patient's left.	Promotes good body mechanics and patient safety.
5 Assist patient into left side-lying (Sims') position with right knee flexed. You can also place children in dorsal recumbent position.	Allows enema solution to flow downward by gravity along natural curve of sigmoid colon and rectum, thus improving retention of solution.

CLINICAL DECISION: *If patient is suspected of having poor sphincter control, position on bedpan. Patient will have difficulty retaining enema solution. Do not administer enema with patient sitting on toilet.*

STEP	RATIONALE
6 Place waterproof pad under hips and buttocks.	Prevents soiling of linen.
7 Cover patient with bath blanket, exposing only rectal area and clearly visualizing anus.	Provides warmth, reduces exposure of body parts, and allows patient to feel more relaxed and comfortable.
8 Place bedpan or commode in easily accessible position. If patient is expelling contents in toilet, ensure that toilet is free. (If patient is getting up to bathroom to expel enema, place his or her slippers and bathrobe in easily accessible position.)	Used in case patient is unable to retain enema solution.
9 Administer enema:	
a. Enema bag	
(1) Add warmed solution to enema bag: warm tap water as it flows from faucet; place saline container in basin of hot water before adding saline to enema bag; check temperature of solution by pouring small amount over inner wrist.	Hot water burns intestinal mucosa. Cold water causes abdominal cramping and is difficult to retain (Holman et al., 2008).
(2) Raise container, release clamp, and allow solution to flow long enough to fill tubing.	Procedure removes air from tubing.
(3) Reclamp tubing.	Reclamping prevents further loss of solution.
(4) Lubricate 6 to 8 cm (2½ to 3 inches) of tip of rectal tube with water-soluble lubricating jelly.	Lubricating allows smooth insertion of rectal tube without risk of irritation or trauma to mucosa.
(5) Gently separate buttocks and locate anus. Instruct patient to relax by breathing out slowly through mouth. Then touch patient's skin next to anus with tip of rectal tube.	Breathing out and touching skin with tube promotes relaxation of external anal sphincter.
(6) Insert end of tubing of enema bag slowly by pointing tip in direction of patient's umbilicus (see illustration). Length of insertion varies: *Adult:* 7.5-10 cm (3-4 inches) *Adolescent:* 7.5-10 cm (3-4 inches) *Child:* 5-7.5 cm (2-3 inches) *Infant:* 2.5-3.75 cm (1-1½ inches)	Careful insertion prevents trauma to rectal mucosa from accidental lodging of tube against rectal wall. Insertion beyond proper limit causes bowel perforation (Pegram et al., 2008).
(7) Hold tubing in rectum constantly until end of fluid instillation.	Bowel contraction causes expulsion of rectal tube.
(8) Open regulating clamp and allow solution to enter slowly with container at patient's hip level.	Rapid instillation stimulates evacuation of rectal tube.
(9) Raise height of enema container slowly to appropriate level above anus: 30-45 cm (12-18 inches) for high enema, 30 cm (12 inches) for regular enema, 7.5 cm (3 inches) for low enema. Instillation time varies with volume of solution you administer.	Proper height allows for continuous, slow instillation of solution. Raising container too high causes rapid instillation and possible painful distention of colon (Pegram et al., 2008). High pressure causes rupture of bowel in infant.
(10) Lower container to decrease flow of solution or clamp tubing if patient experiences cramping or if fluid escapes around rectal tube.	Temporary cessation of instillation prevents cramping, which prevents patient from retaining all fluid, altering effectiveness of enema.
(11) Clamp tubing after all solution is instilled.	Clamping prevents air from entering rectum.

SKILL 46-1 ADMINISTERING A CLEANSING ENEMA—cont'd

STEP	RATIONALE

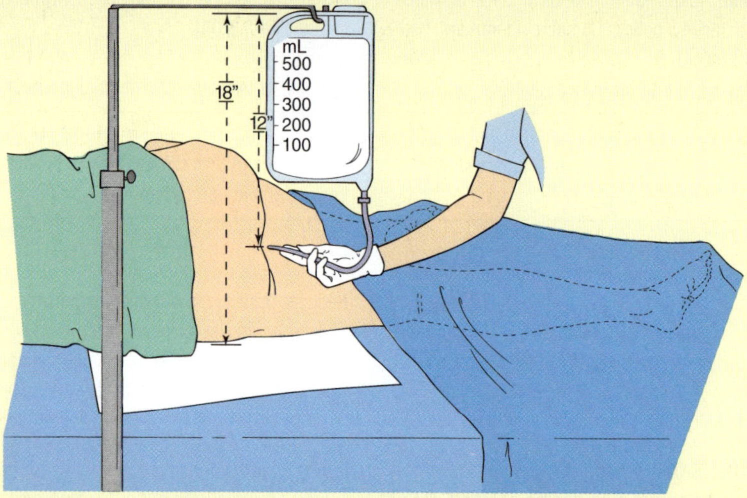

STEP 9a(6) Insertion of enema tube into rectum.

CLINICAL DECISION: *If pain occurs or resistance is felt at any time during procedure, stop and confer with physician. Do not force the tube.*

STEP	RATIONALE
b. Prepackaged disposable container	
(1) Remove plastic cap from rectal tip. Tip is already lubricated, but you can apply more jelly as needed.	Lubrication provides for smooth insertion of rectal tube without causing rectal irritation or trauma.
(2) Gently separate buttocks and locate rectum. Instruct patient to relax by breathing out slowly through mouth.	Breathing out promotes relaxation of external rectal sphincter.
(3) Insert tip of bottle gently into rectum: *Adult:* 7.5-10 cm (3-4 inches) *Adolescent:* 7.5-10 cm (3-4 inches) *Child:* 5-7.5 cm (2-3 inches) *Infant:* 2.5-3.75 cm (1-1½ inches)	Gentle insertion prevents trauma to rectal mucosa.
(4) Squeeze bottle until all of solution has entered rectum and colon. Instruct patient to retain solution until urge to defecate occurs, usually 2 to 5 minutes.	Hypertonic solutions require only small volumes to stimulate defecation. Transient hyperphosphatemia correlates with retention greater than 15 minutes (Jacobson et al., 2010).
10 Place layers of toilet tissue around tube at anus and gently withdraw rectal tube.	Provides patient's comfort and cleanliness.
11 Explain to patient that feeling of distention is normal. Ask patient to retain solution as long as possible while lying quietly in bed. (For infant or young child, gently hold buttocks together for a few minutes.)	Solution distends bowel. Length of retention varies with type of enema and patient's ability to contract rectal sphincter. Longer retention promotes more effective stimulation of peristalsis and defecation (Kyle, 2007b).
12 Discard enema container and tubing in proper receptacle or rinse out thoroughly with warm soap and water if reusing container.	Reduces transmission and growth of microorganisms.
13 Assist patient to bathroom or help to position on bedpan.	Normal squatting position promotes defecation.
14 Assist patient as needed with washing anal area with warm soap and water (if administering perineal care, use gloves).	Fecal contents irritate skin. Hygiene promotes patient's comfort.
15 Remove and discard gloves and perform hand hygiene.	Good hygiene reduces transmission of microorganisms.

EVALUATION

STEP	RATIONALE
1 Evaluate color, consistency, and amount of stool; odor; and fluid passed.	Determines efficacy of enema.
2 Observe abdomen for distention.	Determines if distention is relieved.
3 Ask patient about cramping or discomfort.	Provides information about patient's level of comfort.

CLINICAL DECISION: *When enemas are ordered "until clear," observe contents of solution passed. Return is "clear" when no solid fecal material exists, but the solution sometimes remains discolored.*

UNEXPECTED OUTCOMES AND RELATED INTERVENTIONS

1 Abdomen becomes rigid and distended.
- Stop enema if you are instilling fluid.
- Notify health care provider and obtain vital signs.

2 Abdominal pain or cramping develops.
- Decrease height of enema bag and slow rate of instillation.
- Have patient take slow, deep breaths in through nose and out through mouth.

3 Bleeding occurs.
- Stop enema administration.
- Notify health care provider.
- Obtain vital signs and assess abdomen and rectum.

RECORDING AND REPORTING

- Record type and volume of enema given and characteristics of results.
- Report failure of patient to defecate to health care provider.

HOME CARE CONSIDERATIONS

- For patients who require enemas for bowel preparation at home, instruct family not to exceed recommended fluid volume levels or number of enemas. Instruct family about need for slow administration of warmed fluid.
- Instruct family about the negative side effects of tap water enemas.

SKILL 46-2 INSERTING AND MAINTAINING A NASOGASTRIC TUBE FOR GASTRIC DECOMPRESSION

Delegation Considerations

The skill of inserting and maintaining a nasogastric (NG) tube cannot be delegated to nursing assistive personnel (NAP). Instruct the NAP to:
- Measure and record the drainage.
- Provide oral and nasal hygiene.
- Perform selected comfort measures such as positioning, offering ice chips if allowed.
- Correctly anchor NG tube to patient's gown after changing gown or repositioning patient.

Equipment

- Inserting large-bore tube
  - 14- or 16-Fr NG tube (smaller lumens are not used for decompression in adults because the tube must be able to remove thick secretions)
  - Water-soluble lubricating jelly
  - Clean gloves
  - pH test strips (measure gastric aspirate acidity)
  - Tongue blade
  - Flashlight
  - Emesis basin
  - Asepto bulb or catheter-tipped syringe
  - Normal saline
  - 2.5 cm (1 inch)–wide hypoallergenic tape or commercial fixation device
  - Tincture of benzoin (optional)
  - Safety pin and rubber band
  - Clamp of suction machine and pressure gauge if wall suction is used
  - Towel, facial tissues
  - Glass of water with straw
- Irrigating NG tube
  - Asepto bulb or catheter-tipped syringe
  - Normal saline and basin
  - Clean gloves
- Discontinuing NG tube
  - Towel, facial tissue
  - Clean gloves
  - Soap and water

STEP	RATIONALE
ASSESSMENT	
1 Perform hand hygiene.	Good hygiene reduces transmission of organisms.
2 Inspect condition of patient's nasal and oral cavity.	Baseline condition of nasal and oral cavity determines need for special nursing measures for oral hygiene after tube placement.
3 Ask if patient has had history of nasal surgery and note if deviated nasal septum is present.	You insert tube into **uninvolved** nasal passage. Procedure is often contraindicated if surgery is recent.

SKILL 46-2 INSERTING AND MAINTAINING A NASOGASTRIC TUBE FOR GASTRIC DECOMPRESSION—cont'd

STEP	RATIONALE
4 Auscultate for bowel sounds. Palpate patient's abdomen for distention, pain, and rigidity.	Baseline determination of level of abdominal distention later serves as comparison once tube is inserted. In presence of diminished or absent bowel sounds, auscultate each quadrant for 5 minutes (Seidel et al., 2011).
5 Assess patient's level of consciousness and ability to follow instructions.	Assessment determines patient's ability to assist in procedure.

CLINICAL DECISION: *If patient is confused, disoriented, or unable to follow commands, obtain assistance from another staff member to insert the tube.*

PLANNING

STEP	RATIONALE
1 Identify patient using two identifiers (e.g., Name and birth date or name and account number) according to facility policy. Compare identifiers with information on the patient's medical record.	Ensures correct patient. Complies with a recommended National Patient Safety Goal (TJC, 2011).
2 Explain procedure.	Explanation gains patient's cooperation and lessens possibility that patient will remove tube.
3 Determine if patient had an NG tube insertion in the past and, if so, which naris was used.	Previous experience complements explanations and helps you determine which naris to use.
4 Check medical record for health care provider's order; type of NG tube to be placed; and whether tube is to be attached to suction, gravity, or feeding solution.	Procedure requires health care provider's order. Adequate decompression depends on NG suction.
5 Prepare equipment at bedside. Cut a piece of tape about 10 cm (4 inches) long and split one end in half to form a V or have NG tube fixator device available.	Ensures well-organized procedure. Tape or fixator device is used to hold tube in place after insertion.

IMPLEMENTATION

STEP	RATIONALE
1 Position patient in high-Fowler's position with pillows behind head and shoulders. Raise bed to horizontal level comfortable for nurse.	Promotes patient's ability to swallow during procedure. Positioning of bed prevents strain on nurse.
2 Have patient blow nose. Place bath towel over his or her chest; give him or her facial tissues. Place emesis basin within reach.	Removes existing nasal secretions. Prevents soiling of patient's gown. Tube insertion through nasal passages sometimes causes tearing and coughing with increased salivation.
3 Pull curtain around bed or close room door.	Provides privacy.
4 Stand on patient's right side if right-handed, left side if left-handed.	Allows easiest manipulation of tubing.
5 Perform hand hygiene and apply clean gloves.	Reduces transmission of microorganisms.
6 Instruct patient to relax and breathe normally while occluding one naris. Repeat this action for other naris. Select nostril with greater airflow.	Tube passes more easily through naris that is more patent. Ensures that tube insertion does not obstruct nasal airflow.
7 Measure distance to insert tube: **a.** *Traditional method:* Measure distance from tip of nose to earlobe to xiphoid process (see illustrations) **b.** *Hanson method:* Mark 50-cm (20-inch) point on tube and measure traditionally. Tube insertion is at midway point between 50 cm (20 inches) and traditional mark.	Approximates distance from naris to stomach. Distance varies with each patient (Durston, 2009).

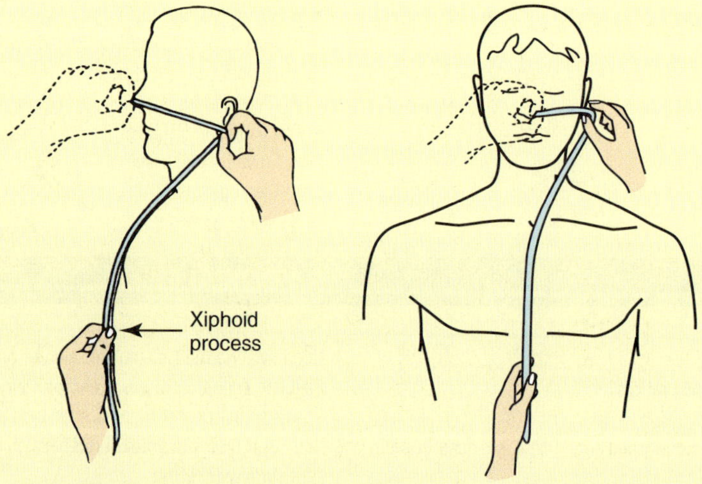

STEP 7a Technique for measuring distance to insert nasogastric tube.

STEP	RATIONALE
8 Mark length of tube to be inserted by placing small piece of tape so it can easily be removed.	Marks amount of tube to be inserted from nares to stomach (Durston, 2009).
9 Curve 10 to 15 cm (4 to 6 inches) of end of tube tightly around index finger and release.	Curving tube tip aids insertion and decreases tube stiffness.
10 Lubricate 7.5 to 10 cm (3 to 4 inches) of end of tube with water-soluble lubricating jelly.	Minimizes friction against nasal mucosa and aids insertion of tube. Water-soluble lubricant is less toxic than oil-based if aspirated.
11 Initially instruct patient to extend neck back against pillow (see illustration); insert tube gently and slowly through naris, aiming end of tube downward.	Facilitates initial passage of tube through naris and maintains clear airway for open naris.

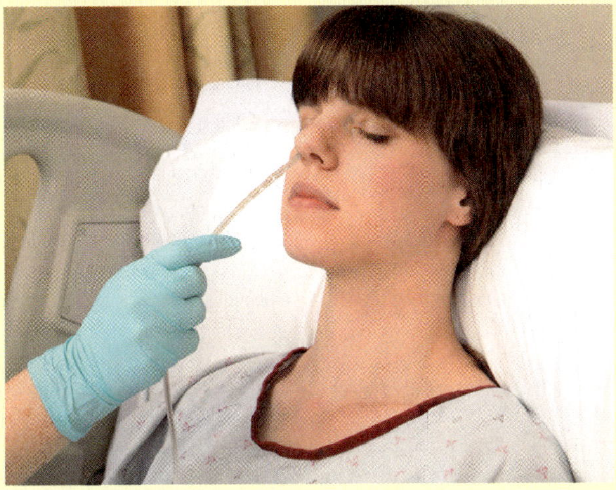

STEP 11 Insert nasogastric tube with curved end pointing downward.

STEP	RATIONALE
12 Continue to pass tube along floor of nasal passage, aiming downward toward patient's ear. If resistance is met, apply gentle downward pressure to advance tube. (Do not force past resistance.)	Minimizes discomfort of tube rubbing against upper nasal turbinates. Resistance is caused by posterior nasopharynx. Downward pressure helps tube curl around corner of nasopharynx.
13 If you meet resistance, try to rotate tube and see if it advances. If still resistant, withdraw tube, allow patient to rest, relubricate tube, and insert into other naris.	Forcing against resistance causes trauma to mucosa (Durai et al., 2009). Helps relieve patient's anxiety.

CLINICAL DECISION: *If unable to insert tube in either naris, stop procedure and notify health care provider.*

STEP	RATIONALE
14 Continue inserting tube until just past nasopharynx by gently rotating it toward opposite nostril and passing it just above oropharynx.	Helps prevent coiling of tube in oropharynx.
a. Stop tube advancement and allow patient to relax, and provide tissues.	Relieves patient's anxiety; tearing is natural response to mucosal irritation, and excessive salivation often occurs because of oral stimulation.
b. Explain to patient that next step requires that he or she swallow. Give patient glass of water unless contraindicated.	Sipping water aids passage of NG tube into esophagus.
15 With tube just above oropharynx, instruct patient to flex head forward, take a small sip of water, and swallow. Advance tube 2.5 to 5 cm (1 to 2 inches) with each swallow of water. If patient is not allowed fluids, instruct to dry swallow or suck air through straw.	Flexed position closes off upper airway to trachea and opens esophagus. Swallowing closes epiglottis over trachea and helps move the tube into the esophagus. Swallowing water reduces gagging or choking. Suction removes water from stomach once it is connected.
16 If patient begins to cough, gag, or choke, withdraw tube slightly (do not remove it) and stop tube advancement. Instruct patient to breathe easily and take sips of water.	Sometimes tube accidentally enters larynx and produces coughing; withdrawal of tube reduces risk of laryngeal entry (Durai et al., 2009). Swallowing water eases gagging. Give water cautiously to reduce risk of aspiration.

CLINICAL DECISION: *If vomiting occurs, help patient clear airway; use oral suctioning if needed. Do not proceed until airway is cleared.*

STEP	RATIONALE
17 If patient continues to gag and cough or complains that tube feels as though it is coiling in back of throat, check back of oropharynx with tongue blade. If tube has coiled, withdraw it until tip is back in oropharynx. Reinsert with patient swallowing.	When tube coils around itself in back of throat, it stimulates gag reflex (Durai et al., 2009).
18 After patient relaxes, continue to advance tube with swallowing until tape or mark is reached. Temporarily anchor tube to patient's cheek with piece of tape until tube placement is verified.	Tip of tube needs to be well within stomach for adequate decompression. Anchor tube before verifying placement.

SKILL 46-2 INSERTING AND MAINTAINING A NASOGASTRIC TUBE FOR GASTRIC DECOMPRESSION—cont'd

STEP	RATIONALE
19 Verify tube placement. Check agency policy for preferred methods for checking NG tube placement.	
a. Inspect posterior pharynx for presence of coiled tube.	Tube is pliable and can coil up in back of pharynx instead of advancing into esophagus (Durai et al., 2009).
b. Attach Asepto or catheter-tipped syringe to end of tube and aspirate gently back on syringe to obtain gastric contents, observing color (see illustration).	Gastric contents are usually cloudy and green but may be off-white, tan, bloody, or brown in color. Aspiration of contents provides means to measure fluid pH and thus determine tube tip placement in gastrointestinal tract (Durai et al., 2009). Other common aspirate colors include the following: duodenal placement (yellow or bile stained), esophagus (may or may not have saliva-appearing aspirate).
c. Measure pH of aspirate with color-coded pH paper with range of whole numbers from 1.0 to 11.0 or greater (see illustration).	Gastric aspirates have decidedly acidic pH values, preferably 5.5 or less, compared with intestinal aspirates, which are usually 6.0 or greater, or respiratory secretions, which are usually alkaline at 7.0 or greater (Durston, 2009). Use only gastric (Gastrocult) pH test and not Hemoccult test.
d. Have ordered x-ray film examination performed of chest/abdomen.	X-ray film is best verification of initial placement of tube (Durai et al., 2009).
e. If tube is not in stomach, advance another 2.5-5 cm (1-2 inches) and repeat Steps 19a-e to check tube position.	Tube must be in stomach to provide decompression.
20 Anchoring tube:	
a. After tube is properly inserted and positioned, either clamp end or connect it to drainage bag or suction source.	Drainage bag is used for gravity drainage. Intermittent low suction is most effective for decompression. Patient going to operating room or for diagnostic test often has tube clamped.
b. Tape tube to nose; avoid putting pressure on nares.	Prevents tissue necrosis. Tape anchors tube securely.
(1) Apply small amount of tincture of benzoin to lower end of nose and allow to dry *(optional)*.	Benzoin prevents loosening of tape if patient perspires.
(2) Apply tape to nose, leaving split ends free. Be sure that top end of tape over nose is secure.	
(3) Carefully wrap two split ends of tape around tube (see illustration).	
(4) *Alternative:* Apply tube fixation device using shaped adhesive patch (see illustration).	
c. Fasten end of NG tube to patient's gown by looping rubber band around tube in slipknot. Pin rubber band to gown (provides slack for movement).	Reduces pressure on nares if tube moves.

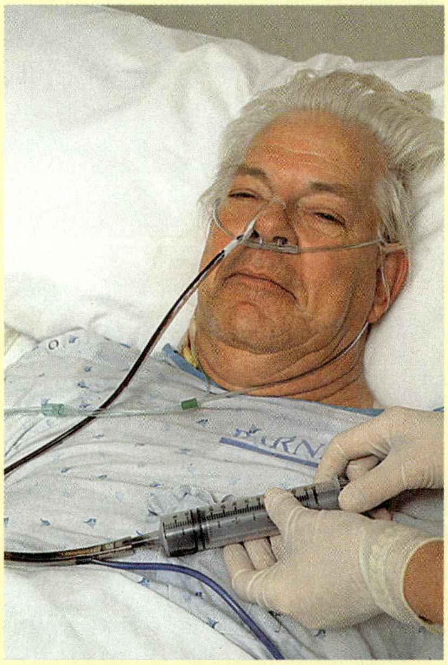

STEP 19b Aspiration of gastric contents.

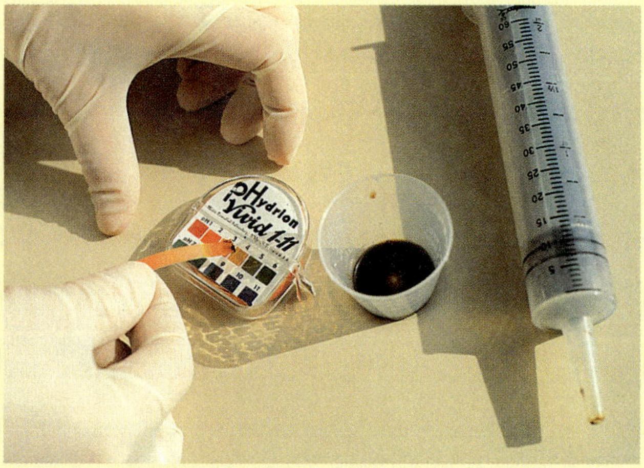

STEP 19c Checking pH of gastric aspirate.

STEP	RATIONALE

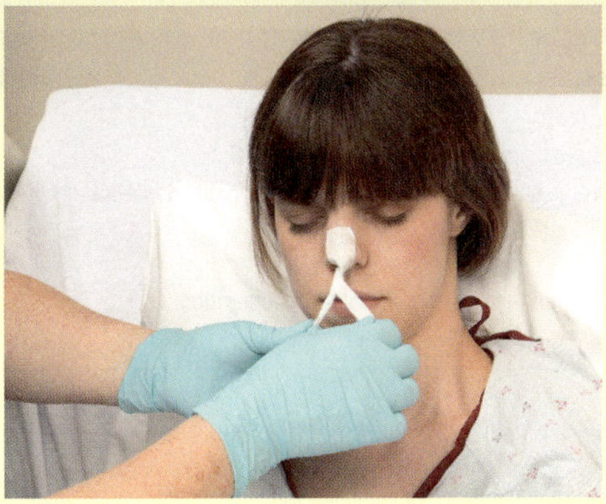

STEP 20b(3) Tape is crossed over and around nasogastric tube.

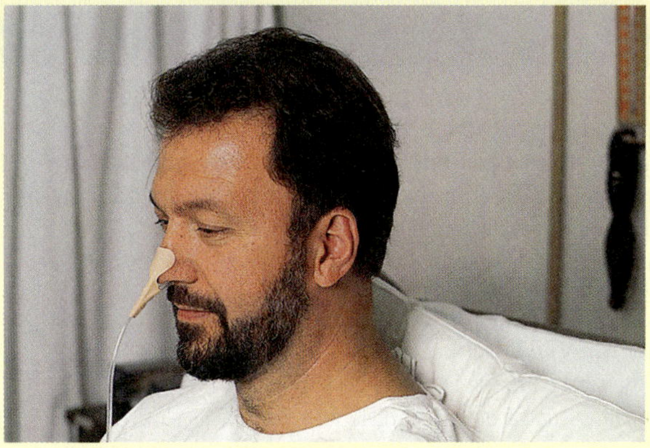

STEP 20b(4) Patient with tube fixation device.

STEP	RATIONALE
21 Unless health care provider orders otherwise, elevate head of bed 30 degrees.	Helps prevent esophageal reflux and minimizes irritation of tube against posterior pharynx (Durai et al., 2009).
22 Once placement is confirmed:	The mark or tube length is to be used as a guide to indicate whether displacement may have occurred.
a. Place red mark on tube to indicate where it exits nose.	
b. Measure tube length from nares to connector as an alternate method.	
c. Document tube length in patient record.	
23 Remove gloves and perform hand hygiene.	Reduces transmission of microorganisms.
24 Tube irrigation:	
a. Perform hand hygiene and apply gloves.	Reduces transmission of microorganisms.
b. Check for tube placement in stomach (see Step 19). Reconnect NG tube to connecting tube.	Prevents accidental entrance of irrigating solution into lungs (Durai et al., 2009).
c. Draw up 30 mL of normal saline into Asepto or catheter-tipped syringe.	Use of saline minimizes loss of electrolytes from stomach fluids.
d. Clamp NG tube. Disconnect from connection tubing and lay end of connection tubing on towel.	Reduces soiling of patient's gown and bed linen.
e. Insert tip of irrigating syringe into end of NG tube. Remove clamp. Hold syringe with tip pointed at floor and inject saline slowly and evenly. Do not force solution.	Position of syringe prevents introduction of air into vent tubing, which could cause gastric distention. Solution introduced under pressure causes gastric trauma. Do not introduce saline through blue "pigtail" air vent of Salem sump tube.
f. If resistance occurs, check for kinks in tubing. Turn patient onto left side. Report repeated resistance to health care provider.	Tip of tube is possibly against stomach lining. Repositioning on left side helps to dislodge tube away from stomach lining. Buildup of secretions causes distention.
g. After instilling saline, immediately aspirate or pull back slowly on syringe to withdraw fluid. If amount aspirated is greater than amount instilled, record difference as output. If amount aspirated is less than amount instilled, record difference as intake.	Irrigation clears tubing; thus stomach remains empty. Fluid remaining in stomach is measured as intake.
h. Reconnect NG tube to drainage or suction. (If solution does not return, repeat irrigation.)	Reestablishes drainage collection; you repeat irrigation or repositioning of tube until NG tube drains properly.
i. Remove gloves and perform hand hygiene.	Reduces transmission of microorganisms.

EVALUATION

1 Determine amount and character of contents draining from NG tube. Ask if patient feels nauseated.	Determines if tube is decompressing stomach of contents.
2 After palpating patient's abdomen, note any distention, pain, and rigidity and auscultate for presence of bowel sounds. Turn off suction while auscultating.	Determines success of abdominal decompression and return of peristalsis. The sound of suction apparatus is transmitted to abdomen and misinterpreted as bowel sounds.
3 Evaluate condition of nares and nose.	Evaluates onset of skin and tissue irritation.
4 Observe position of tubing.	Determines if tension is being applied to nasal structures.
5 Ask if patient feels sore throat or irritation in pharynx.	Evaluates level of patient's discomfort.

DISCONTINUATION OF NASOGASTRIC TUBE

ASSESSMENT

1 Auscultate for presence of bowel sounds.	Serves as baseline for when tube is removed.

SKILL 46-2 INSERTING AND MAINTAINING A NASOGASTRIC TUBE FOR GASTRIC DECOMPRESSION—cont'd

STEP	RATIONALE
PLANNING	
1 Verify order to discontinue NG tube.	Health care provider's order required for procedure.
2 Identify patient using two identifiers (e.g., name and birth date or name and account number) according to facility policy. Compare identifiers with information on the patient's medical record.	Ensures correct patient. Complies with a recommended National Patient Safety Goal (TJC, 2011).
3 Explain procedure to patient and reassure that removal is less distressing than insertion.	Minimizes anxiety and increases patient cooperation.
IMPLEMENTATION	
1 Perform hand hygiene and apply clean gloves.	Reduces transmission of microorganisms.
2 Turn off suction and disconnect NG tube from drainage bag or suction. Remove tape or fixation device from bridge of nose and unpin tube from gown.	Have tube free of all connections before removal.
3 Stand on patient's right side if right-handed, left side if left-handed.	Allows easiest manipulation of tube.
4 Hand patient facial tissue; place clean towel across chest. Instruct patient to take and hold deep breath.	Patient sometimes needs to blow nose after removal of tube. Towel prevents gown from getting soiled. Airway is temporarily obstructed during tube removal.
5 Clamp or kink tubing securely and pull tube out steadily and smoothly into towel held in other hand while patient holds breath.	Clamping prevents tube contents from draining into oropharynx. Reduces trauma to mucosa and minimizes patient's discomfort. Towel covers tube, which is usually an unpleasant sight. Holding breath prevents aspiration.
6 Clean nares and provide mouth care.	Promotes comfort.
7 Dispose of tube and drainage equipment into proper container.	Reduces transmission of microorganisms.
8 Remove gloves and perform hand hygiene.	Reduces transmission of microorganisms.
EVALUATION	
1 After tube removal, auscultate patient's bowel sounds and periodically check for abdominal distention.	Confirms that peristalsis has returned.
2 Measure amount of drainage in container and note character of content.	Provides accurate measure of fluid output.
3 Explain procedure for drinking fluids if not contraindicated.	Requires health care provider's order. Once fluids are allowed, the order usually begins with small amount of ice chips; amount increases as patient is able to tolerate more.

UNEXPECTED OUTCOMES AND RELATED INTERVENTIONS

1 Patient's abdomen becomes distended and/or painful.
- Assess patency of tube and irrigate as needed.
- Verify that suction is on as ordered.

2 Patient complains of sore throat from dry, irritated mucous membranes.
- Increase frequency of oral hygiene.
- Ask health care provider if patient can suck on ice chips or throat lozenges.

3 Patient develops irritation of skin around nares.
- Provide skin care to nares and retape so tube does not press against nares.
- Consider switching tube to other naris.

4 Patient develops signs of pulmonary aspiration: fever, shortness of breath, pulmonary congestion.
- Perform respiratory assessment.
- Notify health care provider; expect order for chest x-ray.

RECORDING AND REPORTING

- Record in nurses' notes time, type, and size of NG tube inserted, patient's tolerance of procedure, confirmation of placement, character of gastric contents, pH value, whether tube is clamped or connected to drainage device, and amount of suction applied.
- Record in nurses' notes and/or flow sheet placement checks and amount and character of contents draining from NG tube every shift, unless ordered more often by health care provider.
- Record in nurse's notes time and date that NG tube was removed, patient's tolerance of procedure, and his or her status following procedure.

SKILL 46-3 POUCHING AN OSTOMY

View Video!

Delegation Considerations

The skill of pouching a newly established ostomy cannot be delegated to nursing assistive personnel (NAP). Pouching an established ostomy can be delegated. Inform NAP about:

- Appropriate pouch and skin barrier.
- The signs of stoma and peristomal skin changes to report to a registered professional nurse.
- Monitoring and reporting characteristics and volume of ostomy output and reporting changes in volume and/or consistency for further assessment.
- Special equipment needed to complete the procedure.

Equipment

- Clear drainable colostomy/ileostomy pouch in correct size for two-piece system or custom cut-to-fit one-piece type with attached skin barrier (Fig. 46-21, *A* and *B*)
- Pouch closure device as needed
- Ostomy measuring guide
- Adhesive remover (optional)
- Clean gloves
- Washcloths
- Towel or disposable waterproof barrier
- Basin with warm tap water
- Scissors/pen
- Skin barrier if not attached to pouching system
- Stoma paste or Stomahesive (optional)
- Tape or ostomy belt (optional)
- Stethoscope

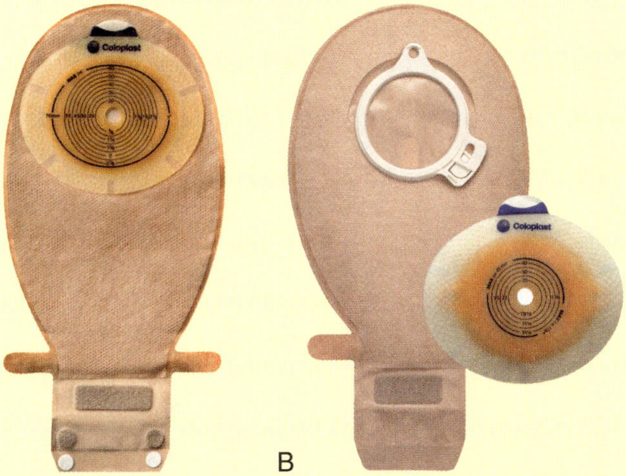

A B

FIG. 46-21 Ostomy pouches and skin barriers. **A,** SenSura® one-piece pouch with Velcro closure. **B,** SenSura® two-piece pouching system with separate skin barrier and attachable pouch. (NOTE: Skin barriers would need to be custom cut according to stoma size.) (Courtesy Coloplast, Minneapolis, Minn)

STEP	RATIONALE
ASSESSMENT	
1 Perform hand hygiene and apply clean gloves.	Reduces transmission of microorganisms.
2 Auscultate for bowel sounds.	Documents presence of peristalsis.
3 Observe skin barrier and pouch for leakage and length of time in place. NOTE: Depending on type of pouching system used (such as with an opaque pouch), remove the pouch to fully observe the stoma. Clear pouches permit viewing of stoma without their removal.	Indicates need for different type of pouch or sealant. Routine observation allows for early detection of potential problems (Dorman, 2009). Leaking often indicates need for different pouch or sealant (Hoeflok et al., 2009). Intact skin barriers with no evidence of leakage do not need to be changed daily and remain in place for 5 to 7 days (Durston, 2009; Richbourg et al., 2008).
4 Observe stoma for color, swelling, trauma, and healing; it is normally moist and reddish-pink. Assess type of stoma. Stoma is flush with skin or budlike protrusion on abdomen (see illustration for a normal bud stoma).	Healthy stomas are pink to brick red in color (WOCN et al., 2010). Notify health care provider immediately if color is blue, brown, or black in color.
5 Observe effluent from stoma and keep record of intake and output. Ask patient about skin tenderness.	Effluent from stoma is caustic; and, if it comes in contact with sensitive peristomal skin, risk of skin breakdown increases (Erwin-Toth et al., 2010).
6 Observe abdominal incision (if present).	Relationship of abdominal incision to stoma determines proper placement of pouch. Presence of pressure areas from pouching system requires a different system (WOCN et al., 2010).
7 Check existing bag for gas accumulation.	If excessive gas accumulation is present, determine need for patient to switch to pouch with vent or filter (WOCN et al., 2010).

SKILL 46-3 POUCHING AN OSTOMY—cont'd

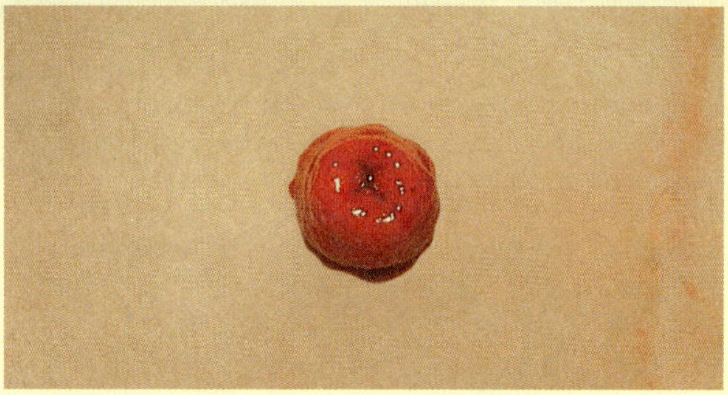

STEP 4 Bud stoma. (Permission to use and/or reproduce this copyrighted photo has been granted by the owner, Hollister Inc.)

STEP	RATIONALE
8 Assess abdomen for best type of pouching system to use. Consider the following: **a.** Contour and peristomal plane **b.** Presence of scars, incisions **c.** Location and type of stoma **d.** Patient's self-care ability	Determines pouching system selection and need for other equipment. For a stoma to have an adequate seal with an ostomy appliance, it needs to be placed within abdominal rectus muscle, away from abdominal creases and folds, away from bony understructures, and surrounded by at least 5 cm (2 inches) of smooth surface on all sides (Rust, 2007). Patients who have difficulty using their hands or limited vision find a one-piece system or a precut pouch and skin barrier more desirable to use (Pearson, 2010). Patients who have mobility problems or spinal cord injuries benefit by using equipment that has a longer pouch, which is easier to empty independently when sitting. For patients who prefer being able to keep the skin barrier in place for several days and change just the pouch, the two-piece system is desirable.

CLINICAL DECISION: *Because of stoma and abdominal characteristics, some patients need their ostomy pouching system to curve outward to avoid leakage (Deitz and Gates, 2010a).*

PLANNING

STEP	RATIONALE
1 Identify patient using two identifiers (e.g., name and birth date or name and account number) according to facility policy. Compare identifiers with information on the patient's medical record.	Ensures correct patient. Complies with a recommended National Patient Safety Goal (TJC, 2011).
2 Explain procedure to patient; encourage patient's interaction and questions.	Lessens patient's anxiety and promotes participation.
3 Assemble equipment and close room curtains or door.	Optimizes use of time; provides privacy.

IMPLEMENTATION

STEP	RATIONALE
1 Position patient either standing or supine and drape, leaving area around stoma exposed. If seated, position patient either on or in front of toilet.	With patient supine there are fewer skin wrinkles, which allows for ease of application of pouching system; maintains patient dignity.
2 Perform hand hygiene and apply gloves.	Reduces transmission of microorganisms.
3 Place towel or disposable waterproof barrier under patient.	Protects bed linen.
4 Gently cleanse peristomal skin with warm water using gauze pads or clean washcloth; do not scrub skin; dry completely by patting with gauze or towel.	Avoid use of soap because it leaves residue on skin that interferes with pouch adhesion. Skin needs to be dry for skin barrier and pouch to adhere. Moisture increases risk for fungal infections. Do not be alarmed if blood appears on gauze pad. Stomas sometimes ooze blood as result of cleansing. Surface of stoma is highly vascular mucous membrane. Bleeding into pouch is abnormal (WOCN et al., 2010).
5 Use adhesive remover to rid remaining portions of skin barrier.	Improper removal of barrier irritates skin, causes skin tears, and results in poor adherence of new pouch (Dorman, 2009; Szymanski et al., 2010).
6 Measure stoma for correct size of pouching system needed using manufacturer measuring guide (see illustration).	Ensures accuracy in determining correct pouch size needed. New stomas shrink up to 6-8 weeks (Deitz, 2010b).
7 Select appropriate pouch based on patient assessment. With custom cut-to-fit pouch, use ostomy guide to cut opening on pouch 0.15 to 0.3 cm ($\frac{1}{16}$ to $\frac{1}{8}$ inch) larger than stoma before removing backing. Prepare pouch by removing backing from barrier and adhesive. With ileostomy, apply thin circle of barrier paste around opening in pouch; allow to dry (see illustration).	Determines correct size equipment. Too large an opening permits fecal drainage to ooze from under appliance, causing skin irritation. Too small an opening causes appliance to cut into stoma (WOCN et al., 2010).

STEP	RATIONALE

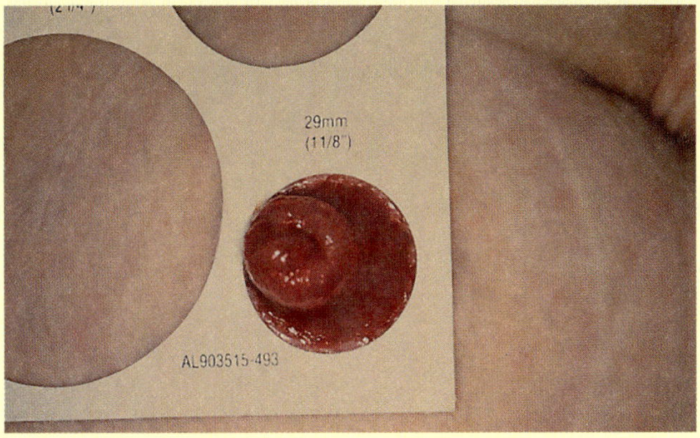

STEP 6 Measuring a stoma.

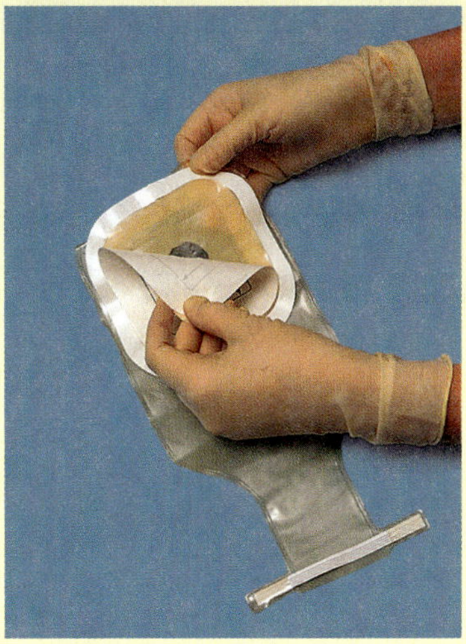

STEP 7 Preparing ostomy pouch.

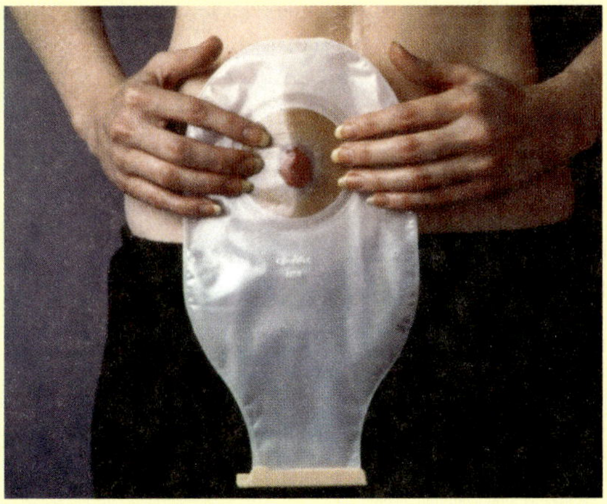

STEP 9a(2) Applying one-piece pouch. (Courtesy ConvaTec, Princeton, NJ.)

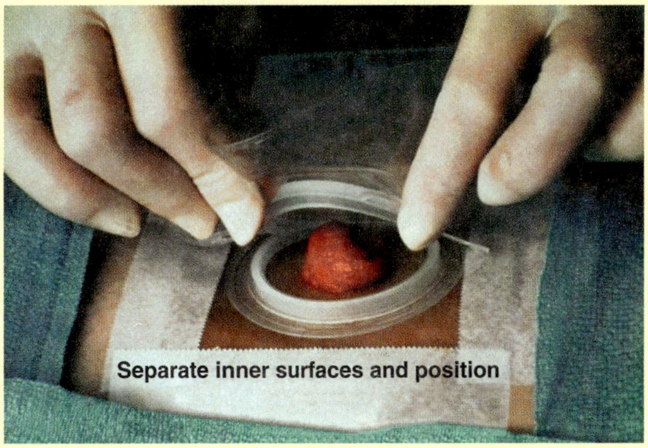

STEP 9b(1) Application of barrier-paste flange. (Courtesy ConvaTec, Princeton, NJ.)

CLINICAL DECISION: *If patient has a large volume of liquid stool from an ileostomy, consider using a "high-output" pouch that contains the volume of effluent and reduces the frequency of pouch emptying.*

STEP	RATIONALE
8 Apply skin barrier and pouch. If creases next to stoma occur, use barrier paste to fill in; let dry 1-2 minutes.	Barrier paste increases adherence of pouch to skin or fills in irregularities (Erwin-Toth et al., 2010).
9 When applying skin barrier to stoma that is close to patient's abdominal incision, trim skin barrier to fit.	Allows for better fit.
a. For one-piece pouching system	
(1) Use skin sealant wipes on skin directly under adhesive skin barrier or pouch; allow to dry. Press adhesive backing of pouch and/or skin barrier smoothly against skin, starting from bottom and working up and around sides.	Ensures smooth, wrinkle-free seal. Be careful of irritated or open areas because skin sealants often contain alcohol (WOCN et al., 2010).
(2) Hold pouch by barrier, center over stoma, and press down gently on barrier; bottom of pouch points toward patient's knees (see illustration).	Different position of pouch is sometimes necessary to allow better gravity flow. For example, patient confined to bed needs to have pouch positioned horizontally over side of abdomen.
(3) Maintain gentle finger pressure 1-2 minutes around barrier.	Gentle pressure and body heat assist in adhesion.
b. For two-piece pouching system	Creates wrinkle-free, secure seal; decreases irritation from adhesive on skin. Some two-piece pouching systems have snapping or clicking sound that occurs when attaching pouch to skin barrier.
(1) Apply barrier-paste flange (barrier with adhesive) as in previous steps for one-piece system. Then snap on pouch and maintain finger pressure (see illustration).	
c. For both pouching systems, gently tug on pouch in downward direction.	Determines that pouch is securely attached.

SKILL 46-3 POUCHING AN OSTOMY—cont'd

STEP	RATIONALE
10 Gently press on pectin or karaya flange to facilitate adhesion.	Skin barriers add to security of keeping pouch system securely attached.
11 Although many ostomy pouches are odor proof, explain to patient not to use "home remedies" to control ostomy odor, which will possibly harm stoma. Do not make pinhole in pouch to relieve odor.	Causes damage to pouch and defeats purpose of odor-proof pouch. **Never add aspirin to ostomy pouch** since it causes stoma bleeding. Making pinhole to remove flatus allows effluent to leak.
12 Fold bottom of drainable open-ended pouches up once. Close using clamp or manufacturer device.	Maintains secure seal to prevent leakage.
13 Properly dispose of old pouch and soiled equipment. Some patients ask to spray air freshener.	Lessens room odor.
14 Remove gloves and perform hand hygiene.	Reduces transmission of microorganisms.
15 Change one- or two-piece pouch every 3-7 days unless leaking. Pouch remains in place for tub bath or shower. After bath pat adhesive dry.	Avoid unnecessary trauma to skin from too-frequent bag changes. Drying ensures adhesion of pouch.

EVALUATION

1 Ask if patient feels discomfort around stoma.	Determines presence of skin irritation.
2 Note appearance of stoma, peristomal skin, and existing incision (if present) while removing pouch and cleansing skin. Observe condition of skin barrier and adhesive. Inspect edges of pouch for "tracking" of effluent under edges.	Determines condition of tissues and progress of healing. Determines presence of leaks.
3 Auscultate bowel sounds and observe characteristics of stool.	Determines status of peristalsis and bowel elimination.
4 Observe patient's nonverbal behaviors while applying the pouch. Ask if patient has any questions about pouching.	Indicates emotional response to stoma and readiness for teaching. Determines level of understanding of procedure.

UNEXPECTED OUTCOMES AND RELATED INTERVENTIONS

1 Patient experiences damage to peristomal skin.
- Assess for and report to health care provider for treatment:
  - Mechanical damage caused by inappropriate skin care, incorrect tape removal.
  - Chemical damage caused by waste coming into contact with peristomal skin or skin reaction to adhesive.
  - Damage caused by a fungal infection (candidiasis), usually caused by persistent moisture on peristomal skin.

2 Stoma becomes necrotic as manifested by purple or black color, dry instead of moist, failure to bleed, or sloughing tissue.
- Assess circulation to stoma and observe for excessive edema or tension on bowel suture line (if present).
- Immediately report this finding to the health care provider.

3 Patient refuses to view stoma or participate in care.
- Allow patient to express feelings.
- Provide information to patient and family about ostomy support groups and ostomy care nurses in the community.

RECORDING AND REPORTING

- Record type of pouch, skin barrier applied, and time; amount and appearance of stool, texture, condition of peristomal skin, and sutures. Record patient teaching.
- Report any of the following to the nurse and/or health care provider:
  - Abnormal appearance of stoma (e.g., bleeding, ulcerations, blue or black in color), suture line, peristomal skin, character of output, absence of bowel sounds
  - No flatus in 24 to 36 hours and no stool by third day
- Document abdominal distention and excessive tenderness, nature of bowel sounds.
- Record patient's level of participation and need for teaching.

HOME CARE CONSIDERATIONS

- Evaluate patient's home toileting facilities. This includes presence of adequate toileting facilities, flushable toilet, and number and location of toilets.
- Caution the patient that most ostomy pouches and barriers cannot be flushed down the toilet; they clog the system. Dispose of used ostomy pouch according to local sanitation regulations.

KEY POINTS

- Mechanical breakdown of food elements, gastrointestinal motility, and selective absorption and secretion of substances by the large intestine influence the character of feces.
- Food high in fiber content and an increased fluid intake keep feces soft.
- Ongoing use of cathartics, laxatives, and enemas affects and delays normal defecation reflexes.
- Vagal stimulation, which slows the heart rate, occurs during straining while defecating, taking rectal temperatures, enemas, and digital removal of impacted stool.
- The greatest danger from diarrhea is development of fluid and electrolyte imbalance.
- The location of an ostomy influences consistency of the stool.
- Focus assessment of elimination patterns on bowel habits, factors that normally influence defecation, recent changes in elimination, and a physical examination.

- Indirect and direct visualization of the lower GI tract requires cleansing of the bowel before the procedure.
- Consider frequency of defecation, fecal characteristics, and effect of foods on GI function when selecting a diet promoting normal elimination.
- Proper positioning on a bedpan allows the patient to assume a position similar to squatting without experiencing muscle strain.
- NG intubation decompresses the gastric contents by removing secretions and gaseous products from the GI tract.
- The purposes of gastric decompression are to keep the GI tract free of secretions, reduce nausea and gas, and decrease the risk of vomiting and aspiration.
- Proper selection and use of an ostomy pouching system is necessary to prevent damage to the skin around the stoma.
- Dangers during digital removal of stool include traumatizing the rectal mucosa and promoting vagal stimulation.
- Skin breakdown occurs after repeated exposure to liquid stool.

CLINICAL APPLICATION QUESTIONS

Preparing for Clinical Practice

A few days after Javier, the home care nurse, visited Larry in his home, Larry became nauseous, bloated, and had abdominal pain. He took an over-the-counter laxative and went to bed. Around 2:00 AM Larry woke with severe abdominal pain. He noticed that his belly was larger than normal, hard, and painful to touch. He felt if he could have a bowel movement, he would feel better. Once Larry was in the bathroom, he began to vomit and passed out from the abdominal pain. His mother heard him and ran to his side, finding him unconscious. She called for an ambulance.

1. Larry arrives in the emergency department of the hospital with vomiting and severe abdominal pain. Which nursing assessment questions does the nurse ask?
2. The nurse receives an order to insert a nasogastric (NG) tube. Once the NG is in place, how does the nurse determine if it is indeed in the stomach?
3. Which additional diagnostic test does the emergency department nurse anticipate that Larry would have?

evolve *Answers to Clinical Application Questions can be found on the Evolve website.*

REVIEW QUESTIONS

Are You Ready to Test Your Nursing Knowledge?

1. During the nursing assessment a patient reveals that he has diarrhea and cramping every time he has ice cream. He attributes this to the cold nature of the food. However, the nurse begins to suspect that these symptoms are associated with:
   1. Food allergy.
   2. Irritable bowel.
   3. Lactose intolerance.
   4. Increased peristalsis.
2. When assessing a 55-year-old patient who is in the clinic for a routine physical, the nurse instructs the patient about the need to obtain a stool specimen for guaiac fecal occult blood testing (gFOBT):
   1. If patient reports rectal bleeding.
   2. When there is a family history of polyps.
   3. As part of a routine examination for colon cancer.
   4. If a palpable mass is detected on digital examination.
3. Which of the following medications listed in a patient's medication history possibly causes gastrointestinal bleeding? (Select all that apply.)
   1. Aspirin
   2. Cathartics
   3. Antidiarrheal opiate agents
   4. Nonsteroidal antiinflammatory drugs (NSAIDs)
4. Nurses discourage patients from straining on defecation primarily because it causes: (Select all that apply.)
   1. Pain.
   2. Impaction.
   3. Hemorrhoids.
   4. Dysrhythmias.
5. A cleansing enema is ordered for a 55-year-old patient before intestinal surgery. The nurse understands that the maximum amount of fluid given is:
   1. 150 to 200 mL.
   2. 200 to 400 mL.
   3. 400 to 750 mL.
   4. 750 to 1000 mL.
6. A patient starts to experience pain while receiving an enema. The nurse notes blood in the return fluid and rectal bleeding. What action does the nurse take first?
   1. Administers pain medication
   2. Slows down the rate of instillation
   3. Tells the patient to breathe slowly and relax
   4. Stops the instillation and obtains vital signs
7. Number the steps to irrigating a nasogastric tube (NG) in correct order:
   1. Slowly aspirate the syringe.
   2. Reconnect the NG tube to suction.
   3. Clamp and disconnect the NG tube.
   4. Perform hand hygiene and apply clean gloves.
   5. Insert tip of syringe into NG tube and slowly inject 30 mL saline.
8. List the correct order in which to apply an ostomy pouch:
   1. Remove the used pouch and skin barrier.
   2. Perform hand hygiene and apply clean gloves.
   3. Assess the stoma for color, swelling, and healing.
   4. Gently cleanse the peristomal skin with warm tap water.
   5. Apply nonallergenic tape around the pectin skin barrier.
   6. Cut an opening on the pouch 0.15-0.3 cm ($\frac{1}{16}$ to $\frac{1}{8}$ inch) larger than the stoma.
   7. Press the adhesive backing of the pouch smoothly against the skin.
9. A patient is admitted for lower gastrointestinal (GI) bleeding. What color of stool does the nurse anticipate the patient to have?
   1. Red
   2. Black
   3. Green
   4. Orange
10. The nurse is caring for a patient with a colostomy. Which intervention is most important?
    1. Cleansing the stoma with hot water
    2. Inserting a deodorant tablet in the stoma bag
    3. Selecting a bag with an appropriate-size stoma opening
    4. Wearing sterile gloves while caring for the stoma
11. The nurse understands that, when comparing nasogastric tubes used for gastric decompression, a Salem sump is specifically designed to:
    1. Minimize the risk of a bowel obstruction.
    2. Ensure drainage of the intestines.

3. Prevent gastric mucosal damage.
4. Promote resting the gut.

12. Before collecting a stool sample for occult blood, the nurse instructs the nursing assistive personnel to:
    1. Ask the patient to void.
    2. Wash the patient's perineum.
    3. Secure a sterile, specimen container.
    4. Plan to collect the first specimen of the day.
13. The nurse is taking a health history of a newly admitted patient with a diagnosis Rule/out bowel obstruction. Which of the following is the priority question to ask the patient?
    1. Describe your bowel movements.
    2. How often do you have a bowel movement?
    3. When was the last time you moved your bowels?
    4. Do you routinely use stool softeners, laxatives, or enemas?
14. The nurse is caring for a 78-year-old man with diarrhea. Of the following problems, which is the most important to consider?
    1. Malnutrition
    2. Dehydration
    3. Skin breakdown
    4. Incontinence
15. The nurse recognizes which patient needs to use a fracture pan for a bowel movement?
    1. The patient who is obese
    2. The patient experiencing confusion
    3. The patient on bed rest
    4. A patient recovering from hip surgery

Answers: **1.** 3; **2.** 3; **3.** 1, 4; **4.** 3, 4; **5.** 4; **6.** 4; **7.** 4, 3, 5, 1, 2; **8.** 2, 1, 4, 3, 6, 7, 5; **9.** 1; **10.** 3; **11.** 3; **12.** 1; **13.** 3; **14.** 2; **15.** 4.

REFERENCES

The American Cancer Society (ACS): *Cancer facts and figures,* 2011a, http://www.cancer.org/acs/groups/content/@epidemiologysurveilance/documents/document/acspc-029771.pdf. Accessed December 3, 2011.

The American Cancer Society (ACS): *Detailed guide: colon and rectum cancer: revised 6/17/2011,* 2011b, http://www.cancer.org/Cancer/ColonandRectumCancer/DetailedGuide/index. Accessed December 3, 2011.

Banning M: Aging and the gut, *Nurs Older People* 20(1):17, 2008.

Calfee D: *Clostridium difficile*: a reemerging pathogen, *Geriatrics* 63(9)10, 2008.

Chien D, Bradway C: Acquired fecal incontinence in community-dwelling adults, *Nurse Pract* 35(1):15, 2010.

Continence Care Position Statement: Role of the wound, ostomy continence nurse or continence care nurse in continence care, *J WOCN* 36(5):529, 2009.

Cronenwett L, et al: Quality and safety education for nurses, *Nurs Outlook* 55(1):122, 2007.

Deitz D, Gates J: Basic ostomy management part 1, *Nursing 2010* 40(2):61, 2010a.

Deitz D, Gates J: Basic ostomy management part 2, *Nursing 2010* 40(5):62, 2010b.

Dixon K: "What really helped me.": a survey of postoperative patients ostomy education needs, *J WOCN* 34(3S): S59, 2007.

Dorman C: Ostomy basics, *RN* 72(7):22, 2009.

Durai R, et al: Nasogastric tubes: insertion technique and confirming the correct position, *Nurs Times* 105(16):12, 2009.

Durston S: Bowel obstruction: backup along the 750, *Nurs Made Incredibly Easy* 7(2):40, 2009.

Erwin-Toth P, et al: Peristomal skin complications, *Am J Nurs* 110(2):43, 2010.

Gordon P: *Principles and practice of surgery for the colon, rectum, and anus,* ed 3, New York, 2007, Informa Healthcare.

Gould D: Prevention and control of *Clostridium difficile* infection, *Nurs Older People* 22(3):29, 2010.

Gray M: Incontinence-related skin damage: essential knowledge, *Ostomy Wound Manage* 53(12):5, 2007.

Gray-Vickrey P: Gathering "pearls" of knowledge for assessing older adults, *Nursing 2010* 40(3):34, 2010.

Grossman S, Mager D: *Clostridium difficile*: implications for nursing, *MedSurg Nurs* 19(3):155, 2010.

Herman A: GI endoscopy: from start to finish, *Nurs Made Incredibly Easy* 8(3):5, 2010.

Holman C, et al: Preventing and treating constipation in later life, *Nurs Older People* 20(5):22, 2008.

Huether S, McCance K: *Understanding pathophysiology,* ed 4, St Louis, 2008, Mosby.

Kyle G: Bowel Care. Part 1: assessment of constipation, *Nurs Times* 103(42)26, 2007a.

Kyle G: Bowel Care. Part 4: administering an enema, *Nurs Times* 103(45)26, 2007b.

Kyle G: Bowel Care. Part 5: a practical guide to digital rectal examination, *Nurs Times* 103(46):28, 2007c.

Lehne R: *Pharmacology for nursing care,* ed 7, St Louis, 2010, Saunders.

Lewis S, et al: *Medical-surgical nursing: assessment and management of clinical problems,* ed 8, St Louis, 2011, Mosby.

McWilliams D: Rectal irrigation for patients with functional bowel disorders, *Nurs Stand* 24(26):42, 2010.

Meiner S: *Gerontologic Nurs,* ed 4, St Louis, 2011, Mosby.

Mengel M: *Family medicine ambulatory care and prevention,* ed 5, New York, 2009, McGraw Hill Lange.

Pagana KD, Pagana TJ: *Mosby's diagnostic and laboratory test reference,* ed 9, St Louis, 2011, Mosby.

Pearson T: Older people should be given practical support to effectively manage their stomas, *Nurs Times* 106(11): 16, 2010.

Pegram A, et al: Safe use of rectal suppositories and enemas with adult patients, *Nurs Stand* 22(38):38, 2008.

Peters D: Colon cancer screening: recommendations and barriers to patient participation, *Nurse Pract* 33(12):15, 2008.

Rust J: Care of patients with stomas: the pouch change procedure, *Nurs Stand* 22(6):43, 2007.

Seidel H, et al: *Mosby's guide to physical examination,* ed 7, St Louis, 2011, Mosby.

Steggall MJ: Digital rectal examination, *Nurs Stand* 22(47): 46, 2008.

Tabloski P: *Gerontological nursing,* Upper Saddle River, NJ, 2009, Pearson Prentice Hall.

The Joint Commission (TJC): *2011 National Patient Safety Goals (NPGs),* 2011, http://www.jointcommission.org/standards_information/npsgs.aspx. Accessed December 3, 2011.

Vonberg R, et al: Infection control measures to limit the spread of *Clostridium difficile, Clin Microbiol Infect* 14 (suppl 5):2, 2008.

Wisniewski A: Acute abdomen: shaking down the suspects. *Nurs Made Incredibly Easy* 8(1):42, 2010.

Wound, Ostomy, and Continence Nurses Society (WOCN): Management of the patient with a fecal ostomy: best practice guideline for clinicians, Mount Laurel, NJ, 2010, Author.

RESEARCH REFERENCES

Griffin K: Biological, psychological and behavioral, and social variables influencing colorectal cancer screening in African Americans, *Nurs Res* 58(5):312, 2009.

Herlufsen P, et al: Study of peristomal skin disorders in patients with permanent stomas, *Brit J Nurs* 15(16):854, 2006.

Hoeflok J, et al: A prospective multicenter evaluation of a moldable stoma skin barrier, *Ostomy/Wound Manage* 55(5):62, 2009.

Jacobson RM, et al: Serum electrolyte shifts following administration of sodium phosphates enema, *Gastroenterol Nurs* 33(3):191, 2010.

Joanna Briggs Institute (JBI): Management of constipation in older adults, *Best Practice* 12(7):1, 2008.

Meurette G, et al: Long-term results of Malone's procedure with antegrade irrigation for severe chronic constipation, *Gastroenterol Clin Biol* 34(3):209, 2010.

Ramirez M, et al: Figuring out sex in a reconfigured body: experiences of female colorectal cancer survivors with ostomies, *Women Health* 49(8):608, 2009.

Ratliff CR, Scarano K, Donovan AM: Descriptive study of peristomal complications, *J Wound Ostomy Continence Nurs* 32(1):33, 2005.

Richbourg L, et al: Ostomy pouch wear time in the United States, *J WOCN* 35(5):504, 2008.

Richbourg L, et al: Difficulties experienced by ostomate after hospital discharge, *J WOCN* 34(1):70, 2007.

Szymanski K, et al: External stoma and peristomal complications following radical cystectomy and ileal conduit diversion: a systematic review, *Ostomy Wound Manage* 56(1):28, 2010.

Thompson H, et al: Matching the skin barrier to the skin type, *Brit J Nurs* 20(16):S27, 2011.

Williams J, et al: Evaluating skin care problems in people with stomas, *Brit J Nurs* 19(17):S6, 2010.

CHAPTER

47

Mobility and Immobility

OBJECTIVES

- Describe the functions of the musculoskeletal (skeleton, skeletal muscles) and nervous systems in the regulation of movement.
- Discuss physiological and pathological influences on body alignment and joint mobility.
- Identify changes in physiological and psychosocial function associated with mobility and immobility.
- Assess for correct and impaired body alignment and mobility.
- Formulate appropriate nursing diagnoses for impaired body alignment and mobility.
- Develop individualized nursing care plans for patients with impaired body alignment and mobility.
- Discuss the importance of no-lift policies for the patient and health care provider.
- Describe equipment needed for safe patient handling and movement.
- Discuss the impact of national patient safety resources, initiatives, and regulations in relation to patient handling and movement.
- Compare and contrast active and passive range-of-motion exercises.
- Evaluate the nursing plan for maintaining body alignment and mobility.

KEY TERMS

Activity tolerance, p. 1139
Anthropometric measurements, p. 1141
Atelectasis, p. 1133
Bed rest, p. 1132
Body alignment, p. 1128
Body mechanics, p. 1127
Chest physiotherapy (CPT), p. 1148
Concentric tension, p. 1129
Disuse osteoporosis, p. 1134
Eccentric tension, p. 1130
Embolus, p. 1142
Exercise, p. 1139
Footdrop, p. 1134
Friction, p. 1128
Gait, p. 1139
Gait belt, p. 1158
Hemiparesis, p. 1158
Hemiplegia, p. 1158
Hypostatic pneumonia, p. 1133
Immobility, p. 1132
Instrumental activities of daily living (IADLs), p. 1157
Isometric contraction, p. 1130
Isotonic contraction, p. 1130
Joint contracture, p. 1134
Leverage, p. 1130
Logroll, p. 1165
Mobility, p. 1127
Muscle atrophy, p. 1131
Muscle tone, p. 1130
Negative nitrogen balance, p. 1132
Orthostatic hypotension, p. 1133
Osteoporosis, p. 1134
Pathological fractures, p. 1128
Posture, p. 1130
Pressure ulcer, p. 1135
Range of motion (ROM), p. 1136
Renal calculi, p. 1134
Shear, p. 1128
Thrombus, p. 1133
Trapeze bar, p. 1153
Trochanter roll, p. 1152
Unossified, p. 1129
Urinary stasis, p. 1134

evolve WEBSITE

http://evolve.elsevier.com/Potter/fundamentals/

- Review Questions
- Video Clips
- Animations
- Concept Map Creator
- Case Study with Questions
- Audio Glossary
- Interactive Learning Activities
- Key Term Flashcards
- Content Updates

People use **mobility** for many purposes (e.g., expression of emotions or satisfaction of basic needs with nonverbal gestures). It is also used to show self-defense, perform activities of daily living (ADLs), and participate in recreational activities. Many functions of the body depend on mobility. Intact musculoskeletal and nervous systems are necessary for optimal physical mobility and functioning.

Clinical nursing practice related to mobility and immobility requires the incorporation of scientific and nursing knowledge and skills to provide competent care. Knowing the movements and functions of muscles in maintaining posture and movement and implementing evidence-based knowledge about safe patient handling are essential to protecting the safety of both the patient and the nurse.

SCIENTIFIC KNOWLEDGE BASE

Nature of Movement

Movement is a complex process that requires coordination between the musculoskeletal and nervous systems. **Body mechanics** is a term used to describe the coordinated efforts of the musculoskeletal and nervous systems. Although nurses need to understand the physics surrounding body mechanics, lifting techniques historically used in nursing practice that emphasize body mechanics often cause debilitating injuries to nursing and other health care staff (de Castro et al., 2006). Today nurses use information about body alignment, balance, gravity, and friction when implementing nursing interventions such as positioning patients, determining the risk of patient falls, and selecting the safest way to move or transfer patients.

Alignment and Balance. The terms *body alignment* and *posture* are similar and refer to the positioning of the joints, tendons, ligaments, and muscles while standing, sitting, and lying. **Body alignment** means that the individual's center of gravity is stable. Correct body alignment reduces strain on musculoskeletal structures, aids in maintaining adequate muscle tone, promotes comfort, and contributes to balance and conservation of energy. Without balance control the center of gravity is displaced, thus creating a risk for falls and subsequent injuries. Balance is enhanced by keeping the center of gravity of the body low with a wide base of support and maintaining correct body posture.

Individuals require balance for maintaining a static position (e.g., sitting) and moving (e.g., walking). Disease, injury, pain, physical development (e.g., age), and life changes (e.g., pregnancy) compromise the ability to remain balanced. Medications that cause dizziness and prolonged immobility also affect balance. Impaired balance is a major threat to physical safety and contributes to a fear of falling and self-imposed restrictions on activity.

Gravity and Friction. Weight is the force exerted on a body by gravity. The force of weight is always directed downward, which is why an unbalanced object falls. Unsteady patients fall if their center of gravity becomes unbalanced because of the gravitational pull on their weight.

To lift safely the lifter has to overcome the weight of the object and know its center of gravity. In symmetrical inanimate objects the center of gravity is at the exact center of the object. However, people are not geometrically perfect; their centers of gravity are usually at 55% to 57% of standing height and are in the midline, which is why only using principles of body mechanics in lifting patients often leads to injury of the nurse or health care professional.

Friction is a force that occurs in a direction to oppose movement. The greater the surface area of the object that is moved, the greater the friction. A larger object produces greater resistance to movement. In addition, the force exerted against the skin while the skin remains stationary and the bony structures move is called **shear.** Unfortunately a common example is when the head of the bed is elevated beyond 60 degrees and gravity pulls the bony skeleton toward the foot of the bed while the skin remains against the sheets. The blood vessels in the underlying tissue are stretched and damaged, resulting in impeded blood flow to the deep tissues. Ultimately pressure ulcers often develop within the undermined tissue; the surface tissue appears less affected. To decrease surface area and reduce friction when patients are unable to assist with moving up in bed, nurses use an ergonomic assistive device such as a full body sling. This sling mechanically lifts the patient off the surface of the bed, thereby preventing friction, tearing, or shearing his or her delicate skin, and protects the nurse and other staff from injury (Nelson et al., 2009).

Physiology and Regulation of Movement

Skeletal System. The skeleton provides attachments for muscles and ligaments and the leverage necessary for movement. Thus the skeleton is the supporting framework of the body and is made up of four types of bones: long, short, flat, and irregular. Long bones contribute to height (e.g., the femur, fibula, and tibia in the leg) and length (e.g., the phalanges of the fingers and toes). Short bones (e.g., the carpal bones in the foot and the patella in the knee) occur in clusters and, when combined with ligaments and cartilage, permit movement of the extremities. Flat bones (e.g., some bones in the skull and the ribs in the thorax) provide structural contour. Irregular bones make up the vertebral column and some bones of the skull such as the mandible.

Bones are further characterized by firmness, rigidity, and elasticity. Firmness results from inorganic salts such as calcium and phosphate that are in the bone matrix. It is related to the rigidity of the bone, which is necessary to keep long bones straight and enables bones to withstand weight bearing. In addition, bones have a degree of elasticity and skeletal flexibility that change with age. For example, the newborn has a large amount of cartilage and is highly flexible but is unable to support weight. The toddler's bones are more pliable than those of an older person and are better able to withstand falls. Older adults, especially women, are more susceptible to bone loss (resorption) and osteoporosis, which increase the risk of fractures.

The skeletal system has several functions. It protects vital organs (e.g., the skull around the brain and the ribs around the heart and lungs) and aids in calcium regulation. Bones store calcium and release it into the circulation as needed. Patients with decreased calcium regulation and metabolism are at risk for developing osteoporosis and **pathological fractures** (fractures caused by weakened bone tissue). In addition, the internal structure of long bones contains bone marrow, participates in red blood cell (RBC) production, and acts as a reservoir for blood. Patients with altered bone marrow function or diminished RBC production fatigue easily because of reduced hemoglobin and oxygen-carrying ability. This fatigue decreases their mobility and increases the risk for falling.

Joints. Joints are the connections between bones. Each joint is classified according to its structure and degree of mobility. There are four classifications of joints: synostotic, cartilaginous, fibrous, and synovial.

The synostotic joint refers to bones jointed by bones. No movement is associated with this type of joint, and the bony tissue that forms between the bones provides strength and stability. The classic example of this type of joint is the skull, where fusion of the joint occurs later in life (Fig. 47-1, *A*).

In the cartilaginous joint, or synchondrosis joint, cartilage unites bony components. This type of joint allows for bone growth while providing stability. When bone growth is complete, the joints ossify. The first sternocostal joint is an example of a synchondrosis joint (Fig. 47-1, *B*).

The fibrous joint, or syndesmosis joint, is a joint in which a ligament or membrane unites two bony surfaces. The fibers of ligaments are flexible and stretch, permitting a limited amount of movement. The paired bones of the lower leg (tibia and fibula) are syndesmotic joints (Huether and McCance, 2008) (Fig. 47-1, *C*).

The synovial joint, or true joint, is a freely movable joint in which contiguous bony surfaces are covered by articular cartilage and connected by ligaments lined with a synovial membrane. Joining of the humeral radius and ulna by cartilage and ligaments forms a pivotal joint (Fig. 47-1, *D*). Other types of synovial joints are the ball-and-socket joints such as the hip joint and the hinge joints such as the interphalangeal joints of the fingers.

Ligaments. Ligaments are white, shiny, flexible bands of fibrous tissue binding joints together and connecting bones and cartilages. Ligaments are elastic and aid joint flexibility and support (Fig. 47-2). In addition, some ligaments have a protective function. For example, ligaments between the vertebral bodies and the ligamentum flavum prevent damage to the spinal cord during movement of the back.

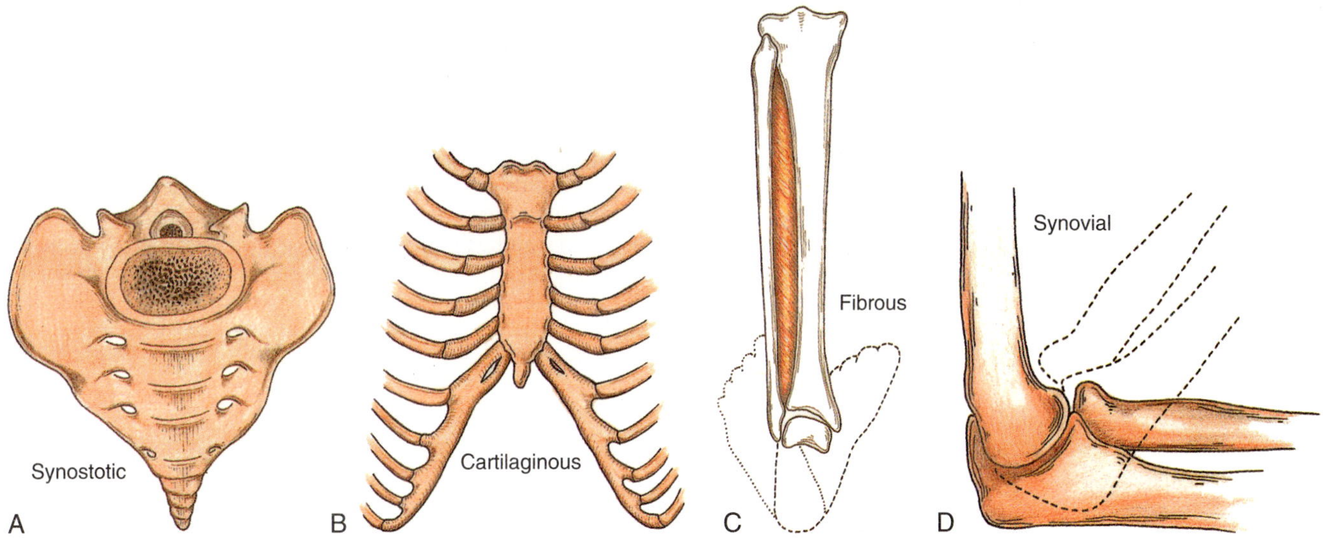

FIG. 47-1 Joint types. **A,** Synostotic. **B,** Cartilaginous. **C,** Fibrous. **D,** Synovial.

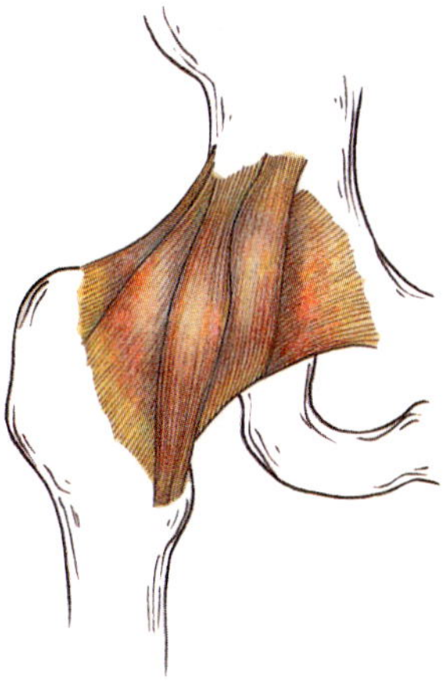

FIG. 47-2 Ligaments of hip joint.

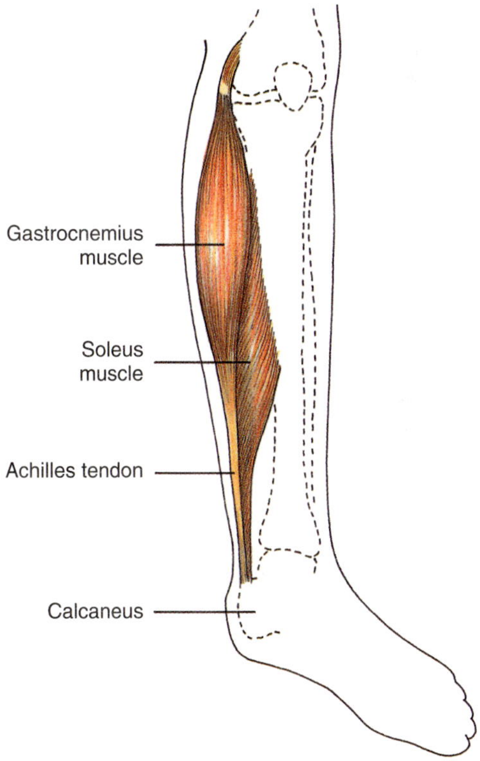

FIG. 47-3 Tendons and muscles of lower leg.

Tendons. Tendons are white, glistening, fibrous bands of tissue that connect muscle to bone. They are strong, flexible, and inelastic; and they occur in various lengths and thicknesses. The Achilles tendon (tendo calcaneus) is the thickest and strongest tendon in the body. It begins near the midposterior of the leg and attaches the gastrocnemius and soleus muscles in the calf to the calcaneal bone in the back of the foot (Fig. 47-3).

Cartilage. Cartilage is nonvascular (without blood vessels) supporting connective tissue located chiefly in the joints and thorax, trachea, larynx, nose, and ear. The fetus has a large amount of temporary cartilage, which is replaced by bone developed during infancy. Permanent cartilage is unossified (not hardened), except in advanced age and diseases such as osteoarthritis.

Joints, ligaments, tendons, and cartilage facilitate strength and flexibility of the skeleton. Strength enables the skeletal system to support the body. A person's flexibility is demonstrated through range of motion (ROM). However, strength and flexibility do not result entirely from these four structures. Adequate skeletal muscle is also necessary.

Skeletal Muscle. Movement of bones and joints involves active processes that are carefully integrated to achieve coordination. Skeletal muscles, because of their ability to contract and relax, are the working elements of movement. Anatomical structure and attachment to the skeleton enhance contractile elements of the skeletal muscle.

Muscles are made of fibers that contract when stimulated by an electrochemical impulse that travels from the nerve to the muscle across the neuromuscular junction. The electrochemical impulse causes the filaments (predominantly protein molecules of myosin and actin) within the fiber to slide past one another, with the filaments changing length.

Muscle contractions are categorized by functional purpose: moving, resisting, or stabilizing body parts. In concentric tension increased muscle contraction causes muscle shortening, resulting in movement such as when a patient uses an overhead trapeze to pull up in bed. **Eccentric tension** helps control the speed and direction of movement. For example, when using an overhead trapeze, the patient slowly lowers himself to the bed. The lowering is controlled when the antagonistic muscles lengthen. Concentric and eccentric muscle actions are necessary for active movement and therefore are referred to as dynamic or **isotonic contraction.** **Isometric contraction** (static contraction) causes an increase in muscle tension or muscle work but no shortening or active movement of the muscle (e.g., instructing the patient to tighten and relax a muscle group, as in quadriceps set exercises or pelvic floor exercises). Voluntary movement is a combination of isotonic and isometric contractions.

Although isometric contractions do not result in muscle shortening, energy expenditure increases. This type of muscle work is comparable to having a car in neutral with the driver continually depressing the accelerator and racing the engine. The driver is not going anywhere but expends a large amount of energy. It is important to understand the energy expenditure (increased respiratory rate and increased work on the heart) associated with isometric exercises because the exercises are sometimes contraindicated in certain patients' illnesses (e.g., myocardial infarction or chronic obstructive pulmonary disease).

Muscle Movement and Posture. Muscles that attach to bones of leverage provide necessary strength to move an object. **Leverage** is an inducing or compelling force and occurs when specific bones such as the humerus, ulna, and radius and the associated joint such as the elbow act together as a lever. Force is applied to one end of the bone to lift a weight as another point rotates the bone in the opposite direction.

Muscles associated primarily with maintaining posture are short and featherlike in appearance because they converge obliquely at a common tendon. Muscles of the lower extremities, trunk, neck, and back are concerned primarily with **posture** (the position of the body in relation to the surrounding space). These muscle groups work together to stabilize and support body weight, and they allow an individual to maintain a sitting or standing posture.

Muscle Regulation of Posture and Movement. Posture and movement depend on the skeleton and the shape and development of skeletal muscles. They also contribute to musculoskeletal function and often reflect personality, discomfort, and mood. For example, a person with a dramatic personality gestures with the hands, a person who is fatigued or depressed may slouch, and a person with abdominal pain may curl into a fetal-like position.

Coordination and regulation of different muscle groups depend on muscle tone and activity of antagonistic, synergistic, and antigravity muscles (see Chapter 38). **Muscle tone,** or tonus, is the normal state of balanced muscle tension. The body achieves tension by alternating contraction and relaxation without active movement of neighboring fibers of a specific muscle group. Muscle tone helps maintain functional positions such as sitting or standing without excess muscle fatigue and is maintained through continual use of muscles. ADLs require muscle action and help maintain muscle tone. When a patient is immobile or on prolonged bed rest, activity level, activity tolerance, and muscle tone decrease.

Nervous System. The nervous system regulates movement and posture. The precentral gyrus, or motor strip, is the major voluntary motor area and is in the cerebral cortex. A majority of motor fibers descend from the motor strip and cross at the level of the medulla. Thus the motor fibers from the right motor strip initiate voluntary movement for the left side of the body, and motor fibers from the left motor strip initiate voluntary movement for the right side of the body.

During voluntary movement impulses descend from the motor strip to the spinal cord. An impulse exits the spinal cord through efferent motor nerves and travels through the nerves. Through a complex process neurotransmitters, or chemicals such as acetylcholine, transfer electric impulses from the nerve across the neuromuscular junction to the muscle. The neurotransmitter reaches a muscle and stimulates it, causing movement. Movement is impaired by disorders that alter neurotransmitter production, transfer of impulses from the nerve to the muscle, or activation of muscle activity. Parkinsonism is an example of such a disorder (see Chapter 38).

Pathological Influences on Mobility

Many pathological conditions affect mobility. Although a complete description of each is beyond the scope of this chapter, an overview of four pathological influences are presented.

Postural Abnormalities. Congenital or acquired postural abnormalities affect the efficiency of the musculoskeletal system and body alignment, balance, and appearance. During assessment observe body alignment and ROM (see Chapter 38). Postural abnormalities can cause pain, impair alignment or mobility, or both. Knowledge about the characteristics, causes, and treatment of common postural abnormalities is necessary for lifting, transfer, and positioning (Table 47-1). Some postural abnormalities limit ROM. Nurses intervene to maintain maximum ROM in unaffected joints and then design interventions to strengthen affected muscles and joints, improve the patient's posture, and adequately use affected and unaffected muscle groups. Referral to and/or collaboration with a physical therapist enhances the nurse's interventions for a patient with a postural abnormality.

Muscle Abnormalities. Injury and disease lead to numerous alterations in musculoskeletal function. For example, the muscular dystrophies are a group of familial disorders that cause degeneration of skeletal muscle fibers. They are the most prevalent of the muscle diseases in childhood. Patients with muscular dystrophy experience progressive, symmetrical weakness and wasting of skeletal muscle groups, with increasing disability and deformity (McCance and Huether, 2009).

Damage to the Central Nervous System. Damage to any component of the central nervous system that regulates voluntary movement results in impaired body alignment, balance, and mobility. Trauma from a head injury, ischemia from a stroke or brain attack (cerebrovascular accident [CVA]), or bacterial infection such as meningitis can damage the cerebellum or the motor strip in the cerebral cortex. Damage to the cerebellum causes problems with balance, and motor impairment is directly related to the amount of destruction of the motor strip. For example, a person with a right-sided cerebral hemorrhage with necrosis has destruction of the right motor strip that results in left-sided hemiplegia. Trauma to the spinal cord also impairs mobility. For example, a complete transection of the spinal cord results in a bilateral loss of voluntary motor control below the level of the trauma because motor fibers are cut.

Direct Trauma to the Musculoskeletal System. Direct trauma to the musculoskeletal system results in bruises, contusions, sprains, and fractures. A fracture is a disruption of bone tissue continuity. Fractures most commonly result from direct external trauma, but they also occur as a consequence of some deformity of the bone (e.g., pathological fractures of osteoporosis, Paget's disease, or osteogenesis imperfecta). Young children are usually able to form new bone more easily than adults and, as a result, have

TABLE 47-1 Postural Abnormalities

ABNORMALITY	DESCRIPTION	CAUSE	POSSIBLE TREATMENTS*
Torticollis	Inclining of head to affected side, in which sternocleidomastoid muscle is contracted	Congenital or acquired condition	Surgery, heat, support, or immobilization, depending on cause and severity, gentle ROM
Lordosis	Exaggeration of anterior convex curve of lumbar spine	Congenital condition Temporary condition (e.g., pregnancy)	Spine-stretching exercises (based on cause)
Kyphosis	Increased convexity in curvature of thoracic spine	Congenital condition Rickets, osteoporosis Tuberculosis of spine	Spine-stretching exercises, sleeping without pillows, using bed board, bracing, spinal fusion (based on cause and severity)
Scoliosis	Lateral "S"- or "C"-shaped spinal column with vertebral rotation, unequal heights of hips and shoulders	Sometimes a consequence of numerous congenital, connective tissue and neuromuscular disorders	Approximately half of children with scoliosis require surgery Nonsurgical treatment is with braces and exercises
Congenital hip dysplasia	Hip instability with limited abduction of hips and occasionally adduction contractures (head of femur does not articulate with acetabulum because of abnormal shallowness of acetabulum)	Congenital condition (more common with breech deliveries)	Maintenance of continuous abduction of thigh so head of femur presses into center of acetabulum Abduction splints, casting, surgery
Knock-knee (genu valgum)	Legs curved inward so knees come together as person walks	Congenital condition Rickets	Knee braces, surgery if not corrected by growth
Bowlegs (genu varum)	One or both legs bent outward at knee, which is normal until 2 to 3 years of age	Congenital condition Rickets	Slowing rate of curving if not corrected by growth With rickets, increase of vitamin D, calcium, and phosphorus intake to normal ranges
Clubfoot	*95%:* Medial deviation and plantar flexion of foot (equinovarus) *5%:* Lateral deviation and dorsiflexion (calcaneovalgus)	Congenital condition	Casts, splints such as Denis Browne splint, and surgery (based on degree and rigidity of deformity)
Footdrop	Inability to dorsiflex and invert foot because of peroneal nerve damage	Congenital condition Trauma Improper position of immobilized patient	None (cannot be corrected) Prevention through physical therapy Bracing with ankle-foot orthotic (AFO)
Pigeon toes	Internal rotation of forefoot or entire foot, common in infants	Congenital condition Habit	Growth, wearing reversed shoes

Data from McCance K, Huether SE: *Pathophysiology: the biologic basis for disease in adults and children,* ed 6, St Louis, 2009, Mosby.
ROM, Range of motion.
*Severity of condition and cause dictate treatment, which is individualized to the patient's needs.

few complications after a fracture. Treatment often includes positioning the fractured bone in proper alignment and immobilizing it to promote healing and restore function. Even this temporary immobilization results in some **muscle atrophy,** loss of muscle tone, and joint stiffness.

NURSING KNOWLEDGE BASE

Fully understanding movement and mobility requires more than an overview of movement and the physiology and regulation of movement by the musculoskeletal and nervous systems. You need to know how to apply these scientific principles in the clinical setting to determine the safest way to move patients and to understand the effect of immobility on the physiological, psychosocial, and developmental aspects of patient care.

Safe Patient Handling

Nurses are exposed to the hazards related to lifting and transferring patients in many settings such as inpatient nursing units, long-term care facilities, and the operating room (de Castro et al., 2006). Manually lifting and transferring patients contributes to the high incidence of work-related musculoskeletal problems and back injuries in nurses and other health care staff (Nelson and Baptiste, 2006). Current evidence shows that many nurses frequently transfer to different positions and leave the profession because of work-related injuries (de Castro et al., 2006). Implementing evidence-based interventions and programs (e.g., lift teams) reduces the number of work-related injuries, which improves the health of the nurse and reduces indirect costs to the health care agency (e.g., workers' compensation and replacing injured workers).

Today many states have laws that mandate safe patient handling in health care agencies. Health care agencies are implementing comprehensive safe patient–handling programs in all parts of the United States. Comprehensive safe patient–handling programs include the following elements: an ergonomics assessment protocol for health care environments, patient assessment criteria, algorithms for patient handling and movement, special equipment kept in convenient locations to help transfer patients, back injury resource nurses, an "after-action review" that allows the health care team to apply knowledge about moving patients safely in different settings, and a no-lift policy (Nelson, 2006).

Factors Influencing Mobility-Immobility

To determine how to move patients safely, assess their ability to move. Mobility refers to a person's ability to move about freely, and **immobility** refers to the inability to do so. Some patients can be mobile or immobile, whereas others experience varying degrees of partial immobility. Think of mobility as a continuum, with mobility on one end, immobility on the other, and varying degrees of partial immobility between the end points. Some patients move back and forth between mobility and immobility, but for others immobility is absolute and continues indefinitely. The terms *bed rest* and *impaired physical mobility* are used frequently when discussing patients on the mobility-immobility continuum.

Bed rest is an intervention that restricts patients to bed for therapeutic reasons. Nurses and health care providers most often prescribe this intervention. Bed rest has many different interpretations among health care professionals. Patients with a wide variety of conditions are placed on bed rest. The duration of bed rest depends on the illness or injury and the patient's prior state of health.

The effects of muscular deconditioning associated with lack of physical activity are often apparent in a matter of days. This cluster of symptoms is often referred to as the "hazards of immobility." The individual of average weight and height without a chronic illness on bed rest loses muscle strength from baseline levels at a rate of 3% a day. Immobility also is associated with cardiovascular, skeletal, and other organ changes. The term *disuse atrophy* describes the tendency of cells and tissue to reduce in size and function in response to prolonged inactivity resulting from bed rest, trauma, casting, or local nerve damage (McCance and Huether, 2009).

Periods of immobility or prolonged bed rest cause major physiological, psychological, and social effects. These effects are gradual or immediate and vary from patient to patient. The greater the extent and the longer the duration of immobility, the more pronounced the consequences. The patient with complete mobility restrictions is continually at risk for the hazards of immobility.

Systemic Effects. All body systems work more efficiently with some form of movement. Exercise has positive outcomes for all major systems of the body. When there is an alteration in mobility, each body system is at risk for impairment. The severity of the impairment depends on the patient's overall health, degree and length of immobility, and age. For example, older adults with chronic illnesses develop pronounced effects of immobility more quickly than do younger patients with the same immobility problem.

Metabolic Changes. Changes in mobility alter endocrine metabolism, calcium resorption, and functioning of the gastrointestinal system. The endocrine system, made up of hormone-secreting glands, maintains and regulates vital functions such as (1) response to stress and injury; (2) growth and development; (3) reproduction; (4) maintenance of the internal environment; and (5) energy production, use, and storage.

When injury or stress occurs, the endocrine system triggers a series of responses aimed at maintaining blood pressure and preserving life. It is important in maintaining homeostasis. Tissues and cells live in an internal environment that the endocrine system helps regulate through maintenance of sodium, potassium, water, and acid-base balance. It also regulates energy metabolism. Thyroid hormone increases the basal metabolic rate (BMR), and energy becomes available to cells through the integrated action of gastrointestinal and pancreatic hormones (McCance and Huether, 2009).

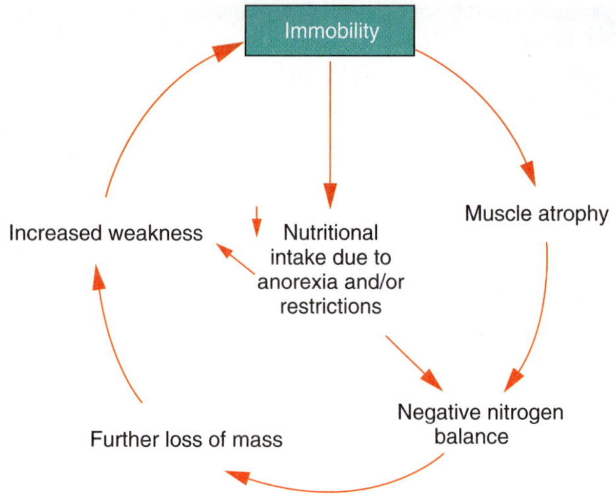

FIG. 47-4 Factors contributing to negative nitrogen balance associated with immobility. (From Gröer MW, Shekleton ME: *Basic pathophysiology: a holistic approach,* ed 3, St Louis, 1989, Mosby.)

Immobility disrupts normal metabolic functioning: decreasing the metabolic rate; altering the metabolism of carbohydrates, fats, and proteins; causing fluid, electrolyte, and calcium imbalances; and causing gastrointestinal disturbances such as decreased appetite and slowing of peristalsis. However, in the presence of an infectious process, immobilized patients often have an increased BMR as a result of fever or wound healing because these increase cellular oxygen requirements (Huether and McCance, 2008).

A deficiency in calories and protein is characteristic of patients with a decreased appetite secondary to immobility. The body is constantly synthesizing proteins and breaking them down into amino acids to form other proteins (see Chapter 41). When the patient is immobile, his or her body often excretes more nitrogen (the end product of amino acid breakdown) than it ingests in proteins, resulting in **negative nitrogen balance** (Fig. 47-4). Weight loss, decreased muscle mass, and weakness result from tissue catabolism (tissue breakdown) (McCance and Huether, 2009).

Another metabolic change associated with immobility is calcium resorption (loss) from bones. Immobility causes the release of calcium into the circulation. Normally the kidneys excrete the excess calcium. However, if the kidneys are unable to respond appropriately, hypercalcemia results. Pathological fractures occur if calcium resorption continues as the patient remains on bed rest or continues to be immobile (Huether and McCance, 2008).

Impairments of gastrointestinal functioning caused by decreased mobility vary. Difficulty in passing stools (constipation) is a common symptom, although pseudodiarrhea often results from a fecal impaction (accumulation of hardened feces). Be aware that this finding is not normal diarrhea, but rather liquid stool passing around the area of impaction (see Chapter 46). Left untreated, fecal impaction results in a mechanical bowel obstruction that partially or completely occludes the intestinal lumen, blocking normal propulsion of liquid and gas. The resulting fluid in the intestine produces distention and increases intraluminal pressure. Over time intestinal function becomes depressed, dehydration occurs, absorption ceases, and fluid and electrolyte disturbances worsen.

Respiratory Changes. Regular aerobic exercise enhances respiratory functioning. Lack of movement and exercise places patients at

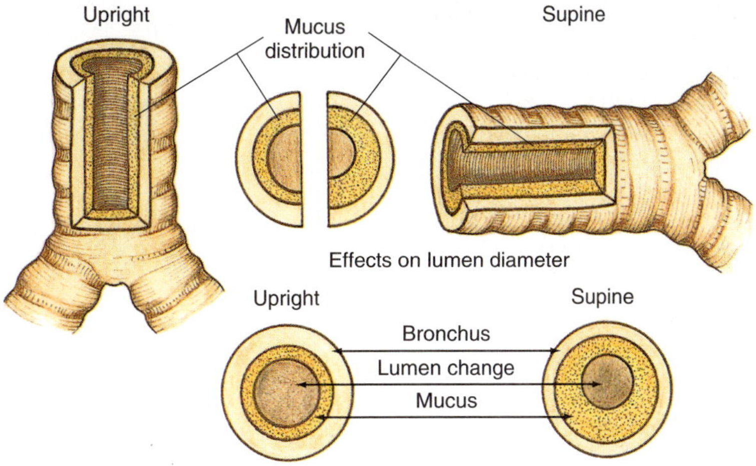

FIG. 47-5 Effect of recumbency and gravity on distribution of respiratory tract and diameter of bronchiolar lumen. (From Gröer MW, Shekleton ME: *Basic pathophysiology: a holistic approach,* ed 3, St Louis, 1989, Mosby.)

higher risk for respiratory complications. Patients who are immobile are at high risk for developing pulmonary complications. The most common respiratory complications are **atelectasis** (collapse of alveoli) and **hypostatic pneumonia** (inflammation of the lung from stasis or pooling of secretions). Both decreased oxygenation and prolonged recovery add to the patient's discomfort (Lewis et al., 2011). In atelectasis secretions block a bronchiole or a bronchus; and the distal lung tissue (alveoli) collapses as the existing air is absorbed, producing hypoventilation. The site of the blockage affects the severity of atelectasis. Sometimes an entire lung lobe or a whole lung collapses. At some point in the development of these complications, there is a proportional decline in the patient's ability to cough productively. Ultimately the distribution of mucus in the bronchi increases, particularly when the patient is in the supine, prone, or lateral position (Fig. 47-5). Mucus accumulates in the dependent regions of the airways (Fig. 47-6). Hypostatic pneumonia frequently results because mucus is an excellent place for bacteria to grow.

Cardiovascular Changes. Immobilization also affects the cardiovascular system. The three major changes are orthostatic hypotension, increased cardiac workload, and thrombus formation.

Orthostatic hypotension is an increase in heart rate of more than 15% and a drop of 15 mm Hg or more in systolic blood pressure or a drop of 10 mm Hg or more in diastolic blood pressure when the patient changes from the supine to standing position (Huether and McCance, 2008). In the immobilized patient decreased circulating fluid volume, pooling of blood in the lower extremities, and decreased autonomic response occur. These are especially evident in the older adult.

As the workload of the heart increases, so does its oxygen consumption. Therefore the heart works harder and less efficiently during periods of prolonged rest. As immobilization increases, cardiac output falls, further decreasing cardiac efficiency and increasing workload.

Patients who are immobile are also at risk for thrombus formation. A **thrombus** is an accumulation of platelets, fibrin, clotting factors, and the cellular elements of the blood attached to the interior wall of a vein or artery, which sometimes occludes the lumen of the vessel (Fig. 47-7). Three factors contribute to venous thrombus formation: (1) damage to the vessel wall (e.g., injury during surgical procedures), (2) alterations of blood flow (e.g., slow blood

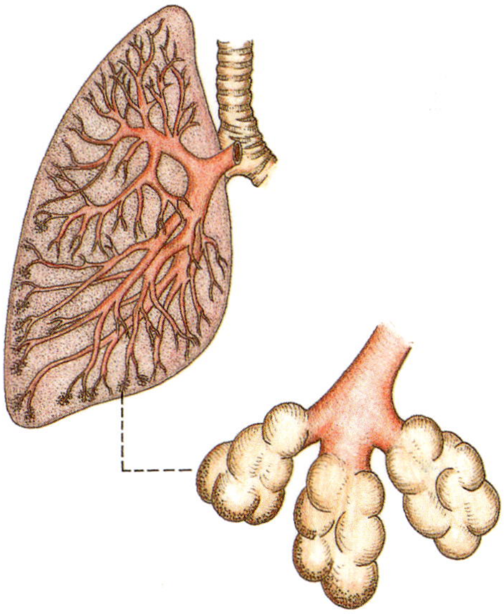

FIG. 47-6 Pooling of secretions in dependent regions of lungs in supine position.

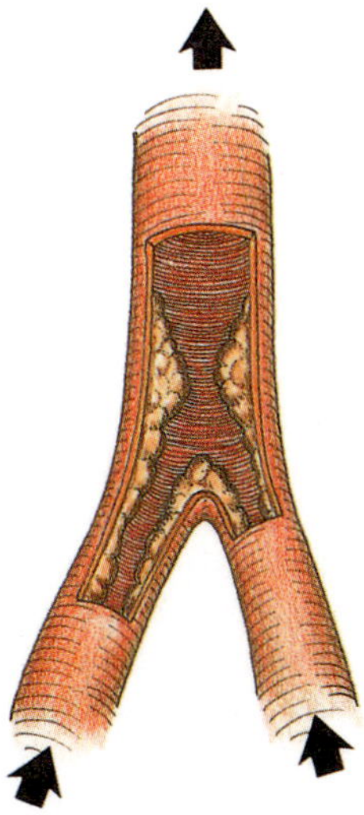

FIG. 47-7 Thrombus formation in a vessel.

flow in calf veins associated with bed rest), and (3) alterations in blood constituents (e.g., a change in clotting factors or increased platelet activity). These three factors are often referred to as *Virchow's triad* (Huether and McCance, 2008).

Musculoskeletal Changes. The effects of immobility on the musculoskeletal system include permanent or temporary impairment or permanent disability. Restricted mobility sometimes results in loss of endurance, strength, and muscle mass and decreased stability and balance. Other effects of restricted mobility affecting the skeletal system are impaired calcium metabolism and joint mobility.

Muscle Effects. Because of protein breakdown, the patient loses lean body mass. The reduced muscle mass is unable to sustain activity without increased fatigue. If immobility continues and the patient does not exercise, there is further loss of muscle mass. Muscle weakness always occurs with immobility, and prolonged immobility often leads to disuse atrophy. Muscle atrophy is a widely observed response to illness, decreased ADLs, and immobilization. Loss of endurance, decreased muscle mass and strength, and joint instability (see Skeletal Effects) put patients at risk for falls (see Chapter 38).

Skeletal Effects. Immobilization causes two skeletal changes: impaired calcium metabolism and joint abnormalities. Because immobilization results in bone resorption, the bone tissue is less dense or atrophied, and **disuse osteoporosis** results. When disuse osteoporosis occurs, the patient is at risk for pathological fractures.

Osteoporosis is a major health concern in this country. The first Surgeon General's report on the topic of bone health stated that one in two Americans over 50 years of age will be at risk for fractures related to osteoporosis by the year 2020. Furthermore, the National Osteoporosis Foundation (2010) reports that 44 million Americans (55% of those over the age of 50) either have osteoporosis or are at risk for developing it. Approximately 80% of people who have osteoporosis are female. Although primary osteoporosis is different in origin from the osteoporosis that results from immobility, it is imperative for nurses to recognize that immobilized patients are at high risk for accelerated bone loss if they have primary osteoporosis.

Immobility can lead to joint contractures. A **joint contracture** is an abnormal and possibly permanent condition characterized by fixation of the joint. It is important to note that flexor muscles for joints are stronger than extensor muscles and therefore contribute to the formation of contractures. Disuse, atrophy, and shortening of the muscle fibers cause joint contractures. When a contracture occurs, the joint cannot achieve full ROM. Contractures sometimes leave a joint or joints in a nonfunctional position, as seen in patients who are permanently curled in a fetal position. Early prevention of contractures is essential; they can begin to form after only 8 hours of immobility in the older adult (Fletcher, 2005).

One common and debilitating contracture is footdrop (Fig. 47-8). When **footdrop** occurs, the foot is permanently fixed in plantar flexion. Ambulation is difficult with the foot in this position because the patient cannot dorsiflex the foot. The patient with footdrop is unable to lift the toes off the ground. Patients who have suffered CVAs or brain attacks with resulting right- or left-sided paralysis (hemiplegia) are at risk for footdrop.

Urinary Elimination Changes. Immobility alters the patient's urinary elimination. In the upright position urine flows out of the renal pelvis and into the ureters and bladder because of gravitational forces. When the patient is recumbent or flat, the kidneys and ureters move toward a more level plane. Urine formed by the

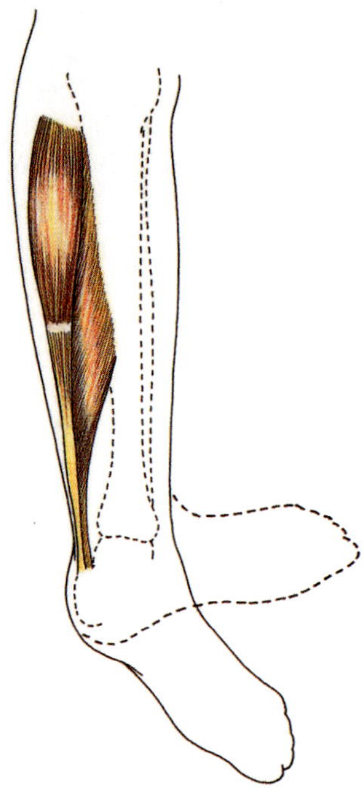

FIG. 47-8 Footdrop. Ankle is fixed in plantar flexion. Normally ankle is able to flex *(dotted line)*, which eases walking.

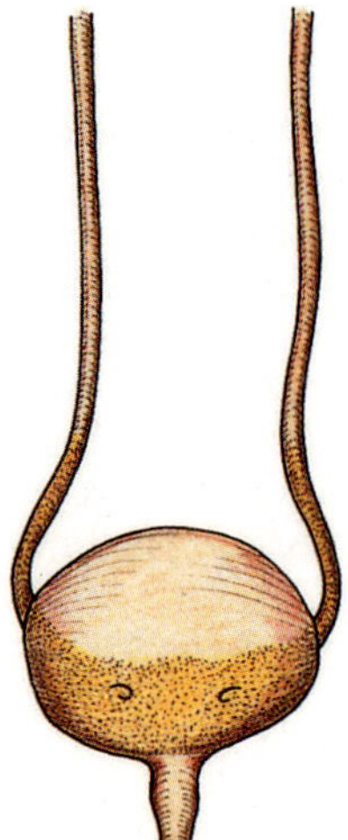

FIG. 47-9 Stasis of urine with reflux to ureters.

kidney needs to enter the bladder unaided by gravity. Because the peristaltic contractions of the ureters are insufficient to overcome gravity, the renal pelvis fills before urine enters the ureters (Fig. 47-9). This condition is called **urinary stasis** and increases the risk of urinary tract infection and renal calculi (see Chapter 45). **Renal calculi** are calcium stones that lodge in the renal pelvis or pass through the ureters. Immobilized patients are at risk for calculi because they frequently have hypercalcemia.

As the period of immobility continues, fluid intake often diminishes. When combined with other problems such as fever, the risk for dehydration increases. As a result, urinary output declines on or about the fifth or sixth day after immobilization, and the urine becomes concentrated. This concentrated urine increases the risk for calculi formation and infection. Inappropriate perineal care after bowel movements, particularly in women, increases the risk of urinary tract contamination by *Escherichia coli* bacteria. Another cause of urinary tract infections in immobilized patients is the use of an indwelling urinary catheter.

Integumentary Changes. The changes in metabolism that accompany immobility add to the harmful effect of pressure on the skin in the immobilized patient. This makes immobility a major risk factor for pressure ulcers. Any break in the integrity of the skin is difficult to heal. Preventing a pressure ulcer is much less expensive than treating one; therefore preventive nursing interventions are imperative (WOCN, 2009).

A **pressure ulcer** is an impairment of the skin as a result of prolonged ischemia (decreased blood supply) in tissues (see Chapter 48). The ulcer is characterized initially by inflammation and usually forms over a bony prominence. Ischemia develops when the pressure on the skin is greater than the pressure inside the small peripheral blood vessels supplying blood to the skin.

Tissue metabolism depends on the supply of oxygen and nutrients to and the elimination of metabolic wastes from the blood. Pressure affects cellular metabolism by decreasing or totally eliminating tissue circulation. When a patient lies in bed or sits in a chair, the weight of the body is on bony prominences. The longer the pressure is applied, the longer the period of ischemia and therefore the greater the risk of skin breakdown. The older adult is especially at risk. For example, an older adult who is immobilized on a backboard following a trauma can develop skin breakdown within 3 hours (Fletcher, 2005).

Psychosocial Effects. Immobilization often leads to emotional and behavioral responses, sensory alterations, and changes in coping. When normal, healthy young men who were part of a National Aeronautics and Space Administration (NASA) study were on bed rest for several weeks, they exhibited signs of sensory deprivation: altered sleep patterns and significant increases in anxiety, hostility, and depression (Fletcher, 2005). Every patient responds to immobility differently.

Patients with restricted mobility may have some depression. Depression is an affective disorder characterized by exaggerated feelings of sadness, melancholy, dejection, worthlessness, emptiness, and hopelessness out of proportion to reality. It results from worrying about present and future levels of health, finances, and family needs. Because immobilization removes the patient from a daily routine, he or she has more time to worry about disability. Worrying quickly increases the patient's depression, causing withdrawal. Withdrawn patients often do not want to participate in their own care.

Developmental Changes

Developmental changes tend to be associated with immobility in the very young and older adults. The immobilized young or middle-age adult who has been healthy experiences few, if any, developmental changes. However, there are exceptions. For example, a mother with complications following birth has to go onto bed rest and as a result cannot interact with her newborn as expected.

Infants, Toddlers, and Preschoolers. The newborn infant's spine is flexed and lacks the anteroposterior curves of the adult (see Chapter 12). As the baby grows, musculoskeletal development permits support of weight for standing and walking. Posture is awkward because the head and upper trunk are carried forward. Because body weight is not distributed evenly along a line of gravity, posture is off balance, and falls occur often. The infant, toddler, or preschooler is usually immobilized because of trauma or the need to correct a congenital skeletal abnormality. Prolonged immobilization delays the child's gross motor skills, intellectual development, or musculoskeletal development.

Adolescents. The adolescent stage usually begins with a tremendous increase in growth (see Chapter 12). Growth is frequently uneven. Prolonged immobilization alters adolescent growth patterns. In addition, adolescents who experience immobility often are behind peers in gaining independence and accomplishing certain skills such as obtaining a driver's license. Social isolation is a concern for this age-group when immobilization occurs.

Adults. An adult who has correct posture and body alignment feels good, looks good, and generally appears self-confident. The healthy adult also has the necessary musculoskeletal development and coordination to carry out ADLs (see Chapter 13). When periods of prolonged immobility occur, all physiological systems are at risk. In addition, the role of the adult often changes with regard to the family or social structure. Some adults lose their jobs, which affects their self-concept (see Chapter 33).

Older Adults. A progressive loss of total bone mass occurs with the older adult. Some of the possible causes of this loss include decreased physical activity, hormonal changes, and bone resorption. The effect of bone loss is weaker bones. Older adults often walk more slowly, take smaller steps, and appear less coordinated. Prescribed medications alter their sense of balance or affect their blood pressure when they change position too quickly, increasing their risk for falls and injuries (see Chapter 14). The outcomes of a fall include not only possible injury but also hospitalization, loss of independence, psychological effects, and quite possibly death (Yeom et al., 2009).

Older adults often experience functional status changes secondary to hospitalization and altered mobility status (Box 47-1). Immobilization of older adults increases their physical dependence on others and accelerates functional losses. Immobilization of some older adults results from a degenerative disease, neurological trauma, or chronic illness. In others it occurs gradually and progressively, and in others—especially those who have had a stroke—immobilization is sudden. When providing nursing care for an older adult, encourage the patient to perform as many self-care activities as possible, thereby maintaining the highest level of mobility. Sometimes nurses inadvertently contribute to a patient's immobility by providing unnecessary help with activities such as bathing and transferring.

BOX 47-1 FOCUS ON OLDER ADULTS

Problems of Nutrition As They Relate to Hospitalized Immobile Older Adults

For many older adults, admission to the hospital often results in functional decline despite the treatment for which they were admitted. Some older adults have problems related to mobility and quickly regress to a dependent state. But keeping in mind their nutritional needs and status is extremely important.

Usual aging is associated with decreased muscle strength and aerobic capacity. This becomes exacerbated when the nutritional state is not assessed properly.

- A nutritional assessment needs to be included in the plan of care for the older adult experiencing immobility.
- Anorexia and insufficient assistance with eating lead to malnutrition, which contributes to the known problems associated with immobility.
- There is a direct relationship between the success of older adults' rehabilitation and their nutritional status.

CRITICAL THINKING

Critical thinking requires the combination of knowledge, experiences, patient data, critical thinking attitudes, and intellectual and professional standards. The needs of the immobile patient are multiple and complex. After conducting a thorough assessment, the nurse identifies appropriate nursing diagnoses and implements effective nursing care.

To understand the impact of immobility on the patient and family, integrate knowledge from nursing and other disciplines, previous experiences, and information gathered from patients. In addition, the use of critical thinking attitudes is necessary when designing a plan of care for successful interventions related to immobility. Professional standards such as those developed by the Agency for Healthcare Research and Quality (AHRQ, 2009) and the Wound, Ostomy and Continence Nurses Society (WOCN, 2009) and intellectual standards such as accuracy provide valuable guides for mobility management (Fig. 47-10). In addition, many agencies have standards for practice related to transferring patients and fall and pressure ulcer prevention.

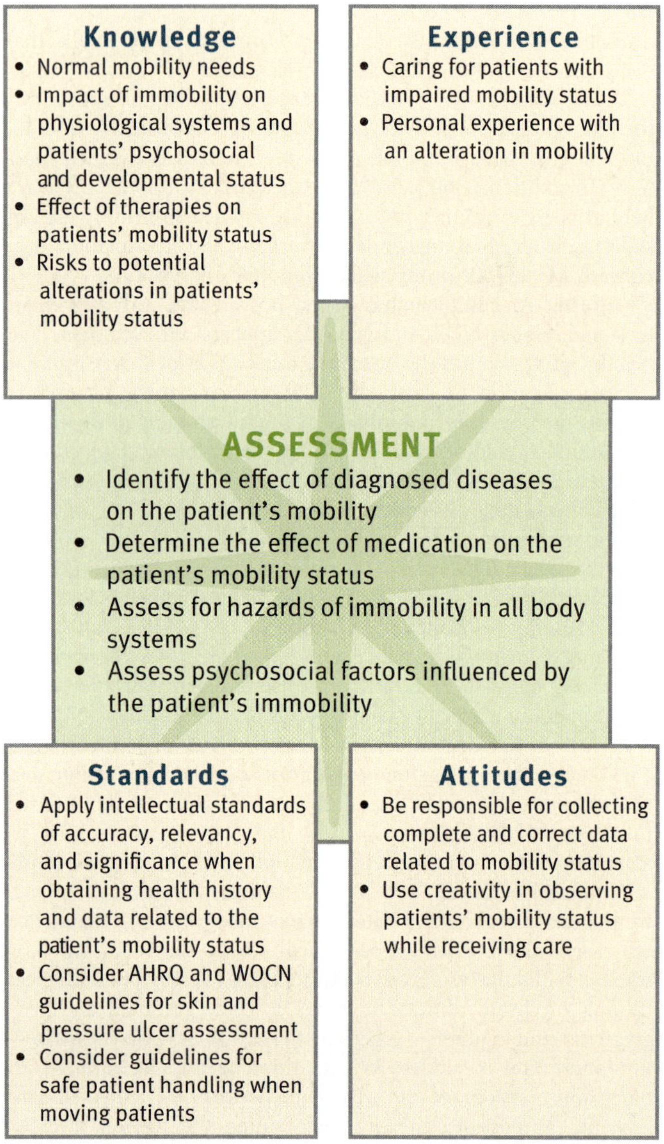

Knowledge
• Normal mobility needs
• Impact of immobility on physiological systems and patients' psychosocial and developmental status
• Effect of therapies on patients' mobility status
• Risks to potential alterations in patients' mobility status
Experience
• Caring for patients with impaired mobility status
• Personal experience with an alteration in mobility
ASSESSMENT
• Identify the effect of diagnosed diseases on the patient's mobility
• Determine the effect of medication on the patient's mobility status
• Assess for hazards of immobility in all body systems
• Assess psychosocial factors influenced by the patient's immobility
Standards
• Apply intellectual standards of accuracy, relevancy, and significance when obtaining health history and data related to the patient's mobility status
• Consider AHRQ and WOCN guidelines for skin and pressure ulcer assessment
• Consider guidelines for safe patient handling when moving patients
Attitudes
• Be responsible for collecting complete and correct data related to mobility status
• Use creativity in observing patients' mobility status while receiving care

FIG. 47-10 Critical thinking model for immobility assessment. *AHRQ,* Agency for Healthcare Research and Quality; *WOCN,* Wound, Ostomy and Continence Nurses Society.

NURSING PROCESS

Apply the nursing process and use a critical thinking approach in your care of patients. The nursing process provides a clinical decision-making approach for you to develop an individualized plan of care. Patients with preexisting mobility impairments and those who are at risk for immobility will *greatly benefit* from your application of the nursing process and the use of your critical thinking skills to design a care plan that improves the patient's functional status, promotes self-care, maintains psychological well-being, and reduces the hazards of immobility.

ASSESSMENT

During the assessment process, thoroughly assess each patient and critically analyze findings to ensure that you make patient-centered clinical decisions required for safe nursing care. Nursing assessment of the patient includes aspects of both mobility and immobility.

Through the Patient's Eyes. Usually the nurse assesses for and asks questions about the patient's degree of both mobility and immobility during physical examination (Box 47-2). Keep in mind that the patient is a full partner in providing information and designing the plan of care. You convey respect for the patient's preferences, values, and needs when implementing the nursing process and designing a plan of care with the patient (Cromwell and Berg, 2006).

Mobility. Assessment of patient mobility focuses on ROM, gait, exercise and activity tolerance, and body alignment. When unsure of the patient's abilities, begin assessment of mobility with the patient in the most supportive position and move to higher levels according to his or her tolerance. Generally the assessment of movement starts while the patient is lying and proceeds to assessing sitting positions in bed, transfers to chair, and finally walking. This helps to protect the patient's safety.

Range of Motion. Range of motion (ROM) is the maximum amount of movement available at a joint in one of the three planes

BOX 47-2 NURSING ASSESSMENT QUESTIONS

Mobility

- Describe any changes you've noticed in your ability to walk and take care of yourself on a daily basis.
- Have you experienced any stiffness, swelling, pain, or difficulty with moving? If so, describe how you felt.
- Have you noticed any shortness of breath?

Immobility

- Describe your normal daily activity. Has this changed recently?
- How have your appetite and diet changed since you've had problems moving around?
- Describe what you eat in a normal day.
- Does your day seem very long?
- Are you sleeping well at night?
- Have you noticed any places on your skin that are reddened or have any open sores?
- Describe any changes you've noticed in urinating and/or in having bowel movements.

of the body: sagittal, transverse, or frontal (Fig. 47-11). The sagittal plane is a line that passes through the body from front to back, dividing it into a left and right side. The frontal plane passes through the body from side to side and divides it into front and back. The transverse plane is a horizontal line that divides the body into upper and lower portions.

Ligaments, muscles, and the nature of the joint limit joint mobility in each of the planes. However, some joint movements are specific to each plane. In the sagittal plane movements are flexion and extension (e.g., fingers and elbows), dorsiflexion and plantar flexion (feet), and extension (e.g., hip). In the frontal plane movements are abduction and adduction (e.g., arms and legs) and eversion and inversion (feet). In the transverse plane movements are pronation and supination (hands) and internal and external rotation (hips).

When assessing ROM, ask questions about and physically examine the patient for stiffness, swelling, pain, limited movement, and unequal movement. Chapter 30 describes specific techniques for measuring the degrees of motion in a joint. Assessment of ROM is important as a baseline measure to compare and evaluate whether loss in joint mobility has occurred. Patients whose mobility is restricted require ROM exercises to reduce the hazards of immobility. Therefore assess the type of ROM exercise that a patient is able to perform. ROM exercises are active (the patient moves all joints through their ROM unassisted), passive (the patient is unable to move independently, and the nurse moves each joint through its ROM), or somewhere in between (Table 47-2). For example,

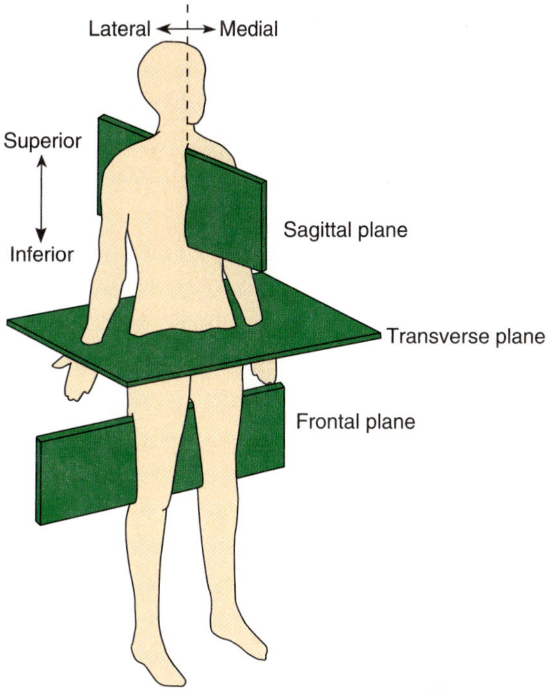

FIG. 47-11 Planes of body.

TABLE 47-2 Range-of-Motion Exercises

BODY PART	TYPE OF JOINT	TYPE OF MOVEMENT	RANGE (DEGREES)	PRIMARY MUSCLES
Neck, cervical spine	Pivotal	*Flexion:* Bring chin to rest on chest.	45	Sternocleidomastoid
		Extension: Return head to erect position.	45	Trapezius
		Hyperextension: Bend head back as far as possible.	10	Trapezius
		Lateral flexion: Tilt head as far as possible toward each shoulder.	40-45	Sternocleidomastoid
		Rotation: Turn head as far as possible in circular movement.	180	Sternocleidomastoid, trapezius
Shoulder	Ball and socket	*Flexion:* Raise arm from side position forward to position above head.	180 45-60	Coracobrachialis, biceps brachii, deltoid, pectoralis major
		Extension: Return arm to position at side of body.	180	Latissimus dorsi, teres major, triceps brachii
		Hyperextension: Move arm behind body, keeping elbow straight.	45-60	Latissimus dorsi, teres major, deltoid
		Abduction: Raise arm to side to position above head with palm away from head.	180	Deltoid, supraspinatus
		Adduction: Lower arm sideways and across body as far as possible.	320	Pectoralis major
		Internal rotation: With elbow flexed, rotate shoulder by moving arm until thumb is turned inward and toward back.	90	Pectoralis major, latissimus dorsi, teres major, subscapularis
		External rotation: With elbow flexed, move arm until thumb is upward and lateral to head.	90	Infraspinatus, teres major, deltoid
		Circumduction: Move arm in full circle (Circumduction is combination of all movements of ball-and-socket joint.)	360	Deltoid, coracobrachialis, latissimus dorsi, teres major
Elbow	Hinge	*Flexion:* Bend elbow so lower arm moves toward its shoulder joint and hand is level with shoulder.	150	Biceps brachii, brachialis, brachioradialis
		Extension: Straighten elbow by lowering hand.	150	Triceps brachii
Forearm	Pivotal	*Supination:* Turn lower arm and hand so palm is up.	70-90	Supinator, biceps brachii
		Pronation: Turn lower arm so palm is down.	70-90	Pronator teres, pronator quadratus

Continued

TABLE 47-2 Range-of-Motion Exercises—cont'd

BODY PART	TYPE OF JOINT	TYPE OF MOVEMENT	RANGE (DEGREES)	PRIMARY MUSCLES
Wrist	Condyloid	*Flexion:* Move palm toward inner aspect of forearm.	80-90	Flexor carpi ulnaris, flexor carpi radialis
		Extension: Move fingers and hand posterior to midline.	80-90	Extensor carpi radialis brevis, extensor carpi radialis longus, extensor carpi ulnaris
		Hyperextension: Bring dorsal surface of hand back as far as possible.	80-90	Extensor carpi radialis brevis, extensor carpi radialis longus, extensor carpi ulnaris
		Abduction: Place hand with palm down and extend wrist laterally toward fifth finger.	Up to 30	Flexor carpi radialis, extensor carpi radialis brevis, extensor carpi radialis longus
		Adduction: Place hand with palm down and extend wrist medially toward thumb.	30-50	Flexor carpi ulnaris, extensor carpi ulnaris
Fingers	Condyloid hinge	*Flexion:* Make fist.	90	Lumbricales, interosseus volaris, interosseus dorsalis
		Extension: Straighten fingers.	90	Extensor digiti quinti proprius, extensor digitorum communis, extensor indicis proprius
		Hyperextension: Bend fingers back as far as possible.	30-60	
		Abduction: Spread fingers apart.	30	Interosseus dorsalis
		Adduction: Bring fingers together.	30	Interosseus volaris
Thumb	Saddle	*Flexion:* Move thumb across palmar surface of hand.	90	Flexor pollicis brevis
		Extension: Move thumb straight away from hand.	90	Extensor pollicis longus, extensor pollicis brevis
		Abduction: Extend thumb laterally (usually done when placing fingers in abduction and adduction).	30	Abductor pollicis brevis
		Adduction: Move thumb back toward hand.	30	Adductor pollicis obliquus, adductor pollicis transversus
		Opposition: Touch thumb to each finger of same hand.		Opponens pollicis, opponens digiti minimi
Hip	Ball and socket	*Flexion:* Move leg forward and up.	90-120	Psoas major, iliacus, sartorius
		Extension: Move back beside other leg.	90-120	Gluteus maximus, semitendinosus, semimembranosus
		Hyperextension: Move leg behind body.	30-50	Gluteus maximus, semitendinosus, semimembranosus
		Abduction: Move leg laterally away from body.	30-50	Gluteus medius, gluteus minimus
		Adduction: Move leg back toward medial position and beyond if possible.	30-50	Adductor longus, adductor brevis, adductor magnus
		Internal rotation: Turn foot and leg toward other leg.	90	Gluteus medius, gluteus minimus, tensor fasciae latae
		External rotation: Turn foot and leg away from other leg.	90	Obturatorius internus, obturatorius externus
		Circumduction: Move leg in circle.		Psoas major, gluteus maximus, gluteus medius, adductor magnus
Knee	Hinge	*Flexion:* Bring heel back toward back of thigh.	120-130	Biceps femoris, semitendinosus, semimembranosus, sartorius
		Extension: Return leg to floor.	120-130	Rectus femoris, vastus lateralis, vastus medialis, vastus intermedius
Ankle	Hinge	*Dorsal flexion:* Move foot so toes are pointed upward.	20-30	Tibialis anterior
		Plantar flexion: Move foot so toes are pointed downward.	45-50	Gastrocnemius, soleus
Foot	Gliding	*Inversion:* Turn sole of foot medially.	10 or less	Tibialis anterior, tibialis posterior
		Eversion: Turn sole of foot laterally.	10 or less	Peroneus longus, peroneus brevis
Toes	Condyloid	*Flexion:* Curl toes downward.	30-60	Flexor digitorum, lumbricalis pedis, flexor hallucis brevis
		Extension: Straighten toes.	30-60	Extensor digitorum longus, extensor digitorum brevis, extensor hallucis longus
		Abduction: Spread toes apart.	15 or less	Abductor hallucis, interosseus dorsalis
		Adduction: Bring toes together.	15 or less	Adductor hallucis, interosseus plantaris

provide support for a weak patient while the patient performs most of the movement. Some patients are able to move some joints actively, whereas the nurse passively moves others. First consider the medical plan of care and if active ROM exercises are appropriate; then assess the patient's ability to engage in active ROM exercises and the need for assistance, teaching, or reinforcement. In general, exercises need to be as active as health and mobility allow. Contractures develop in joints not moved periodically through their full ROM. Assessment data from patients with limited joint movements vary based on the area affected.

Neck. A flexion contracture of the neck is a serious disability because the patient's neck is permanently flexed with the chin close to or actually touching the chest. Assessment reveals altered body alignment, changes in the visual field, and decreased level of independent functioning.

Shoulder. One feature of the shoulder that sets it apart from other joints in the body is that the strongest muscle controlling it, the deltoid, is in complete elongation in the normal position. No other muscle exerts its full strength when in complete elongation. Patients with limited movement in the shoulder have difficulty moving their arms.

Elbow. The elbow functions optimally at an angle of approximately 90 degrees. An elbow fixed in full extension is disabling and limits the patient's independence.

Forearm. Most functions of the hand are best carried out with the forearm in moderate pronation. When the forearm is fixed in a position of full supination, the patient's use of the hand is limited.

Wrist. The primary function of the wrist is to place the hand in slight dorsiflexion, the position of functioning. When the wrist is fixed in even a slightly flexed position, the grasp is weakened.

Fingers and Thumb. The ROM in the fingers and thumb enables the patient to perform ADLs and activities requiring fine-motor skills such as carpentry, needlework, drawing, and painting. The functional position of the fingers and thumb is slight flexion of the thumb in opposition to the fingers.

Hip. Because the lower extremities are concerned chiefly with locomotion and weight bearing, stability of the hip joint is more important than its mobility. For example, if one hip has no mobility but is fixed in a neutral position and fully extended, it is possible to walk without a significant limp. However, contractures often fix the hip in positions of deformity. Excessive abduction makes the affected leg appear too short, whereas excessive adduction makes it appear too long. In either case the patient has limited locomotion and walks with an obvious limp. Internal and external rotation contractures cause an abnormal and unbalanced gait.

Knee. A primary function of the knee is stability, which is achieved by ROM, ligaments, and muscles. However, the knees cannot remain stable under weight-bearing conditions unless there is adequate quadriceps power to maintain the knee in full extension. An immobile knee joint results in serious disability. The degree of disability depends on the position in which the knee is stiffened. If it is fixed in full extension, the person needs to sit with the leg out in front. When the knee is flexed, the person limps while walking. The greater the flexion, the greater is the limp.

Ankle and Foot. Without full ROM of the ankle, gait deviations occur. If the joint is not stable, the person falls. When the person relaxes as in sleep or coma, the foot relaxes and assumes a position of plantar flexion. As a result, it becomes fixed in plantar flexion (footdrop), which impairs the ability to walk.

Toes. Excessive flexion of the toes results in clawing. When this is a permanent deformity, the foot is unable to rest flat on the floor, and the patient is unable to walk properly. Flexion contractures are the most common foot deformity associated with reduced joint mobility.

Gait. The term gait describes a particular manner or style of walking. The gait cycle begins with the heel strike of one leg and continues to the heel strike of the other leg. Assessing a patient's gait allows you to draw conclusions about balance, posture, safety, and ability to walk without assistance. The mechanics of human gait involve coordination of the skeletal, neurological, and muscular systems of the human body.

Exercise and Activity Tolerance. Exercise is physical activity for conditioning the body, improving health, and maintaining fitness. Nurses use it as therapy to correct a deformity or restore the overall body to a maximal state of health. When a person exercises, physiological changes occur in body systems (see Chapter 38).

Assessment of the patient's energy level includes the physiological effects of exercise and activity tolerance. Activity tolerance is the type and amount of exercise or work that a person is able to perform. Assessment of activity tolerance is necessary when planning activity such as walking, ROM exercises, or ADLs. Activity tolerance assessment includes data from physiological, emotional, and developmental domains (see Chapter 38). This assessment is applicable in all clinical settings.

As activity begins, monitor patients for symptoms such as dyspnea, fatigue, chest pain, and/or a change in vital signs. The weak or debilitated patient is unable to sustain even slight changes in activity because of the increased demand for energy. Seemingly simple tasks such as eating and moving in bed often result in extreme fatigue. When the patient experiences decreased activity tolerance, carefully assess how much time he or she needs to recover. Decreasing recovery time indicates improving activity tolerance.

People who are depressed, worried, or anxious are frequently unable to tolerate exercise. Depressed patients tend to withdraw rather than participate. Patients who worry or are frequently anxious expend a tremendous amount of mental energy and often report feeling fatigued. Because of this, they also experience physical and emotional exhaustion.

Developmental changes also affect activity tolerance. As the infant enters the toddler stage, the activity level increases, and the need for sleep declines. The child entering preschool or primary grades expends mental energy in learning and often requires more rest after school or before strenuous play. The adolescent going through puberty requires more rest because much body energy is expended for growth and hormone changes (see Chapter 42).

Changes still occur through the adult years, but many of them are related to work and lifestyle choices. Pregnancy causes fluctuations in a woman's energy tolerance, especially during the first and third trimesters, when she experiences increased fatigue. Hormonal changes and fetal development use body energy, and the woman is sometimes unable or unmotivated to carry out physical activities. During the last trimester fetal development consumes a great deal of the mother's energy; and the size and location of the fetus limit the ability to take a deep breath, resulting in less oxygen being available for physical activities.

As the person grows older, activity tolerance changes. Muscle mass is reduced, and posture and bone composition change. Changes in the cardiorespiratory system such as decreased maximum heart rate and lung compliance, which affect the intensity of exercise, often occur. As age progresses, some older individuals still exercise but do so at a reduced intensity. The more inactive a patient is, the more pronounced are these activity changes.

Body Alignment. Perform assessment of body alignment with the patient standing, sitting, or lying down. This assessment has the following objectives:

- Determining normal physiological changes in body alignment resulting from growth and development for each patient
- Identifying deviations in body alignment caused by incorrect posture
- Providing opportunities for patients to observe their posture
- Identifying learning needs of patients for maintaining correct body alignment
- Identifying trauma, muscle damage, or nerve dysfunction
- Obtaining information concerning other factors that contribute to incorrect alignment such as fatigue, malnutrition, and psychological problems

The first step in assessing body alignment is to put patients at ease so they do not assume unnatural or rigid positions. When assessing the body alignment of an immobilized or unconscious patient, remove pillows and positioning supports from the bed and place the patient in the supine position.

Standing. Characteristics of correct body alignment for the standing patient include the following:

1. The head is erect and midline.
2. When observed posteriorly, the shoulders and hips are straight and parallel.
3. When observed posteriorly, the vertebral column is straight.
4. When observed laterally, the head is erect, and the spinal curves are aligned in a reversed S pattern. The cervical vertebrae are anteriorly convex, the thoracic vertebrae are posteriorly convex, and the lumbar vertebrae are anteriorly convex.
5. When observed laterally, the abdomen is comfortably tucked in, and the knees and ankles are slightly flexed. The person appears comfortable and does not seem conscious of the flexion of knees or ankles.
6. The arms hang comfortably at the sides.
7. The feet are slightly apart to achieve a base of support, and the toes are pointed forward.
8. When viewing the patient from behind, the center of gravity is in the midline, and the line of gravity is from the middle of the forehead to a midpoint between the feet. Laterally the line of gravity runs vertically from the middle of the skull to the posterior third of the foot (Fig. 47-12).

Sitting. Characteristics of correct alignment of the sitting patient include the following:

1. The head is erect, and the neck and vertebral column are in straight alignment.
2. The body weight is distributed evenly on the buttocks and thighs.
3. The thighs are parallel and in a horizontal plane.
4. Both feet are supported on the floor (Fig. 47-13), and the ankles are flexed comfortably. With patients of short stature, use a footstool to ensure that ankles are flexed comfortably.
5. A 2.5- to 5-cm (1- to 2-inch) space is maintained between the edge of the seat and the popliteal space on the posterior surface of the knee. This space ensures that there is no pressure on the popliteal artery or nerve to decrease circulation or impair nerve function.
6. The patient's forearms are supported on the armrest, in the lap, or on a table in front of the chair.

It is particularly important to assess alignment when sitting if the patient has muscle weakness, muscle paralysis, or nerve damage.

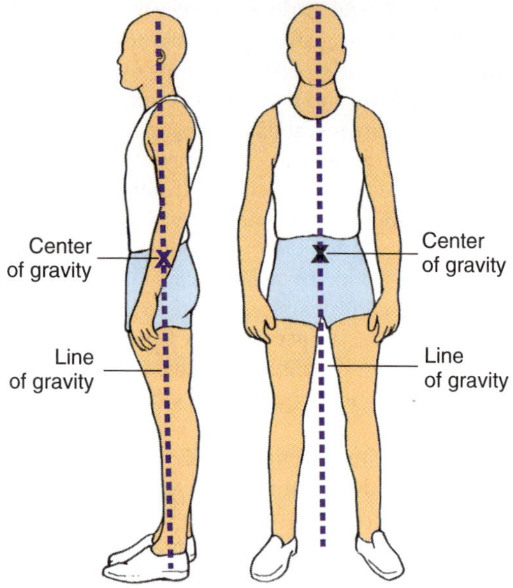

FIG. 47-12 Correct body alignment when standing.

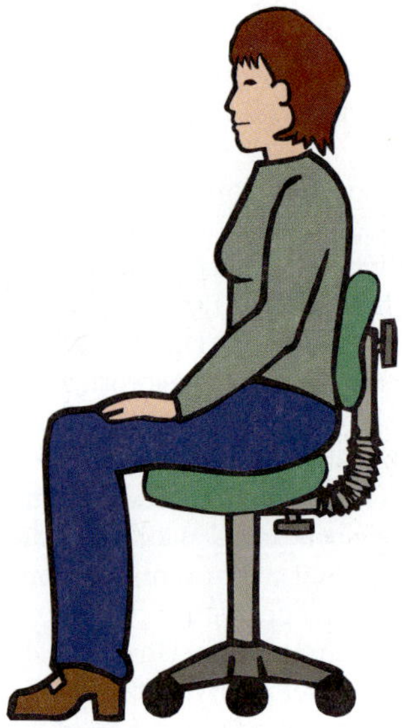

FIG. 47-13 Correct body alignment when sitting.

Patients who have these problems have diminished sensation in the affected area and are unable to perceive pressure or decreased circulation. Proper alignment while sitting reduces the risk of musculoskeletal system damage in such a patient. The patient with severe respiratory disease sometimes assumes a posture of leaning on the table in front of the chair in an attempt to breathe more easily. This is called *orthopnea.*

Lying. People who are conscious have voluntary muscle control and normal perception of pressure. As a result, they usually assume a position of comfort when lying down. Because their ROM, sensation, and circulation are within normal limits, they change positions when they perceive muscle strain and decreased circulation.

Assess body alignment for a patient who is immobilized or bedridden with the patient in the lateral position. Remove all positioning supports from the bed except for the pillow under the head and support the body with an adequate mattress (Fig. 47-14). This

TABLE 47-3 **Assessment of the Physiological Hazards of Immobility**

SYSTEM	ASSESSMENT TECHNIQUES	ABNORMAL FINDINGS
Metabolic	Inspection	Slowed wound healing, abnormal laboratory data
	Inspection	Muscle atrophy
	Anthropometric measurements (mid-upper arm circumference, triceps skinfold measurement)	Decreased amount of subcutaneous fat
	Palpation	Generalized edema
Respiratory	Inspection	Asymmetrical chest wall movement, dyspnea, increased respiratory rate
	Auscultation	Crackles, wheezes
Cardiovascular	Auscultation	Orthostatic hypotension
	Auscultation, palpation	Increased heart rate, third heart sound, weak peripheral pulses, peripheral edema
Musculoskeletal	Inspection, palpation	Decreased range of motion, erythema, increased diameter in calf or thigh
	Palpation	Joint contracture
	Inspection	Activity intolerance, muscle atrophy, joint contracture
Skin	Inspection, palpation	Break in skin integrity
Elimination	Inspection	Decreased urine output, cloudy or concentrated urine, decreased frequency of bowel movements
	Palpation	Distended bladder and abdomen
	Auscultation	Decreased bowel sounds

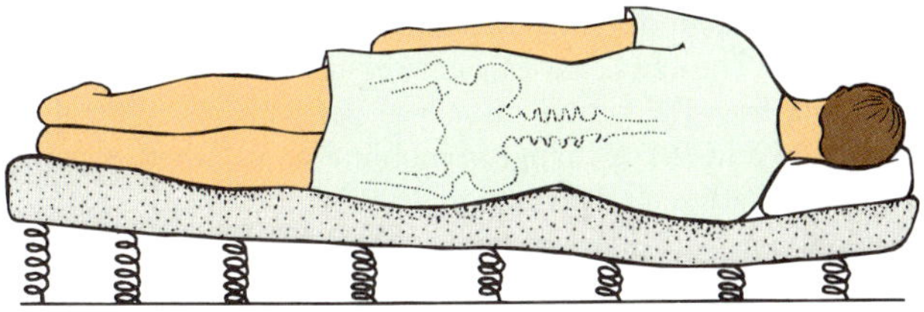
FIG. 47-14 Correct body alignment when lying down.

position allows for full view of the spine and back and helps provide other baseline body alignment data such as whether the patient is able to remain positioned without aid. The vertebrae are aligned, and the position does not cause discomfort. Patients with impaired mobility (e.g., traction or arthritis), decreased sensation (e.g., hemiparesis following a CVA), impaired circulation (e.g., diabetes), and lack of voluntary muscle control (e.g., spinal cord injury) are at risk for damage when lying down.

Immobility. Assess the patient for hazards of immobility by performing a head-to-toe physical assessment (see Chapter 30). In addition, focus on certain physiological areas and the patient's psychosocial and developmental dimensions. Table 47-3 summarizes how to assess for the physiological hazards of immobility.

Metabolic System. When assessing metabolic functioning, use **anthropometric measurements** (measures of height, weight, and skinfold thickness) to evaluate muscle atrophy (see Chapter 30). In addition, analyze intake and output records for fluid balance. Does intake equal output? Intake and output measurements help the nurse determine whether a fluid imbalance exists (see Chapter 41). Dehydration and edema increase the rate of skin breakdown in a patient who is immobilized. Monitoring laboratory data such as levels of electrolytes, serum protein (albumin and total protein), and blood urea nitrogen (BUN) aid the nurse in determining metabolic functioning.

Monitoring food intake and elimination patterns and assessing wound healing help to determine altered gastrointestinal functioning and potential metabolic problems. If the patient has a wound, the rate of healing indicates how well nutrients are delivered to tissues. Normal progression of healing indicates that metabolic needs of injured tissues are being met. Anorexia commonly occurs in patients who are immobilized. Assess the patient's food intake before the meal tray is removed to determine the amount eaten. Assess his or her dietary patterns and food preferences at the onset of immobilization to help prevent nutritional imbalances (see Chapter 44).

Respiratory System. Perform a respiratory assessment at least every 2 hours for patients with restricted activity. Inspect chest wall movements during the full inspiratory-expiratory cycle. If a patient has an atelectatic area, chest movement is often asymmetrical. Auscultate the entire lung region to identify diminished breath sounds, crackles, or wheezes. Focus auscultation on the dependent lung fields because pulmonary secretions tend to collect in these lower regions.

Cardiovascular System. Cardiovascular nursing assessment of the patient who is immobilized includes blood pressure monitoring, evaluation of apical and peripheral pulses, and observation for signs of venous stasis (e.g., edema and delayed wound healing).

Although not all patients experience orthostatic hypotension, nurses monitor their vital signs during the first few attempts at sitting or standing (see Chapter 29). Move the patient gradually during position changes and monitor him or her closely for dizziness while assessing orthostatic blood pressures. The longer the period of immobility, the greater is the risk of hypotension when the patient stands (Huether and McCance, 2008).

Also assess apical and peripheral pulses (see Chapter 30). Recumbent positions increase cardiac workload and result in an increased pulse rate. In some patients, particularly older adults, the heart does not tolerate the increased workload, and a form of cardiac failure develops. A third heart sound, heard at the apex, is an early indication of congestive heart failure. Monitoring peripheral pulses allows the nurse to evaluate the ability of the heart to pump blood. Immediately document and report the absence of a peripheral pulse in the lower extremities to the patient's health care provider, especially if the pulse was present previously.

Edema sometimes develops in patients who have had injury or whose heart is unable to handle the increased workload of bed rest. Because edema moves to dependent body regions, assessment of the patient experiencing immobility includes the sacrum, legs, and feet. If the heart is unable to tolerate the increased workload, peripheral body regions such as the hands, feet, nose, and earlobes are colder than central body regions. To assess for a deep vein thrombosis (DVT), remove the patient's elastic stockings and/or sequential compression devices (SCDs) every 8 hours (or according to agency policy) and observe the calves for redness, warmth, and tenderness. Homans' sign, or calf pain on dorsiflexion of the foot, is contraindicated in patients when a DVT is suspected. It is no longer a reliable indicator in assessing for DVT, and it is present in other conditions (see Chapter 30).

Measure bilateral calf circumference and record it daily as an alternative assessment for DVT. To do this, mark a point on each calf 10 cm (3.9 inches) down from the midpatella. Measure the circumference each day using the mark for placement of the tape measure. Unilateral increases in calf circumference are an early indication of thrombosis. Because DVTs also occur in the thigh, take thigh measurements daily if the patient is prone to thrombosis. A dislodged venous thrombus, called an **embolus,** can travel through the circulatory system to the lungs and impair circulation and oxygenation, resulting in tachycardia and shortness of breath. Venous emboli that travel to the lungs are sometimes life threatening. More than 90% of all pulmonary emboli begin in the deep veins of the lower extremities (Huether and McCance, 2008).

Musculoskeletal System. Major musculoskeletal abnormalities to identify during nursing assessment include decreased muscle tone and strength, loss of muscle mass, and contractures. The anthropometric measurements described previously indicate losses in muscle tone and muscle mass.

Early assessment of ROM is important because it establishes a baseline against which later measurements can be compared to evaluate whether a loss in joint mobility has occurred. Measure ROM with a goniometer (see Fig. 38-9). Physical assessment cannot identify disuse osteoporosis. However, patients on prolonged bed rest, postmenopausal women, patients taking steroids, and people with increased serum and urine calcium levels have a greater risk for bone demineralization. Consider the risk of disuse osteoporosis when planning nursing interventions. Although some falls result in injury, others occur because of pathological fractures secondary to osteoporosis.

Integumentary System. Continually assess the patient's skin for breakdown and color changes such as pallor or redness. Consistently use a standardized tool such as the Braden Scale. This identifies patients with a high risk for impaired skin integrity or early changes in the condition of patients' skin. Early identification allows for early intervention. Observe the skin often during routine care (e.g., when the patient is turned, during hygiene measures, and when providing for elimination needs). At a minimum, skin assessment occurs every 2 hours (see Chapter 48).

Elimination System. Evaluate the patient's elimination status on each shift and total intake and output every 24 hours. Compare the amounts over time. Determine that the patient is receiving the correct amount and type of fluids orally or parenterally (see Chapters 41 and 45). Inadequate intake and output or fluid and electrolyte imbalances increase the risk for renal system impairment, ranging from recurrent infections to kidney failure. Dehydration also increases the risk for skin breakdown, thrombus formation, respiratory infections, and constipation.

Assessment of elimination status includes the adequacy of dietary choices, bowel sounds, and the frequency and consistency of bowel movements (see Chapter 46). Accurate assessment enables the nurse to intervene before constipation and fecal impaction occur.

Psychosocial Assessment. Many alterations in physiological, sociocultural, and developmental functioning are related to immobility. Often these problems are interrelated, and it is imperative that nursing care focuses on all dimensions. Often the focus of immobility is on the easily visible physical problems such as skin impairment, but do not overlook its psychosocial and developmental aspects.

Abrupt changes in personality often have a physiological cause such as surgery, a medication reaction, a pulmonary embolus, or an acute infection. For example, the primary symptom of compromised older patients with an acute urinary tract infection or fever is confusion. Identifying confusion is an important component of the nurse's assessment. Acute confusion in older adults is not normal; a thorough nursing assessment is the priority (Ebersole et al., 2008).

Common reactions to immobilization include boredom and feelings of isolation, depression, and anger. Observe for changes in a patient's emotional status and listen carefully to family if they report emotional changes. Examples of change that indicate psychosocial concerns are a cooperative patient who becomes less cooperative or an independent patient who asks for more help than is necessary. The nurse investigates reasons for such alterations. Identifying how the patient usually copes with loss is vital (see Chapters 35 and 36). A change in mobility status, whether permanent or not, causes a grief reaction. Families are a key resource for information about behavior changes.

Identify and correct unexplained changes in the sleep-wake cycle. Nurses prevent or minimize most stimuli that interrupt the sleep-wake cycle (e.g., nursing activities, a noisy environment, or discomfort). However, some medications such as analgesics, sleeping pills, or cardiovascular drugs also cause sleep disturbances (see Chapter 42).

Because psychosocial changes usually occur gradually, observe the patient's behavior on a daily basis. If behavioral changes occur, determine the cause(s) and evaluate the changes. Identifying the cause helps you to design appropriate nursing interventions.

Developmental Assessment. Include a developmental assessment of patients who are immobilized. When caring for a young child, determine whether he or she is able to meet developmental tasks and is progressing normally. The child's development sometimes regresses or slows because he or she is immobilized. Design nursing interventions that maintain normal development, provide physical and psychosocial stimuli after identifying a child's developmental needs, and assure the parents that developmental delays are usually temporary.

Immobilization of a family member changes family functioning. The family's response to this change often leads to problems, stress, and anxieties. Children, when seeing parents who are immobile, sometimes have difficulty understanding what is occurring and difficulty coping.

Immobility has a significant effect on the older adult's levels of health, independence, and functional status. Nursing assessment enables the nurse to determine the patient's ability to meet needs independently and adapt developmental changes such as declining physical functioning and altered family and peer relationships. A decline in developmental functioning needs prompt investigation to determine why the change occurred and interventions that can return the patient to an optimal level of functioning as soon as possible. Activities that reduce immobility and promote participation in ADLs are vital to preventing functional decline (Kawamoto et al., 2006). Assessment also includes the patient's home and community to identify factors that are risks to his or her mobility and safety (see Chapter 38).

Building Competency in Patient-Centered Care You are caring for Mr. Jason Glynn, 91 years old, in the emergency department (ED). He lives with his wife Eileen of 63 years. Both are competent, active in their community, and not dependent on their two grown children. He was brought to the ED after falling from a ladder while cleaning leaves from the gutters of their home. He has an open fracture of the tibia and fibula of his right leg. He rated his pain as 9 on a scale of 0 to 10 and cannot remember his last tetanus injection. He is scheduled for surgery, an open reduction and internal fixation using plates and screws as soon as the operating room (OR) team is ready. Which assessments must you perform, and what are your priority actions for Mr. Glynn at this time?

Answers to questions can be found on the Evolve website.

NURSING DIAGNOSIS

A patient who is experiencing an alteration in mobility often has one or more nursing diagnoses. The two diagnoses most directly related to mobility problems are *impaired physical mobility* and *risk for disuse syndrome.* The diagnosis of *impaired physical mobility* applies to the patient who has some limitation but is not completely immobile. The diagnosis of *risk for disuse syndrome* applies to the patient who is immobile and at risk for multisystem problems because of inactivity. Beyond these diagnoses, the list of potential diagnoses is extensive, because immobility affects multiple body systems. Other possible nursing diagnoses include the following:

- Ineffective airway clearance
- Ineffective coping
- Risk for injury
- Risk for impaired skin integrity
- Insomnia
- Social isolation

Assessment reveals clusters of data that indicate whether a patient is at risk or if an actual problem exists. The clusters of data include defining characteristics that support the diagnostic label and probable cause of the diagnosis. Locating the probable cause of the diagnosis (based on assessment data) is important to planning patient-centered goals and subsequent nursing interventions that will best help the patient.

Impaired physical mobility related to reluctance to initiate movement requires slightly different interventions than impaired physical mobility related to pain in the left shoulder. Thus it is critical that nursing assessment activities identify and cluster defining characteristics that ultimately support the nursing diagnosis selected (Box 47-3). The diagnosis related to reluctance to initiate movement requires interventions aimed at keeping the patient as mobile as possible and encouraging him or her to perform self-care and ROM. The diagnosis related to pain requires the nurse to assist the patient with comfort measures so he or she is then willing and more able to move. In both situations the nurse explains how activity enhances healthy body functioning.

Often the physiological dimension is the major focus of nursing care for patients with impaired mobility. Thus the psychosocial and developmental dimensions are neglected. Yet all dimensions are important to health. During immobilization some patients experience decreased social interaction and stimuli. These patients frequently use the nurse's call bell to request minor physical attention when their real need is greater socialization. Nursing diagnoses for health needs in developmental areas reflect changes from the patient's normal activities. Immobility leads to a developmental crisis if the patient is unable to resolve problems and continue to mature.

Immobility also leads to multiple complications (e.g., renal calculi, DVT, pulmonary emboli, or pneumonia). If these conditions develop, collaborate with the health care provider or nurse practitioner for prescribed therapy to intervene. Be alert for and prevent these potential complications when possible.

BOX 47-3 NURSING DIAGNOSTIC PROCESS

Impaired Physical Mobility Related to Left Hip/Leg Pain

ASSESSMENT ACTIVITIES	DEFINING CHARACTERISTICS
Measure ROM during exercise of extremities.	Patient has limited ROM in left hip/leg.
Observe patient attempt to move her left leg.	Patient has impaired movement attempting to move her left hip and leg.
Ask patient about perception of pain.	Patient complains of sharp pain in hip and leg when she tries to move it.
Ask patient about endurance and activity tolerance.	Patient reports no muscle strength in left leg. "I can't move it by myself."

ROM, Range of motion.

PLANNING

During planning the nurse synthesizes information from resources such as knowledge of the role of respiratory and physical therapy, standards such as skin care guidelines from the Agency for Healthcare Research and Quality (AHRQ) and Wound, Ostomy and Continence Nurses Society (WOCN), protocols for patients at risk for falls, attitudes such as creativity and perseverance, and past experiences with immobilized patients (Fig. 47-15). Critical thinking ensures that the patient's plan of care integrates all that you know about the individual and key critical thinking elements. Professional standards are especially important to consider when you develop a plan of care. These standards often establish scientifically proven guidelines for selecting effective nursing interventions. Finally, as stated earlier, the patient is a full partner in designing the plan of care, and this input must be reflected when establishing the goals and outcomes.

Goals and Outcomes. Develop an individualized plan of care for each nursing diagnosis (see the Nursing Care Plan). Set realistic expectations for care and include the patient and family when possible. Set goals that are individualized, realistic, and measurable. The goals focus on preventing problems or risks to body alignment and mobility.

Develop goals and expected outcomes to assist the patient in achieving his or her highest level of mobility and reducing the hazards of immobility. For example, a patient who has left-sided paralysis following a stroke has two long-term goals. The first, directed toward improved mobility, is "Patient uses walker to ambulate safely in the home." A parallel goal directed toward the

NURSING CARE PLAN

Impaired Physical Mobility

ASSESSMENT

Ms. Carmella Cavallo, a 97-year-old patient, is admitted to a skilled care unit for rehabilitation 10 days after the surgical procedure of fixation of a fractured left hip. She has a history of smoking but stopped 40 years ago. She has no cardiac problems and no hypertension. She experiences "aches" and "stiffness" in her knees but usually says that she "has no pain" when asked. The three small incisions are clean, dry, and intact. Staples were removed yesterday.

Assessment Activities	*Findings/Defining Characteristics**
Ask Ms. Cavallo to rate her pain on a scale of 0 to 10.	She **rates her pain as a 2** on a scale of 0 to 10 at rest, but it **increases to an 8** with any movement of her left leg.
Assess Ms. Cavallo's ability to transfer.	She is **not able to transfer even** with help from chair to bed.
Ask Ms. Cavallo how her surgery has affected her mobility.	She responds that she wants to get out of bed but, when she moves her left leg, her nonverbal signs indicate that she is in severe pain. She says that it is a "sharp, stabbing pain."

***Defining characteristics** are shown in bold type.

NURSING DIAGNOSIS: Impaired physical mobility related to musculoskeletal impairment from surgery and pain with movement

PLANNING

Goals	*Expected Outcomes†*
	Body Positioning: Self-Initiated
Ms. Cavallo will be able to transfer with assistive device by discharge.	Ms. Cavallo will be able to move from her bed to her chair and back again using her walker and assist ×1 within 5 days. Ms. Cavallo will be able to transfer from her chair to her bedside commode using her walker within 5 days.
	Ambulation
Ms. Cavallo will walk 100 feet using her walker by discharge.	Ms. Cavallo will walk to her door and around her room with her walker within 10 days. Ms. Cavallo will walk 100 feet at a slow pace using her walker 3 times a day in 14 days and will increase the distance that she walks by 100 feet every day after that.

†Nursing outcomes classification from Moorhead S et al., editors: *Nursing outcomes classification (NOC)*, ed 4, St Louis, 2008, Mosby.

INTERVENTIONS‡	**RATIONALE**
Exercise Therapy: Ambulation	
Consult with physical therapist on selection of transfer technique.	Ensures safe transfer technique with less risk of patient injury.
Instruct Ms. Cavallo on safe transfer and ambulation techniques in an environment with few distractions. Provide written materials that reinforce verbal instructions.	Providing instruction in a quiet environment and giving written instructions in large, easy-to-read print enhances learning in the older patient (Mamaril, 2006).
Establish realistic increments for transferring and increasing distance for ambulation.	Gradually increasing physical activity and setting realistic goals for ambulation encourages activity in older adults (Yen, 2005).
Pain Management	
Administer pain medication based on your assessment of Ms. Cavallo's needs and on a schedule rather than prn if patient exhibits signs of being in pain but does not request pain medication and dose is not relieving her pain.	Obtain order to adjust (increase or decrease dose) based on her report of pain severity or her ability to perform activities of daily living (ADLs) (Pasero and McCaffery, 2007).
Observe for overt and covert signs of pain when she is moving or attempting to implement plan from physical therapy (PT) and have prn dose of pain medication ordered if additional pain medication is needed for PT activities.	It is important for you to have "as needed" dose of pain medication for patient in case requires a supplemental dose (APS, 2008).

‡Intervention classification labels from Bulecheck GM, Butcher HK, Dochterman JM: *Nursing interventions classification (NIC)*, ed 5, St Louis, 2008, Mosby.

EVALUATION

Nursing Actions	*Patient Response/Finding*	*Achievement of Outcome*
Ask Ms. Cavallo if her mobility has improved after therapy. Observe her transfer from bed to chair.	Ms. Cavallo is able to transfer from bed to chair using her walker and stand-by assistance of nurse.	Ms. Cavallo has achieved goal of transferring with walker and assistance.
Assess Ms. Cavallo as she walks in the hall; measure how far she walks.	Ms. Cavallo is able to walk 200 feet in the hall with her walker.	Activity level is improving. Continue interventions and continue to encourage ambulation.

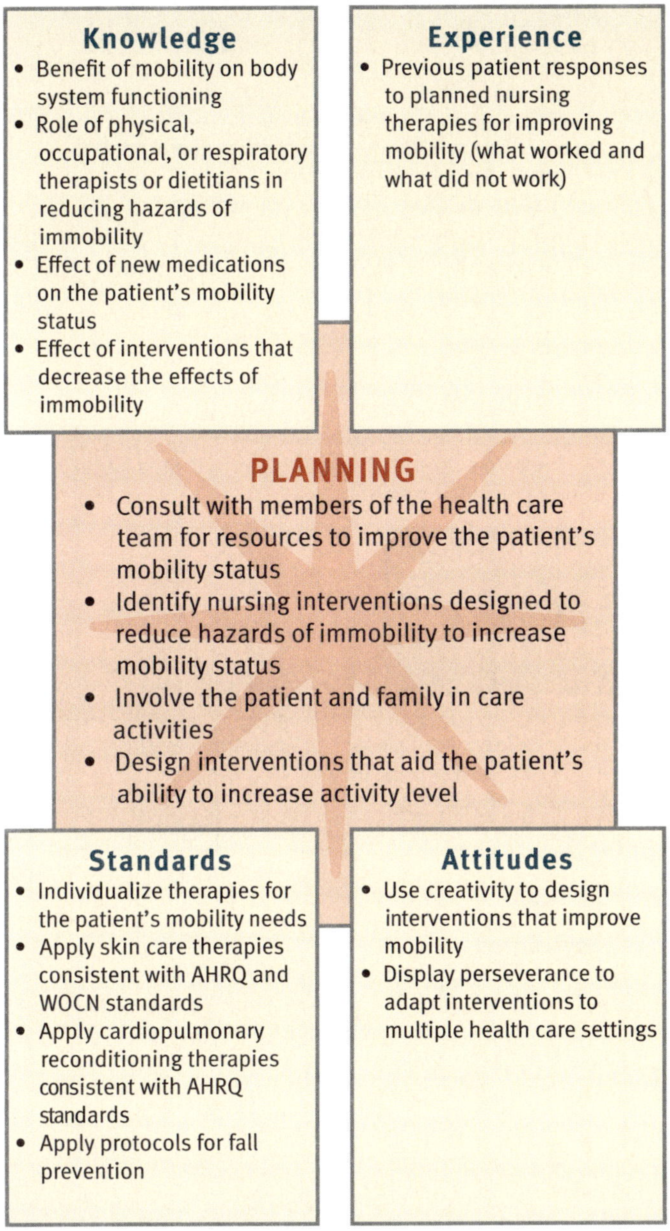
Knowledge
• Benefit of mobility on body system functioning
• Role of physical, occupational, or respiratory therapists or dietitians in reducing hazards of immobility
• Effect of new medications on the patient's mobility status
• Effect of interventions that decrease the effects of immobility
Experience
• Previous patient responses to planned nursing therapies for improving mobility (what worked and what did not work)
PLANNING
• Consult with members of the health care team for resources to improve the patient's mobility status
• Identify nursing interventions designed to reduce hazards of immobility to increase mobility status
• Involve the patient and family in care activities
• Design interventions that aid the patient's ability to increase activity level
Standards
• Individualize therapies for the patient's mobility needs
• Apply skin care therapies consistent with AHRQ and WOCN standards
• Apply cardiopulmonary reconditioning therapies consistent with AHRQ standards
• Apply protocols for fall prevention
Attitudes
• Use creativity to design interventions that improve mobility
• Display perseverance to adapt interventions to multiple health care settings

FIG. 47-15 Critical thinking model for immobility planning. *AHRQ,* Agency for Healthcare Research and Quality; *WOCN,* Wound, Ostomy and Continence Nurses Society.

hazards of immobility is "Patient's skin remains intact." Both of these goals are essential to restoring maximal mobility for this patient. Because there is impaired sensation, both the patient and caregivers need to be aware of the patient's need to have the skin free of pressure. Expected outcomes for the second goal include the following:

- Patient's skin color and temperature return to normal baseline within 20 minutes of position change.
- Patient changes position at least every 2 hours.

Setting Priorities. The effect that problems have on the patient's mental and physical health determines the immediacy of any problem. Set priorities when planning care to ensure that immediate needs are met first. This is particularly important when patients have multiple diagnoses (Fig. 47-16). Plan therapies according to severity of risks to the patient; and individualize the plan according to the patient's developmental stage, level of health, and lifestyle.

It is especially important in priority setting to make sure that you do not overlook potential complications. Many times actual problems such as pressure ulcers and disuse syndrome are addressed only after they develop. Therefore monitor the patient often, reinforcing prevention techniques to both the patient and other caregivers and supervising nursing assistive personnel in carrying out activities aimed at preventing complications of impaired mobility.

Teamwork and Collaboration. Care of the patient experiencing alterations in mobility requires a team approach. Nurses often delegate some interventions to nursing assistive personnel. Nursing assistive personnel can encourage the patient to do leg exercises, use the incentive spirometer, and cough and deep breathe (see Chapter 40). They can turn and position patients and apply elastic stockings. They can also help the nurse measure leg circumferences and height and weight.

Collaborate with other health care team members such as physical or occupational therapists when it is essential to consider mobility needs. Understanding the need for and having open communications with other members of the interdisciplinary care team results in better patient outcomes and hopefully prevents the hazards of immobility. It is through these collaborative efforts and teamwork that patients benefit most. For example, physical therapists are a resource for planning ROM or strengthening exercises, and occupational therapists are a resource for planning ADLs that patients need to modify or relearn. Wound care specialists and respiratory therapists are often involved in patient care, especially with patients who are experiencing complications related to their immobility. Consult a registered dietitian when the patient is experiencing nutritional problems; and refer him or her to a mental health advanced practice nurse, licensed social worker, or psychologist to assist with coping or other psychosocial issues.

Discharge planning begins when a patient enters the health care system. In anticipation of the patient's discharge from an institution, make appropriate referrals or consult a case manager or a discharge planner to ensure that the patient's needs are met at home. Consider the patient's home environment when planning therapies to maintain or improve body alignment and mobility. Referrals to home care or outpatient therapy are often needed.

IMPLEMENTATION

Health Promotion. Health promotion activities include a variety of interventions such as education, prevention, and early detection. Examples of health promotion activities that address mobility and immobility include prevention of work-related injury, fall-prevention measures, exercise, and early detection of scoliosis.

Prevention of Work-Related Musculoskeletal Injuries. The rate of work-related injuries in health care settings has increased in recent years. In 2006 there were 4.4 cases per 100 full-time workers who experienced occupational injury and illness compared with 5 cases per 100 for private industry overall. The rate for nursing homes was 10.1 per 100 workers (USDL, 2007). Most these injuries occurred as a result of overexertion, which resulted in back injuries and other musculoskeletal problems. Back injuries are often the direct result of improper lifting and bending. The most common back injury is strain on the lumbar muscle group, which includes the muscles around the lumbar vertebrae. Injury to these areas affects the ability to bend forward, backward, and from side to side and limits the ability to rotate the hips and lower back. Research has demonstrated that ergonomic programs in health care facilities

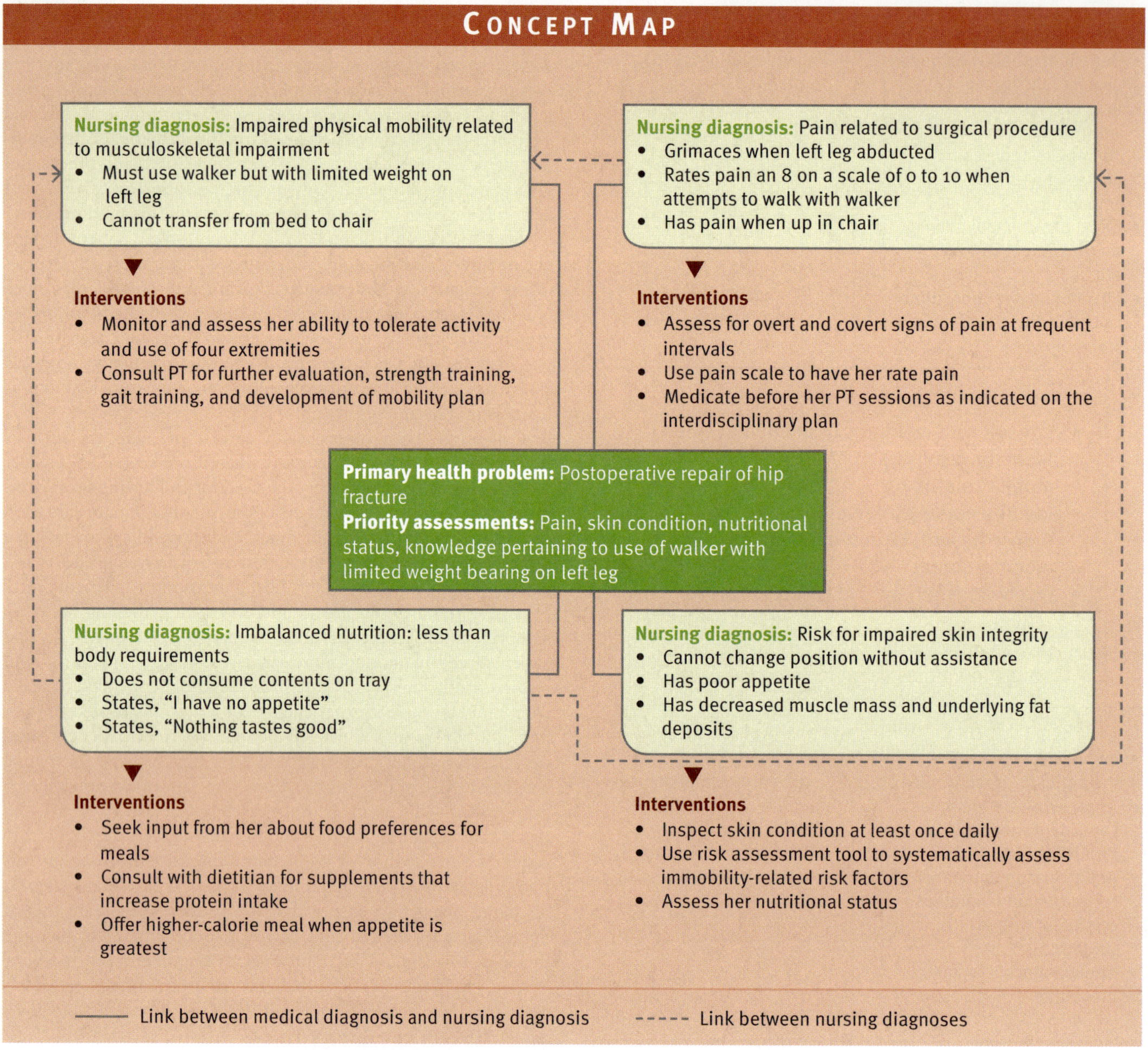
CONCEPT MAP
Nursing diagnosis: Impaired physical mobility related to musculoskeletal impairment
• Must use walker but with limited weight on left leg
• Cannot transfer from bed to chair
Interventions
• Monitor and assess her ability to tolerate activity and use of four extremities
• Consult PT for further evaluation, strength training, gait training, and development of mobility plan
Nursing diagnosis: Pain related to surgical procedure
• Grimaces when left leg abducted
• Rates pain an 8 on a scale of 0 to 10 when attempts to walk with walker
• Has pain when up in chair
Interventions
• Assess for overt and covert signs of pain at frequent intervals
• Use pain scale to have her rate pain
• Medicate before her PT sessions as indicated on the interdisciplinary plan
Primary health problem: Postoperative repair of hip fracture
Priority assessments: Pain, skin condition, nutritional status, knowledge pertaining to use of walker with limited weight bearing on left leg
Nursing diagnosis: Imbalanced nutrition: less than body requirements
• Does not consume contents on tray
• States, "I have no appetite"
• States, "Nothing tastes good"
Interventions
• Seek input from her about food preferences for meals
• Consult with dietitian for supplements that increase protein intake
• Offer higher-calorie meal when appetite is greatest
Nursing diagnosis: Risk for impaired skin integrity
• Cannot change position without assistance
• Has poor appetite
• Has decreased muscle mass and underlying fat deposits
Interventions
• Inspect skin condition at least once daily
• Use risk assessment tool to systematically assess immobility-related risk factors
• Assess her nutritional status
Link between medical diagnosis and nursing diagnosis
Link between nursing diagnoses

FIG. 47-16 Concept map for Ms. Cavallo. *PT,* Physical therapy.

reduce costs, injuries to employees, and missed work days. Matz (2007) noted that patient quality of care is *best* when staff are healthy and they are not experiencing any pain or discomfort.

Nurses and other health care staff are especially at risk for injury to lumbar muscles when lifting, transferring, or positioning immobilized patients. Therefore be aware of agency policies and protocols that protect staff and patients from injury. When lifting, assess the weight you will lift and determine the assistance you will need. Current evidence supports that using mechanical or other ergonomic assistive devices is the safest way to reposition and lift patients who are unable to do these activities themselves (Box 47-4). Many agencies have developed special patient lift teams and have instituted a no-lift policy.

Musculoskeletal injuries among health care workers are not only related to lifting and transferring patients. Nurses spend time in many activities bending and twisting, which also cause injury. Examples of such activities include lifting objects; pushing beds; and bathing, feeding, dressing, and undressing patients (Nelson et al., 2009). Therefore, in addition to knowing how to move patients safely, nurses also need to apply concepts related to body mechanics in the workplace. Before beginning a task, know your individual capabilities for activities such as lifting and moving objects. If providing care (e.g., bathing) to a patient, consider his or her condition and whether or not he or she can assist you. When you cannot safely complete a task (e.g., moving a bed from one room to another), assess the number of people you will need to help you and do not start until the task can be completed safely to prevent injury to you, the other members of the health care team, and the patient. Follow these steps to prevent injury:

1. Keep the weight to be lifted as close to the body as possible; this action places the object in the same plane as the lifter and close to the center of gravity for balance.

BOX 47-4 EVIDENCE-BASED PRACTICE

Reporting Staff Injuries to Reduce Future Injuries and Establish Safe Patient–Handling Policies for ALL Patients

PICO Question: Can the use of the E-OSHA 300 log metric be as effective for health care providers' reporting of injuries acquired while caring for obese patients as those reported while caring for nonobese patients to reduce future injuries to staff?

Evidence Summary

Even though evidence exists that body mechanics do not prevent injuries (Nelson and Baptiste, 2006) and nurses are beginning to report injuries associated with lifting and moving patients in their agencies, there must be a metric to standardize the reporting of these injuries (Randall et al., 2009). Added to the necessity for standardization is the number of individuals who are undergoing bariatric surgery. The evidence collected by the research indicated that the E-OSHA 300 log would provide the data needed to monitor the injuries in a systematic fashion and thereby heighten the awareness of the risks involved in manually handling bariatric patients.

Application to Nursing Practice

- Health care agencies need to provide devices to reduce the risk of injury associated with handling *all* patients (Wanless and Page, 2009).
- Nurses *must stop* using the traditional manual methods when transferring obese patients.
- Use assistive devices according to the assessment performed.
- *Report all injuries* using the E-OSHA 300 log metric for consistency.

E-OSHA, Expanded occupational safety and health administration.

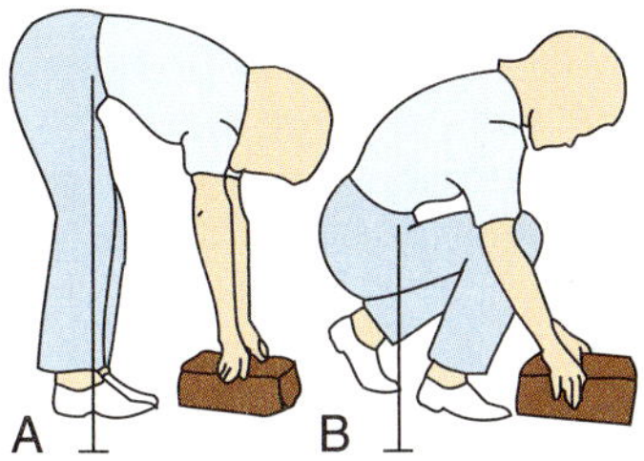

FIG. 47-17 Incorrect **(A)** and correct **(B)** body position for lifting.

2. Bend at the knees; this helps to maintain the center of gravity and uses the stronger leg muscles to do the lifting (Fig. 47-17).
3. Tighten abdominal muscles and tuck the pelvis; this provides balance and helps protect the back.
4. Maintain the trunk erect and knees bent so multiple muscle groups work together in a coordinated manner (see Chapter 38); do not allow the trunk to twist.

Exercise. Although many diseases and physical problems cause or contribute to immobility, it is important to remember that exercise programs enhance feelings of well-being and improve endurance, strength, and health. Exercise reduces the risk of many health problems such as cardiovascular disease, diabetes, and osteoporosis. Help the chronically ill overcome barriers to physical activity. For example, if a patient has a below-the-knee amputation, suggest activities such as lifting soup cans, which capitalize on the patient's strengths and abilities. Encourage hospitalized patients to perform stretching, ROM exercises, and light walking within the limits of their condition (see Chapter 38).

BOX 47-5 CULTURAL ASPECTS OF CARE

Mobility Related to Individuals and Their Cultural Influences

Many activities are specifically linked to culture such as time orientation, health care practices, health promotion, nutrition, religion, family systems, and death. Less attention has been given to the impact of culture on mobility. However, cultural influences have an important role in exercise and physical activity.

Culture influences preferences for activity and exercise. Certain cultures discourage involvement in organized recreational physical activities such as basketball, running, and aerobics. Ethnic dancing is an effective activity that is acceptable in Korean countries. Other cultures emphasize exercise in terms of activities of daily living such as walking, gardening, and prayer/meditation. As an example, people from Bangladesh often view prayer as a structured form of exercise, whereas many Muslims value participation in community activities and consider walking to the mosque a part of their weekly exercise regimen.

A sedentary lifestyle puts a patient at risk for being overweight. Children from many cultures who live in the United States are becoming more sedentary. The number of obese children is especially increasing in Hispanic and Native American populations. One researcher found that older Hispanic women only participated in exercise classes that were required when they were in school. They believed that doing housework and caring for their families met their exercise needs.

Implications for Practice

- Evaluate patterns of daily living and culturally prescribed activities before suggesting specific forms of exercise to patients.
- Help patients plan physical activities that are culturally acceptable.
- Exercise programs need to be flexible and accommodate family and community responsibilities of the culture.
- Encourage culturally specific and individually tailored interventions to facilitate commitment to exercise.
- Educate patients of all ages on the importance of exercise in preserving health and correct any misconceptions.

Nurses contribute to promoting health for many patients by encouraging or starting managed exercise programs. Exercise is a key prescription for health promotion of all patients, regardless of their age. In older adults routine exercise or activity helps maintain ROM and functional mobility and improves balance (Ebersole et al., 2008). Take cultural preferences into consideration when helping patients design exercise plans (Box 47-5).

Bone Health in Patients with Osteoporosis. Patients at risk for or diagnosed with osteoporosis have special health promotion needs. Encourage patients at risk to be screened for osteoporosis and assess their diets for calcium and vitamin D intake. Patients who have lactose intolerance need dietary teaching about alternative sources of calcium.

For patients diagnosed with osteoporosis, early evaluation, consultation, and referral with health care providers, dietitians, and physical therapists are important interventions, especially when they become immobilized. The goal of the patient with osteoporosis is to maintain independence with ADLs. Assistive ambulatory devices, adaptive clothing, and safety bars help the patient maintain independence. Patient teaching needs to focus on limiting the severity of the disease through diet and activity (Box 47-6).

Acute Care. Patients in acute care settings who experience altered physical mobility usually have some problems associated

BOX 47-6 PATIENT TEACHING

Teaching Patients with Osteoporosis

Objective

- Patient will verbalize strategies to prevent or limit the severity of osteoporosis.

Teaching Strategies

- Instruct patient and/or caregiver about common risk factors and how to modify lifestyle (e.g., smoking, caffeine, alcohol, hormone replacement as recommended by health care provider).
- Teach patient and/or caregiver the current recommended dietary allowances for calcium and review foods high in calcium (e.g., milk fortified with vitamin D, leafy green vegetables, yogurt, and cheese).
- Instruct patients and/or caregiver in appropriate types of weight-bearing exercises as recommended by health care provider or physical therapist to prevent injury or fractures.
- Teach patient and/or caregiver about safety, fall prevention, and strategies to create a safe home environment (e.g., remove scatter rugs; ensure that hallways, steps, and rooms are well lit).
- Instruct patient and/or caregiver in self-administration of prescribed medication used to treat osteoporosis.
- Promote positive self-image in patient by providing realistic yet optimistic and positive feedback about changes in appearance and mobility.

Evaluation

- Patient and/or caregiver can verbalize *three lifestyle modifications* such as stopping smoking, reducing caffeine or alcohol intake, or increasing dietary calcium.
- Patient and/or caregiver can verbalize *at least four* foods high in calcium and vitamin D.
- Patient and/or caregiver can *demonstrate appropriate weight-bearing exercises* and plan times for exercise.
- Patient and/or caregiver verbalize *three safety strategies* that they can implement at home to prevent falls.
- Patient and/or caregiver verbalize *specific knowledge* about osteoporosis medications.
- Patient and/or caregiver express positive but realistic feedback regarding effects of disease.

with the hazards of immobility such as impaired respiratory status, orthostatic hypotension, and impaired skin integrity. Therefore design nursing interventions to reduce the impact of immobility on body systems and prepare the patient for the restorative phase of care.

Metabolic System. Because the body needs protein to repair injured tissue and rebuild depleted protein stores, give the immobilized patient a high-protein, high-calorie diet. A high-calorie intake provides sufficient fuel to meet metabolic needs and replace subcutaneous tissue. Also ensure that the patient is taking vitamin B and C supplements when necessary. Supplementation with vitamin C is needed for skin integrity and wound healing; vitamin B complex assists in energy metabolism.

If the patient is unable to eat, nutrition must be provided parenterally or enterally. Total parenteral nutrition refers to delivery of nutritional supplements through a central or peripheral intravenous catheter. Enteral feedings include delivery through a nasogastric, gastrostomy, or jejunostomy tube of high-protein, high-calorie solutions with complete requirements of vitamins, minerals, and electrolytes (see Chapter 44).

Respiratory System. Nursing interventions that support the respiratory system are important. Patients need to frequently reexpand their lungs to maintain their elastic recoil property. In addition, secretions accumulate in the dependent areas of the lungs. Often patients with restricted mobility experience weakness; and, as this progresses, the cough reflex gradually becomes inefficient. All of these factors put the patient at risk of developing pneumonia. The stasis of secretions in the lungs is life threatening for an immobilized patient.

A variety of nursing interventions are available to expand the lungs, dislodge and mobilize stagnant secretions, and clear the lungs. All of these interventions help reduce the risk of pneumonia. Prevention begins with assessment. Assess the patient's respiratory status per agency policy. Assessment findings that indicate pneumonia include productive cough with greenish-yellow sputum; fever; pain on breathing; and crackles, wheezes, and dyspnea. It is essential to implement pulmonary interventions in all patients, even those who do not have pneumonia.

Encourage the patient to deep breathe and cough every 1 to 2 hours. Teach alert patients to deep breathe or yawn every hour or to use an incentive spirometer. Instruct the patient to take in three deep breaths and cough with the third exhalation.

Chest physiotherapy (CPT) (percussion and positioning) is another effective method for preventing pneumonia and keeping the airway clear. CPT helps the patient drain secretions from specific segments of the bronchi and lungs into the trachea so he or she is able to cough and expel them. Respiratory assessment findings identify areas of the lungs requiring CPT (see Chapter 40).

Ensure that patients who are immobile take an adequate fluid intake. Unless there is a medical contraindication, an adult needs to drink at least 1100 to 1400 ml of noncaffeinated fluids daily. This helps keep mucociliary clearance normal. Expect pulmonary secretions to be removed easily with coughing and appear thin, watery, and clear. Without adequate hydration, pulmonary secretions become thick and tenacious and difficult to remove. Offering fluids on a regularly timed schedule also helps with bowel and urine elimination and aids in maintaining circulation and skin integrity.

Cardiovascular System. The effects of bed rest or immobilization on the cardiovascular system include orthostatic hypotension, increased cardiac workload, and thrombus formation. Design nursing therapies to minimize or prevent these alterations.

Reducing Orthostatic Hypotension. When patients who are on bed rest or are immobile move to a sitting or standing position, they often experience orthostatic hypotension. They have an increased pulse rate, a decreased pulse pressure, and a drop in blood pressure. If symptoms become severe enough, the patient can faint (Huether and McCance, 2008). To prevent injury, nurses implement interventions that reduce or eliminate the effects of orthostatic hypotension. Mobilize the patient as soon as the physical condition allows, even if this only involves dangling at the bedside or moving to a chair. This activity maintains muscle tone and increases venous return. Isometric exercises (i.e., activities that involve muscle tension without muscle shortening) have no beneficial effect on preventing orthostatic hypotension, but they improve activity tolerance. When getting an immobile patient up for the first time, assess the situation using a safe patient–handling algorithm (see Fig. 47-21) (Nelson, 2006). This is a precautionary step that protects the nurse and patient from injury and also allows the patient to do as much of the transfer as possible.

Reducing Cardiac Workload. The nurse designs interventions to reduce cardiac workload, which is increased by immobility. A primary intervention is to discourage the patient from using the Valsalva maneuver. The patient holds his or her breath when using this maneuver, such as while straining during defecation or moving up in bed. This increases intrathoracic pressure, which in turn decreases venous return and cardiac output. When the strain is released, venous return and cardiac output immediately increase, and systolic blood pressure and pulse pressure rise. These pressure changes produce a reflex bradycardia and possible decrease in blood pressure that can result in sudden cardiac death in patients with heart disease. Teach the patient to breathe out while moving side-to-side or up in bed.

Preventing Thrombus Formation. The most cost-effective way to address DVT is through an aggressive program of prophylaxis. It begins with identification of patients at risk and continues throughout their immobilization. This is clearly a collaborative role between nurses and health care providers. Use the nursing assessment to identify risk factors. Many interventions reduce the risk of thrombus formation in the immobilized patient. Leg, foot, and ankle exercises; regularly providing fluids; position changes; and patient teaching need to begin when the patient becomes immobile (see Chapter 50).

Common dosage for heparin therapy for DVT prophylaxis is 5000 units given subcutaneously 2 hours before surgery and repeated every 8 to 12 hours until the patient is fully mobile or discharged. Heparin is an anticoagulant, and it suppresses clot formation. Common dosage of enoxaparin (Lovenox) (a low-molecular-weight heparin) in the prophylaxis of DVTs is 30 to 40 mg subcutaneously 2 hours before surgery and continued every 8 to 12 hours throughout the postoperative period. Because bleeding is a potential side effect of these medications, continually assess the patient for signs of bleeding such as hematuria, bruising, coffee ground–like vomitus or GI aspirate, guaiac-positive stools, and bleeding gums.

SCDs and intermittent pneumatic compression (IPC) consist of sleeves or stockings made of fabric or plastic that are wrapped around the leg and secured with Velcro (Box 47-7). Once they are applied, connect the sleeves to a pump that alternately inflates and deflates the stocking around the leg. A typical cycle is inflation for 10 to 15 seconds and deflation for 45 to 60 seconds. Inflation pressures average 40 mm Hg. Use of SCD/IPC on the legs decreases venous stasis by increasing venous return through the deep veins of the legs. For optimal results begin use of SCD/IPC as soon as possible and maintain it until the patient becomes fully ambulatory.

Elastic stockings (sometimes called *antiembolitic stockings)* also aid in maintaining external pressure on the muscles of the lower extremities and thus promote venous return (Box 47-8). To obtain the correct size, measure the patient's calf, thigh, and leg length accurately. When considering applying graded compression stockings, first assess the patient's suitability for wearing them. Do not apply them if he or she has a local condition affecting the leg (e.g., any skin lesion, gangrenous condition, or recent vein ligation) because application compromises circulation. Apply them properly and remove them at least once per shift. Be sure to assess circulation at the toes to ensure that the stockings are not too tight.

Proper positioning reduces the patient's risk of thrombus formation because compression of the leg veins is minimized. Therefore, when positioning patients, use caution to prevent pressure on the posterior knee and deep veins in the lower extremities. Teach patients to avoid the following: crossing the legs, sitting for prolonged periods of time, wearing clothing that constricts the legs or waist, and massaging the legs. Report suspected DVT immediately to the patient's health care provider. Elevate the leg but avoid pressure on the thrombus. Instruct the family, patient, and all health care personnel not to massage the area because of the danger of dislodging the thrombus.

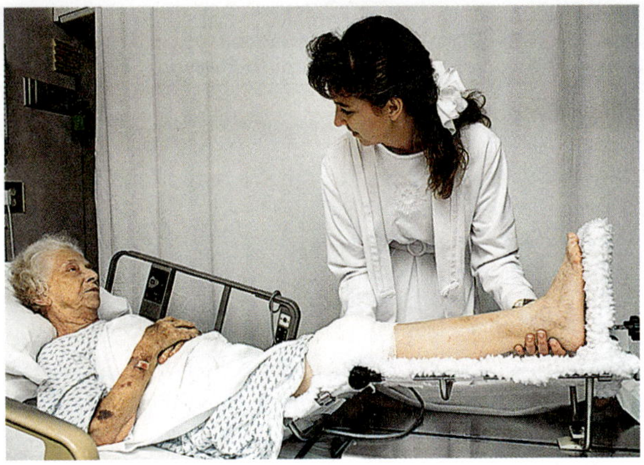

FIG. 47-18 Continuous passive range-of-motion machine.

ROM exercises reduce the risk of contractures and aid in preventing thrombi. Activity causes contraction of the skeletal muscles, which in turn exerts pressure on the veins to promote venous return, thereby reducing venous stasis. Specific exercises that help prevent thrombophlebitis are ankle pumps, foot circles, and knee flexion. Ankle pumps, sometimes called *calf pumps,* include alternating plantar flexion and dorsiflexion. Foot circles require the patient to rotate the ankle. Encourage patients to make the letters of the alphabet with their feet every 1 to 2 hours. Knee flexion involves alternately extending and flexing the knee. These exercises are sometimes referred to as *antiembolic exercises* and need to be done hourly while awake.

Musculoskeletal System. Exercises to prevent excessive muscle atrophy and joint contractures help maintain musculoskeletal function. If the patient is unable to move part or all of the body, perform passive ROM exercises for all immobilized joints while bathing the patient and at least 2 or 3 more times a day. If one extremity is paralyzed, teach the patient to put each joint independently through its ROM. Patients on bed rest need to have active ROM exercises incorporated into their daily schedules. Teach patients to integrate exercises during ADLs.

Some orthopedic conditions require more frequent passive ROM exercises to restore the function of the injured joint after surgery. Patients with such conditions need to use automatic equipment (continuous passive motion [CPM]) for passive ROM exercises) (Fig. 47-18). The CPM machine moves an extremity to a prescribed angle for a prescribed period. Researchers are currently investigating new uses for CPM. In one study patients who had a CVA and received CPM therapy to their affected shoulder had better joint stability than patients who received traditional ROM exercises (Lynch et al., 2005).

Integumentary System. The major risk to the skin from restricted mobility is the formation of pressure ulcers. Early identification of high-risk patients helps prevent pressure ulcers (see Chapter 48). Interventions aimed at prevention include positioning, skin care, and the use of therapeutic devices to relieve pressure. Change the immobilized patient's position according to his or her activity level, perceptual ability, treatment protocols, and daily routines. Although turning every 1 to 2 hours is recommended for preventing ulcers,

BOX 47-7 PROCEDURAL GUIDELINES

Applying Sequential Compression Devices

Delegation Considerations

The skill of applying sequential compression devices (SCDs) can be delegated to NAP. The nurse is responsible for assessing circulation in the extremities. Instruct NAP to notify nurse:

- If patient complains of pain in leg.
- If discoloration develops in extremities.

Equipment

Sequential compression device (SCD) insufflator with air hoses attached, adjustable Velcro compression stockings/SCD sleeve, hygiene supplies

1. Assess patient for need for sequential compression stockings. In some agencies an order is required. Perform hand hygiene.
2. Obtain baseline assessment data about status of circulation, pulse, and skin integrity of patient's lower extremities before initiating sequential compression stockings.
3. Identify patient using two identifiers (i.e., name and birth date or name and account number, according to agency policy). Ask patient to state name.
4. Perform hand hygiene. Provide hygiene to patient's lower extremities as needed.
5. Assemble and prepare equipment.
6. Arrange SCD sleeve under patient's leg according to leg position indicated on inner lining of sleeve (see illustration).
   a. Back of patient's ankle should line up with ankle on inner lining of sleeve.
   b. Position back of the knee with popliteal opening (see illustration).
7. Wrap SCD sleeve securely around patient's leg.
8. Verify fit of SCD sleeves by placing two fingers between patient's leg and sleeve (see illustration).
9. Attach connector of SCD sleeve to plug on mechanical unit. Arrow on compressor lines up with arrow on plug from mechanical unit (see illustration).
10. Turn mechanical unit on. Green light indicates that unit is functioning.
11. Observe functioning of unit for one complete cycle.
12. Reposition patient for comfort and perform hand hygiene.
13. Remove compression stockings at least once per shift.
14. Monitor skin integrity and circulation to patient's lower extremities as ordered or as recommended by SCD manufacturer.

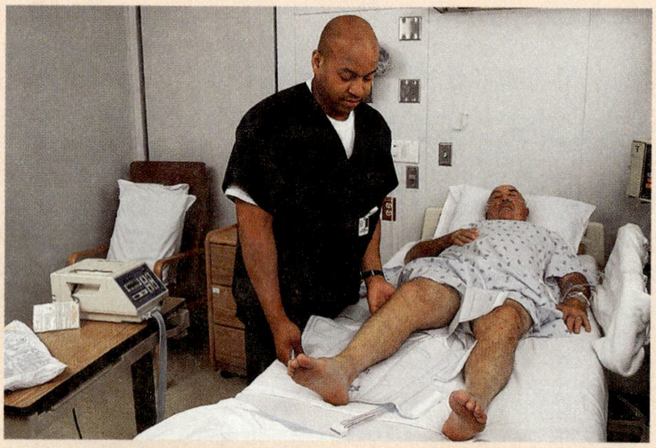

STEP 6 Correct leg position on inner lining.

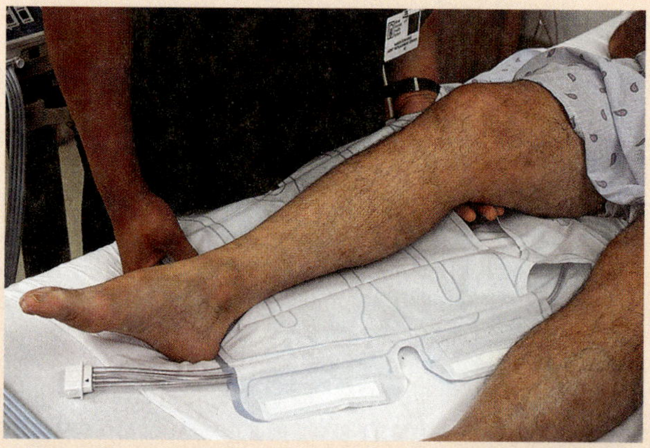

STEP 6b Position back of patient's knee with popliteal opening.

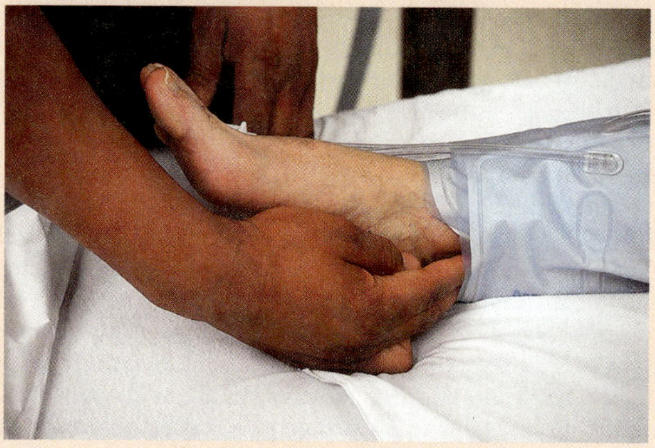

STEP 8 Check fit of SCD sleeve.

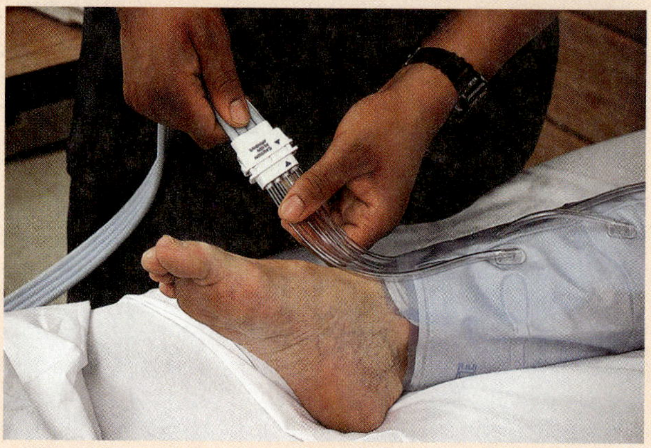

STEP 9 Align arrows when connecting to mechanical unit.

it is sometimes necessary to use devices for relieving pressure. Usually the time that a patient sits uninterrupted in a chair is limited to 1 hour. This interval is shortened in patients who are at very high risk for skin breakdown. Reposition patients frequently because uninterrupted pressure causes skin breakdown. Teach patients to shift their weight every 15 minutes. Chair-bound patients need to have a device for the chair that reduces pressure (AHRQ, 2010).

Elimination System. The nursing interventions for maintaining optimal urinary functioning are directed at keeping the patient well hydrated and preventing urinary stasis, calculi, and infections without causing bladder distention. Adequate hydration (e.g., at

BOX 47-8 **PROCEDURAL GUIDELINES**

View Video!

Applying Antiembolitic Elastic Stockings

Delegation Considerations

The nurse can delegate the skill of applying antiembolitic elastic stockings to nursing assistive personnel (NAP). Before delegation instruct the NAP to inform the nurse:

- If patient complains of leg pain or leg swelling.
- If patient has any skin irritation.

Also instruct the NAP to direct the patient:

- To avoid activities that promote venous stasis (e.g., crossing legs, wearing garters).
- To elevate legs while sitting and before applying stockings to improve venous return.
- Not to massage legs.
- To avoid wrinkles in stocking.

Equipment

Tape measure, elastic support stockings, hygiene supplies

1. Identify patient using two identifiers (i.e., name and birth date or name and account number, according to agency policy). Assess patient for risk factors in Virchow's triad:
   a. *Hypercoagulability:* All patients with clotting disorders, fever, dehydration, pregnancy, and first 6 weeks after delivery if the woman was confined to bed and used oral contraceptive (especially if patient smokes)
   b. *Venous wall abnormalities:* Local trauma, orthopedic surgeries, major abdominal surgery, varicose veins, atherosclerosis
   c. *Blood stasis:* Immobility, obesity, pregnancy
2. Observe for signs, symptoms, and condition of patient skin that contraindicate use of antiembolitic elastic stockings. Signs and symptoms include:
   a. Dermatitis or open skin lesion.
   b. Recent skin graft.
   c. Decreased circulation in lower extremities as evidenced by cyanotic, cool extremities, gangrenous conditions affecting lower limb(s).
3. Assess and document condition of patient's skin and circulation to leg and foot (i.e., presence of popliteal and pedal pulses, edema, and discoloration of skin; temperature; lesions; or abrasions).
4. Obtain physician's or health care provider's order.
5. Assess patient's or caregiver's understanding of application of antiembolitic elastic stockings.

CLINICAL DECISION: Clinical signs of thrombophlebitis vary according to the size and location of the thrombus. Signs and symptoms of superficial thrombosis include palpable veins and surrounding areas being tender to the touch, reddened, and warm. Temperature elevation and edema may or may not be present. Signs and symptoms of deep vein thrombosis (DVT) include swollen extremity; pain; warm, cyanotic skin; and temperature elevation. However, up to 80% of patients are asymptomatic. Homans' sign (pain in the calf on dorsiflexion of the foot) is no longer considered reliable. Less than 20% of patients have a positive Homans' sign (Black and Hawks, 2009).

6. Use tape measure to measure patient's legs to determine proper stocking size.
7. Explain procedure and reasons for applying stockings.
8. Perform hand hygiene. Provide hygiene to patient's lower extremities as needed.
9. Position patient in supine position.
10. Apply elastic stockings:
    a. Turn elastic stocking inside out up to heel. Place one hand into stocking, holding heel. Pull top of stocking with other hand inside out over foot of stocking
    b. Place patient's toes into foot of elastic stocking, making sure that stocking is smooth (see illustration).
    c. Slide remaining portion of stocking over patient's foot, being sure that toes are covered. Make sure that foot fits into toe and heel position of stocking (see illustration).
    d. Slide top of stocking up over patient's calf until stocking is completely extended. Be sure that stocking is smooth and that no ridges or wrinkles are present, particularly behind knee (see illustration).
    e. Instruct patient not to roll stockings partially down.
11. Reposition patient for comfort and perform hand hygiene.
12. Remove stockings at least once per shift.
13. Inspect stockings for wrinkles or constriction.
14. Inspect elastic stockings to determine that there are no wrinkles, rolls, or binding.
15. Observe circulatory status of lower extremities. Observe color, temperature, and condition of skin. Palpate pedal pulses.
16. Observe patient's response to wearing antiembolitic elastic stockings.
17. Observe patient or caregiver applying stockings.

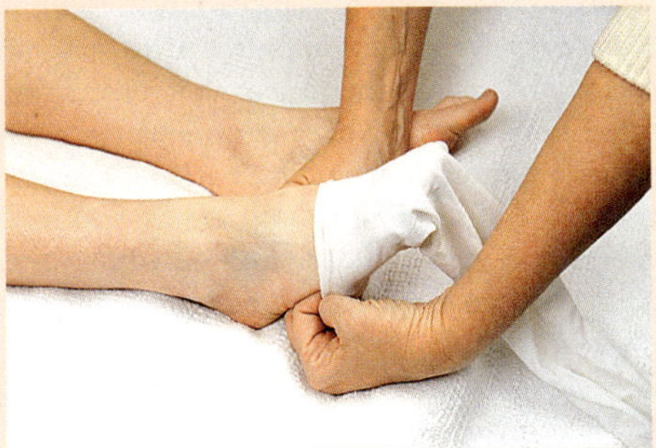

STEP 10b Place toes into foot of stocking.

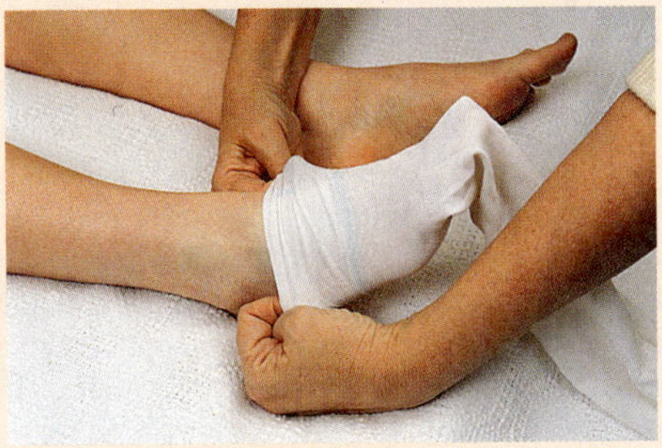

STEP 10c Slide heel of stocking over foot.

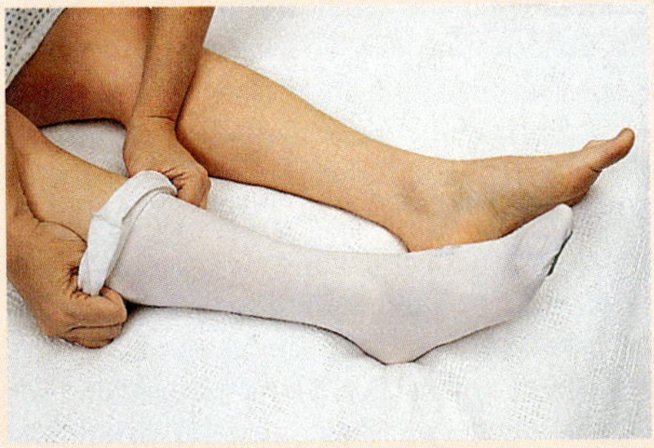

STEP 10d Slide stocking up leg until completely extended.

least 1100 to 1400 mL of noncaffeinated fluids daily) helps prevent renal calculi and urinary tract infections. The well-hydrated patient needs to void large amounts of dilute urine that is approximately equal to fluid intake. Also record the frequency and consistency of bowel movements. Provide a diet rich in fluids, fruits, vegetables, and fiber to facilitate normal peristalsis. If a patient is unable to maintain regular bowel patterns, stool softeners, cathartics, or enemas are sometimes necessary. If the patient is incontinent, modify the care plan to include toileting aids and a hygiene schedule so the increased urinary output does not cause skin breakdown.

Psychosocial Changes. Use assessment data to identify effects of prolonged immobilization. People who have a tendency toward depression or mood swings are at greater risk for developing psychosocial effects during bed rest or immobilization. Many nursing interventions meet the patient's psychosocial needs. Anticipate changes in the patient's psychosocial status and provide routine and informal socialization. Observe the patient's ability to cope with restricted mobility. In institutional health care settings do not schedule nursing care activities between 10:00 PM and 7:00 AM to minimize sleep interruptions. For example, the nurse administers medications and assesses vital signs when the patient is turned or receives special skin care. If the nursing care plan is not improving coping patterns, consult a clinical nurse specialist, counselor, social worker, spiritual adviser, or other health care professional. Incorporate their recommendations into the care plan.

Nurses provide stimuli to maintain a patient's orientation. Plan nursing activities so the patient is able to talk and interact with staff. If possible, place him or her in a room with others who are mobile and interactive. If a private room is required, ask staff members to visit throughout the shift to provide meaningful interaction. A daily newspaper helps the patient keep track of events and time. Bedside conversations at appropriate moments familiarize him or her with nursing activities, meals, and visiting hours. Books help occupy the patient when he or she is alone. The patient can participate in craft activities. Radio, television, and videotapes provide stimulation and help pass the time.

Involve patients in their care whenever possible. For example, encourage the patient to determine when the bed should be made. Some patients rest better during the night when fresh sheets are put on in the evening rather than in the morning. The patient needs to provide as much self-care as possible. Keep hygiene and grooming articles within easy reach. Encourage patients to wear their glasses or artificial teeth and shave or apply makeup. People use these activities to maintain their body image, thus improving their outlook.

Developmental Changes. Ideally immobilized patients continue normal development. Nursing interventions can help. Nursing care needs to provide mental and physical stimulation, particularly for a young child. Incorporate play activities into the care plan. For example, completing puzzles helps a child to develop fine-motor skills, and reading helps him or her to develop cognitively. Encourage parents to stay with a child who is hospitalized. Place a child who is immobilized with children of the same age who are not immobilized unless a contagious disease is present. Allow the child to participate in nursing interventions such as dressing changes, cast care, and care of traction. The nurse needs to recognize significant changes from normal behavioral patterns and consult with a pediatric clinical nurse specialist, counselor, or other health care professional.

Restricted mobility of older patients presents unique nursing problems. Older patients who are frail or have chronic illnesses are often at increased risk for the psychosocial hazards of immobility. Maintaining a calendar and clock with a large dial, conversing about current events and family members, and encouraging visits from significant others reduce the risk of social isolation. Spending time in the room talking and listening to the patient also helps reduce the risk of social isolation.

Nurses need to encourage older immobilized patients to perform as many ADLs as independently as possible. Patients need to continue to perform personal grooming if they did so before their mobility was restricted. This type of activity preserves the patient's dignity and gives him or her a sense of accomplishment.

Positioning Techniques. Patients with impaired nervous, skeletal, or muscular system functioning and increased weakness and fatigability often require help from the nurse to attain proper body alignment while in bed or sitting. Several positioning devices are available for maintaining good body alignment for patients. Pillows are positioning aids and are sometimes readily available. Before using a pillow, determine whether it is the proper size. A thick pillow under the patient's head increases cervical flexion. A thin pillow under body prominences does not protect skin and tissue from damage caused by pressure. When additional pillows are unavailable or if they are an improper size, use folded sheets, blankets, or towels as positioning aids.

Apply positioning boots to prevent footdrop by maintaining the feet in dorsiflexion. Ankle-foot orthotic (AFO) devices also help maintain dorsiflexion. Patients who wear positioning boots or AFOs need to have these removed periodically (e.g., 2 hours on, 2 hours off).

A **trochanter roll** prevents external rotation of the hips when the patient is in a supine position. To form a trochanter roll, fold a cotton bath blanket lengthwise to a width that extends from the greater trochanter of the femur to the lower border of the popliteal space (Fig. 47-19). Place the blanket under the buttocks and roll it counterclockwise until the thigh is in neutral position or inward rotation. When the hip is aligned correctly, the patella faces directly upward. Use sandbags in place of or in addition to trochanter rolls. Sandbags are sand-filled plastic tubes or bags that are shaped to body contours. Hand rolls maintain the thumb in slight adduction and in opposition to the fingers, which maintain a functional

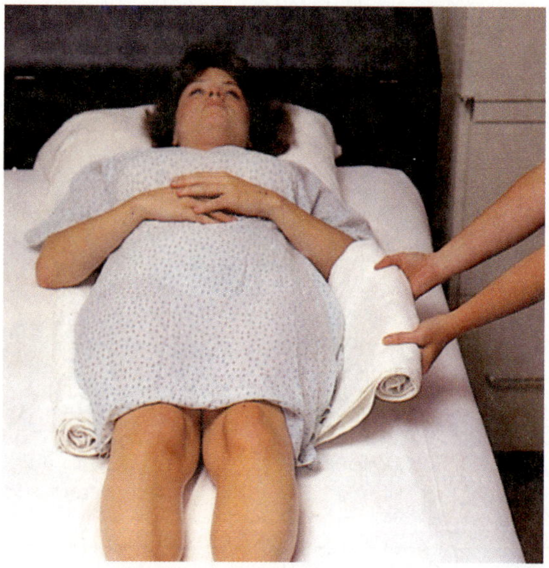

FIG. 47-19 Trochanter roll.

position. Evaluate the hand roll to make sure that the hand is indeed in a functional position. Hand rolls are most often used with patients whose arms are paralyzed or who are unconscious. Do not use rolled washcloths as hand rolls because they do not keep the thumb well abducted, especially in patients who have a spastic paralysis. Hand-wrist splints are individually molded for the patient to maintain proper alignment of the thumb (slight adduction) and wrist (slight dorsiflexion). Use splints only on the patient for whom they were made and follow the splint schedule (e.g., wear for 2 hours, remove for 2 hours).

The **trapeze bar** is a triangular device that hangs down from a securely fastened overhead bar that is attached to the bed frame. It allows the patient to pull with the upper extremities to raise the trunk off the bed, assist in transfer from bed to wheelchair, or perform upper-arm exercises (Fig. 47-20). It increases independence, maintains upper body strength, and decreases the shearing action from sliding across or up and down in bed.

Although each procedure for positioning has specific guidelines, the nurse follows some universal steps for patients who require positioning assistance (Skill 47-1 on pp. 1159-1166). Following the guidelines reduces the risk of injury to the musculoskeletal system when the patient is sitting or lying. When joints are unsupported, their alignment is impaired. Likewise, if joints are not positioned in a slightly flexed position, their mobility is decreased. During positioning also assess for pressure points (see Fig. 48-9). When actual or potential pressure areas exist, nursing interventions involve removal of the pressure, thus decreasing the risk for development of pressure ulcers and further trauma to the musculoskeletal system. In these patients use the 30-degree lateral position.

Supported Fowler's Position. In the supported Fowler's position, the head of the bed is elevated 45 to 60 degrees, and the patient's knees are slightly elevated without pressure to restrict circulation in the lower legs. The patient's illness and overall condition influence the angle of head and knee elevation and the length of time that the patient needs to remain in the supported Fowler's position. Supports need to permit flexion of the hips and knees and proper alignment of the normal curves in the cervical, thoracic, and lumbar vertebrae. The following are common trouble areas for the patient in the supported Fowler's position:

- Increased cervical flexion because the pillow at the head is too thick and the head thrusts forward
- Extension of the knees, allowing the patient to slide to the foot of the bed
- Pressure on the posterior aspect of the knees, decreasing circulation to the feet
- External rotation of the hips
- Arms hanging unsupported at the patient's sides
- Unsupported feet or pressure on the heels
- Unprotected pressure points at the sacrum and heels
- Increased shearing force on the back and heels when the head of the bed is raised greater than 60 degrees

Supine Position. Patients in the supine position rest on their backs. In the supine position the relationship of body parts is essentially the same as in good standing alignment except that the body is in the horizontal plane. Use pillows, trochanter rolls, and hand rolls or arm splints to increase comfort and reduce injury to the skin or musculoskeletal system. The mattress needs to be firm enough to support the cervical, thoracic, and lumbar vertebrae. Shoulders are supported, and the elbows are slightly flexed to control shoulder rotation. A foot support prevents footdrop and maintains proper alignment. The following are some common trouble areas for patients in the supine position:

- Pillow at the head that is too thick, increasing cervical flexion
- Head flat on the mattress
- Shoulders unsupported and internally rotated
- Elbows extended
- Thumb not in opposition to the fingers
- Hips externally rotated
- Unsupported feet
- Unprotected pressure points at the occipital region of the head, vertebrae, coccyx, elbows, and heels

Prone Position. The patient in the prone position lies face or chest down. Often his or her head is turned to the side; but, if a pillow is under the head, it needs to be thin enough to prevent cervical flexion or extension and maintain alignment of the lumbar spine. Placing a pillow under the lower leg permits dorsiflexion of the ankles and some knee flexion, which promote relaxation. If a pillow is unavailable, the ankles need to be in dorsiflexion over the end of the mattress. Although the prone position is seldom used in practice, consider this as an alternative, especially in patients who normally sleep in this position. The prone position also may have some benefits in patients with acute respiratory distress syndrome and acute lung injury (Marklew, 2006). Specialty beds that safely position acutely ill patients in the prone position are available. Assess for and correct any of the following potential trouble points with patients in the prone position:

- Neck hyperextension
- Hyperextension of the lumbar spine
- Plantar flexion of the ankles
- Unprotected pressure points at the chin, elbows, female breasts, hips, knees, and toes

Side-Lying Position. In the side-lying (or lateral) position the patient rests on the side with the major portion of body weight on the dependent hip and shoulder. A 30-degree lateral position is recommended for patients at risk for pressure ulcers (see Chapter 48) (AHRQ, 2010). Trunk alignment needs to be the same as in

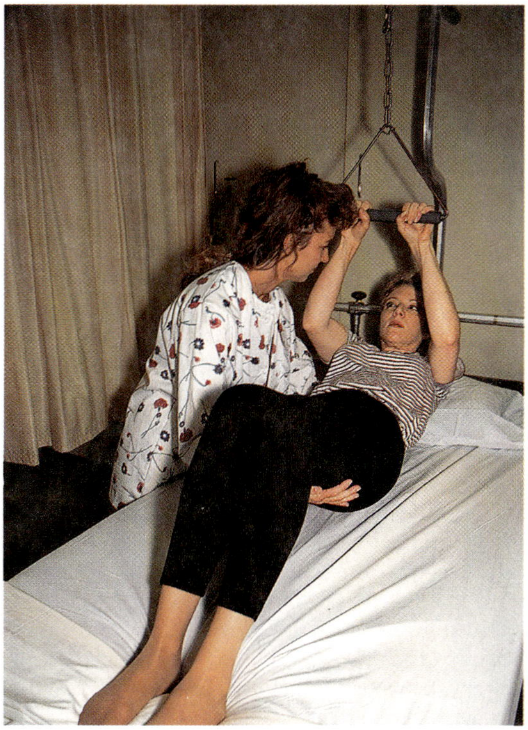

FIG. 47-20 Patient using trapeze bar.

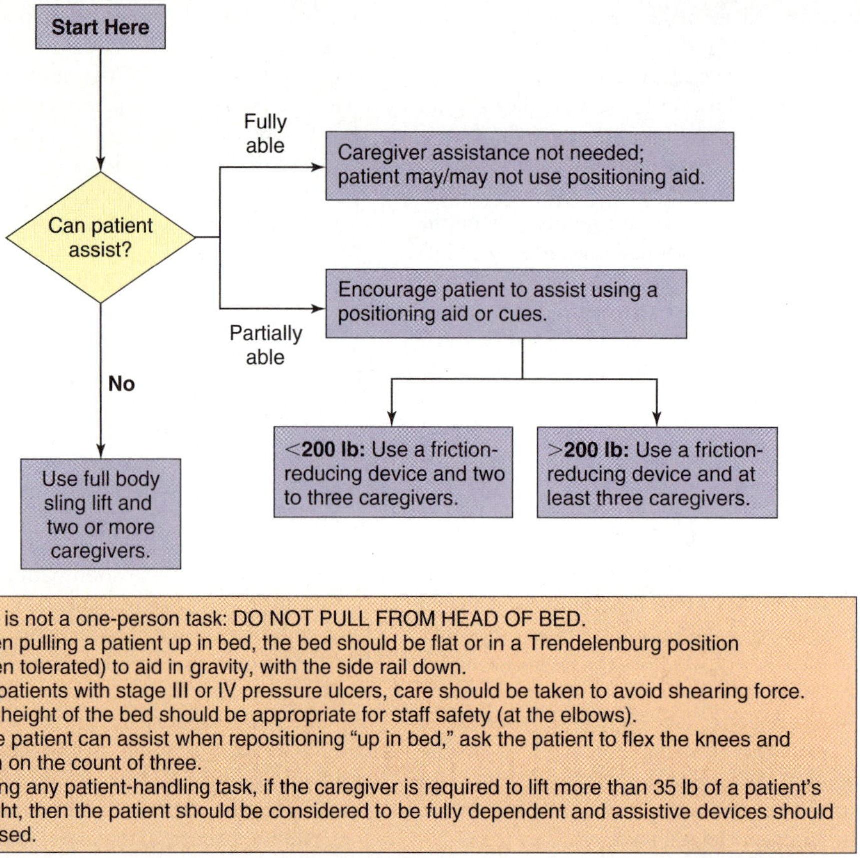

FIG. 47-21 Algorithm used to reposition patient in bed. (From Nelson A: *Safe patient handling and movement algorithms,* 2006, VISN8 Patient Safety Center, http://www.visn8.med.va.gov/patientsafetycenter/SafePtHandling/default.asp.)

standing. The patient needs to maintain the structural curves of the spine, the head needs to be supported in line with the midline of the trunk, and rotation of the spine needs to be avoided. The following trouble points are common in the side-lying position:

- Lateral flexion of the neck
- Spinal curves out of normal alignment
- Shoulder and hip joints internally rotated, adducted, or unsupported
- Lack of foot support
- Lack of protection for pressure points at the ear, shoulder, anterior iliac spine, trochanter, and ankles
- Excessive lateral flexion of the spine if the patient has large hips and a pillow is not placed superior to the hips at the waist

Sims' Position. Sims' position differs from the side-lying position in the distribution of the patient's weight. In Sims' position the patient places the weight on the anterior ileum, humerus, and clavicle. Trouble points common in Sims' position include the following:

- Lateral flexion of the neck
- Internal rotation, adduction, or lack of support to the shoulders and hips
- Lack of foot support
- Lack of protection for pressure points at the ileum, humerus, clavicle, knees, and ankles

Transfer Techniques. Nurses often provide care for immobilized patients whose position must be changed, who must be moved up in bed, or who must be transferred from a bed to a chair or from a bed to a stretcher. As noted earlier, body mechanics alone do not protect the nurse from injury to the musculoskeletal system when moving, lifting, or transferring patients. Although nurses use many transfer techniques, knowledge of ergonomics and safe patient handling is crucial in maintaining caregiver and patient safety.

Assess every situation that involves patient handling and movement to minimize risk of injury. After completing the assessment, nurses use an algorithm (Fig. 47-21) to guide decisions about safe patient handling (Nelson et al., 2009). Use the patient's strength when lifting, transferring, or moving when possible. Involving the patient has the added bonus of increasing participation in self-care, thus promoting a sense of accomplishment. In addition to handling patients safely, nurses need to assume an active role in their workplaces to ensure that a culture of safety exists and that appropriate patient-handling equipment is readily available (Waters et al., 2007).

Moving Patients. A safe transfer is the first priority. Patients require various levels of assistance to move up in bed, move to the side-lying position, or sit up at the side of the bed. For example, a young, healthy woman may need support as she sits at the side of the bed for the first time after childbirth, whereas an older man may need help from two or more nurses to do the same task 1 to 2 days after surgery.

Always ask the patient to help to the fullest extent possible. To determine what the patient is able to do alone and how many people are needed to help move him or her in bed, assess him or

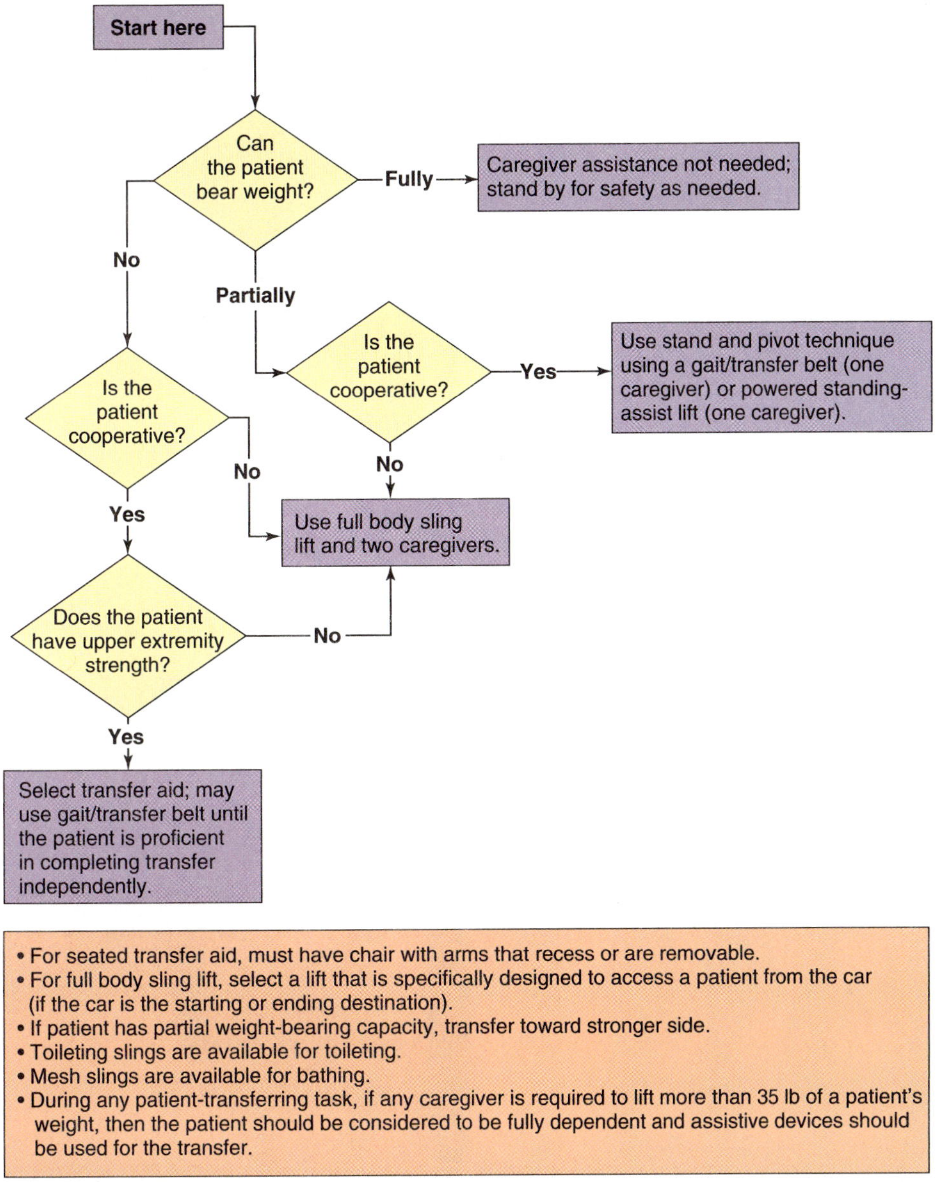
Start here
Can the patient bear weight?
Fully
Caregiver assistance not needed; stand by for safety as needed.
No
Partially
Is the patient cooperative?
Yes
Use stand and pivot technique using a gait/transfer belt (one caregiver) or powered standing-assist lift (one caregiver).
Is the patient cooperative?
No
No
Yes
Use full body sling lift and two caregivers.
Does the patient have upper extremity strength?
No
Yes
Select transfer aid; may use gait/transfer belt until the patient is proficient in completing transfer independently.
• For seated transfer aid, must have chair with arms that recess or are removable.
• For full body sling lift, select a lift that is specifically designed to access a patient from the car (if the car is the starting or ending destination).
• If patient has partial weight-bearing capacity, transfer toward stronger side.
• Toileting slings are available for toileting.
• Mesh slings are available for bathing.
• During any patient-transferring task, if any caregiver is required to lift more than 35 lb of a patient's weight, then the patient should be considered to be fully dependent and assistive devices should be used for the transfer.

FIG. 47-22 Algorithm used to transfer patient to and from bed to chair, chair to toilet, chair to chair, or car to chair. (From Nelson A: *Safe patient handling and movement algorithms,* 2006, VISN8 Patient Safety Center, http://www.visn8.med.va.gov/patientsafetycenter/SafePtHandling/default.asp.)

her to determine whether the illness contradicts exertion (e.g., cardiovascular disease). Next, determine whether the patient comprehends what is expected. For example, a patient recently medicated for postoperative pain is too lethargic to understand instructions; thus to ensure safety, two nurses are necessary to move him or her. Then determine his or her comfort level. It is important to evaluate your personal strength and knowledge of the procedure. Finally determine whether the patient is too heavy or immobile for you to move alone (Nelson et al., 2009). Through assessment tools and patient movement algorithms, you determine the safest method by which to move the patient. Skill 47-1 and Skill 47-2 on pp. 1159-1173 describe the steps commonly used in moving patients in bed and transferring them to a sitting position at the side of the bed.

Transferring a Patient from a Bed to a Chair. Refer to an algorithm when transferring a patient from a bed to a chair (Fig. 47-22). Before beginning, move obstacles out of the way to prepare the environment and ensure that enough help is available. If a caregiver needs to lift more than 35 pounds, use assistive devices for the transfer (Fig. 47-23). Explain the procedure to the patient before the transfer. Place the chair next to the bed.

Next determine if the patient can bear weight. If the patient can bear weight fully, stand near him or her during the transfer as needed for safety reasons. If he or she can only partially bear weight and is cooperative, the transfer requires one caregiver. The nurse either stands and pivots the patient into the chair using a gait or transfer belt or uses a powered standing-assist lift. Two caregivers and a full body sling are needed for transferring uncooperative patients who can bear partial weight and for patients who cannot bear weight and are either uncooperative or do not have upper body strength. A seated transfer aid such as a friction-reducing lateral-assist device is used with or without a gait belt for patients

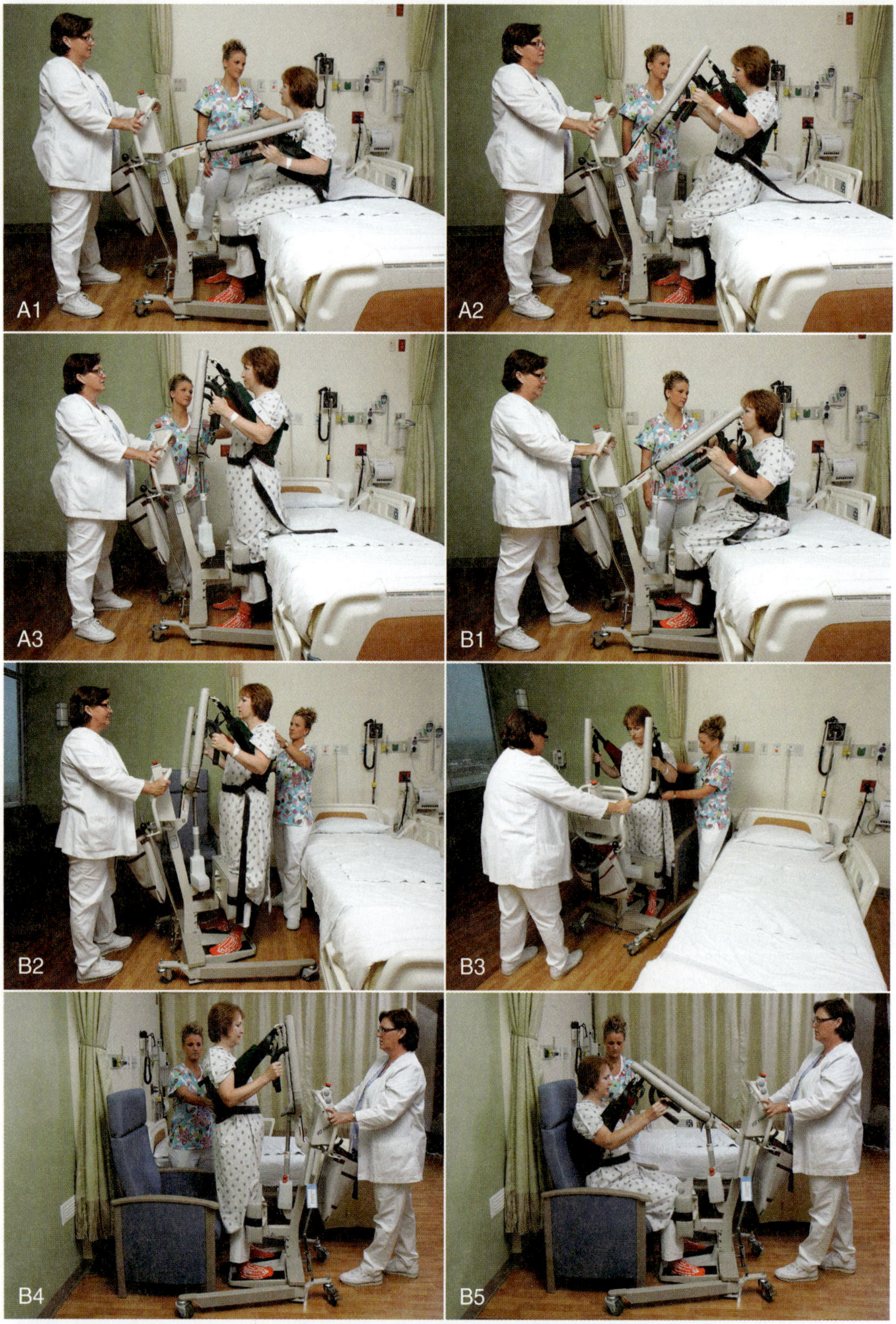

FIG. 47-23 **A1,** Ensure that safety straps are secured appropriately when using motorized lift to help patient move to standing position. **A2,** Patient grasps handles as nurse enables motorized lift. **A3,** Patient is in standing position with feet on floor and is ready to ambulate to chair with nurses' help. **B1,** When patient is unable to walk, secure safety straps and use platform of motorized lift. **B2,** Patient is in upright position. **B3,** Position patient in front of chair. **B4,** Explain to patient need to hold on to handles as motorized lift begins to lower patient into chair. **B5,** Guide patient into chair.

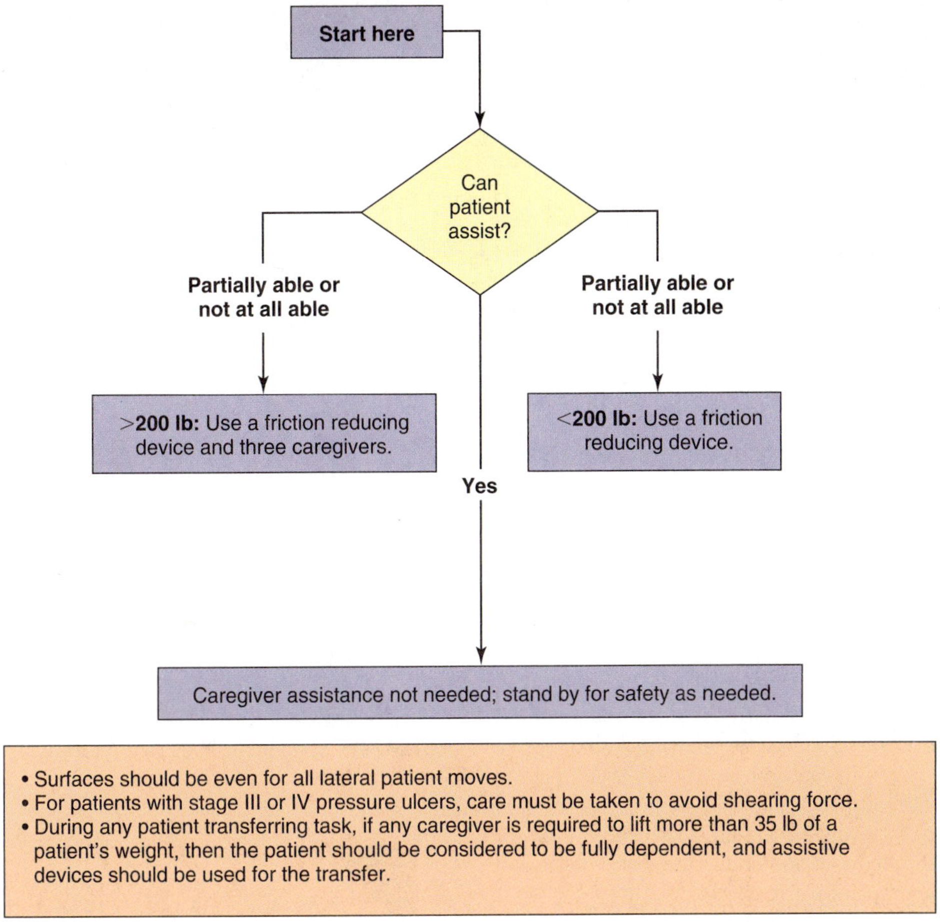

FIG. 47-24 Algorithm used to complete lateral transfer to and from bed to stretcher, trolley. (From Nelson A: *Safe patient handling and movement algorithms,* 2006, VISN8 Patient Safety Center, http://www.visn8.med.va.gov/patientsafetycenter/SafePtHandling/default.asp.)

who cannot bear weight but who are cooperative and have sufficient upper body strength to complete the transfer. If a seated transfer aid is used, the chair needs to have arms that are able to be removed or moved out of the way. Transfer patients who have partial weight bearing toward their stronger side (Baptiste et al., 2006; Nelson et al., 2009).

Transferring a Patient from a Bed to a Stretcher. To transfer a patient from a bed to a stretcher, first consult an appropriate algorithm (Fig. 47-24). Determine if the patient is able to assist in the procedure. Patients who receive opioid pain medications often need additional assistance during the transfer because they may be unable to assist or may have difficulty understanding the caregiver's directions.

Allow patients who can complete the transfer independently to move to the stretcher on their own and stand by to ensure a safe transfer. Determine the patient's weight if he or she can assist partially or cannot assist at all. Use a friction-reducing device for patients who weigh less than 200 pounds. If the patient weighs 200 pounds or more, use a friction-reducing device and three caregivers. Before moving the patient, place the stretcher and the bed side by side to allow him or her to transfer quickly and easily using the friction-reducing device.

Use caution when the patient has or is suspected of having spinal cord trauma. If you have to move the patient, place a transfer board under him or her to maintain spinal alignment before transferring to a stretcher. Prepare the patient for the transfer and ask for help when possible (e.g., by folding the arms over the chest). Make sure that the environment is free from obstacles and remove unnecessary equipment from the bed.

Restorative and Continuing Care. The goal of restorative care for the patient who is immobile is to maximize functional mobility and independence and reduce residual functional deficits such as impaired gait and decreased endurance. The focus in restorative care is not only on ADLs that relate to physical self-care but also on **instrumental activities of daily living (IADLs).** IADLs are activities that are necessary to be independent in society beyond eating, grooming, transferring, and toileting and include such skills as shopping, preparing meals, banking, and taking medications.

The nurse uses many of the same interventions as described in the health promotion and acute care sections, but the emphasis is on working collaboratively with patients and their significant others and with other health care professionals to facilitate the patient's return to maximal functional ability in both ADLs and IADLs.

Intensive specialized therapy such as occupational or physical therapy is common. If the patient is in an institution, he or she likely goes to the therapy department 2 to 3 times a day. The nurse's role is to work collaboratively with these professionals and reinforce exercises and teaching. For example, after a stroke or brain attack, a patient likely receives gait training from a physical therapist; speech rehabilitation from a speech therapist; and help from an occupational therapist for ADLs such as dressing, bathing and toileting, or household chores. The therapy is not always able to restore total functional health, but it often helps the patient adapt to the mobility limitations or complications. Equipment frequently used to help patients adapt to mobility limitations includes walkers, canes, wheelchairs, and assistive devices such as toilet seat extenders, reaching sticks, special silverware, and clothing with Velcro closures.

Range-of-Motion Exercises. To ensure adequate joint mobility, teach the patient about ROM exercises. Walking also increases joint mobility. Patients with restricted mobility are unable to perform some or all ROM exercises independently. Provide ROM exercises to maintain maximum joint mobility. To ensure that patients routinely receive ROM exercises, schedule them at specific times, perhaps with another nursing activity such as during the patient's bath. This enables the nurse to systematically reassess mobility while improving the patient's ROM. In addition, bathing usually requires that extremities and joints are put through complete ROM.

Passive ROM exercises begin as soon as the patient's ability to move the extremity or joint is lost. Carry out movements slowly and smoothly, just to the point of resistance; ROM should not cause pain. Never force a joint beyond its capacity. Each movement needs to be repeated 5 times during the session.

When performing passive ROM exercises, stand at the side of the bed closest to the joint being exercised. Perform passive ROM exercises using a head-to-toe sequence and moving from larger to smaller joints. If an extremity is to be moved or lifted, place a cupped hand under the joint to support it, support the joint by holding the adjacent distal and proximal areas (Fig. 47-25), or support the joint with one hand and cradle the distal portion of the extremity with the remaining arm (Fig. 47-26). See Table 47-2 for detailed ROM for each joint. Appropriate ROM exercises are based on the patient and the affected joint.

Walking. When a patient has a limited ability to walk, assess his or her activity tolerance, tolerance to the upright position (orthostatic hypotension), strength, presence of pain, coordination, and balance to determine the amount of assistance needed. Explain how far the patient should try to walk, who is going to help, when the walk will take place, and why walking is important. In addition, determine with the patient how much independence he or she can assume.

Check the environment to be sure that there are no obstacles in the patient's path. Clear chairs, over-bed tables, and wheelchairs out of the way so the patient has ample room to walk safely. Before starting, establish rest points in case activity tolerance is less than estimated or the patient becomes dizzy. For example, place a chair in the hall for the patient to rest if needed. A nurse who does not have a lot of strength and who is unable to ambulate a patient alone needs to request help and ensure that the patient has an assistive device such as a walker (see Chapter 38). A nurse stands on either side of the patient, and each holds one side of the gait belt.

Provide support at the waist by using a **gait belt** so the patient's center of gravity remains midline. While walking, the patient should not lean to one side because this alters the center of gravity, distorts balance, and increases the risk of falling. Return a patient who at any point appears unsteady or complains of dizziness to a nearby bed or chair. If the patient faints or begins to fall, assume a wide base of support with one foot in front of the other, thus supporting the body weight. Then gently lower the patient to the floor, protecting the head. Although lowering a patient to the floor is not difficult, the nursing student needs to practice this technique with a friend or classmate before attempting it in a clinical setting.

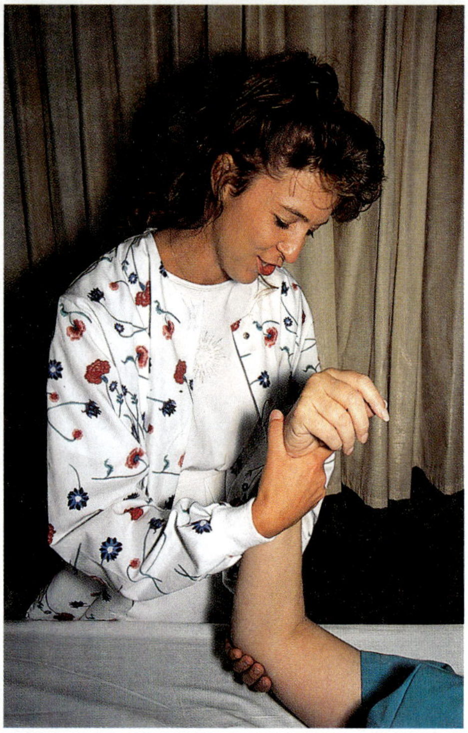

FIG. 47-25 Supporting joint by holding distal and proximal areas adjacent to joint.

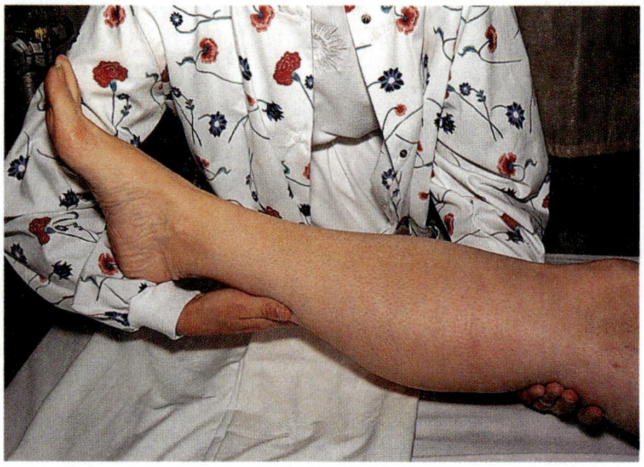

FIG. 47-26 Cradling distal portion of extremity.

Patients with **hemiplegia** (one-sided paralysis) or **hemiparesis** (one-sided weakness) often need assistance with walking. When an assistive device is used, stand on the patient's affected side and support him or her with a gait belt. Providing support by holding the patient's arm is incorrect because the nurse cannot easily support the patient's weight to lower him or her to the floor if he or she faints or falls. In addition, if the patient falls with the nurse holding an arm, a shoulder joint may be dislocated.

EVALUATION

Through the Patient's Eyes. Just as it was important to include the patient during the assessment and planning phase of the care plan, it is essential to have the patient's evaluation of the plan of care. Were the goals met, or is more work required? You must now determine with the patient and others involved with care if the goals or outcomes established with and for the patient have indeed been met; what still needs to be achieved from the patient's perspective; and the construction of a new plan of care. In other words, how have the patient's expectations changed and in what ways?

Patient Outcomes. From your perspective as the nurse, you are to evaluate outcomes and response to nursing care and compare the patient's actual outcomes with the outcomes selected during planning such as his or her ability to maintain or improve body alignment, joint mobility, walking, moving, or transferring. Evaluate the effectiveness of specific interventions designed to promote body alignment, improve mobility, and protect the patient from the hazards of immobility. Evaluate the patient's and family's understanding of all teaching provided as well (Fig. 47-27). The continuous nature of evaluation allows you to determine whether new or revised therapies are required and if new nursing diagnoses have developed.

When outcomes are not met, consider asking the following questions:

- Are there ways we can assist you to increase your activity?
- Which activities are you having trouble completing right now?
- How do you feel about not being able to dress yourself and make your own meals?
- Which exercises do you find most helpful?
- What goals for your activity would you like to set now?

Once these questions have been asked and you have addressed the limited mobility and its associated problems through the patient's eyes, you are prepared to adjust the plan of care to address the remaining clinical problems that your patient is experiencing related to immobility.

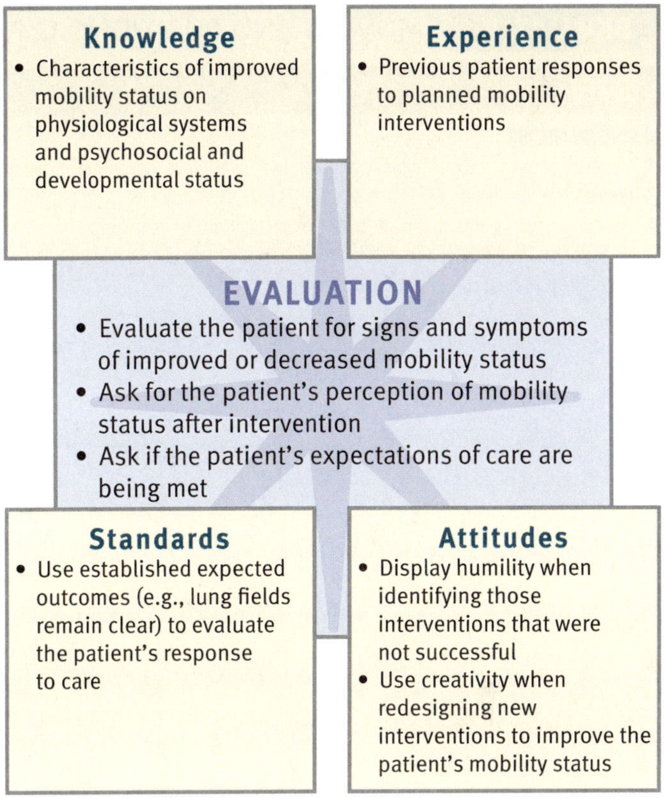
Knowledge
• Characteristics of improved mobility status on physiological systems and psychosocial and developmental status
Experience
• Previous patient responses to planned mobility interventions
EVALUATION
• Evaluate the patient for signs and symptoms of improved or decreased mobility status
• Ask for the patient's perception of mobility status after intervention
• Ask if the patient's expectations of care are being met
Standards
• Use established expected outcomes (e.g., lung fields remain clear) to evaluate the patient's response to care
Attitudes
• Display humility when identifying those interventions that were not successful
• Use creativity when redesigning new interventions to improve the patient's mobility status

FIG. 47-27 Critical thinking model for immobility evaluation.

SAFETY GUIDELINES FOR NURSING SKILLS

Ensuring patient safety is an essential role of the professional nurse. To ensure patient safety, communicate clearly with the members of the health care team, access and incorporate the patient's priorities of care and preferences, and use the best evidence when making decisions about your patient's care. When performing the skills in this chapter, remember the following points to ensure safe, individualized patient-centered care.

- Mentally review the transfer steps before beginning the procedure, this ensures both the patient's and your safety.
- Assess the patient's mobility and strength to determine the assistance that he or she is able to offer during transfer. Stand on patient's weak side when assisting (Pierson and Fairchild, 2008).
- Determine the amount and type of assistance required for safe positioning and transfer, including the type of transfer equipment and the number of personnel to safely transfer and prevent harm to patient and health care providers.
- Raise the side rail on the side of the bed opposite of where you are standing to prevent the patient from falling out of bed on that side.
- Arrange equipment (e.g., intravenous lines, feeding tube, Foley catheter) so it does not interfere with the positioning or transfer process.
- Evaluate the patient for correct body alignment and pressure risks after the transfer.
- Make sure that all personnel understand how equipment functions before it is used.
- Educate patients about how equipment functions to reduce their anxiety and enlist their cooperation.

SKILL 47-1 MOVING AND POSITIONING PATIENTS IN BED

View Video!

Delegation Considerations

The skill of moving and positioning patients in bed can be delegated to nursing assistive personnel (NAP). The nurse is responsible for assessing the patient's level of comfort and for any hazards of immobility. Instruct NAP about:

- Any limitations affecting movement and positioning.
- Scheduled times to reposition patient through the shift.
- When to request assistance (e.g., when the patient is unable to assist the nurse, has a lot of equipment, or is confused.

Equipment

- Pillows
- Therapeutic boots, splints, ankle support devices if needed
- Trochanter roll
- Sandbag
- Hand rolls
- Side rails
- Appropriate safe patient–handling assistive device

SKILL 47-1 MOVING AND POSITIONING PATIENTS IN BED—cont'd

STEP	RATIONALE
ASSESSMENT	
1 Assess patient's body alignment and comfort level while he or she is lying down.	Provides baseline data for later comparisons. Determines ways to improve position and alignment.
2 Assess for risk factors that contribute to complications of immobility:	Increased risk factors require more frequent repositioning.
a. Paralysis, hemiparesis resulting from a cerebrovascular accident (CVA); decreased sensation	Paralysis impairs movement; muscle tone changes; sensation is often affected. Because of difficulty in moving and poor awareness of involved body part, patient is unable to protect and position body part for self (Lewis et al., 2011).
b. Impaired mobility from traction, arthritis, or other contributing disease processes	Traction or arthritic changes of affected extremity result in decreased range of motion (ROM).
c. Impaired circulation	Decreased circulation predisposes patient to pressure ulcers.
d. *Age:* Very young, older adults	Premature and young infants require frequent turning because their skin is fragile. Normal physiological changes associated with aging predispose older adults to greater risks for developing complications of immobility (Butler, 2006; Ebersole et al., 2008).
e. Level of consciousness and mental status.	Comatose or semicomatose patients are unable to verbalize areas of skin pressure, increasing the risk for skin breakdown.
3 Assess patient's physical ability to help with moving and positioning:	Enables nurse to use patient's mobility, coordination, and strength; determines need for additional help. Ensures patient's and nurse's safety (Nelson et al., 2009).
a. Age	Some older adults move more slowly with less strength.
b. Level of consciousness and mental status	Determines need for special aids or devices. Patients with altered levels of consciousness do not always understand instructions and are often unable to help.
c. Disease process	Cardiopulmonary disease requires patient to have head of bed elevated.
d. Strength, coordination	Determines amount of assistance provided by patient during position change.
e. ROM	Limited ROM contraindicates certain positions.
4 Assess patient's height, weight, and body shape.	Devices used for safe patient handling have different weight restrictions; bariatric patients require special beds, lifts, wheelchairs, and toileting and bathing equipment (Nelson et al., 2009).
5 Assess health care provider's orders. Clarify whether any positions are contraindicated because of patient's condition (e.g., spinal cord injury; respiratory difficulties; certain neurological conditions; presence of incisions, drains, and tubing).	Placing patient in an inappropriate position causes injury.
6 Assess for presence of tubes, incisions, and equipment (e.g., traction).	Alters positioning procedure and affects patient's ability to independently change positions.
7 Assess condition of patient's skin.	Provides baseline to determine effects of positioning.
8 Assess ability and motivation of patient, family members, and primary caregiver to participate in moving and positioning patient in bed in anticipation of discharge to home.	Determines ability of patient and caregivers to help with positioning.
PLANNING	
1 Collect appropriate equipment. Get extra help as needed. Close door to room or close bedside curtains.	Having appropriate number of people to position patient prevents patient and nurse injury. Provides for patient privacy.
2 Perform hand hygiene.	Reduces transfer of microorganisms.
3 Verify patient's identity by using at least two patient identifiers (i.e., name and birth date or name and account number) according to facility policy. Compare identifiers with information on the patient's medical record. Explain procedure.	Ensures correct patient. Complies with a recommended National Patient Safety Goal (TJC, 2011). Improves patient safety. In most acute care settings you use the patient's name and identification number on armband and medical record to identify patients. Decreases anxiety and increases patient cooperation.
4 Raise level of bed to comfortable working height. Remove all pillows and devices used for positioning.	Raises work toward nurse's center of gravity. Reduces any interference during positioning.
IMPLEMENTATION	
1 Position patient flat in bed if tolerated. Keep patient aligned.	Repositioning from flat position decreases friction and possible shear on patient's skin.

CLINICAL DECISION: *Before flattening bed, account for all tubing, drains, and equipment to prevent dislodgement or tipping if caught in mattress or bed frame as bed is lowered.*

STEP	RATIONALE
a. Moving patient up in bed (two nurses):	This is not a one-person task. Helping a patient move up in bed without help from other co-workers or without the aid of an assistive device (i.e., friction-reducing pad) is not recommended or considered safe for the patient or nurse (ANA, 2011; CDC, 2009). If the patient is unable to fully assist, then refer to Step 1b.
(1) Remove pillow from under head and shoulders and place it at head of bed.	Prevents striking patient's head against head of bed.
(2) Face head of bed.	Facing direction of movement prevents twisting your body while moving patient.
(3) Each nurse places one arm under patient's head and shoulders and one arm under patient's thighs.	Provides support across length of patient's body.
(4) *Alternate position if patient can assist:* Position one nurse at patient's upper body. Nurse's arm nearest head of bed is under patient's head and opposite shoulder. Position other nurse at patient's lower back and torso.	Prevents trauma to patient's musculoskeletal system by supporting shoulder and hip joints and evenly distributing weight.
(5) Place feet apart, with foot nearest head of bed in front of other foot (forward-backward stance)	Wide base of support increases balance. Stance enables nurse to shift weight as patient moves up in bed, thereby reducing friction, and enables patient to use long muscles for movement.
(6) Before moving patient, instruct him or her to flex knees with feet flat on bed.	Decreases friction and enables patient to use leg muscles during movement.
(7) Also instruct patient to flex neck, tilting chin toward chest.	Prevents hypertension of neck when moving patient up in bed.
(8) Have patient help moving by pushing with feet on bed surface.	Reduces friction. Increases patient mobility. Decreases workload.
(9) Flex your knees and hips, bringing forearms closer to level of bed.	Increases balance and strength by bringing center of gravity of nurse closer to patient. Uses thighs instead of back muscles.
(10) Instruct patient on count of 3 to push heels and elevate trunk while breathing out, thus moving toward head of bed.	Prepares patient for move. Reinforces assistance in moving up in bed. Increases patient cooperation. Breathing out avoids patient performing Valsalva.
(11) On count of 3, rock and shift weight from front to back leg. At the same time patient pushes with heels and elevates trunk.	Rocking enables nurse to improve balance and overcome inertia. Shifting weight counteracts patient's weight and reduces force needed to move load. Patient's assistance reduces friction and workload for nurse.
b. Moving immobile patient up in bed with drawsheet (two nurses):	

CLINICAL DECISION: *Use safe nursing judgment by increasing number of nurses or NAP when moving a larger patient up in bed. If in doubt, acquire more help.*

STEP	RATIONALE
(1) Place drawsheet under patient by turning from side to side. Extend sheet from shoulder to thighs. Return patient to supine position.	Supports patient's body weight and reduces friction during movement.
(2) Position one nurse at each side of patient's hips.	Distributes weight equally between nurses.
(3) Grasp drawsheet firmly near patient.	
(4) Place feet apart, with foot nearest head of bed in front of other, flex your knees and hips, on count of 3 shift weight from front to back leg, and move patient and drawsheet to desired position in bed.	Rocking enables nurse to improve balance and overcome inertia. Shifting weight counteracts patient's weight and reduces force needed to move load.
c. Positioning patient in supported Fowler's position (see illustration):	

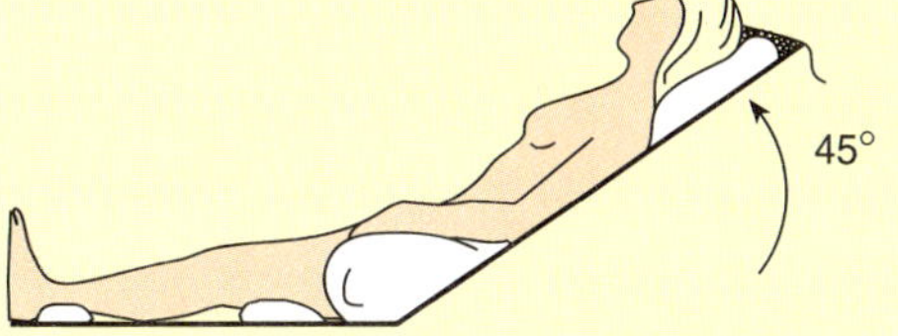

STEP 1c Supported Fowler's position.

STEP	RATIONALE
(1) Elevate head of bed 45 to 60 degrees.	Increases comfort, improves ventilation, and increases patient's opportunity to socialize or relax.
(2) Rest head against mattress or on small pillow.	Prevents flexion contractures of cervical vertebrae.
(3) Use pillows to support arms and hands if patient does not have voluntary control or use of hands and arms.	Prevents shoulder dislocation from effect of downward pull of unsupported arms, promotes circulation by preventing venous pooling, and prevents flexion contractures of arms and wrists.
(4) Position pillow at lower back.	Supports lumbar vertebrae and decreases flexion of vertebrae.
(5) Place small pillow under thigh.	Prevents hyperextension of knee and occlusion of popliteal artery caused by pressure from body weight.
(6) Elevate patient's heel in heel boots or other heel pressure-relief devices.	Heel pressure-relief devices are more effective than pillows for consistently reducing pressure from the mattress on the heels. When pillows are used, they must be repositioned each time the patient moves (Walsh and Plonczynski, 2007).

SKILL 47-1 MOVING AND POSITIONING PATIENTS IN BED—cont'd

STEP	RATIONALE
CLINICAL DECISION: *To keep feet in proper alignment and prevent footdrop, use foot support devices such as ankle or foot boots. In addition, a foot cradle is often used for patients with poor peripheral circulation as a means of reducing pressure on the tips of patient's toes (check agency policy).*	
d. Positioning hemiplegic patient in supported Fowler's position:	
(1) Elevate head of bed 45 to 60 degrees.	Increases comfort, improves ventilation, and increases patient's opportunity to relax.
(2) Position patient in sitting position as straight as possible.	Counteracts tendency to slump toward affected side. Improves ventilation and cardiac output; decreases intracranial pressure. Improves patient's ability to swallow and helps to prevent aspiration of food, liquids, and gastric secretions (Glenn-Molali, 2008).
(3) Position head on small pillow with chin slightly forward. If patient is totally unable to control head movement, avoid hyperextension of neck.	Prevents hyperextension of neck. Too many pillows under head cause or worsen neck flexion contracture.
CLINICAL DECISION: *If the patient has a paralyzed extremity, provide support for involved arm and hand on over-bed table in front of patient. Place arm away from patient's side and support elbow with pillow.* • *Position flaccid hand in normal resting position with wrist slightly extended, arches of hand maintained, and fingers partially flexed; use section of rubber ball cut in half; clasp patient's hands together.* • *Position spastic hand with wrist in neutral position or slightly extended; extend fingers with palm down or leave them in relaxed position palm up. At times it is difficult to position spastic hands without the use of specially made splints for the patient.*	
(4) Flex knees and hips by using pillow or folded blanket under knees.	Ensures proper alignment. Flexion prevents prolonged hyperextension, which possibly impairs joint mobility.
(5) Place trochanter rolls along side of patient's legs.	Reduces external rotation of hip.
(6) Support feet in dorsiflexion with foot support such as ankle or foot boots (check agency policy).	Prevents footdrop by placing ankle in neutral dorsiflexion. Stimulation of ball of foot by firm surface has tendency to increase muscle tone in patient with extensor spasticity of lower extremity.
e. Positioning patient in supine position:	
(1) Be sure that patient is comfortable on back with head of bed flat.	Some patients' physical conditions do not tolerate supine position.
(2) Place small rolled towel under lumbar area of back.	Provides support for lumbar spine.
(3) Place pillow under upper shoulders, neck, or head.	Maintains correct alignment and prevents flexion contractures of cervical vertebrae.
(4) Place trochanter rolls or sandbags parallel to lateral surface of patient's thighs if patient is immobile.	Reduces external rotation of hip.
(5) Position patient's heels in heel boots or other heel pressure-relief device (check agency policy).	Heel pressure-relief devices are more effective than pillows for consistently reducing pressure from the mattress on the heels.
(6) If needed, support feet in dorsiflexion with foot support such as ankle or foot boots (check agency policy).	Prevents footdrop by placing ankle in neutral dorsiflexion. Stimulation of ball of foot by firm surface has tendency to increase muscle tone in patient with extensor spasticity of lower extremity.
(7) Place pillows under pronated forearms, keeping upper arms parallel to patient's body (see illustrations).	Reduces internal rotation of shoulder and prevents extension of elbows. Maintains correct body alignment.

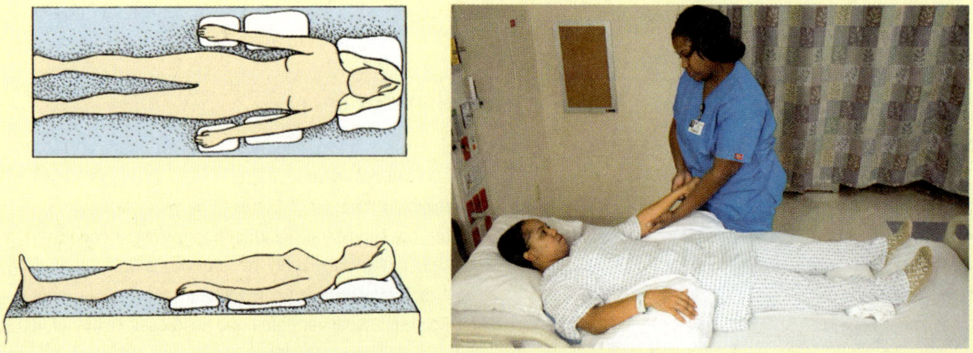

STEP 1e(7) Supine position with supporting pillows.

STEP	RATIONALE
(8) Place firm hand rolls in patient's hands. Consider physical therapy referral for use of hand splints.	Reduces extension of fingers and abduction of thumb. Maintains thumb slightly adducted and in opposition to fingers.

STEP	RATIONALE
f. Positioning hemiplegic patient in supine position:	
(1) Be sure that patient is comfortable on back with head of bed flat.	Some patients' physical conditions do not tolerate supine position.
(2) Place folded towel or small pillow under shoulder of affected side.	Decreases possibility of pain, joint contracture, and subluxation. Maintains mobility in muscles around shoulder to permit normal movement patterns.
(3) Keep affected arm away from body with elbow extended and palm up. (Alternate position is to place arm out to side, with elbow bent and hand toward head of bed.)	Maintains mobility in arm, joints, and shoulder to permit normal movement patterns. (Alternate position counteracts limitation of ability of arm to rotate outward at shoulder [external rotation]. Need external rotation to raise arm overhead without pain.)

CLINICAL DECISION: *Position affected hand in one of the recommended positions for flaccid or spastic hand.*

STEP	RATIONALE
(4) Place folded towel under hip of involved side.	Diminishes effect of spasticity in entire leg by controlling hip position.
(5) Flex affected knee 30 degrees by supporting it on pillow or folded blanket.	Slight flexion breaks up abnormal extension pattern of leg. Extensor spasticity is most severe when patient is supine.
(6) Support patient's heel in heel boots or other heel pressure-relief device (check agency policy).	Prevents footdrop by placing ankle in neutral dorsiflexion. Stimulation of ball of foot by firm surface has tendency to increase muscle tone in patient with extensor spasticity of lower extremity.
g. Positioning patient in prone position:	
(1) With patient supine, place arm on side to be turned alongside the body. Roll patient over the arm positioned close to the body, with elbow straight and hand under hip. Position on abdomen in center of bed.	Positions patient correctly to maintain alignment.
(2) Turn patient's head to one side and support head with small pillow (see illustration).	Reduces flexion or hyperextension of cervical vertebrae.

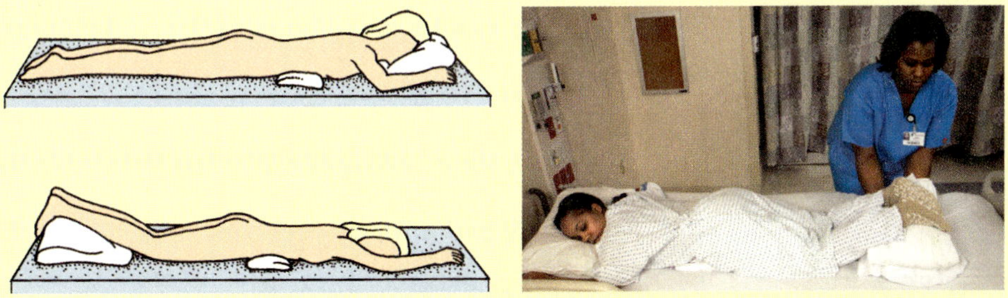

STEP 1g(2) Prone position with supporting pillows.

STEP	RATIONALE
(3) Place small pillow under patient's abdomen below level of diaphragm.	Reduces pressure on breasts of some female patients and decreases hyperextension of lumbar vertebrae and strain on lower back.
(4) Support arms in flexed position level at shoulders.	Maintains proper body alignment. Support reduces risk of joint dislocation.
(5) Support lower legs with pillows to elevate toes.	Prevents footdrop. Reduces external rotation of hips. Eliminates mattress pressure on toes.
h. Positioning hemiplegic patient in prone position:	

CLINICAL DECISION: *Increase frequency of positioning if pressure areas begin to appear; joint mobility becomes impaired or worsened, or patient demonstrates signs of discomfort. Consult with physical and occupational therapists as needed.*

STEP	RATIONALE
(1) Move patient toward unaffected side, with patient remaining supine.	Creates room for proper patient alignment in center of bed when patient rolls onto abdomen.
(2) Place pillow on patient's abdomen.	Prevents sagging of abdomen when patient rolls over; decreases hyperextension of lumbar vertebrae and strain on lower back.
(3) Roll patient onto affected side.	
(4) Roll patient onto abdomen by positioning involved arm close to patient's body, with elbow straight and hand under hip. Roll patient carefully over arm.	Prevents injury to affected side.
(5) Turn head toward involved side.	Promotes development of neck and trunk extension, which is necessary for standing and walking.
(6) Position involved arm out to side, with elbow bent, hand toward head of bed, and fingers extended (if possible).	Counteracts limitation of ability of arm to rotate outward at shoulder (external rotation). External rotation needs to be present to raise arm over head without pain.

SKILL 47-1 MOVING AND POSITIONING PATIENTS IN BED—cont'd

STEP	RATIONALE
(7) Flex knees slightly by placing pillow under legs from knees to ankles.	Flexion prevents prolonged hyperextension, which impairs joint mobility.
(8) Support feet with foot-support devices (e.g., ankle or foot boots) (check agency policy).	Maintains feet in dorsiflexion.
i. Positioning patient in 30-degree lateral (side-lying) position (see illustrations):	
(1) Patient lies supine with head of bed as low as he or she tolerates.	Provides position of comfort for patient and removes pressure from bony prominences on back and buttocks.
(2) Position patient to side of bed. Then move to opposite side of bed toward which patient is to be turned. Use friction-reducing device or mechanical lift per manufacturer guidelines if patient cannot help with moving.	Provides room for patient to turn to side. Use of safe patient–handling equipment reduces workload of caregivers and enhances safety (deCastro et al., 2006).
(3) Prepare to turn patient onto side. Flex his or her knee that is not next to mattress. Place one hand on patient's hip and one hand on patient's shoulder.	Positioning sets up leverage for easy turning.
(4) Roll patient onto side toward nurse.	Decreases trauma to tissues. In addition, patient is positioned so leverage on hip makes turning easy.
(5) Place pillow under patient's head and neck.	Maintains alignment. Reduces lateral neck flexion. Decreases strain on sternocleidomastoid muscle.
(6) Place hands under patient's dependent shoulder and bring shoulder blade forward.	Prevents patient's weight from resting directly on shoulder joint.
(7) Position both arms in slightly flexed position. Support upper arm with pillow level with shoulder; other arm, by mattress.	Decreases internal rotation and adduction of shoulder. Supports both arms in slightly flexed position. Improves ventilation because chest is able to expand.
(8) Place hands under dependent hip and bring hip slightly forward so angle from hip to mattress is approximately 30 degrees	The 30-degree lateral position reduces pressure on trochanter.
(9) Place tuck-back pillow behind patient's back. (Make by folding pillow lengthwise. Smooth area slightly tucked under patient's back.)	Provides support to maintain patient on side.
(10) Place pillow under semiflexed upper leg level at hip from groin to foot.	Maintains leg in correct alignment. Prevents pressure on bony prominence.
(11) Support feet with foot-support devices (e.g., ankle or foot boots) (check agency policy).	Maintains dorsiflexion of feet. Prevents footdrop.
j. Positioning patient in Sims' (semiprone) position (see illustration):	
(1) Be sure that patient is comfortable in supine position.	Provides for proper body alignment while patient is lying down.
(2) Position patient in side-lying position, lying partially on abdomen, with dependent arm straight along his or her body.	Facilitates turning onto side. Avoids injury to arm; semiprone position places less pressure on abdomen.

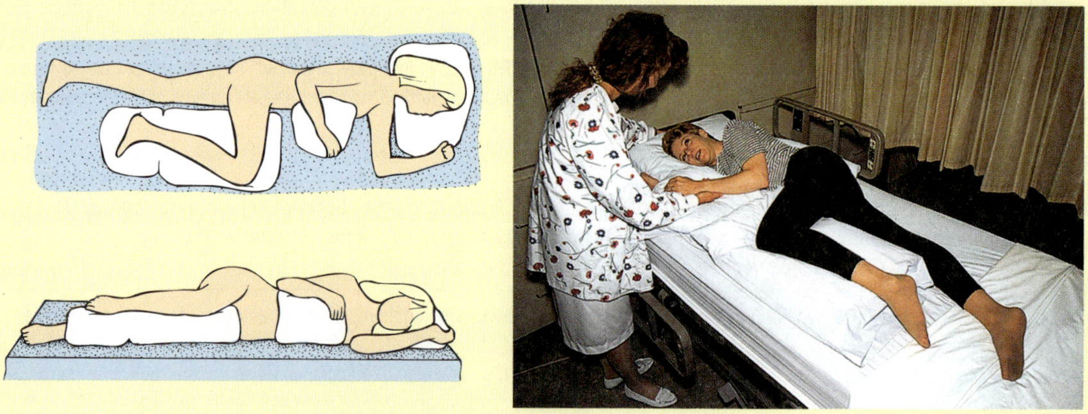

STEP 1i Side-lying position with pillows in place.

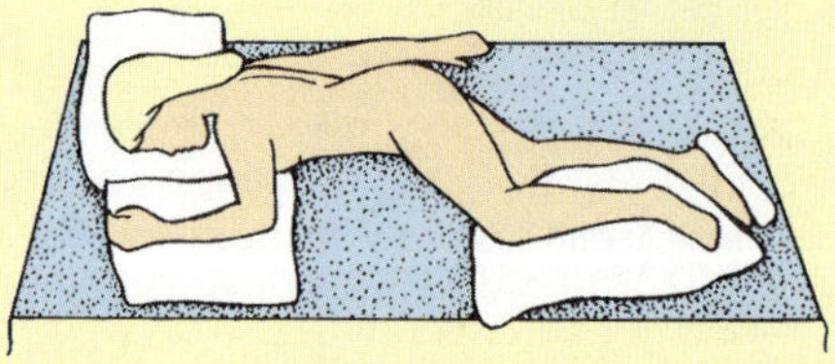

STEP 1j Sims' (semiprone) position with pillows in place.

STEP	RATIONALE
(3) Carefully lift patient's dependent shoulder and bring arm back behind him or her.	
(4) Place small pillow under patient's head.	Patient is rolled only partially on abdomen.
(5) Place pillow under flexed upper arm, supporting arm level with shoulder.	Maintains proper alignment and prevents lateral neck flexion. Prevents internal rotation of shoulder.
(6) Place pillow under flexed upper leg, supporting leg level with hip.	Prevents internal rotation of hip and adduction of leg. Flexion prevents hyperextension of leg. Reduces mattress pressure on knees and ankles.
(7) Support feet with foot-support devices such as ankle or foot boots (check agency policy).	Maintains feet in dorsiflexion. Prevents footdrop.
k. Logrolling patient (three nurses):	

CLINICAL DECISION: *Supervise and aid personnel when there is a health care provider's order to* ***logroll*** *a patient. Patients who have suffered from spinal cord injury or are recovering from neck, back, or spinal surgery often need to keep the spinal column in straight alignment to prevent further injury.*

STEP	RATIONALE
(1) Place pillow between patient's knees.	Prevents tension on spinal column and adduction of hip.
(2) Cross patient's arms on chest.	Prevents injury to arms.
(3) Position two nurses or other staff members on side of bed to which patient will be turned. Position third nurse or staff member on other side of bed (see illustration). If needed, four nurses are used; fourth nurse stands on same side as third nurse.	Distributes weight equally between nurses.
(4) Fanfold or roll drawsheet along side of the patient.	Provides strong handles to grip the drawsheet or pull sheet without slipping.
(5) Move patient as one unit in a smooth, continuous motion on the count of three (see illustration).	This maintains proper alignment by moving all body parts at the same time, preventing tension or twisting of the spinal column.
(6) Nurse on opposite side of bed places pillows along length of patient (see illustration).	Pillows keep patient aligned.
(7) Gently lean patient as a unit back toward pillows for support (see illustration).	Ensures continued straight alignment of spinal column, preventing injury.
2 Perform hand hygiene.	Reduces transmission of microorganisms.

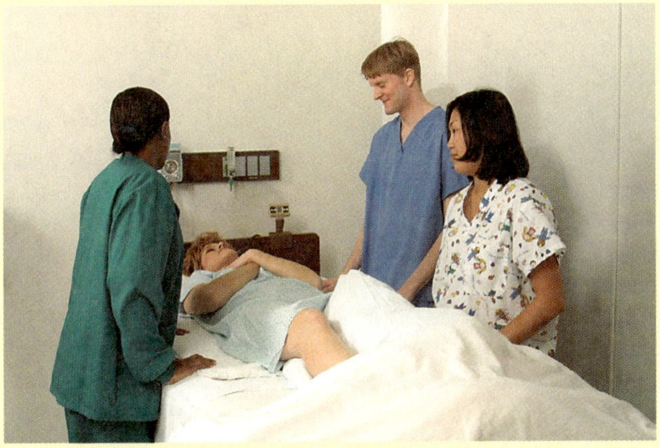

STEP 1k(3) Position nurses on each side of patient.

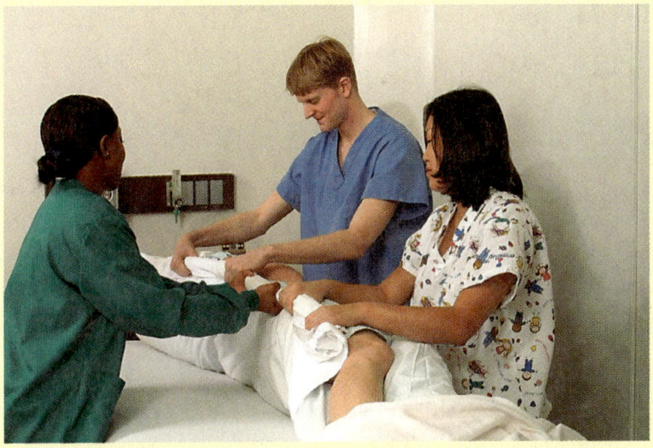

STEP 1k(5) Move patient as a unit, maintaining proper alignment.

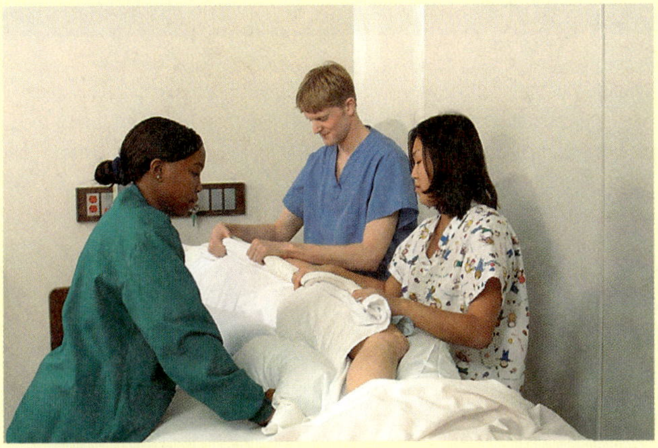

STEP 1k(6) Place pillows along patient's back for support.

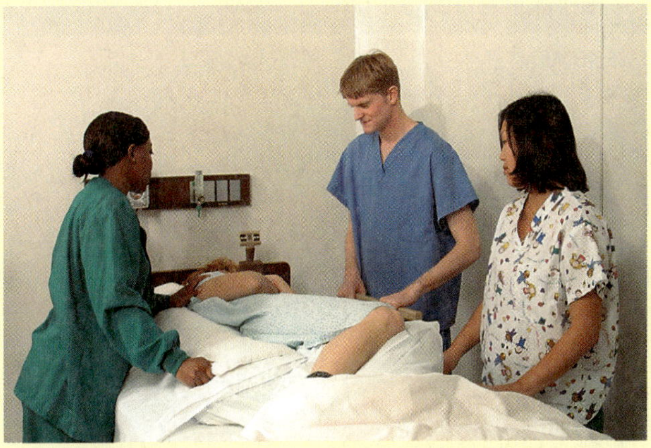

STEP 1k(7) Gently lean patient as a unit against pillows.

SKILL 47-1 MOVING AND POSITIONING PATIENTS IN BED—cont'd

STEP	RATIONALE
EVALUATION	
1 Evaluate patient's body alignment, position, and level of comfort.	Determines effectiveness of positioning. Add or remove supports (e.g., pillows, bath blankets) to promote comfort and correct body alignment.
2 Measure ROM.	Determines if joint contracture is developing.
3 Observe for areas of erythema or breakdown involving skin.	Indicates complications of immobility or improper positioning of body part. Determines if need exists for increasing frequency of repositioning patient.

UNEXPECTED OUTCOMES AND RELATED INTERVENTIONS

1 Joint contractures develop or worsen.
- Consult physical and/or occupational therapy.
- Ensure that activity and ROM orders are implemented consistently.

2 Skin shows areas of erythema and breakdown.
- Increase frequency of turning and repositioning; place turning schedule above patient's bed.
- Consult skin care team.
- Implement other activities per agency skin care policy or protocol (e.g., assess more frequently, consult dietitian, place patient on pressure-relieving mattress).

3 Patient avoids moving.
- Administer pain medications as ordered by a health care provider to ensure patient's comfort before moving if he or she is in pain and allow pain medication to take effect before proceeding.
- Provide patient education about benefits of moving.

RECORDING AND REPORTING

- Document repositioning or turn and observations during procedure (e.g., condition of skin, joint movement, patient's ability to assist with positioning) in nurses' notes.
- Report observations at change of shift.

HOME CARE CONSIDERATIONS

- Teach family how to use safe patient–handling equipment if necessary.
- Teach patient and family about the signs of skin breakdown and the importance of safety during positioning for patients with decreased sensation.

SKILL 47-2 USING SAFE AND EFFECTIVE TRANSFER TECHNIQUES

View Video!

Delegation Considerations

The skill of effective transfer techniques can be delegated to nursing assistive personnel (NAP). Patients who are transferred for the first time after prolonged bed rest, extensive surgery, critical illness, or spinal cord trauma usually require supervision by the nurse. Instruct NAP about:
- Seeking assistance when moving or lifting a patient (e.g., when the patient is overweight or confused).
- Patient limitations (e.g., changes in blood pressure, mobility restrictions) that affect safe transfer techniques

Equipment

- Transfer belt, sling, or lapboard (as needed)
- Nonskid shoes, bath blankets, and pillows
- *Wheelchair:* Position chair at 45-degree angle to bed, lock brakes, remove footrests, lock bed brakes.
- *Stretcher:* Position next to bed, lock brakes on stretcher, lock brakes on bed.
- *Mechanical lift:* Use frame, canvas strips or chains, and hammock or canvas strips.

STEP	RATIONALE
ASSESSMENT	
1 Assess physiological capacity to transfer:	Provides information relative to patient's abilities, physical status, ability to comprehend, and number of individuals needed to provide safe transferring.
a. Muscle strength (legs and upper arms)	Immobile patients have decreased muscle strength, tone, and mass. Affects ability to bear weight or raise body.
b. Joint mobility (range of motion [ROM]) and contracture formation	Immobility or inflammatory processes (e.g., arthritis) sometimes lead to contracture formation and impaired joint mobility.

STEP	RATIONALE
c. Paralysis or paresis (spastic or flaccid)	Patient with central nervous system damage often has bilateral paralysis (requiring transfer by swivel bar, sliding bar, or mechanical lift) or unilateral paralysis, which requires belt transfer to "best" side. Weakness (paresis) requires stabilization of knee while transferring. Flaccid arm needs to be supported with sling during transfer.
d. Risk for orthostatic (postural) hypotension (e.g., previously on bed rest, first time arising from supine position following surgical procedure, history of dizziness when arising)	Determines risk of fainting or falling during transfer. Immobilized patients have decreased ability for autonomic nervous system to equalize blood supply, resulting in drop of 20 mm Hg or more in blood pressure when rising from sitting position (Jarvis, 2008; Monahan et al., 2007).
e. Activity tolerance	Determines ability of patient to assist with transfer.
f. Level of comfort	Pain reduces patient's motivation and ability to be mobile. Pain relief before transfer enhances patient participation.
g. Vital signs	Vital sign changes such as increased pulse and respiration indicate activity intolerance (see Chapter 29).
2 Assess patient's sensory status:	Determine influence of sensory loss on ability to make transfer. Visual field loss decreases patient's ability to see in direction of transfer. Peripheral sensation loss decreases proprioception. Patients with visual and hearing losses need transfer techniques adapted to deficits. Patients with a cerebrovascular accident (CVA) sometimes lose area of visual field, which profoundly affects vision and perception.
a. Adequacy of central and peripheral vision	
b. Adequacy of hearing	
c. Loss of peripheral sensation	

CLINICAL DECISION: *Patients with hemiplegia also often "neglect" one side of the body (inattention to or unawareness of one side of body or environment), which distorts perception of the visual field. If patient experiences neglect of one side, instruct him or her to scan all visual fields when transferring.*

3 Assess patient's cognitive status.	Determines patient's ability to follow directions and learn transfer techniques.

CLINICAL DECISION: *Patients with head trauma or CVA have perceptual cognition deficits that create safety risks. If patient has difficulty comprehending, simplify instructions and maintain consistency.*

4 Assess patient's level of motivation:	Altered psychological states reduce patient's desire to engage in activity.
a. Patient's eagerness versus unwillingness to be mobile	
b. Whether patient avoids activity and offers excuses	
5 Assess previous mode of transfer (if applicable).	Determines mode of transfer and assistance required to provide continuity.
6 Assess patient's specific risk of falling or being injured when transferred (e.g., neuromuscular deficits, motor weakness, calcium loss from bones, cognitive and visual dysfunction, altered balance).	Certain conditions increase risk of falling or potential injury.
7 Assess special transfer equipment needed for home setting. Assess home environment for hazards.	Prior teaching of family and support persons, assessing home for safety risks and functionality, and providing applicable aids greatly enhance transfer ability at home.

PLANNING

1 Gather appropriate equipment.	
2 Determine number of people needed to assist with transfer. Do not start procedure until all caregivers are available.	Ensures safe patient transfer.
3 Perform hand hygiene. Verify that bed brakes are locked.	Reduces transmission of microorganisms. Promotes patient and caregiver safety.
4 Explain procedure to patient.	Increases patient participation.

IMPLEMENTATION

1 Transfer patient

a. Assisting cooperative patient to sitting position in bed:

SKILL 47-2 USING SAFE AND EFFECTIVE TRANSFER TECHNIQUES—cont'd

STEP	RATIONALE

CLINICAL DECISION: *Careful assessment of your patient's ability to assist in the following position technique is extremely important. Consider the use of a mechanical lift. Your role in assisting your patient to a sitting position is a guide and instruction. If patient can bear weight and move to a sitting position independently, allow him or her to do so and offer assistance (Nelson and Baptiste, 2006).*

STEP	RATIONALE
(1) Raise bed to waist level. Place patient in supine position.	Enables nurse to assess patient's body alignment continually.
(2) Face head of bed at a 45-degree angle and remove pillows.	Proper positioning reduces twisting of your body when moving patient. Pillows cause interference when patient is sitting up in bed.
(3) Place feet in wide base of support, with foot closer to bed in front of other foot.	Improves balance and allows transfer of body weight as you move patient to sitting position.
(4) Place hand nearer head of bed under patient's shoulders, supporting his or her head and cervical vertebrae.	Maintains alignment of head and cervical vertebrae and allows for even lifting of patient's upper trunk.
(5) Place other hand on bed surface.	Provides support and balance.
(6) Raise patient to sitting position by shifting weight from front to back leg.	Improves balance, overcomes inertia, and transfers weight in direction in which you move patient.
(7) Push against bed using arm that is placed on bed surface.	Divides activity between arms and legs and protects back from strain. By bracing one hand against mattress and pushing against it as you lift patient, you transfer weight away from your back muscles through your arm onto the mattress.
b. Assisting cooperative patient who can partially bear weight to sitting position on side of bed:	
(1) With bed flat and waist high, turn patient to side, using assistance of another caregiver if necessary. Patient needs to face nurse on side of bed that patient will be sitting (see illustration).	Decreases amount of work needed by nurse and patient.
(2) Raise head of bed 30 degrees.	Facilitates raising patient to sitting position and protects him or her from falling.
(3) Stand opposite patient's hips. Turn diagonally so you face patient and far corner of head of bed.	Places your center of gravity nearer patient. Reduces twisting of your body because you are facing direction of movement.
(4) Place feet apart with foot closest to bed in front of other foot (see illustration).	Increases balance and allows transfer of body weight as you move patient to a sitting position.
(5) Place arm nearer head of bed under patient's shoulders, supporting head and cervical vertebrae.	Maintains alignment of head and cervical vertebrae and allows for even lifting of patient's trunk.

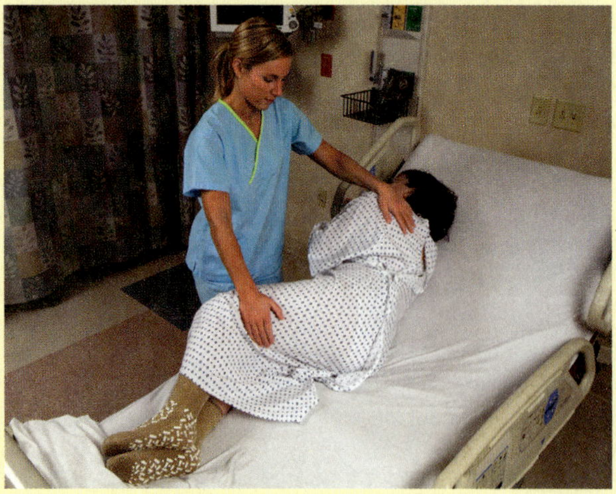

STEP 1b(1) Side-lying position.

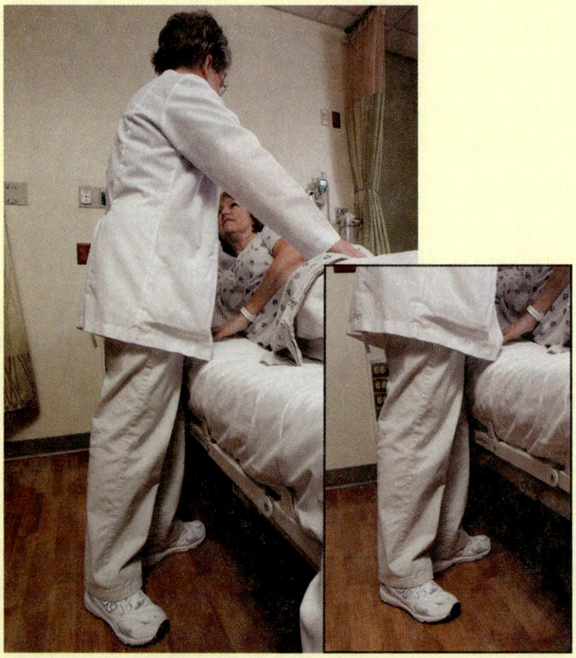

STEP 1b(4) Proper foot placement.

STEP	RATIONALE

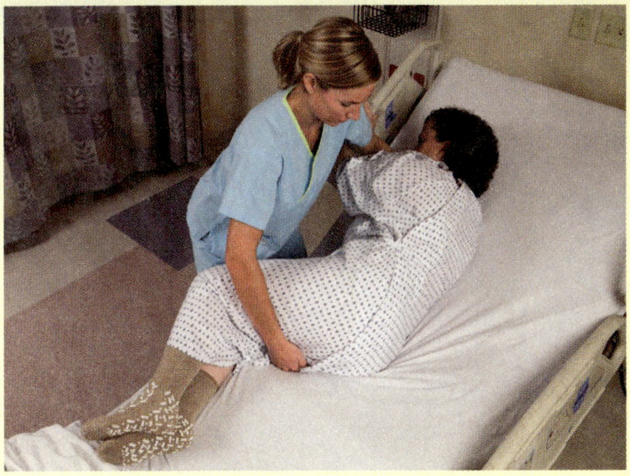

STEP 1b(6) Nurse places arm over patient's thighs.

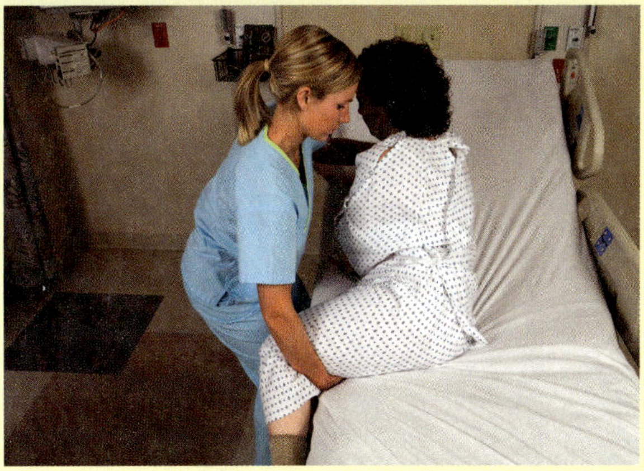

STEP 1b(7) Nurse shifts weight to rear leg and elevates patient.

STEP	RATIONALE
(6) Place other arm over patient's thighs (see illustration).	Supports hip and prevents patient from falling backward during procedure.
(7) Move patient's lower legs and feet over side of bed. Pivot toward rear leg, allowing patient's upper legs to swing downward. At same time shift weight to back leg and elevate patient (see illustration).	Decreases friction and resistance. Weight of patient's legs when off bed allows gravity to lower legs, and weight of legs assists in pulling upper body in sitting position.
c. Transferring cooperative patient who is partially weight bearing from bed to chair:	

CLINICAL DECISION: *Allow patient to transfer independently if able to fully bear weight. Stand by as needed to promote safe transfer (Nelson et al., 2009).*

STEP	RATIONALE
(1) Assist patient to sitting position on side of bed (see Step 1b). Have chair placed next to bed at a 45-degree angle on patient's strong side. Allow patient to sit on side of bed (dangling) for a few minutes before transferring. Ask if patient feels dizzy. Do not leave unattended while dangling.	Positions chair within easy access for transfer. Placing chair on patient's stronger side allows patient to help with transferring. Dangling helps equilibrate blood pressure, reducing risk for dizziness or fainting when standing.
(2) Apply transfer belt or other transfer aids.	Transfer belt maintains stability of patient during transfer and reduces risk for falling (Nelson et al., 2009). Patient's arm needs to be in sling if flaccid paralysis is present.
(3) Ensure that patient has stable nonskid shoes. Weight-bearing or strong leg is forward, with weak foot back.	Nonskid soles decrease risk of slipping during transfer. Always have patient wear shoes during transfer; bare feet increase risk of falls. Patient stands on stronger, or weight-bearing, leg.
(4) Spread feet apart.	Ensures balance with wide base of support.
(5) Flex hips and knees, aligning knees with patient's knees (see illustration).	Flexing knees and hips lowers center of gravity to object to be raised; aligning knees with those of patient allows for stabilization of knees when patient stands.
(6) Grasp transfer belt from underneath along patient's sides.	Provides movement of patient at center of gravity. Never lift patients with upper-extremity paralysis or paresis by or under arms (Nelson et al., 2009).

CLINICAL DECISION: *Use a transfer belt or walking belt with handles in place of the under-axilla technique. The under-axilla technique is physically stressful for nurses and uncomfortable for patients (Owens et al., 1999).*

STEP	RATIONALE
(7) Rock patient up to standing position on count of 3 while straightening hips and legs and keeping knees slightly flexed (see illustration). Unless contraindicated, instruct patient to use hands to push up if applicable.	Rocking motion gives patient's body momentum and requires less muscular effort to lift patient.
(8) Maintain stability of patient's weak or paralyzed leg with knee.	Often patient maintains ability to stand on paralyzed or weak limb with support of knee to stabilize (Pierson and Fairchild, 2008).
(9) Pivot on foot farther from chair.	Maintains support of patient while allowing adequate space for patient to move.
(10) Instruct patient to use armrests on chair for support and ease into chair (see illustration).	Increases patient stability.
(11) Flex hips and knees while lowering patient into chair (see illustration).	Prevents injury to nurse from poor body mechanics.

SKILL 47-2 USING SAFE AND EFFECTIVE TRANSFER TECHNIQUES—cont'd

STEP	RATIONALE

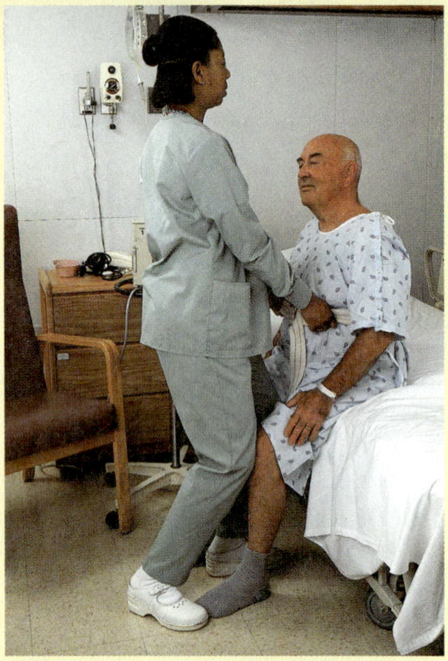

STEP 1c(5) Nurse flexes hips and knees, aligning knees with patient's knees.

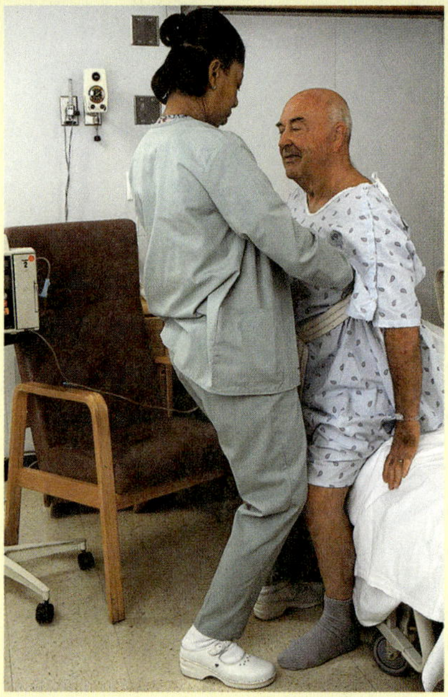

STEP 1c(7) Nurse rocks patient to standing position.

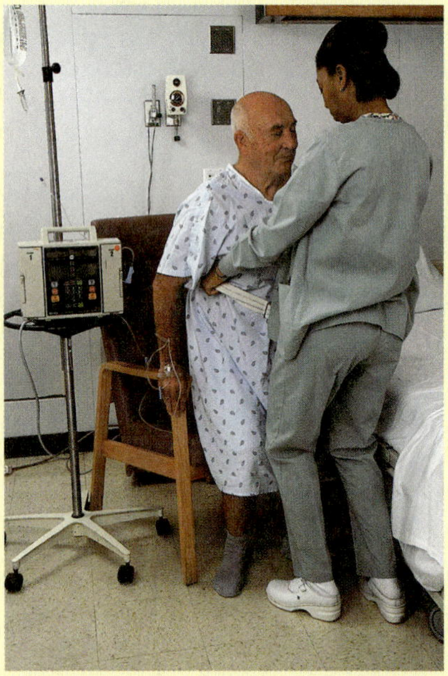

STEP 1c(10) Patient uses armrests for support.

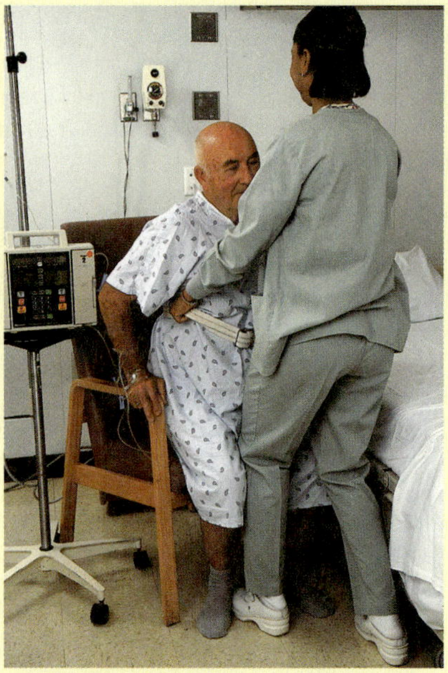

STEP 1c(11) Nurse eases patient into chair.

STEP	RATIONALE
(12) Assess patient for proper alignment for sitting position. Provide support for paralyzed extremities. Lapboard or sling supports flaccid arm. Stabilize leg with bath blanket or pillow.	Prevent injury to patient from poor body alignment.
(13) Praise patient's progress, effort, or performance.	Continued support and encouragement provide incentive for patient perseverance.
d. Using mechanical lift and full body sling to transfer uncooperative patient who can bear partial weight or patient who cannot bear weight and is either uncooperative or does not have upper body strength to move from bed to chair:	
(1) Position lift properly at bedside.	Ensures safe elevation of patient off bed. (Before using lift, be thoroughly familiar with its operation.)
(2) Position chair near bed and allow adequate space to maneuver lift.	Prepares environment for safe use of lift and subsequent transfer.

STEP	RATIONALE
(3) Raise bed to high position with mattress flat. Lower side rail.	Maintains nurses' alignment during transfer.
(4) Keep side rail up on the side opposite from you.	Maintains patient safety.
(5) Roll patient away from you.	Positions patient for use of lift sling.
(6) Place sling under patient. Place lower edge under patient's knees (wide piece) and upper edge under patient's shoulders (narrow piece).	Allows positioning of patient on mechanical/hydraulic sling. Places sling under patient's center of gravity and greatest portion of body weight.
(7) Roll patient to opposite side and pull body sling through.	Completes positioning of patient on mechanical/hydraulic sling.
(8) Roll patient supine onto canvas seat.	Sling needs to extend from shoulders to knees (hammock) to support patient's body weight equally.
(9) Remove patient's glasses if appropriate.	Swivel bar is close to patient's head and can break eyeglasses.
(10) If using a transportable Hoyer lift, place horseshoe-shaped base of lift under side of bed (on side with chair).	Positions lift efficiently and promotes smooth transfer.
(11) Lower upper horizontal bar to sling level following manufacturer directions. Some lifts require valve to be locked.	Positions lift close to patient. Locking valve prevents injury to patient.
(12) Attach hooks on strap to holes in sling. Short straps hook to top holes of sling; longer straps hook to bottom of sling.	Secures hydraulic lift to sling.
(13) Elevate head of bed.	Positions patient in sitting position.
(14) Fold patient's arms over chest.	Prevents injury to paralyzed arms.
(15) Use lift to raise patient off bed (see illustration).	Moves patient off bed.
(16) Use steering handle to pull lift from bed and maneuver to chair.	Moves patient from bed to chair.
(17) Move lift to chair.	Positions lift in front of chair.
(18) Position patient and lower slowly into chair following manufacturer guidelines (see illustration).	Safely guides patient into back of chair as seat descends.
(19) Remove straps and mechanical/hydraulic lift.	Prevents damage to skin and underlying tissues from canvas or hooks.
(20) Check patient's sitting alignment and correct if necessary.	Prevents injury from poor posture.
e. Transferring patient from bed to stretcher (bed at stretcher level):	
(1) Raise bed to height of stretcher.	Bed and stretcher need to be at same level to allow patient to slide from bed to stretcher.
(2) Lower head of bed as much as patient can tolerate. Cross patient's arms on chest. Ensure that bed brakes are locked.	Prevents injury to arms during transfer.
(3) Lower side rails. Two caregivers stand on the side where the stretcher will be; third caregiver stands on other side.	Minimizes caregivers' stretching. Prevents patient from falling out of bed and promotes safety.
(4) Two caregivers help patient roll onto side toward them (use of drawsheet is optional) with smooth, continuous motion.	Positions patient for placing friction-reducing lateral transfer device.
(5) Place slide board under drawsheet or follow manufacturer guidelines (see illustrations). Gently roll patient back onto slide board.	Patient needs to be placed on transfer device properly to allow safe transfer.
(6) Align stretcher along side of bed. Lock wheels of stretcher once it is in place. Instruct patient not to move.	Positions stretcher in correct position for transfer and prevents patient from falling out of bed.
(7) All three caregivers place feet widely apart with one slightly in front of the other and grasp friction-reducing device.	Prepares for transfer. Wide base of support allows nurse to shift weight and minimizes back strain.
(8) On count of three, two caregivers pull drawsheet or patient from bed onto stretcher while third person holds slide board in place. Using friction-reducing device, shift weight from front to back foot (see illustration). Position patient in center of stretcher.	Transfers patient smoothly and efficiently to the stretcher.

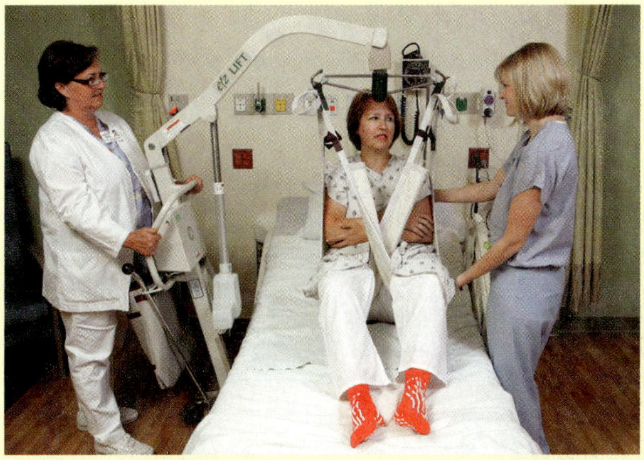

STEP 1d(15) Use mechanical lift to raise patient off bed.

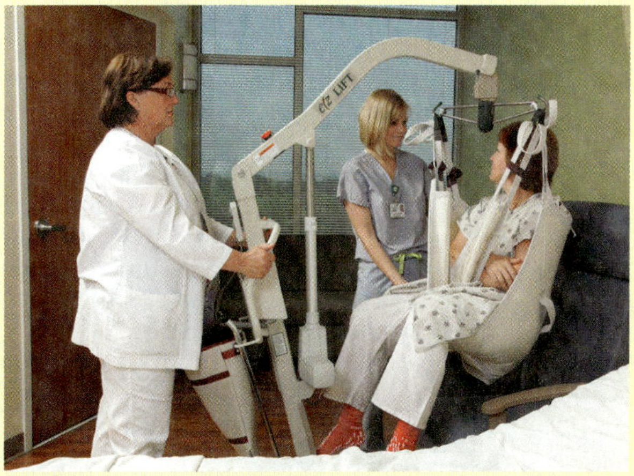

STEP 1d(18) Use mechanical lift to lower patient into chair.

SKILL 47-2 USING SAFE AND EFFECTIVE TRANSFER TECHNIQUES—cont'd

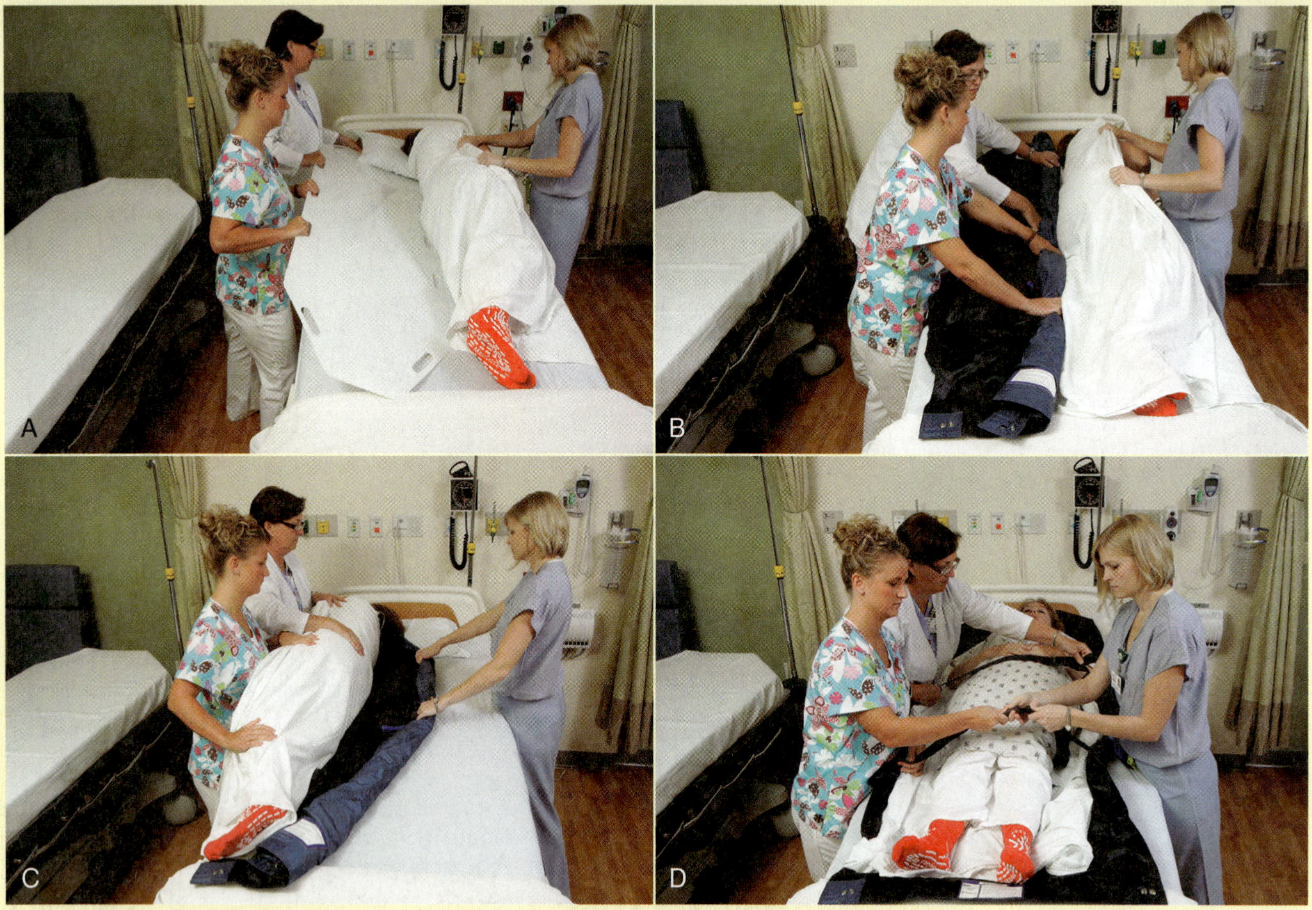

STEP 1e(5) **A,** Two caregivers position sliding board under patient. **B,** Two caregivers place air-assisted device under patient. **C,** Patient rolls to opposite side while other caregiver unrolls air-assisted device. **D,** Secure safety straps.

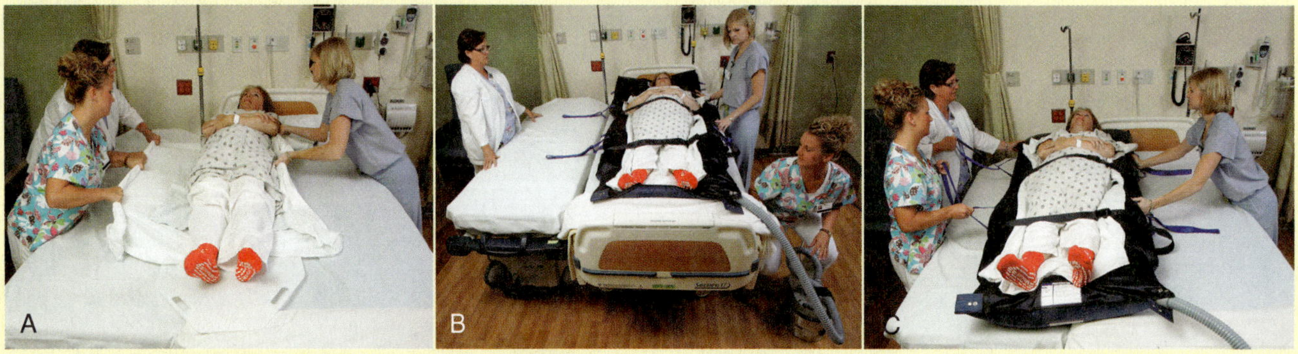

STEP 1e(8) **A,** Transfer of patient from bed to stretcher using sliding board. **B,** Inflating air-assisted transfer device. **C,** Transfer of patient using air-assisted transfer device.

STEP	RATIONALE
(9) Put up side rail of stretcher on side where caregivers are, roll stretcher away from side of bed, and put side rail up on that side.	Side rails prevent patient from falling off stretcher.
(10) Cover patient with sheet or blanket.	Promotes comfort and preserves patient dignity.
(11) Perform hand hygiene.	Reduces transmission of microorganisms.
(12) Following transfer, evaluate patient's body alignment.	Prompt identification of poor alignment reduces risks to patient's skin and musculoskeletal systems.
2 Perform hand hygiene.	Reduces transmission of microorganisms.

STEP	RATIONALE
EVALUATION	
1 Evaluate vital signs. Ask if patient feels fatigued.	Evaluates patient's response to postural changes and activity.
2 Observe for correct body alignment and presence of pressure points on skin.	Minimizes risk for immobility complications.
3 Ask if patient experienced pain during transfer.	Determines need for additional pain control or alteration of technique of transferring.

UNEXPECTED OUTCOMES AND RELATED INTERVENTIONS

1 Patient sustains injury on transfer.
- Evaluate incident that caused injury (e.g., assessment inadequate, change in patient status, improper use of equipment).
- Complete occurrence report according to institution policy.

2 Patient's level of weakness does not permit active transfer.
- Obtain assistance from additional nursing personnel.
- Increase bed activity and exercise to heighten tolerance.

3 Patient continues to bear weight on non–weight-bearing limb.
- Reinforce information about weight-bearing status.

4 Patient transfers well on some occasions, poorly on others.
- Assess patient for factors that affect ability to transfer (e.g., pain, fatigue, confusion) before transfer.
- Allow for a rest period before transferring, medicate for pain if indicated, or reorient patient.

RECORDING AND REPORTING

- Record procedure, including pertinent observations: weakness, ability to follow directions, weight-bearing ability, balance, ability to pivot, number of personnel needed to assist, and amount of assistance (muscle strength) required in nurses' notes.
- Report any unusual occurrence to nurse in charge. Report transfer ability and assistance needed to next shift or other caregivers. Report progress or transfer difficulties to rehabilitation staff (physical therapist or occupational therapist).

HOME CARE CONSIDERATIONS

- Teach family members about safe patient handling and how to use equipment properly. Observe return demonstration of use of equipment.
- Ensure that families have access to appropriate equipment (e.g., transfer belts, mechanical lifts) at home to assist in safe transfer techniques.

KEY POINTS

- Body mechanics are the coordinated efforts of the musculoskeletal and nervous systems as the person moves, lifts, bends, stands, sits, lies down, and completes daily activities.
- Use findings from evidence-based nursing research about safe patient handling to prevent injuries to nurses and patients when moving and transferring.
- Coordination and regulation of muscle groups depend on muscle tone; activity of antagonistic, synergistic, and antigravity muscles; and neural input to muscles.
- Body alignment is the condition of joints, tendons, ligaments, and muscles in various body positions.
- Balance occurs when there is a wide base of support, the center of gravity falls within the base of support, and a vertical line falls from the center of gravity through the base of support.
- Developmental stages influence body alignment and mobility; the greatest impact of physiological changes on the musculoskeletal system is observed in children and older adults.
- The risk of disabilities related to immobilization depends on the extent and duration of immobilization and the patient's overall level of health.
- Immobility presents hazards in the physiological, psychological, and developmental dimensions.
- The nursing process and critical thinking assist in providing care for patients who are experiencing or are at risk for the adverse effects of impaired body alignment and immobility.
- Patients with impaired body alignment require nursing care to maintain correct positioning such as the supported Fowler's, supine, prone, side-lying, and Sims' positions.
- Patient movement algorithms serve as assessment tools and guide safe patient handling and movement.
- Appropriate friction-reducing assistive devices and mechanical lifts need to be used for patient transfers when applicable.
- No-lift policies benefit all members of the health care system: patients, nurses, and administration.

CLINICAL APPLICATION QUESTIONS

Preparing for Clinical Practice

Ms. Cavallo, 97 years of age, has been a resident at the rehabilitation unit for 6 weeks. She has been receiving rehabilitation therapy following the repair of her fractured left hip. The nursing assistive personnel (NAP) tells you that Ms. Cavallo has not been finishing her meals over the past 2 days because of poor appetite. As you enter her room today, she states, "Go away. I'm tired of all of this, and I just want to stay in bed today." You explore why she feels this way. You discover that she is unsure how to use her walker and feels safer in bed. She states, "I'm still afraid that I'm going to fall because I keep forgetting how to use my walker, and I can't fall if I stay in bed, right?"

1. On the basis of these data, you develop a nursing diagnosis of *deficient knowledge* (use of walker and effects of immobility) *related to lack of recall.* Identify one goal, two expected

outcomes, and three related nursing interventions with rationales that will help her meet the identified goal and outcomes.

2. You finish teaching Ms. Cavallo about the hazards of immobility, and you begin your morning assessment. As you are assessing her skin, you notice that she has a 2-cm (0.79-inch) reddened area on her coccyx. The skin in this area is intact, and you find no other reddened areas anywhere else.
   a. How would you document this finding?
   b. Which risk factors contribute to this finding?
3. You convince Ms. Cavallo to get out of bed and sit in her chair for 30 minutes. Describe the decision-making process you use to determine the safest way to transfer her. Include essential assessment data that you need before transferring her into her chair.

evolve *Answers to Clinical Application Questions can be found on the Evolve website.*

REVIEW QUESTIONS

Are You Ready to Test Your Nursing Knowledge?

1. An older adult has limited mobility as a result of a surgical repair of a fracture hip. During assessment you note that the patient cannot tolerate lying flat. Which of the following assessment data support a possible pulmonary problem related to impaired mobility? (Select all that apply.)
   1. B/P = 128/84
   2. Respirations 26 per minute on room air
   3. HR 114
   4. Crackles heard on auscultation
   5. Pain reported as 3 on scale of 0 to 10 after medication
2. A patient has her call bell on and looks frightened when you enter the room. She has been on bed rest for 3 days following a fractured femur. She says, "It hurts when I try to breathe, and I can't catch my breath." Your first action is to:
   1. Call the health care provider to report this change in condition.
   2. Give the patient a paper bag to breathe into to decrease her anxiety.
   3. Assess her vital signs, perform a respiratory assessment, and be prepared to start oxygen.
   4. Explain that this is normal after such trauma and administer the ordered pain medication.
3. The nurse puts elastic stockings on a patient following major abdominal surgery. The nurse teaches the patient that the stockings are used after a surgical procedure to:
   1. Prevent varicose veins.
   2. Prevent muscular atrophy.
   3. Ensure joint mobility and prevent contractures.
   4. Promote venous return to the heart.
4. A nurse is teaching a community group about ways to minimize the risk of developing osteoporosis. Which of the following statements made by a woman in the audience reflects a need for further education?
   1. "I usually go swimming with my family at the YMCA 3 times a week."
   2. "I need to ask my doctor if I should have a bone mineral density check this year."
   3. "If I don't drink milk at dinner, I'll eat broccoli or cabbage to get the calcium that I need in my diet."
   4. "I'll check the label of my multivitamin. If it has calcium, I can save money by not taking another pill."
5. The patient at greatest risk for developing multiple adverse effects of immobility is a:
   1. 1-year-old child with a hernia repair.
   2. 80-year-old woman who has suffered a hemorrhagic cerebrovascular accident (CVA).
   3. 51-year-old woman following a thyroidectomy.
   4. 38-year-old woman undergoing a hysterectomy.
6. An older adult who was in a car accident and fractured his femur has been immobilized for 5 days. Which nursing diagnosis is related to patient safety when the nurse assists this patient out of bed for the first time?
   1. Chronic pain
   2. Impaired skin integrity
   3. Risk for ineffective cerebral tissue perfusion
   4. Risk for activity intolerance
7. A patient had a left-sided cerebrovascular accident 3 days ago and is receiving 5000 units of heparin subcutaneously every 12 hours to prevent thrombophlebitis. The patient is receiving enteral feedings through a small-bore nasogastric (NG) tube because of dysphagia. Which of the following symptoms requires the nurse to call the health care provider immediately?
   1. Pale yellow urine
   2. Unilateral neglect
   3. Slight movement noted on the R side
   4. Coffee ground–like aspirate from the feeding tube
8. A home care nurse is preparing the home for a patient who is discharged to home following a left-sided stroke. The patient is cooperative and can ambulate with a quad-cane. Which of the following must be corrected or removed for the patient's safety? (Select all that apply.)
   1. The rubber mat in the walk-in shower
   2. The three-legged stool on wheels in the kitchen
   3. The braided throw rugs in the entry hallway and between the bedroom and bathroom
   4. The night-lights in the hallways, bedroom, and bathroom
   5. The cordless phone next to the patient's bed
9. The nurse is caring for a patient whose calcium intake must increase because of high risk factors for osteoporosis. The nurse would recommend which of the following menus?
   1. Cream of broccoli soup with whole wheat crackers and tapioca for dessert
   2. Hamburger on soft roll with a side salad and an apple for dessert
   3. Low-fat turkey chili with sour cream and fresh pears for dessert
   4. Chicken salad on toast with tomato and lettuce and honey bun for dessert
10. Before transferring a patient from the bed to a stretcher, which assessment data does the nurse need to gather? (Select all that apply.)
    1. Patient's weight
    2. Patient's level of cooperation
    3. Patient's ability to assist
    4. Presence of medical equipment
    5. 24-hour calorie intake
11. A patient of any age can develop a contracture of a joint when:
    1. The adductors muscles are weakened as a result of immobility.
    2. The muscle fibers become shortened because of disuse.
    3. The calcium-to-phosphorus ratio becomes disrupted.
    4. There is a deficiency in vitamin D.

12. Immobilized patients are at risk for impaired skin integrity. Which of the following interventions would reduce this risk? (Select all that apply.)
    1. Repositioning patient every 1 to 2 hours while awake
    2. Using an objective, valid scale to assess patient's risk for pressure ulcer development
    3. Using a device to relieve pressure when patient is seated in chair
    4. Teaching patient how to shift weight at regular intervals while sitting in a chair
    5. A good rule is: the higher the risk for skin breakdown, the shorter the interval between position changes
13. Which of the following indicates that additional assistance is needed to transfer the patient from the bed to the stretcher?
    1. The patient is 5 feet 6 inches and weighs 120 lbs.
    2. The patient speaks and understands English.
    3. The patient received an injection of morphine 30 minutes ago for pain.
    4. You feel comfortable handling a patient of his size and with his level of cooperation.
14. A patient with left-sided weakness asks his nurse, "Why are you walking on my left side? I can hold on to you better with my right hand." What would be your best therapeutic response?
    1. "Walking on your left side lets me use my right hand to hold on to your arm. In case you start to fall, I can still hold you."
    2. " Would you like me to walk on your right side so you feel more secure?"
    3. "Either side is appropriate, but I prefer the left side. If you like, I can have another nurse walk with you who will hold you on the right side."
    4. "By walking on your left side I can support you and help keep you from injury if you should start to fall. By holding your waist I would protect your shoulder if you should start to fall or faint.
15. Which is an outcome for a patient diagnosed with osteoporosis?
    1. Maintain serum level of calcium.
    2. Maintain independence with activities of daily living (ADLs).
    3. Reduce supplemental sources of vitamin D.
    4. Reverse bone loss through dietary manipulation.

Answers: **1.** 2, 3, 4; **2.** 3; **3.** 4; **4.** 4; **5.** 2; **6.** 4; **7.** 4; **8.** 2, 3; **9.** 1; **10.** 1, 2, 3, 4; **11.** 2; **12.** 2, 3, 4, 5; **13.** 3; **14.** 4; **15.** 2.

REFERENCES

American Nurses Association (ANA): Safe patient handling, 2011, http://www.nursingworld.org/MainMenuCategories/WorkplaceSafety/SafePatient. Accessed January 12, 2012.

American Pain Society (APS): *Principles of analgesics use in acute and chronic pain*, ed 6, Glenview, Ill, 2008, The Society.

Black J, Hawks J: *Medical-surgical nursing: clinical management for positive outcomes*, ed 7, Philadelphia, 2009, Elsevier.

Butler CT: Pediatric skin care: guidelines for assessment, prevention and treatment, *Pediatr Nurs* 32(5):443, 2006.

Centers for Disease Control and Prevention (CDC): Safe patient handling training for schools of nursing: a curricular guide, Bethesda, Md, 2009, Department of Health and Human Services (NIOSH) Pub. no. 2009-127.

de Castro AB, et al: Prioritizing safe patient handling, *J Nurs Admin* 36(7/8):363, 2006.

Ebersole P, et al: *Toward healthy aging: human needs and nursing response*, ed 7, 2008, Mosby.

Fletcher K: Immobility: geriatric self-learning module, *MedSurg Nurs* 14(1):35, 2005.

Glenn-Molali NH: Nourishment and swallowing. In Hoeman SP, editor: *Rehabilitation nursing process, application, and outcomes*, ed 4, St Louis, 2008, Mosby.

Huether SE, McCance K: *Understanding pathophysiology*, St Louis, 2008, Mosby.

Jarvis C: *Physical examination and health assessment*, ed 5, St Louis, 2008, Saunders.

Lewis S, et al: *Medical-surgical nursing*, ed 8, St Louis, 2011, Mosby.

Mamaril ME: Nursing considerations in the geriatric surgical patient: the perioperative continuum of care, *Nurs Clin North Am* 41(2):313, 2006.

Matz M: "Understanding hazards and controls in health care." In Fell-Carlson D, editor: *Working safely in health care: a practical guide*, New York, 2007, Delmar Thomson Learning Publishing.

McCance K, Huether SE: *Pathophysiology*, ed 6, St Louis, 2009, Mosby.

Monahan F, et al: *Phipps's medical surgical nursing*, ed. 8, St Louis, 2007, Mosby.

National Osteoporosis Foundation: *Fast facts*, Washington, DC, 2010, The Foundation, http://www.nof.org/osteoporosis/diseasefacts.htm.

Nelson A: *Safe patient handling and movement algorithms*, Tampa, FL, 2006, VISN8 Patient Safety Center, http://www.visn8.med.va.gov/patientsafetycenter/safePtHandling/default.asp.

Nelson A, et al: *The illustrated guide for safe patient handling and movement*, New York, 2009, Springer Publishing.

Owens B, et al: What are we teaching about lifting and transferring patients? *Res Nurs Health* 22:3, 1999.

Pierson F, Fairchild S: *Principles and techniques of patient care*, ed 4, St Louis, 2008, Saunders.

The Joint Commission (TJC): 2011 National Patient safety Goals (NPGS), 2011, http://www.jointcommission.org/standards_information/npsgs.aspx. Accessed November 6, 2011.

US Department of Labor: *Bureau of Labor Statistics*, 2007, http://www.bls.gov/iif/home.htm. Accessed November 6, 2011.

Waters TR, et al: Patient handling tasks with high risk for musculoskeletal disorders in critical care, *Crit Care Nurs Clin North Am* 19:131, 2007.

Wound, Ostomy and Continence Nurses Society (WOCN): *Pressure ulcer assessment: best practices for clinicians*, Mt Laurel, NJ, 2009, The Society.

Yen PK: Physical activity—the "new" nutrition guideline, *Geriatr Nurs* 26(6):341, 2005.

Yeom HA, et al: Interventions for promoting mobility in community-dwelling older adults, *J Am Acad Nurse Pract* 21 (2):95, 2009.

RESEARCH REFERENCES

Agency for Healthcare Research and Quality (AHRQ): *Pressure ulcer prevention and treatment*, 2010, http://hstat.nlm.nih.gov/hq/Hquest/screen/TextBrowse/t/1049658066834/s/40521. Accessed November 6, 2011.

Baptiste A, et al: Friction-reducing devices for lateral patient transfers, *AAOHN J* 54(4):173, 2006.

Cromwell SL, Berg JA: Lifelong physical activity patterns of sedentary Mexican American women, *Geriatr Nurs* 27(4):209, 2006.

Kawamoto R, et al: Predictors of functional status in Japanese community-dwelling older persons during a 2-year follow up, *Geriatr Gerontol Int* 6(2):116, 2006.

Lynch D, et al: Continuous passive motion improves shoulder joint integrity following stroke, *Clin Rehabil* 19(6):594, 2005.

Marklew A: Body positioning and its effect on oxygenation: a literature review, *Nurs Crit Care* 11(1):16, 2006.

Nelson A, Baptiste AS: Evidence-based practices for safe patient handling and movement, *Orthop Nurs* 25(6):366, 2006.

Pasero C, McCaffery M: Orthopedic postoperative pain management, *J Perianesth Nurs* 22(4):160, 2007.

Randall SB, et al: Expanded occupational safety and health administration 300 log as metric for bariatric patient-handling staff injuries, *Surg Obes Relat Dis* 5(4):463, 2009.

Walsh JS, Plonczynski DJ: Evaluation of a protocol for prevention of facility-acquired heel pressure ulcers, *J Wound Ost Cont Nurs* 34(2):178, 2007.

Wanless S, Page A: Moving and handling education in the community: technology innovations to improve practice, *Br J Commun Nurs* 14(12):530, 2009.

CHAPTER

48

Skin Integrity and Wound Care

OBJECTIVES

- Discuss the risk factors that contribute to pressure ulcer formation.
- Describe the pressure ulcer staging system.
- Discuss the normal process of wound healing.
- Describe the differences of wound healing by primary and secondary intention.
- Describe complications of wound healing.
- Explain the factors that impede or promote wound healing.
- Describe the differences between nursing care of acute and chronic wounds.
- Complete an assessment for a patient with impaired skin integrity.
- List nursing diagnoses associated with impaired skin integrity.
- Develop a nursing care plan for a patient with impaired skin integrity.
- List appropriate nursing interventions for a patient with impaired skin integrity.
- State evaluation criteria for a patient with impaired skin integrity.

KEY TERMS

Abnormal reactive hyperemia, p. 1188
Abrasion, p. 1190
Approximated, p. 1181
Blanching, p. 1177
Collagen, p. 1177
Debridement, p. 1199
Dehiscence, p. 1184
Drainage evacuators, p. 1208
Epithelialization, p. 1183
Eschar, p. 1179
Evisceration, p. 1184
Exudate, p. 1181
Fibrin, p. 1182
Friction, p. 1178
Granulation tissue, p. 1179
Hematoma, p. 1183
Hemorrhage, p. 1183
Hemostasis, p. 1182
Induration, p. 1188
Laceration, p. 1190
Normal reactive hyperemia, p. 1197
Pressure ulcer, p. 1177
Primary intention, p. 1181
Puncture, p. 1190
Purulent, p. 1183
Sanguineous, p. 1190
Secondary intention, p. 1181
Serosanguineous, p. 1190
Serous, p. 1190
Shearing force, p. 1196
Slough, p. 1179
Sutures, p. 1207
Tissue ischemia, p. 1177
Vacuum-assisted closure (V.A.C.), p. 1204
Wound, p. 1181
Wound contraction, p. 1222

evolve WEBSITE

http://evolve.elsevier.com/Potter/fundamentals/

- Review Questions
- Video Clips
- Concept Map Creator
- Case Study with Questions
- Skills Performance Checklists
- Audio Glossary
- Interactive Learning Activities
- Key Term Flashcards
- Content Updates

Skin, the largest organ in the body, constitutes 15% of the total adult body weight (Wysocki, 2012). It is a protective barrier against disease-causing organisms and a sensory organ for pain, temperature, and touch; and it synthesizes vitamin D. Injury to the skin poses risks to safety and triggers a complex healing response. A nurse's most important responsibilities include assessing and monitoring skin integrity; identifying problems; and planning, implementing, and evaluating interventions to maintain skin integrity. Once a wound occurs, it is critical to know the process of normal wound healing to identify the appropriate nursing interventions.

SCIENTIFIC KNOWLEDGE BASE

Skin

The skin has two layers: the epidermis and the dermis (Fig. 48-1). They are separated by a membrane, often referred to as the *dermal-epidermal junction*. The epidermis, or the top layer, has several layers. The stratum corneum is the thin, outermost layer of the epidermis. It consists of flattened, dead, keratinized cells. The cells originate from the innermost epidermal layer, commonly called the *basal layer*. Cells in the basal layer divide, proliferate, and migrate toward the epidermal surface. After they reach the stratum corneum, they flatten and die. This constant movement ensures replacement of surface cells sloughed during normal desquamation or shedding. The thin stratum corneum protects underlying cells and tissues from dehydration and prevents entrance of certain chemical agents. The stratum corneum allows evaporation of water from the skin and permits absorption of certain topical medications.

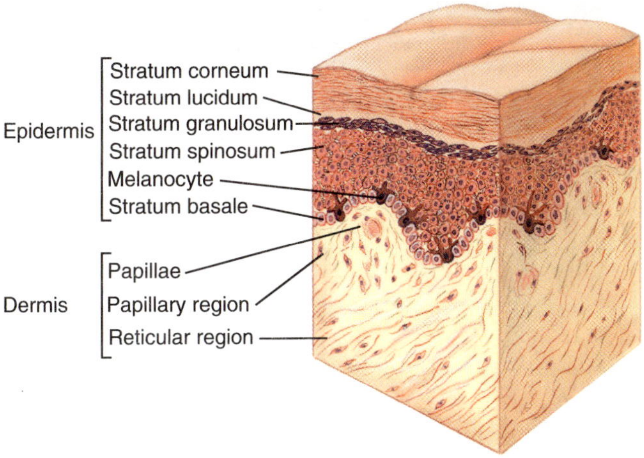

FIG. 48-1 Layers of skin. (From Applegate E: *The anatomy and physiology learning system*, ed 3, St Louis, 2006, Saunders.)

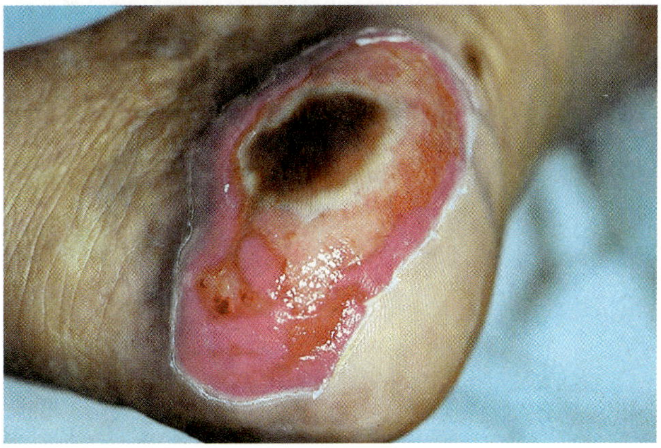

FIG. 48-2 Pressure ulcer with tissue necrosis.

BOX 48-1 FOCUS ON OLDER ADULTS

Skin-Associated Issues

- Age-related changes such as reduced skin elasticity, decreased collagen, and thinning of underlying muscle and tissues cause the older adult's skin to be easily torn in response to mechanical trauma, especially shearing forces (Wysocki, 2012).
- Concomitant medical conditions and polypharmacy, which are common in the older adult, are factors that interfere with wound healing.
- The attachment between the epidermis and dermis becomes flattened in older adults, allowing the skin to be easily torn in response to mechanical trauma (e.g., tape removal).
- Aging causes a diminished inflammatory response, resulting in slow epithelialization and wound healing (Doughty and Sparks-Defriese, 2012).
- The hypodermis decreases in size with age. Older patients have little subcutaneous padding over bony prominences; thus they are more prone to skin breakdown (Wysocki, 2012).
- An identified risk factor for the development of pressure ulcers is malnutrition (Posthauer and Thomas, 2008).

The dermis, the inner layer of the skin, provides tensile strength, mechanical support, and protection to the underlying muscles, bones, and organs. It differs from the epidermis in that it contains mostly connective tissue and few skin cells. **Collagen** (a tough, fibrous protein), blood vessels, and nerves are found in the dermal layer. Fibroblasts, which are responsible for collagen formation, are the only distinctive cell type within the dermis.

Understanding skin structure helps you maintain skin integrity and promote wound healing. Intact skin protects the patient from chemical and mechanical injury. When the skin is injured, the epidermis functions to resurface the wound and restore the barrier against invading organisms while the dermis responds to restore the structural integrity (collagen) and the physical properties of the skin. The normal aging process alters skin characteristics and makes skin more vulnerable to damage. Box 48-1 provides a summary of the changes in aging skin.

Pressure Ulcers

Pressure ulcer, pressure sore, decubitus ulcer, and *bedsore* are terms used to describe impaired skin integrity related to unrelieved, prolonged pressure. The most current terminology is **pressure ulcer** (Fig. 48-2), which is consistent with the recommendations of the pressure ulcer guidelines written by the Wound, Ostomy and Continence Nurses Society (WOCN, 2010). A pressure ulcer is localized injury to the skin and other underlying tissue, usually over a body prominence, as a result of pressure or pressure in combination with shear and/or friction. A number of contributing factors are also associated with pressure ulcers; the significance of these factors is yet to be elucidated (EPUAP and NPUAP, 2009). Any patient experiencing decreased mobility, decreased sensory perception, fecal or urinary incontinence, and/or poor nutrition is at risk for pressure ulcer development.

Many factors contribute to the formation of a pressure ulcer. Pressure is the major cause. Tissues receive oxygen and nutrients and eliminate metabolic wastes via the blood. Any factor that interferes with blood flow in turn interferes with cellular metabolism and the function or life of the cells. Prolonged, intense pressure affects cellular metabolism by decreasing or obliterating blood flow, resulting in tissue ischemia and ultimately tissue death.

Pathogenesis of Pressure Ulcers. Pressure is the major element in the cause of pressure ulcers. Three pressure-related factors contribute to pressure ulcer development: (1) pressure intensity, (2) pressure duration, and (3) tissue tolerance.

Pressure Intensity. A classic research study identified capillary closing pressure as the minimal amount of pressure required to collapse a capillary (e.g., when the pressure exceeds the normal capillary pressure range of 15 to 32 mm Hg) (Burton and Yamada, 1951). Therefore, if the pressure applied over a capillary exceeds the normal capillary pressure and the vessel is occluded for a prolonged period of time, **tissue ischemia** can occur. If the patient has reduced sensation and cannot respond to the discomfort of the ischemia, tissue ischemia and tissue death result.

The clinical presentation of obstructed blood flow occurs when evaluating areas of pressure. After a period of tissue ischemia, if the pressure is relieved and the blood flow returns, the skin turns red. The effect of this redness is vasodilation (blood vessel expansion), called *hyperemia* (redness). Evaluate an area of hyperemia by pressing a finger over the affected area. If it blanches (turns lighter in color) and the erythema returns when you remove your finger, the hyperemia is transient and is an attempt to overcome the ischemic episode, thus called *blanching hyperemia* (Pieper, 2012). However, if the erythematous area does not blanch (nonblanching erythema) when you apply pressure, deep tissue damage is probable.

Blanching occurs when the normal red tones of the light-skinned patient are absent. It does not occur in patients with darkly

BOX 48-2 CHARACTERISTICS OF DARK SKIN WITH IMPAIRED INTEGRITY

Color

- Color remains unchanged when pressure is applied.
- If patient previously has a pressure ulcer, that area of skin may be lighter than original color.

Temperature

- Circumscribed area of intact skin may be warm to touch. As tissue changes color, intact skin feels cool to touch.
- Inflammation is detected by making comparisons to surrounding skin.

Appearance

- Edema may occur with induration and appear taut and shiny.
- Localized area of skin may be purple/blue or violet instead of red.

Adapted from Nix DP: Skin and wound inspection and assessment. In Bryant RA, Nix DP, editors: *Acute and chronic wounds: current management concepts,* ed 4, St Louis, 2012, Mosby.

pigmented skin. The Task Force on the Implications for Darkly Pigmented Intact Skin in the Prediction and Prevention of Pressure Ulcers (Bennett, 1995) defined darkly pigmented skin as skin that "remains unchanged (does not blanch) when pressure is applied over a bony prominence, irrespective of the patient's race or ethnicity." Characteristics of intact dark skin that alert nurses to the potential for pressure ulcers are in Box 48-2.

Pressure Duration. Low pressure over a prolonged period and high-intensity pressure over a short period are two concerns related to duration of pressure. Both types of pressure cause tissue damage. Extended pressure occludes blood flow and nutrients and contributes to cell death (Pieper, 2012). Clinical implications of pressure duration include evaluating the amount of pressure (checking skin for reactive hyperemia) and determining the amount of time that a patient tolerates pressure (checking to be sure after relieving pressure that the affected area blanches).

Tissue Tolerance. The ability of tissue to endure pressure depends on the integrity of the tissue and the supporting structures. The extrinsic factors of shear, friction, and moisture affect the ability of the skin to tolerate pressure: the greater the degree to which the factors of shear, friction, and moisture are present, the more susceptible the skin will be to damage from pressure. The second factor related to tissue tolerance is the ability of the underlying skin structures (blood vessels, collagen) to assist in redistributing pressure. Systemic factors such as poor nutrition, increased aging, hydration status, and low blood pressure affect the tolerance of the tissue to externally applied pressure.

Risk Factors for Pressure Ulcer Development. A variety of factors predispose a patient to pressure ulcer formation. These factors are often directly related to disease such as decreased level of consciousness, the presence of a cast, or secondary to an illness (e.g., decreased sensation following a cerebrovascular accident).

Impaired Sensory Perception. Patients with altered sensory perception for pain and pressure are more at risk for impaired skin integrity than those with normal sensation. Patients with impaired sensory perception of pain and pressure are unable to feel when a portion of their body undergoes increased, prolonged pressure or pain. Thus the patient who can't feel or sense that there is pain or pressure is at risk for the development of pressure ulcers.

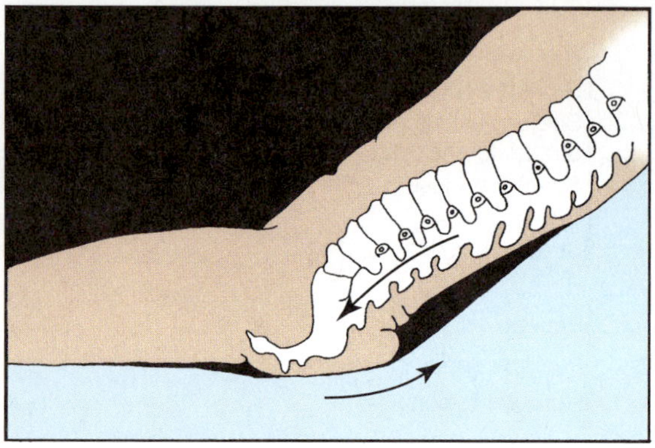

FIG. 48-3 Shear exerted in sacral area.

Impaired Mobility. Patients unable to independently change positions are at risk for pressure ulcer development. For example, patients with spinal cord injuries have decreased or absent motor and sensory impairment and are unable to reposition off bony prominences.

Alteration in Level of Consciousness. Patients who are confused or disoriented and those who have expressive aphasia or other inability to verbalize or changing levels of consciousness are unable to protect themselves from pressure ulcer development. Patients who are confused or disoriented are sometimes able to feel pressure but are not always able to understand how to relieve it or communicate their discomfort. Patients in a coma cannot perceive pressure and are unable to move voluntarily to relieve pressure.

Shear. Shear force is the sliding movement of skin and subcutaneous tissue while the underlying muscle and bone are stationary (Bryant, 2012). For example, shear force occurs when the head of the bed is elevated and the sliding of the skeleton starts but the skin is fixed because of friction with the bed (Fig. 48-3). It also occurs when transferring a patient from bed to stretcher and the patient's skin is pulled across the bed. When shear is present, the skin and subcutaneous layers adhere to the surface of the bed, and the layers of muscle and the bones slide in the direction of body movement. The underlying tissue capillaries are stretched and angulated by the shear force. As a result, necrosis occurs deep within the tissue layers. The tissue damage occurs deep in the tissues, causing undermining of the dermis.

Friction. The force of two surfaces moving across one another such as the mechanical force exerted when skin is dragged across a coarse surface such as bed linens is called **friction** (WOCN, 2010). Unlike shear injuries, friction injuries affect the epidermis or top layer of the skin. The denuded skin appears red and painful and is sometimes referred to as a "sheet burn." A friction injury occurs in patients who are restless, in those who have uncontrollable movements such as spastic conditions, and in those whose skin is dragged rather than lifted from the bed surface during position changes.

Moisture. The presence and duration of moisture on the skin increases the risk of ulcer formation. Moisture reduces the resistance of the skin to other physical factors such as pressure and/or shear force. Prolonged moisture softens skin, making it more susceptible to damage. Immobilized patients who are unable to perform their own hygiene needs depend on the nurse to keep the skin dry and intact. Skin moisture originates from wound drainage, excessive perspiration, and fecal or urinary incontinence.

Classification of Pressure Ulcers

You need to assess pressure ulcers at regular intervals using systematic parameters to evaluate wound healing, plan appropriate interventions, and evaluate progress. Assessment includes depth of tissue involvement (staging), type and approximate percentage of tissue in wound bed, wound dimensions, exudate description, and condition of surrounding skin.

One method for assessment of a pressure ulcer is the use of a staging system. Staging systems for pressure ulcers are based on describing the depth of tissue destroyed. Accurate staging requires knowledge of the skin layers. A major drawback of a staging system is that you cannot stage an ulcer covered with necrotic tissue because the necrotic tissue is covering the depth of the ulcer. The necrotic tissue must be debrided or removed to expose the wound base to allow for assessment.

Pressure ulcer staging describes the pressure ulcer depth at the point of assessment. Thus, once you have staged the pressure ulcer, this stage endures even as it heals. Pressure ulcers do not progress from a stage III to a stage I; rather, a stage III ulcer demonstrating signs of healing is described as a healing stage III pressure ulcer (Pieper, 2012). The EPUAP and NPUAP have developed clinical practice guidelines for pressure ulcers and have advanced the following classification/staging system (EPUAP and NPUAP, 2009):

Stage I: Nonblanchable Redness of Intact Skin. Intact skin presents with nonblanchable erythema of a localized area usually over a bony prominence. Discoloration of the skin, warmth, edema, hardness, or pain may also be present. Darkly pigmented skin may not have visible blanching.

Further description: The area may be painful, firm, soft, warmer, or cooler than adjacent tissue. Stage I may be difficult to detect in individuals with dark skin tones. It may indicate "at-risk" persons (Fig. 48-4, *A*).

Stage II: Partial-thickness Skin Loss or Blister. A partial-thickness loss of dermis presents as a shallow open ulcer with a red-pink wound bed without slough. It may also present as an intact or open/ruptured serum-filled or serosangineous filled blister.

Further description: Stage II presents as a shiny or dry shallow ulcer without slough or bruising. This stage should not be used to describe skin tears, tape burns, incontinence-associated dermatitis, maceration, or excoriation (Fig. 48-4, *B*).

Stage III: Full-thickness Skin Loss (Fat Visible). A stage III ulcer is a full-thickness tissue loss. Subcutaneous fat may be visible; but bone, tendon, or muscle is *not* exposed. Some slough may be present. It *may* include undermining and tunneling.

Further description: The depth of a stage III pressure ulcer varies by anatomical location. The bridge of the nose, ear, occiput, and malleolus do not have (adipose) subcutaneous tissue; and stage III ulcers can be shallow. In contrast, areas of significant adiposity can develop extremely deep stage III pressure ulcers. Bone/tendon is not visible or directly palpable (Fig. 48-4, *C*).

Stage IV: Full-thickness Tissue Loss (Muscle/Bone Visible). A stage IV ulcer is a full-thickness tissue loss with exposed bone, tendon, or muscle. Slough or eschar may be present. It often includes undermining and tunneling.

Further description: The depth of a stage IV pressure ulcer varies by anatomical location. The bridge of the nose, ear, occiput, and malleolus do not have (adipose) subcutaneous tissue; and these ulcers can be shallow. Stage IV ulcers can extend into muscle and/or supporting structures (e.g., fascia, tendon, or joint capsule), making osteomyelitis or osteitis likely to occur. Exposed bone/muscle is visible or directly palpable (Fig. 48-4, *D*).

Unstageable/Unclassified: Full-thickness Skin or Tissue Loss—Depth Unknown. The EPUAP and the NPUAP (2009) developed a definition for an ulcer in which the base of the wound cannot be visualized and a definition of tissue injury in which the depth of injury is unknown. An unstageable ulcer is a full-thickness tissue loss in which actual depth of the ulcer is completely obscured by slough (yellow, tan, gray, green, or brown) and/or eschar (tan, brown, or black) in the wound bed (Fig. 48-4, *E*).

Further description: Until enough slough and/or eschar are removed to expose the base of the wound, the true depth cannot be determined; but it is either a stage III or IV. Stable (dry, adherent, intact without erythema or fluctuance) eschar on the heels serves as "the natural (biological) cover of the body" and should not be removed.

Suspected Deep-Tissue Injury—Depth Unknown. Suspected deep-tissue injury is a purple or maroon localized area of discolored intact skin or blood-filled blister caused by damage of underlying soft tissue from pressure and/or shear (Fig. 48-4, *F*).

Further description: The area may be preceded by tissue that is painful, firm, mushy, boggy, warmer, or cooler than adjacent tissue. Deep-tissue injury may be difficult to detect in individuals with dark skin tones. Evolution may include a thin blister over a dark wound bed. The wound may further evolve and become covered by thin eschar. Evolution may be rapid, exposing additional layers of tissue even with treatment.

In addition, Bennett (1995) suggests that, when assessing patients with darkly pigmented skin, proper lighting is important to accurately assess the skin (see Box 48-2). Either natural light or a halogen light is recommended. This prevents the blue tones that fluorescent light sources produce on darkly pigmented skin, which interferes with accurate assessment. Additional aspects of assessing dark skin are in Box 48-3.

BOX 48-3 CULTURAL ASPECTS OF CARE

Skin Color Impact

Detecting cyanosis and other changes in skin color in patients is an important clinical skill. However, this detection becomes a challenge in dark-skinned patients (Nix, 2012; Rajendran et al, 2006). There are concerns about the inability of practitioners to describe accurately early pressure ulcer or pressure injury in people with darkly pigmented skin (Henderson et al., 1997). Cyanosis is "a slightly bluish-grayish slatelike or dark purple discoloration of the skin caused by the presence of at least 5 g of reduced hemoglobin in arterial blood." Color differentiation of cyanosis varies according to skin pigmentation. In dark-skinned patients, you need to know the individual's baseline skin tone. You should not confuse the normal hyperpigmentation of Mongolian spots that are seen on the sacrum of African, Native American, and Asian patients with cyanosis. Observe the patient's skin in nonglare daylight. The Gaskin's Nursing Assessment of Skin Color (GNASC) is a useful tool for assessment for identifying changes in skin color that increase the patient's risk for pressure ulcers (Gaskin, 1986).

Implications for Practice

- It is difficult but possible to detect cyanosis in the dark-skinned patient.
- Be aware of situations that produce changes in skin tone such as inadequate lighting.
- Examine body sites with the least melanin such as under the arm for underlying color identification.
- Evaluate pigmented skin for color-specific changes in skin tone.

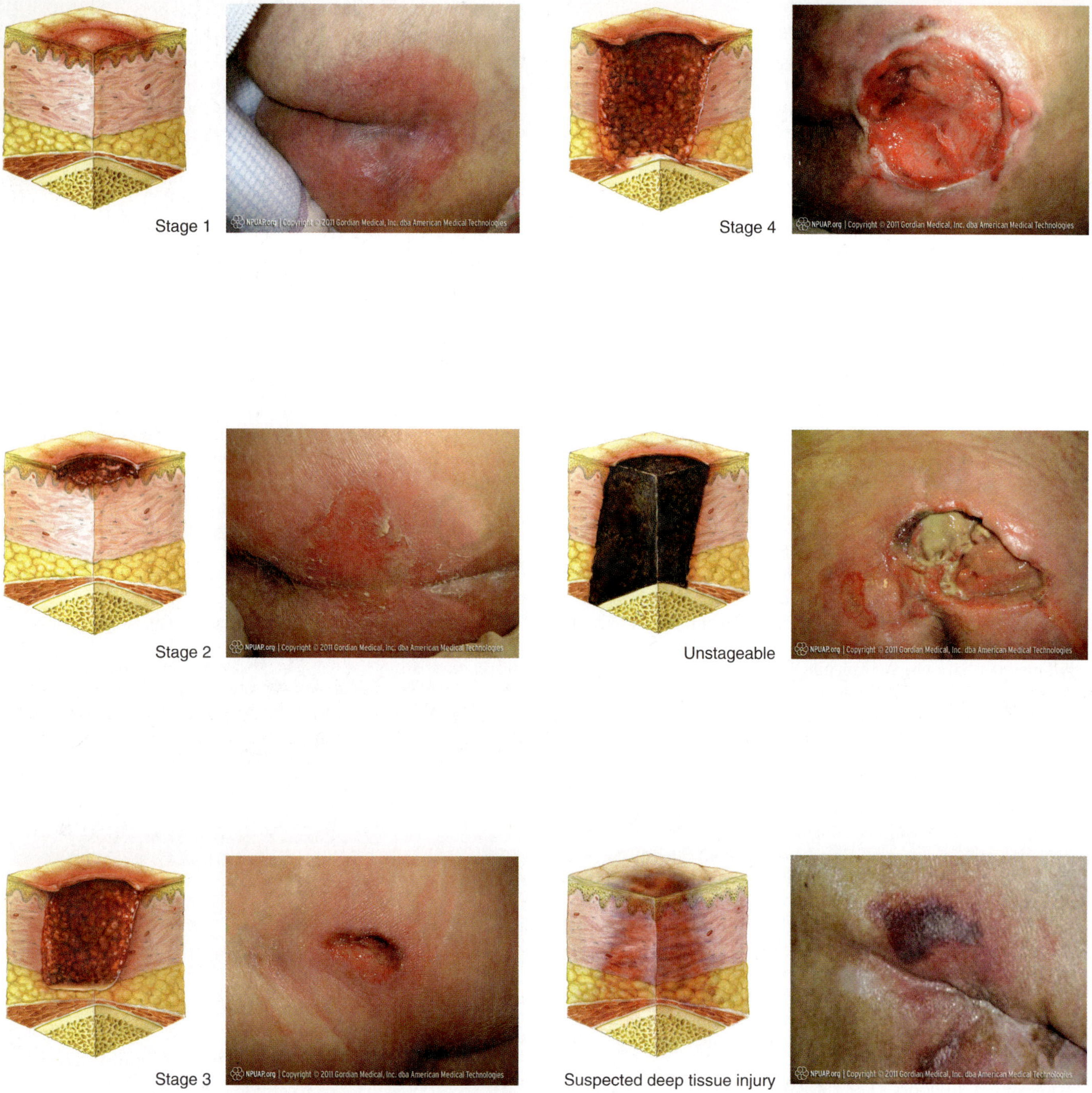

FIG. 48-4 Diagram of stages. **A,** Stage I pressure ulcer. **B,** Stage II pressure ulcer. **C,** Stage III pressure ulcer. **D,** Stage IV pressure ulcer. **E,** Unstageable wound. **F,** Suspected deep tissue injury. (Used with permission of the National Pressure Ulcer Advisory Panel. Copyright © NPUAP.)

You need to assess the type of tissue in the wound base; this information is used to plan appropriate interventions. The assessment of tissue type includes the amount (percentage) and appearance (color) of viable and nonviable tissue. **Granulation tissue** is red, moist tissue composed of new blood vessels, the presence of which indicates progression toward healing. Soft yellow or white tissue is characteristic of **slough** (stringy substance attached to wound bed), and it must be removed by a skilled clinician before the wound is able to heal. Black or brown necrotic tissue is **eschar,** which also needs to be removed before healing can proceed.

The measurement of the size of the wound provides overall changes in size, which is an indicator for wound healing progress (Nix, 2012). Use disposable wound-measuring devices to obtain measurement of width and length. Select a uniform, consistent

TABLE 48-1 **Wound Classification**

DESCRIPTION	CAUSES	IMPLICATIONS FOR HEALING
Onset and Duration		
Acute		
Wound that proceeds through an orderly and timely reparative process that results in sustained restoration of anatomical and functional integrity	Trauma, a surgical incision	Wounds are usually easily cleaned and repaired. Wound edges are clean and intact.
Chronic		
Wound that fails to proceed through an orderly and timely process to produce anatomical and functional integrity	Vascular compromise, chronic inflammation, or repetitive insults to tissue (Doughty and Sparks-Defriese, 2012)	Continued exposure to insult impedes wound healing.
Healing Process		
Primary Intention		
Wound that is closed	Surgical incision, wound that is sutured or stapled	Healing occurs by epithelialization; heals quickly with minimal scar formation.
Secondary Intention		
Wound edges not approximated	Pressure ulcers, surgical wounds that have tissue loss	Wound heals by granulation tissue formation, wound contraction, and epithelialization.
Tertiary Intention		
Wound left open for several days, then wound edges are approximated (see Fig. 48-4, *C*)	Wounds that are contaminated and require observation for signs of inflammation	Closure of wound is delayed until risk of infection is resolved (Doughty and Sparks-Defriese, 2012).

method for measuring wound length and width to facilitate meaningful comparisons of wound measurements across time (EPUAP and NPUAP, 2009). Measure depth by using a cotton-tipped applicator in the wound bed.

Wound **exudate** should describe the amount, color, consistency, and odor of wound drainage and is part of the wound assessment. Excessive exudate indicates the presence of infection. Finally, assess the condition of the skin surrounding the wound for redness, warmth, maceration, or edema (swelling). The presence of any of these factors on the skin surrounding the wound indicates wound deterioration.

The skin around the wound (periwound) should be assessed. Examine the periwound area for redness, warmth, and signs of maceration and palpate the area for signs of pain or induration.

Wound Classifications

A **wound** is a disruption of the integrity and function of tissues in the body (Baharestani, 2008). It is imperative for the nurse to know that *all wounds are not created equal.* Understanding the etiology of a wound is important because the treatment for it varies, depending on the underlying disease process.

There are many ways to classify wounds. Wound classification systems describe the status of skin integrity, cause of the wound, severity or extent of tissue injury or damage, cleanliness of the wound (Table 48-1), or descriptive qualities of the wound tissue such as color (Fig. 48-5). Wound classifications enable a nurse to understand the risks associated with a wound and implications for healing.

Process of Wound Healing. Wound healing involves integrated physiological processes. The tissue layers involved and their capacity for regeneration determine the mechanism for repair for any wound (Doughty and Sparks-Defriese, 2012).

There are two types of wounds: those with loss of tissue and those without. A clean surgical incision is an example of a wound with little tissue loss. The surgical incision heals by **primary intention** (Fig. 48-6, *A*). The skin edges are **approximated,** or closed, and the risk of infection is low. Healing occurs quickly, with minimal scar formation, as long as infection and secondary breakdown are prevented (Doughty and Sparks-Defriese, 2012). In contrast, a wound involving loss of tissue such as a burn, pressure ulcer, or severe laceration heals by **secondary intention.** The wound is left open until it becomes filled by scar tissue. It takes longer for a wound to heal by secondary intention; thus the chance of infection is greater. If scarring from secondary intention is severe, loss of tissue function is often permanent (Fig. 48-6, *B*).

Wound Repair. Partial-thickness wounds are shallow wounds involving loss of the epidermis (top layer) and possibly partial loss of the dermis. These wounds heal by regeneration because epidermis regenerates. An example of this is the repair of a clean surgical wound or an abrasion. Full-thickness wounds extending into the dermis (involving both layers of tissue) heal by scar formation because deeper structures do not regenerate. Pressure ulcers are an example of full-thickness wounds.

Partial-Thickness Wound Repair. Three components are involved in the healing process of a partial-thickness wound: inflammatory response, epithelial proliferation (reproduction) and migration, and reestablishment of the epidermal layers.

Tissue trauma causes the *inflammatory response,* which in turn causes redness and swelling to the area with a moderate amount of serous exudate. This response is generally limited to the first 24 hours after wounding. The epithelial cells begin to regenerate, providing new cells to replace the lost cells. The *epithelial proliferation and migration* start at both the wound edges and the epidermal cells lining the epidermal appendages, allowing for quick resurfacing. Epithelial cells begin to migrate across the wound bed soon after the wound occurs. A wound left open to air can resurface within 6 to 7 days, whereas one that is kept moist can resurface in 4 days. The difference in the healing rate is related to the fact that

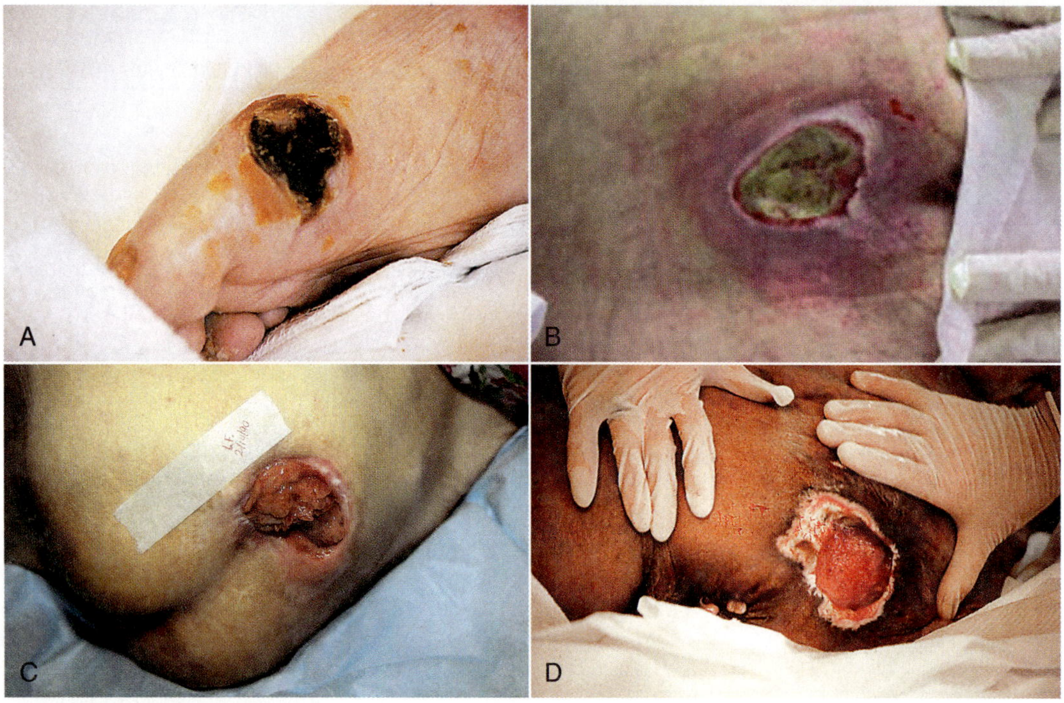

FIG. 48-5 Wounds classified by color assessment. **A,** Black wound. **B,** Yellow wound. **C,** Red wound. **D,** Mixed-color wound. (**A** and **D,** Courtesy Scott Health Care—A Molnlyche Company, Philadelphia, Pa; **B** and **C** from Bryant RA, Nix DP, editors: *Acute and chronic wounds: current management concepts,* ed 4, St Louis, 2012, Mosby.)

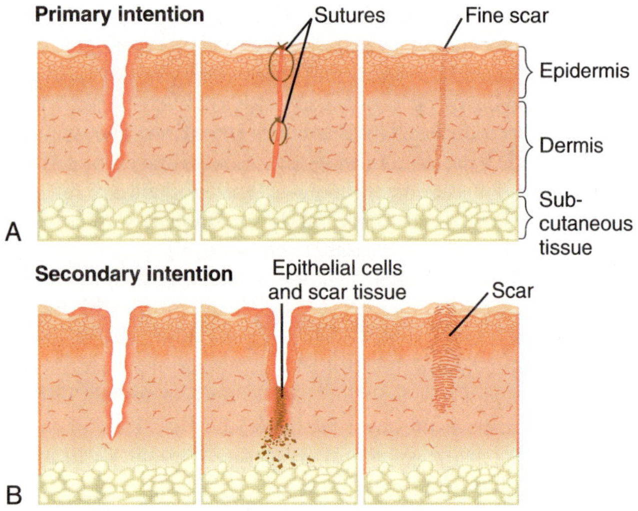

FIG. 48-6 **A,** Wound healing by primary intention such as a surgical incision. Wound healing edges are pulled together and approximated with sutures or staples, and healing occurs by connective tissue deposition. **B,** Wound healing by secondary intention. Wound edges are not approximated, and healing occurs by granulation tissue formation and contraction of the wound edges. (From Black JM, Hawks JH: *Medical-surgical nursing: clinical management for positive outcomes,* ed 8, St Louis, 2009, Mosby.)

epidermal cells only migrate across a moist surface. In a dry wound the cells migrate down into a moist level before migration can occur (Doughty and Sparks-Defriese, 2012). New epithelium is only a few cells thick and must undergo *reestablishment of the epidermal layers.* The cells slowly reestablish normal thickness and appear as dry, pink tissue.

Full-Thickness Wound Repair. The four phases involved in the healing process of a full-thickness wound are hemostasis, inflammatory, proliferative, and remodeling.

Hemostasis. A series of events designed to control blood loss, establish bacterial control, and seal the defect occurs when there is an injury. During **hemostasis** injured blood vessels constrict, and platelets gather to stop bleeding. Clots form a **fibrin** matrix that later provides a framework for cellular repair.

Inflammatory Phase. In the inflammatory stage damaged tissue and mast cells secrete histamine, resulting in vasodilation of surrounding capillaries and exudation of serum and white blood cells into damaged tissues. This results in localized redness, edema, warmth, and throbbing. The inflammatory response is beneficial, and there is no value in attempting to cool the area or reduce the swelling unless the swelling occurs within a closed compartment (e.g., ankle or neck).

Leukocytes (white blood cells) reach the wound within a few hours. The primary-acting white blood cell is the neutrophil, which begins to ingest bacteria and small debris. The second important leukocyte is the monocyte, which transforms into macrophages. The macrophages are the "garbage cells" that clean a wound of bacteria, dead cells, and debris by phagocytosis. Macrophages continue the process of clearing the wound of debris and release growth factors that attract fibroblasts, the cells that synthesize collagen (connective tissue). Collagen appears as early as the second day and is the main component of scar tissue.

In a clean wound the inflammatory phase establishes a clean wound bed. The inflammatory phase is prolonged if too little inflammation occurs, as in a debilitating disease such as cancer or after administration of steroids. Too much inflammation also prolongs healing because arriving cells compete for available nutrients. An example is a wound infection in which the increased metabolic energy requirements present in an infected wound compete for the available calorie intake.

Proliferative Phase. With the appearance of new blood vessels as reconstruction progresses, the proliferative phase begins and lasts from 3 to 24 days. The main activities during this phase are the filling of the wound with granulation tissue, contraction of the wound, and the resurfacing of the wound by **epithelialization.** Fibroblasts are present in this phase and are the cells that synthesize collagen, providing the matrix for granulation. Collagen mixes with the granulation tissue, and this matrix supports the reepithelialization. Collagen provides strength and structural integrity to a wound. During this period the wound contracts to reduce the area that requires healing. Finally the epithelial cells migrate from the wound edges to resurface. In a clean wound the proliferative phase accomplishes the following: the vascular bed is reestablished (granulation tissue), the area is filled with replacement tissue (collagen, contraction, and granulation tissue), and the surface is repaired (epithelialization). Impairment of healing during this stage usually results from systemic factors such as age, anemia, hypoproteinemia, and zinc deficiency.

Remodeling. Maturation, the final stage of healing, sometimes takes place for more than a year, depending on the depth and extent of the wound. The collagen scar continues to reorganize and gain strength for several months. However, a healed wound usually does not have the tensile strength of the tissue it replaces. Collagen fibers undergo remodeling or reorganization before assuming their normal appearance. Usually scar tissue contains fewer pigmented cells (melanocytes) and has a lighter color than normal skin. In dark-skinned individuals the scar tissue may be more highly pigmented than surrounding skin.

Complications of Wound Healing

Hemorrhage. **Hemorrhage,** or bleeding from a wound site, is normal during and immediately after initial trauma. Hemostasis occurs within several minutes unless large blood vessels are involved or the patient has poor clotting function. Hemorrhage occurring after hemostasis indicates a slipped surgical suture, a dislodged clot, infection, or erosion of a blood vessel by a foreign object (e.g., a drain). Hemorrhage occurs externally or internally. For example, if a surgical suture slips from a blood vessel, bleeding occurs internally within the tissues, and there are no visible signs of blood unless a surgical drain is present. A surgical drain may be inserted into tissues beneath a wound to remove fluid that collects in underlying tissues.

You detect internal bleeding by looking for distention or swelling of the affected body part, a change in the type and amount of drainage from a surgical drain, or signs of hypovolemic shock. A **hematoma** is a localized collection of blood underneath the tissues. It appears as a swelling, change in color, sensation, or warmth or mass that often takes on a bluish discoloration. A hematoma near a major artery or vein is dangerous because pressure from the expanding hematoma obstructs blood flow.

External hemorrhaging is obvious. The nurse observes dressings covering the wound for bloody drainage. If bleeding is extensive, the dressing soon becomes saturated, and frequently blood drains from under the dressing and pools beneath the patient. Observe all wounds closely, particularly surgical wounds, in which the risk of hemorrhage is great during the first 24 to 48 hours after surgery or injury.

Infection. Wound infection is the second most common health care–associated infection (nosocomial) (see Chapter 28). According to the Centers for Disease Control and Prevention (CDC) (2001), a wound is infected if purulent material drains from it, even if a culture is not taken or has negative results. A sample of drainage from an infected wound does not always reveal bacteria because of poor culture technique or administration of antibiotics. Positive culture findings do not always indicate an infection because many wounds contain colonies of noninfective resident bacteria. In fact, all chronic dermal wounds are considered contaminated with bacteria. What differentiates contaminated wounds from infected wounds is the amount of bacteria present. It is generally agreed that wounds with more than 100,000 (10^5) organisms per gram of tissue are infected (Stotts, 2012b). The chances of wound infection are greater when the wound contains dead or necrotic tissue, there are foreign bodies in or near the wound, and the blood supply and local tissue defenses are reduced. Bacterial wound infection inhibits wound healing.

Some contaminated or traumatic wounds show signs of infection early, within 2 to 3 days. A surgical wound infection usually does not develop until the fourth or fifth postoperative day. The patient has a fever, tenderness and pain at the wound site, and an elevated white blood cell count. The edges of the wound appear inflamed. If drainage is present, it is odorous and **purulent,** which causes a yellow, green, or brown color, depending on the causative organism (Table 48-2).

TABLE 48-2 Types of Wound Drainage

TYPE	APPEARANCE
Serous	Clear, watery plasma 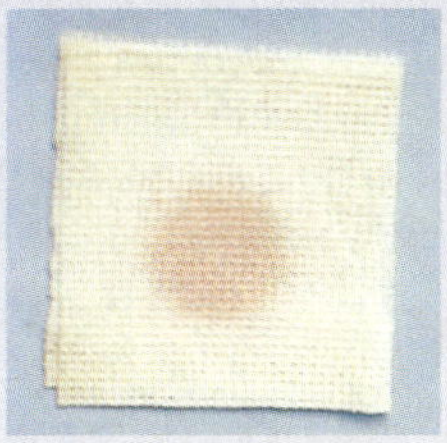
Purulent	Thick, yellow, green, tan, or brown 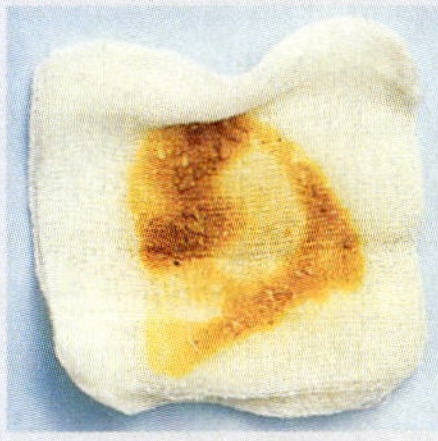
Serosanguineous	Pale, pink, watery; mixture of clear and red fluid 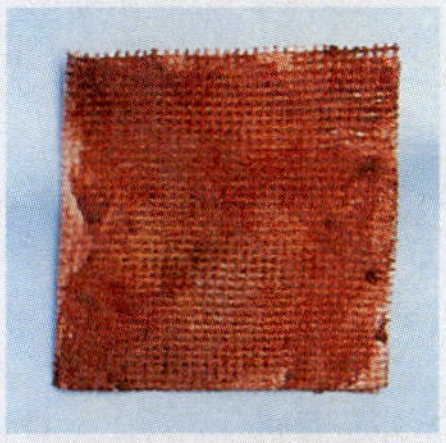
Sanguineous	Bright red; indicates active bleeding 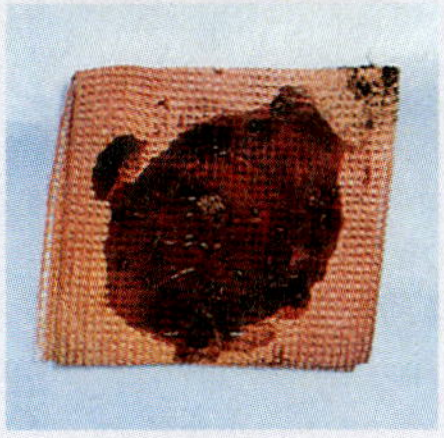

Dehiscence. When a wound fails to heal properly, the layers of skin and tissue separate. This most commonly occurs before collagen formation (3 to 11 days after injury). **Dehiscence** is the partial or total separation of wound layers. A patient who is at risk for poor wound healing (e.g., poor nutritional status, infection, or obesity) is at risk for dehiscence. However, obese patients have a higher risk because of the constant strain placed on their wounds and the poor healing qualities of fat tissue (Camden, 2012). Dehiscence frequently involves abdominal surgical wounds and occurs after a sudden strain such as coughing, vomiting, or sitting up in bed. Patients often report feeling as though something has given way. When there is an increase in serosanguineous drainage from a wound, be alert for the potential for dehiscence. A strategy to prevent dehiscence is to place a folded thin blanket or pillow over an abdominal wound when the patient is coughing. This provides a splint to the area, supporting the healing tissue when coughing increases the intraabdominal pressure.

Evisceration. With total separation of wound layers, **evisceration** (protrusion of visceral organs through a wound opening) occurs. The condition is an emergency that requires surgical repair. When evisceration occurs, the nurse places sterile towels soaked in sterile saline over the extruding tissues to reduce chances of bacterial invasion and drying of the tissues. If the organs protrude through the wound, blood supply to the tissues is compromised. The presence of an evisceration is a surgical emergency. Immediately contact the surgical team, do not allow the patient anything by mouth (NPO), observe him or her for signs and symptoms of shock, and prepare him or her for emergency surgery.

NURSING KNOWLEDGE BASE

Prediction and Prevention of Pressure Ulcers

A major aspect of nursing care is the maintenance of skin integrity. Consistent, planned skin care interventions are critical to ensuring high-quality care. Nurses constantly observe their patients' skin for breaks or impaired skin integrity. Impaired skin integrity occurs from prolonged pressure, irritation of the skin, and/or immobility, leading to the development of pressure ulcers. A pressure ulcer is a localized injury to the skin and/or underlying tissue, usually over a bony prominence, as a result of pressure or pressure in combination with shear and/or friction (EPUAP and NPUAP, 2009).

Risk Assessment. Several instruments are available for assessing patients who are at risk for developing a pressure ulcer. By identifying at-risk patients, you are able to put interventions into place for the at-risk patient and spare patients with little risk for pressure ulcer development the unnecessary and sometimes costly preventive treatment. Prevention and treatment of pressure ulcers are major nursing priorities. The incidence of pressure ulcers in a facility or agency is an important indicator of quality of care. Evidence exists that a program of prevention guided by risk assessment simultaneously reduces the institutional incidence of pressure ulcers by as much as 60% and brings down the costs of prevention at the same time (Braden, 2001). Several risk-assessment scales (Bergstrom et al., 1987; Norton et al., 1962) developed by nurses enable systematic risk assessment of patients. The Braden Scale, a widely used risk-assessment tool, is in the WOCN guidelines (2010) as being a valid tool to use for pressure ulcer risk assessment. The Braden Scale (Table 48-3) was developed based on risk factors in a nursing home population (Bergstrom et al., 1987) and is composed of six subscales: sensory perception, moisture, activity, mobility, nutrition, and friction/shear. The total score ranges from 6 to 23; a lower total score indicates a higher risk for pressure ulcer development (Braden and Bergstrom, 1989). The cutoff score for onset of pressure ulcer risk with the Braden Scale in the general adult population is 18 (Ayello and Braden, 2002). It is highly reliable when used to identify patients at greatest risk for pressure ulcers (Bergstrom et al., 1987; Braden and Bergstrom, 1994). The Braden Scale is the most commonly used assessment scale for pressure ulcer risk.

Prevention. Preventing pressure ulcers is a priority in caring for patients and is not limited to patients with restrictions in mobility. Impaired skin integrity is not usually a problem in healthy, immobilized individuals but is a serious and potentially devastating problem in ill or debilitated patients (WOCN, 2010).

Economic Consequences of Pressure Ulcers. Pressure ulcers are a continual problem in acute and restorative care settings. For adult patients with pressure ulcers, 56.5% were 65 years and older (WOCN, 2010). Paralysis and spinal cord injury are common preexisting conditions among younger adults with primary diagnosis of pressure ulcers. Older adults admitted to acute and long-term facilities are a vulnerable population. Among persons admitted to long-term care, 10.3% to 18.4% had one or more pressure ulcers on admission (Baumgarten et al., 2003; Siem et al., 2003).

When a pressure ulcer occurs, the length of stay in a hospital and the overall cost of health care increase. The actual cost of treatment is difficult to estimate. About 1.6 million patients each year in acute care settings develop pressure ulcers, representing a cost of $11 to $17.2 billion to the U.S. health care system (Pieper, 2012). Adult inpatient hospital stays with a diagnosis of pressure ulcers totaled $11 billion in 2006 (WOCN, 2010). Although it is difficult to get a handle on the exact numbers of pressure ulcers, the number of patients with pressure ulcers, and the cost, the occurrence of pressure ulcers is costly to patients in terms of disability, pain, and suffering and in the costs to institutions and third-party payers. The Centers for Medicare and Medicaid Services (CMS) implemented a policy effective October 1, 2008 whereby hospitals no longer receive additional reimbursement for care related to eight conditions, including stage III and IV pressure ulcers that occur during the hospitalization. This policy was put in place to provide additional incentives for hospitals to improve quality of care. Using guidelines such as the WOCN Guidelines (WOCN, 2010) helps reduce or eliminate the occurrence of pressure ulcers and prevent the expense that will not be reimbursed.

Factors Influencing Pressure Ulcer Formation and Wound Healing

Impaired skin integrity resulting in pressure ulcers is primarily the result of pressure. However, additional factors, including shear force, friction, moisture, nutrition, tissue perfusion, infection, and age, increase the patient's risk for pressure ulcer development and poor wound healing.

Nutrition. For patients weakened or debilitated by illness, nutritional therapy is especially important. A patient who has undergone surgery (see Chapter 50) and is well nourished still requires at least 1500 kcal/day for nutritional maintenance. Alternatives such as enteral feedings (see Chapter 44) and parenteral nutrition (see Chapter 41) are available for patients unable to maintain normal food intake.

Normal wound healing requires proper nutrition (Table 48-4). Deficiencies in any of the nutrients result in impaired or delayed healing (Stotts, 2012a). Physiological processes of wound healing depend on the availability of protein, vitamins (especially A and C), and the trace minerals zinc and copper. Collagen is a protein formed from amino acids acquired by fibroblasts from protein

TABLE 48-3 **Braden Scale for Predicting Pressure Ulcer Risk**

Patient's Name ___________ Evaluator's Name ___________ Date of Assessment ___________

Sensory Perception				
Ability to respond meaningfully to pressure-related discomfort	1. Completely limited Unresponsive (does not moan, flinch, or grasp) to painful stimuli caused by diminished level of consciousness or sedation OR Limited ability to feel pain over most of body surface	2. Very limited Responds only to painful stimuli Cannot communicate discomfort except by moaning or restlessness OR Has sensory impairment that limits ability to feel pain or discomfort over $\frac{1}{2}$ of body	3. Slightly limited Responds to verbal commands but cannot always communicate discomfort or need to be turned OR Has some sensory impairment that limits ability to feel pain or discomfort in one or two extremities	4. No impairment Responds to verbal commands Has no sensory deficit that would limit ability to feel or voice pain or discomfort
Moisture				
Degree to which skin is exposed to moisture	1. Constantly moist Skin kept moist almost constantly by perspiration, urine, etc. Dampness detected every time patient is moved or turned	2. Moist Skin often, but not always, moist Necessary to change linen at least once a shift	3. Occasionally moist Skin occasionally moist, requiring an extra linen change approximately once a day	4. Rarely moist Skin usually dry Required linen changing only at routine intervals
Activity				
Degree of physical activity	1. Bedfast Confined to bed	2. Chairfast Ability to walk severely limited or nonexistent Cannot bear own weight and/or must be assisted into chair or wheelchair	3. Walks occasionally Walks occasionally during day but for very short distances, with or without assistance Spends majority of each shift in bed or chair	4. Walks frequently Walks outside room at least twice a day and inside room at least once every 2 hours during waking hours
Mobility				
Ability to change and control body position	1. Completely immobile Does not make even slight changes in body or extremity position without assistance	2. Very limited Makes occasional slight changes in body or extremity position but unable to make frequent or significant changes independently	3. Slightly limited Makes frequent, although slight, changes in body or extremity position independently	4. No limitations Makes major and frequent changes in position without assistance
Nutrition				
Usual food intake pattern	1. Very poor Never eats a complete meal; rarely eats more than $\frac{1}{3}$ of any food offered; eats 2 servings or less of protein (meat or dairy products) per day Takes fluids poorly; does not take a liquid dietary supplement OR Is NPO and/or maintained on clear liquids or IVs for more than 5 days	2. Probably inadequate Rarely eats a complete meal and generally eats only about $\frac{1}{2}$ of any food offered Protein intake includes only 3 servings of meat or dairy products per day; occasionally takes a dietary supplement OR Receives less than optimum amount of liquid diet or tube feeding	3. Adequate Eats over half of most meals; eats a total of four servings of protein (meat, dairy products) each day Occasionally refuses a meal but usually takes a supplement if offered OR Is on tube feeding or total parenteral nutrition regimen that probably meets most of nutritional needs	4. Excellent Eats most of every meal; never refuses a meal; usually eats a total of four or more servings of meat and dairy products Occasionally eats between meals Does not require supplementation
Friction and Shear				
	1. Problem Requires moderate-to-maximum assistance in moving; complete lifting without sliding against sheets impossible Frequently slides down in bed or chair, requiring frequent repositioning with maximum assistance Spasticity, contractures, or agitation leads to almost constant friction	2. Potential problem Moves feebly or requires minimum assistance; during a move skin probably slides to some extent against sheets, chair, restraints, or other devices Maintains relatively good position in chair or bed most of the time but occasionally slides down	3. No apparent problem Moves in bed and in chair independently and has sufficient muscle strength to lift up completely during move Maintains good position in bed or chair at all times	TOTAL SCORE

IV, Intravenous lines.

TABLE 48-4 **Role of Selected Nutrients in Wound Healing**

NUTRIENT	ROLE IN HEALING	RECOMMENDATIONS	SOURCES
Calories	Fuel for cell energy "Protein protection"	35-40 kcal/kg/day or enough to maintain positive nitrogen balance	
Protein	Fibroplasia, angiogenesis, collagen formation and wound remodeling, immune function	1-1.5 g/kg/day or enough to maintain positive nitrogen balance	Poultry, fish, eggs, beef
Vitamin C (ascorbic acid)	Collagen synthesis, capillary wall integrity, fibroblast function, immunological function, antioxidant	100-1000 mg/day Need long time to develop clinical scurvy from vitamin C deficiency Low toxicity	Citrus fruits, tomatoes, potatoes, fortified fruit juices
Vitamin A	Epithelialization, wound closure, inflammatory response, angiogenesis, collagen formation Can reverse steroid effects on skin and delayed healing	1600-2000 retinol equivalents per day Supplement if deficient 20,000 units × 10 days	Green leafy vegetables (spinach), broccoli, carrots, sweet potatoes, liver
Vitamin E	No known role in wound healing, antioxidant	None	Fish, oysters, liver, dark meat, eggs, legumes
Zinc	Collagen formation, protein synthesis, cell membrane and host defenses	15-30 mg Correct deficiencies No improvement in wound healing with supplementation unless zinc deficient Use with caution—large doses can be toxic May inhibit copper metabolism and impair immune function	Vegetables, meats, legumes
Fluid	Essential fluid environment for all cell function	30-35 mL/kg/day Increase by another 10-15 mL/kg if patient is on an air-fluidized bed	Use noncaffeine, nonalcoholic fluids without sugar Water is best—6-8 glasses/day

Modified from Ayello EA et al.: Nutritional aspects of wound healing, *Home Healthc Nurse* 17(11):719, 1999; and Stotts NA: Nutritional assessment and support. In Bryant RA, Nix DP, editors: *Acute and chronic wounds: current management concepts,* ed 4, St Louis, 2012a, Mosby.

ingested in food. Vitamin C is necessary for synthesis of collagen. Vitamin A reduces the negative effects of steroids on wound healing. Trace elements are also necessary; (i.e., zinc for epithelialization and collagen synthesis and copper for collagen fiber linking).

Calories provide the energy source needed to support the cellular activity of wound healing. Protein needs especially are increased and are essential for tissue repair and growth. A balanced intake of various nutrients (i.e., protein, fat, carbohydrates, vitamins, and minerals) is critical to support wound healing.

Serum proteins are biochemical indicators of malnutrition (Stotts, 2012a). Serum albumin is probably the most frequently measured of these laboratory parameters. Albumin alone is not sensitive to rapid changes in nutritional status. Transferrin also evaluates protein status, but alone it does not determine malnutrition. The best measure of nutritional status is prealbumin, because it reflects not only what the patient has ingested but also what the body has absorbed, digested, and metabolized (Stotts, 2012a).

Tissue Perfusion. Oxygen fuels the cellular functions essential to the healing process; therefore the ability to perfuse the tissues with adequate amounts of oxygenated blood is critical to wound healing (Doughty and Sparks-Defriese, 2012). Patients with peripheral vascular disease are at risk for poor tissue perfusion because of poor circulation. Oxygen requirements depend on the phase of wound healing (e.g., chronic tissue hypoxia is associated with impaired collagen synthesis and reduced tissue resistance to infection).

Infection. Wound infection prolongs the inflammatory phase; delays collagen synthesis; prevents epithelialization; and increases the production of proinflammatory cytokines, which leads to additional tissue destruction (Stotts, 2012b). Indications that a wound infection is present include the presence of purulent drainage; change in odor, volume, or character of wound drainage; redness in the surrounding tissue; fever; or pain.

Age. Increased age affects all phases of wound healing. A decrease in the functioning of the macrophage leads to a delayed inflammatory response, delayed collagen synthesis, and slower epithelialization.

Psychosocial Impact of Wounds. The psychosocial impact of wounds on the physiological process of healing is unknown. The patient's psychological response to any wound is part of the nurse's assessment. Body image changes often impose a great stress on the patient's adaptive mechanisms. They also influence self-concept (see Chapter 33) and sexuality (see Chapter 34). Make sure that the patient's personal and social resources for adaptation are a part of the assessment. Factors that affect the patient's perception of the wound include the presence of scars, drains (drains are often necessary for weeks or even months after certain procedures), odor from drainage, and temporary or permanent prosthetic devices.

CRITICAL THINKING

Successful critical thinking requires a synthesis of knowledge, experience, information gathered from patients, critical thinking attitudes, and intellectual and professional standards. Clinical judgments require the nurse to anticipate the information necessary, analyze the data, and make decisions regarding patient care.

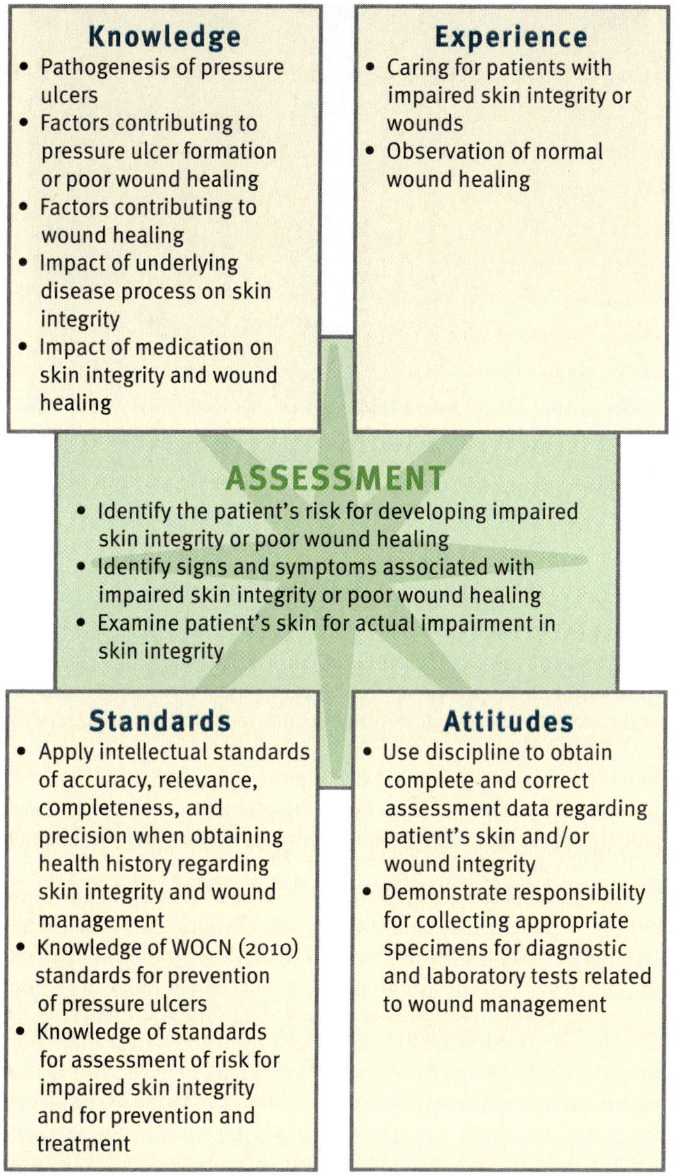

Knowledge
• Pathogenesis of pressure ulcers
• Factors contributing to pressure ulcer formation or poor wound healing
• Factors contributing to wound healing
• Impact of underlying disease process on skin integrity
• Impact of medication on skin integrity and wound healing
Experience
• Caring for patients with impaired skin integrity or wounds
• Observation of normal wound healing
ASSESSMENT
• Identify the patient's risk for developing impaired skin integrity or poor wound healing
• Identify signs and symptoms associated with impaired skin integrity or poor wound healing
• Examine patient's skin for actual impairment in skin integrity
Standards
• Apply intellectual standards of accuracy, relevance, completeness, and precision when obtaining health history regarding skin integrity and wound management
• Knowledge of WOCN (2010) standards for prevention of pressure ulcers
• Knowledge of standards for assessment of risk for impaired skin integrity and for prevention and treatment
Attitudes
• Use discipline to obtain complete and correct assessment data regarding patient's skin and/or wound integrity
• Demonstrate responsibility for collecting appropriate specimens for diagnostic and laboratory tests related to wound management

FIG. 48-7 Critical thinking model for skin integrity and wound care assessment. *WOCN,* Wound, Ostomy, and Continence Nurses Society.

Critical thinking is always changing. During assessment (Fig. 48-7) consider all elements that build toward making appropriate nursing diagnoses.

When caring for patients who have impaired skin integrity and chronic wounds, integrate knowledge from nursing and other disciplines, previous experiences, and information gathered from patients to understand the risk to skin integrity and wound healing. Knowledge of normal musculoskeletal physiology, the pathogenesis of pressure ulcers, normal wound healing, and the pathophysiology of underlying diseases enables you to have a scientific basis for care. The WOCN (2010) has guidelines for assessment of risk for impaired skin integrity, prevention measures, interventions to promote wound healing, and other standards of practice, which you should use in planning care. Past experience with patients at risk for impaired skin integrity or patients with wounds increases the experiential knowledge base helping you to identify interventions. Finally you need to be disciplined during assessment to obtain comprehensive and correct assessment data. You also need to be creative. Because chronic wounds are difficult to heal, be diligent in evaluating nursing interventions and determining which interventions are effective and which need modification.

BOX 48-4 NURSING ASSESSMENT QUESTIONS

Skin Integrity

Sensation
- Do you have decreased feeling in your extremities or any other region?
- Are you sensitive to heat or cold?

Mobility
- Do you have any physical limitations, injury, or paralysis that limits your mobility?
- Can you change your position easily?
- Is movement painful?

Continence
- Do you have any problems with involuntary loss of urine or stool?
- What assistance do you need using the toilet?
- How often do you need to use the toilet? During the day? During the night?

Presence of Wound
- What caused the wound?
- When did the wound occur? What is its location and dimensions?
- When did you receive a tetanus shot?
- What has happened to this wound since it occurred? What were the changes and what caused them?
- Which treatments, activities, or care have slowed or helped the wound-healing process? Are there special needs for this wound to heal?
- Are there associated symptoms such as pain or itching with the wound? How are they being managed, and are the interventions effective?
- What is the goal for the patient, wound, and healing?

NURSING PROCESS

Apply the nursing process and use a critical thinking approach in your care of patients. The nursing process provides a clinical decision-making approach for you to develop and implement an individualized plan of care.

ASSESSMENT

During the assessment process thoroughly assess each patient and critically analyze findings to ensure that you make patient-centered clinical decisions required for safe nursing care. Baseline and continual assessment data provide critical information about a patient's skin integrity and the increased risk for pressure ulcer development. Focusing on specific elements such as a patient's level of sensation, movement, and continence status helps guide the skin assessment (Box 48-4).

Through the Patient's Eyes. When patients have an acute surgical or traumatic wound, the wound sometimes heals promptly and without complications. However, when pressure ulcers or chronic wounds are present, the course of treatment is lengthy and costly. Because the patient and family need to be involved with wound care management, it is important to know the patient's expectations. A patient who has realistic goals and is informed about the length of time for wound healing is more likely to adhere to the specific therapies designed to promote healing and prevent

BOX 48-5 PROCEDURAL GUIDELINES

Skin Assessment

Delegation Considerations

The skill of skin assessment for skin integrity or the presence of skin breakdown cannot be delegated to nursing assistive personnel (NAP). Direct/inform/instruct the NAP to report:

- Any changes in the patient's skin to the nurse immediately.
- Patient's exposure to body fluids (e.g., urine, feces, wound drainage, gastric secretions).

Equipment

Skin assessment documentation record (check agency policy)

1. Observe pressure points. Compression of these areas for prolonged periods of time by bony prominences or external sources causes tissue ischemia and cell death (WOCN, 2010).
   a. Bony prominences—heels, ankles, knees, hips, sacral area, ischial area, spinal area, shoulders, and elbows (see Fig. 48-9)
   b. Cast edges; areas next to nasogastric tubes, drainage tubes, or oxygen tubing
2. When you find reddened areas, gently press the area with a gloved finger to assess the ability of the tissue to blanch. If the area does not blanch, suspect tissue injury.
3. Check perineal area for signs of reddened, irritated skin. Perineal skin is at high risk for skin breakdown in the patient with fecal and/or urinary incontinence.
4. Observe underlying skin areas where tape, tubing, casts, or splints are in contact with skin.
5. Note previous areas of skin breakdown, check for any breaks in skin integrity, or note nonblanching erythema in this area. Areas of previous skin breakdown do not heal to the same strength as intact noninjured skin; therefore these areas are at higher risk for skin breakdown.
6. Determine if potential or actual skin breakdown is present and institute appropriate preventive or treatment protocols.
7. Record findings and the preventive or treatment protocols initiated per agency policy.

further skin breakdown. Therefore it is important to assess the patient's perception of what is occurring with the wound healing interventions. The health care professional wants to determine the patient's and family's understanding of wound assessment; wound interventions; and supportive interventions such as positioning, nutrition, and ambulation.

Skin. A nurse continually assesses the skin for signs of ulcer development (Box 48-5). The neurologically impaired patient; the chronically ill patient in long-term care; the patient with diminished mental status; and the intensive care unit (ICU), oncology, hospice, or orthopedic patient have increased potential for developing pressure ulcers.

Assessment for tissue pressure damage includes visual and tactile inspection of the skin. Perform baseline assessment to determine a patient's normal skin characteristics and any actual or potential areas of breakdown. You need to individualize assessment characteristics of a patient's skin, depending on his or her skin tone (Bennett, 1995; Henderson et al., 1997). Accurate assessment of patients with darker skin pigmentation is an essential skill for all health care providers (Nix, 2012). Assessment characteristics of darkly pigmented skin are in Boxes 48-2 and 48-3.

Pay particular attention to areas located over bony prominences or under casts, traction, splints, braces, collars, or other orthopedic devices. The frequency of pressure checks depends on the schedule

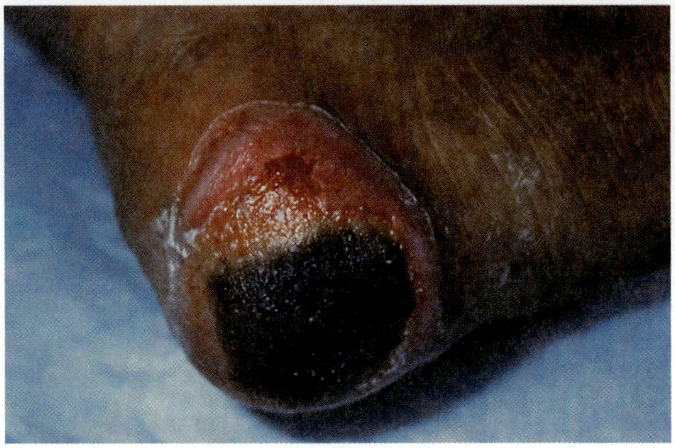

FIG. 48-8 Formation of pressure ulcer on heel resulting from external pressure from mattress of bed. (Courtesy Janice Colwell, RN, MS, CWOCN, FAAN, Clinical Nurse Specialist, University of Chicago Medical Center.)

of appliance application and the response of the skin to the external pressure (Fig. 48-8).

When you note hyperemia, document the location, size, and color and reassess the area after 1 hour. When you suspect **abnormal reactive hyperemia,** outline the affected area with a marker to make reassessment easier. These signs are early indicators of impaired skin integrity, but damage to the underlying tissue is sometimes more progressive. Tactile assessment enables you to use palpation to acquire further data about **induration** and the damage to the skin and underlying tissues.

Gently palpate the reddened tissue, observing for blanching with return to normal skin tones in patients with light-toned skin. In addition, palpate for induration, noting the size in millimeters or centimeters of the induration around the injured area and changes in temperature of the surrounding skin and tissues.

Use visual and tactile inspection over the body areas most frequently at risk for pressure ulcer development (Fig. 48-9). For example, when a patient lies in bed or sits in a chair, he or she places body weight heavily on certain bony prominences. Body surfaces subjected to the greatest weight or pressure are at greatest risk for pressure ulcer formation.

Pressure Ulcers. Pressure ulcers have multiple etiological factors. Assessment for pressure ulcer risk includes using an appropriate predictive measure and assessing a patient's mobility, nutrition, presence of body fluids, and comfort level (Skill 48-1 on pp. 1213-1215).

Predictive Measures. On admission to acute care and rehabilitation hospitals, nursing homes, home care programs, and other health care facilities, assess individuals for risk of pressure ulcer development (WOCN, 2010). Perform pressure ulcer risk assessment systematically (WOCN, 2010). Use an assessment tool such as the Braden scale (see Table 48-3). The interpretation of the meaning of the total numerical scores differs with each risk-assessment scale. Lower numerical scores on the Braden scale indicate that a patient is at high risk for skin breakdown. A benefit of the predictive instruments is to increase a nurse's early detection of patients at greatest risk for ulcer development. Once you identify these patients, institute the appropriate interventions to maintain skin integrity and implement prevention strategies (WOCN, 2010). Perform reassessment for pressure ulcer risk on a scheduled basis.

Mobility. Assessment includes documenting the level of mobility and the potential effects of impaired mobility on skin integrity.

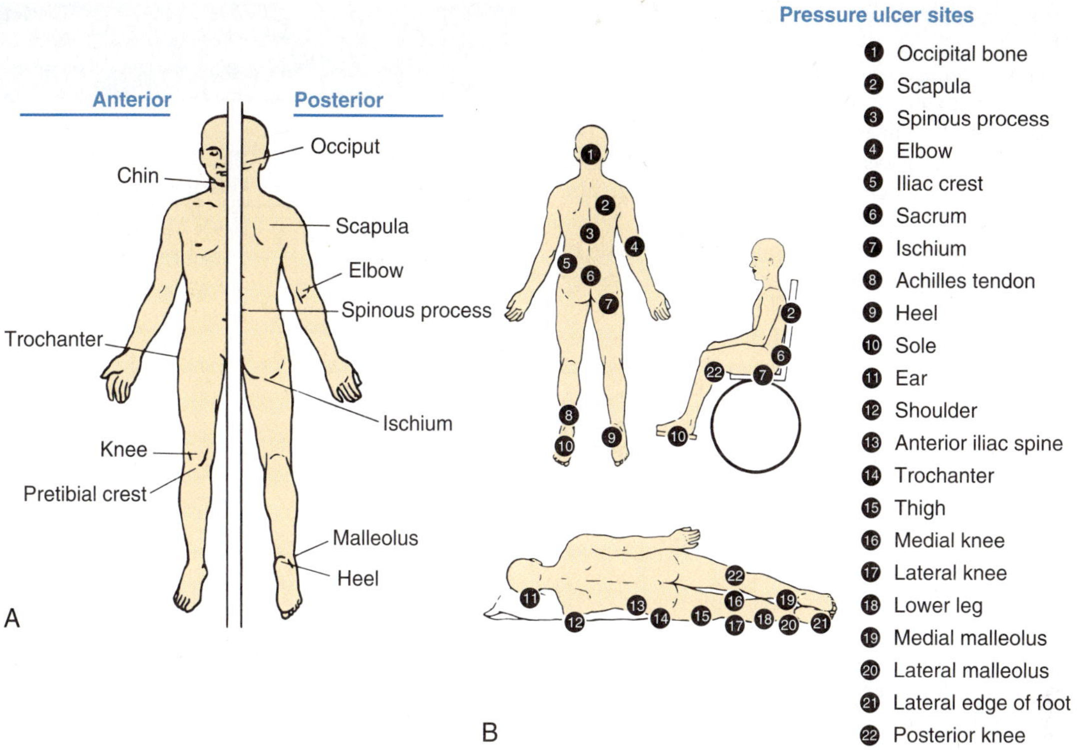

FIG. 48-9 **A,** Bony prominences most frequently underlying pressure ulcer. **B,** Pressure ulcer sites. (Modified from Trelease CC: Developing standards for wound care, *Ostomy Wound Manage* 20:46, 1988.)

Documenting assessment of mobility also includes obtaining data regarding the quality of muscle tone and strength. For example, determine whether the patient is able to lift weight off of the sacral area and roll the body to a side-lying position. Some patients have adequate range of motion to move independently into a more protective position. Finally note the patient's activity tolerance (see Chapter 38).

You must assess mobility as part of baseline data. If a patient has some degree of mobility independence, reinforce the frequency of position changes and measures to relieve pressure. The frequency of position changes is based on ongoing skin assessment; revise it as data change. Be meticulous when assessing pressure sites.

Nutritional Status. An assessment of patients' nutritional status is an integral part of the initial assessment data for patients at risk for impaired skin integrity and wounds (Stotts, 2012a). Malnutrition is a risk factor for pressure ulcer development (Posthauer and Thomas, 2008). A loss of 5% of usual weight, weight less than 90% of ideal body weight, and a decrease of 10 pounds in a brief period are all signs of actual or potential nutritional problems (Stotts, 2012a).

Body Fluids. Continual exposure of the skin to body fluids increases a patient's risk for skin breakdown and pressure ulcer formation (Box 48-6). Some body fluids such as saliva and serosanguineous drainage are not as caustic to the skin, and the risk of skin breakdown from exposure to these fluids is low. However, exposure to urine, bile, stool, ascitic fluid, and purulent wound exudates carries a moderate risk for skin breakdown, especially in patients who have other risk factors such as chronic illness or poor nutrition. Finally exposure to gastric and pancreatic drainage has the highest risk for skin breakdown. Again, it is important to prevent and reduce the patient's exposure to body fluids; and, when exposure occurs, you need to provide meticulous hygiene and skin care.

BOX 48-6 RISK FOR SKIN BREAKDOWN FROM BODY FLUIDS

Low Risk
- Saliva
- Serosanguineous drainage

Moderate Risk
- Bile
- Stool
- Urine
- Ascitic fluid
- Purulent exudate

High Risk
- Gastric drainage
- Pancreatic drainage

Pain. Until recently there has been little research about pain and pressure ulcers. The WOCN (2010) has recommended the assessment and management of pain be included in the care of patients with pressure ulcers (Dallam et al., 2008). Maintaining adequate pain control and patient comfort increases the patient's willingness and ability to increase mobility, which in turn reduces pressure ulcer risk.

Wounds. A nurse often assesses wounds under two conditions: at the time of injury before treatment and after therapy, when the wound is relatively stable. Each condition requires him or her to make different observations and take different actions. Regardless of the setting, it is important that you initially obtain information regarding the cause and history of the wound (see Box 48-4).

Emergency Setting. You see wounds in any setting, including clinics, emergency departments, youth camps, or your own backyard. The type of wound determines the criteria for inspection. For example, you do not need to inspect for signs of internal bleeding after an abrasion, but you should inspect in the event of a puncture wound.

When you judge a patient's condition to be stable because of the presence of spontaneous breathing, a clear airway, and a strong carotid pulse (see Chapters 30 and 40), inspect the wound for bleeding. An **abrasion** is superficial with little bleeding and is considered a partial-thickness wound. The wound often appears "weepy" because of plasma leakage from damaged capillaries. A **laceration** sometimes bleeds more profusely, depending on the depth and location of the wound. For example, minor scalp lacerations tend to bleed profusely because of the rich blood supply to the scalp. Lacerations greater than 5 cm (2 inches) long or 2.5 cm (1 inch) deep cause serious bleeding. **Puncture** wounds bleed in relation to the depth and size of the wound (e.g., a nail puncture does not cause as much bleeding as a knife wound). The primary dangers of puncture wounds are internal bleeding and infection.

Inspect the wound for foreign bodies or contaminant material. Most traumatic wounds are dirty. Soil, broken glass, shreds of cloth, and foreign substances clinging to penetrating objects sometimes become embedded in the wound.

The size of the wound is the next step in assessment. A deep laceration requires suturing. A large, open wound may expose bone or tissue that needs to be protected.

When the injury is a result of trauma from a dirty penetrating object, determine when the patient last received a tetanus toxoid injection. Tetanus bacteria reside in soil and in the gut of humans and animals. A tetanus antitoxin injection is necessary if the patient has not had one within 5 years.

Stable Setting. When a patient's condition is stabilized (e.g., after surgery or treatment), assess the wound to determine progress toward healing. If the wound is covered by a dressing and the health care provider has not ordered it changed, do not directly inspect it unless you suspect serious complications. In such a situation inspect only the dressing and any external drains. If the health care provider prefers to change the dressing, he or she assesses the wound at least daily. When removing dressings, take care to avoid accidental removal or displacement of underlying drains. Because removal of dressings can be painful, consider giving an analgesic at least 30 minutes before exposing a wound.

Wound Appearance. Observe whether wound edges are closed. A surgical incision healing by primary intention should have clean, well-approximated edges. Crusts often form along the wound edges from exudate. A puncture wound is usually a small, circular wound with the edges coming together toward the center. If a wound is open, the edges are separated, and you inspect the condition of tissue at the wound base. Also look for complications such as dehiscence and evisceration. The outer edges of a wound normally appear inflamed for the first 2 to 3 days, but this slowly disappears. Within 7 to 10 days a normally healing wound resurfaces with epithelial cells, and edges close. Table 48-5 lists assessment characteristics for abnormal wound healing in primary and secondary wounds. If infection develops, the area directly surrounding the wound becomes brightly inflamed and swollen.

Skin discoloration usually results from bruising of interstitial tissues or hematoma formation. Blood collecting beneath the skin first takes on a bluish or purplish appearance. Gradually, as the clotted blood is broken down, shades of brown and yellow appear.

TABLE 48-5 Assessment of Abnormal Healing in Primary and Secondary Intention Wounds

PRIMARY INTENTION WOUNDS	SECONDARY INTENTION WOUNDS
Incision line poorly approximated	Pale or fragile granulation tissue, granulation tissue bed excessively dry or moist
Drainage present more than 3 days after closure	Purulent exudate present
Inflammation increased in first 3-5 days after injury	Necrotic or slough tissue present in wound base
No epithelialization of wound edges by day 4	Epithelialization not continuous
No healing ridge by day 9	Fruity, earthy, or putrid odor present Presence of fistula(s), tunneling, undermining

Modified from Stotts NA, Cavanaugh CE: Assessing the patient with a wound, *Home Healthc Nurse* 17(1):27, 1999.

Character of Wound Drainage. Note the amount, color, odor, and consistency of drainage. The amount of drainage depends on the location and extent of the wound. For example, drainage is minimal after a simple appendectomy. In contrast, it is moderate for 1 to 2 days after drainage of a large abscess. When you need an accurate measurement of the amount of drainage within a dressing, weigh the dressing and compare it with the weight of the same dressing when clean and dry. The general rule is that 1 g of drainage equals 1 mL of volume of drainage. Another method of quantifying wound drainage is to chart the number of dressings used and the frequency of change. An increase or decrease in the number or frequency of dressings indicates a relative increase or decrease in wound drainage. The color and consistency of drainage vary, depending on the components. Types of drainage include the following: **serous, sanguineous, serosanguineous,** and purulent (see Table 48-2). If the drainage has a pungent or strong odor, you should suspect an infection. Describe the appearance of the wound according to characteristics observed. An example of accurate recording follows:

Abdominal incision is 5 cm in length in RLQ; edges well approximated without inflammation or exudate. 1.2-cm diameter circle of serous drainage present on one 4 × 4 gauze changed every 8 hours.

Drains. The health care provider inserts a drain into or near a surgical wound if there is a large amount of drainage. Some drains are sutured in place. Exercise caution when changing the dressing around drains that are not sutured in place to prevent accidental removal. A Penrose drain lies under a dressing; at the time of placement a pin or clip is placed through the drain to prevent it from slipping farther into a wound (Fig. 48-10). It is usually the health care provider's responsibility to pull or advance the drain as drainage decreases to permit healing deep within the drain site.

Assess the number of drains, drain placement, character of drainage, and condition of collecting equipment. Observe the security of the drain and its location with respect to the wound. Next note the character of drainage. If there is a collecting device, measure the drainage volume. Because a drainage system needs to be patent, look for drainage flow through and around the tubing.

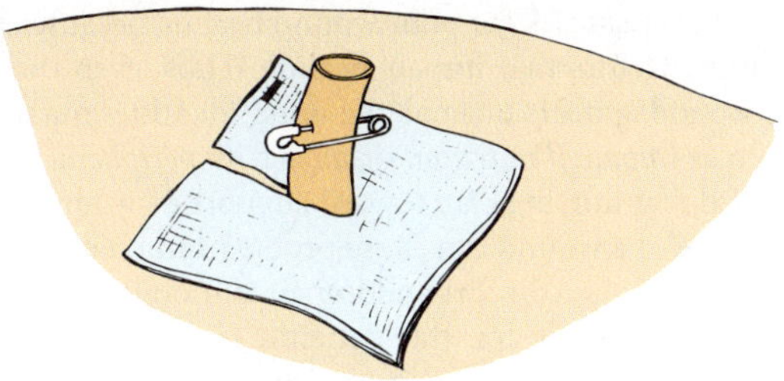

FIG. 48-10 Penrose drain.

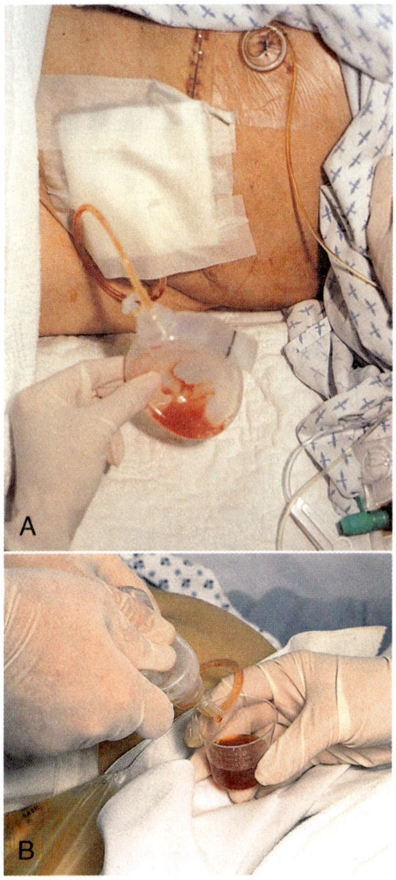

FIG. 48-11 Jackson-Pratt drainage device. **A,** Drainage tubes and reservoir. **B,** Emptying drainage reservoir.

A sudden decrease in drainage through the tubing may indicate a blocked drain, and you need to notify the health care provider. When a drain is connected to suction, assess the system to be sure that the pressure ordered is being exerted. Evacuator units such as a Hemovac or Jackson-Pratt (Fig. 48-11) exert a constant low pressure as long as the suction device (bladder or container) is fully compressed. These types of drainage devices are often referred to as *self-suction*. When the evacuator device is unable to maintain a vacuum on its own, notify the surgeon, who then orders a secondary vacuum system (such as wall suction). If fluid accumulates within the tissues, wound healing does not progress at an optimal rate, and this increases the risk of infection.

Wound Closures. Surgical wounds are closed with staples, sutures, or wound closures. A frequent skin closure is the stainless-steel staple. The staple provides more strength than nylon or silk sutures and tends to cause less irritation to tissue. Look for irritation around staple or suture sites and note whether closures are intact. Normally for the first 2 to 3 days after surgery the skin around sutures or staples is edematous. Continued swelling may indicate that the closures are too tight. The skin can be cut by overly tight suture material, leading to wound separation. Early suture removal reduces formation of defects along the suture line and minimizes chances of unattractive scar formation.

Dermabond is a tissue adhesive that forms a strong bond across apposed wound edges, allowing normal healing to occur below. It can be used to replace small sutures for incisional repair. A vial containing the Dermabond solution is used to apply the product to approximated tissue. The wound edges are held together until the solution dries, providing an adhesive closure. Although generally used for small superficial lacerations, some surgeons use it on larger wounds where subcutaneous sutures are needed (Bruns and Worthington, 2000).

Palpation of Wound. When inspecting a wound, observe swelling or separation of wound edges. While wearing gloves, lightly press the wound edges, detecting localized areas of tenderness or drainage collection. If pressure causes fluid to be expressed, note the character of the drainage. The patient is normally sensitive to palpation of wound edges. Extreme tenderness indicates infection.

Wound Cultures. If you detect purulent or suspicious-looking drainage, obtaining a specimen of the drainage for culture may be necessary (see Chapter 28). Never collect a wound culture sample from old drainage. Resident colonies of bacteria from the skin grow within exudate and are not always the true causative organisms of a wound infection. Clean a wound first with normal saline to remove skin flora. Aerobic organisms grow in superficial wounds exposed to the air, and anaerobic organisms tend to grow within body cavities. Use a different method of specimen collection for each type of organism per agency policy (Box 48-7).

Gram stains of drainage are often performed as well. This test allows the health care provider to order appropriate treatment earlier than when only cultures are done. No additional specimens are usually required. The microbiology laboratory needs only to be notified to perform the additional test.

The gold standard of wound culture is tissue biopsy. A health care provider or wound care specialist with special training obtains the biopsy (Stotts, 2012b).

NURSING DIAGNOSIS

Assessment reveals clusters of data to indicate whether an actual or a risk for *impaired skin integrity* exists. In addition, the assessment data will provide information on the related factor. For example, a postoperative patient has purulent drainage from a surgical wound and reports tenderness around the area of the wound. These data support a nursing diagnosis of *impaired skin integrity related to infection* (Box 48-8). After completing an assessment of a patient's wound, the nurse identifies nursing diagnoses that direct supportive and preventive care. Multiple nursing diagnoses are associated with impaired skin integrity and wounds:

- Risk for infection
- Imbalanced nutrition: less than body requirements
- Acute or chronic pain
- Impaired physical mobility
- Impaired skin integrity
- Risk for impaired skin integrity
- Ineffective peripheral tissue perfusion
- Impaired tissue integrity

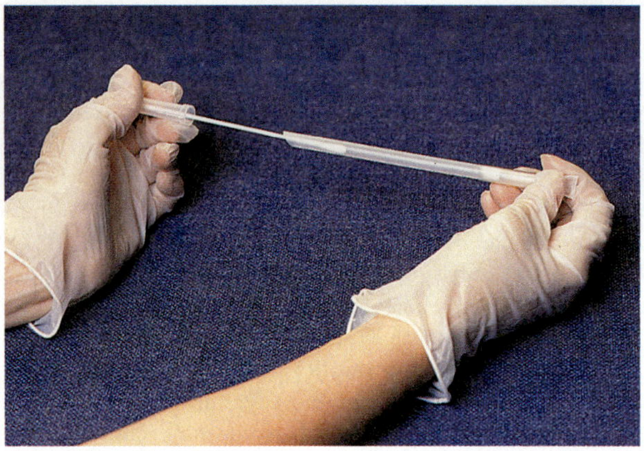

FIG. 48-12 Wound culturette tube.

BOX 48-7 RECOMMENDATIONS FOR STANDARDIZED TECHNIQUES FOR WOUND CULTURES*

Needle Aspiration Procedure

- Clean intact skin with a disinfectant solution. Allow to dry.
- Use a 10-mL disposable syringe with a 22-gauge needle, pulling 0.5 mL of air into the syringe.
- Insert the needle through intact skin next to the wound; withdraw plunger and apply suction to the 10-mL mark.
- Move the needle back and forward at different angles for two to four explorations.
- Remove the needle, expel the excess air, and cap and prepare the syringe for the laboratory (Stotts, 2012b).

Quantitative Swab Procedure

- Clean the wound surface with a nonantiseptic solution.
- Use a sterile swab from a culturette tube (Fig. 48-12).
- Moisten the swab with normal saline.
- Rotate the swab in 1 cm^2 (0.4 in^2) of clean tissue in the open wound. Apply pressure to the swab to elicit tissue fluid (Stotts, 2012b). Insert the tip of the swab into the appropriate sterile container, label, and transport to the laboratory.

Modified from Stotts NA: Wound infection: diagnosis and management. In Bryant RA, Nix DP, editors: *Acute and chronic wounds: current management concepts,* ed 4, St Louis, 2012, Mosby.

*Check agency policy to determine need to obtain health care provider order.

BOX 48-8 NURSING DIAGNOSTIC PROCESS

Impaired Skin Integrity Related to Infection

ASSESSMENT ACTIVITIES	DEFINING CHARACTERISTICS
Inspect surface of skin.	Presence of wound, break in skin integrity Yellow, foul-smelling drainage from wound Edges of wound red and warm, not approximated
Inspect wound for signs of healing.	Brown-red or beige drainage 5 days after surgery Edges of wound not approximated
Obtain patient's temperature, heart rate, white blood cell count, and serum albumin level	Patient febrile, heart rate 125 beats/min, leukocyte (white blood cell) count 12,000/mm^3, serum albumin less than 3.5 g/100 mL

Some patients are at risk for poor wound healing because of previously defined factors that impair healing. Thus, even though the patient's wound appears normal, the nurse identifies nursing diagnoses such as *impaired nutrition* or *ineffective peripheral tissue perfusion* that direct nursing care toward support of wound repair.

The nature of a wound can cause problems unrelated to wound healing. Alteration in comfort and impaired mobility are problems that have implications for the patient's eventual recovery. For example, a large abdominal incision causes enough pain to interfere with the patient's ability to turn in bed effectively.

PLANNING

After identifying nursing diagnoses, develop a plan of care for a patient who has actual or is at risk for *impaired skin integrity*. During planning synthesize information from multiple resources (Fig. 48-13). Critical thinking ensures that a patient's plan of care integrates all that you know about the individual and key critical thinking elements. Professional standards are especially important to consider when you develop a plan of care.

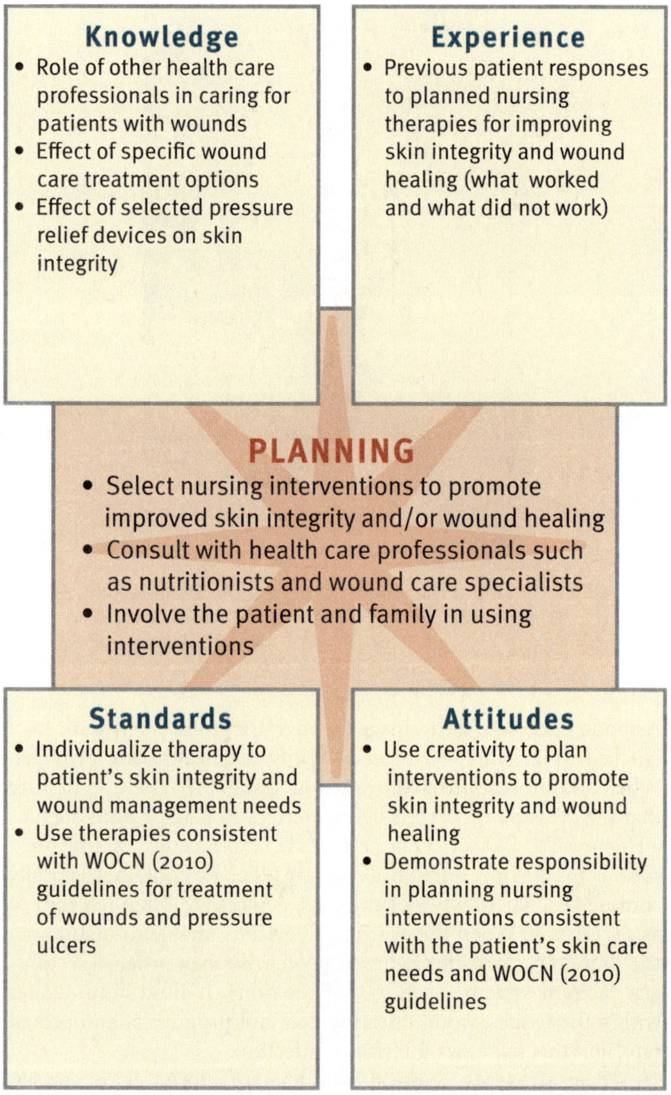
Knowledge
• Role of other health care professionals in caring for patients with wounds
• Effect of specific wound care treatment options
• Effect of selected pressure relief devices on skin integrity
Experience
• Previous patient responses to planned nursing therapies for improving skin integrity and wound healing (what worked and what did not work)
PLANNING
• Select nursing interventions to promote improved skin integrity and/or wound healing
• Consult with health care professionals such as nutritionists and wound care specialists
• Involve the patient and family in using interventions
Standards
• Individualize therapy to patient's skin integrity and wound management needs
• Use therapies consistent with WOCN (2010) guidelines for treatment of wounds and pressure ulcers
Attitudes
• Use creativity to plan interventions to promote skin integrity and wound healing
• Demonstrate responsibility in planning nursing interventions consistent with the patient's skin care needs and WOCN (2010) guidelines

FIG. 48-13 Critical thinking model for skin integrity and wound care planning. *WOCN,* Wound, Ostomy, and Continence Nurses Society.

Patients who have large, chronic wounds or infected wounds have multiple nursing care needs. A concept map helps to individualize care for a patient who has multiple health problems and related nursing diagnoses (Fig. 48-14). This map helps you use critical thinking skills to organize complex patient assessment data into related nursing diagnoses with the patient's chief medical diagnosis. As you identify linkages between the nursing diagnoses and the chief medical diagnosis, the concept map also links potential interventions that apply to the patient's health care needs.

Goals and Outcomes. Nursing care is based on a patient's identified needs and priorities. You establish goals and expected outcomes, and from the goals you plan interventions according to the risk for pressure ulcers or the type and severity of the wound and the presence of any complications such as infection, poor nutrition, peripheral vascular diseases, or immunosuppression that can affect wound healing (see the Nursing Care Plan). A goal frequently identified when working with a patient with a wound is to see wound improvement within a 2-week period. The outcomes of this goal can include the following:

- Higher percentage of granulation tissue in the wound base
- No further skin breakdown in any body location
- An increase in the caloric intake by 10%

These outcomes are reasonable if the overall goal for the patient is to heal the wound. Plan therapies according to the severity and type of wound and the presence of any complicating conditions (e.g.,

NURSING CARE PLAN

Impaired Skin Integrity

ASSESSMENT

Mrs. Stein, who is 76 years of age, is 7 days postoperative for a total hip replacement. She developed redness and oozing of foul-smelling tan-colored drainage from the hip incision on postoperative day 4. Significant medical history includes arthritis and mild hypertension. Because of surgical pain at the incision site, she did not easily transfer from her bed to the chair. Now on day 7 she notes some pain at the incision and complains of a painful, burning sensation in the sacral region. She is continent of urine and stool but continues to "scoot" over to the side of the bed when preparing for bed-to-chair transfers.

Assessment Activities	*Findings/Defining Characteristics**
Obtain an oral temperature.	Patient has **elevated temperature** and is diaphoretic.
Ask Mrs. Stein how the surgical site limits her mobility.	She relates that her hip always aches and the pain increases on movement. She tells you that she prefers to keep the hip immobile to keep the pain level down. Position of comfort is supine, and Mrs. Stein resists position changes.
Perform a total body skin assessment, paying special attention to the surgical incision and sacral area.	Open areas: sacrum and left hip incision.
Sacral area.	Patient has **reactive hyperemia** around the open sacral area; this **area does not blanch on palpation.** There is a **partial-thickness ulcer directly over the sacral area.**
Left hip, surgical incision.	**Small openings** between staples oozing tan foul-smelling fluid. Periwound area red and warm.

***Defining characteristics** are shown in bold type.

NURSING DIAGNOSIS: Impaired skin integrity related to pressure and friction on sacral bony prominence and infection of original wound

PLANNING

Goals	*Expected Outcomes (NOC)*†
	Tissue Integrity: Skin
Injury to Mrs. Stein's skin and underlying tissue resulting from pressure and friction on bony prominence will be reduced within 2 to 4 weeks.	Mrs. Stein will have intact skin integrity in the area of nonblanching erythema. Mrs. Stein's sacral ulcer will show signs of healing. Mrs. Stein will maintain intact skin over other pressure points.
Red area around hip wound and tan-colored drainage will be absent within 5 days.	Left hip wound demonstrates signs of healing.
	Immobility Consequences: Physiological
Mrs. Stein's ability to tolerate position changes and correctly change positions will improve within 2 to 4 weeks.	Reactive hyperemia will be within normal limits at all pressure points. Reactive hyperemia in sacral region will have a decrease in nonblanchable pressure areas.

†Outcome classification labels from Moorhead S et al: *Nursing outcomes classification (NOC),* ed 4, St Louis, 2008, Mosby.

Continued

NURSING CARE PLAN

Impaired Skin Integrity—cont'd

INTERVENTIONS (NIC)‡	RATIONALE
Pressure Management	
Reposition Mrs. Stein every 90 minutes. Offer pain medication as needed. When Mrs. Stein transfers from bed to chair, remind her not to slide over sheets but to pick up pelvis and relocate from one position to another. Be careful not to slide Mrs. Stein on sheets.	Repositioning removes pressure and allows normal hyperemic response. Frequency of turning is based on initial and ongoing assessment (Bryant and Nix, 2012). Sliding patient's skin on sheets causes friction and deteriorates involved area.
Elevate head of bed no more than 30 degrees.	The higher the head of the bed is elevated, the more likely it is that shearing forces are present, adding to pain and deterioration of the skin loss in the sacral area (WOCN, 2010).
Pressure Ulcer Care	
Keep skin dry and clean; avoid rubbing area.	Moisture softens skin and causes a break in skin integrity. Rubbing an area of nonblanching erythema causes further tissue damage (WOCN, 2010).
Use moisture barrier ointment over the ulcer at least 3 times a day to decrease friction and provide moisture to the open tissue.	An ointment covers the area, providing base of ulcer with moisture, which encourages healing. Ointment prevents sheets from rubbing on area, thus decreasing the friction.
Surgical Wound Care	
Irrigate wound with saline solution twice per day per wound care provider's order.	Cleans wound and surrounding area of wound debris and exudate.
Apply dressing (i.e., gauze moistened with antibiotic solution twice a day after irrigation) according to wound care provider's order.	Provides appropriate topical therapy to wound, placing wound in best environment for healing.
At frequent intervals evaluate patient's pain level and offer pain medication as indicated by assessment.	Provides patient with pain reduction/relief, allowing for greater mobility and comfort.

‡Intervention classification labels from Bulechek GM, Butcher HK, and Dochterman JM: *Nursing interventions classification (NIC),* ed 5, St Louis, 2008, Mosby.

EVALUATION

Nursing Actions	*Patient Response/Findings*	*Achievement of Outcome*
Perform daily total body skin and wound assessments. Chart results.	No new skin breakdown noted.	No other areas of pain or discomfort are reported.
	Decreased redness at the sacral area.	Decreased pain at sacral site is reported.
	Presence of reepithelialization in sacral area.	Ulcer in sacral area is healed.
	Reduction in hip wound, periwound redness, and amount of wound drainage.	Surgical incision is no longer open; no drainage and no periwound redness.
Palpate reddened area around sacrum.	Sacral area begins to show signs of normal reactive hyperemia blanching following palpation.	Sacral region is improving; no break in epidermis.
	Other pressure points have normal reactive hyperemia and blanching.	Other pressure points remain intact.

infection, poor nutrition, immunosuppression, and diabetes) that affect wound healing. Other goals of care for patients with wounds include the following: promoting wound hemostasis, preventing infection, promoting wound healing, maintaining skin integrity, gaining comfort, and promoting health.

Setting Priorities. You establish nursing care priorities in wound care based on the comprehensive patient assessment and goals and established outcomes. These priorities also depend on whether the patient's condition is stable or emergent. An acute wound needs immediate intervention; whereas in the presence of a chronic, stable wound the patient's hygiene is more important. When there is a risk for pressure ulcer development, preventive interventions such as skin care practices, elimination of shear, and positioning are high priorities. Promotion of wound healing is a major nursing priority; and the type of wound care administered depends on the type, size, and location of the wound and overall treatment goals.

Other patient factors to consider when establishing priorities include patient preferences, daily activities, and family factors. These factors are important regardless of the setting for health care. The priorities of care may not vary from outpatient, home, acute care, or restorative care settings.

Teamwork and Collaboration. With early discharge from health care settings, it is important to consider a patient's plan for discharge. Anticipating the patient's discharge wound care needs and related equipment and resources such as referral to a home care agency or outpatient wound care clinic helps to improve not only wound healing but also the patient's level of independence. Patients and their families often need to continue the objectives of wound management after discharge (Box 48-9). You need to consider the ability of the caregiver and the amount of time needed to change a particular dressing when selecting a dressing for the patient to use after discharge. For example, in the home setting some caregivers choose more expensive dressing materials

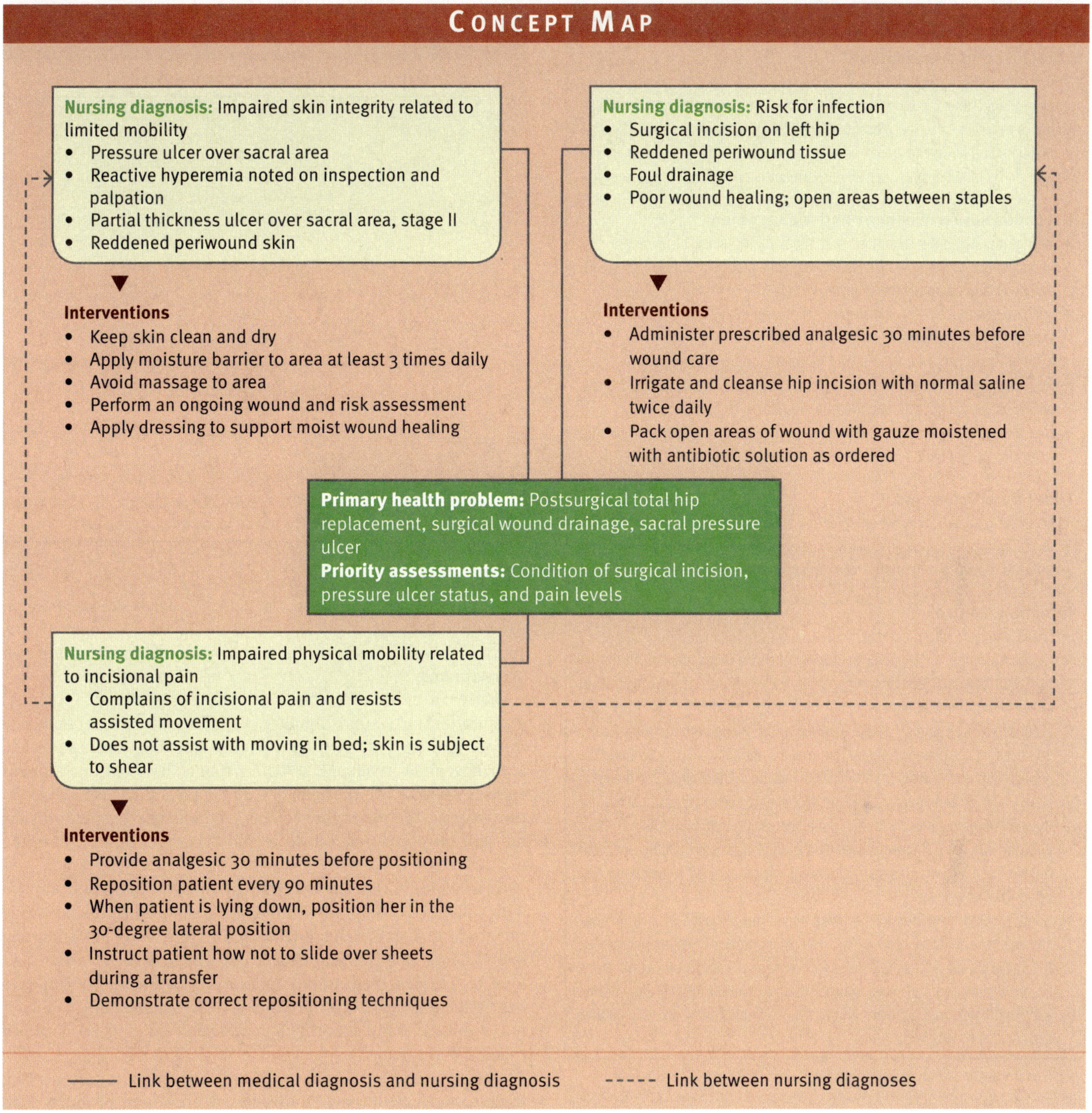
CONCEPT MAP
Nursing diagnosis: Impaired skin integrity related to limited mobility
• Pressure ulcer over sacral area
• Reactive hyperemia noted on inspection and palpation
• Partial thickness ulcer over sacral area, stage II
• Reddened periwound skin
Interventions
• Keep skin clean and dry
• Apply moisture barrier to area at least 3 times daily
• Avoid massage to area
• Perform an ongoing wound and risk assessment
• Apply dressing to support moist wound healing
Nursing diagnosis: Risk for infection
• Surgical incision on left hip
• Reddened periwound tissue
• Foul drainage
• Poor wound healing; open areas between staples
Interventions
• Administer prescribed analgesic 30 minutes before wound care
• Irrigate and cleanse hip incision with normal saline twice daily
• Pack open areas of wound with gauze moistened with antibiotic solution as ordered
Primary health problem: Postsurgical total hip replacement, surgical wound drainage, sacral pressure ulcer
Priority assessments: Condition of surgical incision, pressure ulcer status, and pain levels
Nursing diagnosis: Impaired physical mobility related to incisional pain
• Complains of incisional pain and resists assisted movement
• Does not assist with moving in bed; skin is subject to shear
Interventions
• Provide analgesic 30 minutes before positioning
• Reposition patient every 90 minutes
• When patient is lying down, position her in the 30-degree lateral position
• Instruct patient how not to slide over sheets during a transfer
• Demonstrate correct repositioning techniques
Link between medical diagnosis and nursing diagnosis
Link between nursing diagnoses

FIG. 48-14 Concept map for Mrs. Stein.

to reduce the frequency of dressing changes. The nurse and patient work together to establish ways of maintaining patient involvement in nursing care and promoting wound healing, whether the patient is in the hospital or home.

IMPLEMENTATION

Health Promotion. Perhaps the most effective intervention for problems with skin integrity and wound care is prevention. Prompt identification of high-risk patients and their risk factors helps to prevent pressure ulcers.

Prevention of Pressure Ulcers. When a patient is immobile, the major risk to the skin is the formation of pressure ulcers. Nursing interventions focus on prevention. The first step in prevention is to assess the patient's risk factors for pressure ulcer development (Table 48-6). Plan on reducing or eliminating the identified risk factors.

Early identification of patients at risk and their risk factors helps you prevent pressure ulcers. Prevention minimizes the impact that risk factors or contributing factors have on pressure ulcer development. Three major areas of nursing interventions for prevention of pressure ulcers are: (1) skin care and management of

BOX 48-9 HOME CARE RECOMMENDATIONS

Ulcer/Wound Assessment

Assessment and documentation of a pressure ulcer need to occur at least weekly, unless there is evidence of deterioration, in which case the nurse needs to reassess both the pressure ulcer and the patient's overall management immediately. In the home setting this requires the assistance of the patient and family because weekly assessment is not always feasible.

Psychosocial Assessment and Management

- Assess the patient's resources (e.g., availability and skill of caregivers, finances, equipment). A successful treatment program requires adequate caregiver and equipment resources.
- Evaluate caregivers for their ability to comprehend and implement the treatment requirements.
- Evaluate caregivers for their level of strength and endurance.
- Consider economic factors because they often limit the supply and availability of equipment and opportunities to relieve caregivers.
- Use an approach that focuses on the psychosocial and physical factors affecting wound care

Ulcer Care Dressings

- Consider caregiver time when selecting a dressing.
- In the home setting some caregivers choose dressing materials manufactured to reduce the frequency of dressing changes.

Infection Control

- Clean dressings are most commonly used in the home setting.
- Clean dressings, as opposed to sterile ones, are recommended for home use until research demonstrates otherwise. This recommendation is in keeping with principles regarding nosocomial infections and with past success of clean urinary catheterization in the home setting, and it takes into account the expense of sterile dressings and the dexterity required for application. The caregiver can use the "no-touch" technique for dressing changes. This technique is a method of changing surface dressings without touching the wound or the surface of any dressing that might be in contact with the wound. Adherent dressings should be grasped by the corner and removed slowly, whereas gauze dressings can be pinched in the center and lifted off.
- Contaminated dressings in the home should be disposed of in a manner consistent with local regulations. The Environmental Protection Agency recommends placing soiled dressings in securely fastened plastic bags before adding them to other household trash. However, local regulations vary, and home care agencies and patients need to follow procedures that are consistent with local laws.

Modified from Agency for Health Care Policy and Research, Panel for the Treatment of Pressure Ulcers in Adults: *Treatment of pressure ulcers,* Clinical Practice Guideline No. 15, AHCPR Pub No. 95-0653, Rockville, Md, 1994, Agency for Health Care Policy and Research, Public Health Service, US Department of Health and Human Services.

TABLE 48-6 A Quick Guide to Pressure Ulcer Prevention

RISK FACTOR	NURSING INTERVENTIONS
Decreased sensory perception	Assess pressure points for signs of nonblanching reactive hyperemia. Provide pressure-redistribution surface.
Moisture	Assess need for incontinence management. Following each incontinent episode, clean area with no-rinse perineal cleaner and protect skin with moisture-barrier ointment.
Friction and shear	Reposition patient using drawsheet and lifting off surface. Provide trapeze to facilitate movement. Position patient at a 30-degree lateral turn and limit head elevation to 30 degrees.
Decreased activity/ mobility	Establish and post individualized turning schedule.
Poor nutrition	Provide adequate nutritional and fluid intake; assist with intake as necessary. Consult dietitian for nutritional evaluation.

incontinence; (2) mechanical loading and support devices, which include proper positioning and the use of therapeutic surfaces; and (3) education (WOCN, 2010).

Topical Skin Care and Incontinence Management. You need to perform frequent skin assessment (see Box 48-5) at a minimum on a once-a-day basis. However, high-risk patients have more frequent skin assessments such as every shift. In addition, ensure that the patient's skin is clean and dry.

When you clean the skin, avoid soap and hot water. Use cleaners with nonionic surfactants that are gentle to the skin (WOCN, 2010). Many types of products are available for skin care, and you need to match their use to the specific needs of the patient. After you clean the skin and make sure that it is completely dry, apply moisturizer to keep the epidermis well lubricated but not oversaturated.

Make an effort to control, contain, or correct incontinence, perspiration, or wound drainage. Patients who have fecal incontinence and who are also receiving enteral tube feeding provide a management challenge. When patients have an incontinent episode, gently clean the area, dry, and apply a thick layer of moisture barrier to the exposed areas. A moisture barrier protects the skin from excessive moisture and bacteria found in the urine or stool.

It is helpful to use the expertise of an advanced practice nurse with a focus on wound care or management of incontinence while caring for at-risk patients. Methods for controlling or containing incontinence vary. You can treat urinary incontinence with behavioral techniques, medication, and surgery. Behavioral techniques help patients learn ways to control their bladder and sphincter muscles. Two examples are bladder and habit training, which is also called *timed voiding*.

Consider using absorbent pads and garments only after trying these measures. Although controversial, absorbent products such as absorptive underpads and garments are sometimes part of the treatment plan for an incontinent patient. Use only products that wick moisture away from the patient's skin (WOCN, 2010).

Positioning. Positioning interventions reduce pressure and **shearing force** to the skin. Elevating the head of the bed to 30 degrees or less decreases the chance of pressure ulcer development from shearing forces (WOCN, 2010). Change the immobilized patient's position according to activity level, perceptual ability, and daily routines (Brienza et al., 2008). A standard turning interval of 1½ to 2 hours does not always prevent pressure ulcer development. Patients need repositioning on a schedule of at least every 2 hours if allowed by their overall condition. When repositioning, use positioning devices to protect bony prominences (WOCN, 2010). The WOCN guidelines (2010) recommend a 30-degree lateral position (Fig. 48-15), which should prevent positioning directly over the

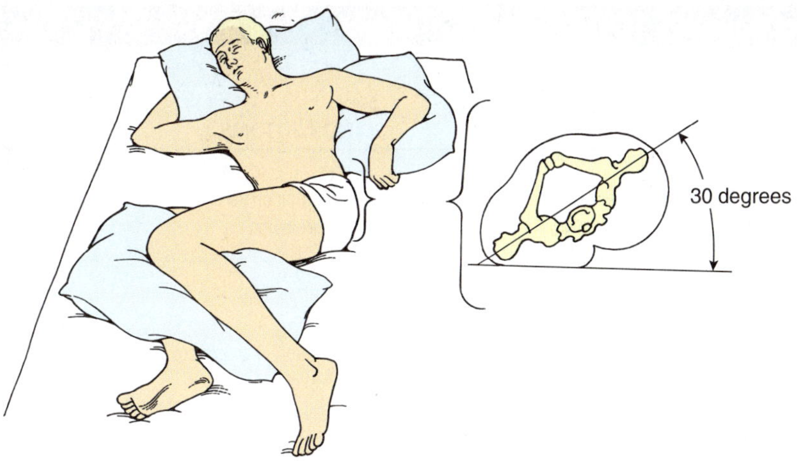

FIG. 48-15 Thirty-degree lateral position at which pressure points are avoided. (Adapted from Bryant RA, Nix DP, editors: *Acute and chronic wounds: current management concepts,* ed 4, St Louis, 2012, Mosby.)

Building Competency in Safety Ms. Willet, a 79-year-old Indian woman, is approximately 300 lb and her height is 5′1″. She has recently undergone a left knee replacement and has an immobilizer on her left knee. The immobilizer makes it difficult for her to assist in movement. There is an order to reposition her every 2 hours as her condition warrants. She is unable to effectively assist in repositioning. What should your considerations be in planning her repositioning schedule?

Answers to questions can be found on the Evolve website.

bony prominence. To prevent shear and friction injuries, use a transfer device to lift rather than drag the patient when changing positions (see Chapter 47).

Some patients are able to sit in a chair. Make sure to limit the total amount of time they sit to 2 hours or less. In the sitting position the pressure on the ischial tuberosities is greater than in the supine position. In addition, teach a mobile patient at risk for skin breakdown in a sitting position to shift weight every 15 minutes (WOCN, 2010). Shifting weight provides short-term relief on the ischial tuberosities. Also have him or her sit on foam, gel, or an air cushion to redistribute weight away from the ischial areas. Rigid and donut-shaped cushions are contraindicated because they reduce blood supply to the area, resulting in wider areas of ischemia (WOCN, 2010).

After repositioning the patient, reassess the skin. Identifying characteristics that indicate early signs of tissue ischemia in darkly pigmented skin are in Boxes 48-2 and 48-3. For patients with light-toned skin, observe for **normal reactive hyperemia** and blanching. Never massage the reddened areas. Massaging reddened areas increases breaks in the capillaries in the underlying tissues and the risk of injury to underlying tissue and pressure ulcer formation (WOCN, 2010).

Support Surfaces (Therapeutic Beds and Mattresses). A support surface is a specialized device for pressure redistribution designed for management of tissue loads, microclimate, and/or other therapeutic functions (i.e., mattresses, integrated bed system, mattress replacement, overlay or seat cushion, or seat cushion overlay) (EPUAP and NPUAP, 2009). A variety of support surfaces, including specialty v and mattresses, reduce the hazards of immobility to the skin and musculoskeletal system. However, none eliminates the need for meticulous nursing care. No single device eliminates the effects of pressure on the skin.

When selecting support surfaces, incorporate the patient's needs. Knowledge about support surface characteristics (Table 48-7) assists you in clinical decision making. In selecting a support surface, know the patient's risks and the purpose for the support surface; a flow chart is often helpful (Fig. 48-16). Teach patients and families the reason for and proper use of the beds or mattresses (Box 48-10). Some common errors with support surfaces are placing the wrong side of the support surface toward the patient, not plugging powered support surfaces into the electrical source,

BOX 48-10 PATIENT TEACHING

Pressure-Redistribution Surfaces

Objective

- Patient and family will describe understanding of the purposes and basic operations of the pressure-redistribution surface.

Teaching Strategies

- Explain the reasons for the pressure-redistribution surface.
- Explain proper body mechanics while using the pressure-redistribution surface.
- Educate in the use and care of the pressure-redistribution surface (WOCN, 2010).
- Explain additional pressure-redistribution measures.

Evaluation

- Patient and family will state basic purposes for the pressure-redistribution surface.
- Patient and family will be able to describe the function of the pressure-redistribution surface.
- Patient and family will be able to demonstrate proper use of the pressure-redistribution surface.

TABLE 48-7 Support Surfaces

CATEGORIES AND DEFINITIONS	MECHANISM OF ACTION	INDICATIONS	EXAMPLES OF MANUFACTURERS' AND PRODUCT NAMES
Low-Air-Loss			
Available as a mattress placed directly on the existing bed frame or an overlay placed directly on top of an existing surface	Pressure redistribution Provides a flow of air to assist in managing the heat and humidity of the skin	Prevention or treatment of skin breakdown	Hill Rom/Flexicair Eclipse, Kinetic Concepts, Inc/First Step Select The ROHO Group/Select Air Mattress
Nonpowered			
Any support surface not requiring or using external sources of energy for operation *Examples:* Foam, interconnected air-filled cells	Pressure redistribution Air moves to and from cells as body position changes	Prevention or treatment of skin breakdown	ROHO/ Dry Flotation Mattress, Gaymar Industries/Sof-Care
Air-Fluidized Beds			
Surfaces that change load distribution properties when powered and when patient is in contact with the surface	Provides pressure redistribution via a fluidlike medium created by forcing air through beads as characterized by immersion and envelopment	Prevention or treatment of skin breakdown May also be used to protect newly flapped or grafted surgical sites and for patients with excessive moisture	Kinetic Concepts, Inc/FluidAir Elite, Hill Rom/Clinitron
Lateral Rotation			
Provides passive motion to promote mobilization of respiratory secretions and provides low-air-loss therapy	A feature of a support surface that provides rotation about a longitudinal axis as characterized by degree of patient turn, duration, and frequency	Treatment and prevention of pulmonary complications associated with immobility	Hill Rom/V-Cue Dynamic Air Therapy, Kinetic Concepts, Inc/ TriaDyne

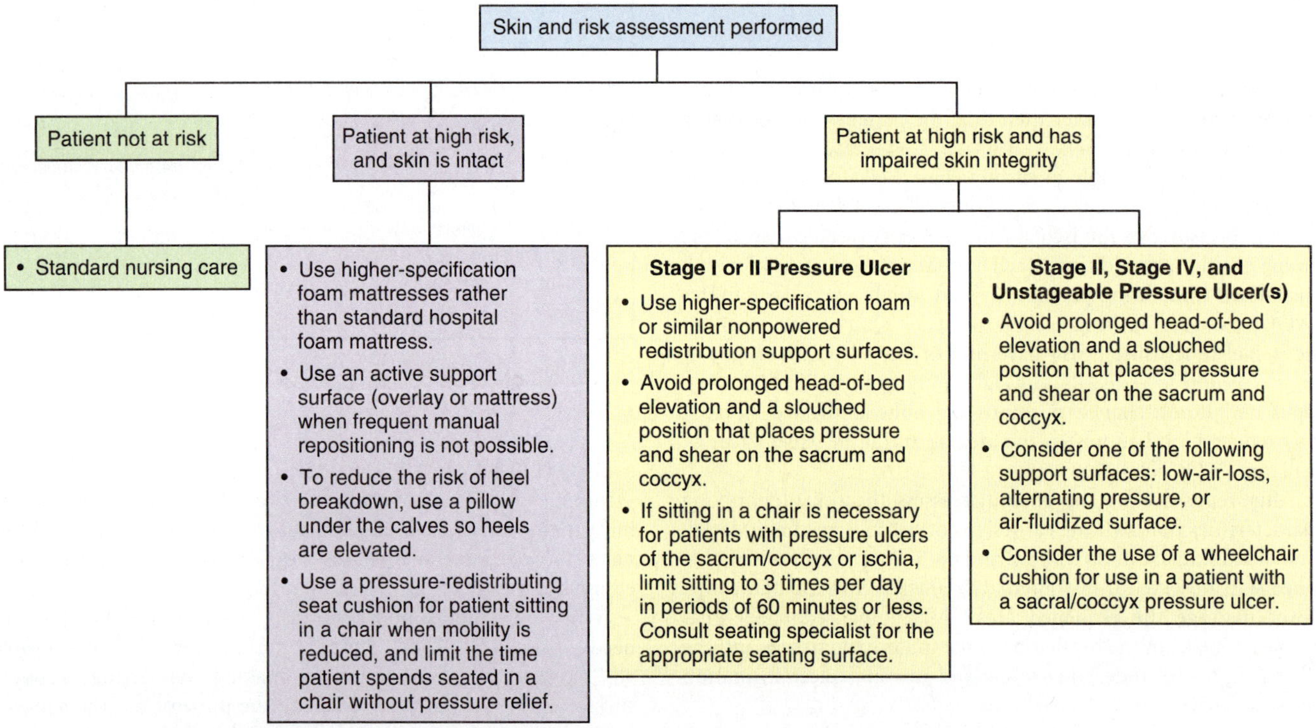

FIG. 48-16 Considerations for choosing the appropriate support surface. (Modified from WOCN: *Guideline for prevention and management of pressure ulcers,* 2010, Mt Laurel, NJ; and National Pressure Ulcer Advisory Panel (NPUAP) and European Pressure Ulcer Advisory Panel (EPUAP): *International guideline for prevention and treatment of pressure ulcers,* Washington DC, 2009, National Pressure Ulcer Advisory Panel.)

not turning on the power source for powered support surfaces, failing to place hand between the metal bed frame and the mattress to determine if patient sinks to the point of touching the bed frame for some support surfaces, and improperly inflating some support surfaces. When used correctly, these support services help reduce pressure ulcers in patients at risk.

Acute Care

Management of Pressure Ulcers. Treatment of patients with pressure ulcers requires a holistic approach that uses the expertise of several multidisciplinary health care professionals (WOCN, 2010). In addition to the nurse, the health care provider, the wound care nurse specialist, physical therapist, occupational therapist, nutritionist, and pharmacist are involved. Aspects of pressure ulcer treatment include local care of the wound and supportive measures such as adequate nutrients and redistribution of pressure (Skill 48-2 on pp. 1215-1217).

When treating a pressure ulcer, reassess the wound for location, stage, size, tissue type and amount, exudate, and surrounding skin condition (Nix, 2012). Acute wounds require close monitoring (every 8 hours). Sometimes chronic wound assessment occurs less frequently. Depending on the topical management system, evaluate the wound with every dressing change, usually not more than 1 time per day.

The use and documentation of a systematic approach to monitor progress of an actual pressure ulcer leads to better decision making and optimum outcomes (Nix, 2012). Several healing and documentation tools are available to document wound assessments over time. Using a tool helps link assessment to outcomes so an evaluation of the plan of care follows objective criteria (Nix, 2012). For example, the Bates-Jensen Wound Assessment Tool (Harris et al., 2010) addresses 15 wound characteristics. You score individual items and calculate the sum total, providing an overall indication of wound status. The scoring assists in evaluating whether the goals of the wound management are effective.

Wound Management. Maintenance of a physiological local wound environment is the goal of effective wound management (Rolstad, Bryant, and Nix, 2012). To maintain a healthy wound environment, you need to address the following principles: prevent and manage infection, clean the wound, remove nonviable tissue, manage exudate, maintain the wound in a moist environment, and protect the wound.

A wound does not move through the phases of healing if it is infected. Preventing wound infection includes cleaning and removing nonviable tissue. Clean pressure ulcers only with noncytotoxic wound cleaners such as normal saline or commercial wound cleaners. Noncytotoxic cleaners do not damage or kill fibroblasts and healing tissue (Rolstad, Bryant, and Nix, 2012). Some commonly used cytotoxic solutions are Dakin's solution (sodium hypochlorite solution), acetic acid, povidone-iodine, and hydrogen peroxide. These **are not** used in clean, granulating wounds.

Irrigation is a common method of delivering a wound-cleaning solution to the wound. Studies have shown that there is an optimal effective range of irrigation pressures that ensures adequate removal of bacteria (Gardner and Frantz, 2008). One method to ensure an irrigation pressure within the correct range is to use a 19-gauge needle or an angiocatheter and a 35-mL syringe that delivers saline to a pressure ulcer at 8 psi (Fig. 48-17).

Debridement is the removal of nonviable, necrotic tissue. Removal of necrotic tissue is necessary to rid the wound of a source of infection, enable visualization of the wound bed, and provide a clean base necessary for healing.

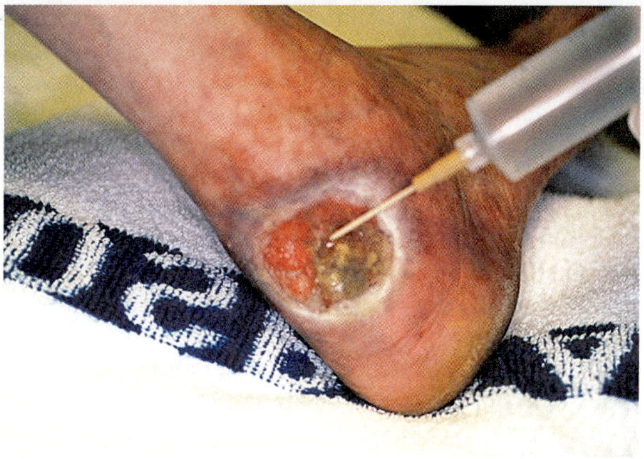

FIG. 48-17 Wound irrigation.

The method of debridement depends on which is most appropriate to the patient's condition and care goals (WOCN, 2010). It is important to remember that during the debridement process some normal wound observations to make include an increase in wound exudate, odor, and size. You need to assess and prevent or effectively manage pain that occurs with debridement (WOCN, 2010).

Methods of debridement include mechanical, autolytic, chemical, and sharp/surgical. One method of mechanical debridement is the use of wet-to-dry saline gauze dressings. Place moistened gauze into the wound and allow the dressing to dry thoroughly before "pulling" the gauze that has adhered to the tissue out of the pressure ulcer. This is a nonselective method of debridement because devitalized and viable tissues are both removed; thus it is not used routinely. Never use this method in a clean, granulating wound. Other methods of mechanical debridement are wound irrigation (high-pressure irrigation and pulsatile high-pressure lavage) and whirlpool treatments (Ramundo, 2012).

Autolytic debridement uses synthetic dressings over a wound to allow the eschar to be self-digested by the action of enzymes that are present in wound fluids. You accomplish this by using dressings that support moisture at the wound surface. If the wound base is dry, use a dressing that adds moisture; if there is excessive exudate, use a dressing that absorbs the excessive moisture while maintaining moisture at the wound bed. Some examples of these dressings are transparent film and hydrocolloid dressings.

You can accomplish chemical debridement with the use of a topical enzyme preparation, Dakin's solution, or sterile maggots. Topical enzymes induce changes in the substrate resulting in the breakdown of necrotic tissue (Ramundo, 2012). Depending on the type of enzyme used, the preparation either digests or dissolves the tissue. These preparations require a health care provider's order. Dakin's solution breaks down and loosens dead tissue in a wound. Apply the solution to gauze and apply to the wound. Sterile maggots are used in a wound because it is thought that they ingest the dead tissue.

Surgical debridement is the removal of devitalized tissue by using a scalpel, scissors, or other sharp instrument. Health care providers and in some states trained advanced practice nurses perform surgical debridement of an ulcer or wound. Nurses should check the Nurse Practice Act for their state to see if surgical debridement is a nursing function. It is the quickest method of debridement. It is usually indicated when the patient has signs of cellulitis or sepsis.

A moist environment supports the movement of epithelial cells and facilitates wound closure. A wound that has excessive exudate (drainage) provides an environment that supports bacterial growth, macerates the periwound skin, and slows the healing process. If excessive wound exudate is present, evaluate the volume, consistency, and odor of the drainage to determine if signs and symptoms of infection are present.

Remember, the wound will not heal unless the contributory factors are controlled or eliminated. Therefore it is critically important for you to address the causative factors (e.g., shear, friction, pressure, and moisture), or it is unlikely that the wound will heal despite topical therapy (Rolstad, Bryant, and Nix, 2012).

The treatment plan needs to be altered as a wound heals. For example, a transparent film dressing is used initially to autolytically debride (liquefy the tissue using body moisture) a necrotic wound. Once the wound is cleaned of necrotic tissue, discontinue the transparent film dressing; and, based on the wound base characteristics, choose a new dressing. A wound with excessive drainage requires a dressing with a high absorptive capacity. Continued reassessment is key to supporting the wound as it moves through the phases of wound healing.

Education. Education of the patient and caregivers is an important nursing function (Rolstad, Bryant, and Nix, 2012). A variety of educational tools, including videotapes and written materials, are available for you to use when teaching patients and caregivers/family to prevent and treat pressure ulcers and care for wounds. The Agency for Health Care Policy and Research (AHCPR, 1992a, 1994) has booklets on pressure ulcer prevention and treatment that are helpful when teaching patients and their caregivers/family. They are available in English and Spanish. Individualize your teaching for each patient, especially older patients.

Understanding and assessing the experience of the patient and support person are also important dimensions in the treatment of people with pressure ulcers (WOCN, 2010). Clinicians are only just now exploring through research the caregiver's perspective of the concerns and issues faced by frail older spouses caring for their loved ones with pressure ulcers. You need to plan interventions to meet the identified psychosocial needs of patients and their support persons (WOCN, 2010).

Nutritional Status. Nutritional assessment and support of the patient with a wound is based on the appreciation that nutrition is fundamental to normal cellular integrity and tissue repair (Stotts, 2012a). Early intervention is necessary to correct inadequate nutrition and support healing. The Joint Commission (2008) recommends nutritional assessment within 24 hours of admission. Reassessments reflect changes in status and effects of interventions (Stotts, 2012a). Box 48-11 defines parameters for clinically significant malnutrition (AHCPR, 1994). Assess the patient's mouth and skin for signs of nutritional deficiencies (see Chapter 44). Give vitamin and mineral supplements if you suspect or know of any deficiencies.

Protein Status. Patients with pressure ulcers who are underweight or losing weight need enhanced caloric and protein supplementation (WOCN, 2010). A patient can lose as much as 50 g of protein per day from an open, weeping pressure ulcer. Although the recommended intake of protein for adults is 0.8 g/kg/day, a higher intake of protein up to 1.8 g/kg/day is necessary for healing. Increased protein intake helps rebuild epidermal tissue. Increased caloric intake helps replace subcutaneous tissue. Vitamin C promotes collagen synthesis, capillary wall integrity, fibroblast function, and immunological function.

Hemoglobin. A low hemoglobin level decreases delivery of oxygen to the tissues and leads to further ischemia. When possible, maintain hemoglobin at 12 g/100 mL.

BOX 48-11 RECOMMENDATIONS FOR NUTRITIONAL ASSESSMENT AND MANAGEMENT OF PRESSURE ULCERS

Assessment of Clinically Significant Malnutrition

- Screen and assess the nutritional status of the patient with a pressure ulcer on admission and with each condition change.
- Assess weight status to determine weight history and significant loss from usual weight (≥5% change in 30 days or ≥10% in 180 days).

Interventions

- Refer patients with pressure ulcers to the dietitian for early intervention for nutritional problems.
- Provide 30-35 calories/kg body weight for individuals under stress with a pressure ulcer.
- Consider nutritional support when oral intake is inadequate.
- Encourage consumption of a balanced diet that includes good sources of vitamins and minerals.

Modified from European Pressure Ulcer Advisory Panel and National Pressure Ulcer Advisory Panel: *Treatment of pressure ulcers: quick reference guide*, Washington, DC, 2009, National Pressure Ulcer Advisory Panel.

First Aid for Wounds. In an emergency setting use first aid measures for wound care. Under stable conditions a variety of interventions ensure wound healing. When a patient suffers a traumatic wound, first aid interventions include stabilizing cardiopulmonary function (see Chapter 40), promoting hemostasis, cleaning the wound, and protecting it from further injury.

Hemostasis. After assessing the type and extent of the wound, control bleeding by applying direct pressure on it with a sterile or clean dressing such as a washcloth. After bleeding subsides, an adhesive bandage or gauze dressing taped over the laceration allows skin edges to close and a blood clot to form. If a dressing becomes saturated with blood, add another layer of dressing, continue to apply pressure, and elevate the affected part. Avoid further disruption of skin layers. Serious lacerations need to be sutured by a health care provider. Pressure dressings used during the first 24 to 48 hours after trauma help maintain hemostasis.

Normally allow a puncture wound to bleed to remove dirt and other contaminants such as saliva from a dog bite. When a penetrating object such as a knife blade is present, *do not remove the object.* The presence of the object provides pressure and controls some bleeding. Removal causes massive, uncontrolled bleeding. Except for skull injuries, apply pressure around the penetrating object but not on it and transport the patient to an emergency facility.

Cleaning. The process of cleaning a wound involves selecting an appropriate cleaning solution and using a mechanical means of delivering that solution without causing injury to the healing wound tissue (WOCN, 2010). Gently cleaning a wound removes contaminants that serve as sources of infection. However, vigorous cleaning using a method with too much mechanical force causes bleeding or further injury. For abrasions, minor lacerations, and small puncture wounds, first rinse the wound with normal saline and lightly cover the area with a dressing. When a laceration is bleeding profusely, only brush away surface contaminants and concentrate on hemostasis until the patient can be cared for in a clinic or hospital.

According to the WOCN guidelines (2010), normal saline is the preferred cleaning agent. It is physiologically neutral and does not harm tissue. Gentle cleaning with normal saline and the application of moist saline dressings are often used in healing wounds. Use saline to maintain the moist surface needed to promote the development and migration of epithelial tissue. Wet-to-dry saline dressings are only for debriding wounds. Never use them in a clean, granulating wound.

Protection. Regardless of whether bleeding has stopped, protect a wound from further injury by applying sterile or clean dressings and immobilizing the body part. A light dressing applied over minor wounds prevents entrance of microorganisms.

Dressings. The more extensive the wound, the larger the dressing required. In the home a clean towel or diaper is often the best secondary dressing. A bulky dressing applied with pressure minimizes movement of underlying tissues and helps immobilize the entire body part. A bandage or cloth wrapped around a penetrating object should immobilize it adequately.

Alternative dressings are available to cover and protect certain types of wounds such as large wounds, wounds with drainage tubes or suction catheters in the wound, and wounds that need frequent changing because of excessive drainage. Pouches or special wound collection systems cover these wounds and collect their drainage. Some of these devices have a plastic door on the front of the wound pouch, allowing you to change the packing without removing the pouch from the skin.

The use of dressings requires an understanding of wound healing. A variety of dressing materials are commercially available. The correct dressing selection facilitates wound healing (Rolstad, Bryant, and Nix, 2012). The dressing type depends on the assessment of the wound and the phase of wound healing. When you identify the objectives for the wound care, the dressing choice becomes clear. A wound that requires infection management requires a different set of dressings than one requiring the removal of nonviable tissue.

For surgical wounds that heal by primary intention, it is common to remove dressings as soon as drainage stops. In contrast, when dressing a wound healing by secondary intention, the dressing material becomes a means for providing moisture to the wound or assisting in debridement.

Purposes of Dressings. A dressing serves several purposes:

- Protects a wound from microorganism contamination
- Aids in hemostasis
- Promotes healing by absorbing drainage and debriding a wound
- Supports or splints the wound site
- Protects patients from seeing the wound (if perceived as unpleasant)
- Promotes thermal insulation of the wound surface
- Provides a moist environment

When the skin is broken, a dressing helps reduce exposure to microorganisms. However, when drainage is minimal, the healing process forms a natural fibrin seal that eliminates the need for a dressing. Wounds with extensive tissue loss always need a dressing.

Pressure dressings promote hemostasis. Applied with elastic bandages, a pressure dressing exerts localized downward pressure over an actual or potential bleeding site. A pressure dressing eliminates dead space in underlying tissues so wound healing progresses normally. Check pressure dressings to be sure that they do not interfere with circulation to a body part. Assess skin color, pulses in distal extremities, the patient's comfort, and changes in sensation. Pressure dressings are not removed routinely.

A primary function of a dressing on a healing wound is to absorb drainage. Most surgical gauze dressings have three layers: a contact or primary layer, an absorbent layer, and an outer protective or secondary layer. The contact dressing covers the incision and part of the adjacent skin. Fibrin, blood products, and debris adhere to its surface. A problem occurs if the wound drainage dries, causing the dressing to stick to the suture line. Improperly removing the dressing causes disruption of the healing epidermal surface. If the dressing is sticking to the surgical incision, lightly moisten it with saline solution. This causes the dressing to become saturated, loosening it from the incisional area and preventing trauma to the incisional area during removal.

The dressing technique varies, depending on the goal of the treatment plan for the wound. For example, if the goal is to maintain a moist environment for a clean granulating wound, it is important to not let the saline-moistened gauze dressing dry and stick to it. This is in direct contrast to the dressing technique that you use if the goal of care is to mechanically debride the wound using a saline wet-to-dry dressing. When wounds such as a necrotic wound require debriding, use a wet-to-dry dressing technique. Place the moist dressing (contact dressing) into the wound and allow it to dry. The contact dressing debrides necrotic tissue and debris. In this case the contact dressing is allowed to dry so it sticks to underlying tissue, and debridement occurs during removal.

Dressings applied to a draining wound require frequent changing to prevent microorganism growth and skin breakdown. Bacteria grow readily in the dark, warm, moist environment under a dressing. Skin surfaces become macerated and irritated. Minimize periwound skin breakdown by keeping the skin clean and dry and reducing the use of tape.

The absorbent dressing layer serves as a reservoir for additional secretions. The wicking action of woven gauze dressings pulls excess drainage into the dressing and away from the wound. The final outer layer of a dressing helps prevent bacteria and other external contaminants from reaching the wound surface. Usually the outer dressing is made of a thicker dressing material. Apply adhesives to this layer to secure the dressings.

A dressing needs to support a moist wound environment if the wound is healing by secondary intention. A moist wound base facilitates the movement of epithelialization, thus allowing the wound to resurface as quickly as possible.

Types of Dressings. Dressings vary by type of material and mode of application (wet or dry) (Skill 48-3 on pp. 1218-1221). They need to be easy to apply, comfortable, and made of materials that promote wound healing. The WOCN guidelines (2010) are helpful when selecting dressings based on the goal of wound treatment (Box 48-12). To avoid causing damage to the periwound skin, it is important that the dressing technique that you use to treat pressure ulcers and other wounds is not excessively moist (Box 48-13).

Most pressure ulcers require dressings. The type of dressing is usually based on the stage of the pressure ulcer, the type of tissue in the wound, and the function of the dressing (Table 48-8). Before placing a dressing on a pressure ulcer, it is important to know the stage of the pressure ulcer; have done a thorough assessment of it; and understand the goal of the treatment, the mechanism of action of the dressing, and principles of wound care.

Gauze sponges are the oldest and most common dressing. They are absorbent and are especially useful in wounds to wick away the wound exudate. Gauze is available in different textures and various lengths and sizes; the 4×4 is the most common size. Gauze can be saturated with solutions and used to clean and pack a wound. When used to pack a wound, the gauze is saturated with the solution (usually normal saline), wrung out, unfolded, and lightly packed into the wound. The purpose of this type of dressing is to

BOX 48-12 DRESSING CONSIDERATIONS

- Clean the wound and periwound area at each dressing change, minimizing trauma to the wound (WOCN, 2010).
- Use a dressing that continuously provides a moist environment.
- Perform wound care using topical dressings as determined by a thorough assessment. No specific studies have proven an optimal dressing type for pressure ulcers (WOCN, 2010).
- Choose a dressing that keeps the surrounding intact (periulcer) skin dry while keeping the ulcer bed moist.
- Choose a dressing that controls exudate but does not desiccate the ulcer bed.
- The type of dressing may change over time as the pressure ulcer heals or deteriorates. The wound should be monitored at every dressing change and regularly assessed to determine whether modifications in the dressing type are needed (WOCN, 2010).
- Consider caregiver time, ease of use, availability, and cost when selecting a dressing.

BOX 48-13 EVIDENCE-BASED PRACTICE

Moisture-Associated Skin Damage

PICO Question: Which interventions can be used to prevent moisture-associated skin damage that can occur around a wound in a patient?

Evidence Summary

Appropriate wound management to support healing is critical for patients with pressure ulcers and other chronic wounds. Advances in wound healing document the benefit of a moist wound environment and the accepted practice of moist wound healing. But when moisture is present in excess and allowed to sit on the periwound skin, it leads to damaging maceration (Woo, Ayello, and Sibald, 2009). Maceration is defined as a softening of tissues by soaking until connective fibers can be teased apart (Gray and Weir, 2007). This condition is classified as moisture-associated skin damage. Interventions that focus on preventive steps include use of a dressing that absorbs excessive moisture while maintaining a moist wound bed (Gray and Weir, 2007), selection of the right dressing and size to absorb the wound exudate, the appropriate frequency of dressing change (Woo, Ayello, and Sibald, 2009), and use of a skin protectant to the periwound skin.

Application to Nursing Practice

- Use of a skin protectant (no-sting film barrier, petrolatum-based or zinc-based protectant) helps to prevent periwound skin maceration.
- Dressing selection needs to be individualized to the type of wound and wound-healing goals.
- Frequency of dressing change should not exceed manufacturer-recommended "wear time" (Woo, Ayello, and Sibald, 2009).
- Assess the effectiveness of the absorbent capacity of the dressing and make changes based on the amount of wound drainage.

provide moisture to the wound yet to allow wound drainage to be wicked into the gauze pad. Unfolding the dressing allows easier wicking action.

Use nonadherent gauze dressings such as Telfa over clean wounds with little or no drainage. Telfa gauze has a shiny, nonadherent surface that does not stick to incisions or wound openings but allows drainage to pass through to the gauze topper.

Another type of dressing is a self-adhesive, transparent film. This type of dressing traps moisture over the wound, providing a moist environment (Fig. 48-18). The transparent film dressing is ideal for small superficial wounds such as partial-thickness wounds or to protect high-risk skin. Use a film dressing as a secondary dressing and for autolytic debridement of small wounds. It has the following advantages:

- Adheres to undamaged skin
- Serves as a barrier to external fluids and bacteria but still allows the wound surface to "breathe" because oxygen passes through the transparent dressing
- Promotes a moist environment that speeds epithelial cell growth
- Can be removed without damaging underlying tissues
- Permits viewing a wound
- Does not require a secondary dressing

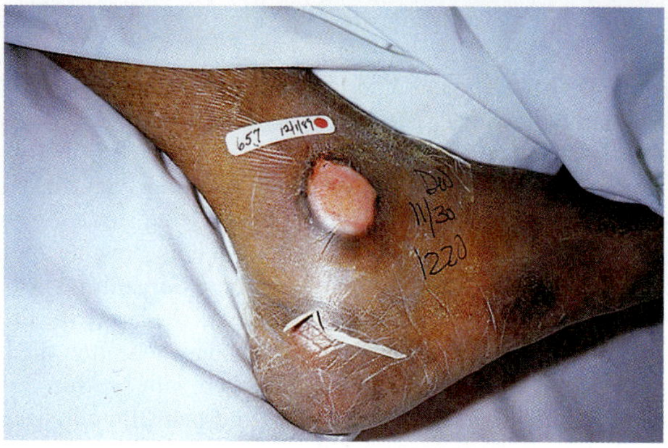

FIG. 48-18 Transparent film dressing.

Hydrocolloid dressings are dressings with complex formulations of colloids, elastomeric, and adhesive components. They are adhesive and occlusive. The wound contact layer of this dressing forms a gel as fluid is absorbed and maintains a moist healing environment. Hydrocolloids support healing in clean granulating wounds and autolytically debride necrotic wounds; they are available in a variety of sizes and shapes. This type of dressing has the following functions:

- Absorbs drainage through the use of exudate absorbers in the dressing
- Maintains wound moisture
- Slowly liquefies necrotic debris
- Is impermeable to bacteria and other contaminants
- Is self-adhesive and molds well
- Acts as a preventive dressing for high-risk friction areas
- May be left in place for 3 to 5 days, minimizing skin trauma and disruption of healing

This type of dressing is most useful on shallow to moderately deep dermal ulcers. Hydrocolloid dressings cannot absorb the amount of drainage from heavily draining wounds, and some are contraindicated for use in full-thickness and infected wounds. Some hydrocolloids leave a residue in the wound bed that is easy to confuse with purulent drainage.

Hydrogel dressings are gauze or sheet dressings impregnated with water- or glycerin-based amorphous gel. This type of dressing hydrates wounds and absorbs some smaller amounts of exudate. Hydrogel dressings are for partial-thickness and full-thickness wounds, deep wounds with some exudate, necrotic wounds, burns, and radiation-damaged skin. They are very useful in painful wounds because they are very soothing to the patient and do not adhere to the wound bed and thus cause little trauma during removal. A disadvantage is that some hydrogels require a secondary

TABLE 48-8 **Dressings by Pressure Ulcer Stage**

PRESSURE ULCER STAGE	PRESSURE ULCER STATUS	DRESSING	COMMENTS*	EXPECTED CHANGE	ADJUVANTS
I	Intact	None	Allows visual assessment	Resolves slowly without epidermal loss over 7-14 days	Turning schedule Support hydration Nutritional support
		Transparent dressing	Protects from shear Not to be used in presence of excessive moisture		
		Hydrocolloid	Does not always allow visual assessment		Pressure-redistribution surface or chair cushion
II	Clean	Composite film	Limits shear	Heals through reepithelialization	Turning schedule Support hydration Nutritional support
		Hydrocolloid	Change when seal of dressing breaks; maximal wear time 7 days		Manage incontinence
		Hydrogel	Provides a moist environment		
III	Clean	Hydrocolloid	Must change when seal of dressing breaks; maximal wear time 7 days	Heals through granulation and reepithelialization	See previous stages; evaluate pressure-redistribution needs
		Hydrogel covered with foam dressing	Applied over wound to protect and absorb moisture		
		Calcium alginate	Used with significant exudate; must cover with secondary dressing		
		Gauze	Used with normal saline or other prescribed solution; must unfold to make contact with wound		
		Growth factors	Used with gauze per manufacturer instructions		
IV	Clean	Hydrogel covered with foam dressing	Applied over wound to protect and absorb moisture	Heals through granulation and reepithelialization	Surgical consultation often necessary for closure (see stages I, II, and III)
		Calcium alginate	Used with significant exudate; must cover with secondary dressing		
		Gauze	Used with normal saline or other prescribed solution; must unfold to make contact with wound; fill all dead space with gauze		
		Growth factors	Used with gauze		
Unstageable	Wound covered with eschar	Adherent film	Facilitates softening of eschar	Eschar lifts at edges as debridement progresses	See previous stages; surgical consultation sometimes considered for debridement
		Gauze plus ordered solution	Delivers solution and wicks wound drainage and softens eschar	Eschar softens	
		Enzymes	Facilitate debridement	Eschar softens	
		None	If eschar is dry and intact, no dressing used, allowing eschar to act as physiological cover; may be indicated for treatment of heel eschar		

*As with all occlusive dressings, wound should *not* be clinically infected.

dressing and you must take care to prevent periwound maceration. Hydrogels come in a sheet dressing or a tube; thus you are able to squirt the gel directly into the wound base.

Hydrogel has the following advantages:

- Is soothing and can reduce wound pain
- Provides a moist environment
- Debrides necrotic tissue (by softening the necrotic tissue)
- Does not adhere to the wound base and is easy to remove

Many other types of dressings are available. Foam and alginate dressings are for wounds with large amounts of exudate and those that need packing. Foam dressings are also used around drainage tubes to absorb drainage. Calcium alginate dressings are manufactured from seaweed and come in sheet and rope form. The alginate forms a soft gel when it comes in contact with wound fluid. These highly absorbent dressings are for wounds with an excessive amount of drainage and do not cause trauma when removed from the wound. *Do not use these in dry wounds, and they require a secondary dressing.* Several manufacturers produce composite dressings, which combine two different dressing types into one dressing. Research is ongoing regarding which type of dressing is best for which type of wound.

Changing Dressings. To prepare for changing a dressing, you need to know the type of dressing, the presence of underlying drains or tubing, and the type of supplies needed for wound care. Poor preparation causes a break in aseptic technique (see Chapter 28) or accidental dislodging of a drain. Your judgment in modifying a dressing change procedure is important during wound care, particularly if the character of a wound changes. Notifying the health care provider of any change is essential.

Sometimes (e.g., with chronic nonsurgical wounds) the nurse uses a clean technique for a dressing change. The clean technique refers to the fact that the nurse maintains medical versus sterile asepsis (Chapter 28). He or she wears clean gloves, but the dressing materials are in sterile packages and are carefully placed over the wound. Deep wounds that require irrigation are usually irrigated with a sterile solution. A complete patient and wound history is essential in determining when a clean dressing technique is appropriate. For example, chronic pressure ulcer wounds use a clean technique. On the other hand, a fresh surgical wound requires sterile technique so as not to introduce microorganisms into a healing wound.

The health care provider's order for changing a dressing indicates the dressing type, the frequency of changing, and any solutions or ointments to be applied to the wound. An order to "reinforce dressing prn" (add dressings without removing the original one) is common right after surgery, when the health care provider does not want accidental disruption of the suture line or bleeding. The medical or operating room record usually indicates whether drains are present and from what body cavity they drain. After the first dressing change, describe the location of drains and the type of dressing materials and solutions to use in the patient's care plan. Follow these guidelines during a dressing change procedure:

- Assessing the skin beneath the tape
- Performing thorough hand hygiene before and after wound care
- Wearing sterile gloves before directly touching an open or fresh wound (see Chapter 28)
- Removing or changing dressings over closed wounds when they become wet or if the patient has signs or symptoms of infection and as ordered

To prepare a patient for a dressing change, do the following:

- Evaluate patient's pain and, if indicated, administer required analgesics so peak effects occur during the dressing change
- Describe steps of the procedure to lessen patient anxiety
- Gather all supplies required for the dressing change
- Recognize normal signs of healing
- Answer questions about the procedure or the wound

Often it is necessary to teach patients how to change dressings in preparation for home care. In this situation, demonstrate dressing changes to the patient and family and then provide an opportunity for them to practice. Usually wound healing has progressed to the point that risks of complications such as dehiscence or evisceration are minimal. The patient needs to be able to change a dressing independently or with assistance from a family member before discharge. Contaminated dressings in the home should be disposed of in a manner consistent with local regulations. Skill 48-3 outlines the steps for changing dry and moist dressings.

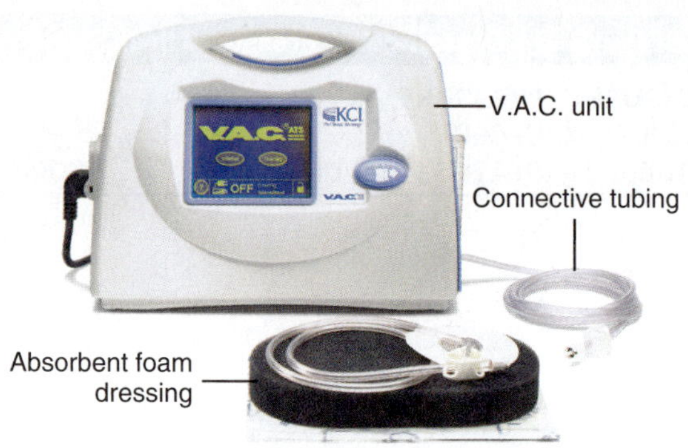

FIG. 48-19 V.A.C. unit. *V.A.C.,* Vacuum-assisted closure. (Courtesy Kinetic Concepts, Inc [KCI], San Antonio, Tex.)

Packing a Wound. The first step in packing a wound is to assess its size, depth, and shape. These characteristics are important in determining the size and type of dressing used to pack a wound. The dressing needs to be flexible and in contact with the entire wound surface. Make sure that the type of material used to pack the wound is appropriate. Many new dressing materials such as alginates are also used for packing. If gauze is the appropriate dressing material, saturate it with the ordered solution, wring out, unfold, and lightly pack into the wound. The entire wound surface needs to be in contact with part of the moist gauze dressing (see Skill 48-3).

It is important to remember not to pack the wound too tightly. Overpacking causes pressure on the tissue in the wound bed. Pack the wound only until the packing material reaches the surface of the wound; there should never be so much packing material that it extends higher than the wound surface. Packing that overlaps onto the wound edges causes maceration of the tissue surrounding the wound.

A treatment modality for wounds is negative-pressure wound therapy (NPWT) or vacuum-assisted closure (one brand name is V.A.C.). NPWT is the application of subatmospheric (negative) pressure of a wound through suction to facilitate healing and collect wound fluid (Netsch, 2012). The **vacuum-assisted closure (V.A.C.)** (Fig. 48-19) is a device that assists in wound closure by applying localized negative pressure to draw the edges of a wound together (Fig. 48-20, *A* and *B*). NPWT supports wound healing by edema reduction and fluid removal, macro deformation and wound contraction, and micro deformation and mechanical stretch perfusion. Secondary effects include angiogenesis, granulation tissue formation, and reduction in bacterial bioburden (Netsch, 2012) (Fig. 48-21). There have been modifications to the V.A.C. The V.A.C. Instill allows intermittent instillation of fluids into the wound, especially those wounds not responding to traditional NPWT (Jerome, 2007).

NPWT is used for treating acute and chronic wounds (Skill 48-4 on pp. 1221-1224). The schedule for changing NPWT dressings varies, depending on the type of wound and amount of drainage. Wear time for the dressing is anywhere from 24 hours to 5 days. As the wound heals, granulation tissue lines its surface. The wound has a stippled or granulated appearance. The surface area sometimes increases or decreases, depending on wound location and the amount of drainage removed by the NPWT system. NPWT is also used to enhance the take of split-thickness skin grafts. It is placed

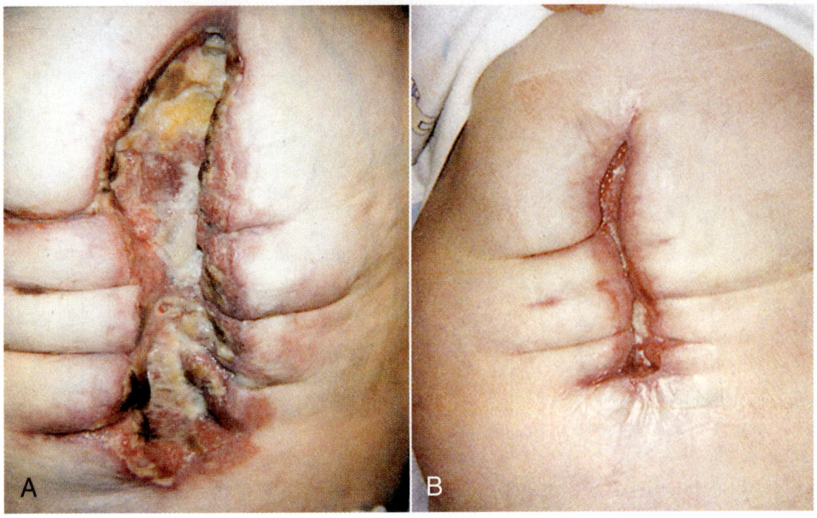

FIG. 48-20 **A,** Dehisced wound before wound V.A.C. therapy. **B,** Dehisced wound after wound V.A.C. therapy. *V.A.C.,* Vacuum-assisted closure. (Courtesy Kinetic Concepts, Inc [KCI], San Antonio, Tex.)

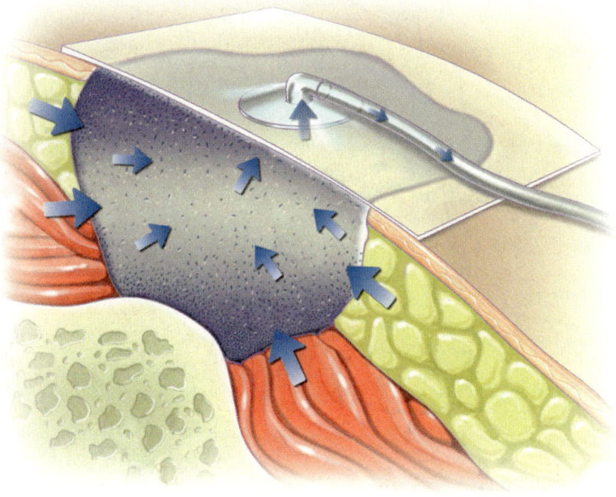

FIG. 48-21 V.A.C. system using negative pressure to remove fluid from area surrounding wound, reducing edema and improving circulation to area. *V.A.C.,* Vacuum-assisted closure. (Courtesy Kinetic Concepts, Inc [KCI], San Antonio, Tex.)

over the graft intraoperatively, decreasing the ability of the graft to shift and evacuating fluids that build up under it (Netsch, 2012; Xie et al., 2010). An airtight seal must be maintained (Box 48-14).

Securing Dressings. Use tape, ties, or a secondary dressing and cloth binders to secure a dressing over a wound site. The choice of anchoring depends on the wound size and location, the presence of drainage, the frequency of dressing changes, and the patient's level of activity.

Most often strips of tape are used to secure dressings if the patient is not allergic to it. Nonallergenic paper and plastic tapes minimize skin reactions. Common adhesive tape adheres well to the surface of the skin, whereas elastic adhesive tape compresses closely around pressure bandages and permits more movement of a body part. Skin sensitive to adhesive tape becomes severely inflamed and denuded and in some cases even sloughs when the tape is removed. It is important to assess skin under tape at each dressing change.

BOX 48-14 MAINTAINING AN AIRTIGHT SEAL

To avoid wound desiccation, the wound needs to stay sealed once therapy is initiated. Problem seal areas include wounds around joints and near the sacrum. The following points assist in maintaining an airtight seal:

- Clip hair around wound.
- Cut transparent film to extend 3 to 5 cm (1.2 to 2 in) beyond wound parameter.
- Avoid wrinkles in transparent film.
- Patch leaks with transparent film.
- Use multiple small strips of transparent film to hold dressing in place before covering it with large piece of transparent film.
- Avoid adhesive remover because it leaves a residue that hinders film adherence.

From Chua PC et al: Vacuum-assisted wound closure, *Am J Nurs* 100(12):45, 2000.

Tape is available in various widths such as 1.3, 2.5, 5 and 7.5 cm (½, 1, 2, and 3 inches). Choose the size that sufficiently secures the dressing. For example, a large abdominal wound dressing needs to remain secure over a large area despite frequent stress from movement, respiratory effort, and possibly abdominal distention. Strips of 7.5-cm (3-inch) adhesive better stabilize such a large dressing so it does not continually slip off. When applying tape, ensure that it adheres to several inches of skin on both sides of the dressing and that it is placed across the middle of the dressing. When securing the dressing, press the tape gently, making sure to exert pressure away from the wound. This way, tension occurs in both directions away from the wound, minimizing skin distortion and irritation. Never apply tape over irritated or broken skin. Protect irritated skin by using a solid skin barrier and applying the tape over the barrier.

To remove tape safely, loosen the ends and gently pull the outer end parallel with the skin surface toward the wound. Apply light traction to the skin away from the wound as the tape is loosened and removed. The traction minimizes pulling of the skin. Adhesive remover also loosens the tape from the skin. If tape covers an area of hair growth, the patient experiences less discomfort if you pull it in the direction of the hair growth.

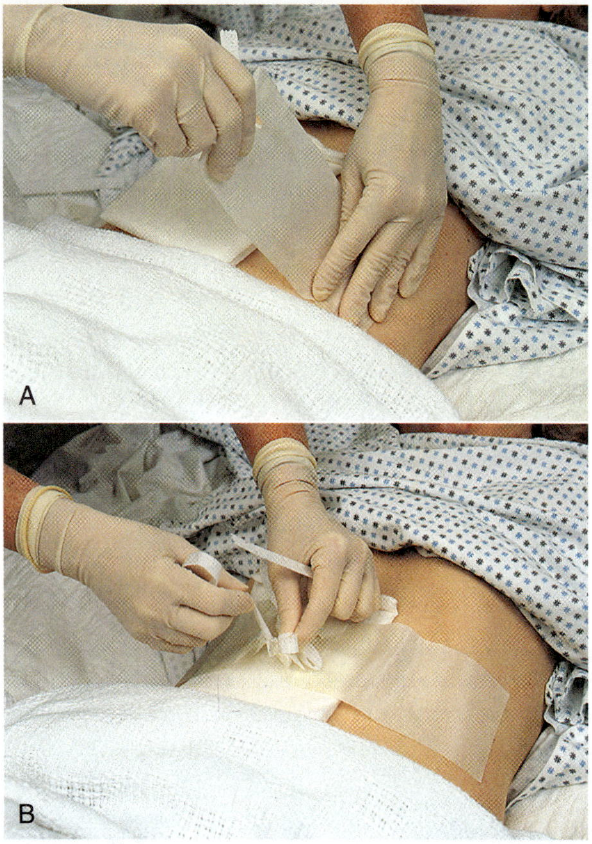

FIG. 48-22 Montgomery ties. **A,** Each tie is placed at side of dressing. **B,** Securing ties encloses dressing.

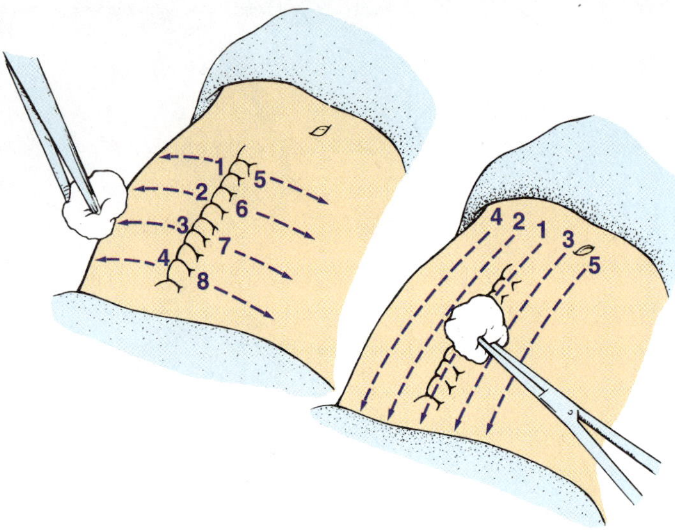

FIG. 48-23 Methods for cleaning a wound site.

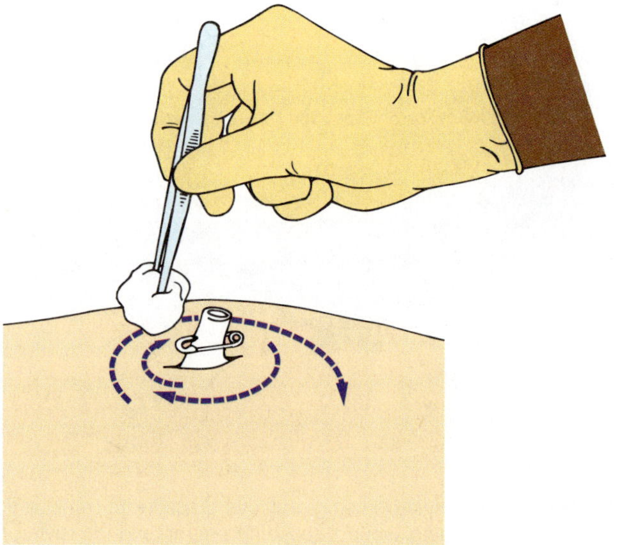

FIG. 48-24 Cleaning a drain site.

To avoid repeated removal of tape from sensitive skin, secure dressings with pairs of reusable Montgomery ties (Fig. 48-22). Each section consists of a long strip; half contains an adhesive backing to apply to the skin, and the other half folds back and contains a cloth tie or a safety pin/rubber band combination that you fasten across a dressing and untie at dressing changes. A large, bulky dressing often requires two or more sets of Montgomery ties. Another method to protect the surrounding skin on wounds that need frequent dressing changes is to place strips of hydrocolloid dressings on either side of the wound edges, cover the wound with a dressing, and apply the tape to the dressing. To provide even support to a wound and immobilize a body part, apply elastic gauze or cloth bandages and binders over a dressing.

Comfort Measures. A wound is often painful, depending on the extent of tissue injury. Use several techniques to minimize discomfort during wound care. Carefully removing tape, gently cleaning wound edges, and carefully manipulating dressings and drains minimize stress on sensitive tissues. Careful turning and positioning also reduce strain on a wound. Administering analgesic medications 30 to 60 minutes before dressing changes (depending on the time of peak action of a drug) also reduces discomfort.

Cleaning Skin and Drain Sites. Although a moderate amount of wound exudate promotes epithelial cell growth, some health care providers order cleaning a wound or drain site if a dressing does not absorb drainage properly or if an open drain deposits drainage onto the skin. Wound cleaning requires good hand hygiene and aseptic techniques (see Chapter 28). You sometimes use irrigation to remove debris from a wound.

Basic Skin Cleaning. Clean surgical or traumatic wounds by applying noncytotoxic solutions with sterile gauze or by irrigation. The following three principles are important when cleaning an incision or the area surrounding a drain:

1. Clean in a direction from the least contaminated area such as from the wound or incision to the surrounding skin (Fig. 48-23) or from an isolated drain site to the surrounding skin (Fig. 48-24).
2. Use gentle friction when applying solutions locally to the skin.
3. When irrigating, allow the solution to flow from the least to most contaminated area (see Skill 48-5).

After applying a solution to sterile gauze, clean away from the wound. Never use the same piece of gauze to clean across an incision or wound twice.

Drain sites are a source of contamination because moist drainage harbors microorganisms. If a wound has a dry incisional area

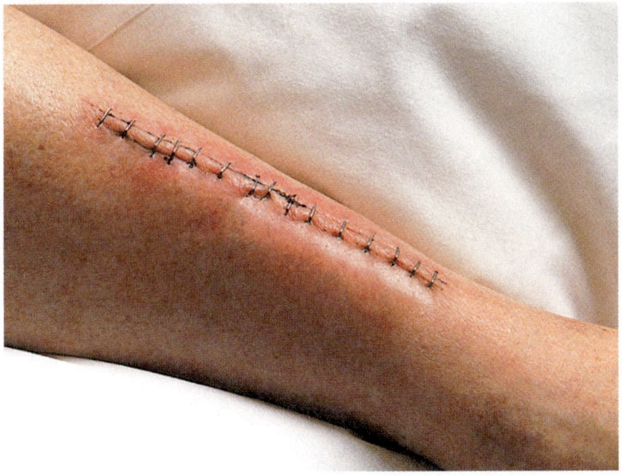

FIG. 48-25 Incision closed with metal staples.

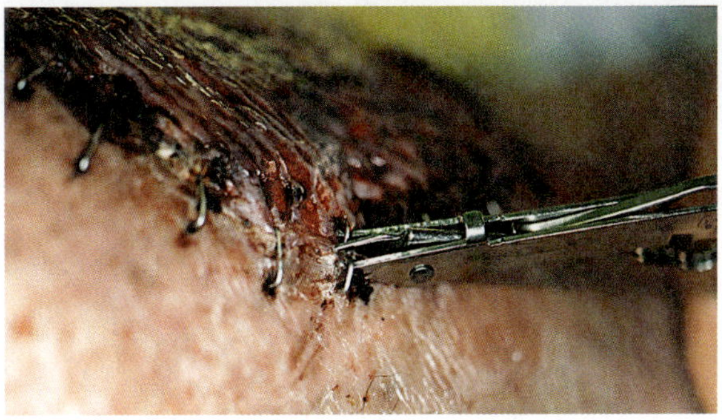

FIG. 48-26 Staple remover.

and a moist drain site, cleaning moves from the incisional area toward the drain. Use two separate swabs or gauze pads, one to clean from the top of the incision toward the drain and one to clean from the bottom of the incision toward the drain. To clean the area of an isolated drain site, clean around the drain, moving in circular rotations outward from a point closest to the drain. In this situation the skin near the site is more contaminated than the site itself. To clean circular wounds, use the same technique as in cleaning around a drain.

Irrigation. Irrigation is a special way of cleaning wounds. Use an irrigating syringe to flush the area with a constant low-pressure flow of solution. The gentle washing action of the irrigation cleans a wound of exudate and debris. Irrigation is particularly useful for open, deep wounds; wounds involving an inaccessible body part such as the ear canal; or when cleaning sensitive body parts such as the conjunctival lining of the eye.

Wound Irrigations. Irrigation of an open wound requires sterile technique. Use a 35-mL syringe with a 19-gauge needle (Rolstad, Bryant, and Nix, 2012) to deliver the solution. This irrigation system has a safe pressure and does not damage healing wound tissue. It is important to never occlude a wound opening with a syringe because this results in the introduction of irrigating fluid into a closed space. The pressure of the fluid causes tissue damage and discomfort. Always irrigate a wound with the syringe tip over but not in the drainage site. Make sure that fluid flows directly into the wound and not over a contaminated area before entering the wound. Skill 48-5 on pp. 1224-1226 lists steps for wound irrigation.

Suture Care. A surgeon closes a wound by bringing the wound edges as close together as possible to reduce scar formation. Proper wound closure involves minimal trauma and tension to tissues with control of bleeding.

Sutures are threads or metal used to sew body tissues together (Fig. 48-25). The patient's history of wound healing, the site of surgery, the tissues involved, and the purpose of the sutures determine the suture material used. For example, if the patient has had repeated surgery for an abdominal hernia, the health care provider can choose wire sutures to provide greater strength for wound closure. In contrast, a small laceration of the face calls for the use of very fine Dacron (polyester) sutures to minimize scar formation.

Sutures are available in a variety of materials, including silk, steel, cotton, linen, wire, nylon, and Dacron. They come with or

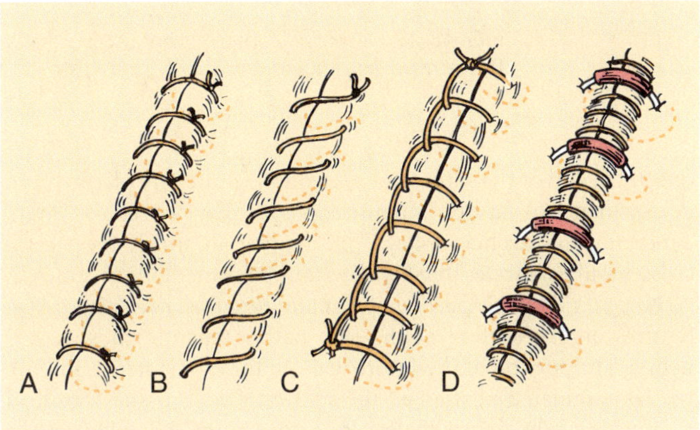

FIG. 48-27 Examples of suturing methods. **A,** Intermittent. **B,** Continuous. **C,** Blanket continuous. **D,** Retention.

without sharp surgical needles attached. Steel staples are a common type of outer skin closure that causes less trauma to tissues than sutures while providing extra strength.

Sutures are placed within tissue layers in deep wounds and superficially as the final means for wound closure. Deep sutures are usually composed of an absorbable material that disappears over time. Sutures are foreign bodies and thus are capable of causing local inflammation. The surgeon tries to minimize tissue injury by using the finest suture possible and the smallest number necessary.

Policies vary within institutions as to who is able to remove sutures. If it is appropriate that the nurse remove them, a health care provider's order is required. An order for suture removal is not written until the health care provider believes that the wound has closed (usually in 7 days). Special scissors with curved cutting tips or special staple removers slide under the skin closures for suture removal (Fig. 48-26). The health care provider usually specifies the number of sutures or staples to remove. If the suture line appears to be healing in certain locations better than in others, some health care providers choose to have only some sutures removed (e.g., every other one).

To remove staples, insert the tips of the staple remover under each wire staple. While slowly closing the ends of the staple remover together, squeeze the center of the staple with the tips, freeing it from the skin (see Fig. 48-26).

To remove sutures, first check the type of suturing used (Fig. 48-27). With intermittent suturing the surgeon ties each individual suture made in the skin. Continuous suturing, as the name implies, is a series of sutures with only two knots, one at the beginning and

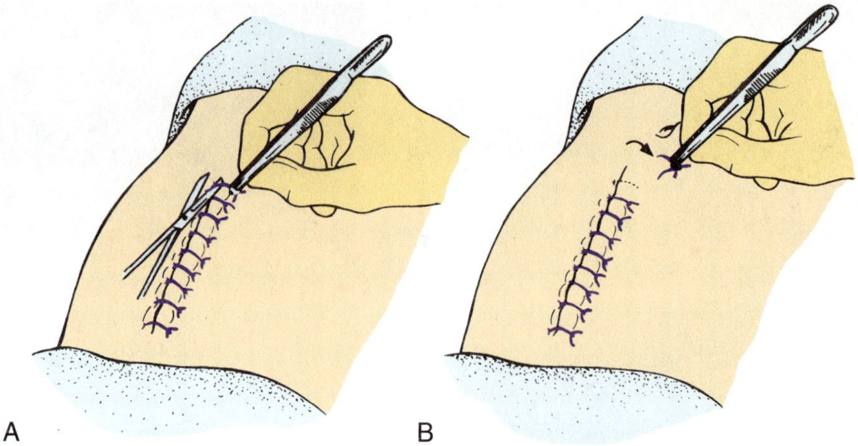

FIG. 48-28 Removal of intermittent suture. **A,** Cut suture as close to skin as possible, away from knot. **B,** Remove suture and never pull contaminated stitch through tissues.

one at the end of the suture line. Retention sutures are placed more deeply than skin sutures, and nurses may or may not remove them, depending on agency policy. The manner in which the suture crosses and penetrates the skin determines the method for removal. *Never pull the visible portion of a suture through underlying tissue.* Sutures on the surface of the skin harbor microorganisms and debris. The portion of the suture beneath the skin is sterile. Pulling the contaminated portion of the suture through tissues can lead to infection. Clip suture materials as close to the skin edge on one side as possible and pull the suture through from the other side (Fig. 48-28).

Drainage Evacuation. When drainage interferes with healing, evacuation is achieved by using either a drain alone or a drainage tube with continuous suction. You may apply special skin barriers, including hydrocolloid dressings similar to those used with ostomies (see Chapter 46), around drain sites. The skin barriers are soft material applied to the skin with adhesive. Drainage flows on the barrier but not directly on the skin. **Drainage evacuators** (Fig. 48-29) are convenient portable units that connect to tubular drains lying within a wound bed and exert a safe, constant, low-pressure vacuum to remove and collect drainage. Ensure that suction is exerted and that connection points between the evacuator and tubing are intact. The evacuator collects drainage. Assess for volume and character every shift and as needed. When the evacuator fills, measure output by emptying the contents into a graduated cylinder and immediately reset the evacuator to apply suction.

Bandages and Binders. A simple gauze dressing is often not enough to immobilize or provide support to a wound. Binders and bandages applied over or around dressings provide extra protection and therapeutic benefits by the following:

1. Creating pressure over a body part (e.g., an elastic pressure bandage applied over an arterial puncture site)
2. Immobilizing a body part (e.g., an elastic bandage applied around a sprained ankle)
3. Supporting a wound (e.g., an abdominal binder applied over a large abdominal incision and dressing)
4. Reducing or preventing edema (e.g., a pressure bandage applied to the lower leg)
5. Securing a splint (e.g., a bandage applied around hand splints for correction of deformities)
6. Securing dressings (e.g., elastic webbing applied around leg dressings after a vein stripping)

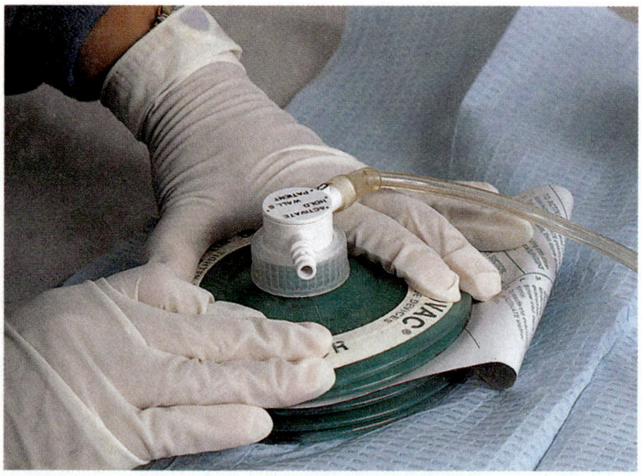

FIG. 48-29 Setting suction on drainage evacuator. *1,* With drainage port open, raise level on diaphragm. *2,* Push straight down on lever to lower diaphragm. *3,* Closure of port prevents escape of air and creates vacuum pressure.

Bandages are available in rolls of various widths and materials, including gauze, elasticized knit, elastic webbing, flannel, and muslin. Gauze bandages are lightweight and inexpensive, mold easily around contours of the body, and permit air circulation to prevent skin maceration. Elastic bandages conform well to body parts but are also for exerting pressure.

Binders are bandages that are made of large pieces of material to fit a specific body part. Most binders are made of elastic or cotton. An abdominal binder and a breast binder are examples.

Principles for Applying Bandages and Binders. Correctly applied bandages and binders do not cause injury to underlying and nearby body parts or create discomfort for the patient. For example, a chest binder should not be so tight as to restrict chest wall expansion. Before applying a bandage or binder, the nurse's responsibilities include the following:

- Inspecting the skin for abrasions, edema, discoloration, or exposed wound edges
- Covering exposed wounds or open abrasions with a sterile dressing
- Assessing the condition of underlying dressings and changing if soiled

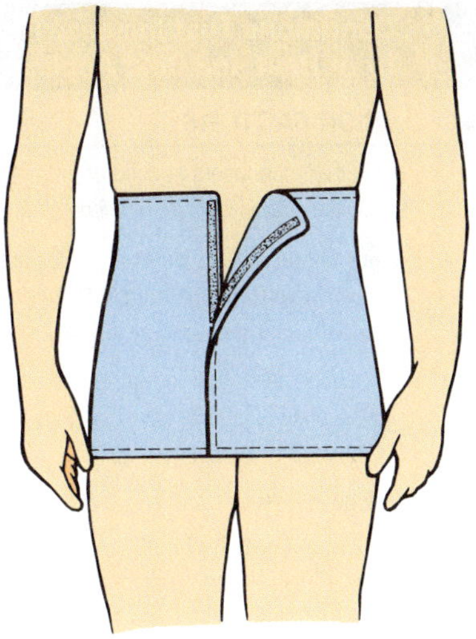

FIG. 48-30 Securing an abdominal binder with Velcro.

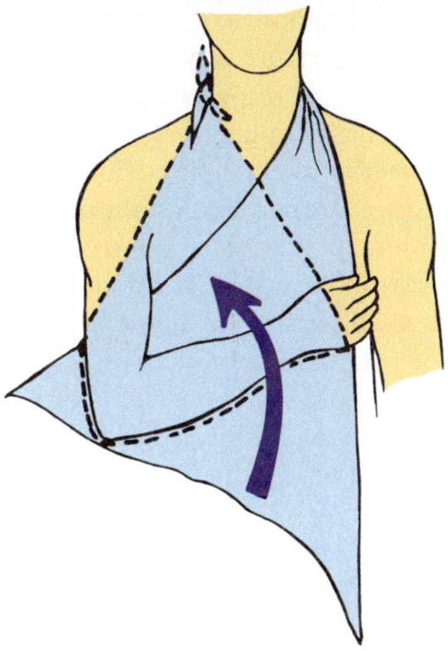

FIG. 48-31 Application of sling.

- Assessing the skin of underlying areas that will be distal to the bandage for signs of circulatory impairment (coolness, pallor or cyanosis, diminished or absent pulses, swelling, numbness, and tingling) to provide a means for comparing changes in circulation after bandage application

After applying a bandage, the nurse assesses, documents, and immediately reports changes in circulation, skin integrity, comfort level, and body function (e.g., ventilation or movement). The nurse who applies a bandage loosens or readjusts it as necessary. He or she needs a health care provider's order before loosening or removing a bandage applied by a health care provider. The nurse explains to the patient that any bandage or binder feels relatively firm or tight. Carefully assess a bandage to be sure that it is applied properly and providing therapeutic benefit and replace any soiled bandages.

Binder Application. Binders are especially designed for the body part to be supported. The most common type of binder is the abdominal binder (Skill 48-6 on pp. 1226-1228). Well-fitting bras are now replacing breast binders. Both provide support after breast surgery or exert pressure to reduce lactation in a woman after childbirth.

Abdominal Binders. An abdominal binder supports large abdominal incisions that are vulnerable to tension or stress as the patient moves or coughs (Fig. 48-30). Secure an abdominal binder with safety pins, Velcro strips, or metal stays.

Slings. Slings support arms with muscular sprains or fractures. A commercially manufactured sling consists of a long sleeve that extends above the elbow with a strap that fits around the neck. In the home patients can use a large triangular piece of cloth. The patient sits or lies supine during sling application (Fig. 48-31). Instruct him or her to bend the affected arm, bringing the forearm straight across the chest. The open sling fits under the patient's arm and over the chest, with the base of the triangle under the wrist and the point of the triangle at his or her elbow. One end of the sling fits around the back of the patient's neck. Bring the other end up and over the affected arm while supporting the extremity. Tie the two ends at the side of the neck so the knot does not press against the cervical spine. Fold the loose material at the elbow evenly around the elbow and pin. Always support the lower arm and hand at a level above the elbow to prevent the formation of dependent edema.

Bandage Application. Rolls of bandage secure or support dressings over irregularly shaped body parts. Each roll has a free outer end and a terminal end at the center of the roll. The rolled portion of the bandage is its body, and its outer surface is placed against the patient's skin or dressing. Skill 48-7 on pp. 1228-1229 describes the steps for applying an elastic bandage. Use a variety of bandage turns, depending on the body part to be bandaged.

Heat and Cold Therapy

Assessment for Temperature Tolerance. Before applying heat or cold therapies, assess the patient's physical condition for signs of potential intolerance to heat and cold. First observe the area to be treated. Assess the skin, looking for any open areas such as alterations in skin integrity (e.g., abrasions, open wounds, edema, bruising, bleeding, or localized areas of inflammation) that increase the patient's risk of injury. Because the health care provider commonly orders heat and cold applications for traumatized areas, the baseline skin assessment provides a guide for evaluating skin changes that can occur during therapy. Include in your assessment the neurological system for sensation (to understand if the patient senses extremes of cold or heat) and the patient's mental status to be sure that he or she can correctly communicate any issues with the hot or cold therapy.

Assessment includes identification of conditions that contraindicate heat or cold therapy. Do not cover an active area of bleeding with a warm application because bleeding will continue. Warm applications are contraindicated when the patient has an acute, localized inflammation such as appendicitis because the heat causes the appendix to rupture. If a patient has cardiovascular problems, it is unwise to apply heat to large portions of the body because the resulting massive vasodilation disrupts blood supply to vital organs.

Cold is contraindicated if the site of injury is already edematous. It further retards circulation to the area and prevents absorption of the interstitial fluid. If the patient has impaired circulation (e.g., arteriosclerosis), it further reduces blood supply to the affected area. Cold therapy is also contraindicated in the presence of neuropathy, because the patient is unable to perceive temperature change and damage resulting from temperature extremes. One other contraindication for cold therapy is shivering. Cold applications sometimes intensify shivering and dangerously increase body temperature.

Assess the patient's response to stimuli. Sensation to light touch, pinprick, and mild temperature variations (see Chapter 30) reveals the ability of the patient to recognize when heat or cold becomes excessive. If a patient has peripheral vascular disease, pay particular attention to the integrity of extremities. For example, if the health care provider's order is to apply a cold compress to a lower extremity, assess circulation to the leg by assessing for capillary refill; observing skin color; and palpating skin temperatures, distal pulses, and edematous areas. If signs of circulatory inadequacy are present, it is important for you to question the order.

Level of consciousness influences the ability to perceive heat, cold, and pain. If a patient is confused or unresponsive, the nurse needs to make frequent observations of skin integrity after therapy begins.

Also assess the condition of equipment being used. Check electrical equipment for cracked cords, frayed wires, damaged insulation, and exposed heating components. Make sure that equipment containing circulating fluids does not have leaks. Check equipment for evenness of temperature distribution.

Local application of heat and cold to an injured body part is sometimes therapeutic. However, before using these therapies, you need to understand normal body responses to local temperature variations, assess the integrity of the body part, determine the patient's ability to sense temperature variations, and ensure proper operation of equipment. You are legally responsible for safe administration of heat and cold applications.

Bodily Responses to Heat and Cold. Exposure to heat and cold causes systemic and local responses. Systemic responses occur through heat-loss mechanisms (sweating and vasodilation) or mechanisms promoting heat conservation (vasoconstriction and piloerection) and heat production (shivering) (see Chapter 30). Local responses to heat and cold occur through stimulation of temperature-sensitive nerve endings within the skin. This stimulation sends impulses from the periphery to the hypothalamus, which becomes aware of local temperature sensations and triggers adaptive responses for maintenance of normal body temperature. If alterations occur along temperature sensation pathways, the reception and eventual perception of stimuli are altered.

The body is able to tolerate wide variations in temperature. The normal temperature of the surface of the skin is 34° C (93.2° F), but temperature receptors usually adapt quickly to local temperatures between 15° and 45° C (59° and 113° F). Pain develops when local temperatures exceed this range. Excessive heat causes a burning sensation. Cold produces a numbing sensation before pain.

The adaptive ability of the body creates the major problem in protecting patients from injury resulting from temperature extremes. A person initially feels an extreme change in temperature but within a short time hardly notices it. This is dangerous because a person insensitive to heat and cold extremes can suffer serious tissue injury. You need to recognize patients most at risk for injuries from heat and cold applications (Table 48-9).

Local Effects of Heat and Cold. Heat and cold stimuli create different physiological responses. The choice of heat or cold therapy depends on local responses desired for wound healing (Table 48-10).

Effects of Heat Application. Heat generally is quite therapeutic, improving blood flow to an injured part. However, if heat is applied for 1 hour or more, the body reduces blood flow by a reflex vasoconstriction to control heat loss from the area. Periodic removal and reapplication of local heat restores vasodilation. Continuous exposure to heat damages epithelial cells, causing redness, localized tenderness, and even blistering.

TABLE 48-9 Conditions That Increase Risk of Injury from Heat and Cold Application

CONDITION	RISK FACTORS
Very young or older patients	Thinner skin layers in children increase risk of burns. Older patients have reduced sensitivity to pain.
Open wounds, broken skin, stomas	Subcutaneous and visceral tissues are more sensitive to temperature variations. They also contain no temperature and fewer pain receptors.
Areas of edema or scar formation	Reduced sensation to temperature stimuli occurs because of thickening of skin layers from fluid buildup or scar formation.
Peripheral vascular disease (e.g., diabetes, arteriosclerosis)	Body extremities are less sensitive to temperature and pain stimuli because of circulatory impairment and local tissue injury. Cold application further compromises blood flow.
Confusion or unconsciousness	Perception of sensory or painful stimuli is reduced.
Spinal cord injury	Alterations in nerve pathways prevent reception of sensory or painful stimuli.
Abscessed tooth or appendix	Infection is highly localized. Application of heat causes rupture with spread of microorganisms systemically.

Effects of Cold Application. The application of cold initially diminishes swelling and pain. Prolonged exposure of the skin to cold results in a reflex vasodilation. The inability of the cells to receive adequate blood flow and nutrients results in tissue ischemia. The skin initially takes on a reddened appearance, followed by a bluish-purple mottling, with numbness and a burning type of pain. Skin tissues freeze from exposure to extreme cold.

Factors Influencing Heat and Cold Tolerance. The response of the body to heat and cold therapies depends on the following factors:

- A person is better able to tolerate short exposure to temperature extremes than prolonged exposure.
- Exposed skin layers and certain areas of the skin (e.g., the neck, inner aspect of the wrist and forearm, and perineal region) are more sensitive to temperature variations. The foot and palm of the hand are less sensitive.
- The body responds best to minor temperature adjustments. If a body part is cool and a hot stimulus touches the skin, the response is greater than if the skin were already warm.
- A person has less tolerance to temperature changes to which a large area of the body is exposed.
- Tolerance to temperature variations changes with age. Patients who are very young or old are most sensitive to heat and cold.
- If a patient's physical condition reduces the reception or perception of sensory stimuli, tolerance to temperature extremes is high, but the risk of injury is also high.
- Uneven temperature distribution suggests that the equipment is functioning improperly.

Application of Heat and Cold Therapies. A prerequisite to using any heat or cold application is a health care provider's order, which includes the body site to be treated and the type, frequency, and duration of application (Box 48-15). Consult agency procedure manual for correct temperatures to use.

TABLE 48-10 Therapeutic Effects of Heat and Cold Applications

PHYSIOLOGICAL RESPONSE	THERAPEUTIC BENEFIT	EXAMPLES OF CONDITIONS TREATED
Heat		
Vasodilation	Improves blood flow to injured body part; promotes delivery of nutrients and removal of wastes; lessens venous congestion in injured tissues	Open wounds, rectal surgery, episiotomy, painful hemorrhoids, muscle tension, vaginal inflammation, wound debridement
Reduced blood viscosity	Improves delivery of leukocytes and antibiotics to wound site	
Reduced muscle tension	Promotes muscle relaxation and reduces pain from spasm or stiffness	
Increased tissue metabolism	Increases blood flow; provides local warmth	
Increased capillary permeability	Promotes movement of waste products and nutrients	
Cold		
Vasoconstriction	Reduces blood flow to injured body part, preventing edema formation; reduces inflammation	Direct trauma (sprains, strains, fractures, muscle spasms), superficial laceration or puncture wound, minor burn, suspected malignancy in area of injury or pain, injections, arthritis and joint trauma
Local anesthesia	Reduces localized pain	
Reduced cell metabolism	Reduces oxygen needs of tissues	
Increased blood viscosity	Promotes blood coagulation at injury site	
Decreased muscle tension	Relieves pain	

BOX 48-15 SAFETY SUGGESTIONS FOR APPLYING HEAT OR COLD THERAPY

- *Do* explain to patient sensations to be felt during the procedure.
- *Do* instruct patient to report changes in sensation or discomfort immediately.
- *Do* provide a timer, clock, or watch so patient can help the nurse time the application.
- *Do* keep the call light within patient's reach.
- *Do* refer to the policy and procedure manual of the institution for safe temperatures.
- *Do not* allow patient to adjust temperature settings.
- *Do not* allow patient to move an application or place hands on the wound site.
- *Do not* place patient in a position that prevents movement away from the temperature source.
- *Do not* leave unattended a patient who is unable to sense temperature changes or move from the temperature source.

BOX 48-16 CHOICE OF DRY OR MOIST APPLICATIONS

Advantages

Moist Applications

- Moist application reduces drying of skin and softens wound exudate.
- Moist compresses conform well to most body areas.
- Moist heat penetrates deeply into tissue layers.
- Warm moist heat does not promote sweating and insensible fluid loss.

Dry Applications

- Dry heat has less risk of burns to skin than moist applications.
- Dry application does not cause skin maceration.
- Dry heat retains temperature longer because evaporation does not occur.

Disadvantages

Moist Applications

- Prolonged exposure causes maceration of skin.
- Moist heat cools rapidly because of moisture evaporation.
- Moist heat creates greater risk for burns to skin because moisture conducts heat.

Dry Applications

- Dry heat increases body fluid loss through sweating.
- Dry applications do not penetrate deep into tissues.
- Dry heat causes increased drying of skin.

Choice of Moist or Dry. You can administer heat and cold applications in dry or moist forms. The type of wound or injury, the location of the body part, and the presence of drainage or inflammation are factors to consider in selecting dry or moist applications. Box 48-16 summarizes advantages and disadvantages of both.

Warm, Moist Compresses. Warm, moist compresses improve circulation, relieve edema, and promote consolidation of purulent drainage. A compress is a piece of gauze dressing moistened in a prescribed warmed solution. A pack is a larger cloth or dressing applied to a larger body area.

Heat from warm compresses dissipates quickly. To maintain a constant temperature, you need to change the compress often or apply a waterproof heating pad over it. Because moisture conducts heat, the temperature setting of any device should be lower for a moist compress than for a dry application. You can also use a layer of plastic wrap or a dry towel to insulate the compress and retain heat. Moist heat promotes vasodilation and evaporation of heat from the surface of the skin. For this reason a patient can feel chilly. Always try to control drafts within the room and keep the patient covered with a blanket or robe.

Warm Soaks. Immersion of a body part in a warmed solution promotes circulation, lessens edema, increases muscle relaxation, and provides a means to apply medicated solution. Sometimes a soak is also accompanied by wrapping the body part in dressings and saturating them with the warmed solution.

Position the patient comfortably, place waterproof pads under the area to be treated, and heat the solution to about 40.5° to 43° C (105° to 110° F). After immersing the body part, cover the container and extremity with a towel to reduce heat loss. It is usually necessary to remove the cooled solution and add heated solution after about 10 minutes. The challenge is to keep the solution at a constant temperature. Never add a hotter solution while the body part remains immersed. After any soak dry the body part thoroughly to prevent maceration.

Sitz Baths. The patient who has had rectal surgery, an episiotomy during childbirth, painful hemorrhoids, or vaginal inflammation benefits from a sitz bath, a bath in which only the pelvic area is immersed in warm or, in some situations, cool fluid. The patient sits in a special tub or chair or a basin that fits on the toilet seat so the legs and feet remain out of the water. Immersing the entire body causes widespread vasodilation and nullifies the effect of local heat application to the pelvic area.

The desired temperature for a sitz bath depends on whether the purpose is to promote relaxation or to clean a wound. It is often necessary to add warm or cool water during the procedure, which normally lasts 20 minutes, to maintain a constant temperature. Agency procedure manuals recommend safe water temperatures. A disposable sitz basin contains an attachment resembling an enema bag that allows gradual introduction of additional water.

Prevent overexposure of the patient by draping bath blankets around his or her shoulders and thighs and controlling drafts. The patient should be able to sit in the basin or tub with feet flat on the floor and without pressure on the sacrum or thighs. Because exposure of a large portion of the body to heat causes extensive vasodilation, assess the pulse and facial color and ask whether the patient feels light-headed or nauseated.

Commercial Hot Packs. Commercially prepared disposable hot packs apply warm, dry heat to an injured area. The chemicals mix and release heat when you strike, knead, or squeeze the pack. Package directions recommend the time for heat application.

Cold, Moist, and Dry Compresses. The procedure for applying cold, moist compresses is the same as that for warm compresses. Apply cold compresses for 20 minutes at a temperature of 15° C (59° F) to relieve inflammation and swelling. You can use clean or sterile compresses.

Commercially prepared cold packs that are similar to the disposable hot packs for dry applications are available. They come in various shapes and sizes to fit different body parts. When using cold compresses, observe for adverse reactions such as burning or numbness, mottling of the skin, redness, extreme paleness, and a bluish skin discoloration.

Cold Soaks. The procedure for preparing cold soaks and immersing a body part is the same as for warm soaks. The desired temperature for a 20-minute cold soak is 15° C (59° F). Control drafts and use outer coverings to protect the patient from chilling. It is often necessary to add cold water during the procedure to maintain a constant temperature.

Ice Bags or Collars. For a patient who has a muscle sprain, localized hemorrhage, or hematoma or who has undergone dental surgery, an ice bag is ideal to prevent edema formation, control bleeding, and anesthetize the body part. Proper use of the bag requires the following steps:

1. Fill the bag with water, secure the cap, invert to check for leaks, and pour out the water.
2. Fill the bag two-thirds full with crushed ice so you are able to easily mold it over a body part.
3. Release any air from the bag by squeezing its sides before securing the cap because excess air interferes with conduction of cold.
4. Wipe off excess moisture.
5. Cover the bag with a flannel cover, towel, or pillowcase.
6. Apply the bag to the injury site for 30 minutes; you can reapply the bag in an hour.

EVALUATION

You evaluate nursing interventions for reducing and treating pressure ulcers by determining the patient's response to nursing therapies and whether he or she achieved each goal. To evaluate outcomes and responses to care, you measure the effectiveness of interventions. The optimal outcomes are to prevent injury to the skin and tissues, reduce injury to the skin and underlying tissues, and possible wound healing with restoration of skin integrity.

Through the Patient's Eyes. It is important to include the patient and caregiver in the evaluation process. Determine what they know about the formation of impaired skin integrity, determine how the patient and caregiver feel about the presence of the wound and the need for wound care, and develop a plan of care to provide education and support. Chronic wounds such as pressure ulcers take time to heal, and it is likely that the patient will be in the home setting with the pressure ulcer.

Patient Outcomes. Because each patient has different risk factors for impaired skin integrity, you need to individualize nursing interventions. Patients with minimal mobility impairments or relatively stable health status need only a few measures. You evaluate nursing interventions for reducing and treating pressure ulcers by determining the patient's response to nursing therapies and whether he or she achieved each goal (Fig. 48-32).

Patients with impaired skin integrity need evaluation on an ongoing basis for factors that contribute to skin breakdown. This includes a comprehensive skin assessment and a wound assessment

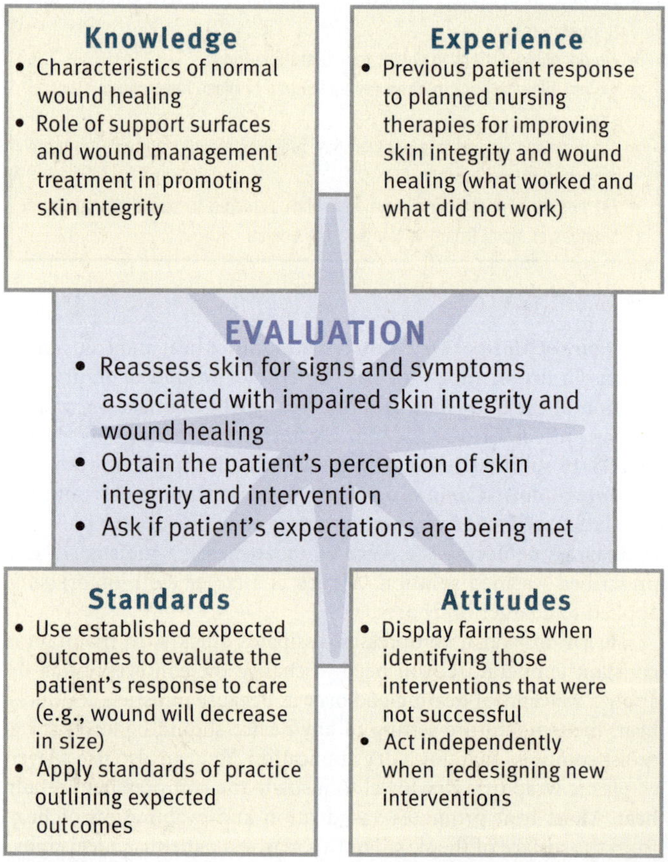
Knowledge
• Characteristics of normal wound healing
• Role of support surfaces and wound management treatment in promoting skin integrity
Experience
• Previous patient response to planned nursing therapies for improving skin integrity and wound healing (what worked and what did not work)
EVALUATION
• Reassess skin for signs and symptoms associated with impaired skin integrity and wound healing
• Obtain the patient's perception of skin integrity and intervention
• Ask if patient's expectations are being met
Standards
• Use established expected outcomes to evaluate the patient's response to care (e.g., wound will decrease in size)
• Apply standards of practice outlining expected outcomes
Attitudes
• Display fairness when identifying those interventions that were not successful
• Act independently when redesigning new interventions

FIG. 48-32 Critical thinking model for skin integrity and wound care evaluation.

using a validated risk-assessment tool. Assessment provides the foundation for the plan of care, and evaluation is critical for monitoring the effectiveness of the plan (Nix, 2012).

If the identified outcomes are not met for a patient with impaired skin integrity, questions to ask include the following:

- Was the etiology of the skin impairment addressed? Were the pressure, friction, shear, and moisture components identified; and did the plan of care decrease the contribution of each of these components?
- Was wound healing supported by providing the wound base with a moist protected environment?
- Were issues such as nutrition assessed and a plan of care developed that provided the patient with the calories to support healing?

Finally, evaluate the need for additional referrals to other experts in wound care and pressure ulcers, such as nurses certified in wound care. Care of patients with a pressure ulcer or wound requires a multidisciplinary team approach.

SAFETY GUIDELINES FOR NURSING SKILLS

Ensuring patient safety is an essential role of the professional nurse. To ensure patient safety, communicate clearly with the members of the health care team, assess and incorporate the patient's priorities of care and preferences, and use the best evidence when making decisions about care. When performing the skills in this chapter, remember the following points to ensure safe, individualized patient-centered care:

- Position patient in a manner that the side rails on the bed are in an upright position to prevent him or her from rolling over the side of the bed.
- When changing wound dressings, keep a plastic bag within reach to discard dressings and prevent cross-contamination. Keep extra gloves within reach to allow a change of gloves if the gloves become soiled.
- If irrigating a wound, use goggles for protection from splashing.
- When applying an elastic bandage, check the extremity where the bandage is applied for temperature or sensation changes.

SKILL 48-1 ASSESSMENT FOR RISK FOR PRESSURE ULCER DEVELOPMENT

View Video!

Delegation Considerations

The skill of assessing patients for risk of pressure ulcers cannot be delegated to nursing assistive personnel (NAP). Direct/inform/instruct the NAP to:

- Report any changes to the patient's skin such as redness, blistering, abrasion, or cuts to the nurse for further nursing assessment.
- Keep the patient's skin dry and provide hygiene following incontinence of urine or stool or exposure to other body fluids.
- Reposition the patient according to the frequency established on the nursing care plan or agency policy.
- Avoid trauma to the patient's skin from tape, pressure, friction, or shear.

Equipment

- Risk assessment tool, Braden Scale
- Documentation record

STEP	RATIONALE
ASSESSMENT	
1 Identify at-risk individuals needing prevention and specific factors placing them at risk.	Determines factors that increase patient's risk for developing pressure ulcers (Braden, 2001).
a. Use validated risk assessment tool such as the Braden Scale.	Ensures consistent, reliable, comparable assessments (WOCN, 2010).
b. Assess patient and obtain risk score on admission to acute care, rehabilitation hospitals, nursing homes, home care programs, and other health care facilities.	Provides baseline assessment.
2 Determine patient's ability to respond meaningfully to pressure-related discomfort (sensory perception).	Patient with complete or partial limited ability to respond to pressure-related discomfort cannot communicate discomfort, has a limitation in ability to feel pain, and thus is at risk for developing pressure ulcers.
3 Apply clean gloves and conduct a systematic skin assessment over bony prominences.	Bony prominences are at high risk of skin breakdown because of high pressures exerted on these areas when patient is immobile. A finding of redness or impairment in skin integrity necessitates planning appropriate interventions.
a. Observe for at-risk areas for skin breakdown, including back of head, shoulders, ribs, hips, sacral region, ischium, inner and outer knees, inner and outer ankles, heels and feet (see Fig. 48-9).	
4 Assess the following potential sites for skin breakdown:	
a. Ears and nares	Cartilage that nasal cannulas or tubing compresses develops pressure necrosis.
b. Lips	Oral airway and endotracheal tubes exert pressure if left in place for prolonged time periods.
c. Tube sites (e.g., gastrostomy or nasogastric tubes, Foley catheters, Jackson-Pratt drains)	Tubes exert pressure if taped snugly against skin or if there is stress at insertion site. If moisture is present around tube insertion sites, leakage of bodily fluids compromises skin integrity.
d. Orthopedic and positioning devices (e.g., casts, braces, cervical collar)	Improperly fitted or applied devices have potential to cause pressure on adjacent skin and underlying tissue.

SKILL 48-1 ASSESSMENT FOR RISK FOR PRESSURE ULCER DEVELOPMENT—cont'd

STEP	RATIONALE
5 Assess all skin surfaces for the following:	
a. Absence of superficial skin layers	Damage of superficial skin layers indicates injury from friction or moisture. The area is moist and sore to the touch.
b. Blisters	Suggests skin damage from friction and/or inappropriate tape removal. Blisters occur when top layer of skin is pulled or rubbed, separating epidermis from dermis.
c. Any loss of epidermis and dermis	Indicates damage to skin. Determine cause of this damage and begin interventions to prevent further damage.
6 Assess degree to which patient's skin is exposed to moisture. Remove gloves and perform hand hygiene.	Exposure to excessive moisture increases risk for skin breakdown (Bryant, 2012).
7 Evaluate patient's activity level.	Patient who is bedfast or chairfast or only walks occasionally is at risk for developing pressure areas because of the degree of physical inactivity (WOCN, 2010).
a. Determine patient's ability to change and control body position (mobility).	Potential for friction and shear increases when patient is completely dependent on others for position change.
b. Determine patient's preferred positions.	Weight of body is on certain bony prominences, and patient resists repositioning off these areas.
8 Assess patient's usual food intake pattern (nutrition).	Patient who rarely or never eats a complete meal is at risk for pressure ulcer formation.
a. Review weight pattern, calorie intake, and nutritional laboratory values (see Box 48-11).	Decreased nutrition status is linked with pressure ulcer formation and poor wound healing (WOCN, 2010).
b. Complete fluid intake assessment.	Fluid imbalance, either dehydration or edema, increases patient's risk for pressure ulcers (Stotts, 2012a).
9 Assess presence of friction and/or shear.	Patient who has a problem moving, requires maximum assistance in moving, or slides against sheets when moved is at an increased risk of skin damage (Bryant, 2012).
PLANNING	
1 Explain procedure to patient.	Promotes patient cooperation and reduces anxiety.
IMPLEMENTATION	
1 Note the score on the risk assessment scale. (NOTE: Numerical values in Steps a through f refer to the Braden Scale.)	The documentation provides a baseline for comparison of increased or decreased risk for development of pressure ulcers and allows planning of interventions.
a. As the Braden Scale scores become lower, predicted risk becomes higher.	*Scores:* 15 to 18, at risk 13 to 14, moderate risk 10 to 12, high risk 9 or below, very high risk
b. Link risk assessment to preventive protocols. Perform hand hygiene and apply gloves.	Protocols target problem areas to assist in prevention of skin breakdown.
(1) Institute at-risk interventions (score of 15 to 18). Consider instituting frequent turning, protecting patient's heels, using a pressure-redistribution surface, and managing moisture.	Decreases risk of skin breakdown.
(2) Institute moderate-risk interventions (score of 13 to 14). Consider protocol of frequent turning; protecting patient's heels; providing pressure-redistribution surface; providing foam wedges for 30-degree lateral positioning; and managing moisture, shear, and friction.	Decreases pressure on bony prominences and reduces the increased risk of skin breakdown.
(3) Institute high-risk interventions (score of 10 to 12). Consider a protocol that increases the frequency of turning; supplements turning with small shifts in position; facilitates maximal remobilization; protects the patient's heels; provides pressure-redistribution surface; provides foam wedges for 30-degree lateral positioning; and manages moisture, friction, and shear. If needed, institute nutritional interventions to reduce risk of pressure ulcer development.	Addresses factors that contribute to skin breakdown and plans for interventions to address causative factors (Bryant, 2012). Nutrition therapy promotes skin healing.
(4) Institute very high–risk interventions (score of 9 or below). Consider protocol that incorporates points for high-risk patients plus uses pressure-redistribution surface if patient has intractable pain or severe pain exacerbated by turning.	Plans interventions to decrease the effects of immobility, decreased sensory perception, moisture, friction, shear, decreased activity, and nutritional issues in a high-risk individual.

STEP	RATIONALE
2 When you note reddened area, check for the following:	
a. Skin discoloration (e.g., redness in light-tone skin; purplish or bluish in darkly pigmented skin) (see Box 48-3)	May indicate that tissue was under pressure.
b. Blanchable erythema	Indicates pressure damage that will resolve. If redness lightens under application of pressure, make sure that vessels are intact and that there is no tissue damage present.
c. Nonblanchable erythema	Indicates potential damage to blood vessels and tissue damage. Once blood vessels are damaged, red area will not lighten in color because tissue and blood vessels are inflamed. Position patient off area.
d. Pallor or mottling	Persistent hypoxia in tissues alters circulation, and pallor or mottling may occur.
3 Remove gloves and perform hand hygiene. Reposition patient.	Reduces transmission of infection.
4 Educate patient and family regarding pressure ulcer risk and prevention.	Helps patients and family understand interventions designed to reduce pressure ulcer risk.
EVALUATION	
1 Observe patient's skin daily, especially areas at risk (check agency policy).	Determines over time patient's response to risk-redistribution interventions.
2 Observe tolerance of patient for positioning.	Frequent change in position further reduces patient's risk for pressure ulcer development.
3 Compare current risk assessment with previous scores.	Documents effectiveness of interventions and assists in providing individualized plan of care.
4 Evaluate food intake and nutrition laboratory values.	Determines success of nutritional supplements in improving nutritional status.

UNEXPECTED OUTCOMES AND RELATED INTERVENTIONS

1 Skin does not blanch when firmly pressed, has purple discoloration, or has significant color change.
- Reassess frequency of turning schedule.
- Implement agency skin care protocols.
- Consider use of pressure-redistribution surface to reduce pressure ulcer risk.

RECORDING AND REPORTING

- Record patient's risk score.
- Record appearance of skin under pressure.
- Describe position, turning intervals, pressure-redistribution devices, and other prevention strategies.
- Report any need for additional consultations for the high-risk patient.

HOME CARE CONSIDERATIONS

- Instruct family caregiver in use of the 30-degree lateral position. This position prolongs the time between position changes, resulting in fewer sleep interruptions for patient and caregiver.
- Individualize pressure-redistribution maneuvers for patient needs and home environment. Provide family with resources for hospital equipment.

SKILL 48-2 TREATING PRESSURE ULCERS

View Video!

Delegation Considerations

The skill of treating pressure ulcers cannot be delegated to nursing assistive personnel (NAP). In some practice settings you can delegate *nonsterile* dressing application for chronic, established wounds when a nurse has evaluated and designated the protocol. The *assessment* of the wound remains within the scope of the nurse even if the dressing change is delegated. Direct/inform/instruct the NAP to:
- Report changes in skin integrity to the nurse immediately.
- Report pain, fever, or wound drainage to the nurse immediately.
- Report any potential contamination to existing dressing (e.g., patient incontinence or other bodily fluids, dressing becomes dislodged).

Equipment

- Clean gloves
- Plastic bag for dressing disposal
- Measuring device
- Cotton-tipped applicators
- Topical cleaning agent
- Dressing of choice (see Table 48-8)
- Hypoallergenic tape (if needed)
- Documentation record
- Scale for assessing wound healing
- Sterile gloves (check agency policy)

STEP	RATIONALE
ASSESSMENT	
1 Identify patient using two identifiers. (i.e., name and birth date or name and account number) according to facility policy. Compare identifiers with information on the patient's medical record.	Ensures correct patient. Complies with a recommended National Patient Safety Goal (TJC, 2011).

SKILL 48-2 TREATING PRESSURE ULCERS—cont'd

STEP	RATIONALE
2 Assess patient's level of comfort using a scale of 0 to 10 and determine need for pain medication.	Patients tolerate dressing change procedure better if pain is controlled.
3 Determine if patient has allergies to topical agents.	Topical agents cause localized skin reactions.
4 Review order for topical agent or dressing and location.	Ensures that you administer proper medication and treatment.
5 Close room door or bedside curtains. Position patient to allow dressing removal. Describe to patient what will be done.	Provides privacy and ensures that area is accessible for dressing change. Decreases patient's anxiety.
6 Perform hand hygiene and apply clean gloves. Remove dressing and place in plastic bag.	Reduces transmission of microorganisms and prevents accidental exposure to body fluids.
7 Assess pressure ulcer(s). All pressure ulcers need individual assessments.	Consistent assessment provides the basis for evaluating wound progress (Nix, 2012).
a. Note color, type, and percentage of tissue type present in wound base.	Tissue type assists in choice of dressing.
b. Measure width and length of ulcer(s). Determine width by measuring dimension from left to right and length from top to bottom (see illustration).	Ulcer size changes as healing progresses; therefore the longest and widest areas of the wound change over time. Measuring the width and length by measuring consistent areas provides a consistent measurement (Nix, 2012).

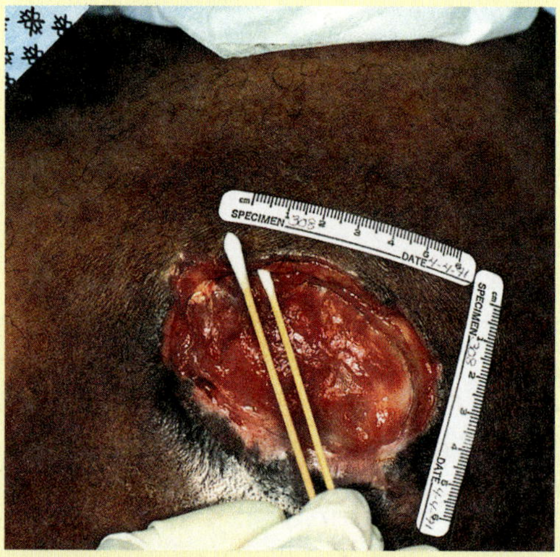

STEP 7b Measuring wound width, length, and undermining.

STEP	RATIONALE
c. Measure depth of pressure ulcer with sterile cotton-tipped applicator or other device that allows measurement of wound depth.	Depth measure is important for determining wound volume. Although surface area adequately represents tissue loss in stage II ulcers, volume more adequately represents tissue loss in stage III and IV wounds.
d. Measure depth of undermining using a cotton-tipped applicator and gently probing under skin edges (see illustration for step 7b).	Undermining represents the loss of the underlying tissue (subcutaneous and muscle) to greater extent than skin. Undermining indicates progressive tissue loss and needs to be accommodated with an appropriate dressing.
8 Assess periwound skin; check for maceration, redness, denuded area.	Deterioration of skin around wound indicates infection, excessive wound exudate, or skin stripping from adhesive removal.

PLANNING

STEP	RATIONALE
1 Explain procedure to patient and family.	Preparatory explanations relieve anxiety, correct any misconceptions about ulcer and its treatment, and offer opportunity for patient and family education.
2 Prepare the following necessary equipment and supplies:	
a. Washbasin, warm water, soap, washcloth, and bath towel	
b. Normal saline or other wound-cleaning agent in sterile solution container	Ulcer surface must be cleaned before application of topical agents and new dressing.

CLINICAL DECISION: *Use only noncytotoxic agents to clean ulcers.*

STEP	RATIONALE
c. Prescribed topical agent (e.g., enzymatic agents, topical antibiotic). Follow manufacturer instruction on package insert carefully.	Enzymes debride dead tissue to clean ulcer surface. Topical antibiotics are used to decrease bioburden of wound and should be considered for use if no healing is noted after 2 to 4 weeks of optimal care (WOCN, 2010).

CLINICAL DECISION: *If using enzymatic debriding agent, do not use wound-cleaning agents with metals.*

STEP	RATIONALE
d. Select appropriate dressing and tape based on pressure ulcer characteristics, purpose for which dressing is intended, and patient care setting (see Table 48-8).	Dressing should maintain a moist environment for wound while keeping surrounding skin dry.
3 Position patient to allow dressing removal and position plastic bag for dressing disposal.	Area should be accessible for dressing change. Proper disposal of old dressing promotes proper handling of contaminated waste.
IMPLEMENTATION	
1 Close room door or bedside curtains. Perform hand hygiene and apply clean gloves. Open sterile packages and topical solution containers as necessary.	Maintains privacy and provides organized access to supplies.
2 Remove bed linen and patient's gown as necessary to expose ulcer and surrounding skin. Keep remaining parts covered.	Prevents unnecessary exposure.
3 Clean ulcer thoroughly with normal saline or cleaning agent. Clean with irrigating syringe for deep ulcers.	Removes wound debris.
4 Remove gloves, perform hand hygiene, and apply clean or sterile gloves.	Aseptic technique must be maintained during cleaning and all phases of pressure ulcer treatment. Check agency policy regarding use of clean or sterile gloves.
5 Apply topical agents as prescribed:	
a. Debriding enzymes	
(1) Apply thin, even layer of ointment over necrotic areas of ulcer only. Do not apply enzyme to surrounding skin. Check manufacturer direction for frequency of application.	Thin layer absorbs and acts more effectively than thick layer. Excess medication irritates surrounding skin (Rolstad, Bryant, and Nix, 2012). Some enzymes cause burning, paresthesia, and dermatitis to surrounding skin.
(2) Apply gauze dressing directly over ulcer.	Protects wound and keeps enzymes in place. Prevents bacteria from entering wound.
(3) Tape securely in place.	Keeps dressing in place.
b. Hydrogel	
(1) Cover surface of ulcer with hydrogel using applicator or gloved hand.	Provides maintenance of moist wound environment.
(2) Apply dry gauze, hydrocolloid, or transparent film dressing over wound and adhere to intact skin.	Covers wound base, maintaining hydrogel wound interface.
c. Calcium alginate	
(1) Pack wound with alginate using applicator or gloved hand.	Provides maintenance of wound moisture while absorbing excess drainage.
(2) Apply dry gauze or foam over alginate. Tape in place.	Holds alginate against wound surface.
6 Reposition patient comfortably off pressure area and other pressure points.	Reduces pressure on existing wound and decreases pressure on at-risk areas.
7 Remove gloves and dispose of soiled supplies. Perform hand hygiene.	Reduces transmission of microorganisms.
EVALUATION	
1 Evaluate pressure ulcer at each dressing change or sooner if wound or patient's condition deteriorates (Nix, 2012). Use agency tool for wound assessment.	Not all patients with wounds demonstrate quick wound healing because of other health care issues. Wound evaluation provides a report of wound healing progress or lack of it.
2 Compare wound findings to identified plan of care; if wound is not progressing toward healing as indicated by an increase in size, increased presence of pain, foul-smelling drainage, or increase in devitalized tissue, discuss findings with health care team.	Ensures that an appropriate plan for wound care is in place.

CLINICAL DECISION: *A clean pressure ulcer should show evidence of some healing within 2 to 4 weeks. Do not use the pressure ulcer staging system to measure healing. System measures depth of wound, not healing (WOCN, 2010).*

UNEXPECTED OUTCOMES AND RELATED INTERVENTIONS

1 Skin surrounding ulcer becomes macerated.
- Reduce exposure of surrounding skin to topical agents and moisture.
- Consider the use of a liquid skin barrier on periwound skin.

2 Ulcer becomes deeper with increased drainage.
- Notify health care provider about possible change in pressure ulcer status.
- Obtain necessary wound cultures.
- Obtain additional consults (e.g., wound care specialist).

RECORDING AND REPORTING

- Complete wound documentation required for one of the wound assessment instruments per agency protocol.
- Record appearance of ulcer; describe type of topical agent, dressing applied, and patient response.
- Report any deterioration in ulcer appearance to nurse in charge or health care provider.

HOME CARE CONSIDERATIONS

- Patients need to dispose of contaminated dressings in the home in a manner consistent with local regulations.
- Discuss need for home pressure-redistribution surface or bed.

SKILL 48-3 APPLYING DRY AND MOIST DRESSINGS

Delegation Considerations

The skill of applying dry and moist dressings to the new acute wound cannot be delegated to nursing assistive personnel (NAP). In some settings aspects of wound care such as changing dressings using *clean* technique for chronic wounds are delegated. The *assessment* of the wound remains within the scope of the nurse even if the dressing change is delegated. Direct the NAP to:

- Report pain, fever, bleeding, or wound drainage to the nurse immediately.
- Report any potential contamination to existing dressing (e.g., patient incontinence or other bodily fluids, dressing becomes dislodged).

Equipment

- Sterile gloves
- Variety of gauze dressings and pads
- Irrigation kit
- Cleaning solution
- Sterile solution
- Clean, disposable gloves
- Tape, ties, or bandage as needed
- Waterproof pad and bag
- Extra gauze dressings, or topper dressing (ABD pads)
- Montgomery ties; elastic net
- Option: Mask or eyewear for risk of splashing

STEP	RATIONALE
ASSESSMENT	
1 Identify patient using two identifiers. (i.e., name and birth date or name and account number) according to facility policy. Compare identifiers with information on the patient's medical record.	Ensures correct patient. Complies with a recommended National Patient Safety Goal (TJC, 2011).
2 Perform hand hygiene. Review medical record for information about size and location of wound.	Reduces transmission of microorganisms. Helps to plan for proper type and amount of supplies needed. Alerts you when assistance is needed to hold dressings in place.
3 Assess patient's level of comfort using a scale of 0 to 10.	Removal of dry dressing is painful; some patients require pain medication.
4 Review orders for dressing change procedure.	Indicates type of dressing or applications to use.
5 Assess patient's and family's knowledge of purpose and steps of dressing change.	Determine specific areas for patient and family teaching.
6 Assess for risk of delayed or poor wound healing (e.g., age, obesity, diabetes, peripheral vascular diseases, poor nutritional status, steroid medications, stress, immunosuppression medications, and radiation therapy).	
PLANNING	
1 Explain procedure to patient and instruct him or her not to touch wound area or sterile supplies.	Decreases anxiety. Sudden, unexpected movement on patient's part results in contamination of wound and supplies.
2 Position patient comfortably and drape with bath blanket to expose only wound site.	Provides access to wound yet minimizes unnecessary exposure.
3 Plan dressing change 30 to 60 minutes following administration of analgesia.	Allows for peak action of medication so patient has optimal level of comfort during dressing change. Patients tolerate dressing changes when their pain is controlled.
IMPLEMENTATION	
1 Close room door or pull bedside curtains. Perform hand hygiene and apply gown, goggles, and mask when risk for spray exists.	Provides privacy and reduces transmission of microorganisms.
2 Position patient comfortably and drape only to expose wound site.	Draping provides access to wound while minimizing unnecessary exposure.
3 Place disposable bag within reach of work area. Fold top of bag to make cuff (see illustration).	Ensures easy disposal of soiled dressings. Prevents soiling of outer surface of bag.
4 *Remove tape:* Pull parallel to skin toward dressing; remove remaining adhesive from skin.	Pulling tape toward dressing reduces stress on suture line or wound edges.
5 With gloved hand carefully remove gauze dressings one layer at a time, taking care not to dislodge drains or tubes.	Removal of one layer at a time reduces chance of accidental removal of underlying drains.
a. If dressing sticks on a wet-to-dry dressing, do not moisten it; instead gently free it and alert patient of potential discomfort.	Wet-to-dry dressing should debride wound (Ramundo, 2012). Do not wet dressing to remove it. It is supposed to be dry so it removes necrotic tissue from wound.
b. If dressing sticks on dry dressing, moisten with saline and then remove.	Prevents tearing of wound edges.

CLINICAL DECISION: *Never use a wet-to-dry dressing in a clean granulating wound. Use only for debridement (Ramundo, 2012).*

STEP	RATIONALE
6 Observe wound for color, edema, drains, and exudates and amount of drainage on dresssing.	Provides estimate of drainage amount and assessment of condition of wound.
7 Fold dressings with drainage contained inside and remove gloves inside out. With small dressings remove gloves inside out over dressing (see illustration). Dispose of gloves and soiled dressings in disposable bag. Perform hand hygiene.	Reduces transmission of microorganisms. Prevents contact of hands with material on gloves.

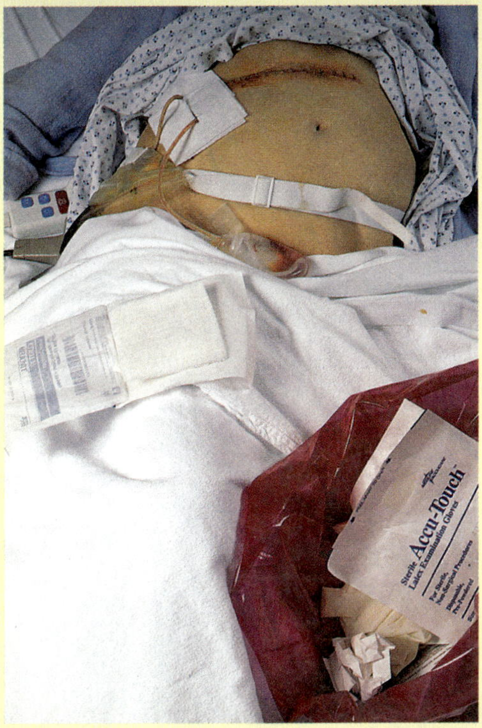

STEP 3 Disposable waterproof bag placed near dressing site.

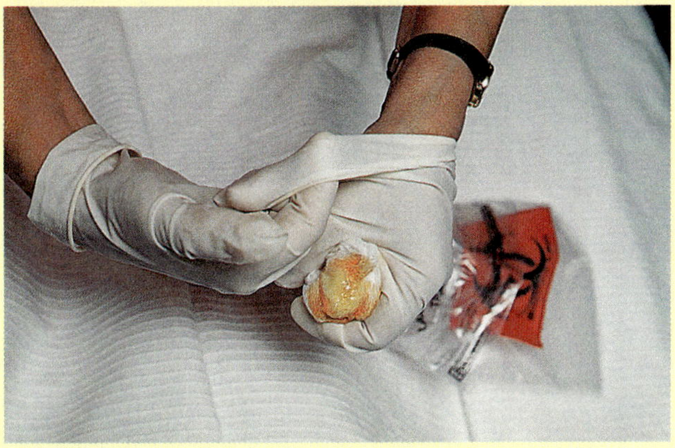

STEP 7 Removal of disposable gloves over contaminated dressing.

STEP	RATIONALE
8 Open sterile dressing tray or individually wrapped sterile supplies. Place on bedside table.	Sterile dressings remain sterile while on or within sterile surface. Preparation of supplies prevents break in technique during dressing change.
9 Clean wound with solution. Clean from least-contaminated area, which is the incision or center of wound, to most-contaminated area, which is outside of incision and surrounding skin. Dry area.	Prevents contamination of previously cleaned area.
10 If ordered, clean or irrigate wound:	Removes drainage containing microorganisms.
a. Pour ordered solution into sterile irrigation container.	
b. Apply clean gloves and protective eyewear. Place waterproof pad under patient. Using syringe, gently allow solution to flow over wound. (Some commercial cleaners come in a spray bottle. Spray wound to loosen debris.)	
c. Continue until irrigation flow is clear.	
d. Dry surrounding skin using gauze pads.	
e. Measure wound.	Measurement of wound size with each dressing change provides data about progression of wound healing.
11 Apply dressing:	
a. Dry dressing	
(1) Apply clean or sterile gloves. Check agency policy.	Some agencies or condition of wounds requires sterile gloves. Allows handling of sterile supplies without contamination.
(2) Inspect wound for appearance, drains, drainage, and integrity.	Indicates status of wound healing.
(3) Apply sterile, loose woven gauze dry dressing, covering wound.	Protects wound from external environment.
(4) Apply topper dressing if indicated.	Topper dressing (e.g., ABD) prevents strike-through of wound drainage and provides a surface to tape the dressing in place.
b. Moist dressing	
(1) Apply sterile gloves (see agency policy).	Allows handling of sterile supplies without contamination.
(2) Assess appearance of surrounding skin (see illustration).	Surrounding skin assessment provides an evaluation of wound management.

SKILL 48-3 APPLYING DRY AND MOIST DRESSINGS—cont'd

STEP	RATIONALE
(3) Moisten gauze with prescribed solution. Gently wring out excess solution. Unfold.	Gauze needs to be moist to allow for absorption of wound debris.
(4) Apply gauze as single layer directly onto wound surface (see illustration). If wound is deep, gently pack dressing into wound base by hand or forceps until all wound surfaces are in contact with gauze. If tunneling is present, use cotton-tipped applicator to place gauze into tunneled area. Be sure that gauze does not touch surrounding skin.	Inner gauze needs to be moist, not dripping wet, to absorb drainage and adhere to debris. Excessively moist dressings result in moisture-associated skin damage (maceration) in periwound skin (Gray and Weir, 2007). Wound needs to be loosely packed to facilitate wicking of drainage into absorbent outer layer of dressing.
(5) Cover with sterile dry gauze and topper dressing.	Topper dressing prevents strike-through of wound drainage and provides surface to tape dressing in place.
12 Secure dressing.	
a. *Tape:* Apply nonallergenic tape to secure dressing in place.	Goal for securing a dressing is to keep dressing in place and intact without causing damage to underlying and surrounding skin.
b. Montgomery ties (see Fig. 48-22)	
(1) Expose adhesive surface of tape on end of each tie.	
(2) Place ties on opposite sides of dressing.	
(3) Place adhesive directly on skin or use skin barrier.	A solid skin barrier protects intact skin from stretch and tension of adhesive tape.
(4) Secure dressing by lacing ties across it.	
c. For dressings on an extremity, secure dressing with rolled gauze or elastic net (see illustration).	Prevents slipping of dressing.

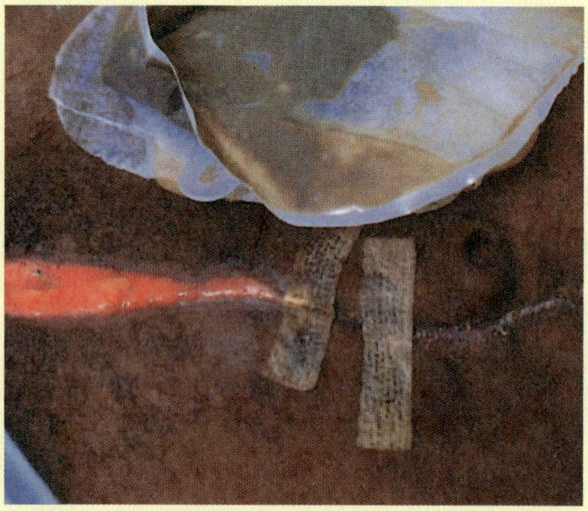

STEP 11b(2) Exposure of wound facilitates assessment of wound and surrounding skin.

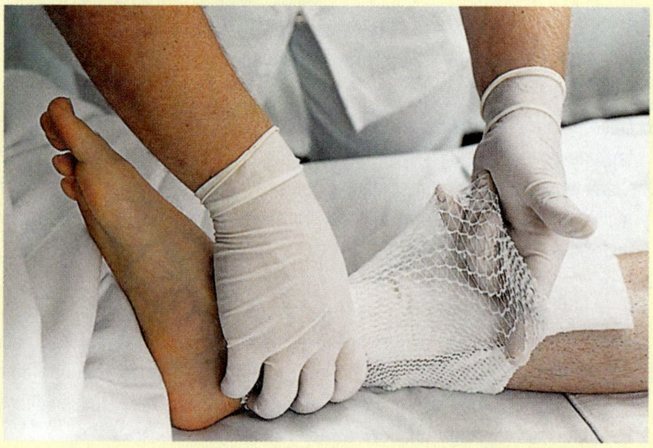

STEP 12c Elastic net securing lower-extremity dressing.

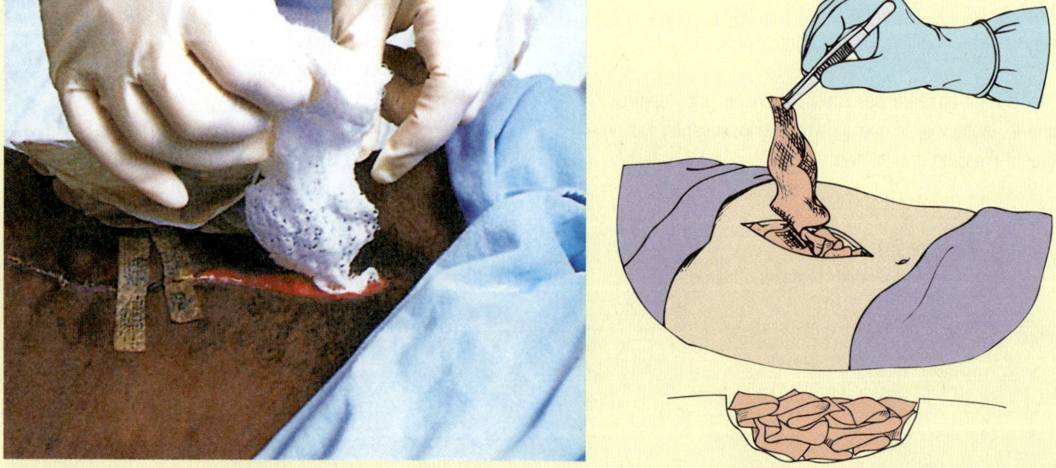

STEP 11b(4) Packing wound with single layer of gauze.

STEP	RATIONALE
12 Remove gloves and dispose of in bag. Remove any mask or eyewear.	Reduces transmission of infection.
13 Write date and time dressing applied on tape in ink (not marker).	
14 Assist patient to comfortable position.	Improves patient comfort.
15 Dispose of supplies and perform hand hygiene.	Reduces transmission of infection.

EVALUATION

1 Inspect condition of wound and any drainage.	Determines rate of healing.
2 Ask patient to rate level of pain during and after procedure.	Pain is early indicator of wound complications or result of dressing material pulling underlying tissue.
3 Inspect condition of dressing and note any observable drainage every shift.	Determines status of wound drainage.
4 Ask patient to describe techniques of dressing change.	Documents patient learning.

UNEXPECTED OUTCOMES AND RELATED INTERVENTIONS

1 Wound appears inflamed, tender, with or without drainage.
- Monitor patient for signs of infection (e.g., increased temperature, white blood cell count).
- Obtain wound culture per order.
- Notify health care provider.

2 Wound drainage increases.
- Increase frequency of dressing changes.
- Notify health care provider, who may consider drain placement to facilitate wound drainage.

3 Wound bleeds during dressing change.
- Observe color. If drainage is bright red and excessive, you need to apply pressure.
- Inspect along dressing and underneath patient to determine amount of bleeding.
- Obtain vital signs as needed.
- Notify health care provider.

4 Patient reports a sensation that "something has given way under the dressing."
- Observe wound for increased drainage or separation of sutures.
- Protect wound. Cover with sterile moist dressing.
- Instruct patient to lie still and place on NPO status.
- Notify health care provider.

RECORDING AND REPORTING

- Report brisk, bright red bleeding, or evidence of wound dehiscence or evisceration to health care provider immediately.
- Report wound and periwound tissue appearance, color, tissue type, presence and characteristics of exudate, type and amount of dressings used, and tolerance of patient to procedure.
- Record patient's level of comfort.

HOME CARE CONSIDERATIONS

- More expensive specialty dressings are sometimes used because they decrease the frequency of dressing changes.
- Clean dressings may also be used in the home setting.
- Patients need to dispose of contaminated dressings in the home in a manner consistent with local regulations.

SKILL 48-4 IMPLEMENTATION OF NEGATIVE-PRESSURE WOUND THERAPY

Delegation Considerations

The assessment for and placement of negative-pressure wound therapy (NPWT) cannot be delegated to nursing assistive personnel (NAP). Direct the NAP to:
- Report to the nurse any change in patient's temperature, level of comfort.
- Change in the pressure in the NPWT unit.
- Any change in the integrity of the dressing.

Equipment

- NPWT unit (For this skill the vacuum-assisted closure (V.A.C.) unit is used for illustration; several other systems are available, and their application may be slightly different; refer to manufacturer directions.) (requires health care provider order) (see Fig. 48-19)
- Foam dressing and transparent dressing
- Tubing for connection between NPWT unit and dressing
- Gloves, clean and sterile
- Scissors (sterile)
- Skin preparation/skin barrier
- Moist washcloth
- Plastic trash bag
- Linen bag
- Stethoscope
- Protective gown, mask, goggles if risk of splashing wound drainage
- Gauze squares

SKILL 48-4 IMPLEMENTATION OF NEGATIVE-PRESSURE WOUND THERAPY—cont'd

STEP	RATIONALE
ASSESSMENT	
1 Identify patient using two identifiers (i.e., name and birth date or name and account number) according to facility policy. Compare identifiers with information on the patient's medical record.	Ensures correct patient. Complies with a recommended National Patient Safety Goal (TJC, 2011).
2 Assess location, appearance, and size of wound to be dressed (see Skill 48-2).	Allows you to gather information regarding status of wound healing, presence of complications, and type of supplies and assistance needed to apply the NPWT dressing.
3 Review health care provider's orders for frequency of dressing change, type of foam to use, and amount of negative pressure to be used.	Health care provider orders frequency of dressing changes and special instructions.
4 Assess patient's level of comfort using a scale of 0 to 10.	Patient who is comfortable during procedure is less likely to move suddenly, causing wound or supply contamination.
5 Assess patient's and family member's knowledge of purpose of dressing.	Identifies patient's learning needs. Prepares patient and family if dressing needs to be changed at home.
PLANNING	
1 Explain to patient what the dressing change involves.	Provides patient with rationale for dressing change and reduces fears. Maintaining patient comfort assists in completing skill smoothly.
2 Administer ordered analgesic 30 minutes before dressing change.	Provides time for pain medication to have optimal effect to reduce or relieve patient's pain at wound site.
3 Perform hand hygiene. Assemble supplies.	Reduces transmission of microorganisms. Organizes procedure.
IMPLEMENTATION	
1 Close room door or cubicle curtains.	Provides privacy.
2 Position patient comfortably and drape to expose only wound site. Instruct patient not to touch wound or sterile supplies.	Draping provides access to wound while minimizing unnecessary exposure.
3 Place disposable waterproof bag within reach of work area with top folded to make a cuff.	Facilitates safe disposal of soiled dressings.
4 Apply clean gloves. If there is a risk for splash or spray, apply protective gown, goggles, and mask.	Reduces exposure to infectious microorganisms.
5 Keep system in "de vac" mode for 30 to 60 minutes before changing dressing.	Found to loosen foam dressing for easier, less painful removal.
6 When NPWT is in place, push therapy on/off button.	
a. Keeping tube connectors with NPWT unit; disconnect tubes from one another to drain fluids into canister.	Deactivates therapy and allows for proper drainage of fluid in drainage tubing.
b. Before lowering, tighten clamp on canister tube.	
7 Gently stretch transparent film horizontally and slowly pull away from skin.	Reduces stress on suture line or wound edges, irritation, and discomfort.
8 Remove old dressing, observing appearance and drainage on dressing. Use caution to avoid tension on any drains that are present. Discard dressing and remove gloves. Perform hand hygiene.	Determines dressings needed for replacement. Avoids accidental removal of drains because they are sometimes sutured in place.
9 Apply sterile or clean gloves (see agency policy). Irrigate wound with normal saline or other solution ordered by health care provider. Blot with gauze to dry.	Irrigation removes wound debris.

CLINICAL DECISION: *When drainage looks purulent, amount or color changes, or it has a foul odor, obtain wound cultures even when they are not ordered for that particular dressing change (Chua et al., 2000; Jerome, 2007).*

STEP	RATIONALE
10 Measure wound as ordered: at baseline, first dressing change, weekly; discharge from therapy. Remove and discard gloves. Perform hand hygiene.	Objectively documents wound healing process in response to NPWT (Nix, 2012).
11 Depending on type of wound, apply new sterile or clean gloves.	Fresh sterile wounds require sterile gloves. Chronic wounds may require clean technique. Never wear same gloves worn to remove old dressing or irrigate wound because cross-contamination may occur.
12 Apply skin protectant/barrier film to skin around wound.	Maintains air-tight seal needed for NPWT and protects periwound skin from maceration.
13 Prepare wound edges with skin preparation to enhance seal and protect the periwound tissue.	Promotes adherence of dressing to site.
14 Prepare foam dressing.	
a. Select appropriate foam.	Black, polyurethane (PU) foam has larger pores and is most effective in stimulating granulation tissue and **wound contraction**. White, polyvinyl alcohol (PVA) soft foam is denser with smaller pores and is used when growth of granulation tissue needs to be restricted (KCI, 2007; Netsch, 2012).

STEP	RATIONALE
b. Using sterile scissors, cut foam to exact wound size with foam height extending ½ inch above skin surface. Dressing must fit size and shape of wound, including tunnels and undermined areas.	Foam will contract to level of skin.

CLINICAL DECISION: *Some patients experience more pain with the black foam because of excessive wound contraction. For this reason they often need to be switched to the PVA soft foam.*

STEP	RATIONALE
15 Gently place foam in wound; be sure that foam is in contact with entire wound base, margins, and tunneled and undermined areas (see illustration).	Maintains negative pressure to entire wound.
16 Apply wrinkle-free transparent dressing over foam and 3 to 5 cm (1.2 to 2 inches) of surrounding healthy skin. Secure tubing to unit (see illustration).	Ensures that wound is properly covered and helps achieve negative-pressure seal (see Box 48-14). Connects negative pressure from the NPWT unit to wound foam.
17 Secure tubing to transparent film, aligning drainage holes to ensure an occlusive seal. Do not apply tension to drape and tubing.	Excessive tension compresses foam dressing and impedes wound healing. It also produces shear force on periwound area (KCI, 2007).
18 Secure tubing several centimeters away from the dressing.	Prevents pull on primary dressing, which causes leaks in negative-pressure system (Chua et al., 2000; KCI, 2007).
19 Once you have completely covered the wound (see illustration), connect tubing from dressing to tubing from canister and NPWT unit.	Intermittent or continuous negative pressure can be administered at 50 to 175 mm Hg, according to health care provider's order and patient comfort. The average is 125 mm Hg (Netsch, 2012).
a. Remove canister from sterile packaging and push into unit until you hear a click. NOTE: An alarm sounds if canister is not engaged properly.	
b. Connect dressing tubing to canister tubing. Make sure that both clamps are open.	
c. Place unit on level surface or hang from foot of bed. NOTE: The unit alarms and deactivates therapy if it is tilted beyond 45 degrees.	
d. Press in green-lit power button and set pressure as ordered.	
20 Discard old dressing materials; remove gloves and perform hand hygiene.	Reduces transmission of microorganisms.
21 Inspect NPWT system to verify that negative pressure is achieved.	Negative pressure is achieved when there is an airtight seal.
a. Verify that display screen reads THERAPY ON.	
b. Be sure that clamps are open and tubing is patent.	
c. Identify air leaks by listening with stethoscope or moving hand around edges of wound while applying light pressure.	
d. If leak is present, use strips of transparent film to patch areas around edges of wound.	

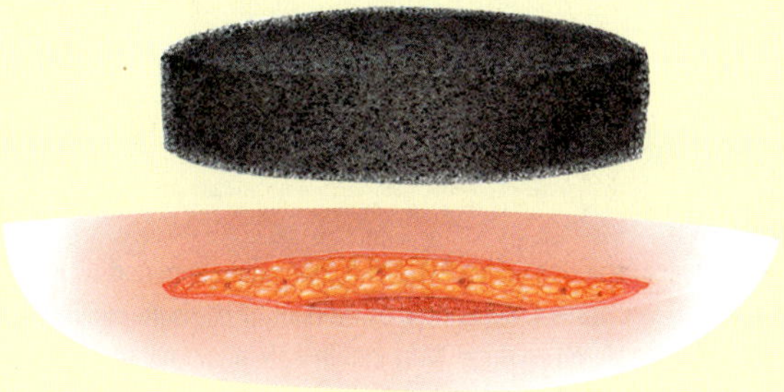

STEP 15 Dressing application. Properly sized foam to cover wound.

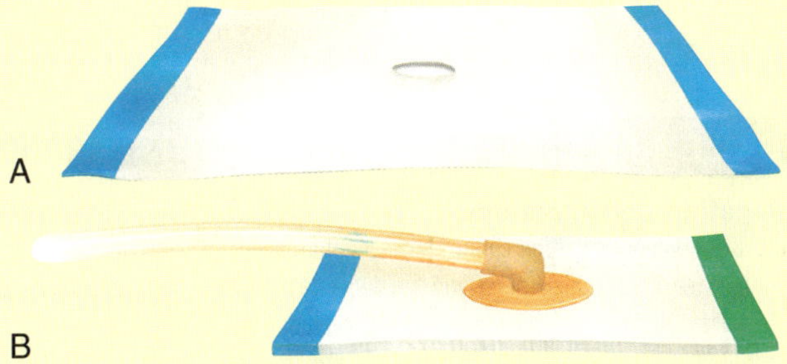

STEP 16 **A,** Wrinkle-free transparent dressing applied over foam. **B,** Secure tubing to foam and transparent dressing. (Courtesy Kinetic Concepts, Inc [KCI], San Antonio, Tex.)

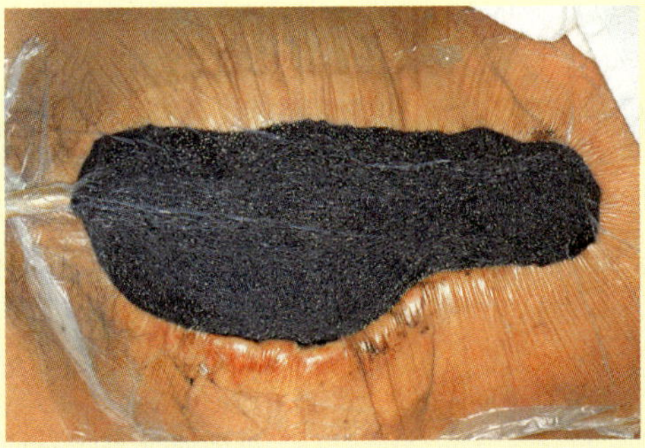

STEP 19 Foam, transparent dressing, and tubing secured over existing wound. (Courtesy Kinetic Concepts, Inc [KCI], San Antonio, Tex.)

SKILL 48-4 IMPLEMENTATION OF NEGATIVE-PRESSURE WOUND THERAPY—cont'd

STEP	RATIONALE
EVALUATION	
1 Inspect condition of wound on an ongoing basis; note drainage and odor.	Determines status of wound healing.
2 Ask patient to rate pain using a scale of 0 to 10.	Determines patient's level of comfort following procedure.
3 Compare wound with baseline wound assessment.	Provides objective documentation of wound healing.
4 Verify airtight dressing seal and proper negative pressure.	To achieve prescribed vacuum level, wound must be covered with airtight seal. This airtight seal and negative pressure promote wound drainage, circulation, and healing.
5 Measure wound drainage in canister on regular basis per agency policy.	Monitors fluid balance and wound drainage.

UNEXPECTED OUTCOMES AND RELATED INTERVENTIONS

1 Wound appears inflamed and tender, drainage has increased, and an odor is present.
- Notify health care provider.
- Obtain wound culture per order.
- Increase frequency of dressing changes.

2 Patient reports increase in pain.
- If using black foam, switch to the PVA foam product.
- Patient sometimes needs more analgesic support when NPWT is initiated.
- Reduce negative pressure.

3 Negative pressure seal has broken.
- *Take preventive measures:* Shave hair around wound, avoid wrinkles in transparent dressing, and avoid use of adhesive remover because it leaves residue that hinders film adherence.
- Reinforce with transparent dressing strips.

RECORDING AND REPORTING

- Record appearance of wound, color, characteristics of any drainage, and presence of wound healing augmentation.
- Record pressure setting of NPWT.
- Record date and time of dressing change.
- Report brisk, bright bleeding; evidence of poor wound healing; and possible wound infection.

HOME CARE CONSIDERATIONS

- Patients can use NPWT in the home safely. Some patients need clinic visits or home care nursing visits to monitor wound healing.
- Provide resources to patient for supplies for NPWT.
- Instruct family and caregiver regarding proper disposal of contaminated product.

SKILL 48-5 PERFORMING WOUND IRRIGATION

View Video!

Delegation Considerations

The skill of wound irrigation cannot be delegated to nursing assistive personnel. In the case of a chronic wound, you can delegate cleaning using *clean* technique. Assessment of any wound, care of acute new wounds, and evaluation of wound irrigation are responsibilities of the nurse and are never delegated. Direct the NAP to:
- Report any change in wound appearance or increased wound drainage to the nurse.
- Use proper clean technique to avoid cross-contamination from irrigation syringes and equipment.

Equipment

- Irrigant/cleaning solution (volume 1.2 to 2 times the estimated wound volume)
- Irrigation delivery system, depending on amount of pressure desired:
- Sterile irrigation 35-mL syringe with sterile soft angio catheter or 19-gauge needle (Rolstad, Bryant, and Nix, 2012)
- Clean gloves and sterile gloves (check agency policy)
- Waterproof underpad, if needed
- Gauze dressing supplies
- Disposable waterproof bag
- Gown, goggles, or mask, if risk of spray

STEP	RATIONALE
ASSESSMENT	
1 Identify patient using two identifiers (i.e., name and birth date or name and account number) according to facility policy. Compare identifiers with information on the patient's medical record.	Ensures correct patient. Complies with a recommended National Patient Safety Goal (TJC, 2011).
2 Assess patient's level of pain. Administer prescribed analgesic 30 to 45 minutes before starting wound irrigation procedure.	Discomfort is related directly to wound or indirectly to muscle tension or immobility. Increased comfort level permits patient to move more easily and be positioned to facilitate wound irrigation.
3 Review medical record for health care provider's prescription for irrigation of open wound and type of solution to be used.	Open wound irrigation requires medical order, including type of solution to use.

STEP	RATIONALE
4 Assess medical record for signs and symptoms related to patient's open wound.	Data provide a baseline to indicate change in condition of wound (Nix, 2012).
a. Extent of impairment of skin integrity, including size of wound (Measure length, width, and depth. Wounds should be measured in centimeters and in the following order: length, width, and depth.)	Assesses volume of irrigation solution needed. Data also used as baseline to indicate change in condition of wound.
b. Drainage from wound (amount and color) (Amount can be measured by part of dressing saturated or in terms of quantity [e.g., scant, moderate, copious].)	Expect amount to decrease as healing takes place. Serous drainage is clear like plasma; sanguineous or bright red drainage indicates fresh bleeding; serosanguineous drainage is pink; purulent drainage is thick and yellow, pale green, or white.
c. Odor (must state whether or not there is odor)	Strong odor indicates infectious process.
d. Wound color	Color represents a balance between necrotic tissue and new scar tissue. Proper selection of wound products based on the color of the wound facilitates removal of necrotic tissue and promotes new tissue growth (Rolstad, Bryant, and Nix, 2007).
e. Consistency of drainage	Type and color of drainage depend on moisture of wound and type of organisms present.
f. Culture reports	Chronic wounds heal by secondary intention, and they are often colonized with bacteria.
g. Condition of dressing: Dry and clean; evidence of bleeding, profuse drainage	Provides an initial assessment of present wound drainage.
PLANNING	
1 Explain procedure of wound irrigation and cleaning.	Information reduces patient's anxiety.
2 Administer prescribed analgesic 30 to 60 minutes before starting wound irrigation procedure.	Promotes pain control and permits patient to move more easily and be positioned to facilitate wound irrigation.
3 Position patient.	
a. Position comfortably so wound is vertical to collection basin, which permits gravitational flow of irrigating solution through wound and into collection receptacle.	Directing solution from top to bottom of wound and from clean to contaminated area reduces spread of infection. Position patient during planning stage, keeping in mind the bed surfaces needed for later preparation of equipment.
b. Place container of irrigant/cleaning solution in basin of hot water to warm solution to body temperature.	Warmed solution increases comfort and reduces vascular constriction response in tissues.
c. Place padding or extra towel in bed.	Protects bedding.
IMPLEMENTATION	
1 Perform hand hygiene.	Reduces transmission of microorganisms.
2 Form cuff on waterproof bag and place it near bed.	Cuffing helps to maintain large opening, thereby permitting placement of contaminated dressing without touching refuse bag itself.
3 Close room door or bed curtains.	Maintains privacy.
4 Apply gown, mask, or goggles if needed.	Protects nurse from splashes or sprays of blood and body fluids.
5 Apply clean gloves and remove soiled dressing and discard in waterproof bag. Discard gloves and perform hand hygiene.	Reduces transmission of microorganisms.
6 Prepare equipment; open sterile supplies.	
7 Put on clean or sterile gloves (check agency policy).	
8 To irrigate wound with wide opening:	
a. Fill 35-mL syringe with irrigation solution.	Flushing wound helps remove debris and facilitates healing by secondary intention.
b. Attach 19-gauge needle or angio catheter (see Fig. 48-17).	Provides ideal pressure for cleaning and removing debris (Gardner and Frantz, 2008).
c. Hold syringe tip 2.5 cm (1 inch) above upper end of wound and over area being cleaned.	Prevents syringe contamination. Careful placement of syringe prevents unsafe pressure of flowing solution.
d. Using continuous pressure, flush wound; repeat Steps 8a, b, and c until solution draining into basin is clear.	Clear solution indicates that you have removed all debris.
9 To irrigate deep wound with very small opening:	
a. Attach soft angio catheter to filled irrigating syringe.	Catheter permits direct flow of irrigant into wound. Expect wound to take longer to empty when opening is small.
b. Lubricate tip of catheter with irrigating solution; then gently insert it into wound and pull out about 1 cm (½ inch).	Removes tip from fragile inner wall of wound.
c. Using slow, continuous pressure, flush wound. **CAUTION:** Splashing sometimes occurs during this step.	Cleans all wound surfaces.
d. Pinch off catheter just below syringe while keeping catheter in place.	Avoids contamination of sterile solution.
e. Remove and refill syringe. Reconnect to catheter and repeat until solution draining into basin is clear.	

SKILL 48-5 PERFORMING WOUND IRRIGATION—cont'd

STEP	RATIONALE
CLINICAL DECISION: *Pulsatile high-pressure lavage may be the irrigation of choice for necrotic wounds. The amount of irrigant depends on the size of the wound. Pressure settings on the device should remain between 8 and 15 psi. Do not use pulsatile high-pressure lavage on exposed blood vessels, muscle, tendon, and bone. This type of irrigation should not be used with graft sites and should be used with caution in patients receiving anticoagulant therapy (Ramundo, 2012).*	
10 Obtain cultures, if needed, after cleaning with nonbacteriostatic saline.	The type of wound culture obtained depends on the resources available in the facility. The three most common types of wound specimens are wound tissue, needle aspirated wound fluid, and swabs (Gardner and Frantz, 2008).
CLINICAL DECISION: *Consider culturing a wound if it has a foul, purulent odor; inflammation surrounds the wound; a nondraining wound begins to drain; or patient is febrile.*	
11 Assess type of tissue in wound bed and periwound skin.	Identifies wound-healing progress and determines type of wound cleaning needed; determines if wound has increased in size.
12 Dry wound edges with gauze.	Prevents maceration of surrounding tissue caused by excess moisture.
13 Apply appropriate dressing (see Skills 48-2 and 48-3).	Maintains protective barrier and healing environment for wound.
14 Remove gloves and, if worn, mask, goggles, and gown.	Prevents transfer of microorganisms.
15 Dispose of equipment and soiled supplies. Perform hand hygiene.	Reduces transmission of microorganisms.
16 Assist patient to comfortable position.	

EVALUATION

1 Inspect dressing periodically.	Determines patient's response to wound irrigation and need to modify plan of care.
2 Determine patient's level of pain.	Patient's pain should not increase as a result of wound irrigation.
3 Observe for presence of retained irrigant.	Retained irrigant is medium for bacterial growth and subsequent infection.

UNEXPECTED OUTCOMES AND RELATED INTERVENTIONS

1 Wound does not appear to heal.
- Obtain wound culture per order.
- Notify health care provider, who may change dressing and or irrigation frequency.

2 Wound drainage increases.
- Apply more absorbent gauze.
- Increase the frequency of irrigation.

RECORDING AND REPORTING

- Record wound irrigation, patient response, and appearance of wound on progress notes.
- Immediately report any evidence of fresh bleeding, sharp increase in pain, retention of irrigant, or signs of shock to attending health care provider.

HOME CARE CONSIDERATIONS

- Teach patient and caregiver how to make normal saline, especially if cost is an issue. You make normal saline by using 8 tsp of salt in 1 gallon of distilled water (Fellows and Cresodina, 2006).

SKILL 48-6 APPLYING AN ABDOMINAL BINDER

Delegation Considerations

The skill of applying an abdominal binder can be delegated to nursing assistive personnel (NAP). The nurse is responsible for wound assessment; the evaluation of wound care interventions and assessment of the patient's ability to breathe deeply, cough effectively, and move independently; and assessment of skin for irritation/abrasion, of incision/wound and dressing, and of comfort level before a binder or sling is applied for the first time. Direct the NAP to:
- Immediately notify the nurse of any change in patient's respiratory status.
- Report any increase in wound drainage to the nurse.
- Report any changes in skin integrity under or adjacent to the binder to the nurse.
- Remove the binder at prescribed intervals.

Equipment

- Gloves if wound drainage is present
- Abdominal binder:
  - Correct size cloth/elastic straight binder
  - Safety pins (unless Velcro closure or metal fasteners are attached): six to eight safety pins are usually adequate for abdominal binders

STEP	RATIONALE
ASSESSMENT	
1 Identify patient using two identifiers (i.e., name and birth date or name and account number) according to facility policy. Compare identifiers with information on the patient's medical record.	Ensures correct patient. Complies with a recommended National Patient Safety Goal (TJC, 2011).
2 Observe patient with need for support of abdomen. Observe ability to breathe deeply and cough effectively.	Baseline assessment determines patient's ability to breathe and cough. Impaired ventilation of lung leads to alveolar atelectasis and inadequate arterial oxygenation.
3 Review medical record if medical order for binder is required and reasons for application.	Application of supportive binders is based on nursing judgment. In some situations health care provider input is required.
4 Inspect skin for actual or potential alterations in integrity. Observe for irritation, abrasion, skin surfaces that rub against one another, or allergic response to adhesive tape used to secure dressing.	Actual impairments in skin integrity sometimes worsen with application of binder. Binders sometimes cause pressure and excoriation.
5 Inspect any surgical dressing.	Dressing replacement or reinforcement precedes application of any binder.
6 Assess patient's comfort level, using analog scale of 0 to 10 (see Chapter 43) and noting any objective signs and symptoms.	Data determines effectiveness of binder placement.
7 Gather necessary data for sizing appropriate binder.	Ensures proper fit of binder.
PLANNING	
1 Explain procedure to patient and family.	Promotes patient's understanding and reduces anxiety.
2 Demonstrate skill to patient or family caregiver.	Reduces anxiety and ensures continuity of care after discharge.
3 Help patient to a comfortable position.	
4 Close room door or bedside curtains.	Provides privacy.
IMPLEMENTATION	
1 Perform hand hygiene and apply gloves (if likely to contact wound drainage).	Reduces transmission of microorganisms.
2 Apply abdominal binder.	
a. Position patient in supine position with head slightly elevated and knees slightly flexed.	Minimizes muscular tension on abdominal organs.
b. Fanfold far side of binder toward midline of binder.	Reduces time patient remains in uncomfortable position.
c. Instruct and help patient to roll onto side away from you and toward raised side rail while firmly supporting abdominal incision and dressing with hands.	Reduces pain and discomfort.
d. Place fan-folded ends of binder under patient.	Permits placement and centering of binder with minimal discomfort.
e. Instruct or assist patient in rolling back over folded ends.	
f. Unfold and stretch ends out smoothly on far side of bed.	Maintains skin integrity and comfort.
g. Instruct patient to roll back into supine position.	Facilitates chest expansion and adequate wound support when binder is closed.
h. Adjust binder so supine patient is centered over it, using symphysis pubis and costal margins as lower and upper landmarks.	Centers support from binder over abdominal structures, which reduces incidence of decreased lung expansion.
CLINICAL DECISION: *Cover any exposed areas of an incision or wound with sterile dressing.*	
i. Close binder. Pull one end of binder over center of patient's abdomen. While maintaining tension on that end of binder, pull opposite end over center and secure with Velcro closure tabs, metal fasteners, or horizontally placed safety pins (see Fig. 48-30).	Provides continuous wound support and comfort.
j. Adjust binder as necessary.	Promotes comfort and chest expansion.
k. Remove and dispose of gloves. Perform hand hygiene.	Reduces transmission of microorganisms.
EVALUATION	
1 Observe site for skin integrity, circulation, and characteristics of wound. (Periodically remove binder and surgical dressing to assess wound characteristics.)	Determines that binder has not resulted in complication to skin, wound, or underlying organs.
2 Evaluate comfort level of patient, using analog scale of 0 to 10 and noting any objective signs and symptoms.	Binders should not increase discomfort.
3 Evaluate patient's ability to ventilate properly, including deep breathing and coughing.	Identifies any impaired ventilation and potential pulmonary complications.
4 Identify patient's need for help with activities such as hair combing, dressing, and ambulating.	Mobility of upper extremities is often limited, depending on severity and location of incision.

SKILL 48-6 APPLYING AN ABDOMINAL BINDER—cont'd

UNEXPECTED OUTCOMES AND RELATED INTERVENTIONS

1 Patient's pain increases.
- Remove binder and assess wound.
- Reapply binder using less pressure.

2 Patient's respiratory rate decreases.
- Remove binder.
- Encourage patient to cough and deep breathe.
- Reapply binder using less pressure.

3 Patient develops impaired skin integrity under binder.
- Remove binder.
- Initiate skin care measure to heal affected site.

RECORDING AND REPORTING

- Report any skin irritation to nurse at between-shift report.
- Record application of binder, condition of skin, circulation, integrity of dressing, and patient's comfort level.

HOME CARE CONSIDERATIONS

- Abdominal binders are washable and placed over a line to dry.
- Instruct caregiver to avoid excessive pressure with binder application.

SKILL 48-7 APPLYING AN ELASTIC BANDAGE

Delegation Considerations

The skill of applying an elastic bandage can be delegated to nursing assistive personnel (NAP). The nurse is responsible for wound assessment and the evaluation of the wound. In addition, the nurse is responsible for assessing for adequate circulation to the extremity distal to the elastic bandage. Direct the NAP to:
- Report any restrictions that the patient has (e.g., unable to independently raise leg or roll over).
- Report any change in the skin color of the patient's injured extremity.
- Report any increases in patient's pain.

Equipment

- Correct width and number of bandages
- Safety pins, clips, or adhesive tape
- Clean gloves if wound drainage is present

STEP	RATIONALE
ASSESSMENT	
1 Identify patient using two identifiers (i.e., name and birth date or name and account number) according to facility policy. Compare identifiers with information on the patient's medical record.	Ensures correct patient. Complies with a recommended National Patient Safety Goal (TJC, 2011).
2 Review medical record for specific orders related to application of elastic bandage. Note area to be covered, type of bandage required, frequency of change, and previous response to treatment.	Specific orders sometimes direct procedure, including factors such as extent of application (e.g., toe to knee, toe to groin) and duration of treatment.
3 Perform hand hygiene and apply gloves if needed. Inspect skin for alterations in integrity as indicated by abrasions, discoloration, chafing, or edema. (Look carefully at bony prominences.)	Altered skin integrity contraindicates the use of elastic bandages.
4 Inspect surgical dressing if present. Remove gloves and perform hand hygiene.	Surgical dressing replacement or reinforcement precedes application of any bandage. Reduces transmission of microorganisms.
5 Observe adequacy of circulation (distal to bandage) by noting surface temperature, skin color, and sensation in body parts to be wrapped.	Comparison of area before and after application of bandage is necessary to ensure continued adequate circulation. Impairment of circulation can result in coolness to touch when compared with opposite side of body, cyanosis, pallor of skin, diminished or absent pulses, edema or localized pooling, and numbness or tingling of part.
6 Assess patient's and family caregiver's present knowledge and level of skill if bandaging will be continued at home.	Ensures that planning and teaching are individualized.

STEP	RATIONALE
PLANNING	
1 Explain each step of procedure to patient.	Increased knowledge promotes cooperation and reduces anxiety.
2 Demonstrate skill to patient and family caregiver.	Helps to ensure continuity of care after discharge.

CLINICAL DECISION: *Apply bandages to lower extremities before patient sits or stands. Elevate dependent extremities for 20 minutes before bandage application to enhance venous return.*

STEP	RATIONALE
IMPLEMENTATION	
1 Close room door or curtains.	Maintains patient's comfort and dignity.
2 Help patient assume comfortable, anatomically correct position.	Maintains alignment. Prevents musculoskeletal deformity.
3 Perform hand hygiene and apply gloves if drainage is present.	Reduces transmission of microorganisms.
4 Hold roll of elastic bandage in dominant hand and use other hand to lightly hold beginning of bandage at distal body part. Continue transferring roll to dominant hand as bandage is wrapped.	Maintains appropriate and consistent bandage tension.

CLINICAL DECISION: *Toes or fingertips need to be visible for follow-up circulatory assessment.*

STEP	RATIONALE
5 Apply bandage from distal point toward proximal boundary using variety of turns to cover various shapes of body parts. A spiral dressing is often used to cover cylindrical body parts such as wrist or upper arms. To apply bandage in an ascending motion, overlapping previous bandage by one-half to two-thirds width of bandage. Use figure-eight dressing to cover joint because snug fit provides excellent immobilization. *To apply:* Overlap turns, alternately ascending and descending over bandaged part; each turn crossing previous one to form figure eight.	Bandage is applied in manner that conforms evenly to body part and promotes venous return.
6 Unroll and very slightly stretch bandage.	Maintains uniform bandage tension.
7 Overlap turns by one-half to two-thirds width of bandage roll.	Prevents uneven bandage tension and circulatory impairment.
8 Secure first bandage with clip or tape before applying additional rolls.	
9 Apply additional rolls without leaving any skin surface uncovered. Secure last bandage applied.	Prevents wrinkling or loose ends.
10 Remove gloves if worn and perform hand hygiene.	Reduces transmission of microorganisms.
EVALUATION	
1 Assess distal circulation when bandage application is complete and at least twice during 8-hour period.	Early detection and management of circulatory impairment ensures healthy neurovascular status.
a. Observe skin color for pallor or cyanosis.	
b. Palpate skin for warmth.	
c. Palpate pulses and compare bilaterally.	
d. Ask if patient is aware of pain, numbness, tingling, or other discomfort.	Neurovascular changes indicate impaired venous return.
e. Observe mobility of extremity.	Determines if bandage is too tight, which restricts movement, or if joint immobility is attained.
2 Have patient demonstrate bandage application.	Return demonstration evaluates learning.

UNEXPECTED OUTCOMES AND RELATED INTERVENTIONS

1 Impaired circulation distal to elastic bandage
- Release bandage.
- Palpate extremity and assess pulse, temperature, and capillary refill.
- Reapply dressing with less pressure.

2 Break in skin under elastic bandage
- Remove bandage.
- Reapply bandage over different area of skin with less pressure.

3 Patient unable to perform dressing change
- Reinstruct patient or family caregiver on bandage application.
- Observe patient or family caregiver apply bandage.

RECORDING AND REPORTING

- Document condition of wound, integrity of dressing, application of bandage, circulation, and patient's comfort level.
- Report any changes in neurological or circulatory status to nurse in charge or health care provider.

HOME CARE CONSIDERATIONS

- Instruct patient or caregiver not to make bandages too tight, which interferes with circulation.
- Elastic bandages that reduce swelling are best applied to the feet and ankles in the morning, before getting out of bed.
- Always remove an elastic bandage daily and inspect skin beneath it.

KEY POINTS

- Pressure ulcers contribute to patient discomfort and decreased functional status, increased length of stay in acute and extended care settings, and increased cost of care.
- Wound assessment scales help measure improvement of a healing pressure ulcer; do not use the staging system for this purpose.
- Evaluate all patients on an ongoing basis for risk factors that contribute to development of impaired skin integrity.
- Alterations in mobility, sensory perception, level of consciousness, and nutrition and the presence of moisture increase the risk for pressure ulcer development.
- The risk of impaired skin integrity related to immobilization depends on the extent and duration of immobilization.
- Pressure, shearing force, and friction are contributing factors to the development of pressure ulcers.
- When the external pressure against the skin is greater than the pressure needed to keep the capillary open, blood flow decreases to the adjacent tissues.
- Meticulous ongoing assessment of the skin and identification of risk factors are important in decreasing the opportunity for pressure ulcer development.
- Preventive skin care is aimed at controlling external pressure on bony prominences and keeping the skin clean, well lubricated and hydrated, and free of excess moisture.
- Proper positioning reduces the effects of pressure and guards against the shearing force.
- Therapeutic beds and mattresses redistribute the effects of pressure; however, base selection on assessment data to identify the best bed for individual needs.
- Cleaning and topical agents used to treat pressure ulcers vary according to the stage of the pressure ulcer and condition of the wound bed. Assessment of the ulcer enables the nurse to select proper skin care agents.
- Direct nutritional interventions at improving wound healing through increasing protein and calorie levels.
- Wound assessment requires a description of the appearance of the wound base, size, presence of exudate, and the periwound skin condition.
- When tissue loss is extensive, a wound heals by secondary intention.
- The chances of wound infection are greater when the wound contains dead or necrotic tissue, when foreign bodies lie on or near the wound, and when the blood supply and tissue defenses are reduced.
- The principles of wound first aid include control of bleeding, cleaning, and protection.
- The layers of a dry dressing absorb drainage and prevent entrance of bacteria.
- A moist environment supports wound healing.
- The wet-to-dry dressing mechanically removes dead tissue and wound exudate to debride the wound.
- When cleaning wounds or drain sites, clean from the least to most contaminated area, away from wound edges.
- Apply a bandage or binder in a manner that does not impair circulation or irritate the skin.
- An acute sprain, closed fracture, or bruise responds best to cold applications.

CLINICAL APPLICATION QUESTIONS

Preparing for Clinical Practice

1. Because of the foul-smelling tan-colored drainage from Mrs. Stein's hip incision, the staples were removed by the health care provider, and an order was written for moist saline gauze dressing to the area 3 times a day. When the dressing is removed, which factors are critical to assess?
2. A head-to-toe skin assessment is done per institutional policy on a daily basis. At the most recent assessment of Mrs. Stein's skin, redness was noted over the sacral area; on direct examination a small area of denuded tissue was noted. The area was assessed and was found to have minimal depth and a red, moist base. How would you describe the impairment in skin integrity in your charting?
3. What will you include in your plan of care for Mrs. Stein to address the impairment in skin integrity in the sacral area?
4. Mrs. Stein will be discharged tomorrow. Which issues must be assessed regarding her care before discharge? Describe why these issues are of importance.

evolve *Answers to Clinical Application Questions can be found on the Evolve website.*

REVIEW QUESTIONS

Are You Ready to Test Your Nursing Knowledge?

1. When repositioning an immobile patient, the nurse notices redness over a bony prominence. What is indicated when a reddened area blanches on fingertip touch?
   1. A local skin infection requiring antibiotics
   2. Sensitive skin that requires special bed linen
   3. A stage III pressure ulcer needing the appropriate dressing
   4. Blanching hyperemia, indicating the attempt by the body to overcome the ischemic episode.
2. Which type of pressure ulcer is noted to have intact skin and may include changes in one or more of the following: skin temperature (warmth or coolness), tissue consistency (firm or soft), and/or pain?
   1. Stage I
   2. Stage II
   3. Stage III
   4. Stage IV
3. When obtaining a wound culture to determine the presence of a wound infection, from where should the specimen be taken?
   1. Necrotic tissue
   2. Wound drainage
   3. Drainage on the dressing
   4. Wound after it has first been cleaned with normal saline
4. After surgery the patient with a closed abdominal wound reports a sudden "pop" after coughing. When the nurse examines the surgical wound site, the sutures are open, and pieces of small bowel are noted at the bottom of the now-opened wound. Which corrective intervention should the nurse do first?
   1. Allow the area to be exposed to air until all drainage has stopped
   2. Place several cold packs over the area, protecting the skin around the wound

3. Cover the area with sterile, saline-soaked towels and immediately notify the surgical team; this is likely to indicate a wound evisceration
4. Cover the area with sterile gauze, place a tight binder over it, and ask the patient to remain in bed for 30 minutes because this is a minor opening in the surgical wound and should reseal quickly

5. Which description best fits that of serous drainage from a wound?
   1. Fresh bleeding
   2. Thick and yellow
   3. Clear, watery plasma
   4. Beige to brown and foul smelling
6. For a patient who has a muscle sprain, localized hemorrhage, or hematoma, which wound care product helps prevent edema formation, control bleeding, and anesthetize the body part?
   1. Binder
   2. Ice bag
   3. Elastic bandage
   4. Absorptive diaper
7. Which skin care measures are used to manage a patient who is experiencing fecal and urinary incontinence?
   1. Keeping the buttocks exposed to air at all times
   2. Using a large absorbent diaper, changing when saturated
   3. Using an incontinence cleaner, followed by application of a moisture-barrier ointment
   4. Frequent cleaning, applying an ointment, and covering the areas with a thick absorbent towel
8. Which of the following describes a hydrocolloid dressing?
   1. A seaweed derivative that is highly absorptive
   2. Premoistened gauze placed over a granulating wound
   3. A debriding enzyme that is used to remove necrotic tissue
   4. A dressing that forms a gel that interacts with the wound surface
9. Which of the following is an indication for a binder to be placed around a surgical patient with a new abdominal wound?
   1. Collection of wound drainage
   2. Reduction of abdominal swelling
   3. Reduction of stress on the abdominal incision
   4. Stimulation of peristalsis (return of bowel function) from direct pressure
10. When is an application of a warm compress indicated? (Select all that apply.)
   1. To relieve edema
   2. For a patient who is shivering
   3. To improve blood flow to an injured part
   4. To protect bony prominences from pressure ulcers
11. What is the removal of devitalized tissue from a wound called?
   1. Debridement
   2. Pressure reduction
   3. Negative pressure wound therapy
   4. Sanitization
12. Name the three important dimensions to consistently measure to determine wound healing.
13. What does the Braden Scale evaluate?
   1. Skin integrity at bony prominences, including any wounds
   2. Risk factors that place the patient at risk for skin breakdown
   3. The amount of repositioning that the patient can tolerate
   4. The factors that place the patient at risk for poor healing
14. On assessing your patient's sacral pressure ulcer, you note that the tissue over the sacrum is dark, hard, and adherent to the wound edge. What is the correct stage for this patient's pressure ulcer?
   1. Stage II
   2. Stage IV
   3. Unstageable
   4. Suspected deep tissue damage
15. Name one intervention and the rationalization to use that intervention to reduce the likelihood of a shear injury to a patient.

Answers: **1.** 4; **2.** 1; **3.** 4; **4.** 3; **5.** 3; **6.** 2; **7.** 3; **8.** 4; **9.** 3; **10.** 1, 3; **11.** 1; **12.** Width, length, and depth; **13.** 2; **14.** 3; **15.** See Evolve.

REFERENCES

Agency for Health Care Policy and Research (AHCPR), Panel for the Prediction and Prevention of Pressure Ulcers in Adults: *Pressure ulcers in adults: prediction and prevention,* Clinical Practice Guideline No. 3, AHCPR Pub No. 92-0047, Rockville, Md, 1992, Agency for Health Care Policy and Research, Public Health Service, US Department of Health and Human Services.

Agency for Health Care Policy and Research (AHCPR), Panel for Treatment of Pressure Ulcers in Adults: *Treatment of pressure ulcers, Clinical Practice Guideline* No. 15, AHCPR Pub No. 95-0653, Rockville, Md, 1994, Agency for Health Care Policy and Research, Public Health Service, US Department of Health and Human Services.

Ayello EA, Braden B: How and why to do pressure ulcer risk assessment, *Adv Skin Wound Care* 15(13):125, 2002.

Baharestani MM: Quality of life and ethical issues. In Baranoski S, Ayello EA, editors: *Wound care essentials: practice principles*, ed 2, Philadelphia, 2008, Lippincott, Williams & Wilkins.

Bennett MA: Report of the Task Force on the Implications for Darkly Pigmented Intact Skin in the Prediction and Prevention of Pressure Ulcers, *Adv Wound Care* 8(6):34, 1995.

Braden BJ: Risk assessment in pressure ulcer prevention. In Krasner DL, Rodeheaver GT, Sibbald RG, editors: *Chronic wound care: a clinical source book for healthcare professionals*, Wayne, Pa, 2001, HMP Communications.

Brienza DM, et al: Pressure redistribution: seating, positioning and support surfaces. In Baranoski S, Ayello EA., editors: *Wound care essentials: practice principles*, ed 2, Philadelphia, 2008, Lippincott, Williams & Wilkins.

Bryant RA: Types of skin damage and differential diagnosis. In Bryant RA, Nix DP, editors: *Acute and chronic wounds: current management concepts*, ed 4, St Louis, 2012, Mosby.

Bryant RA, Nix DP: Developing and maintaining a pressure ulcer prevention program. In Bryant RA, Nix DP, editors: *Acute and chronic wounds: current management concepts*, ed 4, St Louis, 2012, Mosby.

Camden SG: Skin care needs of the obese patient. In Bryant RA, Nix, DP, editors: *Acute and chronic wounds: current management concepts*, ed 4, St Louis, 2012, Mosby.

Centers for Disease Control and Prevention (CDC): Feeding back surveillance data to prevent hospital acquired infections, *Emerg Infect Dis* 7(2):295, 2001.

Chua PC, et al: Vacuum-assisted wound closure, *Am J Nurs* 100(12):45, 2000.

Dallam DE, et al: Pain management and wounds. In Baranoski S, Ayello EA, editors: *Wound care essentials: practice principles*, ed 2, Philadelphia, 2008, Lippincott, Williams & Wilkins.

Doughty DB, Sparks-Defriese B: Wound-healing physiology. In Bryant RA, Nix DP, editors: *Acute and chronic wounds: current management concepts*, ed 4, St Louis, 2012, Mosby.

European Pressure Ulcer Advisory Panel (EPUAP) and National Pressure Ulcer Advisory Panel (NPUAP): *Treatment of pressure ulcers: quick reference guide*, Washington DC, 2009, National Pressure Ulcer Advisory Panel.

Fellows J, Cresodina L: Home prepared saline: a safe, cost effective alternative for wound cleansing in home care, *J Wound Ostomy Continence Nurs* 33(6):606, 2006.

Gardner SE, Frantz RA: Wound bioburden. In Baranoski S, Ayello EA, editors: *Wound care essentials: practice principles*, ed 2, Philadelphia, 2008, Lippincott, Williams & Wilkins.

Gaskin FC: Detection of cyanosis in the person with dark skin, *J Natl Black Nurses Assoc* 1:52, 1986.

Harris C, et al: Bates Jensen wound assessment tool: pictorial guide validation project, *J Wound Ostomy Continence Nurs* 37 (3):253, 2010.

Henderson CT, et al: Draft definition of stage I pressure ulcers: inclusion of persons with darkly pigmented skin, *Adv Wound Care* 10(5):16, 1997.

Jerome D: Advances in negative pressure wound therapy: the V.A.C. Instill, *J Wound Ostomy Continence Nurs* 34(2):191, 2007.

KCI USA: *The V.A.C.: therapy safety information, product information*, San Antonio, 2007, Author.

Netsch DS: Negative-pressure wound therapy. In Bryant RA, Nix DP, editors: *Acute and chronic wounds: current management concepts*, ed 4, St Louis, 2012, Mosby.

Nix D: Skin and wound inspection and assessment. In Bryant RA, Nix DP, editors: *Acute and chronic wounds: current management concepts*, ed 4, St Louis, 2012, Mosby.

Norton D, et al: *An investigation of geriatric nursing problems in hospital*, Edinburgh, 1962, Churchill Livingstone.

Pieper B: Pressure ulcers: impact, etiology, and classification. In Bryant RA, Nix DP, editors: *Acute and chronic wounds: current management concepts*, ed 4, St Louis, 2012, Mosby.

Posthauer ME, Thomas DR: Nutrition and wound care. In Baranoski S, Ayello EA, editors: *Wound care essentials: practice principles*, ed 2, Philadelphia, 2008, Lippincott, Williams & Wilkins.

Rajendran PJ, et al: *Improving the detection of stage I pressure ulcers by enhancing color images*, 2006, Engineering in Medicine and Biology Society, EMBS '06 Annual International Conference of IEEE, New York.

Ramundo JM: Wound debridement. In Bryant RA, Nix DP, editors: *Acute and chronic wounds: current management concepts*, ed 4, St Louis, 2012, Mosby.

Rolstad BS, Bryant RA, Nix DP: Topical management. In Bryant RA, Nix DP, editors: *Acute and chronic wounds: current management concepts*, ed 4, St Louis, 2012, Mosby.

Siem CA, et al: Skin assessment and pressure ulcer care in hospital-based skilled nursing facilities, *Ostomy Wound Manage* 49(6):42, 2003.

Stotts NA: Nutritional assessment and support. In Bryant RA, Nix DP, editors: *Acute and chronic wounds: current management concepts*, ed 4, St Louis, 2012a, Mosby.

Stotts NA: Wound infection: diagnosis and management. In Bryant RA, Nix DP, editors: *Acute and chronic wounds: current management concepts*, ed 4, St Louis, 2012b, Mosby.

The Joint Commission (TJC): *Nutritional, functional and pain assessments and screens*, 2008, http://www.jointcommission.org/standards_information/jcfaqdetails.aspx?StandardsFaqId=208&ProgramId=1. Accessed March 15, 2011.

The Joint Commission (TJC): 2011 *National Patient Safety Goals (NPSG)*, 2011, http://www.jointcommission.org/standards_information/npsgs.aspx. Accessed November 21, 2011.

Thompson G: An overview of negative pressure wound therapy (NPWT), *Wound Care* 6:523, 2008.

Woo KY, Ayello EA, Sibald RG: The skin and periwound skin disorders and management, *Wound Healing S Africa* 2(2):43, 2009.

Wound, Ostomy and Continence Nurses Society: *Guideline for prevention and management of pressure ulcers, Guideline for Prevention and Management of Pressure Ulcers: WOCN Clinical Practice Guideline Series*, Mount Laurel, NJ, 2010, WOCN.

Wysocki AB: Anatomy and physiology of skin and soft tissue. In Bryant RA, Nix DP, editors: *Acute and chronic wounds: current management concepts*, ed 4, St Louis, 2012, Mosby.

RESEARCH REFERENCES

Baumgarten M, et al: Pressure ulcers and the transition to long-term care, *Adv Skin Wound Care* 16:299, 2003.

Bergstrom N, et al: The Braden Scale for predicting pressure sore risk, *Nurs Res* 36(4):205, 1987.

Braden BJ, Bergstrom N: Clinical utility of the Braden Scale for predicting pressure sore risk, *Decubitus* 2(3):50, 1989.

Braden BJ, Bergstrom N: Predictive validity of the Braden Scale for pressure sore risk in a nursing home population, *Res Nurs Health* 17(6):459, 1994.

Bruns TB, Worthington JM: Using tissue adhesive for wound repair: a practical guide to Dermabond, *Am Fam Physician* 61(5):1383, 2000.

Burton AC, Yamada S: Relation between blood pressure and flow in the human forearm, *J Appl Physiol* 4(5):329, 1951.

Gray M, Weir D: Prevention and treatment of moisture-associated skin damage (maceration) in the periwound skin, *J Wound Ostomy Continence Nurs* 34(2):153, 2007.

Xie X, et al: The clinical effectiveness of negative-pressure wound therapy: a systematic review, *J Wound Care* 19(11):490, 2010.

CHAPTER

49

Sensory Alterations

OBJECTIVES

- Differentiate among the processes of reception, perception, and reaction to sensory stimuli.
- Discuss the relationship of sensory function to an individual's level of wellness.
- Discuss common causes and effects of sensory alterations.
- Discuss common sensory changes that normally occur with aging.
- Identify factors to assess in determining a patient's sensory status.
- Identify nursing diagnoses relevant to patients with sensory alterations.
- Develop a plan of care for patients with sensory deficits.
- List interventions for preventing sensory deprivation and controlling sensory overload.
- Describe conditions in a health care agency or patient's home that you can modify to promote meaningful sensory stimulation.
- Discuss ways to maintain a safe environment for patients with sensory deficits.

KEY TERMS

Aphasia, p. 1240
Auditory, p. 1233
Conductive hearing loss, p. 1245
Expressive aphasia, p. 1240
Gustatory, p. 1233
Hyperesthesia, p. 1246
Kinesthetic, p. 1233
Olfactory, p. 1233
Otolaryngologist, p. 1238
Ototoxic, p. 1241
Proprioceptive, p. 1236
Receptive aphasia, p. 1240
Refractive error, p. 1244
Sensory deficit, p. 1234
Sensory deprivation, p. 1234
Sensory overload, p. 1235
Stereognosis, p. 1233
Strabismus, p. 1244
Tactile, p. 1233

evolve WEBSITE

http://evolve.elsevier.com/Potter/fundamentals/

- Review Questions
- Animations
- Concept Map Creator
- Case Study with Questions
- Audio Glossary
- Interactive Learning Activities
- Key Term Flashcards
- Content Updates

Imagine the world without sight, hearing, or the ability to feel objects or sense aromas around you. Human beings rely on a variety of sensory stimuli to give meaning and order to events occurring in their environment. The senses form the perceptual base of our world. Stimulation comes from many sources in and outside the body, particularly through the senses of sight (visual), hearing **(auditory)**, touch **(tactile)**, smell **(olfactory)**, and taste **(gustatory)**. The body also has a **kinesthetic** sense that enables a person to be aware of the position and movement of body parts without seeing them. **Stereognosis** is a sense that allows a person to recognize the size, shape, and texture of an object. The ability to speak is not a sense but it is similar in that some patients lose the ability to interact meaningfully with other human beings. Meaningful stimuli allow a person to learn about the environment and are necessary for healthy functioning and normal development. When sensory function is altered, a person's ability to relate to and function within the environment changes drastically.

Many patients seeking health care have preexisting sensory alterations. Others develop them as a result of medical treatment (e.g., hearing loss from antibiotic use or hearing or visual loss from brain tumor removal) or hospitalization. The health care environment is a place of unfamiliar sights, sounds, and smells and minimal contact with family and friends. If patients feel depersonalized and are unable to receive meaningful stimuli, serious sensory alterations sometimes develop.

As a nurse, you meet the needs of patients with existing sensory alterations and recognize patients most at risk for developing sensory problems. You also help patients who have partial or complete loss of a major sense to find alternate ways to function safely within their environment.

SCIENTIFIC KNOWLEDGE BASE

Normal Sensation

Normally the nervous system continually receives thousands of bits of information from sensory nerve organs, relays the information through appropriate channels, and integrates the information into a meaningful response. Sensory stimuli reach the sensory organs to elicit an immediate reaction or present information to the brain to be stored for future use. The nervous system must be intact for sensory stimuli to reach appropriate brain centers and for an individual to perceive the sensation. After interpreting the significance

TABLE 49-1 Normal Hearing and Vision

FUNCTION	ANATOMY AND PHYSIOLOGY
Ear	
Transmits to the brain an accurate pattern of all sounds received from the environment, the relative intensity of these sounds, and the direction from which they originate	Two ears provide stereophonic hearing to judge sound direction. The external ear canal shelters the eardrum and maintains relatively constant temperature and humidity to maintain elasticity. The middle ear is an air-containing space between the eardrum and oval window. It contains three small bones (ossicles). The eardrum and ossicles transfer sound to the fluid-filled inner ear. Movement of the stapes in the oval window creates vibrations in the fluid that bathes the membranous labyrinth, which contains the end organs of hearing and balance. The union of the vestibular (balance) and cochlear (hearing) portions of the labyrinth explains the combination of hearing and balance symptoms that occur with inner ear disorders. Vibration of the eardrum transmits through the bony ossicles. Vibrations at the oval window transmit in perilymph within the inner ear to stimulate hair cells that send impulses along the eighth cranial nerve to the brain.
Eye	
Transmits to the brain an accurate pattern of light that is reflected from solid objects in the environment and becomes transformed into color and hue	Light rays enter the convex cornea and begin to converge. Fine adjustment of light rays occurs as they pass through the pupil and lens. Change in the shape of the lens focuses light on the retina. The retina has a pigmented layer of cells to enhance visual acuity. The sensory retina contains the rods and cones (i.e., photoreceptor cells sensitive to stimulation from light). Photoreceptor cells send electrical potentials by way of the optic nerve to the brain.

of a sensation, the person is then able to react to the stimulus. Table 49-1 summarizes normal hearing and vision.

Reception, perception, and reaction are the three components of any sensory experience (see Chapter 43). Reception begins with stimulation of a nerve cell called a *receptor,* which is usually for only one type of stimulus such as light, touch, or sound. In the case of special senses, the receptors are grouped close together or located in specialized organs such as the taste buds of the tongue or the retina of the eye. When a nerve impulse is created, it travels along pathways to the spinal cord or directly to the brain. For example, sound waves stimulate hair cell receptors within the organ of Corti in the ear, which causes impulses to travel along the eighth cranial nerve to the acoustic area of the temporal lobe. Sensory nerve pathways usually cross over to send stimuli to opposite sides of the brain.

The actual perception or awareness of unique sensations depends on the receiving region of the cerebral cortex, where specialized brain cells interpret the quality and nature of sensory stimuli. When a person becomes conscious of a stimulus and receives the information, perception takes place. Perception includes integration and interpretation of stimuli based on the person's experiences. A person's level of consciousness influences perception and interpretation of stimuli. Any factors lowering consciousness impair sensory perception. If sensation is incomplete such as blurred vision or if past experience is inadequate for understanding stimuli such as pain, the person can react inappropriately to the sensory stimulus.

It is impossible to react to all stimuli entering the nervous system. The brain prevents sensory bombardment by discarding or storing sensory information. A person usually reacts to stimuli that are most meaningful or significant at the time. However, after continued reception of the same stimulus, a person stops responding, and the sensory experience goes unnoticed. For example, a person concentrating on reading a good book is not aware of background music. This adaptability phenomenon occurs with most sensory stimuli except for those of pain.

The balance between sensory stimuli entering the brain and those actually reaching a person's conscious awareness maintains a person's well-being. If an individual attempts to react to every stimulus within the environment or if the variety and quality of stimuli are insufficient, sensory alterations occur.

Sensory Alterations

The most common types of sensory alterations are sensory deficits, sensory deprivation, and sensory overload. When a patient suffers from more than one sensory alteration, the ability to function and relate effectively within the environment is seriously impaired.

Sensory Deficits. A deficit in the normal function of sensory reception and perception is a **sensory deficit.** A person loses a sense of self with impaired senses. Initially he or she withdraws by avoiding communication or socialization with others in an attempt to cope with the sensory loss. It becomes difficult for the person to interact safely with the environment until he or she learns new skills. When a deficit develops gradually or when considerable time has passed since the onset of an acute sensory loss, a person learns to rely on unaffected senses. Some senses may even become more acute to compensate for an alteration. For example, a blind patient develops an acute sense of hearing to compensate for visual loss.

Patients with sensory deficits often change behavior in adaptive or maladaptive ways. For example, a patient with a hearing impairment turns the unaffected ear toward the speaker to hear better, whereas another patient avoids people because he or she is embarrassed about not being able to understand what other people say. Box 49-1 summarizes common sensory deficits and their influence on those affected.

Sensory Deprivation. The reticular activating system in the brainstem mediates all sensory stimuli to the cerebral cortex; thus patients are able to receive stimuli even while sleeping deeply. Sensory stimulation must be of sufficient quality and quantity to maintain a person's awareness. Three types of **sensory deprivation** are reduced sensory input (sensory deficit from visual or hearing loss), the elimination of patterns or meaning from input (e.g., exposure to strange environments), and restrictive environments (e.g., bed rest) that produce monotony and boredom (Ebersole et al., 2008).

BOX 49-1 COMMON SENSORY DEFICITS

Visual Deficits

Presbyopia: A gradual decline in the ability of the lens to accommodate or focus on close objects. Individual is unable to see near objects clearly.

Cataract: Cloudy or opaque areas in part of the lens or the entire lens that interfere with passage of light through the lens, causing problems with glare and blurred vision. Cataracts usually develop gradually, without pain, redness, or tearing in the eye.

Dry eyes: Result when tear glands produce too few tears, resulting in itching, burning, or even reduced vision.

Glaucoma: A slowly progressive increase in intraocular pressure that, if left untreated, causes progressive pressure against the optic nerve, resulting in peripheral visual loss, decreased visual acuity with difficulty adapting to darkness, and a halo effect around lights.

Diabetic retinopathy: Pathological changes occur in the blood vessels of the retina, resulting in decreased vision or vision loss caused by hemorrhage and macular edema.

Macular degeneration: Condition in which the macula (specialized portion of the retina responsible for central vision) loses its ability to function efficiently. First signs include blurring of reading matter, distortion or loss of central vision, and distortion of vertical lines.

Hearing Deficits

Presbycusis: A common progressive hearing disorder in older adults.

Cerumen accumulation: Buildup of earwax in the external auditory canal. Cerumen becomes hard and collects in the canal and causes conduction deafness.

Balance Deficit

Dizziness and disequilibrium: Common condition in older adulthood, usually resulting from vestibular dysfunction. Frequently a change in position of the head precipitates an episode of vertigo or disequilibrium.

Taste Deficit

Xerostomia: Decrease in salivary production that leads to thicker mucus and a dry mouth. Often interferes with the ability to eat and leads to appetite and nutritional problems.

Neurological Deficits

Peripheral neuropathy: Disorder of the peripheral nervous system, characterized by symptoms that include numbness and tingling of the affected area and stumbling gait.

Stroke: Cerebrovascular accident caused by clot, hemorrhage, or emboli disrupting blood flow to the brain. Creates altered proprioception with marked incoordination and imbalance. Loss of sensation and motor function in extremities controlled by the affected area of the brain also occurs. A stroke affecting the left hemisphere of the brain results in symptoms on the right side such as difficulty with speech. A stroke on the right hemisphere has symptoms on the left side, which includes visual spatial alterations such as loss of half of a visual field or inattention and neglect, especially to the left side.

There are many effects of sensory deprivation (Box 49-2). In adults the symptoms are similar to psychological illness, confusion, symptoms of severe electrolyte imbalance, or the influence of psychotropic drugs. Therefore always be aware of a patient's existing sensory function and the quality of stimuli within the environment.

BOX 49-2 EFFECTS OF SENSORY DEPRIVATION

Cognitive

- Reduced capacity to learn
- Inability to think or problem solve
- Poor task performance
- Disorientation
- Bizarre thinking
- Increased need for socialization, altered mechanisms of attention

Affective

- Boredom
- Restlessness
- Increased anxiety
- Emotional lability
- Panic
- Increased need for physical stimulation

Perceptual

- Changes in visual/motor coordination
- Reduced color perception
- Less tactile accuracy
- Changes in ability to perceive size and shape
- Changes in spatial and time judgment

Modified from Ebersole P et al.: *Toward healthy aging: human needs and nursing response,* ed 7, St Louis, 2008, Mosby.

Sensory Overload. When a person receives multiple sensory stimuli and cannot perceptually disregard or selectively ignore some stimuli, **sensory overload** occurs. Excessive sensory stimulation prevents the brain from responding appropriately to or ignoring certain stimuli. Because of the multitude of stimuli leading to overload, a person no longer perceives the environment in a way that makes sense. Overload prevents meaningful response by the brain; the patient's thoughts race, attention scatters in many directions, and anxiety and restlessness occur. As a result, overload causes a state similar to that produced by sensory deprivation. However, in contrast to deprivation, overload is individualized. The amount of stimuli necessary for healthy function varies with each individual. People are often subject to environmental overload more at one time than another. A person's tolerance to sensory overload varies with level of fatigue, attitude, and emotional and physical well-being.

The acutely ill patient easily experiences sensory overload. The patient in constant pain or who undergoes frequent monitoring of vital signs is at risk. Multiple stimuli combine to cause overload even if the nurse offers a comforting word or provides a gentle back rub. Some patients do not benefit from nursing intervention because their attention and energy are focused on more stressful stimuli. Another example is a patient who is hospitalized in an intensive care unit (ICU), where the activity is constant. Lights are always on. Patients can hear sounds from monitoring equipment, staff conversations, equipment alarms, and the activities of people entering the unit. Even at night an ICU is very noisy.

It is easy to confuse the behavioral changes associated with sensory overload with mood swings or simple disorientation. Look for symptoms such as racing thoughts, scattered attention, restlessness, and anxiety. Patients in ICUs sometimes resort to constantly fingering tubes and dressings. Constant reorientation and control of excessive stimuli become an important part of a patient's care.

NURSING KNOWLEDGE BASE

Factors Influencing Sensory Function

Many factors influence the capacity to receive or perceive stimuli. All are conditions or situations that you manage when delivering care.

Age. Infants and children are at risk for visual and hearing impairment because of a number of genetic, prenatal, and postnatal conditions. A concern with high-risk neonates is that early, intense visual and auditory stimulation can adversely affect visual and auditory pathways and alter the developmental course of other sensory organs (Hockenberry and Wilson, 2011). Visual changes during adulthood include presbyopia and the need for glasses for reading. These changes usually occur from ages 40 to 50. In addition, the cornea, which assists with light refraction to the retina, becomes flatter and thicker. These aging changes lead to astigmatism. Pigment is lost from the iris, and collagen fibers build up in the anterior chamber, which increases the risk of glaucoma by decreasing the resorption of intraocular fluid. Other normal visual changes associated with aging include reduced visual fields, increased glare sensitivity, impaired night vision, reduced depth perception, and reduced color discrimination.

Hearing changes begin at the age of 30. Changes associated with aging include decreased hearing acuity, speech intelligibility, and pitch discrimination. Low-pitched sounds are easiest to hear, but it is difficult to hear conversation over background noise. It is also difficult to discriminate the consonants *(z, t, f, g)* and high-frequency sounds *(s, sh, ph, k)*. Vowels that have a low pitch are easiest to hear. Speech sounds are distorted, and there is a delayed reception and reaction to speech. A concern with normal age-related sensory changes is that older adults with a deficit are sometimes inappropriately diagnosed with dementia (Ebersole et al., 2008).

Gustatory and olfactory changes begin around age 50 and include a decrease in the number of taste buds and sensory cells in the nasal lining. Reduced taste discrimination and sensitivity to odors are common.

Proprioceptive changes common after age 60 include increased difficulty with balance, spatial orientation, and coordination. Older adults cannot avoid obstacles as quickly, and the automatic response to protect and brace oneself when falling is slower. Older adults experience tactile changes, including declining sensitivity to pain, pressure, and temperature secondary to peripheral vascular disease and neuropathies.

Meaningful Stimuli. Meaningful stimuli reduce the incidence of sensory deprivation. In the home meaningful stimuli include pets, music, television, pictures of family members, and a calendar and clock. The same stimuli need to be present in health care settings. Note whether patients have roommates or visitors. The presence of others offers positive stimulation. However, a roommate who constantly watches television, persistently tries to talk, or continuously keeps lights on contributes to sensory overload. The presence or absence of meaningful stimuli influences alertness and the ability to participate in care.

Amount of Stimuli. Excessive stimuli in an environment causes sensory overload. The frequency of observations and procedures performed in an acute health care setting are often stressful. If a patient is in pain or restricted by a cast or traction, overstimulation frequently is a problem. In addition, a room that is near repetitive or loud noises (e.g., an elevator, stairwell, or nurses' station) contributes to sensory overload.

Social Interaction. The amount and quality of social contact with supportive family members and significant others influence sensory function. The absence of visitors during hospitalization or residency in an extended care facility influences the degree of isolation a patient feels. This is a common problem in hospital intensive care settings, where visitation is often restricted. The ability to discuss concerns with loved ones is an important coping mechanism for most people. Therefore the absence of meaningful conversation results in feelings of isolation, loneliness, anxiety, and depression for a patient. Often this is not apparent until behavioral changes occur.

Environmental Factors. A person's occupation places him or her at risk for hearing, visual, and peripheral nerve alterations. Individuals who have occupations involving exposure to high noise levels (e.g., factory or airport workers) are at risk for noise-induced hearing loss and need to be screened for hearing impairments. Hazardous noise is common in work settings and recreational activities. Noisy recreational activities that weaken hearing ability include target shooting and hunting, woodworking, and listening to loud music. Individuals who have occupations involving risk of exposure to chemicals or flying objects (e.g., welders) are at risk for eye injuries and need to be screened for visual impairments. Sports activities and consumer fireworks also place individuals at risk for visual alterations. Occupations that involve repetitive wrist or finger movements (e.g., heavy assembly line work) cause pressure on the median nerve, resulting in carpal tunnel syndrome. Carpal tunnel syndrome alters tactile sensation and is one of the most common industrial or work-related injuries. Patients at risk for carpal tunnel need to be carefully assessed for numbness, tingling, weakness, and pain.

A hospitalized patient is sometimes at risk for sensory alterations as a result of exposure to environmental stimuli or a change in sensory input. Patients who are immobilized by bed rest or who have a chronic disability are unable to experience all of the normal sensations of free movement. Another group at risk includes patients isolated in a health care setting or at home because of conditions such as active tuberculosis (see Chapter 28). These patients stay in private rooms and are often unable to enjoy normal interactions with visitors.

Cultural Factors. Certain sensory alterations occur more commonly in select ethnic groups. Analysis of data from the African Descent and Glaucoma Evaluation study (ADAGES) showed that people of African ethnicity perform significantly worse than people of European descent on tests of visual function (Racette et al., 2010). Cultural disparities in vision impairment are significant, in part because visual impairment may be indirectly associated with an increased risk of suicide through poor self-rated health (Lam et al., 2008). Box 49-3 summarizes additional sensory alterations that are associated with a patient's cultural heritage.

CRITICAL THINKING

Successful critical thinking requires a synthesis of knowledge and information gathered from patients, experience, critical thinking attitudes, and intellectual and professional standards. Clinical judgments require you to anticipate the information necessary, analyze the data, and make decisions regarding patient care. Patients' conditions are always changing. During assessment (Fig. 49-1) consider all critical thinking elements that help you make appropriate nursing diagnoses. In the case of sensory alterations, integrate knowledge of the pathophysiology of sensory deficits, factors that affect sensory function, and therapeutic communication principles. This knowledge enables you to conduct appropriate

BOX 49-3 CULTURAL ASPECTS OF CARE

Disparities in Sensory Alteration

Studies indicate that differences in sensory impairments exist among ethnic groups. Non-Hispanic white and Mexican-American people have a higher prevalence of hearing problems than non-Hispanic black people (Dillon et al., 2010). Latinos have higher rates of developing visual impairment, blindness, diabetic eye disease, and cataracts than non-Hispanic whites (National Eye Institute, 2010a). Whites have a higher incidence of age-related macular degeneration than people of African descent (National Eye Institute, 2010b).

Although early diagnosis and treatment may slow the progression of sensory impairments, patients do not always volunteer information about impairments. They often focus on other symptoms or medical conditions, or they do not think that their primary care physician is the right person to talk to (Rosenberg and Sperazza, 2008).

Implications for Practice

- Encourage patients to discuss sensory impairments by asking a few simple but focused questions.
- Enhance your knowledge of the services available to patients with sensory impairments and educate patients about the organizations that exist to provide assistance.
- Facilitate access to services to promote the early detection and treatment of sensory impairments.
- Identify the patient's preferred method of communication—use an interpreter service if needed.
- Ensure that health information is available in the appropriate language and format (e.g., large print).

assessments, anticipate what to recognize when a patient describes a sensory problem, and make judgments of any abnormalities. For example, knowing the typical symptoms caused by a cataract helps you recognize the pattern of visual changes that a patient with cataracts reports.

Previous experiences in caring for patients with sensory deficits enable nurses to recognize limitations in function in each new patient and how they affect the patient's ability to carry out daily activities. For example, after caring for a patient with a hearing impairment, you are able to conduct a more effective assessment of the next patient by using approaches that promote the patient's ability to hear your questions.

When critical thinking attitudes and standards are applied during assessment, they ensure a thorough and accurate database from which to make decisions. For example, perseverance is necessary to learn details about how visual changes influence a patient's ability to socialize. Evidence-based standards of care and practice such as those from the American Academy of Ophthalmology and the American Speech-Language-Hearing Association provide criteria for screening sensory problems and establishing standards for competent, safe, effective care and practice. Use critical thinking to conduct a thorough assessment and then plan, implement, and evaluate care that enables the patient to function safely and effectively (Box 49-4).

NURSING PROCESS

Apply the nursing process and use a critical thinking approach in your care of patients. The nursing process provides a clinical decision-making approach for you to develop and implement an individualized plan of care for your patients.

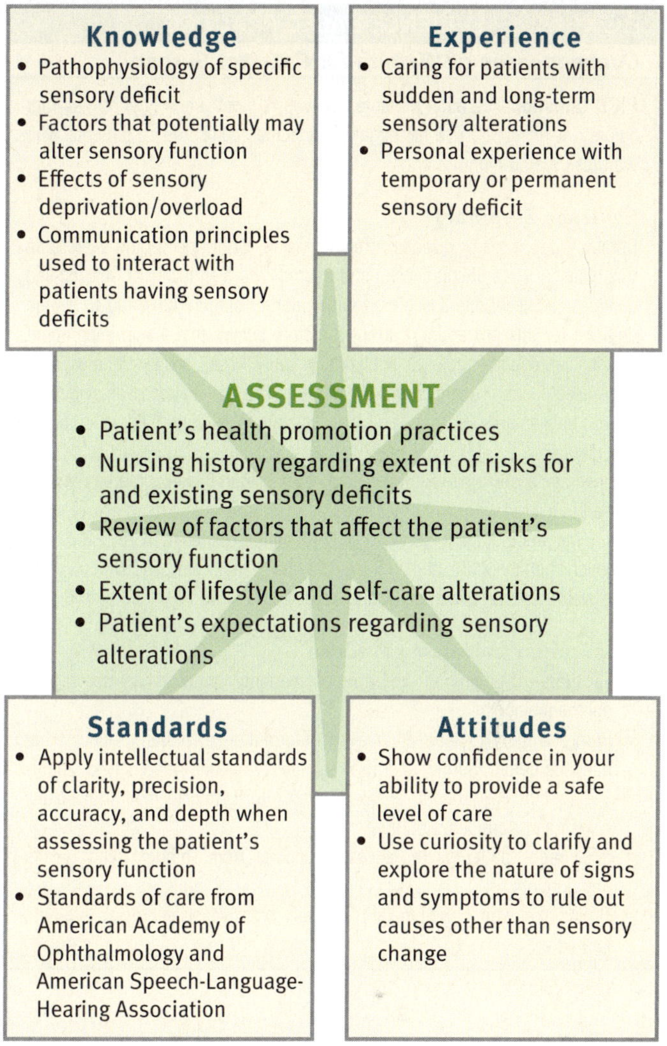

Knowledge
• Pathophysiology of specific sensory deficit
• Factors that potentially may alter sensory function
• Effects of sensory deprivation/overload
• Communication principles used to interact with patients having sensory deficits
Experience
• Caring for patients with sudden and long-term sensory alterations
• Personal experience with temporary or permanent sensory deficit
ASSESSMENT
• Patient's health promotion practices
• Nursing history regarding extent of risks for and existing sensory deficits
• Review of factors that affect the patient's sensory function
• Extent of lifestyle and self-care alterations
• Patient's expectations regarding sensory alterations
Standards
• Apply intellectual standards of clarity, precision, accuracy, and depth when assessing the patient's sensory function
• Standards of care from American Academy of Ophthalmology and American Speech-Language-Hearing Association
Attitudes
• Show confidence in your ability to provide a safe level of care
• Use curiosity to clarify and explore the nature of signs and symptoms to rule out causes other than sensory change

FIG. 49-1 Critical thinking model for sensory alterations assessment.

ASSESSMENT

During the assessment process, thoroughly assess each patient and critically analyze findings to ensure that you make patient-centered clinical decisions required for safe nursing care.

Through the Patient's Eyes. When conducting an assessment, value the patient as a full partner in planning, implementing, and evaluating care. Patients are often hesitant to admit sensory losses. Therefore start gathering information by establishing a therapeutic rapport with the patient. Elicit his or her values, preferences, and expectations with regard to his or her sensory impairment. Many patients have a definite plan as to how they want their care delivered. Some patients expect caregivers to recognize and appropriately manage and adjust their environment to meet their sensory needs. This includes helping the patient learn and adapt to a changed lifestyle based on the specific sensory impairment. Determine from the patient which interventions have been helpful in the past in the management of limitations. Assess the patient's expertise with his or her own health and symptoms. Always remember that patients with sensory alterations have strengthened their other senses and expect caregivers to anticipate their needs (e.g., for safety and security).

BOX 49-4 EVIDENCE-BASED PRACTICE

Consequences of Waiting for Cataract Surgery

PICO Question: Are adult patients who wait 6 months or longer for cataract surgery at increased risk for negative outcomes compared to patients who wait less than 6 months?

Evidence Summary

Cataracts are a major disease affecting vision. With appropriate evaluation this disease is readily diagnosed and treated. The high levels of efficacy and minimal complications associated with cataract surgery have led to a high demand for this procedure. Current literature shows that vision impairment is associated with impaired activities of daily living, social isolation, and decreased function (Lam et al., 2008). Thus the development of evidence-based benchmarks for medically acceptable wait times has significant implications.

Outcomes associated with wait times of less than 6 weeks are better than those associated with wait times more than 6 months. Patients who wait more than 6 months to have cataract surgery typically experience more vision loss, a reduced quality of life, and an increased rate of falls compared with patients who wait less than 6 weeks (Hodge et al., 2007).

Application to Nursing Practice

- Facilitate the prompt referral of patients with cataracts to an ophthalmologist.
- Before surgery provide all relevant information to patients about what happens before, during, and after surgery (Wasfi and Abd-Elsayed, 2008).
- Ensure that all patients receive written information to minimize anxiety (Wasfi and Abd-Elsayed, 2008).
- Encourage patients to access support from others with visual impairments.
- During the wait period help to identify creative strategies to promote self-care.

BOX 49-5 NURSING ASSESSMENT QUESTIONS

Nature of the Problem

- What type of problem are you having with your vision/hearing?
- What have you tried to correct the vision/hearing difficulty?
- Do you use any devices to improve your vision/hearing?

Signs and Symptoms

- Ask a patient with visual alterations: Do you require books with large print or on audiotape? Are you able to prepare a meal or write a check?
- Ask a patient with hearing alterations: What types of sounds or tones do you have difficulty hearing? Do people tell you that they have to "shout" for you to hear them? Do you have a ringing, crackling, or buzzing in your ears?
- Is there pain: sharp, dull, burning, itching?
- Have you noticed any redness, swelling, or drainage? Any signs of infection?

Onset and Duration

- When did you notice the problem? How long has this problem lasted?
- Does it come and go, or is it constant?

Predisposing Factors

- Do you work or participate in any activities that have the potential for vision/hearing injury? If so, how do you protect your hearing and vision?
- Do you have a family history of cataracts, glaucoma, macular degeneration, or hearing loss?
- When was your last vision/hearing examination?

Effect on Patient

- What effect has your vision/hearing problem had on your work, family, or social life?
- Have changes in your vision/hearing affected your feelings of independence?
- How does your vision/hearing problem make you feel about yourself?
- Do you have problems with routine care of glasses, contact lenses, or hearing aids?

When assessing a patient with or at risk for sensory alteration, first consider the pathophysiology of existing deficits and the factors influencing sensory function to anticipate how to approach his or her assessment. For example, if a patient has a hearing disorder, adjust your communication style and focus the assessment on relevant criteria related to hearing deficits. Collect a history that also assesses the patient's current sensory status and the degree to which a sensory deficit affects the patient's lifestyle, psychosocial adjustment, developmental status, self-care ability, health promotion habits, and safety. Also focus the assessment on the quality and quantity of stimuli within the patient's environment.

Persons at Risk. Older adults are a high-risk group because of normal physiological changes involving sensory organs. However, be careful not to automatically assume that a patient's sensory problem is related to advancing age. For example, adult sensorineural hearing loss is often caused by exposure to excess and prolonged noise or metabolic, vascular, and other systemic alterations. Some patients benefit from a referral to an audiologist or **otolaryngologist** if assessment reveals serious hearing problems.

Other individuals at risk for sensory alterations include those living in a confined environment such as a nursing home. Although most quality nursing homes or centers offer meaningful stimulation through group activities, environmental design, and mealtime gatherings, there are exceptions. The individual who is confined to a wheelchair, suffers from poor hearing and/or vision, has decreased energy, and avoids contact with others is at significant risk for sensory deprivation. If the environment creates monotony, the individual is less able to learn and think. Patients who are acutely ill are also at risk because of an unfamiliar and unresponsive environment. This does not mean that all hospitalized patients have sensory alterations. However, you need to carefully assess patients subjected to continued sensory stimulation (e.g., ICU settings, long-term hospitalization, or multiple therapies). Assess the patient's environment within both the health care setting and the home, looking for factors that pose risks or need adjustment to provide safety and more stimulation.

Sensory Alterations History. The nursing history includes assessment of the nature and characteristics of sensory alterations or any problem related to an alteration (Box 49-5). When taking the history, consider the ethnic or cultural background of the patient because certain alterations are higher in some cultural groups.

During the history it is useful to assess the patient's self-rating for a sensory deficit by asking, "Rate your hearing as excellent, good, fair, poor, or bad." Then, based on the patient's self-rating, explore his or her perception of a sensory loss more fully. This provides an in-depth look at how the sensory loss influences the patient's quality of life. In the case of hearing problems, a screening tool such as the Hearing Handicap Inventory for the Elderly

TABLE 49-2 Assessment of Sensory Function

ASSESSMENT ACTIVITIES	BEHAVIOR INDICATING DEFICIT (CHILDREN)	BEHAVIOR INDICATING DEFICIT (ADULTS)
Vision		
Ask patient to read newspaper, magazine, or lettering on menu. Ask patient to identify colors on color chart or crayons. Observe patients performing ADLs.	Self-stimulation, including eye rubbing, body rocking, sniffing or smelling, arm twirling; hitching (using legs to propel while in sitting position) instead of crawling	Poor coordination, squinting, underreaching or overreaching for objects, persistent repositioning of objects, impaired night vision, accidental falls
Hearing		
Assess patient's hearing acuity (see Chapter 30) using spoken word and tuning fork tests. Assess for history of tinnitus. Observe patient conversing with others. Inspect ear canal for hardened cerumen. Observe patient behaviors in a group.	Frightened when unfamiliar people approach, no reflex or purposeful response to sounds, failure to be awakened by loud noise, slow or absent development of speech, greater response to movement than to sound, avoidance of social interaction with other children	Blank looks, decreased attention span, lack of reaction to loud noises, increased volume of speech, positioning of head toward sound, smiling and nodding of head in approval when someone speaks, use of other means of communication such as lip-reading or writing, complaints of ringing in ears
Touch		
Check patient's ability to discriminate between sharp and dull stimuli. Assess whether patient is able to distinguish objects (coin or safety pin) in the hand with eyes closed. Ask whether patient feels unusual sensations.	Inability to perform developmental tasks related to grasping objects or drawing, repeated injury from handling of harmful objects (e.g., hot stove, sharp knife)	Clumsiness, overreaction or underreaction to painful stimulus, failure to respond when touched, avoidance of touch, sensation of pins and needles, numbness Unable to identify object placed in hand
Smell		
Have patient close eyes and identify several nonirritating odors (e.g., coffee, vanilla).	Difficult to assess until child is 6 or 7 years old, difficulty discriminating noxious odors	Failure to react to noxious or strong odor, increased body odor, decreased sensitivity to odors
Taste		
Ask patient to sample and distinguish different tastes (e.g., lemon, sugar, salt). (Have patient drink or sip water and wait 1 minute between each taste.)	Inability to tell whether food is salty or sweet, possible ingestion of strange-tasting things	Change in appetite, excessive use of seasoning and sugar, complaints about taste of food, weight change

ADLs, Activities of daily living.

(HHIE-S) effectively identifies patients needing audiological intervention. The HHIE-S is a 5-minute, 10-item questionnaire that assesses how the individual perceives the social and emotional effects of hearing loss. The higher the HHIE-S score, the greater the handicapping effect of a hearing impairment.

A nursing history also reveals any recent changes in a patient's behavior. Frequently friends or family are the best resources for this information. Ask the family the following questions:

- Has your family member shown any recent mood swings (e.g., outbursts of anger, nervousness, fear, or irritability)?
- Have you noticed the family member avoiding social activities?

Mental Status. Assessment of mental status is valuable when you suspect sensory deprivation or overload. Observation of a patient during history taking, during the physical examination (see Chapter 30), and while providing nursing care offers valuable data about key patient behaviors and his or her mental status. Observe the patient's physical appearance and behavior, measure cognitive ability, and assess his or her emotional status. The Mini-Mental State Examination (MMSE) is a tool you can use to measure disorientation, change in problem-solving abilities, and altered conceptualization and abstract thinking (see Chapter 30). For example, a patient with severe sensory deprivation is not always able to carry on a conversation, remain attentive, or display recent or past memory. An important step toward preventing cognition-related disability is education by nurses about disease process, available services, and assistive devices.

Physical Assessment. To identify sensory deficits and their severity, use physical assessment techniques to assess vision, hearing, olfaction, taste, and the ability to discriminate light touch, temperature, pain, and position (see Chapter 30). Table 49-2 summarizes specific assessment techniques for identifying sensory deficits. You gather more accurate data if the examination room is private, quiet, and comfortable for the patient. In addition, rely on personal observation to detect sensory alterations. Patients with a hearing impairment may seem inattentive to others, respond with inappropriate anger when spoken to, believe people are talking about them, answer questions inappropriately, have trouble following clear directions, and have monotonous voice quality and speak unusually loud or soft.

Ability to Perform Self-Care. Assess patients' functional abilities in their home environment or health care setting, including the ability to perform feeding, dressing, grooming, and toileting activities. For example, assess whether a patient with altered vision is able to find items on a meal tray and read directions on a prescription. Also determine a patient's ability to perform instrumental activities of daily living (IADLs), such as reading bills and writing checks, differentiating money denominations, and driving a vehicle at night. If a patient seems to have a sensory deficit, does he or she show concern for grooming? Does a patient's loss of balance prevent rising from a toilet seat safely? Can a patient recovering from a stroke manipulate buttons or zippers for dressing? If a sensory alteration impairs a patient's functional ability, providing resources within the home is a necessary part of discharge planning. Your findings may indicate the need for an occupational therapy consult.

Health Promotion Habits. Assess the daily routines that patients follow to maintain sensory function. What type of eye and ear care is a part of the patient's daily hygiene? For individuals who participate in sports (e.g., racquetball) or recreational activities (e.g., motorcycle riding) or who work in a setting where ear or eye injury is a possibility (e.g., chemical exposure, welding, glass or stone polishing, or constant exposure to loud noise), determine if they wear safety glasses or hearing protective devices (HPDs). Do patients who use assistive devices such as eyeglasses, contact lenses, or hearing aids know how to provide daily care (see Chapter 39)? Do patients use the devices, and are they in proper working order?

It is also important to assess a patient's adherence with routine health screening. When was the last time the patient had an eye examination or hearing evaluation? For adults routine screening of visual and hearing function is imperative to detect problems early. This is especially true in the case of glaucoma, which, if undetected, leads to permanent visual loss. Recommended screening guidelines usually occur on the basis of age. When a patient begins to show a hearing deficit, incorporate routine screening in regular examinations.

Environmental Hazards. Patients with sensory alterations are at risk for injury if their living environments are unsafe. For example, a patient with reduced vision cannot see potential hazards clearly. A patient with proprioceptive problems loses balance easily. A patient with reduced sensation cannot perceive hot versus cold temperatures. The condition of the home, the rooms, and the front and back entrances are often problematic to the patient with sensory alterations. Assess the patient's home for common hazards, including the following:

- Uneven, cracked walkways leading to front/back door
- Extension and phone cords in the main route of walking traffic
- Loose area rugs and runners placed over carpeting
- Bathrooms without shower or tub grab bars
- Water faucets unmarked to designate hot and cold
- Unlit stairways, lack of handrails

In the hospital environment caregivers often forget to rearrange furniture and equipment to keep paths from the bed and chair to the bathroom and entrance clear. It is helpful to walk into a patient's room and look for safety hazards:

- Is the call light within easy, safe reach?
- Are intravenous (IV) poles on wheels and easy to move?
- Are suction machines, IV pumps, or drainage bags positioned so a patient can rise from a bed or chair easily?

An additional problem faced by patients who are visually impaired is the inability to read medication labels and syringe markings. Ask the patient to read a label to determine if he or she is able to read the dosage and frequency. If a patient has a hearing impairment, check to see whether the sounds of a doorbell, telephone, smoke alarm, and alarm clock are easy to discriminate.

Communication Methods. To understand the nature of a communication problem, you need to know whether a patient has trouble speaking, understanding, naming, reading, or writing. Patients with existing sensory deficits often develop alternate ways of communicating. To interact with the patient and promote interaction with others, understand his or her method of communication (Fig. 49-2). Vision becomes almost a primary sense for people with hearing impairments.

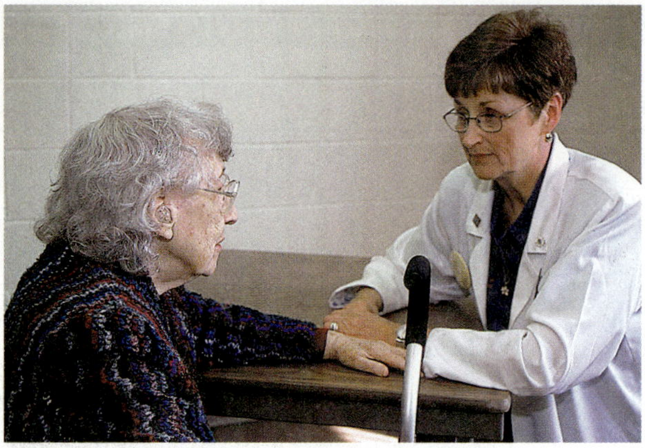

FIG. 49-2 Nurse sits at eye level so patient with hearing impairment can communicate.

Patients with visual impairments are unable to observe facial expressions and other nonverbal behaviors to clarify the content of spoken communication. Instead they rely on voice tones and inflections to detect the emotional tone of communication. Some patients with visual deficits learn to read Braille. Patients with **aphasia** have varied degrees of inability to speak, interpret, or understand language. **Expressive aphasia,** a motor type of aphasia, is the inability to name common objects or express simple ideas in words or writing. For example, a patient understands a question but is unable to express an answer. Sensory or **receptive aphasia** is the inability to understand written or spoken language. A patient is able to express words but is unable to understand questions or comments of others. Global aphasia is the inability to understand language or communicate orally.

The temporary or permanent loss of the ability to speak is extremely traumatic to an individual. Assess a patient's alternate communication method and whether it causes anxiety. Patients who have undergone laryngectomies often write notes, use communication boards or laptop computers, speak with mechanical vibrators, or use esophageal speech. Patients with endotracheal or tracheostomy tubes have a temporary loss of speech. Most use a notepad to write their questions and requests. However, some patients become incapacitated and unable to write messages. Determine whether the patient has developed a sign-language system or symbols to communicate needs.

Social Support. Assess if a patient lives alone and whether family or friends frequently visit. It is important to assess the patient's social skills and level of satisfaction with the support given by family and friends. Is the patient satisfied with the support available? Is he or she able to solve problems with family members? Is there a family caregiver who offers support when the patient requires assistance as a result of a sensory loss? The long-term effects of sensory alterations influence family dynamics and a patient's willingness to remain active in society.

Use of Assistive Devices. Assess the use of assistive devices (e.g., use of a hearing aid or glasses) and the sensory effects for the patient. This includes learning how often the patient uses the devices daily, the patient's or family caregiver's method of cleaning, and the patient's knowledge of what to do when a problem develops. When you identify that the patient has an assistive device, it is important to remember that, just because the individual has the assistive device, it does not mean that it works or that the patient uses it or benefits from it.

BOX 49-6 NURSING DIAGNOSTIC PROCESS

Risk for Injury

ASSESSMENT ACTIVITIES	DEFINING CHARACTERISTICS
Assess patient's visual acuity.	Has reduced ability to see objects clearly; needs brighter light to read; has trouble distinguishing edges of stairs
Visit home setting and inspect for hazards that pose risks to patient.	Lighting in rooms, hallways, and stairwells very dim; carpet in living room old, edges curled up; steps leading up to front entrance of home
Review medical record from clinic visit.	Diagnosis of cataracts in both eyes

Other Factors Affecting Perception. Factors other than sensory deprivation or overload cause impaired perception (e.g., medications or pain). Assess the patient's medication history, which includes prescribed and over-the-counter medications and herbal products. Also gather information regarding the frequency, dose, method of administration, and last time these medications were taken. Some antibiotics (e.g., streptomycin, gentamicin, and tobramycin) are **ototoxic** and permanently damage the auditory nerve, whereas chloramphenicol sometimes irritates the optic nerve. Opioid analgesics, sedatives, and antidepressant medications often alter the perception of stimuli. Conduct a thorough pain assessment (see Chapter 43) when you suspect that pain is causing perceptual problems.

NURSING DIAGNOSIS

After assessment review all available data and look critically for patterns and trends suggestive of a health problem relating to sensory alterations (Box 49-6). Validate findings to ensure accuracy of the diagnosis. Determine the factor that likely causes the patient's health problem. The etiology or related factor of a nursing diagnosis is a condition that nursing interventions can affect. The etiology needs to be accurate; otherwise nursing therapies are ineffective.

Some patients have health care problems for which sensory alteration is the etiology, such as with the diagnosis of *risk for injury.* You select nursing diagnoses by recognizing the way that sensory alterations affect a patient's ability to function (e.g., *self-care deficit*). In addition, most patients present themselves to health care professionals with multiple diagnoses (Fig. 49-3). In the example of the concept map, a patient with a cataract has the nursing diagnoses of *risk for injury, anxiety, fear,* and *risk for falls.* The sensory alteration caused by the cataract is an etiology for both risk for injury and risk for falls. Furthermore, fear occurs as a response to a perceived risk of falling. You need to recognize patterns of data that reveal health problems created by the patient's sensory alteration. Examples of nursing diagnoses that apply to patients with sensory alterations include the following:

- Risk-prone health behavior
- Impaired verbal communication
- Risk for injury
- Impaired physical mobility
- Bathing self-care deficit
- Dressing self-care deficit
- Toileting self-care deficit
- Situational low self-esteem
- Risk for falls
- Social isolation

PLANNING

During planning synthesize information from multiple resources (Fig. 49-4). Reflect on knowledge gained from the assessment and knowledge of how sensory deficits affect normal functioning. In this way you are able to recognize the extent of the patient's deficit and know the type of interventions most likely to be helpful. Also consider the role that health professionals play in planning care and the available community resources that will be useful. Previous experience in caring for patients with sensory alterations is invaluable.

When applying critical thinking to planning care, professional standards are particularly useful. These standards recommend evidence-based interventions for the patient's condition. For example, patients who have visual deficits and are hospitalized are often placed on a fall-prevention protocol that incorporates research-based precautions to ensure patient safety.

Goals and Outcomes. During planning develop an individualized plan of care for each nursing diagnosis (see the Nursing Care Plan). Partner with the patient to develop a realistic plan that incorporates what you know about his or her sensory problems and the extent to which he or she can maintain or improve sensory function. Goals and outcomes need to be realistic and measurable. An example of a goal of care for a patient with an actual or potential sensory alteration is "The patient will achieve improvement in hearing acuity within 2 weeks." Associated outcomes for this goal include the following:

- The patient and family will report using communication techniques to send and receive messages within 2 days.
- The patient will successfully demonstrate correct technique for cleaning a hearing aid within 1 week.
- The patient will self-report improved hearing acuity.

Setting Priorities. You consider the type and extent of sensory alteration affecting a patient when determining priorities of care. For example, a patient who enters the emergency department after experiencing eye trauma has priorities of reducing anxiety and preventing further injury to the eye. In contrast, a patient who is being discharged from an outpatient surgery department following cataract removal has the priority of learning about self-care restrictions. Safety is always a top priority. The patient also helps prioritize aspects of care. For example, a patient wishes to learn ways to communicate more effectively or participate in favorite hobbies given his or her limitation.

Some sensory alterations are short term (e.g., a patient experiencing sensory overload in an ICU). Thus appropriate interventions are likely to be temporary (e.g., frequent reorientation or introduction of pleasant stimuli such as a back rub). Some sensory alterations such as permanent visual loss require long-term goals of care for patients to adapt. Patients who have sensory alterations at the time of entering a health care setting are usually most informed about how to adapt interventions to their lifestyles. For example, allow patients who are blind to control whatever parts of their care they can. Sometimes it becomes necessary for the patient to make major changes in self-care activities,

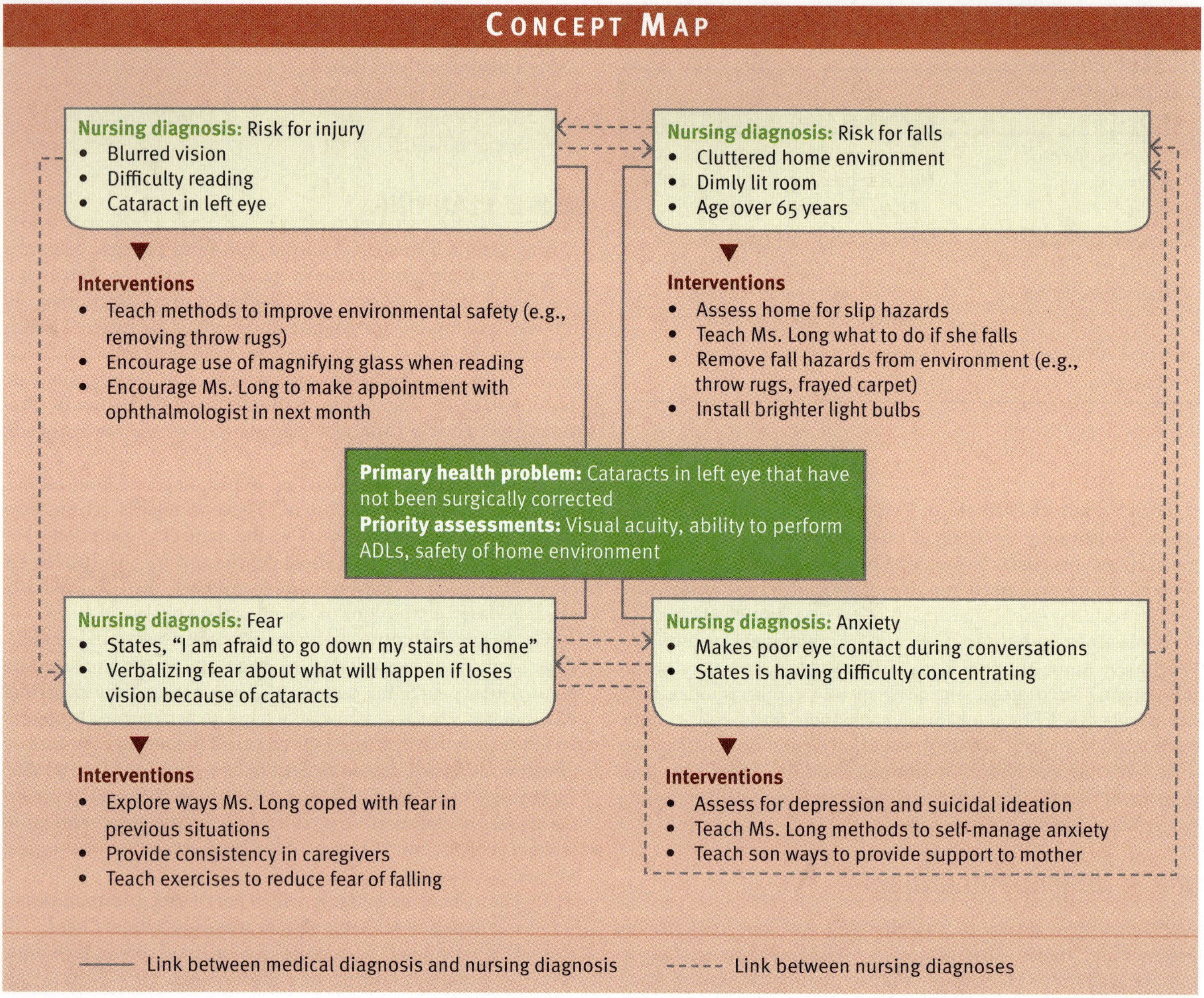
CONCEPT MAP
Nursing diagnosis: Risk for injury
• Blurred vision
• Difficulty reading
• Cataract in left eye
Interventions
• Teach methods to improve environmental safety (e.g., removing throw rugs)
• Encourage use of magnifying glass when reading
• Encourage Ms. Long to make appointment with ophthalmologist in next month
Nursing diagnosis: Risk for falls
• Cluttered home environment
• Dimly lit room
• Age over 65 years
Interventions
• Assess home for slip hazards
• Teach Ms. Long what to do if she falls
• Remove fall hazards from environment (e.g., throw rugs, frayed carpet)
• Install brighter light bulbs
Primary health problem: Cataracts in left eye that have not been surgically corrected
Priority assessments: Visual acuity, ability to perform ADLs, safety of home environment
Nursing diagnosis: Fear
• States, "I am afraid to go down my stairs at home"
• Verbalizing fear about what will happen if loses vision because of cataracts
Interventions
• Explore ways Ms. Long coped with fear in previous situations
• Provide consistency in caregivers
• Teach exercises to reduce fear of falling
Nursing diagnosis: Anxiety
• Makes poor eye contact during conversations
• States is having difficulty concentrating
Interventions
• Assess for depression and suicidal ideation
• Teach Ms. Long methods to self-manage anxiety
• Teach son ways to provide support to mother
Link between medical diagnosis and nursing diagnosis
Link between nursing diagnoses

FIG. 49-3 Concept map for Ms. Long.

communication, and socialization to ensure safe and effective nursing care.

Teamwork and Collaboration. When developing a plan of care, consider all resources available to patients. The family plays a key role in providing meaningful stimulation and learning ways to help the patient adjust to any limitations. Engaging the family or designated surrogate is a fundamental skill of patient-centered care (Cronenwett et al., 2007). You also frequently refer patients to other health care professionals. For example, early referrals to occupational or speech therapists speeds a patient's recovery. If a patient has a major loss of sensory function and is also unable to manage medical needs such as medication self-administration or dressing changes, referral to home care is an option. Valuing intraprofessional and interprofessional collaboration is an essential nurse competency and plays a role in quality patient care (Cronenwett et al., 2007). Numerous community-based resources (e.g., local chapter of the Society for the Blind and Visually Impaired and the Area Agency on Aging) are also available. Try to arrange a volunteer to visit a patient or have printed materials made available that describe ways to cope with sensory problems.

IMPLEMENTATION

Nursing interventions involve the patient and family so the patient is able to maintain a safe, pleasant, and stimulating sensory environment. The most effective interventions enable a patient with sensory alterations to function safely with existing deficits and continue a normal lifestyle. Patients can learn to adjust to sensory impairments at any age with the proper support and resources. Use measures to maintain a patient's sensory function at the highest level possible.

Health Promotion. Good sensory function begins with prevention. When a patient seeks health care, provide education about interventions that reduce the risk for sensory losses. Also recommend relevant visual and hearing guidelines.

Screening. An estimated 80 million people have potentially blinding eye diseases (National Eye Institute, 2010c). Preventable blindness is a worldwide health issue that begins with children and requires appropriate screening. Four recommended interventions are (1) screening for rubella, syphilis, chlamydia, and gonorrhea in women who are considering pregnancy; (2) advocating adequate

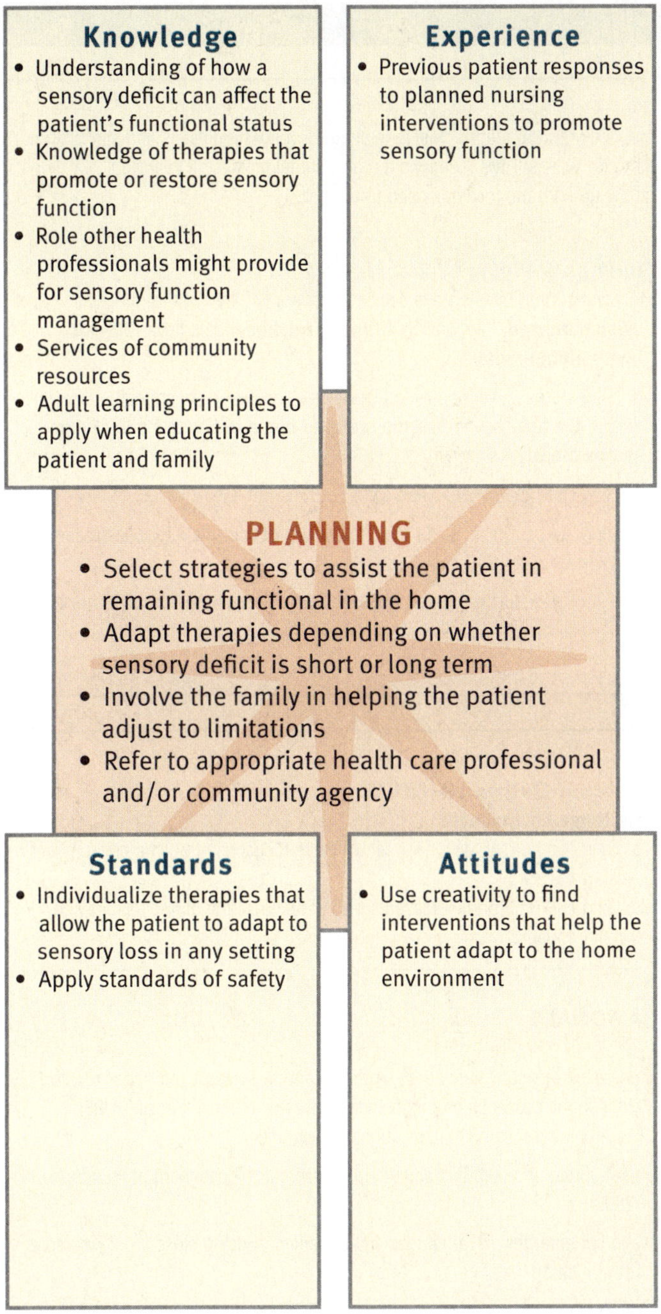
Knowledge
• Understanding of how a sensory deficit can affect the patient's functional status
• Knowledge of therapies that promote or restore sensory function
• Role other health professionals might provide for sensory function management
• Services of community resources
• Adult learning principles to apply when educating the patient and family
Experience
• Previous patient responses to planned nursing interventions to promote sensory function
PLANNING
• Select strategies to assist the patient in remaining functional in the home
• Adapt therapies depending on whether sensory deficit is short or long term
• Involve the family in helping the patient adjust to limitations
• Refer to appropriate health care professional and/or community agency
Standards
• Individualize therapies that allow the patient to adapt to sensory loss in any setting
• Apply standards of safety
Attitudes
• Use creativity to find interventions that help the patient adapt to the home environment

FIG. 49-4 Critical thinking model for sensory alterations planning.

prenatal care to prevent premature birth (with the danger of exposure of the infant to excessive oxygen); (3) administering eye prophylaxis in the form of erythromycin ointment approximately 1 hour after an infant's birth; and (4) periodic screening of all children, especially newborns through preschoolers, for congenital blindness and visual impairment caused by refractive errors and **strabismus** (Hockenberry and Wilson, 2011).

Visual impairments are common during childhood. The most common visual problem is a **refractive error** such as nearsightedness. The nurse's role is one of detection, education, and referral. Parents need to know the signs of visual impairment (e.g., failure to react to light and reduced eye contact from the infant). Instruct parents to report these signs to their health care provider immediately. Vision screening of school-age children and adolescents helps detect problems early. The school nurse is usually responsible for vision testing.

In the United States glaucoma is the second leading cause of blindness in the general population and the primary cause of blindness in African Americans. If left undetected and untreated, it leads to permanent visual loss. The American Academy of Ophthalmology (2010) recommends a regular medical eye examination with measurement of intraocular pressure every 2 years for those over 40 years old. Examinations need to occur every 1 to 2 years if there is a family history of glaucoma or if the patient is of African ancestry, has had a serious eye injury in the past, is taking steroid medications, or is over 65 years of age.

Hearing impairment is one of the most common disabilities in the United States. An estimated 37 million people in the United States are deaf or hard of hearing (CDC, 2008). Children at risk include those with a family history of childhood hearing impairment, perinatal infection (rubella, herpes, or cytomegalovirus), low birth weight, chronic ear infection, and Down syndrome. Advise pregnant women of the importance of early prenatal care, avoidance of ototoxic drugs, and testing for syphilis or rubella.

Children with chronic middle ear infections, a common cause of impaired hearing, need to receive periodic auditory testing. Warn parents of the risks and to seek medical care when the child has symptoms of earache or respiratory infection.

Because aging is associated with degenerative changes in the ear, patients need to have hearing screenings at least every decade through age 50 and every 3 years thereafter (American Speech-Language-Hearing Association, 2011). Once a patient reports a hearing loss, regular testing also becomes necessary. In addition, a patient who works or lives in a high–noise level environment requires an annual screening. Occupational health nurses play a key role in the assessment of the auditory system and the initiation of prompt referrals. The early identification and treatment of problems help older adults be more active and healthy.

Preventive Safety. Trauma is a common cause of blindness in children. Penetrating injury from propulsive objects such as firecrackers or slingshots or from penetrating wounds from sticks, scissors, or toy weapons are just a few examples. Parents and children require counseling on ways to avoid eye trauma such as avoiding use of toys with long, pointed projections and instructing children not to walk or run while carrying pointed objects. Instruct patients that they can find safety equipment in most sports shops and large department stores.

Adults are at risk for eye injury while playing sports and working in jobs involving exposure to chemicals or flying objects. The Occupational Safety and Health Administration (OSHA, 2010) has guidelines for workplace safety. Employers are required to have eye wash stations and to have employees wear eye goggles and/or use equipment such as HPDs to reduce the risk of injury. *Healthy People 2020* (USDHHS, 2009) identifies goals that include reducing new cases of work-related, noise-induced hearing loss. Occupational health nurses reinforce the use of protective devices. In addition, nurses need to routinely assess patients for noise exposure and participate in providing hearing conservation classes for teachers, students, and patients.

Another means of prevention involves regular immunization of children against diseases capable of causing hearing loss (e.g., rubella, mumps, and measles). Nurses who work in health care providers' offices, schools, and community clinics instruct patients

NURSING CARE PLAN

Risk for Injury

ASSESSMENT

Ms. Judy Long is a 70-year-old retired widow who resides in a two-story home with her son. She tells the community health nurse that she is having increased difficulty with night driving and blurry vision. She enjoys reading and sewing; however, her reduced vision limits her ability to participate in these activities. Ms. Long reports that her vision is blurred even with glasses and she is afraid that she will fall. Ms. Long visited an ophthalmologist 1 year ago, but didn't follow up with the recommended treatment.

Assessment Activities	***Findings/Defining Characteristics****
Ask Ms. Long to describe her vision changes.	Ms. Long states, "My left eye seems to have a film over it that makes my **vision blurred.** I am having **difficulty reading.** I also have **difficulty with night driving."**
Ask Ms. Long to describe life changes that have occurred since the change in vision.	Ms. Long states, "I've lost my independence because I can no longer drive at night. **I'm hesitant to use the stairs at home because I can't judge steps clearly**."
Assess Ms. Long's visual acuity.	Ms. Long can't read the Snellen chart with the left eye.
Ask Ms. Long the results of the visit to the ophthalmologist.	Ms. Long states, "I was told I had a **cataract of the left eye,** and surgery was recommended."
Conduct a home hazard assessment.	There is **clutter in the home, dim lighting,** and **stairs without handrails.**

***Defining characteristics** are shown in bold type.

NURSING DIAGNOSIS: Risk for injury

PLANNING

Goal	***Expected Outcomes (NOC)†***
	Safe Home Environment
Ms. Long will maintain independence in a safe home environment.	Ms. Long and her son will make recommended changes to home environment within 4 weeks.
	Ms. Long will report an increased sense of home safety and independence within 4 weeks.

†Outcome classification labels from Moorhead S et al.: *Nursing outcomes classification (NOC),* ed 4, St Louis, 2008, Mosby.

INTERVENTIONS (NIC)‡	**RATIONALE**
Environmental Management	
Teach Ms. Long and her son methods to improve environmental safety such as installing handrails along stairs, securing carpeting, removing throw rugs, and painting stairs.	A decrease in visual acuity and depth perception places a patient at risk for falls in the presence of environmental hazards (Ebersole et al., 2008). Environmental safety modifications reduce injury.
Teach Ms. Long to use a light over the shoulder for reading and sewing.	Good lighting and an adjustable lamp reduce glare (Rosenberg and Sperazza, 2008).
Explain use of a pocket magnifier and offer list of locations where Ms. Long can purchase one.	Magnifier enlarges visual images when reading or doing close work (Ebersole et al., 2008).
Have Ms. Long make appointment with ophthalmologist within the next 4 weeks.	Older adults need a routine eye examination annually or as recommended (Ebersole et al., 2008).
Emotional Support	
Encourage Ms. Long to express feelings regarding loss of vision and lifestyle changes.	Visual impairment often leads to functional disabilities that have adverse effects on quality of life (Hodge et al., 2007).

‡Intervention classification labels from Bulechek GM, Butcher HK, and Dochterman JM: *Nursing interventions classification (NIC),* ed 5, St Louis, 2008, Mosby.

EVALUATION

Nursing Actions	***Patient Response/Finding***	***Achievement of Outcome***
Ask Ms. Long to describe the changes made in the home to reduce environmental hazards.	Ms. Long responds that she has removed the clutter and placed handrails at the entryway. She has also placed lighting behind her chair, and there are 100-watt lights in the living room.	Ms. Long reports feeling safer walking the stairs and moving about in her home. The home hazards have been reduced.
As Ms. Long uses a magnifier, have her read a medication label.	Ms. Long is able to read name of medication and dosage correctly.	Visual acuity has not been further compromised.
Ask Ms. Long if she is able to maintain a degree of independence with the environmental and lifestyle modifications.	Ms. Long states, "I'm more independent at home, and until surgery I don't mind having someone drive for me."	Ms. Long has attained some degree of independence.

BOX 49-7 PATIENT TEACHING

Troubleshooting Hearing Aid Malfunction

Objective

- Patient and family member will identify source of malfunction in hearing aid.

Teaching Strategies

- Show patient and family member locations on hearing aid device where damage (e.g., cracks, fraying) is likely to occur: ear mold or case, earphone, dials, cord, and connection plugs.
- Demonstrate battery replacement: Have extra set of unused batteries available.
- Review method to check volume: Turn dial to maximum gain and check. Is voice clear?
- Consult manufacturer directions for specific care measures for cleaning battery case and ear mold.
- Review factors to report to hearing aid laboratory: static, distortion of sound, poor volume quality.

Evaluation

- Have patient and family member describe types of common malfunctions with hearing aid.
- Have patient and family demonstrate battery removal and cleaning.

about the importance of early and timely immunization. In all populations use caution when administering ototoxic drugs.

Use of Assistive Devices. Patients who wear corrective contact lenses, eyeglasses, or hearing aids need to make sure that they are clean, accessible, and functional (see Chapter 39). It is helpful to have a family member or friend who also knows how to care for and clean an assistive aid (Box 49-7). A contact lens wearer must frequently clean lenses (see Chapter 39) and use the appropriate solutions for cleaning and disinfection. Contact lens wearers are subject to serious eye infections caused by infrequent lens disinfection, contamination of lens storage cases or contact lens solutions, and use of homemade saline. Swimming while wearing lenses also creates a serious risk of infection. Reinforce proper lens care in any health maintenance discussion.

Older adults are often reluctant to use hearing aids. Reasons cited most often include cost, appearance, insufficient knowledge about hearing aids, amplification of competing noise, and unrealistic expectations. Neuromuscular changes in the older adult such as stiff fingers, enlarged joints, and decreased sensory perception also make the handling and care of a hearing aid difficult. Fortunately today there are a wide variety of aids that not only enhance a person's hearing but also are cosmetically acceptable and useful for persons with manual dexterity issues. Chapter 39 summarizes the types of hearing aids available and tips for proper care and use.

Acknowledging a need to improve hearing is a person's first step. Give patients useful information on the benefits of hearing aid use. A person who understands the need for good hearing will likely be influenced to wear hearing aids. It is also important to have a significant other available to assist with hearing aid adjustment. Federal regulations require medical clearance from a health care provider before an individual can purchase a hearing aid. Hearing aids are contraindicated for the following conditions: visible congenital or traumatic deformity of the ear, active drainage in the last 90 days, sudden or progressive hearing loss within the last 90 days, acute or chronic dizziness, unilateral sudden hearing loss within the last 90 days, visible cerumen accumulation or a foreign body in the ear canal, pain or discomfort in the ear, or an audiometric air-bone gap of 15 decibels or greater. A nursing assessment detects the first seven of these conditions during a physical examination. Refer the patient to an otolaryngologist for further counseling (Ebersole et al., 2008).

Promoting Meaningful Stimulation. Life becomes more enriching and satisfying when meaningful and pleasant stimuli exist within the environment. You can help patients adjust to their environment in many ways so it becomes more stimulating. You do this best by considering the normal physiological changes that accompany sensory deficits.

Vision. As a result of the normal changes of aging, the pupil's ability to adjust to light diminishes; thus older adults are often very sensitive to glare. Suggest the use of yellow or amber lenses and shades or blinds on windows to minimize glare. Wearing sunglasses outside obviously reduces the glare of direct sunlight. Other interventions to enhance vision for patients with visual impairment include warm incandescent lighting and colors with sharp contrast and intensity.

The ability to read is important. Therefore allow patients to use their glasses whenever possible (e.g., during procedures and instruction). Some patients with reduced visual acuity need more than corrective lenses. A pocket magnifier helps a patient read most printed material. Telescopic lens eyeglasses are smaller, easier to focus, and have a greater range. Books and other publications are also available in larger print. If a patient has a legal or other important document that he or she wishes to read, standard copying machines have enlarging capabilities. Closed-circuit television magnifying units enlarge written characters up to 45 times (Ebersole et al., 2008).

With aging a person experiences a change in color perception. Perception of the colors blue, violet, and green usually declines. Brighter colors such as red, orange, and yellow are easier to see. Offer suggestions of ways to decorate a room and paint hallways or stairwells so the patient is able to differentiate surfaces and objects in a room.

Hearing. To maximize residual hearing function, work closely with the patient to suggest ways to modify the environment. Patients can amplify the sound of telephones and televisions. An innovative way to enrich the lives of the hearing impaired is recorded music. Some patients with severe hearing loss are able to hear music recorded in the low-frequency sound cycles.

One way to help an individual with a hearing loss is to ensure that the problem is not impacted cerumen. With aging, cerumen thickens and builds up in the ear canal. Excessive cerumen occluding the ear canal causes **conductive hearing loss.** Instilling a softening agent such as 0.5 to 1 mL of warm mineral oil into the ear canal followed by irrigation of a solution of 3% hydrogen peroxide in a quart of warmed water removes cerumen and significantly improves the patient's hearing ability (Ebersole et al., 2008).

Taste and Smell. Promote the sense of taste by using measures to enhance remaining taste perception. Good oral hygiene keeps the taste buds well hydrated. Well seasoned, differently textured food eaten separately heightens taste perception. Flavored vinegar or lemon juice adds tartness to food. Always ask the patient which foods are most appealing. Improving taste perception improves food intake and appetite as well.

Stimulation of the sense of smell with aromas such as brewed coffee, cooked garlic, and baked bread heightens taste sensation. The patient needs to avoid blending or mixing foods because these actions make it difficult to identify tastes. Older persons need to chew food thoroughly to allow more food to contact remaining taste buds.

Improve smell by strengthening pleasant olfactory stimulation. Make a patient's environment more pleasant with smells such as cologne, mild room deodorizers, fragrant flowers, and sachets. Consult with patients to find out which scents they can tolerate. The removal of unpleasant odors (e.g., bedpans or soiled dressings) also improves the quality of a patient's environment.

Touch. Patients with reduced tactile sensation usually have the impairment over a limited portion of their bodies. Providing touch therapy stimulates existing function. If a patient is willing to be touched, hair brushing and combing, a back rub, and touching the arms or shoulders are ways of increasing tactile contact. When sensation is reduced, a firm pressure is often necessary for a patient to feel a nurse's hand. Turning and repositioning also improves the quality of tactile sensation.

If a patient is overly sensitive to tactile stimuli **(hyperesthesia)**, minimize irritating stimuli. Keeping bed linens loose to minimize direct contact with a patient and protecting the skin from exposure to irritants are helpful measures. Physical therapists can recommend special wrist splints for patients to wear to dorsiflex their wrists and relieve nerve pressure when they have numbness and tingling or pain in the hands, as with carpal tunnel syndrome. For patients who use computers, special keyboards and wrist pads are available to decrease the pressure on the median nerve, aid in pain relief, and promote healing.

Establishing Safe Environments. When sensory function becomes impaired, individuals become less secure within their home and workplace. Security is necessary for a person to feel independent. Make recommendations for improving safety within a patient's living environment without restricting independence. During a home visit or while completing an examination in the clinic, offer several useful suggestions for home safety. The nature of the actual or potential sensory loss determines the safety precautions taken.

Adaptations for Visual Loss. When a patient experiences a decrease in visual acuity, peripheral vision, adaptation to the dark, or depth perception, safety is a concern. With reduced peripheral vision a patient cannot see panoramically because the outer visual field is less discrete. With reduced depth perception a person is unable to judge how far away objects are located. This is a special danger when he or she walks down stairs or over uneven surfaces.

Driving is a particular safety hazard for older adults with visual alterations. Reduced peripheral vision prevents a driver from seeing a car in an adjacent lane. A sensitivity to glare creates a problem for driving at night with headlights. Vision is a primary consideration for safety, but there are other factors as well. In the case of older adults, decreased reaction time, reduced hearing, and decreased strength in the legs and arms further compromise driving skills. Some safety tips to share with those who continue to drive include the following: drive in familiar areas, do not drive during rush hour, avoid interstate highways for local drives, drive defensively, use rear-view and side-view mirrors when changing lanes, avoid driving at dusk or night, go slow but not too slow, keep the car in good working condition, and carry a preprogrammed cellular phone.

The presence of visual alterations makes it difficult for a person to conduct normal activities of living within the home. Because of reduced depth perception, patients can trip on throw rugs, runners, or the edge of stairs. Teach patients and family members to keep all flooring in good repair and advise them to use low-pile carpeting. Thresholds between rooms need to be level with the floor. Recommend the removal of clutter to ensure clear pathways for walking and arrangement of furniture so a patient can move about easily without fear of tripping or running into objects. Suggest that stairwells have a securely fastened banister or handrail extending the full length of the stairs.

Front and back entrances to the home, work areas, and stairwells need to be properly lighted. Light fixtures need high-wattage bulbs with wider illumination. A light switch should be located at the top and bottom of stairwells. It is also important to be sure that lighting on the stairs does not cast shadows. Have a family member paint the edge of steps so the patient can clearly see each step, especially the first and last. When possible have patients replace steps inside and outside the home with ramps.

An added consideration is to administer eye medications safely (see Chapter 31). Patients need to closely adhere to regular medication schedules for conditions such as glaucoma. Labels on medication containers need to be in large print. Make sure that a friend or spouse is familiar with dosage schedules in case a patient is unable to self-administer a medication. Patients with visual impairments often have difficulty manipulating eyedroppers.

Adaptations for Reduced Hearing. Patients hear important environmental sounds (e.g., doorbells and alarm clocks) best if they are amplified or changed to a lower-pitched, buzzerlike sound. Lamps designed to turn on in response to sounds such as doorbells, burglar alarms, smoke detectors, and babies crying are also available. Family members and anyone who calls the patient regularly need to learn to let the phone ring for a longer period. Amplified receivers for telephones and telephone communications devices (TCDs) are available that use a computer and printer to transfer words over the telephone for the hearing impaired. Both sender and receiver need to have the special device to complete a call.

Adaptations for Reduced Olfaction. The patient with a reduced sensitivity to odors is often unable to smell leaking gas, a smoldering cigarette, fire, or spoiled food. Advise patients to use smoke detectors and take precautions such as checking ashtrays or placing cigarette butts in water. In addition, teach patients to check food package dates, inspect the appearance of food, and keep leftovers in labeled containers with the preparation date. Pilot gas flames need to be checked visually.

Adaptations for Reduced Tactile Sensation. When patients have reduced sensation in their extremities, they are at risk for injury from exposure to temperature extremes. Always caution these patients on the use of water bottles or heating pads (see Chapter 48). The temperature setting on the home water heater should be no higher than 48.8° C (120° F). If a patient also has a visual impairment, it is important to be sure that water faucets are clearly marked "hot" and "cold," or use color codes (i.e., red for hot and blue for cold).

Communication. A sensory deficit often causes a person to feel isolated because of an inability to communicate with others. It is important for individuals to be able to interact with people around them. The nature of the sensory loss influences the methods and styles of communication that nurses use during interactions with patients (Box 49-8). You also teach communication methods to family members and significant others. For patients with visual deficits or blindness, speak normally, not from a distance, and be sure to have sufficient lighting.

The patient with a hearing impairment is often able to speak normally. To more clearly hear what a person communicates, family and friends need to learn to move away from background noise, rephrase rather than repeat sentences, be positive, and have

BOX 49-8 COMMUNICATION METHODS

Patients with Aphasia
- Listen to the patient and wait for him or her to communicate.
- Do not shout or speak loudly (hearing loss is not the problem).
- If the patient has problems with comprehension, use simple, short questions and facial gestures to give additional clues.
- Speak of things familiar and of interest to the patient.
- If the patient has problems speaking, ask questions that require simple yes or no answers or blinking of the eyes. Offer pictures or a communication board so the patient can point.
- Give the patient time to understand; be calm and patient; do not pressure or tire him or her.
- Avoid patronizing and childish phrases.

Patients with an Artificial Airway
- Use pictures, objects, or word cards so the patient can point.
- Offer a pad and pencil or Magic Slate for the patient to write messages.
- Do not shout or speak loudly.
- Give the patient time to write messages because patients fatigue easily.
- Provide an artificial voice box (vibrator) for the patient with a laryngectomy to use to speak.

Patients with Hearing Impairment
- Get the patient's attention. Do not startle him or her when entering the room. Do not approach a patient from behind. Be sure that he or she knows that you wish to speak.
- Face the patient and stand or sit on the same level. Be sure that your face and lips are illuminated to promote lip-reading. Keep hands away from mouth.
- Be sure that patients keep eyeglasses clean so they are able to see your gestures and face.
- If the patient wears a hearing aid, make sure that it is in place and working.
- Speak slowly and articulate clearly. Older adults often take longer to process verbal messages.
- Use a normal tone of voice and inflections of speech. Do not speak with something in your mouth.
- When you are not understood, rephrase rather than repeat the conversation.
- Use visible expressions. Speak with your hands, your face, and your eyes.
- Do not shout. Loud sounds are usually higher pitched and often impede hearing by accentuating vowel sounds and concealing consonants. If you need to raise your voice, speak in lower tones.
- Talk toward the patient's best or normal ear.
- Use written information to enhance the spoken word.
- Do not restrict the hands of a patient who is deaf. Never have intravenous lines in both of the patient's hands if the preferred method of communication is sign language.
- Avoid eating, chewing, or smoking while speaking.
- Avoid speaking from another room or while walking away.

patience. In a group setting it is better to form a semicircle in front of the patient so he or she can see who is speaking next; this helps foster group involvement. On the other hand, some patients who are deaf have serious speech alterations. Some use sign language or lip reading, wear special hearing aids, write with a pad and pencil, or learn to use a computer for communication. Special communication boards that contain common terms (e.g., *pain, bathroom, dizzy*, or *walk*) help patients express their needs.

Patient education is one aspect of communication. Teaching booklets are available in large print for patients with visual loss. The patient who is blind often requires more frequent and detailed verbal descriptions of information. This is particularly true if there are no instructional booklets written in Braille. Patients with visual impairments can also learn by listening to audiotapes or the sound portion of a televised teaching session. Patients with hearing impairments often benefit from written instructional materials and visual teaching aids (e.g., posters and graphs). Demonstrations by the nurse are very useful. Hospitals are required to make professional interpreters available to read sign language for patients who are deaf.

Acute Care. When patients enter acute care settings for therapeutic management of sensory deficits or as a result of traumatic injury, use different approaches to maximize sensory function existing at the time. Safety is an obvious priority until the patient's sensory status is either stabilized or improved. For example, patients with sensory deficits have a high risk for falls in the acute care environment. It is very important to know the extent of any existing sensory impairment before the acute episode of illness so you are able to reinforce what the patient already knows about self-care or plan for more instruction before and following discharge.

Orientation to the Environment. The patient with recent sensory impairment requires a complete orientation to the immediate environment. Provide reorientation to the institutional environment by ensuring that name tags on uniforms are visible, addressing the patient by name, explaining where the patient is (especially if patients are transported to different areas for treatment), and using conversational cues to time or location. Reduce the tendency for patients to become confused by offering short and simple, repeated explanations and reassurance. Encourage family members and visitors to help orient patients to the hospital surroundings.

Patients with serious visual impairment need to feel comfortable in knowing the boundaries of the immediate environment. Normally we see physical boundaries within a room. Patients who are blind or severely visually impaired often touch the boundaries or objects to gain a sense of their surroundings. The patient needs to walk through a room and feel the walls to establish a sense of direction. Help patients by explaining objects within the hospital room, such as furniture or equipment. It takes time for a patient to absorb room arrangement. He or she often needs to reorient again as you explain the location of key items (e.g., call light, telephone, and chair). Remember to approach the patient from the front to avoid startling him or her.

It is important to keep all objects in the same position and place. After an object is moved even a short distance, it no longer exists for a person who is blind. Simply moving a chair creates a safety hazard. Ask the patient if any item needs to be rearranged to make ambulation easier. Clear traffic patterns to the bathroom. Give the patient extra time to perform tasks. He or she needs a detailed description of how to perform an activity and moves slowly to remain safe.

Patients confined to bed are at risk for sensory deprivation. Normally movement gives an awareness of self through vestibular and tactile stimulation. Movement patterns influence sensory perception. The limited movement of bed rest changes how a person interprets the environment; surroundings seem different, and objects seem to assume shapes different from normal. A person who is on bed rest requires routine stimulation through range-of-motion exercises, positioning, and participation in self-care activities (as appropriate). Comfort measures such as washing the face and hands and providing back rubs improve the quality of stimulation and lessen the chance of sensory deprivation. Planning time to talk with patients is also essential. Explain unfamiliar environmental noises and sensations. A calm, unhurried approach gives you quality time to help reorient and familiarize the patient with care activities. The patient who is well enough to read will benefit from a variety of reading material.

Communication. The most common language disorder following a stroke is aphasia. Depending on the type of aphasia, the inability to communicate is often frustrating and frightening (see Box 49-8). Initially you need to establish very basic communication and recognize that it does not indicate intellectual impairment or degeneration of personality. Explain situations and treatments that are pertinent to the patient because he or she is able to understand the speaker's words. Because a stroke often causes partial or complete paralysis of one side of a patient's body, the patient needs special assistive devices. A variety of communication boards for different levels of disability are available. Sensitive pressure switches activated by the touch of an ear, nose, or chin control electronic communication boards (Ebersole et al., 2008). Make referrals to speech therapists to develop appropriate rehabilitation plans.

In acute care hospitals or long-term care facilities, nurses often care for patients with artificial airways (such as an endotracheal tube) (see Chapter 40). The placement of an endotracheal tube prevents a patient from speaking. In this case the nurse uses special communication methods to facilitate his or her ability to express needs. The patient is sometimes completely alert and able to hear and see the nurse normally. Giving patients time to convey any needs or requests is very important. Use creative communication techniques (e.g., a communication board or laptop computer) to foster and strengthen a patient's interactions with health care personnel, family, and friends.

Controlling Sensory Stimuli. Patients need time for rest and freedom from stress caused by frequent monitoring and repeated tests. Reduce sensory overload by organizing the patient's plan of care. Combining activities such as dressing changes, bathing, and vital sign measurement in one visit prevents him or her from becoming overly fatigued. The patient also needs scheduled time for rest and quiet. Planning for rest periods often requires cooperation from family, visitors, and health care colleagues. Coordination with laboratory and radiology departments minimizes the number of interruptions for procedures. A creative solution to decrease excessive environmental stimuli that prevents restful, healing sleep is to institute "quiet time" in ICUs. Quiet time means dimming the lights throughout the unit, closing the shades, and shutting the doors. Data collected from one hospital that implemented "quiet time" demonstrated significantly lower noise levels and light levels during day-shift quiet time. Patients were also more likely to sleep during daytime quiet hours (Dennis et al., 2010).

Building Competency in Evidence-Based Practice You are the nurse manager of a busy medical intensive care unit (ICU). The administrators of the hospital have reported that patients in the ICU are dissatisfied with noise levels impacting their rest and sleep. They have asked you to determine if implementation of quiet time will have a positive impact on sleep and patient satisfaction. Develop a PICO question (see Chapter 5) that answers the question, and identify each part of the PICO question.

Answers to questions can be found on the Evolve website.

When patients experience sensory overload or deprivation, their behavior is often difficult for family or friends to accept. Encourage the family not to argue with or contradict the patient but to calmly explain location, identity, and time of day. Engaging the patient in a normal discussion about familiar topics assists in reorientation. Anticipating patient needs such as voiding helps reduce uncomfortable stimuli.

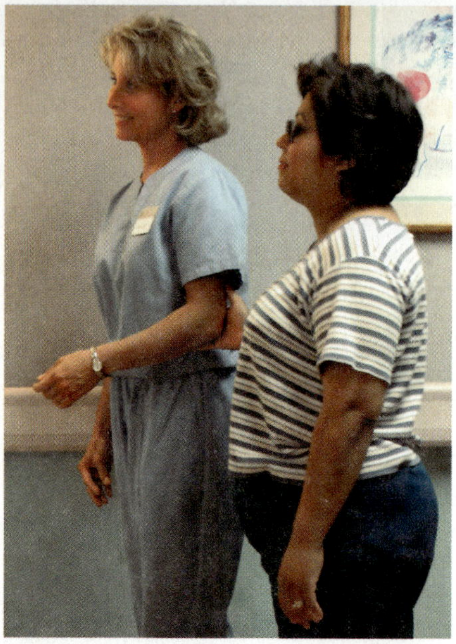

FIG. 49-5 Nurse assists in ambulation of patient with visual impairment. (From Sorrentino SA, Remmert LN: *Mosby's textbook for nursing assistants,* ed 8, St Louis, 2012, Mosby.)

Try to control extraneous noise in and around a patient's room. It is often necessary to ask a roommate to lower the volume on a television or to move the patient to a quieter room. Keep equipment noise to a minimum. Turn off bedside equipment not in use such as suction and oxygen equipment. Avoid making abrupt loud noises such as dropping objects or causing the over-bed table to suddenly adjust to the lowest level. Nursing staff also need to control laughter or conversation at the nurses' station. Allow patients to close their room doors.

When the patient leaves an acute care setting for the home environment, communicate with colleagues in the home care setting about the patient's existing sensory deficits and the interventions that helped the patient adapt to sensory problems. You achieve continuity of care when the patient only has to make minimal changes in the home setting.

Safety Measures. The patient with recent visual impairment often requires help with walking. The presence of an eye patch, frequently instilled eyedrops, and the swelling of eyelid structures following surgery are just a few factors that cause a patient to need more assistance than usual. A sighted guide gives confidence to patients with visual impairments and ensures safe mobility. Ebersole et al. (2008) list three suggestions for a sighted guide:

1. Ask the patient if he or she wants a "sighted guide." If assistance is accepted, offer an elbow or arm. Instruct the patient to grasp your arm just above the elbow (Fig. 49-5). If necessary, physically help the person by guiding his or her hand to your arm or elbow.
2. Go one-half step ahead and slightly to the side of the person. The shoulder of the person needs to be directly behind your shoulder. If the person is frail, place the hand on your forearm.
3. Relax and walk at a comfortable pace. Warn the patient when you approach doorways or narrow spaces.

While walking with the patient, describe the surroundings and ensure that obstacles have been removed. Never leave a patient with a visual impairment standing alone in an unfamiliar area. It is important to teach family members techniques for assisting with ambulation. Nursing staff also need to ensure that the patient knows where the call light is before leaving the patient alone. Place necessary objects in front of the patient to prevent falls caused by reaching over the bedside. Appropriate use of side rails is also an option (see Chapter 38).

Nurses often rely on patients in health care settings to report unusual sounds such as a suction apparatus running improperly or an IV pump alarm. However, the patient with a hearing loss does not always hear these sounds and thus requires more frequent visits by nurses. The patient also benefits from learning to use vision to discover sources of danger. It is wise to note on the intercom system at the nurse's station and in the medical record if the patient is deaf and/or blind. A patient lacking the ability to speak cannot call out for assistance. Patients need to have message boards and call lights close at hand.

Patients with reduced tactile sensation risk injury when their conditions confine them to bed because they are unable to sense pressure on bony prominences or the need to change position. These patients rely on nurses for timely repositioning, moving tubes or devices on which the patient is lying, and turning to avoid skin breakdown. When a patient is less able to sense temperature variations, use extra caution in applying heat and cold therapies (see Chapter 48) and preparing bathwater. Check the condition of the patient's skin frequently.

Restorative and Continuing Care

Maintaining Healthy Lifestyles. After a patient has experienced a sensory loss, it becomes important to understand the implications of the loss and make adjustments needed to continue a normal lifestyle. Sensory impairments need not prevent a person from leading an active, rewarding life. Many of the interventions applicable to health promotion such as adapting the home environment are useful after a patient leaves an acute care setting.

Understanding Sensory Loss. Patients who have experienced a recent sensory loss need to understand how to adapt so their living environments are safe and appropriately stimulating. All family members need to understand the way that a patient's sensory impairment affects normal daily activities. Family and friends are more supportive when they understand sensory deficits and factors that worsen or lessen sensory problems. For example, family and friends need to learn how to communicate with someone who has a hearing loss. Community resources are available to provide information to assist patients with personal management needs. The American Foundation for the Blind, American Red Cross, and National Association for Speech and Hearing offer resource materials and product information.

Socialization. The ability to communicate is gratifying. It tests a person's intellect, opens opportunities, and allows him or her to exchange the feelings that he or she has about others. When sensory alterations hinder interactions, a person feels ineffective and loses self-esteem. When patients feel socially unaccepted, they perceive sensory losses as seriously impairing their quality of life.

Interacting with others becomes a burden for many patients with sensory alterations. They lose the motivation to engage in social situations, resulting in a deep sense of loneliness. Use therapies to reduce loneliness, particularly in older adults (Box 49-9). These principles support the *Healthy People 2020* objective to increase the proportion of adults with disabilities reporting sufficient emotional support. In addition, family members need to learn to focus on a person's ability to interact rather than on his or her disability. For example, do not assume that a person who is hard of hearing does not wish to speak. A person who is blind can still enjoy a walk through a park with a companion describing the sights around them.

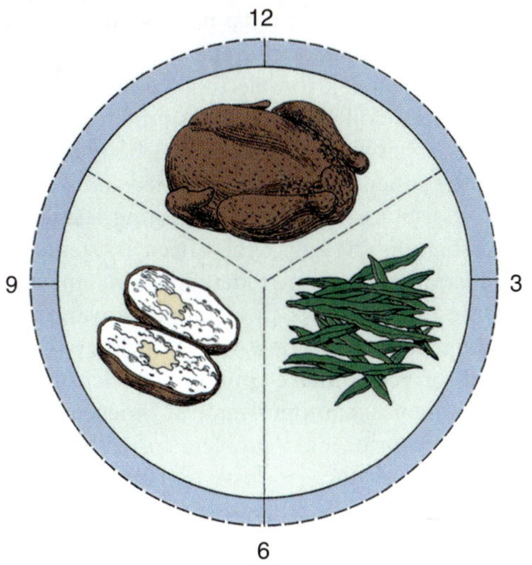

FIG. 49-6 Location of food using clock as frame of reference.

BOX 49-9 FOCUS ON OLDER ADULTS

Principles for Reducing Loneliness

- Spend time with a person in silence or conversation.
- When it is culturally appropriate, use physical contact—holding a hand, embracing a shoulder—to convey caring.
- Recommend alterations in living arrangements if physical isolation is a factor.
- Help older adults keep contact with people important to them.
- Provide information about support groups or groups that provide assistive services.
- Arrange for security escort services as needed.
- Introduce the idea of bringing a companion such as a pet into the home when appropriate
- Link a person with organizations attuned to the social needs of older adults.

Promoting Self-Care. The ability to perform self-care is essential for self-esteem. Frequently family members and nurses believe that persons with sensory impairments require assistance, when in fact they are able to help themselves. To help with meals, arrange food on the plate and condiments, salad, or drinks according to numbers on the face of a clock (Fig. 49-6). It is easy for the patient to become oriented to the items after the nurse or family member explains the location of each item.

Help patients reach toilet facilities safely. Safety bars need to be installed near the toilet. It is often helpful to have the bar a different color than the wall for easier visibility. Never place towels on a safety bar because they interfere with a person's grasp. Toilet paper needs to be within easy reach. Sharply contrasting colors within the room helps the partially sighted and promotes functional independence. General principles for promoting self-care in older adults also include using warm incandescent lighting and controlling glare by using shades and blinds (Ebersole et al., 2008).

If the sense of touch is diminished, the patient can dress more easily with zippers or Velcro strips, pullover sweaters or blouses, and elasticized waists. If a patient has partial paralysis and reduced sensation, the patient dresses the affected side first. Encourage family members responsible for selecting clothing for patients with visual impairments to follow the patient's preferences. Any sensory impairment has a significant influence on body image, and it is important for the patient to feel well groomed and attractive. Some patients need assistance with basic grooming such as brushing, combing, and shampooing hair. Others need assistance with medication administration, clothing identification, and learning to manage routine procedures such as blood pressure and glucose monitoring. An assortment of low-vision devices is now available. It is important for you to make appropriate referrals to allow the patient to maintain a maximum degree of independence.

Patients with proprioceptive problems often lose their balance easily. Make sure that bathrooms have nonskid surfaces in the tub and shower. Install grab bars either vertically or horizontally in tubs and showers, depending on how the patient is able to grasp or hold onto the bar. Instruct family members to supervise ambulation and sitting, make frequent checks to prevent falls, and caution the patient against leaning forward.

EVALUATION

Through the Patient's Eyes. It is important to evaluate whether care measures maintain or improve a patient's ability to interact and function within the environment. The patient is the source for evaluating outcomes. He or she is the only one who knows if sensory abilities are improved and which specific interventions or therapies are most successful in facilitating a change in his or her performance (Fig. 49-7). Collaborate with family members to determine if the patient's ability to function within the home has improved.

If you have successfully developed a good relationship with a patient, notice that subtle behaviors often indicate the level of his or her satisfaction. You may notice that the patient responds appropriately, such as by smiling. However, it is important for you to ask the patient if his or her sensory needs have been met. For example, ask, "Have we done all we can do to help improve your ability to hear?" If the patient's expectations have not been met, ask the patient, "How can the health care team better meet your needs?" Working closely with the patient and family enables you to redefine expectations that can be realistically met within the limits of the patient's condition and therapies. You have been effective when the patient's goals and expectations have been met.

Patient Outcomes. To evaluate the effectiveness of specific nursing interventions, use critical thinking and make comparisons with baseline sensory assessment data to evaluate if sensory alterations have changed. It is your responsibility to determine if expected outcomes have been met. For example, use evaluative data to determine whether care measures improve or at least maintain a patient's ability to interact and function within the environment. The nature of a patient's sensory alterations influences how you evaluate the outcome of care. When caring for a patient with a hearing deficit, use proper communication techniques and then evaluate whether he or she has gained the ability to hear or interact more effectively. When expected outcomes have not been achieved, there is a need to change interventions or alter the patient's environment. If outcomes are not met, it is important to ask questions such as "How are you feeling emotionally?" "Do you feel that you are at risk for injury?"

If you have directed nursing care at improving or maintaining sensory acuity, evaluate the integrity of the sensory organs and the

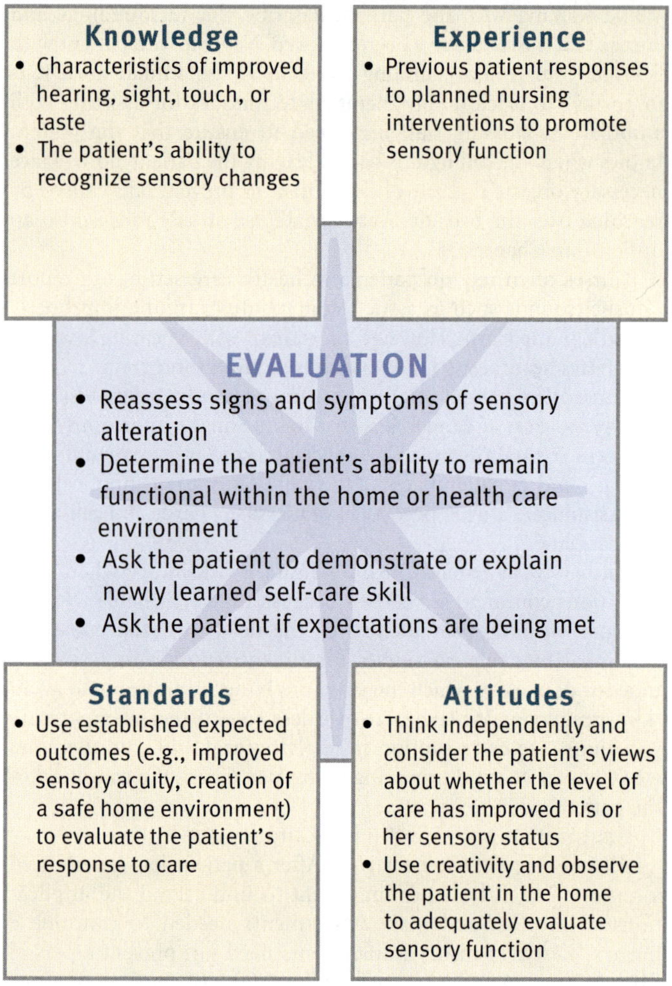
Knowledge
• Characteristics of improved hearing, sight, touch, or taste
• The patient's ability to recognize sensory changes
Experience
• Previous patient responses to planned nursing interventions to promote sensory function
EVALUATION
• Reassess signs and symptoms of sensory alteration
• Determine the patient's ability to remain functional within the home or health care environment
• Ask the patient to demonstrate or explain newly learned self-care skill
• Ask the patient if expectations are being met
Standards
• Use established expected outcomes (e.g., improved sensory acuity, creation of a safe home environment) to evaluate the patient's response to care
Attitudes
• Think independently and consider the patient's views about whether the level of care has improved his or her sensory status
• Use creativity and observe the patient in the home to adequately evaluate sensory function

FIG. 49-7 Critical thinking model for sensory alterations evaluation.

patient's ability to perceive stimuli. Evaluate interventions designed to relieve problems associated with sensory alterations on the basis of the patient's ability to function normally without injury. When you directly or indirectly (through education) alter a patient's environment, evaluate by observing whether the patient makes environmental changes. When designing patient teaching to improve sensory function, it is important to determine whether the patient is following recommended therapies and meeting mutually set goals. Asking the patient to explain or demonstrate self-care skills is an effective evaluative measure. It is often necessary to reinforce previous instruction if learning has not taken place. If outcomes are not met, these are examples of questions to ask:

- "How often do you wear your hearing aids/corrective lenses?"
- "Are you able to participate in a small group discussion?"
- "Are you able to read the newspaper without squinting?"

The results of your evaluation will determine whether to continue the existing plan of care, make modifications, or end the use of select interventions.

KEY POINTS

- Sensory reception involves the stimulation of sensory nerve fibers and the transmission of impulses to higher centers within the brain.

- When sensory function is impaired, the sense of self is impaired and affects one's ability to socialize.
- Sensory deprivation results from an inadequate quality or quantity of sensory stimuli.
- Aging results in a gradual decline of acuity in all senses.
- Patients who are older, immobilized, or confined in isolated environments are at risk for sensory alterations.
- Assessment of a patient's health promotion habits reveals risks for sensory impairment.
- Patients often do not admit to a sensory loss.
- An assessment of hazards in the environment requires the nurse to tour living areas in the home and look for conditions that increase the chances of injury such as falls.
- The plan of care for patients with sensory alterations needs to include participation by family members. The extent of support from family members and significant others influences the quality of sensory experiences.
- Patients with sensory deficits often develop alternate ways of communicating that rely on other senses.
- Care of patients at risk for sensory deprivation includes introducing meaningful and pleasant stimuli for all senses.
- To prevent sensory overload, control stimuli and orient the patient to the environment.
- Patients with artificial airways are able to communicate effectively with communication boards, laptop computers, and written messages.

CRITICAL APPLICATION QUESTIONS

Preparing for Clinical Practice

One month has passed since Ms. Long made an informed decision to have cataract surgery. After surgery she reported improved vision and ability to participate in activities of daily living. Today the community health nurse visits, and Ms. Long reports shortness of breath with activity. After the nurse consults with Ms. Long's health care provider, Ms. Long is admitted to the emergency department with a diagnosis of heart failure exacerbation.

1. Three days after being admitted to the hospital, Ms. Long reports less shortness of breath; however, she is restless and fatigued. She is on a cardiac monitor and continues to receive oxygen. The staff nurse reports that Ms. Long has slept very little since her admission. Her semiprivate room is directly across from a busy central nurses' station, and she frequently calls out for assistance. Identify the sensory alteration Ms. Long is experiencing and identify three strategies that will ensure that she gets enough sleep.
2. Ms. Long was released from the hospital in good health 1 week after admission. Following the recommendation of her health care provider, she regularly attends a heart failure support group. She has asked you to speak with the group regarding age-related visual changes and signs and symptoms that may indicate problems. What information will you share with them to promote healthy vision?
3. Ms. Long is worried about how to communicate with her sister who had a stroke and developed aphasia. What would you teach her to help her communicate more effectively with her sister?

evolve *Answers to Clinical Application Questions can be found on the Evolve website.*

REVIEW QUESTIONS

Are You Ready to Test Your Nursing Knowledge?

1. A patient has been on contact isolation for 4 days because of a gastrointestinal infection. He has had few visitors and few opportunities to leave his room. His ambulation is also still limited. Nursing measures to reduce sensory deprivation include: (Select all that apply.)
   1. Arranging for him to have a roommate.
   2. Turning off the lights and closing the room drapes.
   3. Arranging for peacefulness and frequent rest periods.
   4. Helping him to a chair or bringing a flower into the room.
   5. Sitting down, speaking, touching, and listening to his feelings and perceptions.
2. The home care nurse is instructing a nursing assistant about interventions to facilitate location of items for patients with vision impairment. Which strategy is not effective in enhancing a patient's impaired vision?
   1. Use of fluorescent lighting
   2. Use of warm incandescent lighting
   3. Use of colors with sharp contrast and intensity
   4. Use of yellow or amber lenses to decrease glare
3. A 72-year-old patient with bilateral hearing loss wears a hearing aid in her left ear. Which of the following approaches best facilitate communication with her?
   1. Speak directly into the patient's left ear.
   2. Approach the patient from behind and speak frequently.
   3. Face the patient when speaking; speak slower and in a normal volume.
   4. Face the patient when speaking; use a louder than normal tone of voice.
4. The nurse is caring for an older patient with glaucoma. When developing a discharge plan, which of the priority interventions enables the patient to function safely with existing deficits and continue a normal lifestyle?
   1. Encourage the patient's family to visit him or her once a month.
   2. Suggest to the patient that he or she consider moving to a long-term care facility.
   3. Say nothing because it is most appropriate that the patient identify personal interventions to compensate for a sensory alteration.
   4. Work closely with the patient to identify ways to modify his or her home environment and refer to appropriate community-based resources.
5. A 74-year-old patient who has returned to the nursing home following surgical removal of bilateral cataracts reports feeling a little uncertain about walking by herself. Which of the following approaches do you use to assist her with ambulation?
   1. Walk one-half step behind and slightly to her side.
   2. Have her grasp your arm just above the elbow and walk at a comfortable pace, warning her when you approach obstacles.
   3. Allow her to stand alone in unfamiliar areas to encourage confidence building.
   4. If she requires assistance, place your hand around her waist.
6. Because hearing impairment is one of the most common disabilities among children, a health promotion intervention is to teach parents and children to:
   1. Avoid activities in which there may be crowds.
   2. Delay childhood immunizations until hearing can be verified.

3. Prophylactically administer antibiotics to reduce the incidence of infections.
4. Take precautions when involved in activities associated with high-intensity noises.

7. The nurse is conducting discharge teaching for a patient with diminished tactile sensation. Which of the following statements by the patient would indicate that additional teaching is needed?
   1. "I am at risk for injury from temperature extremes."
   2. "I may be able to dress more easily with zippers or pullover sweaters."
   3. "A home care referral may help me achieve a maximum degree of independence."
   4. "I have right-sided partial paralysis and reduced sensation, so I should dress the left side of my body first."
8. The nurse completes an assessment of a 67-year-old female patient who comes to the clinic for the first time. During the examination the patient's temperature is 99.6° F (37.6° C), heart rate 80 beats/min, respiratory rate 18 breaths/min, and blood pressure 142/84 mm Hg. She is not attentive as the nurse asks questions. At one point, she shouts answers to questions about her diet. However, as the nurse speaks, the patient consistently smiles and nods in agreement. The nurse's assessment indicates:
   1. A visual deficit.
   2. Patient is normal.
   3. A hearing deficit.
   4. Sensory overload.
9. When communicating with a patient who has expressive aphasia, the highest priority for the nurse is:
   1. To ask open-ended questions.
   2. To understand that the patient will be uncooperative.
   3. To coach the patient to respond.
   4. To offer pictures or a communication board so the patient can point.
10. A patient with a history of a hearing deficit comes to the medical clinic for a routine checkup. His wife died 2 years ago, and he admits to feeling lonely much of the time. Interventions the nurse uses to reduce loneliness include: (Select all that apply.)
    1. Reassuring the patient that loneliness is a normal part of aging.
    2. Providing information about local social groups in the patient's neighborhood.
    3. Maintaining distance while talking to avoid overstimulating the patient.
    4. Recommending that the patient consider making living arrangements that will put him closer to family or friends.
11. A nurse is performing an assessment on a patient admitted to the emergency department with eye trauma. The nurse's priority interventions include which of the following? (Select all that apply.)
    1. Conducting a home safety assessment and identifying hazards in the patient's living environment
    2. Reinforcing eye safety at work and in activities that place the patient at risk for eye injury
    3. Placing necessary objects such as the call light and water in front of the patient to prevent falls due to reaching
    4. Orienting the patient to the environment to reduce anxiety and prevent further injury to the eye
12. Which patient is most likely to experience sensory deprivation?
    1. A 79-year-old visually impaired resident of a nursing home who enjoys taking part in different hobbies and activities
    2. A 14-year-old girl isolated in the hospital because of severe immune system suppression
    3. A hearing-impaired 66-year-old woman who lives in an assisted-living facility
    4. A 9-year-old boy who is deaf and uses sign language to communicate with his friends, family, and teachers
13. The medical record of an older adult reveals a stroke affecting the right hemisphere of the brain. Which of these assessment findings should the nurse expect to find? (Select all that apply.)
    1. Visual spatial alterations such as loss of half of a visual field
    2. Loss of sensation and motor function on the right side of the body
    3. Inattention and neglect, especially to the left side
    4. Cloudy or opaque areas in part of the lens or the entire lens
14. A nurse is performing a home care assessment on a patient with a hearing impairment. The patient reports, "I think my hearing aid is broken. I can't hear anything." Which of the following teaching strategies should not be implemented?
    1. Demonstrating hearing aid battery replacement
    2. Reviewing method to check volume on hearing aid
    3. Discussing measures for cleaning battery
    4. Turning dial to minimum setting and, in a louder-than-normal voice, asking the patient, "Is this voice clear?"
15. When assessing a 45-year-old patient's sensory status, which of the following assessment findings does the nurse consider a normal part of aging?
    1. Presbyopia and the need for glasses for reading
    2. Reduced sensitivity to odors
    3. Impaired balance and coordination
    4. Reduced taste discrimination

Answers: 1. 4, 5; 2. 1; 3. 3; 4. 4; 5. 2; 6. 4; 7. 4; 8. 3; 9. 4; 10. 2, 4; 11. 3, 4; 12. 2; 13. 1, 3; 14. 4; 15. 1.

REFERENCES

American Academy of Ophthalmology: *Exam frequency,* 2010, http://www.aao.org. Accessed January 4, 2012.

American Speech-Language-Hearing Association: *Who should be screened for hearing loss?* 2011, http://www.asha.org. Accessed January 4, 2012.

Centers for Disease Control and Prevention (CDC): *Health status and routine physical activities in adults by hearing status,* 2008, http://www.cdc.gov. Accessed January 4, 2012.

Cronenwett L, et al: Quality and safety education for nurses, *Nurs Outlook* 55:122, 2007.

Dillon F, et al: *Vision, hearing, balance, and sensory impairment in Americans aged 70 years and older: United States, 1999-2006, National Center for Health Statistics,* 2010, http://www.cdc.gov. Accessed January 4, 2012.

Ebersole P, et al: *Toward healthy aging: human needs and nursing response,* ed 7, St Louis, 2008, Mosby.

Hockenberry MJ, Wilson D: *Wong's nursing care of infants and children,* ed 9, St Louis, 2011, Mosby.

National Eye Institute: *US Latinos have high rates of developing vision loss and certain eye conditions,* 2010a, http://www.nei.nih.gov. Accessed January 4, 2012.

National Eye Institute: *Facts about age-related macular degeneration,* 2010b, http://www.nei.nih.gov. Accessed January 4, 2012.

National Eye Institute: *Mission and challenges for vision research,* 2010c, http://www.nei.nih.gov. Accessed January 4, 2012.

Occupational Safety and Health Administration (OSHA): *Eye and face protection,* 2010, http://www.osha.gov. Accessed January 4, 2012.

Rosenberg E, Sperazza L: The visually impaired patient, *Am Fam Physician* 77(10):1431, 2008.

US Department of Health and Human Services (USDHHS): *Developing Healthy People 2020, occupational safety and health,* http://www.healthypeople.gov. Accessed January 4, 2012.

RESEARCH REFERENCES

Dennis C, et al: Benefits of quiet time for neuro-intensive care patients, *J Neurosci Nurs* 42(4):217, 2010.

Hodge W, et al: The consequences of waiting for cataract surgery: a systematic review, *CMAJ* 176(9):1285, 2007.

Lam B, et al: Reported visual impairment and risk of suicide: the 1986-1996 national health interview surveys, *Arch Opthalmol* 126(7):975, 2008.

Racette L, et al: African descent and glaucoma evaluation study (ADAGES), *Arch Ophthalmol* 128(5): 551, 2010.

Wasfi EI, Abd-Elsayed AA: Patient satisfaction with cataract surgery, *Intern Arch Med* 1:1, 2008.

CHAPTER 50

Care of Surgical Patients

OBJECTIVES

- Explain the concept of perioperative nursing care.
- Differentiate among classifications of surgery and types of anesthesia.
- Describe the assessment data to collect for a surgical patient.
- Demonstrate postoperative exercises: diaphragmatic breathing, coughing, incentive spirometer use, turning, and leg exercises.
- Design a preoperative teaching plan.
- Prepare a patient for surgery.
- Explain the nurse's role in the operating room.
- Describe the rationale for nursing interventions designed to prevent postoperative complications.
- Explain the differences and similarities in caring for ambulatory versus inpatient surgical patients.

KEY TERMS

evolve WEBSITE

http://evolve.elsevier.com/Potter/fundamentals/

- Review Questions
- Video Clips
- Concept Map Creator
- Case Study with Questions
- Skills Performance Checklists
- Audio Glossary
- Interactive Learning Activities
- Key Term Flashcards
- Content Updates

Perioperative nursing care is nursing care given before (preoperative), during (intraoperative), and after (postoperative) surgery. It takes place in hospitals, surgical centers attached to hospitals, freestanding surgical centers, or health care providers' offices. Perioperative nursing is a fast-paced, changing, and challenging field. It is based on the nurse's understanding of several important principles, including:

- High-quality and patient safety–focused care.
- Multidisciplinary teamwork.
- Effective therapeutic communication and collaboration with the patient, the patient's family, and the surgical team.
- Effective and efficient assessment and intervention in all phases of surgery.
- Advocacy for the patient and the patient's family.
- Understanding of cost containment.

When you work in a perioperative setting, you need to practice strict surgical asepsis, thoroughly document care, and emphasize patient safety in all phases of care. Effective teaching and discharge planning prevent or minimize complications and ensure quality outcomes. The nursing process provides a basis for perioperative nursing, with the nurse individualizing strategies throughout the perioperative period so the patient has a smooth course from admission into the health care system through convalescence. Continuity of care is stressed in the perioperative model.

Care of the patient having surgery has shifted from hospital-based to home-based convalescence, with responsibility shifting to the patient and/or family. As the length of hospital stay decreases, the educational needs of the patient undergoing a surgical procedure increase. Patients return home with complex medical/surgical conditions that require both education and follow-up. Proper patient education is essential to ensuring positive surgical outcomes.

HISTORY OF SURGICAL NURSING

The discipline of surgery progressed as a science in the twentieth century to give physicians the means to treat conditions that were difficult or impossible to manage with medicine alone. In 1956 the

Association of Operating Room Nurses (AORN) was formed to gain knowledge of surgical principles and explore methods to improve nursing care of surgical patients. The organization is now known as the **Association of periOperative Registered Nurses;** however, AORN is still its acronym. AORN is the driving force for the practice of perioperative nursing and has developed standards of nursing practice that outline the scope of responsibility of the perioperative nurse. It was the first nursing organization to develop structure, process, and outcome standards as defined by the American Nurses Association (ANA). Current standards of perioperative professional practice include a patient-centered model of care with focus on (1) clinical practice, (2) professional practice, (3) administrative practice, (4) patient outcomes, and (5) quality improvement (AORN, 2011).

Ambulatory Surgery

During the 1970s the advent of **ambulatory surgery** centers (ASCs), also referred to as *outpatient surgery, short-stay surgery,* or *same-day surgery*, changed the perioperative process. Centers providing these services are hospital-based or freestanding surgical centers. Starting in 1982 Medicare began paying for surgeries performed in ASCs, and now over half of all elective surgical procedures occur on an outpatient basis. This increase is the result of payer changes and advances in medical technology. These procedures include ophthalmic, gastroenterological, gynecological, eye-ear-nose-throat, orthopedic, cosmetic/restorative, and general (Ambulatory Surgery Center Association, 2010). Many patients are discharged the day of surgery following reversal of the anesthetic agent. One-day surgery, in which the patient is admitted the day of surgery and observed overnight (23-hour admission), also occurs.

There are benefits for the patient who has ambulatory surgery. Anesthetic drugs that metabolize rapidly with few aftereffects allow shorter operative times and faster recovery time. Ambulatory surgery also offers cost savings by eliminating the need for hospital stays, thus reducing the possibility of acquiring health care–associated infections (HAIs). For example, many abdominal procedures such as gallbladder removal **(cholecystectomy)** are now performed using **laparoscopic** procedures. Laparoscopic surgery involves the use of minimally invasive techniques with small incisions and cameras or scopes for performance of the surgery as opposed to a large incision required for an open surgery. Because of the small incision, a laparoscopic cholecystectomy involves only a few hours to a 24-hour hospital stay and a recovery period of a week. By contrast, an open cholecystectomy involves a larger abdominal incision with a hospitalization of 1 to 3 days and up to a 4-week recovery period. Advances in medical technology have made laparoscopic procedures more commonplace and less risky. Thus many surgeons use them instead of traditional surgical procedures, thereby decreasing the length of surgery, hospitalization, and associated costs.

SCIENTIFIC KNOWLEDGE BASE

Classification of Surgery

The types of surgical procedures are classified according to seriousness, urgency, and purpose (Table 50-1). Some procedures fall into more than one classification. For example, surgical removal of a disfiguring scar is minor in seriousness, elective in urgency, and reconstructive in purpose. Frequently the classes overlap. An urgent procedure is also major in seriousness. Sometimes the same operation is performed for different reasons on different patients. For example, a gastrectomy may be performed as an emergency procedure to resect a bleeding ulcer or as an urgent procedure to remove a cancerous growth. The classification indicates the level of care a patient requires. The American Society of Anesthesiologists (ASA) assigns classification based on a patient's physiological condition independent of the proposed surgical procedure (Table 50-2). Anesthesia always involves risks even in healthy patients, but certain patients are at higher risk, including those who are volume depleted or who have poor cardiac function (Rothrock, 2007). ASA physical status classes 1 and 2 and also stable class 3 are now acceptable for ambulatory surgery. Classes 4 and 5 require inpatient surgery.

NURSING KNOWLEDGE BASE

Nurses made significant contributions demonstrating the benefit of preoperative education and preparation on positive patient outcomes following surgery. Structured preoperative teaching includes the AORN (2011) standards to prevent pulmonary and circulatory complications. Educating a patient before surgery can lead to increased patient satisfaction and decreased anxiety (Rosen, 2008).

Significant evidence-based knowledge is also available for proper wound care interventions. Nursing research contributes to our knowledge of the characteristics of wound healing and the types of applications most likely to be beneficial after surgery. Chapter 48 describes in detail a variety of interventions used to treat wounds, including surgical wounds.

Within the operating room (OR) setting, nursing knowledge improves the standards for infection control and patient safety. Evidence-based practice changes within the OR improve the quality of care for surgical patients and ultimately patient outcomes.

CRITICAL THINKING

Successful critical thinking synthesizes knowledge, information gathered from patients, previous experience, critical thinking attitudes, and intellectual and professional standards. Clinical judgments require you to anticipate the necessary information, analyze the data, and make decisions about patient care. A patient's condition is always changing. During assessment (Fig. 50-1) consider all of the elements that build toward making appropriate nursing diagnoses.

When caring for the perioperative patient, integrate knowledge from anatomy and physiology, pathophysiology, and the surgical stress response, along with previous experiences in caring for surgical patients. Apply this knowledge using a patient-centered care approach to making clinical decisions. The use of critical thinking attitudes ensures that a plan of care is comprehensive and incorporates evidence-based principles for successful perioperative care (e.g., airway management, infection control, pain management, and discharge planning). The use of professional standards developed by the Agency for Health Care Research and Quality (AHRQ) (http://www.ahrq.gov), AORN (http://www.aorn.org), the **American Society of PeriAnesthesia Nurses (ASPAN)** (http://www.aspan.org), and the **American Society of Anesthesiologists (ASA)** (http://www.asahq.org) provides valuable guidelines for perioperative management and evaluation of process and outcomes. Always review these guidelines within the context of new emerging evidence-based practice, agency policies, and the scope of practice of the state in which you practice.

TABLE 50-1 Classification of Surgical Procedures

TYPE	DESCRIPTION	EXAMPLE
Seriousness		
Major	Involves extensive reconstruction or alteration in body parts; poses great risks to well-being	Coronary artery bypass, colon resection, removal of larynx, resection of lung lobe
Minor	Involves minimal alteration in body parts; often designed to correct deformities; involves minimal risks compared with major procedures	Cataract extraction, facial plastic surgery, tooth extraction
Urgency		
Elective	Performed on basis of patient's choice; is not essential and is not always necessary for health	Bunionectomy, facial plastic surgery, hernia repair, breast reconstruction
Urgent	Necessary for patient's health; often prevents additional problems from developing (e.g., tissue destruction or impaired organ function); not necessarily emergency	Excision of cancerous tumor, removal of gallbladder for stones, vascular repair for obstructed artery (e.g., coronary artery bypass)
Emergency	Must be done immediately to save life or preserve function of body part	Repair of perforated appendix or traumatic amputation, control of internal hemorrhaging
Purpose		
Diagnostic	Surgical exploration that allows health care providers to confirm diagnosis; often involves removal of tissue for further diagnostic testing	Exploratory laparotomy (incision into peritoneal cavity to inspect abdominal organs), breast mass biopsy
Ablative	Excision or removal of diseased body part	Amputation, removal of appendix, cholecystectomy
Palliative	Relieves or reduces intensity of disease symptoms; does not produce cure	Colostomy, debridement of necrotic tissue, resection of nerve roots
Reconstructive/restorative	Restores function or appearance to traumatized or malfunctioning tissues	Internal fixation of fractures, scar revision
Procurement for transplant	Removal of organs and/or tissues from a person pronounced brain dead for transplantation into another person	Kidney, heart, or liver transplant
Constructive	Restores function lost or reduced as result of congenital anomalies	Repair of cleft palate, closure of atrial septal defect in heart
Cosmetic	Performed to improve personal appearance	Blepharoplasty for eyelid deformities; rhinoplasty to reshape nose

TABLE 50-2 Physical Status (PS) Classification of the American Society of Anesthesiologists

CLASS	DESCRIPTION	CHARACTERISTICS
P1	A normal healthy patient	No physiological, biological, organic disturbance
P2	A patient with mild systemic disease	Cardiovascular (CV) disease with minimal restriction on activity
P3	A patient with severe systemic disease	Hypertension (HTN), obesity, diabetes mellitus (DM)
P4	A patient with severe systemic disease that is a constant threat to life	CV or pulmonary disease that limits activity, severe diabetes with systemic complications, history of myocardial infarction (MI), angina pectoris, or poorly controlled HTN
P5	A **moribund** patient who is not expected to survive without the operation	Severe cardiac, pulmonary, renal, hepatic, or endocrine dysfunction
P6	A patient declared brain dead whose organs are being removed for donor purpose	Patients may have a wide variety of dysfunctions that are being managed to optimize blood flow to the heart and organs (e.g., aggressive fluid replacement and blood pressure medications)

Modified from Physical Status (PS) Classification. Reprinted with permission of the American Society of Anesthesiologists, 520 N. Northwest Highway, Park Ridge, Illinois, 60068-2573, http://www.asahq.org/clinical/physicalstatus.htm, 2010.

PREOPERATIVE SURGICAL PHASE

NURSING PROCESS

Apply the nursing process and use a critical thinking approach in your care of patients. The nursing process provides a clinical decision-making approach for you to develop and implement an individualized plan of care.

Patients having surgery enter the health care setting in different stages of health. A patient may enter the hospital or ambulatory surgical center on a predetermined day feeling relatively healthy and prepared to face elective surgery. In contrast, a person in a motor vehicle crash may face emergency surgery with no time to prepare. The ability to establish rapport and maintain a professional relationship with the patient is an essential component of

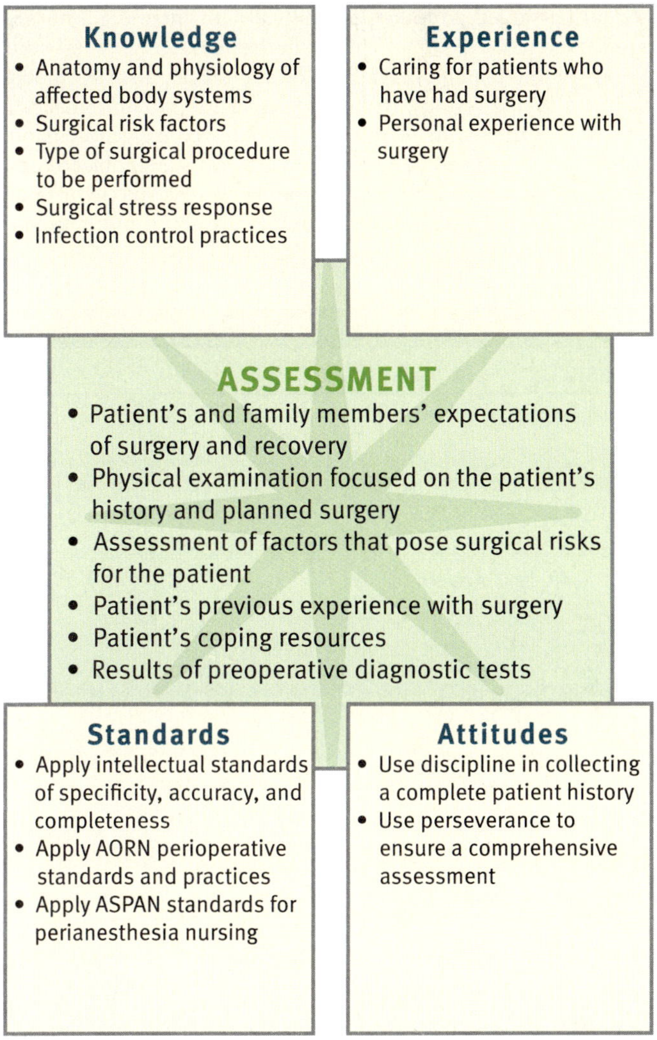
Knowledge
• Anatomy and physiology of affected body systems
• Surgical risk factors
• Type of surgical procedure to be performed
• Surgical stress response
• Infection control practices
Experience
• Caring for patients who have had surgery
• Personal experience with surgery
ASSESSMENT
• Patient's and family members' expectations of surgery and recovery
• Physical examination focused on the patient's history and planned surgery
• Assessment of factors that pose surgical risks for the patient
• Patient's previous experience with surgery
• Patient's coping resources
• Results of preoperative diagnostic tests
Standards
• Apply intellectual standards of specificity, accuracy, and completeness
• Apply AORN perioperative standards and practices
• Apply ASPAN standards for perianesthesia nursing
Attitudes
• Use discipline in collecting a complete patient history
• Use perseverance to ensure a comprehensive assessment

FIG. 50-1 Critical thinking model for surgical patient assessment. *AORN,* Association of periOperative Registered Nurses; *ASPAN,* American Society of PeriAnesthesia Nurses.

the preoperative phase. You must do this quickly, with compassion and effectiveness.

The patient meets many health care personnel, including surgeons, nurse anesthetists, anesthesiologists, surgical technologists, and nurses. All play a role in the patient's care and recovery. Family members attempt to provide support through their presence but face many of the same stressors as the patient. You need to effectively communicate with the patient and family because the nurse-patient relationship is the foundation of care (see Chapter 24). Assess the patient's physical, emotional, and spiritual well-being and cultural heritage; recognize the degree of surgical risk; coordinate diagnostic tests; identify nursing diagnoses and nursing interventions; and establish outcomes in collaboration with the patient and the patient's family. Communicate pertinent data and the plan of care to the surgical team members.

ASSESSMENT

A thorough patient assessment and critical analysis of findings ensure that you make patient-centered clinical decisions required for safe nursing care. The aim of the preoperative assessment is to identify the patient's normal preoperative function to recognize, prevent, and minimize possible postoperative complications. Ambulatory and same-day surgical programs offer challenges in gathering a complete assessment in a short time. A multidisciplinary team approach is essential. Patients are admitted only hours before surgery; thus it is important for you to organize and verify data obtained before surgery and implement a perioperative plan of care. This occurs both in ASCs and with patients who require a hospital stay.

Most assessments begin before admission for surgery—in the health care provider's office, preadmission clinic, or anesthesia clinic or by telephone. Some patients answer a self-report inventory. Other times a health care provider performs a physical examination or orders laboratory tests. Before surgery nurses begin teaching, answer questions, and begin paperwork. This streamlines the care required by the patient on the day of surgery.

So as not to waste time duplicating information from the preoperative examination, focus on key measurements for all body systems to ensure that no one overlooked any obvious problems. Also make sure that the patient understands any previous education. Even though the surgeon screens the patient before scheduling surgery, preoperative assessment occasionally reveals an abnormality that delays or cancels surgery. For example, consider an infection in a patient with a cough and low-grade fever on admission and notify the surgeon immediately.

Through the Patient's Eyes. Individualize each plan of care to be patient centered, including the patient's expectations of surgery and the road to recovery. Does the patient expect full pain relief or simply to have his or her pain reduced? Does the patient expect to be independent immediately after surgery, or does he or she expect to be fully dependent on the nurse or family? These are only a few of the questions that you need to ask to establish a plan of care that matches the patient's needs and expectations. It is important to consider the patient's values as they relate to the nature of surgery. Also be sure to incorporate any of his or her previous experiences with surgery (e.g., pain, ability to advance through postoperative exercises, experience with diet) so your current assessment is accurate and relevant. Findings often reveal patient preferences to postoperative care allowing for a more individualized care approach.

Nursing History. Conduct an initial interview to collect a patient history similar to that described in Chapter 30. If a patient is unable to relate all of the necessary information, rely on family members as resources.

Medical History. A review of the patient's medical history includes past illnesses and surgeries and the primary reason for seeking medical care. The patient's current medical record and medical records from past hospitalizations are excellent sources of data. Preexisting illnesses influence patients' abilities to tolerate surgery and nurses' choices of therapies to help them reach full recovery (Table 50-3). The history of previous surgery influences the level of physical care required after an upcoming surgical procedure. Screen patients scheduled for ambulatory surgery for medical conditions that increase the risk for complications during or after surgery. For example, a patient who has a history of heart failure may experience a further decline in cardiac function during and after surgery. The patient with heart failure in the preoperative period may require beta-blocker medications, intravenous (IV) fluids infused at a slower rate, or administration of a diuretic after blood transfusions. Box 50-1 highlights an example of a focused assessment for a patient with a cardiac history.

Risk Factors. Various conditions and factors increase a person's risk in surgery. Knowledge of risk factors enables you to take necessary precautions in planning care.

Age. Very young and older adults are at risk for complications because of immature or declining physiological status. Mortality rates are higher in very young and very old surgical patients. During surgery nurses and health care providers are especially concerned with maintaining an infant's normal body temperature. The infant has an underdeveloped shivering reflex, and often wide temperature variations occur. Anesthesia adds to the risk because anesthetics often cause vasodilation and heat loss.

During surgery an infant has difficulty maintaining a normal circulatory blood volume. He or she has considerably less total blood volume than an older child or adult. Even a small amount of blood loss is serious. A reduced circulatory volume makes it difficult for the infant to respond to increased oxygen demands during surgery. In addition, the infant is highly susceptible to complications associated with dehydration. However, if blood or fluids are replaced too quickly, overhydration may occur. Other unique

TABLE 50-3 Medical Conditions That Increase Risks of Surgery

TYPE OF CONDITION	REASON FOR RISK
Bleeding disorders (thrombocytopenia, hemophilia)	Increase risk of hemorrhage during and after surgery.
Diabetes mellitus	Increases susceptibility to infection and impairs wound healing from altered glucose metabolism and associated circulatory impairment. Stress of surgery often results in hyperglycemia (Lewis et al., 2011).
Heart disease (recent myocardial infarction, dysrhythmias, heart failure) and peripheral vascular disease	Stress of surgery causes increased demands on myocardium to maintain cardiac output. General anesthetic agents depress cardiac function.
Obstructive sleep apnea	Administration of opioids increases risk of airway obstruction after surgery. Patients desaturate as revealed by drop in oxygen saturation by pulse oximetry.
Upper respiratory infection	Increases risk of respiratory complications during anesthesia (e.g., pneumonia and spasm of laryngeal muscles).
Liver disease	Alters metabolism and elimination of drugs administered during surgery and impairs wound healing and clotting time because of alterations in protein metabolism.
Fever	Predisposes patient to fluid and electrolyte imbalances and may indicate underlying infection.
Chronic respiratory disease (emphysema, bronchitis, asthma)	Reduces patient's means to compensate for acid-base alterations (see Chapter 41). Anesthetic agents reduce respiratory function, increasing risk for severe hypoventilation.
Immunological disorders (leukemia, acquired immunodeficiency syndrome [AIDS], bone marrow depression, and use of chemotherapeutic drugs or immunosuppressive agents)	Increases risk of infection and delayed wound healing after surgery.
Abuse of street drugs	People abusing drugs sometimes have underlying disease (human immunodeficiency virus [HIV], hepatitis) that affects healing.
Chronic pain	Regular use of pain medications often results in higher tolerance. Increased doses of analgesics are sometimes necessary to achieve postoperative pain control.

BOX 50-1 NURSING ASSESSMENT QUESTIONS: CARDIAC HISTORY

Nature of the Problem
- Do you have a history of heart attack, heart failure, angina (chest pain), irregular heartbeat, or valve disease?
- Which medications are you taking?
- Are you taking any vitamins or other supplements?
- Have you had any recent medical testing or procedures on your heart (e.g., cardiac catheterization or echocardiogram)?

Signs and Symptoms
- Are you having any chest pain?
- How do you sleep at night (position, use of pillows, awakened with chest pain)?
- Do your feet swell?
- Are you short of breath or having any difficulty breathing?

Onset and Duration
- How often do you have chest pain, when does it start, how long does it last, what alleviates it?
- When do your feet swell (all the time, end of the day, only after a busy day)?
- When do you become short of breath?

Severity
- On a scale of 0 to 10 (with 0 being no pain and 10 the worst pain), what number do you give your chest pain?
- Describe your usual activity level. Can you climb stairs; can you do housework?
- Do you exercise regularly? What exercise?

Self-Management and Culture
- Have you changed your activity level, sleep amount, diet, or fluid intake recently?
- Are you taking any herbal or over-the-counter medications?

Through the Patient's Eyes
- How are you feeling about your upcoming surgery? Has it affected your symptoms?
- Are you having any additional stress currently?

aspects of a child's surgical care include airway management, management of temperature alterations, and treatment of emergence delirium or delayed emergence from anesthesia.

With advancing age patients have less physical capacity to adapt to the stress of surgery because of deterioration in certain body functions. Perioperative registered nurses (RNs) should recognize the physiological, cognitive/psychological, and sociological changes associated with aging and understand that age alone puts older adults at risk for surgical complications (AORN, 2010). Despite the risk, the majority of patients undergoing surgery are older adults. Table 50-4 summarizes physiological factors that place older patients at risk during surgery.

Nutrition. Before surgery assess if the patient is on a therapeutic diet and if there are any factors influencing food intake such as ability to chew and swallow and the presence of regurgitation after meals. This affects your choice of postoperative foods and liquids. In addition, normal tissue repair and resistance to infection depend on adequate nutrients. Surgery intensifies this need. After surgery a patient requires at least 1500 kcal/day to maintain energy reserves. Increased protein, vitamins A and C, and zinc facilitate wound healing (see Chapters 44 and 48). A patient who is malnourished is prone to poor tolerance to anesthesia, negative nitrogen balance from lack of protein, delayed blood-clotting mechanisms, infection, and poor wound healing. Assess the patient's weight and height to determine body mass index. Many hospitalized patients display some degree of malnutrition. If a patient has elective surgery, attempt to correct nutritional imbalances before surgery. However, if a patient who is malnourished must undergo an emergency procedure, efforts to restore nutrients occur after surgery.

Obesity. Obesity increases surgical risk by reducing ventilatory and cardiac function. Obstructive sleep apnea, hypertension, coronary artery disease, diabetes mellitus, and heart failure are

TABLE 50-4 Physiological Factors That Place the Older Adult at Risk During Surgery

ALTERATIONS	RISKS	NURSING IMPLICATIONS
Cardiovascular System		
Degenerative change in myocardium and valves	Decreased cardiac reserve puts older adults at risk for decreased cardiac output, especially during times of stress (AORN, 2010)	Assess baseline vital signs for tachycardia, fatigue, and arrhythmias (AORN, 2010).
Rigidity of arterial walls and reduction in sympathetic and parasympathetic innervation to the heart	Alterations predispose patient to postoperative hemorrhage and rise in systolic and diastolic blood pressure	Maintain adequate fluid balance to minimize stress to the heart. Ensure that blood pressure level is adequate to meet circulatory demands.
Increase in calcium and cholesterol deposits within small arteries; thickened arterial walls	Predispose patient to clot formation in lower extremities	Instruct patient in techniques of leg exercises and proper turning. Apply elastic stockings or intermittent pneumatic compression (IPC) devices. Administer anticoagulants as ordered by health care provider. Provide education regarding effects, side effects, and dietary considerations.
Integumentary System		
Decreased subcutaneous tissue and increased fragility of skin	Prone to pressure ulcers and skin tears	Assess skin every 4 hours; pad all bony prominences during surgery. Turn or reposition at least every 2 hours.
Pulmonary System		
Decreased respiratory muscle strength and cough reflex (AORN, 2010)	Increased risk for atelectasis	Instruct patient in proper technique for coughing, deep breathing, and use of spirometer. Ensure adequate pain control to allow for participation in exercises.
Reduced range of movement in diaphragm	Residual capacity (volume of air is left in lung after normal breath) increased, reducing amount of new air brought into lungs with each inspiration	When possible, have patient ambulate and sit in chair frequently.
Stiffened lung tissue and enlarged air spaces	Blood oxygenation reduced	Obtain baseline oxygen saturation; measure throughout perioperative period.
Gastrointestinal System		
Gastric emptying delayed	Increases the risk for reflux and indigestion (AORN, 2010)	Position patient with head of bed elevated at least 45 degrees. Reduce size of meals in accordance with ordered diet.
Renal System		
Decreased renal function, with reduced blood flow to kidneys	Increased risk of shock when blood loss occurs; increased risk for fluid and electrolyte imbalance (AORN, 2010)	For patients hospitalized before surgery, determine baseline urinary output for 24 hours.
Reduced glomerular filtration rate and excretory times	Limits ability to eliminate drugs or toxic substances	Assess for adverse response to drugs.
Decreased bladder capacity	Increases the risk for urgency, incontinence, and urinary tract infections (AORN, 2010) (Sensation of need to void often does not occur until bladder is filled)	Instruct patient to notify nurse immediately when sensation of bladder fullness develops. Keep call light and bedpan within easy reach. Toilet every 2 hours or more frequently if indicated.

Continued

TABLE 50-4 Physiological Factors That Place the Older Adult at Risk During Surgery—cont'd

ALTERATIONS	RISKS	NURSING IMPLICATIONS
Neurological System		
Sensory losses, including reduced tactile sense and increased pain tolerance	Decreased ability to respond to early warning signs of surgical complications	Inspect bony prominences for signs of pressure that patient is unable to sense. Orient patient to surrounding environment. Observe for nonverbal signs of pain.
Blunted febrile response during infection (AORN, 2010)	Increased risk of undiagnosed infection	Ensure careful, close monitoring of patient temperature; provide warm blankets; monitor heart function; warm intravenous fluids (AORN, 2010).
Decreased reaction time	Confusion and delirium after anesthesia; increased risk for falls	Allow adequate time to respond, process information, and perform tasks. Perform fall risk screening and institute fall precautions. Screen for delirium with validated tools. Orient frequently to reality and surroundings.
Metabolic System		
Lower basal metabolic rate	Reduced total oxygen consumption	Ensure adequate nutritional intake when diet is resumed but avoid intake of excess calories.
Reduced number of red blood cells and hemoglobin levels	Reduced ability to carry adequate oxygen to tissues	Administer necessary blood products. Monitor blood test results and oxygen saturation.
Change in total amounts of body potassium and water volume	Greater risk for fluid or electrolyte imbalance	Monitor electrolyte levels and supplement as necessary. Provide cardiac monitoring (telemetry) as needed.

common in the **bariatric** (obese) population. Embolus, **atelectasis,** and pneumonia are common postoperative complications in the patient who is obese. He or she often has difficulty resuming normal physical activity after surgery and is susceptible to poor wound healing and wound infection because of the structure of fatty tissue, which contains a poor blood supply. This slows delivery of essential nutrients, antibodies, and enzymes needed for wound healing (see Chapter 48). It is often difficult to close the surgical wound of a patient who is obese because of the thick adipose layer; thus he or she is at risk for dehiscence (opening of the suture line) and evisceration (abdominal contents protruding through surgical incision).

Obstructive Sleep Apnea. **Obstructive sleep apnea (OSA)** is a syndrome of periodic, partial, or complete obstruction of the upper airway during sleep. Patients with diagnosed OSA have an increased incidence of postoperative complications, the most frequent being oxygen desaturation (Liao et al., 2009). Assess for a history of diagnosed OSA and use of continuous positive airway pressure (CPAP), noninvasive positive-pressure ventilation (NIPPV), or apnea monitoring. Instruct patients who use CPAP or NIPPV to bring their machine to the hospital or surgery center. Many patients with OSA are undiagnosed; thus it is becoming standard practice to assess for risk of OSA before surgery. It is necessary to ask the patient and sleep partner about symptoms of OSA such as snoring, apnea during sleep, frequent arousals during sleep, morning headaches, daytime somnolence, and chronic fatigue (ASA, 2006; Seet and Chung, 2010).

Immunocompromise. Patients with conditions that alter immune function are more at risk for developing infection after surgery. Examples include patients with cancer, bone marrow alterations, and those who undergo radiation therapy. Radiation is sometimes given before surgery to reduce the size of a cancerous tumor so it can be removed surgically. It has some unavoidable effects on normal tissue such as excess thinning of skin layers, destruction of collagen, and impaired vascularization of tissue. Ideally the surgeon waits to perform surgery 4 to 6 weeks after completion of radiation treatments. Otherwise the patient may face serious wound-healing problems. In addition, the use of chemotherapeutic drugs for cancer treatment, immunosuppressive medications for preventing rejection after organ transplantation, and steroids for treating a variety of inflammatory or autoimmune conditions increases the risk for infection.

Fluid and Electrolyte Imbalance. The body responds to surgery as a form of trauma. Severe protein breakdown causes a negative nitrogen balance (see Chapter 44) and hyperglycemia. Both of these effects decrease tissue healing and increase the risk of infection. As a result of the adrenocortical stress response, the body retains sodium and water and loses potassium within the first 2 to 5 days after surgery. The severity of the stress response influences the degree of fluid and electrolyte imbalance. Extensive surgery results in a greater stress response. A patient who is hypovolemic or who has serious preoperative electrolyte alterations is at significant risk during and after surgery. For example, an excess or depletion of potassium increases the chance of dysrhythmias during or after surgery. If the patient has preexisting diabetes mellitus or renal, gastrointestinal (GI), or cardiovascular abnormalities, the risk of fluid and electrolyte alterations is even greater.

Pregnancy. The perioperative plan of care addresses not one, but two patients: the mother and the developing fetus. The pregnant patient has surgery only on an emergent or urgent basis. Because all of the mother's major systems are affected during pregnancy, the risk for intraoperative complications is increased. General anesthesia is administered with caution because of the increased risk of fetal death and preterm labor. Psychological assessment of mother and family is essential.

Perceptions and Knowledge Regarding Surgery. A patient's past experience with surgery influences physical and psychological responses to a procedure. Assess the patient's previous experiences with surgery as a foundation for anticipating his or her needs, providing teaching, addressing fears, and clarifying concerns. Ask the patient to discuss the previous type of surgery, level of discomfort, extent of disability, and overall level of care required. Address any complications that the patient experienced. It is also important to assess patients for motion sickness and nausea and vomiting during previous surgeries since these factors increase the risk for aspiration (McCaffrey, 2007). Prior anesthesia records are a useful source of information if previous problems occurred.

The surgical experience affects the family unit as a whole. Therefore prepare both the patient and the family for the surgical experience. Understanding of a patient's and family's knowledge, expectations, and perceptions allows you to plan teaching and provide individualized emotional support measures.

Each patient fears surgery. Some fears are the result of past hospital experiences, warnings from friends and family, or lack of knowledge. Assess the patient's understanding of the planned surgery, its implications, and planned postoperative activities. Ask questions such as "Tell me what you think will happen before and after surgery" or "Explain what you know about surgery." Nurses face ethical dilemmas when patients are misinformed or unaware of the reason for surgery. Confer with the surgeon if the patient has an inaccurate perception or knowledge of the surgical procedure before the patient is sent to the surgical suite. Also determine whether the health care provider explained routine preoperative and postoperative procedures and assess the patient's readiness and willingness to learn. When a patient is well prepared and knows what to expect, reinforce his or her knowledge.

Medication History. Presence of preexisting co-morbid conditions such as hypertension, renal or heart disease, respiratory disorders, and diabetes increases a patient's surgical risk. If a patient regularly uses prescription or over-the-counter medications, the surgeon or anesthesia provider may temporarily discontinue the drugs before surgery or adjust the dosages. Certain medications pose greater risks for surgical complications (Table 50-5). Instruct patients to ask the health care provider if they need to take usual medications the morning of surgery. Also ask them if they take any herbal preparations because many patients do not view herbs as medications and often omit them from their medication history (see Chapter 32). Certain herbs interfere with the action of other medications (consult the pharmacist). For hospitalized patients prescription drugs taken before surgery are automatically discontinued after surgery unless the health care provider reorders them. The use of a medication reconciliation process (see Chapter 31) is common practice to ensure that at the time of a patient's admission a complete list of the medications the patient is taking at home is created and documented. The patient and, as needed, the family needs to be involved to be sure that there is an accurate and current medication list for the patient (TJC, 2011).

Allergies. Assess for patients' allergies to drugs during the perioperative period. Also assess for latex, food, and contact allergies (e.g., to tape, ointments, or solutions). A wide variety of equipment and materials used in the OR contains latex; thus assessment is critical. Patients most at risk for a latex allergy include people with genetic predisposition to latex allergy, children with spina bifida, patients with urogenital abnormalities or spinal cord injury (because of a long history of urinary catheter use), patients with a history of multiple surgeries, health care professionals, and workers who manufacture rubber products. Patients with an allergy to certain foods such as bananas, chestnuts, kiwi fruit, avocadoes, and tomatoes have shown a cross-sensitivity to latex (Sussman and Gold, 2010). Surgical centers provide latex-free environments for patients with known latex allergies.

TABLE 50-5 Drugs with Special Implications for the Surgical Patient

DRUG CLASS	EFFECTS DURING SURGERY
Antibiotics	Potentiate (enhance action of) anesthetic agents. If taken within 2 weeks before surgery, aminoglycosides (gentamicin, neomycin, tobramycin) may cause mild respiratory depression from depressed neuromuscular transmission.
Antidysrhythmics	Medications (e.g., beta blockers) can reduce cardiac contractility and impair cardiac conduction during anesthesia.
Anticoagulants	Medications such as warfarin (Coumadin) or aspirin alter normal clotting factors and thus increase risk of hemorrhaging. Discontinue at least 48 hours before surgery.
Anticonvulsants	Long-term use of certain anticonvulsants (e.g., phenytoin [Dilantin] and phenobarbital) alters metabolism of anesthetic agents.
Antihypertensives	Medications such as beta blockers and calcium channel blockers interact with anesthetic agents to cause bradycardia, hypotension, and impaired circulation. They inhibit synthesis and storage of norepinephrine in sympathetic nerve endings.
Corticosteroids	With prolonged use corticosteroids such as prednisone cause adrenal atrophy, which reduces the ability of the body to withstand stress. Before and during surgery, dosages are often temporarily increased.
Insulin	Patients' need for insulin changes after surgery. Stress response and intravenous (IV) administration of glucose solutions often increase dosage requirements after surgery. Decreased nutritional intake often decreases dosage requirements.
Diuretics	Diuretics such as furosemide (Lasix) potentiate electrolyte imbalances (particularly potassium) after surgery.
Nonsteroidal anti-inflammatory drugs (NSAIDs)	NSAIDs (e.g., ibuprofen) inhibit platelet aggregation and prolong bleeding time, increasing susceptibility to postoperative bleeding.
Herbal therapies: ginger, gingko, ginseng	These herbal therapies have the ability to affect platelet activity and increase susceptibility to postoperative bleeding. Ginseng is reported to increase hypoglycemia with insulin therapy.

Some patients are too young or have not had any exposure to drugs; thus they do not know if they have allergies. The type of allergic response is very important to assess. Allergies are not the same as unpleasant side effects. For example, codeine may cause nausea (a side effect) or hypotension and confusion (an allergy). When asking a patient about allergies, realize that the term *allergy* is confusing for some patients. Asking a patient if he or she has ever "had a problem with a medication or substance" is a helpful approach to questioning. Ensure that you list the patient's allergies appropriately in his or her chart and/or the hospital computer system and any other places designated by institutional policy such as an allergy band.

Smoking Habits. The patient who smokes is at greater risk for postoperative pulmonary complications than a patient who does not (Smetana, 2009). The chronic smoker already has an increased amount and thickness of mucus secretions in the lungs. General anesthetics increase airway irritation and stimulate pulmonary secretions, which the airways retain as a result of reduction in ciliary activity during anesthesia. After surgery the patient who smokes has greater difficulty clearing the airways of mucus secretions and needs to know the importance of postoperative deep breathing and coughing (see Chapter 40).

Alcohol Ingestion and Substance Use and Abuse. Habitual use of alcohol and illegal drugs predisposes the patient to adverse reactions to anesthetic agents. Some patients experience a cross-tolerance to anesthetic agents, necessitating higher-than-normal doses. In addition, the health care provider may need to increase postoperative dosages of analgesics. Patients with a history of excessive alcohol ingestion are often malnourished, which delays wound healing. These patients are also at risk for liver disease, portal hypertension, and esophageal varices (predisposing the patient to bleeding disorders). The patient who habitually uses alcohol and is required to remain in the hospital longer than 24 hours is also at risk for acute alcohol withdrawal and its more severe form, delirium tremens (DTs).

Support Sources. Because a patient's family does not always consist of blood relations, always assess who comprises family and their level of support. The patient usually cannot immediately assume the same level of physical activity enjoyed before surgery. With ambulatory surgery patients and families assume responsibility for postoperative care. The family is an important resource for the patient with physical limitations and provides the emotional support needed to motivate him or her to return to a previous state of health. Sometimes a family member remembers preoperative and postoperative teaching better than the patient. With older adults having ambulatory surgery, it is important to establish before surgery that the patient will receive a postdischarge phone call as a check on recovery progress. Because some older adults are unable to hear or reach a phone after surgery, identify if a family member will be staying with the patient to answer the phone. Another option is an arrangement for the family member to call the surgery center the next day to ensure proper follow-up (Mamaril, 2006).

Ask if family members or friends are able to provide support. Some patients want someone else present when you provide instructions or explanations. Encourage family presence when feasible, especially for patients in the ambulatory setting. Often a family member becomes the patient's coach, offering valuable support during the postoperative period when the patient's participation in care is vital.

Occupation. Surgery often results in physical changes and limits that prevent a person from returning to work or lengthen recovery time before work can be resumed. Assess the patient's occupational history to anticipate the possible effects of surgery on recovery, return to work, and eventual work performance. Explain any restrictions such as lifting, use of the extremities, or climbing stairs before a patient returns to work. When a patient is unable to return to a job, refer him or her to a social worker and/or occupational therapist for job-training programs or to help him or her seek economic assistance.

Preoperative Pain Assessment. Surgical manipulation of tissues, treatments, and positioning on the OR table contribute to postoperative pain. Before surgery conduct a comprehensive pain assessment, including the patient's and family's expectations for pain management following surgery. Ask patients to describe their perceived tolerance to pain, past experiences, and prior successful interventions used. Teaching patients how to score their pain before surgery allows for more effective self-report of pain after surgery (Bond et al., 2005). Use a pain instrument to rate the presence and severity of pain before surgery (see Chapter 43). Frequent pain assessments are necessary to alert nurses to treat the pain and assess the adequacy (outcome) of pain interventions.

Review of Emotional Health. Surgery is psychologically stressful. Patients are often anxious about the surgery and its implications and believe that they are powerless over their situation. Family members may perceive the patient's surgery as a disruption of their lifestyle. Hospitalization and the recovery period at home are sometimes lengthy. The family is usually concerned about the patient returning to a normal, productive life. When the patient has chronic illness, the family is either fearful that surgery will result in further disability or hopeful that it will improve their lifestyle. To understand the impact of surgery on a patient's and family's emotional health, assess the patient's feelings about surgery, self-concept, body image, and coping resources.

It is difficult to assess a patient's feelings thoroughly when ambulatory surgery is scheduled because you have less time to establish a relationship with him or her. You can address these concerns initially with the patient during a home visit or on the telephone before surgery. In a hospital room choose a time for discussion after completing admitting procedures or diagnostic tests. Explain that it is normal to have fears and concerns. For example, patients often have a fear of being "put to sleep" under anesthesia because it causes loss of control. A patient's ability to share feelings partially depends on your willingness to listen, be supportive, and clarify misconceptions. Assure patients of their right to ask questions and seek information.

Self-Concept. Patients with a positive self-concept are more likely to approach surgical experiences appropriately. Assess self-concept by asking patients to identify personal strengths and weaknesses (see Chapter 33). Patients who are quick to criticize or scorn their own personal characteristics may have little self-regard or may be testing your opinion of their character. Poor self-concept hinders the ability to adapt to the stress of surgery and aggravates feelings of guilt or inadequacy.

Body Image. Surgical removal of any diseased body part often leaves permanent disfigurement, alteration in body function, or concern over mutilation. Loss of certain body functions (e.g., with a colostomy or amputation) may compound a patient's fears. Assess for body image alterations that patients perceive will result from surgery. Individuals respond differently, depending on their culture, age, experience in seeing others with alterations, and their own self-concept and self-esteem (see Chapter 33).

Often surgery changes the physical or psychological aspects of patients' sexuality. Excision of breast tissue, an ostomy, hysterectomy, or removal of the prostate gland affects patients' perceptions of their sexuality. Surgery such as hernia repair or cataract extraction forces patients to temporarily refrain from sexual intercourse until they return to normal physical activity. Encourage patients to express concerns about their sexuality. The patient facing even temporary sexual dysfunction requires understanding and support. Hold discussions about the patient's sexuality with his or her sexual partner so the partner gains a shared understanding of how to cope with limitations in sexual function (see Chapter 34).

Coping Resources. Assessment of feelings and self-concept reveals whether the patient is able to cope with the stress of surgery. The physiological effects of stress are well documented. Activation of the endocrine system results in the release of hormones and catecholamines, which increases blood pressure, heart rate, and respiration. Platelet aggregation also occurs, along with many other physiological responses. Be aware of these responses and assist with stress management (see Chapter 37).

Ask the patient about past stress management techniques and behaviors that helped resolve any tension or nervousness. When reviewing the patient's coping resources, ask him or her about specific family members and friends who may provide support. Once identified, include these individuals in any patient teaching and interventions to manage stress and anxiety.

Culture and Religion. Culture is a system of beliefs and values developed over time and passed on through many generations. Patients come from diverse cultural, ethnic, and religious backgrounds, which affect the way each patient perceives and reacts to the surgical experience. An important aspect of patient-centered care is to identify a family's and patient's expectations for relief of pain, discomfort, and suffering (Cronenwett et al., 2007). If you do not acknowledge and plan for cultural, ethnic, and religious differences in the perioperative plan of care, you may not achieve desired surgical outcomes (Box 50-2). The acquisition of knowledge about a patient's cultural and ethnic heritage helps you care for the perioperative patient. Although it is important to recognize and plan for differences based on culture, it is also necessary to recognize that members of the same culture are individuals and do not always hold these shared beliefs.

Physical Examination. Conduct a partial or complete physical examination, depending on the amount of time available and the patient's preoperative condition. Chapter 30 describes physical assessment techniques. Assessment focuses on findings from the patient's medical history and on body systems that the surgery is likely to affect. The nursing assessment complements the surgeon's and anesthesia provider's physical examination (Bray, 2006).

General Survey. Observe the patient's general appearance. Gestures and body movements may reflect weakness caused by illness. Assess the patient for a malnourished appearance. Height, body weight, and history of recent weight loss are important indicators of nutritional status.

Preoperative vital signs, including blood pressure while sitting and standing, and pulse oximetry provide important baseline data with which to compare alterations that occur during and after surgery. Some institutions request that you obtain blood pressure in both arms for comparison. Anxiety and fear commonly cause elevations in heart rate and blood pressure. Preoperative assessment of vital signs is also important to rule out fluid and electrolyte abnormalities (see Chapter 41).

An elevated temperature before surgery is a cause for concern. If the patient has an underlying infection, the surgeon may choose to postpone surgery until the infection has been treated. An elevated body temperature increases the risk of fluid and electrolyte imbalance after surgery. Notify the surgeon immediately if the patient has an elevated temperature.

Head and Neck. The condition of oral mucous membranes is one indicator of the level of hydration. Inspect the area between the gums and cheek, the soft palate, and the nasal sinuses. Sinus drainage indicates respiratory or sinus infection. During the examination of the oral mucosa, identify any loose or capped teeth because they can become dislodged during endotracheal intubation. Note the presence of dentures, prosthetic devices, or piercings so they can be removed before surgery, especially if the patient receives general anesthesia.

Integument. Carefully inspect the skin, especially over bony prominences such as the heels, elbows, sacrum, back of head, and scapula. During surgery patients often lie in a fixed position for several hours, making them at increased risk for pressure ulcers (see Chapter 48) (Walton-Geer, 2009). Chronic use of steroids also increases a patient's susceptibility to skin tears. The overall condition of the skin reveals the patient's level of hydration. An older adult is at high risk for alteration in skin integrity from positioning (pressure forces) and sliding on the OR table (shearing forces).

Thorax and Lungs. Assessment of the patient's breathing pattern and chest excursion measures ventilatory capacity. A decline in ventilatory function places the patient at risk for respiratory complications. Auscultation of breath sounds indicates whether the patient has pulmonary congestion or narrowing of airways. Existing atelectasis or moisture in the airways is aggravated during surgery. Serious pulmonary congestion usually results in postponement of the surgery. Certain anesthetics cause laryngeal muscle spasm. If you auscultate wheezing in the airways before surgery, the patient is at risk for further airway narrowing during surgery and after extubation (removal of the endotracheal tube); therefore notify health care providers of these findings.

Heart and Vascular System. Assess the character of the apical pulse and listen to heart sounds. Assess peripheral pulses, capillary refill, and the color and temperature of extremities. If peripheral pulses are not palpable, use a Doppler instrument for assessment of their presence. Acceptable capillary refill occurs in less than 2 seconds. Measurement of capillary refill and assessment of peripheral pulses are particularly important for the patient having vascular surgery or for a patient who has casts or constricting bandages applied to the extremities after surgery (see Chapter 30).

BOX 50-2 CULTURAL ASPECTS OF CARE

Providing Culturally Sensitive Care for the Patient Having Surgery

Patients' culture, religious group, and country of origin influence their health care beliefs. Your approach to perioperative care should respect patients' cultural values and incorporate them to improve adherence to the care plan (Galanti, 2008). The use of a wide variety of resources within a health care agency, in the literature, and from the Internet helps nurses provide culturally sensitive care.

Implications for Practice

- Preoperative assessment needs to include a cultural assessment with questions such as primary language spoken, feelings regarding surgery and pain, pain management, expectations, support system, and feelings toward self-care with postoperative implications (e.g., Does patient relate to concept of pain? Does patient have feelings about gender of caregiver? Does patient follow custom of giving family members control over decisions? Does patient have religious convictions that affect perioperative care such as opposition to the administration of blood products?).
- Be sensitive about when and who to use as professional interpreters to communicate with non–English-speaking patients because some patients may have difficulty sharing personal health information with people who are younger or of a specific gender.
- Use materials and teaching techniques that are culturally relevant and language appropriate to communicate and assess the non–English-speaking patient regarding factors such as pain, general comfort, temperature, and need to void.
- Provide preoperative and postoperative educational materials in a variety of languages.

TABLE 50-6 Diagnostic Screening for Surgical Patients

MEASUREMENT AND NORMAL VALUES	INTERPRETATION
Complete blood count (CBC) *RBC: Men:* 4.7-6.1 million/mm^3 *Women:* 4.2-5.4 million/mm^3 *Hgb: Men:* 14-18 g/100 mL *Women:* 12-16 g/100 mL *Hct: Men:* 42%-52%; *Women:* 37%-47% *WBC: Adults and children >2 yr:* 5000-10,000/mm^3	Peripheral venous sample of blood may reveal infection, low blood volume, and potential for oxygenation problems. Surgeon may order blood replacement.
Serum electrolytes *Sodium (Na^+):* 136-145 mEq/L (135-145 mmol/L) *Potassium (K^+):* 3.5-5 mEq/L (3.5-5 mmol/L) *Chloride (Cl^-):* 95-105 mEq/L (95-105 mmol/L) *Bicarbonate (HCO_3^-):* 22-26 mEq/L (arterial); 24-30 mEq/L (venous)	Peripheral venous sample of blood may reveal significant fluid and electrolyte imbalances before surgery. Attention is given to Na^+, K^+, and Cl^- levels. IV fluid replacement may be indicated before surgery.
Coagulation studies *PT:* 11-12.5 seconds *INR:* 0.76-1.27 *APTT:* 30-40 seconds *Platelets:* 150,000-400,000/mm^3	PT, INR, APTT, and platelet counts reveal clotting ability of blood and patients at risk for bleeding tendencies and thrombus formation.
Serum creatinine *Men:* 0.6-1.2 mg/100 mL *Women:* 0.5-1.1 mg/100 mL	Ability of kidneys to excrete creatinine, by-product of muscle metabolism, indicates renal function. Elevated level can indicate renal failure.
BUN 10-20 mg/100 mL	Ability of kidneys to excrete urea and nitrogen indicates renal function. BUN becomes elevated if patient is dehydrated. Preoperative IV fluid replacement is often necessary.
Glucose *Fasting:* 70-105 mg/100 mL	Fingerstick or peripheral blood sample. Patients often require treatment of low or high levels before and after surgery.

Modified from Pagana KD, Pagana TJ: *Mosby's diagnostic and laboratory test reference,* ed 10, St Louis, 2011, Mosby.
APTT, Activated partial thromboplastin time; *BUN,* blood urea nitrogen; *Hct,* hematocrit; *Hgb,* hemoglobin; *INR,* international normalized ratio; *IV,* intravenous; *PT,* prothrombin time; *RBC,* red blood cell; *WBC,* white blood cell.

Abdomen. Assess the abdomen for size, shape, symmetry, and presence of distention. Ask how often the patient has regular bowel movements and inquire about the color and consistency of stools. Auscultate bowel sounds.

Neurological Status. Preoperative assessment of neurological status is important for all patients receiving general anesthesia. The baseline neurological status assists with the assessment of ascent from anesthesia. Observe the patient's level of orientation, alertness, mood, and ease of speech, noting whether he or she answers questions appropriately and is able to recall recent and past events. A patient who will have surgery for neurological disease (e.g., brain tumor or aneurysm) sometimes demonstrates an impaired level of consciousness or altered behavior. If the patient is scheduled for spinal anesthesia, preoperative assessment of gross motor function and strength is important. Spinal anesthesia causes temporary paralysis of the lower extremities (see Chapter 43). Be aware of a patient entering surgery with weakness or impaired mobility of the lower extremities and communicate this to the perioperative team so care providers do not become alarmed when full motor function does not return as the spinal anesthetic wears off.

Diagnostic Screening. Patients have a variety of preoperative tests and procedures to confirm or rule out preexisting alterations requiring surgery or that will affect recovery. Usually patients scheduled for ambulatory surgery have tests done several days before surgery. Testing done the day of surgery is usually limited to tests such as glucose monitoring for the patient with diabetes. You need to be familiar with the tests, their purposes, and how to monitor results.

The patient's medical history, physical assessment findings, and surgical procedure determine the type of tests ordered. For example, a type and cross-match are indicated before surgery for procedures in which blood loss is expected (e.g., hip and knee replacements) in case the patient needs a blood transfusion during surgery. The surgeon designates the number of blood units to have available during surgery. Table 50-6 gives the purpose and normal values for common blood tests. If diagnostic tests reveal severe problems, the surgeon will probably cancel surgery until the cause of the problem is identified or the condition stabilizes. You are responsible for preparing patients for diagnostic studies and coordinating completion of the tests. Review diagnostic results as they become available, alert health care providers to findings, and assist with planning appropriate therapy.

If a patient is over the age of 40 or has heart disease, the health care provider often orders a chest x-ray film examination or an electrocardiogram (ECG). The chest x-ray film is an examination of the condition of the heart and lungs. An ECG measures the electrical activity of the heart to determine whether the heart rate, rhythm, and other factors are normal. Pulmonary function testing and occasionally arterial blood gas analysis are conducted on patients with preexisting lung disease. Blood glucose levels are measured before surgery when patients have diabetes.

Autologous infusions are an option for some patients who choose to donate their own blood before surgery to reduce the risk of transfusion-related infections and transfusion reactions (see Chapter 41). The patient makes the donation several weeks before the scheduled surgery. The patient who self-donates sometimes has

BOX 50-3 NURSING DIAGNOSTIC PROCESS

Fear Related to Knowledge Deficit and Previous Surgical Experience

ASSESSMENT ACTIVITIES	DEFINING CHARACTERISTICS
Ask patient to describe previous surgical experiences.	Apprehension over anesthesia and postoperative pain
Ask patient about preoperative education/preparation before admission.	Fear of the unknown, of having complications Unaware of preoperative testing
Observe patient's nonverbal behavior.	Increased tension
Assess vital signs.	Increased heart rate, increased blood pressure

a lower hemoglobin and hematocrit level on the day of surgery. Autotransfusion via a cell-saver device during surgery is possible if health care providers are anticipating large blood loss (e.g., open-heart surgery). Although the cell saver is expensive, it returns washed red blood cells to the patient and decreases the risk of transfusion reactions and blood-related infections by using the patient's own blood (Rothrock, 2007).

NURSING DIAGNOSIS

Cluster patterns of defining characteristics are gathered during the assessment to identify nursing diagnoses for the surgical patient (Box 50-3). The patient with preexisting health problems is likely to have a variety of risk diagnoses. For example, a patient with preexisting bronchitis who has abnormal breath sounds and a productive cough is at risk for *ineffective airway clearance.* The nature of the surgery and assessment of the patient's health status provide defining characteristics and risk factors for a number of nursing diagnoses. For example, because a patient will have a surgical incision and an IV infusion, there is a risk for developing infection at the surgical site or in the bloodstream (sepsis). A diagnosis of *risk for infection* requires your attention from admission through recovery.

The related factors for each diagnosis establish directions for nursing care that is provided during one or all surgical phases. For example, the diagnosis of *ineffective airway clearance related to abdominal pain* requires different interventions than the diagnosis *ineffective airway clearance related to excess mucus.* Preoperative nursing diagnoses allow you to take precautions and actions so care provided during the intraoperative and postoperative phases is consistent with the patient's needs.

Nursing diagnoses made before surgery also focus on the potential risks that a patient may face after surgery. Preventive care is essential so you can manage the surgical patient effectively. The following are some common nursing diagnoses relevant to the patient having surgery:

- Ineffective airway clearance
- Anxiety
- Fear
- Risk for deficient fluid volume
- Risk for perioperative positioning injury
- Deficient knowledge (specify)
- Impaired physical mobility
- Nausea
- Acute pain
- Delayed surgical recovery

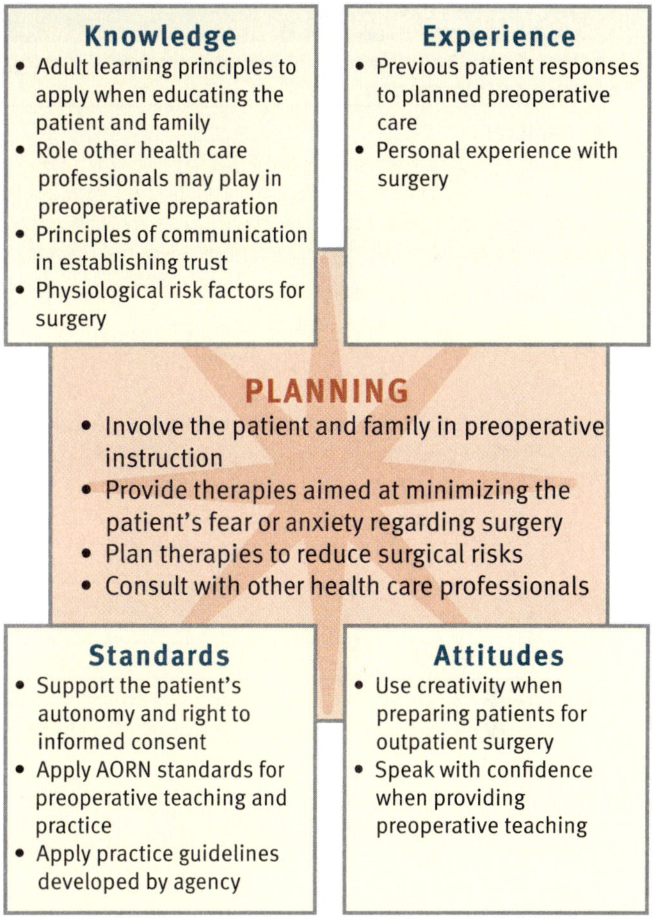
Knowledge
• Adult learning principles to apply when educating the patient and family
• Role other health care professionals may play in preoperative preparation
• Principles of communication in establishing trust
• Physiological risk factors for surgery
Experience
• Previous patient responses to planned preoperative care
• Personal experience with surgery
PLANNING
• Involve the patient and family in preoperative instruction
• Provide therapies aimed at minimizing the patient's fear or anxiety regarding surgery
• Plan therapies to reduce surgical risks
• Consult with other health care professionals
Standards
• Support the patient's autonomy and right to informed consent
• Apply AORN standards for preoperative teaching and practice
• Apply practice guidelines developed by agency
Attitudes
• Use creativity when preparing patients for outpatient surgery
• Speak with confidence when providing preoperative teaching

FIG. 50-2 Critical thinking model for surgical patient planning. *AORN,* Association of periOperative Registered Nurses.

PLANNING

During planning synthesize information to establish a plan of care based on the patient's nursing diagnoses (see the Nursing Care Plan). Apply critical thinking in your selection of nursing interventions (Fig. 50-2). For example, apply knowledge pertaining to adult learning principles, standards for preoperative education (AORN, 2011), and the patient's unique learning needs to formulate a well-designed **preoperative teaching plan** for the diagnosis of *deficient knowledge.* Critical thinking ensures that the patient's plan of care integrates knowledge, previous experiences, critical thinking attitudes, and established standards of practice. Previous experience in caring for surgical patients helps you anticipate how to approach patient care (e.g., complications to prevent and anticipate and methods to reduce anxiety). Professional standards are especially important to consider when selecting interventions for the plan of care. These standards often establish scientifically proven guidelines for preferred nursing interventions.

Successful planning requires involving the surgical patient and family to set realistic expectations for care. Early involvement of the patient when developing the surgical care plan minimizes surgical risks and postoperative complications. A patient informed about the surgical experience is less likely to be fearful and is able to participate in the postoperative recovery phase so expected

NURSING CARE PLAN

Deficient Knowledge Regarding Preoperative and Postoperative Care Requirements Related to Lack of Exposure to Information

ASSESSMENT

Mrs. Campana is an 80-year-old patient scheduled to be admitted in 5 days for elective bowel resection. You are the nurse in the ambulatory surgery center (ASC) preoperative testing area, assigned to prepare Mrs. Campana for surgery. During your initial discussion with Mrs. Campana, you assess that she is alert and oriented. She states she has severely reduced visual acuity but is able to hear your questions clearly. She has had previous surgery, but that was 10 years ago. She lives alone and has a daughter who is coming in town the day of surgery and will stay with her 2 weeks after surgery.

Assessment Activities	*Findings/Defining Characteristics**
Ask Mrs. Campana what she has been told by her surgeon regarding her surgery.	She states that her surgeon explained the procedure with a drawing of the bowel and the location of the part to be removed **but has not described the care she will receive afterward.**
Ask Mrs. Campana what she understands about preoperative preparation and what to expect after surgery.	She verbalizes understanding of medicines to take the morning of surgery, her diet before surgery and when to stop eating, and who to call for questions. **She is unable to explain what to expect after surgery.**
Assess Mrs. Campana's concerns about surgery.	**She appears slightly anxious. She states, "I'm afraid I'll die during my surgery. I don't know what to expect."**

*__Defining characteristics__ are shown in bold type.

NURSING DIAGNOSIS: Deficient knowledge regarding preoperative and postoperative care requirements related to lack of exposure to information

PLANNING

Goals	*Expected Outcomes (NOC)*†
	Knowledge: Treatment Procedures
Mrs. Campana will express understanding of the postoperative routines of surgical care by the day of surgery.	Mrs. Campana will describe the importance of postoperative exercises by the morning of surgery. Mrs. Campana will describe the schedule for activity and diet management following surgery by the first postoperative evening.
Mrs. Campana will participate actively in postoperative recovery activities by postoperative day 1.	Mrs. Campana will successfully perform postoperative exercises (turning, coughing, deep breathing [TCDB], diaphragmatic breathing [DB], incentive spirometry [IS], and leg exercises) on the evening of surgery.

†Outcome classification labels from Moorhead S et al: *Nursing outcomes classification (NOC),* ed 4, St Louis, 2008, Mosby.

INTERVENTIONS (NIC)‡ *Preoperative Teaching*	**RATIONALE**
Before admission to the hospital, provide Mrs. Campana with audiotape program that explains preoperative and postoperative routines. Supply instruction booklet designed for patients with visual impairments. Make a follow-up call 24 hours before surgery to patient encouraging them to ask questions and voice concerns.	Preadmission education often results in less teaching time and better performance of exercises on admission. Education has a beneficial effect in reducing postoperative anxiety (American College of Surgeons, 2006).
On admission to hospital, demonstrate to Mrs. Campana and daughter how to perform postoperative exercises and how to get out of bed with assistance.	Demonstration is an effective method to reinforce instruction.
Coach Mrs. Campana during a return demonstration of postoperative exercises before surgery.	Learning occurs when a patient is actively involved in an education session (Edelman and Mandle, 2009). Evaluates learning and provides opportunity to reinforce instruction.
Correct any unrealistic expectations Mrs. Campana or daughter have regarding surgery.	Unrealistic expectations, when unmet, contribute to patient's anxiety. Psychological preparation for surgery reduces anxiety (American College of Surgeons, 2006).

‡Intervention classification labels from Bulechek GM, Butcher HK, and Dochterman JM: *Nursing interventions classification (NIC),* ed 5, St Louis, 2008, Mosby.

EVALUATION

Nursing Actions	*Patient Response/Finding*	*Achievement of Outcome*
Ask Mrs. Campana to describe activity and diet therapies to expect following surgery.	She is able to verbalize progressive diet from NPO to full liquids but is not sure how quickly she will be expected to ambulate. She states that the booklet and audiotape were both helpful.	Mrs. Campana requires additional discussion of activity and long-term diet plan.

NURSING CARE PLAN

Deficient Knowledge Regarding Preoperative and Postoperative Care Requirements Related to Lack of Exposure to Information—cont'd

EVALUATION—cont'd

Observe Mrs. Campana's demonstration of postoperative exercises.	She correctly demonstrates leg exercises and TCDB but is having difficulty with IS use.	Mrs. Campana demonstrates most postoperative exercises but needs further teaching and practice on IS use.
Explore with Mrs. Campana and daughter if they have any remaining fears or concerns.	Both Mrs. Campana and her daughter deny any fears or concerns at the present time.	Informational and psychological needs of Mrs. Campana and her daughter have been met.

outcomes are met. Establish diagnosis, interventions, and outcomes to ensure recovery or maintenance of the preoperative state.

Goals and Outcomes. Base the goals and outcomes of care on the individualized nursing diagnoses. Review and modify the plan during the intraoperative and postoperative periods. Outcomes established for each goal of care provide measurable behavioral evidence to gauge the patient's progress toward meeting stated goals. As an example, the goal "Patient is able to perform postoperative exercises during postoperative recovery" is measured through the following expected outcomes:

- Patient performs deep-breathing and coughing exercises on awakening from anesthesia.
- Patient performs postoperative leg exercises and early ambulation 24 hours after surgery.
- Patient verbalizes rationale for early ambulation 24 hours after surgery.

Setting Priorities. Use clinical judgment to prioritize nursing diagnoses and interventions based on the unique needs of each patient. Patients requiring emergent surgery often experience changes in their physiological status that require you to reprioritize quickly. For example, if a patient's blood pressure begins to drop; hemodynamic stabilization becomes a priority over education and stress management. Ensure that the approach to each patient is thorough and reflects an understanding of the implications of the patient's age, physical and psychological health, educational level, cultural and religious practices, and stated and/or written wishes concerning advance medical directives.

Teamwork and Collaboration. For patients having ambulatory surgery and those admitted the day of their scheduled surgery, the health care team must collaborate to ensure continuity of care. Preoperative planning ideally occurs days before admission to the hospital or surgical center. The collaboration between the health care provider's office and the surgical center is crucial to preparing the patient for the procedure. Preoperative instruction gives the patient time to think about the surgical experience, make necessary physical preparations (e.g., altering diet or discontinuing medication use), and ask questions about postoperative procedures. The patient having ambulatory surgery usually returns home on the day of surgery. Thus well-planned preoperative care ensures that he or she is well informed and able to be an active participant during recovery. The family or spouse also plays an active supportive role for the patient.

IMPLEMENTATION

Preoperative nursing interventions provide the patient with a complete understanding of the surgery and anticipated postoperative activities and prepare him or her physically and psychologically for surgical intervention.

Informed Consent. Surgery cannot be legally or ethically performed until a patient understands the need for a procedure, the steps involved, risks, expected results, and alternative treatments. Chapter 23 discusses in detail the nurse's responsibilities for **informed consent.** It is the surgeon's responsibility to explain the procedure and obtain the informed consent. After the patient completes the consent form, place it in the medical record. The record goes to the OR with the patient.

Health Promotion. Health promotion activities during the preoperative phase focus on health maintenance, prevention of complications, and anticipation of continued care needed after surgery.

Preoperative Teaching. Patient education is an important aspect of the patient's surgical experience (see Chapter 25). Provided in a systematic and structured format with teaching and learning principles, preoperative teaching regarding a patient's expected postoperative course has a positive influence on the patient's recovery (Kruzik, 2009). Preadmission nurses call patients up to 1 week before surgery to clarify questions and reinforce explanations. Preoperative information and instructions are delivered by telephone calls, mailings from the health care provider's office or hospital, printed preoperative teaching guidelines and checklists, or the use of videotapes or websites. The American College of Surgeons developed a patient education website titled *Partners in Surgical Care,* which provides a supplement to the surgeon's teaching (American College of Surgeons, 2006). Education throughout the perioperative period is essential. The Joanna Briggs Institute (2000) highlights the importance of preoperative teaching for knowledge acquisition and skill performance. It is ideal to attempt perioperative education before admission, during the hospital stay, and after discharge. Including family members in perioperative preparation is advisable. Often a family member is the coach for postoperative exercises when the patient returns from surgery. The family often has better retention of preoperative teaching and will be with the patient and able to help them in their recovery. If anxious relatives do not understand routine postoperative events, it is likely that their anxiety heightens the patient's fears and concerns. Perioperative preparation of family members before surgery lessens anxiety and misunderstanding.

Provide patients with information about sensations typically experienced after surgery. Preparatory information helps them anticipate the steps of a procedure and thus form realistic images of the surgical experience. For example, in the OR the anesthesia provider applies ointment to patients' eyes to prevent corneal damage. Warning patients about sensations of blurred vision reduces their anxiety on awakening from surgery. Other sensations to describe include the expected pain at the surgical site, the tightness of dressings, dryness of the mouth, and the sensation of a sore throat resulting from an endotracheal tube.

Anxiety and fear are barriers to learning, and both emotions heighten as surgery approaches. If the patient is capable of and receptive to learning, present information in a logical sequence, beginning with preoperative events and advancing to intraoperative and postoperative routines. The AORN (2011) has the following standards to demonstrate patient understanding of the surgical experience.

Patient Cites Reasons for Preoperative Instructions and Exercises. When given a rationale for preoperative and postoperative procedures, the patient is better prepared to participate in care. Most preoperative teaching programs include explanation and demonstration of postoperative exercises: diaphragmatic breathing, incentive spirometry, coughing, turning, and leg exercises. These exercises help to prevent postoperative complications (Skill 50-1 on pp. 1287-1292). In addition, if the patient needs graded compression or elastic stockings or intermittent pneumatic compression (IPC) devices, teach about the purposes and the specific nursing care associated with the device (see Chapter 47).

After you explain each exercise, demonstrate it for the patient. Guide him or her through each exercise. For example, assess whether the patient is sitting properly and help him or her place the hands in the proper position during breathing. Allow the patient time for independent practice and return later to evaluate effectiveness before surgery.

Patient States Time of Surgery. Tell the patient and family the approximate time that surgery will begin and when they should arrive at the hospital or ASC. The surgeon informs the patient and family of the anticipated length of surgery. Unanticipated delays occur for many reasons. Make the family aware that delays occur for various reasons and do not necessarily indicate a problem.

Patient States Postoperative Unit and Location of Family During Surgery and Recovery. The unit to which the patient is admitted before surgery is often different from the postoperative unit. The family needs to know where the patient will be after surgery. Also explain where the family can wait and where the surgeon will attempt to find family members after surgery. Many institutions have implemented programs in which the circulating nurse gives periodic reports to the family in the waiting room for surgeries that are expected to be prolonged. If the patient will be taken to a special unit, it helps to orient the patient and family members to the environment of the unit before surgery.

Patient Discusses Anticipated Postoperative Monitoring and Therapies. The patient and family need to know about postoperative events. If they understand the frequency of postoperative vital sign monitoring before surgery occurs, they are less apprehensive when nurses measure vital signs. Also explain whether the patient is likely to have IV lines, monitoring lines, dressings, or drainage tubes or will require ventilator support.

Patient Describes Surgical Procedures and Postoperative Treatment. After the surgeon explains the basic purpose of a surgical procedure, some patients ask you additional questions to clarify information. First clarify with the patient what was discussed with the surgeon. When the patient has little or no understanding about the surgery, notify the surgeon that the patient requires further explanation. You can augment the surgeon's explanations.

Patient Describes Postoperative Activity Resumption. The type of surgery that patients undergo determines how quickly they can resume normal physical activity and regular eating habits. Explain that it is normal to progress gradually in activity and eating. If the patient tolerates activity and diet well, activity levels progress more quickly.

Patient Verbalizes Pain-Relief Measures. Pain is one of the surgical patient's most common fears. The family is also concerned for the patient's comfort. Pain after surgery is expected. Inform the patient and family of interventions available for pain relief (e.g., analgesics, positioning, splinting, and relaxation exercises) (see Chapter 43). The patient needs to know the schedule for analgesic drugs, the route of administration, and their effects.

Some patients avoid taking pain-relief drugs after surgery for fear of becoming dependent on them. Encourage the patient to use analgesics as ordered because, unless the pain is controlled, it is difficult for the patient to participate in postoperative therapy. Encourage the patient to take pain medications at the ordered intervals. Pain relief has been shown to be more effective when analgesics are given around-the-clock (ATC) rather than as needed (prn) (Paice et al., 2005), especially if pain is expected throughout the day. However, prn administration of analgesics after surgery is still very common. Closely assess the patient's pain level, tolerance to activity, and response to pain-relieving interventions. When pain is not regularly addressed, it becomes excruciating, and an analgesic often does not provide relief at the dose ordered. Teach patients who will have patient-controlled analgesia (PCA) how to push the button, the need to push the button when beginning to feel discomfort, and that use of the PCA does not cause overmedication (see Chapter 43). Also explain to the patient the length of time that it takes for the drug to begin working. Information from preoperative pain assessment is helpful when teaching about pain-relief measures (such as positioning and splinting).

Patient Expresses Feelings Regarding Surgery. Some patients feel like part of an assembly line before surgery. Frequent visits by staff, diagnostic testing, and physical preparation for surgery consume time; and the patient has few opportunities to reflect on the experience. Recognize the patient as a unique individual. The patient and family need time to express feelings about surgery and ask questions. The patient's level of anxiety influences the frequency of discussions. While delivering routine care, encourage expression of concerns, be patient and listen attentively. The family may wish to discuss concerns without the patient present so their fears do not frighten the patient and vice versa. Establishing a trusting and therapeutic relationship with the patient and family allows this to happen.

Acute Care. Acute care activities in the preoperative phase focus on the physical preparation of the patient for surgery.

Physical Preparation. The degree of preoperative physical preparation depends on the patient's health status, the planned surgery, and the surgeon's preferences. A seriously ill patient receives more supportive care in the form of medications, IV fluid therapy, and monitoring than the patient facing a minor elective procedure.

Maintaining Normal Fluid and Electrolyte Balance. The surgical patient is vulnerable to fluid and electrolyte imbalances as a result of the stress of surgery, inadequate preoperative intake, and the potential for excessive fluid losses during surgery (see Chapter 41). The American Society of Anesthesiologists Practice Guidelines for Preoperative Fasting (ASA, 2011) reviewed the current fasting practices for elective procedures requiring general anesthesia, regional anesthesia, or sedation. They recommend fasting before nonemergent procedures for the following time periods: do not take clear liquids for 2 hours; do not take breast milk for 4 hours;

and do not take formula, solids, and nonhuman milk for 6 hours. For fatty, fried, and meat sources the recommended fast is for 8 hours. A patient who is at home the evening before surgery needs to understand the importance of the specific fasting period ordered by the health care provider.

Agencies vary regarding these fasting guidelines. One difficulty is that often surgical cases begin before the time they are originally scheduled. When a patient is admitted NPO, remove fluids and solid foods from the patient's bedside and post a sign over the bed to alert hospital personnel and family members about fasting restrictions. Some patients take specific medications (e.g., anticoagulants, cardiovascular medications, anticonvulsants, and antibiotics) with a sip of water as ordered by their health care providers. Although the concept of preoperative fasting has changed over the past 10 years, studies and a systematic review demonstrate that the guidelines are not fully implemented and multidisciplinary improvement processes are necessary (Brady, Kinn, and Stuart, 2003).

Allow patients time to rinse their mouths with water or mouthwash and brush their teeth immediately before surgery as long as they do not swallow water. Notify the surgeon and anesthesia provider if the patient eats or drinks during the fasting period.

During surgery normal mechanisms for controlling fluid and electrolyte balance, including respiration, digestion, circulation, and elimination, are disturbed. Extensive losses of blood and other body fluids sometimes occur. The surgical stress response aggravates any fluid and electrolyte imbalance. Before the day of surgery patients are usually encouraged to eat foods high in protein with sufficient carbohydrates, fat, and vitamins. If a patient cannot eat because of GI alterations or impairments in consciousness, you will probably start an IV route for fluid replacement. The health care provider assesses serum electrolyte levels to determine the type of IV fluids and electrolyte additives to administer during surgery. Patients with severe nutritional imbalances sometimes require supplements with concentrated protein and glucose such as total parenteral nutrition (see Chapter 44).

Reducing Risk of Surgical Site Infection. A surgical site infection is one of the National Quality Forum (NQF)–endorsed patient safety measures that hospitals are encouraged to report (NQF, 2010). As of 2008 the Centers for Medicare and Medicaid Services (2010) no longer pays a higher reimbursement for hospitalizations complicated by certain types of surgical wound infections (e.g., mediastinitis after heart surgery, select orthopedic procedures, and certain bariatric procedures for obesity) if they were not present on admission. Thus there is great emphasis within hospitals for preventing the occurrence of surgical site infections.

The risk of developing a surgical site infection is determined by the amount and type of microorganisms contaminating a wound, susceptibility of the host, and the condition of the surgical wound itself. All three factors interact to cause infection. Antibiotics may be ordered in the preoperative period. A reduction in wound infection rates occurs when an antibiotic is administered 30 to 60 minutes before the surgical incision (Weber et al., 2008). The surgeon orders a specific time before surgery for the oral antibiotic to be taken or an IV antibiotic to be administered.

The skin is a favorite site for microorganisms to grow and multiply. Without proper skin preparation, the risk of postoperative wound infection is high. Many surgeons have patients bathe or shower the evening before surgery. Some health care providers ask patients to bathe or shower more than once, whereas others may have patients use an antibacterial soap to clean the proposed operative site. Depending on the surgical procedure, some patients shower the morning of surgery. If the surgical procedure involves the head, neck, or upper chest area, the patient may also be required to shampoo the hair. Cleaning and trimming fingernails and toenails is sometimes necessary.

The need for hair removal depends on the amount of hair, location of the incision, and surgical procedure planned (AORN, 2011). Hair removal can damage and cause breaks in the patient's skin, which allows for the entry of microorganisms. If required, perform hair removal, preferably with a clipper or shaver, as close to the time of surgery as possible. Short hospital stays reduce the chance of a health care–associated infection (HAI). Patients can also acquire respiratory, urinary tract, and wound infections during hospitalization. One advantage to having ambulatory surgical procedures is that the patient usually returns home after surgery.

Preventing Bowel and Bladder Incontinence. Some patients receive a bowel preparation (e.g., a cathartic or enema) if the surgery involves the lower GI system or lower abdominal organs. Manipulation of portions of the GI tract during surgery results in absence of peristalsis for 24 hours and sometimes longer. Enemas and cathartics such as polyethylene glycol electrolyte solution (GoLytely) clean the GI tract to prevent intraoperative incontinence and postoperative constipation. An empty bowel reduces risk of injury to the intestines and minimizes contamination of the operative wound if a portion of the bowel is incised or opened accidentally or if colon surgery is planned. The surgeon's order reads "give enemas until clear." This means that you administer enemas until the enema return contains no solid fecal material (see Chapter 46). Too many enemas given over a short time can cause serious fluid and electrolyte imbalances (Chapter 41). Most agencies limit the number of enemas (usually three) that a nurse may administer successively. Verify a patient's potassium level following bowel preparation.

Promoting Rest and Comfort. Rest is essential for normal healing. Anxiety about the impending surgery can easily interfere with a patient's ability to relax or sleep. The underlying condition requiring surgery is often painful, further impairing rest. Attempt to make the patient's environment quiet and comfortable. The health care provider may order a sedative-hypnotic or anxiolytic agent for the night before surgery. Sedative-hypnotics (e.g., temazepam [Restoril]) affect and promote sleep. Anxiolytic agents (e.g., alprazolam [Xanax]) act on the cerebral cortex and limbic system to relieve anxiety.

Preparation on the Day of Surgery. Complete several routine procedures before releasing patients for surgery.

Hygiene. Basic hygiene measures provide additional comfort before surgery. If the hospitalized patient is unwilling to take a complete bath, a partial bath is refreshing and removes irritating secretions or drainage from the skin. Because the patient cannot wear personal nightwear to the OR because it is restrictive and is a flammable hazard, provide a clean hospital gown. When the patient is NPO for the last several hours, his or her mouth is often very dry. Offer the patient mouthwash and toothpaste, again cautioning the patient not to swallow water.

Hair and Cosmetics. During surgery with the patient under general anesthesia, his or her head is positioned to introduce an endotracheal tube into the airway (see Chapter 40). This procedure may involve manipulation of the patient's hair and scalp. To avoid injury ask the patient to remove hairpins or clips before leaving for surgery. Electrocautery is frequently used during surgery. Hairpins and clips can become an exit source for the electricity and cause burns. Remove hairpieces or wigs as well. The patient applies a disposable hat before entering the OR.

During and after surgery the anesthesia provider and nurse assess skin and mucous membranes to determine the patient's level of oxygenation and circulation. Therefore remove all makeup (i.e., lipstick, powder, blush, nail polish) to expose normal skin and nail coloring. Pulse oximetry records accurate measurements through most nail polish colors, but removal is still considered good practice. Also remove contact lenses, false eyelashes, and eye makeup. Give the patient's glasses to the family immediately before the patient leaves for the OR. Document this per agency policy.

Removal of Prostheses. It is easy for any type of prosthetic device to become lost or damaged during surgery. The patient needs to remove all prostheses, including partial or complete dentures, artificial limbs, artificial eyes, and hearing aids. If a patient has a brace or splint, check with the health care provider to determine whether it should remain with him or her.

For many patients it is embarrassing to remove dentures, wigs, or other devices that enhance personal appearance. Always offer privacy as the patient removes personal items. Patients are sometimes allowed to keep these until they reach the preoperative area. Place dentures in special containers, labeled with the patient's name and other identification required by the agency, for safekeeping to prevent loss or breakage. In many agencies you document an inventory of all prosthetic devices or personal items and have them locked away. It is also common practice for nurses to give prostheses to family members or to keep the devices at the patient's bedside. Document these actions in the nursing notes, surgical checklist, or per agency policy.

Safeguarding Valuables. If a patient has valuables, give them to family members or secure them for safekeeping. Many hospitals require patients to sign a release to free the institution of responsibility for lost valuables. Valuables are usually stored and locked in a designated location. Often patients are reluctant to remove wedding rings or religious medals. A wedding band can be taped in place, but this is not the preferred practice. If there is a risk that the patient will experience swelling of the hand or fingers (mastectomy, hand surgery, fluid shifts), remove the band. Many hospitals allow patients to pin religious medals to their gowns, although the risk of loss increases. Remove other metal items such as piercings to reduce risk of burns. Document the location of valuables per hospital policy.

Preparing the Bowel and Bladder. Instruct the patient to void just before leaving for the OR and before giving preoperative medications. An empty bladder reduces discomfort during the procedure and reduces the risk of incontinence during surgery. If the patient is unable to void, record this information on the preoperative checklist. A straight urinary catheterization (Chapter 45) may be necessary if a bladder scan reveals large bladder volume, or an indwelling urinary catheter may be placed if the surgery is long or the incision is in the lower abdomen.

Vital Signs. Measure a final preoperative set of vital signs. The anesthesia provider uses these values as a baseline for intraoperative vital signs. If preoperative vital signs are abnormal, surgery may need to be postponed. Notify the surgeon of any abnormalities before sending the patient to surgery.

Documentation. Before the patient goes to the OR, check the contents of the medical record to be sure that pertinent laboratory results are present. Check consent forms for accuracy. A preoperative checklist is a useful tool for ensuring patient safety and completing nursing interventions. Check the nurses' notes to be sure that documentation of care is current. This is especially important if the hospitalized patient experienced unpredicted problems the night before surgery. Send a current medication administration record to the operating room.

Other Procedures. If an IV infusion is not started on the hospital unit, one will be placed in the preoperative holding area. An IV line is essential for establishing a route to deliver medications and fluids during surgery. Some patients need a nasogastric (NG) tube inserted before surgery, but this often occurs in the OR (see Chapter 46).

Administering Preoperative Medications. The advent of ambulatory surgery has reduced the use of preoperative medications. However, the anesthesia provider or surgeon sometimes orders preanesthetic drugs ("on-call medications," "preops") to reduce the patient's anxiety, the amount of general anesthesia required, the risk of nausea and vomiting and resultant aspiration, and respiratory tract secretions. Provide all nursing care measures (e.g., assistance to bathroom) before giving the patient preoperative medications. The patient must sign the consent form before you administer the medications. Because the drugs cause sedation, do not allow the patient to leave the bed or stretcher until surgical personnel arrive to transport him or her to the OR. Warn the patient to expect drowsiness and a dry mouth.

Eliminating Wrong Site and Wrong Procedure Surgery. Because of errors made in the past with patients undergoing the wrong surgery or having surgery performed on the wrong site, The Joint Commission (TJC) instituted Universal Protocol guidelines for preventing such mishaps. The Universal Protocol is now part of TJC ongoing National Patient Safety Goals (TJC, 2011). Implement this protocol whenever an invasive surgical procedure is to be performed no matter the location (e.g., hospital, ASC, or health care provider office). The three principles of the protocol include the following: (1) a preoperative verification that ensures that all relevant documents (e.g., consent forms, allergies, medical history, physical assessment findings) and results of laboratory tests and diagnostic studies are available before the start of the procedure and that the type of surgery scheduled is consistent with the patient's expectations; (2) marking the operative site with indelible ink to mark left and right distinction, multiple structures (e.g., fingers), and levels of the spine; and (3) a "time out" just before starting the procedure for final verification of the correct patient, procedure, site, and any implants (TJC, 2011). All members of the surgical/procedure team perform the time out. This protocol includes active patient or a legally designated representative involvement in the entire process. If the patient refuses a mark, note this on the procedure checklist and notify the surgeon.

Building Competency in Safety You are the nurse in the preoperative holding area and are preparing the patient for the operating room. You completed all preliminary procedures, storing valuables, checking the preoperative checklist, and assisting the patient to the bathroom. You are preparing to perform the Universal Protocol with patient verification. When is the right time to administer the preoperative sedative?

Answers to questions can be found on the Evolve website.

EVALUATION

The admitting nurse and the nurse in the preoperative area evaluate initial patient outcomes (Fig. 50-3). Although limited time is available to evaluate outcomes before surgery, compare the patient's current status with expected outcomes to determine whether new or revised interventions and/or nursing diagnoses need to be implemented.

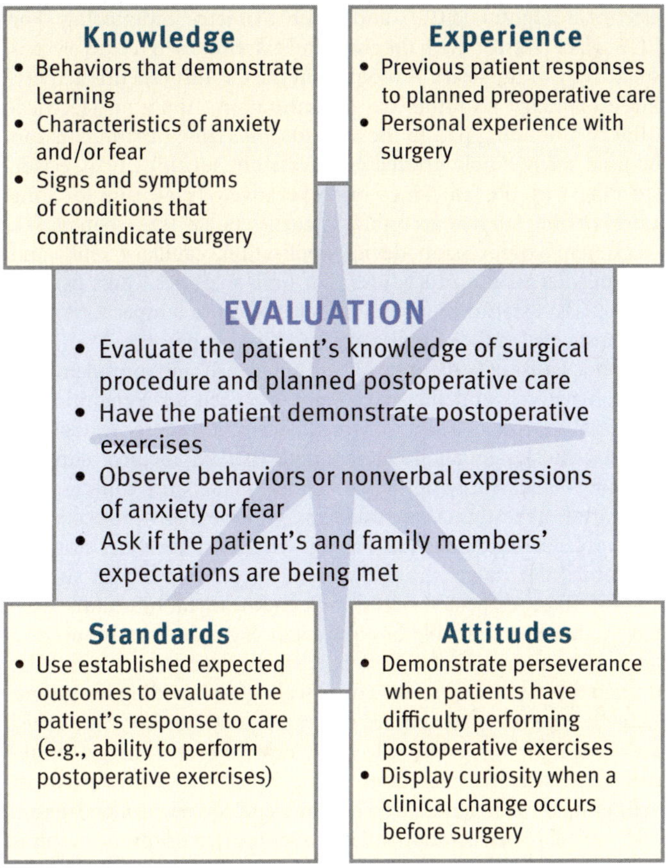
Knowledge
• Behaviors that demonstrate learning
• Characteristics of anxiety and/or fear
• Signs and symptoms of conditions that contraindicate surgery
Experience
• Previous patient responses to planned preoperative care
• Personal experience with surgery
EVALUATION
• Evaluate the patient's knowledge of surgical procedure and planned postoperative care
• Have the patient demonstrate postoperative exercises
• Observe behaviors or nonverbal expressions of anxiety or fear
• Ask if the patient's and family members' expectations are being met
Standards
• Use established expected outcomes to evaluate the patient's response to care (e.g., ability to perform postoperative exercises)
Attitudes
• Demonstrate perseverance when patients have difficulty performing postoperative exercises
• Display curiosity when a clinical change occurs before surgery

FIG. 50-3 Critical thinking model for surgical patient evaluation.

Through the Patient's Eyes. Evaluate whether the patient's expectations were met with respect to surgical preparation. For example, ask patients if they require additional information, if they desire to have their family members more involved, and if they have any unidentified needs. During evaluation, include a discussion of any misunderstandings so patient concerns can be clarified. When patients have expectations about pain control, this is a good time to reinforce how it will be managed after surgery.

Patient Outcomes. You are able to evaluate the patient's response to interventions designed for preoperative nursing diagnoses such as *deficient knowledge*. For example, ask the patient to describe the reason for postoperative exercises and the type of care activities to expect when the patient returns from surgery. Be thorough in your evaluation to determine if further instruction is needed after surgery. Interventions continue during and after surgery; thus the evaluation of many goals and outcomes does not occur until after surgery.

TRANSPORT TO THE OPERATING ROOM

Personnel in the OR notify the nursing unit or ambulatory surgery area when it is time for surgery. In many hospitals a nursing orderly or transporter brings a stretcher for transporting the patient. The transporter checks the patient's identification bracelet for two identifiers (name, birth date, or hospital number) (refer to institutional or agency policy) against the patient's medical record to be sure that the right person is going to surgery. Because some patients receive preoperative sedatives, the nurses and transporter help the patient transfer from bed to stretcher to prevent falls. The ambulatory surgery patient ambulates to the OR if able and not medicated. Provide the family an opportunity to visit before the patient is transported to the OR. Direct the family to a waiting area. In some hospitals the family is allowed to wait with the patient in the OR holding area until he or she is transported into the OR.

INTRAOPERATIVE SURGICAL PHASE

Care of the patient during surgery requires careful preparation and knowledge of the events that occur during the surgical procedure. The nurse usually functions in one of two roles: circulating nurse or scrub nurse. The **circulating nurse** must be an RN. His or her responsibilities include reviewing the preoperative assessment, establishing and implementing the intraoperative plan of care, evaluating the care, and providing for continuity of care after surgery. The circulating nurse assists with procedures such as endotracheal intubation and blood administration as needed. In addition, this nurse positions the patient, monitors sterile technique and a safe OR environment, assists the surgeon and surgical team by operating nonsterile equipment, provides additional supplies, verifies sponge and instrument counts, and maintains accurate and complete written records.

The **scrub nurse** is an RN, a licensed practical nurse, or a surgical technologist. This individual maintains a sterile field during the surgical procedure, assists with applying sterile drapes, hands instruments and other sterile supplies to surgeons, and counts the sponges and instruments.

PREOPERATIVE (HOLDING) AREA

In most hospitals the patient enters a holding area, also known as the preanesthesia care unit or presurgical care unit (PSCU), outside the OR. In the PSCU the nurse explains the steps for preparing the patient for surgery, reviews the preoperative checklist, assesses the patient's readiness both physically and emotionally, and reinforces teaching. Nurses in the PSCU are members of the OR staff and wear surgical scrub suits, hats, and footwear in accordance with infection control policies. In some ambulatory surgical settings a perioperative primary nurse admits the patient, circulates for the operative procedure, and manages the patient's recovery and discharge.

In the PSCU the nurse or anesthesia provider inserts an IV catheter into the arm to establish a route for fluid replacement and IV drugs if not placed previously. A large-bore (18-gauge) IV catheter ensures easy infusion of fluids and blood products if necessary. The nurse monitors vital signs, including pulse oximetry. The anesthesia provider usually performs a patient assessment at this time.

Because of the preoperative medications, the patient begins to feel drowsy. The temperature in the PSCU and adjacent OR suites is usually cool. Offer the patient an extra blanket. Conscious sedation starts at this time. The patient's stay in the PSCU is usually brief.

ADMISSION TO THE OPERATING ROOM

The OR staff transfer the patient to the OR room via a stretcher. The patient is usually still awake and notices nurses and health care providers wearing complete surgical masks, gowns, and eyewear. The staff carefully transfer the patient to the OR table, being sure that the stretcher and table are locked in place. After the patient is on the table, fasten a safety strap around him or her. Support the patient by explaining procedures and encouraging him or her to ask questions. Sights and sounds in the surgical suite are sometimes frightening to patients.

NURSING PROCESS

ASSESSMENT

Thoroughly assess each patient and critically analyze findings to ensure that you make patient-centered clinical decisions required for safe nursing care. For example, typically the nurse in the OR focuses on skin integrity and mobility, identifying any problems that predispose the patient to injury if he or she is not positioned on the OR table correctly. Because patients are not able to speak for themselves while under general anesthesia, this assessment in the OR is very important for their safety. Review the preoperative care plan to establish or revise the intraoperative care plan. Observe the patient's psychological comfort during this assessment as well.

NURSING DIAGNOSIS

Review preoperative nursing diagnoses and modify them to individualize the care plan in the OR. The following are some common nursing diagnoses relevant to the patient intraoperatively:

- Ineffective airway clearance
- Risk for deficient fluid volume
- Risk for perioperative positioning injury
- Risk for impaired skin integrity

PLANNING

Goals and Outcomes. Patient-centered goals and outcomes of preoperative nursing diagnoses extend into the intraoperative phase. For example, a goal for the nursing diagnosis of *risk for impaired skin integrity* is "Skin will remain free of injury through surgical procedure." Expected outcomes for this goal include:

- Patient will have intact skin and show no signs of redness at end of surgery.
- Patient will be free of burns from the grounding pad at end of surgery.

Setting Priorities. The OR nurse uses judgment to provide a safe operative experience for the patient. Providing an aseptic environment and proper use of equipment and instruments are top priorities. If an unsafe practice is occurring, the circulating nurse is integral to ensuring the safety of the patient and operative personnel.

Teamwork and Collaboration. For optimal patient safety the preoperative health care team communicates important assessment findings to the surgical team to ensure a smooth transition in care. For example, alerting the operative team of a latex allergy or risk factors for complications during surgery requires collaboration and timely communication among all team members.

IMPLEMENTATION

A primary focus of intraoperative care is to prevent injury and complications related to anesthesia, surgery, positioning, and equipment use. The perioperative nurse is an advocate for the patient during surgery and protects his or her dignity and rights at all times.

Acute Care

Physical Preparation. After safely securing the patient on the OR table, apply monitoring devices to him or her. Patients receiving general and regional anesthesia undergo continuous electrocardiogram (ECG) and pulse oximetry monitoring. For ECG, place electrodes on the chest and extremities to record electrical activity of the heart. A monitor in the OR displays this activity. Pulse oximetry monitors oxygen saturation. Apply an electrical cautery grounding pad to the skin so cauterizing instruments can be used safely. Apply **graded compression stockings** (e.g., elastic stockings) or IPC stockings intraoperatively (especially for long cases) or after surgery according to agency policy (see Chapter 47). Document compression device application, capillary refill, and patient tolerance to procedures. For limb surgeries assess peripheral pulses distal to the operative site. Measure temperature continuously via bladder, esophageal, or rectal probes.

Latex Sensitivity/Allergy. As the incidence and prevalence of **latex sensitivity** and allergy increase, the need for recognition of potential sources of latex is extremely critical. Federal regulations enacted in September 1998 mandate that all medical supplies contain a label notifying the consumer of the latex content. The OR and postanesthesia care unit (PACU) have many products that contain latex (e.g., gloves, IV tubing, syringes, and rubber stoppers on bottles and vials). It is also present in common objects such as adhesive tape, disposable electrodes, endotracheal tube cuffs, protective sheets, and ventilator equipment. Signs and symptoms of a latex reaction include local effects ranging from urticaria and flat or raised red patches to vesicular, scaling, or bleeding eruptions. Acute dermatitis is sometimes present. Rhinitis and/or rhinorrhea are other common reactions to mild and severe latex allergy. Immediate hypersensitivity reactions are life threatening, with the patient exhibiting focal or generalized urticaria and edema, bronchospasm, and mucus hypersecretion, all of which can compromise respiratory status. Vasodilation compounded by increased capillary permeability can lead to circulatory collapse and eventual death. Because the patient is draped during surgery, blocking visualization of the skin, investigate any unexplained acute deterioration in a previously healthy patient for possible latex allergy.

The AORN (2011) has a guideline for safe and competent care of the patient identified as being at risk for latex allergy. A latex allergy cart needs to be available at all times. All of the contents must be latex free. The American Association of Nurse Anesthetists (AANA) recommends that the patient with a latex allergy be scheduled as the first case of the day in the operating room. The room needs to be cleaned thoroughly, including all equipment, and all unnecessary items removed. The patient can then be safely accommodated by using appropriate latex-free items during the perioperative period and recovery. Box 50-4 lists latex precautions.

Introduction of Anesthesia. Patients undergoing surgical procedures receive one of four types of anesthesia: general, regional, local, or conscious sedation.

General Anesthesia. Modern anesthetic agents are much easier to reverse and allow the patient to recover with fewer negative effects. **General anesthesia** results in an immobile, quiet patient who does not recall the surgical procedure. The patient's amnesia acts as a protective measure from the unpleasant events of the procedure. An anesthesia provider gives general anesthetics by IV infusion and inhalation routes through the three phases of anesthesia: induction, maintenance, and emergence. Surgery requiring general anesthesia involves major procedures with extensive tissue manipulation.

Induction includes the administration of anesthetic agents and endotracheal intubation. The maintenance phase includes positioning the patient, preparing the skin for incision, and the surgical procedure itself. Appropriate levels of anesthesia are maintained during this phase. During emergence anesthetics are decreased, and

BOX 50-4 LATEX AVOIDANCE PRECAUTIONS

1. By touching any latex object, health care workers can transmit the allergen by hand to patients. Caution should be taken to keep the powder from the gloves away from patients because the powder acts as a carrier for the latex protein. Do not snap gloves on and off.
2. Identify latex-sensitive patients. The operating room (OR) should be labeled latex free to avoid having personnel bring rubber products (e.g., wristbands, chart labels) into the room.
3. Develop programs to educate health care workers in the care of latex-sensitive patients. Develop educational programs for patients and their families in the care and precautions that should be taken to prevent latex exposure.

Recommendations for Patient Care (Patients with Latex Allergy or Latex Risk)

The Operating Room

- Notify the OR of potential latex-allergic patients.
- Schedule latex-allergic and/or latex-risk patients as the first case(s) in the morning. This ensures that any latex dust (from the previous day) has been removed by ventilation of the room overnight.
- Remove all latex products from the OR.
- Bring a latex-free cart (if available) into the room.
- Use a latex-free reservoir bag, airways and endotracheal tubes, and laryngeal mask airways.
- Use a nonlatex breathing circuit with plastic mask and bag.
- Place all monitoring devices, cords/tubes (oximeter, blood pressure, electrocardiograph wires) in stockinet and secure with tape to prevent direct skin contact. Items sterilized in ethylene oxide must be rinsed before use. Residual ethylene oxide reacts and can cause an allergic response in a latex-allergic patient.

Intravenous Line Preparation

- Use intravenous (IV) tubing without latex ports; use stopcocks if available.
- If unable to obtain IV tubing without latex ports, cover latex ports with tape.
- Cover all rubber injection ports on IV bags with tape and label as follows: *Do not inject or withdraw fluid through the latex port.* *Note: Pulmonary artery catheters (especially the balloon), central venous catheters, and arterial lines may all contain latex components.*

Operating Room Patient Care

- Use nonlatex gloves. (*Use caution:* Not all substitutes are equally impermeable to bloodborne pathogens; care and investigation should be taken in the selection of substitute gloves.)
- Use nonlatex tourniquets or nonlatex examination gloves or polyvinyl chloride tubing.
- Draw medication directly from opened multidose vials (remove stoppers) if medications are not available in ampules.
- Draw up medications immediately before the beginning of the case or before administration. The rubber allergen could leach out of the plunger of the syringe, causing a reaction. The intensity of this reaction appears to increase over time.
- Use latex-free or glass syringes.
- Use stopcocks to inject drugs rather than latex ports.
- Notify pharmacy and central supply that the patient for whom you are caring is latex sensitive so these departments can use appropriate procedure when preparing medications and instruments. Also notify radiology, respiratory therapy, housekeeping, food service, and postoperative care units so the appropriate precautions can be made to protect the patient.
- Place clear and readily visible signs on the doors of the OR to inform all who enter that the patient has a latex allergy.

Modified from *Perioperative Standards and Recommended Practices: AORN latex guideline,* Denver, 2011, AORN.

the patient begins to awaken. Because of the short half-life of today's medications, emergence often occurs in the OR. The duration of anesthesia depends on the length of surgery. The greatest risks from general anesthesia are the side effects of anesthetic agents, including cardiovascular depression or irritability, respiratory depression, and liver and kidney damage.

Regional Anesthesia. Induction of regional anesthesia results in loss of sensation in an area of the body. The method of induction such as spinal, epidural, or a peripheral nerve block influences the portion of sensory pathways that are anesthetized. No loss of consciousness occurs with regional anesthesia, but the patient is often sedated. The anesthesia provider gives regional anesthetics by infiltration and local application.

Risks are involved with infiltrative anesthetics, particularly in the case of spinal anesthesia. Because the level of anesthesia can rise, which means that the anesthetic agent moves upward in the spinal cord, this can affect breathing. This migration of anesthetic depends on the drug type and amount and patient position. If the level of anesthesia rises, respiratory paralysis can develop, requiring resuscitation. Elevation of the upper body prevents respiratory paralysis. Some patients have a sudden fall in blood pressure, which results from extensive vasodilation caused by the anesthetic block to sympathetic vasomotor nerves and pain and motor nerve fibers. The patient requires careful monitoring during and immediately after surgery.

Because the patient is responsive and capable of breathing voluntarily, it is unnecessary for the anesthesia provider to use an endotracheal tube. OR personnel often gain a false sense of security because of the patient's relative alertness. Remember that burns and other trauma can occur on the anesthetized part of the body without the patient being aware of the injury. It is necessary to frequently observe the position of extremities and the condition of the skin.

Local Anesthesia. Local anesthesia involves loss of sensation at the desired site (e.g., a skin growth or the cornea of the eye). The anesthetic agent (e.g., lidocaine [Xylocaine]) inhibits nerve conduction until the drug diffuses into the circulation. It is injected locally or applied topically. The patient experiences a loss in pain and touch sensation and motor and autonomic activities (e.g., bladder emptying). Local anesthesia is common for minor procedures performed in ambulatory surgery.

Conscious Sedation. Conscious sedation is routinely used for procedures that do not require complete anesthesia but rather a depressed level of consciousness. A patient under conscious sedation must independently maintain a patent airway and adequate ventilation and be able to respond appropriately to verbal stimuli or light tactile stimulation (Rothrock, 2007). Short-acting IV sedatives such as midazolam (Versed) are given.

Advantages of conscious sedation include adequate sedation, reduction of fear and anxiety, amnesia, relief of pain and noxious stimuli, mood alteration, elevation of pain threshold, enhanced patient cooperation, stable vital signs, and rapid recovery. A variety of therapeutic procedures is appropriate for conscious sedation. Nurses assisting with the administration of local anesthesia and conscious sedation need to demonstrate competency in the care of these patients. Knowledge of anatomy, physiology, cardiac dysrhythmias, procedural complications, and pharmacological principles related to the administration of individual agents is essential. You also need to assess, diagnose, and intervene in the event of untoward reactions and demonstrate skill in airway management and oxygen delivery. Resuscitation equipment must be readily available when using local anesthesia or conscious sedation (AORN, 2011).

Positioning the Patient for Surgery. During general anesthesia the nursing personnel and surgeon often do not position the patient until the stage of complete relaxation. The surgical approach usually determines the choice of position. Ideally the patient's position provides good access to the operative site, sustains adequate circulatory and respiratory function, and ensures the patient's safety and skin integrity. It should not impair neuromuscular structures.

An alert person maintains normal range of joint motion by pain and pressure receptors. If a joint is extended too far, pain stimuli provide a warning that muscle and joint strain is too great. In a patient who is anesthetized, normal defense mechanisms cannot guard against joint damage, muscle stretch, and strain. The muscles are so relaxed that it is relatively easy to place the patient in a position the individual normally could not assume while awake. He or she often remains in a given position for several hours. Although it may be necessary to place a patient in an unusual position, try to maintain correct alignment and protect him or her from pressure, abrasion, and other injuries. Special mattresses, use of foam padding, and attachments to the OR table provide protection to extremities and bony prominences. Positioning should not impede normal movement of the diaphragm or interfere with circulation to body parts. If restraints are necessary, pad the skin to prevent trauma.

Documentation of Intraoperative Care. Throughout the surgical procedure, keep an accurate record of patient care activities and procedures performed by OR personnel. Documentation of intraoperative care provides useful data for the patient's postoperative period.

EVALUATION

The circulating nurse conducts an ongoing evaluation to ensure that interventions such as patient position are implemented correctly during the intraoperative phase of surgery.

Through the Patient's Eyes. While a patient is undergoing surgery, it is important to keep the family informed. Hospitals vary on their policies for when and how often families are given an update of the patient's condition. Families expect an estimate of when surgery begins and the length of time it will likely last. When you give an update to a family member, ask if he or she has further questions or concerns.

Patient Outcomes. Evaluate the patient's ongoing clinical status. Continuously monitor vital signs and intake and output (I&O). Measure the patient's body temperature during and at completion of the surgery, with the goal of keeping the patient normothermic. Inspect the skin under the grounding pad and at areas where positioning exerts pressure.

POSTOPERATIVE SURGICAL PHASE

After surgery a patient's care is often complex as a result of physiological changes. The type of anesthesia, nature of surgery, and the patient's previous condition determine the phases of recovery that he or she undergoes and the length of time spent in convalescence on an acute care nursing unit. Typically at the end of surgery the anesthesia provider and the circulating nurse accompany the patient to the PACU and provide a report to the nursing staff.

Patients who undergo general anesthesia are more likely to face complications than those who have only local anesthesia or conscious sedation. The patient who requires general anesthesia usually has extensive surgery and requires close monitoring in the PACU for phase I recovery. This lasts for a few hours. Ultimately the patient returns to the acute care unit for postoperative convalescence, which may last overnight or for several days. In contrast, an ambulatory surgical patient who has had local anesthesia with no sedation or conscious sedation most often only undergoes phase II recovery for a brief time (i.e., 1 to 2 hours). In phase II recovery nursing staff prepare the patient for care in the home or extended care setting (AORN, 2011).

IMMEDIATE POSTOPERATIVE RECOVERY (PHASE I)

Before the patient arrives in the PACU, a PACU nurse obtains data from the surgical team in the OR regarding the patient's general status and need for special equipment and nursing care. Careful planning allows the nursing staff to consider placement of patients in the PACU. For example, patients who undergo spinal anesthesia are aware of their surroundings and benefit from being in a quieter part of the PACU, away from patients needing frequent monitoring. The patient with a serious infection such as tuberculosis is isolated from other patients. Use standard precautions for infection control (see Chapter 28) for all patients.

When the patient is admitted to phase I recovery, personnel notify the nurses on the acute care nursing unit of his or her arrival. This allows the nursing staff to inform family members. Family members usually remain in the designated waiting area so they can be found when the surgeon arrives to explain the patient's condition. *It is the surgeon's responsibility to describe the patient's status, the results of surgery, and any complications that occurred.* You are a valuable resource to the family if complications have arisen in the operative phase and clarifying explanations are necessary.

When the patient enters the PACU, the nurse and members of the surgical team discuss his or her status. A standardized approach or tool for "hand-off" communications assists in providing accurate information about a patient's care, treatment and services, current condition, and any recent or anticipated changes (AORN, 2011; Manser et al., 2010). The hand-off is interactive, multidisciplinary, and done at the patient's bedside, allowing for a communication exchange that gives caregivers the chance to dialogue and ask questions (AORN, 2011). The surgical team's report includes a review of anesthetic agents administered so the PACU nurse is able to anticipate how quickly a patient should regain consciousness and analgesic needs. For example, a report on IV fluids or blood products administered during surgery from the anesthesia provider or perfusionist alerts the nurse to the patient's fluid and electrolyte balance. The surgeon often reports special concerns (e.g., whether the patient is at risk for hemorrhaging or infection). The OR nurse or anesthesia provider discusses whether there were complications during surgery such as excessive blood loss or cardiac irregularities. He or she also reports intraoperative patient positioning and condition of the skin. Frequently this report takes place while PACU nurses are admitting the patient. The PACU nurse attaches the patient to monitoring equipment such as the noninvasive blood pressure monitor, ECG monitor, and pulse oximeter. Patients often receive some form of oxygen in this immediate recovery period.

BOX 50-5 POSTANESTHESIA CARE ASSESSMENT

Parameters to Assess

- Vital signs
- Respiratory adequacy
- Postoperative cardiac status
- Peripheral circulation
- Postoperative neurological status
- Level of consciousness, alertness, lucidity
- Orientation
- Intravenous patency
- Pain level
- Motor abilities
- Return of sensory and motor control
- Skin integrity
- Temperature regulation
- Positioning
- Surgical wound condition
- Presence of nausea and vomiting

Adapted from Association of periOperative Registered Nurses: *Perioperative standards and recommended practices for inpatient and ambulatory settings,* Denver, 2011, AORN.

After receiving hand-off communication from the OR, the PACU nurse conducts a complete systems assessment during the first few minutes of PACU care (AORN, 2011) (Box 50-5). Assessments are performed at least every 15 minutes or more frequently, depending on the patient's condition and unit policy. This assessment usually continues until discharge from the PACU. Perform assessments quickly and thoroughly and target them to the patient's unique needs and type of surgery. In the PACU, nursing interventions focus on monitoring and maintaining airway, respiratory, circulatory, and neurological status and managing pain.

Evaluate a patient's status and eventual readiness for discharge from the PACU on the basis of vital sign stability compared with the preoperative data. Other outcomes for discharge include body temperature control, good ventilatory function and oxygenation status, orientation to surroundings, absence of complications, minimal pain and nausea, controlled wound drainage, adequate urine output, and fluid and electrolyte balance. Patients with more extensive surgery requiring anesthesia of longer duration usually recover more slowly. The Aldrete score is an objective scoring system that helps identify when patients are ready for discharge (Aldrete and Kroulik, 1970). The Aldrete score or the **postanesthesia recovery score (PARS)** is the most widely used scoring tool (Table 50-7). The criteria are assessed on admission; at 5, 15, 30, 45, and 60 minutes; and on discharge from the PACU. The patient must receive a composite score of 8 to 10 before discharge from the PACU (Aldrete, 1998). If the patient's condition is still poor after 2 to 3 hours, the stay lengthens, or the surgeon transfers the patient to an intensive care unit (ICU).

When the patient is discharged from the PACU, another hand-off communication occurs between the PACU nurse and the nurse on the acute nursing unit at the patient's bedside. The nurses verify the patient's identification using two identifiers and the type of surgery performed. The hand-off includes review of vital signs, the type of surgery and anesthesia performed; blood loss; level of consciousness; general physical condition; and presence of IV lines, drainage tubes, and dressings. The PACU nurse's report helps the nurse on the acute nursing unit anticipate special patient needs and obtain necessary equipment. It is important to have uninterrupted time to review the recent pertinent events and ask questions. It is also important at this time for patient's family members to be informed as soon as possible of the patient's transfer plan (AORN, 2011).

The OR staff transport the patient on a stretcher to the nursing unit. Staff members from the unit assist in safely transferring the patient to a bed (see Chapter 38). If the PACU nurse is helping to transport the patient, he or she shows the acute care nurse the recovery room record and reviews the patient's condition and course of care. The PACU nurse also reviews the surgeon's orders that require attention. *Before the PACU nurse leaves the acute care area, the staff nurse assuming care for the patient takes a complete set of vital signs to compare with PACU findings.* Minor vital sign variations normally occur after transporting the patient.

TABLE 50-7 Modified Aldrete Score

CRITERIA	SCORE
Activity	
Able to move four extremities voluntarily or on command	2
Able to move two extremities voluntarily or on command	1
Unable to move extremities voluntarily or on command	0
Respiratory	
Able to breathe deeply and cough freely	2
Dyspnea or limited breathing	1
Apneic	0
Circulation	
BP 20% of preanesthetic level	2
BP 20%-49% of preanesthetic level	1
BP 50% of preanesthetic level	0
Consciousness	
Fully awake	2
Arousable on calling	1
Not responding	0
Oxygen (O_2) Saturation	
Able to maintain O_2 saturation >92% on room air	2
Needs O_2 inhalation to maintain O_2 saturation >92%	1
O_2 saturation <90% even with O_2 supplement	0
TOTALS: Possible score range 0-10	

Modified from Aldrete JA: Modifications to the post anesthesia score for use in ambulatory surgery, *J Perianesth Nurs* 13(3):148, 1998; and Aldrete JA, Kroulik D: A post-anesthetic recovery score, *Anesth Analg* 49:924, 1970.
BP, Blood pressure.

RECOVERY IN AMBULATORY SURGERY (PHASE II)

The thoroughness and extent of postoperative recovery depends on the ambulatory patient's condition, type of surgery, and anesthesia. In some cases the patient goes through both phase I (PACU) and phase II recovery. Assess and care for patients in need of close monitoring in the same fashion as inpatients in phase I. Using the PARS, a score of 8 to 10 determines discharge from the PACU. After patients stabilize and no longer require close monitoring, transfer them to phase II recovery. With new anesthetic agents and techniques, known as *fast-track anesthesia,* patients experience a more rapid awakening in the OR and a quicker recovery (Kranke et al., 2008). Therefore many ambulatory surgery patients are able to bypass phase I.

Phase II recovery consists of a room equipped with medical recliner chairs, side tables, and foot rests. Kitchen facilities for preparing light snacks and beverages are usually located in the area,

TABLE 50-8 **Expanded Postanesthetic Recovery Score for Ambulatory Patients Assessed at 0, 5, 10, 15, 30, 45, and 60 minutes**

INDICES	TASK	SCORE
Activity	Able to move four extremities voluntarily or on command	2
	Able to move two extremities voluntarily or on command	1
	Unable to move extremities voluntarily or on command	0
Respiration	Able to breathe deeply and cough freely	2
	Dyspnea, limited breathing, or tachypnea	1
	Apneic or on mechanical ventilator	0
Circulation	BP 20% of preanesthetic level	2
	BP 20%-49% of preanesthetic level	1
	BP 50% of preanesthetic level	0
Consciousness	Fully awake	2
	Arousable on calling	1
	Not responding	0
O_2 saturation	Able to maintain O_2 saturation >92% on room air	2
	Needs O_2 inhalation to maintain O_2 saturation >92%	1
	O_2 saturation <90% even with O_2 supplement	0
Dressing	Dry and clean	2
	Wet but marked and not increasing	1
	Growing area of wetness	0
Pain	Pain free	2
	Mild pain handled by oral medication	1
	Severe pain requiring parenteral medication	0
Ambulation	Able to stand up and walk straight*	2
	Vertigo when erect	1
	Dizziness when supine	0
Fasting-feeding	Able to drink fluids	2
	Nauseated	1
	Nausea and vomiting	0
Urine output	Has voided	2
	Unable to void but comfortable	1
	Unable to void and uncomfortable	0
TOTALS	**Possible score range 0-20**	

Modified from Aldrete JA: Modifications to the post anesthesia score for use in ambulatory surgery, *J Perianesth Nurs* 13(3):148, 1998; and Aldrete JA, Kroulik D: A post-anesthetic recovery score, *Anesth Analg* 49:924, 1970.

NOTE: Total score must be at least 18 for patient to be discharged to home; lower score allowed if patient unable to walk or move extremities before surgery.

BP, Blood pressure; *O_2,* oxygen.

*May be substituted by Romberg's test, or picking up 12 paper clips in one hand.

along with bathrooms. Aldrete (1998) has added five more areas of functional assessment for the ambulatory surgery patient, which constitute the **postanesthesia recovery score for ambulatory patients (PARSAP)** (Table 50-8). The PARSAP is performed at the same time intervals as the PARS. The phase II environment promotes the patient's and family's comfort and well-being until discharge. Monitor patients but not at the same intensity as during phase I. In phase II recovery initiate postoperative teaching with patients and family members (Box 50-6).

BOX 50-6 **PATIENT TEACHING**

Postoperative Instructions for an Ambulatory Surgical Patient

Objective

- Patient will describe signs and symptoms of postoperative problems to report to health care provider.

Teaching Strategies

- Give instruction sheet with contact information, including health care provider's telephone number, surgery center's number, and follow-up appointment date and time. Allow patient and family to ask questions.
- Explain to family member the signs and symptoms of infection for which to observe.
- Explain name, dose, schedule, and purpose of medications and possible side effects. Provide drug information leaflets.
- Explain activity restrictions, diet progression, wound care guidelines, and the signs of any associated problems. Provide instruction sheet with clear, focused explanations.

Evaluation

- Have patient explain when and how to call health care provider with problems.
- Have patient recite date for follow-up appointment.
- Have patient and family member describe signs and symptoms of infection.
- Have patient verbalize name of drug, dose, when to take, and common side effects.
- Have patient demonstrate proper activity/movement and wound care.

Patients are discharged to home following ambulatory surgery when they meet certain criteria. When you are using the PARSAP, the patient must achieve a score of 18 or higher before being discharged. An exception is allowed if the patient was unable to walk or use extremities before surgery (Aldrete, 1998). Patients with known OSA or at high risk are not discharged from the recovery area to home until they are no longer at risk for postoperative respiratory depression, which may require a longer stay (ASA, 2006). Postoperative nausea and vomiting sometimes occur once the patient is home, even if the symptoms were not present in the surgery center. Options for therapy include the prophylactic use of the drug ondansetron (Zofran) (an orally disintegrating tablet), transcutaneous accupoint electrical stimulation, or a transdermal scopolamine patch (McCaffrey, 2007).

Review written postoperative instructions and prescriptions with the patient and family before releasing the patient and ensure that they verbalize understanding of these instructions. Always discharge the patient to a responsible adult.

POSTOPERATIVE CONVALESCENCE

Inpatients remain in the PACU until their condition stabilizes; they then return to the postoperative nursing unit. Nursing care focuses on returning the patient to a relatively functional level of wellness as soon as possible. The speed of convalescence depends on the type or extent of surgery, risk factors, pain management, and postoperative complications.

NURSING PROCESS

Once a surgical patient is transferred to an acute care nursing unit, ongoing postoperative care is essential to support recovery. Apply the nursing process and use a critical thinking approach in your care of patients.

ASSESSMENT

To assess a patient's postoperative condition, apply critical thinking while relying on information from the preoperative nursing assessment, knowledge regarding the surgical procedure performed, and events occurring during surgery. Critically analyze findings to detect any changes and make clinical decisions about the patient's care. A variation from the patient's norm may indicate the onset of surgically related complications.

Before the patient arrives on the nursing unit, prepare the bed and room for his or her return if he or she is returning to the same nursing unit. You are better prepared to care for the patient after surgery if the room is readied before the patient's return. A postoperative bedside unit should include the following:

1. Sphygmomanometer and/or automated noninvasive blood pressure monitor, stethoscope, and thermometer
2. Emesis basin
3. Clean gown
4. Washcloth, towel, and facial tissues
5. IV pole and infusion pump (if needed)
6. Suction equipment (if needed)
7. Oxygen equipment and oximetry monitor (if needed)
8. Extra pillows for positioning the patient comfortably
9. Bed pads to protect bed linen from drainage
10. Bed raised to stretcher height with bed linens pulled back and furniture moved to accommodate the stretcher and equipment (such as IV lines)

When the patient arrives on the acute care unit, monitor vital signs according to institution policy. Generally he or she is monitored every 15 minutes twice, every 30 minutes twice, hourly for 2 hours, and then every 4 hours or per orders. As the patient's condition stabilizes, he or she usually is monitored once a shift until discharge. Always base the frequency of assessment on the patient's current condition. *Do not assume that further monitoring is unnecessary if the patient appears normal during the initial assessment.* A patient's condition can change rapidly, especially during the postoperative period.

Thoroughly document the assessment, including vital signs, level of consciousness, airway status, condition of dressings and drains, comfort level, IV fluid status, and urinary output measurements. Enter patient data into the medical record on flow sheets, a computerized patient record, or written progress notes. The initial findings provide a baseline for comparing postoperative changes.

Through the Patient's Eyes. When a patient initially returns to the acute care nursing unit, the family and patient have expectations of the patient receiving prompt and attentive care. There is also the expectation that a nurse will explain the patient's immediate status and the plan of care for the next few hours. Seeing the patient return from surgery is a relief in many ways; but, if the patient has had complications or is not responding well, anxiety can easily return. As the patient stabilizes it is important to assess the patient's and family's expectations for recovery and the patient's convalescence once he or she returns home. What do they expect from staff during convalescence? Have you reviewed their expectations for the control of pain and other symptoms? Are family members prepared to assume care at discharge? Make the patient and family partners in your assessment so you can gather information necessary to develop a relevant plan of care. For example, determine the patient's and family's values and beliefs as they pertain to the meaning of the surgical condition and how it will affect the patient's ability to reassume his or her role in the family.

Airway and Respiration. Certain anesthetic agents cause respiratory depression. Thus be alert for shallow, slow breathing and a weak cough. Assess airway patency, respiratory rate, rhythm, depth of ventilation, symmetry of chest wall movement, breath sounds, and color of mucous membranes. If breathing is unusually shallow, place your hand near the patient's nose or mouth to feel exhaled air. Normal pulse oximetry values range between 92% and 100% saturation. Postoperative confusion is frequently secondary to hypoxia, especially in older adults.

An oral or nasal airway (see Chapter 40) may be inserted in the OR or PACU after removal of the endotracheal tube. It maintains a patent airway until patients can protect their airway. As patients awaken, they spit out the airway, or the nurse asks them to spit it out. The ability to do so signifies the return of a normal gag reflex.

One of your greatest concerns is airway obstruction. A number of factors contribute to obstruction, including history of OSA; weak pharyngeal/laryngeal muscle tone from anesthetics; secretions in the pharynx, bronchial tree, or trachea; and laryngeal or subglottic edema. In the postanesthetic patient the tongue causes the majority of airway obstructions. Ongoing assessment of airway patency is crucial. Patients remain in a side-lying position until airways are clear. Continue to assess respiratory status and breath sounds. Older patients, smokers, and patients with a history of respiratory disease are prone to developing complications such as atelectasis or pneumonia. Patients with OSA are often required to have continuous pulse oximetry while receiving IV opioids to detect oxygen desaturation quickly. Also assess the patient for any signs of shortness of breath or difficulty with endurance.

Circulation. The patient is at risk for cardiovascular complications resulting from actual or potential blood loss from the surgical site, side effects of anesthesia, electrolyte imbalances, and depression of normal circulatory-regulating mechanisms and ischemia. Careful assessment of heart rate and rhythm, along with blood pressure, reveals the patient's cardiovascular status. Compare preoperative vital signs with postoperative values. If the patient's blood pressure drops progressively with each check or if the heart rate changes or becomes irregular, notify the health care provider. A rhythm strip of the heart is obtained after surgery, compared with preoperative ECG tracings, and placed in the chart.

Assess circulatory perfusion by noting capillary refill, pulses, and the color and temperature of the nail beds and skin. If the patient has had vascular surgery or has casts or constricting devices that may impair circulation, assess peripheral pulses and capillary refill distal to the site of surgery. For example, after surgery to the femoral artery, assess posterior tibial and dorsalis pedis pulses. In addition, compare pulses in the affected extremity with those in the nonaffected extremity.

A common early circulatory problem is bleeding or hemorrhage. Blood loss may occur externally through a drain or incision or internally. Either type of hemorrhage results in a fall in blood pressure; elevated heart and respiratory rates; thready pulse; cool, clammy, pale skin; and restlessness. Notify the surgeon if these changes occur. Maintain IV fluid infusion. Monitor the patient's vital signs every 15 minutes or more frequently until the patient's condition stabilizes. Continue oxygen therapy. The surgeon may consider medications or volume replacement and order blood counts and coagulation studies.

Temperature Control. The OR and recovery room environments are extremely cool. The patient's anesthetically depressed level of body function results in a lowering of metabolism and fall in body temperature. When patients begin to awaken more fully, they complain of feeling cold and uncomfortable. Older adults and pediatric patients are at higher risk for developing problems associated with hypothermia. The use of forced-air warming units in the PACU is helpful in increasing patient comfort and rewarming the patient.

In rare instances a genetic disorder known as **malignant hyperthermia,** a life-threatening complication of anesthesia, develops. Malignant hyperthermia causes hypercarbia (elevated carbon dioxide), tachypnea, tachycardia, premature ventricular contractions (PVCs), unstable blood pressure, cyanosis, skin mottling, and muscular rigidity. Despite the name, an elevated temperature occurs late. The increased expired carbon dioxide is one of the first signs. Although it often occurs during the induction phase of anesthesia, symptoms can occur after surgery or with repeated exposures to anesthesia (Rothrock, 2007). Without prompt detection and treatment, it is potentially fatal.

Monitor temperature closely in the acute care area. Because an elevated temperature may be the first indication of an infection, assess the patient for a potential source of infection, including the IV site (if present), the surgical incision/wound, and the respiratory and urinary tracts. Notify the health care provider because further evaluation is often necessary.

Fluid and Electrolyte Balance. Because of the surgical patient's risk for fluid and electrolyte abnormalities, assess the hydration status and monitor for signs of electrolyte alterations (see Chapter 41). Monitor and compare laboratory values with the patient's baseline. An important responsibility of the nurse is maintaining patency of IV infusions. The patient's only source of fluid intake immediately after surgery is through IV catheters. Inspect the patient's catheter insertion site to ensure that the catheter is properly positioned within a vein, fluid flows freely, and the site is free of phlebitis or infiltration. Accurate recording of I&O assesses renal and circulatory function. Measure all sources of output, including urine, surgically placed drains, gastric drainage, and wound drainage; note any insensible loss from diaphoresis. Assess daily weight for the first several days after surgery and compare with the preoperative weight. If the patient has a known cardiac history such as heart failure, continue daily weights. It is important to use a consistent scale, amount of clothing, and time of day to obtain accurate weight measurement.

Neurological Functions. In the PACU the patient is often drowsy. As anesthetic agents begin to metabolize, his or her reflexes return, muscle strength is regained, and a normal level of orientation returns. Continue monitoring neurological status on the nursing unit. Ensure that the patient is oriented to self and the hospital and responds to questions appropriately. Assess pupil and gag reflexes, hand grips, and movement of extremities (see Chapter 30). If a patient had surgery involving a portion of the neurological system, conduct a more thorough neurological assessment. For example, if the patient had low back surgery, assess leg movement, sensation, and strength.

Patients with regional anesthesia begin to experience a return in motor function before tactile sensation returns. Check the patient's sensation to touch (see Chapter 30). Knowing where regional anesthesia was introduced helps you check the distribution of the spinal nerves affected. Typically assess sensation by touching the patient bilaterally in the same area (e.g., lower arm on both sides or leg on both sides) and note where the patient feels touch. Test the sense of touch using hand pressure or a gentle pinch of the skin. Extremity strength assessment continues to be important if spinal or epidural anesthesia has been given. However, patients remain in the PACU until sensation and voluntary movement of the lower extremities are reestablished.

Skin Integrity and Condition of the Wound. During recovery and acute postoperative care, assess the condition of the skin, noting pressure areas, rashes, petechiae, abrasions, or burns. A rash often indicates a drug sensitivity or allergy. Abrasions or petechiae may result from a clotting disorder or inappropriate positioning or restraining that injures skin layers. Burns may indicate that an electrical cautery grounding pad was incorrectly placed on the patient's skin. Use an occurrence or adverse event report to document burns or serious injury to the skin according to agency policy (see Chapter 23). Note if the patient is complaining of any burning or pain in the eye that could indicate a corneal abrasion.

After surgery most surgical wounds have dressings that protect the wound site and collect drainage. Observe the amount, color, odor, and consistency of drainage on dressings. It is most common to see serosanguineous drainage immediately after surgery. Estimate the amount of drainage by noting the number of saturated gauze sponges. If drainage appears on the outer surface of a dressing, another way of assessing it is marking the outer perimeter of the drainage with tape or marking it and dating with the time noted. This way you can easily note if drainage is increasing (see Chapter 48). However, this is not the most accurate measure of volume of fluid lost. Reinforce the dressing as needed and call the surgeon if wound drainage is leaking through the dressing.

Many surgeons prefer to change surgical dressings the first time so they can inspect the incisional area. You have the opportunity on the acute care nursing unit to view and thoroughly assess and document the status of the incision/wound at the time of this initial dressing change. Assess if wound edges are approximated and whether there is presence of bleeding or drainage. It is also important to assess the patient's mobility level. If he or she is unable or unwilling to turn, pressure ulcer development is a concern. Institute the use of the Braden scale or another assessment tool to determine the patient's risk of developing pressure ulcers. Institute preventive measures such as a turning schedule and pressure-reduction devices (see Chapter 48).

Metabolism. Researchers have studied glucose control in the postoperative period over the past decade. Normoglycemia or glucose level less than 150 mg/dL in postsurgical patients, while being careful to avoid hypoglycemia, is now recommended as an evidenced-based practice (Lipshutz and Gropper, 2009). Nurses should monitor patient blood glucose levels routinely based on surgeon order or hospital policy.

Genitourinary Function. Depending on the surgery, some patients do not regain voluntary control over urinary function for 6 to 8 hours after anesthesia. An epidural or spinal anesthetic often prevents the patient from feeling bladder fullness. Palpate the lower abdomen just above the symphysis pubis for bladder distention. Another option is to use a bladder scan to assess bladder volume. If the patient has a urinary catheter, there should be a continuous flow of urine of 30 to 50 mL/hr in adults. Observe the color and odor of urine. Surgery involving portions of the urinary tract normally causes bloody urine for at least 12 to 24 hours, depending on the type of surgery.

Gastrointestinal Function. Anesthetics slow GI motility and often cause nausea. Normally during the immediate recovery phase, faint or absent bowel sounds are auscultated in all four quadrants. Inspect the abdomen for distention that may be caused by accumulation of gas. In a patient who has had abdominal surgery, distention develops if internal bleeding occurs; however, this is a late sign of bleeding. Distention also occurs in the patient who develops a **paralytic ileus** (a nonmechanical obstruction caused by lack of intestinal peristalsis) from handling of the bowel in surgery.

In acute care closely monitor the patient's initial oral intake for potential aspiration or the presence of nausea and vomiting. Madsen et al. (2005) implemented a postoperative evidence-based practice project for assessment of bowel function return in patients having abdominal surgery. They found that assessing for the return of flatus and the first postoperative bowel movement as signs of returning bowel function were superior to bowel sound auscultation assessment. Other guidelines may be needed for other types of surgery. If an NG tube is in place, assess the patency of the tube (see Chapter 46) and the color and amount of gastric drainage.

Comfort. As patients awaken from general anesthesia, the sensation of pain becomes prominent. They perceive pain before regaining full consciousness. Acute incisional pain causes them to become restless and may be responsible for temporary changes in vital signs. It is difficult for patients to begin coughing and deep-breathing exercises when they experience pain. The patient who had regional or local anesthesia usually does not experience pain initially because the incisional area is still anesthetized. Ongoing assessment of the patient's discomfort and evaluation of pain-relief therapies are essential throughout the postoperative course. Pain scales are effective for assessing postoperative pain, evaluating the response to analgesics, and objectively documenting pain severity (see Chapter 43). Using preoperative pain assessments as a baseline, evaluate the effectiveness of interventions throughout the patient's recovery.

NURSING DIAGNOSIS

Determine the status of preoperative nursing diagnoses by clustering new postoperative assessment data. Then either revise or resolve preoperative diagnoses and identify relevant new diagnoses after surgery. A previously defined diagnosis such as *impaired skin integrity* may continue as a postoperative problem, particularly if your assessment reveals continued risks such as reduced mobility or excess diaphoresis. It is common to identify new nursing diagnoses after surgery because of the risks or problems associated with surgery. Also consider the assessed needs of a patient's family when you identify nursing diagnoses. In the formulation of nursing diagnoses, be accurate in identifying the related factor. For example, *impaired physical mobility related to reduced lower extremity strength* compared with *impaired physical mobility related to exercise intolerance* requires different nursing interventions. Potential nursing diagnoses for the postoperative patient include the following:

- Ineffective airway clearance
- Anxiety
- Fear
- Risk for infection
- Deficient knowledge (specify)
- Impaired physical mobility
- Nausea
- Acute pain
- Delayed surgical recovery

PLANNING

During the convalescent phase use current physical assessment data and analysis of the preoperative nursing history to plan the patient's care. The surgeon's postoperative orders and surgical team's report of the patient's operative condition also provide valuable data. Typical postoperative orders include:

- Frequency of vital sign monitoring and special assessments.
- Types of IV fluids and rates of infusion.
- Postoperative medications (especially those for pain and nausea).
- Resumption of preoperative medications as condition allows (some oral medications are converted to the IV route with appropriate dose adjustment).
- Fluids and food allowed by mouth.
- Level of activity that the patient is allowed to resume.
- Position that the patient is to maintain while in bed.
- I&O and daily weights.
- Laboratory tests and x-ray film studies.
- Special directions (e.g., surgical drains to suction, tube irrigations, dressing changes).

Goals and Outcomes. Review nursing diagnoses when establishing goals, expected outcomes, and interventions for the individual patient. Measurable outcomes provide specific guidelines for determining a patent's progress toward recovery from surgery. For example, a patient recovering from hip replacement surgery with the diagnosis of *impaired physical mobility related to pain and lower-extremity weakness* has specific outcomes selected that include targeted ambulation (e.g., steps to take and distance down hallway), pain relief, and improved range of joint movement. After meeting each outcome, the patient ultimately achieves the goal of independent ambulation at a preoperative level or better. At times goals and outcomes must extend from the convalescence period into the home setting. Also consider all goals of care established during the preoperative surgical phase that are still relevant. For example, a goal for the diagnosis of *risk for infection* would be "Patient remains free of infection after surgery." Expected outcomes for this goal would include:

- Patient's incision remains closed and intact.
- Patient's incision remains free of infectious drainage.
- Patient remains afebrile.

Setting Priorities. During the convalescent phase of recovery from general anesthesia, priorities for the first 24 hours continue to include maintenance of respiratory, circulatory, and neurological status and pain control. In addition, most surgeons are aggressive in increasing the patient's activity as soon as possible. As the patient progresses, focus priorities on advancement of patient activity (e.g., mobility, diet tolerance) to return the patient to preoperative functioning or better. The patient generally has multiple nursing diagnoses (Fig. 50-4). Reestablish priorities, often quickly, as the status of the patient's health problems change.

Teamwork and Collaboration. During recovery collaborate on the plan of care with respiratory therapy, physical therapy, occupational therapy, dietary, social work, home care, and others. Include family members as much as possible, especially if they will be assuming care responsibilities in the home. The goal of an interdisciplinary approach to care is to help the patient return to the best possible level of functioning with a smooth transition to home, rehabilitation, or long-term care. Acute care settings often have a nurse or social worker in a case manager role to coordinate interdisciplinary care so the most appropriate resources are available to patients.

IMPLEMENTATION

Acute Care. Primary causes for postoperative complications include impaired healing of the surgical wound, the effects of prolonged immobilization during surgery and convalescence, and the influence of anesthesia and analgesics. If a patient has surgical risks before surgery (e.g., increased age [Box 50-7], history of smoking, history of diabetes), the likelihood of complications is greater. Direct your postoperative nursing interventions at preventing complications so the patient returns to the highest level of functioning possible. Failure of the patient to become actively involved in recovery adds to the risk of complications (Table 50-9). Virtually any body system can be affected. Consider the interrelationship of all systems and therapies provided.

Maintaining Respiratory Function. To prevent respiratory complications begin pulmonary interventions early. The benefits of thorough preoperative teaching are reached when patients are able to participate actively in postoperative exercises. When patients awaken from anesthesia, help them maintain a patent airway. Position the patient on one side with the face downward and the neck slightly extended to facilitate a forward movement of the tongue and the flow of mucus secretions out of the mouth. A small folded towel supports the head. Another positioning technique to promote a patent airway involves elevating the head of the bed slightly and extending the patient's neck slightly, with the head turned to the side. In the PACU you sometimes need to perform a jaw thrust maneuver and/or chin lift continuously to maintain the patient's airway. Never position the patient with arms over or across the chest because this reduces maximum chest expansion.

Place patients with known OSA or at risk for OSA in the lateral, prone, or upright position throughout the perioperative period, never the supine position (ASA, 2006). Suction artificial airways and the oral cavity for mucus secretions (see Chapter 40). Avoid continually eliciting the gag reflex, which might cause vomiting.

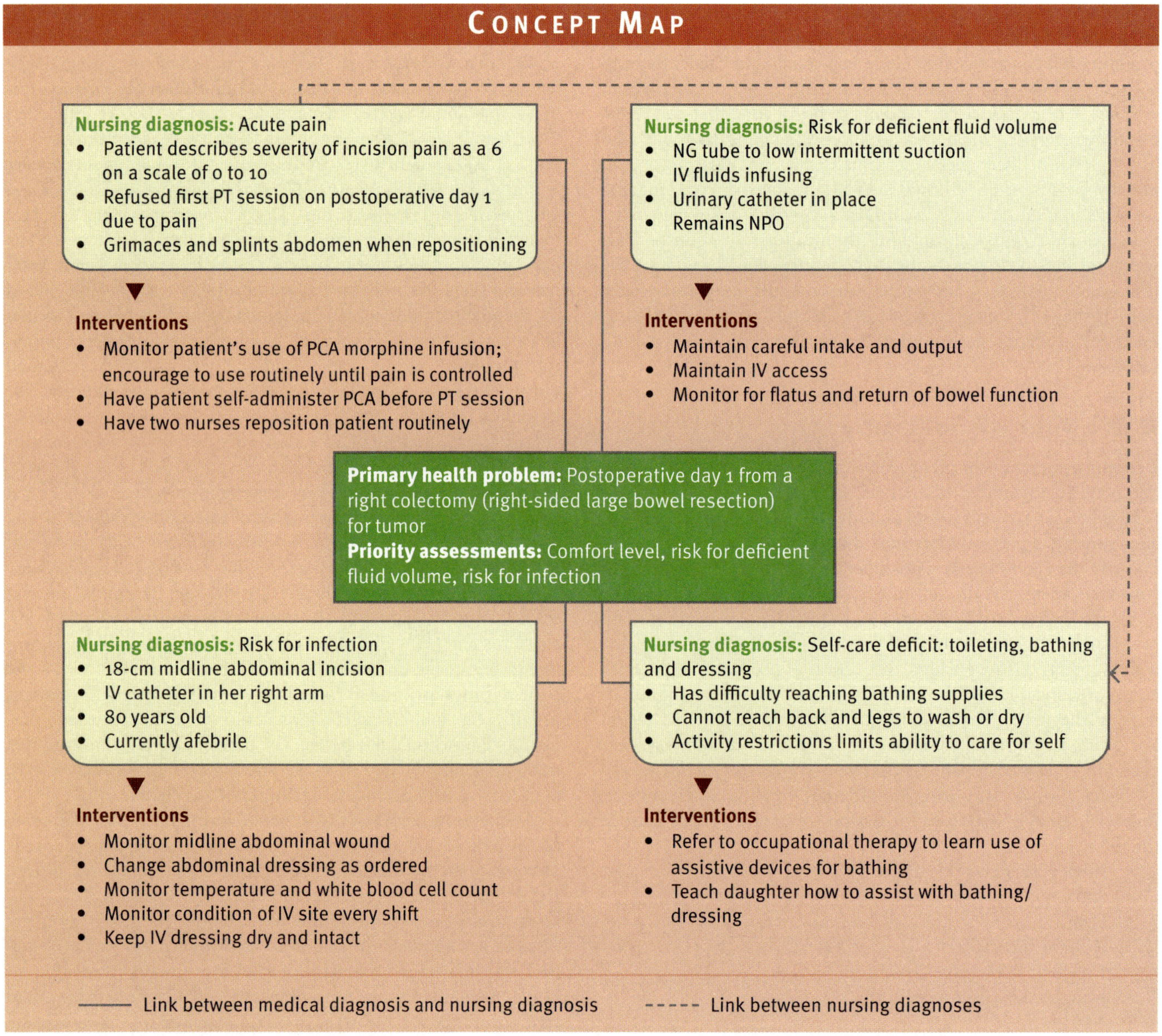
CONCEPT MAP
Nursing diagnosis: Acute pain
• Patient describes severity of incision pain as a 6 on a scale of 0 to 10
• Refused first PT session on postoperative day 1 due to pain
• Grimaces and splints abdomen when repositioning
Interventions
• Monitor patient's use of PCA morphine infusion; encourage to use routinely until pain is controlled
• Have patient self-administer PCA before PT session
• Have two nurses reposition patient routinely
Nursing diagnosis: Risk for deficient fluid volume
• NG tube to low intermittent suction
• IV fluids infusing
• Urinary catheter in place
• Remains NPO
Interventions
• Maintain careful intake and output
• Maintain IV access
• Monitor for flatus and return of bowel function
Primary health problem: Postoperative day 1 from a right colectomy (right-sided large bowel resection) for tumor
Priority assessments: Comfort level, risk for deficient fluid volume, risk for infection
Nursing diagnosis: Risk for infection
• 18-cm midline abdominal incision
• IV catheter in her right arm
• 80 years old
• Currently afebrile
Interventions
• Monitor midline abdominal wound
• Change abdominal dressing as ordered
• Monitor temperature and white blood cell count
• Monitor condition of IV site every shift
• Keep IV dressing dry and intact
Nursing diagnosis: Self-care deficit: toileting, bathing and dressing
• Has difficulty reaching bathing supplies
• Cannot reach back and legs to wash or dry
• Activity restrictions limits ability to care for self
Interventions
• Refer to occupational therapy to learn use of assistive devices for bathing
• Teach daughter how to assist with bathing/dressing
Link between medical diagnosis and nursing diagnosis
Link between nursing diagnoses

FIG. 50-4 Concept map for Mrs. Campana. *IV,* Intravenous; *NG,* nasogastric; *PCA,* patient-controlled analgesia; *PT,* physical therapy.

BOX 50-7 FOCUS ON OLDER ADULTS

The Older-Adult Surgical Patient: Concerns and Nursing Interventions

- Age alone is no longer a factor for determining the benefit that an individual can achieve from a surgical procedure. Consequently nurses are caring for many more surgical patients of advanced age and are required to know the age-related factors that affect a surgical procedure (Eliopoulos, 2005; Turrentine et al., 2006).
- A smaller margin of physiological reserve makes the older adult less able to compensate during the perioperative period for changes that occur as a result of infection, hemorrhage, alterations in blood pressure, and fluid/electrolyte abnormalities. Ongoing, focused assessments are necessary.
- Older patients are at greater risk for postoperative delirium associated with an acute onset. Reduced level of consciousness, reduced ability to maintain attention, perceptual disturbances, and memory impairment characterize the typical presentation (Meiner, 2011).
- Implement individualized measures to help the older-adult surgical patient achieve rest, sleep, and orientation in the postoperative period to reduce the risk of delirium development.
- Altered and unexpected drug responses are often related to different pharmacokinetics in the older adult. Thus the nurse caring for the perioperative older patient needs to be alert to the possibility of a high risk for adverse medication events with the administration of anesthetic agents and postoperative analgesics, especially narcotics (Meiner, 2011). "Start low and go slow" is the guiding principle when medicating older adults because of their slow drug-clearance capability.

Data from Eliopoulos C: *Gerontologic nursing,* ed 6, Philadelphia, 2006, Lippincott; and Meiner SE: *Gerontologic nursing,* ed 4, St Louis, 2011, Mosby.

Before you remove an artificial airway (or the patient removes it), suction the back of the airway so secretions are not retained.

The following measures promote expansion of the lungs:

- Encourage diaphragmatic breathing exercises every hour while patients are awake.
- Administer CPAP or NIPPV to patients who use this modality at home (ASA, 2006).
- Instruct patients to use an incentive spirometer for maximum inspiration. The patient should try to reach the inspiratory target volume achieved before surgery on the spirometer.
- Encourage early ambulation. Walking causes patients to assume a position that does not restrict chest wall expansion and stimulates an increased respiratory rate.
- Help patients who are restricted to bed to turn on their side every 1 to 2 hours while awake and to sit when possible.
- Keep the patient comfortable. A patient who is comfortable is able to participate in deep breathing and coughing. Administer analgesics on time so pain does not become severe.

The following measures promote removal of pulmonary secretions if they are present:

- Encourage coughing exercises every 1 to 2 hours while patients are awake and maintain pain control to promote a deep, productive cough. *For patients who have had eye, intracranial, or spinal surgery, coughing may be contraindicated because of the potential increase in intraocular or intracranial pressure.*

TABLE 50-9 Postoperative Complications

COMPLICATION	CAUSE
Respiratory System	
Atelectasis: Collapse of alveoli with retained mucus secretions. Signs and symptoms include elevated respiratory rate, dyspnea, fever, crackles auscultated over involved lobes of lungs, and productive cough.	Inadequate lung expansion. Anesthesia, analgesia, and immobilized position prevent full lung expansion. There is greater risk in patients with upper abdominal surgery who have pain during inspiration and repress deep breathing.
Pneumonia: Inflammation of alveoli. It may involve one or several lobes of lung. Development in lower dependent lobes of lung is common in immobilized surgical patient. Signs and symptoms include fever, chills, productive cough, chest pain, purulent mucus, and dyspnea.	Poor lung expansion with retained secretions or aspirated secretions. Common resident bacterium in respiratory tract is *Diplococcus pneumoniae,* which causes most cases of pneumonia.
Hypoxemia: Inadequate concentration of oxygen in arterial blood. Signs and symptoms include restlessness, confusion, dyspnea, high or low blood pressure, tachycardia or bradycardia, diaphoresis, and cyanosis.	Anesthetics and analgesics depress respirations. Increased retention of mucus with impaired ventilation occurs because of pain or poor positioning. Patients with OSA are at increased risk for hypoxemia.
Pulmonary embolism: Embolus blocking pulmonary arterial blood flow to one or more lobes of lung. Signs and symptoms include dyspnea, sudden chest pain, cyanosis, tachycardia, and drop in blood pressure.	Same factors lead to formation of thrombus or embolus. Immobilized surgical patient with preexisting circulatory or coagulation disorders is at risk.
Circulatory System	
Hemorrhage: Loss of large amount of blood externally or internally in short period of time. Signs and symptoms include hypotension, weak and rapid pulse, cool and clammy skin, rapid breathing, restlessness, and reduced urine output.	Slipping of suture or dislodged clot at incisional site. Patients with coagulation disorders are at greater risk.
Hypovolemic shock: Inadequate perfusion of tissues and cells from loss of circulatory fluid volume. Signs and symptoms are same as for hemorrhage.	In surgical patient hemorrhage usually causes hypovolemic shock.
Thrombophlebitis: Inflammation of vein often accompanied by clot formation. Veins in legs are most commonly affected. Signs and symptoms include swelling and inflammation of involved site and aching or cramping pain. Vein feels hard, cordlike, and sensitive to touch.	Prolonged sitting or immobilization aggravates venous stasis. Trauma to vessel wall and hypercoagulability of blood increase risk of vessel inflammation.

Continued

TABLE 50-9 Postoperative Complications—cont'd

COMPLICATION	CAUSE
Circulatory System—cont'd	
Thrombus: Formation of clot attached to interior wall of a vein or artery, which can occlude the vessel lumen. Symptoms include localized tenderness along distribution of the venous system, swollen calf or thigh, calf swelling >3 cm (1.2 in) compared to asymptomatic leg, pitting edema in symptomatic leg, and decrease in pulse below location of thrombus (if arterial).	Venous stasis (see discussion of thrombophlebitis) and vessel trauma. Venous injury is common after surgery of hips and legs, abdomen, pelvis, and major vessels. Patients with pelvic and abdominal cancer or traumatic injuries to the pelvis or lower extremities are at high risk for thrombus formation.
Embolus: Piece of thrombus that has dislodged and circulates in bloodstream until it lodges in another vessel (commonly lungs, heart, brain, or mesentery).	Thrombi form from increased coagulability of blood (e.g., polycythemia and use of birth control pills containing estrogen).
Gastrointestinal System	
Paralytic ileus: Nonmechanical obstruction of the bowel caused by physiological, neurogenic, or chemical imbalance associated with decreased peristalsis. Common in initial hours after abdominal surgery.	Handling of intestines during surgery leads to loss of peristalsis for a few hours to several days.
Abdominal distention: Retention of air within intestines and abdominal cavity during gastrointestinal surgery. Signs and symptoms include increased abdominal girth, patient complaints of fullness, and "gas pains."	Slowed peristalsis from anesthesia, bowel manipulation, or immobilization. During laparoscopic surgeries influx of air for procedure causes distention and pain up to shoulders.
Nausea and vomiting: Symptoms of improper gastric emptying or chemical stimulation of vomiting center. Patient complains of gagging or feeling full or sick to stomach.	Abdominal distention, fear, severe pain, medications, eating or drinking before peristalsis returns, and initiation of gag reflex.
Genitourinary System	
Urinary retention: Involuntary accumulation of urine in bladder as result of loss of muscle tone. Signs and symptoms include inability to void, restlessness, and bladder distention. It appears 6-8 hours after surgery.	Effects of anesthesia and narcotic analgesics. Local manipulation of tissues surrounding bladder and edema interfere with bladder tone. Poor positioning of patient impairs voiding reflexes.
Urinary tract infection: An infection of the urinary tract as a result of bacterial or yeast contamination. Signs and symptoms include dysuria, itching, abdominal pain, possible fever, cloudy urine, presence of WBCs and leukocyte esterase positive on urinalysis.	Most frequently a result of catheterization of the bladder.
Integumentary System	
Wound infection: An invasion of deep or superficial wound tissues by pathogenic microorganisms; signs and symptoms include warm, red, and tender skin around incision; fever and chills; purulent material exiting from drains or from separated wound edges. Infection usually appears 3-6 days after surgery.	Infection is caused by poor aseptic technique or contaminated wound or surgical site before surgical exploration. For example, with a bowel perforation the patient is at increased risk for a wound infection because of bacterial contamination from the large intestine.
Wound dehiscence: Separation of wound edges at suture line. Signs and symptoms include increased drainage and appearance of underlying tissues. This usually occurs 6-8 days after surgery.	Malnutrition, obesity, preoperative radiation to surgical site, old age, poor circulation to tissues, and unusual strain on suture line from coughing or positioning cause dehiscence.
Wound evisceration: Protrusion of internal organs and tissues through incision. Incidence usually occurs 6-8 days after surgery.	See discussion of wound dehiscence. Patient with dehiscence is at risk for developing evisceration.
Skin breakdown: Result of pressure or shearing forces. Surgical patients are at increased risk if alterations in nutrition and circulation are present, resulting in edema and delayed healing.	Prolonged periods on the OR table and in the bed after surgery lead to pressure breakdown. Skin breakdown results from shearing during positioning on the OR table and improperly pulling patient up in bed.
Nervous System	
Intractable pain: Pain that is not amenable to analgesics and pain-alleviating interventions.	Intractable pain may be related to the wound or dressing, anxiety, or positioning.
Malignant hyperthermia: Severe hypermetabolic state and rigidity of the skeletal muscles caused by an increase in intracellular calcium ion concentration.	Rare genetic condition triggered with exposure to inhaled anesthetic agents and the depolarizing muscle relaxant succinylcholine.

OR, Operating room; *OSA,* obstructive sleep apnea; *WBCs,* white blood cells.

- Provide oral hygiene to facilitate expectoration of mucus. The oral mucosa becomes dry when patients are NPO or placed on limited fluid intake.
- Initiate orotracheal or nasotracheal suction for patients who are too weak or unable to cough (see Chapter 40).
- Administer oxygen as ordered and monitor oxygen saturation with a pulse oximeter. Continue monitoring oxygen saturations after discharge from the PACU for patients at risk for respiratory compromise from OSA (ASA, 2006). Administer oxygen to patients at risk for or diagnosed with OSA until they are able to maintain their baseline oxygen saturation while breathing room air.

Preventing Circulatory Complications. Measures for preventing circulatory complications avert venous stasis and thrombus formation (Box 50-8). Some patients are at greater risk of venous stasis because of the nature of their surgery or medical history. The following measures promote normal venous return and circulatory blood flow:

- Encourage patients to perform leg exercises at least every hour while awake. Exercise may be contraindicated in an

BOX 50-8 EVIDENCE-BASED PRACTICE

Prevention of Venous Thromboembolism in the Postsurgical Patient

PICO Question: Is mechanical prophylaxis compared with pharmacological prophylaxis the best method to prevent a venous thromboembolism (VTE) in the postsurgical patient?

Evidence Summary

According to the American College of Chest Physicians (ACCP) (Geerts et al, 2008), VTE is a high-risk concern for almost all hospitalized patients and a significant cause of increased hospital morbidity and mortality. It is the second most common complication in patients discharged from acute care hospitals in the United States. Patients have been identified as having higher risk for development of VTE based on varying factors. These risks have been stratified based on surgical procedure (minor, major), age (<40, 40-60, >60) and the presence of risk factors such as cancer or previous VTE (Geerts et al., 2004). Many screening tools are available to perform formal risk assessments on patients, but compliance is often low. Most centers use a simplified risk assessment to determine the method of thromboprophylaxis that increases compliance with prevention strategies.

Mechanical and pharmacological types of prophylaxis are available. Mechanical prevention includes early ambulation, graded compression stockings, intermittent pneumatic compression devices, or venous foot pumps. Mechanical methods are recommended for patients at high risk of bleeding and also in conjunction with pharmacological prevention for high-risk populations. Pharmacological prevention includes administration of low-molecular-weight heparin (LMWH), low-dose unfractionated heparin (LDUH) or fondaparinux (Arixtra). Aspirin alone should not be used for the prevention of VTE. When using LMWH, LDUH or fondaparinux, the target international normalized ratio (INR) should be 2.5 with a range of 2-3, and dosing should be based on renal function and manufacturer recommendations. Certain surgical procedures are associated with increased VTE risk. Patients who have sustained major trauma or spinal cord injury or are undergoing hip or knee arthroplasty or hip fracture surgery are deemed high risk (40%-80%) for VTE. Patients at moderate risk (10%-40% risk) are bed-bound medical patients and patients undergoing most general gynecological and urological surgical procedures. Low-risk patients (<10% risk) include minor surgery on physically mobile patients and active medical patients. Based on the risk of VTE and bleeding, a regimen of either mechanical prophylaxis alone or combined with pharmacological prophylaxis is recommended. Refer to the *ACCP Prevention of VTE Evidence-Based Clinical Practice Guidelines* (Geerts et al., 2008) for more detailed information. General recommendations based on risk are as follows:

- Low risk—Early ambulation, no specific thromboprophylaxis
- Moderate risk—LMWH, LDUH or fondaparinux with mechanical prophylaxis
- High risk—LMWH, fondaparinux, or vitamin K antagonist for prolonged therapy, with an INR goal of 2-3 with mechanical prophylaxis

Application to Nursing Practice

- Level of risk of VTE determines method of prophylaxis prescribed for postsurgical patients.
- Screening methods should be simple and formally applied on all patients.
- Early ambulation and the use of mechanical prophylaxis are recommended in all postsurgical patients.
- Pharmacological prophylaxis should be dosed according to manufacturer suggested dosing guidelines or for a target INR of 2-3. Check all orders carefully.

extremity with a vascular repair or realignment of fractured bones and torn cartilage.

- Apply graded compression stockings or IPC devices as ordered by the health care provider (see Chapter 47). Remove the stockings at least once per shift. Perform a thorough reassessment of the skin of the lower extremities at this time.
- Encourage early ambulation. Most patients ambulate the evening of surgery, depending on the severity of the surgery and their condition. The degree of activity allowed progresses as the patient's condition improves. Encourage ambulation even if a patient has an epidural catheter or PCA device. Before ambulation assess the patient's vital signs. Abnormalities such as hypotension or certain arrhythmias may contraindicate ambulation. If vital signs are at baseline, first help the patient sit on the side of the bed. Patient complaints of dizziness are a sign of postural hypotension. A recheck of blood pressure determines whether ambulation is safe. Assist with ambulation by standing on the patient's strong side and making sure that the patient is able to walk steadily. The first few times out of bed, patients may be able to walk only a few feet. This usually improves each time. Evaluate tolerance to activity by periodically assessing the pulse rate as the patient ambulates and note the rhythm and increase in rate. Know the patient's maximum heart rate achieved during maximum exercise. One simple method to calculate a predicted maximum heart rate is by using this formula (Cleveland Clinic, 2011):

  220 – Patient's age = Predicted maximum heart rate

  Example: A 60-year-old's predicted maximum heart rate is 160 beats/min. However, remember that a patient's acute surgical condition may not allow him or her to reach this rate. Confer with the patient's surgeon or physical therapist about a safe heart rate target. Always ask patients how they feel during exercise and whether they note chest pain or shortness of breath.
- Avoid positioning patients in a manner that interrupts blood flow to extremities. While in bed, patients should not have pillows or rolled blankets placed under the knees. Compression of the popliteal vessels can cause thrombi. When patients sit in chairs, elevate their legs on footstools. Never allow a patient to sit with one leg crossed over the other.
- Administer anticoagulant drugs as ordered. Patients at greatest risk for thrombus formation often receive prophylactic doses of anticoagulants such as heparin. Patients may also receive aspirin, warfarin (Coumadin), or enoxaparin (Lovenox) for anticoagulation.
- Promote adequate fluid intake orally or intravenously. Adequate hydration prevents concentrated accumulation of formed blood elements such as platelets and red blood cells. When the plasma volume is low, these elements gather and form small clots within blood vessels.

Achieving Rest and Comfort. Pain control is a priority to facilitate a surgical patient's recovery. For example, advances have been made in the use of multimodal analgesia, which combines different drug classes delivered through various routes, including use of local anesthetics alone or in combination with other nerve blocks or techniques such as PCA. The goal is to enhance the efficacy of pain control while minimizing side effects of each modality (Costantini et al., 2011).

A patient's pain increases following surgery as the effects of anesthesia diminish. The patient becomes more aware of the surroundings and more perceptive of discomfort. The incisional area is only one source of pain. Irritation from drainage tubes, tight dressings, or casts and the muscular strains caused from positioning on the OR table also cause discomfort.

It is common to administer opioid analgesics (e.g., morphine or fentanyl) immediately after surgery. Initial analgesic doses are usually given by IV infusion in the PACU and titrated to patient comfort. After an anesthetized patient is awake and aware, PCA may be used. This is given by IV infusion, subcutaneous infusion, or an epidural catheter. The PCA system allows patients to administer their own IV analgesics from a specially prepared pump (see Chapter 43). If patients gain a sense of control over their pain, they usually have fewer postoperative problems. Many patients receive regional analgesia such as epidural analgesia continuously throughout the recovery period. Research has shown that epidural PCA provided pain relief and outcomes similar to IV patient-controlled morphine in cardiac surgery patients (Hansdottir et al., 2006). Similarly, Gupta et al. (2006) compared epidural analgesia with patient-controlled IV morphine in patients following radical retropubic prostatectomy and found pain scores to be lower in patients who received epidural analgesia. Epidural techniques are especially useful in patients with OSA who are at increased risk of airway compromise and postoperative complications with the use of systemic opioids after surgery (see Chapter 43). Nonsteroidal antiinflammatory agents are another alternative to systemic opioids in patients with OSA (ASA, 2006). You care for patients with a variety of pain-control techniques. Educate the patient and family regarding the technique and expected response.

If the patient has PCA and is trying to use it more frequently than the amount programmed, contact the health care provider to determine if it is appropriate to increase the amount of medication the patient is able to receive. The PCA provides a useful monitor of the effectiveness of pain medication. As oral intake is tolerated, facilitate changing the patient's pain medication from IV or epidural to oral administration. Do not overlook the importance of nonpharmacological interventions. Assess which care routines contribute to pain and use nonpharmacological measures to treat them. An example is to lower the head of the bed and use a pillow for incisional splinting while turning a patient with recent abdominal surgery. Use other methods of promoting pain relief such as positioning, back rubs, distraction, or imagery. Pain slows recovery. The patient becomes reluctant to cough, breathe deeply, turn, ambulate, or perform necessary exercises. Remember, *do not assume that the patient's pain is incisional.* When the patient without PCA or epidural analgesic asks for pain medication, determine the location, intensity, and character of the pain. Provide analgesics as often as allowed, around the clock the first 24 to 48 hours after surgery to improve pain control. If pain medications are not relieving discomfort, notify the health care provider for additional orders. Recognizing potential complications of analgesics and what to do if they occur is also an important role for the postoperative nurse.

Temperature Regulation. Temperature regulation is important after surgery. Patients are often cool after surgery; the PACU nurse provides warmed blankets immediately. If the temperature is 35.6° C (96° F) or below, use forced air or a convective warming device. Increasing body warmth causes the patient's metabolism to rise and circulatory and respiratory functions to improve.

Shivering is not always a sign of hypothermia but rather a side effect of certain anesthetic agents. Clonidine (Catapres) in small increments can decrease shivering as prescribed by the health care provider. Deep breathing and coughing are performed to help to expel retained anesthetic gases.

Malignant hyperthermia is a potentially lethal condition that can occur in patients receiving various inhaled anesthetic agents and succinylcholine. Suspect this when there is unexpected tachycardia and tachypnea; elevated carbon dioxide levels; jaw muscle rigidity; body rigidity of limbs, abdomen, and chest; or hyperkalemia. Temperature elevation is a late sign (Malignant Hyperthermia Association of the United States, 2010). When malignant hyperthermia develops, immediately administer dantrolene sodium ordered by the health care provider.

Surgical patients are at risk for infection for various reasons. If a patient becomes febrile, be aggressive in providing routine postoperative nursing interventions. For example, deep breathing and coughing, early ambulation, prompt removal of indwelling urinary and IV catheters, and aseptic care of the surgical wound decrease the risk of postoperative infections. Obtain wound and or blood cultures from patients suspected of having infections.

Maintaining Neurological Function. Orientation to the environment is important in maintaining the patient's mental status. Reorient the patient, explain that surgery is completed, and describe procedures and nursing measures. The patient who was properly prepared before surgery is less likely to be anxious during the postoperative period. Report any change in level of consciousness to health care providers.

Maintaining Fluid and Electrolyte Balance. An important nursing responsibility is maintaining patency of IV infusions in the postoperative period. The patient's only source of fluid intake immediately after surgery is through IV catheters. The health care provider orders a prescribed rate for each infusion. As the patient begins to take and tolerate oral fluids, the IV rate is decreased. When an ambulatory surgical patient awakens and is able to tolerate fluids by mouth without GI upset, the health care provider orders removal of the IV catheter. When acute care patients no longer need a continuous IV infusion, the IV line may be saline locked to preserve the site for antibiotics or other use (see Chapter 41). Some patients also receive blood products after surgery, depending on blood loss during surgery.

Promoting Normal Bowel Elimination and Adequate Nutrition. Normally a patient who has had general anesthesia does not receive fluids to drink in the PACU because of bowel sluggishness, the risk of nausea and vomiting, and grogginess from general anesthesia. To minimize nausea, avoid suddenly moving the patient. For patients at high risk for the development of nausea and vomiting or those who must not vomit (e.g., eye surgery), a combination of antiemetics is often more effective than a single agent (McCaffrey, 2007). If the patient has an NG tube, keep it patent by irrigating it as ordered (see Chapter 46). Occlusion of an NG tube results in accumulation of gastric contents within the stomach.

The patient likely begins taking ice chips or sips of fluids when arriving on the acute care unit. If these are tolerated, a clear liquid meal is usually ordered. Interventions for preventing GI complications promote return of normal elimination and faster return of normal nutritional intake. It takes several days for a patient who has had surgery on GI structures (e.g., a colon resection) to resume a normal diet. Normal peristalsis often does not return for 2 to 3 days. In contrast, the patient whose GI tract is unaffected directly by surgery can resume dietary intake after recovering from the effects of anesthesia. The following measures promote return of normal elimination:

- Advance a patient's dietary intake gradually. For the first few hours after surgery he or she receives only IV fluids. Research has shown that the return of flatus and the first postoperative bowel movement are reliable in determining when to begin a normal diet in patients who have undergone abdominal surgery (Madsen, 2005). However, the evidence is limited to one study, and most surgeons rely on the return of flatus or bowel sounds to order a normal diet. Patients usually receive a normal diet the first evening after surgery unless they have undergone surgery on GI structures. Implement diet intake while judging the patient's response. For example, provide clear liquids such as water, apple juice, broth, or tea after nausea subsides. Overloading with large amounts of fluids leads to distention and vomiting. If the patient tolerates liquids without nausea, advance the diet as ordered. Patients who have had abdominal surgery are usually NPO the first 24 to 48 hours. As flatus and peristalsis return, provide clear liquids, followed by full liquids, a light diet of solid foods, and finally a patient's usual diet. Encourage intake of foods high in protein and vitamin C.
- Promote ambulation and exercise. Physical activity stimulates a return of peristalsis. The patient who suffers abdominal distention and "gas pain" may obtain relief while walking.
- Maintain an adequate fluid intake. Fluids keep fecal material soft for easy passage. Fruit juices and warm liquids are especially effective.
- Promote adequate food intake by stimulating the patient's appetite.
- Remove sources of noxious odors and provide small servings of nonspicy foods.
- Assist the patient to a comfortable position during mealtime. Have the patient sit, if possible, to minimize pressure on the abdomen.
- Provide desired servings of food. For example, some patients are more willing to face the first meal when servings are not large.
- Provide frequent oral hygiene. Adequate hydration and cleaning of the oral cavity eliminate dryness and bad tastes.
- Administer fiber supplements, stool softeners, and rectal suppositories as ordered. If constipation or distention develops, the health care provider orders cathartics or enemas to stimulate peristalsis.
- Provide meals when the patient is rested and free from pain. Often a patient loses interest in eating if mealtime has been preceded by exhausting activities such as ambulation, coughing and deep-breathing exercises or extensive dressing changes. When a patient has pain, the associated nausea often causes a loss of appetite.

Promoting Urinary Elimination. The depressant effects of anesthetics and analgesics impair the sensation of bladder fullness. If bladder tone is reduced, the patient has difficulty starting urination. However, patients need to void within 8 to 12 hours after surgery. Because a full bladder is painful and often causes restlessness in recovery, it often becomes necessary to insert a straight catheter. If the patient has an indwelling urinary catheter, the goal is to remove it as soon as possible because of the high risk for the development of an HAI (bladder or urinary tract). To help reduce and eliminate HAIs, evidence-based protocols are often enacted to ensure prompt removal of urinary catheters (Willson et al., 2009).

Patients who undergo surgery of the urinary system frequently have an indwelling urinary catheter inserted to maintain free urinary flow until voluntary control of urination returns. The following measures promote normal urinary elimination (see Chapter 45):

- Check the patient frequently for the need to void. A surgical patient restricted to bed needs assistance in handling and using a bedpan or urinal. Often the patient acquires a sudden feeling of bladder fullness and urgency to void and needs help quickly.
- Assess for bladder distention. If a patient does not void within 8 hours of surgery or bladder distention is present, it may be necessary to insert a straight urinary catheter. A health care provider's order is needed. Continued difficulty in voiding may require an indwelling catheter, although the risk for a urinary tract infection increases. Although the evidence is inconclusive, some centers advocate the use of bladder ultrasound to assess bladder volume and assist in the decision to place a urinary catheter.
- Monitor I&O. If a patient has an indwelling catheter, expect an output of about 30 to 50 mL/hr. Another way to gauge adequacy of output is by determining the patient's weight. An accepted level of urinary output is at least 1 mL/kg/hr for adults. For example, a 132-pound woman (60 kg) would be expected to produce 60 mL of urine hourly. If the urine is dark, concentrated, and low in volume, notify a health care provider. Patients easily become dehydrated as a result of fluid loss from surgical wounds. Measure I&O for several days after surgery until the patient achieves normal fluid intake and urinary output.

Promoting Wound Healing. A surgical wound undergoes considerable stress during convalescence. The stresses of inadequate nutrition, impaired circulation, and metabolic alterations increase the risk for delayed healing (see Chapter 48). A wound also undergoes considerable physical stress. Strain on sutures from coughing, vomiting, distention, and movement of body parts can disrupt the wound layers. Protect the wound and promote healing. A critical time for wound healing is 24 to 72 hours after surgery, after which a seal is established. If a wound becomes infected, it usually occurs 3 to 6 days after surgery. A clean surgical wound usually does not regain strength against normal stress for 15 to 20 days after surgery. Use aseptic technique during dressing changes and wound care (see Chapter 48). Keep surgical drains patent so accumulated secretions can escape from the wound bed. Ongoing observation of the wound identifies early signs and symptoms of infection.

Maintaining/Enhancing Self-Concept. The appearance of wounds, bulky dressings, and extruding drains and tubes threatens a patient's self-concept. The effects of surgery such as disfiguring scars often create permanent changes in a patient's body image. If surgery leads to impairment in body function, the patient's role within the family can change significantly. Observe patients for behaviors reflecting alterations in self-concept. Some patients show revulsion toward their appearance by refusing to look at incisions, carefully covering dressings with bed clothes, or refusing to get out of bed because of tubes and devices. The fear of not being able to return to a functional family role causes some patients to avoid participating in the plan of care.

The family becomes an important part of the efforts to improve the patient's self-concept. Explain the patient's appearance to the family and ways to avoid nonverbal expressions of revulsion or surprise. Encourage the family to accept the patient's needs and support his or her independence. If the condition is permanent, the family learns to help the patient through the grieving process so he or she reaches a stage of acceptance. The following measures help to maintain the patient's self-concept:

- Provide privacy during dressing changes or inspection of the wound. Keep room curtains closed around the bed and drape the patient to expose only the dressing or incisional area.
- Maintain the patient's hygiene. Wound drainage and antiseptic solutions from the surgical skin preparation dry on the surface of the skin and cause irritation. A complete bath the first day after surgery renews the patient. When the gown becomes soiled by wound drainage, offer a clean gown and washcloth. Keep the patient's hair neatly combed and offer frequent oral hygiene. Room deodorizers are useful if the odor from drainage seems particularly troublesome to the patient and family.
- Prevent drainage devices from overflowing. You usually measure contents of drainage collection devices every 8 hours for output recording. The patient sometimes becomes preoccupied with observing the gradual collection of drainage, and some drainage devices leak contents if they become too full. Empty the devices periodically to prevent accidental spills and hampering of the patient's movement.
- Maintain a pleasant environment. Being in pleasant, comfortable surroundings heightens self-concept. Store or remove unused supplies. Keep the patient's bedside orderly and clean.
- Offer opportunities for the patient to discuss feelings about appearance. A patient who avoids looking at an incision may need to discuss fears or concerns. A patient having surgery for the first time is often more anxious than one who has had multiple surgeries. When the patient chooses to look at an incision for the first time, make sure that the area is clean. Eventually he or she will be able to care for the incision site by applying simple dressings or bathing the affected area.
- Provide the family with opportunities to discuss ways to promote the patient's self-concept. Encouraging independence is sometimes difficult for a family member who has a strong desire to help the patient in any way. By knowing about the appearance of a wound or incision, family members can be supportive during dressing changes. The topic or tone of a conversation helps family members distract a patient from dwelling on fears and concerns. Family members do not need to avoid discussing the future. However, they need help to know when it is appropriate to discuss future plans. Then the patient and family can work together to discuss realistic plans for the patient's return home.

Restorative and Continuing Care. In the postoperative period the nurse, patient, and family work to prepare the patient for discharge. Patients often have to continue wound care, follow activity or diet restrictions, continue medication therapy, and observe for signs and symptoms of complications on returning home. Education regarding these activities is specific to the type of surgery and is an ongoing process throughout hospitalization. Pieper et al. (2006) in a study of bariatric surgery patients found that the five most frequently mentioned postdischarge concerns were bowel function, wound pain, looking for wound complications, wound infection, and activity limitations. The higher the amount of perceived information received about incision care, the higher was the patient's knowledge rating. With ambulatory surgery patients, focused education within the limited time frame is essential. Including the family or support system provides a resource for the patient once home (see Box 50-6). With both ambulatory and hospitalized surgical patients, provide a wide variety of written educational materials. For example, offer materials with more pictures and illustrations for patients who do not speak English or have limited reading ability. Ensure that all materials are sensitive to various cultures and religions. Patients receive a copy of signed discharge instructions, and one copy remains in the medical record.

Some patients need home care assistance in the postoperative period after discharge. For example, nurses make referrals to home care for skilled nursing requirements when patients need wound care, ongoing IV therapy, or drain management. In addition, patients who are more physically dependent may require assistance from nursing assistive personnel to provide bathing and hygiene needs. The case coordinator or social worker at the hospital helps with discharge coordination. Encourage patients to show their discharge instructions to any home care provider.

Other patients, especially older adults, sometimes require discharge to a skilled nursing facility after their hospital recovery. During their convalescence in the skilled facility, patients work to gain mobility and recovery of their independent living skills. In addition, nurses provide wound care. A case coordinator or social worker works with the patient, family, and nurse to coordinate transfer to the skilled nursing facility.

EVALUATION

Through the Patient's Eyes. Addressing the ongoing concerns of patients and family members is an important part of evaluation after surgery. Evaluate patients' perceptions of the timeliness of response to their needs such as scheduled times for pain medication and prompt answering of a call light since these factors often influence patient satisfaction This is the opportunity to ask specific questions that address patient expectations and perceptions. For example, "Are you satisfied with the way we are managing your pain?" "Do you feel you have learned enough to be able to follow your diet at home?" "Are you having any ongoing issues, questions, or concerns that we can address for you at this time?" It is important to resolve any concerns or issues that the patient and family have before discharge.

Patient Outcomes. Evaluate the effectiveness of your care on the basis of the patient-centered expected outcomes established after surgery for each nursing diagnosis. Consult with the patient and family to gather evaluation data and remember that evaluation is ongoing. If a patient fails to progress as expected, revise his or her care plan based on evaluation findings and the patient's needs.

Make sure to evaluate for pain relief, using a pain scale. Determine the efficacy of both pharmacological and nonpharmacological measures. Use appropriate evaluative measures; inspect the condition of a wound, measure the distance or number of times that a patient is able to ambulate, and monitor the amount of fluid and food intake.

Part of your evaluation is determining the extent to which the patient and a family caregiver learn self-care measures. Have the patient and caregiver discuss the instructions you have provided so you know that they have the knowledge needed for the patient to return to as healthy and functional a state as possible. If the patient must perform any skill at home such as a dressing change or exercise, evaluate through return demonstration.

A phone call 24 hours after discharge to the patient's home is also helpful for evaluation. At this point the progress of recovery and asking if complications have developed can be addressed. This also is an opportunity to evaluate the patient's understanding of restrictions, wound care, medications, and necessary follow-up.

SAFETY GUIDELINES FOR NURSING SKILLS

Ensuring patient safety is an essential role of the professional nurse. To ensure patient safety, communicate clearly with the members of the health care team, assess and incorporate the patient's priorities of care and preferences, and use the best evidence when making decisions about your patient's care. When performing the skill in this chapter, remember the following points to ensure safe, individualized patient-centered care:

- Coughing and deep breathing may be contraindicated after brain, spinal, head, neck, or eye surgery.
- Bariatric patients may have more improved lung function and vital capacity in the reverse Trendelenburg's position.
- Report any signs of venous thromboembolism such as leg swelling, pain, or redness to the medical team immediately.

SKILL 50-1 DEMONSTRATING POSTOPERATIVE EXERCISES

View Video!

Delegation Considerations

The skill of teaching postoperative exercises cannot be delegated. Nursing assistive personnel (NAP) reinforce and assist patients in performing postoperative exercises. Direct the NAP to:

- Encourage patients to practice exercises regularly following instruction.
- Inform the nurse if patient is unwilling to perform these exercises.

Equipment

- Pillow or wrapped blanket (used to splint surgical incision during coughing)
- Incentive spirometer
- Positive expiratory pressure device

STEP	RATIONALE
ASSESSMENT	
1 Identify patient using two identifiers (i.e., name and birth date or name and account number) according to facility policy. Compare identifiers with information on the patient's medical record.	Ensures correct patient. Complies with a recommended National Patient Safety Goal (TJC, 2011).
2 Assess patient's risk for postoperative respiratory complications. Review medical history to identify presence of chronic pulmonary conditions (e.g., emphysema, asthma), any condition that affects chest wall movement, history of smoking, and presence of reduced hemoglobin.	General anesthesia predisposes patient to respiratory problems because lungs do not fully inflate during surgery, cough reflex is suppressed, and mucus collects within airway passages. After surgery patient may have reduced lung volume and require greater efforts to cough and deep breathe; inadequate lung expansion can lead to atelectasis and pneumonia. Previous chronic lung conditions increase patients' risk for developing respiratory complications (Kaw and Stoller, 2008). Smoking damages ciliary clearance and increases mucus. Reduced hemoglobin leads to inadequate oxygenation.
3 Auscultate lungs.	Establishes baseline for postoperative comparison.
4 Assess patient's ability to cough and deep breathe by having him or her take deep breath and observe movement of shoulders, abdomen, and chest wall. Observe chest excursion during deep breath. Ask patient to cough after taking deep breath.	Reveals maximum potential for chest expansion and ability to cough forcefully; serves as baseline to measure ability to perform exercises after surgery.
5 Assess patient's risk for postoperative venous stasis and thrombus formation (e.g., older patients, primary admitting diagnosis [e.g., trauma, orthopedic fracture, burn], patient's medical history [e.g., active cancer, atrial fibrillation, stroke, dehydration, previous clots], immobilized patients, women over 35 years who smoke and are taking oral contraceptives, position to assume on operating room table) (AORN, 2011).	Venous stasis, hypercoagulability, and vein trauma exist simultaneously for thrombus formation to occur (Geerts et al., 2008, Lewis et al., 2011). After general anesthesia, circulation slows; and when rate of blood flow slows, there is greater tendency for clot formation. Immobilization results in decreased muscular contraction in lower extremities, which promotes venous stasis. Manipulation and positioning during surgery sometimes cause trauma to leg veins.
6 Observe calves for redness, warmth, and tenderness, swollen calf or thigh, calf swelling more than 3 cm (1.2 inches) compared with asymptomatic leg, pitting edema in symptomatic leg, and collateral superficial veins. Compare legs for bilateral equality (Lewis et al., 2011), localized tenderness along distribution of venous system, swollen calf or thigh, calf swelling more than 3 cm (1.2 inches) compared with asymptomatic leg, pitting edema in symptomatic leg, and collateral superficial veins.	Signs of phlebitis and thrombus formation.

CLINICAL DECISION: *If any of the signs of thrombus formation is present, notify the health care provider immediately and do not manipulate extremity further. Surgery will usually be postponed. Graduated compression stockings, intermittent pneumatic compression stockings, and/or coagulation may be ordered.*

STEP	RATIONALE
7 Assess patient's ability to move independently while in bed.	Determines existence of any mobility restrictions.
8 Assess patient's willingness and capability to learn exercises: note attention span, anxiety, level of consciousness, language level. Also assess family members' willingness to learn and support patient after surgery.	Determines ability of patient to learn exercises successfully. Prepares family member to be able to encourage or coach patient in performing exercises after surgery.
9 Assess patient's medical orders before and after surgery.	Some patients require adaptations to performing exercises. In some cases certain exercises may be contraindicated.

SKILL 50-1 DEMONSTRATING POSTOPERATIVE EXERCISES—cont'd

STEP	RATIONALE
PLANNING	
1 Explain postoperative exercises to patient and family caregiver, including importance to recovery and physiological benefits.	Information allows patient to understand significance of exercises and can motivate learning. People tend to learn new skills when they know their benefits.
2 Plan exercises when patient is not in pain.	Decreased pain enhances patient's ability to practice exercises.
3 Prepare the room.	Makes environment conducive to learning.
IMPLEMENTATION	
1 Demonstrate exercises	
a. Diaphragmatic breathing	
(1) Assist patient to comfortable semi-Fowler's position or sitting on side of bed or in chair or standing position.	Upright position facilitates diaphragmatic excursion.
(2) Stand or sit facing patient.	Allows patient to observe breathing exercise.
(3) Instruct patient to place palms of hands across from each other, down and along lower borders of anterior rib cage. Place tips of fingers lightly together (see illustration). Demonstrate for patient.	Position of hands allows patient to feel movement of chest and abdomen as diaphragm descends and lungs expand.

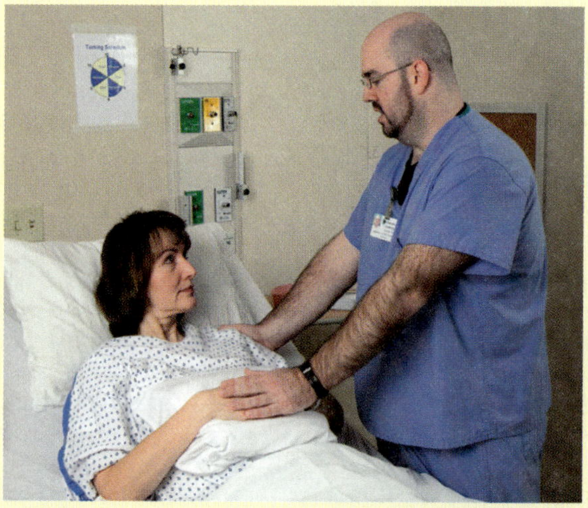

STEP 1a(3) Deep-breathing exercise—placement of hands on upper abdomen during inhalation.

STEP	RATIONALE
(4) Show patient how to take slow, deep breaths, inhaling through nose and pushing abdomen against hands. Have him or her feel middle fingers separate during inhalation. Explain that patient will feel normal downward movement of diaphragm while inhaling and that abdominal organs descend and chest wall expands. Demonstrate again.	Taking slow, deep breaths prevents panting or hyperventilation. Inhaling through nose warms, humidifies, and filters air. Diaphragmatic breathing allows air to pass by, partially obstructing mucus plug, increasing force to expel mucus. Explanation and demonstration focus on normal ventilatory movement of chest wall. Patient learns how diaphragmatic breathing feels.
(5) Instruct patient to avoid using chest and shoulders while inhaling.	Using auxiliary chest and shoulder muscles during breathing wastes energy and does not promote full lung expansion.
(6) Have patient hold slow, deep breath for count of three and then slowly exhale through mouth as if blowing out a candle (through pursed lips). Tell patient that middle fingertips will touch as chest wall contracts during exhalation.	Pursed-lip exhalation allows for gradual expulsion of all air.
(7) Repeat complete breathing exercise 3 to 5 times.	Allows patient to observe slow, rhythmic breathing pattern. Repetition of exercise reinforces learning.
(8) Have patient practice exercise. Instruct him or her to take 10 slow, deep breaths every hour while awake during postoperative period.	Regular deep breathing prevents postoperative complications of atelectasis.
b. Incentive spirometry	
(1) Perform hand hygiene.	Reduces transmission of microorganisms.
(2) Instruct patient to assume semi-Fowler's or high-Fowler's position.	Promotes optimal lung expansion during respiratory maneuver.
(3) For the bariatric patient, consider the reverse Trendelenburg's position.	Bariatric patients are often able to move their diaphragm better in the reverse Trendelenburg's position than in a Fowler's position.

STEP	RATIONALE
(4) Either set or indicate to patient on the incentive spirometer (IS) device scale the volume level to be attained with each breath (a targeted tidal volume). Use manufacturer guidelines to set the volume.	Establishes goal of volume level necessary for adequate lung expansion. Package insert helps determine target based on patient height and age (Pruitt, 2006).
(5) Explain to patient how to place mouthpiece of IS so lips completely cover mouthpiece (see illustration). Have patient demonstrate until position is correct.	Demonstration is reliable technique for teaching psychomotor skill and enables patient to ask questions.
(6) Instruct patient to inhale slowly and maintain constant flow through unit, attempting to reach goal volume. When patient reaches maximal inspiration, have him or her hold breath for 3 to 5 seconds (see illustration) and exhale slowly (Pruitt, 2006). Ensure that number of breaths does not exceed 10 to 12 per minute.	Maintains maximal inspiration and reduces risk of progressive collapse of individual alveoli. Slow breath (less than 12 breaths/min) prevents or minimizes pain from sudden pressure changes in chest.
(7) Instruct patient to breathe normally for short period between each of the 10 breaths on IS.	Prevents hyperventilation and fatigue.
(8) Have patient repeat breaths until goals are achieved.	Ensures correct use of IS.
(9) Have patient end with two coughs after end of 10 IS breaths hourly while awake.	Cough assists with lung secretion mobilization (Pruitt, 2006).
(10) Perform hand hygiene.	Reduces transmission of microorganisms.
c. Positive expiratory pressure therapy and "huff" coughing	
(1) Perform hand hygiene.	Reduces transmission of microorganisms.
(2) Set positive expiratory pressure (PEP) device for setting ordered.	Higher settings require more ventilatory effort.
(3) Instruct patient to assume semi-Fowler's or high-Fowler's position and place nose clip on patient's nose (see illustration).	Promotes optimum lung expansion, enabling patient to expectorate mucus. Clip prevents release of air through nose.
(4) Instruct patient to place lips around mouthpiece or demonstrate placement. Instruct patient to take a full breath and exhale 2 or 3 times longer than inhalation. Repeat pattern for 10 to 20 breaths.	Ensures that patient does all breathing through mouth and uses the device properly.

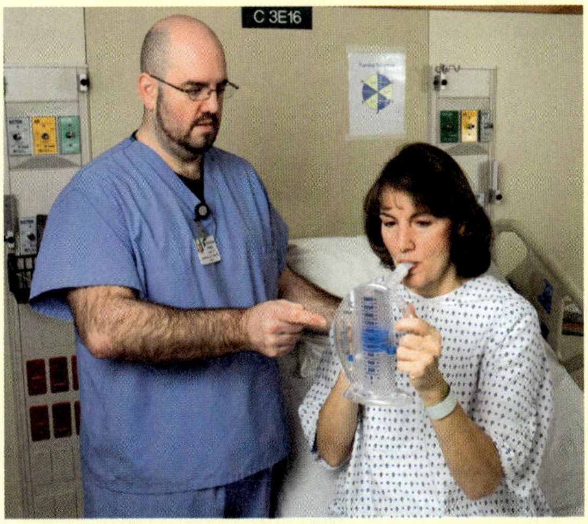

STEP 1b(5) Patient demonstrating incentive spirometry.

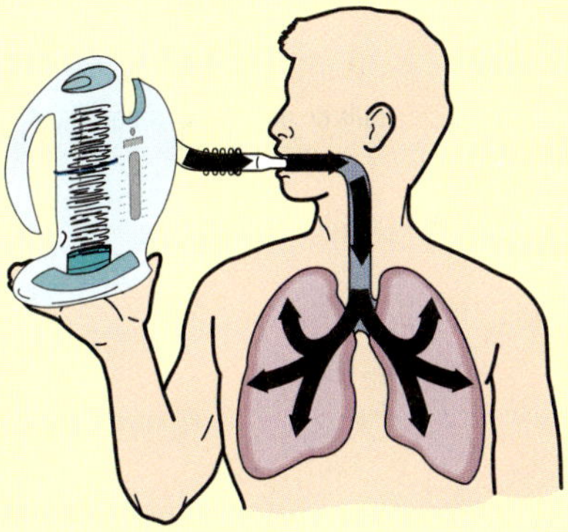
STEP 1b(6) Diagram of use of incentive spirometer.

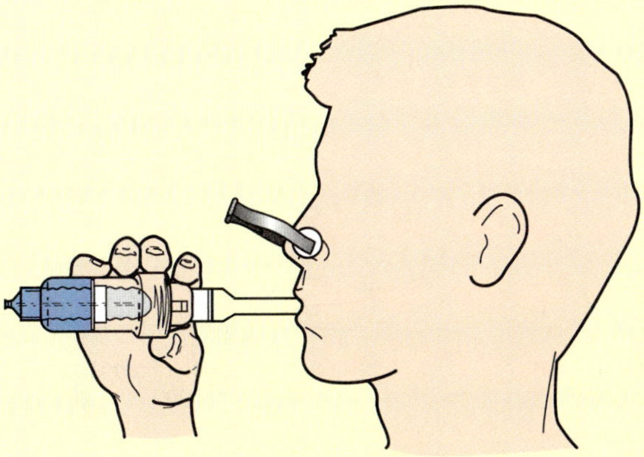
STEP 1c(3) Diagram of use of positive expiratory pressure device.

SKILL 50-1 DEMONSTRATING POSTOPERATIVE EXERCISES—cont'd

STEP	RATIONALE
(5) Have patient remove device from mouth; take a slow, deep breath; and hold for 3 seconds.	Promotes lung expansion before coughing.
(6) Have patient exhale in quick, short, forced "huffs."	"Huff" coughing or forced expiratory technique promotes bronchial hygiene by increasing expectoration of secretions (Fink, 2007).
d. Controlled coughing	
(1) Explain importance of maintaining upright semi-Fowler's or sitting position.	Position facilitates diaphragm excursion and enhances thorax expansion.
(2) If surgical incision will be either abdominal or thoracic, teach patient to place pillow or bath blanket over incisional area and place hands over pillow to splint incision. During breathing and coughing exercises, have patient press gently against incisional area for splinting or support (see illustration).	Surgical incision cuts through muscles, tissues, and nerve endings. Deep breathing and coughing place additional stress on suture line and cause discomfort. Splinting incision with hands or pillow provides firm support and reduces pulling.
(3) Demonstrate coughing. Instruct patient to take two slow, deep breaths, inhaling through nose and exhaling through mouth.	Deep breaths expand lungs fully so air moves behind mucus and facilitates effects of coughing.
(4) Instruct and show how to inhale deeply a third time and hold breath to count of three. Cough fully for two or three consecutive coughs without inhaling between coughs. (Tell patient to push all air out of lungs.)	Consecutive coughs help remove mucus more effectively and completely than one forceful cough.

CLINICAL DECISION: *Coughing is often contraindicated after brain, spinal, head, neck, or eye surgery because of potential increase in intracranial or intraocular pressure.*

STEP	RATIONALE
(5) Caution patient against just clearing throat instead of coughing. Explain that coughing does not cause injury to incision when done correctly.	Clearing throat does not remove mucus from deeper airways. Postoperative incisional pain makes it harder for patient to cough effectively.
(6) Have patient practice coughing exercises, splinting imaginary incision. Instruct patient to cough 2 to 3 times every 2 hours while awake.	Stresses value of deep coughing with splinting to effectively expectorate mucus with less discomfort.
(7) Instruct patient to look at sputum each time for consistency, odor, amount, and color changes and what to report to nurse.	Sputum characteristics indicate presence of pulmonary complication such as pneumonia.
e. Turning (example shows turning to right side)	
(1) Instruct patient to assume supine position and move to side of bed if permitted by surgery. Instruct patient to move by bending knees and pressing heels against mattress to raise and move buttocks (see illustration). Top side rails on both sides of bed should be in up position.	Positioning begins on side of bed so turning to other side does not cause patient to roll toward edge of bed. Buttocks lift prevents shearing force from body movement against sheets.

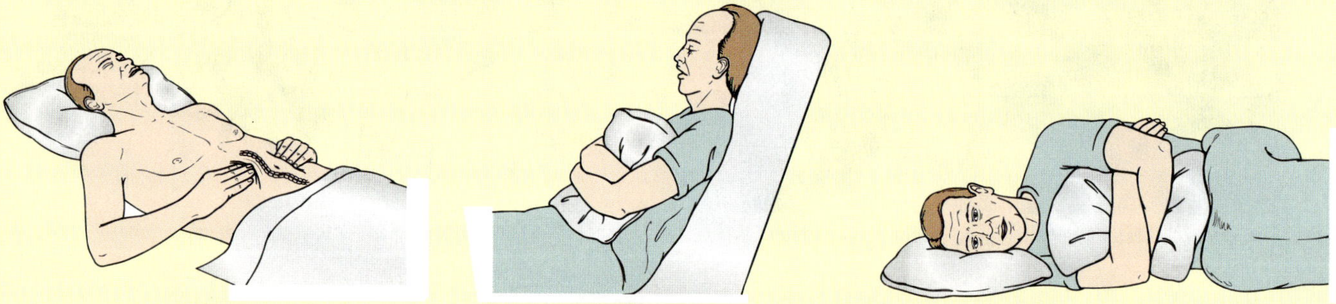

STEP 1d(2) Techniques for splinting incision. (From Lewis S et al: *Medical-surgical nursing: assessment and management of clinical problems,* ed 8, St Louis, 2011, Mosby.)

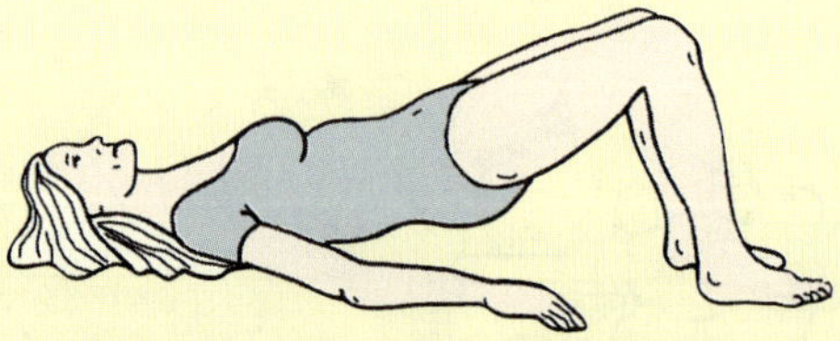

STEP 1e(1) Buttocks lift for moving to side of bed. (From Lowdermilk D, Perry SE: *Maternity and women's health care,* ed 9, St Louis, 2007, Mosby.)

STEP	RATIONALE
(2) Instruct patient to place right hand over incisional area to splint it *(optional)*	Supports and minimizes pulling on suture line during turning.
(3) Instruct patient to keep right leg straight and flex left knee up (see illustration). If back or vascular surgery was performed, patient needs to logroll (see Chapter 47) or requires assistance with turning.	Straight leg stabilizes patient's position. Flexed left leg shifts weight for easier turning.
(4) Have patient grab right side rail with left hand, pull toward right, and roll onto right side.	Pulling toward side rail reduces effort needed for turning.
(5) Instruct patient to turn every 2 hours while awake. Often patients require assistance with turning after surgery.	Reduces risk of vascular and pulmonary complications.
f. Leg exercises	
(1) Have patient assume supine position in bed. Guide through leg exercises by helping him or her perform passive range-of-motion exercises while simultaneously explaining exercise.	Provides normal anatomical position of lower extremities. Depending on surgical procedure and patient status, some of these leg exercises may be contraindicated.
(2) Rotate each ankle in complete circle. Instruct patient to draw imaginary circles with big toe (see illustration). Repeat 5 times.	Leg exercises maintain joint mobility and promote venous return to prevent thrombi.
(3) Alternate dorsiflexion and plantar flexion of both feet. Direct patient to feel calf muscles contract and relax alternately (see illustrations *A* and *B*). Repeat 5 times.	Stretches and contracts gastrocnemius muscles.
(4) Perform quadriceps setting by tightening thigh and bringing knee down toward mattress, then relaxing (see illustration). Repeat 5 times.	Contracts muscles of upper legs, maintains knee mobility, and enhances venous return.
(5) Have patient alternately raise each leg straight up from bed surface, keeping legs straight; have patient bend leg at hip and knee (see illustration). Repeat 5 times.	Promotes contraction and relaxation of quadriceps muscles.

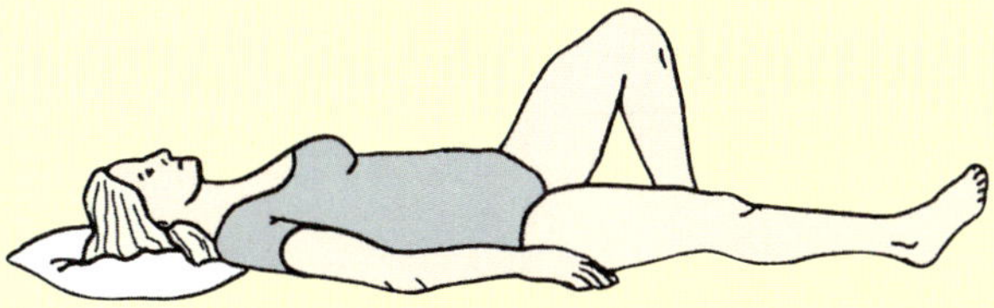

STEP 1e(3) Leg position for turning. (From Lowdermilk D, Perry SE: *Maternity and women's health care,* ed 9, St Louis, 2007, Mosby.)

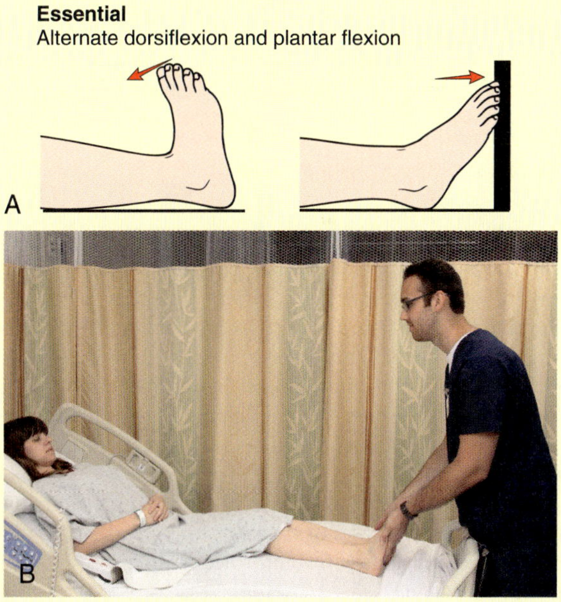

STEP 1f(3) A, Alternate dorsiflexion and plantar flexion. **B,** Patient pushes feet to perform plantar flexion. (**A** From Lewis S et al: *Medical-surgical nursing: assessment and management of clinical problems,* ed 7, St Louis, 2007, Mosby).

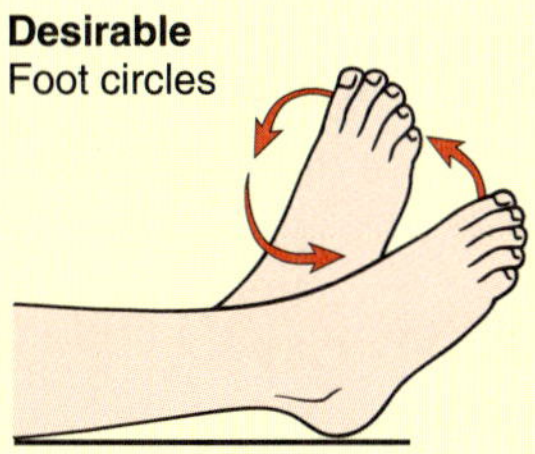

STEP 1f(2) Foot circles. (From Lewis S et al: *Medical-surgical nursing: assessment and management of clinical problems,* ed 7, St Louis, 2007, Mosby.)

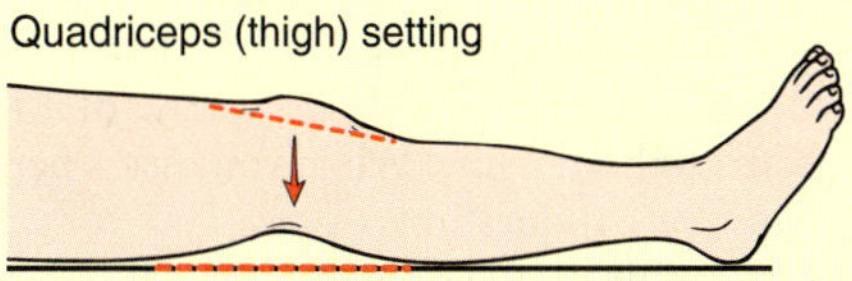

STEP 1f(4) Quadriceps (thigh) setting. (From Lewis S et al: *Medical-surgical nursing: assessment and management of clinical problems,* ed 7, St Louis, 2007, Mosby).

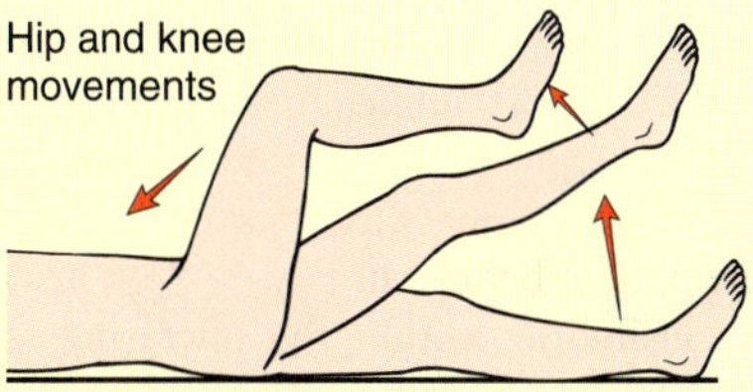

STEP 1f(5) Hip and knee movements. (From Lewis S et al: *Medical-surgical nursing: assessment and management of clinical problems,* ed 7, St Louis, 2007, Mosby).

SKILL 50-1 DEMONSTRATING POSTOPERATIVE EXERCISES—cont'd

STEP	RATIONALE
2 Have patient continue to practice exercises before surgery at least every 2 hours while awake. Teach him or her how to coordinate turning and leg exercises with diaphragmatic breathing, IS, and coughing exercises.	Repetition of exercise sequence reinforces learning. Establishes routine for exercises that develops habit for performance. Sequence of exercises is leg exercises, turning, breathing, and coughing.
EVALUATION	
1 Observe patient perform all five exercises (only IS or PEP, not both) independently.	Provides opportunity for practice and return demonstration. Ensures that patient has learned correct technique.
2 Observe family member coach patient through steps of exercise.	Determines if family member can assist in a positive, appropriate way.

UNEXPECTED OUTCOMES AND RELATED INTERVENTIONS

1 Patient is unable to perform exercises correctly before surgery.
- Assess for the presence of anxiety, pain, and fatigue.
- Teach patient stress reduction techniques and/or pain management strategies.
- Repeat teaching using more demonstration or redemonstration at time when family or friends are present.

2 Patient is unwilling to perform exercises after surgery because of incisional pain of thorax or abdomen (deep breathing, coughing, and turning) or because of surgery involving lower abdomen, groin, buttocks, or legs (leg exercises, turning).
- Instruct patient to ask for pain medication 30 minutes before performing postoperative exercise or to use patient-controlled analgesia (PCA) immediately before exercising.
- Report to surgeon or pain team inadequate pain relief and need to change analgesic or increase dose.

RECORDING AND REPORTING

- Record exercises demonstrated and whether patient is able to perform them independently.
- Report any problems patient has in completing exercises to nurse assigned to patient on next shift for follow-up.

HOME CARE CONSIDERATIONS

- Incorporate teaching of family members to help patient implement postoperative exercises at home.

KEY POINTS

- Surgery is classified by level of severity, urgency, and purpose.
- The preoperative period may be several days or only a few hours long, with some patients assessed in the health care provider's office, preadmission clinic, or anesthesia clinic or by telephone.
- Preoperative assessment of vital signs and physical findings provides an important baseline with which to compare postoperative assessment data.
- Nursing diagnoses for a surgical patient apply to nursing care during one or all phases of surgery.
- Primary responsibility for informed consent rests with the patient's surgeon.
- Structured preoperative teaching positively influences a patient's postoperative recovery.
- The explanation of all preoperative and postoperative routines and demonstration of postoperative exercises are basic to preoperative teaching.
- In ambulatory surgery nurses use the limited time available to educate patients, assess their health status, and prepare them for surgery.
- A routine preoperative safety checklist is a guide for final preparation of the patient before surgery.
- Nurses' responsibilities within the operating room focus on protecting the patient from potential harm.
- All medications taken before surgery are automatically discontinued after surgery unless a health care provider reorders the drugs.
- Family members are important in assisting patients with any physical limitations and providing emotional support during postoperative recovery.
- Care of the postoperative patient centers on the body systems that anesthesia, immobilization, and surgical trauma most likely affect.
- Accurate pain assessment and intervention are necessary for healing.

CLINICAL APPLICATION QUESTIONS

Preparing for Clinical Practice

Mrs. Campana has just been transported to your surgical nursing division from the PACU. She underwent a right colectomy (right-sided large bowel resection) for removal of a tumor. Her vital signs were stable in the postanesthesia care unit (PACU), and her temperature was 36.8° C (98° F). She has an intravenous (IV) line in her right arm, a Foley catheter, a nasogastric (NG) tube, and oxygen at 4 L/min per nasal cannula. She received 10 mg of morphine sulfate intravenously in the PACU and now has morphine patient-controlled analgesia (PCA) with a demand dose of 1 mg every 10 minutes connected to her IV line. When you assess her, she is slow to respond to your verbal questions.

1. Why may Mrs. Campana be slow to respond?
2. In a postoperative patient with decreased responsiveness such as Mrs. Campana, on which key assessments should you focus immediately?

3. Mrs. Campana's daughter enters the room and is very concerned about her mother's slowness to awaken. What do you tell her?

evolve *Answers to Clinical Application Questions can be found on the Evolve website.*

REVIEW QUESTIONS

Are You Ready to Test Your Nursing Knowledge?

1. Obesity places patients at an increased surgical risk because of which of the following factors? (Select all that apply.)
   1. Risk for bleeding is increased.
   2. Ventilatory capacity is reduced.
   3. Fatty tissue has a poor blood supply.
   4. Metabolic demands are increased.
2. The primary reason that family members should be included when the nurse teaches the patient preoperative exercises is so they can:
   1. Coach and encourage the patient after surgery.
   2. Demonstrate to the patient at home.
   3. Relieve the nurse by getting the patient to do the exercises every 2 hours.
   4. Practice with the patient while he or she is waiting to be taken to the operating room.
3. In the postanesthesia care unit (PACU) the nurse notes that the patient is having difficulty breathing and suspects an upper airway obstruction. The nurse would first:
   1. Suction the pharynx and bronchial tree.
   2. Give oxygen through a mask at 4 L/min.
   3. Ask the patient to use an incentive spirometer.
   4. Position the patient on one side with the face down and the neck slightly extended so the tongue falls forward.
4. Because an older adult is at increased risk for respiratory complications after surgery, the nurse should:
   1. Withhold pain medications and ambulate the patient every 2 hours.
   2. Monitor fluid and electrolyte status every shift and vital signs with temperature every 4 hours.
   3. Orient the patient to the surrounding environment frequently and ambulate the patient every 2 hours.
   4. Encourage the patient to turn, deep breathe, and cough frequently and ensure adequate pain control.
5. You are caring for a patient after surgery who underwent a liver resection. His prothrombin time (PT) or an activated partial thromboplastin time (APTT) is greater than normal. He has low blood pressure; tachycardia; thready pulse; and cool, clammy, pale skin, and he is restless. You assess his surgical wound, and the dressing is saturated with blood. Which immediate interventions should you perform? (Select all that apply.)
   1. Notify the surgeon.
   2. Maintain intravenous (IV) fluid infusion and prepare to give volume replacement.
   3. Monitor the patient's vital signs every 15 minutes or more frequently until his condition stabilizes.
   4. Wean oxygen therapy.
   5. Provide comfort through bathing.
6. You are a nurse in the postanesthesia care unit (PACU), and you note that your patient has a heart rate of 130 beats/min and a respiratory rate of 32 breaths/min; you also assess jaw muscle rigidity and rigidity of limbs, abdomen, and chest. What do you suspect, and which intervention is indicated?
   1. *Infection:* Notify surgeon and anticipate administration of antibiotics.
   2. *Pneumonia:* Listen to breath sounds, notify surgeon, and anticipate order for chest radiography.
   3. *Hypertension:* Check blood pressure, notify surgeon, and anticipate administration of antihypertensives.
   4. *Malignant hyperthermia:* Notify surgeon/anesthesia provider immediately, prepare to administer dantrolene sodium (Dantrium), and monitor vital signs frequently.
7. After a surgical patient has been given preoperative sedatives, which safety precaution should a nurse take?
   1. Reinforce to the patient to remain in bed or on the stretcher
   2. Raise the side rails and keep the bed or stretcher in the high position
   3. Determine if the patient has any allergies to latex
   4. Obtain informed consent immediately after sedative administration
8. The operating room (OR) and postanesthesia care unit (PACU) are high-risk environments for patients with a latex allergy. Which safety measures to prevent a latex reaction should the nurse implement? (Select all that apply.)
   1. Screening patients about food allergies known to have a cross-reactivity to latex such as kiwis and bananas
   2. Having a latex allergy cart available at all times
   3. Communicating with the operating room (OR) team as soon as 24 to 48 hours in advance of the surgery when a latex-sensitive patient is identified
   4. Scheduling the latex-sensitive patient for the last operative case of the day
9. A nurse is recovering a patient who received conscious sedation for cosmetic surgery. Which of the following is an advantage that conscious sedation has over general anesthesia?
   1. Loss of sensation at the surgical site
   2. Reduction of fear and anxiety and need for assistance with airway patency and ventilation
   3. Amnesia and relief of pain
   4. Monitoring in phase I recovery
10. You have been given the following postoperative patients to care for on your shift. Based on the information provided, which patient should you see first?
    1. A 75-year-old following hip replacement surgery who is complaining of moderate pain in the surgical site, with a heart rate of 92
    2. A 57-year-old following hip replacement 6 hours earlier who is receiving intravenous patient-controlled analgesia (PCA) with a history of OSA. The pulse oximeter has been alarming and reading 85%
    3. A 36-year-old following bladder neck suspension who is 30 minutes late to receive her postoperative dose of antibiotic
    4. A 48-year-old following total knee replacement who needs help repositioning in bed
11. Hand-off communications that occur between the postanesthesia care unit (PACU) nurse and the nurse on the postoperative nursing unit should be done when a patient returns to the nursing unit. Select appropriate components of a safe and effective hand-off. (Select all that apply.)
    1. Vital signs, the type of anesthesia provided, blood loss, and level of consciousness
    2. Uninterrupted time to review the recent pertinent events and ask questions

3. Verification of the patient using one identifier and the type of surgery performed
4. Review of pertinent events occurring in the operating room (OR) while at the nurses' station

12. A nurse is working in the preoperative holding area and is assigned to care for a patient who is having a prosthetic aortic valve placed. The nurse inserts an intravenous (IV) line and obtains vital signs. The patient has a temperature of 39° C (102° F), heart rate of 120, blood pressure (BP) of 84/50, and an elevated white blood cell (WBC) count. The nurse immediately notifies the surgeon of the patient's vital signs because:
    1. They need to get the patient into the operating room (OR) quickly to start the surgery because of the low blood pressure.
    2. The surgery may need to be delayed to check the patient's WBC count and investigate the source of fever before surgery.
    3. The nurse anticipates the need for a fluid bolus to increase the patient's BP.
    4. The nurse anticipates an order for a sedative to help calm the patient and decrease the heart rate.

13. A nurse is working in an ambulatory care setting and is ready to discharge a patient who is wheelchair dependent. The patient underwent dilation of an esophageal stricture. Her postanesthesia recovery score for ambulatory patients (PARSAP) score is 16. Her family is ready to go and eager to make the long road trip home. In determining if it is safe for the patient to be discharged at this time, the nurse should decide the following:
    1. The PARSAP score must be 18 or higher before being discharged.
    2. The patient's family is capable to care for her, and she understands her discharge instructions; thus the nurse proceeds with discharge.
    3. Since the patient hasn't been drinking much, the nurse is not concerned that she is unable to void and proceeds with discharge.
    4. Since the patient was admitted to the surgical center in a wheelchair, she can be discharged with a lower PARSAP score.

14. A patient is admitted through the emergency department for multisystem trauma following a motorcycle crash with multiple orthopedic injuries. He goes to surgery for repair of fractures. He is postoperative day 3 from an open reduction internal fixation of bilateral femur fractures and external fixator to his unstable pelvic fracture. Interventions that are necessary for prevention of venous thromboembolism in this high-risk postsurgical patient include: (Select all that apply.)
    1. Intermittent pneumatic compression stockings.
    2. Vitamin K therapy.
    3. Subcutaneous heparin or enoxaparin (Lovenox).
    4. Continuous heparin drip with a goal of an international normalized ratio (INR) 5 times higher than baseline.

15. You are caring for a 65-year-old patient 2 days after surgery and helping him walk down the hallway. The surgeon has ordered exercise as tolerated. Your assessment indicates that the patient's heart rate at baseline is 88. After walking approximately 30 yards down the hallway, the heart rate is 110. What should be your next action?
    1. Stop exercise immediately and have him sit in a nearby chair.
    2. Ask him how he feels; determine if there is any discomfort or shortness of breath; and, if not, continue exercise.
    3. Tell him that he needs to walk further to reach a heart rate of 120.
    4. Have him walk slower; he has reached his maximum.

Answers: **1.** 2, 3; **2.** 1; **3.** 4; **4.** 4; **5.** 1, 2, 3; **6.** 4; **7.** 1; **8.** 1, 2, 3; **9.** 3; **10.** 2; **11.** 1, 2; **12.** 2; **13.** 4; **14.** 1, 3; **15.** 2.

REFERENCES

Aldrete JA: Modifications to the post anesthesia score for use in ambulatory surgery, *J Perianesth Nurs* 13(3):148, 1998.

Aldrete JA, Kroulik D: A post-anesthetic recovery score, *Anesth Analg* 49:924, 1970.

Ambulatory Surgery Center Association: 2010, accessed December 4, 2010 from http://www.ascassociation.org.

American College of Surgeons: *Patient education: partners in surgical care*, 2006, http://www.facs.org/patient education/index.html. Accessed November 10, 2011.

American Society of Anesthesiologists (ASA): Practice guidelines for the perioperative management of patients with obstructive sleep apnea: a report by the American Society of Anesthesiologists Task Force on Perioperative Management of Patients with Obstructive Sleep Apnea, *Anesthesiology* 104:1081, 2006.

American Society of Anesthesiologists (ASA): Practice guidelines for preoperative fasting and the use of pharmacologic agents to reduce the risk of pulmonary aspiration: application to healthy patients undergoing elective procedures: an updated report by the American Society of Anesthesiologists Committee on Standards and Practice Parameters, *Anesthesiology* 114:495, 2011.

Association of periOperative Registered Nurses (AORN): *AORN Position statement on care of the older adult in perioperative settings, AORN*, Denver, 2010, AORN. http://www.aorn.org/PracticeResources/AORNPosition Statements/OlderAdult/.

Association of periOperative Registered Nurses (AORN): *Perioperative standards and recommended practices for inpatient and ambulatory setting*, Denver, 2011, AORN.

Bond LM, et al: Effects of preoperative teaching of the use of a pain scale with patients in the PACU, *J Perianesth Nurs* 20(5):333, 2005.

Bray A: Preoperative nursing assessment of the surgical patient, *Nurs Clin North Am* 41(2):130, 2006.

Centers for Medicare and Medicaid Services: *Adverse events in hospitals: public disclosure of information about events*, Washington, DC, 2010, Office of Inspector General, http://oig.hhs.gov/oei/reports/oei-06-09-00360.pdf. Accessed January 25, 2012.

Cleveland Clinic: *Your pulse and your target heart rate*, Miller Family Heart & Vascular Institute at Cleveland Clinic, Preventive Cardiology and Rehabilitation Program, 2011, my.clevelandclinic.org/heart. Accessed August 12, 2011.

Costantini R, et al: Controlling pain in the post-operative setting, *MA Int J Clin Pharmacol Ther* 49(2):116, 2011.

Cronenwett L, et al: Quality and safety education for nurses, *Nurs Outlook* 55(3):122, 2007.

Edelman CL, Mandel CL: *Health promotion throughout the lifespan*, ed 7, St Louis, 2009, Mosby.

Eliopoulos C: *Gerontologic nursing*, ed 6, Philadelphia, 2005, JB Lippincott.

Fink JB: Forced expiratory technique, directed cough and autogenic drainage, *Respir Care* 52(9):1210, 2007.

Galanti GA: *Caring for patients from different cultures*, ed 4, Philadelphia, 2008, University of Pennsylvania Press.

Kaw R, Stoller JK: Pulmonary complications after noncardiac surgery: a review of their frequency and prevention strategies, *Clin Pulmon Med* 15(1):18, 2008.

Kruzik N: Benefits of preoperative education for adult elective surgery patients, *AORN J* 90(3):381, 2009.

Lewis S, et al: *Medical-surgical nursing: assessment and management of clinical problems*, ed 8, St Louis, 2011, Mosby.

Malignant Hyperthermia Association of the United States: *Managing malignant hypertension: clinical update*, online brochure, 2010, http://www.mhaus.org. Accessed September 2010.

Mamaril ME: Nursing consideration in geriatric surgical patient: the perioperative continuum of care, *Nurs Clin North Am* 41:313, 2006.

McCaffrey R: Make PONV prevention a priority, *OR Nurse* 1(2):39, 2007.

Meiner SE: *Gerontologic nursing*, ed 4, St Louis, 2011, Mosby.

National Quality Forum (NQF): *National voluntary consensus standards for public reporting of patient safety event information: a consensus report*, Washington, DC, 2010, NQF.

Pruitt B: Help your patient combat postoperative atelectasis, *Nursing* 36(5):64, 2006.

Rosén S, et al: Calm or not calm: the question of anxiety in the perianesthesia patient, *J Perianesth Nurs* 23(4):237, 2008.

Rothrock JC: *Alexander's care of the patient in surgery*, ed 13, St Louis, 2007, Mosby.
Seet E, Chung F: Obstructive sleep apnea: preoperative assessment, *Anesthesiol Clin* 28(2):199, 2010.
Smetana G: Postoperative pulmonary complications: an update on risk assessment and reduction, *Cleveland Clin J Med* 74(Suppl 4):60, 2009.
Sussman G, Gold M: *Guidelines for the management of latex allergies and safe latex use in health care facilities, American College of Allergy, Asthma and Immunology,* 2010, http://www.acaai.org/patients/resources/allergies/Pages/latex-management-in-healthcare-facilities.aspx. Accessed September 2010.
Turrentine FE, et al: Surgical risk factors, morbidity and mortality in elderly patients, *J Am Coll Surg* 203(6):865, 2006.
The Joint Commission (TJC): *2011 National Patient Safety Goals (NPGS),* 2011, http://www.jointcommission.org/standards_information/npsgs.aspx.
Walton-Geer PS: Prevention of pressure ulcers in the surgical patient, *AORN J* 89(3):538, 2009.

RESEARCH REFERENCES

Brady M, Kinn S, Stuart P: Preoperative fasting for adults to prevent perioperative complications, *Cochrane Database Syst Rev* (4):CD004423, 2003.
Geerts WH, et al: Prevention of venous thromboembolism: The Seventh ACCP Conference on Antithrombotic and Thrombolytic Therapy, *Chest* 126(Suppl): 338S, 2004.
Geerts WH, et al: Prevention of venous thromboembolism: American College of Chest Physicians evidence-based clinical practice guidelines, *Chest* 133:381S, 2008.
Gupta A, et al: Postoperative analgesia after radical retropubic prostatectomy: a double-blind comparison between low thoracic epidural and patient-controlled intravenous analgesia, *Anesthesiology* 105(4):784, 2006.
Hansdottir V, et al: Thoracic epidural versus intravenous patient-controlled analgesia after cardiac surgery: a randomized controlled trial on length of hospital stay and patient-perceived quality of recovery, *Anesthesiology* 104(1):142, 2006.
Joanna Briggs Institute for Evidence Based Nursing and Widwifery: Knowledge retention from pre-operative patient information, *Best Practice* 4(6), 2000.
Kranke P, et al: Pharmacological interventions and concepts of fast-track perioperative medical care for enhanced recovery programs, *Expert Opin Pharmacother* 9(9): 1541, 2008.
Liao P, et al: Postoperative complications in patients with obstructive sleep apnea: a retrospective matched cohort study, *Can J Anaesthiol* 56(11):819, 2009.
Lipshutz AKM, Gropper MA: Perioperative glycemic control an evidence-based review, *Anesthesiology* 110: 408, 2009.
Madsen D, et al: Listening to bowel sounds: an evidence-based practice project, *Am J Nurs* 105(12):40, 2005.
Manser T, et al: Assessing the quality of handoffs at patient care transitions, *Qual Safety Health Care* 19(6):44, 2010.
Paice J, et al: Efficacy and safety of scheduled dosing of opioid analgesics: a quality improvement study, *J Pain* 6(10):639, 2005.
Pieper B, et al: Bariatric surgery: patient incision care and discharge concerns, *Ostomy Wound Manage* 52(6):48, 2006.
Weber WP, et al: The timing of surgical antimicrobial prophylaxis, *Ann Surg* 247(6):918, 2008.
Willson M, et al: Nursing interventions to decrease the risk of catheter-associated urinary tract infection. Part 2: staff education, monitoring and care techniques, *J Wound Ostomy Cont Nurs* 36(2):137, 2009.

GLOSSARY

A

abduction Movement of a limb away from the body.

abrasion Scraping or rubbing away of epidermis; may result in localized bleeding and later weeping of serous fluid.

absorption Passage of drug molecules into the blood. Factors influencing drug absorption include route of administration, ability of the drug to dissolve, and conditions at the site of absorption.

acceptance Fifth stage of Kübler-Ross's stages of grief and dying. An individual comes to terms with a loss rather than submitting to resignation and hopelessness.

accessory muscles Muscles in the thoracic cage that assist with respiration.

accommodation Process of responding to the environment through new activity, thinking, and changing the existing schema or developing a new schema to deal with the new information. For example, a toddler whose parent consistently corrects him when he calls a horse a "doggie" accommodates and forms a new schema for horses.

accountability State of being answerable for one's actions—a nurse answers to himself or herself, the patient, the profession, the employing institution such as a hospital, and society for the effectiveness of nursing care performed.

accreditation Process whereby a professional association or nongovernmental agency grants recognition to a school or institution for demonstrated ability to meet predetermined criteria.

acculturation Process of adapting to and adopting a new culture.

acne Inflammatory, papulopustular skin eruption, usually occurring on the face, neck, shoulders, and upper back.

acromegaly Chronic metabolic condition caused by overproduction of growth hormone and characterized by gradual, marked enlargement and elongation of bones of the face, jaw, and extremities.

active listening Listening attentively with the whole person—mind, body, and spirit. It includes listening for main and supportive ideas; acknowledging and responding; giving appropriate feedback; and paying attention to the other person's total communication, including the content, intent, and feelings expressed.

active range-of-motion (ROM) exercise Exercise to the joint by the patient while doing activities of daily living or during joint assessment.

active strategies of health promotion Activities that depend on the patient's motivation to adopt a specific health program.

active transport Movement of materials across the cell membrane by means of chemical activity that allows the cell to admit larger molecules than would otherwise be possible.

activities of daily living (ADLs) Activities usually performed in the course of a normal day in the patient's life such as eating, dressing, bathing, brushing the teeth, or grooming.

activity tolerance Kind or amount of exercise or work that a person is able to perform.

actual loss Loss of an object, person, body part or function, or emotion that is overt and easily identifiable.

actual nursing diagnosis Judgment that is clinically validated by the presence of major defining characteristics.

acuity recording Mechanism by which entries describing patient care activities are made over a 24-hour period. The activities are then translated into a rating score, or acuity score, that allows for a comparison of patients who vary by severity of illness.

acute care Pattern of health care in which a patient is treated for an acute episode of illness, for the sequelae of an accident or other trauma, or during recovery from surgery.

acute illness Illness characterized by symptoms that are of relatively short duration, are usually severe, and affect the functioning of the patient in all dimensions.

adduction Movement of a limb toward the body.

adolescence Period in development between the onset of puberty and adulthood. It usually begins between 11 and 13 years of age.

adult day care centers Facility for the supervised care of older adults; provides activities such as meals and socialization during specified day hours.

advanced practice registered nurse (APRN) Generally the most independently functioning nurse. An APRN has a master's degree in nursing, advanced education in pathophysiology, pharmacology, and physical assessment; and certification and expertise in a specialized area of practice.

advanced sleep phase syndrome Common in older adults; a disturbance in sleep manifested by early waking in the morning with an inability to get back to sleep. It is thought that this syndrome is caused by advancing of the circadian rhythm of the body.

adventitious sounds Abnormal lung sounds heard with auscultation.

adverse effect Harmful or unintended effect of a medication, diagnostic test, or therapeutic intervention.

adverse reaction Any harmful, unintended effect of a medication, diagnostic test, or therapeutic intervention.

advocacy Process whereby a nurse objectively provides patients with the information they need to make decisions and supports the patients in whatever decisions they make.

afebrile Without fever.

affective learning Acquisition of behaviors involved in expressing feelings about attitudes, appreciation, and values.

afterload Resistance to left ventricular ejection; the work the heart must overcome to fully eject blood from the left ventricle.

age-related macular degeneration Progressive disorder in which the macula (the specialized portion of the retina responsible for central vision) degenerates as a result of aging and loses its ability to function efficiently. First signs include blurring of reading matter, distortion or loss of central vision, sensitivity to glare, and distortion of objects.

agnostic Individual who believes that any ultimate reality is unknown or unknowable.

airborne precautions Safeguards designed to reduce the risk of transmission of infectious agents through the air that a person breathes.

alarm reaction Mobilization of the defense mechanisms of the body and mind to cope with a stressor; the initial stage of the general adaptation syndrome.

aldosterone Mineralocorticoid steroid hormone produced by the adrenal cortex with action in the renal tubule to regulate sodium and potassium balance in the blood.

allergic reactions Unfavorable physiological response to an allergen to which a person has previously been exposed and has developed antibodies.

alopecia Partial or complete loss of hair; baldness.

Alzheimer's disease Disease of the brain parenchyma that causes a gradual and progressive decline in cognitive functioning.

AMBULARM Device used for the patient who climbs out of bed unassisted and is in danger of falling. This device is worn on the leg and signals when the leg is in a dependent position such as over the side rail or on the floor.

amino acid Organic compound of one or more basic groups and one or more carboxyl groups. Amino acids are the building blocks that construct proteins and the end products of protein digestion.

anabolism Constructive metabolism characterized by conversion of simple substances into more complex compounds of living matter.

analgesic Relieving pain; drug that relieves pain.

analogies Resemblances made between things otherwise unlike.

anaphylactic reactions Hypersensitive condition induced by contact with certain antigens.

aneurysm Localized dilations of the wall of a blood vessel; usually caused by atherosclerosis, hypertension, or a congenital weakness in a vessel wall.

anger Second stage of Kübler-Ross's stages of grief and dying. During this stage an individual resists loss by expressing extreme displeasure, indignation, or hostility.

angiotensin Polypeptide occurring in the blood, causing vasoconstriction, increased blood pressure, and the release of aldosterone from the adrenal cortex.

anion gap Difference between the concentrations of serum cations and anions; determined by measuring the concentrations of sodium cations and chloride and bicarbonate anions.

anions Negatively charged electrolytes.

anthropometric measurements Body measures of height, weight, and skinfolds to evaluate muscle atrophy.

anthropometry Measurement of various body parts to determine nutritional and caloric status, muscular development, brain growth, and other parameters.

antibodies Immunoglobulins essential to the immune system that are produced by lymphoid tissue in response to bacteria, viruses, or other antigens.

anticipatory grief Grief response in which the person begins the grieving process before an actual loss.

antidiuretic hormone (ADH) Hormone that decreases the production of urine by increasing the resorption of water by the renal tubules. ADH is secreted by cells of the hypothalamus and stored in the posterior lobe of the pituitary gland.

antiembolic stockings Elasticized stockings that prevent formation of emboli and thrombi, especially after surgery or during bed rest.

antigen Substance, usually a protein, that causes the formation of an antibody and reacts specifically with that antibody.

antipyretic Substance or procedure that reduces fever.

anxiolytics Drugs used primarily to treat episodes of anxiety.

aphasia Abnormal neurological condition in which language function is defective or absent; related to injury to speech center in cerebral cortex, causing receptive or expressive aphasia.

apical pulse Heartbeat as listened to with the bell or diaphragm of a stethoscope placed on the apex of the heart.

apnea Absence of respirations for a period of time.

apothecary system System of measurement. The basic unit of weight is a grain. Weights derived from the grain are the gram, ounce, and pound. The basic measure for fluid is the minim. The fluidram, fluid ounce, pint, quart, and gallon are measures derived from the minim.

approximate To come close together, as in the edges of a wound.

arcus senilis Opaque ring, gray to white in color, that surrounds the periphery of the cornea. The condition is caused by deposits of fat granules in the cornea. Occurs primarily in older adults.

asepsis Absence of germs or microorganisms.

aseptic technique Any health care procedure in which added precautions are used to prevent contamination of a person, object, or area by microorganisms.

assault Unlawful threat to bring about harmful or offensive contact with another.

assertive communication Type of communication based on a philosophy of protecting individual rights and responsibilities. It includes the ability to be self-directive in acting to accomplish goals and advocate for others.

assessment First step of the nursing process. Activities required in the first step are data collection, validation, sorting, and documentation. The purpose is to gather information for health problem identification.

assimilation To become absorbed into another culture and adopt its characteristics.

assisted living Residential living facilities in which each resident has his or her own room and shares dining and social activity areas.

associative play Form of play in which a group of children participates in similar or identical activities without formal organization, direction, interaction, or goals.

atelectasis Collapse of alveoli, preventing the normal respiratory exchange of oxygen and carbon dioxide.

atheist Individual who does not believe in the existence of God.

atherosclerosis Common arterial disorder characterized by yellowish plaques of cholesterol, lipids, and cellular debris in the inner layers of the walls of the large- and medium-size arteries.

atrioventricular (AV) node Part of the cardiac conduction system located on the floor of the right atrium; receives electrical impulses from the atrium and transmits them to the bundle of His.

atrophied Wasted or reduced size or physiological activity of a part of the body caused by disease or other influences.

attachment Initial psychosocial relationship that develops between parents and the neonate.

attentional set Internal state of the learner that allows focusing and comprehension.

auditory Related to or experienced through hearing.

auscultation Method of physical examination; listening to the sounds produced by the body, usually with a stethoscope.

auscultatory gap Disappearance of sound when obtaining a blood pressure; typically occurs between the first and second Korotkoff sounds.

authority Right to act in areas in which an individual has been given and accepts responsibility.

autologous transfusion Procedure in which blood is removed from a donor and stored for a variable period before it is returned to the donor's own circulation.

autonomy Ability or tendency to function independently.

B

back-channeling Active listening technique that prompts a respondent to continue telling a story or describing a situation. Involves use of phrases such as "Go on," "Uh huh," and "Tell me more."

bacteriuria Presence of bacteria in the urine.

balance Position in which the person's center of gravity is correctly positioned so falling does not occur.

bandages Available in rolls of various widths and materials, including gauze, elasticized knit, elastic webbing, flannel, and muslin. Gauze bandages are lightweight and inexpensive, mold easily around contours of the body, and permit air circulation to underlying skin to prevent maceration. Elastic bandages conform well to body parts but can also be used to exert pressure over a body part.

bargaining Third stage of Kübler-Ross's stages of grief and dying. A person postpones the reality of a loss by attempting to make deals in a subtle or overt manner with others or with a higher being.

baridi Condition among the Bena people of Tanzania attributed to disrespectful behavior within the family or transgression of cultural taboos. The person experiences physical and psychological symptoms and is usually treated by a traditional healer, who has the person make a public admission or an apology or who treats the person with herbal remedies.

basal cell carcinoma Malignant epithelial cell tumor that begins as a papule and enlarges peripherally, developing a central crater that erodes, crusts, and bleeds. Metastasis is rare.

basal metabolic rate (BMR) Amount of energy used in a unit of time by a fasting, resting subject to maintain vital functions.

battery Legal term for touching another's body without consent.

bed boards Boards placed under the mattress of a bed that provide extra support to the mattress surface.

bed rest Placement of the patient in bed for therapeutic reasons for a prescribed period.

benchmarking Identifying best practices and comparing them to current organizational practices to improve performance. This process helps to support the claims of quality care delivery by the institution.

beneficence Doing good or actively promoting doing good; one of the four principles of the ethical theory of deontology.

benign breast disease (fibrocystic) Benign condition characterized by lumpy, painful breasts and sometimes nipple discharge. Symptoms are more apparent before the menstrual period. Known to be a risk factor for breast cancer.

bereavement Response to loss through death; a subjective experience that a person suffers after losing a person with whom there has been a significant relationship.

biases and prejudices Beliefs and attitudes associating negative permanent characteristics to people who are perceived as different from oneself.

bi-level positive airway pressure (BiPAP) Ventilatory support used to treat patients with obstructive sleep apnea, patients with congestive heart failure, and preterm infants with underdeveloped lungs.

bilineally Kinship that extends to both the mother's and father's sides of the family.

binders Bandages made of large pieces of material to fit specific body parts.

bioethics Branch of ethics within the field of health care.

biological clock Cyclical nature of body function. Functions controlled from within the body are synchronized with environmental factors; same meaning as biorhythm.

biological half-life Time it takes for the body to lower the amount of unchanged medication by half.

biotransformation Chemical changes that a substance undergoes in the body such as by the action of enzymes.

blanchable hyperemia Redness of the skin caused by dilation of the superficial capillaries. When pressure is applied to the skin, the area blanches, or turns a lighter color.

body image Peoples' subjective concept of their physical appearance.

body mechanics Coordinated efforts of the musculoskeletal and nervous systems to maintain proper balance, posture, and body alignment.

bone resorption Destruction of bone cells and release of calcium into the blood.

borborygmi Audible abdominal sounds produced by hyperactive intestinal peristalsis.

botanica Place that sells religious and herbal remedies.

bradycardia Slower-than-normal heart rate; heart contracts fewer than 60 times/min.

bradypnea Abnormally slow rate of breathing.

bronchospasm Excessive and prolonged contraction of the smooth muscle of the bronchi and bronchioles, resulting in an acute narrowing and obstruction of the respiratory airway.

bruit Abnormal sound or murmur heard while auscultating an organ, gland, or artery.

buccal Of or pertaining to the inside of the cheek or the gum next to the cheek.

buccal cavity Consists of the lips surrounding the opening of the mouth, the cheeks running along the side walls of the cavity, the tongue and its muscles, and the hard and soft palate.

buffer Substance or group of substances that can absorb or release hydrogen ions to correct an acid-base imbalance.

bundle of His Part of the cardiac conduction system that arises from the distal portion of the atrioventricular (AV) node and extends across the AV groove to the top of the intraventricular septum, where it divides into right and left bundle branches.

C

cachexia Malnutrition marked by weakness and emaciation, usually associated with severe illness.

capitation Payment mechanism in which a provider (e.g., health care network) receives a fixed amount of payment per enrollee.

carbohydrates Dietary classification of foods comprising sugars, starches, cellulose, and gum.

carbon monoxide Colorless, odorless, poisonous gas produced by the combustion of carbon or organic fuels.

cardiac index Adequacy of the cardiac output for an individual. It takes into account the body surface area (BSA) of the patient.

cardiac output (CO) Volume of blood expelled by the ventricles of the heart, equal to the amount of blood ejected at each beat multiplied by the number of beats in the period of time used for computation (usually 1 minute).

cardiopulmonary rehabilitation Actively assisting the patient with achieving and maintaining an optimal level of health through controlled physical exercise, nutrition counseling, relaxation and stress management techniques, prescribed medications and oxygen, and compliance.

cardiopulmonary resuscitation (CPR) Basic emergency procedures for life support consisting of artificial respiration and manual external cardiac massage.

care To feel concern for or interest in one who has sorrow or difficulties.

caring Universal phenomenon that influences the way we think, feel, and behave in relation to one another.

carriers People or animals who harbor and spread an organism that causes disease in others but do not become ill themselves.

case management Organized system for delivering health care to an individual patient or group of patients across an episode of illness and/or a continuum of care; includes assessment and development of a plan of care, coordination of all services, referral, and follow-up; usually assigned to one professional.

case management plan Multidisciplinary model for documenting patient care that usually includes plans for problems, key interventions, and expected outcomes for patients with a specific disease or condition.

catabolism Breakdown of body tissue into simpler substances.

cataplexy Condition characterized by sudden muscular weakness and loss of muscle tone.

cataracts Abnormal progressive condition of the lens of the eye characterized by loss of transparency.

cathartics Drugs that act to promote bowel evacuation.

catheterization Introduction of a catheter into a body cavity or organ to inject or remove fluid.

cations Positively charged electrolytes.

center of gravity Midpoint or center of the weight of a body or object.

centigrade Denotes temperature scale in which 0° is the freezing point of water and 100° is the boiling point of water at sea level; also called Celsius.

cerumen Yellowish or brownish waxy secretion produced by sweat glands in the external ear.

chancres Skin lesions or venereal sores (usually primary syphilis) that begin at the site of infection as papules and develop into red, bloodless, painless ulcers with a scooped-out appearance.

change-of-shift report Report that occurs between two scheduled nursing work shifts. Nurses communicate information about their assigned patients to nurses working on the next shift of duty.

channel Method used in the teaching-learning process to present content: visual, auditory, taste, smell. In the communication process a method used to transmit a message: visual, auditory, touch.

charting by exception (CBE) Charting methodology in which data are entered only when there is an exception from that which is normal or expected; reduces time spent documenting in charting. It is a shorthand method for documenting normal findings and routine care.

chest percussion Striking the chest wall with a cupped hand to promote mobilization and drainage of pulmonary secretions.

chest physiotherapy (CPT) Group of therapies used to mobilize pulmonary secretions for expectoration.

chest tube Catheter inserted through the thorax into the chest cavity for removing air or fluid; used after chest or heart surgery or pneumothorax.

Cheyne-Stokes respiration Occurs when there is decreased blood flow or injury to the brainstem.

chronic illness Illness that persists over a long time and affects physical, emotional, intellectual, social, and spiritual functioning.

circadian rhythm Repetition of certain physiological phenomena within a 24-hour cycle.

circulating nurse Assistant to the scrub nurse and surgeon whose role is to provide necessary supplies; dispose of soiled instruments and supplies; and keep an accurate count of instruments, needles, and sponges used.

civil law Statutes concerned with protecting a person's rights.

climacteric Physiological, developmental change that occurs in the male reproductive system between the ages of 45 and 60.

clinical criteria Objective or subjective signs and symptoms, clusters of signs and symptoms, or risk factors.

clinical decision making Problem-solving approach that nurses use to define patient problems and select appropriate treatment.

clinical-decision support systems Computerized programs used within the health care setting to support decision-making.

closed-ended question Form of question that limits a respondent's answer to one or two words.

clubbing Bulging of the tissues at the nail base caused by insufficient oxygenation at the periphery, resulting from conditions such as chronic emphysema and congenital heart disease.

code of ethics Formal statement that delineates a profession's guidelines for ethical behavior. A code of ethics sets standards or expectations for the professional to achieve.

cognitive learning Acquisition of intellectual skills that encompass behaviors such as thinking, understanding, and evaluating.

collaborative interventions Therapies that require the knowledge, skill, and expertise of multiple health care professionals.

collaborative problem Physiological complication that requires the nurse to use nursing- and health care provider–prescribed interventions to maximize patient outcomes.

colloid osmotic pressure Abnormal condition of the kidney caused by the pressure of concentrations of large particles such as protein molecules that will pass through a membrane.

colon Portion of the large intestine from the cecum to the rectum.
colonization Presence and multiplication of microorganisms without tissue invasion or damage.
comforting Acts toward another individual that display both an emotional and physical calm. The use of touch, establishing presence, the therapeutic use of silence, and the skillful and gentle performance of a procedure are examples of comforting nursing measures.
common law One source for law that is created by judicial decisions as opposed to those created by legislative bodies (statutory law).
communicable disease Any disease that can be transmitted from one person or animal to another by direct or indirect contact or by vectors.
communication Ongoing, dynamic series of events that involves the transmission of meaning from sender to receiver.
community health nursing Nursing approach that combines knowledge from the public health sciences with professional nursing theories to safeguard and improve the health of populations in the community.
community-based nursing Acute and chronic care of individuals and families to strengthen their capacity for self-care and promote independence in decision making.
competence Specific range of skills necessary to perform a task.
complete bed bath Bath in which the entire body of a patient is washed in bed.
compress Soft pad of gauze or cloth used to apply heat, cold, or medications to the surface of a body part.
computer-based patient record Comprehensive computerized system used by all health care practitioners to permanently store information pertaining to a patient's health status, clinical problems, and functional abilities.
concentration Relative content of a component within a substance or solution.
concentration gradient Gradient that exists across a membrane, separating a high concentration of a particular ion from a low concentration of the same ion.
concept map Care-planning tool that assists in critical thinking and forming associations between a patient's nursing diagnoses and interventions.
confianza Trust.
confidentiality Act of keeping information private or secret; in health care the nurse only shares information about a patient with other nurses or health care providers who need to know private information about a patient to provide care for him or her; information can only be shared with the patient's consent.
conjunctivitis Highly contagious eye infection. The crusty drainage that collects on eyelid margins can easily spread from one eye to the other.
connectedness Having close spiritual relationships with oneself, others, and God or another spiritual being.
connotative meaning Shade or interpretation of the meaning of a word influenced by the thoughts, feelings, or ideas that people have about the word.
conscious sedation Administration of central nervous system–depressant drugs and/or analgesics to provide analgesia, relieve anxiety, and/or provide amnesia during surgical, diagnostic, or interventional procedures.
constipation Condition characterized by difficulty in passing stool or an infrequent passage of hard stool.
consultation Process in which the help of a specialist is sought to identify ways to handle problems in patient management or in planning and implementing programs.
contact precautions Safeguards designed to reduce the risk of transmission of epidemiologically important microorganisms by direct or indirect contact.
continent urinary diversion (CUR) Surgical diversion of the drainage of urine from a diseased or dysfunctional bladder. Patient uses a catheter to drain the pouch.
continuous positive airway pressure (CPAP) Ventilatory support used to treat patients with obstructive sleep apnea, patients with congestive heart failure, and preterm infants with under developed lungs.
convalescence Period of recovery after an illness, injury, or surgery.
coping Making an effort to manage psychological stress.
core temperature Temperature of deep structures of the body.
cough Sudden, audible expulsion of air from the lungs. The person breathes in, the glottis is partially closed, and the accessory muscles of expiration contract to expel the air forcibly.
counseling Problem-solving method used to help patients recognize and manage stress and enhance interpersonal relationships. It helps patients examine alternatives and decide which choices are most helpful and appropriate.
crackles Fine bubbling sounds heard on auscultation of the lung; produced by air entering distal airways and alveoli, which contain serous secretions.
crime Act that violates a law and that may include criminal intent.
criminal law Concerned with acts that threaten society but may involve only an individual.
crisis Transition for better or worse in the course of a disease, usually indicated by a marked change in the intensity of signs and symptoms.
crisis intervention Use of therapeutic techniques directed toward helping a patient resolve a particular and immediate problem.
critical pathways Tools used in managed care that incorporate the treatment interventions of caregivers from all disciplines who normally care for a patient. Designed for a specific care type, a pathway is used to manage the care of a patient throughout a projected length of stay.
critical period of development Specific phase or period when the presence of a function or reasoning has its greatest effect on a specific aspect of development.
critical thinking Active, purposeful, organized, cognitive process used to carefully examine one's thinking and the thinking of other individuals.
crutch gait Gait achieved by a person using crutches.
cue Information that a nurse acquires through hearing, visual observations, touch, and smell.
cultural and linguistic competence Set of congruent behaviors, attitudes, and policies that come together in a system or agency or among professionals that enables effective work in cross-cultural situations.
cultural assessment Systematic and comprehensive examination of the cultural care values, beliefs, and practices of individuals, families, and communities.
cultural awareness Gaining in-depth awareness of one's own background, stereotypes, biases, prejudices, and assumptions about other people.
cultural care accommodation or negotiation Adapting or negotiating with the patient/families to achieve beneficial or satisfying health outcomes.
cultural care preservation or maintenance Retaining and/or preserving relevant care values so patients are able to maintain their well-being, recover from illness, or face handicaps and/or death.
cultural care repatterning or restructuring Reordering, changing, or greatly modifying a patient's/family's customs for a new, different, and beneficial health care pattern.
cultural competence Process in which the health care professional continually strives to achieve the ability and availability to work effectively with individuals, families, and communities.
cultural encounters Engaging in cross-cultural interactions; refining intercultural communication skills; gaining in-depth understanding of others and avoiding stereotypes; and managing cultural conflict.
cultural imposition Using one's own values and customs as an absolute guide in interpreting behaviors.
cultural knowledge Obtaining knowledge of other cultures; gaining sensitivity to, respect for, and appreciation of differences.
cultural pain Feeling that a patient has after a health care worker disregards the patient's valued way of life.
cultural skills Communication, cultural assessment, and culturally competent care.
culturally congruent care Care that fits people's valued life patterns and sets of meanings generated from the people themselves. Sometimes this differs from the professionals' perspective on care.
culturally ignorant or blind Uneducated about other cultures.
culture Integrated patterns of human behavior that include the language, thoughts, communications, actions, customs, beliefs, values, and institutions of racial, ethnic, religious, or social groups.

culture care theory Leininger's theory that emphasizes culturally congruent care.

culture-bound syndromes Illnesses restricted to a particular culture or group because of its psychosocial characteristics.

culturological nursing assessment Systematic and comprehensive examination of the cultural care values, beliefs, and practices of individuals, families, and communities.

cutaneous stimulation Stimulation of a person's skin to prevent or reduce pain perception. A massage, warm bath, hot and cold therapies, and transcutaneous electrical nerve stimulation are some ways to reduce pain perception.

cyanosis Bluish discoloration of the skin and mucous membranes caused by an excess of deoxygenated hemoglobin in the blood or a structural defect in the hemoglobin molecule.

D

DAR (data, action, patient response) Format used in focus charting for recording patient information.

data analysis Logical examination of and professional judgment about patient assessment data; used in the diagnostic process to derive a nursing diagnosis.

data cluster Set of signs or symptoms that are grouped together in logical order.

database Store or bank of information, especially in a form that can be processed by computer.

debridement Removal of dead tissue from a wound.

decentralized management Organizational philosophy that brings decisions down to the level of the staff. Individuals best informed about a problem or issue participate in the decision-making process.

decision making Process involving critical appraisal of information that results from recognizing a problem and ends with generating, testing, and evaluating a conclusion. Comes at the end of critical thinking.

defecation Passage of feces from the digestive tract through the rectum.

defendant Individual or organization against whom legal charges are brought in a court of law.

defining characteristics Related signs and symptoms or clusters of data that support the nursing diagnosis.

dehiscence Separation of the edges of a wound, revealing underlying tissues.

dehydration Excessive loss of water from the body tissues accompanied by a disturbance of body electrolytes.

delegation Process of assigning another member of the health care team to be responsible for aspects of patient care (e.g., assigning nurse assistants to bathe a patient).

delirium Acute state of confusion that is potentially reversible and often has a physical cause.

dementia Generalized impairment of intellectual functioning that interferes with social and occupational functioning.

denial Unconscious refusal to admit an unacceptable idea.

denotative meaning Meaning of a word shared by individuals who use a common language. The word *baseball* has the same meaning for all individuals who speak English, but the word *code* primarily denotes cardiac arrest to health care providers.

dental caries Abnormal destructive condition in a tooth caused by a complex interaction of food, especially starches and sugars, with bacteria that form dental plaque.

deontology Traditional theory of ethics that proposes to define actions as right or wrong based on the characteristics of fidelity to promises, truthfulness, and justice. The conventional use of ethical terms such as *justice, autonomy, beneficence,* and *nonmaleficence* constitutes the practice of deontology.

depression (1) Reduction in happiness and well-being that contributes to physical and social limitations and complicates the treatment of concomitant medical conditions. It is usually reversible with treatment. (2) Fourth stage of Kübler-Ross's stages of grief and dying. In this stage the person realizes the full impact and significance of the loss.

dermis Sensitive vascular layer of the skin directly below the epidermis; composed of collagenous and elastic fibrous connective tissues that give the dermis strength and elasticity.

determinants of health Many variables that influence the health status of individuals or communities.

detoxify To remove the toxic quality of a substance. The liver acts to detoxify chemicals in drug compounds.

development Qualitative or observable aspects of the progressive changes that one makes in adapting to the environment.

developmental crises Crises associated with normal and expected phases of growth and development (e.g., the response to menopause); same as maturational crises.

diabetic retinopathy Disorder of retinal blood vessels. Pathological changes secondary to increased pressure in the blood vessels of the retina result in decreased vision or vision loss caused by hemorrhage and macular edema.

diagnosis-related group (DRG) Group of patients classified to establish a mechanism for health care reimbursement based on length of stay. Classification is based on the following variables: primary and secondary diagnosis, co-morbidities, primary and secondary procedures, and age.

diagnostic process Mental steps (data clustering and analysis, problem identification) that follow assessment and lead directly to the formulation of a diagnosis.

diagnostic reasoning Process that enables an observer to assign meaning to and classify phenomena in clinical situations by integrating observations and critical thinking.

diaphoresis Secretion of sweat, especially profuse secretion associated with an elevated body temperature, physical exertion, or emotional stress.

diaphragmatic breathing Respiration in which the abdomen moves out while the diaphragm descends on inspiration.

diarrhea Increase in the number of stools and the passage of liquid, unformed feces.

diastolic Pertaining to diastole, or the blood pressure at the instant of maximum cardiac relaxation.

dietary reference intake (DRI) Information on each vitamin or mineral to reflect a range of minimum-to-maximum amounts that avert deficiency or toxicity.

diffusion Movement of molecules from an area of high concentration to one of lower concentration.

digestion Breakdown of nutrients by chewing, churning, mixing with fluid, and chemical reactions.

direct care interventions Treatments performed through interaction with the patient. For example, a patient may require medication administration, insertion of an intravenous infusion, or counseling during a time of grief.

discharge planning Activities directed toward identifying future proposed therapy and the need for additional resources before and after returning home.

discrimination Prejudicial outlook, action, or treatment.

disease Malfunctioning or maladaptation of biological or psychological processes.

disinfection Process of destroying all pathogenic organisms except spores.

disorganization and despair One of Bowlby's four phases of mourning in which an individual endlessly examines how and why the loss occurred.

distress Damaging stress; one of the two types of stress identified by Selye.

disuse osteoporosis Reductions in skeletal mass routinely accompanying immobility or paralysis.

diuresis Increased rate of formation and excretion of urine.

documentation Written entry into the patient's medical record of all pertinent information about him or her. These entries validate the patient's problems and care and exist as a legal record.

dominant culture Customs, values, beliefs, traditions, and social and religious views held by a group of people that prevail over another secondary culture.

dorsiflexion Flexion toward the back.

drainage evacuators Convenient portable units that connect to tubular drains lying within a wound bed and exert a safe, constant, low-pressure vacuum to remove and collect drainage.

droplet precautions Safeguards designed to reduce the risk of droplet transmission of infectious agents.

dysmenorrhea Painful menstruation.

dysphagia Difficulty swallowing; commonly associated with obstructive or motor disorders of the esophagus.

dyspnea Sensation of shortness of breath.

dysrhythmia Deviation from the normal pattern of the heartbeat.

dysuria Painful urination resulting from bacterial infection of the bladder and obstructive conditions of the urethra.

E

ecchymosis Discoloration of the skin or bruise caused by leakage of blood into subcutaneous tissues as a result of trauma to underlying tissues.

ectropion Eversion of the eyelid that exposes the conjunctival membrane and part of the eyeball.

edema Abnormal accumulation of fluid in interstitial spaces of tissues.

egocentric Developmental characteristic wherein a toddler is only able to assume the view of his or her own activities and needs.

electrocardiogram (ECG) Graphic record of the electrical activity of the myocardium.

electrolyte Element or compound that, when melted or dissolved in water or other solvent, dissociates into ions and can carry an electrical current.

electronic health record An electronic record of patient health information generated whenever a patient accesses medical care in any health care delivery setting.

electronic infusion device Piece of medical equipment that delivers intravenous fluids at a prescribed rate through an intravenous catheter.

electronic medical record Part of the electronic health record that contains patient data gathered in a health care setting at a specific time and place.

embolism Abnormal condition in which a blood clot (embolus) travels through the bloodstream and becomes lodged in a blood vessel.

emic worldview Insider or native perspective.

empathy Understanding and acceptance of a person's feelings and the ability to sense the person's private world.

empowered Gave legal authority to or enabled an individual or group; promoted self-actualization of an individual or group.

endogenous infections Infections produced within a cell or organism.

endorphins Hormones that act on the mind such as morphine and opiates and produce a sense of well-being and reducing pain.

endotracheal tube Short-term artificial airways to administer mechanical ventilation, relieve upper airway obstruction, protect against aspiration, or clear secretions.

enema Procedure involving introduction of a solution into the rectum for cleansing or therapeutic purposes.

enteral nutrition (EN) Provision of nutrients through the gastrointestinal tract when the patient cannot ingest, chew, or swallow food but can digest and absorb nutrients.

entropion Condition in which the eyelid turns inward toward the eye.

environment All of the many factors (e.g., physical and psychological) that influence or affect the life and survival of a person.

epidermis Outer layer of the skin that has several thin layers in different stages of maturation; shields and protects the underlying tissues from water loss, mechanical or chemical injury, and penetration by disease-causing microorganisms.

epidural infusion Type of nerve block anesthesia in which an anesthetic is intermittently or continuously injected into the lumbosacral region of the spinal cord.

erythema Redness or inflammation of the skin or mucous membranes that is a result of dilation and congestion of superficial capillaries; sunburn is an example.

eschar Thick layer of dead, dry tissue that covers a pressure ulcer or thermal burn. It may be allowed to be sloughed off naturally, or it may need to be surgically removed.

ethical dilemma Dilemma existing when the right thing to do is not clear. Resolution requires the negotiation of differing values among those involved in the dilemma.

ethical principles Set of guidelines for the expectations a profession and the standards of behavior for its members.

ethics Principles or standards that govern proper conduct.

ethics of care Delivery of health care based on ethical principles and standards of care.

ethnicity Shared identity related to social and cultural heritage such as values, language, geographical space, and racial characteristics.

ethnocentrism Tendency to hold one's own way of life as superior to that of others.

ethnohistory Significant historical experiences of a particular group.

etic worldview Outsider's perspective.

etiology Study of all factors that may be involved in the development of a disease.

eupnea Normal respirations that are quiet, effortless, and rhythmical.

eustress Stress that protects health; one of the two types of stress identified by Selye.

evaluation Determination of the extent to which established patient goals have been achieved.

evidence-based knowledge Knowledge that is derived from the integration of best research, clinical expertise, and patient values.

evidence-based practice Use of current best evidence from nursing research, clinical expertise, practice trends, and patient preferences to guide nursing decisions about care provided to patients.

evisceration Protrusion of visceral organs through a surgical wound.

exacerbations Increases in the gravity of a disease or disorder as marked by greater intensity in signs or symptoms.

excessive daytime sleepiness Extreme fatigue felt during the day. Signs of this include falling asleep at inappropriate times such as while eating, talking, or driving. May indicate a sleep disorder.

excoriation Injury to the surface of the skin caused by abrasion.

exhaustion stage Phase that occurs when the body can no longer resist the stress (i.e., when the energy necessary to maintain adaptation is depleted).

exogenous infection Infection originating outside an organ or part.

exostosis Abnormal benign growth on the surface of a bone.

expected outcomes Expected conditions of a patient at the end of therapy or a disease process, including the degree of wellness and the need for continuing care, medications, support, counseling, or education.

extended care facility Institution devoted to providing medical, nursing, or custodial care for an individual over a prolonged period such as during the course of a chronic disease or the rehabilitation phase after an acute illness.

extension Movement by certain joints that increases the angle between two adjoining bones.

extracellular fluid (ECF) Portion of body fluids composed of the interstitial fluid and blood plasma.

exudate Fluid, cells, or other substances that have been discharged from cells or blood vessels slowly through small pores or breaks in cell membranes.

F

face-saving Way of speaking or acting that preserves dignity.

Fahrenheit Denotes temperature scale in which 32° is the freezing point of water and 212° is the boiling point of water at sea level.

faith Set of beliefs and a way of relating to self, others, and a Supreme Being.

fajita Cotton binder used on a newborn's abdomen among Hispanics and Filipinos to prevent gas and umbilical hernia.

family Group of interacting individuals composing a basic unit of society.

family as context Nursing perspective in which the family is viewed as a unit of interacting members having attributes, functions, and goals separate from those of the individual family members.

family caregiving A family process that occurs in response to an illness and encompasses multiple cognitive, behavioral, and interpersonal processes.

family diversity Unique needs and characteristics of each member in a family.

family durability System of support for a family that includes immediate and extended family members.

family forms Patterns of people considered by family members to be included in the family.

family functioning Processes families use to achieve their goals.

family hardiness Internal strengths and durability of the family unit; characterized by a sense of control over the outcome of life events and hardships, a view of change as beneficial and growth-producing, and an active rather than passive orientation in responding to stressful life events.

family health Determined by the effectiveness of the family's structure, the processes that the family uses to meet its goals, and internal and external forces.

family as patient Nursing approach that takes into consideration the effect of one intervention on all members of a family.

family resiliency Family's ability to cope with expected and unexpected stressors.

family structure Based on organization (i.e., ongoing membership) of the family and the pattern of relationships.

farmacia Place to obtain prescribed medications.

febrile Pertaining to or characterized by an elevated body temperature.

fecal impaction Accumulation of hardened fecal material in the rectum or sigmoid colon.

fecal incontinence Inability to control passage of feces and gas from the anus.

fecal occult blood test (FOBT) Measures microscopic amounts of blood in the feces.

feces Waste or excrement from the gastrointestinal tract.

feedback Process in which the output of a given system is returned to the system.

felony Crime of a serious nature that carries a penalty of imprisonment or death.

feminist ethics Ethical approach that focuses on relationships of those involved in an ethical dilemma rather than traditional abstract principles of deontology.

fever Elevation in the hypothalamic set point so body temperature is regulated at a higher level.

fictive Nonblood kin; considered family in some collective cultures.

fidelity Agreement to keep a promise.

fight-or-flight response Total physiological response to stress that occurs during the alarm reaction stage of the general adaptation syndrome. Massive changes in all body systems prepare a human being to choose to flee or remain and fight the stressor.

filtration Straining of fluid through a membrane.

fistula Abnormal passage from an internal organ to the surface of the body or between two internal organs.

flashback Recollection so strong that the individual thinks that he or she is actually experiencing the trauma again or seeing it unfold before his or her eyes.

flatus Intestinal gas.

flora Microorganisms that live on or within a body to compete with disease-producing microorganisms and provide a natural immunity against certain infections.

flow sheets Documents on which frequent observations or specific measurements are recorded.

Fluid volume deficit (FVD) Fluid and electrolyte disorder caused by failure of bodily homeostatic mechanisms to regulate the retention and excretion of body fluids. The condition is characterized by decreased output of urine, high specific gravity of urine, output of urine that is greater than the intake of fluid in the body, hemoconcentration, and increased serum levels of sodium.

fluid volume excess (FVE) Fluid and electrolyte disorder characterized by an increase in fluid retention and edema, resulting from failure of bodily homeostatic mechanisms to regulate the retention and excretion of body fluids.

focus charting Charting methodology for structuring progress notes according to the focus of the note (e.g., symptoms and nursing diagnosis). Each note includes data, actions, and patient response.

focused cultural assessment Method of evaluating a patient's ethnohistory, biocultural history, social organization, and religious and spiritual beliefs to find issues that are most relevant to the problem at hand.

food poisoning Toxic processes resulting from the ingestion of a food contaminated by toxic substances or bacteria-containing toxins.

food security All members of a household have access to sufficient, safe, nutritious food to maintain a healthy lifestyle.

foot boots Soft, foot-shaped devices designed to reduce the risk of footdrop by maintaining the foot in dorsiflexion.

footdrop Abnormal neuromuscular condition of the lower leg and foot characterized by an inability to dorsiflex, or evert, the foot.

friction Effects of rubbing or the resistance that a moving body meets from the surface on which it moves; a force that occurs in a direction to oppose movement.

functional health illiteracy Inability of an individual to obtain, interpret, and understand basic information about health.

functional health patterns Method for organizing assessment data based on the level of patient function in specific areas (e.g., mobility).

functional nursing Method of patient care delivery in which each staff member is assigned a task that is completed for all patients on the unit.

future orientation Time dimension emphasized by dominant American culture. It is characterized by direct communication and is focused on task achievement, whereas past orientation communication is circular and indirect and is focused on group harmony.

G

gait Manner or style of walking, including rhythm, cadence, and speed.

gastrostomy feeding tube Insertion of a feeding tube through a stoma into the stomach to provide enteral nutrition.

general adaptation syndrome (GAS) Generalized defense response of the body to stress; consists of three stages: alarm, resistance, and exhaustion.

general anesthesia Intravenous or inhaled medications that cause the patient to lose all sensation and consciousness.

genomics Describes the study of all the genes in a person and interactions of those genes with one another and with that person's environment.

geriatrics Branch of health care dealing with the physiology and psychology of aging and the diagnosis and treatment of diseases affecting older adults.

gerontology Study of all aspects of the aging process and its consequences.

gingivae Gums of the mouth; mucous membrane with supporting fibrous tissue that overlies the crowns of unerupted teeth and encircles the necks of teeth that have erupted.

glaucoma Abnormal condition of elevated pressure within an eye caused by obstruction of the outflow of aqueous humor. If untreated, it often results in peripheral visual loss, decreased visual acuity with difficulty adapting to darkness, and a halo effect around lights.

globalization Worldwide scope or application.

glomerulus Cluster or collection of capillary vessels within the kidney involved in the initial formation of urine.

gluconeogenesis Formation of glucose or glycogen from substances that are not carbohydrates such as protein or lipid.

glucose Primary fuel for the body; needed to carry out major physiological functions.

glycogen Polysaccharide that is the major carbohydrate stored in animal cells.

glycogenesis Process for storing glucose in the form of glycogen in the liver.

goals Desired results of nursing actions set realistically by the nurse and patient as part of the planning stage of the nursing process.

Good Samaritan laws Legislation enacted in some states to protect health care professionals from liability in rendering emergency aid unless there is proven willful wrong or gross negligence.

graduated measuring container Receptacle for volume measurement.

granny midwives Amateur health practitioners that assist in labor and delivery.

granulation tissue Soft, pink, fleshy projections of tissue that form during the healing process in a wound not healing by primary intention.

graphic record Charting mechanism that allows for the recording of vital signs and weight in such a manner that caregivers can quickly note changes in the patient's status.

grief Form of sorrow involving the person's thoughts, feelings, and behaviors that occurs as a response to an actual or perceived loss.

grieving process Sequence of affective, cognitive, and physiological states through which the person responds to and finally accepts an irretrievable loss.

grounded Connection between the electric circuit and the ground, which becomes part of the circuit.

growth Measurable or quantitative aspect of an individual's increase in physical dimensions as a result of an increase in number of cells. Indicators of growth include changes in height, weight, and sexual characteristics.

guided imagery Method of pain control in which the patient creates a mental image,

concentrates on that image, and gradually becomes less aware of pain.
gustatory Pertaining to the sense of taste.

H

halal Foods permissible for Muslims to eat.
hand rolls Rolls of cloth that keep the thumb slightly adducted and in opposition to the fingers.
hand-wrist splints Splints individually molded for the patient to maintain proper alignment of the thumb, slight adduction of the wrist, and slight dorsiflexion.
haram Foods prohibited by Muslim religious standards.
health Dynamic state in which individuals adapt to their internal and external environments so there is a state of physical, emotional, intellectual, social, and spiritual well-being.
health belief model Conceptual framework that describes a person's health behavior as an expression of his or her health beliefs.
health beliefs Patient's personal beliefs about levels of wellness that can motivate or impede participation in changing risk factors, participating in care, and selecting care options.
health care–acquired infection Infection that was not present or incubating at the time of admission to a health care setting.
health care problems Any conditions or dysfunctions that the patient experiences as a result of illness or treatment of an illness.
health informatics Application of computer and information science in all basic and applied biomedical sciences to facilitate the acquisition, processing, interpretation, optimal use, and communication of health-related data.
health literacy Patients' reading and mathematics skills, comprehension, ability to make health-related decisions, and successful functioning as a consumer of health care.
health promotion Activities such as routine exercise and good nutrition that help patients maintain or enhance their present level of health and reduce their risk of developing certain diseases.
health promotion model Defines health as a positive, dynamic state, not merely the absence of disease. The health promotion model emphasizes well-being, personal fulfillment, and self-actualization rather than reaction to the threat of illness.
health status Description of health of an individual or community.
heat exhaustion Abnormal condition caused by depletion of body fluid and electrolytes resulting from exposure to intense heat or the inability to acclimatize to heat.
heat stroke Continued exposure to extreme heat that raises the core body temperature to 40.5° C (105° F) or higher.
hematemesis Vomiting of blood, indicating upper gastrointestinal bleeding.
hematoma Collection of blood trapped in the tissues of the skin or an organ.
hematuria Abnormal presence of blood in the urine.
hemolysis Breakdown of red blood cells and release of hemoglobin that may occur after administration of hypotonic intravenous solutions, causing swelling and rupture of erythrocytes.
hemoptysis Coughing up blood from the respiratory tract.
hemorrhoids Permanent dilation and engorgement of veins within the lining of the rectum.
hemostasis Termination of bleeding by mechanical or chemical means or the coagulation process of the body.
hemothorax Accumulation of blood and fluid in the pleural cavity between the parietal and visceral pleurae.
hernia Protrusion of an organ through an abnormal opening in the muscle wall of the cavity that surrounds it.
hilots Amateur health practitioners that assist in labor and delivery among Filipinos.
holistic Of or pertaining to the whole; considering all factors.
holistic health Comprehensive view of the person as a biopsychosocial and spiritual being.
home care Health service provided in the patient's place of residence to promote, maintain, or restore health or minimize the effects of illness and disability.
homeostasis State of relative constancy in the internal environment of the body; maintained naturally by physiological adaptive mechanisms.
hope Confident but uncertain expectation of achieving a future goal.
hospice System of family-centered care designed to help terminally ill people be comfortable and maintain a satisfactory lifestyle throughout the terminal phase of their illness.
Hoyer lift Mechanical device that uses a canvas sling to easily lift dependent patients for transfer.
humidification Process of adding water to gas.
humor Coping strategy based on an individual's cognitive appraisal of a stimulus that results in behavior such as smiling, laughing, or feelings of amusement that lessen emotional distress.
hydrocephalus Abnormal accumulation of cerebrospinal fluid in the ventricles of the brain.
hydrostatic pressure Pressure caused by a liquid.
hyperactive/overactive bladder Common bladder complaint that occurs more frequently with aging and includes the symptoms of urgency, frequency, nocturia, and urge incontinence.
hypercalcemia Greater-than-normal amount of calcium in the blood.
hypercapnia Greater-than-normal amounts of carbon dioxide in the blood; also called hypercarbia.
hyperextension Position of maximal extension of a joint.
hyperglycemia Elevated serum glucose levels.
hypertension Disorder characterized by an elevated blood pressure persistently exceeding 120/80 mm Hg.
hyperthermia Situation in which body temperature exceeds the set point.
hypertonic Situation in which one solution has a greater concentration of solute than another; therefore the first solution exerts greater osmotic pressure.
hypertonicity Excessive tension of the arterial walls or muscles.
hyperventilation Respiratory rate in excess of that required to maintain normal carbon dioxide levels in the body tissues.
hypnotics Class of drug that causes insensibility to pain and induces sleep.
hypostatic pneumonia Pneumonia that results from fluid accumulation as a result of inactivity.
hypotension Abnormal lowering of blood pressure that is inadequate for normal perfusion and oxygenation of tissues.
hypothermia Abnormal lowering of body temperature below 35° C, or 95° F, usually caused by prolonged exposure to cold.
hypotonic Situation in which one solution has a smaller concentration of solute than another; therefore the first solution exerts less osmotic pressure.
hypotonicity Reduced tension of the arterial walls or muscles.
hypoventilation Respiratory rate insufficient to prevent carbon dioxide retention.
hypovolemia Abnormally low circulating blood volume.
hypoxemia Arterial blood oxygen level less than 60 mm Hg; low oxygen level in the blood.
hypoxia Inadequate cellular oxygenation that may result from a deficiency in the delivery or use of oxygen at the cellular level.

I

identity Component of self-concept characterized by one's persisting consciousness of being oneself, separate and distinct from others.
idiosyncratic reaction Individual sensitivity to effects of a drug caused by inherited or other bodily constitution factors.
illness (1) Abnormal process in which any aspect of a person's functioning is diminished or impaired compared with his or her previous condition. (2) The personal, interpersonal, and cultural reaction to disease.
illness behavior Ways in which people monitor their bodies, define and interpret their symptoms, take remedial actions, and use the health care system.
illness prevention Health education programs or activities directed toward protecting patients from threats or potential threats to health and minimizing risk factors.
imam Muslim priest.
immobility Inability to move about freely; caused by any condition in which movement is impaired or therapeutically restricted.
immunity Quality of being insusceptible to or unaffected by a particular disease or condition.
immunization Process by which resistance to an infectious disease is induced or augmented.
implementation Initiation and completion of the nursing actions necessary to help the patient achieve health care goals.

impression management Ability to interpret others' behavior within their own context of meanings and behave in a culturally congruent way to achieve desired outcomes of communication.

incentive spirometry Method of encouraging voluntary deep breathing by providing visual feedback to patients of the inspiratory volume they have achieved.

incident rates Rate of new cases of a disease in a specified population over a defined period of time.

incident report Confidential document that describes any patient accident while the person is on the premises of a health care agency. (See occurrence report.)

independent practice association (IPA) Managed care organization that contracts with physicians or health care providers who usually are members of groups and whose practices include fee-for-service and capitated patients.

indirect care interventions Treatments performed away from the patient but on behalf of the patient or group of patients.

induration Hardening of a tissue, particularly the skin, because of edema or inflammation.

infection Invasion of the body by pathogenic microorganisms that reproduce and multiply.

inference (1) Judgment or interpretation of informational cues. (2) Taking one proposition as a given and guessing that another proposition follows.

infiltration Dislodging an intravenous catheter or needle from a vein into the subcutaneous space.

inflammation Protective response of body tissues to irritation or injury.

informed consent Process of obtaining permission from a patient to perform a specific test or procedure after describing all risks, side effects, and benefits.

infusion pump Device that delivers a measured amount of fluid over a period of time.

infusions Introduction of fluid into the vein, giving intravenous fluid over time.

inhalation Method of medication delivery through the patient's respiratory tract. The respiratory tract provides a large surface area for drug absorption. Inhalation can be through the nasal or oral route.

injections Parenteral administration of medication; four major sites of injection: subcutaneous, intramuscular, intravenous, and intradermal.

insensible water loss Water loss that is continuous and not perceived by the person.

insomnia Condition characterized by chronic inability to sleep or remain asleep through the night.

inspection Method of physical examination by which the patient is visually systematically examined for appearance, structure, function, and behavior.

instillation To cause to enter drop by drop or very slowly.

institutional ethics committee Interdisciplinary committee that discusses and processes ethical dilemmas that arise within a health care institution.

instrumental activities of daily living (IADLs) Activities necessary for independence in society beyond eating, grooming, transferring, and toileting; include such skills as shopping, preparing meals, banking, and taking medications.

integrated delivery network (IDN) Set of providers and services organized to deliver a coordinated continuum of care to the population of patients served at a capitated cost.

interpersonal communication Exchange of information between two persons or among persons in a small group.

interstitial fluid Fluid that fills the spaces between most of the cells of the body and provides a substantial portion of the liquid environment of the body.

interview Organized, systematic conversation with the patient designed to obtain pertinent health-related subjective information.

intracellular fluid Liquid within the cell membrane.

intradermal (ID) Injection given between layers of the skin into the dermis. Injections are given at a 5- to 15-degree angle.

intramuscular (IM) Injections given into muscle tissue. The intramuscular route provides a fast rate of absorption that is related to the greater vascularity of the muscle. Injections are given at a 90-degree angle.

intraocular Method of medication delivery that involves inserting a medication disk similar to a contact lens into the patient's eye.

intrapersonal communication Communication that occurs within an individual (i.e., people "talk with themselves" silently or form an idea in their own mind).

intravascular fluid Fluid circulating within blood vessels of the body.

intravenous Injection directly into the bloodstream. Action of the drug begins immediately when given intravenously.

intravenous fat emulsions Soybean- or safflower oil–based solutions that are isotonic and may be infused with amino acid and dextrose solution through a central or peripheral line.

intubation Insertion of a breathing tube through the mouth or nose into the trachea to ensure a patent airway.

intuition Inner sensing that something is so.

irrigation Process of washing out a body cavity or wounded area with a stream of fluid.

ischemia Decreased blood supply to a body part such as skin tissue or to an organ such as the heart.

isolation Separation of a seriously ill patient from others to prevent the spread of an infection or protect the patient from irritating environmental factors.

isometric exercises Activities that involve muscle tension without muscle shortening, do not have any beneficial effect on preventing orthostatic hypotension, but may improve activity tolerance.

isotonic Situation in which two solutions have the same concentration of solute; therefore both solutions exert the same osmotic pressure.

J

jaundice Yellow discoloration of the skin, mucous membranes, and sclera caused by greater-than-normal amounts of bilirubin in the blood.

jejunostomy tube Hollow tube inserted into the jejunum through the abdominal wall for administration of liquefied foods to patients who have a high risk of aspiration.

joint contracture Abnormality that may result in permanent condition of a joint; is characterized by flexion and fixation; and is caused by disuse, atrophy, and shortening of muscle fibers and surrounding joint tissues.

joints Connections between bones; classified according to structure and degree of mobility.

judgment Ability to form an opinion or draw sound conclusions.

justice Ethical standard of fairness.

K

Kardex Trade name for card-filing system that allows quick reference to the particular need of the patient for certain aspects of nursing care.

karma Asian Indian belief that attributes mental illness to past deeds in one's previous life.

Korotkoff sound Sound heard during the taking of blood pressure using a sphygmomanometer and stethoscope.

Kussmaul respiration Increase in both rate and depth of respirations.

kyphosis Exaggeration of the posterior curvature of the thoracic spine.

L

la cuarantena Period of rest and restricted physical activity after childbirth that usually lasts 40 days.

la dieta Diet.

laceration Torn, jagged wound.

language Code that conveys specific meaning as words are combined.

laryngospasm Sudden uncontrolled contraction of the laryngeal muscles, which in turn decreases airway size.

law Rule, standard, or principle that states a fact or relationship between factors.

laxatives Drugs that act to promote bowel evacuation.

learning Acquisition of new knowledge and skills as a result of reinforcement, practice, and experience.

learning objective Written statement that describes the behavior that a teacher expects from an individual after a learning activity.

left-sided heart failure Abnormal condition characterized by impaired functioning of the left ventricle caused by elevated pressures and pulmonary congestion.

leukoplakia Thick, white patches observed on oral mucous membranes.

licensed practical nurse (LPN) Also known as the licensed vocational nurse (LVN) or in Canada, registered nurse's assistant (RNA); trained in basic nursing skills and the provision of direct patient care.

licensed vocational nurse (LVN) The LVN is the same as a licensed practical nurse (LPN), an individual trained in the United States in basic nursing techniques and direct patient care who practices under the supervision of a registered nurse. The LVN is licensed by a board after completing what is usually a 12-month educational program and passing a licensure examination. In Canada an LVN is called a certified nursing assistant.

lipids Compounds that are insoluble in water but soluble in organic solvents.

lipogenesis Process during which fatty acids are synthesized.

living wills Instruments by which a dying person makes wishes known.

local anesthesia Loss of sensation at the desired site of action.

logroll Maneuver used to turn a reclining patient from one side to the other or completely over without moving the spinal column out of alignment.

lordosis Increased lumbar curvature.

M

maceration Softening and breaking down of skin from prolonged exposure to moisture.

mal de ojo Evil eye.

malignant hyperthermia Autosomal-dominant trait characterized by often fatal hyperthermia in affected people exposed to certain anesthetic agents.

malpractice Injurious or unprofessional actions that harm another.

malpractice insurance Type of insurance to protect the health care professional. In case of a malpractice claim, the insurance pays the award to the plaintiff.

managed care Health care system in which there is administrative control over primary health care services. Redundant facilities and services are eliminated, and costs are reduced. Preventive care and health education are emphasized.

Maslow's hierarchy of needs Model developed by Abram Maslow that is used to explain human motivation.

matrilineal Kinship that is limited to only the mother's side.

maturation Genetically determined biological plan for growth and development. Physical growth and motor development are a function of maturation.

maturational loss Loss, usually of an aspect of self, resulting from the normal changes of growth and development.

Medicaid State medical assistance to people with low incomes, based on Title XIX of the Social Security Act. States receive matching federal funds to provide medical care and services to people meeting categorical and income requirements.

medical asepsis Procedures used to reduce the number of microorganisms and prevent their spread.

medical diagnosis Formal statement of the disease entity or illness made by the physician or health care provider.

medical record Patient's chart; a legal document.

Medicare Federally funded national health insurance program in the United States for people over 65 years of age. The program is administered in two parts. Part A provides basic protection against costs of medical, surgical, and psychiatric hospital care. Part B is a voluntary medical insurance program financed in part from federal funds and in part from premiums contributed by people enrolled in the program.

medication abuse Maladaptive pattern of recurrent medication use.

medication allergy Adverse reaction such as rash, chills, or gastrointestinal disturbances to a medication. Once a drug allergy occurs, the patient can no longer receive that particular medication.

medication dependence Maladaptive pattern of medication use in the following patterns: using excessive amounts of the medication, increased activities directed toward obtaining the medication, or withdrawal from professional or recreational activities.

medication error Any event that could cause or lead to a patient's receiving inappropriate drug therapy or failing to receive appropriate drug therapy.

medication interaction Response that occurs when one drug modifies the action of another drug. The interaction can potentiate or diminish the actions of another drug; or it may alter the way a drug is metabolized, absorbed, or excreted.

melanoma Group of malignant neoplasms, primarily of the skin, that are composed of melanocytes. Common in fair-skinned people having light-colored eyes and those who have been sunburned.

melena Abnormal black, sticky stool containing digested blood that is indicative of gastrointestinal bleeding.

menarche Onset of a girl's first menstruation.

Ménière's disease Chronic disease of the inner ear characterized by recurrent episodes of vertigo; progressive sensorineural hearing loss, which may be bilateral; and tinnitus.

menopause Physiological cessation of ovulation and menstruation that typically occurs during middle adulthood in women.

message Information sent or expressed by sender in the communication process.

metabolic acidosis Abnormal condition of high hydrogen ion concentration in the extracellular fluid caused by either a primary increase in hydrogen ions or a decrease in bicarbonate.

metabolic alkalosis Abnormal condition characterized by the significant loss of acid from the body or increased levels of bicarbonate.

metabolism Aggregate of all chemical processes that take place in living organisms and result in growth, generation of energy, elimination of wastes, and other functions concerned with the distribution of nutrients in the blood after digestion.

metacommunication Dependent not only on what is said but also on the relationship to the other person involved in the interaction. It is a message that conveys the sender's attitude toward self and the message and the attitudes, feelings, and intentions toward the listener.

metastasize Spread of tumor cells to distant parts of the body from a primary site (e.g., lung, breast, or bowel).

metered-dose inhaler (MDI) Device designed to deliver a measured dose of an inhalation drug.

metric system Logically organized decimal system of measurement; metric units can easily be converted and computed through simple multiplication and division. Each basic unit of measurement is organized into units of 10.

microorganisms Microscopic entities such as bacteria, viruses, and fungi that are capable of carrying on living processes.

micturition Urination; act of passing or expelling urine voluntarily through the urethra.

milliequivalent per liter (mEq/L) Number of grams of a specific electrolyte dissolved in 1 L of plasma.

mind mapping Graphic approach to represent the connections between concepts and ideas (e.g., nursing diagnoses) that are related to a central subject (e.g., the patient's health problems).

minerals Inorganic elements essential to the body because of their role as catalysts in biochemical reactions.

minimum data set (MDS) Required by the Omnibus Budget Reconciliation Act of 1987, the MDS is a uniform data set established by the Department of Health and Human Services. It serves as the framework for any state-specified assessment instruments used to develop a written and comprehensive plan of care for newly admitted residents of nursing facilities.

misdemeanor Lesser crime than a felony; the penalty is usually a fine or imprisonment for less than 1 year.

mobility Person's ability to move about freely.

moderate sedation/analgesia/conscious sedation Administration of central nervous system depressant drugs and/or analgesics to provide analgesia, relieve anxiety, and/or provide amnesia during surgical, diagnostic, or interventional procedures. Routinely used for diagnostic or therapeutic procedures that do not require complete anesthesia but simply a decreased level of consciousness.

monosaturated fatty acid Fatty acid in which some of the carbon atoms in the hydrocarbon chain are joined by double or triple bonds. Monounsaturated fatty acids have only one double or triple bond per molecule and are found as components of fats in such foods as fowls, almonds, pecans, cashew nuts, peanuts, and olive oil.

morals Personal conviction that something is absolutely right or wrong in all situations.

motivation Internal impulse that causes a person to take action.

mourning Process of grieving.

murmurs Blowing or whooshing sounds created by changes in blood flow through the heart or abnormalities in valve closure.

muscle tone Normal state of balanced muscle tension.

myocardial contractility Measure of stretch of the cardiac muscle fiber. It can also affect stroke volume and cardiac output. Poor contraction decreases the amount of blood ejected by the ventricles during each contraction.

myocardial infarction Necrosis of a portion of cardiac muscle caused by obstruction in a coronary artery.

myocardial ischemia Condition that results when the supply of blood to the myocardium from the coronary arteries is insufficient to meet the oxygen demands of the organ.

N

NANDA International North American Nursing Diagnosis Association organized in 1973. It formally identifies, develops, and classifies nursing diagnoses.

narcolepsy Syndrome involving sudden sleep attacks that a person cannot inhibit. Uncontrollable desire to sleep may occur several times during a day.

nasogastric (NG) tube Tube passed into the stomach through the nose to empty the stomach of its contents or deliver medication and/or nourishment.

nebulization Process of adding moisture to inspired air by the adding water droplets.

necessary losses Losses that every person experiences.

necrotic Of or pertaining to the death of tissue in response to disease or injury.

negative health behaviors Practices actually or potentially harmful to health such as smoking, drug or alcohol abuse, poor diet, and refusal to take necessary medications.

negative nitrogen balance Condition occurring when the body excretes more nitrogen than it takes in.

negligence Careless act of omission or commission that results in injury to another.

neonate Stage of life from birth to 1 month of age.

nephrons Structural and functional units of the kidney containing renal glomeruli and tubules.

neurotransmitter Chemical that transfers the electrical impulse from the nerve fiber to the muscle fiber.

nociceptors Somatic and visceral free nerve endings of thinly myelinated and unmyelinated fibers. They usually react to tissue injury but may also be excited by endogenous chemical substances.

nocturia Urination at night; can be a symptom of renal disease or may occur in persons who drink excessive amounts of fluids before bedtime.

nonblanchable hyperemia Redness of the skin caused by dilation of the superficial capillaries. The redness persists when pressure is applied to the area, indicating tissue damage.

noninvasive positive-pressure ventilation (NPPV) Used to prevent using invasive artificial airways (endotracheal [ET] tube or tracheostomy) in patients with acute respiratory failure, cardiogenic pulmonary edema, or exacerbation of chronic obstructive pulmonary disease. It has also been used following extubation of an ET tube.

nonmaleficence Fundamental ethical agreement to do no harm. Closely related to the ethical standard of beneficence.

nonrapid eye movement (NREM) sleep Sleep that occurs during the first four stages of normal sleep.

nonshivering thermogenesis Occurs primarily in neonates. Because neonates cannot shiver, a limited amount of vascular brown adipose tissue present at birth can be metabolized for heat production.

nonverbal communication Communication using expressions, gestures, body posture, and positioning rather than words.

normal sinus rhythm (NSR) The wave pattern on an electrocardiogram that indicates normal conduction of an electrical impulse through the myocardium.

numbing One of Bowlby's four phases of mourning. It is characterized by the lack of feeling or feeling stunned by the loss; may last a few days or many weeks.

Nurse Practice Acts Statutes enacted by the legislature of any of the states or the appropriate officers of the districts or possessions that describe and define the scope of nursing practice.

nurse-initiated interventions Response of the nurse to the patient's health care needs and nursing diagnoses. This type of intervention is an autonomous action based on scientific rationale that is executed to benefit the patient in a predicted way related to the nursing diagnosis and patient-centered goals.

nursing diagnosis Formal statement of an actual or potential health problem that nurses can legally and independently treat; the second step of the nursing process, during which the patient's actual and potential unhealthy responses to an illness or condition are identified.

nursing health history Data collected about a patient's present level of wellness, changes in life patterns, sociocultural role, and mental and emotional reactions to illness.

nursing intervention Any treatment based on clinical judgment and knowledge that a nurse performs to enhance patient outcomes.

nursing process Systematic problem-solving method by which nurses individualize care for each patient. The five steps of the nursing process are assessment, diagnosis, planning, implementation, and evaluation.

nursing-sensitive outcomes Outcomes that are within the scope of nursing practice; consequences or effects of nursing interventions that result in changes in the patient's symptoms, functional status, safety, psychological distress, or costs.

nurturant Behavior that involves caring for or fostering the well-being of another individual.

nutrients Foods that contain elements necessary for body function, including water, carbohydrates, proteins, fats, vitamins, and minerals.

O

obesity Abnormal increase in the proportion of fat cells, mainly in the viscera and subcutaneous tissues of the body.

objective data Information that can be observed by others; free of feelings, perceptions, prejudices.

occurrence report Confidential document that describes any patient accident while the person is on the premises of a health care agency. (See incident report.)

olfactory Pertaining to the sense of smell.

oncotic pressure Total influence of the protein on the osmotic activity of plasma fluid.

Open-ended question Form of question that prompts a respondent to answer in more than one or two words.

operating bed Table for surgery.

operating room (1) Room in a health care facility in which surgical procedures requiring anesthesia are performed. (2) Informal: a suite of rooms or an area in a health care facility in which patients are prepared for surgery, undergo surgical procedures, and recover from the anesthetic procedures required for the surgery.

ophthalmic Drugs given into the eye in the form of either eye drops or ointments.

ophthalmoscope Instrument used to illuminate the structures of the eye to examine the fundus, which includes the retina, choroid, optic nerve disc, macula, fovea centralis, and retinal vessels.

opioid Drug substance derived from opium or produced synthetically that alters perception of pain and that, with repeated use, may result in physical and psychological dependence (narcotic).

oral hygiene Condition or practice of maintaining the tissues and structures of the mouth.

orthopnea Abnormal condition in which a person must sit or stand to breathe comfortably.

orthostatic hypotension Abnormally low blood pressure occurring when a person stands.

osmolality Concentration or osmotic pressure of a solution expressed in osmoles or milliosmoles per kilogram of water.

osmolarity Osmotic pressure of a solution expressed in osmoles or milliosmoles per kilogram of the solution.

osmoreceptors Neurons in the hypothalamus that are sensitive to the fluid concentration in the blood plasma and regulate the secretion of antidiuretic hormone.

osmosis Movement of a pure solvent through a semipermeable membrane from a solution with a lower solute concentration to one with a higher solute concentration.

osmotic pressure Drawing power for water, which depends on the number of molecules in the solution.

osteoporosis Disorder characterized by abnormal rarefaction of bone, occurring most frequently in postmenopausal women, sedentary or immobilized individuals, and patients on long-term steroid therapy.

ostomy Surgical procedure in which an opening is made into the abdominal wall to allow the passage of intestinal contents from the bowel (colostomy) or urine from the bladder (urostomy).

otoscope Instrument with a special ear speculum used to examine the deeper structures of the external and middle ear.

ototoxic Having a harmful effect on the eighth cranial (auditory) nerve or the organs of hearing and balance.

outcome Condition of a patient at the end of treatment, including the degree of wellness and the need for continuing care, medication, support, counseling, or education.

outliers Patients with extended lengths of stay beyond allowable inpatient days or costs.

outpatient Patient who has not been admitted to a hospital but receives treatments in a clinic or facility associated with the hospital.

oxygen saturation Amount of hemoglobin fully saturated with oxygen, given as a percent value.

oxygen therapy Procedure in which oxygen is administered to a patient to relieve or prevent hypoxia.

P

pain Subjective, unpleasant sensation caused by noxious stimulation of sensory nerve endings.

palliative care Level of care that is designed to relieve or reduce intensity of uncomfortable symptoms but not to produce a cure. Palliative care relies on comfort measures and use of alternative therapies to help individuals become more at peace during end of life.

pallor Unnatural paleness or absence of color in the skin.

palpation Method of physical examination whereby the fingers or hands of the examiner are applied to the patient's body to feel body parts underlying the skin.

palpitations Bounding or racing of the heart associated with normal emotions or a heart disorder.

Papanicolaou (Pap) smear Painless screening test for cervical cancer. Specimens are taken of squamous and columnar cells of the cervix.

parallel play Form of play among a group of children, primarily toddlers, in which each one engages in an independent activity that is similar to but not influenced by or shared with the others.

paralytic ileus Usually temporary paralysis of intestinal wall that may occur after abdominal surgery or peritoneal injury and that causes cessation of peristalsis; leads to abdominal distention and symptoms of obstruction.

parenteral administration Giving medication by a route other than the gastrointestinal tract.

parenteral nutrition (PN) Administration of a nutritional solution into the vascular system.

parteras Lay midwives.

partial bed bath Bath in which body parts that might cause the patient discomfort if left unbathed (i.e., face, hands, axillary areas, back, and perineum) are washed in bed.

passive range-of-motion (PROM) exercises Range of movement through which a joint is moved with assistance.

passive strategies of health promotion Activities that involve the patient as the recipient of actions by health care professionals.

pathogenicity Ability of a pathogenic agent to produce a disease.

pathogens Microorganisms capable of producing disease.

pathological fractures Fractures resulting from weakened bone tissue; frequently caused by osteoporosis or neoplasms.

patient-centered care Concept to improve work efficiency by changing the way that patient care is delivered.

patient-controlled analgesia (PCA) Drug delivery system that allows patients to self-administer analgesic medications on demand.

patrilineal, patrilineally Kinship that is limited to only the father's side.

pay for performance Quality improvement program that rewards excellence through financial incentives to motivate change to achieve measurable improvements and improve patient care quality and safety.

perceived loss Loss that is less obvious to the individual experiencing it. Although easily overlooked or misunderstood, a perceived loss results in the same grief process as an actual loss.

perception Peoples' mental image or concept of elements in their environment, including information gained through the senses.

percussion Method of physical examination whereby the location, size, and density of a body part is determined by the tone obtained from the striking of short, sharp taps of the fingers.

perfusion (1) Passage of a fluid through a specific organ or an area of the body. (2) Therapeutic measure whereby a drug intended for an isolated part of the body is introduced via the bloodstream. (3) Relates to the ability of the cardiovascular system to pump oxygenated blood to the tissues and return deoxygenated blood to the lungs.

perineal care Procedure prescribed for cleaning the genital and anal areas as part of the daily bath or after various obstetrical and gynecological procedures.

perioperative nursing Refers to the role of the operating room nurse during the preoperative, intraoperative, and postoperative phases of surgery.

peripherally inserted central catheter (PICC) Alternative intravenous access when the patient requires intermediate-length venous access greater than 7 days to 3 months. Intravenous access is achieved by inserting a catheter into a central vein by way of a peripheral vein.

peristalsis Rhythmical contractions of the intestine that propel gastric contents through the length of the gastrointestinal tract.

peritonitis Inflammation of the peritoneum produced by bacteria or irritating substances introduced into the abdominal cavity by a penetrating wound or perforation of an organ in the gastrointestinal or reproductive tract.

PERRLA Acronym for "pupils equal, round, reactive to light, accommodation"; the acronym is recorded in the physical examination if eye and pupil assessments are normal.

personalismo Personalistic.

petechiae Tiny purple or red spots that appear on skin as minute hemorrhages within dermal layers.

pharmacokinetics Study of how drugs enter the body, reach their site of action, are metabolized, and exit from the body.

phlebitis Inflammation of a vein.

physician-initiated interventions Based on the physician's response to a medical diagnosis, the nurse responds to his or her written orders.

PIE note Problem-oriented medical record; the four interdisciplinary sections are the database, problem list, care plan, and progress notes.

placebos Dosage form that contains no pharmacologically active ingredients but may relieve pain through psychological effects.

plaintiff Individual who files formal charges against an individual or organization for a legal offense.

planning Process of designing interventions to achieve the goals and outcomes of health care delivery.

plantar flexion Toe-down motion of the foot at the ankle.

pleural friction rub Adventitious lung sound caused by inflamed parietal and visceral pleura rubbing together on inspiration.

pneumothorax Collection of air or gas in the pleural space.

point of maximal impulse (PMI) Point where the heartbeat can most easily be palpated through the chest wall. This is usually the fourth intercostal space at the midclavicular line.

point of view Way of looking at issues that reflects an individual's culture and societal influences.

poison Any substance that impairs health or destroys life when ingested, inhaled, or absorbed by the body in relatively small amounts.

poison control center One of a network of facilities that provides information regarding all aspects of poisoning or intoxication, maintains records of their occurrence, and refers patients to treatment centers.

polypharmacy Use of a number of different drugs by a patient who may have one or several health problems.

polyunsaturated fatty acid Fatty acid that has two or more carbon double bonds.

population Collection of individuals who have in common one or more personal or environmental characteristics.

positive health behaviors Activities related to maintaining, attaining, or regaining good health and preventing illness. Common positive health behaviors include immunizations, proper sleep patterns, adequate exercise, and nutrition.

postanesthesia care unit (PACU) Area adjoining the operating room to which surgical patients are taken while still under anesthesia.

postmortem care Care of a patient's body after death.

postural drainage Use of positioning along with percussion and vibration to drain secretions from specific segments of the lungs and bronchi into the trachea.

postural hypotension Abnormally low blood pressure occurring when an individual assumes the standing posture; also called orthostatic hypotension.

posture Position of the body in relation to the surrounding space.

power of attorney for health care Person designated by the patient to make health care decisions for the patient if the patient becomes unable to make his or her own decisions.

preadolescence Transitional developmental stage that occurs between childhood and adolescence.

preanesthesia care unit Area outside the operating room where preoperative preparations are completed.

preload Volume of blood in the ventricles at the end of diastole, immediately before ventricular contraction.

preoperative teaching Instruction regarding a patient's anticipated surgery and recovery that is given before surgery. Instruction includes, but is not limited to, dietary and activity restrictions, anticipated assessment activities, postoperative procedures, and pain-relief measures.

presbycusis Hearing loss associated with aging. It usually involves both a loss of hearing sensitivity and a reduction in the clarity of speech.

presbyopia Gradual decline in ability of the lens to accommodate or focus on close objects; reduces ability to see near objects clearly. This condition commonly develops with advancing age.

prescriptions Written directions for a therapeutic agent (e.g., medication, drugs).

presence Deep physical, psychological, and spiritual connection or engagement between a nurse and patient.

present time orientation Time dimension that focuses on what is happening here and now. Communication patterns are circular, and this time orientation is in conflict with the dominant organizational norm in health care that emphasizes punctuality and adherence to appointments.

pressure ulcer Inflammation, sore, or ulcer in the skin over a bony prominence.

presurgical care unit (PSCU) Area outside the operating room where preoperative preparations are completed.

preventive nursing actions Nursing actions directed toward preventing illness and promoting health to avoid the need for primary, secondary, or tertiary health care.

primary appraisal Evaluating an event for its personal meaning related to stress.

primary care First contact in a given episode of illness that leads to a decision regarding a course of action to resolve the health problem.

primary health care Combination of primary and public health care that is accessible to individuals and families in a community and provided at an affordable cost.

primary intention Primary union of the edges of a wound, progressing to complete scar formation without granulation.

primary nursing Method of nursing practice in which the patient's care is managed for the duration by one nurse who directs and coordinates other nurses and health care personnel. When on duty, the primary nurse cares for the patient directly.

primary prevention First contact in a given episode of illness that leads to a decision regarding a course of action to prevent worsening of the health problem.

problem identification One of the steps of the diagnostic process in which the patient's health care problem is recognized as a result of data analysis based on professional knowledge and experience.

problem solving Methodical, systematic approach to explore conditions and develop solutions, including analysis of data, determination of causative factors, and selection of appropriate actions to reverse or eliminate the problem.

problem-oriented medical record (POMR) Method of recording data about the health status of a patient that fosters a collaborative problem-solving approach by all members of the health care team.

productive cough Sudden expulsion of air from the lungs that effectively removes sputum from the respiratory tract and helps clear the airways.

professional standards review organization (PSRO) Focuses on evaluation of nursing care provided in a health care setting. The quality, effectiveness, and appropriateness of nursing care for the patient are the focus of evaluation.

prone Position of the patient lying face down.

proprioception Ability of the body to sense its position and movement in space.

prospective payment system (PPS) Payment mechanism for reimbursing hospitals for inpatient health care services in which a predetermined rate is set for treatment of specific illnesses.

prostaglandins Potent hormonelike substances that act in exceedingly low doses on target organs. They can be used to treat asthma and gastric hyperacidity.

proteins Any of a large group of naturally occurring, complex, organic nitrogenous compounds. Each is composed of large combinations of amino acids containing the elements carbon; hydrogen; nitrogen; oxygen; usually sulfur; and occasionally phosphorus, iron, iodine, or other essential constituents of living cells. Protein is the major source of building material for muscles, blood, skin, hair, nails, and the internal organs.

proteinuria Presence in the urine of abnormally large quantities of protein, usually albumin. Persistent proteinuria is usually a sign of renal disease or renal complications of another disease, hypertension, or heart failure.

protocol Written and approved plan specifying the procedures to be followed during an assessment or in providing treatment.

pruritus Symptom of itching; an uncomfortable sensation leading to the urge to scratch.

psychomotor learning Acquisition of ability to perform motor skills.

ptosis Abnormal condition of one or both upper eyelids in which the eyelid droops; caused by weakness of the levator muscle or paralysis of the third cranial nerve.

puberty Developmental period of emotional and physical changes, including the development of secondary sex characteristics and the onset of menstruation and ejaculation.

public health nursing Nursing specialty that requires the nurse to care for the needs of populations or groups.

public communication Interaction of one individual with large groups of people.

pulmonary hygiene More frequent turning, deep breathing, coughing, use of incentive spirometry, and chest physical therapy (PT) if ordered.

pulse deficit Condition that exists when the radial pulse is less than the ventricular rate as auscultated at the apex or seen on an electrocardiogram. The condition indicates a lack of peripheral perfusion for some of the heart contractions.

pulse pressure Difference between the systolic and diastolic pressures, normally 30 to 40 mm Hg.

Purkinje network Complex network of muscle fibers that spread through the right and left ventricles of the heart and carry the impulses that contract those chambers almost simultaneously.

pursed-lip breathing Deep inspiration followed by prolonged expiration through pursed lips.

pyrexia Abnormal elevation of the temperature of the body above 37° C (98.6° F) because of disease; same as fever.

pyrogens Substances that cause a rise in body temperature, as in the case of bacterial toxins.

Q

QSEN The Quality and Safety in the Education of Nurses (QSEN) initiative is the commitment of nursing to the competencies outlined in the Institute of Medicine report related to nursing education. QSEN encompasses six competencies: patient-centered care, teamwork, collaboration, evidence-based practice, quality improvement, and safety.

quality improvement Monitoring and evaluation of processes and outcomes in health care or any other business to identify opportunities for improvement.

quality indicator Quantitative measure of an important aspect of care that determines whether quality of service conforms to requirements or standards of care.

R

race Common biological characteristics shared by a group of people.

Ramadan Religious observance held during the ninth month of the Islamic calendar year. It involves fasting from sunrise to sunset.

range of motion (ROM) Range of movement of a joint from maximum extension to maximum flexion as measured in degrees of a circle.

rapid eye movement (REM) sleep Stage of sleep in which dreaming and rapid eye movements are prominent; important for mental restoration.

reaction Component of the pain experience that may include both physiological responses such as in the general adaptation syndrome and behavioral responses.

reality orientation Therapeutic modality for restoring an individual's sense of the present.

receiver Person to whom message is sent during the communication process.

reception Neurophysiological components of the pain experience in which nervous system receptors receive painful stimuli and transmit them through peripheral nerves to the spinal cord and brain.

record Written form of communication that permanently documents information relevant to health care management.

recovery Period of time immediately following surgery when the patient is closely observed for effects of anesthesia, changes in vital signs, and bleeding. The area is usually in the postanesthesia care unit.

referent Factor that motivates a person to communicate with another individual.

reflection Process of thinking back or recalling an event to discover the meaning and purpose of that event. Useful in critical thinking.

refractive error Defect in the ability of the lens of the eye to focus light such as occurs in nearsightedness and farsightedness.

regional anesthesia Loss of sensation in an area of the body supplied by sensory nerve pathways.

registered nurse (RN) In the United States a nurse who has completed a course of study at a state-approved, accredited school of nursing and has passed the National Council Licensure Examination (NCLEX-RN).

regression Return to an earlier developmental stage or behavior.

regulatory agencies Local, state, provincial, or national agencies that inspect and certify health care agencies as meeting specified standards. These agencies can also determine the amount of reimbursement for health care delivered.

rehabilitation Restoration of an individual to normal or near-normal function after a physical or mental illness, injury, or chemical addiction.

reinforcement Provision of a contingent response to a learner's behavior that increases the probability of recurrence of the behavior.

related factor Any condition or event that accompanies or is linked with the patient's health care problem.

relaxation Act of being relaxed or less tense.

reminiscence Recalling the past to assign new meaning to past experiences.

remissions Partial or complete disappearances of the clinical and subjective characteristics of chronic or malignant disease; remission may be spontaneous or the result of therapy.

renal calculi Calcium stones in the renal pelvis.

renin Proteolytic enzyme produced by and stored in the juxtaglomerular apparatus that surrounds each arteriole as it enters a glomerulus. The enzyme affects the blood pressure by catalyzing the change of angiotensinogen to angiotensin, a strong repressor.

reorganization Last phase of Bowlby's phases of mourning. During this phase, which sometimes requires a year or more, the person begins to accept unaccustomed roles, acquire new skills, and build new relationships.

reports Transfer of information from the nurses on one shift to the nurses on the following shift. Report may also be given by one of the members of the nursing team to another health care provider (e.g., a physician or therapist).

reservoir Place where microorganisms survive, multiply, and await transfer to a susceptible host.

residual urine Volume of urine remaining in the bladder after a normal voiding; the bladder normally is almost completely empty after micturition.

resistance stage Third stage of the stress response, when the person attempts to adapt to the stressor. The body stabilizes; hormone levels stabilize; and heart rate, blood pressure, and cardiac output return to normal.

resource utilization group (RUG) Method of classification for health care reimbursement for long-term care facilities.

respeto Respectful.

respiration Exchange of oxygen and carbon dioxide during cellular metabolism.

respiratory acidosis Abnormal condition characterized by increased arterial carbon dioxide concentration, excess carbonic acid, and increased hydrogen ion concentration.

respiratory alkalosis Abnormal condition characterized by decreased arterial carbon dioxide concentration and hydrogen ion concentration.

respite care Short-term health services to dependent older adults either in their home or in an institutional setting.

responsibility Carrying out duties associated with a particular role.

restorative care Health care settings and services in which patients who are recovering from illness or disability receive rehabilitation and supportive care.

restraint Device to aid in the immobilization of a patient or patient's extremity.

return demonstration Demonstration after the patient has first observed the teacher and then practiced the skill in mock or real situations.

rhonchi Abnormal lung sound auscultated when the patient's airways are obstructed with thick secretions.

right-sided heart failure Abnormal condition that results from impaired functioning of the right ventricle; characterized by venous congestion in the systemic circulation.

risk factor Any internal or external variable that makes a person or group more vulnerable to illness or an unhealthy event.

risk management Function of hospital or other health facility administration that is directed toward identification, evaluation, and correction of potential risks that could lead to injury of patients, staff members, or visitors and result in property loss or damage.

risk nursing diagnosis Describes human responses to health conditions/life processes that may develop in a vulnerable individual, family, or community.

role performance Way in which a person views his or her ability to carry out significant roles.

root cause analysis Process of data collection and analysis that aids in finding the real cause of the problem and working on dealing with it rather than just dealing with its effects.

S

Sabbath From sundown on Friday to sundown on Saturday, this religious observance is a day of rest and worship for Jews and some Christian sects.

sandbags Sand-filled plastic tubes that can be shaped to body contours. They can immobilize an extremity or maintain body alignment.

saturated fatty acid Fatty acid in which each carbon in the chain has an attached hydrogen atom.

scientific method Codified sequence of steps used in the formulation, testing, evaluation, and reporting of scientific ideas.

scientific rationale Reason why a specific nursing action was chosen based on supporting literature.

scoliosis Lateral spinal curvature.

scrub nurse Registered nurse or operating room technician who assists surgeons during operations.

secondary appraisal Evaluating one's possible coping strategies when confronted with a stressor.

secondary intention Wound closure in which the edges are separated; granulation tissue develops to fill the gap; and, finally, epithelium grows in over the granulation, producing a larger scar than results with primary intention.

secondary prevention Level of preventive medicine that focuses on early diagnosis, use of referral services, and rapid initiation of treatment to stop the progress of disease processes.

sedatives Medications that produce a calming effect by decreasing functional activity, diminishing irritability, and allaying excitement.

segmentation Alternating contraction and relaxation of gastrointestinal mucosa.

self-concept Complex, dynamic integration of conscious and unconscious feelings, attitudes, and perceptions about one's identity, physical being, worth, and roles; how a person perceives and defines self.

self-esteem Feeling of self-worth characterized by feelings of achievement, adequacy, self-confidence, and usefulness.

self-transcendence Sense of authentically connecting to one's inner self.

sender Person who initiates interpersonal communication by conveying a message.

sensible water loss Loss of fluid from the body through the secretory activity of the sweat glands and the exhalation of humidified air from the lungs.

sensory deficits Defects in the function of one or more of the senses, resulting in visual, auditory, or olfactory impairments.

sensory deprivation State in which stimulation to one or more of the senses is lacking, resulting in impaired sensory perception.

sensory overload State in which stimulation to one or more of the senses is so excessive that the brain disregards or does not meaningfully respond to stimuli.

sequential compression stockings Plastic stockings attached to an air pump that inflates and deflates the stockings, applying intermittent pressure sequentially from the ankle to the knee.

serum half-life Time needed for excretion processes to lower the serum drug concentration by half.

sexual dysfunction Inability or difficulty in sexual functioning caused by physiological or psychological factors or both.

sexual orientation Clear, persistent erotic preference for a person of one sex or the other.

sexuality "A function of the total personality . . . concerned with the biological, psychological, sociological, spiritual and culture variables of life . . ." (Sex Information and Education Council of the United States, 1980).

sexually transmitted infection Infectious process spread through sexual contact, including oral, genital, or anal sexual activity.

shear Force exerted against the skin while the skin remains stationary and the bony structures move.

side effect Any reaction or consequence that results from medication or therapy.

side rails Bars positioned along the sides of the length of the bed or stretcher to reduce the patient's risk of falling.

simpatia Friendly.

sinoatrial (SA) node Called the *pacemaker of the heart* because the origin of the normal heartbeat begins at the SA node. The SA node is in the right atrium next to the entrance of the superior vena cava.

situational crisis Unexpected crisis that arises suddenly in response to an external event or a conflict concerning a specific circumstance.

situational loss Loss of a person, thing, or quality resulting from a change in a life situation, including changes related to illness, body image, environment, and death.

sitz bath Bath in which only the hips or buttocks are immersed in fluid.

skilled nursing facility Institution or part of an institution that meets criteria for accreditation established by the sections of the Social Security Act that determine the basis for Medicaid and Medicare reimbursement for skilled nursing care, including rehabilitation and various medical and nursing procedures.

sleep State marked by reduced consciousness, diminished activity of the skeletal muscles, and depressed metabolism.

sleep apnea Cessation of breathing for a time during sleep.

sleep deprivation Condition resulting from a decrease in the amount, quality, and consistency of sleep.

SOAP note Progress note that focuses on a single patient problem and includes subjective and objective data, analysis, and planning; most often used in the problem-oriented medical record (POMR).

socializing Interacting with friends or other people; communicating with others to form relationships and help people feel relaxed.

solute Substance dissolved in a solution.

solution Mixture of one or more substances dissolved in another substance. The molecules of each of the substances disperse homogeneously and do not change chemically. A solution may be a liquid, gas, or solid.

solvent Any liquid in which another substance can be dissolved.

source record Organization of a patient's chart so each discipline (e.g., nursing, medicine, social work, or respiratory therapy) has a separate section in which to record data. Unlike POMR, the information is not organized by patient problems. The advantage of a source record is that caregivers can easily locate the proper section of the record in which to make entries.

sphygmomanometer Device for measuring the arterial blood pressure that consists of an arm or leg cuff with an air bladder connected to a tube, a bulb for pumping air into the bladder, and a gauge for indicating the amount of air pressure being exerted against the artery.

spiritual distress State of being out of harmony with a system of beliefs, a Supreme Being, or God.

spiritual well-being Individual's spirituality that enables a person to love, have faith and hope, seek meaning in life, and nurture relationships with others.

spirituality Spiritual dimension of a person, including the relationship with humanity, nature, and a supreme being.

standard of care Minimum level of care accepted to ensure high-quality care to patients. Standards of care define the types of therapies typically administered to patients with defined problems or needs.

standard precautions Guidelines recommended by the Centers for Disease Control and Prevention (CDC) to reduce risk of transmission of bloodborne and other pathogens in hospitals.

standardized care plans Written care plans used for groups of patients who have similar health care problems.

standing order Written and approved documents containing rules, policies, procedures, regulations, and orders for the conduct of patient care in various stipulated clinical settings.

statutory law Of or related to laws enacted by a legislative branch of the government.

stenosis Abnormal condition characterized by the constriction or narrowing of an opening or passageway in a body structure.

stereotypes Generalizations that are made about individuals without further assessment.

sterilization (1) Rendering a person unable to produce children; accomplished by surgical, chemical, or other means. (2) A technique for destroying microorganisms using heat, water, chemicals, or gases.

stoma Artificially created opening between a body cavity and the surface of the body (e.g., a colostomy formed from a portion of the colon pulled through the abdominal wall).

stress Physiological or psychological tension that threatens homeostasis or a person's psychological equilibrium.

stressor Any event, situation, or other stimulus encountered in a person's external or internal environment that necessitates change or adaptation by the person.

striae Streaks or linear scars that result from rapid development of tension in the skin.

stroke volume (SV) Amount of blood ejected by the ventricles with each contraction. It can be affected by the amount of blood in the left ventricle at the end of diastole (preload), the resistance to left ventricular ejection (afterload), and myocardial contractility.

subacute care Level of medical specialty care provided to patients who need a greater intensity of care than that provided in a skilled nursing facility but who do not require acute care.

subcultures Various ethnic, religious, and other groups with distinct characteristics from the dominant culture.

subcutaneous (sub-Q) Injection given into the connective tissue under the dermis. The subcutaneous tissue absorbs drugs more slowly than those injected into muscle. Injections are usually given at a 45-degree angle.

subjective data Information gathered from patient statements; the patient's feelings and perceptions. Not verifiable by another except by inference.

sublingual Route of medication administration in which the medication is placed underneath the patient's tongue.

Sunrise Model A model developed by Leininger that aids the health care practitioner in designing care decisions and actions in a culturally congruent fashion.

supine Position of the patient in which the patient is resting on his or her back.

suprainfection Secondary infection usually caused by an opportunistic pathogen.

suprapubic catheter Catheter surgically inserted through abdomen into bladder.

surfactant Chemical produced in the lungs to maintain the surface tension of the alveoli and keep them from collapsing.

surgical asepsis Procedures used to eliminate any microorganisms from an area. Also called *sterile technique.*

sympathy Concern, sorrow, or pity felt by the nurse for the patient. Sympathy is a subjective look at another person's world that prevents a clear perspective of all sides of the issues confronting that person.

synapse Region surrounding the point of contact between two neurons or between a neuron and an effector organ.

syncope Brief lapse in consciousness caused by transient cerebral hypoxia.

synergistic effect Effect resulting from two drugs acting synergistically. The effect of the two drugs combined is greater than the effect that would be expected if the individual effects of the two drugs acting alone were added together.

systolic Pertaining to or resulting from ventricular contraction.

T

tachycardia Rapid regular heart rate ranging between 100 and 150 beats/min.

tachypnea Abnormally rapid rate of breathing.

tactile Relating to the sense of touch.

tactile fremitus Tremulous vibration of the chest wall during breathing that is palpable on physical examination.

teaching Implementation method used to present correct principles, procedures, and techniques of health care; to inform patients about their health status; and to refer patients and family to appropriate health or social resources in the community.

team nursing Decentralized system in which the care of a patient is distributed among the members of a team. The charge nurse delegates authority to a team leader, who must be a professional nurse.

teratogens Chemical or physiological agents that may produce adverse effects in the embryo or fetus.

tertiary prevention Activities directed toward rehabilitation rather than diagnosis and treatment.

therapeutic communication Process in which the nurse consciously influences a patient or helps the patient to a better understanding through verbal and/or nonverbal communication.

therapeutic effect Desired benefit of a medication, treatment, or procedure.

thermoregulation Internal control of body temperature.

threshold Point at which a person first perceives a painful stimulus as being painful.

thrill Continuous palpable sensation like the purring of a cat.

thrombus Accumulation of platelets, fibrin, clotting factors, and the cellular elements of the blood attached to the interior wall of a vein or artery, sometimes occluding the lumen of the vessel.

tinnitus Ringing heard in one or both ears.

tissue ischemia Point at which tissues receive insufficient oxygen and perfusion.

tolerance Point at which a person is not willing to accept pain of greater severity or duration.

tort Act that causes injury for which the injured party can bring civil action.

total patient care Nursing delivery of care model originally developed during Florence Nightingale's time. In the model a registered nurse (RN) is responsible for all aspects of care for one or more patients. The RN works directly with the patient, family, physician or health care provider, and health care team members. The model typically has a shift-based focus.

touch To come in contact with another person, often conveying caring, emotional support, encouragement, or tenderness.

toxic effect Effect of a medication that results in an adverse response.

tracheostomy Procedure whereby a surgical incision is made into the trachea and a short artificial airway (a tracheostomy tube) is inserted.

transcendence The belief that there is a force outside of and greater than the person that exists beyond the material world.

transcultural Concept of care extending across cultures that distinguishes nursing from other health disciplines.

transcultural nursing Distinct discipline developed by Leininger that focuses on the comparative study of cultures to understand similarities and differences among groups of people.

transcutaneous electrical nerve stimulation (TENS) Technique in which a battery-powered device blocks pain impulses from reaching the spinal cord by delivering weak electrical impulses directly to the surface of the skin.

transdermal disk Medication delivery device in which the medication is saturated on a waferlike disk, which is affixed to the patient's skin. This method ensures that the patient receives a continuous level of medication.

transfer report Verbal exchange of information between caregivers when a patient is moved from one nursing unit or health care setting to another. The report includes information necessary to maintain a consistent level of care from one setting to another.

transfusion reaction Systemic response by the body to the administration of blood incompatible with that of the recipient.

trapeze bar Metal triangular-shaped bar that can be suspended over a patient's bed from an overhanging frame; permits patients to move up and down in bed while in traction or some other encumbrance.

trimester Referring to one of the three phases of pregnancy.

trochanter roll Rolled towel support placed against the hips and upper leg to prevent external rotation of the legs.

trough The lowest serum concentration of a medication before the next medication dose is administered.

turgor Normal resiliency of the skin caused by the outward pressure of the cells and interstitial fluid.

U

unsaturated fatty acid Fatty acid in which an unequal number of hydrogen atoms are attached and the carbon atoms attach to one another with a double bond.

ureterostomy Diversion of urine away from a diseased or defective bladder through an artificial opening in the skin.

urge incontinence A type of urinary incontinence that results from sudden, involuntary contraction of the muscles of the urinary bladder, resulting in an urge to urinate.

urinal Receptacle for collecting urine.

urinary diversion Surgical diversion of the drainage of urine such as a ureterostomy.

urinary incontinence Inability to control urination.

urinary reflux Abnormal, backward flow of urine.

urinary retention Retention of urine in the bladder; condition frequently caused by a temporary loss of muscle function.

urine hat Receptacle for collecting urine that fits toilet.

urometer Device for measuring frequent and small amounts of urine from an indwelling urinary catheter system.

urosepsis Organisms in the bloodstream.

utilitarianism Ethic that proposes that the value of something is determined by its usefulness. The greatest good for the greatest number of people constitutes the guiding principle for action in a utilitarian model of ethics.

utilization review (UR) committees Physician-supervised committees to review admissions, diagnostic testing, and treatments provided by physicians or health care providers to patients.

V

validation Act of confirming, verifying, or corroborating the accuracy of assessment data or the appropriateness of the care plan.

Valsalva maneuver Any forced expiratory effort against a closed airway such as when an individual holds his or her breath and tightens his or her muscles in a concerted, strenuous effort to move a heavy object or change positions in bed.

value Personal belief about the worth of a given idea or behavior.

valvular heart disease Acquired or congenital disorder of a cardiac valve characterized by stenosis and obstructed blood flow or valvular degeneration and regurgitation of blood.

variances Unexpected event that occurs during patient care and that is different from CareMap predictions. Variances or exceptions are interventions or outcomes that are not achieved as anticipated. Variance may be positive or negative.

variant Differing from a set standard.

vascular access devices Catheters, cannulas, or infusion ports designed for long-term, repeated access to the vascular system.

vasoconstriction Narrowing of the lumen of any blood vessel, especially the arterioles and the veins in the blood reservoirs of the skin and abdominal viscera.

vasodilation Increase in the diameter of a blood vessel caused by inhibition of its vasoconstrictor nerves or stimulation of dilator nerves.

venipuncture Technique in which a vein is punctured transcutaneously by a sharp rigid stylet (e.g., a butterfly needle), a cannula (e.g., an angiocatheter that contains a flexible plastic catheter), or a needle attached to a syringe.

ventilation Respiratory process by which gases are moved into and out of the lungs.

verbal communication Sending of messages from one individual to another or to a group of individuals through the spoken word.

vertigo Sensation of dizziness or spinning.

vibration Fine, shaking pressure applied by hands to the chest wall only during exhalation.

virulence Ability of an organism to rapidly produce disease.

visual Related to or experienced through vision.

vital signs Temperature, pulse, respirations, and blood pressure.

vitamins Organic compounds essential in small quantities for normal physiological and metabolic functioning of the body. With few exceptions, vitamins cannot be synthesized by the body and must be obtained from the diet or dietary supplements.

voiding Process of urinating.

vulnerable populations Collection of individuals who are more likely to develop health problems as a result of excess risks, limits in access to health care services, or being dependent on others for care.

W

wellness Dynamic state of health in which an individual progresses toward a higher level of functioning, achieving an optimum balance between internal and external environments.

wellness education Activities that teach people how to care for themselves in a healthy manner.

wellness nursing diagnosis Clinical judgment about an individual, group, or community in transition from a specific level of wellness to a higher level of wellness.

wheezes, wheezing Adventitious lung sounds caused by a severely narrowed bronchus.

work redesign Formal process used to analyze the work of a certain work group and change the actual structure of the jobs performed.

worldview Cognitive stance or perspective about phenomena characteristic of a particular cultural group.

wound culture Specimen collected from a wound to determine the specific organism that is causing an infectious process.

Y

yearning and searching Second phase of Bowlby's phases of mourning. It is characterized by emotional outbursts of tearful sobbing and acute distress.

Z

Z-track injection Technique for injecting irritating preparations into muscle without tracking residual medication through sensitive tissues.

INDEX

b indicates boxes, *f* indicates illustrations, and *t* indicates tables.

B

SPECIAL FEATURES

Patient Teaching

Concept Maps

Nursing Care Plans